SELDIN AND GIEBISCH'S THE KIDNEY

SELDIN AND GIEBISCH'S THE KIDNEY

PHYSIOLOGY AND PATHOPHYSIOLOGY

FOURTH EDITION

ROBERT J. ALPERN, MD
Yale University School of Medicine
New Haven, Connecticut, USA

STEVEN C. HEBERT, MD
Yale University School of Medicine
New Haven, Connecticut, USA

AMSTERDAM • BOSTON • HEIDELBERG • LONDON • NEW YORK • OXFORD
PARIS • SAN DIEGO • SAN FRANCISCO • SINGAPORE • SYDNEY • TOKYO
Academic Press is an imprint of Elsevier

Academic Press is an imprint of Elsevier
30 Corporate Drive, Suite 400, Burlington, MA 01803, USA
525 B Street, Suite 1900, San Diego, California 92101–4495, USA
84 Theobald's Road, London WCIX 8RR, UK

This book is printed on acid–free paper. ♾

Library of Congress Cataloging-in-Publication Data
2007926491

British Library Cataloging in Publication Data
A catalogue record for this book is available from the British Library.

Set ISBN: 978–0–12–088488–9
Volume 1 ISBN: 978–0–12–088489–6
Volume 2 ISBN: 978–0–12–088490–2

For information on all Elsevier Academic Press publications
visit our Web site at www.books.elsevier.com

Printed in the United States of America
08 09 10 11 12   9 8 7 6 5 4 3 2 1

*To Gerhard Giebisch and Donald Seldin who have served the renal field
as visionary leaders, and who for us have served as
outstanding mentors and close friends.*

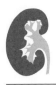

Contents

A selection of color images is located at the back of each volume.

For slides of color images, please visit http://books.elsevier.com/companions/9780120884889

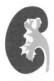

Contributors

Numbers in parentheses indicate the page number(s) on which the contribution begins.

MAURO ABBATE, MD (2563) *Mario Negri Institute for Pharmacological Research, Bergamo, Italy*

DALE R. ABRAHAMSON, PhD (691), *Professor and Chair, Department of Anatomy and Cell Biology, University of Kansas Medical Center, Kansas City, Kansas, USA*

MARCIN ADAMCZAK, MD (2537), *Department of Nephrology, Endocrinology, and Metabolic Diseases, Silesian Medical University, Katowice, Poland*

HORACIO J. ADROGUÉ, MD (1721), *Professor of Medicine, Baylor College of Medicine, Chief, Renal Section, The Methodist Hospital, Houston, Texas, USA*

SETH L. ALPER, MD, PhD (1499), *Professor of Medicine, Harvard Medical School, Molecular and Vascular Medicine Unit and Renal Division, Beth Israel Deaconess Medical Center, Boston, Massachusetts, USA*

ROBERT J. ALPERN, MD (1005, 1539, 1645, 1667), *Dean and Ensign Professor of Medicine, Yale University School of Medicine, New Haven, Connecticut, USA*

THOMAS E. ANDREOLI, MD (849), *Distinguished Professor, Department of Internal Medicine, Department of Physiology and Biophysics, University of Arkansas College of Medicine, Little Rock, Arkansas, USA*

ANITA C. APERIA, MD, PhD (443), *Professor of Pediatrics Karolinska Institutet, Department of Woman and Child Health, Astrid Lindgren Children's Hospital, Stockholm, Sweden*

MATTHEW A. BAILEY (425), *Center for Cardiovascular Science, University of Edinburgh, Edinburgh, United Kingdom*

DANIEL BATLLE, MD, FACP (2113), *Earle, del Greco, and Levin Professor of Nephrology/Hypertension Professor of Medicine Chief, Division of Nephrology/Hypertension, Northwestern University, Feinberg School of Medicine, Chicago, Illinois, USA*

MICHEL BAUM, MD (707), *Professor of Pediatrics and Medicine, University of Texas Southwestern Medical Center, Dallas, Texas, USA*

THERESA J. BERNDT, PhD (1989), *Departments of Internal Medicine, Physiology, and Bioengineering, Division of Nephrology and Hypertension, Mayo Clinic, Rochester, Minnesota, USA*

MARK O. BEVENSEE (1429), *University of Alabama at Birmingham, Birmingham, Alabama, USA*

JÜRG BIBER, PhD (1979), *Institute of Physiology, Centre for Integrative Human Physiology, University Zürich-Irchel, Zürich, Switzerland*

DANIEL G. BICHET, MD, MSc (1225), *Professor of Medicine and Physiology, Hôpital du Sacré-Coeur de Montréal, Université de Montréal, Montréal, Québec, Canada*

RENÉ J.M. BINDELS (1769), *Department of Physiology, Nijmegen Centre for Molecular Life Sciences, Radboud University Nijmegen Medical Center, Nijmegen, The Netherlands*

ROLAND C. BLANTZ, MD (565), *Professor and Head; Division of Nephrology-Hypertension, University of California San Diego and VA San Diego Healthcare System, La Jolla, California, USA*

WALTER F. BORON, MD, PhD (1429, 1481), *Department of Cell and Molecular Physiology, Yale University School of Medicine, New Haven, Connecticut, USA*

D. CRAIG BRATER, MD (2763), *Dean and Walter J. Daly Professor, Indiana University School of Medicine, Indianapolis, Indiana, USA*

JOSEPHINE P. BRIGGS, MD (589), *Senior Scientific Officer, Howard Hughes Medical Institute, Chevy Chase, Maryland, USA*

ALEX BROWN (1803), *Renal Division, Washington University School of Medicine, St. Louis, Missouri, USA*

NIGEL J. BRUNSKILL (979), *Professor of Renal Medicine, Department of Nephrology and Cell Physiology, Leicester General Hospital, University of Leicester, United Kingdom*

GERHARD BURCKHARDT (2045), *Abteilung Vegetative Physiologie und Pathophysiologie, Zentrum Physiologie und Pathophysiologie, Georg-August-Univesilat Göttingen, Göttingen, Germany*

GEOFFREY BURNSTOCK (425), *Department of Anatomy & Developmental Biology, University College London, London, United Kingdom*

LLOYD CANTLEY, MD (297), *Professor of Medicine and Professor of Cellular and Molecular Physiology, Yale University School of Medicine, New Haven, Connecticut, USA*

CHUNHUA CAO, MD, PhD (627), *Department of Medicine, University of Maryland at Baltimore, Baltimore, Maryland, USA*

GIOVAMBATTISTA CAPASSO, MD (979) *Chair of Nephrology, School of Medicine, Second University of Naples, Naples, Italy*

MICHAEL J. CAPLAN, MD, PhD (1, 2283), *Professor, Department of Cell and Molecular Physiology, Yale University School of Medicine, New Haven, Connecticut, USA*

HUGH J. CARROLL, MD (275), *Professor of Medicine, State University of New York, Downstate Medical Center, Brooklyn, New York, USA*

LAURENCE CHAN, MD, DPhil(Oxon), FRCP (1203), *Professor of Medicine, Director, Transplant Nephrology, Division of Renal Diseases and Hypertension, University of Colorado Health Sciences Center, Denver, Colorado, USA*

MOONJA CHUNG-PARK, MD (2399), *Case Western Reserve University, Cleveland, Ohio*

FREDRIC L. COE, MD (1945), *Professor of Medicine and Physiology, Department of Medicine and Physiology, University of Chicago School of Medicine, Chicago, Illinois, USA*

THOMAS M. COFFMAN, MD (343), *James R. Clapp Professor of Medicine, Professor of Cell Biology and Immunology, Chief, Division of Nephrology Duke University and Durham VA Medical Centers, Durham, North Carolina, USA*

WAYNE D. COMPER, PhD, DSc (2081), *Professor, Department of Biochemistry and Molecular Biology, Monash University, Clayton, Victoria, Australia*

KIRK P. CONRAD, MD (2339), *Professor, Departments of Physiology and Functional Genomics, and of Obstetrics and Gynecology, University of Florida College of Medicine, Gainesville, Florida, USA*

STEVEN D. CROWLEY, MD (343), *Division of Nephrology, Duke University and Durham VA Medical Centers, Durham, North Carolina, USA*

NORMAN P. CURTHOYS, PhD (1601), *Professor Laureate, Department of Biochemistry and Molecular Biology, Colorado State University, Fort Collins, Colorado, USA*

PEDRO R. CUTILLAS (979), *Head of Analytical Cell Signaling, Centre for Cell Signaling, Institute of Cancer, Barts and The London, Queen Mary's School of Medicine and Dentistry, Queen Mary, University College London, London, United Kingdom*

THEODORE M. DANOFF, MD, PhD (2477), *Group Director, Clinical Pharmacology and Discovery Medicine, Head, Human Target Validation Laboratory, Cardiovascular and Urogenital Center of Excellence, GlaxoSmithKline Pharmaceuticals, King of Prussia, Pennsylvania, USA*

EDWARD S. DEBNAM (979) *Department of Physiology, University College London, London, United Kingdom*

HENRIK DIMKE, MSc (1095), *The Water and Salt Research Center, Institute of Anatomy, University of Aarhus, Aarhus C, Denmark*

ALAIN DOUCET, PhD (57), *Laboratory of Renal Physiology and Genomics, Centre National de la Recherche Scientifique and Université Pierre et Marie Curie, Paris, France*

RAGHVENDRA K. DUBEY, MS, PhD (413), *Professor, Department of Obstetrics and Gynecology, Clinic for Reproduction-Endocrinology, University Hospital Zurich, Zurich, Switzerland and Associate Professor of Medicine, Center for Clinical Pharmacology, University of Pittsburgh School of Medicine, Pittsburgh, Pennsylvania, USA*

ADRIANA DUSSO, PhD (1803), *Renal Division, Department of Internal Medicine, Washington University School of Medicine, St. Louis, Missouri, USA*

KAI-UWE ECKARDT, MD (2681), *Professor of Medicine, Chief, Department of Nephrology and Hypertension, University of Erlangen-Nuremberg, Erlangen, Germany*

DAVID H. ELLISON, MD (1051), *Head, Division of Nephrology and Hypertension, Oregon Health and Science University, Portland, Oregon, USA*

HITOSHI ENDOU, MD, PhD (185), *Professor Emeritus, Department of Pharmacology and Toxicology, Kyorin University School of Medicine, Tokyo, Japan*

ZOLTÁN HUBA ENDRE (2507), *Professor, Head, Department of Medicine, University of Otago, Christchurch School of Medicine and Health Sciences, Christchurch, New Zealand*

FRANKLIN H. EPSTEIN, MD (1277), *William Applebaum Professor of Medicine, Beth Israel Deaconess Medical Center, Harvard Medical School, Boston, Massachusetts, USA*

ANDREW EVAN, PhD (1945), *Department of Anatomy and Cell Biology, Indiana University, Indianapolis, Indiana, USA*

RONALD J. FALK, MD (2315), *Division of Nephrology and Hypertension, University of North Carolina at Chapel Hill, Chapel Hill, North Carolina, USA*

KAMBIZ FARBAKHSH, MD (2591), *College of Medicine, University of Minnesota, Department of Medicine, Hennepin County Medical Center, Minneapolis, Minnesota, USA*

NICHOLAS R. FERRERI, PhD (359), *Department of Pharmacology, New York Medical College, Valhalla, New York, USA*

PEYING FONG, PhD (769), *Professor, Department of Anatomy and Physiology, Kansas State University, College of Veterinary Medicine, Manhattan, Kansas, USA*

MANASSES CLAUDINO FONTELES, PhD (463), *Reitoria, Universidade Presbiteriana Mackenzie, São Paulo, Brazil*

IAN FORSTER (1979), *Institute of Physiology, University of Zurich-Irchel, Zurich, Switzerland*

LEONARD RALPH FORTE, JR., PhD (463), *Department of Medical Pharmacology and Physiology, The Radiopharmaceutical Sciences Institute, University of Missouri School of Medicine, Senior Research Career Scientist, Truman Memorial VA Hospital, Columbia, Missouri, USA*

HAROLD A. FRANCH, MD (2615), *Renal Division, Emory University School of Medicine, Atlanta, Georgia, USA*

LYNDA A. FRASSETTO, MD (1621), *Associate Clinical Professor, Department of Medicine, University of California, San Francisco, San Francisco, California, USA*

PETER A. FRIEDMAN, PhD (1851), *Department of Pharmacology, University of Pittsburgh School of Medicine, Pittsburgh, Pennsylvania, USA*

JØRGEN FRØKLÆR, MD, DMSc (1095), *Professor, Chief Consultant, Department of Clinical Physiology, Aarhus University Hospital-Skejby, Aarhus, Denmark*

JOHN P. GEIBEL, MD, DSc (1269, 1785), *Department of Surgery and Cellular and Molecular Physiology, Yale University School of Medicine, New Haven, Connecticut, USA*

MICHAEL GEKLE, PhD (2021), *Julius-Bernstein-Institut für Physiologie, Martin-Luther-Universität Halle-Wittenberg, Halle, Germany*

GERHARD GIEBISCH, MD (1301), *Sterling Professor Emeritus Physiology, Department of Cellular and Molecular Physiology, Yale University School of Medicine, New Haven, Connecticut, USA*

PERE GINÈS, MD (2235), *Professor of Medicine, Chairman, Liver Unit, Hospital Clinic, University of Barcelona School of Medicine, Barcelona, Catalunya, Spain*

STEVE A.N. GOLDSTEIN, MD, PhD (1407), *Department of Pediatrics, The Institute for Molecular Pediatric Sciences and Comer Children's Hospital of the University of Chicago Pritzker School of Medicine, Chicago, Illinois, USA*

SIMIN GORAL, MD (2737), *Renal Electrolyte & Hypertension Division, Hospital of the University of Pennsylvania, Philadelphia, Pennsylvania, USA*

SIAN V. GRIFFIN, MD (723), *Consultant Nephrologist, University Hospital of Wales, Heath Park, Cardiff, Wales*

WILLIAM B. GUGGINO, PhD (769), *Professor and Director of Physiology, Professor of Pediatrics, Department of Physiology and Pediatrics, Johns Hopkins University School of Medicine, Baltimore, Maryland, USA*

THERESA A. GUISE, MD (1911), *Gerald D. Aurbach Professor of Endocrinology, Professor of Medicine, Division of Endocrinology and Metabolism, Department of Internal Medicine, University of Virginia, Charlottesville, Virginia, USA*

SUSAN B. GURLEY, MD, PhD (343), *Division of Nephrology, Department of Medicine, Duke University and Durham VA Medical Centers, Durham, North Carolina, USA*

STEPHEN D. HALL, PhD (2763), *Professor of Medicine, Division of Clinical Pharmacology, Department of Medicine, Indiana University School of Medicine, Indianapolis, Indiana, USA*

MITCHELL L. HALPERIN, MD, FRCPC, FRS (1387), *Division of Nephrology, St. Michael's Hospital, Emeritus Professor of Medicine, University of Toronto, Toronto, Ontario, Canada*

L. LEE HAMM, MD (1539), *Huberwald Professor and Chair of Medicine, Tulane University School of Medicine, New Orleans, Louisiana, USA*

STEVEN C. HEBERT, MD (1249, 1785), *C.N. H. Long Professor of Physiology and Medicine and Chair, Department of Cellular and Molecular Physiology, Yale University School of Medicine, New Haven, Connecticut, USA*

MATTHIAS A. HEDIGER, PhD (91), *Director, Institute for Biochemistry and Molecular Biology, University of Bern, Bern, Switzerland*

J. HAROLD HELDERMAN, MD (2737), *Division of Nephrology and Hypertension, Vanderbilt University Medical Center, Nashville, Tennessee, USA*

WILLIAM L. HENRICH, MD, MACP (2193, 2719), *Dean, School of Medicine, Vice President for Medical Affairs, University of Texas Health Science Center at San Antonio, San Antonio, Texas, USA*

AILLEEN HERAS-HERZIG, MD (1911), *Assistant Professor of Research, Division of Endocrinology and Metabolism, University of Virginia, Charlottesville, Virginia, USA*

NATI HERNANDO (1979), *Institute of Physiology, University of Zurich-Irchel, Zurich, Switzerland*

JOOST G.J. HOENDEROP, PhD (1769), *Department of Physiology, Nijmegen Centre for Molecular Life Sciences, Radboud University Nijmegen Medical Center, Nijmegen, The Netherlands*

ULLA HOLTBÄCK, MD, PhD (443), *Associate Professor, Astrid Lindgren Children's Hospital, Karolinska University Hospital, Stockholm, Sweden*

JEAN-DANIEL HORISBERGER, MD (57), *Department of Pharmacology and Toxicology, University of Lausanne, Lausanne, Switzerland*

EDITH HUMMLER (889), *Department of Pharmacology and Toxicology, University of Lausanne School of Medicine, Lausanne, Switzerland*

TRACY E. HUNLEY, MD (385), *Department of Pediatrics, Division of Pediatric Nephrology, Monroe Carell Jr. Children's Hospital at Vanderbilt, Nashville, Tennessee, USA*

EDWIN K. JACKSON, PhD (413), *Professor of Pharmacology and Medicine, Center for Clinical Pharmacology, University of Pittsburgh School of Medicine, Pittsburgh, Pennsylvania, USA*

J. CHARLES JENNETTE, MD (2315), *Brinkhous Distinguished Professor and Chair of Pathology and Laboratory Medicine, Professor of Medicine, University of North Carolina at Chapel Hill, Chapel Hill, North Carolina, USA*

EDWARD J. JOHNS (925), *Department of Physiology, University College Cork, Cork, Republic of Ireland*

JOHN P. JOHNSON (743), *Professor of Medicine and Cell Biology and Physiology, University of Pittsburgh School of Medicine, Pittsburgh, Pennsylvania, USA*

BRIGITTE KAISSLING (479), *Institute for Anatomy, University of Zurich, Zurich, Switzerland*

KAMEL S. KAMEL, MD, FRCP (1387), *Professor of Medicine, Division of Nephrology, St. Michael's Hospital, University of Toronto, Toronto, Ontario, Canada*

S. ANANTH KARUMANCHI, MD (2339), *Associate Professor of Medicine, Beth Israel Deaconess Medical Center & Harvard Medical School, Boston, Massachusetts, USA*

CLIFFORD E. KASHTAN, MD (2447), *Professor of Pediatrics, University of Minnesota School of Medicine, University of Minnesota Children's Hospital-Fairview, Minneapolis, Minnesota, USA*

BERTRAM L. KASISKE, MD (2591), *Department of Medicine, University of Minnesota, Minneapolis, Minnesota, USA*

ADRIAN I. KATZ, MD (1349), *Professor Emeritus of Medicine, Section of Nephrology, University of Chicago, Chicago, Illinois, USA*

BRIAN F. KING (425), *Department of Physiology, University College London, London, United Kingdom*

SAULO KLAHR, MD (2247), *Professor Emeritus, Department of Internal Medicine, Washington University School of Medicine, St. Louis, Missouri, USA*

THOMAS R. KLEYMAN, MD (743), *Chief, Renal-Electrolyte Division, Professor of Medicine, Cell Biology and Physiology, and Pharmacology, University of Pittsburgh, Pittsburgh, Pennsylvania, USA*

HERMANN KOEPSELL, MD (2045), *Professor of Anatomy and Cell Biology, Head of the Department, Institute of Anatomy and Cell Biology of the University of Würzburg, Würzburg, Germany*

VALENTINA KON, MD (385), *Associate Professor, Department of Pediatrics, Division of Pediatric Nephrology, Vanderbilt University School of Medicine, Memphis, Tennessee, USA*

MARTIN KONRAD, MD (1747), *Professor of Pediatric Nephrology, University Children's Hospital, Münster, Germany*

ULLA C. KOPP, PhD (925), *Department of Pharmacology, VA Medical Center, Carver College of Medicine, University of Iowa, Iowa City, Iowa, USA*

RETO KRAPF, MD (1667), *Professor of Medicine, Chief, Department of Medicine, Kantonsspital Bruderholz/University of Basel, Bruderholz/Basel, Switzerland*

WILHELM KRIZ (479), *Institute for Anatomy and Cell Biology, University of Heidelberg, Heidelberg, Germany*

RAJIV KUMAR, MBBS, MACP (1891, 1989), *Ruth and Vernon Taylor Professor, Departments of Internal Medicine, Biochemistry, and Molecular Biology, Mayo Clinic, Rochester, Minnesota, USA*

CHRISTINE E. KURSCHAT (1499), *Department of Nephrology, Internal Medicine IV, University Hospital of Cologne, Cologne, Germany*

ARMIN KURTZ, MD (2681), *Institut für Physiologie der Universität Regensburg, Regensburg, Germany*

TAE-HWAN KWON (1095) *Department of Biochemistry and Cell Biology, School of Medicine, Kyungpook National University, Taegu, Korea*

CHRISTOPHER P. LANDOWSKI (91), *Institute for Biochemistry and Molecular Biology, University of Bern, Bern, Switzerland*

ANTHONY J. LANGONE, MD (2737), *Division of Nephrology and Transplantation, Vanderbilt University Medical Center, Nashville, Tennessee, USA*

FLORIAN LANG, MD (169), *Department of Physiology, University of Tübingen Germany, Tübingen, Germany*

HAROLD E. LAYTON (1143), *Professor of Mathematics, Department of Mathematics, Duke University, Durham, North Carolina, USA*

THU H. LE, MD (343), *Assistant Professor, Division of Nephrology, Department of Medicine, Duke University and Durham VA Medical Centers, Durham, North Carolina, USA*

DANIEL I. LEVY, MD, PhD (1407), *Assistant Professor, Section of Nephrology, Department of Medicine, and The Institute for Molecular Pediatric Sciences, University of Chicago, Chicago, Illinois, USA*

SHIH-HUA LIN, MD (1387), *Professor of Medicine, National Defense Medical Center, Division of Nephrology, Tri-Service General Hospital, Taipei, Taiwan*

MARSHALL D. LINDHEIMER, MD (2339), *Professor (Emeritus) of Medicine, Obstetrics & Gynecology, and Clinical Pharmacology Biological Science Division, Pritzker School of Medicine, University of Chicago, Chicago, Illinois, USA*

CHRISTOPHER Y. LU, MD (2577), *Department of Internal Medicine, Nephrology, The University of Texas Southwestern Medical Center at Dallas, Dallas, Texas, USA*

MICHAEL P. MADAIO, MD (2399), *Chief of Nephrology, Professor of Medicine, Temple University School of Medicine, University of Pennsylvania, Philadelphia, Pennsylvania, USA*

NICOLAOS E. MADIAS, MD (1721), *Chairman, Department of Medicine, Caritas St. Elizabeth's Medical Center, Chief Academic Officer, Caritas Christi Health Care System, Maurice S. Segal, MD, Professor of Medicine, Tufts University School of Medicine, Boston, Massachusetts, USA*

GERHARD MALNIC (1301), *Professor of Physiology, Departamento de Fisiologie e Biofisica, Instituto de Ciencias, Universidade de São Paulo, São Paulo, Brazil*

KARL S. MATLIN, PhD (1), *Laboratory of Epithelial Pathobiology, Department of Surgery, Vontz Center for Molecular Studies, University of Cincinnati College of Medicine, Cincinnati, Ohio, USA*

WILLIAM C. McCLELLAN (2615), *Renal Division, Emory University School of Medicine, Atlanta, Georgia, USA*

JOHN C. MCGIFF, MD (359), *Department of Pharmacology, New York Medical College, Valhalla, New York, USA*

C. CHARLES MICHEL (247), *Emeritus Professor of Physiology and Senior Research Investigator, Department of Bioengineering, Imperial College London, London, United Kingdom*

JEFFREY H. MINER, PhD (691), *Professor of Medicine, Renal Division and of Cell Biology and Physiology, Washington University School of Medicine, St. Louis, Missouri, USA*

WILLIAM E. MITCH, MD (2615), *Gordon A. Cain Chair in Nephrology, Director, Division of Nephrology, Baylor College of Medicine, Houston, Texas, USA*

HIROKI MIYAZAKI, MD, PhD (185), *Institute of Biochemistry and Molecular Medicine, University of Bern, Bern, Switzerland*

ORSON W. MOE, MD (1645), *Professor, Department of Internal Medicine and Physiology, Charles and Jane Pak Center of Mineral Metabolism, University of Texas Southwestern Medical Center, Dallas, Texas, USA*

BRUCE A. MOLITORIS, MD (2143), *Professor of Medicine, Director of Nephrology, Director of The Indiana Center for Biological Microscopy, Indiana University School of Medicine, Indianapolis, Indiana, USA*

R. CURTIS MORRIS, JR., MD (1621), *Professor of Medicine, Pediatrics, and Radiology, University of California, San Francisco, San Francisco, California, USA*

SALIM K. MUJAIS, MD (1349), *Northbrook, Illinois, USA*

HEINI MURER, PhD (1979), *Institute of Physiology, Center for Integrative Human Physiology, University of Zurich, Zurich, Switzerland*

SHIGEAKI MUTO, MD, PhD (1301), *Associate Professor, Department of Nephrology, Jichi Medical School, Shimotsuke, Tochigi, Japan*

EUGENE NATTIE, MD (1587), *Department of Physiology, Dartmouth Medical School, Lebanon, New Hampshire, USA*

ERIC G. NEILSON, MD (2477), *Hugh Jackson Morgan Professor of Medicine and Cell and Developmental Biology Physician-In-Chief, Vanderbilt University Hospital; Chairman, Department of Medicine, Vanderbilt University School of Medicine, Nashville, Tennessee, USA*

SØREN NIELSEN, MD, PhD (1095), *Water and Salt Research Center, Institute of Anatomy, University of Aarhus, Aarhus, Denmark*

SANJAY K. NIGAM, MD (671), *Professor of Pediatrics, Department of Medicine and Cellular and Molecular Medicine, University of California, San Diego, La Jolla, California, USA*

JOSEPH M. NOGUEIRA, MD (2193), *Assistant Professor of Medicine, Division of Nephrology, University of Maryland School Medical System, Baltimore, Maryland, USA*

MAN S. OH, MD (275), *Professor of Medicine, State University of New York, Downstate Medical Center, Brooklyn, New York, USA*

MARK D. OKUSA, MD (1051), *Division of Nephrology, University of Virginia Health System, Charlottesville, Virginia, USA*

TANYA M. OSICKA, PhD (2081), *Research Associate, Department of Medicine, University of Melbourne, Austin Health, Heidelberg, Victoria, Australia*

THOMAS L. PALLONE, MD (627), *Department of Medicine and Nephrology, University of Maryland at Baltimore, Baltimore, Maryland, USA*

BIFF F. PALMER, MD (1005, 2719), *Professor of Internal Medicine, Director Renal Fellowship Training Program, Department of Internal Medicine, Division of Nephrology, University of Texas Southwestern Medical Center, Dallas, Texas, USA*

LAWRENCE G. PALMER, PhD (211), *Professor of Physiology & Biophysics, Weill Medical College of Cornell University, New York, New York, USA*

MARK D. PARKER, PhD (1481), *Department of Cellular and Molecular Physiology, Yale University School of Medicine, New Haven, Connecticut, USA*

JOAN H. PARKS, MBA (1945), *Research Associate (Assistant Professor), Medicine, Department of Medicine, University of Chicago School of Medicine, Chicago, Illinois, USA*

PATRICIA A. PREISIG, PhD (1539), *Professor, Internal Medicine and Cellular and Molecular Physiology, Section of Nephrology, Yale University School of Medicine, New Haven, Connecticut, USA*

GARY A. QUAMME (1747), *Department of Medicine, Vancouver Hospital and Health Science Center Koerner Pavilion, University of British Columbia, Vancouver, British Columbia, Canada*

L. DARRYL QUARLES, MD (2671), *The Kidney Institute and Division of Nephrology, University of Kansas Medical Center, Kansas City, Kansas, USA*

RAYMOND QUIGLEY, MD (707), *Professor of Pediatrics, University of Texas Southwestern Medical Center, Dallas, Texas, USA*

W. BRIAN REEVES, MD (849), *Chief of Nephrology and Professor of Medicine, Division of Nephrology, Penn State College of Medicine, Hershey, Pennsylvania, USA*

GIUSEPPE REMUZZI, MD (2563), *Director, Mario Negri Institute for Pharmacological Research Negri Bergamo Laboratories and Director, Division of Nephrology and Dialysis, Azienda Ospedaliera, Ospedali Riuniti di Bergamo, Bergamo, Italy*

LUIS REUSS, MD (35, 147), *Professor and Chair, Department of Cell Physiology and Molecular Biophysics, Texas Tech University Health Sciences Center, Lubbock, Texas, USA*

DANIELA RICCARDI, PhD (1785), *Reader, Physiology, Cardiff University, Cardiff, Wales*

BRIAN RINGHOFER, MD (2671), *The Kidney Institute and Division of Nephrology, University of Kansas Medical Center, Kansas City, Kansas, USA*

EBERHARD RITZ, MD (2537), *Department of Internal Medicine, Nierenzentrum, Ruperto Carola University, Heidelberg, Germany*

CHRISTOPHER J. RIVARD, PhD (1203), *Assistant Professor of Medicine, Division of Renal Diseases and Hypertension, University of Colorado Health Sciences Center, Denver, Colorado, USA*

GARY L. ROBERTSON, MD (1123), *Professor of Medicine Emeritus, Feinberg Medical School of Northwestern University, Chicago, Illinois, USA*

ROBERT M. ROSA, MD (1277), *Professor of Medicine, Executive Associate Dean for Clinical Affairs, The Feinberg School of Medicine, Northwestern University, Chicago, Illinois, USA*

BERNARD C. ROSSIER, MD (889), *Department of Pharmacology and Toxicology, University of Lausanne School of Medicine, Lausanne, Switzerland*

LEILEATA M. RUSSO, PhD (2081), *Program in Membrane Biology/Division of Nephrology, Massachusetts General Hospital, Harvard Medical School, Boston, Massachusetts, USA*

HENRY SACKIN, PhD (211), *Rosalind Franklin University of Medicine and Science/The Chicago Medical School, North Chicago, Illinois, USA*

HIROYUKI SAKURAI, MD (671), *Associate Project Scientist, Division of Nephrology and Hypertension, Department of Medicine, University of California, San Diego, La Jolla, California, USA*

JEFF M. SANDS, MD (1143), *Juha P. Kokko Professor of Medicine and Physiology, Director, Renal Division, Associate Dean for Clinical and Translational Research, Emory University School of Medicine, Atlanta, Georgia, USA*

LISA M. SATLIN, MD (707), *Professor of Pediatric and Medicine, Mount Sinai School of Medicine, New York, New York, USA*

HEIDI SCHAEFER, MD (2737), *Division of Nephrology and Transplantation, Vanderbilt University Medical Center, Nashville, Tennessee, USA*

JEFFREY R. SCHELLING, MD (2399), *Associate Professor and Nephrology Division Chief, Department of Medicine, Metro Health Medical Center, Department of Physiology and Biophysics, Case Western Reserve University, Cleveland, Ohio, USA*

LAURENT SCHILD (889), *Department of Pharmacology and Toxicology, University of Lausanne School of Medicine, Lausanne, Switzerland*

KARL P. SCHLINGMANN (1747), *Department of Pediatrics, Philipps-University, Marburg, Germany*

JÜRGEN B. SCHNERMANN, *MD (589), Chief, Kidney Disease Branch, National Institute of Diabetes, and Digestive and Kidney Diseases, National Institutes of Health, Bethesda, Maryland, USA*

ROBERT W. SCHRIER, MD (2235), *Professor of Medicine, University of Colorado School of Medicine, Denver, Colorado, USA*

ANTHONY SEBASTIAN, MD (1621), *Department of Medicine, Division of Nephrology, General Clinical Research Center, Special Projects Associate, Clinical and Translational Science, Institute (CTSI), CTSI Strategic Opportunities, Support Center, CTSI Clinical Research Center, University of California, San Francisco, San Francisco, California, USA*

JOHN R. SEDOR, MD (2399), *Kidney Disease Research Center, Rammelkamp Center for Research and Education, MetroHealth System, Case Western Reserve University, Cleveland, Ohio, USA*

YOAV SEGAL, MD, PhD (2447), *Assistant Professor of Medicine, University of Minnesota School of Medicine, Minneapolis VA Medical Center, Minneapolis, Minnesota, USA*

TAKASHI SEKINE, MD (185), *Associate Professor, Department of Pediatrics, Graduate School of Medicine, The University of Tokyo, Tokyo, Japan*

DONALD W. SELDIN, MD (1005, 1645, 1667), *William Buchanan Professor of Internal Medicine, University of Texas Southwestern Medical School, Dallas, Texas, USA*

MARTIN SENITKO, MD (2577), *Nephrology Fellow, Department of Internal Medicine, Division of Nephrology, The University of Texas Southwestern Medical Center at Dallas, Dallas, Texas, USA*

MALATHI SHAH, MD (2113), *Renal Fellow, Division of Nephrology/Hypertension, Northwestern University, Feinberg School of Medicine, Chicago, Illinois, USA*

SUDHIR V. SHAH, MD, FACP (2601), *Division of Nephrology, University of Arkansas School for Medical Sciences, Little Rock, Arkansas, USA*

STUART J. SHANKLAND, MD (723), *Professor of Medicine, Belding H. Scribner Endowed Chair in Medicine, Head, Division of Nephrology, Department of Medicine, University of Washington, Seattle, Washington, USA*

ASIF A. SHARFUDDIN, MD (2143), *Assistant Professor of Clinical Medicine, Division of Nephrology, Indiana University School of Medicine, Indianapolis, Indiana, USA*

KUMAR SHARMA, MD, F.A.H.A. (2215), *Professor of Medicine, Director of Translational Research in Kidney Disease, University of California at San Diego, La Jolla, California, USA*

SHAOHU SHENG, MD (743), *Research Assistant Professor, Department of Medicine, Renal-Electrolyte Division, University of Pittsburgh, Pittsburgh, Pennsylvania, USA*

DAVID G. SHIRLEY (425), *Centre for Nephrology, University College London, London, United Kingdom*

STEFAN SILBERNAGL, PhD (2021), *Department of Physiology, University of Würzburg, Würzburg, Germany*

STEPHEN M. SILVER, MD (1179), *Clinical Associate Professor of Medicine, University of Rochester School of Medicine and Dentistry, Head, Nephrology Unit, Rochester General Hospital, Rochester, New York, USA*

MEL SILVERMAN, MD, FRCP (C) (2007), *Professor of Medicine, University of Toronto and Division of Nephrology University Health Network, Toronto General Hospital, Toronto, Ontario, Canada*

EDUARDO SLATOPOLSKY, MD, FACP (1803), *Joseph Friedman Professor of renal Disease, Department of Medicine, Renal Division, Washington University School of Medicine, Physician Barnes-Jewish Hospital, St. Louis, Missouri, USA*

STEFAN SOMLO, MD, CNH (2283), *Long Professor, Departments of Internal Medicine and Genetics, Section of Nephrology, Yale University School of Medicine, New Haven, Connecticut, USA*

RICHARD H. STERNS, MD (1179), *Professor of Medicine, University of Rochester School of Medicine and Dentistry, Chief of Medicine, Rochester General Hospital, Rochester, New York, USA*

ANDREW K. STEWART (1499), *Department of Medicine, Molecular Medicine and Renal Units, Beth Israel Deaconess Medical Center, Harvard Medical School, Boston, Massachusetts, USA*

YOSHIRO SUZUKI (91), *Institute for Biochemistry and Molecular Biology, University of Bern, Bern, Switzerland*

PETER J. TEBBEN, MD (1891), *Departments of Internal Medicine, Pediatrics, and Adolescent Medicine, Mayo Clinic, Rochester, Minnesota, USA*

SCOTT C. THOMSON, MD (565), *Professor of Medicine, Division of Nephrology-Hypertension, University of California and VA San Diego Healthcare System, San Diego, California, USA*

VICENTE E. TORRES, MD (2283), *Professor of Medicine, Chair, Division of Nephrology and Hypertension, Mayo Clinic College of Medicine, Rochester, Minnesota, USA*

ROBERT J. UNWIN, PhD, FRCP (425, 979), *Renal Physiology and Epithelial Transport Group, Centre for Nephrology and Department of Physiology, Royal Free and University College Medical School, University College London, London, United Kingdom*

FRANÇOIS VERREY (889), *Institute of Physiology, University of Zurich, Zurich, Switzerland*

DAVID L. VESELY, MD, PhD (947), *Professor of Medicine, Molecular Pharmacology and Physiology and Director of University of South Florida Cardiac Hormone Center, Chief of Endocrinology, Diabetes and Metabolism, James A. Haley Veterans Medical Center, Tampa, Florida, USA*

CARSTEN A. WAGNER (1269), *Institute of Physiology, Zurich Center for Integrative Human Physiology, University of Zurich, Zurich, Switzerland*

MERYL WALDMAN, MD (2399), *National Institute of Diabetes and Digestive and Kidney Diseases, National Institutes of Health, Bethesda, Maryland, USA*

ROBERT JAMES WALKER (2507), *Head of Department, Department of Medical and Surgical Sciences, University of Otago, Dunedin School of Medicine, Dunedin, New Zealand*

WEI WANG, MD (1203), *Assistant Professor of Medicine, Department of Medicine, University of Colorado Health Sciences Center, Denver, Colorado, USA*

WEN-HUI WANG, MD (1249), *Professor of Pharmacology, Department of Pharmacology, New York Medical College, Valhalla, New York, USA*

YINGHONG WANG, MD PhD (769), *Department of Medicine, Albany Medical Center, Albany, New York, USA*

ALAN M. WEINSTEIN, MD (793), *Department of Physiology and Biophysics, Cornell University Weill Medical College, New York, New York, USA*

PAUL A. WELLING, MD (325), *Professor, Department of Physiology, University of Maryland School of Medicine, Baltimore, Maryland, USA*

GUNTER WOLF, MD (2215), *Professor of Medicine, Department of Internal Medicine, University Hospital Jena, Jena, Germany*

ELAINE WORCESTER, MD (1945), *Associate Professor of Medicine, Department of Medicine, University of Chicago School of Medicine, Chicago, Illinois, USA*

FUAD N. ZIYADEH, MD (2215), *Professor of Medicine & Biochemistry, Division of Nephrology, Department of Internal Medicine, Acting Chairman, Department of Physiology, Associate Dean for Academic Affairs-Faculty of Medicine, American University of Beirut, Beirut, Lebanon*

CARLA ZOJA, PhD (2563), *Mario Negri Institute for Pharmacological Research, Bergamo, Italy*

Foreword

The first edition of *The Kidney: Physiology and Pathophysiology* was published in 1985. Even at that early period, an abundance of books on kidney disease were in circulation. In general, the principal emphasis was on discrete renal disease, often presented as an isolated phenomenon, independent of the physiologic background generating the disease process. In part, this focus on the descriptive aspects of a disease was the consequence of the lack of basic understanding of the underlying pathophysiologic processes. In large measure, however, the analysis of abnormal kidney function in terms of discreet disease entities was also a conceptual model, derived largely from the triumphs in infectious disease, where a causal root to a disease could be unambiguously identified. The concept of abnormal function as an expression of deranged physiologic regulation was only dimly perceived.

The first edition took cognizance of this orientation and was designed to furnish a broad understanding of the regulatory function of the kidney as the basis for an analysis of renal abnormalities as derangements of regulation. The focus of the early edition was therefore mainly on renal physiology, "conceived broadly as the study of those processes by which the kidney maintains the volume and composition of the body in the face of physiologic demands and pathologic disturbances."

The second edition in 1992 and the third edition in 2000 greatly expanded the treatment of the basic processes underlying exchanges of water and electrolytes and their regulation by the kidney. The advances in structural and molecular biology, immunology, and genetics both deepened and broadened the analytic framework, allowing for a reduction of physiologic processes to very fundamental levels. At the same time the function of physiologic ensembles—the counter-current system, acid-base regulation, homeostatic balance—now characterized at a molecular level, could then be understood as an integrated interactive system.

This fourth edition is now in the editorial hands of two of our colleagues, Robert J. Alpern and Steven C. Hebert. Both are distinguished investigators. Dr. Alpern's principle interest has been the analysis of renal acidification, particularly the mechanisms in the proximal tubule cell which respond to changes in acid-base balance and maintain homeostasis–identifying genes participating in acid-base regulation, characterizing the behavior of transporters involved in acid secretion and bicarbonate efflux, and advancing the appreciation of the role of citrate in response to acid-base changes. These basic studies are accompanied by a deep competence in general renal physiology and clinical medicine that allows for a comprehensive appreciation of overall kidney physiology. His colleague, Steven Hebert, has made fundamental contributions to renal physiology, cloning transporters, characterizing channels, and discovering a system of calcium sensors in the kidney, parathyroid gland, and gastrointestinal tract, which not only participate in the regulation of calcium and sodium balance, but also function as a regulator of overall intestinal absorption and secretion and renal excretion, thereby acting as an internal homeostatic system. Dr. Hebert's interests range widely across the entire area of normal and deranged renal function.

In their hands, this fourth edition has taken on a fresh personality. There is increased emphasis on normal physiologic regulation and its disruption by disease; particularly noteworthy is the detailed attention to the specific mechanisms underlying pathologic changes. By deploying the most fundamental advances in renal physiology—not simply as isolated achievements, but as key ingredients to the understanding of physiologic regulation—this fourth edition constitutes a unique synthesis for the understanding of normal renal regulation and its derangement by disease.

Donald W. Seldin
Gerhard Giebisch

Preface

As described in its preface, the first edition of *The Kidney: Physiology and Pathophysiology,* published in 1985, focused on renal physiology, "conceived broadly as the study of those processes by which the kidney maintains the volume and composition of the body in the face of physiologic demands and pathologic disturbances." Since the publication of the first edition, science has become more reductionist, an evolution that has been reflected in the content of subsequent editions. Dissection of physiologic phenomena at the level of organs and cells was replaced by descriptions of the roles of individual molecules. As this trend in science has continued, so has the present edition continued to evolve in this direction. A complete understanding of physiologic processes must include knowledge of individual molecules—it should also include an integration of how these molecules work together to effect cellular and organ function that ultimately allow the system to address the requisite physiological demands.

The main focus of the **Fourth Edition** is to describe the present state of knowledge from molecules to systems that contribute to normal physiologic function of the kidney and the homeostatic mechanisms subserved by the kidney. The present edition will also concentrate on how these mechanisms malfunction resulting in the diseased state. Again we will address the pathophysiology of disease states from the molecular to the system level. One of the delightful features of nephrology is the ability to understand disease pathophysiology and to appreciate principles of clinical medicine. Thus, the clinician addressing a patient with a fluid and electrolyte disorder need not memorize a list of possible causes, but can deduce them through a thorough understanding of kidney function. As science continues to evolve, our understanding of the pathophysiologic basis of disease can now be applied to a much broader set of ailments. We, therefore, continue to broaden the scope of this book—to place greater emphasis on the mechanisms of disease.

Section One begins with general principles of epithelial and nonepithelial transport and regulation. This extensive section of the book continues a tradition established in the first edition, but builds on it to include a more extensive discussion of transport regulation. *Section Two* describes the organization of the kidney with an emphasis on renal development. *Section Three* follows, describing the mechanisms of fluid and electrolyte regulation and dysregulation. In no other book can one find this subject addressed with the depth and thoroughness found in this textbook. The **Fourth Edition** includes the most in-depth discussion of recently described families of transporters, integrating this information to describe their role in physiologic and pathophysiologic processes.

Section Four, the pathophysiology of renal disease, has been expanded as our knowledge of these processes and their contribution to renal ailments has grown. Of note is a new series of chapters focused on the *mechanisms of renal progression.* Progression of renal disease is a major area in which nephrologists can intervene to ensure that patients with asymptomatic increases in serum creatinine do not continue to lose kidney function, resulting in end stage renal disease. A thorough understanding of the roles of glomerular pressure, proteinuria, inflammation, lipids, and oxidants will allow researchers and clinicians to prevent renal failure, decreasing the need for dialysis and transplant.

The evolution of our understanding of kidney function and dysfunction derives from a series of discoveries made by a myriad of investigators, each benefiting from and building upon the accomplishments of their predecessors. The same can be said for textbooks. This textbook was originally conceived by the vision of two of the greatest renal physiologists of the twentieth century, Donald Seldin and Gerhard Giebisch. Their commitment to science and education created the vision for this book. It is our intent to continue their tradition and to honor them for all that they have contributed to this book, to nephrology, to epithelial physiology, and to science in general.

Robert J. Alpern, MD
Steven C. Hebert, MD

For slides of color images, please visit http://books.elsevier.com/companions/9780120884889

Epithelial and Nonepithelial Transport and Regulation

General Principles of Epithelial and Nonepithelial Transport

CHAPTER **1**

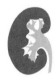 # Epithelial Cell Structure and Polarity

Karl S. Matlin and Michael J. Caplan
University of Cincinnati College of Medicine, Cincinnati, Ohio, USA
Yale University School of Medicine, New Haven, Connecticut, USA

INTRODUCTION

Many of the chapters in this volume are devoted to the mechanisms through which the nephron is able to convert the glomerular filtrate into a concentrated urine that is responsive to the metabolic status of the organism as a whole. The multifactorial nature of this problem necessitates that it be treated at several levels of resolution. A meaningful description of renal tubular function requires an understanding of the nephron's properties as an integrated tissue as well as those of its constituent parts, including the cells and molecules that contribute to its transport functions.

As is detailed elsewhere in this volume, the nephron is a remarkably heterogeneous structure. Throughout its length, the renal tubule is notable for the marked variations in the morphologic and physiologic properties of its epithelial cells, reflecting the numerous and diverse responsibilities that neighboring segments are called on to fulfill. At the tissue level, the function of the kidney is critically dependent on the geometry and topography of the nephron. The precise juxtaposition of various epithelial cell types, which manifest dis-

tinct fluid and electrolyte transport capabilities, in large measure specifies the course of modifications to which the glomerular filtrate is exposed. This dependence on geometry extends as well to renal function at the cellular level.

NATURE AND PHYSIOLOGIC IMPLICATIONS OF EPITHELIAL POLARITY

Despite their variations in form and function, all of the epithelial cells that line the nephron share at least one fundamental characteristic. Like their relatives in other epithelial tissues (including the intestine, lung, liver, etc.), all renal tubular epithelial cell types are polarized. The plasma membranes of polarized epithelial cells are divided into two morphologically and biochemically distinct domains (39, 184, 225, 269, 293). In the case of the nephron, the apical surfaces of the epithelial cells face the tubular lumen. The basolateral surface rests on the epithelial basement membrane and is in contact with the extracellular fluid compartment. The lipid and protein components of these two contiguous plasmalemmal domains are almost entirely dissimilar (39, 184, 225, 269, 293). It is precisely these differences that account for the epithelial cell's capacity to mediate the vectorial transport of solutes and fluid against steep concentration gradients. Thus, the subcellular geometry of renal epithelial cells is critical to renal function.

The principal cell of the collecting tubule provides a useful illustration of the importance of biochemical polarity for renal function. As described in other contributions to this volume, the principal cell is required to resorb sodium against a very steep concentration gradient. It accomplishes this task through the carefully controlled placement of ion pumps and channels (152, 245, 284). The basolateral plasma membrane of the principal cell, like that of most polarized epithelial cells, possesses a large complement of Na^+,K^+-ATPase. This basolateral sodium pump catalyzes the energetically unfavorable transport of three sodium ions out of the cell in exchange for two potassium ions through the consumption of the energy embodied in one molecule of ATP (310). The apical surface of the principal cell lacks a sodium pump, but is equipped with a sodium channel, which allows sodium ions to move passively down their concentration gradients (248). Through the action of the sodium pump the intracellular sodium concentration is kept low and the driving forces across the apical membrane favor the influx of sodium from the tubular fluid through the apical sodium channels. Thus, the combination of a basolateral Na^+,K^+-ATPase and an apical sodium channel lead to the vectorial movement of sodium from the tubule lumen to the interstitial space against its electrochemical gradient. This elegant mechanism is critically dependent on the principal cell's biochemical polarity. If the sodium pump and the sodium channel occupied the same plasmalemmal domain, then the gradients generated by the former could not be profitably exploited by the latter. Thus, the vectorial resorption or secretion of solutes or fluid is predicated on the asymmetric distribution of transport proteins in polarized epithelial cells.

The fact that epithelial cells manifest biochemical polarity implies that they are endowed with the capacity to generate and maintain differentiated subdomains of their cell surface membranes (39, 184, 225, 269, 293). Newly synthesized membrane proteins must be targeted to the appropriate cell surface domain and retained there following their delivery. During tissue development, cell division, and wound healing, plasmalemmal domains must be delimited and their biochemical character established. Clearly, specialized machinery and pathways must exist through which this energetically unfavorable compositional asymmetry can be supported. The nature of these specializations has been the subject of intense study for decades. While firm answers are not yet in, a number of fascinating model systems have been developed and valuable insights have emerged. This chapter will focus on what is known of the processes through which tubular epithelial cells create their polarized geometry.

EPITHELIAL CELL STRUCTURE: MORPHOLOGY AND PHYSIOLOGY

Morphologic Characteristics of Epithelial Polarity

As noted above (as well as in other contributions to this volume), the renal tubular epithelium is composed of a remarkably varied collection of cell types. A detailed delineation of its morphologic diversity is beyond the scope of this discussion. It may be valuable, however, to identify some of the salient structural features of certain renal epithelial subtypes, since they are illustrative of several more or less general aspects of epithelial organization.

Junctional Complex

All epithelial cells, including those of the kidney tubule, are joined together along the lateral surfaces by a series of intercellular junctions first noted by their characteristic ultrastructural appearances and relative locations on the lateral plasma membrane (72). These include the tight junction, or *zonula occludens*, the adherens junction (also known as the *zonula adherens* or intermediate junction), desmosomes, and gap junctions. In most epithelia, the tight junction is located at the apical-most edge of the lateral membrane closely followed by the adherens junction. Desmosomes and gap junctions have less specific locations on the lateral membrane.

Desmosomes are large multiprotein complexes responsible mainly for mechanical attachment between neighboring epithelial cells (286). By transmission electron microscopy they appear as discrete, focal concentrations of dense material in the cytoplasm of adjacent cells as well as in the intercellular space (72). They are composed of both integral membrane proteins of the cadherin family called desmogleins and desmocollins, and peripheral membrane proteins known as desmoplakins, as well as a variety of other protein constituents (286). Adjacent cells adhere to each other through cadherin-mediated interactions. The peripheral components then provide mechanical stability to this interaction via keratin intermediate filaments in the cytoplasm of each cell. Ultrastructurally, these appear as a mass of hair-like protrusions interacting in parallel with each plaque and then splaying out into the cytoplasm (72, 286). In this manner, desmosomes link all cells in the epithelium. While there is evidence that desmosomal components may play an active role in regulating some aspects of cell–cell adhesion and even gene expression (see below) (351), in general their function is considered to be relatively passive.

Gap junctions are so named because of the characteristic 3-nm gap that is evident by transmission electron microscopy between two interacting cells (291). Examination of freeze-fractured specimens reveals the gap junction as a discrete array of intramembranous particles or connexons (291). Each connexon is composed of five identical connexins, a family of transmembrane proteins. Connexons on adjacent cells interact through their extracytoplasmic domains to form a series of low-resistance channels. These permit the passage of small molecules of less than 1 kD, both electrically and metabolically linking neighboring cells in the epithelium. In the kidney, it is likely that gap junctions play important roles during morphogenesis and repair, although their precise functions have not been investigated in detail (290).

Both tight junctions and adherens junctions are essential for establishing and maintaining polarization of epithelial cells, and for the correct physiologic functioning of the epithelium. For this reason, the structure and essential characteristics of each type of junction are extensively described in the next sections, followed by consideration of their roles in polarization.

Tight Junctions

Among the numerous functions subserved by epithelia, perhaps the most important is that of barrier between the intra- and extra-corporeal spaces. In the case of the kidney, the extracorporeal space is defined by the lumen of the renal tubule. The fact that the chemical composition of urine differs substantially from that of the extracellular fluid bathing the epithelial basolateral membranes is evidence that the barrier provided by the tubular epithelium is tight to small molecules. There are two components to this barrier, arranged in parallel (84). The first is comprised of the apical and basolateral plasma membranes of the epithelial cells themselves, which together serve as a pair of series resistances to the flow of solutes across the epithelia. The second barrier is provided by the intercellular junctions that join the epithelial cells to one another. The morphologic manifestation of this second component is the tight junctional ring, or zonula occludens (46, 99, 281, 303, 304).

The zonula occludens defines the border between the apical and basolateral plasma membrane surfaces. In columnar and cuboidal cells of the renal epithelium, it is found at the apical extremity of the lateral membrane and in the plane of the apical surface. Analysis by transmission electron microscopy suggested that the tight junction is actually a zone of partial fusion between the plasmalemmas of adjacent cells (72). When cells that have been treated with osmium are examined at high magnification, their membranes are distinguished by a characteristic pattern. The two leaflets of the lipid bilayer appear as a "unit membrane" defined by a pair of darkly staining parallel lines separated from one another by 5–10 nm (125). In areas corresponding to the tight junction, the four parallel lines representing the two unit membranes of the adjacent epithelial cells are replaced by three lines, which lead to the suggestion that the two outer leaflets contributed by the neighboring cells have in some way merged to form a new trilaminar membrane structure (75).

The putative outer-leaflet fusion suggested by morphologic studies received some support from examinations of lipid mobility in polarized epithelial cells. The mobility of outer-leaflet lipids is restricted by the tight junction (63,

327). Labeled lipid probes inserted into the outer leaflets of epithelial apical or basolateral plasmalemmas have unimpeded mobility within their respective domains but cannot cross the zonula occludens (63, 327). Furthermore, outer-leaflet lipids are unable to diffuse between neighboring epithelial cells through the tight junction. In contrast, inner-leaflet lipids can apparently move freely between the two plasma membrane domains, suggesting that the tight junction presents no barrier to their diffusion. These observations are consistent with a model of the zonula occludens in which the outer leaflets of the lipid bilayer participate in the formation of some junctional structure while the inner leaflet remains unperturbed. These results also suggest that the lipid composition of the apical inner leaflet is necessarily identical to that of the basolateral one, because any difference might be expected to be quickly randomized by diffusion. Thus, the differences in the lipid compositions of the apical and basolateral surfaces alluded to in the introductory paragraphs of this chapter must be entirely contributed by the constituents of the outer leaflet (328, 329).

Electron microscopy has provided further insights relevant to the structure of the zonula occludens. Examination of freeze-fracture replicas of epithelial cells reveals the tight junction to be composed of continuous branching and interwoven strands that surround the entire perimeter of the cell (299). These strands appear as elevations in the P, or cytoplasmic, fracture faces, and are matched by grooves in the E, or external, planes. The strands have a fibrillar appearance, and no discrete subunit structure can be resolved. It is now clear that these strands are composed of proteins known as claudins (90, 325). The claudin family includes more than a dozen members, each of which is a membrane protein that spans the membrane four times (210). Evidence that claudins comprise the principal structural components of the junctional strands derives from heterologous expression studies. Expression of claudins in fibroblast cells leads to the production of strands detectable by freeze fracture electron microscopy that closely resemble those associated with bona fide tight junctions in epithelial cells (87, 89). Claudins also determine the permeability properties of tight junctions (53, 88, 324, 326). In the kidney, the specific paracellular permeability characteristics found in each nephron segment are determined by the inventory of claudins expressed in their resident epithelial cells (292). Finally, it is interesting to note that the number and complexity of the strands seems to be correlated with the capacity of the junction to serve as a barrier (303). The number of parallel strands interposed between the apical and basolateral surfaces has been shown, in some systems, to be a rough indicator of the tightness of the junction as reflected in its electrical resistance.

In addition to the claudins, a large number of membrane and soluble proteins are associated with the zonula occludens (281, 304). The first protein to be identified in highly purified and extracted plasma membrane fractions is a polypeptide with a molecular weight of 225 kD named

ZO-1. In immunocytochemical experiments, antibodies raised against ZO-1 localize it exclusively to the tight junctional region of epithelial cells and to certain nonepithelial cells lacking tight junctions (303–305). Biochemical experiments reveal that ZO-1 is not a transmembrane protein, because it can be removed from plasmalemmal fractions by urea or alkaline extraction. ZO-1 is phosphorylated on serine residues, as well as tyrosine residues under certain circumstances, and is apparently released from the membrane under conditions in which intercellular tight junctions are disrupted (304). Sequencing of ZO-1 revealed that it belongs to a family of proteins known as MAGUK for membrane association and presence of the GUK domain. This family is characterized by the presence of one or more PDZ (PSD-95, discs large, ZO-1) domains, an src homology 3 (SH3) domain, and an area homologous to guanylate kinase (GUK), arranged sequentially on the molecule in the amino- to carboxy-terminal direction 280. Both PDZ and SH3 domains are involved in protein–protein interactions, and PDZ domains, in particular, may play important roles in basolateral localization and cell polarization (see later section). The GUK domain, which is not catalytically active in ZO-1, may also mediate protein–protein contacts. Recently, a splice variant of ZO-1 as well as two shorter homologues, ZO-2 and ZO-3 have been identified and sequenced (111, 120, 142, 304). In renal epithelial cells both ZO-2 and ZO-3 co-immunoprecipitate with ZO-1 and are localized exclusively to tight junctions. Biochemical studies suggest that both associate directly with ZO-1 but not with each other (111, 120, 142, 304). In subconfluent or injured epithelia, ZO-1 migrates to the nucleus, where it interacts with transcription factors to modulate the expression of genes involved in regulating growth control and differentiation (15, 16, 100).

The first transmembrane component of the tight junction identified was the protein occludin. Occludin is a phosphorylated polypeptide of 65 kD that is believed to span the membrane four times with both the amino- and carboxy-termini present on the cytoplasmic side (281, 304). There is in vitro evidence that occludin interacts with ZO-1. Because of its location in the membrane, occludin is believed to mediate cell–cell interactions via at least one of its extracellular loops. Indeed, treatment of cells with peptides corresponding to a loop sequence alters permeability and overexpression of occludin in fibroblasts increases adhesion (281, 304, 346). Recent studies using small interferring RNA technology to knock-down occludin indicate that it may facilitate signals to the actin cytoskeleton to help extrude apoptotic cells from the epithelium (346).

Nevertheless, occludin does not contribute to the interlocking strands of the tight junction because embryonic stem cells in which both occludin alleles have been deleted can still differentiate into epithelial aggregates with morphologically intact and physiologically functional tight junctions (276). In particular, ZO-1 localizes properly in these cells and the pattern of strands and grooves seen by electron microscopy of freeze-fractured specimens appears normal.

At least six other peripheral components of the tight junction have been identified (281, 304). Cingulin, which is homologous to cytoskeletal proteins bearing coiled-coil domains, has been localized further from the junctional membrane than ZO-1. Other notable proteins found at the junctions include small GTP-binding proteins in the rab family, as well as AF-6, which can bind ras, another small GTP-binding protein. Finally, actin, which is certainly not uniquely associated with the tight junction, has been reported to interact directly with ZO-1 in nonepithelial cells. As mentioned earlier, there is evidence that contraction of actin in the terminal web of epithelial cells can substantially alter transepithelial permeability (177, 235, 322).

Adherens Junctions

The adherens junction, or zonula adherens, forms a belt just below the tight junction in most epithelial cells connecting them via extracellular interactions and cytoplasmic linkages to the actin cytoskeleton. In the electron microscope, adherens junctions appear as a dense, somewhat amorphous concentration of submembranous staining, with a mass of impinging actin filaments (72). The major adhesive component of the adherens junction in epithelial cells is E-cadherin (originally called uvomorulin) (343). E-cadherin is a single-pass transmembrane protein that consists of a series of calcium-binding extracellular or EC domains, and a cytoplasmic tail that interacts with a protein called β-catenin. In the membrane, E-cadherin exists as a homodimer, and, while concentrated in the adherens junction, may be distributed over the entire basolateral membrane. β-catenin is homologous to the protein plakoglobin (or α-catenin), that is found mainly in desmosomes but sometimes substitutes for β-catenin in adherens junctions (see below) (343). Both E-cadherin and β-catenin are linked to the actin cytoskeleton through α-catenin, which binds to β-catenin, and is also found to a lesser extent in both tight junctions and desmosomes. In addition to the catenins, there is evidence that a number of other proteins involved in signaling also associate with E-cadherin (343).

In the presence of calcium, epithelial cells adhere to each other initially via E-cadherin. These interactions trigger a number of other events in the cell, some of which are only now beginning to be understood. Formation of tight junctions, for example, is dependent on E-cadherin–mediated linkages, as is the establishment of desmosomes. Cultured epithelial cell lines, for example, will attach to the culture substratum in the near absence of calcium. Under these conditions, not only do adherens junctions fail to form, but neither do tight junctions or desmosomes. As soon as normal concentrations of calcium are added back to the medium, at least adherens junctions and tight junctions rapidly assemble, as demonstrated by the detection of transmonolayer electrical resistance within minutes (231, 330). This hierarchical relationship may be mainly mechanical, with E-cadherin interactions pulling the membranes sufficiently close together to enable the other junctions to form. Alternatively, it is possible that cytoplasmic signals generated by E-cadherin–dependent adhesion somehow activates or initiates assembly of the other junctions.

While the extracellular domain of E-cadherin is intrinsically adhesive, formation of fully functional junctions depends on the cytoplasmic domain and its interaction with the catenins and actin (343). This has been demonstrated in reconstruction experiments in which E-cadherin is expressed in nonepithelial cells (196, 222, 223, 247). While these do not normally form adherens junctions, they still express catenins. Thus, in the presence of exogenous E-cadherin they will adhere to one another, forming a monolayer whose appearance resembles a true epithelium by light microscopy. When E-cadherin mutants lacking the cytoplasmic tail are expressed, some cell–cell adhesion is detected, but it is mechanically unstable and there is no colocalization of catenins or concentration of actin in the region of cell–cell contacts.

In an interesting twist, expression of a chimeric form of E-cadherin fused to α-catenin obviates the need for α-catenin, leading to the formation of fully developed adherens junctions (221). Based on this experiment, one might ask why β-catenin is needed at all as an adapter between E-cadherin and α-catenin. The answer is apparently that β-catenin is an important regulatory molecule of both cell adhesion and gene expression in epithelial cells (343). This conclusion was reached through an amazing confluence of lines of investigation in both cell and cancer biology. Studies of transformed epithelial cells over a number of years demonstrated that transformation in general and invasive behavior in particular seemed to correlate with loss of E-cadherin (17, 20, 112, 351). Originally, this was explained mechanically; clearly, for cells to migrate during invasion of other tissues, cell–cell contacts had to break. Perhaps transformation led to the downregulation of E-cadherin as well as other components of the adherens junction. Independently, other investigators studying the genetics of colon cancer identified a gene for familial adenomatous polyposis coli (APC), which leads to a high frequency of colonic polyps and early incidence of colon cancer (17, 112, 351). The gene product of this APC gene turned out to be a cytoplasmic protein that binds β-catenin and facilitates its proteolytic destruction. In the absence of functional APC, β-catenin not bound to E-cadherin enters the nucleus where it is capable of activating certain genes contributing to carcinogenesis. Recently, it has been found that the degradation of β-catenin captured by the APC protein is negatively regulated by the Wnt/Frz pathway, the mammalian analogue of the wingless/frizzled/disheveled pathway originally described in *Drosophila* (17, 112, 351). When Wnt binds its receptor Frz in the plasma membrane it activates dsh. This in turn inhibits glycogen synthase kinase 3β (GSK3β), a component of the APC-β-catenin complex, preventing its phosphorylation of β-catenin and subse-

quent degradation. In this manner, the available APC protein in the cell becomes saturated with β-catenin, and excess free-cytoplasmic β-catenin enters the nucleus. Thus, β-catenin has three possible fates in the cell. It can bind E-cadherin and facilitate cytoskeletal association with the adherens junction. Alternatively, it can float free in the cytoplasm where it will either bind the APC protein and be proteolytically degraded, or enter the nucleus and activate gene expression (17, 112, 351). As complex as this regulatory pathway seems, the description provided here is undoubtedly oversimplified. APC protein also has a binding site for other proteins, including tubulin and axin (17). Furthermore, how transformation regulates the amount of E-cadherin on the cell surface, one of the original observations that led to the discovery of β-catenin's regulatory role, remains unclear. One possibility is that nuclear β-catenin can affect the expression of E-cadherin, although this remains unproven (17, 112, 351). As will be described in the subsequent section, E-cadherin plays an essential role in epithelial cell polarization. Thus, β-catenin regulation is key to understanding the organization of epithelia.

Apical Microvillar Surface

The apical brush border membrane is perhaps best epitomized by the one that graces the epithelial cells of the proximal tubule. Named for its appearance, the proximal tubular brush border is comprised of densely packed parallel microvilli that rise like the bristles of a brush from the level of the tight junctions to a height of 1 to 1.3 μm. The proximal tubular brush border is far and away the most luxuriant to be found in the nephron; although the apical membranes of other renal epithelial cell types are endowed with small collections of microvilli, much less is known about the structural specializations characteristic of the apical membranes of more distal renal epithelial cells (107).

The functions subserved by apical microvilli are not entirely clear. Certainly their most dramatic and obvious effect on the properties of the apical membrane is manifest as a tremendous amplification of the apical membrane surface area. For the proximal tubule this amplification is on the order of 20-fold (193, 340). As is the case for the epithelia of the small intestine, it is through this redundancy that the proximal tubular epithelial cells markedly increase the efficiency of both their absorptive and degradative functions.

Physiologically, the proximal tubule is responsible for the resorption of ~60% of the filtered load of fluid and solutes (179). Furthermore, it mediates the digestion of essentially all of the polysaccharides and peptides present in the glomerular filtrate, and transports the resultant sugars and amino acids from the lumen to the interstitial fluid space (193). It is apparent, therefore, that the epithelial cells of the proximal tubule must be specially equipped in order to cope efficiently with the comparatively enormous quantities of fluid and substrates that rapidly transit this nephron segment. The presence of an extravagant brush border greatly increases the fraction of the tubular fluid that comes into close contact with the enzymatic and transport systems arrayed on the microvillar surfaces prior to its passage from this tubule segment into the descending loop of Henle. Concomitantly, it proportionally multiplies the number of enzymatic and transport systems available to modify the substrates dissolved in the tubular fluid. Thus, the brush border membrane provides the scaffolding for the relatively massive arsenal of enzymatic and transport machinery required to accomplish the proximal tubule's function as a high capacity and high throughput resorptive system.

Ultrastructurally, a microvillus is composed of a bundle of 20–30 parallel thin filaments that are linked to one another and to the overlying surface membrane by protein cross-bridges (207). The thin filaments extend well beyond the base of the microvillus and are anchored in a dense matrix of fibers oriented parallel to the plane of the membrane. This meshwork, referred to as the terminal web, underlies the entire apical surface and anastomses with the filaments that radiate from the lateral desmosomes and zonulae adherens. The functional implications of these structural arrangements have become clearer as their components have been biochemically identified.

The thin filaments that form the microvillar core are composed of actin (31, 207). Ultrastructural studies employing heavy meromyosin reveal that all of the filaments in the bundle share a single polarity and are oriented with their nucleating end towards the microvillar tip. At their termination in the microvillar tip the filaments are received by an electron-dense cap whose molecular identity has yet to be established (207). As they emerge from the base of the microvillus, the actin filaments are caught up in the fibers of the terminal web. Fodrin, or nonerythroid spectrin, comprises one of the major components of this network (97, 207). It appears to function beneath the brush border as an actin fiber cross-linker. Another of the chief constituents of this fibrillar matrix is a nonmuscle form of myosin II that belongs to the same myosin subfamily as its skeletal muscle counterpart. Bipolar myosin thick filaments appear to interact with the actin filaments as they sweep out of the microvillar sheath to join the terminal web (32, 65, 207). Paired antiparallel myosin filaments cross-link the actin filaments of neighboring microvilli to one another, forming a connection that bears close comparison to the actin–myosin arrangement characteristic of the striated muscle sarcomere. The analogy is strengthened by the presence in the microvillar rootlet of tropomyosin, a protein that functions in skeletal muscle to regulate the interaction between actin and myosin (65, 128).

This marked molecular similarity between the terminal web and the skeletal muscle contractile unit prompted speculation that this arrangement might also be functionally homologous. A number of investigators have postulated that activation of myosin-based contraction at the microvillar base might lead to microvillar shortening (206). Repetitive activation of such a mechanism would lead to a piston-like extension and retraction of these membranous processes, which in turn might stir the surrounding tubular fluid. Such a mixing motion is certainly teleologically appealing, in that it would help to ensure that the tubular fluid is uniformly exposed to the enzymatic and transport systems of the proximal tubular apical membrane surface. No evidence for any such concerted and dynamic properties of microvilli has yet been gathered.

Biochemical studies have shed light on the identities and functional properties of some of the proteins that contribute to the interfibrillar cross-bridges observed in transmission electron micrographic profiles of microvilli. Howe and Mooseker (131) identified a protein of molecular weight 110 kDa that participates in cross-linking the filaments of intestinal microvilli to the plasma membrane. This protein exhibits a high affinity for the calcium-binding protein calmodulin, which participates in the transduction of a number of calcium-regulated phenomena (131). Of further interest was the fact that the 110-kDa protein manifests a myosin-like Mg-ATPase activity (209). Addition of ATP to intact microvilli results in solubilization of the 110-kDa protein and disruption of the cross-links between the actin filaments and the microvillar membrane (56, 188). Thus, attachment of the plasma membrane to the thin filaments may be regulated by ATP and calcium. The degree to which this putative capacity for structural modulation plays a role in microvillar function has yet to be clarified. Subsequent molecular analysis revealed that the brush border 110-kDa protein belongs to the myosin I family of unconventional myosin molecules (92, 130). Unlike skeletal muscle myosin (which is assigned to the myosin II classification), brush border myosin I molecules possess a single globular head group and do not form bipolar filaments (49, 55, 208, 209). Members of the myosin I family, including brush border myosin I, have been found to associate with the membranes of intracellular vesicles, prompting the hypothesis that these motor proteins serve to propel vesicles through the cytoplasm along actin filament tracks (64). Co-localization studies have demonstrated that brush border myosin I and the microtubule-dependent motor protein dynein can be found together on the membranes of post-Golgi vesicles (73). This observation has inspired the hypothesis that apically directed vesicles depart the Golgi along microtubule tracks powered by the action of dynein. Upon their arrival at the actin-rich terminal web, they switch engines and are carried the rest of the way to the brush border by myosin I (74). While brush border myosin I is abundantly expressed in intestinal epithelial cells, it may be present at lower levels in the renal proximal tubule (19). Since the myosin I family is large and diverse, however, it is extremely likely that an as yet unidentified member of this class subserves similar structural and mechanical functions in the epithelial cells of the kidney (58).

Another protein that apparently participates in the organization of the microvillus has a molecular weight of 95 kDa and has been dubbed *villin* (33). A cDNA encoding the villin molecule has been isolated and sequenced (9). It is apparent from this analysis that villin belongs to a large family of actin-binding proteins. Prominent in its structure is a pair of sequence domains that appear to be involved in associations with f-actin. The presence of this tandem repeat justifies the contention that villin mediates the bundling of actin fibers. It is interesting to note that villin is a calcium-binding protein and that interaction with calcium alters its behavior in the presence of actin filaments (189). In experiments carried out with purified villin in solution, it has been found that this protein bundles actin filaments when the free calcium concentration is less than 1 μM. When the calcium concentration rises to 10 μM, villin severs actin filaments into short protofilaments. At intermediate calcium concentrations, villin binds to actin filaments at their growing ends, forming a cap that prevents further elongation. Due to the dynamic nature of the microfilament polymer, this capping results in the formation of shortened filaments. It is not known whether these calcium-dependent activities of villin are manifest in vivo. If villin does indeed sever or shorten actin filaments within the living cell, it would seem likely that perturbations which produce elevations of intracellular calcium concentrations may lead to structurally significant alterations in the organization of the microvillar scaffolding. During embryonic development, villin is expressed throughout the cytoplasm of epithelial cells prior to the elevation of a brush border (265). At later stages, villin becomes localized to the cytosolic surface of the apical membrane and is subsequently incorporated into forming microvilli. This behavior has led to the suggestion that the localization of villin to the apical surface is a watershed event in the biogenesis of microvilli. Interestingly, expression of the cDNA encoding villin in fibroblasts, which normally lack microvillar processes, results in the formation of microvillus-like structures (83). Thus, the formation of interfilamentous bridges presumably mediated by villin may be a critical first step in the organization of the microvillar infrastructure. Supporting this model are the results of experiments in which Caco-2 intestinal epithelial cells were stably transfected with a vector encoding antisense villin mRNA (57). The consequent reduction in villin expression resulted in a loss of the brush border and mis-sorting of a subset of apical microvillar proteins. It must be noted, however, that results from gene knockout experiments argue against a central role for villin in microvillus formation (255). Mice whose villin genes have been disrupted and which produce no villin protein are able nonetheless to generate morphologically and apparently physiologically normal brush borders. Presumably, other components of the microvillar infrastructure can shoulder the cross-linking and organizational duties normally performed by villin. Such functional redundancy is typical of biological systems endowed with architecture as esthetically elegant and complex as that which graces the microvillus.

While villin is limited in its distribution to those cell types endowed with brush borders, another actin-bundling component of the microvillus is present in numerous structures. Fimbrin is a 68-kDa polypeptide associated with the interfilamentous cross-bridges that can also be detected in hair cell stereocilia and in ruffled borders (31). Fimbrin is clearly a multivalent actin-binding protein and participates in the cross-linking of the microvillar actin filament array. The degree to which its role in this process is related to or distinct from that of villin has yet to be established. Several other polypeptides associated with the microvillar core have also been identified. A protein of molecular weight 80 kDa that exhibits homology with a substrate of the epidermal growth factor receptor tyrosine kinase suggests another possible pathway through which microvillar structure and function might be manipulated (104). A 200-kDa protein has been identified which may serve as the transmembrane anchor for the 110-kDa myosin I–like protein discussed above (59). This protein was isolated from porcine intestinal microvilli and may be cleaved to a 140-kDa form during development. In vitro studies suggest that this glycoprotein manifests an affinity for the 110-kDa myosin I polypeptide. It should be noted, however, that studies suggest that the myosin I protein can interact with high affinity with protein-free liposomes composed of negatively charged phospholipids (122). These observations suggest the possibility that myosin I might link actin filaments directly to the lipids of the overlying plasmalemma without any requirement for a transmembrane proteinaceous adapter. Arguing against this possibility are recent results demonstrating that although phospholipid-bound myosin I is active as an ATPase, when attached to membranes in this configuration it loses its capacity to serve as an actin-based motor (354). The nature of all of these interactions remains to be elucidated. Several other proteins have been identified as possible links between microvillar actin filaments and the overlying plasma membrane. Zipper protein is a transmembrane polypeptide that derives its name from a cluster of 27 leucine zipper heptad repeats (25). The C-terminal domain of zipper protein can compete with tropomyosin for binding to actin filaments, suggesting that both polypeptides interact with the same binding site. Zipper protein can also inhibit actin activation of the brush-border myosin I ATPase activity, although it has no effect on the myosin's endogenous ATPase activity. These observations are consistent with the possibility that zipper protein may regulate the association of microvillar actin filaments with molecular motors and other mechanotransducing proteins. Finally, a similar linking function has been ascribed to members of the ezrin-radixin-moesin family of proteins (30). The C-terminal tails of these polypeptides bind to actin filaments, while their N-termini interact with proteins in the membrane. It has also been shown that a number of proteins involved in the generation or regulation of intracellular second messengers associate in macromolecular complexes with ezrin-radixin-moesin family members, suggesting that in addition to functioning as linkers these proteins may also act as scaffolding for the assembly of components involved in signal transduction.

The terminal web mentioned above consists of three morphologically distinguishable domains. In addition to the cytoskeletal fibers that receive the rootlets of the microvilli, fibers that arise from desmosomes and the zonula adherens contribute to this meshwork. The desmosomal fibers consist primarily of 10-nm intermediate filaments composed of keratins (81). At the level of the zonula adherens, the cell is ringed by a complex of randomly polarized actin filaments that also contains myosin and tropomyosin (65). In vitro experiments have demonstrated that this ring has the capacity to contract circumferentially (38). This capacity has led to the speculation that contraction of the zonula adherens ring might contribute to the alterations in tight junctional permeability that have been observed in several epithelial systems in response to certain second messengers and osmotic stress (177). Thus, activation of sodium-coupled glucose uptake in cultured intestinal epithelial cells has been shown to induce a decrease in transepithelial resistance. This effect is dependent on the activity of myosin light-chain kinase (123, 322). It is thought that by shortening in a "purse-string" fashion, these filaments might actually draw neighboring cells away from one another and thus modify the structure and permeability of the occluding junctions. The relevance of this model to the functioning of renal epithelia has yet to be established.

The anisotropy and structural complexity that characterize the filamentous core of the microvillus apparently extend as well to its overlying plasma membrane. The proteins embedded in and associated with the plasmalemma of the proximal tubule brush border are not uniformly distributed over its surface but rather are restricted to specific subdomains. This lateral segregation is epitomized by the behavior of two transmembrane polypeptides, maltase and gp330. The 300-kDa enzyme maltase is distributed over the entire surface of the microvilli themselves, but is absent from the intermicrovillar membrane regions (146, 266). In contrast, the heavily glycosylated gp330 (also known as megalin) is restricted in its distribution to these intermicrovillar regions. The restriction of megalin to the intermicrovillar regions appears to be mediated by its interactions with protein components of the endocytic machinery (224). Ultrastructural examination of the intermicrovillar regions reveals the presence of coated pits. The cytosolic surface of the plasma membrane in these domains is coated with an electron-dense material that biochemical and immunoelectron microscopic studies have demonstrated to be clathrin (266). The presence in these intermicrovillar pits of morphologic and compositional features associated with the process of endocytosis has led investigators to believe that this domain mediates the retrieval of large peptides and proteins from the proximal tubular fluid. The proximal tubular epithelial cells are responsible for capturing and degrading any pro-

teins that pass through the glomerular filtration barrier (193). This function is apparently served by the profusion of coated pits and vesicles that decorate the surfaces of membranes at the microvillar base. The function of gp330/megalin has recently been clearly elucidated. Megalin is a member of the low density lipoprotein (LDL) receptor family and, together with cubulin, serves as receptor that binds to and mediates the uptake of filtered proteins and peptides (27). Megalin knockout mice exhibit low-molecular-weight proteinuria, establishing the critical role for megalin as the proximal tubule's preeminent scavenger (164, 236).

Finally, it is worth noting that most or all of the epithelial cells of the nephron are endowed with a single primary cilium (256). This nonmotile cilium possesses an outer ring of nine microtubules but lacks the central pair of microtubules found in motile cilia. This primary cilium appears to serve sensory functions. Bending the primary cilium, in response to flow or mechanical stimuli, induces calcium signaling in renal epithelial cells (257). Furthermore, the functional integrity of the primary cilium appears to be a prerequisite for the maintenance of normal renal tubular architecture. A number of cystic diseases of the kidney are attributable to mutations in genes encoding proteins found in cilia (170, 172, 205, 345). Similarly, mice in which expression of ciliary proteins has been disrupted develop cysts. The mechanism through which loss of the cilium's mechanosensory functions leads to cystic transformation remains to be established.

Basolateral Plasma Membrane

The rigid subservience of structure to function so elegantly exemplified by the apical brush-border membrane extends as well to the basolateral surface of the epithelial plasma membrane. As was mentioned above, the basolateral membrane possesses the ion pumps that power the transepithelial resorption of solutes and water. The resorptive capacity of a given cell type is thus largely dependent on the quantity of ion pumps embedded within its basolateral plasmalemma. This parameter appears in turn to be roughly proportional to the surface area encompassed by this membrane domain (245). Consequently, renal epithelial cells that participate in the resorption of large quantities of ions and fluid (such as those of the proximal tubule) as well as cells that carry out resorption of ions against steep concentration gradients (such as those of the thick ascending limb of the loop of Henle) are endowed with basolateral plasmalemmas whose surface areas are amplified through massively redundant infoldings.

As was detailed in the discussion of the apical brush border, the lateral distribution of proteins within the plane of the basolateral membrane is not uniform. This fact is most dramatically illustrated by epithelial cell types that lack the deeply invaginated basolateral infoldings discussed above. Studies have demonstrated that the Na^+,K^+-ATPase is concentrated in subdomains of the basolateral membranes of small intestinal epithelial cells (6). The sodium pump is essentially restricted to the lateral membranes of these cells and is absent from the basal surfaces that rest on the basement membrane. Dislodging these cells from the underlying basement membrane produces a redistribution of the sodium pump throughout the entire basolateral plasmalemma. These results suggest that the sodium pump is either actively or passively prevented from entering the basal domain of the plasmalemma in some manner that is dependent on an intact interaction with the basement membrane. The meshwork of cytoskeletal elements associated with those sites at which the epithelial cell is anchored to basement membrane fibrils may be too dense to allow membrane proteins such as the sodium pump to penetrate. Conversely, cytoskeletal restraints whose integrity requires cell attachment to the basement membrane might retain the sodium pump within the lateral subdomains. In each of these scenarios, the cytoskeleton plays an important role in determining the subcellular distribution of a transmembrane protein. Recent research has made it quite clear that the cytoskeleton plays a critical role in defining polarized domains and in determining aspects of their polypeptide compositions (2, 196, 211, 226–229, 231, 249, 264, 277, 336). The role of the cytoskeleton in the generation and maintenance of polarized distributions of membrane proteins will be discussed later in this chapter.

Polarized Distribution of Organelles

The massive complement of ATP driven ion pumps deployed in the basolateral infoldings consumes a significant fraction of the epithelial cell's metabolic energy. It is not surprising, therefore, that the cytosolic spaces between adjacent infoldings are frequently occupied by mitochondria. In the proximal tubule, these mitochondria are oriented parallel to the infoldings. This vertical alignment of the mitochondria associated with the basolateral surface gives rise to this membrane domain's typically striated appearance when examined by light microscopy (318). The mechanism through which mitochondria come to be located in the regions of the cell that are precisely engineered to use energy is entirely unknown. Presumably, this localization is brought about through interactions between the mitochondria and elements of the cytoskeleton such as microtubules. Precedent for mitochondrial–microtubular interaction exists in elegant experiments performed on neuronal axoplasm that demonstrate that mitochondria "crawl" on microtubule tracks with the help of the ATP-driven kinesin motor (323). It is clear that this juxtaposition ensures that energy is delivered to the transport enzymes of the basolateral surface with the smallest possible diffusional losses.

This discussion highlights the fact that the term "polarized," as applied to epithelia, refers not only to the distribution of plasmalemmal proteins, but also to the arrangement of cytosolic structures and organelles. In addition to the nonrandom distribution of mitochondria, epithelial cells are notable for apically disposed Golgi complexes as well as basally positioned nuclei and endoplasmic reticulum (ER) (72). Spe-

cialized, cell-type specific structures are also distributed with polarity. Thus, the apical cytoplasm of α-intercalated cells is populated by acidic endocytic vesicles (285). In contrast, the acidic endosomal vesicles of β-intercalated cells are restricted to cytoplasm in the vicinity of the basolateral plasma membrane (285). Finally, in the absence of antidiuretic hormone stimulation the principal cells of the collecting tubule store transmembrane water channels in vesicles that gather in the apical cytoplasm (118, 167, 333). These examples support the concept that the anisotropy characteristic of epithelia extends to every aspect of their organization. Clearly, epithelial cells organize themselves, both at the molecular and organellar levels, along an axis determined by external stimuli (225, 269). As discussed later in this chapter, it is currently thought that the most important of these external stimuli is contact with the epithelial basement membrane and with adjacent epithelial cells (225, 231, 269, 272, 330, 331, 336). The machinery that transduces and responds to these stimuli includes the integrin family of basement membrane receptors, cell adhesion molecules, and elements of the cytoskeleton with which these families of molecules interact.

BIOGENESIS OF EPITHELIAL POLARITY

In Vitro Systems

The kidney's complicated architecture and cellular heterogeneity renders it a poor substrate for studies designed to examine dynamic cell biologic processes. Over the past three decades, the vast majority of research into the mechanisms through which epithelia generate and maintain their polarized phenotype has made use of several continuous lines of cultured epithelial cells. These cell lines retain many of the differentiated properties of their respective parent tissues in vitro. Thus, LLC-PK1 cells resemble the proximal tubule (although their precise origin is uncertain) (293). Similarly, Caco-2, HT-29, and T84 cells behave like their progenitors, the colonocytes of the large intestine (293). Most importantly for the purposes of this discussion, they manifest in culture the biochemical and morphologic features of the polarized state. Perhaps the best characterized and most heavily used of these culture models is the Madin–Darby canine kidney (MDCK) line. MDCK cells were originally derived from a normal dog kidney in 1959 and grown in culture as a partially transformed line; that is, MDCK cells grow immortally as a monolayer and will not form tumors in nude mice (93, 178). Although their precise point of origin along the nephron is not entirely clear, their physiologic and morphologic properties suggest that they derive from cells of the thick ascending limb, distal tubule, or collecting tubule (127).

The first clues to the polarized nature of the MDCK cell line came from the direct observation of these cells' capacity for vectorial transport. When grown on impermeable substrata, MDCK cells form domes (also called blisters or hemicysts) (165). Physiologic studies have demonstrated that domes develop as a result of the transepithelial transport of solutes from the apical media to the basolateral surface (1). Water that passively follows these solutes results in the generation of fluid-filled blisters. It is fair to say that domes arise in regions where the cells have literally pumped themselves up off the dish. In keeping with this dramatic propensity for unidirectional solute movement, each MDCK cell manifests a polarized distribution of ion-transport proteins, including several routes for sodium entry in its apical membrane and of the order of 10^6 molecules of the Na^+,K^+-ATPase in its basolateral plasmalemma (45). The popularity of MDCK cells for polarity research developed out of the seminal observations of Rodriquez-Boulan and Sabatini in 1978 (268). In studies on the budding of enveloped viruses from MDCK cells, these investigators found that the influenza virus assembles at, and buds from, the apical cell surface (Fig. 1). Of even greater significance was the demonstration that the spike glycoproteins which populate the membranes of these viruses accumulate preferentially at the cell surface from which budding is to occur (267). Thus, the influenza hemagglutinin (HA) protein is predominately on the apical surface of MDCK cells early in infection. Similarly, the G protein of vesicular stomatitis virus (VSV) is almost exclusively basolateral in infected cells. The viral proteins provided investigators with the first experimentally manipulable system for the study of membrane protein sorting. A large number of studies have subsequently elucidated the sorting of many endogenous MDCK cell proteins as well as exogenous proteins expressed from vectors. This system remains the most thoroughly investigated paradigm and, as will be detailed below, has yielded important insights into the nature of the pathways and signals that participate in membrane protein targeting and the overall biogenesis of epithelial polarity.

Recently, investigators have endeavored to develop new cell lines to study particular aspects of renal cell biology. For example, immortalization genes from human papilloma virus or a hybrid between adenovirus and SV40 have been used to create permanent cell lines from human proximal tubule cells (259, 275). These cell lines are of particular interest because of the proclivity of the proximal tubule to suffer injury following ischemic insult. The cell lines retain differentiated characteristics of the proximal tubule, including expression of brush border markers and sodium dependent/phlorizin-sensitive sugar transport. Cultures of cell lines derived in this fashion are not, however, always able to stably maintain the uniform morphology of a simple epithelium, limiting their usefulness for studies of epithelial polarity.

The study of epithelial cell polarization using cell lines has been facilitated by culturing cells in configurations that more closely resemble in vivo conditions. For example, many varieties of epithelial cells can be grown on permeable filter supports (119, 202). Originally, these were designed to mimic the Ussing chamber used for physiologic studies, but

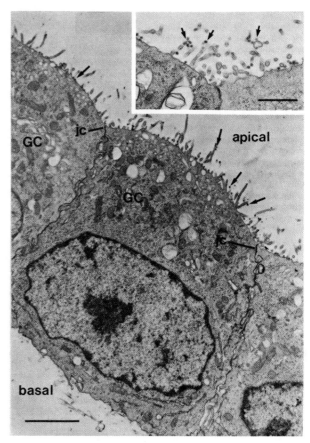

FIGURE 1   The influenza virus buds from the apical surface of MDCK cells. MDCK cells were grown on a hydrated collagen gel, infected with influenza virus for 6 hours, and prepared for electron microscopy. The arrows denote mature virions which assemble at, and bud from, the apical surface. No virus particles are detected at the basal or lateral surfaces. Bar represents 3.0 μm (inset bar represents 1.0 μm). GC, Golgi complex; jc, junctional complex. (Reprinted with permission from Caplan M, Matlin KS. Sorting of membrane and secretory proteins in polarized epithelial cells. In: Matlin KS, Valentich JC, eds. *Functional Epithelial Cells in Culture.* New York: Liss, 1989:71–127.)

later turned out to also be very useful for biochemical and morphologic experiments as well. In their most common configuration, these supports are composed of polycarbonate filters that form the bottom cup (Fig. 2). The cup is then suspended in a plastic well containing media, and media is added to the inner compartment of the cup. Cells are plated on the upper surface of the filter. When a confluent monolayer is formed, it effectively creates a barrier between the two media compartments. The media in the interior of the cup bathes the epithelial apical surface, whereas the basolateral surface communicates with the exterior media compartment through the pores of the filter. As epithelial cells in the kidney and other organs would normally receive most of their nutrition from the basolateral (serosal) surface, permeable supports are in a sense a more natural growth environment than impermeable tissue culture plastic or glass. Indeed, there is some evidence that epithelial cells are more polarized in filter cultures than on solid substrata (86). Fur-

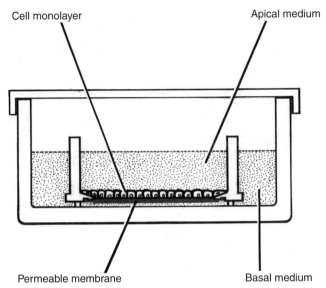

Cell monolayer

Apical medium

Permeable membrane

Basal medium

FIGURE 2 Epithelial monolayers can be grown on permeable filter supports. As depicted in the diagram, a porous filter, composed of cellulose actetate or polycarbonate, forms the bottom of a cylindrical cup. Epithelial cells are plated on top of the filter, and the cup is placed in a well filled with media. When the cells become confluent, the resultant monolayer forms a barrier between the media bathing the apical surface and the media in communication with the basolateral surface. This system thus provides investigators with simultaneous and independent access to both plasmalemmal domains.

thermore, the use of filters for the culture of epithelial cells permits investigators simultaneous and independent access to the apical and basolateral plasmalemmal surfaces (187). This useful capacity has been extensively exploited in the experiments described below.

In addition to permeable supports, a number of investigators have now begun to culture renal and other epithelial cell lines embedded in a gel of collagen I or other extracellular matrix molecules. These are called three-dimensional (3D) cultures to distinguish them from more common two-dimensional (2D) cultures on either solid or permeable culture surfaces (Fig. 3) (238, 352) . As with permeable supports, the idea behind 3D cultures is that placing the epithelial cell in an environment in which it is surrounded by

an interstitium more closely resembles the in vivo environment. While that conclusion is subject to debate, there is no doubt that certain epithelial phenotypes are more readily expressed in 3D than in 2D cultures (238, 352). Nevertheless, these phenotypes are often slow to develop, frequently taking 7 to 10 days, and may occur asynchronously. This, and the inaccessibility of the cultures somewhat limits their usefulness for biochemical studies. With the advent of high-resolution confocal fluorescent microscopy and the wide array of fluorescent proteins and probes, the impact of this limitation is lessened. Most often, individual suspended cells develop into polarized cysts or, when stimulated with certain growth factors, tubules. As will be described below, use of 3D cultures has led to important fundamental observations about epithelial cell polarization (238, 352).

Adhesion Promotes Epithelial Polarization

Morphogenesis of cells into a polarized epithelium depends on signals from the extracellular environment (70, 225, 269, 282, 344). These signals originate from the attachment of cells to each other and to the substratum, which, in most cases, is the extracellular matrix. If the pattern of cell attachments is asymmetric, then the response of the cell is also asymmetric, and a polar phenotype results. The signals are interpreted by the cell hierarchically (225, 269, 282, 344). Cell adhesion leads to restructuring of the cytoskeleton; junction formation, organization of the cytoplasm and organelles, and sorting of membrane components to the apical and basolateral plasma membrane domains then follow. Although the outline of this complex series of events has been known for some time, until recently only a few of the molecules involved in the process had been identified. As described previously, cell–cell contacts are mediated primarily via E-cadherin and its associated proteins. Cell substratum interactions, on the other hand, are mainly accomplished through integrins interacting with specific extracellular matrix molecules. Following adhesion, signals are generated within the cell that are translated into reorganization of the cytoskeleton, expression of new proteins, and positioning of these proteins into locations within the cell such that their

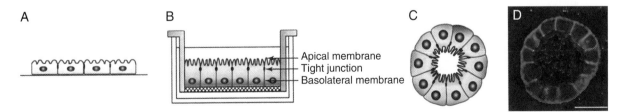

A   B   Apical membrane — Tight junction — Basolateral membrane   C   D

FIGURE 3 Two- and three-dimensional cultures of polarized epithelial cells. Epithelial cell lines may be grown on conventional impermeable substrata such as plastic or glass (A), or on permeable supports (B). In both cases, the provision of a flat, two-dimensional surface may provide spatial signals that normally would be generated by the cells themselves in vivo. In this regard, three-dimensional culture of cells in collagen gels, where a polarized cyst develops over 7 to 10 days (C), may more accurately represent the in vivo environment. In (D), an MDCK cell cyst is fluorescently labeled with antibodies to β-catenin to highlight the basolateral surface. (Reprinted with permission from Zegers MM, O'Brien LE, Yu W, Datta A, Mostov KE. Epithelial polarity and tubulogenesis in vitro. *Trends Cell Biol* 2003;13:169–176.)

function first creates and then maintains the polarized state. Recent research suggests that the mechanisms for generating cell asymmetry are shared by all eukaryotic cells, including simple microorganisms such as yeast and nonepithelial cells such as fibroblasts. What is unique in epithelial cells is not that an axis of polarity is set up within the cell, but that this axis is oriented identically in all interacting cells in the epithelium and is stable as long as the epithelium is not disrupted.

The following sections will summarize current knowledge of the mechanisms of epithelial polarization. As with the polarization hierarchy itself, the presentation will proceed from the proximal adhesive events to signals generated by adhesion and subsequent organization of specific protein complexes believed to be essential for polarization.

Integrins and Other Extracellular Matrix Receptors

The integrins are a superfamily of cell adhesion molecules found in nearly all cells (124, 138, 139). Each integrin consists of a heterodimer of α and β subunits, both of which are transmembrane glycoproteins. A total of 18 α and 8 β subunits are now known in mammals, resulting in at least 24 heterodimers (138). Although integrins are known to be receptors for a variety of extracellular matrix proteins, they may also participate in cell–cell adhesion (124, 138, 139). Epithelial cells of the kidney and other organs typically express an array of integrins including multiple forms with the β1 subunit as well as some with the β3 or β5 subunits (157). The former are most often receptors for collagens and laminins, while the latter are receptors for interstitial or serum proteins such as fibronectin or vitronectin. Many epithelial cells also express integrin α6β4, a laminin receptor (138, 157). The β4 subunit is uniquely found in epithelial cells, and, unlike most other integrins, mediates adhesion through cytokeratins rather than the actin cytoskeleton. The MDCK cell line, for example, expresses α2β1, α3β1, α6β4, and αVβ3 (283). The β1 integrins are receptors for collagens and laminins in these cells, while α6β4 is a receptor for the laminin-5 (LN5) isoform and possibly other laminins (157). Integrin αVβ3 mediates attachment to ligands containing arginine-glycine-aspartate (RGD) sequences such as fibronectin and vitronectin. Recent expression analysis also suggests that integrins containing both the β5 and β6 subunits are also expressed (A. Manninen, University of Oulu, Oulu, Finlar, personal communication, 2006). The complement of integrins expressed varies along the nephron, as does the expression of their extracellular matrix ligands, underlining their involvement not only in cell adhesion but also differentiation (157).

In adherent cells, most integrins mediate adhesion through dynamic interactions with the actin cytoskeleton (94, 348–350). Linkage to actin is mediated by adapter protein complexes that bind to integrin cytoplasmic tails and then to actin. Proteins found in these complexes include talin, which binds directly to integrins and activates their adhesive properties, paxillin, α-actinin, and vinculin (94,

348–350). Studies of migrating cells suggest that initial adhesive interactions occur through small "focal complexes" that form on leading lamellipodia and are linked to polymerizing actin through the action of the small signaling GTPase of the rho family Rac. As the cell moves over these contacts, they mature into larger "focal adhesions" that associate with robust actin stress fibers (at least in culture) controlled by another GTPase Rho and its effectors (94, 348–350). While the general elements of this model have been somewhat validated in epithelial cells during wound healing, the status of focal complexes and focal adhesions in mature polarized epithelia of the kidney and elsewhere, as well as their functions in adhesion and polarization, remain, for the most part, unexplored.

In addition to their role in mechanical adhesion, focal complexes and focal adhesions are also platforms for signaling (94, 348–350). A variety of kinases including, notably, focal adhesion kinase (FAK) and members of the src family of tyrosine kinases, associate with integrin adhesion complexes and are activated by binding to the extracellular matrix. Subsequent signals then activate downstream serine/threonine kinases such as integrin-linked kinase (ILK) and mitogen-activated protein (MAP) kinases such as ERK, as well as members of the rho-GTPase family including RhoA, Rac, and Cdc42. Indeed, at least 50 different cytoskeletal, adapter, and signaling proteins are known to be associated with integrin adhesion complexes, depending on the cell type and circumstances (348, 349).

In addition to the integrins, other membrane proteins are involved in epithelial cell adhesion to the extracellular matrix including dystroglycan, a laminin receptor, and possibly a membrane-bound form of the Lutheran antigen (199, 200). In addition, there is evidence that glycolipids may also serve as transient laminin receptors (169, 353). While not proven that any of these receptors play a direct role in epithelial polarization, they may act indirectly by affecting assembly of the basal lamina (see below) (169).

Cell Adhesion and Development of Primordial Kidney Tubular Epithelium

The developing kidney provides an example of the collaborative roles of cell–cell and cell–substratum interactions in the formation of a polarized epithelium. In the developing kidney, the initial extracellular signal that leads to cell polarization and differentiation of the tubular epithelium arises from mesenchyme following induction by the ureteric bud. The inductive event itself, for which the molecular basis is not understood (232), is isotropic in the sense that is does not impart any spatial information to the differentiation process. The first morphologic indication of differentiation is the formation of multicellular aggregates or condensates. These condensates are spatially differentiated: cells at the peripheries of the condensates have both a "free" plasma membrane domain facing the outside of the condensates and the undifferentiated mesenchyme and an "attached" plasma membrane domain in contact with other cells of the condensate (Fig. 4). Following this rudimentary polarization, the adherent mesenchymal cells in the condensate become more polarized, eventually reorganizing into a simple epithelium attached to a basal lamina and facing a lumen (Fig. 4). Although cell adhesion molecules are expressed in the undifferentiated mesenchyme, the appearance of the epithelial-specific adhesion molecule E-cadherin coincides with condensation (70, 166, 332). As described earlier, E-cadherin is a member of a family of calcium-dependent cell adhesion molecules found concentrated at the zonula adherens just below the tight junction (312). E-cadherin is present throughout the mesenchyme distributed at the sites of cell–cell contact (70, 332). Despite its coincident expression at the time of condensation, it is unclear whether it plays a key role in the differentiation process. Antibodies against E-cadherin, which disrupt cell–cell contacts in cultured cells, fail to disaggregate or block formation of the epithelium in organ cultures of kidney mesenchyme (332). These results suggest that other cell adhesion molecules of greater significance may await identification.

At a later stage of differentiation, it is likely that the extracellular matrix protein laminin is important in formation of the kidney epithelium from condensate. Laminins are a family of large heterotrimeric glycoproteins found together with collagen type IV, proteoglycans, and other proteins in the basal lamina underlying all epithelia (199, 200, 317). Laminin-1 (LN1), the prototypical molecule of the family, consists of three chains (α1, β1, γ1) associated in a cross-like configuration by disulfide bonding. Although laminin βl chains are expressed in the primitive mesenchyme and in later developmental stages, laminin α1 is first detected following condensation (70, 151, 168, 199). Expression is localized to the periphery of the condensate, suggesting that the crude polarization caused by condensation may have led to polarized secretion of laminin. Antibodies to laminin α1 block formation of the epithelium (151). Thus, assembly of

basal lamina containing LN1 around the condensate is essential for differentiation of a polarized epithelium.

Recent results derived from a variety of other experimental systems generally support the conclusion that laminins and their integrin receptors play a role in epithelial polarization (168). Mutations in either integrin or laminin subunits lead to disruption of epithelial differentiation and polarization in the nematode *Caenorhabditis elegans* and the fruit fly *Drosophila* (168). In the mouse embryo, expression of laminin generally coincides with development of epithelial tissues. In embryoid bodies derived from cultures of aggregated embryonic stem (ES) cells, a LN-1-containing basement membrane forms between the endoderm and the polarizing inner cell mass cells. When ES cells deleted of both laminin γ1 alleles are aggregated into embryoid bodies, the inner cell mass forms but does not polarize (168).

The primary receptors for laminins are integrins (157, 197, 199, 200). It is likely that integrins play an important role in morphogenesis and differentiation of the kidney (157). In both the developing and adult kidneys, βl integrins are expressed in a characteristic, cell-type–dependent pattern (147, 154, 157). In uninduced mesenchyme, only the α1 subunit is expressed. As condensates form and epithelialization commences, α6β1, a laminin receptor, appears. Function-blocking antibodies against the α6 subunit inhibit epithelial differentiation in organ cultures of induced mesenchyme, suggesting that this integrin plays a key role. Upon the development of the S-shaped nephron precursor, other α subunits (presumably as heterodimeric complexes with β1) are expressed in a pattern that is retained in the adult (154, 157). Thus, α1 is observed in mesangial cells and the endothelium, α2 is observed in glomerular endothelium and distal tubules, and α3 is observed in podocytes, Bowman's capsule, and distal tubules (154, 157). The α6 subunit is expressed transiently in podocytes during development and basally throughout the tubules from then on (154, 157). Additional evidence for the key roles of integrins in kidney morphogenesis comes from mouse knockouts. Deletion of both α8 (another partner of βl) and α3 integrin subunits affects kidney development (156, 157, 218). Surprisingly, knockout of α6 has no effect on kidney development despite its apparent role in epithelial differentiation in organ culture and its ubiquitous expression in the adult kidney (95). This finding no doubt implies functional redundancy among integrin subunits.

Adhesion and Renal Epithelial Polarization In Vitro

The role of cell adhesion in epithelial polarization is even more clearly indicated through studies with kidney cell lines (269). MDCK cells cultured in a single cell suspension lack polarized plasma membrane domains. Upon attachment to a substratum, cells quickly make cell–cell contacts, forming small islands (230). Under these conditions, apical proteins are restricted to the free or apical surface whereas basolateral proteins are distributed over the entire plasma membrane

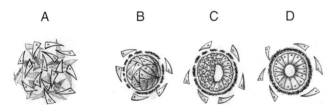

A   B   C   D

FIGURE 4 Development of the kidney epithelium from induced mesenchyme. The kidney epithelium develops *in vivo* following induction of the metanephric mesenchyme by the ureteric bud. The initial stages of differentiation from mesenchymal to epithelial cells may also be followed *in vitro* by organ culture. In this schematic view, induced mesenchymal cells are initially randomly oriented and show little cell–cell adhesion (A). Some mesenchymal cells adhere closely to each other and begin to produce a basement membrane at the periphery of the condensate (B). The cells of the condensate begin to reorganize into an epithelium and form a lumen as the basement membrane becomes more extensive (C). Finally, formation of the pretubular renal vesicle consisting of a polarized epithelium is complete (D). (Redrawn with permission from Ekblom P. Developmentally regulated conversion of mesenchyme to epithelium. *FASEB J* 1989;3:2141–2150.)

(270, 330). As the cells reach confluency, forming a true epithelium, basolateral proteins also become completely polarized (14, 230).

The effects of cell–cell and cell–substratum interactions can be dissected by culturing MDCK cells in medium containing reduced amounts of calcium (231, 330, 331). If cells are cultured on collagen in medium with less than 5 μM calcium, then they attach to the substratum, but formation of cell–cell contacts is inhibited (231, 330, 331). Cells assume a rounded morphology with no appreciable lateral membrane. In this situation, an immature apical surface forms. Microvilli are decreased in number, and expression of apical proteins on the cell surface, although reduced in quantity, remains polarized to the free surface (330). It has also been reported that intracellular concentrations of apical (but not basolateral) proteins, called "vacuolar apical compartments" (VACs), are also present (331). Basolateral proteins, in contrast, are not polarized in medium containing low calcium concentrations. When the calcium concentration is raised to normal values (1.8 mM), then cell–cell contacts rapidly form, VACs exocytose, and basolateral proteins polarize.

The culturing of MDCK cells as multicellular aggregates also permits the effects of cell–cell and cell–substratum interactions to be independently examined (336). Under these conditions, aggregated cells gradually form cysts with central lumina. In the absence of recognizable cell–substratum contact, both apical and basolateral polarization occurs, with the apical surface facing the outside of the cell aggregate. At this time, the tight junctional protein ZO-1 is found distributed over the lateral membrane, where cell–cell contacts occur. As the lumen forms, the cells secrete and deposit type IV collagen and laminin. Interaction with this extracellular matrix then triggers redistribution of ZO-1 to the point of intersection between the apical and lateral membranes (336). The observations with MDCK cells suggest that cell–cell and cell–substratum interactions have somewhat independent, though complementary, effects on cell polarization. In the absence of cell–cell contacts, as in medium with reduced calcium concentrations, cell–substratum interactions are sufficient to induce a degree of apical polarity. Formation of cell–cell contacts then consolidates apical polarity and promotes polarization of basolateral proteins. Conversely, cell–cell contacts in the absence of interaction of cells with a substratum are enough to cause polarization of both apical and basolateral proteins in suspended cell aggregates. The appearance of a collagen substratum, however, affects the localization of tight junctions.

Laminin has also been implicated in the polarization of renal MDCK cells. A monoclonal antibody that blocks MDCK cell adhesion to LN-1, but not collagen, prevents complete polarization (353). Because this particular antibody was directed against a neutral glycolipid Forssman antigen, the significance of this observation was initially uncertain. However, recent results implicating glycolipids

in laminin assembly into a basal lamina may help to explain these findings (237, 347). When MDCK cells are cultured in 3D collagen gels for 7–10 days, they form polarized cysts with the apical surface facing the lumen and the basal surface facing the extracellular matrix. Under these conditions, the cells secrete laminin and assemble it into a discrete basal lamina adjacent to the outer surface of the cyst. When MDCK cells are either treated with a function-blocking anti-β1 integrin antibody or express a dominant-negative mutant of the small GTPase Rac1, the laminin-containing basal lamina does not form properly, although the laminin is secreted, and the cells display an inverted and somewhat disorganized polarity (237, 347). Addition of excess exogenous LN-1 to the collagen gel partially rescues both basal lamina assembly and correct polarization, possibly by driving laminin assembly adjacent to the basal plasma membrane (237, 347). The conclusion from these experiments is that the primary defect caused by both the function-blocking anti-β1 antibody and dominant-negative Rac1 is in the laminin assembly, and that an assembled, laminin-containing basal lamina is essential for polarization of MDCK cells in 3D culture.

In summary, the experiments with MDCK cell cysts suggest that a "serpentine" signaling pathway snakes its way from the extracellular matrix in and out of MDCK cells to first signal laminin assembly and then polarization (Fig. 5). The first step in this pathway is interaction of MDCK cells with either the collagen gel or some other matrix molecule through a β1 integrin. Ligation of the integrin then activates Rac1, which then, in a manner that is unclear, leads to laminin assembly on the cell surface. The assembled laminin is then recognized by an integrin or other matrix receptor that in turn signals polarization. As stated earlier, the evidence for this pathway is that both anti-β1 integrin and dominant-negative Rac1 block laminin assembly and polarization, but also that the effects of anti-β1 can be neutralized by overexpression of constitutively active Rac1, and the effects of dominant-negative Rac1 overcome by excess LN-1. While instructive, this pathway is still fragmentary and many questions remain. In MDCK cells, the laminin isoform that makes up the critical basal lamina is likely LN-10 (α5β1γ1), a close cousin of LN-1 (347). However, MDCK cells also synthesize and secrete LN5 (α3β3γ2), a truncated laminin that cannot assemble properly (Mak G, et al., submitted. University of Cincinatti College of Medicine, Cincinatti, Ohio). Whether this molecule plays any role in either basal lamina assembly or polarization in 3D culture is unclear. Furthermore, evidence from 3D cultures of mammary epithelial cells suggests that the epithelial-specific integrin α6β4 may also be involved in polarization (339). However, polarization of MDCK cells, which also express this integrin, are unaffected by function-blocking anti-α6 antibodies (347). Finally, the nature of the polarization signal that apparently depends on the spatial organization of the basal lamina is completely unknown.

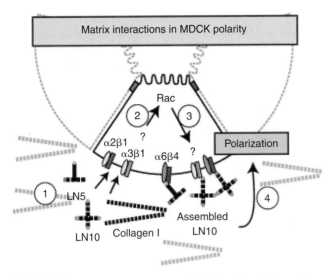

FIGURE 5 Determination of the apical–basal axis in polarizing epithelial cells may depend on a "serpentine" signaling pathway from the extracellular matrix substratum in and out and into the cell. MDCK cells suspended in a three-dimensional collagen gel interact with the collagen, and/or various laminin isoforms via a β1 integrin. This association activates Rac which, in some manner, leads to the assembly of a laminin basal lamina. Signals from this assembled matrix then cause the cells to polarize with the apical plasma membrane in the interior of the cyst and the basal surface on the outside. (From data in O'Brien LE, Jou TS, Pollack AL, Zhang Q, Hansen SH, Yurchenco P, Mostov KE. Rac1 orientates epithelial apical polarity through effects on basolateral laminin assembly. *Nat Cell Biol* 2001;3:831–838; Yu W, Datta A, Leroy P, O'Brien LE, Mak G, Jou TS, Matlin KS, Mostov KE, Zegers MM. Beta1-integrin orients epithelial polarity via Rac1 and laminin. *Mol Biol Cell* 2005;16:433–445; and Mak G, et al., submitted University of Cincinatti College of Medicine, Cincinatti, Ohio.)

Effects of Cell–Cell and Cell–Substratum Interactions on Cytoskeleton

While it is evident that adhesion between epithelial cells and the extracellular matrix substratum elicits both mechanical effects and activates a variety of signaling proteins and intermediates, it is unclear how this information is translated into the formation of the apical–basal axis orthogonal to the adherent surface. Such an axis is essential for establishing the unique identities of the basolateral and apical plasma membrane that define epithelial cell polarity as well as proper assembly and placement of junctional complexes necessary for integrity of the epithelium and its permeability barrier. One possibility is that cortical actin interacts with the microtubule cytoskeleton to affect cell organization. Because of the arrangement of α and β tubulin, microtubules are inherently polar structures. Although microtubule growth may occur from both ends, it occurs faster from the "plus" ends; the "minus" ends associate with microtubule organizing centers (MTOCs) (150). In many cell types, the centrosome is the major MTOC. How the structural polarity of microtubules might be used to translate signals at the cell periphery into asymmetric morphogenesis is suggested by the dynamic instability model of Kirschner and Mitchison (Fig. 6) (150). According to this model, microtubules growing from initiation sites (MTOCs) spontaneously and suddenly disassem-

ble. As the microtubule extend and contract, each transient configuration represents a potential cell morphology that is only realized if factors are present that stabilize particular microtubule configurations and prevent disassembly. Candidates for such stabilization factors are MAPs, including capping proteins that might bind the "plus" ends and MAPs that associate with the sides of the microtubules (150). If such factors bind to a particular locale within the cell cortex, then microtubules extending to this region will be stabilized and preserved (Fig. 6). A line extending along the stable microtubules from the point of capping in the cortex to the point of initiation at the MTOC would represent a primitive axis around which cell polarity might develop (Fig. 6).

Microtubule dynamics in MDCK cells are certainly consistent with this model. The microtubule cytoskeleton in MDCK cells undergoes dramatic rearrangement and stabilization as cultures progress from subconfluency to confluency and cells become more polarized (Fig. 7) (13, 28). In subconfluent cultures, the microtubules originate primarily from the juxtanuclear centrosome (Fig. 7). As the cells form contacts and become more confluent, the centrosome moves first to the periphery of the cell (where it no longer organizes microtubules) and ultimately resides in the center of apical surface (where it may act as a basal body for central cilium) (Fig. 7). At the same time, the microtubule cytoskeleton becomes polarized along the emerging apical-to-basal axis (Fig. 7) (13, 28). When the cells are fully polarized, microtubules are organized into a dense apical cap and also run along the length of the cell, with their minus ends apical and their plus ends basal (Fig. 7) (13). A network of tubules is also found on the basal surface (13, 262). Several lines of evidence also suggest that the microtubules found in fully developed monolayers are also greatly stabilized (28, 29). Furthermore, observations in fibroblast cell lines suggest

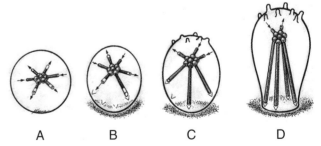

A   B   C   D

FIGURE 6 Morphogenesis of a polarized epithelial cell through stabilization of particular microtubules. Microtubules nucleated by a central microtubule organizing center (MTOC) grow and contract spontaneously, as if testing different configurations (A). Association of the cell with basal lamina (B) leads to the binding of factors (*V*) to the cell cortex in the region where adhesion occurs. When microtubules growing toward the region of substratum contact encounter the factors, they are stabilized and an axis perpendicular to the substratum is created, which leads to morphogenesis of polarized cell (D). The polarity of microtubules seen in MDCK cells is consistent with the model (see Fig. 7). (Redrawn with permission from Kirschner M, Mitchison T. Beyond self-assembly: from microtubules to morphogenesis. *Cell* 1986;45:329–342.)

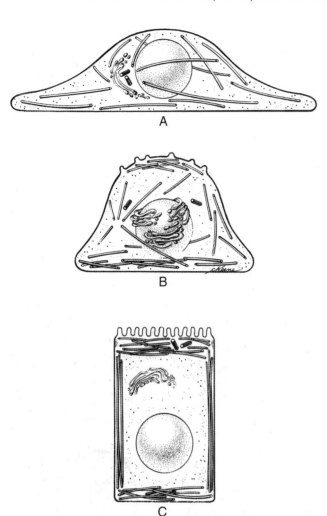

FIGURE 7 Reorganization of microtubules in MDCK cells. In sparsely confluent cultures of MDCK cells, microtubules are nucleated by a juxtanuclear centrosome lying near the Golgi complex (A). As the cultures mature the microtubule organization is no longer nucleated from the centrosome. The centrioles split and move toward the apical lateral borders of the cell. At the same time, the microtubules begin to form an apical cap (B). When fully confluent and polarized, the centrioles are positioned under the apical plasma membrane, where they may serve as a basal body for central cilium. The microtubules are highly organized with a dense apical cap and vertical microtubules running along the lateral borders. Some microtubules are also found on the basal surface (C). The orientation of the vertical microtubules is with the minus-end apical and the plus-end basal, suggesting that organizing centers are found in the apical region. Note also that movement of the Golgi complex from the juxtanulear location to the apical cytoplasm (compare B and C). (From results Bacallao R, Antony C, Dotti C, Karsenti E, Stelzer EHK, Simons K. The subcellular organization of Madin–Darby canine kidney cells during formation of a polarized epithelium. *J Cell Biol* 1989;109:2817–2832; and Bre MH, Kreis TE, Karsenti E. Control of microtubule nucleation and stability in Madin–Darby canine kidney cells: the occurrence of noncentrosomal, stable detyrosinated microtubules. *J Cell Biol* 1987;105:1283–1296.)

that focal adhesions may be a site where growing microtubules are captured and stabilized (145).

Work over the past few years has identified a number of proteins involved in the capping and organization of microtubules in polarized epithelial cells. Chief among these is

APC, the protein also known as a regulator of Wnt signaling and β-catenin degradation described previously (203, 262). Careful studies by Näthke and others in highly polarized epithelial cells from the inner ear, which possess bundles of microtubules oriented along the apical–basal axis, clearly established that APC is found exclusively localized to the basal surface under these conditions, near the plus ends of microtubules (203). APC interacts with microtubules directly through a C-terminal–binding site, but also probably interacts indirectly at its N-terminus through armadillo repeats that bind a kinesin-associated protein (KAP3) (203, 262). The N-terminus of APC also binds Asef, a Rac-GEF, that may facilitate APC association with the basal actin cortex (203, 262). This could provide a potential linkage between basal adhesion complexes and microtubules. Other plus-end microtubule-binding proteins, such as EB-1 and p150^{Glued}, associate also with the sides of microtubules, as does APC, and influence microtubule dynamics in the basal cortex (262). All of these proteins may also help link microtubules via actin to the lateral plasma membrane as epithelial cells polarize, facilitating development of the fully polarized cell. Despite these intriguing and relevant observations, involvement of dynamic microtubules in the establishment of the apical–basal axis is far from proven. In cultured epithelial cells such as MDCK and Caco-2, the relationship between an oriented microtubule cytoskeleton and localization of key microtubule-binding proteins such as APC is far from strict (110, 203). It is likely that microtubule dynamics represent but one of many redundant mechanisms responsible for establishing the epithelial apical–basal axis in what must, by necessity, be a very robust process.

While the microtubule cytoskeleton may help to establish the apical–basal axis, cell–cell adhesion clearly affects organization of the cortical cytoskeleton on the lateral plasma membrane. How this may occur may be inferred from studies of the submembranous cytoskeleton composed of fodrin, ankyrin, and actin (226). Fodrin is an analogue of erythroid spectrin found in many nonerythroid cell types (22). In polarized kidney cells, fodrin is associated exclusively with the cytoplasmic side of the basolateral surface (65, 230). In MDCK cells, fodrin forms a complex with ankyrin and Na$^+$,K$^+$-ATPase (211, 227). This suggests that the organization of the fodrin-based cytoskeleton in epithelial cells might resemble that seen in the erythrocyte, where ankyrin acts to link the network of spectrin and actin to the membrane by associating with both spectrin and the anion transport–protein band 3 (22, 66). In polarized MDCK cells, fodrin is found in a metabolically stable and biochemically insoluble state (62, 230). In contrast, fodrin is diffusely distributed in the cytoplasm of newly plated MDCK cells, and in cells cultured in medium containing reduced calcium concentrations, basolateral polarity is lacking (62, 230, 231). Under these conditions, fodrin exists in metabolically unstable complexes that are extractable with nonionic detergent (62, 230, 231). In addition to fodrin, ankyrin, and Na$^+$,K$^+$-ATPase, these complexes also contain E-cadherin (228). Because of this, it has been postulated that upon cell–cell contact, E-cadherin induces assembly of the fodrin cytoskeleton (227, 228, 269). In this manner, the fodrin cytoskeleton would form only on regions of the membrane where cell–cell contacts occur, namely, the lateral plasma membrane domain. Polarization of membrane proteins might then come about either by ankyrin-mediated redistribution or by endocytosis and degradation of proteins misplaced to the incorrect domain. Elements of this hypothesis are supported by the observation that expression of E-cadherin in nonpolar cells causes endogenous fodrin and Na$^+$,K$^+$-ATPase to be localized exclusively to the membranes involved in E-cadherin expression, suggesting that more than one molecular mechanism may be important in the development of the basolateral domain (196).

Par Proteins and Establishment of Apical and Basolateral Membrane Identity

Although the importance of cell adhesion and epithelial polarization is clear, the detailed mechanisms by which this occurs are undoubtedly very complex. Studies of early development in the model organisms *C. elegans* and *Drosophila* identified a number of genes responsible for the asymmetric partitioning of cell fate determinants during cell division and establishment of the anterior–posterior axis (176, 225). In some cases, these genes controlled the orientation of the axis of cell division, which is clearly related to epithelial polarity where cell division may either yield two identical epithelial daughter cells or one epithelial cell and a new cell type. Mutants in such genes were termed "PAR" for partition defective. Of the six genes originally identified in *C. elegans*, five along with the small GTPase Cdc42 and an atypical isoform of protein kinase-C (aPKC) have been implicated in polarization of mammalian epithelial cells (176, 225). These include PAR1 (in mammals also called MARK/CTAK/KP78/EMK), PAR3 (Bazooka in *Drosophila*), PAR4 (in mammals LKB1/STK11), PAR5 (in mammals an isoform of the phosphoserine-binding protein 14-3-3), and PAR6.

Based on work primarily in *Drosophila*, some PAR proteins appear to associate with other proteins into three complexes that function together to establish apical and basolateral membrane domains and properly position junctional complexes, while others function independently (26). These are PAR3, PAR6, and aPKC (Baz or Par complex), Crumbs, PATJ, and Stardust (PALS) (Crb complex), and lethal giant larva (LGL), Scribble, and discs large (DLG) (Scrib complex). Each of these complexes has at least one component with a PDZ domain that presumably facilitates their association with the junctional region. In *Drosophila*, the Baz complex initiates apical polarity after being recruited to the adherens junction. The Scrib complex binds to the basolateral membrane and represses apical identity in this region, while the Crb complex, recruited apically by the

Baz complex, antagonizes Scrib and reinforces the "apicalization" effects of Baz (26).

How these protein complexes may function in mammalian epithelial cells is currently under intensive investigation (176). The small GTPase Cdc42 is of particular interest because it has long been implicated in polarized functions such as bud site selection in yeast and in establishment of transient polarity during neutrophil chemotaxis (176). Furthermore, Cdc42 has also been implicated with PAR6 in directional migration of astrocysts and wounded endothelial cell monolayers (176). How it might function in the context of epithelial polarization is not clear. Evidence from both *Drosophila* and MDCK cells suggests that aPKC, PAR1 (also serine/threonine kinase), and PAR5 (14-3-3) might function together to restrict certain protein complex functions to the apical membrane (26, 176). In particular, phosphorylation of PAR1 by aPKC generates a binding site for 14-3-3 that restricts its location to the basolateral surface (23, 136, 137, 308, 309). PAR1 may then phosphorylate PAR3 to also create a 14-3-3 binding site that prevents its association with PAR6, thereby limiting its the activity of the PAR3/PAR6 complex to the nascent apical surface.

Despite these clues, other observations hint at the complexity of the polarization process and possible differences between mammals and invertebrates. PAR3 is essential for epithelial polarization in *Drosophila*, for example (26, 176). Knockdown of PAR3 in MDCK cells using RNA interference, however, significantly affects tight junction formation but not necessarily polarity (47, 48). Furthermore, this function of PAR3 in MDCK cells is apparently independent of its interaction with PAR6 or aPKC. Suppression of PAR3, at the same time, constitutively activates Rac, and a Rac-dominant negative mutant rescues tight junction formation (47, 48). Similarly, PAR4, a serine/threonine kinase, was implicated in polarization in *C. elegans* and *Drosophila*. When the mammalian PAR4 homologue LKB1 is activated in an intestinal cell line by inducible-expression of the adapter STRAD, individual cells form an apical surface and localize junctional proteins adjacent to this surface in the absence of any cell–cell contacts, despite the fact that LKB1 itself is not distributed in a polarized fashion (12). Thus, some as yet undefined markers of asymmetry remain to be identified that are critical in initiating the cascade of events leading to polarization.

SORTING PATHWAYS

One of the first, and perhaps most easily addressed questions presented by the phenomenon of epithelial polarity relates to where, within the cell, sorting occurs. The membrane proteins that populate the apical and basolateral plasmalemmal domains are all synthesized in association with the membranous elements of the rough ER (335). It has further been shown that after their cotranslational insertion into the membranes of the rough ER, apically and basolaterally directed proteins share the same cisternae of the Golgi complex as they transit the secretory pathway en route to their respective sites of ultimate functional residence (85, 263). Immunoelectron microscopic studies performed on MDCK cells doubly infected with the VSV and influenza viruses revealed, through double labeling, that the influenza HA protein and the VSV G protein could be colocalized throughout the cisternae of the Golgi complex (263).

This observation was confirmed and extended through a series of elegant biochemical studies. It had previously been shown that when cells are incubated at 20°C newly synthesized membrane proteins accumulate in the trans-most cisterna of the Golgi complex (186, 278). Elevating the temperature to 37°C relieves this block and allows the proteins to proceed to the cell surface (108). By examining the nature of the complex N-linked glycosylation associated with the VSV G protein, it was demonstrated that sialic acid residues are added in the 20°C compartment (85). These investigators took advantage of the fact that, in addition to the HA protein, the membrane of the influenza virus contains a neuraminidase in their efforts to determine whether segregation of the apically directed influenza proteins from the basolaterally targeted VSV G protein occurs before or after the 20°C block compartment. They found that in singly infected cells incubated at 20°C, the VSV G protein became heavily sialylated. In contrast, when cells that had been doubly infected with both the VSV and influenza viruses were incubated at 20°C, little if any sialic acid could be detected on the newly synthesized VSV G protein. These results demonstrate that as late as the 20°C block compartment, which corresponds to the trans-most cisterna of the Golgi complex, the newly synthesized apical neuraminidase and basolateral VSV G protein are still intermingled and capable of physical interaction. The segregation of these two classes of proteins from one another must, therefore, occur at or after this subcellular locus. It is interesting to note that immunoelectron microscopic studies of endocrine cells reveal that proteins destined for packaging in secretory granules are separated from those bound for constitutive delivery to the cell surface in the trans-most cisterna of the Golgi complex (246, 319, 320). Observations such as these have prompted investigators to speculate that this compartment, which is also referred to as the trans-Golgi network (TGN), might be the site of several intracellular sorting events (109). More recently it has been shown that sorting may occur as well at the level of the recycling endosome. Loading endosomes with HRP (horseradish peroxidase)-conjugated transferrin and subsequently disrupting endosome function through the deposition of peroxidase reaction product prevents the surface delivery of newly synthesized basolateral membrane proteins (7).

Three pathways for this sorting process can be imagined (Fig. 8) (39, 184, 269, 293). In the direct model, sorting would take place prior to cell surface delivery. Segregation of basolateral from apical proteins would be completed intracellularly and proteins would never appear, even tran-

Sorting pathways

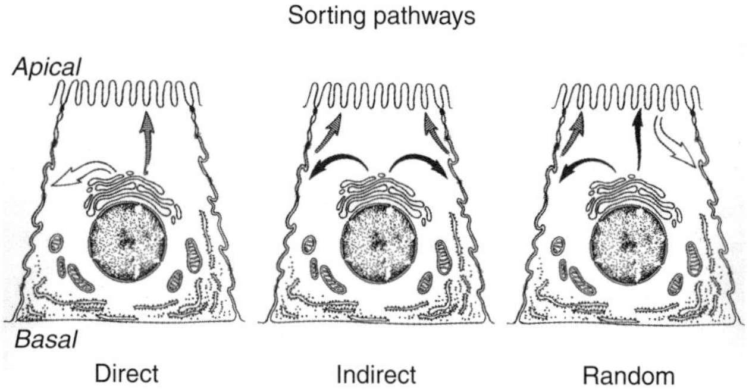

FIGURE 8   Three putative pathways for the sorting of membrane proteins in polarized epithelial cells. In the vectorial sorting scheme, apical and basolateral membrane proteins are separated from one another intracellularly and prior to plasmalemmal delivery (left). The indirect, or obligate, misdelivery model predicts that all newly synthesized plasma membrane proteins are carried together to cone–cell surface domain. Proteins destined for the opposite surface are then internalized and transported to their appropriate destinations (middle). Finally, random sorting is defined by a complete lack of intracellular segregation. Apical and basolateral proteins are delivered without preference to both surfaces and are subsequently redistributed by endocytosis and transcellular transport (right). Clear arrows represent vesicles carrying only basolateral proteins, hatched arrows denote vesicles carrying only apical proteins, and black arrows indicate vesicles carrying intermixed apical and basolateral membrane proteins. (Reprinted with permission from Caplan M, Matlin KS. Sorting of membrane and secretory proteins in polarized epithelial cells. In: Matlin KS, Valentich JC, eds. *Functional Epithelial Cells in Culture*. New York: Liss, 1989:71–127.)

siently, in the inappropriate membrane domain. The random sorting scheme dictates that no separation of apical from basolateral proteins occurs prior to arrival at the cell surface. Following their insertion into the plasmalemma, proteins that find themselves in the wrong surface domain would be removed by endocytosis and either transcytosed to the proper surface (185) or degraded. Finally, the indirect paradigm predicts that all newly synthesized plasmalemmal proteins initially appear together either at either the apical or basolateral membrane. The proteins for which this delivery is correct would be retained in that membrane domain, while those that had been mis-delivered would be internalized and transcytosed to their sites of ultimate functional residence.

These three models, although perhaps somewhat simplistic, are valuable for the relative ease with which they can be experimentally distinguished. Over the past two decades a great deal of effort has been invested in identifying which of these routes is, in fact, operational. The rather surprising answer appears to indicate that the sorting pathway pursued varies among different cell types and even among different proteins within the same cell type.

Technical Approaches

Much of the early research into the nature of epithelial sorting pathways was carried out on MDCK cells that have been infected with the VSV or influenza viruses. The infected cells produce massive quantities of viral proteins and retain their polarized distribution throughout at least the initial stages of the infection. These properties greatly facilitate the detection of cohorts of newly synthesized membrane proteins in the pulse chase protocols generally employed to monitor the polarity of cell surface delivery. Pulse labeling experiments demonstrated that the VSV G protein is not accessible to apically added antibodies at any point during its postsynthetic processing (253). In the case of the influenza HA protein, the converse is true. Proteases (187) or antibody probes (201) added to the media compartment bathing the basolateral surfaces of MDCK cells grown on filters cannot cleave or interact with this polypeptide during its journey to the apical cell surface. From these results it was concluded that the direct model of sorting applies for at least these two proteins in MDCK cells.

Other labeling tools have also been brought to bear on the study of sorting pathways. The N-hydroxysuccinimidyl (NHS) derivative of biotin is a membrane-impermeable molecule that will covalently combine with the ϵ-amino groups of exposed lysine residues (279). Proteins thus modified are substrates for precipitation or detection with avidin-conjugated secondary reagents. These tools can be used to follow the fate of large numbers of membrane proteins that have been exposed at one or the other cell surface to the NHS biotin compound. Using such a protocol, it has been demonstrated that several MDCK-cell apical and basolateral membrane proteins are directly targeted to their appropriate membrane domains (162, 174). Similar results have been gathered for an adenocarcinoma cell line (161).

Sodium Pump Targeting

Further support for the vectorial paradigm in MDCK cells came from studies on the sorting of the endogenous Na$^+$,K$^+$-ATPase (40, 41). Filter-grown MDCK cells that had been pulse-labeled with [35S]-methionine were exposed to the N-azidobenzoyl (NAB) derivative of ouabain at either their apical or basolateral surfaces during the course of a 90-minute chase. NAB-ouabain will bind to catalytically active sodium pumps with high affinity and, following UV photolysis, will become covalently incorporated into the protein backbone of the Na$^+$,K$^+$-ATPase's α subunit (42, 79, 80). By analyzing immunoprecipitates prepared from these cells using an anti-ouabain antibody, it was possible to demonstrate that no sodium pump in a state competent to bind ouabain ever appears at the apical surface.

Another investigation of sodium pump sorting in a different clonal line of MDCK cells made use of the NHS biotin surface-labeling technique and arrived at a conclusion diametrically opposed to the one described above. The results of this study indicated that the Na$^+$,K$^+$-ATPase is randomly delivered to the apical and basolateral plasmalemmal surfaces (116). The authors further suggested that stabilizing interactions with cytoskeletal elements that underlie the basolateral but not the apical cell surface (211, 227, 231) result in a much longer residence time for pump inserted into the basolateral domain. These studies are thus consistent with a model in which the sodium pump is not sorted intracellularly, but instead achieves its basolateral distribution through a mechanism based on random delivery followed by differential stabilization.

The experiments of Hammerton et al. (116) made use of NHS biotin as the membrane-impermeable covalent tag (279) with which to monitor the cell surface delivery of the newly synthesized sodium pump. Using this approach, these investigators found that newly synthesized Na$^+$,K$^+$-ATPase labeled during a 1-hour pulse was available to biotinylation from both the apical and basolateral surfaces in roughly equal proportions. This experiment was subsequently repeated employing a similar protocol with minor modifications and using the same clone of MDCK cells as had been used in the NAB-ouabain study. Newly synthesized Na$^+$,K$^+$-ATPase could be detected at the basolateral surface as early as the 30-minute chase point. Less than 5% of the total radiolabelled sodium pump was biotinylatable from the apical surface at any of the chase intervals employed in this study (102). E-cadherin, another basolateral membrane protein (228), was also found to appear exclusively at the basolateral surface. In contrast, a 114-kDa apical protein (14) could only be biotinylated from the apical surface at each time point, demonstrating that the NHS-biotin reagent does, in fact, have access to this cell surface domain. Thus, these results demonstrate that newly synthesized Na$^+$,K$^+$-ATPase is sorted intracellularly and targeted directly to the basolateral surface. This observation is consistent with the previous studies employing NAB-ouabain (41) and was corroborated by the similar studies performed on thyroid epithelial cells (356). Finally, it is important to note that subsequent studies have made use of the NHS-biotin technique to compare the delivery of Na$^+$,K$^+$-ATPase to the cell surface in the two different MDCK cell clones alluded to above (195). This study found that the cell line associated with random delivery once again produced this result, whereas the cell line in which vectorial delivery had been detected once again exhibited vectorial delivery. Thus, the apparent discrepancy among these studies appears to be attributable to differences in the pathways and processes through which these closely related cell lines achieve the polarized distribution of the Na$^+$,K$^+$-ATPase. While one line targets the pump directly to its basolateral destination, the other delivers it randomly and depends on cytoskeletal interactions to stabilize only the basolateral pool. Clearly, therefore, while cytoskeletal interactions may be sufficient to localize the Na$^+$,K$^+$-ATPase to the basolateral surface, they are clearly not the sole mechanism involved in producing the sodium pump's anisotropic distribution. Instead, they may act as a failsafe mechanism to back up and reinforce the initial biosynthetic sorting of the Na$^+$,K$^+$-ATPase to ensure that its polarized distribution is attained and maintained.

The preceding discussion suggests that the direct scheme cannot be applied to all epithelia or even to all MDCK cell clones. An alternate system has been shown to apply to the liver, for example. Cell fractionation studies performed on liver by Bartles et al. (18) reveal that several apical membrane proteins appear in the fraction corresponding to the hepatocyte basolateral plasma membrane prior to being delivered to the apical surface. This route has been especially well documented for the polymeric immunoglobulin receptor (pIgR) expressed by hepatocytes. This 120-kDa polypeptide serves to carry dimeric IgA from the blood to the lumena of the bile canaliculi. During its biosynthesis, the pIgR is transported directly from the TGN to the basolateral cell surface where it is available to bind dimeric IgA (129, 311). Independent of any interaction with IgA, the receptor becomes phosphorylated in the basolateral plasmalemma, and the phosphorylated form is internalized and carried by a transcytotic vesicle to the apical, or canalicular, surface (159). Following its insertion into the apical plasma membrane the ectodomain of the pIgR is cleaved and released into the bile as an 80-kDa protein referred to as secretory component (129, 311). Association with the secretory component helps to protect the bound IgA from intestinal proteases. Coupled with other results (14), the behavior of pIgR in hepatocytes supports the contention that apical membrane proteins arrive at their site of ultimate functional residence via obligate mis-delivery to the basolateral domain. This paradigm may not apply to all apical proteins in hepatocytes. Studies of the trafficking of apical members of the multidrug-resistance family of transport proteins indicate that these polytopic membrane proteins do not make an appearance at the basolateral surface en route to the apical membrane (149, 334). Thus, within a single polarized cell type, multiple trafficking routes can be employed to target different proteins to the same place.

A combination of the direct and indirect paradigms seems to be involved in membrane protein delivery in cultured intestinal cells. The Caco-2 line of human colon carcinoma cells can be grown on filters and subjected to the NHS-biotin labeling protocol described above. Such experiments reveal that the basolateral protein followed is vectorially targeted (190). Analysis of the apical polypeptides produced a somewhat more complicated picture. A fraction of these proteins appeared to transit through the basolateral plasmalemma prior to their apical delivery. The remainder of the apical proteins studied in this sampling were sorted intracellularly and inserted directly at the apical domain. Related and somewhat more complicated results have been gathered from studies on the biogenesis of brush border hydrolases by colonocytes in situ (2, 121, 182).

To complete this already confusing picture it is necessary to return to a discussion of targeting studies in MDCK cells. A cDNA encoding the pIgR has been expressed by transfection in this cell line. Remarkably, the sorting pathway pursued by this protein in the cultured renal epithelium is apparently identical to the rather baroque scheme that characterizes its route in hepatocytes (214). From the TGN the pIgR travels to the basolateral surface, from which it is internalized and subsequently transcytosed to the apical pole or recycled to the basolateral side. These observations demonstrate that an obligate mis-delivery pathway is either created or simply revealed in MDCK cells expressing the pIgR.

This apparent diversity of sorting pathways is perhaps not as surprising as it first appears. The relative flow of membranous vesicles from the Golgi complex to the two plasmalemmal surfaces in different epithelial cell types is likely to reflect a cell's biologic mission as well as the nature of the environment in which it functions. It appears, for example, that although hepatocytes produce copious quantities of secretory proteins, none are released directly into the bile (132). It has been proposed that newly synthesized membrane proteins depart the Golgi in the same transport vesicles that carry proteins destined for constitutive secretion (132, 293). Were this the case, then cells that do not produce a secretory content targeted for one or another membrane domain may also lack direct traffic of membrane vesicles directed from the Golgi to that domain. The full complement of plasmalemmal proteins might thus be forced by default to share the same carrier out of the Golgi and to be sorted by transcytosis subsequent to cell surface delivery. Some hepatic apical membrane proteins may transit through the basolateral surface because there is very little nonstop cargo traveling from the TGN to the apical domain in this particular cell type. The apparent multiplicity of sorting pathways available to different proteins within the same cell type may reflect specializations relevant to these proteins' functions. Diversity may also arise from nature of the signals and mechanisms that mediate these proteins' polarized distribution. The potential contribution of this latter influence will be referred to again in sections to follow. The lack of a single answer or unifying solution to the problem of sorting pathways is a theme that carries through the entire study of epithelial polarity. A number of equally effective mechanisms appear to have evolved for segregating membrane proteins into distinct domains. It remains to be determined how these differing approaches benefit their respective tissues and contribute to the maintenance of their unique functions.

Sorting Signals

Rodriguez-Boulan and Sabatini's 1978 observation that viral spike glycoproteins are targeted to opposite domains of polarized epithelial cells (267, 268) gave rise to the hypothesis that sorting signals—that is, the information required to direct a protein or proteins to a given subcellular location—might be wholly contained within the structure of the sorted proteins themselves. Evidence in favor of this contention has come from studies examining the distribution of viral membrane proteins expressed by transfection (rather than infection) in polarized cultured cells. A number of investigators have shown that the influenza HA protein, the VSV G protein and related viral spike glycoproteins are sorted correctly in the absence of any other proteins encoded by viral genomes (103, 144, 271, 302). It is apparent, therefore, that all of the addressing information necessary to produce the polarized distributions of these polypeptides must be embodied within the proteins themselves. It has further been shown that this information is almost certainly associated with the protein backbone rather than with any post-translational modification. Cells whose capacity to add asparagine-linked sugar residues has been impaired, either through mutation or via treatment with tunicamycin (106, 272), are nonetheless able to correctly target the viral spike proteins. Observations such as these have sparked an intensive search for the actual molecular information that specifies localization and for the machinery that acts on this information. It must be stated at the outset, however, that despite the rather confident and declarative tone of this section's heading, the identification and characterization of epithelial-sorting signals and mechanisms is still in its infancy.

Several distinct classes of signals have been found to specify basolateral sorting. Perhaps the best characterized of these are short motifs that contain tyrosine residues and resemble or overlap with sequences involved in endocytosis. Work from a number of groups has suggested that sequences in the cytosolic tail of membrane proteins determine the rates at which these proteins are internalized. The presence of a tyrosine residue appears to be a critical determinant of the efficacy of an endocytosis signal (62). The rapid endocytosis of both the LDL receptor and the transferrin receptor, for example, is dependent on the presence of short, tyrosine-containing sequences in these proteins' cytoplasmic tails. Mutation of this tyrosine residue to any other amino acid vastly reduces the rates at which both of these proteins are internalized. The apically sorted influenza HA protein is normally endocytosed extremely slowly. Addition of a tyrosine residue to the cytosolic tail of the influenza HA protein causes it to behave like the LDL receptor or transferrin receptor with respect to endocytosis—that is, it is rapidly internalized and recycled (160). When this altered form of the HA protein is expressed in MDCK cells, it is detected predominantly at the basolateral plasma membrane (35). It would appear, therefore, that a signal which is permissive for endocytosis is also competent to mediate basolateral accumulation.

Studies of the VSV G protein reveal that its basolateral sorting is also driven by a tyrosine-containing motif (314, 315). Uptake measurements suggest, however, that the VSV G protein is internalized relatively slowly, suggesting that its tyrosine-based motif confers basolateral targeting but not rapid endocytosis. Mutagenesis studies of the tyrosine-modified influenza HA protein as well as several other basolateral membrane proteins indicate that while internalization signals and basolateral sorting signals can share the same critical tyrosine residues, they are not identical (171). Altering residues near the tyrosine can produce apically sorted influenza HA protein that is rapidly endocytosed and basolateral HA protein that is internalized only slowly. Thus, basolateral and endocytosis signals can overlap, sharing one or more residues, but are clearly distinguishable

from one another. Presumably, therefore, they must be interpreted by distinct cellular machinery.

Data pointing to a similar conclusion have been gathered for Fc receptors (135). One of the Fc receptor isoforms includes a di-leucine sequence in its cytoplasmic tail. This sequence has been shown to function as an endocytosis signal and it also appears to confer basolateral targeting when the protein is expressed in polarized cells. Once again, alteration of residues flanking the di-leucine motif demonstrates that the sequence requirements for basolateral sorting are distinct from those that specify internalization (133, 192).

Tyrosine-containing basolateral sorting signals that are entirely distinct from recognizable endocytosis motifs have also been detected. The LDL receptor depends on a basolateral sorting signal that bears no sequence resemblance to any known internalization motif (134, 192). Although this motif includes a tyrosine residue, mutation of that tyrosine to phenylalanine still permits basolateral localization. A distinct tyrosine-containing motif appears to mediate the internalization of the LDL receptor (191). In the absence of the primary basolateral signal, this endocytosis motif can mediate a basolateral sorting function. Once again, however, with the exception of the tyrosine residue, the amino acids that contribute to the basolateral and endocytic aspects of this signal are distinct from one another.

Several basolateral sorting signals unrelated to tyrosine residues have also been reported. The well-characterized tyrosine-based endocytosis motif of the transferrin receptor is completely distinct from this protein's basolateral targeting signal, which resides in a different portion of the cytoplasmic tail. The peptide-processing enzyme furin cycles between the trans-Golgi network and the basolateral plasmalemma (239). Its trafficking to the basolateral surface appears to be driven by residues that are associated with a casein kinase-II phosphorylation site (143, 289). The invariant chain of the major histocompatibility class I1 complex is sorted to the basolateral membrane by virtue of the dihydrophobic sequence Met-Leu (240). Once again, endocytic internalization of this molecule is conferred by a similar dihydrophobic sequence, Leu-Ile, which is present at another position on the cytoplasmic tail. All of the basolateral sorting motifs discussed thus far function in the context of membrane proteins that span the bilayer once. As will be discussed below, a completely different cadre of molecular sequences appears to mediate the targeting of ion transporters and other multispanning membrane proteins. The list of identified basolateral sorting signals is considerably more extensive than the inventory of characterized apical-membrane protein-sorting signals. Perhaps the best studied member of this latter roster is not, in fact, a protein-based signal at all, but is instead constituted entirely of phospholipid. Glycophospholipid (GPI)-linked proteins are synthesized as transmembrane polypeptides that are cotranslationally inserted into the membrane of the rough ER (61). While still associated with the ER, the GPI-linked protein's ectodomain is proteolytically removed and transferred to a preassembled structure composed of a complex glycan tethered to the membrane through its attachment to a molecule of phospholipid (frequently phosphotidylinositol). Previous work has shown that in polarized epithelial cells, essentially all of the GPI-linked proteins reside in the apical plasmalemma (173, 174). Interestingly, the apical surface also plays host to the cell's full complement of glycolipid (327). Investigators prepared a construct in which the VSV G ectodomain was wedded to the transmembrane tail of Thy-1, which carries a signal for glycophospholipidation (37). The resultant GPI-linked G protein is sorted to the apical membrane. Similar results have been gathered by another group using a different construct. The results of these and related experiments have generally been interpreted to indicate that a strong apical sorting signal is embodied in some component of the GPI linkage itself. The transmembrane domains of several single-spanning apical membrane proteins appear to carry information important for apical targeting. The transmembrane domains of the influenza virus neuraminidase and HA proteins, for example, are sufficient to mediate sorting to the apical surface when they are included in constructs expressed by transfection in MDCK cells (158, 220). As will be discussed below, the same mechanisms that are thought to be involved in recognizing the GPI tail as an apical sorting motif may also interpret signals embedded in transmembrane domains. Furthermore, transmembrane domain sorting signals may be important not only in the localization of single spanning membrane proteins, but may also determine the distributions of polytopic ion pumps such as the Na^+, K^+ and H^+, K^+-ATPases (see below). It should also be noted that the extracytoplasmic, or ecto domains of several apical proteins appear to incorporate directional signals. Roth et al. (273) have shown that the ectodomain of the influenza HA protein is sufficient to specify apical targeting. When a cDNA construct encoding an anchor-minus form of the HA protein, which lacks both the cytosolic and transmembrane segments, is expressed in polarized cells, it is secreted exclusively into the apical medium compartment. This is true as well for the polymeric immunoglobulin receptor (212). These results suggest that a signal involved in apical sorting resides in the lumenal portion of the HA molecule and that this signal remains interpretable when it is presented as a soluble protein or in association with portions of a basolateral membrane polypeptide. Finally, recent evidence suggests that N-linked sugar groups, which are also present on the extracytoplasmic domains of membrane proteins, can in some circumstances contribute apical sorting information (280). It is logical to conclude from this discussion that machinery necessary to read and interpret this putative ectodomain apical sorting information must be exposed at the lumenal surface of the organellar compartments involved in the segregation and targeting of newly synthesized membrane proteins.

As discussed above in the section on sorting pathways, not all of the plasma membrane proteins expressed by polarized epithelial cells pursue a direct course to their sites of ultimate functional residence. The polymeric immunoglobulin receptor (pIgR) for example, when examined in its native liver (129, 215, 311) or in transfected MDCK cells (214), travels first to the basolateral surface and subsequently to the apical pole. A number of studies have examined the contributions that various portions of pIgR molecule may make to this complicated sorting behavior. Anchor-minus ectodomain constructs of the pIgR are secreted apically from transfected MDCK cells (212). Furthermore, deletion of the pIgR cytosolic tail results in a membrane protein that travels directly to the apical surface without ever appearing at the basolateral side (213). These observations have led to the suggestion that the ectodomain of the pIgR receptor contains an apical sorting signal and that this protein's cytosolic tail embodies information that is required for its initial appearance at the basolateral plasma membrane. Extensive mutational analysis reveals that a trio of amino acids in the sequence his, arg, Val, is primarily responsible for the vectorial targeting of the newly synthesized pIgR protein to the basolateral plasmalemma. This motif constitutes yet another addition to the growing collection of distinct amino acid sequences that can encode basolateral sorting (8, 261).

During its tenure at the basolateral membrane, the pIgR's cytosolic tail becomes phosphorylated on a serine residue. The phosphorylation event occurs both in liver (159) and in transfected MDCK cells (44). Intriguing experiments demonstrated that the addition of this phosphate group acts as a switch that allows the apical sorting signal to predominate and results in the protein's transcytosis to the apical side. Site-directed mutagenesis has been performed on the cDNA encoding the pIgR in order to convert the serine of interest into either an alanine or an aspartate residue (44). When expressed in MDCK cells, the wildtype as well as the two mutant forms, are all initially targeted to the basolateral surface and all three undergo endocytosis and recycling at similar rates. Interestingly, however, while the wildtype receptor undergoes fairly rapid transcytosis, the alanine form remains largely associated with the basolateral plasma membrane. In contrast, the aspartate form is transcytosed at a rate that exceeds that characteristic of the nonmutant form. These observations suggest that the negative charge associated with the phosphate and aspartate residues permits or activates the incorporation of the pIgR into transcytotic vesicles and thus initiates the protein's delivery to the apical surface. The mechanism through which this signal is detected and interpreted remains unclear.

The recognition and segregation of pIgR destined for transcytosis probably occurs in an endosome following internalization from the basolateral surface. The second sorting event involved in the targeting of the pIgR is thus almost certainly completed at a subcellular location distinct from the TGN. This behavior suggests that, once again, the sorting of apical from basolateral proteins need not occur exclusively on the exocytic pathway. The endosome or an endosome-related compartment appears competent to sense and act on the sorting signals that are necessary for the pIgR's apical localization. It remains to be determined whether signals detected in the endosome correspond to the same ectodomain-associated information that mediates the apical secretion of an anchor-minus form of the pIgR. The segregation of this secretory form to the apical pathway almost certainly occurs during its passage through the Golgi and is not likely to involve elements of the endocytic apparatus.

Most ion transport proteins and receptors span the membrane several times and many are composed of multiple subunits. Their intricate structures complicate the search for sorting signals and increase the likelihood that multiple independent or hierarchical signals might be present. This is clearly the case for the gastric H^+,K^+-ATPase. Acid secretion in the stomach is mediated by the gastric H^+,K^+-ATPase. This dimeric ion pump is stored within an intracellular population of membranous vesicles known as tubulovesicular elements (TVEs) in gastric parietal cells. Stimulation of acid secretion by secretagogues induces the TVEs to fuse with the parietal-cell apical plasma membrane, resulting in the formation of deeply invaginated secretory canaliculi rich in H^+,K^+-ATPase. The cessation of acid secretion involves the retrieval of the H^+,K^+-ATPase from the cell surface and the regeneration of the TVE storage compartment (342). Both the α and β subunits of the H^+,K^+-ATPase belong to the large P-type ATPase gene family (126). Their closest cousins in this collection are the corresponding α and β subunits of the Na^+,K^+-ATPase. Interestingly, while the H^+,K^+-ATPase functions at the apical surface of gastric parietal epithelial cells, the Na^+,K^+-ATPase is restricted in its distribution to the basolateral plasmalemma in this and most other epithelial cell types (40). The homology relating these ATPase functions has permitted the creation of chimeric ion pumps, whose subunits are composed of complementary portions of the H^+,K^+ and Na^+,K^+-ATPase α and β polypeptides. By expressing these constructs in cultured polarized epithelial cells it has been possible to determine the molecular domains of the ion-pump subunit proteins that are responsible for their sorting. Through this analysis it has become clear that both the α- and β-subunit polypeptides of the H^+,K^+-ATPase contain molecular signals that can contribute to the targeting of the holo-enzyme (101, 220). Expression of a large number of progressively more refined α-subunit chimeras reveals that an eight amino acid sequence within the α subunit of the H^+,K^+-ATPase is sufficient to specify apical sorting (68). This domain is predicted to reside within a transmembrane helix, thus suggesting that protein-lipid or protein–protein interactions within the plane of the membrane are responsible for pump sorting.

The β subunit of the H^+,K^+-ATPase contains a tyrosine-based sorting signal that functions to internalize the pump complex from the surface of the gastric parietal cell and return it to an intracellular regulated storage compartment (60, 101). This internalization is responsible for the cessation of gastric acid secretion following the removal of secretagogue stimulation. This was demonstrated by generating a transgenic mouse that expresses an H^+,K^+-ATPase β subunit lacking this endocytosis signal (60). These animals are unable to re-internalize H^+,K^+-ATPase from the apical surfaces of their gastric parietal cells. Consequently, they produce elevated gastric acid secretion during the interdigestive period. Mice carrying the mutant β-subunit develop gastritis and gastric ulcerations with histologic features that are essentially identical to those found in human disease. Examination of renal potassium clearance in these animals reveals that the same β-subunit sorting signal regulates active potassium resorption in the collecting tubule (338).

Several other studies have begun to define other signals employed in the polarized sorting of polytopic membrane proteins. Recently, for example, a novel motif has been identified in the cytoplasmic tail of rhodopsin, the seven-membrane span receptor that mediates this protein's apical sorting when it is expressed in MDCK cells (51, 316). Another member of the seven transmembrane G protein–coupled receptor family, the P2Y2 receptor, manifests an apical sorting signal in one of its extracellular loops (258). Furthermore, studies of neurotransmitter re-uptake systems have demonstrated that the four members of the highly homologous GABA transporter gene family are differentially sorted in epithelial cells and in neurons (3, 254). The GAT1 and GAT3 isoforms, which are restricted to axons when expressed endogenously or by transfection in neurons, are sorted to the apical membranes of epithelial cells. The GAT2 and betaine transporters, which are 50%–67% identical to GAT1 and GAT3, behave as basolateral proteins in epithelia and are restricted to dendrites when expressed in neurons. Production of chimeric and deletion constructs have permitted the identification of very short amino acid sequences at the extreme C-terminal tails of these transporters that manifest targeting information. The nature of these sequences suggests that they may interact with polypeptides containing PDZ-type protein–protein interaction domains, raising the possibility that this newly characterized association may play a direct role in the sorting of ion transport proteins (219). A similar PDZ-dependent mechanism also appears to mediate the apical trafficking of CFTR (50, 198, 216, 217).

Cell Type–Specific Sorting Patterns

The message encoded within a membrane protein's sorting signal is dependent not only on its own specific biochemical composition, but also the cellular context in which it is expressed. Several examples of membrane proteins that are differentially targeted in distinct epithelial cell types have been documented. The vacuolar H^+-ATPase, for example, accumulates at the apical surfaces of α-type intercalated cells but at the basolateral plasmalemmas of β-type intercalated cells in the renal collecting duct (4). Similarly, the Na$^+$,K$^+$-ATPase is basolateral in most epithelia, but behaves as an apical protein in cells derived from the neural crest, such as the choroid plexus and retinal pigment epithelium (5, 113). Targeting of particular proteins or classes of proteins can also vary as a function of the differentiation states of epithelial cells. For example, the sorting of well-characterized polarity markers expressed in *Drosophila* via germ-line transformation was followed in the developing *Drosophila* embryo. Human placental alkaline phosphatase (PLAP) is a glycosylphosphatidyl inositol (GPI)–linked protein that accumulates at the apical membranes of mammalian epithelial cells. A chimeric construct composed of the transmembrane and cytosolic portions of the vesicular stomatitis virus (VSV) G protein coupled to the ectodomain of PLAP has been found to behave as a basolateral protein when expressed in the MDCK cell system (37). The subcellular distributions of these proteins were examined in the epithelial tissues of transgenic *Drosophila* embryos that expressed these proteins under the control of a heat shock promoter (287). In the surface ectoderm both PLAP and PLAPG were restricted to the basolateral membranes throughout development. Internal epithelia derived from the surface ectoderm accumulated PLAP at their apical surfaces, while PLAPG retained its basolateral distribution. The redistribution of PLAP from the basolateral to the apical plasma membrane was found to be coincident with the invagination of the surface epithelium to form internal structures, suggesting that the sorting pathways that function in the epithelium of the *Drosophila* embryo are developmentally regulated. More recent studies demonstrated that various lines of renal epithelial cells can interpret differently a specific, defined sorting motif. When expressed by itself in LLC-PK1, cells, the gastric H$^+$,K$^+$-ATPase β subunit accumulates at the apical plasmalemma. As noted previously, the amino acid sequence of the gastric H$^+$,K$^+$-ATPase β subunit reveals that its cytoplasmic tail contains a 4–amino-acid motif, YXRF, which has been shown to function as an endocytosis motif for the holoenzyme in gastric parietal cells in situ (54, 60, 96, 101). Since tyrosine-containing endocytosis motifs have been shown to be sufficient to ensure basolateral targeting of membrane proteins in MDCK cells (34, 135, 163, 192, 315), it is perhaps surprising that the H$^+$,K$^+$ β behaves as an apical protein in LLC-PK1 cells. To further examine the H$^+$,K$^+$-ATPase β-subunit's sorting signal, MDCK cells were stably transfected with the rabbit gastric H$^+$,K$^+$-ATPase β-subunit cDNA (274). Examination of this protein's distribution by surface immunofluorescence and cell surface biotinylation indicated that it was restricted to the basolateral plasma membrane.

Mutagenesis experiments support the hypothesis that sorting information is contained within the cytoplasmic tail and, more specifically, within the tyrosine-based sorting motif of the H$^+$,K$^+$-ATPase β-subunit. These data suggest that sorting and internalization motifs are, as a class, differentially interpreted in the MDCK and LLC-PK1 cell lines (251). A possible molecular basis for this sort of disparate behavior has recently emerged. While MDCK cells express the μ1b subunit of the AP1 adapter complex, this protein is not found in LLC-PK1 cells (242). As will be discussed in the next section on sorting mechanisms, it is now established that μ1b expression can ensure the basolateral targeting of membrane proteins bearing tyrosine-based sorting motifs (78). While this μ1b-dependent mechanism appears to be sufficient to account for the sorting behaviors of a number of proteins that are differentially sorted by MDCK and LLC-PK1 cells, it appears not to explain the distribution of the H$^+$,K$^+$-ATPase β subunit in these two cell types (67).

In light of both the multiplicity of sorting signals presented in the preceding section and the apparent potential for heterogeneity in their interpretation discussed above, it is natural to wonder whether any logic or consistency governs nature's solution to the deceptively simple problem of apportioning proteins among two separate membrane domains. Upon further reflection, however, the complexity and degeneracy of the "sorting code" can be seen as a tremendous virtue. Two different epithelial cell types may need to target a given membrane protein to opposite surfaces of their respective plasma membranes in order to fulfill their unique physiologic functions. These same functions may also require, however, that other membrane proteins occupy the same surface distributions in both cellular contexts. Thus, while the sodium pump occupies the apical membranes of the cells of the choroid plexus and the basolateral membranes of renal epithelial cells, receptors for basement membrane components are present at the basolateral surfaces of both cell types. If only a single class of basolateral sorting signal and a single class of apical sorting signal existed, then it would not be possible for a cell to selectively alter the distribution of one set of plasmalemmal proteins without simultaneously altering the distributions of the entire population of the plasma membrane. In order to target the sodium pump to the apical surface, choroid plexus epithelial cells would be forced to target basement membrane receptors there as well. This would obviously constitute a wasteful compromise. In order to endow each epithelial cell type with the capacity to select individualized complements of proteins for its apical and basolateral domains, a dizzying multitude of sorting signals has evolved. Cells can thus customize the distributions of proteins among their plasmalemmal domains without the constraints that would be imposed by a limited number of sorting signals. According to this interpretation, sorting signals do not specify a specific destination such as apical or basolateral. Instead, they specify classes of proteins whose members are always sorted together. The membrane domain to which any one of these classes is sorted will depend on the cellular context in which it is expressed, and will be determined by the idiosyncratic array of sorting machinery and pathways present in each individual epithelial cell type.

Sorting Mechanisms

It is safe to say that we are just beginning to understand the mechanisms through which the sorting signals discussed above exert their effects and ensure the polarized delivery of newly synthesized plasma-membrane proteins. The strong evidence for the existence of sorting signals leads quite naturally to the postulate that sorting receptors must exist that are capable both of recognizing these signals and of transducing their messages to the relevant cellular machinery. Such receptors have, in fact, been demonstrated in the case of lysosomal enzyme sorting. Targeting of a newly synthesized hydrolase to the lysosome is mediated by the interaction between the enzyme's mannose-6-phosphate (man-6-P) recognition marker and one of two receptors that bind man-6-P–bearing ligands in the Golgi and mediate their segregation to prelysosomal endosomes (155). Binding of newly synthesized lysosomal enzymes to the man-6-P receptors is pH dependent. At the relatively neutral pH of the Golgi, ligands are tightly bound, whereas in the acid environment of the prelysosomal endosome they are rapidly released. No such well-characterized receptor systems have yet emerged to explain the sorting behavior of secretory and membrane proteins in polarized cells. While sorting receptors for secretory proteins remain to be identified definitively, some progress has been made in understanding how such receptors might function. Lysosomotropic amines, such as NH_4Cl and chloroquine, elevate the lumenal pH of acidic organelles (194). The resulting neutralization of acidic compartments can have profound effects on sorting. In the case of lysosomal enzyme targeting, addition of NH_4Cl raises the pH of the prelysosomal endosome and thus prevents the acid-dependent unbinding of newly synthesized hydrolases from the man-6-P receptor (155). In the continued presence of the drug, the Golgi becomes depleted of receptors available to complex with free ligand. Newly synthesized enzymes bearing the man-6-P recognition marker are thus secreted constitutively and by default. Experiments on cultured polarized epithelial cells suggest that a similar pH-dependent mechanism may function in the sorting of basolateral secretory proteins (43).

Laminin and heparan sulfate proteoglycan are constituents of epithelial basement membranes (181, 200). Studies of permeable-filter–grown MDCK cells supports revealed that both of these proteins are normally secreted predominantly into the basolateral medium compartment (43). When secretion from cells treated with NH_4Cl was monitored, it was found that both proteins were released into both media compartments in roughly equal proportions. Removal of the drug reversed this effect and restored normal basolateral secretion. As mentioned above, studies have demonstrated that the secretory default pathway for MDCK cells—that is, the route pursued by soluble proteins that lack any means of interacting with the cellular sorting machinery—is apical and basolateral (43, 103, 153). It appears, therefore, that targeting of these two basolateral secretory proteins requires the participation of an intracellular acidic compartment. Elevation of the lumenal pH of this compartment reversibly blocks laminin and HSPG (heparan sulfate proteoglycans) sorting and results in their apical and basolateral default secretion.

Although the nature of the dependence of this sorting event on acidic compartments remains unknown, it is interesting to speculate that a mechanism similar to that which functions in lysosomal enzyme sorting may also be involved in routing basolateral secretory proteins. In such a model, binding or unbinding of laminin and HSPG from a sorting receptor would require the participation of an acidic organellar pH. Confirmation of this hypothesis will await the identification of such a pH-dependent–binding protein with affinity for these and other basolaterally targeted proteins (52). Finally, it is worth noting that the basolateral sorting of the Na^+,K^+-ATPase and the apical sorting of the influenza HA protein and a complex of secretory polypeptides occur normally in the presence and absence of NH_4Cl (41, 43, 183). It would appear, therefore, that different mechanisms are brought to bear in ushering different classes of proteins to their sites of ultimate functional residence.

Tyrosine-Based Motifs and Adapters

Recent studies suggest that several different classes of soluble proteins may regulate the subcellular distributions of proteins bearing tyrosine-based signals. Perhaps the best understood of these are the adaptins (252). The adaptins comprise a group of peripheral membrane proteins that mediate the interaction between transmembrane proteins and the clathrin skeletons of coated pits and vesicles. Adaptins recognize and bind to tyrosine-containing coated pit localization sequences and link the proteins bearing these motifs to the clathrin coat (21, 241, 250-252). Adaptins can thus be considered to be among the most proximal elements of the endocytic sorting machinery—they recognize polypeptides endowed with endocytosis signals and ensure that they are incorporated into the specified internalization pathway. Distinct classes of adaptins function in the segregation of proteins into the coated structures associated with the trans-Golgi network and into cell surface coated pits (252). While AP2 adapters mediate internalization of proteins from the cell surface, AP1 adapter complexes participate in trafficking proteins out of the TGN. The μ subunits of adapter complexes appear to be responsible for interacting with tyrosine-based motifs (241). Two isoforms of μ subunits are found in AP-1 complexes. The μ1a protein is ubiquitously expressed and is found in both polarized and nonpolar cell types. The μ1b protein is instead found in only a subset of polarized cell types (242). As noted above, proteins bearing tyrosine-based motifs are basolaterally sorted in MDCK cells but accumulate apically in LLC-PK1 cells (274). It was noted that MDCK cells express μ1b, whereas this protein is absent from LLC-PK1 cells. Remarkably, expression of μ1b in LLC-PK1 cells at least partially "normalizes" their sorting properties, so that many (but not all) membrane proteins containing tyrosine-based signals are directed to the basolateral surface (78). Thus, μ1b constitutes perhaps the best characterized component of the sorting machinery. It is clearly capable of recognizing a class of sorting signals and acting on the instructions that they convey.

It is interesting to note that recent studies demonstrate that different proteins bind to and interpret the messages encoded by tyrosine-based and di-leucine endocytosis motifs. Over expression of tyrosine-motif–containing proteins can inhibit the endocytosis of other proteins carrying a similar endocytosis signal, presumably by competing for limited quantities of the adapter proteins that cluster proteins bearing these signals into clathrin-coated pits. This intervention does not affect, however, the internalization of proteins endowed with di-leucine motifs, indicating that they must be recognized and interpreted by a different class of polypeptides (180). It appears that the β subunits of adapter complexes interact with di-leucine motifs (260). Finally, a very different type of protein has been shown to interact with a tyrosine-based proline-rich sequence in the C-terminal tails of epithelial sodium channel (ENaC) subunits. The Nedd-4 protein possesses an ubiquitin ligase domain, and through its interaction with the ENaC tails may lead to downregulation of these channels through degradation (300).

The association of basolateral membrane proteins such as the Na^+,K^+-ATPase with elements of the subcortical cytoskeleton (211, 229) has led to the speculation that this interaction may play a role in targeting. Evidence in support of this proposition was found in the studies, described above, which suggested that, at least in one MDCK cell clone, the Na^+,K^+-ATPase may be delivered in equal proportions to the apical and basolateral surface (117). Apically delivered material may be rapidly degraded, whereas the basolateral sodium pump would be stabilized through interaction with the cytoskeleton and consequently turn over very slowly. The pump's polarized distribution would thus be the product of differential susceptibility to degradation rather than sorting at the level of the Golgi. The degree to which stabilization through interaction with the cytoskeleton contributes to the polarized distribution of the sodium pump or any other proteins remains to be established.

The observation that all of the glycolipids and GPI-linked proteins associated with epithelial cells tend to be found in the apical plasmalemmal domain has led to the proposal that lipids may play a role in membrane protein sorting (294). Since glycolipids and GPI-linked proteins are only associated with the outer leaflet of the plasma membrane, these molecules will be exposed at the lumenal face of the organelles of the biosynthetic pathway. Any sorting machinery that interacts with glycolipids, therefore, must do so either at the lumenal surface or within the plane of the membrane itself. These constraints have suggested to some investigators the possibility that lipid–lipid interactions are sufficient to segregate apically directed glycolipids and GPI-linked proteins into distinct patches during their residence in the Golgi. These self-assembled patches could then serve as the nuclei from which apically directed vesicles would bud. The biophysical properties of these patches might be involved in ensnaring other apically directed proteins as well as the components necessary to appropriately target the resultant transit vesicle (295). While evidence of lipid patches exists in both in vitro and in vivo systems (10, 327), their precise role in the sorting process remains to be elucidated. Independent of its applicability, however, this model is extremely interesting. It is a useful reminder that forces other than simple receptor–ligand interactions are likely to be involved in generating and maintaining the anisotropic protein distributions that define the polarized state.

As noted above, several proteins are targeted to the apical membrane by virtue of signals embedded within their transmembrane domains. The fact that the amino acid residues of a transmembrane domain may be in direct contact with lipid molecules suggests the possibility that they may mediate apical sorting through interactions with glycosphingolipid-rich membrane domains. According to this hypothesis, the composition of its transmembrane domain may permit a protein to partition into glycosphingolipid-rich patches and thus to become concentrated in a region of the membrane that will give rise to an apically directed transport vesicle. GPI-linked proteins that have become associated with glycosphingolipid-rich membrane domains are insoluble in 1% Triton X-100 at 4°C. When a cell lysate prepared in this fashion is fractionated on a sucrose gradient, insoluble proteins are found near the top of the gradient, whereas soluble proteins remain in the heavier fractions (10). Interestingly, the transmembrane domain of the apical protein influenza neuraminidase carries apical sorting information and also enables the protein to incorporate into insoluble.

Glycosphingolipid-Rich Membrane Domains

Evidence suggests that the basolateral sorting of the Na^+,K^+-ATPase might occur as the result of exclusion from glycosphingolipid-rich membrane regions. MDCK cells treated with the drug fumonisin, which prevents sphingolipid synthesis, randomly deliver newly synthesized Na^+,K^+-ATPase to both cell surface domains. In light of the observation that H^+,K^+ and Na^+,K^+-ATPase targeting appears to be mediated by a transmembrane sequence, it is tempting to hypothesize that their differential distributions are determined by their differing abilities to partition into glycosphingolipid-rich membrane regions. This possibility has been examined by determining the detergent solubility of apically-directed pump chimeras. When epithelial cells expressing an apically targeted pump chimera are lysed on ice with 1% Triton X-100, the endogenous GPI-linked alkaline phosphatase migrates to the top of a sucrose floatation gradient. The endogenous Na^+,K^+-

ATPase on the other hand, appears in the heavier fractions, a pattern typical for detergent-soluble membrane proteins. If the chimera containing the fourth transmembrane span of the gastric H⁺,K⁺-ATPase partitions into insoluble glycolipid patches, it should codistribute with the GPI-linked alkaline phosphatase. However, the chimera is found in the same fractions as the Na⁺,K⁺-ATPase, and is completely absent from the fractions containing alkaline phosphatase activity. Thus, an apically located chimera containing the fourth transmembrane domain of the H⁺,K⁺-ATPase exhibits no difference in its detergent solubility characteristics as compared with the basolaterally located Na⁺,K⁺-ATPase. This result suggests that mechanisms other than lipid association may be responsible for the sorting function of at least one transmembrane domain localization signal.

As discussed above, the C-terminus of GABA transporter GAT-3 appears to be important for its apical localization in MDCK cells (219). The final residues of this C-terminal tail, threonine, histidine, and phenylalanine (THF), are reminiscent of the sequences present at the extreme C-terminal tails of proteins known to associate with members of the membrane associated guanylate kinase (MAGUK) family. The MAGUK proteins incorporate one or more copies of the PDZ domain, which is named for three of the proteins in which the sequence homology defining this protein–protein interaction motif were first identified: PSD-95/SAP90, Dlg, and ZO1. Interactions between the PDZ domain of a MAGUK protein and the extreme cytoplasmic tail of an integral membrane polypeptide appear to be important in organizing the surface distributions of intrinsic membrane proteins (71, 297).

Observations obtained from a number of experimental systems provide further evidence for the involvement of PDZ domain–containing polypeptides in epithelial membrane protein sorting (148). The LET23 receptor tyrosine kinase is localized to the basolateral cell surfaces of vulvar epithelial cells in *C. elegans*. Genetic studies reveal that at least three proteins contribute to the generation or maintenance of this distribution. Mutation of the lin2, lin7, or lin10 genes leads to loss of LET-23 basolateral polarity. Each of the proteins encoded by these genes includes one or more PDZ domains. A mutation in the *Drosophila* discs lost protein, which contains multiple PDZ domains, also leads to the mis-localization of several apical and basolateral proteins in the epithelial structures of affected embryos (24). It would appear, therefore, that PDZ domain–containing proteins may play a direct role in the polarized sorting of at least some membrane proteins or may be required for the generation or definition of polarized domains. These observations may be especially relevant to physiologic function of polarized renal epithelial cells, since a number of important ion transport proteins, including CFTR and NHE3, appear to interact with cytoplasmic proteins containing PDZ domains (115, 288, 337). It seems likely that these interactions may play a role in establishing these proteins' distributions and

hence determining their capacity to participate in vectorial ion transport.

Finally, it is important to note that once proteins have been sorted into the vesicles that will carry them to the appropriate cell surface domain, these vesicles need to themselves be targeted appropriately. Presumably, the vesicular membranes include proteins that ensure that the vesicles will interact and fuse with only the proper domain of the epithelial plasmalemma. This recognition machinery is likely to include components of the membrane fusion machinery, such as vesicular SNARE (soluble NSF attachment receptor) proteins (76). SNARE proteins present in both vesicular and target membranes form complexes that appear to be necessary for most normal cellular fusion processes. The extent to which different members of the SNARE family impart specificity to intracellular vesicular fusion events remains to be established (140, 141, 175). Interestingly, however, a newly identified component of the machinery involved in vesicular targeting in yeast has recently been identified in mammalian cells (114). This Sec 6/8 complex appears to play a role specifically in the fusion of basolaterally directed, but not apically directed post-Golgi carrier vesicles in epithelial cells (98). It is likely that the number of "destination-specific" vesicular and plasma membrane proteins important for directing vesicular traffic in polarized cells will continue to grow.

EPITHELIAL CELL POLARITY AND RENAL DISEASE

Because kidney function is dependent on the polarity of tubular epithelial cells, any condition that compromises this polarity will lead to renal failure (77, 301). In general, this may occur through neoplastic processes, cell injury due to ischemia or nephrotoxicity, or inherited genetic effects (77, 282). Each of these may affect the tubular epithelial cells, their surrounding environment including the basal lamina and interstitial compartment, or both.

Carcinogenesis

During neoplastic growth it can be appreciated on the basis of morphology alone that the changes in cell and tissue organization wrought by tumorigenesis are likely to affect cell polarity (282). Model studies confirm this suspicion. When MDCK cells, which are not normally tumorigenic, are oncogenically transformed by introduction of the v-Ki-*ras* oncogene, they are converted from a simple epithelium to a multilayer, with great heterogeneity in overall cell morphology (282). Ultrastructural examination of these cells suggests that apical–basal polarity is severely compromised (282). Microvilli are diminished from the cells at the top layer, and organization of the cytoplasm is scrambled. Golgi complexes and centrosomes, which normally reside in an apical supranuclear location, are now found randomly positioned (282). Despite this apparent high degree of disorganization, immunocytochemical localization of specific antigens and physiologic measurements suggests that polarity is not totally disrupted. Basolateral proteins, including Na$^+$,K$^+$-ATPase and the cell-adhesion molecule E-cadherin, are restricted to regions of cell–cell contact, as in normal polarized MDCK cells (282). Apical proteins, on the other hand, are randomly localized to the free surface of the multilayered epithelial as well as to areas of cell–cell contact in cells throughout the multilayer (282). The tight junctional antigen ZO-1 is found typically at the point where the free and adherent surfaces of the uppermost cell layer meet as well as at a number of sites within the multilayer (282). The latter may be intercellular lumina or canaliculi connected to the upper surface. This localization probably reflects the presence of functional tight junctions, because the multilayer is both electrically tight and impermeable to inulin. Disruption of polarity of this type might have significant implications for net ion flow. For example, redistribution of a sodium channel normally found on the apical surface to both the apical and basolateral domains might occur as a result of the oncogenic process (77). If tight junctions remain intact and the Na$^+$,K$^+$-ATPase is retained on the basolateral surface under these circumstances, then sodium transport would be short-circuited, making it much less efficient. It is also interesting to note that recent studies demonstrate that proteins encoded by tumor suppressor genes may function as key regulators of polarity. Mutations in the gene encoding the LKB1 protein kinase are responsible for Peutz–Jaeger syndrome, an inherited form of tumor susceptibility associated with the development of numerous hamartomas. As mentioned previously, epithelial cells expressing LKB1 that is constitutively activated are able to form polarized domains in the absence of cell–cell and cell–substratum contact (12). Thus, proteins that participate in epithelial polarization may function as tumor suppressors by virtue of their capacity to control the growth and morphogenesis of the cells in which they are expressed.

Ischemic Injury

Other alterations in cell polarity may come about through the effect of renal ischemia on the tubular epithelium (69, 243, 244, 296, 313). Ischemic episodes of less than 1 hour often do not lead to tubular necrosis but may, nevertheless, cause diminished sodium and water uptake by the proximal tubule (204). Such brief ischemia compromises the polarity of tubular cells, resulting in the redistribution of a fraction of the Na$^+$,K$^+$-ATPase from the basolateral domain to the apical domain, preventing net sodium uptake by the tubule (204, 298). At the same time, leucine aminopeptidase moves from the apical to the basolateral domain and also becomes intracellular, presumably through endocytosis. At later times, Na$^+$,K$^+$-ATPase and leucine aminopeptidase are randomly

distributed on the plasma membrane of tubular epithelial cells remaining attached to the basement membrane or exfoliated into the lumenal space. The mechanism leading to this loss of polarity is not known. It is possible that ischemia, which is known to affect mitochondria and other organelles and to possibly alter the permeability of the plasma membrane, may result in increased cytoplasmic calcium concentrations (69, 296, 313). This, in turn, could disrupt elements of the cytoskeleton, perhaps affecting the maintenance of polarity. In fact, tubular epithelial cells have been observed by electron microscopy to develop basal densities following ischemia (296). These may represent disruption or perturbation of the cortical actin cytoskeleton. In support of this, in vitro studies with renal epithelial cell lines demonstrate that ATP depletion causes redistribution of actin from its normal locations in the cell cortex, terminal web, and microvilli to perinuclear cytoplasmic aggregates. Such alterations might affect transduction of spatial signals from the extracellular matrix to the polarization machinery along the lines previously discussed.

During reperfusion following renal ischemia, tubular epithelial cells detach from the basement membrane and accumulate in the lumen. It has been postulated that ischemia-induced depolarization of integrins from basal to apical domains of the plasma membrane contributes not only to cell detachment but also to cell aggregation and tubular obstruction. According to this hypothesis, at early times postischemia, redistribution of integrins would loosen attachment of cells from the basal lamina, allowing some of them to detach (91, 98, 234). Released cells would then aggregate and adhere to remaining tubular epithelial cells via their integrins. These would either bind directly to each other by homotypic interactions, or associate through bridging matrix molecules. Collections of such aggregates would obstruct the tubules, causing oliguria and destruction of renal tissue (91, 98, 234). In support of this hypothesis, integrins were observed to redistribute apically in oxidatively injured epithelial cell lines (91). Even more compelling was the observation that infusion of RGD peptides, which block some integrin-matrix interactions, appeared to ameliorate the effects of ischemia induced by clamping of the renal artery (233, 234). Recent in vivo findings using a rat model of renal ischemia do not, however, support this hypothesis, at least with regard to β1 integrins (355). Soon after reperfusion, β1 integrins were redistributed from a strictly basal to basolateral location in cells of the S3 segment of the proximal tubule, but did not appear on the apical plasma membrane at this time (355). Surprisingly, β1 integrins could not be detected by immunofluorescence in cells released from the basal lamina into the tubular lumen, precluding the possibility that they were mediating either cell aggregation or attachment of exfoliated cells to the residual tubular epithelium. Apical β1 integrins only appeared at later times postischemia as cells lost polarity in the process of regeneration (355).

Polycystic Kidney Disease

The progressive formation of renal cysts, which characterizes autosomal dominant polycystic kidney disease (ADPKD), has also been suggested to occur as a result of polarity defects. ADPKD is the most common potentially lethal dominant genetic human disease. Approximately 85% of all cases are linked to mutations in the PKD1 gene with another 10% linked to PKD2 (321). While the specific functions of the proteins encoded by these genes are the focus of intense study, the behavior of cyst epithelial cells in situ and in culture is consistent with a role for the PKD proteins in directing epithelial differentiation. Whereas renal tubular epithelial cells normally mediate fluid and electrolyte absorption, cyst epithelial cells carry out net secretion (105, 307). It has been suggested that the proximal cause of renal cyst formation in polycystic kidney disease may be the mis-targeting of Na^+,K^+-ATPase to the apical plasmalemma. According to this model, the presence of sodium pump at the apical surface leads to active apical ion secretion and the accumulation of lumenal cyst fluid (11, 341). Other studies suggest that mislocalization of Na^+,K^+-ATPase can not be the primary driving force for cyst fluid accumulation. When examined in cyst cells in culture or in situ, the Na^+,K^+-ATPase was found to be exclusively basolateral (36). Instead, the secretion appears to be driven by intracellular chloride accumulation via a basolateral $Na^+,K^+,2Cl^-$ cotransporter and apical chloride exit through the CFTR protein (36). A similar mechanism is responsible for fluid secretion by the poorly differentiated epithelial cells lining the crypts of the small intestine. As these crypt cells migrate up the intestinal villus they mature functionally, metamorphosing from secretory into resorptive epithelial cells (82). It has been suggested that the secretory phenotype is characteristic of immature epithelial cells, while more highly developed epithelial cells acquire the capacity to absorb fluid and electrolytes (306). The physiologic similarities relating cyst and crypt epithelial cells has prompted the hypothesis that loss of appropriate PKD function results in the dedifferentiation of mature resorptive renal tubular epithelial cells into more primitive secretory cells. The precise mechanisms through the PKD1 and PKD2 mutations produce the dramatic pathology associated with ADPKD, and the potential role of epithelial differentiation and sorting pathways, remain to be determined.

Acknowledgments

Work in our respective laboratories was supported by the National Institutes of Health (NIH DK46768 and NIH DK068568 [KSM], DK072614 and DK17833 [MJC]). We also thank our laboratory colleagues for helpful discussions, and Corryn Morris for assistance with organization of the authors and the manuscript.

References

1. Abaza NA, Leighton J, Schultz SG. Effects of ouabain on the function and structure of a cell line (MDCK) derived from canine kidney. *In Vitro* 1974;10:172–183.
2. Achler C, Filmer D, Merte C, Drenckhahn D. Role of microtubules in polarized delivery of apical membrane proteins to the brush border of the intestinal epithelium. *J Cell Biol* 1989;109:179–189.
3. Ahn J, Mundigl O, Muth TR, Rudnick G, Caplan MJ. Polarized expression of GABA transporters in Madin–Darby canine kidney cells and cultured hippocampal neurons. *J Biol Chem* 1996;271:6917–6924.
4. Al-Awqati Q. Plasticity in epithelial polarity of renal intercalated cells: targeting of the H-ATPase and band 3. *Am J Physiol* 1996;270:C1571–C1580.
5. Alper SL, Stuart-Tilley A, Simmons CF, Brown D, Drenckhahn D. The fodrin-ankyrin cytoskeleton of choroid plexus preferentially colocalizes with apical Na1K(1)-ATPase rather than with basolateral anion exchanger AE2. *J Clin Invest* 1994;93:1430–1438.
6. Amerongen HM, Mack JA, Wilson JM, Neutra MR. Membrane domains of intestinal epithelial cells: distribution of Na,K-ATPase and the membrane skeleton in adult rat intestine during fetal development and after epithelial isolation. *J Cell Biol* 1989;109:21219–22138.
7. Ang AL, Taguchi T, Francis S, Folsch H, Murrells LJ, Pypaert M, Warren G, Mellman I. Recycling endosomes can serve as intermediates during transport from the Golgi to the plasma membrane of MDCK cells. *J Cell Biol* 2004;167:531–543.
8. Areoti B, Kosen PA, Kuntz ID, Cohen FE, Mostov KE. Mutational and secondary structural analysis of the basolateral sorting signal of the polymeric immunoglobulin receptor. *J Cell Biol* 1993;123:1149–1160.
9. Arpin M, Pringault E, Finidori J, Garcia A, Jeltsch J-M, Vandekerckhove J, Louvard D. Sequence of human villin: a large duplicated domain homologous with other actin-severing proteins and a unique small carboxy-terminal domain related to villin specificity. *J Cell Biol* 1988;107:1759–1766.
10. Arreaza G, Melkonian KA, Bernt-LaFevre M, Brown DA. Triton X-100 membrane complexes from cultured kidney epithelial cells contain the Src family protein tyrosine kinase p62^{yes}. *J Biol Chem* 1994;269:19123–19127.
11. Avner ED, Sweeney WE, Nelson WJ. Abnormal sodium pump distribution during renal tubulogenesis in congenital murine polycystic kidney disease. *Proc Natl Acad Sci U S A* 1992; 89:7447–7451.
12. Baas AF, Kuipers J, van der Wel NN, Batlle E, Koerten HK, Peters PJ, Clevers HC. Complete polarization of single intestinal epithelial cells upon activation of LKB1 by STRAD. *Cell* 2004;116:457–466.
13. Bacallao R, Antony C, Dotti C, Karsenti E, Stelzer EHK, Simons K. The subcellular organization of Madin–Darby canine kidney cells during formation of a polarized epithelium. *J Cell Biol* 1989;109:2817–2832.
14. Balcarova-Stander J, Pfeiffer SE, Fuller SD, Simons K. Development of cell surface polarity in the epithelial Madin–Darby canine kidney (MDCK) cell line. *EMBO J* 1984;3:2687–2694.
15. Balda MS, Garrett MD, Matter K. The ZO-1–associated Y-box factor ZONAB regulates epithelial cell proliferation and cell density. *J Cell Biol* 2003;160:423–432.
16. Balda MS, Matter K. The tight junction protein ZO-1 and an interacting transcription factor regulate ErbB-2 expression. *EMBO J* 2000;19:2024–2033.
17. Barth AI, Nathke IS, Nelson WJ. Cadherins, catenins and APC protein: interplay between cytoskeletal complexes and signaling pathways. *Curr Opin Cell Biol* 1997;9:683–690.
18. Bartles JR, Feracci HM, Stieger B, Hubbard AL. Biogenesis of the rat hepatocyte plasma membrane in vivo: comparison of the pathways taken by apical and basolateral proteins using subcellular fractionation. *J Cell Biol* 1987;105:1241–1251.
19. Barylko B, Wagner MC, Reizes O, Albanesi JP. Purification and characterization of a mammalian myosin 1. *Proc Natl Acad Sci U S A* 1992;89:490–494.
20. Behrens J, Vakaet L, Friis R, Winterhager E, Vanroy F, Mareel MM, Birchmeier W. Loss of epithelial differentiation and gain of invasiveness correlates with tyrosine phosphorylation of the E-cadherin/beta-catenin complex in cells transformed with a temperature-sensitive v-SRC gene. *J Cell Biol* 1993;120:757–766.
21. Beltzer JP, Spiess M. In vitro binding of the asialoglycoprotein receptor to the b adaptin of plasma membrane coated vesicles. *EMBO J* 1991;10:3735–3742.
22. Bennett V. The membrane skeleton of human erythrocytes and its implications for more complex cells. *Annu Rev Biochem* 1985;54:273–304.
23. Benton R, St Johnston D. Drosophila PAR-1 and 14-3-3 inhibit Bazooka/PAR-3 to establish complementary cortical domains in polarized cells. *Cell* 2003;115:691–704.
24. Bhat MA, Izaddoost S, Lu Y, Cho KO, Choi KW, Bellen HJ. Discs lost, a novel multi-PDZ domain protein, establishes and maintains epithelial polarity. *Cell* 1999;96:833–845.
25. Bikle DD, Munson S, Komuves L. Zipper protein, a B-G protein with the ability to regulate actin/myosin 1 interactions in the intestinal brush border. *J Biol Chem* 1996;271:9075–9083.
26. Bilder D, Schober M, Perrimon N. Integrated activity of PDZ protein complexes regulates epithelial polarity. *Nat Cell Biol* 2003;5:53–58.
27. Birn H, Fyfe JC, Jacobsen C, Mounier F, Verroust PJ, Orskov H, Willnow TE, Moestrup SK, Christensen EI. Cubilin is an albumin binding protein important for renal tubular albumin reabsorption. *J Clin Invest* 2000;105:1353–1361.
28. Bre MH, Kreis TE, Karsenti E. Control of microtubule nucleation and stability in Madin–Darby canine kidney cells: the occurrence of noncentrosomal, stable detyrosinated microtubules. *J Cell Biol* 1987;105:1283–1296.
29. Bre M-H, Pepperkok R, Hill AM, Levilliers N, Ansorge W, Stelzer EHK, Karsenti E. Regulation of microtubule dynamics and nucleation during polarization in MDCK II cells. *J Cell Biol* 1990;111:3013–3021.
30. Bretscher A, Reczek D, Berryman M. Ezrin: a protein requiring conformational activation to link microfilaments to the plasma membrane in the assembly of cell surface structures. *J Cell Sci* 1997;110:3011–3018.
31. Bretscher A, Weber K. Fimbrin: a new microfilament-associated protein present in microvilli and other cell surface structures. *J Cell Biol* 1980;86:335–343.

32. Bretscher A, Weber K. Localization of actin and microfilament-associated proteins in the microvilli and terminal web of the intestinal brush border by immunofluorescent microscopy. *J Cell Biol* 1978;79:839–845.

33. Bretscher A, Weber K. Villin. The major microfilament-associated protein of the intestinal microvillus. *Proc Natl Acad Sci U S A* 1979;76:2321–2325.

34. Brewer CB, Roth MG. A single amino acid change in the cytoplasmic domain alters the polarized delivery of influenza virus hemagglutinin. *J Cell Biol* 1991;114:413–421.

35. Brewer CB, Thomas D, Roth MG. A signal for basolateral sorting of proteins in MDCK cells. *J Cell Biol* 1990;111:327a.

36. Brill S, Ross KE, Davidow CJ, Grantham JJ, Caplan MJ. Immunolocalization of ion transport proteins in human autosomal dominant polycystic kidney epithelial cells. *Proc Natl Acad Sci U S A* 1996;93:10206–10211.

37. Brown DA, Crise B, Rose JK. Mechanism of membrane anchoring affects polarized expression of two proteins in MDCK cells. *Science* 1989;245:1499–1501.

38. Burgess DR. Reactivation of intestinal epithelial cell brush border motility. ATP dependent contraction via a terminal web contractile ring. *J Cell Biol* 1982;95.

39. Caplan M, Matlin KS. Sorting of membrane and secretory proteins in polarized epithelial cells. In: Matlin KS, Valentich JC, eds. *Functional Epithelial Cells in Culture*. New York: Liss; 1989:71–127.

40. Caplan MJ. Biosynthesis and sorting of the sodium, potassium-ATPase. In: Reuss L, Russell JM, Szabo G, eds. *Regulation of Potassium Transport Across Biological Membranes*. Austin: University of Texas Press; 1990:77–101.

41. Caplan MJ, Anderson HC, Palade GE, Jamieson JD. Intracellular sorting and polarized cell surface deliver of (Na1,K1) ATPase, and endogenous component of MDCK cell basolateral plasma membranes. *Cell* 1986;46:623–631.

42. Caplan MJ, Forbush B, Palade GE, Jamieson JD. Biosynthesis of the Na,K-ATPase in Madin–Darby canine kidney cells. Activation and cell surface delivery. *J Biol Chem* 1990;265:3528–3534..

43. Caplan MJ, Stow JL, Newman AP, Madri J, Anderson HC, Farquhar MG, Palade GE, Jamieson JD. Dependence on pH of polarized sorting of secreted proteins. *Nature* 1987;329:632–635.

44. Casanova JE, Breitfeld PP, Ross SA, Mostov KE. Phosphorylation of the polymeric immunoglobulin receptor required for its efficient transcytosis. *Science* 1990;248:742–745.

45. Cereijido M, Ehrenfeld J, Fernandez-Castelo S, Meza I. Fluxes, junctions, and blisters in cultured monolayers of epithelioid cells (MDCK). *Ann N Y Acad Sci* 1981;372:422–440.

46. Cereijido M, Ponce A, Gonzalez-Mariscal L. Tight junctions and apical/basolateral polarity. *J Membr Biol* 1989;110:1–9.

47. Chen X, Macara IG. Par-3 controls tight junction assembly through the Rac exchange factor Tiam1. *Nat Cell Biol* 2005;7:262–269.

48. Chen X, Macara IG. Par-3 mediates the inhibition of LIM kinase 2 to regulate cofilin phosphorylation and tight junction assembly. *J Cell Biol* 2006;172:671–678.

49. Cheney RE, Mooseker MS. Unconventional myosins. *Curr Opin Cell Biol* 1992;4:27–35.

50. Cheng J, Moyer BD, Milewski M, Loffing J, Ikeda M, Mickle JE, Cutting GR, Li M, Stanton BA, Guggino WB. A Golgi-associated PDZ domain protein modulates cystic fibrosis transmembrane regulator plasma membrane expression. *J Biol Chem* 2002;277: 3520–3529.

51. Chuang JZ, Sung CH. The cytoplasmic tail of rhodopsin acts as a novel apical sorting signal in polarized MDCK cells. *J Cell Biol* 1998;142:1245–1256.

52. Chung K-N, Walter P, Aponte G, Moore H-PH. Molecular sorting in the secretory pathway. *Science* 1989;243:192–197.

53. Colegio OR, Van Itallie CM, McCrea HJ, Rahner C, Anderson JM. Claudins create charge-selective channels in the paracellular pathway between epithelial cells. *Am J Physiol Cell Physiol* 2002;283:C142–147.

54. Collawn JF, Stangel M, Kuhn LA, Esekogwu V, Jing S, Trowbridge IS, Tainer JA. Transferrin receptor internalization sequence YXRF implicates a tight turn as the structural recognition motif for endocytosis. *Cell* 1990;63:1061–1072.

55. Coluccio LM. Myosin I. *Am J Physiol* 1997;273:C347–C359.

56. Coluccio LM, Bretscher A. Reassociation of the microvillar core proteins: making a microvillar core in vitro. *J Cell Biol* 1989;108:495–502.

57. Costa de Beauregard MA, Pringault E, Robine S, Louvard D. Suppression of villin expression by antisense RNA impairs brush border assembly in polarized epithelial intestinal cells. *EMBO J* 1995;14:1409–1421.

58. Coudrier E, Kerjaschki D, Louvard D. Cytoskeletal organization and submembranous interactions in intestinal and renal brush borders. *Kidney Int* 1988;34:309–320.

59. Coudrier E, Reggio H, Louvard D. Characterization of an integral membrane glycoprotein associated with the microfilaments of pig intestinal microvilli. *EMBO J* 1983;2: 469–475.

60. Courtois-Coutry N, Roush DL, Rajendran V, McCarthy JB, Geibel J, Kashgarian M, Caplan MJ. A tyrosine-based signal targets H/K-ATPase to a regulated compartment and is required for the cessation of gastric acid secretion. *Cell* 1997;90:501–510.

61. Cross GAM. Eukaryotic protein modification and membrane attachment via phosphatidylinositol. *Cell* 1987;48:179–181.

62. Davis CG, Lehrman MA, Russell DW, Anderson RGW, Brown MS, Goldstein JL. The J.D. Mutation in familial hypercholesterolemia: amino acid substitution in cytoplasmic domain impedes internalization of LDL receptors. *Cell* 1986;45:15–24.

63. Dragsten PR, Blumenthal R, Handler JS. Membrane asymmetry in epithelia: is the tight junction a barrier to diffusion in the plasma membrane? *Nature* 1981;294:718–722.

64. Drenckhahn D, Demietzel R. Organization of the actin filament cytoskeleton in the intestinal brush border: a quantitative and qualitative immunoelectron microscope study. *J Cell Biol* 1988;107:1037–1048.

65. Drenckhahn D, Groschel-Stewart U. Localization of actin, myosin and tropomyosin in rat intestinal epithelium: immunohistochemical studies at the light and electron microscope levels. *J Cell Biol* 1980;86:475–482.

66. Drenckhahn D, Schlüter KS, Allen DP, Bennett V. Colocalization of band III with ankyrin and spectrin at the basal membrane of intercalated cells in the rat kidney. *Science* 1985;230:1287–1289.

67. Duffield A, Folsch H, Mellman I, Caplan MJ. Sorting of H,K-ATPase beta-subunit in MDCK and LLC-PK cells is independent of mu 1B adaptin expression. *Traffic* 2004;5:449–461.

68. Dunbar LA, Roush DL, Courtois-Coutry N, Muth TR, Gottardi CJ, Rajendran V, Geibel J, Kashgarian M, Caplan MJ. Sorting and regulation of ion pumps in polarized epithelial cells. *Acta Physiol Scand Suppl* 1998;643:289–295.

69. Edelstein CL, Ling H, Schrier RW. The nature of renal cell injury. *Kidney Int* 1997;51: 1341–1351.

70. Ekblom P. Developmentally regulated conversion of mesenchyme to epithelium. *FASEB J* 1989;3:2141–2150.

71. Fanning AS, Anderson JM. PDZ domains and the formation of protein networks at the plasma membrane. *Curr Top Microbiol Immunol* 1998;228:209–233.

72. Farquhar MG, Palade GE. Junctional complexes in various epithelia. *J Cell Biol* 1963;17:375–412.

73. Fath KR, Burgess DR. Golgi-derived vesicles from developing epithelial cells bind actin filaments and possess myosin-i as a cytoplasmically oriented peripheral membrane protein. *J Cell Biol* 1993;120:117–127.

74. Fath KR, Trimbur GM, Burgess DR. Molecular motors are differentially distributed on Golgi membranes from polarized epithelial cells. *J Cell Biol* 1994;126:661–675.

75. Fawcett DW. *Bloom and Fawcett: A Textbook of Histology*. Philadelphia: W.B. Saunders, 1986.

76. Ferro-Novick S, Jehn R. Vesicle fusion from yeast to man. *Nature* 1994;370:191–193.

77. Fish EM, Molitoris BA. Alterations in epithelial polarity and the pathogenesis of disease. *N Eng J Med* 1994;267:1580–1588.

78. Folsch H, Ohno H, Bonifacino JS, Mellman I. A novel clathrin adaptor complex mediates basolateral targeting in polarized epithelial cells. *Cell* 1999;99:189–198.

79. Forbush BI, Hoffman JF. Evidence that ouabain binds to the same large polypeptide chain of dimer Na,K-ATPase that is phosphorylated from Pi. *Biochemistry* 1979;18:2308–2315.

80. Forbush IB, Kaplan JH, Hoffman JF. Characterization of a new photoaffinity derivative of oubain: labelling of the large polypeptides and of a proteolipid component of the Na, K-ATPase. *Biochemistry* 1978;17:3667–3675.

81. Franke WW, Winter S, Grund C, Schmid E, Schiller DL, Jarasch ED. Isolation and characterization of desmosome associated tonofilaments from rat intestinal brush border. *J Cell Biol* 1981;90:116–127.

82. Freeman TC. Parallel patterns of cell-specific gene expression during enterocyte differentiation and maturation in the small intestine of the rabbit. *Differentiation* 1995;59:179–192.

83. Friedreich E, Huet C, Arpin M, Louvard D. Villin induces microvilli growth and actin redistribution in transfected fibroblasts. *Cell* 1989;59:461–475.

84. Frompter E, Diamond JM. Route of passive ion permeation in epithelia. *Nat New Biol (London)* 1972;235:9–13.

85. Fuller SD, Bravo R, Simons K. An enzymatic assay reveals that proteins destined for apical or basolateral domains of an epithelial cell line share the same late Golgi compartments. *EMBO J* 1985;4:297–307.

86. Fuller SD, Simons K. Transferrin receptor polarity and recycling accuracy in "tight" and "leaky" strains of Madin–Darby canine kidney cells. *J Cell Biol* 1986;103:1767–1779.

87. Furuse M, Fujita K, Hiiragi T, Fujimoto K, Tsukita S. Claudin-1 and -2: novel integral membrane proteins localizing at tight junctions with no sequence similarity to occludin. *J Cell Biol* 1998;141:1539–1550.

88. Furuse M, Furuse K, Sasaki H, Tsukita S. Conversion of zonulae occludentes from tight to leaky strand type by introducing claudin-2 into Madin–Darby canine kidney I cells. *J Cell Biol* 2001;153:263–272.

89. Furuse M, Sasaki H, Fujimoto K, Tsukita S. A single gene product, claudin-1 or -2, reconstitutes tight junction strands and recruits occludin in fibroblasts. *J Cell Biol* 1998;143:391–401.

90. Furuse M, Tsukita S. Claudins in occluding junctions of humans and flies. *Trends Cell Biol* 2006;16:181–188..

91. Gailit J, Colflesh D, Rabiner I, Simone J, Goligorsky MS. Redistribution and dysfunction of integrins in cultured renal epithelial cells exposed to oxidative stress. *Am J Physiol* 1993;264: F149–F157.

92. Garcia A, Coudrier E, Carboni J, Anderson J, Vanderkerkhove J, Mooseker M, Louvard D, Arpin M. Partial deduced sequence of the 110-kD–calmodulin complex of the avian intestinal microvillus shows that this mechanoenzyme is a member of the myosin I family. *J Cell Biol* 1989;109:2895–2903.

93. Gausch CR, Hard WL, Smith TF. Characterization of an established line of canine kidney epithelial cells (MDCK). *Proc Soc Exp Biol Med* 1966;122:931–935.

94. Geiger B, Bershadsky A. Assembly and mechanosensory function of focal contacts. *Curr Opin Cell Biol* 2001;13:584–592.

95. George-Labouesse E, Messaddeq, Yehia G, Cadalbert L, Dierich A, Le Meur M. Absence of integrin a6 leads to epidermolysis bullosa and neonatal death in mice. *Nat Genet* 1996;13:370–373.

96. Girones N, Alvarez E, Seth A, Lin IM, Latour DA, Davis RJ. Mutational analysis of the cytoplasmic tail of the human transferrin receptor: identification of a sub-domain that is required for rapid endocytosis. *J Biol Chem* 1991;266:19006–19012.

97. Glenney JR, Glenney P. Fodrin is the general spectrin-like protein found in most cells whereas spectrin and the TW protein have a restricted distribution. *Cell* 1983;34:503–512.

98. Goligorsky MS, Lieberthal W, Racusen L, Simon EE. Integrin receptors in renal tubular epithelium: new insights into pathphysiology of acute renal failure. *Am J Physiol* 1993;264: F1–F8.

99. Gonzalez-Mariscal L, Chavez de Ramirez B, Cereijido M. Tight junction formation in cultured epithelial cells (MDCK). *J Membr Biol* 1985;86:113–125.

100. Gottardi CJ, Arpin M, Fanning AS, Louvard D. The junction-associated protein, zonula occludens-1, localizes to the nucleus before the maturation and during the remodeling of cell–cell contacts. *Proc Natl Acad Sci U S A* 1996;93:10779–10784.
101. Gottardi CJ, Caplan MJ. An ion-transporting ATPase encodes multiple apical localization signals. *J Cell Biol* 1993;121:283–293.
102. Gottardi CJ, Caplan MJ. Vectorial targeting of newly synthesized Na,K-ATPase in polarized epithelial cells. *Science* 1993;260:552–554.
103. Gottlieb TA, Beaudry G, Rizzolo L, Colman A, Rindler M, Adesnik M, Sabatini DD. Secretion of endogenous and exogenous proteins from polarized MDCK cell monolayers. *Proc Natl Acad Sci U S A* 1986;83:2100–2104.
104. Gould KL, Cooper JA, Bretscher A, Hunter T. The protein-tyrosine kinase substrate p81 is homologous to a chicken microvillar core protein. *J Cell Biol* 1986;102:660–669.
105. Grantham JJ. Fluid secretion, cellular proliferation and the pathogenesis of renal epithelial cysts. *J Am Soc Nephrol* 1993;3:1843–1857.
106. Green RF, Meiss HK, Rodriguez-Boulan E. Glycosylation does not determine segregation of viral envelope proteins in the plasma membrane of epithelial cells. *J Cell Biol* 1981;89: 230–239.
107. Griffith LD, Bulger RE, Trump BF. Fine structure and staining of mucosubstances on "intercalated cells" from rat distal convoluted tubule and collecting duct. *Anat Rec* 1968;160:643–662.
108. Griffiths G, Pfeiffer S, Simons K, Matlin K. Exit of newly synthesized membrane proteins from the trans cisterna of the Golgi complex to the plasma membrane. *J Cell Biol* 1985;101:949–964.
109. Griffiths G, Simons K. The *trans* Golgi network: sorting at the exit site of the Golgi complex. *Science* 1986;234:438–443.
110. Grindstaff KK, Bacallao RL, Nelson WJ. Apiconuclear organization of microtubules does not specify protein delivery from the trans-Golgi network to different membrane domains in polarized epithelial cells. *Mol Biol Cell* 1998;9:685–699.
111. Gumbiner B, Lowenkopf T, Apatira D. Identification of a 160-kD polypeptide that binds to the tight junction protein ZO-1. *Proc Natl Acad Sci U S A* 1991;88:3460–3464.
112. Gumbiner BM. Carcinogenesis: a balance between beta-catenin and APC. *Curr Biol* 1997;7: R443–R446.
113. Gunderson D, Orlowski J, Rodriguez-Boulan E. Apical polarity of Na,K-ATPase in retinal pigment epithelium is linked to reversal of ankyrin-fodrin submembrane cytoskeleton. *J Cell Biol* 1991;112:863–872.
114. Guo W, Roth D, Walch-Solimena C, Novick P. The exocyst is an effector for Sec4p, targeting secretory vesicles to sites of exocytosis. *EMBO J* 1999;18:1071–1080.
115. Hall RA, Ostedgaard LS, Premont RT, Blitzer JT, Rahman N, Welsh MJ, Lefkowitz RJ. A C-terminal motif found in the beta2-adrenergic receptor, P2Y1 receptor and cystic fibrosis transmembrane conductance regulator determines binding to the Na,H exchanger regulatory factor family of PDZ proteins. *Proc Natl Acad Sci U S A* 1998;95:8496–8501.
116. Hammerton RW, Krzeminski KA, Mays RW, Ryan TA, Wollner DA, Nelson WJ. Mechanism for regulating cell surface distribution of Na^1, K^1-ATPase in polarized epithelial cells. *Science* 1991;254:847–850.
117. Hammerton RW, Nelson WJ. Development of cell surface polarity of Na,K-ATPase of MDCK cells. *J Cell Biol* 1990;111:458a.
118. Handler JS. Antidiuretic hormone moves membranes. *Am J Physiol* 1988;255:F375–F382.
119. Handler JS, Preston AS, Steele RE. Factors affecting the differentiation of epithelial transport and responsiveness to hormones. *Federation Proc* 43:2221–2224.
120. Haskins J, Gu L, Wittchen ES, Hibbard J, Stevenson BR. ZO-3, a novel member of the MAGUK protein family found at the tight junction, interacts with ZO-1 and occludin. *J Cell Biol* 1998;141:199–208.
121. Hauri H-P, Quaroni A, Isselbacher KJ. Biogenesis of intestinal plasma membrane: posttranslational route and cleavage of sucrase-isomaltase. *Proc Natl Acad Sci U S A* 1979;76:5183–5186.
122. Hayden SM, Wolenski JS, Mooseker MS. Binding of brush border myosin I to phospholipid vesicles. *J Cell Biol* 1990;111:443–451.
123. Hecht G, Pestic L, Nikcevic G, Koutsouris A, Tripuraneni J, Lorimer DD, Nowak G, Guerriero V, Elson EL, Lanerolle PD. Expression of the catalytic domain of myosin light chain kinase increases paracellular permeability. *Am J Physiol* 1996;271:C1678–C1684.
124. Hemler ME. VLA proteins in the integrin family: structures, functions, and their role in leukocytes. *Annu Rev Immunol* 1990;8:365–400.
125. Hendler RW. Biological membrane ultrastructure. *Phys Rev* 1971;51:1–66.
126. Hersey SJ, Sachs G. Gastric acid secretion. *Phys Rev* 1995;75:155–189.
127. Herzlinger DA, Easton TG, Ojakian GK. The MDCK epithelial cell line expresses a cell surface antigen of the kidney distal tubule. *J Cell Biol* 1982;93:269–277.
128. Hirokawa N, Keller TCS, Chasan R, Mooseker MS. Mechanism of brush border contractility studied by the quick-freeze-deep-etch method. *J Cell Biol* 1983;96:1325–1336.
129. Hoppe CA, Connolly TP, Hubbard AL. Transcellular transport of polymeric IgA in the rat hepatocyte: biochemical and morphological characterization of the transport pathway. *J Cell Biol* 1985;101:2113–2123.
130. Hoshimaru M, Nakanishi N. Identification of a new type of mammalian myosin heavy chain by molecular cloning. *J Biol Chem* 1987;262:14625–14632.
131. Howe CL, Mooseker MS. Characterization of the 110 kilodalton actin-, calmodulin- and membrane-binding protein from microvilli of intestinal epithelial cells. *J Cell Biol* 1983;97:974–985.
132. Hubbard AL, Stieger B. Biogenesis of endogenous plasma membrane proteins in epithelial cells. *Annu Rev Physiol* 1989;51:755–770.
133. Hunziker W, Fumey C. A di-leucine motif mediates endocytosis and basolateral sorting of macrophage IgG Fc receptors in MDCK cells. *EMBO J* 1994;13:2963–2967.
134. Hunziker W, Harter C, Matter K, Mellman I. Basolateral sorting in MDCK cells requires a distinct cytoplasmic domain determinant. *Cell* 1991;66:907–920.
135. Hunziker W, Mellman I. Expression of macrophage-lymphocyte Fc receptors in Madin–Darby canine kidney cells: polarity and transcytosis differ for isoforms with or without coated pit localization domains. *J Cell Biol* 1989;109:3291–3302.
136. Hurd TW, Fan S, Liu CJ, Kweon HK, Hakansson K, Margolis B. Phosphorylation-dependent binding of 14-3-3 to the polarity protein Par3 regulates cell polarity in mammalian epithelia. *Curr Biol* 2003;13:2082–2090.
137. Hutterer A, Betschinger J, Petronczki M, Knoblich JA. Sequential roles of Cdc42, Par-6, aPKC, and Lgl in the establishment of epithelial polarity during Drosophila embryogenesis. *Dev Cell* 2004;6:845–854.
138. Hynes RO. Integrins: bidirectional, allosteric signaling machines. *Cell* 2002;110:673–687.
139. Hynes RO. Integrins: versatility, modulation, and signaling in cell adhesion. *Cell* 1992;69:11–25.
140. Ikonen E, Tagaya M, Ullrich O, Montecucco C, Simons K. Different requirements for NSF, SNAP, and Rab proteins in apical and basolateral transport in MDCK cells. *Cell* 1995;81: 571–580.
141. Inoue T, Nielsen S, Mandon B, Terris J, Kishore BK, Knepper MA. SNAP-23 in rat kidney: colocalization with aquaporin-2 in collecting duct vesicles. *Am J Physiol* 1998;275:F752–F760.
142. Jesaitis LA, Goodenough DA. Molecular characterization and tissue distribution of ZO-2, a tight junctional protein homologous to ZO-1 and the Drosophila discs–large tumor suppressor protein. *J Cell Biol* 1994;124:949–961.
143. Jones BG, Thomas L, Molloy SS, Thulin CD, Fry MD, Walsh KA, Thomas G. Intracellular trafficking of furin is modulated by the phosphorylation state of a casein kinase II site in its cytoplasmic tail. *EMBO J* 1995;14:5869–5883.
144. Jones LV, Compans RW, Davis AR, Bos TJ, Nayak DP. Surface expression of influenza virus neuraminidase, an aminoterminally anchored viral membrane glycoprotein, in polarized epithelial cells. *Mol Cell Biol* 1985;5:2181–2189.
145. Kaverina I, Rottner K, Small JV. Targeting, capture, and stabilization of microtubules at early focal adhesions. *J Cell Biol* 1998;142:181–190.
146. Kerjaschki D, Noronha-Blob L, Saktor B, Farquhar MG. Microdomains of distinctive glycoprotein composition in the kidney proximal tubule brush border. *J Cell Biol* 1984;98:1505–1513.
147. Kerjaschki D, Ojha PP, Susani M, Horvat R, Binder S, Hovorka A, Hillemanns P, Pytela R. A b_1-integrin receptor for fibronectin in human kidney glomeruli. *Am J Pathol* 1989;134:481–489.
148. Kim SK. Polarized signaling: basolateral receptor localization in epithelial cells by PDZ-containing proteins. *Curr Opin Cell Biol* 1997;9:853–859.
149. Kipp H, Arias IM. Trafficking of canalicular ABC transporters in hepatocytes. *Annu Rev Physiol* 2002;64:595–608.
150. Kirschner M and Mitchison T. Beyond self-assembly: from microtubules to morphogenesis. *Cell* 1986;45:329–342.
151. Klein G, Langegger M, Timpl R, Ekblom P. Role of the laminin A chain in the development of epithelial cell polarity. *Cell* 1988;55:331–341.
152. Koeppen BM, Giebisch GH. Mineralocorticoid regulation of sodium and potassium transport by the cortical collecting duct. In: Graves JS, ed. *Regulation and Development of Membrane Transport Processes*. New York: John Wiley & Sons, 1985:89–104.
153. Kondor-Koch C, Bravo R, Fuller SD, Cutler D, Garoff H. Exocytotic pathways exist to both the apical and the basolateral cell surface of the polarized epithelial cell MDCK. *Cell* 1985;43:297–306.
154. Korhonen M, Ylanne J, Laitinen L, Virtanen I. The a1–a6 subunits of integrins are characteristically expressed in distinct segments of developing and adult human nephron. *J Cell Biol* 1990;111:1245–1254.
155. Kornfeld S. Trafficking of lysosomal enzymes. *FASEB J* 1987;1:462–468.
156. Kreidberg JA, Donovan MJ, Goldstein SL, Rennke H, Shepherd K, Jones RC, Jaenisch R. Alpha 3 beta 1 integrin has a crucial role in kidney and lung organogenesis. *Development* 1996;122:3537–3547.
157. Kreidberg JA, Symons JM. Integrins in kidney development, function, and disease. *Am J Physiol Renal Physiol* 2000;279:F233–242.
158. Kundu A, Avalos RT, Sanderson CM, Nayak DP. Transmembrane domnain of influenza virus neuraminidase, a type II protein, possesses an apical sorting signal in polarized MDCK cells. *J Virol* 1996;70:6508–6515.
159. Larkin JM, Sztul ES, Palade GE. Phosphorylation of the rat hepatic polymeric IgA receptor. *Proc Natl Acad Sci U S A* 1986;83:4759–4763.
160. Lazorovits J, Roth M. A single amino acid change in the cytoplasmic domain allows the influenza virus hemeagglutinin to be endocytosed through coated pits. *Cell* 1988;53:743–752.
161. Le Bivic A, Real FX, Rodriguez-Boulan E. Vectorial targeting of apical and basolateral plasma membrane proteins in a human adenocarcinoma epithelial cell line. *Proc Natl Acad Sci U S A* 1989;86:9313–9317.
162. Le Bivic A, Sambuy Y, Mostov K, Rodriguez-Boulan E. Vectorial targeting of an endogenous apical membrane sialoglycoprotein and uvomorulin in MDCK cells. *J Cell Biol* 1990;110:1533–1539.
163. Le Bivic A, Sambuy Y, Patzak A, Patil N, Chao M, Rodriguez-Boulan E. An internal deletion in cytoplasmic tail reverses apical localization of human GF receptor in transfected MDCK cells. *J Cell Biol* 1991;115:607–618.
164. Leheste JR, Rolinski B, Vorum H, Hilpert J, Nykjaer A, Jacobsen C, Aucouturier P, Moskaug JO, Otto A, Christensen EI, Willnow TE. Megalin knockout mice as an animal model of low molecular weight proteinuria. *Am J Pathol* 1999;155:1361–1370.
165. Leighton J, Brada Z, Estes LW, Justh G. Secretory activity and oncogenicity of a cell line (MDCK) derived from canine kidney. *Science* 163:472–473, 1969.
166. Lelongt B, Ronco P. Role of extracellular matrix in kidney development and repair. *Pediatr Nephrol* 2003;18:731–742.
167. Lencer WI, Verkman AS, Arnaout MA, Ausiello DA, Brown D. Endocytic vesicles from renal papilla which retrieve the vasopressin-sensitive water channel do not contain a functional H1-ATPase. *J Cell Biol* 1990;111:379–389.
168. Li S, Edgar D, Fassler R, Wadsworth W, Yurchenco PD. The role of laminin in embryonic cell polarization and tissue organization. *Dev Cell* 2003;4:613–624.

169. Li S, Liquari P, McKee KK, Harrison D, Patel R, Lee S, Yurchenco PD. Laminin-sulfatide binding initiates basement membrane assembly and enables receptor signaling in Schwann cells and fibroblasts. *J Cell Biol* 2005;169:179–189.
170. Lin F, Hiesberger T, Cordes K, Sinclair AM, Goldstein LS, Somlo S, Igarashi P. Kidney-specific inactivation of the KIF3A subunit of kinesin-II inhibits renal ciliogenesis and produces polycystic kidney disease. *Proc Natl Acad Sci U S A* 2003;100:5286–5291.
171. Lin S, Naim HY, Roth MG. Tyrosine-dependent basolateral sorting signals are distinct from tyrosine-dependent internalization signals. *J Biol Chem* 1997;272:26300–26305.
172. Lina F, Satlinb LM. Polycystic kidney disease: the cilium as a common pathway in cystogenesis. *Curr Opin Pediatr* 2004;16:171–176.
173. Lisanti MP, Caras IW, Davitz MA, Rodriguez-Boulan E. A glycophospholipid membrane anchor acts as an apical targeting signal in polarized epithelial cells. *J Cell Biol* 1989;109:2145–2156.
174. Lisanti MP, Le Bivic A, Saltiel AR, Rodriguez-Boulan EJ. Preferred apical distribution of glycosyl-phosphatidylinositol (GPI) anchored proteins: a highly conserved feature of the polarized epithelial cell phenotype. *J Membr Biol* 1990;113:155–167.
175. Low SH, Chapin SJ, Wimmer C, Whiteheart SW, Komuves LG, Mostov KE, Weimbs T. The SNARE machinery is involved in apical plasma membrane trafficking in MDCK cells. *J Cell Biol* 1998;141:1503–1513.
176. Macara IG. Parsing the polarity code. *Nat Rev Mol Cell Biol* 2004;5:220–231.
177. Madara JL, Hecht G. Tight (occluding) junctions in cultured (and native) epithelial cells. In: Matlin KS, Valentich JD, eds. *Functional Epithelial Cells in Culture.* New York: Liss, 1989:131–164.
178. Madin SH, Darby NB. *American Type Culture Collection Catalogue of Strains II.* Rockville, MD: American Type Culture Collection, 1975.
179. Mandel LJ, Balaban RS. Stoichiometry and coupling of active transport to oxidative metabolism in epithelial tissues. *Am J Physiol* 1981;240:F357–F371.
180. Marks MS, Woodruff L, Ohno H, Bonifacino JS. Protein targeting by tyrosine- and dileucine-based signals: evidence for distinct saturable components. *J Cell Biol* 1996;135:341–354.
181. Martin GR, Timpl R. Laminin and other basement membrane components. *Annu Rev Cell Biol* 1987;3:57–86.
182. Massey D, Feracci H, Gorvel J-P, Soulie JM, Maroux S. Evidence for the transit of aminopeptidase N through the basolateral membrane before it reaches the brush border of enterocytes. *J Membr Biol* 1987;96:19–25.
183. Matlin KS. Ammonium chloride slows transport of the influenza virus hemagglutinin but does not cause mis-sorting in a polarized epithelial cell line. *J Biol Chem* 1986;261:15172–15178.
184. Matlin KS. The sorting of proteins to the plasma membrane in epithelial cells. *J Cell Biol* 1986;103.
185. Matlin KS, Bainton DF, Pesonen M, Louvard D, Genty N, Simons K. Transepithelial transport of a viral membrane glycoprotein implanted into the apical plasma membrane of MDCK cells. I. Morphological evidence. *J Cell Biol* 1983;97:627–637.
186. Matlin KS, Simons K. Reduced temperature prevents transfer of a membrane glycoprotein to the cell surface but does not prevent terminal glycosylation. *Cell* 1983;34:233–243.
187. Matlin KS, Simons K. Sorting of an apical plasma membrane glycoprotein occurs before it reaches the cell surface in cultured epithelial cells. *J Cell Biol* 1984;99:2131–2139.
188. Matsudaira PT, Burgess DR. Identification and organization of the components in the isolated microvillus cytoskeleton. *J Cell Biol* 1979;83:667–673.
189. Matsudaira PT, Burgess DR. Partial reconstruction of the microvillus core bundle: characterization of villin as a Ca-dependent, actin bundling/depolymerizing protein. *J Cell Biol* 1982;92:648–656.
190. Matter K, Brauchbar M, Bucher K, Hauri HP. Sorting of endogenous plasma membrane proteins occurs from two sites in cultured human intestinal epithelial cells (Caco-2). *Cell* 1990;60:429–437.
191. Matter K, Hunziker W, Mellman I. Basolateral sorting of LDL receptor in MDCK cells—the cytoplasmic domain contains 2 tyrosine-dependent targeting determinants. *Cell* 1992;71:741–753.
192. Matter K, Yamamoto EM, Mellman I. Structural requirements and sequence motifs for polarized sorting and endocytosis of LDL and Fc receptors in MDCK cells. *J Cell Biol* 1994;126:991–1004.
193. Maunsbach AE. Cellular mechanism of tubular protein transport. *Int Rev Physiol* 2:145–167.
194. Maxfield FR. Weak bases and ionophores rapidly and reversibly raise the pH of endocytic vesicles in cultured mouse fibroblasts. *J Cell Biol* 1982;95:676–681.
195. Mays RW, Siemers KA, Fritz BA, Lowe AW, van Meer G, Nelson WJ. Hierarchy of mechanisms involved in generating Na/K-ATPase polarity in MDCK epithelial cells. *J Cell Biol* 1995;130:1105–1115.
196. McNeil H, Ozawa M, Kemler R, Nelson WJ. Novel function of the cell adhesion molecule uvomorulin as an inducer of cell surface polarity. *Cell* 1990;62:309–316.
197. Mercurio AM. Laminin receptors: achieving specificity through cooperation. *Trends Cell Biol* 1995;5:419–423.
198. Milewski MI, Mickle JE, Forrest JK, Stafford DM, Moyer BD, Cheng J, Guggino WB, Stanton BA, Cutting GR. A PDZ-binding motif is essential but not sufficient to localize the C terminus of CFTR to the apical membrane. *J Cell Sci* 2001;114:719–726.
199. Miner JH. Renal basement membrane components. *Kidney Int* 1999;56:2016–2024.
200. Miner JH and Yurchenco PD. Laminin functions in tissue morphogenesis. *Annu Rev Cell Dev Biol* 2004;20:255–284.
201. Misek DE, Bard E, Rodriguez-Boulan EJ. Biogenesis of epithelial cell polarity: intracellular sorting and vectorial exocytosis of an apical plasma membrane glycoprotein. *Cell* 1984;39:537–546.
202. Misfeldt DS, Hamamoto ST, Pitelka DR. Transepithelial transport in cell culture. *Proc Natl Acad Sci U S A* 73:1212–1216.
203. Mogensen MM, Tucker JB, Mackie JB, Prescott AR, Nathke IS. The adenomatous polyposis coli protein unambiguously localizes to microtubule plus ends and is involved in establishing parallel arrays of microtubule bundles in highly polarized epithelial cells. *J Cell Biol* 157:1041–1048.
204. Molitoris BA, Chan LK, Shapiro JI, Conger JD, Falk SA. Loss of epithelial polarity: a novel hypothesis for reduced proximal tubule Na1 transport following ischemic injury. *J Membr Biol* 1989;107:119–127.
205. Mollet G, Silbermann F, Delous M, Salomon R, Antignac C, Saunier S. Characterization of the nephrocystin/nephrocystin-4 complex and subcellular localization of nephrocystin-4 to primary cilia and centrosomes. *Hum Mol Genet* 2005;14:645–656.
206. Mooseker MS. Brush border motility: microvillar contraction in triton-treated brush border isolated from intestinal epithelium. *J Cell Biol* 71:417–432.
207. Mooseker MS. Organization, chemistry and assembly of the cytoskeletal apparatus of the intestinal brush border. *Annu Rev Cell Biol* 1985;1:209–241.
208. Mooseker MS and Cheney RE. Unconventional myosins. *Annu Rev Cell Dev Biol* 1995;11:633–675.
209. Mooseker MS, Coleman TR. The 110-kD protein-calmodulin complex of the intestinal microvillus (brush border myosin I) is a mechanoenzyme. *J Cell Biol* 1989;108:2395–2400.
210. Morita K, Furuse M, Fujimoto K, Tsukita S. Claudin multigene family encoding four-transmembrane domain protein components of tight junction strands. *Proc Natl Acad Sci U S A* 1999;96:511–516.
211. Morrow JS, Cianci CD, Ardito T, Mann AS, Kashgarian M. Ankyrin links fodrin to the alpha subunit of Na,K-ATPase in Madin–Darby canine kidney cells and in intact renal tubule cells. *J Cell Biol* 1989;108:455–465.
212. Mostov KE, Breitfeld P, Harris JM. An anchor-minus form of the polymeric immunoglobulin receptor is secreted predominantly apically in Madin–Darby canine kidney cells. *J Cell Biol* 1987;105:2031–2036.
213. Mostov KE, de Bruyn Kops A, Deitcher DL. Deletion of the cytoplasmic domain of the polymeric immunoglobulin receptor prevents basolateral localization and endocytosis. *Cell* 1986;47:359–364.
214. Mostov KE, Deitcher DL. Polymeric immunoglobulin receptor expressed in MDCK cells transcytoses IgA. *Cell* 1986;46:613–621.
215. Mostov KE, Simister NE. Transcytosis. *Cell* 1985;43:389–390.
216. Moyer BD, Denton J, Karlson KH, Reynolds D, Wang S, Mickle JE, Milewski M, Cutting GR, Guggino WB, Li M, Stanton BA. A PDZ-interacting domain in CFTR is an apical membrane polarization signal. *J Clin Invest* 1999;104:1353–1361.
217. Moyer BD, Duhaime M, Shaw C, Denton J, Reynolds D, Karlson KH, Pfeiffer J, Wang S, Mickle JE, Milewski M, Cutting GR, Guggino WB, Li M, Stanton BA. The PDZ-interacting domain of cystic fibrosis transmembrane conductance regulator is required for functional expression in the apical plasma membrane. *J Biol Chem* 2000;275:27069–27074.
218. Muller U, Wang D, Denda S, Meneses JJ, Pedersen RA, Reichardt LF. Integrin a8b1 is critically important for epithelial–mesenchymal interactions in kidney morphogenesis. *Cell* 1997;88:603–613.
219. Muth TR, Ahn J, Caplan MJ. Identification of sorting determinants in the C-terminal cytoplasmic tails of the g-aminobutyric acid transporters GAT-2 and GAT-3. *J Biol Chem* 1998;273:25616–25627.
220. Muth TR, Gottardi CJ, Roush DL, Caplan MJ. A dominant basolateral sorting signal is encoded in the a-subunit of the Na,K-ATPase. *Am J Physiol* 1998;274:C688–C696.
221. Nagafuchi A, Ishihara S, Tsukita S. The roles of catenins in the cadherin-mediated cell adhesion: functional analysis of E-cadherin-a-catenin fusion molecules. *J Cell Biol* 1994;127:235–245.
222. Nagafuchi A, Takeichi M. Cell binding function of E-cadherin is regulated by the cytoplasmic domain. *EMBO J* 1988;7:3679–3684.
223. Nagafuchi A, Takeichi M. Transmembrane control of cadherin- mediated adhesion: a 94-kDa protein functionally associated with a specific region of the cytoplasmic domain of E-cadherin. *Cell Regul* 1989;1:37–44.
224. Nagai M, Meerloo T, Takeda T, Farquhar MG. The adaptor protein ARH escorts megalin to and through endosomes. *Mol Biol Cell* 2003;14:4984–4996.
225. Nelson WJ. Adaptation of core mechanisms to generate cell polarity. *Nature* 2003;422:766–774.
226. Nelson WJ. Development and maintenance of epithelial polarity: a role for the submembranous cytoskeleton. In: Matlin KS, Valentich JD, eds. *Functional Epithelial Cells in Culture.* New York: Liss; 1989:3–42.
227. Nelson WJ, Hammerton RW. A membrane-cytoskeletal complex containing Na,K-ATPase, ankyrin, and fodrin in Madin–Darby canine kidney (MDCK) cells: implications for the biogenesis of epithelial cell polarity. *J Cell Biol* 1989;108:893–902.
228. Nelson WJ, Shore EM, Wang AZ, Hammerton RW. Identification of a membrane-cytoskeletal complex containing the cell adhesion molecule uvomorulin (E-cadherin), ankyrin and fodrin in Madin-Darby canine kidney epithelial cells. *J Cell Biol* 1990;110:349–357.
229. Nelson WJ, Veshnock PJ. Ankyrin binding to Na,K-ATPase and implications for organization of membrane domains in polarized cells. *Nature* 1987;328:533–536.
230. Nelson WJ and Veshnock PJ. Dynamics of membrane-skeleton (fodrin) organization during development of polarity in Madin–Darby canine kidney epithelial cells. *J Cell Biol* 1986;103:1751–1765.
231. Nelson WJ, Veshnock PJ. Modulation of fodrin (membrane skeleton) stability by cell–cell contacts in Madin–Darby canine kidney epithelial cells. *J Cell Biol* 1987;104:1527–1537.
232. Nishinakamura R, Takasato M. Essential roles of Sall1 in kidney development. *Kidney Int* 2005;68:1948–1950.
233. Noiri E, Gailit J, Sheth D, Magazine H, Gurrath M, Muller G, Kessler H, Goligorsky MS. Cyclic RGD peptides ameliorate ischemic acute renal failure in rats. *Kidney Int* 1994;46:1050–1058.
234. Noiri E, Romanov V, Czerwinski G, Gailit J, DiBona GF, Som P, Oster Z, Goligorsky MS. Adhesion receptors and tubular obstruction in acute renal failure. *Ren Fail* 1996;18:513–515.

235. Nusrat A, Giry M, Turner JR, Colgan SP, Parkos CA, Carnes D, Lemichez E, Boquet P, Madara JL. Rho protein regulates tight junctions and perijunctional actin organization in polarized epithelia. *Proc Natl Acad Sci U S A* 1995;92:10629–10633.
236. Nykjaer A, Dragun D, Walther D, Vorum H, Jacobsen C, Herz J, Melsen F, Christensen EI, Willnow TE. An endocytic pathway essential for renal uptake and activation of the steroid 25-(OH) vitamin D3. *Cell* 1999;96:507–515.
237. O'Brien LE, Jou TS, Pollack AL, Zhang Q, Hansen SH, Yurchenco P, Mostov KE. Rac1 orientates epithelial apical polarity through effects on basolateral laminin assembly. *Nat Cell Biol* 2001;3:831–838.
238. O'Brien LE, Zegers MM, Mostov KE. Opinion: building epithelial architecture: insights from three-dimensional culture models. *Nat Rev Mol Cell Biol* 2002;3:531–537.
239. Odorizzi G, Pearse A, Domingo D, Trowbridge IS, Hopkins CR. Apical and basolateral endosomes of MDCK cells are interconnected and contain a polarized sorting mechanism. *J Cell Biol* 1996;135:139–152.
240. Odorizzi G, Trowbridge IS. Structural requirements for basolateral sorting of the human transferrin receptor in the biosynthetic and endocytic pathways of Madin–Darby canine kidney cells. *J Cell Biol* 1997;137:1255–1264.
241. Ohno H, Stewart J, Fournier MC, Bosshart H, Rhee I, Miyatake S, Saito T, Gallusser A, Kirchhausen T, Bonifacino JS. Interaction of tyrosine based sorting signals with clathrin associated proteins. *Science* 1995;269:1872–1875.
242. Ohno H, Tomemori T, Nakatsu F, Okazaki Y, Aguilar RC, Foelsch H, Mellman I, Saito T, Shirasawa T, Bonifacino JS. Mu1B, a novel adaptor medium chain expressed in polarized epithelial cells. *FEBS Lett* 1999;449:215–220.
243. Oliver J. Correlations of structure and function and mechanisms of recovery in acute tubular necrosis. *Am J Med* 1953;15:535–557.
244. Oliver J, MacDowell M, Tracy A. The pathogenesis of acute renal failure associated with traumatic and toxic injury. Renal ischemia, nephrotoxic damage and the ischemuric episode. *J Clin Invest* 1951;30:1307–1351.
245. O'Neil RG. Adrenal steroid regulation of potassium transport. *Curr Trends Membr Trans* 1987;28:185–206.
246. Orci L, Ravazzola M, Amherdt M, Perrelet A, Powell SK, Quinn DL, Moore H-PH. The *trans*-most cisternae of the Golgi complex: a compartment for sorting of secretory and plasma membrane proteins. *Cell* 1987;51:1039–1051.
247. Ozawa M, Baribault H, Kemler R. The cytoplasmic domain of the cell adhesion molecule uvomorulin associates with three independent proteins structurally related in different species. *EMBO J* 1989;8:1711–1717.
248. Palmer LG, Frindt G. Amiloride-sensitive Na channels from the apical membrane of the rat cortical collecting tubule. *Proc Natl Acad Sci U S A* 1986;83:2767–2770.
249. Parczyk K, Haase W, Kondor KC. Microtubules are involved in the secretion of proteins at the apical cell surface of the polarized epithelial cell, Madin–Darby canine kidney. *J Biol Chem* 1989;264:16837–16846.
250. Pearse BMF. Assembly of the mannose-6-phosphate receptor onto reconstituted clathrin coats. *EMBO J* 1985;4:2457–2460.
251. Pearse BMF. Receptors compete for adaptors found in plasma membrane coated pits. *EMBO J* 1988;7:3331–3336.
252. Pearse BMF, Robinson MS. Clathrin, adaptors and sorting. *Annu Rev Cell Biol* 1990;6: 151–171.
253. Pfeiffer S, Fuller SD, Simons K. Intracellular sorting and basolateral appearance of the G protein of vesicular stomatitis virus in MDCK cells. *J Cell Biol* 1985;101:470–476.
254. Pietrini G, Suh YJ, Edelmann L, Rudnick G, Caplan MJ. The axonal GABA transporter is sorted to the apical membranes of polarized epithelial cells. *J Biol Chem* 1994;269:4668–4674.
255. Pinson KI, Dunbar L, Samuelson L, Gumucio DL. Targeted disruption of the mouse villin gene does not impair the morphogenesis of microvilli. *Dev Dynam* 1998;211:109–212.
256. Praetorius HA, Spring KR. A physiological view of the primary cilium. *Annu Rev Physiol* 2005;67:515–529.
257. Praetorius HA, Spring KR. The renal cell primary cilium functions as a flow sensor. *Curr Opin Nephrol Hypertens* 2003;12:517–520.
258. Qi AD, Wolff SC, Nicholas RA. The apical targeting signal of the P2Y2 receptor is located in its first extracellular loop. *J Biol Chem* 2005;280:29169–29175.
259. Racusen LC, Monteil C, Sgrignoli A, Lucskay M, Marouillat S, Rhim JG, Morin JP. Cell lines with extended in vitro growth potential from human renal proximal tubule: characterization, response to inducers, and comparison with established cell lines. *J Lab Clin Med* 1997;129:318–329.
260. Rapoport I, Chen YC, Cupers P, Shoelson SE, Kirchhausen T. Dileucine-based sorting signals bind to the beta chain of AP-1 at a site distinct and regulated differently from the tyrosine-based motif-binding site. *EMBO J* 1998;17:2148–2155.
261. Reich V, Mostov K, Areoti B. The basolateral sorting signal of the polymeric immunoglobulin receptor contains two functional domains. *J Cell Sci* 1996;109:2133–2139.
262. Reilein A, Nelson WJ. APC is a component of an organizing template for cortical microtubule networks. *Nat Cell Biol* 2005;7:463–473.
263. Rindler MJ, Ivanov IE, Plesken H, Rodriguez-Boulan EJ, Sabatini DD. Viral glycoproteins destined for the apical or basolateral plasma membrane domains traverse the same Golgi apparatus during their intracellular transport in double infected Madin–Darby canine kidney. *Cells J Cell Biol* 1984;98:1304–1319.
264. Rindler MJ, Ivanov IE, Sabatini DD. Microtubule-acting drugs lead to the nonpolarized delivery of the influenza hemagglutinin to the cell surface of polarized Madin–Darby canine kidney cells. *J Cell Biol* 1987;104:231–241.
265. Robine S, Huet C, Moll R, Sahuquillo-Merino C, Coudrier E, Zweibaum A, Louvard D. Can villin be used to identify malignant and undifferentiated normal digestive epithelial cells? *Proc Natl Acad Sci U S A* 1986;82:8488–8492.
266. Rodman JS, Seidman L, Farquhar MG. The membrane composition of coated pits, microvilli, endosomes and lysosomes is distinctive in the rat kidney proximal tubule cell. *J Cell Biol* 1986;5:77–87.
267. Rodriguez Boulan E, Pendergast M. Polarized distribution of viral envelope proteins in the plasma membrane of infected epithelial cells. *Cell* 1980;20:45–54.
268. Rodriguez-Boulan E, Sabatini DD. Asymmetric budding of viruses in epithelial monolayers: a model system for study of epithelial polarity. *Proc Natl Acad Sci U S A* 1978;75:5071–5075.
269. Rodriguez-Boulan E, Nelson WJ. Morphogenesis of the polarized epithelial cell phenotype. *Science* 1989;245:718–725.
270. Rodriguez-Boulan E, Paskiet KT, Sabatini DD. Assembly of enveloped viruses in MDCK cells: polarized budding from single attached cells and from clusters of cells in suspension. *J Cell Biol* 1983;96:866–874.
271. Roth MG, Compans RW, Giusti L, Davis AR, Nayak DP, Gething M, Sambrook J. Influenza virus hemagglutinin expression is polarized in cells infected with recombinant SV40 viruses carrying cloned hemagglutinin DNA. *Cell* 1983;33:435–443.
272. Roth MG, Fitzpatrick JP, Compans RW. Polarity of influenza and vesicular stomatitis virus maturation in MDCK cells: lack of requirement for glycosylation of viral glycoproteins. *Proc Natl Acad Sci U S A* 1979;76:6430–6434.
273. Roth MG, Gunderson D, Patil N, Rodriguez-Boulan EJ. The large external domain is sufficient for the correct sorting of secreted or chimeric influenza virus hemeagglutinins in polarized monkey kidney cells. *J Cell Biol* 1987;104:769–782.
274. Roush DL, Gottardi CJ, Naim HY, Roth MG, Caplan MJ. Tyrosine-based membrane protein sorting signals are differentially interpreted by polarized MDCK and LLC-PK1 epithelial cells. *J Biol Chem* 1998;273:26862–26869.
275. Ryan MJ, Johnson G, Kirk J, Fuerstenberg SM, Zager RA, Torok SB. HK-2: an immortalized proximal tubule epithelial cell line from normal adult human kidney. *Kidney Int* 1994;45:48–57.
276. Saitou M, Fujimoto K, Doi Y, Itoh M, Fujimoto T, Furuse M, Takano H, Noda T, Tsukita S. Occludin-deficient embryonic stem cells can differentiate into polarized epithelial cells bearing tight junctions. *J Cell Biol* 1998;141:397–408.
277. Salas PJ, Vega-Salas DE, Hochman J, Rodriguez-Boulan EJ, Edidin M. Selective anchoring in the specific plasma membrane domain: a role in epithelial cell polarity. *J Cell Biol* 1988;107:2363–2373.
278. Saraste J, Kuismanen E. Pre- and post-Golgi vacuoles operate in the transport of Semliki Forest virus membrane glycoproteins to the cell surface. *Cell* 1984;38:535–549.
279. Sargiacomo M, Lisanti M, Graeve L, Le Bivic A, Rodriguez-Boulan E. Integral and peripheral protein composition of the apical and basolateral domains in MDCK cells. *J Membr Biol* 1989;107:277–286.
280. Scheiffele P, Peranen J, Simons K. N-glycans as apical sorting signals in epithelial cells. *Nature* 1995;378:96–98.
281. Schneeberger EE, Lynch RD. The tight junction: a multifunctional complex. *Am J Physiol Cell Physiol* 2004;286:C1213–1228.
282. Schoenenberger C-A, Matlin KS. Cell polarity and epithelial oncogenesis. *Trends Cell Biol* 1991;1:87–92.
283. Schoenenberger CA, Zuk A, Zinkl GM, Kendall D, Matlin KS. Integrin expression and localization in normal MDCK cells and transformed MDCK cells lacking apical polarity. *J Cell Sci* 1994;107(Pt 2):527–541.
284. Schultz SG. Cellular Models of epithelial ion transport. In: Andreoli TE, Hoffman JF, Fanestil DD, Schultz SG, eds. *Physiology of Membrane Disorders*. New York: Plenum, 1986:519–534.
285. Schwartz GJ, Al-Awqati Q. Regulation of transepithelial H1 transport by exocytosis and endocytosis. *Annu Rev Physiol* 1986;48:153–161.
286. Schwarz MA, Owaribe K, Kartenbeck J, Franke WW. Desmosomes and hemidesmosomes: constitutive molecular components. *Annu Rev Cell Biol* 1990;6:461–491.
287. Shiel MJ, Caplan MJ. Developmental regulation of membrane protein sorting in Drosophila embryos. *Am J Physiol* 1995;269:C207–C216.
288. Short DB, Trotter KW, Reczek D, Kreda SM, Bretscher A, Boucher R, Stutts MJ, Milgram SL. An apical PDZ protein anchors the cystic fibrosis transmembrane conductance regulator to the cytoskeleton. *J Biol Chem* 1998;273:19797–19801.
289. Simmen T, Nobile M, Bonifacino JS, Hunziker W. Basolateral sorting of furin in MDCK cells requires a phenylalanine-isoleucine motif together with an acidic amino acid cluster. *Mol Cell Biol* 1999;19:3136–3144.
290. Simon AM. Gap junctions: more roles and new structural data. *Trends Cell Biol* 1999;9:169–170.
291. Simon AM, Goodenough DA. Diverse functions of vertebrate gap junctions. *Trends Cell Biol* 1998;8:477–483.
292. Simon DB, Lu Y, Choate KA, Velazquez H, Al-Sabban E, Praga M, Casari G, Bettinelli A, Colussi G, Rodriguez-Soriano J, McCredie D, Milford D, Sanjad S, Lifton RP. Paracellin-1, a renal tight junction protein required for paracellular Mg21 resorption. *Science* 1999; 285:103–106.
293. Simons K, Fuller SD. Cell surface polarity in epithelia. *Annu Rev Cell Biol* 1985;1:243–288.
294. Simons K, Wandinger-Ness A. Polarized sorting in epithelia. *Cell* 1990;62:207–210.
295. Skibbens JE, Roth MG, Matlin KS. Differential extractability of the influenza virus hemagglutinin during intracellular transport in polarized epithelial cells and nonpolar fibroblasts. *J Cell Biol* 1989;108:821–832.
296. Solez K. Acute renal failure ("Acute tubular necrosis," infraction, and cortical necrosis). In: Heptinstall RH, ed. *Pathology of the Kidney*. 3rd ed. Boston/Toronto: Little, Brown and Company; 1980:1069–1148.
297. Songyang Z, Fanning AS, Fu C, Xu J, Marfatia SM, Chishti AH, Crompton A, Chan AC, Anderson JM, Cantley LC. Recognition of unique carboxyl-terminal motifs by distinct PDZ domains. *Science* 1997;275:73–77.
298. Spiegel DM, Wilson PD, Molitoris BA. Epithelial polarity following ischemia: a requirement for normal cell function. *Am J Physiol* 1989;256:F430–F436.
299. Staehlin LA. Further observations on the fine structure of freeze cleaved tight junctions. *J Cell Sci* 13:768–786, 1973.

300. Staub O, Dho S, Henry PC, Correa J, Ishikawa T, McGlade J, Rotin D. WW domains of Nedd4 bind to the proline rich PY motifs in the epithelial Na channel deleted in Liddle's syndrome. *EMBO J* 1996;15:2371–2380.

301. Stein M, Wandinger-Ness A, Roitbak T. Altered trafficking and epithelial cell polarity in disease. *Trends Cell Biol* 2002;12:374–381.

302. Stephens EB, Compans RW, Earl P, Moss B. Surface expression of viral glycoproteins is polarized in epithelial cells infected with recombinant vaccinia viral vectors. *EMBO J* 1986;5:237–245.

303. Stevenson BR, Anderson JM, Bullivan S. The epithelial tight junction: structure, function and preliminary biochemical characterization. *Mol Cell Biochem* 1988;83:129–145.

304. Stevenson BR, Keon BH. The tight junction: morphology to molecules. *Annu Rev Cell Biol* 1998;14:89–109.

305. Stevenson BR, Siliciano JD, Mooseker MS, Goodenough DA. Identification of ZO-1: a high-molecular weight polypeptide associated with the tight junction (zonula occludens) in a variety of epithelia. *J Cell Biol* 1986;103:755–766.

306. Sullivan LP, Grantham JJ. Mechanisms of fluid secretion by polycystic epithelia. *Kidney Int* 1996;49:1586–1591.

307. Sullivan LP, Wallace DP, Grantham JJ. Epithelial transport in polycystic kidney disease. *Phys Rev* 1998;78:1165–1191.

308. Suzuki A, Hirata M, Kamimura K, Maniwa R, Yamanaka T, Mizuno K, Kishikawa M, Hirose H, Amano Y, Izumi N, Miwa Y, Ohno S. aPKC acts upstream of PAR-1b in both the establishment and maintenance of mammalian epithelial polarity. *Curr Biol* 2004;14:1425–1435.

309. Suzuki A, Ohno S. The PAR-aPKC system: lessons in polarity. *J Cell Sci* 2006;119:979–987.

310. Sweadner KJ, Goldin SM. Active transport of sodium and potassium. *N Engl J Med* 1980;302:777–783.

311. Sztul ES, Howell KE, Palade GE. Biogenesis of polymeric IgA receptor in rat hepatocytes. II. Localization of its intracellular forms by cell fractionation studies. *J Cell Biol* 1985; 100:1255–1261.

312. Takeichi M. Cadherins: a molecular family important in selective cell–cell adhesion. *Annu Rev Biochem* 1990;59:237–252.

313. Thadhani R, Pascual M, Bonventre JV. Acute renal failure. *N Engl J Med* 1996;334:1448–1460.

314. Thomas DC, Brewer CB, Roth MG. Vesicular stomatitis virus glycoprotein contains a dominant cytoplasmic basolateral sorting signal critically dependent upon a tyrosine. *J Biol Chem* 1993;268:3313–3320.

315. Thomas DC, Roth MG. The basolateral targeting signal in the cytoplasmic domain of glycoprotein G from vesicular stomatitis virus resembles a variety of intracellular targeting motifs related by primary sequence but having diverse targeting activities. *J Biol Chem* 1994;269:15732–15739.

316. Timpl R. Structure and biological activity of basement membrane proteins. *Eur J Biochem* 1989;180:487–502.

317. Timpl R, Brown JC. The laminins. *Matrix Biol* 1994;14:275–281.

318. Tischer CC, Bulger RE, Trump BF. Human renal ultrastructure I. Proximal tubule of healthy individuals. *Lab Invest* 1966;15:1357–1364.

319. Tooze J, Tooze SA, Fuller SD. Sorting of progeny coronavirus from condensed secretory proteins at the exit from the trans Golgi network of AtT 20 cells. *J Cell Biol* 1987;105:1215–1226.

320. Tooze SA, Huttner WB. Cell-free protein sorting to the regulated and constitutive secretory pathways. *Cell* 1990;60:837–847.

321. Torres VE. New insights into polycystic disease and its treatment. *Curr Opin Nephron Hypertens* 1998;7:159–169.

322. Turner JR, Rill BK, Carlson SL, Carnes D, Kerner R, Mrsny RJ, Madara. JL. Physiological regulation of epithelial tight junctions is associated with myosin light-chain phosphorylation. *Am J Physiol* 1997;273:C1378–C1385.

323. Vale RD. Intracellular based transport using microtubule based motors. *Annu Rev Cell Biol* 1987;3:347–378.

324. Van Itallie C, Rahner C, Anderson JM. Regulated expression of claudin-4 decreases paracellular conductance through a selective decrease in sodium permeability. *J Clin Invest* 2001;107:1319–1327.

325. Van Itallie CM, Anderson JM. Claudins and epithelial paracellular transport. *Annu Rev Physiol* 2006;68:403–429.

326. Van Itallie CM, Anderson JM. The molecular physiology of tight junction pores. *Physiology (Bethesda)* 2004;19:331–338.

327. van Meer G. Polarity and polarized transport of membrane lipids in a cultured epithelium. In: Matlin KS, Valentich JD, eds. *Functional Epithelial Cells in Culture.* New York: Liss, 1989:43–69.

328. van Meer G, Simons K. The function of tight junctions in maintaining differences in lipid composition between the apical and the basolateral cell surface domains of MDCK cells. *EMBO J* 1986;5:1455–1464.

329. Van Meer G, Simons K. The tight junction does not allow lipid molecules to diffuse from one epithelial cell to the next. *Nature* 1986;322:639–641.

330. Vega-Salas DE, Salas PJI, Gundersen D, Rodriguez-Boulan E. Formation of the apical pole of epithelial (Madin–Darby kidney) cells: polarity of an apical protein is independent of tight junctions while segregation of a basolateral marker requires cell–cell interactions. *J Cell Biol* 1987;104:905–916.

331. Vega-Salas DE, Salas PJI, Rodriguez-Boulan E. Modulation of the expression of an apical plasma membrane protein of madin-darby canine kidney epithelial cells: cell–cell interactions control the appearance of a novel intracellular storage compartment. *J Cell Biol* 1987;104: 1249–1259.

332. Vestweber D, Kemler R, Ekblom P. Cell-adhesion molecule uvomorulin during kidney development. *Dev Biol* 1985;112:213–221.

333. Wade JB, Stetson B, Lewis SA. ADH action: evidence for a membrane shuttle mechanism. *Ann N Y Acad Sci U S A* 1981;372:106–117.

334. Wakabayashi Y, Lippincott-Schwartz J, Arias IM. Intracellular trafficking of bile salt export pump (ABCB11) in polarized hepatic cells: constitutive cycling between the canalicular membrane and rab11-positive endosomes. *Mol Biol Cell* 2004;15:3485–3496.

335. Walter P, Lingappa VR. Mechanism of protein translocation across the endoplasmic reticulum membrane. *Annu Rev Cell Biol* 1986;2:499–516.

336. Wang AZ, Ojakian GK, Nelson WJ. Steps in the morphogenesis of a polarized epithelium. II. Disassembly and assembly of plasma membrane domains during reversal of epithelial polarity in multicellular epithelial cysts. *J Cell Biol* 1990;95:153–156.

337. Wang S, Raab RW, Schatz PJ, Guggino WB, Li M. Peptide binding consensus of the NHE-RF-PDZ1 domain matches the C-terminal sequence of cystic fibrosis transmembrane conductance regulator (CFTR). *FEBS Lett* 1998;427:103–108.

338. Wang T, Courtois-Coutry N, Giebisch G, Caplan MJ. A tyrosine-based signal regulates H,K-ATPase-mediated potassium reabsorption in the kidney. *Am J Physiol* 1998;275:F818–F826.

339. Weaver VM, Lelievre S, Lakins JN, Chrenek MA, Jones JC, Giancotti F, Werb Z, Bissell MJ. beta4 integrin-dependent formation of polarized three-dimensional architecture confers resistance to apoptosis in normal and malignant mammary epithelium. *Cancer Cell* 2002;2:205–216.

340. Welling LW, Welling DJ. Surface areas of brush border and lateral cell walls in the rabbit proximal nephron. *Kidney Int* 1975; 8:343–351.

341. Wilson PD, Sherwood AC, Palla K, Du J, Watson R, Norman JT. Reversed polarity of Na,K-ATPase: mislocation to apical plasma membranes in polycystic kidney disease. *Am J Physiol* 1991;260:F420–F430.

342. Wolosin JM, Forte JG. Stimulation of oxyntic cell triggers K1 and Cl- conductances in apical H1-K1-ATPase membrane. *Am J Physiol* 1984;246:C537–C5345.

343. Yap AS, Brieher WM, Gumbiner BM. Molecular and functional analysis of cadherin-based adherens junctions. *Annu Rev Cell Biol* 1997;13:119–146.

344. Yeaman C, Grindstaff KK, Nelson WJ. New perspectives on mechanisms involved in generating epithelial cell polarity [review]. *Physiol Rev* 1999;79:73–98.

345. Yoder BK, Mulroy S, Eustace H, Boucher C, Sandford R. Molecular pathogenesis of autosomal dominant polycystic kidney disease. *Expert Rev Mol Med* 2006;8:1–22.

346. Yu AS, McCarthy KM, Francis SA, McCormack JM, Lai J, Rogers RA, Lynch RD, Schneeberger EE. Knockdown of occludin expression leads to diverse phenotypic alterations in epithelial cells. *Am J Physiol Cell Physiol* 2005;288:C1231–1241.

347. Yu W, Datta A, Leroy P, O'Brien LE, Mak G, Jou TS, Matlin KS, Mostov KE, Zegers MM. Beta1-integrin orients epithelial polarity via Rac1 and laminin. *Mol Biol Cell* 2005;16:433–445.

348. Zamir E, Geiger B. Components of cell–matrix adhesions. *J Cell Sci* 2001;114:3577–3579.

349. Zamir E, Geiger B. Molecular complexity and dynamics of cell–matrix adhesions. *J Cell Sci* 2001;114:3583–3590.

350. Zamir E, Katz BZ, Aota S, Yamada KM, Geiger B, Kam Z. Molecular diversity of cell–matrix adhesions. *J Cell Sci* 1999;112(Pt 11):1655–1669.

351. Ze'ev A, Geiger B. Differential molecular interactions of b-catenin and plakoglobin in adhesion, signaling, and cancer. *Curr Opin Cell Biol* 1998;10:629–639.

352. Zegers MM, O'Brien LE, Yu W, Datta A, Mostov KE. Epithelial polarity and tubulogenesis in vitro. *Trends Cell Biol* 2003;13:169–176.

353. Zinkl GM, Zuk A, van der Bijl P, van Meer G, Matlin KS. An antiglycolipid antibody inhibits Madin–Darby canine kidney cell adhesion to laminin and interferes with basolateral polarization and tight junction formation. *J Cell Biol* 1996;133:695–708.

354. Zot HG. Phospholipid membrane-associated brush border myosin-I activity. *Cell Motil Cytoskeleton* 1995;30:26–37.

355. Zuk A, Bonventre JV, Brown D, Matlin KS. Polarity, integrin, and extracellular matrix dynamics in the postischemic rat kidney. *Am J Physiol* 1998;275:C711–C731.

356. Zurzolo C, Rodriguez-Boulan E. Delivery of Na1(K1)-ATPase in polarized epithelial cells. *Science* 1993;260:550–552.

CHAPTER 2

Mechanisms of Ion Transport Across Cell Membranes and Epithelia

Luis Reuss
Texas Tech University Health Sciences Center, Lubbock, Texas, USA

INTRODUCTION

Ion transport by cell membranes serves two large purposes in pluricellular organisms, the maintenance of the volume and composition of the intracellular fluid and the preservation and regulation of the volume and composition of the extracellular fluid. The first process involves fluxes between the cell interior and its surrounding medium ("homocellular transport," 92), whereas the second one occurs because of transport across epithelial and endothelial cell layers (transcellular or "heterocellular" transport, 92). In addition, ion transport across intracellular membranes, which surround the nucleus and cytoplasmic organelles, are essential to generate and maintain ion concentration gradients between those organelles and the cytosol.

Needless to say, the narrowly regulated volume and ionic composition—inorganic cations ($Na^+, K^+, H^+, Ca^{2+}, Mg^{2+}$) and anions ($Cl^-$, phosphate, bicarbonate)—is essential for cell survival, and for the cell's normal functions. A similar argument can be made for the extracellular fluid compartments, that is, whole-body balances of water and the ions listed above are essential for the survival, growth, and development of the organism.

Our main focus in this chapter will be on the molecular mechanisms of ion transport by the plasma membranes of cells. The cell membrane is a phospholipid bilayer doped with abundant proteins. This structure is both a barrier between the cytoplasm and the extracellular fluid and the pathway for ion and water transport between the two compartments. For most ions, the lipid bilayer is the barrier and membrane transport proteins are the pathway for these fluxes.

The Cell Interior and Extracellular Fluid Have Different Ionic Compositions

A crucial property of living cells is their capacity to maintain an internal (intracellular or cytosolic) composition different from that of the surrounding (extracellular) medium. As all other ionic solutions, the cytosol and the extracellular fluid obey the principle of macroscopic (or bulk) electroneutrality, that is, the sum of cationic and anionic charges are the same in each compartment. As discussed below, there is a microscopic deviation from this principle at the membrane surfaces when there is a difference in electrical potential across the membrane, but the actual difference in ion concentrations is extremely small.

The maintenance of ionic asymmetry between intracellular and extracellular compartments is based on the existence of the cell membrane (or plasma membrane), which separates the cell interior from its surroundings. As shown schematically in Fig. 1, the membrane is a phospholipid bilayer ~4 nm thick, with high protein content. Membrane proteins can be tightly bound to the phospholipid bilayer (integral proteins, some of which span the membrane, known as transmembrane proteins) or can be loosely associated with the membrane surface (peripheral proteins). Transmembrane proteins perform many functions, including translocation of ions, nonelectrolytes, and water across the membrane (transport function, the main theme of this chapter); sensing and early transduction of extracellular events (signaling function); and attachment to components of the extracellular matrix or to adjacent cells (adhesion function).

Two properties of the cell membrane have been demonstrated to generate and maintain the intracellular ion composition essential for life: the barrier function and the transport function. This distinction is didactically convenient, although both functions are clearly linked. By the barrier function, the cell membrane prevents the flux of certain molecules; by the transport function, it translocates certain molecules. These two functions bring about a steady state in which cell volume and composition are kept constant and appropriate for cell survival. Relative to the extracellular fluid, some substances are maintained at high concentrations (e.g., K^+ and ATP), whereas others are maintained at low concentrations (e.g., Ca^{2+} and Cl^-) inside the cell.

The cell interior is not homogeneous, but rather a complex medium including a highly structured cytoplasm (cytosol and cytoskeleton) and numerous organelles. The latter are separated from the cytosol by their own membranes. Exchanges between each organelle and the cytosol occur in ways similar to those described for the plasma membrane

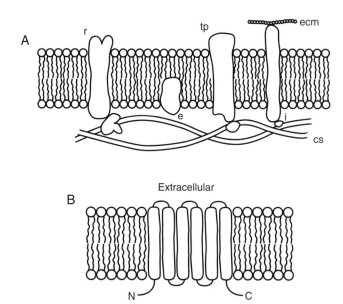

FIGURE 1   A. Structure of the plasma membrane. This 2D representation of the plasma membrane is based on the fluid-mosaic model of Singer and Nicholson (98), modified according to recent observations (115). The membrane is a lipid bilayer that contains integral and peripheral membrane proteins. The bilayer is largely made of phospholipids that have polar heads and hydrophobic tails. The hydrophobic tails face each other, while the polar head groups face the aqueous solutions (extracellular fluid and cytosol). In addition, the membrane contains glycolipids and cholesterol (not shown). The phospholipid compositions of the two leaflets differ; phosphatidyl inositol (PI) is more abundant in the inner leaflet. Additionally, certain areas of the membrane form *lipid rafts* (see text). A small fraction of the membrane surface area is occupied by either strongly-bound proteins (integral membrane proteins), some crossing the membrane one or more times (transmembrane proteins) or loosely attached (peripheral) membrane proteins. Some membrane proteins are attached to components of the cytoskeleton or the exoskeleton, directly or via other proteins. Integral membrane proteins can associate forming oligomers, as well as macromolecular complexes (not shown). Symbols: r, receptor; e, enzyme (e.g., protein kinase C); tp, transport protein (pore, channel, carrier or pump); i, integrin; cs, cytoskeleton; ecm, extracellular matrix. B. Diagrammatic representation of a transmembrane protein of an animal cell. *N* and *C*: N-terminal and C-terminal domains, whose localization can be intra- or extra-cellular. The *transmembrane domain* of the protein is formed by α-helices (shown as rectangles), joined by intra- and extra-cellular *loops*. When the number of transmembrane helices is even, both N- and C-terminal domains are on the same side of the membrane; when the number is odd, N- and C-terminal domains are on opposite sides of the membrane. The amino acid residues in the transmembrane α-helices can face aqueous medium (e.g., pore of an ion channel), lipid (bilayer), or amino acids from another helix. The grouping of the transmembrane helices is referred to as helix packing. (Modified with permission from Reuss L. Ussing's two-membrane hypothesis: the model and half a century of progress. *J Membr Biol* 2001;184: 211–217.)

vis-à-vis the cytosol and the extracellular fluid. In this chapter I will not address organelle membrane function.

The Plasma Membrane: Structure Related to Function

In the fluid-mosaic membrane model (99, 100), biological membranes are two-dimensional viscous phospholipid bilayers in which integral membrane proteins are dissolved and free to rotate and diffuse laterally. Although this model has been very valuable and continues to explain many membrane phenomena, recent studies suggest that many membrane proteins cluster with others in microdomains in which the lipid composition may differ from that of the bulk bilayer. These clusters are maintained by intramembrane lipid–lipid, protein–protein, and protein–lipid interactions, as well as interactions with intracellular molecules (cytoskeletal proteins) and extracellular components (extracellular matrix proteins and membrane proteins of adjacent cells). In addition to lateral differences in lipid composition within a monolayer, it is clear that the two monolayers also differ in composition. Lipid rafts in membranes are domains in the submicron range that consist of cholesterol and sphingolipids in the external leaflet and cholesterol and phospholipids with saturated fatty acids in the internal leaflet of the plasma membrane. The surrounding bilayer is abundant in unsaturated fatty acids and more fluid than that in the raft (53). Rapid changes in composition and location in the membrane are essential for the role that lipid rafts play in signaling processes (e.g., receptor tyrosine kinases).

This new notion of the structure of the plasma membrane (115) is based on results of biophysical studies, including fluorescence recovery after photo-bleaching, single-particle tracking techniques, optical trapping by laser tweezers, and fluorescence correlation spectroscopy. These methods, applied to cell membranes, have yielded quantitative dynamic information on the distribution, mobility, and compartmentalization of membrane proteins (115). Biochemical, molecular, and physiological studies indicate that membrane transport proteins are not randomly distributed, but that they undergo homo- and hetero-associations (53), and that these associations may have functional significance. A case in point is the proposed proximity between plasma membrane Ca^{2+} channels and Ca^{2+}-sensitive proteins, including Ca^{2+}-activated channels: Ca^{2+} entry results in a large, but highly localized increase in intracellular $[Ca^{2+}]$, because of effective cytosolic buffering, and thus its signaling effects may be quite local (71).

In summary, the current view of the structure of the plasma membrane is that of a compartmentalized two-dimensional structure, mosaic-like, with less fluidity than proposed by the Singer–Nicolson model. Free diffusion of membrane proteins may be restricted by the structure of the lipid domain, interactions with cytoskeletal proteins, or other cytoplasmic components, and/or homo- and hetero-associations with other integral membrane proteins. Future studies of membrane-transport proteins along these lines are likely to reveal important aspects of their function and regulation in health and disease.

The Plasma Membrane Is Selectively Permeable

The barrier and transport functions of the plasma membrane are determined by its composition, that is, phospholipids and integral transmembrane proteins (for membrane structure, see 53, 99, 100, 115; for a review of membrane proteins, see 105). When the membrane is *permeable* to a specific molecule, then that molecule can cross the membrane. *Permeability* is a property of a specific membrane for a specific molecule. The amount of substance that crosses the membrane per unit of time and membrane area is the *flux*. Using radioactive techniques unidirectional fluxes can be measured (e.g., in case of a cell, influx and efflux); the *net flux* is the difference between the two unidirectional fluxes. A finite net flux denotes the presence of a driving force across the membrane.

Permeation of a specific molecule can take place through the lipid phase (i.e., *solubility-diffusion*) and/or through membrane proteins (i.e., *mediated transport*). Solubility-diffusion always results in equilibrating transport, dissipating differences in concentration or electrochemical potential (see Diffusion and Electrodiffusion section below). In contrast, mediated transport can either dissipate or generate differences in chemical or electrochemical potentials across the membrane. An example of mediated transport is the operation of the sodium pump, that is, the Na^+, K^+-ATPase.

The lipid phase of the plasma membrane is hydrophobic, and therefore has high permeability for lipophilic molecules and low permeability for hydrophilic molecules. Thus, a protein-free phospholipid membrane has a high permeability for nonpolar small molecules such as O_2 and CO_2, a much lower permeability for uncharged small polar substances such as water, urea, and glycerol, and an extremely low permeability for ions and for larger uncharged polar molecules, such as glucose. Most molecules are measurably permeable across plasma membranes. However, the diffusive permeability coefficients range over several orders of magnitude. It is thought that many molecules permeate the membrane bilayer because the thermal motion of the phospholipid molecules causes transient kinks in the bilayer structure.

Transport proteins can be classified in four groups, namely pores, channels, carriers (also referred to as transporters) and pumps (see next section). The expression of some transport proteins can be specific to tissue, cell, and sometimes membrane domain. Others are expressed in most, if not all cell membranes. The functional significance of transport proteins is apparent in two realms. Some are primarily related to the establishment and maintenance of cellular composition (intracellular "homeostasis"), such as the Na^+, K^+-ATPase and K^+ channels in most animal cells. Others are primarily related to specific cell functions, such as excitability (e.g., the tetrodotoxin-sensitive, voltage-activated Na^+ channel in nerve and muscle), and transepithelial Na^+ transport (e.g., the amiloride-sensitive, voltage-insensitive Na^+ channel in the apical membrane of certain epithelial cells).

A *pore* is an aqueous communication between both sides of the membrane, accessible to both sides at all times—that is, it is always "open" (permeable). A *channel* is also an aqueous communication between the two sides of the membrane, but it opens and closes stochastically by changes in conformation called *gating*; when open, a channel is accessible from both sides of the membrane; when closed, it is impermeable to ions. A *carrier* is a membrane-transport protein

that is not simultaneously accessible to both sides of the membrane, but to one side at a time; changes in conformation change the orientation of the carrier, moving the transported ion to the other side; an appropriate simplified description is that a carrier has two gates and they are never open at the same time. Finally, a *pump* has the properties of a carrier, but in addition it is coupled to a metabolic energy source, that is, hydrolysis of ATP.

MECHANISMS OF ION TRANSPORT

Ion Transport Can Be Active or Passive

The definitions of active and passive transport are thermodynamic. Passive transport occurs in the direction expected for the existing driving force, which in the case of ions involves the chemical gradient (given by the difference in concentration between the sides of the membrane) and the electrical gradient (given by the transmembrane electrical potential difference or membrane voltage). In other words, passive transport is energetically downhill. In contrast, active transport takes place in the absence of or against the prevailing electrochemical gradient. In other words, active transport is energetically uphill and therefore requires an energy input. Depending on the origin of this energy, one can distinguish two types of active transport.

Primary active transport is characterized by the direct use of metabolic energy, supplied by light, redox potential, or ATP hydrolysis. In most cases of plasma-membrane primary active transport in eukaryotic organisms, the energy is provided by the hydrolysis of ATP, a process catalyzed by the same molecule that performs the transport. Hence, in this case the transporter is also an ATP hydrolase (ATPase). Transporters responsible for primary active transport are referred to as pumps. In plasma membranes of most animal cells there can be expression of one or more of four ion-transporting ATPases. These are the Na^+,K^+-ATPase, H^+-ATPase, H^+,K^+-ATPase, and Ca^{2+}-ATPase.

Secondary active transport is characterized by the indirect use of metabolic energy. The energy stored in the electrochemical gradient for one substrate is utilized to transport actively another species (ion or molecule). In animal cells, including those from epithelia, secondary active transport is most frequently linked to Na^+ transport. The Na^+,K^+-ATPase establishes an electrochemical potential gradient for Na^+ across the plasma membrane, which includes chemical (high extracellular and low intracellular $[Na^+]$) and electrical components (cell electrically negative to the extracellular compartment), both contributing to a net driving force favoring Na^+ entry into the cell. This gradient is then utilized to transport other substrates, by coupling at the molecular level their translocation to that of Na^+.

Depending on the directions of the fluxes, there are two kinds of secondary active transport: First is *cotransport* (or *symport*) in which the substrates move in the same direction, such as downhill for Na$^+$ and uphill for the cotransported substrate (e.g., Na$^+$–glucose cotransport). Second is *counter-transport* (also *antiport* or *exchange*) in which the fluxes are in opposite directions (e.g., Na$^+$–H$^+$ exchange). In most instances, secondary active transport involves only two species (Na$^+$ and another substrate), but in some cases there are three: an example is the Na$^+$–K$^+$–2Cl$^-$ cotransporter, an electroneutral symporter that is expressed principally in epithelial cells. This transporter accounts for uphill Cl$^-$ uptake, a step necessary for Cl$^-$ absorption (e.g., in the apical membrane of cells of the thick ascending limb of the loop of Henle) or Cl$^-$ secretion (e.g., in the basolateral membrane of crypt cells in the intestine and epithelial cells in the airway). For quantitative analyses of membrane transport processes, see Läuger (62), Macey and Moura (67), and Stein (104).

Active and Passive Transport Processes Can Be Evaluated by Considering Direction of Electrochemical Potential Difference (Driving Force)

As stated above, passive transport is energetically downhill, that is, driven by the preexisting driving force. This force depends on the chemical or the electrochemical gradient, for uncharged and charged solutes, respectively. Under isothermal conditions the driving force encompasses differences in concentration, electrical potential, and/or pressure across the membrane. Under these conditions, the electrochemical potential difference ($\Delta\bar{\mu}_j$) for the *j*th ion is given by Eq. 1:

$$\Delta\bar{\mu}_j = z_j V_m F + RT \ln\left(\frac{C_j^i}{C_j^o}\right) + \Delta P \bar{V}_j \quad (1)$$

where z is the valence, V_m is the membrane voltage, F is the Faraday constant, R is the gas constant, T is the absolute temperature, C is the concentration, *i* and *o* refer to the two sides of the membrane (inside and outside, respectively), ΔP is the transmembrane hydrostatic pressure difference, and $\bar{V}$ is the ion's partial molar volume. The electrochemical potential has the three components defined above, given by the three terms on the right side of the equation. Across animal cell membranes, steady-state hydrostatic or osmotic pressure differences are small or nil (see Chapter 5), and therefore the third term of Eq. 1 is eliminated, yielding:

$$\Delta\bar{\mu}_j = z_j V_m F + RT \ln\left(\frac{C_j^i}{C_j^o}\right) \quad (2)$$

This equation is used to evaluate the driving force for ion transport under isobaric conditions. In the case of nonelectrolytes, $z = 0$ and the first term of Eq. 2 can be eliminated as well, yielding:

$$\Delta\mu_j = RT \ln\left(\frac{C_j^i}{C_j^o}\right) \quad (3)$$

where $\Delta\mu_j$ denotes the chemical potential difference. This equation describes the driving force for nonelectrolyte transport.

From Eq. 2 (under isobaric and isothermal conditions), Ussing (112) derived the flux-ratio equation, a fundamental expression which provides a thermodynamic test for active or passive transport:

$$J_{in}/J_{out} = (C_i/C_o)\exp(zV_m F/RT) \quad (4)$$

where J is flux (the subscripts *i* and *o* denote influx and efflux, respectively). The test proceeds as follows: the ratio of unidirectional fluxes (J_{in}/J_{out}) is determined experimentally, and the driving forces are measured; if the ratio deviates from the prediction given by Eq. 4, which evaluates the passive driving forces, then active transport should be suspected. Deviations from the flux-ratio equation can also result from the presence of exchange diffusion and single-file diffusion, as discussed by Schultz (91).

Pathways and Mechanisms of Passive Transport

Passive transport can be via the lipid bilayer (solubility-diffusion) or via transmembrane proteins (mediated). Solubility-diffusion is a permeation process that involves the movement of a molecule dissolved in the aqueous solution bathing one side of the membrane into the lipid phase of the membrane, then across the membrane, and then from the membrane lipid into the solution bathing the opposite side. Clearly, two processes are involved. The first one ("solubility") governs the fluxes at the solution–membrane interfaces, and depends on the relative solubility of the molecule in lipid and water, which can be quantified by the oil–water partition coefficient, β, a coefficient equal to the ratio of the molecule's steady-state concentrations in lipid and water. The second process ("diffusion") governs the solute translocation within the membrane lipid, which depends largely on the mass and shape of solute molecules. The lipid solubility of the molecule is the main factor determining its permeability via the lipid moiety of the membrane.

Mediated transport is the mode of transmembrane transport of substances with very low solubility in phospholipids, that is, charged and polar substances. The transport proteins provide a hydrophilic path across the membrane, through which the solute permeates.

DIFFUSION AND ELECTRODIFFUSION

Diffusion and electrodiffusion are the main processes of passive solute transport across homogeneous phases (e.g., lipid membranes or aqueous pores) by independent motion of the solute molecules. Diffusion applies to uncharged particles and electrodiffusion to ions. Although diffusion does not strictly apply to ion transport, its analysis is simpler and helps in understanding electrodiffusion.

Diffusion of a solute in aqueous solution is the result of the random thermal motion of solute molecules. Disregarding convection, if there are differences in concentration between different sectors of the solution, then random solute motion will tend to make its distribution homogeneous (equilibrating transport). All solute particles move randomly at uniform average velocities, dependent on the solution temperature. Hence, more particles will tend to move from regions of high concentration to sectors of low concentration than in the opposite direction, simply because there are more particles per unit volume in the high-concentration regions. In other words, differences in concentration cause unequal unidirectional fluxes in a regime of diffusion because of differences in the number of particles flowing in each direction per unit of time, not because of different velocities of individual particles flowing in one direction or the other. In diffusion, the molecules move independently of each other and of other particles present in the solution, that is, there is no flux coupling. This is the *independence principle*.

Diffusion of a nonelectrolyte in solution is described by Fick's first law (25):

$$J_s = -D_s \frac{dC_s}{dx} \qquad (5)$$

where J_s is the solute flux (moles·cm^2·sec^{-1}), D_s is the solute diffusion coefficient (cm^2·sec^{-1}) and dC_s/dx is the concentration gradient. The negative sign denotes the direction of the flux.

Fick's second law of diffusion considers the time course of the process:

$$\frac{dC}{dt} = D_s \frac{d^2C_s}{dx^2} \qquad (6)$$

where dC/dt is the rate of change in solute concentration and x denotes distance.

The average time required by diffusing particles to cover a given distance is inversely proportional to the diffusion coefficient and directly proportional to the square of the traveled distance. Einstein approximated the second law of diffusion with $\lambda = (D_s t)^{1/2}$, where λ is the traveled distance in the x-axis. The dependence of t on the square of the distance makes diffusion a very slow transport process for long distances. For a typical $D_s = 10^{-5}$ cm^2·sec^{-1}, it takes 1 millisecond for the solute to diffuse 1 μm, but it takes 1000 seconds (~16.7 minutes) to diffuse 1 mm. Convective flow (see Chapter 9) is a much more effective mass transport mechanism for long distances.

Now we consider a thin lipid membrane of thickness δ_m separating two aqueous compartments (Fig. 2). The solutions on both sides are well stirred, so that the solute concentrations are homogeneous in both. Inserting the solute partition coefficient (β_s) to denote its lipid solubility relative to its water solubility, at the steady state, the following expression is obtained for the solute flux:

$$J_s = -\frac{D_s \beta_s}{\delta_m} \Delta C_s \qquad (7)$$

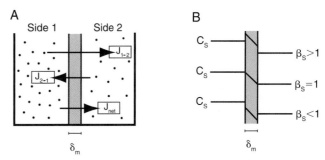

FIGURE 2 Diffusion across a membrane. **A:** A membrane separates two aqueous solutions (1 and 2). The dots represent molecules of a solute to which the membrane is permeable; the solute concentration (Cs) is greater in solution 1. Solute molecules move randomly in each solution and collide with the membrane with a probability proportional to the concentration. Solutes collide, dissolve in and diffusing across the membrane. The unidirectional fluxes ($J_{1\to2}$ and $J_{2\to1}$) are proportional to the solute concentrations in sides 1 and 2, respectively; the net flux (J_{net}) is proportional to the concentration difference. The concentration difference does not accelerate the molecules, and hence it is not a force, although it is usually referred to as the *chemical driving force*. Diffusion is passive, equilibrating transport, i.e., net transport ceases when the concentrations on both sides of the membrane are equal. **B:** Lines denote solute concentration profiles in the solutions and the membrane depending on the partition coefficient (β_s). When $\beta_s = 1$, solute concentration in the membrane boundaries are identical to those in the adjacent solutions; concentrations in the membrane are greater or smaller than those in the adjacent solution if β_s is greater or smaller than unity, respectively.

where ΔC_s is the solute concentration difference between the two solutions. Defining the solute permeability (P_s) as $P_s = D_s \beta_s / \delta_m$, Eq. 7 reduces to:

$$J_s = -P_s \Delta C_s \qquad (8)$$

The diffusive permeability coefficient of the membrane relates the flux to the driving force and denotes the ease with which the membrane permits mass transfer of a particular species. Its units are centimeters per tenth of a second, that is, those of velocity. In the simple case of a nonelectrolyte, under isothermal and isobaric conditions, the permeability (P) of solute s is given by a rearrangement of Eq. 8: $P_s = -J_s/\Delta C_s$. This is the phenomenological, experimentally determined permeability, calculated by dividing the steady-state solute flux by the difference between the solute concentrations of well-stirred bathing solutions. The other definition of diffusive permeability is mechanistic and considers the factors involved in solubility-diffusion, D_s, β_s, and δ_m, as described above.

The preceding discussion considers the specific case of solubility-diffusion, but the phenomenological definition of permeability can be applied in principle to any transport mechanism. Of course, its interpretation varies. An important case is that of the permeation of certain hydrophilic nonelectrolytes through aqueous pores in the membrane. If the lipid bilayer is impermeable to the solute, then diffusive transport is entirely via the pores. The permeable area of this membrane (S_p) is only a fraction of the total membrane area, given (for 1 cm^2 of membrane) by $S_p = n\pi r^2$, where n is the density of homogeneous pores of radius r. The partition coefficient is unity (the solute is dissolved in water both inside and outside of the pore) and is hence eliminated from the equation:

$$P_s = n\pi r^2 D_s / L \qquad (9)$$

where L is the pore length (about equivalent to membrane thickness).

ELECTRODIFFUSION

Electrodiffusion is the main mechanism of passive transport of ions in homogeneous media, that is, bulk aqueous solution or relatively large water-filled pores. Electrodiffusive transmembrane ion transport is a mediated transport process, but it is better discussed at this point for continuity with diffusion. In large-diameter pores, electrodiffusion theory explains ion permeation very well. In ion channels, which have smaller diameter than pores and are highly selective, there are significant interactions between the ions and the permeation pathway. For this reason, simple electrodiffusion theory is not entirely applicable to ion channels, but is nevertheless a useful approximation. For ion transport across a membrane, two factors determine the flux: the chemical potential difference (difference in concentration across the membrane) and the electrical potential difference (membrane voltage). The net ion flux (J_i) is given by the Nernst–Planck equation (see 44). If a constant electrical field is assumed in the membrane and other assumptions are made, the Nernst–Planck equation can be solved, yielding the Goldman-Hodgkin-Katz (GHK) equation (35, 45):

$$J_i = -P_i \frac{z_i V_m F}{RT} \left[\frac{C_i^o - C_i^i \exp(V_m F / RT)}{1 - \exp(V_m F / RT)} \right] \qquad (10)$$

where R, T, z, and F have their usual meanings, P is permeability, V_m is membrane voltage, C is concentration, the subscript i denotes the ith ion and the superscripts i and o denote the two sides of the membrane.

Under zero-current conditions, the GHK flux equation yields the membrane voltage as a function of the permeabilities and concentrations of all permeant ions. For the case of three monovalent permeant ions (Na^+, K^+, and Cl^-), the equation (GHK voltage equation) is:

$$V_m = -\frac{RT}{F} \ln \frac{P_{Na}[Na^+]_i + P_K[K^+]_i + P_{Cl}[Cl^-]_o}{P_{Na}[Na^+]_o + P_K[K^+]_o + P_{Cl}[Cl^-]_i} \qquad (11)$$

where the brackets denote concentrations. Note that if the fraction including permeability coefficients and ion concentrations is inverted, then the sign of the right side of the equation is also inverted. I prefer the notation given here because it gives the intracellular potential minus the extracellular potential, the convention used in electrophysiology. This also applies to the Nernst equation below.

Note that if only one ion is permeable, e.g., if P_{Na} and P_{Cl} are 0 in Eq. 11, then the membrane voltage becomes equal to the equilibrium potential for that ion, in this example K^+. The equilibrium potential is given by the Nernst equation (76):

$$V_m = -\frac{RT}{F} \ln \frac{[K^+]_i}{[K^+]_o} \qquad (12)$$

Under these conditions, the two compartments separated by the membrane are at a *steady state* (the amounts of K^+ on each side remain constant with time) but also at *equilibrium*, which means that the net driving force on K^+ is zero, and hence the unidirectional fluxes are equal (Fig. 3). In the case of cells, one frequently observes a steady-state K^+ distribution without equilibrium: the net efflux through channels is exactly balanced by influx via the Na^+,K^+-ATPase.

Another interesting point is that the Nernst equation indicates that if only one ion is permeable, then the membrane voltage is determined by the concentration ratio for the ion, not its absolute concentrations. In addition, the membrane voltage is independent of the absolute value of the ion permeability. As shown by the GHK voltage equation, in the case of a membrane permeable to more than one ion, the membrane voltage depends on the absolute concentrations and permeability coefficients of all permeant ions. The Nernst equation can be derived more directly from the definitions of electrochemical potential (Eq. 1) and equilibrium ($\Delta\bar{\mu}_i = 0$).

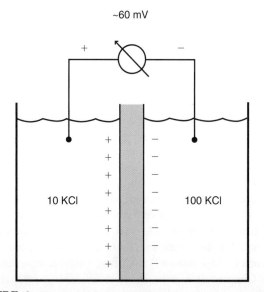

FIGURE 3 Electrochemical equilibrium. A membrane permeable to K^+ and impermeable to Cl^- separates two KCl solutions of concentrations, 10 mM and 100 mM, respectively. Because of the difference in concentrations, there is a chemical driving force for K^+ and Cl^- fluxes from left to right. While the impermeant Cl^- cannot move, the permeant K^+ moves across the membrane, and in doing so creates a difference in electrical potential across the membrane. The membrane becomes electrically charged by a tiny excess of K^+ ions on the left and a tiny excess of Cl^- ions on the right. This difference in electrical potential (the *transmembrane voltage*) opposes further K^+ flux and a state is reached at which the chemical driving force and the electrical driving force for K^+ movement are equal and opposite. This condition, described by the Nernst equation (Eq. 12), is electrochemical equilibrium.

The most important points concerning electrodiffusion are that ion fluxes across membranes are determined by both permeability and driving force, and that the driving force has chemical and electrical components. Hence, these three elements must be known to predict the direction and magnitude of the flux. For example, knowledge of the K^+ concentrations inside and outside a cell is insufficient to decide whether the ion is at equilibrium across the membrane or whether there is a passive driving force inwardly or outwardly directed. To establish this simple point, it is necessary to know the membrane voltage. However, knowledge of the electrochemical gradient is insufficient to predict the magnitude of the K^+ flux expected for this gradient; the K^+ permeability of the membrane must be known as well.

MEDIATED TRANSPORT

This expression means that translocation across the membrane is not via the lipid bilayer, but via membrane transport proteins, that is, pores, channels, carriers, or pumps. Mediated transport is the process by which ions and polar nonelectrolytes undergo passive transport across the cell membrane. Hence, this mechanism is complementary of that provided by solubility-diffusion, in that it is specialized for hydrophilic solutes, whereas solubility-diffusion is more effective for lipophilic solutes. For certain solutes, both mechanisms may operate. Even for solutes with very low permeability across the phospholipid moiety of the membrane, a significant contribution of the diffusive flux may exist because of the large fractional area covered by phospholipids, in particular if there is also a low level of expression of the relevant transporters.

In mediated transport, specialized proteins spanning the membrane provide an aqueous environment that allows for the transmembrane flux of particles that are virtually insoluble in phospholipids. Recent advances in molecular biology have permitted the molecular identification of many of these proteins, as well as the genes that encode them. In addition to providing an aqueous environment for solute translocation, these molecules may undergo conformational changes during or related to the substrate translocation. The transport proteins underlying mediated transport can be classified in four groups: pores, channels, carriers, and pumps.

THERMODYNAMICS OF MEDIATED PASSIVE TRANSPORT

Pores, channels, and carriers are membrane-transport proteins that can only perform *overall* passive transport, meaning that the total energy employed in the transport is equal or less than the energy available in the electrochemical gradients (see Secondary Active Transport section below). Carriers and channels do not use a metabolic energy supply for solute translocation. Some channels are activated by ATP binding and hydrolysis, but once they become permeable, ion translocation is passive and does not use metabolic energy. Some carriers are able to transport more than one solute in the same cycle. In this case, the energy stored in the electrochemical gradient for one of these solutes (accessory) can be employed

for uphill transport of another (principal) solute, a process known as secondary active transport. Nevertheless, the total energy change is dissipative, that is, the energy stored in the accessory solute's electrochemical gradient is always greater than that used to actively transport the principal solute.

KINETICS OF MEDIATED PASSIVE TRANSPORT

The dependences of the transport rates on solute concentration are different in solubility-diffusion and carrier-mediated transport. As shown in Fig. 4, in diffusion the flux increases linearly with the concentration, whereas in carrier-mediated transport it saturates. This is explained because transport occurs via a finite number of carrier molecules that can also operate at a finite rate. The simplest case of carrier-mediated transport can be described by the Michaelis–Menten equation; the two kinetic parameters are the maximum flux (J_{max}) and K_m (the concentration at which the flux is half-maximal (see Fig. 4):

$$J_s = -\frac{C_s J_{max}}{C_s + K_m} \tag{13}$$

where J_s is the solute flux and C_s its concentration.

MODES OF COUPLED TRANSPORT

Coupled transport denotes the linked translocation of two or more species (ions and/or molecules) through a barrier. One can distinguish two coupling modes. *Molecular* coupling denotes carrier- or pump-mediated transport of more than one species by the same molecule. Examples shown in Fig. 5A are the Na^+ and glucose fluxes via the Na^+–glucose cotransporter and the Na^+ and K^+ fluxes via the Na^+,K^+-ATPase. In addition, there is *thermodynamic* coupling. In this case, the fluxes of two or more species occur through different molecules, but are related to each other by electrochemical driving forces. For example, transepithelial Na^+ transport via cell

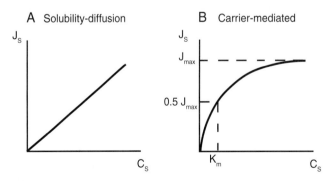

FIGURE 4 Kinetics of diffusion and mediated transport. Both graphs depict solute flux (J_s) as a function of solute concentration (C_s). In A, the mechanism of translocation across the membrane is diffusion, which does not involve chemical reactions between solute and membrane. In B, the mechanism of translocation is mediated (i.e., it involves reaction of the solute with transport proteins in the membrane). In A, the flux is linear with the concentration, whereas in B it saturates, because of occupation of a finite number of sites by a solute that moves at a finite velocity. In the simplest case, the relationship in B is described by the Michaelis–Menten equation (Eq. 13).

membranes (apical-membrane Na$^+$ channel in series with basolateral-membrane Na$^+$ pump) can produce a transepithelial electrical-potential difference responsible for a passive Cl$^-$ flux via the intercellular (junctional) pathway. In this instance, the coupling is not obligatory (if the potential difference is abolished, Cl$^-$ transport ceases while Na$^+$ transport continues), and does not involve the Na$^+$-transport molecules. Instead, it corresponds to the parallel operation of two transporters linked by a driving force (Fig. 5B). This apparently simple point has been a source of confusion in the transport literature (in particular of epithelial cells), where on occasion it has been incorrectly implied that all coupling is molecular.

Pathways and Mechanisms of Active Transport

PRIMARY ACTIVE TRANSPORT

Primary active transport occurs in the absence of or against the existing electrochemical gradient, and is powered by metabolic energy, such as that originated by the exergonic hydrolysis of ATP (Fig. 6). Ion pumps are the only molecules capable of performing primary active transport. Most ion pumps of interest to us are transport ATPases, that is, they are bifunctional molecules that both hydrolyze ATP and perform the translocation of the substrate against the prevailing electrochemical gradient. The Na$^+$,K$^+$-ATPase, Na$^+$-K$^+$ pump, or Na$^+$ pump, was the first enzyme demonstrated to be an active ion transporter (reviewed in 101, 102). It is likely that the energy-consuming steps are the conformational changes of the pump protein required for the substrate translocation, that is, for making the substrate first inaccessible to the cis side and then accessible to the trans side of the membrane.

SECONDARY ACTIVE TRANSPORT

Secondary active transport is characterized by the indirect use of metabolic energy. The electrochemical gradient drives a downhill substrate flux, and part of this energy is utilized for the uphill flux of another substrate (Fig. 6). The coupling between the two fluxes occurs in the transport protein—that is, it is molecular coupling.

In animal cells, secondary active transport is most frequently linked to Na$^+$ transport. The Na$^+$,K$^+$-ATPase establishes an electrochemical potential gradient for Na$^+$ across the plasma membrane, which includes a chemical (higher extracellular [Na$^+$]) and an electrical component (cell electrically negative to the extracellular compartment), both contributing to a net driving force (electrochemical gradient) favoring Na$^+$ entry into the cell. This energy is utilized to transport other substrates by coupling translocation to that of Na$^+$ at the molecular level.

Depending on the directions of the fluxes, there are two kinds of secondary active transport: *cotransport* (or *symport*), in which the substrates move in the same direction, such as downhill for Na$^+$ and uphill for the cotransported substrate

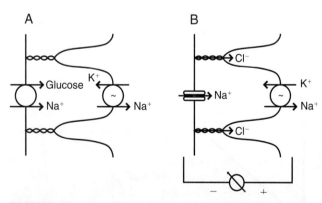

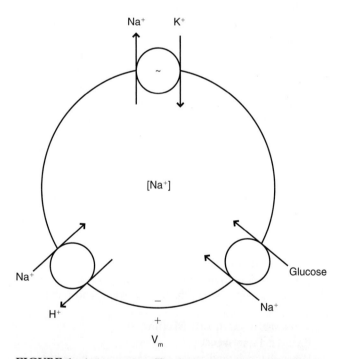

FIGURE 5 Modes of coupled transport. A. Molecular coupling: glucose-absorbing epithelial cell (e.g., renal proximal tubule). Two cases of molecular coupling are depicted: the Na$^+$–glucose cotransporter (SGLT) at the apical membrane and the Na$^+$,K$^+$-ATPase at the basolateral membrane. In both instances, the transport of two substrates occurs obligatorily in the same transport molecule. B. Thermodynamic coupling: the epithelial cell depicted absorbs Na$^+$ by an electrogenic process that generates a lumen-negative transepithelial voltage. This voltage drives a paracellular, electrodiffusive Cl$^-$ flux. The Na$^+$ and Cl$^-$ fluxes occur via different pathways, and linked by the driving force, not by the operation of a single molecule. The secretion of K$^+$ and the absorption of Na$^+$ by the principal cells of the cortical collecting duct is another example of thermodynamic coupling of ion fluxes.

FIGURE 6 Active transport. The diagram represents a cell expressing three membrane transporters. Top: Primary-active transport of Na$^+$ and K$^+$ via the Na$^+$,K$^+$-ATPase. The energy for active transport is provided by the hydrolysis of ATP. The flux coupling is 3Na$^+$:2K$^+$ per ATP molecule hydrolyzed. Bottom: Two mechanisms of secondary active transport. In both cases, the Na$^+$ electrochemical gradient (oriented inwards) is the driving force for the uphill movement of the other solute (glucose or H$^+$). On the right, Na$^+$–glucose cotransport via SGLT, the stoichiometry (Na$^+$:glucose) is 1:1 (SGLT2) or 2:1 (SGLT1). On the left, Na$^+$–H$^+$ exchange via NHE; the stoichiometry is 1:1. Note that the Na$^+$ driving forces operative in the two cases are different. Since Na$^+$–H$^+$ is electroneutral, the driving force depends only on the difference in Na$^+$ concentrations. Since Na$^+$–glucose cotransport is electrogenic, the driving force involves both the Na$^+$ chemical gradient and the membrane voltage. For a quantitative analysis, see text.

(e.g., glucose), and *countertransport* (also *antiport* or *exchange*) in which the fluxes are in opposite directions. Secondary active transport may involve two substrates (Na^+ and another substrate) or more (e.g., the Na^+–K^+,–$2Cl^-$ cotransporter). Sodium–glucose cotransport was the first secondary active transport mechanism studied experimentally, giving rise to the *Na^+ gradient hypothesis* (13).

Transport by Na^+–glucose cotransporters and Na^+–Ca^{2+} exchangers is electrogenic, that is, there is net translocation of charge across the membrane in each cycle. The concentration ratios (intracellular/extracellular) for glucose and Ca^{2+}, respectively, depend on both the Na^+ concentration ratio and the membrane voltage (V_m). The equation describing the maximum substrate concentration ratio that can be obtained by cotransport is:

$$\frac{S_i}{S_o} = \left[\frac{A_o}{A_i}\right]^n e - \frac{nzFV_m}{RT} \qquad (14)$$

where S is the main substrate (glucose); A is the accessory substrate (Na^+); the subscripts i and o denote intra- and extra-cellular concentrations, respectively; n is the transport stoichiometry (number of A molecules/number of S molecules); z is the valence of the translocated species per cycle ($z = zA - zS$); V_m is the membrane voltage; and R, T, and F have their usual meanings. Changing to decimal power notation and inserting appropriate values for the constants, the exponent becomes ~$nzV_m/60$. Hence, in the case of glucose transport via SGLT1 ($n = 2$), for $V_m = -60$ mV and Na^+ concentration ratio is 10, the maximum glucose concentration ratio (cell/lumen) is 10^4.

A similar equation describes the minimum concentration ratio of main substrate that can be achieved by countertransport:

$$\frac{S_i}{S_o} = \left[\frac{A_o}{A_i}\right]^n e - \frac{nzFV_m}{RT} \qquad (15)$$

where the symbols are the same as for Eq. 14. The difference is that the concentration ratios for A are inverted in these equations, denoting that in one case S and A are transported in the same direction, and in the other case they are transported in opposite directions. For the example of Na^+–Ca^{2+} exchange with $V_m = -60$ mV and Na^+ concentration ratio is 10, the minimum Ca^{2+} concentration ratio (cell/extracellular) is 10^{-6} for $n = 4$, the most likely stoichiometry.

ION TRANSPORT PROTEINS

Ion transport proteins are best classified in four groups: pores, channels, carriers (also called *transporters*), and pumps. Ion pores and channels are integral membrane proteins that when "open" communicate the aqueous solutions adjacent to the membrane and permit ion flux in a direction determined by the electrochemical gradient. The permeant ion interacts little with the pore or channel, and thus the number of ions translocated per unit time (turnover number) is very high, typically 10^6–10^8 s^{-1}. Whereas pores are always open (ion-conductive), ion channels undergo "gating," that is, transitions between open (conductive) and close (nonconductive) states. The part of the protein thought to move during the gating is called the *gate* or *gating particle*. Gating can be elicited by physical factors (changes in membrane voltage or mechanical stretch), or chemical factors (such as neurotransmitters or second messengers).

Carriers are also integral membrane proteins. In contrast with channels, the function of carrier proteins involves a chemical interaction with the transported ion, namely ion binding, which elicits a series of conformational changes in the carrier eventually resulting in the translocation of the ion across the membrane. Because of these interactions between the carrier and the transported ion, the transport rate is much slower than that of channels, typically 10^2–10^4 s^{-1}. The net ion flux through carriers is also determined by the electrochemical gradient, as in channels, but in a more complex fashion, because certain carriers can transport several ions in the same cycle.

Pumps are similar to carriers in that there are ion-binding and conformational changes that cause ion translocation, but differ in that a metabolic energy source, such as ATP hydrolysis, is necessary for their function. Pumps have low turnover numbers, similar to those of carriers.

Many ion transport proteins associate with so-called adapter proteins (21) that appear to have two roles: to determine the subcellular location of the transport protein and to facilitate its interaction with signal transduction components, including receptors, second messenger-producing enzymes, and protein kinases. These adapter proteins often contain a specific protein–protein interaction domain called the *PDZ domain* (77). Adapter proteins therefore contribute to the formation of macromolecular complexes of which ion-transport proteins are important components.

The phospholipid composition of the plasma membrane has been recently recognized to play a regulatory role in the function of many ion transport proteins by specific binding of phosphatidylinositol 4,5-bisphosphate (PIP$_2$). Localized changes in synthesis or degradation of PIP$_2$ may exert rapid effects on transporter activity. The regulation by PIP$_2$ may be stimulatory or inhibitory and affects a large number of membrane-transport proteins (43). Certainly, being a dielectric is not the only function of the phospholipid moiety of the cell membrane.

Pores

Pores are wide conduits across biological membranes that do not gate, that is, they are permanently open (Fig. 7A). The best studied examples are those formed by bacterial porins, but they are also present in animal cells, that is, in mitochondria (porins) and in lymphocytes (perforin, a secretory product). It is also possible that aquaporins are pores (see Chapters 5 and 38).

Channels

For a detailed discussion of ion channels, see Chapter 4. In addition, excellent treatments of ion channels in general can be found in the book by Hille (44) and the review articles by Catterall (11) and Dawson (14). There are also several excellent recent reviews on ion-channel structure–function relationships (17, 18, 69), and on ion channels in renal epithelial cells (12, 39, 46, 50). Chapters 28, 29, 44, 62 cover renal Na^+, Cl^-, K^+, and Ca^{2+} channels, "respectively.

Like pores, channels have the property of being accessible to both sides of the membrane at the same time, but this occurs only part of the time. Channels open and close by the gating process. Gating may be determined by physical or chemical processes (see below), both requiring a sensing mechanism. In the open channel there is ion permeation with a characteristic selectivity for one or more ion species. Hence, the functional "fingerprint" of a channel includes gating, sensing mechanism, permeation, and selectivity.

In channels, the main transport-related conformational change is the gating between open and closed states (Fig. 7B). The gate is the portion of the channel protein that "moves" to cause channel opening and closure. When the channel is closed, it is impermeable, that is, nonconductive. When it is open, it is permeable or conductive, and allows ion fluxes, with a net flux that can also be expressed as the current carried by the ions. The flux and

hence the current are determined by the permeability of the channel and the driving force, that is, the electrochemical gradient for the permeant ion. The channel persists in the open state for a given time and allows ion permeation without additional conformational changes during the opening. Hence, one conformational change (gating) allows for transport of a large number of ions with no other necessary chemical reactions. The open channel constitutes a membrane pore, that is, a water-filled conduit that perforates the lipid bilayer, communicating the two solutions separated by the membrane. The interior of the open channel is accessible from both solutions at the same time. Channel turnover numbers are high, typically 10^6–10^8 per second. The large number of ions that cross a channel per unit of time causes a measurable electrical current. This fact allows investigators to measure net ion movement across individual molecules, that is, single-channel events, either in situ, using the patch-clamp technique (89), or reconstituting purified channels and incorporating them in artificial planar bilayers (72). The two channel conformations underlie the discrete levels observed in current records.

The total current (which denotes ion flux) via a population of channels of one kind in a plasma membrane is given by:

$$I = N \times P_o \times g \times \left(V_m - E_i\right) \tag{16}$$

where I is the current, N is the number of functional channels in the membrane, P_o is the channel open probability (time open/total time), g is the single channel conductance (conductance is the reciprocal of resistance), V_m is the membrane voltage, and E_i is the permeant ion's equilibrium po-

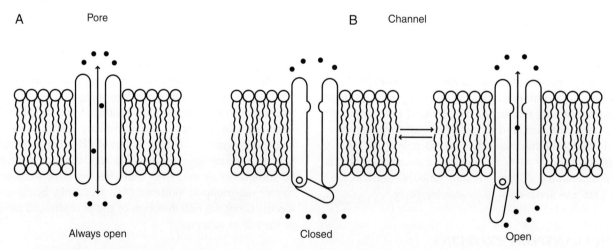

FIGURE 7 Pores and channels. A. A pore is a transmembrane protein that forms an aqueous conduit across the membrane that is always accessible from both sides and never closed. Pores are generally of large diameter and thus permit passive transport of small ions as well as larger hydrophilic solutes, driven by the electrochemical gradient across the membrane. B. A channel is also a transmembrane protein that forms an aqueous conduit across the membrane. However, in contrast with a pore, it can have two conformations, closed and open. The change in conformation is depicted in the figure by a swiveling portion of the molecule, the gate. Gating is the process by which the channels open and close. When the channel is open, it is permeable (conductive) and its interior is accessible to both sides. When the channel is closed, it is impermeable. Channels are generally of smaller radius than pores and exhibit varying degrees of ion selectivity. As in the case of pores, ion fluxes through channels are driven by the electrochemical gradient across the membrane.

tential. Note that the term $g (V_m - E_i)$ denotes i, the single-channel current. Equation 16 encompasses all mechanisms of channel-function regulation: number of copies, open probability (gating), conductance, and electrochemical driving force.

Whereas carriers can be uniporters, symporters, or antiporters, channels can be only uniporters. There can be ion–ion interactions in channels, such as single-file diffusion (27, 44), but molecular flux coupling, such as observed in carriers, does not occur. As is the case with carriers, channels exhibit substrate selectivity, typical pharmacological inhibition, and transport saturation, although the latter is more evident in carriers.

Certain channels are highly selective for specific ions, whereas others discriminate less among different ions. The bases of selectivity are ion size and charge. It has been well established that the Na^+, K^+, and Ca^{2+} channels of excitable membranes, as well as the epithelial Na^+ channel, K^+ channels, and Cl^- channels, are highly selective, that is, the permeability ratios between two ions of the same charge and similar size can be 100 or more. As explained in more detail below, the structural basis of high-selectivity channels is a very narrow region in the pore, called the *selectivity filter*, in which the dehydrated permeant ion is coordinated by dipoles (69). Other ion channels are less selective. For example, gap-junction channels, which communicate with adjacent cells, have cation–anion permeability ratios ranging from about 1 to about 10, values similar to those of tight junctions of leaky (high-permeability) epithelia. These channels are wider, the ions permeate in the hydrated state, and the cation–anion selectivity is probably governed by fixed charges facing the pore.

Carriers

Carrier-mediated transport is covered in Chapter 4. The reader is also referred to LeFevre (64), Schultz (91), and Stein (104) for quantitative treatments of carrier-mediated transport. Some specific carriers are well covered in recent reviews by Abramson et al. (1), Hediger et al. (41), Tanner (106), and Zachos et al. (117).

Carriers are transporters that perform transmembrane translocation of solute (and perhaps water; see Chapter 5) by a process thought to involve three basic steps. First, binding of the transported substrate to the carrier facing one side of the membrane; second, change in conformation of the carrier, involving translocation of the substrate (and the binding site) to the opposite side of the membrane; and third, release of the substrate. It is thought that access to the binding site from either bathing solution is by diffusion (or electrodiffusion) in porelike regions of the carrier molecule (57). Hence, two such steps could be added to the simplified scheme above.

In the operation of some carriers, there is a state in which the binding site and the substrate are inaccessible from either side of the membrane (56). The existence of this state, called *occlusion*, is one of many arguments supporting the idea of conformational change in carrier function. Carriers behave like enzymes in that the substrate binds to the protein; however, instead of chemical transformation of the substrate, the carrier performs its translocation. Carriers contain substrate-binding domains accessible from one side of the membrane at a time. In contrast with channels, they never form a conduit that communicates the two bathing solutions. Instead, they undergo conformational changes that alter the "sidedness" of the substrate-binding site, that is, substrate binds on one side, the conformation of the carrier protein changes, the binding site is translocated (with substrate) to the other side of the membrane, and the substrate is then released. In comparison with a channel, which has one gate, a carrier may be considered to have two gates, as illustrated in Fig. 8.

The notion of a carrier protein as a "ferryboat" binding the substrate at a membrane–solution interface and carrying it to the other side, where the solute is released to the other solution, is inconsistent with current knowledge of the biochemistry and molecular biology of carriers. Nevertheless, kinetic schemes based on the ferryboat model remain very useful to explain carrier function at a phenomenological level.

Substrate transport by carriers is inherently slow because each substrate molecule (or group of molecules in cases of coupled transport; see below) must undergo an independent binding reaction, followed by the conformational change of the carrier molecule. This is the explanation of the low turnover number of carriers, similar to the rate of most instances of enzymatic catalysis, that is, $10^2–10^3$ per second (104).

Most carriers have exquisite substrate selectivity (e.g., the glucose carrier GLUT1 transports D-glucose, but not L-glucose) and can also exhibit quite specific pharmacological inhibition. At low substrate concentration, the substrate flux increases linearly with the concentration, and can be confused with simple diffusion, but at high substrate concentration it saturates, as expected from occupancy of a limited number of slowly turning binding sites. The low turnover number, high substrate selectivity and saturation of carriers, and to some extent the mechanisms of pharmacological inhibition, also support the notions of substrate binding and conformational change during the transport cycle.

Carrier-mediated transport can be classified in three types depending on the number of substrates and the transport directions (Fig. 9). When the carrier transports only one substrate the process is called *facilitated diffusion* or *uniport*; the carrier is a uniporter. Other carriers transport two or more substrates. When all substrates are transported in the same direction, the process is called *cotransport* or *symport*; the carrier is a *cotransporter* or *symporter*. When there is substrate transport in opposite directions, the process is called *countertransport*, *exchange*, or *antiport*; the carrier is a *countertransporter*, *exchanger*, or *antiporter*. Uniporters can only perform passive transport. The overall transport via a symporter or an antiporter is downhill. There is always passive translocation of at least one substrate and there can be secondary active translocation of one or more additional substrates. For example, in the case of two substrates, all the energy employed in uphill

One gate open   Both gates closed   Other gate open

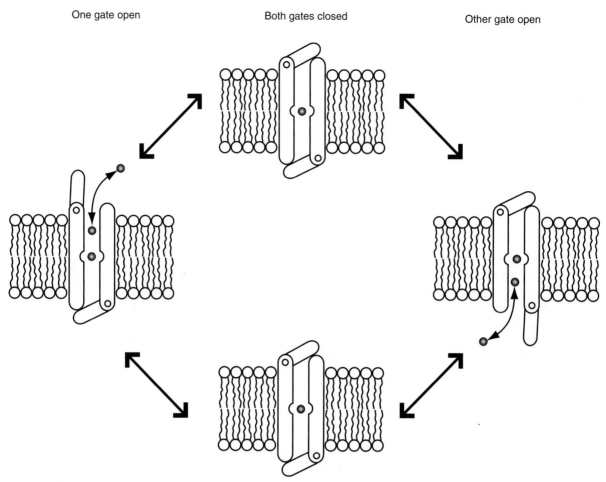

FIGURE 8 Carriers. A carrier can be understood as a membrane-transport protein with two gates and one or more binding sites for the substrate. The figure depicts the transport stages for a uniporter, the simplest kind of carrier molecule. From left to right: the substrate binds to the carrier at a site available to only one side of the membrane (first gate open, second gate closed); this closes the second gate and the substrate is occluded (both gates closed); the second gate opens and the binding site and the substrate become accessible to the other side of the membrane, and the substrate is then released. The transport process is passive. The unidirectional and net fluxes are determined by the chemical or electrochemical potential difference, for uncharged and charged substrates, respectively. (Modified with permission from Gadsby DC. Ion transport: spot the difference. *Nature* 2004;427:795–797.)

translocation of one species derives from the passive transport of the other one, so that no metabolic energy is directly used.

Pumps

Ion pumps are discussed in Chapter 3. Other reviews of ion pumps are Apell (4, 5), Facciotti et al. (23), Fambrough and Inesi (24), Finbow and Harrison (26), Horisberger (48, 49), Läuger (63), and Sachs et al. (87).

Ion pumps can be classified according to the source of metabolic energy. Pumps in general can be driven by light, redox state, or ATP hydrolysis. Animal-cell plasma membrane ATPases belong to the P type, which is characterized by the formation of a phosphorylated intermediary (Na^+,K^+-, H^+,K^+-, and Ca^{2+}-ATPase), or to the V type (vacuolar H^+-ATPase). In intracellular membranes, there is expression of the vacuolar-type H^+ pump, as well as F-type (or F_1- or F_0-type) ATPases, that is, the ATP synthase expressed in the inner mitochondrial membrane. ATP synthases are also ex-

pressed in purple bacteria and in green plants. Their function can be outlined as follows. Multimeric protein complexes (respiratory-chain complex in mitochondria, bacteriorhodopsin in purple bacteria, photosynthetic reaction center in chloroplasts) generate a H^+ electrochemical gradient from the redox potential of NADPH (mitochondria) or light energy (others). The transmembrane H^+ electrochemical gradient is then used by ATP synthases to synthesize ATP from ADP and PI. Hence, the function of these proteins is to synthesize ATP, dissipating the ion gradient in the process. However, they are reversible, that is, under appropriate conditions they will hydrolyze ATP and generate an electrochemical ion gradient. Similarly, the Na^+,K^+-ATPase normally hydrolyzes ATP to transport actively Na^+ and K^+, but under certain conditions can operate in a reverse mode, that is, downhill ion fluxes coupled to the synthesis of ATP.

The ion pumps present in plasma membranes of epithelial cells are the Na^+,K^+-ATPase, Ca^{2+}-ATPase, H^+-ATPase, and H^+,K^+-ATPase. Other pumps have been suggested to

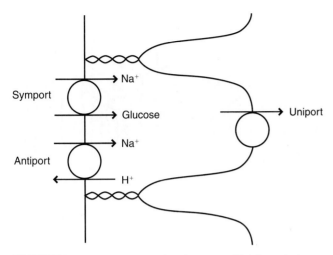

FIGURE 9 Types of carrier-mediated transport. The figure depicts an epithelial cell (e.g., renal proximal tubule) expressing different kinds of carriers, classified according to the number of substrates and the directions of the net fluxes. *Uniporter* is a carrier that transports only one substrate in a complete cycle; the process is known as facilitated diffusion or uniport, and is always passive. Shown in the figure is a glucose uniporter at the basolateral membrane. *Symporter* is a carrier that transports at least two substrates in the same direction in each cycle. The process is known as cotransport or symport; the overall transport process is downhill, but the electrochemical gradient of one substrate can be used to transport the other one actively (a form of secondary active transport). Shown in the figure is a Na^+–glucose symporter at the apical membrane. *Antiporter* is a carrier that transports at least two substrates in opposite directions in each cycle. The process is known as countertransport, exchange, or antiport; the overall transport process is downhill, but again the electrochemical gradient of one substrate can be used to translocate the other one actively (secondary active transport). Shown in the figure is a Na^+/H^+ antiporter at the apical membrane. See also Fig. 6.

exist in these tissues, but they are either unique to certain epithelia or controversial. The molecular structures of these pumps have been identified and significant progress has been made in understanding their function, but much work remains to be done in this area. Ion occlusion is a well-known stage during the pump cycle (34). As is the case with carrier function, occlusion denotes that the conformational change necessary for transport does change the accessibility of the substrate-binding sites to the solutions bathing the membrane.

The Na^+,K^+-, H^+,K^+-, and Ca^{2+}-ATPase are all of the P type, which is characterized by the phosphorylation of an aspartic acid residue (in the sequence DKTG) during the pump catalytic cycle. The Na^+,K^+-ATPase is a ubiquitous pump in epithelial cells. In each cycle, one ATP molecule is hydrolyzed, three Na^+ are transported from the cytoplasm to the interstitial fluid, and two K^+ are transported in the opposite direction. In each cycle there is thus a net transfer of charge across the membrane (one net charge is extruded), and hence the pump is electrogenic, tending to hyperpolarize the cell. Its turnover number is in the range of values for carriers, that is, less than 10^2 s^{-1}. The catalytic cycle of P-type ATPases is shown in Fig. 10.

The Na^+,K^+-ATPase is expressed in most, if not all, vertebrate epithelial cells. It is generally targeted to the basolateral membrane. In the choroid plexus and the retinal pigment epithelium, the pump is located at the apical membrane and cell polarity appears inverted vis-à-vis other epithelia. The pump consists of α and β subunits in a 1:1 stoichiometry (probably $\alpha 2\beta 2$). The α subunit has four isoforms (apparent molecular mass of 120 kDa) and the β subunit has two isoforms (1 and 2) with apparent molecular mass of 50 kDa. The α subunit is responsible for both ion transport and ATP activity, and contains the Na^+,K^+ (and ouabain)-binding sites, as well as the phosphorylation site. The β subunit (three isoforms) appears to be required for assembly and plasma membrane targeting of the protein. The pump isoforms are tissue-specific and change during organ development.

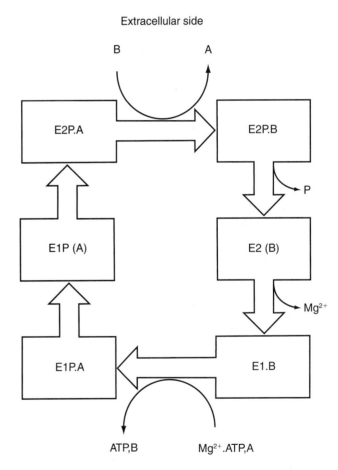

FIGURE 10 Catalytic cycle for P-type ATPases modeled as countertransport pumps exchanging Na^+ (*A*) for K^+ (*B*), Ca^{2+} (*A*) for H^+ (*B*) and H^+ (*B*) for K^+ (*A*) (Na^+,K^+-, Ca^{2+}- and H^+,K^+-ATPase, respectively). E1, conformation with ion-binding sites accessible from cytoplasm; E2, conformation with ion-binding sites accessible from the extracellular face; E(A) or E(B), ion "occluded" in the protein. (Modified with permission from Saier MH Jr. A functional-phylogenetic classification system for transmembrane solute transporters. *Microbiol Mol Biol Rev* 2000;64: 354–411.)

Structure–Function Correlations of Ion-Transport Proteins

During the last decade, atomic-resolution structures have been obtained by x-ray crystallography for bacterial pores (15, 95), prototypical bacterial ion channels (19, 22), the lac-permease of *Escherichia coli* carrier (1, 2), and the mammalian sarcoplasmic-reticulum Ca^{2+} pump (108, 109). These studies have provided detailed insight into the mechanism of the function of these specific transport proteins, as well as a framework in which to analyze other proteins. An example is the modeling of the Na^+,K^+-ATPase based on the structure of the SERCA (sarcoplasmic and endoplasmic reticulum ATPase) pump (78).

PORES

Bacterial pores formed by the transmembrane proteins called *porins* are radically different from animal membrane proteins in that the transmembrane domains, instead of α helices, are β sheets. For a discussion of porin structures, see Delcour (15) and Schulz (95).

CHANNELS

All known K^+ channels belong to a single protein family, characterized by the highly conserved K^+ channel signature sequence (42), which forms the selectivity filter. K^+ channels display high selectivity and high conduction rates. X-ray crystallographic studies performed in recent years have revealed the atomic structures of several K^+ channels. Roderick MacKinnon was awarded the 2003 Nobel Prize for Chemistry for this work. In this section, I summarize the current understanding of K^+ channel selectivity and conduction derived from structural studies. For a discussion of the gating process, see MacKinnon (69).

The K^+ channel is formed by four subunits arranged around a central pore (17, 120). Each subunit consists of two transmembrane α helices (inner and outer, relative to the pore), and the pore helix, which is tilted and penetrates only half of the membrane thickness. Near the center of the membrane the pore forms a water-filled cavity that contains a hydrated K^+ (120). As shown in Fig. 11, the selectivity filter, formed by the signature-sequence amino acids, is located between the central cavity and the extracellular solution. The filter consists of four layers of carbonyl oxygen atoms and a layer of threonine hydroxyl oxygen atoms, creating four K^+ binding sites (one to four from the extracellular side). Thus, each dehydrated K^+ is surrounded by eight oxygen atoms, four "above" and four "below." The selectivity filter thus mimics the arrangement of the K^+ hydration shell, in which a single K^+ is surrounded on average by eight water molecules. The K^+ ions are "transferred" by diffusion from water to the selectivity filter, the hydration energy being compensated by the binding energy in the filter. Sodium ions do not enter the selectivity filter (119, 120) because the selectivity-filter binding energy cannot compensate for the higher hydra-

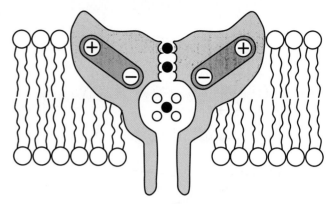

FIGURE 11 Diagram representing the structure of the KcsA channel. Two of the four subunits are depicted, with the extracellular side on top. The narrow portion is the selectivity filter, in which there are four possible positions for dehydrated K^+ ions (filled circles). Because of electrostatic repulsion, only two of these positions can be simultaneously occupied (first and third as shown, or second and fourth). The selectivity filter communicates with a larger cavity that can accommodate hydrated K^+ (four water molecules—open circles—are depicted). In the tetramer, each K^+ in the selectivity filter is coordinated by eight oxygens, and in the cavity each K^+ is surrounded by eight water molecules. Oriented helices point their carboxyl ends (relatively negative) toward the cavity, helping stabilize K^+ ions inside the membrane. (Modified with permission from Doyle DA, Morais Cabral J, Pfuetzner RA, Kuo A, Gulbis JM, Cohen SL, Chait BT, MacKinnon R. The structure of the potassium channel: molecular basis of K^+ conduction and selectivity. *Science* 1998;280:69–77. Copyright 1998 by the American Association for the Advancement of Science.)

tion energy. The small distances between the four K^+ binding sites cause electrostatic repulsion, so only two sites (one and three, or two and four) are thought to be occupied at any time (74). The electrostatic repulsion tends to balance the binding forces, thus ensuring a high turnover number (69).

CARRIERS

The largest family of secondary active transporters, the major facilitator superfamily (MFS), comprises 25% of all transport proteins (88). MFS proteins are expressed from bacteria to vertebrates. They range from 400 to 600 amino acids in size, have 12 transmembrane helices, and N- and C-termini are located on the cytoplasmic side. These proteins transport numerous substrates and may be uniporters, symporters, or antiporters. The atomic structures of two bacterial members of the MFS were obtained in 2003: the H^+-lactose cotransporter (LacY) or lac-permease (2) and the PI/glycerol-3-phosphate antiporter (GlpT) (52). In both structures the transmembrane helices form two domains, N- and C-termini (each consisting of a six-helix bundle) with a pseudo-twofold symmetry. A large cavity was detected in both structures, open to the cytoplasm and closed to the periplasm, suggesting that the crystals correspond to the inward-facing conformation.

In lac-permease, the cavity is formed by helices I, II, IV, and V of the N-terminal domain, and helices VII, VIII, X, and XI of the C-terminal domain. Helices III, VI, IX, and

XII are not exposed to the pore. The sugar-binding pocket is formed by helices I, IV, and V of the N-terminal domain and helices VII and XI of the C-terminal domain. Proton translocation involves Glu325 (helix X) and Arg302 (helix IX), and the coupling of substrate binding and proton translocation involves His322 (helix X) and Glu269 (helix VIII). Thus, the proton translocation site does not interact directly with the sugar-binding site.

Substrate translocation must involve a conformational change generating an outward-facing conformation open to the periplasmic side. It has been suggested (1) that the conformational change is a rotation between the N- and C-termini domains around the sugar-binding site, but there is no structural proof of this hypothesis. A more clear understanding of the mode of operation of lac-permease and other carrier proteins will require crystal structures under additional experimental conditions.

PUMPS

The Ca^{2+}-ATPase from rabbit skeletal muscle sarcoplasmic reticulum (SERCA1a) is not a plasma–membrane protein, but is a good prototype for P-type ion-transporting ATPases. The mass of SERCA1a is 110 kDa, it has 10 transmembrane helices (M1–M10), three cytoplasmic domains (A [actuator or anchor], N [nucleotide-binding], and P [phosphorylation]), and small SR-lumen loops. SERCA1a transports, against the electrochemical gradient across the SR membrane, two Ca^{2+} per ATP hydrolyzed, reducing $[Ca^{2+}]$ in the cytosol and accumulating it in the SR lumen. Two or three H^+ are exchanged for the Ca^{2+} in each cycle (107). As is the case with other P-ATPases, primary active ion transport is thought to result from a conformational change of the pump (from E1 to E2). In E1, the Ca^{2+} ions bind with high affinity and face the cytoplasm; in E2, the affinity is low and Ca^{2+} ions face the SR lumen. The Ca^{2+} translocation would take place between E1P and E2P, two states of the phosphorylated pump. Similar states exist in the operation of the Na^+,K^+-ATPase (see Chapter 3).

The structure of SERCA1 has been determined by x-ray crystallography with and without Ca^{2+} binding as well as with and without exposure to the inhibitor thapsigargin (see 110 for a review). The atomic structure (108, 109) revealed that the transmembrane helices 4, 5, and 6 contain the amino acid residues that bind the two Ca^{2+} ions transported per cycle. However, neither the permeation pathway, nor the gates have been identified yet.

The Na^+,K^+-ATPase has not been crystallized yet, but a homology model based on the structure of the Ca^{2+} pump (78) suggests that the homologous helices 4, 5, and 6 of the alpha subunit contain the amino acid residues that would bind two of the three Na^+ and the two K^+ that are translocated in each cycle; the third Na^+ would be coordinated in a pocket formed by transmembrane helices 6, 8, and 9. As in the case of the SERCA pump, the ion translocation pathway and the identity of the gates remain unknown.

Differences between the structures in various biochemical conditions revealed that SERCA1 Ca^{2+} binding and dissociation elicit large conformational changes in the transmembrane domains mechanically linked to similar changes in the cytoplasmic domains. Homology modeling revealed that the cation-binding sites of the Ca^{2+}- and Na^+,K^+-ATPases are virtually the same (78). A critical movement of transmembrane helix 4 causes the release of a cation (Ca^{2+} or Na^+) and the binding of the other cation (H^+ or K^+) at a displaced position with respect to the membrane, thus preventing competition between the cations.

COMMON, BASIC ION-TRANSPORT MOLECULE?

The marine toxin palitoxin (PTX) is a ~3000-Da molecule that consists of a chain of over 100 carbons with a complex variety of organic side groups (32). The mechanism of the toxic effect of PTX it to convert the Na^+,K^+-ATPase from a cation pump into a nonselective cation channel that dissipates the Na^+ and K^+ gradients between the cell and the extracellular fluid. This could be explained if the effect of PTX were to open the two gates necessary for the normal operation of the pump, thus revealing the ion translocation pathway. PTX was shown to interact with the pump in excised membrane patches, and this interaction was dependent of the presence of ATP on the inside of the membrane, and was modulated by extracellular K^+, indicating that the PTX-dependent channel function shares properties of the native pump (6, 7). In other studies, the permeation pathway was mapped using the technique known as cysteine-scanning mutagenesis, in which the accessibility of amino acid sites to small hydrophilic thiol reagents is assessed after mutating those sites to Cys. Residues in transmembrane domains 4, 5, and 6 became accessible by exposure to PTX (36, 37, 51), consistently with the structural studies described above. These interesting studies suggest that ion channels and pump, and likely carriers as well, share a basic molecular architecture (see 21 for a discussion). Further support for this notion was obtained by the demonstration that bacterial homologues of the mammalian ClC channels function as antiporters (3). In sum, and as illustrated in Fig. 12, the simplest ion transport protein would be a pore (no gate), followed by a pore with one gate (channel), a pore with two gates (carrier), and finally a pore with two gates coupled to a metabolic-energy source (pump).

ION TRANSPORT ACROSS EPITHELIA

Epithelia are two-dimensional sheets of cells joined together by a network of tight junctions. Epithelia can be monolayered or multilayered, and they can be planar, or form tubes or acini. Epithelia line external surfaces of the body (skin, gastrointestinal, respiratory, and urinary tracts) and also separate fluid compartments inside the body (choroid plexus, inner ear epithelia). The vascular endothelium, which lines

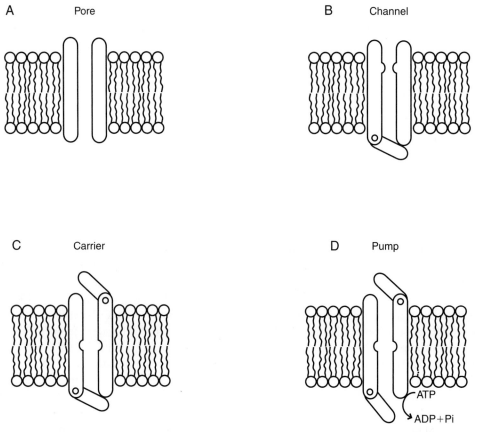

FIGURE 12   A simplified view of structure–function correlations in ion-transport proteins. A. Pore, the simplest transmembrane protein, is a transmembrane aqueous conduit with no gates, accessible to both sides of the membrane at all times (always open). B. Channel, a pore with a gate whose position determines whether the channel is open or closed. The open channel is accessible to both sides of the membrane. C. Carrier, a transmembrane protein with two gates that are never open at the same time. Thus, the carrier interior may be accessible to only one side of the membrane; when both gates are closed, the substrate is occluded (inaccessible to either side). D. Pump, a carrier that is directly coupled to a metabolic energy source, that is, hydrolysis of ATP.

the inside of blood vessels, shares structural and functional features with epithelia.

Epithelial Structure–Function Relationships

Transepithelial transport may be transcellular and/or paracellular (intercellular). Transcellular transport requires substrate translocation across one cell membrane, diffusion in the cell interior, and translocation across the opposite membrane. Paracellular transport involves substrate translocation across the junctional complex and diffusion/convection along the lateral intercellular spaces. Transcellular transport rates can be quite high. In the mammalian proximal tubule, during fluid reabsorption total cell water is completely replaced six times per minute (103). Paracellular transport is a passive phenomenon, that is, it is always energetically downhill, driven by the gradients developed by primary and secondary active transport events in the transcellular pathway.

Transcellular transport can be active or passive. In most instances it involves an active step at one membrane and a passive step at the other one. In such a case, one refers to the overall process as active. Transcellular transport is possible because membrane-transport proteins in transporting epithelia are polarized, that is, they are expressed differentially in apical and basolateral membrane domains (21, 22) (see Chapter 1). The mechanisms of establishment and maintenance of cell polarity are not fully understood, but involve targeting of newly synthesized transport proteins and retention of these proteins once they are inserted in the correct membrane domain. Retention occurs because the tight junction is a barrier to lateral diffusion of transmembrane proteins between the two domains (20) and also because, following their insertion in the membrane, the proteins can bind to the cytoskeleton (8). The existence of cell polarity permits specific transporters to operate in series, allowing for *vectorial*, that is, directional, net transport across the epithelium. Depending on its direction, transepithelial transport can be called *absorption* (in the renal tubule, *reabsorption*), when it occurs *toward* the extracellular fluid compartment, or secretion, when it occurs *from* the extracellular fluid. The main theme of this section is how specific molecules are organized in the two membrane domains of the epithelial cell to perform transepithelial transport. Several such systems are discussed elsewhere in this book (see Chapters 1, 5, 8, 30, 47).

Two Types of Epithelia

Ion-transporting epithelia exposed in vitro to aqueous solutions of identical compositions may develop a large transepithelial voltage (V_t), whereas other epithelia transport ions at the same or even at a higher rate in the presence of a nil or very small V_t. In this kind of experiment, V_t is related to transepithelial transport and ultimately depends on active transport processes, because it occurs in the absence of transepithelial electrochemical driving forces. The V_t is generated by the transcellular pathway, where active transport takes place. Because epithelia consist of two cell membranes in series, and these are in turn in parallel with the paracellular pathway, the origin of V_t is complex (see Chapter 8). High-V_t epithelia perform electrogenic transport, that is, there is independent movement of the transported ion(s) and have low paracellular ion permeability (high paracellular electrical resistance). Low-V_t epithelia usually perform electroneutral ion transport and have high paracellular ion permeability (low electrical resistance). Depending on the relationship between the paracellular and transcellular electrical resistances (R_p and RC, respectively), epithelia have been classified in tight (high R_p/P_c) and leaky (low R_p/P_c), a concept introduced by Diamond (16). In general, leaky epithelia have low V_t and tight epithelia generate a high V_t.

The Two-Membrane Hypothesis

Ussing and colleagues proposed a simple and elegant mechanism for active Na^+ transport by the frog epidermis, the *two-membrane hypothesis* (Fig. 13) (55). Transepithelial active Na^+ transport occurs by passive (electrodiffusive) influx across the apical cell membrane and active (pump-mediated) efflux across the basolateral membrane. The two ion-transport proteins responsible for influx and efflux are the epithelial Na^+channel (ENaC) and the Na^+,K^+-ATPase, respectively. ENaC has a high Na^+/K^+ selectivity, and the Na^+ pump catalyzes the exit of $3Na^+$ and the entry of $2K^+$ per molecule of ATP hydrolyzed. The net operation of the pump is to lower intracellular $[Na^+]$ and raise intracellular $[K^+]$, making V_m more negative. The Na^+ concentration gradient and the membrane voltage provide an electrochemical gradient favoring Na^+ influx. The ion composition of the epithelial cells is maintained during transport because Na^+ influx and efflux are equal, and the K^+ taken up by the pump recycles to the basolateral solution via K^+ channels.

Experimentally, using identical salt solutions on both sides of the epithelium, an electric current can be passed across the isolated frog-skin epithelium to abolish the V_t generated by Na^+ transport. Under these conditions, the current (*short-circuit current*) is virtually identical to net Na^+ transport (113), and thus provides an accurate measurement with excellent time resolution. Without current application (*open-circuit conditions*), Na^+ transport generates a V_t (apical-solution negative) that tends to oppose further transport of the cation. However, the frog epidermis has a high paracel-

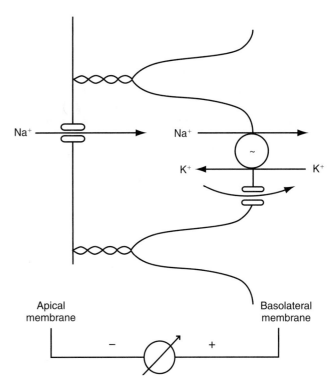

FIGURE 13 Basic mechanism of Na^+ transport in Na^+-absorptive epithelia. The figure summarizes Ussing's two-membrane hypothesis for Na^+-absorbing tight epithelia (55). At the apical cell membrane, Na^+ entry is via a Na^+ channel that is blockable by low concentrations of the diuretic amiloride. At the basolateral cell membrane, extrusion of Na^+ is mediated by the Na^+,K^+-ATPase, inhibitable by cardiac steroids such as ouabain. K^+ recycles across the basolateral cell membrane via a K^+-channel. (Modified with permission from Reuss L, Cotton CU. Volume regulation in epithelia: transcellular transport and cross-talk. In: Strange K, ed. *Cellular and Molecular Physiology of Cell Volume Regulation.* Boca Raton Press, FL: CRC, 1994:31–48.)

lular Cl^- permeability, so that Cl^- is passively reabsorbed (driven by V_t), decreasing the transepithelial voltage generated by Na^+ transport.

The essential idea in the two-membrane hypothesis (or two-membrane model) is that transcellular ion transport results from the concerted operation of an active transporter ("pump") in one membrane, in series with a passive transporter ("leak") in the other membrane. The pump, via its effects on intracellular ion concentration and/or membrane voltage, generates the driving force for ion flux across the leak. With appropriate modifications, this model can be applied to most if not all cases of epithelial ion transport (82). The pump-leak model is an important concept in cell physiology. It applies to both epithelial and nonpolar cells (47).

Does Two-Membrane Model Apply to Other Epithelia?

Another case of electrogenic transepithelial ion transport involves absorption of one ion and secretion of another one of the same charge. Such is the case with Na^+ absorption and

K$^+$ secretion by the principal cells of the renal cortical collecting duct. The Na$^+$-transporting mechanism is the same as in the frog skin, but the K$^+$ channels expressed in the apical membrane permit K$^+$ secretion: primary active K$^+$ influx at the basolateral membrane (via the Na$^+$ pump) and passive efflux across apical-membrane K$^+$ channels (Fig. 14).

Studies of other epithelia revealed other electrogenic transport processes than Na$^+$ absorption, such as Cl$^-$ secretion (Fig. 15) (96, 118). The mechanism is still a pump-leak system like the two-membrane model applied to Na$^+$ transport. Influx is via the pump and efflux is via the leak (Cl$^-$ channels). The "pump" is complex, involving the concerted operation of three transport proteins, the Na$^+$ pump, the Na$^+$–K$^+$–2Cl$^-$ cotransporter (66) and the K$^+$ channel. The Cl$^-$ influx is secondary active, not primary active.

In most leaky (low-V$_t$) epithelia, ion influx is mediated by carriers, such as Na$^+$–Cl$^-$ or Na$^+$–K$^+$–2Cl$^-$ cotransporters, and Na$^+$–H$^+$ and Cl$^-$–HCO$_3^-$ exchangers operating in parallel. In these epithelia, the mechanism of the low V$_t$ is dual:

electroneutral transport at one membrane (Fig. 16) and "shunting" by the paracellular pathway of potential differences created by the transcellular pathway. The efflux mechanism at the basolateral membrane of electroneutral Na$^+$-transporting epithelia is the same as in electrogenic epithelia. In contrast, Cl$^-$ transport is not paracellular, but transcellular, by Cl$^-$ channels (79) and/or the K$^+$-Cl$^-$ cotransporter (80).

The Paracellular Pathway

In normal epithelia, the paracellular pathway is intercellular, that is, it consists of the tight junctions in series with the lateral intercellular spaces (see Chapter 1). Electrophysiological (30, 116) and morphological (68) studies in renal-tubule and gallbladder epithelia demonstrated a high ion permeability of the junctions. The notions of "tight" and "leaky" epithelia (16), discussed above, derived from this work.

The composition of tight junctions was recently ascertained by Tsukita et al. (111). The main components are four

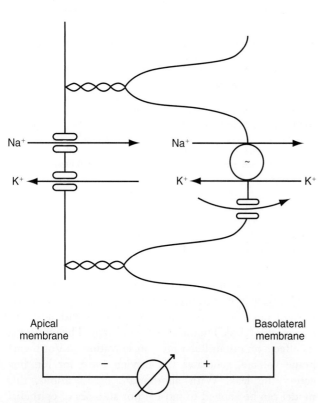

FIGURE 14 Basic mechanisms of Na$^+$ and K$^+$ transport in Na$^+$-absorptive and K$^+$-secretory epithelia. A single transport protein (an apical-membrane K$^+$ channel) is added to the simpler model depicted in Fig. 13. K$^+$ is above electrochemical equilibrium because of the operation of the Na$^+$,K$^+$-ATPase; further, the membrane voltage across the apical membrane is less than that across the basolateral membrane, because of the contribution of Na$^+$ channels at the former. The K$^+$ taken up by the pump will in part be secreted across the apical membrane and in part recycle across the basolateral membrane. The relative rates of these fluxes will depend on the K$^+$ conductances of both membranes and on the driving forces. Higher Na$^+$ permeability or higher [Na$^+$] in the lumen will increase the driving force for K$^+$ secretion.

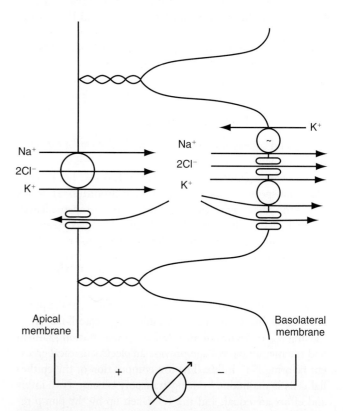

FIGURE 15 Basic mechanism of Cl$^-$ transport in Cl$^-$-absorptive epithelia. Intracellular [Cl$^-$] is maintained above electrochemical equilibrium by electroneutral Na$^+$–K$^+$–2Cl$^-$ cotransport across the apical cell membrane. The main driving force for this secondary active Cl$^-$ influx is the low intracellular [Na$^+$], maintained by the operation of the Na$^+$,K$^+$-ATPase expressed in the basolateral membrane; the K$^+$ influx across the apical membrane is largely balanced by efflux via K$^+$ channels in the same membrane (K$^+$ recycling). Basolateral-membrane Cl$^-$ efflux proceeds through Cl$^-$ channels and the KCl cotransporter. This Cl$^-$ transport model applies to the thick ascending limb of Henle's loop, a Cl$^-$-absorptive epithelium. (Modified with permission from Reeves WB, Andreoli TE. Renal epithelial chloride channels. *Annu Rev Physiol* 1992;54:29–50. Copyright 1992 by Annual Reviews.)

transmembrane-segment proteins named occludin and claudins. Claudins are always present in tight junctions and their expression is necessary and sufficient to form junctional strands. Occludin by itself does not form complete strands, but may contribute to the regulation of tight-junction permeability and to cytoskeletal architecture and the phenotype of epithelial cells (see ref. 90 for a review).

The paracellular pathway is thought to participate in transepithelial transport of ions and water. In tight epithelia, the paracellular path is essentially a barrier, whereas in leaky epithelia it is a conduit. In leaky epithelia, the paracellular pathway acts as a shunt, electrically coupling the two cell membranes. Because of the dominant basolateral membrane K^+ conductance, there is an intraepithelial current loop that hyperpolarizes the apical membrane (see Chapter 8), increasing the driving force for entry of cationic solutes. This mechanism is prominent in the renal proximal tubule and the small intestine, where it facilitates organic solute entry via Na^+–glucose and Na^+–amino acid cotransporters. A second function of the paracellular pathway is electrodiffusive ion transport. The V_t generated by electrogenic transcellular transport drives ion transport via the paracellular pathway. An example is the thick ascending segment of the loop of Henle: the lumen-positive V_t causes paracellular reabsorption of Na^+, Ca^{2+}, and Mg^{2+} (see Chapters 31 and 65). In contrast, in frog epidermis, the V_t generated by Na^+ transport drives Cl^- via the paracellular pathway. Tight junctions are ion selective depending on expression of specific claudin isoforms (114). The paracellular transport of Ca^{2+} and Mg^{2+} by the thick ascending loop of Henle results from the expression of claudin-16 (or paracellin-1), the protein that confers the high permeability for divalent cations to the tight junctions (98). Mutations of this protein cause a genetic disease with excessive loss of Ca^{2+} and Mg^{2+} in the urine. Finally, water transport may be another important function of the paracellular pathway, both in terms of solute-coupled transport and solvent drag (Chapter 5).

The preceding discussion serves to emphasize that highly preserved cell polarity (see Chapter 1) is the essential feature underlying the capacity of epithelial cells to perform vectorial transport. Two pathological conditions in which renal tubule cells appear to lose or reverse their polarity are meta-

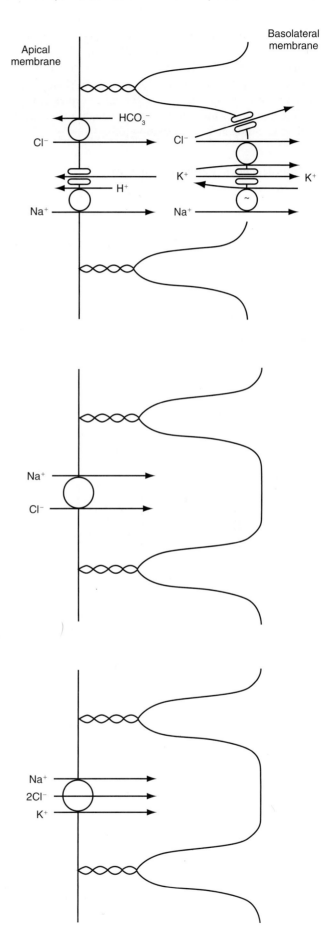

FIGURE 16 Ion-transport mechanisms in leaky Na-Cl absorbing epithelia. A. Na^+ and Cl^- influxes across apical cell membrane via exchanges with H^+ and HCO_3^-, respectively. Cl^- exit across basolateral cell membrane is via Cl^- channels and/or via K^+–Cl^- cotransport. Na^+ extrusion is mediated by Na^+,K^+-ATPase. K^+ recycles via channels (basolateral or both cell membranes). This model accounts for NaCl transport in most "leaky" NaCl-absorptive epithelia. B. The mechanism of salt entry is Na^+-Cl^- cotransport (demonstrated for flounder urinary bladder and mammalian renal distal tubule). Basolateral transport mechanisms as in top diagram. C. Mechanism of salt entry is Na^+–K^+–$2Cl^-$ cotransport (demonstrated for flounder intestine). Basolateral transport mechanisms as in top diagram. (Modified with permission from Reuss L, Cotton CU. Volume regulation in epithelia: transcellular transport and cross-talk. In: Strange K, ed. *Cellular and Molecular Physiology of Cell Volume Regulation*. Boca Raton, FL: CRC Press, 1994:31–48.)

bolic injury during acute renal failure and polycystic kidney disease, respectively. In the first condition, the loss of polar expression of the Na^+,K^+-ATPase may contribute to the reduction in proximal tubule salt and water reabsorption (73). In polycystic kidney disease, the apical expression of a CFTR-like Cl^- channel in the cysts is thought to play a role in fluid secretion and cyst dilatation (38).

Interdependence of Epithelial–Cell Transport Processes

The preservation of ion transport electroneutrality, as well as the volume and composition of transporting epithelial cells, depend on fine adjustments between the rates of ion transport by various membrane proteins. These adjustments can occur at the same membrane and/or at the opposite membranes.

There are many examples of adjustments of ion fluxes across transport proteins expressed in the same membrane. For example, in $NaCl^-$ absorptive epithelia, the steady-state rates of Na^+ entry and Cl^- entry across the apical membrane are the same. This was interpreted to indicate Na^+-Cl^- cotransport (29), but later studies showed that in most $NaCl^-$ transporting epithelia, entry is instead by the parallel operation of Na^+–H^+ and Cl^-–HCO_3^- exchangers (65, 81). The fluxes can be transiently dissociated but are equivalent in the steady state, being modulated by changes in intracellular pH (81). A second example of flux adjustment at the same membrane is so-called *pump-leak parallelism* (94). The intracellular ATP concentration couples the rate of the Na^+,K^+-ATPase (K^+ influx) to the open probability of basolateral K^+ channels (K^+ efflux), both expressed in the basolateral membrane, thus matching their fluxes.

Adjustments of fluxes between the opposite membranes have been called *cross-talk mechanisms* (59, 85, 92, 93). These processes involve a primary change in the ion-transport rate at one membrane, a signaling event in the cell, sensing and transduction of the signal, and a change in transporter activity at the opposite membrane. Cross-talk has been demonstrated in numerous epithelia, starting with the frog epidermis, where Na^+-pump inhibition decreased the apical-membrane Na^+ permeability (70). The underlying mechanism may involve changes in intracellular $[Ca^{2+}]$ and/or pH_i (see 82 for a review). Experiments in cortical-collecting duct cells showed directly that intracellular pH and $[Ca^{2+}]$ modulate the open probability of ENaC in the right directions to account for the cross-talk mechanism (28, 97). Another example of cross-talk involves leaky epithelia such as the small intestine and renal proximal tubule. Cotransport of Na^+ and organic solute (e.g., glucose) is electrogenic, depolarizes the apical membrane, and reduces the ratio of cell–membrane electrical resistances (apical–basolateral) because of the added conductance via the Na^+–glucose carrier. After this response, the membrane voltage and the membrane resistance ratio return to normal in the continued presence of glucose. The mechanism is an increase in basolateral-membrane K^+ conductance resulting

from solute influx via the apical membrane, and likely mediated by cell swelling (60, 93).

No single signaling mechanism accounts for epithelial cross-talk. The available data suggest changes in cell volume and intracellular ion concentrations as the initial signals. Cell volume changes may influence membrane-transport proteins by physical and/or biochemical factors, such as membrane tension and dilution of intracellular mediators, respectively. Changes in intracellular $[Ca^{2+}]_i$ or pH, as well as protein phosphorylation, may be part of the signaling mechanism. It is likely that both the signals and the transduction mechanisms operative in epithelial cross-talk are multiple and interactive.

References

1. Abramson J, Iwata S, Kaback HR. Lactose permease as a paradigm for membrane transport proteins. *Mol Membr Biol* 2004;21:227–236.
2. Abramson J, Smirnova I, Kasho V, Verner G, Kaback HR, Iwata S. Structure and mechanism of the lactose permease of *Escherichia coli*. *Science* 2003;301:610–615.
3. Accardi A, Miller C. Secondary active transport mediated by a prokaryotic homologue of ClC Cl^- channels. *Nature* 2004;427:803–807.
4. Apell HJ. Structure-function relationship in P-type ATPases—a biophysical approach. *Rev Physiol Biochem Pharmacol* 2003;150:1–35.
5. Apell HJ. How do P-type ATPases transport ions? *Bioelectrochemistry* 2004;63:149–56.
6. Artigas P, Gadsby DC. Na^+/K^+ pump ligands modulate gating of palytoxin-induced ion channels. *Proc Natl Acad Sci U S A* 2003;100:501–505.
7. Artigas P, Gadsby DC. Large diameter of palytoxin-induced Na^+/K^+ pump channels and modulation of palytoxin interaction by Na^+/K^+ pump ligands. *J Gen Physiol* 2004;123:357–376.
8. Beck KA, Nelson WJ. The spectrin-based membrane skeleton as a membrane protein-sorting machine. *Am J Physiol* 1996;270:C1263–C1270.
9. Caplan MJ. Ion pumps in epithelial cells: sorting, stabilization, and polarity. *Am J Physiol* 1997;272:G1304–G1313.
10. Caplan MJ, Rodríguez-Boulan E. Epithelial cell polarity: challenges and methodologies. In: Hoffman JF, Jamieson JD, eds. *Handbook of Physiology. Section 14: Cell Physiology*. New York: Oxford University Press, 1997:665–688.
11. Catterall WA. Structure and function of voltage-gated ion channels. In: Schultz SG, Andreoli TE, Brown AM, Fambrough DM, Hoffman JF, Welsh MJ, eds. *Molecular Biology of Membrane Transport Disorders*. New York: Plenum Press, 1996:129–145.
12. Chen TY. Structure and function of ClC channels. *Annu Rev Physiol* 2005;67:809–839.
13. Crane RK. Intestinal absorption of sugars. *Physiol Rev* 1960;40:789–825.
14. Dawson DC. Permeability and conductance in ion channels: a primer. In: Schultz SG, Andreoli TE, Brown AM, Fambrough DM, Hoffman JF, Welsh MJ, eds. *Molecular Biology of Membrane Transport Disorders*. New York: Plenum Press, 1996:87–110.
15. Delcour AH. Solute uptake through general porins. *Front Biosci* 2003;8:d1055–d1071.
16. Diamond JM. Tight and leaky junctions of epithelia: a perspective on kisses in the dark. *Federal Proc* 1974;33:2220–2224.
17. Doyle DA. Molecular insights into ion channel function. *Mol Membr Biol* 2004;21:221–225.
18. Doyle DA. Structural changes during ion channel gating. *Trends Neurosci* 2004;27:298–302.
19. Doyle DA, Morais Cabral J, Pfuetzner RA, Kuo A, Gulbis JM, Cohen SL, Chait BT, MacKinnon R. The structure of the potassium channel: molecular basis of K^+ conduction and selectivity. *Science* 1998;280:69–77.
20. Dragsten PR, Blumenthal R, Handler JS. Membrane asymmetry in epithelia: is the tight junction a barrier to diffusion in the plasma membrane? *Nature* 1981;294:718–722.
21. Dubyak GR. Ion homeostasis, channels, and transporters: an update on cellular mechanisms. *Adv Physiol Educ* 2004;28:143–154.
22. Dutzler R, Campbell EB, Cadene M, Chait BT, MacKinnon R. X-ray structure of a ClC chloride channel at 3.0 Å reveals the molecular basis of anion selectivity. *Nature* 2002;415:287–294.
23. Facciotti MT, Rouhani-Manshadi S, Glaeser RM. Energy transduction in transmembrane ion pumps. *Trends Biochem Sci* 2004;29:445–451.
24. Fambrough DM, Inesi G. Cation transport ATPases. In: Schultz SG, Andreoli TE, Brown AM, Fambrough DM, Hoffman JF, Welsh MJ, eds. *Molecular Biology of Membrane Transport Diseases*. New York: Plenum Press, 1996:223–241.
25. Fick A. Ueber diffusion. *Ann Phys Chem* 1855;94:59–86.
26. Finbow ME, Harrison MA. The vacuolar H^+-ATPase: a universal proton pump of eukaryotes. *Biochem J* 1997;324:697–712.
27. Finkelstein A, Rosenberg PA. Single-file transport: Implications for ion and water movement through gramicidin A channels. In: Stevens CF, Tsien RW, eds. *Membrane Transport Processes*. New York: Raven Press, 1979:73–88.
28. Frindt G, Silver RB, Windhager EE, Palmer LG. Feedback regulation of Na channels in rat CCT. II. Effects of inhibition of Na entry. *Am J Physiol* 1993;264:F565–F574.

29. Frizzell RA, Dugas MC, Schultz SG. Sodium chloride transport by rabbit gallbladder. Direct evidence for a coupled NaCl influx process. *J Gen Physiol* 1975;65:769–795.

30. Frömter E, Diamond J. Route of passive ion permeation in epithelia. *Nature New Biol* 1972;235:9–13.

31. Gadsby DC. Ion transport: spot the difference. *Nature* 2004;427:795–797.

32. Hilgemann DW. From pump to a pore: how palytoxin opens the gates. *Proc Natl Acad Sci U S A* 2003;100:386–388.

33. Gillen CM, Brill S, Payne JA, Forbush BI. Molecular cloning and functional expression of the K-Cl cotransporter from rabbit, rat, and human. *J Biol Chem* 1996;271:16237–16244.

34. Glynn IM, Hoffman JF. Nucleotide requirements for sodium-sodium exchange catalysed by the sodium pump in human red cells. *J Physiol* 1971;218:239–256.

35. Goldman DE. Potential, impedance, and rectification in membranes. *J Gen Physiol* 1943; 27:37–60.

36. Guennoun S, Horisberger JD. Structure of the 5th transmembrane segment of the Na, K-ATPase a subunit: a cysteine-scanning mutagenesis study. *FEBS Lett* 2000;482:144–148.

37. Guennoun S, Horisberger JD. Cysteine scanning mutagenesis study of the 6th transmembrane segment of the Na, K-ATPase a subunit: a cysteine-scanning mutagenesis study. *FEBS Lett* 2002;513:277–288.

38. Hanaoka K, Devuyst O, Schwiebert EM, Wilson PD, Guggino WB. A role for CFTR in human autosomal dominant polycystic kidney disease. *Am J Physiol* 1996;270:C389–C399.

39. Hebert SC, Desir G, Giebisch G, Wang W. Molecular diversity and regulation of renal potassium channels. *Physiol Rev* 2005;85:319–371.

40. Hediger MA, Kanai Y, You G, Nussberger S. Mammalian ion-coupled solute transporters. *J Physiol* 1995;482:7S–17S.

41. Hediger MA, Romero MF, Peng JB, Rolfs A, Takanaga H, Bruford EA. The ABCs of solute carriers: physiological, pathological and therapeutic implications of human membrane transport proteins. *Pflügers Arch* 2004;447:465–468.

42. Heginbotham L, Lu Z, Abramson T, MacKinnon R. Mutations in the K+ channel signature sequence. *Biophys J* 1994;66:1061–1067.

43. Hilgemann DW, Feng S, Nasuhoglu C. The complex and intriguing lives of PIP₂ with ion channels and transporters. *Science-STKE* 2001;111:1–8.

44. Hille B. *Ionic Channels of Excitable Membranes*. 3rd ed. Sunderland: Sinauer, 2001.

45. Hodgkin AL, Katz B. The effect of sodium ions on the electrical activity of the giant axon of the squid. *J Physiol (London)* 1949;108:37–77.

46. Hoenderop JG, Nilius B, Bindels RJ. Calcium absorption across epithelia. *Physiol Rev* 2005;85:373–422.

47. Hoffmann EK. The pump and leak steady-state concept with a variety of regulated leak pathways. *J Membr Biol* 2001;184:321–330.

48. Horisberger JD. *The Na, K-ATPase: Structure-Function Relationship*. Boca Raton, FL: CRC Press, 1994:1–20.

49. Horisberger JD. Recent insights into the structure and mechanism of the sodium pump. *Physiology (Bethesda)* 2004;19:377–387.

50. Horisberger JD, Chraibi A. Epithelial sodium channel: a ligand-gated channel? *Nephron Physiol* 2004;96:37–41.

51. Horisberger JD, Kharoubi-Hess S, Guennoun S, and Michielin O. The fourth transmembrane segment of the Na, K-ATPase a subunit-a systematic mutagenesis study. *J Biol Chem* 2004; 279:29542–29550.

52. Huang Y, Lemieux MJ, Song J, Aue, M., Wang DN. Structure and mechanism of the glycerol-3-phosphate transporter from *Escherichia coli*. *Science* 2003;301:616–620.

53. Jacobson K, Dietrich C. Looking at lipid rafts? *Trends Cell Biol* 1999;9:87–91.

54. Jacobson K, Sheets ED, Simson R. Revisiting the fluid mosaic model of membranes. *Science* 1995;268:1441–1442.

55. Koefoed-Johnsen V, Ussing HH. The nature of the frog skin potential. *Acta Physiol Scand* 1958;42:298–308.

56. Krarup T, Jensen BS, Hoffmann EK. Occlusion of K+ in the Na+/K+/2Cl− cotransporter of Ehrlich ascites tumor cells. *Biochim Biophys Acta* 1996;1284:97–108.

57. Krämer R. Functional principles of solute transport systems: concepts and perspectives. *Biochim Biophys Acta* 1994;1185:1–34.

58. Kusumi A, Nakada C, Ritchie K, Murase K, Suzuki K, Murakoshi H, Kasai RS, Kondo J, Fujiwara T. Paradigm shift of the plasma membrane concept from the two-dimensional continuum fluid to the partitioned fluid: high-speed single-molecules tracking of membrane molecules. *Annu Rev Biophys Biomol Struct* 2004;34:351–378.

59. Lapointe J, Garneau L, Bell PD, Cardinal J. Membrane crosstalk in the mammalian proximal tubule during alterations in transepithelial sodium transport. *Am J Physiol* 1990;258: F339–F345.

60. Lau KR, Hudson RL, Schultz SG. Cell swelling induces a barium-inhibitable potassium conductance in the basolateral membrane of *Necturus* small intestine. *Proc Natl Acad Sci U S A* 1984;81:3591–3594.

61. Läuger P. A channel mechanism for electrogenic ion pumps. *Biochim Biophys Acta* 1979;552:143–161.

62. Läuger P. Dynamics of ion transport systems in membranes. *Physiol Rev* 1987;67: 1296–1331.

63. Läuger P. *Electrogenic Ion Pumps*. Sunderland: Sinauer, 1991.

64. LeFevre PG, Bronner F, Kleinzeller A. The present state of the carrier hypothesis. *Curr Top Membr Transport* 1975;7:109–251.

65. Liedtke, C.M., Hopfer, U. Mechanism of Cl− translocation across small intestinal brush-border membrane. I. Absence of Na+-Cl− cotransport. *Am J Physiol* 1982;242:G263–G271.

66. Lytle C., Forbush B, III. The Na-K-Cl cotransport protein of shark rectal gland. II. Regulation by direct phosphorylation. *J Biol Chem* 1992;267:25438–25443.

67. Macey RI, Moura TF. Basic principles of transport. In: Hoffman JF, Jamieson JD, eds. *Handbook of Physiology. Section 14: Cell Physiology*. New York; Oxford: Oxford University Press, 1997:181–260.

68. Machen TE, Erlij D, Wooding FBP. Permeable junctional complexes. The movement of lanthanum across rabbit gallbladder and intestine. *J Cell Biol* 1972;54:302–312.

69. MacKinnon R. Potassium channels. *FEBS Lett* 2003;555:62–65.

70. MacRobbie EAC, Ussing HH. Osmotic behavior of the epithelial cells of frog skin. *Acta Physiol Scand* 1961;53:348–365.

71. Macrez N, Mironneau J. Local Ca²⁺ signals in cellular signaling. *Curr Mol Med* 2004;4: 263–275.

72. Miller C. *Ion Channel Reconstitution*. New York: Plenum Press, 1986.

73. Molitoris BA, Wagner MC. Surface membrane polarity of proximal tubular cells: alterations as a basis for malfunction. *Kidney Int* 1996;49:1592–1597.

74. Morais-Cabral JH, Zhou Y, MacKinnon R. Energetic optimization of ion conduction rate by the K+ selectivity filter. *Nature* 2001;414:37–42.

75. Nellans HN, Frizzell RA, Schultz SG. Coupled sodium-chloride influx across the brush border of rabbit ileum. *Am J Physiol* 1973;225:467–475.

76. Nernst W. Zur Kinetik der in Lösung befindlichen Körper: Theorie der Diffusion. *Z Phys Chem* 1888;2:613–637.

77. Noury C, Grant SGN, Borg JP. PDZ domain proteins: plug and play! *Science-STKE* 2003;179(RE7):1–12.

78. Ogawa H, Toyoshima C. Homology modeling of the cation binding sites of the Na+,K+-ATPase. *Proc Natl Acad Sci U S A* 2002;99:15977–15982.

79. Reeves WB, Andreoli TE. Renal epithelial chloride channels. *Annu Rev Physiol* 1992;54: 29–50.

80. Reuss L. Basolateral KCl co-transport in a NaCl-absorbing epithelium. *Nature (London)* 1983;305:723–726.

81. Reuss L. Independence of apical membrane Na+ and Cl− entry in *Necturus* gallbladder epithelium. *J Gen Physiol* 1984;84:423–445.

82. Reuss L. Epithelial transport. In: Hoffman JF, Jamieson JD, eds. *Handbook of Physiology. Section 14: Cell Physiology*. New York; Oxford: Oxford University Press, 1997:309–388.

83. Reuss L. Basic mechanisms of ion transport. In: Seldin DW, Giebisch G, eds. *The Kidney, Physiology and Pathophysiology*. 3rd ed. Philadelphia: Lippincott, Williams & Wilkins, 2000:85–106.

84. Reuss L. Ussing's two-membrane hypothesis: the model and half a century of progress. *J Membr Biol* 2001;184:211–217.

85. Reuss L, Cotton CU. Volume regulation in epithelia: transcellular transport and cross-talk. In: Strange K, ed. *Cellular and Molecular Physiology of Cell Volume Regulation*. Boca Raton, FL: CRC Press, 1994:31–48.

86. Sachs G, Munson K. Mammalian phosphorylating ion-motive ATPases. *Curr Opin Cell Biol* 1991;3:685–694.

87. Sachs G, Shin JM, Bamberg K, Prinz C. Gastric acid secretion: the H,K-ATPase and ulcer disease. In: Schultz SG, Andreoli TE, Brown AM, Fambrough DM, Hoffman JF, Welsh MJ, eds. *Molecular Biology of Membrane Transport Disorders*. New York: Plenum Press, 1996; 469–484.

88. Saier MH Jr. A functional-phylogenetic classification system for transmembrane solute transporters. *Microbiol Mol Biol Rev* 2000;64:354–411.

89. Sakmann B, Neher E. *Single-Channel Recording*. New York: Plenum Press, 1995.

90. Schneeberger EF, Lynch RD. The tight junction: a multifunctional complex. *Am J Physiol Cell Physiol* 2004;286:C1213–C1228.

91. Schultz, SG. *Basic Principles of Membrane Transport*. Cambridge: Cambridge University Press, 1980.

92. Schultz SG. Homocellular regulatory mechanisms in sodium-transporting epithelia: avoidance of extinction by "flush-through." *Am J Physiol* 1981;241:F579–F590.

93. Schultz SG. Membrane cross-talk in sodium-absorbing epithelial cells. In: Seldin DW, Giebisch G, eds. *The Kidney: Physiology and Pathophysiology*. New York: Raven Press, 1992:287–299.

94. Schultz SG, Dubinsky WP. Sodium absorption, volume control and potassium channels: in tribute to a great biologist. *J Membr Biol* 2001;184:255–261.

95. Schulz GE. The structure of bacterial outer membrane proteins. *Biochim Biophys Acta* 2002;1565:308–317.

96. Silva P, Stoff J, Field M, Fine L, Forrest JN, Epstein FH. Mechanism of active chloride secretion by shark rectal gland: role of Na-K-ATPase in chloride transport. *Am J Physiol* 1977;233: F298–F306.

97. Silver RB, Frindt G, Windhager EE, Palmer LG. Feedback regulation of Na channels in rat CCT. I. Effects of inhibition of Na pump. *Am J Physiol* 1993;264:F557–F564.

98. Simon DB, Lu Y, Choate KA, Velazquez H, Al-Sabban E, Praga M., Casari G, Bettinelli A, Coluissi G, Rodriguez-Soriano JMD, Milford D, Sanjad S, Lifton RP. Paracellin-1, a renal tight junction protein required for paracellular Mg²¹ resorption. *Science* 1999;285:103–106.

99. Singer SJ. The structure and function of membranes–a personal memoir. *J Membr Biol* 1992;129:3–12.

100. Singer SJ, Nicolson GL. The fluid mosaic model of the structure of cell membranes. *Science (Washington DC)* 1972;175:720–731.

101. Skou JC. The Na-K pump. *News Physiol Sci* 1992;7:95–100.

102. Skou JC, Esmann M. The Na,K-ATPase. *J Bioenerg Biomembr* 1992;24:249–261.

103. Spring KR. Mechanism of fluid transport by epithelia. In: Schultz SG, Field M, Frizzell RA, eds. *Handbook of Physiology: Section 6. The Gastrointestinal System*. Bethesda, MD: American Physiological Society, 1991;195–207.

104. Stein WD. *Channels, Carriers, and Pumps. An Introduction to Membrane Transport*. San Diego: Academic Press, 1990.

105. Tanford C, Reynolds JA. Membrane structure/proteins. In: Hoffman JF, Jamieson JD, eds. *Handbook of Physiology. Section 14: Cell Physiology*. New York: Oxford University Press, 1997:59–74.

106. Tanner MJA. The structure and function of band 3 (AE1): recent developments. *Membr Biol* 1997;14:155–165.

107. Toyoshima C, Inesi G. Structural basis of ion pumping by Ca²⁺-ATPase of sarcoplasmic reticulum. *Annu Rev Biochem* 2004;73:269–292.

108. Toyoshima C, Nakasake M, Nomura H, Ogawa H. Crystal structure of the calcium pump of sarcoplasmic reticulum at 2.6 Å resolution. *Nature* 2000;405:647–655.

109. Toyoshima C, Nomura H. Structural changes in the calcium pump accompanying dissociation of calcium. *Nature* 2002;418:605–611.
110. Toyoshima C, Nomura H, Sugita Y. Structural basis of ion pumping by Ca^{2+}-ATPase of sarcoplasmic reticulum. *FEBS Lett* 2003;555:106–110.
111. Tsukita S, Furuse M, Itoh M. Multifunctional strands in tight junctions. *Nat Rev Mol Cell Biol* 2001;2:285–293.
112. Ussing HH. The distinction by means of tracers between active transport and diffusion. *Acta Physiol Scand* 1949;19:43–56.
113. Ussing HH, Zerahn K. Active transport of sodium as the source of electric current in the short-circuited isolated frog skin. *Acta Physiol Scand* 1951;23:110–127.
114. Van Itallie CM, Fanning AS, Anderson JM. Reversal of charge selectivity in cation or anion-selective epithelial lines by expression of different claudins. *Am J Physiol* 2003;285:F1078–1084.
115. Vereb G, Szöllösi J, Matkó J, Nagy P, Farkas T, Vigh L, Mátyus L, Waldmann TA, Damjanovich S. Dynamic, yet structured: the cell membrane three decades after the Singer–Nicolson model. *Proc Natl Acad Sci U S A* 2003;100:8053–8058.
116. Windhager EE, Boulpaep EL, Giebisch G. Electrophysiological studies in single nephrons. In: Schreiner GE, ed. *Proceedings of the Third International Congress on Nephrology.* Vol. 1. Washington, DC; New York: Karger 1967:35–47.
117. Zachos NC, Tse M, Donowitz M. Molecular physiology of intestinal Na^+/H^+ exchange. *Annu Rev Physiol* 2005;67:411–443.
118. Zadunaisky JA. Active transport of chloride in frog cornea. *Am J Physiol* 1966;211:506–512.
119. Zhou Y, MacKinnon R. The occupancy of ions in the K^+ selectivity filter: charge balance and coupling of ion binding to a protein conformational change underlie high conduction rates. *J Mol Biol* 2003;333:965–975.
120. Zhou Y, Morais-Cabral JH, Kaufman A, MacKinnon R. Chemistry of ion coordination and hydration revealed by a K^+ channel-Fab complex at 2.0 Å resolution. *Nature* 2001;414:43–48.

CHAPTER **3**

Renal Ion-Translocating ATPases: The P-Type Family

Jean-Daniel Horisberger and Alain Doucet

University of Lausanne, Lausanne, Switzerland
Université Pierre et Marie Curie, Paris, France

P-TYPE ATPASES

Ion Motive ATPASES

The active transport of solutes across membranes against their concentration or electrochemical gradient requires energy. This process is in fact an exchange between two forms of energy—the energy contained in the electrochemical gradient across the membrane and another form of energy such as light, redox potential, mechanical work, or the chemical energy provided by ATP hydrolysis. Such energy conversion mechanisms are essential to the most fundamental processes in all living cells. The molecular machines that are able to perform energy conversion between the ion electrochemical gradient and the ATP/ADP ratio are called *ion-motive ATPases*. Three main types of ion-motive ATPases are known: F-type, V-type, and P-type. The F-type ATPases, or ATP synthases, are present in bacteria, in the thylakoid membrane of the chloroplast of green plants, and in the inner mitochondrial membrane of eukaryotic cells, and are responsible for the generation of ATP using the energy of the proton gradient created by the respiratory chain or the photosynthetic complex. The V-type ATPases are mostly present in intracellular organelles (lysosomes, vacuoles, secretory vesicles, etc.), and are responsible for the vesicular acidification by transport of protons from the cytoplasm to the lumen of these organelles. V-ATPases are also present in the plasma membrane of some epithelial cells and are described in more detail in the chapter about proton transport (see Chapter 51). Although F- and V-ATPases usually work in opposite directions (ATP synthesis at the expense of proton entry vs. proton extrusion at the expense of ATP hydrolysis, respectively), they share a common general architecture with a large number of subunits (242), both catalyze the transport of protons (although Na^+-transporting F-ATPases are also known in bacteria) and, most probably, function according to the same general principle.

The P-type ATPases (P-ATPases for short, also earlier called E1,E2-ATPases) form the third group of ion-motive ATPases.

P-Type ATPASES Gene Family

There is a large variety of P-ATPases that perform either unidirectional transport or exchange transport of a variety of monovalent (H^+, Na^+, K^+) or divalent (Ca^{++}, Cu^{++}, Mg^{++}, and others) cations or perhaps organic molecules as well. The family draws its name from the fact that the γ phosphate of ATP is transiently attached to an aspartate residue of the ATPase protein during the transport cycle. The members of this family share a common general architecture that is completely different from the F- and V-type ATPases. As shown in Fig. 1, the protein, or in the case of heteromeric proteins, the major subunit of the protein, consists of a series of hairpins formed by pairs of transmembrane segments linked by short extracellular loops. Two large intracellular loops make the connection between the first, second, and third hairpins. The part common to all P-ATPases consists of three pairs of transmembrane segment and the two large intracellular loops between them. The largest cytoplasmic loop contains the main elements specific to P-ATPases, namely the phosphorylation site, located in a short motif of highly conserved amino acids close to the beginning of the large cytoplasmic loop and the ATP-binding domain. Sequences of highly conserved amino acids are found in the two main cytoplasmic loops and in the transmembrane segment just preceding the large cytoplasmic loop of all P-ATPases (see Fig. 1). These conserved motifs are now used to identify proteins belonging to this family. Some members of the family are probably active as a single polypeptide, while in other cases, the main polypeptide is associated with one or several other subunits. In the heteromeric P-ATPases, the main subunit is named the *catalytic subunit* because it carries the domains responsible for binding and hydrolysis of ATP.

With the systematic sequencing of the whole genome of several organisms and of expressed RNA (expressed sequence tags [ESTs]), the number of proteins presenting the P-ATPase "signature sequences" is growing rapidly. However, little or nothing is known about the physiology or the functional role of most of the corresponding proteins.

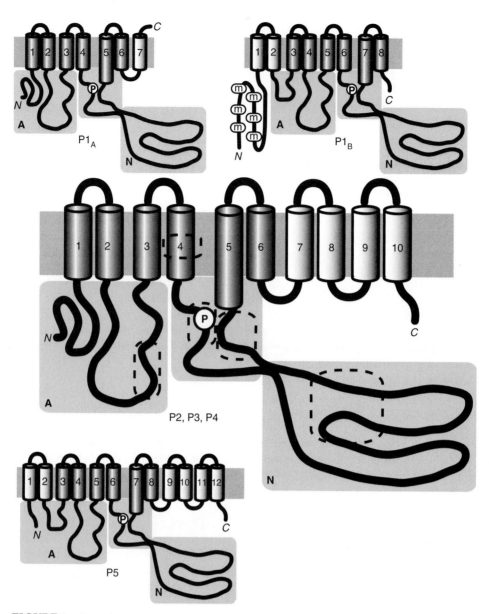

FIGURE 1 General structure and conserved motifs of P-ATPases. The four schemes show the general architecture of the main catalytic subunit of the large groups of P-ATPases. The large scheme in the center corresponds to the common general structure of the P2, P3, and P4 subfamilies. The two smaller schemes on the top illustrate the structure of the bacterial KDP-B potassium transport ATPase (P1$_A$ subfamily, left) and the universal metal ion transport ATPases (P1$_B$ subfamily, right) in which the large N terminal domain that contains a number (usually 6) cysteine rich metal-binding domains (m). The small scheme at the bottom left illustrates the putative structure of the P5 ATPase. The 6 transmembrane segments that are common to all P-ATPase together with the two main intracellular domains form the core of the ion translocation engine are shaded in a darker gray. The positions of highly conserved motives common to all P-ATPases are circled by a dashed line. The cytoplasmic part of the protein is divided into three A, P, and N main functional domains according to Toyoshima et al. (396). The circled P indicates the location of the phosphorylation site. The N- and C-termini are indicated by the italicized *N* and *C*.

P-ATPASE GENERAL CLASSIFICATION

A general classification of the P-ATPases has been proposed by Axelsen and Palmgren (23) on the basis of protein sequence comparison. This classification establishes five main groups and a number of subgroups that are described graphically as a phylogenetic tree in Fig. 2. A more detailed presentation of this classification can be found in an internet site maintained by K. B. Axelsen (http://www.patbase.kvl.dk/).

P-ATPases exist in all three main branches of living organisms: bacteria, archaea, and eukaryotes. This indicates that P-ATPases must have been a constituent of the very first forms of living cells that existed before the separation into the three main branches of the tree of life, even though

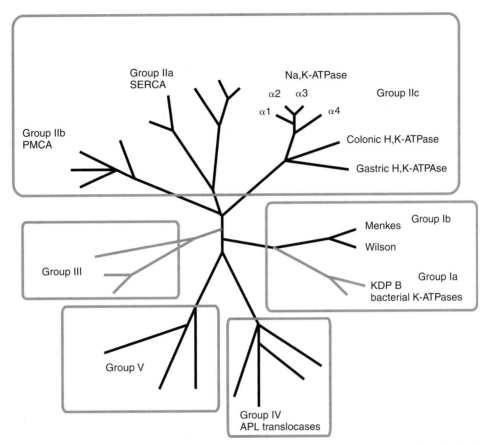

FIGURE 2 Phylogenetic tree of the P-type ATPases. This schematic phylogenetic tree is drawn by hand from indications found in several references (92, 296, 379) and several sequence alignments. The length of the branches does not represent exactly computed divergences distances; more quantitative phylogenetic tree can be found in cited references (92, 379). This scheme indicates qualitatively the relationship between the various groups of the P-ATPases. For groups II and I_B, the branches correspond effectively to the genes identified in the human genome. Groups I_A and III, which do not have homologues in vertebrates, are drawn in gray. APL-translocases stands for amino-phospho-lipid translocase, which is the putative function of this group of protein found in protozoa, yeast, and mammals (see main text for references).

a number of bacteria seem to possess no genes for a P-type ATPase (see http://www.patbase.kvl.dk/). Table 1 indicates the number of P-ATPase genes identified in a variety of organisms whose genome has been completely sequenced. The structure and function of only a few of these proteins has been characterized as described below but very little or nothing is known about most of the others.

Type-1 P-ATPases are characterized by the presence of a large N-terminal domain and a reduced set of C-terminal transmembrane segments. A first subgroup, type I_A, is composed of potassium-activated ATPases found only in bacteria. The KDP system of *Escherichia coli* is the best characterized (8). A second group, type I_B, includes a large number of ATPases that have been characterized in plants and bacteria as factors of resistance to the presence of toxic cations such as cadmium or copper, and are thought to perform the extrusion of toxic divalent cations (370). These proteins have been studied mostly in bacteria but are also found in animals and plants. In mammals, this group comprises two ATPases involved in the transport of copper ions (see below).

Type-2 P-ATPases have a general structure comprising a shorter N-terminal domain and four transmembrane segments before the large cytoplasmic loop and usually six transmembrane segments in the C-terminal part. This

TABLE 1 Example of Distribution of P-Type ATPase Genes Identified in Various Species

	P1	**P2**	**P3**	**P4**	**P5**	**Total**
Halobacterium	4	0	0	0	0	4
E. coli	3	0	1	0	0	4
S. cerevisiae	2	5	2	5	2	16
A. thaliana	8	15	12	12	1	48
D. melanogaster	1	6	0	6	1	14
C. elegans	1	10	0	6	4	21
Human	2	15	0	14	5	36

P1 to P5 indicate the main types of P-ATPase according to the classification by Palmgren and Axelsen (23). Examples are given for Archea (*Halobacterium* sp.), Bacteria (*Escherichia coli*), yeast (*Saccharomyces cerevisiae*), green plants (*Arabidopsis thaliana*), nematode (*Caenorhabditis elegans*), arthropod (*Drosophila melanogaster*), and vertebrate (human).

group contains the best characterized proteins of the P-ATPase family, namely, Na,K- and H,K-ATPases, the various forms of Ca-ATPase of animal cells, and the H-ATPase found in yeast, plants, and protozoa.

Type 3 comprises a large group of proton-exporting ATPases expressed in yeast, protozoa, or plants (type 3_A). The yeast H-pump has been studied extensively and a high-resolution structure obtained by electron microscopy is available (253). A smaller group (type 3_B) of magnesium-transporting ATPases exclusively expressed in bacteria is involved in the regulated uptake of Mg^{++} (297).

The classification of the other P-ATPase genes, of mostly unknown function, is awaiting more information. Some of these may actually perform other functions than cation transport: a possible role in aminophospholipid translocation has been proposed for a group of P-ATPases (type 4) found in protozoa and mammals (388). Finally, a subfamily of P-ATPase has tentatively been designed as type 5 (92), until sufficient functional data allow a more comprehensive and meaningful classification.

P-ATPases of Animal Cells

Most of P-type ATPases that have been studied in mammals belong to type P2. This group is composed of the *sarco/endoplasmic reticulum ATPase* (SERCA), which forms the subgroup 2_A together with the related secretory pathway calcium ATPase, the *plasma membrane calcium ATPases* (PMCA, type 2_B), and *Na,K- and H,K-ATPases* (subgroup 2_C).

SERCA

The SERCA is found, as indicated by its name, in the membranes of intracellular organelles related to the endoplasmic reticulum. It is extremely abundant in the sarcoplasmic reticulum of cardiac and skeletal muscle cells, and most functional or structural studies have been performed with enzymes from these tissues. Three genes coding for isoforms of SERCA are known: SERCA1 in fast-twitch skeletal muscle; SERCA2 in slow-twitch skeletal muscle, and heart and smooth muscle cells; and SERCA3 in the endoplasmic reticulum of blood, endothelial, and epithelial cells. The functional role of SERCA is to perform the reuptake of calcium ions from the cytoplasm into the sarcoplasmic reticulum after calcium has been released from intracellular stores. It acts therefore as a signal terminator in the excitation–contraction coupling process in muscle or in the excitation–secretion coupling in neurons or other secretory cells. The high density of this enzyme in heart and skeletal muscle is necessary to remove calcium from the cytoplasm swiftly enough to allow for repeated high-frequency signaling.

Extensive structure–function studies that have been performed with SERCA (280), and a high-resolution structure of this protein has been obtained under several conformations (377, 395–398). The knowledge of this structure is extremely important because it allows predictions by homology

of the molecular structure of other related P-ATPases such as Na,K- or H,K-ATPases. (See the section "Gene and Structure" for discussion of molecular structure.)

The calcium pumps encoded by two other closely related genes are expressed in the membranes of the secretory pathway Ca^{2+}-ATPase (SPCA), and are involved in the accumulation of calcium in the Golgi complex in relation with its role of intracellular calcium store (436).

PMCA

The PMCA is expressed at the cell surface of most animal cells. It carries out control of intracellular calcium by extruding this cation out of the cell. With the sodium–calcium exchanger, PMCA is responsible for regulation of the whole-cell calcium balance (in contrast with SERCA, which instead controls cytosolic calcium activity by acting on the balance of calcium between cytosolic and intracellular stores). A structural feature that distinguishes PMCA from the other P-ATPases is the presence of a long C-terminal intracellular domain, which is involved in the regulation of calcium pump activity. This C-terminal domain interacts with the catalytic site (large cytoplasmic loop) keeping the enzyme inactive. This autoinhibition mechanism can be released by binding of calcium-loaded calmodulin to a specific site on the C-terminus, providing an obvious feedback control loop: when calcium activity rises in the cytosol, it binds to calmodulin, which can then interact with the C-terminal domain of PMCA, releasing the autoinhibition and thus activating the Ca pump. Calcium extrusion by the active PMCA results in a decrease of the cytosolic calcium activity to a value low enough to allow dissociation of calcium from calmodulin, release of calmodulin, and finally resulting in auto-inhibition of PMCA by its free C-terminal domain (88). Auto-inhibition can also be released by phosphorylation of a threonine in the C-terminal domain by protein kinase C. A similar mechanism exists for the regulation of SERCA, but the inhibition is provided by a small associated protein, phospholamban, which plays a role equivalent to that of the C-terminal domain of PMCA. Phosphorylation of phospholamban by protein kinase C results in releasing the SERCA inhibition (279).

Four PMCA genes are presently known, with multiple splicing variants for each gene, resulting in the existence of about 20 isoforms. The expression of PMCA1 and PMCA4 is ubiquitous, while PMCA2 and PMCA3 are restricted to neurons, brain, muscle, and kidney. A more complete description of isoforms, splicing variants, and their general distribution can be found in Carafoli (88). The distribution of PMCA isoforms mRNA has been examined in the kidney (281). PMCA1 is most abundant in the glomerulus. PMCA2 and PMCA4 are present in all tubular segments, while PMCA3 is found exclusively in the thin descending loop of Henle (89). The role of PMCA in the renal tubular reabsorption of calcium is discussed in Chapter 65.

COPPER-ATPASES

Only two type-1 P-ATPases are known in mammalian cells and both belong to the P1$_B$ subgroup. Both are copper-transport ATPases that have been discovered as genes responsible for hereditary diseases of copper metabolism in human, the Menkes and Wilson diseases (75, 350, 415). Their characteristic structural feature is a large N-terminal intracellular domain containing six cysteine motifs assumed to be part of copper-binding sites (277).

AMINOPHOSPHOLIPID TRANSLOCASES

Although there are a large number of genes belonging to group IV in mammalian genomes, only a single member of this group has been studied in mammals (bovine). The function attributed to this protein was the translocation of aminophospholipid from one leaflet of the membrane to the other (flippase) (388), but this role needs to be confirmed by more detailed functional studies.

Na,K- AND H,K-ATPASE FAMILY

Genes and Structure

All members of the Na,K- and H,K-ATPase family are heteromeric proteins made of a main, catalytic subunit, α subunit, and a second, smaller glycosylated subunit, the β subunit. Na,K-ATPase activity, ouabain binding, or cation transport activities have been demonstrated by coexpression of α and β subunits in several artificial expression systems, mammalian cells, *Xenopus* oocytes (217), baculovirus-infected insect cells (125), and even yeast (323, 351, 351). The Na- (or H-) and K-activated ATPase activity and the cation transport function (i.e., uphill cation pumping driven by ATP hydrolysis) characteristic of Na,K- or H,K-ATPases have been demonstrated only in the presence of both α and β subunits. Expression of the α subunit alone in transfected insect cells (58) resulted in the expression of Mg^{++}-dependent ATPase activity, but this activity was not specifically activated by Na$^+$ and K$^+$. In other systems, when α subunits are expressed alone they are rapidly degraded and do not reach the cell surface in significant amount (185). An unresolved question concerns the exact stoichiometry of the minimal functional unit. Na,K-ATPase activity is associated with solubilized αβ protomers (424) and cross-linking experiments do not show evidence for a close interaction between α subunits (284). However kinetic evidence indicating the presence of two interacting ATP-binding sites would require that a diprotomer $(\alpha\beta)_2$ is the active form (324).

A third type of subunit, the γ subunit can be associated with the αβ complex. The γ subunit belongs to a recently identified family of small proteins with a single transmembrane segment designated as "FXYD" proteins because they all contain the conserved motif F-X-Y-D (phenylalanine-any residue-tyrosine-aspartic acid) (387). As described below, several FXYD proteins have been shown to associate with Na,K-ATPase.

CATALYTIC α SUBUNIT: ISOFORMS

Until now, six different genes of α subunit have been identified in mammals. They are usually named as the α1, α2, α3, and α4 isoforms of the α subunit of Na,K-ATPase, the α subunit of the gastric H,K-ATPase, and the α subunit of the colonic H,K-ATPase. As explained below, these names may not reflect the present state of knowledge about function and distribution of these proteins. We will, however, keep this nomenclature and use the following abbreviations: α1, α2, α3, α4, αHKg, and αHKc, respectively. Related isoforms have been identified outside the mammalian class: α1, α2, and α3 in birds (chicken), α1 and αHKg (*Xenopus laevis*), and the *Bufo marinus* bladder H,K-ATPase related to αHKc in amphibian. On the other hand, Na,K-ATPase sequences known from the nematode *Caenorhabditis elegans* or from the fly *Drosophila melanogaster* do not show close similarity with any specific branch of this group. This suggests that the divergence between the α subunit genes of Na,K- and H,K-ATPase group predates the divergence of mammalian, amphibian, and birds, but has occurred early in vertebrate evolution.

All isoforms of Na,K-ATPase are involved in the maintenance of the Na$^+$ and K$^+$ gradients across the cell membrane. These cation gradients are essential for many functions of the cells. The large inwardly directed electrochemical gradient for Na$^+$ is used by numerous secondary active transport systems for "housekeeping" functions: maintenance of intracellular pH (through Na–H exchangers); extrusion of calcium (through Na–Ca exchanger); control of cell volume (through Na–K–2Cl symport and other coupled transport systems); and import of amino acids, nucleotides, and other nutriments or osmolytes through various Na$^+$-coupled cotransport systems (see Chapters 2 and 4). The outwardly directed electrochemical gradient for potassium is responsible for the intracellular negative membrane potential because positively charged K$^+$ ions are allowed to flow out of the cell together through the K$^+$ selective channels active in most cells. In addition to these ubiquitous housekeeping functions, the gradients of Na$^+$ and K$^+$ across the cell membrane are essential for many specialized function of differentiated cells, such as the generation and propagation of action potentials in excitable cells, the reuptake of neurotransmitters through Na$^+$- and K$^+$-coupled transport systems, or the reabsorptive and secretory transcellular transport of solutes and water by epithelial cells. Some complex transport systems use the chemical gradient for both Na$^+$ and K$^+$ to energize the extrusion or uptake of other solutes such as the Na$^+$–K$^+$–Ca^{++} exchanger found in photoreceptors or the glutamate reuptake system in neurons and glial cells (438, 438, 445).

The α1 isoform is the most abundant and ubiquitous isoform (149, 270, 270, 385, 385). It is usually considered as responsible for the maintenance of the whole-cell Na$^+$ and K$^+$ gradients necessary for the housekeeping functions. In addition, because it is the most abundant, if not the only isoform present in many epithelial cells, it is also considered the main provider of the driving force for transepithelial solute and water transport. Its essential role in the kidney will be described in detail in the Na,K-ATPase in the Kidney section of this chapter.

The α2 subunit is found in skeletal and heart muscle and the nervous system (neurons and glial cells) (188, 188, 270). The α3 isoform is essentially a neuronal isoform (364), and is the dominant form in the pineal gland (365). It has, however, also recently been identified in other cell types, such as blood cells or macrophages (380, 407).

The distribution of α1, α2, and α3 isoforms in the nervous system is complex and developmentally regulated. This topic is beyond the scope of this chapter, but relevant information can be found in Peng et al. (325) and Sweadner (383).

The α4 isoform is found mainly in the testes (360), and its sequence is clearly more closely related to the α1, α2, and α3 than to the αHKg or αHKc. Artificial expression of this protein indicated that it is indeed a ouabain-sensitive Na$^+$- and K$^+$-activated ATPase (435). Its expression in sperm and a critical role in sperm motility have recently been demonstrated (434).

The αHKg is abundantly expressed in the parietal cells of the gastric gland. It is the primary motor of proton secretion by gastric glands (212). Under resting conditions, it is mainly located in the membranes of an intracellular network of vesicles and tubules. After a secretory stimulus, the membranes of the tubular-vesicular system fuse with the apical membrane, and the H,K-pump can then actively transport protons from the cell to the gastric gland lumen in exchange for potassium (212). The evidence supporting the expression of αHKg in the kidney and its potential role in this organ will be discussed in the H,K-ATPases in the Kidney section.

The αHKc has been first identified in the rat colon (119), but a closely related sequence (ATPAL1) has also been cloned from human skin (201). A protein with a related sequence has been identified in the urinary bladder of the toad *Bufo marinus* (226). These sequences are sufficiently similar to suggest that they are homologous proteins. In the rat, the αHKc is expressed mostly in the distal colon, but also in the kidney and uterus, and at a lower level in heart (119). Its distribution and role in the kidney will also be discussed in H,K-ATPases in the Kidney section.

STRUCTURE OF α SUBUNIT

Na,K- and H,K-ATPase α-subunit peptides range in length from about 1000 to 1040 amino acids. Their primary structure is characteristic of type II P-ATPase with a first group of four transmembrane segments, a large cytoplasmic loop, and a second group of six transmembrane segments (see Figs. 1 and 3). The relatively high degree of homology with SERCA suggests that Na,K- and H,K-ATPases have the general structure of 10 transmembrane segments now known for the calcium pump (215). Strong experimental support for this architecture is available for the α1 (171, 196, 237) and the

αHKg (26, 57). In the following, the putative membrane-spanning segments will be designated by *M1* to *M10*.

The three-dimensional (3D) structure of Na,K-ATPase is not known at high resolution, but the general architecture of the molecule is consistent with the predictions drawn from the primary structure. About one-third of the mass of the protein is in the membrane, about two-thirds are in a large cytoplasmic domain, and only a small portion is exposed to the extracytoplasmic side of the membrane (374).

As stated earlier, the molecular structure of Na,K- and H,K-ATPases can be inferred from the high-resolution structure of SERCA, which has been now obtained by X-ray crystallography under several different conformations (377, 395–398). The homology of sequence between SERCA and Na,K- and H,K-ATPases is high enough to allow safe structural prediction, at least for the general architecture of the molecule and for large domains in which homology is the highest. Structural predictions are also hampered by the presence of additional subunits in Na,K- and H,K-ATPases. The structure of the N-terminal domain, several extracellular loops, and the transmembrane segments M7 to M10, for which there are large differences in the primary structure, is still conjectural. Several structural models obtained by homology have been published recently (76, 249, 312, 318, 338, 386). The main features of the structure, for which most models agree, are presented in Fig. 3.

β–SUBUNIT GENES AND STRUCTURE

As stated earlier, the β subunit seems to be an essential constituent of a functional ion pump in this Na,K- and H,K-ATPase group. The α subunit can reach a mature and functional conformation and be translocated from the endoplasmic reticulum to the plasma membrane only when associated with a coexpressed β subunit (39, 184, 287). Therefore, the β subunit is a limiting component for the expression of functional Na,K-ATPases, and the rate of synthesis of the β subunit may be the factor regulating the Na,K-pump density in several tissues (182).

Five different genes encoding similar proteins are known in the mammalian genomes: β1, β2, β3, βHK, and βm. Four genes are also known in amphibians, and they can be considered as homologous to the four mammalian genes based on recognition of the isoform first named β$_{bladder}$, when it was cloned from the urinary bladder of the toad (227) is the homologous of the β2 isoform of mammals as suggested by sequence comparison. Sequence comparison also indicates that the chick β isoform initially described as β2 is in fact homologous to the mammalian and amphibian β3. β1, β2, and β3 are clearly isoforms of the Na,K-ATPase β subunit. βHK is coexpressed with the gastric H,K-ATPase in the stomach. βm (m for muscle from its known tissue expression in skeletal and cardiac muscle) shares sufficient sequence similarity to be classified in the same family, but it does not associate with any known α subunit (111). Its role remains to be determined.

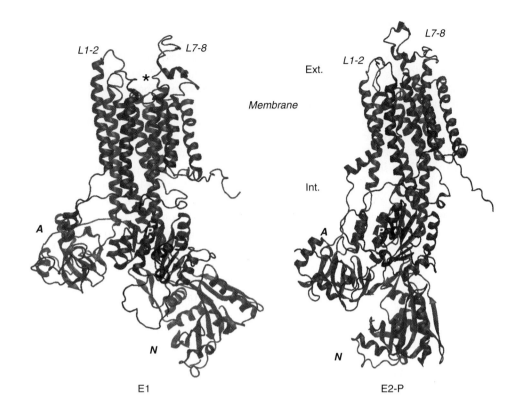

FIGURE 3 Structure of the α subunit. Two conformations of Na,K-ATPase are shown: E1 and E2-P, resulting from homology modeling using MODELLER (344) with the E1-2Ca and E2-MgF$_4^{2-}$ high-resolution structures of SERCA (PDB code 1SU4 and 1WPG), respectively (396, 398). The A, N, and P intracellular domains are indicated as well as the L1-2 short extracellular loop linking M1 and M2 and the L7-8 long extracellular loop linking M7 and M8. One site of interaction between the α and β subunit is located in this L7-8 loop. Binding sites for inhibitors (*) of the Na,K- and H-K-ATPase are located in the groove between the extracellular loop L1-2 and L3-4 on one side and L7-8-L9-10 on the other side. Comparison of the two conformations shows the large movements of the (translations and rotations) of the A and N domains. The downward movement (toward the cell interior) of the first hairpin (M1 and M2) and the kink in M1 are also obvious in E2.

The β1 isoform is usually described as ubiquitous, but it appears to be absent, or at most only a minor component, in several tissues such as liver (18) or red blood cells (380). The β2 isoforms were initially identified in glial cells (193), but are also present in other cell types, including neurons, blood cells, and epithelial cells (94, 154, 285, 380, 425). The β3 isoform, initially identified in the nervous system of the frog (199) or rat neurons (282) also has a wider distribution, and appears to be most abundant as a protein in testes, liver, and lungs, but it is also present in significant amounts in skeletal muscle and the kidney (18).

The β-subunit peptides range in length from 288 to 315 amino acids, and show a lower degree of homology (about 30%–40% identity between isoforms) than the α subunits. In contrast with the α subunit, no high-resolution structure of a homologous protein is available. Our knowledge of the β-subunit structure is therefore limited to predictions based on the primary structure and some low-resolution 3D structure of the α/β complex, where the presence of a β subunit is apparent as density in the extracellular part of the protein (210). The primary structure allows prediction of a single transmembrane segment, preceded by a ∼35–amino-acid, N-terminal domain, and followed by a large extracellular domain containing three to seven glycosylation sites, depending on the isoform, and six cysteine residues that form three disulfide bridges (245). Both glycosylation and the formation of the disulfide bonds appear to be necessary for the β subunit to reach a conformation that is able to fully assemble with the α subunit and produce functional Na,K pumps at the cell surface. However, mutant β subunits in which all glycosylation sites had been removed allowed the expression of a low number of Na,K pumps with unaltered physiological characteristics (41).

β-SUBUNIT FUNCTIONAL ROLE AND INTERACTION WITH α/β SUBUNIT

The isoform of the β subunit has been shown to confer different physiological characteristics to the whole enzyme in several expression systems (115, 134, 228). It has been proposed that some of the functional differences observed among various tissues in Na,K-ATPase activity, differences that cannot be explained by difference in α subunit composition, may be due to the specific β subunit (18, 380, 392).

Except for the gastric αHK and the βHK, which are most abundantly expressed in a single cell type (parietal cells of the gastric glands), there is no obvious common pattern of distribution between α isoforms and β isoforms that would define preferential physiological associations. The nature of the β subunit that is physiologically associated with the αHKc is still a matter of debate. Each of the β isoforms is able to associate with αHKc in some expression system. Recent colocalization studies favor the association of αHKc with the β1 isoform, at least in the prostate, where this complex is expressed at high density (326). Other indirect evidence has supported the assembly with the βHK, β2, or β3 isoform (181, 186, 346).

The β1 isoform is found in abundance in tissues in which the α1 isoform is largely predominant, such as the kidney, strongly suggesting that the α1β1 dimer is the predominant physiological association in such tissues. The existence (or nonexistence) and physiological relevance of other possible associations are more difficult to demonstrate. The difficulty comes from the fact that, in artificial expression systems, practically all four β subunits are able to form functional complexes with all six α subunits (151, 228, 267, 353), with the exception of αHKg/β1, which does not seem to associate significantly (230), and α1/βHKg, which is generally poorly expressed (228). Some cells are known to express as many as three α isoforms and at least two β isoforms, creating the possibility of numerous associations, unless the formation of specific dimers is favored or repressed by some as yet unknown mechanisms. But the fact that a functional dimer can be formed under conditions of artificial expression (i.e., under conditions of very high expression level for both subunits) does not mean that this dimer exists at a physiologically relevant level in natural tissues. Some degree of specificity between α1 and β1 and between α2 and β2, evidenced by resistance to detergent-mediated dissociation, has been demonstrated (353).

The *association between the α and the β subunit*s has been studied in detail. For both the Na,K- and the H,K-ATPase, the extracellular loop connecting the M7 and M8 transmembrane segment has been shown to be essential for the α/β interaction (266, 363). The two-hybrid system has demonstrated that a conserved 4–amino-acid segment (SYGQ) of this region was crucial for the α/β subunit association and that the interacting domain of the β subunit was the stretch immediately following the transmembrane segment (104). However, assembly of α/β dimer also involves other domains of the β subunit—the transmembrane segment (230) and a hydrophobic domain formed by the 10 most C-terminal amino acids (40). In addition, the extracellular carbohydrate moiety of the β subunit seems to be required for a correct isoform-specific assembly of the two subunits (353).

FXYD PROTEINS

Evidence for the existence of a third protein component closely associated to Na,K-ATPase came first from copurification and photolabeling of a small peptide with renal Na,K-ATPase (103, 173, 174). Cloning and sequencing this first associated subunit known as the γ *subunit* revealed a short, 57–amino-acid peptide with a single predicted transmembrane segment (291). Analysis of mRNA indicated that this small protein is abundantly expressed in the kidney and at a low level in other epithelial organs (skin, stomach) (291). However, significant amounts of the γ subunit protein could be detected only in the kidney by Western blot analysis (390). The orientation of the γ subunit in the membrane was shown to be with an extracellular N-terminus and a cytoplasmic C-terminus (46). Coexpression studies in *Xenopus* oocytes showed that the γ subunit is stabilized by association with α/β Na,K-ATPase dimer and reaches the cell surface only when associated with a α/β dimer. This association is specific since coexpression with αβ H,K-ATPase, the α subunit alone, the β subunit alone of the Na,K-ATPase, or other membrane proteins did not allow observing surface expression of the γ subunit. In addition, evidence supporting a 1:1:1 stoichiometry of the α/β/γ complex has been provided (46). The level of active enzyme at the cell surface was, however, not modified by the presence of the γ subunit, indicating that the γ subunit is not required for expression of functional Na,K pumps.

More recently, a gene family of similar small-membrane proteins was identified (387). Alignment of these proteins show that they share a conserved motif FXYD (phenylalanine, any amino acid, and tyrosine, aspartic acid) in the extracellular N-terminal domain just before the transmembrane helix, two glycine residues in the transmembrane segment, and one serine at the beginning of the intracellular C-terminal domain. In addition to the γ subunit, this gene family includes four known proteins (phospholemman, MAT-8, CHIF, and RIC), and two novel proteins. The seven FXYD proteins are presented in Table 2. Also indicated in Table 2 is the association of five members of this family with α/β Na,K-ATPase, and the effects on apparent affinity for intracellular Na^+ (Na^+_i) and extracellular K^+ (K^+_e) that have been reported.

The distribution and role of FXYD proteins in the kidney are discussed in the Na,K-ATPase in Kidney section of this chapter.

PHYSIOLOGICAL AND PHARMACOLOGICAL PROPERTIES OF NA,K- AND H,K-ATPASES

PHYSIOLOGICAL ROLE

Gene inactivation studies have shown that Na,K-ATPase is essential for life. Absence of expression of Na,K-ATPase α1 gene is developmentally lethal (229), even though the $α1^{-/-}$ embryos develop beyond the blastocyst stage (28). In contrast, $α2^{-/-}$ animals are born alive but die soon after birth, most probably as the result of respiratory trouble related to dysfunction of neuronal circuit involved in respiration control (222, 301), or of the diaphragmatic muscle. Heterozygous animal tissues for α1 or α2 genes inactivation display mostly cardiac phenotype, and support an important role of the α2 isoform in the intracellular homeostasis of

TABLE 2   FXYD Protein Family

| | Other name | Distribution | Effect on Apparent Affinity | | References |
			Na_i	K_e	
FXYD1	Phospholemman	Heart, skeletal muscle, liver	↓↓	↓	(112, 176)
FXYD2	Na,K-ATPase γ subunit	Kidney, brain (hippocampus)	↓	=	(46, 390)
FXYD3	Mat-8	Uterus, stomach, colon, skin	↓	↓	(116)
FXYD4	CHIF	Colon epithelium, collecting duct	↑↑	↓↓	(43, 180)
FXYD5	RIC				
FXYD6					
FXYD7		Neurons	=	↓↓	(44)

An experimentally demonstrated association with Na,K-ATPase was found for FXYD1–4 and FXYD7. The References column cites the published evidence for a function association between Na,K-ATPase and FXYD proteins. A more complete set of references can be found in Crambert and Geering (113) and Geering (183).

calcium, particularly in heart, vascular smooth muscle, and glial tissues (129, 300, 361). Gene inactivation of the α3 and α4 isoforms has not been reported. Inactivation of the colonic H,K-ATPase affects mostly potassium homeostasis in the colon and kidney as discussed in the H,K-ATPases in Kidney section.

Only two human genetic diseases are known to be related to Na,K-ATPase gene. A familial form of hemiplegic migraine has been associated with mutations in the α2 gene (120) (OMIM #602481). These mutations appear to abolish or greatly reduce the function of the α2 isoform of Na,K-ATPase (86). Rapid-onset dystonia parkinsonism has been associated with inactivating mutation of the α3 gene (2) (OMIM #128235). In both cases, the mode of inheritance is dominant, suggesting that the disease is due to haploinsufficiency of the α2 and α3 isoform, respectively.

TRANSPORT CHARACTERISTICS AND DIFFERENCES AMONG ISOFORMS

Under physiological conditions, Na,K-ATPase transports three Na^+ ions out of the cell in exchange for two K^+ in the cell and uses one ATP during each transport cycle (9, 215, 216). Therefore, the transport activity of the Na,K pump is the source of an outward current of one net charge per cycle (a current of the order of 20 to 100 charges per second or about 10^{-5} pA, that is, orders of magnitude lower than the current carried by ion channels). The outward current generated by the activity of the Na,K pump tends to hyperpolarize the cell membrane, although the contribution of this electrogenic activity to the cell membrane potential amounts to only a few millivolts under steady-state conditions (the main part of the −50 to −80 mV resting-membrane potential is due to the flow of K^+ ions through selective channel, which is also related to the activity of the Na,K pump because the high intracellular K^+ concentration is maintained by the Na,K pump). Although the $3Na^+,2K^+$-1ATP stoichiometry has not been demonstrated formally for all isoforms of the Na,K pump, the similarity of the transport

properties suggests that it holds at least for the Na,K pumps made of the α1, α2, and α3 isoforms (218) (little is known about the transport carried out by the α4 isoform), and does not depend on the type of associated β subunit. Under some experimental conditions, a different stoichiometry can be observed (62) and it has also been shown that proton can substitute for Na^+ or K^+ (331).

The apparent affinities for the activating cations Na^+ and K^+ are highly dependent on experimental conditions (cation concentrations on each sides of the membrane, membrane potential, ATP concentration, etc.); but under physiological circumstances, intracellular Na^+ activates the Na,K pump with a half-activation constant $K_{1/2}$ of about 10 to 20 mM, a Hill coefficient between 2 and 3; extracellular K^+ has a $K_{1/2}$ of about 1 mM with a Hill coefficient between 1 and 2 (216).

The difference in physiological transport properties between α Na,K-ATPase isoforms has been the subject of many studies, but the question is not entirely resolved. Initial studies comparing enzymes isolated from tissues of known isoform composition (kidney for α1, brain for predominantly α2 and α3) or using ouabain sensitivity for discriminating between α1 and α2/α3 usually indicated a higher affinity of the α2/α3 isoforms for Na^+ (365, 371, 384). More recent studies comparing isoforms artificially expressed in the same expression system showed a Na^+ affinity slightly lower for α2 (about 20 mM) and much lower for α3 (30–70 mM) for Na^+ (307), but other studies have found much smaller differences between various isoforms (114, 218, 392, 443). Factors other than the α subunit isoform seem to be involved in the determination of the transport properties of Na,K-ATPase, in particular the type of associated FXYD protein; still other factors remain to be determined (392).

TRANSPORT CHARACTERISTICS OF H,K-ATPASES

The gastric H,K-ATPase appears to carry nonelectrogenic transport, indicating that a symmetrical number of H^+ and K^+ ions are translocated across the membrane during each transport cycle (337). The exact stoichiometry of the transport probably depends on experimental conditions: under high, close to neutral pH, the stoichiometry is $2H^+, 2K^+$-1ATP, while it shifts to $1H^+, 1K^+$-1ATP under physiological conditions, namely with a very low extracellular pH (306).

Transport properties of the "nongastric" or colonic H, K-ATPases (rat colonic H,K-ATPase, human ATP1AL1, and *Bufo* bladder H,K-pump) are not yet completely defined. In all three cases, expression in artificial systems has demonstrated inward transport of K^+ (as assayed by rubidium fluxes) and outward transport of protons (as assayed either by intracellular alcalinization or extracellular acidification) (107, 226, 295), and these results provided the reason to name these enzymes "H,K-ATPase." However, more recent data obtained in experiments with expressed ATPAL1 in which fluxes of K^+ and proton were measured and compared, suggest that another cation is transported, most probably sodium (200). Indeed, expression of the rat or *Bufo* H,K-ATPase has been shown to lower intracellular Na^+, indicating that Na^+ ions may also be transported by these enzymes (106). According to these findings, these enzymes would carry out the exchange of K^+ ions against Na^+ or H^+ ions. As the activity of this transport ATPase has been shown to be nonelectrogenic (77), the transport stoichiometry can be assumed to be an exchange of 2 cations (Na^+ or H^+) for two K^+. The physiological role of this isoform will be discussed in detail in the "H,K-ATPases in Kidney" section of this chapter.

ION TRANSLOCATION MECHANISM

The mechanism of the active translocation of cations has been studied in a very large number of experiments using a variety of technical approaches and preparations: kinetics of cation-dependent phosphorylation reaction, kinetics of cation transport under various conditions, kinetics of cation binding and release, measurements of steady-state current, transient charge translocation or charge movement in the membrane. Most of these experiments were performed with the predominantly α1 kidney Na,K-ATPase, but others were obtained with brain, heart, or oocyte preparation. Extensive exploration of the cation transport mechanism has also been performed for the Ca-ATPase (280, 296). These experiments, performed over the decades since the first identification of Na,K-ATPase in the 1950s (372), cannot easily be summarized (see reviews in 9, 194, 296, 342, 373), but a few central points can be made, which are illustrated in Fig. 4.

First, Na,K-ATPase exists under two main conformations E1 and E2, and transport activity is performed by a transport cycle in which the protein is transiently phosphorylated and alternately adopts the E1 and the E2 conformation. Second, these two conformations differ in their apparent affinity for Na^+ and K^+; the E1 form has high affinity sites for Na^+ exposed to the intracellular side of the membrane while the E2 conformation has high affinity sites for extracellular K^+. Third, three Na^+ and two K^+ ions are

alternately bound to the enzyme and then "occluded," that is, tightly bound inside the protein.

Figure 4 presents a general model of the functional cycle of the Na,K pump that is compatible with most of the available experimental data. This model is based on the principles proposed by Albers (7) and Post et al. (332) and on the "alternating access" model of the ion pump (263), and is also compatible with information gained by research on the structure of the main conformations of the SERCA calcium pump (394).

STRUCTURE–FUNCTION RELATIONSHIP: MECHANISM OF CATION TRANSPORT

The molecular mechanics that allow the coupling of ATP hydrolysis to the forward running of the cation transport cycle is not yet completely understood, but the structure–function model provides the conceptual framework to understand the ion pumping mechanism, and several elements of this model can be considered as established.

The ATP-binding site has been precisely located by covalent binding of ATP analogues or other molecules and site-directed mutagenesis experiments (148, 152, 294, 322, 399), and is now well defined by homology with SERCA, for which structures with bound ATP analogues are known (377, 395). Considering the very high degree of sequence similarity in this domain between the different proteins of the family, it is assumed that the ATP-binding site is common to all P-ATPases. In addition, the structure of the isolated N (nucleotide binding) domain of Na,K-ATPase and the effect of nucleotide binding on this structure have been obtained via nuclear magnetic resonance (213).

The study of the structure responsible for cation translocation by site-directed mutagenesis has been rendered difficult because the ion transport is the result of a complex sequence of cation binding or release steps and conformational changes. Alteration in the kinetics of any single step has effects on the entire cycle, and may influence the apparent kinetic parameters of other steps in the cycle; hence, a change in the apparent affinity for a ligand usually cannot be simply interpreted as due to modification of a binding site (422).

According to the functional model illustrated in Fig. 4, the pump must provide a cation-binding pocket, the cation occlusion site, and access pathways to this pocket alternately from each side of the membrane. There is strong evidence supporting the location of the cation occlusion site(s) in the membrane part of the Na,K-ATPase, and the fact that this pocket must be formed by the transmembrane segments. Indeed, the ion occlusion phenomenon can be observed in a modified enzyme, in which most of the intracellular mass of the protein has been removed by proteolytic digestion, the so-called "19-KD membranes" preparation (238), which consists of the transmembrane segments of the α and β subunits, the short extracellular loops, and the three last intracellular loops of the α subunit. This indicates that the peptides of the "19-KD membranes" are able to form by themselves a rather stable structure, with the presence of associated cations (359).

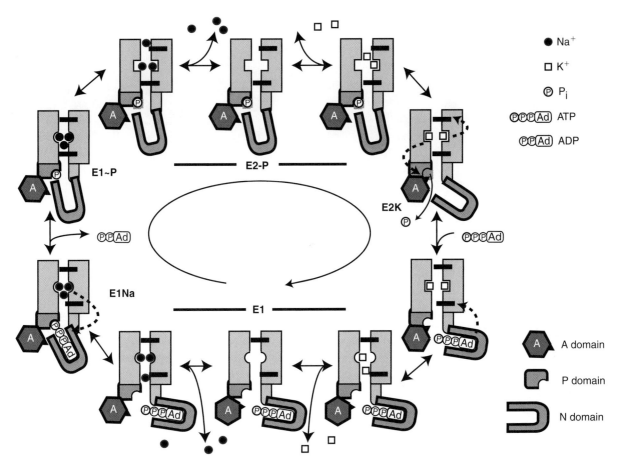

FIGURE 4 Na,K-ATPase transport cycle. This cartoon illustrates the principle of the "alternating access" model of transport of Na,K-ATPase. The Na$^+$ ions are indicated by the small filled circles and K$^+$ ions by the small open squares. Starting from the E$^+$ conformation with ATP present in its binding site, three Na$^+$ ions enters from the intracellular site through the open internal gate and reach their occlusion site (E1Na state). Na$^+$ binding induces (dotted arrow) a movement of the N domain resulting in positioning of the γ phosphate close to the phosphorylation site, phosphorylation of the α subunit by transfer of the γ phosphate to Asp351, release of ADP, and closure of the internal gate, which results in the occlusion of the 3Na$^+$ ions in the E1~P state. The following conformational change to the E2-P state results in the opening of the extracellular gate and a change in the structure of the cation-binding site resulting and a large decrease of their affinity for Na$^+$ and increase affinity for K$^+$, followed by release of Na$^+$ to extracellular side and loading of two K$^+$ ions. K$^+$ binding has two major consequences (dotted arrows), closing the external gate resulting in K$^+$ occlusion and dephosphorylation of D$_{351}$ (E2K state), which is catalyzed by a conserved motif (TGES, small black triangle) of the A domain brought in contact with the phosphorylation site by a rotation of this domain. There is also a movement of the N domain, the result of which is then accessible (with a low affinity) to ATP. Binding of ATP results then in the opening of the intracellular gate (back to E1 conformation) and allows the release of K$^+$ ions to the intracellular side. This last step can also occur in the absence of ATP, but at a much reduced rate. A more complete description of this scheme is given in Horisberger (215).

The results of fast-charge-movement measurement have shown that the translocation of three Na$^+$ ions is associated with the movement of one charge in the same direction, while the translocation of two K$^+$ ions was electroneutral (308). Assuming the simplest structural model, in which Na$^+$ and K$^+$ ions are alternately occluded in the same pocket, these results suggested that the cation-binding site should comprise two negative charges. Two of the three Na$^+$ ions, or the two K$^+$ ions bind to these negative charges and move with them across the membrane electrical field, allowing the movement of two cations to appear electrically silent. A number of experiments aiming at the identification of these negative charges have been performed, using either site-directed mutagenesis or the covalent chemical modification of specific residues in the transmembrane domains. These experiments have demonstrated the critical role of two aspartyl residues in the M6 segment (254, 323); the presence of negatively charged residues in these positions was required to observe any effect of K$^+$ ions. Modification of other charged amino acids in the transmembrane segments also had significant effects on transport functions or cation binding, although cation transport with modified kinetics could still be observed (12, 160, 197, 232, 255, 402, 408–410). All these results are largely confirmed by the structural model of the cation-binding sites that has been established by homology modeling with SERCA (312). The contribution of residues in transmembrane segments 4, 5, 6, 8, and 9 to the cation-binding sites are illustrated in Fig. 5. The core structure of the cation-binding sites is made of the three

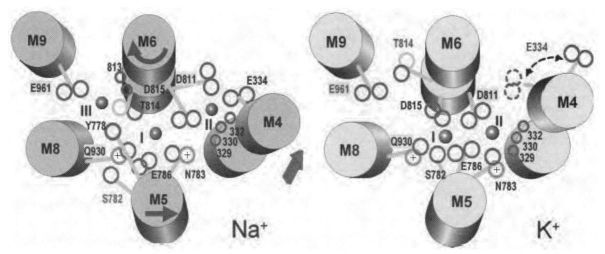

FIGURE 5   Cation-binding sites in Na,K-ATPase. This schematic shows the contribution of the M4, M5, M6, M8, and M9 transmembrane helices to the putative structure of the three Na^+-binding sites I, II, and III (E1 conformation at left with three Na^+ ions indicated by the gray spheres) and two K^+-binding sites (E2 conformation, right with two K^+ ions indicated by the gray spheres). The large empty circles represent side-chain oxygen atoms, small empty circles represent oxygen atoms of the backbone carbonyl, and circles with a plus sign (+) indicate nitrogen atoms. The proposed position for Na^+ site III has received recent experimental support (268). (Adapted with permission from Ogawa H, Toyoshima C. Homology modeling of the cation binding sites of the Na^+K^+-ATPase. *Proc Natl Acad Sci U S A* 2002;99:15977–15982.)

transmembrane segments M4, M5, and M6. A first site (I) is located between the transmembrane segments M5 and M6, and a second site (II) is mostly made by an unwound part of the fourth transmembrane helix. Additional contributions are provided by one or two residues of segments M8 and M9.

The mechanism and structure responsible for the *coupling* between ATP hydrolysis and ion transport are less well understood. But observation of the movements of the intracellular domains in SERCA, particularly domain A, and the effects of these movements on the relative positions of the transmembrane segments, allows researchers to propose hypotheses such as the closure of an internal gate by the formation of a cluster of hydrophobic residues between M1 and M2 during the E1-to-E2 conformation change (377) or the opening of an external ion pathway in the E2 conformation (398).

PHYSIOLOGICAL REGULATION OF EXPRESSION AND ACTIVITY

The activity of an enzyme that is of such paramount importance for many cellular and organ functions must obviously be well regulated. Thus, physiological regulation of Na,K-ATPase activity is complex and occurs at several levels. First, the density of Na,K pumps at the cell surface may be controlled by the *rate of synthesis*, at transcriptional and post-transcriptional levels, or by the *degradation rate* of the protein, or by the *distribution between the active site at the cell surface and intracellular pools*. Second, for short-term regulation, the activity of the Na,K pump present at the cell surface can be regulated by post-translational modification such as phosphorylation. Third, the activity of Na,K-ATPase is dependent

on its three substrates, Na^+, K^+, and ATP. Finally, there is some evidence for direct "hormonal" regulation of Na,K-ATPase activity by an extracellular ligand, that is, a circulating inhibitor. Because the nature of this inhibitor is related to well-known pharmacological agents, the cardiac glycosides, this subject will be discussed in the "Pharmacology and Toxicology" section of this chapter.

Regarding direct *activation by substrates*, intracellular sodium is thought to be the most physiologically relevant. The interaction of intracellular Mg-ATP with Na,K-ATPase is complex and involves a high- and a low-affinity site (63). As concentrations of intracellular ATP are normally maintained largely above the half-activation constant ($K_{1/2}$), even that of the low-affinity site, ATP is not considered a limiting factor for the activity of the Na,K pump under physiological conditions. However, it has to be recognized that not much is known about subcellular local concentrations of ATP even in cells as simple as red blood cells (214). Obviously, ATP may become rate limiting under pathological conditions with decreased production such as ischemia. The normal concentration of extracellular K^+ (3.5–4.5 mM) is also above the measured $K_{1/2}$, and thus variations in this normal range are not expected to have a strong influence on Na,K-ATPase activity, although severe hypokalemia could result in a significant decrease of the Na^+ and K^+ transport activity. In contrast, intracellular Na^+ concentration is usually below, or close to, the $K_{1/2}$ measured in many preparations, and, considering the steep concentration–activity relationship with a measured Hill coefficient between 2 and 3, it is expected that Na,K-ATPase operates far from its maximal rate with regard to intracellular Na^+ (51). Thus, even small variations in intracellular Na^+ should be instantaneously followed by parallel variations in Na,K-pump activity. By this mechanism, the activity of the Na,K pump tends to maintain a constant intracellular Na^+ concentration, and the extrusion of Na^+ through the Na,K pump tends to closely match the rate of Na^+ entry into the cell. This has an important consequence for the study of mechanisms of regulation of the Na,K-pump activity: to demonstrate a direct effect on Na,K-ATPase activity, measurements have to be made either at saturating intracellular Na^+ concentrations, or at a well-controlled, constant level of intracellular Na^+ activity, a condition often difficult to realize.

The intracellular Na^+ and extracellular K^+ concentrations do not only stimulate the Na,K-pump activity by direct substrate activation, but can also have a long-term effect on the density of Na,K pump. The influence of the extracellular K^+ balance on the expression of the $\alpha 2$ isoform has been well demonstrated in skeletal muscle (393). In hypokalemia, the $\alpha 2$ isoform is downregulated, allowing some release of K^+ from the large muscular intracellular pool and the fine regulation of K^+ homeostasis in the small extracellular pool. Similarly, chronic increase in intracellular Na^+ leads to increased expression of the Na,K pump (246) (see also the "Na,K-ATPase in Kidney" section in this chapter for data obtained on kidneys).

Besides the transient autophosphorylation of the aspartate residue that occurs during each catalytic cycle, Na,K-ATPase α subunits can be phosphorylated by several protein kinases. Present knowledge about α-subunit phosphorylation and its potential effects in general is presented here, while effects studied in the kidney are discussed in the section titled "Regulation of Na,K-ATPase in Proximal Tubule by Protein Kinases" in this chapter. Site-directed mutagenesis studies have permitted determination of the sites of phosphorylation by protein kinase A (PKA) and protein kinase C (PKC). PKA phosphorylates a serine residue (S_{943}) (42, 172) conserved in all members of the Na,K- and H,K-ATPase family and located in the short intracellular loop joining the M8 and M9 transmembrane segments. Activation of PKC also results in the phosphorylation of the α subunit on two residues located in the intracellular N-terminal domain (S_{16} and S_{27} in the rat $\alpha 1$, T_{15}, and S_{16} in the *Bufo* $\alpha 1$). This last site is not considered a classical PKC phosphorylation motif, and is conserved only in $\alpha 1$ isoforms (42, 45). Most of these studies have been performed on kidney preparation or in artificial expression systems on the $\alpha 1$ subunit. The $\alpha 2$ and $\alpha 3$ subunits are much poorer substrates for PKC, or are not phosphorylated at all (45). In the heart, protein kinase A can be activated by β-adrenergic receptor simulation of, for instance, phosphorylate residues in the intracellular domain of the associated FXYD1 protein (phospholemman), and this phosphorylation results in an increased affinity for intracellular Na^+ and thus an increased Na,K-pump activity (124).

The physiological significance of α-subunit phosphorylation has been more difficult to establish. First, both PKC and PKA have been described to increase or to decrease Na,K-pump activity in various cell types or expression systems (56, 345, 403, 404). Although the effects of protein kinase activation on Na,K-ATPase activity are obvious in several tissues or whole-cell preparations (320) (see also "Na,K-ATPase in Kidney" section), few results support an effect directly mediated by α-subunit phosphorylation. The removal of the PKC phosphorylation site of the α-subunit N-terminus appeared to modify the response to PKC when mutant rat $\alpha 1$ subunits were transfected in COS cells (48), but not when mutant *Bufo* $\alpha 1$ subunits were expressed in A6 cells (50). Previous in vivo activation of PKC does not modify ATPase activity measured in permeabilized cells, even though Na, K-ATPase is indeed phosphyorylated (170).

In summary, the α subunit (at least the $\alpha 1$ subunit) can be phosphorylated in vitro and in vivo by both protein kinases A and C, and kinase stimulation is followed by changes in Na,K-ATPase activity in intact cells. However, the evidence for a causal relationship between these two observations has been often negative or weak.

As the α/β subunit stoichiometry is fixed, regulation through control of the rate of synthesis must involve both subunits. Hormonal control by glucocorticoids, mineralocorticoids, and thyroid hormones has been well demonstrated. Thyroid hormones have been shown to regulate the synthesis of both subunits, but the mechanism of this regulation is complex and different in various organs. Transcriptional control, with increase of α and β subunit has been described in the heart for all three α isoforms and for the β subunit (211, 236), with the larger effect on the $\alpha 2$ isoform (190, 317). A thyroid-hormone response element has been found in the 5' flanking region of the human $\beta 1$ gene (159). In skeletal muscle, thyroid hormones have a strong transcriptional effect on $\alpha 2$ and $\beta 2$ isoforms, but no effect on $\alpha 1$ or $\beta 1$ (24). In the liver, triiodothyronine (T3) produced a coordinate augmentation of $\alpha 1$ and $\beta 1$ mRNA (189), and in renal cells, T3 potentiates the effect of aldosterone on Na,K-ATPase activity (31). On the other hand, in heart and skeletal muscle, the hypothyroid state was shown to decrease mainly the translation rate of $\alpha 1$ and $\alpha 2$ subunits with little effect on mRNA levels (219). Glucocorticoids stimulate the transcription of mostly β-subunit mRNA in the lungs, but α and β proteins are both increased, which indicates complex transcriptional and post-transcriptional control (33, 223). The effect of mineralocorticoids on Na,K-ATPase in the kidney will be discussed in the "Na,K-ATPase in Kidney" section.

PHARMACOLOGY AND TOXICOLOGY

A group of natural compounds found in plants or animals are toxic because of their potent inhibitory effect on Na,K-ATPase. These compounds are known as "cardiac steroids" because they include a steroid nucleus to which a lactone ring is attached, and because of their principal medical use for the treatment of congestive heart failure (376). Natural cardiac steroids are found as glycosides (and are therefore often designated as "cardiac glycosides"), but cardiac steroids are also active in the absence of their sugar moiety. Besides their still important clinical use, interest in these inhibitors has been revived by observations suggesting that one or several endogenous related compounds may act as hormonal agents to control the activity of Na,K-ATPase.

The interactions of cardiac steroids, in particular ouabain, with Na,K-ATPase have been studied in great detail. The observation of sequence differences between isoforms with various ouabain affinities, and then the study of numerous mutants obtained by site-directed or random mutagenesis, have allowed researchers to define a number of extracellular domains of the protein that are important for ouabain binding (for reviews see 82, 272).

The mechanism of ouabain binding and Na,K-ATPase inhibition is complex (173) and not fully understood. The association rate constant (K_{on}) depends mostly on the conformation of the enzyme, and thus on the presence of cations Na^+ and K^+, and somewhat on the size of the ligand (slower for glycosides). The dissociation rate constant (K_{off}) is determined mainly by two factors. First, the constant is dependent on the receptor isoform (ouabain K_{off} ranges from <0.5 hour^{-1} for sensitive isoforms to >60 hours^{-1} for resistant isoforms), as if the main determinant of the dissociation rate was not the ligand–protein interaction, but rather a receptor-isoform–dependent conformational change. Second, the dissociation rate depends on the presence of a sugar group linked to the cardiac steroid: the glycosides have a K_{off} about 50 times slower that the aglycone. The isoforms or mutants that have been studied show a similar ratio (in the order of 20:50) between glycoside and aglycone affinity (81, 355).

Large differences in sensitivity to ouabain are found among species. The α1 isoform, that is, the ubiquitous and dominant kidney isoform, is notably ouabain resistant in the rat, mouse, and toad *Bufo marinus*, while it is more sensitive in the human, rabbit, sheep, or *Xenopus* (216). The α2 and α3 isoforms (or the tissue known to contain these isoforms) are usually more sensitive than the α1 isoform (59, 231). However, in the case of humans, which is considered a "sensitive" species, little difference of equilibrium binding is found among the α1, α2, and α3 isoforms, except for a slightly higher K_I for the α2 isoform; there was, however, a marked difference in the kinetics of ouabain binding the α2 isoforms, showing faster association and dissociation rate constant than the α1 and α3 isoforms (114). The "resistant" phenotype of rat, mouse, or *Bufo marinus* could be attributed to the presence of charged amino acids in the first extracellular loop, located between M1 and M2 (333). Extensive site-directed or random mutagenesis experiments have allowed researchers to demonstrate the involvement of other domains of the α subunit, namely, a cysteine located in the outer third of M1, two positions in the M3–M4 loop, two other positions in the M5–M6 loop, and two positions in the beginning of the M7–M8 loop (271). Detailed analysis

of the first extracellular loop of the human Na,K-ATPase showed that two residues in this loop are responsible for the differences in the kinetics of ouabain binding (118).

Using chimerical constructs between H,K- and Na,K-ATPase, de Pont and collaborators demonstrated a crucial role of the second (transmembrane segments 3 and 4) and third (transmembrane segments 5 and 6) hairpins in the ouabain-binding site (248), and identified two residues in the outer part of transmembrane segments M5 and M6 that probably make direct contact with the ouabain molecule (336).

Finally, molecular "docking" with binding-site structure that is obtained by homology modeling has recently allowed researchers to propose a precise position of ouabain in its binding site (319).

In summary it appears that the cardiac steroids make close contact with the extracellular part of the M5–M6 loop, similarly to the gastric H,K-ATPase inhibitors (306), but that access to this site is controlled by several elements of the extracellular part of the Na,K-ATPase, in particular, the first extracellular loop, which seems to be involved in the control of the access of the binding site.

Gastric H,K-ATPase has been found totally insensitive to ouabain (286), that is, absence of detectable effects of millimolar concentrations of ouabain. The nongastric H,K-ATPases, expressed in *Xenopus* oocytes, show, however, some sensibility to ouabain. Inhibitory constants (K_I) between 10 and 100 μM have been measured in the presence of K^+ for *Bufo* bladder, human ATPAL1, or rat colon H,K-ATPase (107, 226, 295). These values are close to those observed for the α1 Na,K-ATPase in the "ouabain-resistant" species.

The hormonal control of the activity of one or the other isoforms of the Na,K pump by an endogenous circulating inhibitor ("endo-ouabain") could be of a great physiological significance due to its effects on renal tubular sodium reabsorption or on the level of intracellular sodium and calcium in cardiac and vascular smooth muscle cells. This mechanism has been implicated in the pathogenesis of conditions such as arterial hypertension or heart failure (60, 61, 309, 310). The presence of "endo-ouabains" has been demonstrated by their effect on ATPase activity, rubidium uptake, or by detection of immunoreactivity to antibodies raised against known cardiac glycosides (206). The precise molecular identification of these compounds has, however, proven difficult. Without a well-identified substance, it has been very difficult to assess the selectivity of endo-ouabains toward each Na,K-ATPase isoform, although there is some indication that it might be different from ouabain (168). Some investigators have reported the presence of a substance that could not be distinguished from ouabain, which had to be ouabain itself or an isomer (206), while other investigators identified different compounds (269, 401) or even presented data that excluded the presence of ouabain (447). Endo-ouabain has been found concentrated in the adrenal gland, and release from this tissue to the blood has been described (68, 276). In contrast, other authors could show an increase in endo-ouabain activity in adrenalectomized rats exposed to a high-salt diet (265). Considering the lack of agreement concerning the nature of the substance itself, the absence of a definitive demonstration of a controlled synthesis (in contrast with accumulation) in the organism and the widespread presence of related compounds in the normal food of animals and humans (341), it is not currently possible to exclude the possibility that at least some of these compounds are ingested with food or are metabolites of food components. In spite of several indications of modulation by extracellular fluid volume expansion or other conditions such as heart failure (207), the physiological and pathophysiological significance of the regulation of Na,K-ATPase activity still needs to be established. In summary, although the presence of circulating inhibitors of Na,K-ATPase is well demonstrated, their precise chemical nature needs to be clarified, the control of their synthesis and release must be better understood, and their specific effects more precisely described, before the hypothesis of hormonal control of Na,K-ATPase activity can be considered as established.

Two types of inhibitor are known for the gastric H,K-pump. First, the compound SCH-28080 is a reversible inhibitor acting in competition with extracellular K^+ (343, 419). Recent studies with Na,K-/H,K-ATPase chimeras (278) have shown that introduction of only 11 amino acids of the αHKg M1 domain in Na,K-ATPase produced a chimera that was sensitive to both cardiac steroids and SCH 28080; this indicates that the first transmembrane segment of the H,K-ATPase is essential for SCH-28080 binding even though this site appears to be located close to that of cardiac steroids. Second, substituted benzimidazole compounds irreversibly inhibit the gastric H,K-ATPase by formation of a covalent (disulfide) bond between the sulfonamide form of the compound and the thiol group of a surface cysteine, C_{813}, located in the short loop connecting the M5 and M6 of the α subunit (57, 343). The sulfonamide form is produced when these substances are exposed to strongly acid pH. The substance is therefore not active at physiological pH, but becomes active when accumulated in an acid compartment such as the tubulovesicular system of the gastric gland principal cells, where it can bind and inhibit the gastric H,K-ATPase. Extensive site-directed mutagenesis experiments coupled with molecular modeling analysis have yielded a reliable model for the binding site of the two types of H,K-ATPase inhibitor (306).

Palytoxin is a potent nonprotein toxin produced by the marine coelenterate *Palythoa*. Palytoxin inhibits Na,K-ATPase and induces a cation conductance in the plasma membrane of animal cells (205). In addition, palytoxin is known as a tumor promoter, an effect related to its ability to increase intracellular sodium (256). The effects of palytoxin can be observed only in membranes containing active Na,K-ATPases and can be prevented by previous treatment with ouabain (305, 440). Demonstration that the effects of palytoxin can be induced by transfection of

Na,K-ATPase in yeast cells (340) or can be restored after ouabain inhibition by expression of a ouabain-resistant isoform (421) strongly supports the hypothesis that palytoxin associates with Na,K-ATPase and transforms it into a cation channel. In addition, mutagenesis experiments have shown that the pathway opened by palytoxin is constituted, at least in part, by the same elements that comprise the cation-binding site in the normal Na,K-pump cycle (202, 203). The kinetics of the interaction between the Na,K pump and palytoxin have been studied in detail by Artigas and Gadsby (15, 16); these results showed that palytoxin seems to act by altering the control of one or both of the two gates of the ion translocation mechanism, while preserving some aspects of this control by intracellular (ATP) or extracellular (K^+) ligands.

Na,K-ATPase IN THE KIDNEY

The renal, tubular epithelial cell layer separates the serosal compartment (characterized by a remarkable constancy in composition), in equilibrium with blood plasma, and the mucosal compartment (characterized by composition that greatly varies from one nephron segment to another and with time). Tubular epithelial cells are characterized by their functional polarity. In particular, Na,K-ATPase is exclusively located in the basolateral membrane (356), the infoldings of which are closely surrounded by mitochondria. In contrast, the sodium gradient generated by Na,K-ATPase between intra- and extra-cellular compartments is mainly dissipated across the apical membrane. A net reabsorption of sodium results from this architectural organization, and the main role of Na,K-ATPase in the kidney is to energize sodium reabsorption. In humans, kidneys reabsorb over 500 g of sodium per day, and utilize over 2 kg of ATP to fuel Na,K-ATPase for this purpose. In relation to this enormous transport capacity, the kidney is one of the richest sources of Na,K-ATPase, and it has been used for purification of the pump and for studying its general properties.

Although renal Na,K-ATPase also energizes secondary active transport of other solutes, its main function, and therefore its principal regulation, is related to sodium transport and to the maintenance of sodium balance. We have therefore focused in this chapter on the role of renal Na,K-ATPase in the maintenance of sodium balance. The purpose of this chapter is twofold: analyze the distribution of Na,K-ATPase along the nephron in relation to sodium transport capacity of the successive nephron segments, and review the parameters and mechanisms that control renal Na,K-ATPase. This last part has been restricted to the proximal tubule because it is the site of more than 60% of sodium reabsorption, and the collecting duct because it is the site of the final adjustment of sodium excretion and therefore that of minute control of Na,K-ATPase.

Expression of Na,K-ATPASE Along Mammalian Nephron

Although the role of Na,K-ATPase in tubular ion transport was demonstrated long ago, its exact contribution to various transport processes was made possible only with the development of tubular microdissection methods and of microenzymatic assays to measure hydrolytic activity as well as other indications of the presence of Na,K-ATPase (ion transport, ouabain binding, etc.) at the level of discrete nephron segments.

AXIAL HETEROGENEITY OF NA,K-ATPASE EXPRESSION ALONG NEPHRON

Measurements in microdissected segments of nephron from different mammalian species (179, 240, 354) indicate that Na,K-ATPase activity (at V_{max}) is high in the thick ascending limb of Henle's loop and the distal convoluted tubule, intermediate in the proximal tubule and the collecting duct, and vanishingly low in the thin segments of Henle's loop. In proximal tubules and collecting ducts, Na,K-ATPase activity declines from the kidney cortex (proximal convoluted tubule [PCT] and cortical collecting duct [CCD]) toward the outer medulla (proximal straight tubule [PST] and outer medullary collecting duct [OMCD]) and inner medulla (inner medullary collecting duct [IMCD]) (179, 240, 389). This distribution profile is confirmed by immunocytochemistry on kidney sections (239) and by quantification of the number of pump units in isolated nephron segments determined by ^{3}H-ouabain binding (144) or by Western blotting of α_1 and β_1 subunits (288). Immunohistochemistry on kidney sections (239) and measurement of ^{3}H-ouabain binding in immunodissected CCD cells (158) indicate that Na,K-ATPase is much higher in principal than in intercalated cells.

In contrast, quantification of Na,K-ATPase subunits mRNAs along the rat nephron does not confirm the axial heterogeneity of distribution, at least for α and β subunits (Table 3). This suggests the presence of segment-specific control mechanisms of the translation and/or degradation of Na,K-ATPase.

TABLE 3   Distribution Profile of Na,K-ATPase Subunits mRNAs Along Rat Nephron Determined by Quantitative RT-PCR on Microdissected Nephron Segments (1000 mRNAs/mm ± SE)

α and β	α_1	β_1	γ
PCT	137 ± 13 (3)	200 ± 13 (3)	5.7 ± 2.4 (4)
PST	92 ± 33 (3)	118 ± 23 (3)	7.6 ± 1.5 (4)
MTAL	198 ± 43 (3)	245 ± 91 (3)	39.8 ± 6.0 (4)
CTAL	155 ± 17 (3)	194 ± 38 (3)	33.0 ± 10.0 (4)
CCD	120 ± 13 (4)	309 ± 52 (3)	6.8 ± 1.2 (4)
OMCD	66 ± 12 (3)	164 ± 51 (3)	1.4 ± 0.4 (4)

The number of mRNA copies encoding the three subunits of Na,K-ATPase was quantitated by RT-PCR using specific mutant cRNA as internal standards (72). Results are means ± standard error from several animals (number in parentheses).

FUNCTIONAL PROPERTIES OF TUBULAR NA,K-ATPASE

Quantification of ^{3}H-ouabain binding in nephron segments demonstrates the very high level of expression of Na,K-ATPase in renal tubular cells, with 3 to 50 million pumps per cell (144). The hydrolytic activity (at V_{max}) and the number of catalytic units of Na,K-ATPase are used to calculate a maximal molecular activity of ~2,000 cycles/ouabain-binding site^{-1}/minute^{-1}. A much higher figure has been reported for the purified renal enzyme: 10,000 cycles/ouabain-binding site^{-1}/minute^{-1} (235). This apparent discrepancy reveals the presence of cellular components that downregulate the pump activity. Comparison of ^{3}H-ouabain binding with high levels of mRNA shows that there are 20,000 to 60,000 Na,K-ATPase units per α-subunit mRNA, which suggests a slow turnover rate of the protein.

As expected from its central role in sodium transport, Na,K-ATPase activity is correlated with the transtubular Na^+ reabsorption capacity in the various nephron segments. In the rabbit nephron, there is a linear relationship between Na,K-ATPase activity and sodium transport as determined by in vitro microperfusion, and the ratio of the number of sodium ions transported per ATP molecule hydrolyzed is 1.8 (177). The difference between this experimental stoichiometry and the theoretical 3Na/1ATP stoichiometry (see Na,K- and H,K-ATPase section in this chapter) is accounted for by three factors that may have opposite effects. First, although all transepithelial Na^+ reabsorption is primarily energized by Na,K-ATPase, part of Na^+ ions reabsorbed is not directly mediated by Na,K-ATPase (e.g., paracellular Na^+ reabsorption in the thick ascending limb of Henle or Na^+/HCO_3^- cotransport in the basolateral membrane of PCT). Second, part of Na^+ reabsorbed through Na,K-ATPase may back-diffuse toward the luminal fluid, driven by the apical, negative transepithelial voltage. Third, and more importantly, Na,K-ATPase activity is determined under saturating Na^+ concentration (V_{max}) whereas sodium transport is determined under rate-limiting intracellular Na^+ conditions.

The actual activity of Na,K-ATPase in intact cells and under V_{max} conditions was evaluated for rat nephron segments by the rate of ouabain-sensitive rubidium uptake determined either in intact cells and in sodium-loaded cells. Comparison with the V_{max} of Na,K-ATPase hydrolytic activity shows that the Rb/ATP stoichiometry is 0.4–0.7 and 1.8–2.0 (i.e., the admitted stoichiometry) (see Na,K- and H,K-ATPase Family section in this chapter) under these two conditions, respectively (95). The comparison indicates that under normal conditions, restricted intracellular sodium limits tubular Na,K-ATPase activity to approximately 20%–35% of its V_{max}.

In another study, the dependency of Na,K-ATPase transport capacity on intracellular Na^+ concentration was directly determined on rabbit CCD (65). For this purpose, the tubular segments were first preloaded in the cold with ^{22}Na, and then the rate of ^{22}Na efflux induced by rewarming was monitored. Because Na^+ entry was blocked during this second phase, the intracellular concentration of Na^+ could be determined from the tubular volume and the difference between the initial intracellular and the cumulative exit of radioactivity. This study shows a sigmoid activation of Na^+ efflux by Na,K-ATPase as a function of intracellular Na^+ concentration. Half-maximal and maximal transports are observed with approximately 45 mM and 80 mM intracellular Na^+, respectively. Again, this demonstrates the large reserve of transport capacity of Na,K-ATPase that can be triggered by intracellular Na^+ increase.

ISOFORMS OF NA,K-ATPASE IN KIDNEY

Northern and RT-PCR analysis demonstrated that Na,K-ATPase α_1- and β_1-subunit mRNAs are abundantly expressed in the kidney (149, 154, 188, 275), indicating that the $\alpha_1\beta_1$ holoenzyme is the main form of Na,K-ATPase expressed in the kidney. This conclusion is also supported by transcriptome analysis of human nephron segments (93) (Table 4), RT-PCR in single nephron segments (94, 101, 400), in situ hybridization (4, 153, 154), ribonuclease protection assay (101), and Western blotting on whole kidney (366) or microdissected nephron segments (288, 400, 400).

Alpha Subunit More controversial are results concerning the presence of a2 and a3 isoforms of the Na,K-ATPase catalytic subunit in the nephron. In the rat kidney, several authors failed to detect a2 and a3 mRNAs and/or proteins in whole-kidney preparations and in microdissected nephron segments (94, 188, 288, 366). Using the same methods (Northern analysis, RT-PCR, in situ hybridization, ribonuclease protection assay, or Western analysis), others were successful (4, 101, 149, 274, 400). When compared, however, the level of expression of a2 and a3 mRNAs was less than 1% that of a1 mRNAs (273), suggesting that the contribution of a2 and a3 subunits to the whole renal Na,K-ATPase is negligible. In contrast, a2 and/or a3 isoforms are expressed in the kidney of other species. Table 4 shows that a3 mRNA tags, but not a2, are detected at significant level along the whole human nephron, and a3 has been immunopurified from in pig and human kidney (21). Also, Western blotting revealed that a2 and a3 account for approximately 15% of the whole Na,K-ATPase in pig and mink kidneys (208).

Beta Subunit There is a general consensus for the expression of Na,K-ATPase b2-subunit mRNAs along the rat nephron (4, 101, 154, 400), but the b2 protein has not been detected (147). In human nephron transcriptome, b2 subunit-specific tag is almost undetectable (Table 4), and accordingly, b2 subunit is not detected in the human kidney except in two specific circumstances. In early to mid-gestation, the human metanephric kidney expresses both b1 and

TABLE 4 Expression of Na,K-ATPase and H,K-ATPase Subunits and FXYD Protein mRNAs Along Human Nephron

Gene	Glom	PCT	PST	MTAL	CTAL	DCT	CCD	OMCD
Na,K-ATPase α_1 subunit (*ATP1A1*)	5	10	6	53	93	29	7	10
Na,K-ATPase α_2 subunit (*ATP1A2*)	0	0	1	0	0	0	0	0
Na,K-ATPase α_3 subunit (*ATP1A3*)	2	1	1	0	1	1	0	1
Na,K-ATPase β_1 subunit (*ATP1B1*) long variant transcript	20	51	28	111	138	132	57	58
Na,K-ATPase β_1 subunit (*ATP1B1*) short variant transcript	7	9	13	34	31	33	11	16
Na,K-ATPase β_2 subunit (*ATP1B2*)	0	0	1	0	0	0	0	0
Na,K-ATPase β_3 subunit (*ATP1B3*) long variant transcript	1	0	0	1	1	0	1	1
Na,K-ATPase β_3 subunit (*ATP1B3*) short variant transcript	3	0	0	2	2	2	5	1
FXYD 1 (phospholemman) (*FXYD1*)	1	0	0	0	0	0	0	0
FXYD 2 (Na,K-ATPase γ subunit) (*FXYD2, ATP1G1*)	0	50	44	115	83	156	7	7
FXYD 3 (Mat-8) (*FXYD3*)	0	1	0	2	0	0	0	1
FXYD 4 (CHIF) (*FXYD4, CHIF*)	0	2	27	1	0	4	191	348
FXYD 5 (*FXYD5*)	0	0	1	0	1	0	1	2
FXYD 6 (*FXYD6*)	3	0	0	0	0	0	0	1
FXYD 7 (*FXYD7*)	0	0	0	0	0	0	0	0
Gastric H,K-ATPase α subunit (*ATP4A*)	0	0	0	0	0	0	0	0
Gastric H,K-ATPase β subunit (*ATP4B*)	0	0	0	0	0	0	0	0
Nongastric H,K-ATPase α subunit (ATP1AL1) (*ATP12A*)	0	0	0	0	0	1	0	0

Abundance of transcript-specific tags for Na,K-ATPase α_{1-3} and β_{1-3} subunits and FXYD1–7 in SAGE libraries made from glomerulus (Glom) and various segments of the human nephron. Figures indicate tag occurrence numbers in a total 50,000 tags sequenced in each library. At this level of analysis, there is 95% confidence for detecting a transcript expressed at a level of 18 copies per cell; an occurrence number of 1 corresponds to transcript quantity of 6 copies per cell. Note that two variant transcripts with the same ORF encode Na,K-ATPase β_1 and β_3 subunits. PCT and PST, proximal convoluted and straight tubule; MTAL and CTAL, medullary and cortical thick ascending limb of Henle's loop; DCT, distal convoluted tubule; CCD and OMCD, cortical and outer medullary collecting duct. (Data from Chabardes-Garonne D, Mejean A, Aude JC, et al. A panoramic view of gene expression in the human kidney. *Proc Natl Acad Sci U S A* 2003;100:13710–13715.)

b2 Na,K-ATPase subunit mRNAs, but only the b2 protein is detected (78). The b2 protein is also expressed in the kidneys from patients with autosomal dominant polycystic kidney disease (430), a genetic disorder characterized by cystic dilatation of tubules associated with abnormal fluid and solute secretion. It is noteworthy that under these two circumstances, Na,K-ATPase is mispolarized to the apical membrane, suggesting that overexpression of the b2 subunit may account for the mistargeting of Na,K-ATPase in epithelial cells. Expression of b3 Na,K-ATPase subunit mRNA is also detected in the kidney (282) (Table 4) but the corresponding protein is detected at vanishingly low levels (18).

FXYD Subunit   At least five of the seven members of the FXYD protein family (FXYD1–4 and FXYD7) can associate with Na,K-ATPase and modulate its activity (see Table 2), and therefore be considered as a third subunit. Transcriptome analysis (93) indicates that mRNAs for all FXYD proteins except FXYD7 are detected in the human nephron, some in a highly segment-specific manner (Table 4).

FXYD1, or phospholemman, is mainly expressed in heart, liver, and skeletal muscle, but also at lower levels in the juxtaglomerular apparatus (429) where its function has not been investigated. FXYD1-deficient mice show decreased cardiac Na,K-ATPase activity (233), but no renal phenotype has been described.

FXYD2, or the Na,K-ATPase γ subunit, is predominantly expressed in the kidney (291, 390). FXYD2 mRNAs are expressed at high levels in the human proximal tubule, thick ascending of Henle's loop, and distal convoluted tubule, and at much lower levels in the cortical and outer medullary collecting duct (Table 4). FXYD exists as two splice variants (FXYD2a and FXYD2b or γa and γb) that differ in their N-terminal domains (257) and segment-specific distribution.

Despite some discrepancies between reports (20 and 334 vs. 330 and 428), the following generally accepted distribution of the two splice variants has emerged. Both FXYD2a and FXYD2b are expressed in proximal tubules and medullary thick ascending limbs. Only FXYD2a is expressed in CCD principal cells, intercalated cells of initial IMCD, and IMCD cells of terminal IMCD. In contrast, FXYD2b is expressed in cortical thick ascending limb, distal convoluted tubule, and connecting tubule. No variant of FXYD is detected in the OMCD. In all positive cells, FXYD2a and/or FXYD2b colocalize with Na,K-ATPase at the basolateral membrane.

FXYD2 induces complex functional effects on Na,K-ATPase, which may depend on post-translational modifications. FXYD2 increases or decreases the apparent affinity of Na,K-ATPase for potassium at high or less negative membrane voltages respectively. The first effect is independent of sodium whereas the second is only observed in the presence of extracellular sodium (43). FXYD2 also increases the affinity of Na,K-ATPase for ATP (390, 391). Finally, FXYD2 decreases the affinity of Na,K-ATPase for sodium (19, 43). Although FXYD2a and FXYD2b do not have the same intramembrane localization, and therefore associate to distinct pools of Na,K-ATPase (169), their

functional effects on Na,K-ATPase, when compared, are similar (43, 334). Post-translational modifications abolish the effect of FXYD2a but not of FXYD2b on the apparent affinity of Na,K-ATPase for sodium, whereas modifications of FXYD2b are necessary to induce changes in potassium affinity of Na,K-ATPase (17).

The physiological role of FXYD2 was addressed in FXYD2-deficient mice, which are viable. FXYD2-deficient mice show Na,K-ATPase with increased apparent affin-ity for sodium (234), which confirms the main effect of FXYD2 observed in artificial systems. However, FXYD2-deficient mice do not exhibit any alteration of their renal function (234), suggesting that changes in sodium affinity are fully compensated. In humans, however, a dominant-negative mutation of the codon of a conserved glycine residue in the transmembrane domain of FXYD2 is associated with dominant renal hypomagnesaemia in a family (289) (OMIM #154020). Although it was initially proposed that the mutation provoked a defective routing of Na,K-ATPase to the plasma membrane (289), further studies showed that it abolished the association of FXYD2 with Na,K-ATPase but did not alter cell surface expression of the pump (117, 335). In the human nephron, FXYD2 is expressed in the main sites of calcium and magnesium transport, which are the thick ascending limb of Henle's loop and the distal convoluted tubule (Table 4). However, the dissociation between Na,K-ATPase and FXYD2 by the mutation should increase the sodium affinity of Na,K-ATPase, and thereby its activity. In turn, increased Na,K-ATPase activity is expected to increase, rather than decrease, the reabsorption of divalent cations. Thus, the FXYD2 mutation observed in these patients may induce the hypermagnesiuria and hypocalciuria independently of its effect on Na,K-ATPase.

In cultured murine inner-medullary collecting duct cells (IMCD3), hypertonicity induces the synthesis and membrane targeting of FXYD2. This effect is mediated by activation of cJun N-terminal kinase 2 (JNK2) and phosphatidylinositol 3-kinase (PI3K) (83, 329). JNK2 and PI3K control expression of FXYD2 at the transcriptional and translational level, respectively (84). Hypertonicity-induced overexpression of FXYD2 is dependent on chloride, whereas that of Na,K-ATPase α subunit is dependent on sodium (85). However, because medullary hypertonicity cannot be made by sodium independently of chloride, and reciprocally, it is recognized that hypertonicity induces the overexpression of both α and γ subunits. Under such conditions, the beneficial effect of α-subunit overexpression on sodium transport may be abrogated in part by γ-subunit–induced reduction in sodium affinity. Thus, the functional relevance of γ-subunit overexpression might not be related to sodium transport but to some other effect of the γ subunit. Interestingly, blocking hypertonicity-induced FXYD2 synthesis decreases cell survival (83), whereas expression of FXYD2 is associated with decreased rate of cell proliferation (17, 427). Control of FXYD2 expression in the kidney medulla by tonicity may therefore be related to protection against stress rather than to the modulation of sodium balance.

FXYD3, or Mat-8, was initially identified in breast tumors (299). Its mRNA expression was detected at very low levels in the human proximal tubule, thick ascending limb, and collecting duct (Table 4), and its protein expression has not been investigated in the kidney yet. When coexpressed in *Xenopus* oocyte, FXYD3 modulates the glycosylation of Na,K-ATPase β subunit and also decreases the apparent affinity of the pump for both sodium and potassium (116). FXYD3 might therefore reduce the pump activity in vivo.

FXYD4 or corticosteroid hormone–induced factor (CHIF) is coexpressed with Na,K-ATPase in the distal colon and the kidney. By in situ hybridization, expression of CHIF mRNAs was detected along the collecting duct, from the deeper part of the CCD to the IMCD (87). However, transcriptome analysis of the human nephron also revealed its expression in the proximal straight tubule (Table 4). The CHIF protein was detected in principal cells of the collecting duct and in IMCD cells (155, 330, 362). In the collecting duct, CHIF is expressed in the cells that do not express FXYD2.

CHIF induces a marked increase in the affinity of Na, K-ATPase for sodium (43, 180), which might increase the activity of the pump in vivo. Also, expression of high sodium-affinity pump in the terminal segment of the nephron appears as a relevant physiological property to mediate final sodium reabsorption even at low luminal sodium concentration. Changes in sodium affinity of Na,K-ATPase were confirmed in CHIF-deficient mice (6). However, this defect is fully compensated and the CHIF-deficient mice do not display abnormal handling of electrolyte under basal conditions nor in response to dietary sodium or potassium restriction (6, 195).

Aldosterone and sodium restriction markedly increase the expression of CHIF in the distal colon, whereas they have no or only modest effects on CHIF expression in the distal nephron (69, 87, 416). Metabolic acidosis is the only known condition that markedly increases the expression of CHIF in the distal nephron (87), but the physiological significance of this effect is not known.

FXYD4 and FXYD5 mRNAs are detected at low levels in the human nephron (Table 4). However, it is not known whether these two proteins associate with Na,K-ATPase and modulate its activity. FXYD7 associates with Na,K-ATPase and modulates its activity (44), but it is exclusively expressed in the brain, and accordingly its mRNAs are not detected in the human nephron (Table 4).

In conclusion, although the functional consequences on Na,K-ATPase properties of the cell-specific expression of different isoforms of α and β subunits with or without specific FXYD proteins has been established during the past decade, the relevance in renal physiology and the potential pathophysiological role of various heterodi(tri)mers of Na,K-ATPase subunits remain to be established. In particular, one might question whether specific α and β

isoforms or FXYD proteins might be responsible for the fact that (1) Na,K-ATPase displays a higher sensitivity to ouabain and to Na+ in the collecting duct than in more proximal nephron segments of the rabbit nephron (29, 30, 130), and (2) each segment of nephron contains two subpopulations of Na,K-ATPase characterized by different sensitivities to ouabain (162).

Regulation of Na,K-ATPASE in Proximal Tubule by Protein Kinases

As discussed previously, Na,K-ATPase catalytic subunits (mainly the α_1 isoform) can be phosphorylated by serine/threonine and tyrosine protein kinases. The functional consequence of such phosphorylations on pump activity and membrane expression appears to be highly tissue specific. Extensive study of the regulation of Na,K-ATPase by protein kinases in the proximal tubule and proximal tubule OK cell line illustrates that even in a same cellular model, phosphorylation of Na,K-ATPase may have opposite functional effects, depending on the experimental/environmental conditions.

INSULIN INCREASES NA,K-ATPASE AFFINITY FOR SODIUM VIA TYROSINE PHOSPHORYLATION

In vitro addition of insulin to isolated rat nephron segments increases ouabain-sensitive rubidium uptake along the proximal tubule (165) without changing its V_{max}, but rather by increasing its affinity for Na+, and thereby by increasing the efficiency of each preexisting unit (163). Stimulation of Na,K-ATPase by insulin in the PCT likely participates to the stimulation of Na+ reabsorption described in this nephron segment (35). Activation of receptor tyrosine kinase by epidermal growth factor (EGF) also stimulates Na,K-ATPase. The effects of insulin and EGF are not additive; they are abolished by tyrosine kinase inhibition and they are mimicked by tyrosine phosphatase inhibition (164). This suggests that a tyrosine phosphorylation process controls Na,K-ATPase activity in the rat PCT. As a matter of fact, insulin increases the tyrosine phosphorylation level of the Na,K-ATPase catalytic subunit with the same time course and dose dependence as the stimulation of rubidium uptake, suggesting that tyrosine phosphorylation of the pump might be responsible for its activation (162). However, the causal relationship between tyrosine phosphorylation of Na,K-ATPase and increased sodium affinity still remains to be demonstrated directly. Insulin also reduces the inhibitory effect of dopamine on Na,K-ATPase (see next section) (27), and this effect may also participate in its overall stimulatory effect.

DOPAMINE INDUCES NA,K-ATPASE ENDOCYTOSIS VIA PKC ACTIVATION

Dopamine is produced from L-dopa by proximal tubules and its synthesis is increased by high sodium intake, making it a putative modulator of sodium and fluid handling in this nephron segment. As a matter of fact, dopamine decreases fluid and sodium reabsorption in the in vitro microperfused rabbit proximal tubule (36, 47). Accordingly, dopamine decreases the V_{max} of Na,K-ATPase in proximal tubules (53, 220, 10, 53, 55, 357) as well as in OK cells (98). Although dopamine also increases the apparent affinity of proximal tubule Na,K-ATPase for sodium (10, 220), the overall resulting effect in intact cells is inhibition of Na,K-ATPase (357, 375).

The mechanism of dopamine-induced decrease in V_{max} of Na,K-ATPase has been extensively studied in rat proximal tubules and in OK cells. Inhibition of Na,K-ATPase results from the activation of both dopamine DA_1 and DA_2 dopamine receptors (10, 53), but it is independent of PKA-dependent phosphorylation of the protein phosphatase 1 regulators DARPP-32 (11). Rather, dopamine-induced inhibition of Na,K-ATPase is mediated by PKC (97, 100), and more specifically by PKCζ (135).

Within minutes, dopamine induces a redistribution of Na,K-ATPase units from the plasma membrane toward intracellular compartments: the decreased number of Na,K-ATPase units expressed at the basolateral membrane (99) is associated with the sequential increase in Na,K-ATPase abundance in clathrin-coated pits (1 minute), early endosomes (2.5 minutes), and late endosomes (5 minutes) (97, 99). The inhibitory effect of dopamine is dependent on PKC-mediated phosphorylation of the Na,K-ATPase α subunit, which is achieved within 2.5 minutes (99). As a matter of fact, dopamine-induced internalization of Na,K-ATPase is abolished in OK cells expressing a truncated rat α_1 Na,K-ATPase subunit lacking the first 31 amino acids that include the two PKC phosphorylation sites (Ser-11 and Ser-18) (99). Although both Ser-11 and Ser-18 are phosphorylated in response to dopamine, only phosphorylation of Ser-18 is involved in the endocytosis of Na,K-ATPase (98). Interestingly, ERK-dependent phosphorylation of Ser-11 promotes endocytosis of Na,K-ATPase in response to PTH (243). Following endocytosis, the Na,K-ATPase α subunit is dephosphorylated in the late endosome compartment (99).

Dopamine-induced endocytosis of Na,K-ATPase is also associated with activation of phosphatidylinositol 3-kinase (PI3K), a critical enzyme for membrane traffic (100). However, dopamine-induced activation of PI3K is not secondary to its phosphorylation. Rather, Ser-18 phosphorylation of Na,K-ATPase α subunit serves as an anchor signal for the sequential recruitment of 14-3-3 protein (138) and of PI3K (442) to the membrane. In turn, activation of PI3K generates the local production of phosphatidylinositol 3-phosphate, which allows binding of Na,K-ATPase with adaptor protein-2 (AP2), recruitment of clathrin, and endocytosis of Na,K-ATPase. Tyr 537 of the Na,K-ATPase α subunit appears essential for binding AP2 (128). Concomitantly, dopamine activates protein phosphatase 2A that dephosphorylates dynamin 2 and allows its plasma membrane recruitment at the site of Na,K-ATPase endocytosis (139).

PHORBOL ESTERS INDUCE NA,K-ATPASE EXOCYTOSIS VIA PKC ACTIVATION

Under certain experimental conditions (see below), direct stimulation of PKC by the phorbol ester phorbol 12-myristate 13-acetate (PMA) activates Na,K-ATPase (161, 320, 321). Physiologically, PKC-dependent stimulation of proximal tubule Na,K-ATPase occurs in response to α-adrenergic agonists (25, 37) and likely participates to the antinatriuretic action of these catecholamines.

PMA-induced stimulation of Na,K-ATPase is mediated by PKCβ (135). PMA induces the phosphorylation of both Ser-11 and Ser-18, and experiments with α subunit mutants indicated that phosphorylation of the two residues is required for PMA action (136). Ouabain binding and biotin labeling of cell membrane proteins indicate that PMA increases the plasma membrane quantity of Na,K-ATPase. The recruitment of Na,K-ATPase is mediated by clathrin-coated vesicles, and results from PMA-induced interaction of Na,K-ATPase with adaptor protein-1 (AP-1). The functional effect of phorbol ester on Na,K-ATPase V_{max} through recruitment to the basolateral membrane may be amplified by a phorbol ester-induced increase in the affinity of the pump for intracellular sodium (161).

Under specific conditions, phorbol ester–induced activation of PKC inhibits Na,K-ATPase in proximal tubules. In a comparative study, phorbol 12,13 dibutyrate (PDBu) was shown to either inhibit or stimulate ouabain-sensitive rubidium uptake in rat proximal tubules under low or high O_2 conditions, respectively (161). While the stimulatory effect of PDBu is directly related to the phosphorylation level of the Na,K-ATPase catalytic subunit (90), the inhibitory effect is mediated by the PLA_2/monooxygenase pathway triggered in these cells in response to PKC stimulation (54). Activation of the phospholipase A_2/cytochrome P450-dependent monooxygenase pathway leads to the synthesis of arachidonic acid derivatives (20 HETE, 12(R)-HETE, and 11,12 DHT) that directly inhibit the pump activity (315, 349). Besides oxidative status, sodium also controls phorbol ester effect. PMA activates Na,K-ATPase at basal intracellular sodium concentration, whereas PMA inhibits Na,K-ATP when sodium concentration is higher than 16 mM (137). A similar dual action of PKC stimulation is also observed in response to the serotonin agonist (71).

PKA-MEDIATED REGULATION OF NA,K-ATPASE

In rat PCT, activation of the PKA pathway either has no effect or stimulates Na,K-ATPase activity. In one study, stimulation of adenylyl cyclase/PKA pathway by forskolin or by a cAMP analogue did not alter Na,K-ATPase activity (53). However, the same group had previously reported that irreversible activation of the protein G_s-adenylyl cyclase complex by cholera toxin stimulated Na,K-ATPase activity (52). Forskolin and cAMP analogues also stimulate the functional activity of Na,K-ATPase in the rabbit proximal tubule, independently of Na^+ availability (38, 70). cAMP analogues and forskolin also increase the phosphorylation level of Na,K-ATPase α subunit and stimulate ouabain sensitive rubidium uptake (91), two effects that are blocked by inhibition of PKA. Phosphorylation and stimulation of Na,K-ATPase displayed similar time courses and dose dependencies, strongly suggesting that stimulation of the pump resulted from the phosphorylation of its catalytic subunit. Thus, in proximal tubules, PKA activation likely stimulates Na,K-ATPase-mediated transport under physiological conditions.

PKA-dependent stimulation of Na,K-ATPase in proximal tubule seems paradoxical in view of the physiological action of parathyroid hormone (PTH) which is the main physiologic stimulus of the adenylyl cyclase/PKA pathway in the proximal tubule. Indeed, PTH primarily inhibits phosphate and bicarbonate reabsorption and secondarily reduces fluid reabsorption (reviewed in 298). In proximal tubules, however, the involvement of changes in Na,K-ATPase activity in these effects is difficult to predict since in proximal tubules, only part of the active transport of Na^+ across the basolateral membrane is directly mediated by Na,K-ATPase, with the remaining occurring via a Na^+–HCO_3^- cotransport (439). Because this latter pathway is abolished secondarily to PTH-induced inhibition of bicarbonate reabsorption, Na,K-ATPase might not be inhibited by PTH despite the observed decrease in water and solute reabsorption. Alternatively, PTH was proposed to inhibit proximal tubule Na,K-ATPase via PKC and not PKA (315). Thus, the PKA-mediated stimulation of Na,K-ATPase by PTH might be opposed by the inhibitory PKC-mediated pathway.

Control of Na,K-ATPase in Collecting Duct

The mammalian connecting tubules and collecting ducts are the main sites of the fine-tuning of sodium reabsorption that permits adjusting daily urinary sodium excretion to dietary intake. In these nephron segments, apical sodium entry is mediated by amiloride-sensitive sodium channels (ENaC). It has long been admitted that ENaC was the main regulated step of sodium transport, and that the activity of Na,K-ATPase was secondarily adapted through changes in intracellular sodium concentration brought about by changes in ENaC activity. However, it is now clearly established that the regulation of sodium transport results from the intimate regulation of both ENaC and Na,K-ATPase. In this chapter, we focus on aldosterone and sodium, the main factors that control sodium transport in the connecting duct and collecting tubule. We also consider the mechanism of sodium retention in nephrotic syndrome because it is a rare example of defective renal sodium handling resulting from a primary dysregulation of Na,K-ATPase. In recent years, this research field has profited from development of collecting-duct principal cell lines sensitive to most physiological regulatory factors, and in particular the mouse mpkCCD$_{Cl4}$ cell line (49), which facilitated addressing the mechanism of regulation.

REGULATION OF NA,K-ATPASE BY ALDOSTERONE

Within 4–5 days, adrenalectomy decreases Na,K-ATPase activity (V_{max}) by ~70% in collecting ducts (131, 146, 179, 304), and this effect is prevented by administration of aldosterone (303). Symmetrically, administration of either pharmacological or high physiological doses of mineralocorticoid (i.e., doses that increase the plasma aldosterone level up to that observed in response to sodium restriction) to adrenal-intact rats increases Na,K-ATPase activity in the collecting duct (142, 177, 302, 311). This time-dependent increase appears after a 24-hour latency and culminates after approximately 6 days. Administration of aldosterone to adrenalectomized animals (143, 146, 328) or in vitro addition of aldosterone to nephron segments isolated from adrenalectomized animals (31, 339) also increases the V_{max} of Na,K-ATPase activity in the collecting duct, but this effect is much more rapid than in adrenal-intact animals, as it is observed as early as 1 hour and reaches its maximum after only 2–3 hours (339). These early data indicate that aldosterone controls Na,K-ATPase activity in the collecting duct in both adrenal-intact and adrenalectomized animals, but with different time-courses: the lower the initial plasma aldosterone and CCD Na,K-ATPase activity are, the faster the stimulatory response (209). This suggests that different mechanisms account for aldosterone action in aldosterone-deplete and -replete animals.

The mechanism of aldosterone action on Na,K-ATPase in aldosterone-deplete animals was further investigated in CCDs from adrenalectomized animals or in collecting-duct principal cell lines starved of mineralocorticoids beforehand. Increased V_{max} of Na,K-ATPase observed in CCDs shortly after administration of aldosterone to adrenalectomized animals or in vitro addition of aldosterone to CCDs isolated from adrenalectomized animals is paralleled by an increase of Na,K-ATPase abundance (31). In mpkCCD$_{C14}$ cells, 2 hours treatment with aldosterone markedly increases cell surface expression of Na,K-ATPase through recruitment of a latent pool of pumps (382). Although cell fractionation and cell-surface labeling studies suggest that the latent pool of Na,K-ATPase is intracellular (97, 198), its exact intracellular localization is not yet established. All reports except one (328) concluded that this short-term stimulation of Na,K-ATPase occurs independently of the effect of aldosterone on apical ENaC and sodium entry (31, 187, 382). In both CCDs from adrenalectomized rats and mpkCCD$_{C14}$ cells, the stimulatory effect of aldosterone is fully abolished by inhibitors of transcription and translation (31, 382). Experiences in Xenopus oocytes coexpressing exogenous Na,K-ATPase and the serum and glucocorticoid-regulated kinase-1 (SGK1), an early aldosterone-induced gene, demonstrated that SGK1 increased the activity and cell surface expression of Na,K-ATPase (358, 444). This suggests that the short-term effect of aldosterone on recruitment of a latent pool of Na,K-ATPase may be mediated induction of SGK1. The early recruitment of latent Na,K-ATPase is followed by transcriptional stimulation of pump synthesis. As a matter of fact, in A6 cells, a cell line deriving from *Xenopus laevis* kidney, aldosterone induces an early (6-hour) increase in the abundance of mRNAs for both α_1 and β_1 subunits of Na,K-ATPase. The transcription rate of these mRNAs, determined by nuclear run-on assay, increases as soon as 15 minutes (406). Here again, this effect is blocked by inhibition of protein synthesis (406), suggesting that it might also be mediated by SGK1. Experiments in mp-kCCD$_{C14}$ cells transfected with human α_1–α_3 Na,K-ATPase isoforms indicate that only α_1 Na,K-ATPase is a target of aldosterone (381).

Fewer studies have addressed the mechanism of the delayed response to aldosterone observed in aldosterone-replete animals. Although long-term aldosterone is supposed to induce the synthesis of Na,K-ATPase, adrenalectomy and aldosterone administration to adrenal-intact animals induce only mild variation (for α_1) or no variation (for β_1) of the number of mRNAs (150, 154) in the CCD. It should be stressed, however, that (1) transcriptional upregulation of α_1 mRNAs may be sufficient to increase the rate of Na,K-ATPase synthesis if the α-subunit mRNA abundance is the limiting step, which may be proposed since β_1-subunit mRNAs are over twofold greater than α_1 subunit mRNAs in the CCD (Table 3); and (2) as discussed above, given the apparent high efficiency of the translational/post-translational process in Na,K-ATPase synthesis, a modest variation in mRNA quantity may lead to a higher relative increase in protein quantity. Finally, it should be mentioned that although aldosterone has no short-term effect (a few hours) on the V_{max} of Na,K-ATPase in the collecting duct of adrenal-intact rats, it does increase ouabain-sensitive rubidium uptake within 2 hours (175). This stimulation of the pump is likely accounted for by an aldosterone-induced increase of its affinity for Na$^+$, as observed in A6 cells (51).

REGULATION OF NA,K-ATPASE BY SODIUM AVAILABILITY

Acute increases in intracellular Na$^+$ concentration with sodium ionophores in cortical collecting ducts not only activates Na,K-ATPase activity through a substrate effect, but also rapidly increases the V_{max} and the number of active Na,K-ATPase units (32, 66). Because this rapid stimulation occurs independently of protein synthesis, it was proposed that increased intracellular Na$^+$ concentration triggers the recruitment of a latent pool of Na,K-ATPase units preexisting in the cells. The size of this pool is controlled by corticosteroids, as it decreases after adrenalectomy. Physiologically, an acute increase in intracellular sodium concentration and recruitment of Na,K-ATPase can be brought by vasopressin, through its V_2 receptors and cAMP and protein kinase–A signaling (109, 122, 198), and by hypotonicity-induced cell swelling (110). The vasopressin/cAMP-recruitable pool of Na,K-ATPase might be located in the trans-Golgi network (198), and its recruitment is mediated by activation of serine/threonine phosphatase-2A activity (67) and dephosphorylation of the Na,K-ATPase α subunit (126). Sodium ionophore and hypotonicity induce the recruitment of the same pool of Na,K-ATPase secondarily to increased Na$^+$ entry

and activation of protein kinase A, but this effect is independent of cAMP (411, 412). cAMP-independent activation of PKA results from the dissociation of a complex between NFκB, IκB and the catalytic subunit of PKA (413).

Long-term alteration of apical sodium entry also controls expression of Na,K-ATPase, but at transcriptional level. Thus, in a rat collecting-duct cell line, treatment with vasopressin increased the expression of Na,K-ATPase α-subunit mRNA (127). Conversely, a decrease in apical Na$^+$ entry in αENaC-deficient mice is associated with reduced Na,K-ATPase α-subunit mRNA expression, despite high plasma aldosterone (64).

The Na$^+$ load delivered to the various nephron segments was proposed very early as a factor modulating the regulation of Na,K-ATPase biosynthesis (241). Teleologically, the higher the Na$^+$ load the higher Na,K-ATPase is a satisfactory concept. The Na$^+$ load delivered to the collecting duct is specifically increased by inhibition of Na$^+$ reabsorption in the thick ascending limb by loop diuretics. Accordingly, the stimulatory effect of chronic administration of furosemide on collecting-duct Na,K-ATPase (145, 352) was initially attributed to increased Na$^+$ delivery, independently of aldosterone. However, administration of equidiuretic doses of piretanide, another loop diuretic acting on the same molecular target as furosemide, does not alter collecting-duct Na,K-ATPase (74). This study showed that the stimulatory effect of furosemide on collecting-duct Na,K-ATPase was curtailed by the of angiotensin-converting enzyme enalapril, but not by clamping changes in plasma aldosterone or by blocking angiotensin-1 receptors. In contrast, it is mimicked by inhibitors of bradykinin B2 receptors. The lack of stimulation observed in response to piretanide results from the dual effect of the diuretic that increases sodium delivery to the collecting duct (stimulatory signal) and increases circulating bradykinin (inhibitory signal). In contrast, furosemide only triggers the stimulatory response (74).

INDUCTION OF NA,K-ATPASE IS RESPONSIBLE FOR SODIUM RETENTION IN NEPHROTIC SYNDROME

Interstitial edema is a clinical expression of nephrotic syndrome. It is secondary to the accumulation of sodium in the extracellular compartment brought about by an imbalance between dietary sodium intake and urinary sodium output, along with alterations of fluid transfer across the capillary endothelial barrier. The intrarenal site and the mechanism of sodium retention have been investigated in the model of puromycin aminonucleoside (PAN)–induced nephrotic syndrome in the rat.

Both in vivo and in vitro studies demonstrated that the cortical collecting duct is the main site of increased sodium reabsorption in PAN nephrotic rats (123, 221). The hydrolytic and transport activities of Na,K-ATPase are increased twofold in the cortical collecting duct of PAN nephrotic rats (166, 414). The time course of Na,K-ATPase stimulation, which culminates at day 6 following PAN administration, is parallel to that of the decrease in urinary sodium excretion and the development of a positive sodium balance (121). Moreover, a linear inverse correlation between urinary sodium excretion and collecting-duct Na,K-ATPase activity is observed in three different experimental models of nephrotic syndrome (121). Stimulation of Na,K-ATPase activity is paralleled by increased abundance of α and β Na,K-ATPase subunits mRNAs and Na,K-ATPase protein at the basolateral membrane (122).

Induction of Na,K-ATPase is also associated with overexpression of ENaC at the apical border of collecting duct cells (244). However, a recent study indicates that induction of Na,K-ATPase is independent of ENaC stimulation. As a matter of fact, when PAN-induced hyperaldosteronemia is clamped, activation of ENaC is abolished whereas induction of Na,K-ATPase is not altered. Moreover, in response to PAN, aldosterone-clamped rats develop sodium retention and ascites with the same time course and efficiency as adrenal-intact rats. This demonstrates that induction of collecting-duct Na,K-ATPase is the primary cause of sodium retention in nephrotic syndrome, and that the sole induction of Na,K-ATPase, in the absence of ENaC activation, is sufficient to induce sodium retention and ascites.

Primary stimulation of Na,K-ATPase and of sodium transport, independently of ENaC, is also observed in the collecting duct in response to activation of the $ERK_{1,2}$ pathway (292).

In summary, the studies mentioned in the preceding paragraphs outline the complexity of the regulation of kidney Na,K-ATPase through phosphorylation/dephosphorylation of its catalytic subunit and at the transcriptional level. They demonstrate that (1) hormonal triggering of intracellular signaling pathways can rapidly alter the V_{max} of Na,K-ATPase and/or modulate its affinity for Na^+; (2) these changes are true regulatory mechanisms independent of the changes in apical Na^+; and (3) they are usually accompanied by concomitant regulation of apical pathways for Na^+ entry. Thus, these short-term regulatory mechanisms of Na,K-ATPase contribute to the control of whole-body sodium balance and to the maintenance of intracellular Na^+ homeostasis during the rapid changes in Na^+ reabsorption that characterize kidney function. Finally, primary alterations of Na,K-ATPase expression or function are of etiological relevance in pathophysiology.

H,K-ATPASES IN KIDNEY

The concept of H,K-ATPase has emerged from confronting the functional properties of acid secretion in the gastric mucosa based on knowledge of the archetypal Na,K-ATPase. Gastric H,K-ATPase can be defined on the basis of enzymatic, functional, pharmacological, molecular, and pathophysiological criteria (165), which include: ATP hydrolyzing activity stimulated by submillimolar concentrations of K^+ in the absence of Na, active electroneutral exchange of intracel-

lular H against extracellular K, sensitivity to vanadate, omeprazole and Sch 28080, and insensitivity to bafilomycin and ouabain. All these properties are found both in the native stomach tissue and in cells artificially coexpressing the cloned gastric H,K-ATPase α and β subunits (αHKg and βHKg).

The involvement of H,K-ATPase in the kidney has first emerged from the description of a primary active K^+ reabsorption process (191) and of a H,K-ATPase-like activity in the mammalian distal nephron (21, 25). After the first cloning of gastric and colonic H,K-ATPase α subunits, further evidence came from the demonstration that mRNAs coding these two ATPases are expressed in the kidney. During the following two decades, attempts were made to establish causal relationships between H,K-ATPase-like activities, K-dependent K^+ and H^+ transport, and expression of αHKg and αHKc in the kidney. However, these studies often provided controversial results. Possible reasons for discrepancies include, first, that physiological species differences, in particular the renal adaptation of rabbits and rodents to K^+ depletion, have not always been considered. Next, in contrast to gastric H,K-ATPase, the functional and pharmacological properties of colonic H,K-ATPase characterized in artificial systems are likely different from those expressed in native tissue. The β subunit associated with αHKc in native kidney tissue, which has not yet been identified, and putatively, the FXTD protein, may account in part for the differences. Finally, there is a functional redundancy in transport processes that account for proton and potassium transport in the distal tubule, making it difficult to determine the functional relevance of these individual processes.

However, recent studies in mice genetically deficient in either αHKg or αHKc have helped to delineate the roles of these two H,K-ATPases in renal function. In this chapter, we shall try to determine the specific inference of gastric and colonic H,K-ATPases in kidney H,K-ATPase-mediated events. Special attention will be given to studies carried out in K^+-replete and K^+-deplete animals when considering gastric and colonic H,K-ATPases, respectively. Indeed, kidney expression of αHKc is very low, or absent, in K^+-replete animals, whereas it is markedly induced in response to K^+ depletion. In addition, we consider separately studies in rabbits and in rodents.

Gastric H,K-ATPase

RENAL EXPRESSION OF GASTRIC H,K-ATPASE
Measurement of Na^+-independent, K^+-activated ATPase activity in isolated nephron segments (132, 178) was the first, although indirect, piece of evidence suggesting the presence of gastric H,K-ATPase in the kidney. Activity of this ATPase, referred to as type I K-ATPase, was evidenced in CCD and OMCD of normal rats (132), in CNT, CCD, and OMCD of normal rabbits (132, 178), and in CCD and OMCD of normal mice (125a). Functional pieces of evidence show that type I K-ATPase originates from α- and β- intercalated cells

in rat CCD and OMCD (260). Type I K-ATPase differs from ubiquitous Na,K-ATPase not only by its independence to sodium but also by its insensitivity to ouabain (up to 1 mM). Type I K-ATPase is inhibited by vanadate, a common feature of all P-type ATPases, and by more specific inhibitors of gastric H,K-ATPase such as omeprazole and the imidazopyridine Sch 28080. Thus, type I K-ATPase shares the kinetic and pharmacological properties of gastric H,K-ATPase in both gastric mucosa and artificial systems (247, 286). Type I K-ATPase is not detected in collecting ducts of mice genetically deficient in αHKg (125a), which directly demonstrates that type I K-ATPase activity is actually accounted for by gastric H,K-ATPase.

Except for two controversial studies that failed to detect the expression of αHKg mRNA in rat kidneys and rat collecting ducts (96, 119), most studies have concluded that it is present. In normal rats, moderate expression of αHKg mRNAs is demonstrated by Northern analysis in whole-kidney (133) and kidney-cortex preparations (3, 5). Expression of αHKg mRNAs is also evidenced in CCD and IMCD by RT-PCR (3). In situ hybridization reveals the presence of αHKg mRNAs in CNT, CCD, OMCD, and IMCD, and, to a lesser extent, in PST, CTAL, and DCT (3). This study also indicates that intercalated cells are more intensely labeled than principal cells in CNT and CCD. Expression of βHK mRNA was demonstrated by in situ hybridization in intercalated cells of CNT, CCD, and OMCD as well as principal cells of OMCD (inner stripe), and IMCD cells of normal rat kidney (80). Tags for αHKg and βHKg were not detected in transcriptomes from the different segments of the human nephron (Table 4), indicating that the mRNA-expression level of gastric H,K-ATPase subunits is very low in the human nephron.

Western blot reveals low amounts of a protein of the expected molecular weight for αHKg in the rat kidney (251, 313). Immunohistochemistry confirms the presence of αHKg immunoreactive material in the kidney, and localizes it in CCD and OMCD intercalated cells in the rat, rabbit, and human kidney (250, 432). In the human kidney, a faint staining is also observed in principal cells (250). In the rat kidney, based on the percentage of stained cells, it was proposed that only α-intercalated cells express αHKg. Another study, however, revealed that all intercalated cells of rat CCD, OMCD, and initial IMCD are stained (34), whereas the principal cells as well as terminal IMCD cells are not. Furthermore, double labeling with an anti–V-type H-ATPase antibody demonstrated the intracellular colocalization of H,K-ATPase and H-ATPase immunoreactivity (34). Thus, αHKg is present at the apical and basolateral poles of α- and β-intercalated cells, respectively. Western blot demonstrates immunoreactive material with the expected molecular weight for βHK in the rat, rabbit, mouse, and pig kidney (79). The localization of βHK along the nephron and in different cell types has not been investigated.

Altogether, these results indicate that mainly intercalated cells of the mammalian connecting tubule and collecting duct express the gastric H,K-ATPase, which accounts for type I K-ATPase activity. Given its cellular localization, gastric H,K-ATPase is supposed to participate in the acid–base handling by the distal tubule.

RENAL FUNCTION OF GASTRIC H,K-ATPASE

The functional contribution of H,K-ATPase to H^+–HCO_3^- transport has been evaluated along the collecting duct of the normal rat by in vitro microperfusion (192). Reabsorption of HCO_3^- is inhibited by luminal (but not peritubular) addition of Sch 28080 in the OMCD and initial IMCD, but not in the CCD. However, peritubular addition of Sch 28080 reduces HCO_3^- secretion induced by in vivo alkalosis in the CCD. These results suggest the involvement of apical H,K-ATPase in OMCD α-intercalated cells and in the basolateral membrane of CCD β-intercalated cells, at least during metabolic alkalosis. Involvement of H,K-ATPase in intracellular pH recovery after acidification in the terminal IMCD of the rat was also demonstrated in primary cultures of IMCD (316).

The functional role of collecting-duct H,K-ATPase has been more extensively studied in normal rabbits. In vitro microperfusion of rabbit OMCD indicated that HCO_3^- reabsorption is markedly reduced by luminal addition of Sch 28080, as well as nonpermeant inhibitors of gastric H,K-ATPase, and by removal of luminal K^+ (13, 14, 431). Further analysis was performed at the level of individual cells by measuring the rate of pH recovery after intracellular acidification. These studies reveal a Sch 28080–sensitive, K-dependent mechanism of H^+ extrusion in α- and β-intercalated cells of CCD (105, 293, 368, 426), and in OMCD, likely in α-intercalated cells (258). In both CCD and OMCD, H,K-ATPase-dependent transports are insensitive to ouabain (368, 431), as expected from the involvement of gastric H,K-ATPase. In rabbit OMCD, inhibition of apical K^+ conductance by Ba^{2+} reduces HCO_3^- reabsorption to the same extent as inhibition of H,K-ATPase by removal of luminal K^+ (13). This strongly suggests that K^+ ions accumulated within the cells by H,K-ATPase recycle across the apical membrane through K^+ channels, meaning that H,K-ATPase does not participate to transepithelial K^+ transport in the rabbit collecting duct.

The role of gastric H,K-ATPase in ion transport was also addressed using transgenic mice. The cytoplasmic domain of βHK contains a tyrosine-based signal that controls the endocytosis of the gastric holoenzyme (108). Transgenic mice expressing a mutant βHK in which the endocytosis signal has been disabled display constitutive hypersecretion of gastric acid and constitutive expression of H,K-ATPase at the apical membrane of stomach parietal cells (108). They also display constitutively active renal K^+ reabsorption (420), suggesting that gastric H,K-ATPase participates in K^+ reabsorption in the mouse kidney, at least when it is overexpressed at the apical membrane.

Thus, it appears surprising that transgenic mice deficient for αHKg do not display any alteration of the renal handling of proton and potassium (378), and that the rate of K-dependent proton secretion is similar in CCD-intercalated cells from wildtype and αHKg-deficient mice (327). However, K-dependent proton secretion is sensitive to Sch 28080 in wildtype mice, in agreement with the involvement of gastric H,K-ATPase, whereas it is insensitive to Sch 28080 in αHKg-deficient mice (327). This suggests that αHKg is involved in K-dependent proton secretion in mouse collecting duct but that its genetic deficiency is functionally compensated by expression of an other, yet unidentified, K-dependent proton transporter.

Altogether, these studies indicate that gastric H,K-ATPase expressed in collecting-duct intercalated cells from the normal rat, rabbit, and mouse kidney mainly participates in urinary acidification and/or HCO_3^- reabsorption, and that its contribution to a K^+-reabsorption process is weak unless it is artificially overexpressed.

REGULATION OF GASTRIC H,K-ATPASE IN KIDNEY

Although the involvement of gastric H,K-ATPase from collecting ducts in H^+–HCO_3^- transport has been suggested very early, only a few studies evaluated its adaptation to disorders of the acid–base balance. On the one hand, type I K-ATPase activity is increased in rat CCD and OMCD during hypercapnia-induced respiratory acidosis, whereas it is reduced by hypocapnia (141). On the other hand, chronic metabolic acidosis does not alter the expression of αHKg mRNAs in rat kidney (133), although it increases H,K-ATPase-mediated H^+ secretion by intercalated cells of the rabbit CCD (369). This suggests that regulation of gastric H,K-ATPase in metabolic acidosis occurs via a post-transcriptional mechanism.

Post-transcriptional control of gastric H,K-ATPase in rat collecting ducts is demonstrated by the in vitro stimulatory effects of calcitonin and isoproterenol on type I K-ATPase (260), two hormones that stimulate proton secretion and reabsorption in α- and β-intercalated cells, respectively (367). Stimulation of type I K-ATPase by calcitonin in α-intercalated cells is mediated by activation of $ERK_{1,2}$ by a cAMP-dependent and protein kinase A–independent mechanism. In this pathway, cAMP activates the guanine-nucleotide exchange factor Epac 1 (262). Stimulation of type I K-ATPase by isoproterenol in β-intercalated cells is also secondary to the activation of $ERK_{1,2}$, but through a protein kinase A–dependent activation of the Ras/Raf1 pathway (261).

The late distal tubule and the collecting duct of animals chronically submitted to dietary K^+ restriction no longer secrete potassium but reabsorb it by an active mechanism (167, 258, 314, 448). Based on the increase in K-ATPase activity observed in the collecting duct of K^+-depleted animals (132, 178), it was initially proposed that gastric H,K-ATPase was involved in renal K^+ reabsorption and was upregulated by K^+ restriction. However, later

studies indicated that (1) gastric H,K-ATPase is likely not involved in transepithelial transport of potassium in the collecting duct (see preceding discussion), and (2) expression of αHKg mRNAs and protein in the collecting duct is not altered in K^+-restricted animals (133, 251, 423). The apparent discrepancy between the stimulation of K-ATPase activity during K^+ depletion on the one hand, and the absence of involvement of gastric H,K-ATPase in K^+ reabsorption on the other, was resolved when it was shown that increased K-ATPase activity in the collecting duct of K-depleted rats is not accounted for by type I K-ATPase but by a type III ATPase that is sensitive to both Sch 28080 and ouabain (73, 441). Also, in vitro microperfusion of collecting ducts shows that H,K-ATPase-dependent reabsorption of bicarbonate and/or potassium is sensitive to ouabain in K-depleted rabbits (448) and rats (418), and therefore is not accounted for by gastric H,K-ATPase. Gastric H,K-ATPase is not stimulated by K-depletion; it is even inhibited since type I K-ATPase activity disappears in the collecting duct of K-depleted rats (73). This post-transcriptional inhibition of gastric H,K-ATPase might be related to the metabolic alkalosis that develops during K depletion.

Colonic H,K-ATPase

PHARMACOLOGICAL PROPERTIES OF COLONIC H,K-ATPASE EXPRESSED IN ARTIFICIAL SYSTEMS AND IN NATIVE KIDNEY TISSUE

Nongastric H,K-ATPase was initially cloned by Crowson and Shull (119) from the rat colon (and thus is known as colonic H,K-ATPase) and by Jaisser et al. (226) in the urinary bladder of the toad *B. marinus* (226). When coexpressed in the *Xenopus* oocyte with a toad β subunit, the *B. marinus* ATPase exchanges intracellular H^+ against extracellular K^+ in a ouabain- and Sch 28080–sensitive manner (226). The pharmacological properties of these ATPases were determined in different expression systems. Despite some discrepancies among reports, which apparently can be attributed neither to the different expression systems used nor to the different origin of the coexpressed β subunits, data summarized in Table 5 show that there is now a consensus that rat colonic H,K-ATPase is insensitive to Sch 28080 and moderately sensitive to ouabain (same order of sensitivity as the low-sensitivity Na,K-ATPase forms) when expressed in artificial systems. In contrast, ATP1AL1, the presumed human orthologue of rat colonic H,K-ATPase, is sensitive to both ouabain and Sch 28080 (Table 5).

Type III K-ATPase activity is detected in the collecting duct of K^+-depleted rats but not of normal rats. It was initially considered to be the functional counterpart of expressing colonic H,K-ATPase because both type III K-ATPase activity and αHKc mRNAs and protein abundance are increased during K^+ depletion. However, although its pharmacological profile is similar to that of amphibian nongastric H,K-ATPase and of human ATP1AL1, it proved to

TABLE 5   Pharmacological Properties of Colonic H,K-ATPase Expressed in Different Systems

Expression system	Subunit		Sensitivity to		Reference
	α	β	Ouabain	Sch 28080	
Xenopus oocyte	*Bufo m.* αHK	*Bufo m.* β2	25 μM (K$^+$ = 5 mM)	230 μM (K$^+$ = 5 mM)	226
Xenopus oocyte	Rat αHKc	*Bufo m.* β	970 μM (K$^+$ = 5 mM) 70 μM (K$^+$ = 0.2 mM)	Insensitive (0.5 mM) (K$^+$ = 5 mM)	107
Xenopus oocyte	Rat αHKc	Rat βHKg	390 μM (K$^+$ = 1 mM)	Insensitive (0.5 mM) (K$^+$ = 1 mM)	102
Xenopus oocyte	Rat αHKc	Rat β	640 μM (K$^+$ = 1 mM)	Insensitive (0.5 mM) (K$^+$ = 1 mM)	102
Sf9 cells	Rat αHKc	None	Insensitive (1 mM) (K$^+$ = 25 mM)	18% inhibition (0.1 mM) (K$^+$ = 1 mM)	264
HEK-293 cells	Rat αHKc	Rat βHKc or rat β	Insensitive (1 mM) (K$^+$ = 5 mM)	Insensitive (0.5 mM) (K$^+$ = 5 mM)	347
HEK-293 cells	Pig αHKc	Rabbit βHKg or torpedo β1	52 μM (K$^+$ = 13 mM)	8% inhibition (0.1 mM) (K$^+$ = 15 mM)	22
HEK-293 cells	Human ATP1AL1	Rabbit βHKg	42 μM (K$^+$ = 5 mM)	131 μM (K$^+$ = 5 mM)	200
Xenopus oocyte	Human ATP1AL1	Rabbit βHKg	13 μM (K$^+$ = 0.5 mM)	70% inhibition (0.5 mM) (K$^+$ = 0.5 mM)	295
Sf21 cells	Human ATP1AL1	Rabbit βHKg	84 μM (K$^+$ = 0 mM)	93 μM (K$^+$ = 0 mM)	1

The table lists the cells that were transfected with exogenous ATPase subunits (column 1), the nature and origin of transfectants (columns 2 and 3 for α and β subunits, respectively), and sensitivity to ouabain and Sch 28080 (columns 4 and 5). The nomenclature for ATPase subunits is the same as in the text except for the following: *Bufo marinus* αHK refers to a αP ATPase subunit cloned from *Bufo marinus*, rat βHKc refers to a β subunit cloned from rat colon, and ATP1AL1 is considered to be the human orthologue of αHKc. Sensitivities to drugs are indicated as (1) the concentration inducing 50% inhibition of the ATPase; (2) insensitive, which means that no significant inhibition was observed at the inhibitor concentration indicated in parentheses; or (3) percentage inhibition observed at inhibitor concentration indicated in parentheses. In all circumstances, the concentration of K$^+$ in the assay is indicated in parenthesis because K$^+$ behaves as a competitor of both ouabain and Sch 28080.

be clearly different from that of rat colonic H,K-ATPase, in that it is sensitive to both Sch 28080 (IC50 ≈ 1 μM) and ouabain (IC50 ≈ 20 μM) (73). Nonetheless, recent studies in αHKc-deficient mice demonstrated that type III K-ATPase activ-ity is accounted for by expression of colonic H,K-ATPase. Indeed, type III K-ATPase activity present in both CCD and OMCD of K$^+$-depleted wildtype mice is absent from collecting ducts of K$^+$-depleted αHKc-deficient mice (125a). This suggests that local factors specifically expressed in collecting duct cells are able to modify the pharmacological profile of the colonic H,K-ATPase α subunit.

RENAL EXPRESSION OF COLONIC H,K-ATPASE

With only one exception (224), all reports demonstrate that αHKc mRNAs are expressed in the kidney of normal rats (5, 133, 348): αHKc mRNAs are detected along the entire distal nephron, from MTAL to IMCD (5, 283). However, the expression level is low, at less than one mRNA copy per cell (283). The same holds for the human nephron in which the occurrence of the ATP1AL1-specific tag is very low (Table 5). In K$^+$-depleted rats, all studies report expression of αHKc mRNAs in the kidney (5, 133, 225, 252, 283), and when compared, the level of expression is higher in K$^+$-depleted rats than in normal ones (5, 133, 283); Northern analysis indicates a fivefold increase in the outer and inner medulla but no change in the cortex (5). Quantitative RT-PCR demonstrates a marked increase of expression in the OMCD of K$^+$-depleted rats (from 25 to >10,000 copies per millimeter of tubule length), but also in the CCD (from 200 to 5000 copies/mm) (283). Finally, in situ hybridization provided contradictory results regarding the cellular localization of αHKc mRNAs. In one study, only intercalated cells of OMCD and initial IMCD were labeled (5), whereas only OMCD principal cells were labeled in two other reports (225, 259).

In the normal rat, a protein of the expected size for αHKc is found in microsome-enriched kidney fractions (251), and immunohistochemistry reveals the labeling of the apical membrane of OMCD principal cells (348). Renal expression of αHKc is markedly increased in K$^+$-depleted rats, both at the whole kidney level (251, 348, 423) and in apical membrane of principal cells in OMCD. Curiously, K$^+$ depletion does not reveal labeling of CCD principal cells (348), although increased expression of αHKc also concerns the kidney cortex (423), and CCD from K$^+$-depleted rats displays increased mRNA expression (283) and increased type III K-ATPase activity (73).

In the normal rabbit kidney, αHKc mRNAs are expressed in CNT cells and in all three cell types of CCD and OMCD (156, 158). Immunohistochemistry reveals the presence of the αHKc protein at the apical pole of CNT cells (157, 405) and of the three cell types present in CCD and OMCD (405).

In transgenic mice carrying an insertional αHKc promoter–EGFP reporter gene construct, the transgene is specifically expressed in collecting duct principal cells (446).

Altogether, these studies demonstrate a specific expression of αHKc at the apical pole of principal cells of the rat and mouse collecting duct, and this expression is markedly increased in response to K⁺ depletion. This localization of αHKc in principal cells is consistent with the functional localization of type III K-ATPase (260). In the rabbit kidney, αHKc is also present in connecting tubule cells as well as intercalated cells of the collecting duct. This differential profile of expression of αHKc along the rabbit nephron on the one hand and the mouse and rat nephron on the other may be related to the different dietary behaviors (herbivorous vs. omnivorous) of these two groups of mammals and the associated differences in dietary potassium load.

RENAL FUNCTION OF COLONIC H,K-ATPASE

Given its major induction during K⁺ depletion, that is, a condition in which collecting ducts reabsorb rather than secrete potassium, and its location at the apical pole of principal cells, colonic H,K-ATPase was proposed as the motor for potassium reabsorption in the collecting duct of K⁺-depleted rats and mice. In the rabbit distal nephron, it may also participate to proton transport in intercalated cells.

Using in vitro microperfusion, Wingo and colleagues provided the first evidence for H,K-ATPase–dependent reabsorption of potassium and bicarbonate in the OMCD from K⁺-deprived rabbits (433, 448, 449, 450). In OMCD, Sch 28080–sensitive rubidium lumen-to-bath flux was inhibited more than 50% by 100 µM of ouabain (448), consistent with the involvement of colonic H,K-ATPase. H,K-ATPase–mediated proton transport was shown to originate in intercalated and not principal cells of OMCD from K⁺-depleted rabbits (258), but the cellular origin of K⁺ reabsorption has not been determined.

Sch 28080–sensitive K⁺ reabsorption also occurs in distal tubules accessible to in vivo micropuncture in K⁺-depleted rats but not in normal rats (314). In addition, part of bicarbonate reabsorption is inhibited by both ouabain and Sch 28080 in the inner medullary collecting duct of K⁺-depleted rats (417).

Surprisingly, αHKc-deficient mice do not display any renal phenotype, even when fed a K⁺-depleted diet (290). This indicates that an alternative transport mechanism functionally compensates for the deficiency in colonic H,K-ATPase, the nature and properties of which have not been investigated.

In artificial expression systems, colonic H,K-ATPase exchanges either protons or sodium against potassium (see previous discussion). Whether this also occurs in the kidney, and if so, the functional relevance of an apical colonic Na,K-ATPase in collecting duct principal cells, remain unaddressed questions.

REGULATION OF COLONIC H,K-ATPASE IN KIDNEY

As discussed above, dietary K⁺ restriction is a major inducing factor for expression of colonic H,K-ATPase in the kidney. Because chronic dietary K⁺ restriction induces met-

abolic alkalosis and reduces plasma aldosterone level, the question raises whether changes in the expression of collecting duct H,K-ATPase are directly related to K⁺ balance or are secondary to the associated changes in circulating corticosteroids and/or in acid–base balance.

The role of mineralocorticoids on the dietary control of H,K-ATPase was investigated in collecting ducts of rats clamped at no aldosterone, or physiological or high-plasma aldosterone (140). Results indicate that K⁺ depletion increased H,K-ATPase activity whatever the aldosterone status was, and that aldosterone had no effect per se (140). In the same line, adrenalectomy, aldosterone administration to adrenalectomized rats, as well as feeding a Na⁺-depleted diet to normal rats did not alter the expression of αHKc mRNAs in the kidney medulla (225, 348). Thus, aldosterone does not control the expression of H,K-ATPase in the collecting duct and does not intervene in its regulation by K⁺ balance. Similarly, increased expression of αHKc mRNAs in the kidney during K⁺ depletion is likely not related to alkalosis since it is observed in the absence of significant changes in plasma acid–base parameters (133). Also, low K⁺ upregulates H,K-ATPase-mediated H⁺ transport in a cell line derived from mouse OMCD, whereas low pH does not (204). Overexpression of αHKc mRNAs by dietary K⁺ restriction is under the control of pituitary hormones, since it is abolished in hypophysectomized rats (423).

Although metabolic alkalosis does not intervene in the response of colonic H,K-ATPase in the collecting duct, it does induce per se the expression of αHKc mRNAs in rabbit CCD (158). In contrast, metabolic acidosis does not alter αHKc mRNA expression in the rat kidney (133). Nonetheless, a decrease in intracellular pH brought about by increasing pCO₂ results in increased H,K-ATPase–mediated potassium and bicarbonate reabsorption in the CCD of K⁺-depleted rabbits (450, 451), demonstrating post-transcriptional regulation of colonic H,K-ATPase during acidosis.

Post-transcriptional regulation of colonic H,K-ATPase also occurs in the CCD of K⁺–depleted rats in response to vasopressin, which increases type III ATPase activity in a protein-kinase-A–dependent manner (260). In the long term, cyclic AMP also controls the expression of αHKc through binding to cAMP-responsive elements present on the proximal αHKc promoter (437).

In conclusion, gastric H,K-ATPase is expressed in intercalated cells of the distal nephron where, along with other systems, it participates to the transport of proton and the regulation of acid–base balance. Colonic H,K-ATPase is also expressed in the distal nephron, but in principal cells where it energizes potassium reabsorption, especially in case of dietary K⁺ restriction. None of these two ATPases appears essential for animal survival or even for maintenance of acid–base and potassium balance under all experimental conditions studied so far. Compensatory transport systems are able to palliate the genetic absence of either gastric or colonic H,K-ATPase in the kidney. The characterization of these compensatory mechanisms, and in particular whether they rely on the activity of yet unidentified ATPases, remains to be determined.

References

1. Adams G, Tillekeratne M, Yu CL, Pestov NB, Modyanov NN. Catalytic function of nongastric H,K-ATPase expressed in Sf-21 insect cells. *Biochemistry* 2001;40:5765–5776.

2. Agular PD, Sweadner KJ, Penniston JT, et al. Mutations in the Na$^+$/K$^+$-ATPase alpha 3 gene ATP1A3 are associated with rapid-onset dystonia parkinsonism. *Neuron* 2004;43: 169–175.

3. Ahn KY, Kone BC. Expression and cellular localization of mRNA encoding the gastric isoform of H$^+$-K$^+$-ATPase alpha-subunit in rat kidney. *Am J Physiol Renal Fluid Electrolyte Physiol* 1995;37:F99–F109.

4. Ahn KY, Madsen KM, Tisher CC, Kone BC. Differential expression and cellular distribution of mRNAs encoding a- and b-isoforms of Na$^+$-K$^+$-ATPase in rat kidney. *Am J Physiol Renal Fluid Electrolyte Physiol* 1993;265:F792–F801.

5. Ahn KY, Park KY, Kim KK, Kone BC. Chronic hypokalemia enhances expression of the H$^+$-K$^+$-ATPase alpha(2)-subunit gene in renal medulla. *Am J Physiol Renal Fluid Electrolyte Physiol* 1996;40:F314–F321.

6. Aizman R, Asher C, Fuzesi M, et al. Generation and phenotypic analysis of CHIF knockout mice. *Am J Physiol Renal Physiol* 2002;283:F569–F577.

7. Albers RW. Biochemical aspects of active transport. *Ann Rev Biochem* 1967;36:727–756.

8. Altendorf K, Siebers A, Epstein W. The KDP ATPase of *Escherichia coli*. *Ann N Y Acad Sci* 1992;671:228–243.

9. Apell H-J. Electrogenic properties of the Na,K pump. *J Membr Biol* 1989;110:103–114.

10. Aperia A, Bertorello A, Seri I. Dopamine causes inhibition of Na$^+$-K$^+$-ATPase activity in rat proximal convoluted tubule segments. *Am J Physiol* 1987;252:F39–F45.

11. Aperia A, Fryckstedt J, Svensson L, et al. Phosphorylated M_r 32,000 dopamine- and cAMP-regulated phosphoprotein inhibits Na$^+$,K$^+$-ATPase activity in renal tubule cells. *Proc Natl Acad Sci U S A* 1991;88:2798–2801.

12. Argüello JM, Peluffo RD, Feng JN, Lingrel JB, Berlin JR. Substitution of glutamic 779 with alanine in the Na,K-ATPase alpha sub-unit removes voltage dependence of ion transport. *J Biol Chem* 1996;271:24610–24616.

13. Armitage FE, Wingo CS. Luminal acidification in K-replete OMCD$_i$: contributions of H-K-ATPase and bafilomycin-A$_1$-sensitive H-ATPase. *Am J Physiol Renal Fluid Electrolyte Physiol* 1994;267:F450–F458.

14. Armitage FE, Wingo CS. Luminal acidification in K-replete OMCDi: inhibition of bicarbonate absorption by K removal and luminal Ba. *Am J Physiol* 1995;269:F116–F124.

15. Artigas P, Gadsby DC. Na$^+$/K$^+$-ligands modulate gating of palytoxin-induced ion channels. *Proc Natl Acad Sci U S A* 2003;100:501–505.

16. Artigas P, Gadsby DC. Large diameter of palytoxin-induced Na/K pump channels and modulation of palytoxin interaction by Na/K pump ligands. *J Gen Physiol* 2004;123: 357–376.

17. Arystarkhova E, Donnet C, Asinovski NK, Sweadner KJ. Differential regulation of renal Na,K-ATPase by splice variants of the gamma subunit. *J Biol Chem* 2002;277:10162–10172.

18. Arystarkhova E, Sweadner KJ. Tissue-specific expression of the Na,K-ATPase beta-3 subunit—the presence of beta-3 in lung and liver addresses the problem of the missing subunit. *J Biol Chem* 1997;272:22405–22408.

19. Arystarkhova E, Wetzel RK, Asinovski NK, Sweadner KJ. The g subunit modulates Na$^+$ and K$^+$ affinity of the renal Na,K-ATPase. *J Biol Chem* 1999;274:33183–33185.

20. Arystarkhova E, Wetzel RK, Sweadner KJ. Distribution and oligomeric association of splice forms of Na$^+$-K$^+$-ATPase regulatory gamma-subunit in rat kidney. *Am J Physiol Renal Fluid Electrolyte Physiol* 2002;282:F393–F407.

21. Arystarkhova EA, Lakhtina OE, Modyanov NN. Immunodetection of Na,K-ATPase alpha 3-isoform in renal and nerve tissues. *FEBS Lett* 1999;250:545–548.

22. Asano S, Hoshina S, Nakaie Y, et al. Functional expression of putative H$^+$-K$^+$-ATPase from guinea pig distal colon. *Am J Physiol Cell Physiol* 1998;44:C669–C674.

23. Axelsen KB, Palmgren MG. Evolution of substrate specificities in the P-type ATPase superfamily. *J Mol Evol* 1998;46:84–101.

24. Azuma KK, Hensley CB, Tang M-J, McDonough AA. Thyroid hormone specifically regulates skeletal muscle Na$^+$-K$^+$-ATPase a2- and b2-isoforms. *Am J Physiol* 1993;265:C680–C687.

25. Baines AD, Drangova R, Ho P. Role of diacylglycerol in adrenergic-stimulated ^{86}Rb uptake by proximal tubules. *Am J Physiol* 1990;258:F1133–F1138.

26. Bamberg K, Sachs G. Topological analysis of H$^+$,K$^+$-ATPase using in vitro translation. *J Biol Chem* 1994;269:16909–16919.

27. Banday AA, Asghar M, Hussain T, Lokhandwala MF. Dopamine-mediated inhibition of renal Na,K-ATPase is reduced by insulin. *Hypertension* 2003;41:1353–1358.

28. Barcroft LC, Moseley AE, Lingrel JB, Watson AJ. Deletion of the Na/K-ATPase alpha 1-subunit gene (Atp1a1) does not prevent cavitation of the preimplantation mouse embryo. *Mech Dev* 2004;121:417–426.

29. Barlet-Bas C, Arystarkhova E, Cheval L, et al. Are there several isoforms of Na,K-ATPase a subunit in the rabbit kidney? *J Biol Chem* 1993;268:11512–11515.

30. Barlet-Bas C, Cheval L, Khadouri C, Marsy S, Doucet A. Difference in the Na affinity of Na$^+$-K$^+$-ATPase along the rabbit nephron: modulation by K. *Am J Physiol Renal Fluid Electrolyte Physiol* 1990;259:F246–F250.

31. Barlet-Bas C, Khadouri C, Marsy S, Doucet A. Sodium-independent in vitro induction of Na$^+$,K$^+$-ATPase by aldosterone in renal target cells: permissive effect of triiodothyronine. *Proc Natl Acad Sci U S A* 1988;85:1707–1711.

32. Barlet-Bas C, Khadouri C, Marsy S, Doucet A. Enhanced intracellular sodium concentration in kidney cells recruits a latent pool of Na-K-ATPase whose size is modulated by corticosteroids. *J Biol Chem* 1990;265:7799–7803.

33. Barquin N, Ciccolella DE, Ridge KM, Sznajder JI. Dexamethasone upregulates the Na-K-ATPase in rat alveolar epithelial cells. *Am J Physiol Lung Cell Mol Physiol* 1997;17:L825–L830.

34. Bastani B. Colocalization of H-ATPase and H,K-ATPase immunoreactivity in the rat kidney. *J Am Soc Nephrol* 1995;5:1476–1482.

35. Baum M. Insulin stimulates volume absorption in the rabbit proximal convoluted tubule. *J Clin Invest* 1987;79:1104–1109.

36. Baum M, Quigley R. Inhibition of proximal convoluted tubule transport by dopamine. *Kidney Int* 1998;54:1593–1600.

37. Beach RE, Schwab SJ, Brazy PC, Dennis VW. Norepinephrine increases Na$^+$-K$^+$-ATPase and solute transport in rabbit proximal tubules. *Am J Physiol* 1987;252:F215–F220.

38. Beck JS, Marsolais M, Noël J, Breton S, Laprade R. Dibutyryl cyclic adenosine monophosphate stimulates the sodium pump in rabbit renal cortical tubules. *Renal Physiol Biochem* 1995;18:21–26.

39. Beggah A, Mathews P, Béguin P, Geering K. Degradation and endoplasmic reticulum retention of unassembled alpha- and beta-subunits of Na,K-ATPase correlate with interaction of bip. *J Biol Chem* 1996;271:20895–20902.

40. Beggah AT, Béguin P, Jaunin P, Peitsch MC, Geering K. Hydrophobic C-terminal amino acids in the b-subunit are involved in the assembly with a-subunit of Na,K-ATPase. *Biochemistry* 1993;32:14117–14124.

41. Beggah AT, Jaunin P, Geering K. Role of glycosylation and disulfide bond formation in the b subunit in the folding and functional expression of Na,K-ATPase. *J Biol Chem* 1997;272:10318–10326.

42. Béguin P, Beggah AT, Chibalin AV, et al. Phosphorylation of the Na,K-ATPase a-subunit by protein kinase A and C in vitro and in intact cells. Identification of a novel motif for PKC-mediated phosphorylation. *J Biol Chem* 1994;269:24437–24445.

43. Béguin P, Crambert G, Guennoun S, et al. CHIF, a member of the FXYD protein family, is a regulator of Na,K-ATPase distinct from the gamma-subunit. *EMBO J* 2001;20:3993–4002.

44. Béguin P, Crambert G, Monnet-Tschudi F, et al. FXYD7 is a brain-specific regulator of Na,K-ATPase alpha 1-beta isozymes. *EMBO J* 2002;21:3264–3273.

45. Béguin P, Peitsch MC, Geering K. a1 but not a2 or a3 isoforms of Na,K-ATPase are efficiently phosphorylated in a novel protein kinase C motif. *Biochemistry* 1996;35:14098–14108.

46. Béguin P, Wang XY, Firsov D, et al. The g subunit is a specific component of the Na, K-ATPase and modulates its transport function. *EMBO J* 1997;16:4250–4260.

47. Belloreuss E, Higashi Y, Kaneda Y. Dopamine decreases fluid reabsorption in straight portions of rabbit proximal tubule. *Am J Physiol* 1982;242:F634–F640.

48. Belusa R, Wang ZM, Matsubara T, et al. Mutation of the protein kinase C phosphorylation site on rat alpha-1 Na$^+$,K$^+$-ATPase alters regulation of intracellular Na$^+$ and pH and influences cell shape and adhesiveness. *J Biol Chem* 1997;272:20179–20184.

49. Bens M, Vallet V, Cluzeaud F, et al. Corticosteroid-dependent sodium transport in a novel immortalized mouse collecting duct principal cell line. *J Am Soc Nephrol* 1999;10:923–934.

50. Beron J, Forster I, Béguin P, Geering K, Verrey F. Phorbol 12-myristate 13-acetate down-regulates Na,K-ATPase independent of its protein kinase C site—decrease in basolateral cell surface area. *Mol Biol Cell* 1997;8:387–398.

51. Beron J, Mastroberardino L, Spillmann A, Verrey F. Aldosterone modulates sodium kinetics of Na,K-ATPase containing an alpha-1 subunit in A6 kidney cell epithelia. *Mol Biol Cell* 1995;6:261–271.

52. Bertorello A, Aperia A. Regulation of Na$^+$-K$^+$-ATPase activity in kidney proximal tubules: involvement of GTP binding proteins. *Am J Physiol* 1989;256:F57–F62.

53. Bertorello A, Aperia A. Inhibition of proximal tubule Na$^+$-K$^+$-ATPase activity requires simultaneous activation of DA$_1$ and DA$_2$ receptors. *Am J Physiol Renal Fluid Electrolyte Physiol* 1990;259:F924–F928.

54. Bertorello A, Aperia A. Na$^+$-K$^+$-ATPase is an effector protein for protein kinase C in renal proximal tubule cells. *Am J Physiol* 1989;256:F370–F373.

55. Bertorello A, Hokfelt T, Goldstein M, Aperia A. Proximal tubule Na+-K+-ATPase activity is inhibited during high-salt diet: evidence for DA-mediated effect. *Am J Physiol* 1988;254: F795–F801.

56. Bertorello AM, Aperia A, Walaas SI, Nairn AC, Greengard P. Phosphorylation of the catalytic subunit of Na$^+$,K$^+$-ATPase inhibits the activity of the enzyme. *Proc Natl Acad Sci U S A* 1991;88:11359–11362.

57. Besancon M, Simon A, Sachs G, Shin JM. Sites of reaction of the gastric H,K-ATPase with extracytoplasmic thiol reagents. *J Biol Chem* 1997;272:22438–22446.

58. Blanco G, DeTomaso AW, Koster J, Xie ZJ, Mercer RW. The a-subunit of the Na,K-ATPase has catalytic activity independent of the b-subunit. *J Biol Chem* 1994;269:23420–23425.

59. Blanco G, Xie ZJ, Mercer RW. Functional expression of the a2 and a3 isoforms of the Na,K-ATPase in baculovirus-infected insect cells. *Proc Natl Acad Sci U S A* 1993;90: 1824–1828.

60. Blaustein MP. Endogenous ouabain—role in the pathogenesis of hypertension. *Kidney Int* 1996;49:1748–1753.

61. Blaustein MP, Hamlyn JM. Pathogenesis of essential hypertension: a link between dietary salt and high blood pressure. *Hypertension* 1991;18(Suppl 3):III184–III195.

62. Blostein R. The influence of cytoplasmic sodium concentration on the stoichiometry of the sodium pump. *J Biol Chem* 1983;258:12228–12232.

63. Blostein R, Wilczynska A, Karlish SJD, Argüello JM, Lingrel JB. Evidence that ser(775) in the alpha subunit of Na,K-ATPase is a residue in the cation binding pocket. *J Biol Chem* 1997;272:24987–24993.

64. Blot-Chabaud M, Djelidi S, Courtois-Coutry N, et al. Coordinate control of Na,K-ATPase mRNA expression by aldosterone, vasopressin and cell sodium delivery in the cortical collecting duct. *Cell Mol Biol* 2001;47:247–253.

65. Blot-Chabaud M, Jaisser F, Gingold M, Bonvalet J-P, Farman N. Na$^+$-K$^+$-ATPase-dependent sodium flux in cortical collecting tubule. *Am J Physiol* 1988;255:F605–F613.

66. Blot-Chabaud M, Wanstok F, Bonvalet J-P, Farman N. Cell sodium-induced recruitment of Na$^+$-K$^+$-ATPase pumps in rabbit cortical collecting tubules is aldosterone-dependent. *J Biol Chem* 1990; 265:11676–11681.

67. Blot-Chabaud M, Coutry N, Laplace M, Bonvalet JP, Farman N. Role of protein phosphatase in the regulation of Na$^+$-K$^+$-ATPase by vasopressin in the cortical collecting duct. *J Membr Biol* 1996;153:233–239.

68. Boulanger BR, Lilly MP, Hamlyn JM, et al. Ouabain is secreted by the adrenal gland in awake dogs. *Am J Physiol Endocrinol Metab* 1993;264:E413–E419.

69. Brennan FE, Fuller PJ. Acute regulation by corticosteroids of channel-inducing factor gene messenger ribonucleic acid in the distal colon. *Endocrinology* 1999;140:1213–1218.

70. Breton S, Beck JS, Laprade R. cAMP stimulates proximal convoluted tubule Na$^+$-K$^+$-ATPase activity. *Am J Physiol Renal Fluid Electrolyte Physiol* 1994;266:F400–F410.

71. Budu CE, Efendiev R, Cinelli AM, Bertorello AM, Pedemonte CH. Hormonal-dependent recruitment of Na$^+$,K$^+$-ATPase to the plasmalemma is mediated by PKC beta and modulated by [Na$^+$]$_{(i)}$. *Br J Pharmacol* 2002;137:1380–1386.

72. Buffin-Meyer B, Verbavatz JM, Cheval L, et al. Regulation of Na$^+$, K$^+$-ATPase in the rat outer medullary collecting duct during potassium depletion. *J Am Soc Nephrol* 1998;9:538–550.

73. Buffin-Meyer B, Younes-Ibrahim M, Barlet-Bas C, et al. K depletion modifies the properties of SCH-28080-sensitive K-ATPase in rat collecting duct. *Am J Physiol Renal Fluid Electrolyte Physiol* 1997;41:F124–F131.

74. Buffin-Meyer B, Younes-Ibrahim M, El Mernissi G, et al. Differential regulation of collecting duct Na$^+$,K$^+$-ATPase and K$^+$ excretion by furosemide and piretanide: role of bradykinin. *J Am Soc Nephrol* 2004;15:876–884.

75. Bull PC, Thomas GR, Rommens JM, Forbes JR, Cox DW. The Wilson disease gene is a putative copper transporting P-type ATPase similar to the Menkes gene. *Nat Genet* 1993;5:327–337.

76. Burnay M, Crambert G, Kharoubi-Hess S, Geering K, Horisberger J-D. Electrogenicity of Na,K- and H,K-ATPase activity and presence of a positively charged amino acid in the fifth transmembrane segment. *J Biol Chem* 2003;278:19237–19244.

77. Burnay M, Geering K, Horisberger J-D. The *Bufo marinus* bladder H,K-ATPase carries out electroneutral ion transport. *Am J Physiol* 2001;281:F869–F874.

78. Burrow CR, Devuyst O, Li XH, et al. Expression of the beta 2-subunit and apical localization of Na$+$-K$+$-ATPase in metanephric kidney. *Am J Physiol Renal Fluid Electrolyte Physiol* 1999;46:F391–F403.

79. Callaghan JM, Tan SS, Khan MA, et al. Renal expression of the gene encoding the gastric H$^+$-K$^+$-ATPase beta-subunit. *Am J Physiol Renal Fluid Electrolyte Physiol* 1995;37:F363–F374.

80. Campbell-Thompson ML, Verlander JW, Curran KA, et al. In situ hybridization of H-K-ATPase beta-subunit mRNA in rat and rabbit kidney. *Am J Physiol* 1995;269:F345–F354.

81. Canessa CM, Horisberger J-D, Louvard D, Rossier BC. Mutation of a cysteine in the first transmembrane segment of Na-K-ATPase a subunit confers ouabain resistance. *EMBO J* 1992;11:1681–1687.

82. Canessa CM, Jaisser F, Horisberger J-D, Rossier BC. Structure–function relationship of Na,K-ATPase: the digitalis receptor. In: Caplan M, ed. *Cell Biology and Membrane Transport Processes*. San Diego: Academic Press, 1994:71–85.

83. Capasso JM, Rivard C, Berl T. The expression of the gamma subunit of Na-K-ATPase is regulated by osmolality via C-terminal Jun kinase and phosphatidylinositol 3-kinase-dependent mechanisms. *Proc Natl Acad Sci U S A* 2001;98:13414–13419.

84. Capasso JM, Rivard CJ, Berl T. Synthesis of the Na-K-ATPase gamma-subunit is regulated at both the transcriptional and translational levels in IMCD3 cells. *Am J Physiol Renal Physiol* 2005;288:F76–F81.

85. Capasso JM, Rivard CJ, Enomoto LM, Berl T. Chloride, not sodium, stimulates expression of the gamma subunit of Na/K-ATPase and activates JNK in response to hypertonicity in mouse IMCD3 cells. *Proc Natl Acad Sci U S A* 2003;100:6428–6433.

86. Capendeguy O, Horisberger J-D. Functional effects of Na$^+$,K$^+$-ATPase gene mutations linked to familial hemiplegic migraine. *Neuromol Med* 2005;6:105–116.

87. Capurro C, Coutry N, Bonvalet JP, et al. Cellular localization and regulation of CHIF in kidney and colon. *Am J Physiol Cell Physiol* 1996;40:C753–C762.

88. Carafoli E. Biogenesis: plasma membrane calcium ATPase—15 years of work on the purified enzyme. *FASEB J* 1994;8:993–1002.

89. Caride AJ, Chini EN, Yamaki M, Dousa TP, Penniston JT. Unique localization of mRNA encoding plasma membrane Ca^{2+} pump isoform 3 in rat thin descending loop of Henle. *Am J Physiol* 1995;269:F681–F685.

90. Carranza ML, Féraille E, Favre H. Protein kinase C-dependent phosphorylation of Na$^+$-K$^+$-ATPase alpha-subunit in rat kidney cortical tubules. *Am J Physiol Cell Physiol* 1996;40:C136–C143.

91. Carranza ML, Féraille E, Kiroytcheva M, Rousselot M, Favre H. Stimulation of ouabain-sensitive Rb-86(+) uptake and Na$+$,K$+$-ATPase alpha-subunit phosphorylation by a cAMP-dependent signalling pathway in intact cells from rat kidney cortex. *FEBS Lett* 1996;396:309–314.

92. Catty P, Dexaerde AD, Goffeau A. The complete inventory of the yeast saccharomyces cerevisiae P-type transport ATPases. *FEBS Lett* 1997;409:325–332.

93. Chabardes-Garonne D, Mejean A, Aude JC, et al. A panoramic view of gene expression in the human kidney. *Proc Natl Acad Sci U S A* 2003;100:13710–13715.

94. Cheval L, Barlet-Bas C, Doucet A. Characterization of the molecular isoforms of Na$^+$/K$^+$-ATPase subunits along the rat nephron by polymerase chain reaction. In: Bamberg E, Schoner W, eds. *The Sodium Pump*. Darmstadt: Steinkopff, 1994:704–709.

95. Cheval L, Doucet A. Measurement of Na-K-ATPase-mediated rubidium influx in single segments of rat nephron. *Am J Physiol Renal Fluid Electrolyte Physiol* 1990;259:F111–F121.

96. Cheval L, Elalouf JM, Doucet A. Re-evaluation of the expression of the gastric H,K-atpase alpha subunit along the rat nephron. *Pflügers Arch* 1997;433:539–541.

97. Chibalin AV, Katz AI, Berggren PO, Bertorello AM. Receptor-mediated inhibition of renal Na$^+$-K$^+$-ATPase is associated with endocytosis of its alpha- and beta-subunits. *Am J Physiol Cell Physiol* 1997;42:C1458–C1465.

98. Chibalin AV, Ogimoto G, Pedemonte CH, et al. Dopamine-induced endocytosis of Na$^+$, K$^+$-ATPase is initiated by phosphorylation of ser-18 in the rat alpha subunit and is responsible for the decreased activity in epithelial cells. *J Biol Chem* 1999;274:1920–1927.

99. Chibalin AV, Pedemonte CH, Katz AI, et al. Phosphorylation of the catalytic alpha-subunit constitutes a triggering signal for Na$^+$,K$^+$-ATPase endocytosis. *J Biol Chem* 1998;273:8814–8819.

100. Chibalin AV, Zierath JR, Katz AI, Berggren PO, Bertorello AM. Phosphatidylinositol 3-kinase-mediated endocytosis of renal Na$^+$,K$^+$-ATPase alpha subunit in response to dopamine. *Mol Biol Cell* 1998;9:1209–1220.

101. Clapp WL, Bowman P, Shaw GS, Patel P, Kone BC. Segmental localization of mRNAs encoding Na$^+$-K$^+$-ATPase a- and b-subunit isoforms in rat kidney using RT-PCR. *Kidney Int* 1994;46:627–638.

102. Codina J, Kone BC, Delmasmata JT, Dubose TD. Functional expression of the colonic H$^+$,K$^+$-ATPase alpha-subunit—pharmacologic properties and assembly with X$^+$,K$^+$-ATPase beta-subunits. *J Biol Chem* 1996;271:29759–29763.

103. Collins JH, Forbush B3, Lane LK, et al. Purification and characterization of an (Na$^+$ + K$^+$)-ATPase proteolipid labeled with a photoaffinity derivative of ouabain. *Biochim Biophys Acta* 1982;686:7–12.

104. Colonna TE, Huynh L, Fambrough DM. Subunit interactions in the Na,K-ATPase explored with the yeast two-hybrid system. *J Biol Chem* 1997;272:12366–12372.

105. Constantinescu A, Silver RB, Satlin LM. H-K-ATPase activity in pna-binding intercalated cells of newborn rabbit cortical collecting duct. *Am J Physiol Renal Fluid Electrolyte Physiol* 1997;41:F167–F177.

106. Cougnon M, Bouyer P, Planelles G, Jaisser F. Does the colonic H,K-ATPase also act as an Na,K-ATPase? *Proc Natl Acad Sci U S A* 1998;95:6516–6520.

107. Cougnon M, Planelles G, Crowson MS, et al. The rat distal colon P-ATPase alpha subunit encodes a ouabain- sensitive H$^+$,K$^+$-ATPase. *J Biol Chem* 1996;271:7277–7280.

108. Courtois-Coutry N, Roush D, Rajendran V, et al. A tyrosine-based signal targets H/K-atpase to a regulated compartment and is required for the cessation of gastric acid secretion. *Cell* 1997;90:501–510.

109. Coutry N, Farman N, Bonvalet JP, Blotchabaud M. Synergistic action of vasopressin and aldosterone on basolateral Na$^+$-K$^+$-ATPase in the cortical collecting duct. *J Membr Biol* 1995;145:99–106.

110. Coutry N, Farman N, Bonvalet J-P, Blot-Chabaud M. Role of cell volume variations in Na$^+$-K$^+$-ATPase recruitment and/or activation in cortical collecting duct. *Am J Physiol Cell Physiol* 1994;266:C1342–C1349.

111. Crambert G, Béguin P, Pestov NB, Modyanov NN, Geering K. bm, a structural member of the X,K-ATPase beta subunit family, resides in the ER and does not associate with any known X,K-ATPase alpha subunit. *Biochemistry* 2002;41:6723–6733.

112. Crambert G, Fuzesi M, Garty H, Karlish SJD, Geering K. Phospholemman (FXYD1) associates with Na,K-ATPase and regulates its transport properties. *Proc Natl Acad Sci U S A* 2002; 99:11476–11481.

113. Crambert G, Geering K. FXYD proteins: new tissue-specific regulators of the ubiquitous Na,K-ATPase. *Sci STKE* 2003;(166):RE1.

114. Crambert G, Hasler U, Beggah AT, et al. Transport and pharmacological properties of nine different human Na,K-ATPase isozymes. *J Biol Chem* 2000;275:1976–1986.

115. Crambert G, Horisberger J-D, Modyanov NN, Geering K. Human nongastric H$^+$-K$^+$-ATPase: transport properties of ATP1al1 assembled with different beta-subunits. *Am J Physiol Cell Physiol* 2002;283:C305–C314.

116. Crambert G, Li CM, Claeys D, Geering K. FXYD3 (Mat-8), a new regulator of Na, K-ATPase. *Mol Biol Cell* 2005;16:2363–2371.

117. Crambert G, Li CM, Swee LK, Geering K. FXYD7, mapping of functional sites involved in endoplasmic reticulum export, association with and regulation of Na,K-ATPase. *J Biol Chem* 2004;279:30888–30895.

118. Crambert G, Schaer D, Roy S, Geering K. New molecular determinants controlling the accessibility of ouabain to its binding site in human Na,K-ATPase alpha isoforms. *Mol Pharmacol* 2004;65:335–341.

119. Crowson MS, Shull GE. Isolation and characterization of a cDNA encoding the putative distal colon H$^+$,K$^+$-ATPase. Similarity of deduced amino acid sequence to gastric H$^+$,K$^+$-ATPase and Na$^+$,K$^+$-ATPase and mRNA expression in distal colon, kidney, and uterus. *J Biol Chem* 1992;267:13740–13748.

120. De Fusco M, Marconi R, Silvestri L, et al. Haploinsufficiency of ATP1A2 encoding the Na$^+$/K$^+$ pump alpha 2 subunit associated with familial hemiplegic migraine type 2. *Nat Genet* 2003;33:192–196.

121. Deschenes G, Doucet A. Collecting duct Na$^+$/K$^+$-ATPase activity is correlated with urinary sodium excretion in rat nephrotic syndromes. *J Am Soc Nephrol* 2000;11:604–615.

122. Deschenes G, Gonin S, Zolty E, et al. Increased synthesis and AVP unresponsiveness of Na,K-ATPase in collecting duct from nephrotic rats. *J Am Soc Nephrol* 2001;12:2241–2252.

123. Deschenes G, Wittner M, Di Stefano A, Jounier S, Doucet A. Collecting duct is a site of sodium retention in PAN nephrosis: a rationale for amiloride therapy. *J Am Soc Nephrol* 2001;12:598–601.

124. Despa S, Bossuyt J, Han F, et al. Phospholemman-phosphorylation mediates the b-adrenergic effects on Na/K pump function in cardiac myocytes. *Circ Res* 2005;97:252–259.

125. DeTomaso AW, Jian Xie Z, Liu G, Mercer RW. Expression, targeting, and assembly of functional Na,K-ATPase polypeptides in baculovirus -infected insect cells. *J Biol Chem* 1993;268:1470–1478.

125a. Dherbecourt O, Cheval L, Bloch-Faure M, Meneton P, Doucet A. Molecular identification of Sch28080-sensitive K-ATPase activities in the mouse kidney. *Pflügers Arch* 2006;451(6):769–775.

126. Djelidi S, Beggah A, Courtois-Coutry N, et al. Basolateral translocation by vasopressin of the aldosterone-induced pool of latent Na-K-ATPases is accompanied by alpha 1 subunit dephosphorylation: Study in a new aldosterone-sensitive rat cortical collecting duct cell line. *J Am Soc Nephrol* 2001;12:1805–1818.
127. Djelidi S, Fay M, Cluzeaud F, et al. Transcriptional regulation of sodium transport by vasopressin in renal cells. *J Biol Chem* 1997;272:32919–32924.
128. Done SC, Leibiger IB, Efendiev R, et al. Tyrosine 537 within the Na^+,K^+-ATPase alpha-subunit is essential for AP-2 binding and clathrin-dependent endocytosis. *J Biol Chem* 2002;277:17108–17111.
129. Dostanic I, Paul RJ, Lorenz JN, et al. The alpha(2)-isoform of Na-K-ATPase mediates ouabain-induced hypertension in mice and increased vascular contractility in vitro. *Am J Physiol Heart Circ Physiol* 2005;288:H477–H485.
130. Doucet A, Barlet-Bas C. Evidence for differences in the sensitivity to ouabain of Na-K-ATPase along the nephrons of rabbit kidney. *J Biol Chem* 1986;261:993–995.
131. Doucet A, Katz AI. Short-term effect of aldosterone on Na-K-ATPase in single nephron segments. *Am J Physiol* 1981;241:F273–F278.
132. Doucet A, Marsy S. Characterization of K-ATPase activity in distal nephron: stimulation by potassium depletion. *Am J Physiol* 1987;253:F418–F423.
133. Dubose TD, Codina J, Burges A, Pressley TA. Regulation of H^+-K^+-ATPase expression in kidney. *Am J Physiol Renal Fluid Electrolyte Physiol* 1995;38:F500–F507.
134. Eakle KA, Kabalin MA, Wang S-G, Farley RA. The influence of b subunit structure on the stability of Na^+/K^+-ATPase complexes and interaction with K^+. *J Biol Chem* 1994;269: 6550–6557.
135. Efendiev R, Bertorello AM, Pedemonte CH, et al. PKC-beta and PKC-zeta mediate opposing effects on proximal tubule Na^+,K^+-ATPase activity. *FEBS Lett* 1999;456:45–48.
136. Efendiev R, Bertorello AM, Pressley TA, et al. Simultaneous phosphorylation of Ser11 and Ser18 in the alpha-subunit promotes the recruitment of Na^+,K^+-ATPase molecules to the plasma membrane. *Biochemistry* 2000;39:9884–9892.
137. Efendiev R, Bertorello AM, Zandomeni R, Cinelli AR, Pedemonte CH. Agonist-dependent regulation of renal Na^+,K^+-ATPase activity is modulated by intracellular sodium concentration. *J Biol Chem* 2002;277:11489–11496.
138. Efendiev R, Chen ZP, Krmar RT, et al. The 14-3-3 protein translates the Na^+,K^+-ATPase alpha(1)-subunit phosphorylation signal into binding and activation of phosphoinositide 3-kinase during endocytosis.*J Biol Chem* 2005;280:16272–16277.
139. Efendiev R, Yudowski GA, Zwiller J, et al. Relevance of dopamine signals anchoring dynamin-2 to the plasma membrane during Na^+,K^+-ATPase endocytosis. *J Biol Chem* 2002;277:44108–44114.
140. Eiam-Ong S, Kurtzman NA, Sabatini S. Regulation of collecting tubule adenosine triphosphatases by aldosterone and potassium. *J Clin Invest* 1993;91:2385–2392.
141. Eiam-Ong S, Laski ME, Kurtzman NA, Sabatini S. Effect of respiratory acidosis and respiratory alkalosis on renal transport enzymes. *Am J Physiol* 1994;267:F390–F399.
142. El Mernissi G, Charbades D, Doucet A, et al. Changes in tubular basolateral membrane markers after chronic treatment. *Am J Physiol* 1983;245:F100–F109.
143. El Mernissi G, Doucet A. Short-term effect of aldosterone on renal sodium transport and tubular Na-K-ATPase in the rat. *Pflügers Arch* 1983;399:139–146.
144. El Mernissi G, Doucet A. Quantification of (3H)ouabain binding and turnover of Na-K-ATPase along the rabbit nephron. *Am J Physiol* 1984;247:F158–F167.
145. El Mernissi G, Doucet A. Stimulation of Na-K-ATPase in the rat collecting tubule by two diuretics: furosemide and amiloride. *Am J Physiol* 1984;247:F485–F490.
146. El Mernissi G, Doucet A. Short-term effects of aldosterone and dexamethasone on Na-K-ATPase along the rabbit nephron. *Pflügers Arch* 1983;399:147–151.
147. Eleno N, DiezPanero LM, Rodriguez-Lopez A, et al. Expression of the beta-isoforms of Na,K-ATPase in the renal cortex of rats. *Exp Nephrol* 1997;5:82–87.
148. Ellis-Davies GCR, Kaplan JH. Modification of lysine 501 in Na,K-ATPase reveals coupling between cation occupancy and changes in the ATP binding domain. *J Biol Chem* 1993;268: 11622–11627.
149. Emanuel JR, Garetz S, Stone L, Levenson R. Differential expression of Na^+, K^+-ATPase alpha- and beta-subunit mRNAs in rat tissues and cell lines. *Proc Natl Acad Sci U S A* 1987;84: 9030–9034.
150. Escoubet B, Coureau C, Bonvalet JP, Farman N. Noncoordinate regulation of epithelial Na channel and Na pump subunit mRNAs in kidney and colon by aldosterone. *Am J Physiol Cell Physiol* 1997;41:C1482–C1491.
151. Fambrough DM, Lemas MV, Hamrick M, et al. Analysis of subunit assembly of the Na-K-ATPase. *Am J Physiol Cell Physiol* 1994;266:C579–C589.
152. Farley RA, Tran CM, Carilli CT, Hawke D, Shively JE. The amino acid sequence of a fluorescein-labeled peptide from the active site of (Na, K)-ATPase. *J Biol Chem* 1984;259:9532–9535.
153. Farman N, Corthésy-Theulaz I, Bonvalet JP, Rossier BC. Localization of a-isoforms of Na^+-K^+-ATPase in rat kidney by in situ hybridization. *Am J Physiol Cell Physiol* 1991;260: C468–C474.
154. Farman N, Coutry N, Logvinenko N, et al. Adrenalectomy reduces a_1 and not b_1 Na^+-K^+-ATPase mRNA expression in rat distal nephron. *Am J Physiol Cell Physiol* 1992;263: C810–C817.
155. Farman N, Fay M, Cluzeaud F. Cell-specific expression of three members of the FXYD family along the renal tubule. *Ann N Y Acad Sci* 2003;986:428–436.
156. Fejes-Tóth G, Naray FT, Velazquez H, et al. Intrarenal distribution of the colonic H, K-ATPase mRNA in rabbit. *Kidney Int* 1999;56:1029–1036.
157. Fejes-Tóth G, Naray-Fejes-Toth A. Immunohistochemical localization of colonic H-K-ATPase to the apical membrane of connectingtubule cells. *Am J Physiol Renal Physiol* 2001; 281:F318–F325.
158. Fejes-Tóth G, Rusvai E, Longo KA, Narayfejestoth A. Expression of colonic H-K-ATPase mRNA in cortical collecting duct—regulation by acid/base balance. *Am J Physiol Renal Fluid Electrolyte Physiol* 1995;38:F551–F557.
159. Feng J, Orlowski J, Lingrel JB. Identification of a functional thyroid hormone response element in the upstream flanking region of the human Na, K-ATPase b1 gene. *Nucleic Acids Res* 1993;21:2619–2626.
160. Feng JN, Lingrel JB. Functional consequences of substitutions of the carboxyl residue glutamate 779 of the Na,K-ATPase. *Cell Mol Biol Res* 1995;41:29–37.
161. Féraille E, Carranza ML, Buffin-Meyer B, et al. Protein kinase C-dependent stimulation of Na^+-K^+-ATPase in rat proximal convoluted tubules. *Am J Physiol Cell Physiol* 1995;37: C1277–C1283.
162. Féraille E, Carranza ML, Rousselot M, Caverzasio J, Favre H. Insulin stimulates Na, K-ATPase through tyrosine phosphorylation of its a subunit in rat cortical collecting tubules. *J Am Soc Nephrol* 1995;6:336.
163. Féraille E, Carranza ML, Rousselot M, Favre H. Insulin enhances sodium sensitivity of Na-K-ATPase in isolated rat proximal convoluted tubule. *Am J Physiol* 1994;267:F55–F62.
164. Féraille E, Carranza ML, Rousselot M, Favre H. Modulation of Na^+,K^+-atpase activity by a tyrosine phosphorylation process in rat proximal convoluted tubule. *J Physiol (London)* 1997;498:99–108.
165. Féraille E, Marsy S, Cheval L, et al. Sites of antinatriuretic action of insulin along rat nephron. *Am J Physiol* 1992;263:F175–F179.
166. Féraille E, Vogt B, Rousselot M, et al. Mechanism of enhanced Na-K-ATPase activity in cortical collecting duct from rats with nephrotic syndrome. *J Clin Invest* 1993;91:1295–1300.
167. Fernandez R, Lopes MJ, De Lira RF, et al. Mechanism of acidification along cortical distal tubule of the rat. *Am J Physiol Renal Fluid Electrolyte Physiol* 1994;266:F218–F226.
168. Ferrandi M, Minotti E, Salardi S, et al. Ouabainlike factor in Milan hypertensive rats. *Am J Physiol Renal Fluid Electrolyte Physiol* 1992;263:F739–F748.
169. Ferrandi M, Molinari I, Barassi P, et al. Organ hypertrophic signaling within caveolae membrane subdomains triggered by ouabain and antagonized by PST 2238. *J Biol Chem* 2004;279:33306–33314.
170. Feschenko MS, Sweadner KJ. Phosphorylation of Na,K-atpase by protein kinase C at ser(18) occurs in intact cells but does not result in direct inhibition of ATP hydrolysis. *J Biol Chem* 1997;272:17726–17733.
171. Fiedler B, Scheiner-Bobis G. Transmembrane topology of alpha- and beta-subunits of Na^+, K^+-ATPase derived from beta-galactosidase fusion proteins expressed in yeast. *J Biol Chem* 1996;271:29312–29320.
172. Fisone G, Cheng SXJ, Nairn AC, et al. Identification of the phosphorylation site for cAMP-dependent protein kinase on Na^+,K^+-ATPase and effects of site-directed mutagenesis. *J Biol Chem* 1994;269:9368–9373.
173. Forbush B3. Cardiotonic steroid binding to Na,K-ATPase. *Curr Top Membr Transport* 1983;19:167–201.
174. Forbush B3, Kaplan JH, Hoffman JF. Characterization of a new photoaffinity derivative of ouabain: labeling of the large polypeptide and of a proteolipid component of the Na, K-ATPase. *Biochemistry* 1978;17:3667–3676.
175. Fujii Y, Takemoto F, Katz AI. Early effects of aldosterone on Na-K pump in rat cortical collecting tubules. *Am J Physiol Renal FluidElectrolyte Physiol* 1990;259:F40–F45.
176. Fuller W, Parmar V, Eaton P, Bell JR, Shattock MJ. Cardiac ischemia causes inhibition of the Na/K ATPase by a labile cytosolic compound whose production is linked to oxidant stress. *Cardiovasc Res* 2003;57:1044–1051.
177. Garg LC, Knepper MA, Burg MB. Mineralocorticoid effects on Na-K-ATPase in individual nephron segments. *Am J Physiol* 1981;240:F536–F544.
178. Garg LC, Narang N. Ouabain-insensitive K-adenosine triphosphatase in distal nephron segments of the rabbit. *J Clin Invest* 1988;81:1024–1028.
179. Garg LC, Narang N, Wingo CS. Glucocorticoid effects on Na-K ATPase in rabbit nephron segments. *Am J Physiol* 1985;248:F487–F491.
180. Garty H, Lindzen M, Scanzano R, et al. A functional interaction between CHIF and Na-K-ATPase: implication for regulation by FXYD proteins. *Am J Physiol Renal Physiol* 2002;283:F607–F615.
181. Geering K. The functional role of beta subunits in oligomeric P-type ATPases. *J Bioenerg Biomembr* 2001;33:425–438.
182. Geering K. Na,K-ATPase. *Curr Opin Nephrol Hypertens* 1997;6:434–439.
183. Geering K. FXYD proteins: new regulators of Na,K-ATPase. *Am J Physiol Am J Physiol Renal Physiol* 2005;290:F241–F250.
184. Geering K. The functional role of the b-subunit in the maturation and intracellular transport of Na,K-ATPase. *FEBS Lett* 1991;285:189–193.
185. Geering K, Beggah A, Good P, et al. Oligomerization and maturation of Na,K-ATPase—functional interaction of the cytoplasmic NH2 terminus of the beta subunit with the alpha subunit. *J Cell Biol* 1996;133:1193–1204.
186. Geering K, Crambert G, Yu CL, et al. Intersubunit interactions in human X,K-ATPases: role of membrane domains M9 and M10 in the assembly process and association efficiency of human, nongastric H,K-ATPase alpha subunits (ATP1al1) with known beta subunits. *Biochemistry* 2000;39:12688–12698.
187. Geering K, Girardet M, Bron C, Kraehenbühl J-P, Rossier BC. Hormonal regulation of (Na^+,K^+)-ATPase biosynthesis in the toad bladder. Effect of aldosterone and 3,5,3'-triiodo-L-thyronine. *J Biol Chem* 1982;257:10338–10343.
188. Gick GG, Hatala MA, Chon D, Ismail-Beigi F. Na,K-ATPase in several tissues of the rat: tissue-specific expression of subunit mRNAs and enzyme activity. *J Membr Biol* 1993;131: 229–236.
189. Gick GG, Ismail-Beigi F. Thyroid hormone induction of Na^+-K^+-ATPase and its mRNAs in a rat liver cell line. *Am J Physiol Cell Physiol* 1990;258:C544–C551.
190. Gick GG, Melikian J, Ismail-Beigi F. Thyroidal enhancement of rat myocardial Na,K-ATPase: preferential expression of a2 activity and mRNA abundance. *J Membr Biol* 1990; 115:273–282.
191. Giebisch G. Renal potassium transport. In: Giebisch G, Tosteson DC, Ussing HH, eds. *Membrane Transport in Biology*. Volume IV A. Berlin: Springer Verlag, 1979:215–298.

192. Gifford JD, Rome L, Galla JH. H+-K+-ATPase activity in rat collecting duct segments. *Am J Physiol Renal Fluid Electrolyte Physiol* 1992;262:F692–F695.

193. Gloor S, Antonicek H, Sweadner KJ, et al. The adhesion molecule on glia (AMOG) is a homologue of the b subunit of the Na,K-ATPase. *J Cell Biol* 1990;110:165–174.

194. Glynn IM. "All hands to the sodium pump." *J Physiol (London)* 1993;462:1–30.

195. Goldschmidt I, Grahammer F, Warth R, et al. Kidney and colon electrolyte transport in CHIF knockout mice. *Cell Physiol Biochem* 2004;14:113–120.

196. Goldshleger R, Tal DM, Karlish SJD. Topology of the alpha-subunit of Na,K-ATPase based on proteolysis—lability of the topological organization. *Biochemistry* 1995;34:8668–8679.

197. Goldshleger R, Tal DM, Moorman J, Stein WD, Karlish SJD. Chemical modification of Glu-953 of the a chain of Na+, K+-ATPase associated with inactivation of cation occlusion. *Proc Natl Acad Sci U S A* 1992;89:6911–6915.

198. Gonin S, Deschenes G, Roger F, et al. Cyclic AMP increases cell surface expression of functional Na,K-ATPase units in mammalian cortical collecting duct principal cells. *Mol Biol Cell* 2001;12:255–264.

199. Good PJ, Richter K, Dawid IB. A nervous system-specific isotype of the b subunit of Na+, K+-ATPase expressed during early development of *Xenopus laevis. Proc Natl Acad Sci U S A* 1990;879088–9092.

200. Grishin AV, Bevensee MO, Modyanov NN, et al. Functional expression of the cDNA encoded by the human ATP1AL1 gene. *Am J Physiol Renal Fluid Electrolyte Physiol* 1996;40: F539–F551.

201. Grishin AV, Sverdlov VE, Kostina MB, Modyanov NN. Cloning and characterization of the entire cDNA encoded by ATP1AL1—a member of the human Na,K/H,K-ATPase gene family. *FEBS Lett* 1994;349:144–150.

202. Guennoun S, Horisberger J-D. Cysteine-scanning mutagenesis study of the sixth transmembrane segment of the Na,K-ATPase a subunit. *FEBS Lett* 2002;513:277–281.

203. Guennoun S, Horisberger J-D. Structure of the 5th transmembrane segment of the Na, K-ATPase a subunit: a cysteine-scanning mutagenesis study. *FEBS Lett* 2000;482:144–148.

204. Guntupalli J, Onuigbo M, Wall S, et al. Adaptation to low-K+ media increases H+-K+-ATPase but not H+-ATPase-mediated pHi recovery in OMCD1 cells. *Am J Physiol* 1997;273: C558–C571.

205. Habermann E. Palytoxin acts through Na+,K+-ATPase. *Toxicon* 1989;27:1171–1187.

206. Hamlyn JM, Blaustein MP, Bova S, et al. Identification and characterization of a ouabain-like compound from human plasma. *Proc Natl Acad Sci U S A* 1991;88:6259–6263.

207. Hamlyn JM, Manunta P. Ouabain, digitalis-like factors and hypertension. *J Hypertens* 1992;10(Suppl 7):S99–S111.

208. Hansen O. Heterogeneity of Na,K-ATPase from kidney. *Acta Physiol Scand* 1992;146: 229–234.

209. Hayhurst RA, O'Neil RG. Time-dependent actions of aldosterone and amiloride on Na+-K+-ATPase of cortical collecting duct. *Am J Physiol* 1988;254:F689–F696.

210. Hebert H, Purhonen P, Thomsen K, Vorum H, Maunsbach AB. Renal Na,K-ATPase structure from cryo-electron microscopy of two-dimensional crystals. *Ann N Y Acad Sci* 2003;986:9–16.

211. Hensley CB, Azuma KK, Tang M-J, McDonough AA. Thyroid hormone induction of rat myocardial Na+-K+-ATPase: a1-, a2-, and b1-mRNA and -protein levels at steady state. *Am J Physiol Cell Physiol* 1992;262:C484–C492.

212. Hersey SJ, Sachs G. Gastric acid secretion. *Physiol Rev* 1995;75:155–189.

213. Hilge M, Siegal G, Vuister GW, et al. ATP-induced conformational changes of the nucleotide-binding domain of Na,K-ATPase. *Nat Struct Biol* 2003;10:468–474.

214. Hoffman JF. ATP compartmentation in human erythrocytes. *Curr Opin Hematol* 1997;4: 112–115.

215. Horisberger J-D. Recent insights into the structure and mechanism of the sodium pump. *Physiology* 2004;19:377–387.

216. Horisberger J-D. *The Na,K-ATPase: Structure-Function Relationship.* Austin, TX: Landes, 1994.

217. Horisberger J-D, Jaunin P, Good PJ, Rossier BC, Geering K. Coexpression of a1 with putative b3 subunits results in functional Na-K-pumps in *Xenopus* oocyte. *Proc Natl Acad Sci U S A* 1991;88:8397–8400.

218. Horisberger J-D, Kharoubi-Hess S. Functional differences between a subunit isoforms of the rat Na,K-ATPase expressed in *Xenopus* oocytes. *J Physiol (London)* 2002;539:669–680.

219. Horowitz B, Hensley CB, Quintero M, et al. Differential regulation of Na, K-ATPase alpha 1, alpha 2, and beta subunit mRNA and protein levels by thyroid hormone. *J Biol Chem* 1990;265:14308–14314.

220. Ibarra F, Aperia A, Svensson L-B, Eklöf A-C, Greengard P. Bidirectional regulation of Na+,K+-ATPase activity by dopamine and an a-adrenergic agonist. *Proc Natl Acad Sci U S A* 1993;90:21–24.

221. Ichikawa I, Rennke HG, Hoyer JR, et al. Role for intrarenal mechanisms in the impaired salt excretion of experimental nephrotic syndrome. *J Clin Invest* 1983;71:91–103.

222. Ikeda K, Onimaru H, Yamada J, et al. Malfunction of respiratory-related neuronal activity in Na+,K+-ATPase alpha 2 subunit–deficient mice is attributable to abnormal Cl− homeostasis in brainstem neurons. *J Neurosci* 2004;24:10693–10701.

223. Ingbar DH, Duvick S, Savick SK, et al. Developmental changes of fetal rat lung Na-K-ATPase after maternal treatment with dexamethasone. *Am J Physiol Lung Cell Mol Physiol* 1997;16: L665–L672.

224. Jaisser F, Coutry N, Farman N, Binder HJ, Rossier BC. A putative H,K-ATPase is selectively expressed in surface epithelial cells of rat distal colon. *Am J Physiol* 1993;265:C1080–C1089.

225. Jaisser F, Escoubet B, Coutry N, et al. Differential regulation of putative K+-ATPase by low-K+ diet and corticosteroids in rat distal colon and kidney. *Am J Physiol Cell Physiol* 1996;39:C679–C687.

226. Jaisser F, Horisberger J-D, Geering K, Rossier BC. Mechanisms of urinary K+ and H+ excretion: primary structure and functional expression of a novel H,K-ATPase. *J Cell Biol* 1993;123:1421–1429.

227. Jaisser F, Horisberger J-D, Rossier BC. Primary sequence and functional expression of a novel b subunit of the P-ATPase gene family. *Pflügers Arch* 1993;425:446–452.

228. Jaisser F, Jaunin P, Geering K, Rossier BC, Horisberger J-D. Modulation of the Na,K-pump function by the b-subunit isoforms. *J Gen Physiol* 1994;103:605–623.

229. James PF, Grupp IL, Grupp G, et al. Identification of a specific role for the Na,K-ATPase alpha 2 isoform as a regulator of calcium in the heart. *Mol Cell* 1999;3:555–563.

230. Jaunin P, Jaisser F, Beggah AT, et al. Role of the transmembrane and extracytoplasmic domain of b-subunits in subunit assembly, intracellular transport and functional expression of Na,K-pumps. *J Cell Biol* 1993;123:1751–1759.

231. Jewell EA, Lingrel JB. Comparison of the substrate dependence properties of the rat Na, K-ATPase a1, a2, and a3 isoforms expressed in HeLa cells. *J Biol Chem* 1991;266:16925–16930.

232. Jewell-Motz EA, Lingrel JB. Site-directed mutagenesis of the Na,K-ATPase: consequences of substitutions of negatively-charged amino acids localized in the transmembrane domains. *Biochemistry* 1993;32:13523–13530.

233. Jia LG, Donnet C, Bogaev RC, et al. Hypertrophy, increased ejection fraction, and reduced Na-K-ATPase activity in phospholemman-deficient mice. *Am J Physiol Heart Circ Physiol* 2005;288:H1982–H1988.

234. Jones DH, Li TY, Arystarkhova E, et al. Na,K-ATPase from mice lacking the gamma subunit (FXYD2) exhibits altered Na+ affinity and decreased thermal stability. *J Biol Chem* 2005;280:19003–19011.

235. Jorgensen PL. Sodium and potassium ion pump in kidney tubules. *Physiol Rev* 1980;60: 864–917.

236. Kamitani T, Ikeda U, Muto S, et al. Regulation of Na,K-ATPase gene expression by thyroid hormone in rat cardiocytes. *Circ Res* 1992;71:1457–1464.

237. Karlish SJD, Goldshleger R, Jorgensen PL. Location of Asn[831] of the a chain of Na/K-ATPase at the cytoplasmic surface. Implication for topological models. *J Biol Chem* 1993;268:3471–3478.

238. Karlish SJD, Goldshleger R, Stein WD. A 19-kDa C-terminal tryptic fragment of the a chain of Na/K-ATPase is essential for occlusion and transport of cations. *Proc Natl Acad Sci U S A* 1990;87:4566–4570.

239. Kashgarian M, Biemesderfer D, Caplan M, Forbush B. Monoclonal antibody to Na-K-ATPase: immunocytochemical localization along nephron segments. *Kidney Int* 1985;28: 899–913.

240. Katz AI, Doucet A, Morel F. Na-K-ATPase activity along the rabbit, rat, and mouse nephron. *Am J Physiol* 1979;237:114–120.

241. Katz AI, Epstein FH. The role of sodium-potassium-activated adenosine triphosphatase in the reabsorption of sodium by the kidney. *J Clin Invest* 1967;46:1999–2011.

242. Kawasaki-Nishi S, Nishi T, Forgac M. Proton translocation driven by ATP hydrolysis in V-ATPases. *FEBS Lett* 2003;545:76–85.

243. Khundmiri SJ, Bertorello AM, Delamere NA, Lederer ED. Clathrin-mediated endocytosis of Na+,K+-ATPase in response to parathyroid hormone requires ERK-dependent phosphorylation of Ser-11 within the alpha(1)-subunit. *J Biol Chem* 2004;279:17418–17427.

244. Kim SW, Wang WD, Nielsen J, et al. Increased expression and apical targeting of renal ENaC subunits in puromycin aminonucleoside-induced nephrotic syndrome in rats. *Am J Physiol Renal Physiol* 2004;286:F922–F935.

245. Kimura H, Mujais SK. Cortical collecting duct Na-K pump in obstructive nephropathy. *Am J Physiol Renal Fluid Electrolyte Physiol* 1990;258:F1320–F1327.

246. Kirtane A, Ismail-Beigi N, Ismail-Beigi F. Role of enhanced Na+ entry in the control of Na,K-ATPase gene expression by serum. *J Membr Biol* 1994;137:9–15.

247. Klaassen CHW, Van Uem TJF, De Moel MP, et al. Functional expression of gastric H, K-ATPase using the baculovirus expression system. *FEBS Lett* 1993;329:277–282.

248. Koenderink JB, Hermsen HPH, Swarts HGP, Willems PHGM, De Pont JJHHM. High-affinity ouabain binding by a chimeric gastric H+,K+-ATPase containing transmembrane hairpins M3-M4 and M5-M6 of the alpha(1)-subunit of rat Na+,K+-ATPase. *Proc Natl Acad Sci U S A* 2000;97:11209–11214.

249. Koenderink JB, Swarts HGP, Willems PHGM, Krieger E, De Pont JJHHM. A conformation specific interhelical salt bridge in the K+-binding site of gastric H,K-ATPase. *J Biol Chem* 2004;279:16417–16424.

250. Kraut JA, Helander KG, Helander HF, et al. Detection and localization of H+-K+-ATPase isoforms in human kidney. *Am J Physiol Renal Physiol* 2001;281:F763–F768.

251. Kraut JA, Hiura J, Besancon M, et al. Effect of hypokalemia on the abundance of HK alpha 1 and HK alpha 2 protein in the rat kidney. *Am J Physiol* 1997;272:F744–F750.

252. Kraut JA, Starr F, Sachs G, Reuben M. Expression of gastric and colonic H+-K+-ATPase in the rat kidney. *Am J Physiol Renal Fluid Electrolyte Physiol* 1995;37:F581–F587.

253. Kuhlbrandt W, Zeelen J, Dietrich J. Structure, mechanism, and regulation of the neurospora plasma membrane H+-ATPase. *Science* 2002;297:1692–1696.

254. Kuntzweiler TA, Argüello JM, Lingrel JB. Asp(804) and asp(808) in the transmembrane domain of the Na,K-ATPase alpha subunit are cation coordinating residues. *J Biol Chem* 1996;271:29682–29687.

255. Kuntzweiler TA, Wallick ET, Johnson CL, Lingrel JB. Glutamic acid 327 in the sheep alpha-1 isoform of Na+,K+-ATPase stabilizes a K+-induced conformational change. *J Biol Chem* 1995;270:2993–3000.

256. Kuroki DW, Minden A, Sanchez I, Wattenberg EV. Regulation of a c-Jun amino-terminal kinase/stress-activated protein kinase cascade by a sodium-dependent signal transduction pathway. *J Biol Chem* 1997;272:23905–23911.

257. Kuster B, Shainskaya A, Pu HX, et al. A new variant of the gamma subunit of renal Na,K-ATPase—identification by mass spectrometry, antibody binding, and expression in cultured cells. *J Biol Chem* 2000;275:18441–18446.

258. Kuwahara M, Fu WJ, Marumo F. Functional activity of H-K-ATPase in individual cells of OMCD—localization and effect of K+ depletion. *Am J Physiol Renal Fluid Electrolyte Physiol* 1996;39:F116–F122.

259. Laroche-Joubert N, Helies-Toussaint C, Marsy S, Doucet A. Cellular origin of H,K-ATPase in the colleting duct of normal and K-depleted rats. *J Am Soc Nephrol* 1997;8:37A.

260. Laroche-Joubert N, Marsy S, Doucet A. Cellular origin and hormonal regulation of K$^+$-ATPase activities sensitive to Sch-28080 in rat collecting duct. *Am J Physiol Renal Fluid Electrolyte Physiol* 2000;279:F1053–F1059.

261. Laroche-Joubert N, Marsy S, Luriau S, Imbert-Teboul M, Doucet A. Mechanism of activation of ERK and H-K-ATPase by isoproterenol in rat cortical collecting duct. *Am J Physiol Renal Physiol* 2003;284:F948–F954.

262. Laroche-Joubert N, Marsy S, Michelet S, Imbert-Teboul M, Doucet A. Protein kinase A–independent activation of ERK and H,K-ATPase by cAMP in native kidney cells—role of Epac I. *J Biol Chem* 2002;277:18598–18604.

263. Läuger P. A channel mechanism for electrogenic ion pumps. *Biochim Biophys Acta* 1979;552:143–161.

264. Lee JS, Rajendran VM, Mann AS, Kashgarian M, Binder HJ. Functional expression and segmental localization of rat colonic K-adenosine triphosphatase. *J Clin Invest* 1995;96:2002–2008.

265. Leenen FHH, Harmsen E, Yu H, Yuan B. Dietary sodium stimulates ouabainlike activity in adrenalectomized spontaneously hypertensive rats. *Am J Physiol Heart Circ Physiol* 1993;265:H421–H424.

266. Lemas MV, Hamrick M, Takeyasu K, Fambrough DM. 26 amino acids of an extracellular domain of the Na,K-ATPase a-subunit are sufficient for assembly with the Na,K-ATPase b-subunit. *J Biol Chem* 1994;269:8255–8259.

267. Lemas MV, Yu H-Y, Takeyasu K, Kone B, Fambrough DM. Assembly of Na,K-ATPase a-subunit isoforms with Na,K-ATPase b-subunit isoforms and H,K-ATPase b-subunit. *J Biol Chem* 1994;269:18651–18655.

268. Li C, Capendeguy O, Geering K, Horisberger J-D. A third Na$^+$ binding site in the sodium pump. *Proc Natl Acad Sci U S A* 2005;102:12706–12711.

269. Lichtstein D, Samuelov S, Gati I, et al. Identification of 11,13-dihydroxy-14-octadecaenoic acid as a circulating Na$^+$/K$^+$-ATPase inhibitor. *J Endocrinol* 1991;128:71–78.

270. Lingrel JB. Na,K-ATPase: Isoform structure, function, and expression. *J Bioenerg Biomembr* 1992;24:263–270.

271. Lingrel JB, Argüello JM, Van Huysse J, Kuntzweiler TA. Cation and cardiac glycoside binding sites of the Na,K-ATPase. *Ann N Y Acad Sci* 1998;834:194–206.

272. Lingrel JB, Van Huysse J, O'Brien W, et al. Structure-function studies of the Na,K-ATPase. *Kidney Int Suppl* 1994;44:S32–S39.

273. Lucking K, Nielsen JM, Pedersen PA, Jorgensen PL. Na-k-ATPase isoform (alpha3, alpha2, alpha1) abundance in rat kidney estimated by competitive rt-PCR and ouabain binding. *Am J Physiol Renal Fluid Electrolyte Physiol* 1996;40:F253–F260.

274.

275.

276. Ludens JH, Clark MA, Robinson FG, DuCharme DW. Rat adrenal cortex is a source of a circulating ouabainlike compound. *Hypertension* 1992;19:721–724.

277. Lutsenko S, Tsivkovskii R, Walker JM, Cooper MJ. The multifaceted role of the N-terminal domain in regulation of the Wilson's disease protein (WNDP), a human copper-transporting ATPase. *FASEB J* 2002;16:A462–A462.

278. Lyu RM, Farley RA. Amino acids val(115)-ile(126) of rat gastric H$^+$-K$^+$-ATPase confer high affinity for sch-28080 to Na$^+$-K$^+$-ATPase. *Am J Physiol Cell Physiol* 1997;41:C1717–C1725.

279. Maclennan DH, Kranias EG. Phospholamban: a crucial regulator of cardiac contractility. *Nature Rev Mol Cell Biol* 2003;4:566–577.

280. Maclennan DH, Rice WJ, Green NM. The mechanism of Ca^{2+} transport by sarco(endo)plasmic reticulum Ca^{2+}-ATPases. *J Biol Chem* 1997;272:28815–28818.

281. Magocsi M, Yamaki M, Penniston JT, Dousa TP. Localization of mRNAs coding for isozymes of plasma membrane Ca(2+)-ATPase pump in rat kidney. *Am J Physiol* 1992;263:F7–F14.

282. Malik N, Canfield VA, Beckers MC, Gros P, Levenson R. Identification of the mammalian Na,K-ATPase beta-3 subunit. *J Biol Chem* 1996;271:22754–22758.

283. Marsy S, Elalouf JM, Doucet A. Quantitative rt-PCR analysis of mRNAs encoding a colonic putative H,K-ATPase alpha subunit along the rat nephron—effect of K$^+$ depletion. *Pflügers Arch* 1996;432:494–500.

284. Martin DW, Sachs JR. Cross-linking of the erythrocyte (Na$^+$,K$^+$)-ATPase. Chemical cross-linkers induce a-subunit-band 3 heterodimers and do not induce a-subunit homodimers. *J Biol Chem* 1992;267:23922–23929.

285. Martin-Vasallo P, Dackowski W, Emanuel JR, Levenson R. Identification of a putative isoform of the Na,K-ATPase b subunit. Primary structure and tissue-specific expression. *J Biol Chem* 1989;264:4613–4618.

286. Mathews PM, Claeys D, Jaisser F, et al. Primary structure and functional expression of the mouse and frog a-subunit of the gastric H$^+$-K$^+$-ATPase. *Am J Physiol Cell Physiol* 1995;37:C1207–C1214.

287. McDonough AA, Geering K, Farley RA. The sodium pump needs its b subunit. *FASEB J* 1990;4:1598–1605.

288. McDonough AA, Magyar CE, Komatsu Y. Expression of Na$^+$-K$^+$-ATPase a- and b-subunits along rat nephron: isoform specificity and response to hypokalemia. *Am J Physiol Cell Physiol* 1994;267:C901–C908.

289. Meij IC, Koenderink JB, van Bokhoven H, et al. Dominant isolated renal magnesium loss is caused by misrouting of the Na$^+$,K$^+$-ATPase gamma-subunit. *Nat Genet* 2000;26:265–266.

290. Meneton P, Schultheis PJ, Greeb J, et al. Increased sensitivity to K$^+$ deprivation in colonic H,K-ATPase-deficient mice. *J Clin Invest* 1998;101:536–542.

291. Mercer RW, Biemesderfer D, Bliss DP, Jr., Collins JH, Forbush B3. Molecular cloning and immunological characterization of the gamma polypeptide, a small protein associated with the Na,K-ATPase. *J Cell Biol* 1993;121:579–586.

292. Michlig S, Mercier A, Doucet A, et al. ERK1/2 controls Na,K-ATPase activity and transepithelial sodium transport in the principal cell of the cortical collecting duct of the mouse kidney. *J Biol Chem* 2004;279:51002–51012.

293. Milton AE, Weiner ID. Intracellular pH regulation in the rabbit cortical collecting duct a-type intercalated cell. *Am J Physiol Renal Fluid Electrolyte Physiol* 1997;42:F340–F347.

294. Minh Tran C, Scheiner-Bobis G, Schoner W, Farley RA. Identification of an amino acid in the ATP binding site of Na$^+$/K$^+$-ATPase after photochemical labeling with 8-azido-ATP. *Biochemistry* 1994;33:4140–4147.

295. Modyanov NN, Mathews PM, Grishin AV, et al. Human ATP1al1 gene encodes a ouabain-sensitive H-K-ATPase. *Am J Physiol Cell Physiol* 1995;38:C992–C997.

296. Moller JV, Juul B, Lemaire M. Structural organization, ion transport, and energy transduction of ATPases. *Biochim Biophys Acta* 1996;1286:1–51.

297. Moncrief MBC, Maguire ME. Magnesium transport in prokaryotes. *J Biol Inorg Chem* 1999;4:523–527.

298. Morel F, Doucet A. Hormonal control of kidney functions at the cell level. *Physiol Rev* 1986;66:377–468.

299. Morrison BW, Moorman JR, Kowdley GC, et al. Mat-8, a novel phospholemman-like protein expressed in human breast-tumors, induces a chloride conductance in *Xenopus* oocytes. *J Biol Chem* 1995;270:2176–2182.

300. Moseley AE, Huddleson JP, Bohanan CS, et al. Genetic profiling reveals global changes in multiple biological pathways in the hearts of Na,K-ATPase alpha 1 isoform haploinsufficient mice. *Cell Physiol Biochem* 2005;15:145–158.

301. Moseley AE, Lieske SP, Wetzel RK, et al. The Na,K-ATPase alpha 2 isoform is expressed in neurons, and its absence disrupts neuronal activity in newborn mice. *J Biol Chem* 2003;278:5317–5324.

302. Mujais SK, Chekal A, Jones WJ, Hayslett JP, Katz AI. Modulation of renal sodium-potassium-adenosine triphosphatase by aldosterone. *J Clin Invest* 1985;76:170–176.

303. Mujais SK, Chekal MA, Jones WJ, Hayslett JP, Katz AI. Regulation of renal Na-K-ATPase in the rat. Role of the natural mineralo- and gluco-corticoid hormones. *J Clin Invest* 1984;73:13–19.

304. Mujais SK, Chekal MA, Lee S-M, Katz AI. Relationship between adrenal steroids and renal Na-K-ATPase. *Pflügers Arch* 1984;402:48–51.

305. Mullin JM, Snock KV, McGinn MT. Effects of apical vs. basolateral palytoxin on LLC-PK$_1$ renal epithelia. *Am J Physiol Cell Physiol* 1991;260:C1201–C1211.

306. Munson K, Garcia R, Sachs G. Inhibitor and ion binding sites on the gastric H,K-ATPase. *Biochemistry* 2005;44:5267–5284.

307. Munzer JS, Daly SE, Jewell-Motz EA, Lingrel JB, Blostein R. Tissue- and isoform-specific kinetic behavior of the Na,K-ATPase. *J Biol Chem* 1994;269:16668–16676.

308. Nakao M, Gadsby DC. Voltage dependence of the Na translocation by the Na/K pump. *Nature* 1986;323:628–630.

309. Nicholls MG, Richards AM, Lewis LK, Yandle TG. Welcome to ouabain—a new steroid hormone. *Lancet* 1991;338:543–544.

310. Nicholls MG, Richards AM, Lewis LK, Yandle TG. Ouabain—a new steroid hormone. *Lancet* 1995;346:1381–1382.

311. O'Neil RG, Hayhurst RA. Sodium-dependent modulation of the renal Na-K-ATPase: influence of mineralocorticoids on the cortical collecting duct. *J Membr Biol* 1986;85:169–179.

312. Ogawa H, Toyoshima C. Homology modeling of the cation binding sites of the Na$^+$ K$^+$-ATPase. *Proc Natl Acad Sci U S A* 2002;99:15977–15982.

313. Okusa MD, Gottardi CJ, Rajendran VM, Binder HJ, Caplan MJ. Expression of a protein in rat kidney and distal colon that is related to the gastric H,K-ATPase. *Cell Physiol Biochem* 1995;5:1–9.

314. Okusa MD, Unwin RJ, Velazquez H, Giebisch G, Wright FS. Active potassium absorption by the renal distal tubule. *Am J Physiol* 1992;262:F488–F493.

315. Ominato M, Satoh T, Katz AI. Regulation of Na-K-ATPase activity in the proximal tubule—role of the protein kinase c pathway and of eicosanoids. *J Membr Biol* 1996;152:235–243.

316. Ono S, Guntupalli J, Dubose TD. Role of H$^+$-K$^+$-ATPase in pH(i) regulation in inner medullary collecting duct cells in culture. *Am J Physiol Renal Fluid Electrolyte Physiol* 1996;39:F852–F861.

317. Orlowski J, Lingrel JB. Thyroid and glucocorticoid hormones regulate the expression of multiple Na,K-ATPase genes in cultured neonatal rat cardiac myocytes. *J Biol Chem* 1990;265:3462–3470.

318. Patchornik G, Munson K, Goldshleger R, et al. The ATP-Mg^{2+} binding site and cytoplasmic domain interactions of Na$^+$,K$^+$-ATPase investigated with Fe^{2+}-catalyzed oxidative cleavage and molecular modeling. *Biochemistry* 2002;41:11740–11749.

319. Paula S, Tabet MR, Ball WJ. Interactions between cardiac glycosides and sodium/potassium-ATPase: three-dimensional structure-activity relationship models for ligand binding to the E-2-P-i form of the enzyme versus activity inhibition. *Biochemistry* 2005;44:498–510.

320. Pedemonte CH, Pressley TA, Cinelli AR, Lokhandwala MF. Stimulation of protein kinase C rapidly reduces intracellular Na$^+$ concentration via activation of the Na$^+$ pump in OK cells. *Mol Pharmacol* 1997;52:88–97.

321. Pedemonte CH, Pressley TA, Lokhandwala MF, Cinelli AR. Regulation of Na,K-ATPase transport activity by protein kinase C. *J Membr Biol* 1997;155:219–227.

322. Pedersen PA, Rasmussen JH, Jorgensen PL. Consequences of mutations to the phosphorylation site of the alpha-subunit of Na,K-atpase for ATP binding and E(1)-E(2) conformational equilibrium. *Biochemistry* 1996;35:16085–16093.

323. Pedersen PA, Rasmussen JH, Nielsen JM, Jorgensen PL. Identification of asp(804) and asp(808) as Na$^+$ and K$^+$ coordinating residues in alpha-subunit of renal Na,K-ATPase. *FEBS Lett* 1997;400:206–210.

324. Peluffo RD, Garrahan PJ, Rega AF. Low affinity superphosphorylation of the Na,K-ATPase by ATP. *J Biol Chem* 1992;267:6596–6601.

325. Peng L, Martin-Vasallo P, Sweadner KJ. Isoforms of Na,K-ATPase alpha and beta subunits in the rat cerebellum and in granule cell cultures. *J Neurosci* 1997;17:3488–3502.

326. Pestov NB, Korneenko TV, Radkov R, et al. Identification of the beta-subunit for nongastric H-K-ATPase in rat anterior prostate. *Am J Physiol Cell Physiol* 2004;286:C1229–C1237.

327. Petrovic S, Spicer Z, Greeley T, Shull GE, Soleimani M. Novel Schering and ouabain-insensitive potassium-dependent proton secretion in the mouse cortical collecting duct. *Am J Physiol Renal Fluid Electrolyte Physiol* 2002;282:F133–F143.

328. Petty KJ, Kokko JP, Marver D. Secondary effect of aldosterone on Na-K-ATPase activity in the rabbit cortical collecting tubule. *J Clin Invest* 1981;68:1514–1521.
329. Pihakaski-Maunsbach K, Tokonabe S, Vorum H, et al. The gamma-subunit of Na-K-ATPase is incorporated into plasma membranes of mouse IMCD3 cells in response to hypertonicity. *Am J Physiol Renal Physiol* 2005;288:F650–F657.
330. Pihakaski-Maunsbach K, Vorum H, Locke EM, et al. Immunocytochemical localization of Na,K-ATPase gamma subunit and CHIF in inner medulla of rat kidney. *Ann N Y Acad Sci* 2003;986:401–409.
331. Polvani C, Blostein R. Protons as substitutes for sodium and potassium in the sodium pump reaction. *J Biol Chem* 1988;263:16757–16763.
332. Post RL, Hegyvary C, Kume S. Activation by adenosine triphosphate in the phosphorylation kinetics of sodium and potassium ion transport adenosine triphosphatase. *J Biol Chem* 1972;247:6530–6540.
333. Price EM, Rice DA, Lingrel JB. Structure-function studies of Na,K-ATPase. Site-directed mutagenesis of the border residues from the H1-H2 extracellular domain of the a subunit. *J Biol Chem* 1990;265:6638–6641.
334. Pu HX, Cluzeaud F, Goldshleger R, et al. Functional role and immunocytochemical localization of the gamma(a) and gamma(b) forms of the Na,K-ATPase gamma subunit. *J Biol Chem* 2001;276:20370–20378.
335. Pu HX, Scanzano R, Blostein R. Distinct regulatory effects of the Na,K-ATPase gamma subunit. *J Biol Chem* 2002;277:20270–20276.
336. Qiu LY, Koenderink JB, Swarts HGP, Willems PHGM, De Pont JJHHM. Phe(783), Thr(797), and Asp(804) in transmembrane hairpin M5-M6 of Na^+,K^+-ATPase play a key role in ouabain binding. *J Biol Chem* 2003;278:47240–47244.
337. Rabon EC, Reuben MA. The mechanism and structure of the gastric H,K-ATPase. *Annu Rev Physiol* 1990;52:321–344.
338. Rakowski RF, Sagar S. Found: Na^+ and K^+ binding sites of the sodium pump. *News Physiol Sci* 2003;18:164–168.
339. Rayson BM, Lowther SO. Steroid regulation of Na^+-K^+-ATPase: differential sensitivities along the nephron. *Am J Physiol* 1984;246:F656–F662.
340. Redondo J, Fiedler B, Scheiner-Bobis G. Palytoxin-induced Na^+ influx into yeast cells expressing the mammalian sodium pump is due to the formation of a channel within the enzyme. *Mol Pharmacol* 1996;49:49–57.
341. Ridker PM. Toxic effects of herbal teas. *Arch Environ Health* 1987;42:133–136.
342. Robinson JD, Pratap PR. Indicators of conformational changes in the Na^+/K^+-ATPase and their interpretation. *Biochim Biophys Acta* 1993;1154:83–104.
343. Sachs G, Shin JM, Briving C, Wallmark B, Hersey S. The pharmacology of the gastric acid pump—the H^+,K^+ ATPase. *Annu Rev Pharmacol Toxicol* 1995;35:277–305.
344. Sali A, Blundell TL. Comparative protein modelling by satisfaction of spatial restraints. *J Mol Biol* 1993;234:779–815.
345. Sampson SR, Brodie C, Alboim SV. Role of protein kinase C in insulin activation of the Na-K pump in cultured skeletal muscle. *Am J Physiol Cell Physiol* 1994;266:C751–C758.
346. Sangan P, Kolla SS, Rajendran VM, Kashgarian M, Binder HJ. Colonic H-K-ATPase b-subunit: identification in apical membranes and regulation by dietary K depletion. *Am J Physiol Cell Physiol* 1999;45:C350–C360.
347. Sangan P, Thevananther S, Sangan S, Rajendran VM, Binder HJ. Colonic H-K-ATPase a- and b-subunits express ouabain-insensitive H-K-ATPase. *Am J Physiol Cell Physiol* 2000;278:C182–C189.
348. Sangan PC, Rajendran VM, Mann AS, Kashgarian M, Binder HJ. Regulation of colonic H-K-ATPase in large intestine and kidney by dietary Na-depletion and dietary K depletion. *Am J Physiol Cell Physiol* 1997;41:C685–C696.
349. Satoh T, Cohen HT, Katz AI. Different mechanism of renal Na,K-ATPase regulation by protein kinases in proximal and distal nephron. *Am J Physiol* 1993;265:F399–F405.
350. Schaefer M, Gitlin JD. Genetic disorders of membrane transport. IV. Wilson's disease and Menkes disease. *Am J Physiol Gastrointest Liver Physiol* 1999;276:G311–G314.
351. Scheiner-Bobis G, Farley RA. Subunit requirements for expression of functional sodium pumps in yeast cells. *Biochim Biophys Acta* 1994;1193:226–234.
352. Scherzer P, Wald H, Popovtzer MM. Enhanced glomerular filtration and Na^+-K^+-ATPase with furosemide administration. *Am J Physiol* 1987;252:F910–F915.
353. Schmalzing G, Ruhl K, Gloor SM. Isoform-specific interactions of Na,K-ATPase subunits are mediated via extracellular domains and carbohydrates. *Proc Natl Acad Sci U S A* 1997; 94:1136–1141.
354. Schmidt U, Dubach UC. Activity of (Na^+K^+)-stimulated adenosintriphosphatase in the rat nephron. *Pflügers Arch* 1969;306:219–226.
355. Schultheis PJ, Lingrel JB. Substitution of transmembrane residues with hydrogen-bonding potential in the a subunit of Na,K-ATPase reveals alterations in ouabain sensitivity. *Biochemistry* 1993;32:544–550.
356. Schwartz IL, Shlatz LJ, Kinnesaf E, Kinne R. Target-cell polarity and membrane phosphorylation in relation to mechanism of action of antidiuretic-hormone. *Proc Natl Acad Sci U S A* 1974;71:2595–2599.
357. Seri I, Kone BC, Gullans SR, et al. Locally formed dopamine inhibits Na^+-K^+-ATPase activity in rat renal cortical tubule cells. *Am J Physiol* 1988;255:F666–F673.
358. Setiawan I, Henke G, Feng YX, et al. Stimulation of *Xenopus* oocyte Na+,K(+)ATPase by the serum and glucocorticoid-dependent kinase sgk1. *Pflügers Arch* 2002;444: 426–431.
359. Shainskaya A, Karlish SJD. Evidence that the cation occlusion domain of Na/K-ATPase consists of a complex of membrane-spanning segments. Analysis of limit membrane-embedded tryptic fragments. *J Biol Chem* 1994;269:10780–10789.
360. Shamraj OI, Lingrel JB. A putative fourth Na^+,K^+-ATPase a-subunit gene is expressed in testis. *Proc Natl Acad Sci U S A* 1994;91:12952–12956.
361. Shelly DA, He SW, Moseley A, et al. Na+ pump alpha 2-isoform specifically couples to contractility in vascular smooth muscle: evidence from gene-targeted neonatal mice. *Am J Physiol Cell Physiol* 2004;286:C813–C820.
362. Shi HK, Holzman RL, Cluzeaud F, Farman N, Garty H. Membrane topology and immunolocalization of CHIF in kidney and intestine. *Am J Physiol Renal Fluid Electrolyte Physiol* 2001;280:F505–F512.
363. Shin JM, Sachs G. Identification of a region of the H,K-ATPase a subunit associated with the b subunit. *J Biol Chem* 1994;269:8642–8646.
364. Shull GE, Greeb J, Lingrel JB. Molecular cloning of three distinct forms of the Na^+, K^+-ATPase alpha-subunit from rat brain. *Biochemistry* 1986;25:8125–8132.
365. Shyjian AW, CeñV, Klein DC, Levenson R. Differential expression and enzymatic properties of the Na^+,K^+-ATPase a3 isoenzyme in rat pineal glands. *Proc Natl Acad Sci U S A* 1990; 87:1178–1182.
366. Shyjian AW, Levenson R. Antisera specific for the a1, a2, a3, and b subunits of the Na, K-ATPase: differential expression of a and b subunits in rat tissue membranes. *Biochemistry* 1989;28:4531–4535.
367. Siga E, Houillier P, Mandon B, Moine G, Derouffignac C. Calcitonin stimulates H^+ secretion in rat kidney intercalated cells. *Am J Physiol Renal Physiol* 1996;40:F1217–F1223.
368. Silver RB, Frindt G. Functional identification of H-K-ATPase in intercalated cells of cortical collecting tubule. *Am J Physiol Renal Fluid Electrolyte Physiol* 1993;264:F259–F266.
369. Silver RB, Mennitt P, Satlin LM. Stimulation of apical H-K-ATPase in intercalated cells of cortical collecting duct with chronic metabolic acidosis. *Am J Physiol Renal Fluid Electrolyte Physiol* 1996;39:F539–F547.
370. Silver S. Bacterial resistances to toxic metal ions—a review. *Gene* 1996;179:9–19.
371. Skou JC. Preparation from mammalian brain and kidney of the enzyme system involved in active transport of Na^+ and K^+. *Biochim Biophys Acta* 1962;58:314–325.
372. Skou JC. The influence of some cations on an adenosinetriphosphatase from peripheral nerves. *Biochim Biophys Acta* 1957;23:394–401.
373. Skou JC, Esmann M. The Na,K-ATPase. *J Bioenerg Biomembr* 1992;24:249–261.
374. Skriver E, Kavéus U, Hebert H, Maunsbach AB. Three-dimensional structure of Na, K-ATPase determined from membrane crystals induced by cobalt-tetrammine-ATP. *J Struct Biol* 1992;108:176–185.
375. Slobodyansky E, Aoki Y, Gaznabi AKM, et al. Dopamine and protein phosphatase activity in renal proximal tubules. *Am J Physiol Renal Physiol* 1995;37:F279–F284.
376. Smith TW. Digitalis: mechanisms of action and clinical use. *N Engl J Med* 1988;318:358–365.
377. Sorensen TLM, Moller JV, Nissen P. Phosphoryl transfer and calcium ion occlusion in the calcium pump. *Science* 2004;304:1672–1675.
378. Spicer Z, Miller ML, Andringa A, et al. Stomachs of mice lacking the gastric H,K-ATPase alpha-subunit have achlorhydria, abnormal parietal cells, and ciliated metaplasia. *J Biol Chem* 2000;275:21555–21565.
379. Stangeland B, Fuglsang AT, Malmström S, et al. P-type H^+- and Ca^{2+}-ATPases in plant cells. *Ann N Y Acad Sci* 1997;834:77–87.
380. Stengelin MK, Hoffman JF. Na,K-ATPase subunit isoforms in human reticulocytes—evidence from reverse transcription-pcr for the presence of alpha-1, alpha-3, beta-2, beta-3, and gamma. *Proc Natl Acad Sci U S A* 1997;94:5943–5948.
381. Summa V, Camargo SMR, Bauch C, Zecevic M, Verrey F. Isoform specificity of human Na^+,K^+-ATPase localization and alclosterone regulation in mouse kidney cells. *J Physiol (London)* 2004;555:355–364.
382. Summa V, Mordasini D, Roger F, et al. Short-term effect of aldosterone on Na,K-ATPase cell surface expression in kidney collecting duct cells. *J Biol Chem* 2001;276:47087–47093.
383. Sweadner KJ. Overlapping and diverse distribution of Na-K ATPase isozymes in neurons and glia. *Can J Physiol Pharmacol* 1992;70(Suppl):S255–S259.
384. Sweadner KJ. Enzymatic properties of separated isozymes of Na,K-ATPase. *J Biol Chem* 1985;260:11508–11513.
385. Sweadner KJ. Isozymes of the Na^+/K^+-ATPase. *Biochim Biophys Acta* 1989;988:185–220.
386. Sweadner KJ, Donnet C. Structural similarities of Na,K-ATPase and SERCA, the Ca^{2+}-ATPase of the sarcoplasmic reticulum. *Biochem J* 2001;356:685–704.
387. Sweadner KJ, Rael E. The FXYD gene family of small ion transport regulators or channels: cDNA sequence, protein signature sequence, and expression. *Genomics* 2000;68:41–56.
388. Tang XJ, Halleck MS, Schlegel RA, Williamson P. A subfamily of P-type ATPases with aminophospholipid transporting activity. *Science* 1996;272:1495–1497.
389. Terada Y, Knepper MA. Na^+-K^+-ATPase activities in renal tubule segments of rat inner medulla. *Am J Physiol* 1989;256:F218–F223.
390. Therien AG, Goldshleger R, Karlish SJD, Blostein R. Tissue-specific distribution and modulatory role of the gamma subunit of the Na,K-ATPase. *J Biol Chem* 1997;272:32628–32634.
391. Therien AG, Karlish SJD, Blostein R. Expression and functional role of the g subunit of the Na,K-ATPase in mammalian cells. *J Biol Chem* 1999;274:12252–12256.
392. Therien AG, Nestor NB, Ball WJ, Blostein R. Tissue-specific versus isoform-specific differences in cation activation kinetics of the Na,K-ATPase. *J Biol Chem* 1996;271:7104–7112.
393. Thompson CB, McDonough AA. Skeletal muscle Na,K-ATPase alpha and beta subunit protein levels respond to hypokalemic challenge with isoform and muscle type specificity. *J Biol Chem* 1996;271:32653–32658.
394. Toyoshima C, Inesi G. Structural basis of ion pumping by Ca^{2+}-ATPase of the sacroplasmic reticulum. *Annu Rev Biochem* 2004;73:269–292.
395. Toyoshima C, Mizutani T. Crystal structure of the calcium pump with a bound ATP analogue. *Nature* 2004;430:529–535.
396. Toyoshima C, Nakasako M, Nomura H, Ogawa H. Crystal structure of the calcium pump of sarcoplasmic reticulum at 2.6 A resolution. *Nature* 2000;405:647–655.
397. Toyoshima C, Nomura H. Structural changes in the calcium pump accompanying the dissociation of calcium. *Nature* 2002;418:605–611.
398. Toyoshima C, Nomura H, Tsuda T. Lumenal gating mechanism revealed in calcium pump crystal structures with phosphate analogues. *Nature* 2004;432:361–368.
399. Tran CM, Huston EE, Farley RA. Photochemical labeling and inhibition of Na,K-ATPase by 2-azido-ATP. Identification of an amino acid located within the ATP binding site. *J Biol Chem* 1994;269:6558–6565.

400. Tumlin JA, Hoban CA, Medford RM, Sands JM. Expression of Na- K-ATPase a- and b-subunit mRNA and protein isoforms in the rat nephron. *Am J Physiol Renal Fluid Electrolyte Physiol* 1994;266:F240–F245.

401. Tymiak AA, Norman JA, Bolgar M, et al. Physicochemical characterization of a ouabain isomer isolated from bovine hypothalamus. *Proc Natl Acad Sci U S A* 1993;90:8189–8193.

402. Van Huysse JW, Jewell EA, Lingrel JB. Site-directed mutagenesis of a predicted cation binding site of Na,K-ATPase. *Biochemistry* 1993;32:819–826.

403. Vasilets LA, Schmalzing G, Madefessel K, Haase W, Schwarz W. Activation of protein kinase C by phorbol ester induces downregulation of the Na+/K(+)-ATPase in oocytes of *Xenopus laevis*. *J Membr Biol* 1990;118:131–142.

404. Vasilets LA, Schwarz W. Regulation of endogenous and expressed Na+/K+ pumps in *Xenopus* oocytes by membrane potential and stimulation of protein kinases. *J Membr Biol* 1992;125:119–132.

405. Verlander JW, Moudy RM, Campbell WG, Cain BD, Wingo CS. Immunohistochemical localization of H-K-ATPase alpha(2c)-subunit in rabbit kidney. *Am J Physiol Renal Physiol* 2001;281:F357–F365.

406. Verrey F, Kraehenbühl J-P, Rossier BC. Aldosterone induces a rapid increase in the rate of Na,K-ATPase gene transcription in cultured kidney cells. *Mol Endocrinol* 1989;3:1369–1376.

407. Vignery A, Wang F, Qian H-Y, Benz EJ Jr, Gilmore-Hebert M. Detection of the Na+-K+-ATPase a3-isoform in multinucleated macrophages. *Am J Physiol Renal Fluid Electrolyte Physiol* 1991;260:F704–F709.

408. Vilsen B. Glutamate 329 located in the fourth transmembrane segment of the a-subunit of the rat kidney Na+,K+-ATPase is not an essential residue for active transport of sodium and potassium ions. *Biochemistry* 1993;32:13340–13349.

409. Vilsen B. A Glu329->Gln variant of the a-subunit of the rat kidney Na+,K+-ATPase can sustain active transport of Na+ and K+ and Na+,K+-activated ATP hydrolysis with normal turnover number. *FEBS Lett* 1993;333:44–50.

410. Vilsen B. Mutant Glu781Ala of the rat kidney Na+,K+-ATPase displays low cation affinity and catalyzes ATP hydrolysis at a high rate in the absence of potassium ions. *Biochemistry* 1995;34:1455–1463.

411. Vinciguerra M, Arnaudeau S, Mordasini D, et al. Extracellular hypotonicity increases Na,K-ATPase cell surface expression via enhanced Na+ influx in cultured renal collecting duct cells. *J Am Soc Nephrol* 2004;15:2537–2547.

412. Vinciguerra M, Deschenes G, Hasler U, et al. Intracellular Na+ controls cell surface expression of Na,K-ATPase via a cAMP-independent PKA pathway in mammalian kidney collecting duct cells. *Mol Biol Cell* 2003;14:2677–2688.

413. Vinciguerra M, Hasler U, Mordasini D, et al. Cytokines and sodium induce protein kinase A–dependent cell-surface Na,K-ATPase recruitment via dissociation of NF-kB/IkB/protein kinase A catalytic subunit complex in collecting duct principal cells. *J Am Soc Nephrol* 2005;16:2576–2585.

414. Vogt B, Favre H. Na+,K+-Atpase activity and hormones in single nephron segments from nephrotic rats. *Clin Sci* 1991;80:599–604.

415. Vulpe C, Levinson B, Whitney S, Packman S, Gitschier J. Isolation of a candidate gene for Menkes disease and evidence that it encodes a copper-transporting ATPase. *Nat Genet* 1993;3:7–13.

416. Wald H, Goldstein O, Asher C, Yagil Y, Garty H. Aldosterone induction and epithelial distribution of CHIF. *Am J Physiol Renal Fluid Electrolyte Physiol* 1996;40:F322–F329.

417. Wall SM, Mehta P, DuBose TD Jr. Dietary K+ restriction upregulates total and Sch-28080-sensitive bicarbonate absorption in rat tIMCD. *Am J Physiol Renal Physiol* 1998;275:F543–F549.

418. Wall SM, Mehta P, Dubose TD. Dietary K+ restriction upregulates total and Sch-28080-sensitive bicarbonate absorption in rat tIMCD. *Am J Physiol Renal Fluid Electrolyte Physiol* 1998;44.

419. Wallmark B, Briving C, Fryklund J, et al. Inhibition of gastric H+,K+-ATPase and acid secretion by SCH 28080, a substituted pyridyl(1,2a)imidazole. *J Biol Chem* 1987;262:2077–2084.

420. Wang T, Courtois-Coutry N, Giebisch G, Caplan MJ. A tyrosine-based signal regulates H-K-ATPase-mediated potassium reabsorption in the kidney. *Am J Physiol Renal Fluid Electrolyte Physiol* 1998;44:F818–F816.

421. Wang X, Horisberger J-D. Palytoxin effects through interaction with the Na,K-ATPase in *Xenopus* oocyte. *FEBS Lett* 1997;409:391–395.

422. Wang X, Jaisser F, Horisberger J-D. Role in cation translocation of the N-terminus of the a-subunit of the Na+,K+-pump of *Bufo*. *J Physiol (London)* 1996;491:579–594.

423. Wang Z, Baird N, Shumaker H, Soleimani M. Potassium depletion and acid-base transporters in rat kidney: differential effect of hypophysectomy. *Am J Physiol* 1997;272:F736–F743.

424. Ward DG, Cavieres JD. Solubilized ab Na,K-ATPase remains protomeric during turnover yet shows apparent negative cooperativity toward ATP. *Proc Natl Acad Sci U S A* 1993;90:5332–5336.

425. Watts AG, Sanchez-Watts G, Emanuel JR, Levenson R. Cell-specific expression of mRNAs encoding Na+,K+-ATPase a- and b-subunit isoforms within the rat central nervous system. *Proc Natl Acad Sci U S A* 1991;88:7425–7429.

426. Weiner ID, Milton AE. H+-K+-ATPase in rabbit cortical collecting duct b-type intercalated cell. *Am J Physiol Renal Fluid Electrolyte Physiol* 1996;39:F518–F530.

427. Wetzel RK, Pascoa JL, Arystarkhova E. Stress-induced expression of the gamma subunit (FXYD2) modulates Na,K-ATPase activity and cell growth. *J Biol Chem* 2004;279:41750–41757.

428. Wetzel RK, Sweadner KJ. Immunocytochemical localization of Na-K-ATPase alpha- and gamma-subunits in rat kidney. *Am J Physiol Renal Physiol* 2001;281:F531–F545.

429. Wetzel RK, Sweadner KJ. Phospholemman expression in extraglomerular mesangium and afferent arteriole of the juxtaglomerular apparatus. *Am J Physiol Renal Physiol* 2003;285:F121–F129.

430. Wilson PD, Devuyst O, Li XH, et al. Apical plasma membrane mispolarization of NaK-ATPase in polycystic kidney disease epithelia is associated with aberrant expression of the beta 2 isoform. *Am J Pathol* 2000;156:253–268.

431. Wingo CS, Armitage F E. Rubidium absorption and proton secretion by rabbit outer medullary collecting duct via H-K-ATPase. *Am J Physiol Renal Fluid Electrolyte Physiol* 1992;263:F849–F857.

432. Wingo CS, Madsen KM, Smolka A, Tisher CC. H-K-ATPase immunoreactivity in cortical and outer medullary collecting duct. *Kidney Int* 1990;38:985–990.

433. Wingo CS, Straub SG. Active proton secretion and potassium absorption in the rabbit outer medullary collecting duct. Functional evidence for proton-potassium-activated adenosine triphosphatase. *J Clin Invest* 1989;84:361–365.

434. Woo AL, James PF, Lingrel JB. Roles of the Na,K-ATPase alpha 4 isoform and the Na+/H+ exchanger in sperm motility. *Mol Reprod Dev* 2002;62:348–356.

435. Woo AL, James PF, Lingrel JB, et al. Characterization of the fourth alpha isoform of the Na,K-ATPase. *J Membr Biol* 1999;169:39–44.

436. Wuytack F, Raeymaekers L, Missiaen L. PMR1/SPCA Ca2+ pumps and the role of the Golgi apparatus as a Ca2+ store. *Pflügers Arch* 2003;446:148–153.

437. Xu XY, Zhang WZ, Kone BC. CREB trans-activates the murine H+-K+-ATPase alpha(2)-subunit gene. *Am J Physiol Cell Physiol* 2004;287:C903–C911.

438. Yau KW, Nakatani K, Tamura T. Sodium-calcium exchange and phototransduction in retinal photoreceptors. *Ann N Y Acad Sci* 1991;639:275–284.

439. Yoshitomi K, Burckhardt BC, Fromter E. Rheogenic sodium-bicarbonate cotransport in the peritubular cell membrane of rat renal proximal tubule. *Pflügers Arch* 1985;405:360–366.

440. Yoshizumi M, Ishimura Y, Masuda Y, et al. Inhibition by ouabain of palytoxin-induced catecholamine secretion and calcium influx into cultured bovine adrenal chromaffin cells. *Biochem Pharmacol* 1994;48:1047–1049.

441. Younes-Ibrahim M, Barlet-Bas C, Buffin-Meyer B, et al. Ouabain-sensitive and -insensitive k-ATPases in rat nephron—effect of K depletion. *Am J Physiol Renal Fluid Electrolyte Physiol* 1995;37:F1141–F1147.

442. Yudowski GA, Efendiev R, Pedemonte CH, et al. Phosphoinositide–3 kinase binds to a proline-rich motif in the Na+,K+-ATPase alpha subunit and regulates its trafficking. *Proc Natl Acad Sci U S A* 2000;97:6556–6561.

443. Zahler R, Zhang ZT, Manor M, Boron WF. Sodium kinetics of Na,K-ATPase a isoforms in intact transfected Hela cells. *J Gen Physiol* 1997;110:201–213.

444. Zecevic M, Heitzmann D, Camargo SMR, Verrey F. SGK1 increases Na,K-ATP cell-surface expression and function in *Xenopus laevis* oocytes. *Pflügers Arch* 2004;448:29–35.

445. Zerangue N, Kavanaugh MP. Flux coupling in a neuronal glutamate transporter. *Nature* 1996;383:634–637.

446. Zhang WZ, Xia XF, Zou L, et al. In vivo expression profile of a H+-K+-ATPase alpha(2)-subunit promoter-reporter transgene. *Am J Physiol Renal Physiol* 2004;286:F1171–F1177.

447. Zhao N, Lo LC, Berova N, et al. Na,K-ATPase inhibitors from bovine hypothalamus and human plasma are different from ouabain—nanogram scale CD structural analysis. *Biochemistry* 1995;34:9893–9896.

448. Zhou X, Wingo CS. H-K-ATPase enhancement of Rb efflux by cortical collecting duct. *Am J Physiol Renal Fluid Electrolyte Physiol* 1992;263:F43–F48.

449. Zhou X, Wingo CS. Mechanisms of rubidium permeation by rabbit cortical collecting duct during potassium restriction. *Am J Physiol Renal Fluid Electrolyte Physiol* 1992;263:F1134–F1141.

450. Zhou XM, Lynch IJ, Xia SL, Wingo CS. Activation of H+-K+-ATPase by CO2 requires a basolateral Ba2+-sensitive pathway during K restriction. *Am J Physiol Renal Physiol* 2000;279:F153–F160.

451. Zhou XM, Nakamura S, Xia SL, Wingo CS. Increased CO2 stimulates K/Rb reabsorption mediated by H-K-ATPase in CCD of potassium-restricted rabbit. *Am J Physiol Renal Physiol* 2001;281:F366–F373.

CHAPTER **4**

The Mammalian Transporter Families

Christopher P. Landowski, Yoshiro Suzuki, and Matthias A. Hediger
University of Bern, Bern, Switzerland

INTRODUCTION

To maintain cellular biological homeostatis, molecules must be delivered into and removed from cells and organelles. This critical task is performed by transport proteins that reside in plasma and intracellular membranes. Transport proteins facilitate the movement of vital biological molecules such as sugars, amino acids, vitamins, and nucleotides across cellular membranes along or against their electrochemical gradients. In the past, determining the molecular identity of the transporters responsible for various cellular activities has been a difficult challenge due to their hydrophobic and membrane-bound nature. Expression cloning made it possible to more rapidly identify transporters belonging to various functional classes, and greatly expanded the transporter field (669). Genome sequencing advanced the field further, by significantly facilitating the identification and characterization of many "missing" transporters and transporter families. Sequencing the human genome has uncovered approximately 2000 transporter related genes (5%–10% of the genome), underscoring their biological significance and role in cellular homeostasis. The solute carrier (SLC) families represent over 300 transporters and new ones are constantly being identified.

Transporters mediate transmembrane substrate flux via either passive or active mechanisms. Passive transporters facilitate diffusion of solutes such as glucose, amino acid, and urea across membranes down their electrochemical gradients. Active carriers mediate uphill transport of solutes and use various energy-coupling mechanisms. For instance, glucose transport across the intestinal brush border membrane is coupled to sodium cotransport to allow active accumulation of glucose in the enterocytes. Classically it was thought that active cotransporters in mammals were mainly coupled to sodium gradients, as illustrated by the intestinal Na^+–glucose cotransporter SGLT1 (307). However, later on, it was shown that proton gradients can also provide a driving force for mammalian solute transport, as demonstrated by the peptide transporter PEPT1 (197) and the divalent metal-ion transporter DMT1 (285).

Numerous inherited or acquired human diseases are caused by faulty transporter proteins or dysregulation of their expression (Table 1). A list of transporters and their involvement in human diseases can be found at the Website http://www.bioparadigms.org/slc/menu.asp. This chapter provides minisummaries for all the mammalian SLC transporter families. The SLC series comprises genes that encode passive transporters, ion-coupled transporters, and exchangers. Human gene symbols approved by the Human Gene Nomenclature Committee (http://www.gene.ucl.ac.k/nomenclature) are listed on the Bioparadigms Website. The database currently contains 43 different SLC transporter families (Table 1). In general, the genes are numbered numerically using the root abbreviation SLC (e.g., SLC1, solute carrier family 1), followed by the letter A and the number of the individual transporter (e.g., SLC1A2). A transporter has been assigned to a specific family if it has at least 20%–25% amino acid sequence identity to other members of that family.

GLUTAMATE–NEUTRAL AMINO ACID TRANSPORTER FAMILY (SLC1)

SLC1 family members provide cells with amino acids for metabolic function and play a critical role in the termination of synaptic transmission. In the kidney, glutamate transporters reabsorb filtered acidic amino acids, regulate ammonia and bicarbonate production, and protect cells from osmotic stress. This family contains five high-affinity glutamate transporters EAAC1 (SLC1A1), GLT-1 (SLC1A2), GLAST (SLC1A3), EAAT4 (SLC1A6), and EAAT5 (SLC1A7) and two neutral (alanine, serine, threonine, and cysteine) amino acid transporters, ASCT1 (SLC1A4) and ASCT2 (SLC1A5) (20). The glutamate transporters exhibit 44%–55% amino acid sequence identity with each other. ASCT1 and ASCT2 are 57% identical and show 40%–44% sequence identity to glutamate transporters.

These transporters are integral plasma membrane proteins that are predicted to have eight transmembrane domains, a large glycosylated loop between domains 3 and 4, and a predicted loop structure that extends into the "translocation pore" between domains 7 and 8 (276, 277). Many of these predicted features are observed in the recent crystal structure produced from a glutamate transporter homologue, Glt_Ph from *Pyrococcus horikoshii*, which reveals the

TABLE 1 Solute Carrier Family Series

	Number of Genes	Linked Disease
SLC1: High-affinity glutamate and neutral amino acid transporter family	7	Dicarboxylic amino aciduria (SLC1A1), amyotrophic lateral sclerosis (SLC1A2)
SLC2: Facilitative GLUT transporter family	14	Fanconi-Bickel syndrome (SLC2A2), non–insulin-dependent diabetes mellitus (SLC2A2,A4), hypoglycorrhachia (SLC2A1)
SLC3: Heavy subunits of heteromeric amino acid transporters	2	Type I cystinuria (SLC3A1)
SLC4: Bicarbonate transporter family	10	Hemolytic anemia (SLC4A1), distal renal tubular acidosis (SLC4A1), permanent proximal renal tubular acidosis (SLC4A4)
SLC5: Sodium–glucose cotransporter family	12	Glucose-glactose malabsorption (SLC5A1), familial renal glucosuria (SLC5A2), thyroid hormonogenesis (SLC5A5)
SLC6: Sodium- and chloride-dependent neurotransmitter transporter family	16	Epilepsy (SLC6A1), schizophrenia (SLC6A1), autism (SLC6A4), parkinsonism (SLC6A3), depression (SLC6A2)
SLC7: Cationic amino acid transporter/glycoprotein-associated family	13	Lysinuric protein intolerance (SLC7A7), type B cystinuria (SLC7A9)
SLC8: Na^+–Ca^{2+} exchanger family	3	—
SLC9: Na^+–H^+ exchanger family	9	—
SLC10: Sodium bile salt cotransport family	6	Primary bile acid malabsorption (SLC10A2)
SLC11: Proton-coupled metal ion transporter family	2	Hereditary hemochromatosis (SLC11A2)
SLC12: Electroneutral cation–Cl cotransporter family	9	Bartter's syndrome type I (SLC12A1), Gitelman's syndrome (SLC12A3), peripheral neuropathy (SLC12A6)
SLC13: Human Na^+-sulfate–carboxylate cotransporter family	5	—
SLC14: Urea transporter family	2	Kidd antigen (SLC14A1), orthostatic hypotension (SLC14A2)
SLC15: Proton oligopeptide cotransporter family	4	—
SLC16: Monocarboxylate transporter family	14	Exercise intolerance (SLC16A1)
SLC17: Vesicular glutamate transporter family	8	Sialic acid storage disease (SLC17A5)
SLC18: Vesicular amine transporter family	3	—
SLC19: Tolate/thiamine transporter family	3	Thiamine-responsive megaloblastic anemia (SLC19A2)
SLC20: Type III Na^+–phosphate cotransporter family	2	—
SLC21/SLCO: Organic anion transporting family	20	—
SLC22: Organic cation/anion/zwitterion transporter family	18	Primary systemic carnitine deficiency (SLC22A5), idiopathic renal hypouricemia (SLC22A12)
SLC23: Na^+-dependent, ascorbic acid transporter family	4	—
SLC24: $Na^+/(Ca^{2+}$-$K^+)$ exchanger family	5	—
SLC25: Mitochondrial carrier family	29	Citrullinemia type II (SLC25A13), HHH syndrome (SLC25A15), Amish microcephaly (SLC25A9), AdPEO (SLC25A4), Senger syndrome (SLC25A4), CAC deficiency (SLC25A20)
SLC26: Multifunctional anion exchanger family	11	Chondrodysplasias (SLC26A2), Pendred syndrome (SLC26A4)
SLC27: Fatty-acid transport protein family	6	—
SLC28: Na^+-coupled nucleoside transport family	3	—
SLC29: Facilitative nucleoside transporter family	4	—
SLC30: Zinc efflux family	9	—
SLC31: Copper transporter family	2	—
SLC32: Vesicular inhibitory amino acid transporter family	1	—
SLC33: Acetyl-CoA transporter family	1	—
SLC34: Type II Na^+–phosphate cotransporter family	3	X-linked hypophosphatemia (SLC34A1), autosomal-dominant hypophosphatemic rickets (SLC34A1), oncogenic hypophosphatemic osteomalacia (SLC34A1)
SLC35: Nucleoside–sugar transporter family	23	Leukocyte adhesion deficiency type II (SLC35C1), congenital disorder of glycosylation IIc (SLC35C1)
SLC36: Proton-coupled amino acid transporter family	4	—
SLC37: The sugar-phosphate/phosphate exchanger family	4	Glycogen storage disease non-1a (SLC37A4)
SLC38: System A and N, sodium-coupled, neutral amino acid transporter family	6	—
SLC39: Metal ion transporter family	14	Acrodermatitis enteropathica (SLC39A4)
SLC40: Basolateral iron transporter family	1	Type IV hemochromatosis (SLC40A1)
SLC41: MgtE-like magnesium transporter family	3	—
SLC42: Rh ammonium transporter family	3	Rh_{null}-regulator, Rh_{mod} (SLC42A1)
SLC43: Na^+-independent, system-L–like amino acid transporter family	3	—
Total	321	—

molecular structure of glutamate transporters (905). The Glt$_{Ph}$ protein shares 37% amino acid identity with excitatory glutamate transporter GLT-1 (SLC1A2) and has homology to other SLC1 transporters. Glt$_{Ph}$ forms a bowl-shaped trimer containing an aqueous basin facing the extracellular solution, which extends halfway through the membrane bilayer. Each monomer contains eight transmembrane domains, TMs, and two helical hairpins, HPs. The first six transmembrane domains form a distorted N-terminal cylinder, whose outer surface arbitrates the intersubunit contacts in the trimer. The TM7, TM8, HP1, and HP2 domains, implicated in substrate transport, are contained within the N-terminal cylinder, which suggests that each monomer may function independently. Reaching from opposite sides of the membrane, HP1 and HP2 meet at the bottom of the basin where the glutamate binding site is proposed to occur, near the interface between HP1 and HP2. Based on the crystal structure, HP2 is speculated to provide the extracellular gate and HP1 forms the intracellular gate directly under the binding pocket (905).

While SLC1 transporters have a similar predicted structure, they demonstrate distinct functional properties based on a common transport mechanism. Cellular glutamate uptake must occur against a steep electrochemical gradient. To accomplish this, glutamate transporters couple glutamate uptake to organic ion transport, thereby using the electrochemical potential stored in ion gradients as free energy to drive glutamate transport. Glutamate transport is accompanied by intracellular acidification (371) and driven by the pH gradient (558, 908). Electrogenic transport occurs when three Na^+ ions and one H^+ are cotransported and 1 K^+ is countertransported with each glutamate molecule, resulting in the net translocation of two positive charges per transport cycle (37, 84, 379, 844, 908). The glutamate transport mechanism has been demonstrated to be an ordered process in which Na^+ and K^+ are moved through discrete steps. First the three Na^+ ions bind followed by loading the glutamate carrier with glutamate$^-$/H^+, which leads to translocation of these substrate across the plasma membrane and release inside the cell. To complete the transport cycle, one K^+ binds to the inner side of the carrier and is transported outward (373, 378, 618). Additionally, glutamate transporters can mediate an uncoupled chloride ion flux, induced by glutamate in a sodium-dependent manner (194, 843). Therefore this suggests a link between gating of anion conductance and glutamate permeation. The physiological role of this anion conductance is not completely understood, but it has been suggested that this mechanism for enhancing chloride permeability may change neuronal excitability (194).

The GLT-1 glutamate transporter (SLC1A2) is expressed in astrocytes found in various brain regions, predominantly the cerebral cortex and hippocampus (805). GLT-1 knockout mice have lethal, spontaneous epileptic seizures, and behavioral patterns similar to those after NMDA-induced seizures (788). In humans, reduction in GLT-1 transporter function, due to aberrant RNA processing, has been implicated in amyotrophic lateral sclerosis (459), temporal lobe epilepsy (323), and Alzheimer's disease (506, 913). The GLT-1 transporter has been purified and was functionally reconstituted by Kanner and colleagues (148, 618). It was found to account for 90% of all glutamate uptake in the brain, while only representing approximately 0.6% of the protein in crude synaptosomal fractions.

The glutamate transporter GLAST (SLC1A3) is particularly abundant in Bergmann glia of the cerebellum and expressed at moderate levels in astrocytes and ependymal cells throughout the central nervous system (675, 760). GLAST knockout mice develop normally, but demonstrate motor discoordination when performing difficult tasks, consistent with a cerebellum irregularity (862). GLAST contributes approximately 5%–10% to all glutamate uptake capacity in the brain. Outside the brain, GLAST mRNA has been found in the heart, skeletal muscle, placenta, and in the urinary surface epithelium in the kidney, ureter, and bladder.

The glutamate transporter EAAC1 (SLC1A1) was identified through expression cloning in *Xenopus* oocytes (371). EAAC1 is expressed in neurons found in the hippocampus, cerebral cortex, olfactory bulb, striatum, superior colliculus, and thalamus, in various kidney segments, as well as in other organs (47, 350, 675, 723). In situ hybridization and immunocytochemistry of rat kidney sections revealed that EAAC1 is predominantly expressed in the apical membrane of the proximal tubule S2 and S3 segments (723). This evidence supports the idea that the EAAC1 is responsible for reabsorption of glutamate that escaped the earlier segment of the proximal tubule. EAAC1 knockout mice exhibit dicarboxylic aminoaciduria, in addition to associated behavioral abnormalities (604) and seizures (674), which confirms the role of EAAC1 in glutamate reabsorption.

The kidney also appears to contain a Na^+- and K^+-dependent, low-affinity glutamate transporter (19, 562, 867). In the rat kidney, microperfusion and free-flow micropuncture studies showed that greater than 90% of filtered acidic amino acids are reabsorbed within the first third of the proximal convolution (S1 segments) (735, 736). The low-affinity transporter would be expected to account for the glutamate reabsorption in early proximal tubule segments; however, its molecular identity remains elusive.

Two sodium-dependent neutral amino acid transporters were identified based on their sequence homology to glutamate transporters (47, 370, 391, 675, 719, 821). ASCT1 (SLC1A4) is a ubiquitously expressed neutral amino acid transporter that stereoselectively accepts L-alanine, L-serine, L-cysteine, and L-threonine. Similar to glutamate transporters, ASCT1-mediated transport is associated with chloride conductance. ASC transporters can thus behave like ligand-gated anion channels (88, 908). However, in contrast to glutamate transporters that require K^+ to fulfill their relocation step, ASC transporters are not coupled to K^+ countertransport and appear not to be coupled to H^+ transport (88, 908). Instead, ASCT1 (SLC1A4) functions exclusively as a sodium-dependent, amino acid exchanger. The functional properties of ASCT1 suggest that it may function to equilibrate different pools of neutral amino acids and to provide a mechanism to link amino-acid concentration gradients (908). ASCT2 (SLC1A5) is also a sodium-dependent, neutral amino acid exchanger, but has a broader substrate range than ASCT1. In addition to the typical ASC substrates, ASCT2 transports glutamine and asparagines, as well as other amino acids including glutamate with low affinity (88, 821). ASCT2 is mainly expressed in the kidney, large intestine, lung, skeletal muscle, testis, and adipose tissue (821). In the kidney ASCT2 was shown to be present in the brush border membranes of the proximal tubule (27).

FACILITATED GLUCOSE TRANSPORTER FAMILY (SLC2)

The kidneys play a major role in regulating plasma glucose homeostasis. Over a 24-hour period, the kidneys filter approximately 180 g of glucose through the proximal tubules, leading to approximately 90% of glucose reabsorption. Due to the hydrophilic nature of glucose, cellular glucose must be taken up by glucose transporters. Glucose transporters are divided into two families: the facilitated-diffusion glucose transporters (GLUT family), and the Na^+-dependent glucose transporters (SGLT family; see SLC5). Glucose influx into kidney tissue occurs through apical SGLT cotransporters that reabsorb glucose and concentrate glucose in tubules. Glucose efflux follows through basolateral GLUT transporters. There are currently 14 facilitated-diffusion glucose-transporter family members. This family contains 12 facilitated glucose transporters (SLC2A1-A4 [GLUT1-4], SLC2A6-A12 [GLUT6-12], SLC2A14 [GLUT14]), 1 fructose transporter (SLC2A5 [GLUT5]), and 1 *myo*-inositol transporter (SLC2A13 [HMIT, GLUT13]).

The GLUT1-5 were identified through expression cloning and cDNA library screening techniques, while GLUT6-14 were identified by screening genome databases. The transporters all contain 12 transmembrane domains with both amino and carboxy-terminal ends located on the cytosolic side and a unique N-linked oligosaccharide side chain on either the first or fifth extracellular loop (545). Expressed in every cell of the body, the GLUT transporters facilitate the movement of various hexoses, fructose, and *myo*-inositol across the plasma membrane in the direction determined by its electrochemical gradient. However, much remains to be uncovered about the substrate specificity and function of the recently discovered isoforms (GLUT6-14).

GLUT1 (SLC2A1) is a high-affinity glucose transporter found in almost every tissue with varying expression levels in different cell types. GLUT1 is critical for glucose transport across the blood–brain barrier. In rat kidneys, GLUT1 was found in the basolateral membrane of cells forming the proximal straight tubules (S3 segments) (801), due to its likely involvement in transepithelial glucose transport and delivery for energy production through glycolysis.

The low-affinity glucose transporter, GLUT2 (SLC2A2), is the major facilitated glucose transporter in hepatocytes. In addition, GLUT2 is the primary glucose transporter expressed in the basolateral membranes of intestinal and renal absorptive epithelial cells (800). In these epithelial cells it transports glucose in coordination with the apically expressed sodium-dependent glucose transporters SLGT1 and SLGT2. GLUT2 is present in the plasma membrane of pancreatic β cells where it maintains normal glucose homeostasis as well as the function and development of the endocrine pancreas. GLUT2 knockout mice display symptoms characteristic of non–insulin-dependent diabetes and abnormal postnatal pancreatic islet development (281). In humans, mutations that inactivate the GLUT2 (SLC2A2) gene cause Fanconi–Bickel syndrome (690). In the GLUT3 (SLC2A3), a high-affinity glucose transporter, mRNA is nearly ubiquitously expressed in humans, although its protein expression is limited to brain neurons, spermatozoa in the testis (287, 550), and skeletal muscle (762).

GLUT4 (SLC2A4) is an insulin-responsive glucose transporter (229), which after insulin stimulation is recruited from intracellular vesicles and translocated to the plasma membrane to increase glucose influx by myocytes and adipocytes (771). GLUT5 (SLC2A5) was identified as a facilitated fructose transporter localized to the apical membrane of epithelial cells. It is expressed primarily in the jejunal segment of small intestine where it plays an important role in fructose absorption. Lower expression levels have also been found in the kidney, skeletal muscle, adipose tissue, brain, and spermatozoa (93, 390, 498). GLUT6 (SLC2A6) was found to be expressed in the brain, spleen, and peripheral leucocytes, but its function is still unclear (461). GLUT7 (SLC2A7) has been identified by a genomic homology search (364), and recently has been characterized (456). In *Xenopus* oocytes, it demonstrated the ability to facilitate high-affinity transport of glucose and fructose. The mRNA expression showed that GLUT7 is present in the human small intestine, colon, testis, and prostate. Protein expression was confirmed in the rat small intestine, and indicated that the transporter was predominantly expressed in the brush-border membrane of the enterocyte.

GLUT8 (SLC2A8, previously called GLUTX1) was the first SLC2 isoform to be identified by database mining and functional expression. When expressed in oocytes or mammalian cells, it is retained in intracellular membranes. GLUT8 is expressed in the brain (cerebellum), adrenal gland, liver and spleen, brown adipose tissue, and lung (339). It is also expressed in blastocytes where it may function as a glucose transporter responsible for insulin-stimulated glucose uptake (104). In mice, GLUT8 was localized to glomerular podocytes and tubular epithelial cells in the distal nephron. In vivo, GLUT8 (SLC2A8) expression in the kidney was affected by plasma glucose levels, suggesting that it may contribute to serum glucose maintenance (648, 160, 701). Yet, the exact physiological role of GLUT8 is still unclear.

With respect to GLUT9 (SLC2A9), its high homology to GLUT5 suggests that it may function as a fructose transporter. However, to date no functional data have been published supporting this activity. Its mRNA expression is almost exclusively present in the kidney and liver (611). The GLUT9 protein was localized to the proximal tubules in human kidney. Subcellular fractionation revealed the presence of GLUT9 protein in plasma membranes and high-density microsomal membranes (23). Based on *Xenopus*-oocyte expression studies, GLUT10 (SLC2A10) is a glucose transporter, and it is expressed in the heart, lung, brain, liver, and skeletal muscle. Interestingly, its chromosomal localization is at a loci associated with type 2 diabetes (518). GLUT11 (SLC2A11) is expressed in skeletal muscle and heart (885), and GLUT12 (SLC2A12) in the heart, skeletal muscle, brown adipose tissue, prostate, and mammary gland (484). When expressed in *Xenopus* oocytes, GLUT12 demonstrated functional glucose transport activity (664), and was shown to be expressed in human breast and prostate cancer but not in the corresponding benign tissues, suggesting a role in cancer development (111, 665). GLUT14 (SLC2A14) is an alternatively spliced duplicon of GLUT3 that is expressed only in the testis (883). HMIT (SLC2A13) is a *myo*-inositol transporter expressed in the brain where it may play an important role in controlling inositol metabolism (820).

SLC3 FAMILY: ACTIVATORS OF CYSTINE, AND DIBASIC AND NEUTRAL AMINO ACID TRANSPORT

The SLC3 family includes type II–membrane glycoproteins that are required for functional expression of the SLC7 family amino acid transporters. This family is comprised of two proteins: rBAT (SLC3A1) and 4F2hc (SLC3A2). These type II glycoproteins are predicted to have only one transmembrane domain where the C-terminus localizes outside the cell, an unusual structure for a membrane transport protein. The carboxy-terminal extracellular domains of SLC3A1 and SLC3A2 are significantly homologous to a family of carbohydrate-metabolizing enzymes including α-amylases and α-glucosidases. However, the biological relevance of such carbohydrate-metabolizing activities is unclear (868).

Heteromeric amino acid transporters (HATs) are functionally active when a light glycosylated and a nonglycosylated heavy subunit dimerize and are held together in the endoplasmic reticulum by a disulfide bond or noncovalent interactions. The SLC3 "heavy subunits" dimerize with the "light" SLC7 transporter to generate functional amino acid transporter. The heavy subunit rBAT (SLC3A1), for ex-

ample, dimerizes with the amino acid transporter SLC7A9 to form the functional amino acid transporter b$^{0,+}$, which is the main transporter system responsible for apical reabsorption of cystine in the kidney (Fig. 1). A defect in cystine reabsorption causes cystinuria, a common primary inherited aminoaciduria. This condition results in cystine excretion into the urine and consequently the lower solubility of cystine in urine leads to kidney stone formation (50). Mutations in SLC3A1 frequently cause type I cystinuria, the most common form of the disease (100, 586, 625, 682). Many are mis-sense mutations that affect the glucosidase-like extracellular domain of the SLC3A1 protein. All cystinuria-specific rBAT mutations functionally assessed demonstrate trafficking defects, in agreement with its role in routing rBAT/b$^{0,+}$ AT to the plasma membrane. Mutational analysis of SLC3 and SLC7 genes in patients with cystinuria revealed that mutations in the SLC3A1-gene case type I cystinuria, whereas mutations in SLC7A9 cause non–type I cystinuria (see section on SLC7). The main difference between type I non–type I cystinuria is that in type I, the heterozygotes exhibit normal urinary amino acid excretion, whereas in non–type I (i.e., type II or type III), cystine and lysine excretion are above normal levels. This indicates that the reduced activity of SLC3A1 in type I heterozygotes is sufficient to fully activate the SLC7 cystine transporters, whereas reduced activity of the SLC7 transporter in non–type I heterozygotes results in increased urinary amino acid excretion.

Screening the rat renal cDNA library for clones capable of inducing ^{14}C-cystine uptake in oocytes originally resulted in the identification of kidney- and intestine-specific clones that encode the SLC3A1 protein in the rat (868) and rabbit (53). Based on *Xenopus* oocytes expression studies, SLC3A1 induced the Na$^+$-independent high-affinity transport of cystine, dibasic amino acids, and, surprisingly, neutral amino acids. SLC3A1 is localized in the rat brush-border membranes of proximal S3 tubule segments in the kidney and of the intestine (375, 539).

Interestingly, the SLC3A1 amino acid sequence shows significant sequence identity (29%) to the heavy chain of the SLC3A2/4F2 cell surface antigen (CD98). The CD98 antigen is a 125-kDa disulfide-linked heterodimer composed of a glycosylated heavy chain (85 kDa) and a nonglycosylated light chain (41 kDa). The SLC3A2/4F2 is a ubiquitously expressed multifunctional protein involved in such activities as cell adhesion (202), T-cell activation (258), and tumor cell growth (731, 894). Unlike SLC3A1, mutations in SLC3A2/4F2 have not been associated with disease, because these mutations are believed to be lethal. SLC3A2 is the heavy subunit of several amino acid transporters (system L, y$^+$L, x$_c^-$, and asc) and is involved in various other cellular functions. The SLC3A2 heterodimeric amino acid transporters are sorted to the basolateral membrane, whereas SLC3A1 amino acid transporters sort to the apical membrane (40, 41). Expression of human SLC3A2 heavy chains in oocytes stimulated the uptake of dibasic and neutral

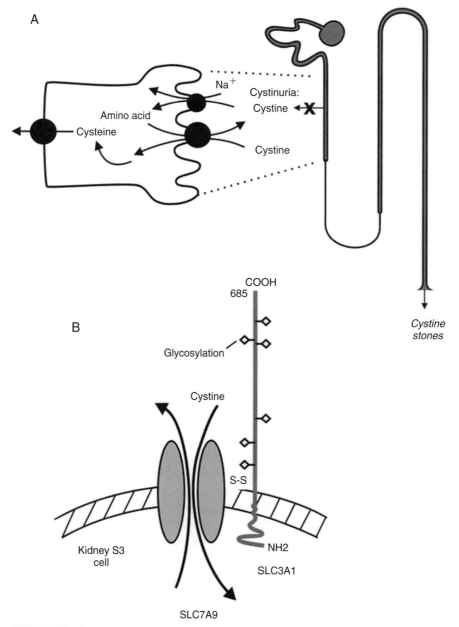

FIGURE 1   Cystine reabsorption in the kidney and cystinuria. A. Cystine reabsorption occurs through the heterodimeric amino acid transporter SLC7A9/SLC3A1 in exchange for intracellular neutral amino acids. The free energy for cystine uptake is provided by coupling neutral amino acid uptake to the inwardly directed sodium gradient. Cytoplasmic cystine is rapidly reduced to cysteine, which thus exits the cell via SLC7A8 in the basolateral membrane. B. SLC3A1 and SLC7A8 are covalently linked through a disulfide bridge as well by noncovalent interactions. SLC3A1 is N-glycosylated, and is required for apical membrane expression of the nonglycosylated SLC7A8 transporter. Mis-sense mutations in the C-terminal portion of SLC3A1 are the cause of type I cystinuria. Genetic mutations that occur in SLC7A8 are the cause of non–type I cystinuria (i.e., type II or type III cystinuria).

amino acids but notably not cystine (53, 869). In contrast to SLC3A1, SLC3A2 induced Na⁺-dependent uptake of neutral but not dibasic amino acids (869). Thus, SLC3A1- and SLC3A2-induced amino acid transport in oocytes has significantly different substrate specificities and Na⁺ dependences, because they induce the expression of different oocyte transporters.

ANION EXCHANGERS–BICARBONATE COTRANSPORTER FAMILY (SLC4)

The SLC4 cotransporter family includes 10 human genes. This solute carrier family can be subdivided into two major subfamilies based on function: anion exchangers (AEs) and sodium coupled bicarbonate cotransporters (NBCs). Transporters in this family carry bicarbonate and/or carbonate. Structurally SLC4 transporters have 10 to 14 putative transmembrane domains and extracellular loops that are N-glycosylated.

Anion Exchangers

Four SLC4 anion exchangers have been identified: AE1 (SLC4A1), AE2 (SLC4A2), AE3 (SLC4A3), and AE4 (SLC4A9) (154, 415, 416). Overall, these anion exchangers share 60%–70% of sequence homology (789). The first three human AEs (AE1-3) have been characterized as electroneutral exchangers, which carry one monovalent anion in exchange for a second monovalent anion. The AEs predominately transport HCO_3^- and Cl^-, but can also carry OH^- as a substrate. Additionally, AE1 (SLC4A1) has been shown to mediate a low rate of SO_4^{2-} plus H^+ exchange for Cl^-. However, physiologically the most relevant activity is Cl^- exchange for HCO_3^-. In most cell types there is an inward flux of Cl^- and an efflux of HCO_3^-, but this can reverse depending on existing chemical gradients. This electroneutral transport process is inhibited by stilbene disulfonate derivatives such as SITS and DIDS.

AE1 (SLC4A1) represents 25% of all membrane protein and is the most abundant membrane glycoprotein in erythrocytes (416). In blood cells, AE1 (SLC4A1) plays a critical role in the movement of CO_2 from the systemic tissues to the lungs. Structurally, the 404-amino acid N-terminal domain is located in cytoplasm, where cytoskeleton components, hemoglobin, or glycolytic enzymes can attach. The membrane-associated portion carries out the anion exchange function, while the remaining C-terminal, cytoplasmic tail contains a binding site for carbonic anhydrase II (835). It is also reported that carbonic anhydrase IV binds one of the AE1 (SLC4A1) extracellular loops (757).

In addition to blood cells, AE1 is also expressed in other tissues including hepatocytes, lung, and brain. In the kidney, the N-terminal variant of AE1 (kAE1) is the major isoform. This variant is derived from an alternative promoter site that results in a unique transcript that lacks the first 65 amino acids of erythroid hAE1 (91). AE1 (SLC4A1) is localized to the basolateral membrane of the intercalated cells of collecting duct (822), where it serves to reabsorb HCO_3^-. This AE1 exchange activity is important to counter the net H^+ efflux into the tubular lumen.

Mutations in AE1 (SLC4A1) that affect its function cause diseases affecting either erythrocyte or kidney distal tubule function (10, 722). When the conserved arginines in the membrane domain are altered, decreased membrane association of the transporter occurs, and results in hereditary spherocytosis characterized by sphere-shaped red blood cells and chronic hemolytic anemia (356). Mis-sense mutations in kidney AE1 (SLC4A1) are associated with autosomal-dominant distal tubular acidosis, which is characterized by malfunctioning urinary acidification (357). In Southeast Asians, autosomal recessive distal tubular acidosis is related

to deletions or mutations in the AE1 transmembrane region (10). Recently, the mechanisms of renal tubular acidosis caused by AE1 (SLC4A1) mutation have been reported. Many mutations (R589H, R589C, R589S, G609R, R901X) caused mistrafficking of the transporter (157), but others (G701D and S773S) resulted in AE1 misfolding (405). Those effects are in the kidney, but interestingly, a zebrafish mutation of AE1 causes diserythropoiesis, suggesting that the erythroid AE1 isoform is involved in red blood cell development (599).

Knocking out AE2 (SLC4A2) in mice caused achlorhydria, indicating that AE2 was essential for generating stomach acid (Cl^- excretion for stomach acid) (239). AE2 (SLC4A2) knockout (KO) mice also indicated an inhibition of spermatogenesis (519), which suggests that AE2 plays an important role in maintaining extracellular bicarbonate concentration and pH environment for sperm formation in the testis.

Sodium Bicarbonate Transporters

The kidney manages HCO_3^- levels in blood by regulating H^+ secretion into the lumen of various tubule segments, modulating HCO_3^- absorption and synthesis and absorption of new HCO_3^-. On the apical membrane of the renal proximal tubule cell sodium proton exchangers and proton pumps transport protons into the tubule lumen where they can be used to titrate filtered HCO_3^-. The resulting protonated form, H_2CO_3, is then transformed into CO_2 by luminal carbonic anhydrase IV. The CO_2 rapidly permeates the proximal tubule cell where carbonic anhydrase II reconverts it back into HCO_3^-. Intracellular HCO_3^- then exits the basolateral membrane into the blood via electrogenic $Na^+HCO_3^-$ cotransport mediated by the sodium bicarbonate transporter, NBC1 (SLC4A4).

The sodium bicarbonate transporters, NBCs, are the second major group of SLC4 transporters, and play a vital role in acid–base movement in most cell and tissue types including blood cells, stomach, pancreas, intestine, kidney, heart, liver, reproductive systems, and central nervous system. There are two varieties of NBCs: electrogenic cotransporters such as SLC4A4 and SLC4A5, and the electroneutral sodium-coupled transporters SLC4A7, SLC4A8, and SLC4A10. The electrogenic cotransporters move one Na^+ and either two or three HCO_3^- molecules in a single transport cycle.

The first Na^+ bicarbonate cotransporter identified (NBC1, NBCe1, SLC4A4) is 30% identical at the amino acid sequence level to the SLC4 anion exchangers (3, 95, 126, 667, 668). Three NBC1 (SLC4A4) isoforms are known; similar to AE1, the kidney expresses a unique NBC1 isoform (kNBC1, NBCe1-A, SLC4A4a) that is derived from a discrete promoter site in intron 3 (4). However, the second NBC1 isoform (pNBC1, SLC4A4b) is the most widespread splice variant (3, 126) and accounts for NBC1 transport activity in the gut, heart, and brain (666). The third isoform (SLC4A4c) is found almost exclusively in the brain (56). The kidney splice variant, localized to the basolateral membrane of the renal proximal tubule (703), carries one Na^+ ion with three HCO_3^- ions from inside the tubule cell to the blood and thus completes the reabsorption of HCO_3^-. Thus far it appears that the SLC4A4b and -c isoforms have similar physiology as kidney NBC1. Protein localization studies found NBC1 expressed also in astrocytes and some neurons in the brain (702), intestine, lung, and epididymus (358). Four naturally occurring mutations in SLC4A4 have been reported (340, 341), all of which result in severe and continual proximal renal tubular acidosis (pRTA) and ocular pathologies (bilateral cataracts, bilateral glaucoma, and bandkeratopathy). When kNBC1 was truncated due to mutation, the transporter protein could not reach the plasma membrane suggesting mistrafficking of kNBC1 in those patients (343)

A second electrogenic Na^+–HCO_3^- cotransporter (NBC4, NBCe2, SLC4A5) has been characterized and encodes a protein of greater than 1000 amino acids (633, 691, 837). RNA transcript levels are highest in the liver, testis, and spleen, with reduced levels in the heart, lung, and kidney. Six SLC4A5 isoforms (SLC4A5a-f) are reported, but five of the six variants may be cloning artifacts (633, 634, 891). The only variant known to function as an electrogenic transporter is SLC4A5c. NBC4c (SLC4A5c) expressed in *Xenopus* oocytes demonstrates electrogenic cotransport with an apparent stoichiometry (Na^+:HCO_3^-) of 1:2 (837); however, when expressed in the mPCT renal cell line, the stoichiometry is 1:3 (691). The SLC4A5f isoform has been characterized as an electroneutral Na^+–HCO_3^- cotransporter (891). A cohort study provided information that the NBC4 is implicated in hypertension (38).

One group of sodium bicarbonate transporters is characterized by electroneutral Na^+ and HCO_3^- cotransport. In this group, NBCn1 (SLC4A7) was the first reported electroneutral Na^+–HCO_3^- cotransporter (125, 632), of which there are four known isoforms (A–D). Normally, NBCn1 cotransports one Na^+ and one HCO_3^- across the plasma membrane. Isoform B (NBCn1-B) has unequivocally been shown to mediate electroneutral transport (125), is found in mTAL, and is upregulated by metabolic acidosis (433). However, NBCn1-D is localized to a subset of intercalated cells in the CCD (635), and is not modulated by acidosis (433). Unlike other SLC4 family members, the NBCn1-D isoform is not sensitive to stilbenes, but instead ethylisopropyl amiloride (EIPA) (632). In the CCD, NBCn1 colocalizes with the vacuolar H^+ pump at the apical membrane (635). But recent data indicated that NBCn1 was highly expressed in the basolateral membrane of choroid plexus epithelial cells. Since the basolateral membrane of choroid plexus has a function like the apical membrane of kidney tubule cells, this result suggested that NBCn1 had a key role in Na^+ transport for CSF formation (624). SLC4A7 (NBCn1) knockout mice phenotypically display blindness and auditory impairment (71). Since SLC4A7 was highly expressed in photoreceptor cells of the retina, it may have a role in intracellular Ca^{2+} homeostasis coupling with the plasma membrane Ca^{2+}-ATPases in sensory neurons.

The electroneutral SLC4 transporter NDCBE (SLC4A8) mediates activity that is equivalent to the electroneutral exchange of $NaHCO_3$ for HCl. This Na^+ driven Cl^-–HCO_3^- exchanger (NDCBE, SLC4A8) is highly expressed in the brain and testis and moderately present in the kidney and ovary (266). A second Na^+-dependent Cl^-–HCO_3^- exchanger (NCBE, SLC4A10) appears not to require Cl^-, although the Cl^- dependence is controversial (124, 848). The data thus far are consistent with the hypothesis that NCBE is an electroneutral Na^+–HCO_3^- cotransporter. Renal localization has not been reported for NCBE, but it is expressed on the basolateral membrane in brain choroid-plexus epithelial cells (624).

Two additional SLC4 gene family members have recently been revealed through genome sequencing and analysis of EST databases. Two novel NBC-like splice variants were from rabbit kidney and characterized as a Na^+-independent Cl^-,HCO_3^- exchangers (AE4, SLC4A9) (810). The SLC4A9 protein localized to the apical membrane of b-intercalated cells of the CCD (810). But another report showed that AE4 was a DIDS-sensitive exchanger in the basolateral membrane of a-intercalated cells, which suggested that AE4 was related to HCO_3^- secretion in the collecting duct (410). Finally, Parker et al. (596) identified a unique SLC4 member, bicarbonate transporter–related protein (BTR1, SLC4A11), which is found in the kidney.

THE SODIUM–GLUCOSE COTRANSPORTER FAMILY (SLC5)

The sodium–glucose cotransporters comprise an ancient gene family that contains 12 known members in the human genome. These proteins have diverse, multiple functions including active transport, channeling, and glucose sensing in neurons. Eleven transporters have been characterized using heterologous expression systems. These studies concluded that eight are Na^+–substrate cotransporters for glucose, *myo*-inositol, monocarboxylates, and iodine; one is a Na^+–Cl^-–choline cotransporter; one is an anion transporter; one is a putative glucose activated ion channel. In addition to their expected function, unanticipated properties have also emerged from these expression studies. Although the major function of these proteins is secondary active transport in epithelia, they can also behave as sodium uniporters, urea and water channels, and urea and water cotransporters.

Glucose absorption from the diet and the glomerular filtrate is a critical process that is mediated by Na^+–glucose cotransporters. The SLC5 family includes the high-affinity Na^+-glucose transporter SGLT1 (SLC5A1) (307), the three low-affinity isoforms SGLT2 (SLC5A2) (372), SGLT3 (SLC5A4, SAAT1) (486), and SGLT4 (SLC5A9) (794); two inositol transporters SMIT1 (SLC5A3) (432) and SGLT6 (SMIT2, SLC5A11) (137); one iodide transporter NIS (SLC5A5) (146); the vitamin transporter SMVT

(SLC5A6) (627); a choline transporter CHT1 (SLC5A7) (16, 573); two monocarboxylate transporters SMCT1 (SLC5A8) (136) and SMCT2 (SLC5A12) (751); and the incompletely characterized Na$^+$ cotransporter SLGT5 (SLC5A10).

The intestinal sodium-coupled glucose transporter SGLT1 (SLC5A1) was identified by expression cloning using *Xenopus laevis* oocytes (307). The SGLT1 protein has 662 amino acid residues corresponding to a 74-kDa molecular weight and up to 14 transmembrane domains (816). Functional characterization identified this clone as the high-affinity glucose transporter (D-glucose K$_m$ is 0.3 mM in rabbit and 0.8 mM in human). SGLT1 is primarily expressed in the brush border membrane of mature enterocytes in the small intestine where it absorbs dietary glucose and galactose from the intestinal lumen (882). In the kidney, D-glucose is freely filtered at the glomerulus and then almost completely extracted from the urine in the proximal tubule and returned to the blood. Approximately 90% of the filtered glucose is assumed to be reabsorbed in the early S1 segment of the proximal tubule by a second low-affinity transporter, named SGLT2 (K$_m$ for D-glucose ~2 mM) (881). The high-affinity SGLT1 transporter located later in the proximal tubule S3 segments absorbs any glucose that escapes the S1 segment. For SGLT1 (SLC5A1), the Na$^+$-to-glucose coupling ratio is 2:1, which is consistent with its role in sugar absorption against a large concentration gradient. In contrast, the low-affinity transporter, SGLT2 (SLC5A2), has Na$^+$-to-glucose coupling ratios of 1:1, and consequently has a much lower concentrating capacity than SGLT1.

Unlike some of its better-known family members, SGLT3 (SLC5A4) is incapable of sugar transport. While SGLT3 (SLC5A4) was found to be expressed in small intestine, upon closer inspection microscopy indicated that it was expressed in cholinergic neurons in the submucosal and myenteric plexuses but not in the enterocytes. Additionally, SGLT3 was found located in skeletal muscle plasma membrane associated with nicotinic acetylcholine receptors at the neuromuscular junctions. Electrophysiology studies demonstrate that glucose induces SGLT3 to depolarize the plasma membrane in a saturable, Na$^+$-dependent, phlorizin-sensitive manner (159). Thus, it is probably not a sugar transporter per se, but instead appears to be a glucose-gated ion channel. These data suggest a role for SGLT3 as a glucose sensor regulating the activity of smooth and skeletal muscles. SGLT4 (SLC5A9) appears to be expressed mainly in the intestine and kidney, but also widely at lower levels in the liver, lung, and brain (794). SGLT5 (SLC5A10) appears to be restricted to the kidney. Functional studies suggest that SGLT4 (SLC5A9) is a low-affinity transporter for sugars including mannose, glucose, and fructose (794), but no functional data are available for SGLT5 (SLC5A10).

The significance of Na$^+$–glucose cotransport as the major glucose absorptive pathway in the intestinal brush border membrane is demonstrated when defects occur in SGLT1 (SLC5A1) function, which lead to glucose–galactose malabsorption (GGM). The inability to absorb dietary sugars results in an accumulation of intestinal sugars and subsequent reversal of osmotic flow that causes severe diarrhea unless glucose and galactose are removed from the diet. Most mutants occur in the coding region and produce truncated proteins (505). Similar genetic evidence from a patient with autosomal recessive renal glycosuria suggests that SGLT2 (SLC5A2) is the key transporter involved in glucose reabsorption from the glomerular filtrate (823). Increased Na$^+$ and glucose reabsorption by the renal Na$^+$–glucose cotransporters SGLT1 and SGLT2 may contribute significantly to the kidney pathology observed in diabetes (308).

In the intestinal brush border membrane, Na$^+$-coupled solute transporters such as SGLT1 also facilitate fluid absorption. Sodium that enters epithelial cells through Na$^+$-coupled transport is pumped into the blood by the Na$^+$, K$^+$-ATPase, resulting in a transepithelial Na$^+$ flux that generates an osmotic gradient and drives fluid absorption. The presence of luminal glucose and galactose stimulates transepithelial salt and water absorption. Recent studies have indicated that SGLT1 itself is capable of transporting water, indicating that Na$^+$-coupled sugar transport directly contributes to water absorption (521).

The sodium–*myo*-inositol cotransporter SMIT (SLC5A3) is a plasma membrane protein responsible for concentrative accumulation of *myo*-inositol in various tissues. The *myo*-inositol is an essential component in phosphoinositide synthesis and, as an osmolyte, contributes to cell volume regulation. In renal and brain cells, hypertonicity causes an increase in SMIT message levels in order to raise the cellular concentration of *myo*-inositol. Renal medullary cells maintain high concentrations of *myo*-inositol, sorbitol, betaine, and glycerophosphocholine. Accumulating these organic osmolytes helps these cells regulate their osmolarity in response to high extracellular osmolality that occurs in situations such as concentrating urine. Multiple tonicity-responsive enhancers in the upstream promoter regulate SMIT (SLC5A3) at the transcriptional level (657). Hypertonicity leads to increased transcription, SMIT protein levels, and transport. A second *myo*-inositol transporter, SMIT2 (SLC5A11), was recently characterized (137) after the sequence was identified over 10 years ago (318). This transporter is widely expressed in the brain, heart, kidney, and liver (318). SMIT2 (SLC5A11) has similar affinity for *myo*-inositol and Na$^+$ as SMIT (SLC5A3), but its activity is distinctive in that it transports *chiro*-inositol and D-glucose and is not inhibited by L-fructose (137).

Iodide (I$^-$) is an essential component of the thyroid hormones T$_3$ and T$_4$, and is actively accumulated by the thyroid gland. The Na$^+$–iodide cotransporter (NIS, SLC5A5), mainly found in the thyroid gland, is responsible for this iodide accumulation. Biophysically, NIS (SLC5A5) transports 2 Na$^+$: 1 anion (I$^-$) and thus is electrogenic (188). Patients who are lacking iodine transport do not accumulate iodine in their thyroids, often resulting in severe hypothyroidism. A single amino acid substitution in NIS (T354P) was identified as the cause of this condition in two independent patients (452). NIS expression, mRNA, and protein are upregulated during lactation and in breast cancers (795). The closest relative to NIS is AIT (SLC5A8), which is also expressed in the thyroid but is located in the apical membrane (663). Preliminary studies imply that AIT (SLC5A8) can function as a ClO_4^- sensitive I^- transporter involved in efflux of iodide from the thyrocyte into lumen of the gland. Additionally, SLC5A8 (SMCT1, AIT) mediates the Na^+-coupled and electrogenic transport of monocarboxylates including short-chain fatty acids, lactate, and nicotinate with variable Na^+- monocarboxylate stoichiometry, depending on the substrate (2:1 for L-lactate and 4:1 for propionate) (136, 254, 255, 535). Being expressed abundantly in the colon, ileum, and kidney, SLC5A8 is assumed to play a role in the absorption of short-chain fatty acids, lactate, and nicotinate. Butyrate is produced in the colonic lumen at high levels due to bacterial fermentation of dietary fiber. Due to its ability to inhibit histone deacetylases, it is known to induce apoptosis in several tumors including colonic tumors. Consequently, butyrate transport into colonic epithelial cells via SLC5A8 may explain the potential tumor suppressor function of this transporter (237). The newly identified SLC5A12 (SMCT2) mRNA is expressed in the kidney, small intestine, and skeletal muscle. The mouse SMCT2 induces electrogenic and Na^+-dependent transport of lactate, nicotinate, propionate, and butyrate (751). The substrate specificity is similar to that of SLC5A8, although the substrate affinities of SLC5A12 are much lower.

The sodium-dependent multivitamin cotransporter SMVT (SLC5A6) was the first vitamin transporter cloned from mammalian tissue (627). It transports pantothenate, biotin, and lipoate, and has a widespread distribution. The final member of the SLC5 family is a Na^+- and Cl^--dependent choline transporter (CHT1, SLC5A7) (16, 573). Consistent with its assumed role in support of ACh synthesis, CHT1 is expressed in spinal cord and medulla and appears to be immunolocalized to the cell bodies and presynaptic terminals of cholinergic neurons. CHT immunoreactivity is visible at the presynaptic terminal plasma membrane, although the greatest density was surprisingly found associated with intracellular vesicles (205).

GABA TRANSPORTER FAMILY (SLC6)

This family comprises transporters for a diverse range of amino acid-related substrates, including the inhibitory neurotransmitters GABA (γ-aminobutyric acid) and glycine; the aminergic transmitters norepinephrine, serotonin, and dopamine; the osmolytes betaine and taurine; and the neutral amino acids plus proline. In the nervous system, these transporters function primarily in regulating neuronal signaling via sequestering extracellular neurotransmitters. Consistent with the assorted roles of this family, these

transporters are also found in non-neuronal tissue such as testis, intestine, and kidney, where, for example, they can control osmotic balance.

The SLC6 transporters act to regulate neurotransmission by mediating the neurotransmitter uptake from the synaptic clefts in neurons and glial cells and thereby controlling receptor activation during synaptic transmission. In the brain, the neurotransmitter GABA is the predominant inhibitory neurotransmitter that is carried by the SLC6 family. The molecular characterization of the SLC6 family began with the pioneering work of Kanner and colleagues who first purified and cloned a high-affinity GABA transporter from rat brain (GAT-1, SLC6A1) (280). Subsequently, two additional mammalian GABA transporter isoforms were isolated (GAT-2 and GAT-3; SLC6A13 and SLC6A11, respectively). GAT-1 has a specific neuronal distribution (483, 641), whereas GAT-2 and GAT-3 have a primarily glial distribution in the brain. GAT-2 is also expressed in the liver and kidney. These GABA transporter isoforms show distinct pharmacological properties.

Structurally, members of this family are predicted to have 12 membrane-spanning domains and consensus sites for N-glycosylation localized in the extracellular loop between transmembrane helices III and IV (557). These transporters are all Na^+ cotransporters and some members additionally cotransport Cl^-. The Na^+ coupling is an absolute necessity since the Na^+ gradient provides the energy for uphill neurotransmitter transport. The role of Cl^- is less clear, but it may enhance Na^+ binding affinity (78, 474). In general, members of the GABA transporter family are coupled to the cotransport of one or two Na^+ ions and one Cl^- ion. One member of the human SLC6 family (the serotonin transporter SERT, SLC6A4) requires the K^+ for countertransport (680). Electrophysiological analyses of the currents associated with GABA transporter family members showed that they also exhibit "leak currents" that are not stoichiometrically linked to substrate movement. This supports the emerging concept that transporters share properties with ionic channels (234, 745).

Following the identification of GABA transporter cDNAs, expression cloning and homology screening approaches led to the isolation of clones corresponding to additional neurotransmitter transporters such as norepinephrine (NET1, SLC6A2), dopamine (DAT1, SLC6A3), serotonin (SERT, SLC6A4), proline (PROT, SLC6A7), and glycine (GLYT1, SLC6A9) (220, 223, 249, 321, 396, 464, 465, 720, 729). The monoamine transporters NET1 (SLC6A2), DAT1 (SLC6A3), and SERT (SLC6A4) are the primary sites of action for many drugs that have both therapeutic and abuse potential. Drugs that block monoamine transport have powerful behavioral and physiological actions. For example, the serotonin transporter is inhibited by antidepressant drugs such as fluoxetine (Prozac®) (231). The tricyclic antidepressant drug, desipramine, inhibits norepinephrine transport and is also used to treat depression (656). Inhibition of the dopamine transporter has been closely linked to the euphoric and reinforcing properties of psychomotor stimulants such as cocaine and amphetamines.

In this family, two proline transporters have been identified and characterized. The first proline transporter, PROT (SLC6A7), was isolated from rat and human brain (223, 720). It is specific for L-proline and shows exclusive expression in the brain. While the function of proline in the central nervous system (CNS) is not yet clearly understood, PROT potentially plays a role in regulating excitatory synaptic transmission. It is also not clear whether this transporter corresponds to the imino system expressed in the intestinal and renal brush border membrane (758). Rather, it appears that the second proline transporter, the recently identified SIT1 (SLC6A20), is a more likely candidate. The human and rat transporter SIT1 exhibits properties of the classical system IMINO, defined as the Na$^+$-dependent proline transport activity that escapes inhibition by alanine (781). When expressed in *Xenopus* oocytes, rat SIT1 mediated the uptake of imino acids such as proline ($K_{0.5} \oplus 0.2$ mM) and pipecolate, as well as *N*-methylated amino acids such as *N*-methylaminoisobutyrate and sarcosine. Rat SIT1 mRNA expression was found in the intestinal epithelial cells of duodenum, jejunum, ileum, stomach, cecum, colon, and kidney proximal tubule S3 segments. SIT1 mRNA was also detected in the choroid plexus, microglia, and meninges of the brain and in the ovary.

In contrast to proline, the role of the amino acid glycine in neurotransmission is much clearer as it acts as an inhibitory neurotransmitter in the caudal mammalian brain. For the transporting glycine two main types of GLYT isoforms are known, GLYT-1 and GLYT-2 (SLC6A9 and SLC6A5, respectively) (76, 400, 464, 465). GLYT1 is the predominant glial glycine transporter and has multiple splice variants. Three different N-terminal splice variants exist for GLYT-1 in human: GLYT-1a, GLYT-1b and GLYT-1c (400) and two C-terminal GLYT-1d and GLYT-1e (769). GLYT-1 transporters appear to be exclusively expressed in the brain, whereas GLYT-2 is expressed in the brain as well as in macrophages and mast cells. GLYT-2 is predominantly localized to neurons at the glycinergic nerve terminals.

Additional SLC6 family members include a taurine transporter TAUT (SLC6A6), a betaine transporter BGT1 (SLC6A12), and two creatine transporters, CT1 and CT2 (SLC6A8 and SLC6A10, respectively). Taurine and betaine transporters have been identified in both the brain and kidney (817, 896). In the renal medulla, betaine and taurine are important osmolytes used for volume regulation (294). Handler and colleagues have shown that *cis*- and *trans*-acting factors regulate the transcription of the BGT1 (SLC6A12) gene in response to hypertonicity (530). The abundance of taurine in the brain and the general importance of taurine and betaine as nonperturbing osmolytes suggest similar TAUT and BGT1 functions in the CNS. CT1 (SLC6A8) is a widely expressed creatine transporter (284), consistent with a general metabolic role of creatine

as a precursor for phosphocreatine biosynthesis, which is critical in maintaining ATP homeostasis. CT2 (SLC6A10) is a creatine transporter isoform mainly expressed in the testis.

The neutral and cationic amino acid transporter, ATB$^{0,+}$ (SLC6A14) also belongs to the SLC6 family even though it transports a wide array of amino acids in a Na$^+$-dependent manner. This transport system is most similar to the glycine and proline transporters and is expressed in many non-neural tissues including intestine, pituitary, and lung (824). Not all SLC6 members have identified substrates or functional roles. Accordingly, the orphan transporters v7-3 (SLC6A15) and NTT5 (SLC6A16) have not been functionally characterized.

AMINO ACID PERMEASE FAMILY (SLC7)

Members of the amino acid permease family primarily mediate the Na$^+$-independent transport of amino acids across cell membranes. They are either simple facilitated transporters or obligate exchangers that transport either neutral amino acids or basic amino acids and sometimes both. In some cells the CATs may regulate NO synthesis by controlling L-arginine uptake. With some isoforms, neutral amino acid transport requires Na$^+$-binding to substitute the positive charge of basic amino acids. This family can be further divided into two subgroups, the cationic amino acid transporters (CATs, SLC7A1-4) (156, 398) and the *glycoprotein-associate amino acid transporters* (gpaATs, SLC7A5-11), also commonly referred to as catalytic light chains of the heterodimeric amino acid transporters (HATs) (92, 374, 507, 552). The identities between members of the CAT and gpaATs are 20%–30%. The identities within the CAT family are ~60% and those within the gpaATs ~40%–55%.

Cationic Amino Acid Transporters

The CAT subfamily mediates the transport cationic amino acids by facilitated diffusion. Four CAT isoforms—CAT-1, CAT-2, CAT-3, and CAT-4 (SLC7A1-A4)—have been identified. They have 14 putative transmembrane segments that are glycosylated (133, 156). The gpaATs have two transmembrane segments less and are not glycosylated. Therefore, the gpaATs need to associate with a SLC3 glycoprotein (4F2hc or rBAT) to provide surface expression. CAT-1 (SLC7A1) and CAT-2 (SLC7A2) correspond to mammalian system y$^+$ and are both facilitated transporters, which accept predominantly cationic amino acids. CAT-1 is expressed in most tissues except in the liver, whereas CAT-2a is a low-affinity homologue expressed in hepatocytes (134). The CAT-1 (SLC7A1) gene is induced in response to hormones such as insulin and glucocorticoids, and partial hepatectomy (26). CAT-1 appears to be the most essential y$^+$ transporter in most cells. Homozygous knockout mice normally die within 1 day of birth (606). CAT-2b, an alternative splice product of CAT-2a, has different kinetic properties (135). In mouse,

CAT-2a and CAT-2b differ by an internal domain of 41 amino acids and are expressed in cells derived from different tissues. In most cell types, significant CAT-2b expression is only detected after cytokine or lipopolysaccharide stimulation. For example, lymphocytic activation induces CAT-2b expression and is often induced together with NO synthase. Activating the CAT-2b transport system results in the accumulation of intracellular arginine, which correlates with an increased need for nitric oxide as an immune response regulator (82, 156, 389).

CAT transporters mediate the uptake of important amino acids such as arginine, lysine, and ornithine. Arginine, synthesized in the kidney and liver, is the precursor for nitric oxide; lysine is a precursor for the synthesis of trimethyllysine and carnitine, which supply long chain fatty acids through β-oxidation (58); and ornithine is required for polyamine production needed during cell proliferation and tissue growth (355). In most cells CAT-1 (SLC7A1) or CAT-2 (SLC7A2) also serve to transport cationic amino acids into cells in order to allow leucine uptake in exchange for cationic amino acids via system y^+L. Subsequently, leucine inside the cell is used to allow the uptake of other essential amino acids in exchange for leucine via system L.

CAT-3 (SLC7A3) is a high-affinity, brain-specific, cationic amino acid transporter (324). There is no apparent correlation between CAT-3 expression and the neuronal NOS production. The CAT-4 (SLC7A4) isoform is only ~40% identical to CAT1-3. CAT-4 (SLC7A4) is abundantly expressed in the brain, testis, and placenta. The CAT-4 gene was mapped to human chromosome 22q11.2, the commonly deleted region of the velocardiofacial syndrome (VCFS, Shprintzen syndrome) (750). In a patient affected by VCFS, deletion of CAT-4 was demonstrated.

Glycoprotein–Associate Amino Acid Transporters

The gpaAT subfamily includes nine members, SLC7A5 to SLC7A11, and two newly identified members, Asc-2 and AGT1. These proteins display homology to bacterial and yeast amino acid permeases and therefore belong to the "APC" (amino acid, polyamine, choline) superfamily (655). These gpaATs proteins require association with type II membrane proteins such rBAT and 4F2hc (see SLC3) for expression on the membrane surface. Of these known light chains, six are known to associate with 4F2hc and result in basolateral sorting of the transporter complex in the kidney and intestine epithelia. The light chains SLC7A1 (LAT1, also known as ASUR4b and E16), SLC7A6 (y^+LAT2), SLC7A7 (y^+LAT1), SLC7A8 (LAT2), SLC7A10 (asc-1), and SLC7A11 (xCT) associate with the 4F2 heavy chain (SLC3A2) to allow functional expression of the transporter (374, 507, 806). The light, nonglycosylated chain SLC7A9 ($b^{0,+}$AT) presumably complexes in the ER with the glycosylated SLC3A1 type II membrane glycoprotein via a disulfide bridge followed by expression in the apical membrane of the epithelial cells in the kidney proximal tubule and small intestine. The exact mechanism of the process, however, is still unclear.

LAT1 (SLC6A5) corresponds to the classically characterized amino acid transport system L (sodium-independent uptake of neutral amino acids), which plays an important role in growing cells, including tumor cells (374, 507). LAT1-4F2hc is an obligatory neutral amino acid exchanger that is strongly trans-stimulated by intracellular amino acids and has an exchange stoichiometry of 1:1 (520). LAT1 facilitates the cellular uptake of amino acid in exchange of amino acids that have been taken up by other transporters (i.e., ion-coupled transporters). LAT1-4F2hc does not mediate net amino acid uptake, but instead functions to equilibrate various amino acid levels in the cell.

y^+LAT2 (SLC7A6) is widely expressed in epithelial and nonepithelial tissues (643), in contrast to y^+LAT1 (89). It mediates Na^+-independent uptake of cationic amino acids as well as the Na^+-dependent uptake of neutral amino acids. Expression of 4F2 heavy chain (SLC3A2) in *Xenopus* oocytes along with SLC7A6 results in y^+LAT2 activity (869). The heterodimer complex mediates the obligatory exchange of neutral and cationic amino acids with a 1:1 stoichiometry. However, the efflux of cationic amino acids is far more efficient than the transport of neutral ones (89).

Based on homology to LAT1, y^+LAT1 (SLC7A7) was identified and has been shown to mediate neutral amino acid uptake in the presence of Na^+ in exchange for cationic amino acids that are effluxed from the cell (system y^+L) (608, 806). y^+LAT2 (SLC7A6) is expressed in the basolateral membrane of kidney proximal tubule cells (i.e., S1 segments). Its expression in the kidney proximal tubule and ability to efflux cationic amino acids suggested it may be involved in the hereditary disease lysinuric protein intolerance (LPI). Subsequently it was shown that genetic defects in SLC7A6 cause LPI, which results in hypersecretion of cationic amino acids but not cystine (807).

LAT2 (SLC7A8) is a system L-type transporter (616, 642, 673). It is similar to LAT1 but has a broader substrate range, accepting smaller amino acids as well. In the kidney proximal tubule S1 segments and in the intestine, it mediates neutral amino acid exchange across the basolateral membranes. It also mediates basolateral efflux of cysteine following apical uptake of cystine, which is reduced intracellularly.

$b^{0,+}$ AT (SLC7A9) corresponds to the $b^{0,+}$ transport system originally described in mouse blastocysts that transport neutral and cationic amino acids and cystine in the kidney proximal tubule (110, 643). This transporter requires association with D2/rBAT (SLC3A1) for functional expression and is found in the brush border membrane of the early proximal tubule and the upper intestine (Fig. 1). This is demonstrated when endogenous SLC7A9 activity is induced in *Xenopus* oocytes following expression of D2/rBAT (SLC3A1) (868). Under physiological conditions in the kidney proximal tubule (i.e., S3 segments) and in the intestine, the SLC7A9 transporter mediates Na^+-independent uptake of luminal cystine, arginine, and ornithine in exchange for neutral amino acids, which are effluxed from the cell. Genetic defects in SLC7A9 cause non–type I cystinuria (201) (see SLC3 family).

Asc-1 (SLC7A10) is activated by 4F2 heavy chain (SLC3A2) and mediates Na^+-independent transport of small neutral amino acids including glycine, alanine, serine, and cystine (228). It prefers to function in exchange mode, but not exclusively. Asc-1 mRNA was detected in the brain, lung, and small intestine. The exact physiological roles of this transporter have not yet been elucidated.

The xCT (SLC7A11) transporter delivers cystine into cells in exchange for glutamate. Intracellular cystine is rapidly degraded to cysteine and used for glutathione synthesis (693). This transporter corresponds to system X_{-c}. The expression of SLC7A10 is highest in cells that require glutathione to scavenge free radicals such as in activated macrophages, neurons, and glial cells.

Two additional members of the SLC7 family have been recently identified, Asc-2 (109) and AGT1 (509). They exhibit low sequence similarity to the other light-chain proteins. These transporters are not linked to activation by 4F2hc or rBAT and may require other, as yet unknown, type II glycoproteins for expression in the plasma membrane. However, when Asc-2 was expressed as a fusion protein with 4F2hc or rBAT, these complexes demonstrated functions similar to the Na^+-independent transport system asc but are more stereoselective. Asc-2 expression was found in the collecting ducts of the kidney, placenta, lung, spleen, and also in skeletal muscle. AGT1 (aspartate–glutamate transporter 1) is 48% identical to Asc-2 (509). Fusion proteins made with the heavy-chain proteins provide functional activity capable of transporting anionic amino acids, but distinct from xCT. Unlike xCT it does not transport cystine or homocysteate and demonstrates high affinity for aspartate and glutamate. AGT1 expression is mainly found in the proximal tubule and distal convoluted tubules in the kidney.

SODIUM–CALCIUM EXCHANGER FAMILY (SLC8)

Plasma membrane Na^+–Ca^{2+} exchangers are vital for controlling cytosolic calcium concentrations in many tissues, particularly in excitable cells. There are two distinct families of Na^+–Ca^{2+} exchangers, the NCX (SLC8) family and the NCKX (SLC24) family. The NCX family prototype is the sodium–calcium exchanger from dog heart (NCX1), which catalyzes the electrogenic exchange of three sodium ions for one calcium ion (565).

NCX1 (SLC8A1) is the most plentifully and broadly expressed Na^+–Ca^{2+} exchanger gene, with products present in almost every tissue and present at particularly high levels in the heart, brain, and kidney. NCX1 is the primary Ca^{2+} extrusion mechanism in cardiac myocytes; therefore, it has a central role in regulating myocardial contractility. Ischemia can easily reverse cellular ion gradients so that NCX1 pathologically increases cellular Ca^{2+}. In the kidney, NCX mediates basolateral Ca^{2+} absorption in the distal and connecting tubule. NCX1 (SLC8A1) was originally isolated by Philipson and colleagues using the polyclonal antibodies (565). Two additional mammalian Na^+–Ca^{2+} exchangers, NCX2 (SLC8A2) and NCX3 (SLC8A3), are expressed primarily in the brain and skeletal muscle, respectively (398, 564, 565). All three Na^+–Ca^{2+} exchangers are predicted to have 11 putative transmembrane domains with a large intracellular loop that is over 500 amino acids in length. The intracellular loop participates in regulatory responses and has a binding site for Ca^{2+} and a XIP regulatory sequence (510). NCX1 (SLC8A1) contains a signal sequence and one membrane span clipped by post-translational modification (64).

NCX1 (SLC8A1) is extensively alternatively spliced, primarily in exons of the intracellular loop, generating four tissue-specific variants (638). Both NCX2 (SLC8A2) and NCX3 (SLC8A3) have a deletion of 37 amino acids in this variable region of the intracellular loop. NCX3 (SLC8A3) differs from the other NCXs in its sensitivity to inhibition by Ni^{2+}, Co^{2+}, and the isothiourea derivative KB-R7943 (353). Recently, arterial-specific transgenic mice of NCX1 indicated that NCX1 was involved in salt-sensitive hypertension. NCX1 is related to the Ca^{2+} intake pathway in vascular smooth muscle cell for regulating vascular tone (352). The brain isoform of the Na^+–Ca^{2+} exchanger, NCX2, is implicated in learning and memory. The NCX2 (SLC8A2) knockout mice demonstrated hyperactive behavior, suggesting that NCX2 was related to the LTP–LTD process of neurons (359). NCX3 (SLC8A3) knockout mice showed necrosis of skeletal muscle fibers as well as defects of neuromuscular junction. Those suggested that NCX3 played an important role in intracellular Ca^{2+} regulation of the neuromuscular junction (743).

SODIUM–HYDROGEN EXCHANGER FAMILY (SLC9)

The Na^+–H^+ exchangers (NHEs) perform essential functions in transepithelial salt, base and acid transport, intracellular and extracellular pH regulation, and cell volume regulation. The SLC9 family contains ten family members that differ in their transport characteristics, tissue distribution, membrane targeting, and pharmacology. Membrane topology predicted by hydropathy analysis places the N-terminal and C-terminal domains in the cytoplasm, with a central core of 12 transmembrane (TM) domains. Homology among members is most distinct in the region between TM3 to TM12, which is thought to participate directly in cation exchange (578). The Na^+ affinity of the NHEs for which functional data are available ranges from 2 to 50 mM (578). Cation selectivity is variable, such that some of the family members may function primarily as K^+–H^+ exchangers (569). They are pharmacological targets for the diuretic amiloride and its analogues, with the following order of sensitivity for those expressed at the plasma membrane: NHE1 ≥ NHE2 > NHE5 > NHE3 (394).

The NHE protein tissue distribution ranges from ubiquitous (NHE1) to relatively tissue-specific as with NHE5. NHE1 (SLC9A1) and NHE4 (SLC9A4) are expressed at the basolateral membrane of renal epithelia (620), where as NHE2 (SLC9A2), NHE3 (SLC9A3), and NHE8 (SLC9A8) are found at the apical membrane (60, 260). NHE6 (SLC9A6), NHE7 (SLC9A7), and NHE9 (SLC9A9) are unique in that these proteins target to the membrane of intracellular organelles, NHE6 is located in early recycling endosome, NHE7 is in TGN, and NHE9 is in late recycling endosome (553). The physiological role of these intracellular NHEs is still unknown, but they most probably function to regulate organellar pH.

NHE1 has progressively more recognized roles in intracellular pH regulation, cell proliferation, cell survival, cell migration, and cytoskeletal organization (636). NHE1 (SLC9A1)-deficient mice exhibit a seizure disorder and ataxia (142), attributed to decreased neuronal pH (900) and selective neuronal death (142). Its transport activity is enhanced by growth factors, suggesting a role in cellular proliferation. Expressing NHE1, NHE2, or NHE3 in NHE-deficient fibroblasts increases cell proliferation (381) that is dependent on intact H^+ transport, but not on interactions with the cytoskeleton (155). NHE1 is targeted by multiple signaling pathways in response to growth factors and other stimuli. Significant progress has been made in defining the phosphorylation sites and regulatory interactions involved in NHE1 regulation (636). Interestingly, NHE1 has been shown to interact directly with the cytoskeleton through members of the ERM (*e*zrin-*r*adixin-*m*oesin) family, which bind to a positively charged region within the C-terminal domain (155). This interaction has been shown to be critical for the association between actin filaments and the cytoskeleton, such that cells with a disruption of the NHE1-ERM complex have abnormal cell shape and impaired adhesion (155).

One of the novel findings regarding NHE1 is that it appears to be involved in the regulation of HCO_3^- transport in the thick ascending limb of Henle's loop in the kidney. Curiously, NHE1 KO mice demonstrated a loss in HCO_3^- reabsorption, although it occurred in the opposite direction because NHE1 was thought to be expressed in the basolateral membrane (252). Some reports indicated that NHE1 activity in the basolateral membrane was, at least in part, linked to the NHE3 activity in the apical membrane (252). The inhibition of NHE1 activity in basolateral membrane caused decrease of NHE3 activity in apical membrane, resulting in decrease activity of HCO_3^- transporters.

NHE2 (SLC9A2) may play a compensatory role for NHE3, because in NHE2 knockout mice the NHE3 expression was twice higher than normal mice in colonic crypts (31). In the kidney of NHE3 (SLC9A3) KO mice, H^+ secretion was compensated by distal tubular H^+ secretion mediated by NHE2 (34). Thus, NHE2 may be involved in luminal pH regulation like NHE3.

NHE3 activity is critical for salt and fluid transport in both the intestine and kidney. Apical salt absorption via the proximal tubule (PT) is thought to be accomplished through coordinated actions of Na^+–H^+ exchange and Cl^--formate or Cl^--base exchange, and/or Na^+ SO_4^{2-} cotransport and Cl^--oxalate exchange (18, 855). Salt absorption by the intestine also involves cooperation between NHE3 and a Cl^--base exchanger, most likely encoded by the SLC26A3 gene (322, 522). NHE3 -/- mice are thus moderately volume depleted due to both intestinal fluid loss and impaired proximal tubular fluid absorption (476, 707). The increase in proximal chloride absorption induced by luminal perfusion with formate is abolished in NHE3 -/- mice, while preserving the stimulatory effect of oxalate (856); presumably since oxalate induces Na^+ reabsorption through the apical Na^+-SO_4^{2-} cotransporter (855). Despite the quantitative importance of NHE3 in transepithelial transport, evidence from knockout mice deficient in both NHE2 and NHE3 reveals residual Na^+–H^+ exchange or Na^+–HCO_3^- cotransport (127), potentially mediated by NHE8 (260). The NHE3 -/- mice also have a proximal renal tubular acidosis due to impaired proximal reabsorption of filtered HCO_3^- (707). Apical NHE3 is furthermore thought to play a role in bicarbonate absorption by the thick ascending limb, where the exchanger is upregulated in response to metabolic acidosis (435).

NHE3 (SLC9A3) activity in the renal proximal tubule is dynamically controlled through multiple hormones, although prominently by angiotensin II and dopamine. Angiotensin II activates apical Na^+–H^+ exchange in the proximal tubule (683), thereby increasing both HCO_3^- and Na^+–Cl^- absorption from the glomerular ultrafiltrate (462, 463, 708). Dopamine, a prominent natriuretic hormone, inhibits apical Na^+–H^+ exchange in the proximal tubule by inducing NHE3 endocytosis from clathrin-coated pits through a protein kinase A–dependent mechanism (328). The biochemical interaction between NHE3 and megalin (59), a key component of coated pits in the proximal tubule (451), is especially intriguing in this regard. Protein kinase A–mediated inhibition of NHE3 in the proximal tubule also requires the presence of two PDZ-domain accessory proteins, now denoted NHERF-1 and NHERF-2 (NHE regulatory factor-1 and -2) (865, 907). NHE3 and other transport proteins interact with NHERFs through a type I PDZ interaction motif (748) at the extreme C-terminal end of the protein. The NHERFs also bind to ezrin (650), which functions as an anchoring protein for protein kinase A, bringing the kinase into close proximity to NHE3 and other transport proteins (164, 767). The entire tripartite complex of NHE3–NHERF–ezrin appears to be required for full inhibition of epithelial Na^+–H^+ exchange by cyclic AMP (866). However, there is clear evidence for direct interactions between the PDZ domains of NHERFs and C-terminal PDZ interaction motifs in hormone receptors, including the β_2-adrenergic receptor (292), PTH receptor (491), and PDGF receptor (511). With the β_2-adrenergic receptor, receptor stimulation by hormone may bypass or even abrogate the inhibitory effect of PKA and NHERF (292).

In contrast, NHE4 (SLC9A4) plays a critical role in H^+ secretion in the stomach. NHE4 KO mice are hypochlorhydric, indicating that NHE4 was one of dominant transporters for stomach acid formation (238).

SODIUM–BILE ACID COTRANSPORTER FAMILY (SLC10)

Bile acids facilitate intestinal digestion and absorption of lipid-soluble vitamins (i.e., A, D, E, and K), xenobiotics, and heavy metals, and are essential for cholesterol homeostasis. They are synthesized from cholesterol in the liver mostly as bile salts, secreted into the gallbladder for storage, and delivered to the intestine in response to a meal. Bile acids are absorbed from the small intestine, particularly from the ileum, and returned to the liver via the portal vein. Intestinal bile absorption requires Na^+-coupled bile acid transporters in the intestinal brush border membrane and the sinusoidal membrane of hepatocytes. In the plasma, most bile acids are bound to proteins. Free bile acids are filtered in the kidney and are reabsorbed by renal proximal tubules. Intestinal bile acid absorption is critical for maintaining enterohepatic circulation, which thereby affects liver cholesterol synthesis because the rate-limiting enzyme of hepatic bile acid synthesis, cholesterol 7α-hydroxylase, is inhibited by the bile acids. Disrupting bile acid synthesis, biliary secretion, and enterohepatic circulation can lead to major defects in hepatic and gastrointestinal physiology. In particular, reduced bile acid reabsorption leads to both reduced absorption of fat and vitamins as well as reduced blood cholesterol levels.

There are two well-characterized SLC10 members and three orphan transporters in this family. The two sodium-dependent bile acid transporters ASBT (SLC10A2) (143) and Na^+/taurocholate cotransporting polypeptide (NTCP, SLC10A1) (288) are vital for maintaining enterohepatic circulation of bile salts. NTCP accounts for the majority of the Na^+-dependent bile salt uptake in hepatocytes (370). It is located on the basolateral (sinusoidal) membrane of hepatocytes where it can proficiently extract bile acids from the portal blood. ASBT is expressed in the brush border members of intestine (mainly in the ileum) and kidney tubules (143, 877), where it actively absorbs bile salts from the intestinal lumen and delivers them back to the portal circulation. Mutations in the human ASBT gene were found to cause congenital primary bile acid malabsorption (PBAM) (570), confirming the importance of ASBT in intestinal reclamation of bile acids. Both cotransport systems are electrogenic and carry two Na^+ with one bile acid. The Na^+ gradient needed is provided by the basolateral Na^+–K^+ ATPase and a negative intracellular potential. While both transporters mediate uptake of conjugated and unconjugated bile salts, ASBT has narrower substrate specificity than NTCP.

Other than their tissue distribution, not much is known about the three orphan members of this family. P3 (SLC10A3) has a wide tissue distribution and is thought to have housekeeping functions. It shares 27% of sequence identity with ASBT and NTCP. The hypothetical protein MGC29802 (SLC10A4, P4) shares 37% of sequence identity with NTCP and appears to be expressed mostly in neuroblastomas. The fifth SLC10 member (SLC10A5, P5) is expressed in the fetal brain. Functional characterization of P6 (SLC10A6, SOAT) has revealed that this gene encodes a sodium-dependent organic anion transporter (SOAT), which transports estrone-3-sulfate and dehydroepiandrosterone sulfate (DHEAS), but not taurocholate, estradiol-17β-glucuronide, ouabain, estrone, dehydroepiandrosterone (DHEA), or digoxin (244). SLC10A6 mRNA is expressed in the heart, lung, liver, spleen, testis, adrenal gland, small intestine, colon, and placenta.

PROTON–METAL-ION COTRANSPORTER FAMILY (SLC11)

Metal ions are important in many catalytic functions and physiological processes. A variety of human diseases are related to disturbances in metal ion homeostasis, including anemia (311, 840), hemochromatosis (196), Menke's disease (117, 524), and neurodegenerative diseases including Alzheimer's disease (253, 637), Parkinson's disease (316), and Friedreich's ataxia (28). The divalent-cation transporter family SLC 11 has two mammalian members: NRAMP1 (SLC11A1) (216) and DMT1 (SLC11A2) (285).

NRAMP1 (natural resistance-associated macrophage protein 1, SLC11A1) was identified by positional cloning in mice susceptible to infections of various mycobacteria and other intracellular parasites (739). Not surprisingly, NRAMP1 is expressed almost exclusively in macrophages (832, 833), or macrophage-derived cells and neurons (189). Its expression can be stimulated by mycobacterial infection in the peritoneal macrophages (845) and RAW264.7 macrophages (259).

The amino acid sequence was predicted to result in a protein with 12 transmembrane domains. The NRAMP1 protein was localized to late endosomal compartments of macrophages and to phagosomal membranes during phagocytosis (272). NRAMP1 (SLC11A1) might confer resistance to infections by depleting Fe^{2+} or Mn^{2+}, or other essential metal ions from the phagosome, thereby preventing the propagation of the bacteria (257, 546). NRAMP1 can transport several divalent cations including Mn^{2+}, Fe^{2+}, and Co^{2+}. Although the NRAMP1 mechanism of action is still not fully understood, NRAMP1 and DMT1 (SLC11A2) appear to transport iron via a common H^+/metal-ion cotransport mechanism (218, 614).

In an attempt to identify a mammalian iron transporter, expression cloning with *Xenopus* oocytes resulted in the identification of the DMT1 (SLC11A2) transporter (285). DMT1-mediated absorption of iron is electrogenic, voltage-dependent and H^+-coupled with an H^+ to Fe^{2+} coupling ratio of 1:1. Further studies under voltage clamp conditions revealed that DMT1 also transports Zn^{2+}, Mn^{2+}, Cu^{2+}, Co^{2+}, Cd^{2+}, and Pb^{2+}, with similar affinities. In the small intestine, DMT1 is absent from the iron-sensing crypt cells, although it is expressed at high levels along the duodenal crypt-to-villus axis, and also in other tissues such as kidney, brain, liver, bone marrow, and thymus. The acidic environment in the duodenal segment provides an H^+ electrochemical gradient sufficient for driving Fe^{2+} uptake into the enterocytes. The functional properties of DMT1 show the need for an acidic environment, as found in the early part of the duodenum of the intestine, as well as in the lumen of endosomes, where DMT1 is required for iron absorption via transferrin receptor–mediated endocytosis, allowing H^+-coupled transfer of iron from the acidic endosomal lumen into the cytosol.

Microcytic anemia (mk) mice display a characteristic intestinal defect in iron absorption and a defect in erythroid iron utilization. Andrews and colleagues (216) found that the mk locus coincides with the NRAMP2/DMT1 gene described earlier (271). The studies showed that the mk mice possess a single point mutation in DMT1 substituting arginine for glycine (G185R) (216). This mutation occurs in a transmembrane region (transmembrane domain 4), and results in a loss of function, consistent with the phenotype of the mk/mk mouse (132). Similar to mk mice, the Belgrade (b) rats have a severe hypochromic microcytic anemia that is associated with defects in erythroid iron utilization and intestinal iron uptake in the apical membrane of the enterocytes. Interestingly, the b rats also have the G185R mutation in transmembrane domain 4 (215). It is possible that a subset of human patients with congenital anemia also harbor mutations in DMT1. Indeed, isolated families have been described with apparently autosomal, recessively inherited iron-deficiency anemia, which is unresponsive to iron therapy (297), with an overall phenotype similar to that of the b rat and mk mouse.

ELECTRONEUTRAL CATION–CHLORIDE-COUPLED COTRANSPORTER FAMILY (SLC12)

The cation–chloride cotransporters perform electroneutral cotransport of Na^+ and/or K^+. These cotransporters are always accompanied by Cl^- in a 1:1 stoichiometry; therefore, they produce no change in membrane potential (153, 286, 444, 542). The family is composed of seven well-characterized membrane proteins including one thiazide-sensitive Na^+-Cl^- cotransporter, two bumetanide-sensitive Na^+-K^+-$2Cl^-$ cotransporters, and four K^+-Cl^- cotransporters. These cotransporters are involved in various physiological functions such as ion absorption and excretion, cell volume regulation, and regulating intracellular Cl^- concentrations. Some members of this family are pharmacologically significant because they are targets for thiazide-like diuretics and loop diuretics such as bumetanide, commonly used to treat high blood pressure and reduce the amount of water in the body. Inactivating mutations in three SLC12 cotransporters result in inherited human diseases, such as Bartter's syndrome type 1 and Gitelman's syndrome.

The founding member of the SLC12 family was the thiazide-sensitive Na^+-Cl^- cotransporter cloned from the *Pseudopleuronectes americanus* (winter flounder fish) urinary bladder (235). The human SLC12A3 was originally identified in an effort to study Gitelman's syndrome (737), and was simultaneously reported by Mastroianni et al. (508) after isolating it from a human kidney cDNA library. The NCC (SLC12A3) transporter is expressed almost exclusively in the kidney, specifically in the apical membrane of the distal convoluted tubule, but variably extends into the connecting segment in many species (32, 623, 471, 61). When expressed in *Xenopus* oocytes, NCC promotes thiazide-sensitive Cl^--dependent Na^+ uptake with a 1:1 stoichiometry (235, 536). The ions are proposed to bind in a random order, but binding of the first ion facilitates subsequent binding of the counterion. NCC (SLC12A3) cotransport of Na^+-Cl^- is the major sodium reabsorption pathway along the distal convoluted tubule, particularly in the early segment where it is the only pathway (102, 140, 179, 470). NCC is the major target for clinically useful thiazide diuretics such as bendroflumethiazide and hydrochlorothiazide, which inhibit NCC activity.

Magnesium and calcium reabsorption are also regulated by NCC. Inhibiting NCC with thiazides increases Ca^{2+} reabsorption, while increased activity or expression reduces Ca^{2+} reabsorption (140). This calcium-reabsorption modulating effect is the basis for using thiazides in the treatment of calcium stone disease and may explain their protective effects in osteoporosis (646, 706, 861). The fundamental role of SLC12A3 in preserving extracellular fluid volume and divalent cation homeostasis has been affirmed by identification of mutations in SLC12A3 that disrupt NCC function, which are the cause of Gitelman's syndrome, an autosomal recessive salt-wasting disorder (738, 429).

The NKCC2 (SLC12A1) gene encodes a renal specific Na^+-K^+-$2Cl^-$ cotransporter that is exclusively expressed in the apical membrane of thick ascending limb of Henle and macula densa cells (380, 566). This cotransporter is loop diuretic–sensitive and has been shown to mediate Na^+-K^+-$2Cl^-$ cotransport in an electroneutral manner (265, 303, 304). NKCC2 is not only has a critical role in NaCl reabsorption, but also in the production and maintenance of the countercurrent mechanism essential for urine concentration. The critical importance of NKCC2 in salt reabsorption in the thick ascending limb is supported by the identification of inactivating mutations in the SLC12A1 gene that cause Bartter's syndrome type I (737, 827). Knocking out SLC12A1 in mice replicates much of the Bartter's phenotype, although with a much greater defect in urinary concentrating ability (153, 777). NKCC2 (SLC12A1) is also important in cardiovascular and renal pharmacology, since it is the main target of loop diuretics such as furosemide and bumetanide used to treat clinical conditions including acute pulmonary edema and edema associated with chronic renal insufficiency.

The bumetanide-sensitive $Na^+-K^+-2Cl^-$ cotransporter NKCC1 (SLC12A2) is ubiquitously expressed in both epithelial and nonepithelial cells. In epithelial cells, expression is confined to the basolateral membrane, with exception to the choroid plexus, where it is found in the apical membrane (622). In the kidney, it is found in glomerular and extraglomerular mesangial cells and renin-positive juxtaglomerular cells, as well as at the basolateral membrane of the IMCD (380). At the cellular level the major role of SLC12A2 is in cell volume regulation, mainly as part of volume-increasing mechanisms induced upon cell shrinkage (440). In epithelial cells, where it is polarized to the basolateral membrane, the $Na^+-K^+-2Cl^-$ cotransporter is critically important to providing the cell with Cl^- that will be secreted from the apical membrane (153, 246). No human disease has been linked to mutations in SLC12A2, but targeted deletion in mice has revealed important roles for NKCC1 in hearing, spermatogenesis, salivation, and sensory perception (152, 190, 768). Interesting phenotypes include deafness, frequent loss of balance, male infertility, reduction in saliva production, and growth retardation.

The K^+-Cl^- cotransport mechanism was first described as a swelling-activated K^+ efflux pathway in red blood cells (170, 446). The cotransport of K^+ and Cl^- in red blood cells is interdependent, occurring with a 1:1 stoichiometry and low affinity (443). Red blood cell KCCs mediate K^+-Cl^- efflux under most conditions, whereas neuronal KCCs can promote efflux as well as influx. The four K^+-Cl^- cotransporters in the SLC12 family were molecularly identified in the gene database based on their homology to the Na^+-dependent cation–chloride cotransporters (245, 543, 601).

The K^+-Cl^- cotransporter KCC1 (SLC12A4) is a ubiquitously expressed membrane protein that appears to play an essential role in cell volume regulation. The K^+-Cl^- cotransport activity in erythrocytes has been predominately attributed to KCC1, which can be activated by cell swelling (245, 447, 523). K^+-Cl^- efflux from red cells has been speculated to be an important mechanism for cell size reduction occurring with maturation (445). However, the global physiological role of KCC1 remains elusive due to lack of knockout data.

KCC2 (SLC12A5) transport protein is unique among the KCCs since it is restricted to neurons in the central nervous system (601) and retina (826, 839). KCC2 is also unique in its ability to mediate isotonic K^+-Cl^- cotransport (600, 746, 761), a property that may be conferred via this cytoplasmic KCC2-specific domain. KCC2 has surfaced as a crucial component in regulating neuronal excitability and neuronal development via direct effects on neuronal chloride concentration and downstream modulation of the response to GABA and other neurotransmitters (527). KCC2 is essential in CNS physiology since KCC2 null mice experience early neonatal death caused by apneic respiratory failure, which is attributed to a defect in motor neuron regulation (334). GABA and glycine were inhibitory in wildtype neurons but excitatory in KCC2 null mice, consistent with KCC2 being necessary to switch GABA responses from excitatory to inhibitory. Mice deficient in KCC2 lived longer after birth but display a profound seizure disorder, partly due to a loss in the inhibitory effect of GABA (879). These animal studies are evidence for the involvement of KCC2 (SLC12A5) in regulating neuronal excitability and suggest a role for KCC2 in human epilepsy.

The KCC3 (SLC12A6) transcript is plentiful in many tissues, including muscle, brain, spinal cord, kidney, heart, pancreas, and placenta (313, 543, 640). KCC3 is expressed in most brain regions, including cerebellum, brain stem, cerebral cortex, and hypothalamus and in the spinal cord (602). The presence of KCC3 at the base of the choroid plexus suggests a potential function in cerebrospinal fluid K^+ reabsorption. Mutations in SLC12A6 leading to loss of function in KCC3 cause a rare neurological illness known as hereditary motor and sensory neuropathy associated with agenesis of the corpus callosum, also known as peripheral neuropathy associated with agenesis of the corpus callosum or Anderman's disease (327). This disease provides a unique example of a genetic defect producing clinical manifestations resulting from developmental and neurodegenerative problems involving both the central and the peripheral nervous systems. Most neurological problems seen in Anderman's disease can be reproduced in a SLC12A6 knockout mouse model (70, 327). However, despite genetic and functional evidence involving SLC12A6, the pathobiology of this disorder is not yet clear. KCC3 also has an important role in development and function of the inner ear, since knockout mice are not deaf at birth but become so during their first year due to cochlea degeneration.

The KCC4 K^+-Cl^- cotransporter isoform is widely distributed in the body. KCC4 knockout mice are normal at birth and exhibit no obvious nervous system dysfunction (69). Within the first few weeks the hearing in these mice is normal, but rapidly deteriorates until the mice are completely deaf. This observation is associated with complete loss of outer hair cells of the basal cochlea, potentially due to impaired K^+ uptake by supporting Deiter's cells (69). KCC4 may thus have a role in K^+ recycling in the cochlear as does KCC3. In the kidney, KCC4 (SLC12A7) has been identified at the basolateral membrane of type A intercalated cells and at the proximal tubule (69). KCC4-deficient mice develop renal tubular acidosis caused by defective acid secretion by intercalated cells (69), suggesting the involvement of KCC4 in basolateral Cl^- recycling required for H^+ secretion in the collecting duct.

In addition to the seven well-characterized SLC12 members, two orphan transporters exist in the cation–chloride cotransporter family. CCC9 (SLC12A8) was identified in a region of chromosome 3q21 linked to psoriasis susceptibility (312). SLC12A8 is ubiquitously expressed and has a unique predicted membrane topology compared to other SLC12 members. CCC9 is a short protein (714 amino acids) lacking predicted extracellular loops within the central core and is predicted to contain a glycosylated extracellular C-terminal tail. The transport function of SLC12A8 is not yet known. The final member, named the cation–chloride cotransporter interacting protein (CIP, SLC12A9), inhibits NKCC1 function when coexpressed (105). CIP may have a transport function of its own but the substrates are as yet unknown.

SODIUM CARBOXYLATE–SULFATE COTRANSPORTER FAMILY (SLC13)

The five proteins in this family can be divided into two functional groups: the Na^+–carboxylate cotransporters (NaC) and the Na^+–sulphate cotransporters (NaS). The SLC13 family includes the renal Na^+-dependent inorganic-sulfate transporter NaS1 (SLC13A1, NaSi1), the Na^+-dependent dicarboxylate transporter NaC1 (SLC13A2, SDCT1), the NaC3 (SLC13A3, SDCT2), the sulfate transporter-1 NaS2 (SLC13A4, SUT1), and the Na^+-coupled citrate transporter NaC2 (SLC13A5, NaCT). In general these proteins are proposed to produce membrane proteins with 8–13 transmembrane domains. While they have a wide tissue distribution, expression is most concentrated in epithelial tissues of the kidney and intestine. SLC13 members are Na^+-coupled symporters (Na^+/anion ratio of 3:1) and have a strong preference for divalent anions such as tetraoxyanions (via NaS) or Krebs cycle intermediates such as mono-, di-, and tri-carboxylates (via NaC).

The Na^+-carboxylate cotransporters in the intestine provide an absorption pathway for dietary dicarboxylates, like citrate and Krebs cycle intermediates, and NaCs in the kidney reabsorb dicarboxylates from the circulating plasma. Absorbed citrate is mainly utilized in the liver and kidney; less is known about citrate metabolism in other organ systems (293). In the proximal tubule of the kidney, di- and tri-carboxylates are taken up from both the tubular and peritubular side through Na^+-coupled transport systems, thus allowing maintenance of intracellular concentrations three- to fourfold higher than in the plasma. The Krebs cycle intermediates transported from tubular plasma membranes are incorporated into the intramitochondrial tricarboxylic acid cycle, which accounts for 10%–15% of oxidative metabolism in the kidney. Intracellular dicarboxylate accumulation also provides a driving force for the counterexchange of organic anions in the basolateral membrane that allows a variety of organic anions to be secreted including xenobiotics from the kidney (630). Citrate reabsorption from the tubule lumen is an important determinant of urinary citrate concentration, which is closely related to kidney stone formation (585). In hepatocytes, dicarboxylate transport plays a role in hepatic glutamine and ammonia metabolism and cooperates with the organic anion–dicarboxylate exchanger (OAT2; see SLC22A7) to facilitate exit of organic anions and drugs into the blood (68).

Three mammalian NaC cotransporters have been identified: NaC1 (SLC13A2), NaC2 (SLC13A5), and NaC3 (SLC13A3). These DIDS-insensitive cotransporters mediate electrogenic dicarboxylate transport with a Na^+ to substrate stoichiometry of 3:1 or 4:1 (for NaC2). The mechanisms are believed to be ordered, with the Na^+ binding to the transporter first, followed by the anion (583). Human NaC1 displays low-affinity, pH-independent (pH 6–8) transport of the anions succinate and citrate ($K_m = 7$ mM at pH 7.5) (582, 563). NaC3 is a pH-dependent, high-affinity Na^+-dicarboxylate cotransporter (717) that has a preference for the anions succinate, dimethylsuccinate, citrate, and N-acetyl-aspartate (119, 333). NaC2 encodes a pH-dependent, low-affinity cotransporter that can transport citrate, but not succinate or malate.

The NaC1 (SLC13A2) transporter displays a relatively wide tissue distribution that includes kidney, intestine, lung, and liver (581). The NaC2 (SLC13A5) transporter is expressed most predominately in the liver, while it has weaker expression in the brain and testis (346). NaC3 (SLC13A3) is primarily expressed in the placenta, kidney, liver, and brain, as well as other tissues (851). In the kidney, NaC1 and NaC3 mRNA transcripts are localized exclusively in S3 proximal tubule segments. This localization for NaC1 was confirmed by immunochemical analysis revealed that NaC1 is expressed in the apical membrane of the proximal tubule cells (584, 717). However, microperfusion studies have shown that the bulk of filtered citrate or α-ketoglutarate is reabsorbed in the convoluted S1–S2 segments of the proximal tubule (83, 207). Whether the putative citrate transporter in S1–S2 segments, which displays low-affinity (K_m ⊕ 6–7 mM) and high-capacity characteristics, corresponds to NaC1 or another transporter remains to be determined. The functional characteristics of NaC3 revealed that it corresponds to the basolateral transporter. Thus, in proximal tubule S3 segments, Krebs cycle intermediates, such as citrate, succinate, and α-ketoglutarate are actively absorbed from both from the glomerular filtrate and the peritubular capillaries by NaC1 in the apical and NaC3 in the basolateral plasma membrane. In the liver, the NaC2 transporter is suggested to facilitate uptake of circulating citrate for the production of metabolic energy and provide for the synthesis of cholesterol and fatty acids (345, 346).

Hypocitraturia is a common cause of nephrolithiasis. About 50% of patients with frequent kidney stones exhibit low urinary citrate excretion. In these patients, hypocitraturia is often the result of metabolic acidosis. Chronic metabolic acidosis increases proximal tubule citrate absorption. Consistent with this, it has been shown that this increase is associated with increased expression of NaC1 (21). These data suggested that the changes in blood bicarbonate and pH signal the increase in NaC1.

Sulfate transporters play an important role in the body's sulfate homeostasis. Two sulfate transporters have been identified thus far: NaS1 (SLC13A1) and NaS2 (SLC13A4). Urinary excretion of sulfate is ~10% of the filtered loadm and sulfate is reabsorbed in the proximal tubule by the Na^+-coupled sulfate transporter NaS1. This transporter has at least eight putative membrane-spanning regions and undergoes electrogenic pH-insensitive Na^+–sulfate cotransport with a stoichiometry of $\sim$3:1 (502, 97). It favors the anions sulphate, thiosulphate, and selenate, and the cation sodium as substrates (97, 502). NaS2 also mediates sulfate uptake, but no kinetics has been determined thus far (248).

The NaS1 (SLC13A1) transporter was found localized to the apical/brush border membrane of the epithelial cells of the renal proximal tubule and intestine (501). Due to its localization and special regulation, NaS1 is suggested to be the most critical protein in the regulation of serum sulfate levels (55, 501). NaS1 is sensitive to inhibition by heavy metals such as mercury, lead, and chromium; thus, blockage may be responsible for sulfaturia following heavy metal intoxication. The NaS2 (SLC13A4) expression has been predominately found in the placenta with lesser expression evident in the heart and testis (248). Its presence in the placenta potentially provides sulfate exchange between the mother and fetus.

UREA TRANSPORTER FAMILY (SLC14)

In mammals, urea is the major end product of nitrogen metabolism, and its absorption in the kidney is essential for urinary concentration. Urea formed in the liver via the urea cycle enters the circulation and is mostly excreted by the kidneys. Carrier-mediated transport allows swift urea movement, which aids in the urinary concentration process in the kidney and for rapid urea equilibrium in nonrenal tissues. Urea transporters are separated into two categories: the renal tubular/testicular type (UT-A1–A5) derived from the SLC14A2 gene and the erythrocyte UTB1 transporter encoded by SLC14A1 (575, 577, 726, 740, 812, 906).

The human SLC14A2 gene encodes at least four unique isoforms (UTA1, UTA2, UTA3, and UTA6), which arise from alternative splicing. UTA4 has been identified only in the rat and mouse while the UTA5 is only present in the mouse (203, 382). The proposed urea transporter structure contains two hydrophobic membrane-spanning domains and an extracellular glycosylated-connecting loop. UTA1, derived from gene duplication, consists of two internally homologous UTA1 units connected by a hydrophilic segment. UTA3 is identical to the N-terminal half of UTA1 and UTA2 is identical to the carboxy terminal half of UTA1. In the rat kidney, UTA1 is expressed in the apical membrane of the inner medullary collecting duct (IMCD) cells, with the highest concentration found in the terminal portion (Fig. 2). It corresponds to the vasopressin-regulated apical urea transporter involved in the majority of urea reabsorption in the terminal IMCD, and is activated by stimulation of protein kinase A through vasopressin.

UTA2 expression is found on the apical membrane in the late, thin descending limbs of the short loops and in the inner medullary part of the long loops of Henle where it is involved in "urea recycling" to limit the escape of urea from the hyper-

tonic renal medulla (724). The UTA3 urea transporter can also be found in the kidney within the apical IMCD membrane (798). There is less known about UTA4. It appears to be present in the inner medulla, but the protein has not been characterized (382). UTA-5 is expressed in the testis and may be involved in spermatogenesis (203). The UTA-6 isoform, a 235-amino acid protein isolated from colonic mucosa, promotes urea transport that can be inhibited by phloretin (741). It has been suggested that all UTA isoforms are expressed in tissues other than the kidney, including colon, heart, brain, liver, and testis (166, 204, 406, 906).

Unlike UTA isoforms, the UTB1 transporter has broad tissue distribution, including kidney and extrarenal tissue. UTB1 is expressed in many tissues, including erythrocytes, kidney inner and outer medulla, testis, brain, and spleen. In humans, UTB1 corresponds to the Kidd (JK) blood type antigen (576). In the kidney, UTB1 is expressed not in nephron segments but instead in the descending vasa recta, the papillary surface epithelium, and the transitional epithelium of the ureters. UTB1 expression in blood vessels allows countercurrent urea exchange between ascending and descending vasa recta, a process that enhances the corticopapillary osmolality gradient. Mice lacking the UTB1 transporter are unable to concentrate urea in the renal medulla, resulting in a urea-selective urinary concentrating defect that leads to higher blood urea and lower urine urea concentrations (897). UTB1 is also expressed in astrocytes and ependymal cells in the rat brain and in Sertoli cells in seminiferous tubules of the testis (49). In the brain and testis, the presence of UTB1 may be a mechanism to control urea formation during polyamine synthesis. Polyamines are positively charged molecules that are critically involved in cell division and proliferation. They are primarily synthesized from ornithine, thus generating urea as a byproduct. UTB1 expression in astrocytes may be involved in the regulation and dispersal of high urea levels in the brain. Similarly, UTB1 expression by Sertoli cells in the testis may allow the exit of urea from these cells during polyamine synthesis.

The regulation of UTA1 and UTA2 allows the kidney to adapt to physiologic stresses such as dehydration and starvation, and to maintain appropriate fluid and body nitrogen homeostasis. Quick responses can occur through vasopressin stimulation and can rapidly increase rat IMCD urea permeability after several minutes. UTA1 in the inner medulla is downregulated in response to increased vasopressin levels, as occurs during dehydration, nephritic syndrome, or exogenous administration (206, 725, 797) and upregulated conditions that lead to reduced urinary concentration. However, each isoform responds differently to the regulatory stimuli. While UTB1 protein expression is downregulated like UTA1 after vasopressin stimulation (798), UTA2 and UTA3 levels increase after dehydration-induced vasopressin release.

UTA1 and UTA2 have been shown to be regulated at the transcriptional level in response to changes in the hydration state and dietary protein intake (811). During a 1-week low-protein diet, UTA2 mRNA upregulates in the base of the rat

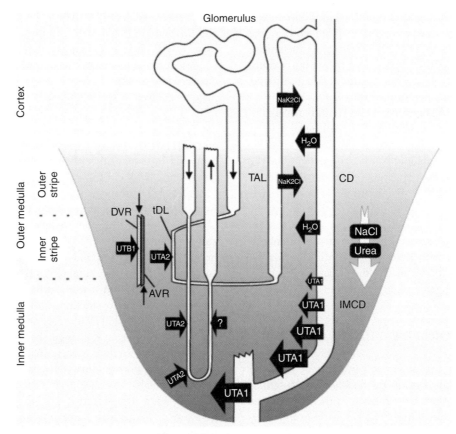

FIGURE 2   Urea transporter distribution and the urinary concentrating mechanism. The distribution of urea transporters in the inner medullary collecting duct (IMCD), descending thin limb of short loop (tdl-s), long loop (tdl-l), and descending vasa recta (DVR) are shown. The terminal part of the IMCD also expresses UT-A3 and possibly UT-A4 (not shown). AVR, ascending vasa recta; CD, collecting duct; TAL, thick ascending limb.

kidney inner medulla, but returns to normal levels after 2 weeks (22). Dehydration in Sprague–Dawley rats following 3-day water restriction resulted in a large increase in UTA2 mRNA levels, while the UTA1 mRNA level in the kidney inner medulla was not elevated. A similar increase in UTA2 mRNA was also seen in Brattleboro rats after continuous infusion with vasopressin for 1 week. The functional role of UTA2 transcript upregulation in this region has not been clearly defined, although it is likely a mechanism to maintain high levels of urea and increased hypertonicity in the inner medulla during water restriction.

PROTON–OLIGOPEPTIDE COTRANSPORTER FAMILY (SLC15)

The dietary proteins broken down in the gastrointestinal tract by brush border membrane-bound peptidases and pancreatic enzymes can result in as many as 400 different dipeptides and 8000 tripeptides. Therefore, peptide transporters adapted to accommodate a vast array of substrates. Di- and tri-peptides are subsequently absorbed by proton-coupled peptide transporters oriented in the brush border membrane. Similarly, the kidney has an analogous transport system for reabsorption of di- and tri-peptides in the proximal tubules. Additionally, in the brain, peptide transporters are involved in the clearance of degraded neuropeptides and xenobiotics. There are currently four members of the SLC15 transporter family: PEPT1 (SLC15A1), PEPT2 (SLC15A2), PHT1 (SLC15A4), and PHT2 (SLC15A3) (5, 79, 466, 688, 895). The PEPTs have been extensively studied, whereas less is known about the PHTs (SLC15A3 and SLC15A4).

The PEPT transporters have 12 putative transmembrane domains with both N- and C-termini facing the cytosol. PEPT1 is expressed predominantly in the brush border membrane of intestinal enterocytes, to a lesser degree in kidney proximal-tubule S1 segments (742), and in bile duct epithelial cells (409, 571). PEPT1 is a low-affinity, high-capacity cotransporter functioning in bulk uptake of dietary peptides. PEPT2, which has 50% sequence identity to PEPT1, has a wider tissue distribution, but is predominately found in the apical membranes of renal S2 and S3 proximal tubules, in brain astrocytes, and in epithelial cells of the choroid plexus (48, 799). While these two transporters share similar substrate specificities, PEPT2 demonstrates high-affinity, low-capacity transport for many substrates, and appears to differentially recognize certain antibiotics compared to PEPT1. PEPT2 in the kidney proximal tubule is well suited as a high-affinity transporter for reabsorption of oligopeptides and peptidomimetics compounds. In contrast, PEPT2 expressed in the choroid plexus epithelium plays an efflux role, as it appears to be responsible for neuropeptide clearance into the cerebrospinal fluid (727, 733). To drive peptide transport, these transporters undergo proton-coupled cotransport, which is accomplished in coordination with ion exchangers and channels in the epithelial cell (Fig. 3). PEPT1 transports one proton along with one neutral or one cationic dipeptide. However, when anionic dipeptides are carried as a charged species, two protons are required, whereas in neutral form only one is needed (418, 485, 756). PEPT2 utilizes two protons per neutral substrate (120), although charged substrates have more variable coupling ratios.

To assess the role and importance of peptide transport in animal models, two PEPT2-deficient mouse models have been developed and characterized in recent reports (678, 733). These animals were viable and displayed no noticeable kidney or brain abnormalities. However, functional ability of the choroid plexus cells to transport dipeptide was nearly

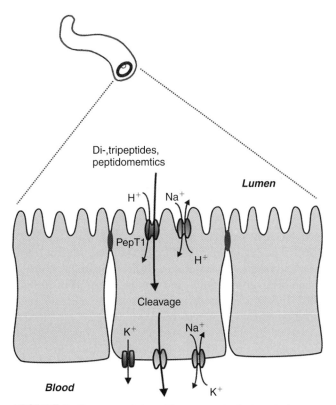

FIGURE 3 Proton-coupled peptide transport in the intestinal enterocyte. The proton-coupled transport of peptides and peptidomimetics is accomplished with the cooperation of ion exchangers and ion channels that provide a proton gradient into the epithelial cell. In the intestinal enterocyte, PEPT1 mediates the active uptake process, whereas in the kidney, PEPT2 reabsorbs the majority of peptides and peptideometics.

eliminated and renal reabsorption of model dipeptides was diminished. In humans, there have been no clear reports of peptide transporter–related pathology, although it has been suggested that PEPT1 may be involved in the inflammatory process related to inflamed colon tissues. PEPT1 has been shown to be expressed in these inflamed colonic tissues, while it is not normally expressed in healthy colon. PEPT1 expression may be linked to this condition because it has been shown to mediate uptake of bacteria-derived chemotactic peptides such as fMLP (525), which seems to mediate intestinal inflammation (98).

The capacity of PEPT1 and PEPT2 to transport almost any di- and tri-peptide, regardless of their charge, size, and composition is a unique property of these transporters. Single amino acids and larger oligopeptides (more than four mers) are excluded. A detailed analysis of the structural requirements for PEPT1 and PEPT2 transport using hundreds of compounds led to many insights (35). Bulky hydrophobic side chains and free amino- and carboxy-termini are preferred, since modifying these positions greatly reduces binding affinity. A terminal carboxyl group is not essential, although if present the sterical location is most critical. The transporters are partially stereoselective since peptides containing L-amino acids show greater affinity than D-amino acids. Proton-coupled peptide transporters also mediate the transport of many biologically active and therapeutically important peptidomimetics. Many orally active antibiotics (e.g., amino-penicillin, cyclacillin, amino-cephalosporins, cephradine, and cefadroxil) possess structural features similar to those of physiologic oligopeptide substrates. Several β-lactam antibiotics that lack protonatable amino groups (e.g., cefixime and cefdinir) are also transported. The peptide transporters also mediate the uptake of other active peptides such as angiotensin-converting enzyme inhibitors (e.g., captopril) and anticancer agents (e.g., bestatin). Based on the relatively flexible substrate requirements, rational drug design is possible to improve the oral bioavailability of drug compounds by routing them for uptake via PEPT1 in the intestine. The prodrug concept has produced several anticancer and antiviral prodrugs such as amino acid esters of acyclovir, ganciclovir, gemcitabine, and floxuridine (236, 439, 747). Intestinal transporters are important for more than improving drug bioavailability; peptidomimetic compounds would also have the potential to be substrates for the PEPT2 carrier expressed in the renal tubules. Renal reabsorption could reduce the renal clearance of the compounds, and thus may positively improve the drug pharmacokinetics.

The two newly identified transporters, PHT1 and PHT2, are 22%–27% identical to PEPT1/2 at the amino acid sequence level. They are unique from the PEPTs because they are able to transport the amino acid histidine, in addition to certain di- and tri-peptides. However, the PHT transport driving force, transport mechanism, and substrate specificity have not been extensively investigated. PHT1 (SLC15A4) is abundantly expressed in neurons and glial cells of rat brain and in the eye where it may be involved in the removal of degraded neuropeptides. When the rPHT1 was expressed in *Xenopus* oocytes, it was capable of transporting histidine and carnosine in a pH-dependent manner (895). rPHT2 is abundant in the lung, spleen, and lymphatic tissue, but is also found in the brain, liver, and heart, as well as in trace amounts in the kidney (688). The human PHT2 (SLC15A3) appears to function as a lysosomal histidine and histidyl-leucine transporter. These PHT transporters have yet to be detected on the plasma membrane, but instead have been reported to be present on the lysosomal membrane where they are thought to salvage histidine and dipeptide from lysosomal degradation by transporting them back into the cytosol.

PROTON–MONOCARBOXYLATE COTRANSPORTER FAMILY (SLC16)

The monocarboxylate cotransporter (MCT) family encompasses up to 14 members, but less than half have been functionally characterized. MCT1–MCT4 (SLC16A1, SLC16A7, SLC16A8, and SLC16A3) have demonstrated the ability to mediate H^+-coupled transport of metabolically significant monocarboxylates such as lactate, pyruvate, and ketone bodies. Not all MCTs transport monocarboxylates. However, it is surprising that a member of this family, MCT8 (SLC16A2), is a specific thyroid hormone transporter (225). Another exception is TAT1, which is a Na^+-coupled transporter of aromatic amino acids. Interestingly, TAT1 does not accept monocarboxylates (397).

Lactic acid is an important metabolite and substantial amounts are utilized or produced by almost all mammalian cells. Under hypoxic conditions, cells become glycolytic, and lactic acid export becomes particularly important. In muscle, however, MCT4 (SLC16A3) displays a low affinity for lactic acid, presumably to prevent systemic acidosis during prolonged exercise (366). Hepatocytes and kidney cells, in contrast, absorb lactic acid for metabolic purposes such as gluconeogenesis (291). In the heart, muscle, and brain (neurons), lactate is used source of metabolic energy (51, 73). In the brain, glial cells export lactic acid via MCT1 (SLC16A1) and MCT4 (SLC16A3), and thereby taken up by neurons via MCT1 or MCT2 (SLC16A7) to be used for oxidative metabolism (51). In the human colon, MCT1 expression was localized to the apical membrane of cells along the crypt to villus axis. Analysis of carcinoma samples revealed reduced levels of MCT1 and an increase in the high-affinity glucose transporter, GLUT1, suggesting a switch from lactate/butyrate to glucose as an energy source in colonic epithelia during the transition to malignancy (438).

Each MCT isoform has a unique tissue distribution and also appears to possess different transport preferences (628). For example, MCT1 (SLC16A1) is abundant in erythrocytes, cardiac muscle, basolateral membrane of intestinal epithelium and brain glial limiting membranes, and brain endothelial cells. MCT1 and MCT4 are expressed in glial cells where they contribute in the transport of brain fuels and metabolites between neurons and glia (241). MCT1 mediates the net transport of either one monocarboxylate with one proton or can exchange one carboxylate for another. The transporter has the ability to carry short-chain, unbranched aliphatic monocarboxylates such as acetate, propionate, lactate, pyruvate, and ketone bodies, but requires a type I auxiliary protein, CD147, for functional membrane expression (402). CD147 knockout mice exhibit abnormal ERG (electroretinogram), suggesting that decreased MCT-1 and -4 expression on the surfaces of Müller and photoreceptor cells may impair energy metabolism in the outer retina, leading to irregular photoreceptor cell function and degeneration (612).

Similarly MCT2 (SLC16A7) transports monocarboxylates along with a proton (74). Like MCT1 it transports a range of monocarboxylates, but with more affinity. The MCT2 expression in major human tissues is poor (628). MCT3 (SLC16A8) has a unique basolateral distribution, being expressed in retinal pigment epithelial cells and choroid plexus epithelium, suggesting that MCT3 regulates lactate levels in CSF (613). MCT4 (SLC16A3) is broadly expressed but especially strong expression is found in glycolytic tissues such as the skeletal muscle, astrocytes, and white blood cells. Additionally, CD147 is known to transport lactate, pyruvate, and ketone bodies, and may be important in the placenta for lactic acid export from fetal circulation (628). Several other MCTs with known expression patterns include MCT5 (SLC16A4) in the kidney, ovary, and placenta; MCT6 (SLC16A5) in kidney muscle and placenta; and MCT7 (SLC16A6) in the brain, pancreas, and heart. However, no functional data are available for these isoforms.

Two MCT family members have rather unique substrate preferences. The newly characterized transporter MCT8 (SLC16A2) appears to play a role in thyroid hormone metabolism. It has been shown to induce uptake of the thyroid hormones thyroxine (T4), 3,3',5-triiodothyronine (T3), 3,3',5'-triiodothyronine (rT3), and 3,3'-diiodothyronine, and is most predominately expressed in the liver, kidney, brain, and heart (225). The transporter TAT1 (SLC16A10) cannot carry monocarboxylates; instead it mediates uptake of aromatic amino acids in a sodium- and proton-independent manner (397). It has strong basolateral expression in the intestine and can also be found in muscles and the kidney.

Several human disorders are associated with the MCT family. A defect in MCT1 has been implicated in cryptic exercise intolerance, suggesting that the potential MCT1 dysfunction may be related to a lack of lactate efflux (213). In the patients of Allan–Herndon–Dudley syndrome and severe X-linked psychomotor retardation, MCT8 mutations have been found (226). Since those patients have high serum T3 concentration, loss of function of MCT8 (SLC16A2) thyroid hormone transporter may cause impaired T3 action and metabolism (709).

VESICULAR GLUTAMATE–ORGANIC ANION–PHOSPHATE TRANSPORTER FAMILY (SLC17)

Phosphate cotransporters have been divided into three gene families: NPT-type I (SLC17, this family), PIT (SLC20), and NPT type II (SLC34). The SLC17 family facilitates the transmembrane movement of organic anions, such as phosphate and sialic acid. Phosphate is an important component of bone, nucleic acids, and regulatory proteins. The founding member of the SLC17 gene family is NaPI1, a type I transporter (NPT1) (871) that functions as a Na^+–phosphate cotransporter, although the NPT2 knockout mouse has revealed that NaPI1 is not important for the proximal tubule as a renal phosphate transporter (42). The role of the NPT–type I transporters in phosphate movement remains unclear; however, as it is apparent that this family facilitates the transport of organic anions involved in various cellular processing including vesicular glutamate storage and glycoprotein metabolism.

In addition to the NPT type-I phosphate transporters, the SLC17 gene family includes vesicular glutamate transporters (VGLUT1–3) and the sialic acid transporter (sialin). Currently, there are eight SLC17 members: four Na^+–phosphate cotransporters, including NPT1 (NaPI1, SLC17A1) (871), NPT3 (SCL17A2), NPT4 (SLC17A3), and KAIA2138 (SLC17A4) (679); a lysosomal H^+–sialic acid cotransporter sialin (AST, SLC17A5) (829); and three vesicular H^+–glutamate exchangers VGLUT1 (DNPI, SLC17A7) (46, 224), VGLUT2 (BNPI, SLC17A6) (8, 224), and VGLUT3 (SLC17A8) (696, 780).

When expressed in *Xenopus* oocytes, rabbit kidney NPT1 (SLC17A1) increased inorganic phosphate uptake up to sixfold with a $K_m \oplus 1$ mM (871), while the human form has a slight higher affinity, $K_m = 0.3$ mM (534). However, when phosphate transport is measured in native tissues the affinity appears much higher, which suggests other carriers. This high-affinity transport appears to result from the type II– and type III–phosphate transporter families. While NPT1 may not be the primary transporter mediating phosphate uptake (548), it may play a more important role in transporting organic anions such as benzylpenicillin. The anion transport is electrogenic, but the endogenous substrates remain unclear. Interestingly, expression in *Xenopus* oocytes reveals an associated Cl^- conductance (90, 96). Type I–phosphate transporters have a narrow tissue distribution. NPT1 is expressed in the brush border membrane of the kidney proximal tubule and at reduced levels in the sinusoidal membrane of hepatocytes (57, 145, 871, 892). The other type I–phosphate transporters are also found in the kidney. Additionally, NPT3 (SLC17A2) mRNA has been found in high levels in the heart and muscle, NPT4 (SLC17A3) expression can be identified as well in the small intestine and testis, and SLC17A4 in the liver, pancreas, small intestine, and colon. Yet, no functional characterization has been performed with SLC17A2–4.

The degradation of glycosylated membrane proteins in lysosomes leads to production of free sialic acid, which can be recovered via carrier mediated export. The carrier responsible for sialic acid recovery is the lysosomal sialic acid transporter (SLC17A5) (495). This transport activity is pH dependent, showing highest transport levels at low extralumenal pH (302, 494). In addition to sialic acid, this carrier mediates transport of monocarboxylic acids, including lactate, gluconate, and glucuronic acid. When sialic acid efflux is disrupted, this material can accumulate in lysosomes and cause disorders such as sialic acid storage disorders, Salla disease, and infantile sialic acid storage disease (ISSD) (25). As many as 16 disease causing mutations have been identified in sialic transporter genes, often producing variable phenotypes (24).

VGLUT1 (SLC17A7) and VGLUT2 (SLC17A6), as initially characterized, mediate Na^+–phosphate cotransport activity when expressed in *Xenopus* oocytes (7, 561). Yet, all three isoforms have been shown to also transport glutamate, all with similar affinity for glutamate ($K_m \oplus 1$ mM). This transport process is driven by a proton electrochemical gradient across the vesicular membrane. Like NPT1, when VGLUT1 acts as a glutamate transporter it is also associated with Cl^- transport (46). The transporters VGLUT1–3 are all found at the termini of glutamanergic neurons where they are thought to concentrate glutamate into neurosecretory vesicles for subsequent release. VGLUT3 (SLC17A8) is the most recently characterized isoform and is distinct from VGLUT1 and VGLUT2, because it is expressed in neurons not classically considered glutamatergic. VGLUT3 is present in both excitatory and inhibitory neurons, cholinergic neurons, monoamine neurons, and glia. It is also expressed in the kidney and liver, suggesting that it may function in the peripheral glutamatergic nervous system (222).

Thus, rather than being a "phosphate transporter" family, the major physiological role of the SLC17 transporters appear to be organic anion transport/exchange. Knockouts and further physiology experiments will highlight the dominant role of this gene family.

VESICULAR MONOAMINE (ACETYLCHOLINE) TRANSPORTER FAMILY (SLC18)

This family includes two vesicular monoamine transporters, SLC18A1 and SLC18A2 (VMAT1 and VMAT2, respectively) (186, 770), and a vesicular acetylcholine transporter, SLC18A3 (VAChT) (186). These transporters function in accumulating acetylcholine and biogenic amines into secretory vesicles used during neurotransmission. The transport of these positively charged amines is coupled to the countertransport of protons. At the expense of the proton gradient maintained by a vacuolar ATPase, one amine is accumulated per two translocated protons. Remarkably, these transporters are able to concentrate substrates in vesicles up to final concentrations of up to 500 mM, which is 100-fold higher than the cytosolic acetylcholine concentration and 10,000-fold higher than the typical biogenic amine concentration (597).

VMAT1 (SLC18A1) is exclusively expressed in neuro-endocrine cells, including adrenal chromaffin and entero-chromaffin cells, which can be found in tissues such as the adrenal gland, sympathetic ganglia, skin, and intestine. VMAT2 (SLC18A2) is expressed in chromaffin cells as well as in central, peripheral, and enteric neurons located in various tissues including the brain, intestine, and pancreas, and in enterochromaffin-like cells in the oxyntic mucosa of stomach. These proteins are expressed as integral membrane proteins in the membrane of the secretory vesicles. VMAT1 and VMAT2 have different affinities for catecholamines (dopamine, adrenaline, noradrenaline), serotonin, and histamine, and they show different inhibitory profiles for some drugs (187). The vesicular monoamine transporters are the action sites for important pharmacologic agents such as reserpine and tetrabenazine (186). Malfunctions of these transporters are thought to be implicated in severe neuropsychiatric disorders. Homozygous knockouts of VMAT2 are lethal in mice, while heterozygous animals show only half the dopamine, norepinephrine, and serotonin in the brain (217, 778, 858). Human polymorphisms in the SLC18A2/VMAT2 were proposed to lead to alterations in drug response and vulnerability to drug addiction (819).

The VAChT gene (SLC18A3) is located within the first intron of the gene for choline acetyltransferase (ChAT), the enzyme required for acetylcholine biosynthesis in the peripheral and central cholinergic nervous systems. The transcription of VAChT and ChAT mRNA from promoters within the same regulatory locus represents a unique mechanism for the coordinated regulation of the two proteins whose expression is required to establish a mammalian neuronal phenotype. VAChT can be found expressed in neurons in many tissues, including the brain, peripheral nervous system, and intestine, where it transports acetylcholine into synaptic vesicles. VAChT is a distinctive marker for cholinergic synapses and neuroeffector junctions.

FOLATE AND THIAMINE TRANSPORTER FAMILY (SLC19)

This family includes a reduced folate transporter RFT (SLC19A1) and two thiamine transporters, ThTr1 (SLC19A2) and ThTr2 (SLC19A3), which are responsible for transporting two important water-soluble vitamins, folate and thiamine. These transporters are members of a large, phylogenetically distributed transporter superfamily, called "major facilitator superfamily" (MFS) (595). Members of this superfamily are involved in functions such as sugar uptake, drug efflux, and oligosaccharide–H^+ symport. SLC19 members are rather ubiquitously expressed in many tissues, but can be particularly highly expressed in absorptive tissues (intestine, kidney, and placenta) on either the apical or basolateral membranes. All three transporters utilize a transmembrane pH gradient to drive transport, although by different mechanisms.

Folate and its derivative compounds can be transported into cells either via a receptor-mediated pathway or a simple carrier-mediated mechanism (123). The carrier-mediated mechanism can internalize both natural folates and their cytotoxic analogues in tumor and normal proliferative tissues. RFT (SLC19A1) has 12 transmembrane domains and was the first vitamin transporter to be cloned in human (123, 560, 626, 874, 878, 898). RFT mediates the cellular uptake of reduced folates such as 5-methyltetrahydrofolate, and is inhibited by stilbenedisulfonate derivatives in a pH-dependent manner. It shows a greater affinity for reduced folates such as N^5-methyltetrahydrofolate and methotrexate compared to folate (734). At physiological pH all the RFT substrates exist as anions, and their transport is sensitive to the classical organic anion inhibitor, probenecid. Transport appears to be coupled to the symport of protons into the cell or antiport of hydroxide ions (645).

RFT (SLC19A1) is expressed in all human tissues but at higher levels in intestinal epithelial cells, especially the upper half of the villi, placenta, and kidney. In the intestine, it is expressed in the apical membrane where it mediates the uptake of dietary folates (857). In the placenta, it is located on the basal membrane of the syncytiotrophoblast where it delivers folates into fetal circulation. Subcellularly it is also been found on the mitochondrial membranes where it appears to traffic folate derivatives from the cytoplasm to the mitochondrial matrix (808). RFT is also expressed in tumor cells and transports cytotoxic folate analogues such as the chemotherapeutic agent methotrexate. Mutations in the SLC19A1 gene can cause resistance to antifolates. Gene knockout studies revealed that in the absence of RFT (SLC19A1) function, neonatal animals die because hematopoietic organs fail (909).

The widely expressed ThTr1 (SLC19A2) and ThTr2 (SLC19A3) carriers mediate the specific transport of thiamine, possibly by countertransporter with H^+ (172). ThTr1 proteins are both the plasma membrane and intracellular membranes (214). Deletion of ThTr1 in mice results in diabetes, sensorineural deafness, and megaloblastosis when the animals were kept on a thiamin-deficient diet (572). The animals recovered after dietary thiamin repletion. Similar to rats, mutations in human ThTr1 result in the thiamine-responsive megaloblastic anemia (TRMA) with diabetes and deafness (158, 269, 434, 647). Erythrocytes and cultured skin fibroblasts from TRMA patients exhibited a defect in the plasma membrane transport of thiamine and dietary supplementation of thiamine ameliorates the disease. The more recently identified thiamine transporter, ThTr2, most likely transports thiamine through an antiport process involving protons (644) and is also widely expressed in human tissues. Nutritional thiamine deficiency is normally associated with cardiovascular and neurological problems but is not seen in human TRMA patients or in ThTr1 knockout mice. Therefore, ThTr2 or some other thiamine transporters may be sufficient to compensate for the loss of ThTr1.

PIT PHOSPHATE COTRANSPORTER FAMILY (SLC20)

The two members of SLC20 were originally identified as cell surface receptors for gibbon ape leukemia virus 1 (GLVR1) and rat amphotropic leukemia virus (Ram-1, GLVR2) (388, 875). However, their normal physiological function is phosphate transport; therefore, they are now classified as type III sodium phosphate cotransporters. These SLC20 transporters include the two isoforms, PIT1 (SLC20A1) and PIT2 (SLC20A2) (369, 825). Phosphate transport via PIT is sodium dependent and electrogenic, and is inhibited by viral infection. PIT1 and PIT2 transporters have three- or fourfold higher affinity for phosphate than the renal type II NaPI Na^+–phosphate cotransporters of the SLC34 family. Both PIT1 and PIT2 have wide but distinct tissue distributions that include the kidney, brain, heart, liver, muscle, and bone marrow, and their expression is increased by phosphate deprivation. Their physiological function may be to regulate cellular phosphate homeostasis, rather than phosphate reabsorption.

In the parathyroid gland, the expression of PIT1 was shown to be upregulated by 1,25-dihydroxyvitamin D_3 and dietary phosphate deprivation, the predominant factors that downregulate PTH secretion in parathyroid cells (790). Therefore, it was proposed that PIT1 functions such as an inorganic phosphate sensor regulate the secretion of PTH in response to circulating 1,25-dihydroxyvitamin D_3 and phosphate levels (531, 533, 790). In renal failure, inorganic phosphate retention (hyperphosphatemia) and low rates of 1,25-dihydroxyvitamin D_3 synthesis in the kidney result in increased PTH secretion and hyperparathyroidism. It is likely that PIT1 is responsible for the beneficial effect of dietary phosphate restriction on hyperparathyroidism in patients with renal failure.

Both PIT transporters are expressed in the kidney along with two other sodium–phosphate cotransport systems. PIT1 and PIT2 mRNA expression levels in the kidney are only 0.5% the total content relative to the other phosphate transporter systems, which are type I (15%) and type II (85%) (796). The type II system has also been shown to be the major phosphate transport system in the renal cortex (532). While, type II expression is found mostly in the proximal tubules, PIT1 was found expressed throughout the kidney. In NaP_i-IIa null mice, the expression of the PITs increased, but the mice fail to show the ability to increase renal phosphate transport even though serum phosphate levels decreased (320). Such data suggest that PIT transporters function very little in overall renal phosphate reabsorption.

In the intestine, 1,25-dihydroxyvitamin D_3 treatment of vitamin D_3–deficient rats resulted in the increased NaP_i transport in apical membrane vesicles, which appears to correspond to the increase in PIT2 expression (386). These results suggest that PIT2 may be involved in the regulation of intestinal phosphate absorption.

ORGANIC ANION TRANSPORTER FAMILY (SLC21)

The organic anion transporter protein (OATP) SLC21 family contains 11 verified human genes. The OATPs are sodium-independent systems that transport substrates via anion exchange, coupling the cellular uptake of organic compounds with the efflux of bicarbonate, glutathione, or glutathione-S-conjugates (454, 455, 692, 728). The exchange activity seems to be pH-dependent and electroneutral. In general, SLC21 substrates are anionic, amphipathic compounds with high molecular weight (>450), and are highly albumin bound. Most Oatps/OATPs have extensive substrate overlap and mediate the transport of a wide array of amphipathic organic compounds such as bile salts, hormones, and their conjugates (e.g., estrogen, T_3, T_4), eicosanoids, drugs (e.g., ouabain, digoxin, methotrexate, fexofenadine), organic anions (e.g., bilirubin derivatives), and toxins (microcystin and phalloidin) (289). Other known substrates are endothelin-receptor antagonist BQ-123, the thrombin inhibitor CRC-220, the opioid receptor agonists [D-penicillamine 2,5]enkephalin (DPDPE) and deltorphin II, the angiotensin-converting enzyme inhibitors enalapril and temocaprilat, the HMG-CoA reductase inhibitor pravastatin, and the antihistamine fexofenadine (289). This broad specificity for most members of the OATP1A and OATP1B subfamilies suggests that they play a key role, in conjunction with multidrug resistance proteins, in drug absorption and drug disposition.

While some OATPs are selectively or preferentially expressed in the liver (e.g., OATP1B1 and OAT1B3), there are also many in the brain, kidney, and intestine. All liver OATPs are expressed on the basolateral membrane of the hepatocyte. However, the membrane localization depends on the tissue. In the rat choroid plexus, renal proximal tubule, and intestinal epithelial cells, the Oatp1a1 and Oatp1a5 can be found expressed on apical membranes. In contrast, Oatp1a4 exhibits a constant basolateral presence on polarized epithelial cells (289).

The traditional SLC21/SLC21 classification system did not permit the subclassification of the Oatp/OATP superfamily into families and subfamilies. Therefore, a new "SLCO" symbol for gene classification and the "OATP" symbol for the corresponding protein were introduced to provide unequivocal and species-independent identification of genes and proteins. All Oatps/OATPs are newly classified within the SLCO/OATP superfamily and subdivided into families, subfamilies, individual genes, and proteins according to phylogenetic relationships and identification chronology. OATPs in the same family share ~40% amino acid sequence identity and are assigned as follows: OATP1, OATP2, OATP3, OATP4, OATP5, and OATP6. Within the subfamilies, the Oatps/OATPs share ~60% sequence identity, and are assigned by letters: OATP1A, OATP1B, OATP1C, OATP2A, OATP2B, OATP3A, and so on. The individual proteins within each subfamily are numbered based on the chronology of identification, as in OATP1A1, OATP1A2, OATP1A3, and so on. The new SLC gene symbol is written by replacing "OATP" with "SLCO," where the "O" in SLCO comes from the first letter in OATP. Hence, the new gene symbol for OATP1A1 would simply be SLCO1A1.

The OATP1A subfamily contains a single human transporter, OATP1A2 (OATP-A, SLC21A3, SLCO1A2), which is 670 amino acid glycoprotein that shares up to 77% identity with its rodent orthologues (289, 425). It is present at high levels in the brain and at lower levels in the liver and kidney. Functionally it has the widest substrate profile of any human OATP (426). These substrates include bile salts, steroid hormone conjugates, thyroid hormones, prostaglandin E2, the thrombin inhibitor CRC-220, fexofenadine, some magnetic resonance imaging agents, and the cyanobacteria toxin microcystin (289). The predominate expression of OATP1A at the blood–brain barrier advocates suggests that it may function either to deliver neuropeptides and drugs to the brain or removal of organic metabolites.

The transporters OATP1B1 and OATP1B3 are human members of the OATP1B subfamily. They share 80% sequence identity with each other, but only ~65% with their rodent orthologue Oatp1b2. OATP1B1 (OATP-C, SLC21A6, SLCO1B1) is restricted to expression on the basolateral membrane of hepatocytes where it is assumed to function in the clearance of albumin-bound organic compounds. Its substrate range is similarly wide compared to OATP1A members (426). Genetic polymorphisms in the OATP1B1 gene have been associated with significantly reduced transport function (526, 568, 803). The liver transcription factor HNF-1a regulates the basal expression of OATP1B1 (367). Additionally, transcription is markedly reduced (50%) in patients with primary sclerosing cholangitis, a disease causing inflammation and scarring of the bile ducts inside and outside the liver (579).

The OATP1B3 (OATP8, SLC21A8, SLCO1B3) transporter shares many similarities with OATP1B1, including a restricted expression in hepatocytes and a wide substrate selectivity. OAT1B3 has also been shown to be expressed in multiple cancer cell lines derived from gastric, colon, pancreas, gallbladder, lung, and brain cancers (2), but the pathological significance of this finding has yet to be determined. Its somewhat unique transport properties are that it can carry the intestinal peptide cholecystokinin 8 (351), the opioid peptide deltorphin II, and the cardiac glycosides digoxin and ouabain (426). The transcription is controlled by HNF1a, as well as the bile acid nuclear receptor FXR/BAR (368).

The OATP1C subfamily contains one human member OATP1C1 (OATP-F, SLC21A14, SLCO1C1), which on the RNA level is expressed in the brain and testis. Although it belongs to the OATP1 family, which is typically known for transporters with a wide substrate range, OATP1C1 has a limited substrate spectrum (619). It has high affinity for transporting the thyroid hormones thyroxine (T_4) and reverse tri-iodothyronine (rT_3), and some limited ability to transport the thyroid hormone T_3, estrone-3-sulfate, estradiol-17β-glucuronide, and bromosulfophthalein (BSP). These characteristics suggest that it may play a role in thyroid hormone delivery to brain and testis.

The OATP2A subfamily contains the human OATP2A1 (also know as PGT, SLC21A2, SLCO2A1). PGT transports a variety of prostaglandins, and in particular prostaglandin E2 and F2a as well as thromboxane B_2. PGT is thought to play a role in the transport and metabolic clearance of prostaglandins in diverse human tissues. PGT mRNA transcripts are ubiquitously with highest levels being found in the heart, skeletal muscle, and pancreas. In the kidney, PGT is expressed in the proximal tubules (479). The OATP2B1 (OATP-B, SLC21A9, SLCO2B1) transporter is highly expressed in the liver and spleen, although it was originally cloned from the brain (551). In the liver it localizes to the basolateral membrane of the hepatocytes along with OATP1B1 and OATP1B3. Functionally, OATP2B1 has few substrates, including BSP, estrone-3-sulfate, and dehydroepiandrosterone-sulfate (785).

The OATP3A1 (OATP-D, SLC21A11, SLCO3A1) transporter is the only human member of the OATP3 subfamily. Messenger RNA analysis indicates that it is ubiquitously expressed, demonstrating the widest distribution of all OATPs (785). Although its transport properties have not been studied extensively, it has been shown to carry estrone-3-sulfate, PGE_2, and benzylpenicillin.

OATP4A1 (OATP-E, SLC21A12, SLCO4A1) is also ubiquitously expressed, with the strongest presence in the liver, heart, placenta, and pancreas (227). In the placenta, protein expression was localized to the apical surface of the syncytiotrophoblast (694). It too appears to have limited substrates, carrying only thyroid hormones (T_3, T_4, and rT_3), steroid conjugates, PGE_2, and benzylpenicillin (785).

For the remaining human transporters OATP4C1 (OATP-H, SLC21A20, SLCO4A1), OATP5A1 (OATP-J, SLC21A15, SLCO4A1), and OATP6A1 (OATP-I, GST, SLC21A19, SLCO6A1) very little information is currently available.

ORGANIC CATION–ANION TRANSPORTER FAMILY (SLC22)

Most SLC22 members are polyspecific transporters that carry multiple organic and xenobiotic substrates, including drugs, toxins, hormones, neurotransmitters, and cellular metabolites. The family can be divided into subgroups based on substrates and mechanism: the organic cation transporters (OCTs) (412), the organic anion transporters (OATs) (716), and the zwitterion–cation transporters (OCTNs) (786). Transporters in this family function as uniporters that facilitate transport in both directions (OCTs), anion exchange (OAT1, OAT3, URAT1), and Na$^+$–carnitine cotransport (OCTN2). Most SLC22 transporters are expressed in the liver, kidney, and intestine where they function in absorption and/or excretion of xenobiotics and endogenous compounds. SLC22 transporters can also be found in the placenta (108), choroid plexus (774, 775), and testis (184, 786).

The three OCT subtypes 1–3 translocate organic cations and weak bases by mechanisms that are electrogenic, potential-sensitive, Na^+-independent, and reversible with respect to direction. The organic cation transporter OCT1 (SLC22A1) was the first SLC22 member molecularly identified (273). OCT1 is basolaterally localized in the liver, intestine, and kidney. Most OCT1 substrates are organic cations, as well as some weak bases including tetraethylammoniun (TEA) (362); N-methylquinine; drugs such as acyclovir (783), metformin (849), and cimetidine (165); and endogenous compounds such as serotonin (393). OCT1 knockout mice exhibited a reduction in hepatic uptake and intestinal excretion of TEA (362). There is a broad overlap of substrate and inhibitor specificities of OCT1, compared to OCT2 (SLC22A2) (275). OCT1 is also coexpressed with OCT1 at the basolateral membrane of the S2 and S3 segments of the proximal tubule (383). OCT2 targeted disruption had little effect on TEA pharmacokinetics, but OCT1/OCT2 double knockout mice showed complete disruption of renal TEA secretion, suggesting that OCT1 and OCT2 cooperatively work on the renal excretion of small organic cations (363). OCT3 (SLC22A3) is predominately expressed in human muscle, liver, placenta, kidney, heart, and brain, and has substrate specificities similar to OCT1 and OCT2 (413). OCT3 is expressed and appears to function in neurons of the superior cervical ganglion (421). Although, OCT3 knockout mice display no obvious physiological defects or imbalance of noradrenalin or dopamine. However, these animals exhibited impaired extraneuronal uptake-2 activity (914), as well as increased ingestion of hypertonic saline under thirst and salt appetite conditions, suggesting that OCT3 is important in salt-intake regulation (830). In addition, OCT3 may mediate antiarrhythmic drug transport (298). A reduction of OCT3 expression using antisense oligonucleotides produced behavioral changes in methamphetamine-induced locomotor activity analysis (404).

The second SLC22 subgroup of transporters function as either an organic cation uniporter or H^+–organic cation antiporter (OCTN1), or as a uniporter for organic cations or Na^+–carnitine cotransporter (OCNT2). The human OCTN1 (SLC22A4) is polyspecific and transports monovalent cations like TEA and verapamil and the zwitterion carnitine (787). Human OCTN1 is expressed in tissues including kidney, skeletal muscle, placenta, prostate, and heart, and displays significant species differences (413, 884). A recent study indicated that an endogenous substrate of OCTN1 was ergothioneine (274). It has been suggested that ergothioneine has a role in the protection of monocytes and/or macrophages and may be involved in chronic inflammatory disorders. In the kidney proximal tubule, hOCNT1 is involved in secretion of organic cations, and since it can function bidirectionally it may also participate in reabsorption (893).

The OCTN1 (SLC22A4) gene is associated with chronic inflammatory diseases, rheumatoid arthritis, and Crohn's disease (605, 804).

OCTN2 (SLC22A5) is also widely expressed in tissues including kidney, heart, and brain. OCNT2 has been localized to the apical membrane of the proximal tubule and syncytiotrophoblasts of the placenta (270, 784). OCTN2 functions as a high-affinity Na^+–carnitine cotransporter, but alternatively can function as a polyspecific, Na^+-independent organic cation uniporter (786). This transporter is important for the concentrative reabsorption of L-carnitine after glomerular filtration in the kidney and may also have a role in carnitine transport in the placenta (436). Mutations in SLC22A5 that cause loss of function have been reported in primary systemic carnitine deficiency in both mice (478, 912) and humans (559). Carnitine deficiency is characterized by cardiomyopathy and muscle weakness, hyperammonemia, and hypoglycemia. The mOCTN3 transporter is limited in its tissue distribution being predominately expressed in the mouse testis (786), but also in the rat small intestine along the villus on the basolateral membrane (171). Unlike the other OCTNs, OCNT3 mediates Na^+-independent carnitine transport and does not transport the organic cation tetraethylamonium (786).

The six OAT subfamily members are critical players in the excretion and detoxification of various pharmaceutical drugs, toxins, hormones, and neurotransmitter metabolites. The first organic anion transporter, OAT1, was independently cloned by several groups from rat, mouse, and flounder kidneys (475, 718, 776, 876). OAT1 (SLC22A6) is strongly expressed in the kidney, with transcripts also found in the brain and placenta (94). Immunohistochemistry indicates that OAT1 localizes to the basolateral membrane of the proximal tubule in the rat and humans (325, 414). Characterization of rOAT1 function revealed dose-dependent cis-inhibition and trans-stimulation of p-aminohippurate uptake by glutarate, a substitute for α-ketoglutarate (630, 718, 776). This physiological profile indicates that OAT1 functions as an organic anion–dicarboxylate exchanger, using an outward directed gradient of α-ketoglutarate or glutarate to provide the driving force for organic anion uptake (716). Working in parallel with OAT2 (SLC22A7) and OAT3 (SLC22A8) on the basolateral membrane, OAT1 (SLC22A6) helps mediate the renal excretion of a wide array of drugs such as antibiotics, diuretics, and antineoplastics, as well as a variety of endogenous substrates such as cyclic nucleotides and uric acid.

The human OAT2 (SLC22A7) is expressed in the liver and at reduced levels in the kidney. The rOAT2 localized to the apical surface of the medullary thick ascending limb of Henle's loop and the collecting duct (414), while the human OAT2 was found on the basolateral membrane of the proximal tubule (183). The human OAT2 is a sodium-independent, multispecific, organic anion–dimethyldicarboxylate exchanger. Fumarate and succinate, but not glutarate, trans-stimulate transport of organic compounds (411).

Similar to OAT1, the OAT3 (SLC22A8) functions as an organic anion–dicarboxylate exchanger responsive to Na^+-dependent *trans*-stimulation by glutarate (36). Predominately, hOAT3 is expressed in the basolateral membrane of proximal tubules in the kidney as well as skeletal muscle and choroid plexus of the brain (107). OAT3 knockout mice showed impaired renal transport of *p*-aminohippurate and other anions (775). OAT3-deficient mice also showed a reduction of organic anion uptake in the apical membrane of choroid plexus, suggesting OAT3 involvement in an excretion of toxins from brain to blood (775). OAT4 (SLC22A11) is abundantly expressed in the kidney like the other OATs, but hOAT4 is unique since it is the only OAT known to be expressed in the placenta (775), where it may have a role in fetal-derived, steroid uptake (818). In the apical membrane of proximal tubule, it is thought that it may mediate reabsorption of OAs from the tubular fluid driven by the outwardly directed α-ketoglutarate gradient (30, 177).

Urate accumulation has been proposed to have beneficial effects, since it is a potent antioxidant (11, 43). The transporter that reabsorbs urate has been identified as the urate exchanger URAT1 (SLC22A12) (538), expressed in the apical membrane of proximal tubule cells (182) (Fig. 4). Urate transported across the apical membrane of the proximal tubule cells, in exchange for anions that enter cells either by Na^+-coupled transporters in the apical membrane or by organic anion transporters in the basolateral membrane (182, 307, 661, 662). However, the transporter(s) responsible for moving urate across the basolateral membrane into the blood is still unknown. "Uricosuric" drugs (e.g., probenecid, furosemide, and losartan), used to treat inflammation or high blood pressure, block uric acid reabsorption, and "antiuricosuric" drugs (e.g., pyrazinoic acid and nicotinate) enhance it. Uricosuric compounds directly inhibit URAT1 from the apical side, whereas antiuricosuric drugs serve as the exchanging anion from inside tubule cells, thereby stimulating reabsorption (182).

Urate has beneficial benefits, but in conjunction with genetic or environmental factors it can cause significant health problems. URAT1 mutations that cause loss of function were identified in patients with idiopathic renal hypouricemia, thus demonstrating the importance of URAT1 in regulating serum uric acid levels (182). The roles of URAT1 in gout, nephrolithiasis (420), hyperten-

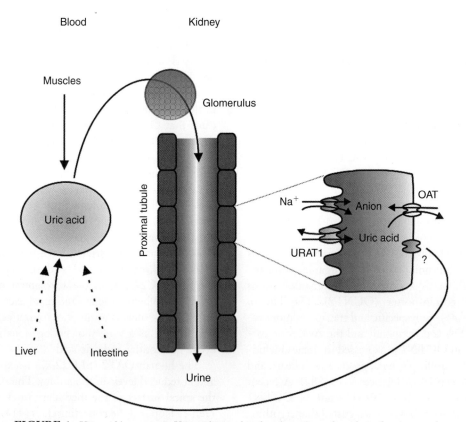

FIGURE 4   Uric acid homeostasis. Uric acid is produced as the major end-product of purine metabolism in the liver and can be produced by muscle during exercise. While the uric acid is a weak acid with a pK_a of 5.8, the urate ion is much more soluble than the nonionized molecule. This metabolic byproduct enters the blood because urate can efficiently be reabsorbed in the kidney. Urate is reabsorbed via URAT1 in exchange for anions that enter the epithelial cell via apically located, sodium-coupled transporters or basolaterally located, organic anion transporters.

sion (513, 514), and hyperuricemic nephropathy (752, 759) are also under consideration.

Na$^+$–VITAMIN C TRANSPORTER FAMILY (SLC23)

Vitamin C (L-ascorbic acid) is required as a cofactor in enzymatic reactions such as biosynthesis of collagen or noradrenalin and α-amidation of neuropeptides. In these reactions, it serves to maintain prosthetic metal ions in their reduced forms, such as Fe^{2+} and Cu^{2+} (181, 580). Additionally, vitamin C is an effective antioxidant and free radical scavenger that helps protect cells from oxidative damage (670). To provide the necessary vitamin C for cellular functions, there exist two vitamin C transporters, SVCT2 (SLC23A1) and SVCT2 (SLC23A2), and two orphan transporters, SVCT3 (SLC23A3) and SVCT4 (SLC23A4). SVCT1 and SVCT2 display similar functional properties, including high affinity for vitamin C, but are distributed differently in the body. SVCT1 expression is limited to epithelial tissues involved in absorption including the intestine, kidney, and liver, while SVCT2 functions in specialized cells and tissues such as neurons, the eye, the lung, and endothelial tissues.

The two Na$^+$-dependent vitamin C transporter family isoforms, SVCT1 and SVCT2, share 65% of amino acid sequence identity (814). All SLC23 members show weak sequence homology (20%–30% identity) with nucleobase transporters in bacteria, yeast, and plants, but not with any other known mammalian transporter family (193). SVCT1 was identified by expression cloning, that is, screening a rat kidney cDNA library for Na$^+$-dependent L-[^{14}C]-ascorbic acid transport activity in RNA-injected *Xenopus* oocytes. Subsequent PCR-based homology screening yielded a related cDNA (6.5 kb, from rat brain), SVCT2. Both SVCT1 and SVCT2 are Na$^+$-coupled, high-affinity vitamin C transporters with the following substrate preference: L-ascorbic acid > D-isoascorbic acid > dehydroascorbic acid. Even though there is some sequence similarity to nucleobase transporters, no SVCT transporter has yet exhibited nucleobase transport activity. SVCT1 is mainly confined to bulk-transporting epithelial systems (intestine, kidney, liver), whereas SVCT2 is expressed in many different tissues such as the brain, eye, pituitary, adrenal gland, pancreas, testis, bone, thymus, spleen, and lung. SVCT1 expression suggests a primary role in dietary L-ascorbic acid absorption and renal reabsorption. Human polymorphisms in the SVCT1 gene have yet to be identified, suggesting that mutations which lead to loss in SVCT1 function might be lethal. No mouse knockouts are yet available. In contrast to humans, mice are able to generate their own vitamin C, and therefore phenotypic changes in a SVCT1 knockout mouse may be minor. Among many possible roles for SVCT2, it seems to function in providing L-ascorbic acid to tissues that require the most protection from oxidative stress caused

by high metabolic activity, particularly neurons of the brain and retina (814). SVCT2 is also critical for sustaining enzyme activity, since vitamin C is required to maintain metal ions in their reduced state. The drastic effects of knocking out SVCT2 in mice are discussed below.

No substrates for SVCT3 and SVCT4 have been identified yet. However, it is known that SVCT3 does not transport vitamin C, DHA, sugar derivatives, or nucleobases and nucleotides (Hediger and colleagues, unpublished data). It has also been shown that SVCT1 and SVCT2 together account for all the L-ascorbic acid transport in the intestine, kidney, and adrenal gland (814), suggesting that the two orphan transporters may transport different substrates. In the mouse, SVCT3 is expressed in the kidney and placenta (193, 283), and SVCT4 seems to be present in human kidney tumors.

Plasma vitamin C concentrations are tightly maintained at 10–160 μM, and any excess over 160 μM will lead to kidney excretion. In contrast, it is accumulated at levels at least 100 times higher in tissues that require the vitamin for biochemical reactions, such as the adrenal glands, pituitary gland, thymus, corpus luteum, retina, and cornea. Therefore, vitamin C needs to be delivered in a regulated manner into organs at the appropriate concentration, and this requires specific, concentrative transport processes such as SVCT2. Interestingly, humans and certain other species have lost their ability to synthesize vitamin C due to a nonfunctional gene for the enzyme L-gulono-γ-lactone oxidase, the last step of ascorbate synthesis. However, regardless of whether the vitamin is derived from dietary absorption or synthesis in the liver (certain mammals) or kidneys (reptiles), specific transport mechanisms are required to distribute vitamin C into the tissues. In humans severe vitamin C deficiency leads to the disease scurvy. This disease produces muscle weakness, swollen and bleeding gums, loss of teeth, bleeding under the skin, and impaired wound healing. Many of these symptoms are related to inhibition of collagen synthesis for which vitamin C is essential. Impaired collagen synthesis is believed to be responsible for the connective tissue and hemorrhagic manifestations of scurvy.

To study whether the lack of SVCT2 results in scurvy-like symptoms, Nussbaum and colleagues established SVCT2 knockout mice (749). Loss of SVCT2 function had a dramatic effect since these mice died within a few minutes of birth, displaying respiratory failure and extensive intracerebral hemorrhage. The vitamin-C tissue levels in the brain, adrenal gland, pituitary, and pancreas of the SVCT -/- mice were undetectable (749) and to some extent also in heterozygous (SVCT2 +/-) adults, compared to wildtype. The observed intracerebral hemorrhage in SVCT2 null mice further confirms the significance of vitamin C and SVCT2 in protecting the brain from free radical damage. The respiratory failure shows that vitamin C and SVCT2 play a previously unrecognized role during the transition to extrauterine life requirements, and changes of the fetal lung to enable postnatal gas exchange. Once again, it is possible that the toxic accumulation of free radicals is the cause for the respiratory failure. The studies also showed that SVCT2 is required for appropriate transfer of vitamin C across the placenta.

SODIUM–CALCIUM–POTASSIUM EXCHANGER FAMILY (SLC24)

Early studies on retinal rod photoreceptors led to the conclusion that sodium–calcium exchange was critical for their function. The Na^+–Ca^{2+}–K^+ exchange activity was first described in the outer segments of the vertebrate rod receptors (ROS), where it appears to be the only mechanism for removing Ca^{2+} that enters the ROS through light-sensitive and cGMP-gated channels. There are two families of sodium–calcium exchangers: the SLC8 family of sodium–calcium exchangers (NCXs) and the SLC24 family of potassium-dependent sodium–calcium exchangers (NCKX). In the SLC24 family there are now five members: NCKX1 (SLC24A1) (653, 815), NCKX2 (SLC24A2) (809), NCKX3 (SLC24A3) (419), NCKX4 (SLC24A4) (457), and NCKX5 (SLC24A5). The overall structures of the NCX and NCKX proteins appear to be similar, since both have two clusters of five and six hydrophobic helices separated by a central large cytoplasmic loop. However, there is no significant overall sequence homology between the two families (653), except for two short stretches in hydrophobic helix clusters that may provide the ion-binding pocket required for transport activity (563, 710).

Extensive in situ characterization has only been carried out for NCKX1 (SLC24A1). Heterologous studies with NCKX1 and NCKX2 transporters revealed that they both have similar basic functional characteristics. Transport stoichiometry is four sodium ions in exchange for one calcium and one potassium ion, resulting in electrogenic calcium exit (809). Normally these transporters efflux calcium from the cells, but when the transmembrane gradient is reversed they can also carry calcium into the cell. These isoforms are presumed to be expressed in cells with high plasma membrane calcium flux and where calcium homeostasis must be maintained in the face of a dramatically reduced membrane potential and sodium gradient. NCKX1 and NCKX2 may also operate in a cellular environment in which calcium concentrations must be kept extremely low. Only an exchanger of the NCKX type could harness sufficient thermodynamic driving force to achieve such levels.

NCKX1 (SLC24A1) appears to have the most restricted tissue distribution of the SLC24 family, being expressed in retinal rod outer segments, brain neurons (653), and platelets (401). A clear functional role for NCKX1 has only been established in retinal rod and cone photoreceptors. Calcium influx across the plasma membrane of rod and cone outer segments generated by cGMP-gated channels due to darkness is balanced by calcium efflux via NCKX1. Coupling transport to a potassium gradient allows NCKX1 to control calcium levels in rods even when the membrane potential and sodium gradient are diminished in darkness (652, 704, 705).

NCKX2 (SLC24A2) is primarily expressed in brain neurons, retinal ganglion cells, and cone photoreceptors (809). Interestingly, the expression of NCKX1 and NCKX2 in brain overlaps in some areas (cerebral cortex, hippocampus) but not in others (503), suggesting potential functional differences between the two isoforms. The newest SLC24 members NCKX3 and NCKX4 have qualitatively similar physiologic activity as NCKX1-2 (419, 457, 482). NCKX3 (SLC24A3) mRNA appears to be the most widespread, with expression in the brain, smooth muscle tissues (such as aorta, uterus, and intestine), and skeletal muscle (419), while only trace levels of SLC24A3 are detected in the liver and kidney. Post-translational processing can result in the loss of the N-terminus and the M0 transmembrane span. The N-terminal region is not essential for expression, but increases functional activity at least 10-fold and may represent a cleavable signal sequence (419). NCKX3 is predominantly expressed in mast cells, suggesting that NCKX3 is involved in Ca^{2+} signaling for mast cell activation by antigens (15).

The NCKX4 (SLC24A4) transporter is most similar to NCKX3. The SLC24A4 transcript is expressed in the brain, as well as in the aorta, lung, thymus and at reduced levels in the kidney (457). There are two NCKX4 isoforms that differ due to a 19–amino acids insertion, with the shorter transcript being more abundant. The cellular localization, especially in the kidney, is still unknown. The localization of NCKX4 in the kidney will allow a better understanding of renal cellular physiology. The NCKX5 (SLC24A5) sequence is present in GeneBank, but remains uncharacterized. The six members of the SLC24 family, identified from GeneBank, encode a 585-amino acid plasma membrane protein that exhibited K^+-dependent Na^+–Ca^{2+} exchange activity (99). NCKX6 (SLC24A6) transcripts were ubiquitously expressed in all tissues, suggesting that it may function in maintaining cellular Ca^{2+} homeostasis in a broad range of tissues and cell types.

MITOCHONDRIAL CARRIER FAMILY (SLC25)

The primary function of the mitochondria is to produce energy for the cell. The mitochondria oxidize fatty acids and pyruvate and subsequently release the energy stored in the high-energy electron carriers, NADH and $FADH_2$, by oxidative phosphorylation to generate ATP. Although their primary function is to convert organic materials into cellular energy in the form of ATP, mitochondria play an important role in many important metabolic tasks such as regulating the cellular redox state, heme synthesis, steroid synthesis, amino acid synthesis, and detoxifying ammonia. To sustain these many functions, a wide variety of substrates must be allowed to enter and exit the mitochondria. This essential link across the inner mitochondrial membrane is facilitated by at least 29 mitochondrial carriers (MCs) embedded in the inner membrane.

All the SLC25 members have a similar ~30-kDa molecular mass and share 23%–34% amino acid sequence identity. They contain three tandemly repeated homologous domains, each about 100 amino acid residues in length. Each domain is folded into two transmembrane helices joined by a hydrophilic extramembrane loop, yielding 6 total transmembrane segments (587). The majority of MCs that have been isolated are homodimers, based on numerous studies including cross-linking (62, 492), molecular weight determinations (417, 460), and neutron scattering (65). The recently crystallized bovine ADP/ATP carrier (SLC25 family) confirms many of these structural features, but surprisingly no dimer structures were found in the crystals (603).

The tricarboxylate carrier (CIC, CTP, SLC25A1) (250) mediates electroneutral exchange of tricarboxylate (e.g., citrate, isocitrate) across the inner membrane in exchange for a tricarboxylate, a dicarboxylate (e.g., malate), or phosphoenolpyruvate (PEP) (337). CIC accepts only the single protonated form of citrate (H-citrate^{2-}) and the unprotonated malate^{2-}; thus, exchange is electroneutral. CIC is expressed in many tissues, including the liver, testis, ovary, and gut, and also in the fetal brain, lung, liver, and kidney. The citrate export from the mitochondria to the cytosol is required for fatty acid and sterol biosynthesis. The gene for CIC has been localized to an area on chromosome 22q11 that is missing in patients with the DiGeorge syndrome or the velocardiofacial syndrome (250, 310). Similarly to CIC, the oxoglutarate/malate carrier (OGC, SLC25A11) mediates oxoglutarate transport into the mitochondrial matrix by an electroneutral exchange for malate or some other dicarboxylic acid (162, 338, 681). OGC transcripts have been found in the heart, liver, kidney, and brain. This carrier is involved in both the malate-aspartate and the oxoglutarate-isocitrate shuttles, as well as in nitrogen metabolism and gluconeogenesis.

Two ornithine carriers, ORC1 (SLC25A15) and ORC2 (SLC25A2), have been identified in humans (101). In a reconstituted system, both ORC isoforms demonstrate the ability to carry the basic amino acids ornithine, lysine, or arginine in exchange for citrulline plus H$^+$. This electroneutral exchange reaction can be inhibited by spermine and spermidine (101). While they have many transport properties in common, they differ in several respects. ORC2 additionally transports L- and D-histidine, L-homoarginine, and the D-isomers of ornithine, lysine, and arginine with equal efficiency as the L-isomers. ORC2 has higher affinity for lysine and arginine, but lower affinity for ornithine and citrulline compared to ORC1. Overall, ORC2 is threefold less active than ORC1. The final difference is that ORC1 expression levels are generally higher in all human tissues examined thus far. For the cell, the exchanging cytosolic ornithine for intramitochondrial citrulline is essential for maintaining the urea cycle. Loss-of-function mutations in the ORC1 gene cause hyperammonemia, hyperornithinemia, and homocitrullinuria in human patients with HHH syndrome (101). Most patients suffering from this disorder display episodes of coma when fed high-protein diets, growth retardation, and phases of lethargy, ataxia, and myclonic seizures. ORC1 expression restores ornithine metabolism in fibroblasts from patients with HHH syndrome. The ORC carriers are also important for delivering the amino acids lysine, arginine, and histidine to the mitochondria for protein synthesis.

In the terminal steps of oxidative phosphorylation, the electrochemical energy from protons flowing across the mitochondrial inner matrix is used to synthesize ATP for the cell. For this process the membrane-bound enzyme, ATP synthetase, must be supplied with inorganic phosphate and ADP. Phosphate is also required by the mitochondria for enzymatic reactions and allows other exchangers to uptake other metabolites. In humans the phosphate carrier (PIC, SLC25A3) has been identified; it catalyzes phosphate transport into the mitochondrial matrix in exchange for OH$^-$, or in cotransport with H$^+$ (161). Two distinct isoforms have been identified (A and B). PIC-A is present only in muscles, while PIC-B is ubiquitous (209); the two also differ in their kinetic properties, as PIC-A has three times more affinity for phosphate but a one-third slower V$_{max}$.

ATP production also requires a ready supply of ADP, which enters the mitochondrial matrix via ADP/ATP carriers (AAC1, AAC2, and AAC3). Three highly homologous AAC isoforms have been found in humans: AAC1 (SLC25A4) is abundant in the heart and skeletal muscle (453); AAC2 (SLC25A5) is present in the liver, kidney, brain, heart, and skeletal muscle (118, 422, 699); and AAC3 (SLC25A6) was cloned from the human liver but is also found in brain, kidney, and muscle tissue (326, 700). AAC1 is the most abundant protein in the mitochondria, which underscores its important role. This exchange mechanism moves ATP into the cytosol while at the same time providing ADP to the mitochondria. AAC1 knockout mice are viable, but display a severe intolerance to exercise and lactic acidosis (263). This also suggests that AAC2 and AAC3 are sufficient for survival. The human diseases autosomal-dominant, progressive external ophthalmoplegia (adPEO) and Sengers syndrome are thought be caused by defective AAC1 (365, 387, 556).

An additional adenine nucleoside carrier exists as well, but it is localized to the peroxisomal membrane (838), in contrast to the other carriers in the SLC25 family. The adenine nucleoside carrier (ANC, SLC25A17) is homologous to the yeast protein Ant1p, which is essential for yeast growth on fatty acids (589). Ant1p transports ATP, ADP, AMP, and corresponding deoxynucleotides, although less efficiently. Ant1p is different from the AACs due to its ability to carry AMP and its insensitivity to AAC inhibitors. The human ANC carrier is assumed to be required for activation of branched and very long fatty acids that are oxidized in the peroxisomes.

Being less specific than the ATP/ADP carriers, the deoxynucleotide carrier (DNC, SLC25A19) transports all deoxynucleoside diphosphates (dNDPs), and deoxynucleoside triphosphates (dNTPs) (less efficiently), in exchange for

ATP or ADP. The enzyme ribonucleotide reductase is located in the cytosol; therefore, the completed deoxynucleotides need to be transported into the mitochondria to provide for mtDNA synthesis. In the mitochondria the dNDPs are converted into dNTPs and added into mtDNA. Interestingly, DNC also transports dideoxynucleotides more efficiently than the corresponding deoxy form, suggesting that it may transport certain antiviral nucleoside analogues into the mitochondria and cause toxicity by interfering with mtDNA synthesis. Loss in DNC transport activity in humans, due to mutation, causes Amish microcephaly (671). The disorder is characterized by individuals with smaller head circumferences, immature brain, and premature death.

The mitochondrial uncoupling proteins (UCPs) are responsible for the proton transport that is not coupled to oxidative phosphorylation. Activation of the UCPs leads to the uncoupled passage of protons and heat generation as well as the control of oxygen radical production. Expression and activation are usually mediated by the sympathetic nervous system, and are directly controlled by norepinephrine as part of the adaptive response to cold temperatures. Five UCPs have been identified: UCP1–5 (SLC25A7, SLS25A8, SLC25A9, SLC25A27, and SLC25A14, respectively). UCP1 is specific to human brown adipose tissue (80, 106). UCP1-null mice are sensitive to cold, but do not become obese. In comparison to UCP1, UCP2 has a greater uncoupling effect on the mitochondrial membrane. UCP2 is widely expressed in adult human tissues, including tissues rich in macrophages, and it is upregulated in white fat in response to fat feeding. UCP2 plays a role in the altered metabolism in diabetes and obesity. UCP3 is expressed in skeletal muscle and the heart (77, 834). UCP2 or UPC3 knockout mice are not cold-sensitive, show no weight gain, but overproduce oxygen radicals. UCP4 and UCP5 (originally, brain mitochondrial carrier protein-1) are predominantly expressed in the brain (689).

The dicarboxylate carrier DIC (SLC25A10) plays a role in gluconeogenesis, urea synthesis, and sulfur metabolism by transporting dicarboxylates such as malate and succinate across the inner mitochondrial membrane in exchange for phosphate, sulfate, sulfite, or thiosulfate. DIC is strongly expressed in the liver, and with less abundance in the heart and the brain (211). Knockout yeast cells suggest that the primary role for DIC is to provide the mitochondria with dicarboxylates (590).

Another distinct dicarboxylate carrier is also present in mitochondria. The oxodicarboxylate carrier (ODC, SLC25A21) has the greatest preference for 2-oxoadipate and 2-oxoglutarate (210). The countersubstrate for 2-oxoadipate uptake most likely is 2-oxoglutarate. However, unlike the oxoglutarate carrier, ODC cannot transport malate, succinate, or maleate. ODC functions to provide 2-oxoglutarate to the mitochondria for catabolism of lysine, hydroxylysine, and tryptophan. This role suggests that ODC may be involved in the disease 2-oxoadipate acidemia. This disorder is marked by accumulation and secretion of 2-oxoadipate, 2-aminoadipate, and 2-hydroxyadipate in urine, with clinical symptoms including mental retardation and learning disability (210).

Two additional mitochondrial carriers, AGC1 (SLC25A12) and AGC2 (SLC25A13), possess unique structures that contain a carboxyl-terminal domain that resembles the mitochondrial carriers and an amino-terminal domain that contains four Ca^{2+}-binding domains (151, 863). The binding of cytosolic Ca^{2+} on the external side of the inner mitochondrial membrane stimulates transport activity (588). AGCs transport aspartate, glutamate, and cysteinesulphinate via an obligatory 1:1 exchange mechanism. Aspartate and cysteinesulphinate are carried as anions, while glutamate is cotransported with a proton. Therefore, aspartate/glutamate and cysteinesulphinate/glutamate exchanges are electrogenic, but aspartate/cysteinesulphinate is not (588). AGC1 is found mainly in excitable tissues and AGC2 is abundant in the liver. Mutations in AGC2 cause type II citrullinemia, characterized by hyperammonemia and neuropsychiatric symptoms, commonly leading to rapid death (687). ASCs play an important role in several processes such as the malate–aspartate shuttle, urea synthesis, purine and pyrimidine syntheses, protein synthesis, and gluconeogenesis from lactate.

Glutamate can also be transported by the carriers GC1 (SLC25A22) and GC2 (SLC25A18). Both isoforms mediate L-glutamate transport along with H^+ or in exchange for OH^-, but carry the structurally similar amino acids aspartate, glutamate, and homocysteinesulphinate (212). The two isoforms differ in their kinetics, where GC2 has the highest affinity ($K_m = 0.2$ mM) but the lower V_{max}. The predominant role for these transporters is to import glutamate from the cytosol into the mitochondria to feed the urea cycle. GCs may also operate in reverse to limit accumulation of glutamate. Both GC isoforms are distributed rather ubiquitously, with GC1 being more abundant than GC2 in all tissues, except in the brain. GC1 is particularly expressed at high levels in the pancreas, where glutamate may serve as an intracellular messenger involved in insulin secretion (489).

The carnitine–acylcarnitine carrier (CAC, SLC25A20) is an antiporter that mediates mitochondrial uptake of acylcarnitine in exchange for carnitine. The carrier thus supplies the mitochondrial matrix with acyl groups for fatty acid oxidation (344). β-oxidation of long-chain fatty acids provides the majority of energy during long fasts, and is particularly important in generating energy in the cardiac and skeletal muscles during exercise. CAC deficiency, caused by numerous loss-of-function mutations in the CAC gene, was detected in several patients with impaired long-chain fatty acid oxidation (85). This disease is characterized episodes of coma induced by fasting, hypoketosis, hypoglycemia, hyperammonemia, variable dicarboxylic aciduria, and fatty hepatomegaly, as well as cardiac symptoms and muscle weakness. CAC is expressed in various tissues, but is especially high in the heart, skeletal muscle, and liver.

Graves' disease carrier (GDC, SLC25A16) was cloned from a human thyroid cDNA library derived from Graves' disease patients. However, despite its name, GDC is not likely to be involved directly in the disease (631). Functionally, it is thought to mediate the mitochondrial import of coenzyme A or a precursor, but this has not been directly confirmed.

Recently, three ATP-Mg–P_i transporter isoforms, APC1 (SLC25A23), APC2 (SLC25A24) and APC3 (SLC25A25), have been identified that correspond to one of the previously "missing" MCs (208). The transport activity involving ATP-Mg transport in exchange for phosphate activity had previously been observed in mitochondria and thoroughly investigated but no protein had been associated with the activity. These APCs have a characteristic structure contains mitochondrial carrier structural features in the C-terminus and three EF-hand Ca^{2+}-binding domains in the N-terminal domain. The Ca^{2+}-binding motifs in the N-terminal domains suggest Ca^{2+} regulation, but this could not be confirmed in the most recent study. As suspected these carriers mediate the reversible exchange of ATP-Mg^{2-} for P_i, but were found to also carry ADP, AMP, related nucleotides, and pyrophosphate. Phosphate transported by the APCs recycles through the phosphate carrier; therefore, these three APCs are most likely accountable for the net uptake or efflux of adenine nucleotides into or out of the mitochondria. APC1 was expressed highest in the testis, APC2 was most abundant in the skeletal muscles and brain, and APC3 was most prevalent in the lung, brain, and testis.

The mitochondrial transporter for S-adenosylmethionine (SAM) was also among the "missing" MCs until it was recently identified by Agrimi et al. (6). SAM is the methyl group donor used for nearly all enzymatic methylation reactions; in the mitochondria SAM is necessary for DNA, RNA, and protein methylation. The SAM transport activity now can be associated with the mitochondrial-localized SAM carrier (SAMC, SLC25A26), which is ubiquitously expressed in human tissue. SAMC mediates countertransport of SAM in exchange for S-adenosylhomocysteine, S-adenosylcysteine, or adenosylornithine.

ANION EXCHANGER FAMILY (SLC26)

The SLC26 gene family encodes multifunctional anion exchangers with roles in normal physiology as well as in human pathophysiology. These exchangers are important in a variety of processes including renal bicarbonate excretion (677), Na^+–Cl^- transport (322, 407, 886), and thyroid hormone synthesis (192). The monovalent and divalent anions transported by the 11 SLC26 family members include sulphate (SO_4^{2-}), chloride (Cl^-), iodide (I^-), formate, oxalate, hydroxyl ion (OH^-), and bicarbonate (HCO_3^-) (63, 360, 385, 540, 695, 712). The ion specificity differs considerably among family members. For example, SLC26A3 and SLC26A6 transport most if not all these ions (360, 886). SLC26A1 cannot transport Cl^- or formate, but is capable of transporting SO_4^{2-} and oxalate. SLC26A4 mediates transport of the monovalent anions Cl^-, I^-, and formate, but not the divalent anions SO_4^{2-} and oxalate (712, 713). Most

uniquely in this family, SLC26A5 has not been shown to mediate vectorial transport of anions across membranes, but appears instead to function as a "voltage sensor" (574).

Sat 1 (SLC26A1) was identified as a sodium-independent, SO_4^{2-}–oxalate exchanger through expression cloning from rat liver (63). The basolateral membrane localization of Sat 1 in the proximal tubule, where it is suggested to be involved in sulfate reabsorption and oxalate secretion (385). Its role as a hepatic canalicular sulfate-anion exchanger is not completely clear. In the mouse and rat it has been demonstrated that SO_4^{2-} uptake can be significantly increased by extracellular Cl^- and essentially absent without Cl^- (448, 695). Further, it has been shown that other halides, formate, lactate, and oxalate also stimulate SO_4^{2-} uptake. Sulfate exchange is also significantly stimulated by an acid–outside pH gradient (886). The physiological or mechanistic significance of this activation effect is unknown.

DTDST (SLC26A2) was discovered through positional cloning of a gene for diastrophic dysplasia, a rare skeletal dysplasia that results in short limb stature and other skeletal defects (299). It mediates SO_4^{2-} transport that can be inhibited by Cl^- or oxalate. SLC26A2 is found in most tissues, although most abundantly in the intestine and cartilage. The L483P loss-of-function mutation, detected in an achondrogenesis 1B patient, resulted in reduced sulfate uptake in fibroblasts and chondrocytes. Additionally, there was drastic reduction in sulfation of cartilage proteoglycans, which thereby decreases the response to matrix-dependent developmental cues such as fibroblast growth factor (672). Therefore, it is not surprising to see irregularities in skeletal development due to loss of SLC26A2 function.

SLC26A3 (DRA, CLD) was initially recognized as a possible tumor suppressor gene that downregulated in adenoma (711), but expressed at particularly high levels in the duodenum and colon (354). In the brush border membrane of differentiated colonic epithelial cells (290), it is thought to function in Cl^--base exchange in coordination with Na^+–H^+ exchange via NHE3 (540, 707). Recessive loss-of-function mutations (540) in the SLC26A3 gene produce severe congenital diarrhea, indicating that SLC26A3 is critical for Na^+–Cl^- absorption in the colon (322).

SLC26A4 was identified by positional characterization of the gene that causes Pendred syndrome. Loss of function in SLC26A4 is an autosomal recessive disease characterized by sensorineural deafness and an enlarged thyroid, sometimes accompanied by hypothyroidism (649). SLC26A4 protein is found on the apical membrane of thyroid follicles facing the colloid lumen, where it appears to function as a Cl^-–I^- exchanger to deliver iodide into the follicular lumen for organification of thyroglobulin (676, 713). It appears to be selective for monovalent anions, but can also transport formate. It has also been demonstrated that SLC26A4 is a Cl^-–base exchanger (410, 744). These functional characteristics can be associated with its role in the thyroid and kidney, both tissues with high SLC26A4 expression levels. Defects in SLC26A4 function often result in goiter and

Pendred syndrome; however, mice deficient in SLC26A4 do not display thyroid structure or function abnormalities (191). Targeted deletion of SLC26A4 results in profound deafness and variable deficits in vestibular function, with endolymphatic dilatation in the inner ear. Within the kidney, SLC26A4 is expressed at the apical membrane of type-B intercalated cells, where it functions in renal bicarbonate secretion (677). The "molecular motor" responsible for cochlear amplification in the inner ear was identified to be prestin (SLC26A5) (910). Thus, the targeted disruption of mouse SLC26A5 causes deafness (458). It is suggested that prestin is the motor protein of the inner hair cells and that Cl^- and HCO_3^- inside these cells act as a voltage sensor for prestin (574).

PAT-1 (SLC26A6, CFEX) is a widely expressed anion exchanger that is particularly abundant in tissues such as the kidney, intestine, pancreas, and heart (407, 472, 846). Immunolocalization studies have found that SLC26A6 is localized to the apical membrane of the kidney proximal tubule (407) and the villi of the duodenum (859). When expressed in vitro SLC26A6 has demonstrated the ability to mediate multiple anion exchange activities such as Cl^-–HCO_3^-, Cl^-–oxalate, SO_4^{2-}–oxalate, SO_4^{2-}–Cl^-, Cl^-–OH^-, and Cl^-–formate (360, 407, 472, 859, 886). Studies conducted in SLC26A6-null mice demonstrate major defects in apical Cl^-–base exchange activity and oxalate-stimulated NaCl absorption in the kidney proximal tubule. In the duodenum, SLC26A6-null mice display a significant reduction in HCO_3^- secretion, a pathway necessary to protect against acid injury (860). The Cl^-–HCO_3^- exchange mediated by SLC26A6 is electrogenic, coupling the transport of 1 Cl^- to at least two HCO_3^-. Removal of extracellular Cl^- in the presence of HCO_3^- hyperpolarized oocytes expressing SLC26A6 while generating an outward directed current. In the same study it was also shown that the cystic-fibrosis, transmembrane conductance regulator (CFTR) is able to activate SLC26A6-mediated Cl^-–base exchange by five- to sixfold (410). A recent study by Ko et al. (410) demonstrated that SLC26A6 stimulation activated CFTR by increasing its overall open probability when coexpressed in vitro. However, studies in SLC26A6-null mice indicate that SLC26A6 does not play an important role in forskolin-activated CFTR in the murine duodenum (860).

Functionally the SLC26A7-9 exchangers have been shown to transport chloride, sulfate, and oxalate (473), whereas SLC26A11 seems to only transport sulfate. Some of the newer SLC26 family members have tissue-specific expression patterns: SLC26A7 exclusive to the kidney, SLC26A8 to the testis, and SLC26A9 to the lung and stomach (886, 890), while SLC26A11 is widely expressed in many tissues (836). SLC26A7 has recently been identified as a basolateral Cl^-–HCO_3^- exchanger in intercalated cells of the outer medullary collecting duct, where it may play an important role in bicarbonate reabsorption in the medullary collecting duct (607). When expressed in *Xenopus* oocytes or HEK293 cells, it has been reported that SLC26A7 functions as a $pH_{(i)}$–regulated Cl^- channel, while displaying minimal OH^-–HCO_3^- permeability (399). SLC26A9 is expressed on the apical membrane of gastric surface epithelial cells. Functional studies in HEK293 cells indicate that SLC26A9 mediates Cl^-–HCO_3^- exchange, Cl^--independent HCO_3^- extrusion, and, unlike other anion exchangers, it is inhibited by NH_4^+ (886). Isolated from high endothelial venules endothelial cells, SLC26A11 is cell surface expressed, and exhibits Na^+-independent sulfate transport activity that is sensitive to the anion exchanger inhibitor 4,4'-diisothiocyanostilbene-2,2'-disulfonic acid (836).

FATTY ACID TRANSPORTER FAMILY (SLC27)

Long-chain fatty acids (LCFAs) are not only important as an energy source for many tissues, but they are also essential in signaling pathways that lead to the activation of protein kinase C (PKC) and nuclear transcription factors such as peroxisome proliferator-activated receptors (PARPs). To function in cells they must first cross the plasma membrane, which can occur either by passive diffusion or carrier-mediated transport. It has been estimated that about 90% of LCFA uptake into tissues like adipose takes place by saturable, active transport (764). Active LCFA transport is mediated via members of the fatty acid transport protein (FATP) family (697). The SLC27 contains six highly homologous carriers, FATP1–6, which are found in fatty acid–utilizing tissues such as the liver, heart, intestine, and adipose. Irregularities in fatty acid uptake and metabolism have been suggested to be involved in type 2 diabetes, acute liver failure, and heart disease; thus, faulty FATPs may be responsible.

FATP1 (SLC27A1), an integral membrane protein with six predicted membrane-spanning regions, was originally isolated from cultured mouse adipocytes by expression cloning, and is the most well-studied FATP in this family. Screening the EST database using the mouse FATP1 protein sequence led to the identification of four additional FATP isoforms (315). Human homologues and an additional sixth human gene were also isolated. FATP1 is found ubiquitously throughout the body but the highest levels are in skeletal muscle, heart, and adipose tissue. FATP1 is the major FATP in human adipose tissue (753). In adipocytes, insulin promotes intracellular stores of the transporter to be moved to the plasma membrane, thereby providing increased LCFA uptake. Undoubtedly, regulating these transporters is important when maintaining energy homeostasis.

FATP2 (SLC27A2) is expressed exclusively in the liver and the kidney cortex (315). FATP3 (SLC27A3) displays a broad expression distribution, but especially high levels in the lung, liver, and testis (754). Lung pneumocytes require LCFAs to produce lung surfactant, a phospholipid–protein complex to sustain alveoli structures (361). FATP4 (SLC27A4) is expressed in the heart, brain, lung, liver, and kidney. It is also the only FATP present in the intestine, where it is assumed to absorb dietary fatty acids (755).

FATP5 (SLC27A5) is restricted to the liver (315). FATP6 (SLC27A6) is mainly expressed in the heart where it is the major fatty acid transporter present. The uptake mechanisms by which long-chain fatty acids enter cardiac myocytes are not well understood but appear to occur predominantly by protein-mediated transport. In the heart muscle, much of the oxidative metabolism comes from the β-oxidation of fatty acids (247). The transport protein localizes to the sarcolemma of cardiac myocytes where it appears on the plasma membrane in areas juxtaposed to small blood vessels (247). In these membrane domains, FATP6 also colocalizes with another molecule involved in LCFA uptake, CD36.

The FATPs, like glucose transporters, may differ in their substrate specificity and uptake kinetics. The function of the FATP gene family is conserved throughout evolution, as the FATPs contain several regions that are unusually well conserved (>90% at the amino acid level) from mycobacteria to humans. The mechanism of FATP-mediated transport is poorly understood, and there are no obvious similarities between the FATPs to other transporters. One model for LCFA uptake involves protein complexes containing FATP, fatty-acid binding proteins (FABP), and long-chain fatty acyl-CoA synthetase (LACS). LCFA may first be gathered on the plasma membrane by proteins, such as CD36, and then translocated into the cell by FATPs. To trap the fatty acids and prevent efflux, the internalized LCFAs are coupled to coenzyme A via LACS. The unloading of the transporters and synthetases may be assisted by FABP and acyl-CoA–binding proteins, which would act as intracellular fatty acid buffers (408). The most detailed substrate studies are available for FATP1 (697, 753) and FATP4 (755). The studies indicate that fatty acids shorter than 10 carbons are not transported by FATP1, but its ability to carry long fatty acids such as oleate is strong. FATP4 demonstrates the ability to transport saturated and unsaturated long and very long chain fatty acids, but not fatty acid esters or lipid-soluble vitamins.

Many factors have been reported to regulate FATP expression, such as diet and hormones. FATP mRNA levels are downregulated by insulin in cultured 3T3-L1 adipocytes and upregulated by nutrient depletion in murine adipose tissue (493). Further, the fatty acid levels in the blood are insulin-dependent, and are dysregulated in diseases such as non–insulin-dependent diabetes and obesity (66). Thus, hormonal modulated changes in FATP expression may be involved in the regulation of free fatty-acid concentrations in the blood. Mouse FATP have been shown to be positively regulated by ligands that activate either peroxisome proliferator–activated receptor (PPAR)–retinoid X receptor (RXR) heterodimers in the liver and intestine (504, 541). A PPAR binding site has been found in the mouse FATP1 (SLC27A1) promoter; therefore, fatty acid derivatives such as prostaglandins and PPAR ligands, may help regulate FATP expression through a feedback loop.

SODIUM NUCLEOSIDE COTRANSPORTER FAMILY (SLC28)

Nucleosides are important biological molecules that function as signaling molecules and as precursors to nucleotides needed for DNA and RNA synthesis. Synthetic nucleoside analogues are used clinically to treat a range of cancers and viral infections. Given that these molecules are usually hydrophilic molecules, nucleoside transporters are necessary for cellular uptake. Concentrative nucleoside transporters play a vital role in the absorption and reabsorption of exogenous physiological nucleosides, and at the cellular level mediate transmembrane movement of nucleosides and analogues. Most cells are able to synthesize new nucleosides. However, it is energetically cheaper to recycle them using salvage pathways that involve transport proteins. Nucleoside transporters are divided into sodium-dependent, concentrative nucleoside transporters (CNTs, SLC28), and sodium-independent, equilibrative nucleoside transporters (ENTs, SLC29). The CNTs and ENTs share no sequence homology and represent separate families.

At least three different CNT activities have been identified based on their substrate specificity, sensitivity to inhibitors, and tissue distribution. Two of these, CNT1 and CNT2, have been cloned in the rat and humans. CNT1 (SLC28A1) has a preference for pyrimidine nucleosides and additionally accepts adenosine (195, 332, 659), whereas CNT2 (SLC28A2, SPNT) prefers purine nucleosides but also transports uridine (116, 853). CNT3 (SLC28A3) has broad purine and pyrimidine specificity (331). Both CNT1 and CNT2 have 14 putative membrane-spanning domains, and mediate an electrogenic nucleoside uptake with a 1:1 Na^+/nucleoside stoichiometry. CNT1 and CNT2 are apical nucleoside transporters in the intestine, and are also found in the liver and brain (12, 200). CNT1 is also strongly expressed in the kidney. While CNTs are localized to the apical membrane of epithelial cells, they work in coordination with ENTs that are expressed on the basolateral membrane (437, 496, 497). CNT3 is expressed at high levels in the pancreas, mammary gland, trachea, and bone marrow (658). CNT3-mediated transport is coupled to two Na^+ ions in contrast to the 1:1 ratio used by CNT1 and CNT2 (621, 658). CNT2 transports a number of anticancer nucleoside analogues (658).

There are no known diseases associated with CNTs, but due to their tissue distribution these transporters influence the pharmacokinetics and pharmacodynamics of anticancer and antiviral therapeutics. Many purine analogues are substrates for CNT1, including the antiviral therapeutics zidovudine, lamivudine, and zalcitabine (264, 659, 903); and the cytotoxic cytidine analogues cytarabine and gemcitabine, which used for treatment of various leukemias, breast cancer, non–small cell lung cancer, and pancreatic cancer (477, 488). The drug substrates for CNT2 are mostly limited to the antiviral compounds didanosine and ribavirin (243, 598, 660). The wide substrate selectivity of CNT3 allows it to transport numerous anticancer drugs including cladrabine, gemcitabine, 5dU, 5-fluorouridine, fludarabine, and zebularine (658). As expected, it can also carry the antiviral compounds AZT, ddC, and ddI.

FACILITATED NUCLEOSIDE TRANSPORTER FAMILY (SLC29)

Similar to SLC28 transporters, the SLC29 nucleoside carriers are important for the nucleoside and nucleobase uptake for salvage pathways, as well as for uptake of nucleoside analogues used for viral and cancer treatment. In the kidney and intestinal epithelial cells, ENT1 and ENT2—located on the basolateral membrane—are important for cellular exit of nucleosides. Additionally, they control cellular adenosine levels that are necessary for regulating coronary blood flow, inflammation, and neurotransmission (732). The SLC29 family contains four equilibrative (or facilitated) nucleoside transport proteins, including the NBMPR (nitrobenz-ylmercaptopurine riboside)-sensitive nucleoside transporter SLC29A1 (ENT1) (267), the NBMPR-insensitive nucleoside transporter SLC29A2 (ENT2) (144), ENT3 (336), and ENT4 (268, 901). ENT1, ENT2, and ENT3 contain 11 predicted transmembrane domains, and they have a broad selectivity for purine and pyrimidines. Less is known about ENT4, but it appears to be able to transport adenosine.

ENT1 is the major equilibrative carrier in most cells, as it has been shown to be nearly ubiquitously expressed in human tissues. In the rat kidney cortex, ENT1 is located on the basolateral membrane of the tubular epithelial cells, in contrast to the apical expression of the CNTs (901). These two transport systems appear to work together to mediate transepithelial nucleoside absorption. It is able to transport purine and pyrimidine nucleosides, with exceptions to the pyrimidine base uracil (267). Antiviral compounds such as ddC and ddI are only poor substrates for ENT1 (903). The nucleoside transporter ENT2 can transport purine and pyrimidine nucleosides but, in general, with less affinity as ENT1. ENT2 further differs from ENT1 it has the capability to also efficiently carry a wide range of purine and pyrimidine nucleobases (144, 904). ENT2 is widely distributed in tissues including adult ovary and ovarian tumors, fetal brain, and heart (268). It appears to be an important ENT transporter for cellular uptake of the HIV antivirals AZT, ddC, and ddI, due to its greater capacity to transport these substrates over ENT1. The expression of ENT1 and ENT2 in the heart is of pharmacological interest, since adenosine is critically involved in regulating the myocardial oxygen supply (544) and has beneficial cardioprotective effects in the ischemic/reperfused myocardium (442). They are important enough that ENT1 is the target for coronary vasodilator drugs such as dipyridamole and dilazep (45).

ENT3 and ENT4 have not been fully characterized. Preliminary work has suggested that ENT3 has substrate specificity similar to ENT2, and that it is widely distributed throughout the body (336). Even less is known about ENT4, which appears to transport adenosine.

ZINC TRANSPORTER FAMILY (SLC30)

Maintaining zinc homeostasis in the cell and within intracellular compartments is accomplished, in part, through the SLC30 zinc transporter family. Members of this family mediate zinc efflux from the cytosol across the plasma membrane or facilitate zinc transport from the cytosol into intracellular compartments such as synaptic vesicles, endosomes, and Golgi network (Fig. 5). Countering the SLC30 transporters, the SLC39 family transports zinc into the cell to help maintain proper levels of cellular zinc. The SLC30 family possesses nine zinc transporters, known as ZNT1 through ZNT9. All, with the exception of ZNT5, are thought to have six membrane-spanning regions, and most have a histidine-rich intracellular loop between transmembrane domains 4 and 5.

ZNT1 (594) is ubiquitously expressed throughout the body, where it mediates cellular zinc efflux and protects cells from zinc toxicity. In the intestine, ZNT1 (SLC30A1) is abundantly expressed on the basolateral side of enterocytes lining the villi of duodenum and jejunum (517). Dietary zinc supplementation elevates intestinal ZNT1 mRNA by ~50% (517), indicating that ZNT1 (SLC30A1) transcription is regulated b y dietary zinc intake. ZNT1 is also thought to be important for zinc secretion from the pancreas (468) for maintaining total-body zinc homeostasis. ZNT1 (SLC30A1) knockout mice exhibited embryonic death, suggesting that ZNT1 is vital in placental zinc transfer from mother to fetus (13). At the cellular level, ZNT1 plays a dominant role in regulating intracellular free zinc levels (591).

In contrast to ZNT1, ZNT2 (SLC30A2) works to increase the cellular accumulation of zinc by transporting zinc in endosomes, lysosomes, or vacuoles in the intestine, kidney, and testis (592). Likewise, ZNT3 (SLC30A3) is involved in zinc uptake into synaptic vesicles in glutamatergic neurons and possibly into testis cells (593, 870). In the brain of ZNT3-null mice, there is a complete lack of zinc within synaptic vesicles but the mice appear normal (138). Like ZNT1, ZNT3 may have a role in pancreatic zinc secretion from acinar cells (468). ZNT4 (SLC30A4) is highly expressed in the brain and mammary gland, where it presumably functions to facilitate zinc accumulation in secretory vesicles (329). Nonfunctional mouse ZNT4 results in zinc-deficient milk, which fails to support growth of nursing pups (604). ZNT4 was dominantly expressed in mast cells and localized in apical granules (319). Since Zn^{2+} is thought to be a caspase inhibitor, it suggested that ZNT4 might be involved in regulating apoptosis in mast cells. ZNT5 (SLC30A5) is involved in the maturation of osteoblasts in bone tissue and in the maintenance of normal cardiac conduction in the heart (345). ZNT5 (SLC30A5)-null mice develop hunched backs and osteopenia

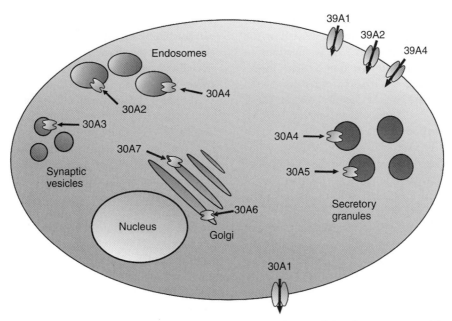

FIGURE 5 Zinc transporter subcellular localization. SLC30A1 is a cellular efflux transporter, while the SLC39 family transporters counter this movement by providing zinc influx. All the other members of the SLC30 family function to accumulate zinc in various intracellular compartments.

from the reduced osteoblastic activity. Additionally, ZNT5 and ZNT7 are necessary for activation of alkaline phosphatase (772). Potentially, ZNT6 (SLC30A6) and ZNT7 (SLC30A7) may play a role in zinc transport from the cytosol to Golgi network (403, 772). No functional data are available for ZNT8 (SLC30A8), but it appears to be localized in insulin-secretory granules in pancreatic β cells. Lastly, this family includes additional orphan transporter ZNT9 (SLC30A9), which has not yet been characterized.

COPPER TRANSPORTER FAMILY (SLC31)

Copper is an essential cofactor of many biological processes including mitochondrial oxidative phosphorylation, neurotransmitter synthesis, pigment formation, peptide biogenesis, antioxidant defense and iron metabolism. The copper transporter family includes CTR1 (SLC31A1) and CTR2 (SLC31A2), which mediate cellular copper uptake. hCTR1 was isolated by complementation of the yeast high-affinity copper-uptake mutant ctr1 by expre ssing a HeLa cDNA library (911). The structure of these transporters is of interest since they appear to have only three transmembrane domains, an uncommon feature for transporters. Crosslinking studies recently showed that hCTR1 exists as a homotrimer at the plasma membrane in mammalian cells (449).

CTR1 (SLC31A1) is thought to be a major uptake transporter of Cu uptake into mammalian cells. Studies done in yeast provided information about the major copper entry mechanisms, and revealed that the SLC31A1 gene was required for high-affinity copper transport into yeast

(149, 150). Functional studies of human CTR1 expressed in SF9 and HEK293 cells were performed using either ^{64}Cu or ^{67}Cu. The studies revealed that CTR1 mediates saturable copper uptake with a K_m of approximately 3.5 μM (176, 449). The transporter was found to be copper-specific, energy-independent, and stimulated by extracellular acidic pH and high K$^+$ concentrations. In the mouse, mCtr1 is essential for development because targeted deletion results in a prenatally lethal phenotype (430, 450). Heterozygous animals showed reduced brain copper content and reduced activities in the copper-dependent enzymes. It is possible that CTR1 copper uptake into cells provides a supply of copper to the metallochaperone-mediated copper delivery pathways (450). CTR2 might be a low-affinity copper transporter that closely resembles the yeast CTR-2, but this transport activity has yet to be demonstrated. Based on its similarity to yCtr-2, CTR2 may function inside the cell for mobilizing stored copper to the cytoplasm (911). Both CTR1 and CTR2 are expressed ubiquitously, but the highest levels of CRT1 are found in the liver.

VESICULAR GABA TRANSPORTER FAMILY (SLC32)

The vesicular inhibitory amino acid transporter (VIAAT, SLC32A1), also known as vesicular GABA transporter (VGAT) (684), is the only known SLC32 family member (515). VIAAT belongs to a eukaryotic superfamily of H$^+$-coupled transporters that also includes the SLC36 (H$^+$-proton coupled amino acid transporters) and SLC38 (Na$^+$-coupled system A and N amino acid transporters) families.

While VIAAT has no sequence similarity to the vesicular monoamine and acetylcholine transporters (SLC18) or the vesicular glutamate transporters (SLC17), it functions to transport GABA and glycine into synaptic vesicles in exchange for protons. Whereas the transport mediated by the SLC18 family relies primarily on the chemical component of the proton gradient across the vesicular membrane, VIAAT depends more equally on both chemical and electrical components of this gradient. The vacuolar-type H^+-ATPase acidifies the secretory vesicles, thereby providing the driving force for neurotransmitter uptake. The uptake of GABA can be inhibited by glycine, which appears to be also a substrate. The antiepileptic drug vigabatrin inhibits VIAAT, and thus shows affinity similar to that of GABA (515). Vigabatrin treatment leads to increased GABA levels in the brain and higher vesicular GABA content; therefore, the VIAAT activity does not seem to be affected by low doses of the drug (180).

The expression of VIAAT is restricted to the brain. Immunoreactivity for VIAAT has been shown on synaptic vesicles in GABAergic and glycinergic neurons (113), suggesting that VIAAT is responsible for the uptake of these neurotransmitters into synaptic vesicles before exocytotic release into the synaptic cleft. Rat VIAAT expression has also been detected in pancreatic islet cells (122), pituitary (512), and pineal glands (651). The islet cell localization is consistent with previous observations that there is storage of the inhibitory amino acid GABA in microvesicles within the pancreatic islet.

ACETYL-CoA TRANSPORTER FAMILY (SLC33)

This family consists of a single member, the acetyl-CoA transporter (ACATN, SLC33A1). It was originally identified in humans by expression cloning (376) and then subsequently in the rat and mouse (75, 721). The transporter is a multitransmembrane protein found in the endoplasmic reticulum that delivers acetyl-CoA synthesized in the cytosol to the lumen of the Golgi apparatus. There, the acetate donor is used for *O*-acetylation of sialoglycan chains to modify the terminal sialic acid of glycoproteins and gangliosides. *O*-acetylatation of gangliosides is though to play an important role in tissue development and organization during the early embryonic stages. Even though acetylated gangliosides are highly tissue specific, ACATN is ubiquitously expressed in the human tissues. In humans no diseases related to ACATN (SLC33A1) function have been reported.

Na$^+$-COUPLED PHOSPHATE COTRANSPORTER FAMILY (SLC34)

There are two major divisions of the Na$^+$-coupled phosphate cotransporters: the PIT families (SLC20) and the NPT type-II (SLC34) family. As indicated in previous sec-

tions, phosphate is an essential component of the skeletal system, enzymes, cofactors, nucleic acids, regulatory proteins, and so on. Bone is the major store for phosphate, especially as calcium and magnesium phosphate. Phosphate levels are typically controlled at ~1 mM in plasma. Phosphate plays an important role in the kidney as a titratable acid that can be secreted. This process allows the kidney to secrete H^+ generated from daily metabolism.

Type II transporters are apically located in intestinal and renal epithelia and are the major transporters for inorganic phosphate absorption and reabsorption. Both sites control extracellular phosphate concentrations, although it is predominately controlled by renal reabsorption of inorganic phosphate from urine. There are three isoforms of type II transporters (549): type IIa (NaPi-IIa, NaPi-3, SLC34A1) (490), type IIb (NaPi-IIb, SLC34A2) (198, 887), and type IIc (NaPi-IIc, SLC34A3) (714). Both NaPi-IIa (SLC34A1) and NaPi-IIc (SLC34A3) are found in the kidney brush border membranes of proximal tubules. NaPi-IIa is exclusively expressed in the convoluted part (S1/S2 segments) of kidney proximal tubules. NaPi-IIc is highly expressed in weaning rats in superficial and juxtamedullary nephrons, but only in juxtamedullary nephrons of adults. NaPi-IIb is dominant in the lung and intestine.

The type II transporters exhibit the known characteristics of brush border Na$^+$–Pi cotransport. SLC34A1 and SLC34A2 have a stoichiometry of 3 Na$^+$:1 HPO$_4^{2-}$, and both HPO$_4^{2-}$ and H$_2$PO$_4$– can be transported (219). However, NaPi-IIc (SLC34A3) exhibits electroneutral Na$^+$–Pi cotransport, although this transport is still pH dependent (684). The importance of NaPi-IIa in renal Pi uptake was evident when knocking out *Napi2* (NaPi-IIa) in mice resulted in severe hypophosphatemia. This phenotype is explained by an increase in fractional Pi excretion and ~70% decrease in brush border Na$^+$–Pi cotransport (42). The residual transport capacity has been attributed to NaPi-IIc. Thus, for the adult NaPi-IIa seems the major route of Pi absorption.

NaPi-IIa (SLC34A1) and NaPi-IIc (SLC34A3) renal type II transporters are regulated by numerous hormonal and metabolic signals (548, 714). Their regulation in the proximal tubule involves affecting the amount of transporter protein on the brush border membrane. For NaPi-IIa (SLC34A1) this process occurs via regulated endocytosis, while less is currently known about NaPi-IIc (SLC34A3). Parathyroid hormone (PTH) is a potent inhibitor of proximal tubule NaPi cotransport and leads to transporter retrieval from the brush border membrane due to activation of adenylate cyclase and phospholipase C. This retrieval is followed by lysosomal degradation; therefore, recovery from PTH-induced inhibition requires synthesis of new transporter molecules (610, 611). Recently, both PK-G and the ERK/MAPK pathways were also contributors to this regulatory process (549).

NaPi-IIa is thought to be involved in inherited disorders associated with hypophosphatemia (128, 162). Studies related to X-linked hypophosphatemia, autosomal-dominant hypophosphatemic rickets, and oncogenic hypophosphatemic osteomalacia suggest that the genes PHEX and FGF23 affect the abundance of NaPi-IIa in the renal proximal tubule (230, 428). FGF23, part of the fibroblast growth factor family, was found elevated in phosphaturia (139). Treatment of mice with FGF-23 decreases serum Pi levels while increasing Pi excretion (730). Additionally, two human mutants of NaPi-IIa were identified to be linked to cases of renal phosphate wasting disorders (629).

In the small intestine, NaPi-IIb isoform appears to be involved in phosphate absorption (301, 386, 888). Dietary signals such as 1,25-$(OH)_2$-vitamin D_3 and phosphate levels are involved in controlling NaPi-IIb protein abundance. When these signals induce NaPi-IIb upregulation, the mechanism appears not to be transcriptional, but instead seems to increase protein abundance. Other hormones such as EGF, glucocorticoids, and thyroid hormone have also been reported to regulate this transporter (17, 33, 889).

NUCLEOTIDE–SUGAR TRANSPORTER FAMILY (SLC35)

Protein and lipid glycosylation in the endoplasmic reticulum (ER) and the Golgi compartment is vital for proper function in many biological processes. The glycotransferases in these organelles require raw material in the form of nucleotide sugars in order to elongate the carbohydrate chains of glycoproteins, glycolipids, and polysaccharides. Nucleotide sugars made in the cytosol and nucleus cannot passively permeate through the lipid bilayers. Therefore, they require nucleotide sugar transporters (NTSs) to reach their destination and to deliver specific nucleotide sugars pooled in the cytosol into the lumen of the Golgi compartment and/or the ER. Currently there are at least 23 nucleoside sugar transporters in the SLC35 family, but most have not yet been uncharacterized. The family is broadly divided into five subfamilies (A through E) based on their amino acid similarity.

Evidence for specific nucleoside sugar transporters was identified through studies of lactose synthesis in microsomes from mammary glands of lactating rats (424). The search for transporters that deliver UDP-galactose to the ER and Golgi led to the identification of related nucleotide sugar transporters: a CMP-sialic acid transporter (SLC35A1) (174, 175, 348), a UDP-galactose transporter (SLC35A2) (529), a UDP-GlcNAc transporter (SLC35A3) (282, 349, 350), and a UDP-glucuronic acid transporter (SLC35D1) (547). These transporters are antiporters that transport nucleotide sugars in exchange for the corresponding nucleoside monophosphate, such as UMP-galactose for UDP-galactose. The transporters SLC35A1, SLC35A2, and SLC35A3 are localized in the Golgi membrane where they provide substrates utilized in the synthesis of N-linked oligosaccharides and glycolipids. CMP-sialic acid transporter malfunction may be linked to hereditary-inclusion body

myopathy type II (adult muscular dystrophy) (175). A defect in the UDP-Gal transporter in murine Had-1 cells was shown to result in severe impairment of glycosylation of glycoproteins and glycolipids (296). In addition to transporting UDP-galactose, SLC35A2 also can carry UDP-GalNAc (715). The human UDP-GlcNAc transporter expressed in yeast has demonstrated its specificity for UDP-GlcNAc (68-77).

Currently available information is even more limited regarding subfamilies B through E. Through the analysis of the human-disease leukocyte adhesion type II, some functional information can be derived for SLC35C1 (GDP-fucose transporter) (480, 481). An impairment in fucose transport caused by SLC35C1 mutations leads to a loss in fucosylated glycoconjugates, including sialyl Lewis x, on the leukocyte surface, which results in immunodeficiency (240, 317). The subfamily D member, SLC35D1 (UGTrel7), translocates both UDP-glucuronic acid and UDP-N-acetylgalactosamine from the cytosol into the ER. It is thought to participate in glucuronidation and/or chondroitin sulfate biosynthesis (547).

Malignant transformations are known to be associated with irregular carbohydrate antigens and glycolipids. Kumamoto et al. (427) showed that SLC35A2 expression is increased in human colon cancer tissues compared with nonmalignant mucosa tissues. In contrast, the expression of SLC35A1 and SLC35A3 was not altered. The data indicated that increased expression of the SLC35A2 UDP-Gal transporter in colon cancers results in enhanced expression of cancer-associated carbohydrate determinants such as Thomsen–Friedenreich and sialyl Lewis A/X antigens. Such determinants serve as ligands for the adhesion molecule E-selectin expressed in vascular endothelial cells, and therefore facilitate hematogenous metastasis of colon cancer cells (377).

LYSOSOMAL–PROTON-COUPLED AMINO ACID TRANSPORTER FAMILY (SLC36)

While sodium is the most common driving force for plasma-membrane amino acid transport, brush border–membrane vesicle studies revealed proton-dependent amino acid transporters in the mammalian small intestine and kidney (251, 802). The first member of this transporter type, PAT1 (LYAAT1, SLC36A1), was identified as a lysosomal amino acid transporter mediating export of proteolysis products back into the cytosol (685). The SLC36 family now includes two characterized members, PAT1 and PAT2, and two orphan members, PAT3 and PAT4. Expression of PAT1 (SLC36A1) mRNA was found in all rat tissues tested except testis and muscle, with the highest levels of expression in the brain. The tissue distribution of two mouse orthologues, PAT1 and PAT2, was studied in detail (mouse SLC36A1 and A2, respectively). The highest expression of PAT1 was found in the kidney, small intestine, brain, and colon, and PAT2 (SLC36A2) is highly expressed in the lung, and heart (72). In the rat brain, PAT1 was localized to lysosomes of glutamatergic neurons (685). In contrast, when murine PAT2 was expressed in HeLa cells, it localized to the plasma membrane and perinuclear regions, but only at low levels in lysosomal organelles (72).

The two transport proteins also exhibit functional differences. PAT1 transports small neutral α-amino acids (glycine, alanine, proline), as well as GABA, α-alanine and the D-isomers of alanine, proline, and serine (72, 121, 685). PAT2 demonstrates more specificity for its substrates, and transports small amino acid substrates with more affinity than PAT1. GABA, β-alanine, and D-amino acids are poor substrates for PAT2. The PAT transporters were the first H^+–amino acid symporters identified in mammals. Under the voltage clamp of *Xenopus* oocytes expressing PAT1 or PAT2, the transporters exhibited inward substrate–evoked currents (72). Experiments in tissue culture with PAT1 revealed H^+–amino acid cotransport activity that was independent of extracellular sodium or chloride levels (685). The H^+–amino acid symport occurs with a 1:1 stoichiometry ratio and therefore is electrogenic. Membrane potential changes can also modify the transport rate, which may be an important feature for functioning in neurons where there is no significant pH gradient (880).

Given its transport capabilities and tissue distribution, it seems that PAT1 plays several different roles. Its lysosomal localization in brain neurons indicates that it functions to export amino acids from the lysosome into the cytosol (685). However, in the small intestine it is likely to be involved in dietary amino acid absorption. The acidic climate in the intestine generated via the NHE3 sodium–proton exchanger presumably provides the necessary driving for PAT1-mediated transport. The physiological role of PAT2 is still unknown, but it has been suggested to play a role in myelination of peripheral nerves (52).

GLYCEROL 3–PHOSPHATE PERMEASE FAMILY (SLC37)

In an effort to identify genes on chromosome 21 that might be related to Down syndrome, exon trapping experiments were preformed, and subsequently led to the identification of a human homologue (SLC37A1) of the bacterial glycerol 3-phosphate permease genes, called the "glpTs" (39). SLC37A1 shares 30% of sequence identity with the bacterial transporter glpT, which is fairly well studied (441). The SLC37 family consists of four poorly characterized sugar transporters. The human SLC37A1 gene (SPX1, G3PP), located on 21q22.3, exists in up to three splice variants, all of which were found to be coexpressed in all tissues tested. Particularly high mRNA expression levels were detected in the adult kidney, bone marrow, liver, spleen, small intestine, and several fetal tis-

sues, especially the liver, brain, and spleen. At this time no functional or cellular localization data are available for the human gene. However, sequence homology with glpT suggests that SPX1 (SLC37A1) is likely inorganic phosphate–dependent and antiporter specific for glycerol 3-phosphate. SPX1 (SLC37A1) does contain a mitochondrial leader sequence, and is expressed in tissues that undergo extensive gluconeogenesis, evidence that is in agreement with its proposed function.

Analysis of polymorphisms excluded SLC37A1 as the gene responsible for diseases related to glycerol kinase deficiency syndromes without mutations in the glycerol kinase gene (39). Furthermore, SLC37A1 could be excluded as gene deficient in autosomal recessive deafness (DFNB10), although it is located in the vicinity of the critical region at chromosome 21q22.3. Whether the gene is dysregulated in Down syndrome is still unknown.

The human SLC37A2 (SPX2) gene maps to chromosomal position 11q24.2, which encodes a 501–amino acid protein. SLC37A2 shares 90% identity with its mouse homologue, SLC37A2, which is slightly better studied. The mouse SLC37A2 is strongly upregulated by cAMP in RAW264 macrophages (779). High levels of mRNA transcript are found in mouse bone marrow and at lower levels in the spleen. Very little is known about SLC37A3 (SPX3), but its mRNA transcripts are widely expressed and appear to be highest in breast and stomach tissue.

In contrast, there is more known about SLC37A4 (G6PT1) (242). Mutations in G6PT1 were identified in human patients with glycogen-storage disease type Ib (GSD Ib). These patients are unable to use glucose that is stored as glycogen; therefore, glycogen accumulates in tissues such as liver and muscle. The main symptoms of this disease are hepathomegaly, nephromegaly, recurrent infections, and neutropenia. As would be expected, the highest expression levels are found in the liver, kidney, and hematopoietic progenitor cells (342). The SLC37A4 (G6PT1) transporter allows glucose 6-phosphate (G6P) to pass into the ER lumen, where the G6P is dephosphorylated to yield inorganic phosphate and glucose. Mutant G6PT1s, corresponding to the clinically identified mutants, have been shown in vitro to have a significantly reduced ability to transport G6P (314).

SODIUM-COUPLED AMINO ACID TRANSPORTER FAMILY (SLC38)

The classically described system A and system N transport activities are represented by this family of sodium-coupled neutral amino acid transporters (SNAT). Currently there are three system A members, two system N members, and one orphan family member (SLC38A6, NAT-1). System A is widely expressed in mammalian cells where it mediates Na^+-coupled cellular uptake of small aliphatic amino acids, and in particular, alanine, serine, and glutamine (130). In the intestine and proximal tubule of the kidney, system A is localized to the basolateral membrane where it absorbs amino acids from the blood for metabolic requirements (309). In the intestine, alanine is used for the generation of α-ketoglutarate, the preferred metabolic fuel of enterocytes over glucose. Alanine is a particularly important nitrogen donor via alanine aminotransferase in peripheral tissues, such as the liver and skeletal muscle and in the brain (872). In the liver, system A transports alanine to provide carbon atoms for gluconeogenesis and nitrogen for urea production (129, 199). System A is subject to regulation by environmental conditions and hormonal signals. System A in the liver is known to be upregulated by glucagon and insulin, facilitating the conversion of amino acids to glucose and stimulating urea nitrogen production (131). In the heart and muscle, system A, together with the glutamine transport system N (see below), likely plays an important role in the synthesis of oxidative fuel.

At least three system A subtypes exist: SLC38A1 (SNAT1), SLC38A2 (SNAT2), and SLC38A4 (SNAT4) (765, 766, 899). The existence of several subtypes is important given the varied roles that system-A substrates play in different tissues, and the various factors that regulate system A (185, 335, 899).

SNAT1 (SLC38A1) is most abundant in the brain, retina, placenta, and heart tissues (115, 279, 828, 852). In the rat brain and spinal cord, SNAT1 (SLC38A1) is expressed in the central glutamatergic and GABAergic neurons (828). Additionally, it is found in dopaminergic neurons of the substantia nigra, cholinergic motor neurons, and in retinal ganglion cells (279, 487). SNAT1 (SLC38A1) shows the highest preference for transporting glutamate, alanine, asparagine, cysteine, histidine, and serine (9, 115), but can mediate transport of all zwitterionic, aliphatic amino acids to some degree. Amino acid transport is unidirectional and coupled to a sodium gradient with a 1:1 stoichiometry (487). Curiously, it also displays a nonsaturable cation leak property that might be involved in neuronal excitability (487).

SNAT2 (SLC38A2) operates by a similar mechanism and has substrate preferences similar to SNAT1. One distinguishing feature is that it is more widely distributed and its mRNA has been found in every tissue tested. It is detectable in glutamatergic neurons, spinal motor neurons, glial cells, and the blood–brain barrier (654, 782, 899). SNAT4 (SLC38A4) is more dissimilar in that it is more liver specific in its localization, although mRNA can also be found in skeletal muscle, the kidney, and pancreas (278, 300). Interestingly, glutamine is not a preferred substrate as with other system A members.

System N is Na^+ coupled and specific for neutral amino acids. It has a more restricted tissue distribution than systems A, and is expressed in the liver, muscle, and CNS. In the liver, system N is involved in the transport of glutamine, asparagines, and histidine, and it plays an important role in glutamine metabolism (395). There are two system N subtypes: SNAT3 (SLC38A3) and SNAT5 (SLC38A5) (371).

While the system A transporters mainly were expressed in neurons, SNAT3 (SLC38A3) is instead found largely in astrocytes throughout the brain and retina (81). In the rat kidney, the SNAT3 transporter was shown to be part of an important adaptation to chronic metabolic acidosis in rats. Under normal conditions, renal uptake of glutamine from the blood is minimal but during chronic metabolic acidosis renal uptake of glutamine increases markedly via upregulation of the SNAT3 (SLC38A3) transporter (384). As part of this metabolic acidosis response, skeletal muscle increases the release of glutamine, the kidney becomes the major site of glutamine consumption, and intracellular acidosis triggers alterations in renal glutamine utilization. As a consequence, glutamine, produced during metabolic acidosis in muscle tissue, is utilized by kidney proximal tubules to form bicarbonate, which enters the blood through the basolateral bicarbonate cotransporter NBC, as well ammonium, which enters the lumen via the sodium–proton exchanger NHE3 (305). Excretion of ammonium serves to effectively eliminate protons while the bicarbonate replenishes the plasma alkaline reserve during metabolic acidosis. Thus, the production of bicarbonate and ammonium serves to counteract the reduced plasma pH during metabolic acidosis.

Functionally, system N is distinguished from system A in that amino acid uptake is coupled to the exchange of protons (87, 112, 114). The mechanism of coupling for SNAT3 (SLC38A3) involves one Na^+ and one glutamate in exchange for one H^+. There is also evidence that SNAT3 can mediate cellular efflux of glutamate when the proton gradient is reversed. SNAT5 (SLC38A5) also performs Na^+–amino acid cotransport and countertransport of protons, which differs in its substrate preference (87). While SNAT3 only transports glutamate and histidine, SNAT5 additionally accepts serine and asparagines. SNAT5 (SLC38A5) appears also to be more widely expressed as it can be detected in multiple brain regions, lung, colon, small intestine, and kidney (554).

In the CNS, these two systems work together since the system A and N transporters are involved in the glutamate/glutamine cycle (115). Following glutamate release at glutamatergic synapses, glutamate is taken up by astrocytes and converted into glutamine. Glutamine then exits the astrocytes via the SNAT3 (SLC38A3) transporter and enters neurons via one of the system A transporters (e.g., SNAT2 [SLC38A2]) where it is required by neurons to resynthesize glutamate.

METAL ION TRANSPORTER FAMILY (SLC39)

The SLC39 transporters are involved in increasing cytoplasmic zinc (and other metal ions) concentration by promoting extracellular and, perhaps, vesicular zinc transport into the cytoplasm (232). Some SLC39 transports appear also be involved in organellar metal efflux into the cytoplasm. The SLC39 transporters are members of the ZIP family, a large metal ion transporter family that is widely distributed in the plant and animal kingdoms. The designation ZIP refers to "Zrt-Irt–like Protein," where Zrt stands for zinc transporters and Irt for iron transporters. In total there are 14 human members, including several orphan transporters. Characteristically, ZIP transporters are predicted to possess eight transmembrane domains and similar predicted topology.

ZIP1 (ZIRTL, SLC39A1) displays a wide tissue distribution and is a major zinc uptake transporter for zinc accumulation in prostate cells (221). Prostate cells contain high zinc concentrations since zinc is thought to act as an inhibitor of mitochondrial aconitase, which leads to accumulation and secretion citrate into prostatic fluid. When expressed in some cell lines such as the prostate cancer cell line PC3, ZIP1 mainly localizes to the ER (528). The in vitro overexpression of human or mouse ZIP1 leads to enhanced Zn uptake (168, 221, 233). K_m values reported in these investigations ranged from 1.7 to 7 μM, which is higher than the intracellular concentration (low nanomolar range or less) of free Zn^{2+} in plasma or in cells. The mechanism responsible for transport has not been extensively studied. However, there is some evidence that it is energy independent (232, 233). The expression of the SLC39A1 gene is repressed after zinc treatment and induced by prolactin (141).

ZIP2 (SLC39A2) is similar to ZIP1 in that it also appears to be involved in cellular zinc uptake and that its expression is zinc regulated (103, 232). hZIP2-induced Zn uptake could be inhibited by Mn^{2+} and Co^{2+}, metals that do not significantly affect hZIP1-induced Zn uptake (233). Zn uptake mediated by hZIP2 appears to be stimulated by HCO_3^-, non–ATP dependent, and sensitive to N-ethylmaleimide (232). The tissue distribution of ZIP2 is less extensive, as it is found in fewer tissues including the prostate, uterus, and monocytes. ZIP3 (SLC39A3) plays a role in zinc uptake in mammary epithelial cells and, like ZIP1, is regulated by prolactin (392). Overexpression of the mZIP3 homologue in HEK293 cells increased Zn uptake similarly to mZIP1 and mZIP2, but the mZIP3 was shown to be less specific for zinc (168).

ZIP4 (SLC39A4) plays an important role in dietary zinc absorption in the intestine and reabsorption in the kidney. SLC39A4 expression in human tissue is limited to the small intestine and kidney (106). SLC39A4 was shown to be present on the apical membrane in the mouse small intestine (854). Expression of SLC39A4 increased in the small intestine when adult nonpregnant mice were fed a zinc-deficient diet, and decreased after zinc supplementation (169).

Additional supporting evidence for this role is based on genetic defects of ZIP4 that have been linked to the autosomal recessive disease, acrodermatitis enteropathica. This disease is characterized by defective zinc absorption, confirming the role of ZIP4 in transepithelial zinc transport (431, 854).

The majority of the remaining SLC39 family members appear to be widely expressed in many tissues. Besides expression data, limited functional information is available. Overexpressing the ZIP genes SLC39A6, SLC39A7, and SLC39A8 in CHO cells promotes increased zinc accumulation (44, 791, 792). ZIP5 (SLC39A5) expression is lim-

ited to a few tissues including the kidney, intestine, and pancreas. Additionally, when expressed in MDCK cells it is targeted into the basolateral membrane (850). The role of ZIP5 may include removal of excess zinc from the blood via the pancreas and intestine (167). SLC39A6 (LIV-1, ZIP6) has been found as a breast cancer–associated protein that appears to be related to tumor progression (698). ZIP7 (SLC39A7) may be involved in zinc homeostasis of the Golgi apparatus (330), while ZIP8 (SLC39A8) is related to cadmium-induced toxicity in the testis. Zinc accumulation mediated by ZIP8 causes cell death (147). Recently, ZIP14 (SLC39A14) has been identified and is thought to be involved in hypozincemia during acute inflammation (469). Overexpressed in CHO cells, SLC39A14 has been shown to mediate cellular zinc accumulation (793). There are no published reports concerning SLC39A9–SLC39A13.

BASOLATERAL IRON TRANSPORTER FAMILY (SLC40)

This family consists of a single member, SLC40A1. SLC40A1 encodes an iron efflux transporter, called ferroportin (also known as ferroportin, IREG1 and MTP1), which was independently identified by three different groups (1, 163, 516). SLC40A1 is highly expressed in duodenal enterocytes, placental syncytiophoblasts, and in spleen and liver macrophages. In the enterocytes of the proximal intestine, iron (Fe^{2+}) is first taken up by the divalent metal ion transporter DMT1 (SLC11A2), and then exits via ferroportin across the basolateral membrane (14, 257, 615). Another protein, called hephaestin, has also been shown to be required for transepithelial iron export at the basolateral membrane. While ferroportin is a multitransmembrane transport protein, hephaestin is a membrane-bound multi–copper oxidase with a single transmembrane domain and high homology to the non–membrane-bound serum protein ceruloplasmin (841). The current concept is that, as soon as Fe^{2+} arrives at the extracellular surface, it donates an electron to the multi–copper oxidase hephaestin to become Fe^{3+} prior to its release from the transporter molecule. Fe^{3+} iron then binds apotransferrin in the plasma to form the diferric transferring complex, which is the major form of iron present in the blood. Currently there are no data regarding the SLC40A1 iron transport mechanism, the role of other ions, or the transport energy source.

In macrophages, ferroportin plays an important role in recycling iron from the hemoglobin of senescent erythrocytes. Iron from the breakdown of heme is transported out of the macrophage into the plasma via ferroportin. This process of recycling iron from dead red blood cells accounts for 30 mg/day, which is 30 times more than the amount absorbed per day. SLC40A1 mutations have been described in patients with type IV hemochromatisis, a condition that results in iron accumulation in macrophages resident in the liver Kupffer cells (371, 567, 537, 847). This observation supports the role of IREG1 as the main regulator of iron recycling in macrophages.

MgtE-LIKE MAGNESIUM TRANSPORTER FAMILY (SLC41)

Intracellular magnesium plays fundamental roles in cellular processes, but very little is known about how magnesium is transported and controlled inside cells. Based on homology with the prokaryotic MgtE magnesium transporter, the first human homologue, SLC41A1, was identified and subsequently characterized. Currently the SLC41 family includes three members—SLC41A1–A3—two of which have been characterized. SLC41A1 transcript levels demonstrate tissue-specific expression, with the highest levels detected in the heart and testis (842). When expressed in *Xenopus* oocytes, SLC41A1 mediates Mg^{2+} transport that is rheogenic, voltage dependent, and not coupled to Na^+ or Cl^-. In addition to Mg^{2+}, SLC41A1 also transport various other divalent cations: Sr^{2+}, Zn^{2+}, Cu^{2+}, Fe^{2+}, Co^{2+}, Ba^{2+}, Cd^{2+}, but not Ca^{2+}, Mn^{2+}, or Ni^{2+} (261). Mice maintained on a low-magnesium diet for 5 days upregulated expression of SLC41A1 in kidney cortical tissue, while mRNA levels of SLC41A2 did not change (262).

SLC41A2 also functions as a divalent metal transporter when expressed in oocytes but has a different substrate selectivity profile. It mediates voltage-dependent and saturable uptake of Mg^{2+}, Ba^{2+}, Ni^{2+}, Co^{2+}, Fe^{2+}, and Mn^{2+}, but not Zn^{2+}, Cu^{2+}, or Ca^{2+} (262). The third member, SLC41A3, has yet to be functionally characterized. The transporters in the SLC41 family appear to be involved with cellular magnesium homeostasis, but further studies are needed to confirm this role.

Rh AMMONIUM TRANSPORTER FAMILY (SLC42)

Rhesus (Rh) glycoproteins are best known for their presence on human blood cells and role in immunity. These Rh proteins are expressed on the surface of the red blood cell in a complex consisting of one D subunit, one CE subunit, and two Rh-associated glycoproteins (RhAG) subunits. This Rh complex has important antigenic properties, but is also thought to provide stability and structure to the blood cell. Two new non–blood cell Rh proteins, RhCG and RhBG, were cloned from mice and humans, which are expressed in tissues including the kidney and liver (499). Beyond their assumed classical roles, recent studies have revealed new functions for the Rh proteins as ammonium transporters. On this evidence, a new family SLC42 was formed to include three membrane proteins RhAG (SLC42A1), RhBG (SLC42A2), and RhCG (SLC42A3).

The human RhAG glycoprotein is best known as a blood cell antigen, but it was the first Rh family member linked to NH_3–NH_4+ transport through homology with the yeast MEP/Amt transporters (499, 500). When RhAG was expressed in yeast mutants deficient in endogenous NH_4+ transporters (MEPs), it was shown to restore some growth. When expressed in oocytes, RhAG demonstrated electroneutral countertransport of the radioactive analogue of ammonium [^{14}C]methylamine coupled to proton efflux (873). Methylamine uptake was also significantly inhibited by ammonia ($K_i = 1.14$ mM).

RhCG shares 50% sequence identity to RhAG, but is not expressed on red blood cells. Instead, it is abundantly expressed in the kidney, brain, testis, placenta, pancreas, and prostate (178, 467, 830). Detailed studies of the rat kidney show apical labeling of RhCG in the cortex, outer medullar, and upper part of the inner medulla. It is also expressed in all cells in the cortical collecting duct, intercalated cells of the outer medullary collecting duct, and inner medullary collecting duct. Limited functional studies have revealed that RhCG promotes electrogenic transport of NH_4+ (295, 499).

RhBG has a more limited tissue distribution than RhCG, with significant expression only in the kidney and liver. In contrast to RhCG, RhBG is basolaterally expressed in a majority of cells in the connecting segment and cortical collecting duct, and intercalated cells in the outer and inner medullary collecting duct (639, 830). In many cell types, both RhCG and RhBG are coexpressed, but with distinct apical and basolateral localizations. In the mouse liver, RhBG was found on the basolateral membrane of hepatocytes around the central veins (864). When RhBG is expressed in *Xenopus* oocytes, this transporter mediates the electrogenic, saturable uptake of NH^+ (555). The transport characteristics for ammonium uptake strongly suggest that RhBG is unlikely to be a NH_4+–H^+ exchanger or a NH_3 transporter. The functional properties and localization of these newly found proteins, RhBG and RhCG, provide support for the existence for renal-specific NH_4+ transporters.

Na$^+$-INDEPENDENT, SYSTEM-L–LIKE AMINO ACID TRANSPORTER FAMILY (SLC43)

Sodium-independent transport of large neutral amino acids is mediated by system-L amino acid transporters (LATs). It represents the major pathway to provide cells with aromatic and branched amino acids. Basolaterally expressed LATs play an important role in intestinal and renal proximal tubule absorption. The LAT1 and LAT2 transporters are part of the SLC7 family, while the SLC43 family includes LAT3 (SLC43A1), LAT4 (SLC43A2), and EEG1 (SLC43A3). However, the SLC43 members are structurally distinct from SLC7 members because they function without the type II glycoprotein subunits (SLC3A1 and SLC3A2), serve as facilitated diffusion transporters, exhibit two-component kinetics, and show narrower substrate selectivities. When expressed in *Xenopus* oocytes, LAT3 (SLC43A1) mediated Na^+-independent transport of neutral amino acids such as leucine, isoleucine, valine, and phenylalanine, and was inhibited by 2-aminobicyclo[2.2.1]heptane-2-carboxyl acid (29). In addition to amino acids, LAT3 also recognized amino acid alcohols. LAT3 (SLC43A1)-mediated leucine transport was saturable, but Eadie–Hofstee plots were curvilinear and fit to a two-component kinetic model. The leucine transport demonstrated by LAT3 (SLC43A1) is very different from the properties of the typical amino acid exchangers LAT1 (SLC7A5) and y$^+$LAT1 (SLC7A7). LAT3 transport was electroneutral, not dependent on Na$^+$, Cl$^-$, or H$^+$, which suggest that this process is not coupled to inorganic ions. Therefore, it appears that transport occurs via facilitated diffusion rather than exchange of amino acids. The highest LAT3 (SLC43A1) transcript expression levels are found in the pancreas and liver.

LAT4 (SLC43A2) shares 57% sequence identity to LAT3, as well as many functional characteristics such as sodium, chloride, pH independence, narrow substrate preference, and two-component kinetics (67). The transport activities can be distinguished because *N*-ethylmaleimide strongly inhibits LAT3, but only moderately blocks LAT4 activity. The biggest difference may be in the tissue distribution since LAT4 (SLC43A2) was found highly expressed in the placenta, PCT kidney cells, kidney, and intestine. LAT4 activity in the PCT cells was detected from the basolateral membrane, suggesting such localization in epithelial tissues. Localization studies show LAT4 (SLC43A2) restricted to the distal tubule and collecting duct epithelial cells in the kidney where it may function to mediate basolateral movement of neutral amino acids during recycling. In the intestine, it is predominately located in the crypt cells.

Lastly, there are no functional data for the orphan SLC43 member EEG1 (SLC43A3), but it shares ~30% identity to LAT3 and LAT4. Available expression data reveal that EEG1 (SLC43A3) is expressed in the fetal liver, lung, placenta, and kidney, where it may be involved in nutrient transport in developing tissues (763).

References

1. Abboud S, Haile DJ. A novel mammalian iron-regulated protein involved in intracellular iron metabolism. *J Biol Chem* 2000;275:19906–19912.
2. Abe T, et al. LST-2, a human liver–specific organic anion transporter, determines methotrexate sensitivity in gastrointestinal cancers. *Gastroenterology* 2001;120:1689–1699.
3. Abuladze N, et al. Molecular cloning, chromosomal localization, tissue distribution, and functional expression of the human pancreatic sodium bicarbonate cotransporter. *J Biol Chem* 1998;273:17689–17695.
4. Abuladze N, et al. Structural organization of the human NBC1 gene: kNBC1 is transcribed from an alternative promoter in intron 3. *Gene* 2000;251:109–122.
5. Adibi SA. The oligopeptide transporter (Pept-1) in human intestine: biology and function. *Gastroenterology* 1997;113:332–340.
6. Agrimi G, et al. Identification of the human mitochondrial S-adenosylmethionine transporter: bacterial expression, reconstitution, functional characterization and tissue distribution. *Biochem J* 2004;379:183–190.
7. Aihara Y, et al. Molecular cloning of a novel brain-type Na(+)-dependent inorganic phosphate cotransporter. *J Neurochem* 2000; 74:2622–2625.
8. Aihara Y, et al. Assignment of SLC17A6 (alias DNPI), the gene encoding brain/pancreatic islet-type Na$^+$-dependent inorganic phosphate cotransporter to human chromosome 11p14. *Cytogenet Cell Genet* 2001;92:167–169.
9. Albers A, et al. Na$^+$ transport by the neural glutamine transporter ATA1. *Pflugers Arch* 2001;443:92–101.
10. Alper SL. Genetic diseases of acid-base transporters. *Annu Rev Physiol* 2002;64:899–923.
11. Ames BN, et al. Uric acid provides an antioxidant defense in humans against oxidant- and radical-caused aging and cancer: a hypothesis. *Proc Natl Acad Sci U S A* 1981;78:6858–6862.
12. Anderson CM, et al. Demonstration of the existence of mRNAs encoding N1/cif and N2/cit sodium/nucleoside cotransporters in rat brain. *Brain Res Mol Brain Res* 1996;42:358–361.
13. Andrews GK, et al. Mouse zinc transporter 1 gene provides an essential function during early embryonic development. *Genesis* 2004;40:74–81.
14. Andrews NC. A genetic view of iron homeostasis. *Semin Hematol* 2002;39:227–234.
15. Aneiros E, et al. Modulation of Ca2+ signaling by Na$^+$/Ca2+ exchangers in mast cells. *J Immunol* 2005;174:119–130.
16. Apparsundaram S, et al. Molecular cloning of a human, hemicholinium-3-sensitive choline transporter. *Biochem Biophys Res Commun* 2000;276:862–867.
17. Arima K, et al. Glucocorticoid regulation and glycosylation of mouse intestinal type IIb Na-P(i) cotransporter during ontogeny. *Am J Physiol Gastrointest Liver Physiol* 2002;283:G426–G434.
18. Aronson PS, Giebisch G. Mechanisms of chloride transport in the proximal tubule. *Am J Physiol* 1997;273:F179–F192.
19. Arriza JL, et al. Excitatory amino acid transporter 5, a retinal glutamate transporter coupled to a chloride conductance. *Proc Natl Acad U S A* 1997;94:4155–4160.
20. Arriza JL, et al. Functional comparisons of three glutamate transporter subtypes cloned from human motor cortex. *J Neurosci* 1994;14:5559–5569.
21. Aruga S, et al. Chronic metabolic acidosis increases NaDC-1 mRNA and protein abundance in rat kidney. *Kidney Int* 2000;58:206–215.
22. Ashkar ZM, et al. Urea transport in initial IMCD of rats fed a low-protein diet: functional properties and mRNA abundance. *Am J Physiol* 1995;268:F1218–F1223.
23. Augustin R, et al. Identification and characterization of human glucose transporter-like protein-9 (GLUT9): alternative splicing alters trafficking. *J Biol Chem* 2004;279:16229–16236.
24. Aula N, et al. The spectrum of SLC17A5-gene mutations resulting in free sialic acid-storage diseases indicates some genotype–phenotype correlation. *Am J Hum Genet* 2000;67:832–840.
25. Aula P, Gahl WA. *Disorders of Free Sialic Acid Storage*. Scriver CR, et al., eds. New York: McGraw-Hill, 2001:5109–5120.
26. Aulak KS, et al. Molecular sites of regulation of expression of the rat cationic amino acid transporter gene. *J Biol Chem* 1996;271:29799–29806.
27. Avissar NE, et al. Na(+)-dependent neutral amino acid transporter ATB(0) is a rabbit epithelial cell brush-border protein. *Am J Physiol Cell Physiol* 2001;281:C963–C971.
28. Babcock M, et al. Regulation of mitochondrial iron accumulation by Yfh1p, a putative homolog of frataxin. *Science* 1997;276:1709–1712.
29. Babu E, et al. Identification of a novel system L amino acid transporter structurally distinct from heterodimeric amino acid transporters. *J Biol Chem* 2003;278:43838–43845.
30. Babu E, et al. Role of human organic anion transporter 4 in the transport of ochratoxin A. *Biochim Biophys Acta* 2002;1590:64–75.
31. Bachmann O, et al. The Na$^+$/H+ exchanger isoform 2 is the predominant NHE isoform in murine colonic crypts and its lack causes NHE3 upregulation. *Am J Physiol Gastrointest Liver Physiol* 2004;287:G125–G133.
32. Bachmann S, et al. Expression of the thiazide-sensitive Na-Cl cotransporter by rabbit distal convoluted tubule cells. *J Clin Invest* 1995;96:2510–2514.
33. Bacic D, et al. Regulation of the renal type IIa Na/Pi cotransporter by cGMP. *Pflugers Arch* 2001;443:306–313.
34. Bailey MA, et al. NHE2-mediated bicarbonate reabsorption in the distal tubule of NHE3 null mice. *J Physiol* 2004;561:765–775.
35. Bailey PD, et al. How to make drugs orally active: a substrate template for peptide transporter PepT1. *Angew Chem Int Ed Engl* 2000;39:505–508.
36. Bakhiya A, et al. Human organic anion transporter 3 (hOAT3) can operate as an exchanger and mediate secretory urate flux. *Cell Physiol Biochem* 2003;13:249–256.
37. Barbour B, Brew H, Attwell D. Electrogenic glutamate uptake in glial cells is activated by intracellular potassium. *Nature* 1988;335:433–435.
38. Barkley RA, et al. Positional identification of hypertension susceptibility genes on chromosome 2. *Hypertension* 2004;43:477–482.
39. Bartoloni L, et al. Cloning and characterization of a putative human glycerol 3-phosphate permease gene (SLC37A1 or G3PP) on 21q22.3: mutation analysis in two candidate phenotypes, DFNB10 and a glycerol kinase deficiency. *Genomics* 2000;70:190–200.
40. Bauch C, et al. Functional cooperation of epithelial heteromeric amino acid transporters expressed in Madin–Darby canine kidney cells. *J Biol Chem* 2003;278:1316–1322.
41. Bauch C, Verrey F. Apical heterodimeric cystine and cationic amino acid transporter expressed in MDCK cells. *Am J Physiol Renal Physiol* 2002;283:F181–F189.
42. Beck L, et al. Targeted inactivation of Npt2 in mice leads to severe renal phosphate wasting, hypercalciuria, and skeletal abnormalities. *Proc Natl Acad Sci U S A* 1998;95:5372–5377.
43. Becker BF. Towards the physiological function of uric acid. *Free Radic Biol Med* 1993;14:615–631.
44. Begum NA, et al. Mycobacterium bovis BCG cell wall and lipopolysaccharide induce a novel gene, BIGM103, encoding a 7-TM protein: identification of a new protein family having Zn-transporter and Zn-metalloprotease signatures. *Genomics* 2002;80:630–645.
45. Belardinelli L, Linden J, Berne RM. The cardiac effects of adenosine. *Prog Cardiovasc Dis* 1989;32:73–97.
46. Bellocchio EE, et al. Uptake of glutamate into synaptic vesicles by an inorganic phosphate transporter. *Science* 2000;289:957–960.
47. Berger UV, Hediger MA. Comparative analysis of glutamate transporter expression in rat brain using differential double in situ hybridization. *Anat Embryol (Berl)* 1998;198:13–30.
48. Berger UV, Hediger MA. Distribution of peptide transporter PEPT2 mRNA in the rat nervous system. *Anat Embryol (Berl)* 1999;199:439–449.
49. Berger UV, Tsukaguchi H, Hediger MA. Distribution of mRNA for the facilitated urea transporter UT3 in the rat nervous system. *Anat Embryol (Berl)* 1998;197:405–414.
50. Bergeron M, Scriver CR. *Pathophysiology of Renal Hyperaminoacidurias and Glucosuria*. Seldin DW, Giebisch G, eds. New York: Raven Press, 1992:2947–2969.

51. Bergersen L, Rafiki A, Ottersen OP. Immunogold cytochemistry identifies specialized membrane domains for monocarboxylate transport in the central nervous system. *Neurochem Res* 2002;27:89–96.
52. Bermingham JR Jr, et al. Identification of genes that are downregulated in the absence of the POU domain transcription factor pou3f1 (Oct-6, Tst-1, SCIP) in sciatic nerve. *J Neurosci* 2002;22:10217–10231.
53. Bertran J, et al. Stimulation of system y(+)-like amino acid transport by the heavy chain of human 4F2 surface antigen in Xenopus laevis oocytes. *Proc Natl Acad Sci U S A* 1992;89: 5606–5610.
54. Bertran J, et al. Expression cloning of a cDNA from rabbit kidney cortex that induces a single transport system for cystine and dibasic and neutral amino acids. *Proc Natl Acad Sci U S A* 1992; 89:5601-5605.
55. Besseghir K, Roch-Ramel F. Renal excretion of drugs and other xenobiotics. *Ren Physiol* 1987;10:221–241.
56. Bevensee MO, et al. An electrogenic Na(+)-HCO(-)(3) cotransporter (NBC) with a novel COOH- terminus, cloned from rat brain. *Am J Physiol Cell Physiol* 2000;278: C1200–C1211.
57. Biber J, et al. Localization of NaPi-1, a Na/Pi cotransporter, in rabbit kidney proximal tubules. II. Localization by immunohistochemistry. *Pflugers Arch* 1993;424:210–215.
58. Bieber LL. Carnitine. *Annu Rev Biochem* 1988;57:261–283.
59. Biemesderfer D, et al. Specific association of megalin and the Na^+/H+ exchanger isoform NHE3 in the proximal tubule. *J Biol Chem* 1999;264:17518–17524.
60. Biemesderfer D, et al. NHE3: a Na^+/H+ exchanger isoform of renal brush border. *Am J Physiol* 1993;265:736–742.
61. Biner HL, et al. Human cortical distal nephron: distribution of electrolyte and water transport pathways. *J Am Soc Nephrol* 2002;13:836–847.
62. Bisaccia F, et al. The formation of a disulfide cross-link between the two subunits demonstrates the dimeric structure of the mitochondrial oxoglutarate carrier. *Biochim Biophys Acta* 1996;1292:281–288.
63. Bissig M, et al. Functional expression cloning of the canalicular sulfate transport system of rat hepatocytes. *J Biol Chem* 1994;269:3017–3021.
64. Blaustein MP, Lederer WJ. Sodium/calcium exchange: its physiological implications. *Physiol Rev* 1999;79:763–854.
65. Block MR, et al. Small angle neutron scattering of the mitochondrial ADP/ATP carrier protein in detergent. *Biochem Biophys Res Commun* 1982;109:471–477.
66. Boden G Role of fatty acids in the pathogenesis of insulin resistance and NIDDM. *Diabetes* 1997;46:3–10 (erratum: *Diabetes* 1997;46:536).
67. Bodoy S, et al. Identification of LAT4, a novel amino acid transporter with system L activity. *J Biol Chem* 2005;280:12002–12011.
68. Boelsterli UA, Zimmerli B, Meier PJ. Identification and characterization of a basolateral dicarboxylate/cholate antiport system in rat hepatocytes. *Am J Physiol* 1995;268:G797–G805.
69. Boettger T, et al. Deafness and renal tubular acidosis in mice lacking the K-Cl co-transporter Kcc4. *Nature* 2002;416:874–878.
70. Boettger T, et al. Loss of K-Cl co-transporter KCC3 causes deafness, neurodegeneration and reduced seizure threshold. *EMBO J* 2003; 22:5422–5434.
71. Bok D, et al. Blindness and auditory impairment caused by loss of the sodium bicarbonate cotransporter NBC3. *Nat Genet* 2003;34:313–319.
72. Boll M, et al. Functional characterization of two novel mammalian electrogenic proton-dependent amino acid cotransporters. *J Biol Chem* 2002;277:22966–22973.
73. Bonen A. The expression of lactate transporters (MCT1 and MCT4) in heart and muscle. *Eur J Appl Physiol* 2001;86:6–11.
74. Bonen A, et al. Isoform-specific regulation of the lactate transporters MCT1 and MCT4 by contractile activity. *Am J Physiol Endocrinol Metab* 2000;279:E1131–E1138.
75. Bora RS, et al. cDNA cloning of putative rat acetyl-CoA transporter and its expression pattern in brain. *Cytogenet Cell Genet* 2000;89:204-208.
76. Borowsky B, Mezey EE, Hoffman BJ. Two glycine transporter variants with distinct localization in the CNS and peripheral tissues are encoded by a common gene. *Neuron* 1993;10:851–863.
77. Boss O, et al. Uncoupling protein-3: a new member of the mitochondrial carrier family with tissue-specific expression. *FEBS Lett* 1997;408:39–42.
78. Bossi E, et al. Role of anion-cation interactions on the pre-steady-state currents of the rat Na(+)-Cl(-)-dependent GABA cotransporter rGAT1. *J Physiol* 2002;541:343–350.
79. Botka CW, et al. Human proton/oligopeptide transporter (POT) genes: identification of putative human genes using bioinformatics. *AAPS Pharm Sci* 2000;2:E16.
80. Bouillaud F, et al. Detection of brown adipose tissue uncoupling protein mRNA in adult patients by a human genomic probe. *Clin Sci* 1988;75:21–27.
81. Boulland JL, et al. Cell-specific expression of the glutamine transporter SN1 suggests differences in dependence on the glutamine cycle. *Eur.J Neurosci* 2002;15:1615–1631.
82. Boyd CA, Crawford DH. Activation of cationic amino acid transport through system y+ correlates with expression of the T-cell early antigen gene in human lymphocytes. *Pflugers Arch* 1992;422:87–89.
83. Brennan S, Hering-Smith K, Hamm L. Effect of pH on citrate reabsorption in the proximal convoluted tubule. *Am J Physiol* 1988;255:F301–F306.
84. Brew H, Attwell D. Electrogenic glutamate uptake is a major current carrier in the membrane of axolotl retinal glial cells. *Nature* 1987;327:707–709 (erratum: *Nature* 987;328:742).
85. Brivet M, et al. Diagnosis of carnitine acylcarnitine translocase deficiency by complementation analysis. *J Inherit Metab Dis* 1994;17:271–274.
86. Deleted in proof.
87. Broer A, et al. Regulation of the glutamine transporter SN1 by extracellular pH and intracellular sodium ions. *J Physiol* 2002;539:3–14.
88. Broer A, et al. Neutral amino acid transporter ASCT2 displays substrate-induced Na^+ exchange and a substrate-gated anion conductance. *Biochem J* 2000;346:705–710.
89. Broer A, et al. The heterodimeric amino acid transporter 4F2hc/y+LAT2 mediates arginine efflux in exchange with glutamine. *Biochem J* 2000;349:787–795.
90. Broer S, et al. Chloride conductance and Pi transport are separate functions induced by the expression of NaPi-1 in Xenopus oocytes. *J Membr Biol* 1998;164:71–77.
91. Brosius FC III, et al. The major kidney band 3 gene transcript predicts an amino-terminal truncated band 3 polypeptide. *J Biol Chem* 1989;264:7784–7787.
92. Brown D, Hirsch S, Gluck S. Localization of a proton-pumping ATPase in rat kidney. *J Clin Invest* 1988;82:2114–2126.
93. Burant CF, et al. Fructose transporter in human spermatozoa and small intestine is GLUT5. *J Biol Chem* 1992;267:14523–14526.
94. Burckhardt BC, Burckhardt G. Transport of organic anions across the basolateral membrane of proximal tubule cells. *Rev Physiol Biochem Pharmacol* 2003;146:95–158.
95. Burnham CE, et al. Cloning and functional expression of a human kidney Na^+:HCO_3^- cotransporter. *J Biol Chem* 1997;272:19111–19114.
96. Busch AE, et al. Expression of a renal type I sodium/phosphate transporter (NaPi-1) induces a conductance in Xenopus oocytes permeable for organic and inorganic anions. *Proc Natl Acad Sci U S A* 1996;93:5347–5351.
97. Busch AE, et al. Electrogenic cotransport of Na^+ and sulfate in Xenopus oocytes expressing the cloned Na^+SO4(2-) transport protein NaSi-1. *J Biol Chem* 1994;269:12407–12409.
98. Buyse M, et al. PepT1-mediated fMLP transport induces intestinal inflammation in vivo. *Am J Physiol Cell Physiol* 2002;283:C1795–C1800.
99. Cai X, Lytton J. Molecular cloning of a sixth member of the K+-dependent Na^+/Ca2+ exchanger gene family, NCKX6. *J Biol Chem* 2004;279:5867–5876.
100. Calonge MJ, et al. Genetic heterogeneity in cystinuria: the SLC3A1 gene is linked to type I but not to type III cystinuria. *Proc Natl Acad U S A* 1995;92:9667–9671.
101. Camacho JA, et al. Hyperornithinaemia-hyperammonaemia-homocitrullinuria syndrome is caused by mutations in a gene encoding a mitochondrial ornithine transporter. *Nat Genet* 1999;22:151–158.
102. Campean V, et al. Localization of thiazide-sensitive Na(+)-Cl(-) cotransport and associated gene products in mouse DCT. *Am J Physiol Renal Physiol* 2001;281:F1028–F1035.
103. Cao J, et al. Effects of intracellular zinc depletion on metallothionein and ZIP2 transporter expression and apoptosis. *J Leukoc Biol* 2001;70:559–566.
104. Carayannopoulos MO, et al. GLUT8 is a glucose transporter responsible for insulin-stimulated glucose uptake in the blastocyst. *Proc Natl Acad Sci U S A* 2000;97:7313–7318.
105. Caron L, et al. Cloning and functional characterization of a cation-Cl- cotransporter–interacting protein. *J Biol Chem* 2000;275:32027–32036.
106. Cassard AM, et al. Human uncoupling protein gene: structure, comparison with rat gene, and assignment to the long arm of chromosome 4. *J Cell Biochem* 1990;43:255–264.
107. Cha SH, et al. Identification and characterization of human organic anion transporter 3 expressing predominantly in the kidney. *Mol Pharmacol* 2000;59:1277–1286.
108. Cha SH, et al. Molecular cloning and characterization of multispecific organic anion transporter 4 expressed in the placenta. *J Biol Chem* 2000;275:4507–4512.
109. Chairoungdua A, et al. Identification and characterization of a novel member of the heterodimeric amino acid transporter family presumed to be associated with an unknown heavy chain. *J Biol Chem* 2001;276:49390–43999.
110. Chairoungdua A, et al. Identification of an amino acid transporter associated with the cystinuria-related type II membrane glycoprotein. *J Biol Chem* 1999;274:28845–28848.
111. Chandler JD, et al. Expression and localization of GLUT1 and GLUT12 in prostate carcinoma. *Cancer* 2000;97:2035–2042.
112. Chaudhry FA, et al. Coupled and uncoupled proton movement by amino acid transport system N. *EMBO J* 2001;20:7041–7051.
113. Chaudhry FA, et al. The vesicular GABA transporter, VGAT, localizes to synaptic vesicles in sets of glycinergic as well as GABAergic neurons. *J Neurosci* 1998;18:9733–9750.
114. Chaudhry FA, et al. Molecular analysis of system N suggests novel physiological roles in nitrogen metabolism and synaptic transmission. *Cell* 1999;99:769–780.
115. Chaudhry FA, et al. Glutamine uptake by neurons: interaction of protons with system a transporters. *J Neurosci* 2002;22:62–72.
116. Che M, Ortiz DF, Arias IM. Primary structure and functional expression of a cDNA encoding the bile canalicular, purine-specific Na(+)-nucleoside cotransporter. *J Biol Chem* 1995;270:13596–13599.
117. Chelly J, et al. Isolation of a candidate gene for Menkes disease that encodes a potential heavy metal binding protein. *Nat Genet* 1993;3:14–19.
118. Chen ST, et al. A human ADP/ATP translocase gene has seven pseudogenes and localizes to chromosome X. *Somat Cell Mol Genet* 1990;16:143–149.
119. Chen X, et al. Molecular and functional analysis of SDCT2, a novel rat sodium-dependent dicarboxylate transporter. *J Clin Invest* 1999;103:1159–1168.
120. Chen XZ, et al. Stoichiometry and kinetics of the high-affinity H+-coupled peptide transporter PepT2. *J Biol Chem* 1999;274:2773–2779.
121. Chen Z, et al. Structure, function and immunolocalization of a proton-coupled amino acid transporter (hPAT1) in the human intestinal cell line Caco-2. *J Physiol* 2003;546: 349–361.
122. Chessler SD, et al. Expression of the vesicular inhibitory amino acid transporter in pancreatic islet cells: distribution of the transporter within rat islets. *Diabetes* 2002;51:1763–771.
123. Chiao JH, et al. RFC-1 gene expression regulates folate absorption in mouse small intestine. *J Biol Chem* 1997;272:11165–11170.
124. Choi I, et al. Functional characterization of "NCBE," a Na/HCO3 cotransporter. *FASEB J* 2002;16:A796.
125. Choi I, et al. An electroneutral sodium/bicarbonate cotransporter NBCn1 and associated sodium channel. *Nature* 2000;405:571–575.
126. Choi I, et al. Cloning and characterization of a human electrogenic Na^+-HCO_3^- cotransporter isoform (hhNBC). *Am J Physiol* 1999;276:C576–C584.
127. Choi JY, et al. Novel amiloride-sensitive sodium-dependent proton secretion in the mouse proximal convoluted tubule. *J Clin Invest* 2000;105:1141–1146.
128. Chong SS, et al. Cloning, genetic mapping, and expression analysis of a mouse renal sodium-dependent phosphate cotransporter. *Am J Physiol* 1995;268:F1038–F1045.
129. Christensen HN. Interorgan amino acid nutrition. *Physiol Rev* 1982;62:1193–1233.

130. Christensen HN. Role of amino acid transport and countertransport in nutrition and metabolism. *Physiol Rev* 1990;70:43–77.
131. Christensen HN, Kilberg M. Hepatic amino acid transport primary to the urea cycle in regulation of biologic neutrality. *Nutr Rev* 1995;53:74–76.
132. Chua AC, Morgan EH. Manganese metabolism is impaired in the Belgrade laboratory rat. *J Comp Physiol* 1997;167:361–369.
133. Closs E. CATs, a family of three distinct cationic amino acid trasnporters. *Amino Acids* 1996;11:193–208.
134. Closs EI, et al. Identification of a low affinity, high capacity transporter of cationic amino acids in mouse liver. *J Biol Chem* 1993;268:7538–7544.
135. Closs EI, et al. Characterization of the third member of the MCAT family of cationic amino acid transporters. Identification of a domain that determines the transport properties of the MCAT proteins. *J Biol Chem* 1993;268:20796–20800.
136. Coady MJ, et al. The human tumour suppressor gene SLC5A8 expresses a Na^+-monocarboxylate cotransporter. *J Physiol* 2004;557:719–731.
137. Coady MJ, et al. Identification of a novel Na^+/myo-inositol cotransporter. *J Biol Chem* 2002; 277:35219–35224.
138. Cole TB, et al. Elimination of zinc from synaptic vesicles in the intact mouse brain by disruption of the ZnT3 gene. *Proc Natl Acad Sci U S A* 1999;96:1716–1721.
139. Consortium, ADHR. Autosomal dominant hypophosphataemic rickets is associated with mutations in FGF23. The ADHR Consortium. *Nat Genet* 2000;26:345–348.
140. Costanzo LS. Localization of diuretic action in microperfused rat distal tubules: Ca and Na transport. *Am J Physiol* 1985;248:F527–F535.
141. Costello LC, et al. Evidence for a zinc uptake transporter in human prostate cancer cells which is regulated by prolactin and testosterone. *J Biol Chem* 1999;274:17499–17504.
142. Cox GA, et al. Sodium/hydrogen exchanger gene defect in slow-wave epilepsy mutant mice. *Cell* 1997;91:139–148.
143. Craddock AL, et al. Expression and transport properties of the human ileal and renal sodium-dependent bile acid transporter. *Am J Physiol* 1998;274:G157–169.
144. Crawford CR, et al. Cloning of the human equilibrative, nitrobenzylmercaptopurine riboside (NBMPR)-insensitive nucleoside transporter ei by functional expression in a transport-deficient cell line. *J Biol Chem* 1998;273:5288–5293.
145. Custer M, et al. Localization of NaPi-1, a Na-Pi cotransporter, in rabbit kidney proximal tubules. I. mRNA localization by reverse transcription/polymerase chain reaction. *Pflugers Arch* 1993;424:203–209.
146. Dai G, Levy O, Carrasco N. Cloning and characterization of the thyroid iodide transporter. *Nature* 1996;379:458–460.
147. Dalton T P, et al. Identification of mouse SLC39A8 as the transporter responsible for cadmium-induced toxicity in the testis. *Proc Natl Acad Sci U S A* 2005;102:3401–3406.
148. Danbolt NC, Storm-Mathisen J, Kanner BI. An [Na^+ + K+]coupled L-glutamate transporter purified from rat brain is located in glial cell processes. *Neuroscience* 1992;51:295–310.
149. Dancis A, et al. The Saccharomyces cerevisiae copper transport protein (Ctr1p). Biochemical characterization, regulation by copper, and physiologic role in copper uptake. *J Biol Chem* 1994;269:25660–25667.
150. Dancis A, et al. Molecular characterization of a copper transport protein in S. cerevisiae: an unexpected role for copper in iron transport. *Cell* 1993;76:393–402.
151. del Arco A, Satrustegui J. Molecular cloning of Aralar, a new member of the mitochondrial carrier superfamily that binds calcium and is present in human muscle and brain. *J Biol Chem* 1998;273:23327–23334.
152. Delpire E, et al. Deafness and imbalance associated with inactivation of the secretory Na-K-2Cl co-transporter. *Nat Genet* 1999;22:192–195.
153. Delpire E, Mount DB. Human and murine phenotypes associated with defects in cation-chloride cotransport. *Annu Rev Physiol* 2002;64 803–843.
154. Demuth DR, et al. Cloning and structural characterization of a human non-erythroid band 3–like protein. *EMBO J* 1986;5:1205–1214.
155. Denker SP, et al. Direct binding of the Na—H exchanger NHE1 to ERM proteins regulates the cortical cytoskeleton and cell shape independently of H(+) translocation. *Mol Cell* 2000;6:1425–1436.
156. Deves R, Boyd CA. Transporters for cationic amino acids in animal cells: discovery, structure, and function. *Physiol Rev* 1998;78:487–545.
157. Devonald MA, et al. Non-polarized targeting of AE1 causes autosomal dominant distal renal tubular acidosis. *Nat Genet* 2003;33:125–127.
158. Diaz G A, et al. Mutations in a new gene encoding a thiamine transporter cause thiamine-responsive megaloblastic anaemia syndrome. *Nat Genet* 1999;22:309–312.
159. Diez-Sampedro A, et al. A glucose sensor hiding in a family of transporters. *Proc Natl Acad Sci U S A* 2003;100:11753–11758.
160. Doege H, et al. GLUT8, a novel member of the sugar transport facilitator family with glucose transport activity. *J Biol Chem* 2000;275:16275–16280.
161. Dolce V, et al. The sequences of human and bovine genes of the phosphate carrier from mitochondria contain evidence of alternatively spliced forms. *J Biol Chem* 1994;269:10451–10460.
162. Dolce V, et al. Cloning and sequencing of the rat cDNA encoding the mitochondrial 2-oxoglutarate carrier protein. *DNA Seq* 1994;5:103–109.
163. Donovan A, et al. Positional cloning of zebrafish ferroportin1 identifies a conserved vertebrate iron exporter. *Nature* 2000;403:776–781.
164. Dransfield DT, et al. Ezrin is a cyclic AMP-dependent protein kinase anchoring protein. *EMBO J* 1997;16:35–43.
165. Dresser MJ, Leabman MK, Giacomini KM. Transporters involved in the elimination of drugs in the kidney: organic anion transporters and organic cation transporters. *J Pharm Sci* 2001;90:397–421.
166. Duchesne R, et al. UT-A urea transporter protein in heart: increased abundance during uremia, hypertension, and heart failure. *Circ Res* 2001;89:139–145.
167. Dufner-Beattie J, et al. The adaptive response to dietary zinc in mice involves the differential cellular localization and zinc regulation of the zinc transporters ZIP4 and ZIP5. *J Biol Chem* 2004;279:49082–49090.
168. Dufner-Beattie J, et al. Structure, function, and regulation of a subfamily of mouse zinc transporter genes. *J Biol Chem* 2003;278:50142–50150.
169. Dufner-Beattie J, et al. The acrodermatitis enteropathica gene ZIP4 encodes a tissue-specific, zinc-regulated zinc transporter in mice. *J Biol Chem* 2003;278:33474–3481.
170. Dunham PB, Stewart GW, Ellory JC. Chloride-activated passive potassium transport in human erythrocytes. *Proc Natl Acad Sci U S A* 77:1711–1715.
171. Duran JM, et al. OCTN3: A Na^+-independent L-carnitine transporter in enterocytes basolateral membrane. *J Cell Physiol* 2005;202:929–935.
172. Dutta B, et al. Cloning of the human thiamine transporter, a member of the folate transporter family. *J Biol Chem* 1999;274:31925–31929.
173. Eckhardt M, Gerardy-Schahn R. Molecular cloning of the hamster CMP-sialic acid transporter. *Eur J Biochem* 1997;248:187–192.
174. Eckhardt M, et al. Expression cloning of the Golgi CMP-sialic acid transporter. *Proc Natl Acad U S A* 1996;93:7572–7576.
175. Eisenberg I, et al. The UDP-N-acetylglucosamine 2-epimerase/N-acetylmannosamine kinase gene is mutated in recessive hereditary inclusion body myopathy. *Nat Genet* 2001;29: 83–87.
176. Eisses JF, Kaplan JH. Molecular characterization of hCTR1, the human copper uptake protein. *J Biol Chem* 2002;277:29162–29171.
177. Ekaratanawong S, et al. Human organic anion transporter 4 is a renal apical organic anion/dicarboxylate exchanger in the proximal tubules. *J Pharmacol Sci* 2004;94:297–304.
178. Eladari D, et al. Expression of RhCG, a new putative NH(3)/NH(4)(+) transporter, along the rat nephron. *J Am Soc Nephrol* 2002;13:1999–2008.
179. Ellison DH, Velazquez H, Wright FS. Thiazide-sensitive sodium chloride cotransport in early distal tubule. *Am J Physiol* 1987;253:F546–F554.
180. Engel D, et al. Plasticity of rat central inhibitory synapses through GABA metabolism. *J Physiol* 2001;535:473–482.
181. Englard S, Seifter S. The biochemical functions of ascorbic acid. *Annu Rev Nutr* 1986;6: 365–406.
182. Enomoto A, et al. Molecular identification of a renal urate anion exchanger that regulates blood urate levels. *Nature* 2002;417:447–452.
183. Enomoto A, et al. Interaction of human organic anion transporters 2 and 4 with organic anion transport inhibitors. *J Pharmacol Exp Ther* 2002;301:797–802.
184. Enomoto A, et al. Molecular identification of a novel carnitine transporter specific to human testis. Insights into the mechanism of carnitine recognition. *J Biol Chem* 2002;277: 36262–36271.
185. Ensenat D, et al. Transforming growth factor-beta 1 stimulates vascular smooth muscle cell L-proline transport by inducing system A amino acid transporter 2 (SAT2) gene expression. *Biochem J* 2001;360:507–512.
186. Erickson JD, Eiden LE, Hoffman BJ. Expression cloning of a reserpine-sensitive vesicular monoamine transporter. *Proc Natl Acad U S A* 1992;89:10993–10997.
187. Erickson JD, et al. Distinct pharmacological properties and distribution in neurons and endocrine cells of two isoforms of the human vesicular monoamine transporter. *Proc Natl Acad Sci U S A* 1996;93:5166–5171.
188. Eskandari S, et al. Thyroid Na^+/I- symporter. Mechanism, stoichiometry, and specificity. *J Biol Chem* 1997;272:27230–27238.
189. Evans CA, et al. Nramp1 is expressed in neurons and is associated with behavioural and immune responses to stress. *Neurogenetics* 2001;3:69–78.
190. Evans RL, et al. Severe impairment of salivation in Na^+/K+/2Cl- cotransporter (NKCC1)–deficient mice. *J Biol Chem* 2000; 275:26720–26726.
191. Everett LA, et al. Targeted disruption of mouse Pds provides insight about the inner-ear defects encountered in Pendred syndrome. *Hum Mol Genet* 2001;10:153–161.
192. Everett LA, et al. Pendred syndrome is caused by mutations in a putative sulphate transporter gene (PDS). *Nat Genet* 1997;17:411–422.
193. Faaland CA, et al. Molecular characterization of two novel transporters from human and mouse kidney and from LLC-PK1 cells reveals a novel conserved family that is homologous to bacterial and Aspergillus nucleobase transporters. *Biochim Biophys Acta* 1998;1442:353–360.
194. Fairman WA, et al. An excitatory amino-acid transporter with properties of a ligand-gated chloride channel. *Nature* 1995;375:599–603.
195. Fang X, et al. Functional characterization of a recombinant sodium-dependent nucleoside transporter with selectivity for pyrimidine nucleosides (cNT1rat) by transient expression in cultured mammalian cells. *Biochem J* 1996;317:457–465.
196. Feder JN, et al. A novel MHC class I-like gene is mutated in patients with hereditary haemochromatosis. *Nat Genet* 1996;13:399–408.
197. Fei YJ, et al. Expression cloning of a mammalian proton-coupled oligopeptide transporter. *Nature* 1994;368:563–566.
198. Feild JA, et al. Cloning and functional characterization of a sodium-dependent phosphate transporter expressed in human lung and small intestine. *Biochem Biophys Res Commun* 1999;258:578–582.
199. Felig P. Amino acid metabolism in man. *Annu Rev Biochem* 1975;44:933–955.
200. Felipe A, et al. Na^+-dependent nucleoside transport in liver: two different isoforms from the same gene family are expressed in liver cells. *Biochem J* 1998;330:997–1001.
201. Feliubadalo L, et al. Non-type I cystinuria caused by mutations in SLC7A9, encoding a subunit (bo,+AT) of rBAT. International Cystinuria Consortium. *Nat Genet* 1999;23:52–57.
202. Fenczik CA, et al. Complementation of dominant suppression implicates CD98 in integrin activation. *Nature* 1997;390:81–85.
203. Fenton RA, et al. Molecular characterization of a novel UT-A urea transporter isoform (UT-A5) in testis. *Am J Physiol Cell Physiol* 2000;279:C1425–C1431.
204. Fenton RA, et al. Characterization of mouse urea transporters UT-A1 and UT-A2. *Am J Physiol Renal Physiol* 2002;283:F817–F825.
205. Ferguson SM, et al. Vesicular localization and activity-dependent trafficking of presynaptic choline transporters. *J Neurosci* 2003;23:9697–9709.
206. Fernandez-Llama P, et al. Impaired aquaporin and urea transporter expression in rats with adriamycin-induced nephrotic syndrome. *Kidney Int* 1998;53:1244–1253.

207. Ferrier B, Martin M, Baverel G. Reabsorption and secretion of alpha-ketoglutarate along the rat nephron: a micropuncture study. *Am J Physiol* 1985;248:F404–F412.
208. Fiermonte G, et al. Identification of the mitochondrial ATP-Mg/Pi transporter. Bacterial expression, reconstitution, functional characterization, and tissue distribution. *J Biol Chem* 2004;279:30722–30730.
209. Fiermonte G,Dolce V, Palmieri F. Expression in Escherichia coli, functional characterization, and tissue distribution of isoforms A and B of the phosphate carrier from bovine mitochondria. *J Biol Chem* 1998;273:22782–22787.
210. Fiermonte G, et al. Identification of the human mitochondrial oxodicarboxylate carrier. Bacterial expression, reconstitution, functional characterization, tissue distribution, and chromosomal location. *J Biol Chem* 2001;276:8225–8230.
211. Fiermonte G, et al. The sequence, bacterial expression, and functional reconstitution of the rat mitochondrial dicarboxylate transporter cloned via distant homologs in yeast and Caenorhabditis elegans. *J Biol Chem* 1998;273:24754–24759.
212. Fiermonte G, et al. Identification of the mitochondrial glutamate transporter. Bacterial expression, reconstitution, functional characterization, and tissue distribution of two human isoforms. *J Biol Chem* 2002;277:19289–19294.
213. Fishbein WN. Lactate transporter defect: a new disease of muscle. *Science* 1986;234: 1254–1256.
214. Fleming JC, et al. Characterization of a murine high-affinity thiamine transporter, Slc19a2. *Mol Genet Metab* 2001;74:273–280.
215. Fleming MD, et al. Nramp2 is mutated in the anemic Belgrade (b) rat: evidence of a role for Nramp2 in endosomal iron transport. *Proc Natl Acad U S A* 1998;95:1148–1153.
216. Fleming MD, et al. Microcytic anaemia mice have a mutation in Nramp2, a candidate iron transporter gene. *Nat Genet* 1997;16:383–386.
217. Fon EA, et al. Vesicular transport regulates monoamine storage and release but is not essential for amphetamine action. *Neuron* 1997;19:1271–1283.
218. Forbes JR, Gros P. Iron, manganese, and cobalt transport by Nramp1 (Slc11a1) and Nramp2 (Slc11a2) expressed at the plasma membrane. *Blood* 2003;102:1884–1892.
219. Forster I, et al. The voltage dependence of a cloned mammalian renal type II Na^+/Pi cotransporter (NaPi-2). *J Gen Physiol* 1998;112:1–18.
220. Forster IC, et al. Electrophysiological characterization of the flounder type II Na^+/Pi cotransporter (NaPi-5) expressed in Xenopus laevis oocytes. *J Membr Biol* 1997;160:9–25.
221. Franklin RB, et al. Human ZIP1 is a major zinc uptake transporter for the accumulation of zinc in prostate cells. *J Inorg Biochem* 2003;96:435–442.
222. Fremeau RT Jr, et al. The identification of vesicular glutamate transporter 3 suggests novel modes of signaling by glutamate. *Proc Natl Acad Sci U S A* 2002;99:14488–14493.
223. Fremeau RT Jr, Caron MG, Blakely RD. Molecular cloning and expression of a high affinity L-proline transporter expressed in putative glutamatergic pathways of rat brain. *Neuron* 1992;8:915–926.
224. Fremeau RT Jr, et al. The expression of vesicular glutamate transporters defines two classes of excitatory synapse. *Neuron* 2001;31:247–260.
225. Friesema EC, et al. Identification of monocarboxylate transporter 8 as a specific thyroid hormone transporter. *J Biol Chem* 2003;278:40128–40135.
226. Friesema EC, et al. Association between mutations in a thyroid hormone transporter and severe X-linked psychomotor retardation. *Lancet* 2004;364:1435–1437.
227. Fujiwara K, et al. Identification of thyroid hormone transporters in humans: different molecules are involved in a tissue-specific manner. *Endocrinology* 2001;142:2005–2012.
228. Fukasawa Y, et al. Identification and characterization of a Na(+)-independent neutral amino acid transporter that associates with the 4F2 heavy chain and exhibits substrate selectivity for small neutral D- and L-amino acids. *J Biol Chem* 2000;275:9690–9698.
229. Fukumoto H, et al. Cloning and characterization of the major insulin-responsive glucose transporter expressed in human skeletal muscle and other insulin-responsive tissues. *J Biol Chem* 264:7776–7779.
230. Fukumoto S, Yamashita T. Fibroblast growth factor-23 is the phosphaturic factor in tumor-induced osteomalacia and may be phosphatonin. *Curr Opin Nephrol Hypertens* 2002;11: 385–389.
231. Fuller RW. Uptake inhibitors increase extracellular serotonin concentration measured by brain microdialysis. *Life Sci* 1994;55:163–167.
232. Gaither LA, Eide DJ. Functional expression of the human hZIP2 zinc transporter. *J Biol Chem* 2000;275:5560–5564.
233. Gaither LA, Eide DJ. The human ZIP1 transporter mediates zinc uptake in human K562 erythroleukemia cells. *J Biol Chem* 2001;276:22258–22264.
234. Galli A, et al. Drosophila serotonin transporters have voltage-dependent uptake coupled to a serotonin-gated ion channel. *J Neurosci* 1997;17:3401–3411.
235. Gamba G, et al. Primary structure and functional expression of a cDNA encoding the thiazide-sensitive, electroneutral sodium-chloride cotransporter. *Proc Natl Acad U S A* 1993; 90: 2749–2753.
236. Ganapathy ME, et al. Valacyclovir: a substrate for the intestinal and renal peptide transporters PEPT1 and PEPT2. *Biochem Biophys Res Commun* 1998;246:470–475.
237. Ganapathy V, et al. Biological functions of SLC5A8, a candidate tumour suppressor. *Biochem Soc Trans* 2005;33:237–240.
238. Gawenis LR, et al. Impaired gastric acid secretion in mice with a targeted disruption of the NHE4 $Na^+/H+$ exchanger. *J Biol Chem* 2005;280:12781–12789.
239. Gawenis LR, et al. Mice with a targeted disruption of the AE2 Cl-/HCO_3^- exchanger are achlorhydric. *J Biol Chem* 2004;279:30531–30539.
240. Gerardy-Schahn R, Oelmann S, Bakker H. Nucleotide sugar transporters: biological and functional aspects. *Biochimie* 2001;83:775–782.
241. Gerhart DZ, et al. Expression of the monocarboxylate transporter MCT2 by rat brain glia. *Glia* 1998;22:272–281.
242. Gerin I, et al. Sequence of a putative glucose 6-phosphate translocase, mutated in glycogen storage disease type Ib. *FEBS Lett* 1997;419:235–238.
243. Gerstin KM, Dresser MJ, Giacomini KM. Specificity of human and rat orthologs of the concentrative nucleoside transporter, SPNT. *Am J Physiol Renal Physiol* 2002;283:F344–F349.
244. Geyer J, Godoy JR, Petzinger E. Identification of a sodium-dependent organic anion transporter from rat adrenal gland. *Biochem Biophys Res Commun* 2004;316:300–306.
245. Gillen CM, et al. Molecular cloning and functional expression of the K-Cl cotransporter from rabbit, rat, and human. A new member of the cation-chloride cotransporter family. *J Biol Chem* 1996;271:16237–16244.
246. Gillen CM, Forbush B III. Functional interaction of the K-Cl cotransporter (KCC1) with the Na-K-Cl cotransporter in HEK-293 cells. *Am J Physiol* 1999;276:C328–C336.
247. Gimeno RE, et al. Characterization of a heart-specific fatty acid transport protein. *J Biol Chem* 2003;278:16039–16044.
248. Girard JP, et al. Molecular cloning and functional analysis of SUT-1, a sulfate transporter from human high endothelial venules. *Proc Natl Acad Sci U S A* 1999;96:12772–12777.
249. Giros B, et al. Cloning and functional characterization of a cocaine-sensitive dopamine transporter. *FEBS Lett* 1991;295:149–154.
250. Goldmuntz E, et al. Cloning, genomic organization, and chromosomal localization of human citrate transport protein to the DiGeorge/velocardiofacial syndrome minimal critical region. *Genomics* 1996;33:271–276.
251. Gonska T, Hirsch JR, Schlatter E. Amino acid transport in the renal proximal tubule. *Amino Acids* 2000;19:395–3407.
252. Good DW, et al. Transepithelial HCO_3^- absorption is defective in renal thick ascending limbs from $Na^+/H+$ exchanger NHE1 null mutant mice. *Am J Physiol Renal Physiol* 2004; 287:F1244–F1249.
253. Good PF, et al. Evidence of neuronal oxidative damage in Alzheimer's disease. *Am J Pathol* 1996;149:21–28.
254. Gopal E, et al. Sodium-coupled and electrogenic transport of B-complex vitamin nicotinic acid by slc5a8, a member of the Na/glucose co-transporter gene family. *Biochem J* 2005; 388:309–316.
255. Gopal E, et al. Expression of slc5a8 in kidney and its role in Na(+)-coupled transport of lactate. *J Biol Chem* 2004;279:44522–44532.
256. Goswami T, et al. Natural-resistance-associated macrophage protein 1 is an H+/bivalent cation antiporter. *Biochem J* 2001;354:511–519.
257. Goswami T, Rolfs A, Hediger MA. Iron transport: emerging roles in health and disease. *Biochem Cell Biol* 2002;80:679–689.
258. Gottesdiener KM, et al. Isolation and structural characterization of the human 4F2 heavy-chain gene, an inducible gene involved in T-lymphocyte activation. *Mol Cell Biol* 8:3809–3819.
259. Govoni G, et al. Cell-specific and inducible Nramp1 gene expression in mouse macrophages in vitro and in vivo. *J Leukoc Biol* 1997;62:277–286.
260. Goyal S, Vanden Heuvel G, Aronson PS. Renal expression of novel $Na^+/H+$ exchanger isoform NHE8. *Am J Physiol Renal Physiol* 2003;284:467–473.
261. Goytain A, Quamme GA. Functional characterization of human SLC41A1, a Mg2+ transporter with similarity to prokaryotic MgtE Mg2+ transporters. *Physiol Genomics* 2005;21:337–342.
262. Goytain A, Quamme GA. Functional characterization of the human solute carrier, SLC41A2. *Biochem Biophys Res Commun* 2005;330:701–705.
263. Graham BH, et al. A mouse model for mitochondrial myopathy and cardiomyopathy resulting from a deficiency in the heart/muscle isoform of the adenine nucleotide translocator. *Nat Genet* 1997;16:226–234.
264. Graham KA, et al. Differential transport of cytosine-containing nucleosides by recombinant human concentrative nucleoside transporter protein hCNT1. *Nucleosides Nucleotides Nucleic Acids* 2000;19:415–434.
265. Greger R, Schlatter E, Lang F. Evidence for electroneutral sodium chloride cotransport in the cortical thick ascending limb of Henle's loop of rabbit kidney. *Pflugers Arch* 396:308–314.
266. Grichtchenko II, et al. Cloning, characterization, and chromosomal mapping of a human electroneutral Na(+)-driven Cl-HCO_3^- exchanger. *J Biol Chem* 2001;276:8358–8363.
267. Griffiths M, et al. Cloning of a human nucleoside transporter implicated in the cellular uptake of adenosine and chemotherapeutic drugs [see comments]. *Nat Med* 1997;3:89–93.
268. Griffiths M, et al. Molecular cloning and characterization of a nitrobenzylthioinosine-insensitive (ei) equilibrative nucleoside transporter from human placenta. *Biochem J* 1997; 328:739–743.
269. Gritli S, et al. A novel mutation in the SLC19A2 gene in a Tunisian family with thiamine-responsive megaloblastic anaemia, diabetes and deafness syndrome. *Br J Haematol* 2001; 113:508–513.
270. Grube M, et al. Expression, localization, and function of the carnitine transporter octn2 (slc22a5) in human placenta. *Drug Metab Dispos* 2005;33:31–37.
271. Gruenheid S, et al. Identification and characterization of a second mouse Nramp gene. *Genomics* 1995;25:514–525.
272. Gruenheid S, et al. Natural resistance to infection with intracellular pathogens: the Nramp1 protein is recruited to the membrane of the phagosome. *J Exp Med* 1997;185:717–730.
273. Grundemann D, et al. Drug excretion mediated by a new prototype of polyspecific transporter. *Nature* 1994;372:549–552.
274. Grundemann D, et al. Discovery of the ergothioneine transporter. *Proc Natl Acad Sci U S A* 2005;102:5256–5261.
275. Grundemann D, et al. Transport of monoamine transmitters by the organic cation transporter type 2, OCT2. *J Biol Chem* 1998;273:30915–30920.
276. Grunewald, Bendahan A, Kanner BI. Biotinylation of single cysteine mutants of the glutamate transporter GLT-1 from rat brain reveals its unusual topology. *Neuron* 1998;21:623–632.
277. Grunewald M, Kanner BI. The accessibility of a novel reentrant loop of the glutamate transporter GLT-1 is restricted by its substrate. *J Biol Chem* 2000;275:9684–9689.
278. Gu S, et al. A novel human amino acid transporter, hNAT3: cDNA cloning, chromosomal mapping, genomic structure, expression, and functional characterization. *Genomics* 2001; 74:262–272.
279. Gu S, et al. Characterization of an N-system amino acid transporter expressed in retina and its involvement in glutamine transport. *J Biol Chem* 2001;276:24137–24144.
280. Guastella J, et al. Cloning and expression of a rat brain GABA transporter. *Science* 1990;249:1303–1306.

281. Guillam MT, et al. Early diabetes and abnormal postnatal pancreatic islet development in mice lacking Glut-2. *Nat Genet* 1997;17:327–330 (errata: *Nat Genet* 1997;17:503, 1998;18:88).

282. Guillen E, Abeijon CC, Hirschberg CB. Mammalian Golgi apparatus UDP-N-acetylglucosamine transporter: molecular cloning by phenotypic correction of a yeast mutant. *Proc Natl Acad Sci U S A* 1998;95:7888–7892.

283. Guimaraes MJ, et al. A new approach to the study of haematopoietic development in the yolk sac and embryoid bodies. *Development* 1995;121:3335–3346.

284. Guimbal C, Kilimann MW. A Na(+)-dependent creatine transporter in rabbit brain, muscle, heart, and kidney. cDNA cloning and functional expression. *J Biol Chem* 1993;268:8418–8421.

285. Gunshin H, et al. Cloning and characterization of a mammalian proton-coupled metal-ion transporter. *Nature* 1997;388:482–488.

286. Haas M, Forbush B. The Na-K-Cl cotransporters. *J Bioenerg Biomembr* 1998;30:161–172.

287. Haber RS, et al. Tissue distribution of the human GLUT3 glucose transporter. *Endocrinology* 1993;132:2538–2543.

288. Hagenbuch B, Meier PJ. Molecular cloning, chromosomal localization, and functional characterization of a human liver Na^+/bile acid cotransporter. *J Clin Invest* 1994;93:1326–1331.

289. Hagenbuch B, Meier PJ. The superfamily of organic anion transporting polypeptides. *Biochim Biophys Acta* 2003;1609:1–18.

290. Haila S, et al. SLC26A2 (diastrophic dysplasia sulfate transporter) is expressed in developing and mature cartilage but also in other tissues and cell types. *J Histochem Cytochem* 2001; 49:973–982.

291. Halestrap AP, Price NT. The proton-linked monocarboxylate transporter (MCT) family: structure, function and regulation. *Biochem J* 1999;343:281–299.

292. Hall RA, et al. The beta2-adrenergic receptor interacts with the Na^+/H+-exchanger regulatory factor to control Na^+/H+ exchange. *Nature* 1998;392:626–630.

293. Hamm LL. Renal handling of citrate. *Kidney Int* 1990;38:728–735.

294. Handler JS, Kwon HM. Regulation of renal cell organic osmolyte transport by tonicity. *Am J Physiol* 1993;265:C1449–C1455.

295. Handlogten ME, et al. Apical ammonia transport by the mouse inner medullary collecting duct cell (mIMCD-3). *Am J Physiol Renal Physiol* 2005;289:F347–F358.

296. Hara T, et al. Elucidation of the phenotypic change on the surface of Had-1 cell, a mutant cell line of mouse FM3A carcinoma cells selected by resistance to Newcastle disease virus infection. *J Biochem (Tokyo)* 1989;106:236–247.

297. Hartman KR, Barker JA. Microcytic anemia with iron malabsorption: an inherited disorder of iron metabolism. *Am J Hematol* 1996;51: 269–275.

298. Hasannejad H, et al. Human organic cation transporter 3 mediates the transport of antiarrhythmic drugs. *Eur J Pharmacol* 2004;499:45–51.

299. Hastbacka J, et al. The diastrophic dysplasia gene encodes a novel sulfate transporter: positional cloning by fine-structure linkage disequilibrium mapping. *Cell* 1994;78:1073–1087.

300. Hatanaka T, et al. Evidence for the transport of neutral as well as cationic amino acids by ATA3, a novel and liver-specific subtype of amino acid transport system A. *Biochim Biophys Acta* 2001;1510:10–17.

301. Hattenhauer O, et al. Regulation of small intestinal Na-P(i) type IIb cotransporter by dietary phosphate intake. *Am J Physiol* 1999;277:G756–G762.

302. Havelaar AC, et al. Purification of the lysosomal sialic acid transporter. Functional characteristics of a monocarboxylate transporter. *J Biol Chem* 1998;273:34568–34574.

303. Hebert SC, Culpepper RM, Andreoli TE. NaCl transport in mouse medullary thick ascending limbs. I. Functional nephron heterogeneity and ADH-stimulated NaCl cotransport. *Am J Physiol* 1981;241:F412–F431.

304. Hebert SC, Culpepper RM, Andreoli TE. NaCl transport in mouse medullary thick ascending limbs. II. ADH enhancement of transcellular NaCl cotransport; origin of transepithelial voltage. *Am J Physiol* 1981;241:F432–F442.

305. Hediger MA. Glutamate transporters in kidney and brain. *Am J Physiol* 1999;277: F487–F492.

306. Hediger MA. Kidney function: gateway to a long life? *Nature* 2002;417:393, 395.

307. Hediger MA, et al. Expression cloning and cDNA sequencing of the Na^+/glucose cotransporter. *Nature* 1987;330:379–381.

308. Hediger MA, Rhoads DB. Molecular physiology of sodium-glucose cotransporters. *Physiol Rev* 1994;74:993–1026.

309. Hediger MA, Welbourne TC. Introduction: glutamate transport, metabolism, and physiological responses. *Am J Physiol* 1999;277:F477–F480.

310. Heisterkamp N, et al. Localization of the human mitochondrial citrate transporter protein gene to chromosome 22Q11 in the DiGeorge syndrome critical region. *Genomics* 1995; 29:451–456.

311. Hershko C, Link G, Cabantchik I. Pathophysiology of iron overload. *Ann N Y Acad Sci* 1998;850:1191–1201.

312. Hewett D, et al. Identification of a psoriasis susceptibility candidate gene by linkage disequilibrium mapping with a localized single nucleotide polymorphism map. *Genomics* 2002;79:305–314.

313. Hiki K, et al. Cloning, characterization, and chromosomal location of a novel human K+-Cl- cotransporter. *J Biol Chem* 1999;274:10661–10667.

314. Hiraiwa H, et al. Inactivation of the glucose 6-phosphate transporter causes glycogen storage disease type 1b. *J Biol Chem* 1999;274:5532–5536.

315. Hirsch D, Stahl A, Lodish HF. A family of fatty acid transporters conserved from mycobacterium to man. *Proc Natl Acad Sci U S A* 1998;95:8625–8629.

316. Hirsch EC. Biochemistry of Parkinson's disease with special reference to the dopaminergic systems. *Mol Neurobiol* 1994;9:135–142.

317. Hirschberg CB. Golgi nucleotide sugar transport and leukocyte adhesion deficiency II. *J Clin Invest* 2001;108:3–6.

318. Hitomi K, Tsukagoshi N. cDNA sequence for rkST1, a novel member of the sodium ion-dependent glucose cotransporter family. *Biochim Biophys Acta* 1994;1190:469–472.

319. Ho LH, et al. Labile zinc and zinc transporter ZnT4 in mast cell granules: role in regulation of caspase activation and NF-kappaB translocation. *J Immunol* 2004;172:7750–7760.

320. Hoag HM, et al. Effects of Npt2 gene ablation and low-phosphate diet on renal Na(+)/phosphate cotransport and cotransporter gene expression. *J Clin Invest* 1999;104:679–686.

321. Hoffman BJ, Mezey E, Brownstein MJ. Cloning of a serotonin transporter affected by antidepressants. *Science* 1991;254:579–580.

322. Hoglund P, et al. Mutations of the Down-regulated in adenoma (DRA) gene cause congenital chloride diarrhoea. *Nat Genet* 1996; 14:316–319.

323. Hoogland G, et al. Alternative splicing of glutamate transporter EAAT2 RNA in neocortex and hippocampus of temporal lobe epilepsy patients. *Epilepsy Res* 2004;59:75–82.

324. Hosokawa H, et al. Cloning and characterization of a brain-specific cationic amino acid transporter. *J Biol Chem* 1997;272:8717–8722.

325. Hosoyamada M, et al. Molecular cloning and functional expression of a multispecific organic anion transporter from human kidney. *Am J Physiol* 1999;276:F122–F128.

326. Houldsworth J, Attardi G. Two distinct genes for ADP/ATP translocase are expressed at the mRNA level in adult human liver. *Proc Natl Acad Sci U S A* 85:377–381.

327. Howard HC, et al. The K-Cl cotransporter KCC3 is mutant in a severe peripheral neuropathy associated with agenesis of the corpus callosum. *Nat Genet* 2002;32:384–392.

328. Hu MC, et al. Dopamine acutely stimulates Na^+/H+ exchanger (NHE3) endocytosis via clathrin-coated vesicles: dependence on protein kinase A-mediated NHE3 phosphorylation. *J Biol Chem* 2001;276:26906–26915.

329. Huang L, Gitschier J. A novel gene involved in zinc transport is deficient in the lethal milk mouse. *Nat Genet* 1997;17:292–297.

330. Huang L, et al. The ZIP7 gene (Slc39a7) encodes a zinc transporter involved in zinc homeostasis of the Golgi apparatus. *J Biol Chem* 2005;280:15456–15463.

331. Huang QQ, et al. Functional expression of Na(+)-dependent nucleoside transport systems of rat intestine in isolated oocytes of Xenopus laevis. Demonstration that rat jejunum expresses the purine-selective system N1 (cif) and a second, novel system N3 having broad specificity for purine and pyrimidine nucleosides. *J Biol Chem* 1993;268: 20613–20619.

332. Huang QQ, et al. Cloning and functional expression of a complementary DNA encoding a mammalian nucleoside transport protein. *J Biol Chem* 1994;269:17757–17760.

333. Huang W, et al. Transport of N-acetylaspartate by the Na(+)-dependent high-affinity dicarboxylate transporter NaDC3 and its relevance to the expression of the transporter in the brain. *J Pharmacol Exp Ther* 2000;295:392–403.

334. Hubner CA, et al. Disruption of KCC2 reveals an essential role of K-Cl cotransport already in early synaptic inhibition. *Neuron* 2001;30:515–524.

335. Hyde R Peyrollier K, Hundal HS. Insulin promotes the cell surface recruitment of the SAT2/ATA2 system A amino acid transporter from an endosomal compartment in skeletal muscle cells. *J Biol Chem* 2002;277:13628–13634.

336. Hyde RJ, et al. The ENT family of eukaryote nucleoside and nucleobase transporters: recent advances in the investigation of structure/function relationships and the identification of novel isoforms. *Mol Membr Biol* 2001;18:53–63.

337. Iacobazzi V, Lauria G, Palmieri F. Organization and sequence of the human gene for the mitochondrial citrate transport protein. *DNA Seq* 1997;7:127–139.

338. Iacobazzi V, et al. Sequences of the human and bovine genes for the mitochondrial 2-oxoglutarate carrier. *DNA Seq* 1992;3:79–88.

339. Ibberson M, Uldry M, Thorens B. GLUTX1, a novel mammalian glucose transporter expressed in the central nervous system and insulin-sensitive tissues. *J Biol Chem* 2000;275:4607–4612.

340. Igarashi T, et al. Mutations in SLC4A4 cause permanent isolated proximal renal tubular acidosis with ocular abnormalities. *Nat Genet* 1999;23:264–266.

341. Igarashi T, et al. Novel nonsense mutation in the Na^+/HCO_3^- cotransporter gene (*SLC4A4*) in a patient with permanent isolated proximal renal tubular acidosis and bilateral glaucoma. *J Am Soc Nephrol* 2001;12:713–718.

342. Ihara K, et al. Quantitative analysis of glucose-6-phosphate translocase gene expression in various human tissues and haematopoietic progenitor cells. *J Inherit Metab Dis* 2000;23: 583–592.

343. Inatomi J, et al. Mutational and functional analysis of SLC4A4 in a patient with proximal renal tubular acidosis. *Pflugers Arch* 2004;448:438–444.

344. Indiveri C, et al. The mitochondrial carnitine carrier protein: cDNA cloning, primary structure and comparison with other mitochondrial transport proteins. *Biochemistry J* 997;321:713–719.

345. Inoue K, et al. Osteopenia and male-specific sudden cardiac death in mice lacking a zinc transporter gene, Znt5. *Hum Mol Genet* 2005;11:1775–1784.

346. Inoue K, Zhuang L, Ganapathy V. Ganapathy. Human Na^+-coupled citrate transporter: primary structure, genomic organization, and transport function. *Biochem Biophys Res Commun* 2002; 299:465–471.

347. Inoue K, et al. Structure, function, and expression pattern of a novel sodium-coupled citrate transporter (NaCT) cloned from mammalian brain. *J Biol Chem* 2002;277:39469–39476.

348. Ishida N, et al. Functional expression of human golgi CMP-sialic acid transporter in the Golgi complex of a transporter-deficient Chinese hamster ovary cell mutant. *J Biochem (Tokyo)* 1998;124:171–178.

349. Ishida N, et al. Molecular cloning and characterization of a novel isoform of the human UDP-galactose transporter, and of related complementary DNAs belonging to the nucleotide-sugar transporter gene family. *J Biochem (Tokyo)* 1996;120:1074–1078.

350. Ishida N, et al. Molecular cloning and functional expression of the human Golgi UDP-N-acetylglucosamine transporter. *J Biochem (Tokyo)* 1999;126:68–77.

351. Ismair MG, et al. Hepatic uptake of cholecystokinin octapeptide by organic anion-transporting polypeptides OATP4 and OATP8 of rat and human liver. *Gastroenterology* 2001;121:1185–1190.

352. Iwamoto T, et al. Salt-sensitive hypertension is triggered by Ca2+ entry via Na^+/Ca2+ exchanger type-1 in vascular smooth muscle. *Nat Med* 2004;10:1193–1199.

353. Iwamoto T, Shigekawa M. Differential inhibition of Na^+/Ca2+ exchanger isoforms by divalent cations and isothiourea derivative. *Am J Physiol* 1998;275:C423–C430.

354. Jacob P, et al. Down-regulated in adenoma mediates apical Cl-/HCO_3^- exchange in rabbit, rat, and human duodenum. *Gastroenterology* 2002;122:709–724.

355. Janne J, Alhonen L, Leinonen P. Polyamines: from molecular biology to clinical applications. *Ann Med* 1991;23:241–259.
356. Jarolim P, et al. Mutations of conserved arginines in the membrane domain of erythroid band 3 lead to a decrease in membrane-associated band 3 and to the phenotype of hereditary spherocytosis. *Blood* 1995;85:634–640.
357. Jarolim P, et al. Autosomal dominant distal renal tubular acidosis is associated in three families with heterozygosity for the R589H mutation in the AE1 (band 3) Cl^-/HCO_3^- exchanger. *J Biol Chem* 1998;273:6380–6388.
358. Jensen LJ, et al. Localization of sodium bicarbonate co-transporter (NBC) protein and mRNA in rat epididymis. *Biol Reprod* 1999;60:573–579.
359. Jeon D, et al. Enhanced learning and memory in mice lacking Na^+/Ca2+ exchanger 2. *Neuron* 2003;38:965–976.
360. Jiang Z, et al. Specificity of anion exchange mediated by mouse Slc26a6. *J Biol Chem* 2002;277:33963–33967.
361. Jobe A. An in vivo comparison of acetate and palmitate as precursors of surfactant phosphatidylcholine. *Biochim Biophys Acta* 1979;572:404–412.
362. Jonker JW, et al. Reduced hepatic uptake and intestinal excretion of organic cations in mice with a targeted disruption of the organic cation transporter 1 (Oct1 [Slc22a1]) gene. *Mol Cell Biol* 2001; 21:5471–5477.
363. Jonker JW, et al. Deficiency in the organic cation transporters 1 and 2 (Oct1/Oct2 [Slc22a1/Slc22a2]) in mice abolishes renal secretion of organic cations. *Mol Cell Biol* 2003;23: 7902–7908.
364. Joost HG, Thorens B. The extended GLUT-family of sugar/polyol transport facilitators: nomenclature, sequence characteristics, and potential function of its novel members (review). *Mol Membr Biol* 2001;18:247–256.
365. Jordens EZ, et al. Adenine nucleotide translocator 1 deficiency associated with Sengers syndrome. *Ann Neurol* 2002;52:95–99.
366. Juel C, Halestrap AP. Lactate transport in skeletal muscle—role and regulation of the monocarboxylate transporter. *J Physiol* 1999;517:633–642.
367. Jung D, et al. Character ization of the human OATP-C (SLC21A6) gene promoter and regulation of liver-specific OATP genes by hepatocyte nuclear factor 1 alpha. *J Biol Chem* 2001;276:37206–37214.
368. Jung D, et al. Human organic anion transporting polypeptide 8 promoter is transactivated by the farnesoid X receptor/bile acid receptor. *Gastroenterology* 2002;122:1954–1966.
369. Kaelbling M, et al. Localization of the human gene allowing infection by gibbon ape leukemia virus to human chromosome region 2q11-q14 and to the homologous region on mouse chromosome 2. *J Virol* 1991;65:1743–1747.
370. Kanai Y, et al. Neuronal high-affinity glutamate transport in the rat central nervous system. *Neuroreport* 1995;6:2357–2362.
371. Kanai Y, Hediger MA. Primary structure and functional characterization of a high-affinity glutamate transporter. *Nature* 1992;360:467–471.
372. Kanai Y, et al. The human kidney low affinity Na^+/glucose cotransporter SGLT2. Delineation of the major renal reabsorptive mechanism for D- glucose. *J Clin Invest* 1994;93:397–404.
373. Kanai Y, et al. Electrogenic properties of the epithelial and neuronal high affinity glutamate transporter. *J Biol Chem* 1995;270:16561–16568.
374. Kanai Y, et al. Expression cloning and characterization of a transporter for large neutral amino acids activated by the heavy chain of 4F2 antigen (CD98). *J Biol Chem* 1998;273:23629–23632.
375. Kanai Y, et al. Expression of mRNA (D2) encoding a protein involved in amino acid transport in S3 proximal tubule. *Am J Physiol* 1992;263:F1087–F1092.
376. Kanamori A, et al. Expression cloning and characterization of a cDNA encoding a novel membrane protein required for the formation of O-acetylated ganglioside: a putative acetyl-CoA transporter. *Proc Natl Acad Sci U S A* 1997;94:2897–2902.
377. Kannagi R Carbohydrate-mediated cell adhesion involved in hematogenous metastasis of cancer. *Glycoconj J* 1997;14:577–584.
378. Kanner BI, Bendahan A. Binding order of substrates to the sodium and potassium ion coupled L- glutamic acid transporter from rat brain. *Biochemistry* 1982;21:6327–6330.
379. Kanner BI, Sharon I. Active transport of L-glutamate by membrane vesicles isolated from rat brain. *Biochemistry* 1978;17:3949–3953.
380. Kaplan MR, et al. Apical localization of the Na-K-Cl cotransporter, rBSC1, on rat thick ascending limbs. *Kidney Int* 1996;49:40–47.
381. Kapus A, et al. Functional characterization of three isoforms of the Na^+/H+ exchanger stably expressed in Chinese hamster ovary cells. ATP dependence, osmotic sensitivity, and role in cell proliferation. *J Biol Chem* 1994;269:23544–23552.
382. Karakashian A, et al. Cloning and characterization of two new isoforms of the rat kidney urea transporter: UT-A3 and UT-A4. *J Am Soc Nephrol* 1999;10:230–237.
383. Karbach U, et al. Localization of organic cation transporters OCT1 and OCT2 in rat kidney. *Am J Physiol Renal Physiol* 2000;279:679–687.
384. Karinch AM, et al. Regulation of expression of the SN1 transporter during renal adaptation to chronic metabolic acidosis in rats. *Am J Physiol Renal Physiol* 2002;283:F1011–F1019.
385. Karniski L P, et al. Immunolocalization of sat-1 sulfate/oxalate/bicarbonate anion exchanger in the rat kidney. *Am J Physiol* 1999;275:F79–F87.
386. Katai K, et al. Regulation of intestinal Na^+-dependent phosphate co-transporters by a low-phosphate diet and 1,25-dihydroxyvitamin D3. *Biochem J* 1999;343:705–7012.
387. Kaukonen J, et al. Role of adenine nucleotide translocator 1 in mtDNA maintenance. *Science* 2000;289:782–785.
388. Kavanaugh MP, et al. Cell-surface receptors for gibbon ape leukemia virus and amphotropic murine retrovirus are inducible sodium-dependent phosphate symporters. *Proc Natl Acad Sci U S A* 1994; 91:7071–7075.
389. Kavanaugh MP, et al. Control of cationic amino acid transport and retroviral receptor functions in a membrane protein family. *J Biol Chem* 1994;269:15445–15450.
390. Kayano T, et al. Human facilitative glucose transporters. Isolation, functional characterization, and gene localization of cDNAs encoding an isoform (GLUT5) expressed in small intestine, kidney, muscle, and adipose tissue and an unusual glucose transporter pseudogene-like sequence (GLUT6). *J Cell Biol* 1990;265:13276–13282.
391. Kekuda R, et al. Cloning of the sodium-dependent, broad-scope, neutral amino acid transporter Bo from a human placental choriocarcinoma cell line. *J Biol Chem* 1996;271:18657–8661.
392. Kelleher SL B Lonnerdal. Zip3 plays a major role in zinc uptake into mammary epithelial cells and is regulated by prolactin. *Am J Physiol Cell Physiol* 2005;288:C1042–C1047.
393. Kerb R, et al. Identification of genetic variations of the human organic cation transporter hOCT1 and their functional consequences. *Pharmacogenetics* 2002;12:591–595.
394. Khadilkar A P Iannuzzi, and J. Orlowski. Identification of sites in the second exomembrane loop and ninth transmembrane helix of the mammalian Na^+/H+ exchanger important for drug recognition and cation translocation. *J Biol Chem* 2001;276:43792–43800.
395. Kilberg MS, Handlogten ME, Christensen HN. Characteristics of an amino acid transport system in rat liver for glutamine, asparagine, histidine, and closely related analogs. *J Biol Chem* 1980;255:4011–4019.
396. Kilty JE, Lorang D, Amara SG. Cloning and expression of a cocaine-sensitive rat dopamine transporter. *Science* 1991;254:578–579.
397. Kim DK, et al. Expression cloning of a Na^+-independent aromatic amino acid transporter with structural similarity to H+/monocarboxylate transporters. *J Biol Chem* 2001;276:17221–17228.
398. Kim JW, et al. Transport of cationic amino acids by the mouse ecotropic retrovirus receptor. *Nature* 1991;352:725–728.
399. Kim KH, et al. SLC26A7 is a Cl- channel regulated by intracellular pH. *J Biol Chem* 2005;280:6463–670.
400. Kim KM, et al. Cloning of the human glycine transporter type 1: molecular and pharmacological characterization of novel isoform variants and chromosomal localization of the gene in the human and mouse genomes. *Mol Pharmacol* 1994;45:608–617.
401. Kimura M, et al. Physiological and molecular characterization of the Na^+/Ca2+ exchanger in human platelets. *Am J Physiol* 1999;277:H911–H917.
402. Kirk P, et al. CD147 is tightly associated with lactate transporters MCT1 and MCT4 and facilitates their cell surface expression. *EMBO J* 2000;19:3896–3904.
403. Kirschke CP, Huang L. ZnT7, a novel mammalian zinc transporter, accumulates zinc in the Golgi apparatus. *J Biol Chem* 2003;278:4096–4102.
404. Kitaichi K, et al. Behavioral changes following antisense oligonucleotide-induced reduction of organic cation transporter-3 in mice. *Neurosci Lett* 2005;382:195–200.
405. Kittanakom S, et al. Trafficking defects of a novel autosomal recessive distal renal tubular acidosis mutant (S773P) of the human kidney anion exchanger (kAE1). *J Biol Chem* 2004;279:40960–40971.
406. Klein JD, et al. UT-A urea transporter protein expressed in liver: upregulation by uremia. *J Am Soc Nephrol* 1999;10:2076–2083.
407. Knauf F, et al. Identification of a chloride-formate exchanger expressed on the brush border membrane of renal proximal tubule cells. *Proc Natl Acad Sci U S A* 2001;98:9425–9430.
408. Knudsen J. Acyl-CoA-binding protein (ACBP) and its relation to fatty acid-binding protein (FABP): an overview. *Mol Cell Biochem* 1990;98:217–223.
409. Knutter I, et al. H+-peptide cotransport in the human bile duct epithelium cell line SK-ChA-1. *Am J Physiol Gastrointest Liver Physiol* 2002;283:G222–G229.
410. Ko SB, et al. A molecular mechanism for aberrant CFTR-dependent HCO(3)(-) transport in cystic fibrosis. *EMBO J* 2002;21:5662–5672.
411. Kobayashi Y, et al. Transport mechanism and substrate specificity of human organic anion transporter 2 (hOat2 [SLC22A7]). *J Pharm Pharmacol* 2005;57:573–578.
412. Koepsell H, et al. Polyspecific cation transporters in the proximal tubule. *Nephrol Dial Transplant* 2000;15(Suppl 6):3–4.
413. Koepsell H, Schmitt BM, Gorboulev V. Organic cation transporters. *Rev Physiol Biochem Pharmacol* 2003;150:36–90.
414. Kojima R, et al. Immunolocalization of multispecific organic anion transporters, OAT1, OAT2, and OAT3, in rat kidney. *J Am Soc Nephrol* 2002;13:848–857.
415. Kopito RR, et al. Regulation of intracellular pH by a neuronal homolog of the erythrocyte anion exchanger. *Cell* 1989;59:927–937.
416. Kopito RR, Lodish HF. Primary structure and transmembrane orientation of the murine anion exchange protein. *Nature* 1985;316:234–238.
417. Kotaria R, et al. Oligomeric state of wild-type and cysteine-less yeast mitochondrial citrate transport proteins. *J Bioenerg Biomembr* 1999;31:543–549.
418. Kottra G A Stamfort, and H. Daniel. PEPT1 as a paradigm for membrane carriers that mediate electrogenic bidirectional transport of anionic, cationic, and neutral substrates. *J Biol Chem* 2002;277:32683–32691.
419. Kraev A, et al. Molecular cloning of a third member of the potassium-dependent sodiumcalcium exchanger gene family, NCKX3. *J Biol Chem* 2001;276:23161–23172.
420. Kramer HM, Curhan G. The association between gout and nephrolithiasis: the National Health and Nutrition Examination Survey III, 1988–1994. *Am J Kidney Dis* 2002;40:37–42.
421. Kristufek D, et al. Organic cation transporter mRNA and function in the rat superior cervical ganglion. *J Physiol* 2002;543:117–134.
422. Ku D H, et al. The human fibroblast adenine nucleotide translocator gene. Molecular cloning and sequence. *J Biol Chem* 1990;265:16060–16063.
423. Deleted in proof.
424. Kuhn NJ, White A. Evidence for specific transport of uridine diphosphate galactose across the Golgi membrane of rat mammary gland. *Biochem J* 1976;154:243–244.
425. Kullak-Ublick GA, et al. Molecular and functional characterization of an organic anion transporting polypeptide cloned from human liver. *Gastroenterology* 1995;109:1274–1282.
426. Kullak-Ublick GA, et al. Organic anion-transporting polypeptide B (OATP-B) and its functional comparison with three other OATPs of human liver. *Gastroenterology* 2001;120:525–533.
427. Kumamoto K, et al. Increased expression of UDP-galactose transporter messenger RNA in human colon cancer tissues and its implication in synthesis of Thomsen–Friedenreich antigen and sialyl Lewis A/X determinants. *Cancer Res* 2001;61:4620–4627.
428. Kumar R. New insights into phosphate homeostasis: fibroblast growth factor 23 and frizzled-related protein-4 are phosphaturic factors derived from tumors associated with osteomalacia. *Curr Opin Nephrol Hypertens* 2002;11:547–553.
429. Kunchaparty S, et al. Defective processing and expression of thiazide-sensitive Na-Cl co-transporter as a cause of Gitelman's syndrome. *Am J Physiol* 1999;277:F643–F649.

430. Kuo YM, et al. The copper transporter CTR1 provides an essential function in mammalian embryonic development. *Proc Natl Acad Sci U S A* 2001;98:6836–6841.
431. Kury S, et al. Identification of SLC39A4, a gene involved in acrodermatitis enteropathica. *Nat Genet* 2002;31:239–240.
432. Kwon HM, et al. Cloning of the cDNa for a Na^+/myo-inositol cotransporter, a hypertonicity stress protein. *J Biol Chem* 1992; 267:6297–6301.
433. Kwon TH, et al. Chronic metabolic acidosis upregulates rat kidney Na-HCO cotransporters NBCn1 and NBC3 but not NBC1. *Am J Physiol Renal Physiol* 2002;282:F341–F351.
434. Labay V, et al. Mutations in SLC19A2 cause thiamine-responsive megaloblastic anaemia associated with diabetes mellitus and deafness. *Nat Genet* 1999;22:300–304.
435. Laghmani K, et al. Chronic metabolic acidosis enhances NHE-3 protein abundance and transport activity in the rat thick ascending limb by increasing NHE-3 mRNA. *J Clin Invest* 1997;99:24–30.
436. Lahjouji K, et al. L-Carnitine transport in human placental brush-border membranes is mediated by the sodium-dependent organic cation transporter OCTN2. *Am J Physiol Cell Physiol* 2004;287:C263–C269.
437. Lai Y, Bakken AH, Unadkat JD. Simultaneous expression of hCNT1-CFP and hENT1-YFP in Madin-Darby canine kidney cells. Localization and vectorial transport studies. *J Biol Chem* 2002;277:37711–37717.
438. Lambert DW, et al. Molecular changes in the expression of human colonic nutrient transporters during the transition from normality to malignancy. *Br J Cancer* 2002;86:1262–1269.
439. Landowski CP, et al. Targeted delivery to PEPT1-overexpressing cells: acidic, basic, and secondary floxuridine amino acid ester prodrugs. *Mol Cancer Ther* 2005;4:659–667.
440. Lang F, et al. Functional significance of cell volume regulatory mechanisms. *Physiol Rev* 1998;78:247–306.
441. Larson TJ, Schumacher G, Boos W. Identification of the glpT-encoded sn-glycerol-3-phosphate permease of Escherichia coli, an oligomeric integral membrane protein. *J Bacteriol* 1982;152:1008–1021.
442. Lasley RD, Mantzer RM Jr. Protective effects of adenosine in the reversibly injured heart. *Ann Thorac Surg* 1995;60:843–846.
443. Lauf PK. Kinetic comparison of ouabain-resistant K:Cl fluxes (K:Cl [Co]-transport) stimulated in sheep erythrocytes by membrane thiol oxidation and alkylation. *Mol Cell Biochem* 1988;82:97–106.
444. Lauf PK, Adragna NC. K-Cl cotransport: properties and molecular mechanism. *Cell Physiol Biochem* 2000;10:341–354.
445. Lauf PK, et al. Erythrocyte K-Cl cotransport: properties and regulation. *Am J Physiol* 1992;263:C917–C932.
446. Lauf PK, Theg BE. A chloride dependent K+ flux induced by N-ethylmaleimide in genetically low K+ sheep and goat erythrocytes. *Biochem Biophys Res Commun* 1980;92:1422–1428.
447. Lauf PK, et al. K-Cl co-transport: immunocytochemical and functional evidence for more than one KCC isoform in high K and low K sheep erythrocytes. *Comp Biochem Physiol A Mol Integr Physiol* 2001;130:499–509.
448. Lee A L, Beck D, Markovich D. The mouse sulfate anion transporter gene Sat1 (Slc26a1): cloning, tissue distribution, gene structure, functional characterization, and transcriptional regulation thyroid hormone. *DNA Cell Biol* 2003;22:19–31.
449. Lee J, et al. Biochemical characterization of the human copper transporter Ctr1. *J Biol Chem* 2002;277:4380–4387.
450. Lee J, Prohaska JR, Thiele DJ. Essential role for mammalian copper transporter Ctr1 in copper homeostasis and embryonic development. *Proc Natl Acad Sci U S A* 2001;98: 6842–6847.
451. Leheste JR, et al. Hypocalcemia and osteopathy in mice with kidney-specific megalin gene defect. *FASEB J* 2003;17:247–249.
452. Levy O, et al. Identification of a structural requirement for thyroid Na^+/I- symporter (NIS) function from analysis of a mutation that causes human congenital hypothyroidism. *FEBS Lett* 1998;429:36–40.
453. Li K, et al. A human muscle adenine nucleotide translocator gene has four exons, is located on chromosome 4, and is differentially expressed. *J Biol Chem* 1989;264:13998–4004.
454. Li L, et al. Identification of glutathione as a driving force and leukotriene C4 as a substrate for oatp1, the hepatic sinusoidal organic solute transporter. *J Biol Chem* 1998;273: 16184–16191.
455. Li L, Meier PJ, Ballatori N. Oatp2 mediates bidirectional organic solute transport: a role for intracellular glutathione. *Mol Pharmacol* 2000;58:335–340.
456. Li Q, et al. Cloning and functional characterization of the human GLUT7 isoform SLC2A7 from the small intestine. *Am J Physiol Gastrointest Liver Physiol* 2004;287:G236–G242.
457. Li XF, Kraev A, Lytton J. Molecular cloning of a fourth member of the potassium-dependent sodium-calcium exchanger gene family. *J Biol Chem* 2003;276:48410–48417.
458. Liberman MC, et al. Prestin is required for electromotility of the outer hair cell and for the cochlear amplifier. *Nature* 2002;419:300–304.
459. Lin CL, et al. Aberrant RNA processing in a neurodegenerative disease: the cause for absent EAAT2, a glutamate transporter, in amyotrophic lateral sclerosis. *Neuron* 1998;20:589–602.
460. Lin CS, Hackenberg H, Klingenberg EM. The uncoupling protein from brown adipose tissue mitochondria is a dimer. A hydrodynamic study. *FEBS Lett* 1980;113:304–306.
461. Lisinski I, et al. Targeting of GLUT6 (formerly GLUT9) and GLUT8 in rat adipose cells. *Biochem J* 2001;358:517–522.
462. Liu FY, Cogan MG. Angiotensin II stimulation of hydrogen ion secretion in the rat early proximal tubule. Modes of action, mechanism, and kinetics. *J Clin Invest* 1988;82:601–607.
463. Liu FY, Cogan MG. Angiotensin II stimulates early proximal bicarbonate absorption in the rat by decreasing cyclic adenosine monophosphate. *J Clin Invest* 1989;84:83–91.
464. Liu QR, et al. Cloning and expression of a spinal cord- and brain-specific glycine transporter with novel structural features. *J Biol Chem* 1993;268:22802–22808.
465. Liu QR, et al. Cloning and expression of a glycine transporter from mouse brain. *FEBS Lett* 1992;305:110–114.
466. Liu W, et al. Molecular cloning of PEPT 2, a new member of the H+/peptide cotransporter family, from human kidney. *Biochim Biophys Acta* 1995;1235:461–466.
467. Liu Z, et al. Characterization of human RhCG and mouse Rhcg as novel nonerythroid Rh glycoprotein homologues predominantly expressed in kidney and testis. *J Biol Chem* 2000;275:25641–25651.
468. Liuzzi JP, et al. Responsive transporter genes within the murine intestinal-pancreatic axis form a basis of zinc homeostasis. *Proc Natl Acad Sci U S A* 2004;101:14355–14360.
469. Liuzzi JP, et al. Interleukin-6 regulates the zinc transporter Zip14 in liver and contributes to the hypozincemia of the acute-phase response. *Proc Natl Acad Sci U S A* 2005;102:6843–6848.
470. Loffing J, Kaissling B. Sodium and calcium transport pathways along the mammalian distal nephron: from rabbit to human. *Am J Physiol Renal Physiol* 2003;284:F628–F643.
471. Loffing J, et al. Distribution of transcellular calcium and sodium transport pathways along mouse distal nephron. *Am J Physiol Renal Physiol* 2001;281:F1021–F1027.
472. Lohi H, et al. Mapping of five new putative anion transporter genes in human and characterization of SLC26A6, a candidate gene for pancreatic anion exchanger. *Genomics* 2000;70:102–112.
473. Lohi H, et al. Functional characterization of three novel tissue-specific anion exchangers SLC26A7, -A8, and -A9. *J Biol Chem* 2002;277:14246–14254.
474. Loo DD, et al. Role of Cl- in electrogenic Na^+-coupled cotransporters GAT1 and SGLT1. *J Biol Chem* 2000;275:37414–37422.
475. Lopez-Nieto CE, et al. Molecular cloning and characterization of NKT, a gene product related to the organic cation transporter family that is almost exclusively expressed in the kidney. *J Biol Chem* 1997;272:6471–6478.
476. Lorenz JN, et al. Micropuncture analysis of single-nephron function in NHE3-deficient mice. *Am J Physiol* 1999;277:F447–F453.
477. Lostao MP, et al. Electrogenic uptake of nucleosides and nucleoside-derived drugs by the human nucleoside transporter 1 (hCNT1) expressed in Xenopus laevis oocytes. *FEBS Lett* 2000;481:137–140.
478. Lu K, et al. A missense mutation of mouse OCTN2, a sodium-dependent carnitine cotransporter, in the juvenile visceral steatosis mouse. *Biochem Biophys Res Commun* 1998;252:590–594.
479. Lu R, et al. Cloning, in vitro expression, and tissue distribution of a human prostaglandin transporter cDNA(hPGT). *J Clin Invest* 1996;98:1142–1149.
480. Lubke T, et al. Complementation cloning identifies CDG-IIc, a new type of congenital disorders of glycosylation, as a GDP-fucose transporter deficiency. *Nat Genet* 2001;28:73–76.
481. Luhn K, et al. The gene defective in leukocyte adhesion deficiency II encodes a putative GDP-fucose transporter. *Nat Genet* 2001;28:69–72.
482. Lytton J, et al. K+-dependent Na^+/Ca2+ exchangers in the brain. *Ann N Y Acad Sci* 2002;976:382–393.
483. Mabjeesh NJ, et al. Neuronal and glial gamma-aminobutyric acid+ transporters are distinct proteins. *FEBS Lett* 1992;299:99–102.
484. Macheda ML, et al. Expression and localisation of GLUT1 and GLUT12 glucose transporters in the pregnant and lactating rat mammary gland. *Cell Tissue Res* 2003;311:91–97.
485. Mackenzie B, et al. The human intestinal H+/oligopeptide cotransporter hPEPT1 transports differently-charged dipeptides with identical electrogenic properties. *Biochim Biophys Acta* 1996;1284:125–128.
486. Mackenzie B, et al. SAAT1 is a low affinity Na^+/glucose cotransporter and not an amino acid transporter. A reinterpretation. *J Biol Chem* 1994;269:22488–22491.
487. Mackenzie B, et al. Functional properties and cellular distribution of the system A glutamine transporter SNAT1 support specialized roles in central neurons. *J Biol Chem* 2003;278: 23720–23730.
488. Mackey JR, et al. Gemcitabine transport in xenopus oocytes expressing recombinant plasma membrane mammalian nucleoside transporters. *J Natl Cancer Inst* 1991;91:1876–1881.
489. Maechler P, Wollheim CB. Mitochondrial signals in glucose-stimulated insulin secretion in the beta cell. *J Physiol* 2000;529:49–56.
490. Magagnin S, et al. Expression cloning of human and rat renal cortex Na/Pi cotransport. *Proc Natl Acad Sci U S A* 1993;90:5979–5983.
491. Mahon MJ, et al. Na(+)/H(+) exchanger regulatory factor 2 directs parathyroid hormone 1 receptor signalling. *Nature* 2002;417:858–861.
492. Majima E, et al. Translocation of loops regulates transport activity of mitochondrial ADP/ATP carrier deduced from formation of a specific intermolecular disulfide bridge catalyzed by copper-o-phenanthroline. *J Biol Chem* 1995;270:29548–29554.
493. Man MZ, et al. Regulation of the murine adipocyte fatty acid transporter gene by insulin. *Mol Endocrinol* 1996;10:1021–1028.
494. Mancini GM, et al. Functional reconstitution of the lysosomal sialic acid carrier into proteoliposomes. *Proc Natl Acad Sci U S A* 1992;89:6609–6613.
495. Mancini GM, et al. Characterization of a proton-driven carrier for sialic acid in the lysosomal membrane. Evidence for a group-specific transport system for acidic monosaccharides. *J Biol Chem* 1989;264:15247–15254.
496. Mangravite LM, et al. Localization of GFP-tagged concentrative nucleoside transporters in a renal polarized epithelial cell line. *Am J Physiol Renal Physiol* 2001;280:F879–F885.
497. Mangravite L M. G Xiao, and K. M. Giacomini. Localization of human equilibrative nucleoside transporters, hENT1 and hENT2, in renal epithelial cells. *Am J Physiol Renal Physiol* 2003;284:F902–F910.
498. Mantych GJ, James DE, Devaskar SU. Jejunal/kidney glucose transporter isoform (Glut-5) is expressed in the human blood–brain barrier. *Endocrinology* 1993;132:35–40.
499. Marini AM, et al. The human Rhesus-associated RhAG protein and a kidney homologue promote ammonium transport in yeast. *Nat Genet* 2000;26:341–344.
500. Marini AM, et al. The Rh (rhesus) blood group polypeptides are related to NH4+ transporters. *Trends Biochem Sci* 1997;22:460–461.
501. Markovich D. Physiological roles and regulation of mammalian sulfate transporters. *Physiol Rev* 2001;81:1499–1533.
502. Markovich D, et al. Expression cloning of rat renal $Na^+/SO_4(^{2-})$ cotransport. *Proc Natl Acad Sci U S A* 1993;90:8073–8077.
503. Marlier LN, et al. Regional distribution in the rat central nervous system of a mRNA encoding a portion of the cardiac sodium/calcium exchanger isolated from cerebellar granule neurons. *Brain Res Mol Brain Res* 1993;20:21–39.

504. Martin G, et al. Coordinate regulation of the expression of the fatty acid transport protein and acyl-CoA synthetase genes by PPARalpha and PPARgamma activators. *J Biol Chem* 1997;272:28210–28217.
505. Martin MG, et al. Defects in Na^+/glucose cotransporter (SGLT1) trafficking and function cause glucose-galactose malabsorption. *Nat Genet* 1996;12:216–220.
506. Masliah E, et al. Deficient glutamate transport is associated with neurodegeneration in Alzheimer's disease. *Ann Neurol* 1996;40:759–766.
507. Mastroberardino L, et al. Amino-acid transport by heterodimers of 4F2hc/CD98 and members of a permease family. *Nature* 1998;395:288–291.
508. Mastroianni N, et al. Molecular cloning, expression pattern, and chromosomal localization of the human Na-Cl thiazide-sensitive cotransporter (SLC12A3). *Genomics* 1996;35: 486–493.
509. Matsuo H, et al. Identification of a novel Na^+-independent acidic amino acid transporter with structural similarity to the member of a heterodimeric amino acid transporter family associated with unknown heavy chains. *J Biol Chem* 2002;277:21017–21026.
510. Matsuoka S, et al. Regulation of cardiac Na(+)-Ca2+ exchanger by the endogenous XIP region. *J Gen Physiol* 1997;109:273–286.
511. Maudsley S, et al. Platelet-derived growth factor receptor association with Na(+)/H(+) exchanger regulatory factor potentiates receptor activity. *Mol Cell Biol* 2000;20:8352–8363.
512. Mayerhofer A, et al. Gamma-aminobutyric acid (GABA): a para- and/or autocrine hormone in the pituitary. *FASEB J* 2001;15:1089–1091.
513. Mazzali M, et al. Elevated uric acid increases blood pressure in the rat by a novel crystal-independent mechanism. *Hypertension* 2001;38:1101–1106.
514. Mazzali M, et al. Hyperuricemia induces a primary renal arteriolopathy in rats by a blood pressure-independent mechanism. *Am J Physiol Renal Physiol* 2002;282:991–997.
515. McIntire SL, et al. Identification and characterization of the vesicular GABA transporter. *Nature* 1997;389:870–876.
516. McKie AT, et al. A novel duodenal iron-regulated transporter, IREG1, implicated in the basolateral transfer of iron to the circulation. *Mol Cell* 2000;5:299–309.
517. McMahon RJ, Cousins RJ. Regulation of the zinc transporter ZnT-1 by dietary zinc. *Proc Natl Acad Sci U S A* 1998;95:4841–4846.
518. McVie-Wylie AJ, Lamson DR, Chen YT. Molecular cloning of a novel member of the GLUT family of transporters, SLC2a10 (GLUT10), localized on chromosome 20q13: a candidate gene for NIDDM susceptibility. *Genomics* 2001;72:113–117.
519. Medina JF, et al. Anion exchanger 2 is essential for spermiogenesis in mice. *Proc Natl Acad Sci U S A* 2003;100:15847–15852.
520. Meier C, et al. Activation of system L heterodimeric amino acid exchangers by intracellular substrates. *EMBO J* 2002;21:580–589.
521. Meinild A, et al. The human Na^+-glucose cotransporter is a molecular water pump. *J Physiol (Lond)* 1998;508:15–21.
522. Melvin JE, et al. Mouse down-regulated in adenoma (DRA) is an intestinal Cl(-)/HCO(3)(-) exchanger and is up-regulated in colon of mice lacking the NHE3 Na(+)/H(+) exchanger. *J Biol Chem* 1999;247:22855–22861.
523. Mercado A, et al. Functional comparison of the K+-Cl- cotransporters KCC1 and KCC4. *J Biol Chem* 2000;275:30326–30334.
524. Mercer JF, et al. Isolation of a partial candidate gene for Menkes disease by positional cloning. *Nat Genet* 1993;3:20–25.
525. Merlin D, et al. hPepT1-mediated epithelial transport of bacteria-derived chemotactic peptides enhances neutrophil–epithelial interactions. *J Clin Invest* 1998;102:2011–2018.
526. Michalski C, et al. A naturally occurring mutation in the SLC21A6 gene causing impaired membrane localization of the hepatocyte uptake transporter. *J Biol Chem* 2002;277: 43058–43063.
527. Miles R Neurobiology. A homeostatic switch. *Nature* 397:215–216.
528. Milon B, et al. Differential subcellular localization of hZip1 in adherent and non-adherent cells. *FEBS Lett* 2001;507:241–246.
529. Miura N, et al. Human UDP-galactose translocator: molecular cloning of a complementary DNA that complements the genetic defect of a mutant cell line deficient in UDP-galactose translocator. *J Biochem (Tokyo)* 1996;120:236–241.
530. Miyakawa H, et al. Cis- and trans-acting factors regulating transcription of the BGT1 gene in response to hypertonicity. *Am J Physiol* 1998;274:F753–F761.
531. Miyamoto K, et al. Secondary hyperparathyroidism and phosphate sensing in parathyroid glands. *J Med Invest* 2000;47:118–122.
532. Miyamoto K, et al. Relative contributions of Na^+-dependent phosphate co-transporters to phosphate transport in mouse kidney: RNase H-mediated hybrid depletion analysis. *Biochem J* 1997; 327:735–739.
533. Miyamoto K, et al. Regulation of PiT-1, a sodium-dependent phosphate co-transporter in rat parathyroid glands. *Nephrol Dial Transplant* 1999;(Suppl 1):73–75.
534. Miyamoto K, et al. Cloning and functional expression of a Na(+)-dependent phosphate co-transporter from human kidney: cDNA cloning and functional expression. *Biochem J* 1995; 305:81–85.
535. Miyauchi S, et al. Functional identification of SLC5A8, a tumor suppressor down-regulated in colon cancer, as a Na(+)-coupled transporter for short-chain fatty acids. *J Biol Chem* 2004;279:13293–13296.
536. Monroy A, et al. Characterization of the thiazide-sensitive Na(+)-Cl(-) cotransporter: a new model for ions and diuretics interaction. *Am J Physiol Renal Physiol* 2000;279: F161–F169.
537. Montosi G, et al. Autosomal-dominant hemochromatosis is associated with a mutation in the ferroportin (SLC11A3) gene. *J Clin Invest* 2001;108:619–623.
538. Mori K, et al. Kidney-specific expression of a novel mouse organic cation transporter-like protein. *FEBS Lett* 1997;417:371–374.
539. Mosckovitz R, et al. Characterization of the rat neutral and basic amino acid transporter utilizing anti-peptide antibodies. *Proc Natl Acad Sci U S A* 1993;90:4022–4026.
540. Moseley RH, et al. Downregulated in adenoma gene encodes a chloride transporter defective in congenital chloride diarrhea. *Am J Physiol* 1999;276:G185–G192.
541. Motojima K, et al. Expression of putative fatty acid transporter genes are regulated by peroxisome proliferator-activated receptor alpha and gamma activators in a tissue- and inducer-specific manner. *J Biol Chem* 1998;273:16710–16714.
542. Mount DB, et al. The electroneutral cation-chloride cotransporters. *J Exp Biol* 1998;201:2091–2102.
543. Mount DB, et al. Cloning and characterization of KCC3 and KCC4, new members of the cation-chloride cotransporter gene family. *J Biol Chem* 1999;274:16355–16362.
544. Mubagwa K, Mullane K, Flameng W. Role of adenosine in the heart and circulation. *Cardiovasc Res* 1996;32:797–813.
545. Mueckler M. Facilitative glucose transporters. *Eur J Biochem* 1994;219:713–725.
546. Mulero V, et al. Solute carrier 11a1 (Slc11a1; formerly Nramp1) regulates metabolism and release of iron acquired by phagocytic, but not transferrin-receptor- mediated, iron uptake. *Biochem J* 2002; 363:89–94.
547. Muraoka M, Kawakita M, Ishida N. Molecular characterization of human UDP-glucuronic acid/UDP-N- acetylgalactosamine transporter, a novel nucleotide sugar transporter with dual substrate specificity. *FEBS Lett* 2001;495:87–93.
548. Murer H, et al. Proximal tubular phosphate reabsorption: molecular mechanisms. *Physiol Rev* 2000;80:1373–1409.
549. Murer H, et al. Regulation of Na/Pi transporter in the proximal tubule. *Annu Rev Physiol* 2003;65:531–542.
550. Nagamatsu S, et al. Glucose transporter expression in brain. cDNA sequence of mouse GLUT3, the brain facilitative glucose transporter isoform, and identification of sites of expression by in situ hybridization. *J Biol Chem* 1992;267:467–472.
551. Nagase T, et al. Prediction of the coding sequences of unidentified human genes. IX. The complete sequences of 100 new cDNA clones from brain which can code for large proteins in vitro. *DNA Res* 1998;5:31–39.
552. Nagase T, et al. Prediction of the coding sequences of unidentified human genes. VI. The coding sequences of 80 new genes (KIAA0201-KIAA0280) deduced by analysis of cDNA clones from cell line KG-1 and brain. *DNA Res* 1996;3:321–354.
553. Nakamura N, et al. Four Na^+/H+ exchanger isoforms are distributed to Golgi and post-Golgi compartments and are involved in organelle pH regulation. *J Biol Chem* 2005;280: 1561–1572.
554. Nakanishi T, et al. Structure, function, and tissue expression pattern of human SN2, a subtype of the amino acid transport system N. *Biochem Biophys Res Commun* 2001;281:1343–1348.
555. Nakhoul NL, et al. Characteristics of renal Rhbg as an NH4(+) transporter. *Am J Physiol Renal Physiol* 2005;288:F170–F181.
556. Napoli L, et al. A novel missense adenine nucleotide translocator-1 gene mutation in a Greek adPEO family. *Neurology* 2001;57:2295–2298.
557. Nelson N The family of Na^+/Cl- neurotransmitter transporters. *J Neurochem* 1998;71: 1785–1803.
558. Nelson PJ, et al. Hydrogen ion cotransport by the renal brush border glutamate transporter. *Biochemistry* 1983;22:5459–5463.
559. Nezu J, et al. Primary systemic carnitine deficiency is caused by mutations in a gene encoding sodium ion-dependent carnitine transporter. *Nat Genet* 1999;21:91–94.
560. Nguyen TT, et al. Human intestinal folate transport: cloning, expression, and distribution of complementary RNA. *Gastroenterology* 1997;112:783–7891.
561. Ni B, et al. Molecular cloning, expression, and chromosomal localization of a human brain–specific Na(+)-dependent inorganic phosphate cotransporter. *J Neurochem* 1996;66:2227–2238.
562. Nicoletti F, et al. Metabotropic glutamate receptors: a new target for the therapy of neurodegenerative disorders? *Trends Neurosci* 1996;19:267–271.
563. Nicoll DA, et al. Mutation of amino acid residues in the putative transmembrane segments of the cardiac sarcolemmal Na^+-Ca2+ exchanger. *J Biol Chem* 1996;271:13385–3391.
564. Nicoll DA, Longoni S, Philipson KD. Molecular cloning and functional expression of the cardiac sarcolemmal $Na(^+)$-Ca^{2+} exchanger. *Science* 1990;250:562–565.
565. Nicoll DA, et al. Cloning of a third mammalian Na^+-Ca^{2+} exchanger, NCX3. *J Biol Chem* 1996;271:24914–24921.
566. Nielsen S, et al. Ultrastructural localization of Na-K-2Cl cotransporter in thick ascending limb and macula densa of rat kidney. *Am J Physiol* 1998;275:F885–F893.
567. Njajou OT, et al. A mutation in SLC11A3 is associated with autosomal dominant hemochromatosis. *Nat Genet* 2001;28:213–214.
568. Nozawa T, et al. Genetic polymorphisms of human organic anion transporters OATP-C (SLC21A6) and OATP-B (SLC21A9): allele frequencies in the Japanese population and functional analysis. *J Pharmacol Exp Ther* 2002;302:804–813.
569. Numata M, Orlowski J. Molecular cloning and characterization of a novel (Na^+,K+)/H+ exchanger localized to the trans-Golgi network. *J Biol Chem* 2001;276:17387–17394.
570. Oelkers P, et al. Primary bile acid malabsorption caused by mutations in the ileal sodium-dependent bile acid transporter gene (SLC10A2). *J Clin Invest* 1997;99:1880–1887.
571. Ogihara H, et al. Immuno-localization of H+/peptide cotransporter in rat digestive tract. *Biochem Biophys Res Commun* 1996;220:848–852.
572. Oishi K, et al. Targeted disruption of Slc19a2, the gene encoding the high-affinity thiamin transporter Thtr-1, causes diabetes mellitus, sensorineural deafness and megaloblastosis in mice. *Hum Mol Genet* 2002;11:2951–2960.
573. Okuda T, et al. Identification and characterization of the high-affinity choline transporter. *Nat Neurosci* 2000;3:120–125.
574. Oliver D, et al. Intracellular anions as the voltage sensor of prestin, the outer hair cell motor protein. *Science* 2001;292:2340–2343.
575. Olives B, et al. Molecular characterization of a new urea transporter in the human kidney. *FEBS Lett* 1996;386:156–160.
576. Olives B, et al. Kidd blood group and urea transport function of human erythrocytes are carried by the same protein. *J Biol Chem* 1995;270:15607–15610.
577. Olives B, et al. Cloning and functional expression of a urea transporter from human bone marrow cells. *J Biol Chem* 1994;269:31649–31652.
578. Orlowski J, Grinstein SS. Na^+/H+ exchangers of mammalian cells. *J Biol Chem* 997;272:22373–22376.

579. Oswald M, et al. Expression of hepatic transporters OATP-C and MRP2 in primary sclerosing cholangitis. *Liver* 2001;21:247–253.

580. Padh H. Vitamin C: newer insights into its biochemical functions. *Nutr Rev* 1991;49:65–70.

581. Pajor AM. Molecular cloning and functional expression of a sodium- dicarboxylate cotransporter from human kidney. *Am J Physiol* 1996;270:F642–F648.

582. Pajor AM. Sodium-coupled transporters for Krebs cycle intermediates. *Annu Rev Physiol* 1999;61:663–682.

583. Pajor AM. Molecular properties of sodium/dicarboxylate cotransporters. *J Membr Biol* 2000;175:1–8.

584. Pajor AM, Sun N. Characterization of the rabbit renal Na(+)-dicarboxylate cotransporter using antifusion protein antibodies. *Am J Physiol* 1996;271:C1808–C1816.

585. Pak CY. Citrate and renal calculi. *Miner Electrolyte Metab* 1987;13:257–266.

586. Palacin M, Borsani G, Sebastio G. The molecular bases of cystinuria and lysinuric protein intolerance. *Curr Opin Genet Dev* 2001;11:328–335.

587. Palmieri F, et al. Mitochondrial metabolite transporters. *Biochim Biophys Acta* 1996;1275:127–132.

588. Palmieri L, et al. Citrin and aralar1 are Ca(2+)-stimulated aspartate/glutamate transporters in mitochondria. *EMBO J* 2001;20:5060–5069.

589. Palmieri L, et al. Identification and functional reconstitution of the yeast peroxisomal adenine nucleotide transporter. *EMBO J* 2001; 20:5049–5059.

590. Palmieri L, et al. The mitochondrial dicarboxylate carrier is essential for the growth of Saccharomyces cerevisiae on ethanol or acetate as the sole carbon source. *Mol Microbiol* 1999;31:569–577.

591. Palmiter RD. Protection against zinc toxicity by metallothionein and zinc transporter 1. *Proc Natl Acad Sci U S A* 2004;101:4918–4923.

592. Palmiter RD, Cole TB, Findley SD. ZnT-2, a mammalian protein that confers resistance to zinc by facilitating vesicular sequestration. *EMBO J* 1996;15:1784–791.

593. Palmiter RD, et al. ZnT-3, a putative transporter of zinc into synaptic vesicles. *Proc Natl Acad U S A* 1996;93:14934–14939.

594. Palmiter RD, Findley SD. Cloning and functional characterization of a mammalian zinc transporter that confers resistance to zinc. *EMBO J* 1995;14:639–649.

595. Pao SS, Paulsen IT, Saier MH Jr. Major facilitator superfamily. *Microbiol Mol Biol Rev* 1998;62:1–34.

596. Parker MD, Ourmozdi EP, Tanner MJ. Human BTR1, a new bicarbonate transporter superfamily member and human AE4 from kidney. *Biochem Biophys Res Commun* 2001;282:1103–1109.

597. Parsons SM. Transport mechanisms in acetylcholine and monoamine storage. *FASEB J* 2000;14:2423–2434.

598. Patil SD, et al. Intestinal absorption of ribavirin is preferentially mediated by the Na+-nucleoside purine (N1) transporter. *Pharm Res* 1998;15:950–952.

599. Paw BH, et al. Cell-specific mitotic defect and dyserythropoiesis associated with erythroid band 3 deficiency. *Nat Genet* 2003;34:59–64.

600. Payne JA. Functional characterization of the neuronal-specific K-Cl cotransporter: implications for [K+]o regulation. *Am J Physiol* 1997;273:C1516–C1525.

601. Payne JA, Stevenson TJ, Donaldson F. Molecular characterization of a putative K-Cl cotransporter in rat brain. A neuronal-specific isoform. *J Biol Chem* 1996;271:16245–16252.

602. Pearson MM, et al. Localization of the K(+)-Cl(-) cotransporter, KCC3, in the central and peripheral nervous systems: expression in the choroid plexus, large neurons and white matter tracts. *Neuroscience* 2001;103:481–491.

603. Pebay-Peyroula E, et al. Structure of mitochondrial ADP/ATP carrier in complex with carboxyatractyloside. *Nature* 2003;426:39–44.

604. Peghini P, Janzen J, Stoffel W. Glutamate transporter *EAAC-1*-deficient mice develop dicarboxylic aminoaciduria and behavioral abnormalities but no neurodegeneration. *EMBO J* 1997;16:3822–3832.

605. Peltekova VD, et al. Functional variants of OCTN cation transporter genes are associated with Crohn disease. *Nat Genet* 2004;36:471–475.

606. Perkins CP, et al. Anemia and perinatal death result from loss of the murine ecotropic retrovirus receptor mCAT-1. *Genes Dev* 1997;11:914–925.

607. Petrovic S, et al. SLC26A7: a basolateral Cl-/HCO3⁻ exchanger specific to intercalated cells of the outer medullary collecting duct. *Am J Physiol Renal Physiol* 2004;286:F161–F169.

608. Pfeiffer R, et al. Amino acid transport of y+L-type by heterodimers of 4F2hc/CD98 and members of the glycoprotein-associated amino acid transporter family. *EMBO J* 1999;18:49–57.

609. Pfister MF, et al. Parathyroid hormone-dependent degradation of type II Na+/Pi cotransporters. *J Biol Chem* 1997;272:20125–20130.

610. Pfister MF, et al. Parathyroid hormone leads to the lysosomal degradation of the renal type II Na/Pi cotransporter. *Proc Natl Acad Sci U S A* 1998;95:1909–1914.

611. Phay JE, Hussain HB, Moley JF. Cloning and expression analysis of a novel member of the facilitative glucose transporter family, SLC2A9 (GLUT9). *Genomics* 2000;66:217–220.

612. Philp NJ, et al. Loss of MCT1, MCT3, and MCT4 expression in the retinal pigment epithelium and neural retina of the 5A11/basigin-null mouse. *Invest Ophthalmol Vis Sci* 2003;44:1305–1311.

613. Philp NJ, Yoon H, Lombardi L. Mouse MCT3 gene is expressed preferentially in retinal pigment and choroid plexus epithelia. *Am J Physiol Cell Physiol* 2001;280:C1319–C1326.

614. Picard V, et al. Nramp 2 (DCT1/DMT1) expressed at the plasma membrane transports iron and other divalent cations into a calcein-accessible cytoplasmic pool. *J Biol Chem* 2000; 275:35738–35745.

615. Pietrangelo A. Physiology of iron transport and the hemochromatosis gene. *Am J Physiol Gastrointest Liver Physiol* 2002;282:G403–G414.

616. Pineda M, et al. Identification of a membrane protein, LAT-2, that co-expresses with 4F2 heavy chain, an L-type amino acid transport activity with broad specificity for small and large zwitterionic amino acids. *J Biol Chem* 1999;274:19738–19744.

617. Pines G, et al. Cloning and expression of a rat brain L-glutamate transporter. *Nature* 1992;360:464–467.

618. Pines G, Kanner BI. Counterflow of L-glutamate in plasma membrane vesicles and reconstituted preparations from rat brain. *Biochemistry* 1990;29:11209–11214.

619. Pizzagalli F, et al. Identification of a novel human organic anion transporting polypeptide as a high affinity thyroxine transporter. *Mol Endocrinol* 2002;16:2283–2296.

620. Pizzonia JH, et al. Immunochemical characterization of Na+/H+ exchanger isoform NHE4. *Am J Physiol* 1998;275:510–517.

621. Plagemann PG, Aran JM. Characterization of Na(+)-dependent, active nucleoside transport in rat and mouse peritoneal macrophages, a mouse macrophage cell line and normal rat kidney cells. *Biochim Biophys Acta* 1990;1028:289–298.

622. Plotkin MD, et al. Expression of the Na(+)-K(+)-2Cl- cotransporter BSC2 in the nervous system. *Am J Physiol* 272:C173–C183.

623. Plotkin MD, et al. Expression of the BSC2 Na-K-Cl cotransporter in adult and postnatal developing rat brain. *J Am Soc Nephrol* 1996;7:1288.

624. Praetorius J, Nejsum LN, Nielsen S. A SCL4A10 gene product maps selectively to the basolateral plasma membrane of choroid plexus epithelial cells. *Am J Physiol Cell Physiol* 2004;286:C601–C610.

625. Pras E, et al. Mutations in the SLC3A1 transporter gene in cystinuria. *Am J Hum Genet* 1995;56:1297–1303.

626. Prasad PD, et al. Molecular cloning of the human placental folate transporter. *Biochim Biophys Res Commun* 1995;206:681–687.

627. Prasad PD, et al. Cloning and functional expression of a cDNA encoding a mammalian sodium-dependent vitamin transporter mediating the uptake of pantothenate, biotin, and lipoate. *J Biol Chem* 1998;273:7501–7506.

628. Price NT, Jackson VN, Halestrap AP. Cloning and sequencing of four new mammalian monocarboxylate transporter (MCT) homologues confirms the existence of a transporter family with an ancient past. *Biochem J* 1998;329:321–328.

629. Prie D, et al. Nephrolithiasis and osteoporosis associated with hypophosphatemia caused by mutations in the type 2a sodium-phosphate cotransporter. *N Engl J Med* 2002;347:983–991.

630. Pritchard JB, Miller DS. Mechanisms mediating renal secretion of organic anions and cations. *Physiol Rev* 1993;73:765–796.

631. Prohl C, et al. The yeast mitochondrial carrier Leu5p and its human homologue Graves' disease protein are required for accumulation of coenzyme A in the matrix. *Mol Cell Biol* 2001;21:1089–1097.

632. Pushkin A, et al. Cloning, tissue distribution, genomic organization, and functional characterization of NBC3, a new member of the sodium bicarbonate cotransporter family. *J Biol Chem* 1999;274:16569–16575.

633. Pushkin A, et al. Cloning, characterization and chromosomal assignment of NBC4, a new member of the sodium bicarbonate cotransporter family. *Biochim Biophys Acta* 2000;1493:215–218.

634. Pushkin A, et al. Two C-terminal variants of NBC4, a new member of the sodium bicarbonate cotransporter family: cloning, characterization, and localization. *IUBMB Life* 2000;50:13–19.

635. Pushkin A, et al. NBC3 expression in rabbit collecting duct: colocalization with vacuolar H+-ATPase. *Am J Physiol* 1999;277:F974–F981.

636. Putney LK, Denker SP, Barber DL. The changing face of the Na+/H+ exchanger, NHE1: structure, regulation, and cellular actions. *Annu Rev Pharmacol Toxicol* 2002;42:527–552.

637. Qian ZM, Wang Q. Expression of iron transport proteins and excessive iron accumulation in the brain in neurodegenerative disorders. *Brain Res Brain Res Rev* 1998;27:257–267.

638. Quednau BD, Nicoll DA, Philipson KD. Tissue specificity and alternative splicing of the Na+/Ca2+ exchanger isoforms NCX1, NCX2, and NCX3 in rat. *Am J Physiol* 1997;272:C1250–C1261.

639. Quentin F, et al. RhBG and RhCG, the putative ammonia transporters, are expressed in the same cells in the distal nephron. *J Am Soc Nephrol* 2003;14:545–554.

640. Race JE, et al. Molecular cloning and functional characterization of KCC3, a new K-Cl cotransporter. *Am J Physiol* 1999;277:C1210–C1219.

641. Radian R, et al. Immunocytochemical localization of the GABA transporter in rat brain. *J Neurosci* 1990;10:1319–1330.

642. Rajan DP, et al. Cloning and functional characterization of a Na(+)-independent, broad-specific neutral amino acid transporter from mammalian intestine. *Biochim Biophys Acta* 2000;1463:6–14.

643. Rajan DP, et al. Cloning and expression of a b(0,+)-like amino acid transporter functioning as a heterodimer with 4F2hc instead of rBAT. A new candidate gene for cystinuria. *J Biol Chem* 1999;274:29005–29010.

644. Rajgopal A, et al. SLC19A3 encodes a second thiamine transporter ThTr2. *Biochim Biophys Acta* 2001;1537:175–178.

645. Rajgopal A, et al. Expression of the reduced folate carrier SLC19A1 in IEC-6 cells results in two distinct transport activities. *Am J Physiol Cell Physiol* 2001;281:C1579–C1586.

646. Ray WA, et al. Long-term use of thiazide diuretics and risk of hip fracture. *Lancet* 1989;1:687–690.

647. Raz T, et al. The spectrum of mutations, including four novel ones, in the thiamine-responsive megaloblastic anemia gene SLC19A2 of eight families. *Hum Mutat* 2000;16:37–42.

648. Reagan LP, et al. GLUT8 glucose transporter is localized to excitatory and inhibitory neurons in the rat hippocampus. *Brain Res* 2002;932:129–134.

649. Reardon W, et al. Prevalence, age of onset, and natural history of thyroid disease in Pendred syndrome. *J Med Genet* 1999;36:595–598.

650. Reczek D, Berryman M, Bretscher A. Identification of EBP50: a PDZ-containing phosphoprotein that associates with members of the ezrin-radixin-moesin family. *J Cell Biol* 1997;139:169–179.

651. Redecker P, et al. Evidence for microvesicular storage and release of glycine in rodent pinealocytes. *Neurosci Lett* 2001;299:93–96.

652. Reeves JP, Sutko JL. Competitive interactions of sodium and calcium with the sodium-calcium exchange system of cardiac sarcolemmal vesicles. *J Biol Chem* 1983;258:3178–3182.

653. Reilander H, et al. Primary structure and functional expression of the Na/Ca,K-exchanger from bovine rod photoreceptors. *EMBO J* 1992;11:1689–1695.

654. Reimer RJ, et al. Amino acid transport system A resembles system N in sequence but differs in mechanism. *Proc Natl Acad Sci U S A* 2000;97:7715–7720.

655. Reizer J, et al. Mammalian integral membrane receptors are homologous to facilitators and antiporters of yeast, fungi, and eubacteria. *Protein Sci* 1993;2:20–30.

656. Richelson E, Pfenning M. Blockade by antidepressants and related compounds of biogenic amine uptake into rat brain synaptosomes: most antidepressants selectively block norepinephrine uptake. *Eur J Pharmacol* 1984;104:277–286.

657. Rim JS, et al. Transcription of the sodium/myo-inositol cotransporter gene is regulated by multiple tonicity-responsive enhancers spread over 50 kilobase pairs in the 5'-flanking region. *J Biol Chem* 1998;273:20615–20621.

658. Ritzel MW, et al. Molecular identification and characterization of novel human and mouse concentrative Na+-nucleoside cotransporter proteins (hCNT3 and mCNT3) broadly selective for purine and pyrimidine nucleosides (system cib). *J Biol Chem* 2001;276:2914–2927.

659. Ritzel MW, et al. Molecular cloning and functional expression of cDNAs encoding a human Na+-nucleoside cotransporter (hCNT1). *Am J Physiol* 1997;272:C707–C714.

660. Ritzel MW, et al. Molecular cloning, functional expression and chromosomal localization of a cDNA encoding a human Na+/nucleoside cotransporter (hCNT2) selective for purine nucleosides and uridine. *Mol Membr Biol* 1998;15:203–211.

661. Roch-Ramel F, Guisan B. Renal transport of urate in humans. *News Physiol Sci* 1999;14:80–84.

662. Roch-Ramel F, Guisan B, Schild. Indirect coupling of urate and p-aminohippurate transport to sodium in human brush-border membrane vesicles. *Am J Physiol* 1996;270:61–68.

663. Rodriguez AM, et al. Identification and characterization of a putative human iodide transporter located at the apical membrane of thyrocytes. *J.Clin.Endocrinol Metab* 2002;87:3500–3503.

664. Rogers S, et al. Glucose transporter GLUT12-functional characterization in Xenopus laevis oocytes. *Biochem Biophys Res Commun* 2003;308:422–426.

665. Rogers S, et al. Differential expression of GLUT12 in breast cancer and normal breast tissue. *Cancer Lett* 2003;193:225–233.

666. Romero MF. The electrogenic Na+/CO3- cotransporter, NBC. *J Pancreas (Online)* 2001;2(Suppl 4):182–191.

667. Romero MF, et al. Cloning and functional expression of rNBC, an electrogenic Na(+)-HCO3- cotransporter from rat kidney. *Am J Physiol* 1998;274:F425–F432.

668. Romero MF, et al. Expression cloning and characterization of a renal electrogenic Na+/HCO3- cotransporter. *Nature* 1997;387:409–413.

669. Romero MF, et al. Expression cloning using Xenopus laevis oocytes. *Methods Enzymol* 1998;296:17–52.

670. Rose RC, Bode AM. Biology of free radical scavengers: an evaluation of ascorbate. *FASEB J* 1993;7:1135–1142.

671. Rosenberg MJ, et al. Mutant deoxynucleotide carrier is associated with congenital microcephaly. *Nat Genet* 2002;32:175–179.

672. Rossi A, et al. Undersulfation of proteoglycans synthesized by chondrocytes from a patient with achondrogenesis type 1B homozygous for an L483P substitution in the diastrophic dysplasia sulfate transporter. *J Biol Chem* 1996;271:18456–18464.

673. Rossier G, et al. LAT2, a new basolateral 4F2hc/CD98-associated amino acid transporter of kidney and intestine. *J Biol Chem* 1999;274:34948–34954.

674. Rothstein JD, et al. Knockout of glutamate transporters reveals a major role for astroglial transport in excitotoxicity and clearance of glutamate. *Neuron* 1996;16:675–686.

675. Rothstein JD, et al. Localization of neuronal and glial glutamate transporters. *Neuron* 1994;13:713–725.

676. Royaux IE, et al. Pendrin, the protein encoded by the Pendred syndrome gene (PDS), is an apical porter of iodide in the thyroid and is regulated by thyroglobulin in FRTL-5 cells. *Endocrinology* 2000;141:839–845.

677. Royaux IE, et al. Pendrin, encoded by the Pendred syndrome gene, resides in the apical region of renal intercalated cells and mediates bicarbonate secretion. *Proc Natl Acad Sci U S A* 2001;98:4221–4226.

678. Rubio-Aliaga I, et al. Targeted disruption of the peptide transporter Pept2 gene in mice defines its physiological role in the kidney. *Mol Cell Biol* 2003;23:3247–3252.

679. Ruddy DA, et al. A 1-Mb transcript map of the hereditary hemochromatosis locus. *Genome Res* 1997;7:441–456.

680. Rudnick G, Clark J. From synapse to vesicle: the reuptake and storage of biogenic amine neurotransmitters. *Biochim Biophys Acta* 1993; 1144:249–263.

681. Runswick MJ, et al. Sequence of the bovine 2-oxoglutarate/malate carrier protein: structural relationship to other mitochondrial transport proteins. *Biochemistry* 1990;29:11033–11040.

682. Saadi I, et al. Molecular genetics of cystinuria: mutation analysis of SLC3A1 and evidence for another gene in type I (silent) phenotype. *Kidney Int* 1998;54:48–55.

683. Saccomani G, Mitchell KD, Navar LG. Angiotensin II stimulation of Na(+)-H+ exchange in proximal tubule cells. *Am J Physiol* 1990;258:F1188–F1195.

684. Sagawa K, et al. Glucocorticoid-induced alterations of renal sulfate transport. *J Pharmacol Exp Ther* 2000;294:658–663.

685. Sagne C, et al. Identification and characterization of a lysosomal transporter for small neutral amino acids. *Proc Natl Acad Sci U S A* 2001;98:7206–7211.

686. Sagne C, et al. Cloning of a functional vesicular GABA and glycine transporter by screening of genome databases. *FEBS Lett* 1997; 417:177–183.

687. Saheki T, Kobayashi K. Mitochondrial aspartate glutamate carrier (citrin) deficiency as the cause of adult-onset type II citrullinemia (CTLN2) and idiopathic neonatal hepatitis (NICCD). *Hum Genet* 2002;47:333–341.

688. Sakata K, et al. Cloning of a lymphatic peptide/histidine transporter. *Biochem J* 2001;356:53–60.

689. Sanchis D, et al. BMCP1, a novel mitochondrial carrier with high expression in the central nervous system of humans and rodents, and respiration uncoupling activity in recombinant yeast. *J Biol Chem* 1998;273:34611–34615.

690. Santer R, et al. The mutation spectrum of the facilitative glucose transporter gene SLC2A2 (GLUT2) in patients with Fanconi–Bickel syndrome. *Hum Genet* 2002;110:21–29.

691. Sassani P, et al. Functional characterization of NBC4: a new electrogenic sodium- bicarbonate cotransporter. *Am J Physiol Cell Physiol* 2002;282:C408–C416.

692. Satlin LM, Amin V, Wolkoff AW. Organic anion transporting polypeptide mediates organic anion/HCO3- exchange. *J Biol Chem* 1997;272:26340–26345.

693. Sato H, et al. Cloning and expression of a plasma membrane cystine/glutamate exchange transporter composed of two distinct proteins. *J Biol Chem* 1999;274:11455–11458.

694. Sato K, et al. Expression of organic anion transporting polypeptide E (OATP-E) in human placenta. *Placenta* 2003;24:144–148.

695. Satoh H, et al. Functional analysis of diastrophic dysplasia sulfate transporter. Its involvement in growth regulation of chondrocytes mediated by sulfated proteoglycans. *J Biol Chem* 1998;273:12307–12315.

696. Schafer MK, et al. Molecular cloning and functional identification of mouse vesicular glutamate transporter 3 and its expression in subsets of novel excitatory neurons. *J Biol Chem* 2002;277:50734–50748.

697. Schaffer JE, Lodish HF. Expression cloning and characterization of a novel adipocyte long chain fatty acid transport protein. *Cell* 1994;79:427–436.

698. Schaner ME, et al. Gene expression patterns in ovarian carcinomas. *Mol Biol Cell* 2003; 14:4376–4386.

699. Schiebel K, et al. Localization of the adenine nucleotide translocase gene ANT2 to chromosome Xq24-q25 with tight linkage to DXS425. *Genomics* 1994;24:605–606.

700. Schiebel K, et al. A human pseudoautosomal gene, ADP/ATP translocase, escapes X-inactivation whereas a homologue on Xq is subject to X-inactivation. *Nat Genet* 1993; 3:82–87.

701. Schiffer M, et al. Localization of the GLUT8 glucose transporter in murine kidney and regulation in vivo in non-diabetic and diabetic conditions. *Am J Physiol Renal Physiol* 2005;289:F186–F193.

702. Schmitt BM, et al. Na/HCO3 cotransporters in rat brain: expression in glia, neurons, and choroid plexus. *J Neurosci* 2000;20:6839–6848.

703. Schmitt BM, et al. Immunolocalization of the electrogenic Na+-HCO3- cotransporter in mammalian and amphibian kidney. *Am J Physiol* 1992;276:F27–F38.

704. Schnetkamp PP. Na-Ca or Na-Ca-K exchange in rod photoreceptors. *Prog Biophys Mol Biol* 1989;54:1–29.

705. Schnetkamp PP. Calcium homeostasis in vertebrate retinal rod outer segments. *Cell Calcium* 1995;18:322–330.

706. Schoofs MW, et al. Thiazide diuretics and the risk for hip fracture. *Ann Intern Med* 2003;139:476–482.

707. Schultheis PJ, et al. Renal and intestinal absorptive defects in mice lacking the NHE3 Na+/H+ exchanger. *Nat Genet* 1998;19:282–285.

708. Schuster VL, Kokko, Jacobson HR. Angiotensin II directly stimulates sodium transport in rabbit proximal convoluted tubules. *J Clin Invest* 1984;73:507–515.

709. Schwartz CE, et al. Allan–Herndon–Dudley syndrome and the monocarboxylate transporter 8 (MCT8) gene. *Am J Hum Genet* 2005;77:41–53.

710. Schwarz EM, Benzer S. Calx, a Na–Ca exchanger gene of Drosophila melanogaster. *Proc Natl Acad Sci U S A* 1997;94:10249–10254.

711. Schweinfest CW, et al. Identification of a colon mucosa gene that is down-regulated in colon adenomas and adenocarcinomas. *Proc Natl Acad Sci U S A* 1993;90:4166–4170.

712. Scott DA, Karniski LP. Human pendrin expressed in Xenopus laevis oocytes mediates chloride/formate exchange. *Am J Physiol Cell Physiol* 2000;278:C207–C211.

713. Scott DA, et al. The Pendred syndrome gene encodes a chloride-iodide transport protein. *Nat Genet* 1999;21:440–443.

714. Segawa H, et al. Growth-related renal type II Na/Pi cotransporter. *J Biol Chem* 2002; 277:19665–19672.

715. Segawa H, Kawakita M, Ishida N. Human and Drosophila UDP-galactose transporters transport UDP-N-acetylgalactosamine in addition to UDP-galactose. *Eur J Biochem* 2002; 269:128–138.

716. Sekine T, Cha SH, Endou H. The multispecific organic anion transporter (OAT) family. *Pflugers Arch* 2000;440:337–350.

717. Sekine T, et al. Cloning, functional characterization, and localization of a rat renal Na+-dicarboxylate transporter. *Am J Physiol* 1998;275:F298–F305.

718. Sekine T, et al. Expression cloning and characterization of a novel multispecific organic anion transporter. *J Biol Chem* 1997; 272:18526–18529.

719. Shafqat S, et al. Cloning and expression of a novel Na(+)-dependent neutral amino acid transporter structurally related to mammalian Na+/glutamate cotransporters. *J Biol Chem* 1993; 268:15351–15355.

720. Shafqat S, et al. Human brain-specific L-proline transporter: molecular cloning, functional expression, and chromosomal localization of the gene in human and mouse genomes. *Mol Pharmacol* 1995;48:219–229.

721. Shashidharan P, et al. Neuron-specific human glutamate transporter: molecular cloning, characterization and expression in human brain. *Brain Res* 1994;662:245–250.

722. Shayakul C, Alper SL. Inherited renal tubular acidosis. *Curr Opin Nephrol Hypertens* 2000;9:541–546.

723. Shayakul C, et al. Localization of the high-affinity glutamate transporter EAAC1 in rat kidney. *Am J Physiol* 1997;273:F1023–F1029.

724. Shayakul C, et al. Segmental localization of urea transporter mRNAs in rat kidney. *Am J Physiol* 1997;272:F654–F660.

725. Shayakul C, et al. Long-term regulation of urea transporter expression by vasopressin in Brattleboro rats. *Am J Physiol Renal Physiol* 2000;278:F620–F627.

726. ShayakulC, Steel A, Hediger MA. Molecular cloning and characterization of the vasopressin-regulated urea transporter of rat kidney collecting ducts. *J Clin Invest* 1996;98:2580–2587.

727. Shen H, et al. Targeted disruption of the PEPT2 gene markedly reduces dipeptide uptake in choroid plexus. *J Biol Chem* 2003;278:4786–4791.

728. Shi X, et al. Stable inducible expression of a functional rat liver organic anion transport protein in HeLa cells. *J Biol Chem* 1995; 270:25591–25595.

729. Shimada S, et al. Cloning and expression of a cocaine-sensitive dopamine transporter complementary DNA. *Science* 1991;254:576–578 (erratum: *Science* 1992;255:1195).

730. Shimada T, et al. Cloning and characterization of FGF23 as a causative factor of tumor-induced osteomalacia. *Proc Natl Acad Sci U S A* 2001;98:6500–6505.

731. Shishido T, et al. Transformation of BALB3T3 cells caused by over-expression of rat CD98 heavy chain (HC) requires its association with light chain: mis-sense mutation in a cysteine residue of CD98HC eliminates its transforming activity. *Int J Cancer* 2000;87:311–316.

732. Shryock JC, Belardinelli L. Adenosine and adenosine receptors in the cardiovascular system: biochemistry, physiology, and pharmacology. *Am J Cardiol* 1997;79:2–10.

733. Shu C, et al. Role of PEPT2 in peptide/mimetic trafficking at the blood-cerebrospinal fluid barrier: studies in rat choroid plexus epithelial cells in primary culture. *J Pharmacol Exp Ther* 2002;301:820–829.

734. Sierra EE, Goldman ID. Recent advances in the understanding of the mechanism of membrane transport of folates and antifolates. *Semin Oncol* 1999;26(Suppl 6):11–23.

735. Silbernagl S. Kinetics and localization of tubular resorption of "acidic" amino acids. A microperfusion and free flow micropuncture study in rat kidney. *Pflugers Arch* 1983;396:218–224.

736. Silbernagl S, Volkl H. Molecular specificity of the tubular resorption of "acidic" amino acids. A continuous microperfusion study in rat kidney in vivo. *Pflugers Arch* 1983;396:225–230.

737. Simon DB, et al. Bartter's syndrome, hypokalaemic alkalosis with hypercalciuria, is caused by mutations in the Na-K-2Cl cotransporter NKCC2. *Nat Genet* 1996;13:183–188.

738. Simon DB, et al. Gitelman's variant of Bartter's syndrome, inherited hypokalaemic alkalosis, is caused by mutations in the thiazide-sensitive Na-Cl cotransporter. *Nat Genet* 1996;12:24–30.

739. Skamene E. The Bcg gene story. *Immunobiology* 1994;191:451–460.

740. Smith CP, et al. Cloning and regulation of expression of the rat kidney urea transporter (rUT2). *J Clin Invest* 1995;96:1556–1563.

741. Smith CP, et al. Characterization of a human colonic cDNA encoding a structurally novel urea transporter, hUT-A6. *Am J Physiol Cell Physiol* 2004;287:C1087–C1093.

742. Smith DE, et al. Tubular localization and tissue distribution of peptide transporters in rat kidney. *Pharm Res* 1998;15:1244–1249.

743. Sokolow S, et al. Impaired neuromuscular transmission and skeletal muscle fiber necrosis in mice lacking Na/Ca exchanger 3. *J Clin Invest* 2004;113:265–273.

744. Soleimani M, et al. Pendrin: an apical Cl-/OH-/HCO$_3^-$ exchanger in the kidney cortex. *Am J Physiol Renal Physiol* 2001;280:F356–F364.

745. Sonders M S, et al. Multiple ionic conductances of the human dopamine transporter: the actions of dopamine and psychostimulants. *J Neurosci* 1997;17:960–974.

746. Song L, et al. Molecular, functional, and genomic characterization of human KCC2, the neuronal K-Cl cotransporter. *Mol Brain Res* 2002;103:91–105.

747. Song X, et al. Amino acid ester prodrugs of the anticancer agent gemcitabine: synthesis, bioconversion, metabolic bioevasion, and hPEPT1-mediated transport. *Mol Pharm* 2005;2:157–167.

748. Songyang Z, et al. Recognition of unique carboxyl-terminal motifs by distinct PDZ domains. *Science* 1997;275:73–77.

749. Sotiriou S, et al. Ascorbic-acid transporter Slc23a1 is essential for vitamin C transport into the brain and for perinatal survival. *Nat Med* 2002;8:514–517.

750. Sperandeo MP, et al. The gene encoding a cationic amino acid transporter (SLC7A4) maps to the region deleted in the velocardiofacial syndrome. *Genomics* 1998;49:230–236.

751. Srinivas SR, et al. Cloning and functional identification of slc5a12 as a sodium-coupled low-affinity transporter for monocarboxylates (SMCT2). *Biochem J* 2005;392:655–664.

752. Stacey JM, et al. Genetic mapping studies of familial juvenile hyperuricemic nephropathy on chromosome 16p11-p13. *J Clin Endocrinol Metab* 2003;88:464–470.

753. Stahl A, et al. Insulin causes fatty acid transport protein translocation and enhanced fatty acid uptake in adipocytes. *Dev Cell* 2002;2:477–488.

754. Stahl A, et al. Fatty acid transport proteins: a current view of a growing family. *Trends Endocrinol Metab* 2001;12:266–273.

755. Stahl A, et al. Identification of the major intestinal fatty acid transport protein. *Mol Cell* 1999;4:299–308.

756. Steel A, et al. Stoichiometry and pH dependence of the rabbit proton-dependent oligopeptide transporter PepT1. *J Physiol (Lond)* 1997;498:563–569.

757. Sterling D, Alvarez BV, Casey JR. The extracellular component of a transport metabolon. Extracellular loop 4 of the human AE1 Cl-/HCO$_3^-$ exchanger binds carbonic anhydrase IV. *J Biol Chem* 2002;277:25239–25246.

758. Stevens BR, Ross HJ, Wright EM. Multiple transport pathways for neutral amino acids in rabbit jejunal brush border vesicles. *J Membr Biol* 1982;66:213–225.

759. Stiburkova B, et al. Familial juvenile hyperuricemic nephropathy: localization of the gene on chromosome 16p11.2- and evidence for genetic heterogeneity. *Am J Hum Genet* 2000;66:1989–1994.

760. Storck T, et al. Structure, expression, and functional analysis of a Na(+)-dependent glutamate/aspartate transporter from rat brain. *Proc Natl Acad U S A* 1992;89:10955–10959.

761. Strange K, et al. Dependence of KCC2 K-Cl cotransporter activity on a conserved carboxy terminus tyrosine residue. *Am J Physiol Cell Physiol* 2000;279:C860–C867.

762. Stuart CA, Wen G, Jiang J. GLUT3 protein and mRNA in autopsy muscle specimens. *Metabolism* 1999;48:876–880.

763. Stuart RO, et al. EEG1, a putative transporter expressed during epithelial organogenesis: comparison with embryonic transporter expression during nephrogenesis. *Am J Physiol Renal Physiol* 2001;281:F1148–F1156.

764. Stump DD, Fan X, Berk PD. Oleic acid uptake and binding by rat adipocytes define dual pathways for cellular fatty acid uptake. *J Lipid Res* 2001;42:509–520.

765. Sugawara M, et al. Cloning of an amino acid transporter with functional characteristics and tissue expression pattern identical to that of system A. *J Biol Chem* 2000;275:16473–16477.

766. Sugawara M, et al. Structure and function of ATA3, a new subtype of amino acid transport system A, primarily expressed in the liver and skeletal muscle. *Biochim Biophys Acta* 2000;1509:7–13.

767. Sun F, et al. Protein kinase A associates with cystic fibrosis transmembrane conductance regulator via an interaction with ezrin. *J Biol Chem* 2000; 275:14360–14366.

768. Sung KW, et al. Abnormal GABAA receptor-mediated currents in dorsal root ganglion neurons isolated from Na-K-2Cl cotransporter null mice. *J Neurosci* 2000;20:7531–7538.

769. Supplisson S, Roux MJ. Why glycine transporters have different stoichiometries. *FEBS Lett* 2002;529:93–101.

770. Surratt CK, et al. A human synaptic vesicle monoamine transporter cDNA predicts posttranslational modifications, reveals chromosome 10 gene localization and identifies TaqI RFLPs. *FEBS Lett* 1993; 318:325–330.

771. Suzuki K, Kono T. Evidence that insulin causes translocation of glucose transport activity to the plasma membrane from an intracellular storage site. *Proc Natl Acad Sci U S A* 1980; 77:2542–2545.

772. Suzuki T, et al. Zinc transporters, ZnT5 and ZnT7, are required for the activation of alkaline phosphatases, zinc-requiring enzymes that are glycosylphosphatidylinositol-anchored to the cytoplasmic membrane. *J Biol Chem* 2005;280:637–643.

773. Deleted in proof.

774. Sweet DH, Miller DS, Pritchard JB. Ventricular choline transport: a role for organic cation transporter 2 expressed in choroid plexus. *J Biol Chem* 2001;276:41611–41619.

775. Sweet DH, et al. Impaired organic anion transport in kidney and choroid plexus of organic anion transporter 3 (Oat3 (Slc22a8)) knockout mice. *J Biol Chem* 2002;277:26934–26943.

776. Sweet DH, Wolff NA, Pritchard JB. Expression cloning and characterization of ROAT1. The basolateral organic anion transporter in rat kidney. *J Biol Chem* 1997;272:30088–30095.

777. Takahashi N, et al. Uncompensated polyuria in a mouse model of Bartter's syndrome. *Proc Natl Acad Sci U S A* 2000;97:5434–5439.

778. Takahashi N, et al. VMAT2 knockout mice: heterozygotes display reduced amphetamine-conditioned reward, enhanced amphetamine locomotion, and enhanced MPTP toxicity. *Proc Natl Acad Sci U S A* 1997;94:9938–9943.

779. Takahashi Y, et al. Identification of cAMP analogue inducible genes in RAW264 macrophages. *Biochim Biophys Acta* 2000;1492:385–394.

780. Takamori S, et al. Molecular cloning and functional characterization of human vesicular glutamate transporter 3. *EMBO Rep* 2002;3:798–803.

781. Takanaga H, Mackenzie B, Hediger MA. Sodium-dependent ascorbic acid transporter family SLC23. *Pflugers Arch* 2003;447:677–682.

782. Takanaga H, et al. ATA2 is predominantly expressed as system A at the blood–brain barrier and acts as brain-to-blood efflux transport for L-proline. *Mol Pharmacol* 2002;61:1289–1296.

783. Takeda M, et al. Human organic anion transporters and human organic cation transporters mediate renal antiviral transport. *J Pharmacol Exp Ther* 2002;300:918–924.

784. Tamai I, et al. Na(+)-coupled transport of L-carnitine via high-affinity carnitine transporter OCTN2 and its subcellular localization in kidney. *Biochim Biophys Acta* 2001;1512:273–284.

785. Tamai I, et al. Molecular identification and characterization of novel members of the human organic anion transporter (OATP) family. *Biochem Biophys Res Commun* 2000;273:251–260.

786. Tamai I, et al. Molecular and functional characterization of organic cation/carnitine transporter family in mice. *J Biol Chem* 2000; 275:40064–40072.

787. Tamai I, et al. Cloning and characterization of a novel human pH-dependent organic cation transporter, OCTN1. *FEBS Lett* 1997;419:107–111.

788. Tanaka K, et al. Epilepsy and exacerbation of brain injury in mice lacking the glutamate transporter GLT-1. *Science* 1997;276:1699–1702.

789. Tanner MJ. Molecular and cellular biology of the erythrocyte anion exchanger (AE1). *Semin Hematol* 1993;30:34–57.

790. Tatsumi S, et al. Molecular cloning and hormonal regulation of PiT-1, a sodium-dependent phosphate cotransporter from rat parathyroid glands. *Endocrinology* 1998;139:1692–1699.

791. Taylor KM, et al. Structure-function analysis of LIV-1, the breast cancer–associated protein that belongs to a new subfamily of zinc transporters. *Biochem J* 2003;375:51–59.

792. Taylor KM, et al. Structure-function analysis of HKE4, a member of the new LIV-1 subfamily of zinc transporters. *Biochem J* 2004;377:131–139.

793. Taylor KM, et al. Structure-function analysis of a novel member of the LIV-1 subfamily of zinc transporters, ZIP14. *FEBS Lett* 2005;579:427–432.

794. Tazawa S, et al. SLC5A9/SGLT4, a new Na$^+$-dependent glucose transporter, is an essential transporter for mannose, 1,5-anhydro-D-glucitol, and fructose. *Life Sci* 2005;76:1039–1050.

795. Tazebay UH, et al. The mammary gland iodide transporter is expressed during lactation and in breast cancer. *Nat Med* 2000;6:871–878.

796. Tenenhouse HS, et al. Differential expression, abundance, and regulation of Na$^+$-phosphate cotransporter genes in murine kidney. *Am J Physiol* 1998;275:F527–F534.

797. Terris J, et al. Long-term regulation of renal urea transporter protein expression in rat. *J Am Soc Nephrol* 1998;9:729–736.

798. Terris JM, Knepper MA, Wade JB. UT-A3: localization and characterization of an additional urea transporter isoform in the IMCD. *Am J Physiol Renal Physiol* 2001;280:F325–F332.

799. Teuscher NS, et al. Functional evidence for presence of PEPT2 in rat choroid plexus: studies with glycylsarcosine. *J Pharmacol Exp Ther* 2000;294:494–499.

800. Thorens B, et al. Liver glucose transporter: a basolateral protein in hepatocytes and intestine and kidney cells. *Am J Physiol* 1990;259:C279–C285.

801. Thorens B, Lodish HF, Brown D. Differential localization of two glucose transporter isoforms in rat kidney. *Am J Physiol* 1990;259:C286–C294.

802. Thwaites DT, Stevens BC. H+-zwitterionic amino acid symport at the brush-border membrane of human intestinal epithelial (CACO-2) cells. *Exp Physiol* 1999;84:275–284.

803. Tirona RG, et al. Polymorphisms in OATP-C: identification of multiple allelic variants associated with altered transport activity among European- and African-Americans. *J Biol Chem* 2001;276:35669–35675.

804. Tokuhiro S, et al. An intronic SNP in a RUNX1 binding site of SLC22A4, encoding an organic cation transporter, is associated with rheumatoid arthritis. *Nat Genet* 2003;35:341–348.
805. Torp R, et al. Differential expression of two glial glutamate transporters in the rat brain: an in situ hybridization study. *Eur J Neurosci* 1994;6:936–942.
806. Torrents D, et al. Identification and characterization of a membrane protein (y+L amino acid transporter-1) that associates with 4F2hc to encode the amino acid transport activity y+L. A candidate gene for lysinuric protein intolerance. *J Biol Chem* 1998;273:32437–32445.
807. Torrents D, et al. Identification of SLC7A7, encoding y+LAT-1, as the lysinuric protein intolerance gene. *Nat Genet* 1999;21:293–296.
808. Trippett TM, et al. Localization of a human reduced folate carrier protein in the mitochondrial as well as the cell membrane of leukemia cells. *Cancer Res* 2001;61:1941–1947.
809. Tsoi M, et al. Molecular cloning of a novel potassium-dependent sodium–calcium exchanger from rat brain. *J Biol Chem* 1998;273:4155–4162.
810. Tsuganezawa H, et al. A new member of the HCO3(-) transporter superfamily is an apical anion exchanger of beta-intercalated cells in the kidney. *J Biol Chem* 2001;276:8180–8189.
811. Tsukaguchi H, et al. Urea transporters in kidney: molecular analysis and contribution to the urinary concentrating process. *Am J Physiol* 1998;275:F319–F324.
812. Tsukaguchi H, et al. Cloning and characterization of the urea transporter UT3: localization in rat kidney and testis. *J Clin Invest* 1997;99:1506–1515.
813. Deleted in proof.
814. Tsukaguchi H, et al. A family of mammalian Na^+-dependent L-ascorbic acid transporters. *Nature* 1999;399:70–75.
815. Tucker JE, et al. cDNA cloning of the human retinal rod Na-Ca + K exchanger: comparison with a revised bovine sequence. *Invest Ophthalmol Vis Sci* 1998;39:435–440.
816. Turk E, Wright EM. Membrane topology motifs in the SGLT cotransporter family. *J Membr Biol* 1997;159:1–20.
817. Uchida S, et al. Molecular cloning of the cDNA for an MDCK cell Na(+)- and Cl(−)-dependent taurine transporter that is regulated by hypertonicity *Proc Natl Acad Sci U S A* 1993;90:7424 (erratum). *Proc Natl Acad U S A* 1992;89:8230–8234.
818. Ugele B, et al. Characterization and identification of steroid sulfate transporters of human placenta. *Am J Physiol Endocrinol Metab* 2003;284:E390–E398.
819. Uhl G R, et al. The VMAT2 gene in mice and humans: amphetamine responses, locomotion, cardiac arrhythmias, aging, and vulnerability to dopaminergic toxins. *FASEB J* 2000;14: 2459–2465.
820. Uldry M, et al. Identification of a mammalian H(+)-myo-inositol symporter expressed predominantly in the brain. *EMBO J* 2001; 20:4467–4477.
821. Utsunomiya-Tate N, Endou H, Kanai Y. Cloning and functional characterization of a system ASC-like Na^+-dependent neutral amino acid transporter. *J Biol Chem* 1996;271:14883–14890.
822. van Adelsberg JS, Edwards JC, al-Awqati Q. The apical Cl/HCO3 exchanger of beta intercalated cells. *J Biol Chem* 1993;268:11283–11289.
823. van den Heuvel LP, et al. Autosomal recessive renal glucosuria attributable to a mutation in the sodium glucose cotransporter (SGLT2). *Hum Genet* 2002;111:544–547.
824. Van Winkle LJ. Amino acid transport regulation and early embryo development. *Biol Reprod* 2001;64:1–12.
825. van Zeijl M, et al. A human amphotropic retrovirus receptor is a second member of the gibbon ape leukemia virus receptor family. *Proc Natl Acad U S A* 1994;91:1168–1172.
826. Vardi N, et al. Evidence that different cation chloride cotransporters in retinal neurons allow opposite responses to GABA. *J Neurosci* 2000;20:7657–7663.
827. Vargas-Poussou R, et al. Novel molecular variants of the Na-K-2Cl cotransporter gene are responsible for antenatal Bartter syndrome. *Am J Hum Genet* 1998;62:1332–1340.
828. Varoqui H, et al. Cloning and functional identification of a neuronal glutamine transporter. *J Biol Chem* 2000;275:4049–4054.
829. Verheijen FW, et al. A new gene, encoding an anion transporter, is mutated in sialic acid storage diseases. *Nat Genet* 1999;23:462–465.
830. Verlander JW, et al. Localization of the ammonium transporter proteins RhBG and RhCG in mouse kidney. *Am J Physiol Renal Physiol* 2003;284:F323–F337.
831. Vialou V, et al. Organic cation transporter 3 (Slc22a3) is implicated in salt-intake regulation. *J Neurosci* 2004;24:2846–2851.
832. Vidal S, Gros P, Skamene E. Natural resistance to infection with intracellular parasites: molecular genetics identifies Nramp1 as the Bcg/Ity/Lsh locus. *J Leukoc Biol* 1995;58: 382–390.
833. Vidal SM, et al. Natural resistance to infection with intracellular parasites: isolation of a candidate for Bcg. *Cell* 1993;73:469–485.
834. Vidal-Puig A, et al. UCP3: an uncoupling protein homologue expressed preferentially and abundantly in skeletal muscle and brown adipose tissue. *Biochem Biophys Res Commun* 1997;235:79–82.
835. Vince JW, Reithmeier RA. Carbonic anhydrase II binds to the carboxyl terminus of human band 3, the erythrocyte C1-/HCO_3^- exchanger. *J Biol Chem* 1998;273:28430–28437.
836. Vincourt JB, et al. Molecular and functional characterization of SLC26A11, a sodium-independent sulfate transporter from high endothelial venules. *FASEB J* 2003;17:890–892.
837. Virkki LV, et al. Functional characterization of human NBC4 as an electrogenic Na+-HCO cotransporter (NBCe2). *Am J Physiol Cell Physiol* 2002;282:C1278–C1289.
838. Visser WF, et al. Identification of human PMP34 as a peroxisomal ATP transporter. *Biochem Biophys Res Commun* 2002;299:494–497.
839. Vu TQ, Payne JA, Copenhagen DR. Localization and developmental expression patterns of the neuronal K-Cl cotransporter (KCC2) in the rat retina. *J Neurosci* 2000;20:1414–1423.
840. Vulpe C, Gitschier J. Ironing out anaemia. *Nat Genet* 1997;16:319–320.
841. Vulpe CD, et al. Hephaestin, a ceruloplasmin homologue implicated in intestinal iron transport, is defective in the sla mouse. *Nat Genet* 1999;21:195–199.
842. Wabakken T, et al. The human solute carrier SLC41A1 belongs to a novel eukaryotic subfamily with homology to prokaryotic MgtE Mg2+ transporters. *Biochem Biophys Res Commun* 2003;306:718–724.
843. Wadiche JI, Amara SG, Kavanaugh MP. Ion fluxes associated with excitatory amino acid transport. *Neuron* 1995;15:721–728.
844. Wadiche JI, et al. Kinetics of a human glutamate transporter. *Neuron* 1995;14:1019–1027.
845. Waheed A, et al. Association of HFE protein with transferrin receptor in crypt enterocytes of human duodenum. *Proc Natl Acad Sci U S A* 1999;96:1579–1584.
846. Waldegger S, et al. Cloning and characterization of SLC26A6, a novel member of the solute carrier 26 gene family. *Genomics* 2001;72:43–50.
847. Wallace DF, et al. Novel mutation in ferroportin1 is associated with autosomal dominant hemochromatosis. *Blood* 2002;100:692–694.
848. Wang CZ, et al. The Na^+-driven Cl-/HCO_3^- exchanger: cloning, tissue distribution, and functional characterization. *J Biol Chem* 2000;275:35486–35490.
849. Wang DS, et al. Involvement of organic cation transporter 1 in hepatic and intestinal distribution of metformin. *J Pharmacol Exp Ther* 2002;302:510–515.
850. Wang F, et al. The mammalian Zip5 protein is a zinc transporter that localizes to the basolateral surface of polarized cells. *J Biol Chem* 2004;279:51433–51441.
851. Wang H, et al. Structure, function, and genomic organization of human Na(+)-dependent high-affinity dicarboxylate transporter. *Am J Physiol Cell Physiol* 2000;278:C1019–C1030.
852. Wang H, et al. Cloning and functional expression of ATA1, a subtype of amino acid transporter A, from human placenta. *Biochem Biophys Res Commun* 2000;273:1175–1179.
853. Wang J, et al. Na(+)-dependent purine nucleoside transporter from human kidney: cloning and functional characterization. *Am J Physiol* 1997;273:F1058–F1065.
854. Wang K, et al. A novel member of a zinc transporter family is defective in acrodermatitis enteropathica. *Am J Hum Genet* 2002;71:66–73.
855. Wang T, et al. Mechanisms of stimulation of proximal tubule chloride transport by formate and oxalate. *Am J Physiol* 1996;271:446–550.
856. Wang T, et al. Essential role of NHE3 in facilitating formate-dependent NaCl absorption in the proximal tubule. *Am J Physiol Renal Physiol* 2001;281:288–292.
857. Wang Y, et al. Localization of the murine reduced folate carrier as assessed by immunohistochemical analysis. *Biochim Biophys Acta* 2001;1513:49–54.
858. Wang YM, et al. Knockout of the vesicular monoamine transporter 2 gene results in neonatal death and supersensitivity to cocaine and amphetamine. *Neuron* 1997;19:1285–1296.
859. Wang Z, et al. Identification of an apical Cl(-)/HCO3(-) exchanger in the small intestine. *Am J Physiol Gastrointest Liver Physiol* 2002;282:G573–G579.
860. Wang Z, et al. Renal and intestinal transport defects in Slc26a6-null mice. *Am J Physiol Cell Physiol* 2005;288:C957–C965.
861. Wasnich R, et al. Effect of thiazide on rates of bone mineral loss: a longitudinal study. *BMJ* 1990;301:1303–1305.
862. Watase K, et al. Motor discoordination and increased susceptibility to cerebellar injury in GLAST mutant mice. *Eur J Neurosci* 1998;10:976–988.
863. Weber FE, et al. Molecular cloning of a peroxisomal Ca2+-dependent member of the mitochondrial carrier superfamily. *Proc Natl Acad Sci U S A* 1997;94:8509–8514.
864. Weiner ID, Miller RT, Verlander JW. Localization of the ammonium transporters, Rh B glycoprotein and Rh C glycoprotein, in the mouse liver. *Gastroenterology* 2003;124: 1432–1440.
865. Weinman EJ, Steplock D, Shenolikar S. Acute regulation of NHE3 by protein kinase A requires a multiprotein signal complex. *Kidney Int* 2001;60:450–44.
866. Weinman EJ, et al. Ezrin binding domain-deficient NHERF attenuates cAMP-mediated inhibition of Na(+)/H(+) exchange in OK cells. *Am J Physiol Renal Physiol* 2001;281:374–380.
867. Weiss SD, et al. Glutamine and glutamic acid uptake by rat renal brushborder membrane vesicles. *J Membr Biol* 1978;43:91–105.
868. Wells RG, Hediger MA. Cloning of a rat kidney cDNA that stimulates dibasic and neutral amino acid transport and has sequence similarity to glucosidases. *Proc Natl Acad U S A* 1992; 89:5596–5600.
869. Wells RG, et al. The 4F2 antigen heavy chain induces uptake of neutral and dibasic amino acids in *Xenopus* oocytes. *J Biol Chem* 1992;267:15285–15288.
870. Wenzel HJ, et al. Ultrastructural localization of zinc transporter-3 (ZnT-3) to synaptic vesicle membranes within mossy fiber boutons in the hippocampus of mouse and monkey. *Proc Natl Acad Sci U S A* 1997;94:12676–12681.
871. Werner A, et al. Cloning and expression of cDNA for a Na/Pi cotransport system of kidney cortex. *Proc Natl Acad U S A* 1991;88:9608–9612.
872. Westergaard N, et al. Uptake, release, and metabolism of alanine in neurons and astrocytes in primary cultures. *J Neurosci Res* 1993;35:540–445.
873. Westhoff CM, et al. Identification of the erythrocyte Rh blood group glycoprotein as a mammalian ammonium transporter. *J Biol Chem* 2002;277:12499–12502.
874. Williams FM, Flintoff WF. Isolation of a human cDNA that complements a mutant hamster cell defective in methotrexate uptake. *J Biol Chem* 1995;270:2987–2992.
875. Wilson CA, et al. The dual-function hamster receptor for amphotropic murine leukemia virus (MuLV), 10A1 MuLV, and gibbon ape leukemia virus is a phosphate symporter. *J Virol* 1995;69:534–537.
876. Wolff NA, et al. Express ion cloning and characterization of a renal organic anion transporter from winter flounder. *FEBS Lett* 1997; 417:287–291.
877. Wong MH, Oelkers P, Dawson PA. Identification of a mutation in the ileal sodium-dependent bile acid transporter gene that abolishes transport activity. *J Biol Chem* 1995;270:27228–27234.
878. Wong SC, et al. Isolation of human cDNAs that restore methotrexate sensitivity and reduced folate carrier activity in methotrexate transport-defective Chinese hamster ovary cells. *J Biol Chem* 1995; 270:17468–17475.
879. Woo NS, et al. Hyperexcitability and epilepsy associated with disruption of the mouse neuronal-specific K-Cl cotransporter gene. *Hippocampus* 2002;12:258–268.
880. Wreden CC, et al. The H+-coupled electrogenic lysosomal amino acid transporter LYAAT1 localizes to the axon and plasma membrane of hippocampal neurons. *J Neurosci* 2003;23:1265–1275.
881. Wright EM. Renal Na(+)-glucose cotransporters. *Am J Physiol Renal Physiol* 2001;280: F10–F18.

882. Wright EM, et al. Intestinal sugar transport. In: Johnson LR, ed. *Physiology of Gastrointestinal Tract.* 3rd ed. New York: Raven Press, 1994: 1751–1772.

883. Wu X, Freeze HH. GLUT14, a duplicon of GLUT3, is specifically expressed in testis as alternative splice forms. *Genomics* 2002;80:553–557.

884. Wu X, et al. Structural and functional characteristics and tissue distribution pattern of rat OCTN1, an organic cation transporter, cloned from placenta. *Biochim Biophys Acta* 2000; 1466:315–327.

885. Wu X, et al. Cloning and characterization of glucose transporter 11, a novel sugar transporter that is alternatively spliced in various tissues. *Mol Genet Metab* 2002;76:37–45.

886. Xie Q, et al. Molecular characterization of the murine Slc26a6 anion exchanger: functional comparison with Slc26a1. *Am J Physiol Renal Physiol* 2002;283:F826–F838.

887. Xu H, et al. Molecular cloning, functional characterization, tissue distribution, and chromosomal localization of a human, small intestinal sodium- phosphate (Na$^+$-Pi) transporter (SLC34A2). *Genomics* 1999;62:281–284.

888. Xu H, et al. Age-dependent regulation of rat intestinal type IIb sodium-phosphate cotransporter by 1,25-(OH)(2) vitamin D(3). *Am J Physiol Cell Physiol* 2002;282:C487–C493.

889. Xu H, et al. Regulation of the human sodium-phosphate cotransporter NaP(i)-IIb gene promoter by epidermal growth factor. *Am J Physiol Cell Physiol* 2001;280:C628–C636.

890. Xu J, et al. SLC26A9 is expressed in gastric surface epithelial cells, mediates Cl-/HCO$_3^-$ exchange, and is inhibited by NH4+. *Am J Physiol Cell Physiol* 2005;289:C493–C505.

891. Xu J, et al. Expression of the Na$^+$-HCO$_3^-$ cotransporter NBC4 in rat kidney and characterization of a novel NBC4 variant. *Am J Physiol Renal Physiol* 2004;284:F41–F50.

892. Yabuuchi H, et al. Hepatic sinusoidal membrane transport of anionic drugs mediated by anion transporter Npt1. *J Pharmacol Exp Ther* 1998;286:1391–1396.

893. Yabuuchi H, et al. Novel membrane transporter OCTN1 mediates multispecific, bidirectional, and pH-dependent transport of organic cations. *J Pharmacol Exp Ther* 1999;289:768–773.

894. Yagita H, Masuko TT, Hashimoto Y. Inhibition of tumor cell growth in vitro by murine monoclonal antibodies that recognize a proliferation-associated cell surface antigen system in rats and humans. *Cancer Res* 1986;46:1478–1484.

895. Yamashita T, et al. Cloning and functional expression of a brain peptide/histidine transporter. *J Biol Chem* 1997;272:10205–10211.

896. Yamauchi A, et al. Cloning of a Na(+)- and Cl($^-$)-dependent betaine transporter that is regulated by hypertonicity. *J Biol Chem* 1992;267:649–652.

897. Yang B, et al. Urea-selective concentrating defect in transgenic mice lacking urea transporter UT-B. *J Biol Chem* 2002;277:10633–10637.

898. Yang-Feng TL, et al. Assignment of the human folate transporter gene to chromosome 21q22 by somatic cell hybrid analysis and in situ hybridization. *Biochem Biophys Res Commun* 1995;210:874–879.

899. Yao D, et al. A novel system A isoform mediating Na$^+$/neutral amino acid cotransport. *J Biol Chem* 2000;275:22790–22797.

900. Yao H, et al. Intracellular pH regulation of CA1 neurons in Na(+)/H(+) isoform 1 mutant mice. *J Clin Invest* 1999;104:637–645.

901. Yao SY, et al. Molecular cloning and functional characterization of nitrobenzylthioinosine (NBMPR)-sensitive (es) and NBMPR-insensitive (ei) equilibrative nucleoside transporter proteins (rENT1 and rENT2) from rat tissues. *J Biol Chem* 1997;272:28423–28430.

902. Deleted in proof.

903. Yao SY, et al. Transport of antiviral 3'-deoxy-nucleoside drugs by recombinant human and rat equilibrative, nitrobenzylthioinosine (NBMPR)-insensitive (ENT2) nucleoside transporter proteins produced in Xenopus oocytes. *Mol Membr Biol* 2001;18:161–167.

904. Yao SY, et al. Functional and molecular characterization of nucleobase transport by recombinant human and rat equilibrative nucleoside transporters 1 and 2. Chimeric constructs reveal a role for the ENT2 helix 5-6 region in nucleobase translocation. *J Biol Chem* 2002; 277:24938–24948.

905. Yernool D, et al. Structure of a glutamate transporter homologue from Pyrococcus horikoshii. *Nature* 2004;431:811–818.

906. You G, et al. Cloning and characterization of the vasopressin-regulated urea transporter. *Nature* 1993;365:844–847.

907. Yun CH, et al. cAMP-mediated inhibition of the epithelial brush border Na$^+$/H+ exchanger, NHE3, requires an associated regulatory protein. *Proc Natl Acad Sci U S A* 1997; 94:3010–3015.

908. Zerangue N, Kavanaugh MP. ASCT-1 is a neutral amino acid exchanger with chloride channel activity. *J Biol Chem* 1996;271:27991–27994.

909. Zhao R, et al. Rescue of embryonic lethality in reduced folate carrier-deficient mice by maternal folic acid supplementation reveals early neonatal failure of hematopoietic organs. *J Biol Chem* 2001;276:10224–10228.

910. Zheng J, et al. Prestin is the motor protein of cochlear outer hair cells. *Nature* 2000;405: 149–155.

911. Zhou B, Gitschier J. hCTR1: a human gene for copper uptake identified by complementation in yeast. *Proc Natl Acad Sci U S A* 1997; 94:7481–7486.

912. Zhu Y, et al. Genomic interval engineering of mice identifies a novel modulator of triglyceride production. *Proc Natl Acad Sci U S A* 2000;97:1137–1142.

913. Zoia C, et al. Glutamate transporters in platelets: EAAT1 decrease in aging and in Alzheimer's disease. *Neurobiol Aging* 2004;25:149–157.

914. Zwart R, et al. Impaired activity of the extraneuronal monoamine transporter system known as uptake-2 in Orct3/Slc22a3-deficient mice. *Mol Cell Biol* 2001;21:4188–4196.

CHAPTER **5**

Mechanisms of Water Transport Across Cell Membranes and Epithelia

Luis Reuss
Texas Tech University Health Sciences Center, Lubbock, Texas, USA

The main purpose of this chapter is to review the basic aspects of water transport mechanisms across cell membranes and epithelia. In the first section, I will discuss biophysical principles and definitions, with the aim of providing a theoretical framework useful for the analysis of experimental observations. In the second section, I will address general issues pertaining to water transport across cell membranes, focusing on intracellular water and the pathways and mechanism for osmotic water flow. In the third section, I discuss water transport by epithelia, focusing on pathways and mechanisms, in particular the role of solute–solvent coupling. I intend this chapter to serve as both an overview and an introduction to chapters covering specific aspects of water transport (Chapters 6, 9, 38, 40). The three sections of the chapter are to a certain extent independent from each other and can be studied separately.

The field of water transport across biological membranes has made a recent major transition with the discovery and characterization of the aquaporins. Aquaporins are integral membrane proteins, most of which are highly specific water pores and that are expressed in plants and animals, from bacteria to humans. The discovery of the aquaporins confirmed a long-held prediction for the existence of these pores, emanating from biophysical studies in red blood cells (79) and renal proximal tubules (122).

BASIC PRINCIPLES

This section is largely based on the excellent water transport treaty by Finkelstein (25). Other sources are House (47), Reuss and Cotton (88), Dawson (20), Hallows and Knauf (37), and Macey and Moura (66). Derivations of the equations can be found in Finkelstein (25). Deliberately, this section has been kept simple and qualitative explanations have been superimposed on a succinct quantitative analysis. The reason for this is to make these ideas accessible to readers with various backgrounds and tastes.

The main mechanism of *net water transport* in animal cells is osmosis, that is, net water flow driven by differences in water chemical potential, in turn dependent on differences in solute concentrations. Concerning water flow across a cell membrane, an important issue is whether water moves through the phospholipid bilayer and/or through specialized water-conducting pores. The mechanisms involved in water permeation via these two pathways constitute the main content of this first section. Hence, we start with osmosis.

Osmotic Equilibrium Is a Balance of Osmotic and Hydrostatic Forces

The principle of *osmotic equilibrium* can be illustrated by considering a simple system, that is, a semipermeable membrane separating two aqueous phases: pure water and a solution that contains a nondissociating solute (Fig. 1). The membrane is permeable to water and impermeable to the solute (hence the term *semipermeable*). At thermodynamic equilibrium the net water flow across the membrane is zero. (In the case of water, flow can be expressed in molar terms [moles of water per unit area and unit time] or volume terms [volume of water per unit area and unit time]. For conversion to volume flow, the molar flow must be multiplied by $\bar{V}_w$ (partial molar volume, a constant equal to 18 cm^3/mole].) This is the result of the equality of two forces: an osmotic force favoring water flow into the solution and an opposing hydrostatic force resulting, for instance, from the difference in height of the fluid compartments generated by the osmotic water flow. For dilute solutions, osmotic equilibrium is approximately described by Van't Hoff's law (110):

$$\Delta P = \pi = RTC_s \qquad (1)$$

where ΔP (atm) is the hydrostatic pressure difference between the two compartments ($P' - P''$), R (cm^3·atm·mol^{-1}·K^{-1}) and T [K] are the gas constant and the absolute temperature, respectively, C_s (mol·cm^{-3}) is the molar concentration of the solute, and π (atm) is the *osmotic pressure* of the solution. The latter is conveniently defined as the hydrostatic pressure in the solution compartment (relative to the pressure in the water compartment) needed to abolish water flow across the membrane.

When the semipermeable membrane separates two solutions, equilibrium is described by a slightly different equation:

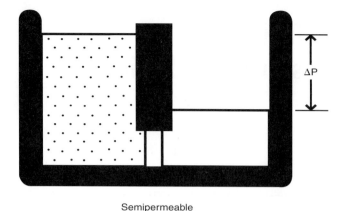

Semipermeable
membrane

FIGURE 1 Osmotic equilibrium. A semipermeable membrane (clear section of middle partition) separates two aqueous compartments: a solution containing impermeable solute (left) and pure water (right). If the heights of both compartments are initially equal, then water will flow from right to left until equilibrium is established. At equilibrium, the water flow across the membrane is zero, and is described by Eq. 1, that is, ΔP and πP cancel each other.

$\Delta P = \Delta \pi = RT\Delta C_s$, where $\Delta \pi$ is the difference in osmotic pressure ($\pi' - \pi''$) and ΔC_s is the solute concentration difference ($C_s' - C_s''$).

The osmotic pressure depends on the molar concentration (C_s) and on the degree of dissociation of the solute, that is, the number of particles that each molecule yields in solution (n). Ideally, the osmolality of a solution, in osmol/kg of water, is given by $Osm = nC_s$, where C_s is in mol·l^{-1}. However, the effect of solute on the activity of the solvent is generally nonideal, that is, it may depend on the nature of the solute. The correction term for this effect is the osmotic coefficient, ϕ_s, where the subscript denotes the solute. For physiological concentration ranges, the osmotic coefficient is closer to unity than the activity coefficient, but it can be significantly greater than 1 for macromolecules (37). For the sake of simplicity, the osmotic coefficient will be neglected in this discussion.

A 1-Osm solution at room temperature exerts an osmotic pressure of about 24.6 atm, which is equivalent to about 18,700 mm Hg. In a mammal, a 1% change in extracellular fluid osmolality ($\sim$3 mosmol/kg) is equivalent, as a driving force for water flow, to a hydrostatic pressure of 56 mm Hg. In animal cells, changes in osmolality cause large water fluxes across the plasma membrane, whereas hydrostatic pressure changes do not. Osmolality is a measure of concentration of particles, not of osmotic pressure, but it is frequently used to denote the latter.

The generation of ΔP in the presence of impermeant solute on one side can be explained (70) on the basis of changes in the water chemical potential (μ_w), which is given by:

$$\mu_w = \mu_w^o + RT \ln X_w + P\bar{V}_w \qquad (2)$$

where μ_w^o is the standard chemical potential, X_w is the water mole fraction (moles of water/[moles of water + moles of solute]), and $\bar{V}_w$ is the partial molar volume of water. A solute addition to one side (at constant total volume) reduces the water chemical potential in that side (μ_w') because the water is "diluted" by the solute (and X_w falls). The difference in water chemical potential thus generated ($\Delta\mu_w = \mu_w' - \mu_w''$) is the "driving force" for water flow toward the side of higher osmolality (and lower μ_w). If both compartments are open and of appropriate dimensions, then a ΔP will result from changes in height (Fig. 1). If a compartment is closed, then its pressure will change in proportion to the water flux, with a proportionality constant dependent on compliance of the compartment.

Osmotic Water Flows Across Lipid and Porous Membranes have Different Properties

Near equilibrium, the volume flow is linearly related to the driving force:

$$J_v = L_p (\Delta P - \Delta \pi) \qquad (3)$$

where J_v is the volume flow (volume·area^{-1}·time^{-1}), L_p is the *hydraulic permeability coefficient* of the membrane, and ΔP and $\Delta \pi$ are the differences in hydrostatic and osmotic pressure, respectively. The L_p can be expressed in cm·sec^{-1}·(osmol/kg)$^{-1}$. In most cases, a *filtration* (P_f) or *osmotic permeability coefficient* (P_{os}; $P_f = P_{os}$) is used instead of L_p. The P_{os} (cm·sec^{-1}) is related to L_p by $P_{os} = L_p RT / \bar{V}_w$.

The above discussion underscores the fact that ΔP and $\Delta \pi$ are equivalent as "driving forces" in causing osmotic water flow. The mechanism of this equivalence can be understood if one considers the nature of the membrane and the mechanism of osmotic water transport, as explained below.

Osmotic Water Flow across Lipid Membranes

Osmotic water flow across lipid membranes occurs by *solubility diffusion*. Water molecules move from one aqueous solution into the lipid and then into the other solution by independent, random motion. When $\Delta P = \Delta \pi$ (0 net driving force) there are two diffusive water fluxes of equal magnitude and opposite direction, with no net water flow across the membrane. In the presence of a net driving force ($\Delta P - \Delta \pi \neq 0$), a net flux arises. To examine the mechanism of water flow, let us consider the effects of ΔC_s and ΔP on the water chemical potential in the two compartments.

A net diffusive water flow requires a difference in water chemical potential across the membrane. In a homogeneous membrane, a steady flux denotes a constant chemical potential gradient throughout the membrane thickness. If there is a difference in osmotic pressure between the two solutions, then the water mole fractions (and therefore the water concentrations) at the two sides, *just inside* the membrane, must differ. It is commonly assumed that water transport across the membrane–solution interfaces is faster than water diffusion in the membrane itself. It follows that the water chemical potential just inside the membrane is very close to that in the adjacent layer of solution; therefore, water is near equilibrium across the interfaces. Finally, since μ_w is inversely related to C_s, a gradient of water concentration must exist across the membrane. This intramembrane gradient is the direct consequence of the differences in impermeant solute concentrations in the adjacent aqueous phases.

When $\Delta\pi = 0$, but $\Delta P \neq 0$, the chemical potentials of water in the two solutions differ (see Eq. 2). If $P' > P''$, then the water flux from side $'$ is greater than that from side $''$, creating an intramembrane gradient of water concentration and chemical potential.

The osmotic water permeability coefficient of a lipid membrane is given by:

$$P_{os} = \frac{D_w^m \beta_w \bar{V}_w}{\delta_m \bar{V}_{oil}} \qquad (4)$$

where D_w^m is the diffusion coefficient of water in the membrane, β_w is the partition coefficient of water in the membrane (oil/water), δ_w is the thickness of the membrane,

and $\bar{V}_{oil}$ is the partial molar volume of the membrane lipid.

OSMOTIC WATER FLOW ACROSS A POROUS MEMBRANE

Let us consider a membrane made of a rigid, water-impermeable material. The pore density (number of pores per unit area) is n. Each pore is a water-filled cylinder of length L and radius r, and cannot be penetrated by the solute. The mechanism of water flow in this situation depends on pore radius. In large pores there is viscous water flow that can be described by Newtonian mechanics. In pores of molecular dimensions there is no appropriate theoretical treatment, but if the pores are so small that there is single-file water transport (i.e., water molecules in the pore cannot slip past each other), then there is a surprisingly simple solution.

Large Pores In large pores water flow driven by a hydrostatic pressure is described by Poiseuille's law, which was derived for water flow in thin capillaries:

$$J_v = n\frac{(\Pi)r^4}{8L\eta}\Delta P \qquad (5)$$

where η is the water viscosity and Π denotes 3.1415... (do not confuse with π, which is osmotic pressure). This

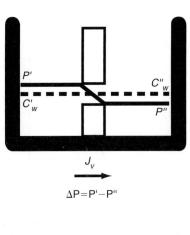

J_v

$\Delta P = P' - P''$

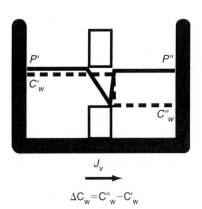

J_v

$\Delta C_w = C''_w - C'_w$

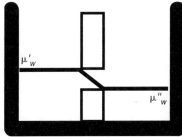

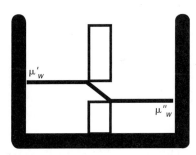

FIGURE 2 Water flow across a porous membrane. *Top left.* Driving force is a hydrostatic-pressure difference ($P' - P''$), continuous line. Same water concentrations on both side ($C'_w = C'_w$), segmented line. *Top right.* Driving force is a difference in osmotic pressure. Same pressures on both sides, but the water concentrations differ. *Bottom.* The steady-state water chemical potential gradients (μ_w, proportional to the sum of hydrostatic and osmotic pressure) are the same for both conditions. (Modified with permission from Reuss L. General principles of water transport. In: Seldin DW, Giebisch G, eds. *The Kidney: Physiology and Pathophysiology.* New York: Raven Press, 2000:321–340.)

law is valid for steady-state flow and neglects pore-access effects. Under these conditions, the pressure gradient along the pore (dP/dL) has a constant value (Fig. 2A). From Eq. 4 and the definition of P_{os}, the P_{os} for a membrane containing large homogeneous cylindrical pores is $n(\Pi)r^4RT/8L\eta \, \overline{V}_w$.

If the only driving force is osmotic, then the mechanism of water flow involves the development of a hydrostatic pressure gradient within the pore. Initially, the water concentrations in the pore and in the water-filled compartment are the same, but at the other interface the solution has lower water concentration than the pore. If water transport across the membrane interfaces is faster than within the membrane, then the water chemical potentials just inside the pore are equal to those in the adjacent solutions. At the pore end facing the water compartment there is no difference in hydrostatic pressure, but at the end facing the solution compartment the pressure inside the pore falls, because the lower water concentration in the solution elicits a water efflux from the pore. If $\Delta\mu_w$ is zero across the opening, then the difference in water concentration between solution and pore is exactly balanced by a drop in the pore pressure (70). In the steady state, the pressure gradient in the pore is constant (Fig. 2B).

The analysis presented above holds for pores of r equal to or greater than 15 nm (7). For pores smaller than 15 nm, several corrections have been attempted, but the underlying assumptions are questionable (25). Regardless of the lack of a satisfactory theory, it has been suggested that Poiseuille's law is a reasonable approximation for water diffusion and convection in small pores (61).

Single-File Pore The P_{os} of a single-file pore is given by (25, 26):

$$P_{os} = n\frac{\overline{v}_w kTN}{\gamma L^2} \tag{6}$$

where $\overline{V}_w$ is the volume of a water molecule, k is the Boltzmann constant (gas constant/molecule, equal to R/N_A where N_A is Avogadro's number), N is the number of water molecules inside the pore, and γ is the friction coefficient per water molecule. Assuming that the water densities in the pore and in the bulk solution are equal, and recalling that $kT/\gamma = D_w$:

$$P_{os} = n\frac{(\Pi)r^2 D_w}{L} \tag{7}$$

which is the result expected for osmotic water flow through a single-file pore if it can be described as a diffusive flux.

Comparison of Diffusion and Osmotic Permeability Coefficients Reveals Whether Water Permeates Lipid Bilayer or Pores

Now we consider a membrane exposed to solutions of identical composition, except that water is partially replaced with tracer water at a concentration C_w^* (Fig. 3). There are

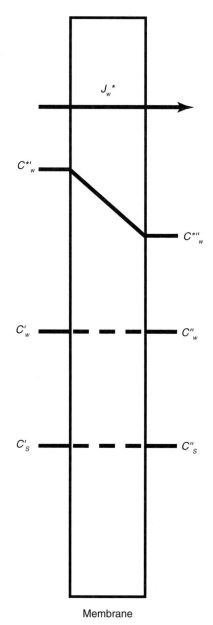

Membrane

FIGURE 3   Tracer water diffusion across a lipid membrane separating solutions of identical compositions ($C'w = C'w$, $C's = C's$, as shown by the two lines at the bottom). At the steady state (constant flux, J_w), the tracer concentration gradient in the membrane (second line from top) is also constant. Arbitrarily, the oil/water partition coefficient (β) of tracer water is 1.0. If β were smaller, the tracer water concentrations inside the membrane would be less than in the respective solutions. (Modified with permission from Reuss L. General principles of water transport. In: Seldin DW, Giebisch G, eds. *The Kidney: Physiology and Pathophysiology.* New York: Raven Press, 2000:321–340.)

no other differences in composition or pressure between the two compartments. Both contain solutions of infinite volume and ideally mixed (C_w^* at the membrane surface = C_w^* in the bulk). The tracer water flux is given by:

$$J_w^* = P_{dw}\Delta C_w^* \tag{8}$$

where P_{dw} is the diffusive water permeability coefficient and ΔC_w^* is the difference in concentration of tracer water

$(C_w^{*\prime} - C_w^{*\prime\prime})$. The cases of a lipid membrane and a porous membrane are discussed below.

LIPID MEMBRANE

The tracer-water flux is by solubility diffusion; hence:

$$P_{dw} = \frac{D_w^m \beta_w \bar{V}_w}{d\bar{V}_{oil}} \qquad (9)$$

This expression is identical to that for P_f (or P_{os}) for a lipid membrane (Eq. 7). Therefore, for a lipid membrane, $P_{os} = P_{dw}$.

POROUS MEMBRANE

If the pores obey Poiseuille's law, the diffusive water flux via the pores is:

$$J_w^* = \frac{n(\Pi)r^2 D_w}{L}\Delta C_w^* \qquad (10)$$

where the pore cross-sectional area $[n(\Pi)r^2]$ is available for water diffusion and is the water self-diffusion coefficient (tracer water traverses the membrane via the aqueous pores). P_{dw} is $n(\Pi)r^2 D_w/L$. Hence, the ratio between and for a porous membrane is:

$$P_{os}/P_{dw} = \frac{RT}{8\eta D_w \bar{V}_w}r^2 + 1 \qquad (11)$$

where the second term on the right (= 1) denotes the diffusive water flow via the pores. The equivalent pore radius can be estimated from the experimental values of and using Eq. 11; at 25°C, the value of $[RT/(8\eta D_w \bar{V}_w)]$ is 8.04×10^{-14} cm^{-2}.

For single-file pores, the diffusive water flux is $J_w^* = nP_{dw}\Delta n^*$, where Δn^* is the tracer-water concentration difference (molecules per unit volume). P_{dw} is given by:

$$P_{dw} = \frac{n\bar{v}_w kT}{dL^2} \qquad (12)$$

and the ratio P_{os}/P_{dw}, from Eqs. 6 and 12, equals the number of water molecules in the pore: $P_{os}/P_{dw} = N$.

Water movement in single-file pores is not independent of the movement of neighboring water molecules: For a tracer molecule to cross the pore, other water molecules must cross as well.

Unstirred Layers Are a Major Source of Artifacts in Water Permeability Measurements

Unstirred layers are static layers of fluid at membrane-solution interfaces, that is, they are not mixed by convection. Unstirred-layer solute concentrations are entirely determined by diffusion, can differ from that of the bulk solutions, and are position dependent. Unstirred layers introduce errors in the experimental determination of P_{dw} and P_{os}.

These errors can lead to incorrect conclusions about the existence of aqueous pores. For an excellent treatment of unstirred layers, see Barry and Diamond (6).

UNSTIRRED-LAYER EFFECTS ON MEASUREMENT OF P_{DW}

In the system illustrated in Fig. 4, tracer water encounters three barriers to diffusion between the two solutions, namely the membrane and the two unstirred layers (of width δ_1 and δ_2, respectively). These three barriers are in series. The *observed* (experimentally determined) diffusive water permeability of the system differs from the true diffusive water permeability of the membrane (P_{dw}) according to:

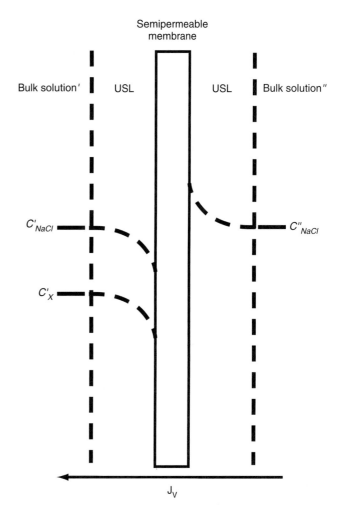

FIGURE 4 Unstirred-layer effects on the measurement of $P_{os} \cdot C_{NaCl}$ and C_x, concentrations of NaCl and the osmotic solute, respectively. Both are assumed impermeant for simplicity. The osmotic water flow ($J_w = J_v$) "dilutes" both solutes on the hyperosmotic side (solution′) and "concentrates" the NaCl on the hyposmotic side (solution″). The net result is a reduction in the concentration gradient of the osmotic solute (reduced ΔC_x), and the creation of an opposing ΔC_{NaCl} at the membrane boundaries. Hence, the driving force for J_v is diminished. (Modified with permission from Reuss L. General principles of water transport. In: Seldin DW, Giebisch G, eds. *The Kidney: Physiology and Pathophysiology.* New York: Raven Press, 2000:321–340.)

$$\frac{1}{P_{dw}^o} = \frac{1}{P_{dw}} + \frac{1}{D_w/\delta_1} + \frac{1}{D_w/\delta_2} \qquad (13)$$

where P_{dw}^o is the observed value. Inasmuch as D_w has a finite value, P_{dw} and P_{dw}^o are equal only when $\delta_1 = \delta_2 = 0$. For typical permeability and unstirred-layer-thickness values, P_{dw} can be easily underestimated by 50% or more.

UNSTIRRED-LAYER EFFECTS ON THE MEASUREMENT OF P_{OS}

In the experiment depicted in Fig. 5, a semipermeable membrane separates equal NaCl solutions; then, a second solute is added to one side ($C'_s > C''_s$, eliciting osmotic water flow. The NaCl concentration in the unstirred layers

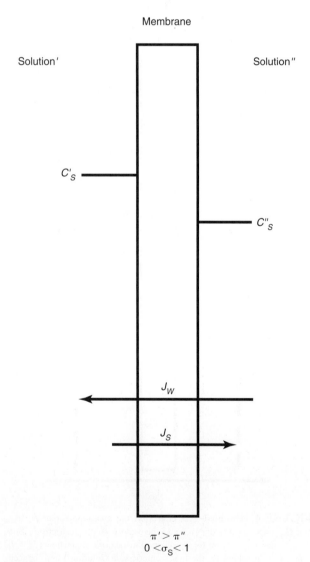

FIGURE 5 Volume flow (J_v) between solutions containing different concentrations of a permeant solute ($0 < \sigma_s < 1$). C_s is the solute concentration. J_v is the difference between the net water flow (J_w) to the left, and the net solute flow (J_s) to the right (i.e., $J_v = J_w - J_s$). (Modified with permission from Reuss L. General principles of water transport. In: Seldin DW, Giebisch G, eds. *The Kidney: Physiology and Pathophysiology.* New York: Raven Press, 2000:321–340.)

changes because of the water flow, rising in the right side and falling in the left side, relative to the bulk-solution concentrations. The added solute qualitatively behaves like the NaCl present on the same side. Water flow tends to accentuate the changes described, whereas solute diffusion in the solution has the opposite effect. At the steady state, the effects of osmotic water flow and solute diffusion balance each other and the unstirred-layer concentration profiles remain constant. At the surface of the membrane:

$$C_m = C_b \exp\left(\pm v\delta/D_s\right) \qquad (14)$$

where the sign of the exponent is $(-)$ for the left ("diluted") side and $(+)$ for the right ("concentrated") side, and denote solute concentrations (membrane surface and bulk solution, respectively), v is the water flow velocity (normal to the membrane), and D_s is the solute diffusion coefficient in water.

The ratio between P_{os}^o (observed value) and P_{os} (true value) is $-v\delta/D_s$, that is, the magnitude of the error in estimating P_{os} is directly proportional to v and inversely proportional to D_s. In planar membranes, for small v (low water flux and flow velocity) the exponential term approaches 1. In folded membranes, where there can be water "funneling" (microvilli, lateral intercellular spaces), v can be much larger than in a planar membrane and can be seriously underestimated (6).

The above analysis is limited to the effect of J_v on impermeant solute concentration. If permeant solutes are present as well, they must be considered, making the analysis more complex (6).

Solute Reflection Coefficients Denote Effective Osmolality of a Solution vis-à-vis a Membrane

The situation is more complicated than the preceding analysis if the solute is permeant (Fig. 6). In this case, J_v will be described by:

$$J_v = L_p(\Delta P - \sigma_s\Delta\pi) \qquad (15)$$

where σ_s is the reflection coefficient of the solute. If $\sigma_s < 1$, then J_v will be less than if the same osmotic gradient is elicited with an impermeable solute. The value of σ_s is specific for each combination of membrane and solute, and depends on both permeabilities and partial molar volumes of water and solute (see below). In general, the value of σ_s varies between 0 (solute as permeable as water) and 1 (solute impermeable).

LIPID MEMBRANE

It can be shown that the solute reflection coefficient of a lipid membrane is (25):

$$\sigma_s = 1 - \frac{P_{ds}\bar{V}_s}{P_{dw}\bar{V}_w} \qquad (16)$$

As expected, $\sigma_s = 1$ when $P_{ds} = 0$, $\sigma_s = 0$ when $P_{ds}V_s = P_{dw}V_w$, and $\sigma_s < 0$ when $P_{ds}V_s > P_{dw}V_w$. In other words, σ_s de-

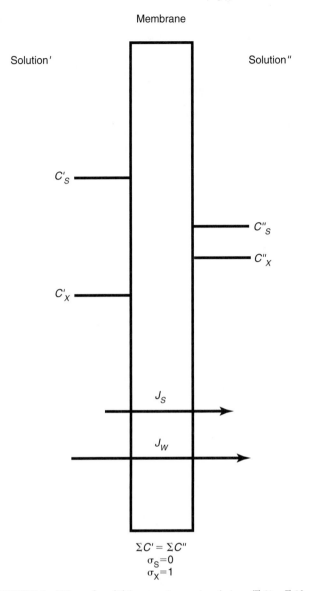

$$\Sigma C' = \Sigma C''$$
$$\sigma_S = 0$$
$$\sigma_X = 1$$

FIGURE 6   Volume flow (J_v) between isosmotic solutions ($\Sigma C' = \Sigma C''$). Solutes s and x have of the same magnitude and opposite direction. Since the reflection coefficients differ, the effective osmolalities also differ, and there is a net J_v toward the side containing impermeant solute (i.e., $J_v = J_w + J_s$). (Modified with permission from Reuss L. General principles of water transport. In: Seldin DW, Giebisch G, eds. *The Kidney: Physiology and Pathophysiology.* New York: Raven Press, 2000:321–340.)

pends on the solute permeability and partial molar volume compared with those of water. If the products are the same for solute and water, then the reflection coefficient is zero: solute addition to one side causes no transmembrane volume flow because the water flux toward the solute is of the same magnitude as the solute flux in the opposite direction. A solute with a negative σ_s will elicit a net volume flow in the opposite direction to the water flow ("negative osmosis") (25).

PROUS MEMBRANE

For a quantitative analysis of this complicated problem, see Anderson and Malone (3) and Finkelstein (25). For

large pores and solute particles larger than water particles, the solute is excluded from the periphery of the pore, that is, from a region slightly wider than the solute radius. In the pore axis, C_s is maximum (equal to the concentration in the bulk solution) and C_w is less than at the pore periphery (where the solute is excluded). This generates a radial water concentration gradient within the pore. At equilibrium, this gradient is balanced by a fall in hydrostatic pressure in the periphery of the pore (see Eq. 4). In addition, there is a solute concentration gradient along the pore length, because of the transmembrane difference in C_s. These two gradients combine to generate a longitudinal hydrostatic pressure gradient along the pore's periphery, which causes water flow toward the high-concentration side. The thickness of the ring subjected to this regime is directly proportional to the molecular size of the solute. When the solute is so large that it cannot enter the pore, J_v is maximum and $\sigma_s = 1$. When the solute has the same size as water, its distribution within the pore is identical to that of water, no pressure gradient develops, the water and solute net fluxes are purely diffusive and of equal magnitude and opposite direction, and $J_v = 0$. When the solute is smaller than water, J_v is in the same direction as J_s, because water is now excluded from the periphery of the pore, and the pressure gradient within the pore drives solute in the opposite direction.

We consider now the case of single-file pores; the solution is dilute enough so that the number of solute molecules inside a pore can be only 0 or 1. Two pore populations will exist at any given time: pores containing water only, through which there is water flow toward the high-C_s side, and pores containing solute, in which solute and water are transported toward the low-C_s side by single file diffusion. When both water and solute permeation are single file, σ_s is (25, 62):

$$\sigma_s = 1 - \frac{P_{ds}\bar{V}_p^s}{P_{dw}\bar{V}_p} \qquad (17)$$

where $\bar{V}_p$ denotes pore molar volume, solute-containing (superscript s) and solute-free (no superscript). Compare with Eq. 16.

In a system with more than one solute there can be net water and/or volume flows between solutions with the same total solute concentrations (and osmolalities). This will occur if the specific C_s values on the two sides of the membrane and the reflection coefficients differ. As shown in Fig. 6, if, $\Delta C_s = -\Delta C_x$, $\sigma_s = 0$, and $\sigma_x = 1$, then there will be a net volume flow towards the right, although the solutions have equal total osmolalities. If the hydrostatic pressures are the same on both sides, then $J_v = L_p RT (\sigma_x \Delta C_x - \sigma_s \Delta C_s)$. Expressions such as σRTC denote "effective osmolality," in contrast with the "total osmolality" given by RTC. Effective osmolality is also referred to as *tonicity*. In epithelia, active transepithelial solute transport can generate asymmetries in the composition of the adjacent solutions. These asymmetries may in principle drive net water transport without differences in the total osmolalities of the bulk solutions, because of differences in the solute reflection coefficients.

Solvent Drag Can Account for Uphill Solute Transport

When there is net water flow (filtration and/or osmosis) across a porous membrane and a pore-permeant solute is present, there is a solute flux in the same direction as the water flow. This flux reflects water-solute frictional interaction within the pores. In the case of large pores, if $C_s' = C_s'' = C_s$, and J_v is elicited by a hydrostatic pressure gradient or an asymmetrical addition of impermeant solute, the solute flux due to solvent drag is given by:

$$J_s = J_v C_s (1 - \sigma_s) \qquad (18)$$

Uphill solute transport (i.e., transport in the absence of or against the prevailing electrochemical gradient) can be demonstrated, which is always in the same direction as the water flow. The energy is provided by the water flow and conveyed to the solute by frictional interaction.

Demonstration of solvent drag is in principle a clear-cut argument for the existence of pores in membranes. However, many such demonstrations have been proven to be experimental artifacts. If there are unstirred layers, J_v will produce changes in solute concentrations at the membrane-solution interfaces; if the membrane is permeable to the solute, then a diffusive solute flux will occur (see Eq. 14). This phenomenon is called "pseudo-solvent drag" (6). Putative demonstrations of pore-mediated water transport based on the observation of "solvent drag" must consider this possibility.

WATER TRANSPORT ACROSS THE CELL MEMBRANE

In this section I will first address some general issues pertinent to intracellular water and then discuss in some detail the pathways and mechanisms for water transport across the cell membrane. Cell volume regulation is the subject of Chapter 6 and will not be addressed here.

Intracellular Water Behaves Similar to Free Solution

The best direct assessment of the state of intracellular water was obtained from nuclear magnetic resonance (NMR) studies, which indicate that only a small fraction of cell water (~5%) behaves as if it were immobilized (99). However, indirect arguments suggest that this may be an underestimation (37). A related issue is whether the cytosol is a near-ideal aqueous solution or a gel, as suggested by numerous observations (60). If this is the case, its higher viscosity may have a strong effect on enzymatic rates and on the dependence of enzymatic activities on the total concentration of macromolecules (macromolecular crowd-

ing) (74). In any event, the behavior of water fluxes in cells supports the idea that most of the intracellular water behaves as in free solution.

The Osmotic Behavior of Cells Is Not Ideal

Consider a cell at steady state (constant volume) in suspension; then, the external concentration of an impermeant solute (and hence the external osmolality) are suddenly changed. If the cell is permeable to water, then water will flow until its osmolality becomes equal to the new medium osmolality. Numerically, $V_0 \cdot \pi_0' = V_t \cdot \pi_t'$, where V is cell water volume and π' is total solute concentration (or osmolality), and the subscripts 0 and t denote steady-state values before and after the solution change. The above equation assumes that there is no change in the amount of cell solute between 0 and t, and defines ideal ("osmometric") behavior of cells. However, not all cells behave ideally. Nonideal behavior can result from loss or gain of solute between times 0 and t (e.g., some cell solutes are permeable) or from changes in the osmotic coefficient of intracellular solute(s) secondary to the water flux. This appears to be the case in red blood cells, because of concentration dependence of the osmotic coefficient of hemoglobin. This and other issues relevant to nonideal osmotic behavior of cells have been discussed by Hallows and Knauf (37).

Another important point in quantifying cell volume changes in response to alterations in extracellular osmolality is the fact that although most of the cell volume is solvent water ("osmotically sensitive"), a fraction is nonsolvent volume (also referred to as "solids"). If one considers this factor, then the above equation becomes:

$$(V_0 - b)\pi_0' = (V_t - b)\pi_t' \qquad (19)$$

where b is the nonsolvent volume. This is a modified form of the Boyle-Van't Hoff equation, and is very useful to interpret changes in cell volume. The plot of Eq. 19 is shown in Fig. 7.

In experimental osmotic studies, the behavior of cells or membrane vesicles may not be linear for the reasons given above. For instance, if the amount of cell solute changes during the experiment, then the slope will not be a constant.

Net Water Transport Across Membranes of Animal Cells Is Osmotic

In plant cells, which have rigid walls, the intracellular hydrostatic pressure can vary over a considerable range. In animal cells, which have compliant plasma membranes, hydrostatic pressure differences are small. In contrast, small differences in concentration of impermeable or low-permeability solutes across the cell membrane can result in sizable water flows by osmotic mechanisms. The water flow under these conditions can be via the phospholipid bilayer (solubility diffusion, driven by the difference in

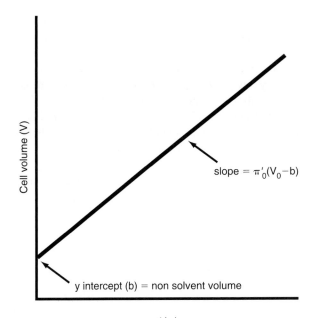

FIGURE 7 Boyle–Van't Hoff plot for a theoretical cell. The equation plotted is $V = (1/\pi')[\pi_0(V_0 - b)] + b$ (see Eq. 19). The y-axis intercept is b, the nonsolvent volume, and the slope is $)[\pi_0(V_0 - b)$, that is, the amount of water-dissolved solutes in the cell. (Copyright 1994 by CRC Press, Inc. From Hallows KR, Knauf PA. *Principles of Cell Volume Regulation.* Boca Raton FL: CRC Press, 1994. Reproduced with permission of Routledge/ Taylor & Francis Group, LLC.)

water chemical potential across the membrane) or via pores, driven by a hydrostatic pressure gradient inside the pore. This pressure gradient is caused by the difference between the water chemical potentials inside the pore and in the external solution (see Fig. 2). It is generally assumed that under steady-state conditions in vivo, the osmolalities of the intracellular and extracellular compartments are equal. There is some experimental evidence supporting this (69), but based on rather indirect estimations of intracellular osmolality. Also, it has been argued that, in order to balance a 1-mosmol/kg difference in osmolality (cell higher), the cell hydrostatic pressure would have to be ~19 mm Hg higher than the extracellular pressure, something that a soft-tissue cell membrane is extremely unlikely to support (68). However, mechanical support of the cell membrane by the cytoskeleton and/or the exoskeleton may allow for the maintenance of transmembrane hydrostatic pressure gradients (37). Strictly speaking, this issue is unresolved, but it is unlikely that in the steady state large gradients of osmotic or hydrostatic pressure exist across plasma membranes.

Quantitative treatment of water transport across the plasma membrane usually involves another assumption, namely that the cytoplasm behaves as a free solution, similar to the interstitial fluid. However, it is far more likely that the cytoplasm is a gel, as discussed above (60). This problem is also unresolved.

The fact that animal cells lack rigid walls and do not develop sizeable transmembrane hydrostatic pressure differences determines that the only means to maintain or regulate cell volume is to change the cell content of osmotically active solutes. This is the main theme of the next section.

Cell Volume Is Determined by Amount of Cell Solute and Extracellular Osmolality

With the questionable exception of water cotransport, net water transport between intracellular and extracellular compartments is the result of differences in effective osmotic pressure between these compartments. The effective osmotic pressure, in turn, is proportional to the total number of particles in solution and also to the reflection coefficients of these particles. Hence, at the same total osmotic pressure, impermeant particles are more effective than permeable particles in generating water flow toward the side in which they are contained. This can be demonstrated experimentally by exposing cells to solutions of identical osmolalities but different tonicities, by using solutes having different permeabilities. Depending on the relative permeabilities of the plasma membrane to water and the solute, cell volume can remain constant, increase, or decrease. This phenomenon can be explained by the effect of the solute reflection coefficient on osmotic water flow.

A solution is defined as isotonic when exposure of cells to this solution results in no change in cell volume; hypertonic and hypotonic solutions elicit decreases and increases in cell volume, respectively. Therefore, a hypertonic solution has a greater effective osmolality and a hypotonic solution a lower effective osmolality than the isotonic solution. Because of the role of the solute reflection coefficient in determining the effective osmolality, the terms hypertonic and hypotonic are not equivalent to hyperosmotic or hyposmotic; the latter expressions denote the total osmolality of the solutions, disregarding the reflection coefficients. The osmolalities of biological fluids are largely determined by their total salt concentrations, because low-molecular-weight salts are the solutes at highest concentrations, expressed as number of particles relative to water mass. Hence, the extracellular fluid osmolality is largely determined by Na^+ salts, mainly chloride and bicarbonate, and the intracellular osmolality is mostly determined by K^+ salts.

Under most physiological and pathophysiological conditions, the intracellular and extracellular compartments can be treated as two closed compartments separated by a semipermeable membrane (i.e., a membrane permeable to water and impermeable to the solute). This simplification is valid because, in the short term, solute gains or losses by the whole system and solute fluxes between the compartments are slow relative to potential water fluxes. It follows that(1) the amount of solute in each compartment can be considered constant, and

(2) the steady-state osmolalities of both compartments must be equal. Therefore, the amount of cell water is inextricably related to the amount of cell solute and to the extracellular osmolality:

$$V_w^c = \frac{S^c}{Osm_{ec}} \qquad (20)$$

where V_w^c is the cell-water volume (l), S^c is the amount of cell solute (mosmol) and Osm_{ec} is the extracellular osmolality (mosmol/kg water); 1 liter of water is ~1 kg.

It follows from Eq. 20 that cell volume can change by two mechanisms, namely changes in the amount of cell solute or in the extracellular osmolality. From a homeostasis point of view, if pure water is added to the extracellular compartment, reducing its tonicity, then part of the water will flow across the cell membrane into the intracellular compartment, until the osmolalities are again equal. If pure water is lost from the extracellular compartment, then water will flow from the intracellular compartment until the osmolalities become equal. In contrast, if isotonic solution is added to or lost from the extracellular compartment, there will be no water flow across the cell membrane, because no osmotic pressure difference has been established, and in the body the ensuing changes in hydrostatic pressure will be very small. This analysis is rather qualitative; knowledge or assumption of the initial conditions allows for a highly quantitative analysis, essential for understanding the pathogenesis and planning the treatment of water and electrolyte disorders.

Water Permeability of Plasma Membrane Varies Considerably Among Cell Types

Cell membranes are endowed with highly variable osmotic water permeability coefficients, ranging from practically zero (apical membrane of thick-ascending loop of Henle cells) to 400–600 $\mu m \cdot s^{-1}$ in red blood cells and renal proximal tubules. Most nonepithelial cells display quite high osmotic water permeabilities. The best-studied case is that of the mammalian red blood cell, whose P_{os} is in the range of 50–400 $\mu m \cdot s^{-1}$ (28). In artificial lipid bilayers, P_{os} ranges from <1 to ~100 $\mu m \cdot s^{-1}$, depending on the lipid composition. Bilayers of higher fluidity are more permeable to water and sterol content decreases the bilayer water permeability. Recent studies have shown that certain biological membranes that are highly water permeable contain water-selective pores (aquaporins).

The structural bases for the extremely low P_{os} of some cell membranes were recently discovered; others remain unknown. As detailed in Chapter 2, lipid rafts in membranes are domains in the submicron range that are rich in cholesterol and sphingolipids in the external leaflet and cholesterol and phospholipids with saturated fatty acids in the internal leaflet of the membrane. The surrounding bilayer is abundant in unsaturated fatty acids and considerably more fluid than that in the raft (50). Membrane rafts have low fluidity and hence a low diffusional water permeability.

Apical membranes of certain tight epithelia have an extremely low permeability to water. A case in point is the apical membrane of the urothelium, that is, the epithelium that lines the renal calices, pelvis, ureters, urinary bladder, and urethra. The apical membranes of the epithelial cells of the urothelium are covered by rigid plaques consisting of hexagonal arrays of particles (9, 44, 115). The plaques contain four-transmembrane-domain proteins named uroplakins, of which there are four isoforms (63, 126, 128). It has been suggested that uroplakins could influence the passive permeability of the apical membrane of the urothelium (43), but evidence was lacking until the permeabilities of urinary bladders of normal mice and mice in which the gene encoding uroplakin III (UPIII) was ablated were compared (48). The normal mouse bladder has high transepithelial electrical resistance and low water permeability. The bladder from UPIII-deficient mice maintained the high transepithelial resistance, but its water permeability was 20-fold higher than in controls. These results strongly suggest that the low permeability of the tight junctions and the apical membrane to ions are preserved in the knockout mice, whereas the water permeability of the apical membrane is increased. This is the first instance in which expression of a transmembrane protein has been shown to decrease the permeability of a biological membrane.

The thick ascending limb of the loop of Henle also has an extremely low permeability to water (91), necessary for the operation of the urine concentration mechanism (see Chapter 40). The biophysical reasons for this low permeability are not entirely clear. Certainly there is no expression of water pores (AQP) in this domain (see Chapter 38), and the surface area is small relative to the basolateral membrane (91), but whether the composition of the membrane has a role is yet to be determined.

Pathways for Water Transport Across Cell Membranes

As explained above, water transport across biological membranes can be across the lipid phase of the membrane (solubility diffusion) or across membrane proteins. The aquaporin family consists of about 20 members that form water pores and are expressed in the plasma membranes of numerous cell types. Their important role in water transport across cell membranes is unquestionable. It has also been suggested that other transport proteins may transport water in addition to its substrates. Such suggestions have been made for both ion channels and carriers. We will discuss first aquaporins and then these membrane proteins in the context of water transport across cell membranes. The accepted water transport pathways across the cell membrane are illustrated in Fig. 8.

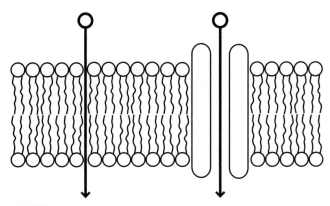

FIGURE 8 Water transport pathways across plasma membranes. Left arrow: Solubility diffusion across the phospholipid bilayer. The water permeability is directly proportional to the fluidity of the membrane. Right arrow: Permeation via pores. The water flux obeys Pouiseuille's law in wide pores, and occurs by single-file diffusion in narrow pores such as the aquaporins.

WATER PORES DETERMINE HIGH CELL-MEMBRANE WATER PERMEABILITY

The existence of water pores was first deduced from biophysical studies (reviewed in Macey [65] and Verkman [111]) and then elegantly confirmed by biochemical, molecular-biological, and structural studies (reviewed in Agre [1] and King et al. [53]). Over the years, several criteria were developed to ascertain the presence of water pores in membranes. The principal ones are discussed below.

High P_{os}/P_d If the membrane contains pores, then osmotic water flow does not occur via a diffusion-like mechanism, which obeys the independence principle. Instead, it involves some form of interaction between water molecules, either Poiseuille-like (viscous) flow in thin capillaries or single-file transport. As discussed previously, in both cases the flow of individual water molecules depends on the flow of other water molecules. It follows that the value of P_{os}/P_d is significantly greater than unity (the ratio is proportional to the square of the pore radius in case of viscous flow and equal to the number of water molecules contained in the case of single-file transport). However, unstirred-layer effects can cause a disproportionately large underestimation of P_d relative to P_{os}, with the end result of an artifactually large ratio. This error can be prevented by measuring the unstirred-layer equivalent thickness and making appropriate corrections for P_{os} and P_d (25). In conclusion, a correctly obtained $P_{os}/P_d >$ 1 is strong evidence for water transport via pores. The value of P_{os}/P_d can denote either the pore radius or the number of water molecules in the pore. Resolving this issue requires additional experimental work, such as permeation studies with solutes of varying sizes to estimate the pore radius.

Low Arrhenius Activation Energy The activation energies (E_a) for water permeation via aqueous pores and for water self-diffusion are about the same (<5 kcal mol^{-1}), that is, much lower than the E_a for water permeation by solubility diffusion across a lipid membrane ($\sim$12 kcal mol^{-1}). This can be established by measuring the water permeability at different temperatures.

Sensitivity to Hg Water transport via proteinaceous pores is inhibited by HgCl$_2$ and organic mercurial compounds, an effect suggestive of a critical SH group in the protein underlying the pore function (66). This was corroborated when the protein was identified (82).

Flux Interactions In the case of large pores with finite solute permeability, there is frictional interactions between water and solutes (see above), with the end result of solvent drag and/or electrokinetic phenomena. Although this has been demonstrated for some membrane pores, it does not seem to take place with aquaporins, the water-selective pores in animal cell membranes. This suggests that these pores are impermeable to most solutes, and hence too narrow for solvent drag or electrokinetic phenomena.

Among cell membranes from epithelia, the best studied from a water-pore viewpoint is the apical membrane of the mammalian renal proximal tubule. In this instance, the above criteria have been clearly satisfied (124). Water pores have been identified in numerous organs and cell types. In the renal proximal tubule the pores are constitutively active; in contrast, in the collecting duct under resting conditions they exist in a cytoplasmic vesicular pool, and are inserted in the apical membrane after stimulation by vasopressin (10, 11).

CELL-MEMBRANE WATER PORES ARE AQUAPORINS

The existence of water pores on cell membranes was demonstrated in red cells and renal tubules by the biophysical approaches described above (for reviews see Macey [65] and Verkman [111]). The molecular identification of the pores occurred by the discovery of that the red-cell membrane protein first named CHIP28 (21, 82), and now aquaporin 1 or AQP1 when expressed in amphibian oocytes or purified and reconstituted in liposomes forms Hg^{2+}-sensitive water pores with low activation energy, and no ion conductance (reviewed in Agre [2], Engel et al. [24], Heymann [42], King et al. [53]). Later studies have shown three important facts: (1) AQPs are expressed in plant and animal cells, in both simple and complex organisms; (2) AQPs are expressed in the plasma and intracellular membranes of most cells, not just red cells and renal epithelial cells; and (3) there are at least 11 AQP isoforms in mammals, which have unique cellular and subcellular distributions (53). Aquaporins are present in most cell types in the body, and there is reason to suspect that they are the predominant pathway for water transport across cell membranes (53). In this section I will discuss aquaporins largely from a molecular point of view. Aquaporins in the kidney are treated in Chapter 38 and aquaporins in other organs by King et al. (53). For excellent recent reviews on AQPs, see Agre (1) and King et al. (53). Peter Agre received the 2003 Nobel Prize in Chemistry for his work on aquaporins.

The AQP family consists of two groups: aquaporins, most of which are permeated only by water (isoforms 0, 1, 2, 4,

5, 6, 8), and aquaglyceroporins (isoforms 3, 7, 9, 10), which are permeated by both water and small solutes, and in particular glycerol. The AQPs are assembled as tetramers (with one subunit N-glycosylated) in the cell membrane (51, 98), with each monomer containing a water pore. The AQP1 monomer is a 28-kDa protein with intracellular N- and C-termini, and consists of tandem repeats, each with three bilayer-spanning a-helices. In each repeat the TM2–TM3 loops are highly conserved and include the Asp-Pro-Ala (NPA) signature motif. The mercury sensitivity of water transport is conferred by a specific cysteine residue (Cys189) (100). The predicted topology of AQP1 and mutagenesis experiments led to the "hourglass model," in which the six membrane-spanning helices

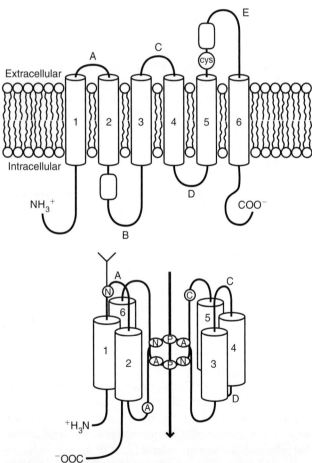

FIGURE 9 Membrane topology and structure of AQP1. **A:** Predicted secondary structure: AQP consists of two repeats of three transmembrane helices (1, 2, and 3; 4, 5, and 6). Amino and carboxyl termini are on the cytoplasmic side. Loops B and E contain Asn-Pro-Ala motifs, which possibly form part of the water pore. Loop E contains Cys189, responsible for Hg sensitivity. **B:** Hypothetical structure of the water pore. Loops B and E form the thin barrier accounting for water selectivity. The α helices form the surrounding wall. The monomer shown is functional per se, but AQP1 assembles into tetramers. (Modified with permission from Preston GM, Agre P. Isolation of the cDNA for erythrocyte integral membrane protein of 28 kilodaltons: member of an ancient channel family. *Proc Natl Acad Sci U S A* 1991;88:11110–11114; and Jung JS, Preston GM, Smith BL, Guggino WB, Agre P. Molecular structure of the water channel through aquaporin CHIP: the tetrameric-hourglass model. *J Biol Chem* 1994;269:14648–14654.)

surround the pore (lined by the two NPA-containing loops), which enter the membrane from the opposite surfaces and form a ring at the junction of the NPA motifs (82). The hourglass model was confirmed by cryoelectron microscopy of human AQP1 from red blood cells (75, 84, 116, 117) and the x-ray atomic structures of GlpF (30) and of bovine AQP1 (104). A schema of this structure is shown in Fig. 9.

MECHANISM OF WATER PERMEATION IN AQP1

The high selectivity of AQP1 for water—excluding even proton permeation—is consistent with the minimum width of the pore (2.8 Å), which limits the size of permeant molecules. A conserved arginine contributes a fixed positive charge at this site. Other members of the family, including the *Escherichia coli* GlpF channel, allow permeation of small solutes; in the case of GlpF, the minimum diameter of the pore is ~3.8 Å, allowing passage of glycerol. In addition, the water molecules inside the pore interact with dipoles formed by the NPA motifs, and thus cannot form hydrogen bonds with adjacent water molecules. In other words, similar to what happens to K^+ permeating K^+-selective channels, the water molecules in the AQP1 pore lose contact with other molecules. One could say that the water becomes "dehydrated" and permeates in single file. The lack of hydrogen bonding of water molecules inside the pore prevents proton conduction via "water wires" (104, 106).

CERTAIN AQUAPORINS ARE PERMEABLE TO SOLUTES

As shown in Table 1, 5 of the 11 AQP isoforms have been shown to display solute permeability in addition to water permeability. It has also been claimed that AQP1 has ion-channel activity when stimulated by cGMP, but this is unclear at this time (see below). With this possible exception and AQP6, which has anion permeability, other isoforms are permeable to small, neutral, hydrophilic solutes. Of these, needless to say, urea is critical for renal function (see Chapters 38 and 40).

REGULATION OF AQP-MEDIATED WATER PERMEABILITY

In principle, the water permeability of a cell membrane via AQP depends, analogously to the conductance of an ion channel, on the number of functional pores (N per cell or membrane surface area), the single-pore water permeability, and the pore open probability (the fraction of the time that it is water permeable). Changes in N have been clearly demonstrated to regulate AQP-mediated water permeability. The most striking example of this mechanism is the effect of vasopressin on the insertion of AQP2 in the luminal membrane of the cortical collecting duct (see Chapter 42). As discussed below, certain solutes decrease the water permeability of AQP pores, but there is no evidence for a regulatory role of pore "gating" in the sense that this expression is used in ion channel function (see Chapter 2).

TABLE 1 Permeability Characteristics and Predominant Distribution for Known
Mammalian Aquaporin (AQP) Homologues

Isoform	Permeability	Tissue Distribution	Subcellular Distribution[a]
AQP0	Water (low)	Lens	Plasma membrane
AQP1	Water (high)	Red blood cell, kidney lung, vascular endothelium, brain, eye	Plasma membrane
AQP2	Water (high)	Kidney, vas deferens	Apical membrane, intracellular
AQP3	Water (high), glycerol (high), urea (moderate)	Kidney, skin, lung, eye, colon	Basolateral membrane
AQP4	Water (high)	Brain, muscle, kidney, lung, stomach, small intestine	Basolateral membrane
AQP5	Water (high)	Salivary gland, lacrimal gland, sweat gland, lung, cornea	Apical membrane
AQP6	Water (low), anions (NO_3^- > Cl^-)	Kidney	Intracellular
AQP7	Water (high), glycerol (high), urea (high), arsenite	Adipose tissue, kidney, testis	Plasma membrane
AQP8[b]	Water (high)	Testis, kidney, liver, pancreas, small intestine, colon	Plasma membrane, intracellular
AQP9	Water (low), glycerol (high), urea (high), arsenite	Liver, leukocytes, brain, testis	Plasma membrane
AQP10	Water (low), glycerol (high) urea (high)	Small intestine	Intracellular

[a]Homologues that are present primarily in either the apical or basolateral membrane are noted as residing in one of these membranes, whereas homologues that are present in both of these membranes are described as having a plasma-membrane distribution.

[b]AQP8 might be permeated by water and urea.

From King LS, Kozono D, Agre P. From structure to disease: the evolving tale of aquaporin biology. *Nat Rev Mol Cell Biol* 2004;5:687–698, with permission of authors and *Nature*.

The permeability of several AQP isoforms is modulated by the composition of the extracellular solution. The water permeability of AQP0 expressed in *Xenopus* oocytes was reported to be increased by lowering external pH and $[Ca^{2+}]$ (77). Both effects require His40, which is present in the pore, as determined by x-ray crystallography (32). In another study, the water permeability of AQP3, also expressed in oocytes, was found to be reduced by external acidification, whereas AQP0, AQP1, AQP2, AQP4, and AQP5 were found to be pH-insensitive (132), in contrast with the study quoted above. In oocytes or LLC-PK1 cells expressing heterologous AQP4, PKC agonists were reported to reduce cell-membrane water permeability (38, 129), an effect abolished by deletion of Ser180 (129). However, when purified AQP4 was reconstituted in liposomes, its phosphorylation by PKC did not affect the water permeability (quoted in King et al. [53]). In addition to a water pore, AQP6 is an acidification-induced anion channel, with a high selectivity for NO_3^- over Cl^- (49). Finally, *Xenopus* oocytes expressing AQP1 develop an ion current after injection of cGMP, whereas this agent had no effect on oocytes expressing AQP5 (4). Further, the effect is dependent on specific charged residues in the C-terminal domain of AQP1 (8). It is not clear, however, that the pathways for water permeation and ion fluxes are the same: When the experiment is carried out with AQP1 reconstituted in planar bilayers, an organic mercurial compound inhibited water permeability, but not cGMP-induced ion conductance (96). Further, the ratio of ion permeability to water permeability was extremely small, suggesting that only a minute fraction of AQP1 molecules would form cGMP-activated ion channels (96). In conclusion, contrary to statements in the literature, there is no evidence that the AQP water pore is gated, that is, opens and closes stochastically as an ion channel. The available information is consistent with modulatory effects, such as by pH or divalent cations that could simply block the water permeation pathway. It is also clear that the finding that expression of a membrane protein results in water and ion permeability does not mean that they occur through the same pathway.

A very interesting issue is whether AQPs are permeable to gases, in particular CO_2. It was reported that AQP1 expression in *Xenopus* oocytes elicits an almost twofold, Hg^{2+} sensitive increase in plasma-membrane CO_2 permeability (15, 76), and an even larger effect (also Hg^{2+}-sensitive) was obtained in *E. coli* membrane vesicles expressing AQP1 (81). However, the CO_2 permeabilities of red blood cells and alveolar epithelium of mice in which *Aqp1* was deleted were found to be not different from those of wildtype mice (127). The differences between these sets of studies remain unresolved (see 16, 112).

OTHER MEMBRANE PROTEINS MAY CONTRIBUTE TO WATER TRANSPORT

Water permeation through narrow ion channels has been studied by molecular-dynamics simulations based in the atomic structure of the KcsA channel (92) (see also Chapter 2). In the narrow part of the pore (selectivity filter), K^+ is transported in single file; two adjacent ions are separated by a water molecule; therefore, the molar flux ratio (K^+/water) is unity. For "near-isosmotic" water transport, the flux of 1 ion would be coupled to that of 157 water molecules. Therefore, direct coupling between ion and water transport in narrow ion channels contributes only a minute fraction of the water flux expected to be produced by the changes in the osmolality of the solutions adjacent to the membrane produced by the ion flux.

One would expect that wider ion channels, in which the ions permeate in a hydrate state would result in larger water fluxes coupled to the ion flow, and perhaps also in water permeation in the absence of a net ion flux. No atomic structure of large channels in mammalian cells is available, but it was recently shown that blocking the volume-regulated anion channel (VRAC) decreased significantly the water permeability of endothelial cells (78). This result suggests that these channels constitute a significant pathway for osmotic water flow in these cells.

DO COTRANSPORTERS PERFORM ACTIVE WATER TRANSPORT?

Experiments in the choroid plexus epithelium of *Necturus maculosus* (130) and retinal pigment epithelium of frog (131) suggested that water transport and solute transport (KCl and lactate, respectively) are directly coupled. Under energetically favorable conditions, water would move uphill in the direction of the net ion flux and by the same pathway, implying molecular coupling (in the carrier molecule) between the solute and water fluxes. If this is correct, then the water is cotransported, that is, transported uphill by a secondary active mechanism. Several cotransporters have been suggested to perform this function when expressed in *Xenopus* oocytes: Na^+-glucose (59, 71), Na^+-glutamate (64), Na^+-dicarboxylate (72), and others (see 56). The rate of water transport via these carriers would range between 50 and 400 molecules per cycle. The water/solute coupling ratio in the case of the human Na^+-glucose cotransporter (71) indicates that the transported fluid would be hyperosmotic, instead of near-isosmotic. Hence, near-isosmolality could result from the parallel operation of transcellular osmosis. The critical experimental result supporting the water cotransport hypothesis is that solute transport via a cotransporter is associated with a water flux much larger than that observed with a similar solute flux via ion channels (58), an argument that would rule out the alternative explanation that the cotransporter-mediated solute flux increases the osmolality in the plane adjacent to the membrane, and that the resultant generated osmotic gradient is responsible for water flux across the plasma membrane (55, 56), not necessarily the cotransporter itself. A careful study of water fluxes in *Xenopus* oocytes expressing heterologous Na^+-glucose cotransporters, glucose transporters, or the K^+ channel ROMK2, permitted another group to relate solute accumulation in the oocytes to water flow. Their conclusion is that the glucose accumulation quantitatively accounts for the water flux by simple osmosis, and therefore that there would be no need to postulate water cotransport (31). A critical factor in the solute accumulation in these studies is the intracellular solute diffusion coefficient, which in the oocytes is about one-fifth of that in free solution (14).

Summary and Conclusions

In conclusion, the osmotic behavior of cells is not ideal, because of the presence of cell solids; water transport across the cell membrane occurs by osmosis; and the determinants of cell volume are the intracellular solute content and the extracellular osmolality. Water permeation across the plasma membrane occurs via AQP pores and/or the phospholipid bilayer. Other pathways contribute at most a small fraction of the water flow.

WATER TRANSPORT IN EPITHELIA

Two modalities of transepithelial water transport occur in renal tubules in situ: (1) net transport between isosmotic (or near-isosmotic) fluids (e.g., water reabsorption in the proximal tubule), and (2) net transport in the direction of a pre-existing osmotic gradient (e.g., water reabsorption in the collecting duct). Although other mechanisms have been proposed, the dominant view is that water transport is passive and driven by osmotic forces. Pinocytosis has also been suggested, but is considered highly unlikely (124). Solute–water cotransport, discussed in the previous section, is also unlikely given recent experimental results (31). Electro-osmosis (95) and mechano-osmosis (93) have also been proposed, largely on the basis of neglecting the presence of unstirred layers in theoretical or experimental analyses. The reader interested in these hypotheses should consult the references cited previously.

Characteristics of Transepithelial Water Transport

The main consequence of water transport across cell membranes of epithelial cells is to contribute to transepithelial transport, that is, fluid absorption or secretion. In addition, similar to most other cells, epithelial cells are endowed with mechanisms of maintenance and regulation of their own volume. Physiologic regulation of transepithelial transport may involve changes in solute transport rate at one of the two cell membranes. This causes an instantaneous imbalance between the transport rates of apical and basolateral membranes, and therefore a change in cell solute and water content. In most epithelial cells, there is a rapid readjustment of the transport rate by a complex process called intermembrane "cross-talk" (97, 98) (see Chapter 2).

Epithelia Have Very Different Water Permeabilities

Epithelia differ widely in their osmotic water permeabilities (Table 2). From the points of view of magnitude and regulation of their osmotic permeability coefficient, epithelia can be classified in the following three groups:

(1) *High constitutive osmotic water permeability.* In these epithelia the P_{os} is permanently high. This group includes most leaky epithelia (epithelia with high paracellular permeability relative to the transcellular permeability), such asrenal proximal tubule, descending limb of the loop of Henle, small intestine, gallbladder, and choroid plexus. The high value of P_{os} is in large part (or exclusively) attributable to high per-

TABLE 2 Osmotic Water Permeability of Epithelial Cell Membranes

Epithelium	Apical	Basolateral	Transepithelial	Reference
ADH-insensitive				
Rabbit PST	4500	5000	4280	13
Necturus gallbladder	640	460	350	17
Rabbit/rat TALH	—	—	0–20[a]	83
ADH-sensitive				
Rabbit CCD (−) ADH	70	450	—	103
(+) ADH	310	490	—	
Rabbit IMCD (−) ADH	70	480	—	27
(+) ADH	260	390	—	

P_f values are rounded and expressed in $\mu m \cdot s^{-1}$, without correction for membrane folding factors; that is, they are referred to "idealized" epithelial surface. For P_f values considering membrane folding, see Tripathi and Boulpaep (107).

[a]Range of several studies.

ADH, antidiuretic hormone (vasopressin); PST, proximal straight tubule; TALH, thick ascending limb of loop of Henle; CCD, cortical collecting duct; IMCD, inner medullary collecting duct.

meabilities of both cell membranes (apical and basolateral). The cell membranes express water pores, so that water is likely to permeate both by solubility diffusion (via the lipid bilayer) and osmosis (via the pores). It is also possible that part of the water flow is intercellular (or paracellular), as discussed below.

(2) *Low constitutive osmotic water permeability.* In mammals the only epithelia with this property are the ascending limb of the loop of Henle and urinary-tract epithelia. The P_{os} is extremely low and insensitive to hormonal action (antidiuretic hormone). Both the apical membranes and the junctional complexes are low-permeability barriers. In the thick ascending loop of Henle, the basolateral membrane has a high water permeability, so that changes in peritubular fluid osmolality result in rapid cell volume changes (41, 105), whereas changes in luminal (apical) solution osmolality are ineffective. The transepithelial P_{os} is low, although there is a high junctional ionic permeability. This lack of correlation between permeability to ions and water is not unexpected. As discussed in the context of cell-membrane water permeability, ion channels permeate little water, and their expression level is quite low, so they do not increase P_{os} by a large amount. The molecular explanations for the low P_{os} of the apical membranes and junctions of the ascending limb of loop of Henle cells are unknown. In the case of urinary tract epithelia, there appears to be a major role of apical membrane uroplakins (see previous discussion and Hu et al. [48]).

(3) *Variable (regulated) water permeability.* The renal collecting duct and the anuran urinary bladder and epidermis have low baseline P_{os} values, which are elevated when plasma osmolality rises, by a mechanism involving secretion ofantidiuretic hormone (in mammals, vasopressin) by the neurohypophysis. Vasopressin binds to the basolateral V2

receptor and activates a signaling mechanism that involves an increase in intracellular cAMP, resulting in insertion and then retrieval of preformed water pores in the apicalmembrane by exocytosis and endocytosis, respectively. The cytoplasmic pool of pores is contained in subapical tubulovesicles (11, 39, 40, 111, 113, 114).

Two Types of Transepithelial Water Transport

It is not difficult to understand the mechanisms of water reabsorption in either the cortical or the medullary collecting duct (CCD and MCD, respectively) under the influence of vasopressin. The tubule fluid at the end of the distal tubule is hyposmotic to plasma (and to the renal-cortex interstitial fluid). Hence, if the CCD is water permeable, then water will be reabsorbed down the osmotic gradient. A similar situation occurs in the MCD, where the entering lumen fluid is at most isosmotic to plasma and the osmolality of the surrounding interstitial fluid ranges in humans, from 300 at the cortico-medullary junction to 1200 mosmol/kg at the papilla (Chapter 40). In the frog epidermis, water reabsorption occurs from the pond (osmolality <10) to the frog's extracellular fluid (~250 mosmol/kg). Thus, in these three epithelia there is a pre-existing osmotic force, and whether water is absorbed or not depends on the P_{os} of the apical membrane of the epithelial cells. As discussed previously, P_{os} at this membrane is regulated by insertion and retrieval of AQP2 water pores, in response to changes in extracellular osmolality, a process mediated by secretion of vasopressin (see also Chapters 38, 39, 40).

In the renal proximal tubule, small intestine, gallbladder, and other epithelia, the fluids bathing the epithelium are usually isosmotic or near-isosmotic and transepithelial water transport can take place in the absence of a measurable driving force between the bulk solutions. Further, early experimental observations showed that water absorption can occur against the transepithelial osmotic gradient, that is, from the concentrated to the diluted solution (19). This occurs both in small intestine and renal proximal tubule, and unquestionably demonstrates uphill water transport (see Whittembury and Hill [123] and Whittembury and Reuss [124] for detailed discussions). Of course, this does not necessarily mean that there is a "water pump" (primary or secondary active water transporter) in the system. Studies in small intestine epithelium revealed that uphill water absorption occurs only together with net solute absorption and in the same direction, suggesting some form of "coupling" between water and solute fluxes (19, 119, 120). Over the next 50 years, these puzzling observations elicited a great amount of experimental and theoretical work, which resulted in successive proposals to explain: (1) water transport between isosmotic bulk solutions, (2) uphill water transport, and (3) the nature of the coupling between solute and water flow.

Solute–Solvent Coupling

Passive mechanisms may exist that would couple salt to water absorption or secretion. Intuitively, active salt absorption by an epithelium (see Chapter 2) will create, at both apical and basolateral membranes, differences in the concentration of salt, with the side from which the salt is transported becoming "dilute" and the side toward which the salt is transported becoming "concentrated." The magnitude of the concentration changes in the fluids adjacent to the epithelial cells will depend on whether they are mixed (by convection) with the bulk solutions, and on the rates of solute diffusion into or away from these areas. Clearly, changes in concentration must be created inside the cell, in the surfaces immediately adjacent to the membranes, where the cytosol is not well mixed and the diffusion rates are much smaller than in free solution. In addition, in the extracellular surfaces adjacent to the cell membranes the solutions are not well mixed with the bulk, for two reasons: the existence of unstirred layers (see above) and the existence of anatomic restricted spaces in which good mixing cannot occur. In the case of the basolateral cell membrane of an epithelium, the histology indicates that there can be no good mixing with the extracellular solution, because of the complex architecture of the lateral intercellular spaces, the basal membrane infoldings, and the presence of the basement membrane, which is a barrier for hydraulic flow. At the apical membrane surface, fluid mixing is easier, but is also not ideal if there are microvilli. Hence, in a fluid-transporting epithelium at the steady state one would expect a solute concentration profile in which there are salt concentration gradients across the apical membrane, with the lumen fluid diluted with respect to the cell interior, and across the basolateral membrane with the cell diluted with respect to the extracellular solution.

The central points in this analysis of solute–solvent coupling in epithelia will be two. First, the functional anatomy of epithelia determines the existence of compartments (i.e., spaces that are "unstirred"); in these spaces osmotic coupling occurs, explaining the relationship (coupling) between salt and water transport. Second, the water permeability of the cell membranes is so high that the osmotic gradients required for near-isosmotic coupling are very small, and detectable only under rather artificial experimental conditions. This view is not universally accepted. As we discuss the details below, I will point out criticisms and alternative positions.

THREE-COMPARTMENT MODELS DEFINE THE PROBLEM

An epithelial monolayer and the surrounding fluid compartments can be modeled as a three-compartment system with two barriers. The essence of these models is that the specific properties of the barriers and the compartments can account for solute–water flux coupling and explain apparently active water transport. Two proposals were developed based on this idea, namely the three-compartment model of Curran and MacIntosh (18) and the standing-gradient hypothesis of Diamond and Bossert (23).

In the three-compartment model, illustrated in Fig. 10, water transport occurs from cis solution (A) to trans solution (B) against the osmotic pressure difference between these two solutions $[C_s(B) > C_s(A)]$. The cis solution and trans solution are separated from the middle compartment (M) by barriers with different properties—semipermeable and porous, respectively. Active salt transport into an unstirred intraepithelial compartment renders it hyperosmotic to the cis solution (hyperosmotic middle compartment). Water then flows from A to M by osmosis (the membrane is semiperme-

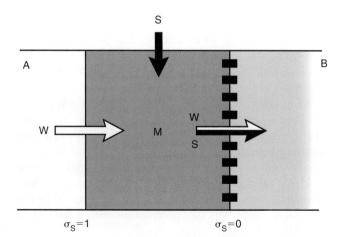

FIGURE 10 Three-compartment model of Curran and MacIntosh (18). Solute entry (s, solid arrow) $C_s(M) > C_s(A)$ into the middle compartment (compartment M) causes osmotic *water* flow (w, open arrow) from compartment A to compartment M. The elevation of the hydrostatic pressure in compartment M causes *solution* flow from compartment M into compartment B (w/s open/solid arrow). Hence, there is water flux from A to B, although $C_s(B) > C_s(A)$. See text.

able), and, as the hydrostatic pressure rises in M, solution flows from the M into B by bulk flow (the membrane is porous). The equivalent of this system in an absorptive epithelium would be as follows: The semipermeable membrane is constituted by the two cell membrane domains (apical and basolateral) in series, and the porous membrane by the distal end of the lateral intercellular spaces and the basement membrane, also in series. Compartment A is the lumen, compartment B the basolateral (interstitial) solution, and compartment M the lateral intercellular space. Water can be transported uphill (against the osmotic gradient between A and B) only while the middle compartment is hyperosmotic to the cis compartment. In addition, for this model to operate the absorbed fluid must be hyperosmotic to the cis solution. Experimental studies showed that the emerging fluid was virtually isosmotic with the cis solution (22), requiring revision of the above theory. This resulted in the formulation of the standing-gradient hypothesis, explained below.

STANDING-GRADIENT HYPOTHESIS EXPLAINS NEAR-ISOSMOTIC FLUID TRANSPORT, BUT IS DIFFICULT TO RECONCILE WITH CURRENT EXPERIMENTAL KNOWLEDGE

The standing-gradient hypothesis of Diamond and Bossert (23) is depicted in Fig. 11. It is based on the following definitions and assumptions: (1) The lateral intercellular space is the hyperosmotic middle compartment. (2) The junctional complexes are impermeable to both solute and water. (3) Solute transport from the cell to the trans solution takes place across the lateral membranes near the apical poles of the cells. (4) In contrast, secondary (osmotic) water flow occurs across the entire lateral membrane. (5) The lateral intercellular space solution is unstirred. (6) Solute diffusion along the length of the lateral intercellular spaces is restricted by their geometry (the spaces are long and narrow). Under these conditions, the solution of the complicated mathematical model describing the system yields a continuously decreasing osmolality from the apical (blind) to the basolateral (open) end of the space. Also, the emerging solution is more likely to be near-isosmotic when the following conditions hold: long and narrow spaces, small solute diffusion coefficient, and high cell-membrane P_{os} relative to the solute transport rate.

Direct and indirect observations demonstrated that some of the above assumptions are not correct. (1) In many instances the junctions have high permeability to ions (29, 46, 121, 125) and perhaps to water (122, 124). (2) The Na^+,K^+-ATPase is distributed homogeneously in the lateral cell membrane (73), not restricted to the apical region. (3) Both morphometric studies and electrophysiological computations yield short times for lateral-space solute diffusion (45, 52, 94, 116, 119), making longitudinal concentration gradients unlikely. (4) Realistic calculations based on geometry predict that the transported fluid must be hyperosmotic (94), that is, that the spaces are not sufficiently long and narrow. (5) The hypothesis predicted sizable hyperosmolality in the lateral intercellular spaces, because the early estimations of transepithelial P_{os} were in error due to unstirred-layer artifacts (6, 47). (6) Measurements of transepithelial voltage changes elicited by changes in solution osmolality revealed that the lateral intercellular spaces are in virtual osmotic equilibrium with the cell (89, 90).

An important point in this discussion is that for a constant fluid transport rate, the magnitude of the osmotic gradient and of the hyperosmolality of the transported fluid is inversely proportional to the effective P_{os} of the osmotic barriers. In fact, many of the above problems were solved with the development of methods to measure the osmotic water permeability of the cell membranes of leaky epithelia, which was demonstrated to be very large. On these bases, some of the above notions must be discarded because they were based on incorrect experimental data and a simpler mechanism of transepithelial water transport has emerged.

NEAR-ISOSMOTIC FLUID TRANSPORT MODEL SOLVES THE DIFFICULTIES OF THREE-COMPARTMENT MODELS

Measurements of P_{os} in high-water-permeability membranes give values ranging from 100 to 400 $\mu m \cdot s^{-1}$, that is, 10- to 100-fold greater than early estimates (124). Hence, instead of a needed osmolality difference of about 20

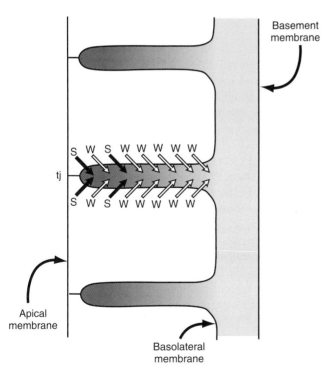

FIGURE 11 Standing-gradient hypothesis of Diamond and Bossert (23). Solute transport (s, solid arrows) into the channel (lateral intercellular space) causes a local increase in osmolality; water flows osmotically across the bounding membranes (w, open arrows), "diluting" the solution in the channel. Transport toward the open end is by bulk flow and diffusion. See text.

mosmol·kg^{-1}, as predicted from the standing-gradient hypothesis, a very small difference in osmolality, of only 1–2 mosmol·kg^{-1}, quantitatively accounts for the measured water-transport rates (17, 80, 124). As explained previously, the primary event in transepithelial water transport is active salt transport. Inasmuch as solute is removed from the cis side and added to the trans side, there must be a decrease in cis fluid and an increase in trans fluid osmolality in the immediate vicinity of the respective membranes, as well as opposite changes in osmolality at the intracellular surface of the two membranes: an increase at the apical membrane and a decrease at the basolateral membrane. The magnitude of these changes will depend on the transport rate and geometry of the systems, and can be generally expected to be quite small. Measurements in fluid samples from isolated, perfused renal tubules reveal small differences, supporting this view (5, 34). In conclusion, recent studies support the notion that so-called isosmotic transepithelial water transport is not truly isosmotic, but near-isosmotic. Further, the osmotic driving forces required to account for water transport are quite small, and hence difficult to determine in situ, and substantial hyperosmotic compartments or sizable longitudinal standing gradients probably do not exist (86, 101, 124) (see Fig. 12).

SOLUTE RECIRCULATION IN THE PARACELLULAR PATHWAY IN THEORY EXPLAINS TRULY ISOSMOTIC TRANSEPITHELIAL FLUID TRANSPORT

Truly isosmotic transepithelial water transport (108, 109) may occur, in theory, if there is solute recirculation across the epithelium. In other words, it is argued that an epithelium cannot perform transepithelial truly isosmotic transport if it is bathed by identical solutions on both sides and there are no differences in electrical potential or hydrostatic pressure, unless part of the transported solute recirculates to the solution of origin. In frog skin glands, there is transcellular Cl$^-$ secretion (secondary active uptake at the basolateral membrane, channel-mediated downhill Cl$^-$ extrusion across the apical membrane) and paracellular Na$^+$ secretion (driven by the lumen-negative transepithelial voltage generated by Cl$^-$ transport). As such, this transport mechanism would cause secretion of a hyperosmotic fluid, but it was proposed that this fluid can become truly isosmotic. Larsen and coworkers (57) developed an interesting mathematical model for solute recirculation in the epithelium of the small intestine. The essential points are as follows: the primary transport event is active Na$^+$ transport across the lateral cell membrane (by the Na$^+$,K$^+$-ATPase). Water follows osmotically across the lateral cell membranes and the tight junctions. With appropriate geometric and transport parameters, the solution in the lateral intercellular spaces would be hyperosmotic by a small amount. The transported fluid would become isosmotic by uptake (recirculation) of salt across the basal membrane, via Na$^+$-K$^+$-2Cl$^-$ cotransport. This model has been criticized (102) on two main grounds: the use of experimental measurements

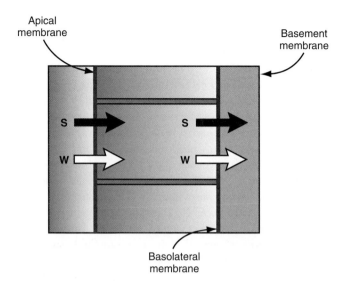

FIGURE 12   Near-isosmotic transport model. Because of the high osmotic water permeability of the cell membranes, the differences in solution osmolality (C$_s$) needed to account for fluid transport are small, probably localized at epithelium–solution interfaces. Salt transport causes dilution of solution on cis side and concentration of the solution on trans side at the two cell membranes. In the case of fluid absorption, at the apical membrane the intracellular solution is hyperosmotic to the lumen solution; at the basolateral membrane, the intracellular solution is hyposmotic to the extracellular solution. These small differences in osmolality, denoted in the figure by shades in gray (hyperosmotic solution being darker), cause osmotic water flow into the cell across the apical membrane and out of the cell across the basolateral membrane. The magnitude of the paracellular water flow is uncertain. Because of the high surface area of the lateral membranes and the small volume of the lateral intercellular spaces, the space osmolality is "clamped" by the cell osmolality, making longitudinal osmotic gradients in the spaces small at most.

of the Cs$^+$ flux ratio to assess transcellular and paracellular Na$^+$ fluxes and the energetic cost of recirculation, namely the fact that about half of the pump work would be wasted. Both sides agree that the model is amenable to further experimental testing (57, 102).

IN CERTAIN EPITHELIA ASYMMETRIES IN SOLUTE COMPOSITION PLAY SIGNIFICANT ROLES

It is possible that factors other than the total osmolalities of the solutions on either side of the epithelium contribute to transepithelial water transport. Three possibilities should be considered (see Whittembury and Hill [123] for a more detailed discussion). First is a colloid-osmotic force: Transepithelial differences in protein concentration can result in colloid-osmotic pressure differences that can be significant in the case of epithelia with high permeability to water and small solutes. In the renal proximal tubule, this factor accounts for a small portion of water reabsorption (36). Second is a difference in the effective osmolalities of the solutions: If the epithelium is exposed to solutions containing solutes of different reflection coefficients, then there could be transepithelial effective osmolality gradients even if the solutions have the same total osmolality. Under the conditions described there will be osmotic water flow toward the side containing the higher concentration of low-permeability (high-reflection-coefficient) solutes (35). This has been proposed to occur in the late renal proximal tubule because of reabsorption of organic solutes and preferential reabsorption of HCO_3^-. Both have been claimed to have higher reflection coefficients than Cl^-. However, the notion of low reflections coefficients in epithelial cells has been recently disputed and attributed to errors caused by uncorrected unstirred-layer effects (113). Third is hydrostatic pressure differences: Under most conditions, these differences are small and hence do not contribute significantly to water flow.

Pathways for Transepithelial Water Transport Are Also Controversial

Is water transport transcellular and/or paracellular? Epithelial transport pathways can be in series or in parallel. The cells consist of pathways in series (apical membrane, cytoplasm, and basolateral membrane) as does the intercellular (paracellular) pathway (junction in series with lateral intercellular space). In turn, the transcellular pathway and the paracellular pathway are in parallel with each other. A major problem in the phenomenological description of transepithelial transport has been to ascertain the portions of ion and water fluxes occurring across each pathway. In the case of ions, it has been clearly shown that in some epithelia most passive permeation is paracellular (leaky epithelia), whereas in others most passive permeation is transcellular (tight epithelia) (see Reuss [86] for a review). In the case of water, there is convincing experimental evidence demonstrating transcellular transport but paracellular transport is controversial.

TRANSCELLULAR OSMOTIC WATER TRANSPORT IS SUPPORTED BY HIGH CELL-MEMBRANE P_{os}

In high water-permeability epithelia (mammalian renal proximal tubule, *Necturus* gallbladder), apical and basolateral membrane P_{os} values range from ~500 to 5000 $\mu m \cdot s^{-1}$ (renal tubule [12–14, 33, 124]; gallbladder [17, 80]). In both membrane domains, there can be considerable "amplification," by the presence of microvilli at the apical membrane and infoldings at the basolateral membrane. Hence, the P_{os} values expressed per unit surface area of membrane are much smaller than those relative to the idealized geometry of the tissue. Regardless of this, the water permeability of these epithelia is high and attributable to the expression of water pores.

PARACELLULAR OSMOTIC WATER TRANSPORT IS SUPPORTED BY INDIRECT ARGUMENTS

The paracellular P_{os} can be estimated in principle from the transepithelial and cell membrane P_{os}. Given that the transcellular and paracellular pathways are in parallel:

$$P_{os}^t = P_{os}^c + P_{os}^p \tag{21}$$

where P_{os} denotes osmotic permeability, and the superscripts t, c, and p refer to transepithelial, cellular, and paracellular path-

ways, respectively. In the proximal tubule, P_{os}^t appears to be significantly higher than P_{os}^c, suggesting that P_{os}^c is sizable (124). The problems with these calculations are the errors involved in the measurements of transepithelial and cell-membrane P_{os} values.

Paracellular water transport is also supported by quantitative assessments of the effect of organomercurial compounds, presumed to be specific pore blockers, on P_{os}^t and P_{os}^c. An agent such as pCMBS inhibits P_f^c by more than 90%, but P_{os}^t is reduced by only 50%, which strongly suggests a finite parallel water-permeation pathway (124). These calculations imply a single site of action of pCMBS and other effects are in principle possible.

Another argument suggesting paracellular water flow is the observation of solvent drag and electrokinetic phenomena. If osmotic water flow takes place across large pores, which are also permeable to solute, then there will be a frictional interaction between water and solute and the water flow will cause a solute flow in the same direction. This solute flux can occur in the absence of a favorable solute electrochemical gradient between the solutions. It is usually demonstrated using hydrophilic nonelectrolytes (e.g., small sugars such as mannitol); the mannitol and water fluxes correlate linearly, as predicted by Eq. 18. Results suggesting solvent drag have been reported for several epithelia (124). The simplest electrokinetic phenomenon to study is the streaming potential produced when, in the absence of a favorable electrochemical gradient, the solute is a permeant ion that flows in the same direction as water. This occurs if the water permeation pathway is ion-selective, that is, more permeable to that ion than to the counterion. The observation of this phenomenon has been interpreted as supportive of solute–water coupling in the paracellular pathway (reviewed in Tripathi and Boulpaep [107]).

The main problem with experiments purporting to demonstrate solvent drag or streaming potentials is the complication introduced by unstirred layers. Water transport in such a system causes changes in solute concentrations next to the membrane surfaces, raising the concentration on the cis side and lowering it on the trans side. Therefore, even if the concentrations of a given solute are the same in the bulk solution, there will be a concentration gradient at the membrane surfaces (unstirred-layer polarization), which explains the apparent solvent drag (pseudo-solvent drag). Pseudo-streaming potentials can be similarly caused by ion concentration changes elicited by the water flux. It is possible to distinguish true from apparent streaming potentials by comparing the time courses of the transepithelial voltage changes caused by the addition of nonelectrolyte or by a unilateral ionic substitution (85, 89, 90). This criterion could help confirm or rule out the legitimacy of claimed true streaming potentials.

In sum, the cellular pathway is certain to contribute to transepithelial osmotic water transport and there are suggestions of a significant paracellular contribution. However, the latter is based on indirect evidence and questionable because of possible unstirred-layer artifacts. This problem will be definitively solved only by direct measurements of transcellular and paracellular water flows, which is a daunting task. Recent elegant fluorescence microscopy studies (54) suggest that there is no significant water flow across tight junctions of MDCK monolayers, relative to the transcellular flow. However, in these experiments the rate of transepithelial water flux was much smaller than observed in native epithelia. Sachar-Hill and Hill (93) have argued, on the basis of analyses of hydrophilic probe and water fluxes, that the paracellular water flux of several epithelia is quite high. However, the problem of unstirred layers was neglected in their analysis.

Summary and Conclusions

Water transport in leaky epithelia occurs in the same direction as solute transport and in near-isosmotic proportions. The available experimental evidence supports the view that the coupling between solute and water transport is not molecular, but thermodynamic, that is, osmotic. Solute transport by pumps, carriers, and/or channels elicits differences in solute concentration at the membrane surfaces, with a decrease in concentration on the cis side and an increase on the trans side. The establishment of osmotic gradients is favored because of the architecture of epithelia, which contain compartments that do not mix well with the surrounding fluids. The magnitude of the osmotic gradients is small and difficult to measure, but sufficient to account for the measured rates of fluid transport. Osmotic water flow takes place predominantly across the cell membranes, via both AQP pores and the phospholipid bilayer, with a small or nil contribution of other proteins. It is possible that part of the water flow is paracellular via the tight junctions, but this is likely to be relatively small.

References

1. Agre P. Aquaporin water channels (Nobel Lecture). *Angew Chem Int Ed Engl* 2004;43:4278–4290.
2. Agre P, Preston GM, Smith BL, Jung JS, Raina S, Moon C, Guggino WB, Nielsen S. Aquaporin CHIP: the archetypal molecular water channel. *Am J Physiol* 1993;265:F463–F476.
3. Anderson JL, Malone DM. Mechanism of osmotic flow in porous membranes. *Biophys J* 1974;14:957–982.
4. Anthony TL, Brooks HL, Boassa D, Leonov S, Yanochko GM, Regan JW, Yool AJ. Cloned human aquaporin-1 is a cyclic GMP-gated ion channel. *Mol Pharm* 2000;57:576–588.
5. Barfuss DW, Schafer JA. Hyperosmolarity of absorbate from isolated rabbit proximal tubules. *Am J Physiol* 1984;247:F130–F139.
6. Barry PH, Diamond JM. Effects of unstirred layers on membrane phenomena. *Physiol Rev* 1984;64:763–873.
7. Bean CP. The physics of porous membranes—neutral pores. In: Eisenman G, ed. *Membranes I. Macroscopic Systems and Models.* New York: Dekker, 1972:1–54.
8. Boassa D, Yool AJ. Single amino acids in the carboxyl terminal domain of aquaporin-1 contribute to cGMP-dependent ion channel activation. *BMC Physiol* 2003;3:12.
9. Brisson A, Wade RH. Three-dimensional structure of luminal plasma membrane protein from urinary bladder. *J Mol Biol* 1983;166:21–36.
10. Brown D. Membrane recycling and epithelial cell function. *Am J Physiol* 1989;256:F1–F12.
11. Brown D. Structural–functional features of vasopressin-induced water flow in the kidney collecting duct. *Semin Nephrol* 1991;11:478–501.
12. Carpi-Medina P, González E, Whittembury G. Cell osmotic water permeability of isolated rabbit proximal convoluted tubules. *Am J Physiol* 1984;244:F554–F563.
13. Carpi-Medina P, Whittembury G. Comparison of transcellular and transepithelial water osmotic permeabilities in the isolated proximal straight tubule of the rabbit kidney. *Pflügers Arch* 1988;412:66–74.
14. Charron F, Lapointe JY. Slow ionic diffusion in oocytes and the water cotransport hypothesis. *FASEB J* 2005;19:A1156.
15. Cooper GJ, Boron WF. Effect of PCMBS on CO_2 permeability of *Xenopus* oocytes expressing aquaporin-1 or its C189S mutant. *Am J Physiol* 1998;275:C1481–C1486.
16. Cooper GJ, Zhou Y, Bouyer P, Grichtchenko II, Boron WF. Transport of volatile solutes through AQP1. *J Physiol* 2002;542:17–29.
17. Cotton CU, Weinstein AM, Reuss L. Osmotic water permeability of Necturus gallbladder. *J Gen Physiol* 1989;93:649–679.
18. Curran PF, MacIntosh JR. A model system for biological water transport. *Nature (Lond)* 1962;193:347–348.
19. Curran PF, Solomon AK. Ion and water fluxes in the ileum of rats. *J Gen Physiol* 1957;41:143–168.
20. Dawson DC. Water transport. In: Seldin DW, Giebisch G, eds. *The Kidney: Physiology and Pathophysiology.* New York: Raven Press, 1992:301–316.
21. Denker BM, Smith BL, Kuhajda FP, Agre P. Identification, purification, and partial characterization of a novel M, 28,000 integral membrane protein from erythrocytes and renal tubule. *J Biol Chem* 1988;263:14634–15642.
22. Diamond JM. The mechanism of water transport by the gall-bladder. *J Physiol (Lond)* 1962;161:503–527.
23. Diamond JM, Bossert WH. Standing-gradient osmotic flow: a mechanism for coupling of water and solute transport in epithelia. *J Gen Physiol* 1967;50:2061–2083.
24. Engel A, Walz T, Agre P. The aquaporin family of membrane water channels. *Curr Opin Struct Biol* 1994;4:545–553.
25. Finkelstein, A. *Water Movement Through Lipid Bilayers, Pores and Plasma Membranes: Theory and Reality.* New York: John Wiley & Sons, 1986.
26. Finkelstein A, Rosenberg PA. Single-file transport: implications for ion and water movements through gramicidin A channels. In: Stevens CF, Tsien RW, eds. *Membrane Transport Processes.* Vol. 3. Copenhagen: Munksgaard, 1979:107–119.
27. Flamion B, Spring KR. Water permeability of apical and basolateral cell membranes of rat inner medullary collecting duct. *Am J Physiol* 1990;259:F986–F999.
28. Forster RE. The transport of water in erythrocytes, In: Bronner F, Kleinzeller A, eds. *Current Topics in Membranes and Transport.* Vol. 2. New York: Academic Press, 1971:41–98.
29. Frömter E. The route of passive ion movement through the epithelium of Necturus gallbladder. *J Membr Biol* 1972;8:259–301.
30. Fu D, Libson A, Miercke LJ, Weitzman C, Nollert P, Krucinski J, Stroud RM. Structure of a glycerol-conducting channel and the basis for its selectivity. *Science* 2000;290:481–486.
31. Gagnon MP, Bissonnette P, Deslandes LM, Wallendorff B, Lapointe JY. Glucose accumulation can account for the initial water flux triggered by Na1/glucose cotransport. *Biophys J* 2004;86:125–133.
32. Gonen T, Sliz P, Kistler J, Cheng Y, Walz T. Aquaporin-0 membrane junctions reveal the structure of a closed water pore. *Nature* 2004;429:193–197.
33. González E, Carpi-Medina P, Whittembury G. Cell osmotic water permeability of isolated rabbit proximal straight tubules. *Am J Physiol* 1982;242:F321–F330.
34. Green R, Giebisch G. Luminal hypotonicity: a driving force for fluid absorption from the proximal tubule. *Am J Physiol* 1984;246:F167–F174.
35. Green R, Giebisch G. Reflection coefficients and water permeability in rat proximal tubule. *Am J Physiol* 1989;257:F658–F668.
36. Green R, Windhager EE, Giebisch G. Protein osmotic pressure effects on proximal tubule fluid movement in the rat. *Am J Physiol* 1974;226:267–276.
37. Hallows KR, Knauf PA. Principles of cell volume regulation. In: Strange K, ed. *Cellular and Molecular Physiology of Cell Volume Regulation.* Boca Raton FL: CRC Press, 1994:3–29.
38. Han H, Wax MB, Patil RV. Regulation of aquaporin-4 water channels by phorbol ester-dependent protein phosphorylation. *J Biol Chem* 1998;273:6001–6004.
39. Handler JS. Antidiuretic hormone moves membranes. *Am J Physiol* 1988;255:F375–F382.
40. Harris HW, Handler JS. The role of membrane turnover in the water permeability response to antidiuretic hormone. *J Membr Biol* 1988;103:207–216.
41. Hebert SC. Hypertonic cell volume regulation in mouse thick limbs. I. ADH dependency and nephron heterogeneity. *Am J Physiol* 1986;250:C907–C919.
42. Heymann JB, Agre P, Engel A. Progress on the structure and function of aquaporin 1. *J Struct Biol* 1998;121:191–206.
43. Hicks RM. The mammalian urinary bladder: an accommodating organ. *Biol Rev Camb Philos Soc* 1975;50:215–246.
44. Hicks RM, Ketterer B. Hexagonal lattice of subunits in the thick luminal membrane of the rat urinary bladder. *Nature* 1969;224:1304–1305.
45. Hill AE. Solute-solvent coupling in epithelia: a critical examination of the standing-gradient osmotic flow theory. *Proc R Soc Lond Biol* 1975;190:99–114.
46. Hoshi T, Sakai F. A comparison of the electrical resistances of the surface cell membrane and cellular wall in the proximal tubule of the newt kidney. *Jpn J Physiol* 1967;17:627–637.
47. House CR. *Water Transport in Cells and Tissues.* London: Arnold, 1974.
48. Hu P, Meyers S, Liang FX, Deng FM, Kachar B, Zeidel ML, Sun TT. Role of membrane proteins in permeability barrier function: uroplakin ablation elevates urothelial permeability. *Am J Physiol Renal Physiol* 2002;283:F1200–1207.
49. Ikeda M, Beitz E, Kozono D, Guggino WB, Agre P, Yasui M. Characterization of aquaporin-6 as a nitrate channel in mammalian cells. *J Biol Chem* 2002;277:39873–39879.
50. Jacobson K, Dietrich C. Looking at lipid rafts? *Trends Cell Biol* 1999;9:87–91.
51. Jung JS, Preston GM, Smith BL, Guggino WB, Agre P. Molecular structure of the water channel through aquaporin CHIP: the tetrameric-hourglass model. *J Biol Chem* 1994;269:14648–14654.
52. King-Hele JA. Approximate analytical solutions for water and solute flow in intercellular spaces with a leaky tight junction. *J Theor Biol* 1979;80:451–465.
53. King LS, Kozono D, Agre P. From structure to disease: the evolving tale of aquaporin biology. *Nat Rev Mol Cell Biol* 2004;5:687–698.
54. Kovbasnjuk O, Leader JP, Weinstein AM, Spring KR. Water does not flow across the tight junctions of MDCK cell epithelium. *Proc Natl Acad Sci U S A* 1998;95:6526–6520.

55. Lapointe Jy, Gagnon M, Poirier S, Bissonnette P. The presence of local osmotic gradients can account for the water flux driven by the Na^1-glucose cotransporter. *J Physiol* 2002;542:61–62.

56. Lapointe JY, Gagnon MP, Gagnon DG, Bissonnette P. Controversy regarding the secondary active water transport hypothesis. *Biochem Cell Biol* 2002;80:525–533.

57. Larsen EH, Sørensen JB, Sørensen JN. Analysis of the sodium recirculation theory of solute-coupled water transport in small intestine. *J Physiol* 2002;542:33–50.

58. Loo DD, Wright EM, Zeuthen T. Water pumps. *J Physiol* 2002; 542:53–60.

59. Loo DD, Zeuthen T, Chandy G, Wright EM. Cotransport of water by the Na^1/glucose cotransporter. *Proc Natl Acad Sci U S A* 1996; 93:13367–13370.

60. Lechène C. Cellular volume and cytoplasmic gel. *Biol Cell* 1985; 55:177–180.

61. Levitt DG. Kinetics of diffusion and convection in 3-X pores. Exact solution by computer simulation. *Biophys J* 1973;13:186–206.

62. Levitt DG. A new theory of transport for cell membrane pores. I. General theory and application to red cell. *Biochim Biophys Acta* 1974; 373:115–131.

63. Lin, JH, Wu XR, Kreibich G, Sun TT. Precursor sequence, processing, and urothelium-specific expression of a major 15-kDa protein subunit of asymmetric unit membrane. *J Biol Chem* 1994;269:1775–1784

64. MacAulay N, Gether U, Klaerke DA, Zeuthen T. Water transport by the human Na^1-coupled glutamate cotransporter expressed in *Xenopus* oocytes. *J Physiol* 2001;530:367–378.

65. Macey RI. Transport of water and urea in red blood cells. *Am J Physiol* 1984;246:C195–C203.

66. Macey RI, Farmer REI. Inhibition of water and solute permeability in human red cells. *Biochim Biophys Acta* 1970;211:104–106.

67. Macey RI, Moura TF. Basic principles of transport. In: Hoffman JD, Jamieson JD. *Handbook of Physiology*. New York: Oxford University Press, 1997:181–259.

68. Macknight ADC. Principles of cell volume regulation. *Renal Physiol Biochem* 1988;11:114–148.

69. Maffly RH, Leaf A. The potential of water in mammalian tissues. *J Gen Physiol* 1959;42:1257–1275.

70. Mauro A. The role of negative pressure in osmotic equilibrium and osmotic flow. In: Ussing HH, Bindslev N, Lassen NA, Sten-Knudsen O, eds. *Water Transport across Epithelia. Barriers, Gradients and Mechanisms*. Copenhagen: Munksgaard, 1981:107–119.

71. Meinild A-K, Klaerke D, Loo DDF, Wright EM, Zeuthen T. The human Na^1/glucose cotransporter is a molecular water pump. *J Physiol* 1998;508:15–21.

72. Meinild AK, Loo DD, Pajor AM, Zeuthen T, Wright EM. Water transport by the renal Na^1-dicarboxylate cotransporter. *Am J Physiol Renal Physiol* 2000;278:F777–F783.

73. Mills JW, DiBona DR. Distribution of Na^1 pump sites in the frog gallbladder. *Nature (Lond)* 1978;271:273–275.

74. Minton AP, Colclasure GC, Parker JC. Model for the role of macromolecular crowding in regulation of cellular volume. *Proc Natl Acad Sci U S A* 1992;89:10504–10506.

75. Murata K, Mitsuoka K, Hirai T, Walz T, Agre P, Heymann JB, Engel A, Fujiyoshi Y. Structural determinants of water permeation through aquaporin-1. *Nature* 2000;407:599–605.

76. Nakhoul NL, Davis BA, Romero MF, Boron WF. Effect of expressing the water channel aquaporin-1 on the CO_2 permeability of *Xenopus* oocytes. *Am J Physiol* 1988;45:C543–C548.

77. Nemeth-Cahalan KL, Hall JE. pH and calcium regulate the water permeability of aquaporin 0. *J Biol Chem* 2000;275:6777–6782.

78. Nilius B. Is the volume-regulated anion channel VRAC a "water-permeable" channel? *Neurochem Res* 2004;29:3–8.

79. Paganelli CV, Solomon AK. The rate of exchange of tritiated water across the human red cell membrane. *J Gen Physiol* 1957;41: 259–277.

80. Persson BE, Spring KR. Gallbladder epithelial cell hydraulic water permeability and volume regulation. *J Gen Physiol* 1982;79:481–505.

81. Prasad GV, Coury LA, Fin F, Zeidel ML. Reconstituted aquaporin 1 water channels transport CO_2 across membranes. *J Biol Chem* 1998;273:33123–33126.

82. Preston GM, Agre P. Isolation of the cDNA for erythrocyte integral membrane protein of 28 kilodaltons: member of an ancient channel family. *Proc Natl Acad Sci U S A* 1991;88:11110–11114.

83. Reeves WB, Andreoli E. Sodium chloride transport in the loop of Henle. In: Seldin DW, Giebisch G. *The Kidney: Physiology and Pathophysiology*. New York: Raven Press, 1992: 1975–2001.

84. Ren G, Reddy VS, Cheng A, Melnyk P, Mitra AK. Visualization of a water-selective pore by electron crystallography in vitreous ice. *Proc Natl Acad Sci U S A* 2001;98:1398–1403.

85. Reuss L. Pathways for osmotic water transport in gallbladder epithelium. In: Ussing HH, Fischbarg J, Sten-Knudsen O, Larsen EH, Willumsen NJ, eds. *Isotonic Transport in Leaky Epithelia*. Alfred Benzon Symposium 34. Copenhagen: Munksgaard, 1993:181–200.

86. Reuss L. Epithelial transport. In: Hoffman JE, Jamieson, eds. *Handbook of Physiology: Cell Physiology*. New York: Oxford University Press, 1997:309–338.

87. Reuss L. General principles of water transport. In: Seldin DW, Giebisch G, eds. *The Kidney: Physiology and Pathophysiology*. New York: Raven Press, 2000:321–340.

88. Reuss L, Cotton CU. Isosmotic fluid transport across epithelia. *Contemp Nephrol* 1988;4:1–37.

89. Reuss L, Simon B, Cotton CU. Pseudo-streaming potentials in Necturus gallbladder epithelium. II. The mechanism is a junctional diffusion potential. *J Gen Physiol* 1992;99:317–338.

90. Reuss L, Simon B, Xi Z. Pseudo-streaming potentials in Necturus gallbladder epithelium. I. Paracellular origin of the transepithelial voltage changes. *J Gen Physiol* 1992;99:297–316.

91. Rivers R, Blanchard A, Eladari D, Leviel F, Paillard M, Podevin RA, Zeidel ML. Water and solute permeabilities of medullary thick ascending limb apical and basolateral membranes. *Am J Physiol* 1998;274:F453–F462.

92. Roux B, Schulten K. Computational studies of membrane channels. *Structure (Camb)* 2004;12:1343–1351.

93. Sachar-Hill B, Hill AE. Paracellular fluid transport by epithelia. *Int Rev Cytol* 2002;215: 319–350.

94. Sackin H, Boulpaep EL. Models for coupling of salt and water transport. Proximal tubular reabsorption in Necturus kidney. *J Gen Physiol* 1975;66:671–733.

95. Sánchez JM, Li Y, Rubanshkin A, Iserovich P, Wen Q, Ruberti JW, Smith RW, Rittenband D, Kuang K, Diecke FPJ, Fischbarg J. Evidence for a central role for electro-osmosis in fluid transport by corneal endothelium. *J Membr Biol* 2002;187:37–50.

96. Saparov SM, Kozono D, Rothe U, Agre P, Pohl P. Water and ion permeation of aquaporin-1 in planar lipid bilayers. *J Biol Chem* 2001;276:31515–31520.

97. Schultz SG. Homocellular regulatory mechanisms in sodium-transporting epithelia: avoidance of extinction by "flush-through." *Am J Physiol* 1981;241: F579–F590.

98. Schultz SG, Hudson RL. Biology of sodium-absorbing epithelial cells: dawning of a new era. In: Schultz SG, Field M, Frizzell RA, eds. *Handbook of Physiology. The Gastrointestinal System*. New York: Oxford University Press, 1991:45–81.

99. Shporer M, Civan MM. Structuring of water and immobilization of ions within the intracellular fluids: the contribution of NMR spectroscopy. *Curr Topics Membr Trans* 1977;9:1–69.

100. Smith BL, P Agre. Erythrocyte M$_r$ 28,000 transmembrane protein exists as a multisubunit oligomer similar to channel proteins. *J Biol Chem* 1991;266:6407–6415.

101. Spring KR. Mechanism of fluid transport by epithelia. In: Schulz SG, Field M, Frizzell RA, eds. *Handbook of Physiology. The Gastrointestinal System*. New York: Oxford University Press, 1991:195–207.

102. Spring KR. Solute recirculation. *J Physiol* 2002;542:51.

103. Strange K, Spring KR. Cell membrane permeability of rabbit cortical collecting duct. *J Membr Biol* 1987;96:27–43.

104. Sui H, Han BG, Lee JK, Walian P, Jap BK. Structural basis of water-specific transport through the AQP1 water channel. *Nature* 2001;414:872–878.

105. Sun AM, Saltzbert SN, Kikeri D, Hebert. SC. Mechanisms of cell volume regulation by the mouse medullary thick ascending limb of Henle. *Kidney Int* 1990;38:1019–1029.

106. Tajkhorshid E, Nollert P, Jensen MO, Miercke LJ, O'Connell J, Stroud RM, Schulten K. Control of the selectivity of the aquaporin water channel family by global orientational tuning. *Science* 2002;296:525–530.

107. Tripathi S, Boulpaep EL. Mechanisms of water transport by epithelial cells. *Q J Exp Physiol* 1989;74:385–417.

108. Ussing HH, Eskesen K. Mechanism of isotonic water transport in glands. *Acta Physiol Scand* 1989;136:443–454.

109. Ussing HH, Lind F, Larsen EH. Ion secretion and isotonic transport in frog skin glands. *J Memb Biol* 1996;152:101–110.

110. vant'Hoff JH. Die Rolle des osmotischen Druckes in der Analogie zwischen Lösungen und Gasen. *Z Physik Chemie* 1887;1:481–493.

111. Verkman AS. Mechanisms and regulation of water permeability in renal epithelia. *Am J Physiol* 1989;257:C837–C850.

112. Verkman, A. S. Does aquaporin 1 pass gas? An opposing view. *J Physiol* 2002;542:31.

113. Verkman AS, van Hoek AN, Ma T, Frigeri A, Skach WR, Mitra A, Tamarappoo BK, Farinas J. Water transport across mammalian cell membranes. *Am J Physiol* 1996;270:C12–C30.

114. Wade JB. Role of membrane traffic in the water and Na^1 responses to vasopressin. *Semin Nephrol* 1994;14:322–332.

115. Walz T, Haner M, Wu XR, Henn C, Engel A, Sun TT, Aebi U. Towards the molecular architecture of the asymmetric unit membrane of the mammalian urinary bladder epithelium: a closed "twisted ribbon" structure. *J Mol Biol* 1995;248:887–900.

116. Walz T, Hirai T, Murata K, Heymann JB, Mitsuoka K, Fujiyoshi Y, Smith BL, Agre P, Engel A. The three-dimensional structure of aquaporin-1. *Nature* 1997;387:624–626.

117. Walz T, Smith BL, Agre P, Engel A. The 3-D structure of human erythrocyte aquaporin CHIP. *EMBO J* 1994;13:2985–2993.

118. Weinstein AM, Stephenson JL. Electrolyte transport across a simple epithelium. Steady-state and transient analysis. *Biophys J* 1979;27:165–186.

119. Weinstein AM, Stephenson JL. Coupled water transport in standing gradient models of the lateral intercellular space. *Biophys J* 1981; 35:167–191.

120. Weinstein AM, Stephenson JL. Models of coupled salt and water transport across leaky epithelia. *J Membr Biol* 1981;60:1–20.

121. Whittembury G, Rawlins FA. Evidence of a paracellular pathway for ion flow in the kidney proximal tubule: electron microscopic demonstration of lanthanum precipitate in the tight junction. *Pflügers Arch* 1971;330:302–309.

122. Whittembury G, Carpi-Medina P, Gonzalez E, Linares H. Effect of parachloromercuribenzene sulfonic acid and temperature on cell water osmotic permeability of proximal straight tubules. *Biochim Biophys Acta* 1984;775:365–373.

123. Whittembury G, Hill A. Coupled transport of water and solute across epithelia. In: Seldin DW, Giebisch G, eds. *The Kidney: Physiology and Pathophysiology*. New York: Raven Press, 2000:341–362.

124. Whittembury G, Reuss L. Mechanisms of coupling of solute and solvent transport in epithelia. In: Seldin DW, Giebisch G, eds. *The Kidney: Physiology and Pathophysiology*. New York: Raven Press, 1992:317–360.

125. Windhager EE, Boulpaep EL, Giebisch G. Electrophysiological studies in single nephrons. In: Schreiner GE, ed. *Proceedings of the Third International Congress on Nephrology*. New York: Karger, 1967:35–47.

126. Wu XR, Manabe M, Yu J, Sun TT. Large scale purification and immunolocalization of bovine uroplakins I, II, and III. Molecular markers of urothelial differentiation. *J Biol Chem* 1990;265:19170–19179.

127. Yang B, Fukuda N, van Hoek A, Matthay MA, Ma T, Verkman AS. Carbon dioxide permeability of aquaporin-1 measured in erthrocytes and lung of aquaporin-1 null mice and in reconstituted liposomes. *J Biol Chem* 2000;275:2686–2692.

128. Yu J, Manabe M, Wu XR, Xu C, Surya B, Sun TT. Uroplakin I: a 27-kD protein associated with the asymmetric unit membrane of mammalian urothelium. *J Cell Biol* 1990;111:1207–1216.

129. Zelenina M, Zelenin S, Bondar AA, Brismar H, Aperia A. Water permeability of aquaporin-4 is decreased by protein kinase C and dopamine. *Am J Physiol* 2002;283:F309–F318.

130. Zeuthen T. Cotransport of K^1, Cl^2 and H_2O by membrane proteins from choroid plexus epithelium of Necturus maculosus. *J Physiol (Lond)* 1994;478:203–219.

131. Zeuthen T, Hamann S, La Cour M. Cotransport of H^1, a lactate and H_2O by membrane proteins in retinal pigment epithelium of bullfrog. *J Physiol* 1996;497:3–17.

132. Zeuthen T, Klaerke DA. Transport of water and glycerol in aquaporin 3 is gated by H^1. *J Biol Chem* 1999;274:21631–21636.

CHAPTER **6**

Cell Volume Control

Florian Lang

University of Tübingen, Tübingen, Germany

Cells have to avoid gross alterations of volume in order to survive. Obviously, excessive cell swelling will jeopardize the integrity of the cell membrane, and both cell swelling and cell shrinkage will interfere with cytoskeletal architecture. Moreover, cellular function critically depends on the hydration of cytosolic proteins. Proteins and protein-bound water occupy a large portion of the cell interior (macromolecular crowding) leaving only a small fraction of cellular volume to free water (21, 68, 75, 158, 160, 168). Abstraction or addition of only a few percentage points of cellular water thus has profound effects on protein function and cellular performance.

In most mammalian cells, the plasma membrane is highly permeable to water (45, 152). In theory, driving forces for movement of water include hydrostatic andosmotic pressure gradients. However, the cell membrane is too fragile to withstand significant hydrostatic pressure gradients, and if extension of the cell is not prevented by extracellular constraints the movement of water is governed almost exclusively by osmotic gradients (79, 82, 116, 185). Thus, to avoid swelling or shrinkage, a cell has to achieve osmotic equilibrium across the cell membrane (Fig. 1). At excessive intracellular osmolarity, water will enter following its osmotic gradient and the cell will swell. Conversely, at excessive extracellular osmolarity water will leave and the cell will shrink. As outlined in this chapter, a wide variety of factors modify intra- or extra-cellular osmolarity, and thus challenge osmotic equilibrium across the cell membrane.

For maintenance of volume constancy, cells employ a number of mechanisms including metabolism and altered transport across the cell membrane. These mechanisms not only serve the maintenance of cell volume constancy, but may also participate in the regulation of cell function. Hormones and mediators may influence cell volume regulatory mechanisms and thus manipulate cell volume. Alterations of cell volume will in turn modify other cell volume–sensitive functions. The interplay among cell volume regulatory mechanisms, cell hydration, and cell function does not only contribute to physiological regulation of cellular function, but also participates in the pathophysiology of a wide variety of diseases.

In this chapter a description of cell volume regulatory mechanisms will be followed by a synopsis of factors challenging cell volume constancy and a discussion on the impact of cell volume regulatory mechanisms on physiology and pathophysiology of cellular function. Due to space constraints, many excellent original papers on cell volume regulation could not be quoted and the reader is referred to reviews instead. For more detailed analysis of the pertinent original literature, the reader is encouraged to consult previous reviews on cell volume regulation (22, 24, 26, 72, 89, 93, 100, 119, 124, 130, 132, 133, 157, 177, 178, 204, 205, 230).

CELL VOLUME REGULATORY MECHANISMS

Cell volume constancy is constantly challenged by alterations of extracellular osmolarity, by intracellular metabolic generation of osmotically active solutes and transport across the cell membrane (132). To counteract those challenges, cells employ a variety of cell volume regulatory mechanisms (133). Following cell swelling, these mechanisms decrease intracellular osmolarity and cell volume, thus accomplishing regulatory cell volume decrease (RVD). Upon cell shrinkage the mechanisms increase intracellular osmolarity and cell volume, thereby accomplishing regulatory cell volume increase (RVI).

The most powerful mechanisms of cell volume regulation are ion transporters in the cell membrane (133). As outlined below, uneven ion composition of intracellular and extracellular fluid is one prerequisite for the establishment of osmotic equilibrium across the cell membrane. Furthermore, several ion transport systems in the cell membrane are modified upon alterations of cell volume. Following cell swelling they mediate cellular ion release; upon cell shrinkage they allow cellular ion accumulation to reestablish osmotic equilibrium across the cell membrane.

However, the use of ions in cellular osmoregulation is limited, since high inorganic ion concentrations interfere with the stability of proteins (159). Beyond that, altered ion gradients across the cell membrane interfere with the function of gradient-driven transporters. For instance, an increase

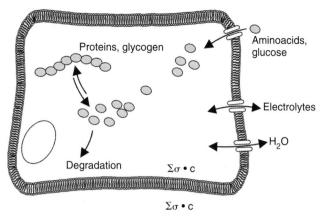

FIGURE 1 Determinants of cell volume. Water moves according to osmotic gradients across the cell membranes, that is, differences between intracellular and extracellular $\Sigma\sigma \cdot c$, where σ is the reflection coefficient and c the concentration of each solute on either side. Even at constant extracellular $\Sigma\sigma \cdot c$, an osmotic gradient is generated by transport of osmotically active solutes across the cell membrane and by metabolic generation or disposal of intracellular solutes.

of intracellular Na^+ activity decreases the chemical gradient for Na^+ across the cell membrane and reduces the driving force for Ca^{++} extrusion via the Na^+Ca^+ exchanger, which increases intracellular Ca^{++} activity. To avoid excessive alterations of intracellular ion concentration, cells also utilize organic osmolytes for osmoregulation (25, 72). Moreover, cells adapt a variety of metabolic functions, and thus modify the cellular generation or disposal of osmotically active organic substances.

It should be pointed out that a single cell does not usually employ all cell volume regulatory mechanisms described in the following. In most cases, it is not clear why a given cell selects a certain set of ion transporters and osmolytes without using other mechanisms. Presumably, the large repertoire of cell volume regulatory transporters and osmolytes available enables any given cell to regulate its volume with relatively little impairment of cellular function.

Cell Volume Regulatory Ion Transport

To counterbalance the intracellular osmolarity due to osmotically active organic solutes, such as amino acids and carbohydrates, cell volume regulatory mechanisms have to maintain intracellular concentrations of inorganic ions below extracellular ion concentrations. In addition, cell volume regulatory ion transport systems are employed to counteract alterations of cell volume by appropriate transport of ions across the cell membrane.

IONS IN CELL VOLUME MAINTENANCE

To compensate for the cellular accumulation of organic solutes, cells maintain a low intracellular Cl^- concentration (132). In most cells Cl^- may move across the cell membrane through Cl^- channels. Cl^- movement through those channels is governed by the cell's negative potential

across the cell membrane, which is built up by asymmetric cation gradients (152): The cells extrude Na^+ in exchange for K^+ by the Na^+, K^+-ATPase. The cell membrane is, on average, less permeable to Na^+ than to K^+. K^+ tends to leave the cell through K^+ channels following its chemical gradient. The exit of K^+ generates a cell-negative potential difference across the cell membrane, and thus establishes the driving force for the exit of anions such as Cl^-. At a cell membrane potential of some -18 mV, for instance, Cl^- is in equilibrium at a chemical gradient of 1:2. Accordingly, at an extracellular Cl^- concentration of 110 mmol/L, the intracellular Cl^- concentration is in electrochemical equilibrium at 55 mmol/L. In theory, such a Cl^- distribution would allow the excess accumulation of 55 mmol/L of organic solutes. In most cells the potential difference across the cell membrane is higher (more negative) than -18 mV, and intracellular Cl^- is even lower than 55 mmol/L.

As long as the cell membrane is perfectly impermeable to Na^+, cell membrane potential, cytosolic Cl^- concentration, and cell volume could be maintained constant without continued expenditure of energy. Maintenance of the asymmetric cation distribution requires, however, that any Na^+ entering the cell is subsequently extruded by Na^+, K^+-ATPase, an ATP-consuming process.

ION RELEASE FOLLOWING CELL SWELLING

Ion transport is not only crucial for the establishment of osmotic equilibrium across the cell membrane, but accomplishes rapid correction of any osmotic imbalance across the cell membrane. Following cell swelling, cells have to release ions to decrease their osmolarity. Most cells release ions by activation of K^+ channels and/or anion channels (Fig. 2). Cell volume regulation requires the operation of both ion channel types, since neither K^+ nor anions can leave the cells without the respective counterion. Several cell volume regulatory ion channels have been identified at the molecular level, including the K^+ channels Kv1.3 (51), Kv1.5 (56), IsK (28, 29), TWIK1 (48), TASK2 (7), MaxiK (228), and the anion channels ClC-2 (81, 108, 109, 151, 213) and ClC-3 (110). The role of other ion channels in cell volume regulation, such as I_{Cln} (32, 170, 179), P-glycoprotein (MDR) (88, 98, 111, 112) and CFTR (40, 222), has been a matter of controversy. Clearly, many different ion channels are likely to contribute to cell volume regulation in various tissues, and the molecular identity of most of those channels is still elusive. Some anion channels do not only allow the exit of Cl^-, but also HCO_3^-, organic anions, and noncharged osmolytes (37, 107, 114, 120, 121, 166, 182, 206).

Swelling of some cells activates unspecific cation channels (133, 184, 185). Since the electrochemical gradient favors entry rather than exit of cations, these channels cannot directly serve cell volume regulation. Instead, the channels allow the entry of Ca^{++}, which in turn activates Ca^{++}-sensitive K^+ channels and/or Cl^- channels.

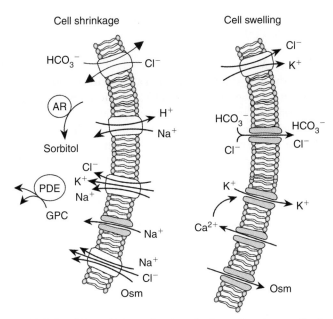

Cell shrinkage   Cell swelling

FIGURE 2 Most widely employed mechanisms of regulatory cell volume regulation. Left: Mechanisms of regulatory cell volume decrease. Cell swelling leads to activation of KCl cotransport, anion channels, K⁺ channels, cation channels, and channels releasing organic osmolytes such as sorbitol, inositol, taurine, and betaine. The cation channels do not directly serve cell volume regulatory decrease but rather increase of cytosolic Ca⁺ activity that triggers activation of Ca⁺⁺ sensitive K⁺ channels. Right: Mechanisms of cell volume increase. Cell shrinkage leads to parallel activation of Na⁺H⁺ exchanger and Cl⁻HCO₃- exchanger, Na⁺K⁺2Cl- cotransport, Na⁺ channels, and Na⁺-coupled accumulation of inositol, taurine, and betaine. Furthermore, cell shrinkage leads to cellular accumulation of glycerophosphorylcholine by inhibition of phosphodiesterase (PDE) and of sorbitol by activation of aldosereducase (AR).

Besides ion channels, the most important mechanism contributing to regulatory cell volume decrease is KCl cotransport (14, 143–145, 171, 214), which allows coupled cellular release of both ions.

Some cells release cellular KCl via parallel activation of K⁺–H⁺ exchange and Cl⁻–HCO₃⁻ exchange (16, 34). The H⁺ and HCO₃⁻ thus taken up in exchange for KCl react via H_2CO_3 to CO_2, which can easily leave the cell again.

Ion Uptake upon Cell Shrinkage

Cell shrinkage activates the ubiquitously expressed Na⁺–K⁺–2Cl⁻ cotransport NKCC2 (52, 77, 97), and/or the Na⁺–H⁺ exchangers NHE1 (226), NHE2 (49), or NHE4 (17) parallel to the Cl⁻–HCO₃⁻ exchanger AE1 (6, 80, 178). The parallel activation of Na⁺–H⁺ exchangers and Cl⁻–HCO₃⁻ exchangers leads to uptake of NaCl, while the H⁺ and HCO₃⁻ lost in exchange for NaCl are replenished in the cell from CO_2 via H_2CO_3 (Fig. 2). The Na⁺ ions accumulated by either Na⁺–K⁺–2Cl⁻ cotransport or Na⁺–H⁺ exchange are extruded by Na⁺, K⁺-ATPase in exchange for K⁺. Accordingly, the transporters eventually lead to cellular KCl uptake.

Several cells activate Na⁺ channels or unspecific cation channels following cell shrinkage (33, 38, 136, 225, 229, 231). The resulting depolarization drives Cl⁻ into the cell so that the net effect is cellular accumulation of NaCl. Other cells inhibit K⁺ and/or Cl⁻ channels to avoid cellular ion loss (133).

Osmolytes

The most important osmolytes are polyols such as sorbitol and myoinositol, methylamines such as betaine and glycerophosphorylcholine, as well as amino acids including taurine (25, 72, 75, 124, 169, 230). In contrast to inorganic ions, organic osmolytes do not destabilize proteins but rather stabilize them. They counteract the destabilizing effects of inorganic ions, some organic ions (e.g., spermidine) and urea (26, 75). The stabilizing potency of the diverse organic osmolytes is not identical. The destabilizing effects of urea are counteracted most efficiently by betaine and glycerophosphorylcholine and less efficiently by myoinositol (26). The stabilizing effects of osmolytes may protect proteins against excessive ion concentrations, as well as against heat shock, freezing, desiccation, and presumably radiation (3, 35, 192, 202, 212).

Osmolyte Accumulation by Metabolism

Sorbitol is generated from glucose under the catalytic action of aldose reductase (9, 60, 74). Stimulation of the transcription rate of the aldose reductase during osmotic cell shrinkage leads to cellular accumulation of sorbitol. The expression of the protein takes many hours and the appropriate increase of sorbitol concentration requires hours to days (71).

Glycerophosphorylcholine (GPC) is produced from phosphatidylcholine under the catalytic action of a phospholipase A₂, which is distinct from the arachidonyl selective enzyme (72, 73). GPC is degraded by a phosphodiesterase to glycerol-phosphate and choline. Inhibition of the phosphodiesterase during cell shrinkage leads to cellular accumulation of GPC (221).

Osmolyte Accumulation by Transport

Myoinositol (inositol) (11, 86, 124, 125, 235), betaine (27, 210, 233) and taurine (220) are taken up by specific Na⁺-coupled transporters SMIT (inositol), BGT (betaine), and NCT (tautine), respectively. The carriers accumulate Na⁺, the respective organic osmolyte, and in the case of BGT and NCT, Cl⁻ as well. Movement of excess positive charge by the carriers depolarizes the cell membrane, thus favoring entry of Cl⁻ via anion channels. The transporters thus mediate uptake of NaCl parallel to organic osmolytes. The transcription rate of the transporters and the cellular accumulation of the respective osmolytes are stimulated by osmotic cell shrinkage. Expression of the transporters is slow, and full adaptation requires hours to days. Moreover, volume regulation by activation of transport systems depends on the availability of osmolytes in the extracellular fluid.

Analogous to osmolytes, some amino acids are accumulated by cell volume–sensitive, Na^+-coupled transport (39, 201, 234). In addition, amino acids could be generated by autophagic proteolysis, as discussed in the next section.

OSMOLYTE RELEASE

Cell swelling stimulates the rapid release of GPC (118, 119), sorbitol (4, 76, 232), inositol (69, 119), betaine (69, 119), and taurine (13, 121, 128, 190). The mechanisms mediating osmolyte release are still poorly understood. Clearly, several mechanisms are simultaneously operative. At least some of the release mechanisms are thought to be anion channels.

Metabolic Pathways Sensitive to Cell Volume

Alterations of cell volume influence a variety of metabolic pathways. The effects of cell volume on metabolism are accomplished in part by activation and inhibition and in part by altered expression of enzymes (132).

PROTEIN AND GLYCOGEN METABOLISM

Cell shrinkage stimulates the breakdown of proteins to amino acids and of glycogen to glucosephosphate (10, 84, 90, 91, 93). Moreover, cell shrinkage inhibits protein and glycogen synthesis (90, 91). The sum of amino acids generated during proteolysis is osmotically more active than the osmolarity of the respective protein. Thus, net formation of macromolecules decreases cellular osmolarity. Cell swelling stimulates protein and glycogen synthesis and inhibits proteolysis and glycogenolysis, thus decreasing the intracellular concentration of amino acids and glucosephosphate.

GLUCOSE AND AMINO ACID METABOLISM

In addition to affecting protein and glycogen metabolism, alterations of cell volume influence several pathways of glucose and amino acid metabolism (91). Cell swelling inhibits glycolysis, stimulates flux through the pentose phosphate pathway, and favors lipogenesis from glucose, effects reversed by cell shrinkage (91, 187). Transcription of phosphoenolpyruvate carboxykinase, a key enzyme for gluconeogenesis, is decreased by cell swelling. Cell swelling stimulates glycine and alanine oxidation and glutamine breakdown, as well as formation of NH_4^+ and urea from amino acids; these effects are reversed by cell shrinkage (91)

OXIDATIVE METABOLISM

The stimulation of flux through the pentose phosphate pathway during cell swelling enhances NADPH production, which favors the formation of glutathione (GSH) (91, 187). Cell shrinkage decreases NADPH production and GSH formation. Accordingly, cell swelling increases and cell shrinkage decreases cellular resistance to oxidative stress. On the other hand, cell shrinkage decreases the activity of NADPH-oxidase, and thus impedes cellular O_2^- formation. Accordingly, leukocyte oxidative burst, and thus immune

response, is blunted by the high osmolarity of kidney medulla (106, 115).

OTHER METABOLIC PATHWAYS

Cell swelling stimulates ketoisocaproate oxidation, acetyl CoA carboxylase, and lipogenesis, and inhibits carnitine palmitoyltransferase I. It decreases cytosolic ATP and phosphocreatine concentrations and increases respiration. Cell swelling stimulates RNA and DNA synthesis. All of these effects are reversed by cell shrinkage (132).

Cell Volume–Sensitive Genes

Cell volume influences the expression of a wide variety of genes (25, 132). Many of those genes are related to cell volume regulation. Accordingly, cell shrinkage stimulates expression of enzymes or transporters engaged in cellular formation or accumulation of osmolytes, such as aldose reductase, and the Na^+-coupled transporters for betaine (BGT), taurine (NCT), inositol (SMIT), and amino acids, as well as $Na^+,K^+,2Cl^-$ cotransport (see above). Moreover, cell shrinkage upregulates the expression of the ATPase α1 subunit (62).

The products of other genes may be involved in the signaling of cell volume regulatory mechanisms, such as the kinases ERK1, ERK2, and JNK-1, which are expressed during cell swelling (1044), or the serum and glucocorticoid inducible kinase SGK1 (65, 227) and cyclooxygenase-2 (238), which are preferably expressed in shrunken cells (132).

Heat shock proteins serve to stabilize proteins, and their expression in shrunken cells may counteract the destabilizing effects of accumulated ions (2, 8, 44, 199, 211). Several genes expressed in response to altered cell volume do not have obvious roles in cell volume regulation. Cell swelling stimulates the expression of the cytoskeletal elements β-actin and tubulin, the immediate early gene c-jun and c-fos, the enzymes ornithine decarboxylase and the cytokine TNF-α (64, 186, 237).

Cell shrinkage stimulates the expression of the channels CIC-K1, the transporter P-glycoprotein, the immediate early genes Egr-1 and c-fos, the GTPase inhibitor α1-chimaerin, the CDβ antigen, the enzymes phosphoenolpyruvate carboxykinase (PEPCK), arginine succinate lyase, tyrosine aminotransferase, tyrosine hydroxylase, dopamine β-hydroxylase, matrix metalloproteinase 9, and tissue plasminogen activator, as well as matrix proteins including biglycan and laminin B_2 (132). Cell shrinkage stimulates both expression and release of ADH, which serves to eliminate water and thus increase extracellular osmolarity (162).

The mechanisms mediating the altered gene expression are beginning to be understood. The promoter region of the genes encoding aldose reductase, BGT, TAUT, and SGK1 have been described to contain osmolarity responsive (ORE), tonicity responsive– (TonE), or cell volume–responsive (CVE) elements, which are required for osmolarity or cell volume–sensitive expression of the respective genes (59, 60,

183). TonE has been shown to bind a tonicity-responsive, element-binding protein TonEBP for stimulation of expression (61, 78, 103, 104, 126, 147, 150, 208). Recent evidence indicates that TonEBP is regulated by ataxia teleangiectasia-mutated (ATM) kinase (103).

Signaling of Cell Volume Regulation

The stimulation of effectors of cell volume regulation requires that alterations of cell volume or osmolarity are perceived and trigger a signaling cascade eventually leading to stimulation of cell volume regulatory mechanisms.

Little is known about sensors of cell size and hydration. Circumstantial evidence points to the ability of cells to determine cellular protein content or macromolecular crowding (23). It has been speculated that a serine/threonine kinase sensitive to macromolecular crowding directly or indirectly regulates the activity of cell volume regulatory KCl^- and $Na^+–K^+–2Cl^-$ cotransport (132). Alternatively, alterations of cell size are thought to impose stretch on the cytoskeleton and/or cell membrane, again leading directly or indirectly to activation of cell volume regulatory mechanisms (85, 102, 132).

A multitude of signaling pathways link the alterations of cell volume and cell volume regulatory mechanisms. Similar to cell volume regulatory mechanisms, the respective signaling may vary considerably between different cells or a given cell in different functional states.

INTRACELLULAR Ca^{++}

Cell swelling increases intracellular Ca^{++} activity in many but not all cells. Ca^{++} enters through Ca^{++} channels in the plasma membrane and/or is released from intracellular stores triggered by 1,4,5-inositol-trisphosphate. Ca^{++} in turn activates some cell volume regulatory K^+ channels and Cl^- channels (156, 217). In addition to its involvement in regulatory cell volume decrease, intracellular Ca^{++} may mediate some of the functional consequences of cell shrinkage.

CYTOSKELETON

Alterations of cell volume modify the architecture of the cytoskeleton and the expression of cytoskeletal proteins (47, 95, 167, 209). Both microtubules (47) and actin filaments (95) have been implicated in cell volume regulation. In several cells, disruption of actin filaments and/or the microtubule network has been shown to interfere with cell volume regulation (132).

PROTEIN PHOSPHORYLATION

Cell swelling and cell shrinkage have both been shown to modify the phosphorylation of a variety of proteins. Kinases reported to be activated during cell swelling include tyrosine kinases (58, 148, 163, 216; 224), protein kinase-C (176, 180), phosphoinositol-3 (PI3) kinase (215), protein kinase-C (176, 180), Jun-kinase, and extracellular signal–regulated kinases ERK-1 and ERK-2 (1, 70, 87, 105, 164, 186, 196,

216), as well as focal adhesion kinase (p121[FAK]) (215). In Jurkat lymphocytes, for instance, cell swelling leads to activation of the src-like kinase lck[56], which in turn activates the cell volume regulatory Cl^- channel ORCC (148).

Osmotic cell shrinkage has been shown to trigger several MAP (mitogen-activated protein) kinase cascades, leading to activation of SAPK, p38 kinase, and myosin light-chain kinase (MLCK) (12, 57, 94, 99, 161, 181). The latter kinase may modulate the cytoskeleton and thus cell volume regulatory ion transport. Moreover, the kinase cascades lead to activation of transcription factors governing expression of cell volume regulated genes (132). Hyperosmolarity activates the tyrosine kinase Fyn–dependent phosphorylation of caveolin (191), which in turn inhibits volume-sensitive Cl^- channels (219).

PHOSPHOLIPASE A_2 AND EICOSANOIDS

Cell swelling activates phospholipase A_2 and subsequently stimulates the formation of the 15-lipoxygenase product hepoxilin A_3 and the 5-lipoxygenase product leukotriene LTD_4 (127). In some cells these eicosanoids stimulate cell volume regulatory K^+, Cl^- channels, and/or taurine release (127). Enhanced formation of leukotrienes parallels decreased formation of PGE_2 with subsequent decrease of Na^+ channel activity (127, 129). Conversely, osmotic cell shrinkage may stimulate formation of PGE_2 with subsequent activation of PGE_2-sensitive Na^+ channels (141). In other cells PGE_2 may activate volume regulatory K^+ channels (42). In erythrocytes, activation of phospholipase A_2 by hyperosmotic shock leads to release of platelet-activating factor PAF, which in turn activates a sphingomyelinase, thus stimulating ceramide formation (142).

pH OF ACIDIC CELLULAR COMPARTMENTS

In all cells studied thus far, swelling alkalinizes and cell shrinkage acidifies acidic cellular compartments, presumably including endosomes, lysosomes, and secretory granules (31, 132). This effect is apparently mediated by the microtubules since it is abolished by disrupture of the microtubule network. The alkalinization of the acidic cellular compartments may contribute to the antiproteolytic action of cell swelling, since the pH optimum of lysosomal proteases is in the acidic range, and lysosomal alkalinization has indeed been shown to inhibit proteolysis (30).

CHALLENGES AND FUNCTIONS AFFECTING CELL VOLUME

A wide variety of factors alters extracellular and/or intracellular osmolarity, and thus challenge cell volume constancy. Due to the exquisite sensitivity of cell function to even minor alterations of cell volume, those factors may modify a multitude of physiological functions and participate in several pathophysiological conditions.

Alterations of Extracellular Fluid Osmolarity and Composition

In mammals, most cells are usually bathed in well-controlled extracellular fluid. However, both extracellular osmolarity and composition could vary to an extent challenging cell volume regulation.

OSMOLARITY

Excessive alterations of extracellular osmolarity are only encountered in kidney medulla, where extracellular osmolarity may approach 1400 mosmol/L in humans (see Chapter 40). Renal medullary cells are exposed to this excessive extracellular osmolarity during antidiuresis, and have to cope with rapid changes of extracellular osmolarity during transition from antidiuresis to diuresis. Blood cells passing the kidney medulla experience high medullary osmolarity and subsequent return to isoosmolarity within seconds (see Chapter 40).

During intestinal absorption, intestinal cells are exposed to anisosmotic luminal fluid and liver cells to minor alterations of portal blood osmolarity. Other tissues are exposed to anisotonic extracellular fluid during deranged regulation of extracellular osmolarity (see Chapters 41 and 42). As Na^+ salts (mainly NaCl) contribute normally more than 90% to extracellular osmolarity, hypernatremia is necessarily paralleled by increase of extracellular osmolarity (see Chapter 42). During hypernatremia, extracellular osmolarity is always enhanced, and cells avoid cell shrinkage by triggering regulatory cell volume increase involving cellular accumulation of osmolytes. Owing to cell volume regulation, cell volume may become normal despite enhanced extracellular osmolarity. Rapid correction of chronically enhanced osmolarity may then lead to deleterious cell swelling since the organic osmolytes accumulated during hyperosmolarity cannot be rapidly released. The most serious consequence is cerebral edema.

Hyponatremia cannot be equated with hypoosmolarity but may occur in isoosmolar or even hyperosmolar states, as in hyperglycemia of uncontrolled diabetes mellitus and ethanol poisoning (see Chapter 41). When hyponatremia reflects a decreased extracellular osmolarity the cells must undergo regulatory cell volume decrease to escape cell swelling. Among other mechanisms cells release organic osmolytes. Upon rapid correction of hyponatremia, cells are unable to rapidly accumulate the osmolytes, and the iatrogenic cell shrinkage may prove more harmful than the untreated hypoosmolarity.

Hypoosmolar hyponatremia is observed following burns, pancreatitis, and crush syndrome, which are generally paralleled by cell shrinkage (93). In those conditions, the primary event may be cell shrinkage leading to ADH release with subsequent renal water retention and to cellular catabolism with enhanced release of organic solutes to the extracellular fluid.

EXTRACELLULAR K^+ CONCENTRATION

The potential difference across the cell membrane is maintained by K^+ flux through K^+ channels, which in turn depends on the electrochemical driving force for K^+. An increase of extracellular K^+ concentration decreases the chemical gradient for K^+ ions, impedes K^+ efflux, depolarizes the cell membrane and thus favors Cl^- entry into the cell. The cellular accumulation of KCl eventually leads to cell swelling. Conversely, a decrease of extracellular K^+ may lead to cell shrinkage secondary to cellular loss of KCl (132).

H^+ AND HCO_3^- CONCENTRATION

Upon increase of extracellular HCO_3^- concentration, cellular HCO_3^- release through anion channels and Na^+–HCO_3^- cotransport is blunted or even reversed, and the decreased efflux of negative charge hyperpolarizes the cell membrane and thus decreases the electrochemical gradient for K^+ efflux. As a result, the cell may swell due to accumulation of K^+ and HCO_3^- (173).

An increasing extracellular pH favors the cellular H^+ elimination through the Na^+–H^+ exchanger, and the resulting cellular Na^+ accumulation may lead to cell swelling (223). During hyperkapnea, cellular CO_2 dissociates to form H^+, which is subsequently extruded by the Na^+–H^+ exchanger. Again, cellular Na^+ accumulation is paralleled by cell swelling. Due to sensitivity of the Na^+–H^+ exchanger to intracellular pH, cellular acidification favors cell swelling whereas cellular alkalinization has the opposite effect (189).

ORGANIC ACIDS

Some organic anions, such as acetate, lactate, and proprionate, may enter cells as unionized acids. Intracellular dissociation of the acids then leads to intracellular acidification, stimulation of Na^+–H^+ exchange, accumulation of Na^+ and organic anions, and subsequent cell swelling (132). Isotonic replacement of Cl^- with impermeant gluconate, on the other hand, leads to cell shrinkage due to cellular loss of Cl^- (132)

UREA, DRUGS, AND TOXINS

Urea readily passes cell membranes and does not usually create osmotic gradients across them. On the other hand, it has been shown that urea destabilizes proteins, and thus shifts the cell volume regulatory set point towards smaller cell volumes. Through activation of some cell volume regulatory mechanisms such as KCl cotransport, urea shrinks cells, as shown for erythrocytes, hepatocytes, renal cells, and vascular smooth muscle cells (132). Beyond these mechanisms, cell volume is influenced by a wide variety of drugs and toxins, interfering with cell volume regulatory mechanisms (132). For instance, inhibition of K^+ channels leads to cell swelling, and inhibition of Na^+–K^+–$2Cl^-$ cotransport and/or Na^+–H^+ exchanger leads to to cell shrinkage.

Functional States Affecting Cell Volume Control

Even at normal extracellular osmolarity and composition osmotic gradients across the cell membrane could arise from unbalanced transport across the cell membrane and from intracellular generation or disposal of osmotically active solutes. Cellular conditions and functions affecting intracellular osmolarity thus impact on cell volume control (Fig. 3).

ENERGY DEPLETION

Impairment of Na$^+$,K$^+$-ATPase function, such as during pharmacological inhibition, energy depletion, or decrease of ambient temperature, eventually leads to cell swelling due to cellular Na$^+$ accumulation, dissipation of the K$^+$ gradient, depolarization, and subsequent accumulation of Cl$^-$ (132). In some cells, the swelling is preceded by transient cell shrinkage (36, 55, 200). The increase of intracellular Na$^+$ concentration reverses the driving force for the Na$^+$–Ca^{++} exchanger; the increase of intracellular Ca^{++} activity in turn leads to activation of Ca^{++}-sensitive K$^+$ channels and/or Cl$^-$ channels as well as contraction of cytoskeletal elements.

TRANSPORT

Most epithelial cells are faced with large transcellular fluxes of osmotically active substances (see Chapter 2). To cope with transcellular transport, the cells have to coordinate the various transport systems at the apical and basolateral cell membranes. In both reabsorbing and secreting epithelia, cell volume participates in the coupling of those transport processes.

In proximal renal tubules (137) and intestine (197), for instance, Na$^+$-coupled transport of substrates such as amino acids or glucose across the luminal cell membrane leads to cellular accumulation of Na$^+$ and substrate. Moreover, the entry of excess positive charge leads to depolarization impeding exit of Cl$^-$ and HCO$_3^-$ and thus favoring cell swelling. In Na$^+$ reabsorbing epithelia such as renal collecting duct and colon, entry of Na$^+$ via Na$^+$ channels similarly challenges cell volume constancy. Limitation of cell swelling during stimulated Na$^+$ transport requires the operation of cell volume regulatory mechanisms including activation of K$^+$ channels, which in turn maintain the electrical driving force for Na$^+$ entry into the cell (137, 197). Activation of Cl$^-$ and/or K$^+$ channels in several Cl$^-$ secreting epithelia is paralleled by decrease of intracellular Cl$^-$ activity and cell shrinkage, which in turn stimulate Na$^+$–K$^+$–2Cl$^-$ cotransport and/or Na$^+$–H$^+$ exchanger with Cl$^-$–HCO$_3^-$ exchanger (66, 101, 154, 155).

The influence of Na$^+$-coupled transport on cell volume is not limited to epithelials cells. In several epithelial and nonepithelial cells, concentrative uptake of substrates such as amino acids, glucose, taurine, and taurocholate increases cell volume (132).

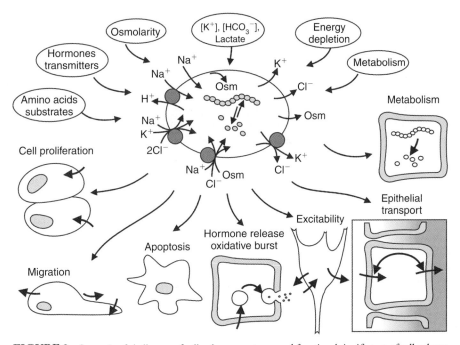

FIGURE 3 Synopsis of challenges of cell volume constancy and functional significance of cell volume regulatory mechanisms. Cell volume is altered by concentrative uptake of amino acids and additional substrates, alterations of ion transport by hormones and transmitters, changes of extracellular osmolarity, alterations of extracellular K$^+$, HCO$_3$- and organic acid concentrations, energy depletion, and metabolic generation or disposal of osmolarity. Altered cell volume as well as cell volume regulatory transport and metabolism participate in the regulation of cell proliferation, migration, apoptosis, hormone release and oxidative burst, neuromuscular excitability, epithelial transport, and metabolism.

Deranged transport participates in disordered function of erythrocytes in sickle cell disease. In this disorder a point mutation of hemoglobin (HbS) favors polymerization of desoxyhemoglobin, dramatically decreasing erythrocyte deformability and increasing blood viscosity (113). The depolymerization of hemoglobin is critically dependent on cell volume. Cell shrinkage due to enhanced ambient osmolarity, activation of KCl cotransport by urea, or activation of Ca^{++}-sensitive K^+ channels by rise of intracellular Ca^{++} activity potentiates polymerization of HbS. The high osmolarity and urea concentration in kidney medulla thus contribute to the particular vulnerability of this tissue to ischemia in sickle cell anemia. Cell shrinkage and subsequent triggering of erythrocyte scramblase (see previous discussion) presumably participate in accelerated erythrocyte turnover of various anemic conditions (138).

INFLUENCE OF HORMONES AND TRANSMITTERS ON CELL VOLUME

A wide variety of hormones and other mediators have been shown to alter cell volume (132). Insulin swells liver cells by activation of both Na^+–H^+ exchange and Na^+–K^+–$2Cl^-$ cotransport, and glucagon shrinks hepatocytes, presumably by activation of ion channels (131). The effect of these hormones on cell volume accounts for several of their metabolic effects (Fig. 4). Notably, the swelling effect of insulin accounts for the antiproteolytic effect, and the shrinking effect of glucagon accounts for the proteolytic effect of the hormones (194, 195).

Virtually all known growth factors increase cell volume by stimulation of Na^+–H^+ exchange, and in some cases of Na^+–K^+–$2Cl^-$ cotransport. As amplified below, an increase of cell volume appears to be required for cell proliferation (177).

Several excitatory neurotransmitters, such as glutamate, activate Na^+ channels or nonselective cation channels, the entry of Na^+ and depolarization then favor cell swelling (41, 172, 193). Other neurotransmitters, such as GABA, activate K^+ channels and/or anion channels, and thus induce cell shrinkage (5).

Mediators and hormones regulating epithelial transport, such as ADH, adrenaline, or acetylcholine, may either swell or shrink epithelial cells, depending on their effect on ion transport (132). Stimulation of Na^+–H^+ exchange, Na^+–K^+–$2Cl^-$ cotransport or Na^+ channels tends to swell epithelial cells, whereas prevailing stimulation of Cl^- and/or K^+ channels shrinks epithelial cells.

Cell volume may in turn affect hormone and transmitter release. In a variety of cells, swelling stimulates and cell shrinkage inhibits the release of hormones (207).

NEUROMUSCULAR EXCITABILITY

Cell volume could affect neuronal excitability by affecting ionic gradients, ion channel activity, or cell volume regulatory release of neurotransmitters (132). Dehydration enhances the neuronal expression of SGK1, which in turn regulates channels that are transporters relevant for neuroexcitability (15). Moreover, glial cell swelling may

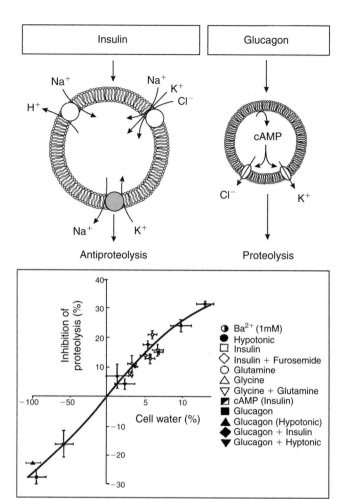

FIGURE 4 Cell volume in the regulation of metabolism by hormones. Insulin swells cells by KCl uptake via activation of Na^+–H^+ exchange, Na^+–K^+–$2Cl^-$ cotransport and Na^+,–K^+-ATPase. Glucagon shrinks cells by activation of K^+ and anion channels. The cell volume changes participate in the the signaling of hormone action. Cell swelling stimulates protein synthesis and cell shrinkage stimulates proteolysis. The diagram at the bottom illustrates the correlation between inhibition of proteolysis and hydration of hepatocytes. Cell swelling was induced by inhibition of K^+ channels (Ba^+) decrease of extracellular osmolarity (hypotonic), insulin ± Na^+–K^+–$2Cl^-$ cotransport inhibitor furosemide, or concentrative uptake of amino acids (glutamine ± glycine). Cell swelling was counteracted or shrinkage accomplished by (additional) application of glucagon or cyclic AMP. The cell volume changes fully account for the effect of both hormones on proteolysis and contribute to the other effects on macromolecule metabolism such as protein synthesis as well as glycogen formation and breakdown. (Modified from Haussinger D, Lang F. Cell volume: a "second messenger" in the regulation of metabolism by amono acids and hormones. *Cell Physiol Biochem* 1991;1:121–130.)

impede glial cell function (117). In liver insufficiency, for instance, formation of urea is impaired leading to accumulation of NH_3. NH_3 enters the brain and is taken up by glial cells, which then stimulates cellular formation and accumulation of glutamine resulting eventually in glial cell swelling (46, 165). To counteract swelling, glial cells release inositol, a mechanism, however, limited by the availability of inositol (92, 123). Inhibition of glutamine synthase has indeed been shown to protect against hepatic encephalopathy (96).

METABOLISM

Any reaction resulting in an increase of osmotically active solutes, such as degradation of proteins to amino acids, glycogen to glucose phosphate, or triglycerides to glycerol and fatty acids, is expected to create intracellular osmolarity (132). The degradation of the substrates to CO_2 and H_2O then decreases intracellular osmolarity.

Enhanced glycolysis as it occurs during forced exercise, for instance, leads to cellular accumulation of lactate and H^+, subsequent activation of Na^+–H^+ exchanger, and cell swelling (188). Metabolic pathways may influence cell volume indirectly through alteration of transport across the cell membrane. A decrease of cellular ATP could activate ATP-sensitive K^+ channels and thus shrink susceptible cells (132). Similarly, cellular formation of peroxides may shrink cells through activation of K^+ channels, as shown for hepatocytes, pancreatic β cells and vascular smooth muscle cells (132). In endothelial cells, peroxides inhibit Na^+–K^+–$2Cl^-$ cotransport, an effect similarly expected to shrink the cells (54). On the other hand, oxidation leads to inhibition of n-type K^+ channels in lymphocytes and IsK K^+ channels in a variety of tissues, effects that tend to favor cell swelling (132).

In several hypercatabolic states, such as burns, acute pancreatitis, severe injury, and liver carcinoma, a decrease of muscle cell volume is observed that correlates with urea excretion, an indicator of protein degradation (93). Since cell shrinkage is known to stimulate proteolysis, this correlation points to a causal role of altered cell volume in these hypercatabolic states. Conversely, hypercatabolism can be reversed by glutamine, which is known to swell cells by Na^+-coupled cellular accumulation (93).

Diabetic ketoacidosis may be paralleled by cell swelling due to cellular accumulation of organic acids and enhanced Na^+–H^+ exchange activity in response to cellular acidosis (20, 43, 122, 223, 236). Furthermore, the excessive glucose concentrations of hyperglycemia stimulate cellular formation and accumulation of sorbitol through aldose reductase (24). As an attempt to counteract swelling, cells decrease other osmolytes such as myoinositol, an effect that can be reversed by inhibition of aldose reductase with sorbinil (53, 63, 218). On the other hand, hyperglycemia is paralleled by hyperosmolarity, and intriguing evidence has been gathered pointing to cell shrinkage in hyperosmolar diabetes mellitus, which increases cellular Ca^{++} concentration and thus induces cell injury (50, 135). Obviously, more experimental information is needed to clarify the role of cell volume changes in the pathophysiology of diabetic complications.

In uremia, extracellular osmolarity is usually enhanced due to accumulation of urea which interferes with protein stability and thus cell volume regulation (see previous discussion). The high urea concentrations in uremia stimulate the formation of methylamines, which counteract the per-

turbing effect of urea (146). Rapid alterations of urea concentration, such as during dialysis, presumably do not allow full adjustment of osmolyte concentration, and are thus expected to disturb the balance of stabilizing osmolytes and destabilizing urea (67). Alterations of cell volume may participate in the progression of renal failure: TGF-β1 has been postulated to accelerate renal fibrosis by inhibition of proteolysis and stimulation of protein synthesis, which both lead to enhanced deposition of matrix proteins (135, 149).

CELL PROLIFERATION

Mitogenic factors are known to stimulate Na^+–H^+ exchange and Na^+–K^+–$2Cl^-$ cotransport (177). As shown in ras oncogene–expressing cells, activation of those carriers leads to a shift of the set point for cell volume regulation toward greater volumes (Fig. 5). In addition, activation of Na^+–H^+ exchange leads to cellular alkalinization. Apparently, the increase of cell volume is one of the prerequisites for cell proliferation, which is impeded by pharmacological inhibition of Na^+–H^+ exchanger and Na^+–K^+–$2Cl^-$ cotransport as well as osmotic cell shrinkage (132).

MIGRATION

Locomotion of cells requires alterations of cell shape and thus of cytoskeletal architecture. At the leading edge, actin filaments are polymerized and at the rear they are depolymerized (203). The movement of cells is paralleled by movements of water that is driven by osmotic gradients. Na^+–H^+ exchange and Na^+–K^+–$2Cl^-$ cotransport drive water entry at the leading edge, and the activity of K^+ channels and anion channels allow water extrusion at the rear (132, 198). Activation of cell volume regulatory mechanisms during migration is similar to that of cell proliferation (Fig. 6). However, the elements are polarized, and cells undergo cell volume regulatory increase at the leading edge and cell volume regulatory decrease at the rear (132).

APOPTOTIC CELL DEATH

Cell shrinkage is one of the hallmarks of apoptotic cell death and marked osmotic cell shrinkage (>30%) has been shown to trigger apoptotic cell death (181). Apoptotic cell shrinkage requires the participation of cell volume regulatory mechanisms (Fig. 6). Apoptotic death of Jurkat T-lymphocytes following CD95 triggering is indeed paralleled by inhibition of the Na^+–H^+ exchanger as well as activation of the anion channel ORCC and osmolyte release (134). The release of ions and subsequent cell shrinkage are apparently a prerequisite for induction of apoptosis (18, 19, 153). On the other hand, at an early stage of CD95 triggering, the cell volume–regulatory K^+ channel Kv1.3 is inhibited and a moderate decrease of cell volume (<30%) has been shown to blunt receptor (CD95)–triggered apoptotic cell death (83). The cellular mechanisms triggered by moderate osmotic cell shrinkage apparently interfere with the signaling of the CD95 receptor, such as cellular O_2-formation.

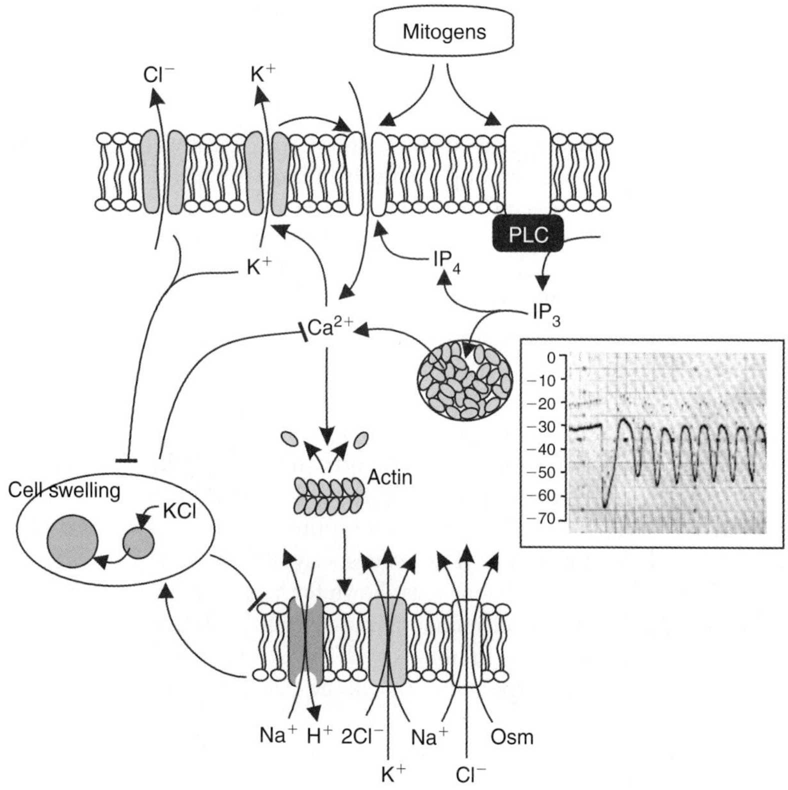

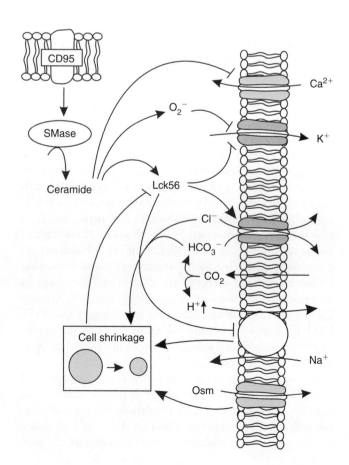

FIGURE 5   Cell volume regulatory transport in regulation of cell proliferation. The case of Ras oncogene expressing cells. Application of mitogenic factors in cells overexpressing Ras oncogene triggers intracellular Ca^+ release and Ca^+ entry, leading to oscillations of cytosolic Ca^+ activity and cell membrane potential (insert). Increased cytosolic Ca^+ activity stimulates Ca^+-sensitive K^+ channels and triggers initial cell shrinkage. Ca^+ further leads to depolymerization of the microfilaments, which disinhibits the Na^+-H^+ exchanger and $Na^+-K^+-2Cl^-$ cotransporter. The activation of these carriers eventually leads to cell swelling, a prerequisite for cell proliferation. (From Lang F, Busch GL, Ritter M, Volkl H, Waldegger S, Gulbins E, Haussinger D. Functional significance of cell volume regulatory mechanisms. *Physiol Rev* 1998;78(1):247-306.)

FIGURE 6   Cell volume regulatory ion transport during CD95-induced apoptosis of lymphocytes. CD95-induced apoptosis of Jurkat T-lymphocytes is paralleled by inhibition of the Na^+-H^+ exchanger as well as activation of the anion channel ORCC and osmolyte release. The altered transport leads eventually to cytosolic acidification and cell shrinkage. Initially, CD95 stimulation leads to inhibition of the cell volume regulatory K^+ channel Kv1.3, thus preventing early cell shrinkage. At a later stage (not shown), additional activation of K^+ channels leads to apoptotic cell shrinkage. (From Lang F, Lepple-Wienhues A, Paulmichi M, Szabo I, Siemen D, Gulbins E. Ion channels, cell volume, and apoptotic cell death. *Cell Physiol Biochem* 1998;8(6):285-292.)

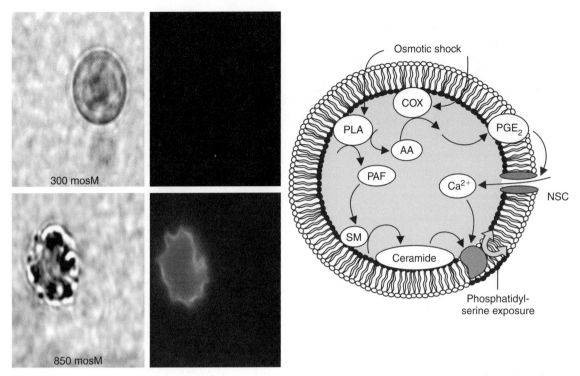

FIGURE 7 Stimulation of erythrocyte death by osmotic cell shrinkage. Osmotic shock activates a phospholipase A_2 leading to formation of platelet activating factor (PAF) on the one hand and of arachidonic acid on the other. PAF stimulates a sphingomyelinase leading to formation of ceramide, arachidonic acid is converted by cyclooxygenase (COX) to PGE2 which activates a Ca^+ and Na^+ permeable cation channel. Ca^+ entering through the cation channels activates a scramblase leading to phosphatidylserine exposure at the cell surface (left), a typical feature of apoptotic cells. Ceramide sensitizes the scramblase for Ca^+ and thus contributes to the activation of this enzyme. (From Lang KS, Lang PA, Bauer C, Duranton C, Wieder T, Huber SM, Lang F. Mechanisms of suicidal erythrocyte death. *Cell Physiol Biochem* 2005;15:195–202.) See color insert.

The triggering of cell death by hyperosmotic shock has been attributed to upregulation or clustering and subsequent activation of apoptosis-inducing receptors such as CD95 or TNFα-receptor (174, 175, 181), or to formation of their ligands such as TNFα (139). In erythrocytes, hyperosmotic shock stimulates a phospholipase A_2 with subsequent formation of PGE_2 (141) and PAF (142). PGE_2 stimulates a cation channel allowing the entry of Ca^+ and subsequent activation of a Ca^+-sensitive scramblase (141). PAF stimulates a sphingomyelinase that leads to formation of ceramide, which sensitizes the erythrocyte scramblase for Ca^+ (142). Activation of the scramblase leads to breakdown of phosphatidylserine asymmetry and exposure of phosphatidylserine at the outer surface of the cell membrane, a typical feature of apoptotic cells (Fig. 7). Whether or not similar mechanisms are triggered in nucleated cells remains to be determined.

NECROTIC CELL DEATH

As pointed out above, energy depletion impairs the function of the Na^+, K^+-ATPase, dissipates the Na^+ and K^+ gradients, depolarizes the cell membrane, and leads to cellular accumulation of Cl^- (132). During ischemia, the cell membrane is further depolarized by increasing extracellular K^+ concentrations. Cellular Na^+ and Cl^- accumulation eventually leads to cell swelling. Moreover, the excessive formation

and reduced clearance of lactate during ischemia induces cellular acidosis and enhanced Na^+–H^+ exchange activity, compounding cell swelling. In the brain, the depolarization triggers the release of glutamate, which activates unspecific cation channels and thus induces further cell swelling (132).

References

1. Agius L, Peak M, Beresford G, al Habori M, Thomas TH. The role of ion content and cell volume in insulin action. *Biochem Soc Trans* 1994;22:516–522.
2. Alfieri R, Petronini PG, Urbani S, Borghetti AF. Activation of heat-shock transcription factor 1 by hypertonic shock in 3T3 cells. *Biochem J* 1996;319(Pt 2):601–606.
3. Back JF, Oakenfull D, Smith MB. Increased thermal stability of proteins in the presence of sugars and polyols. *Biochemistry* 1979;18:5191–5196.
4. Bagnasco SM, Murphy HR, Be dford JJ, Burg MB. Osmoregulation by slow changes in aldose reductase and rapid changes in sorbitol flux. *Am J Physiol* 1988;254:C788–C792.
5. Ballanyi K, Grafe P. Cell volume regulation in the nervous system. *Ren Physiol Biochem* 1988;11:142–157.
6. Barone S, Amlal H, Xu J, Kujala M, Kere J, Petrovic S, Soleimani M. Differential regulation of basolateral Cl-/HCO$_3$- exchangers SLC26A7 and AE1 in kidney outer medullary collecting duct. *J Am Soc Nephrol* 2004;15:2002–2011.
7. Barriere H, Belfodil R, Rubera I, Tauc M, Lesage F, Poujeol C, Guy N, Barhanin J, Poujeol P. Role of TASK2 potassium channels regarding volume regulation in primary cultures of mouse proximal tubules. *J Gen Physiol* 2003;122:177–190.
8. Beck FX, Grunbein R, Lugmayr K, Neuhofer W. Heat shock proteins and the cellular response to osmotic stress. *Cell Physiol Biochem* 2000;10:303–306.
9. Bedford JJ, Bagnasco SM, Kador PF, Harris HW Jr, Burg MB. Characterization and purification of a mammalian osmoregulatory protein, aldose reductase, induced in renal medullary cells by high extracellular NaCl. *J Biol Chem* 1987;262:14255–14259.
10. Berneis K, Ninnis R, Haussinger D, Keller U. Effects of hyper- and hypoosmolality on whole body protein and glucose kinetics in humans. *Am J Physiol* 1999;276:E188–E195.
11. Berry GT, Mallee JJ, Kwon HM, Rim JS, Mulla WR, Muenke M, Spinner NB. The human osmoregulatory Na+/ myo-inositol cotransporter gene (SLC5A3): molecular cloning and localization to chromosome 21. *Genomics* 1995;25:507–513.

12. Bode JG, Gatsios P, Ludwig S, Rapp UR, Haussinger D, Heinrich PC, Graeve L. The mitogen-activated protein (MAP) kinase p38 and its upstream activator MAP kinase kinase 6 are involved in the activation of signal transducer and activator of transcription by hyperosmolarity. *J Biol Chem* 1999;274:30222–30227.
13. Boese SH, Wehner F, Kinne RK. Taurine permeation throughswelling-activated anion conductance in rat IMCD cells in primary culture. *Am J Physiol* 1996;271:F498–F507.
14. Boettger T, Rust MB, Maier H, Seidenbecher T, Schweizer M, Keating DJ, Faulhaber J, Ehmke H, Pfeffer C, Scheel O, Lemcke B, Horst J, Leuwer R, Pape HC, Volkl H, Hubner CA, Jentsch TJ. Loss of K-Cl co-transporter KCC3 causes deafness, neurodegeneration and reduced seizure threshold. *EMBO J* 2003;22:5422–5434.
15. Bohmer C, Philippin M, Rajamanickam J, Mack A, Broer S, Palmada M, Lang F. Stimulation of the EAAT4 glutamate transporter by SGK protein kinase isoforms and PKB. *Biochem Biophys Res Commun* 2004;324:1242–1248.
16. Bonanno JA. K(+)-H+ exchange, a fundamental cell acidifier in corneal epithelium. *Am J Physiol* 1991;260:C618–C625.
17. Bookstein C, Musch MW, DePaoli A, Xie Y, Villereal M, Rao MC, Chang EB. A unique sodium-hydrogen exchange isoform (NHE-4) of the inner medulla of the rat kidney is induced by hyperosmolarity. *J Biol Chem* 1994;269:29704–29709.
18. Bortner CD, Cidlowski JA. Caspase independent/dependent regulation of K(+), cell shrinkage, and mitochondrial membrane potential during lymphocyte apoptosis. *J Biol Chem* 1999;274:21953–21962.
19. Bortner CD, Hughes FM Jr, Cidlowski JA. A primary role for K+ and Na+ efflux in the activation of apoptosis. *J Biol Chem* 1997;272:32436–32442.
20. Brizzolara A, Barbieri MP, Adezati L, Viviani GL. Water distribution in insulin-dependent diabetes mellitus in various states of metabolic control. *Eur J Endocrinol* 1996;135:609–615.
21. Brown GC. Total cell protein concentration as an evolutionary constraint on the metabolic control distribution in cells. *J Theor Biol* 1991;153:195–203.
22. Burg MB. Molecular basis of osmotic regulation. *Am J Physiol* 1995;268:F983–F996.
23. Burg MB. Macromolecular crowding as a cell volume sensor. *Cell Physiol Biochem* 2000; 10:251–256.
24. Burg MB, Kador PF. Sorbitol, osmoregulation, and the complications of diabetes. *J Clin Invest* 1988;81:635–640.
25. Burg MB, Kwon ED, Kultz D. Osmotic regulation of gene expression. *FASEB J* 1996; 10:1598–1606.
26. Burg MB, Kwon ED, Peters EM. Glycerophosphocholine and betaine counteract the effect of urea on pyruvate kinase. *Kidney Int Suppl* 1996;57:S100–S104.
27. Burnham CE, Buerk B, Schmidt C, Bucuvalas JC. A liver-specific isoform of the betaine/GABA transporter in the rat: cDNA sequence and organ distribution. *Biochim Biophys Acta* 1996;1284:4–8.
28. Busch AE, Maylie J. MinK channels: a minimal channel protien with a maximal impact. *Cell Physiol Biochem* 1993;3:270–276.
29. Busch AE, Varnum M, Adelman JP, North RA. Hypotonic solution increases the slowly activating potassium current IsK expressed in xenopus oocytes. *Biochem Biophys Res Commun* 1992;184:804–810.
30. Busch GL, Schreiber R, Dartsch PC, Volkl H, Vom Dahl S, Haussinger D, Lang F. Involvement of microtubules in the link between cell volume and pH of acidic cellular compartments in rat and human hepatocytes. *Proc Natl Acad Sci U S A* 1994;91:9165–9169.
31. Busch GL, Lang HJ, Lang F. Studies on the mechanism of swelling-induced lysosomal alkalinization in vascular smooth muscle cells. *Pflugers Arch* 1996;431(5):690–696.
32. Buyse G, de Greef C, Raeymaekers L, Droogmans G, Nilius B, Eggermont J. The ubiquitously expressed pICln protein forms homomeric complexes in vitro. *Biochem Biophys Res Commun* 1996;218:822–827.
33. Cabado AG, Vieytes MR, Botana LM. Effect of ion composition on the changes in membrane potential induced with several stimuli in rat mast cells. *J Cell Physiol* 1994;158:309–316.
34. Cala PM. Volume regulation by Amphiuma red blood cells: strategies for identifying alkali metal/H+ transport. *Fed Proc* 1985;44:2500–2507.
35. Carpenter JF, Crowe JH. The mechanism of cryoprotection of proteins by solutes. *Cryobiology* 1988;25:244–255.
36. Chacon E, Reece JM, Nieminen AL, Zahrebelski G, Herman B, Lemasters JJ. Distribution of electrical potential, pH, free Ca2+, and volume inside cultured adult rabbit cardiac myocytes during chemical hypoxia: a multiparameter digitized confocal microscopic study. *Biophys J* 1994;66:942–952.
37. Chan HC, Fu WO, Chung YW, Huang SJ, Chan PS, Wong PY. Swelling-induced anion and cation conductances in human epididymal cells. *J Physiol* 1994;478(Pt 3):449–460.
38. Chan HC, Nelson DJ. Chloride-dependent cation conductance activated during cellular shrinkage. *Science* 1992;257:669–671.
39. Chen JG, Klus LR, Steenbergen DK, Kempson SA. Hypertonic upregulation of amino acid transport system A in vascular smooth muscle cells. *Am J Physiol* 1994;267:C529–C536.
40. Cho WK, Siegrist VJ, Zinzow W. Impaired regulatory volume decrease in freshly isolated cholangiocytes from cystic fibrosis mice: implications for cystic fibrosis transmembrane conductance regulator effect on potassium conductance. *J Biol Chem* 2004;279: 14610–14618.
41. Choi DW, Rothman SM. The role of glutamate neurotoxicity in hypoxic-ischemic neuronal death. *Annu Rev Neurosci* 1990;13:171–182.
42. Civan MM, Coca-Prados M, Peterson-Yantorno K. Pathways signaling the regulatory volume decrease of cultured nonpigmented ciliary epithelial cells. *Invest Ophthalmol Vis Sci* 1994;35:2876–2886.
43. Clements RS Jr, Blumenthal SA, Morrison AD, Winegrad AI. Increased cerebrospinal-fluid pressure during treatment of diabetic ketosis. *Lancet* 1971;2:671–675.
44. Cohen DM, Wasserman JC, Gullans SR. Immediate early gene and HSP70 expression in hyperosmotic stress in MDCK cells. *Am J Physiol* 1991;261:C594–C601.
45. Colombe BW, Macey RI. Effects of calcium on potassium and water transport in human erythrocyte ghosts. *Biochim Biophys Acta* 1974;363:226–239.
46. Cordoba J, Gottstein J, Blei AT. Glutamine, myo-inositol, and organic brain osmolytes after portocaval anastomosis in the rat: implications for ammonia-induced brain edema. *Hepatology* 1996;24:919–923.
47. Cornet M, Lambert IH, Hoffmann EK. Relation between cytoskeleton, hypo-osmotic treatment and volume regulation in Ehrlich ascites tumor cells. *J Membr Biol* 1993;131:55–66.
48. Decressac S, Franco M, Bendahhou S, Warth R, Knauer S, Barhanin J, Lazdunski M, Lesage F. ARF6-dependent interaction of the TWIK1 K+ channel with EFA6, a GDP/GTP exchange factor for ARF6. *EMBO Rep* 2004;5:1171–1175.
49. Demaurex N, Grinstein S. Na+/H+ antiport: modulation by ATP and role in cell volume regulation. *J Exp Biol* 1994;196:389–404.
50. Demerdash TM, Seyrek N, Smogorzewski M, Marcinkowski W, Nasser-Moadelli S, Massry SG. Pathways through which glucose induces a rise in [Ca2+]i of polymorphonuclear leukocytes of rats. *Kidney Int* 1996;50:2032–2040.
51. Deutsch C, Chen LQ. Heterologous expression of specific K+ channels in T lymphocytes: functional consequences for volume regulation. *Proc Natl Acad Sci U S A* 1993;90:10036–10040.
52. Dunham PB, Jessen F, Hoffmann EK. Inhibition of Na-K-C1 cotransport in Ehrlich ascites cells by antiserum against purified proteins of the cotransporter. *Proc Natl Acad Sci U S A* 1990;87:6828–6832.
53. Edmands S, Yancey PH. Effects on rat renal osmolytes of extended treatment with an aldose reductase inhibitor. *Comp Biochem Physiol C* 1992;103:499–502.
54. Elliott SJ, Schilling WP. Oxidant stress alters Na+ pump and Na(+)-K(+)-Cl- cotransporter activities in vascular endothelial cells. *Am J Physiol* 1992;263:H96–102.
55. Faff-Michalak L, Reichenbach A, Dettmer D, Kellner K, Albrecht J. K(+)-, hypoosmolarity-, and NH4(+)-induced taurine release from cultured rabbit Muller cells: role of Na+ and Cl- ions and relation to cell volume changes. *Glia* 1994;10:114–120.
56. Felipe A, Snyders DJ, Deal KK, Tamkun MM. Influence of cloned voltage-gated K+ channel expression on alanine transport, Rb+ uptake, and cell volume. *Am J Physiol* 1993;265: C1230–C1238.
57. Feranchak AP, Berl T, Capasso J, Wojtaszek PA, Han J, Fitz JG. p38 MAP kinase modulates liver cell volume through inhibition of membrane Na+ permeability. *J Clin Invest* 2001;108:1495–1504.
58. Feranchak AP, Kilic G, Wojtaszek PA, Qadri I, Fitz JG. Volume-sensitive tyrosine kinases regulate liver cell volume through effects on vesicular trafficking and membrane Na+ permeability. *J Biol Chem* 2003;278:44632–44638.
59. Ferraris JD, Williams CK, Jung KY, Bedford JJ, Burg MB, Garcia-Perez A. ORE, a eukaryotic minimal essential osmotic response element. The aldose reductase gene in hyperosmotic stress. *J Biol Chem* 1996;271:18318–18321.
60. Ferraris JD, Williams CK, Martin BM, Burg MB, Garcia-Perez A. Cloning, genomic organization, and osmotic response of the aldose reductase gene. *Proc Natl Acad Sci U S A* 1994;91:10742–10746.
61. Ferraris JD, Williams CK, Persaud P, Zhang Z, Chen Y, Burg MB. Activity of the TonEBP/OREBP transactivation domain varies directly with extracellular NaCl concentration. *Proc Natl Acad Sci U S A* 2002;99:739–744.
62. Ferrer-Martinez A, Casado FJ, Felipe A, Pastor-Anglada M. Regulation of Na+,K(+)-ATPase and the Na+/K+/Cl- co-transporter in the renal epithelial cell line NBL-1 under osmotic stress. *Biochem J* 1996;319(Pt 2):337–342.
63. Finegold D, Lattimer SA, Nolle S, Bernstein M, Greene DA. Polyol pathway activity and myo-inositol metabolism. A suggested relationship in the pathogenesis of diabetic neuropathy. *Diabetes* 1983;32:988–992.
64. Finkenzeller G, Newsome W, Lang F, Haussinger D. Increase of cjun mRNA upon hypo-osmotic cell swelling of rat hepatoma cells. *FEBS Lett* 1994;340:163–166.
65. Firestone GL, Giampaolo JR, O'Keeffe BA. Stimulus-dependent regulation of the serum and glucocorticoid inducible protein kinase (Sgk) transcription, subcellular localization and enzymatic activity. *Cell Physiol Biochem* 2003;13:1–12.
66. Foskett JK, Wong MM, Sue AQ, Robertson MA. Isosmotic modulation of cell volume and intracellular ion activities during stimulation of single exocrine cells. *J Exp Zool* 1994;268: 104–110.
67. Friedrich B, Alexander D, Aicher WK, Duszenko M, Schaub T, Passlick-Deetjen J, Waldegger S, Wolf S, Risler T, Lang F. Influence of standard haemodialysis on transcription of human serum- and glucocorticoid-inducible kinase SGK1 and taurine transporter TAUT in blood leukocytes. *Nephrol Dialysis Transpl* 2005;20:768–774.
68. Fulton AB. How crowded is the cytoplasm? *Cell* 1982;30:345–347.
69. Furlong TJ, Moriyama T, Spring KR. Activation of osmolyte efflux from cultured renal papillary epithelial cells. *J Membr Biol* 1991; 123:269–277.
70. Galcheva-Gargova Z, Derijard B, Wu IH, Davis RJ. An osmosensing signal transduction pathway in mammalian cells. *Science* 1994;265:806–808.
71. Garcia-Perez A, Ferraris JD. Aldose reductase gene expression and osmoregulation in mammalian renal cells. In Strange K, ed. *Cellular and Molecular Physiology of Cell Volume Regulation*. Boca Raton, FL: CRC Press, 1994:373–382.
72. Garcia-Perez A, Burg MB. Renal medullary organic osmolytes. *Physiol Rev* 1991;71: 1081–1115.
73. Garcia-Perez A, Burg MB. Role of organic osmolytes in adaptation of renal cells to high osmolality. *J Membr Biol* 1991;119:1–13.
74. Garcia-Perez A, Martin B, Murphy HR, Uchida S, Murer H, Cowley BD Jr, Handler JS, Burg MB. Molecular cloning of cDNA coding for kidney aldose reductase. Regulation of specific mRNA accumulation by NaCl-mediated osmotic stress. *J Biol Chem* 1989;264:16815–16821.
75. Garner MM, Burg MB. Macromolecular crowding and confinement in cells exposed to hypertonicity. *Am J Physiol* 1994;266:C877–C892.
76. Garty H, Furlong TJ, Ellis DE, Spring KR. Sorbitol permease: an apical membrane transporter in cultured renal papillary epithelial cells. *Am J Physiol* 1991;260:F650–F656.
77. Geck P, Pfeiffer B. Na+ + K+ + 1 2Cl- cotransport in animal cells—its role in volume regulation. *Ann N Y Acad Sci* 1985;456:166–182.

78. Go WY, Liu X, Roti MA, Liu F, Ho SN. NFAT5/TonEBP mutant mice define osmotic stress as a critical feature of the lymphoid microenvironment. *Proc Natl Acad Sci U S A* 2004;101:10673–10678.
79. Graf J, Haddad P, Haeussinger D, Lang F. Cell volume regulation in liver. *Ren Physiol Biochem* 1988;11:202–220.
80. Grinstein S, Clarke CA, Rothstein A. Activation of Na+/H+ exchange in lymphocytes by osmotically induced volume changes and by cytoplasmic acidification. *J Gen Physiol* 1983;82:619–638.
81. Grunder S, Thiemann A, Pusch M, Jentsch TJ. Regions involved in the opening of CIC-2 chloride channel by voltage and cell volume. *Nature* 1992;360:759–762.
82. Guharay F, Sachs F. Stretch-activated single ion channel currents in tissue-cultured embryonic chick skeletal muscle. *J Physiol* 1984;352:685–701.
83. Gulbins E, Welsch J, Lepple-Wienhuis A, Heinle H, Lang F. Inhibition of Fas-induced apoptotic cell death by osmotic cell shrinkage. *Biochem Biophys Res Commun* 1997;236:517–521.
84. Hallbrucker C, Vom Dahl S, Lang F, Haussinger D. Control of hepatic proteolysis by amino acids. The role of cell volume. *Eur J Biochem* 1991;197:717–724.
85. Hamill OP, Martinac B. Molecular basis of mechanotransduction in living cells. *Physiol Rev* 2001;81:685–740.
86. Hammerman MR, Sacktor B, Daughaday WH. myo-Inositol transport in renal brush border vesicles and it inhibition by D-glucose. *Am J Physiol* 1980;239:F113–F120.
87. Han J, Lee JD, Bibbs L, Ulevitch RJ. A MAP kinase targeted by endotoxin and hyperosmolarity in mammalian cells. *Science* 1994; 265:808–811.
88. Hardy SP, Goodfellow HR, Valverde MA, Gill DR, Sepulveda V, Higgins CF. Protein kinase C–mediated phosphorylation of the human multidrug resistance P-glycoprotein regulates cell volume-activated chloride channels. *EMBO J* 1995;14:68–75.
89. Haussinger D, Lang F. Cell volume: a "second messenger" in the regulation of metabolism by amono acids and hormones. *Cell Physiol Biochem* 1991;1:121–130.
90. Haussinger D, Lang F, Bauers K, Gerok W. Control of hepatic nitrogen metabolism and glutathione release by cell volume regulatory mechanisms. *Eur J Biochem* 1990;193: 891–898.
91. Haussinger D, Lang F, Gerok W. Regulation of cell function by the cellular hydration state. *Am J Physiol* 1994;267:E343–E355.
92. Haussinger D, Laubenberger J, Vom Dahl S, Ernst T, Bayer S, Langer M, Gerok W, Hennig J. Proton magnetic resonance spectroscopy studies on human brain myo-inositol in hypo-osmolarity and hepatic encephalopathy. *Gastroenterology* 1994;107:1475–1480.
93. Haussinger D, Roth E, Lang F, Gerok W. Cellular hydration state: an important determinant of protein catabolism in health and disease. *Lancet* 1993;341:1330–1332.
94. Haussinger D, Schliess F, Dombrowski F, Vom Dahl S. Involvement of p38MAPK in the regulation of proteolysis by liver cell hydration. *Gastroenterology* 1999;116:921–935.
95. Haussinger D, Stoll B, Vom Dahl S, Theodoropoulos PA, Markogiannakis E, Gravanis A, Lang F, Stournaras C. Effect of hepatocyte swelling on microtubule stability and tubulin mRNA levels. *Biochem Cell Biol* 1994;72:12–19.
96. Hawkins RA, Jessy J, Mans AM, De Joseph MR. Effect of reducing brain glutamine synthesis on metabolic symptoms of hepatic encephalopathy. *J Neurochem* 1993;60:1000–1006.
97. Hebert SC, Mount DB, Gamba G. Molecular physiology of cation-coupled Cl- cotransport: the SLC12 family. *Pflugers Arch* 2004; 447:580–593.
98. Higgins CF. Volume-activated chloride currents associated with the multidrug resistance P-glycoprotein. *J Physiol* 1995;482:31S–36S.
99. Hoffmann EK. Intracellular signalling involved in volume regulatory decrease. *Cell Physiol Biochem* 2000;10:273–288.
100. Hoffmann EK, Dunham PB. Membrane mechanisms and intracellular signalling in cell volume regulation. *Int Rev Cytol* 1995;161:173–262.
101. Hoffmann EK, Ussing HH. Membrane mechanisms in volume regulation in vertebrate cells and epithelia. In: Giebisch GH, Schafer JA, Ussing HH, Kristensen P, eds. *Membrane Transport in Biology*. Heidelberg: Springer-Verlag, 1992:317–399.
102. Ingber DE. Tensegrity: the architectural basis of cellular mechanotransduction. *Annu Rev Physiol* 1997;59:575–599.
103. Irarrazabal CE, Liu JC, Burg MB, Ferraris JD. ATM, a DNAdamage-inducible kinase, contributes to activation by high NaCl of the transcription factor TonEBP/OREBP. *Proc Natl Acad Sci U S A* 2004; 101:8809–8814.
104. Ito T, Fujio Y, Hirata M, Takatani T, Matsuda T, Muraoka S, Takahashi K, Azuma J. Expression of taurine transporter is regulated through the TonE (tonicity-responsive element)/TonEBP (TonE-binding protein) pathway and contributes to cytoprotection in HepG2 cells. *Biochem J* 2004;382:177–182.
105. Itoh T, Yamauchi A, Imai E, Ueda N, Kamada T. Phosphatase toward MAP kinase is regulated by osmolarity in Madin–Darby canine kidney (MDCK) cells. *FEBS Lett* 1995;373:123–126.
106. Iyer SS, Pearson DW, Nauseef WM, Clark RA. Evidence for a readily dissociable complex of p47phox and p67phox in cytosol of unstimulated human neutrophils. *J Biol Chem* 1994;269:22405–22411.
107. Jackson PS, Strange K. Volume-sensitive anion channels mediate swelling-activated inositol and taurine efflux. *Am J Physiol* 1993;265:C1489–C1500.
108. Jentsch TJ. Molecular physiology of anion channels. *Curr Opin Cell Biol* 1994;6:600–606.
109. Jentsch TJ. Chloride channels: a molecular perspective. *Curr Opin Neurobiol* 1996;6:303–310.
110. Jin NG, Kim JK, Yang DK, Cho SJ, Kim JM, Koh EJ, Jung HC, So I, Kim KW. Fundamental role of ClC-3 in volume-sensitive Cl- channel function and cell volume regulation in AGS cells. *Am J Physiol Gastrointest Liver Physiol* 2003;285:G938–G948.
111. Jirsch J, Deeley RG, Cole SP, Stewart AJ, Fedida D. Inwardly rectifying K+ channels and volume-regulated anion channels in multidrug-resistant small cell lung cancer cells. *Cancer Res* 1993;53:4156–4160.
112. Jirsch JD, Loe DW, Cole SP, Deeley RG, Fedida D. ATP is not required for anion current activated by cell swelling in multidrug-resistant lung cancer cells. *Am J Physiol* 1994;267: C688–C699.
113. Joiner CH. Cation transport and volume regulation in sickle red blood cells. *Am J Physiol* 1993;264:C251–C270.
114. Junankar PR, Kirk K. Organic osmolyte channels: a comparative view. *Cell Physiol Biochem* 2000;10:355–360.
115. Kataoka S, Fujita Y. [Basal experiments of active oxygen generation in urinary polymorphonuclear leukocytes]. *Nippon Hinyokika Gakkai Zasshi* 1991;82:16–23.
116. Kelly SM, Macklem PT. Direct measurement of intracellular pressure. *Am J Physiol* 1991;260: C652–C657.
117. Kimelberg HK. Current concepts of brain edema. Review of laboratory investigations. *J Neurosurg* 1995;83:1051–1059.
118. Kinne RK. The role of organic osmolytes in osmoregulation: from bacteria to mammals. *J Exp Zool* 1993;265:346–355.
119. Kinne RK, Czekay RP, Grunewald JM, Mooren FC, Kinne-Saffran E. Hypotonicity-evoked release of organic osmolytes from distal renal cells: systems, signals, and sidedness. *Ren Physiol Biochem* 1993;16: 66–78.
120. Kinne RK, Tinel H, Kipp H, Kinne-Saffran E. Regulation of sorbitol efflux in different renal medullary cells: similarities and diversities. *Cell Physiol Biochem* 2000;10:371–378.
121. Kirk K, Ellory JC, Young JD. Transport of organic substrates via a volume-activated channel. *J Biol Chem* 1992;267:23475–23478.
122. Krane EJ, Rockoff MA, Wallman JK, Wolfsdorf JI. Subclinical brain swelling in children during treatment of diabetic ketoacidosis. *N Engl J Med* 1985;312:1147–1151.
123. Kreis R, Ross BD, Farrow NA, Ackerman Z. Metabolic disorders of the brain in chronic hepatic encephalopathy detected with H-1 MR spectroscopy. *Radiology* 1992;182:19–27.
124. Kwon HM, Handler JS. Cell volume regulated transporters of compatible osmolytes. *Curr Opin Cell Biol* 1995;7:465–471.
125. Kwon HM, Yamauchi A, Uchida S, Preston AS, Garcia-Perez A, Burg MB, Handler JS. Cloning of the cDNa for a Na+/myo-inositol cotransporter, a hypertonicity stress protein. *J Biol Chem* 1992;267:6297–6301.
126. Lam AK, Ko BC, Tam S, Morris R, Yang JY, Chung SK, Chung SS. Osmotic response element-binding protein (OREBP) is an essential regulator of the urine concentrating mechanism. *J Biol Chem* 2004;279:48048–48054.
127. Lambert IH. Eicosanoids and cell volume regulation. In: Strange K, ed. *Cellular and Molecular Physiology of Cell Volume Regulation*. Boca Raton, FL: CRC Press, 1994:279–298.
128. Lambert IH, Hoffmann EK. Regulation of taurine transport in Ehrlich ascites tumor cells. *J Membr Biol* 1993;131:67–79.
129. Lambert IH, Hoffmann EK, Christensen P. Role of prostaglandins and leukotrienes in volume regulation by Ehrlich ascites tumor cells. *J Membr Biol* 1987;98:247–256.
130. Lang F. *Cell Volume Regulation*. Basel: Karger, 1998.
131. Lang F, Busch G, Völkl H, Häussinger D. Cell volume: a second message in regulation of cellular function. *News Physiol Sci* 1995;10:18–22.
132. Lang F, Busch GL, Ritter M, Völkl H, Waldegger S, Gulbins E, Häussinger D. Functional significance of cell volume regulatory mechanisms. *Physiol Rev* 1998;78:247–306.
133. Lang F, Busch GL, Volkl H. The diversity of volume regulatory mechanisms. *Cell Physiol Biochem* 1998;8:1–45.
134. Lang F, Gulbins E, Szabo I, Lepple-Wienhues A, Huber SM, Duranton C, Lang KS, Lang PA, Wieder T. Cell volume and the regulation of apoptotic cell death. *J Mol Recognit* 2004;17:473–480.
135. Lang F, Klingel K, Wagner CA, Stegen C, Warntges S, Friedrich B, Lanzendorfer M, Melzig J, Moschen I, Steuer S, Waldegger S, Sauter M, Paulmichl M, Gerke V, Risler T, Gamba G, Capasso G, Kandolf R, Hebert SC, Massry SG, Broer S. Deranged transcriptional regulation of cell-volume-sensitive kinase hSGK in diabetic nephropathy. *Proc Natl Acad Sci U S A* 2000; 97:8157–8162.
136. Lang F, Lang KS, Wieder T, Myssina S, Birka C, Lang PA, Kaiser S, Kempe D, Duranton C, Huber SM. Cation channels, cell volume and the death of an erythrocyte. *Pflugers Arch* 2003;447:121–125.
137. Lang F, Rehwald W. Potassium channels in renal epithelial transport regulation. *Physiol Rev* 1992;72:1–32.
138. Lang KS, Lang PA, Bauer C, Duranton C, Wieder T, Huber SM, Lang F. Mechanisms of suicidal erythrocyte death. *Cell Physiol Biochem* 2005;15:195–202.
139. Lang KS, Fillon S, Schneider D, Rammensee HG, Lang F. Stimulation of TNF alpha expression by hyperosmotic stress. *Pflugers Arch* 2002;443:798–803.
140. Lang KS, Myssina S, Brand V, Sandu C, Lang PA, Berchtold S, Huber SM, Lang F, Wieder T. Involvement of ceramide in hyperosmotic shock-induced death of erythrocytes. *Cell Death Differ* 2004;11:231–243.
141. Lang PA, Kempe DS, Tanneur VBC, Eisele K, Klarl BA, Myssina S, Jendrossek V, Ishii S, Shimizu T, Waidmann M, Hessler G, Huber SM, Lang F, Weider T. PGE2 in the regulation of programmed erythrocyte death. *Cell Death Diff* 2005;.
142. Lang PA, Kempe DS, Tanneur V, Eisele K, Klarl BA, Myssina S, Jendrossek V, Ishii S, Shimizu T, Weidmann M, Huber SM, Lang F, Wieder T. Stimulation of erythrocyte ceramide formation by platelet activating factor. *J Cell Sci* 2005;118:1233–1243.
143. Lauf PK. K:Cl cotransport: emerging molecular aspects of a ouabain-resistant, volume-responsive transport system in red blood cells. *Ren Physiol Biochem* 1988;11:248–259.
144. Lauf PK, Adragna NC. K-Cl cotransport: properties and molecular mechanism. *Cell Physiol Biochem* 2000;10:341–354.
145. Lauf PK, Erdmann A, Adragna NC. K-Cl cotransport, pH, and role of Mg in volume-clamped low-K sheep erythrocytes: three equilibrium states. *Am J Physiol* 1994;266:C95–C103.
146. Lee JA, Lee HA, Sadler PJ. Uraemia: is urea more important than we think? *Lancet* 1991;338:1438–1440.
147. Lee SD, Colla E, Sheen MR, Na KY, Kwon HM. Multiple domains of TonEBP cooperate to stimulate transcription in response to hypertonicity. *J Biol Chem* 2003;278:47571–47577.
148. Lepple-Wienhues A, Szabo I, Laun T, Kaba NK, Gulbins E, Lang F. The tyrosine kinase p56lck mediates activation of swelling-induced chloride channels in lymphocytes. *J Cell Biol* 1998;141:281–286.

149. Ling H, Vamvakas S, Busch G, Dammrich J, Schramm L, Lang F, Heidland A. Suppressing role of transforming growth factor-beta 1 on cathepsin activity in cultured kidney tubule cells. *Am J Physiol* 1995;269:F911–F917.

150. Lopez-Rodriguez C, Antos CL, Shelton JM, Richardson JA, Lin F, Novobrantseva TI, Bronson RT, Igarashi P, Rao A, Olson EN. Loss of NFAT5 results in renal atrophy and lack of tonicity-responsive gene expression. *Proc Natl Acad Sci U S A* 2004;101:2392–2397.

151. Lorenz C, Pusch M, Jentsch TJ. Heteromultimeric CLC chloride channels with novel properties. *Proc Natl Acad Sci U S A* 1996;93:13362–13366.

152. Macknight AD. Principles of cell volume regulation. *Ren Physiol Biochem* 1988;11:114–141.

153. Maeno E, Ishizaki Y, Kanaseki T, Hazama A, Okada Y. Normotonic cell shrinkage because of disordered volume regulation is an early prerequisite to apoptosis. *Proc Natl Acad Sci U S A* 2000;97:9487–9492.

154. Manganel M, Turner RJ. Agonist-induced activation of Na+/H+ exchange in rat parotid acinar cells is dependent on calcium but not on protein kinase C. *J Biol Chem* 1990;265:4284–4289.

155. Manganel M, Turner RJ. Rapid secretagogue-induced activation of Na+H+ exchange in rat parotid acinar cells. Possible interrelationship between volume regulation and stimulus-secretion coupling. *J Biol Chem* 1991;266:10182–10188.

156. McCarty NA, O'Neil RG. Calcium signaling in cell volume regulation. *Physiol Rev* 1992;72:1037–1061.

157. McManus ML, Churchwell KB, Strange K. Regulation of cell volume in health and disease. *N Engl J Med* 1995;333:1260–1266.

158. Minton AP. Excluded volume as a determinant of macromolecular structure and reactivity. *Biopolymers* 1981;20:2093–2120.

159. Minton AP. Influence of macromolecular crowding on intracellular association reactions: possible role in volume regulation. In: Strange K, ed. *Cellular and Molecular Physiology of Cell Volume Regulation*. Boca Raton, FL: CRC Press, 1994:181–190.

160. Minton AP. Macromolecular crowding and molecular recognition. *J Mol Recognit* 1993;6:211–214.

161. Moriguchi T, Kawasaki H, Matsuda S, Gotoh Y, Nishida E. Evidence for multiple activators for stress-activated protein kinase/c-Jun amino-terminal kinases. Existence of novel activators. *J Biol Chem* 1995;270:12969–12972.

162. Murphy D, Carter D. Vasopressin gene expression in the rodent hypothalamus: transcriptional and posttranscriptional responses to physiological stimulation. *Mol Endocrinol* 1990;4:1051–1059.

163. Nilius B, Eggermont J, Droogmans G. The endothelial volume-regulated anion channel, VRAC. *Cell Physiol Biochem* 2000;10:313–320.

164. Noe B, Schliess F, Wettstein M, Heinrich S, Haussinger D. Regulation of taurocholate excretion by a hypo-osmolarity-activated signal transduction pathway in rat liver. *Gastroenterology* 1996;110:858–865.

165. Norenberg MD, Bender AS. Astrocyte swelling in liver failure: role of glutamine and benzodiazepines. *Acta Neurochir Suppl (Wien)* 1994; 60:24–27.

166. Okada SF, O'Neal WK, Huang P, Nicholas RA, Ostrowski LE, Craigen WJ, Lazarowski ER, Boucher RC. Voltage-dependent anion channel-1 (VDAC-1) contributes to ATP release and cell volume regulation in murine cells. *J Gen Physiol* 2004;124:513–526.

167. Papakonstanti EA, Vardaki EA, Stournaras C. Actin cytoskeleton: a signaling sensor in cell volume regulation. *Cell Physiol Biochem* 2000;10:257–264.

168. Parker JC. In defense of cell volume? *Am J Physiol* 1993;265:C1191–C1200.

169. Pasantes-Morales H, Franco R, Torres-Marquez ME, Hernandez-Fonseca K, Ortega A. Amino acid osmolytes in regulatory volume decrease and isovolumetric regulation in brain cells: contribution and mechanisms. *Cell Physiol Biochem* 2000;10:361–370.

170. Paulmichl M, Li Y, Wickman K, Ackerman M, Peralta E, Clapham D. New mammalian chloride channel identified by expressioncloning. *Nature* 1992;356:238–241.

171. Perry PB, O'Neill WC. Swelling-activated K fluxes in vascular endothelial cells: volume regulation via K-Cl cotransport and K channels. *Am J Physiol* 1993;265:C763–C769.

172. Polischuk TM, Andrew RD. Real-time imaging of intrinsic optical signals during early excitotoxicity evoked by domoic acid in the rat hippocampal slice. *Can J Physiol Pharmacol* 1996;74:712–722.

173. Poronnik P, Schumann SY, Cook DI. HCO3(-)-dependent ACh-activated Na+ influx in sheep parotid secretory endpieces. *Pflugers Arch* 1995;429:852–858.

174. Reinehr R, Becker S, Hongen A, Haussinger D. The Src family kinase Yes triggers hyperosmotic activation of the epidermal growth factor receptor and CD95. *J Biol Chem* 2004;279:23977–23987.

175. Reinehr R, Gorg B, Hongen A, Haussinger D. CD95-tyrosine nitration inhibits hyperosmotic and CD95 ligand-induced CD95 activation in rat hepatocytes. *J Biol Chem* 2004;279:10364–10373.

176. Richter EA, Cleland PJ, Rattigan S, Clark MG. Contraction-associated translocation of protein kinase C in rat skeletal muscle. *FEBS Lett* 1987;217:232–236.

177. Ritter M, Woell E. Modification of cellular ion transport by the ha-ras oncogene: steps towards malignant transformation. *Cell Physiol Biochem* 1996;6:245–270.

178. Ritter M, Fuerst J, Woll E, Chwatal S, Gschwentner M, Lang F, Deetjen P, Paulmichl M. Na(+)/H(+)exchangers: linking osmotic dysequilibrium to modified cell function. *Cell Physiol Biochem* 2001;11:1–18.

179. Ritter M, Ravasio A, Jakab M, Chwatal S, Furst J, Laich A, Gschwentner M, Signorelli S, Burtscher C, Eichmuller S, Paulmichl M. Cell swelling stimulates cytosol to membrane transposition of ICln. *J Biol Chem* 2003;278:50163–50174.

180. Rosales OR, Sumpio BE. Changes in cyclic strain increase inositol trisphosphate and diacylglycerol in endothelial cells. *Am J Physiol* 1992;262:C956–C962.

181. Rosette C, Karin M. Ultraviolet light and osmotic stress: activation of the JNK cascade through multiple growth factor and cytokine receptors. *Science* 1996;274:1194–1197.

182. Roy G, Banderali U. Channels for ions and amino acids in kidney cultured cells (MDCK) during volume regulation. *J Exp Zool* 1994;268:121–126.

183. Ruepp B, Bohren KM, Gabbay KH. Characterization of the osmotic response element of the human aldose reductase gene promoter. *Proc Natl Acad Sci U S A* 1996;93:8624–8629.

184. Sachs F. Mechanical transduction by membrane ion channels: a mini review. *Mol Cell Biochem* 1991;104:57–60.

185. Sackin H. Stretch-activated ion channels. In: Strange K, ed. *Cellular and Molecular Physiology of Cell Volume Regulation*. Boca Raton, FL: CRC Press, 1994:215–240.

186. Sadoshima J, Qiu Z, Morgan JP, Izumo S. Tyrosine kinase activation is an immediate and essential step in hypotonic cell swelling-induced ERK activation and c-fos gene expression in cardiac myocytes. *EMBO J* 1996;15:5535–5546.

187. Saha N, Stoll B, Lang F, Haussinger D. Effect of anisotonic cell-volume modulation on glutathione-S-conjugate release, t-butylhydroperoxide metabolism and the pentose-phosphate shunt in perfused rat liver. *Eur J Biochem* 1992;209:437–444.

188. Sakai H, Kakinoki B, Diener M, Takeguchi N. Endogenous arachidonic acid inhibits hypotonically-activated Cl- channels in isolated rat hepatocytes. *Jpn J Physiol* 1996;46:311–318.

189. Saltin B, Sjogaard G, Strange S, Juel C. Redistribution of K+ in the human body during muscular exercise: its role to maintain whole body homeostasis. In Shiraki KYMK, ed. *Man in Stressful Environments: Thermal and Work Physiology*. Springfield, IL: Thomas, 1987:247–267.

190. Sanchez-Olea R, Morales-Mulia M, Moran J, Pasantes-Morales H. Inhibition by polyunsaturated fatty acids of cell volume regulation and osmolyte fluxes in astrocytes. *Am J Physiol* 1995;269:C96–C102.

191. Sanguinetti AR, Cao H, Corley MC. Fyn is required for oxidative- and hyperosmotic-stress-induced tyrosine phosphorylation of caveolin-1. *Biochem J* 2003;376:159–168.

192. Santoro MM, Liu Y, Khan SM, Hou LX, Bolen DW. Increased thermal stability of proteins in the presence of naturally occurring osmolytes. *Biochemistry* 1992;31:5278–5283.

193. Saransaari P, Oja SS. Excitatory amino acids evoke taurine release from cerebral cortex slices from adult and developing mice. *Neuroscience* 1991;45:451–459.

194. Schliess F, Haussinger D. Call volume and insulin signaling. *Int Rev Cytol* 2003;225:187–228.

195. Schliess F, Reissmann R, Reinehr R, Vom Dahl S, Haussinger D. Involvement of integrins and Src in insulin signaling toward autophagic proteolysis in rat liver. *J Biol Chem* 2004;279:21294–21301.

196. Schliess F, Sinning R, Fischer R, Schmalenbach C, Haussinger D. Calcium-dependent activation of Erk-1 and Erk-2 after hypo-osmotic astrocyte swelling. *Biochem J* 1996;320 (Pt 1):167–171.

197. Schultz SG. Homocellular regulatory mechanisms in sodium-transporting epithelia: avoidance of extinction by "flush-through." *J PhysiolAm J Physiol* 1981;241:F579–F590.

198. Schwab A. Function and spatial distribution of ion channels and transporters in cell migration. *Am J Physiol Renal Physiol* 2001;280:F739–F747.

199. Sheikh-Hamad D, Garcia-Perez A, Ferraris JD, Peters EM, Burg MB. Induction of gene expression by heat shock versus osmotic stress. *Am J Physiol* 1994;267:F28–F34.

200. Smith TW, Rasmusson RL, Lobaugh LA, Lieberman M. Na+/K+ pump inhibition induces cell shrinkage in cultured chick cardiac myocytes. *Basic Res Cardiol* 1993;88:411–420.

201. Soler C, Felipe A, Casado FJ, McGivan JD, Pastor-Anglada M. Hyperosmolarity leads to an increase in derepressed system A activity in the renal epithelial cell line NBL-1. *Biochem J* 1993;289(Pt 3):653–658.

202. Storey KB, Storey JM. Freeze tolerance in animals. *Physiol Rev* 1988;68:27–84.

203. Stossel TP. On the crawling of animal cells. *Science* 1993;260:1086–1094.

204. Strange K. *Cellular and Molecular Physiology of Cell Volume Regulation*. Boca Raton, FL: CRC Press, 1994.

205. Strange K. Cellular volume homeostasis. *Adv Physiol Educ* 2004; 28:155–159.

206. Strange K, Jackson PS. Swelling-activated organic osmolyte efflux: a new role for anion channels. *Kidney Int* 1995;48:994–1003.

207. Strbak V, Greer MA. Regulation of hormone secretion by acute cell volume changes: Ca(2+)-independent hormone secretion. *Cell Physiol Biochem* 2000;10:393–402.

208. Stroud JC, Lopez-Rodriguez C, Rao A, Chen L. Structure of a TonEBP-DNA complex reveals DNA encircled by a transcription factor. *Nat Struct Biol* 2002;9:90–94.

209. Szaszi K, Grinstein S, Orlowski J, Kapus A. Regulation of the epithelial Na(+) /H(+) exchanger isoform by the cytoskeleton. *Cell Physiol Biochem* 2000;10:265–272.

210. Takenaka M, Bagnasco SM, Preston AS, Uchida S, Yamauchi A, Kwon HM, Handler JS. The canine betaine gamma-amino-n-butyric acid transporter gene: diverse mRNA isoforms are regulated by hypertonicity and are expressed in a tissue-specific manner. *Proc Natl Acad Sci U S A* 1995;92:1072–1076.

211. Tanaka K, Jay G, Isselbacher KJ. Expression of heat-shock andglucose-regulated genes: differential effects of glucose starvation and hypertonicity. *Biochim Biophys Acta* 1988;950:138–146.

212. Taneja S, Ahmad F. Increased thermal stability of proteins in the presence of amino acids. *Biochem J* 1994;303(Pt 1):147–153.

213. Thiemann A, Grunder S, Pusch M, Jentsch TJ. A chloride channel widely expressed in epithelial and non-epithelial cells. *Nature* 1992;356:57–60.

214. Thornhill WB, Laris PC. KCl loss and cell shrinkage in the Ehrlich ascites tumor cell induced by hypotonic media, 2-deoxyglucose and propranolol. *Biochim Biophys Acta* 1984;773:207–218.

215. Tilly BC, Edixhoven MJ, Tertoolen LG, Morii N, Saitoh Y,Narumiya S, de Jonge HR. Activation of the osmo-sensitive chloride conductance involves P21rho and is accompanied by a transient reorganization of the F-actin cytoskeleton. *Mol Biol Cell* 1996;7:1419–1427.

216. Tilly BC, van den BN, Tertoolen LG, Edixhoven MJ, de Jonge HR. Protein tyrosine phosphorylation is involved in osmoregulation of ionic conductances. *J Biol Chem* 1993;268:19919–19922.

217. Tinel H, Kinne-Saffran E, Kinne RK. Calcium signalling during RVD of kidney cells. *Cell Physiol Biochem* 2000;10:297–302.

218. Tomlinson DR, Stevens EJ, Diemel LT. Aldose reductase inhibitors and their potential for the treatment of diabetic complications. *Trends Pharmacol Sci* 1994;15:293–297.

219. Trouet D, Carton I, Hermans D, Droogmans G, Nilius B, Eggermont J. Inhibition of VRAC by c-Src tyrosine kinase targeted to caveolae is mediated by the Src homology domains. *Am J Physiol Cell Physiol* 2001;281:C248–C256.

220. Uchida S, Kwon HM, Yamauchi A, Preston AS, Marumo F, Handler JS. Molecular cloning of the cDNA for an MDCK cell Na(+)- and Cl(-)-dependent taurine transporter that is regulated by hypertonicity. *Proc Natl Acad Sci U S A* 1992;89:8230–8234.

221. Ullrich KJ. Glycerylphosphorylcholinumsatz und Glycerylphosphorylcholindiesterase in der Säugetier-Niere. *Biochem Z* 1959;331:98–102.

222. Valverde MA, Vazquez E, Munoz FJ, Nobles M, Delaney SJ,Wainwright BJ, Colledge WH, Sheppard DN. Murine CFTRchannel and its role in regulatory volume decrease of small intestine crypts. *Cell Physiol Biochem* 2000;10:321–328.

223. Van der Meulen JA, Klip A, Grinstein S. Possible mechanism for cerebral oedema in diabetic ketoacidosis. *Lancet* 1987;2:306–308.

224. van der Wijk T, Tomassen SF, de Jonge HR, Tilly BC. Signalling mechanisms involved in volume regulation of intestinal epithelial cells. *Cell Physiol Biochem* 2000;10:289–296.

225. Volk T, Fromter E, Korbmacher C. Hypertonicity activates nonselective cation channels in mouse cortical collecting duct cells. *Proc Natl Acad Sci U S A* 1995;92:8478–8482.

226. Wakabayashi S, Shigekawa M, Pouyssegur J. Molecular physiology of vertebrate Na+/H+ exchangers. *Physiol Rev* 1997;77:51–74.

227. Waldegger S, Barth P, Raber G, Lang F. Cloning and characterization of a putative human serine/threonine protein kinase transcriptionally modified during anisotonic and isotonic alterations of cell volume. *Proc Natl Acad Sci U S A* 1997;94:4440–4445.

228. Wang SX, Ikeda M, Guggino WB. The cytoplasmic tail of large conductance, voltage- and Ca2+-activated K+ (MaxiK) channel is necessary for its cell surface expression. *J Biol Chem* 2003;278:2713–2722.

229. Wehner F, Bohmer C, Heinzinger H, van den BF, Tinel H. Thehypertonicity-induced Na(+) conductance of rat hepatocytes: physiological significance and molecular correlate. *Cell Physiol Biochem* 2000;10:335–340.

230. Wehner F, Olsen H, Tinel H, Kinne-Saffran E, Kinne RK. Cell volume regulation: osmolytes, osmolyte transport, and signal transduction. *Rev Physiol Biochem Pharmacol* 2003;148:1–80.

231. Wehner F, Sauer H, Kinne RK. Hypertonic stress increases the Na+ conductance of rat hepatocytes in primary culture. *J Gen Physiol* 1995;105:507–535.

232. Wiesinger H, Thiess U, Hamprecht B. Sorbitol pathway activity and utilization of polyols in astroglia-rich primary cultures. *Glia* 1990; 3:277–282.

233. Yamauchi A, Kwon HM, Uchida S, Preston AS, Handler JS. Myo-inositol and betaine transporters regulated by tonicity are basolateral in MDCK cells. *Am J Physiol* 1991;261:F197–F202.

234. Yamauchi A, Miyai A, Yokoyama K, Itoh T, Kamada T, Ueda N,Fujiwara Y. Response to osmotic stimuli in mesangial cells: role of system A transporter. *Am J Physiol* 1994;267:C1493–C1500.

235. Yamauchi A, Sugiura T, Ito T, Miyai A, Horio M, Imai E, Kamada T. Na+/myo-inositol transport is regulated by basolateral tonicity in Madin–Darby canine kidney cells. *J Clin Invest* 1996;97:263–267.

236. Young E, Bradley RF. Cerebral edema with irreversible coma in severe diabetic ketoacidosis. *N Engl J Med* 1967;276:665–669.

237. Zhang F, Warskulat U, Haussinger D. Modulation of tumor necrosis factor-alpha release by anisoosmolarity and betaine in rat liver macrophages (Kupffer cells). *FEBS Lett* 1996;391:293–296.

238. Zhang F, Warskulat U, Wettstein M, Schreiber R, Henninger HP, Decker K, Haussinger D. Hyperosmolarity stimulates prostaglandin synthesis and cyclooxygenase-2 expression in activated rat liver macrophages. *Biochem J* 1995;312(Pt 1):135–143.

CHAPTER 7

Solute Transport, Energy Consumption, and Production in the Kidney

Takashi Sekine, Hiroki Miyazaki, and Hitoshi Endou

The University of Tokyo, Tokyo, Japan
University of Bern, Bern, Switzerland
Kyorin University School of Medicine, Tokyo, Japan

INTRODUCTION

The kidney must reabsorb more than 99% of approximately 180 liters of water and 25,000 mmoles of Na^+ daily. To do this, the kidney consumes a large amount of energy. Although the kidney is only 0.5% of total body weight, it utilizes approximately 7% of the oxygen consumed by the body (272). In fact, the kidney is second only to the heart in terms of the rate of energy consumption (272). In this chapter, we describe the energy consumption and production processes in the kidney, along with their mutual relationships. We also refer to the pathophysiological states in which renal energy production is inhibited.

ENERGY CONSUMPTION

Na Transport and Energy Consumption

NA^+ TRANSPORT AND O_2 CONSUMPTION

The energy utilized in the kidney is primarily for the active reabsorption of Na^+ from the glomerular filtrate (Fig. 1). This seems rational considering that the amount of Na^+ reabsorbed by the kidney is much higher than that of HCO_3^- (4,800 mmole/day), Ca^{2+} (210 mmole/day), other electrolytes, and organic substances. The active Na^+ transport also energizes the reabsorption of water and other solutes via the osmotic gradient generated by Na^+ transport, and by the electrochemical gradient of Na^+ across the plasma membrane.

With regard to the energy production, the kidney generates approximately 95% of the ATP produced via aerobic mechanism (245), while in some nephron segments anaerobic metabolism also occurs efficiently. This is reasonable because of highly efficient ATP production via mitochondrial oxidative phosphorylation compared to anaerobic glycolysis. Thirty-six moles of ATP generated by the mitochondrial oxidative phosphorylation of 1 mole of glucose, whereas only 2 moles of ATP are produced via glycolysis in the absence of O_2. Thus, his-

torically the relationship between Na transport and O_2 consumption (QO_2) (Fig. 1) in renal tissues has been extensively investigated.

Prior to investigations in renal epithelia, Zerahn measured QO_2 and the short-circuit current of Na^+ in frog skin, and demonstrated a linear relationship between Na^+ transport and QO_2 with a stoichiometry of $17{\sim}18\ Na^+/O_2$ (300, 301). Assuming that oxidative phosphorylation provides six ATP molecules through the oxidation of one molecule of O_2, an $18\ Na^+/O_2$ stoichiometry indicated by the ratio of $3\ Na^+/ATP$ in sodium transport, which is now recognized as the 3:1 stoichiometry for $Na^+{:}ATP$ in Na^+, K^+ ATPase. This calculation by Zerahn was correctly performed before the discovery of Na^+, K^+ ATPase by Skou. This $18\ Na^+/O_2$ stoichiometry in sodium transport was also confirmed in the toad urinary bladder (197).

Thereafter, several investigators examined the Na^+/O_2 stoichiometry in the kidney (57, 144, 261). Thurau demonstrated a linear relationship between Na^+ transport and QO_2 with a ratio of $28\ Na^+/O_2$ in the whole dog kidney (261) (Fig. 2). This stoichiometry is equal to the ratio of 4.6 for Na^+/ATP, which indicates more efficient transport in the kidney compared to that in the frog skin and toad bladder. The discrepancy has been studied by many investigators and is attributed to factors described in the following (175).

First, there are alternative pathways for Na^+ transport in the nephron. In the leaky epithelia such as proximal tubule (PT), paracellular Na^+ transport occurs, while only transepithelial transport is possible in the tight epithelia in cortical collecting duct (CCD) cells. Second, coupling of Na^+ transport to that of other solutes occurs, such as bicarbonate transport in PT and Na^+–K^+–$2Cl^-$ transport via NKCC2 in the thick ascending limb of Henle (TAL). These two mechanisms produce more efficient Na^+ transport in certain nephron segments compared to that observed in frog skin and toad bladder, where only cellular transport of Na^+ driven by Na^+,K^+-ATPase occurs. The different $Na^+/O_2/ATP$ stoichiometry among individual nephron segments will be described in a subsequent section.

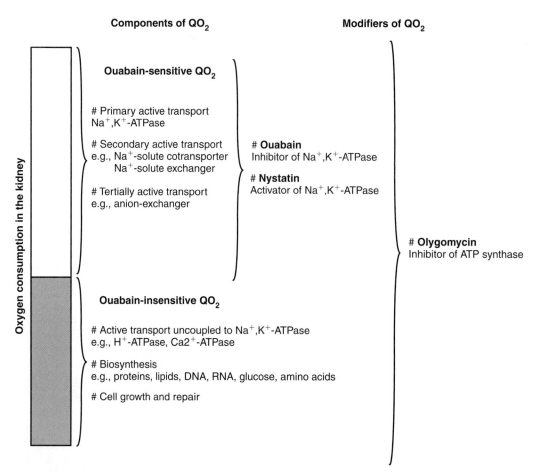

Components of QO₂

Modifiers of QO₂

Oxygen consumption in the kidney

Ouabain-sensitive QO₂

\# Primary active transport
Na⁺,K⁺-ATPase

\# Secondary active transport
e.g., Na⁺-solute cotransporter
Na⁺-solute exchanger

\# Tertially active transport
e.g., anion-exchanger

\# **Ouabain**
Inhibitor of Na⁺,K⁺-ATPase

\# **Nystatin**
Activator of Na⁺,K⁺-ATPase

\# **Olygomycin**
Inhibitor of ATP synthase

Ouabain-insensitive QO₂

\# Active transport uncoupled to Na⁺,K⁺-ATPase
e.g., H⁺-ATPase, Ca2⁺-ATPase

\# Biosynthesis
e.g., proteins, lipids, DNA, RNA, glucose, amino acids

\# Cell growth and repair

FIGURE 1   Cellular components of oxygen consumption (QO₂). Cellular QO₂ is divided primarily into two components. The first is ouabain-sensitive QO₂, which is identical to the sum of Na⁺,K⁺-ATPase, and secondary active and tertiary active transport coupled to the Na⁺ gradient. The other is an ouabain-insensitive portion, which is related to transport processes uncoupled to Na⁺,K⁺-ATPase (e.g., H⁺-ATPase and Ca²⁺-ATPase) and catabolic processes (e.g., biosynthesis and cell growth and repair). Ouabain-sensitive QO₂ is markedly different among nephron segments. In the proximal convoluted tubule, 60% of QO₂ is ouabain-sensitive, whereas in OMCD, only 8% of QO₂ is ouabain-sensitive. These differences reflect the activities of Na⁺,K⁺-ATPase among nephron segments.

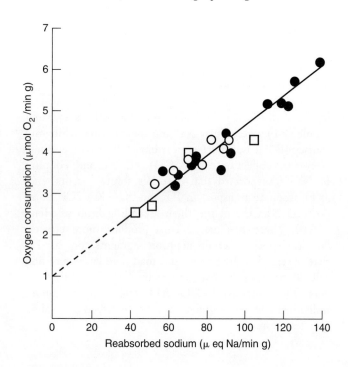

FIGURE 2   Oxygen consumption as a function of net sodium reabsorption in whole dog kidneys. (Adapted with permission from Thurau K. Renal Na-reabsorption and O2-uptake in dogs during hypoxia and hydrochlorothiazide infusion. *Proc Soc Exp Biol Med* 1961;106:714–717.)

The data... in Fig. 2 indicate... Extrapolatio... the basal o... energy used... and was esti... studies indi... in the kidne...

HETERO...
ALONG...

PROXIM...
In the P... responding... the PT (S...

(99), resulting in a rise in the luminal Cl^- concentration termed as the axial anionic asymmetry (9, 224) (Fig. 3). In the basolateral membrane of proximal tubular cells, a Na^+-bicarbonate cotransporter (NBC) extrudes Na^+ with HCO_3^- (243) with a stoichiometry of 1:2~3 (102). The electrochemical gradient of HCO_3^- across the plasma membrane in the PT cells, which is generated by the coordinated function of carbonic anhydrase and H^+–ATPase or the Na^+–H^+ exchanger, drives Na^+ efflux via NBC. Because PT is more permeable to Cl^- than to HCO_3^-, a driving force for isotonic fluid transport develops. It was suggested that 30% (145) to 50% (84) of Na^+ transport in the PT is passive, and not directly related to ATP consumption. In addition, in the early part of the PT, glucose, amino acids, and phosphate are actively reabsorbed via the Na^+.

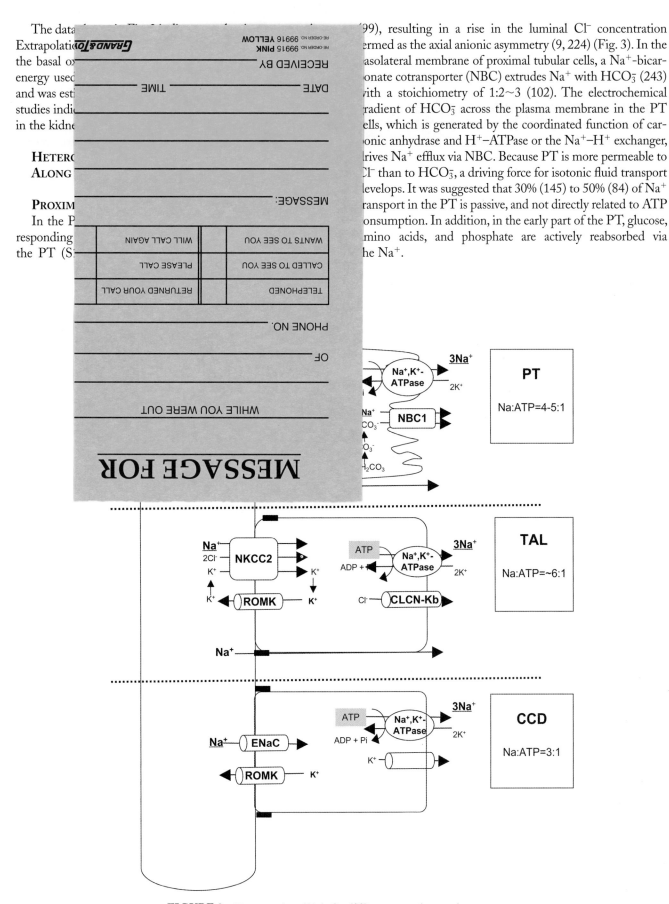

FIGURE 3 Heterogeneity of Na^+–O_2–ATP transsport along nephron segments.

Cotransport mechanism, thereby rapidly reducing their concentration in the lumen. This luminal hypotonicity also contributes to the solvent drag, which involves Na^+. Thus, in the PT, more than three Na^+ could be transported via the hydrolysis of 1 mole of ATP.

Thick Ascending Limb of Henle In the TAL, the most efficient sodium transport occurs with the Na^+–K^+–$2Cl^-$ cotransporter (NKCC2) playing an important role. The transport by NKCC2 is electrically neutral, and the K^+ reabsorbed by NKCC2 in the TAL is back leaked into the tubular lumen via the ROMK channel in the apical membrane. This K^+ leakage results in a positive electrical potential difference in the lumen, which drives paracellular transport of Na^+ from the lumen to the plasma. Although no direct measurement has been made of the $Na^+/O_2/ATP$ stoichiometry in the TAL, results obtained in the rectal gland (236) and tracheal epithelium (287) indicated that the Na^+/ATP ratio could theoretically be up to 6 in the TAL.

Cortical Collecting Duct In the CCD, the efficiency of Na^+ transport is the lowest among the nephron segments. In this segment, the junction between the epithelia is very tight and paracellular transport is minimal. In addition, Na^+ entry from the luminal side into CCD cells is mediated only by ENaC, which is not associated with any coupled transport other than that of Na^+. Thus, the Na^+/ATP ratio in the CCD is estimated to be 3.

Energy Cost of Primary Active Transport

The cellular transport of electrolytes and organic substances is classified into three types, namely, primary active, secondary active, and tertiary active. Primary active transport refers to that which directly utilizes ATP hydrolysis energy to accomplish transepithelial transport. The primary active transporter in the plasma membrane of mammalian cells is further subdivided into three subtypes: P-type-ATPase, V-type-ATPase, and ABC transporter. The secondary active transporters utilize the Na^+ gradient across the plasma membrane generated by the Na^+,K^+-ATPase. Na^+-coupled cotransporters (e.g., Na^+-glucose cotransporter, Na^+-amino acid cotransporter) carry substrates with Na^+ in the same direction, while Na^+ exchangers (e.g., the Na^+–H^+ exchanger [NHE]) transport substrate and Na^+ in opposite directions. In addition, there are tertiary active transporters. One example is anion exchangers (AE) (Cl^-–HCO_3^- exchanger). The proton gradient generated by the coordinated function of Na^+,K^+-ATPase (primary active transporter) and NHE (secondary active transporter) is used as the driving force for the exchange of Cl^- and HCO_3^- via AE (tertiary active transporter).

The energy used by the secondary and tertiary active transport processes is attributed to the active transport via Na^+,K^+-ATPase, which alone is accompanied by hydrolysis of ATP. Primary active transporters other than Na^+,K^+-ATPase are also related to energy consumption processes in the kidney. In general, the expression level of ATPases along

the nephron segments has correlated well with the transport activity of each solute.

P-Type ATPases

P-type-ATPases, including Na^+,K^+-ATPase, H^+,K^+-ATPase, and Ca^{2+}-ATPase, share several common features: (1) they possess a 7-amino acid motif with aspartate to which ATP binds, (2) they are transiently phosphorylated during the cation transport cycle (the term P-type derives from this transient phosphorylation), and (3) they catalyze cation transport between E_1 and E_2 conformations (P-type-ATPase was previously called E_1-E_2-ATPase). The transport activity of P-type-ATPases is commonly inhibited by vanadate.

Na^+,K^+-ATPase Na^+,K^+-ATPase extrudes three Na^+ and takes up two K^+ across the plasma membranes through the hydrolysis of one ATP molecule in the presence of Mg^{2+}. Na^+,K^+-ATPase generates an inward-directed Na^+ gradient and inside negative electrical gradient. Na^+,K^+-ATPase accounts for approximately half of the total Na^+ reabsorption in the kidney (219).

Na^+,K^+-ATPase is a heterodimeric integral membrane protein, with a minimal composition of α- and β-subunits. The α-subunit possesses 10 membrane-spanning domains with a molecular mass of approximately 100 kDa. The β-subunit is a glycosylated type II membrane protein with a molecular weight of approximately 55 kDa (138). In mammalian genomes, four α-subunits and at least three β-subunits of Na^+,K^+-ATPase have been identified (21, 130). In addition, a γ-subunit, a member of the FXYD family of type II transmembrane proteins, constitutes a Na^+,K^+-ATPase (251). In the kidney, two γ-subunit isoforms are expressed (21, 130). The combination of each isoform comprises a number of Na^+,K^+-ATPase isozymes that are expressed in a tissue- and cell-specific manner to evolve distinct properties to respond to cellular requirements (21). In the kidney, α1β1 is predominantly expressed (16, 76, 130).

The α-subunit is the catalytic subunit of the Na^+,K^+-ATPase, and α1, α2, and α3 isoforms differ in their affinities for ATP, Na^+, and K^+ (228). β-subunits are suggested to facilitate the correct membrane integration and packing of the α-subunit, and β-subunits also participate in the determination of the intrinsic transport properties of Na^+,K^+-ATPase (91). The γ-subunit was shown to be a specific regulator of renal α1β1 isozymes (92). A putative dominant-negative mutation in the gene encoding the γ-subunit (FXYD2) that leads to defective routing of the protein in a family with dominant renal hypomagnesemia indicates the physiological importance of the γ-subunit (186). The overall structure of the α-subunit of Na^+,K^+-ATPase determined by electron crystallography using two-dimensional crystals is similar to the xray structure of Ca^{2+}-ATPase (117, 131).

The pump activity of Na^+,K^+-ATPase has been investigated using direct measurement of hydrolysis activity, and axial heterogeneity in the nephron segments was demonstrated (62, 66, 85, 142, 143) (Fig. 4). Na^+,K^+-ATPase hy-

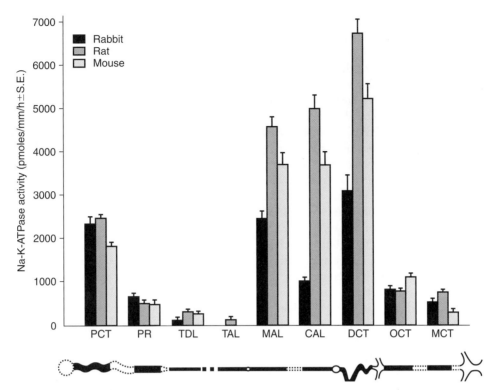

FIGURE 4 Na$^+$,K$^+$-ATPase activity in individual nephron segments measured using hydrolysis activity. (Adapted with permission from Katz AI, Doucet A, Morel F. Na-K-ATPase activity along the rabbit, rat, and mouse nephron. *Am J Physiol* 1979;237:F114–F120.)

drolysis activity was high in the TAL, distal convoluted tubule (DCT), and proximal convoluted tubule (PCT), and low in the pars recta (PST) and collecting tubule (CT) (62, 66, 85, 142, 143). Ouabain-binding studies show the highest density of Na$^+$,K$^+$-ATPase (20–30 fmol/mm length of tubule) in the DCT and medullary thick ascending limb (MTAL), intermediate density (10 fmol/mm) in the PCT and connecting tubule (CNT), and lowest density (2–7 fmol/mm) in the PST, cortical thick ascending limb (CTAL), and CT (71). The pump activity was proportional to the number of catalytic units. α1β1 has a maximum turnover rate of 7700/min (129). The measurement of Na$^+$,K$^+$-ATPase hydrolytic activity at V$_{max}$ and initial rates of ouabain-sensitive Rb uptake indicated that in intact cells the pump works at approximately 20–30% of its V$_{max}$ (51). Western blotting analysis (185, 265), RT-PCR using microdissected nephron segments (265), in situ hybridization (3, 76), and immunohistochemical analysis (141, 210, 289) demonstrated similar intranephron heterogenetic localization of Na$^+$,K$^+$-ATPase consistent with those observed in the studies on pump activity.

Regulation of Na$^+$,K$^+$-ATPase by dexamethasone (64), deoxycorticosterone (257), intracellular Na concentration (278), cAMP (147), potassium depletion (38), aldosterone, and vasopressin (78, 79) was demonstrated. Many of these modulations influence the cell surface expression of Na$^+$,K$^+$-ATPase (78, 79), while MEK1/2 inhibitors changed the intrinsic activity rather than cell surface expression (189).

Ca^{2+}-ATPase Renal calcium transport is comprised of two processes: a paracellular, passive process that predominates in most nephron segments, and a transcellular, energy-dependent step in the DCT. Transcellular calcium transport involves (1) entry into the DCT cell via a Ca^{2+} channel (ECaC) across the luminal membrane, (2) intracellular Ca movement facilitated by the presence of the vitamin D-dependent calcium-binding protein (calbindin D), and (3) extrusion by the Ca^{2+}-ATPase located at the basolateral membrane (31). The extrusion of Ca^{2+}, the final step in the transcellular transport of Ca^{2+}, is mediated by the plasma membrane Ca^{2+}-ATPase (PMCA) which is a P-type-ATPase.

PMCA is a monomeric protein consisting of approximately 1,220 amino acids with a molecular mass of 140 kDa (173, 276). The sequence contains the calmodulin-binding domain, and two domains resembling calmodulin, one of which may play a role in the binding of Ca^{2+} (276). There are at least four isoforms of PMCA, and isoforms 1 and 4 are more widely distributed than 2 and 3 (206, 246, 247). The activity of renal PMCA showed two saturable components: a high-affinity component with a Km of 33 μM ATP and a low-affinity component with a Km of 0.63 mM ATP (36). PMCA is regulated by calmodulin (206), estrogen and dihydrotestosterone (58), protein kinase C or A (206), extracellular ATP (213), and pathophysiologic states such as hypercalciuria (42). RT-PCR (41, 172), immunohistochemical analysis (171), and Western blot analysis (173) demonstrated high expression of PMCA in the DCT. PMCA was also detected in Madin–Darby canine kidney (MDCK) cells (146). Doucet and coworkers ex amined sodium azide–insensitive plasma membrane Ca^{2+}-ATPase activity. The Ca^{2+}-ATPase was maximally activated via Ca^{2+} concentrations with an apparent Km of 0.3–0.4 µM. Ca^{2+}-ATPase activity was found in all segments of the nephron: activity was highest in the DCT and CCT, intermediate in the PCT and MTAL, and lowest in the PST, CTAL, and MCT (63).

In addition to PMCA, there exists another distinct Ca^{2+}-ATPase, the sarco/endoplasmic reticulum Ca^{2+}-ATPase (SERCA), which belongs also to the P-type-ATPase. The SERCA family includes three gene products: SERCA1 (ATP2A1), SERCA2 (ATP2A2), and SERCA 3 (ATP2A3) (180), which function for the removal of free cytosolic Ca^{2+} into the sarco/endoplasmic reticulum. Although thapsigarigin is known to be a specific inhibitor of the endoplasmic reticulum Ca^{2+} pump (260), no study has been reported on the relative energy consumption rate of SERCA in the kidney.

H^+,K^+-ATPase H^+,K^+-ATPase was originally characterized in a study of gastric mucosa. The gastric H^+,K^+-ATPase is located in the apical membrane of stomach parietal cells and mediates electroneutral exchange of K^+ and H^+. The gastric H^+,K^+-ATPase activity is independent of extracellular sodium, and inhibited by vanadate (67).

Molecular cloning identified two types of H^+,K^+-ATPase: gastric and colonic type H^+,K^+-ATPase. H^+,K^+-ATPase is comprised of α and β subunits. The catalytic α-subunit of gastric H^+,K^+-ATPase shows structural similarity to that of Na^+,K^+-ATPase, and the greatest homology occurs in the phosphorylation site region and in domains presumably involved in nucleotide binding and energy transduction (232). The α-subunit of colonic H^+,K^+-ATPase exhibits 63% amino acid identity to that of the gastric H^+,K^+-ATPase (53). The β-subunit of H^+,K^+-ATPase shows 41% amino acid sequence identity to the β2 subunit of Na^+,K^+-ATPase in the rat (40).

In the kidney, the existence of both gastric H^+,K^+-ATPase (232) and colonic H^+,K^+-ATPase (53) was demonstrated. Gastric H^+,K^+-ATPase is expressed constitutively along the length of the collecting duct and is responsible for H^+ secretion and K^+ reabsorption under normal conditions; it may be stimulated with acid–base perturbations and/or K^+ depletion (237). The level of expression of colonic H^+,K^+-ATPase is much lower in the kidney than in the distal colon (53).

Using in vitro microperfusion, Wingo and colleagues provided evidence of the existence of omeprazole-sensitive acidification and a K^+-absorptive mechanism in OMCD in rabbits (291). By enzymatic analysis, Doucet (65) and Garg (88) quantified the K^+-stimulated, Na-insensitive ATPase activity in nephron segments. K^+-stimulated ATPase activity was identified in the CNT, CCT, and MCT, although the activities were very low compared to those of other P-type-ATPases in the kidney (88). The renal K^+-ATPase had a high affinity for K^+ (Km 0.2~0.4 mM) and was inhibited by vanadate, omeprazole, and SCH 28080, specific

inhibitors of gastric H^+,K^+-ATPase, but was insensitive to ouabain (65, 88). A correlation between the magnitude of enzymatic activity and the percentage of intercalated cells in a given segment suggested that K^+-ATPase activity originates in intercalated cells (65).

Immunohistochemical analysis revealed H^+,K^+-ATPase in intercalated cells in the CCD and OMCD. In all segments studied, except for the CCD, the percentage of H^+,K^+-ATPase-immunoreactive cells corresponded to the percentage of intercalated cells (292). The RT-PCR technique demonstrated the gastric H^+,K^+-ATPase α-subunit in the CCD and IMCD, and a specific hybridization signal for the gastric H^+,K^+-ATPase α-subunit cDNA was demonstrated (4). The colonic H^+,K^+-ATPase α-subunit is specifically expressed in the CCD and OMCD in K^+-depleted rats (179). An increase in H^+,K^+-ATPase activity (65) and enhanced expression of gastric H^+,K^+-ATPase α-subunit (5) and colonic H^+,K^+-ATPase (237) in K^+ depletion suggest the physiological adaptation of renal H^+,K^+-ATPase.

V-TYPE-ATPASES

V-type (vacuolar) ATPases represent the second family of ATP-dependent ion pumps. Vacuolar H^+-ATPase is primarily responsible for the acidification of intracellular compartments such as endosomes, lysosomes, Golgi apparatus and clathrin-coated vesicles. H^+-ATPase is also expressed in the plasma membrane, and functions in acid/base transport in epithelia. In the kidney, vacuolar H^+-ATPase mediates H^+ secretion mainly in the PT and CCD (94, 279).

H^+-ATPase is a multisubunit complex composed of two functional domains (80, 103). The V(1) domain is a 570-kDa peripheral complex composed of eight subunits of molecular mass ranging from 73 to 14 kDa (subunits A–H) that is responsible for ATP hydrolysis. The V(o) domain is a 260-kDa integral complex composed of five subunits of molecular mass ranging from 100 to 17 kDa (subunits a, d, c, c′, and c″) that is responsible for proton translocation.

H^+-ATPase is insensitive to vanadate or ouabain, but is inhibited by bafilomycin A, N,N′-dicyclohexylcarbodiimide (DCCD) (Ki = 50 µM), and N-ethylmaleimide (NEM) (Ki = 20 µM). Physiological experiments indicated the existence of H^+-ATPase in the PT. DCCD caused a 15% fall in CO_2 absorption during eucapnia, and a 30% fall during acute hypercapnia in the PT (15). In other experiments, the S_3 segment was shown to possess a plasma membrane H^+-ATPase activity (156).

The relative contribution of H^+-ATPase to the ATP consumption by the kidney was examined by Noel et al. (200). In dog proximal tubules incubated under control conditions, 81% of the respiration was directly related to oligomycin-sensitive ATP synthesis, and 29% of this amount was inhibited by bafilomycin A. In rabbit and hamster PT, the bafilomycin-insensitive ATP requirement involves only 5 and 10%, respectively, of the total ATP turnover. Thus, the metabolic cost of H⁺-ATPase in PT varies significantly among species.

Ait-Mohamed et al. (6) examined the localization of NEM-sensitive ATPase in all segments of the rat nephron: its activity was highest in the PCT; intermediate in the PST, TAL, and CCT; and lowest in the OMCD. Immunocytochemical analysis demonstrated localization of rat H⁺-ATPase in the PCT, the initial part of the thin descending limb, TAL, DCT, and CT (32) consistent with the aforementioned H⁺-ATPase activity.

Garg and coworkers examined the effect of acid–base balance (86, 89, 90) and aldosterone (87) on NEM-sensitive ATPase activity, and demonstrated the modulation of NEM-sensitive ATPase activity by metabolic acidosis and administration of aldosterone, and these effects were observed mainly in the CT.

The significance of H⁺-ATPase in final urinary acidification along the collecting system has been confirmed by hereditary defects in H⁺-ATPase. Mutations in the gene encoding the B1 subunit of H⁺-ATPase cause distal renal tubular acidosis with sensorineural deafness, and defects in the 116-kDa subunit ATP6N1B cause recessive distal renal tubular acidosis with preserved hearing (140, 241, 249).

ABC SUPERFAMILY

The third subgroup of primary active transporters is the ABC (ATP-binding cassette) transporter family. The prototype ABC transporter is the P-glycoprotein (P-gp) encoded by the MDR gene. P-gp was originally isolated as a drug extrusion pump in cancer cells that confers multiresistance to antineoplastic drugs (8, 98). Later, P-gp was also shown to be expressed in normal tissues such as the kidney, intestine, and the brain capillary cells, where it acts as a functional barrier to xenobiotics by extruding them from the tissues. Then, a subfamily of ABC transporters,

the MRP (multidrug-resistance-associated protein) family, was identified and the number of its isoforms is expanding rapidly (113).

The common molecular structure of ABC transporters is as follows: they possess two transmembrane (TM) domains, each with six TM segments, and two nucleotide-binding domains, both of which can hydrolyze ATP (122). The stoichiometry of two ATPs hydrolyzed per molecule of drug transported was proposed (8).

Although the molecular properties of the members of ABC transporters, such as tissue distribution and substrate selectivity, have been extensively characterized, their significance in energy consumption in the kidney remains to be investigated, and to date no information is available.

COMPARISON OF ION-TRANSPORTING ATPASE ACTIVITIES AND QO₂ ALONG THE NEPHRON

In Fig. 5, a comparison of the ion-transporting ATPase activities is shown (from Gullans and Mandel [111] with permission).

METABOLIC BASIS

Energy Production Pathway

ATP synthesis in the kidney is mainly performed via mitochondrial oxidative phosphorylation, and a variety of energy fuels, such as glucose, fatty acids, and ketone bodies, are metabolized. Anaerobic glycolysis also occurs in certain nephron segments. Because of its heterogeneity in structural and functional properties, metabolic pathways and preferred substrates are distinct among the nephron segments. In this section, the metabolic bases in the kidney and individual nephron segments are described.

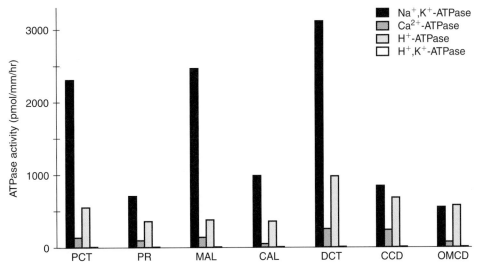

FIGURE 5 Comparison of ATPase activities employed from representative studies. (Adapted with permission Gullans SR, Mandel LJ. Coupling of energy to transport in proximal and distal nephron. In: Seldin DW, Giebisch G, eds. *The Kidney: Physiology and Pathophysiology.* 3rd ed. New York: Raven Press, 2000:443–482.)

MITOCHONDRIAL OXIDATIVE PHOSPHORYLATION

Mitochondrial oxidative phosphorylation is comprised of the following three steps: (1) production of reduced equivalents, that is, NADH and $FADH_2$, mostly by the TCA cycle in the mitochondria matrix; (2) electron transfer via the mitochondrial respiratory chain in the inner membrane of mitochondria, associated with proton extrusion across the inner membrane of mitochondria; and (3) ATP production by F_0F_1-ATPase using the proton gradient generated (116) (Figs. 6 and 7). The mitochondrial respiratory chain catalyzes electron transfer via four large multimeric integral membrane protein complexes (complex I to IV), ATP synthase (alternatively called complex V), and two relatively small hydrophobic proteins, that is, ubiquinone (Q: Coenzyme Q) and cytochrome c (Figure 6).

NADH:ubiquinone oxidoreductase (complex I) is the first and largest complex in the electron transport chain of mitochondria consisting of at least 42 different subunits with a molecular mass of approximately 890 kDa in cattle (101). Complex I possesses an L-shaped appearance comprising a thin, stalk region linking the membrane-bound globular arm with the intrinsic membrane domain (101).

Complex I oxidizes NADH and transfers electrons to ubiquinone (Q). The free energy released by this reaction is utilized for extrusion of three to five protons from the mitochondrial matrix by complex I. Complex II (succinate:ubiquinone oxidoreductase) oxidizes succinate to fumarate and passes the electrons directly to Q. Complex II serves as the sole direct link between activity in the TCA cycle and electron transport in the mitochondrial membrane (1). Complex II does not transport protons during the oxidation of succinate. Ubiquinol-cytochrome c oxidoreductase (Complex III), alternatively called the cytochrome bc complex, transfers one electron from reduced Q (QH2) to cytochrome c, and extrudes four protons (20). Thereafter, cytochrome c oxidase (CCO: Complex IV) catalyzes the reduction of molecular oxygen to water, a process in which four electrons, four protons, and one oxygen molecule are consumed. The reaction by CCO is coupled to the pumping of 3 to 4 protons across the membrane (188). Thus, through electron transfer between NADH or FADH2 to O_2, proton extrusion continues, and a steep proton gradient with a 200- to 230-mV membrane potential is generated across the mitochondrial inner membrane (191). Finally, ATP synthase (F_0F_1-ATPase)

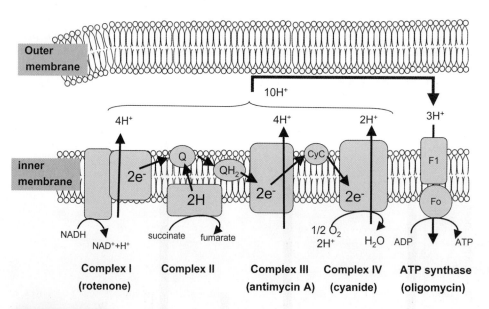

FIGURE 6 Schematic representation of mitochondrial oxidative phosphorylation. In the inner membrane of the mitochondria, four large multimeric membrane proteins complexes (Complexes I, II, III, and IV) catalyze electron transfer and proton extrusion. Two relatively small mobile proteins (Q and CytC) also mediate electron transport. Finally, ATP synthase produces ATP using the electrochemical gradient generated across the inner membrane of the mitochondria. Rotenone, antimycin A, cyanide, and oligomycin are representative inhibitors for the Complexes I, III, and IV, and ATP synthase, respectively.

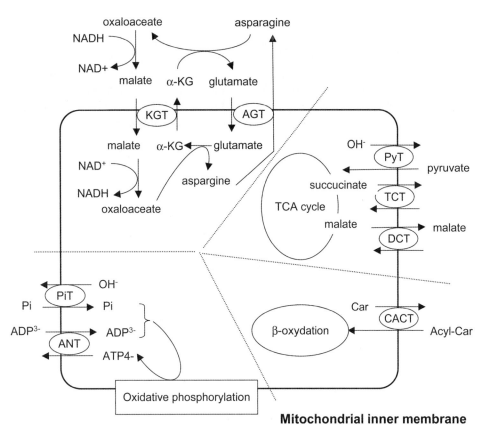

Mitochondrial inner membrane

FIGURE 7 Mitochondrial solute transporters located in mitochondrial inner membrane. These transporters are divided into four groups from the functional viewpoints. The lower left part indicates the interchange of ADP, Pi, and ATP between the inner membrane by ANT and PiT. The left upper part indicates the malate-asparagine shuttle transports the reducing potential from the cytosol to the matrix. The right upper part indicates the transport of substrates of the TCA cycle. The right lower part indicates the acyl-CoA transport to the mitochondrial matrix. Acyl-CoA is used for β-oxidation. In this figure, the ornithine transport system is not depicted.

catalyzes the following reaction: ADP + Pi, then $nH_p^+ \rightleftharpoons$ ATP + H_2O + nH_N^+. Here, the number of H^+ required to produce one ATP molecule is considered to be three to four (26, 27).

The mitochondrial inner membrane is impermeable to ionic substances, and there exist several transporters encoded by the *SLC25* gene family that shuttle metabolites across the mitochondrial inner membrane (139, 205). All mitochondrial transporters with known function are composed of three tandemly related segments of about 100 amino acids with six transmembrane domains (205). They probably function as homodimers. The driving force of each transporter is the chemical gradient of individual solutes, and electrical gradients (inside alkaline and negative).

The mitochondrial transporters essential for energy production and catabolism are divided into several groups (Fig. 7). The first group is comprised of the ADP/ATP translocase (ANT) and the Pi–OH exchanger (PiT), which facilitates interchange between cytosolic ADP and Pi, and intramitochondrial ATP. The rate of transport of the ATP/ADP exchanger is critical in determining the respiration rate of mitochondria (163). The second group, malate-aspartate shuttle proteins, consists of the α-ketoglutarate–malate exchanger (KGT) and the glutamate–aspartate exchanger. The malate-aspartate shuttle transports reduced equivalents into mitochondria to fulfill the oxidative respiration because the mitochondrial inner membrane is impermeable to NADH. This system is very active in the kidney, liver, and brain. The third group consists of pyruvate–OH^- exchanger (PyT), tricarboxylate exchanger (TCT), and dicarboxylate exchanger (DCT). PyT (121) transports pyruvate into mitochondrial matrix using the proton gradient across the inner membrane. DCT and TCT exchange tricarboxylate and dicarboxylate, respectively. Malate transported by DCT, and citrate by TCT from the matrix to the cytosol, are used for synthesis of fatty acids and glucose (gluconeogenesis), respectively. The fourth group is the carnitine/acylcarnitine translocase (CACT), which transports acylcarnitines into mitochondria in exchange for free carnitine; therefore, it is essential for fatty acid β-oxidation (125). All of these mitochondrial membrane transporters are essential for energy production processes.

TRICARBOXYLIC ACID CYCLE

The tricarboxylic acid (TCA) cycle is present in all mammalian cells, except those lacking mitochondria such as mature red blood cells. The TCA cycle oxidizes acetyl CoA derived from carbohydrates, fatty acids, amino acids, and ketone bodies, and produces NADH and $FADH_2$. In addition, the TCA cycle provides intermediates that are utilized for the formation of glucose, lipids, and amino acids. Thus, the TCA cycle is central for metabolism, and is regulated to meet a variety of cellular metabolic demands.

Le Hir and Dubach (160) assayed three TCA cycle enzymes—oxoglutarate dehydrogenase, citrate synthase, and isocitrate dehydrogenase—in dissected rat nephron segments. The activities of the enzymes were higher in distal segments (TAL and DCT) than in the PT. The distal versus proximal ratios of activities were about 1.5, 2.5, and 2 for oxoglutarate dehydrogenase, citrate synthase, and isocitrate dehydrogenase, respectively. Oxoglutarate dehydrogenase showed the lowest activity along entire nephron segments and appeared to catalyze the rate-limiting step of the TCA cycle. Marver and Schwartz (181) determined citrate synthase levels in isolated rabbit nephron segments. The order of relative citrate synthase activities in normal rabbit nephron segments (per kilogram of dry tissue) was as follows: DCT > PCT > CTAL > CCD > PST. The activity in CCD was regulated by aldosterone.

β-OXIDATION OF FATTY ACIDS

Fatty acid is a major energy fuel in the kidney. β-oxidation of short-, medium- and long-chain fatty acids occurs in mitochondria, and that of very long–chain fatty acids in peroxisomes. The 3-hydroxyacyl-CoA dehydrogenase activity, which represents mainly the mitochondrial β-oxidation pathway, is similarly distributed in all cortical proximal and distal segments and is much lower in glomeruli and collecting ducts (Fig. 8). The peroxisomal

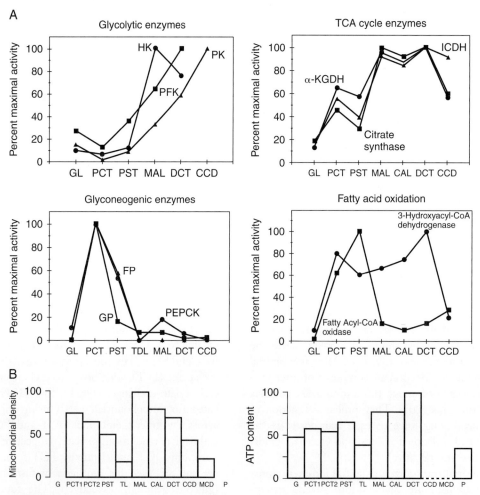

FIGURE 8   A. Distribution of enzymes involved in four major metabolic pathways: (1) TCA cycle, (2) β-oxidation of fatty acids, (3) glycolysis, and (4) gluconeogenesis. (Adapted with permission from Gullans SR, Mandel LJ. Coupling of energy to transport in proximal and distal nephron. In: Seldin DW, Giebisch G, eds. *The Kidney: Physiology and Pathophysiology*. 3rd ed. New York: Raven Press, 2000:443–482.) B. Mitochondrial density distribution and ATP content along nephron segments. (Adapted with permission from Soltoff SP. ATP and the regulation of renal cell function. *Annu Rev Physiol* 1986;48:9–31.)

fatty acyl-CoA oxidase is restricted to the PT with a capacity comparable to that in liver cells (161).

KETONE BODY METABOLISM

The kidney, as well as the muscle and brain, utilizes ketone bodies as metabolic fuel, while the liver cells do not. Acetoacetate and β-hydroxybutyrate are converted to acetyl CoA in the mitochondrial matrix. In this process, three enzymes, that is, D-3-hydroxybutyrate dehydrogenase, 3-ketoacyl CoA transferase (3-oxoacid CoA-transferase), and acetoacetyl CoA thiorase, are involved.

Guder and co-workers (105) measured 3-oxoacid CoA-transferase and D-3-hydroxybutyrate dehydrogenase in mouse nephron. The activities of these enzymes were high in TAL and DCT, but decreased to nearly 20% in the CCD. In the PCT and PST, the 3-oxoacid CoA-transferase activity was almost equal, while the 3-hydroxybutyrate dehydrogenase activity was fivefold higher in PST than in PCT. In glomeruli and thin descending limbs of Henle's loop, the enzymatic activities were markedly low. These results indicate that 3-hydroxybutyrate and acetoacetate can be metabolized in all mouse nephron segments with different capacities. The enzymatic activities for ketone bodies oxidation mirror the distribution of mitochondria along the nephron segment.

GLYCOLYSIS

The role of glycolysis as a metabolic pathway is different among cells and the state of oxygen supply. In the kidney, glycolysis occurs primarily from glucose since the storage of glycogen is minimal (225). The hexokinase activity in single microdissected rabbit nephron segments was the lowest in the PCT, and increased along the nephron segments (Fig. 8). It was the highest activity in the CNT (273). The activities of phosphofructokinase and pyruvate kinase in the rat nephron were 10-fold higher in the distal nephron than in the proximal portion (226). Thus, the glycolytic activity in the kidney is mostly distributed along the distal part of the nephron. Lactate production from glucose with and without antimycin A was investigated in the rat nephron (10). PT produced no lactate, and the distal segments all produced lactate. Antimycin A, an inhibitor of mitochondrial oxidation, increased lactate production significantly in all of the distal segments. The increase was the largest in the MTAL (1400%) and cortical (798%) and outer medullary collecting ducts (357%). Increments were smaller in the CTAL (98%) and DCT (98%), and were the lowest in the IMCD (28%). Thus, anaerobic glycolysis is important, particularly in the distal segments of the nephron.

GLUCONEOGENESIS

The capacity of the kidney to conduct gluconeogenesis was demonstrated in 1963. Actually, the glucose synthesis rate of the kidney is higher than that of the liver when compared using the same tissue amount (154) (Fig. 8). The release of glucose by the kidney has been reported to account for ~20% of all glucose released into the circulation in postabsorptive healthy humans (187). Sustained hypoglycemia enhances the renal extraction of circulating precursors for gluconeogenesis, and stimulates renal glucose production, which may represent an important additional component of the body's defense mechanism against hypoglycemia in humans (43, 44).

Among the nephron segments, the PT is the only site where net glucose synthesis occurs (111, 174). The gluconeogenic enzyme PEPCK was exclusively found in the PT, and the PST exhibited 50% of the enzyme activity in the PCT (273). All other renal structures exhibited only a negligible PEPCK activity (273). Thus, the activities of glycolysis and gluconeogenesis are a mirror image. Meyer et al. (187) demonstrated that lactate is the most important precursor in renal gluconeogenesis, which exceeded the sum of renal gluconeogenesis from glycerol, glutamine, and alanine. Gluconeogenesis from these substrates accounts for ~90% of renal glucose release.

Kondou et al. (149) demonstrated that renal gluconeogenesis is stimulated by short-term ischemia (149). They suggested that such stimulating gluconeogenesis supplies an energy fuel for further regeneration in nephron segments other than the PT.

There are several studies indicating a reciprocal relationship between Na^+ transport and gluconeogenesis. When ouabain inhibited Na^+,K^+-ATPase, gluconeogenesis was stimulated (83, 109, 194). In contrast, the stimulation of Na^+,K^+-ATPase by nystatin- and monesin-inhibited gluconeogenesis (109, 275). Silva et al. (234, 235) suggested that under certain circumstances, gluconeogenesis competes with Na^+ reabsorption in an intact kidney.

METABOLIC PARAMETERS ALONG NEPHRON SEGMENTS

As described, aerobic and anaerobic metabolisms are different among the nephron segments. This difference is in accordance with the distribution of mitochondria along the nephron. Pfaller and colleagues (207, 208) investigated the density of mitochondrial volume (mitochondrial volume per unit volume of cytoplasm) by stereoscopic analysis, and demonstrated PCT (33%), PST (22%), thin limb (6%–8%), MTAL (44%), DCT (33%), CCD (20%), and MCD (10%) (Fig. 8).

Intracellular ATP contents in various nephron segments were measured by several investigators (10, 39, 267). Uchida and Endou (267) demonstrated that the cellular ATP content is largely dependent on the exogenous substrates available (Fig. 9). When appropriate exogenous substrates are present, the cellular ATP content is high in the PT, MTAL DT, and CCD, whereas it is low in glomerulus, CTAL, and MCD.

Preference of Metabolic Substrates in Nephron Segments

SUBSTRATE PREFERENCE ALONG NEPHRON SEGMENTS

Ever since Gyoergy et al. (112) identified metabolism differences between the renal cortex and medulla in 1928, numerous studies have identified various metabolic profiles along the nephron (Fig. 10A, B). In the previous section, the

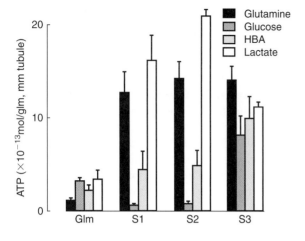

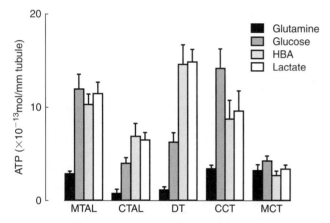

FIGURE 9   ATP content in nephron segments in the presence of several metabolic substrates. (Adapted with permission from Uchida S, Endou H. Substrate specificity to maintain cellular ATP along the mouse nephron. *Am J Physiol* 1988;255:F977–F983.)

activities of metabolic enzymes in the nephron were described. However, preferred substrates for each segment do not always correlate well with the distribution of specific enzymes. The substrate preference in a specific nephron segment depends on several factors other than enzymatic activities, such as the cellular uptake systems for substrates, oxygen supply, hormonal stimuli, and the demand for metabolic end products.

Knowledge of the preferred substrates for each segment has accumulated, especially from studies using microdissected nephrons. The determination of $^{14}CO_2$ production from distinct labeled substrates in conjunction with the effects of the substrate on cellular ATP level, QO2, redox state (NADH fluorescence), and active ion transports, provide evidence that a variety of metabolic fuels, such as lactate, glucose, pyruvate, fatty acids, ketone bodies, amino acids, and TCA cycle intermediates are involved in cellular metabolisms.

In this section, we briefly summarize the data on the substrate preference in each nephron segment.

PROXIMAL TUBULE

Numerous studies examined the metabolic profiles of the PT, and consistently indicated that the PT metabolizes a variety of substrates, such as fatty acids, ketone bodies, lactate, pyruvate, glutamine, glutamate, and TCA cycle intermediates. One notable exception is glucose: the PT, especially the proximal convoluted tubule (PCT), poorly metabolizes glucose.

Glucose PT poorly metabolizes glucose, and there exists a difference in the utilization of glucose between PCT and the proximal straight tubule (PST). $^{14}CO_2$ production from glucose in the PT was low (148, 222, 283), and glucose was poorly converted to lactate under both aerobic and anaerobic conditions (10). Uchida and Endou (267) measured cellular ATP contents in mouse nephron segments in the presence of several exogenous substrates. When solely glucose was supplied to the PT, the cellular ATP content significantly decreased in the S1 and S2 segments, while it was sustained in the S3 segment (PST) (267). A study using rabbit PCT or PST suspensions demonstrated a similar metabolic profile for glucose: the addition of glucose to the rabbit PCT did not increase QO2, whereas adding it to the rabbit PST increased it by 57% (222). The differences in glucose utilization do not correlate with the distribution of glycolytic enzymes between the PCT and PST (106), suggesting that a metabolic regulation mechanism other than that by glycolytic enzymes may determine the ability of each segment to utilize glucose. It should be noted that the gluconeogenic activity is high in the PT.

Fatty Acids Short-chain fatty acids are important fuels in the PT. Balaban and Mandel (13) examined the effects of various short-chain fatty acids, carboxylic acids, and amino acids on NADH fluorescence and QO2 in the rabbit PT. The short-chain fatty acids (butyrate, valerate, and heptanoate) were the most effective in increasing NADH fluorescence and QO2, followed by the carboxylic acids and amino acids. Butyrate supported mitochondrial respiration to a greater degree than lactate, glucose, and alanine when the Na^+,K^+-ATPase activity was maximally stimulated by nystatin (115). Butyrate was also shown to enhance the volume regulation of the isolated nonperfused PST under hypoosmotic conditions by activating Na^+–Cl^- transport (218). Ruegg et al. (222) demonstrated that PT exhibits maximal QO2 and ATP content when incubated in culture medium with 2 mM of heptanoate. In contrast, palmitate oxidation occurs minimally in the PCT (148). Thus, short-chain fatty acids are one of the best substrates, especially when active sodium transport is stimulated.

TCA Cycle Intermediates The PCT demonstrated marked $^{14}CO_2$ production from labeled succinate, 2-oxoglutarate, glutamate, glutamine, and malate (approximately 10–45 pmoles/mm/hr) and moderate $^{14}CO_2$ production from citrate (approximately 3 pmoles/ml/hr) (148). Gullans et al. demonstrated that succinate stimulates gluconeogenesis, and the hyperpolarization of the plasma membrane potential, and promotes intracellular K^+ without altering Na^+,K^+-ATPase

A

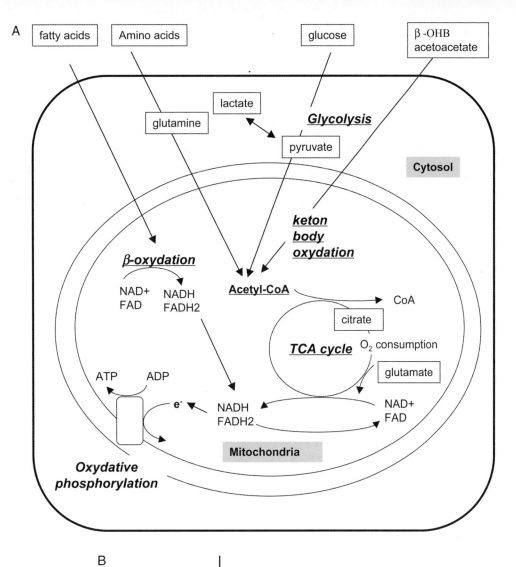

fatty acids | Amino acids | glucose | β -OHB acetoacetate

glutamine | lactate | **Glycolysis**

pyruvate

Cytosol

keton body oxydation

β-oxydation

NAD+ FAD → NADH FADH2

Acetyl-CoA → CoA

citrate

TCA cycle O₂ consumption

glutamate

ATP ADP

e⁻ NADH FADH2 ← NAD+ FAD

Oxydative phosphorylation

Mitochondria

B		Preferred substrates
PT	Lactate	Glutamine
	Glutamine	Pyruvate
	Citrate	Acetate
	Fatty acids	Ketone bodies
TAL	Glucose	Lactate
	Fatty acids	Ketone bodies
	Acetate	
DCT	Glucose	Lactate
	β-OHB	
CCD	Glucose	Lactate
	Pyruvate	Fatty acids
	β-OHB	
OMCD	Glucose	Lactate
	Glutamine	β-OHB
IMCD	Glucose	Lactate

FIGURE 10   A. Metabolic pathways and substrates used to fuel renal transport. Boxed substances are typical substrates used in nephron segments. B. Substrate preference of each nephron segment.

activity (110). Since TCA cycle intermediates are highly hydrophilic substances, cellular metabolisms of TCA cycle intermediates require specific transporters in the plasma membrane. The sodium-dicarboxylate cotransporters, NADCs encoded by the *SLC13* family, are expressed in both the luminal and basolateral membrane of the PT (178, 204, 229, 269).

Ketone Bodies Guder et al. (107) reported that ketone bodies, that is, acetoacetate and β-hydroxybutyrate, are presumably the most preferred substrate as kidney fuel. In a study using kidney slices (283), acetoacetate was estimated to support up to 80% of renal energy demands. β-hydroxybutyrate supported ATP levels to the same extent as lactate and glutamine in isolated mouse S3, while S1 and S2 had a low capacity to metabolize β-hydroxybutyrate. These results correlate with the high enzyme activities for ketone bodies such as 3-hydroxybutylate dehydrogenase in this segment (111).

Lactate Lactate is also a preferred substrate for the PT. Goldstein et al. (95) investigated the extraction of substrates from the blood by the rat kidney in normal, acidotic, and diabetic ketoacidotic conditions, and demonstrated that lactate accounts for 78% of the total amount of substrates extracted in normal control rats. Exogenous lactate maintained the cellular ATP content in the mouse PT (267). However, Kline et al. (148) indicated that a negligible amount of $^{14}CO_2$ was released from the labeled lactate as well as glucose in the rat PCT.

Thus, the proximal tubule metabolizes a wide range of substrates. This seems to be, at least in part, due to the existence of cellular transport systems for various substrates in the PT. PT cells possess Na-dependent transport systems for most of the nutrients across the luminal membrane. There exist also nutrient transporters in the basolateral membrane of the PT. Recent molecular studies have revealed the exclusive distribution of these transporters in the PT.

In the rat PT, preferred substrates are ketone bodies, short-chain fatty acids, lactate, and TCA cycle intermediates. However, there exist species differences: the rabbit PT has a limited capacity to oxidize ketone bodies (13).

The PT normally conducts transport work at 50%–60% of its maximal respiratory capacity, and has significant amounts of endogenous fuels, probably neutral lipids, which support about half of the energy in the absence of exogenous substrates. Metabolism of endogenous fuel is suppressed when there is an adequate supply of exogenous substrates. The preferred substrates differ under various physiological conditions (95).

THIN DESCENDING LIMB OF LOOP OF HENLE

The data available regarding the metabolic profile of the thin descending limb (TDL) is insufficient. The mitochondrial density of this segment is low, and its oxidative metabolism is limited. Jung and Endou (134) measured the cellular ATP content in the rat short loop of TDL (SDL) and the rat long loop of TDL (LDL) in the presence of alanine, glucose, glutamine, β-HBA, lactate, and pyruvate. They demonstrated that the substrate preference in SDL is pyruvate = glucose > glutamine = lactate = β-HBA >

alanine, and that in the LDL is pyruvate = glucose = glutamine > alanine = β-HBA = lactate. They also demonstrated that ATP is depleted when the TDL is incubated in the absence of exogenous substrate, indicating a limited store of endogenous fuels in this segment.

CORTICAL THICK ASCENDING LIMB OF LOOP OF HENLE

In the TAL, the rate of Na^+ transport and QO_2 are high, and the mitochondria are enriched, suggesting active oxidative metabolism in this segment. Klein et al. (148) measured $^{14}CO_2$ production from ^{14}C-labeled substrates in the rat MTAL and CTAL. MTAL and CTAL oxidized glucose, 2-oxoglutarate, lactate, glutamate, and glutamine, but not malate, succinate, and citrate. Palmitate oxidation occurred in MTAL and CTAL (148). Lactate production from glucose in the rat nephron indicated that the distal segments produce a significant amount of lactate from glucose, and under anaerobic conditions (with antimycin A), lactate production increased significantly in all of the distal segments. The increase was the largest in the MTAL (1400%), CCD (798%), and OMCD (357%), whereas increments were smaller in CTAL (98%) and DCT (98%), and were the lowest in the IMCD (28%) (10). Thus, CTAL possesses modest anaerobic glycolysis capacity. The ATP content in the mouse CTAL is maintained in the presence of glucose, β-OHB, or lactate, but not with glutamine (267).

Wittner et al. (293) investigated substrate preference by measuring the short-circuit current (Isc) in the isolated rabbit CTAL perfused in vitro (293). Additionally, they examined the side—luminal or basolateral—that the substrates were taken up. Isc rapidly decreased to 50% after 3 minutes and to 27% after 10 minutes without any exogenous substrates, indicating that Na^+ transport is strictly related to the presence of substrates in CTAL segments (293). When substrates were added from the luminal side, only butyrate sustained Isc, while all other substrates tested (pyruvate, acetate, β-OHB, D-glucose, and L-lactate) showed a marked decrease in Isc. When the substrates were added from the basolateral side, D-glucose, D-mannose, butyrate, β-OHB, acetoacetate, L-lactate, acetate, and pyruvate sustained the Isc, but citrate, α-etoglutarate, succinate, glutamate, glutamine, propionate, caprylate, and oleate did not. This study clearly indicates that the cellular uptake system is an important determinant in the substrate metabolisms in the CTAL. In the CTAL, most substrates, except for butyrate, are taken up by basolateral nutrient transporters. In fact, cytochalasin B and phloretin—inhibitors of the facilitated glucose transporters (GLUTs)—inhibited sustaining the Isc by glucose (293).

Regarding fatty acids, the CTAL possesses mitochondrial β-oxidation activity (3-hydroxyacyl-CoA dehydrogenase) (161), and $^{14}CO_2$ is produced from palmitate (148), while oleate (C-18) does not sustain Isc in the CTAL (293). Taken together, glucose, lactate, pyruvate, ketone bodies, and fatty acids are the preferred exogenous substrates for the CTAL.

MEDULLARY THICK ASCENDING LIMB OF LOOP OF HENLE

Chamberlin and Mandel measured QO_2 in MATL suspensions (47). In the absence of exogenous substrates, the control QO_2 decreased only by 15%. Torikai et al. demonstrate a similar result in the rat MTAL (262). These results indicate that endogenous substrates support most of the energy required for the MTAL under normal conditions. However, nystatin-stimulated QO_2 was inhibited by 36% in the absence of exogenous substrates, indicating that the oxidation of endogenous substrates cannot meet ATP demand when Na^+ transport is fully stimulated. They also investigated the role of endogenous substrates in the MTAL. The inhibitors of fatty acid, carbohydrate, or amino acid metabolisms further inhibited QO_2, revealing that endogenous fatty acids, glycogen, and amino acids (or proteins) contribute to energy production in the MTAL. The addition of fatty acids or acetoacetate increased QO_2 in 10 mM of glucose, indicating that the MTAL oxidizes exogenous fatty acids and ketones in addition to glucose. In the MTAL, organic acids failed to enhance QO_2, possibly due to the absence of transport systems for organic acids. The rat MAL generated $^{14}CO_2$ from glucose, lactate, palmitate, glutamate, glutamine, and α-ketoglutarate. $^{14}CO_2$ from succinate, citrate, and malate was minimal. Glucose, β-hydroxybutyrate, and lactate maintained the intracellular ATP content, whereas the effect of glutamine on ATP content was partial (267). The tight coupling of Na transport and QO_2 was demonstrated in the MTAL. Furosemide inhibited oxygen consumption by 43% and ouabain inhibited it by 42% (46): 50% of the oxygen consumption of the MTAL cells is related to the transport of Na^+ and Cl^- (75).

In the MTAL, anaerobic glycolysis is also an important energy source (48). Ten minutes of anoxia led to only a 15% decrease in potassium content in the rabbit MTAL, and an anaerobic metabolism maintained 73% of cellular ATP during 10 minutes of anoxia. The exposure of anoxic tubules to iodoacetate produced a 57% decrease in the ATP level and a 33% decrease in potassium content. Lactate production was remarkably enhanced in the MTAL (1400%) under anaerobic conditions with antimycin A (10).

DISTAL CONVOLUTED TUBULE

Although studies have examined the metabolic and transport properties in DCT, such as the mitochondrial density, Na^+,K^+-ATPase activity and enzymatic activities, data regarding its substrate preference are limited. The ATP content of the DCT was maximal in the presence of β-OHB or lactate, and somewhat lower in the presence of glucose. Glutamine did not increase the ATP content in the DCT (267). The lactate production rates from glucose under aerobic conditions was comparable to that observed in the CTAL, whereas under anoxic conditions, the glycolytic lactate production rate was increased twofold as observed in CTAL (10). These results indicate that DCT utilizes both oxidative metabolisms and anaerobic glycolysis.

CORTICAL COLLECTING DUCT

Torikai (262) demonstrated that substrate deprivation for 30 minutes does not change the cellular ATP content in the rat CCD and OMCD. However, a marked decrease in the PT and the medullary TDL, and a slight decrease in CTAL and MTAL were observed, suggesting that CCD and OMCD possess sufficient amount of endogenous fuels (262). Hering-Smith et al. (120) demonstrated the dependence of CCD on oxidative metabolisms in the Na^+ reabsorption and bicarbonate transport in the rabbit CCD. There was no significant glycolysis, or a difference of substrate dependence of solute transport in the CCD. Na^+ reabsorption was optimally supported by a mixture of basolateral metabolic substrates (glucose, acetate, and fatty acid), whereas bicarbonate secretion was fully supported by either glucose or acetate. This result indicates that principal cells and intercalated cells differ not only in their morphology and function, but also in their metabolism. Alanine was not effective in the CCD. Nonaka and Stokes (201) examined the effects of substrates on Na^+ transport in the rabbit CCD, and concluded that the majority of the energetic support of Na^+ transport appears to come from an oxidative metabolism. Glucose supports transport better than the other substrates tested, and lactate, pyruvate, and some organic acids also provide near maximal support.

The CCD synthesized modest amounts of lactate from glucose under aerobic conditions, which increased eight times under anaerobic conditions (10). The addition of glucose, β-hydroxybutyrate, or lactate, but not glutamine, restored the cellular ATP content, and glucose was the best substrate in CCD for maintaining the ATP level (267). Natke (195) showed that the rabbit nonperfused CCD regulates the cellular volume against extracellular hypertonic solution when exogenous butyrate is available, although rat CCD possesses a relatively low enzymatic activity for β-oxidation.

OUTER MEDULLARY COLLECTING DUCT

The OMCD cells play an important role in the final acidification of the urine, which is mediated by apical H^+-ATPase (32). The OMCD has a relatively low QO_2, which is inhibited only by 8% by ouabain (297). Several studies indicated the importance of anaerobic glycolysis in this segment. The ATP content in the OMCD did not significantly change by the addition of antimycin A (262). Lactate production from glucose was significantly increased in the OMCD (357%) under anaerobic conditions (10). Under aerobic conditions, the ATP content was supported equally well by glucose, glutamine, lactate, or β-hydroxybutyrate. Thus, glucose appears to be a preferred substrate for this segment, particularly under hypoxic of anoxic conditions, but other alternative substrates, such as glutamine, lactate, or β-hydroxybutyrate, can be metabolized under aerobic conditions. The uptake of glucose by the OMCD as well as that by the TAL cells, is mainly through facilitated basolateral diffusion (277). Studies on H^+ transport (298) and ATP contents (267) also indicated the existence of a significant amount of endogenous fuel, most likely glycogen in OMCD.

INNER MEDULLARY COLLECTING DUCT

Substrate metabolism in the inner medullary collecting duct (IMCD) cells has not been sufficiently analyzed. QO_2 in IMCD is lower than those in other nephron segments (104, 248, 299). The glycolysis under aerobic and anaerobic condition was investigated by several researchers. Addition of glucose to IMCD cells stimulates both QO_2 and lactate production, indicating that glucose can be readily metabolized to both CO_2 and lactate under aerobic conditions (10, 104, 150, 248). Lactate production in the IMCD under aerobic conditions was three- to fivefold greater than that in other nephron segments in the outer medulla, such as the TAL or OMCD (10).

To evaluate the relative contributions of aerobic and anaerobic metabolisms in the IMCD, the effects of specific inhibitors of mitochondrial oxidative phosphorylation and glycolysis were examined. Stokes et al. (248) examined metabolism in rat renal papillary collecting duct cells, that is, IMCD cells. In the presence of rotenone, glycolysis increased by 56% and maintained the cellular ATP level at 65% of the control. Without any exogenous substrates, IMCD respired normally and had a nearly normal ATP content, but lactate production was markedly decreased. At normal PO_2 and in the presence of D-glucose, the IMCD cells showed a substantial amount of aerobic glycolysis, although their mitochondrial respiration was not rate limiting. In the absence of glucose, the cells acquired the majority of their energy from an endogenous substrate (248). Kone and coworkers (150) showed that the addition of glucose to IMCD cells results in the accumulation of 12% more intracellular K^+ even in the presence of lactate and glutamine. The data indicate that glucose is a preferred substrate in IMCD.

COUPLING OF TRANSPORT AND METABOLISM

As described in the first section, Na transport and QO_2 show a linear relationship in the kidney. The nature of the cellular mechanism linking active transport to energy production is a fundamental physiological question. Alterations in the rate of active transport cause changes in the mitochondrial state and/or concentrations of adenine nucleotides in epithelia (175). Conversely, the cellular respiration rate and/or ATP concentration affects active transport. This chapter focuses on the coupling mechanism of transport and energy production in the kidney.

The Effect of Active Transport on Metabolism

WHITTAM MODEL: INTRACELLULAR SIGNALING BETWEEN TRANSPORT AND ENERGY PRODUCTION

Whittam and coworkers primarily proposed a simple model indicating the coupling of active transport and mitochondrial respiration (23, 290) (Fig. 11). In this model, active cation transport is a pacemaker for cellular respiration in

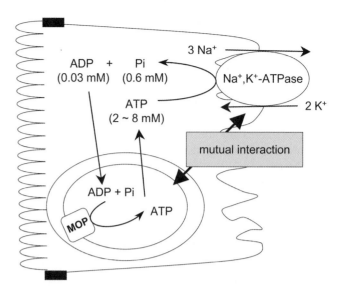

FIGURE 11 Schematic representation of Whittam model. MOP, mitochondrial oxidative phosphorylation.

the renal cells: increased ATP hydrolysis and elevated cytosolic levels of ADP and Pi by Na^+,K^+-ATPase activity would activate mitochondrial oxidative phosphorylation and oxygen consumption. Conversely, decreased Na^+,K^+-ATPase activity would induce the opposite result.

The validity of this model has been examined by (1) direct measurement of ATP, ADP, Pi, and/or (2) monitoring of the mitochondrial redox state in various states of transport. Early investigations on the intracellular nucleotide concentration failed to detect change in the intracellular ATP levels (215, 271). This was probably due to rapid ATP turnover in the renal cortex; the half-life of ATP in the anoxic state was estimated to be as low as 3.3 seconds (196). Balaban et al. (12) measured the cellular ATP/ADP concentrations and the QO_2 of a rabbit cortical tubule suspension under ideally designed conditions. They demonstrated that (1) ouabain caused a 54% inhibition of QO_2 and a 30% increase in the ATP/ADP ratio, and (2) the addition of K^+ (5 mM) to K^+-depleted tubules caused an initial 127% stimulation of QO_2 followed by a new steady-state QO_2 50% above the control, and a 47% decrease in the cellular ATP/ADP ratio.

The monitoring of the redox state by optical measurements also demonstrated appropriate "mitochondrial state of transition." Stimulation of Na^+,K^+-ATPase activity stimulated QO_2 and decreased NADH fluorescence (in whole kidney and proximal tubules). Inhibition of Na^+,K^+-ATPase with ouabain decreased QO_2 and increased NADH. Addition of rotenone to proximal tubules decreased QO_2, ATP content and net fluid transport with increase of NADH fluorescence (12).

REGULATION OF MITOCHONDRIAL RESPIRATION

The precise mechanisms by which the rate of mitochondrial oxidative phosphorylation is regulated are of a major interest in the field. There is much evidence suggesting the importance of cytosolic ADP concentration. Chance and Williams first proposed that the availability of ADP determines the mitochondrial respiration rate (49, 127, 158). The respiratory state of mitochondria was classified into five states according to the supply of ADP, Pi, substrates, and O_2 (49, 175). The addition of ADP to the mitochondria with a sufficient amount of substrates and O_2 induces the maximal rate of respiration called *state 3 (active)* respiration. When all of the ADP is phosphorylated to ATP, QO_2 and ATP production decrease (the phase called "state 4 resting" respiration). The ratio of QO_2 in state 3 and state 4 is called the *respiratory control index*. This change in respiration was also demonstrated in proximal tubules permeabilized to ADP by digitonin, in which QO_2 was stimulated four- to five-fold by the addition of ADP (114). Nevertheless, the predominant parameter (e.g., only [ADP] itself, [ATP]/[ADP] ratio, or [ATP]/[ADP][Pi] ratio) should be determined by further studies using mitochondria, and two conflicting hypotheses on mitochondrial phosphorylation have been proposed.

The first hypothesis indicated that the [ATP]/[ADP] ratio is the rate-limiting step in oxidative phosphorylation (240). This hypothesis is founded on kinetic considerations of adenine nucleotide translocase. Addition of atractyloside, an inhibitor of ATP/ADP translocase, caused inhibition of ADP influx into the mitochondrial matrix and oxidative respiration (163). However, the data from intact tissues with high oxidative phosphorylation capacities, that is, heart, brain, and kidney, indicated that the cytosolic concentration of ADP and Pi do not change significantly with work (14).

The second hypothesis, called the *near-equilibrium theory*, stated that oxidative phosphorylation is dependent on phosphorylation potential (73, 74). This hypothesis suggested that oxidative phosphorylation is regulated thermodynamically by four factors: (1) [ATP]/[ADP][Pi] ratio, (2) intramitochondrial [NAD$^+$]/[NADH] ratio, (3) respiratory chain components, especially cytochrome c oxidase, and (4) oxygen concentration. This theory was partially correct; however, oxidative phosphorylation is not always close to equilibrium, at least in isolated mitochondria (33).

Furthermore, both of these hypotheses should be reevaluated by determination of the cytosolic concentration of ATP, ADP, and Pi by nuclear magnetic resonance (NMR) spectroscopy. In NMR spectroscopy, the radiofrequency signal of specific molecules (P, N, C, and H) in a strong magnetic field can be recorded and quantified. There are particular features of this technology that can be applied to the measurement of biological events as follows: (1) the ability to define the chemical nature of phosphorus-containing molecules and follow their transition in time, (2) completely nondestructive and repeated determination is possible, (3) rapid determination over a few seconds, and (4) wide application from isolated mitochondria to intact kidney in vivo (81, 294). Freeman et al. (82) quantified inorganic phosphate (Pi) and high-energy phosphates in the isolated, functioning perfused rat kidney. Compared

with enzymatic analysis, 100% of ATP, but only 25% of ADP and 27% of Pi were visible by NMR spectroscopy (82), indicating that a large proportion of both ADP and Pi are bound to proteins in the intact kidney. The data obtained by NMR spectroscopy along with biochemical assays estimated the free concentration of cytosolic ADP as approximately 30 μM (82, 274) and Pi as 0.6 mM (82). As a consequence, the [ATP]/[ADP][Pi] ratio (phosphorylation potential) and [ATP]/[ADP] ratio should be at least one order of magnitude higher than previously estimated values.

There are several other theories on the regulation of mitochondrial respiration. One claimed that the interplay of all aspects of oxidative phosphorylation affects respiration control (28). Another new hypothesis implies the regulation of respiration and ATP synthesis via allosteric modification of respiratory chain complexes, in particular of cytochrome c oxidase via metabolites, cofactors, ions, hormones, and membrane potential (136, 137). At the moment, there seems no simple answer to the question "What controls respiration." The answer varies with (1) size of the system examined (mitochondria, cells, or organs), (2) conditions (rate of ATP use, level of hormonal stimulation), and (3) the particular organ examined (33).

Effect of Metabolism on Active Transport

INTRACELLULAR ATP AND CATION TRANSPORT

The intracellular ATP content was reported 2~8 mM (7, 12, 209, 227, 244, 270), and the Km value of α-subunits for ATP was estimated at 0.1–0.4 mM (54) (Fig. 12). Therefore, Na$^+$,K$^+$-ATPase should be saturated for ATP under physiological conditions. However, intact renal cells normally function at almost half of their maximal respiratory capacity (176). Harris et al. (115) measured cellular QO_2 during stimulation and inhibition of the Na$^+$,K$^+$-ATPase in mitochondria released from rabbit renal tubules by digitonin shock. In the presence of NADH-linked substrates and fats, isolated renal cells respired at 50%–60% of the maximum occurring in state 3 respiration, and addition of ouabain resulted in a decline in respiration to 25%–30%. Stimulation of the Na$^+$,K$^+$-ATPase by nystatin resulted in increased respiration with increased oxygen consumption (115). Gullans et al. (108) demonstrated that partial inhibition of oxidative metabolism with rotenone caused proportional reduction in QO_2, ATP content, and absorption rates of fluid and phosphate (108). The effect of inhibition of oxidative metabolism on transport systems was also demonstrated using arsenate, which uncouples oxidative phosphorylation (29).

This inconsistency was explained in a study by Soltoff and Mandel (244). In the membrane fraction of the PT, Na$^+$,K$^+$-ATPase hydrolytic activity showed saturated kinetics with a Km value of 0.4 mM for ATP. In contrast, Na$^+$,K$^+$-ATPase activity was demonstrated to have a linear, nonsaturating dependence on the ATP concentration in the

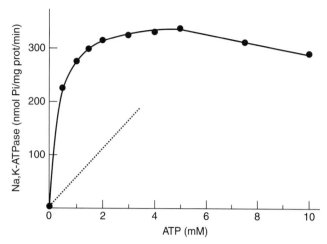

FIGURE 12   Dependence of Na$^+$,K$^+$ ATPase activity of proximal tubule membranes (solid line) and that of intact proximal tubules (dashed line) on ATP concentration. (Adapted with permission from Uchida S, Endou H. Substrate specificity to maintain cellular ATP along the mouse nephron. *Am J Physiol* 1988;255:F977–F983.)

intact proximal cells (Fig. 12) (244). The authors speculated that unknown cytosolic factors in the intact renal cell, such as local concentration of ADP, Pi, and Mg in the vicinity of Na$^+$,K$^+$-ATPase may be different, which might account for the discrepancy between the two measurements. In contrast to Na$^+$,K$^+$-ATPase, decreased concentration of cytosolic ATP does not significantly alter the Ca^{2+}-ATPase activity, probably due to its relatively high affinity for ATP (96).

Other Factors Linking Transport and Cellular Metabolism

ATP-SENSITIVE CATION CHANNELS

ATP-sensitive K$^+$ channels (K$^+$-ATP channels), the activity of which are inhibited by micromolar to millimolar concentrations of ATP, contribute to the potassium balance by coupling cellular metabolism with K$^+$ transport (118, 190, 282). Tsuchiya of the Welling laboratory identified K$^+$-ATP channel activity at the basolateral membrane in the PT, which is a major determinant of macroscopic K conductance (264). The open probability of the K$^+$-ATP channel determined by intracellular ATP concentration altered the extent of K recycling: A decrease in intracellular ATP by stimulation of Na$^+$,K$^+$-ATPase activity increased macroscopic K conductance, and intracellular ATP loading uncoupled the response. Wang and Giebisch (281) demonstrated the effect of ATP on the small-conductance potassium channel in the CCD apical membrane using the patch-clamp technique (281). A dual effect of ATP was observed: Low concentrations of ATP (0.05–0.1 mM) restored channel activity in the presence of cAMP-dependent PKA, while high concentrations of ATP (1 mM) and ADP (1.2 mM) blocked it completely. The dual effect of ATP was explained by assuming (1) ATP-dependent PKA-mediated phosphorylation of the potassium channel under physiological conditions, and

(2) direct inhibitory action of high concentrations of ATP on the channel activity. ATP-sensitive K$^+$ channels, the open probability of which was downregulated by ATP concentrations greater than 0.1 mmol/L, were also identified in the TAL (22). These studies indicate that ATP acts as a coupling modulator between cellular metabolism and K$^+$-ATP channel activity and regulates the transepithelial transport of K$^+$. Tsuboi and coworkers (263) investigated the molecular effect of ATP on a Kir6.2, a K$^+$-ATP channel. ATP inhibits the channel activity by binding to a specific site formed by the N- and C-termini of the pore-forming subunit. The structural changes associated with the interaction of ATP with Kir6.2 follow: (1) the interaction between the N- and C-terminal domains was altered, (2) both intrasubunit and intersubunit interactions were probably involved, (3) ligand binding and not channel gating was affected, and (4) these effects occurred in intact cells when subplasmalemmal ATP concentrations change in the millimolar range (263).

The regulation of cation transport by intracellular ATP was also identified in a stretch-activated nonselective cation channel in the basolateral membrane of the PT (124). This cation channel is primarily regulated by stretching (membrane deformation), depolarization, and hypotonic swelling. In addition, intracellular ATP reversibly blocks this cation channel (Ki ∼0.48 mM). Thus, this cation channel activity is coupled to the metabolic state of the cell, particularly when intracellular ATP is depleted, as occurs during increased transepithelial transport or ischemia.

PURINERGIC RECEPTORS

ATP and its metabolites, ADP, UTP, and UDP, act as extracellular signaling molecules via purinergic P2 receptors (162, 214, 268). ATP is readily released from epithelial cells across their luminal membrane when the cells are damaged by ischemia or toxic effects of exogenous compounds. ATP released from the cells is metabolized by ecto-nucleotidases, and thereby acts on the epithelial cells as paracrine and autocrine regulators. Mammalian P2 receptors are subdivided into P2Y (G-protein–coupled) and P2X (ligand-gated) channels. In the kidneys, P2 receptors are expressed both in the basolateral and luminal membranes, and induce a variety of biological effects. In the distal nephron, luminal nucleotides inhibit Ca^{2+} and Na$^+$ absorption and K$^+$ secretion via the P2Y$_2$ receptor. In steroid-sensitive cells, luminal ATP/UTP inhibits epithelial Na$^+$ channel–mediated Na$^+$ absorption. Adenosine generated by ecto-nucleotidases may introduce further effects on ion transport, often opposite of those caused by ATP. Bailey (11) demonstrated that activation of the P2Y$_1$ receptor impairs acidification in the PT through inhibiting the reabsorption of bicarbonate (11). In addition to having effects on solute transport, P2 receptors also modulate cellular metabolism. Cha and Endou (45) demonstrated that renal gluconeogenesis was increased via P2Y stimulation. The suggested functions of luminal P2 receptors include (1) an epithelial "secretory" defense, (2) the regulation of cell volume when transcellular solute transport is out of balance, and (3) autocrine/paracrine regulators mediating cellular protection and regeneration after ischemic cell damage (162).

Nephrons are also equipped with adenosine/P1 receptors, which have been further subdivided into four subtypes—A1, A2A, A2B, and A3—all of which couple to G proteins (214). Adenosine is produced by biochemical reactions, and by the extracellular cAMP-adenosine pathway, in which cAMP effluxed from cells is converted to adenosine by the serial actions of ecto-phosphodiesterase and ecto-5′-nucleotidase (126). Adenosine modulates Na^+,K^+-ATPase via A1 and A2 adenosine receptors (288).

NITRIC OXIDE

In the kidney, nitric oxide (NO) participates in several regulatory processes, including those for the glomerular and medullary hemodynamics, tubuloglomerular feedback, renin release, and extracellular fluid volume (151, 202). NO is formed from L-arginine by NO synthases (NOSs), a family of related enzymes encoded by separate unlinked genes. Three isoforms of NOS—that is, nNOS (or NOS I), eNOS (or NOS III), and iNOS (or NOS III)—were shown to be expressed in the kidney with distinct localization (151, 258). NO affects transporters and channels, such as Na^+,K^+-ATPase, NHE3, NKCC2, H^+-ATPase, and K^+-channels, in a segment-specific manner (202). For example, NO inhibited Na^+,K^+-ATPase in PT cells, while it did not change Na^+,K^+-ATPase activity in the TAL and CCD (202). NO also affects mitochondrial QO_2. Granger and Lehninger initially observed an inhibition of mitochondrial electron transport in a murine cell line exposed to endotoxin-stimulated macrophages (100), and subsequently NO was suggested to mediate this phenomenon (250). NO inhibits QO_2 (231), and conversely nitro-L-arginine, a NO synthesis inhibitor, increases QO_2 (230). The inhibitory effect of NO on QO_2 appears to occur reversibly through the direct inhibition of the mitochondrial electron transport chain (34, 35). Adler et al. (2) investigated the effects of renal NO production on QO_2 using eNOS knockout (KO) mice (2). Basal QO_2 in the renal cortex was higher in eNOS KO mice than in the heterozygous control mice. NO production stimulated by bradykinin or ramiprilat decreased QO_2 to a lesser extent in eNOS KO mice than the control mice. These results indicate that NO production via eNOS regulates renal QO_2. Laycock and colleagues (159) indicated that NO plays a role in maintaining a balance between QO_2 and sodium reabsorption in the dog (159). The administration of nitro-L-arginine decreased sodium reabsorption and increased renal QO_2.

BOLD MRI

Recently, a technique called the blood oxygen level–dependent (BOLD) MRI method has been applied to renal physiology. The BOLD MRI method measures blood deoxyhemoglobin and indirectly estimates intrarenal oxygenation in a noninvasive fashion, allowing sequential measurements in humans as well as animals in response to a variety of physiological or pharmacological stimuli, with high reproducibility (165, 212). The effects of diuretics on renal oxygenation were investigated using the BOLD method. Furosemide, but not acetazolamide, increased medullary oxygenation by inhibiting active transport and QO_2 in the MTAL, consistent with their separate sites of action in the nephron (211). The effect of furosemide on medullary oxygenation was absent or slight in an elderly human population (72). Moreover, the BOLD method was applied to changes in intrarenal oxygenation in a variety of pathophysiological states, such as an acute reduction in RBF (132), the diabetic state (216), and the administration of NO synthase inhibitor (164). BOLD contrast imaging appears to predict the tissue at risk from ischemia by revealing information on the balance between tubular workload and delivery of oxygen (216). Refined methods with improved visualization and more precise quantification have been developed (303).

PATHOPHYSIOLOGICAL STATES IN ENERGY PRODUCTION

Pathophysiological states, in which energy production is inhibited, lead to significant alterations in renal function. In this final section, we focus on these pathophysiological states.

Mitochondrial Cytopathies

Mitochondrial cytopathies are metabolic diseases caused by mutations in nuclear DNA or mitochondrial DNA encoding the proteins involved in the mitochondrial oxidative chain. These genetic lesions alter mitochondrial oxidative phosphorylation, with a reduction in energy produced for cell activity (37). The manifestation of mitochondrial cytopathies occurs in tissues where the energy requirement is high, such as skeletal muscle and the brain. Given the high energy utilization in the kidney, it is not surprising that mitochondrial cytopathies cause dysfunction of renal transport, and various renal involvements in mitochondrial diseases have been reported.

In most cases of Fanconi syndrome, a generalized dysfunction of proximal tubular cells results in glucosuria, aminoaciduria, and phosphaturia (157, 192, 198, 199, 221, 280). In patients manifesting Fanconi syndrome, defects in complex IV (CCO) activities are most commonly detected (198). Bartter syndrome (97), acute renal failure (123), chronic renal failure (295), and chronic tubulointerstitial nephritis (220, 252) were also reported. The renal tubule in patients with mitochondrial disease may be susceptible to renal hypoxic injury and acute renal failure. In the renal tissues of patients with mitochondrial cytopathies, giant and degenerated mitochondria are observed by electron microscopy (93, 302). Glomerular involvement was occasionally reported (50, 61, 128, 155, 192, 223).

Renal Ischemia

Ischemia-induced renal dysfunction involves multifactorial events, and there are two effects regarding tubular damage due to ischemia: effects that occur during ischemia, and the other is those occurring during reperfusion (reoxygenation), although these two factors are not always separable (59). If the ischemic damage is severe, tubular cells undergo necrosis and/or apoptosis.

Necrosis is characterized by the progressive loss of cytoplasmic membrane integrity, rapid influx of Na^+, Ca^{2+}, and water due to the disturbance of several ATP-dependent ion channels, which results in cytoplasmic swelling, disruption of the actin cytoskeleton, nuclear pyknosis, and eventual collapse of the cells (17, 203). Necrosis is considered to be mediated by ATP depletion (169), redistribution of Na^+,K^+-ATPase (193), increase in free cytosolic Ca^{2+} (70), reactive oxygen species generation (259), and activation of several enzymes, such as proteases, phospholipases, and endonucleases. Apoptosis is a highly coordinated process mediated by active intrinsic mechanism or extrinsic factors (203).

Both apoptosis and necrosis occur simultaneously in acute renal failure (ARF) (55), and the relative contribution of the two mechanisms depends on the severity of the injury and the cell type (166). Lieberthal et al. investigated the effect of graded ATP depletion ranging from 2% to 70% of control levels induced by either antimycin or 2-deoxyglucose in mouse PT cells (168). The cells subjected to ATP depletion of less than 15% of the control level developed necrosis uniformly. In contrast, the cells subjected to ATP depletion of 25% to 70% of control levels developed apoptosis. A narrow range of ATP depletion exists (15%–25% of control level), representing a threshold that determines whether cells die by necrosis or apoptosis. The degree of cellular GTP depletion also plays a crucial role in determining the mode of cell death (167).

ATP Depletion During Acute Ischemia and Its Consequence

After 1 minute of ischemia, whole kidney ATP content decrease by 70% (119), and during 10 minutes, renal ischemia ATP levels fall quickly to less than 10% of control values (233). During ischemia, tubular cells should maintain ATP content by anaerobic metabolisms, and vulnerability of each nephron segment depends partly on the glycolytic properties. The S3 (PST) segment of the PT is extremely susceptible to ischemic injury, because of its low glycolytic capacity, and severe ATP depletion leads to necrotic cell death in this segment. In the rabbit PT, hypoxia (1% O_2) induced lactate production, whereas anoxia (0% O_2) failed to stimulate glycolysis. The addition of ouabain during rotenone treatment reduced lactate production by 50%, indicating that glycolytic ATP can be used to fuel the Na^+,K^+-ATPase when mitochondrial ATP production is inhibited. In addition, this study suggested that mitochondrial inhibition is not obligatorily linked to the activation of glycolysis (60).

Weinberg and colleagues investigated anaerobic metabolism other than glycolysis in the PT during ischemia (285, 286). A severe mitochondrial energy deficit in the PT subjected to hypoxia/reoxygenation was prevented and reversed by supplementation with α-ketoglutarate (α-KG) and aspartate. The anaerobic metabolism of α-KG and aspartate generated ATP, and maintained the mitochondrial membrane potential. Malate and fumarate were also effective singly or in combination with α-KG, while succinate showed a protective effect only during reoxygenation. In other studies, Weinberg and coworkers further demonstrated that the events upstream of complex I are important for the energetic deficit in the PT during hypoxia (77).

The TAL possesses a relatively greater glycolytic capacity than the PT, and is less vulnerable to ischemic injury (24, 25). In a suspension of rabbit MTAL under anoxic conditions, anaerobic metabolism maintained 73% of cellular ATP during 10 minutes of anoxia, and exposure of anoxic tubules to iodoacetate, an inhibitor of glycolysis, resulted in a 57% decline in ATP levels, indicating that glycolysis is an important pathway in supplying energy during anaerobiosis in MTAL (48). Cellular damage of TAL by ischemia is influenced by cellular transport. The TAL develops a specific structural lesion during perfusion of the isolated rat kidney. The fraction of TAL showing severe damage was reduced by furosemide but not by acetazolamide, and the lesion was also eliminated by perfusion with ouabain or by preventing glomerular filtration (30).

Mitochondrial Injury During Reperfusion

It is known that cell death following ischemia-reperfusion is closely related to functional changes in the mitochondria. Liu et al. revealed that apoptotic programmed death is associated with the release of cytochrome c (cyt c) due to caspase (cysteinyl aspartate–specific proteinase) activity (170). Cyt c release is dependent on the site and the type of mitochondrial injury. Isolated mouse PT was subjected to mitochondrial oxidative phosphorylation inhibitors, rotenone and antimycin A, or hypoxia. Antimycin A caused a significantly higher level of cyt c release from the PT than rotenone or hypoxia (296). The efflux of cyt c and other apoptosis-related compounds, such as apoptosis-inducing factor (AIF) and pro-caspases-2, -3, and -9, is mediated by the disrupted mitochondrial membrane or MPT (mitochondrial permeability transition) (153). Although the precise molecular mechanism of MPT remains to be elucidated, MPT occurs by a multiprotein channel composed of a voltage-dependent anion channel (VDAC), which comprises a nonselective channel for any substances with a molecular mass less than 15 kDa (256), and adenine nucleotide translocase (ANT).

ATP depletion causes an increase in cellular free Ca^{2+} (184, 242, 284), and this phenomenon causes mitochondrial injury and apoptosis in renal tubular cells. Tanaka and colleagues demonstrated that voltage-dependent Ca^{2+} channels are involved in cellular and mitochondrial accumulation of Ca^{2+} due to ATP depletion (254).

CHRONIC ISCHEMIA

Accumulating evidence emphasizes the effects of chronic hypoxia on the renal structure and function (69). In the advanced stage of renal dysfunction with tubulointerstitial damage, peritubular capillaries are lost, and the development of interstitial fibrosis decreases oxygen diffusion to tubules. As a consequence, nephron segments are exposed to chronic hypoxia, and this in turn exacerbates renal insufficiency. Diffuse cortical hypoxia was demonstrated in the puromycin aminonucleoside-induced nephrotic syndrome and focal and segmental hypoxia in a remnant kidney model (253).

When cells are exposed to hypoxia, the activation of hypoxia-inducible factor-1 (HIF-1) occurs, which is a primary defensive mechanism against hypoxia (177, 183). HIF-1 transcriptionally regulates many factors associated with hypoxia, such as the increased expression of VDGF (19), erythropoietin (18), a glucose transporter (Glut-1) (68), and PGK (217); thus, chronic hypoxia alters the cellular transport and metabolism via HIF-1 activation. It is suggested that the induction of the HIF signal, which adapts the renal cells to hypoxia, may be a therapeutic option against the development of renal dysfunction.

Nephrotoxicants

Several nephrotoxic drugs, such as certain cephalosporins (266), tacrolimus and sirolimus (239), cadmium metallothionein (255), probenecid (182), prednisolone and azathioprine (238), and cyclosporine A (135), were shown to impair mitochondria and cellular metabolism. Ochratoxin A, a mycotoxin, also inhibits mitochondrial oxidative phosphorylation in the PT (133). In contrast, enalapril and losartan attenuate mitochondrial dysfunction (56).

CONCLUSIONS

Most of the energy produced in the kidney is primarily utilized for the active reabsorption of Na^+, which further drives the cellular and paracellular transport of water and solutes. Renal metabolism for energy production is regulated by transport activity, and conversely, transport is affected by cellular energy status. The intracellular adenine nucleotide level is an important regulatory factor for metabolism and transport; however, the interactions of these two processes are diverse and complex. Other regulators, such as ATP-sensitive cation channels, NO, and purinergic receptors, should be involved in these processes. Future studies are required to elucidate the fine regulatory mechanisms for renal transport and cellular metabolisms. Recent molecular information on renal solute transporters and metabolizing enzymes, in conjunction with novel methodologies, such as BOLD MRI, will provide progress in this field.

From pathophysiological viewpoints, the susceptibility of the kidney to ischemia and agents affecting energy production are critical clinical issues. The roles of acute ischemia and chronic ischemia in the kidney are currently considered to be novel research subjects.

Acknowledgment

The authors are grateful to Dr. Steven R. Gullans for his critical reading of this chapter.

References

1. Ackrell BA. Progress in understanding structure-function relationships in respiratory chain complex II. *FEBS Lett* 2000;466:1–5.
2. Adler S, Huang H, Loke KE, et al. Endothelial nitric oxide synthase plays an essential role in regulation of renal oxygen consumption by NO. *Am J Physiol Renal Physiol* 2001;280: F838–843.
3. Ahn KY, Madsen KM, Tisher CC, et al. Differential expression and cellular distribution of mRNAs encoding alpha- and beta-isoforms of Na(+)-K(+)-ATPase in rat kidney. *Am J Physiol* 1993;265:F792–F801.
4. Ahn KY, Kone BC. Expression and cellular localization of mRNA encoding the "gastric" isoform of H(+)-K(+)-ATPase alpha-subunit in rat kidney. *Am J Physiol* 1995;268: F99–109.
5. Ahn KY, Turner PB, Madsen KM, et al. Effects of chronic hypokalemia on renal expression of the "gastric" H(+)-K(+)-ATPase alpha-subunit gene. *Am J Physiol* 1996;270: F557–F566.
6. Ait-Mohamed AK, Marsy S, Barlet C, et al. Characterization of N-ethylmaleimide-sensitive proton pump in the rat kidney. Localization along the nephron. *J Biol Chem* 1986;261: 12526–12533.
7. Akerboom TP, Bookelman H, Tager JM. Control of ATP transport across the mitochondrial membrane in isolated rat-liver cells. *FEBS Lett* 1977;74:50–54.
8. Ambudkar SV, Kimchi-Sarfaty C, Sauna ZE, et al. P-glycoprotein: from genomics to mechanism. *Oncogene* 2003;22:7468–7485.
9. Andreoli TE, Schafer JA. Effective luminal hypotonicity: the driving force for isotonic proximal tubular fluid absorption. *Am J Physiol* 1979;236:F89–F96.
10. Bagnasco S, Good D, Balaban R, et al. Lactate production in isolated segments of the rat nephron. *Am J Physiol* 1985;248:F522–526.
11. Bailey MA. Inhibition of bicarbonate reabsorption in the rat proximal tubule by activation of luminal P2Y1 receptors. *Am J Physiol Renal Physiol* 2004;287:F789–F796.
12. Balaban RS, Mandel LJ, Soltoff SP, et al. Coupling of active ion transport and aerobic respiratory rate in isolated renal tubules. *Proc Natl Acad Sci U S A* 1980;77:447–451.
13. Balaban RS, Mandel LJ. Metabolic substrate utilization by rabbit proximal tubule. An NADH fluorescence study. *Am J Physiol* 1988;254:F407–F416.
14. Balaban RS. Regulation of oxidative phosphorylation in the mammalian cell. *Am J Physiol* 1990;258:C377–C389.
15. Bank N, Aynedjian HS, Mutz BF. Evidence for a DCCD-sensitive component of proximal bicarbonate reabsorption. *Am J Physiol* 1985;249:F636–F644.
16. Barlet-Bas C, Arystarkhova E, Cheval L, et al. Are there several isoforms of Na,K-ATPase alpha subunit in the rabbit kidney? *J Biol Chem* 1993;268:11512–11515.
17. Barros LF, Hermosilla T, Castro J. Necrotic volume increase and the early physiology of necrosis. *Comp Biochem Physiol A Mol Integr Physiol* 2001;130:401–409.
18. Bernaudin M, Marti HH, Roussel S, et al. A potential role for erythropoietin in focal permanent cerebral ischemia in mice. *J Cereb Blood Flow Metab* 1999;19:643–651.
19. Bernaudin M, Tang Y, Reilly M, et al. Brain genomic response following hypoxia and reoxygenation in the neonatal rat. Identification of genes that might contribute to hypoxia-induced ischemic tolerance. *J Biol Chem* 2002;277:39728–39738.
20. Berry EA, Guergova-Kuras M, Huang LS, et al. Structure and function of cytochrome bc complexes. *Annu Rev Biochem* 2000;69:1005–1075.
21. Blanco G, Mercer RW. Isozymes of the Na-K-ATPase: heterogeneity in structure, diversity in function. *Am J Physiol* 1998;275:F633–F650.
22. Bleich M, Schlatter E, Greger R. The luminal K^+ channel of the thick ascending limb of Henle's loop. *Pflügers Arch* 1990;415:449–460.
23. Blond DM, Whittam R. The regulation of kidney respiration by sodium and potassium ions. *Biochem J* 1964;92:158–167.
24. Bonventre JV. Mechanisms of ischemic acute renal failure. *Kidney Int* 1993;43:1160–1178.
25. Bonventre JV Weinberg JM. Recent advances in the pathophysiology of ischemic acute renal failure. *J Am Soc Nephrol* 2003;14:2199–2210.
26. Boyer PD. The ATP synthase—a splendid molecular machine. *Annu Rev Biochem* 1997;66:717–749.
27. Boyer PD. Toward an adequate scheme for the ATP synthase catalysis. *Biochemistry (Mosc)* 2001;66:1058–1066.
28. Brand MD, Murphy MP. Control of electron flux through the respiratory chain in mitochondria and cells. *Biol Rev Camb Philos Soc* 1987;62:141–193.
29. Brazy PC, Balaban RS, Gullans SR, et al. Inhibition of Renal Metabolism. Relative effects of arsenate on sodium, phosphate, and glucose transport by the rabbit proximal tubule. *J Clin Invest* 1980;66:1211–1221.
30. Brezis M, Rosen S, Silva P, et al. Transport activity modifies thick ascending limb damage in the isolated perfused kidney. *Kidney Int* 1984;25:65–72.
31. Bronner F. Renal calcium transport: mechanisms and regulation—an overview. *Am J Physiol* 1989;257:F707–F711.

32. Brown D, Hirsch S, Gluck S. Localization of a proton-pumping ATPase in rat kidney. *J Clin Invest* 1988;82:2114–2126.

33. Brown GC. Control of respiration and ATP synthesis in mammalian mitochondria and cells. *Biochem J* 1992;284(Pt 1):1–13.

34. Brown GC, Cooper CE. Nanomolar concentrations of nitric oxide reversibly inhibit synaptosomal respiration by competing with oxygen at cytochrome oxidase. *FEBS Lett* 1994;356: 295–298.

35. Brown GC. Nitric oxide regulates mitochondrial respiration and cell functions by inhibiting cytochrome oxidase. *FEBS Lett* 1995;369:136–139.

36. Brunette MG, Mailloux J, Chan M, et al. Characterization of the high and low affinity components of the renal Ca2(+)–Mg2+ ATPase. *Can J Physiol Pharmacol* 1990;68: 718–726.

37. Buemi M, Allegra A, Rotig A, et al. Renal failure from mitochondrial cytopathies. *Nephron* 1997;76:249–253.

38. Buffin-Meyer B, Verbavatz JM, Cheval L, et al. Regulation of Na+, K(+)-ATPase in the rat outer medullary collecting duct during potassium depletion. *J Am Soc Nephrol* 1998;9: 538–550.

39. Burch HB, Choi S, Dence CN, et al. Metabolic effects of large fructose loads in different parts of the rat nephron. *J Biol Chem* 1980;255:8239–8244.

40. Canfield VA, Okamoto CT, Chow D, et al. Cloning of the H,K-ATPase beta subunit. Tissue-specific expression, chromosomal assignment, and relationship to Na,K-ATPase beta subunits. *J Biol Chem* 1990;265:19978–19884.

41. Caride AJ, Chini EN, Homma S, et al. mRNA encoding four isoforms of the plasma membrane calcium pump and their variants in rat kidney and nephron segments. *J Lab Clin Med* 1998;132:149–156.

42. Caride AJ, Chini EN, Penniston JT, et al. Selective decrease of mRNAs encoding plasma membrane calcium pump isoforms 2 and 3 in rat kidney. *Kidney Int* 1999;56:1818–1825.

43. Cersosimo E, Garlick P, Ferretti J. Renal glucose production during insulin-induced hypoglycemia in humans. *Diabetes* 1999;48: 261–266.

44. Cersosimo E, Garlick P, Ferretti J. Renal substrate metabolism and gluconeogenesis during hypoglycemia in humans. *Diabetes* 2000; 49:1186–1193.

45. Cha SH, Jung KY, Endou H. Effect of P2Y-purinoceptor stimulation on renal gluconeogenesis in rats. *Biochem Biophys Res Commun* 1995;211:454–461.

46. Chamberlin ME, Le Furgey A, Mandel LJ. Suspension of medullary thick ascending limb tubules from the rabbit kidney. *Am J Physiol* 1984;247:F955–964.

47. Chamberlin ME, Mandel LJ. Substrate support of medullary thick ascending limb oxygen consumption. *Am J Physiol* 1986;251:F758–F763.

48. Chamberlin ME, Mandel LJ. Na+-K+-ATPase activity in medullary thick ascending limb during short-term anoxia. *Am J Physiol* 1987;252:F838–F843.

49. Chance B, Williams GR. The respiratory chain and oxidative phosphorylation. *Adv Enzymol Relat Subj Biochem* 1956;17:65–134.

50. Cheong HI, Chae JH, Kim JS, et al. Hereditary glomerulopathy associated with a mitochondrial tRNA(Leu) gene mutation. *Pediatr Nephrol* 1999;13:477–480.

51. Cheval L, Doucet A. Measurement of Na-K-ATPase-mediated rubidium influx in single segments of rat nephron. *Am J Physiol* 1990;259:F111–F121.

52. Cohen JJ, Kamm DE. *Renal Metabolism: Relation to Renal Function*. Philadelphia: Saunders, 1976.

53. Crowson MS, Shull GE. Isolation and characterization of a cDNA encoding the putative distal colon H+,K(+)-ATPase. Similarity of deduced amino acid sequence to gastric H+,K(+)-ATPase and Na+,K(+)-ATPase and mRNA expression in distal colon, kidney, and uterus. *J Biol Chem* 1992;267:13740–13748.

54. Daly SE, Lane LK, Blostein R. Functional consequences of amino-terminal diversity of the catalytic subunit of the Na,K-ATPase. *J Biol Chem* 1994;269:23944–23948.

55. De Broe ME. Apoptosis in acute renal failure. *Nephrol Dial Transplant* 2001;16(Suppl 6):23–26.

56. de Cavanagh EM, Piotrkowski B, Basso N, et al. Enalapril and losartan attenuate mitochondrial dysfunction in aged rats. *FASEB J* 2003;17:1096–1098.

57. Deetjen P. Measurement of metabolism during renal work. *Int J Biochem* 1980;12:243–244.

58. Dick IM, Liu J, Glendenning P, et al. Estrogen and androgen regulation of plasma membrane calcium pump activity in immortalized distal tubule kidney cells. *Mol Cell Endocrinol* 2003;212:11–18.

59. Dickman KG, Jacobs WR, Mandel LJ. Renal metabolism and acute renal failure. *Pediatr Nephrol* 1987;1:359–366.

60. Dickman KG, Mandel LJ. Differential effects of respiratory inhibitors on glycolysis in proximal tubules. *Am J Physiol* 1990;258:F1608–1615.

61. Doleris LM, Hill GS, Chedin P, et al. Focal segmental glomerulosclerosis associated with mitochondrial cytopathy. *Kidney Int* 2000;58:1851–1858.

62. Doucet A, Morel F, Katz AI. Microdetermination of Na-K-ATPase in single tubules: its application for the localization of physiologic processes in the nephron. *Int J Biochem* 1980;12:47–52.

63. Doucet A, Katz AI. High-affinity Ca-Mg-ATPase along the rabbit nephron. *Am J Physiol* 1982;242:F346–F352.

64. Doucet A, Hus-Citharel A, Morel F. In vitro stimulation of Na-K-ATPase in rat thick ascending limb by dexamethasone. *Am J Physiol* 1986;251:F851–F857.

65. Doucet A, Marsy S. Characterization of K-ATPase activity in distal nephron: stimulation by potassium depletion. *Am J Physiol* 1987;253:F418–F423.

66. Doucet A. Function and control of Na-K-ATPase in single nephron segments of the mammalian kidney. *Kidney Int* 1988;34:749–760.

67. Doucet A. H+, K(+)-ATPASE in the kidney: localization and function in the nephron. *Exp Nephrol* 1997;5:271–276.

68. Ebert BL, Firth JD, Ratcliffe PJ. Hypoxia and mitochondrial inhibitors regulate expression of glucose transporter-1 via distinct Cis-acting sequences. *J Biol Chem* 1995;270:29083–29089.

69. Eckardt KU, Rosenberger C, Jurgensen JS, et al. Role of hypoxia in the pathogenesis of renal disease. *Blood Purif* 2003;21:253–257.

70. Edelstein CL, Ling H, Schrier RW. The nature of renal cell injury. *Kidney Int* 1997;51: 1341–1351.

71. El Mernissi G, Doucet A. Quantitation of [3H]ouabain binding and turnover of Na-K-ATPase along the rabbit nephron. *Am J Physiol* 1984;247:F158–F167.

72. Epstein FH, Prasad P. Effects of furosemide on medullary oxygenation in younger and older subjects. *Kidney Int* 2000;57:2080–2083.

73. Erecinska M, Wilson DF, Nishiki K. Homeostatic regulation of cellular energy metabolism: experimental characterization in vivo and fit to a model. *Am J Physiol* 1978;234: C82–C89.

74. Erecinska M, Wilson DF. Regulation of cellular energy metabolism. *J Membr Biol* 1982;70: 1–14.

75. Eveloff J, Bayerdorffer E, Silva P, et al. Sodium-chloride transport in the thick ascending limb of Henle's loop. Oxygen consumption studies in isolated cells. *Pflügers Arch* 1981;389: 263–270.

76. Farman N, Corthesy-Theulaz I, Bonvalet JP, et al. Localization of alpha-isoforms of Na(+)-K(+)-ATPase in rat kidney by in situ hybridization. *Am J Physiol* 1991;260:C468–C474.

77. Feldkamp T, Kribben A, Roeser NF, et al. Preservation of complex I function during hypoxia-reoxygenation-induced mitochondrial injury in proximal tubules. *Am J Physiol Renal Physiol* 2004;286:F749–F759.

78. Feraille E, Doucet A. Sodium-potassium-adenosinetriphosphatase–dependent sodium transport in the kidney: hormonal control. *Physiol Rev* 2001;81:345–418.

79. Feraille E, Mordasini D, Gonin S, et al. Mechanism of control of Na,K-ATPase in principal cells of the mammalian collecting duct. *Ann N Y Acad Sci* 2003;986:570–578.

80. Forgac M. Structure, mechanism and regulation of the clathrin-coated vesicle and yeast vacuolar H(+)-ATPases. *J Exp Biol* 2000; 203:71–80.

81. Foxall PJ, Nicholson JK. Nuclear magnetic resonance spectroscopy: a non-invasive probe of kidney metabolism and function. *Exp Nephrol* 1998;6:409–414.

82. Freeman D, Bartlett S, Radda G, et al. Energetics of sodium transport in the kidney. Saturation transfer 31P-NMR. *Biochim Biophys Acta* 1983;762:325–336.

83. Friedrichs D, Schoner W. Stimulation of renal gluconeogenesis by inhibition of the sodium pump. *Biochim Biophys Acta* 1973;304:142–160.

84. Fromter E, Rumrich G, Ullrich KJ. Phenomenologic description of Na+, Cl− and HCO3− absorption from proximal tubules of rat kidney. *Pflügers Arch* 1973;343:189–220.

85. Garg LC, Knepper MA, Burg MB. Mineralocorticoid effects on Na-K-ATPase in individual nephron segments. *Am J Physiol* 1981;240:F536–F544.

86. Garg LC, Narang N. Stimulation of an N-ethylmaleimide-sensitive ATPase in the collecting duct segments of the rat nephron by metabolic acidosis. *Can J Physiol Pharmacol* 1985;63: 1291–1296.

87. Garg LC, Narang N. Effects of aldosterone on NEM-sensitive ATPase in rabbit nephron segments. *Kidney Int* 1988;34:13–17.

88. Garg LC, Narang N. Ouabain-insensitive K-adenosine triphosphatase in distal nephron segments of the rabbit. *J Clin Invest* 1988; 81:1204–1208.

89. Garg LC, Narang N. Decrease in N-ethylmaleimide-sensitive ATPase activity in collecting duct by metabolic alkalosis. *Can J Physiol Pharmacol* 1990;68:1119–1123.

90. Garg LC, Narang N. Changes in H-ATPase activity in the distal nephron segments of the rat during metabolic acidosis and alkalosis. *Contrib Nephrol* 1991;92:39–45.

91. Geering K. The functional role of beta subunits in oligomeric P-type ATPases. *J Bioenerg Biomembr* 2001;33:425–438.

92. Geering K, Beguin P, Garty H, et al. FXYD proteins: new tissue- and isoform-specific regulators of Na,K-ATPase. *Ann N Y Acad Sci* 2003;986:388–394.

93. Gilbert RD, Emms M. Pearson's syndrome presenting with Fanconi syndrome. *Ultrastruct Pathol* 1996;20:473–475.

94. Gluck SL, Underhill DM, Iyori M, et al. Physiology and biochemistry of the kidney vacuolar H+-ATPase. *Annu Rev Physiol* 1996; 58:427–445.

95. Goldstein L. Renal substrate utilization in normal and acidotic rats. *Am J Physiol* 1987;253: F351–357.

96. Goligorsky MS, Hruska KA. Hormonal modulation of cytoplasmic calcium concentration in renal tubular epithelium. *Miner Electrolyte Metab* 1988;14:58–70.

97. Goto Y, Itami N, Kajii N, et al. Renal tubular involvement mimicking Bartter syndrome in a patient with Kearns-Sayre syndrome. *J Pediatr* 1990;116:904–910.

98. Gottesman MM, Fojo T, Bates SE. Multidrug resistance in cancer: role of ATP-dependent transporters. *Nat Rev Cancer* 2002;2:48–58.

99. Gottschalk CW, Mylle M. Micropuncture study of the mammalian urinary concentrating mechanism: evidence for the countercurrent hypothesis. *Am J Physiol* 1959;196:927–936.

100. Granger DL, Lehninger AL. Sites of inhibition of mitochondrial electron transport in macrophage-injured neoplastic cells. *J Cell Biol* 1982;95:527–535.

101. Grigorieff N. Three-dimensional structure of bovine NADH:ubiquinone oxidoreductase (complex I) at 22 A in ice. *J Mol Biol* 1998; 277:1033–1046.

102. Gross E, Hawkins K, Pushkin A, et al. Phosphorylation of Ser(982) in the sodium bicarbonate cotransporter kNBC1 shifts the HCO(3)(−): Na(+) stoichiometry from 3:1 to 2:1 in murine proximal tubule cells. *J Physiol* 2001;537:659–665.

103. Gruber G. Introduction: A close look at the vacuolar ATPase. *J Bioenerg Biomembr* 2003; 35:277–280.

104. Grunewald RW, Kinne RK. Sugar transport in isolated rat kidney papillary collecting duct cells. *Pflügers Arch* 1988;413:32–37.

105. Guder WG, Purschel S, Wirthensohn G. Renal ketone body metabolism. Distribution of 3-oxoacid CoA-transferase and 3-hydroxybutyrate dehydrogenase along the mouse nephron. *Hoppe Seylers Z Physiol Chem* 1983;364:1727–1737.

106. Guder WG, Ross BD. Enzyme distribution along the nephron. *Kidney Int* 1984;26: 101–111.

107. Guder WG, Wagner S, Wirthensohn G. Metabolic fuels along the nephron: pathways and intracellular mechanisms of interaction. *Kidney Int* 1986;29:41–45.

108. Gullans SR, Brazy PC, Soltoff SP, et al. Metabolic inhibitors: effects on metabolism and transport in the proximal tubule. *Am J Physiol* 1982;243:F133–140.

109. Gullans SR, Brazy PC, Dennis VW, et al. Interactions between gluconeogenesis and sodium transport in rabbit proximal tubule. *Am J Physiol* 1984;246:F859–869.
110. Gullans SR, Harris SI, Mandel LJ. Glucose-dependent respiration in suspensions of rabbit cortical tubules. *J Membr Biol* 1984;78:257–262.
111. Gullans SR, Mandel LJ. Coupling of energy to transport in proximal and distal nephron. In: Seldin DW, Giebisch G, eds. *The Kidney: Physiology and Pathophysiology*. 3rd ed. New York: Raven Press, 2000:443–482.
112. Gyoergy P, Keller W, Brehme TH. Nierestoffwechsel und Nierenentwicklung. *Biochem Zeitschr* 1928;200:356–366.
113. Haimeur A, Conseil G, Deeley RG, et al. The MRP-related and BCRP/ABCG2 multidrug resistance proteins: biology, substrate specificity and regulation. *Curr Drug Metab* 2004;5: 21–53.
114. Harris SI, Balaban RS, Mandel LJ. Oxygen consumption and cellular ion transport: evidence for adenosine triphosphate to O2 ratio near 6 in intact cell. *Science* 1980;208: 1148–1150.
115. Harris SI, Balaban RS, Barrett L, et al. Mitochondrial respiratory capacity and Na^+- and K^+-dependent adenosine triphosphatase-mediated ion transport in the intact renal cell. *J Biol Chem* 1981;256:10319–10328.
116. Hatefi Y. The mitochondrial electron transport and oxidative phosphorylation system. *Annu Rev Biochem* 1985;54:1015–1069.
117. Hebert H, Purhonen P, Thomsen K, et al. Renal Na,K-ATPase structure from cryo-electron microscopy of two-dimensional crystals. *Ann N Y Acad Sci* 2003;986:9–16.
118. Hebert SC, Desir G, Giebisch G, et al. Molecular diversity and regulation of renal potassium channels. *Physiol Rev* 2005;85:319–371.
119. Hems DA, Brosnan JT. Effects of ischaemia on content of metabolites in rat liver and kidney in vivo. *Biochem J* 1970;120:105–111.
120. Hering-Smith KS, Hamm LL. Metabolic support of collecting duct transport. *Kidney Int* 1998;53:408–415.
121. Hildyard JC, Halestrap AP. Identification of the mitochondrial pyruvate carrier in Saccharomyces cerevisiae. *Biochem J* 2003;374:607–611.
122. Hrycyna CA, Ramachandra M, Ambudkar SV, et al. Mechanism of action of human P-glycoprotein ATPase activity. Photochemical cleavage during a catalytic transition state using orthovanadate reveals cross-talk between the two ATP sites. *J Biol Chem* 1998;273: 16631–16634.
123. Hsieh F, Gohh R, Dworkin L. Acute renal failure and the MELAS syndrome, a mitochondrial encephalomyopathy. *J Am Soc Nephrol* 1996;7:647–652.
124. Hurwitz CG, Hu VY, Segal AS. A mechanogated nonselective cation channel in proximal tubule that is ATP sensitive. *Am J Physiol Renal Physiol* 2002;283:F93–F104.
125. Iacobazzi V, Naglieri MA, Stanley CA, et al. The structure and organization of the human carnitine/acylcarnitine translocase (CACT1) gene2. *Biochem Biophys Res Commun* 1998;252: 770–774.
126. Jackson EK Raghvendra DK. The extracellular cyclic AMP-adenosine pathway in renal physiology. *Annu Rev Physiol* 2004;66:571–599.
127. Jacobus WE, Moreadith RW, Vandegaer KM. Mitochondrial respiratory control. Evidence against the regulation of respiration by extramitochondrial phosphorylation potentials or by [ATP]/[ADP] ratios. *J Biol Chem* 1982;257:2397–2402.
128. Jansen JJ, Maassen JA, van der Woude FJ, et al. Mutation in mitochondrial tRNA(Leu(UUR)) gene associated with progressive kidney disease. *J Am Soc Nephrol* 1997;8:1118–1124.
129. Jorgensen PL. Structure, function and regulation of Na,K-ATPase in the kidney. *Kidney Int* 1986;29:10–20.
130. Jorgensen PL. Aspects of gene structure and functional regulation of the isozymes of Na, K-ATPase. *Cell Mol Biol (Noisy-le-grand)* 2001;47:231–238.
131. Jorgensen PL, Hakansson KO, Karlish SJ. Structure and mechanism of Na,K-ATPase: functional sites and their interactions. *Annu Rev Physiol* 2003;65:817–849.
132. Juillard L, Lerman LO, Kruger DG, et al. Blood oxygen level–dependent measurement of acute intra-renal ischemia. *Kidney Int* 2004;65:944–950.
133. Jung KY, Endou H. Nephrotoxicity assessment by measuring cellular ATP content. II. Intranephron site of ochratoxin A nephrotoxicity. *Toxicol Appl Pharmacol* 1989;100:383–390.
134. Jung KY, Endou H. Cellular adenosine triphosphate production and consumption in the descending thin limb of Henle's loop in the rat. *Ren Physiol Biochem* 1990;13:248–258.
135. Justo P, Lorz C, Sanz A, et al. Intracellular mechanisms of cyclosporin A-induced tubular cell apoptosis. *J Am Soc Nephrol* 2003;14:3072–3080.
136. Kadenbach B. Regulation of respiration and ATP synthesis in higher organisms: hypothesis. *J Bioenerg Biomembr* 1986;18:39–54.
137. Kadenbach B. Intrinsic and extrinsic uncoupling of oxidative phosphorylation. *Biochim Biophys Acta* 2003;1604:77–94.
138. Kaplan JH. Biochemistry of Na,K-ATPase. *Annu Rev Biochem* 2002;71:511–535.
139. Kaplan RS. Structure and function of mitochondrial anion transport proteins. *J Membr Biol* 2001;179:165–183.
140. Karet FE, Finberg KE, Nelson RD, et al. Mutations in the gene encoding B1 subunit of H^+-ATPase cause renal tubular acidosis with sensorineural deafness. *Nat Genet* 1999;21: 84–90.
141. Kashgarian M, Biemesderfer D, Caplan M, et al. Monoclonal antibody to Na,K-ATPase: immunocytochemical localization along nephron segments. *Kidney Int* 1985;28:899–913.
142. Katz AI, Doucet A, Morel F. Na-K-ATPase activity along the rabbit, rat, and mouse nephron. *Am J Physiol* 1979;237:F114–F120.
143. Katz AI. Distribution and function of classes of ATPases along the nephron. *Kidney Int* 1986;29:21–31.
144. Kiil F, Aukland K, Refsum HE. Renal sodium transport and oxygen consumption. *Am J Physiol* 1961;201:511–516.
145. Kiil F, Sejersted OM, Steen PA. Energetics and specificity of transcellular NaCl transport in the dog kidney. *Int J Biochem* 1980;12:245–250.
146. Kip SN, Strehler EE. Characterization of PMCA isoforms and their contribution to transcellular Ca^{2+} flux in MDCK cells. *Am J Physiol Renal Physiol* 2003;284:F122–F132.
147. Kiroytcheva M, Cheval L, Carranza ML, et al. Effect of cAMP on the activity and the phosphorylation of Na^+,K(+)-ATPase in rat thick ascending limb of Henle. *Kidney Int* 1999;55:1819–1831.
148. Klein KL, Wang MS, Torikai S, et al. Substrate oxidation by isolated single nephron segments of the rat. *Kidney Int* 1981;20:29–35.
149. Kondou I, Nakada J, Hishinuma H, et al. Alterations of gluconeogenesis by ischemic renal injury in rats. *Ren Fail* 1992;14:479–483.
150. Kone BC, Kikeri D, Zeidel ML, et al. Cellular pathways of potassium transport in renal inner medullary collecting duct. *Am J Physiol* 1989;256:C823–C830.
151. Kone BC. Nitric oxide in renal health and disease. *Am J Kidney Dis* 1997;30:311–333.
152. Kone BC. The metabolic basis of solute transport. In: Brenner BM, ed. *The Kidney*. 7th ed. Philadelphia: Saunders, 2004:231–260.
153. Kowaltowski AJ, Castilho RF, Vercesi AE. Mitochondrial permeability transition and oxidative stress. *FEBS Lett* 2001;495:12–15.
154. Krebs HA. Renal Gluconeogenesis. *Adv Enzyme Regul* 1963;17:385–400.
155. Kurogouchi F, Oguchi T, Mawatari E, et al. A case of mitochondrial cytopathy with a typical point mutation for MELAS, presenting with severe focal-segmental glomerulosclerosis as main clinical manifestation. *Am J Nephrol* 1998;18:551–556.
156. Kurtz I. Apical Na^+/H^+ antiporter and glycolysis-dependent H^+-ATPase regulate intracellular pH in the rabbit S3 proximal tubule. *J Clin Invest* 1987;80:928–935.
157. Kuwertz-Broking E, Koch HG, Marquardt T, et al. Renal Fanconi syndrome: first sign of partial respiratory chain complex IV deficiency. *Pediatr Nephrol* 2000;14:495–498.
158. Lardy HA, Wellman H. Oxidative phosphorylations; role of inorganic phosphate and acceptor systems in control of metabolic rates. *J Biol Chem* 1952;195:215–224.
159. Laycock SK, Vogel T, Forfia PR, et al. Role of nitric oxide in the control of renal oxygen consumption and the regulation of chemical work in the kidney. *Circ Res* 1998;82: 1263–1271.
160. Le Hir M, Dubach UC. Activities of enzymes of the tricarboxylic acid cycle in segments of the rat nephron. *Pflügers Arch* 1982;395:239–243.
161. Le Hir M, Dubach UC. Peroxisomal and mitochondrial beta-oxidation in the rat kidney: distribution of fatty acyl-coenzyme A oxidase and 3-hydroxyacyl-coenzyme A dehydrogenase activities along the nephron. *J Histochem Cytochem* 1982;30:441–444.
162. Leipziger J. Control of epithelial transport via luminal P2 receptors. *Am J Physiol Renal Physiol* 2003;284:F419–432.
163. Lemasters JJ, Sowers AE. Phosphate dependence and atractyloside inhibition of mitochondrial oxidative phosphorylation. The ADP-ATP carrier is rate-limiting. *J Biol Chem* 1979;254:1248–1251.
164. Li L, Storey P, Kim D, et al. Kidneys in hypertensive rats show reduced response to nitric oxide synthase inhibition as evaluated by BOLD MRI. *J Magn Reson Imaging* 2003;17: 671–675.
165. Li LP, Storey P, Pierchala L, et al. Evaluation of the reproducibility of intrarenal R2* and DeltaR2* measurements following administration of furosemide and during waterload. *J Magn Reson Imaging* 2004; 19:610–616.
166. Lieberthal W, Levine JS. Mechanisms of apoptosis and its potential role in renal tubular epithelial cell injury. *Am J Physiol* 1996;271:F477–F488.
167. Lieberthal W, Koh JS, Levine JS. Necrosis and apoptosis in acute renal failure. *Semin Nephrol* 1998;18:505–518.
168. Lieberthal W, Menza SA, Levine JS. Graded ATP depletion can cause necrosis or apoptosis of cultured mouse proximal tubular cells. *Am J Physiol* 1998;274:F315–F327.
169. Lieberthal W, Nigam SK. Acute renal failure. I. Relative importance of proximal vs. distal tubular injury. *Am J Physiol* 1998;275:F623–F631.
170. Liu X, Kim CN, Yang J, et al. Induction of apoptotic program in cell-free extracts: requirement for dATP and cytochrome c. *Cell* 1996;86:147–157.
171. Loffing J, Loffing-Cueni D, Valderrabano V, et al. Distribution of transcellular calcium and sodium transport pathways along mouse distal nephron. *Am J Physiol Renal Physiol* 2001;281: F1021–F1027.
172. Magosci M, Yamaki M, Penniston JT, et al. Localization of mRNAs coding for isozymes of plasma membrane Ca(2+)-ATPase pump in rat kidney. *Am J Physiol* 1992;263:F7–F14.
173. Magyar CE, White KE, Rojas R, et al. Plasma membrane Ca^{2+}-ATPase and NCX1 Na^+/Ca^{2+} exchanger expression in distal convoluted tubule cells. *Am J Physiol Renal Physiol* 2002;283:F29–F40.
174. Maleque A, Endou H, Koseki C, et al. Nephron heterogeneity: gluconeogenesis from pyruvate in rabbit nephron. *FEBS Lett* 1980;116:154–156.
175. Mandel LJ Balaban RS. Stoichiometry and coupling of active transport to oxidative metabolism in epithelial tissues. *Am J Physiol* 1981;240:F357–F371.
176. Mandel LJ. Primary active sodium transport, oxygen consumption, and ATP: coupling and regulation. *Kidney Int* 1986;29:3–9.
177. Manotham K, Tanaka T, Ohse T, et al. A biologic role of HIF-1 in the renal medulla. *Kidney Int* 2005;67:1428–1439.
178. Markovich D, Murer H. The SLC13 gene family of sodium sulphate/carboxylate cotransporters. *Pflügers Arch* 2004;447:594–602.
179. Marsy S, Elalouf JM, Doucet A. Quantitative RT-PCR analysis of mRNAs encoding a colonic putative H, K-ATPase alpha subunit along the rat nephron: effect of K^+ depletion. *Pflügers Arch* 1996; 432:494–500.
180. Martin V, Bredoux R, Corvazier E, et al. Three novel sarco/endoplasmic reticulum Ca^{2+}-ATPase (SERCA) 3 isoforms. Expression, regulation, and function of the membranes of the SERCA3 family. *J Biol Chem* 2002;277:24442–24452.
181. Marver D, Schwartz MJ. Identification of mineralocorticoid target sites in the isolated rabbit cortical nephron. *Proc Natl Acad Sci U S A* 1980;77:3672–3676.
182. Masereeuw R, van Pelt AP, van Os SH, et al. Probenecid interferes with renal oxidative metabolism: a potential pitfall in its use as an inhibitor of drug transport. *Br J Pharmacol* 2000;131:57–62.
183. Maxwell P. HIF-1: an oxygen response system with special relevance to the kidney. *J Am Soc Nephrol* 2003;14:2712–2722.

184. McCoy CE, Selvaggio AM, Alexander EA, et al. Adenosine triphosphate depletion induces a rise in cytosolic free calcium in canine renal epithelial cells. *J Clin Invest* 1988;82:1326–1332.

185. McDonough AA, Magyar CE, Komatsu Y. Expression of Na(+)-K(+)-ATPase alpha- and beta-subunits along rat nephron: isoform specificity and response to hypokalemia. *Am J Physiol* 1994;267:C901–C908.

186. Meij IC, Koenderink JB, van Bokhoven H, et al. Dominant isolated renal magnesium loss is caused by misrouting of the Na(+),K(+)-ATPase gamma-subunit. *Nat Genet* 2000;26:265–266.

187. Meyer C, Stumvoll M, Dostou J, et al. Renal substrate exchange and gluconeogenesis in normal postabsorptive humans. *Am J Physiol Endocrinol Metab* 2002;282:E428–E434.

188. Michel H. Cytochrome c oxidase: catalytic cycle and mechanisms of proton pumping—a discussion. *Biochemistry* 1999;38:15129–15140.

189. Michlig S, Mercier A, Doucet A, et al. ERK1/2 controls Na,K-ATPase activity and transepithelial sodium transport in the principal cell of the cortical collecting duct of the mouse kidney. *J Biol Chem* 2004;279:51002–51012.

190. Misler S, Giebisch G. ATP-sensitive potassium channels in physiology, pathophysiology, and pharmacology. *Curr Opin Nephrol Hypertens* 1992;1:21–33.

191. Mitchell P, Moyle J. Estimation of membrane potential and pH difference across the cristae membrane of rat liver mitochondria. *Eur J Biochem* 1969;7:471–484.

192. Mochizuki H, Joh K, Kawame H, et al. Mitochondrial encephalomyopathies preceded by de-Toni–Debre–Fanconi syndrome or focal segmental glomerulosclerosis. *Clin Nephrol* 1996;46:347–352.

193. Molitoris BA. Na(+)-K(+)-ATPase that redistributes to apical membrane during ATP depletion remains functional. *Am J Physiol* 1993;265:F693–F697.

194. Nagami GT, Lee P. Effect of luminal perfusion on glucose production by isolated proximal tubules. *Am J Physiol* 1989;256:F120–F127.

195. Natke E, Jr. Cell volume regulation of rabbit cortical collecting tubule in anisotonic media. *Am J Physiol* 1990;258:F1657–F1665.

196. Needleman P, Passonneau JV, Lowry OH. Distribution of glucose and related metabolites in rat kidney. *Am J Physiol* 1968;215:655–659.

197. Nellans HN, Finn AL. Oxygen consumption and sodium transport in the toad urinary bladder. *Am J Physiol* 1974;227:670–675.

198. Niaudet P, Rotig A. Renal involvement in mitochondrial cytopathies. *Pediatr Nephrol* 1996;10:368–373.

199. Niaudet P. Mitochondrial disorders and the kidney. *Arch Dis Child* 1998;78:387–390.

200. Noel J, Vinay P, Tejedor A, et al. Metabolic cost of bafilomycin-sensitive H+ pump in intact dog, rabbit, and hamster proximal tubules. *Am J Physiol* 1993;264:F655–F661.

201. Nonaka T, Stokes JB. Metabolic support of Na+ transport by the rabbit CCD: analysis of the use of equivalent current. *Kidney Int* 1994;45:743–752.

202. Ortiz PA, Garvin JL. Role of nitric oxide in the regulation of nephron transport. *Am J Physiol Renal Physiol* 2002;282:F777–F784.

203. Padanilam BJ. Cell death induced by acute renal injury: a perspective on the contributions of apoptosis and necrosis. *Am J Physiol Renal Physiol* 2003;284:F608–627.

204. Pajor AM. Sodium-coupled transporters for Krebs cycle intermediates. *Annu Rev Physiol* 1999;61:663–682.

205. Palmieri F. The mitochondrial transporter family (SLC25): physiological and pathological implications. *Pflügers Arch* 2004;447:689–709.

206. Penniston JT, Enyedi A. Modulation of the plasma membrane Ca2+ pump. *J Membr Biol* 1998;165:101–109.

207. Pfaller W, Rittinger M. Quantitative morphology of the rat kidney. *Int J Biochem* 1980;12:17–22.

208. Pfaller W. Structure function correlation on rat kidney. Quantitative correlation of structure and function in the normal and injured rat kidney. *Adv Anat Embryol Cell Biol* 1982;70:1–106.

209. Pfaller W, Guder WG, Gstraunthaler G, et al. Compartmentation of ATP within renal proximal tubular cells. *Biochim Biophys Acta* 1984;805:152–157.

210. Piepenhagen PA, Peters LL, Lux SE, et al. Differential expression of Na(+)-K(+)-ATPase, ankyrin, fodrin, and E-cadherin along the kidney nephron. *Am J Physiol* 1995;269:C1417–C1432.

211. Prasad PV, Edelman RR, Epstein FH. Noninvasive evaluation of intrarenal oxygenation with BOLD MRI. *Circulation* 1996;94:3271–3275.

212. Prasad PV, Priatna A. Functional imaging of the kidneys with fast MRI techniques. *Eur J Radiol* 1999;29:133–148.

213. Qi Z, Murase K, Obata S, et al. Extracellular ATP-dependent activation of plasma membrane Ca(2+) pump in HEK-293 cells. *Br J Pharmacol* 2000;131:370–374.

214. Ralevic V, Burnstock G. Receptors for purines and pyrimidines. *Pharmacol Rev* 1998;50:413–492.

215. Rea C, Segal S. ATP content of rat kidney cortex slices: relation to alpha-aminoisobutyric acid uptake. *Kidney Int* 1972;2:101–106.

216. Ries M, Basseau F, Tyndal B, et al. Renal diffusion and BOLD MRI in experimental diabetic nephropathy. Blood oxygen level-dependent. *J Magn Reson Imaging* 2003;17:104–113.

217. Rodriguez H, Drouin R, Holmquist GP, et al. A hot spot for hydrogen peroxide-induced damage in the human hypoxia-inducible factor 1 binding site of the PGK 1 gene. *Arch Biochem Biophys* 1997;338:207–212.

218. Rome L, Grantham J, Savin V, et al. Proximal tubule volume regulation in hyperosmotic media: intracellular K+, Na+, and Cl. *Am J Physiol* 1989;257:C1093–V1100.

219. Ross B, Leaf A, Silva P, et al. Na-K-ATPase in sodium transport by the perfused rat kidney. *Am J Physiol* 1974;226:624–629.

220. Rotig A, Goutieres F, Niaudet P, et al. Deletion of mitochondrial DNA in patient with chronic tubulointerstitial nephritis. *J Pediatr* 1995;126:597–601.

221. Rotig A. Renal disease and mitochondrial genetics. *J Nephrol* 2003;16:286–292.

222. Ruegg CE, Mandel LJ. Bulk isolation of renal PCT and PST. II. Differential responses to anoxia or hypoxia. *Am J Physiol* 1990;259:F176–F185.

223. Scaglia F, Vogel H, Hawkins EP, et al. Novel homoplasmic mutation in the mitochondrial tRNATyr gene associated with atypical mitochondrial cytopathy presenting with focal segmental glomerulosclerosis. *Am J Med Genet A* 2003;123:172–178.

224. Schafer JA, Patlak CS, Andreoli TE. Fluid absorption and active and passive ion flows in the rabbit superficial pars recta. *Am J Physiol* 1977;233:F154–F167.

225. Schlender KK. Regulation of renal glycogen synthase. Interconversion of two forms in vitro. *Biochim Biophys Acta* 1973;297:384–398.

226. Schmid H, Mall A, Scholz M, et al. Unchanged glycolytic capacity in rat kidney under conditions of stimulated gluconeogenesis. Determination of phosphofructokinase and pyruvate kinase in microdissected nephron segments of fasted and acidotic animals. *Hoppe Seylers Z Physiol Chem* 1980;361:819–827.

227. Schwenke WD, Soboll S, Seitz HJ, et al. Mitochondrial and cytosolic ATP/ADP ratios in rat liver in vivo. *Biochem J* 1981;200:405–408.

228. Segall L, Daly SE, Blostein R. Mechanistic basis for kinetic differences between the rat alpha 1, alpha 2, and alpha 3 isoforms of the Na,K-ATPase. *J Biol Chem* 2001;276:31535–31541.

229. Sekine T, Cha SH, Hosoyamada M, et al. Cloning, functional characterization, and localization of a rat renal Na+-dicarboxylate transporter. *Am J Physiol* 1998;275:F298–F305.

230. Shen W, Xu X, Ochoa M, et al. Role of nitric oxide in the regulation of oxygen consumption in conscious dogs. *Circ Res* 1994;75:1086–1095.

231. Shen W, Hintze TH, Wolin MS. Nitric oxide. An important signaling mechanism between vascular endothelium and parenchymal cells in the regulation of oxygen consumption. *Circulation* 1995;92:3505–3512.

232. Shull GE, Lingrel JB. Molecular cloning of the rat stomach (H+ + K+)-ATPase. *J Biol Chem* 1986;261:16788–16791.

233. Siegel NJ, Avison MJ, Reilly HF, et al. Enhanced recovery of renal ATP with postischemic infusion of ATP-MgCl2 determined by 31P-NMR. *Am J Physiol* 1983;245:F530–F534.

234. Silva P, Ross B, Spokes K. Competition between sodium reabsorption and gluconeogenesis in kidneys of steroid-treated rats. *Am J Physiol* 1980;238:F290–F295.

235. Silva P, Hallac R, Spokes K, et al. Relationship among gluconeogenesis, QO2, and Na+ transport in the perfused rat kidney. *Am J Physiol* 1982;242:F508–F513.

236. Silva P, Myers MA. Stoichiometry of sodium chloride transport by rectal gland of Squalus acanthias. *Am J Physiol* 1986;250:F516–F519.

237. Silver RB, Soleimani M. H+-K+-ATPases: regulation and role in pathophysiological states. *Am J Physiol* 1999;276:F799–F811.

238. Simon N, Zini R, Morin C, et al. Prednisolone and azathioprine worsen the cyclosporine A-induced oxidative phosphorylation decrease of kidney mitochondria. *Life Sci* 1997;61:659–666.

239. Simon N, Morin C, Urien S, et al. Tacrolimus and sirolimus decrease oxidative phosphorylation of isolated rat kidney mitochondria. *Br J Pharmacol* 2003;138:369–376.

240. Slater EC, Rosing J, Mol A. The phosphorylation potential generated by respiring mitochondria. *Biochim Biophys Acta* 1973;292:534–553.

241. Smith AN, Skaug J, Choate KA, et al. Mutations in ATP6N1B, encoding a new kidney vacuolar proton pump 116-kD subunit, cause recessive distal renal tubular acidosis with preserved hearing. *Nat Genet* 2000;26:71–75.

242. Snowdowne KW, Freudenrich CC, Borle AB. The effects of anoxia on cytosolic free calcium, calcium fluxes, and cellular ATP levels in cultured kidney cells. *J Biol Chem* 1985;260:11619–11626.

243. Soleimani M, Burnham CE. Na+:HCO(3−) cotransporters (NBC): cloning and characterization. *J Membr Biol* 2001;183:71–84.

244. Soltoff SP, Mandel LJ. Active ion transport in the renal proximal tubule. III. The ATP dependence of the Na pump. *J Gen Physiol* 1984;84:643–662.

245. Soltoff SP. ATP and the regulation of renal cell function. *Annu Rev Physiol* 1986;48:9–31.

246. Stauffer TP, Hilfiker H, Carafoli E, et al. Quantitative analysis of alternative splicing options of human plasma membrane calcium pump genes. *J Biol Chem* 1993;268:25993–26003.

247. Stauffer TP, Guerini D, Carafoli E. Tissue distribution of the four gene products of the plasma membrane Ca2+ pump. A study using specific antibodies. *J Biol Chem* 1995;270:12184–12190.

248. Stokes JB, Grupp C, Kinne RK. Purification of rat papillary collecting duct cells: functional and metabolic assessment. *Am J Physiol* 1987;253:F251–F262.

249. Stover EH, Borthwick KJ, Bavalia C, et al. Novel ATP6V1B1 and ATP6V0A4 mutations in autosomal recessive distal renal tubular acidosis with new evidence for hearing loss. *J Med Genet* 2002;39:796–803.

250. Stuehr DJ, Nathan CF. Nitric oxide. A macrophage product responsible for cytostasis and respiratory inhibition in tumor target cells. *J Exp Med* 1989;169:1543–1555.

251. Sweadner KJ, Rael E. The FXYD gene family of small ion transport regulators or channels: cDNA sequence, protein signature sequence, and expression. *Genomics* 2000;68:41–56.

252. Szabolcs MJ, Seigle R, Shanske S, et al. Mitochondrial DNA deletion: a cause of chronic tubulointerstitial nephropathy. *Kidney Int* 1994;45:1388–1396.

253. Tanaka T, Miyata T, Inagi R, et al. Hypoxia in renal disease with proteinuria and/or glomerular hypertension. *Am J Pathol* 2004; 165:1979–1992.

254. Tanaka T, Nangaku M, Miyata T, et al. Blockade of calcium influx through L-type calcium channels attenuates mitochondrial injury and apoptosis in hypoxic renal tubular cells. *J Am Soc Nephrol* 2004;15:2320–2333.

255. Tang W, Shaikh ZA. Renal cortical mitochondrial dysfunction upon cadmium metallothionein administration to Sprague–Dawley rats. *J Toxicol Environ Health A* 2001;63:221–235.

256. Tatton WG, Olanow CW. Apoptosis in neurodegenerative diseases: the role of mitochondria. *Biochim Biophys Acta* 1999;1410:195–213.

257. Terada Y, Knepper MA. Na+-K+-ATPase activities in renal tubule segments of rat inner medulla. *Am J Physiol* 1989;256:F218–F223.

258. Terada Y, Tomita K, Nonoguchi H, et al. Polymerase chain reaction localization of constitutive nitric oxide synthase and soluble guanylate cyclase messenger RNAs in microdissected rat nephron segments. *J Clin Invest* 1992;90:659–665.

259. Thadhani R, Pascual M, Bonventre JV. Acute renal failure. *N Engl J Med* 1996;334:1448–1460.

260. Thastrup O, Cullen PJ, Drobak BK, et al. Thapsigargin, a tumor promoter, discharges intracellular Ca^{2+} stores by specific inhibition of the endoplasmic reticulum Ca2(+)-ATPase. *Proc Natl Acad Sci U S A* 1990;87:2466–2470.

261. Thurau K. Renal Na-reabsorption and O_2-uptake in dogs during hypoxia and hydrochlorothiazide infusion. *Proc Soc Exp Biol Med* 1961;106:714–717.

262. Torikai S. Dependency of microdissected nephron segments upon oxidative phosphorylation and exogenous substrates: a relationship between tubular anatomical location in the kidney and metabolic activity. *Clin Sci (Lond)* 1989;77:287–295.

263. Tsuboi T, Lippiat JD, Ashcroft FM, et al. ATP-dependent interaction of the cytosolic domains of the inwardly rectifying K^+ channel Kir6.2 revealed by fluorescence resonance energy transfer. *Proc Natl Acad Sci U S A* 2004;101:76–81.

264. Tsuchiya K, Wang W, Giebisch G, et al. ATP is a coupling modulator of parallel Na, K-ATPase-K-channel activity in the renal proximal tubule. *Proc Natl Acad Sci U S A* 1992;89:6418–6422.

265. Tumlin JA, Hoban CA, Medford RM, et al. Expression of Na-K-ATPase alpha- and beta-subunit mRNA and protein isoforms in the rat nephron. *Am J Physiol* 1994;266: F240–F245.

266. Tune BM, Hsu CY. Toxicity of cephalosporins to fatty acid metabolism in rabbit renal cortical mitochondria. *Biochem Pharmacol* 1995;49:727–734.

267. Uchida S, Endou H. Substrate specificity to maintain cellular ATP along the mouse nephron. *Am J Physiol* 1988;255:F977–F983.

268. Unwin RJ, Bailey MA, Burnstock G. Purinergic signaling along the renal tubule: the current state of play. *News Physiol Sci* 2003;18:237–241.

269. Unwin RJ, Capasso G, Shirley DG. An overview of divalent cation and citrate handling by the kidney. *Nephron Physiol* 2004;98:15–20.

270. Urbaitis BK, Kessler RH. Concentration of adenine nucleotide compounds in renal cortex and medulla. *Nephron* 1969;6:217–234.

271. Urbaitis BK, Kessler RH. Actions of inhibitor compounds on adenine nucleotides of renal cortex and sodium excretion. *Am J Physiol* 1971;220:1116–1123.

272. Valtin H. *Renal Function: Mechanisms Preserving Fluid and Solute Balance in Health.* Boston: Little, Brown, 1983.

273. Vandewalle A, Wirthensohn G, Heidrich HG, et al. Distribution of hexokinase and phosphoenolpyruvate carboxykinase along the rabbit nephron. *Am J Physiol* 1981;240:F492–F500.

274. Veech RL, Lawson JW, Cornell NW, et al. Cytosolic phosphorylation potential. *J Biol Chem* 1979;254:6538–6547.

275. Veiga JA, Carpenter CA, Saggerson ED. Effect of the Na^+ ionophore monensin on basal and noradrenaline stimulated gluconeogenesis in rat renal tubule fragments. *FEBS Lett* 1981;134:183–184.

276. Verma AK, Filoteo AG, Stanford DR, et al. Complete primary structure of a human plasma membrane Ca^{2+} pump. *J Biol Chem* 1988;263:14152–14159.

277. Vinay P, Senecal J, Noel J, et al. Basolateral glucose transport in distal segments of the dog nephron. *Can J Physiol Pharmacol* 1991;69:964–977.

278. Vinciguerra M, Deschenes G, Hasler U, et al. Intracellular Na^+ controls cell surface expression of Na,K-ATPase via a cAMP-independent PKA pathway in mammalian kidney collecting duct cells. *Mol Biol Cell* 2003;14:2677–2688.

279. Wagner CA, Finberg KE, Breton S, et al. Renal vacuolar H+-ATPase. *Physiol Rev* 2004;84:1263–1314.

280. Wang LC, Lee WT, Tsai WY, et al. Mitochondrial cytopathy combined with Fanconi's syndrome. *Pediatr Neurol* 2000;22:403–406.

281. Wang W, Giebisch G. Dual effect of adenosine triphosphate on the apical small conductance K^+ channel of the rat cortical collecting duct. *J Gen Physiol* 1991;98:35–61.

282. Wang W. Renal potassium channels: recent developments. *Curr Opin Nephrol Hypertens* 2004;13:549–555.

283. Weidemann MJ, Krebs HA. The fuel of respiration of rat kidney cortex. *Biochem J* 1969;112:149–166.

284. Weinberg JM, Davis JA, Trivedi B. Calcium compartmentation in isolated renal tubules in suspension. *Biochem Med Metab Biol* 1988;39:234–245.

285. Weinberg JM, Venkatachalam MA, Roeser NF, et al. Mitochondrial dysfunction during hypoxia/reoxygenation and its correction by anaerobic metabolism of citric acid cycle intermediates. *Proc Natl Acad Sci U S A* 2000;97:2826–2831.

286. Weinberg JM, Venkatachalam MA, Roeser NF, et al. Anaerobic and aerobic pathways for salvage of proximal tubules from hypoxia-induced mitochondrial injury. *Am J Physiol Renal Physiol* 2000;279:F927–F943.

287. Welsh MJ. Energetics of chloride secretion in canine tracheal epithelium. Comparison of the metabolic cost of chloride transport with the metabolic cost of sodium transport. *J Clin Invest* 1984;74:262–268.

288. Wengert M, Berto C, Jr., Kaufman J, et al. Stimulation of the proximal tubule Na+-ATPase activity by adenosine A(2A) receptor. *Int J Biochem Cell Biol* 2005;37:155–165.

289. Wetzel RK, Sweadner KJ. Immunocytochemical localization of Na-K-ATPase alpha- and gamma-subunits in rat kidney. *Am J Physiol Renal Physiol* 2001;281:F531–F545.

290. Whittam R. Active cation transport as a pace-maker of respiration. *Nature* 1961;191: 603–604.

291. Wingo CS. Active proton secretion and potassium absorption in the rabbit outer medullary collecting duct. Functional evidence for proton-potassium-activated adenosine triphosphatase. *J Clin Invest* 1989;84:361–365.

292. Wingo CS, Madsen KM, Smolka A, et al. H-K-ATPase immunoreactivity in cortical and outer medullary collecting duct. *Kidney Int* 1990;38:985–990.

293. Wittner M, Weidtke C, Schlatter E, et al. Substrate utilization in the isolated perfused cortical thick ascending limb of rabbit nephron. *Pflügers Arch* 1984;402:52–62.

294. Wong GG, Ross BD. Application of phosphorus nuclear magnetic resonance to problems of renal physiology and metabolism. *Mineral Electrolyte Metab* 1983;9:282–289.

295. Yanagihara C, Oyama A, Tanaka M, et al. An autopsy case of mitochondrial encephalomyopathy with lactic acidosis and stroke-like episodes syndrome with chronic renal failure. *Intern Med* 2001;40:662–665.

296. Zager RA, Johnson AC, Hanson SY. Proximal tubular cytochrome c efflux: determinant, and potential marker, of mitochondrial injury. *Kidney Int* 2004;65:2123–2134.

297. Zeidel ML, Seifter JL, Lear S, et al. Atrial peptides inhibit oxygen consumption in kidney medullary collecting duct cells. *Am J Physiol* 1986;251:F379–F383.

298. Zeidel ML, Silva P, Seifter JL. Intracellular pH regulation in rabbit renal medullary collecting duct cells. Role of chloride-bicarbonate exchange. *J Clin Invest* 1986;77:1682–1688.

299. Zeidel ML. Hormonal regulation of inner medullary collecting duct sodium transport. *Am J Physiol* 1993;265:F159–F173.

300. Zerahn K. Oxygen consumption and active sodium transport in the isolated and short-circuited frog skin. *Acta Physiol Scand* 1956;36:300–318.

301. Zerahn K. Oxygen consumption and active transport of sodium in the isolated, short-circuited frog skin. *Nature* 1956;177:937–938.

302. Zsurka G, Ormos J, Ivanyi B, et al. Mitochondrial mutation as a probable causative factor in familial progressive tubulointerstitial nephritis. *Hum Genet* 1997;99:484–487.

303. Zuo CS, Rofsky NM, Mahallati H, et al. Visualization and quantification of renal R2* changes during water diuresis. *J Magn Reson Imaging* 2003;17:676–682.

CHAPTER **8**

Electrophysiological Analysis of Transepithelial Transport

Henry Sackin and Lawrence G. Palmer

Rosalind Franklin University of Medicine and Science/The Chicago Medical School, North Chicago, Illinois, USA
Weill Medical College of Cornell University, New York, New York, USA

INTRODUCTION

In this chapter we discuss electrophysiological approaches to the study of renal function. The purpose is to provide an overview of the available techniques, with particular emphasis on what can be learned using the latest methods. However, the chapter is neither a technical manual nor a comprehensive review of the literature. For this, we refer the reader to other sections of the book that deal with specific nephron segments and transport mechanisms. Finally, we will not derive mathematical equations from first principles. Equations that are essential to the text are provided in the main body of the chapter, while the more detailed formulae are described in the appendices.

We have arbitrarily divided the field of epithelial electrophysiology into three major sections. The first describes measurements of transepithelial electrical properties. The second section focuses on the use of intracellular microelectrodes to discriminate apical and basolateral membrane properties. The final section deals with the technique of patch clamping to investigate the functional characteristics of individual ion channels.

The interpretation of electrical signals from epithelia is complicated by the geometry of the tissues. At least three structures within an epithelium contribute to its electrical properties: the apical plasma membrane, basolateral plasma membrane, and paracellular pathway. The individual cell membrane properties will in turn be determined by various conductive pathways, including those of passive or dissipative pathways, through which ions flow driven by their own electrochemical potential differences, and active transport, which can use metabolic energy to drive ions against these potential differences. The paracellular pathway, in turn, consists of the tight junctions connecting the epithelial cells and the lateral interspaces between the cells.

The electrical properties of this complex structure can be most easily understood in terms of equivalent circuits. A comprehensive equivalent circuit of a generic reabsorbing epithelium is illustrated in Fig. 1. Electrolyte diffusion across the apical membrane can be separated into its con-

stituent ionic pathways as shown by the expanded view of the apical membrane in Fig. 1. Each ionic pathway is associated with an electromotive force (EMF) or battery representing the chemical potential for each ion. Electrogenic carriers such as the Na–glucose cotransporter can also be represented by an additional resistor (R_{glu}) and EMF (E_{glu}) in parallel with the diffusional elements. All of the batteries and resistors can be lumped, respectively, into a single apical EMF (E_{ap}) and a single resistance R_{ap} as shown in the center diagram. The basal membrane has a similar set of elements, R_b and E_b, which represent a dissipative ion pathway in parallel with an active transport pathway, represented by a resistor (R_p) and an EMF (E_p).

Thus:

$$E_x = -\frac{RT}{z_i F} Ln \left[\frac{X_1}{X_2} \right] \quad (1)$$

where $[X_1]$ and $[X_2]$ are the concentrations of ion X on the two sides of the membrane and z_i is the charge on the ion. The weighting factor for each ion is the transference number, t_x, which expresses the fraction of membrane conductance that is attributable to that particular ion, as in:

$$t_x = \frac{g_x}{g_{tot}} \quad (2)$$

where g represents the conductance of the individual ion pathways and g_{tot} is the total ionic conductance of the membrane. In most cases g_{tot} will simply be the sum of the Na, K, and Cl conductances of the barrier. Hence the total EMF can be generally expressed by the following equation:

$$E = t_{Na}E_{Na} + t_K E_K + t_{Cl}E_{Cl} = -\frac{RT}{F} \sum_{x=Na,K,Cl} \frac{t_x}{z_x} Ln \left[\frac{X_1}{X_2} \right] \quad (3)$$

The overall goal of classical electrophysiology, described in the first two sections of this chapter, is to evaluate the various elements of this equivalent circuit, to quantify the various resistances and EMFs, and to describe the extent to which they

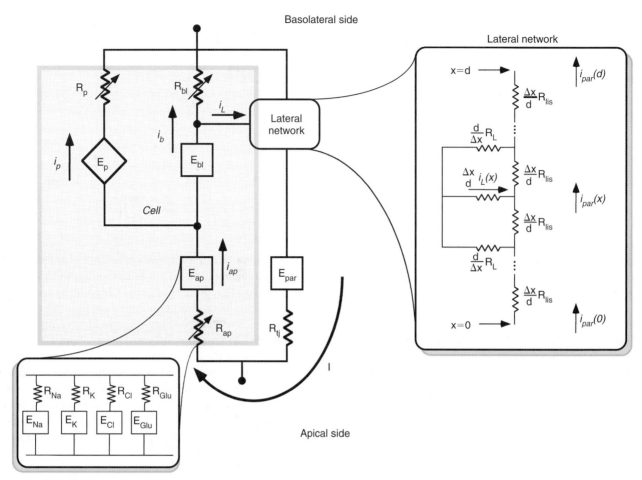

FIGURE 1   Electrical equivalent circuit for a general epithelium. Each membrane or barrier is associated with an electromotive force (E) that represents the weighted average of the ionic diffusion potentials at that barrier. Electrogenic carriers (such as the apical Na–glucose cotransporter) and electrogenic pumps (such as the basolateral Na,K-ATPase) can also be formally represented by a series resistor and an associated electromotive force. The lateral network takes into account the nonzero electrical resistance of the lateral intercellular spaces.

change during regulation. To this end, it has often been desirable to use reductions of the main equivalent circuit of Fig. 1, and to work under conditions in which these reduced circuits are applicable. Such simplifications are discussed in more detail in the following sections: Transepithelial Measurements and Intracellular Measurements. Finally, the section entitled Measurements of Individual Ion Channels describes application of the patch clamp technique to epithelia and permits a description of ion transport in more molecular terms.

The rationale for representing the pump by a resistance and an EMF is discussed further in the Intracellular Measurements section. Briefly, the E_p represents the maximum amount of energy that the pump derives from splitting ATP or, alternatively, the maximum electrochemical potential difference against which the pump can operate. The pump pathway must also include a nonzero internal resistance. The magnitude of this internal resistance is determined by the actual current–voltage relation for the membrane-bound Na,K-ATPase. To maintain generality, all membrane resistances are shown as variable resistors to include the possibility of intrinsic or extrinsic regulation of ion channels.

Although the paracellular pathway is not a membrane barrier, it can also be modeled by resistive (R_{tj}) and electromotive elements (E_{par}). A lateral network (indicated to the right of the main circuit) is also included in the model. This network takes into consideration the finite resistance of fluid in the lateral spaces. This aspect of the circuit becomes important for calculation of individual membrane resistances from voltage deflection experiments (see Intracellular Measurements section).

TRANSEPITHELIAL MEASUREMENTS

Measurements of transepithelial electrical properties are by far the simplest to perform and the most difficult to interpret. They are easy to carry out because they are noninvasive; only extracellular electrodes are employed. They are difficult to interpret because the parameters that can be measured reflect in most cases a combination of many of the circuit elements shown in Fig. 1. In this chapter we will describe how transepithelial techniques are used to measure three basic parameters that characterize an epithelium: transepithelial voltage, transepithelial resistance, and short-circuit current. We will then discuss a number of special extracellular approaches that have been employed to gain additional insights into epithelial properties.

Measurement of Transepithelial Voltage

Methods of measuring transepithelial voltage (V_{te}) are conceptually simple. In principle, the potential difference between two electrodes placed on either side of the epithelium is simply determined with an appropriate electrometer. With flat epithelia that can be mounted in Ussing chambers, the transepithelial electrodes are placed in the two bathing compartments (131). In cylindrical epithelia like the renal nephron, classical measurements of transepithelial potential have been performed in vivo using micropuncture techniques. In this technique, a pipette filled with electrolyte is introduced into the lumen of the tubule and voltage is measured relative to another electrode placed in a capillary. If the nephron segment can be isolated and perfused in vitro, the perfusion and/or collection pipette can be used to monitor the intraluminal voltage with respect to the bath potential. This is illustrated in Fig. 2.

Measurement of Transepithelial Resistance

For measurements of transepithelial resistance (R_{te}), current must be injected across the epithelium to perturb V_{te}. This is most easily accomplished when the epithelium can be mounted

in Ussing chambers, where current flow and voltage changes are assumed to be uniform in the plane of the tissue. Resistance can then be computed from Ohm's law as the ratio of the change in V_{te} to the amount of current passed:

$$R_{te} = \frac{\Delta V_{te}}{\Delta I} \tag{4}$$

Epithelia can be studied in the open-circuited or voltage-clamped conditions. In open circuit the tissue is allowed to maintain its spontaneous transepithelial voltage. In this case the resistance is determined from the change in voltage produced by passing a known amount of current. Under voltage-clamp conditions a current is passed across the epithelium to maintain the transepithelial voltage at a predetermined level. The case in which this level is zero, so that the transepithelial voltage is abolished, is called the "short-circuited" state. If the epithelium is voltage clamped, resistance is determined from the change in current produced by a controlled voltage step. In open-circuited tubular epithelia, transepithelial current flow is not constant along the length of the tubule. In this case, cable analysis must be used to estimate the transepithelial resistance (see the next section).

Measurement of Transepithelial Resistance in Open-Circuited Renal Tubules

The measurement of overall transepithelial resistance, R_{te}, in renal tubules under open-circuit conditions is best carried out with a double-barreled perfusion pipette system similar

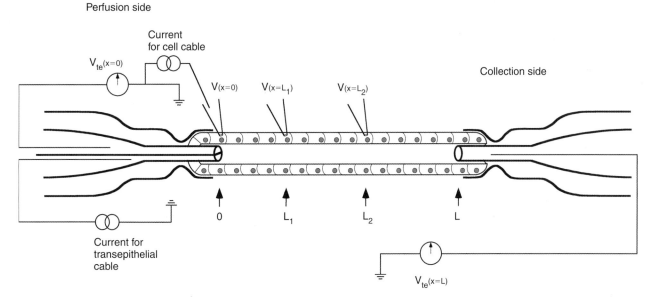

FIGURE 2 Experimental apparatus for determining electrophysiological properties of renal epithelia. The segment of isolated renal tubule is held at both ends by constriction pipettes. The tubule perfusion pipette is fabricated from *theta* glass, and has separate pathways for both current injection and transepithelial measurement, $V_{te}(x=0)$. The transepithelial potential, $V_{te}(x = L)$, can also be determined at the collection side of the tubule. For determination of cell membrane resistance, current is passed into the cell layer via the microelectrode at location $x = 0$ and the resultant voltage deflections are measured by intracellular microelectrodes at locations $x = 0$, L_1, and L_2.

to the one illustrated in Fig. 2. In this technique, the tubule is cannulated at both the perfusion and collection ends. The double-barreled perfusion pipette, fabricated from *theta* glass (39, 49, 119), creates separate pathways for current flow and voltage recording. An alternative technique uses the same single-barreled pipette for both current injection and voltage measurement. This is not nearly as accurate as the double-barreled technique because the voltage deflection arising from the internal resistance of the perfusion pipette must be nulled with a bridge circuit. The external microelectrodes in Fig. 2 are for evaluation of individual cell membrane resistances. This will be discussed in the Intracellular Measurements section.

A thin fluid-exchange tubing (not shown) can be inserted into one barrel of the perfusion pipette of Fig. 2 to permit rapid exchange of the perfusion solution while measuring the transepithelial potential $V_{te}(x = 0)$. Current is passed from a chlorided silver wire glued into the other barrel of the pipette. The transepithelial length constant of the tubule λ_{te} is determined from the voltage deflections at the perfusion, $\Delta V_{te}(x = 0)$, and collection, $\Delta V_{te}(x = L)$, sides of the tubule, resulting from a transepithelial current pulse, I_{te}, through the current side of the perfusion pipette. For a doubly cannulated, isolated tubule of length L, λ_{te} is given by Eq. 5 from Sackin and Boulpaep (120):

$$\frac{L}{\lambda_{te}} = cosh^{-1}\left[\frac{\Delta V_{te}(x = 0)}{\Delta V_{te}(x = L)}\right] \qquad (5)$$

The transepithelial resistance R_{te} in ohms centimeters squared is given by Eq. 6:

$$R_{te} = 2\sqrt{\pi\lambda_{te}^3 R_{in} R_i}\sqrt{tanh(L/\lambda_{te})} \qquad (6)$$

In this equation, R_{in} is the input resistance measured in ohms. It is operationally defined as the voltage deflection at the perfusion end $\Delta V_{te}(x = 0)$ divided by the total injected current I_{te}. Typical injected currents for proximal tubules are 100nA pulses of 1- to 5-second duration. Ideally, none of the current injected into the lumen from the perfusion pipette enters the compressed region of tubule within the holding pipette, which presumably acts like an electrical insulator when compared to the relatively low resistance of the tubule. However, artifacts may still arise from current leaks at either the perfusion or collection ends of the tubule. These can be detected by a "mismatch" between the calculated electrical radius (r_e) of the tubule and its measured optical radius (r_o):

$$r_e = \frac{2R_i\lambda_{te}^2}{R_{te}} \qquad (7)$$

Use of a double-barreled perfusion pipette (Fig. 2) eliminates much of the uncertainty in R_{in}. If a single pipette is used for both current injection and voltage recording small variations in perfusion pipette resistance greatly affect the value of $\Delta V_{te}(x = 0)$, as determined with a bridge circuit. Double-barreled perfusion pipettes have the addi-

tional advantage that R_{te} can be measured during changes in the perfusion solution. This is practically impossible with a single-barreled perfusion pipette because the bridge circuit is unstable during solution changes. Finally, the term R_i (ohms-centimeter) is the volume resistivity of the perfusion solution, as measured with a standard conductivity meter.

Although transepithelial cable measurements provide no direct information about individual membrane properties, they are generally more reliable than cellular cable measurements since potential deflections are recorded with macroscopic perfusion and collection pipettes that are completely devoid of tip potential artifacts (see Intracellular Measurements section). Furthermore, the cell layer remains undamaged since measurements are made only at the open ends of the tubule.

Measurement of Transepithelial Resistance in Voltage-Clamped Renal Tubules

There have been a number of early attempts to elucidate the electrical properties of renal tubules using voltage-clamp techniques similar to those originally developed for flat epithelia. The basis of these methods is to isolate a segment of tubule (usually with oil droplets) that is short enough to permit a uniform current distribution across the epithelium. To accomplish this, metallic axial electrodes have directly inserted into the lumen of the tubule (126). These axial electrodes can also be used for alternating current impedance analysis (50). However, one important problem with metal electrodes is the release of ions into a restricted space during continuous current flow.

More recent techniques have employed segments of isolated, perfused tubules that have been shortened to such an extent that the current distribution within the lumen is virtually homogeneous (58). In this case, R_{te} is essentially determined from the input resistance calculated in the following expression:

$$R_{te} = 2\pi r_o L \cdot R_i \qquad (8)$$

where r_o is the optical radius, and R_{te} has units of ohms-centimeter squared.

Typical Results

Measurements of V_{te} and R_{te} in some representative epithelia are shown in Table 1. The range of both these parameters is large, with values of V_{te} ranging from ± 2 mV in the proximal tubule to as much as -60 to -80 mV in the CCT. R_{te} values vary from less than 10 Ωcm^2 in proximal tubule to more than 5000 Ωcm^2 in urinary bladder. Despite the range of values observed, transepithelial voltages in all cases reflect two factors: conductance of the epithelium to the major ions and the active transport of ions. In general, a high value of V_{te} indicates that active transport is taking place across a high-resistance epithelium, whereas low val-

TABLE 1   Transepithelial Properties of Renal Epithelia

Tissue	V_{te} (mV)	R_{te} (Ωcm^2)	R_{par} (Ωcm^2)	$(P_{Na}/P_{Cl})_{par}$	Reference
Amphibians					
Proximal tubule (*Ambystoma*)	−10	70	70	0.25	119
Diluting segment (*Amphiuma*, frog)	+10	290	306	4–5	43
Collecting duct (*Amphiuma*)	−24	160	200	0.84	63
Urinary bladder (*Toad*)	−94	8,900	50,000	—	18
Mammals					
Proximal tubule (rabbit)	−2 to +2	5	5		28
TALH (rabbit)	+3 to +10	10–35	10 to 50	2–4	40
CCD (rabbit)	0 to −60 (rabbit)	110	160	0.8	72
Urinary bladder (rabbit)	−20 to −75	13,000–23,000	>78,000	—	79

CCD, cortical collecting duct; TALH, thick ascending limb of Henle's loop.

ues of V_{te} can reflect either a low R_{te} or a low rate of active transport.

Traditionally, epithelia have been divided into the categories "tight" and "leaky" according to their transepithelial resistances. In leaky epithelia the low value of R_{te} is thought to largely reflect the low resistance of the tight junctions, which constitute the major electrical resistance of the paracellular pathway between the epithelial cells (27). In tight epithelia the tight junctional resistance, and therefore the transepithelial resistance, is much higher. However, the resistance above which an epithelium is considered "tight" is not precisely defined (29). Even though the amphibian proximal tubule and the mammalian collecting duct have similar absolute values of paracellular resistance, the proximal tubule is considered a leaky epithelium, whereas the collecting duct is usually referred to as "tight." Thus, a better definition of a leaky epithelium is one in which the paracellular resistance is low relative to that of the cell membranes. For example, in leaky proximal tubules R_{te} is virtually equal to R_{par}, which is small compared the parallel transcellular resistance R_c (Table 1). In tight epithelia R_{par} is significantly larger than R_{te}. This implies that R_{par} is of the same order of magnitude as R_c, or even much larger in the case of the urinary bladder. Another feature of a tight epithelium is its ability to separate two fluid compartments with very different ion compositions. High-resistance tight junctions slow the "back leak" of ions and other solutes down their concentration gradients. Thus, in a tight epithelium it is harder to dissipate the ion gradients established by active transport processes.

Interpretation of V_{te} and R_{te} Measurements

As discussed previously, transepithelial measurements of voltage and resistance are difficult to interpret because they lump together information from many different electrical pathways arranged in parallel. To analyze such data, it is often useful to use a simplified equivalent electrical circuit (Fig. 3).

The terms R_c and E_c represent the resistance and electromotive forces across the transcellular pathway, whereas R_{tj} and E_{par} are, respectively, the resistance and electromo-

tive forces across the paracellular pathway. If the potential differences V_{te}, E_c, and E_{par} are all defined with respect to the bath or serosal side, the overall measured transepithelial values R_{te} and V_{te} are related to this circuit by Eqs. 9 and 10:

$$R_{te} = \frac{R_{tj}R_c}{R_{tj} + R_c} \tag{9}$$

$$V_{te} = \frac{E_c R_{tj} + E_{par} R_c}{R_{tj} + R_c} \tag{10}$$

The dissection of the measured parameters into the appropriate contributions from cellular and paracellular pathways can sometimes be accomplished by using maneuvers that affect only one of the pathways, or cause one pathway to dominate the other. Some of these perturbations and special conditions will be discussed in the section: Estimation of Membrane Parameters from Transepithelial Measurement.

Contribution of Active Transport to V_{te}

The major effect of the pump is to establish transmembrane ionic gradients, that is, to keep cell Na low and cell K high. As was first pointed out by Koefoed-Johnsen and Ussing in their classic paper of 1958 (68), the permeability properties of the apical and basolateral membranes of frog skin are quite different. Since the apical membrane is selectively permeable to Na and the driving force for this ion is inward, the entry of Na will tend to make the cell voltage positive with respect to the

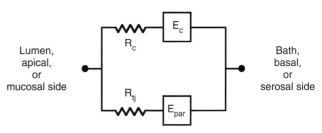

FIGURE 3   Simplified equivalent electrical circuit for an epithelium.

mucosal solution. Conversely, the basolateral membrane is selectively permeable to K. This ion will tend to flow out of the cell, making the cell voltage negative with respect to that of the serosal fluid. The EMFs E_{ap} ($RT/F \Delta\ln[Na]$) and E_{bl} ($RT/F \Delta\ln[K]$) will be in the same direction with respect to the epithelium and the transepithelial EMF, and hence V_{te} will reflect their sum (Fig. 4).

Although the Na–K ATPase is ultimately responsible for the transepithelial potential in many Na-reabsorptive epithelia, the magnitude of V_{te} does not correlate with the magnitude of active transport when various tissues are compared. In general, the effect of active ion transport will be shunted by paracellular resistance. This shunting is lowest in the tight epithelia like frog skin and toad urinary bladder, where V_{te} can be over 100 mV. In leaky epithelia such as the proximal tubule, the shunting is considerable and the values of V_{te} are much lower.

In most epithelia, E_{par} will be much smaller than E_c (Fig. 4) since ion gradients across the tight junction are relatively small. In addition, $R_{tj} > R_c$ for tight epithelia, so that the term $E_{par}R_c$ will be small compared to E_cR_{tj}, and Eq. 10 becomes:

$$V_{te} = \frac{E_c}{1 + R_c / R_{tj}} \qquad (11)$$

The implication of Eq. 11 is that if $R_{tj} >> R_c$, V_{te} will approach E_c, a quantity that is limited by the EMF of the Na pump. In general V_{te} will be reduced according to the ratio R_c/R_{tj}. The contribution of active transport to cell membrane potential is discussed in the section, Estimation of Renal Na/K Pump Current and Electrogenic Potential.

The mammalian TALH, and its amphibian counterpart the diluting segment, have lumen *positive* V_{te} despite the fact that they are also Na-reabsorbing epithelia (Table 1) (Fig. 4). This turns out to be the exception that proves the rule. As discussed in detail by Greger (40), Na does not enter the TALH cell through a conductive mechanism, as in the frog skin and other epithelia, but through an electrically neutral cotransport system along with K and Cl. Consequently, Na entry does not contribute to a lumen-negative voltage, and in fact the membrane is more permeable to K than to Na. Furthermore, the basolateral membrane has a rather high permeability to Cl. This makes the lumped EMF E_{ap} less negative than E_{bl}, and the potential difference between the cell and the blood side is less negative than the potential difference between the cell and the lumen. Hence, the mechanism for the lumen positive potential in the TALH is accounted for by the different permeability properties of the two membranes, just as in frog skin.

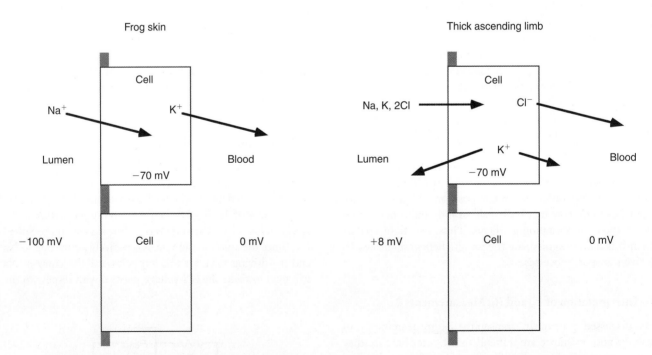

FIGURE 4   Contribution of transcellular potentials to the transepithelial potential. On the left is a tight epithelium such as the frog skin or cortical collecting duct. Influx of Na across the apical membrane and efflux of K across the basolateral membrane create a lumen-negative voltage that is not significantly shunted because of the high tight-junctional resistance. Consequently, most of the transepithelial potential arises from diffusion potentials for Na and K that are established across the cell membranes by active transport and various ion selectivities of the apical and basolateral membranes. The figure on the right is a model of a TALH cell. Here Na entry across the luminal membrane is electrically silent. The dominant electrodiffusive ion movements are K efflux across both apical and basolateral membranes, and Cl efflux across the basolateral membrane. The basolateral Cl conductance makes the cell less negative relative to interstitial fluid versus luminal fluid.

Contribution of Diffusion Potentials to V_{te}

Paracellular diffusion potentials can contribute significantly to the overall transepithelial potential, especially when V_{te} is small. For example, in the mammalian proximal tubule the early portion of the segment has a lumen-negative V_{te} in vivo, which is thought to reflect active Na reabsorption. Farther down the nephron, however, the lumen becomes positive with respect to the blood. Preferential luminal reabsorption of HCO_3^- relative to Cl^- establishes opposing gradients for Cl^- and HCO_3^- across the tight junction (Fig. 5). This results in a lumen positive potential since Cl^- diffuses more rapidly across the junctions than HCO_3^- (28).

Diffusion potentials may also contribute to the normal lumen-positive V_{te} in the mammalian TALH (Table 1). In this segment NaCl is reabsorbed but water is not, leading to a dilution of the luminal fluid. Since the tight junctions of the mammalian TALH are cation-selective, Na diffuses back more rapidly than the Cl, contributing to a lumen-positive diffusion potential (40) (Fig. 5).

Contribution of Circulating Current to V_{te}

The various equivalent EMFs at the apical and basolateral sides of the cell produce circulating current (I), which traverses both cell membranes in series and returns via the paracellular shunt (Fig. 1). The magnitude of this current depends on the relative resistances of paracellular versus cell pathways as well as the active transport rate for the particular epithelium (5, 7). For example, in renal proximal tubules, the low shunt resistance (compared to transcellular resistance) characterizes this nephron segment as a leaky epithelia with large circulating current (28, 44). On the other hand, tight epithelia like the urinary bladder or the frog skin have shunt resistances comparable to or larger than the transcellular resistance, so that the circulating current is small in comparison with that in the proximal tubule (139).

The effect of circulating current on renal transepithelial potentials can be understood qualitatively by considering the electrical profiles depicted in Fig. 6. In this figure the serosal or blood side of the epithelium is considered at ground and the voltage at any point is displayed as a function of distance from mucosa to serosa. For the sake of simplicity, we have assumed that the apical membrane is primarily selective to sodium, the basolateral membrane is primarily selective to potassium, and the interior of the cell is isopotential. Therefore, in the absence of circulating current, there is a "staircase" voltage profile through the epithelium determined by the respective diffusion potentials across the mucosal (or apical) membrane and across the serosal (or basolateral) membrane (Fig. 6A). Under these conditions the measured

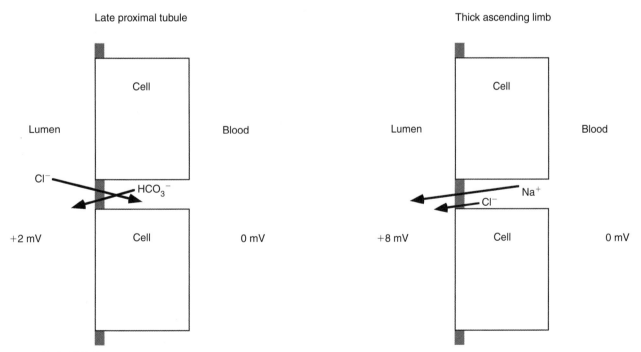

FIGURE 5 Contribution of paracellular potentials to the transepithelial potential. The figure on the left corresponds to the late proximal tubule. Preferential reabsorption of HCO_3^- in the early proximal tubule produces opposite gradients for Cl^- and HCO_3^- across the tight junction of late proximal tubule. Since the junctions are more permeable to Cl^- than to HCO_3^-, a lumen-positive diffusion potential develops. The paracellular contribution in the TALH is illustrated on the right. Here, reabsorption of NaCl across the water-impermeable epithelium results in an accumulation of NaCl within the interspaces between the cells, producing a similar gradient for both Na^+ and Cl^- across the tight junction. Since the junctions in this epithelium are more permeable to Na^+ than to Cl^-, a lumen-positive diffusion potential develops.

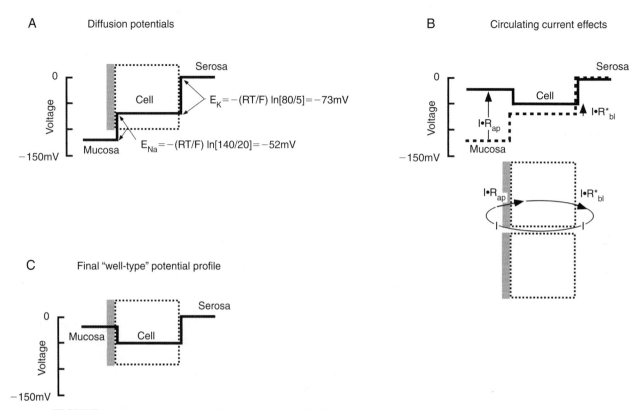

A Diffusion potentials

$E_K = -(RT/F) \ln[80/5] = -73\text{mV}$

$E_{Na} = -(RT/F) \ln[140/20] = -52\text{mV}$

B Circulating current effects

$I \cdot R_{ap}$ $I \cdot R^*_{bl}$

C Final "well-type" potential profile

FIGURE 6   Electrical potential profiles across a simple epithelium. A. In the absence of circulating currents, the electrical potential from serosal to mucosal sides would be largely determined by the Na diffusion potential at the apical membrane and the K diffusion potential at the serosal membrane. B. Circulating currents that arise from a net (open-circuit) EMF produce additional voltage drops across both the apical membrane ($I \cdot R_{ap}$) and across the basolateral membrane ($I \cdot R_{bl}$). C. This changes the "staircase" potential profile to a "well-type" potential, where the cell is more negative than either the mucosal or serosal sides.

V_{te} (mucosa minus serosa) would actually be more negative than the basolateral cell membrane potential (E_K).

In most epithelia, the diffusion potential steps of Fig. 6A would be modified by the effect of circulating current (I) across the resistance of the mucosal and serosal barriers. Specifically, the mucosal-to-cell step will be raised by an amount $I \cdot R_{ap}$ due to the circulating current crossing the mucosal membrane resistance (Fig. 6B). The same current crossing the basolateral side of the cell will decrease the size of the cell-to-serosal step by $I \cdot R^*_{bl}$, where R^*_{bl} is the effective basolateral resistance. The final values of V_{te} and V_{bl} can be calculated by considering the complete equivalent circuit (Appendix 1).

In most epithelia, the resistance of the apical membrane is larger than the resistance of the basolateral membrane and the effect of the circulating current is to transform the staircase potential (Fig. 6A) into a "well-type" potential (Fig. 6C), where the intracellular region is the most negative space and V_{te} is directly dependent on the magnitude of the current and the tightness of the epithelial cell layer. In some tight epithelia (*Necturus* urinary bladder) with high paracellular resistance and low circulating current, the "staircase" potential profile is still maintained despite "IR drops" at both membranes (55).

Short-Circuit Current

It is also possible to measure transepithelial currents while controlling the transepithelial voltage. A special case of this voltage-clamp approach is the short-circuit current technique (131) in which V_{te} is maintained at zero. If the solutions on both sides of the epithelium are identical, there is no net movement of ions through the paracellular spaces, since both electrical and chemical driving forces are reduced to zero. The current across the tissue, which must also pass through the external circuit and can thus be readily measured, results only from active transport processes (defined as those that take place against an electrochemical activity gradient). Thus this current, called the short-circuit current, will equal the sum of all active ion transport processes.

The particular ion being actively transported can be identified rigorously by measuring net fluxes at the same time as the short-circuit current. For some cases, such as the frog skin and toad bladder (78, 131) the short-circuit current can be accounted for by the active transport of only one ion species, namely Na (Table 2). In general the short-circuit current will represent the sum of the net transport of Na, K, H, and Cl. Another way to identify actively

TABLE 2 Equivalence of Net Na$^+$ Fluxes and Short-circuit Current in Model Epithelia, Transepithelial fluxes (nEq/cm^2/min)

Type of Epithelium	Mucosal to Serosal	Serosal to Mucosal	Net	Short-circuit Current
Frog skin	24.6	1.5	23.1	23.6
Toad urinary bladder	35.7	9.5	26.2	26.8

Data for frog skin from Ussing HH, Zerahn K. Active transport of sodium as the source of electric current in the short-circuited isolated frog skin. *Acta Physiol Scand* 1951;23:110–127; and for toad bladder, Leaf A, Anderson J, Page LB. Active sodium transport by the isolated toad bladder. *J Gen Physiol* 1958;41:657–668.

transported ions is to eliminate them from the bathing media and measure the resulting effects on short-circuit current. This approach is often experimentally much simpler but it is less rigorous since changing the external environment of the tissue can lead to secondary changes in cell composition and volume. In any case, once the transported species have been identified, the technique becomes a very convenient way to analyze the regulation of the active transport systems.

An important limitation of the short-circuit current technique is that it often requires nonphysiological conditions. For example, short circuiting high-resistance epithelia like frog skin will reduce the normally large V_{te} to values near zero. This will necessarily affect the transmembrane voltage of one or both cell membranes, which may in turn affect the ionic conductances of those membranes.

The short-circuit technique also involves bathing the apical side of the tissue with a solution that has an electrolyte composition close to that of the blood. This is a highly nonphysiological condition for many tight epithelia like the frog skin, which is normally in contact with pond water, and the toad bladder, which is normally in contact with dilute urine. Another important problem with short-circuit experiments is that short-circuited tissues do not have to maintain electroneutrality of the transported species. For example, in Na-transporting epithelia such as the frog skin Na ions can be reabsorbed only if another cation (e.g., K, H) is secreted or if an anion (Cl) is also reabsorbed. Under physiological conditions these other ionic pathways can be rate-limiting for Na reabsorption.

Finally, the uniform current distribution required by the short-circuit technique has largely restricted its use to flat epithelia, which can be mounted in Ussing chambers. However, in some cases it has been possible to voltage-clamp large-diameter amphibian tubules (57). Attempts have also been made to circumvent these technical problems by defining an "equivalent short-circuit current" for renal epithelia. In this method, the current at $V_{te} = 0$ is estimated by dividing the spontaneous value of V_{te} by the transepithelial resistance R_{te}. This approach assumes that R_{te} is constant; that

is, that the current voltage relation of the epithelium is linear. Even when this conditions is satisfied, it is not always possible to attribute the equivalent short-circuit current to specific ion species, since net fluxes of the ions must be measured under true short-circuited conditions.

Technical Problems

For epithelia that can be studied as flat sheets in vitro, the major technical problem in transepithelial measurements is avoiding edge damage to the tissues, particularly when these tissues are mounted in Ussing chambers (18, 53). On the other hand, for renal micropuncture experiments performed in situ, the major technical problem is localization of the microelectrode tip within the tubular lumen (28).

The most important general problem in the measurement of transepithelial resistance is the choice of the magnitude and duration of the applied perturbations. Currents (or voltage changes) that are too large can result in changes in the electrical properties of the membranes due to voltage-dependent ion conductances. Perturbations that are either too large or too long can lead to redistribution of ions across the cell membranes, which can also alter electrical properties. For example, in toad urinary bladder modest changes in V_{te} on the order of 10 mV under voltage-clamp conditions can result in time-dependent changes in the tissue resistance (137). On the other hand, if perturbations are too small they are difficult to measure accurately, and if they are applied for too short a time the capacitive, as well as the resistive properties of the epithelium will affect the response. There are no generally accepted rules for determining the size and duration of the perturbations.

Estimation of Membrane Parameters from Transepithelial Measurements

Measurement of transepithelial electrical properties does not, in general, give any direct, quantitative information about the circuit elements of greatest interest, namely the conductances of individual membranes to specific ions. As emphasized throughout this section, R_{te} is a lumped parameter determined by R_{ap}, R_b, R_{tj}, and in some cases R_{lis} (see Fig. 1). V_{te} is determined by all the Rs and EMFs in the circuit. Clearly, measuring two parameters are insufficient to determine seven or eight unknowns.

However, in some cases, it has been possible to either use conditions that simplify the equivalent circuit or to use experimental perturbations that selectively change only one electrical parameter. These methods have provided a good deal of information about epithelial properties from purely transepithelial measurements. Some examples follow.

PARACELLULAR RESISTANCE AND SELECTIVITY

When the paracellular (tight junction) resistance is low compared to the transcellular resistance the transepithelial resistance is dominated by the resistance of the paracellular pathway. This happens in a leaky epithelium like the proximal tubule. This condition can also be produced in some tight epithelia by blocking the major conductive pathways at the apical membrane. The most frequently used blockers are amiloride, for the Na conductance, and Ba, for the K conductance. In both of these cases the paracellular resistance can then be estimated from transepithelial measurements (Table 1), although intracellular recordings are usually required to prove that the transcellular resistance is high.

The ion selectivity of the paracellular pathway can also be evaluated under these circumstances. This involves measurement of the transference numbers for various ions across the tight junction (see Eq. 12). The most important ions in this case are Na and Cl, and their transference numbers can be estimated by reducing the concentration of NaCl on one side of the junction by diluting one of the bathing solutions. If the transcellular resistance is sufficiently high (i.e., $R_{ap} >> R_{tj}$; see Eq. A2.3 in Appendix 2) and is unaffected by the dilution, the measured change in V_{te} will approximately reflect the change in E_{par} where:

$$\Delta E_{par} = -\frac{RT}{F}(t_{Na} - t_{Cl})Ln\frac{[NaCl]_1}{[NaCl]_2} \qquad (12)$$

If sodium and chloride are the only conducting ions in the external solutions, the absolute transference numbers can be calculated from Eq. 12 and the requirement that $t_{Na} + t_{Cl} = 1$.

Some measurements of paracellular selectivity in renal epithelia are listed in Table 1. This parameter is of considerable physiological interest. The results range from a significant selectivity for anions (Cl) over cations (Na) in the amphibian proximal tubule to a cation selectivity in the thick ascending limb of Henle's loop or its count-erpart, the diluting segment, in the amphibian kidney. If ions moved through the tight junctions as if they were in free solution, a permeability ratio P_{Na}/P_{Cl} of 0.8 would be expected.

MEMBRANE SELECTIVITY

If the paracellular or tight junction resistance is much greater than the transcellular resistance, it is possible to determine the ion selectivity of the individual cell membranes. Specifically, if R_{tj} is very large compared to $R_{ap} + R_{bl}$, there will be negligible current through either the paracellular pathway or the cell pathway under open-circuited conditions. Under these conditions, the circuit of Fig. 1 predicts that changes in E_{ap} will parallel changes in V_{ap}, which in turn can be estimated from the measured changes in transepithelial potential ΔV_{te} (see Eqs. A1.8 and A1.11–A1.13 in Appendix 1). Such a situation was studied by Koefoed-Johnsen and Ussing (68) in their classic paper on the frog skin, where pre-treatment of the skins with low concentrations of Cu^{+2} produced very high values of R_{te} and V_{te}.

This permits evaluation of individual membrane selectivities from transepithelial measurements alone if the concentra-

tion of just one ion on one side of the epithelium is replaced with an impermeant species and the conditions associated with Eq. A1.13 (Appendix 1) are satisfied. If this is the case and Na is partially replaced on the apical side, then:

$$\Delta V_{te} = \Delta E_{ap} = -\frac{RT}{F}t_{Na}Ln\frac{[Na]_{ap}^{exp}}{[Na]_{ap}^{con}} \text{ for } R_{tj} >> R_{ap} + R_{bl}^* \quad (13)$$

where the change in potential is measured as experimental minus control. $[Na]^{exp}$ and $[Na]^{con}$ represent the concentrations of Na under experimental and control conditions, that is, after and before the solution change.

Koefoed-Johnsen and Ussing (68) found that changes in mucosal Na produced changes in V_{te} close to those that would be expected if $t_{Na} = 1$. From this they inferred that the apical membrane was primarily conductive to Na ions. Similarly, changes in serosal K concentration produced changes consistent with the idea that the basolateral membrane conducted only K. The elegant conclusions of this study depended upon the rather unusual conditions achieved, namely a very high paracellular resistance, and the absence of other "leak" pathways due to other cell types. Except for the case of the urinary bladder, such conditions are difficult to achieve in renal epithelia where paracellular pathways are usually leakier than in the frog skin.

Selectivity of the epithelial basolateral membrane has also been studied by using pore-forming polyene antibiotics to reduce apical membrane resistance (80) so that V_{te} becomes a reasonable estimate of the basolateral potential V_{bl} (Eq. A1.16 in Appendix 1). For example, in the turtle colon, Germann et al. (33) were able to characterize two different conductances for K across the basolateral membrane using the amphotericin-B permeabilized epithelium. This approach has also been used mostly in flat epithelia rather than renal tubules.

IMPEDANCE ANALYSIS

Impedance analysis permits estimation of the electrical properties of individual membranes using transepithelial measurements (11). In principle, transepithelial impedance can be measured from the time course of the response to any electrical perturbation. In practice, it is usually obtained either under "current-clamp" conditions, using sine wave current perturbations at different frequencies, or under voltage-clamp conditions by applying voltage perturbations. Since the apical and basolateral membranes will each have an associated complex impedance that depends on frequency, it is possible to distinguish contributions from the two membranes if they have very different time constants ($\tau = RC$, where R is the resistance and C the capacitance).

Typically four parameters (consisting of the amplitudes and time constants of the two membrane components) are measured to fit a circuit with five parameters (resistance and capacitance of apical and basolateral membranes and the paracellular resistance). To fully solve the system one model parameter (e.g., the paracellular resistance) usually must be determined independently.

Impedance analysis has also been used to derive detailed information about the paracellular pathway, including the distribution of resistance across tight junctions and along intercellular spaces. In this regard, it has been used to estimate individual resistances and capacitances of the apical and basolateral membranes of flat epithelial sheets obtained from frog skin, amphibian and mammalian urinary bladder, colon, and cultured epithelial cells (2, 10, 133, 140). The elegance of the technique is that it is noninvasive, yielding information about individual membranes without the need for intracellular probes or electrodes. Because of the requirement of uniform currents or voltage fields, its application to renal tubules has been very limited (50, 127). A complete discussion is beyond the scope of this chapter.

Conclusions

Many important epithelial properties can be determined from transepithelial measurements alone. In fact, the original Koefoed-Johnsen/Ussing model for Na transport by the frog skin was based entirely on transepithelial electrical and flux measurements and the ingenious use of special simplifying conditions. Even though microelectrodes are now routinely used to characterize many cell parameters, a number of important physical and thermodynamic properties of epithelia are still estimated from transepithelial measurements, particularly in renal tissues. These include the magnitude and selectivity of the paracellular shunt pathway, the ion selectivity of cell membranes (qualitatively in most instances) and the currents and EMFs associated with active transepithelial transport. On the other hand, the quantitative description of membrane properties requires detailed intracellular measurements to specifically characterize the apical and basolateral membrane components as well as the contribution of the paracellular pathway. These measurements will be discussed in the next section.

INTRACELLULAR MEASUREMENTS

Intracellular measurements with voltage-sensitive and ion-sensitive microelectrodes permit a more detailed evaluation of individual membrane parameters than do transepithelial measurements. This has been essential to our understanding of ion transport in epithelia. Three important membrane characteristics that are amenable to study with intracellular techniques are (1) ionic selectivity, (2) membrane conductance, and (3) estimation of pump current. Although there are significant differences in the methodology of these measurements depending on the particular tissue involved, much of the underlying theory is similar in both flat epithelia and renal tubules. The emphasis of this section will be on describing the simplest and most straightforward methods for evaluation of single-membrane parameters with emphasis on renal epithelia, although much of the theory is applicable to flat epithelia as well. In this regard, no attempt

is made to provide an exhaustive historical review of the many procedures that have been used over the years. The techniques described represent what the authors perceive as the most practical methodology for evaluation of *macroscopic* membrane parameters.

Cell Membrane Potentials in Epithelia

An epithelium is a sheet of polarized cells joined together to function as a selective barrier between two compartments. Epithelia not only structurally define two compartments, but also maintain the composition of those compartments via the specific transport of electrolytes, nonelectrolytes and water. The electrical voltage measured across either the apical or basolateral membrane of an epithelium is the sum of the ionic diffusion potentials across the membrane and the voltage drops arising from current flow across the resistance of that membrane. This current flow (depicted by the thick arrow in Fig. 1) arises in part from the differences in membrane ionic diffusion potentials and the sum of epithelial barrier electrical resistances (Appendix 1).

In practice, cell membrane potentials are determined by impaling the cell with fine-tipped glass microelectrodes, filled with a highly conductive electrolyte solution (1 M or 3 M KCl). Uniform filling is often accomplished by starting with glass tubing that contains a thin glass filament, allowing solution to flow smoothly from the back to the tip of the finished electrode. The microelectrode is then mounted on a stable micromanipulator. Given the elasticity of most cell membranes, impalement usually requires a rapid forward movement of the tip that can be accomplished either mechanically or with piezoelectric headstage. Sometimes a high-frequency alternating current is briefly applied to the tip to permit entry into the cell with minimum damage.

A major technical problem with microelectrode measurements is the damage to the cell that may be produced by impalement. For a discussion of this topic see Higgins et al. (55) and Nelson et al. (96). Cell damage can be minimized by utilizing epithelia with large cells (e.g., *Necturus* and *Amphiuma*), and by recording from the basolateral rather than the apical membrane. This will result in less electrical shunting of the membrane potential since in many cases the basolateral membrane has a much lower resistance than the apical membrane and an additional leak conductance at the basal side will have a smaller overall effect (55). Furthermore, epithelia like the proximal tubule, whose cells are electrically coupled, are less sensitive to impalement artifact since the effective cell membrane area is larger. Finally, the use of very fine-tipped micropipettes can minimize membrane damage during intracellular measurements.

Use of microelectrodes to measure cell potential may result in KCl leakage into the cell. Although these tips are extremely small (<0.2 μm), the use of concentrated KCl in the electrode to minimize liquid junction potentials can lead to KCl influx into the cell, alterations in cell composition, and cell swelling (96). Thus, the choice of a filling solution is a trade-off between a concentrated KCl solution, which yields low tip potentials but possible KCl leakage, versus a low-salt pipette solution that results in higher tip potentials but less salt leakage into the cytoplasm.

Intracellular potential can also be measured with relatively large diameter patch-clamp pipettes. In a "whole-cell clamp" experiment, a high-resistance seal is formed between the pipette and the cell membrane. This permits direct electrical contact between the recording electrode and the cell interior with negligible impalement damage. If the amplifier is used in the voltage-clamp mode, the holding potential that reduces the membrane current to zero becomes a good measure of the cell potential. One disadvantage of using the whole-cell clamp to measure cell potential is that the cell is dialyzed with the pipette solution (45). This can sometimes be useful for studying cell regulatory processes, but the exchange of vital cell constituents with the pipette solution may alter both the intracellular ion composition and the normal cell membrane permeabilities.

Evaluation of Individual Membrane Resistances from an Equivalent Circuit Analysis

The simplest technique for determining individual cell membrane resistance is to measure intracellular and transepithelial potential during an experimental maneuver that produces only a single perturbation in the parameters of the equivalent circuit. These techniques have been particularly useful in mammalian proximal tubules where multiple microelectrode impalements are difficult or in nephron segments that are not electrically coupled.

When only one microelectrode is used, the circuit of Fig. 1 must be simplified to permit an indirect evaluation of the cell membrane resistances. This type of reduction is illustrated in Fig. 7 and is permissible when most of the paracellular resistance is contributed by the tight junction resistance (i.e., when $R_{par} \approx R_{tj}$), which is equivalent to the assumption that R_{tj} is much greater than lateral interspace resistance (R_{lis}). This is particularly appropriate for mammalian proximal tubule where basal interdigitations of adjacent cells greatly reduce the lateral space resistance and most of the paracellular resistance is contributed by the tight junction resistance.

The circuit of Fig. 7A can be further reduced to the simpler form of Fig. 7B by defining an effective basolateral EMF (E_{bl}^*) and an effective basolateral resistance (R_{bl}^*) as described in Appendix 1. Although the electromotive forces or EMFs (E_{ap}, E_{bl}, E_{par}) in the circuit cannot be measured directly, the potential differences across each barrier can be measured with intracellular or transepithelial electrodes. These are defined as transepithelial potential (lumen to bath), V_{te}; apical cell membrane potential (lumen to cell), V_{ap}; and basolateral potential (cell to bath), V_{bl}.

An important consequence of the circulating epithelial current in Fig. 7 is that alterations in any of the electrical parameters on one side of the cell will produce changes in the measured electrical potentials on the contralateral side.

This actually provides an indirect method for evaluating those resistances that remain constant during a change in loop current, I. Individual cell membrane resistances R_{bl}^* and R_{ap} can be evaluated by any experimental maneuver that changes only the parameters at one membrane. For example, rapid addition of amiloride or glucose to the apical solution presumably alters only the resistance and/or the EMF of the apical membrane by blocking Na channels or stimulating Na–glucose cotransport, respectively.

Amiloride causes a hyperpolarization of V_{bl} by both increasing the measured apical resistance (R_{ap}) and decreasing the contribution of the Na gradient to the value of E_{ap} (see Eq. A1.7 in Appendix 1). On the other hand, addition of glucose to the luminal solution depolarizes V_{bl} by stimulating Na–glucose cotransport, which effectively increases both the apical Na conductance and the relative contribution of the Na gradient to the apical diffusion potential. Since the primary effect of both amiloride and glucose occurs at the apical membrane, the ratio of basolateral to apical resistance is directly related to the measured ratio of basolateral to transepithelial voltage deflections according to Eq. 14, which applies for addition of either apical-side amiloride or apical-side glucose.

$$\frac{R_{bl}^*}{R_{tj}} = -\frac{\Delta V_{bl}}{\Delta V_{te}} = \beta \qquad (14)$$

This equation implicitly assumes that neither glucose nor amiloride affect the paracellular pathway and that the potential measurements can be performed before any changes in cell composition have occurred that would affect E_{ap}, E_{bl}, and R_{bl}.

Similarly, measurement of the ratio of apical to transepithelial potential change following addition of barium to the basolateral solution permits estimation of the apical membrane resistance via Eq. 15.

$$\frac{R_{ap}}{R_{tj}} = -\frac{\Delta V_{ap}}{\Delta V_{te}} = \frac{\Delta V_{bl}}{\Delta V_{te}} - 1 \equiv \alpha \qquad (15)$$

Again, it has been assumed that basolateral application of barium has no effect on the paracellular pathway and that the measurement can be performed rapidly enough to avoid changes in cell composition.

Finally, in cases where it is feasible to make changes on only one side of the epithelium, the voltage divider ratio can be used instead of either Eq. 14 or 15. When current is injected into the tubule lumen via the perfusion pipette, a certain fraction of that current will cross the apical and basolateral cell membrane in series, producing voltage deflections ΔV_{ap} and ΔV_{bl}. If the lateral and basal resistances of Fig. 1 are combined into a single effective resistance R_{bl}^* (defined in Appendix 1, Eq. A1.4), the ratio of apical to basolateral resistance during transepithelial injection of current is given by the following equation:

$$\gamma = \frac{R_{ap}}{R_{bl}^*} = \frac{\Delta V_{ap}}{\Delta V_{bl}} = \frac{\Delta V_{te}}{\Delta V_{bl}} - 1 \qquad (16)$$

A

B

Basolateral side

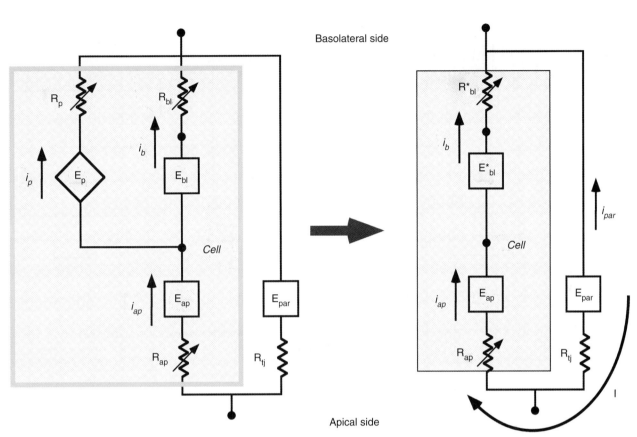

Apical side

FIGURE 7 A. Reduced form of the general equivalent circuit, where the lateral resistive network has been neglected because most of the paracellular resistance is assumed to reside at the tight junction (i.e., $R_{tj} >> R_{lis}$). This situation applies in a number of epithelia and greatly simplifies the equivalent circuit. B. Reduced circuit in which the parallel diffusive and active transport paths across the basolateral membrane have been combined into an effective basolateral EMF (E_{bl}^*) and an effective basolateral resistance (R_{bl}^*). I direction of positive net circulating current under open-circuit conditions.

The term γ is sometimes referred to as the voltage divider ratio. An alternative to Eq. 16 is to define the "fractional resistance" of the apical (fR_{ap}) or basolateral membranes (fR_{bl}), according to Eqs. 17a and 17b.

$$fR_{ap} = \frac{R_{ap}}{R_{ap} + R_{bl}^*} = 1 - \frac{\Delta V_{bl}}{\Delta V_{te}} \qquad (17a)$$

$$fR_{bl}^* = \frac{R_{bl}^*}{R_{ap} + R_{bl}^*} = \frac{\Delta V_{bl}}{\Delta V_{te}} \qquad (17b)$$

Since γ, α, β, and R_{te} are all measured quantities, the individual resistances , R_{ap}, and R_{tj}, can be evaluated by using any three of the following four expressions: Eqs. 14–16 and A1.5.

An example of these methods is illustrated by the experiment depicted in Fig. 8 (3). In this experiment, changes in transepithelial (V_{te}) and basolateral potential (V_{bl}) are shown during addition of 1 mM barium to the bath (Fig.

8A), followed by addition of 8 mM glucose to the lumen (Fig. 8B). The superimposed smaller deflections are due to periodic current injection for evaluating γ from Eq. 16.

In both these experiments, ΔV_{bl} and ΔV_{te} were taken as the initial changes in voltage resulting from a particular maneuver. For example, in the barium experiment, only changes in V_{bl} and R_{bl}^* were presumed to occur, and ΔV_{bl} was taken as the difference between the baseline V_{bl} and the V_{bl} at the inflection point (asterisk). The origin of the slow secondary depolarization of V_{bl} in Fig. 8A is not known.

The methods described here have been used to determine individual cell membrane resistance in mammalian proximal tubule. Some of these results are summarized in Table 3. Although there are some differences in the absolute values of cell resistances, there is general agreement that in proximal tubule the resistance of the cellular pathway is between 20 and 30 times higher than the resistance of the shunt pathway. This factor is even higher in amphibian proximal tubule.

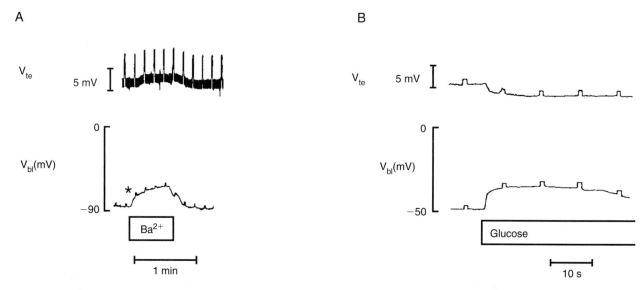

FIGURE 8   Effect of barium and glucose on membrane voltages in rabbit proximal convoluted tubule. A. Reversible depolarization of both the transepithelial (V_{te}) and the basolateral membrane potential (V_{bl}) produced by addition of barium to the basolateral side of isolated proximal tubules. B. Simultaneous depolarization of the transepithelial (V_{te}) and hyperpolarization of the basolateral membrane potential (V_{bl}) produced by addition of glucose to the apical side of isolated proximal tubules. In both panels, the superimposed periodic voltage deflections were produced by current pulses injected through the perfusion pipette. (From Bello-Reuss E. Cell membrane and paracellular resistances in isolated renal proximal tubules from rabbit and *Ambystoma J Physiol* 1986;370:25–38.)

TABLE 3   Cell Membrane Resistances in Mammalian Tubules (Ωcm^2 Epithelium)

Segment	Apical Resistance	Basolateral Resistance	Shunt Resistance	Method	Species	Reference
PCT	238	68	16	Apical glucose Basal Ba[21] Voltage divider	Rabbit (PCT)	3
PCT	118	39	8	Apical glucose Voltage divider	Rabbit (PCT)	76
PCT	255	92	5	Apical glucose Voltage divider	Rat	26
TALH	88	47	47	Apical high K^+, Ba^{2+} Voltage divider	Rabbit	41
TALH	57	21	37	Apical Ba^{2+} Voltage divider	Mouse	40
CCD	149	123	166	Apical Ba^{2+} Voltage divider	Rabbit	99
CCD	57	80	230	Apical amiloride, Ba^{2+} Voltage divider	Rabbit	70
OMCD	707	176	393	Apical glucose Voltage divider	Rabbit	69, 71
Urinary bladder	3,700–154,000	5,000–10,300	6,500–38,000	Apical amiloride Voltage divider Cell cable	Rabbit	81

CCD, cortical collecting duct; OMCD, outer medullary collecting duct; PCT, proximal convoluted tubule; TALH, thick ascending limb of Henle's loop.

Adapted from Koeppen B. Electrophysiology of ion transport in renal tubule epithelia. *Semin Nephrol* 1987;7:37–47.

Determination of individual membrane parameters from Eqs. 14–16 involves certain practical problems. These methods require measurement of ΔV_{te} and ΔV_{bl} in the same tubule at the same axial distance along its length. As indicated in Fig. 8, the small magnitude of the change in transepithelial potential renders the two ratios α and β in Eqs. 14 and 15 particularly susceptible to errors in ΔV_{te}. Measurements of ΔV_{te} obtained by advancing a microelectrode into the lumen are unreliable because damage to the epithelium can produce artificially low values of ΔV_{te}. Since transepithelial potential is measured only at the perfusion or collection ends of the tubule, the value of ΔV_{te} must be calculated from the electrotonic voltage spread along the tubule using a terminated cable analysis (see Transepithelial Measurements section).

Evaluation of Individual Membrane Resistances Using Multiple Intracellular Recordings

In the relatively large cells of amphibian proximal tubule (30 μm diameter), direct electrical measurement of cell membrane resistance is possible. Exploiting the property of electrical coupling between adjacent proximal cells (44), it is possible to pass current from an intracellular microelectrode through an annular syncytium, with an outer specific resistance of R_{bl}^* and an inner specific resistance of R_{ap}. This cannot be done in nephron segments like the collecting duct where adjacent cells are not electrically coupled (24).

In practice, a segment of isolated tubule is cannulated at both the perfusion and collection sides. External Sylgard pipettes are unnecessary for electrical isolation if the perfusion and constriction pipettes are carefully matched to produce a tight electrical seal. Elimination of the Sylgard insulation system permits a significant length of tubule to rest firmly on the bottom of the chamber (119). This is essential for long-term microelectrode recording from individual cells. Mechanical stability during the recording can be further enhanced by using an optically transparent biological adhesive (Cell-Tak, BD Biosciences Labware, Bedford, MA) to attach the tubule to the bottom of the chamber (121).

The use of cellular cable analysis to evaluate the individual resistances R_{bl}^*, R_{ap}, and R_{tj} still depends on the definition of transepithelial resistance (Eq. A1.5) and the "voltage-divider" ratio (Eq. 16); both were discussed in the Cell Membrane Potentials in Epithelia section. However, instead of relying on the ratio $\Delta V_{bl}/\Delta V_{te}$, obtained during application of barium or amiloride, the parallel resistance of the cell layer (R_z) is computed directly from the electrotonic voltage spread along the double core cable, where R_z is defined by Eq. 18:

$$1/R_z = 1/R_{ap} + 1/R_{bl}^* \qquad (18)$$

In practice, R_z is evaluated by injecting current I_o into the cell layer at $x = 0$ via a microelectrode and measuring the voltage deflection ΔV_x at two or more locations x, downstream from the injection site. The arrangement of microelectrodes is illustrated in Fig. 2. If x is at least twice the

diameter of the tubule, the electrotonic voltage spread along the cable will be given by Eq. 19, where λ_c is the cellular length constant of the tubule (120):

$$Ln[\Delta V_x] = Ln\left[\frac{R_z I_o}{4\pi r \lambda_c}\right] - \frac{1}{\lambda_c}x \qquad (19)$$

The best fit for the two unknown parameters λ_c and R_z is determined by evaluating Eq. 19 at a number of locations along the tubule. The radius of the tubule, r_o, is measured with an optical micrometer. Combining Eqs. 16, 18, and A1.5, the individual membrane resistances R_{ap}, R_{bl}^*, and R_{tj} are uniquely determined by the two parameters R_z and γ, and the measured value of R_{te} according to Eqs. 20–22:

$$R_{ap} = R_z\left[1 + \gamma\right] \qquad (20)$$

$$R_{bl}^* = R_z\left[1 + \frac{1}{\gamma}\right] \qquad (21)$$

$$R_{tj} = \frac{R_{te}[R_{bl}^* + R_{ap}]}{R_{ap} + R_{bl}^* - R_{te}} \qquad (22)$$

The transepithelial resistance of the tubule, R_{te}, is determined by passing current and measuring voltage through a doubled barreled perfusion pipette according to the methods described in the section Transepithelial Measurements and Fig. 2.

In amphibian proximal tubule, most measurements of individual cell resistances have been performed using a cellular cable analysis with two or more intracellular microelectrodes. On the other hand, in mammalian tubules, the method of relative voltage deflections (Eqs. 14 and 15) has been used exclusively. However, in *Ambystoma* proximal tubule, a direct comparison of the two methods has been made under similar conditions. These results are summarized in the first two rows of Table 4. As indicated, the absolute values of resistance are quite close considering the propagation of errors that occur with both types of measurements. The remaining rows of Table 4 summarize additional resistances measurements in amphibian renal epithelia.

As with the mammalian proximal tubule, the ratio of shunt to cell resistance clearly establishes the amphibian proximal tubule as a "leaky" epithelium. In contrast, the *Necturus* urinary bladder (a "tight" epithelium) possesses a shunt resistance that is several times larger than the cell resistance pathway. Neither the diluting segment nor the collecting tubule of the *Amphiuma* fall neatly into the "tight" or "leaky" category since both of these segments have cellular and paracellular resistances that are on the same order of magnitude. Interestingly, both the diluting segment and collecting duct have higher shunt resistances and lower cellular resistances than the corresponding membrane of the proximal tubule. Mammalian collecting ducts and diluting segments also have higher shunt resistances than mammalian proximal tubules although differences in cell resistance are less dramatic along the mammalian nephron.

TABLE 4   Cell Membrane Resistances in Amphibian Tubules ($\Omega\,cm^2$ Epithelium)

Segment	Apical Resistance	Basolateral Resistance	Shunt Resistance	Method	Species	Reference
Proximal tubule	2509	683	71	Apical glucose Basal barium Voltage divider	*Ambystoma*	3
Proximal tubule	2305	591	53	2 electrode Cable analysis	*Ambystoma*	90, 120
Proximal tubule	6957	2399	267	2 electrode Cable analysis	*Necturus*	44
Proximal tubule	2700	1900	—	2 electrode Cable analysis	Frog	92
Proximal tubule	1350	2100	166	2 electrode Cable analysis	*Triturus*	62
Dilute segment[a]	550	219	306	2 electrode Cable analysis	*Amphiuma*	100
Collecting tubule	154	192[b]	454	Voltage clamp Voltage divider	*Amphiuma*	58, 59
Urinary bladder	9000–65,000	1000–7000	100,000	Apical amiloride Voltage divider	*Necturus*	30

[a]These measurements assumed that the *Amphiuma* diluting segment has only one cell type.

[b]The basolateral conductance of this segment is strongly inward rectifying and quoted value applies only at a membrane potential of –60mV.

The resistances quoted for the *Amphiuma* diluting segment in Table 4 assumed a single cell type throughout the cable analysis (100). This greatly simplified the calculation of membrane resistance. Unfortunately, subsequent experiments indicated that this nephron segment actually consists of two cell types with dissimilar conductive properties (42). One cell type has a high basal K and Cl conductance (HBC), whereas the other cell type (LBC) has a low basolateral conductance for both ions (42). There is also some evidence that mammalian TALH may exhibit a certain amount of cell heterogeneity as well (41). Since it is unlikely that various cell types in the same nephron segment are directly coupled to each other, a unique value of cell membrane resistance cannot be determined from cable analysis on these nephron segments unless all recordings are made from the same cell type.

The cellular cable equations (Eqs. 18 and 19) were originally derived for in situ proximal tubules, in which the cables are effectively infinite in length (44). However, they should be reasonably valid for isolated perfused tubules as long as the voltage-recording microelectrodes are several tubule diameters from either end of the tubule. Under these conditions the electrotonic voltage spread would be effectively the same as for an infinite cable. The problem of "cross-talk" or interactions between the transepithelial and cellular cables has been suggested as a source of error in these measurements (1). The complication of cable–cable interactions would only be significant if current injected into the cell layer leaks into the lumen and then re-enters the cell layer at some point downstream. A thorough analysis by Guggino et al. (44) for *Necturus* proximal tubule suggests that cross talk will be negligible if intracellular voltage deflections ΔV_x are recorded at locations where $x > \lambda_c$.

Evaluation of cell membrane resistance via Eqs. 14–16 is only as accurate as the equivalent circuit of Fig. 7. An important aspect of this electrical model is the assumption that the tight junction constitutes the principal resistance of the paracellular pathway, or $R_{par} \oplus R_{tj}$. This is probably true in tight epithelia like the urinary bladder, where the lateral intercellular space has a negligible resistance compared to that of the tight junction. However, the low transepithelial resistance of the proximal tubule raises the possibility that the resistivity of free solution in the lateral space contributes significantly to overall shunt resistance. In this case, evaluation of the divider ratio is complicated by the lateral resistive network shown in Fig. 1. Current flow through a distributed network of this kind will cause the measured value of $\Delta V_{ap}/\Delta V_{bl}$ to *underestimate* the actual value of R_{ap}/R_{bl}^* by an amount that depends on the ratio of lateral space resistance, R_{lis}, to paracellular resistance, R_{par} (see Fig. 9).

As illustrated in Fig. 9, the larger the contribution of the fluid-filled interspace to the total paracellular resistance (i.e., the larger the ratio R_{lis}/R_{par}), the more the measured voltage ratio will underestimate the actual resistance ratio, γ. In epithelia where the paracellular resistance is essentially determined by the resistance of the tight junction and $R_{lis}/R_{par} < 0.01$, the resistance ratio (γ) will be correctly given by Eq. 16. On the other hand, if the lateral interspace is long and narrow and constitutes a non-negligible electrical resistance, R_{par} will be related to R_{te} according to a complicated function (see Eqs. 31–40 in Boulpaep and Sackin [6] with $R_3 = R_{par}$). As can be seen in the figure, significant deviations from Eq. 16 occur even if R_{lis} is as little as 10% of R_{par}. A detailed analysis regarding the effect of lateral resistive networks on measurement of cell membrane resistance has been has also been presented by Weber and Frömter (136).

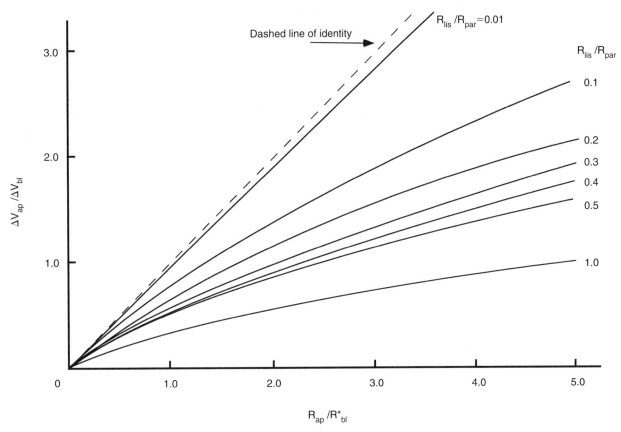

FIGURE 9   Relationship between the measured voltage divider ratio ($\Delta V_{ap}/\Delta V_{bl}$) and the actual ratio of apical to basolateral resistance (R_{ap}/R_{bl}) at different values of fractional interspace resistance (R_{lis}/R_{par}). Negligible values of R_{lis} result in the voltage divider ratio being a good measure of R_{ap}/R_{bl} (line of identity). In epithelia where R_{lis} is a significant fraction of the paracellular resistance, the voltage divider ratio is not a good measure of the apical to basal resistance ratio. (From Boulpaep EL, Sackin H. Electrical analysis of intraepithelial barriers. *Curr Top Membr Transp* 1980;13:169–197.).

Determination of individual cell membrane resistances involves a number of technical difficulties. In addition to those indicated previously, positioning of the intracellular electrodes is particularly tedious. If the first cell voltage electrode is within one cell length constant of the cell current electrode, there may be significant cross talk between cell and luminal cables. If the second cell voltage electrode is too far from the current injection electrode, the size of the deflection will be immeasurably small. Use of a third voltage recording electrode gives a better definition of the electrotonic voltage spread but is often impractical. If sequential voltage impalements are used, the first recording should be made at the farthest distance from the current electrode. In this manner intracellular recording at $x = L_1$ will be insignificantly affected by cell damage at $x = L_2$, as long as $L_2 > L_1$, and the current electrode is maintained at $x = 0$ (see Fig. 2).

A significant source of error in cellular cable measurements arises from voltage-dependent membrane conductances. Patch-clamp experiments have indicated that a number of renal channels are voltage-gated. The specific magnitude and type of gating varies with each nephron segment. Since the current injections used for determination of cell membrane resistance often produce 10- to 15-mV voltage deflections across the basolateral membrane, the conductance could be affected by the process of measurement. One solution to this difficulty has been to take the average value of ΔV_{bl} determined from both positive and negative going currents.

Estimates of Basolateral Membrane Resistance from Voltage Clamping

The isolated perfused tubule of Fig. 2 can (in principle) be shortened to a length that results in a homogeneous current flow across the epithelium during a transepithelial voltage clamp. If, at the same time, a microelectrode is also inserted into one of the cells, the resulting basolateral voltage can be recorded as a function of transcellular current. This provides a simple method for determination of basolateral resistance from the current voltage (I–V) relation of the membrane. Transcellular current at any voltage is calculated as the difference between the total transepithelial current and the current remaining after block of the apical membrane conductance. This method would be difficult to use with leaky epithelia since most of the current injected into the lumen from the perfusion pipette would traverse the paracellular path. Transcellular current would then be the difference between two large currents (total minus paracellular) and small errors in either of these quantities would have a profound effect on the calculated transcellular current.

In the amphibian collecting tubule, amiloride has been used to identify transcellular current as the amiloride-sensitive component of the epithelial current. Under these conditions, an inward rectifying *I–V* relation was obtained for the basolateral membrane of *Amphiuma* collecting tubule (58). At cell potentials between −50 mV and −80 mV, the resulting specific resistance of the basolateral membrane was 151 Ωcm^2 in this preparation. In addition to the problem that transcellular current is determined as the difference between two large numbers, effects of the lateral resistive network of Fig. 1 become more significant at the high current densities required in these experiments. During voltage clamp, an unknown fraction of the amiloride-insensitive current could re-enter the cell from the interspace via the lateral network and contribute to the observed basolateral voltage. This might distort the measured *I–V* relation of the basolateral membrane. The technical difficulty of voltage clamping individual nephron segments may explain why it has only been attempted in few instances (50, 57, 126).

EVALUATION OF ION SELECTIVITIES FROM ION SUBSTITUTION EXPERIMENTS

One of the most important membrane properties that can be determined from electrophysiological measurements is membrane selectivity. The basic equation that defines the transference number of the membrane for ion *x* is obtained by rearranging Eq. 3 to yield the following expression:

$$t_x = -\frac{\Delta E}{\dfrac{RT}{z_x F} Ln\left[\dfrac{[X^{expt}]}{[X^{con}]}\right]} \tag{23}$$

Equation 23 can then be used to evaluate the ion selectivity of the individual epithelial membranes from changes in the total EMF ΔE (experimental [expt] − control [con]) produced by replacement of a specific *apical* ion *X* by an impermeant ion. In Eq. 23, X^{expt} and X^{con}, respectively, refer to the extracellular ion concentration of the apical solution under expt or con conditions. If ΔE is produced by a change in *basolateral* composition, the transference numbers would be calculated from the negative of Eq. 23. As indicated in Fig. 7B, the circulating current, *I*, prevents a simple equivalence between the measured change in potential difference (ΔV) and the actual change in the EMF of the membrane (ΔE). The effects of circular current flow on the actual changes in EMF resulting from ion substitution, ΔE are described in detail in Appendix 2. These equations are essential for the evaluating membrane selectivities from ion substitution experiments.

The partial conductance of the membrane for any ion *x* (G_x) can be determined from the transference number for the membrane and the total ionic conductance of that membrane (G_{tot}), according to the following expression:

$$G_x = t_x \cdot G_{tot} \tag{24}$$

There is no simple relation between the partial ionic *conductance* and the *permeability* of the membrane to a particular ion. However, it is possible to develop a general relation between the conductance and the permeability of a particular ion (*X*). This is given by Eq. 25, where $\langle X \rangle$ is a weighted average of the concentrations of *X* on both sides of the membrane. Its value depends on the particular assumptions about ion permeation across the membrane.

$$G_x \approx P_x \frac{z^2 F^2}{RT} \langle X \rangle \tag{25}$$

In the constant field assumption, $\langle X \rangle$ is a complicated function of both the membrane potential and the ion concentrations on both sides of the membrane. Explicit forms of Eq. 25 are discussed in Appendix 3. However, if the membrane is assumed to be permeant to only three ions—Na, K, and Cl—the permeability ratios P_{Na}/P_K and P_{Cl}/P_K can be evalua-ted from a two-parameter fit to the general form of the Goldman–Hodgkin–Katz equation (139). This procedure has not been used extensively for renal epithelia because of uncertainties in a simultaneous evaluation of P_{Na}/P_K and P_{Na}/P_{Cl}.

On the other hand, if the membrane is primarily selective to two rather than three ions, a closed form expression can be obtained for the permeability ratio, as follows:

$$\frac{P_K}{P_{Na}} = \frac{[Na]_O - [Na]_i \exp\left(\dfrac{E_{rev}}{RT/F}\right)}{[K]_i \exp\left(\dfrac{E_{rev}}{RT/F}\right) - [K]_O} \tag{26}$$

In Eq. 26 the term, E_{rev}, is the potential difference, inside (*i*) minus outside (*o*), associated with zero current across the membrane. The principal disadvantage of Eq. 26 for kidney tubules is that determination of E_{rev} requires voltage clamping the individual cell membranes of the epithelium. So far this has really only been accomplished for the *Amphiuma* collecting tubule (57).

Since the specific conductance of a membrane for ion *X* is generally a function of the concentration of that ion (Eq. 25), the values of t_x obtained from Eq. 23 only apply to the concentration range over which the ion replacement is actually performed. Consequently, any determination of normal transference numbers requires that the ionic replacement $X^{con} - X^{expt}$ be as small as possible but still produce a measurable ΔE. On the other hand, the permeability ratio of Eq. 26 should (in theory) be less dependent on external ion concentrations.

Estimation of Renal Na/K Pump Current and Electrogenic Potential

The 3Na/2K stoichiometry and electrogenic nature of the Na/K pump has been demonstrated in a number of nonepithelial tissues (15, 35). Most studies on red cells (32, 112), squid axon (114) and Purkinje fibers (16) indicate a fairly consistent Na/K coupling ratio of 3/2 for the Na,K-ATPase. This electrogenicity not only causes the pump to contribute to total membrane potential but also requires that the pump itself be dependent on membrane potential.

Mullins and Noda (95) and Ascher (cited in Thomas [129]) have derived an expression for the electrogenic contribution to the membrane potential of nerve and muscle cells, which predicts a steady-state contribution of no larger than about 11 mV. This theory depends on the observation that electroneutrality conditions on symmetric cells require that there be no net macroscopic current under open-circuit, steady-state conditions. The estimate of 11 mV maximal electrogenic hyperpolarization also depends on the assumption that the membrane permeabilities are voltage independent, which is somewhat of an approximation, even for nonexcitable tissues.

In epithelial tissues, where current circulates around a cellular and paracellular path (see Fig. 7), the electrogenic contribution to the membrane potential may be larger than in symmetric cells, but it is also more difficult to quantify. Early estimates of pump current and electrogenic potential in epithelial tissues were determined by comparing the observed change in basolateral potential ΔV_{bl} to the potential changes predicted from the measured ion gradients and electrical resistances, during rapid return of K to the basolateral solution (120) or application of cardiac glycosides (57, 59). These experiments clearly demonstrated net transfer of charge by the pump, but uncertainty about the potassium concentration in unstirred layers outside the cell made it difficult to determine pump stoichiometry from these types of experiments.

In general, the calculation of the electrogenic potential in epithelial tissues requires explicit knowledge of both membrane and pump resistances, which may themselves be a function of pump activity (see Appendix 4). This significantly complicates the situation, and the electrogenicity of the pump is better characterized by evaluating its I–V relation than by evaluating its contribution to the open-circuit potential.

Since electrogenicity requires that pump current be sensitive to membrane potential, the I–V relation for the pump must intersect the voltage axis at some reversal potential E_p. Intuitively, the reversal potential of the pump should correspond to the membrane potential against which the pump can no longer translocate a net charge (i.e., 3 Na for 2 K). The value of E_p can be calculated from Eq. 27 using estimates of the free energy of ATP hydrolysis (E_{ATP}) and the concentration work involved in moving m sodium ions (mE_{Na}) and n potassium ions (nE_K) per molecule of ATP split (14). Thus:

$$E_p = EMF_{pump} = \frac{E_{ATP} + mE_{Na} - nE_K}{m - n} \quad (27)$$

where E_{ATP} is the free energy of ATP hydrolysis (about -600 mV for $m - n = 1$, from DeWeer [14]), and E_{Na} and E_K, are, respectively, the Na and K Nernst potentials across the membrane. For amphibian tubules, E_{Na} is about 55 mV and E_K is about -80 mV at room temperature. According to Eq. 27, the predicted value of E_p is about -275 mV for a net translocation of one ($m - n$) positive charge. This value of E_p corresponds to the reversal potential of the current-voltage relation for the pump.

The existence of a pump reversal potential defined by Eq. 27 provides no information about the sensitivity of pump current to membrane voltage. This sensitivity is determined by the specific shape of the current-voltage $(I$–$V)$ relation of the pump. For example, if the pump I–V relation exhibits a low angle slope in the region of normal membrane potential, the pump would be best represented as a (Norton equivalent) constant current source. On the other hand, if the I–V relation is linear between zero voltage and the pump reversal potential, the pump would be best represented as a (Thevenin equivalent) constant voltage source (Figs. 1 and 7). Four examples of I–V relations for the Na,K-ATPase are illustrated in Fig. 10.

These pump current-voltage relations were determined by measuring either the strophanthidin (A, C) or the ouabain (B, D)-sensitive currents at different voltages. Figures 10A and B are I–V relations from symmetric cell preparations whereas Figs. 10C and D were measured in renal epithelia. In both isolated guinea-pig ventricular myocytes (31) and *Xenopus* oocytes (113), pump current is linearly dependent on membrane voltage with a reversal potential of at least -150 mV. Saturation of current, with decreasing slope, was only evident at positive membrane potentials.

On the other hand, voltage-clamp studies in amphibian (*Amphiuma*) collecting tubules (57) indicate a curvilinear I–V relation (Fig. 10C), which would imply that (in this tissue) the Na/K pump behaves as a constant current source at normal membrane potentials (-20 mV to -75 mV). Differences in the I–V curves of Fig. 10A through C, may indicate true distinctions between Na pumps of various preparations, or may simply reflect differences in experimental technique. The final I–V relation (Fig. 10D) indicates that the pump current in the CCD, like that of symmetric cells, is sensitive to voltage in the physiological range.

The variability in the shape of the I–V relations for the Na,K-ATPase (Fig. 10) implies some uncertainty as to whether the Na pump of a particular tissue behaves more like a constant current or a constant voltage source. Nonetheless, we have chosen to represent the Na pump in the equivalent circuits of Figs. 1 and 7 as a voltage source (E_p) in series with an internal resistance (R_p), because this is a somewhat more general form than a constant-current source.

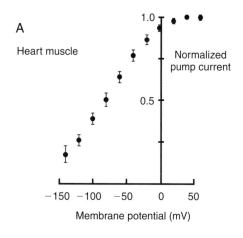

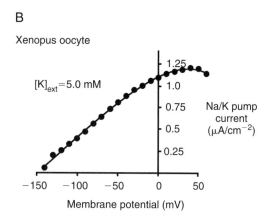

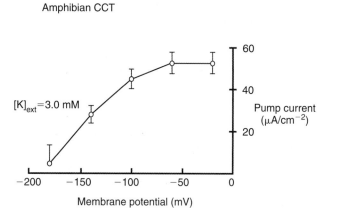

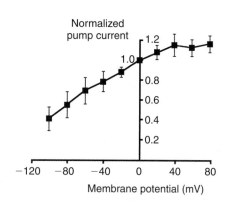

FIGURE 10   A. Current–voltage relation of the cardiac Na,K-ATPase as determined from the strophanthidin-sensitive pump current in a whole-cell recording from a single isolated ventricular myocyte. Dissipative current pathways were blocked with Cs, Cd, TEA, and Ba. (From Gadsby D, Nakao M. The steady-state current-voltage relationship of the Na/K pump in guinea pig ventricular myocytes. *J Gen Physiol* 1989;94:511–537.) B. Current–voltage relation for the Na/K pump of *Xenopus* oocytes, bathed in a 90-mM Na, 5-mM K solution. Pump current was determined as the difference between current measured at 5 mM external K and current measured in K-free solutions. (From Rakowski RF, Vasilets LA, LaTona J, Schwarz W. A negative slope in the current-voltage relationship of the Na/K pump in *Xenopus* oocytes produced by reduction of external [K]. *J Membr Biol* 1991;121:177–187.) C. Current–voltage relation of the basolateral Na pump of *Amphiuma* collecting tubule as determined from the strophanthidin-sensitive current in short segments of voltage-clamped tubules. (From Horisberger JD, Giebisch G. Intracellular Na and K activities and membrane conductances in the collecting tubule of *Amphiuma*. *J Gen Physiol* 1988;92:643–665.) D. Current–voltage relation of the rat principal cell Na-K ATPase. Ouabain-sensitive currents were normalized to their values at 0 mV. (From Palmer LG, Antonian L, Frindt G. Regulation of the Na-K pump of the rat cortical collecting tubule by aldosterone. *J Gen Physiol* 1993;102:43–57.)

Conclusions

With the use of microelectrodes to record intracellular voltages and voltage changes, it has been possible to characterize renal epithelia according to the equivalent circuit in Fig. 1. Overall conductance of apical and basolateral membranes can be computed, and the contribution of various ions to these conductances can be estimated. Our understanding of the major nephron segments at this level is fairly secure. In the next section we discuss how measurements at the single-channel level have yielded a more detailed description of renal ion transport processes.

PATCH-CLAMP AND SINGLE-CHANNEL ANALYSIS

Defining a Channel

The ability to measure currents through individual ion channels in small "patches" of biological membranes has over the course of the past 25 years increased enormously the type of information that can be gleaned about ion channels and the details of our knowledge of how these transport proteins work. With this technique we can find out how many different types of channels there are in a membrane and how many of each type is present without the need for specific pharmacological agents. It is possible to determine what gene produces a given membrane conductance by comparing the properties of the channels in that membrane with those of the gene product when it is heterologously expressed in another cells type. In other cases a gene can be specifically deleted using genetic techniques and the disappearance of a channel type from the membrane can be followed. The patch-clamp technique can also be very useful to determine what agents or second messengers directly or indirectly regulate ion channels.

An ion channel is defined in physical terms as a membrane protein that forms a continuous pathway for the diffusion of an ion from one side of the membrane to the other. In contrast to active transporters, the direction of movement of the ion is determined by the electrochemical energy difference across the membrane. Unlike more complex "carriers" (including facilitated transporters and co- and countertransporters) a conformation change in the channel protein is not required for the translocation of the ions. This permits ions to move quite quickly through the channels. While cotransporters or exchangers generally have maximal turnover rates of about 10^5/sec, and metabolically driven pumps are even slower, channels can achieve rates of 10^8/sec or more through individual units (56).

Most channels exhibit gating; they switch between distinct open and closed states producing abrupt transitions in current under voltage-clamp conditions. Patch-clamp recording can generally resolve currents of around 10^6/sec or 0.15 pA. Thus the ability to see an individual transport unit using the patch-clamp is a reasonably good operating definition of a channel. Although the appearance of current transitions is a good operational definition of channel activity, this is actually too restrictive since some channels may have a low turnover rate. Nevertheless the definition is a useful one, and most channels that we know about have currents large enough—at least under optimal conditions—to be seen by patch clamp.

Most biologically important channels will also have a density high enough to be observed frequently. For a moderate membrane conductance of 1 mS/cm^2, a single-channel conductance of 40 pS and an open probability of 0.5, the density of channels will be 5×10^7/cm^2 or 0.5/μm^2. If a patch contains 5 μm^2 it will have on the average two to three channels. This simple calculation illustrates that a patch pipette of average diameter will usually contain at least one channel, making this technique a highly efficient method for studying the characteristics of individual ion channels.

High-resolution patch-clamp recording was developed in the early 1980s by Neher, Sackmann, and colleagues (45). The patch methodology consists of four major configurations, three of which can be used to study single channels. As illustrated in Fig. 11, the cell-attached patch consists simply of forming a seal on the surface of a cell and studying the resulting piece of membrane in situ. This is obviously the most physiological condition. The same patch can be excised from the cell membrane forming an inside-

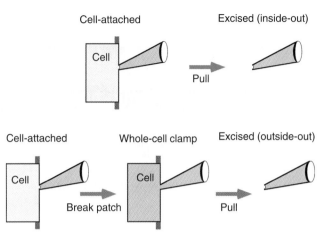

FIGURE 11 Schematic of the patch-clamp technique, applied to the apical membrane of an epithelium. Patch-clamping the basolateral membrane involves a similar procedure. In a cell-attached recording, the cell retains its original composition. Formation of a (conventional) whole-cell clamp causes most of the cell contents to be replaced by pipette solution. Withdrawal of the pipette from the whole-cell configuration often produces an excised, outside-out patch.

out patch in which the cytoplasmic surface of the membrane now faces the bathing medium. This is useful for studying the effects of second messengers and other cytoplasmic components that can be added back to the medium to test for their ability to regulate the channels. A cell-attached patch can also be broken with suction, to form a whole-cell voltage clamp. This is a very convenient method for studying the total current from the entire cell membrane. It is usually not possible to resolve single-channel events in this configuration, although noise analysis of whole-cell recordings can give information about single-channel properties (see Noise Analysis). Finally, withdrawing the pipette from the cell under the whole-cell condition often gives rise to the outside-out configuration in which a new patch is formed with the former extracellular surface of the membrane facing the bath. This can be used to study the effects of hormones, drugs and other ligands that interact with the external face of the channel.

Parameters Measured on Single Channels

SINGLE-CHANNEL CURRENT

The simplest measure of channel electrical activity is the single-channel current (Fig. 12). This is the change in current under voltage-clamp conditions that occurs when a channel opens or closes (Fig. 12A). It is generally quite reproducible for a given set of conditions but varies with ion concentration, temperature and voltage. It is common to characterize channels by their single-channel conductance. This is defined as the slope of the current versus voltage relationship (Fig. 12B). For some channels this conductance is roughly independent of voltage. Many others, however, have highly nonlinear current-voltage relationships. In the

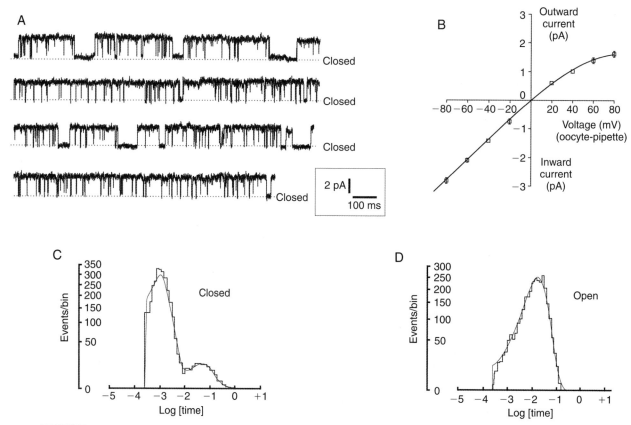

FIGURE 12 Example of single-channel current records and associated analysis. ROMK2 was expressed in *Xenopus* oocytes, and currents were recorded from a single channel in a cell-attached patch. The oocyte membrane potential was reduced close to zero by 100 mM of KCl in the bath. The patch pipette also contained 100 mM of KCl. Neither divalent ions nor specific chelating agents like EDTA were added to the pipette. A. Currents recorded with the membrane potential clamped at −80 mV (cytoplasm relative to pipette). Upward deflections from the closed state correspond to inward K currents. B. Current voltage relation for ROMK2, constructed by recording currents at different (clamped) membrane potentials. C. Closed time distribution at −80 mV, showing two discrete closed states with time constants of 1.2 msec and 47 msec. D. Open time distribution at −80 mV, with mean open time of 19 msec. (From Chepilko S, Zhou H, Sackin H, Palmer LG. Permeation and gating properties of a cloned renal K+ channel. *Am J Physiol* 1995;268: C389–C401.)

latter case, the voltage at which the conductance was measured must always be specified.

Normally, the lowest single channel conductance that can be reliably measured is in the neighborhood of 1pS. This would correspond to measuring a 0.1 pA current at an electrical driving force of 100 mV. Most channels can conduct much larger currents; an upper limit of about 33 pA has been estimated from limitations of diffusion rates (56). Eukaryotes have channels with conductances up to about 400 pS.

Some channels have more than one conducting state. Usually the largest one is chosen as the characteristic conductance and smaller ones are referred to as "sub-conductance" states. Presumably these reflect different conformations of the channel protein. In one special case of the Cl channel CLC-0, the channel has two conductance states with one being precisely half of the other (93). The interpretation of these results was that two identical conducting pores are linked together such that they can close either separately or together. The "full" conductance state represents both pores conducting simultaneously, and the "sub" conductance state

reflects the opening of just one of them. In general, the structural basis of subconductance states—which can have any fraction of the full conductance—is not well understood.

Channel Selectivity

In addition to conductance, the ionic selectivity of the channel can also be determined from single-channel *I–V* plots under appropriate conditions. As in the case of macroscopic currents discussed in the last section, the selectivity of an individual ion channel can be defined and measured in various ways. Inside-out and outside-out patches are particularly well suited for measurements of permeability ratios since the ions on both sides of the membrane can be set to known concentrations.

The ionic transference numbers for a channel can be evaluated using the same relationships discussed previously (see Eq. 23). However, instead of perturbing the concentration of an ion across the membrane, it is simpler in a patch-clamp experiment to change the transmembrane voltage (see Eq. 26). The reversal potential (E_{rev}) is then defined as the voltage at which current flow through the channel changes direction. Measurement of E_{rev} is easiest to interpret in excised patches, where ionic concentrations can be precisely controlled. For measurement of cation versus anion selectivity, dilution conditions are normally used, with a single salt at various concentrations (S_1 and S_2) on both sides of the membrane. For the case of a monovalent salt:

$$E_{rev} = (t_+ - t_-) \frac{RT}{F} Ln \frac{S_1}{S_2} \qquad (28)$$

where t_+ and t_- are the transference numbers for ion movement through the individual pore, and S_1 and S_2 are the salt concentrations on either side of the membrane. This is equivalent to Eq. 12. Thus, if a channel has perfect selectivity for cations (or for anions) the reversal potential will shift by 59 mV for a 10-fold concentration gradient (at 25°C).

The permeability ratio is a common measure of the selectivity among ions of the same charge. In general, the permeability ratio can be computed from a constant-field equation similar to Eq. 26. This equation reduces to a particularly simple and useful form under bi-ionic conditions, with two different salts at the same concentration on either side of the membrane (e.g., NaCl and KCl for an exclusively cation-selective channel):

$$E_{rev} = \frac{RT}{F} Ln \frac{P_x}{P_y} \qquad (29)$$

where P_x and P_y represent the permeabilities of the two ions x and y. A selectivity (permeability ratio) of 10 will give rise to a reversal potential of 59 mV at 25°C. Note that Eq. 29 does not involve the actual salt concentration as long as the concentration of salt X on one side is the same as the concentration of salt Y on the other side.

The relative permeability of a channel to different ions can be measured in cell-attached patches, even when the intracellular ion composition is not precisely known, from changes in the single-channel reversal potential associated with various patch-pipette solutions. When the highly selective renal K channel, ROMK2, is expressed in K-depolarized *Xenopus* oocytes, the single-channel (cell-attached) *I–V* curve intersects the origin at a reversal potential of zero (solid line, Fig. 13). When the same experiment is performed with Rb (rather than K) in the patch pipette, the single-channel *I–V* relation becomes less steep, and the reversal potential shifts in a negative direction by 14 mV (dashed line, Fig. 13). Using Eq. 29, this change in reversal potential implies a permeability ratio, $P_{Rb}/P_K = 0.63$ for ROMK2, expressed in *Xenopus* oocytes.

Ionic selectivity can also be estimated from single-channel conductance ratios determined under various ionic condi-

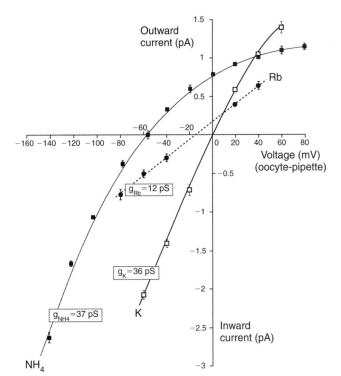

FIGURE 13 Differences between relative conductances and relative permeabilities. When Rb replaces K as the permeating cation of ROMK2, there is a shift in both the reversal potential (x intercept) and single-channel conductance (slope) of the *i–V* relation. The Rb/K permeability ratio calculated from the change in reversal potential was 0.63, which is significantly larger than the Rb/K conductance ratio of 0.36 determined from the inward slopes of the *i–V* curves. Similarly, the NH$_4$/K permeability ratio calculated from the change in reversal potential was 0.12, compared to a NH$_4$/K inward conductance ratio of unity. (From Chepilko S, Zhou H, Sackin H, Palmer LG. Permeation and gating properties of a cloned renal K$^+$ channel. *Am J Physiol* 1995;268:C389–C401.)

tions. These can be compared with selectivity ratios derived from the permeability ratios described previously. In general, the conductance ratio will differ from the permeability ratio, derived from reversal potentials and Eq. 29. For example, using the data of Fig. 13, the ratio of inward Rb conductance to inward K conductances is $g_{Rb}/g_K = 0.36$. This differs significantly from the permeability ratio, $P_{Rb}/P_K = 0.63$ determined from reversal potentials. The discrepancy is even larger when the selectivity of K versus NH$_4$ is considered. Here the shift in reversal potential implies $P_{NH_4}/P_K = 0.1$. However the conductance to NH$_4$ at large negative potentials is equal to or higher than that to K at voltages driving inward currents, giving $g_{NH_4}/g_K > 1$ (9, 105). Discrepancies of this kind may indicate an interaction between the permeant ions and the channel. Rb may bind tightly a particular site within the pore, thus passing slowly through the channel. However this binding will displace K from the channel, also reducing K conductance. The permeability ratio will reflect the relative affinity of the binding site for the two ions. Conversely, NH$_4$ may bind less tightly than K within the conduction pathway.

Open Probability

A second fundamental parameter of an ion channel that can be measured directly using single-channel recording is the open probability (P_o) or the fraction of time the channel spends in the open state. If there is only a single channel in the patch, P_o is determined by dividing the amount of time spent in the open state by the total recording time. P_o can also be measured in patches with more than one channel, provided that the number of channels (N) is known. This requires identification of the states with all channels open and with all channels closed, as discussed in the next section.

A useful measure of overall channel activity in multichannel patches is the mean number of open channels, defined by the next equation:

$$NP_o = \sum_{n=1}^{N} nP_n \qquad (30)$$

where P_n equals (the dwell time with n channels open)/(total time); and N is the total number of channels in the patch. Single channel open probability (P_o) can be readily determined from Eq. 30, if the number (N) of channels in the patch is known. One caveat is that channels whose kinetics are very slow relative to the recording time may not be counted by Eq. 30.

An alternative method for estimating open probability is to compare the total macroscopic current (I) resulting from N channels to the single-channel current (i), using Eq. 31, assuming that the number of channel proteins (N^*) can be measured independently. Under these conditions, the open probability would be given by (P_o^*) as follows:

$$P_o^* = I/N^*i \qquad (31)$$

In *Xenopus* oocytes expressing ENaC channels, P_o^* was estimated to be 0.05 with Eq. 31 (Table 5). This is an order of magnitude lower than the P_o of about 0.5 that was determined by conventional electrical methods (21). Presumably, this difference reflects a large number of silent channels that are electrically invisible and therefore do not contribute to patch-clamp determinations of P_o. Equations 30 and 31

TABLE 5 Open Probability of Na Channels Expressed in *Xenopus* Oocytes

Direct measurement: $P_o = 0.42$	Patch clamp
Macroscopic current: $I = 0.94\ \mu A$ (100 mV)	TEVC
Single-channel current: $i = 0.60$ (−100 mV)	Patch clamp
channel number $N^* = 1.7 \times 10^8$/cell	Ab binding (assume 4 subunits/channel)
Open probability: $P_o^* = I/N^*i = 0.04$	

Data from Firsov D, Schild L, Gautschi I, Merillat AM, Schneeberger E, Rossier BC. Cell surface expression of the epithelial Na channel and a mutant causing Liddle syndrome: a quantitative approach. *Proc Natl Acad Sci U S A* 1996;93(26):15370–15375.

yield comparable estimates of P_o only for the special case where all channels in the membrane are active during the electrical measurements.

For a particular ion X, macroscopic currents (I_x) and conductances (G_x) are related to single channel currents (i_x) and conductances (g_x) according to equations 32 and 33:

$$I_x = NP_o \cdot i_x \qquad (32)$$

$$G_x = NP_o \cdot g_x \qquad (33)$$

Number of Channels

The number of channels in a patch (N) divided by the area of the patch will reflect, on average, the density of channels in the membrane. In principle, N can be observed. In practice not all the possible current levels will be visited during the lifetime of the recording. This is particularly troublesome when the P_o of the channels is either very low or very high. Furthermore, it is not always possible to know if all the states have been visited. Sometimes this problem can be mitigated by maximally activating or deactivating channels at the end of a recording by applying voltage or chemical regulators, but this is not always possible.

If the properties of all channels are identical and are independent of each other, then the percentage of time spent in each state (e.g., one channel open, two channels open, etc.) should follow the binomial distribution. Fitting the measured distribution of times with a binomial function can then be used to estimate channel number (107). This method is less biased than that of counting current levels, as the latter will always be an underestimate. However, the assumption that channels have identical kinetics is probably not always valid.

In some cases the kinetics of the channels can be used to estimate N. If all channels have a high P_o such that the state with all channels open is clearly defined, and a reproducible mean open time t_{open} (see next section) then the mean time that an ensemble of N channels will stay in the all-open state will be t_{open}/N. Therefore, N can be estimated even if the current level with all channels closed is never directly identified (108). A similar procedure can be used on channels with a low P_o if the mean closed time is reproducible. This procedure works only if the channels have a single open (or closed) state (see next section).

The area of patches is also difficult to quantify precisely. When the membrane patch can be seen in the light microscope, it often appears to be drawn a considerable distance into the patch-clamp pipette by the process of seal formation. A typical patch geometry might correspond to a membrane area of about 5 μm^2. Areas estimated from electrical capacitance measurements varied from about 1 μm^2 to over 15 μm^2 (123). The area will depend on both the size of the micropipette and the cell type. Perhaps the surest way of estimating channel density is to combine single channel measurements with a macroscopic measurement. For example, the number of Na channels in the apical membrane

TABLE 6 Computation of Na-Channel Density
in Rat Cortical Collecting Duct

Macroscopic conductance: $I_{Na} = 510$ pA/cell ($V_m = -100$ mV)	Whole-cell clamp
Apical membrane area: $A = 185$ μm^2/cell	Morphological studies
Single channel conductance: $i_{Na} = 0.81$ pA ($V_m = -100$ mV)	Patch clamp
Open probability: $P_o = 0.5$	Patch clamp
Channel density $N = I_{Na}/[A \cdot i_{Na} \cdot P_o]$ $N = 1260$/cell $= 6.8/\mu m^2$	

Data from Frindt G, Masilamani S, Knepper MA, Palmer LG. Activation of epithelial Na channels during short-term Na deprivation. *Am J Physiol* 2001;280:F112–F118; Pácha J, Frindt G, Antonian L, Silver R, Palmer LG. Regulation of Na channels of the rat cortical collecting tubule by aldosterone. *J Gen Physiol* 1993;102:25–42; and Palmer LG, Sackin H, Frindt G. Regulation of Na channels by luminal Na in rat cortical collecting tubule. *J Physiol (Lond)* 1998;509:151–162.

of the rat CCD has been estimated from the whole-cell, amiloride-sensitive conductance and the average single-channel conductance and open probability measured under similar conditions (Table 6).

Open and Closed Times

All channels that open and close can be characterized not only by the percentage of time in the open state (P_o), but also by the mean times spent in these states or, equivalently, the rates of transition between them. The mean lifetimes of the open and closed states can range from less than 1 millisecond to more than 1 second. The lifetimes of a given state are presumed to be exponentially distributed, similar to those of radioactive isotopes. The transition rates can be estimated by plotting the number of open (or closed) events of a given duration as a function of that duration.

In the simplest kinetic scheme, a channel that has just one open and one closed state can be diagrammed as follows:

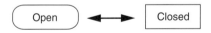

This will result in open- and closed-time histograms that are monotonically decreasing functions of interval length and which can be fitted by a single exponential decay curve.

In practice, the kinetic parameters of a particular channel are usually estimated by fitting the open and closed dwell time distributions with multiple exponential components. In this regard, it has proved most useful to generate event histograms with a logarithmic time axis and a square root transformation of the ordinate. This greatly simplifies interpretation and fitting of distributions that contain multiple exponential components. Examples of two such fitted distributions are shown in Fig. 12C and Fig. 12D, respectively, for the closed and open times of single ROMK2 channels, ex-

pressed in *Xenopus* oocytes. In this type of representation, the peaks of each of the skewed, bell-shaped curves correspond to time constants for the open and closed states of the channel.

Even after the number and duration of closed and open states have been determined, the exact kinetic scheme for the channel may still be ambiguous. Both of the models depicted below are consistent with two closed states and one open state. The first model corresponds to transitions between a single open state and a long-lived closed state (closed 2) that can only be reached by passage through a short-lived closed state (closed 1). In the second model, both the short and long-lived closed states are accessible from the open state. Even with this modest degree of complexity these two patterns cannot readily be distinguished, and the rate constants among the states cannot always be unequivocally derived.

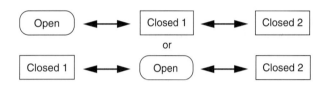

Channels can have multiple open states as well as multiple closed states. In Ca-activated BK channels, for example, models with 50 different states are required to portray channel kinetics (12). As the number of possible open and closed states increases, the difficulty of the analysis increases as well, making it difficult to assign values to individual rate constants or to distinguish alternative kinetic schemes.

The situation can be even more complicated if the channel exhibits bursts of activity that are themselves part of a larger pattern of activity. This behavior requires even more states. Alternatively, a kinetic scheme based on fractals has been proposed (83) on the basis that a burst within a burst pattern will continue to be observed as the time domain over which measurements are made becomes smaller or larger. The relative merits of fractal models as opposed to the more conventional discrete-state models are discussed in detail elsewhere (73, 91, 94). Although the fractal approach is mathematically elegant, it is rarely used in practice since discrete-state models more closely correspond to the simple physical picture of a channel protein having several alternative conformations. It emphasizes, however, that the kinetic models are based on measurable time scales determined by technical limitations. Events of less than 0.1 milliseconds duration are difficult to resolve with current instrumentation. On the other side of the spectrum, it is difficult to record a sufficient number of events of duration more than 10 seconds to analyze accurately.

In some cases multiple gating "modes" have been distinguished from various kinetic states (54, 61). Here a channel will shift abruptly from one pattern of gating to another. This can be thought of as preserving the same open and closed states but changing the rate constants for moving from one state to another. In some cases, changes in gating mode could reflect a chemical modification of a channel, such as a change in the phosphorylation state. However, reversible mode switches have also been observed with channels reconstituted into planar lipid bilayers (98). In these cases the modes must be intrinsic to the channel proteins themselves.

Channel Pharmacology

Another defining characteristic of a channel type is its response to pharmacological agents, usually those which block the channel. If a specific blocker can be identified, it is also quite useful to compare single channel data with macroscopic currents, similar to what was done previously for estimation of channel density. Amiloride is a commonly used blocker for Na channels, whereas Ba, tetraethylammonium (TEA), Cs, quinidine, and lidocaine block K channels. The dihydropyridines and certain divalent cations such as Cd^{+2} block Ca-selective channels, disulfonic stilbenes as

well as a variety of organic anions block Cl channels, and gadolinium inhibits stretch-activated cation channels.

Channel blockers can affect either the open probability of the channel or its (apparent) single-channel conductance. The effect depends on the rates of association and dissociation of the blocker with the channel. In particular, if the off-rate is *slow* relative to the bandwidth of the recording device and the duration of the spontaneous open and closed states the blocking action will be revealed as a new long-lived closed state. Block of the maxi-K channel by Ba^{+2} on the cytoplasmic side is an example of this type of interaction (Fig. 14A). On the other hand, if the blocking action is *fast* relative to the bandwidth it will show up as a decrease in the apparent single channel conductance. Block of the maxi-K channel by extracellular TEA is a good example of this (Fig. 14B).

Often the on-rates for blocking ions are diffusion limited, that is, very roughly in the range of 10^8 sec^{-1} M^{-1}. In this case, the rates of unblocking are inversely related to the affinities of block. For blockers with affinities in the nanomolar range the off-rate will be 10^{-1}/sec. This is a slow block with a mean lifetime of the blocked state of 10 sec-

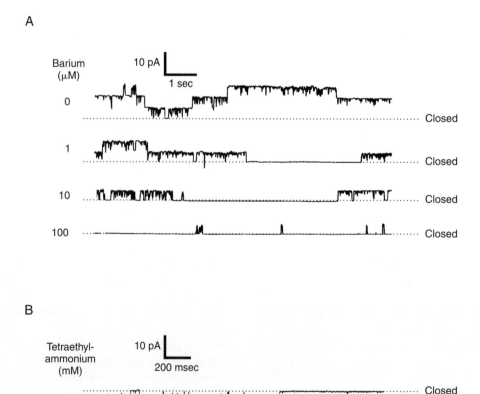

FIGURE 14 Comparison of block of maxi-K channels by a slow blocker, barium, which is effective at micromolar concentrations and reduces the open probability, with block by tetraethylammonium, which is effective at millimolar concentrations and reduces the apparent single-channel conductance. (From Frindt G, Palmer LG. Ca-activated K channels in apical membrane of mammalian CCT, and their role in K secretion. *Am J Physiol* 1987;252:F458–F467.)

onds. For blockers with affinities in the micromolar range the mean lifetime could be 10 milliseconds, corresponding to an intermediate blocking speed in which the blocking events are readily observed in patch-clamp recordings. For blockers with affinities in the millimolar range the mean lifetime of the closed state would be 10 microseconds, too fast to be resolved under most conditions.

There are at least two basic mechanisms of block, regardless of the blocking kinetics. In one, the blocker enters the pore part way and sticks there by binding to a site within the pore. This type of block is usually voltage dependent, particularly if the blocker is charged, since the transmembrane electric field will tend to either pull it into the pore or push it out. Voltage dependence may also arise if the blocker displaces permeant ions from the electric field. Examples of this type of block include those of Mg^{+2} and polyamines in inward-rectifier channels (87), Ba^{+2} on several types of K channels (77) and amiloride on the epithelial Na channel. Another type of block involves an allosteric interaction with the channel protein. This changes the conformation of the protein to one in which the pore is closed or stabilizing a spontaneously occurring closed conformation. A well-studied example of this type of block is that of dihydropyridines on voltage-dependent Ca channels (54). The second type of block may be voltage independent. However, a voltage-dependence could arise if the conformational change involves a movement of charge on the channel protein with respect to the electric field across the membrane.

Application to Epithelia

One of the major difficulties in the application of the patch clamp technique to renal epithelia has been gaining access to the plasma membranes. Different methods have been used for both apical and basolateral membranes.

APICAL MEMBRANES

One successful approach to gaining access to the apical membrane is to split the tubules mechanically and flatten them onto their basolateral surfaces (19, 64). The use of a transparent, nontoxic, molluscan adhesive (Cell-Tak, BD Biosciences Labware, Bedford, MA) has greatly improved attachment of the basement membrane to the bottom of the chamber and increased the stability of the patch-clamp recording (19, 118). An example of a split, flattened proximal tubule from *Necturus maculosus* is shown in Fig. 15. Absence of staining with Trypan blue, except around the edge of the tissue, indicates viability of most of the hexagonal cells. Gigaohm seals can be formed on the apical surface of this preparation (shadow of a patch pipette can be seen near the center of the field). Although splitting individual nephron segments works best in large, amphibian tubules (19, 117, 118, 121), it has also been successfully used in rat CCD and TALH (64, 106, 135).

A second approach to patch-clamping the apical surface of renal tubules has been to insert a micropipette into

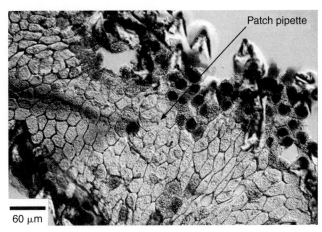

FIGURE 15 Light micrograph of split-open *Necturus* proximal tubule (apical side up), viewed from below with modulation contrast optics. The tissue was attached with Cell-Tak. Nuclei of damaged cells at the periphery are readily identified by their uptake of Trypan blue. Undamaged cells are approximately hexagonal in shape and exhibit well-defined boundaries with a diagonal diameter of about 30 μm. The tip and shadow of a patch pipette are visible at the left.

the open lumen of a perfused tubule (37). This has the advantage of maintaining the tubule in the perfused state, and theoretically permits independent control of the solution on both sides of the tubule. However, this technique significantly increases the complexity of the patch-clamp procedure and decreases cell visibility, making it difficult or impossible to be absolutely sure which cell type is actually being studied within a given nephron segment. Another technique that preserves the separation of apical and basolateral solutions entails the eversion of the entire tubule, which can then be perfused with the luminal surface on the outside (17, 128). This approach has the advantage of maintaining the integrity of the entire tubule, but is technically demanding and has so far been applied only to amphibian tubules.

Finally, renal cells can be studied in culture, taking advantage of the tendency of epithelial cells to attach to a suitable substrate with their basolateral side down, leaving the apical membranes facing up and accessible for patch clamping. Both continuous cell lines (46, 75, 97) and primary cultures of renal tubules (34, 84, 86) have been used. A problem with this approach is the difficulty of preserving the properties of the original cells in culture. One cell line that does appear to closely resemble native epithelial cells from the distal nephron is the A6 line from *Xenopus* kidney (48). This has been a particularly useful preparation for studying epithelial Na channels (46, 88, 89, 102).

BASOLATERAL MEMBRANES

Basolateral channels are more difficult to study than apical channels because the basolateral surface is covered with a basement membrane that must be removed to allow access to the plasma membrane. With isolated amphibian tubules it has been possible to gain access to the basolateral membrane by manually removing a small segment of basement membrane (67, 121). This process has also been applied to the mammalian collecting tubule (124). However, most patch-clamp studies on mammalian basolateral membranes have required pre-treatment of the tubules with a collagenase solution to remove enough of the basement membrane to permit formation of a high-resistance patch-clamp seal (65, 110, 111, 124, 130).

In an effort to circumvent the possible problems associated with enzymatic digestion, the lateral cell membranes of mammalian nephron segments have been patch-clamped either on the open end of a perfused tubule (36) or by mechanically removing an adjacent cell in an otherwise intact epithelium. The latter method was used to study basolateral channels on the lateral membrane of principal cells of rat CCD (134). Here a suction pipette is used to remove an entire intercalated cell from a split-open rat collecting tubule. This exposes a clean, lateral surface of an adjacent principal cell on which a high-resistance seal can be formed with a standard patch pipette (Fig. 16).

ISOLATED CELLS

Another way of gaining access to either the apical or basolateral cell membranes is to use isolated, polarized cells, derived by a brief collagenase or trypsin treatment of the epithelium. This weakens the basement membrane sufficiently so that individual, undamaged cells can be obtained by moderate mechanical agitation. A number of studies have been carried out using isolated cell preparations of proximal tubules since these cells often retain their polarity for extended periods (8, 20, 66, 116, 125). Detailed cytochemical studies on isolated cells of this type have confirmed the stability of markers normally associated with either the apical or basolateral membranes of

intact epithelia (125). An example of an isolated amphibian proximal tubule cell is illustrated in Fig. 17 (20, 125). These cells maintain their polarity by assuming a bi-spherical, minimum energy, configuration. In this picture the apical surface, with brush border, is clearly visible as the smaller hemisphere, whereas the larger spherical surface consists of basolateral membrane (Fig. 17).

Noise Analysis

Noise or fluctuation analysis provides an alternative approach to obtaining information at the level of single channels. In this technique, both the mean current level as well as the variations about the mean are used to infer single-channel properties. The principle behind the measurement is that random openings and closures of channels within a population will give rise to appreciable fluctuations in the overall number of open channels. The amplitudes of the fluctuations depend on the number channels, their open probability and the single-channel current (see below). For a given mean current level, the fluctuations will be larger for small number of channels (with large single-channel currents) than for a large number of channels (with smaller single-channel currents), since opening or closing one channel will produce a larger change in the mean current. A major disadvantage of this approach versus that of patch-clamp is that the single-channel events are not observed directly but need to be extracted from the data using kinetic models, Fourier transforms and curve fitting. A second drawback is that information on variations in channel behavior may be lost, and only the mean properties of an ensemble of the

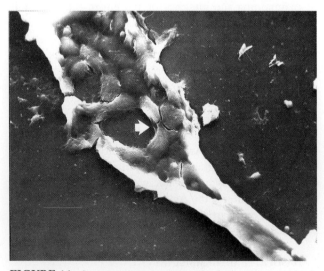

FIGURE 16 Scanning electron micrograph of split-open cortical collecting duct. Arrow shows lateral membrane of a principal cell. The intercalated cell adjacent to the principal cell was removed by mechanical suction, leaving the principal cell intact. (From Wang W, McNicholas CM, Segal AS, Giebisch G. A novel approach allows identification of K channels in the lateral membrane of rat CCD. *Am J Physiol* 1994;266:F813–F822.)

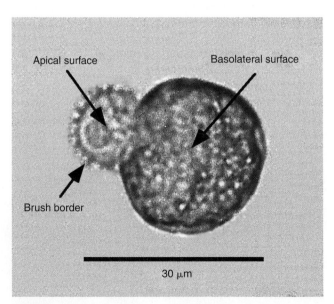

FIGURE 17 Isolated *Necturus* proximal tubule cell. The cell is bi-spherical in shape and about 30 μm in diameter. Evidence of a brush border is apparent on the smaller apical sphere. The larger spherical side of the cell consists of basolateral membrane. Isolated amphibian proximal tubule cells retain their polarity much longer than mammalian isolated epithelial cells. Patch-clamp recordings from both apical and basal surfaces indicate channel types similar to those found in native tubules.

channels are obtained. This loss of information can sometimes be a blessing in disguise, particularly when the overall performance of the whole population of channels needs to be assessed, by focusing attention on the quantitatively important aspects of channel function. Another advantage is that the sampling of channel properties is not biased by those of a few "good" patches that may be easy to analyze but not necessarily representative. A third advantage of noise analysis over direct recording of single-channel events is that it can resolve smaller single-channel currents. For example, the inward-rectifier K channel Kir7.1 has a single-channel conductance of ~50 fS estimated from noise analysis (74). Single-channel openings and closings associated with this conductance would be impossible to see using patch-clamp recordings.

Like single-channel recordings, noise analysis depends on abrupt changes in currents that occur when channels open or close, giving rise to fluctuations. Although it is possible to analyze noise due to spontaneous opening and closing, in practice most uses of noise analysis in epithelia have made use of blocker-induced noise in which the fluctuations are promoted by addition of blocking ions to the medium. This has two advantages. First, if the blockers interact with the channel through a first-order process, the kinetic scheme is particularly simple, as seen in the following diagram:

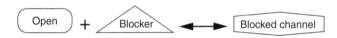

In the frequency domain, such a scheme predicts fluctuations which follow the form of a simple Lorentzian equation (85), that is:

$$S = S_o/(1 + (f/f_c)^2) \qquad (34)$$

where S is the power associated with a given frequency f, S_o is the plateau power approached at low frequencies and f_c is a constant called the corner frequency and is the frequency at which the power is reduced to half that of the plateau (Fig. 18). Furthermore, f_c is determined by the kinetics of the blocking interaction:

$$2\pi f_c = [B]k_{on} + k_{off} \qquad (35)$$

where $[B]$ is the blocker concentration, and k_{on} and k_{off} are the on and off rate constants, respectively, for the blocking reaction.

A second advantage of studying blocker-induced noise is that both the blocker and its concentration can be chosen to optimize the frequency of the fluctuations. This is important because technical problems can often limit the frequencies over which the noise can be reliably measured. For example, although amiloride-induced noise was originally used to study properties of epithelial Na channels (85), recordings could be improved by using a lower-affinity analogue that produced fluctuations at higher frequencies (52).

The simplest piece of information that can be extracted from the noise analysis is the single-channel current (85), as follows:

$$i = S_o 2\pi f_c / 4IF_B \qquad (36)$$

where F_B represents the fraction of blocked channels and I is the total (mean) current through the ensemble of channels measured in the presence of the blocker. F_B can be determined from the ratio of k_{on}/k_{off}, noting that $F_B = 1/(1 + k_{off}/k_{on} \cdot [B])$. F_B can also be estimated from the macroscopic dose–response curve (Fig. 18A), although this may give different results if the blocker increases the number of channels contributing to the noise. The quantity N_o (mean number of open plus blocked channels) can be calculated as follows:

$$N_o = I/[i (1 - F_B)] \qquad (37)$$

In general, N_o will be smaller than the total number of active channels N since closed channels are not included. Helman and colleagues have made use of this discrepancy and the finding that N_o increases as the concentration of blocker is increased to assess P_o, the open probability of unblocked channels. This was analyzed in terms of the following three-state model (52).

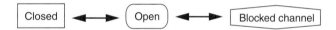

Assuming that closed channels cannot be blocked, the number of open plus blocked channels is increased by the blocker through the principle of mass action.

A second approach to estimate P_o is to measure the fluctuations associated with the spontaneous opening and closing (13). Again a simple model is assumed, as follows:

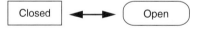

in which the variance (σ^2) of the current is given by the next expression (56).

$$\sigma^2 = Ni^2P_o(1 - P_o) = I(1 - P_{i_o})i \qquad (38)$$

Therefore, the three measurements of blocker-induced noise, mean current, and variance in the absence of blocker can be used to estimate the three variables i, N, and P_o.

Most noise-analysis studies have used flat epithelia in which the transepithelial voltage is clamped. Both native tissues (82, 85, 132, 138) and cultured cells (4, 51) have been successfully studied. In these instances blockers have been added to the apical side of the epithelia to measure properties of Na channels (using amiloride or its analogues as blockers) or K channels (using Ba^{+2}). More recently, fluctuation analysis has been applied to whole-cell recordings of renal epithelia, particularly the CCD, where the cells are not electrically coupled to each other (24). Na channel fluctuations similar to those of flat epithelial can be measured in this way (13).

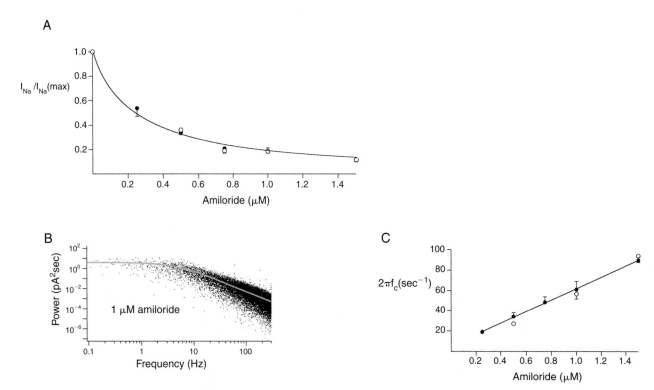

FIGURE 18   Noise analysis of whole-cell currents in a principal cell of the mouse cortical collecting duct. The power-density spectrum was obtained with 1 μM amiloride in the bath. The line represents a fit to a Lorentzian function with S_o = 3.06 pA^2 seconds and f_c = 3.8 Hz. (From Dahlmann A, Pradervand S, Hummler E, Rossier BC, Frindt G, Palmer LG. Mineralocorticoid regulation of epithelial Na$^+$ channels is maintained in a mouse model of Liddle's syndrome. *Am J Physiol* 2003;285:F310–F318.)

Another application involved characterization of basolateral K channels, which as described in a previous section, are difficult to study directly (38). Similar techniques were also used to examine cell-attached patches in which channel density was too high to resolve single-channel events directly (25).

Conclusions

The patch-clamp approach has made it possible to study renal ion channels one molecule at a time. Insights into ion transport mechanisms that have emerged from these studies have greatly expanded the information that was previously available from equivalent circuit analysis. Although single-channel measurements provide details about how ion *channels* work, they do not provide complete information about how an *epithelium* works. Achieving this goal requires measurements of transepithelial, intracellular, and single-channel properties.

APPENDIX 1

Basic Equations for General Equivalent Circuit

The lateral resistive network in the circuit of Fig. 1 makes it difficult to obtain a closed form solution for the electrical parameters of interest. However, if the lateral network is

neglected, Fig. 1 reduces to the simpler circuit of Fig. 7A that can be evaluated as described here.

Since the pump and diffusional EMFs are in parallel, the effective EMF of the cellular pathway is the sum of the individual EMFs weighted by their relative conductances:

$$E_{bl}^* = \frac{R_{bl}}{R_p + R_{bl}} E_p + \frac{R_p}{R_p + R_{bl}} E_{bl} \qquad (A1.1)$$

where E_p is the reversal potential of the pump and E_{bl} is the total ionic diffusion potential across the basolateral membrane, as given either by the mosaic membrane equation (Eq. A1.2) or the constant field equation (Eq. A1.3).

$$E_{bl} = -\frac{RT}{F}\left[t_{Na} Ln\frac{[Na]_c}{[Na]_b} + t_K Ln\frac{[K]_c}{[K]_b} + t_{Cl} Ln\frac{[Cl]_b}{[Cl]_c} \right]$$
$$(A1.2)$$

$$E_{bl} = -\frac{RT}{F} Ln\frac{P_{Na}[Na]_c + P_K[K]_c + P_{Cl}[Cl]_b}{P_{Na}[Na]_b + P_K[K]_b + P_{Cl}[Cl]_c} \qquad (A1.3)$$

The effective basolateral resistance R_{bl}^* is the parallel sum of pump resistance (R_p) and the passive resistive elements of the membrane (R_{bl}):

$$R_{bl}^* = \frac{R_p \cdot R_{bl}}{R_p + R_{bl}} \qquad (A1.4)$$

Transepithelial resistance (R_{te}) is a function of the other resistances in the network as defined by:

$$\frac{1}{R_{te}} = \frac{1}{R_{tj}} + \frac{1}{R_{ap} + R_{bl}^*} \quad \text{(A1.5)}$$

Considering the circuit of Fig. 7B, the total circulating current (I) can be calculated from the total EMF of the circuit divided by the total resistance according to the following equation:

$$I = \frac{-E_{bl}^* - E_{ap} + E_{par}}{R_{bl}^* + R_{ap} + R_{tj}} \text{ where } E_{bl}^* \text{ and } E_{ap} < 0 \quad \text{(A1.6)}$$

Under these conditions, the measured basolateral potential will be given by:

$$V_{bl} = E_{bl}^* + I \cdot R_{bl}^* = \frac{E_{bl}^*(R_{ap} + R_{tj}) + R_{bl}^*(E_{par} - E_{ap})}{R_{bl}^* + R_{ap} + R_{tj}} \quad \text{(A1.7)}$$

The measured apical membrane potential will be given by:

$$V_{ap} = E_{ap} + I \cdot R_{ap} = \frac{E_{ap}(R_{bl}^* + R_{tj}) + R_{ap}(E_{par} - E_{bl}^*)}{R_{bl}^* + R_{ap} + R_{tj}} \quad \text{(A1.8)}$$

and the measured transepithelial potential will be given by:

$$V_{te} = E_{par} - I \cdot R_{par} = \frac{E_{par}(R_{ap} + R_{bl}^*) + R_{tj}(E_{ap} + E_{bl}^*)}{R_{bl}^* + R_{ap} + R_{tj}} \quad \text{(A1.9)}$$

Equations A1.7–A1.9 can be evaluated for the limiting cases of very tight and very leaky epithelia. In the case where the cell (rather than the interspace) is the primary conductive pathway:

$$Lim \ V_{bl} = E_{bl}^* \text{ for } R_{tj} >> R_{ap} + R_{bl}^*$$
$$\text{(very tight epithelium)} \quad \text{(A1.10)}$$

and

$$Lim \ V_{ap} = E_{ap} \text{ for } R_{tj} >> R_{ap} + R_{bl}^*$$
$$\text{(very tight epithelium)} \quad \text{(A1.11)}$$

If perturbations are confined to the apical membrane, the additional limiting case is sometimes useful when only transepithelial measurements can be performed as follows:

$$Lim \ \Delta V_{ap} = \Delta E_{ap} = \Delta V_{te} \text{ for } R_{tj} >> R_{ap} + R_{bl}^*$$
$$\text{(very tight epithelium)} \quad \text{(A1.12)}$$

since:

$$Lim \ V_{te} = E_{ap} + E_{bl}^* \text{ for } R_{tj} >> R_{ap} + R_{bl}^*$$
$$\text{(very tight epithelium)} \quad \text{(A1.13)}$$

At the other extreme, if the paracellular pathway has a much higher conductance than the cellular pathway:

$$Lim \ V_{te} = E_{par} \text{ for } R_{ap} + R_{bl}^* >> R_{tj}$$
$$\text{(very leaky epithelium)} \quad \text{(A1.14)}$$

Finally, two other limiting cases of the general circuit equations permit determination of cell membrane properties from transepithelial measurements under special conditions. First, application of a high K solution to the serosal side of an epithelium having a predominantly K selective basolateral membrane reduces both R_{bl}^* and E_{bl}^* to values close to zero. Under these conditions, Eqs. A1.8 and A1.9 imply the following simple relation between V_{ap} and V_{te}:

$$V_{ap} = V_{te} = \frac{R_{tj}}{R_{ap} + R_{tj}} E_{ap} + \frac{R_{ap}}{R_{ap} + R_{tj}} E_{par}$$
$$\text{(K depolarized tissue)} \quad \text{(A1.15)}$$

Second, protocols that involve selective permeabilization of the apical membrane reduce both R_{ap} and E_{ap} to values near zero, and Eqs. A1.7 and A1.9 imply a simple relation between V_{bl} and V_{te} as follows:

$$V_{bl} = V_{te} = \frac{R_{tj}}{R_{bl}^* + R_{tj}} E_{bl}^* + \frac{R_{bl}^*}{R_{bl}^* + R_{tj}} E_{par}$$
$$\text{(permeabilized apical membrane)} \quad \text{(A1.16)}$$

APPENDIX 2

Relation Between Real Change in EMF and Measured Change in Potential

Circular current flow in polarized epithelial cells produces important discrepancies between the real change in EMF at a particular barrier, ΔE, and the change in voltage, ΔV, that can actually be measured with electrodes (see Fig. 7). In order to evaluate individual ion selectivities, some assumption must be made about the equivalent circuit of the epithelium. In the simple model of Fig. 7A, luminal replacement of Na, K, or Cl with an impermeant ion will produce changes in the measured basolateral ΔV_{bl} and transepithelial potentials ΔV_{te} that are related to the change in apical membrane EMF according to:

$$\Delta E_{ap} = \Delta V_{te} - \Delta V_{bl}\left[1 + \frac{R_{ap}}{R_p} + \frac{R_{ap}}{R_{bl}}\right] \quad \text{(A2.1)}$$

where R_{ap}, R_{bl}, and R_p, respectively, refer to the apical membrane resistance, the lumped basolateral membrane resistance, and the intrinsic resistance of the basolateral Na/K pump. In Eqs. A2.1–A2.3, it is assumed that the external ion replacements are performed rapidly enough so that the resistance ratios (R_{ap}/R_p, R_{ap}/R_{bl}) are constant, and the ion composition of the cell is essentially unchanged. The equations were derived by noting that the total current entering the cell across the apical membrane must equal the total current leaving the cell across the basolateral membrane.

Basolateral replacement of Na, K, or Cl with an impermeant ion yields the following analogous expression for the relation between the change in basolateral EMF and the measured potentials ΔV:

$$\Delta E_{bl} = \Delta V_{bl}\left[1+\frac{R_{bl}}{R_p}+\frac{R_{bl}}{R_{ap}}\right]-\frac{R_{bl}}{R_{ap}}\Delta V_{te} \qquad (A2.2)$$

Finally, the paracellular EMF would be given by Eq. A2.3 for experiments involving basolateral replacement of Na, K, or Cl by an impermeant ion.

$$\Delta E_{par} = \Delta V_{te}\left[1+\frac{R_{tj}}{R_{ap}}\right]-\frac{R_{tj}}{R_{ap}}\Delta V_{bl} \qquad (A2.3)$$

Equations A2.1–A2.3 would be used together with Eq. 23 of the text to evaluate the ionic transference numbers of the apical, basolateral and paracellular barriers.

APPENDIX 3

Equations for Partial Ionic Conductance

Specific expressions for the partial conductance G_x can be obtained by differentiating the Goldman–Hodgkin–Katz flux equation with respect to voltage, as follows:

$$G_x = \frac{\partial I_x}{\partial V}$$

$$= \frac{\partial}{\partial V}\left\{P_x\frac{z^2F^2}{RT}V\cdot\left[\frac{[X]_o-[X]_i\,e^{zFV/RT}}{(1-e^{zFV/RT})}\right]\right\} \quad (A3.1)$$

In the limiting case of zero membrane potential, the complicated form of Eq. A3.1 reduces to the arithmetic average of the concentrations on both sides of the membrane. The following equation does not depend on the ion being distributed near its electrochemical equilibrium:

$$G_x \approx P_x\frac{z^2F^2}{RT}\frac{1}{2}(X_o+X_i) \qquad (A3.2)$$

At large negative membrane potentials, positive ions will be driven from outside to inside and the limiting conductance will be:

$$G_x \approx P_x\frac{z^2F^2}{RT}X_o \qquad (A3.3)$$

Conversely, at large positive potentials, negative ions will be driven from inside to outside and the limiting conductance will be:

$$G_x \approx P_x\frac{z^2F^2}{RT}X_i \qquad (A3.4)$$

Although the relations presented here reduce the complicated general equation (Eq. A3.1) to a manageable form, neither the assumption of zero membrane potential (Eq. A3.2) nor the assumption of very large membrane potentials (Eqs. A3.3 and A3.4) are very physiologically credible.

For ions like K and Cl, which are often distributed close to their electrochemical equilibrium, it is possible to simplify the algebraic form of the $\langle X \rangle$ term in Eq. 25 of the text. Under these conditions, the conductance would be given by the following equation:

$$G_x \approx P_x\frac{z_x^2F^2}{RT}\left(\frac{[X]_i[X]_o}{[X]_o-[X]_i}\right)\mathrm{Ln}\frac{[X]_o}{[X]_i} \qquad (A3.5)$$

If more than one ion (X and Y) are distributed close to equilibrium across the membrane, the ratios of transference numbers, conductances and permeabilities are given by the following equation:

$$\frac{t_x}{t_y}=\frac{G_x}{G_y}\approx\frac{P_x}{P_y}\cdot\frac{[X]_o}{[Y]_i}=\frac{P_x}{P_y}\cdot\frac{[X]_i}{[Y]_o} \qquad (A3.6)$$

APPENDIX 4

Contribution of Electrogenic Na/K Pump to Membrane Potential

The contribution of the Na/K pump to the cell membrane potential of epithelial tissues is different than its contribution to the membrane potential of symmetric cells. The existence of circulating currents in the open-circuited state places a different set of constraints on the magnitude of the cell potential. This can be derived from the reduced equivalent circuit of Fig. 7B. In this circuit, the electrogenic and diffusive ion pathways are combined into an effective EMF of the basolateral membrane (E_{bl}^*) and an effective basolateral resistance (R_{bl}^*). These lumped quantities are directly related to the individual parameters of the pump and the basolateral diffusion potential according to standard equations of linear circuit theory, as follows:

$$R_{bl}^* = \frac{R_{bl}\cdot R_p}{R_{bl}+R_p} \qquad (A4.1)$$

$$E_{bl}^* = \frac{R_{bl}}{R_{bl}+R_p}E_p+\frac{R_p}{R_{bl}+R_p}E_{bl} \qquad (A4.2)$$

If the circulating currents of Fig. 7B are also considered, the measured membrane potential (V_{bl}) can be described by Eq. A4.3, which indicates the specific contribution of the electrogenic pump (E_p), the ionic diffusion potential (E_{bl}), and the apical and paracellular diffusion potentials (E_{ap}, E_{par}).

$$V_{bl} = f\left[\frac{R_{bl}}{R_{bl}+R_p}\right]E_p$$

$$+f\left[\frac{R_p}{R_{bl}+R_p}\right]E_{bl} + h\left[E_{par}-E_{ap}\right] \quad (A4.3)$$

In Eq. A4.3, the factors f and h arise from the circulating current I in the model of Fig. 7B, as follows:

$$f = \frac{R_{ap}+R_{tj}}{R_{bl}^*+R_{ap}+R_{tj}} \quad (A4.4)$$

$$h = \frac{R_{bl}^*}{R_{bl}^*+R_{ap}+R_{tj}} \quad (A4.5)$$

Equations A4.3–A4.5 are the general equations for the relative contributions of the electrogenic pump (denoted by E_p), ionic diffusion (denoted by E_{bl}), and circulating current (denoted by $E_{par}-E_{ap}$) to the observed basolateral membrane potential (V_{bl}). As indicated by Eq. A4.3, the membrane potential depends critically on the relative magnitude of the pump resistance (R_p) versus the diffusion resistance of the membrane.

The term R_{bl}^* can be determined from cable analysis (as described in the text). This value can then be used to calculate (R_{bl}) from Eq. A4.1, assuming that the internal resistance of the pump (R_p) can be estimated from its I–V relation (see Fig. 10).

If the internal pump resistance (R_p) is high compared to the ionic resistance (R_{bl}), the ratio $R_{bl}/(R_{bl}+R_p)$ will be low and the measured membrane potential V_{bl} (given by Eq. A4.3) will be dominated by the diffusional EMF term involving E_{bl}. Conversely, if the internal pump resistance is low, V_{bl} will be dominated by the pump term involving E_p.

References

1. Anagnostopoulos T, Velu E. Electrical resistance of cell membranes in *Necturus* kidney. *Pflügers Arch* 1974;346:327–339.
2. Awayda M, Van Driessche W, Helman SI. Frequency-dependent capacitance of the apical membrane of frog skin: dielectric relaxation processes. *Biophys J* 1999;76:219–232.
3. Bello-Reuss E. Cell membrane and paracellular resistances in isolated renal proximal tubules from rabbit and *Ambystoma*. *J Physiol* 1986;370:25–38.
4. Blazer-Yost BL, Helman SI. The amiloride-sensitive epithelial Na+ channel: binding sites and channel densities. *Am J Physiol* 1997;272(3):C761–C769.
5. Boulpaep E. Electrical phenomena in the nephron. *Kidney Int* 1976;9:88–102.
6. Boulpaep EL, Sackin H. Electrical analysis of intraepithelial barriers. *Curr Top Membr Transp* 1980;13:169–197.
7. Boulpaep EL, Sackin H. Equivalent electrical circuit analysis and rheogenic pumps in epithelia. *Fed Proc* 1979;38:2030–2036.
8. Cemerikic D, Sackin H. Substrate activation of mechanosensitive, whole cell currents in renal proximal tubule. *Am J Physiol* 1993;264:F707–F714.
9. Chepilko S, Zhou H, Sackin H, Palmer LG. Permeation and gating properties of a cloned renal K+ channel. *Am J Physiol* 1995;268:C389–C401.
10. Clausen C, Lewis SA, Diamond JM. Impedance analysis of a tight epithelium using a distributed resistance model. *Biophys J* 1979;26:291–317.
11. Clausen C, Wills NK. Impedance analysis in epithelia. In: Schultz SG, ed. *Ion Transport by Epithelia: Recent Advances.* New York: Raven Press, 1981:79–92.
12. Cox DHaA, R.W. Role of the beta1 subunit in large-conductance Ca²⁺-activated K⁺ channel gating energetics. Mechanisms of enhanced Ca²⁺ sensitivity. *J Gen Physiol* 2000;116:411–432.
13. Dahlmann A, Pradervand S, Hummler E, Rossier BC, Frindt G, Palmer LG. Mineralocorticoid regulation of epithelial Na⁺ channels is maintained in a mouse model of Liddle's syndrome. *Am J Physiol* 2003;285:F310–F318.
14. DeWeer P. Cellular sodium-potassium transport. In: Seldin DW, Giebisch G, eds. *The Kidney: Physiology and Pathophysiology.* New York: Raven Press, 1985:31–48.
15. DeWeer P. Electrogenic pumps: theoretical and practical considerations. In: Blaustein M, Lieberman M, eds. *Electrogenic Transport: Fundamental Principles and Physiological Implications.* New York: Raven Press, 1984:1–15.
16. Eisner DA, Lederer WJ, Vaughan-Jones RD. The dependence of sodium pumping and tension on intracellular sodium activity in voltage-clamped sheep Purkinje fibres. *J Physiol (Lond)* 1981;317:163–187.
17. Engbretson BG, Beyenbach KW, Stoner LC. The everted renal tubule: a methodology for direct assessment of apical membrane function. *Am J Physiol* 1988;255:F1276–F1280.
18. Erlij D. Basic electrical properties of tight epithelia determined with a simple method. *Pflügers Arch* 1976;364:91–93.
19. Filipovic D, Sackin H. A calcium-permeable stretch-activated cation channel in renal proximal tubule. *Am J Physiol* 1991;260:F119–F129.
20. Filipovic D, Sackin H. Stretch- and volume-activated channels in isolated tubule cells. *Am J Physiol* 1992;262:F857–F870.
21. Firsov D, Schild L, Gautschi I, Merillat AM, Schneeberger E, Rossier BC. Cell surface expression of the epithelial Na channel and a mutant causing Liddle syndrome: a quantitative approach. *Proc Natl Acad Sci U S A* 1996;93(26):15370–15375.
22. Frindt G, Masilamani S, Knepper MA, Palmer LG. Activation of epithelial Na channels during short-term Na deprivation. *Am J Physiol* 2001;280:F112–F118.
23. Frindt G, Palmer LG. Ca-activated K channels in apical membrane of mammalian CCT, and their role in K secretion. *Am J Physiol* 1987;252:F458–F467.
24. Frindt G, Sackin H, Palmer LG. Whole-cell currents in rat cortical collecting tubule: low-Na diet increases amiloride-sensitive conductance. *Am J Physiol* 1990;258:F562–F567.
25. Frindt G, Silver RB, Windhager EE, Palmer LG. Feedback regulation of Na channels in rat CCT. III. Response to cAMP. *Am J Physiol* 1995;268:F480–F489.
26. Frömter E. Electrophysiological analysis of rat renal sugar and amino acid transport. I. Basic phenomena. *Pflügers Arch* 1982;393:179–189.
27. Frömter E. The route of passive ion movement through the epithelium of *Necturus* gallbladder. *J Membr Biol* 1972;8:259–301.
28. Frömter E. Viewing the kidney through microelectrodes. *Am J Physiol* 1984;247:F695–F705.
29. Frömter E, Diamond JM. Route of passive ion permeation in epithelia. *Nat New Biol* 1972;235:9–13.
30. Frömter E, Gebler B. Electrical properties of amphibian urinary bladder epithelia III. The cell membrane resistances and the effect of amiloride. *Pflügers Arch* 1977;371:99–108.
31. Gadsby D, Nakao M. The steady-state current-voltage relationship of the Na/K pump in guinea pig ventricular myocytes. *J Gen Physiol* 1989;94:511–537.
32. Garrahan PJ, Glynn IM. The stoichiometry of the sodium pump. *J Physiol (Lond)* 1967;192:217–235.
33. Germann WJ, Lowy ME, Ernst SA, Dawson DC. Differentiation of two distinct K conductances in the basolateral membrane of turtle colon. *J Gen Physiol* 1986;88:237–251.
34. Gitter AH, Beyenbach KW, Christine C, Gross P, Minuth WW, Frömter E. High conductance K+ channel in apical membranes of principal cells cultured from rabbit renal cortical collecting duct anlagen. *Pflügers Arch* 1987;408:282–290.
35. Glynn IM. The electrogenic sodium pump. In: Blaustein MP, Lieberman M, ed. New York: Raven Press, 1984:33–48.
36. Gögelein H, Greger R. Properties of single K channels in the basolateral membrane of rabbit proximal straight tubules. *Pflügers Arch* 1987;410:288–295.
37. Gögelein H, Greger R. Single channel recordings from basolateral and apical membranes of renal proximal tubules. *Pflügers Arch* 1984;401:424–426.
38. Gray DA, Frindt G, Zhang YY, Palmer LG. Basolateral K+ conductance in principal cells of rat CCD. *Am J Physiol* 2004;288:F493–F504.
39. Greger R. Cation selectivity of the isolated perfused cortical thick ascending limb of Henle's loop of rabbit kidney. *Pflügers Arch* 1981;390:30–37.
40. Greger R. Ion transport mechanisms in thick ascending limb of Henle's loop of mammalian nephron. *Physiol Rev* 1985;65:760–797.
41. Greger R, Schlatter E. Properties of the lumen membrane of the cortical thick ascending limb of Henle's loop of rabbit kidney: a model for secondary active chloride transport. *Pflügers Arch* 1983;396:315–324.
42. Guggino WB. Functional heterogeneity in the early distal tubule of the *Amphiuma* kidney: evidence for two modes of Cl and K transport across the basolateral cell membrane. *Am J Physiol* 1986;250:F430–F440.
43. Guggino WB, Oberleithner H, Giebisch G. The amphibian diluting segment. *Am J Physiol* 1988;254:F615–F627.
44. Guggino WB, Windhager EE, Boulpaep EL, Giebisch G. Cellular and paracellular resistances of the *Necturus* proximal tubule. *J Membr Biol* 1982;67:143–154.
45. Hamill OP, Marty A, Neher E, Sakmann B, Sigworth FJ. Improved patch clamp techniques for high resolution current recording from cells and cell-free membrane patches. *Pflügers Arch* 1981;391:85–100.
46. Hamilton KL, Eaton DC. Single channel recordings from amiloride-sensitive epithelial sodium channel. *Am J Physiol* 1985;249:C200–C207.
47. Deleted in proof.
48. Handler JS, Preston AS, Perkins FM, Matsumura M. The effect of adrenal steroid hormones on epithelia formed in culture by A6 cells. *Ann N Y Acad Sci* 1981;372:442–454.
49. Hebert SC, Friedman PA, Andreoli TE. Effect of antidiuretic hormone on cellular conductive pathways in mouse medullary thick ascending limbs of Henle. I. ADH increases transcellular conductive pathways. *J Membr Biol* 1984;80:201–219.

50. Hegel U, Boulpaep EL. Studies of electrical impedance of kidney proximal tubular epithelium in *Necturus*. Proceedings of 6th International Congress of Nephrology, 1975:45(abstr.).
51. Helman IS, Baxendale LM, Sariban-Sohraby S, Benos DJ. Blocker-induced noise of Na^+ channels in cultured A6 epithelia. *Fed Proc* 1986;45:516(abstr.).
52. Helman SI, Baxendale LM. Blocker-related changes of channel density. Analysis of a three-state model for apical Na channels of frog skin. *J Gen Physiol* 1990;95:647–678.
53. Helman SI, Miller DA. In vitro techniques for avoiding edge damage in studies of the frog skin. *Science* 1971;173:146–148.
54. Hess P, Lansman JB, Tsien RW. Different modes of Ca channel gating behaviour favored by dihydropyridine Ca agonists and antagonists. *Nature* 1984;311:538–544.
55. Higgins JT, Gebler B, Frömter E. Electrical properties of amphibian urinary bladder epithelia II. The cell potential profile in *Necturus* maculosus. *Pflügers Arch* 1977;371:87–97.
56. Hille B. *Ionic Channels of Excitable Membranes*. 3rd ed. Sunderland, MA: Sinauer Associates, 2001.
57. Horisberger J-D, Giebisch G. Na/K pump currents in the *Amphiuma* collecting tubule. *J Gen Physiol* 1989;94:493–510.
58. Horisberger J-D, Giebisch G. Voltage dependence of the basolateral membrane conductance in the *Amphiuma* collecting tubule. *J Membr Biol* 1988;105:257–263.
59. Horisberger JD, Giebisch G. Intracellular Na and K activities and membrane conductances in the collecting tubule of *Amphiuma*. *J Gen Physiol* 1988;92:643–665.
60. Deleted in proof.
61. Horn R, Vandenbert C, Lange K. Statistical analysis of single sodium channels. Effects of N-bromoacetamide. *Biophys J* 1984;45:323–335.
62. Hoshi T, Kawahara K, Yokoyama R, Suenga K. Change in membrane resistances of renal proximal tubule induced by cotransport of sodium and organic solutes. In: Takacs L, ed. *Advances in Physiological Science (Kidney and Body Fluids)*. Budapest: Pergamon Press and Akademiai Kiado, 1981.
63. Hunter M, Horisberger J-D, Stanton BA, Giebisch G. The collecting tubule of Amphiuma I. Electrophysiological characterization. *Am J Physiol* 1987;253:1263–1272.
64. Hunter M, Lopes AG, Boulpaep E, Giebisch G. Single channel recordings of calcium-activated potassium channels in the apical membrane of rabbit cortical collecting tubule. *Proc Natl Acad Sci U S A* 1984;81:4237–4239.
65. Hurst AM, Beck J, Laprade R, Lapointe J-Y. Na pump inhibition downregulates an ATP-sensitive K channel in rabbit proximal tubule. *Am J Physiol* 1993;264:F760–F764.
66. Kawahara K. A stretch-activated K+ channel in the basolateral membrane of *Xenopus* kidney proximal tubule cells. *Pflügers Arch* 1990;415:624–629.
67. Kawahara K, Hunter M, Giebisch G. Potassium channels in *Necturus* proximal tubule. *Am J Physiol* 1987;253:F488–F494.
68. Koefoed-Johnsen V, Ussing HH. On the nature of the frog skin potential. *Acta Physiol Scand* 1958;42:298–308.
69. Koeppen B. Electrophysiology of ion transport in renal tubule epithelia. *Semin Nephrol* 1987;7:37–47.
70. Koeppen B, Giebisch G. Cellular electrophysiology of potassium transport in the mammalian cortical collecting tubule. *Pflügers Arch* 1985;405(Suppl 1): S143–S146.
71. Koeppen BM. Conductive properties of the rabbit outer medullary collecting duct: outer stripe. *Am J Physiol* 1986;250:F70–F76.
72. Koeppen BM, Biagi BA, Giebisch G. Intracellular microelectrode characterization of the rabbit cortical collecting duct. *Am J Physiol* 1983;244:F35–F47.
73. Korn SJ, Horn R. Statistical discrimination of fractal and Markov models of single-channel gating. *Biophys J* 1988;54:871–877.
74. Krapininsky G, Medina I, Eng L, Krapivinsky L, Yang Y, Clapham D. A novel inward rectifier K^+ channel with unique pore properties. *Neuron* 1998;20:995–1005.
75. Lang F, Friedrich F, Paulmilch M, Schobersberger W, Jungwirth A, Ritter M, Steidl M, Weiss H, Woll E, Tschernko E, Paulmilch R, Hallbrucker C. Ion channels in Madin–Darby canine kidney cells. *Ren Physiol Biochem* 1990;13:82–93.
76. Lapointe JY, Laprade R, Cardinal J. Transepithelial and cell membrane electrical resistances of the rabbit proximal convoluted tubule. *Am J Physiol* 1984;247:F637–F649.
77. Latorre R, Miller C. Conduction and selectivity in potassium channels. *J Membr Biol* 1983;71:11–30.
78. Leaf A, Anderson J, Page LB. Active sodium transport by the isolated toad bladder. *J Gen Physiol* 1958;41:657–668.
79. Lewis SA, Diamond JM. Na^+ transport by rabbit urinary bladder, a tight epithelium. *J Membr Biol* 1976;28:1–40.
80. Lewis SA, Eaton DC, Clausen C, Diamond JM. Nystatin as a probe for investigating the electrical properties of a tight epithelum. *J Gen Physiol* 1977;70:427–440.
81. Lewis SA, Eaton DC, Diamond JM. The mechanism of Na+ transport by rabbit urinary bladder. *J Membr Biol* 1976;28:41–70.
82. Li JH-Y, Palmer LG, Edelman IS, Lindemann B. The role of the sodium channel density in the natriferic response of the toad urinary bladder to an antidiuretic hormone. *J Membr Biol* 1982;64:79–89.
83. Liebovitz LS, Fischbarg J, Koniarek JP. Ion channel kinetics: a model based on fractal scaling rather than multistate Markov processes. *Math Biosci* 1987;84:37–68.
84. Light DB, McCann FV, Keller TM, Stanton BA. Amiloride-sensitive cation channel in apical membrane of inner medullary collecting duct. *Am J Physiol* 1988;255:F278–F286.
85. Lindemann B, Van-Driessche W. Sodium specific membrane channels in frog skin are pores: current fluctuations reveal high turnover. *Science* 1977;195:292–294.
86. Ling BN, Hinton CF, Eaton DC. Amiloride-sensitive sodium channels in rabbit cortical collecting tubule primary cultures. *Am J Physiol* 1991;261:F933–F944.
87. Lopatin AN, Makhina EN, Nichols CG. The mechanism of inward rectification of potassium channels: "long-pore plugging" by cytoplasmic polyamines. *J Gen Physiol* 1995;106:923–956.
88. Ma HP, Li L, Zhou ZH, Eaton DC, Warnock DG. ATP masks stretch activation of epithelial sodium channels in A6 distal nephron cells. *Am J Physiol* 2002;282:F501–F505.
89. Marunaka Y, Eaton DC. Effects of vasopressin and cAMP on single amiloride-blockable Na channels. *Am J Physiol* 1991;260:C1071–C1084.
90. Maunsbach AB, Boulpaep EL. Quantitative ultrastructure and functional correlates in proximal tubules of *Ambystoma* and *Necturus*. *Am J Physiol* 1984;246:F710–F724.
91. McManus OB, Weiss DS, Spivak CE, Blatz AL, Magleby KL. Fractal models are inadequate for the kintics of four different ion channels. *Biophys J* 1988;45:859–870.
92. Messner G, Wang W, Paulmichl M, Oberleithner H, Lang F. Ouabain decreases apparent potassium-conductance in proximal tubules of the amphibian kidney. *Pflügers Arch* 1985;404:131–137.
93. Miller C. Open-state substructure of single chloride channels from *Torpedo* electroplax. *Phil Trans R Soc Lond B* 1982;299:401–411.
94. Millhauser GL, Salpeter EE, Oswald RE. Diffusion models of ion-channel gating and the origin of power-law distributions from single channel recordings. *Proc Natl Acad Sci U S A* 1988;85:1503–1507.
95. Mullins LJ, Noda K. The influence of sodium-free solutions on the membrane potential of frog muscle fibers. *J Gen Physiol* 1963;47:117–139.
96. Nelson DJ, Ehrenfeld J, Lindemann B. Volume changes and potential artifacts of epithelial cells of frog skin following impalement with microelectrodes filled with 3M KCl. *J Membr Biol* 1978;40(special issue):91–119.
97. Nelson DJ, Tang JM, Palmer LG. Single-channel recordings of apical membrane chloride conductance in A6 epithelial cells. *J Membr Biol* 1984;80:81–89.
98. O'Connell AM. *Modal Gating Behavior of Batrachotoxin-Modified Sodium Channels*. Ithaca, NY: Cornell University Medical College, 1992.
99. O'Neil RG, Sansom SC. Electrophysiological properties of cellular and paracellular conductive pathways of the rabbit cortical collecting duct. *J Membr Biol* 1984;82:281–295.
100. Oberleithner H, Guggino W, Giebisch G. Resistance properties of the diluting segment of *Amphiuma* kidney: influence of K adaptation. *J Membr Biol* 1985;88:139–147.
101. Oh YK, Na KY, Han JS, Lee JS, Joo KW, Earm J-H, Knepper MA, Kim G-H. Chronic hydrochlorothiazide infusion alters the abundance of collecting duct epithelial sodium channel and H^+-ATPase protein in rat kidney. *J Am Soc Nephrol* 2001;12:38A.
102. Ohara A, Matsunaga H, Eaton DC. G protein activation inhibits amiloride-blockable highly selective sodium channels in A6 cells. *Am J Physiol* 1993;264(2pt1):C352–360.
103. Pácha J, Frindt G, Antonian L, Silver R, Palmer LG. Regulation of Na channels of the rat cortical collecting tubule by aldosterone. *J Gen Physiol* 1993;102:25–42.
104. Palmer LG, Antonian L, Frindt G. Regulation of the Na-K pump of the rat cortical collecting tubule by aldosterone. *J Gen Physiol* 1993;102(1):43–57.
105. Palmer LG, Choe H, Frindt G. Is the secretory K channel in the rat CCT ROMK? *Am J Physiol* 1997;273:F404–F410.
106. Palmer LG, Frindt G. Amiloride-sensitive Na^+ channels from the apical membrane of the rat cortical collecting tubule. *Proc Natl Acad Sci U S A* 1986;83:2767–2770.
107. Palmer LG, Frindt G. Conductance and gating of epithelial Na^+ channels from rat cortical collecting tubule. Effects of luminal Na and Li. *J Gen Physiol* 1988;92:121–138.
108. Palmer LG, Frindt G. Regulation of apical K channels in rat cortical collecting tubule during changes in dietary K intake. *Am J Physiol* 1999;277:F805–F812.
109. Palmer LG, Sackin H, Frindt G. Regulation of Na channels by luminal Na in rat cortical collecting tubule. *J Physiol (Lond)* 1998;509:151–162.
110. Parent L, Cardinal J, Sauvé R. Single-channel analysis of a K channel at basolateral membrane of rabbit proximal convoluted tubule. *Am J Physiol* 1988;254:F105–F113.
111. Paulais M, Teulon J. cAMP-activated chloride channel in the basolateral membrane of the thick ascending limb of the mouse kidney. *J Membr Biol* 1990;113:253–260.
112. Post RL, Jolly PC. The linkage of sodium, potassium and ammonium active transport across the human erthrocyte membrane. *Biochim Biophys Acta* 1957;25:118–128.
113. Rakowski RF. Charge movement by the Na/K pump in *Xenopus* oocytes. *J Gen Physiol* 1993;101:117–144.
114. Rakowski RF, Gadsby DC, DeWeer P. Stoichiometry and voltage dependence of the sodium pump in voltage-clamped, internally dialyzed squid giant axon. *J Gen Physiol* 1989;93:903–941.
115. Rakowski RF, Vasilets LA, LaTona J, Schwarz W. A negative slope in the current-voltage relationship of the Na/K pump in *Xenopus* oocytes produced by reduction of external [K]. *J Membr Biol* 1991;121:177–187.
116. Robson L, Hunter M. Volume regulatory responses infrog isolated proximal tubules. *Pflügers Arch* 1994;428:60–68.
117. Sackin H. A stretch-activated K^+ channel sensitive to cell volume. *Proc Natl Acad Sci U S A* 1989;86:1731–1735.
118. Sackin H. Stretch-activated potassium channels in renal proximal tubules. *Am J Physiol* 1987;253:F1253–F1262.
119. Sackin H, Boulpaep EL. Isolated perfused salamander proximal tubule: methods, electrophysiology, and transport. *Am J Physiol* 1981;241:F39–F52.
120. Sackin H, Boulpaep EL. Rheogenic transport in the renal proxima l tubule. *J Gen Physiol* 1983;82:819–851.
121. Sackin H, Palmer LG. Basolateral potassium channels in renal proximal tubule. *Am J Physiol* 1987;253:F476–F487.
122. Deleted in proof.
123. Sakmann B, Neher E. *Single-Channel Recording*. 2nd ed. New York: Plenum Press, 1995.
124. Sansom SC, La B-Q, Carosi SL. Potassium and chloride channels of the basolateral membrane (BLM) of the rabbit cortical collecting duct (CCD). *Kidney Int* 1990;37:570.
125. Segal A, Boulpaep EL, Maunsbach AB. A novel preparation of dissociated renal proximal tubule cells that maintain epithelial polarity in suspension. *Am J Physiol (Cell)* 1996;270: C1843–C1863.
126. Spring K. Insertion of an axial electrode into renal proximal tubule. *Yale J Biol Med* 1972;45:426.
127. Spring KR. Current-induced voltage transients in *Necturus* proximal tubule. *J Membr Biol* 1973;13:299–322.
128. Stoner LC, Viggiano SC. Environmental KCl causes an upregulation of apical membrane maxi K and ENaC channels in everted *Ambystoma* collecting tubule. *J Membr Biol* 1998;162:107–116.

129. Thomas RC. Electrogenic sodium pump in nerve and muscle cells. *Physiol Rev* 1972;52: 563–594.
130. Tsuchiya K, Wang W, Giebisch G, Welling PA. ATP is a coupling modulator of parallel Na/K ATPase K channel activity in the renal proximal tubule. *Proc Natl Acad Sci U S A* 1992;89:6418–6422.
131. Ussing HH, Zerahn K. Active transport of sodium as the source of electric current in the short-circuited isolated frog skin. *Acta Physiol Scand* 1951;23:110–127.
132. Van Driessche W, Zeiske W. Ba2+-induced conductance fluctuations of spontaneously fluctuating K+ channels in the apical membrane of frog skin (*Rana temporaria*). *J Membr Biol* 1980;56:31–42.
133. Van-Driessche W, Erlij D. Cyclic AMP increases electrical capacitance of apical membrane of toad urinary bladder. *Arch Int Physiol Biochim Biophys* 1991;99(6):409–11.
134. Wang W, McNicholas CM, Segal AS, Giebisch G. A novel approach allows identification of K channels in the lateral membrane of rat CCD. *Am J Physiol* 1994;266:F813–F822.
135. Wang W, White S, Geibel J, Giebisch G. A potassium channel in the apical membrane of rabbit thick ascending limb of Henle's loop. *Am J Physiol* 1990;258:F244–F253.
136. Weber GH, Frömter E. Influence of lateral intercellular spaces on current propagation in tubular epithelia as estimated by a multi-cable model. *Pflügers Arch* 1988;411:153–159.
137. Weinstein FC, Rosowski JJ, Peterson K, Delalic Z, Civan MM. Relationship of transient electrical properties to active sodium transport by toad urinary bladder. *J Membr Biol* 1980;52:25–35.
138. Wills NK, Alles WP, Sandle GI, Binder HJ. Apical membrane properties and amiloride binding kinetics of the human descending colon. *Am J Physiol* 1984;247: G749–G757.
139. Wills NK, Eaton D, Lewis SA, Ifshin M. Current-voltage relationship of the basolateral membrane of a tight epithelium. *Biochim Biophys Acta* 1979;555:519–523.
140. Wills NK, Purcell RK, Clausen C. Na+ transport and impedance properties of cultured renal (A6 and 2F3) epithelia. *J Membr Biol* 1992;125(3):273–285.

CHAPTER **9**

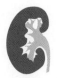

Exchange of Fluid and Solutes Across Microvascular Walls

C. Charles Michel

Imperial College, London, London, United Kingdom

INTRODUCTION

Transfer of water and solutes through microvascular walls is both the initial and final step of their transport by circulation. In most tissues, microvascular exchange is a passive process. Lipophilic molecules and small water-soluble molecules and ions can diffuse between the capillary blood and the surrounding interstitial fluid (ISF) but microvascular walls are a barrier to macromolecules, impeding their exchange. The small differences in macromolecular concentration across microvascular walls are responsible for differences in osmotic pressure, which were identified over a century ago to play an essential role in the balance of fluid between the circulating blood and the tissues (135).

Although small hydrophilic molecules can exchange rapidly between the blood and the tissues, it is wrong to assume that microvascular walls are no barrier to them. The rate at which changes in concentration of a solute in the blood can be reflected as changes in ISF concentration depends on the blood flow to the capillary beds as well as the permeability of the capillary walls to the solute. It is often assumed that for small molecules only blood flow is important, but once flow has exceeded a certain minimum range of values, the rate of equilibration of blood and ISF become limited by permeability.

There is a wide range of values for the permeability to water and small hydrophilic solutes in various capillary beds. Although absolute values cover a range of three orders of magnitude, these values are related by general principles; this chapter is focused on such principles. Not discussed here are the very low permeabilities of the microvessels of the central nervous system. The exchange of solutes between the blood and the brain and spinal cord is achieved by a series of specialized transport mechanisms that are characteristic of tight epithelia. For this reason, they are not considered in this chapter.

Whereas useful generalizations of microvascular exchange are physiological principles, microvascular permeability itself has an ultrastructural basis, which is considered first in this chapter. Next is a discussion of microvascular permeability

starting with the principles of passive transport through membranes that define the permeability coefficients and then considers the ultrastructural basis of permeability. Finally, the physiological process of fluid and solute exchange through microvascular walls is reviewed with a brief summary of current ideas of how permeability might change.

ULTRASTRUCTURE OF MICROVASCULAR WALLS

Light microscopy in the second half of the 19th century revealed that capillary walls were made of a single layer of flattened endothelial cells. In certain places these fine tubes were reinforced on the outside by pericytes, and the further upstream to the arterioles, the greater the density of the spiral of smooth muscle cells. The lines of contact between the endothelial cells could be stained with silver salts, an observation that led to the idea that they were held together by "cement-like substance" (22).

Electron microscopy of capillary walls revealed that the endothelium is of two distinct types that have been called "continuous" and "fenestrated" (Fig. 1). Continuous endothelium is found in microvessels of skin, muscle, lung, and connective tissues. Here, the endothelial cells are joined together by tight junctions to form a continuous layer surrounded by a continuous basement membrane. The plasmalemmal membranes of the continuous endothelia retain their integrity, even in areas where the cells are flattened, which reduces their thickness to less than 0.1 µm, the distinct luminal and abluminal membranes are separated by a thin layer of cytoplasm.

Fenestrated endothelium is found in microvessels associated with secretory and absorptive epithelia, such as the villus capillaries of the intestinal mucosae, and glomerular and peritubular capillaries of the kidney. The walls of fenestrated microvessels are also made of a single continuous layer of endothelial cells joined by tight junctions and surrounded by a continuous basement membrane, but in these vessels attenuated areas of cells appear to be penetrated by circular openings 40–70 nm in diameter. These are the fenestrae (or

A

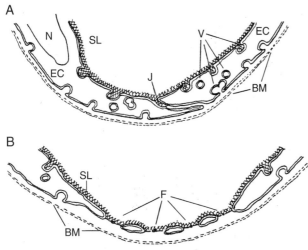

B

FIGURE 1 Diagrams showing the ultrastructural features of microvascular walls in transverse section. **A.** Vessel with continuous endothelium. **B.** Vessel with fenestrated endothelium. The basement membrane forms a continuous layer around the outside of both vessel types, and the luminal surfaces of both endothelia are covered with a negatively charged glycocalyx (SL). BM, basement membrane; EC, endothelial cell; F, fenestration (fenestra); J, junction.

fenestrations), and in most cases the fenestrations are closed by a thin electron-dense diaphragm, which appears to be arranged as a series of broad spokes with central "hub" (14) (Fig. 2).

Although both continuous and fenestrated endothelia have been found to contain the various inclusions common to most cells (e.g., mitochondria, rough and smooth endoplasmic reticulum), the dominating ultrastructural feature seen in transmission electron micrography is the large number of small endoplasmic vesicles or caveolae (Fig. 3). Before 1980, each vesicle was considered to be a separate entity that moved within the cell and occasionally fused with another vesicle or with the luminal or abluminal membrane where they formed flask-like pits (intracellular caveolae) (16). Differential staining (19) and reconstruction from serial ultrathin sections (37) showed that the majority of vesicles are arranged in fused clusters that communicate with caveolae on either the luminal or abluminal surfaces of the cells. Chains of fused vesicles forming channels that pass through endothelial cells (133) appear to be relatively rare occurrences in unstimulated endothelium but are a feature of endothelium activated by certain mediators (35, 36). The small (70-nm diameter) vesicles were originally believed to be uncoated, in contrast to the clathrin-coated (rough) endocytic vesicles, which are also found in endothelial cells. Structural evidence of a coat for these vesicles was followed by the identification of caveolin as one of the principal components of the coat (101, 124). Subsequent isolation of small vesicles from rat lung endothelium (57) has shown a variety of proteins are located in caveolae membranes, such as Ca ATPase, IP3 receptors, GTPases including dynamin, aquaporin 1, vesicle-associated membrane protein 2 (VAMP-2), soluble NSF-

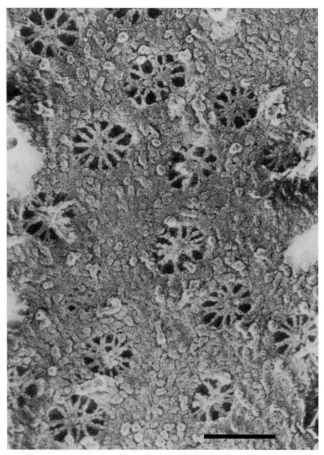

FIGURE 2 En face view of fenestrated endothelium of peritubular capillary of the kidney in a rapid-freeze deep-etch preparation. Scale bar = 0.1 μm. (From Bearer EL, Orci L. Endothelial fenestral diaphragms: a quick freeze deep etch study. *J Cell Biol* 1985;100:418–428.)

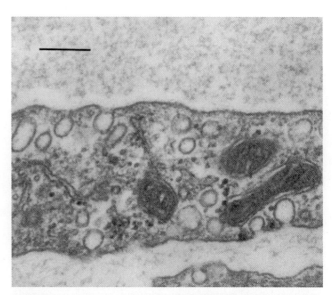

FIGURE 3 Electron micrograph of microvascular endothelium of frog. There are three mitochondria in the central part of the cell and large numbers of plasmalemmel vesicles. Scale bar = 0.2 μm. (Electron micrograph by H. Moffitt.)

sensitive protein (SNAP), as well as NO synthase, which is also found in other regions of the endothelial plasmalemmal membrane (128, 129).

In addition to caveolae, endothelial cells also contain vacuoles and as noted earlier, clathrin-coated vesicles. In the endothelium of vessels supplying tumors and in venular endothelium of skin and muscle, clusters of caveolae are often associated with larger vacuoles. These composite structures have been named *vesico-vacuolar organelles* (VVOs) (34). There are reasons to believe that VVOs play an important part in the regulation of microvascular permeability (34, 35).

The endothelial cytoskeleton is less conspicuous than the vesicles in conventional electron micrographs. It is made up of three types of supporting fiber: (1) extensive systems of polymerized actin, (2) microtubules formed from tubulin, and (3) intermediate filaments. The actin fibers are present in three forms. First, there is the cortical web, which consists of a network of fine actin fibers beneath the cell surface membranes. Second, stress fibers, which are multistranded cables of actin, tend to be aligned in the direction of the shearing force. Third, there are junctional associated filaments (JAF), which lie within the cell close to the intercellular junctions (32). Like stress fibers, the JAF are made of multistranded cables of actin filaments and both these forms of the actin cytoskeleton can be readily visualized using light microscopy and appropriate staining techniques. Studies using these methods have demonstrated the dynamic nature of the endothelial actin cytoskeleton. Stress fibers that are normally absent from cultured endothelial cells in vitro can be induced by subjecting the cells to shear (33). Breaks in the JAF are seen to occur in venular endothelial cells exposed to histamine (139).

The microtubules are fibers that can resist compression, and it has been suggested that many short-term mechanical responses of endothelium can be accounted for if changes in cell shape are determined by contractile fibers that generate isometric tension by compressing microtubular structures.

Thus, changes in cell shape and the transmission of mechanical forces across a cell may be determined by changes in the supporting structures (opposing tension) in regions of the cell rather than by generation of additional tension (56). This "tensegrity" model of endothelial cell shape may account for the rounding up of endothelial cells when their attachments have been lost.

Endothelial cells are attached through α/β integrins on their abluminal surfaces to focal adhesion sites on the basement membranes. The integrins connect via "linker" molecules (e.g., α-actinin, vinculin, talin) to fibers of the cytoskeleton. The cells are also linked to each other in the junctional region. The detailed ultrastructure of the intercellular junctions is of great importance in understanding microvascular permeability. In conventional electron micrographs of both continuous and fenestrated endothelia, there is a cleft between adjacent endothelial cells, and for most of its length, it is 15–20 nm wide. At one or more points along its length, however, the cleft is narrowed and the outer leaflets of the adjacent cell membranes appear to fuse (Fig. 4). These points of apposition appear to prevent the diffusion of lanthanum ions within the clefts. Reconstructions from serial sections (4, 5, 18) show that the tight regions extend as lines or strands of molecules along the cleft roughly parallel to the luminal surface. These strands are equivalent to rows of membrane particles that run as discontinuous branching ridges in freeze-fracture preparations of intercellular clefts. Lanthanum ions can diffuse through occasional breaks in the strands, indicating that these breaks are a pathway for small hydrophilic solutes through the endothelial barrier (5).

Cytoplasmic aspects of the membranes in the tight junctions are linked to the cytoskeleton through the cadherin and catenin groups of proteins. The role of the cytoskeleton in regulating the tight region of the clefts is a subject of much speculation. In work on the regulation of tight junctions in epithelial cells, there is evidence to suggest that

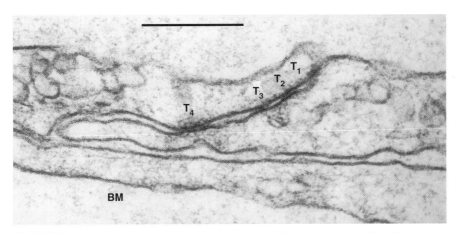

FIGURE 4 Electron micrograph of intercellular junction of frog mesenteric capillary. Note how the outer leaflets of the adjacent cells appear to touch and fuse at four points (T1–T4). Scale bar = 0.2 μm. (With permission, from Mason JC, Curry FE, White IF, Michel CC. The ultrastructure of frog mesenteric capillaries of known filtration coefficient. *Q J Exp Physiol* 1979;64:217–224.) BM, basement membrane.

tyrosine phosphorylation of the β catenins may trigger a cascade of events that opens the tight junction (2).

Another ultrastructural feature of importance in microvascular permeability is the glycocalyx of the endothelium (Fig. 5). This layer of glycosylated protein covers the luminal surface (including the fenestrae) and in electron micrographs appears to extend for 30–50 nm beyond the outer plasmalemmal leaflet into the vessel lumen. In vivo observations using confocal microscopy suggest that it may extend even further, being up to 1.0 μm in microvessels and up to 3 μm in larger (100-μm diameter) arterioles (142, 143). The layer was originally demonstrated by electron microscopy using cationic stains such as ruthenium red and alcian blue, but has since been shown by a range of other methods (122, 123, 134). Although a variety of molecules of the glycocalyx have been identified, until recently there has been little experimental evidence for its general organization. Luft's hypothesis (69) that it might act as a molecular filter was supported by observation of exclusion of native ferritin molecules from the luminal caveolae (23, 68, 131), and led to the fiber matrix theory of permeability (30). A consequence of this quantitative theory was that a network of filamentous molecules would act as a more efficient filter if the spaces within it were of uniform size (76, 77). This implies a regularity of structure and recent image analysis of electron micrographs of glycocalyx prepared using a range of different techniques show a quasiperiodic structure consistent with this prediction (134). Some of the specimens used in this study were prepared by rapid freeze-deep etch in the absence of chemical fixatives. Squire et al. (134) have proposed that the glycocalyx is made up of regular arrays of either large globular proteins linked by short filamentous chains or a lattice of large-diameter (12 nm) cylindrical molecules (Fig. 6).

Microvascular Permeability

The barrier nature of microvascular walls can be demonstrated in vivo by inspecting the microcirculation of a suitably illuminated tissue after intravascular injection of macromolecules labeled with dyes or fluorescent tracers. If the macromolecules are larger than serum albumin, the labeled molecules are retained within the microcirculation for tens of minutes after their injection into the blood. By contrast, if the tracer is not bound to macromolecules and itself has a low molecular weight, it leaks out of the microcirculation into the tissues within minutes or less. Observations of this kind have been made with varying degrees of sophistication for more than 100 years. They are still used for detecting increases in vascular permeability to macromolecules when increases in the net transport of macromolecules into tissues are assumed to indicate increases in permeability. This assumption is valid only when such experiments are carefully controlled, because blood flow, mean microvascular pressure, and the number of perfused exchange vessels in a tissue may vary, alone or together, and may have large effects on net transport.

The functional measurements that can be related directly to permeability itself are the permeability coefficients. These arise from the general principles of passive transport of fluids and solutes through porous membranes, and it is useful to define them in this context.

Passive Transport and Permeability Coefficients of Porous Membranes

Net transport of fluid and solutes through a membrane is said to be passive when the transport is driven by the differences in the potential energy of the solutions on each

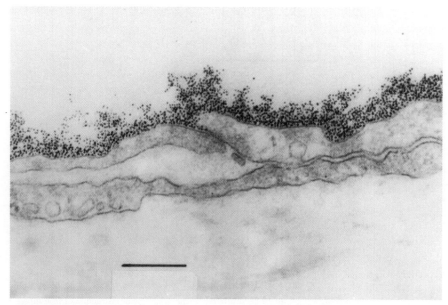

FIGURE 5   Transverse section of microvessel with cationized ferritin binding to the glycocalyx on the luminal endothelial surface. Scale bar = 0.5 μm. (Electron micrograph by Dr. G. Clough.)

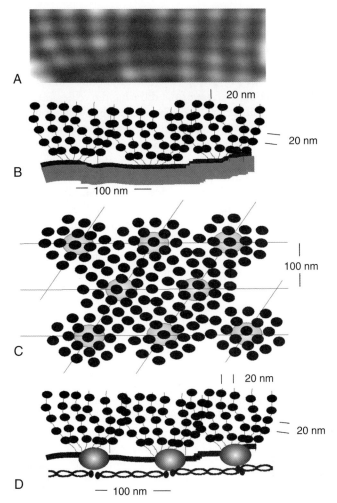

FIGURE 6 Models of glycocalyx based on image analysis of electron micrographs. (a) An autocorrelation function of the glycocalyx indicating the underlying regularity of structure with a periodicity of approximately 20 nm both parallel and perpendicular to the cell membrane. (b) A molecular interpretation of (a) informed by results of Rostgaard and Qvortrup (123). It consists of clusters of fibrous strands projecting perpendicular to the luminal cell membrane with the 20-nm periodicity along the strand provided by equally spaced globular proteins. It is suggested that adjacent clusters are separated by approximately 100 nm (consistent with a longer range periodicity), where they are linked to the cortical cytoskeleton of the cell. Parts (c) and (d) show luminal surface and saggital views of proposed structure. (From Squire JM, Chew M, Nnije G, Neal C, Michel CC. Quasi-`periodic substructure in the microvessel endothelial glycocalyx: possible explanation for molecular filtering? *J Struct Biol* 2002;136:239–255.)

side of the membrane, and no energy is supplied to the transport process within the membrane. Across microvascular walls, differences in potential energy between the plasma and interstitial fluid arise from differences in the local hydrostatic pressures and solute concentrations. The mechanisms of transport are convection and diffusion. Convection is equivalent to bulk flow of solutions and the solutes within them. Thus, if a solution flows from a reservoir A at a high pressure to a second reservoir, B, at a lower pressure, there is bulk flow of the solution and transport of

the solutes by convection. If J_V is the rate at which the solution flows from A to B (in milliliters per second), it is proportional to the difference in hydrostatic pressure, ΔP, between A and B as follows:

$$J_V = K\Delta P \tag{1}$$

where K is the conductance of the system between A and B.

If A and B are separated by a porous membrane, K is proportional to the area of the membrane, A_m, through which fluid can flow. Thus:

$$J_V = L_P A_m \Delta P \tag{2}$$

where L_P is the hydraulic conductivity or hydraulic permeability of the membrane. L_P is a permeability coefficient of the membrane. It describes the ease with which fluid flows through a unit area of membrane by a unit difference in pressure. It can be thought of as describing the frictional interactions between the membrane molecules and the molecules of the solution (principally water). If small water-filled pores penetrate the membrane, L_P is proportional to the number of pores per unit area of membrane, to the fluid viscosity, and to a function of pore dimensions. This function depends on the size and shape of the pores and the nature of flow through them.

The rate of solute transport, J_S, by convection through the membrane from A to B depends on J_V and the hindrance that the solute molecules encounter relative to the water molecules as the solution flows through the membrane. If the membrane hinders the flow of water and solute to an equal extent, then J_S is equal to $J_V C$ (in moles per second), where C is the solute concentration in the solution (in moles per milliliter). Under these conditions the solution flowing out of the membrane into B has the same concentration as that entering the membrane from A. If, however, the flow of solute molecules through the membrane is hindered to a greater extent than water, then the solution emerging from the membrane into B will have a lower solute concentration than that entering the membrane at A. Under these conditions a fraction of the solute molecules can be considered to be rejected or reflected by the membrane. The degree of reflection or rejection of a solute is described by a second permeability coefficient, the reflection coefficient, σ_f. Convective transport of solute through the membrane is now described by the relation:

$$J_S = J_V(1 - \sigma_f)C \tag{3}$$

where C now refers to concentration entering the membrane from A. Rearrangement of Eq. 3 provides a definition of σ_f:

$$\sigma_f = 1 - \frac{J_S}{J_V C} \tag{4}$$

A second mechanism of transport through porous membranes is diffusion. This is the most important mechanism for the transport of small molecules across microvascular walls. In contrast to the stately progression of molecules by convection, diffusion results from the random jostling of all molecules in a solution that represents their thermal energy. Diffusion is a mixing process, and where there are differences in concentration in a solution, diffusion is responsible for the spontaneous net transport of solute from regions of high to regions of low concentration. On a macroscopic scale, Fick's first law of diffusion describes net transport of solute by diffusion as follows:

$$J_S = DA\left(\frac{-dC}{dx}\right) \qquad (5)$$

where D is the diffusion coefficient of the solute in the solution, A is the area through which diffusion occurs and the derivative $(-dC/dx)$, is the concentration gradient of solute down which diffusion occurs. The negative sign of the derivative is to indicate that diffusion occurs from a region of high concentration (low value of x) to a region of lower concentration (higher value of x).

Diffusion coefficients of solutes in aqueous solutions reflect the ability of solute molecules to slip past adjacent molecules of water. They are measured and defined in terms of net movements of solute under conditions in which there is no overall movement of the solution. Thus, diffusion in solution is a displacement process whereby the displacement of a solute molecule in one direction is accompanied by the displacement of an equal volume of water in the opposite direction. Because the rate at which displacement occurs is dependent on the thermal energy of the solution, the diffusion coefficient is directly proportional to temperature. It is also inversely proportional to the frictional interactions between the solute and water molecules.

When diffusion of a solute occurs through a thin porous membrane, the diffusional permeability of the membrane to the solute, P_d, is defined in terms of the net solute flux, J_S, the solute concentration difference across the membrane, ΔC, and the membrane area, A_m, under conditions where there is no volume flow through the membrane. Thus:

$$P_d = \left(\frac{J_S}{A_m \Delta C}\right)_{J_V = 0} \qquad (6)$$

P_d has units of velocity (cm sec^{-1}) and like L_P and σ_f, it has meaning in terms of the interactions between the solute molecules, the molecules of the membrane, and the water within the membrane. Such interactions depend critically on the ultrastructure of the pathways for solute and water through the membrane, particularly when the width of the pathways is comparable to the diameters of the diffusing molecules.

Diffusional permeability coefficients are defined under conditions where there is no net volume flow through the membrane ($J_V = 0$). In measuring P_d of microvascular walls, it is often convenient to use radioactive isotopes or fluores-

cent tracers because their fluxes can be detected when their concentration differences are in the micromolar range. Larger differences in concentration may set up significant differences in osmotic pressure which may complicate the estimation of P_d by giving rise to net fluid flows in the opposite direction to those of the diffusing molecules.

The magnitude of the osmotic pressure that is set up by a solute concentration difference across a membrane is related not only to the concentration difference itself but also to the osmotic reflection coefficient, σ_d, of the membrane to the diffusing solute. For an "ideal" solute, σ_d is equal to σ_f. Some insight to this equality is gained by considering that only those molecules that are reflected at the membrane during ultrafiltration can exert an osmotic pressure across it. Thus, the osmotic pressure difference, $\Delta\Pi$, is related to the concentration difference, ΔC, through the universal gas constant, R, and the absolute temperature, T, as follows:

$$\Delta\Pi = \sigma_d RT\Delta C$$

and

$$\sigma_d = \frac{\Delta\Pi}{RT\Delta C} \qquad (7)$$

Reflection coefficients have maximum values of 1.0 (100% reflection) and minimum values for hydrophilic solutes of zero. Negative values of reflection coefficient are possible and represent situations where the solute can cross the membrane more rapidly than the solvent. If the only pathway for both water and solutes through the membrane is a population of equally sized channels, σ_d and σ_f are determined only by the ratio of the dimensions of the solute molecules to those of the channels, and are independent of the number of channels per unit area of membrane.

At microvascular walls, macromolecules such as plasma proteins have high values of σ_d and σ_f (0.8–0.999), whereas small ions (e.g., Na$^+$, K$^+$, Cl$^-$) and small hydrophilic molecules (e.g., glucose, lactic acid, amino acids, urea) have σ values of less than 0.2 in most vessels.

Permeability Coefficients in Different Microvascular Beds

Most of the early quantitative estimates of microvascular permeability were based on fluxes of solutes and fluid into whole tissues and organs. Even though the fluxes themselves could be measured with accuracy, the pressure and concentration differences across the walls of the exchange vessels, although estimated by a range of ingenious techniques, were averages. The permeability coefficients derived from them could therefore be no more than average properties of hundreds of thousands of individual exchange vessels in a particular organ or tissue. A further uncertainty lies in estimates of the area of the exchange vessel walls through which the measured fluxes had occurred. This was once again an average based on the histology of the tissue. Despite these limitations, a clear picture of the general properties of microvascular permeability emerged and this picture has been confirmed and extended by studies on single microvessels (79, 80, 85).

From the point of view of solute permeability, solutes can be divided into three groups: lipophilic solutes, small hydrophilic solutes, and macromolecules. The permeability of each group is considered in the following sections.

PERMEABILITY TO LIPOPHILIC SOLUTES

Solutes that can dissolve to a significant extent in lipids have high cell membrane permeabilities and very high microvascular permeabilities. It is assumed that these molecules diffuse directly through the entire microvascular wall. This group of solutes includes gas molecules, including O_2 and CO_2 as well as N_2, the inert gases and molecules of general anesthetics.

Lipophilic solutes can cross microvascular walls so rapidly that, under physiological conditions, their transport between the blood and the tissues is always limited by their rate of delivery or clearance by blood flow through the microcirculation. This has made it impossible to estimate their microvascular permeability coefficients with accuracy. Perl et al. (100) investigated the transport of a series of amides and diols in the microcirculation of dog lungs, and concluded that these molecules had permeability coefficients in the range of 12 to 50×10^{-5} cm sec^{-1} but these values may underestimate their true values by an order of magnitude or more. Microvascular walls appear to be no more of a barrier to the exchange of the lipophilic molecules than the surrounding tissue, and this is usually assumed to be so in calculations of gradients of O_2 and CO_2 concentration (or partial pressure) in tissues.

Microvascular permeability to lipophilic molecules is sensitive to temperature. Renkin (107) showed that antipyrene, which is fat soluble at body temperature, could exert substantial osmotic pressures across the walls of capillaries in cat hind limbs when the tissue was cooled to 15°C, but not when the tissue was at 37°C. A similar phenomenon has been demonstrated by Curry (25) in single mesenteric capillaries.

PERMEABILITY TO SMALL HYDROPHILIC SOLUTES

The division of hydrophilic solutes into small and large may seem arbitrary, but it has an important physiological basis. If permeability coefficients to hydrophilic molecules of different molecular sizes are determined for a given type of microvessel, it is found that those for the small molecules decline steeply as molecular size increases up to the size of the serum albumin molecule. For larger molecules, it is found that permeability coefficients decline much less rapidly as molecular size increases. This is shown in Fig. 7, which is based on data for microvessels in the limbs of dogs and cats where the endothelium is continuous. Values of P_d have been plotted on a logarithmic scale so that a full range of values can be displayed. Log P_d falls almost linearly until molecular diameter reaches 71 Å

(7.1 nm), which is the molecular diameter of serum albumin. From this point onward, P_d declines much less rapidly. This two-component relation between P_d and molecular diameter is seen in nearly all microvascular beds, and suggests that different mechanisms or pathways are available to small molecules and large molecules through microvascular walls.

Some of the early rapid decline of P_d with increasing molecular size can be accounted for by the decrease in diffusion coefficient of hydrophilic molecules in aqueous solutions (D) with increasing molecular diameter. But P_d declines far more rapidly than D as molecular diameter increases. This difference is regarded as evidence for *restricted diffusion*, such as would occur if the solutes were diffusing through water-filled channels whose width was comparable to the diameters of the diffusing molecules (97). If the channels are cylindrical pores or rectangular slits, the radius of the pore or width of the slit can be calculated from the degree of restricted diffusion, assuming that all the channels have the same dimensions (97).

While the pattern of declining P_d with molecular diameter is seen in all microvessels where it has been sought, the absolute values of P_d for the smaller molecules vary considerably in exchange vessels of one tissue compared with those in another. Thus, the permeability of mesenteric capillaries to Na^+ and K^+ ions is 20 to 30 times greater than that of capillaries in skeletal muscle even though both types of vessel have walls of continuous endothelium, which appear to be very similar in conventional electron micrographs.

The wide range of values of P_d to the smaller hydrophilic solutes is correlated with the range of values of hydraulic permeability (L_p) in different microvascular beds. This is shown in Fig. 8, where each point represents the mean value of L_p plotted against the mean value of P_d to Na^+ or K^+ in the same microvessel or microvascular bed, with points representing values for vessels in various tissues. The data have been plotted on logarithmic scales so that values covering two orders of magnitude can be compared. The slope that has been drawn through the points has been given a value of unity to indicate that direct proportionality is a reasonable description of the relationship. The correlation is strong, circumstantial evidence for believing that the same pathways through the endothelium serve both for the rapid exchange of small hydrophilic solutes and for most of net fluid movements. Furthermore, because Na^+ ions are likely to follow an extracellular route, it seems likely that this shared pathway is extracellular. This line of reasoning is greatly strengthened by the demonstration of similar linear correlations between L_P and P_d values for other extracellular solutes such as sucrose and inulin (85) in different microvascular beds.

Although most of the net movements of fluid do occur through the same channels as those used for exchanges of small hydrophilic molecules, some water may also cross microvascular walls of continuous endothelium by channels not available to solutes. In the last decade, this additional route

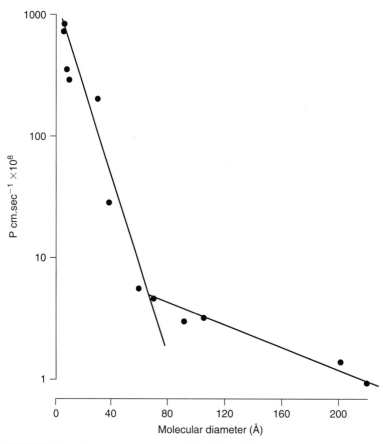

FIGURE 7 Relations between permeability (P) of dog hind-limb microvessels to hydrophilic solutes and the molecular diameter of the solutes. The endothelium of these vessels is continuous, and P has been calculated assuming that the vessels have a surface area for exchange of 7000 cm² 100g⁻¹ of tissue. Note that P, which has been plotted on a logarithmic scale, declines sharply as molecular diameter increases up to 70 Å (7 nm), which is approximately the diameter of serum albumin. A less steep relation is seen for larger molecules. (With permission from Michel CC, Clough GF. Capillary permeability and transvascular fluid balance. In: Sleight P, Vann Jones J, eds. *Scientific Foundations of Cardiology.* London: Heinemann, 1983:25–30.)

has been identified as channels formed by the membrane protein aquaporin-1, AQP-1, (7). Evidence for a "water only" pathway was first demonstrated by Yudilevich and Alvarez (154) who found that the rate of diffusional exchange of triated water through dog heart capillaries was greater than that for Na⁺ by a factor that was too large to be accounted for by the difference in their diffusion coefficients in water. Curry et al. (29) showed that in single perfused capillaries, the values of reflection coefficients to small hydrophilic solutes did not extrapolate to zero as their molecular size decreased to that of a water molecule. They concluded that this could be accounted for if 5%–10% of the net fluid movements occurred through channels that were unavailable to small solutes. More recently, Turner and Pallone (140) have shown that a similar proportion of the L_P of descending vasa recta of rat kidney is accounted for by "water only" channels. Here, Pallone and colleagues (95) have demonstrated water flow through this pathway can be inhibited by mercurial compounds (which block AQP channels), and

that the magnitude of this pathway is directly proportional to the density of AQP-1 molecules in endothelial cells. It is worth emphasizing that although fluid movements through AQP-1 channels of the descending vasa recta are of physiological importance, the channels contribute no more than 5%–10% to the total L_P of these vessels. Although it has been suggested that AQP-1 channels might contribute to as much as 30% of the L_P of skeletal muscle capillaries (151), the strong correlation between P_d and L_P shown in Fig. 8 indicates that the contribution of AQP-1 channels to the L_P of most exchange vessels is small.

Although absolute values of L_P and P_d to small hydrophilic solutes vary greatly from one microvascular bed to another, the reflection coefficients to large molecules are remarkably similar in different vessels when the tissues are undamaged (or unstimulated). This is shown in Fig. 9, where the mean values of σ to serum albumin have been plotted against the mean value of L_P for various tissues. Whereas L_P varies over three orders of magnitude, σ to al-

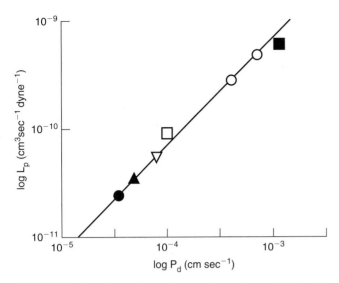

FIGURE 8 Variations in L_P and P_d to small ions (Na^+ and K^+) in different microvascular beds. The scales are logarithmic to include values covering two orders of magnitude and the line has a slope of 1.0, indicating direct proportionality. Each point represents the value for L_P and P_d for one vascular bed; where several values of P_d are available, the largest has been used to minimize errors resulting from flow-limited transport. (With permission from Michel CC. Review lecture–capillary permeability and how it may change. *J Physiol* 1988; 404:1–29.) O, frog mesentery; ▽ frog muscle; ●, mammalian skeletal muscle; □, mammalian heart muscle; ▲, dog lung; ■, cat salivary gland.

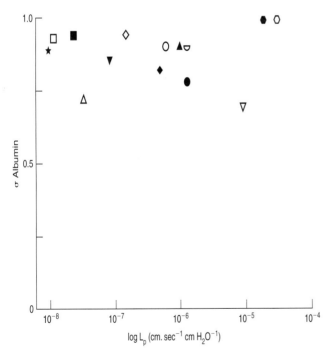

FIGURE 9 Relation between the reflection coefficient to serum albumin (σ) and the LP in various microvascular beds. Each point represents a mean value for one vascular bed. (Based on Michel CC. Review lecture—capillary permeability and how it may change. *J Physiol* 1988;404:1–29 with permission, with more recent additions.) *, dog paw; □, dog skeletal muscle; ■, rat skeletal muscle; △, dog lung; ▼, rabbit heart muscle; ◇, rat mesentery; ♦, frog mesentery; O, cat salivary gland; ▲, rat descending vasa recta; ▽, cat small intestine; ●, rabbit synovium; ▽, rat ascending vasa recta; ◕, dog renal glomerulus; O, rat renal glomerulus.

bumin is usually in the range of 0.8 to 1.0. There is no trend in the relation between $\sigma_{albumin}$ and L_P. Vessels with high values of L_P have mean values of $\sigma_{albumin}$ that are as high if not higher than those in vessels with low values of L_P. This strongly suggests that the channels or pores that are largely responsible for the L_P of vessels in different tissues all restrict the passage of albumin to a similar extent. The differences in the values of L_P and P_d for small molecules are the result of differences in the number of channels per unit area of microvascular wall rather than variations in the size or structure of individual pores or channels.

Ultrastructural Basis of Permeability to Water and Small Hydrophilic Molecules

The vessels with the five highest values of L_P in Fig. 9 have walls of fenestrated endothelia. By contrast, all but one of the other vessels in Fig. 9 have walls of continuous endothelia. The inference that the fenestrae were responsible for the high values of L_P of fenestrated endothelia was greatly strengthened by a quantitative analysis of Levick and Smaje (67). These authors found that variations in L_P and P_d to small hydrophilic solutes in fenestrated vessels can be correlated with the number of fenestrations per unit area of endothelium. They were able estimate the L_P of a single fenestration with a 60-nm diameter at 0.6–2.5 cm sec^{-1} cm H_2O^{-1}. Although in conventionally prepared transmission electron micrographs, fenestrations appear as pores passing through the endothelium, the fenestrations themselves are much too large to account for the sieving of macromolecules and their consequent high reflection coefficients. Molecular sieving is achieved by the endothelial glycocalyx with significant contributions to the hydraulic resistance from the fenestral diaphragms and the basement membrane.

While the variations in L_P of fenestrated vessels may result from variations in the number of fenestrae per unit area of vessel wall, why do vessels with continuous endothelia have L_P values that vary so much from tissue to tissue? It has been widely believed for many years that pathways through continuous endothelium for water and small water-soluble solutes are located in the intercellular clefts. Nearly all the ultrastructural evidence reported before 1993 was qualitative and open to debate and controversy. While electron opaque tracers, such as microperoxidase, myoglobin, and horseradish peroxidase, could be injected into the blood of an experimental animal and subsequently found to be labeling the intercellular clefts of microvessels, this labeling could be observed consistently only if several minutes elapsed between the injection of the tracer and the sampling of the tissue. The failure of the intercellular clefts to label consistently led to doubts that the pathways were located here particularly when tracer could be seen in the small vesicles by this time (132). Simionescu et al. (133) proposed that the channels through the endothelial cells were formed by chains of fused vesicles. These, however, are hard to find in continuous endothelium and there is now evidence to suggest that they might be associated with endothelial cell activation (35).

One of the problems of merely looking for the presence or absence of tracer in the intercellular cleft is that only a fraction of the cleft needs to be open to account for the permeability of most capillaries with continuous endothelium. As early as 1970, calculations had indicated that the permeability of muscle capillaries to Cr-EDTA (which has the same molecular diameter as sucrose) could be accounted for if only 5%–10% of the intercellular clefts were open (63). Wissig and Williams (150) first provided ultrastructural evidence that only a fraction of the intercellular cleft was available for paracellular transport in mouse diaphragm capillaries. From an analysis of the passage of microperoxidase and freeze-fracture images of the junctions, these authors suggested that small solutes followed a tortuous route through breaks in the tight junctions. Convincing support for this idea was subsequently published by Bundgaard (18). Reconstructing the intercellular clefts of mouse heart capillaries from serial sections, he showed that occasional breaks in the tight junctions allowed a tortuous path to be followed through the cleft from vessel lumen to basement membrane. Bundgaard (18), however, suggested that this tortuous path was not the principal route for small solutes and water because at no point did it appear narrow enough to hinder the passage of macromolecules. Throughout wide regions of the cleft, adjacent endothelial cells are separated by a distance of approximately 18 to 20 nm, and Bundgaard found a similar separation was present at the breaks in the tight junctions. Because these sites could not act as appropriate molecular filters, Bundgaard looked elsewhere for the small solute pathway. In occasional ultrathin sections, he observed that in the region of the tight junction the two outer leaflets of the adjacent endothelial cells were not fused but separated by a difference of 4 nm. He suggested that these openings in the tight junction were the "small pores" which constituted the principal hydrophilic pathway through the vessel wall, and that macromolecules were filtered from plasma here.

A few years later, Ward and colleagues (146) showed that electron microscopic examination of the tight junctions in microvascular endothelium on a tilting stage revealed that the outer leaflets of adjacent cells are always separated by a gap of 2 to 5 nm (5, 146). In spite of the apparent pathway indicated by this gap, the tight junctions are impermeable to lanthanum ions although these ions pass freely through the breaks. Adamson and Michel (5) found that these breaks in the tight junctional strands extended for 0.15–0.17 μm in frog mesenteric capillaries, and occurred only once every 2 to 3 μm along the length of the cleft. Using a mathematical model developed by Parker and colleagues (98), Adamson and Michel (5) went on to show that the frequency and dimensions of these breaks were sufficient for a pathway to account for a hydraulic permeability that was two to three times greater than their measurements in these same frog mesenteric capillaries. They concluded that this route was the principal pathway for water and small hydrophilic solutes

through the walls of microvessels with continuous endothelium. The mathematical model provided rigorous arguments for believing that a small break in the junctional strands has a much greater effect on L_P than its size might suggest. The pressure gradient driving fluid flow through the intercellular cleft is steepest across the tiny distance through the break in the strand, and is much greater than that calculated for the entire cleft. More detailed mathematical models have been developed by Weinbaum and colleagues (39, 55, 148), and more recently, Adamson et al. (4) have shown the fine structure of the tight junction in intercellular clefts of rat mesenteric venules is very similar to that seen in frog vessels.

The L_P of mesenteric vessels is approximately three times greater than the L_P of heart muscle capillaries, which is approximately three times greater than the L_P of capillaries in skeletal muscle. These differences in permeability appear to correlate with the complexity of the pathway through the tight junction in these various types of capillary. Reconstruction of the junctions of both frog and rat mesenteric vessels show that although there may be two or more junctional strands for variable distances along the intercellular cleft, only one of these forms a continuous barrier (4, 5). Breaks in this strand offer a more or less direct pathway through the cleft (Fig. 10). The arrangement of junctional strands in heart capillaries appears to be more complex with usually two or more strands running along its entire length (18). A pathway through breaks in these strands is likely to be more tortuous, and thus the permeability of these vessels is lower. Yet more complicated arrangements of junctional strands are found in skeletal muscle capillaries (Fig. 11). It seems most probable that the wide variations in permeability to fluid and small hydrophilic solutes that is found in microvessels with continuous endothelium are determined by the complexity of the tight junctional architecture within the intercellular clefts.

While the detailed examination of the intercellular clefts in continuous capillaries revealed a pathway through the ves-

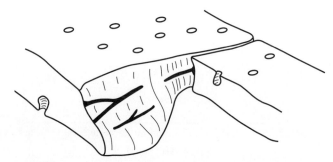

FIGURE 10 Diagram of the ultrastructure of an intercellular cleft based on reconstructions from serial ultrathin sections (5). Part of the cell in the foreground has been removed to expose the interior of the cleft showing the junctional strands (heavy lines), which correspond to points of close apposition between the cells (tight junctions) in single sections. Lanthanum ions cannot diffuse through the junctional strands but pass through breaks in the strands. Because there is usually only one continuous strand in the junctions of mesenteric microvessels, each break provides a direct pathway through the cleft.

A   B   C

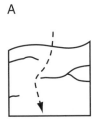 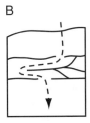 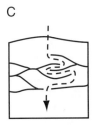

FIGURE 11 Variations in the complexity of junctional strands arrangement in intercellular clefts of microvessels with different hydraulic permeabilities. The dashed lines with arrows indicate potential pathways through the breaks in the strands. A. Mesenteric capillary. (Based on Adamson RH, Michel CC. Pathways through the intercellular clefts of frog mesenteric capillaries. *J Physiol* 1993;466:303–327.) B. Cardiac muscle capillary. (Based on Bundgaard M. The three dimensional organization of tight junctions in a capillary endothelium as revealed by serial section electron microscopy. *J Ultrastruct Res* 1984;88:1–17.) C. Skeletal muscle capillary. (Based on Wissig S, Williams MC. The permeability of muscle capillaries to microperoxidase. *J Cell Biol* 1978;76:341–359.)

sel walls, it did not reveal structures that could act as a barrier to macromolecules and thus be responsible for the ultrafiltration. Adamson and Michel (5) suggested that the glycocalyx on the luminal surface of the endothelium was the ultrafilter as proposed in the fiber matrix model of permeability by Curry and Michel (30). Earlier, Adamson (1) had shown that the L_P of single vessels was doubled by brief perfusions of pronase that disrupt the glycocalyx without having any other detectable effects on endothelial ultrastructure. More recently, Vink, Duling, and colleagues (53, 142, 143) reported observations consistent with the exclusion of macromolecules by the glycocalyx in vivo and loss of this exclusion after perfusion with hyaluronidase (53). More direct evidence comes from the recent analysis of electron micrographs of glycocalyx (134). Examining very differently prepared specimens including some made by the rapid-freeze deep-etch technique in the absence of chemical fixatives, Squire et al. (134) have concluded that the glycocalyx may be regarded as a regular cubic lattice with side length of 20 nm and a cubic internal space of side length 8 nm (Fig. 6). The dimensions of this internal space are consistent with the glycocalyx acting as the molecular filter in microvascular walls.

In summary, the main permeability pathways through microvascular walls to water and small hydrophilic solutes are located in the fenestrations of fenestrated endothelium and through the intercellular clefts in vessels with continuous endothelium. In both types of endothelia, the molecular filter that forms the barrier to macromolecules at most microvascular walls is in the luminal glycocalyx of the endothelial cells.

Permeability to Macromolecules

PERMEABILITY COEFFICIENTS AND THEIR MEASUREMENTS

Apart from the sinusoids of the liver and spleen, microvascular walls have high reflection coefficients and low permeabilities to macromolecules, permeability properties

that are essential if the circulating blood is to be retained within the vascular system. Although their permeabilities are low, macromolecules do cross the walls of all microvessels at slow but finite rates. Table 1 compares estimates of σ and P_d made from the transport of macromolecules between blood and lymph in the dog paw and the cat intestine. Although it is possible that the values given in this table are actually overestimates of the permeability coefficient of macromolecules (see below), there are three important points to note here. First, the values of P_d for serum albumin are more than 3000 times less than the permeabilities of the same vessels to Na^+ and urea. The diffusion coefficient of albumin in aqueous solutions is only 20 times less than those of Na^+ and urea. This means that the diffusion of albumin molecules through microvascular walls is hindered 150 times more than the diffusion of Na^+ ions or urea molecules. Second, compared with the changes seen for small molecules, there is a relatively small decrease in P_d and a rise in σ with increases in molecular size. The third point is the similarity of the values of σ and P_d to the same molecule at the continuous endothelium of the dog paw capillaries and at the predominantly fenestrated endothelium of vessels in the small intestine. The values of L_P and P_d to small hydrophilic solutes in these two microvascular beds differ by nearly two orders of magnitude. This would seem to be further evidence supporting the belief that the transport pathways through microvascular walls for macromolecules are different from those responsible for water small hydrophilic solutes.

Before discussing the possible transport mechanisms for macromolecular transport through endothelium, let us consider the various methods that have been used to estimate the permeability coefficients to macromolecules and differing values that are obtained from them. Much of the quantitative evidence concerning macromolecular transport, like the data shown in Table 1, has been acquired by studying the transport of macromolecules between the blood and the lymph. This approach, first used by Grotte (46) to study the relations between permeability and molecular size in a wide range of dextran polymers, was greatly refined by Renkin (109, 112, 114) and Taylor (136, 137) and colleagues. Because of their work, the importance of raising the filtration rate to high levels in order to estimate the convective and nonconvective components of macromolecular transport came to be appreciated and sophisticated methods of analysis were developed. There are, however, difficulties in interpreting the transport of macromolecules from plasma to lymph.

To yield valid information about transport processes occurring across microvascular walls, most analyses assume that a steady state is established between the newly formed ultrafiltrate just outside the microvessels within the tissue and lymph that is leaving the tissue. This means that the flow of the lymph is assumed to equal the filtration of fluid through microvascular walls and its composition to be that of the newly formed ultrafiltrate. Simple calculations

TABLE 1 Reflection Coefficients (σ) and Permeability Coefficients (P_d) to Macromolecules of Selected Molecular Radii (a_{ES}, nm) in Microvascular Beds of Dog Paw and Cat Ileum

Molecule	a_{ES} (nm)	Dog Paw		Cat Ileum	
		σ	$P_d \times 10^8$ (cm sec^{-1})	σ	$P_d \times 10^8$ (cm sec^{-1})
Serum albumin	3.55	0.89	1.0–4.7	0.9	3.0
Transferrin	4.3	0.89	6.3	—	—
Haptoglobin	4.6	0.91	3.1	—	1.4
Immunoglobulin	5.6	0.91	3.3	0.95	—
Fibrinogen	10.0	0.94	1.6	0.98	0.7

Renkin EM. Transport pathways and processes. In: Simionescu N, Simionescu M, eds. *Endothelial Cell Biology.* New York: Plenum Publishing, 1988:51–68.

suggest that in some tissues, the time taken to reach a steady state after a change in microvascular filtration rate can be many hours (82). This can be understood by considering the events that follow an increase in microvascular filtration. A rise in filtration rate is accompanied by a rise in lymph flow and a fall in the concentrations of macromolecules in the newly formed interstitial fluid. It may, however, take several hours before the lymph has the same composition as this new filtrate, and if the lymph is sampled prematurely, its concentration of macromolecules will be greater than that in the ultrafiltrate. The lymph flow, however, may reach its new steady-state level before the lymph concentration of macromolecules; if flux of macromolecules is estimated from values for the product of lymph flow and lymph concentration of macromolecules at this stage, its value will exceed the real rate of transport into the tissue. Not only is macromolecular transport overestimated, but the mean concentration differences across the microvascular walls are also underestimated. Consequences of these errors are (1) macromolecular permeability of the vessels is overestimated, and (2) the convective component of macromolecular transport is also overestimated. In most studies of macromolecular transport between plasma and lymph, increased microvascular fluid filtration does increases blood to tissue transport of macromolecules. Because it seems likely that a new steady state was not established in many these studies, it is possible that the permeability values estimated on these occasions were overestimates.

Since 1990, much work has been conducted on the passage of macromolecules through monolayers of cultures endothelial cells. In many of these studies, changes in permeability to macromolecules have been investigated and relative rather than absolute values of permeability coefficients have been reported. The permeability of monolayers of cultured endothelial cells to albumin, however, is in the range of 10^{-6} cm sec^{-1}, about 100 times greater than the values of P_d to albumin at microvascular walls in situ (8). The reasons for this difference are not understood at present. Although studies on cultured endothelial cells have provided essential

information of intracellular processes, conclusions from them relating to macromolecular permeability should be viewed with caution.

Although molecular size is the principal characteristic that determines how rapidly a hydrophilic solute may penetrate microvascular walls, molecular charge is also important as the molecule becomes larger. Evidence for the charge-selective nature of ultrafiltration in the renal glomerular capillaries is well known but in other microvessels, charge selectivity has been investigated in less detail. Areekul (9) first provided evidence for charge selectivity in systemic capillaries. Working on the isolated perfused rabbit ear, he showed that σ_d to sulfated dextran (which is negatively charged) was always greater than σ_d to neutral dextran of the same molecular weight. Work on single perfused capillaries (3) and on microvascular beds in rat hind limbs also supported the view that of microvascular walls as a negatively charged barrier.

This picture was temporarily confused by studies on the transport of charged macromolecules between plasma and lymph. Negatively charged macromolecules appeared more rapidly in the lymph and at higher concentrations than positively charged molecules, suggesting a positively charged barrier. It was then appreciated that the large number of fixed anionic sites in the interstitium (see Gyenge [50]) would reduce the volume of distribution of the negatively charged molecules relative to cationic or neutral molecules of the same molecular size. Parker and co-workers (98) showed that the greater volume of distribution of neutral and cationic molecules increased the time for these molecules to reach a steady-state concentration in the interstitial fluid. This delay accounted for the apparently more rapid transport of the anionic molecules, a conclusion reinforced by the 2003 study of Gyenge and coworkers (50) on albumin distribution in skin and muscle tissue. With this point clarified, the evidence once again supports the concept of a negatively charged barrier at microvascular walls hindering the transport of negatively charged macromolecules greater than 3.0 nm in diameter.

PATHWAYS FOR MACROMOLECULAR PERMEABILITY

Just how macromolecules cross the walls of small blood vessels remains a controversial subject. Two apparently conflicting hypotheses emerged from very different lines of evidence more than 40 years ago, and the question of which is more correct has not been finally resolved. On the one hand, a purely functional approach led to the proposal that microvascular walls were penetrated by a small number of "large pores" (40–80 nm in diameter) and macromolecules passed through these from plasma to ISF (46). The large pores were estimated to occur so infrequently that their contribution to the P_d of small hydrophilic solutes would be negligible, although they might make a 5%–10% contribution to L_P. The large pores, however, would be entirely responsible for the permeability of macromolecules, and transport through them would be largely by convection. The alternative view, which arose from electron microscopy of microvascular walls (16, 17, 21), suggested that macromolecules crossed endothelium through vesicles. After electron opaque macromolecules had been injected into the blood, they could be found labeling caveolae and small vesicles of the endothelia. Initially it was suggested that the vesicles acted as ferries. Equilibrating with plasma when they opened as caveolae at the luminal surface, the small vesicles then budded off to travel across the cell where they fused with the abluminal surface of the endothelium and equilibrated with the ISF. In the absence of evidence for active transport of macromolecules through microvascular walls, it was suggested that equal fluxes of macromolecules occurred in opposite directions across the cells and the vesicles moved as a result of Brownian motion (21). A detailed examination of the labeling of vesicles with ferritin molecules, led to a more complicated model in which neighboring vesicles transiently fused with each other long enough for their contents to equilibrate (23). It was also shown that cooling the tissue inhibited the labeling of vesicles with ferritin (24).

The fusion–fission hypothesis was consistent with the detailed structural analysis showing the vesicles to be arranged in fused clusters communicating with caveolae at either the luminal or the abluminal cell membranes (19, 37). One extreme form of the fusion–fission hypothesis is for the joined vesicles to form channels through the endothelium. Evidence for such vesicular channels has been reported (133) and these could act as large pores.

Because it is widely believed that vesicular transport is not affected by fluid filtration through microvascular walls or by raised microvascular pressure, observations of increased macromolecular transport following increases in microvascular pressure accompanied by increased filtration have been interpreted as evidence in favor of the large pore hypothesis. Much of this evidence has come from studies investigating transport between blood and lymph where it is possible that the failure to reach a steady state might have suggested convective transport incorrectly (116). The strongest evidence for the large pore hypothe-

sis, however, comes from experiments that are free from this criticism (119).

Rippe and colleagues (119) investigated the effects of various factors on the accumulation of labeled albumin in skeletal muscle of an isolated, perfused, rat hind-limb preparation. Defining the clearance of tracer from the blood flowing into the tissue as the rate of its accumulation divided by the perfusate concentration, they not only showed that clearance of albumin increased linearly with fluid filtration into the tissues but also that cooling the tissue from 36°C to 14°C reduced albumin clearance by only 40%. This was similar to the reduction of the apparent hydraulic permeability of the microvessels. The results of this classic experiment are shown in Fig. 12. A 40% reduction in L_P would be expected because the flow of filtrate through the water-filled channels in the vessel walls is inversely proportional to fluid viscosity and the viscosity of water at 36°C is approximately 60% of that at 14°C. Because albumin transport is proportional to filtration rate and is reduced in parallel to J_V as the viscosity of water is increased, Rippe and colleagues (119) concluded that albumin is transported through water-filled channels in the microvascular walls. Figure 12 shows that the clearance of albumin from plasma to tissue is significant when fluid filtration is zero. Rippe and colleagues (119) accounted for this by pointing out that, because the hydrostatic pressure difference across microvascular walls is greater than zero under these conditions, there would still be fluid filtration through the large pores and consequent transport of albumin because σ_d to plasma proteins here is low. This filtration through the large pores would not be detected in whole tissue because it would be balanced by an equal and opposite uptake of fluid through the "small pores" where σ_d to plasma proteins is high. Rippe, Haraldsson, and colleagues (117, 118) have extended this work since the early 1980s, and building on the work of Renkin, Taylor, and others, have developed an elegant quantitative description of macromolecular permeability in terms of flow and diffusion through two populations of pores, small pores (radii of 4–6 nm) and large pores (radii of 20–40 nm) (118).

Direct evidence for transport through vesicles of normal endothelium has been reported by Wagner and Chen (144) who used reconstructions from electron micrographs of serial sections. A series of papers by Schnitzer and colleagues (126–130) seemed to bolster the idea of vesicular shuttling or fusion–fission as an important mechanism of macromolecular transport through endothelium. These investigators made use of two agents, filipin and N-ethylmaleimide (NEM), which interfere with the formation and fusion of caveolae. The cholesterol scavenger, filipin, removes caveolae in cultured endothelial cells, and was found to have a similar effect in microvessels of the isolated perfused rat lung where it also appeared to reduce the clearance of albumin from perfusate to tissue quite significantly. NEM inhibits fusion processes of vesicles and vacuoles in yeast, in

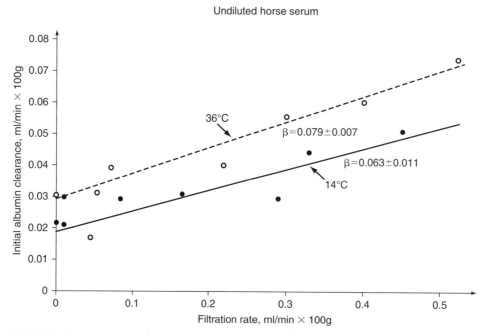

FIGURE 12   The clearance of serum albumin from perfusate into tissues of rat skeletal muscle at different filtration rates in experiments conducted at 36°C and 13°–15°C. β is the slope of the relation. (With permission, from Rippe B, Kamiya A, Folkow B. Transcapillary passage of albumin, effects of tissue cooling and of increases in filtration and plasma colloid osmotic pressure. *Acta Physiol Scand* 1979;105:171–187.)

synaptic vesicles, and in transport vesicles operating between the Golgi stacks and the endoplasmic reticulum. Palade's group and Schnitzer's group reported that NEM inhibited transendothelial transport of macromolecules in microvessels of mouse heart (103) and rat lung (127). Schnitzer and colleagues (130) have also reported that endothelial caveolae from rat lung capillaries can bud away from their anchorage in the presence of GTP and cytosol extracts.

Critical studies by Rippe and colleagues, however, have cast serious doubt on these findings (20, 121). They have found that in the isolated perfused rat lung, both filipin and NEM increased albumin transport. NEM was also found to reduce σ to albumin. Reducing the tissue temperature from 35°C to 22°C, however, lowered both albumin clearance and L_PS in rough proportion to increased water viscosity. Rippe, Carlsson, and colleagues (20) found that NEM also increased both albumin clearance and L_PS in the microcirculation of rat muscle. In both rat lung and rat muscle, NEM was found to increase precapillary vascular resistance. The authors suggested that increased resistance would reduce microvascular perfusion and this could account for the earlier studies where NEM appeared to reduce albumin clearance. Rippe and colleagues reviewed the controversy in 2002 (120).

Rippe's arguments for large pores are convincing. There are two possible criticisms. The first is that the experiments are based on albumin transport, and a different picture might emerge if larger test molecules were investigated. The second criticism is that the values they report for albumin clearance in their perfused tissues are greater, and those for σ_d are less, than have been reported for the same tissues in experiments carried out on intact animals (104, 115). This raises the question of whether the large pores are induced in the microcirculation during, or as a result of, the preparation of isolated perfused tissues. At present, however, the weight of the evidence strongly favors the large-pore hypothesis, which is a reversal of the view accepted in the late-1990s. As mentioned already, it could be that large pores are transendothelial channels which formed the fusion of vesicles. At normal tissue temperatures they might be continually forming and reforming, so accounting for the progressive labeling of the vesicle system with tracer macromolecules. On cooling the tissues, the open channels would remain open but new channels would form, accounting for effects of cooling on albumin transport. It could also be that handling of tissues could increase the frequency of these large pores in the microcirculation.

The question of whether macromolecules are transported mainly by convection through large pores in the walls of microvessels in normal healthy tissue has implications for our understanding of fluid exchange between blood and tissues. It could be that the question of the quantitative importance of convective and nonconvective transport of macromolecules in healthy tissues may be resolved in the course of future investigations of fluid exchange.

FORMATION OF INTERSTITIAL FLUID BY CONVECTION AND DIFFUSION THROUGH MICROVASCULAR WALLS

Coupling of Fluid and Solute Transport During Ultrafiltration

In most tissues, ISF is formed by the ultrafiltration of plasma, a process driven by the greater hydrostatic pressure inside the microvessels than in the surrounding tissues. As fluid begins to be filtered through the vessel walls, its composition is determined by the rates at which the various plasma solutes can move with the filtrate by convection and diffusion. If one considers the transport of a solute past a point at distance x cm along a pathway within the microvascular wall of cross-sectional area, A, the net flux of solute, J_S, can be described by adding together the contributions of convection and diffusion. Thus, from Eqs. 3–5:

$$J_S = J_V \left(1 - \sigma_f\right) C + D' A \left(-dC / dx\right) \qquad (8)$$

where C is the solute concentration of the solute at x, D' is solute diffusion coefficient and $(-dC/dx)$ is the concentration gradient in the direction plasma to ISF. The first term on the right side of Eq. 8 is the convective component of transport, and the second term is the diffusive component. The concentration gradient that is responsible for net transport by diffusion is equal to the solute concentration difference between the plasma and the ISF divided by the length of the pathway through the wall only when fluid filtration is zero and there is no convection of solute. When net fluid movements are present, they distort the concentration gradients in the channels within the vessel walls. Once a steady state is established so the solute flux, J_S, is the same at all points along the diffusion pathway (i.e., the rate of solute entry equals the rate of its exit from the channels), then the extent of the distortion can be inferred by integrating Eq. 8. This leads to a form of the Patlak expression (99), which here relates J_S through an area of vessel wall, A_m, to the plasma concentration of solute, C_p, and the concentration emerging from the vessel walls into the peri-capillary ISF, C_i, as follows:

$$\frac{J_S}{A_m} = \frac{J_V}{A_m} \left(1 - \sigma_f\right) \frac{\left(C_p - C_i e^{-Pe}\right)}{\left(1 - e^{-Pe}\right)} \qquad (9)$$

where

$$Pe = \frac{J_V \left(1 - \sigma_f\right)}{P_d A_m}$$

Pe is a dimensionless number called the Peclet number and expresses the ratio of convective to unidirectional diffusive transport of solute, with P_d being the diffusional permeability coefficient. Curry (26) recast Eq. 9 in a form that allows the convective and diffusive components of transport to be recognized:

$$\frac{J_S}{A_m} = \frac{J_V}{A_m} \left(1 - \sigma_f\right) C_p + P_d \left(C_p - C_i\right) \left(\frac{Pe}{e^{Pe} - 1}\right) \qquad (10)$$

Equation 10 is analogous to Eq. 8 with the first term on the right side describing convective transport and the second term describing diffusion. The expression $Pe/(e^{Pe} - 1)$ describes the effects of solute convection on the mean concentration gradient within the diffusion pathway by convective flow in the same direction as net diffusion.

Earlier it was noted that ultrafiltration through microvascular walls is driven by the hydrostatic pressure difference, ΔP, between the plasma inside the vessels and the surrounding ISF. If all the solutes were initially at the same concentration in plasma and ISF, the filtration rate per unit area of vessel wall (J_V) is $L_P Am\Delta P$ as in Eq. 2. The process of ultrafiltration, however, soon leads to differences in solute concentration between the plasma and the newly formed ISF as a consequence of the differences in σ and the Peclet numbers of the different solutes. These concentration differences give rise to osmotic pressure differences that oppose ΔP. In this way, the rate of fluid filtration per unit area of vessel wall becomes the product of L_P and the difference between ΔP and the sum of all the osmotic pressures opposing it. Thus:

$$\frac{J_V}{A} = L_P \left(\Delta P - \sum_n \sigma_{d_n} \Delta \Pi_n \right) \qquad (11)$$

where $\sigma_{d_n}\Pi_n$ is the effective osmotic pressure set up across the vessel wall by the nth solute.

Equation 9 can be used to calculate the contribution of different plasma solutes to the osmotic term in Eq. 11. When filtration rate is steady, C_i becomes equal to the ratio of the rate of solute transport to the filtration rate, that is, $C_i = J_S/J_V$. Combining this relation with Eq. 9 leads to the following expressions for C_i and $C = C_p - C_i$:

$$C_i = \frac{J_S}{J_V} = C_P \frac{\left(1 - \sigma_f\right)}{\left(1 - \sigma_f e^{-Pe}\right)} \qquad (12)$$

and

$$\Delta C = C_p - C_i = C_p \sigma_f \frac{\left(1 - e^{-Pe}\right)}{\left(1 - \sigma_f e^{-Pe}\right)} \qquad (13)$$

Differences in concentration (and hence differences in osmotic pressure) can only be sustained for those solutes that have low permeabilities. If permeability is high, concentration gradients are dissipated by diffusion. Equation 13 is more precise and indicates that for differences of concentration and osmotic pressure to be maintained, both the reflection coefficient and Peclet number must be high. The implication of this is that when Pe is zero (e.g., when $J_V = 0$), the concentration differences will dissipate even for those solutes that have very low permeabilities.

The message of Eq. 13 can be appreciated by evaluating Pe for urea and serum albumin during slow filtration (at a rate of 2×10^{-7} cm^3 cm^{-2} sec^{-1}) through the walls of skeletal muscle capillaries. For urea, P_d is 2.7×10^{-5} cm sec^{-1} and σ is 0.1, so that Pe is 0.0074; for serum albumin with P_d at 10^{-8} cm sec^{-1} and σ at 0.95, Pe is 1. Thus, C_i would be more than 99.9% C_p for urea, and ΔC is therefore 0.1% C_p so that urea makes a negligible contribution to (about 0.1 cm H$_2$O). For serum albumin, however, C_i is only 7.6% of C_p and ΔC is 92.4% C_p accounting for the major contribution of albumin to $\sigma_{d_n}\Delta\Pi$ (about 19 cm H$_2$O). Similar calculations can be made for microvessels in most other tissues (the exception being those of the brain), and it is therefore the osmotic pressure of the macromolecules that constitutes the pressure difference which acts as a break on fluid filtration and holds the plasma in the vascular system. The osmotic pressure of the macromolecules of plasma and other body fluids is often referred to as the *oncotic pressure*. Equations 12 and 13 indicate the close coupling between microvascular fluid exchange and microvascular solute permeability. The concentration of plasma proteins in the ISF (and hence the ISF oncotic pressure) is almost an inverse function of the ultrafiltration rate. This relation is of considerable significance in interpreting microvascular fluid exchange, and its consequences are discussed further below.

The principle that fluid in the vascular system is a balance of hydrostatic and oncotic pressures across capillary walls was recognized over a century ago by Ernest Starling (135). Since then it has been demonstrated to apply in a large number of vascular beds in various animals including humans, using a variety of techniques. It remains the basis for understanding fluid exchange between blood and tissues (81, 83).

Fluid Movements Through Microvascular Walls

GENERAL APPROXIMATION: STARLING FORCES

For most purposes, Eq. 11 can be written in a simplified form in which the effective osmotic pressure term becomes the effective oncotic pressure difference across microvascular walls, $\sigma_m(\Pi_c - \Pi_i)$, that is,

$$\frac{J_V}{A} = L_P\left(\Delta P - \sigma_m \Delta\Pi\right) = L_P\left[\left(P_c - P_i\right) - \sigma_m\left(\Pi_p - \Pi_i\right)\right]$$

(14)

The reflection coefficient, σ_m, refers to the mean (or effective) reflection coefficient of microvascular walls to macromolecules and P_c, P_i, Π_c, and Π_i are often referred to as the *Starling pressures*.

Equation 14 is a clear statement of Starling's principle of transcapillary fluid movements. Under suitable experimental conditions, it is possible to compare fluid movements through microvascular walls when ΔP is varied as $\Delta\Pi$ is held constant. This has been achieved most unambiguously in single perfused microvessels (e.g., Fig. 13). Essentially similar results have been obtained by less direct methods in perfused vascular beds (96) (see Michel [83] for review).

Experiments such as that shown in Fig. 13 reveal several general features of the permeability of microvascular walls. The linearity of the relation between fluid flux and pressure suggests that the pathways conducting fluid through the vessel walls are not stretched or deformed over this range of pressures. If the channels were stretched and widened, their conductivity, L_P, would be raised, and this would be seen as an increase in the slope of the relation between J_V/A and ΔP (which is L_P) with increasing pressure. Furthermore, the value of L_P is the same during fluid absorption (negative values of J_V/A) as it is during filtration, indicating that there is no significant rectification of flow within the conducting channels. (With less careful experimental design, however, rectification of flow may appear to occur.) A third feature of importance is the effect of changing the concentration of macromolecules in the perfusate. The consequent change in oncotic pressure results in a parallel shift of the relation between J_V/A and fluid pressure. The magnitude of the displacement is equivalent to 70% of the perfusate oncotic pressure as measured in a membrane osmometer. This suggests that σ_d is greater than or at least equal to 0.7 in this vessel. Overall, the experiment reveals that the permeability coefficients L_P and σ_m can be regarded as independent of the Starling forces. Although permeability can

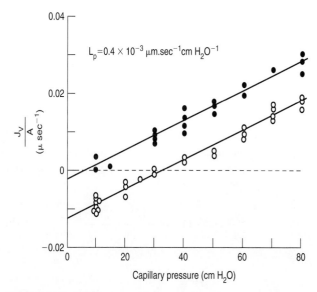

FIGURE 13 Relation between net fluid movement per unit area of microvascular wall (J_V/A) and capillary pressure in a single frog mesenteric capillary perfused with Ringer's solution containing high (O) and low (●) concentrations of serum albumin. Positive values of J_V/A indicate fluid filtration from vessel to tissue, and negative values show movement from tissue into vessel. (With permission, from Michel CC. In: Ussing HH, Bindslev N, Lassen NA, et al., eds. *Water Transport across Epithelia.* Copenhagen: Munksgaard, 1981:268–279.)

be and is modulated, a background of constant permeability provides a basis to discuss fluid movements that occur physiologically as a result of changes in the Starling pressures.

CHANGES IN MICROVASCULAR PRESSURE

Although textbooks often assert that P_c has a mean value that approximates to plasma oncotic pressure, this is true only for systemic microvessels of small mammals and for systemic pressures at the heart level in larger mammals. In the pulmonary microcirculation of all mammals investigated, mean P_c is more often closer to a third of the value of plasma oncotic pressure. In larger mammals such as humans, mean P_c varies with the vertical height between the vessel and the heart. When a human subject lies horizontally, mean P_c in most systemic microcirculations may approximate plasma oncotic pressure, but as soon as the subject sits or stands, P_c in vessels below the heart increases and that in vessels above the heart decreases. The changes in P_c above and below the heart are not symmetrical; the decrease in P_c in vessels in the upper parts of the body is checked as the local venous pressure falls below atmospheric and the veins collapse. Measurements of P_c in skin suggest that once this happens, P_c becomes independent of position (61). Below the heart, arterial and venous pressures increase in proportion to their vertical distance from the heart, providing that the subject remains still and mean P_c in the feet also increases but to a lesser extent than arterial and venous pressures. Movements of the legs increase venous return from the feet, reducing the local venous pressures and P_c.

The smaller increase in P_c than arterial and venous pressure in tissues below heart level (Fig. 14) suggests how P_c may be regulated. For blood to flow through a vascular bed, there must be a lower pressure in the veins than in the capillaries and in the capillaries than in the arteries. The fall in pressure from arteries to capillaries, $P_a - P_c$, is the product of blood flow from arteries to capillaries and the resistance of vessels between them (i.e., the precapillary resistance, r_a). Similarly the fall in pressure between the capillaries to the veins, $P_c - P_v$, is the product of blood flow and postcapillary resistance, r_v. Given that the flow of blood into the microcirculation equals the outflow, P_c can be related to P_a and P_v through r_a and r_v as follows:

$$\frac{\left(P_a - P_c\right)}{\left(P_c - P_v\right)} = \frac{r_a}{r_v}$$

which can be rearranged in the form derived by Pappenheimer and Soto-Rivera (96):

$$P_c = \frac{P_a + P_v\left(r_a / r_v\right)}{1 + r_a / r_v} \qquad (15)$$

Equation 15 reveals how the value of P_c between P_a and P_v is determined by the ratio of r_a / r_v, and since local blood flow is regulated in most vascular beds by alterations in r_a, it also suggests how P_c might be regulated. Even if P_a and

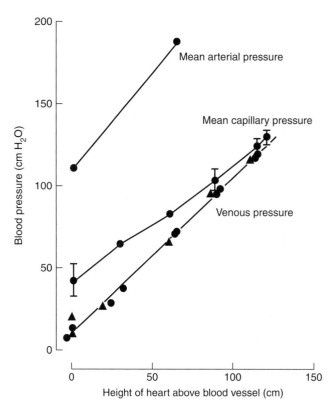

FIGURE 14 Relation between the local blood pressure in the feet and the height of the heart above the feet in two normal subjects in supine, sitting, and standing positions. Mean values for capillary pressure were based on direct measurements (by micropuncture) of capillary loops in the nail fold of the great toe. (With permission, from Levick JR, Michel CC. The effects of position and temperature on the capillary pressures in the fingers and toes. *J Physiol* 1978;274:97–109.)

P_v remain constant, arteriolar vasodilatation, which reduces r_a/r_v, increases P_c and enhances fluid filtration. Arteriolar vasoconstriction, which increases r_a/r_v, reduces P_c and thus reduces fluid filtration and promotes fluid absorption from the tissues. The rapid shift of fluid from ISF to blood that follows hemorrhage (or blood donation) is a consequence of vasoconstriction, which increases r_a/r_v largely in skin and muscle (94).

In most tissues a local increase in P_v is associated with constriction of the local arterioles, increasing r_a/r_v and tending to minimize the increase in P_c. This phenomenon has been called the veno-arteriolar response and appears to be a local response dependent on the presence but not the central connections of the sympathetic nerves (52). It is largely responsible for the smaller increase in P_c than either P_z or P_v in the skin of the human foot as the subject moves from a supine to a standing position (Fig. 14). Although P_c has to remain above P_v, it approaches P_v very closely when the subject is standing still. As soon as the subject moves, the picture changes. With an efficient muscle pump acting on the veins in the leg, P_v may be reduced from 120 to 130 cm H_2O to less than 30 cm H_2O within a few seconds and P_c presumably is reduced with it.

Landis (62) argued that P_c was the most variable of the Starling pressures in human subjects, drawing attention to the large changes in its value that followed changes in posture. It could also be argued that P_c is the one Starling pressure that can be regulated in parallel with the local blood flow. It is not known whether the changes in r_a/r_v that regulate blood flow have also evolved to regulate P_c. It is known, however, that the changes they induce minimize the loss of fluid from the circulation and lead to fluid shifts between the circulation and the ISF that appear to improve the chances of the organism's survival.

PLASMA ONCOTIC PRESSURE

Although reduced levels of circulating plasma proteins may be associated with edema, the steady-state relations between edema formation and plasma protein concentration are complicated by adjustments of microvascular pressures and of ISF hydrostatic and oncotic pressures (93). There is evidence to suggest that the ISF oncotic pressure may be adjusted by atrial natriuretic peptide regulating the transport of proteins from plasma to ISF (141).

In normal healthy subjects, oncotic pressure of the arterial plasma may be regarded as constant in the short term. The plasma oncotic pressure, however, may increase considerably as blood flows through the microcirculation under conditions where the filtration rate becomes a significant fraction of the plasma flow. In most microvascular beds, L_P is too low for this to be significant, but it does occur in the renal glomerular capillaries (15), where L_P is higher than in any other type of microvessel and filtration fraction is 20% or more, and in the microcirculation of the feet of human subjects during prolonged standing or sitting, when P_c is high and plasma flow is very low (41, 90, 92). In the glomerular capillaries, it underlies the dependence of glomerular filtration rate on renal blood flow (see Chapter 21).

INTERSTITIAL HYDROSTATIC PRESSURE

Before 1963, P_i was believed to approximate to atmospheric pressure in nonedematous tissues, and that steady fluid filtration, which expanded ISF volume, was thought to increase P_i proportionately. In this way, it was thought that the increase in P_i would reduce the difference in hydrostatic pressure across microvascular walls and so limit the rate of filtration protecting the tissues from edema.

The pioneering work of Guyton and colleagues showed that P_i of subcutaneous and many other tissues was 4 to 7 mm Hg below atmospheric pressure (47, 49). After much controversy, subatmospheric or negative vales for P_i in nonedematous tissues have been confirmed using a series of techniques. There is some variation from tissue to tissue, the most negative values being found in the lung, and the most positive values being found in the kidney with the subcutaneous tissues of many mammals being in the range of −0.5 to −2.0 mm Hg (10).

At an early stage in his investigations, Guyton (48) showed that expansion of the ISF by filtration from the microvasculature quickly raised P_i to atmospheric pressure. Further expansion of the ISF volume, however, was accompanied by little change of P_i in most tissues. These relations between P_i and ISF volume have been extended and confirmed by others (149) (Fig. 15). Whereas there have been minor differences in some of the absolute values reported by investigators, the general picture of a steep relation between P_i and ISF volume (low interstitial compliance) at normal and at low ISF volumes and a flat relation between P_i and ISF volume (high compliance) when ISF volume is slightly expanded and P_i has risen to atmospheric pressure, has been widely confirmed (Fig. 15). The renal interstitium appears to be an exception to this general pattern. In the kidney, P_i is +4 to +6 mm Hg and increases and decreases linearly with ISF volume (42). It has been argued that, in the kidney, P_i does fulfill the role of limiting the expansion of ISF volume and promotes the uptake of fluid and solutes (including macromolecules) by the microcirculation (11, 70, 71).

INTERSTITIAL ONCOTIC PRESSURE

Measurements of ISF oncotic pressure are usually global values for a particular tissue. The values of importance for microvascular fluid exchange, however, are those for the newly formed ISF in contact with the abluminal surface of the ultrafilter within walls of the microvessels. Here we have to be guided by theory. Equations 12 and 13 argue that if microvascular permeability of a solute is finite, the concentration of that solute in the ISF ultimately depends on its permeability and the rate of fluid filtration through the microvascular walls.

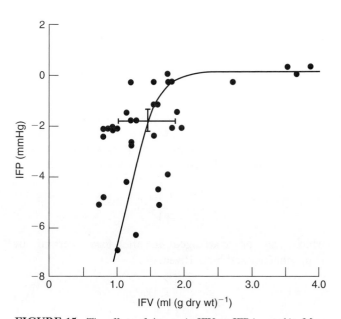

FIGURE 15 The effects of changes in IFV on IFP in cat skin. Mean and standard deviations represent control values. IFV was varied by intravenous infusion of saline or by peritoneal dialysis. (With permission from Wiig H, Reed RK. Interstitial compliance and transcapillary Starling pressures in cat skin and skeletal muscle. *Am J Physiol* 1985;248:H666–H673.) IFP, interstitial fluid pressure; IFV, interstitial fluid volume.

It means that the differences in oncotic pressure across microvascular walls are ultimately dependent on low levels of fluid filtration from plasma into the tissues (Fig. 16). Accordingly, a state of fluid balance between the circulating plasma and the tissues can only be a transient phenomenon. In the absence of fluid filtration, the protein concentration in ISF will increase, raising Π_i so that the oncotic pressure term, $\sigma_m(\Pi_c - \Pi_i)$ on the right side of Eq. 14 falls below the hydrostatic pressure term, $(P_c - P_i)$, and filtration resumes. A steady state can only be achieved in the presence of a steady rate of fluid filtration.

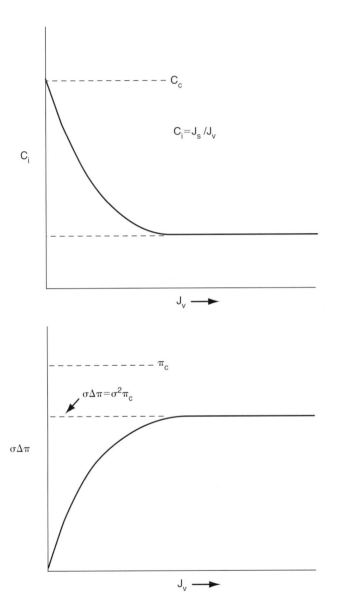

FIGURE 16 Steady-state relations between the concentration of proteins (C_i) in capillary ultrafiltrate and the capillary filtration rate, J_V. The limiting value of C_i is $C_c(1 - \sigma)$ where C_c is the microvascular concentration of protein (upper graph). Steady-state relations between the effective oncotic pressure across the walls of the microvessel ($\sigma\Pi$) consequent to changes in C_i and J_V. The oncotic pressure of the plasma, Π_c, is indicated as is the maximum value of $\sigma\Delta\Pi$ (bottom graph). (With permission from Michel CC. Starling: the formulation of his hypothesis of microvascular fluid exchange and its significance after 100 years. *Exp Physiol* 1997;82:1–30.)

The uptake of fluid from the tissues into the blood is also an ephemeral process, which diminishes with time as Π_i increases. In addition to its effects on Π_i, fluid uptake from ISF to blood is limited because it also reduces P_i, and so increases ΔP. Using Eq. 13 to estimate the changes in oncotic pressure, the steady-state relations between J_V/A and ΔP have been calculated (78, 87) and they predict a strikingly nonlinear relation. This bears a strong resemblance to data collected in experiments on perfused capillary beds of the lung, the intestine, and the limbs.

Figure 17 compares nonlinear steady-state relations (when $\Delta\Pi$ is set by J_V/A) with values for J_V/A and P_c obtained in the same single vessel under transient conditions in which $\Delta\Pi$ would have the same value for all estimates of J_V/A (88). Not only are the results consistent with the theoretical picture, but analysis of the steady-state data also allows estimates to be made for both σ_m and P_d (the macromolecular permeability), which agree quantitatively with other determinations (88). The linear portion of the steady-state relation at high values of ΔP has a slope of L_P and is described by the following expression:

$$\frac{J_V}{A} = L_P\left(\Delta P - \sigma_m^2\Pi_c\right) \tag{16}$$

Strictly speaking, the term σ_m^2 should be $\sigma_f\sigma_d$ because it expresses the fact that at high J_V/A, C_i is $(1 - \sigma_f)C_C$. It also draws attention to the fact that a decrease in σ leads to a proportionately larger decrease in $\sigma\Pi$ because $\sigma_f\sigma_d\Pi_c$ is the maximum steady-state value of $\sigma_d\Delta\Pi$ (88).

One surprising observation made during the measurement of the steady-state relations on single mesenteric capillaries was the relatively short time (2–5 minutes) required for a new steady state to be established after capillary pressure had been changed (88). This drew attention the importance of the value of Π_i in the small volume of ISF in microvessel contact and the relative lack of importance of the value of Π_i for the ISF of the entire tissue.

STEADY-STATE FLUID MOVEMENTS ACROSS MICROVASCULAR WALLS

Figure 18 summarizes the transient and steady-state changes in fluid filtration and absorption in a microvessel of constant permeability, perfused at a rate sufficient to keep the plasma oncotic pressure constant. If P_c initially has a value, A, which is less than the plasma oncotic pressure, and remains constant for long enough for a steady state to be established (point T), a subsequent increase in P_c from A to B leads to a rapid increase in filtration ($T \rightarrow W$). J_V then attenuates (to X) as Π_i is reduced and P_i increases. If P_c is then returned to A, fluid uptake from the tissues occurs ($X \rightarrow S$) and the rate of absorption diminishes as Π_i increases returning J_V to its initial level of T.

In pulmonary microcirculation, mean values of P_c are usually well below Π_c and fluid movements fluctuate around a point halfway along the flat part of the steady-state

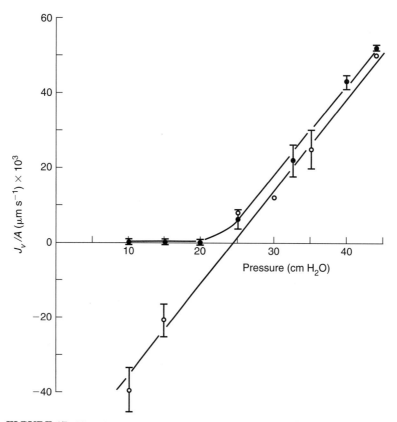

FIGURE 17 The relations between fluid filtration and absorption (J_v/A) and microvascular pressure in a single frog mesenteric microvessel under transient (O) and steady-state (●) conditions. Perfusate oncotic pressure was 32 cm H_2O. The oncotic pressure difference was the same at all values of J_v/A under transient conditions, but varied with J_v/A in the steady state in the way indicated in Fig. 16 (bottom graph). Note that absorption of fluid from the tissues is seen only under transient conditions. (With permission, from Michel CC, Phillips ME. Steady state fluid filtration at different capillary pressures in frog mesenteric capillaries. *J Physiol* 1987;388:421–435.)

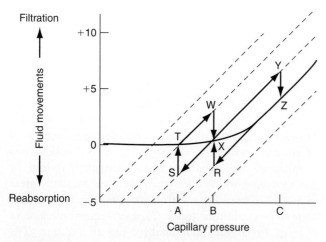

FIGURE 18 Transient and steady-state relations between fluid movements and microvascular (capillary) pressure. The dashed lines have slopes equal to L_P. The arrowed straight line shows the transient changes in fluid movements with changes in pressure. The curve, OTXZ (heavy line), represents the steady-state relation between J_v/A and capillary pressure. (With permission, from Michel CC, Moyses C. The measurement of fluid filtration in human limbs. In: Tooke JE, Smaje LH, eds. *Clinical Investigation of the Microcirculation.* Boston: Martinus Nijhoff, 1986:103–126.)

relationship. Small changes in P_c lead to changes in filtration or absorption that are rapidly checked as a new steady state is established. So long as $P_c - P_i$ is greater than $\Pi_c - \Pi_i$, there is a low level of fluid filtration into the tissues that is balanced by lymph drainage.

The steady-state analysis predicts that when the exchange vessels are finitely permeable to macromolecules and there is no source of ISF other than the ultrafiltrate from these vessels, fluid absorption from the tissues is transient, and low levels of fluid filtration from blood to the tissues maintain the differences in oncotic pressures between the plasma and the ISF. The sustained levels of fluid filtration are matched by lymphatic drainage from the tissue so that ISF volume remains approximately constant. Providing that the time-averaged mean P_c in most tissues approximates to the plasma oncotic pressure, this picture is consistent with blood–tissue fluid balance. It is not consistent, however, with the popular representation of the Starling principle, which depicts fluid being filtered into the tissues from the arterial end of a capillary and absorbed from the tissues at its venous end. Quite apart from the lack of evidence for this picture, the steady-state analysis predicts that rising concentrations of macromolecules around the venular regions of the vessel would bring absorption to a halt. The experimental and theoretical arguments against this textbook picture of the filtering-absorbing capillary have been forcefully expressed in a series of publications by Levick (64, 65).

Continuous uptake of fluid into the microcirculation does occur in tissues such as intestinal mucosa, the postglomerular capillaries of the renal cortex, and the ascending vasa recta of the renal medulla. In these tissues, however, the bulk of the ISF is not formed by filtration from the capillaries but by the secretion of protein free fluid from the adjacent epithelia. In intestinal mucosa and in renal cortex, the large fluid uptake from the ISF into the blood capillaries is accompanied by a very much smaller flow of ISF into the lymphatics (43, 44). Although only a fraction of the fluid absorbed from the ISF, the lymph flow is sufficient to clear proteins and keep their ISF concentrations low.

The renal medulla, however, has no lymphatics and special mechanisms appear to operate here. The continuous addition of protein-free fluid into the medullary ISF is matched by the uptake of fluid into the ascending vasa recta (AVR). The AVR have a relatively low σ to plasma proteins (0.7 to albumin). This allows the absorbed fluid to carry protein from the ISF into the blood. The uptake of labeled proteins from medullary ISF into the blood has been demonstrated directly (138) and estimates of P_c, P_i, Π_c, and Π_i, in and around the AVR indicate that these favor fluid uptake (71). Theoretical studies have supported this "bootstraps" mechanism, whereby plasma proteins are carried up their own concentration gradient by the osmotic flow that arises from that same gradient (71, 145, 155). In addition, unusual structural features of the ascending vasa recta and the low compliance of the renal interstitium ensure that fluid uptake is maintained even if Π_i increases. The low compliance means that P_i is high and rises if ISF volume expands to levels that may equal or even exceed the pressure in the ascending vasa recta. When this occurs the vessels do not collapse as there are fine projections from their endothelial cells, which are inserted into the basal laminae of neighboring vessels and tubules, holding them open (70). Because L_P of these fenestrated vessels is very high, an increment of P_i over P_c of only 1.0 to 2.5 cm H$_2$O is sufficient to account for the clearance of all fluid entering the medullary ISF from the loops of Henle and collecting ducts (70). A more detailed discussion of the special features of the extraglomerular renal microcirculation is given elsewhere in this volume.

Starling Pressures and Local Lymph Flow

In most tissues, ISF volume is maintained by a low level of filtration from the microcirculation being matched by an equal efflux of fluid from the tissue in the lymph. From this, one would anticipate that the magnitude of the lymph flow from a tissue could be estimated from the mean Starling pressures, the L_P, and the exchange surface area of the microcirculation. In an incisive review, Levick (64) pointed out that where the mean Starling pressures have been measured, they predict much greater filtration rates than the lymph flow and the lymph protein concentration would indicate. From 15 sets of data, he estimated P_0, the net pressure opposing filtration from the following relation:

$$P_0 = \sigma_m \left(\Pi_c - \Pi_i \right) + P_i \qquad (17)$$

When values of P_0 are compared with direct measurements of pressure in postcapillary venules, P_{Vc}, it is found that P_{Vc} is nearly always greater than P_0 and in several cases P_{Vc} exceeds P_0 by 5 to 10 mm Hg (Table 2). Net driving pressures for filtration of this magnitude would be expected to result in high lymph flows but in most of the tissues concerned (e.g., subcutaneous tissue, muscle, and mesentery), the basal lymph flows are so low that they are difficult to measure.

To account for these discrepancies, Levick (64) suggested that vasomotion, the spontaneous contraction and relaxation of arteriolar smooth muscle, might be responsible for large variations in P_c, and that P_c measurements tended to be made in vessels where there was brisk flow and a higher-than-average P_c. The few direct estimates of P_c during vasomotion, however, suggest that the fluctuations are relatively small.

An alternative hypothesis was put forward by Michel (83) and Weinbaum (147). Independently, both realized that if the filtrate leaving the small pores was uncontaminated by fluid containing the higher concentration of macromolecules, the effective σΔΠ opposing filtration may approximate to that across the small pores. This would be considerably greater than that calculated from global values of Π_i and would increase the force opposing filtration (P_0), reducing filtration rates to levels consistent with basal rates of lymph flow. The significant deviations between P_0 and P_{Vc} reported by Levick (64) are found in microvessels with continuous endothelium where the small pores are the interstices of the glycocalyx lying above the intercellular clefts. The downstream side of the microvascular ultrafilter is therefore the abluminal surface of the glycocalyx, which is separated from the ISF immediately outside the microvessel by the intercellular cleft with its tortuous pathway through the tight junctions. The pathway for macromolecules (the large pores) is either through the endothelial cell vesicles (via channels or by a fission–fusion mechanism) or by the very occasional leaky intercellular cleft. For the high protein concentration of this large pore filtrate to mix with that emerging from the small pores, protein molecules would have to diffuse back through the intercellular clefts to the site of ultrafiltration at the glycocalyx. Although this pathway is short, diffusion has to occur against the flow of fluid from the vessel lumen. The velocity of this filtrate is increased 10-fold or more as it passes through the breaks in the tight junctions. Rough calculations (83) and a detailed mathematical model (55) both indicate that even with filtration rates driven by pressure differences across the

TABLE 2   Starling Pressures in Muscle, Mesentery, and Subcutaneous
Tissues at Heart Level

Species and Tissue	Π_c	Π_i	P_i	P_o	P_c	$P_c - P_o$
Dog, skeletal muscle	26.0	11.0	−2.0	13.0	12–20	−1−+7
Cat, mesentery	19.1	6.1	0	13.0	23.5	10.5
Human, chest subcutis	26.8	15.6	−1.5	9.7	>15.0	>5.3

P_o is calculated from Eq. 17 assuming that $\sigma = 1$ and thus an overestimate. P_c is based on direct measurements in venules or venular capillaries, and is therefore an underestimate of mean P_c. The difference $(P_c - P_o)$ is consequently the minimum difference based on available data.

(From Levick JR. Capillary filtration–absorption balance reconsidered in light of dynamic extravascular factors. *Exp Physiol* 1991;76:825–85.)

glycocalyx as small as 1–2 cm H_2O, fluid velocity through the breaks in the tight junctions imposes a major barrier to the diffusion of proteins through the clefts in the luminal direction. These levels of filtration, nevertheless, are consistent with basal rates of lymph flow.

The hypothesis has been examined experimentally in single frog mesenteric capillaries (54) and more recently in rat mesenteric venules (4). In these studies, it was found that even when the interstitial concentration of serum albumin in contact with the outside wall of a vessel was the same as that in the perfusate, fluid movements through the vessel wall were opposed by oncotic pressures much greater than those estimated from global values of Π_i. The authors concluded that these observations were consistent with the theory that oncotic pressures opposing fluid filtration are those exerted across the glycocalyx and the global values of Π_i do not determine fluid exchange directly. Some of the authors' data are shown in Fig. 19.

Microvascular Blood Flow and Solute Transport

The rate of delivery of molecules and the rate of their clearance to and from a tissue depends on both microvascular blood flow and microvascular permeability. Where permeability is very high, transport depends on blood flow alone and is said to be "flow limited." Where solute permeability is low, increasing blood flow increases transport to a progressively smaller extent and when further increases in blood flow no longer increase transport, transport is said to be "diffusion limited" or "permeability limited." Renkin set out the general principles of blood–tissue exchange in a series of papers between 1955 and 1970 (107, 108, 110, 111). Figure 20, which is based on Renkin's work, illustrates flow-limited and permeability-limited transport for two solute molecules, antipyrene and urea, which are usually considered to have high permeabilities. As flow increases, however, the transport of urea becomes independent of

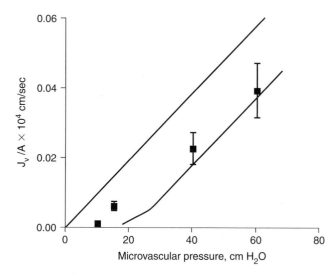

FIGURE 19 Steady-state relations between microvascular filtration (J_V/A) and pressure in single rat microvessels when the interstitial oncotic pressure is varied by superfusion. The vessel is perfused with a 5% serum albumin solution ($\Pi_c = 21.25$ cm H_2O). The points are mean values from four experiments in which the interstitial fluid concentration of albumin in contact with the outside of the vessel was equal to the perfusate concentration. The linear relation on the left is that predicted by the "classical Starling relation" when the interstitial concentration of albumin in contact with vessel is the same as the perfusate concentration; the curve on the right is predicted from steady-state theory for conditions when no albumin is added to the superfusate. Note that at high P_c, the observed values of J_V/A approximate to the prediction that no albumin is present outside the vessel. Only at low J_V/A when P_c is less than Π_c, does Π_i appear to influence the steady state. (Data points from Adamson RH, Lenz JF, X Zhang, et al. Oncotic pressures opposing filtration across nonfenestrated rat microvessels. *J Physiol* 2004;557:889–907.)

flow. This maximum level of transport is determined by the product of P_d to urea and the surface area of the exchange vessels. Antipyrene is lipid soluble and has a much higher permeability than urea. Its transport remains proportional to flow over the range investigated.

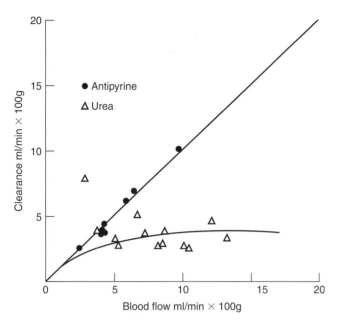

FIGURE 20 Relations between blood–tissue clearance and blood flow for a small lipid-soluble solute (antipyrene) and a small hydrophilic solute (urea) in skeletal muscle. Whereas the clearance of antipyrene is limited only by blood flow over the range of flows investigated, clearance of urea is limited by its microvascular permeability and is independent of flow when this exceeds 5 ml/min^{-1}/100 g^{-1} tissue. (With permission, re-plotted from Renkin EM. Blood flow and transcapillary exchange in skeletal and cardiac muscle. In: Marchetti G, Taccardi B, eds. *International Symposium on Coronary Circulation*. Basel: Karger, 1967:18–30.)

Insight into the relations between blood flow and solute transport can be gained by considering the plasma or blood concentrations of a diffusible solute as it flows along an exchange vessel. If the Peclet number for the solute is low, its unidirectional transport through the vessel wall from a small volume, ΔV, flowing along the vessel (Fig. 21) is proportional to the product of its concentration, C, in that volume and its permeability, P_d. It is also proportional to the surface area, ΔA, with which ΔV makes contact as it flows along the vessel (Fig. 21). The changes in C resulting from unidirectional loss of solute from ΔV are given by the following equation:

$$-\Delta V \frac{dC}{dt} = P_d \Delta A . C \qquad (18)$$

For a cylindrical vessel the ratio of $\Delta A/\Delta V$ is constant, and is equal to the ratio of surface area to volume for the entire vessel, A/V. Thus:

$$C_{(t)} = C_0 \exp\left(\frac{-P_d A . t}{V}\right) \qquad (19)$$

where $C_0 = C$ at time $= 0$, that is, the concentration of solute at the point of entry to the vessel, and this would usually be the arterial concentration, C_a. When t is equal to τ, the transit time through the vessel, $C = C_v$, the venous concentration of the solute. Furthermore, V/τ is equivalent

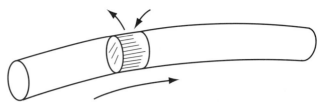

FIGURE 21 Model illustrating the principles of diffusion and flow in microvascular exchange. Exchange of solute is considered to occur from a small volume as it flows along a cylindrical microvessel.

to the flow through the vessel, F, so that Eq. 19 can be re-written as:

$$C_V = C_a e^{-P_d A/F} \qquad (20)$$

The net transport of solute from blood to tissue, J_S, is equal to the product of the blood flow through the tissue, F, and the arteriovenous concentration difference of the solute. Thus:

$$J_S = F\left(C_a - C_v\right) = FC_a \left(1 - e^{-P_d A/F}\right) \qquad (21)$$

Since the clearance of solute from blood to tissue is J_S/C_a:

$$\text{Clearance} = F\left(1 - e^{-P_d A/F}\right) \qquad (22)$$

Renkin used expressions such as Eq. 22 to describe data such as those shown in Fig. 20.

Equation 19 can be used to give additional insight in to the nature of flow-limited and permeability-limited transport. In Fig. 22, Eq. 19 has been used to calculate the changes in concentration that occur in a bolus of blood flowing along a single vessel. The three curves represent the concentrations for three solutes that have different values of P_d. It is assumed that the flow is constant so that distance and time are directly proportional to one another. The three curves start from a single point, C_a, and finish at three different points, the venous concentrations. From Eq. 21, the net transport of solute from blood to tissue, J_S, for each solute is $F(C_a - C_v)$. F varies inversely with τ so that if F is doubled, τ is halved. Because solute A reaches its end capillary concentration before it has spent half its residence time in the vessel, doubling F will not change $(C_a - C_v)$. Doubling F will therefore double J_S, and the relation between clearance and blood flow is linear so that transport is flow limited and over this range of flows will resemble that for antipyrene in Fig. 20. By contrast, for solute C, halving τ almost halves $(C_a - C_v)$, so that the product, $F(C_a - C_v)$, remains almost constant as flow is increased. Transport is now "permeability limited," and the relation between clearance and flow resembles that shown for urea high blood flows in Fig. 20. In theory, the transport of all solutes is limited by permeability if blood flow is high enough. In practice, the permeability of microvascular walls to some substances is so high that transport is always flow limited.

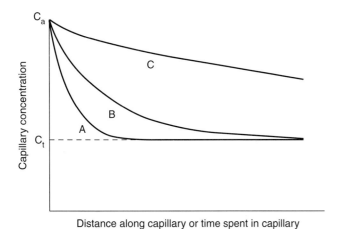

FIGURE 22   Decrease in plasma concentration of three solutes as they equilibrate with the tissues during their passage along a microvessel. The vessel is more permeable to A than to B and more permeable to B then to C. Because equilibration is achieved for A and B before the blood leaves the vessel, net transport for these substances can only be increased by increasing the flow (see curve for antipyrene in Fig. 20). Substance C does not equilibrate and its transport is said to be permeability or diffusion limited (cf. with curve for urea in Fig. 20). (With permission, from Michel CC. Flows across the capillary wall. In: Bergel DH, ed. *Cardiovascular Fluid Dynamics* 2nd ed. New York: Academic Press, 1972:241–298.)

Although thus far we have discussed only solute transport from blood to tissue, equivalent expressions describe the clearance of substances from tissues to blood so long as the barrier to diffusion through microvascular walls is greater than the resistance to diffusion through the tissues. The latter is certainly not true when the clearance of highly diffusible lipid-soluble solutes is being considered. For these molecules, transport between blood and tissues is determined more by the gradients of their concentration in the tissues.

The Renkin expressions (e.g., Eqs. 20 and 22) have provided the basis of understanding blood tissue exchange, but Renkin himself has drawn attention to their limitations (111). Considerations of heterogeneity of microvascular flow and permeability in diverse vessels in a microvascular bed have led to sophisticated models for the analysis of blood tissue exchange in intact tissues (13, 111). These models may well have to be revised in the light of recent observations on relations between flow and transport of small hydrophilic solutes in single capillaries in situ. Indications that P_d may itself vary with flow (153) have been confirmed and greatly extended in series of measurements on single mesenteric microvessels of frogs and rats (58, 59, 89). The increase in P_d with flow can be inhibited in rat vessels with NO-synthase blockers and by procedures that raise intracellular cAMP levels. The effects of flow on P_d are largest for small ions and small hydrophilic molecules. They appear to involve a pathway more selective than the traditional small pores and therefore make little contribution to fluid exchange (89).

The implications of these findings for blood–tissue transport in the intact animal have yet to be assessed, but

they could mean that increases in P_dA, which in the past have been interpreted as the consequence of increases in A, are the result of changes in P_d, and a common set of control mechanisms regulate the permeability and perfusion of the microcirculation.

Increased Microvascular Permeability

The increased microvascular permeability that characterizes inflammation has been studied most intensively over the past few years. Although the majority of recent studies have been carried out on monolayers of cultured endothelial cells, very important conclusions have been reached from investigations on intact microvessels both in situ and in vitro.

In 1961, Majno and Palade (72) showed that classical mediators of acute inflammation (e.g., histamine, serotonin) increased vascular permeability by opening gaps in endothelium of the postcapillary venules. The openings, which may exceed 1 μm in width, were believed to lie between the endothelial cells, and Majno (7) went on to suggest that they were formed by the contraction of adjacent endothelial cells away from each other, a view that is shared by many current investigators. This view has remained controversial and continues to be so.

Since the mid-1990s, reconstructions of the openings in venular endothelium have been made from electron micrographs of ultrathin serial sections of venules exposed to a range of mediators to increase their permeability. Whereas with some stimuli, the openings are predominantly paracellular with other stimuli, they pass through the body of one cell close to the intercellular cleft but clearly separate from it (36, 91). The origin of these transcellular openings is not understood, but Neal and Michel (91) suggested that they might be derived from vesicles or vacuoles in the endothelium. Similar findings have been reported by the Dvoraks and colleagues (36, 91). Initially, the Dvoraks group identified fused clusters of vesicles and vacuoles (VVOs) in the highly permeable vessels of tumors as transcellular pathways for ferritin molecules (34). Subsequent work by the same group on venular endothelium in normal skin and muscle of rats, mice, and guinea pigs led them to conclude that VVOs were present but did not form a pathway for macromolecules until the tissues were stimulated by mediators such as histamine, serotonin, or vascular endothelial growth factor (VEGF) (35).

A more quantitative picture of the changes in permeability of venules in response to histamine is shown in Fig. 23. As might be anticipated with the development of gaps in the endothelium, L_P increases and σ to macromolecules falls (86). The increased permeability induced by exposure to a constant concentration of histamine is relatively short-lived, reaching a peak at 5–10 minutes and starting to decline after 10–15 minutes, with permeability coefficients being restored to their basal values within 30–40 minutes. A similar short-lived increase in vascular permeability characterizes the first

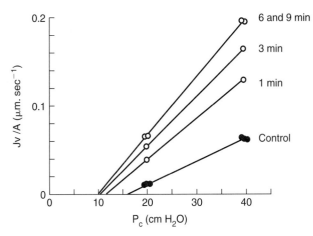

FIGURE 23 Changes in fluid filtration following addition of histamine to the solution washing a single venule in rat mesentery. Note how the slope of the relation between J_V/A and P_c (L_P) increases rapidly and the intercept with the P_c axis $(\sigma\Delta\Pi)$ falls over the first 6 minutes of exposure to histamine when it reaches a maximum. (From Michel CC, Kendall S. Differing effects of histamine and serotonin on microvascular permeability in anaesthetized rats. *J Physiol* 1997;501:657–662.)

phase of acute inflammation (where histamine is a mediator), although this is usually followed by a second phase in which increased permeability is long-lasting and induced by different agonists.

Most recent work has focused on the signaling events between the binding of an agonist with its receptor on the venular endothelial cell and the appearance of openings in the vessel wall (27, 28). From studies both in cultured endothelial cells and in intact vessels, it is clear that the early stages of signaling involve a steep rise in the intracellular activity of free Ca^{2+}. The agonist molecules such as histamine and ATP bind to endothelial cell membrane receptors linked to G proteins, which then activate phospholipases (particularly β and γ isoforms of phospholipase-C) that release inositol triphosphate (IP_3) and diacylglyceric acid (DAG) from the membrane lipids. IP_3 releases Ca^{2+} from intracellular Ca^{2+} stores and this in turn leads to the opening of Ca^{2+} channels in the cell membrane so that the Ca^{2+} activity of the cytosol is rapidly raised by the combined influx of Ca^{2+} from both the stores and ISF (for review see Curry [28]). Agonists such as VEGF bind to a tyrosine kinase receptor that phosphorylates PLC-γ, and activate a DAG signal that opens membrane Ca^{2+} channels directly (102). With VEGF, the rise in cytosolic Ca^{2+} is achieved entirely by influx from the ISF and is independent of its release from intracellular Ca^{2+} stores.

As of January 2005, the sequence of events that followed the rise of cytosolic Ca^{2+} activity was less clear. Studies on monolayers of cultured endothelium have focused on the contraction of cells to form intercellular gaps. Some years ago before actin and myosin were shown to be present in endothelium at the borders of an opening (125), it was shown that when suitably activated, cultured endothelium can exert ten-

sion on the surface to which it adheres (60). In most of the recent studies aimed at defining the signaling cascade, thrombin has been used as an agonist and this enzyme opens very large gaps between the cultured cells. These thrombin-induced gaps appear to be the result of actin–myosin contraction, which is principally regulated by the phosphorylation of myosin light-chain kinase (MLCK) and myosin light-chain phosphatase (MLCP).

While inhibition of key steps in the regulation of actin–myosin interaction prevents increases in permeability in endothelial monolayers, Adamson et al. (6) have found it does not diminish the increased permeability induced in intact venules by bradykinin, ATP, and PAF (platelet activation factor). Furthermore, thrombin does not increase permeability in intact and hitherto unstimulated venules (31). Several studies have shown that, in intact venules, cascade involves NO and cGMP downstream from the initial peak of intracellular Ca^{2+} activity (12, 152). The increased microvascular permeability induced by histamine, bradykinin, ATP, PAF, and VEGF are prevented or greatly attenuated if the enzymes of the NO-synthase–cGMP cascade are blocked (51, 152). In smooth muscle and other cells, cGMP induces relaxation rather than contraction; thus far, no mechanism has been described that suggests how cGMP might stimulate contraction of actin–myosin complexes in venular endothelium. Some investigators are therefore examining mechanisms of increasing microvascular permeability by means other than endothelial contraction. One possibility is that cGMP regulates the adherens junctions that are known to determine the formation of the tight junctions in epithelial cells. Such a mechanism might account for the modulation of intercellular openings, but it is not clear how it might be involved when openings pass through the endothelial cells.

It should be noted that in addition to its role as an intracellular signal increasing microvascular permeability, NO also has a role as scavenger of free radicals (40). Scavenging of free radicals seems to be the most likely explanation of reports that NO donors may lower permeability when permeability is raised.

Whereas thrombin does not appear to increase the permeability of "healthy" unstimulated venules, it does increase the permeability of these same vessels several hours after their permeability has been increased by some other agent (31). It appears that after stimulation by the primary agonist, the endothelium requires a latent period of several hours before it will respond to thrombin. This finding is significant in several respects. It suggests that for permeability studies, cultured endothelial cells cannot be regarded as representing the normal unstimulated endothelium of intact vessels and the high permeability of confluent monolayers to macromolecules (e.g., P_d to albumin being 100 times greater than in intact vessels) is reflected in differences in their phenotype. While this means that studies on cultured endothelium may not be relevant to the mechanisms responsible for the initial increase in permeability in acute inflammation, they may well reflect the changes in the endothelium of chronically inflamed tissues. It is reasonable to hope that a much clearer picture of the mechanisms of increased permeability in inflammation will be available by the time that the fifth edition of *The Kidney* is published.

An increase in microvascular permeability alone cannot account for the very rapid fluid filtration into tissues that causes blistering after stings and burns. Reed and colleagues (105, 106) have shown that in these types of injury, P_i decreases rapidly and this, combined with a rise in P_c that results from vasodilatation of the local arterioles, greatly increases the pressures driving fluid from blood to tissues. The decrease in P_i is related to the breaking of attachments between integrin molecules on cell membranes with fibers of the interstitial matrix. Treating tissues with antibodies to specific integrins can simulate it. The largest changes in P_i have been observed after burns to the skin of anaesthetized rats.

While the mechanisms responsible for increased permeability in acute inflammation are the focus of much current investigation, it is possible that more subtle changes in permeability are involved in normal physiological responses. Two examples, already referred to in this chapter, are the increase in permeability to small hydrophilic solutes with increases in flow velocity and the regulation of macromolecule permeability in responses to changes in blood volume. Thus, although the general principles of microvascular exchange are understood, we have barely started to appreciate how it may be regulated physiologically by variations in microvascular permeability and the contribution that this regulation makes to the integration of cardiovascular function in the maintenance of homeostasis.

References

1. Adamson RH. Permeability of frog mesenteric capillaries after partial pronase digestion of the endothelial glycocalyx. *J Physiol* 1990;428:1–13.
2. Adamson RH. Protein tyrosine phosphorylation modulates microvessel permeability in frog mesentery. *Microcirculation* 1996;3:245–247.
3. Adamson RH, Huxley VH, Curry FE. Single capillary permeability to proteins having similar size but different charge. *Am J Physiol* 1988;254:H304–H312.
4. Adamson RH, Lenz JF, Zhang X, Adamson GN, Weinbaum S, Curry FE. Oncotic pressures opposing filtration across non-fenestrated rat microvessels. *J Physiol* 2004;557:889–907.
5. Adamson RH, Michel CC (appendix by Parker KH, Phillips CG, Wang W). Pathways through the intercellular clefts of frog mesenteric capillaries. *J Physiol* 1993;466:303–327.
6. Adamson RH, Zeng M, Adamson GN, et al. PAF- and bradykinin-induced hyperpermeability of rat venules is independent of actin myosin contraction. *Am J Physiol* 2003;285:H406–H417.
7. Agre P, Brown D, Nielsen S. Aquaporin water channels: unanswered questions and unresolved controversies. *Curr Opin Cell Biol* 1995;7:472–483.
8. Albelda SM, Sampson PM, Haselton FR, et al. Permeability characteristics of cultures endothelial cell monolayers. *J Appl Physiol* 1988;64:308–322.
9. Areekul S. Reflection coefficients of neutral and sulphate-substituted dextran molecules in capillaries of the isolated perfused ear. *Acta Societatis Medicorum Uppsaliensis* 1969;74:129–138.
10. Aukland K. Interstitial fluid balance in experimental animals and man. In: Staub NC, Hogg JC, Hargens AR, eds. *Interstitial-Lymphatic Liquid and Solute Movement.* Basel: Karger, 1987:110–123.
11. Aukland K, Bogusfky RT, Renkin EM. Renal cortical interstitium and fluid absorption by peritubular capillaries. *Am J Physiol* 1994;266:F175–F184.
12. Bates DO, Curry FE. Vascular endothelial growth factor increases microvascular permeability via Ca^{2+}-dependent pathway. *Am J Physiol* 1997;273:H687–H694.
13. Bass L. Flow dependence of first-order uptake of substances by heterogeneous perfused organs. *J Theor Biol* 1980;86:365–376.
14. Bearer EL, Orci L. Endothelial fenestral diaphragms: a quick freeze, deep etch study. *J Cell Biol* 1985;100:418–428.
15. Brenner BM, Baylis C, Deen WM. Transport of molecules across renal glomerular capillaries. *Physiol Rev* 1976;56:502–534.
16. Bruns RR, Palade GE. Studies on blood capillaries I. General organization of blood capillaries in muscle. *J Cell Biol* 1968;37:244–276.
17. Bruns RR, Palade GE. Studies on blood capillaries II. Transport of ferritin molecules across the wall of muscle capillaries. *J Cell Biol* 1968;37:277–299.
18. Bundgaard M. The three dimensional organization of tight junctions in a capillary endothelium as revealed by serial section electron microscopy. *J Ultrastruct Res* 1984;88:1–17.
19. Bundgaard M, Frokjaer-Jensen J, Crone C. Endothelial plasmalemmal vesicles as elements in a system of branching invaginations from the cell surface. *Proc Natl Acad Sci* 1979;76:6439–6442.
20. Carlsson O, Rosengren B-I, Rippe B. Transcytosis inhibitor N-ethylmaleimide increases microvascular permeability in rat muscle. *Am J Physiol* 2001;281:H1728–1733.
21. Casley-Smith JR. The Brownian movements of pinocytotic vesicles. *J Microscopy* 1963;82:257.
22. Chambers R, Zweifach BW. Intercellular cement and capillary permeability. *Physiol Rev* 1947;27:436–463.
23. Clough G, Michel CC. The role of vesicles in the transport of ferritin across frog endothelium. *J Physiol* 1981;315:127–142.
24. Clough G, Michel CC. The effects of temperature on ferritin transport by endothelial cell vesicles in capillaries of frog mesentery. *Int J Microcirc Clin Exp* 1982;1:29–39.
25. Curry FE. Antipyrine and aminopyrine permeability of individually perfused frog capillaries. *Am J Physiol* 1981;240:H597–H605.
26. Curry FE. Mechanics and thermodynamics of transcapillary exchange. In: Renkin EM, Michel CC, eds. *Handbook of Physiology.* Vol. IV. Washington, DC: American Physiological Society, 1984:309–374.
27. Curry FE. Modulation of venular microvessel permeability by calcium influx into endothelial cells. *FASEB J* 1992;6:2456–2466.
28. Curry FE. Microvascular injury: mechanisms and modulation. *Int J Angiol* 2002;11:1–6.
29. Curry FE, Mason JC, Michel CC. Osmotic reflection coefficients of capillary walls to low molecular weight hydrophilic solutes measured in single perfused capillaries of the frog mesentery. *J Physiol* 1976;261:319–336.
30. Curry FE, Michel CC. A fiber matrix model of capillary permeability. *Microvasc Res* 1980;20:96–99.
31. Curry FE, Zeng M, Adamson RH. Thrombin increases permeability only in venules exposed in inflammatory conditions. *Am J Physiol* 2003;285:H2446–H2453.
32. Drenckhahn D, Ness W. The endothelial contractile cytoskeleton. In: Born GVR, Schwarz CJ, eds. *Vascular Endothelium: Physiology, Pathology and Therapeutic Opportunities.* Stuttgart: Schattauer, 1997:1–25.
33. Drenckhahn D, Wagner J. Stress fibers in the splenic endothelium in situ: molecular structure, relationship to the extracellular matrix and contractility. *J Cell Biol* 1986;102:1738–1747.
34. Dvorak AM, Kohn S, Morgan ES et al. The vesiculo-vacuolar organelle (VVO): a distinct endothelial cell structure that provides a transcellular pathway for macromolecular extravasation. *J Leukoc Biol* 1996;59:100–115.
35. Feng D, Nagy JA, Hipp J, et al. Vesiculo-vacuolar organelles and the regulation of venule permeability to macromolecules by vascular permeability factor, histamine and serotonin. *J Exp Med* 1996;183:1981–1986.
36. Feng D, Nagy JA, Hipp, et al. Reinterpretation of endothelial cell gaps induced by vasoactive mediators in guinea pig, mouse and rat: many are transcellular pores. *J Physiol* 1997;504:747–761.
37. Frøkjaer-Jensen J. Three dimensional organization of plasmalemmal vesicles in endothelial cell: an analysis based on serial sectioning of frog mesenteric capillaries. *J Ultrastruct Res* 1980;73:9–20.
38. Frøkjaer-Jensen J. Permeability of single capillaries to potassium ions. *Microvasc Res* 1982;24:168–183.
39. Fu BM, Weinbaum S, Tsay RY, Curry FE. A junction-orifice-fiber entrance layer model for capillary permeability: application to frog mesenteric capillaries. *J Biomechan Eng* 1994;116:502–513.
40. Gaboury J, Woodman RC, Granger DN, Reinhardt P, Kubes P. Nitric oxide prevents leukocyte adherence role of superoxide. *Am J Physiol* 1993;265:H862–H867.
41. Gamble J, Christ F, Gartside IB. The effect of passive tilting on microvascular parameters in the human calf: a strain gauge plethysmographic study. *J Physiol* 1997;498:541–552.
42. Garcia-Estan J, Roman RJ. Role of interstitial hydrostatic pressure in the pressure diuresis response. *Am J Physiol* 1989;256:F63–F70.
43. Gore R, Bohlen HG. Microvascular pressures in rat intestinal smooth muscle and mucosal villi. *Am J Physiol* 1978;233:H685–H693.
44. Granger DN, Kvietys PR, Premen AJ. Microcirculation of the intestinal mucosa. In: Schultz SG, Woods JD, eds. *Handbook of Physiology.* Vol. 1. Bethesda, MD: American Physiological Society, 1989;1405–1474.
45. Granger DN, Mortillaro NA, Kvietys PR, et al. Role of interstitial matrix during intestinal absorption. *Am J Physiol* 1980;238:G183–G189.
46. Grotte G. Passage of dextran molecules across the blood–lymph barrier. *Acta Chir Scand Suppl* 1956;211:1–84.
47. Guyton AC. A concept of negative interstitial pressure based on pressures in implanted perforated capsules. *Circ Res* 1963;12:399–415.
48. Guyton AC. Interstitial fluid pressure, II: pressure volumes curves of the interstitial space. *Circ Res* 1965;16:452–460.
49. Guyton AC, Granger HJ, Taylor AE. Interstitial fluid pressure. *Physiol Rev* 1971;51:527–563.
50. Gyenge CC, Tenstad O, Wiig H. In vivo determination of steric and electrostatic exclusion of albumin in rat skin and skeletal muscle. *J Physiol* 2003;552:907–916.

51. He P, Zeng M, Curry FE. cGMP modulates basal and activated microvascular permeability independently of [Ca^{2+}]$_i$. *Am J Physiol* 1998;274:H1865–H1874.

52. Henriksen O. Local sympathetic reflex mechanism in regulation of blood flow in human subcutaneous adipose tissue. *Acta Physiol Scand* 1977;450(Suppl.):7–48.

53. Henry CBS, Duling BR. Permeation of the luminal capillary glycocalyx is determined by hyaluronan. *Am J Physiol* 1999;277:H508–H514.

54. Hu X, Adamson RH, Lui B, et al. Starling forces that oppose filtration after tissue oncotic pressure is increased. *Am J Physiol* 2000;279:H1724–H1736.

55. Hu X, Weinbaum S. A new view of Starling's hypothesis at the microstructural level. *Microvasc Res* 1999;58:281–304.

56. Ingber DE. Cellular tensegrity: designing new rules of biological design that govern the cytoskeleton. *J Cell Sci* 1993;104:613–627.

57. Jacobsen BS, Schnitzer JE, McCaffery M, Palade GE. Isolation and partial characterization of the luminal plasmalemma of microvascular endothelium of rat lungs. *Eur J Cell Biol* 1992;58:296–306.

58. Kajimura M, Head SD, Michel CC. The effects of flow on the transport of potassium ions through the walls of single perfused frog mesenteric capillaries. *J Physiol* 1998;511:707–718.

59. Kajimura M. Michel CC. Flow modulates the transport of K$^+$ through the walls of single perfused mesenteric venules in anaesthetized rats. *J Physiol* 1999;521:665–667.

60. Kolodney MS, Wysolmerski RB. Isometric contraction by fibroblasts and endothelial cells in tissue culture: a quantitative study. *J Cell Biol* 1992;117:73–82.

61. Landis EM. Micro-injection studies of capillary blood pressure in human skin. *Heart* 1930;15:209–228.

62. Landis EM. Capillary pressure and capillary permeability. *Physiol Rev* 1934;14:404–481.

63. Lassen NA, Trap-Jensen J. Examination of the fraction of the inter-endothelial slit which must be open in order to account for observed transcapillary exchange of small hydrophilic molecules in skeletal muscle in man. In: Crone C, Lassen NA, eds. *Capillary Permeability*. Proceedings of the Second Alfred Benzon Symposium. Copenhagen: Munksgaard, 1970:647–653.

64. Levick JR. Capillary filtration–absorption balance reconsidered in the light of extravascular factors. *Exp Physiol* 1991;76:825–857.

65. Levick JR. *An Introduction to Cardiovascular Physiology*. 4th ed. London: Arnold, 2003:170–198.

66. Levick JR, Michel CC. The effects of position and skin temperature on the capillary pressure in the fingers and toes. *J Physiol* 1978;274:97–109.

67. Levick JR, Smaje LH. An analysis of the permeability of a fenestra. *Microvasc Res* 1987;33:233–256.

68. Loudon MF, Michel CC, White IF. The labeling of vesicles in frog endothelial cells with ferritin. *J Physiol* 1979;296:97–112.

69. Luft JH. Fine structure of the capillary and endo-capillary layer as revealed by ruthenium red. *Fed Proc* 1966;25:1773–1783.

70. Macphee PJ, Michel CC. Sub-atmospheric closing pressures in individual microvessels of rats and frogs. *J Physiol* 1995;486:183–187.

71. Macphee PJ, Michel CC. Fluid uptake from the renal medulla into the ascending vasa recta of anaesthetized rats. *J Physiol* 1995;487:169–183.

72. Majno G, Palade GE. Studies on inflammation I. The effects of histamine and serotonin on vascular permeability. An electron microscopic study. *J Biophy Biochem Cytol* 1961;11:571–605.

73. Majno G, Shea S, Leventhal M. Endothelial contraction induced by histamine type mediators. An electron microscopic study. *J Cell Biol* 1969;42:647–672.

74. Mason JC, Curry FE, White IF, et al. The ultrastructure of frog mesenteric capillaries of known filtration coefficient. *Q J Exp Physiol* 1979;64:217–224.

75. Michel CC. Flows across the capillary wall. In: Bergel DH, ed. *Cardiovascular Fluid Dynamics* 2nd ed. New York: Academic Press, 1972: 241–298.

76. Michel CC. The flow of water through the capillary wall. In: Ussing HH, Bindslev N, Lassen NA, et al., eds. *Water Transport across Epithelia*. Copenhagen: Munksgaard, 1981:268–279.

77. Michel CC. The effects of certain proteins on capillary permeability to fluid and macromolecules. In: Lambert PP, Bergmann P, Beauwens R, eds. *Pathogenicity of Cationic Proteins*. New York: Raven Press, 1983:125–140.

78. Michel CC. Fluid movements through capillary walls. In: Renkin EM, Michel CC, eds. *Handbook of Physiology*. Vol. 4. Bethesda, MD: American Physiological Society, 1984:375–409.

79. Michel CC. The Malpighi Lecture—vascular permeability: the consequence of Malphighi's hypothesis. *Int J Microcirc Clin Exp* 1985;4:265–284.

80. Michel CC. Review lecture–capillary permeability and how it may change. *J Physiol* 1988;404:1–29.

81. Michel CC. One hundred years of Starling's hypothesis. *News Physiol Sci* 1996;11:229–237.

82. Michel CC. Transport of macromolecules through microvascular walls. *Cardiovasc Res* 1996;32:644–653.

83. Michel CC. Starling: the formulation of his hypothesis of microvascular fluid exchange and its significance after 100 years. *Exp Physiol* 1997;82:1–30.

84. Michel CC, Clough GF. Capillary permeability and transvascular fluid balance. In: Sleight P, Vann Jones J, eds. *Scientific Foundations of Cardiology*. London: Heineman, 1983:25–30.

85. Michel CC, Curry FE. Microvascular permeability. *Physiol Rev* 1999;79:703–761.

86. Michel CC, Kendall S. Differing effects of histamine and serotonin on microvascular permeability in anaesthetized rats. *J Physiol* 1997;501:657–662.

87. Michel CC, Moyses C. The measurement of fluid filtration in human limbs. In: Tooke JE, Smaje LH, eds. *Clinical Investigation of the Microcirculation*. Boston: Nijhoff, 1986:103–126.

88. Michel CC, Phillips ME. Steady state filtration at different capillary pressures in perfused frog mesenteric capillaries. *J Physiol* 1987;388: 421–435.

89. Montermini D, Winlove CP, Michel CC. Effects of perfusion rate on permeability of frog and rat microvessels to sodium fluorescein. *J Physiol* 2002;543:959–975.

90. Moyses C, Cederholm-Williams SA, Michel CC. Haemoconcentration and accumulation of white cells in the feet during venous stasis. *Int J Microcirc Clin Exp* 1987;5:311–320.

91. Neal CR, Michel CC. Transcellular gaps in microvascular walls of frog and rat when permeability is increased by perfusion with the ionophore A23187. *J Physiol* 1995;488:427–437.

92. Noddeland H, Aukland K, Nicolaysen G. Plasma colloid osmotic pressure in venous blood from the human foot in orthostasis. *Acta Physiol Scand* 1981;113:447–454.

93. Noddeland H, Riisnes SM, Fadnes HO. Interstitial fluid colloid osmotic pressure and hydrostatic pressure in subcutaneous tissue of patients with nephritic syndrome. *Scand J Clin Lab Invest* 1982;42:139–146.

94. Öberg B. Effects of cardiovascular reflexes on net capillary fluid transfer. *Acta Physiol Scand* 1964;62(Suppl):229.

95. Pallone TL, Kishore BK, Nielsen S, et al. Evidence the aquaporin-1 mediates NaCl induced water flux across the descending vasa recta. *Am J Physiol* 1997;272:F587–F596.

96. Pappenheimer JR, Soto-Rivera A. Effective osmotic pressure of the plasma proteins and other quantities associated with the capillary circulation in the hind limbs of cats and dogs. *Am J Physiol* 1948;152:471–491.

97. Pappenheimer JR, Renkin EM, Borrero LM. Filtration, diffusion and molecular sieving through peripheral capillary membranes. A contribution to the pore theory of capillary permeability. *Am J Physiol* 1951;167:13–46.

98. Parker JC, Gilchrist S, Cartledge JT. Plasma-lymph exchange and interstitial distribution volumes of charged macromolecules in the lung. *Am J Physiol* 1985;59:1128–1136.

99. Patlak CS, Goldstein DA, Hoffman JF. The flow of solute and solvent across a two-membrane system. *J Theoret Biol* 1963;5:426–442.

100. Perl W, Silverman F, Delea AC, et al. Permeability of dog lung endothelium to sodium, diols, amides and water. *Am J Physiol* 1976;230:1708–1721.

101. Peters K-R, Carley WW, Palade GE. Endothelial plasmalemmal vesicles have a characteristic striped bipolar surface structure. *J Cell Biol* 1985;101:2233–2238.

102. Pocock TM, Foster RR, Bates DO. Evidence for a role for TRPC channels in VEGF-mediated increased vascular permeability in vivo. *Am J Physiol* 2004;286:H1015–1026.

103. Predescu D, Horvat R, Predescu S, et al. Transcytosis in the continuous endothelium of the myocardial microvasculature is inhibited by N-ethylamide. *Proc Natl Acad Sci U S A* 1994; 91:3014–3018.

104. Reed RK. Transcapillary albumin extravasation in rat skin and muscle: effect of increased venous pressure. *Acta Physiol Scand* 1988;134:375–382.

105. Reed RK. Interstitial fluid pressure. In: Reed RK, McHale NG, Bert JL, et al., eds. *Interstitium, Connective Tissue and Lymphatics*. London: Portland Press, 1995:85–100.

106. Reed RK, Rodt SÅ. Increased negativity of interstitial fluid pressure during the onset of inflammatory edema in rat skin. *Am J Physiol* 1991;260:H1985–H1991.

107. Renkin EM. Capillary permeability to lipid soluble molecules. *Am J Physiol* 1952;168:538–545.

108. Renkin EM. Transport of potassium-42 from blood to tissue in isolated mammalian skeletal muscle. *Am J Physiol* 1959;197:1205–1210.

109. Renkin EM. Transport of large molecules across capillary walls. *Physiologist* 1964;7:13–28.

110. Renkin EM. Blood flow and transcapillary exchange in skeletal and cardiac muscle. In: Marchetti G, Taccardi B, eds. *International Symposium on Coronary Circulation*. Basel: Karger, 1967:18–30.

111. Renkin EM. Control of microcirculation and blood tissue exchange. In: Renkin EM, Michel CC, eds. *Handbook of Physiology. The Cardiovascular System*. Vol. IV. Washington, DC: American Physiological Society, 1984:627–687.

112. Renkin EM. Capillary transport of macromolecules: pores and other endothelial pathways. *J Appl Physiol* 1985;58:315–325.

113. Renkin EM. Transport pathways and processes. In: Simionescu N, Simionescu M, eds. *Endothelial Cell Biology*. New York: Plenum Publishing, 1988:51–68.

114. Renkin EM, Joyner WL, Sloop CH, et al. The influence of venous pressure on plasma lymph transport in the dog's paw. Convection and dissipative mechanisms. *Microvasc Res* 1977;14:191–204.

115. Renkin EM, Gustafson-Sgro M, Sibley L. Coupling of albumin flux to volume flow in skin and muscles of anaesthetized rats. *Am J Physiol* 1988;255:H458–H466.

116. Renkin EM, Tucker VL. Measurements of microvascular transport parameters of macromolecules in tissues and organs of intact animals. *Microcirculation* 1998;5:139–152.

117. Rippe B, Haraldssson B. Fluid and protein fluxes across small and large pores in the microvasculature. Application of two pore equations. *Acta Physiol Scand* 1987;131:411–428.

118. Rippe B, Haraldsson B. Transport of macromolecules across microvascular walls: two pore theory. *Physiol Rev* 1994;74:163–219.

119. Rippe B, Kamiya A, Folkow B. Transcapillary passage of albumin, effects of tissue cooling and of increases in filtration and plasma colloid osmotic pressure. *Acta Physiol Scand* 1979;105:171–187.

120. Rippe B, Rosengren B-I, Carlsson O, et al. Transendothelial transport: the vesicle controversy. *J Vasc Res* 2002;39:375–390.

121. Rippe B, Taylor AE. NEM and filipin increase albumin transport in lung microvessels. *Am J Physiol* 2001;280:H34–H41.

122. Rostgaard J, Qvortrup K, Poulsen SS. Improvements in the technique of vascular perfusion-fixation employing a fluorocarbon containing perfusate and a peristaltic pump controlled by pressure feedback. *J Microsc* 1993;172:137–151.

123. Rostgaard J, Qvortrup K. Electron microscopic demonstrations of filamentous molecular sieve plugs in capillary fenestrae. *Microvasc Res* 1997;53:1–13.

124. Rothberg JG, Heuser JE, Donzell WC, et al. Caveolin: a protein component of caveola membrane coats. *Cell* 1992;68:673–682.

125. Schnittler HJ, Wilke A, Gress T, et al. Role of actin and myosin in the control of paracellular permeability in pig, rat and human vascular endothelium. *J Physiol* 1990;431:379–401.

126. Schnitzer J, Oh P, Pinney E, et al. Filipin sensitive caveolae-mediated transport in endothelium: reduced transcytosis, scavenger endocytosis and capillary permeability of select macromolecules. *J Cell Biol* 1994; 127:1217–1232

127. Schnitzer J, Allard J, Oh P. NEM inhibits transcytosis, endocytosis and capillary permeability: implication of caveolae fusion in endothelia. *Am J Physiol* 1995;268:H48–H55.

128. Schnitzer J, Oh P, Jacobson BS, et al. Caveolae from luminal plasmalemma of rat lung endothelium: microdomains enriched in caveolin, Ca^{2+}-ATPase and IP3 receptor. *Proc Natl Acad Sci U S A* 1995;92:1759–1763.

129. Schnitzer J, Lui J, Oh P. Endothelial caveolae have the molecular transport machinery for vesicle budding, docking and fusion including VAMP, NSF, SNAP, annexins and GTPases. *J Biol Chem* 1995;270:14399–14404.

130. Schnitzer J, Oh P, McIntosh DP. Role of GTP hydrolysis in fission of caveolae directly from plasma membranes. *Science* 1996;274:239–242.

131. Shirahama T, Cohen AS. The role of mucopolysaccharides in vesicle architecture and endothelial transport. *J Cell Biol* 1972;52:198–205.

132. Simionescu N, Simionescu M, Palade GE. Permeability of muscle capillaries to exogenous myoglobin. *J Cell Biol* 1973;57:424–452.

133. Simionescu N, Simionescu M, Palade GE. Permeability of muscle capillaries to small heme-peptides. *J Cell Biol* 1975;64:586–607.

134. Squire JM, Chew M, Nneji G, et al. Quasi-periodic substructure in the microvessel endothelial glycocalyx: a possible explanation for molecular filtering? *J Struct Biol* 2001;136:239–255.

135. Starling EH. On the absorption of fluids from connective tissue spaces. *J Physiol* 1896;19:312–326.

136. Taylor AE, Granger DN. Exchange of macromolecules across the microcirculation. In: Renkin EM, Michel CC, eds. *Handbook of Physiology. Microcirculation.* Vol. IV. Washington, DC: American Physiological Society, 1984:467–520.

137. Taylor AE, Granger DN, Brace RA. Analysis of lymphatic protein flux data. I. Estimation of reflection coefficient and permeability surface product for total proteins. *Microvasc Res* 1977;13:297–313.

138. Tenstad O, Heyeraas KJ, Wiig H, Aukland K. Drainage of plasma proteins from the renal medullary interstitium in rats. *J Physiol* 2001;536:533–539.

139. Thurston G, Baldwin A, Wilson LM. Changes in endothelial actin cytoskeleton at leakage sites in the rat mesenteric microvasculature. *Am J Physiol* 1995;266:H316–H329.

140. Turner MR, Pallone TL. Hydraulic and diffusional permeabilities of isolated outer medullary descending vasa recta from the rat. *Am J Physiol* 1997;272:H392–H400.

141. Tucker VL, Simanok KE, Renkin EM. Tissue specific effects of physiological ANP infusion on blood tissue albumin transport. *Am J Physiol* 1992;63: R945–R953.

142. Van Haaren PMA, VanBavel E, Vink H, Spaan JAE. Localization of the permeability barrier to solutes in isolated arteries by confocal microscopy. *Am J Physiol* 2003;285:H2848–H2856.

143. Vink H, Duling BR. Identification of distinct luminal domains for macromolecules, erythrocytes and leukocytes within mammalian capillaries. *Circ Res* 1996;79:581–589.

144. Wagner RC, Chen SC. Transcapillary transport of solute by the endothelial vesicular system: evidence from serial section analysis. *Microvasc Res* 1991;42:139–150.

145. Wang W, Michel CC. Modeling exchange of plasma proteins between microcirculation and interstitium of renal medulla. *Am J Physiol* 2000;279:F334–F344.

146. Ward BJ, Baumann KF, Firth JA. Interendothelial junctions of cardiac capillaries in rats: their structure and permeability properties. *Cell Tissue Res* 1988;252:57–66.

147. Weinbaum S. Distinguished lecture. Models to solve the mysteries in biomechanics at a cellular level. A new view of fiber matrix layers. *Ann Biomed Eng* 1998;26:627–643.

148. Weinbaum S, Tsay R, Curry FE. A three-dimensional junction-pore matrix model for capillary permeability. *Microvasc Res* 1992;44:85–111.

149. Wiig H, Reed RK. Interstitial compliance and transcapillary pressures in cat skin and skeletal muscle. *Am J Physiol* 1985;248:H666–H673.

150. Wissig S, Williams MC. The permeability of muscle capillaries to microperoxidase. *J Cell Biol* 1978;76:341–359.

151. Wolf MB, Watson PD. Measurement of osmotic reflection coefficient for small molecules in cat hind limbs. *Am J Physiol* 1989;256:H282–H290.

152. Wu HM, Huang Q, Yuan Y, Granger HJ. VEGF induces NO-dependent hyperpermeability in coronary venules. *Am J Physiol* 1996;271:H2735–H2739.

153. Yuan Y, Granger HJ, Zawieja, et al. Flow modulates coronary venular permeability by a nitric oxide related mechanism. *Am J Physiol* 1992;263:H641–H646.

154. Yudilevich DL, Alvarez OA. Water, sodium and thiourea transcapillary diffusion in the dog heart. *Am J Physiol* 1967;213:308–314.

155. Zhang W, Edwards A. Transport of plasma proteins across vasa recta in the renal medulla. *Am J Physiol* 2001;281:F478–F492.

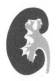

CHAPTER 10

External Balance of Electrolytes and Acids and Alkali

Man S. Oh and Hugh J. Carroll
State University of New York, Downstate Medical Center, Brooklyn, New York, USA

INTRODUCTION

Prolonged imbalance between input and output of any quantifiable element in a living organism is incompatible with life. The duration of imbalance varies, but eventually balance must be achieved if the subject is to survive. This rule applies to any quantifiable element. Red cell destruction equals red cell production. Oxygen uptake equals oxygen utilization. Sodium intake must equal sodium output, and water input must match water loss. However, transient discrepancies occur regularly between input and output, and between synthesis and breakdown, but given sufficient time, balance is always achieved, because permanent imbalance is theoretically impossible.

WHY IS BALANCE ALWAYS RESTORED?

It is often stated that salt intake is always equal to salt output, water intake is always equal to water output, and so on. The statement is both true and false. The statement is false because accurate measurement will show that daily salt intake is never exactly equal to daily salt output, and daily water input is never exactly equal to daily water output. Some discrepancy will always occur no matter how well the kidney functions and no matter how sensitively the kidney is tuned. On the other hand, the statement is true, because the long-term balance is always attained between salt intake and salt output and between water input and water output. It is obvious that even a minor imbalance—for example, 100 ml of discrepancy in water balance per day for a protracted period—will be inevitably fatal. The restoration of balance is achieved even when the regulating system is dysfunctional as in chronic renal failure or primary hyperaldosteronism. The fact that a person with chronic renal failure or primary hyperaldosteronism can survive for a prolonged period without medical intervention is proof that balance is restored.

Eventual restoration of balance in all control systems suggests the universal existence of a foolproof mechanism. What is the nature of such a mechanism in any control system, particularly in a biological system? For example, how is

salt balance achieved? Could this be achieved by the presence of a receptor that accurately counts the quantity of salt entering the body? Or is there a sensor that counts the total salt content in the body accurately. Suppose that salt balance were achieved by a sensor that counts salt entry into the body and the sensor's accuracy were nearly perfect, but miscounted the entry of salt by mere 5 mmol/day. The error may not be fatal for months, even for a year. But if it remained uncorrected for a longer period, it would ultimately lead to death either by volume depletion or by volume overload.

The mechanism that allows eventual restoration of balance must be perfect and foolproof. For the restoration and achievement of balance of fluid and electrolytes, the kidney clearly is a central player, but the smartness of the kidney is not the reason for perfect balance. The kidney is merely using a principle ubiquitous in nature. The kidney merely accelerates the process, but does not determine the ultimate outcome. The most crucial element of the control system that results in ultimate balance between input and output is that discrepancy between intake and output of an element inevitably leads to a change in total content of the element in the system, and the uncorrected balance leads to a cumulative change in the overall content of the element, either progressive increase or progressive decrease. The principles that allow inevitable balance between input and output have the following three characteristics:

- Control of balance involves a quantifiable element
- The quantity of the element in a compartment has an influence on either input into or output out of the compartment
- The compartment has a finite size

The following is the sequence of events in the control system. A certain amount of an element is contained in a compartment. If input of the element into the compartment exceeds its output or the output exceeds the input, the content of the element in the compartment increases or decreases. The resulting change in content of the element affects either output or input of the element, and thereby reduces discrepancy between input and output. But as long as any discrepancy between input and output remains, the cumulative change in the content of the element becomes increasingly larger. The influence of these changes on input or output also becomes increasingly larger. As long as imbalance remains, the cumulative change in the content of the element will persist. The cumulative change stops only when input equals output (Fig. 1).

Restoration of sodium balance will be used as an example. A person in a state of sodium balance ingests 100 mEq per day and excretes 100 mEq per day. Now assume that diuretic therapy is started on this person. On the first day of diuretic therapy, sodium output is 200 mEq per day, resulting in a net loss of 100 mEq of sodium. The next day, although the patient is still receiving the same dosage of diuretic, sodium excretion decreases to 150 mEq a day because the reduction in effective vascular volume caused by the previous day's net sodium loss activates sodium-retaining mechanisms such as the renin-angiotensin-aldosterone system and the sympathetic system. At the same time, the production of salt-losing hormones such as natriuretic peptides is reduced. All these changes jointly oppose the sodium-excreting effect of the diuretic. However, the overall result is an additional negative balance of 50 mEq of sodium. Although the negative balance of sodium is less on the second day than the first day, the cumulative loss is now 150 mEq, a larger amount than the amount on the first day, and the effective vascular volume

decreases further. Influenced by the effects of the lower effective volume, the kidney reduces sodium output further on the third day—for example, to 120 mEq per day—resulting in an additional negative balance of 20 mEq of sodium, and the overall cumulative loss of sodium of 170 mEq. As long as the sodium output remains greater than sodium intake (100 mEq per day), the cumulative sodium loss becomes larger and larger, albeit less steeply than before. Cumulative sodium loss stops becoming larger only when sodium output is equal to sodium intake, that is, 100 mEq per day. Indefinite salt loss is theoretically impossible because the continued sodium loss will ultimately cause such severe volume depletion that the person will become hypotensive, and eventually go into circulatory collapse. At this point, sodium excretion would be zero. Of course, long before the state of volume depletion becomes clinically apparent, renal excretion of sodium would decrease to 100 mEq per day. At this point, renal sodium excretion equals sodium intake. Hence, a new steady state is achieved, and no further reduction in effective vascular volume occurs. In the example given, restoration of balance is not caused by the smartness of kidney or cleverness of humoral mechanisms. For instance, the sodium balance would still be restored in the absence of aldosterone, in which case the person could be quite sick with severe volume depletion when the balance is finally attained. Sodium balance will

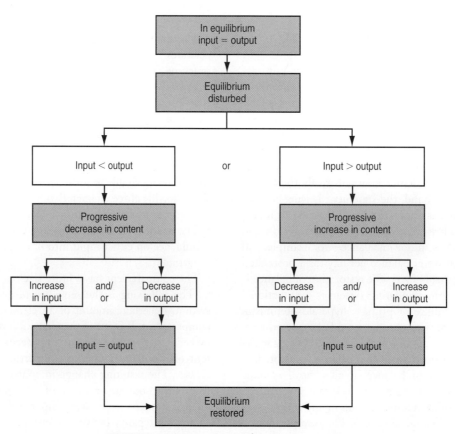

FIGURE 1   Mechanisms by which balance is restored.

be restored in the presence of renal insufficiency, in which case volume depletion will be less severe when balance is restored.

The same control mechanism explains why urinary excretion of potassium does not remain greater than intake in patients with primary hyperaldosteronism. If a person develops the disease, initially K output will exceed K intake. The resulting negative K balance causes hypokalemia, which in turn tends to reduce urine K excretion. However, as long as K excretion exceeds K intake, cumulative K loss will become larger and larger, and serum K will decrease progressively until K excretion finally equals K intake. Rarely, a patient dies of a cardiac arrhythmia before balance is attained. In the vast majority of cases, however, balance is achieved before the patient succumbs to ventricular fibrillation.

SPEED OF BALANCE RESTORATION

In a living organism, the speed of restoration of balance is teleologically determined. If an organism can tolerate protracted imbalance of a particular element without death or severe disability, balance need not be restored promptly. If quick restoration of balance is vital for survival, a mechanism for rapid restoration of balance is necessarily acquired in the process of evolution. Thus, the acceptable duration of discrepancy, or alternatively, rapidity with which restoration of balance is achieved, depends on the importance of maintaining the content of an element within a narrow range in order to prevent the demise or serious disability of the organism. Three main factors influence the speed of balance restoration:
- Magnitude of flux
- Basal store
- Capacity for additional storage

For example, an adult of average size has about 40 liters of total body water, and daily intake and output of water are about 5% of the body water content, 2 liters each. It is obvious that water output exceeding water intake by a mere liter a day would lead to fatal dehydration within 2 weeks. Conversely, water intake exceeding water output by the same magnitude would lead to water intoxication and death in the same period. An opposite example is calcium homeostasis. The total body calcium content of an average adult is 1,200,000 mg (600,000 mEq), and net daily external flux is about 150 mg (7.5 mEq). A daily negative balance of calcium of 100 mg for 1 year would reduce total body calcium by 36,500 mg, only 3% of total body calcium content. Obviously, a negative calcium balance of such a magnitude, even for a protracted period, is not incompatible with life. Indeed during the period of development of osteoporosis, a substantial negative balance of calcium for a protracted period of time is a common occurrence. Similarly, a positive caloric balance of 500 calories a day for a year will result in a total positive balance of 182,500 calories ($500 \times 365 = 182,500$).

This amount would result in an increase in adipose tissue weight of some 50 lb, a situation uncomfortable and undesirable but not incompatible with life. Consequently, protracted positive caloric balance is not uncommon.

All control mechanisms are activated by introduction of a new influence into a system that results in imbalance between input and output of an element causing a quantifiable disturbance in some parameter of the element in the system. In biological systems, parameters that are most often disturbed are concentrations of elements in the plasma. Other parameters that may be disturbed include pressure, volume, temperature, and body weight. Alterations in the parameter affect either input or output of the element, which in turn affects the parameter directly or indirectly. Examples of an element that is directly responsible for a change in a parameter are the balance of potassium (element) affecting plasma potassium concentration (parameter), the balance of magnesium (element) affecting the plasma magnesium concentration (parameter). Examples of an element that is indirectly responsible for a change in parameter include the balance of sodium (element) affecting the effective vascular volume (parameter), and the balance of calories (element) affecting the body weight (parameter). Compensation mechanisms restore the balance between input and output.

The degree of deviation of the parameter from the baseline value when the balance between input and output is restored depends on the effectiveness of the compensation mechanism. A poor compensation mechanism will restore the balance with the parameter greatly deviated from the baseline value. When urea production doubles, eventually renal excretion will increase to equal the increased production rate, but at equilibrium the plasma urea concentration will be twice the baseline value. This is an example of a poor compensation mechanism. In contrast, when salt intake is doubled, renal excretion of salt will eventually double, but at this point the effective vascular volume would be very slightly higher than the baseline. This is an example of an excellent compensation mechanism. Only when the compensation mechanism utilizes the infinite gain control mechanism (which will be discussed in the next section), is the abnormality completely corrected.

INFINITE GAIN CONTROL MECHANISM

The purpose of feedback control is to correct an abnormality caused by introduction of a new variable. Most control mechanisms partially correct abnormalities. The infinite gain control mechanism is unique in that abnormality is completely corrected. This type of compensation mechanism was first recognized by Guyton, who presented the concept in his discussion of the regulation of arterial blood pressure (26–29). He boldly predicted that in the absence of an altered state of renal excretion of salt, no abnormality will sustain hypertension chronically. This prediction was made on the basis of the observation that arterial blood pressure was normally a powerful regulator of renal salt excretion, and that a minute increase in blood pressure results in a large increase in salt excretion, which would continue until the blood pressure returns to normal (27). Suppose hypertension develops as a result of increased systemic vascular resistance, while the responsiveness of the kidney to changes in blood pressure to influence salt output (i.e., renal function curve in response to blood pressure) remains unchanged. Increased salt output caused by a higher blood pressure in the absence of commensurate increase in salt intake would lead to a net negative salt balance. The negative salt balance would reduce effective vascular volume, circulating blood volume, and eventually cardiac output. A lower cardiac output will reduce blood pressure to a lower level, but as long as the blood pressure is still higher than the baseline, salt output will remain greater than the basal salt output. The salt output in excess of salt intake progressively reduces the salt content of the body. Only when the blood pressure returns to the original baseline value, will the salt output return to the baseline value. At this point, balance is restored between the salt intake and salt output, and the abnormality in blood pressure has completely dissipated (Fig. 2).

In Guyton's use, the term "gain" is defined as the fraction of abnormality that has been corrected divided by the fraction yet to be corrected (29). For example, if an abnormality causes an increase in blood pressure, and a control system brings it back halfway to the original value, the feedback gain is one. Gain is zero if a control system does not correct at all. Gain is infinite if the abnormality is almost all corrected with virtually nothing left to be corrected, because division of a number by an infinitely small number results in an infinitely large number.

Why does abnormality disappear completely in the infinite gain control mechanism, but not in other control mechanisms? The main difference is the nature of the influence that causes disturbances in the system. When the disturbance introduced affects either input or responsiveness of the system to change in a parameter (function curve) for the output, abnormality in the parameter will not be corrected completely, and the compensation mechanism does not involve the infinite gain control mechanism. On the other hand, when the disturbance introduced is not one of these two kinds, the compensation mechanism is an infinite gain control mechanism. Examples of the control that do not involve infinite gain are: (1) an increase in salt intake or increase in potassium intake will result in increase in effective vascular volume or increase in plasma K when balance is restored, and (2) a reduced rate of renal sodium excretion by a kidney disease or primary hyperaldosteronism (i.e., a change in function curve of renal sodium excretion) will result in increased effective vascular volume until increase in effective vascular volume is sufficiently great to restore the amount of sodium excreted to equal the intake of sodium.

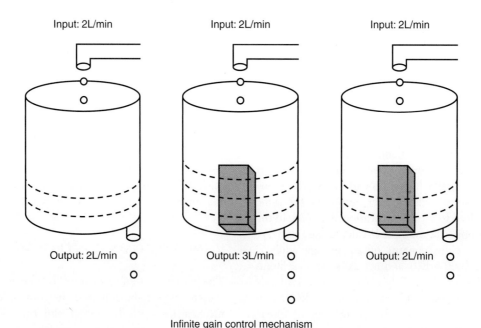

Infinite gain control mechanism

FIGURE 2 Infinite gain control mechanism. Water input and water output determine the balance, but water output is determined by the size of the hole at the bottom and the height of water column. If water input and the size of the hole at the bottom remain unchanged, any change in the capacity of the tank will alter the water column height only temporarily. For example, putting a brick into the tank reduces the capacity of the tank instantly, which will increase water column height. A higher level of the water column with the same size of the outlet hole will increase the water output in excess of water input. Only when the water column height returns to the original level is a balance restored between input and output.

The following example will clarify the concept better than an abstract description of the mechanism. Assume that a person produces 10 g of urea daily, and has urea clearance of 100 liters/24 hours. Serum urea concentration will be stable when equilibrium is reached between urea excretion and urea production. Since urea production is 10 g per day, urea excretion would have to be 10 g per day at equilibrium. In order to excrete 10 g of urea per day with a urea clearance of 100 liters per day, the plasma concentration would have to be 100 mg/liter (10 mg/dl); 100 liters/day $\times$ 100 mg/liter = 10,000 mg (10 g) per day. At this point we will introduce a disturbance by doubling the total body water of this person, leaving both urea production and urea clearance unchanged. Initially, dilution will reduce plasma urea concentration to 50 mg/liter (5 mg/dl). Urea excretion will decrease, because urea concentration is lower but the clearance is the same. Initially the urea excretion rate will decrease to 5 g per day (50 mg/liter $\times$ 100 = 5000 mg = 5 g). Since urea production (10 g) exceeds urea excretion (5 g), plasma urea concentration will increase to a higher level. As plasma urea increases to, for example, 70 mg/liter (7 mg/dl), the urea excretion rate will be 7 g per day. At this rate, urea excretion is still less than the production, and urea accumulation continues and serum urea concentration rises. The process will continue, as long as serum urea is under 100 mg/liter. Only when the urea concentration reaches 100 mg/liter, will urea excretion be 10 g per day, equaling the urea production rate. When a new balance is achieved, no further increase in urea concentration is needed. At this point, urea concentration is exactly at the original level, although total body water remains at twice the usual value.

Infinite gain control mechanisms are responsible for restoring the effective vascular volume to the original value when the volume is reduced by edema formation in congestive heart failure, ascites formation in liver disease, or edema formation due to hypoalbuminemia. The infinite gain control mechanism works in these conditions, because in all of them the initial disturbances that led to reduction in effective vascular volume (parameter) affect neither the intake of sodium (element) nor the output function of sodium, namely, the renal function curve for the sodium excretion. Detailed explanation of the compensation mechanisms for these conditions will be discussed subsequently in this chapter.

MODELS OF EXTERNAL BALANCE

The pattern of establishment of new balance for control of various elements in the human body is broadly classified into three models. The main source of input for most electrolytes in the body is oral intake, and the main output is renal excretion, with some small additional output through the gastrointestinal (GI) tract for certain substances.

Model A

This model is depicted in Fig. 3 as a cylinder filled with water. Water enters from a faucet into the cylinder, and leaves it through a hole at the side bottom. The height of the water column depends on water input and water output, and water output in turn depends on the size of the hole at the bottom and hydrostatic pressure. Hydrostatic pressure in turn depends on the height of the water column. Under these conditions, two factors can change the height of the water column permanently: the rate of water input and the size of the hole. If the size of the outlet hole is kept constant, and the rate of water input doubled, soon water output will have to double when balance is restored.

Since the outlet hole size remains unchanged, doubling of water output would require doubling of hydrostatic pressure, which in turn requires doubling of the water column height. A rise in water column height occurs because water input exceeds water output. The progressive rise in water column height gradually increases the hydrostatic pressure, and therefore water output. Hence, the discrepancy between water input and water output gradually lessens. However, as long as water input remains greater than water output, water level will keep rising, and the rise will halt only when water output equals water input, which occurs when water column height is exactly doubled, doubling the hydrostatic pressure at the bottom hole.

Conversely, decreasing the size of the outlet hole to half with unchanged water input will initially reduce water output to half. The ensuing imbalance between water output and water input causes a gradual rise in water column. A higher hydrostatic pressure resulting from a rise in the water column allows more water to come out through a narrower hole. Thus, when the outlet hole size is the half of the original value, doubling of the water column height will restore the water output to the baseline value. At this point, a new balance is restored between input and output.

The main characteristic of this type of compensation is that the alteration in content or concentration of a substance caused by a disturbance is directly or inversely proportionate to the magnitude of the alteration in input or output function. For example, if the input of a substance is doubled, the content or concentration of the substance will be doubled when the balance is restored. If input is increased threefold, the content or concentration will be tripled. Similarly, if the output function is halved, the content or concentration will be doubled when balance is restored. If the output function is reduced to one-tenth of the baseline, the content or concentration will be increased 10-fold when balance is restored.

Many substances in the body follow this pattern of compensation mechanism in order to achieve a new balance. When a substance follows this pattern of compensation, the body must have a high degree of tolerance for a large deviation in body content or concentration for the substance. For example, if creatinine clearance diminishes to half of

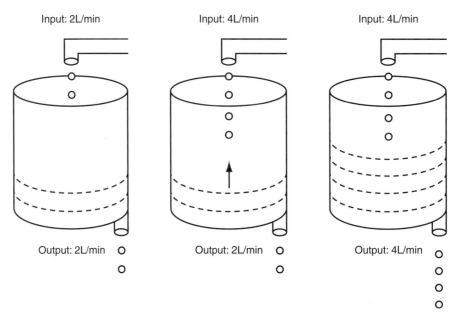

FIGURE 3   Model A. The input and output determines the balance, but the output changes in proportion to the water column height. When the water input doubles with the size of the output hole remaining unchanged, the only way for the output to increase to the same level as the input is to double the water column height. At this point, a new balance is struck between input and output. For example, if creatinine production doubles while creatinine clearance remains unchanged, serum creatinine concentration will be doubled when a new balance is achieved between creatinine production and creatinine excretion.

the baseline value with unchanged creatinine production, serum creatinine concentration will double in order to achieve balance between creatinine production and renal excretion. Similarly, if creatinine production is reduced to half of the original value with unchanged renal function, serum creatinine concentration will be half of the original value. Likewise, if urea production is doubled with unchanged kidney function, serum urea concentration is doubled when balance is restored.

Model B

In this model, the cylinder has a wedge-shaped slit on its side instead of a bottom hole (Fig. 4). Water enters into the cylinder from a faucet, and leaves it through the slit. As in Model A, water output depends on the height of water column. But, because of the wedge-shaped slit, a rise in water level increases water output exponentially. Therefore, when water intake doubles, doubling of water output, which is needed to match the intake, does not require doubling of the height of water column. Depending on the shape of the slit, the water level may rise only slightly before a new balance is restored. In other words, an increase in water output in response to a change in the height of the water column is magnified in this system. Furthermore, unlike Model A, when water level drops below the lowest part of the slit, water output stops altogether.

The regulation of the body content or plasma concentration of most electrolytes and other essential body elements utilizes this type of compensation. For example, when potas-

sium intake is increased fivefold, plasma potassium concentration does not increase fivefold when balance between input and output is restored. In the presence of normal renal function and normal aldosterone response, plasma potassium concentration will increase only slightly. Likewise, a fivefold increase in sodium intake causes only a slight increase in the body sodium content or plasma sodium concentration. When sodium intake is greatly reduced, the body sodium content decreases only slightly before renal sodium excretion ceases.

Model C

The pattern of water excretion in Model C (Fig. 5) is similar to Model A, but in this model two cylinders, one big (A) and one small (B), are joined together at the bottom, and each has a hole at the bottom. Water enters only cylinder A, but once it enters it equilibrates with cylinder B. Ordinarily, cylinder A has a bigger hole than cylinder B. Hence, the water level is determined primarily by water input and the size of hole A. However, as the size of hole A decreases, the role of hole B in the regulation of the water level increases. When water input is doubled, the height of the water column will have to be doubled in order to permit establishment of a new steady state. On the other hand, when the size of hole A is decreased by one-half, the height of water column will be less than doubled when balance is restored, provided that the size of hole B is unchanged.

When the excretion rate through hole A decreases, the excretion through hole B becomes more important. The

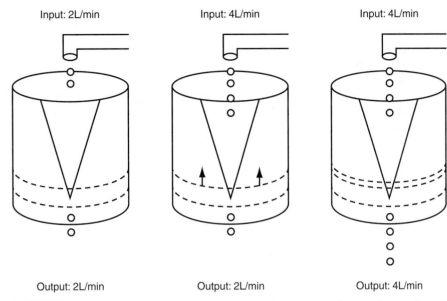

Input: 2L/min   Input: 4L/min   Input: 4L/min

Output: 2L/min   Output: 2L/min   Output: 4L/min

FIGURE 4   Model B. As in Model A, input and output determine the balance, and output depends on the water column height. However, unlike Model A, a change in water output by the change in the height of water column is magnified. When the water column height increases slightly, water output increases greatly, and a decrease in height reduces water output markedly. Furthermore, when the water column height decreases below a certain level, output ceases completely. Thus, doubling of input from 2 liters/min to 4 liters/min requires increases in water level only slightly before output also increases to 4 liters/min.

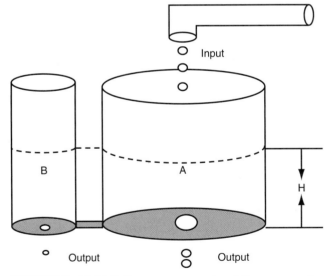

Input

B   A

H

Output   Output

FIGURE 5   Model C. Two compartments A and B are connected to each other, and each has an outlet hole. Water output from both compartments depends on the height of water column. Because the size of hole A is much larger than that of hole B, normally the bulk of water output occurs through hole A, but when hole A becomes smaller, output through hole B plays a greater role in water output. Elimination of uric acid and creatinine through the kidney (similar to hole A) and the colon (similar to hole B) follows this pattern of excretion.

regulation of plasma concentration of uric acid follows the pattern in Model C. In the case of uric acid, it is cleared by the kidney and is also cleared metabolically by colonic bacteria. The renal clearance of uric acid is normally about

8 liters per day, and the colonic clearance about 4 liters per day. Thus, two-thirds of the uric acid produced is cleared by the kidney and one-third by the colon (74). Thus, if the plasma concentration of uric acid is 5 mg/dl (50 mg/liter), renal excretion of uric acid would be 400 mg per day, and the amount cleared by the colonic bacteria would be 200 mg, with a total uric acid removal rate of 600 mg per day. If chronic renal disease reduces the renal clearance of uric acid to 4 liters a day (half of normal) with the same rate of production (600 mg/day), plasma uric acid concentration will not double if the colonic clearance remains unchanged.

The regulation of plasma creatinine concentration follows the same type of compensation as shown in Model C. Normally, creatinine is cleared mainly by the kidney with a daily clearance of about 180 liters, but the colonic bacteria also remove a small amount of creatinine, providing about 3 liters of creatinine clearance per day (17). Thus, normally the colonic clearance, which constitutes less than 2% of total creatinine clearance, has little impact on the plasma concentration of creatinine. However, in the presence of advanced renal failure, which does not diminish the colonic clearance of creatinine, it could have a substantial impact on plasma concentration of creatinine. For example, a person who has 5 ml/min of renal creatinine clearance (7.2 liters per day), 3 liters of colonic clearance would now represent about 30% of the total creatinine clearance. For these reasons, the rate of increase in serum creatinine in advanced renal failure is not exactly inversely proportionate to the reduction in renal clearance of creatinine.

Basic Rules Concerning External Balance

The cumulative net loss of a substance from the body cannot exceed the total amount of that substance contained in the body (Table 1). For example, one can conclude with certainty that a person who has total body sodium content of 3500 mEq could not have been in daily negative balance of sodium by 30 mEq per day for 1 year, since the total loss of 10,950 mEq (30 × 365 = 10,950) would exceed the total body store of sodium.

Even before exceeding total body content, a physiological limit of deficit for the substance cannot be exceeded. For example, potassium loss in excess of a third of the body store (3000 mEq) is usually fatal. Hence, you would reject a claim that a patient with Conn's tumor has been losing 20 mEq of potassium daily for 3 months, since loss of such an amount (20 × 30 × 3 = 1800 mEq) would be surely lethal. In contrast, the body can tolerate a greater fraction of sodium loss. A person who loses half of body sodium would be gravely ill, but still alive.

While the total stored amount sets the absolute upper limit on losses, the amount that can be gained depends on additional storage capacity, which varies widely with electrolytes. In the case of sodium, the storage capacity for additional Na^+ in the body is enormous. In certain edema-forming states, the Na^+ content may increase by 300% of the basal amount. Caloric balance is another example. In an average (healthy) adult, calories stored in fat and protein total about 130,000. At the caloric consumption rate of 1200 calories per day, about 50% of the stored calories would be consumed in 55 days. In contrast, a person can gain 500 lb of fat, which could provide 4,500,000 calories, about 35 times the normal caloric storage.

COMMON MISCONCEPTIONS AND NEW INSIGHTS

A series of topics discussed in the following sections deals with widespread misconceptions regarding principles related to restoration of balance states.

Is There a Set Point for Renal Sodium Excretion?

Hollenberg, citing earlier writing on the same subject by Straus and colleagues (32), proposed a hypothesis for the existence of a set point for the regulation of body sodium content by the kidney. The set point is defined in his writings as the level of sodium content in the body that the kidney tries to maintain as the normal and desirable level (32). Henceforth, this hypothesis will be called the *set point hypothesis*, which is based on the following line of evidence.

First, when sodium intake is suddenly reduced, the rate of decrease in urine sodium excretion is exponential. The exponential decline was considered thermodynamically unsound if the reduction in urine sodium excretion were in response to volume depletion. If it were in response to progressive volume depletion, the author argued, the decline should be accelerating, not declining exponentially.

Second, when a patient in sodium balance on a low-sodium diet (10 mEq/day) was given a small amount of extra sodium (e.g., 30 mEq), the extra sodium was promptly excreted. The set point hypothesis holds that if the patient had been volume depleted at the time, he should not have excreted the extra sodium.

Finally, when a patient who was volume depleted by chronic diuretic therapy was given sodium, no sodium diuresis occurred until the body sodium content was brought back to the level achieved on zero sodium intake.

On the basis of these observations, the set point for renal sodium excretion was defined as the amount of sodium in the body when the subject is in balance on a salt-free diet. Accordingly, most humans are in a state of sodium excess, and a sodium-free diet starts the unloading of excess sodium, and diminishes the stimulus for sodium diuresis, and thus, exponential decrease in renal sodium excretion. It was further argued that the absence of a set point would lead to chaos, and that a control system without a reference point is unimaginable. The possibility of a set point being higher or lower than the level defined above was dismissed; the exponential decrease in sodium excretion on a salt-free diet is considered to be evidence against

TABLE 1   Total Body Contents of Main Elements and Daily Turnover for Average Adult Male

Body Elements	Total Body Content	Usual Daily Turnover (%)	Days for 50% Turnover
Na	3500 mEq	4.0	12
K	3000 mEq	2.3	22
Ca	60,000 mEq	0.01	2700
Mg	2000 mEq	0.5	100
P	18,000 mmol	0.17	290
Water	40 liters	5.0	10
Alkali	28,000 mEq	0.2	250
Calories	130,000 kcal	1.5	33
Creatinine	400 mg	.400	0.12
Urea-N	4000 mg	250	0.2

a higher set point, whereas the absence of sodium diuresis upon salt administration in patients pretreated with a diuretic was thought to be evidence against the existence of a lower set point.

The set point hypothesis has been debated in public forum previously (7, 75), but the novelty of the current argument against the hypothesis is that it is advanced by use of counterexamples. The counterexamples presented below are directed mainly against the following argument.

Argument: The authors of the set point hypothesis state that the exponential decline in renal salt excretion on a salt-free diet is inconsistent with the position that the salt content of the body on usual salt intake is normal. They argue that if the volume were normal at the usual salt intake, reduction in salt output on a salt-free diet should accelerate as the subject becomes more and more volume depleted. They further argue that on a salt-free diet, renal salt excretion declines exponentially because salt excess is declining exponentially.

Counterexample 1. A counterexample to this argument is the pattern of urine water output on zero water intake. With increasing water deficit on zero water intake, urine output declines exponentially, not accelerating, despite progressive water deficit and progressive activation of the water-conserving mechanism with each passing moment.

Counterexample 2. When a patient is on a potassium-free diet, urinary excretion of potassium declines exponentially, and does not accelerate despite a progressive increase in potassium deficit.

Counterexample 3. In a patient with metabolic acidosis, the arterial pCO_2 declines exponentially with increasing severity of the acidosis.

The finding that urinary sodium declines exponentially neither supports nor disproves the existence of a set point as previously defined. When sodium intake is stopped, urine sodium decreases progressively because effective vascular volume declines progressively with the result that sodium reabsorption mechanisms in the kidney are activated progressively. Whether the body sodium content at usual sodium intake is normal or excessive is not a question that can be decided by the pattern of renal sodium excretion, just as we cannot decide the normal plasma potassium concentration by the pattern of renal potassium output in response to a change in potassium intake.

In an attempt to define a normal value in the set point hypothesis, a special meaning has been attached to the pattern of renal sodium excretion. However, it is our opinion that normalcy of any physiological values must ultimately be decided by their relation to morbidity and mortality. Given the well-known effects of body salt content on blood pressure, it may be more advantageous to have a salt content that is achieved on a near salt-free diet than the content attained on usual salt intake. The fact the body sodium content attained on a near salt-free diet is more advantageous to human health is, in our opinion, pure chance, but it probably contributed to the set point hypothesis. At different times in human history, a slight excess in sodium content might have been beneficial to survival when salt was not readily available in many parts of the world and salt loss was a common occurrence from gastroenteritis and sweating. This scenario seems more plausible when one realizes that the main adverse effect of excess salt content in the body is increase in blood pressure, and hypertension was not the main cause of death when the average life span was 30 to 40 years. Normally, urine sodium excretion decreases when effective vascular volume declines. Thus, the relationship between effective vascular volume and renal sodium excretion can be summed up in one sentence: The lower the effective vascular volume, the lower the renal sodium output, and the higher the effective vascular volume, the higher the renal sodium output.

As explained in Model B, the relationship between renal sodium excretion and effective vascular volume is not continuous; below a certain level of effective vascular volume, renal sodium output virtually disappears, and this happens before any overt signs of clinical dehydration. When effective vascular volume decreases further, renal sodium excretion cannot decrease further because renal sodium excretion cannot be a negative number even though the sodium-retaining mechanisms are even more active. Administration of sodium in such a state would not cause sodium diuresis until effective vascular volume increases to a higher level. The proponent of the set point hypothesis asks the question, "If a subject is volume depleted on a 10-mEq-per-day sodium diet, why would he excrete the administered sodium?" The simple answer would be "because he is less volume depleted now."

The central core of the set point hypothesis is that the kidney stops excreting sodium at the set point—that is, the salt content attained at near zero sodium intake—in order to preserve the most desirable value of body sodium content. However, that is not the consistent behavior of the kidney. Urine output never becomes zero until the kidney is completely shut off despite progressive water-deficit and clear clinical evidence of dehydration. Likewise, renal potassium output does not cease on a zero potassium intake despite clinically evident hypokalemia (68).

Does Salt Excretion Exceed Salt Intake in Salt-Losing Nephropathy?

An often-cited diagnostic criterion for salt-losing nephropathy is urine sodium excretion in excess of sodium intake (71). This is obviously impossible on a chronic basis, just as chronic diuretic therapy cannot produce persistent net sodium loss. Overall, salt intake must equal salt output in the long run, but transient imbalance is possible and often occurs. Salt output exceeds intake while volume depletion develops, but the reverse occurs when volume depletion is being corrected. If a patient with salt-losing nephropathy who had been on a high-salt diet reduces salt intake because of an illness, the patient will develop volume depletion as urine salt output exceeds salt intake. Measurement during this period would show a negative salt balance. On the other hand, it is obvious that when the same patient resumes her usual salt intake or receives intravenous fluid, salt balance will be positive during the period of recovery. Thus, salt balance will be positive if it is measured while the volume-depleted patient with salt losing nephropathy is being treated with intravenous saline solution. On the other hand, salt balance would be negative even in a normal person if the measurement were made when sodium intake was suddenly reduced. The diagnosis of salt-losing nephropathy requires documentation of inappropriate urinary salt excretion in the presence of volume depletion.

Mechanism of Low Urea Nitrogen Concentration in Liver Disease

It is often stated that serum urea nitrogen level is usually very low in chronic liver disease because urea is produced in the liver and the diseased liver cannot produce urea at the normal rate (49). It is obvious that a low serum urea concentration without increased urea clearance must be due to reduced production, but the reason for reduced production is not impaired liver function. Once ingested protein is broken down to individual amino acids and absorbed into the bloodstream, it has three metabolic pathways: (1) metabolism to urea and its eventual excretion in urine, (2) metabolism to nonurea nitrogen compounds, and their eventual excretion in urine, and (3) protein synthesis. Patients with chronic liver disease are not in a state of net protein synthesis, that is, they are not in an anabolic state. Nonurea nitrogen compounds normally excreted in urine include ammonia, amino acids, creatinine, and uric acid, and urinary excretion of these compounds is not increased in chronic liver diseases. One might suggest that nitrogen could accumulate as ammonia in the blood as the metabolic conversion of ammonia to urea is impaired in liver disease. In severe liver disease, ammonia concentration in plasma is indeed increased, but the total amount of nitrogen that can accumulate in the body in the form of ammonia without fatal consequences is negligible. The concentrations of ammonia in plasma are in micrograms whereas those of urea in milligrams. Accumulation of ingested nitrogen as ammonia instead of its conversion to urea would lead to fatal hyperammonemia within hours.

The only logical explanation for low urea production therefore is reduced protein intake. Chronic alcoholics often have persistently low protein ingestion, and these patients have low plasma urea nitrogen. However, any normal person ingesting a low-protein diet will also have low urea nitrogen production, and therefore low plasma urea nitrogen. A strict vegetarian often has a low urea nitrogen concentration for these reasons. When a patient with a liver disease has a GI hemorrhage, serum urea nitrogen concentration rises promptly indicating that the diseased liver can produce urea rapidly when the substrate is available. If a person with severe liver disease ingests a normal amount of protein, urea production will be normal, but plasma ammonia will be higher.

It is a general rule that an impaired metabolic pathway does not reduce the output of its metabolic product unless there is another pathway to which the precursor of the product can be shunted. In the absence of another pathway, the concentration of the precursor will be increased at equilibrium, and the rate of output of the metabolic product will return to the baseline. The situation is analogous to the quantity of creatinine excretion in chronic renal failure. When the kidney function is impaired, the amount of creatinine excreted in the urine does not decrease as long as the creatinine production remains unchanged. The amount excreted will decrease at the onset of renal failure, but at equilibrium, it will return to the baseline. No one would suggest measurement of the rate of urinary creatinine excretion as a means of determining renal function; instead, serum creatinine concentration is examined. Likewise, the rate of production of urea by the liver does not offer any clue about the level of liver function, but the serum ammonia level does.

Renal Sodium Excretion Alone, Without Knowledge of Sodium Intake, Is the Best Predictor of Effective Vascular Volume

The assessment of effective vascular volume by urinary sodium excretion is a widely used and useful clinical tool. Most physicians, however, believe that knowledge of both sodium intake and urine sodium output provides a better clue to the status of effective vascular volume. The following example explains why this belief is in error.

Question. Two subjects, A and B, have been admitted to the hospital with unknown status of their effective vascular volume. Subject A was given a sodium intake of 100 mEq per day, and Subject B a sodium intake of 20 mEq per day. Subject A was found to excrete 60 mEq of sodium per day, and Subject B 40 mEq per day in 24-hour urine samples. On the basis of this information, who do you believe has a higher effective vascular volume? You should assume that neither subject has any renal or hormonal disorder that would affect renal sodium excretion.

Answer and discussion. Most people predict that A has lower effective vascular volume than B. The reason for the choice follows: Subject A is in positive sodium balance because he is volume depleted, whereas Subject B is in negative sodium balance because volume expansion compels her to excrete the excess sodium. It is true that the balance data indicates that A is in a state of sodium retention and B in a state of sodium loss. However, sodium retention need not indicate the presence of volume depletion, and sodium loss not does necessarily prove the state of expanded volume. The following examples will make these points obvious.

Example 1. If a person in salt balance while ingesting 100 mEq of sodium per day suddenly increased sodium intake to 200 mEq per day, and excreted only 150 mEq the first day, the result is also a positive sodium balance. However, the positive sodium balance in this instance would not be labeled renal sodium retention, since the positive balance is due to increased intake, not reduced excretion. Furthermore, despite a positive sodium balance, the effective vascular volume on the first day of increased sodium intake would be higher than the previous day, which is the reason for the high rate of urinary sodium excretion.

Example 2. A patient with intractable heart failure was ingesting 50 mEq of sodium per day and excreting only 10 mEq/day. He is retaining sodium avidly, and hence the term renal sodium retention would be appropriate in this setting. The sodium retention is due to low effective vascular volume. Now he is given a salt-free diet, and urine sodium drops further to 5 mEq/day. At this point, his overall sodium balance is negative by 5 mEq/day. Can we say, then, that his effective vascular volume is no longer diminished since he is no longer retaining sodium?

Sodium intake itself has no direct effect on renal sodium output. Any influence of sodium intake on renal sodium output is always mediated through effective vascular volume because sodium intake, along with sodium output, determines effective vascular volume. If we think of renal sodium output in terms of Model B (Fig. 4), the height of the water column represents effective vascular volume. Just as the only factor that influences water output in Model B is the height of the water column, the only factor that influences renal sodium excretion directly is effective vascular volume. Thus, renal sodium output reflects effective vascular volume, just as water output reflects water column height in Model B. The higher the urine sodium, the higher the effective vascular volume; the lower the urine sodium, the lower the effective vascular volume. Once this relationship is understood, the answer to the question regarding Subjects A and B is easy: Subject A has higher effective vascular volume, because he is excreting more sodium in urine than Subject B.

The reason for the widespread confusion in the use of sodium intake and output as a predictor of effective vascular volume is likely to be in the misuse of the term renal sodium retention. The train of logic goes as follows. First, sodium intake in excess of sodium output represents sodium retention. Second, sodium retention is most often due to reduced renal excretion of sodium, and is rarely due to increased intake. Third, reduced renal excretion of sodium is most often due to low effective vascular volume. Fourth, sodium retention, therefore, is most often due to low effective vascular volume. Finally, any sodium retention, that is, positive sodium balance, signifies low effective vascular volume. Although the fatal error in reasoning is in the final step, the major mistake occurred in thinking that sodium retention is always due to reduced renal sodium output, instead of thinking that it is usually due to reduced renal sodium output (56).

Does Evidence Exist for the "Overflow Mechanism" in Ascites Formation?

The overflow theory of ascites formation states that an important mechanism of sodium retention in ascites formation in cirrhosis of the liver is primary renal sodium retention due to a diseased liver. The argument is based on data from drug-induced cirrhosis of the liver in dogs, which developed ascites and salt retention in the absence of signs of reduced effective vascular volume such as elevated plasma renin activity and plasma aldosterone concentration. On the basis of these observations, the authors of the study concluded that renal sodium retention could not have been a response to volume depletion caused by loss of fluid to the peritoneal cavity (i.e., underfilling), and therefore renal salt retention was a primary event that led to increased effective vascular volume resulting in the ascites formation (i.e., overflow) (11, 47). Two major lines of error were made in this conclusion.

The first error was the assumption that the proof of salt retention (i.e., positive salt balance) due to the underfilling mechanism requires the presence of overt volume depletion. The following example will demonstrate how effective vascular volume could remain within a normal range during slow ascites formation by an underfilling mechanism. Assume that a person who has been in salt balance while ingesting 15 g of salt/day and excreting 15 g/day, develops chronic diarrhea and loses 5 g of salt in the stool daily. The net GI absorption of salt after subtracting the amount lost in stool would then be 10 g/day, and she would excrete 10 g of salt in the urine per day. Effective vascular volume during diarrhea will be lower than it was before the start of diarrhea, but not lower than that of a person without diarrhea ingesting 10 g of salt. Likewise, if a person ingesting 15 g of salt per day develops ascites slowly, and sequesters 5 g of salt daily in the peritoneal space, her effective vascular volume would not be lower than a person who ingests 10 g of salt a day without developing ascites. In both cases, ingestion of 15 g of salt, in the absence of abnormal salt loss, would have resulted in excretion of 15 g of salt. With the advent of ascites formation or diarrhea, the kidney excretes 10 g instead of 15 g, because the effective vascular volume is now slightly lower than that without ascites formation or diarrhea. In both cases, the reduction in renal sodium output clearly was in response to "underfilling," even though there would be no discernible volume depletion. In both examples, effective vascular volume was maintained sufficiently high to allow renal excretion of 10 g of salt per day. If plasma renin activity were measured during the period of sodium retention in these examples, it would have been normal. The absence of apparent volume depletion in any edema-forming conditions does not prove that the kidney did not retain sodium in response to a volume stimulus.

The second error is the failure to recognize that the infinite gain control mechanism operates in ascites formation by the underfilling mechanism. Thus, if salt intake and the function curve for the renal salt output remain unchanged, the effective vascular volume will return to the baseline when steady state is achieved. The sequence of events would be as follows. Ascites formation by the transudation of fluid from the vascular space into the peritoneal cavity would reduce the effective vascular volume, and this reduces renal salt output. Normal salt intake with reduced renal salt output causes net salt retention, which would tend to increase the effective vascular volume. However, as long as the effective vascular volume remains lower than the baseline value, renal salt output will remain lower than the baseline, and the positive salt balance will continue. Only when the effective vascular volume returns to the baseline will renal salt output return to the baseline and the salt retention stop. Thus, at equilibrium the effective vascular volume in any patient with ascites would be normal unless treated with a low-salt diet or a diuretic.

Is Primary Renal Salt Retention More Important Than Low Oncotic Pressure in Nephrotic Edema?

Primary renal salt retention is commonly thought to play a more important role in the formation of nephrotic edema than low oncotic pressure, which would cause secondary renal salt retention (22). This belief is based on the observation that nephrotic patients often have low plasma renin activity. The reasoning goes this way: If low oncotic pressure is the primary cause of edema, transudation of fluid from the vascular space into the interstitial space would cause reduction in effective vascular volume, which would increase plasma renin activity; the suppressed plasma renin activity therefore is evidence for the dominant role of primary salt retention in the pathogenesis of nephrotic edema.

The flaw of this reasoning lies in the same type of the faulty assumption as in the mechanism of ascites formation, that is, edema due to low oncotic pressure must be accompanied by low effective vascular volume. The truth is that nephrotic edema entirely due to low oncotic pressure would not be persistently associated with the low effective vascular volume, unless the patient is treated with salt restriction or a diuretic, because the compensatory mechanism for the low effective vascular volume in such situations would be the infinite gain control mechanism.

Imagine a patient in a Third World country developing nephrotic syndrome. The patient is not treated with a diuretic, and he continues to ingest a diet that contains the same usual amount of salt, but almost invariably his renal salt output returns to the baseline and salt retention stops. Otherwise, the patient would develop relentless sodium retention, progressive edema, and death in a relatively short period. Since a slight reduction in effective vascular volume diminishes renal sodium excretion to virtually zero, restoration of renal sodium excretion to a usual normal value is proof that the effective vascular volume has been restored to normal. Plasma-renin activity at this point would be normal.

If a patient now develops a renal disease that results in primary renal salt retention, edema will worsen, effective vascular volume will be greater than a usual normal value, and plasma renin activity will now be suppressed. When the natriuretic effect of the increased effective vascular volume is sufficient to counterbalance the sodium-retaining effect of the renal disease, renal sodium output will again increase to a level that equals intake. A new steady state is achieved between sodium intake and sodium output, and edema will not progress any further. The presence of suppressed plasma renin activity in a patient with nephrotic syndrome is a strong indication for the presence of primary renal sodium retention, but it does not argue against the importance of low oncotic pressure in edema formation. Indeed, primary renal Na retention alone, such as in acute glomerulonephritis, rarely causes as edema as severe as that found in nephrotic syndrome. On the other hand, a low oncotic pressure by causes other than urinary loss of protein, such as malnutrition, also results in severe edema.

EXPLANATION OF DISEASE MANIFESTATIONS IN SELECTED TOPICS

The following discussion deals with a few selected topics that require clear understanding of the principles of external balance in order to explain certain manifestations of disease states.

Sodium Delivery to Cortical Collecting Duct Is Increased in Hyperaldosteronism and Decreased in Hypoaldosteronism

According to the principles outlined at the beginning of this chapter, in the steady state, urinary sodium excretion is equal to sodium intake in all normal and abnormal states including both primary and secondary hyperaldosteronism. One might therefore conclude that sodium delivery to the cortical collecting duct could also return to baseline once a steady state is achieved. However, that is not the case. The principles discussed in earlier sections predict that total sodium output must equal intake in the long run; they do not indicate that sodium reabsorption at any particular nephron site cannot remain chronically altered. That the delivery of sodium to the collecting duct will not return to what it had been before the start of diuretic therapy or the onset of primary hyperaldosteronism is apparent from the following considerations.

The steady-state principle predicts that sodium excretion will equal sodium intake in the long run. Thus, a patient receiving chronic diuretic therapy or one with primary hyperaldosteronism will excrete the same amount of sodium as was excreted before the abnormalities developed if the intake remains the same. In both states, however, a greater amount of sodium must be reabsorbed at the collecting duct because of the increased aldosterone effect, but the amount excreted in the final urine cannot remain increased or reduced. To satisfy both conditions, it is necessary to deliver an increased amount of sodium to the collecting duct. The sequence of events will be as follows with primary hyperaldosteronism as an example.

The initial abnormality in primary hyperaldosteronism is increased salt reabsorption at the cortical collecting duct. At the beginning, this would cause net salt retention and reduced renal salt excretion. The resulting positive salt balance increases effective vascular volume, which inhibits the proximal salt reabsorption, resulting in increased delivery of salt to the cortical collecting duct. Despite the increased delivery of salt, the amount of salt that escapes into urine is more than at the beginning, but still less than the intake because of increased salt reabsorption caused by increased aldosterone activity. As long as the urinary excretion of salt is less than the intake, net positive salt retention continues, causing further increase in effective vascular volume. The higher effective vascular volume further increases proximal inhibition of salt reabsorption, causing even greater increase in the distal delivery of salt. The process will continue with further increase in salt excretion. Only when the renal excretion of salt increases sufficiently to match the intake, will net positive balance of salt stop. At equilibrium, salt output equals salt intake, but the quantity of salt delivered to the collecting duct remains increased.

In the case of chronic therapy with a loop diuretic or a thiazide diuretic, initially salt delivery to the collecting duct would be greatly increased resulting in negative salt balance. The ensuing volume depletion activates salt-retaining mechanisms in the proximal tubule and also stimulates aldosterone secretion causing increased reabsorption of salt in the cortical collecting duct. On the second day, the increased salt reabsorption by the proximal tubule will partially negate the diuretic effect, so that a somewhat smaller amount of salt would be delivered to the collecting duct. With the reduced delivery of salt and increased reabsorption due to secondary hyperaldosteronism, urinary salt excretion will be reduced further. But as long as the amount excreted exceeds the salt intake, the effective vascular volume will continue to decline, and salt-retaining mechanisms for the proximal tubule and stimulation of aldosterone secretion will further intensify. Only when renal salt output equals the intake, will further reduction in volume cease and a new balance be achieved. A key point is that despite increased salt reabsorption in the proximal tubule that opposes the natriuretic effect of the diuretic, delivery of salt to the collecting duct must be increased when balance is restored. If the salt delivery were back to the baseline value or reduced below the baseline, renal salt output would not be equal to the intake since salt reabsorption in the collecting duct is increased to a level greater than the baseline. For the same reasons as described above, the sodium delivery to the cortical collecting duct remains chronically reduced in states of hypoaldosteronism.

Mechanism of Chronic Volume Expansion in Syndrome of Inappropriate Secretion of ADH

Ample evidence exists that patients with SIADH (syndrome of inappropriate secretion of ADH) are volume expanded when chronic hyponatremia is present. As evidence for ex-panded volume status, these patients have increased clearances of creatinine, urea, and uric acid (21, 36). However, the persistence of chronic volume expansion in SIADH would seem paradoxical, since these patients do not have a reason for primary renal sodium retention such as primary hyperaldosteronism or a renal disorder. In the absence of such disorders, would not the normal kidney promptly increase renal salt excretion until the volume is restored to the usual normal value?

The explanation for the persistence of volume expansion in SIADH lies in the antinatriuretic effect of hyponatremia (8, 65). The sequence of events is as follows. Initially, water retention causes hyponatremia and volume expansion. Volume expansion causes sodium diuresis resulting in further reduction in serum sodium. But as serum sodium declines, the antinatriuretic effect of hyponatremia opposes the natriuretic effect of volume expansion. When these two opposing effects are about equal, the renal salt excretion returns to the baseline value, and a new balance is established, with renal salt excretion equaling salt intake. In other words, when renal salt excretion returns to the baseline, the effective vascular is still somewhat expanded.

Effective Vascular Volume is Low in Chronic Hypernatremia Despite Adequate Salt Intake

In the presence of normal renal function, chronic hypernatremia is always accompanied by reduced effective vascular volume, and the degree of reduction in effective vascular volume is proportionate to the level of serum sodium (1, 55). Exceptions are chronic hypernatremia in renal failure, or hypernatremia that develops as a result of chronic administration of a large amount of sodium. Even in the latter condition, the effective vascular volume would be lower with high serum sodium than with normal serum sodium for the same amount of sodium administered. Although some authors still postulate that the effective vascular volume is normal in essential hypernatremia (55), this rule applies even to essential hypernatremia. The following analysis will show why the effective vascular volume is low in all states of chronic hypernatremia, including essential hypernatremia.

As stated earlier, hyponatremia is antinatriuretic. Likewise, hypernatremia is natriuretic (9, 37). For this reason, renal sodium excretion will be increased in normovolemic hypernatremia as long as kidney function is normal. Increased renal sodium excretion with the usual intake of sodium would reduce effective vascular volume. Volume depletion would then tend to oppose the natriuretic effect of hypernatremia and to reduce renal sodium excretion, but as long as the renal sodium excretion exceeds sodium intake, volume depletion will become progressively greater. Only when volume depletion is sufficiently great to exactly oppose the natriuretic effect of hypernatremia, does renal sodium excretion return to the baseline and thus equals intake. At this point, a new sodium balance is attained, but at the expense of maintenance of volume depletion. Since the natriuretic effect of hypernatremia is proportionate to the degree of hypernatremia, the volume depletion needed to counterbalance the natriuretic effect of hypernatremia must also be proportionately great to match the degree of hypernatremia when the new sodium balance is achieved. In other words, the greater the severity of hypernatremia, the greater the volume depletion in a steady state.

It has been suggested that patients with essential hypernatremia are euvolemic because hypernatremia in this condition is a result of the resetting of the osmostat (55). Resetting means that the osmostat is regulated normally but at higher than usual serum sodium concentrations. The more recent evidence indicates that essential hypernatremia is caused by defects in the osmoreceptors, not the resetting of the osmostat (64). However, regardless of its pathogenetic mechanism, chronic volume depletion is inevitable in essential hypernatremia if renal function is normal. Since hypernatremia is natriuretic, sodium balance will occur only when the natriuretic effect of hypernatremia is counterbalanced by the antinatriuretic effect of volume depletion. Mild volume depletion can escape detection even by careful physical examination. For example, a small amount of a diuretic, such as 50 mg of hydrochlorothiazide, can reduce effective vascular volume sufficiently for the kidney to sense a reduction in volume, and thereby reduce clearances of urea, creatinine, and uric acid. Yet, a careful physical examination by an astute physician will not detect signs of dehydration without the help of laboratory tests, such as a higher serum urate. Indeed, it has been shown that most patients with essential hypernatremia have laboratory evidence of volume depletion when the data are carefully analyzed (1).

EXTERNAL BALANCE OF PROTONS

Determination of external balance of most univalent ions such as sodium, potassium, and chloride is straightforward; intestinal absorption is complete and they are eventually eliminated from the body since these ions are not metabolized. Balance of polyvalent inorganic ions such as calcium, magnesium, and phosphate is more complicated because of their incomplete intestinal absorption. External balance of acids and bases is even more complicated than that of polyvalent ions because of uncertainties in their intestinal absorption and variations in their metabolism after absorption.

In the steady state, hydrogen ion enters the body through ingestion of acid and endogenous creation of acid through metabolism. The pH of food offers no guidance to its character as a donor of acid or alkali. Most fruit juices have low pH because of their organic acid contents, but overall they are contributors of alkali. Sulfur-containing amino acids are neutral until they are metabolized to produce sulfuric acid, but the amount of acid produced cannot be predicted accurately from the sulfur content, because some of the sulfur follows different metabolic pathways.

The intestinal absorption of the dietary acid and alkali is incomplete, and until recently it was thought that the amount excreted in the stool has to be known in order to determine net intestinal absorption.

Under steady-state conditions, net acid production must equal net acid excretion, and the traditional view on the external acid–base balance has been as follows. Acids are produced from three main sources: sulfuric acid derived from the metabolism of sulfur-containing amino acids, incompletely metabolized organic acids, and acid (or alkali) of diet absorbed in the intestine (44, 57, 63). Acids are excreted either in the form of ammonium or titratable acid, while a small amount of alkali is lost in the urine as bicarbonate. Hence, the total acid excretion measured as the sum of urine ammonium and titratable acid minus bicarbonate is called net acid excretion. However, this traditional view of the acid–base balance must be re-evaluated in light of conceptual uncertainties of this approach and methodological limitations in the measurement of parameters of acid–base balance by the conventional techniques (57). The following discussion is intended to shed some light on these uncertainties and limitations.

MEASUREMENT OF NET ACID EXCRETION

The concept of titratable acid is straightforward. The pH of urine following glomerular ultrafiltration is the same as that of plasma, but decreases progressively due to addition of H^+ by tubular secretion. Most of the secreted H^+ is buffered by HCO_3^-, and this results in indirect reabsorption of HCO_3^-. As urine pH falls further with tubular secretion of H^+, other urinary buffers are titrated to retard a fall in urine pH. The addition of alkali to the urine until its pH is the same as that of the plasma measures the titratable acid. This back-titration of urine releases all the H^+ titrated by nonbicarbonate buffers except those in the form of NH_4^+, which is not titrated because of its high pK (9.2), and thus is measured separately.

It is our contention that the measurement of titratable acid, ammonium, and bicarbonate does not accurately reflect net acid excretion by the kidney for the following reasons. First, there is a technical problem with the measurement of titratable acid (41). The addition of alkali to the urine causes partial precipitation of urine calcium with HPO_4^{2-}. Selective depletion of HPO_4^{2-} causes conversion of some $H_2PO_4^-$ to HPO_4^{2-} with liberation of protons, leading to overestimation of titratable acid. Furthermore, titration of urine to the plasma pH results in titration of 1/64th of urinary ammonium (calculated with the pKa of ammonium of 9.2) and causes further overestimation of titratable acid; this error is usually negligible, but would be substantial when the urine contains a large amount of ammonium.

A potentially more serious source of error is the presence of buffers other than ammonium that are not titrated when urine pH is increased to 7.4 (58). The original assumption that ammonium is the only urinary buffer that escapes titration during the measurement of titratable acid has not been fully proven. Normal urine contains various amines such as ethanolamine, phosphoethanolamine, methylamine, and dimethylamine, and urinary excretion of these substances would represent acid excretion as does the excretion of ammonium. However, titration of urine to pH 7.4 does not detect the presence of such substances. The individual urine concentration of each of these substances appears to be quite low individually, but the amount might be substantial collectively.

SOURCES OF ACID

Sulfuric Acid

The metabolism of sulfur-containing amino acids produces sulfuric acid as follows:

$$RN\text{-}S \rightarrow CO_2 + Urea + H_2SO_4$$

The resulting H_2SO_4 is buffered by body alkali, mainly HCO_3^-. Since with ordinary diet virtually all urinary sulfates originate from sulfur-containing amino acids, urinary sulfate fairly accurately represents the production rate of sulfuric acid. However, the metabolism of sulfur-containing amino acids does not result in an equimolar production of sulfuric acid (34, 43), because some of the sulfur is excreted in a neutral form such as cystine or taurine. Furthermore, a substantial amount of sulfate is consumed in sulfate conjugation, most notably in the conjugation of both endogenous and exogenous phenolic compounds (4, 24, 38), and such reaction would reduce the acid load achieved by complete sulfur oxidation as explained below. Each millimole of H_2SO_4 produces 2 mEq of protons in the following reaction:

$$H_2SO_4 \rightarrow SO_4^= + 2H^+$$

On the other hand, the sulfate conjugation reaction consumes a proton; the result is net production of only 1 mol of protons for each mole of sulfur oxidized:

$$R\text{-}OH + SO_4^= + H^+ \rightarrow R\text{-}O\text{-}SO_3\text{-}$$

Sulfate conjugation reaction is an important detoxification mechanism, and the reactions are regulated by various enzymes such as phenol sulfotransferase (4, 24, 38). The rate of sulfate conjugation reaction seems to depend, in part, on the availability of inorganic sulfate, and it can also be saturated depending on the availability of enzymes. For these reasons, the fraction of sulfur contained in amino acids that is oxidized to sulfuric acid might vary with individuals and also with the amount of protein intake. In one study, urinary sulfate recovered following ingestion of methionine was shown to be 85% to 90% of the sulfur content of the ingested amino acid (34). On the other hand, urinary excretion of sulfate esters has been shown to be as much as 17% of total urinary sulfur excretion (3), and this amount might be higher in certain situations such as renal insufficiency, in which plasma sulfate concentrations are higher (69, 72).

The sulfur content of proteins in different food sources varies greatly, and depends on the content of methionine and cysteine (15). For example, the sulfur content of human milk protein is only half of that of most cereal proteins. The sulfur content of beef is less than that of pork or lamb. In general, with the exception of grains, proteins of vegetable origin have lower sulfur content than do proteins of animal sources (15).

In conclusion, the proper way of determining the contribution of sulfuric acid to the endogenous acid production would require the measurement of both sulfate and sulfate esters in the urine as described below:

Acid production from sulfur oxidation (mEq) = Urine sulfate (millimoles) $\times$ 2 + Urine sulfate esters.

Sulfate is multiplied by 2 because it is divalent, while sulfate esters are monovalent.

Organic Acid

Production of organic acid results in consumption of HCO_3^- in the reaction:

$$RH + HCO_3^- \rightarrow R^- + H_2CO_3\text{-}$$

If the organic anion is retained in the body, and is subsequently metabolized to HCO_3^-, there is no net loss of alkali. When the organic anion is not metabolized or is not metabolizable (e.g., urate), or escapes metabolism because it is excreted in the urine (e.g., citrate), this represents a net loss of alkali. The nature of many of these organic anions excreted in the urine is not known (13, 14, 40), and therefore total organic acid production cannot be determined by measuring individual components. Instead, they are measured collectively by titration of urine. However, the titration method used most widely is that of Van Slyke and Palmer (73), which contains many potential sources of error, some of which result in underestimation and some in overestimation (18, 59).

When a metabolizable organic anion cannot be excreted because of renal failure, it is eventually metabolized. Hence, renal function is an important consideration in the overall contribution of organic acids to acid production. In the absence of renal excretion, only nonmetabolizable organic acids would accumulate. It is not known what fraction of organic acids normally excreted in urine is metabolizable, and what fraction nonmetabolizable. To the extent that metabolizable organic anions are not excreted, patients in renal failure would have reduced net acid production as shown in patients treated with maintenance hemodialysis (70). On the other hand, net organic acid production is greatly increased during hemodialysis procedures as a large amount of organic anions are lost into the dialysate during dialysis (70).

Net organic acid production can also be regulated by the blood pH (10, 33, 39). The regulation of net production of organic acids occurs in two ways. One way is the regulation of its production, which is pH dependent. It has been shown that acidic systemic pH decreases production of both keto acid and lactic acid, while alkaline pH promotes their production (33). Another mechanism of net organic acid production by systemic pH is the regulation of renal excretion. This effect is mediated mainly by the proximal tubular cell pH. An acidic pH of the proximal tubular cell increases reabsorption of organic anions, and thereby reduces urinary excretion, while an alkaline pH has the opposite effects (39). Usually the proximal cell pH parallels the blood pH, but sometimes the two are dissociated. In proximal renal tubular acidosis and type IV RTA, the systemic pH is low, but the proximal tubular cell pH is not, and hence organic anion excretion remains normal. On the other hand, in K^+ depletion, the tubular cell pH tends to be low (as H^+ enters the cell in exchange for K^+), and therefore organic anion loss is reduced, contributing to the genesis of metabolic alkalosis.

Phosphoric Acid

Phosphate is ingested as inorganic phosphate and organic phosphate. Phosphates in milk and other dairy products are mostly inorganic. Inorganic phosphates in food usually have neutral pH, and hence their influence on the acid–base balance depends mainly on the absorption of phosphate relative to its accompanying cation, calcium (46). To the extent that phosphate absorption exceeds calcium absorption, acid will be added to the body.

Organic phosphates are ingested in food as components of intracellular organic compounds. These include creatine phosphate, ATP, ADP, AMP, cyclic AMP, phospholipids in the cell membrane, nucleic acid in DNA and RNA, and phosphoproteins. Their eventual fate either as acid or alkali depends on the number of nonmetabolizable cations that balance the phosphate anions. If the total number of nonmetabolizable cations is 1.8 times the number of phosphate anions, the compound would be neutral. This prediction is based on the fact that the average balance of phosphate at pH 7.4 is 1.8. When the sum of all nonmetabolizable cations in milliequivalents is greater than 1.8 times, the number of phosphates in millimoles, the compound is an alkali, and when it is lower than 1.8, it would be an acid. For example, each molecule of ATP has three molecules of phosphate (which has 5.4 negative charge equivalents when metabolized completely) balanced by four cationic charges, two of which are usually provided by magnesium. Hence, the metabolic breakdown of ATP results in production of acid. Likewise, metabolism of ADP (three cationic charges for 3.6 P) and cyclic AMP (one cationic charge for 1.8 P) produces acid, while breakdown of AMP (two cationic charges for 1.8 P) would produce alkali (Fig. 6). Metabolism of phospholipids and nucleic acids in DNA and RNA produces acid, whereas metabolism of phosphoproteins and creatine phosphate produces alkali (Table 2).

Another way of determining the fate of phosphate as acid or alkali is to examine the number of ester bonds. Phosphate has a total of three anionic sites when it is fully dissociated. As

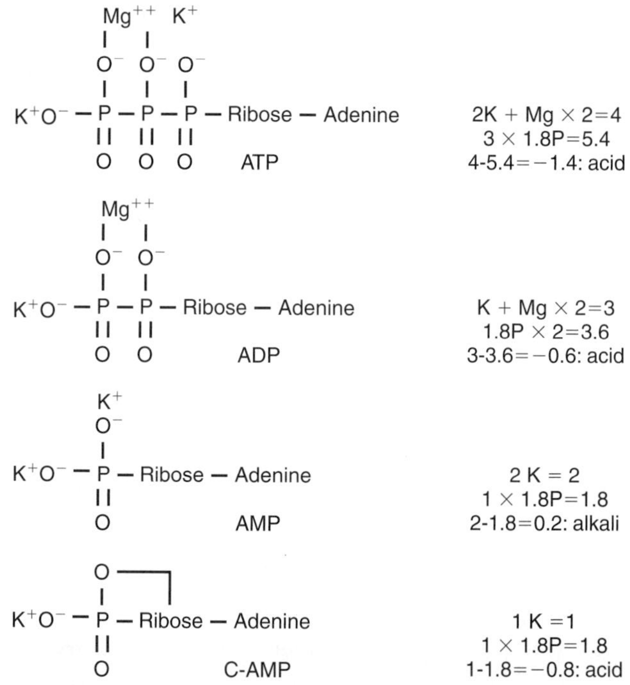

FIGURE 6 Net charge difference between nonmetabolizable cation (K 1 Mg) and nonmetabolic anion (P) on different types of adenosine phosphates. When the total K plus Mg charge exceeds that of P, alkali will be formed when they are metabolized. When P charges exceed K plus Mg charges, acid will be produced upon metabolism. In the calculation, the average balance of P is assumed to be 1.8, and that of Mg to be 2.

phosphate forms an ester bond with an organic substance, the number of anionic sites is reduced and hence the requirement for the number of nonmetabolizable cations such as potassium to balance the anion is also reduced. Thus, when phosphate forms two ester bonds (diester), it has only one anionic site remaining to be balanced by a cation. Phosphates in ATP, ADP, nucleic acids in the DNA and RNA, and phospholipids all form diester bonds. That explains why metabolism of AMP results in production of alkali, whereas metabolism of cyclic AMP and cyclic GMP (both are diesters) results in production of acid. In the case of ATP, the first two phosphates form diester bonds, and the third phosphate has monoester bond. As with inorganic phosphate, the relative GI absorption of organic phosphate must be considered before its contribution to the acid–base balance is ascertained (Fig. 6).

The fraction of phosphate absorbed depends greatly on the type of cation that accompanies phosphate. When phosphate is ingested from the usual diet, about two-thirds are absorbed from the intestine because food contains calcium and calcium binds phosphate to form brushite ($CaHPO_4$), which is rapidly precipitated and excreted in stool as such.

TABLE 2   Production of Acid and Alkali
from Organic Phosphates

Acid production: ATP, ADP, nucleic acid, phospholipids, cyclic AMP
Alkali production: AMP, creatinine P, and phosphoproteins

On the other hand, phosphate ingested as Na or K phosphate is nearly completely absorbed because sodium and potassium are completely absorbed, as long as the amount ingested does not exceed the capacity of the sodium-phosphate transporter (52, 53, 62). When a large amount of sodium phosphate is ingested, the excess amount causes diarrhea. In summary, the contribution of phosphate to net acid production cannot be determined from dietary intake or urinary excretion of phosphate, but is included as part of the net GI alkali absorption, which will be discussed separately later in this chapter.

Amino Acids

The contribution of sulfur-containing amino acids has already been discussed. Other proteins are also potential sources of acid or alkali depending mainly on their relative contents of basic amino acids and acidic amino acids. Metabolism of cationic amino acids, arginine and lysine, produces acid as follows:

$$Arginine^+ Cl^- \rightarrow Urea + CO_2 + HCl$$

On the other hand, metabolism of aspartic acid and glutamic acid results in production of alkali:

$$Na^+ glutamate^- + H_2CO_3 \rightarrow NaHCO_3 + CO_2 + Urea$$

The imidazole group of histidine is present in two forms: neutral or cationic. Metabolism of the cationic histidine results in the production of acid, whereas metabolism of neutral histidine has no effect on acid balance. The ratio of the neutral histidine to cationic histidine depends on the pK of the imidazole group in the molecule and the pH of the solution in which histidine is dissolved. However, the pK of histidine varies widely between 5 and 8, depending on the nature of the molecule with which histidine is associated (31). The pK is 6.21 in L-histidine, but carnosine, a dipeptide composed of β alanine and histidine, which is an important intracellular buffer in the muscle of many vertebrates, has a pK of 7.01. When histidine is a part of a protein molecule, its pK depends on the adjacent amino acid. Next to an acidic group, the pK rises to a level between 7 to 8, and next to a basic group, the pK decreases to a level between 5 to 6. Histidine content of hemoglobin is particularly high, which explains the excellent buffering capacity of hemoglobin. Oxygenation of hemoglobin at the lung reduces the pK of the imidazole group, i.e., it makes it a stronger acid. The acid reacts with bicarbonate to create more CO_2, which is eliminated by ventilation.

Even in the case of the basic and acidic amino acids, their eventual acidity or alkalinity depends on the nature of the counterions balancing the respective amino or carboxyl groups. When these groups are balanced by noncombustible ions such as Na^+, K^+, Cl^-, or phosphate, their metabolism results in a net gain of acid or alkali. If the counterions are organic, the metabolism of the amino acid does not result in a net gain of

acid or alkali. In most foods the total number of nonmetabolizable cations exceeds that of nonmetabolizable anions (30), and therefore, apart from the contribution of sulfuric acid production, their metabolism would produce alkali.

Organic Acids in Meat

A substantial amount of organic anions, especially lactate, has been found in meat, and it has been suggested that a role for lactic acid be included in the overall calculation of dietary net acid production (5). However, most of the lactate present in meat is produced after the death of the animal. Initially, lactic acid is formed, and reacts with cellular alkali. When the meat is digested and absorbed during the process of lactate metabolism, the same amount of protons as released during the lactic acid production is consumed. In the end, the net alkali or acid content of the body is unaffected by the production of lactic acid. By analogy, addition of acetic acid in the form of vinegar to food would produce acetate but would not alter its net acid or the alkali value of the food. As long as the content of noncombustible cations and anions remains the same, the net acid or alkali of meat would not change.

Gastrointestinal Absorption of Acids and Alkali

The normal diet contains large quantities of alkali, potential alkali, acids, and potential acids, but their ultimate impact on the body's acid–base balance depends primarily on their absorption. The pattern of absorption depends not only on the nature of the substance, but also on its interaction with other chemicals, both endogenous and exogenous (20, 45). In general, the amount absorbed is nearly equal to the amount ingested if the substance is soluble and is readily absorbed. Examples include $NaHCO_3$, Na^+ citrate, K^+ citrate, and NH_4Cl. An insoluble substance such as $CaCO_3$ must react with gastric acid or acid in food to become soluble and absorbable. In some cases, only the anionic part is absorbable (e.g., Cl^- in cholestyramine chloride); in other cases, only the cationic part (e.g., Na^+ sodium polystyrene sulfonate). The overall effects of these substances on the body's acid–base balance are complex, and are often unrelated to the acidity or alkalinity of the substance. The following section describes two major categories of chemical substances and the effects of their ingestion on acid–base balance.

INGESTION OF NONABSORBABLE OR POORLY ABSORBABLE CATION ACCOMPANIED BY ABSORBABLE ANION

Intravenous $CaCl_2$ is neutral, but ingested $CaCl_2$ is an acidifying agent. When ingested, virtually all of the Cl^- but only a fraction of the Ca^{++} is absorbed. The excess Ca^{++} remaining in the gut is excreted in the stool after combining with $CO_3^=$, organic anions, or $HPO_4^=$. The type of anionic exchange determines the effect on acid–base balance. Typically, ingested $CaCl_2$ reacts with $NaHCO_3$ as follows:

$$CaCl_2 + 2NaHCO_3 \rightarrow 2NaCl + CaCO_3 + H_2CO_3$$

NaCl is absorbed and the insoluble $CaCO_3$ is excreted in stool, resulting in net loss of $NaHCO_3$. Thus, the net effect of oral ingestion of $CaCl_2$ is loss of 2 mol of alkali for each mole of Ca ingested. When $CaCl_2$ reacts with Na_2HPO_4, NaCl is absorbed and $CaHPO_4$ is excreted in the stool:

$$CaCl_2 + Na_2HPO_4 \rightarrow 2NaCl + CaHPO_4$$

The loss of 1 mol of Na_2HPO_4 changes the ratio of Na_2HPO_4/NaH_2PO_4 from 4:1 to 3:1. In order to reestablish the ratio of Na_2HPO_4/NaH_2PO_4 at 4:1, 0.2 mol of NaH_2PO_4 must be converted to 0.2 mol of Na_2HPO_4, which would release of 0.2 mol of H^+, which would consume 0.2 mol of alkali. Thus, the net effect is the loss of 0.2 mol of alkali for each mol of $CaCl_2$ ingested. The absorbed $CaCl_2$ would have no effect on the acid–base balance. Since $SO_4^=$ is more readily absorbed than Mg^{++}, the overall effect of $MgSO_4$ ingestion would be similar to that of ingestion of $CaCl_2$. Similarly, $FeSO_4$ could result in net gain of acid to the extent that more SO_4^{2-} than Fe^{2+} is absorbed.

When a person ingests salts consisting of a nonabsorbable or poorly absorbable cation, accompanied by an absorbable and metabolizable anion (e.g., $CaCO_3$, $Al(OH)_3$, calcium acetate, and calcium citrate), the amount of alkali gained depends on the absorption of anions, either with the accompanying cations, or in exchange for nonmetabolizable anion such as phosphate. Absorption of $CaCO_3$ is facilitated when it reacts with HCl in the stomach or acid in food because $CaCO_3$ is poorly soluble. The reaction in the stomach follows:

$$CaCO_3 + 2HCl \rightarrow CaCl_2 + H_2CO_3$$

The fate of $CaCl_2$ thus formed will be the same as that of $CaCl_2$ ingested as such. Absorption of Ca as $CaCO_3$ represents alkali gain. Exchange of $CO_3^=$ for $HPO_4^=$ also represents a gain of alkali. Loss of $CaCO_3$ in stool, of course, has no effect on acid–base balance. Ingestion of Ca organic salts such as calcium citrate, calcium lactate, calcium gluconate, and calcium acetate also results in similar gain of alkali. As with calcium carbonate, an alkali gain occurs when these organic anions are absorbed either with calcium or in exchange with phosphate. The overall alkalinizing effect of various calcium antacids depends more on the ability of calcium to bind phosphate than on the absorption of calcium, because the amount of Ca^{++} absorbed is usually much less than the amount bound to phosphate to be excreted in the stool. Phosphate-binding ability depends in part on availability of soluble calcium (67). This might explain why the amount of phosphate bound by calcium when calcium is ingested as $CaCl_2$ is comparable to that bound by aluminum ingested as $Al(OH)_3$ (35), whereas calcium carbonate salt removes only half as much phosphate for the same amount of calcium because of its poor solubility. Despite poor absorption of aluminum, net gain of alkali is greater with $Al(OH)_3$ than with $CaCO_3$,

because aluminum is a more effective binder of phosphate than calcium.

Anion exchange resins are additional examples of nonreabsorbable cations accompanied by absorbable anions (35). As with calcium salts, they have either an acidifying or alkalinizing effect depending on whether the accompanying anion is metabolizable or not. When the counterion is nonmetabolizable, such as chloride (e.g., cholestyramine), its absorption in exchange for organic anions, carbonate, or bicarbonate represents loss of alkali. When chloride is exchanged for phosphate, it represents 0.2 mEq of alkali loss for each mole of phosphate lost as HPO_4. When the counterion is metabolizable (e.g., acetate), a net gain of alkali occurs when the metabolizable anion is absorbed in exchange for chloride or phosphate. Exchange of a metabolizable anion with organic anions, carbonate, or bicarbonate is a neutral process (Table 3).

INGESTION OF NONABSORBABLE OR POORLY ABSORBABLE ANION ACCOMPANIED BY ABSORBABLE CATION

An example is ingestion of Na^+ or K^+ phosphate. Ordinarily, intestinal absorption of Na^+ and K^+ is nearly complete as long as the accompanying anion can also be readily absorbed. Absorption of phosphate on the other hand is limited for two reasons. First, absorption of phosphate is achieved by sodium–phosphate cotransporter (52, 53, 62), which has a limited capacity. When the intake of phosphate is in excess of the transporter's capacity, unabsorbed phosphate is excreted in stool. Second, some of the ingested phosphate can form an insoluble complex with calcium, which is precipitated and excreted in stool. Na^+ or K^+, balanced by the anion that is left behind by the precipitated calcium, will be absorbed. If the anion that is absorbed with sodium or potassium is an organic anion or carbonate, the result will be net gain of alkali:

$$Na_2HPO_4 + CaCO_3 \rightarrow Na_2CO_3 \text{ (absorbed after conversion to } NaHCO_3) + CaPO_4 \text{ (excreted in stool)}$$

Ingestion of a cation-exchange resin results in net gain of alkali by a similar mechanism. The nonabsorbable anion in a cation exchange resin is usually sulfonate attached to a polystyrene skeleton balanced by an exchangeable and absorbable cation, such as Na^+ in sodium polystyrene sulfonate (Kayexalate). When Na^+ exchanges for K^+, it has no

TABLE 3   Effect on Acid–Base Balance by Ingestion of AER

AER-metabolizable anion exchanged with nonmetabolizable anion → Gain of alkali

AER-metabolizable anion exchanged with metabolizable anion → Neutral process

AER-nonmetabolizable anion exchanged with metabolizable anion → Gain of acid

AER-nonmetabolizable anion exchanged with nonmetabolizable anion → Neutral process

AER, anion exchange resin

effect on acid–base balance. Exchange of Na^+ for NH_4^+ or H^+ results in alkali gain. When it exchanges with Ca^{++}, the net effect is also alkali gain, because normally the bulk of Ca^{++} excreted in stool is insoluble calcium carbonate, which represents loss of alkali (51, 66). When Ca^{++} in calcium carbonate is exchanged for Na^+ in sodium polystyrene sulfonate, Na_2CO_3 is formed and then absorbed; at physiological pH, Na_2CO_3 will quickly react with H_2CO_3, and two molecules of $NaHCO_3$ will form. This effect is more pronounced when the resin is administered with calcium salts (51, 66), aluminum salts, or magnesium salts. Exchange between Na^+ and Al^{+++} or Mg^{++} results in formation of $NaOH$ or $NaCO_3$, which is readily absorbable directly or indirectly:

$$Na_2\text{-PSS} + CaCO_3 \rightarrow Ca\text{-PSS (excreted in stool)} + Na_2CO_3 \text{ (absorbed after conversion to } NaHCO_3)$$

where PSS is polystyrene sulfonate.

If the drug is ingested along with $Al(OH)_3$, the following reaction will occur:

$$Na_3\text{-PSS} + Al(OH)_3 \rightarrow Al\text{-PSS (excreted in stool)} + 3NaOH \text{ (absorbed after conversion to } 3NaHCO_3)$$

CALCULATION OF NET ALKALI CONTENT IN COMPLEX MIXTURE OF SUBSTANCES

Ingestion of 20 mmol of K^+ citrate, which is completely absorbable and metabolized to $KHCO_3$ in the body, would result in a net gain of 20 mEq of alkali. On the other hand, ingestion of 10 mmol of arginine chloride would result in net gain of 10 mEq of acid. If a food contained both, the net gain of alkali would be 10 mEq. Food contains numerous chemicals, and their absorption depends not only on the type of chemicals ingested but also on interactions with gastric acid and other chemicals in simultaneously ingested food or drugs. Thus, prediction of the effect of food ingestion on acid–base balance is nearly impossible. Measurements are made, instead, by analyzing net alkali content of food and feces. The difference between these two represents net alkali absorbed.

Net alkali content of food and feces is estimated by the electrolyte balance technique, that is, the sum of noncombustible cations ($Na^+ + K^+ + Ca^{++} + Mg^{++}$) minus the sum of noncombustible anions ($Cl^- + 1.8 P$) (63). The assumption here is that when nonmetabolizable cations are accompanied by metabolizable anions, their subsequent absorption and metabolism of their anions would result in gain of alkali, and that ingestion and absorption of nonmetabolizable anions accompanied by metabolizable cations would lead to acid gain. Hence, the difference between the two represents a net gain of alkali (44,45). The concentrations of all of the electrolytes are expressed in milliequivalents, except phosphate, which is expressed in millimoles and then multiplied by the factor 1.8, the average valence of phosphate. The pH of food or feces is not a determinant in the calculation of valency of phosphate, since that pH is relevant only in reference to the blood pH.

For the calculation of net alkali content of food and feces, the only nonmetabolizable ions presumed to be present are Na^+, K^+, Ca^{++}, Mg^{++}, Cl^-, and P, because no other ions in food are present in a significant amount. Urinary excretion of sulfate is substantial, but originates almost exclusively from sulfur-containing amino acids, and is separately measured (34). Some organic anions found in food (e.g., tartarate) are poorly metabolized by the human body, and such anions would result in a falsely increased estimation of net GI alkali absorption. On the other hand, all organic anions excreted in urine estimated by the titration method are assumed to originate from organic acids produced in the body, and this assumption results in a falsely increased measurement of organic acid generation by the same extent. Usually, these two errors cancel each other out. Furthermore, it has been shown that the bulk of ingested tartarate in humans is metabolized by colonic bacteria, and only about 14% of ingested tartarate appears in urine unchanged (12). Choline is an example of an incompletely absorbable cation, but choline is also metabolized by colonic bacteria (19).

The measurement of GI absorption of alkali by the analysis of food and feces is difficult and prone to inaccuracies for obvious technical reasons. Measurements can be made only in inpatient settings with controlled diet, and consequently no study has measured net GI absorption of alkali on a normal diet in an outpatient setting.

In a simplified technique, net GI absorption of alkali is estimated as urinary noncombustible cations minus urinary noncombustible anions (54):

$$\text{Net GI alkali absorption} = \text{Urine } (Na^+ + K^+ + Ca^{++} + Mg^{++}) - \text{Urine } (Cl^- + P \times 1.8)$$

The method is based on the assumption that the difference between the amounts of noncombustible cations and noncombustible anions absorbed from the gut equals the difference between the amounts excreted in the urine under stable conditions. The validity of this assumption is supported by empirical as well as theoretical evidence. Theoretically, the amount of noncombustible ions absorbed must equal the amount excreted for the following reasons. The total extracellular content of divalent ions is small (about 45 mEq of Ca^{++}, 30 mEq of Mg^{++}, and 30 mEq of P), and their daily net flux with bone is negligible (57). Hence, the amount of divalent ions excreted in the urine is quite close to the amount absorbed from the GI tract. Furthermore, in the steady state the amounts of Na^+, K^+, and Cl^- excreted in the urine are nearly equal to the amounts absorbed from the GI tract. Urinary Na^+ and Cl^- content in a given 24-hour period may be different from the amounts absorbed from the GI tract during the same period, because the extracellular volume tends to fluctuate, especially with varying salt intake. However, daily fluctuations in Na^+ and Cl^- excretion would not affect the calculation of net GI absorption of alkali as long as both ions are retained or lost together, and that is usually the case. The amount of alkali absorbed on a usual diet is about 30 mEq/day (57).

Bone Buffering in Chronic Metabolic Acidosis

It was once widely believed that bone was very important in maintaining stable serum HCO_3^- in chronic metabolic acidosis. Studies have shown that patients with chronic renal acidosis are able to maintain a stable serum HCO_3^- despite estimated retention of 12–19 mEq of acid daily, with an average duration of acidosis of 6 years. Because bone is known to have a large alkali reserve, the maintenance of a stable serum HCO_3^- in such settings has been attributed to the release of alkali from bone (25, 42).

However, there has been little direct evidence for substantial bone buffering of acids in acidosis of long duration. The best evidence against any substantial role of bone in chronic renal acidosis is the lack of significant calciuria (48). Addition of alkali to the body from Ca^{++} release occurs only when Ca^{++} is excreted in urine. Redeposition of Ca^{++} salts in tissues or excretion in the stool as alkaline Ca^{++} salts will reclaim alkali released from bone (16). In fact, if all of the released calcium is lost in stool as $CaCO_3$, there might be slight net loss of alkali by the process. Each mole of calcium hydroxyapatite releases 10 mol of Ca and 9.2 mEq of alkali. When 10 mol of calcium bind 10 mol of $CO_3^=$ and excreted in stool, it is removing 20mEq of alkali from the body. Hence, the net alkali loss would be 10.8mEq. If calcium from bone is released as $CaCO_3$, and excreted in stool as $CaCO_3$, there will be no loss or gain of alkali. Furthermore, the total amount of alkali reserve in bone is insufficient to account for the buffering of acid for such a protracted period. Assuming total bone content of Ca^{++} at 60,000 mEq, the total alkali content of bone is estimated to be about 25,000 mEq. At the rate of 19 mEq of acid buffering per day, the bone alkali store would be exhausted in 3.6 years (57, 60).

Bone Buffering in Acute Metabolic Acidosis

It is also widely believed that bone plays an important role in buffering in superacute acidosis, but the available evidence is not convincing. Fraley and Adler showed that rats and dogs with total thyroparathyroidectomy developed a much more severe metabolic acidosis than those with intact organs within 5 hours of acute acid loading (23). The authors concluded that without intact parathyroid glands, nonextracellular buffers titrated only 3% and 22% of the administered acid in rats and dogs respectively. They concluded that the difference in buffering capacity was due to the difference in bone buffering. Arruda et al. (2), concurred with Fraley and Adler (23) that PTH significantly affected the overall buffering (2), but the data of Madias et al., did not show any difference in buffering capacity after thyroparathyroidectomy (50). Buffering of acid by bone could occur in three different ways: (1) release of cations such as Na^+, K^+, Ca^{++}, and Mg^{++} accompanied by alkali such as carbonate or hydroxide or phosphate; (2) exchange of bone carbonate for extracellular phosphate, and (3) deposition in bone of extracellular nonmetabolizable anion such as Cl^-

along with an H^+. The third mechanism has not been shown to exist.

For the first mechanism to operate, a cation must be released from bone, and only Ca^{++} could play that role. Mg^{++} does not participate in acid buffering of bone. Release of bone K^+ cannot play a quantitatively significant role, because the entire bone content of K^+ in adult humans is a mere 20 mEq (61). Evidence for Na^+ release from bone exists in acute metabolic acidosis, but the magnitude is not very substantial. Bettice and Gamble (6) showed that the bone content of exchangeable Na^+ decreased by about 5% in 5 hours following acute acid loading in dogs. Since about 40% of the bone Na^+ is exchangeable, the total exchangeable Na^+ in bone is about 480 mEq, and the 5% represents a mere 24 mEq (480 × 0.05 = 24). The following considerations make it highly improbable that bone contributes substantially to the buffering in superacute metabolic acidosis (acidosis within a few hours).

Release of Ca^{++} from bone is an important mechanism of bone buffering in subacute metabolic acidosis, when urinary excretion of Ca^{++} can increase by as much as 80 mEq per day. If the entire amount came from Ca^{++} carbonate, the amount of calcium released would be accompanied by release of 80 mEq of alkali. If the same amount of Ca^{++} originated from hydroxyapatite, alkali release would be equivalent to 36.8 mEq of alkali. Increased excretion of Ca^{++} in metabolic acidosis reaches maximal a few days after the start of acid load (42).

The likely explanation for the appearance of impaired buffering in animals with thyroparathyroidectomy is tissue underperfusion due to circulatory shock. Since the blood flow to the muscle in humans is only about 700 ml/min, it is obvious that buffering by skeletal muscle would not be complete in 30 minutes in a resting state. Reduced blood flow by circulatory shock would further delay the buffering by both intra- and extra-cellular fluid of the muscle, and could have given the impression that cell buffering was virtually absent in this setting.

In conclusion, bone is not an important source of alkali in chronic metabolic acidosis of several years duration. In an acute acidosis, contribution of bone to acid buffering could be substantial, but its contribution in superacute acidosis (that of several hours duration) is negligible.

APPENDIX

Endogenous Sources of Acid/Alkali

1. Production of sulfuric acid from metabolism of sulfur-containing amino acids:

$$RN\text{-}S \rightarrow CO_2 + Urea + H_2SO_4$$

   a. Production of sulfuric acid:

$$H_2SO_4 \rightarrow SO_4^= + 2\,H^+ \text{ (production of 2 mol of acid for each mole of sulfur oxidized)}$$

   b. Production of sulfuric acid and then subsequent sulfate ester formation:

$R\text{-}OH + H_2SO_4 \rightarrow R\text{-}O\text{-}SO_3^- + H^+ + H_2O$ (production of 1 mol of acid for each mole of sulfur oxidized)

2. Production of organic acids:

$$R\text{-}HOH + 1/2\ O_2 \rightarrow R\text{-}OOH + H_2O$$

$$R\text{-}OOH \rightarrow R\text{-}OO^- + H^+$$

Renal excretion of organic anions ($R\text{-}OO^2$) results in a permanent net gain of acid, hence a net loss of alkali. Metabolism of organic anions results in regeneration of alkali that is lost in the titration by the acid.

3. The effect of metabolism of amino acids on acid–base balance:
   a. Metabolism of cationic amino acids:

$$ArginineCl \rightarrow Arginine + HCl \ (gain\ of\ acid)$$

$$LysineCl \rightarrow Lysine + HCl \ (gain\ of\ acid)$$

   b. Metabolism of anionic amino acids:

$$Na\ glutamate \rightarrow Glutamic\ acid + NaHCO_3$$
$$(gain\ of\ alkali)$$

$$Na\ aspartate \rightarrow Aspartic\ acid + NaHCO_3$$
$$(gain\ of\ alkali)$$

4. Metabolism of adenosine phosphates:
   a. Adenosine-P_3-Mg-K_2 (ATP) + 3 H_2O (6 H) → Adenosine (1 H) + $MgHPO_4$ (1 H) + 1.4 $KHPO_4$ (1.4 H) + 0.6 KH_2PO_4 (1.2 H) + 1.4 H^+ (net gain of acid)
   b. Adenosine-P_2-Mg-K (ADP) + 2 H_2O (4 H) → Adenosine (1 H) + $MgHPO_4$ (1 H) + 0.6 HPO_4 (0.6 H) + 0.4 KH_2PO_4 (0.8 H) + 0.6 H^+ (net gain of acid)
   c. Adenosine-P-K_2 (AMP) + H_2O (2 H) → Adenosine (1 H) + 0.8 $KHPO_4$ (0.8 H) + 0.2 KH_2PO_4 (0.4 H) − 0.2 H^+ (net loss of acid)
   d. Cyclic AMP-K + 2 H_2O (4 H) → Adenosine (2 H) + 0.8 HPO_4 (0.8H) + 0.2 KH_2PO_4 (0.4) + 0.8 H^+ (net gain of acid)
   Because cyclic AMP has two ester bonds, the break of the ester bonds results in consumption of 2 H molecules for each adenosine molecule.

5. Metabolism of phospholipids:

$$Phosphotidyl\text{-}K\text{-}choline + 2\ H_2O\ (4\ H) \rightarrow$$
$$Adenosine\ (H) + Choline\ (1\ H) +$$
$$0.8\ HPO_4\ (0.8\ H) + 0.2\ KH_2PO_4\ (0.4) + 0.8\ H^+\ (net$$
$$gain\ of\ acid)$$

6. Metabolism of creatine phosphate:

$$Creatine\text{-}P\text{-}K_2 + H_2O\ (2\ H) \rightarrow Creatine\ (1\ H) + 0.8$$
$$KHPO_4\ (0.8\ H) + 0.2\ KH_2PO_4\ (0.4\ H) -$$
$$0.2\ H^+\ (net\ loss\ of\ acid)$$

Note 1: The numbers before H shown in parentheses represent the number of H molecules that are added from water and the number of H atoms that are consumed in the production of new products when ester bonds are broken.

Note 2: The estimation of the effects of metabolisms of phosphate containing chemicals on acid–base balance can be made more quickly from the difference between the total number of nonmetabolizable cations and nonmetabolizable anions (phosphate in this case) than from detailed calculations as illustrated above. For example, each mole of ATP contains 4 equivalents of nonmetabolizable cations (a mole of Mg with 2 equivalents and 2 mol of K with 2 equivalents), while it contains 3 mol of phosphate with 1.8 equivalents for each phosphate (the mean valence of P is 1.8). Thus, the net alkali content of ATP = 1 Mg × 2 + 2K × 1 − 3P × 1.8 = 4 − 5.4 = −1.4.

Calculation of Net Amount of GI Alkali Absorbed: Net GI Alkali

$$Net\ GI\ alkali = Net\ alkali\ content\ of\ food - Net\ alkali$$
$$content\ of\ feces = Food\ [(Na + K + Ca + Mg) -$$
$$(Cl + 1.8\ P)] - Fecal\ [(Na + K + Ca + Mg) -$$
$$(Cl + 1.8\ P)]$$

Alternative method for net GI alkali:

$$Net\ GI\ alkali = urine\ [(Na + K + Ca + Mg) -$$
$$(Cl + 1.8\ P)]$$

Whole Body Acid–Base Balance

1. Net acid excretion:

$$NH_4^+ + Titratable\ acid - Bicarbonate$$

2. Net acid production

$$Urinary\ organic\ anions + Sulfate - Net\ GI\ alkali$$

References

1. Alford FP, Scoggins BA, Wharton C. Symptomatic essential hypernatremia. *Am J Med* 1973;54:359
2. Arruda JA, Alla V, Rubinstein H, et al. Metabolic and hormonal factors influencing extrarenal buffering of an acute acid load. *Miner Electrolyte Metab* 1982;8:36–43.
3. Baldetorp L, Martensson J. Urinary excretion of inorganic sulfate, ester sulfate, total sulfur and taurine in cancer patients. *Acta Med Scand* 1980;208:293–295.
4. Banoglu E. Current status of the cytosolic sulfotransferases in the metabolic activation of promutagens and procarcinogens. *Curr Drug Metab* 2000;1:1–30.
5. Berlyne GM, Adler AJ, Barth RH. Perspectives on acid–base balance in advanced chronic renal failure. *Contrib Nephrol* 1992;100:105–117.
6. Bettice JA, Gamble JL Jr. Skeletal buffering of acute metabolic acidosis. *Am J Physiol* 1975;229:1618–1624.
7. Bonventre JV, Leaf A. Sodium homeostasis: steady states without a set point. *Kidney Int* 1982;21:880–883.
8. Boonjaren S, Stein J, Baehlr R, et al. Effect of plasma sodium concentration on diluting segment sodium reabsorption. *Kidney Int* 1974;5:1.
9. Bresler EH, Nielson KT. Miller MC, et al. Renal tubular reabsorptive response to hypernatremia. *Am J Physiol* 1976;231:642.
10. Brown JC, Packer RK, Knepper MA. Role of organic anions in renal response to dietary acid and base loads. *Am J Physiol* 1989;257:F170–F176.
11. Cardenas A, Arroyo V. Mechanisms of water and sodium retention in cirrhosis and the pathogenesis of ascites. *Best Pract Res Clin Endocrinol Metab* 2003;17:607–22.
12. Chadwick VS, Vince A, Killingley M, Wrong OM. The metabolism of tartrate in man and the rat. *Clin Sci Mol Med* 1978;54:273–281.

13. Chalmers RA, Healy MJ, Lawson AM, Watts RW. Urinary organic acids in man. II. Effects of individual variation and diet on the urinary excretion of acidic metabolites. *Clin Chem* 1976;22:1288–1291.
14. Chalmers RA, Healy MJ, Lawson AM, et al. Urinary organic acids in man. III. Quantitative ranges and patterns of excretion in a normal population. *Clin Chem* 1976;22:1292–1298.
15. Ciba-Geigy Ltd. Composition of foods. In: *Geigy Scientific Tables*. Vol. 1. Basel, Switzerland: Ciba-Geigy, 1981:241–266.
16. Contiguglia SR, Alfrey AC, Miller NL, et al. Nature of soft tissue calcification in uremia. *Kidney Int* 1973;4:229–235.
17. Costello JF, Smith M, Stolarski C, Sadovnic MJ. Extrarenal clearance of oxalate increases with progression of renal failure in the rat. *J Am Soc Nephrol* 1992;3:1098–1104.
18. Dawson J, Dempsey E, Bartter F, et al. Evidence for the presence of an amphoteric electrolyte in the urine of patients with "renal tubular acidosis." *Metabolism* 1953;2:225–237.
19. De La Huerga J, Gyorgy P, Waldstein D, et al. The effects of antimicrobial agents upon choline degradation in the intestinal tract. *J Clin Invest* 1953;32:1117–1120.
20. de Strihou C van Y. Importance of endogenous acid production in the regulation of acid-base equilibrium: the role of the digestive tract. *Adv Nephrol* 1980;9:367–385.
21. Decaux G, Genette F, Mokel J. Hypoutremia in the syndrome of inappropriate secretion of antidiuretic hormone. 1968;93:716–717.
22. Dorhout EJ, Roos JC, Boer P, et al. Observations on edema formation in the nephrotic syndrome in adults with minimal lesions. *Am J Med* 1979;67:378–84.
23. Fraley DS, Adler S. An extrarenal role for parathyroid hormone in the disposal of acute acid loads in rats and dogs. *J Clin Invest* 1979;63:985–997.
24. Glatt H. Sulfotransferases in the bioactivation of xenobiotics. *Chem Biol Interact* 2000 1;129:141–170.
25. Goodman AD, Lemann J Jr, Lennon EJ, et al. Production, excretion and net balance of fixed acid in patients with renal acidosis. *J Clin Invest* 1965;44:495–506.
26. Guyton AC. Control of blood pressure. *Am J Med* 1972;52:584–592.
27. Guyton AC. Abnormal renal function and autoregulation in essential hypertension. *Hypertension* 1991;18(Suppl 5):III49–III53.
28. Guyton AC. The surprising kidney-fluid mechanism for pressure control—its infinite gain! *Hypertension* 1990;16:725–730.
29. Guyton AC, Hall JE, Lohmeier TE, et al. Blood pressure regulation: basic concepts. *Fed Proc* 1981;4:2252–2256.
30. Halperin ML, Jungas RL. Metabolic production and renal disposal of hydrogen ions. *Kidney Int* 1983;24:709–713.
31. Hochachka PW, Somero GN. *Biochemical Adaptations*. Princeton, NJ: Princeton University Press, 1984:337–348.
32. Hollenberg NK. Set point for sodium homeostasis: surfeit, deficit and their implications. *Kidney Int* 1980;17:423–429.
33. Hood VL, Tannen RL. Protection of acid-base balance by pH regulation of acid production. *N Engl J Med* 1998;339:819–826.
34. Hunt JN. The influence of dietary sulphur on the urinary output of acid in man. *Clin Sci* 1956;15:119–134.
35. Hurst PE, Morrison RB, Timoneer J, et al. The effect of oral anion exchange resins on faecal anions. Comparison with calcium salts and aluminium hydroxide. *Clin Sci* 1963;24:187–200.
36. Jaenike JR, Waterhouse C. The renal response to sustained administration of water and vasopressin in man. *J Clin Endocrinol Metab* 1961;21:231.
37. Kamm DE, Levinsky NG. Inhibition of renal tubular sodium reabsorption by hypernatremia. *J Clin Invest* 1965;44:1144.
38. Kauffman FC. Sulfonation in pharmacology and toxicology. *Drug Metab Rev* 2004;36:823–843.
39. Kaufman AM, Brod-Miller C, Kahn T. Role of citrate excretion in acid–base balance in diuretic-induced alkalosis in the rat. *Am J Physiol* 1985;248:F796–F803.
40. Lawson AM, Chalmers RA, Watts RW. Urinary organic acids in man. I. Normal patterns. *Clin Chem* 1976;22:1283–1287.
41. Lemann J Jr, Lennon EJ, Brock J. A potential error in the measurement of urinary titratable acid. *J Lab Clin Med* 1966;67:906–913.
42. Lemann J Jr, Litzow JR, Lennon EJ. The effects of chronic acid loads in normal man: further evidence for the participation of bone mineral in the defense against chronic metabolic acidosis. *J Clin Invest* 1966;45:1608–1614.
43. Lemann J Jr, Relman AS. The relation of sulfur metabolism to acid–base balance and electrolyte excretion: the effects of DL-methionine in normal man. *J Clin Invest* 1959;38:2215–2223.
44. Lennon EJ, Lemann J Jr, Litzow JR. The effects of diet and stool composition on the net external acid balance of normal subjects. *J Clin Invest* 1966;45:1601–1607.
45. Lennon EJ, Lemann J Jr. Influence of diet composition on endogenous fixed acid production. *Am J Clin Nutr* 1968; 21(5):451–456.
46. Lennon EJ, Lemann J Jr, Relman AS. The effects of phosphoproteins on acid balance in normal subjects. *J Clin Invest* 1962;41:637–645.
47. Levy M, Wexler MJ. Renal sodium retention and ascites formation in dogs with experimental cirrhosis but with portal hypertension or increased splanchnic vascular capacity. *J Lab Clin Med* 1978;91:520.
48. Litzow JR, Lemann J Jr, Lennon EJ. The effect of treatment of acidosis on calcium balance in patients with chronic azotemic renal disease. *J Clin Invest* 1967;46:280–286.
49. Lum G, Leal-Khouri S. Significance of low serum urea nitrogen concentrations. *Clin Chem* 1989;35:639–640.
50. Madias NE, Johns CA, Homer SM. Independence of the acute acid-buffering response from endogenous parathyroid hormone. *Am J Physiol* 1982;243:F141–F149.
51. Madias NE, Levey AS. Metabolic alkalosis due to absorption of "nonabsorbable" antacids. *Am J Med* 1983;74:155–158.
52. Murer H, Forster I, Biber J. The sodium phosphate cotransporter family SLC34. *Pflugers Arch* 2004;447:763–767.
53. Murer H, Hernando N, Forster L, Biber J. Molecular mechanisms in proximal tubular and small intestinal phosphate reabsorption (plenary lecture). *Mol Membr Biol* 2001;18:3–11.
54. Oh MS, Carroll HJ. A new method for the measurement of net GI absorption of alkali. *Kidney Int* 1989;36:915–917.
55. Oh MS, Carroll HJ. Essential hypernatremia: is there such a thing? *Nephron*;1994;67:144–147.
56. Oh MS, Carroll HJ. Salt output in relation to salt intake vs salt output alone: which is a better predictor of effective vascular volume? *Nephron* 1992;61:7–9.
57. Oh MS, Carroll HJ. Whole body acid-base balance. *Contrib Nephrol* 1992;100:89–104.
58. Oh MS, Kim MJ, Tan C, et al. Untitrated titratable acid in urine. *Proc Am Soc Nephrol* 1992;.
59. Oh MS, Rakesh V, Carroll HJ. A new method for measurement of organic anions in urine. *Proc Am Soc Nephrol* 1993;.
60. Oh MS. Irrelevance of bone buffering to acid-base homeostasis in chronic metabolic acidosis. *Nephron* 1991;59:7–10.
61. Pellegrino ED, Biltz RM. The composition of human bone in uremia. Observations on the reservoir functions of bone and demonstration of a labile fraction of bone carbonate. *Medicine (Baltimore)* 1965;44:397–418.
62. Quamme GA, Shapiro RJ. Membrane controls of epithelial phosphate transport. *Can J Physiol Pharmacol* 1987;65:275–284.
63. Relman AS, Lennon EJ, Leman J Jr. Endogenous production of fixed acid and the measurement of the net balance of acid in normal subjects. *J Clin Invest* 1961;40;1621–1630.
64. Robertson GL, Aycinena P, Zerbe RL. Neurogenic disorders of osmoregulation. *Am J Med* 1982;72:339–353.
65. Schrier RW, Fein FL, McNeil TS, et al. Influence of interstitial fluid volume expansion and plasma sodium concentration on the natriuresis response to volume expansion in dogs. *Clin Sci* 1969;36:371.
66. Schroeder ET. Alkalosis resulting from combined administration of a "nonsystemic" antacid and a cation-exchange resin. *Gastroenterology* 1969;56:868–874.
67. Sheikh MS, Maguire JA, Emmett M, Santa Ana CA, Nicar MJ, Schiller LR, Fordtran JS. Reduction of dietary phosphorus absorption by phosphorus binders. A theoretical, in vitro, and in vivo study. *J Clin Invest* 1989;83:66–73.
68. Squires RD, Huth EJ. Experimental potassium depletion in normal human subjects. Relation of ion intake to the renal conservation of potassium. *J Clin Invest* 1959:38:1134–1148.
69. Uribarri J, Buquing J, Oh MS. Acid–base balance in chronic peritoneal dialysis patients. *Kidney Int* 1995;47:269–273.
70. Uribarri J, Douyon H, Oh MS. A re-evaluation of the urinary parameters of acid production and excretion in patients with chronic renal acidosis. *Kidney Int* 1995;47:624–627.
71. Uribarri J, Oh MS, Carroll HJ. Salt-losing nephropathy. Clinical presentation and mechanisms. *Am J Nephrol* 1983;3:193–198.
72. Uribarri J, Zia M, Mahmood J, et al. Acid production in chronic hemodialysis patients. *J Am Soc Nephrol* 1998;9:114–120.
73. Van Slyke DD, Palmer WW. Studies of acidosis. XVI. Titration of organic acids in urine. *J Biol Chem* 1920;41:567–569.
74. Vaziri ND, Freel RW, Hatch M. Effect of chronic experimental renal insufficiency on urate metabolism. *J Am Soc Nephrol* 1995;6:1313–1317.
75. Walser M. Phenomenological analysis of sodium and potassium homeostasis. *Kidney Int* 1985;217:837–841.

Transport Regulation

CHAPTER **11**

Principles of Cell Signaling

Lloyd Cantley

Yale University School of Medicine, New Haven, Connecticut, USA

INTRODUCTION

The successful transition from single cells to complex multicellular organisms has required the development of mechanisms for cells to communicate with each other so as to act in concert during processes such as nutrient acquisition, motility, and defense. The most basic of these are cell–cell junctions that serve as structural organizers, but also provide information that individual cells can utilize to orient themselves in relation to the remainder of the organism. In larger species that contain multiple layers of cells, the need to communicate information regarding the external and internal environment over long distances has led to the development of diffusible factors that are secreted by one cell and travel to distant cells. These factors can be delivered via the circulation (e.g., hormones and cytokines) or via the nervous system (e.g., neurotransmitters), and are recognized by the appropriate cell surface receptor on the recipient cell. The complex nature of the numerous signals presented to the cell at any given point in time has led to the development of an intricate array of receptor-activated intracellular second messengers that, by undergoing a coordinated series of interactions and enzymatic alterations, can transduce the information presented on the cell surface to effector molecules that mediate the appropriate cellular response.

The kidney serves to protect the internal milieu of higher organisms from perturbations due to the accumulation of metabolic products as well as those resulting from fluctuations in the intake or loss of water and various salts. To perform this intricate function, the body must continuously monitor the composition and quantity of the extracellular fluid and then signal the nephron to appropriately regulate glomerular filtration and tubular cell function in response to

changes in these parameters. Regulation of these exquisitely precise events requires that the cells of the kidney are able to respond to signals emanating from distant sites and then efficiently communicate in an intercellular and intracellular manner to coordinate the response. This chapter will provide an overview of several of the most common receptors and intracellular second messenger pathways that are utilized in this process.

CELL SURFACE RECEPTORS

In the best-studied pathway of cell signaling, a first messenger is secreted by one group of cells and travels either to distant cells (endocrine factors) or local cells (autocrine or paracrine factors) where it binds to a specific receptor. The first messengers in these classic pathways are generally either proteins (growth factors, cytokines), catecholamines (epinephrine, dopamine), or steroids (mineralocorticoids, sex hormones), although receptors have been identified for multiple circulating factors including lipids (e.g., lysophosphatidic acid), ions (e.g., calcium), eicosanoids (e.g., prostaglandin E_2), sugars (e.g., glucose), nucleosides (e.g., ATP), and gases (e.g., nitric oxide). Most of these receptors are located on the cell surface and have an extracellular region (domain) that recognizes and binds to the specific ligand. This ligand-binding domain is connected via one or more transmembrane segments to the intracellular (cytosolic) domain that undergoes a change in conformation or activity in response to ligand binding, and thus initiates the activation and/or modification of intracellular second messengers. In contrast to these cell surface receptors, steroid receptors, which are discussed later in the chapter, are typically located in the cytoplasm. The lipophilic steroid ligands are capable of crossing the cell membrane and binding the receptor, which then initiates signaling events by translocating into the nucleus where the ligand–receptor complex can regulate gene transcription.

Based on their structure, the type of ligand that they bind, and the principal second messengers that they activate, classical cell surface receptors can be grouped into G-protein–coupled receptors, receptor tyrosine kinases (RTKs), serine/threonine kinase receptors, and receptor-like phosphatases. However, it has become increasing clear that other surface proteins serve as signaling initiators to transduce information about the environment surrounding the cell. Thus, cell–cell and cell–matrix adhesion molecules initiate signaling cascades that regulate cell shape, differentiation, proliferation, and survival. The following section will provide a brief overview of these various signaling initiators focused on those presently considered to be important in regulating normal renal development and maintaining adult kidney homeostasis.

G-Protein–Coupled Receptors

The receptor subtype that is responsible for mediating the signaling responses of the greatest number of ligands in the kidney is probably the G-protein–coupled receptor (GPCR). GPCRs make up the largest family of cell surface receptors, with over 1000 members predicted from the sequence of the human genome (reviewed in Miura et al. [131]). GPCRs are transmembrane proteins with their amino terminus on the cell exterior, seven transmembrane α-helical segments, and the carboxyl terminus in the cell interior (Fig. 1). This ar-

rangement results in three extracellular loops and three intracellular loops joining the transmembrane segments. They bind to extracellular ligands such as epinephrine, dopamine, angiotensin II, adenosine, vasopressin, calcium, and parathyroid hormone, and mediate their intracellular actions.

The extracellular loops serve as the primary binding site for the specific GPCR ligand, with the amino terminus also contributing to the binding site for some ligands. The intracellular loops, most critically the 5–6 loop, serve as the binding site for the principal GPCR intracellular effectors, the heterotrimeric G proteins. These small GDP/GTP-binding protein complexes are made up of α, β, and γ subunits, with the α subunit serving as the GDP/GTP-binding site, and the βγ subunits acting both as regulators of α subunit localization and independently as intracellular signaling effectors. The existence of multiple different α, β, and γ subunits allows for hundreds of potential combinations of heterotrimeric G proteins, and thus imparts specificity of response to the individual GPCR and its ligand.

In the absence of receptor activation, the α subunit is bound to GDP and associates with the βγ subunits at the membrane. However, following ligand binding to the extracellular surface of the GPCR, a conformational change of the receptor results in disassociation of GDP and binding of GTP to the α subunit. The binding of GTP stimulates disassociation of the α subunit from the βγ subunits and the receptor. The GTP-loaded α subunit can then associate with its intermediary effectors (such as adenylyl cyclase and phospholipase), while the βγ subunits can associate with and regulate independent effectors such as ion channels

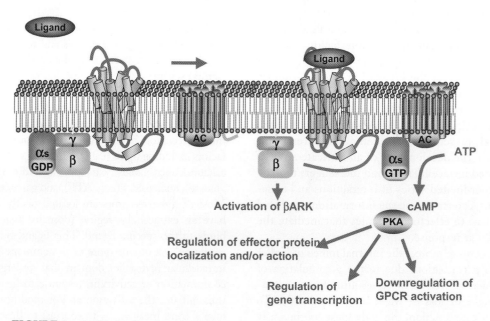

FIGURE 1 GPCR signaling through adenylate cyclase. Binding of the extracellular ligand to the GPCR results in the exchange of GTP for GDP on Gα, and its disassociation from the αβγ heterotrimer. βγ can then associate with and activate downstream effectors such as the β-adregeneric receptor kinase (BARK), while the GTP-loaded α subunit can bind and regulate effectors, including adenylate cyclase (AC). In the example shown, Gsα activates AC to convert ATP to cAMP and thus stimulates downstream PKA signaling.

and the β-adrenergic receptor kinase (βARK) (reviewed in Malbon [120] and Strock and Diverse-Pierluissi [193]).

The protein products of the 16 mammalian genes encoding Gα subunits have been grouped into 4 classes, the $G_{s\alpha}$ (stimulatory for adenylyl cyclase), $G_{i\alpha}$ (inhibitory for adenylyl cyclase), $G_{q/11\alpha}$ (regulators of phospholipase Cβ [PLCβ]), and $G_{12\alpha}$ (regulators of RhoGEF). Binding of the appropriate GTP-loaded Gα subunit to its primary effector results in the activation or inhibition of effector function. For example, adenylyl cyclase catalyzes the cyclation of ATP to form 3′,5′-cyclic AMP (cAMP), an intracellular second messenger that can then bind and activate downstream signaling proteins such as protein kinase A (PKA). This reaction is activated by GTP-$G_{s\alpha}$ binding to adenylyl cyclase and inhibited by GTP-$G_{i\alpha}$ binding. In addition, βγ binding to adenylyl cyclase can augment its activation by GTP-$G_{s\alpha}$.

An important concept in all forms of signal transduction is the ability of the cell to carefully control the site, size, and duration of the signal. Signal amplification is the process whereby the cell can regulate the size of the signal. For example, a single GPCR can generate between tens and hundreds of GTP-coupled Gα subunits that can subsequently bind to and activate similar numbers of adenylyl cyclase enzymes, which in turn generate multiple copies of cAMP. The number and availability of the intracellular effector enzymes and substrates thus determines the level of signal amplification following the activation of relatively few receptors on the cell surface.

Just as important as signal amplification is the ability of the cell to downregulate the signaling pathway once the desired response has been initiated. For GPCRs, this occurs in several ways. First, the α subunit is itself a GTPase, meaning that it hydrolyzes GTP to form GDP and inorganic phosphate. This hydrolysis occurs spontaneously following GTP binding to Gα, but can be augmented by the association of specific RGS proteins (regulators of G-protein signaling) with the GDP/Gα complex, as this interaction stabilizes the inactivated state. Once the Gα subunit is in the GDP bound state, it can associate again with the βγ subunit to regenerate the inactive heterotrimeric G protein.

In addition, many GPCRs are themselves inactivated by a process called homologous desensitization. As noted above, the βγ subunits can associate with the cytosolic protein βARK. βARK, also known as GRK2, is a member of the G-protein–coupled receptor kinases (GRKs) that, following association with $G_{\beta\gamma}$, phosphorylate the intracellular loops and/or C terminus of ligand-associated GPCRs on serine and/or threonine residues. This phosphorylation results in the association of β-arrestin with the receptor, mediating the uncoupling of the ligand–receptor complex from the heterotrimeric G proteins, and thus diminishing its activity. Binding of β-arrestin has also been shown to target the receptor–ligand complexes to clathrin-coated pits on the cell surface, followed by internalization and either lysosomal degradation or recycling of the inactivated receptor to the cell surface (100).

The downstream effector adenylyl cyclase is also subject to phosphorylation-dependent inhibition. As noted above, activated adenylyl cyclase catalyzes the formation of cAMP, which in turn associates with and activates PKA. This enzyme, an intracellular serine/threonine kinase, has multiple phosphorylation substrates within the cell. Phosphorylation of these substrates can regulate their activity, cellular localization, and/or their interaction with other proteins. One phosphorylation substrate is adenylyl cyclase itself, resulting in inhibition of cAMP production. A second substrate is the GPCR. In a process known as heterologous desensitization, activation of PKA by a non-GPCR signal can result in phosphorylation of the GPCR and subsequent inhibition of ligand-mediated GPCR activation (206).

RECEPTORS FOR DOPAMINE AND AVP ARE GPCRS THAT REGULATE ADENYLYL CYCLASE

The dopamine receptors are a prototypic family of GPCRs in the kidney. There are five dopamine receptors presently described (D_1–D_5), and they are further subclassified into D_1-like (D_1 and D_5) or D_2-like (D_2–D_4). The D_1-like receptors are associated with $G_{s\alpha}$ and therefore activate adenylyl cyclase, whereas the D_2-like receptors inhibit adenylyl cyclase activity (reviewed in Jose et al. [82] and Missale et al. [130]). In the kidney, D_1-like and D_2-like receptors are expressed throughout the tubules. The net effect of activating these receptors is the induction of a diuresis, although by different mechanisms in the various tubular segments. For example, dopamine-mediated activation of D_1 receptors in the proximal tubule results in activation of adenylyl cyclase, leading to cAMP-dependent inhibition of the activity of NHE-3, NaPi-2, and the Na,K-ATPase, thus inhibiting proximal sodium reabsorption. In contrast, activation of the D_2-like receptor D_4 in the cortical collecting duct leads to a water diuresis by preventing vasopressin-stimulated adenylyl cyclase activation. Dopamine receptors also mediate renal vasodilatation and appear to regulate renin secretion. Due to these effects, defects in dopamine receptor function in mice are associated with salt retention, vasoconstriction, and increased blood pressure (83, 228).

Arginine vasopressin (AVP, also known as antidiuretic hormone [ADH]) binds to three GPCRs, the $G_{q/11\alpha}$-linked V1a and V1b receptors, and the $G_{s\alpha}$-linked V2 receptor. V1 receptors are located on several cell types, including smooth muscle cells of blood vessels, and mediate the vasoconstrictive ("pressor") response of vasopressin, while V2 receptors are located on epithelial cells in the collecting duct and mediate water reabsorption. Binding of vasopressin to the V2 receptor stimulates adenylyl cyclase–mediated cAMP production, which in turn causes insertion of vesicles containing the water-channel aquaporin-2 into the apical membrane of collecting duct cells. By inhibiting adenylyl cyclase activation in these cells, dopamine can partially counteract this water-reabsorptive effect of vasopressin.

GPCRs Can Also Signal Through Phospholipase C and MAPK

An example of a GPCR that is coupled to PLCβ signaling is the type 1 receptor for angiotensin II (AT$_{1A}$R) (Fig. 2). Angiotensin II is the 8-amino-acid peptide product of the angiotensin-converting enzyme (ACE)–mediated cleavage of angiotensin I. Angiotensin II is capable of binding to and activating two distinct G-protein–coupled receptors, the type 1 receptor (AT$_{1A}$R) and the type 2 receptor. The predominant actions of angiotensin in the kidney and adrenal gland are mediated by the AT$_{1A}$R, including vasoconstriction, smooth muscle growth, sodium retention, and aldosterone secretion. Most data presently support the idea that the type 2 receptor acts as an antagonist to AT$_{1A}$R signaling (18), possibly by forming a heterodimeric complex with AT$_{1A}$R (131).

The AT$_{1A}$R is in the G$_{q/11\alpha}$ family of GPCRs, meaning that binding of angiotensin II to the receptor stimulates GTP loading of G$_{q\alpha}$, which in turn associates with and activates phospholipase Cβ (PLCβ). The active form of PLCβ mediates the hydrolysis of phosphotidylinositol 4,5 bisphosphate (PI$_{4,5}$P$_2$) in the membrane to produce diacylglycerol (DAG) and inositol trisphosphate (IP$_3$). IP$_3$ is hydrophilic and enters the cytoplasm where it activates the IP$_3$ receptor on the surface of the endoplasmic reticulum, thereby stimulating calcium release from internal stores. The simultaneous production of DAG at the membrane and local release of stored calcium leads to the recruitment and activation of the classic, calcium-dependent protein kinases C (PKCs). Activation of PKC appears to be required for angiotensin II–mediated, renal efferent arteriole vasoconstriction (136), Na,K-ATPase recruitment to the membrane in proximal tubule cells (resulting in increased proximal so-

dium reabsorption) (38, 158), and stimulation of aldosterone secretion by adrenal zona glomerulosa cells (44).

In addition to activation of PLCβ, a second signaling pathway that is activated by the AT$_{1A}$R is the mitogen-activated protein kinase (MAPK) pathway. As mentioned earlier, phosphorylation of GPCRs by βARK results in the recruitment of β-arrestin to the receptor complex and subsequent receptor internalization. β-arrestin has been found to act as a binding scaffold for the core components of the MAPK pathway, including Raf, MEK, and ERK (see Intracellular Signaling Pathways section), resulting in the activation of this pathway that mediates cell growth and proliferation (90, 221). Activation of these signaling pathways appears to play an important role during kidney development since newborn mice null for the type 1 angiotensin receptor, or in which angiotensin signaling has been inhibited, have significant renal developmental abnormalities, including renal arterial hypertrophy and papillary atrophy (20, 207).

A second means by which GPCRs can activate MAPK signaling was discovered when the levels of β-arrestin were depleted using small interfering RNA (siRNA). Under these conditions, angiotensin II was still able to activate MAPK, although to a lesser degree. These experiments uncovered a β-arrestin–independent pathway of angiotensin II–dependent MAPK stimulation that occurs via activation of a second cell surface receptor, a process known as receptor transactivation. As noted above, stimulation of G$_{q\alpha}$ by the AT$_{1A}$R leads to activation of PKC. PKC, in addition to regulating processes such as ion transport, can activate a cell surface protein called heparin-binding epidermal growth factor (HB-EGF). HB-EGF is one of the ligands for a separate cell surface receptor, the epidermal growth factor

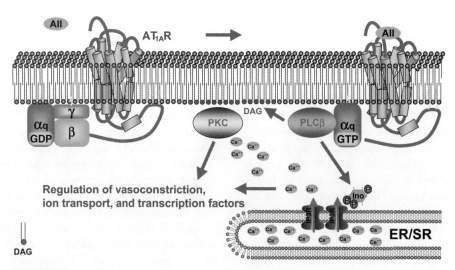

FIGURE 2 Signaling by the angiotensin II (AII) receptor. Binding of AII results in GTP-loading of the associated Gqα subunit of the αβγ heterotrimer, which in turns activates phospholipase C β (PLCβ). Activated PLCβ - stimulates th-e hydrolysis of PI$_4$,5P$_2$ in the membrane to form IP$_3$ and diacylglycerol (DAG). IP$_3$ can then bind to its receptor on the endoplasmic or sarcoplasmic reticulum, activating calcium release. The increase in cytosolic calcium can stimulate multiple cellular responses including activation of PKC (which associates with DAG at the membrane), influx of extracellular calcium via channels at the cell surface, and contraction via actin–myosin coupling.

receptor (EGFR), and binding of HB-EGF to the EGFR results in the stimulation of multiple signaling events including MAPK activation (see Intracellular Signaling Pathways section) (44).

LOCALIZATION AND TIMING OF PATHWAY ACTIVATION PROMOTES DIVERSE CELL-TYPE–SPECIFIC RESPONSES

These two independent pathways for activating MAPK signaling provide an example of how scaffolding proteins can compartmentalize signaling within the cell. The β-arrestin–mediated ERK activation is sustained for several hours and occurs in the cytoplasm, whereas the $G_{q\alpha}$/PKC-dependent ERK activation appears to be more transient and primarily within the nucleus. This ability to localize activated ERK in different cellular compartments allows the cell to differentially regulate specific effector proteins, and thus direct distinct cellular outcomes. In the heart, for example, $AT_{1A}R$-mediated $G_{q\alpha}$/PKC-dependent transactivation of the EGFR and ultimately MAPK nuclear signaling is believed to at least partially mediate angiotensin-stimulated cardiac hypertrophy (39, 202).

Many GPCRs can activate multiple Gα subunits, depending on cellular location and availability. For example, the parathyroid hormone (PTH) receptor can potentially activate $G_{s\alpha}$ (thus activating adenylate cyclase and PKA), $G_{q\alpha}$ (activating PLCβ and PKC), and G_i (inhibiting adenylate cyclase). PTH is an 84-amino-acid peptide hormone secreted by the parathyroid gland that acts on bone to increase calcium and phosphate release into the circulation, as well as on the proximal and distal tubules of the kidney to inhibit phosphate reabsorption and stimulate calcium reabsorption, respectively. PTH binds to and activates the PTH receptor, a class B GPCR (defined by the six conserved cysteine residues that form disulfide bonds in the large extracellular amino terminal domain) (50). Expression of a mutant form of the receptor that selectively fails to activate $G_{q\alpha}$-dependent PLCβ signaling in mice results in abnormalities in bone ossification without a change in serum calcium (56). The normal serum calcium in these animals suggests that renal tubular calcium handling in these mice is dependent on $G_{s\alpha}$- or G_i-regulated adenylate cyclase signaling, while bone ossification appears to require $G_{q\alpha}$-PLCβ signaling. In support of this hypothesis, complete loss of PTH receptor signaling results in hypocalcemia in addition to the bone abnormalities (99, 105). In humans this is recapitulated by an autosomal recessive mutation in the receptor in patients with Blomstrand chondrodysplasia, a lethal disorder characterized by excessive bone maturation and mineralization (80).

Kinase Receptors

A second class of transmembrane receptors are the kinase receptors. These proteins typically contain an extracellular ligand-binding domain at the amino terminus, a single membrane-spanning domain, and an intracellular carboxy-terminus that includes the kinase domain. In most cases, binding of the ligand to the receptor results in homodimerization of two receptor molecules, bringing the intracellular kinase domains into close proximity where they phosphorylate substrate residues on the adjacent receptor. This phosphorylation step generates binding sites for the recruitment of intracellular signaling molecules, as well as further activating the kinase domain so that nonreceptor substrates recruited to the complex can be phosphorylated as well.

TYROSINE KINASE RECEPTORS

The largest class of kinase receptors are the tyrosine kinase receptors, also known as receptor tyrosine kinases (RTKs) (Fig. 3). These molecules frequently serve as receptors for extracellular growth factors, which are circulating proteins that stimulate cell growth and division. Examples of ligand–receptor combinations in this family include epidermal growth factor (EGF) and its receptors ErbB1 (or EGFR) and ErbB2, platelet-derived growth factor (PDGF) and the PDGF receptor, insulin and the insulin receptor, and vascular endothelial growth factor and its receptors VEGFR1 and VEGFR2 (also called Flt1 and Flk1).

Once the growth factor has bound to and activated the receptor, newly phosphorylated tyrosine residues on the intracellular carboxy-terminus of the receptor serve as binding sites for cytosolic or membrane-associated proteins that contain phosphotyrosine-binding domains. The best characterized of these domains are the src-homology 2 (SH2) domains that share characteristic features first described in the phosphotyrosine-binding region of the cytosolic tyrosine kinase Src. SH2 domains are approximately 100 amino acids in length and provide specificity of interaction in two ways. First, the interaction of the binding pocket of the SH2 domain and the tyrosine residue is only stabilized when the tyrosine residue is phosphorylated. Second, the amino acids immediately flanking the phosphorylated tyrosine residue determine which SH2 domain interaction is preferred. For example, the SH2 domain on the p85 adaptor protein, a subunit of the lipid enzyme phosphoinositide 3-kinase (PI 3-K; see Intracellular Signaling Pathways section), strongly prefers to bind to phosphotyrosine with a methionine residue at the +3 position (189). Thus, receptors containing the sequence pTyr-X-X-Met (where X can be almost any amino acid) specifically recruit and activate the PI 3-K.

In the kidney, tyrosine kinase receptors have been implicated in controlling development, mediating hypertrophy, regulating the balance between repair and fibrosis after injury, and promoting the growth of renal carcinomas. During development, glial–derived neurotrophic factor (Gdnf) is made by the embryonic metanephric mesenchyme and activates the c-Ret tyrosine kinase receptor that is expressed on the epithelial cells of the adjacent Wolffian duct. The activation of Ret is somewhat unusual since Gdnf does not directly bind to Ret, but rather binds to a third membrane protein, Gfrα, that mediates dimerization of Ret in response

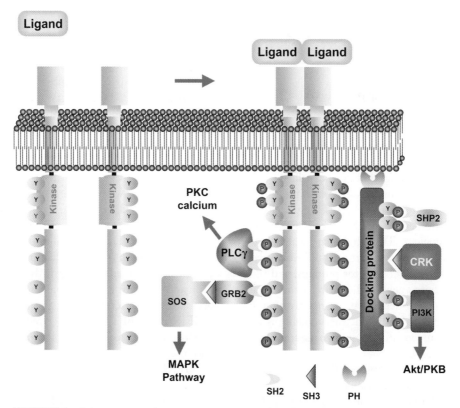

FIGURE 3   Schematic view of a receptor tyrosine kinase (RTK). In the inactive state the receptor is primarily in monomeric form. Following binding of the extracellular ligand, the receptor dimerizes, bringing the kinase domains in close proximity where they cross-phosphorylate each other. This activates the receptor and leads to phosphorylation of tyrosine residues outside the kinase domain, which in turn become binding sites for proteins that contain SH2 domains. In this manner, downstream signaling pathways can be regulated by recruitment to the receptor. This recruitment can occur via direct association of the effector protein with the receptor (as is the case for phospholipase Cγ [PLCγ]), via association with small adaptor proteins such as Grb2 (as is the case for the guanine exchange factor Sos), or via association with a larger docking protein such as Gab1 or Nck that mediate the association of multiple proteins with the receptor (as can be seen with the phosphoinositide 3-kinase (PI 3-K) or the tyrosine phosphatase SHP2). Some of these proteins are additionally stabilized at the membrane via lipid-binding domains such as the pleckstrin homology (PH) domain on Gab1. In addition to SH2 domain interactions, multiple other protein–protein interactions occur and regulate the recruitment of proteins into the complex, including interactions between SH3 domains and proline-rich regions in interacting partners. In this manner, multiple signaling effectors are brought into close proximity where they can interact with each other, be phosphorylated or dephosphorylated (thereby altering their activity or interacting partners), or regulate processes at the cell membrane. See color insert.

to association with Gdnf (reviewed in Sariola and Saarma [173]). Activation of Ret in this manner results in the activation of multiple intracellular signaling pathways, including the Erk-MAPK pathway, the PI 3-K pathway, members of the Src family of nonreceptor tyrosine kinases, and phospholipase Cγ (PLCγ). Activation of the MAPK and Src pathways (see Intracellular Signaling Pathways section) have been found to be critical for the outgrowth and branching of the ureteric bud from the Wolffian duct, the first step in formation of the metanephric kidney (30).

Many growth factor receptors are expressed in the mature kidney and are believed to be critical for maintenance of normal tubule architecture and for regulating the cellular response to injury. Renal tubular epithelial cells express EGF receptors as well as the c-Met receptor for hepatocyte

growth factor (HGF). These tyrosine kinase receptors directly bind their respective ligands via their extracellular amino terminal domains, followed by homodimerization and activation of intracellular signaling. A major mediator of the intracellular signaling mediated by EGF and HGF is the Gab1 docking protein (65). Docking (also referred to as scaffolding) proteins are typically large intracellular proteins that contain numerous protein–protein interaction domains as well as amino acid residues that are targets for tyrosine and/or serine/threonine kinases. Thus, recruitment of Gab1 to c-Met or the EGFR results in its phosphorylation on multiple tyrosine residues and subsequent association with p85, PLCγ, Grb2, a second adaptor protein known as Crk, and the protein tyrosine phosphatase SHP2 (222). Following acute renal injury, the level of HGF increases in the kidney, resulting in activation of c-Met, thereby mediating MAPK, PI 3-K, and PLC signaling (73, 79). These pathways in turn are believed to be important for inhibition of apoptosis (the PI 3-K pathway), and stimulation of cell migration and proliferation during the repair process (PI 3-K, MAPK, and PLC pathways) (74, 124, 127).

SERINE/THREONINE KINASE RECEPTORS

A second group of transmembrane kinase receptors are the serine-threonine kinase receptors. Like the nonreceptor kinases PKA and PKC, these receptors catalyze the phosphorylation of serine or threonine residues in their substrate molecules. Perhaps the best studied of these receptors in the kidney is the receptor for transforming growth factor β (TGFβ), a member of the TGFβ superfamily of secreted factors that also includes the bone morphogenic proteins (BMPs) and activin (219) (Fig. 4). TGFβ-like proteins signal into the cell via a heterotetrameric complex comprised of two subclasses of serine/threonine kinase receptors, the type I receptor and the type II receptor (116). Like the tyrosine kinase receptors, these proteins have an extracellular ligand recognition domain, a single transmembrane-spanning domain, and an intracellular kinase domain. The various TGFβ-like ligands utilize distinct type I and II receptor combinations. For example, TGFβ1–3 signal via the combination of the type II receptor TβR-II and the type I receptors activin receptor-like

kinase 1 (ALK-1) or ALK-5 (145, 177), while BMPs signal through the type II receptors ActR-II or BMPR-II and the type I receptors ALK-3 or ALK-6 (200).

TGFβ receptor signaling begins when the ligand binds to the extracellular domain of its cognate type II receptor. The kinase domain of type II receptors is constitutively active, and binding to the extracellular ligand results in the recruitment of the appropriate type I receptor into the complex, where the type I receptor is phosphorylated and activated by the type II receptor. In this manner, the TGFβ1-dependent association of ALK-5 with TβR-II allows the constitutively active TβR-II to phosphorylate ALK-5 and activate its intracellular serine/threonine kinase domain. The specificity of signaling by TGFβ family members is further regulated by the presence in many cells of the accessory receptors betaglycan and endoglin. These transmembrane proteins lack intracellular kinase domains, and appear to regulate the affinity of TGFβ proteins for the various type II receptors, as well as modifying intracellular signaling by the ligand–receptor complex (110, 172).

As opposed to tyrosine kinase receptors that signal primarily via recruitment of SH2 domain–containing proteins to activate pathways such as MAPK and PI 3-K, TGFβ receptors signal via a distinct signaling pathway, the Smad proteins. Smads are small cytoplasmic proteins that contain a DNA-binding domain and a TβR-I/Smad4 interacting

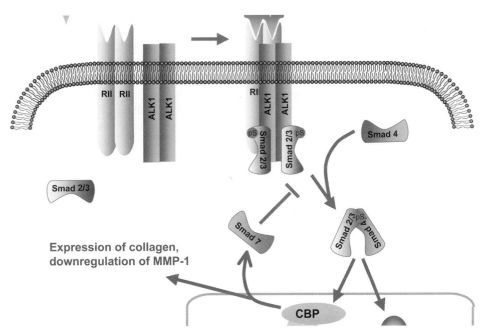

FIGURE 4 Signaling by the TGFβ family of serine/threonine kinase receptors. Binding of the TGF ligand to the constitutively active, type II receptor results in association of RII with the appropriate type I receptor (in this case ALK-1), which is phosphorylated and activated. The activated type I receptor can then phosphorylate the appropriate Smad protein, which then disassociates from the receptor complex, associates with Smad 4, and translocates into the nucleus. In the nucleus, the Smad complex can regulate RNA transcription by binding directly to the appropriate DNA Smad response elements (SRE) or by binding to and regulating transcriptional regulators such as the cAMP response element (CRE)–binding protein (CBP). One of the DNA targets regulated by Smad activation is the inhibitory Smad, Smad7. Increased expression of Smad7 inhibits TβR signaling, providing a negative feedback to prevent sustained activation of the pathway.

domain. Based on their structure and function, Smads have been divided into three groups—the receptor-activated Smads (Smad1, 2, 3, 5, 8), a regulatory Smad (Smad4), and the inhibitory Smads (Smad6, 7). Upon activation of TβR-I, the appropriate receptor-activated Smads (e.g., Smad2 and 3 for ALK-5) are phosphorylated on regulatory serine residues in the TβR-I/Smad4 interacting domain resulting in their disassociation from the receptor and association with Smad4. This Smad2/Smad4 complex then translocates to the nucleus where the Smad DNA-binding domain can mediate direct association with Smad-binding elements (SBE) in the DNA of the promoter region of target genes as well as association with other transcriptional regulators.

One of the transcriptional targets regulated by Smad2/4 signaling is another member of the Smad family, Smad7. Smad7 is an inhibitory Smad that can bind to TβR-I and prevent Smad2 or Smad3 from associating and being activated. In this manner, TGFβ stimulation of Smad7 transcription provides a negative feedback loop that acts to prevent sustained Smad2 and Smad3 activation by the TGFβ receptor (138).

TGFβ Signaling in Kidney Studies in mice that have undergone genetic inactivation of various TGFβ family members demonstrate that Bmp4 has an important role in normal kidney development. In the mouse embryo, Bmp4 is expressed in the metanephric mesenchyme (the region that will differentiate into the glomerulus and proximal portions of the nephron through the connecting segment) while the Bmp receptors Alk3 and Alk6 are expressed on the invading ureteric bud (the epithelial structure that will branch to form the entire collecting system of the kidney) (132). While complete loss of Bmp4 results in embryonic lethality before kidney development (106), mice that are heterozygous for loss of Bmp4 expression exhibit multiple defects in the collecting system of the kidney, including doubling of the collecting system, hydroureter, and dysplastic kidneys (132). Thus, it appears that Bmps normally act to inhibit ureteric bud branching and overgrowth during development. This idea is supported by experiments showing that mice expressing a constitutively active form of the Bmp4 receptor Alk3 have decreased ureteric bud branching and develop medullary cysts (67).

In addition to their role in kidney development, TGFβ proteins have been shown to play a major role in regulating fibrotic responses of the adult kidney by both increasing new matrix deposition and inhibiting matrix degradation (11, 219). In vitro studies have shown that TGFβ-dependent Smad3/Smad4 nuclear signaling can induce the expression of multiple collagen isoforms (214, 217), and activated Smad3 has been found to mediate decreased transcription of the gene for matrix metalloproteinase-1 (*MMP-1*) (58). In support of an important role for the TGFβ-Smad signaling pathway in the development and progression of renal fibrosis in vivo, genetic overexpression of TGFβ in the rat has been shown to induce glomerulosclerosis due to increased extracellular matrix deposition (70), while mice lacking Smad3 demonstrate less fibrosis following ureteral obstruction (174).

Receptor-Like Phosphatases

Much attention has been focused in the field of signal transduction on the role of substrate phosphorylation by receptor kinases in regulating protein–protein interactions or altering the activity of effector proteins. However, a second class of proteins, the phosphatases, are emerging as equally important signaling regulators in determining cellular responses. Similar to kinases, phosphatases can be grouped into transmembrane receptor-like phosphatases and intracellular (cytosolic) phosphatases (to be discussed below). The receptor-like phosphatases that have been identified to date are protein tyrosine phosphatases (PTPs) with an extracellular domain, single transmembrane-spanning segment, and intracellular phosphatase domain. Unlike receptor tyrosine kinases however, the ligands for the receptor-like PTPs have been difficult to identify.

The first receptor-like PTP to be cloned and sequenced was the T- and B-cell antigen CD45. This protein was found to be necessary for normal activation of T cells following engagement of the T-cell receptor (reviewed in Mustelin and Tasken [135]). While the extracellular ligand that regulates CD45 remains to be determined, one critical intracellular substrate that has been identified is the cytosolic tyrosine kinase Lck. Lck, like the related tyrosine kinase Src, is normally maintained in the inactive state by the association of phosphotyrosine 505 near the carboxy-terminus with its own SH2 domain closer to the amino terminus of the protein (227). This interaction results in folding of Lck and thereby prevents the intervening tyrosine kinase domain from recognizing or phosphorylating its substrates. Dephosphorylation of phosphotyrosine 505 by CD45 following antigen presentation by a nearby dendritic cell allows Lck to unfold and activates the kinase domain (134). The resultant phosphorylation of the ζ chain of the T-cell receptor by activated Lck is necessary for recruitment of a second cytosolic tyrosine kinase, ZAP70, to the complex and subsequent T-cell activation (78) (Fig. 5). The administration of monoclonal antibodies that prevent activation of CD45 has been shown to markedly diminish the occurrence of acute rejection in a rodent model of kidney transplantation (107).

In contrast to CD45, the receptor-like protein tyrosine phosphatase PTPζ/β is expressed on epithelial cells and has been found to bind to several putative extracellular ligands, including contactin, neural cell adhesion molecule (NCAM), and pleiotrophin (118, 153). Rather than activating PTPζ/β, as is typical of most ligand–receptor interactions, the association of pleiotrophin with PTPζ/β inhibits the phosphatase activity of PTPζ/β (126). In the kidney, pleiotrophin has been shown to markedly increase branching by the explanted ureteric bud, and thus is believed to play a significant role in determining the number of nephrons that form during kidney development (171). One substrate for PTPζ/β is the cytosolic protein Git1 (88), a multifunction adaptor protein that can regulate the

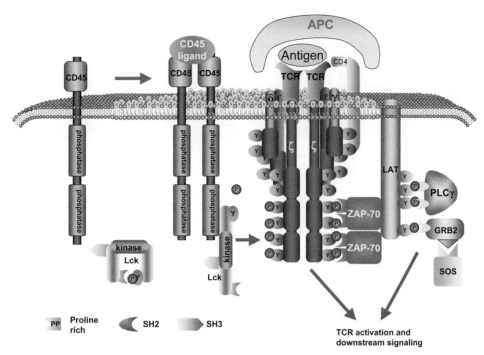

FIGURE 5 Signaling by the CD45 receptor phosphatase. CD45 is a single membrane–spanning receptor phosphatase that is activated by an unknown extracellular ligand. Ligand binding activates the intracellular phosphatase domains, possibly by clustering of the receptors, which dephosphorylate the carboxy-terminal tyrosine residue on the cytosolic nonreceptor tyrosine kinase Lck. This allows a conformational change in Lck that exposes the kinase domain and facilitates phosphorylation of the ζ chain of the multimeric T-cell receptor. This phosphorylation, in conjunction with antigen presentation by an antigen-presenting cell (APC) to the extracellular domain of the TCR, results in recruitment of a second tyrosine kinase, ZAP70, to the complex via binding of the ZAP70 SH2 domains to the phosphorylated receptor. ZAP70 recruitment and activation are required for normal TCR activation and for phosphorylation of the adaptor protein, linker for activation of T cells (LAT). LAT in turn serves as the site for recruitment of multiple signaling pathways involved in the T-cell immune response, including PLCγ (for activation of PKC and calcium signaling) and Grb2-Sos (for MAPK signaling). See color insert.

signaling pathways that control actin cytoskeletal rearrangement (121). Dephosphorylation of Git1 by PTPζ/β is therefore proposed to play an important role in the regulation of cell adhesion and migration, as well as cytosolic vesicle trafficking (46).

Receptors Activated by Proteolytic Cleavage

The previously described receptors bind to their respective ligands and then signal into the cell via activation of substrate protein phosphorylation or dephosphorylation, thus regulating cytosolic signaling pathways that in turn mediate the activation or inhibition of downstream effectors. In contrast, cleavage-activated receptors such as Notch, signal directly to the nucleus to regulate gene transcriptional events (Fig. 6). Notch is a cell surface protein that contains an extracellular ligand-binding domain, a single transmembrane-spanning segment, and an intracellular domain capable of binding and activating nuclear transcriptional factors (reviewed in Fortini [43]). The Notch ligands, such as Jagged, are also transmembrane proteins that contain extracellular EGF-like repeats and a unique domain for binding Notch. When Jagged on one cell engages Notch on an ad-

jacent cell, a cleavage site is exposed on the extracellular side of Notch near the membrane, and Notch is cleaved by a member of the a disintegrin and metalloproteinase (ADAM) family of proteases (14). The remaining transmembrane/intracellular portion of Notch then becomes a target for further cleavage by presenilin (a member of the γ-secretase complex) at a conserved site in the intramembranous domain of Notch (29).

This final cleavage event releases the cytosolic domain of Notch that translocates to the nucleus where it can directly bind and regulate transcription factors. In mammals, Notch can control transcriptional regulation by the DNA-binding protein CSL, which in turn regulates transcriptional expression of members of the hairy and enhancer of split (HES) and hairy-related transcription factor (HRT) family of transcription factors. These nuclear proteins control the expression of genes that are critical for regulating normal development. In the kidney, Notch signaling has been specifically implicated in the specification of the proximal tubule and in podocyte formation (22, 23, 181).

As the Notch/γ-secretase pathway has been investigated during the past 10 years, it has become clear that receptor

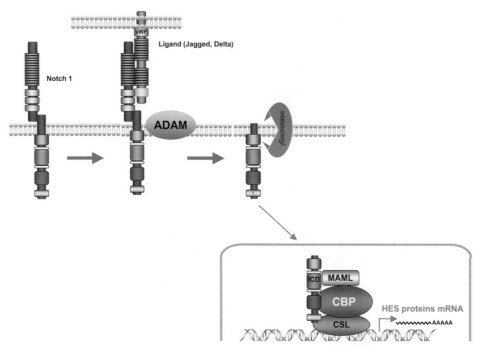

FIGURE 6   Notch signaling as an example of regulated intramembranous proteolysis (Rip). It is believed that Notch is proteolytically processed in the endoplasmic reticulum (site 1 cleavage) and expressed on the cell surface as a disulfide-linked dimer of the extracellular domain and the transmembrane-intracellular domain. Binding of the extracellular domain to a Notch ligand (such as Jagged-1) on an adjacent cell exposes a juxtamembrane cleavage site (site 2) for a member of the ADAM family of extracellular proteases. This second cleavage allows the γ-secretase complex (containing presenilin) to cleave the remaining carboxy-terminus at a site within the membrane (site 3 cleavage), releasing the intracellular domain (ICD), which translocates to the nucleus. In the nucleus, the ICD of Notch can bind to members of the CSL family of transcriptional repressors, and in the presence of CSL-binding protein (CBP) and mastermind-like protein-1 (MAML), activate transcription of the HES family of genes.

activation by regulated cleavage plays a role in signaling by other cell surface proteins. For example, the γ-secretase complex has been shown to cleave the EGF tyrosine kinase receptor ErbB4 and the adherens junction protein E-cadherin (143). In the case of ErbB4, this cleavage event is required for the normal proapoptotic effects of receptor activation, arguing that some cell outcomes previously ascribed to activation of tyrosine kinase cascades may in fact be due to receptor cleavage and subsequent direct regulation of nuclear transcriptional events (215). While the nuclear targets of some of these cleaved receptors remain to be determined, the likely importance of this pathway in normal cell signaling is emphasized by the finding that the HGF receptor c-Met undergoes a similar cleavage event that regulates cell survival signaling (208) and that the proximal tubule brush border protein megalin can undergo ligand-dependent γ-secretase–mediated cleavage (239).

Receptors That Signal Cell Location

One of the most important roles of cell signaling is to determine whether a given cell is directed to act as a terminally differentiated cell with a highly specialized function (such as the increase in sodium transporters in the brush border of a proximal tubule cell in response to angiotensin

II signals mediated by volume depletion [104]) or is to undergo processes such as cell division and migration (e.g., during development of the embryonic kidney or recovery of the adult kidney from acute renal failure). While these widely divergent responses are primarily mediated by receptor–ligand interactions such as those mentioned above, cells also have surface proteins that provide important clues regarding cell location and density, and thus establish their level of differentiation, polarity, and responsiveness to these outside signals.

CELL–MATRIX INTERACTIONS CAN SIGNAL CELL LOCATION

The cells of the nephron reside on a complex basement membrane that provides specific clues regarding cell location. In the glomerulus this structure is highly specialized to not only support epithelial cell attachment (the podocyte), but also endothelial cell attachment, and to serve as a significant component of the glomerular filtration barrier. The basement membrane of the kidney has been shown to be composed of multiple matrix proteins, including collagen, laminin, perlecan, nidogen, nephronectin, and entactin. The specific isoforms and relative contributions of these proteins vary during the course of renal development as well as along the length of the adult nephron (reviewed in Miner

[128]). These matrix proteins interact with members of a large family of specific cell surface receptors, the heterodimeric αβ integrins (Fig. 7).

In the kidney, $\alpha_1\beta_1$, $\alpha_2\beta_1$, $\alpha_3\beta_1$, $\alpha_6\beta_4$, $\alpha_8\beta_1$, and $\alpha_V\beta_3$ have been found to be highly expressed in developing and/or adult renal tubular cells (reviewed in Pozzi and Zent [154]). The binding of the heterodimeric integrin complex to its matrix ligand in the basement membrane (e.g., $\alpha_2\beta_1$ integrin and type IV collagen) results in clustering of the integrins on the basal surface of the cell at contact sites known as focal contacts or adhesions, and the concomitant accumulation of a large group of intracellular signaling proteins at these sites known as the focal adhesion complex. This complex typically includes the focal adhesion scaffolding proteins paxillin and HEF1, the nonreceptor kinases Src, PI 3-K, integrin-linked kinase (ILK) and focal adhesion kinase (FAK), the small G-protein–regulated signaling proteins PIX and PAK, and actin-binding proteins such as vinculin, talin, and actopaxin (reviewed in Turner [209] and Zheng and McKeown-Longo [238]). Signaling through this complex can occur in a traditional "outside-in" manner in which integrin binding to matrix results in formation and activation of the signaling complex, or in an "inside-out" manner in which signals from other sites, such as activated growth factor receptors, can regulate the affinity of the integrin complex for its matrix ligand, such as during growth factor–stimulated cell adhesion and/or migration.

Signals emanating from focal adhesions provide critical clues regarding cell location, establishment of cell polarity, regulation of cell proliferation, and determination of cell differentiation. The recruitment of actin-binding proteins into the focal adhesion complex provides important clues for cell polarity, while the regulation of small G-proteins such as Rac and Cdc42 is critical for regulating cell differentiation and directed migration (25). Focal adhesion signaling through Src, FAK, and the PI 3-K is required to normally activate the ERK MAPK pathway in response to proliferative growth factor stimuli, and thus promote entry into the cell cycle and subsequent cell proliferation (180). In the event that cell–matrix adhesion is lost, such as can occur in proximal tubule cells following ischemic renal injury, growth factor signaling is muted, the cells enter cell cycle arrest, and eventually undergo anoikis (programmed cell death induced by cell detachment) due to activation of the JNK MAPK pathway (see Intracellular Signaling Pathways section) (45).

The importance of providing the right matrix environment for normal kidney development and function has been demonstrated in mice lacking specific matrix proteins and/or integrin receptors. For example, failure to express laminin-10 results in severe abnormalities in glomerular development, as does loss of expression of the laminin-10 receptor $\alpha_3\beta_1$ integrin (101, 129). In contrast, mice lacking integrin α_1 expression demonstrate normal kidney development (49), but have increased fibrosis after glomerular

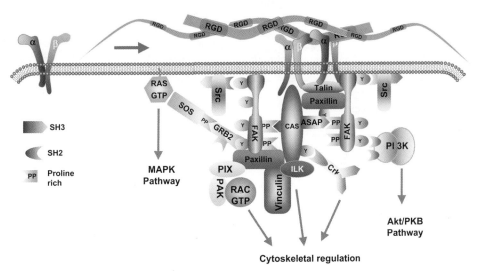

FIGURE 7 Integrin signaling at the cell–matrix interface. The αβ integrin heterodimers on the cell surface bind to specific sequences in the subcellular matrix (e.g., RGD domains in collagen), triggering a conformational change in the integrin and the subsequent recruitment of a large number of cytosolic and membrane-associated proteins (the focal adhesion complex). These proteins include the adaptor and scaffolding proteins p130Cas, Paxillin, Crk, and Grb2. These adaptor proteins in turn mediate the interaction of large numbers of signaling proteins, including tyrosine kinases such as Src, which can phosphorylate and activate other proteins in the complex (including the EGF receptor), and FAK, which activates turnover of the focal adhesion so that cells can migrate. The formation of this complex also activates cell survival and proliferation signals, including the PI 3-kinase and MAPK pathways, and regulators of the actin cytoskeleton such as vinculin, talin, integrin-linked kinase (ILK), and Rac. See color insert.

injury due to an increase in reactive oxygen species (ROS) generation (19).

CELL–CELL INTERACTIONS SUCH AS ADHERENS JUNCTIONS AND GAP JUNCTIONS CAN SIGNAL CELL DENSITY AND ALLOW CELLS TO ACT IN CONCERT

A second means by which cells obtain clues about their immediate environment is via cell–cell interactions. Of the many types of cell–cell interactions, at least two, the adherens junction and the gap junction, appear to play important roles in cell signaling. Adherens junctions form at the lateral border of adjacent cells due to the intercellular interactions of cadherins, a family of cell-type specific transmembrane proteins (reviewed in Gumbiner [55]). There are multiple cadherin family members, including the classic epithelial cell member E-cadherin, the endothelial cell cadherin VE-cadherin, and the renal tubule associated cadherin Ksp-cadherin (203). The extracellular portion of cadherins contains five repeat sequences, known as EC repeats, that can interact in a homophilic, calcium-dependent manner with the EC repeats present on cadherins present in adjacent cells. This interaction is important for providing cell sorting signals during tissue development (191).

The intracellular domain of the cadherins associates with a group of cytoplasmic proteins known as the catenins. One of these proteins, β-catenin, has a dual role in the cell. It directly binds to cadherins and thus participates in the formation of cell–cell junctions, but also can disassociate from adherens junctions and translocate to the nucleus where it regulates signaling events involved in cell differentiation and proliferation (Fig. 8). Originally it was believed that the direct interaction of cadherins with β-catenin created a stable binding site for the actin-binding protein α-catenin, thus generating a static site for lateral attachment of the actin cytoskeleton.

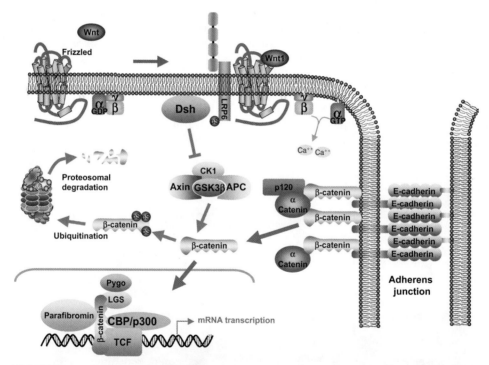

FIGURE 8 β-Catenin signaling. Formation of stable cell–cell adherens junctions in mature epithelia occurs due to the lateral interactions of cadherins on adjacent cells. This results in the formation of an intracellular complex of proteins comprised of β-catenin, α-catenin, and p120. α-Catenin can interact with the actin cytoskeleton and the adherens junction complex in a dynamic manner and thus serve as a nidus for actin cytoskeletal arrangement along the lateral border of the cell. β-Catenin can be sequestered in the adherens junction, or at times of dedifferentiation or during development, released into the cytosol where it is capable of translocating to the nucleus and activating the transcription of multiple genes involved in cell proliferation and dedifferentiation. In mature, nonproliferating cells, cytosolic β-catenin levels are maintained at low levels because phosphorylation by GSK-3β targets β-catenin for ubiquitination and degradation in the proteosome. GSK-3β is found in a complex that includes the regulatory/targeting proteins axin and APC. The kinase activity of GSK-3β can be inhibited following activation of several growth factor receptors. In the best-studied pathway, stimulation of the Wnt receptor Frizzled leads to phosphorylation of the membrane-spanning protein Lrp6, which in turn causes the cytosolic protein Disheveled (Dsh) to inhibit GSK-3β. The resultant increase in cytosolic levels of β-catenin leads to its translocation to the nucleus, where it serves as a scaffold for the association of a complex of proteins that bind and activate RNA polymerase II, leading to gene transcription. There are data supporting a second signaling pathway downstream of Frizzled in which GTP loading of the $G_{\alpha i}$ subunit of the heterotrimeric G protein results in release of the βγ subunit, which in turn activates phosphoinositide hydrolysis and downstream calcium release.

However, more recent studies have demonstrated that this protein complex is a dynamic structure that can support actin filament rearrangement during the movement of cells while maintaining cell–cell junctional integrity (35).

β-Catenin Signaling Can Regulate Cell Differentiation and Proliferation   As noted, β-catenin can leave the adherens junction and enter the nucleus where it acts as a transcriptional regulator by binding to the TCF/Lef transcriptional complex (133). Genes that are induced downstream of β-catenin typically lead to increased cell proliferation and inhibition of differentiation, processes that are important during normal development but that are typically downregulated in the adult. This transcriptional activity of β-catenin is tightly regulated by controlling the free cytosolic pool of β-catenin that is available for translocation into the nucleus. In the adult renal tubule, the extensive array of intercellular adherens junctions that forms in the confluent monolayer of epithelial cells results in sequestration of the majority of β-catenin with cadherin. To further ensure that free β-catenin levels remain low in the cytosol, a serine/threonine kinase, glycogen synthase kinase-3β (GSK-3β), phosphorylates cytosolic β-catenin and targets it for degradation by the proteosomal pathway (40). GSK-3β is associated with the adenomatous polyposis coli (APC) protein, and mutations in this complex that prevent β-catenin phosphorylation and degradation lead to increased nuclear β-catenin signaling, cell proliferation, and subsequent tumor formation (97).

During organ development, and following some types of organ injury, β-catenin nuclear signaling is activated by destabilization of adherens junctions (thereby releasing β-catenin into the cytoplasm) and coincident inhibition of GSK-3β kinase activity. The classic developmental regulator that has been found to activate β-catenin signaling in this manner is the growth factor Wnt and its receptor Frizzled (Fz) (224). Frizzled is a member of the GPCR family of seven membrane-spanning cell surface receptors, and has been proposed to signal, at least in part, by activation of heterotrimeric G proteins (183). However, in the canonical Wnt signaling pathway, binding of Wnt to Fz leads to the phosphorylation of a second membrane-spanning protein, the low-density lipoprotein receptor–related protein 6 (LRP6), which in turn mediates the activation of the cytosolic protein disheveled (Dsh) (237). Dsh, by a mechanism that is not presently understood, inhibits GSK-3β–dependent phosphorylation of β-catenin and thus prevents β-catenin degradation (218). In the developing kidney, Wnt signaling has been shown to be critical for regulating ureteric bud branching as well as for mesenchymal-epithelial transformation during formation of the proximal nephron (91, 119). In addition, several Wnt family members are upregulated in tubular cells following acute ischemic renal injury, suggesting that Wnt signaling may play a role in regulating the dedifferentiation and/or proliferative response of surviving tubular cells that is believed to be required for nephron repair (196, 201).

Gap Junctions Promote Rapid Signaling Between Clusters or Sheets of Cells   A second type of cell–cell interaction that is important for cell signaling is the gap junction. These junctions are formed by the alignment of hemichannels on the lateral borders of two adjacent cells to establish a direct cytoplasmic link between the cells, thus allowing the rapid movement of small molecules and electrical charge through multiple cells within a specified region of the organ (111). Gap junctions are primarily composed of a family of proteins known as connexins, and have traditionally been studied for their ability to rapidly transmit contraction signals through muscles. Investigation of gap junction function within the kidney has demonstrated that mesangial cells contain large numbers of gap junctions comprised of connexin 43 (Cx43), and that these are critical for mediating intercellular calcium-dependent coordinated mesangial contraction (229). In addition, tubular epithelial cells maintain intercellular gap junctions that can be regulated by growth factors as well as ischemic injury (212, 216), although the precise role of these channels in normal tubule function is presently not well understood.

Cilia as a Signaling Structure

Many cells of the body, including renal epithelial cells, have a surface structure known as the primary cilium. Cilia are elongated membrane protrusions that surround a central core of microtubules arising from a microtubule organizing center known as the basal body (reviewed in Davenport and Yoder [28] and Praetorius and Spring [155]). Cells that express cilia with a microtubular arrangement of 9+2 (9 microtubule doublets arranged in a cylinder around a core of 2 microtubule singlets), such as those lining the trachea, are motile and can act to facilitate directional movement of fluid (reviewed in Afzelius [1]). In other cells, such as those lining the renal tubules, cilia have a 9+0 arrangement, are nonmotile, and were previously believed to be rudimentary structures. However, the finding that genetic mutations that interrupt cilia formation can result in cystic kidney diseases in rodents (66, 199), along with the recent discovery that the two predominant gene products known to cause human autosomal dominant polycystic kidney disease, polycystin-1 (Pc-1) and polycystin-2 (Pc-2), localize to cilia, has resulted in intense investigations of the role of nonmotile cilia as renal epithelial mechanosensors (141, 233).

These studies have demonstrated that Pc-2 acts as a cation channel and that regulation of this channel activity can be mediated by its interaction with Pc-1 (17, 53, 59). In vitro studies have demonstrated that Pc-1 and Pc-2 colocalize on the primary cilium of the apical cell membrane in renal epithelial cells, and that physiological levels of fluid shear stress, such as that created by urine flow in the renal tubule, may be sufficient to stimulate cilia-dependent Pc-1/Pc-2–mediated calcium signaling (113, 140, 233). It is presently hypothesized that failure of this signaling pathway can result in abnormal rates of cell proliferation and thus lead to cyst formation.

INTRACELLULAR SIGNALING PATHWAYS

As is clear from the preceding section, activation of cell surface receptors results in the regulation of multiple intracellular signaling pathways. Although numerous studies since the mid-1990s have emphasized the vast amount of cross-talk among the proteins involved in these pathways, it remains useful to identify core signaling cascades that can transduce signals from the receptor to effector proteins that mediate specific cellular responses. Several of these signaling cascades, including the heterotrimeric G-protein-adenylate cyclase-cAMP-PKA pathway, the TGFβ-Smad pathway, and the Wnt-Fz-Dsh-GSK-3β-β-catenin pathways, are described in some detail in the Cell Surface Receptors section. This section focuses on several other signaling cascades that are believed to be fundamental regulators of cell survival and function in the kidney, including the PLC-Ca-PKC pathway, the MAPK pathway, and the PI 3-kinase pathway.

Phospholipase C Pathway Regulates Intracellular Calcium Release and Activates PKC Signaling

Phospholipase C (PLC) is an enzyme that catalyzes the hydrolysis of the membrane lipid phosphoinositide 4,5 bisphosphate ($PI_{4,5}P_2$) to generate diacylglycerol (DAG) in the membrane and release inositol trisphosphate (IP_3) into the cytoplasm (reviewed in Rhee [161]) (Fig. 9). DAG provides a binding site to recruit protein kinase C (PKC) to the membrane, while IP_3 binds to its receptor on the endoplasmic reticulum that mediates the intracellular release of stored calcium. Thus activation of PLC regulates both PKC-dependent and calcium-dependent intracellular signaling.

In mammals, there are four known families of phospholipases C, PLCβ, PLCγ, PLCδ, and PLCε. While all four groups share the catalytic X and Y lipase domains, the regulatory domains are widely divergent, allowing activation by distinct upstream receptors. For example, PLCβ is activated following stimulation of certain GPCRs because it has a carboxy-terminal domain that recognizes and binds GTP-loaded $G_{q\alpha}$ as well as the free βγ heterodimer (148, 149) (see G-Protein–Coupled Receptors section). In contrast, PLCγ family members lack the Gα- and βγ-binding re-

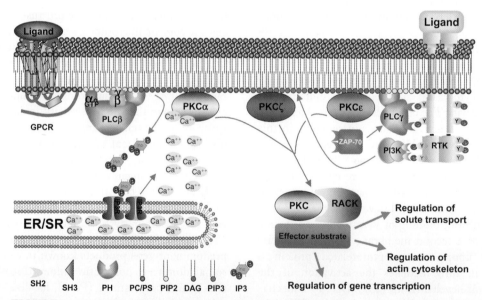

FIGURE 9   Phospholipase C-protein kinase C signaling. Activation of G-protein–coupled receptors coupled to $G_{\alpha q}$ can recruit PLCβ to the membrane and activate its phospholipase activity via interactions with the GTP-loaded α subunit as well as the free βγ subunit. PLCγ is classically activated via binding of its SH_2 domains to phosphotyrosine residues on RTKs, although PLCγ can also be activated by the nonreceptor tyrosine kinase ZAP70. Both PLCβ and PLCγ are stabilized at the membrane via their lipid-binding PH domain where they hydrolyze $PI_{4,5}P_2$ (PIP_2) to generate DAG and IP_3. DAG serves as a binding site at the membrane for both conventional PKCs (such as PKCα) and novel PKCs (such as PKCε). While novel PKCs are activated as a consequence of this membrane recruitment, conventional PKCs also require calcium binding for full activation. This calcium signal comes from IP_3 -mediated calcium release from intracellular stores. A third family of PKCs, the atypical PKCs such as PKCζ, lack the DAG-binding domain and are recruited to the membrane and activated by binding to phosphatidyl serine (PS) as well as the lipid product of the PI 3-kinase (PI 3-K), $PI_{3,4,5}P_3$ (PIP_3). Specificity of signaling for this diverse family of serine/threonine kinases is provided by association of activated C kinase (RACK), which target the activated PKC isoform to the correct effector protein (such as the α subunit of the Na,K-ATPase in renal tubular cells). See color insert.

gions but instead encode two SH2 domains and one SH3 domain that mediate their recruitment and activation by receptor tyrosine kinases (RTKs) such as the PDGF receptor, vascular endothelial growth factor (VEGF) receptor, and HGF receptor (211). Interestingly, PLCγ can also be phosphorylated and activated by nonreceptor-protein tyrosine kinases such as Src family members. In this manner, PLCγ can be secondarily activated in immune cells downstream of T-cell receptor activation (Fig. 5), as well as following activation of certain GPCRs such as the angiotensin II receptor (57). Activation of PLCδ and PLCε are poorly understood, although current results suggest that PLCδ may be activated in a calcium-dependent fashion, whereas PLCε has a Ras-binding domain and appears to be activated by associating with GTP-loaded Ras (3, 89).

For PLC to hydrolyze $PI_{4,5}P_2$, it must be recruited to the membrane. Members of both the PLCβ and PLCγ families have pleckstrin homology (PH) domains at their amino termini that promote membrane association by binding to select membrane phospholipids such as $PI_{4,5}P_2$ and $PI_{3,4,5}P_3$ (8). PLCβ family members are further stabilized at the membrane because their PH domain can also interact with the membrane-bound βγ G-protein heterodimer, while the SH2 domains of PLCγ proteins enhance membrane association by mediating recruitment to cell surface receptors. In this manner, PLC is recruited to specific sites at the membrane in the vicinity of the activating receptor, allowing the cell to selectively upregulate DAG and IP_3 production in that area.

PLC-dependent generation of DAG provides a membrane-binding site for recruitment and activation of several members of the protein kinase C (PKC) family of nonreceptor serine/threonine kinases. PKCs are a large group of proteins that are subdivided into conventional PKCs, novel PKCs, and atypical PKCs. The conventional PKCs (PKCα, PKCβ, PKCγ) are activated in a calcium-dependent fashion following recruitment to the cell membrane by binding to DAG and phospholipids such as phosphatidylserine (PS). The novel PKCs (PKCδ, PKCε, PKCη, and PKCθ) are also recruited to the membrane by binding to DAG and membrane phospholipids, but do not require calcium for activation. The atypical PKCs (PKCλ, PKCζ, PKCμ, and PKCι) lack both the DAG and calcium-binding sites and instead appear to be associated with the membrane and activated solely via their association with membrane phospholipids (reviewed in Ron and Kazanietz [165]). In addition to PS, it has been found that the 3-phosphorylated lipid products of the PI 3-K (such as $PI_{3,4}P_2$ and $PI_{3,4,5}P_3$) can bind and activate both novel and atypical PKCs (205).

Once activated, PKCs have multiple potential phosphorylation targets in the cell. The determination of which targets are phosphorylated is dependent on cell type, the isoform of PKC that is activated, and targeting proteins that specify subcellular localization of the activated PKC. Proteins that are not phosphorylation substrates of PKC but serve only to target specific PKCs to select sites in the cell

are collectively termed RACKs (receptors of activated C kinase). For example, the cell polarity protein Par6 associates with atypical PKCs such as PKCζ and specifically targets them to epithelial tight junctions on renal tubular cells (81). In this location, PKCζ has been shown to regulate tight junction assembly, although the exact phosphorylation targets of PKCζ have yet to be identified (48).

Recent studies have demonstrated that PKC localization to the basolateral membrane can regulate Na,K-ATPase activity in the renal tubule as well. Several phosphorylation sites for classical PKCs (such as PKCα) have been identified in the amino terminus of the Na,K-ATPase α subunit, and phosphorylation of these sites appears to increase cellular sodium pump activity by increasing membrane localization of the enzyme (37, 152). Interestingly, activation of PKC downstream of the D_1-type dopamine receptors appears to have the opposite effect, inhibiting sodium pump activity as part of the overall effect of D_1 receptor on inhibiting tubular sodium reabsorption (52). Exploration of this response has demonstrated that novel PKCs such as PKCθ and PKCε are likely to mediate this Na,K-ATPase inhibitory effect (230). It is unknown whether these PKCs phosphorylate different sites on the sodium pump than does PKCα, or act indirectly via phosphorylation of intermediate proteins.

Another group of PKC regulatory targets are transcription factors. PKC isoforms such as PKCδ, PKCε, and PKCθ have been found to regulate the activity of multiple transcription factors including NFκB (involved in immune and inflammatory responses), signal transducers and activators of transcription (STATs, regulators of inflammatory responses, cell proliferation, and differentiation), and Jun N-terminal kinase (JNK, involved in cell stress response and survival) (reviewed in Steinberg [192]). By acting upstream of JNK as well as the Raf-MEK-ERK pathway (see subsequent discussion), PKC isoforms can cooperate to mediate increased activity of the immediate early-response genes Jun and Fos (188).

An interesting example of convergence of PKC with other signaling pathways is seen during the activation of T cells. The rise in intracellular calcium following T-cell stimulation results in the activation of calmodulin and binding of the calcium–calmodulin complex to the nonreceptor serine/threonine phosphatase calcineurin (also known as protein phosphatase 2B, or PP2B). Activated calcineurin dephosphorylates and activates the nuclear translocation of another protein, nuclear factor of activated T cells, or NFAT (reviewed in Isakov and Altman [71] and Schulz and Yutzey [179]). While originally described in T cells, NFATs are expressed in multiple cell types and control the expression of genes such as Il-2, GM-CSF, interferon-γ, TNFα, and Cox2 that regulate processes as diverse as T- and B-cell proliferation in response to antigen stimulation, cardiac myocyte differentiation and hypertrophy, and sodium channel expression (reviewed in Kobayashi et al. [93] and Macian et al. [117]). However, the DNA-binding sites of many of these gene targets contain nearby AP-1 promoter sites and are only upregulated in an efficient manner following the concerted actions of NFAT and the AP-1-binding elements Jun and Fos. Thus, concerted activation of PKC (to activate Jun and Fos) and calcineurin (to activate NFAT) leads to maximal gene expression and cellular response. The importance of calcineurin in mediating immune cell activation has led to the extensive use of calcineurin inhibitors such as cyclosporine and tacrolimus for the prevention of transplant rejection.

Mitogen-Activated Protein Kinase Pathway Regulates Cell Survival, Proliferation, and Morphology

The mitogen-activated protein kinase (MAPK) pathway provides an excellent example of the way in which various extracellular signals can converge on the regulation of a single intracellular signaling pathway, and demonstrates how targeting of that pathway to specific sites in the cell via scaffolding proteins can determine which effector proteins are regulated and what cell responses are affected. As the name implies, this protein cascade was originally identified based on its activation downstream of pro-proliferative growth factors such as insulin and EGF (13). In the classic MAPK cascade, binding of the growth factor to its receptor tyrosine kinase (RTK) initiates a series of protein–protein interactions that ultimately result in activation of the cytosolic serine/threonine kinase ERK, which can phosphorylate and regulate diverse effector substrates including transcription factors in the nucleus, focal adhesion proteins at the cell surface, and contractile proteins in the cytosol (92, 114, 223).

The core proteins of this classic MAPK cascade are three kinases—Raf, MEK, and ERK (Fig. 10). Raf-1 (also called MEK kinase [MEKK] or MAPK kinase kinase [MAP-KKK]) is a serine/threonine kinase that phosphorylates and activates two closely related MEK isoforms, MEK1 and 2. These isoforms are dual specificity (tyrosine as well as serine/threonine) kinases that phosphorylate ERK1 and 2 on a highly conserved amino-acid motif, Thr-Glu-Tyr, contained in the activation loop of the protein (26). The efficient activation of ERK in this cascade requires that the three proteins (Raf, MEK, and ERK) are brought into close proximity on a single scaffolding protein. Present studies indicate that several different proteins can serve this scaffolding function, including β-arrestin, IQGAP, kinase suppressor of Ras (KSR), and paxillin (75, 142, 168, 221). The location of the scaffolding protein and the regulation of Raf/MEK/ERK association appear to determine which effector proteins are likely to be regulated (reviewed in Kolch [95]).

The core module of Raf, MEK, and ERK can be activated following binding of receptor tyrosine kinases to their extracellular ligands. The initial step in RTK-mediated MAPK activation is the recruitment of the GRB2 adaptor protein to the tyrosine phosphorylated receptor. GRB2 is a small molecule that is composed of one SH2 domain and two SH3 domains (115). As noted previously, proteins containing SH2 domains interact with other proteins that contain phosphorylated tyrosine residues flanked by the appro-

priate amino acids. The GRB2 SH2 domain preferentially binds to phosphotyrosine residues with an asparagine at the +2 position, such as tyrosine 1096 in the activated c-Ret receptor (pYA*N*W) or tyrosine 1356 in activated c-Met (pYV*N*V). In contrast, SH3 domains typically mediate constitutive association with short proline-rich sequences in target proteins. The guanine nucleotide exchange factor (GEF) Sos contains such a sequence and associates with the GRB2 SH3 domain in a constitutive fashion. Sos acts as a GEF for the membrane-associated small GTP-binding protein Ras (10).

Ras is structurally similar to the α subunit of the αβγ heterotrimer that associates with GPCRs. However, Ras is activated by non-GPCR GEFs such as Sos, and, in the GTP-bound state, associates with and activates Raf rather than adenylyl cyclase. This activation step appears to involve the Ras-dependent dephosphorylation of Raf by PP2A, a nonreceptor protein phosphatase (102). Thus, RTK activation results in recruitment of the GRB2-Sos complex to the membrane where it mediates GTP loading of Ras, and activation of the Raf-MEK-ERK signaling pathway.

In addition to this classic model of GRB2-Sos-Ras-dependent MAPK activation mediated by RTKs, several alternative mechanisms of MAPK pathway activation have now been elucidated. For example, as described in the G-Protein–Coupling Receptors section, the recruitment of β-arrestin to GPCRs can result in activation of β-arrestin as a scaffold for Raf-MEK-ERK association and thus facilitate ERK activation. Another pathway of MAPK activation is that of PKC-mediated Raf activation. As noted previously, PKCs are activated downstream of GPCRs, RTKs and nonreceptor kinases (such as the PI 3-K) by associating with DAG and/or phospholipids at the cell membrane. Once activated, one of the potential PKC phosphorylation targets is Raf (182), leading to Raf activation and the downstream activation of MEK and ERK even in the absence of GTP-loaded Ras (96).

ERK Activation Is Regulated by Cross-Talk of Multiple Signaling Pathways

Classically, activated ERK has been shown to regulate gene transcription factors involved in promoting cell survival and inducing cell proliferation. Careful control of these events is fundamental to normal organ physiology, so it is not surprising that ERK activation is regulated by a complex series of signals derived from extracellular stimuli such as growth factors and cell–matrix interactions. It has long been known that adherent cells such as endothelial cells and epithelial cells can proliferate when attached to the proper basement membrane, but undergo anoikis when they lose their attachment. This type of cell death is common in detached tubular epithelial cells following acute renal injury, and it is believed that the loss of anoikis contributes to the metastatic spread of tumor cells (144, 151, 157). As described earlier, the sites of cell attachment to the basement

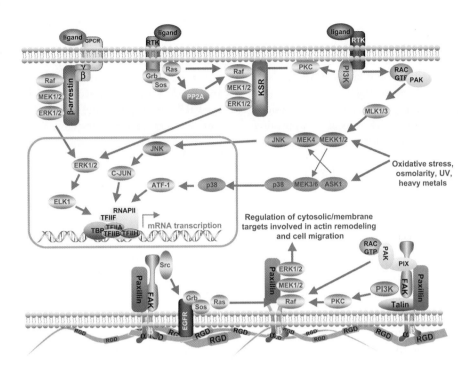

FIGURE 10 MAPK signaling. The prototypic MAPK pathway involves the growth factor–stimulated activation of the small G-protein Ras at the membrane, followed by Ras binding and activation of the serine/threonine kinase Raf (a MAPK kinase kinase or MAPKKK). This process involves dephosphorylation of Raf at an inhibitory site by the serine/threonine phosphatase PP2A. In addition, Raf can be activated by PKC-dependent phosphorylation, or by recruitment to the GPCR scaffolding protein β-arrestin. The MAPK pathway can also be activated in a growth factor–independent fashion via focal adhesion signaling when cells attach to the basement membrane. Activation of Raf results in phosphorylation and activation of the downstream kinases MEK and ERK. Depending on the site of ERK activation, it can translocate to the nucleus where it phosphorylates and activates transcription factors such as Elk1, or it can remain in the cytoplasm where it phosphorylates and regulates proteins involved in actin cytoskeletal rearrangement and cell migration such as myosin light-chain kinase (MLCK) and paxillin. Two other MAPK pathways present in most cells are the stress-activated protein kinases (SAPK) p38 and JNK. Multiple factors have been shown to activate p38 and JNK, including oxidative or osmolar stress, heavy metals, cytokines, and growth factors such as EGF and TGFβ. These stimuli induce the activation of a group of MAPKKKs, including apoptosis signal-regulating kinase-1 (ASK1), transforming growth factor–β activated kinase-1 (TAK1), MEKK1/2, and MEKK4. Activation of MAPKKK results in phosphorylation of the appropriate dual-specificity MAPKK (MEK), such as MEK3, MEK4, and MEK6, which in turn phosphorylate and activate JNK and p38. Small G proteins such as Rac and Cdc42 can also activate the p38 and JNK pathways via binding and activating intermediate kinases such as the mixed lineage kinase (MLK) family of serine/threonine kinases. There is considerable cross-talk between these pathways resulting in simultaneous activation of JNK and p38 under many conditions. Like ERK, activated JNK and p38 translocate into the nucleus where they phosphorylate regulatory transcription factors such as c-Jun, ATF-1, Elk-1, and Sap1. These in turn regulate the RNA polymerase transcription initiation complex to activate the transcription of multiple genes including prosurvival and proapoptotic factors, matrix proteins, heat shock factors, and so on. See color insert.

membrane are known as focal adhesions, and they provide the nidus for the aggregation of multiple signaling proteins on the cytosolic face of the attachment. Among the many proteins involved in this complex are the MAPK scaffolding protein paxillin, the Rac-activated protein p21–associated kinase (PAK), the EGF receptor, and the nonreceptor tyrosine kinases Src and FAK.

Attachment of the cell to a subcellular matrix can activate MAPK signaling even in the absence of extracellular growth factor or cytokine stimulation. One mechanism for this activation is that attachment-dependent activation of

FAK results in the recruitment and activation of the PI 3-kinase, which leads to the local production of $PI_{3,4,5}P_3$. As noted earlier, $PI_{3,4,5}P_3$ binds and activates PKC, which in turn can phosphorylate and activate Raf (194). Furthermore, the EGF receptor localizes to focal contacts in adherent cells and can be phosphorylated and transactivated by the nonreceptor tyrosine kinase Src even in the absence of extracellular EGF, thus mediating ERK activation via the classical Grb2-Sos-Ras pathway. In addition to the ability of focal adhesions to directly activate MAPK signaling, these signaling structures are also required for growth factors to efficiently stimulate MAPK signaling (5). Although the exact mechanism of this is not presently understood, recent studies suggest that activation of the focal adhesion–associated serine/threonine kinase PAK leads to phosphorylation of Raf that is required for the efficient activation of Raf by GTP-Ras (36). Thus, focal adhesions serve as sites to directly activate ERK as well as supporting ERK activation downstream of proliferative stimuli.

ERK REGULATES BOTH NUCLEAR AND CYTOSOLIC PROTEIN ACTIONS

Translocation of activated ERK to the nucleus has been found to signal both pro-proliferative and antiapoptotic responses. In the nucleus, ERK phosphorylates and activates transcription factors such as Elk-1 and RUNX2, which in turn regulate the mRNA expression of the cell cycle proteins cyclin D1 and p21^{WAF1} (51, 156, 197) (reviewed in Roovers and Assoian [166]). Furthermore, ERK activation can down-regulate the expression of proapoptotic proteins such as Bim1, a process that is believed to be critical for ERK-dependent inhibition of anoikis (160). These effects of ERK depend on both the amplitude and the duration of ERK activation. For example, transient high-level ERK activation in renal tubular cells treated with the growth factor HGF results in activation of focal complex signaling and Rac-dependent cell migration, but does not result in significant cell proliferation (75). In contrast, sustained low-level ERK activation appears to be required for cell cycle entry (leading to proliferation) and the antiapoptotic effects of ERK (24, 125, 204). For this reason, the degree of ERK activation is tightly regulated by a series of phosphorylation and dephosphorylation steps at the level of Raf (reviewed in Dhillon and Kolch [32]).

Activation of ERK can also lead to the phosphorylation of substrate proteins in the cytoplasm. ERK has been shown to phosphorylate and activate myosin light-chain kinase (MLCK), resulting in stimulation of cell motility (92). In addition, ERK activation at focal adhesions in renal epithelial cells can mediate phosphorylation of paxillin and subsequent FAK and PI 3-K activation (74). This process plays a regulatory role in the local activation of another family of small GTP-binding proteins, Rho, Rac, and Cdc42. These proteins are regulators of actin cytoskeletal remodeling, and by binding to their respective effector proteins (such as the Rho-kinase for Rho), mediate the cytoskeletal changes required for cell spreading, lamellipodia formation, and migration (reviewed in Schmitz et al. [176]). Besides activation downstream of ERK and the PI 3-K, focal adhesion signaling can also activate Rho family members by stimulating the guanine nucleotide exchange factors Vav and/or PIX (reviewed in DeMali et al. [31]). In the kidney, regulated activation of Rac and Rho are fundamental for the morphogenic changes involved in developmental tubulogenesis (163), and Rho activation appears to be required for angiotensin II–dependent regulation of glomerular arteriolar tone (137).

In addition to the classic ERK MAPK pathway, two other well conserved MAPK pathways, the JNK and p38 pathways, have been extensively studied and found to play important roles in regulating cell survival (reviewed in Roux and Blenis [167] and Zarubin and Han [236]). Similar to the ERK pathway, p38 and JNK signaling are mediated by a core complex of three proteins, including a MEK kinase, which when activated phosphorylates a MEK family member (MEK3 or 6 in the p38 pathway, MEK4 or 7 in the JNK pathway), which in turn phosphorylates the effector kinase p38 or JNK, respectively. Activated p38 or JNK can then translocate to the nucleus where they phosphorylate and regulate transcription factors such as ATF-1, ATF-2, c-Jun, and STAT-3.

Activation of the p38 and JNK signaling cascades occurs in response to cell stress signals, including UV irradiation, ischemia, and hypoxia, as well as following cytokine stimulation (IL-1 and TNFα) and certain growth factors (EGF, TGFβ) (21, 175). Based on in vitro studies demonstrating increased extracellular matrix production following p38 activation, it has been proposed that p38 may play an important role in the development of renal fibrosis following injury. In support of this, in vivo studies using p38 inhibitors in rodents have demonstrated that activation of p38 stimulates the progressive renal tubular fibrosis seen in models of chronic ureteral obstruction (190). Similarly, mice that overexpress TGFβ exhibit p38-dependent glomerular podocyte apoptosis, an early component of the progression to glomerulosclerosis (175), and p38 activation may be required for the development of proteinuria following acute glomerular injury (98). Activation of the ERK, p38, and JNK pathways occurs during the oxidative stress of renal ischemia/reperfusion. Under these conditions, JNK activation appears to mediate the tubular cell apoptotic response while ERK activation can be protective (6, 68, 150).

Phosphoinositide 3-Kinase Pathway Regulates Diverse Events Such as Glucose Metabolism, Cell Migration, Cell Survival, and Proliferation

Another major intracellular signaling pathway is activated by a lipid kinase known as the phosphoinositide 3-kinase (PI 3-K) (7). This enzyme is composed of two subunits, the p85 adapter protein and the p110 catalytic subunit. Recruitment of the p85/p110 complex to the membrane occurs when p85 binds via its SH2 domains to tyrosine phosphorylated receptors (such as the PDGF receptor) or docking proteins (such as the EGF receptor–associated protein Gab1 or the insulin receptor associated protein IRS-1). The p110 enzymatic subunit is activated by this translocation and phosphorylates target lipids, such as $PI_{4,5}P_2$ (PIP_2), to form the 3-phosphorylated derivative $PI_{3,4,5}P_3$ (PIP_3). PIP_3 then serves as a membrane-binding site for multiple proteins that contain lipid-binding domains such as the pleckstrin homology (PH) domain, the PTB domain, and FYVE domains (reviewed in Balla [9]).

As described previously, several PKC family members are recruited to the membrane and activated by binding to PIP$_3$, as are the docking protein DOCK180 and the guanine nucleotide exchange factor Vav (94, 146). However, the best-described targets of PIP$_3$ are the PH-domain–containing proteins 3-phosphoinositide-dependent kinase-1 (PDK1) and its major substrate enzyme Akt (also known as protein kinase B [PKB]). The generation of PIP$_3$ at the membrane results in recruitment and activation of PDK1, which in turn phosphorylates and activates Akt (4). In addition to Akt, activated PDK1 can phosphorylate and activate IKK, the upstream regulator of the NF-κB transcription factor, as well as the p70 and p90 ribosomal S6 kinases, and several PKC isoforms (2, 198) (Fig. 11).

Akt is a serine/threonine kinase that regulates multiple intracellular events including protein ubiquitination/degradation, glucose metabolism, nitric oxide generation, cell survival, and cell proliferation. To regulate these disparate processes, Akt associates with and phosphorylates multiple cytosolic protein targets (reviewed in Woodgett [225]). One of these targets is the constitutively active cytosolic enzyme glycogen synthase kinase-3β (GSK-3β), described previously for its role as a regulator of β-catenin ubiquitination and degradation downstream of the Wnt signaling pathway (27, 169). Similar to the effects of Wnt and its downstream effetor disheveled (Dsh), phosphorylation of GSK-3β by Akt causes an inhibition of the GSK-3β kinase activity, leading to an increase in free cytosolic β-catenin levels. β-Catenin can then translocate into the nucleus where it regulates the transcriptional expression of genes involved in stimulating cell proliferation and dedifferentiation. In addition to β-catenin, GSK-3β has also been shown to phosphorylate several other cellular substrates that regulate cell proliferation as well as cell

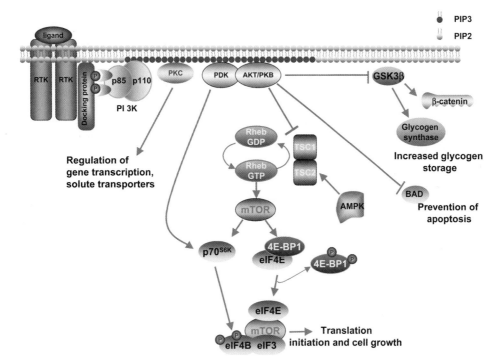

FIGURE 11   Signaling through the PI 3-kinase/Akt pathway. The activation of growth factor receptors results in the recruitment of the p85/p110 PI 3-kinase heterodimer to the membrane via binding of the SH2 domains of p85 to phosphotyrosine residues on the receptor or an associated docking protein such as IRS-1. Activation of the lipid kinase activity of p110 occurs, resulting in generation of PI$_{3,4,5}$P$_3$ (PIP$_3$) at the inner leaflet of the membrane. PIP$_3$ serves as a binding site for proteins that contain lipid-binding domains, including several PKC family members, docking proteins, and the serine/threonine kinase, phosphoinositide-dependent kinase (PDK). PDK has several targets in the cell including the protein translation activator p70 S6kinase and the cytosolic serine/threonine kinase protein kinase B (PKB), also known as Akt. Akt phosphorylates multiple substrates in the cell (typically resulting in inhibition of their action) that promote cell growth and survival. Thus, phosphorylation of the tuberosis sclerosis complex (TSC1 and TSC2) inhibits their GTPase activity, leading to accumulation of GTP Rheb and activation of mTOR. mTOR in turn activates p70 S6kinase and phosphorylates 4E-BP, resulting in its disassociation from eukaryotic initiation factor 4E (eIF4E), and cumulatively stimulating increased protein translation. During times of ATP depletion and AMP accumulation, mTOR activity is inhibited by the AMP-activated kinase AMPK. AMPK phosphorylates and activates the TSC complex, thus converting GTP Rheb to GDP Rheb and inactivating mTOR. Activated Akt also phosphorylates and inhibits proapoptotic factors such as BAD and caspase 9, and inhibits degradation of intracellular proteins such as glycogen synthase by phosphorylating and inhibiting GSK-3β.

survival. For example, GSK-3β can enter the nucleus where it phosphorylates the cell cycle protein cyclin D1, thus targeting it for rapid degradation (33). In addition, phosphorylation of translation initiation factor eIF2B by GSK-3β inhibits protein translation, leading to initiation of apoptosis and ultimately cell death (147). Thus, activation of the PI 3-K/Akt pathway, by inhibiting GSK-3β, results in increased cyclin D1 levels and eIF2B activation, promoting entry into the cell cycle and preventing apoptosis.

Besides these indirect effects of Akt on preventing cell apoptosis, Akt activation directly inhibits apoptotic responses by phosphorylating and inhibiting the pro-apoptotic factors BAD and caspase 9, as well as the fork-head transcription factor FKHRL1 (15). In addition, Akt activation can stimulate protein synthesis and cell growth via its effects on mTOR, the mammalian target of rapamycin (reviewed in Fingar and Blenis [41]). mTOR is a serine/threonine kinase that phosphorylates and activates the ribosomal protein translation initiators S6 kinase and 4EBP, leading to increased protein translation and promoting cell growth and division. Rapamycin, by inhibiting mTOR, prevents protein translation and inhibits cell division, leading to its use to suppress tumor growth and as an immune suppressant (due to inhibition of T- and B-cell expansion).

The kinase activity of mTOR is activated by binding to the small GTP-binding protein Rheb. Like Ras, Rac, and Gα, Rheb is active when in the GTP-bound state and inactive when in the GDP-bound state. Conversion of GTP-Rheb to GDP-Rheb is mediated by a GTPase complex made up of two proteins, tuberin and hammartin. The GTPase activity of these proteins, which are mutated in many patients with tuberous sclerosis, is in turn negatively regulated by phosphorylation of tuberin by activated Akt (123). In this manner, activation of Akt downstream of the PI 3-K results in stabilization of Rheb in the GTP-bound state, thereby activating mTOR and accelerating cell growth and division.

In addition to its fundamental role in regulating cell survival and proliferation, another major physiological process regulated by the PI 3-K/Akt pathway is insulin-dependent glucose metabolism (reviewed in Katso et al. 87]). Binding of insulin to its receptor tyrosine kinase results in the tyrosine phosphorylation of a docking protein, insulin receptor substrate (IRS), which in turn activates multiple intracellular signaling pathways including the PI 3-K. Activation of the PI 3-K has been shown to regulate insulin-dependent glucose uptake, glycogen synthesis, and lipolysis. Glucose uptake is mediated by the transport protein GLUT4. In the absence of insulin, GLUT4 is located in intracellular vesicles, but fuses with the plasma membrane following insulin stimulation. This translocation of GLUT4-containing vesicles to the membrane is mediated by $PI_{3,4,5}P_3$-dependent activation of both PKCζ and Akt (reviewed in Ishiki and Klip [76]).

Once glucose enters the cell, it is rapidly sequestered by conversion into glycogen via the actions of the enzyme gly-cogen synthase. In quiescent cells, the constitutively active form of GSK-3β normally phosphorylates glycogen synthase, keeping it in the inactive state. By stimulating the PI 3-kinase, insulin can increase Akt activation, thereby inhibiting GSK-3β activity and increasing glycogen synthase–dependent incorporation of glucose into glycogen (195).

EXAMPLES OF SIGNALING EFFECTORS IN THE KIDNEY

The extraordinarily complex interactions that initiate, regulate, and terminate intracellular second messenger pathways such as those described above ultimately lead to the change in location, function, or amount of effector proteins that actually mediate the cellular response to the initial signal. These effector proteins regulate fundamental cellular events such as division, programmed cell death, migration, and differentiation that are required for the development, maintenance, and repair of all tissues. In the kidney, signaling pathways are also critical for the precise regulation of glomerular filtration and for alteration of tubular-cell channel function in response to changes in the internal milieu.

One of the principal environmental stimuli that the kidney must respond to is variations in extracellular volume. For example, a decline in extracellular volume leads to a fall in renal perfusion that would be expected to be reflected in a concomitant fall in glomerular filtration rate (GFR). While a decreased GFR would be beneficial from the standpoint of limiting the further loss of fluid and salt by the kidney, it would also limit the clearance of the waste products of metabolism. Therefore, the kidney responds to decreases in circulating volume by coordinately increasing the fraction of the blood that is filtered at the glomerulus (thus minimizing the fall in GFR), while also increasing the fraction of the filtrate that is reabsorbed by the tubule (limiting further fluid and electrolyte loss). While more detailed descriptions of these regulatory events are presented in the appropriate chapters of the text, examples of several specific effector proteins are presented here in order to provide general paradigms of the ways in which signaling pathways can regulate effector protein function in the kidney.

Regulation of Glomerular Vascular Tone

Maintenance of GFR in the face of falling renal perfusion is achieved by the regulation of afferent and efferent vascular tone, with a confluence of signals resulting in relative dilation of the afferent arteriole and constriction of the efferent arteriole. Arteriolar tone is mediated by contraction or relaxation of the smooth muscle in the wall of the arteriole. Smooth muscle contraction is a complex process that begins with an increase in intracellular calcium that leads to the activation of the calcium-binding protein calmodulin. In smooth muscle, calcium-loaded calmodulin binds and activates myosin light-chain kinase (MLCK), which in turn phosphorylates and activates the regulatory light chain of smooth muscle myosin-II, leading to actin–myosin coupling and muscle contraction. The phosphorylation sites on the myosin light chain are targets for dephosphorylation by another regulatory molecule, myosin light-chain phosphatase (MLCP, also known as myosin phosphatase). In addition to binding and activating MLCK, sustained increases in intracellular calcium can lead to calmodulin–calcineurin interactions and subsequent activation of gene transcription factors such as NFAT involved in promoting muscle cell hypertrophy (reviewed in Im and Rao [69]).

In the efferent arteriole of the glomerulus, stimulation of smooth muscle contraction by angiotensin II requires the coordinated regulation of both MLCK and MLCP (reviewed in Kanaide et al. [86] and Woodsome et al. [226]). Activation of the AT1 receptor on the efferent arteriole results in activation of $G_{\alpha q}$ and the downstream second messenger PLCβ. As noted previously, the hydrolysis of PIP_2 by PLCβ results in the formation of DAG and the release of IP_3. In smooth muscle cells, IP_3 binds to its receptor on the sarcoplasmic reticulum, stimulating intracellular calcium release, which can in turn activate calcium entry from outside of the cell. The resultant rise in intracellular calcium leads to activation of calmodulin, which binds to and activates MLCK (Fig. 12).

In concert with its activation of MLCK, activation of the AT1 receptor stimulates two pathways that lead to inhibition of MLCP (reviewed in Ito et al. [77]). First, the formation of DAG in the membrane, coupled with the rise in intracellular calcium, leads to recruitment and activation of both conventional and novel PKCs. One of the phosphorylation targets of activated PKC in the smooth muscle cell is CPI-17, and in the phosphorylated state CPI-17 associates with and inhibits MLCP via binding to the PP1Cδ catalytic subunit. A second phosphorylation target of PKC are the matrix metalloproteinases (42). These proteins are involved in cleaving and shedding cell surface proteins including the cell-attached growth factor HB-EGF. Shedding of HB-EGF leads to activation of the EGF receptor, with stimulation of downstream signaling including the PI 3-kinase.

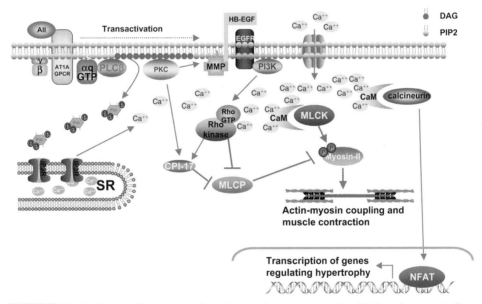

FIGURE 12 Angiotensin II regulation of vascular smooth muscle contraction. Binding of angiotensin II to the AT1A receptor results in activation of PLCβ and subsequent generation of IP_3 and DAG. DAG production at the membrane can mediate the recruitment and activation of PKC, while IP_3 binding to the IP_3 receptor in the sarcoplasmic reticulum stimulates calcium release. Angiotensin II may also stimulate extracellular calcium entry via cell surface calcium channels. Binding of the calcium to calmodulin (CaM) results in calmodulin-dependent activation of myosin light-chain kinase (MLCK), which phosphorylates myosin II to initiate actin–myosin contraction. Myosin II is dephosphorylated by myosin light-chain phosphatase (MLCP) to end the contraction. However, during the period immediately after AT1A stimulation, myosin II phosphorylation is maximized because MLCP is inhibited by PKC-dependent phosphorylation of the MLCP inhibitory binding protein CPI-17. In addition, GPCR activation can stimulate transactivation of nearby growth factor receptors (such as EGFR), which in turn can activate the PI 3-K. One mechanism of transactivation is the PKC-dependent activation of matrix metalloproteinases (MMPs), which cause shedding of the cell-attached protein HB-EGF that binds and activates EGFR. The resultant PI 3-K activation mediates GTP loading of the small G protein Rho and subsequent activation of Rho kinase. Rho kinase can directly phosphorylate MLCP at an inhibitory site, and can phosphorylate CPI-17 and thus increase its inhibitory effect on MLCP. Sustained contractile stimuli result in the calmodulin-dependent activation of calcineurin. Calcineurin is a phosphatase that binds to and dephosphorylates the nuclear factor of activated T cells (NFAT), resulting in NFAT-dependent transcriptional regulation of genes involved in smooth muscle cell hypertrophy.

This process of GPCR-dependent activation of a nearby growth factor receptor is termed transactivation.

In smooth muscle cells, one target of the activated PI 3-kinase is the Rho GEF leukemia-associated Rho guanine nucleotide exchange factor (LARG) (232). Activation of LARG converts Rho to the GTP-bound state, mediating its association with Rho kinase. This activation of Rho kinase can inhibit MLCP activity both by direct phosphorylation of MLCP at an inhibitory site, and via phosphorylation of CPI-17 in conjunction with PKC. By simultaneously increasing the phosphorylation of the light chain of myosin II via activation of MLCK and inhibiting its dephosphorylation via inactivation of MLCP, angiotensin II can greatly augment myosin II coupling with actin and subsequent smooth muscle contraction.

Regulation of Ion Transport Channels

The regulation of GFR by controlling afferent and efferent vascular tone must be coordinated with appropriate changes in solute reabsorption along the nephron. Typically this regulation occurs in one of three ways: regulation of the amount of the transporter in the cell, regulation of the location of the transporter, or regulation of the active state of the transporter at the membrane. In most cases, more than one of these regulatory steps is utilized, allowing both short-term and long-term regulation of transporter function.

SODIUM REABSORPTION IN COLLECTING DUCT CAN BE REGULATED BY CONTROLLING CELLULAR LEVELS OF ENaC

The epithelial sodium channel ENaC is expressed on the apical membrane of principal cells of the collecting duct. Regulation of ENaC function is one of the major ways in which the kidney controls the amount of sodium that is excreted in the urine each day. ENaC is comprised of three subunits that are synthesized in the ER and then transported to the Golgi for proteolytic cleavage and activation followed by trafficking to the apical membrane. ENaC channels present in the membrane can then be internalized where they are either degraded or maintained in a submembranous pool available for rapid recycling back to the membrane. The principal factors that regulate the synthesis, location, and degradation of ENaC are aldosterone and, to a lesser degree, AVP (Fig. 13).

Steroid Hormones Such as Aldosterone Bind to Cytoplasmic Receptors and Regulate Nuclear Transcription Events Aldosterone is a steroid hormone that binds and activates the mineralocorticoid receptor (MR). This receptor is expressed in the principal cell as well as other cell types, including intestinal epithelial cells, neuronal cells, and cardiac myocytes. The MR is a member of the steroid/thyroid family of ligand-inducible transcription factors that includes the vitamin D receptor, glucocorticoid receptor, thyroid receptor, and retinoic acid receptor (reviewed in Rogerson et al. [164]). Unlike the transmembrane receptors

discussed in the Cell Surface Receptors section, these receptors reside in the cytoplasm. The ligand, such as thyroid hormone or aldosterone, can cross the cell membrane where it binds to the receptor in the cytoplasm. The receptor-hormone complex then translocates into the nucleus and binds to specific DNA sequences known as steroid response elements (SRE). In the case of aldosterone, these regulatory sequences are found in the promoter regions of target genes such as *SCNN1A* (the ENaC α-subunit gene) and *Sgk-1* (encodes SGK, serum, and glucocorticoid-induced kinase).

In the principal cell, the β and γ subunits of ENaC are produced in excess, but do not traffic efficiently to the cell surface until the α subunit is made (reviewed in Snyder [185]). The increase in ENaC α-subunit protein expression that occurs following stimulation with aldosterone leads to ER assembly of αβγ into a complex with the predicted stoichiometry of 2α:β:γ and its subsequent proteolytic activation in the Golgi. In this manner aldosterone directly increases the total number of active ENaC transporters available in the cell, leading to an increase in sodium reabsorptive capacity.

A second way in which aldosterone can increase the number of ENaC channels available to reabsorb sodium is by inhibiting ENaC degradation. This is mediated by the transcriptional regulation of SGK expression (139). SGK is a serine/threonine kinase that phosphorylates and inactivates Nedd4-2, a ubiquitin-protein ligase that can associate with ENaC and stimulate its internalization and degradation (187). By increasing SGK expression, aldosterone mediates an inhibition of Nedd4-2 function and thereby increases the amount of ENaC present on the cell surface. Mutations in ENaC that prevent its association with Nedd4-2 lead to sustained increases in sodium reabsorption due to increased ENaC expression, resulting in the progressive hypertension seen in Liddle's syndrome (60).

In addition to inhibitory phosphorylation by SGK, Nedd4-2 can be phosphorylated at the same sites by PKA, again leading to inhibition of the Nedd4–2/ENaC association (186). Based on this observation, as well as prior evidence that vasopressin can increase sodium reabsorption in a PKA-dependent manner (178), it has been proposed that AVP-mediated stimulation of the G-protein–coupled V2 receptors on collecting duct cells leads to cAMP production and PKA activation, thereby inhibiting Nedd4–2/ENaC association. The subsequent increase in ENaC surface expression is thus believed to partially mediate the observed increase in sodium reabsorption following AVP treatment.

Finally, there is evidence to suggest that ENaC function can be regulated by trafficking of submembranous pools of the channel to the membrane. In cultured renal tubular cells, it has been shown that cAMP, presumably via activation of PKA, can stimulate the insertion of ENaC from a pool of internalized channels into the membrane, providing a means for rapid increases in the sodium reabsorptive capacity of the collecting duct in response to vasopressin stimulation (16, 184).

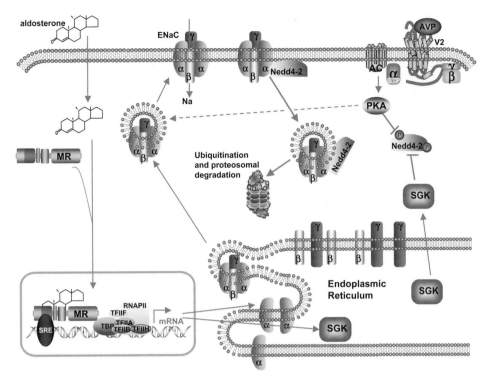

FIGURE 13 Regulation of ENaC. Aldosterone is a steroid hormone that can cross the cell membrane and bind to the mineralocorticoid receptor (MR) in the cell cytoplasm. The aldosterone–MR complex translocates into the nucleus where it binds to steroid response elements in genes such as *SCNN1A* encoding the α subunit of ENaC and *Sgk-1* encoding a cytosolic serine threonine kinase. Synthesis of the α subunit of ENaC promotes formation of the complete ENaC multimer in the endoplasmic reticulum and its translocation to the cell surface. At the membrane, the ubiquitin ligase Nedd4-2 can bind to ENaC, targeting it for internalization and proteosomal degradation. Nedd4-2 function is inhibited following phosphorylation by SGK, further increasing ENaC expression at the cell membrane and therefore sodium reabsorptive capacity. Vasopressin (AVP), acting through the V2 GPCR, can also increase collecting-duct sodium reabsorption. V2 activation leads to cAMP production and subsequent PKA activation. Like SGK, PKA can phosphorylate and inhibit Nedd4-2. It also appears that PKA can stimulate membrane insertion of ENaC-containing vesicles. See color insert.

REGULATION OF WATER REABSORPTION IN COLLECTING DUCT IS ACHIEVED BY TRAFFICKING OF AQUAPORIN-2

The regulation of channel amount by altering rates of synthesis and/or degradation is a relatively slow process that typically takes hours to days to accomplish and is believed to be most relevant in the adaptive responses to long-standing volume depletion or volume excess. In contrast, regulation of channel location provides a way to rapidly alter channel function in the cell. Aquaporins, transmembrane channels that provide a conduit for water movement across cell membranes, are one of the proteins that can be regulated in this fashion. In the kidney, aquaporin-2 (AQP2) is expressed in cells of the collecting duct and its ability to mediate water movement is regulated by AVP (reviewed in Valenti et al. [210]). In contrast, AQP1 (present in the proximal tubule and thin descending limb [170]) and AQP3 (present on the basolateral side of collecting duct cells [72]) are relatively insensitive to AVP.

In the absence of AVP, AQP2 is present primarily in submembranous vesicles in the collecting duct. Stimulation of V2 receptors by AVP results in the fusion of these vesicles with the apical membrane of the collecting duct cell. Mutations in either the V2 receptor or AQP2 itself result in nephrogenic diabetes insipidus due to failure of the collecting duct to increase water reabsorption in response to AVP. The translocation of AQP2 vesicles to the cell membrane is dependent on AVP-stimulated production of cAMP and the subsequent activation of PKA. Activated PKA is targeted to AQP2-containing vesicles via association with A kinase–anchoring proteins (AKAPs). AKAPs comprise a large family of proteins that localize activated PKA to specific sites within the cell, thus providing specificity and compartmentalization of PKA signaling. Recently, AKAP18δ, PKA, and AQP2 were copurified from vesicles isolated from the cytosol of inner medullary collecting-duct cells, suggesting that this AKAP may be important for facilitating the interaction of PKA and AQP2 (64).

Activated PKA is capable of directly phosphorylating serine 256 in the carboxy-terminus of AQP2. Phosphorylation of this site correlates with membrane translocation of AQP2-containing vesicles, and AQP2 mutant proteins in which this site cannot be phosphorylated fail to insert in the membrane (103). Interestingly, phosphorylation of serine 256 following activation of cGMP by nitric oxide or atrial natriuretic peptide (ANP) can induce translocation of AQP2 to the membrane in an AVP-independent manner (12). How phosphorylation of serine-256 in AQP2 mediates vesicle fusion with the membrane is not yet fully understood. Based on present studies, it appears likely that membrane targeting involves the association of SNARE proteins (such as syntaxin-4) on the AQP2-containing vesicles with SNAP partners (such as SNAP23) at the cell membrane (54, 122).

Similar to the data demonstrating that ENaC function is regulated by several signaling events, AQP2 can be regulated by mechanisms besides trafficking to the membrane. In the setting of continuous stimulation by AVP, total cellular levels of AQP2 message and protein increase, demonstrating that AVP can induce transcription of the AQP2 gene. In vitro experiments have suggested that this is due to transcriptional activation of AQP2 mRNA expression via a cyclic AMP response element (CRE) in the AQP2 promoter (231). Activation of multiple intracellular serine/threonine kinases, including PKA, can stimulate phosphorylation and activation of the CRE-binding protein (CREB), which in turn binds CRE and activates transcription of the appropriate target gene, in this case AQP2. Sustained exposure to hypertonicity can also increase AQP2 mRNA expression in cultured collecting duct cells, independent of AVP-mediated PKA activation (61).

TRANSPORTERS SUCH AS ROMK CAN BE REGULATED BY CHANGES IN THEIR ACTIVE STATE

A third way in which transporters can be regulated is via alteration of the active state of the protein. For membrane channels this typically means a change in the open probability (P_o) of the channel (the time that the channel spends in the open configuration). ROMK (also known as Kir1.1) is an apical membrane potassium channel in thick ascending limb cells and principal cells that is required for potassium recycling in the TAL and potassium secretion in the collecting duct (reviewed in Wang [220]). One of the major determinants of P_o for ROMK is the concentration of PIP$_2$ in the membrane in the vicinity of the channel, an effect that appears to be due to an extensive series of interactions between the basic amino acids in the carboxy-terminus of ROMK and the negatively charged head groups of the membrane phospholipids (reviewed in Hebert et al. [63]). PIP$_2$ is produced by lipid kinases such as PI(4)P$_5$ kinase and degraded by phospholipases such as PLA$_2$ and PLC (reviewed in Doughman et al. [34] and Heath et al. [62]). Thus, it is speculated that signals that enhance PIP$_2$ production or inhibit its degradation will increase ROMK activity at the membrane.

Alterations in the P_o for ROMK have also been found to be due to direct phosphorylation of the channel by PKA (reviewed in Hebert et al. [63]). In vitro studies have demonstrated three PKA phosphorylation sites in ROMK, and phosphorylation of two of those sites (serine 219 and 313)

causes an increase in P_o for the channel without changing the number of the channels at the membrane. As with other PKA effectors, the presence of the appropriate AKAP is required to target activated PKA to ROMK at the membrane. Although the precise mechanism by which PKA phosphorylation regulates P_o in ROMK has yet to be determined, it appears that at least part of the effect is due to an increased affinity of ROMK for PIP$_2$, thus reducing the concentration of PIP$_2$ needed to support the channel in the open state (112). Based on these studies, it is presently believed that the AVP-stimulated increase in thick ascending-limb potassium recycling is due to V2-dependent activation of PKA and subsequent phosphorylation and activation of ROMK (159).

Similar to the regulation of aquaporin-2 and ENaC, ROMK can also be regulated by altering channel location or synthesis. Several kinases have been implicated in regulating the trafficking of ROMK including PKA, SGK and a recently described kinase WNK (with no K [lysine]). As noted above, there are three PKA phosphorylation sites on ROMK. While two of the sites directly regulate channel open probability, phosphorylation of the third residue (serine 44) increases the number of channels present on the cell membrane. In addition to PKA, SGK can phosphorylate ROMK on serine 44 and increase channel activity in the oocyte expression system (235). This appears to occur in concert with a scaffolding protein, NHERF2, which increases trafficking of ROMK to the membrane via its interaction with the carboxy-terminal PDZ-binding motif (234). Thus, the increased expression of SGK following aldosterone stimulation can lead to sustained increases in ROMK-dependent potassium excretion via increased numbers of channels on the cell membrane.

Recently another family of serine/threonine kinases, the WNKs, have been found to play an important role in regulating the activity of diverse ion channels in the kidney (reviewed in Gamba [47]). To date there have been four WNK kinases described in humans, all sharing the unusual substitution of a cysteine residue for the more typical lysine in β strand three of the kinase domain (213). Of these four, WNK1, WNK3, and WNK4 have been directly implicated in regulation of tubular ion transport, including the sodium-potassium-chloride cotransporter in the TAL (NKCC2), the sodium-chloride cotransporter in the distal convoluted tubule (NCC), ROMK, and the tight junctional proteins claudin1–4 that regulate paracellular chloride flux. Mutations of WNK1 and WNK4 have been shown to cause pseudohypoaldosteronism II (PHAII), a syndrome consisting of increased sodium reabsorption, hypertension and hyperkalemia (108, 109, 162) (reviewed in Kahle et al. [85]). Interestingly, it has been demonstrated that WNK4 normally inhibits ROMK trafficking to the cell membrane and that mutations that cause PHAII are gain-of-function in this respect, and thus result in increased ROMK inhibition (84). Similarly, the mutations in WNK1 that have been found in patients with PHAII result in overexpression of the long form of

WNK1, which has been found to stimulate ROMK endocytosis (108). Thus, the hyperkalemia observed in PHAII appears to be due to trafficking defects that result in less ROMK present at the membrane. The precise mechanism of these trafficking defects, and how WNK activity is regulated, remain to be elucidated.

References

1. Afzelius BA. Cilia-related diseases. *J Pathol* 2004;204:470–477.
2. Alessi DR, Kozlowski MT, Weng QP, Morrice N, Avruch J. 3-Phosphoinositide–dependent protein kinase 1 (PDK1) phosphorylates and activates the p70 S6 kinase in vivo and in vitro. *Curr Biol* 1998;8:69–81.
3. Allen V, Swigart P, Cheung R, Cockcroft S, Katan M. Regulation of inositol lipid–specific phospholipase cdelta by changes in Ca2+ ion concentrations. *Biochem J* 1997;327:545–552.
4. Andjelkovic M, Maira SM, Cron P, Parker PJ, Hemmings BA. Domain swapping used to investigate the mechanism of protein kinase B regulation by 3-phosphoinositide–dependent protein kinase 1 and Ser473 kinase. *Mol Cell Biol* 1999;19:5061–5072.
5. Aplin AE, Juliano RL. Integrin and cytoskeletal regulation of growth factor signaling to the MAP kinase pathway. *J Cell Sci* 1999;112:695–706.
6. Arany I, Megyesi JK, Kaneto H, Tanaka S, Safirstein RL. Activation of ERK or inhibition of JNK ameliorates H(2)O(2) cytotoxicity in mouse renal proximal tubule cells. *Kidney Int* 2004;65:1231–1239.
7. Auger KR, Serunian LA, Soltoff SP, Libby P, Cantley LC. PDGF-dependent tyrosine phosphorylation stimulates production of novel polyphosphoinositides in intact cells. *Cell* 1989;57:167–175.
8. Bae YS, Cantley LG, Chen CS, Kim SR, Kwon KS, Rhee SG. Activation of phospholipase C-gamma by phosphatidylinositol 3,4,5-trisphosphate. *J Biol Chem* 1998;273:4465–4469.
9. Balla T. Inositol–lipid binding motifs: signal integrators through protein–lipid and protein–protein interactions. *J Cell Sci* 2005;118:2093–2104.
10. Bonfini L, Karlovich CA, Dasgupta C, Banerjee U. The son of sevenless gene product: a putative activator of Ras. *Science* 1992;255:603–606.
11. Border WA, Noble NA. TGF-beta in kidney fibrosis: a target for gene therapy. *Kidney Int* 1997;51:1388–1396.
12. Bouley R, Breton S, Sun T, McLaughlin M, Nsumu NN, Lin HY, Ausiello DA, Brown D. Nitric oxide and atrial natriuretic factor stimulate cGMP-dependent membrane insertion of aquaporin 2 in renal epithelial cells. *J Clin Invest* 2000;106:1115–1126.
13. Boulton TG, Yancopoulos GD, Gregory JS, Slaughter C, Moomaw C, Hsu J, Cobb MH. An insulin-stimulated protein kinase similar to yeast kinases involved in cell cycle control. *Science* 1990;249:64–67.
14. Brou C, Logeat F, Gupta N, Bessia C, LeBail O, Doedens JR, Cumano A, Roux P, Black RA, Israel A. A novel proteolytic cleavage involved in Notch signaling: the role of the disintegrin-metalloprotease TACE. *Mol Cell* 2000;5:207–216.
15. Brunet A, Bonni A, Zigmond MJ, Lin MZ, Juo P, Hu LS, Anderson MJ, Arden KC, Blenis J, Greenberg ME. Akt promotes cell survival by phosphorylating and inhibiting a forkhead transcription factor. *Cell* 1999;96:857–868.
16. Butterworth MB, Edinger RS, Johnson JP, Frizzell RA. Acute ENaC stimulation by cAMP in a kidney cell line is mediated by exocytic insertion from a recycling channel pool. *J Gen Physiol* 2005;125:81–101.
17. Cai Y, Maeda Y, Cedzich A, Torres VE, Wu G, Hayashi T, Mochizuki T, Park JH, Witzgall R, Somlo S. Identification and characterization of polycystin-2, the PKD2 gene product. *J Biol Chem* 1999;274:28557–28565.
18. Carey RM. Update on the role of the AT2 receptor. *Curr Opin Nephrol Hypertens* 2005;14:67–71.
19. Chen X, Moeckel G, Morrow JD, Cosgrove D, Harris RC, Fogo AB, Zent R, Pozzi A. Lack of integrin alpha1beta1 leads to severe glomerulosclerosis after glomerular injury. *Am J Pathol* 2004;165:617–630.
20. Chen Y, Lasaitiene D, Friberg P. The renin-angiotensin system in kidney development. *Acta Physiol Scand* 2004;181:529–535.
21. Chen Z, Gibson TB, Robinson F, Silvestro L, Pearson G, Xu B, Wright A, Vanderbilt C, Cobb MH. MAP kinases. *Chem Rev* 2001;101:2449–2476.
22. Cheng HT, Kopan R. The role of Notch signaling in specification of podocyte and proximal tubules within the developing mouse kidney. *Kidney Int* 2005;68:1951–1952.
23. Cheng HT, Miner JH, Lin M, Tansey MG, Roth K, Kopan R. Gamma-secretase activity is dispensable for mesenchyme-to-epithelium transition but required for podocyte and proximal tubule formation in developing mouse kidney. *Development* 2003;130:5031–5042.
24. Collins NL, Reginato MJ, Paulus JK, Sgroi DC, Labaer J, Brugge JS. G1/S cell cycle arrest provides anoikis resistance through Erk-mediated Bim suppression. *Mol Cell Biol* 2005;25:5282–5291.
25. Cox EA, Sastry SK, Huttenlocher A. Integrin-mediated adhesion regulates cell polarity and membrane protrusion through the Rho family of GTPases. *Mol Biol Cell* 2001;12:265–277.
26. Crews CM, Alessandrini A, Erikson RL. The primary structure of MEK, a protein kinase that phosphorylates the ERK gene product. *Science* 1992;258:4784–4780.
27. Cross DA, Alessi DR, Cohen P, Andjelkovich M, Hemmings BA. Inhibition of glycogen synthase kinase-3 by insulin mediated by protein kinase B. *Nature* 1995;378:785–789.
28. Davenport JR, Yoder BK. An incredible decade for the primary cilium: a look at a once-forgotten organelle. *Am J Physiol Renal Physiol* 2005;289:F1159–F1169.
29. De Strooper B, Annaert W, Cupers P, Saftig P, Craessaerts K, Mumm JS, Schroeter EH, Schrijvers V, Wolfe MS, Ray WJ, Goate A, Kopan R. A presenilin-1–dependent gamma-secretase-like protease mediates release of Notch intracellular domain. *Nature* 1999;398:518–522.
30. Degl'Innocenti D, Arighi E, Popsueva A, Sangregorio R, Alberti L, Rizzetti MG, Ferrario C, Sariola H, Pierotti MA, Borrello MG. Differential requirement of Tyr1062 multidocking site by RET isoforms to promote neural cell scattering and epithelial cell branching. *Oncogene* 2004;23:7297–7309.
31. DeMali KA, Wennerberg K, Burridge K. Integrin signaling to the actin cytoskeleton. *Curr Opin Cell Biol* 2003;15:572–582.
32. Dhillon AS, Kolch W. Untying the regulation of the Raf-1 kinase. *Arch Biochem Biophys* 2002;404:3–9.
33. Diehl JA, Cheng M, Roussel MF, Sherr CJ. Glycogen synthase kinase-3beta regulates cyclin D1 proteolysis and subcellular localization. *Genes DevGenes Dev* 1998;12:3499–3511.
34. Doughman RL, Firestone AJ, Anderson RA. Phosphatidylinositol phosphate kinases put PI4,5P(2) in its place. *J Membr Biol* 2003;194:77–89.
35. Drees F, Pokutta S, Yamada S, Nelson WJ, Weis WI. Alpha-catenin is a molecular switch that binds E-cadherin–beta-catenin and regulates actin-filament assembly. *Cell* 2005;123:903–915.
36. Edin ML, Juliano RL. Raf-1 serine 338 phosphorylation plays a key role in adhesion-dependent activation of extracellular signal-regulated kinase by epidermal growth factor. *Mol Cell Biol* 2005;25:4466–4475.
37. Efendiev R, Bertorello AM, Pressley TA, Rousselot M, Feraille E, Pedemonte CH. Simultaneous phosphorylation of Ser11 and Ser18 in the alpha-subunit promotes the recruitment of Na(+),K(+)-ATPase molecules to the plasma membrane. *Biochemistry* 2000;39:9884–9892.
38. Efendiev R, Budu CE, Cinelli AR, Bertorello AM, Pedemonte CH. Intracellular Na+ regulates dopamine and angiotensin II receptors availability at the plasma membrane and their cellular responses in renal epithelia. *J Biol Chem* 2003;278:28719–28726. Epub May 20, 2003.
39. Eguchi S, Numaguchi K, Iwasaki H, Matsumoto T, Yamakawa T, Utsunomiya H, Motley ED, Kawakatsu H, Owada KM, Hirata Y, Marumo F, Inagami T. Calcium-dependent epidermal growth factor receptor transactivation mediates the angiotensin II–induced mitogen-activated protein kinase activation in vascular smooth muscle cells. *J Biol Chem* 1998;273:8890–8896.
40. Fagotto F, Guger K, Gumbiner BM. Induction of the primary dorsalizing center in *Xenopus* by the Wnt/GSK/beta-catenin signaling pathway, but not by Vg1, Activin or Noggin. *Development* 1997;124:453–460.
41. Fingar DC, Blenis J. Target of rapamycin (TOR): an integrator of nutrient and growth factor signals and coordinator of cell growth and cell cycle progression. *Oncogene* 2004;23:3151–1571.
42. Flannery PJ, Spurney RF. Transactivation of the epidermal growth factor receptor by angiotensin ii in glomerular podocytes. *Nephron Exp Nephrol* 2006;103:e109–e118.
43. Fortini ME. Gamma-secretase–mediated proteolysis in cell-surface –receptor signalling. *Nat Rev Mol Cell Biol* 2002;3:673–684.
44. Foster RH. Reciprocal influences between the signalling pathways regulating proliferation and steroidogenesis in adrenal glomerulosa cells. *J Mol Endocrinol* 2004;32:893–902.
45. Frisch SM, Vuori K, Kelaita D, Sicks S. A role for Jun-N-terminal kinase in anoikis; suppression by bcl-2 and crmA. *J Cell Biol* 1996; 135:1377–1382.
46. Fujikawa A, Shirasaka D, Yamamoto S, Ota H, Yahiro K, Fukada M, Shintani T, Wada A, Aoyama N, Hirayama T, Fukamachi H, Noda M. Mice deficient in protein tyrosine phosphatase receptor type Z are resistant to gastric ulcer induction by VacA of Helicobacter pylori. *Nat Genet* 2003;33:375–381. Epub Feb 24, 2003.
47. Gamba G. Role of WNK kinases in regulating tubular salt and potassium transport and in the development of hypertension. *Am J Physiol Renal Physiol* 2005;288:F245–F252.
48. Gao L, Joberty G, Macara IG. Assembly of epithelial tight junctions is negatively regulated by Par6. *Curr Biol* 2002;12:221–225.
49. Gardner H, Kreidberg J, Koteliansky V, Jaenisch R. Deletion of integrin alpha 1 by homologous recombination permits normal murine development but gives rise to a specific deficit in cell adhesion. *Dev Biol* 1996;175:301–313.
50. Gensure RC, Gardella TJ, Juppner H. Parathyroid hormone and parathyroid hormone-related peptide, and their receptors. *Biochem Biophys Res Commun* 2005;328:666–678.
51. Gille H, Kortenjann M, Thomae O, Moomaw C, Slaughter C, Cobb MH, Shaw PE. ERK phosphorylation potentiates Elk-1–mediated ternary complex formation and transactivation. *EMBO J* 1995;14:951–962.
52. Gomes P, Soares-da-Silva P. Role of cAMP-PKA-PLC signaling cascade on dopamine-induced PKC-mediated inhibition of renal Na(+)-K(+)-ATPase activity. *Am J Physiol Renal Physiol* 2004;F1084–F1096.
53. Gonzalez-Perrett S, Kim K, Ibarra C, Damiano AE, Zotta E, Batelli M, Harris PC, Reisin IL, Arnaout MA, Cantiello HF. Polycystin-2, the protein mutated in autosomal dominant polycystic kidney disease (ADPKD), is a Ca2+-permeable nonselective cation channel. *Proc Natl Acad Sci U S A* 2001;98:1182–1187.
54. Gouraud S, Laera A, Carmosino M, Procino G, Rossetto O, Mannucci R, Rosenthal W, Svelto M, Valenti G. Functional involvement of VAMP/synaptobrevin-2 in cAMP-stimulated aquaporin 2 translocation in renal collecting duct cells. *J Cell Sci* 2002; 115:3667–3674.
55. Gumbiner BM. Regulation of cadherin-mediated adhesion in morphogenesis. *Nat Rev Mol Cell Biol* 2005;6:622–634.
56. Guo J, Chung UI, Kondo H, Bringhurst FR, Kronenberg HM. The PTH/PTHrP receptor can delay chondrocyte hypertrophy in vivo without activating phospholipase C. *Dev Cell* 2002;3:183–194.
57. Haendeler J, Yin G, Hojo Y, Saito Y, Melaragno M, Yan C, Sharma VK, Heller M, Aebersold R, Berk BC. GIT1 mediates Src-dependent activation of phospholipase Cgamma by angiotensin II and epidermal growth factor. *J Biol Chem* 2003;278:49936–49944. Epub Sep 30, 2003.
58. Hall MC, Young DA, Waters JG, Rowan AD, Chantry A, Edwards DR, Clark IM. The comparative role of activator protein 1 and Smad factors in the regulation of Timp-1 and MMP-1 gene expression by transforming growth factor–beta 1. *J Biol Chem* 2003;278:10304–10313. Epub Jan 13, 2003.

59. Hanaoka K, Qian F, Boletta A, Bhunia AK, Piontek K, Tsiokas L, Sukhatme VP, Guggino WB, Germino GG. Co-assembly of polycystin-1 and -2 produces unique cation-permeable currents. *Nature* 2000; 408:990–994.
60. Hansson JH, Nelson-Williams C, Suzuki H, Schild L, Shimkets R, Lu Y, Canessa C, Iwasaki T, Rossier B, Lifton RP. Hypertension caused by a truncated epithelial sodium channel gamma subunit: genetic heterogeneity of Liddle syndrome. *Nat Genet* 1995;11:76–82.
61. Hasler U, Vinciguerra M, Vandewalle A, Martin PY, Feraille E. Dual effects of hypertonicity on aquaporin-2 expression in cultured renal collecting duct principal cells. *J Am Soc Nephrol* 2005;16:1571–1582. Epub Apr 20, 2005.
62. Heath CM, Stahl PD, Barbieri MA. Lipid kinases play crucial and multiple roles in membrane trafficking and signaling. *Histol Histopathol* 2003;18:989–998.
63. Hebert SC, Desir G, Giebisch G, Wang W. Molecular diversity and regulation of renal potassium channels. *Physiol Rev Physiol Rev* 2005;85:319–371.
64. Henn V, Edemir B, Stefan E, Wiesner B, Lorenz D, Theilig F, Schmitt R, Vossebein L, Tamma G, Beyermann M, Krause E, Herberg FW, Valenti G, Bachmann S, Rosenthal W, Klussmann E. Identification of a novel A-kinase anchoring protein 18 isoform and evidence for its role in the vasopressin-induced aquaporin-2 shuttle in renal principal cells. *J Biol Chem* 2004;279:26654–26665. Epub Mar 22, 2004.
65. Holgado-Madruga M, Emlet DR, Moscatello DK, Godwin AK, Wong AJ. A Grb2–associated docking protein in EGF- and insulin-receptor signalling. *Nature* 1996;379:560–564.
66. Hou X, Mrug M, Yoder BK, Lefkowitz EJ, Kremmidiotis G, D'Eustachio P, Beier DR, Guay-Woodford LM. Cystin, a novel cilia-associated protein, is disrupted in the cpk mouse model of polycystic kidney disease. *J Clin Invest* 2002;109:53 3–5340.
67. Hu MC, Piscione TD, Rosenblum ND. Elevated SMAD1/sbeta-catenin molecular complexes and renal medullary cystic dysplasia in ALK3 transgenic mice. *Development* 2003; 130:2753–2766.
68. Hung CC, Ichimura T, Stevens JL, Bonventre JV. Protection of renal epithelial cells against oxidative injury by endoplasmic reticulum stress preconditioning is mediated by ERK1/2 activation. *J Biol Chem* 2003;278:29317–29326. Epub May 8, 2003.
69. Im SH, Rao A. Activation and deactivation of gene expression by Ca2+/calcineurin-NFAT–mediated signaling. *Mol Cells* 2004;18:1–9.
70. Isaka Y, Fujiwara Y, Ueda N, Kaneda Y, Kamada T, Imai E. Glomerulosclerosis induced by in vivo transfection of transforming growth factor-beta or platelet-derived growth factor gene into the rat kidney. *J Clin Invest* 1993;92:2597–2601.
71. Isakov N, Altman A. Protein kinase C(theta) in T cell activation. *Annu Rev Immunol* 2002;20:761–794.
72. Ishibashi K, Sasaki S, Fushimi K, Uchida S, Kuwahara M, Saito H, Furukawa T, Nakajima K, Yamaguchi Y, Gojobori T, et al. Molecular cloning and expression of a member of the aquaporin family with permeability to glycerol and urea in addition to water expressed at the basolateral membrane of kidney collecting duct cells. *Proc Natl Acad Sci U S A* 1994;91:6269–6273.
73. Ishibashi K, Sasaki S, Sakamoto H, Hoshino Y, Nakamura T, Marumo F. Expressions of receptor gene for hepatocyte growth factor in kidney after unilateral nephrectomy and renal injury. *Biochem Biophys Res Commun* 1992;187:1454–1459.
74. Ishibe S, Joly D, Liu ZX, Cantley LG. Paxillin serves as an ERK-regulated scaffold for coordinating FAK and Rac activation in epithelial morphogenesis. *Mol Cell* 2004;16: 257–267.
75. Ishibe S, Joly D, Zhu X, Cantley LG. Phosphorylation-dependent paxillin-ERK association mediates hepatocyte growth factor–stimulated epithelial morphogenesis. *Mol Cell* 2003; 12:1275–1285.
76. Ishiki M, Klip A. Minireview: recent developments in the regulation of glucose transporter-4 traffic: new signals, locations, and partners. *Endocrinology* 2005;146:5071–5078. Epub Sep 8, 2005.
77. Ito M, Nakano T, Erdodi F, Hartshorne DJ. Myosin phosphatase: structure, regulation and function. *Mol Cell Biochem* 2004;259–:197–209.
78. Iwashima M, Irving BA, van Oers NS, Chan AC, Weiss A. Sequential interactions of the TCR with two distinct cytoplasmic tyrosine kinases. *Science* 1994;263:1136–1139.
79. Joannidis M, Spokes K, Nakamura T, Faletto D, Cantley LG. Regional expression of hepatocyte growth factor/c-met in experimental renal hypertrophy and hyperplasia. *Am J Physiol* 1994;267:F231–F236.
80. Jobert AS, Zhang P, Couvineau A, Bonaventure J, Roume J, Le Merrer M, Silve C. Absence of functional receptors for parathyroid hormone and parathyroid hormone-related peptide in Blomstrand chondrodysplasia. *J Clin Invest* 1998;102:34–40.
81. Joberty G, Petersen C, Gao L, Macara IG. The cell-polarity protein Par6 links Par3 and atypical protein kinase C to Cdc42. *Nat Cell Biol* 2000;2:531–539.
82. Jose PA, Eisner GM, Felder RA. Renal dopamine and sodium homeostasis. *Curr Hypertens Rep* 2000;2:174–183.
83. Jose PA, Eisner GM, Felder RA. Role of dopamine receptors in the kidney in the regulation of blood pressure. *Curr Opin Nephrol Hypertens* 2002;11:87–92.
84. Kahle KT, Gimenez I, Hassan H, Wilson FH, Wong RD, Forbush B, Aronson PS, Lifton RP. WNK4 regulates apical and basolateral Cl- flux in extrarenal epithelia. *Proc Natl Acad Sci U S A* 2004;101:2064–2069. Epub Feb 9, 2004.
85. Kahle KT, Wilson FH, Lifton RP. Regulation of diverse ion transport pathways by WNK4 kinase: a novel molecular switch. *Trends Endocrinol Metab* 2005;16:98–103.
86. Kanaide H, Ichiki T, Nishimura J, Hirano K. Cellular mechanism of vasoconstriction induced by angiotensin II: it remains to be determined. *Circ Res* 2003;93:1015–1017.
87. Katso R, Okkenhaug K, Ahmadi K, White S, Timms J, Waterfield MD. Cellular function of phosphoinositide 3-kinases: implications for development, homeostasis, and cancer. *Annu Rev Cell Dev Biol* 2001;17:615–675.
88. Kawachi H, Fujikawa A, Maeda N, Noda M. Identification of GIT1/Cat-1 as a substrate molecule of protein tyrosine phosphatase zeta /beta by the yeast substrate-trapping system. *Proc Natl Acad Sci U S A* 2001;98:6593–6598. Epub May 29, 2001.
89. Kelley GG, Reks SE, Ondrako JM, Smrcka AV. Phospholipase C(epsilon): a novel Ras effector. *EMBO J* 2001;20:743–754.
90. Kim J, Ahn S, Ren XR, Whalen EJ, Reiter E, Wei H, Lefkowitz RJ. Functional antagonism of different G protein-coupled receptor kinases for beta-arrestin–mediated angiotensin II receptor signaling. *Proc Natl Acad Sci U S A* 2005;102:1442–1447. Epub 2005 Jan 25.
91. Kispert A, Vainio S, McMahon AP. Wnt-4 is a mesenchymal signal for epithelial transformation of metanephric mesenchyme in the developing kidney. *Development* 1998;125: 4225–4234.
92. Klemke RL, Cai S, Giannini AL, Gallagher PJ, de Lanerolle P, Cheresh DA. Regulation of cell motility by mitogen-activated protein kinase. *J Cell Biol* 1997;137:481–492.
93. Kobayashi H, Shiraishi S, Yanagita T, Yokoo H, Yamamoto R, Minami S, Saitoh T, Wada A. Regulation of voltage-dependent sodium channel expression in adrenal chromaffin cells: involvement of multiple calcium signaling pathways. *Ann N Y Acad Sci* 2002;971:127–134.
94. Kobayashi S, Shirai T, Kiyokawa E, Mochizuki N, Matsuda M, Fukui Y. Membrane recruitment of DOCK180 by binding to PtdIns(3,4,5)P3. *Biochem J* 2001;354:73–78.
95. Kolch W. Coordinating ERK/MAPK signalling through scaffolds and inhibitors. *Nat Rev Mol Cell Biol* 2005;6:827–837.
96. Kolch W, Heidecker G, Kochs G, Hummel R, Vahidi H, Mischak H, Finkenzeller G, Marme D, Rapp UR. Protein kinase C alpha activates RAF-1 by direct phosphorylation. *Nature* 1993;364:249–252.
97. Korinek V, Barker N, Morin PJ, van Wichen D, de Weger R, Kinzler KW, Vogelstein B, Clevers H. Constitutive transcriptional activation by a beta-catenin-Tcf complex in APC−/−colon carcinoma. *Science* 1997;275:1784–1787.
98. Koshikawa M, Mukoyama M, Mori K, Suganami T, Sawai K, Yoshioka T, Nagae T, Yokoi H, Kawachi H, Shimizu F, Sugawara A, Nakao K. Role of p38 mitogen-activated protein kinase activation in podocyte injury and proteinuria in experimental nephrotic syndrome. *J Am Soc Nephrol* 2005;16:2690–701. Epub June 29, 2005.
99. Kovacs CS, Lanske B, Hunzelman JL, Guo J, Karaplis AC, Kronenberg HM. Parathyroid hormone-related peptide (PTHrP) regulates fetal-placental calcium transport through a receptor distinct from the PTH/PTHrP receptor. *Proc Natl Acad Sci U S A* 1996;93:15233–15238.
100. Krasel C, Bunemann M, Lorenz K, Lohse MJ. Beta-arrestin binding to the beta2–adrenergic receptor requires both receptor phosphorylation and receptor activation. *J Biol Chem* 2005;280:9528–9535. Epub Jan 5, 2005.
101. Kreidberg JA, Donovan MJ, Goldstein SL, Rennke H, Shepherd K, Jones RC, Jaenisch R. Alpha 3 beta 1 integrin has a crucial role in kidney and lung organogenesis. *Development* 1996;122:3537–3547.
102. Kubicek M, Pacher M, Abraham D, Podar K, Eulitz M, Baccarini M. Dephosphorylation of Ser-259 regulates Raf-1 membrane association. *J Biol Chem* 2002;277:7913–7919.
103. Kuwahara M, Fushimi K, Terada Y, Bai L, Marumo F, Sasaki S. cAMP-dependent phosphorylation stimulates water permeability of aquaporin-collecting duct water channel protein expressed in *Xenopus* oocytes. *J Biol Chem* 1995;270:10384–10387.
104. Kwon TH, Nielsen J, Kim YH, Knepper MA, Frokiaer J, Nielsen S. Regulation of sodium transporters in the thick ascending limb of rat kidney: response to angiotensin II. *Am J Physiol Renal Physiol* 2003;285:F152–F165. Epub Mar 25, 2003.
105. Lanske B, Karaplis AC, Lee K, Luz A, Vortkamp A, Pirro A, Karperien M, Defize LH, Ho C, Mulligan RC, Abou-Samra AB, Juppner H, Segre GV, Kronenberg HM. PTH/PTHrP receptor in early development and Indian hedgehog–regulated bone growth. *Science* 1996;273:663–666.
106. Lawson KA, Dunn NR, Roelen BA, Zeinstra LM, Davis AM, Wright CV, Korving JP, Hogan BL. Bmp4 is required for the generation of primordial germ cells in the mouse embryo. *Genes Dev* 1999;13:424–436.
107. Lazarovits AI, Poppema S, Zhang Z, Khandaker M, Le Feuvre CE, Singhal SK, Garcia BM, Ogasa N, Jevnikar AM, White MH, Singh G, Stiller CR, Zhong RZ. Prevention and reversal of renal allograft rejection by antibody against CD45RB. *Nature* 1996;380: 717–720.
108. Lazrak A, Liu Z, Huang CL. Antagonistic regulation of ROMK by long and kidney-specific WNK1 isoforms. *Proc Natl Acad Sci U S A* 2006;103:1615–620. Epub Jan 20, 2006.
109. Leng Q, Kahle KT, Rinehart J, Macgregor GG, Wilson FH, Canessa CM, Lifton RP, Hebert SC. WNK3, a kinase related to genes mutated in hereditary hypertension with hyperkalemia, regulates the K+ channel ROMK1 (Kir1.). *J Physiol* 2005;15:15.
110. Letamendia A, Lastres P, Botella LM, Raab U, Langa C, Velasco B, Attisano L, Bernabeu C. Role of endoglin in cellular responses to transforming growth factor-beta. A comparative study with betaglycan. *J Biol Chem* 1998;273:33011–33019.
111. Li H, Liu TF, Lazrak A, Peracchia C, Goldberg GS, Lampe PD, Johnson RG. Properties and regulation of gap junctional hemichannels in the plasma membranes of cultured cells. *J Cell Biol* 1996;134:1019–1030.
112. Liou HH, Zhou SS, Huang CL. Regulation of ROMK1 channel by protein kinase A via a phosphatidylinositol 4,5–bisphosphate-dependent mechanism. *Proc Natl Acad Sci U S A* 1999;96:5820–5825.
113. Liu W, Murcia NS, Duan Y, Weinbaum S, Yoder BK, Schwiebert E, Satlin LM. Mechanoregulation of intracellular Ca2+ concentration is attenuated in collecting duct of monocilium-impaired orpk mice. *Am J Physiol Renal Physiol* 2005;289:F978–F988. Epub Jun 21, 2005.
114. Liu ZX, Yu CF, Nickel C, Thomas S, Cantley LG. Hepatocyte growth factor induces ERK-dependent paxillin phosphorylation and regulates paxillin-focal adhesion kinase association. *J Biol Chem* 2002;277:10452–10458. Epub Jan 9, 2002.
115. Lowenstein EJ, Daly RJ, Batzer AG, Li W, Margolis B, Lammers R, Ullrich A, Skolnik EY, Bar-Sagi D, Schlessinger J. The SH2 and SH3 domain-containing protein GRB2 links receptor tyrosine kinases to ras signaling. *Cell* 1992;70:431–442.
116. Luo K, Lodish HF. Signaling by chimeric erythropoietin-TGF-beta receptors: homodimerization of the cytoplasmic domain of the type I TGF-beta receptor and heterodimerization with the type II receptor are both required for intracellular signal transduction. *EMBO J* 1996;15:4485–4496.
117. Macian F, Lopez-Rodriguez C, Rao A. Partners in transcription: NFAT and AP-1. *Oncogene* 2001;20:2476–489.

118. Maeda N, Nishiwaki T, Shintani T, Hamanaka H, Noda M. 6B4 proteoglycan/phosphacan, an extracellular variant of receptor-like protein-tyrosine phosphatase zeta/RPTPbeta, binds pleiotrophin/heparin-binding growth-associated molecule (HB-GAM). *J Biol Chem* 1996;271:21446–1452.
119. Majumdar A, Vainio S, Kispert A, McMahon J, McMahon AP. Wnt11 and Ret/Gdnf pathways cooperate in regulating ureteric branching during metanephric kidney development. *Development* 2003;130:3175–185.
120. Malbon CC. G proteins in development. *Nat Rev Mol Cell Biol* 2005;6:689–6701.
121. Manabe R, Kovalenko M, Webb DJ, Horwitz AR. GIT1 functions in a motile, multimolecular signaling complex that regulates protrusive activity and cell migration. *J Cell Sci* 2002; 115:1497–1510.
122. Mandon B, Chou CL, Nielsen S, Knepper MA. Syntaxin-4 is localized to the apical plasma membrane of rat renal collecting duct cells: possible role in aquaporin-2 trafficking. *J Clin Invest* 1996;98:906–913.
123. Manning BD, Cantley LC. United at last: the tuberous sclerosis complex gene products connect the phosphoinositide 3-kinase/Akt pathway to mammalian target of rapamycin (mTOR) signalling. *Biochem Soc Trans* 2003;31:573–578.
124. Maroun CR, Naujokas MA, Holgado-Madruga M, Wong AJ, Park M. The tyrosine phosphatase SHP-2 is required for sustained activation of extracellular signal-regulated kinase and epithelial morphogenesis downstream from the met receptor tyrosine kinase. *Mol Cell Biol* 2000;20:8513–8525.
125. Marshall CJ. Specificity of receptor tyrosine kinase signaling: transient versus sustained extracellular signal-regulated kinase activation. *Cell* 1995;80:179–185.
126. Meng K, Rodriguez-Pena A, Dimitrov T, Chen W, Yamin M, Noda M, Deuel TF. Pleiotrophin signals increased tyrosine phosphorylation of β-catenin through inactivation of the intrinsic catalytic activity of the receptor-type protein tyrosine phosphatase β/ζ. *Proc Natl Acad Sci U S A* 2000;97:2603–2608.
127. Miller SB, Martin DR, Kissane J, Hammerman MR. Hepatocyte growth factor accelerates recovery from acute ischemic renal injury in rats. *Am J Physiol* 1994;266:F129–F134.
128. Miner JH. Renal basement membrane components. *Kidney Int* 1999;56:2016–2024.
129. Miner JH, Li C. Defective glomerulogenesis in the absence of laminin alpha5 demonstrates a developmental role for the kidney glomerular basement membrane. *Dev Biol* 2000;217:278–289.
130. Missale C, Nash SR, Robinson SW, Jaber M, Caron MG. Dopamine receptors: from structure to function. *Physiol Rev* 1998;78:189–225.
131. Miura S, Saku K, Karnik SS. Molecular analysis of the structure and function of the angiotensin II type 1 receptor. *Hypertens Res* 2003; 26:937–943.
132. Miyazaki Y, Oshima K, Fogo A, Hogan BL, Ichikawa I. Bone morphogenetic protein 4 regulates the budding site and elongation of the mouse ureter. *J Clin Invest* 2000;105:863–873.
133. Molenaar M, van de Wetering M, Oosterwegel M, Peterson-Maduro J, Godsave S, Korinek V, Roose J, Destree O, Clevers H. XTcf-3 transcription factor mediates beta-catenin–induced axis formation in *Xenopus* embryos. *Cell* 1996;86:391–399.
134. Mustelin T, Coggeshall KM, Altman A. Rapid activation of the T-cell tyrosine protein kinase pp56lck by the CD45 phosphotyrosine phosphatase. *Proc Natl Acad Sci U S A* 1989;86:6302–6306.
135. Mustelin T, Tasken K. Positive and negative regulation of T-cell activation through kinases and phosphatases. *Biochem J* 2003;371:15–27.
136. Nagahama T, Hayashi K, Ozawa Y, Takenaka T, Saruta T. Role of protein kinase C in angiotensin II–induced constriction of renal microvessels. *Kidney Int* 2000;57:215–223.
137. Nakamura A, Hayashi K, Ozawa Y, Fujiwara K, Okubo K, Kanda T, Wakino S, Saruta T. Vessel- and vasoconstrictor-dependent role of rho/rho-kinase in renal microvascular tone. *J Vasc Res* 2003;40:244–251.
138. Nakao A, Afrakhte M, Moren A, Nakayama T, Christian JL, Heuchel R, Itoh S, Kawabata M, Heldin NE, Heldin CH, ten Dijke P. Identification of Smad7, a TGFbeta-inducible antagonist of TGF-beta signalling. *Nature* 1997;389:631–635.
139. Naray-Fejes-Toth A, Fejes-Toth G. The sgk, an aldosterone-induced gene in mineralocorticoid target cells, regulates the epithelial sodium channel. *Kidney Int* 2000;57:1290–1294.
140. Nauli SM, Alenghat FJ, Luo Y, Williams E, Vassilev P, Li X, Elia AE, Lu W, Brown EM, Quinn SJ, Ingber DE, Zhou J. Polycystins 1 and 2 mediate mechanosensation in the primary cilium of kidney cells. *Nat Genet* 2003;33:129–137. Epub Jan 6, 2003.
141. Nauli SM, Zhou J. Polycystins and mechanosensation in renal and nodal cilia. *Bioessays* 2004;26:844–856.
142. Nguyen A, Burack WR, Stock JL, Kortum R, Chaika OV, Afkarian M, Muller WJ, Murphy KM, Morrison DK, Lewis RE, McNeish J, Shaw AS. Kinase suppressor of Ras (KSR) is a scaffold which facilitates mitogen-activated protein kinase activation in vivo. *Mol Cell Biol* 2002;22:3035–3045.
143. Ni CY, Murphy MP, Golde TE, Carpenter G. gamma-Secretase cleavage and nuclear localization of ErbB-4 receptor tyrosine kinase. *Science* 2001;29454:2179–2181. Epub Oct 25, 2001.
144. Nony PA, Schnellmann RG. Mechanisms of renal cell repair and regeneration after acute renal failure. *J Pharmacol Exp Ther* 2003;304:905–912.
145. Oh SP, Seki T, Goss KA, Imamura T, Yi Y, Donahoe PK, Li L, Miyazono K, ten Dijke P, Kim S, Li E. Activin receptor-like kinase 1 modulates transforming growth factor-beta 1 signaling in the regulation of angiogenesis. *Proc Natl Acad Sci U S A* 2000;97:2626–2631.
146. Palmby TR, Abe K, Der CJ. Critical role of the pleckstrin homology and cysteine-rich domains in Vav signaling and transforming activity. *J Biol Chem* 2002;277:39350–39359. Epub Aug 12, 2002.
147. Pap M, Cooper GM. Role of translation initiation factor 2B in control of cell survival by the phosphatidylinositol 3–kinase/Akt/glycogen synthase kinase 3beta signaling pathway. *Mol Cell Biol* 2002;22:578–586.
148. Park D, Jhon DY, Lee CW, Lee KH, Rhee SG. Activation of phospholipase C isozymes by G protein beta gamma subunits. *J Biol Chem* 1993;268:4573–4576.
149. Park D, Jhon DY, Lee CW, Ryu SH, Rhee SG. Removal of the carboxyl-terminal region of phospholipase C-beta 1 by calpain abolishes activation by G alpha q. *J Biol Chem* 1993;68:3710–3714.
150. Park KM, Kramers C, Vayssier-Taussat M, Chen A, Bonventre JV. Prevention of kidney ischemia/reperfusion-induced functional injury, MAPK and MAPK kinase activation, and inflammation by remote transient ureteral obstruction. *J Biol Chem* 2001;277:2040–2049. Epub Nov 5, 2001.
151. Park MY, Lee RH, Lee SH, Jung JS. Apoptosis induced by inhibition of contact with extracellular matrix in mouse collecting duct cells. *Nephron* 1999;83:341–351.
152. Pedemonte CH, Pressley TA, Lokhandwala MF, Cinelli AR. Regulation of Na,K-ATPase transport activity by protein kinase C. *J Membr Biol* 1997;155:219–227.
153. Peles E, Nativ M, Campbell PL, Sakurai T, Martinez R, Lev S, Clary DO, Schilling J, Barnea G, Plowman GD, Grumet M, Schlessinger J. The carbonic anhydrase domain of receptor tyrosine phosphatase beta is a functional ligand for the axonal cell recognition molecule contactin. *Cell* 1995;82:251–260.
154. Pozzi A, Zent R. Integrins: sensors of extracellular matrix and modulators of cell function. *Nephron Exp Nephrol* 2003;94:e77–e84.
155. Praetorius HA, Spring KR. A physiological view of the primary cilium. *Annu Rev Physiol* 2005;67:515–529.
156. Qiao M, Shapiro P, Kumar R, Passaniti A. Insulin-like growth factor–1 regulates endogenous RUNX2 activity in endothelial cells through a phosphatidylinositol 3-kinase/ERK-dependent and Akt-independent signaling pathway. *J Biol Chem* 2004;279:42709–42718. Epub Aug 9, 2004.
157. Racusen LC, Fivush BA, Li YL, Slatnik I, Solez K. Dissociation of tubular cell detachment and tubular cell death in clinical and experimental "acute tubular necrosis." *Lab Invest* 1991;64:546–556.
158. Rangel LB, Caruso-Neves C, Lara LS, Lopes AG. Angiotensin II stimulates renal proximal tubule Na(+)-ATPase activity through the activation of protein kinase C. *Biochim Biophys Acta* 2002;1564:310–316.
159. Reeves WB, McDonald GA, Mehta P, Andreoli TE. Activation of K+ channels in renal medullary vesicles by cAMP-dependent protein kinase. *J Membr Biol* 1989;109:65–72.
160. Reginato MJ, Mills KR, Paulus JK, Lynch DK, Sgroi DC, Debnath J, Muthuswamy SK, Brugge JS. Integrins and EGFR coordinately regulate the pro-apoptotic protein Bim to prevent anoikis. *Nat Cell Biol* 2003;5:733–740.
161. Rhee SG. Regulation of phosphoinositide-specific phospholipase C. *Annu Rev Biochem* 2001;70:281–312.
162. Rinehart J, Kahle KT, de Los Heros P, Vazquez N, Meade P, Wilson FH, Hebert SC, Gimenez I, Gamba G, Lifton RP. WNK3 kinase is a positive regulator of NKCC2 and NCC, renal cation-Cl- cotransporters required for normal blood pressure homeostasis. *Proc Natl Acad Sci U S A* 2005;102:16777–167782. Epub Nov 7, 2005.
163. Rogers KK, Jou TS, Guo W, Lipschutz JH. The Rho family of small GTPases is involved in epithelial cystogenesis and tubulogenesis. *Kidney Int* 2003;63:1632–1644.
164. Rogerson FM, Brennan FE, Fuller PJ. Mineralocorticoid receptor binding, structure and function. *Mol Cell Endocrinol* 2004;217:203–212.
165. Ron D, Kazanietz MG. New insights into the regulation of protein kinase C and novel phorbol ester receptors. *FASEB J* 1999;13:1658–1676.
166. Roovers K, Assoian RK. Integrating the MAP kinase signal into the G1 phase cell cycle machinery. *Bioessays* 2000;22:818–826.
167. Roux PP, Blenis J. ERK and p38 MAPK-activated protein kinases: a family of protein kinases with diverse biological functions. *Microbiol Mol Biol Rev* 2004;68:320–344.
168. Roy M, Li Z, Sacks DB. IQGAP1 is a scaffold for mitogen-activated protein kinase signaling. *Mol Cell Biol* 2005;25:7940–7952.
169. Rubinfeld B, Albert I, Porfiri E, Fiol C, Munemitsu S, Polakis P. Binding of GSK3beta to the APC-beta-catenin complex and regulation of complex assembly. *Science* 1996;272:1023–1026.
170. Sabolic I, Valenti G, Verbavatz JM, Van Hoek AN, Verkman AS, Ausiello DA, Brown D. Localization of the CHIP28 water channel in rat kidney. *Am J Physiol* 1992;263:C1225–Ç1233.
171. Sakurai H, Bush KT, Nigam SK. Identification of pleiotrophin as a mesenchymal factor involved in ureteric bud branching morphogenesis. *Development* 2001;128:3283–3293.
172. Sankar S, Mahooti-Brooks N, Centrella M, McCarthy TL, Madri JA. Expression of transforming growth factor type III receptor in vascular endothelial cells increases their responsiveness to transforming growth factor beta 2. *J Biol Chem* 1995;270:13567–13572.
173. Sariola H, Saarma M. Novel functions and signalling pathways for GDNF. *J Cell Sci* 2003;116:3855–3862.
174. Sato M, Muragaki Y, Saika S, Roberts AB, Ooshima A. Targeted disruption of TGF-beta1/Smad3 signaling protects against renal tubulointerstitial fibrosis induced by unilateral ureteral obstruction. *J Clin Invest* 2003;112:1486–1494.
175. Schiffer M, Bitzer M, Roberts IS, Kopp JB, ten Dijke P, Mundel P, Bottinger EP. Apoptosis in podocytes induced by TGF-beta and Smad7. *J Clin Invest* 2001;108:807–816.
176. Schmitz AA, Govek EE, Bottner B, Van Aelst L. Rho GTPases: signaling, migration, and invasion. *Exp Cell Res* 2000;261:1–12.
177. Schnaper HW, Hayashida T, Hubchak SC, Poncelet AC. TGF-beta signal transduction and mesangial cell fibrogenesis. *Am J Physiol Renal Physiol* 2003;284:F243–F252.
178. Schnizler M, Mastroberardino L, Reifarth F, Weber WM, Verrey F, Clauss W. cAMP sensitivity conferred to the epithelial Na^+ channel by alpha-subunit cloned from guinea-pig colon. *Pflugers Arch* 2000; 439:579–587.
179. Schulz RA, Yutzey KE. Calcineurin signaling and NFAT activation in cardiovascular and skeletal muscle development. *Dev Biol* 2004;266:1–16.
180. Schwartz MA, Assoian RK. Integrins and cell proliferation: regulation of cyclin-dependent kinases via cytoplasmic signaling pathways. *J Cell Sci* 2001;114:2553–2560.
181. Sharma M, Fopma A, Brantley JG, Vanden Heuvel GB. Coexpression of Cux-1 and Notch signaling pathway components during kidney development. *Dev Dyn* 2004;231: 828–838.
182. Siegel JN, Klausner RD, Rapp UR, Samelson LE. T cell antigen receptor engagement stimulates c-raf phosphorylation and induces c-raf–associated kinase activity via a protein kinase C-dependent pathway. *J Biol Chem* 1990;265:18472–18480.
183. Slusarski DC, Corces VG, Moon RT. Interaction of Wnt and a Frizzled homologue triggers G-protein–linked phosphatidylinositol signalling. *Nature* 1997;390:410–413.

184. Snyder PM. Liddle's syndrome mutations disrupt cAMP-mediated translocation of the epithelial Na(+) channel to the cell surface. *J Clin Invest* 2000;105:45–53.

185. Snyder PM. Minireview: regulation of epithelial Na⁺ channel trafficking. *Endocrinology* 2005;146:5079–5085. Epub Sep 8, 2005.

186. Snyder PM, Olson DR, Kabra R, Zhou R, Steines JC. cAMP and serum and glucocorticoid-inducible kinase (SGK) regulate the epithelial Na(+) channel through convergent phosphorylation of Nedd4-2. *J Biol Chem* 2004;279:45753–45758. Epub Aug 24, 2004.

187. Snyder PM, Olson DR, Thomas BC. Serum and glucocorticoid-regulated kinase modulates Nedd4-2-mediated inhibition of the epithelial Na⁺ channel. *J Biol Chem* 2002;277:5–8. Epub Nov 5, 2001.

188. Soh JW, Lee EH, Prywes R, Weinstein IB. Novel roles of specific isoforms of protein kinase C in activation of the c-fos serum response element. *Mol Cell Biol* 1999;19:1313–1324.

189. Songyang Z, Blechner S, Hoagland N, Hoekstra MF, Piwnica-Worms H, Cantley LC. Use of an oriented peptide library to determine the optimal substrates of protein kinases. *Curr Biol* 1994;4:973–982.

190. Stambe C, Atkins RC, Tesch GH, Masaki T, Schreiner GF, Nikolic-Paterson DJ. The role of p38alpha mitogen–activated protein kinase activation in renal fibrosis. *J Am Soc Nephrol* 2004;15:370–379.

191. Steinberg MS, Takeichi M. Experimental specification of cell sorting, tissue spreading, and specific spatial patterning by quantitative differences in cadherin expression. *Proc Natl Acad Sci U S A* 1994;91:206–209.

192. Steinberg SF. Distinctive activation mechanisms and functions for protein kinase Cdelta. *Biochem J* 2004;384:449–459.

193. Strock J, Diverse-Pierluissi MA. Ca2+ channels as integrators of G protein–mediated signaling in neurons. *Mol Pharmacol* 2004;66:1071–1076. Epub Jul 21, 2004.

194. Subauste MC, Pertz O, Adamson ED, Turner CE, Junger S, Hahn KM. Vinculin modulation of paxillin–FAK interactions regulates ERK to control survival and motility. *J Cell Biol* 2004;165:371–381.

195. Summers SA, Kao AW, Kohn AD, Backus GS, Roth RA, Pessin JE, Birnbaum MJ. The role of glycogen synthase kinase 3beta in insulin-stimulated glucose metabolism. *J Biol Chem* 1999;274:17934–17940.

196. Surendran K, Simon TC. CNP gene expression is activated by Wnt signaling and correlates with Wnt4 expression during renal injury. *Am J Physiol Renal Physiol* 2003;284:F653–F662. Epub Dec 10, 2002.

197. Talarmin H, Rescan C, Cariou S, Glaise D, Zanninelli G, Bilodeau M, Loyer P, Guguen-Guillouzo C, Baffet G. The mitogen-activated protein kinase kinase/extracellular signal-regulated kinase cascade activation is a key signalling pathway involved in the regulation of G(1) phase progression in proliferating hepatocytes. *Mol Cell Biol* 1999;19:6003–6011.

198. Tanaka H, Fujita N, Tsuruo T. 3-Phosphoinositide-dependent protein kinase-1–mediated IkappaB kinase beta (IkkB) phosphorylation activates NF-kappaB signaling. *J Biol Chem* 2005;280:40965–40973. Epub Oct 5, 2005.

199. Taulman PD, Haycraft CJ, Balkovetz DF, Yoder BK. Polaris, a protein involved in left-right axis patterning, localizes to basal bodies and cilia. *Mol Biol Cell* 2001;12:589–599.

200. ten Dijke P, Yamashita H, Sampath TK, Reddi AH, Estevez M, Riddle DL, Ichijo H, Heldin CH, Miyazono K. Identification of type I receptors for osteogenic protein-1 and bone morphogenetic protein-4. *J Biol Chem* 1994;269:16985–16988.

201. Terada Y, Tanaka H, Sasaki S. Wnt-4 and Ets-1 signaling pathways for regeneration after acute renal failure. *Kidney Int* 2005;68:1969.

202. Thomas WG, Brandenburger Y, Autelitano DJ, Pham T, Qian H, Hannan RD. Adenoviral-directed expression of the type 1A angiotensin receptor promotes cardiomyocyte hypertrophy via transactivation of the epidermal growth factor receptor. *Circ Res* 2002;90:135–142.

203. Thomson RB, Igarashi P, Biemesderfer D, Kim R, Abu-Alfa A, Soleimani M, Aronson PS. Isolation and cDNA cloning of Ksp-cadherin, a novel kidney-specific member of the cadherin multigene family. *J Biol Chem* 1995;270:17594–17601.

204. Thrane EV, Schwarze PE, Thoresen GH, Lag M, Refsnes M. Persistent versus transient map kinase (ERK) activation in the proliferation of lung epithelial type 2 cells. *Exp Lung Res* 2001;27:387–400.

205. Toker A, Meyer M, Reddy KK, Falck JR, Aneja R, Aneja S, Parra A, Burns DJ, Ballas LM, Cantley LC. Activation of protein kinase C family members by the novel polyphosphoinositides PtdIns-3,4-P2 and PtdIns-3,4,5-P3. *J Biol Chem* 1994;269:32358–32367.

206. Tran TM, Friedman J, Qunaibi E, Baameur F, Moore RH, Clark RB. Characterization of agonist stimulation of cAMP-dependent protein kinase and G protein-coupled receptor kinase phosphorylation of the beta2-adrenergic receptor using phosphoserine-specific antibodies. *Mol Pharmacol* 2004;65:196–206.

207. Tsuchida S, Matsusaka T, Chen X, Okubo S, Niimura F, Nishimura H, Fogo A, Utsunomiya H, Inagami T, Ichikawa I. Murine double nullizygotes of the angiotensin type 1A and 1B receptor genes duplicate severe abnormal phenotypes of angiotensinogen nullizygotes. *J Clin Invest* 1998;101:755–760.

208. Tulasne D, Deheuninck J, Lourenco FC, Lamballe F, Ji Z, Leroy C, Puchois E, Moumen A, Maina F, Mehlen P, Fafeur V. Proapoptotic function of the MET tyrosine kinase receptor through caspase cleavage. *Mol Cell Biol* 2004;24:10328–10339.

209. Turner CE. Paxillin and focal adhesion signalling. *Nat Cell Biol* 2000;2:E231–E236.

210. Valenti G, Procino G, Tamma G, Carmosino M, Svelto M. Minireview: aquaporin 2 trafficking. *Endocrinology* 2005;146:5063–5070. Epub Sep 8, 2005.

211. Van Lint J, Ni Y, Valius M, Merlevede W, Vandenheede JR. Platelet-derived growth factor stimulates protein kinase D through the activation of phospholipase Cgamma and protein kinase C. *J Biol Chem* 1998;273:7038–7043.

212. Vergara L, Bao X, Cooper M, Bello-Reuss E, Reuss L. Gap-junctional hemichannels are activated by ATP depletion in human renal proximal tubule cells. *J Membr Biol* 2003;196:173–184.

213. Verissimo F, Jordan P. WNK kinases, a novel protein kinase subfamily in multi-cellular organisms. *Oncogene* 2001;20:5562–5569.

214. Verrecchia F, Chu ML, Mauviel A. Identification of novel TGF-beta/Smad gene targets in dermal fibroblasts using a combined cDNA microarray/promoter transactivation approach. *J Biol Chem* 2001; 276:17058–17062. Epub Mar 8, 2001.

215. Vidal GA, Naresh A, Marrero L, Jones FE. Presenilin-dependent gamma-secretase processing regulates multiple ERBB4/HER4 activities. *J Biol Chem* 2005;280:19777–19783. Epub Mar 3, 2005.

216. Vikhamar G, Rivedal E, Mollerup S, Sanner T. Role of Cx43 phosphorylation and MAP kinase activation in EGF induced enhancement of cell communication in human kidney epithelial cells. *Cell Adhes Commun* 1998;5:451–460.

217. Vindevoghel L, Lechleider RJ, Kon A, de Caestecker MP, Uitto J, Roberts AB, Mauviel A. SMAD3/4-dependent transcriptional activation of the human type VII collagen gene (COL7A promoter by transforming growth factor beta. *Proc Natl Acad Sci U S A* 1998; 95:14769–14774.

218. Wallingford JB, Habas R. The developmental biology of Dishevelled: an enigmatic protein governing cell fate and cell polarity. *Development* 2005;132:4421–4436.

219. Wang W, Koka V, Lan HY. Transforming growth factor-beta and Smad signalling in kidney diseases. *Nephrology (Carlton)* 2005;10:48–56.

220. Wang WH. Regulation of ROMK (Kir1.1) channels: new mechanisms and aspects. *Am J Physiol Renal Physiol* 2006;290:F14–F19.

221. Wei H, Ahn S, Shenoy SK, Karnik SS, Hunyady L, Luttrell LM, Lefkowitz RJ. Independent beta-arrestin 2 and G protein-mediated pathways for angiotensin II activation of extracellular signal-regulated kinases 1 and 2. *Proc Natl Acad Sci U S A* 2003;100:10782–10787.

222. Weidner KM, Di Cesare S, Sachs M, Brinkmann V, Behrens J, Birchmeier W. Interaction between Gab1 and the c-Met receptor tyrosine kinase is responsible for epithelial morphogenesis. *Nature* 1996;384:173–176.

223. Whitmarsh AJ, Shore P, Sharrocks AD, Davis RJ. Integration of MAP kinase signal transduction pathways at the serum response element. *Science* 1995;269:403–407.

224. Wodarz A, Nusse R. Mechanisms of Wnt signaling in development. *Annu Rev Cell Dev Biol* 1998;14:59–88.

225. Woodgett JR. Recent advances in the protein kinase B signaling pathway. *Curr Opin Cell Biol* 2005;17:150–157.

226. Woodsome TP, Polzin A, Kitazawa K, Eto M, Kitazawa T. Agonist- and depolarization-induced signals for myosin light chain phosphorylation and force generation of cultured vascular smooth muscle cells. *J Cell Sci* 2006;119:1769–1780. Epub Apr 11, 2006.

227. Yamaguchi H, Hendrickson WA. Structural basis for activation of human lymphocyte kinase Lck upon tyrosine phosphorylation. *Nature* 1996;384:484–489.

228. Yang Z, Sibley DR, Jose PA. D5 dopamine receptor knockout mice and hypertension. *J Recept Signal Transduct Res* 2004;24:149–164.

229. Yao J, Morioka T, Li B, Oite T. Coordination of mesangial cell contraction by gap junction–mediated intercellular Ca(2+) wave. *J Am Soc Nephrol* 2002;13:2018–1026.

230. Yao LP, Li XX, Yu PY, Xu J, Asico LD, Jose PA. Dopamine D1 receptor and protein kinase C isoforms in spontaneously hypertensive rats. *Hypertension* 1998;32:1049–1053.

231. Yasui Z, Zelenin SM, Celsi G, Aperia A. Adenylate cyclase–coupled vasopressin receptor activates AQP2 promoter via a dual effect on CRE and AP1 elements. *Am J Physiol* 1997;272: F443–F450.

232. Ying L, Jin L, Palmer T, Webb RC. Angiotensin II up-regulates leukemia-associated rho guanine nucleotide exchange factor (LARG), a RGS domain containing rhoGEF, in vascular smooth muscle cells. *Mol Pharmacol* 2005;14:14.

233. Yoder BK, Hou X, Guay-Woodford LM. The polycystic kidney disease proteins, polycystin-1, polycystin-2, polaris, and cystin, are co-localized in renal cilia. *J Am Soc Nephrol* 2002; 13:2508–2516.

234. Yoo D, Flagg TP, Olsen O, Raghuram V, Foskett JK, Welling PA. Assembly and trafficking of a multiprotein ROMK (Kir 1.1) channel complex by PDZ interactions. *J Biol Chem* 2003;279:6863–6873. Epub Nov 5, 2003.

235. Yoo D, Kim BY, Campo C, Nance L, King A, Maouyo D, Welling PA. Cell surface expression of the ROMK (Kir 1. channel is regulated by the aldosterone-induced kinase, SGK-1, and protein kinase A. *J Biol Chem* 2003;278:23066–23075. Epub Apr 8, 2003.

236. Zarubin T, Han J. Activation and signaling of the p38 MAP kinase pathway. *Cell Res* 2005;15:11–18.

237. Zeng X, Tamai K, Doble B, Li S, Huang H, Habas R, Okamura H, Woodgett J, He X. A dual-kinase mechanism for Wnt co-receptor phosphorylation and activation. *Nature* 2005;438:873–877.

238. Zheng M, McKeown-Longo PJ. Regulation of HEF1 expression and phosphorylation by TGF-beta 1 and cell adhesion. *J Biol Chem* 2002;277:39599–39608. Epub Aug 19, 2002.

239. Zou Z, Chung B, Nguyen T, Mentone S, Thomson B, Biemesderfer D. Linking receptor-mediated endocytosis and cell signaling: evidence for regulated intramembrane proteolysis of megalin in proximal tubule. *J Biol Chem* 2004;279:34302–34310.

CHAPTER 12

Scaffolding Proteins in Transport Regulation

Paul A. Welling
University of Maryland School of Medicine, Baltimore, Maryland, USA

INTRODUCTION

The construction and maintenance of architecture require scaffolds to situate the proper assemblage of trades and tools to the right sites at ideal times. Cells are no different. In recent years, there has been an explosion of discovery about proteins that function as molecular scaffolds, working to dynamically assemble appropriate components of signal transduction cascades with their effectors within different subcellular locales at precise physiologic times. Many of these molecular scaffolds control the assembly, trafficking, subcellular location, and activity of epithelial transport proteins and their regulators and, thus, are critical determinants of epithelial transport modulation. This chapter provides a review of the present state of knowledge about the two major classes of molecular scaffolds, PDZ-proteins and AKAPs, and their role in epithelial transport.

PDZ-PROTEINS

PDZ domains (also known as DHR domains or GLGF repeats) are ~ 90–amino acid, protein–protein interaction modules that bind short amino-acid motifs (four to five residues) generally found at the extreme COOH-terminus of target proteins (161). More rarely, PDZ domains recognize internal sequences that fold into a beta finger conformation and mimic the canonical COOH-terminal PDZ binding motif (61, 67). The term *PDZ* is derived from the names of the three proteins that the structure was originally identified: **P**SD 95, a postsynaptic density protein, **D**lg (*Drosophila d*isc large tumor suppressor), and **Z**O-1 (zona occludens, the tight junction protein). Since its discovery as a region of sequence homology in these few proteins (28), the PDZ domain has become recognized as one of the most common interaction modules in the genome, present in nearly 500 human proteins. Interestingly, the structure is evolutionarily conserved, emerging largely in metazoans, perhaps to accommodate the increased signaling needs of multicellular organisms (62).

PDZ-domain–containing proteins usually possess multiple protein–protein recognition modules. Because the domains usually act independently and allow concurrent recruitment of different binding targets, PDZ proteins function as molecular scaffolds. Indeed, PDZ proteins facilitate multiprotein complex formation and organize expression of target proteins on specific membrane domains for a wide range of physiological processes. As an ever-growing body of work has strongly implicated PDZ proteins in targeting and clustering various receptors, channels, transporters, and signal transduction elements at specific plasma membrane domains in neurons (153), muscle (2), and the *Drosophila* visual system (190), it has also become evident that PDZ proteins play important roles in epithelial transport processes.

Classes of PDZ Domains

PDZ domains are conventionally divided into three different classes, categorized by the chemical nature of their ligands (161). Different ligand classes are distinguished by differences in the penultimate binding residues found at the extreme COOH of target proteins (Fig. 1). Type I domains recognize the sequence, $X-S/T-X-\Phi^*$ (where X= any amino acid, Φ = hydrophobic amino acid, * COOH terminus). Type II domains bind to ligands with the sequence $X-\Phi-X-\Phi^*$. Type III domains interact with sequences with $X-X-C^*$ (15, 115). Binding specificity within each domain class can be conferred by the variant (X) residues as well as residues outside the canonical binding motif. Moreover, a few PDZ domains do not fall into any of these specific classes (62).

Structural Basis for PDZ Interaction

In recent years, the structures of different PDZ domains have been solved at atomic resolution. Like many protein–protein recognition modules, PDZ domains are small globular structures. Composed of six beta strands ($\beta A-\beta F$) and two alpha helices (αA and αB), PDZ domains fold into a six-stranded beta sandwich (21, 43) (Fig. 1). The peptide ligand inserts into a binding cleft, created by the βB strand and the αB helix, effectively forming an additional antiparallel beta strand. An extensive network of hydrogen bonds and hydrophobic interactions stabilizes binding of the peptide. For instance, the conserved glycine-leucine-glycine-phenylalanine-alanine (GLGF) motif contained with in $\beta A-\beta B$ linker provides a cradle of main chain amides and confers recognition of the terminal carboxylate group of the peptide (43). A hydrophobic

A

	(X-P$_{-2}$-X-P$_0$)
Type I	X-S/T-X-Φ-COOH
Type II	X-Φ-X-Φ-COOH
Type III	X-X-C-COOH

B

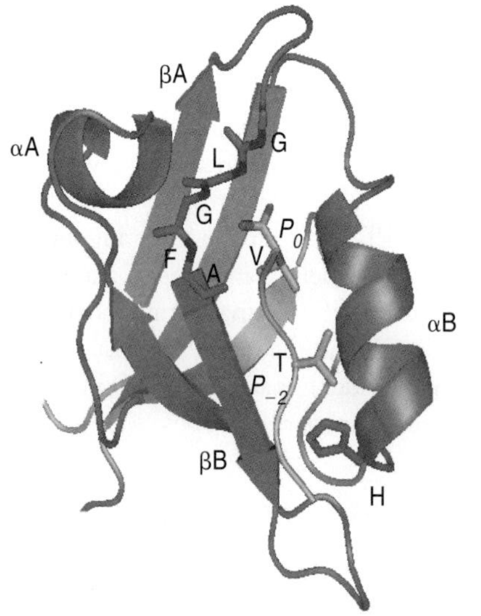

FIGURE 1   PDZ binding classes and structures. **A.** PDZ binding motifs of the three different PDZ ligand classes are shown. X, any amino acid; Φ, hydrophobic amino acid. Residues in PDZ ligands are conventionally numbered from the final amino acid at the extreme COOH terminus, the so-called P0 position. **B.** Structure of a type 1 PDZ domain (*black*) with its ligand (*light gray*) (third PDZ domain of PSD-95 is shown (PDB,1BFE) (43). The conserved GLGF motif in βA-βB linker provides a cradle of main chain amides for interaction with the terminal carboxylate group of the P$_0$ residue. A hydrophobic pocket accommodates the hydrophobic P$_0$ side chain. The first residue of the αB helix, a conserved histidine, forms hydrogen bonds with the P$_{-2}$ threonine residue in the target protein. See color insert.

pocket accommodates the hydrophobic COOH-terminal residue, thereby accounting for preferential interaction with proteins ending with a hydrophobic residue (the so-called P$_0$ position).

Binding specificity among the different binding classes is largely determined by interactions of P$_{-2}$ residue of the target protein COOH-terminal peptide with the first residue of the αB helix (43). In class I PDZ domains, a conserved histidine residue forms hydrogen bonds with the invariant P$_{-2}$ serine or threonine residue in the target protein. In class II PDZ domains, this position of the PDZ domain and the P$_{-2}$ residue of the target protein are both occupied by a hydrophobic amino acid (37).

Binding specificity within each domain class is also observed. At least two factors account for this. First, unique PDZ domain residues that are within or adjacent to the peptide-binding groove can interact with residues other than the penultimate P$_{-2}$ and P$_0$ residues (43, 82, 170). For example, the side chain of the P$_{-2}$ target protein residue usually points away from the invariant interaction surface but can bond with residues that are unique to particular PDZ domains (82). Structural data also indicate that the P$_{-3}$ side chain directly contacts unique residues in the interaction groove and is, therefore, a determinant of ligand specificity. Sites proximal to the archetypal, 4–amino-acid binding motif can also interact with regions outside the canonical binding site, and thereby contribute to binding specificity and affinity (12). Second, because interacting residues in PDZ domains can undergo large ligand-dependent conformational changes (83), it is likely that differences in ligand binding preferences within a PDZ binding class can also be determined by variations in binding pocket flexibility. Such a mechanism has been proposed to explain the different binding specificity of the two highly homologous PDZ domains in NHERF-1, which have almost identical binding clefts (97).

Regulation of PDZ binding

PDZ interactions can be dynamically regulated to control the composition and stoichiometry of different multimeric complexes. Phosphorylation of the binding target is the most common mechanism. This is explained by the fact that the COOH-termini of many type I PDZ targets contain a canonical serine/threonine kinase motif in which the penultimate binding residue, the P$_{-2}$ serine or threonine, is the substrate for phosphorylation. In these cases, phosphorylation of the residue creates an energetically unfavorable PDZ ligand and consequently abrogates PDZ interaction. For example, phosphorylation of the COOH-terminal site in the Kir 2.3 channel by protein kinase A inhibits its interaction with the synaptic PDZ protein, PSD-95 (33), presumably altering channel regulation (68). Likewise, phosphorylation of the P$_{-2}$ serine in the β2 adrenergic receptor uncouples the receptor from the NHERF-1 PDZ protein, and, disrupts receptor recycling in the postendocytic pathway (23).

Phosphorylation of sites within PDZ proteins is emerging as an additional mechanism for modulating PDZ binding. Evidence for this was first provided by observations that the interaction of a PDZ protein, NHERF-1 (see following paragraphs), with CFTR is negatively regulated by phosphorylation of a residue in the second PDZ domain (140). Phosphorylation of sites that are involved in PDZ–PDZ protein oligomerization has also been observed (101). This is believed to modulate the extent to which some PDZ proteins can form higher order scaffolding complexes.

Polarized Expression of PDZ Proteins in Epithelial cells

A number of PDZ proteins are preferentially expressed at polarized membrane domains or within critical sorting compartments (Fig. 2) where they perform retention/sorting

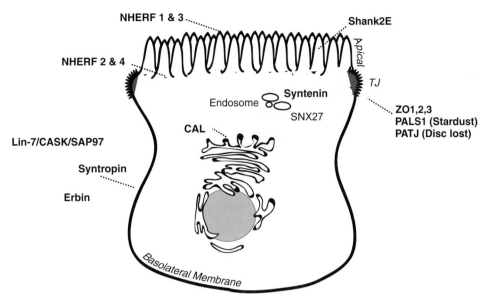

FIGURE 2   Major PDZ proteins in epithelial cells. PDZ-domain–containing proteins differentially localize to epithelial cell brush borders, subapical domains, endosomes, tight junctions, and basolateral membranes.

operations and organize local signaling complexes at polarized locales (22). Examples of PDZ proteins that predominately reside at the basolateral membrane of certain intestinal and renal epithelia include syntrophin (77) (see Dystrophin-Associated Protein Complex); Lin-7 (136, 163) (See Lin-7/CASK/SAP97); the ErbB interacting protein, ERBIN (13); and certain members of the membrane associated guanylate kinase family of PDZ proteins, such as CASK (32), PSD-93 (171), and SAP97 (also known as discs large homolog 1; 187). Other PDZ proteins, including the sodium hydrogen exchange regulator factors (see NHERF), Shank2E (120), and PSD-95 (171), are chiefly expressed on or near the apical membrane. Some PDZ proteins, such as zonula occludens, PALS1 (Stardust), and PATJ (Disc lost) (144), play important roles in the generation and maintenance of the tight junction. Still others, like CAL, which is primarily located in the Golgi (27), or SNX27 (76) and syntenin (48, 158), which are found in endosomes, reside in biosynthetic or endocytotic sorting compartments.

As would be predicted if PDZ proteins directly affect polarized sorting or retention of proteins that interact with them, a PDZ-binding motif appears to be necessary for polarized expression of a variety of different membrane proteins in epithelial cells. One of the first examples evolved from studies aimed at identifying polarized sorting signals in the GABA transporters or GATs (3); deletion of the PDZ binding motif from the apical isoform, GAT-3, caused the transporter to localize randomly to apical and basolateral membranes (125). Basolateral membrane expression of several membrane proteins has also been found to require a PDZ binding motif. For instance ERBB receptors, which play crucial roles in morphogenesis and oncogenesis, interact with a basolateral PDZ protein, called ERBIN, and require a PDZ binding motif for basolateral membrane expression

(13). Efficient basolateral membrane expression of a number of transporters that interact with the basolateral PDZ protein Lin-7, also require intact PDZ binding sites.

MAGUKs, the Archetypal PDZ Scaffolds

Members of the MAGUK (*m*embrane *a*ssociated *g*uanylate *k*inase) family of PDZ proteins are the archetypal PDZ scaffolds. Characterized by one to three PDZ domains, an SRC homology 3 domain (SH3), and a catalytically inactive guanylate kinase–like (GK) domain, MAGUK proteins are equipped to assemble large molecular complexes. In addition to the PDZ domains, the GK and the SH3 domains function as independent protein–protein interaction modules; GK domains recruit scaffold adaptor molecules called guanylate kinase–associated proteins or GKAPs (87), while SH3 domains have been shown to coordinate interaction with at least one nonreceptor tyrosine kinase (149). The SH3 and GK domains can also interact with one another, forming a composite SH3-GK structure (117, 167) that acts as an additional intermolecular protein–protein interaction domain with a binding specificity that is distinct from either SH3 or GK domains (34).

The PSD-95 family, encoded by four genes *(PSD-95/SAP90, PSD-93/Chapsyn-110, SAP102,* and *SAP97),* exemplifies MAGUK proteins. Two of these, *PSD-93* (171) and *SAP97* (see subsequent sections), are expressed in renal epithelial cells. However, the best characterized member, *PSD-95,* is largely expressed in excitable tissues and plays central roles in maintaining and modulating the strength and structure of glutamatergic synapses (88). Its general properties and functions are likely to be applicable to the other MAGUKs, including those expressed in the kidney.

Like many scaffolds, PSD-95 not only contains multiple protein–protein interaction modules, it also assembles into multimers, creating an extended platform for efficient scaffolding (30, 71). These qualities, combined with palmitoylation-dependent membrane tethering and synaptic localization signals (45), make PSD-95 ideally designed to cluster ion channels, receptors, trafficking proteins, and signal transduction machinery at the postsynaptic membrane. In doing so, PSD-95 influences trafficking, endocytosis, and activities of target proteins at the synapse (88). Organizing local signaling complexes is one of the most important clustering functions of PSD-95. For example, the PDZ domains in PSD-95 independently interact with the calcium/calmodulin-activated nitric oxide synthase, nNOS, and NMDA (*N*-methyl-D-aspartate) receptors to form a ternary complex (16, 29). The organization is thought to be important for regulated synthesis of nitric oxide, a diffusible transmitter that influences synaptic transmission and excitotoxicity. Because NMDA receptors are permeable to calcium, the physical linkage of nNOS with the excitatory receptors is believed to allow nitric oxide production to be efficiently coupled to receptor activation, calcium influx, and local changes in intracellular calcium (116). Significantly, disruption of NMDAR interaction with PSD-95 dissociates the receptors from downstream neurotoxic signaling without blocking synaptic activity or calcium influx (1).

Local signaling complexes that control the production of NOS in the kidney have been proposed (96). One may involve PSD-93, the predominate MAGUK in renal epithelial cells (171). Similar to PSD-95, PSD-93 associates with the plasmalemma via palmitoylation-dependent tethering signals (46) where it recruits and clusters various target proteins, including nNOS (17). In the kidney, PSD-93 is largely expressed along the basolateral membrane of the thick ascending limb, macula densa cells, and the distal nephron (171). In the macula densa, PSD-93 colocalizes with the pool of nNOS that is associated with intracellular vesicles and the basolateral membrane (171). It remains to be tested if PSD-93 interaction with nNOS in the macula densa coordinates regulated NO production in the manner that is observed with PSD-95 at the excitatory synapse.

FORM AND FUNCTION OF PDZ PROTEIN FAMILIES IN THE KIDNEY

Apical Membrane PDZ Protein Complexes

NHERF

The *Na/H* *e*xchange *r*egulator *f*actor PDZ proteins, NHERF, are highly expressed in the kidney and small intestine where they act as molecular scaffolds, associating with a number of transporters, channels, signaling proteins, transcription factors, and receptors to regulate apical membrane

transport processes (156, 180). Sequence similarity modeling reveals a family of four related NHERF proteins encoded by separate genes (42, 168) (Fig. 3). Originally known by many disparate names, a unifying nomenclature has been proposed (42, 168), designating the genes as *NHERF-1* (181, 184) (also known as ezrin binding protein-50, EBP-50 (142); *NHERF-2* (also known as NHE-3 kinase A (E3KARP) (198), tyrosine kinase activator-1 (TKA-1), and sex-determining region of the Y chromosome (SRY-1)- interacting protein (139); *NHERF-3* (also called PDZK1(93), Cap70 (176), DiPHOR, or *NaPi-Cap1* (55); and *NHERF-4* (also called IKEPP [148] DIPHOR-2, and NaPi-Cap2 [55]). Each member of the NHERF family of proteins is believed to play important roles in the regulation of transport processes within the proximal tubule as well as other sites along the nephron, acting by three different but not mutually exclusive mechanisms. Present evidence indicates that the NHERFs function to (1) organize local signaling complexes, often called transducisomes or signalosmomes; (2) control apical membrane trafficking; and (3) couple apical membrane transport proteins with other PDZ-binding targets.

Like other scaffolding proteins, the functions of the NHERFs are made possible by the presence of their multiple protein–protein interaction domains. NHERF-1 and NHERF-2 contain two PDZ domains and a COOH-terminal Ezrin/Radixin/Mosein/Merlin (ERM)–binding domain. The latter coordinates interaction with the ERM family of actin binding and A-kinase anchoring proteins to direct linkage with the actin cytoskeleton (18) and signal transduction machinery (44). By contrast, NHERF-3 and NHERF-4 contain four PDZ domains but no ERM domain (Fig. 3).

NHERF proteins can also interact with one another, presumably forming higher order protein networks. Indeed, NHERF-1 and NHERF-2 associate as homodimers and heterodimers (49, 54, 101, 154). Interestingly, oligomerization of NHERF-1, but not NHERF-2, is highly regulated by association with other proteins and by phosphorylation (101). NHERF-3 has been reported to interact with NHERF-1 and NHERF-2 to form an extensive heteromeric complex (54).

NHERF in epithelial transport. A growing body of evidence indicates each NHERF isoform has individual and specialized activities in the kidney. In some cases, specific roles of several NHERF proteins may converge and act cooperatively to regulate target proteins. Here we review the state of knowledge about each NHERF isoform.

NHERF-1 organizes local signaling complexes. NHERF-1 was originally discovered as a cofactor necessary for cAMP-kinase–dependent phosphorylation and inhibition of NHE-3, a brush border a Na1/H1 exchanger (181, 184). Biochemical studies and work in heterologous expression systems established a likely mechanism whereby NHERF-1 organizes a local PKA signaling complex, using its PDZ domains and the ERM binding domain (Fig. 3B). The second PDZ domain of NHERF-1 directly interacts

A

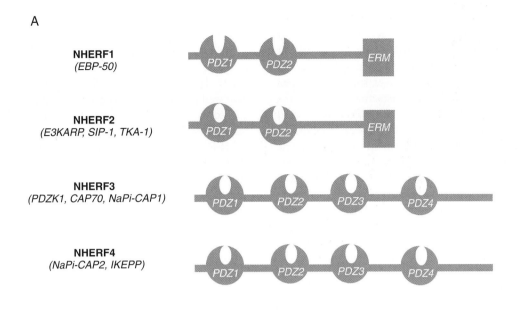

B

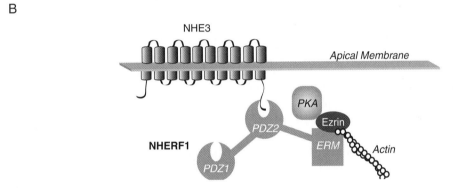

FIGURE 3 NHERF. (**A**) Domain architecture of NHERF family members. NHERF-1 and NHERF-2 contain two PDZ domains and an ERM-binding domain. NHERF-3 and NHERF-4 contain four PDZ domains but no ERM-binding domain. (**B**) The protein–protein interaction modules in NHERF-1 allow it to assemble a multiprotein complexes, consisting of PDZ-binding targets (such as NHE-3, shown), erzrin, and protein kinase A.

with NHE-3 (185) while the ERM binding domain simultaneously engages ezrin (99). By acting as an A-kinase anchor protein (AKAP) (44), ezrin recruits the regulatory subunit of PKA II (99) to the NHERF-1 complex. Consequently, NHERF-1 juxtaposes PKA with NHE-3 for efficient phosphorylation of the transporter and inhibition of Na1/H1 exchange. Consistent with the model, removal of the ERM binding domain in NHERF-1 disrupts formation of NHERF-1–ezrin signal complex and attenuates the inhibitory effect of cAMP on NHE-3 activity (183).

Direct evidence that the NHERF-1 signal complex is required for phosphoregulation of NHE-3 has been provided by studies in NHERF-1 gene knockout mice (155). In this model, activation of PKA fails to phosphorylate and inhibit NHE-3 activity in the proximal tubule, contrasting the robust response in wild-type mice (182). The response appears to be specific to NHERF-1 removal. Indeed, the

other proximal tubule NHERF isoforms are not affected by NHERF-1 gene ablation. Moreover, the inhibitory effect of PTH-receptor activation and PKA can be completely restored in NHERF-1-null proximal tubule cells upon adenoviral-mediated delivery of wild-type NHERF-1 (36).

The PKA coupling function of NHERF-1 is believed to be widespread with an emerging body of work indicating that NHERF-1 can act as a nexus of signaling complex assembly for efficient phosphorylation and regulation of a variety of transporters, channels, and receptors (reviewed in [177]). For example, NHERF-1 (as well as NHERF-2 [58] binds to CFTR [157, 175] though a PDZ interaction to potentiate PKA phosphorylation-dependent CFTR Cl⁻ currents (164) in an ezrin-AKAP–dependent manner.

Simultaneous PDZ-dependent recruitment of G-protein–coupled receptors by NHERF proteins can further focus local signaling around NHE-3 and other transport proteins (180).

For instance, studies in heterologous systems reveal that NHERF binds to the β_2-adrenergic receptor (BAR2) by means of a PDZ-domain–mediated interaction to recruit NHE-3 and the receptor into a local signaling complex for efficient receptor-mediated regulation of sodium-hydrogen exchange. Removal of the PDZ interaction motif in the BAR2 disrupts receptor interaction with NHERF-1 and markedly reduces β_2-adenergic receptor-mediated regulation of NHE-3 without altering activation of adenylyl cyclase (59). Likewise, NHERF-1 facilitates the assembly of a complex containing the β_2-adenergic receptor, ezrin, PKA, and CFTR at the apical membrane of epithelial cells for compartmentalized and specific signaling of the channel (126). Other examples have been extensively reviewed (180).

The tandem PDZ domains in NHERF-1 also provide a structural framework to link PDZ-binding transport proteins with PDZ-binding signal transduction machinery. Indeed, several different kinases (60, 121), phospholipase C isoforms (166), and the receptor for activated C kinase, RACK (109), have been identified as NHERF-1 PDZ binding targets. Characterization of consensus-binding sequences of isolated NHERF-1 PDZ domains by phage-display, affinity selection techniques revealed that the two PDZ domains have different ligand binding specificities with distinct preferences for residues at the 0, 1, and 3 positions of type I PDZ ligands (175). Thus NHERF-1 has a biochemical capacity to tether different PDZ binding targets on a single molecule. In addition, because NHERF-1 interacts with itself and links with the actin cytoskeleton, formation of an extended network of NHERF-1 molecules may join different PDZ-interacting proteins to the same locale. Such a mechanism has been proposed to explain NHERF-1 dependent coupling of phospholipase C with the TRP4 channel (166).

In some cases, the PDZ domains in NHERF-1 can support simultaneous interaction of two identical proteins. The best-characterized example is CFTR, which interacts with both PDZ domains in NHERF-1, albeit with different binding affinities (141). In this case, NHERF-1 has been reported to induce a high open probability conformation of CFTR by cross-linking the C-terminal tails of a CFTR dimer. Because CFTR binds to the two PDZ domains with different kinetics and affinities, channel gating is profoundly sensitive to alterations in NHERF-1 abundance. Moreover, the composition and stoichiometry of NHERF-CFTR interactions can be dynamically regulated. Phosphorylation of NHERF-1 has been found to specifically disrupt CFTR interaction with the second PDZ domain, uncoupling the tethered C-terminal tails and inducing a low open-probability conformation (140). A similar PDZ-dependent cross-linking mechanism to potentiate CFTR channel activity has been described with NHERF-3 (176).

NHERF-1–dependent apical membrane trafficking. In addition to co-localizing key components of signal transduction pathways, NHERF-1 can also regulate cell surface expression and localization of some of its binding targets. It appears to function by controlling trafficking operations in the postendocytic recycling pathway (23, 165) as well as by anchoring target proteins on the plasma membrane (65, 157).

Regulation of the Na-dependent phosphate transporter, Na P_i -IIa, in the proximal tubule provides a salient example. It is well known that factors that regulate proximal tubule P_i reabsorption and P_i homeostasis do so by altering the density of type IIa cotransporters at the apical membrane. NHERF-1 plays an important role in this process. Indeed, NHERF-1 gene ablation has been reported to cause diminished expression of NaP_i-IIa at the apical membrane and renal phosphate wasting (155). In the NHERF-1 knockout model, the NaP_i-IIa transporter is misrouted into a subapical, intracellular compartment (155, 178), indicative of a trafficking defect.

Studies in model systems have begun to cast light on the underlying mechanism. NaP_i-IIa binds to first PDZ domain of NHERF-1 via a type I interaction, requiring the last three amino acids of the cotransporter (55). These residues are also necessary for efficient apical expression of NaP_i-IIa (65, 66, 81), suggesting that apical targeting and/or anchoring are specified by direct NHERF-1 interaction. Apical localization of the cotransporter can be blocked by ectopic expression of truncated NHERF-1 proteins, which contain the first PDZ domain and are able to interact with the transporter but lack the ERM-binding domain. Thus, it is likely that NHERF-1 coordinates localization of the cotransporter by tethering NaP_i-IIa with the actin cytoskeleton through the ERM-binding domain (65).

Exciting recent studies reveal that PTH-induced internalization and lysosomal degradation of NaP_i-IIa in the proximal tubule are coincident with phosphorylation of NHERF-1 and disruption of NaP_i-IIa/NHERF-1 interaction (39). These observations strongly suggest that NaPi-IIa-NHERF-1 interactions are physiologically regulated to control NaPi-II apical surface density for maintenance of calcium and phosphate metabolism. Combined with the studies described in the previous section, the results indicate that NHERF-1 physiologically regulates apical expression of NaP_i-IIa by a trafficking mechanism, involving brush border retention and/or endocytic recycling. The latter mechanism would be consistent with observations that NHERF-1 mediates recycling of CFTR (165) and internalized G-protein–coupled receptors (23, 160).

NHERF-2 NHERF-2 appears to have different functions than NHERF-1 in the kidney (42, 179) even though the two PDZ proteins share a common domain structure and NHERF-2 is equally effective as NHERF-1 in mediating cAMP inhibition of NHE-3 in heterologous systems (198). Unlike NHERF-1, which is exclusively expressed in the human, rat, and mouse proximal tubule, expression of NHERF-2 in the proximal tubule is species-specific. Found only in the mouse proximal tubule, NHERF-2 predominately localizes to a subapical, intermicrovillar compartment that is distinct from NHERF-1 in the brush border (173). Importantly, NHERF-2 does not support phosphorylation-dependent inhibition of NHE-3 or apical localization of NaPi-IIa in the NHERF-1 knockout model, indicating that NHERF-2 does not share physiologically redundant functions with NHERF-1 in the proximal tubule (179).

The functions of NHERF-2 are better understood at sites outside the proximal tubule. In the kidney, NHERF-2 is predominately expressed in the glomerulus, vas recta, and collecting duct (174). Physiologically important PDZ binding partners have been identified in each of these locales. In the glomerulus, NHERF-2 interacts with podocalyxin, possibly functioning to retain podocalyxin at the apical surface of the podocyte and provide a mechanism for linking this important surface sialomucin to the actin cytoskeleton (108). NHERF-2 associates with the TRPC4 channel in the descending vasa recta where it has been suggested to control $Ca2^+$ signaling (104) similar to the way that the INAD PDZ protein controls TRP in the *Drosophila* eye (122). In the collecting duct, NHERF-2 co-localizes and interacts with the ROMK channel. Studies in heterologous expression systems indicate that NHERF-2 couples accessory proteins and signal transduction machinery to ROMK for efficient channel regulation and trafficking (193).

The PDZ binding specificity of NHERF-2 also undoubtedly contributes to its unique functions as compared to NHERF-1. While NHERF-2 shares many of the same PDZ binding partners as NHERF-1, with nearly 60 having been identified (156), it also interacts with several proteins that NHERF-1 does not. These include α-actinin-4 (89); cGMP kinase I and II (26); a putative Cl/HCO3 exchanger downregulated in adenoma (98); podocalyxin (108); human Y-linked testis determining gene binding factor (139); serum glucocorticoid stimulated kinase, SGK-1 (196); and transcriptional coactivation with PDZ-binding motif, TAZ (80).

By organizing these unique partners into protein complexes, NHERF-2 can affect functions that are distinct from NHERF-1. NHERF isoform–specific regulation of NHE-3 in heterologous systems provides an excellent illustration. For example, NHERF-2 uniquely confers $Ca2^+$-dependent inhibition on NHE-3 (103) by scaffolding the exchanger to PKCα and α-actinin-4 (42). NHERF-1 does not support this activity, presumably because it is not capable of interacting with α-actinin-4. Likewise, by acting as a unique protein kinase G–anchoring protein, NHERF-2 specifically confers cGMP inhibition on NHE-3 (26). Finally activation of NHE-3 by dexamethasone requires NHERF-2 rather than NHERF-1 (196). In this case, the first PDZ domain of NHERF-2 uniquely recruits the serum- and glucocorticoid-induced protein kinase, SGK-1, into a complex with NHE-3 to phosphorylate and enhance exchanger activity. Such a mechanism may offer an explanation for glucocorticoid stimulation of sodium absorption in ileum, proximal colon, and renal proximal tubule (196).

NHERF-2-dependent scaffolding of SGK-1 may also play an important role in the collecting duct for the regulation of the potassium secretory channel, ROMK (194, 197).

Reportedly, NHERF-2 can synergize with SGK-1 to augment cell surface expression of ROMK in oocyte expression experiments (197). Biochemical studies indicate that NHERF-2 has the capacity to recruit ROMK and SGK-1 into a ternary complex by preferentially binding to channel with the first PDZ domain (193) while simultaneously recruiting the kinase by preferred interaction with the second PDZ domain (196). Formation of such a complex would allow efficient phosphorylation of a residue that is required for delivery of the channel to the cell surface. Indeed, SGK-1 directly phosphorylates serine 44 (194) in ROMK1, creating a forward trafficking signal (192) that overrides an endoplasmic reticulum localization signal (132, 192). Together the observations suggest a potential molecular mechanism for the regulation of ROMK density by dietary potassium, whereby the NHERF-2 scaffold juxtaposes the SGK-1 with ROMK for efficient phosphorylation-dependent trafficking to the apical membrane.

NHERF-3 NHERF-3 was first discovered as PDZK1, a PDZ domain–containing protein that is upregulated in carcinomas and abundantly expressed in the proximal tubule brush border (54, 93, 94). Significantly, the four PDZ domains of NHERF-3 support interaction with many proximal tubule apical membrane transporter proteins, including NaPi-IIa, the solute carrier SLC17A1 (NaPi-I), NHE-3, the organic cation transporter (OCTN1), chloride-formate exchanger (CFEX), and the urate-anion exchanger (URAT1) (54) as well as a protein kinase A–anchoring protein, D-AKAP2 (53). Based on the observations and findings that NHERF-1 also can interact with NHERF-3, NHERF-3 and NHERF-1 may form an extended scaffolding network in brush borders of proximal tubular cells for the regulation of transport.

Although the NHERF-3–NHERF-1 scaffolding network concept is an attractive hypothesis, it should be pointed out that targeted disruption of the NHERF-3 gene by homologous recombination does not cause global alterations in the expression or localization of most of its interacting transport proteins in the proximal tubule (95, 169). Instead, the major effects of NHERF-3 gene disruption appear to be specific, confined largely to one interacting protein. Only a selective reduction in the abundance and functional activity of the chloride–formate exchanger, CFEX, at the proximal tubule brush broader is observed in the NHERF-3–null animals (169). A minor role of NHERF-3 in NaP$_i$-IIa regulation can be provoked by physiological perturbations; while NHERF-3 null animals on a normal or low-phosphate diet do not exhibit alterations in NaP$_i$-IIa abundance or function, high dietary phosphate unmasks a modest attenuation of NaP$_i$-IIa levels at the proximal tubule brush border (24). It remains to be directly tested whether these modest effects of NHERF-3 removal simply reflect compensatory or redundant activities served by other PDZ proteins such as NHERF-1, which shares many interacting partners with NHERF-3.

NHERF-4 This member of the NHERF family was originally identified in independent screens for PDZ binding partners of the NaPi-IIa transporter (55) and the receptor guanylyl cyclase (148). First dubbed as NaPi Cap-2 or IKEPP (intestinal and kidney-enriched PDZ protein), it was subsequently reclassified as NHERF-4 on the basis of sequence homology modeling (168). In the proximal tubule where it is abundantly expressed, NHERF-4 localizes to a subapical region, much like NHERF-2, which is distinct from the brush border and NHERF-1 (55). Little is known about the function of NHERF-4 except that it inhibits heat–stable, toxin–induced cGMP synthesis (148) by a mechanism suggested to involve PDZ-dependent recruitment of inhibitory factors (168). Based on its structural similarities with other NHERF forms and the site of expression in the kidney (168), it seems likely that NHERF-4 also modulates apical membrane transport and cell signaling in the proximal tubule.

Shank (SH3 Domain and Ankyrin Repeating Proteins: Proline-Rich Synapse-Associated Protein-1/Cortactin Binding Protein 1 (ProSAP1/CortBP1) Members of the Shank (*S*H3 domain and *ank*yrin repeating proteins) family of proteins have recently emerged as another class of apical membrane–associated scaffolds in epithelial cells, extending their function beyond their established role as master scaffolds at the post synaptic density (152). The three known Shank genes (Shank1, Shank2, and Shank3) are expressed in a tissue-specific manner. Shank1 is almost exclusively expressed in the brain; products of the Shank2 gene are found in brain, kidney, and liver; and Shank3 is most abundantly expressed in the heart (110). The prototypical Shank, Shank1, is a relatively large protein (>200 KDa) containing multiple ankyrin repeats (124), an SH3 domain, a PDZ domain, and a long proline repeat domain. A self-oligomerization domain, called a *sterile alpha motif* (SAM), assembles the scaffolds into head-to-tail helical sheets, likely forming an extensive Shank network

for protein complex assembly (10). Multiple splice variants of each gene have been identified that contain different combinations of protein-protein interaction domains (Fig. 4). For example, Shank2E, a form that is predominately expressed in epithelial cells (120), contains ankyrin repeats whereas the Shank2 splice form found in the brain does not.

Extensive studies in the brain provide models for Shank function in epithelial cells. It is well established that Shank family members localize to the postsynaptic density of excitatory synapses where they act as master scaffolds along with PSD-95 (152). Here, the Shanks physically couple the two major receptor complexes, *N*-methyl-D-aspartate receptors (NMDARs) and metabotropic glutamate receptors (mGluRs), and recruit associated signaling proteins. They do so by concurrently engaging two different adaptors through distinct protein–protein interaction domains. The Shank PDZ domain associates with the GUK-associated protein, GKAP, which, in turn, interacts with the PSD-95 complex, containing NMDA receptors (152). At the same time, the proline-rich domain of Shank interacts withanother adaptor protein, called Homer, to link with metabotropic glutamate receptors. Proline-rich domains often serve as binding sites for SH3 (SrC homology), WW (conserved two-tryptophan domain), and EVH1 domains (enabled/vasodilator-stimulated phosphoprotein homology 1) (84). A single EVH1 domain in Homer directly interacts with a PPXXF motif in the Shank proline-rich domain as well as with similar proline motifs in group 1 mGluR and other proteins, such as the IP3 receptor (188). Because Homer proteins self-associate in a head-to-tail fashion, two EVH1 domains per dimer are available to bridge Shank with group 1 mGluRs. Consequently, Shank cross-links Homer and PSD-95 complexes in the PSD, presumably to couple signaling transduction pathways emanating from NMDAR and mGluR.

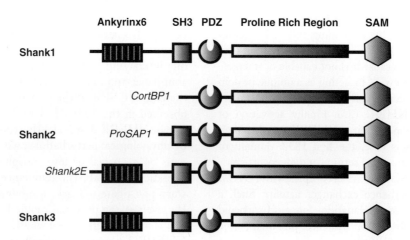

FIGURE 4 Shank family members. Domain architectures of Shank1, 2, 3, and Shank2 splice variants are shown. The major epithelial form, Shank2E, contains six ankyrin repeats, an SH3 domain, a PDZ domain, a proline-rich domain, and a self-oligomerization region called a SAM domain.

More recently, Shank2 forms have been implicated in the modulation of apical membrane transport processes. In the kidney, Shank2E is concentrated at the apical membrane of proximal tubule cells were it interacts with NHE-3 and NaPi-IIa, similar to NHERF-1. Present evidence indicates that Shank2 and NHERF may control the activity of these transport proteins in divergent manners, however. Studies with NHE-3 in heterologous expression systems, for example, revealed that Shank2 positively regulates NHE-3 membrane expression and blunts the cAMP-dependent inhibition of NHE-3 as if it antagonizes the action of NHERF-1. Likewise, in pancreatic duct cells, Shank2E associates with CFTR at the apical membrane and inhibits Cl channel activity (90), contrasting the positive effects of NHERF-1 and NHERF-2 on CFTR.

Shank2E appears to regulate NaP$_i$-IIa differently than NHERF-1. In the proximal tubule, increased extracellular Pi triggers internalization and degradation of Shank2E and NaP$_i$-2a in parallel but has no effect on NHERF-1 localization or abundance (119). Combined with observations that regulated endocytosis of NaP$_i$-IIa is associated with disruption of NaP$_i$-IIa/NHERF-1 interaction at the brush border (39), one might speculate that internalization of NaP$_i$-IIa involves a NHERF-1–to-Shank2E interaction switch. Importantly, Shank interacts with dynamin II, a GTPase that is critical for endocytic vesicle formation, via proline-rich domain interaction (134). Thus, Shank2E is especially poised to facilitate NaP$_i$-IIa endocytosis and/or lysosomal trafficking, contrasting the apparent membrane-retention and/or recycling function of NHERF-1. The molecular mechanisms underlying the function of Shank2E in the proximal tubule remain to be firmly established, however. It will be interesting to learn if the activities of Shank2E depend on scaffold adaptors, such as Homer and GKAP, as have been shown in excitatory synapses.

Basolateral Membrane PDZ Protein Complexes

THE LIN-7/CASK/PSD-97 SYSTEM

Lin-7 and CASK (Lin-2) are components of an evolutionarily conserved basolateral membrane scaffolding complex, important for polarized targeting and controlling cell surface density of their PDZ binding partners. They were discovered along with another PDZ protein, Lin-10 (Lin, from abnormal cell *lin*eage), in a genetic screen for components of the LET-23 receptor tyrosine kinase signaling pathway in *Caenorhabditis elegans* vulva progenitor cells (VPCs) (78). These molecules form a tripartite protein complex in VPC that interacts with a receptor tyrosine kinase, LET-23, to coordinate receptor expression on the basolateral membrane (78, 145, 159). Indeed, null mutations in *Lin-7, Lin-2,* or *Lin-10* cause the Let-23 receptor to become mislocalized to the apical membrane and consequently disrupt LET-23 signaling and VPC development.

Orthologues of the *C. elegans* PDZ protein complex have been identified in mammalian tissues (Lin-7 = mLin7/Veli/ MALS; Lin-2 = CASK; Lin-10 = Mint-1/X11) (14, 20, 135, 163). In the mammalian kidney, a partially conserved complex, consisting of mLin-7 and CASK but not Lin-10 (14), localizes to the basolateral membrane (136, 163) where it coordinates polarized expression of mLin-7 binding partners (Fig. 5). Indeed, it has been implicated in basolateral expression of the epithelial GABA transporter, BGT-1 (138), the strong inward-rectifying potassium channels, Kir 2.X (105, 106, 135), and the EGF-like receptor, ErbB-2/Her2 (151). Present evidence suggests that the mLin-7/CASK complex may offer a general mechanism for polarized expression of basolateral membrane proteins containing type 1 PDZ–binding motifs.

According to the current understanding, Lin-7 acts as the upstream scaffolding molecule, binding directly to target

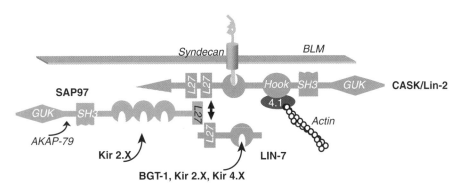

FIGURE 5 Lin-7/CASK/SAP-97 complex at the basolateral membrane (BLM). Lin-7 recruits PDZ binding targets, such as the BGT-1 transporter and the inwardly rectifying potassium channels, Kir 2.X and Kir 4.X, to the basolateral membrane by interacting with CASK through an L27 domain interaction. CASK acts as the master anchor; it not only interacts with Lin-7 it also binds to extracellular matrix receptors, such as syndecan, through a type II PDZ interaction while simultaneously engaging the actin cytoskeleton through a hook domain interaction with 4.1 proteins. CASK also recruits SAP-97 to the basolateral membrane through an L27 interaction. SAP-97 has the capacity to recruit PDZ binding targets as well as proteins that interact with the guanylate kinase (GK) and SH3 domains, such as AKAP-79.

molecules through a type 1 PDZ interaction while simultaneously engaging CASK via another protein–protein interaction module (102, 163), called a L27 domain (from *Lin-2,Lin-7*) (40). L27 domains, present in a number of related PDZ proteins (see PALS), are helical bundle structures (47, 107) that mediate heterotypic assembly, important for polymerization of different scaffolds. In fact, basolateral membrane localization of Lin-7 and its PDZ binding partners is afforded by the L27 domain and CASK interaction (163).

CASK associates with the basolateral membrane through a web of interactions to function as the master basolateral membrane attachment factor. As a member of the MAGUK family, CASK contains multiple protein–protein interactions sites, allowing it to simultaneously bind to Lin-7, extracellular matrix receptors, adhesion molecules, the actin cytoskeleton 4.1 binding proteins (32) and another MAGUK protein, SAP-97 (102). The mLin-7 and SAP-97 L27 domains separately assemble with two L27 domains of CASK, possibly as a dimer of L27 heterodimers (47, 107), to form a mLin-7/SAP97/CASK complex (102, 106). By linking extracellular matrix receptors and the cytoskeleton, the Lin-7/CASK/SAP97 complex has the capacity to act as a stable anchor to retain Lin-7 interacting proteins on the basolateral membrane.

The mammalian counterpart of Lin-10 is actually encoded by a family of proteins called the Mints or X11s (133). Although all three members of the Mint family share C-terminal PDZ and PTB domains, only Mint-1, contains a CASK interaction domain (14). In neuronal tissues and the heart, which express the complete Lin-7/CASK/Mint-1 complex, Mint-1 has been suggested to provide an additional membrane trafficking function. Mint-1 interacts with microtubule motors and has been reported to transport NMDA-type receptor vesicles along microtubules (150). In addition, Mint-1 interacts with Munc-18 docking machinery (14, 20, 63). Importantly, mammalian epithelial cells do not express Mint-1. In its absence, the Lin-2/CASK system looses the obvious link to microtubule-mediated trafficking and fusion, suggesting that Lin-7/CASK plays a major role in a retention rather than directed-delivery in renal epithelia.

Consistent with this notion, present evidence indicates that Lin-7/CASK primarily functions to retain target proteins at the basolateral membrane of mammalian epithelia. For example, Perego et al. (138) found that removing the PDZ ligand in BGT-1 disrupted Lin-7 association in MCDK cells and dramatically increased the internalization of the transporter from the plasmalemma. Observations that Lin-7 is sufficient to stabilize the Kir 2.3 channel on the cell surface provide direct evidence for Lin-7 as a retention factor (135). Moreover, expression of a dominant negative CASK construct, which contains both L27 domains but no basolateral membrane localization determinants, causes a related mLin-7 binding partner, Kir 2.2, to mislocalize into a vesicular compartment in MDCK cells (106).

Although Lin-7 primarily operates as a component of a basolateral membrane retention machine in mammalian epithelial cells, it should be pointed out that disruption of Lin-7 interactions can produce a wide range of mislocalization phenotypes, depending on the Lin-7 binding partner and the types of sorting signals embedded within them. For instance, mutant BGT transporters, lacking their PDZ binding motif, are predominately localized on the basolateral membrane. In this case, BGT-1 transporters are presumably directed to the basolateral membrane by non-PDZ dependent sorting signals (137). On the other hand, mutant Kir2.3 channels, lacking the PDZ binding motif, are largely directed to an endosomal compartment rather than the basolateral membrane (135), consistent with strong endosomal targeting signals. An apical-missorting phenotype is produced by removing the PDZ-binding site from a chimeric LET-23/nerve growth factor receptor protein (162). In this case, Lin-7 interaction may stabilize the receptor on the basolateral membrane or limit post-endocytic trafficking in such a way that it prevents transcytosis to the apical membrane.

At present, it is not known if the Lin-7/CASK/SAP97 scaffold also participates in signal complex localization and organization at the basal membrane in the way that has been described for the NHERF proteins at the apical membrane. SAP97 has been shown to recruit AKAP proteins to related PDZ protein complexes in neurons (34) and the Drosophila CASK Orthologue, Camguk, protein functionally modulates Ether-a-go-go potassium channels by a phosphorylation-dependent mechanism (114). However, it remains to be established if similar mechanisms are in place at the basolateral membrane of renal epithelial cells, which express the Lin-7/CASK/SAP97 complex.

LIN 7 ISOFORMS (VELI/MALS) AND PALS (*P*ARTNERS OF *LIN* 7) IN THE KIDNEY

Three different Lin-7 isoforms, encoded by separate genes, have been identified. In mammalian systems, these are often called Veli/MALS 1, 2, 3 (*Ve*rtebrate *Lin*-7 or *Ma*mmalian *Lin* *S*even). Each MALS/Veli isoform is expressed in the kidney, being differentially localized along the nephron (136). MALS/Veli 1 is predominately expressed in the glomerulus, the thick ascending limb (TAL) of Henle loop, and the distal convoluted tubule (DCT). MALS/Veli 2 is exclusively expressed in the vasa recta. MALS/Veli 3 is largely located in the DCT and collecting duct. The subcellular localization of MALS/Veli proteins can vary, depending on the isoform and the cell-type. In contrast to the predominate basolateral location of MALS/Veli 1 in the TAL and DCT and MALS/Veli 3 in the DCT, MALS/Veli 1 is found diffusely throughout the cytosol of intercalated cells. In the collecting duct, MALS/Veli 3 is chiefly located on the basal membrane. Collectively, these results suggest that different MALS/Veli isoforms may carry out cell-type–specific functions. MALS/Veli 1 and 2 isoforms in the thick ascending limb and distal segments appear to have the most significant capacity for a basolateral membrane targeting mechanism.

The disparate subcellular localization patterns of MALS/Veli isoforms are likely to arise from at least two different factors. First, differences in the primary structures provide reason to suspect that the MALS/Velis may have specific binding preferences. In contrast to the nearly identical PDZ domains amongst the MALS/Veli isoforms, the extreme NH2- and COOH-termini are highly divergent. Most importantly, the region believed to direct MALS/Veli subcellular localization, the L27 interaction module, exhibit only 57% amino acid identity between isoforms, raising the possibility that different isoforms preferentially bind to different L27 domain proteins. Secondly, cell-specific expression of Lin-7 binding partners may account for differences in isoform localization in different nephron segments and cell types. A group of CASK-like MAUGK proteins, called PALS (*Partners of Lin-7*), that contain L27 hetero-oligomerization domains, have been identified as potential partners of Lin-7 (79). The different PALS might substitute for CASK under certain circumstances, forming MALS/Veli complexes with different subcellular locations and disparate functions. For instance, PALS1 targets Lin-7 to the tight junction (143), contrasting the basolateral membrane location of the CASK/Lin-7 complex.

DYSTROPHIN-ASSOCIATED PROTEIN COMPLEX

The dystrophin-associated protein complex (DPC) is a transmembrane scaffolding machine that is expressed in a variety of tissues. Extensive studies in skeletal muscle have revealed that the DPC serves structural and cell signaling functions (100). In epithelia, the DPC localizes to the basolateral membrane (Fig. 6), where it is organized in a manner similar to the skeletal muscle complex, functioning to compartmentalize and tether signaling and transport proteins.

In the sarcolemma, the DPC is nucleated by dystrophin, a flexible rodlike cytoplasmic protein containing multiple spectrinlike repeats. Dystrophin directly interacts with the transmembrane protein, β-dystroglycan, via a C-terminal cysteine-rich region, and connects the complex to lammin through α-dystroglycan (Fig. 6). Because dystrophin also binds actin, it effectively links the extracellular matrix with the cytoskeleton, offering an architecture that protects the sarcolemma from shearing forces of contraction. This point is underscored by the link to disease. Specific mutations in the X-linked dystrophin have been identified that disrupt dystrophin and consequently destabilize DGC elements at the sarcolemma, producing Duchenne muscular dystrophy, the milder Becker muscular dystrophy, and X-linked dilated cardiomyopathy (reviewed in [100]).

Dystrophin also interacts with the scaffolding molecules dystrobrevin, and three isoforms of syntrophin (α1, β1, and β2), to organize local signaling complexes in muscle. The syntrophrins contain several protein–protein interaction domains, including two pleckstrin homology domains and a PDZ domain. The PDZ domains recruit a variety of proteins to the DPC, including voltage-gated sodium channels (52, 147) and nNOS (67). α-Dystrobrevin directly interacts with dystrophin via coiled-coil domains while simultaneously binding to the syntrophins through an independent binding site (56).

The basolateral membrane–associated DRC in renal epithelial cells exhibits the same basic design as in skeletal

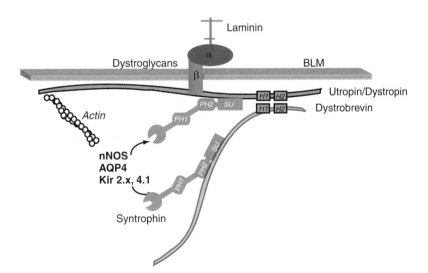

FIGURE 6 The dystrophin-associated protein complex (DPC) at the basolateral membrane. The PDZ protein, syntrophin, is recruited to the basolateral membrane via its interaction with utropin and possibly dystrobrevin, requiring one of its pleckstrin homology (PH2) domains and the syntrophin unique (SU) domain. This leaves the syntrophin PDZ domain free to recruit basolateral membrane proteins such as the AQP4 water channel, potassium channels, Kir 2.X and Kir 4.X, as well as nNOS. Utropin/dysropin interacts with actin via N-terminal spectrin repeats, with β-dystroglycan via a C-terminal cysteine-rich region and with dystrobrevin via coiled-coiled domains (H₁, H₂).

muscle but differs somewhat in molecular composition (57, 111). An autosomal homolog of dystrophin, called utrophin, along with less abundant C-terminal dystrophin isoforms, Dp71 and Dp140 (100), takes the place of the longer muscle-specific dystrophin in renal epithelia. In addition, differential expression of dystrobrevin and three syntrophin isoforms along the nephron give rise to nephron-segment–specific DPCs with distinct molecular properties (57). In the connecting segment and the cortical collecting duct where the DPC is especially enriched, the DPC includes utrophin, β1-/β2-syntrophin, dystrobrevin and β-dystroglycan (57).

Like dystrophin in muscle, utrophin directly interacts with the actin cytoskeleton in epithelial cells (85) while associating with laminin in the extracellular matrix via the basolateral dystroglycans (74) (Fig. 6). Thus, utrophrin is poised to provide a secure anchoring point for polarized expression of syntrophin. Consistent with this notion, it has been reported that basolateral membrane localization of β2-syntrophin depends on its utrophin-binding activity, requiring one of its pleckstrin homology domains and the syntrophin unique (SU) domain (77). Moreover, utrophin knockout mice exhibit a selective reduction of β2-syntrophin at renal epithelial basolateral membrane domains (57). Syntrophins also interact with dystrobrevin via the PH and SU domains, allowing recruitment of additional syntrophin molecules to the same DPC (128).

Importantly, the association of syntrophin with dystrobrevin, utrophin and the basolateral membrane occurs independently of the syntrophin PDZ domain (77). This leaves the type 1 PDZ domain free to interact with proteins containing a syntrophin PDZ recognition motif. Basolateral membrane proteins such as the inward rectifying channel proteins, Kir 2.X (105) and Kir 4.X (35), the AQP4 water channel (127), and nNOS, have been shown to interact with the syntrophin PDZ binding domain. The functional relevance of these interactions in the kidney is not well understood.

Several clues about the roles of transport protein interaction with syntrophin and the DPC are provided by studies in other tissues. In astrocytes, for example, α-syntrophin is required for the polarized expression of AQP4 (127) and Kir 4.1 (35) at end-feet membranes adjacent to blood vessels for efficient water and potassium siphoning (7, 8). It will be interesting to learn if genetic ablation of β2-syntrophin, the prevalent form in the kidney, has similar effects on AQP4 in the proximal straight tubule (131) and Kir 4.1 in the distal nephron (73).

Utrophin knockout animals have been generated (38). Unfortunately, expression of the shorter C-terminal dystrophin forms in the kidney compensate for the utrophin ablation, making it difficult to precisely define the functional role of the renal DPC by a genetic approach. Double utrophin/dystrophin knockout mice exhibit a fragile phenotype with complete disintegration of the DPC and premature death (57). It will be important to determine how much of the phenotype can be attributed to impaired kidney function.

AKAP

AKAPs are a diverse group of molecules that function as cell signaling scaffolds. Specifically, AKAPs dynamically organize and juxtapose protein kinase A (PKA) with specific substrates and other signaling machinery at specific cellular locales. In doing so, AKAP proteins can precisely control where and when second messengers will act on select cellular effectors. Since the first discovery of an AKAP, a microtubule anchoring protein that binds to the regulatory subunit of PKA with high affinity (112), more than 50 AKAP proteins have been identified. Many of them control phosphorylation of channels, receptors, and membrane transport proteins (50). Several are suspected to modulate renal tubule transport processes.

Common Properties of AKAP Proteins

AKAP proteins are structurally diverse, related only by general signaling functions and three common properties. First, classification as an AKAP protein requires the presence of a PKA-anchoring domain. Second, AKAPs contain cellular localization signals, allowing spatial organization of second-messenger cascades at specific subcellular compartments. Third, AKAPs possess other protein–protein interaction domains, which specify interaction with select effectors and/or other signaling molecules. Although all AKAPs have these common properties, they each have distinct targeting signals and different scaffolding motifs. Consequently, they have specialized functions, modulating distinct intracellular signaling events.

AKAPs bind PKA by means of a small anchoring domain, comprising a short (13-18 amino acid), amphipathic α-helix. Nuclear magnetic resonance (NMR) solution structures reveal that the hydrophobic side of the amphipathic helix makes numerous hydrophobic contacts within a hydrophobic surface of a four-helix bundle formed by the N-terminal domains of the PKA regulatory subunit homodimer (9, 129, 130). Consequently, the AKAP–PKA interaction occurs with relatively high affinity (~1-10 nM). Although most AKAPs interact with the RII isotypes of the PKA regulatory subunit, several AKAPs have been identified, D-AKAP1 (72) and D-AKAP2 (72), which also interact with the RI form. Importantly, AKAP function can be disrupted by exogenous expression of a peptide mimic of the amphipathic helix (6). Regulatory subunit–isotype specific competitors have been developed (19).

Specialized targeting sequences on anchoring proteins specifically compartmentalize different AKAPs to distinct subcellular compartments, including plasma membrane microdomains, intracellular vesicles, nuclei, mitochondria, microtubules, and the actin cytoskeleton (186). Certain AKAPs contain polarized trafficking signals, directing asymmetric localization in epithelia cells. AKAP2 (AKAP-KL), for example, is compartmentalized on the apical membrane (41) by its PDZ–binding motif, which specifies interaction with NHERF-3 (55). Similarly ezrin, a low RII affinity AKAP, localizes to the apical membrane through a protein–protein recognition domain that directs interaction with NHERF-1 (123). In many cases, different splice products of the same AKAP gene can be differentially targeted to different compartments. Splice forms of the AKAP18 gene, for instance, are expressed on opposite plasma membrane domains in epithelial cells; AKAP18-α is targeted to basolateral membranes, whereas AKAP18-β localizes the apical membrane. In this case, a unique 23–amino acid insert in AKAP18-β acts as an apical membrane targeting determinant (172).

As multivalent scaffolds, AKAPs can juxtapose the right combination of enzymes with their substrates. Consequently, AKAPs not only synchronize signal transduction processes but they can also orchestrate signal termination events. The archetypal example is provided by the AKAP75/150 family, which influences the phosphorylation state of several different channels and transporters, including the NaP$_i$-IIa cotransporter (86), L-type calcium channels (51), M-type potassium channels (70), and AMPA-type glutatamate receptors (25, 146). AKAP75 not only contains a binding site for PKA, it also directly interacts with PKC and the calcium-calmodulin–dependent phosphatase, PP2B (calcineurin) (31, 91). Consequently, the same AKAP scaffold can coordinate signal transduction processes by phosphorylation and dephosphorylation. Thus, AKAPs can influence the balance of signal transduction and termination by differentially tethering different signaling components and effectors (69).

Function of AKAPS in Kidney Transport Processes

AKAP-Dependent AQP2 Water Channel Shuttling

A critical role for AKAPs in water channel trafficking is strongly suggested by observations that cAMP-dependent AQP2 translocation to the cell surface can be inhibited with a synthetic peptide mimic of the AKAP amphipathic helix, which prevents binding of AKAPs to the PKA RII subunit (92). Several different AKAPs appear to be associated with endosomal structures containing AQP2. Biochemical characterization of inner medullary collecting duct (IMCD) heavy endosomes, containing AQP2, revealed the presence of an associated multiprotein-signaling complex, composed of a 90-kD AKAP, PKA, and protein phosphatase 2a (75). Although the precise molecular identity of the 90-kD AKAP is still not certain, a smaller anchoring protein, AKAP18-δ, was subsequently discovered (64). In the kidney, AKAP18-δ is mainly expressed in IMCD principle cells, where it appears to be confined to intracellular vesicles containing AQP2 and PKA. Observations that vasopressin recruits AKAP18-δ with AQP2 to the plasma membrane suggest that this AKAP is specifically involved in the PKA phosphorylation-dependent AQP2 translocation process. Reminiscent of the multifactoral roles of AKAP75 (see above), the AKAP-signaling

complex in IMCD endosomes also contains PP2B (75) and phosphodiesterases (118). Thus, the endosomal AKAPs in the collecting duct are also likely to participate in maintaining AQP2 in a quiescent dephosphorylated conformation in water diuresis.

AKAPs in the Proximal Tubule Apical Membrane Scaffolding Complex

Two different AKAPs, D-AKAP2 and AKPA79, have been implicated in the modulation of proximal tubule sodium phosphate transport. AKAP2 has been shown to interact with a PDZ scaffolding protein, NHERF-3, at the apical membrane where it has been suggested to play an important role in the parathyroid hormone (PTH)-mediated regulation of NaPi-IIa, involving PKA compartmentalization (53). In a proximal tubule model, OK cells, PTH-dependent regulation of NaP$_i$-IIa can be uncoupled with a synthetic peptide mimic of the AKAP amphipathic helix, indicating that an AKAP is required for PKA-dependent modulation of NaP$_i$-IIa regulation. In this system, AKAP79 was shown to associate with the NaP$_i$-IIa transporter, PKA, and the parathyroid hormone receptor (86). Because AKAP 79 also has the capacity to interact with PDZ proteins in neuronal systems (34), it may interact with the NaP$_i$-IIa cotransporter and the PTH receptor through its interaction with the apical NHERF complex.

AKAP Control of the Potassium Secretory Channel ROMK (Kir 1.1)

Studies on the renal potassium secretory channel, ROMK, in heterologous expression systems have suggested a potential role for AKAPs in the physiological regulation of potassium secretion. Because open channel gating and cell surface expression of the ROMK require direct phosphorylation by PKA (113, 191) and other kinases (194), a critical role of an AKAP has been an attractive idea. In fact, it has been reported that maximal activation of ROMK in Xenopus oocytes by forskolin and/or 8-bromo-cAMP–dependent kinase requires co-expression of an AKAP (4). High basal phosphorylation of the channel in this expression system makes the effects of AKAPs modest. Nevertheless, the response appears to be AKAP specific, being dependent on AKAP-75 but not AKAP18, AKAP-2 (KL) (5). AKAP-75 is not expressed with ROMK in the thick ascending limb or collecting duct, however, so the AKAP in the kidney that interacts with ROMK still remains to be determined. Given observations that ROMK interacts with NHERF-1 and 2 (see above), the ERM proteins (44) are obvious AKAP candidates.

SUMMARY

Exciting discoveries in recent years have cast light onto the molecular mechanisms of epithelial transport modulation. The discovery of proteins that bring together physiologically appropriate assemblages of cell signaling and trafficking proteins with transport molecules for efficient regulation has been especially insightful. The molecular identifies and functions of many these scaffolding molecules in the kidney have now begun to come in focus. The field is still its infancy, however, with much more to be learned. For example, observations that some transport protein such as NHE1, the housekeeping sodium–hydrogen exchanger (11), and the Na,K-ATPase (189, 195), might act as scaffolding proteins is emerging as an intriguing possibility that we certainly will hear more about in the future. Also, with the application of powerful new tools in cell biology, genomics, and proteomics, it is likely that more scaffolding candidates will be identified. As they are, it will be important not only to continue probing into the mechanistic basis of function in model systems but also to rigorously explore how they these fascinating molecules work in their native cellular environments. There are many hints in the field that a single transport protein can interact with different scaffolding proteins, depending on its natural history and the physiological setting. It will be very important determine how this is accomplished.

References

1. Aarts M, Liu Y, Liu L, Besshoh S, Arundine M, Gurd JW, Wang YT, Salter MW, Tymianski M. Treatment of ischemic brain damage by perturbing NMDA receptor- PSD-95 protein interactions. *Science* 2002;298 (5594):846–850.

2. Adams ME, Mueller HA, Froehner SC. In vivo requirement of the alpha-syntrophin PDZ domain for the sarcolemmal localization of nNOS and aquaporin-4. *J Cell Biol* 2001;155: 113–122.

3. Ahn J, Mundigl O, Muth TR, Rudnick G, Caplan MJ. Polarized expression of GABA transporters in Madin-Darby canine kidney cells and cultured hippocampal neurons. *J Biol Chem* 1996;271:6917–6924.

4. Ali S, Chen X, Lu M, Xu JZ, Lerea KM, Hebert SC, Wang WH. The A kinase anchoring protein is required for mediating the effect of protein kinase A on ROMK1 channels. *Proc Natl Acad Sci U S A* 1998; 95:10274–10280.

5. Ali S, Wei Y, Lerea KM, Becker L, Rubin CS, Wang W. PKA-induced stimulation of ROMK1 channel activity is governed by both tethering and non-tethering domains of an A kinase anchor protein. *Cell Physiol Biochem* 2001;11(3):135–142.

6. Alto NM, Soderling SH, Hoshi N, Langeberg LK, Fayos R, Jennings PA, Scott JD. Bioinformatic design of A-kinase anchoring protein-in silico: a potent and selective peptide antagonist of type II protein kinase A anchoring. *Proc Natl Acad Sci U S A* 2003;100(8):4445–4450.

7. Amiry-Moghaddam M, Otsuka T, Hurn PD, Traystman RJ, Haug FM, Froehner SC, Adams ME, Neely JD, Agre P, Ottersen OP, Bhardwaj A. An alpha-syntrophin-dependent pool of AQP4 in astroglial end-feet confers bidirectional water flow between blood and brain. *Proc Natl Acad Sci U S A* 2003;100(4):2106–2111.

8. Amiry-Moghaddam M, Williamson A, Palomba M, Eid T, de Lanerolle NC, Nagelhus EA, Adams ME, Froehner SC, Agre P, Ottersen OP. Delayed K+ clearance associated with aquaporin-4 mislocalization: phenotypic defects in brains of alpha-syntrophin-null mice. *Proc Natl Acad Sci U S A* 2003;100(23):13615–13620.

9. Banky P, Newlon MG, Roy M, Garrod S, Taylor SS, Jennings PA. Isoform-specific differences between the type Ialpha and IIalpha cyclic AMP-dependent protein kinase anchoring domains revealed by solution NMR. *J Biol Chem* 2000;275(45):35146–35152.

10. Baron MK, Boeckers TM, Vaida B, Faham S, Gingery M, Sawaya MR, Salyer D, Gundelfinger ED, Bowie JU. An architectural framework that may lie at the core of the postsynaptic density. *Science* 2006; 311(5760):531–535.

11. Baumgartner M, Patel H, Barber DL. Na(+)/H(+) exchanger NHE1 as plasma membrane scaffold in the assembly of signaling complexes. *Am J Physiol Cell Physiol* 2004;287(4): C844–850.

12. Birrane G, Chung J, Ladias JA. Novel mode of ligand recognition by the Erbin PDZ domain. *J Biol Chem* 2003;278(3):1399–1402.

13. Borg JP, Marchetto S, Le Bivic A, Ollendorff V, Jaulin-Bastard F, Saito H, Fournier E, Adelaide J, Margolis B, Birnbaum D. ERBIN: a basolateral PDZ protein that interacts with the mammalian ERBB2/HER2 receptor. *Nat Cell Biol* 2000;2:407–414.

14. Borg JP, Straight SW, Kaech SM, de Taddeo-Borg M, Kroon DE, Karnak D, Turner RS, Kim SK, Margolis B. Identification of an evolutionarily conserved heterotrimeric protein complex involved in protein targeting. *J Biol Chem* 1998;273:31633–31636.

15. Borrell-Pages M, Fernandez-Larrea J, Borroto A, Rojo F, Baselga J, Arribas J. The carboxy-terminal cysteine of the tetraspanin L6 antigen is required for its interaction with SITAC, a novel PDZ protein. *Mol Cell Biol* 2000;11:4217–4225.

16. Brenman JE, Chao DS, Gee SH, McGee AW, Craven SE, Santillano DR, Huang F, Xia H, Peters MF, Froehner SC, Bredt DS. Interaction of nitric oxide synthase with the postsynaptic density protein PSD-95 and alpha-1 syntrophin mediated by PDZ motifs. *Cell* 1996;84:757–767.

17. Brenman JE, Christopherson KS, Craven SE, McGee AW, Bredt DS. Cloning and characterization of postsynaptic density 93, a nitric oxide synthase interacting protein. *J Neurosci* 1996;16(23):7407–7415.

18. Bretscher A, Edwards K, Fehon RG. ERM proteins and merlin: integrators at the cell cortex. *Nat Rev Mol Cell Biol* 2002;3(8):586–599.

19. Burns-Hamuro LL, Ma Y, Kammerer S, Reineke U, Self C, Cook C, Olson GL, Cantor CR, Braun A, Taylor SS. Designing isoform-specific peptide disruptors of protein kinase A localization. *Proc Natl Acad Sci U S A* 2003;100(7):4072–4077.

20. Butz S, Okamoto M, Sudhof TC. A tripartite protein complex with the potential to couple synaptic vesicle exocytosis to cell adhesion in brain. *Cell* 1998;94:773–782.

21. Cabral JH, Petosa C, Sutcliffe MJ, Raza S, Byron O, Poy F, MarfatiaSM., Chishti AH, Liddington RC. Crystal structure of a PDZ domain. *Nature* 1996;382:649–652.

22. Campo C, Mason A, Maouyo D, Olsen O, Yoo D, Welling PA. Molecular mechanisms of membrane polarity in renal epithelial cells. *Rev Physiol Biochem Pharmacol* 2005;153:47–99.

23. Cao TT, Deacon HW, Reczek D, Bretscher A, von Zastrow M. A kinase-regulated PDZ-domain interaction controls endocytic sorting of the beta2-adrenergic receptor. *Nature* 1999;401:286–290.

24. Capuano P, Bacic D, Stange G, Hernando N, Kaissling B, Pal R, Kocher O, Biber J, Wagner CA, Murer H. Expression and regulation of the renal Na/phosphate cotransporter NaPi-IIa in a mouse model deficient for the PDZ protein PDZK1. *Pflugers Arch* 2005;449(4):392–402.

25. Carr DW, Stofko-Hahn RE, Fraser ID, Bishop SM, Acott TS, Brennan RG, Scott JD. Interaction of the regulatory subunit (RII) of cAMP-dependent protein kinase with RII-anchoring proteins occurs through an amphipathic helix binding motif. *J Biol Chem* 1991;266 (22):14188–14192.

26. Cha B, Kim JH, Hut H, Hogema BM, Nadarja J, Zizak M, Cavet M, Lee-Kwon W, Lohmann SM, Smolenski A, Tse CM, Yun C, de Jonge HR, Donowitz M. cGMP inhibition of Na+/H+ antiporter 3 (NHE-3) requires PDZ domain adapter NHERF-2, a broad specificity protein kinase G-anchoring protein. *J Biol Chem* 2005;280(17): 16642–16650.

27. Cheng J, Moyer BD, Milewski M, Loffing J, Ikeda M, Mickle JE, Cutting GR, Li M, Stanton BA, Guggino WB. A Golgi-associated PDZ domain protein modulates cystic fibrosis transmembrane regulator plasma membrane expression. *J Biol Chem* 2002;277:3520–3529.

28. Cho KO, Hunt CA, Kennedy MB. The rat brain postsynaptic density fraction contains a homolog of the Drosophila discs-large tumor suppressor protein. *Neuron* 1992;9(5): 929–942.

29. Christopherson KS, Hillier BJ, Lim WA, Bredt DS. PSD-95 assembles a ternary complex with the N-methyl-D-aspartic acid receptor and a bivalent neuronal NO synthase PDZ domain. *J Biol Chem* 1999;274(39):27467–27473.

30. Christopherson KS, Sweeney NT, Craven SE, Kang R, El-Husseini Ael D, Bredt DS. Lipid- and protein-mediated multimerization of PSD-95: implications for receptor clustering and assembly of synaptic protein networks. *J Cell Sci* 2003;116(Pt 15):3213–3219.

31. Coghlan VM, Perrino BA, Howard M, Langeberg LK, Hicks JB, GallatinWM., Scott JD. Association of protein kinase A and protein phosphatase 2B with a common anchoring protein. *Science* 1995;267:108–111.

32. Cohen AR, Woods DF, Marfatia SM, Walther Z, Chishti AH, Anderson JM, Wood DFW. Human CASK/LIN-2 binds syndecan-2 and protein 4.1 and localizes to the basolateral membrane of epithelial cells [published erratum appears in *J Cell Biol* 1998 Aug 24;142(4): following 1156]. *J Cell Biol* 1998;142:129–138.

33. Cohen NA, Brenman JE, Snyder SH, Bredt DS. Binding of the inward rectifier K channel Kir2.3 to PSD-95 is regulated by protein kinase A phosphorylation. *Neuron* 1996;17: 759–767.

34. Colledge M, Dean RA, Scott GK, Langeberg LK, Huganir RL, Scott JD. Targeting of PKA to glutamate receptors through a MAGUK-AKAP complex. *Neuron* 2000;27(1):107–119.

35. Connors NC, Adams ME, Froehner SC, Kofuji P. The potassium channel Kir4.1 associates with the dystrophin-glycoprotein complex via alpha-syntrophin in glia. *J Biol Chem* 2004;279(27):28387–28392.

36. Cunningham R, Steplock D, Wang F, Huang H, E X, Shenolikar S, Weinman EJ. Defective parathyroid hormone regulation of NHE-3 activity and phosphate adaptation in cultured NHERF-1-/- renal proximal tubule cells. *J Biol Chem* 2004;279(36):37815–37821.

37. Daniels DL, Cohen AR, Anderson JM, Brunger AT. Crystal structure of the hCASK PDZ domain reveals the structural basis of class II PDZ domain target recognition. *Nat Struct Biol* 1998;5:317–325.

38. Deconinck AE, Potter AC, Tinsley JM, Wood SJ, Vater R, Young C, Metzinger L, Vincent A, Slater CR, Davies KE. Postsynaptic abnormalities at the neuromuscular junctions of utrophin-deficient mice. *J Cell Biol* 1997;136(4):883–894.

39. Deliot N, Hernando N, Horst-Liu Z, Gisler SM, Capuano P, Wagner CA, Bacic D, O'Brien S, Biber J, Murer H. Parathyroid hormone treatment induces dissociation of type IIa Na+-P(i) cotransporter-Na+/H+ exchanger regulatory factor-1 complexes. *Am J Physiol Cell Physiol* 2005;289(1):C159–167.

40. Doerks T, Bork P, Kamberov E, Makarova O, Muecke S, Margolis B. L27, a novel heterodimerization domain in receptor targeting proteins Lin-2 and Lin-7. *Trends Biochem Sci* 2000;25:317–318.

41. Dong F, Feldmesser M, Casadevall A, Rubin CS. Molecular characterization of a cDNA that encodes six isoforms of a novel murine A kinase anchor protein. *J Biol Chem* 1998;273(11): 6533–6541.

42. Donowitz M, Cha B, Zachos NC, Brett CL, Sharma A, Tse CM, Li X. NHERF family and NHE-3 regulation. *J Physiol* 2005;567(Pt 1):3–11.

43. Doyle DA, Lee A, Lewis J, Kim E, Sheng M, MacKinnon R. Crystal structures of a complexed and peptide-free membrane protein-binding domain: molecular basis of peptide recognition by PDZ. *Cell* 1996;85:1067–1076.

44. Dransfield DT, Bradford AJ, Smith J, Martin M, Roy C, Mangeat PH, Goldenring JR. Ezrin is a cyclic AMP-dependent protein kinase anchoring protein. *EMBO J* 1997;16:35–43.

45. El-Husseini AE, Craven SE, Chetkovich DM, Firestein BL, Schnell E, Aoki C, Bredt DS. Dual palmitoylation of PSD-95 mediates its vesiculotubular sorting, postsynaptic targeting, and ion channel clustering. *J Cell Biol* 2000;148:159–172.

46. El-Husseini AE, Topinka JR, Lehrer-Graiwer JE, Firestein BL, Craven SE, Aoki C, Bredt DS. Ion channel clustering by membrane-associated guanylate kinases. Differential regulation by N-terminal lipid and metal binding motifs. *J Biol Chem* 2000;275(31):23904–23910.

47. Feng W, Long JF, Fan JS, Suetake T, Zhang M. The tetrameric L27 domain complex as an organization platform for supramolecular assemblies. *Nat Struct Mol Biol* 2004;11:475–480.

48. Fialka I, Steinlein P, Ahorn H, Bock G, Burbelo PD, Haberfellner M, Lottspeich F, Paiha K, Pasquali C, Huber LA. Identification of syntenin as a protein of the apical early endocytic compartment in Madin-Darby canine kidney cells. *J Biol Chem* 1999;274:26233–22629.

49. Fouassier L, Yun CC, Fitz JG, Doctor RB. Evidence for ezrin-radixin-moesin-binding phosphoprotein 50 (EBP50) self-association through PDZ-PDZ interactions. *J Biol Chem* 2000;275:25039–25045.

50. Fraser ID, Scott JD. Modulation of ion channels: a "current" view of AKAPs. *Neuron* 1999;23(3):423–426.

51. Gao T, Yatani A, Dell'Acqua ML, Sako H, Green SA, Dascal N, Scott JD, Hosey MM. cAMP-Dependent regulation of cardiac L-type Ca2+ channels requires membrane targeting of PKA and phosphorylation of channel subunits. *Neuron* 1997;19:185–196.

52. Gee SH, Madhavan R, Levinson SR, Caldwell JH, Sealock R, Froehner SC. Interaction of muscle and brain sodium channels with multiple members of the syntrophin family of dystrophin-associated proteins. *J Neurosci* 1998;18(1):128–137.

53. Gisler SM, Madjdpour C, Bacic D, Pribanic S, Taylor SS, Biber J, Murer H. PDZK1: II. an anchoring site for the PKA-binding protein D-AKAP2 in renal proximal tubular cells. *Kidney Int* 2003;64(5):1746–1754.

54. Gisler SM, Pribanic S, Bacic D, Forrer P, Gantenbein A, Sabourin LA, Tsuji A, Zhao ZS, Manser E, Biber J, Murer H. PDZK1: I. a major scaffolder in brush borders of proximal tubular cells. *Kidney Int* 2003;64:1733–1745.

55. Gisler SM, Stagljar I, Traebert M, Bacic D, Biber J, Murer H. Interaction of the type IIa Na/Pi cotransporter with PDZ proteins. *J Biol Chem* 2001;276:9206–9913.

56. Grady RM, Grange RW, Lau KS, Maimone MM, Nichol MC, Stull JT, Sanes JR. Role for alpha-dystrobrevin in the pathogenesis of dystrophin-dependent muscular dystrophies. *Nat Cell Biol* 1999;1(4):215–220.

57. Haenggi T, Schaub MC, Fritschy JM. Molecular heterogeneity of the dystrophin-associated protein complex in the mouse kidney nephron: differential alterations in the absence of utrophin and dystrophin. *Cell Tissue Res* 2005;319(2):299–313.

58. Hall RA, Ostedgaard LS, Premont RT, Blitzer JT, Rahman N, Welsh MJ, Lefkowitz RJ. A C-terminal motif found in the beta2-adrenergic receptor, P2Y1 receptor and cystic fibrosis transmembrane conductance regulator determines binding to the Na+/H+ exchanger regulatory factor family of PDZ proteins. *Proc Natl Acad Sci U S A* 1998;95:8496–8501.

59. Hall RA, Premont RT, Chow CW, Blitzer JT, Pitcher JA, Claing A, Stoffel RH, Barak LS, Shenolikar S, Weinman EJ, Grinstein S, Lefkowitz RJ. The beta2-adrenergic receptor interacts with the Na+/H+-exchanger regulatory factor to control Na+/H+ exchange. *Nature* 1998;392:626–630.

60. Hall RA, Spurney RF, Premont RT, Rahman N, Blitzer JT, Pitcher JA, Lefkowitz RJ. G protein-coupled receptor kinase 6A phosphorylates the Na(+)/H(+) exchanger regulatory factor via a PDZ domain-mediated interaction. *J Biol Chem* 1999;274:24328–24348.

61. Harris BZ, Hillier BJ, Lim WA. Energetic determinants of internal motif recognition by PDZ domains. *Biochimica et Biophysica Acta* 2001;40:5921–5530.

62. Harris BZ, Lim WA. Mechanism and role of PDZ domains in signaling complex assembly. *J Cell Sci* 2001;114(Pt 18):3219–3231.

63. Hata Y, Slaughter CA, Sudhof TC. Synaptic vesicle fusion complex contains unc-18 homologue bound to syntaxin. *Nature* 1993;366:347–351.

64. Henn V, Edemir B, Stefan E, Wiesner B, Lorenz D, Theilig F, Schmitt R, Vossebein L, Tamma G, Beyermann M, Krause E, Herberg FW, Valenti G, Bachmann S, Rosenthal W, Klussmann E. Identification of a novel A-kinase anchoring protein 18 isoform and evidence for its role in the vasopressin-induced aquaporin-2 shuttle in renal principal cells. *J Biol Chem* 2004;279(25): 26654–26665.

65. Hernando N, Deliot N, Gisler SM, Lederer E, Weinman EJ, Biber J, Murer H. PDZ-domain interactions and apical expression of type IIa Na/P(i) cotransporters. *Proc Natl Acad Sci U S A* 2002;99:11957–11962.

66. Hernando N, Karim-Jimenez Z, Biber J, Murer H. Molecular determinants for apical expression and regulatory membrane retrieval of the type IIa Na/Pi cotransporter. *Kidney Int* 2001;60:431–445.

67. Hillier BJ, Christopherson KS, Prehoda KE, Bredt DS, Lim WA. Unexpected modes of PDZ domain scaffolding revealed by structure of nNOS-syntrophin complex. *Science* 1999;284: 812–885.

68. Horio Y, Hibino H, Inanobe A, Yamada M, Ishii M, Tada Y, Satoh E, Takai Y, Kurachi Y. Clustering and enhanced activity of an inwardly rectifying potassium channel, Kir4.1, by an anchoring protein, PSD-95/SAP90. *J Biol Chem* 1997;272:12885–12888.

69. Hoshi N, Langeberg LK, Scott JD. Distinct enzyme combinations in AKAP signalling complexes permit functional diversity. *Nat Cell Biol* 2005;7(11):1066–1073.

70. Hoshi N, Zhang JS, Omaki M, Takeuchi T, Yokoyama S, Wanaverbecq N, Langeberg LK, Yoneda Y, Scott JD, Brown DA, Higashida H. AKAP150 signaling complex promotes suppression of the M-current by muscarinic agonists. *Nat Neurosci* 2003;6(6):564–571.

71. Hsueh YP, Kim E, Sheng M. Disulfide-linked head-to-head multimerization in the mechanism of ion channel clustering by PSD-95. *Neuron* 1997;18(5):803–814.

72. Huang LJ, Wang L, Ma Y, Durick K, Perkins G, Deerinck TJ, Ellisman MH, Taylor SS. NH2-Terminal targeting motifs direct dual specificity A-kinase-anchoring protein 1 (D-AKAP1) to either mitochondria or endoplasmic reticulum. *J Cell Biol* 1999;145(5): 951–959.

73. Ito M, Inanobe A, Horio Y, Hibino H, Isomoto S, Ito H, Mori K, Tomoike H, Kurachi Y. Immunolocalization of an inwardly rectifying K+ channel, K(AB)-2 (Kir4.1), in the basolateral membrane of renal distal tubular epithelia. *FEBS Lett* 1996;388:11–15.

74. James M, Nuttall A, Ilsley JL, Ottersbach K, Tinsley JM, Sudol M, Winder SJ. Adhesion-dependent tyrosine phosphorylation of (beta)-dystroglycan regulates its interaction with utrophin. *J Cell Sci* 2000;113(Pt 10):1717–1726.

75. Jo I, Ward DT, Baum MA, Scott JD, Coghlan VM, Hammond TG, Harris HW. AQP2 is a substrate for endogenous PP2B activity within an inner medullary AKAP-signaling complex. *Am J Physiol Renal Physiol* 2001;281(5):F958–965.

76. Joubert L, Hanson B, Barthet G, Sebben M, Claeysen S, Hong W, Marin P, Dumuis A, Bockaert J. New sorting nexin (SNX27) and NHERF specifically interact with the 5-HT4a receptor splice variant: roles in receptor targeting. *J Cell Sci* 2004;117(Pt 22):5367–5379.

77. Kachinsky AM, Froehner SC, Milgram SL. A PDZ-containing scaffold related to the dystrophin complex at the basolateral membrane of epithelial cells. *J Cell Biol* 1999;145:391–402.

78. Kaech SM, Whitfield CW, Kim SK. The LIN-2/LIN-7/LIN-10 complex mediates basolateral membrane localization of the C. elegans EGF receptor LET-23 in vulval epithelial cells. *Cell* 1998;94:761–771.

79. Kamberov E, Makarova O, Roh M, Liu A, Karnak D, Straight S, Margolis B. Molecular cloning and characterization of Pals, proteins associated with mLin-7. *J Biol Chem* 2000;275:11425–11431.

80. Kanai F, Marignani PA, Sarbassova D, Yagi R, Hall RA, Donowitz M, Hisaminato A, Fujiwara T, Ito Y, Cantley LC, Yaffe MB. TAZ: a novel transcriptional co-activator regulated by interactions with 14-3-3 and PDZ domain proteins. *EMBO J* 2000;19(24):6778–6791.

81. Karim-Jimenez Z, Hernando N, Biber J, Murer H. Molecular determinants for apical expression of the renal type IIa Na+/Pi-cotransporter. *Pflugers Archiv* 2001;442:782–790.

82. Karthikeyan S, Leung T, Ladias JA. Structural basis of the Na+/H+ exchanger regulatory factor PDZ1 interaction with the carboxyl-terminal region of the cystic fibrosis transmembrane conductance regulator. *J Biol Chem* 2001;276:19683–19696.

83. Karthikeyan S, Leung T, Ladias JA. Structural determinants of the Na+/H+ exchanger regulatory factor interaction with the beta 2 adrenergic and platelet-derived growth factor receptors. *J Biol Chem* 2002;77:18973–18978.

84. Kay BK, Williamson MP, Sudol M. The importance of being proline: the interaction of proline-rich motifs in signaling proteins with their cognate domains. *FASEB J* 2000;14:231–241.

85. Keep NH, Winder SJ, Moores CA, Walke S, Norwood FL, Kendrick-Jones J. Crystal structure of the actin-binding region of utrophin reveals a head-to-tail dimer. *Structure* 1999;7(12):1539–1546.

86. Khundmiri SJ, Rane MJ, Lederer ED. Parathyroid hormone regulation of type II sodium-phosphate cotransporters is dependent on an A kinase anchoring protein. *J Biol Chem* 2003;278(12):10134–10141.

87. Kim E, Naisbitt S, Hsueh YP, Rao A, Rothschild A, Craig AM, Sheng M. GKAP, a novel synaptic protein that interacts with the guanylate kinase-like domain of the PSD-95/SAP90 family of channel clustering molecules. *J Cell Biol* 1997;136:669–678.

88. Kim E, Sheng M. PDZ domain proteins of synapses. *Nat Rev Neurosci* 2004;5(10):771–781.

89. Kim JH, Lee-Kwon W, Park JB, Ryu SH, Yun CH, Donowitz M. Ca(2+)-dependent inhibition of Na+/H+ exchanger 3 (NHE-3) requires an NHE-3-E3KARP-alpha-actinin-4 complex for oligomerization and endocytosis. *J Biol Chem* 2002;277(26):23714–23724.

90. Kim JY, Han W, Namkung W, Lee JH, Kim KH, Shin H, Kim E, Lee MG. Inhibitory regulation of cystic fibrosis transmembrane conductance regulator anion-transporting activities by Shank2. *J Biol Chem* 2004;279(11):10389–10396.

91. Klauck TM, Faux MC, Labudda K, Langeberg LK, Jaken S, Scott JD. Coordination of three signaling enzymes by AKAP79, a mammalian scaffold protein. *Science* 1996;271(5255): 1589–1592.

92. Klussmann E, Maric K, Wiesner B, Beyermann M, Rosenthal W. Protein kinase A anchoring proteins are required for vasopressin-mediated translocation of aquaporin-2 into cell membranes of renal principal cells. *J Biol Chem* 1999;274(8):4934–4938.

93. Kocher O, Comella N, Gilchrist A, Pal R, Tognazzi K, Brown LF, Knoll JH. PDZK1, a novel PDZ domain-containing protein up-regulated in carcinomas and mapped to chromosome 1q21, interacts with cMOAT (MRP2), the multidrug resistance-associated protein. *Lab Invest* 1999;79(9):1161–1170.

94. Kocher O, Comella N, Tognazzi K, Brown LF. Identification and partial characterization of PDZK1: a novel protein containing PDZ interaction domains. *Lab Invest* 1998;78(1): 117–125.

95. Kocher O, Pal R, Roberts M, Cirovic C, Gilchrist A. Targeted disruption of the PDZK1 gene by homologous recombination. *Mol Cell Biol* 2003;23:1175–1180.

96. Kone BC, Kuncewicz T, Zhang W, Yu ZY. Protein interactions with nitric oxide synthases: controlling the right time, the right place, and the right amount of nitric oxide. *Am J Physiol Renal Physiol* 2003;285(2):F178–190.

97. Ladias JA. Structural Insights into the CFTR-NHERF Interaction. *J Mol Biol* 2003;192: 79–88.

98. Lamprecht G, Heil A, Baisch S, Lin-Wu E, Yun CC, Kalbacher H, Gregor M, Seidler U. The down regulated in adenoma (dra) gene product binds to the second PDZ domain of the NHE-3 kinase A regulatory protein (E3KARP), potentially linking intestinal Cl−/HCO3− exchange to Na+/H+ exchange. *Biochemistry* 2002;41:12336–12342.

99. Lamprecht G, Weinman EJ, Yun CH. The role of NHERF and E3KARP in the cAMP-mediated inhibition of NHE-3. *J Biol Chem* 1998;273:29972–29978.

100. Lapidos KA, Kakkar R, McNally EM. The dystrophin glycoprotein complex: signaling strength and integrity for the sarcolemma. *Circ Res* 2004;94(8):1023–1031.

101. Lau AG, Hall RA. Oligomerization of NHERF-1 and NHERF-2 PDZ domains: differential regulation by association with receptor carboxyl-termini and by phosphorylation. *Biochemistry* 2001;40:8572–8580.

102. Lee S, Fan S, Makarova O, Straight S, Margolis B. A novel and conserved protein-protein interaction domain of mammalian Lin-2/CASK binds and recruits SAP97 to the lateral surface of epithelia. *Mol Cell Biol* 2002;22:1778–1791.

103. Lee-Kwon W, Kim JH, Choi JW, Kawano K, Cha B, Dartt DA, Zoukhri D, Donowitz M. Ca2+-dependent inhibition of NHE-3 requires PKC alpha which binds to E3KARP to decrease surface NHE-3 containing plasma membrane complexes. *Am J Physiol Cell Physiol* 2003;285(6):C1527–1536.

104. Lee-Kwon W, Wade JB, Zhang Z, Pallone TL, Weinman EJ. Expression of TRPC4 channel protein that interacts with NHERF-2 in rat descending vasa recta. *Am J Physiol Cell Physiol* 2005;288(4):C942–949.

105. Leonoudakis D, Conti LR, Anderson S, Radeke CM, McGuire LM, Adams ME, Froehner SC, Yates JR, Vandenberg CA. Protein trafficking and anchoring complexes revealed by proteomic analysis of inward rectifier potassium channel (Kir2.x)-associated proteins. *J Biol Chem* 2004;279:22331–22346.
106. Leonoudakis D, Conti LR, Radeke CM, McGuire LM, Vandenberg CA. A multiprotein trafficking complex composed of SAP97, CASK, Veli, and Mint1 is associated with inward rectifier Kir2 potassium channels. *J Biol Chem* 2004;279:19051–19063.
107. Li Y, Karnak D, Demeler B, Margolis B, Lavie A. Structural basis for L27 domain-mediated assembly of signaling and cell polarity complexes. *EMBO J* 2004;23(14):2723–2733.
108. Li Y, Li J, Straight SW, Kershaw DB. PDZ domain-mediated interaction of rabbit podocalyxin and Na(+)/H(+) exchange regulatory factor-2. *Am J Physiol Renal Physiol*.2004;282: F1129–F1139.
109. Liedtke CM, Yun CH, Kyle N, Wang D. Protein kinase C epsilon-dependent regulation of cystic fibrosis transmembrane regulator involves binding to a receptor for activated C kinase (RACK1) and RACK1 binding to $Na^+/H+$ exchange regulatory factor. *J Biol Chem* 2002;277:22925–22933.
110. Lim S, Naisbitt S, Yoon J, Hwang JI, Suh PG, Sheng M, Kim E. Characterization of the Shank family of synaptic proteins. Multiple genes, alternative splicing, and differential expression in brain and development. *J Biol Chem* 1999;274(41):29510–29518.
111. Loh NY, Newey SE, Davies KE, Blake DJ. Assembly of multiple dystrobrevin-containing complexes in the kidney. *J Cell Sci* 2000;113(Pt 15):2715–2724.
112. Lohmann SM, DeCamilli P, Einig I, Walter U. High-affinity binding of the regulatory subunit (RII) of cAMP-dependent protein kinase to microtubule-associated and other cellular proteins. *Proc Natl Acad Sci U S A* 1984;81(21):6723–6727.
113. MacGregor GG, Xu JZ, McNicholas CM, Giebisch G, Hebert SC. Partially active channels produced by PKA site mutation of the cloned renal K+ channel, ROMK2 (kir1.2). *Am J Physiol* 1998;275:F415–F422.
114. Marble DD, Hegle AP, Snyder ED, 2nd, Dimitratos S, Bryant PJ, Wilson GF. Camguk/CASK enhances Ether-a-go-go potassium current by a phosphorylation-dependent mechanism. *J Neurosci* 2005;25(20):4898–4907.
115. Maximov A, Sudhof TC, Bezprozvanny I. Association of neuronal calcium channels with modular adaptor proteins. *J Biol Chem* 1999;274:24453–24456.
116. McGee AW, Bredt DS. Assembly and plasticity of the glutamatergic postsynaptic specialization. *Curr Opin Neurobiol* 2003;13(1):111–118.
117. McGee AW, Dakoji SR, Olsen O, Bredt DS, Lim WA, Prehoda KE. Structure of the SH3-guanylate kinase module from PSD-95 suggests a mechanism for regulated assembly of MAGUK scaffolding proteins. *Mol Cell* 2001;8(6):1291–1301.
118. McSorley T, Stefan E, Henn V, Wiesner B, Baillie GS, Houslay MD, Rosenthal W, Klussmann E. Spatial organisation of AKAP18 and PDE4 isoforms in renal collecting duct principal cells. *Eur J Cell Biol* 2006;85:673–678.
119. McWilliams RR, Breusegem SY, Brodsky KF, Kim E, Levi M, Doctor RB. Shank2E binds NaP(i) cotransporter at the apical membrane of proximal tubule cells. *Am J Physiol Cell Physiol* 2005;289(4):C1042–1051.
120. McWilliams RR, Gidey E, Fouassier L, Weed SA, Doctor RB. Characterization of an ankyrin repeat-containing Shank2 isoform (Shank2E) in liver epithelial cells. *Biochem J* 2004;380(Pt 1):181–191.
121. Mohler PJ, Kreda SM, Boucher RC, Sudol M, Stutts MJ, Milgram SL. Yes-associated protein 65 localizes p62(c-Yes) to the apical compartment of airway epithelia by association with EBP50. *J Cell Biol* 1999;147:879–890.
122. Montell C. TRP trapped in fly signaling web. *Curr Opin Neurobiol* 1998;8(3):389–397.
123. Morales FC, Takahashi Y, Kreimann EL, Georgescu MM. Ezrin-radixin-moesin (ERM)-binding phosphoprotein 50 organizes ERM proteins at the apical membrane of polarized epithelia. *Proc Natl Acad Sci U S A* 2004;101(51):17705–17710.
124. Mosavi LK, Cammett TJ, Desrosiers DC, Peng ZY. The ankyrin repeat as molecular architecture for protein recognition. *Protein Sci* 2004;13(6):1435–1448.
125. Muth TR, Ahn J, Caplan MJ. Identification of sorting determinants in the C-terminal cytoplasmic tails of the gamma-aminobutyric acid transporters GAT-2 and GAT-3. *J Biol Chem* 1998;273:25616–25627.
126. Naren AP, Cobb B, Li C, Roy K, Nelson D, Heda GD, Liao J, Kirk KL, Sorscher EJ, Hanrahan J, Clancy JP. A macromolecular complex of beta 2 adrenergic receptor, CFTR, and ezrin/radixin/moesin-binding phosphoprotein 50 is regulated by PKA. *Proc Natl Acad Sci U S A* 2003;100:342–346.
127. Neely JD, Amiry-Moghaddam M, Ottersen OP, Froehner SC, Agre P, Adams ME. Syntrophin-dependent expression and localization of Aquaporin-4 water channel protein. *Proc Natl Acad Sci U S A* 2001;98(24):14108–14113.
128. Newey SE, Benson MA, Ponting CP, Davies KE, Blake DJ. Alternative splicing of dystrobrevin regulates the stoichiometry of syntrophin binding to the dystrophin protein complex. *Curr Biol* 2000;10(20):1295–1298.
129. Newlon MG, Roy M, Morikis D, Carr DW, Westphal R, Scott JD, Jennings PA. A novel mechanism of PKA anchoring revealed by solution structures of anchoring complexes. *EMBO J* 2001;20(7):1651–1662.
130. Newlon MG, Roy M, Morikis D, Hausken ZE, Coghlan V, Scott JD, Jennings PA. The molecular basis for protein kinase A anchoring revealed by solution NMR. *Nat Struct Biol* 1999;6(3):222–227.
131. Nielsen S, Frokiaer J, Marples D, Kwon TH, Agre P, Knepper MA. Aquaporins in the kidney: from molecules to medicine. *Physiol Rev* 2002;82:205–244.
132. O'Connell AD, Leng Q, Dong K, MacGregor GG, Giebisch G, Hebert SC. Phosphorylation-regulated endoplasmic reticulum retention signal in the renal outer-medullary K+ channel (ROMK). *Proc Natl Acad Sci U S A* 2005;102(28):9954–9959.
133. Okamoto M, Sudhof TC. Mints, Munc18-interacting proteins in synaptic vesicle exocytosis. *J Biol Chem* 1997;272:31459–31464.
134. Okamoto PM, Gamby C, Wells D, Fallon J, Vallee RB. Dynamin isoform-specific interaction with the shank/ProSAP scaffolding proteins of the postsynaptic density and actin cytoskeleton. *J Biol Chem* 2001;276(51):48458–48465.
135. Olsen O, Liu H, Wade JB, Merot J, Welling PA. Basolateral membrane expression of the Kir 2.3 channel is coordinated by PDZ interaction with Lin-7/CASK complex. *Am J Physiol Cell Physiol* 2002;282:C183–C195.
136. Olsen O, Wade JB, Morin N, Bredt DS, Welling PA. Differential localization of mammalian Lin-7 (MALS/Veli) PDZ proteins in the kidney. *Am J Physiol Renal Physiol* 2005;288(2): F345–352.
137. Perego C, Bulbarelli A, Longhi R, Caimi M, Villa A, Caplan MJ. Sorting of two polytopic proteins, the gamma-aminobutyric acid and betaine transporters, in polarized epithelial cells. *J Biol Chem* 1997;272:6584–6592.
138. Perego C, Vanoni C, Villa A, Longhi R, Kaech SM, Frohli E, Hajnal A, Kim SK, Pietrini G. PDZ-mediated interactions retain the epithelial GABA transporter on the basolateral surface of polarized epithelial cells. *EMBO J* 1999;18:2384–2393.
139. Poulat F, Barbara PS, Desclozeaux M, Soullier S, Moniot B, Bonneaud N, Boizet B, Berta P. The human testis determining factor SRY binds a nuclear factor containing PDZ protein interaction domains. *J Biol Chem* 1997;272(11):7167–7172.
140. Raghuram V, Hormuth H, Foskett JK. A kinase-regulated mechanism controls CFTR channel gating by disrupting bivalent PDZ domain interactions. *Proc Natl Acad Sci U S A* 2003;100:9620–9625.
141. Raghuram V, Mak DD, Foskett JK. Regulation of cystic fibrosis transmembrane conductance regulator single-channel gating by bivalent PDZ-domain-mediated interaction. *Proc Natl Acad Sci U S A* 2001;98:1300–1305.
142. Reczek D, Berryman M, Bretscher A. Identification of EBP50: A PDZ-containing phosphoprotein that associates with members of the ezrin-radixin-moesin family. *J Cell Biol* 1997;139:169–179.
143. Roh MH, Makarova O, Liu CJ, Shin K, Lee S, Laurinec S, Goyal M, Wiggins R, Margolis B. The Maguk protein, Pals1, functions as an adapter, linking mammalian homologues of Crumbs and Discs Lost. *J Cell Biol* 2002;157:161–172.
144. Roh MH, Margolis B. Composition and function of PDZ protein complexes during cell polarization. *Am J Physiol Renal Physiol* 2003;285(3):F377–387.
145. Rongo C, Whitfield CW, Rodal A, Kim SK, Kaplan JM. LIN-10 is a shared component of the polarized protein localization pathways in neurons and epithelia. *Cell* 1998;94:751–759.
146. Rosenmund C, Carr DW, Bergeson SE, Nilaver G, Scott JD, Westbrook GL. Anchoring of protein kinase A is required for modulation of AMPA/kainate receptors on hippocampal neurons. *Nature* 1994;368(6474):853–856.
147. Schultz J, Hoffmuller U, Krause G, Ashurst J, Macias MJ, Schmieder P, Schneider-Mergener J, Oschkinat H. Specific interactions between the syntrophin PDZ domain and voltage-gated sodium channels. *Nat Struct Biol* 1998;5(1):19–24.
148. Scott RO, Thelin WR, Milgram SL. A novel PDZ protein regulates the activity of guanylyl cyclase C, the heat-stable enterotoxin receptor. *J Biol Chem* 2002;277:22934–22941.
149. Seabold GK, Burette A, Lim IA, Weinberg RJ, Hell JW. Interaction of the tyrosine kinase Pyk2 with the N-methyl-D-aspartate receptor complex via the Src homology 3 domains of PSD-95 and SAP102. *J Biol Chem* 2003;278(17):15040–15048.
150. Setou M, Nakagawa T, Seog DH, Hirokawa N. Kinesin superfamily motor protein KIF17 and mLin-10 in NMDA receptor-containing vesicle transport. *Science* 2000;288:1796–1802.
151. Shelly M, Mosesson Y, Citri A, Lavi S, Zwang Y, Melamed-Book N, Aroeti B, Yarden Y. Polar expression of ErbB-2/HER2 in epithelia. Bimodal regulation by Lin-7. *Dev Cell* 2003;5:475–486.
152. Sheng M, Kim E. The Shank family of scaffold proteins. *J Cell Sci* 2000;113(Pt 11): 1851–1856.
153. Sheng M, Sala C. PDZ domains and the organization of supramolecular complexes. *Neuroscience* 2001;24:1–29.
154. Shenolikar S, Minkoff CM, Steplock DA, Evangelista C, Liu M, Weinman EJ. N-terminal PDZ domain is required for NHERF dimerization. *FEBS Lett* 2001;489(2-3):233–236.
155. Shenolikar S, Voltz JW, Minkoff CM, Wade JB, Weinman EJ. Targeted disruption of the mouse NHERF-1 gene promotes internalization of proximal tubule sodium-phosphate cotransporter type IIa and renal phosphate wasting. *Proc Natl Acad Sci U S A* 2002;99:11470–11475.
156. Shenolikar S, Weinman EJ. NHERF: targeting and trafficking membrane proteins. *Am J Physiol Renal Physiol* 2001;280:F389–F395.
157. Short DB, Trotter KW, Reczek D, Kreda SM, Bretscher A, Boucher RC, Stutts MJ, Milgram SL. An apical PDZ protein anchors the cystic fibrosis transmembrane conductance regulator to the cytoskeleton. *J Biol Chem* 1998;273:19797–19801.
158. Simonsen A, Gaullier JM, D'Arrigo A, Stenmark H. The Rab5 effector EEA1 interacts directly with syntaxin-6. *J Biol Chem* 1999;274:28857–2860.
159. Simske JS, Kaech SM, Harp SA, Kim SK. LET-23 receptor localization by the cell junction protein LIN-7 during *C. elegans* vulva induction. *Cell* 1996;85:195–204.
160. Sneddon WB, Syme CA, Bisello A, Magyar CE, Rochdi MD, Parent JL, Weinman EJ, Abou-Samra AB, Friedman PA. Activation-independent parathyroid hormone receptor internalization is regulated by NHERF-1 (EBP50). *J Biol Chem* 2003;278(44):43787–43796.
161. Songyang Z, Fanning AS, Fu C, Xu J, Marfatia SM, Chishti AH, Chan AC, Anderson JM, Cantley LC. Recognition of unique carboxyl-terminal motifs by distinct PDZ domains. *Science* 1997;275:73–77.
162. Straight SW, Chen L, Karnak D, Margolis B. Interaction with mLin-7 alters the targeting of endocytosed transmembrane proteins in mammalian epithelial cells. *Mol Biol Cell* 2001;12:1329–1140.
163. Straight SW, Karnak D, Borg JP, Kamberov E, Dare H, Margolis B, Wade JB. mLin-7 is localized to the basolateral surface of renal epithelia via its NH(2) terminus. *Am J Physiol Renal Physiol* 2000;278:F464–F475.
164. Sun F, Hug MJ, Lewarchik CM, Yun CH, Bradbury NA, Frizzell RA. E3KARP mediates the association of ezrin and protein kinase A with the cystic fibrosis transmembrane conductance regulator in airway cells. *J Biol Chem* 2002;275:29539–29546.
165. Swiatecka-Urban A, Duhaime M, Coutermarsh B, Karlson KH, Collawn J, Milewski M, Cutting GR, Guggino WB, Langford G, Stanton BA. PDZ domain interaction controls the endocytic recycling of the cystic fibrosis transmembrane conductance regulator. *J Biol Chem* 2002;277:40099–40105.

166. Tang Y, Tang J, Chen Z, Trost C, Flockerzi V, Li M, Ramesh V, Zhu MX. Association of mammalian trp4 and phospholipase C isozymes with a PDZ domain-containing protein, NHERF. *J Biol Chem* 2000;275:37559–37564.

167. Tavares GA, Panepucci EH, Brunger AT. Structural characterization of the intramolecular interaction between the SH3 and guanylate kinase domains of PSD-95. *Mol Cell* 2001;8(6): 1313–1325.

168. Thelin WR, Hodson CA, Milgram SL. Beyond the brush border: NHERF-4 blazes new NHERF turf. *J Physiol* 2005;567(Pt 1):13–19.

169. Thomson RB, Wang T, Thomson BR, Tarrats L, Girardi A, Mentone S, Soleimani M, Kocher O, Aronson PS. Role of PDZK1 in membrane expression of renal brush border ion exchangers. *Proc Natl Acad Sci U S A* 2005;102(37):13331–13336.

170. Tochio H, Zhang Q, Mandal P, Li M, Zhang M. Solution structure of the extended neuronal nitric oxide synthase PDZ domain complexed with an associated peptide. *Nat Struct Biol* 1999;6:417–421.

171. Tojo A, Bredt DS, Wilcox CS. Distribution of postsynaptic density proteins in rat kidney: relationship to neuronal nitric oxide synthase. *Kidney Int* 1999;55:1384–1394.

172. Trotter KW, Fraser ID, Scott GK, Stutts MJ, Scott JD, Milgram SL. Alternative splicing regulates the subcellular localization of A-kinase anchoring protein 18 isoforms. *J Cell Biol* 1999;147(7):1481–1492.

173. Wade JB, Liu J, Coleman RA, Cunningham R, Steplock DA, Lee-Kwon W, Pallone TL, Shenolikar S, Weinman EJ. Localization and interaction of NHERF isoforms in the renal proximal tubule of the mouse. *Am J Physiol Cell Physiol* 2003;285(6):C1494–1503.

174. Wade JB, Welling PA, Donowitz M, Shenolikar S, Weinman EJ. Differential renal distribution of NHERF isoforms and their colocalization with NHE-3, ezrin, and ROMK. *Am J Physiol Cell Physiol* 2001;280:C192–C18.

175. Wang S, Raab RW, Schatz PJ, Guggino WB, Li M. Peptide binding Consesus of the NHE-RF-PDZ1 doamin matches the C-terminal sequence of CFTR. *FEBS Lett* 1998;427: 103–108.

176. Wang S, Yue H, Derin RB, Guggino WB, Li M. Accessory protein facilitated CFTR-CFTR interaction, a molecular mechanism to potentiate the chloride channel activity. *Cell* 2001;103:169–179.

177. Weinman EJ. New functions for the NHERF family of proteins. *J Clin Invest* 2001;108: 185–160.

178. Weinman EJ, Boddeti A, Cunningham R, Akom M, Wang F, Wang Y, Liu J, Steplock D, Shenolikar S, Wade JB. NHERF-1 is required for renal adaptation to a low-phosphate diet. *Am J Physiol Renal Physiol* 2003;285:F1225–F1232.

179. Weinman EJ, Cunningham R, Wade JB, Shenolikar S. The role of NHERF-1 in the regulation of renal proximal tubule sodium-hydrogen exchanger 3 and sodium-dependent phosphate cotransporter 2a. *J Physiol* 2005;567(Pt 1):27–32.

180. Weinman EJ, Hall RA, Friedman PA, Liu-Chen LY, Shenolikar S. The association of NHERF adaptor proteins with G protein-coupled receptors and receptor tyrosine kinases. *Annu Rev Physiol* 2005.

181. Weinman EJ, Steplock D, Shenolikar S. CAMP-mediated inhibition of the renal brush border membrane Na$^+$-H+ exchanger requires a dissociable phosphoprotein cofactor. *J Clin Invest* 1993;92:1781–1176.

182. Weinman EJ, Steplock D, Shenolikar S. NHERF-1 uniquely transduces the cAMP signals that inhibit sodium-hydrogen exchange in mouse renal apical membranes. *FEBS Lett* 2003;536(1-3):141–144.

183. Weinman EJ, Steplock D, Wade JB, Shenolikar S. Ezrin binding domain-deficient NHERF attenuates cAMP-mediated inhibition of Na(+)/H(+) exchange in OK cells. *Am J Physiol Renal Physiol* 2001;281 (2):F374–380.

184. Weinman EJ, Steplock D, Wang Y, Shenolikar S. Characterization of a protein cofactor that mediates protein kinase A regulation of the renal brush border membrane Na(+)-H+ exchanger. *J Clin Invest* 1995;95:2143–2219.

185. Weinman EJ, Wang Y, Wang F, Greer C, Steplock D, Shenolikar S. A C-terminal PDZ motif in NHE-3 binds NHERF-1 and enhances cAMP inhibition of sodium-hydrogen exchange. *Biochemistry* 2003;42(43):12662–12668.

186. Wong W, Scott JD. AKAP signalling complexes: focal points in space and time. *Nat Rev Mol Cell Biol* 2004;5(12):959–970.

187. Wu H, Reuver SM, Kuhlendahl S, Chung WJ, Garner CC. Subcellular targeting and cytoskeletal attachment of SAP97 to the epithelial lateral membrane. *J Cell Sci* 1998;111:2365–2276.

188. Xiao B, Tu JC, Worley PF. Homer: a link between neural activity and glutamate receptor function. *Curr Opin Neurobiol* 2000;10(3):370–374.

189. Xie Z. Molecular mechanisms of Na/K-ATPase-mediated signal transduction. *Ann N Y Acad Sci* 2003;986:497–503.

190. Xu XZ, Choudhury A, Li X, Montell C. Coordination of an array of signaling proteins through homo- and heteromeric interactions between PDZ domains and target proteins. *J Cell Biol* 1998;142:545–555.

191. Xu ZC, Yang Y, Hebert SC. Phosphorylation of the ATP-sensitive, inwardly rectifying K+ channel, ROMK, by cyclic AMP-dependent protein kinase. *J Biol Chem* 1996;271: 9313–9319.

192. Yoo D, Fang L, Mason A, Kim BY, Welling PA. A phosphorylation-dependent export structure in ROMK (Kir 1.1) channel overrides an endoplasmic reticulum localization signal. *J Biol Chem* 2005;280(42):35281–35290.

193. Yoo D, Flagg TP, Olsen O, Raghuram V, Foskett JK, Welling PA. Assembly and Trafficking of a Multiprotein ROMK (Kir 1.1) Channel Complex by PDZ Interactions. *J Biol Chem* 2000;279:6863–6873.

194. Yoo D, Kim BY, Campo C, Nance L, King A, Maouyo D, Welling PA. Cell surface expression of the ROMK (Kir 1.1) channel is regulated by the aldosterone-induced kinase, SGK-1, and protein kinase A. *J Biol Chem* 2003;278:23066–23075.

195. Yuan Z, Cai T, Tian J, Ivanov AV, Giovannucci DR, Xie Z. Na/K-ATPase tethers phospholipase C and IP3 receptor into a calcium-regulatory complex. *Mol Biol Cell* 2005;16 (9):4034–4045.

196. Yun CC, Chen Y, Lang F. Glucocorticoid activation of Na(+)/H(+) exchanger isoform 3 revisited. The roles of SGK1 and NHERF-2. *J Biol Chem* 2002;277:7676–7783.

197. Yun CC, Palmada M, Embark HM, Fedorenko O, Feng Y, Henke G, Setiawan I, Boehmer C, Weinman EJ, Sandrasagra S, Korbmacher C, Cohen P, Pearce D, Lang F. The serum and glucocorticoid-inducible kinase SGK1 and the Na(+)/H(+) exchange regulating factor NHERF-2 synergize to stimulate the renal outer medullary K(+) channel ROMK1. *J Am Soc Nephrol* 2002;13:2823–2830.

198. Yun CH, Oh S, Zizak M, Steplock D, Tsao S, Tse CM, Weinman EJ, Donowitz M. cAMP-mediated inhibition of the epithelial brush border Na$^+$/H+ exchanger, NHE-3, requires an associated regulatory protein. *Proc Natl Acad Sci U S A* 1997;94:3010–3015.

CHAPTER **13**

The Renin-Angiotensin System

Thu H. Le, Steven D. Crowley, Susan B. Gurley, and Thomas M. Coffman
Duke University and Durham VA Medical Centers, Durham, North Carolina, USA

Highly conserved through phylogeny, the renin-angiotensin system (RAS) is an essential regulator of blood pressure and fluid balance. This biological system is a multi-enzymatic cascade in which angiotensinogen, its major substrate, is processed in a two-step reaction by renin and angiotensin-converting enzyme (ACE), resulting in the sequential generation of angiotensin I and angiotensin II (Fig. 1). Along with its importance in maintaining normal circulatory homeostasis, abnormal activation of the RAS can contribute to the development of hypertension and target organ damage.

The importance of the RAS in clinical medicine is highlighted by two sets of observations. First are associations between polymorphisms of genes encoding RAS components and cardiovascular disease (17, 28, 142, 273, 283, 297). Second and perhaps more compelling is the impressive efficacy of pharmacological agents that inhibit the synthesis or activity of angiotensin II. For example, ACE inhibitors are very effective and well-tolerated antihypertensive agents (129). Along with their ability to lower blood pressure, these agents effectively prevent or ameliorate morbidity and mortality associated with cardiovascular diseases. In this regard, large clinical trials have demonstrated that ACE inhibitors improve survival in patients with congestive heart failure (136, 137) and in patients with risk factors for coronary artery disease (298). They also slow the progression of a variety of kidney diseases, including diabetic nephropathy (169). Angiotensin-receptor blockers (ARBs), which block AT_1 receptors, are similarly effective for treating these disorders (32, 58, 168).

The purpose of this chapter is to provide an overview of the major physiological features of the RAS, focusing on its role in the kidney.

THE COMPONENTS OF THE RENIN-ANGIOTENSIN SYSTEM

Renin

The aspartyl protease renin was first isolated from the kidney by Tigerstedt more than a century ago. Renin is synthesized as a precursor protein, prorenin, containing an additional 43 amino acids at the N-terminus that block the enzyme's active site (59). Active renin is generated by removal of this N-terminal peptide fragment, presumably by proteases in the juxtaglomerular cells of the kidney. Whether intact prorenin has a distinct physiological role remains to be determined; however, there is accumulating evidence suggesting specific contributions of the prorenin molecule in some normal and disease states (64, 177, 220, 280).

Active renin specifically cleaves the 10 amino acids from the N-terminus of angiotensinogen to form angiotensin I. A substantial excess of angiotensinogen is present in serum and ACE is ubiquitous in the endothelium and plasma (218). Accordingly, in the bloodstream, the amount of renin is a key rate-limiting step determining the level of angiotensin II and thus the activity of the system. The primary source of renin in the circulation is the kidney, where its expression and secretion are tightly regulated at the juxtaglomerular apparatus by two distinct mechanisms: a renal baroreceptor (26, 39) and sodium chloride delivery to the macula densa (16, 175, 176). Through these sensing mechanisms, levels of renin in plasma can be incrementally titrated in response to changes in blood pressure and salt balance. These regulatory principles provide a basis for many of the physiological characteristics of the RAS and regulation of renin release in the kidney will be discussed in detail subsequent sections.

In addition to its protease activity, renin may also bind specifically to other proteins or putative receptors (1, 200, 220, 278). This binding may induce physiologically significant intracellular signaling (200). It has been suggested that the mannose-6-phosphate receptor (M6P-R), also known as insulin-like growth factor II receptor, binds renin and prorenin leading to internalization and degradation (1). Recently, Nguyen et al. (200) reported cloning a receptor from human kidney expression library that binds renin and prorenin specifically and with high affinity. Binding of the putative ligands causes a conformational change of the enzymes that leads to increased catalytic activity. Furthermore, binding of renin to this receptor induces a rapid and sustained activation of ERK1/ERK2 without affecting concentrations of calcium or cAMP (200). Although the physiological significance of this putative renin/prorenin receptor is not clear, it has been

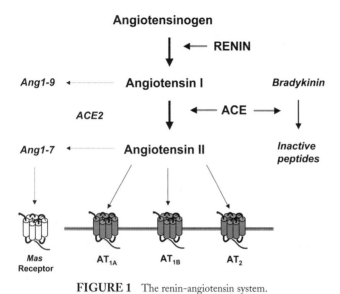

FIGURE 1   The renin-angiotensin system.

suggested that it may mediate angiotensin II–independent effects of renin and might also indicate a functional role of prorenin (201).

Angiotensinogen

Angiotensinogen, the substrate for renin, is the source of all angiotensin peptides. Angiotensinogen in the circulation is derived primarily from synthesis in the liver. In humans, plasma concentrations of angiotensinogen are typically near the half maximal activity (Km) of renin (100) so that changes in plasma concentration may influence the rate of angiotensin I generation at any given level of renin. In human hypertensive siblings, Jeunemaitre et al. (142) showed that a specific variant of the human angiotensinogen gene, *M235T*, was linked to hypertension and was associated with a modestly elevated plasma angiotensinogen concentration, about 120% of normal. They proposed that this variant of the *AGT* gene leads to an increase in plasma angiotensinogen levels and thereby eventually to increased blood pressure. However, because amino acid 235 is in a nonconserved portion of the angiotensinogen protein and variation of this amino acid does not affect protein stability, a mechanism to explain the physiological consequences of the mutation was not clear. An apparent explanation came later, when the M235T variant was found to be in linkage disequilibrium with another variant in the 5′ untranslated region of the *AGT* gene (135). This second variant, a single nucleotide substitution in the promoter of the *AGT* gene, was associated with increased transcriptional activity of the gene (135). Higher levels of *AGT* mRNA were found in patients carrying the variant allele (135). The causal capacity of alterations in plasma angiotensinogen level to affect blood pressure was demonstrated in studies of mice engineered to carry from zero to four copies of the *Agt* gene (146). In these animals, there was a positive correlation

between the number of *Agt* gene copies, plasma levels of angiotensinogen, and blood pressure.

In addition to its synthesis by the liver, angiotensinogen is also produced by other tissues including the brain, immune system, and kidney (68). In the kidney, synthesis of angiotensinogen in proximal tubules has been well documented (134), and proximal tubule synthesis may be regulated in part by the end product, angiotensin II (151). Along with angiotensinogen, the kidney expresses all of the other components of the RAS. Accordingly, it has been suggested that regulation and functioning of autonomous "tissue" RAS in the kidney, as well as other organs, may contribute to the physiological functions of the system, especially in disease states (72). This hypothesis has been used to explain additional complexity of the system whereby the apparent activity of the RAS is not reflected by measured plasma levels of it major components. For example, in the broad population of patients with hypertension, diabetes, and cardiovascular disease, pharmacological antagonists of the RAS lower blood pressure and prevent end-organ damage even in the absence of overt elevation of plasma renin levels. However, the precise nature and physiological contributions of these tissue systems have been difficult to define experimentally.

Angiotensin-Converting Enzyme

ACE is a carboxypeptidase that generates the vasoactive peptide angiotensin II by cleaving two amino acids from the c-terminus of the inactive precursor angiotensin I (53). There are two distinct forms of ACE, somatic and testicular, both generated by alternative splicing of a single gene (76, 128, 161). Somatic ACE is expressed as an ectoenzyme on the surface of endothelial cells throughout the body and is particularly abundant in lung, intestine, choroid plexus, placenta, and on brush border membranes in the kidney. A soluble form of ACE that circulates in plasma is formed by enzymatic cleavage of tissue-bound ACE at its transmembrane domain (15). As with other components of the RAS, molecular variants of *ACE* have been proposed as candidate genes in hypertension, cardiovascular, and kidney diseases (242). Insertion (I) and deletion (D) polymorphisms of the human *ACE* gene are common and have been associated with altered levels of ACE in plasma (229, 282). In some cohorts but not others, these *ACE* gene variants have been linked to differing susceptibilities to hypertension and cardiovascular and renal diseases (242, 263).

In addition to angiotensin I, other biologically active peptides are substrates for ACE. Perhaps the most important of these is bradykinin (179). ACE degrades bradykinin into an inactive peptide, representing a significant biological pathway for bradykinin metabolism in vivo (36); in older literature, ACE was referred to as kininase II. Since bradykinin has vasodilator and natriuretic properties (179), it has been suggested that one mechanism of blood pressure reduction with ACE inhibition is blockade of this kininase activity. This was clearly demonstrated by Brown and associates, who showed that the antihypertensive efficacy of ACE inhibitors is attenuated by simultaneous administration of a bradykinin receptor antagonist (91).

Using genome-based strategies, homologs of ACE have been identified (69, 272, 300). One of these, ACE2, exhibits more than 40% identity at the protein level with the catalytic domain of ACE (69, 272). Similar to ACE, ACE2 is expressed on the surface of certain endothelial cell populations. However, compared to the ubiquitous distribution of ACE, the expression pattern of ACE2 is more limited with most abundant expression in kidney followed by heart and testis (69, 272). Their substrate specificities also differ; ACE2 hydrolyzes angiotensin II with high efficiency, but has much lower activity against angiotensin I (69, 281). Hydrolysis of angiotensin II by ACE2 generates another peptide with putative biological actions: angiotensin 1–7 (281). Accumulating evidence indicates that this peptide causes vasodilation and natriuresis and may promote reduced blood pressures (79) via the Mas receptor (239). It has been further suggested that ACE2 may be a major pathway for synthesis of angiotensin 1–7 (80). Thus, the functions of ACE2 may be determined by its distinct actions to metabolize angiotensin II and to generate angiotensin 1–7.

Although the precise physiological role of ACE2 is not clear, it was originally identified and cloned from a cDNA library prepared from ventricular tissue of a patient with heart failure (69). Studies in ACE2-deficient mice have suggested a role for ACE2 in cardiac function (56) and in blood pressure regulation (103). A third member of the ACE gene family, collectrin, was identified as a gene that is upregulated in the subtotal nephrectomy model of chronic kidney disease (300, 301). Collectrin is highly homologous to the transmembrane portion of ACE2, but lacks the carboxypeptidase domain (300). Its physiological functions have not yet been clearly defined.

Angiotensin Receptors

The biological actions of angiotensin II are mediated by cell surface receptors that belong to the large family of seven transmembrane receptors (129, 271). The angiotensin receptors can be divided into two pharmacological classes: type 1 (AT_1) and type 2 (AT_2), based on their differential affinities for various nonpeptide antagonists. Studies using these antagonists suggested that most of the classically recognized functions of the RAS are mediated by AT_1 receptors (271). Gene-targeting studies have confirmed these conclusions (268).

AT_1 receptors from a number of species have been cloned (133, 196, 240) and two subtypes, designated AT_{1A} and AT_{1B}, have been identified in rat (140, 143, 238) and mouse (241). In the classical view, AT_1 receptors signal through $G_{\alpha q}$-linked signaling pathways involving phospholipase C, IP3, and increases in intracellular calcium (63). However, the AT_1 receptor has also been linked to JAK/STAT activation (180) and β-arrestin–dependent pathways linked to ERK activation (4, 249). In addition, recent studies have shown that the AT1 receptor has the capacity to transactivate the EGF receptor (75). This pathway may contribute to chronic kidney injury (162).

The murine AT_1 receptors are products of separate genes and share substantial sequence homology (35, 141, 143). AT_{1A} receptors predominate in most organs, except the adrenal gland and regions of the central nervous system (CNS), where AT_{1B} expression may be more prominent (35, 92, 174). A single report has suggested that AT_{1B} receptors might also exist in man (153), but this has not been confirmed in the unpublished work of several independent groups and the consensus view is that there is no human counterpart to the murine AT_{1B} receptor. Thus, the AT_{1A} receptor is considered the closest murine homologue to the single human AT_1 receptor.

The binding signatures of the AT_{1A} and AT_{1B} receptors are virtually identical (47) and it was difficult to discriminate their in vivo functions pharmacologically. Experiments using gene targeting have provided insights into the discrete functions of the two AT_1 receptor genes (205, 206). Although the AT_{1B} receptor has a unique role to mediate thirst responses in the CNS (62), AT_{1A} receptors have the predominant role in determining the level of blood pressure (138, 185, 260) and in mediating vasoconstrictor responses (138, 205). The phenotype of markedly reduced blood pressures and profound sodium sensitivity in mice lacking the AT_{1A} receptor (138, 207) underscores its importance in blood pressure control.

Pharmacological and genetic studies have confirmed that virtually all of the classically recognized functions of the RAS are mediated by AT_1 receptors. Until recently, little was known about the physiological role of AT_2 receptors. AT_2 receptors are found in abundance during fetal development (101, 189) but their expression generally falls after birth (201a). However, persistent AT_2 receptor expression can be detected in several adult tissues including the kidney, adrenal gland, and brain, and absolute levels of AT_2 receptor expression may be modulated by angiotensin II and certain growth factors (132). AT_2 receptors appear to signal by coupling to $G_{\alpha i2}$ and $G_{\alpha i3}$ proteins (19). Using site-directed mutagenesis, the intermediate portion of the third intracellular loop of the AT_2 receptor was found to be necessary for normal receptor signaling (117, 164). Moreover, it has been suggested that activation of AT_2 receptors stimulates bradykinin, nitric oxide, and guanosine cyclic 3′,5′-monophosphate (cGMP) (40, 254), and these pathways may mediate actions of the receptor to promote natriuresis and blood pressure lowering. Finally, there is also evidence to support HETEs as second messengers for AT_2 receptors in the kidney, leading to ERK1/2 phosphorylation (70).

Targeted disruption of the mouse *Agtr2* gene did not cause a dramatically abnormal phenotype. These animals clearly manifest increased sensitivity to the pressor actions of angiotensin II (121, 131). One of the AT_2-deficient lines manifested increased baseline blood pressure and heart rate (121). Interestingly, behavioral changes were also observed in AT_2-deficient mice. They had decreased spontaneous movements and rearing activity (121, 131) and impaired drinking response to water deprivation (131). Transgenic mice that overexpress the AT_2-receptor gene under control of a cardiac-specific promoter have decreased sensitivity to AT_1-mediated pressor and chronotropic actions (182). Moreover, the pressor actions of angiotensin II are significantly attenuated in these transgenic mice. This attenuation was completely reversed following pretreatment with a specific AT_2 receptor antagonist. Taken together, these data suggest that a primary function of the AT_2 receptor may be to negatively modulate the actions of the AT_1 receptor.

Aldosterone

Aldosterone is a steroid hormone synthesized in the zona glomerulosa (ZG) of the adrenal gland. The two dominant regulators of aldosterone synthesis and release are angiotensin II and the level of serum potassium (3). The RAS-dependent component of aldosterone regulation is triggered by binding of angiotensin II to AT_1 receptors in the ZG (3). Stimulation of aldosterone release by angiotensin II contributes to enhanced sodium reabsorption and antinatriuresis. Independently of angiotensin II, hyperkalemia can control the release of aldosterone through a process that involves the membrane depolarization of ZG cells (203, 227). In addition, adrenocorticotropic hormone (ACTH) can stimulate aldosterone via its G-protein–coupled receptor (227). Elevations in ACTH influence aldosterone production only during short-term stress as this response is attenuated with persistent exposure to ACTH. In contrast, angiotensin II and potassium can both exert a chronic, sustained stimulation of aldosterone generation by the ZG (2).

The classically recognized effects of aldosterone to influence sodium handling in the distal nephron are mediated by aldosterone binding to the mineralocorticoid receptor (MR). The MR is a 107-kD protein that acts as a transcription factor to regulate gene expression in target tissues. The molecular mechanisms used by the MR to drive epithelial sodium channel (ENaC) function in the collecting tubule have been reviewed recently (90). Cortisol actually exhibits a higher affinity for the mineralocorticoid receptor than aldosterone, but locally expressed 11β-hydroxysteroid dehydrogenase type 2 "protects" the MR by converting cortisol to cortisone, which does not activate the MR (230). The binding of aldosterone to the MR in the principle cell of the collecting tubule epithelium induces transcription of the α subunit and the multimeric coupling of the α, β, and γ subunits of the ENaC and the translocation of the ENaC complex to the luminal surface of the tubule (8, 183).

Along with these transcriptional effects, aldosterone further enhances ENaC activity by upregulating serum- and glucocorticoid-regulated kinase 1 (sgk1) (20, 31, 197). Sgk1 in turn phosphorylates Nedd4-2 causing ENaC proteins to remain in the apical membrane of the principal cell (186, 277). Once inserted into the luminal membrane of the principal cell, ENaC permits cellular uptake of intraluminal sodium generating an electronegative potential in the distal tubular lumen which favors secretion of potassium from the principal cell into the urinary filtrate via the renal outer medullary potassium channel (ROMK). Sgk1 may also phosphorylate ROMK similarly increasing its apical density, further facilitating the kaliuresis induced by aldosterone (296). In addition, aldosterone appears to directly increase ROMK expression (12). Through this pathway, the MR regulates sodium and potassium transport within the mineralocorticoid-responsive segments of the distal nephron.

Recent human phenotyping studies and animal studies using gene-targeting strategies have confirmed the contribution of the MR to tubular function and salt balance. For example, in humans with a mutation leading to a constitutively active MR, early-onset hypertension develops (94), whereas heterozygosity for an inactivating mutation of the MR leads to salt-wasting, hypotension, metabolic acidosis, and hyperkalemia (95). Mice genetically deficient for the MR similarly develop severe salt-wasting that leads to neonatal death (18). Mutations that activate the ENaC may cause hypertension (81, 170, 264), whereas global inactivation of the subunits of the ENaC in mice causes sodium wasting, potassium retention, and early mortality and in humans it causes pseudohypoaldosteronism type 1 with severe salt-wasting (235). In contrast, inactivation of the α-ENaC gene only in the collecting duct does not impair sodium and potassium balance (237), suggesting that the regulation by aldosterone of ENaC in the more distal regions of the distal convoluted tubule and/or the connecting tubule may also contribute to sodium and fluid homeostasis (21).

Integrated Actions of the RAS in the Kidney

The important role of the kidney in regulation of blood pressure has been long recognized (104a), and the relationship between alterations in systemic blood pressure and changes in renal sodium excretion is well documented (7). For example, an elevation in perfusion pressure in the renal artery results in a rapid increase in sodium and water excretion by the kidney, so-called pressure natriuresis (7). Based on such observations, Guyton and coworkers suggested that whenever arterial pressure is elevated, activation of this pressure-natriuresis mechanism will cause sufficient excretion of sodium and water to return systemic pressures to normal (104). They further hypothesized that the substantial capacity for sodium excretion by the kidney provides a compensatory system of virtually infinite gain to oppose processes, including increases in peripheral vascular resistance, which would tend to increase blood pressure (Fig. 2). It follows that defects in renal excretory function would therefore be a prerequisite for sustaining a chronic increase in intra-arterial pressure.

The RAS has potent actions to modulate pressure–natriuresis relationships in the kidney (107, 111) and these actions shape the characteristics of RAS-dependent blood pressure regulation in normal physiology and in disease states. For example, as depicted in Fig. 2B, chronic infusion of angiotensin II causes a shift of the pressure natriuresis curve to the right, suggesting that when the RAS is activated, higher pressures are required to excrete an equivalent sodium load (108). Conversely, administration of ACE inhibitors or ARBs shifts the curve to the left, meaning that natriuresis is facilitated at lower levels of blood pressure (Fig. 2B). The basic features of endogenous control of the RAS are consistent with these homeostatic functions. As shown in Fig. 2A, the system is activated at low levels of salt intake stimulating renal sodium reabsorption and conservation of body fluid volumes and blood pressure. In contrast, with high sodium intake, the system is suppressed, facilitating natriuresis.

REGULATION OF RENIN

As discussed in the preceding paragraphs, the concentration of renin in plasma is a key rate-limiting step in the production of angiotensin II. Accordingly, the activity of the RAS in the circulation is largely determined by the factors that regulate renin. The kidney is the major source of renin where its generation and secretion are primarily controlled by the activity of the sympathetic nervous system, renal perfusion pressure, and luminal delivery of sodium chloride to the macula densa in the distal nephron. The major features of these regulatory processes are described in the sections that follow.

Sources of Renin

The major source of renin in the circulation is the kidney. Following bilateral nephrectomy, plasma levels of renin and angiotensin II fall precipitously (37). In the kidney, renin is primarily found in granular cells, which are modified smooth muscle cells within the juxtaglomerular apparatus (JGA). The JGA is located in the region where the afferent arteriole enters the glomerulus (9, 265). As shown in Fig. 3, the JGA is a highly organized structure composed of three distinct anatomical parts: granular cells, the macula densa, and the extraglomerular mesangial cells (279). The macula densa is a specialized tubular area that marks the transition from the ascending loop of Henle to the distal tubule lying in direct contact with the vascular pole of the glomerulus from which it originated (279). By light microscopy, the unique characteristics of the macula densa epithelial cells can be discerned by their narrow, columnar shape and apparent accumulation of nuclei distinguishing them from cells in the adjacent parts of the distal tubule. (9). By electron microscopy, the basement membrane of the macula densa appears to be fused with the vacular component and continuous with the basement membranes surrounding the granular and agranular cells in the extraglomerular mesangium (9). As described in the following paragraphs, the macula densa acts as a sensor of chloride concentration in the distal tubule, providing signals that are important for control of renin (279). The anatomical organization of the JGA facilitates the regulation of renin secretion in response to critical environmental cues.

Although JG cells are clearly the primary source of renin in the kidney, studies by Lalouel and associates (231) suggest that renin is also present in the connecting tubule, at least in the mouse kidney. Moreover, their studies indicate that renin expression in the connecting tubule may be regulated by sodium intake. Although its physiological role is unclear, it has been suggested that renin expressed in the distal

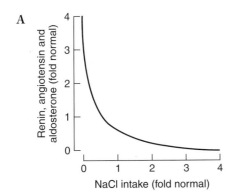
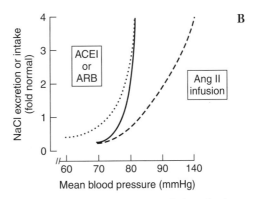

FIGURE 2 Idealized, steady-state relationships between (A) dietary sodium intake and plasma levels of renin, angiotensin II, or aldosterone and (B) sodium excretion or intake and blood pressure in a healthy individual *(solid line)*, during chronic infusion of angiotensin II *(dashed line)*, and with administration of an ACE inhibitor (ACEI) or angiotensin receptor blocker (ARB) *(dotted line)*. (From Wilcox in Greenberg et al. *Primer on Kidney Diseases*. Philadelphia: Elsevier Saunders; 2001:556–561.)

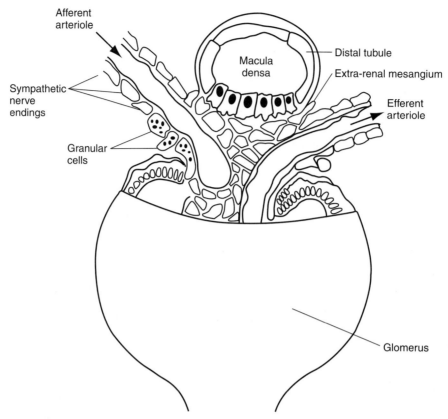

FIGURE 3 The juxtaglomerular apparatus (JGA). Integration of the regulated secretion of renin is carried out at the JGA. Three major pathways regulate the secretion of renin by granular cells at the JGA: the baroreceptor, the macula densa mechanism, and direct stimulation by the sympathetic nervous system. The renal baroreceptor monitors renal perfusion pressure and signals an increase in renin when renal perfusion pressure falls. In the macula densa mechanism, macula densa cells sense the decrease in chloride ions in the filtrate in the distal tubule, thereby stimulating release of renin. Increased activity of renal sympathetic nerves directly stimulates renin release via activation of β-adrenergic receptors. Sympathetic innervation also modulates both the baroreceptor and macula densa mechanisms.

nephron may contribute to regulation of angiotensin peptide concentrations in the tubular lumen.

Expression of renin outside the kidney has also been documented. Levi and associates have recently shown that mast cells express renin mRNA and contain large quantities of renin protein, apparently within the secretory granules (252). Mast cell–derived renin can efficiently convert angiotensinogen to angiotensin I after mast cell degranulation (252). Moreover, release of renin by cardiac mast cells can be triggered by ischemia, producing pathophysiological consequences such as release of norepinephrine and generation of cardiac arrhythmias (178). Taken together, this work has suggested that resident mast cells in the heart and perhaps other organs, with appropriate stimulation, are capable of generating ample quantities of renin to activate the RAS locally and thereby affect organ function. Furthermore, it appears the factors controlling renin release from mast cells will be quite different from those that regulate JG cells and are likely to involve signals associated with inflammation and injury (163). Nonetheless, it re-

mains to be determined whether this alternative pathway for RAS activation plays any major role in physiology or disease pathogenesis.

Baroreceptor Regulation of Renin Release

The baroreceptor theory was developed to explain observations that renin secretion is directly stimulated by reduced renal perfusion. This theory was first developed in the context of experimental observations that granularity of the JG cells was inversely correlated with the magnitude of renal perfusion pressure (274). Since then, numerous studies have shown that renin secretion is inversely related to renal perfusion pressure or pulse amplitude (26, 105, 148, 202, 255). This relationship is preserved in denervated kidneys (23, 24) and in isolated perfused kidneys with a non-functioning macula densa mechanism (85, 123, 276). Thus, the baroreceptor is an independent mechanism for controlling renin, residing within the kidney and clearly separate from regulation by the sympathetic nervous system (105). In renovascular hypertension, the baroreceptor is the primary mechanism for stimulating renin release. In the presence of a critical stenosis of the renal artery, renal perfusion pressure drops, stimulating renin and generating hypertension (234).

Although the independent nature of the baroreceptor mechanism and its localization to the kidney has been clearly established, identification of its precise nature has been elusive. Various models have been proposed to explain the mechanism for pressure sensing and consequent signal transduction including direct stretch of the JG cells due to transmural pressure across the afferent arteriole (39, 84) or indirect pathways involving secondary release of autocoids (211). Some of these candidate soluble factors include nitric oxide (150, 157, 219), prostanoids (60, 96), which are stimulatory, or endothelins, which are inhibitory (195).

Gene targeting in the mouse has been used to examine the role of some of these mediators in the baroreceptor response. In one study, genetic deletion of endothelial nitric oxide synthase (eNOS) had no effect on renin release in response to change in renal perfusion pressure, suggesting that eNOS-derived nitric oxide is not a mediator of the baroreceptor-renin coupling (14). On the other hand, the absence of the IP receptor, the single known receptor for PGI$_2$ (prostacyclin) conferred substantial resistance to hypertension and hyperreninemia after unilateral renal artery stenosis (88). This suggests an absolute requirement for PGI$_2$ in triggering of renin release after baroreceptor activation. However, a number of questions remain concerning the nature and location of the pressure sensor, the mechanism and cell lineages controlling synthesis of key mediators such as prostacyclin, and the cellular targets for these mediators affecting renin release (83).

Macula Densa Mechanism for Renin Regulation

The second major pathway for physiological regulation of renin is the so-called macula densa mechanism whereby cells at the macula densa sense a reduction in chloride ions in the filtrate of the distal tubule, triggering renin release (176). In this circumstance, release of renin, and the consequent generation of angiotensin II, is believed to serve as a mechanism for enhancing renal sodium reabsorption in states of fluid volume depletion. The anatomical association of the macula densa with the JG cells stimulated the first speculation by Goormaghtigh of its physiological function (99). As discussed previously, the macula densa comprises specialized epithelial cells at the terminal portion of the thick ascending limb. Their basolateral membrane is in contact with glomerular mesangial cells, which, in turn, are contiguous with granular cells in the JGA (16). The role of the macula densa in renin regulation was initially hypothesized by Vander in 1967 (279) and there is now general consensus that this mechanism provides a control of renin secretion that is directly determined by

sodium chloride delivery to the distal nephron (256, 270). Moreover, several studies indicate that chloride flux through the Na-K-2CL transporter (NKCC2) regulates the signaling pathways linked to renin secretion (181, 243). Increased chloride delivery to the MD inhibits, whereas reduced chloride delivery stimulates, renin release (154, 176, 245).

Several candidate signaling pathways linking distal tubule solute concentration to control of renin have been proposed, including adenosine, nitric oxide, and prostanoids (49). The most compelling evidence suggests that MD stimulation of renin involves activation of cyclooxygenase (COX)-2 (114) constitutively expressed at high levels in the macula densa, generating the prostanoid PGE$_2$ (247, 248). PGE$_2$ then activates an EP receptor (probably EP4) on granular cells in the JGA to stimulate renin release (247). The capacity for prostaglandins to directly stimulate renin secretion has been long recognized (13, 285). Moreover, studies using specific inhibitors and COX-2–deficient mice have clearly demonstrated the importance of COX-2 in the macula densa pathway (46, 112). In addition, the activity of various components of this system has been demonstrated in the isolated perfused macula densa segments (221) and JG cell lines (294). However, at least one study (88) has failed to confirm a nonredundant role for individual EP receptors for PGE$_2$ in furosemide-stimulated renin release in vivo.

Initial evidence suggesting a role for adenosine in MD signaling came from studies using the selective A1AR antagonist 8-cyclopentyl-1,3-dipropylxanthine. The major effect of the inhibitor was to attenuate the actions of increasing luminal NaCl concentrations to inhibit renin release (287). Later studies using A1AR-deficient mice confirmed that the role of adenosine is primarily restricted to the arm mediating inhibition of renin release. In A1AR-deficient mice, renin-inhibitory actions of enhanced sodium chloride delivery to the macula densa are blocked, whereas stimulation of renin secretion caused by reduced sodium chloride transport at the macula densa is unaffected (147).

Macula densa cells express high levels of neuronal nitric oxide synthase (nNOS) (194, 290). The role of NO in regulation of renin was first tested using nonselective inhibitors of nitric oxide synthesis, which attenuated renin release stimulated by reduced luminal sodium chloride concentrations (120, 267). The specific roles of the individual NOS isoforms have been examined using mice with targeted deletion of nNOS or eNOS. In these studies, activation of the macula densa pathway was achieved by administration of NKCC2-blocking loop diuretics in vivo and in isolated perfused mouse kidneys. Deficiency of either nNOS or eNOS alone did not significantly affect macula densa–dependent renin secretion (43), whereas nonspecific NOS blockade attenuated renin stimulation by loop diuretics. This suggests that nitric oxide plays a permissive rather than a primary role in the macula densa control of renin release (43).

Short Loop Feedback: Regulation of Renin by Angiotensin II

Angiotensin II also contributes to the regulatory pathways for renin and may control its own synthesis by activating AT_1 receptors, highly expressed at the JGA, thereby suppressing renin release (208, 250). Evidence supporting the existence of this so-called short-loop feedback mechanism includes studies in the isolated perfused kidney where infusion of angiotensin II suppresses renin release (105). Administration of ACE inhibitors and angiotensin receptor blockers increase renin mRNA expression and cause JGA hypertrophy (98). Similarly, mice lacking AT_{1A} receptors also develop marked JGA hypertrophy (185, 208). However, in *Agtr1a*$^{-/-}$ chimeric mice (185) and in kidney cross-transplantation experiments (57), JGA hypertrophy correlated with blood pressure, but not with the absence of AT_1 receptors at the JGA, indicating a significant role for baroreceptor mechanisms in this response. Nonetheless, a role for the short-loop feedback mechanism to alter the sensitivity of baroreceptor or MD mechanisms would be consistent with current data.

Role of Sympathetic Nerve Activity

The capacity for sympathetic nerve activation to stimulate renin has been long recognized. For example, β-adrenoceptors are abundant in the JGA of kidneys from various species (167). Furthermore, numerous studies have demonstrated that administration of β-adrenergic agonists is sufficient to stimulate renin release (144). The β-adrenergic receptor signals via G_s-proteins, increasing intracellular concentration of cAMP, which is a key pathway stimulating renin release in the juxtaglomerular cell (see following sections). Chronic renal nerve activation also stimulates renin (124, 125) along with its affects to modulate renal blood flow and tubular function. In experiments controlling for these factors, a clear relationship between increasing renal sympathetic nerve activity and renin secretion is maintained (66, 149). Accordingly, it has been suggested that inhibition of β-adrenergic effects on renin release is one mechanism explaining the antihypertensive efficacy of β-blockers in patients with hypertension. Although β-adrenergic activation is sufficient to trigger renin release, renal denervation does not abolish the capacity of the baroreceptor (22, 24) or macula densa mechanisms to stimulate renin release (85, 123, 276).

Regulation of Cellular Release of Renin

At the JGA, renin is stored in cytoplasmic granules within granular cells. In response to activating stimuli, renin is released into the circulation by exocytosis. This process of renin secretion is carried out by fusion events between the secretory granules and cell membrane of afferent arterioles (87). Furthermore, the extent of secretory activity or exocytosis can be assessed using electrophysiological tech-

niques that directly measure cell membrane capacitance of single mouse JG cells (86). The control mechanisms for renin, described previously, act by triggering this exocytotic pathway. Compared with the relative wealth of available information about physiological regulation of renin, much less is known about the precise intracellular pathways involved in renin secretion and how these mechanisms are controlled in the granular cell. The general consensus is that the environmental signals regulating renin act through a limited number of intracellular second messengers including calcium and cyclic AMP (cAMP) (51, 248).

The cAMP pathway appears to be the major trigger for cellular release of renin. In a variety of experimental models, maneuvers causing an elevation of intracellular concentrations of cAMP cause rapid stimulation of renin secretion (51, 156). In this regard, most of the documented secretagogues for renin including PGE_2, PGI_2, dopamine, and β-adrenoreceptor act via seven trans-membrane receptors linked to G_s proteins that increase cAMP levels in JG cells (156). The specific biochemical pathways by which cAMP acts to stimulate renin secretion are unclear, but likely involve protein kinase A, since inhibition of protein kinase A attenuates the stimulatory effect of β-adrenoreceptors on renin secretion (157).

By contrast, increases in intracellular calcium levels may inhibit renin release. For example, experimental maneuvers that reduce intracellular calcium concentration stimulate renin release (51). Moreover, several mediators with putative actions to inhibit renin release, such as angiotensin II, α-receptor agonist, vasopressin, and endothelin, have receptors that couple to G_q proteins and activation of these receptors by ligand increases intracellular calcium concentrations in JG cells (51, 248). The inhibitory effect of calcium on renin release appears to be mediated by protein kinase C because stimulation of protein kinase C inhibits renin secretion (48, 50, 155) whereas blockade of protein kinase C attenuates the inhibitory effect on renin secretion (48, 50, 157). There is also evidence that the effects of calcium on renin release are mediated in part by a calmodulin-dependent process, since inhibition of calmodulin activity stimulates renin secretion (65, 215). Antagonistic interactions between the cAMP and intracellular calcium may ultimately determine the final consequences of extracellular signals upon renin release (51, 228).

Regulation of Renin Gene Expression

The steady-state activity of the RAS is generally reflected by renin mRNA levels in the kidney. During chronic stimulation of the RAS, for example, upregulation of renin gene expression is required to sustain over time the enhanced release of renin protein by the JGA. Understanding of tissue-specific control of renin gene expression has been complicated by difficulty in developing tractable cell culture preparations derived from JG cells. Thus, transgenic mice have been used extensively to assess in vivo regulation of renin gene expression (89, 251). Using this approach, minimal segments of the human renin gene sufficient to recapitulate temporal- and cell-specific patterns of gene expression have been identified (89, 251).

There is strong sequence conservation of 5′ proximal promoter regions between the renin genes of the human, rat, and mouse (214). This region contains a cyclic AMP (cAMP) response element (CRE) (29, 216, 257), which is required for cAMP stimulation of transcription (29, 193). In addition, there are at least seven transcription factor binding sites within the proximal promoter, including a binding site for HOX proteins that play critical roles in specifying positional information along embryonic axes (214). The renin promoter is relatively weak in isolation (29, 193, 295), but is strengthened up to 80-fold by a distal enhancer element (97, 223). This enhancer contains at least 11 transcription factor binding sites responsive to a variety of signal transduction pathways (213). Inhibitory factors including endothelin-1, angiotensin II, mechanical stretch, and inflammatory cytokines may act through target sequences within the enhancer (213).

Post-transcriptional mechanisms also play a key role in determining steady-state renin mRNA levels. cAMP appears to be a critical mediator in this process. For example, in cell systems, cAMP has only a modest effect on inducing renin gene transcription of the renin gene, but nonetheless causes marked induction of renin mRNA levels (160). This augmentation is associated with enhanced stability of renin mRNA (44). cAMP also increases levels of RNA-binding proteins targeting the 3′ UTR of the human renin gene (192), suggesting a potential mechanism for its effects to promote renin mRNA stability.

Control of Renal Hemodynamics by the RAS

Angiotensin II, acting via its AT_1 receptor, is a potent vasoconstrictor. Stimulation of AT_1 receptors in vascular smooth muscle cells initiates a signaling cascade including increased intracellular calcium concentration and alterations in cytoskeleton, inducing contraction with consequent increases in vascular resistance (102). Studies in mice deficient in the AT_{1A} and AT_{1B} receptor isoforms have confirmed the importance of AT1 receptors in this response (138, 206). The pressor response to acute angiotensin II infusion is completely abolished in these double-knockout animals (206); whereas response to another pressor agent, epinephrine, is not affected. These vasoconstrictor actions of angiotensin II play a central role in maintaining circulatory homeostasis in a number of tissues, including the kidney. In the kidney, the hemodynamic actions of angiotensin II impact renal blood flow, glomerular filtration rate, excretion of salt and water, and progression of renal damage in disease states.

GLOMERULAR MICROCIRCULATION

The coordinated regulation of resistances in the afferent and efferent arterioles plays a critical role in determining and maintaining the glomerular filtration rate (GFR). The RAS has potent effects on glomerular hemodynamics. Angiotensin II causes constriction of the afferent and efferent arterioles. However, high levels of angiotensin II induce a more profound constriction of the efferent arteriole (25, 71, 198). The reasons for this disproportionate effect of angiotensin II on the efferent arteriole is not clear, but may include differences in levels of AT_1 receptor expression (187), modulating actions of vasodilators such as prostaglandins and nitric oxide on pre-glomerular vessels (139, 209), or differences in calcium responses to angiotensin II in the afferent versus efferent arterioles (41, 42, 82). In mice, the AT_{1A} and AT_{1B} receptor isoforms have distinct actions in the glomerular circulation. Both AT_{1A} and AT_{1B} receptors contribute to the afferent arteriolar response to angiotensin II, whereas the efferent arteriolar response is mediated exclusively by AT_{1A} receptors (116).

The overall effect of angiotensin II on glomerular hemodynamics is a predominant increase in postglomerular resistance, resulting in an increase in glomerular hydrostatic pressure. These actions serve to protect GFR in states of intravascular volume depletion. Because angiotensin II also simultaneously reduces renal blood flow, there will be a coincident increase in filtration fraction and a decrease in peritubular capillary pressure (55), promoting an increase in sodium reabsorption in the proximal tubule (73, 74). The importance of angiotensin II in maintaining GFR when renal perfusion is threatened is illustrated by the effect of ACE inhibitors in patients with critical bilateral renal artery stenosis or critical stenosis in the renal artery of a single functioning kidney. When blood pressures in such patients are reduced to equivalent levels with a non-specific vasodilator such as nitroprusside compared to an ACE inhibitor, the ACE inhibitor causes a much more marked deterioration in GFR (126, 266).

The glomerular hemodynamic responses to angiotensin II may be modified significantly by other circulating factors. For example, the vasoconstrictor actions of angiotensin II may be substantially augmented in the presence of elevated adenosine levels (106, 190, 191, 258, 292). This can occur in pathological states including malignant hypertension, renal artery stenosis, and some experimental models of renal ischemia (184, 212, 293). When angiotensin II and adenosine are present at high concentrations, there is a dramatic increase in preglomerular resistance that does not occur with either agent alone. Other mediators such as prostanoids (225) and nitric oxide may also modulate the actions of angiotensin II in the glomerular microcirculation. In angiotensin II–induced hypertension, for example, nitric oxide attenuates afferent arteriolar constriction (130).

In kidney disease, abnormal activation of the RAS and coincident increases in glomerular hydrostatic pressure might contribute to progressive renal injury (188, 299). For example, in the remnant kidney model of chronic kidney disease, postglomerular resistances are increased and this is associated with increased glomerular hydrostatic pressures (6, 253). This abnormal glomerular hemodynamic pattern is reversed with RAS blockade. These observations formed the basis of the rationale for using ACE inhibitors or angiotensin receptor blockers in chronic kidney diseases. Reduction of glomerular hemodynamic pressure may be a key mechanism explaining the renoprotective effects of these agents in diseases such as diabetic nephropathy (32, 168, 169).

Renal Medullary Circulation

Along with its effects on the glomerular circulation, angiotensin II acting through AT$_1$ receptors has important regulatory functions in the renal circulation in general. In the mouse, regulation of renal blood flow by angiotensin II is primarily mediated by AT$_{1A}$ receptors (236). Moreover, effects of AT$_1$ receptors to modulate blood flow in the medulla significantly impact the kidney's excretory capacity for sodium (78). In this regard, it has been suggested that regulation of medullary blood flow by angiotensin II represents a critical pathway for modulating the pressure–natriuresis response discussed earlier in the chapter (54, 104). Thus, regulation of medullary blood flow by the RAS is likely to be a key pathway used by the kidney to maintain blood pressure homeostasis.

The mechanisms controlling medullary blood flow in the kidney are complex. As in the glomerulus, vasodilator effects of mediators such as nitric oxide and prostanoids act to counterbalance the actions of angiotensin II. For example, a subpressor dose of angiotensin II, which by itself has a negligible effect on the medullary circulation, significantly reduces medullary blood flow when combined with the NO inhibitor L-NAME (302). Cortical blood flow is unaffected in this circumstance. Nitric oxide also protects medullary blood flow during chronic infusion of angiotensin II (262). In the outer medulla, angiotensin II stimulates NO production by tubular epithelium, potentially as a compensatory mechanism, and this may be an example of *tubulo–vascular cross-talk,* whereby effects of angiotensin II on tubular epithelium may modify its vasoconstrictor actions (67). Similarly, renal prostaglandins also appear to modulate pressure natriuresis by altering renal medullary hemodynamics (232). These hemodynamic changes from the inhibition of prostaglandin production lead to increased chloride reabsorption in the loop of Henle and collecting duct (122, 233).

Alterations in the balance of angiotensin II and NO in the medulla may have significant consequences on systemic blood pressure regulation. For example, angiotensin II–stimulated NO production is impaired in Dahl-sensitive hypertensive rats (44, 45, 261), and attenuated generation of NO in kidneys of these animals is associated with reduced medullary blood flow (119, 127). In contrast to intravenous infusion, delivery of L-arginine directly into the renal medulla of Dahl salt-sensitive rats reverses the hypertensive actions of angiotensin II (261).

Renal Epithelial Actions of the RAS

Along with its hemodynamic actions, angiotensin II may modulate fluid and solute excretion through two distinct pathways: (1) an indirect pathway involving stimulation of aldosterone release from the adrenal gland and (2) direct effects of AT$_1$ receptors expressed by renal epithelia (111).

In the adrenal cortex, activation of AT$_1$ receptors stimulates the release of aldosterone (3) that in turn promotes sodium reabsorption by binding to mineralocorticoid receptors in the mineralocorticoid-responsive segments of the distal nephron (183). The biology of the aldosterone system is described elsewhere and historically was thought to be the major effector system used by the RAS to control renal sodium handling (90). Direct actions of angiotensin II in the kidney were defined later using isolated perfused tubules (93, 152, 222, 246, 275, 288) and micropuncture studies (10, 52, 166, 284). Using these approaches, renal epithelial responses to angiotensin II were documented in several nephron segments. However, it has been difficult, in the intact animal, to separate effects of AT$_1$ receptors in renal epithelium from other renal and systemic effects of angiotensin II and to determine their contribution to integrated control of blood pressure. Nonetheless, recent studies using renal cross-transplantation clearly indicate significant, non-redundant contributions of AT$_1$ receptors within the kidney to determining the level of blood pressure (57). In the next section, we will provide an overview of tubular actions of the RAS.

TUBULAR EFFECTS OF ANGIOTENSIN II

Proximal Tubule Direct actions of angiotensin II in the proximal tubule are perhaps the best characterized. These actions were first implied in whole animal studies (108, 109, 210) and then were specifically defined using in vitro-perfused proximal tubules (246) and micropuncture studies (52). Taken together, these studies suggest that angiotensin II acting through AT$_1$ receptors on the basolateral surface of proximal tubules promotes sodium reabsorption by coordinately stimulating the sodium–proton antiporter on the luminal membrane along with the sodium–potassium ATPase on the basolateral surface (52, 93, 246). These actions result in enhanced basolateral sodium bicarbonate flux (93). The capacity for proximal tubular actions of the RAS to influence blood pressure was demonstrated in elegant experiments by Sigmund and associates (61). In these studies, isolated co-expression of human renin and angiotensinogen in the proximal tubule caused hypertension without any detectable increase in circulating angiotensin II levels.

AT$_1$ receptors are also present on the luminal brush border of the proximal tubular epithelium (33, 34, 115). Moreover, angiotensin II is secreted into the proximal tubular lumen where its levels may not correlate with plasma angiotensin II levels (30, 199). Control of angiotensin II generation in this luminal compartment might provide separate regulation of epithelial function that is independent of the systemic RAS (226). Moreover, activation of AT$_1$ receptors on the luminal membrane of the proximal tubular cell can promote sodium reabsorption, in part through a G$_i$-protein–mediated reduction in cAMP (52,

246). There is some evidence of an independent regulation of luminal concentrations of angiotensin II. For example, although both whole-kidney and proximal tubular angiotensin II levels are elevated in response to reduced renal perfusion (27), angiotensin II levels in proximal tubular fluid are not suppressed with acute volume expansion and may even increase in this setting (27, 269).

The net effect of angiotensin II on bicarbonate handling in the proximal tubule appears to be neutral. Coordinate with its stimulation of the apical membrane sodium–proton exchanger, angiotensin II enhances activity of the sodium–bicarbonate cotransporter on the basolateral surface of the early proximal tubule (93, 246). As such, angiotensin II acts as a potent stimulus for proximal acidification coupled to reclamation of bicarbonate from the early proximal tubule (93, 171, 172). Nevertheless, the resulting reduction in delivery of bicarbonate to the late proximal tubule leads to less bicarbonate reabsorption in that segment such that the bicarbonate concentration in the urinary filtrate reaching the distal convoluted tubule is not altered by angiotensin II stimulation (173). Thus, the contribution of the RAS to acid-base regulation is primarily mediated by aldosterone in the distal nephron (11, 113, 118, 259, 289).

Loop of Henle Compared with the proximal tubule, the functions of angiotensin II in the medullary thick ascending limb (MTAL) are not as well-characterized. AT_1 receptors are expressed on the luminal and basolateral membranes of the MTAL epithelium (217, 224). In vitro studies addressing the role of angiotensin II in MTAL ion transport suggest that cellular responses may differ depending on the local concentrations of angiotensin II (5, 165). At lower concentrations of angiotensin II, inhibition of the sodium–potassium–chloride cotransporter (NKCC2) may be seen (5, 165), whereas stimulation of NKCC2 can be seen at higher concentrations (5). In vivo microperfusion experiments have also demonstrated physiological consequences of angiotensin II in the MTAL including increased bicarbonate transport out of the urinary filtrate (38). This heightened bicarbonate flux is likely due to an increase in sodium–hydrogen exchange as has been observed in the proximal tubule, suggesting that angiotensin II increases sodium reabsorption from the MTAL. These data are consistent with the finding that in vivo administration of angiotensin II leads to heightened expression of both the NHE3 sodium–hydrogen exchanger and NKCC2 in the MTAL (159).

Distal Nephron Solute Transport Although angiotensin II indirectly influences distal and collecting tubular function through the generation of aldosterone, more recent studies have demonstrated that angiotensin II also has direct effects to modulate ion flux along the distal nephron. As in other nephron segments, all the elements of the RAS are present along the distal nephron, and relatively high concentrations of angiotensin II can be detected in the tubular fluid of these segments (115, 199, 231). Angiotensin II acting via AT_1 receptors stimulates sodium–hydrogen exchange in the cortical distal tubule leading to an increase in bicarbonate reabsorption (10, 166). On the apical membrane of the principal cells in the cortical collecting duct (CCD), luminal angiotensin II stimulates amiloride-sensitive sodium transport by increasing activity of the epithelial sodium channel (ENaC) through an AT_1 receptor-dependent mechanism (222, 284). Furthermore, activation of AT_1 receptors on the basolateral membrane of CCD cells stimulates the activity of potassium channels via a nitric oxide-dependent pathway (286). As the distal nephron ultimately determines urine flow and composition, actions of angiotensin II to modulate sodium handling at this site may impact blood pressure homeostasis (110, 222).

Water Handling Recent studies suggest a role for the RAS in the control of urinary concentrating mechanisms and free water handling. For example, the complete absence of angiotensinogen, ACE, or AT_{1A}/AT_{1B} receptors in mice is associated with atrophy of the renal papilla and a marked urinary concentrating defect (77, 145, 208). Mice lacking AT_{1A} receptors are also unable to generate maximally concentrated urine, despite having apparently normal renal papillae (204). These animals generate vasopressin normally in response to water restriction but are resistant to 1-desamino-8-d-arginine vasopressin (DDAVP) (204). Administration of an AT_1 receptor–antagonist to wild-type mice recapitulates this urinary concentrating defect (204). Similarly, AT_1 receptor blockade also blunts the maximal urine concentrating capacity in DDAVP-challenged rats and this effect is associated with reduced expression of aquaporins-1 and -2 (158). In cells isolated from the inner medullary collecting duct (IMCD), angiotensin II upregulates gene expression for the V_2 vasopressin receptor and the aquaporin-2 channel (291). These effects are mediated through a protein kinase A–dependent pathway (291). Thus, direct effects of angiotensin II on expression of water channels ands perhaps vasopressin receptors may contribute to its actions on renal water handling.

References

1. Admiraal PJ, et al. Uptake and proteolytic activation of prorenin by cultured human endothelial cells. *Hypertension* 1999;17(5):621–629.
2. Aguilera G. Factors controlling steroid biosynthesis in the zona glomerulosa of the adrenal. *J Steroid Biochem Mol Biol* 1993;45(1-3):147–151.
3. Aguilera G. Role of angiotensin II receptor subtypes on the regulation of aldosterone secretion in the adrenal glomerulosa zone in the rat. *Mol Cell Endocrinol* 1992;90(1):53–60.
4. Ahn D, et al. Collecting duct-specific knockout of endothelin-1 causes hypertension and sodium retention. *J Clin Invest* 2004;114(4):504–511.
5. Amlal H, et al. ANG II controls Na(1)-K1(NH41)-2Cl- cotransport via 20-HETE and PKC in medullary thick ascending limb. *Am J Physiol* 1998;274(4 Pt 1):C1047–1056.
6. Anderson S, et al. Control of glomerular hypertension limits renal injury in rats with reduced renal mass. *J Clin Invest* 1985;76:612–619.
7. Aperia AC, Broberger CG, Soderlund S. Relationship between renal artery perfusion pressure and tubular sodium reabsorption. *Am J Physiol* 1971;220(5):1205–1212.
8. Asher C, et al. Aldosterone-induced increase in the abundance of Na1 channel subunits. *Am J Physiol* 1996;271(2 Pt 1):C605–611.
9. Barajas L. Anatomy of the juxtaglomerular apparatus. *Am J Physiol* 1979;237(5):F333–343.
10. Barreto-Chaves ML, Mello-Aires M. Effect of luminal angiotensin II and ANP on early and late cortical distal tubule HCO3- reabsorption. *Am J Physiol* 1996;271(5 Pt 2):F977–984.
11. Batlle DC, Segmental characterization of defects in collecting tubule acidification. *Kidney Int* 1986;30(4):546–554.

12. Beesley AH, Hornby D, White SJ. Regulation of distal nephron K1 channels (ROMK) mRNA expression by aldosterone in rat kidney. *J Physiol* 1998;509 (Pt 3):629–634.

13. Beierwaltes WH, et al. Renin release selectively stimulated by prostaglandin I2 in isolated rat glomeruli. *Am J Physiol* 1982;243(3):F276–283.

14. Beierwaltes WH, Potter DL, Shesely EG. Renal baroreceptor-stimulated renin in the eNOS knockout mouse. *Am J Physiol Renal Physiol* 2002;282(1):F59–64.

15. Beldent V, et al. Proteolytic release of human angiotensin-converting enzyme. Localization of the cleavage site. *J Biol Chem* 1993;268(35):26428–26434.

16. Bell PD, et al. Macula densa cell signaling involves ATP release through a maxi anion channel. *Proc Natl Acad Sci U S A* 2003; 100(7):4322–4327.

17. Benetos A, et al. Angiotensin-converting enzyme inhibitors: Influence of angiotensin-converting enzyme and angiotensin II type 1 receptor gene polymorphisms on aortic stiffness in normotensive and hypertensive patients. *Circulation* 1996;94:698–703.

18. Berger S, et al. Mineralocorticoid receptor knockout mice: Pathophysiology of Na1 metabolism. *PNAS* 1998;95(16):9424–9429.

19. Berry C, et al. Angiotensin receptors: signaling, vascular pathophysiology, and interactions with ceramide. *Am J Physiol Heart Circ Physiol* 2001;281(6):H2337–2365.

20. Bhargava A, et al. The serum- and glucocorticoid-induced kinase is a physiological mediator of aldosterone action. *Endocrinology* 2001;142(4):1587–1594.

21. Biner HL, et al. Human cortical distal nephron: distribution of electrolyte and water transport pathways. *J Am Soc Nephrol* 2002;13(4):836–847.

22. Blaine EH, Davis JO, Prewitt RL. Evidence for a renal vascular receptor in control of renin secretion. *Am J Physiol* 1971;220(6):1593–1597.

23. Blaine EH, Davis JO, Witty RT. Renin release after hemorrhage and after suprarenal aortic constriction in dogs without sodium delivery to the macula densa. *Circ Res* 1970;27(6):1081–1089.

24. Blaine EH, Davis JO. Evidence for a renal vascular mechanism in renin release: new observations with graded stimulation by aortic constriction. *Circ Res* 1971;28(5):Suppl 2:118–126.

25. Blantz RC, Konnen KS, Tucker BJ. Angiotensin II effects upon the glomerular microcirculation and ultrafiltration coefficient of the rat. *J Clin Invest* 1976;57(2):419–434.

26. Bock HA, et al. Pressure dependent modulation of renin release in isolated perfused glomeruli. *Kidney Int* 1992;41(2):275–280.

27. Boer WH, et al. Effects of reduced renal perfusion pressure and acute volume expansion on proximal tubule and whole kidney angiotensin II content in the rat. *Kidney Int* 1997;51(1):44–49.

28. Bonnardeaux A, et al. Angiotensin II type 1 receptor gene polymorphisms in human essential hypertension. *Hypertension* 1994;24:63–69.

29. Borensztein P, et al. Cis-regulatory elements and trans-acting factors directing basal and cAMP-stimulated human renin gene expression in chorionic cells. *Circ Res* 1994;74(5):764–773.

30. Braam B, et al. Proximal tubular secretion of angiotensin II in rats. *Am J Physiol* 1993;264(5 Pt 2):F891–898.

31. Brennan FE, Fuller PJ. Rapid upregulation of serum and glucocorticoid-regulated kinase (sgk) gene expression by corticosteroids *in vivo*. *Mol Cell Endocrinol* 2000;166(2):129–136.

32. Brenner BM, et al. Effects of losartan on renal and cardiovascular outcomes in patients with type 2 diabetes and nephropathy. *N Engl J Med* 2001;345(12):861–869.

33. Brown GP, Douglas JG. Angiotensin II binding sites on isolated rat renal brush border membranes. *Endocrinology* 1982;111(6):1830–1836.

34. Brown GP, Douglas JG. Angiotensin II-binding sites in rat and primate isolated renal tubular basolateral membranes. *Endocrinology* 1983;112(6):2007–2014.

35. Burson JM, et al. Differential expression of angiotensin receptor 1A and 1B in mouse. *Am J Physiol* 1994;267(2 Pt 1):E260–267.

36. Campbell DJ, et al. Effect of reduced angiotensin-converting enzyme gene expression and angiotensin-converting enzyme inhibition on angiotensin and bradykinin peptide levels in mice. *Hypertension* 2004;43(4):854–859.

37. Campbell DJ. Extrarenal renin and blood pressure regulation: an alternative viewpoint. *Am J Hypertens* 1989;2(4):266–275.

38. Capasso G, et al. Bicarbonate transport along the loop of Henle. II. Effects of acid-base, dietary, and neurohumoral determinants. *J Clin Invest* 1994;94(2):830–838.

39. Carey RM, et al. Biomechanical coupling in renin-releasing cells. *J Clin Invest* 1997;100(6):1566–1574.

40. Carey RM, Wang ZQ, Siragy HM. Role of the angiotensin type 2 receptor in the regulation of blood pressure and renal function. *Hypertension* 2000;35(1 Pt 2):155–163.

41. Carmines PK, Morrison TK, Navar LG. Angiotensin II effects on microvascular diameters of *in vitro* blood-perfused juxtamedullary nephrons. *Am J Physiol* 1986;251(4 Pt 2):F610–618.

42. Carmines PK, Navar LG. Disparate effects of Ca channel blockade on afferent and efferent arteriolar responses to ANG II. *Am J Physiol* 1989;256(6 Pt 2):F1015–1020.

43. Castrop H, et al. Permissive role of nitric oxide in macula densa control of renin secretion. *Am J Physiol Renal Physiol* 2004;286(5):F848–857.

44. Chen M, et al. Cyclic AMP selectively increases renin mRNA stability in cultured juxtaglomerular granular cells. *J Biol Chem* 1993; 268(32):24138–24144.

45. Chen PY, Sanders PW. L-arginine abrogates salt-sensitive hypertension in Dahl/Rapp rats. *J Clin Invest* 1991;88(5):1559–1567.

46. Cheng H, Harris R. Angiotensin converting enzyme inhibitor-mediated increases in renal renin expression are not seen in cyclooxygenase-2 knockout mice. *J Am Soc Nephrol* 1999; 10:343A.

47. Chiu A, et al. Characterization of angiotensin AT1A receptor isoform by it ligand binding signature. *Regul Pept* 1993;44:141–147.

48. Churchill MC, Churchill PC. 12-0-Tetradecanoylphorbol 13-acetate inhibits renin secretion of rat renal cortical slices. *J Hypertension* 1984;2(1):25–28.

49. Churchill PC, Churchill MC. A1 and A2 adenosine receptor activation inhibits and stimulates renin secretion of rat renal cortical slices. *J Pharmacol Exp Ther* 1985;232(3):589–594.

50. Churchill PC, et al. Effect of melittin on renin and prostaglandin E2 release from rat renal cortical slices. *J Physiol* 1990;428:233–241.

51. Churchill PC, Second messengers in renin secretion. *Am J Physiol Renal Physiol* 1985;249(2):F175–184.

52. Cogan MG. Angiotensin II: a powerful controller of sodium transport in the early proximal tubule. *Hypertension* 1990;15(5):451–458.

53. Corvol P, Williams TA, Soubrier F. Peptidyl dipeptidase A: angiotensin I-converting enzyme. *Methods Enzymol* 1995;248:283–305.

54. Cowley AW Jr, Roman RJ. The role of the kidney in hypertension. *JAMA* 1996;275(20):1581–1589.

55. Cowley AW, et al. Effect of renal medullary circulation on arterial pressure. *J Hypertens Suppl* 1992;10(7):S187–193.

56. Crackower MA, et al. Angiotensin-converting enzyme 2 is an essential regulator of heart function. *Nature* 2002;417(6891):822–828.

57. Crowley SD, et al. Distinct roles for the kidney and systemic tissues in blood pressure regulation by the renin-angiotensin system. *J Clin Invest* 2005;115(4):1092–1099.

58. Dahlof B, et al. Cardiovascular morbidity and mortality in the Losartan Intervention For Endpoint reduction in hypertension study (LIFE): a randomised trial against atenolol. *Lancet* 2002;359(9311):995–1003.

59. Danser AH, Deinum J. Renin, prorenin and the putative (pro)renin receptor. *Hypertension* 2005;46(5):1069–1076.

60. Data JL, et al. The prostaglandin system. A role in canine baroreceptor control of renin release. *Circ Res* 1978;42(4):454–458.

61. Davisson R, et al. Novel mechanism of hypertension revealed by cell-specific targeting of human angiotensinogen in transgenic mice. *Physiol Genomics* 1999;1:3–9.

62. Davisson RL, et al. Divergent functions of angiotensin II receptor isoforms in the brain. *J Clin Invest* 2000;106(1):103–106.

63. de Gasparo M, et al. International union of pharmacology. XXIII: the angiotensin II receptors. *Pharmacol Rev* 2000;52(3):415–472.

64. Deinum J, et al. Increase in serum prorenin precedes onset of microalbuminuria in patients with insulin-dependent diabetes mellitus. *Diabetologia* 1999;42(8):1006–1010.

65. Della Bruna R, et al. Calmodulin antagonists stimulate renin secretion and inhibit renin synthesis *in vitro*. *Am J Physiol* 1992;262(3 Pt 2):F397–402.

66. DiBona GF. Neural regulation of renal tubular sodium reabsorption and renin secretion. *Fed Proc* 1985;44(13):2816–2822.

67. Dickhout JG, Mori T, Cowley AW Jr. Tubulovascular nitric oxide crosstalk: buffering of angiotensin II-induced medullary vasoconstriction. *Circ Res* 2002;91(6):487–493.

68. Dickson ME, Sigmund CD. Genetic basis of hypertension: revisiting angiotensinogen. *Hypertension* 2006;48(1):14–20.

69. Donoghue M, et al. A novel angiotensin-converting enzyme-related carboxypeptidase (ACE2) converts angiotensin I to angiotensin 1-9; *Circ Res* 2000;87(5):E1–9.

70. Dulin NO, et al. Phospholipase A2-mediated activation of mitogen-activated protein kinase by angiotensin II. *Proc Natl Acad Sci U S A* 1998;95(14):8098–8102.

71. Dworkin LD, Ichikawa I, Brenner BM. Hormonal modulation of glomerular function. *Am J Physiol* 1983;244(2):F95–104.

72. Dzau VJ, et al. A comparative study of the distributions of renin and angiotensinogen messenger ribonucleic acids in rat and mouse tissues. *Endocrinology* 1987;120(6):2334–2338.

73. Earley LE, Friedler RM. Changes in renal blood flow and possibly the intrarenal distribution of blood during the natriuresis accompanying saline loading in the dog. *J Clin Invest* 1965;44:929–941.

74. Earley LE, Friedler RM. The effects of combined renal vasodilatation and pressor agents on renal hemodynamics and the tubular reabsorption of sodium. *J Clin Invest* 1966;45(4):542–551.

75. Eguchi S, et al. Calcium-dependent epidermal growth factor receptor transactivation mediates the angiotensin II-induced mitogen-activated protein kinase activation in vascular smooth muscle cells. *J Biol Chem* 1998;273(15):8890–8896.

76. Ehlers MR, et al. Molecular cloning of human testicular angiotensin-converting enzyme: the testis isozyme is identical to the C-terminal half of endothelial angiotensin-converting enzyme. *Proc Natl Acad Sci U S A* 1989;86(20):7741–7445.

77. Esther C, et al. Mice lacking angiotensin converting enzyme have low blood pressure, renal pathology, and reduced male fertility. *Lab Invest* 1996;74:953–965.

78. Faubert PF, Chou SY, Porush JG. Regulation of papillary plasma flow by angiotensin II. *Kidney Int* 1987;32(4):472–478.

79. Ferrario C, et al. Angiotensin-(1-7): a new hormone of the angiotensin system. *Hypertension* 1991;18:III-126–133.

80. Ferrario CM, Trask AJ, Jessup JA. Advances in biochemical and functional roles of angiotensin-converting enzyme 2 and angiotensin-(1-7) in regulation of cardiovascular function. *Am J Physiol Heart Circ Physiol* 2005;289(6):H2281–2290.

81. Firsov D, et al. Cell surface expression of the epithelial Na channel and a mutant causing Liddle syndrome: a quantitative approach. *PNAS* 1996;93(26):15370–15375.

82. Fleming JT, Parekh N, Steinhausen M. Calcium antagonists preferentially dilate preglomerular vessels of hydronephrotic kidney. *Am J Physiol* 1987;253(6 Pt 2):F1157–1163.

83. Francois H, Coffman TM. Prostanoids and blood pressure: which way is up? *J Clin Invest* 2004;114(6):757–759.

84. Fray JC. Regulation of renin secretion by calcium and chemiosmotic forces: (patho) physiological considerations. *Biochim Biophys Acta* 1991;1097(4):243–262.

85. Fray JC. Stretch receptor model for renin release with evidence from perfused rat kidney. *Am J Physiol* 1976;231(3):936–944.

86. Friis UG, et al. Direct demonstration of exocytosis and endocytosis in single mouse juxtaglomerular cells. *Circ Res* 1999;84(8):929–936.

87. Friis UG, et al. Exocytosis and endocytosis in juxtaglomerular cells. *Acta Physiol Scand* 2000;168(1):95–99.

88. Fujino T, et al. Decreased susceptibility to renovascular hypertension in mice lacking the prostaglandin I2 receptor IP. *J Clin Invest* 2004; 114(6):805–812.

89. Fukamizu A, et al. Human renin in transgenic mouse kidney is localized to juxtaglomerular cells. *Biochem J* 1991;278(Pt 2):601–603.

90. Fuller PJ, Young MJ. Mechanisms of mineralocorticoid action. *Hypertension* 2005;46(6):1227–1235.
91. Gainer JV, et al. Effect of bradykinin-receptor blockade on the response to angiotensin-converting-enzyme inhibitor in normotensive and hypertensive subjects. *N Engl J Med* 1998;339(18):1285–1292.
92. Gasc JM, et al. Tissue-specific expression of type 1 angiotensin II receptor subtypes. An in situ hybridization study. *Hypertension* 1994;24(5):531–537.
93. Geibel J, Giebisch G, Boron WF. Angiotensin II stimulates both Na(1)-H1 exchange and Na1/HCO3- cotransport in the rabbit proximal tubule. *Proc Natl Acad Sci U S A* 1990;87(20): 7917–7920.
94. Geller DS, et al. Activating mineralocorticoid receptor mutation in hypertension exacerbated by pregnancy. *Science* 2000;289(5476):119–123.
95. Geller DS, et al. Mutations in the mineralocorticoid receptor gene cause autosomal dominant pseudohypoaldosteronism type I. *Nat Genet* 1998;19(3):279–281.
96. Gerber JG, Keller RT, Nies AS. Prostaglandins and renin release: the effect of PGI2, PGE2, and 13,14-dihydro PGE2 on the baroreceptor mechanism of renin release in the dog. *Circ Res* 1979;44(6):796–799.
97. Germain S, et al. A novel distal enhancer confers chorionic expression on the human renin gene. *J Biol Chem* 1998;273(39):25292–25300.
98. Gomez RA, et al. Recruitment of renin gene-expressing cells in adult rat kidneys. *Am J Physiol* 1990;259(4 Pt 2):F660–665.
99. Goormaghtigh NJ. Facts in favour of an endocrine function of the renal arterioles. *J Pathol Bacteriol* 1945;57:392–404.
100. Gould AB, Green D. Kinetics of the human renin and human substrate reaction. *Cardiovasc Res* 1971;5(1):86–89.
101. Grady E, et al. Expression of AT2 receptors in the developing rat fetus. *J Clin Invest* 1991; 88:921–933.
102. Griendling KK, et al. Angiotensin II signaling in vascular smooth muscle: new concepts. *Hypertension* 1997;29(1 Pt 2):366–373.
103. Gurley SB, et al. Altered blood pressure responses and normal cardiac phenotype in ACE2-null mice. *J Clin Invest* 2006;116(8):2218–2225.
104. Guyton AC, et al. Arterial pressure regulation: overriding dominance of the kidneys in long-term regulation and in hypertension. *Am J Med* 1972;52(5):584–594.
104a. Guyton AC. Blood pressure control—special role of the kidneys and body fluids. *Science* 1991; 252:1813–1816.
105. Hackenthal E, et al. Morphology, physiology, and molecular biology of renin secretion. *Physiol Rev* 1990;70(4):1067–1116.
106. Haddy FJ, Scott JB. Metabolically linked vasoactive chemicals in local regulation of blood flow. *Physiol Rev* 1968;48(4):688–707.
107. Hall JE, Brands MW, Henegar JR. Angiotensin II and long-term arterial pressure regulation: the overriding dominance of the kidney. *J Am Soc Nephrol* 1999;10 Suppl 12:S258–265.
108. Hall JE, et al. Blood pressure and renal function during chronic changes in sodium intake: role of angiotensin. *Am J Physiol Renal Physiol* 1980;239(3):F271–280.
109. Hall JE, et al. Control of glomerular filtration rate by renin-angiotensin system. *Am J Physiol* 1977;233(5):F366–372.
110. Hall JE, Granger JP. Adenosine alters glomerular filtration control by angiotensin II. *Am J Physiol* 1986;250(5 Pt 2):F917–923.
111. Hall JE. Control of sodium excretion by angiotensin II: intrarenal mechanisms and blood pressure regulation. *Am J Physiol* 1986;250(6 Pt 2):R960–972.
112. Harding P, et al. Cyclooxygenase-2 mediates increased renal renin content induced by low-sodium diet. *Hypertension* 1997;29(1 Pt 2):297–302.
113. Harrington JT, et al. Mineralocorticoid-stimulated renal acidification: the critical role of dietary sodium. *Kidney Int* 1986;30(1):43–48.
114. Harris RC, Breyer MD. Physiological regulation of cyclooxygenase-2 in the kidney. *Am J Physiol Renal Physiol* 2001;281(1):F1–11.
115. Harrison-Bernard LM, et al. Immunohistochemical localization of ANG II AT1 receptor in adult rat kidney using a monoclonal antibody. *Am J Physiol* 1997;273(1 Pt 2):F170–177.
116. Harrison-Bernard LM, Monjure CJ, Bivona BJ. Efferent arterioles exclusively express the subtype 1A angiotensin receptor: functional insights from genetic mouse models. *Am J Physiol Renal Physiol* 2006;290(5):F1177–1186.
117. Hayashida W, Horiuchi M, Dzau VJ. Intracellular third loop domain of angiotensin II type-2 receptor. Role in mediating signal transduction and cellular function. *J Biol Chem* 1996;271(36):21985–21992.
118. Hays SR, Mineralocorticoid modulation of apical and basolateral membrane H1/OH-/HCO3-transport processes in the rabbit inner stripe of outer medullary collecting duct. *J Clin Invest* 1992;90(1):180–187.
119. He H, et al. Dietary L-arginine supplementation normalizes regional blood flow in DahlIwai salt-sensitive rats. *Am J Hypertens* 1997;10(5 Pt 2):89S–93S.
120. He XR, et al. Effect of nitric oxide on renin secretion, II: studies in the perfused juxtaglomerular apparatus. *Am J Physiol* 1995;268(5 Pt 2):F953–959.
121. Hein L, et al. Behavioural and cardiovascular effects of disrupting the angiotensin II type-2 receptor in mice. *Nature* 1995;377(6551):744–747.
122. Higashihara E, et al. Cortical and papillary micropuncture examination of chloride transport in segments of the rat kidney during inhibition of prostaglandin production: possible role for prostaglandins in the chloruresis of acute volume expansion. *J Clin Invest* 1979;64(5):1277–1287.
123. Hofbauer KG, et al. Function of the renin-angiotensin system in the isolated perfused rat kidney. *Circ Res* 1974:I1193–I202.
124. Holdaas H, DiBona GF, Kiil F. Effect of low-level renal nerve stimulation on renin release from nonfiltering kidneys. *Am J Physiol* 1981;241(2):F156–161.
125. Holdaas H, et al. Mechanism of renin release during renal nerve stimulation in dogs. *Scand J Clin Lab Invest* 1981;41(7):617–625.
126. Hricik DE, Captopril-induced renal insufficiency and the role of sodium balance. *Ann Intern Med* 1985;103(2):222–223.
127. Hu L, Manning RD Jr., Role of nitric oxide in regulation of long-term pressure-natriuresis relationship in Dahl rats. *Am J Physiol* 1995;268(6 Pt 2):H2375–2383.
128. Hubert C, et al. Structure of the angiotensin I-converting enzyme gene. Two alternate promoters correspond to evolutionary steps of a duplicated gene. *J Biol Chem* 1991;266(23):15377–15383.
129. Husain A, Graham R. *Drugs, Enzymes and Receptors of the Renin-Angiotensin System: Celebrating a Century of Discovery*. Sidney: Harwood Academic, 2000.
130. Ichihara A, et al. Interactive nitric oxide-angiotensin II influences on renal microcirculation in angiotensin II-induced hypertension. *Hypertension* 1998;31(6):1255–1260.
131. Ichiki T, et al. Effects on blood pressure and exploratory behaviour of mice lacking angiotensin II type-2 receptor. *Nature* 1995;377(6551):748–750.
132. Ichiki T, Kambayashi Y, Inagami T. Multiple growth factors modulate mRNA expression of angiotensin II type-2 receptor in R3T3 cells. *Circ Res* 1995;77(6):1070–1076.
133. Inagami T, et al. Cloning, expression and regulation of angiotensin II receptors. *J Hypertens* 1992;10(8):713–716.
134. Ingelfinger JR, et al. In situ hybridization evidence for angiotensinogen messenger RNA in the rat proximal tubule. An hypothesis for the intrarenal renin angiotensin system. *J Clin Invest* 1990;85(2):417–423.
135. Inoue I, et al. A nucleotide substitution in the promoter of human angiotensinogen is associated with essential hypertension and affects basal transcription *in vitro*. *J Clin Invest* 1997;99(7):1786–1797.
136. Investigators TS. Effect of enalapril on mortality and the development of heart failure in asymptomatic patients with reduced left ventricular ejection fractions. The SOLVD Investigators. *N Engl J Med* 1992;327:725–727.
137. Investigators TS. Effect of enalapril on survival in patients with reduced left ventricular ejection fractions and congestive heart failure. The SOLVD Investigators. *N Engl J Med* 1991. 325:293–302.
138. Ito M, et al. Regulation of blood pressure by the type 1A angiotensin II receptor gene. *Proc Natl Acad Sci U S A* 1995;92(8):3521–3525.
139. Ito S, Johnson CS, Carretero OA. Modulation of angiotensin II-induced vasoconstriction by endothelium-derived relaxing factor in the isolated microperfused rabbit afferent arteriole. *J Clin Invest* 1991;87(5):1656–1663.
140. Iwai N, et al. Differential regulation of rat AT1a and AT1b receptor mRNA. *Biochem Biophys Res Commun* 1992;188(1):298–303.
141. Iwai N, Inagami T. Identification of two subtypes in the rat type I angiotensin receptor. *FEBS Lett* 1992;298:257–2560.
142. Jeunemaitre X, et al. Molecular basis of human hypertension: role of angiotensinogen. *Cell* 1992;71(1):169–80.
143. Kakar S, Riel K, Neill J. Differential expression of angiotensin II receptor subtype mRNAs (AT-1A and AT-1B) in the brain. *Biochem Biophys Res Comm* 1992;185:688–692.
144. Keeton TK, Campbell WB. The pharmacologic alteration of renin release. *Pharmacol Rev* 1980;32(2):81–227.
145. Kihara M, et al. Genetic deficiency of angiotensinogen produces an impaired urine concentrating ability in mice. 1998;53(3):548.
146. Kim HS, et al. Genetic control of blood pressure and the angiotensinogen locus. *Proc Natl Acad Sci U S A* 1995;92(7):2735–2739.
147. Kim SM, et al. Adenosine as a mediator of macula densa-dependent inhibition of renin secretion. *Am J Physiol Renal Physiol* 2006;290(5):F1016–1023.
148. Kirchheim H, Ehmke H. Physiology of the renal baroreceptor mechanism of renin release and its role in congestive heart failure. *Am J Cardiol* 1988;62(8):68E–71E.
149. Kirchheim HR, et al. Autoregulation of renin release and its modification by renal sympathetic nerves in conscious dogs. *Kidney Int* 1981;20:152.
150. Knoblich PR, Freeman RH, Villarreal D. Pressure-dependent renin release during chronic blockade of nitric oxide synthase. *Hypertension* 1996;28(5):738–742.
151. Kobori H, Harrison-Bernard LM, Navar LG. Expression of angiotensinogen mRNA and protein in angiotensin II-dependent hypertension. *J Am Soc Nephrol* 2001;12(3):431–439.
152. Komlosi P, et al. Angiotensin I conversion to angiotensin II stimulates cortical collecting duct sodium transport. *Hypertension* 2003;42:195–199.
153. Konishi H, et al. Novel subtype of human angiotensin II type 1 receptor: cDNA cloning and expression. *Biochem Biophys Res Commun* 1994;199(2):467–474.
154. Kotchen TA, Galla JH, Luke RG. Failure of NaHCO3 and KHCO3 to inhibit renin in the rat. *Am J Physiol* 1976;231(4):1050–1056.
155. Kurtz A, et al. Role of protein kinase C in inhibition of renin release caused by vasoconstrictors. *Am J Physiol* 1986;250(4 Pt 1):C563–571.
156. Kurtz A, Wagner C. Cellular control of renin secretion. *J Exp Biol* 1999;202(Pt 3):219–225.
157. Kurtz A, Wagner C. Role of nitric oxide in the control of renin secretion. *Am J Physiol* 1998;275(6 Pt 2):F849–862.
158. Kwon T-H, et al. Angiotensin II AT1 receptor blockade decreases vasopressin-induced water reabsorption and AQP2 levels in NaCl-restricted rats. *Am J Physiol Renal Physiol* 2005; 288(4):F673–684.
159. Kwon TH, et al. Regulation of sodium transporters in the thick ascending limb of rat kidney: response to angiotensin II. *Am J Physiol Renal Physiol* 2003;285(1):F152–165.
160. Lang JA, et al. Transcriptional and posttranscriptional mechanisms regulate human renin gene expression in Calu-6 cells. *Am J Physiol* 1996;271(1 Pt 2):F94–100.
161. Langford KG, et al. Transgenic mice demonstrate a testis-specific promoter for angiotensin-converting enzyme. *J Biol Chem* 1991;266(24):15559–15562.
162. Lautrette A, et al. Angiotensin II and EGF receptor cross-talk in chronic kidney diseases: a new therapeutic approach. *Nat Med* 2005;11(8):867–874.
163. Le TH, Coffman TM. A new cardiac MASTer switch for the renin-angiotensin system. *J Clin Invest* 2006;116(4):866–869.
164. Lehtonen JY, et al. Analysis of functional domains of angiotensin II type 2 receptor involved in apoptosis. *Mol Endocrinol* 1999;13(7):1051–1060.
165. Lerolle N, et al. Angiotensin II inhibits NaCl absorption in the rat medullary thick ascending limb. *Am J Physiol Renal Physiol* 2004;287(3):F404–410.

166. Levine DZ, et al. Role of angiotensin II in dietary modulation of rat late distal tubule bicarbonate flux *in vivo*. *J Clin Invest* 1996;97(1):120–125.
167. Lew R, Summers RJ. The distribution of beta-adrenoceptors in dog kidney: an autoradiographic analysis. *Eur J Pharmacol* 1987;140(1):1–11.
168. Lewis EJ, et al. Renoprotective effect of the angiotensin-receptor antagonist irbesartan in patients with nephropathy due to type 2 diabetes. *N Engl J Med* 2001;345(12):851–860.
169. Lewis EJ, et al. The effect of angiotensin-converting-enzyme inhibition on diabetic nephropathy. The Collaborative Study Group. *N Engl J Med* 1993;329(20):1456–62.
170. Lifton R. Genetic determinants of human hypertension. *PNAS* 1995;92(19):8545–8551.
171. Liu FY, Cogan MG. Angiotensin II stimulation of hydrogen ion secretion in the rat early proximal tubule: modes of action, mechanism, and kinetics. *J Clin Invest* 1988;82(2):601–607.
172. Liu FY, Cogan MG. Angiotensin II: a potent regulator of acidification in the rat early proximal convoluted tubule. *J Clin Invest* 1987;80(1):272–275.
173. Liu FY, Cogan MG. Role of angiotensin II in glomerulotubular balance. *Am J Physiol* 1990;259(1 Pt 2):F72–79.
174. Llorens-Cortes C, et al. Tissular expression and regulation of type 1 angiotensin II receptor subtypes by quantitative reverse transcriptase-polymerase chain reaction analysis. *Hypertension* 1994;24(5):538–548.
175. Lorenz JN, et al. Effects of adenosine and angiotensin on macula densa-stimulated renin secretion. *Am J Physiol* 1993;265(2 Pt 2):F187–194.
176. Lorenz JN, et al. Renin release from isolated juxtaglomerular apparatus depends on macula densa chloride transport. *Am J Physiol* 1991;260(4 Pt 2):F486–493.
177. Luetscher JA, et al. Increased plasma inactive renin in diabetes mellitus: a marker of microvascular complications. *N Engl J Med* 1985;312(22):1412–1417.
178. Mackins CJ, et al. Cardiac mast cell-derived renin promotes local angiotensin formation, norepinephrine release, and arrhythmias in ischemia/reperfusion. *J Clin Invest* 2006;116(4):1063–1070.
179. Margolius HS, Kallikreins and kinins: molecular characteristics and cellular and tissue responses. *Diabetes* 1996;45 Suppl 1:S14–19.
180. Marrero M, et al. Direct stimulation of Jak/STAT pathway by the angiotensin II AT_1 receptor. *Nature* 1995;375:247–250.
181. Martinez-Maldonado M, et al. Role of macula densa in diuretics-induced renin release. *Hypertension* 1990;16(3):261–268.
182. Masaki H, et al. Cardiac-specific overexpression of angiotensin II AT2 receptor causes attenuated response to AT1 receptor-mediated pressor and chronotropic effects. *J Clin Invest* 1998;101(3):527–535.
183. Masilamani S, et al. Aldosterone-mediated regulation of ENaC alpha, beta, and gamma subunit proteins in rat kidney. *J Clin Invest* 1999;104(7):R19–23.
184. Mason J. The pathophysiology of ischaemic acute renal failure. A new hypothesis about the initiation phase. *Ren Physiol* 1986;9(3):129–147.
185. Matsusaka T, et al. Chimeric mice carrying 'regional' targeted deletion of the angiotensin type 1A receptor gene. Evidence against the role for local angiotensin in the *in vivo* feedback regulation of renin synthesis in juxtaglomerular cells. *J Clin Invest* 1996;98(8):1867–1877.
186. McCormick JA, et al. SGK1: a rapid aldosterone-induced regulator of renal sodium reabsorption. *Physiology (Bethesda)* 2005;20:134–139.
187. Mendelsohn F, et al. Angiotensin II receptors in the kidney. *Fed Proc* 1986;45:1420–1425.
188. Meyer TW, et al. Reversing glomerular hypertension stabilizes established glomerular injury. *Kidney Int* 1987;31(3):752–759.
189. Millan M, et al. Novel sites of expression of functional angiotensin II receptors in the late gestation fetus. *Science* 1989;244:1340–1342.
190. Miller WL, et al. Adenosine production in the ischemic kidney. *Circ Res* 1978;43(3):390–397.
191. Miyamoto M, et al. Effects of intrarenal adenosine on renal function and medullary blood flow in the rat. *Am J Physiol* 1988;255(6 Pt 2):F1230–1234.
192. Morris BJ, et al. cAMP controls human renin mRNA stability via specific RNA-binding proteins. *Acta Physiol Scand* 2004;181(4):369–373.
193. Morris BJ, et al. Function of human renin proximal promoter DNA. *Kidney Int* 1994;46(6):1516–1521.
194. Mundel P, et al. Expression of nitric oxide synthase in kidney macula densa cells. *Kidney Int* 1992;42(4):1017–1019.
195. Munter K, Hackenthal E. The effects of endothelin on renovascular resistance and renin release. *J Hypertens Suppl* 1989;7(6):S276–277.
196. Murphy TJ, et al. Isolation of a cDNA encoding the vascular type-1 angiotensin II receptor. *Nature* 1991;351(6323):233–236.
197. Naray-Fejes-Toth A. Sgk: a new player (star?) in the early action of aldosterone. *News Physiol Sci* 1999;14:274–275.
198. Navar LG, et al. Paracrine regulation of the renal microcirculation. *Physiol Rev* 1996;76(2):425–536.
199. Navar LG, et al. Tubular fluid concentrations and kidney contents of angiotensins I and II in anesthetized rats. *J Am Soc Nephrol* 1994;5(4):1153–1158.
200. Nguyen G, et al. Pivotal role of the renin/prorenin receptor in angiotensin II production and cellular responses to renin. *J Clin Invest* 2002;109(11):1417–1427.
201. Nguyen G. Renin/prorenin receptors. *Kidney Int* 2006;69(9):1503–1506.
201a. Nio Y et al. Regulation of gene transcription of angiotensin II receptor subtypes in myocardial infarction. *J Clin Invest* 1995;95:46–54.
202. Nobiling R, et al. Influence of pulsatile perfusion upon renin release from the isolated perfused rat kidney. *Pflugers Arch* 1990;415(6):713–717.
203. Okubo S, et al. Angiotensin-independent mechanism for aldosterone synthesis during chronic extracellular fluid volume depletion. *J Clin Invest* 1997;99(5):855–860.
204. Oliverio MI, et al. Abnormal water metabolism in mice lacking the type 1A receptor for ANG II. *Am J Physiol Renal Physiol* 2000;278(1):F75–82.
205. Oliverio MI, et al. Angiotensin II responses in AT1A receptor-deficient mice: a role for AT1B receptors in blood pressure regulation. *Am J Physiol* 1997;272(4 Pt 2):F515–520.
206. Oliverio MI, et al. Reduced growth, abnormal kidney structure, and type 2 (AT2) angiotensin receptor-mediated blood pressure regulation in mice lacking both AT1A and AT1B receptors for angiotensin II. *Proc Natl Acad Sci U S A* 1998;95(26):15496–15501.
207. Oliverio MI, et al. Regulation of sodium balance and blood pressure by the AT(1A) receptor for angiotensin II. *Hypertension* 2000;35(2):550–554.
208. Oliverio MI, et al. Renal growth and development in mice lacking AT1A receptors for angiotensin II. *Am J Physiol* 1998;274(1 Pt 2):F43–50.
209. Olsen ME, et al. Interaction between renal prostaglandins and angiotensin II in controlling glomerular filtration in the dog. *Clin Sci (Lond)* 1987;72(4):429–436.
210. Olsen ME, et al. Mechanisms of angiotensin II natriuresis and antinatriuresis. *Am J Physiol* 1985;249(2 Pt 2):F299–307.
211. Osborn JL, et al. Interactions among renal nerves, prostaglandins, and renal arterial pressure in the regulation of renin release. *Am J Physiol* 1984;247(5 Pt 2):F706–713.
212. Osswald H, Schmitz HJ, Kemper R. Tissue content of adenosine, inosine and hypoxanthine in the rat kidney after ischemia and postischemic recirculation. *Pflugers Arch* 1977;371(1-2):45–49.
213. Pan L, Gross KW. Transcriptional regulation of renin: an update. *Hypertension* 2005;45(1):3–8.
214. Pan L., et al. Enhancer-dependent inhibition of mouse renin transcription by inflammatory cytokines. *Am J Physiol Renal Physiol* 2005;288(1):F117–124.
215. Park CS, et al. Involvement of calmodulin in mediating inhibitory action of intracellular Ca21 on renin secretion. *Am J Physiol* 1986;251(6 Pt 2):F1055–1062.
216. Paul M, et al. Tissue specificity of renin promoter activity and regulation in mice. *Am J Physiol* 1992;262(5 Pt 1):E644–650.
217. Paxton WG, et al. Immunohistochemical localization of rat angiotensin II AT1 receptor. *Am J Physiol* 1993;264(6 Pt 2):F989–995.
218. Peach MJ. Renin-angiotensin system: biochemistry and mechanisms of action. *Physiol Rev* 1977;57(2):313–370.
219. Persson PB, et al. Endothelium-derived NO stimulates pressure-dependent renin release in conscious dogs. *Am J Physiol* 1993;264(6 Pt 2):F943–947.
220. Peters J, et al. Functional significance of prorenin internalization in the rat heart. *Circ Res* 2002;90(10):1135–1141.
221. Peti-Peterdi J, et al. Luminal NaCl delivery regulates basolateral PGE2 release from macula densa cells. *J Clin Invest* 2003;112(1):76–82.
222. Peti-Peterdi J, Warnock DG, Bell PD. Angiotensin II directly stimulates ENaC activity in the cortical collecting duct via AT(1) receptors. *J Am Soc Nephrol* 2002;13(5):1131–1135.
223. Petrovic N, et al. Role of proximal promoter elements in regulation of renin gene transcription. *J Biol Chem* 1996;271(37):22499–22505.
224. Poumarat JS, et al. The luminal membrane of rat thick limb expresses AT1 receptor and aminopeptidase activities. *Kidney Int* 2002;62(2):434–445.
225. Purdy KE, Arendshorst WJ. Prostaglandins buffer ANG II-mediated increases in cytosolic calcium in preglomerular VSMC. *Am J Physiol* 1999;277(6 Pt 2):F850–858.
226. Quan A Baum M. Endogenous production of angiotensin II modulates rat proximal tubule transport. *J Clin Invest* 1996;97(12):2878–2882.
227. Quinn SJ, Williams GH. Regulation of aldosterone secretion. *Annu Rev Physiol* 1988;50:409–426.
228. Rasmussen H, Barrett PQ. Calcium messenger system: an integrated view. *Physiol Rev* 1984;64(3):938–984.
229. Rigat B, et al. An insertion/deletion polymorphism in the angiotensin I-converting enzyme gene accounting for half the variance of serum enzyme levels. *J Clin Invest* 1990;86(4):1343–1346.
230. Rogerson FM, Fuller PJ. Mineralocorticoid action. *Steroids* 2000;65(2):61–73.
231. Rohrwasser A, et al. Elements of a paracrine tubular renin-angiotensin system along the entire nephron. *Hypertension* 1999;34(6):1265–1274.
232. Roman RJ, Kauker ML. Renal effect of prostaglandin synthetase inhibition in rats: micropuncture studies. *Am J Physiol* 1978;235(2):F111–118.
233. Roman RJ, Lianos E. Influence of prostaglandins on papillary blood flow and pressure-natriuretic response. *Hypertension* 1990;15(1):29–35.
234. Romero JC, et al. New insights into the pathophysiology of renovascular hypertension. *Mayo Clin Proc* 1997;72(3):251–260.
235. Rossier BC, et al. Epithelial sodium channel and the control of sodium balance: interaction between genetic and environmental factors. *Annu Rev Physiol* 2002;64:877–897.
236. Ruan X, et al. Renal vascular reactivity in mice: AngII-induced vasoconstriction in AT1A receptor null mice. *J Am Soc Nephrol* 1999;10(12):2620–2630.
237. Rubera I, et al. Collecting duct-specific gene inactivation of alphaENaC in the mouse kidney does not impair sodium and potassium balance. *J Clin Invest* 2003;112(4):554–565.
238. Sandberg K, et al. Cloning and expression of a novel angiotensin II receptor subtype. *J Biol Chem* 1992;267(14):9455–9458.
239. Santos RA, et al. Angiotensin-(1-7) is an endogenous ligand for the G protein-coupled receptor Mas. *Proc Natl Acad Sci U S A* 2003;100(14):8258–8263.
240. Sasaki K, et al. Cloning and expression of a complementary DNA encoding a bovine adrenal angiotensin II type-1 receptor. *Nature* 1991;351(6323):230–233.
241. Sasamura H, et al. Cloning, characterization, and expression of two angiotensin receptor (AT-1) isoforms from the mouse genome. *Biochem Biophys Res Commun* 1992;185(1):253–239.
242. Sayed-Tabatabaei FA, et al. ACE polymorphisms. *Circ Res* 2006;98(9):1123–1133.
243. Schlatter E, et al. Macula densa cells sense luminal NaCl concentration via furosemide sensitive Na12Cl-K1 cotransport. *Pflugers Arch* 1989;414(3):286–290.
244. Schnermann J, Homer W. Smith Award lecture. The juxtaglomerular apparatus: from anatomical peculiarity to physiological relevance. *J Am Soc Nephrol* 2003;14(6):1681–1694.
245. Scholz H, et al. Differential effects of extracellular anions on renin secretion from isolated perfused rat kidneys. *Am J Physiol* 1994;267(6 Pt 2):F1076–1081.
246. Schuster VL, Kokko JP, Jacobson HR. Angiotensin II directly stimulates sodium transport in rabbit proximal convoluted tubules. *J Clin Invest* 1984;73(2):507–515.
247. Schweda F, et al. Stimulation of renin release by prostaglandin E2 is mediated by EP2 and EP4 receptors in mouse kidneys. *Am J Physiol Renal Physiol* 2004;287(3):F427–433.

248. Schweda F, Kurtz A. Cellular mechanism of renin release. *Acta Physiol Scand* 2004;181(4): 383–390.

249. Lefkowitz RJ, Shenoy SK. Transduction of receptor signals by β-arrestins. *Science* 2005; 308:512–517.

250. Shricker K, et al. The role of angiotensin II in the feedback control of renin gene expression. *Pflugers Arch* 1997;434(2):166–172.

251. Sigmund CD, et al. Regulated tissue- and cell-specific expression of the human renin gene in transgenic mice. *Circ Res* 1992;70(5):1070–1079.

252. Silver RB, et al. Mast cells: a unique source of renin. *Proc Natl Acad Sci USA* 2004;101(37):13607–13612.

253. Simons JL, et al. Pathogenesis of glomerular injury in the fawn-hooded rat: effect of unilateral nephrectomy. *J Am Soc Nephrol* 1993;4(6):1362–1370.

254. Siragy HM, Carey RM. The subtype-2 (AT2) angiotensin receptor regulates renal cyclic guanosine 3′, 5′-monophosphate and AT1 receptor-mediated prostaglandin E2 production in conscious rats. *J Clin Invest* 1996;97(8):1978–1982.

255. Skinner SL, McCubbin JW, Page IH. Control of renin secretion. *Circ Res* 1964;15:64–76.

256. Skott O, Briggs JP. Direct demonstration of macula densa-mediated renin secretion. *Science* 1987;237(4822):1618–1620.

257. Smith DL, et al. Identification of cyclic AMP response element in the human renin gene. *Biochem Biophys Res Commun* 1994;200(1):320–329.

258. Spielman WS, Thompson CI. A proposed role for adenosine in the regulation of renal hemodynamics and renin release. *Am J Physiol* 1982;242(5):F423–435.

259. Stone DK, et al. Mineralocorticoid modulation of rabbit medullary collecting duct acidification. A sodium-independent effect. *J Clin Invest* 1983;72(1):77–83.

260. Sugaya T, et al. Angiotensin II type 1a receptor-deficient mice with hypotension and hyperreninemia. *J Biol Chem* 1995;270(32):18719–18722.

261. Szentivanyi M Jr, et al. Renal medullary nitric oxide deficit of Dahl S rats enhances hypertensive actions of angiotensin II. *Am J Physiol Regul Integr Comp Physiol* 2002;283(1):R266–272.

262. Szentivanyi M Jr, Maeda CY, Cowley AW Jr. Local renal medullary L-NAME infusion enhances the effect of long-term angiotensin II treatment. *Hypertension* 1999;33(1 Pt 2): 440–445.

263. Takahashi N, Smithies O. Human genetics, animal models and computer simulations for studying hypertension. *Trends Genet* 2004;20(3):136–145.

264. Tamura H, et al. Liddle disease caused by a missense mutation of beta subunit of the epithelial sodium channel gene. *J Clin Invest* 1996; 97(7):1780–1784.

265. Taugner C, et al. Immunocytochemical localization of renin in mouse kidney. *Histochemistry* 1979;62(1):19–27.

266. Textor SC, et al. Regulation of renal hemodynamics and glomerular filtration in patients with renovascular hypertension during converting enzyme inhibition with captopril. *Am J Med* 1984;76(5B):29–37.

267. Tharaux PL, et al. Activation of renin synthesis is dependent on intact nitric oxide production. *Kidney Int* 1997;51(6):1780–1787.

268. Tharaux P-L, Coffman TM. Transgenic mice as a tool to study the renin-angiotensin system. *Contrib Nephrol* 2001;135:72–91.

269. Thomson SC, et al. An unexpected role for angiotensin II in the link between dietary salt and proximal reabsorption. *J Clin Invest* 2006; 116(4):1110–1116.

270. Thurau K, et al. Composition of tubular fluid in the macula densa segment as a factor regulating the function of the juxtaglomerular apparatus. *Circ Res* 1967;21(1):Suppl 2:79–90.

271. Timmermans PB, et al. Angiotensin II receptors and angiotensin II receptor antagonists. *Pharmacol Rev* 1993;45(2):205–251.

272. Tipnis SR, et al. A human homolog of angiotensin-converting enzyme. Cloning and functional expression as a captopril-insensitive carboxypeptidase. *J Biol Chem* 2000;275(43):33238–33243.

273. Tiret L, et al. Synergistic effects of angiotensin converting enzyme and angiotensin II type I receptor polymorphisms on risk of myocardial infarction. *Lancet* 1994;344:910–913.

274. Tobian L, Tomboulian A, Janecek J. The effect of high perfusion pressures on the granulation of juxtaglomerular cells in an isolated kidney. *J Clin Invest* 1959;38(4):605–610.

275. Tojo A, Tisher CC, Madsen KM. Angiotensin II regulates H(1)-ATPase activity in rat cortical collecting duct. *Am J Physiol* 1994;267(6 Pt 2):F1045–1051.

276. Tokumori Y, et al. Biphasic renin release from perfused rat kidney. *Horm Metab Res* 1983;15(6):310–311.

277. Vallon V, et al. Role of Sgk1 in salt and potassium homeostasis. *Am J Physiol Regul Integr Comp Physiol* 2005;288(1):R4–10.

278. van Kesteren CAM, et al. Mannose 6-phosphate receptor-mediated internalization and activation of prorenin by cardiac cells. *Hypertension* 1997;30(6):1389–1396.

279. Vander AJ. Control of renin release. *Physiol Rev* 1967;47(3):359–382.

280. Veniant M, et al. Vascular damage without hypertension in transgenic rats expressing prorenin exclusively in the liver. *J Clin Invest* 1996;98(9):1966–1970.

281. Vickers C, et al. Hydrolysis of biological peptides by human angiotensin-converting enzyme-related carboxypeptidase. *J Biol Chem* 2002;277(17):14838–14843.

282. Villard E, et al. Identification of new polymorphisms of the angiotensin I-converting enzyme (ACE) gene, and study of their relationship to plasma ACE levels by two-QTL segregation-linkage analysis. *Am J Hum Genet* 1996;58(6):1268–12678.

283. Wang J, Staessen J. Genetic polymorphisms in the renin-angiotensin system: relevance for susceptibility to cardiovascular disease. *Eur J Pharmacol* 2000;410:289–302.

284. Wang T, Giebisch G. Effects of angiotensin II on electrolyte transport in the early and late distal tubule in rat kidney. *Am J Physiol* 1996;271(1 Pt 2):F143–149.

285. Webber PC, et al. Stimulation of renin release from rabbit renal cortex by arachidonic acid and prostaglandin endoperoxides. *Circ Res* 1976;39(6):868–874.

286. Wei Y, Wang W. Angiotensin II stimulates basolateral K channels in rat cortical collecting ducts. *Am J Physiol Renal Physiol* 2003;284(1):F175–181.

287. Weihprecht H, et al. Effect of adenosine1-receptor blockade on renin release from rabbit isolated perfused juxtaglomerular apparatus. *J Clin Invest* 1990;85(5):1622–1628.

288. Weiner I, et al. Regulation of luminal alkalinization and acidification in the cortical collecting duct by angiotensin II. *Am J Physiol* 1995;38:F730–F738.

289. Weiner ID, Hamm LL. Regulation of intracellular pH in the rabbit cortical collecting tubule. *J Clin Invest* 1990;85(1):274–281.

290. Wilcox CS, Welch WJ. Macula densa nitric oxide synthase: expression, regulation, and function. *Kidney Int Suppl* 1998;67:S53–57.

291. Wong NL, Tsui JK. Angiotensin II upregulates the expression of vasopressin V2 mRNA in the inner medullary collecting duct of the rat. *Metabolism* 2003;52(3):290–205.

292. Woodcock EA, et al. Demonstration of RA-adenosine receptors in rat renal papillae. *Biochem Biophys Res Commun* 1984;121(2):434–440.

293. Yagil Y, Miyamoto M, Jamison RL. Inner medullary blood flow in postischemic acute renal failure in the rat. *Am J Physiol* 1989;256(3 Pt 2):F456–461.

294. Yang T, et al. Renin expression in COX-2-knockout mice on normal or low-salt diets. *Am J Physiol Renal Physiol* 2000;279(5):F819–825.

295. Ying L, Morris BJ, Sigmund CD. Transactivation of the human renin promoter by the cyclic AMP/protein kinase A pathway is mediated by both cAMP-responsive element binding protein-1 (CREB)-dependent and CREB-independent mechanisms in Calu-6 cells. *J Biol Chem* 1997;272(4):2412–2420.

296. Yoo D, et al. Cell surface expression of the ROMK (Kir 1.1) channel is regulated by the aldosterone-induced kinase, SGK-1, and protein kinase. *Am J Biol Chem* 2003;278(25):23066–23075.

297. Yoshida H, Kon V, Ichikawa I. Polymorphisms of the renin-angiotensin system genes in progressive renal diseases. *Kidney Int* 1996;50:732–744.

298. Yusuf S, et al. Effects of an angiotensin-converting-enzyme inhibitor, ramipril, on cardiovascular events in high-risk patients. The Heart Outcomes Prevention Evaluation Study Investigators. *N Engl J Med* 2000;342(3):145–53.

299. Zatz R, et al. Prevention of diabetic glomerulopathy by pharmacological amelioration of glomerular capillary hypertension. *J Clin Invest* 1986;77:1925–1930.

300. Zhang H, et al. Collectrin, a collecting duct-specific transmembrane glycoprotein, is a novel homolog of ACE2 and is developmentally regulated in embryonic kidneys. *J Biol Chem* 2001;276(20):17132–17139.

301. Zhang H, et al. Screening for genes up-regulated in 5/6 nephrectomized mouse kidney. *Kidney Int* 1999;56(2):549–558.

302. Zou AP, Wu F, Cowley AW Jr., Protective effect of angiotensin II-induced increase in nitric oxide in the renal medullary circulation. *Hypertension* 1998;31(1 Pt 2):271–276.

CHAPTER **14**

Eicosanoids and the Kidney.

John C. McGiff and Nicholas R. Ferreri

New York Medical College, Valhalla, New York, USA

IN PRINCIPIO

In his welcoming address to the first symposium dedicated to prostaglandins, held in Stockholm in 1966, U. S. von Euler, one of the founding fathers of this research area stated:

> *...we have indeed in prostaglandin a unique hormone...its scope of action is still wider, however, and it may well be that the prostaglandins represent a group of compounds which are involved in a variety of actions ranging from effects on the central nervous system to intricate metabolic actions, thus justifying their very special chemical configuration".* (219)

These predictions were fulfilled in less than a decade.

The progression of renal eicosanoid studies can be divided into several phases. As with all eicosanoid studies, they had their inception in the primordial/classical studies of Bergström performed in the late 1950s at the Karolinska Institute, culminating in the structural identification of prostaglandin (PG) E_1 and $PGF_{2\alpha}$ isolated in pure crystalline form from Icelandic sheep prostatic glands (10). The origin of renal eicosanoid studies can be traced to the seminal studies of Lee and colleagues (106), who reported in 1967 on the isolation of three prostaglandins in the rabbit renal medulla: PGE_2, $PGF_{2\alpha}$, and PGA_2 (Fig. 1). PGA_2 was proposed to fill the role of the long-sought "renal antihypertensive factor." PGA_2, unlike PGE_2 and $PGF_{2\alpha}$, was not degraded by the lungs (125); that is, PGA_2, on release into renal venous blood, passed unmetabolized across the lungs to enter the systemic circulation, a property shown later to be shared with PGI_2 (prostacyclin) (233). PGA_2 was named medullin, and stirred a great deal of interest (105), spurred by the development of a spurious RIA that addressed "circulating" PGA_2 (260). However, in the original study of Lee et al., PGA_2 was suggested to arise from dehydration of PGE_2 during preparation of renal tissue and blood samples for analyses (106). This interpretation was later validated by GC-MS analyses of plasma samples (62) and PGA_2 passed into history as an experimental artifact. PGE_2, on the other hand, assumed a position of prominence in prostaglandin-related renal mechanisms.

The labile cyclooxygenase (COX) products, thromboxane (TxA_2) (64) and prostacyclin (PGI_2) (18), were initially identified in perfusates/incubates by the ingenious application of the principle of parallel pharmacological assays developed by John Vane (50) (Fig. 2). Bioassay tissues were arranged in a cascade and superfused with organ perfusates or circulating blood (the superfusion or blood bathed organ assays). Selection of tissues was based on specificity of responses to targeted eicosanoids (e.g., TxA_2 contracts rabbit aorta). Six years before the chemical structure of TxA_2 was announced, in response to antigen challenge of the sensitized guinea pig lung, TxA_2 was detected in pulmonary effluents by its ability to contract the rabbit aorta (155). This property occasioned its being designated RCS (*r*abbit aorta *c*ontracting *s*ubstance in studies performed at the *Royal College of Surgeons*). RCS was the fingerprint that identified TxA_2, a labile eicosanoid having a half life in body fluids of ~30 seconds. The biological activity of TxA_2 would otherwise have been lost in an extraction procedure of even short duration. Further, tracking the biological activity of TxA_2 during isolation and purification of TxA_2 from tissues/plasma assisted in the chemical structural identification (64, 185).

The labile vascular hormone, PGI_2, having a half-life of approximately 2 minutes, was also "discovered through the inspired use of bioassay methods" (18); namely, the superfusion bioassay system for detection and for biological characterization: (1) vascular strips (PGI_2 relaxes blood vessels) and (2) platelet aggregometry (PGI_2 inhibits platelet aggregation). These discoveries of TxA_2 and PGI_2 (Fig. 1) in biological fluids and tissue perfusates by Piper and Vane (155) and Vane and colleagues (18), respectively, represented the triumph of intellect over technology. They depended on the application of established bioassay methods to the detection of highly labile active substances in plasma and organ effluents within seconds of their production. Further, the biological activities of TxA_2 (RCS) and PGI_2 (PGX) provided the fingerprints for tracking their isolation and ultimate chemical identification.

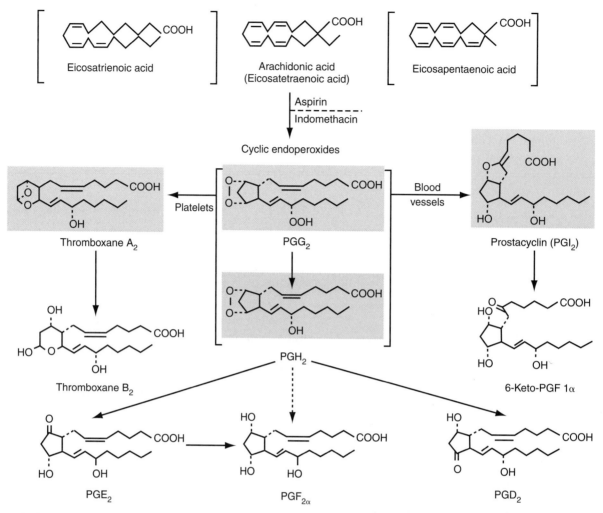

FIGURE 1   Metabolism of arachidonic acid to form prostaglandins and thromboxanes. The more unstable products are indicated by shading. Eicosatrienoic and eicosapentaenoic acids, bracketed at the top of the figure, give rise to products (not shown) having one and three double bonds, respectively. (From McGiff JC. Protaglandins, prostacyclin, and thromboxanes. *Ann Rev Pharmacol Toxicol* 1981;21:479-509. Annual Review of Pharmacology and Toxicology, Volume 21 ©1981 by Annual Reviews www.annualreviews.org.)

RENAL PROSTAGLANDINS: THE EARLY DAYS

Prostaglandin-dependent renal mechanisms operating within either the whole kidney or renal zones (juxtamedullary, medullary, and cortical) occupied studies for most of the first two decades of renal eicosanoid research with notable exceptions (e.g., cultured mesangial cells [205] and isolated glomeruli [67]). The nephron and its segments were passed over, with the exception of the collecting ducts (11). Key nephron segments, proximal tubules and thick ascending limbs (TALs), had undetectable or minimal prostaglandin synthetic capabilities that could be accounted for by vascular contamination (200). Mapping the distribution of COX by immunofluorescence within the nephron, pointed to the medullary collecting ducts as the principle site of renal tubular prostaglandin synthesis. The loop of Henle was identified as the major source of urinary prostanoids (54). In 1966, Orloff and Grantham proposed that PGE_1 dampened the

effects of vasopressin on water permeability of collecting ducts by preventing vasopressin-induced elevation of cyclic AMP (cAMP) (150). This study identified a principle property of prostaglandins, their acting as modulators of vasoactive hormones in mechanisms regulating blood flow and salt and water metabolism. It should be viewed as the classical progenitor of studies designed to define renal eicosanoid-related mechanisms.

Either angiotensin II (ANG II) (121) or bradykinin (124) given into the renal artery produced a large efflux of prostaglandins. The response of renal prostaglandins to functional perturbations produced by vasoactive hormones is initiated by hormonal activation of phospholipases with release of arachidonic acid (AA) that is cyclized by COX to form PGG_2, which, in turn, is acted upon by the intrinsic endoperoxide peroxidase of COX to form PGH_2 (198) (Fig. 1). The endoperoxide PGH_2 is transformed to end products: PGE_2, PGI_2, $PGF_{2\alpha}$, PGD_2, or TxA_2 that vary according to experimental conditions (e.g., high vs low salt intake) and su-

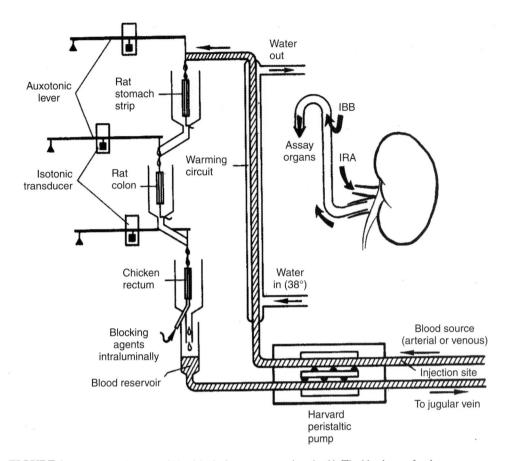

FIGURE 2 Schematic diagram of blood-bathed organ system (one bank). The blood-superfused organ system schematized for one bank of organs (three banks of organs were used). Blood was withdrawn at the rate of 10 to 15 mL/min by a pump. After traversing a constant-temperature circuit, the blood cascaded over three assay organs arranged in series. Changes in the length of the assay organs were transduced and recorded on a multichannel recorder. The blood was collected in a reservoir and returned at a constant rate to the animal. Selective blockade of assay organs is possible by direct intraluminal application of a blocking agent. A major use of this method is shown by the schematized kidney on the right. Thus, a substance may be given into the renal artery (IRA) and its effects on assay organs compared with its direct effects on administration into the extracorporeal circuit (IBB, into the bathing blood) indicated by *injection site* in the diagram of the assay system. Indirect effects of hormones may thereby be determined (e.g., release of intrarenal substances by angiotensin II). (From McGiff JC, Crowshaw K, Terragno NA, et al. Prostaglandin-like substances appearing in canine renal venous blood during renal ischemia. *Circ Res* 1970;27:765-782, with permission.)

perimposed experimental diseases (e.g., streptozotocin-induced diabetes [98,162]). The expression/activity of the transforming enzymes—prostaglandin and thromboxane synthases/isomerases—is determined by the physiological/pathophysiological status of the animal/subject. For example, renal TxA_2 synthesis is increased in patients with severe congestive heart failure (31). In response to oral administration of picotamide, a TxA_2 synthase and TxA_2/PGH_2 (TP) receptor inhibitor, renal plasma flow and glomerular filtration rate (GFR) increased (filtration fraction decreased) associated with natriuresis and decreased excretion of TxB_2, the hydrolysis product of TxA_2. Extracellular fluid depletion with contraction of intravascular volume produced by diuretic therapy or reduced salt intake evokes co-expression of COX-2 and the inducible membranal PGE_2 isomerase (mPGES-1) in preglomerular microvessels (PGMVs) (36, 186). PGH_2 may act also untransformed, in which case its effects are transduced by

TxA_2/PGH_2 (TP) receptors, thereby reproducing the actions of TxA_2 (163). The final products of the intrarenal eicosanoid biosynthetic pathways are reflected in eicosanoids exiting via venous and ureteral effluents (167).

COX ISOFORMS AND METABOLISM OF AA

Two isoforms of prostaglandin H (PGH) synthase, commonly referred to as COX-1 and COX-2, are encoded by two separate genes (199, 235). The present phase of eicosanoid studies commenced with the discovery of COX-2 reported by Simmons and colleagues in 1991 (235) that eventuated in the delineation of the distinctive roles of eicosanoids in health and disease, indicating the pervasive involvement of eicosanoid-dependent mechanisms in human physiology and pathophysiology. Identification of COX-2 opened up areas of research to those of us in the field that exceeded the wildest predictions of the founders of eicosanoid studies only three decades earlier.

COX-1 and COX-2 share a high degree of sequence identity, are structurally similar, and contain highly conserved residues that account for the comparable catalytic activities (199, 235). Both isoforms are homodimers, contain heme, and exhibit a long substrate channel and a stretch of hydrophobic residues that anchor the enzymes to the inner surface of endoplasmic reticulum and nuclear envelope. They catalyze the same reactions (i.e., AA is converted to PGG_2, followed by a peroxidase reaction in which the 15-hydroperoxyl group of PGG_2 is reduced to the 15-hydroxyl group of PGH_2).

Specific isomerases metabolize the COX product PGH_2 in a cell-specific manner. Subtypes of isomerases, for instance mPGES-1 and cytosolic PGE synthase, may be preferentially linked to COX-1 or COX-2 to form PGE_2 in collecting tubules and medullary interstitial cells (186). Constitutive expression of COX-1 is evident in many tissues whereas constitutive expression of COX-2 is restricted to the kidney and central nervous system (CNS) when compared to other organs (199). COX-1 and COX-2 are associated with distinct cellular activities and are essential components in mechanisms that participate in physiological and pathophysiological processes within the renal and cardiovascular systems as COX-2 in inflammation and neoplasia.

Prostaglandin Metabolism

Unlike the arachidonate products of the cytochrome P450 monooxygenase pathway (CYP), epoxyeicosatrienoic acids (EETs) and hydroxyeicosatetraenoic acids (HETEs) (23, 89), prostaglandins are not stored, with the exception in seminal fluid. Under normal conditions, prostaglandins are rapidly degraded locally, thereby restricting their primary area of action to the site of synthesis (231). There is an abundance of the principle prostaglandin catabolizing enzyme, 15-hydroxy-prostaglandin dehydrogenase (15-OH PGDH) in the kidney that inactivates prostaglandins (232). PGI_2 is rapidly catabolized by 15-OH PGDH in arteries and veins to an inactive product, 6,15-diketo $PGF_{1\alpha}$ (234). Further, metabolism of PGI_2 in vivo is initiated by 15-OH PGDH: Several urinary metabolites of injected tritiated PGI_2 in rats possess a keto group at position C-15, strongly suggesting the primacy of 15-OH PGDH in the metabolism of PGI_2. (126).

The urinary excretory rate of 2,3 dinor 6-keto $PGF_{1\alpha}$ (PGI-M), a PGI_2 metabolite, has been used to estimate changes in systemic PGI_2 production (117). Unmetabolized PGI_2, on the other hand, is excreted as the hydrolysis product, 6-keto $PGF_{1\alpha}$, and is considered to represent production of PGI_2 within the kidney (158). The effect of 15-OH PGDH activity on underestimating renal prostaglandin production is rarely, if ever, considered when calculating renal prostaglandin production that is based on

urinary excretion of unmetabolized prostaglandins. Moreover, genetic and drug-induced variations in the activity of renal 15-OH PGDH have been described in rat strains (New Zealand) (4) and in response to loop diuretics (37,146), which will affect urinary excretory rates of unmetabolized prostaglandins. Renal venous and ureteral efflux of unmetabolized prostaglandins indicates that significant amounts of renal prostaglandins evade local catabolism. As noted, the largest component of urinary prostaglandins enters the tubular fluid from the loop of Henle (54). Prostaglandins of renal origin entering the vena cava by the renal venous route are destined for catabolism in the lung, PGI_2 excepted (231). The free passage of PGI_2 across the lung is a function of PGI_2 having low affinity for the lung uptake mechanism, which is the obligatory step for catabolism by cytosolic 15-OH PGDH. When lung uptake is eliminated by adding PGI_2 to lung homogenates, PGI_2 is rapidly metabolized by cytosolic 15-OH PGDH to the inactive product, 6,15-diketo, to $PGF_{1\alpha}$ (209). The lung can produce PGI_2 in relatively large quantities, a function which has salutary circulatory implications by delivering into the general circulation biologically significant amounts of PGI_2, the antiproliferative anti-thrombotic-vasodilator prostanoid.

PROSTAGLANDINS SERVE RENAL ADAPTIVE/PROTECTIVE MECHANISMS

In response to diverse stimuli (e.g., hormones, antigen challenge, and thrombin) prostaglandins are rapidly synthesized, showing many-fold increases from low basal levels within a few minutes, and either subsiding to basal levels on withdrawal of the stimulus, or maintaining levels, above basal, in response to altered physiological states (e.g., pregnancy and congestive heart failure). These changes in prostaglandin levels are in keeping with a primary adaptive/protective function of prostaglandins as exemplified in (1) their cytoprotective role in the gastrointestinal tract (172); (2) the gestational adjustments of the maternal and fetal circulations (213); (3) the compensatory response of the renal circulation to cardiovascular (31), hepatic (182), and kidney diseases, ischemic injury, and depletion of extracellular volume such as produced by diuretic therapy (146); and (4) renal ontogeny: Expression of COX-2 in the fetus and neonate is essential for tubular and glomerular morphogenesis (251).

Destabilizing procedures such as general anesthesia and laparotomy evoked a renal prostaglandin response as reflected in a five-fold increase in PGE concentrations in the renal vein (212) that, in view of recent findings, is dependent on expression of COX-2 (186). COX-2 and mPGES-1 act in concert to synthesize PGE_2, having been induced concordantly in response to renal functional changes produced by disease, salt depletion, and ischemia (237) or, as in the example cited previously, the stress of general anesthesia and surgery. Either glucocorticoid treatment or COX-2 inhibi-

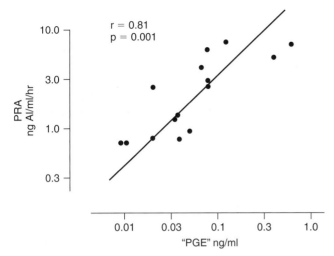

FIGURE 3 The relationship between plasma renin activity (PRA) (*ordinate*) and the log of the concentration (*abscissae*) of prostaglandin E–like substances (PGE) in renal venous blood of conscious and anesthetized surgically stressed dogs. (From Terragno NA, Terragno DA, McGiff JC. Contribution of prostaglandins to the renal circulation in conscious, anesthetized, and laparotomized dogs. *Circ Res* 1977;40:590-595, with permission.)

tion will block expression/activity of COX-2 and mPGES-1 (135). The vital contribution of this prostaglandin mechanism to the maintenance of renal blood flow (RBF) in dogs subject to surgical stress was uncovered by the administration of a nonsteroidal anti-inflammatory drug (NSAID), indomethacin; namely, RBF and PGE concentrations in renal venous blood declined sharply with elevation of blood pressure. Under basal conditions, indomethacin did not affect canine RBF and blood pressure (212). The negative renal hemodynamic effects of cyclosporine A (CsA) have also been related to suppression of COX-2 expression (71) consequent to inhibition by CsA of the nuclear factor of activated T cells (NFAT), a transcription factor that regulates COX-2 expression (1). Activity of COX-2 is critically related to production of vasodilator, diuretic and antipressor prostaglandins, PGE_2 and PGI_2 (159); failure of COX-2–dependent vascular and tubular mechanisms would severely compromise renal functional responses to stress and injury (236, 238).

A key factor in the differential renal functional responses to inhibition of COX in resting versus anesthetized, surgically stressed dogs was increased activity of the renin angiotensin aldosterone system (RAAS) as reflected in the plasma renin activity (PRA) (212) in stressed dogs. The renal venous concentrations of PGE_2 varied over a 100-fold range

and were positively correlated with levels of PRA and, by extrapolation, to circulating levels of ANG II (Fig. 3). Vasoactive hormones have long been recognized as a potent stimulus to renal PGE_2 production (121).

As levels of ANG II increase, ANG II acts in a negative feedback mechanism that regulates expression of COX-2 and consequently renin production and ANG II generation (34). In line with the important observation that high concentrations of ANG II inhibit expression of COX-2 (Schema 1) (and, thereby, synthesis of renin and formation of ANG II), were the effects on COX-2 expression of strategies designed to prevent ANG II negative feedback regulation of COX-2 expression/activity and, thereby, augment COX-2 expression (34). This was accomplished in one of two ways: (1) reducing the levels of ANG II by inhibiting angiotensin-converting enzyme (ACE) or (2) preventing the inhibitory action of ANG II on COX-2 expression by AT_1 receptor blockade. Both interventions produced greatly increased cortical COX-2 expression in rats. Under these conditions, selective inhibition of COX-2 prevented the heightened increase in PRA induced by ACE inhibition, thus providing additional evidence that increased COX-2 activity (in conjunction with increased PGI_2 synthesis) was responsible for elevating PRA.

Renal Functional Responses to Selective COX-2 Inhibition

The development of COX-1– and COX-2–selective inhibitors enabled distinguishing the individual contributions of each isozyme to the renal functional response to challenges such as activation of the RAAS by low-salt (LS) intake. In conscious dogs on either normal salt (NS) or high-salt (HS) intake, inhibition of COX-2 with nimesulide produced an early transient decline in Na^+ excretion and reduced RBF. Only with LS intake did nimesulide produce a modest decrease in GFR as well as in RBF (173). *However, when nitric oxide synthase (NOS) and COX-2 were inhibited simultaneously, a precipitous decline in GFR was produced even in dogs on HS intake* (175). The reduction in GFR (20%–40%), produced by combined inhibition of NOS and COX-2, was sustained during the entire 8-day study. Interactions between NO and eicosanoids may explain these findings:

1. NO augments COX-2 catalytic activity (93) that will increase PGE_2 and PGI_2 synthesis (159). Further, peroxynitrite formed from the interaction of superoxide and NO can activate COX by reacting directly with it (61).

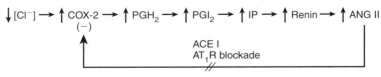

SCHEMA 1. [Cl^-], Cl^- concentration in tubular fluid at the level of the macula densa; IP, prostacyclin receptor; ACEI, angiotensin converting enzyme inhibition)

2. NO exerts a tonic inhibitory effect on 20-HETE synthesis and consequently prevents 20-HETE enhancement of vascular tone and vascular reactivity (153, 208). Thus, inhibition of NO synthesis can be expected to reduce synthesis of vasodilator prostaglandins while increasing synthesis of 20-HETE, resulting in depressed GFR and RBF (153).

COX-2 inhibition decreased PRA and increased plasma potassium concentration to the greatest degree under conditions of LS intake (175). However, plasma aldosterone was unaffected by COX-2 inhibition. The latter finding is in conflict with the generally accepted cause of hyperkalemia in response to NSAIDs, namely, decreased aldosterone synthesis resulting from reduced ANG II generation (154) (Fig. 4). To

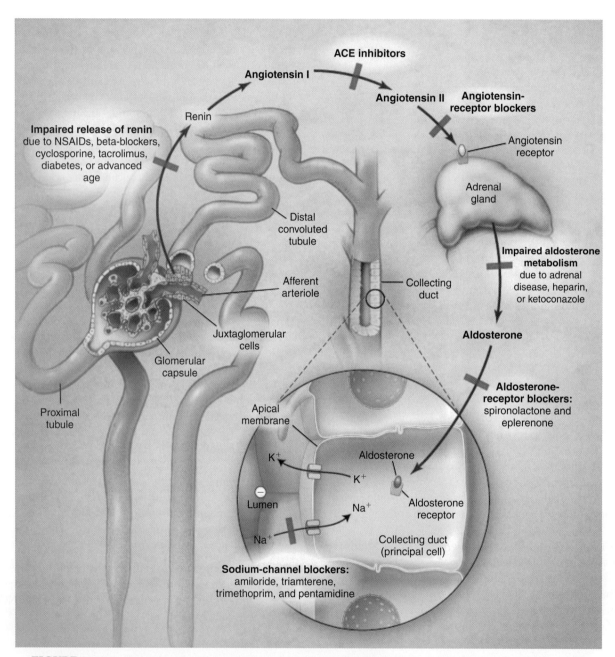

FIGURE 4   The renin-angiotensin-aldosterone system and regulation of potassium excretion in the kidney. Aldosterone binds to a cytosolic receptor in the principle cell and stimulates sodium reabsorption across the luminal membrane through a well-defined sodium channel. As sodium is reabsorbed, the electronegativity of the lumen increases, thereby providing a more favorable driving force for the secretion of potassium through an apically located potassium channel. The permeability of the anion that accompanies sodium also influences the secretion of potassium, with less permeable anions having a greater stimulatory effect on this secretion. Disease states or drugs that interfere at any point along this system can impair the secretion of potassium in the kidney and increase the risk of hyperkalemia when angiotensin-converting enzyme (ACE) inhibitors or angiotensin-receptor blockers are used. In many patients, this risk is magnified because of disturbances at multiple points in this system. NSAIDs, nonsteroidal anti-inflammatory drugs. (From Palmer BF. *N Engl J Med* 2004;351:585–592, with permission.)

$$NSAID \rightarrow \downarrow COX\text{-}2 \rightarrow \downarrow PGH_2 \rightarrow \downarrow PGI_2 \rightarrow IP \rightarrow \downarrow \underset{plasma}{Renin} \rightarrow \downarrow ANG\ II \rightarrow \downarrow ALDO \rightarrow \downarrow K^+\ secretion \rightarrow \uparrow K^+$$

SCHEMA 2. Effects of NSAIDs on K^+ homeostasis; IP, prostacyclin receptor.

summarize: Hyperkalemia produced by NSAID treatment results from a sequence of related effects beginning with inhibition of COX-2 that blocks production of PGH_2, the precursor to the renin secretagogue PGI_2, and inhibits PGI_2 synthesis with an attendant diminished secretion of renin and reduction of circulating levels of ANG II, resulting in decreased synthesis of aldosterone and reduced secretion of K^+ into tubular fluid (154) (Schema 2). In a study in older persons (aged 60–80 years) receiving a LS diet, the effects of COX-2 inhibition on renal function did not differ from those produced by nonselective COX inhibitors. Older persons demonstrate an insidious decline in renal function as seen in rising serum creatinine and reduced levels of aldosterone that increases the risk of hyperkalemia when treated with drugs that negatively affect the RAAS axis: NSAIDs, ACE inhibitors, aldosterone antagonists (8). The principle change in response to either nonselective COX inhibitors or selective COX-2 antagonists, was decreased GFR (210).

RENAL ZONAL REGULATIONS OF COX-2 DIFFER

The negative feedback mechanism activated by ANG II that inhibits COX-2 applies only to regulating expression of COX-2 in cortical structures such as the macula densa and PGMVs. In the renal medulla and papilla, COX-2 expression was increased by HS and decreased by LS intake, changes opposite to those occurring in the cortex. Thus, COX-2 is regulated in a zone-specific manner in response to changes in salt intake (238), indicating that COX-2 subserves different functions in the cortex (vascular resistance) and in the medulla (salt and water homeostasis). In contrast to the primary hemodynamic effects of cortical COX-2 expression mediated via PGE_2 and PGI_2 production, COX-2 expression in the renal papilla/medulla affects principally salt and water excretion and the adaptation of medullary interstitial cells and collecting tubules (ducts) to altered medullary tonicity (128).

COX-2 in the renal medulla was also increased in response to hypercalcemia, an effect inhibited by blockade of AT_1 receptors whereas AT_1-receptor blockade in the renal cortex produced additional increases in the elevated COX-2 of the rat, reaffirming the basic differences in the regulation of COX-2 in the renal cortex compared to the medulla. (114). These findings can be brought into sharper focus by examining the effects of Ca^{2+} on oxygenase activity in a key nephron segment in the medulla having well-defined Ca^{2+} receptors, the medullary (m)TAL (222). Activation of mTAL Ca^{2+}-sensing receptors by raising ionized calcium (1.2 → 2.0 mM) in the short term

(<15 minutes), increased synthesis of 20-HETE, the major product of AA metabolism in the mTAL. However, long-term exposure (2–3 hours) of the cells of the mTAL to elevated Ca^{2+} caused expression of COX-2 and synthesis of PGE_2 (220).

An additional mechanism, having negative effects on COX-2 expression in the TAL, is mediated by glucocorticoids that act tonically to suppress COX-2 in the mTAL (217) (Fig. 5). Adrenalectomy produced a florid expression of COX-2 in the TAL, beginning in proximity to the macula densa and extending linearly into the medulla. This extensive expression of COX-2 in the TAL was reversed by glucocorticoid treatment and recalls the pivotal role of COX-2 in renal morphogenesis in embryonic and perinatal life that required suppression of glucocorticoid synthesis for activation (68, 251).

COX-2 and Renal Differentiation and Development

The fetal kidney is a rich source of COX-2–derived prostaglandins. They are essential for differentiation and development of the kidney that has its onset about the 16th embryonic day in the rat and peaks in the first 2 postnatal weeks (251), coinciding with a marked decline in plasma levels of glucocorticoids (68). COX-2 knockout mice (130), in contrast to COX-1 knockout mice (102), exhibited small kidneys with few functional nephrons and immature glomeruli. Uremic death followed within several months. Do these findings apply to primates? Pregnant Rhesus monkeys, given NSAIDs chronically, demonstrated similar renal lesions to those of COX-2 knockout mice (142). Mothers taking indomethacin throughout pregnancy have given birth to anuric infants who died in the neonatal period (215).

MACULA DENSA: COX-2-/PGI$_2$-DEPENDENT ACTIVATION OF THE RAAS

Endothelial cells, macrophages, and fibroblasts coordinately upregulate COX-2 and the inducible membranal PGE_2 isomerase (mPGES-1) in response to proinflammatory factors, a response blocked by glucocorticoids (186). A similar mechanism, one that also involves both COX-2 and mPGES-1 is activated by low $[Cl^-]$ in tubular fluid and is housed in the macula densa, the specialized cells of the cTAL in apposition to the afferent arteriole at its point of entry into the glomerulus (237). COX-2 is also expressed in PGMVs as is ω/ω-1-hydroxylase; the expression and activity of each is increased in rats on LS diets (36).

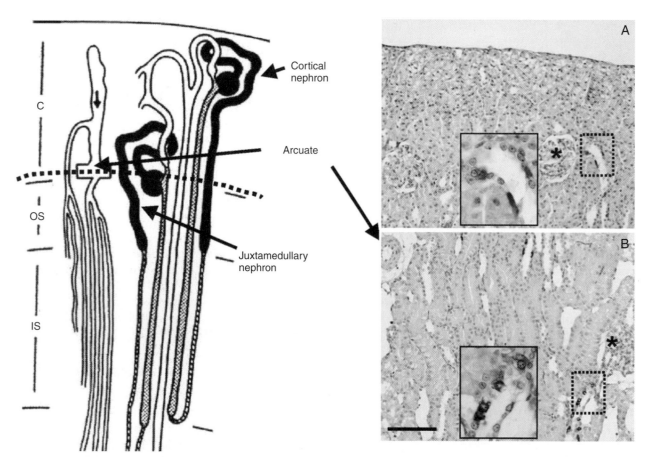

FIGURE 5   Immunohistochemical localization of COX-2 in renal sections. Note the small number of thick ascending limb (TAL) cells containing COX-2 (darkened cells within the boxed areas in panels A and B). TAL belonging to cortical and juxtamedullary nephrons expresses COX-2. The division of cortex and outer medulla is identified by the presence of the arcuate artery (*arrow;* B). The illustration shows the anatomy of the medulla and the length of the TAL between the cortical and juxtamedullary nephrons (B). The dotted line indicates the outer medulla, which is composed mainly of mTAL cells. The inserts show high magnification of TAL cells containing COX-2. *glomeruli. Scale bar = 100 μm. (From Rodriguez JA, Vio CP, Pedraza PL, et al. Bradykinin regulates cyclooxygenase-2 in rat renal thick ascending limb cells. *Hypertension* 2004;44:230-235,with permission.) See color insert.

Release of renin with activation of the RAAS in response to salt depletion or renal ischemia is mediated by the coordinate activities of COX-2 and PGI_2 synthase acting through the prostacyclin (IP) receptor via increased cAMP formation (55) and operating within the macula densa and granular cells of the afferent arteriole, which, together with contiguous cells of the extraglomerular mesangium, comprise the juxtaglomerular apparatus (JGA) (187). Under basal conditions in the adult rat kidney, COX-2 is restricted to a few cTAL cells adjacent to the macula densa, the medullary interstitial cells, the PGMVs and, perhaps, to low levels in the macula densa itself (36, 65, 218). This quiescent phase is succeeded by manifest COX-2 expression in the macula densa and adjacent cTAL with activation of the RAAS in response to either reduced salt intake or salt depletion produced by diuretic therapy (116, 237). Furosemide-induced natriuresis, which stimulates COX-2 expression (115), is blunted by selective inhibition of COX-2 in human (206).

Macula Densa as Cl^- Sensor and Stimulation of PGE_2 and PGI_2 Synthesis

The macula densa senses changes in $[Cl^-]$ in tubular fluid for which function the macula densa is optimally located at the tubular-luminal interface (237). At this site in the cortical segment of the TAL, tubular fluid NaCl concentration is most reflective of the state of total body NaCl balance (187). The macula densa sensor is thus positioned to link changes in tubular NaCl concentration to altering the activity of the RAAS and producing changes in GFR and adjustments in NaCl reabsorption by key nephron segments, thereby stabilizing NaCl excretion. Low NaCl concentration in the tubular fluid in contact with the macula densa cells that "act as receptors of luminal NaCl concentration" (187) stimulates prostacyclin synthesis that activates IP receptor to increase renin mRNA, renin synthesis and release, elevating PRA and producing increased formation of ANG II (55). (Schema 3):

$$\downarrow[Cl^-]: Phospholipids \rightarrow AA \rightarrow PGH_2 \rightarrow PGI_2 \rightarrow IP \rightarrow Renin \rightarrow ANG\ II \rightarrow PAC$$
$$PLA_2 \qquad\qquad COX\text{-}2 \qquad PGI_2\text{-}S$$

SCHEMA 3. PLA_2 = phospholipase A_2; PGI_2-S = prostacyclin synthase; IP = prostacyclin receptor; PAC = plasma aldosterone concentration.

Low $[Cl^-]$ in the macula densa induces phosphorylation of MAP kinases (ERK 1/2 and p38) resulting in COX-2 expression (237) with release of renin via the intervening mediation of COX-2 linkage to PGI_2 synthase producing PGI_2, the mediator ultimately responsible for activation of the RAAS by stimulating the IP to increase synthesis and release of renin (55). MAP kinases also activate cytosolic PLA_2 (70), the first step in the initiation of the activity of macula densa COX-2 by providing AA for metabolism by COX-2, forming PGH_2 that is metabolized within the JGA by synthases generating PGE_2 (modulates transport and moderates pressor hormones) and PGI_2 (activates the RAAS and maintains the integrity of the endothelium of PGMVs), respectively. A similar mechanism operating via MAP kinases causes induction of COX-2 expression in collecting duct cells (236).

Salt depletion increases expression of both COX-2 and mPGES-1 in the macula densa (57) and in PGMVs (36). Additional evidence that COX-2 is linked to mPGES-1 in the macula densa rather than the constitutive membranal PGE_2 synthase (mPGES-2) is based on studies of the PGE_2 synthetic capabilities of human embryonic kidney (HEK) 293 cells cotransfected with COX-2 and mPGES-1 versus those cotransfected with human COX-2 and mPGES-2 (136). Large increases in PGE_2 were produced only in HEK 293 cells cotransfected with COX-2 and mPGES-1 in response to stimulation of phospholipase with a calcium ionophore.

Modulation of 20-HETE by COX-2

COX-2 linkage to mPGES-1 also provides a mechanism to modulate the renal actions of high levels of ANG II (and pressor hormones generally) by generating PGE_2 to attenuate the intensity of the renal vasoconstrictor-antidiuretic effects of the pressor agent (121). COX-2 linkage to mPGES-1 has an additional function; namely, metabolism of 20-HETE (Schema 4), the principle eicosanoid of PGMVs, to a prostaglandin analog, 20-OH PGE_2, with loss of the vasoconstrictor activity of 20-HETE (vide infra), thereby lessening the tone and reactivity of PGMVs, particularly the afferent arteriole (36, 81) (Fig. 6). This mechanism serves a

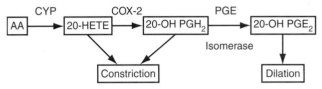

FIGURE 6 Schematic showing transformation of the vasoconstrictor, 20-HETE, by COX-2 and prostaglandin E_2 isomerase to 20-OH PGE2, which produces vasodilation.

defensive role under conditions of either salt restriction or in response to diseases that activate the RAAS producing ANG II, which stimulates synthesis of microvascular 20-HETE by activating AT_2 receptors (39). In turn, 20-HETE can be metabolized by the PGE_2 isomerase to 20-OH PGE_2 depending on the status of salt and water homeostasis. Untransformed 20-HETE released by ANG II would, presumably, increase tone and reactivity of PGMVs to a degree having deleterious effects on renal function, particularly when vascular volume is altered by salt depletion or disease. This possibility becomes a reality when NSAIDs are given to elderly people, as noted, a group that is subject to insidious decline in renal function (8). It is of particular concern in those individuals, both elderly as well as others having activation of the RAAS secondarily to congestive heart failure (31), hepatic cirrhosis with ascites (182), and compromised renal function (154).

TUBULOGLOMERULAR FEEDBACK: EICOSANOID MEDIATED

Tubuloglomerular feedback (TGF) regulates afferent arteriolar tone and reactivity, the effector unit in the mechanism that controls filtrate delivery to the renal tubules (17). TGF is housed in the JGA, as is the mechanism regulating renin synthesis and release; it is activated by high $[Cl^-]$ in tubular fluid producing constriction of the afferent arteriole. These two functions of the JGA have been notably described by Schnermann (187), whose studies of the past three decades have penetrated the shrouds that enveloped the JGA. TGF and renin release "are related to Na^+ balance in a temporally sequential manner, with control of afferent arteriolar tone being the major JGA function in the short term and control of renin secretion being its dominant role in the long term" (187). The 20-HETE is a candidate second messenger mediating TGF (259) by constricting PGMVs evoked by ATP, the purinoceptor $(P)_2$ agonist, acting through the P_2X receptor (253). It is at this site that 20-HETE also mediates autoregulation of RBF (78).

$$AA \rightarrow 20\text{-HETE} \rightarrow 20\text{-OH PGH}_2 \rightarrow 20\text{-OH PGE}_2$$
$$\omega\text{-hydroxylase} \quad COX\text{-}2 \qquad\qquad mPGES\text{-}1$$

SCHEMA 4. COX-2-dependent transformation of 20-HETE.

HYPERCHLOREMIA ACTIVATES COX- AND CYP-DEPENDENT VASCULAR MECHANISMS: THE TGF CONNECTION

The involvement of eicosanoid-dependent mechanisms in the renal hemodynamic and excretory changes produced by hyperchloremia (. 103 mM Cl^-) underscores the critical role of $[Cl^-]$ in tubular fluid as sensed by the macula densa that initiates the signals that regulate the activities of both the RAAS ($\downarrow[Cl^-]$) and TGF ($\uparrow[Cl^-]$) (187). *The analysis that follows identifies 20-OH PGH_2, an endoperoxide analog of 20-HETE, a product of the concerted actions of v-hydroxylase and COX-2 that activates the TxA_2/PGH_2 (TP) receptor as the candidate mediator of the renal functional response to systemic hyperchloremia. The 20-OH PGH_2 also fulfills major criteria to serve as the mediator of TGF* (Schema 5).

This schema depicts key elements in TGF that regulate the rate of filtrate delivery (GFR) to the nephron as determined by variations in intake of dietary salt. The rationale for the hypothesis that a product of CYP-AA metabolism via a COX transformation step stimulates TP receptor is based on the following: (1) COX inhibition abolishes TGF (188); (2) a TxA_2 mimetic enhances TGF (228); (3) 20-HETE is the principle AA metabolite of PGMVs and the afferent arteriole (39, 81); and (4) inhibition of NO synthesis potentiates TGF (214, 230). As NO exerts a braking action on 20-HETE synthesis (2), inhibition of NO synthesis will enhance 20-HETE formation and potentiate TGF (153).

The renal response to changes in $[Cl^-]$ acting independently of Na^+ concentration (maintained as a constant) was examined in the rat isolated kidney thereby excluding systemic hormonal and nervous inputs (5). The renal functional effects of COX inhibition were determined in the presence of high (117 mM) and low (87 mM) $[Cl^-]$ in the renal perfusate with Na^+ held constant (143 mM) as was osmolality. Inhibition of COX with NSAIDs (nonselective COX inhibitors), in most experimental settings, produces renal vasoconstriction and fluid retention by eliminating vasodilator prostaglandins (14). However, renal vasodilation and natriuresis will occur in response to NSAIDs if the pressor eicosanoids, TxA_2 and PGH_2, predominate as in ANG II–dependent hypertension (127) as well as in response to elevated $[Cl^-]$ in the blood/perfusate entering the kidney.

High $[Cl^-]$ decreased GFR and produced antinatriuresis that was prevented by COX inhibition and by the less selective antagonist (SQ29548) of the TP receptor but not by the highly selective TP receptor antagonist (BMS 180291). This difference can be accounted for by the ability of SQ 29548 to attenuate vasoconstriction produced by $PGF_{2\alpha}$, 20-HETE, and the isoprostane 8-epi-$PGF_{2\alpha}$ in addition to TxA_2 and PGH_2 (144). These results argue against either TxA_2 or PGH_2 mediating the negative renal functional effect of hyperchloremia as the highly selective TP antagonist (BMS 180291) was without effect on high $[Cl^-]$-induced depression of GFR and Na^+ retention. Thus, a product of COX that is inhibited by blockade of the TP receptor by SQ 29548, specifically the 20-HETE analog of PGH_2, 20-OH PGH_2, is the most likely mediator of the renal functional response to systemic hyperchloremia and of TGF.

The candidacy of 20-OH PGH_2 received additional support from the studies of Escalante and Schwartzman (48,192) who came to the same conclusion, showing that vasoactivity of 20-HETE was dependent on metabolism by COX forming 20-OH PGH_2 (Fig. 7), which was inhibited either by COX blockade or by TP receptor blockade with the less selective TP antagonist (SQ 29548). Support of this hypothesis was also obtained from two findings: (1) hyperchloremia increased by twofold 20-HETE release from the rat kidney and (2) the renal vasoconstrictor response to 20-HETE given into the renal artery was inhibited both by indomethacin and by blockade of TP receptors, indicating rapid conversion of 20-HETE by COX to a product that stimulates the TP receptor; namely, 20-OH PGH_2 (5). The latter conclusion to be validated requires (1) demonstrating increased production by the JGA of 20-OH PGH_2, a labile compound, in response to high $[Cl^-]$; and (2) reproducing the renal hemodynamic effects of high $[Cl^-]$ by administering authentic 20-OH PGH_2.

MACULA DENSA: $PGI_2 \rightarrow$ RENIN $\rightarrow$ RENOVASCULAR HYPERTENSION

The critical role of PGI_2, the renin secretagogue in the pathogenesis of renovascular hypertension, was highlighted in mice lacking PGI_2 receptors ($IP^{-/-}$) (55). These mice did not secrete renin in response to salt depletion, whereas mice lacking the four PGE_2 receptors (EP_{1-4}) responded appropriately to salt deprivation by increasing renin secretion, which invalidated the proposed role of PGE_2 as a primary renin secretagogue. In addition, IP receptor deletion suppressed development of renovascular hypertension by preventing renin release when mice were challenged with renal ischemia produced by constriction of the renal artery.

$\uparrow[Cl^-]$: PL $\longrightarrow$ AA $\longrightarrow$ PGH_2 $\longrightarrow$ 20-OH PGH_2 $\longrightarrow$ TP $\longrightarrow$ aa constriction
      PLase COX-2 ω-hydroxylase

SCHEMA 5. $[Cl^-]$, Cl^- concentration in tubular fluid; PL, phospholipids; PLase, phospholipase; TP, TxA_2/PGH_2 receptor; AA, afferent arteriole.

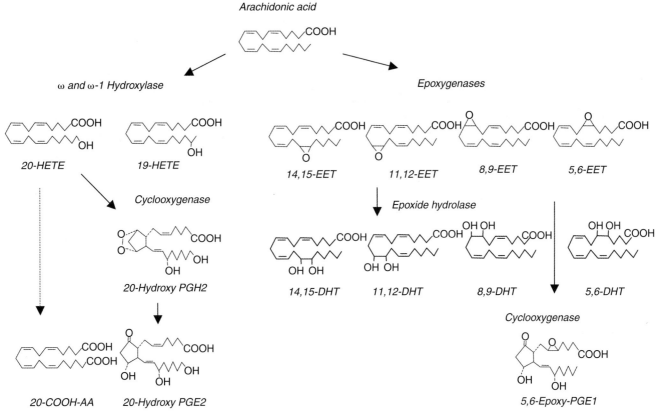

FIGURE 7   Arachidonic acid (AA) metabolism by cytochrome P450-dependent mono-oxygenases to ω- and ω-1 hydroxyeicosa-tetraenoic acids (HETEs), epoxyeicosatrienoic acids (EETS), and dihydroxyeicosatrienoic acids (DHTs). The 20-HETE and 5,6-EET can be converted by cyclooxygenase to analogs of prostaglandins. (From the American Physiological Society. *Am J Physiol* 1999;277: R607-R623, with permission.)

The role of COX in the development of renovascular hypertension was initially defined by Jackson, Oates, and Branch (86). In a rat model of renovascular hypertension produced by ligation of the aorta between the origin of renal arteries, indomethacin decreased PRA and lowered blood pressure. In human renovascular hypertension, an aspirin compound also reduced blood pressure and decreased the elevated PRA (75). In contrast to the blood pressure–lowering effects of aspirin compounds in renovascular hypertension, inhibition of COX produced additional elevations of blood pressure in human essential hypertension that can be accounted for by the demonstrated properties of aspirin-like drugs to retain salt and water (14).

In view of the essential role of COX-2 in regulating renin release, selective inhibition of COX-2 was hypothesized to lower blood pressure in renovascular hypertension whereas a selective COX-1 inhibitor should be ineffectual. Confirmation of the hypothesis was obtained in a rat model of renovascular hypertension; namely, selective inhibition of COX-2, not COX-1, lowered the elevated blood pressure and decreased production and release of renin (224) (Schema 6).

$$AA \xrightarrow[\text{COX-2}]{\overset{\text{NSAID}}{\centernot\longrightarrow}} \downarrow PGH_2 \rightarrow \underset{PGI_2\text{-}S}{\downarrow PGI_2} \rightarrow IP \rightarrow \downarrow Renin \rightarrow \downarrow ANG\,II$$

SCHEMA 6. PGI_2-S = PGI_2 synthase.

On the other hand, intrarenal arterial infusion of PGE_2 produced hypertension in conscious dogs (72), an apparent paradox as PGE_2 has prominent antipressor properties including antagonism of pressor hormones, promotion of salt and water excretion and renal vasodilatation. This anomalous prohypertensive response to PGE_2, however, can be rationalized in terms of activation of either EP receptors (EP_1 and EP_3) that may increase renal vascular resistance (RVR) (159) and/or stimulation of renin release by PGE_2 acting through an indirect mechanism, i.e., bypassing the IP receptor (88) (Schema 7).

ENLARGEMENT OF THE AA CASCADE

The field of eicosanoid research was thought to be entering a quiescent phase in the early 1980s. The 1982 Nobel Prize in Medicine and Physiology had been awarded to the prime movers of prostaglandin research, Bergstrom,

$$\downarrow[Cl^-] \rightarrow \uparrow COX\text{-}2 \rightarrow \uparrow PGH_2 \rightarrow \uparrow PGI_2 \rightarrow TP \rightarrow \uparrow Renin\ PRA \rightarrow \uparrow ANG\ II$$
$$PGI_2 - S$$

SCHEMA 7.

Samuelsson, and Vane, usually a sign that a field has concluded the logarithmic phase of its development. However, several papers were published in the early 1980s that were to usher in the second phase of eicosanoid research; namely, arachidonate metabolism via CYP, which had been considered to be primarily, if not exclusively, directed to drug metabolism (22, 131, 145). This discovery of the third pathway of AA metabolism reopened Pandora's box and emptied the magician's hat; for it eventuated in a flood of novel AA products generated by the CYP system that influenced all aspects of renal function (176, 203). The CYP-derived AA metabolites possess wide-ranging biological properties: vasoactivity, mitogenicity, profibrinolytic, and pro- and anti-atherogenesis. They promote apoptosis, are anti-inflammatory and antiproliferative, and affect blood pressure, both elevating and reducing blood pressure (122, 203, 204). The principle products of the two branches of this AA pathway, 20-HETE and 11,12-EET, exhibit opposing effects as in the autoregulatory response of RBF (78), the result of their antagonism at the Ca^{2+}-activated K^+ (K_{Ca}) channel (21, 256). The liver, which contains the largest components of the CYP-dependent mixed-function oxidase system, is surpassed by the kidney in terms of specific activity of CYP-related AA metabolism (191); the highest activity in the renal outer medulla and cortex is several-fold that of the liver.

The Third Pathway of AA Metabolism

CYP has been designated the third pathway of AA metabolism (190) (Fig. 7) as it was the last to be discovered yet overtaking the second pathway, lipoxygenases, in scope, having ramifications involving all mammalian biological systems. CYP arachidonate metabolites are essential components in basic mechanisms in blood vessels and transporting epithelia (176) that govern vascular tone and reactivity, salt and water balance, and the response to injury and inflammation (123, 140, 176). These studies have redefined basic renal mechanisms in terms of the "missing eicosanoid" (122). For example, within the renal microcirculation, 20-HETE is the effector molecule of renal circulatory autoregulation (258) and participates in pressure natriuresis (77); within the nephron, 20-HETE modulates the Na^+-K^+-$2Cl^-$ cotransporter (46) and the 70 pS K^+ channel in the TAL (110) and inhibits the Na^+ pump (143) and the Na^+-H^+ exchanger (NHE_3) in the proximal tubules. In the collecting duct, 11,12-EET participates in the regulation of Na^+ reabsorption by modulating the activity of the ENaC (227).

Epoxides (EETs), which are synthesized by PGMVs in response to adenosine activation of the A_{2A} receptor (35), are the agents of adaptation evoked by an adenosine mechanism that responds to renal ischemia, hypoxia, and oxidative stress (66). Adenosine has been aptly named the *retaliatory molecule*. This designation now takes on added dimension as adenosine has been linked to the remarkable range of activities of EETs: anti-inflammatory, anti-migratory, profibrinolytic, vasodilator, and natriuretic (203, 204, 245).

THE TWO BRANCHES OF CYP-AA METABOLISM:

HETE synthesis: ω-hydroxylases (20-HETE) and subterminal hydroxylases produce HETEs (16-, 17-, 18-, and 19) of which 20-HETE predominates because of (1) properties highly relevant to renal functional adaptation/maladaptation in health and in disease: vasoactivity, mitogenicity, and ion transport regulation (122); and (2) formation by key renal structures: PGMVs, particularly the afferent arteriole (39), glomerulus (176), proximal tubules (49), and TAL (28). Subterminal HETEs, 16-,17-, 18-, and 19-HETEs, are produced in the kidney but have received little attention (with the exception of 19-HETE) despite their ability to antagonize some of the key actions of 20-HETE on vascular reactivity and Na^+ transport (25, 160, 248, 249). An interesting development, having therapeutic implications, relates to alcohol upregulation of the liver enzyme 2E1, which generates 18- and 19-HETEs (100). The subterminal HETEs are candidate mediators of the advantageous antihypertensive effect of moderate alcohol consumption by antagonizing 20-HETE related increases in vascular reactivity (247). A high degree of specificity for the 18-(R) and 19-(R) stereoisomers in producing these antagonistic effects was observed.

Epoxygenases generate 5,6-EET, 8,9-EET, 11,12-EET, and 14,15-EET. The 11,12-EET opposes the renal vasoconstrictor action of 20-HETE (78) and may serve as the long-sought endothelial derived hyperpolarizing factor (EDHF) in the coronary circulation (21, 53, 161). The 5,6-EET, as reflected in urinary excretion of 5,6-(DHT), is a major component together with 11,12-EET of the epoxide-dependent mechanism that moderates elevation of blood pressure in response to salt loading (113) and like 11,12-EET, possesses many of the requisite properties to serve as an EDHF (56). Stimulation of EDHF (EET) synthesis via a kinin mechanism is an additional therapeutic benefit of treatment with ACE inhibitors as they enhance kinin levels by preventing kinin degradation, which promotes release of endothelial-derived EETs (164).

Several key products of the CYP pathway interact with COX, forming metabolites that differ in their biological profile from the parent compound. An example, already cited, is the transforming effect of the coordinate activities of COX-2-mPGES-1 on the vasoconstrictor action of 20-HETE, forming 20-OH PGE$_2$, a vasodilator prostaglandin analog of 20-HETE in PGMVs (36). The potential versatility of 20-HETE as a vascular hormone was underscored by Hill, Fitzpatrick, and Murphy who demonstrated that human platelets rapidly metabolized 20-HETE via both COX and 12-LOX pathways to TxA$_2$ and 12-HETE analogs of 20-HETE (69). Further, 20-HETE blocked platelet aggregation produced by most agonists (thrombin excepted), an effect associated with inhibition of platelet TxA$_2$ production.

Vasoactivity of 5,6-EET

A wide range of biological responses to 5,6-*cis*-EET has been reported: modulation of renal tubular transport (179), epithelial growth factor signaling (20), somatostatin release (90), and prolactin secretion (30). Of the epoxides, only 5,6-EET can undergo cyclization to form endoperoxide intermediates and prostaglandin analogs (24). The 8,9-EET is converted by COX to a noncyclized product (250). 5,6-EET is unique in its vascular actions (56, 181), having dilator as well as constrictor activities with variable COX-dependency that is vascular bed (e.g., renal vs mesenteric) and species specific (24, 80). The 5,6-EET was the only EET that dilated the rat caudal artery (29), an effect abolished by either removal of the endothelium or inhibition of COX (26). The 5,6-EET metabolites, 5,6-DHT and 5,6-γ-lactone, lack vasoactivity as is the case for DHTs in most studies (203); a notable exception is the reported potency of DHTs on canine isolated coronary arterioles (147).

The rat arcuate artery, representative of the reactivity of PGMVs to agonists, dilated in response to nM concentrations of 5,6-EET and 11,12-EET (35). The vasodilator effect to 5,6-EET was abolished by inhibition of COX whereas 11,12-EET–induced vasodilatation was unaffected. The vasodilator action of 5,6-EET in the rabbit kidney was also dependent on COX as it was inhibited by aspirin-like drugs (27); 5,6-EET has two prostaglandin components: the release of vasodilator prostaglandins, PGE$_2$ and PGI$_2$, and metabolism of 5,6-EET by COX and PGE$_2$ synthase to form the vasodilator prostaglandin analog, 5,6-epoxy-PGE$_1$ (24) (Fig. 7).

INTERACTION OF THE TWO BRANCHES OF CYP-DEPENDENT-AA METABOLISM TAKES TWO FORMS:

Functional

The 20-HETE as the agent of renal autoregulation (258) contracts PGMVs and is opposed by the dilator action of 11,12-EET (78). The availability of specific inhibitors of the ω-hydroxylase and epoxygenase pathways, through the extraordinary synthetic capabilities of Dr. J. R. Falck, has

sharpened our discrimination of the individual contributions of each pathway to vascular and transport mechanisms. Inhibition of 20-HETE synthesis abrogated the renal autoregulatory response to increased perfusion pressure (78). Contrarily, inhibition of EET synthesis enhanced autoregulatory-related vasoconstriction, underscoring the antagonistic actions of 20-HETE versus EETs operating at the afferent arteriole of PGMVs. Vascular EETs may also serve as EDHFs as has been proposed for the rat coronary and renal vasculatures (53, 161) at which sites vascular 20-HETE interacts with EETs, attenuating their relaxant effects. The demonstration that 20-HETE antagonized EDHF-mediated relaxation of small coronary arteries is consistent with an EET–20-HETE interaction (164). The mechanism involved activation of protein kinase C (PKC) by 20-HETE producing inhibition of Na$^+$,K$^+$-ATPase, a mechanism identical to that involving 20-HETE inhibition of Na$^+$ transport in the proximal tubules (49, 143).

Biochemical

Capdevila and colleagues (38) etched a significant addition to those mechanisms activating the nuclear receptor PPARα by identifying *a novel mechanism, the hydroxylation of EETs by CYP 4A isoforms, forming hydroxyepoxyeicosatrienoic acids (HEETs) that bind to PPARα with high affinity.* The four 4A isoforms exhibit differential preferences for EETs: 4A1 prefers 8,9-EET, forming 20,8,9-HEET; 4A2, 4A3, and 4A8 prefer 11,12-EET, forming 20-, 11,12-HEET. *HEETs are also synthesized by CYP 2C23–dependent epoxygenation of 20-HETE (133)* (Schema 8).

These studies provide evidence that HEETs regulate the transcriptional activities of the PPARα receptor that targets renal 4A hydroxylase isoforms and 2C23 epoxygenase (38). Thus, a novel class of PPARα activators, the HEETs, is generated by the interaction of the two branches of CYP 450-AA metabolism, epoxygenases and ω-hydroxylases. HEETs, by activating PPARα regulate expression of the CYP 4A1, 2 and 3 isoforms of ω/ω-1- hydroxylases. The fourth isoform of the rat CYP 4A gene subfamily, CYP4A8, is regulated by testosterone (137), first demonstrated in mice following deletion of the mouse homolog of the rat 4A2 gene, which, via an obscure mechanism, increased androgen levels that induced expression of the mouse 4A12 isoform with increased formation of 20-HETE and hypertension in male mice. Castration prevented the induction of the 4A12 isozyme and abolished the hypertension, each of which was restored by androgen replacement (73). Treatment of rats with 5α-dihydrotestosterone produced upregulation of vascular CYP 4A8 mRNA and increased 20-HETE

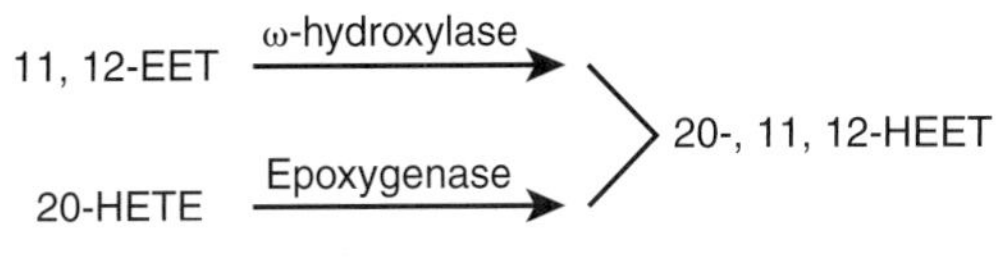

SCHEMA 8.

synthase activity by fourfold with production of hypertension in male and female rats. These findings should contribute to the development of a rationale for the predisposition of the male to more severe forms of hypertension (165).

Increased EET hydroxylation reduced EET levels in rat liver and plasma; the principle plasma EETs, 8,9- and 14,15- EETs showing a 40%–50% decline from plasma levels of 4.0 and 9.0 ng/ml, respectively (38). The rate of ω/ω-1-hydroxylation of EETs exceeded that of AA, suggesting that the preferred substrates for ω/ω-1-hydroxylases are EETs, not AA. These findings identified a mechanism, hydroxylation of EETs, that affects steady state levels of EETs in body tissues and fluids in addition to several well-defined mechanisms: enzymatic hydration of EETs by sEH (33, 129), forming dihydroxyeicosatrienoic acids (DHTs), ω-oxidation, and storage by incorporation of EETs into phospholipids (89, 203); the biological activities of HEETs, in addition to activation of PPARα, remain to be defined.

EETS ARE ANTI-INFLAMMATORY AGENTS

The anti-inflammatory properties of EETs were strikingly demonstrated in rats overexpressing human renin and angiotensinogen genes, the double-transgenic rats (dTGRs) (133). These rats are severely hypertensive and demonstrate rapidly developing inflammatory end-organ damage, most striking in the kidney. They are an excellent model to test the ameliorative effects of interventions designed to activate anti-inflammatory systems such as that represented by epoxygenases. Untreated dTGRs die by 8 weeks of age from cardiac and renal failure; they exhibit downregulation of the 2C23 epoxygenase. The latter is the principal renal epoxygenase isoform and is co-expressed with ω-hydroxylase 4A isoforms in "cortical and outer medullary" tubules and in renal microvessels. Fenofibrate, which activates 2C23 via a PPARα mechanism, prevented the renal damage and reversed the hypertension in dTGRs. Reduction of blood pressure without affecting ANG II generation did not prevent end-organ injury. The candidate EET responsible for these anti-inflammatory effects is 11,12-EET, the principle product of 2C23 and the EET possessing the greatest anti-inflammatory potency (140). The 11,12-EET inhibits cytokine-induced activation of the nuclear transcription factor, NFκB, preventing inflammation at an early phase in its development.

In constructing a schema for regulation of the levels, metabolism and activities of 11,12-EET, the starting point is the principle 11,12-EET synthesizing enzyme 2C23 (74) (Fig. 8). The 11,12-EET undergoes transformation by ω-hydroxylase isoforms to 20-, 11,12-HEET that stimulates EET production via activating the PPARα nuclear receptor that targets both the 2C23 epoxygenase and ω/ω-1-hydroxylase isoforms (38). Additional features of

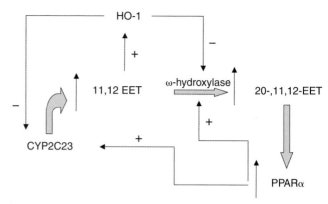

FIGURE 8 Feedback mechanisms that regulate CYP2C23 and ω-1 hydroxylase: Formation of 11,12-EET via CYP2C23 increases 20-, 11,12-EET synthesis, which provides a PPARα-dependent positive feedback signal for CYP2C23 and ω-hydroxylase activity. Heme oxygenase-1 (HO-1), induced by 11,12-EET, contributes to a negative regulatory mechanism via inhibition of CYP2C23 and ω-hydroxylase activity.

the effects of 11,12-EET and its hydroxylation product, 20-, 11,12-EET, are (1) the regulation of 11,12-EET levels by their metabolism via ω/ω-1-hydroxylases; and (2) induction of heme oxygenase (HO)-1 by 11,12-EET. HO-1 inhibits CYP-AA metabolism by catabolyzing the breakdown of the heme moiety that contains the catalytic component of the CYP enzyme complex. Induction of HO-1 by 11,12-EET represents a negative feedback mechanism that regulates the activity of CYP-AA metabolism and, thereby, EET formation (Fig. 8).

EETS: ANTIPRESSOR, ANTI-INFLAMMATORY AND RELEASE BY ADENOSINE

EETs Are Antihypertensive: Prevention of Pressor Response to High-Salt Intake

EETs have beneficial vascular effects that make their increased production a therapeutic target for regulating blood pressure (156, 242). In a landmark study, Capdevila and colleagues established the importance of renal EETs to blood pressure regulation (113). In rats maintained on a HS diet, which by itself did not increase blood pressure, inhibition of epoxygenases produced elevation of blood pressure (i.e., rendered rats salt-sensitive). The blood pressure of age-matched rats receiving standard laboratory chow was unaffected by epoxygenase inhibition with clotrimazole. CYP 2C23 has been identified in the rat kidney as (1) the major 2C arachidonate epoxygenase and (2) the isoform of the 2C family that is subject to regulation by dietary salt (74). CYP2C23 is downregulated by ANG II in combination with a HS diet (254), a finding that can explain the failure to contain/prevent tissue damage in rats produced by ANG II infusion;

namely, deficient synthesis of the anti-inflammatory epoxide, 11,12-EET, by the 2C23 epoxygenase. Fenofibrate stimulation of the nuclear receptor PPARα activated CYP 2C23 and greatly reduced ANG II–related renal injury: it normalized blood pressure, decreased albuminuria and renal leukocyte infiltration and reduced activity of NFκβ (133).

Adenosine A_{2A} Receptors are Coupled to Epoxygenase Activity

The demonstration of hypertension in mice lacking the adenosine A_{2A} receptor (104) and the finding that renal adenosine A_{2A} receptors are affected by Na^+ intake (195) occasioned testing the *hypothesis that salt loading evokes an antipressor purinoceptor mechanism activated by adenosine with stimulation of the A_{2A} receptor and release of EETs (107).* In rats fed a HS diet that increases 2C23 expression, kidneys were isolated and perfused at an elevated pressure of 200 mm Hg (phenylephrine induced). Stimulation of renal adenosine receptors with 2-chloro-adenosine produced a sharp decline in RVR; EET release in response to 2-chloro-adenosine was fourfold greater in HS fed rats than in rats on a NS diet. A selective epoxygenase inhibitor, MS-PPOH, produced a diminished renal efflux of EETs by 70% and blocked the reduction in RVR produced by A_{2A} receptor stimulation (107).

THE DAHL SALT-SENSITIVE RAT: 20-HETE AND EET DEFICIENCY

Deficiency of mTAL 20-HETE may contribute to the development of hypertension in the Dahl salt-sensitive (DS) rat by increasing NaCl reabsorption in the mTAL consequent to increased activity of the luminal Na^+,K^+-$2Cl^-$ cotransporter (83). As noted, the expression and activity of several isoforms of ω-hydroxylase are regulated by the transcription factor, PPARα, which is activated by fibrates (38,133). Administration of clofibrate corrected the deficiency of 20-HETE in the mTAL, which restored inhibitory modulation of the Na^+,K^+-$2Cl^-$ cotransporter, reduced NaCl reabsorption, and normalized blood pressure (177).

Evidence supporting the role of EETs in addition to that of 20-HETE in moderating the pressor response to salt loading was obtained in the DS rat, a "model of genetic salt-dependent hypertension" (83). DS rats exhibit a deficiency of both 20-HETE and EETs; they respond to salt loading by an increase in blood pressure associated with failure to increase production of EETs (113). The Dahl salt-resistant (DR) rats, on the other hand, increased excretion of EETs in response to salt loading and maintained normal blood pressure. *These separate lines of evidence—obtained from (1) a rat model of genetic hypertension, the DS rat, and (2) induction*

of hypertension by epoxygenase inhibition in salt loaded normal rats—converge on a shared renal antipressor mechanism, one mediated by renal CYP-derived EETs. An underlying common mechanism that prevents hypertension in the DR and in the salt-loaded normal rat may be related to the ability of 11,12-EET to inhibit ENaC in the cortical collecting ducts. A deficiency of 11,12-EET would increase Na^+ reabsorption at this site, with an attendant expansion of extracellular fluid volume and elevation of blood pressure. The importance of the ENaC to blood pressure control has been underscored by Lifton: "ENaC activity is absolutely required for normal salt homeostasis" (108). Lesions that produce increased activity of ENaC have been linked to genetically determined hypertension as in Liddle syndrome.

These studies have pointed to the therapeutic possibilities of manipulating EETs in hypertension and cardiovascular diseases. Another potentially important therapeutic target is cytosolic (soluble) epoxide hydrolase (sEH), which hydrates EETs, forming DHTs. Inhibition of sEH decreased blood pressure in the SHR (243) and disruption of the gene coding for sEH produced hypotension in mice (194) by increasing tissue/plasma levels of EETs. Several studies have supported the renal protective and blood pressure lowering properties of EETs in rats, by fenofibrate stimulating their production via PPARα activation with induction of 2C23 activity (133) and by decreasing EET conversion via sEH to DHTs (194).

EICOSANOID SEGMENTAL ANALYSIS: NEPHRON AND MICROVESSELS

The third phase of renal eicosanoid studies was based on segmental analysis of the nephron and microcirculation in terms of lipid mediators and modulators that targeted key enzymes/transporters in the nephron and in the renal vasculature and microcirculation.

Tubular Targets

1. 20-HETE: The sodium-hydrogen exchanger (NHE$_3$) (6, 42) and the Na^+ pump (Na^+,K^+-ATPase) in the proximal tubule (143).
2. 20-HETE: The Na^+,K^+-$2Cl^-$ cotransporter and intermediate conductance 70-pS K^+ channel in the TAL (46, 225).
3. 11,12-EET: The Na^+ channel (ENaC) in the collecting ducts (227).

Vascular Targets

1. 20-HETE and 11,12-EET: Ca^{2+}-activated K channels (K_{Ca}) in vascular smooth muscle (VSM) (43,257).
2. 20-HETE: L-type Ca^{2+} channels in VSM (240).

Eicosanoids and Renal Blood Vessels

The renal (micro) vasculature has been fractionated/segmented, as has the nephron, to define variations in oxygenase activity and eicosanoid product formation. The preglomerular vascular elements (PGMVs = arcuate − interlobular − afferent arterioles) command primary attenion because of their strategic importance as the effector component of autoregulation of RBF and TGF (176) and, thereby, control of glomerular filtration. The renal vasculature has been examined in terms of longitudinal distribution of oxygenases and synthases: COX-1 and COX-2 and their linkages to prostaglandin synthases; 12-LOX (12(S)-HPETE) and ω/ω-1-hydroxylase and epoxygenases (76, 139). The relative abundance of the CYP enzymes generating 20- and 19-HETEs peaks in PGMVs—arcuate, interlobular and afferent arterioles (39). Medium and large arteries (interlobar-main artery and its bifurcation) are less well endowed with 20-HETE and EET synthesizing capabilities than PGMVs (36).

COX-2 is expressed under physiological conditions, by cyclical variations in vascular wall tension (i.e., pulsatile flow that generates hemodynamic forces that influence vascular wall biology and endothelial function) (60). COX-2, the endothelial isoform of NOS, and manganese-dependent superoxide dismutase (Mn-SOD) represent products a set of genes that are expressed "in a sustained fashion by steady laminar shear stress, but not by turbulent shear stress." The encoded enzymes exert effects and/or generate products that are vasoprotective as for example, the coupling of COX-2 to PGI_2 synthase, forming PGI_2, the antiplatelet, antithrombotic and anti-atherogenic eicosanoid. These studies, particularly that of FitzGerald and colleagues (117) linking PGI_2 synthesis to endothelial COX-2, provided the rationale for the increased risk of myocardial infarction in patients treated with selective COX-2 inhibitors (12). Namely, COX-2 inhibition decreases vascular PGI_2 synthesis as reflected in reduced excretion of a PGI_2 metabolite while sparing platelet COX-1–derived synthesis of TxA_2. This results in unopposed platelet aggregatory—prothrombotic effects of TxA_2 at the blood–endothelial interface of atherosclerotic blood vessels. Thus, clinical validation was obtained for the therapeutic construct first suggested by the study of Bunting, Gryglewski, Moncada, and Vane regarding production of an anti-platelet vascular hormone PGX that characterized the principle biological activity (inhibition of platelet clumping) generated by rabbit fresh arterial tissue. Later structural analysis of arterial extracts revealed the labile PGI_2 to be the anti-aggregatory vasodilator agent. With extraordinary insight into future therapeutic developments, they predicted that: "Formation of PGX could be the underlying mechanism which actively prevents, under normal conditions, the accumulation of platelets on the vessel wall" (18). This served as the impetus to develop the paradigm ripe with therapeutic implications, viz., imbalance of platelet COX-1–derived TxA_2 (unaffected) relative to vascular

$$COX\text{-}2 \xrightarrow[\text{inhibitor}]{\text{COX-2}} \!\!\!\!/\!\!\!\!\longrightarrow TxA_2 / \downarrow PGI_2 \rightarrow \text{Platelet clumping} \rightarrow \text{Thrombus}$$

SCHEMA 9.   COX-2 selective inhibition favors platelet aggregation: $\downarrow PGI_2$, unaffected TxA_2.

COX-2–derived PGI_2 (decreased), predisposes to vascular thrombosis and atherogenesis (19) (Schema 9).

This formulation gave impetus to therapeutic interventions such as low-dose aspirin that reduces prothrombotic TxA_2 production while sparing the antiplatelet, antithrombotic, vascular hormone, PGI_2.

When blood vessels are viewed cross-sectionally, the endothelium occupies a dominant role as the site of generation of multiple factors affecting vasoactivity, thrombosis, VSM proliferation and vascular architecture as described in the catch phrase, "vascular remodeling." The generation of EETs by the endothelium can account for many of the salutary properties of the endothelium by affecting the expression/activity of enzymes, mediators and modulators governing endothelial integrity (204) and vascular resistance to deformation by atherogenesis. For example, endothelial 11,12-EET increases tissue plasminogen activator (t-PA) protein, a profibrinolytic factor (141). Prostacyclin and EETs are synthesized predominantly in the endothelium; the capacity to synthesize 20-HETE, considered to be restricted to VSM, has also been identified in the endothelium (255).

The Hepatorenal Syndrome and 20-HETE

The localization of 20-HETE biosynthesis in PGMVs (36), particularly in the afferent arteriole (256), and the ability of 20-HETE to constrict arterioles-arteries by increasing vascular tone and reactivity to pressor hormones (248), earmarked 20-HETE as a candidate agent mediating the intense constriction of the renal vasculature (without organic nephropathy) that characterizes the hepatorenal syndrome (45). The posited contribution of 20-HETE to the development of the hepatorenal syndrome was evaluated in patients with cirrhosis (182). Incubation of urine with β-glucuronidase was required to free 20-HETE, which is excreted as a glucuronide conjugate in humans (157); urinary free 20-HETE was measured by gas chromatography–mass spectrometry (vide infra). Excretion of 20-HETE was eightfold greater in patients with cirrhosis and ascites than in healthy subjects and two- to threefold greater than in cirrhotic patients without ascites. Moreover, excretion of HETEs (16-, 17-, and 18-HETEs) other than 20-HETE was not increased. The excretory rate of 20-HETE exceeded excretion of prostaglandins and thromboxane by a factor of three or more. To validate the proposed critical role of 20-HETE as a prime agent in the pathogenesis of the hepatorenal syndrome requires demonstrating reversal of the renal functional changes by treatment with either a specific inhibitor of ω-hydroxylase or antagonist of 20-HETE, interventions presently precluded in humans. The 20-HETE agonists and antagonists have been used to evaluate the contribution of 20-HETE to vascular mechanisms evoked by both physiological and pathophysiological conditions (223, 241).

Analysis of the Distribution of Oxygenase Products in the Renal Vasculature

The pre-eminence of an oxygenase and its eicosanoid biosynthetic capabilities in renal and other regional vascular studies is dependent on disease, species, age, sex, the specific vascular segment and experimental conditions (e.g., blood vs. artificial perfusate and isolated vs. in situ kidneys). The contribution of eicosanoids to the renal vascular actions of endothelins required clarification (151). Endothelins share effects on eicosanoid production with ANG II (e.g., release of renal prostaglandins and 20-HETE) (39,152). As the renovascular responses to ANG II are well defined in terms of oxygenase (COX, LOX, CYP) interactions (76,139), they served as the standard to which those of endothelin (ET)-1 were compared. An inhibitor of all pathways of AA metabolism, ETYA produced a similar decrease in the vasoconstrictor response of the intact kidney to ET-1 and ANG II (60%–70%) (151). The COX contribution (indomethacin inhibitable) to the renal vasoconstrictor responses of the intact kidney produced by ET-1 and ANG II, disclosed a similar prostaglandin component of approximately 30%. However, inhibition of LOX enzymes (12- LOX and 5-LOX) produced a cleavage: the constrictor effect of ANG II on the intact kidney was reduced by 40%–60% whereas the constrictor action of ET-1 was unaffected. For the afferent arteriole, the constrictor actions of ET-1 and ANG II were affected similarly by superoxide ion produced by peptide activation of NADPH oxidase (221). Each peptide demonstrated an enhanced vasoconstrictor effect that was greatly inhibited by a free radical scavenger.

As the 12-LOX product 12-HPETE inhibits PGI_2 synthesis, the antihypertensive effect of inhibition of 12-LOX on ANG II-induced hypertension was examined in terms of the contribution of increased PGI_2 to the blood pressure lowering response to LOX inhibition (184). In rats made hypertensive by a 2-week infusion of ANG II, the participation of PGI_2 in the antipressor response to LOX inhibition was identified by the almost complete restoration of the pressor action of ANG II on eliminating PGI_2 by giving anti-PGI_2 antibodies (211). Support for this interpretation was based on evidence of increased synthesis of PGI_2 in rats treated with a 12-LOX inhibitor before administration of antibodies; namely, increased conversion of PGH_2 to PGI_2 in vascular rings obtained from hypertensive rats and increased concentration of PGI_2 in the blood and elevated renal excretion of the PGI_2 hydrolysis product, 6-keto-$PGF_{1\alpha}$ in hypertensive rats.

A similar disparity was noted relative to inhibition of ω/ω-1-hydroxylases with DBDD in the intact kidney; ET-1 induced renal vasoconstriction was decreased by DBDD treatment whereas that to ANG II was unaffected despite the ability of ANG II to release 20-HETE from PGMVs

(39). ANG II in nanomolar concentrations increased release of 20- and 19-HETEs from isolated PGMVs by two- to threefold above basal levels in a ratio of 4:1::20-HETE:19-HETE, and in significantly lesser quantities from interlobar and large arteries. Unexpectedly, 20-HETE release by ANG II was inhibited by AT_2 receptor blockade and was linked to activation of phospholipase C. Thus, eicosanoids produced by specific vascular segments (microvessels) can be overlooked if the analysis is based on the vascular responses of the whole kidney to the hormone.

Pre- and Postglomerular Tone: 12(S)-HETE

Examination of the 12-LOX component in the response of the isolated afferent arteriole to ANG II disclosed a significant 12(S)-HETE contribution by activation of L-type Ca^{2+} channels (240). 20-HETE is a major determinant of the constrictor responses of the afferent arteriole (256) and probably represents the principle eicosanoid acting under physiological conditions as 12-LOX expression/activity has been associated with the development of tissue injury (111). For example, 12-LOX activation in diabetes contributes decisively to the development of accelerated atherogenesis (138). VSM hypertrophy and matrix gene expression produced by ANG II was shown to be mediated by 12(S)-HETE through activation of Ras and MAPK (166).

The three pathways of AA metabolism—COX, LOX, CYP—converge on the PGMVs and can be activated either singly or in combination by vasoactive hormones and by AA. However, the role of AA metabolites in the regulation of efferent arteriolar tone is uncertain (79). Glomerular eicosanoids can participate in the regulation of efferent arteriolar tone (169). For example, bradykinin releases 20-HETE of glomerular origin that antagonizes the "downstream" efferent arteriolar release of EETs by bradykinin. Bradykinin also releases a COX-1–derived vasodilator prostaglandin from the glomerulus that synergizes with the dilator action of EETs on the efferent arteriole.

The Glomerulus: A Target of Inflammation

The morphological responses to inflammatory diseases of the kidney are manifest in the glomerulus and renal interstitium, associated with alterations of glomerular hemodynamics and tubular transport that are, in part, produced by immune cell–derived mediators (e.g., macrophage release of cytokines with production of leukotrienes and TxA_2) (189). The localization of expression of 5-, 12-, and 15-LOX and leukotriene receptors in the rat glomerulus and along the nephron has also identified the glomerulus as a major source and target for 5- and 12-HETEs and leukotrienes (168). In a model of antibody-induced mesangial cell injury in the rat, the fall in GFR was produced by a marked decline in the ultrafiltration coefficient (K_f) mediated by TxA_2 and products of 5-LOX (15). In experimental diabetes, characterized by accumulation of glomerular extracellular matrix and mesangial cell hypertrophy, mediation by 12(S)-HPETE, particularly through its interactions with the cytokine TFG-β family, producing amplification of the injurious response, has been advanced as a principle factor in the pathogenesis of diabetic nephropathy (94). Leukotriene (LT) A_4 hydrolase, forming LTB_4 is found in all nephron segments. The collecting ducts are major sources of 15-HPETE that may serve a cytoprotective function as transfection of the rat kidney with human 15-LOX (possibly acting through lipoxin generation) suppressed inflammation and preserved renal function in experimental glomerulonephritis (134).

Fulfilling the universal dictum that every action begets a countervailing reaction, LOX pathways are also involved in limiting tissue injury through the generation of lipoxins (acronym for *lipox*ygenase *in*teraction product*s*). Platelet 12-LOX and epithelial cell 15-LOX and their products, 12- and 15- HPETE, interact with 5-LOX of neutrophils and its product, LTA_4, forming lipoxins that contain and resolve renal injury as shown in experimental models of acute renal failure and glomerulonephritis (92).

THE MEDULLA: TONICITY, COX-2, AND PGE_2

Among the earliest studies on renal PGs were those of Larsson and Angaard (103) and Muirhead and associates (41) who identified a gradient of zonal PGE_2 production: papilla and inner medulla > outer medulla > cortex. This gradient of renal PGE_2 synthesis resembled the gradient of mPGES-1 in the rabbit kidney (186). Delineating the zonal distribution of prostaglandins was prelude to the structural localization of PGE_2 synthesis; viz., medullary interstitial cells, thin loops of Henle, macula densa, and the cortical and medullary collecting ducts have relatively high rates of PGE_2 synthesis as can be demonstrated by salt deprivation (cortical structures) or salt excess (medullary structures) (238). PGE_2 , the principle vasodepressor lipid in the renal medulla, increases medullary blood flow (84), inhibits NaCl transport in the mTAL (207), and modulates the hydro-osmotic response to arginine vasopressin in collecting ducts (196) to name the chief PGE_2 actions in the medulla.

Medullary tonicity is subject to wide swings occasioned by large changes in fluid intake as affected by environmental factors, work, exercise, and the effect of diseases and drugs on extracellular fluid volume regulation. This is of particular concern with increased NaCl concentration producing hypertonic conditions in the medullary interstitium that evokes corresponding increases in accumulation of "intracellular small organic solutes" (128), the compatible osmolytes that are essential for survival of medullary cells under hypertonic conditions. This adaptive response to hypertonic stress is dependent on MAPK mediation of COX-2 expression and activity in medullary cells that increase intracellular osmo-

lyte concentration (236). COX-2 inhibition in the face of hypertonic stress produced cell apoptosis and cell death. These findings raise the question and perhaps answer it, as to whether a similar COX-2-dependent mechanism, when inhibited, is responsible for analgesic nephropathy (95).

The vasodilator effects of PGE_2 are coupled to activation of EP_2 and EP_4 receptors that increase cAMP (16). The EP_2 receptor modulates vascular reactivity; EP_2 receptor gene knockout mice demonstrate salt-sensitive hypertension (91). Activation of EP_1 and EP_3 receptors expressed in collecting ducts and TAL (EP_3) contribute to the diuretic–natriuretic response to PGE_2. EP_1 stimulation inhibits Na^+ and water reabsorption in the collecting ducts linked to an increase in cytosolic Ca^{2+}. These actions of PGE_2, when prevented by inhibition of COX, are the primary basis for the retention of salt and water and elevation of blood pressure produced by NSAIDs (14).

The Renal Antihypertensive Hormone

The medullary interstitial cells were identified by Muirhead as the source of an antipressor lipid and named "the renal antihypertensive hormone" (132). The positive effect of salt excess on medullary COX-2 expression and PGE_2 production (238) has prompted studies directed toward selective inhibition or gene deletion of COX- 1 and COX-2 to determine functional consequences of each enzyme on salt and water homeostasis and blood pressure regulation. COX-2 generates vasodilator, antipressor prostaglandins as COX-2 inhibition or gene knockout greatly enhanced pressor responses to ANG II whereas COX-1 inhibition or gene knockout attenuated the pressor response to the peptide (159). COX-2 inhibition, but not inhibition of COX-1, reduced medullary blood flow, urine volume, and Na^+ excretion, additional evidence of the antipressor basis for COX-2–dependent renal effects. The contribution of COX-2 to the antipressor function of the renal medulla was demonstrated by the pressor response produced by medullary interstitial infusion of a selective COX-2 inhibitor in rats maintained on increased salt intake (246). Clinical studies also support COX-2-dependent promotion of salt and water excretion (14). Acute Na^+ retention in response to selective COX-2 inhibition was shown in healthy older adults (32).

DISTRIBUTION OF PROSTAGLANDIN SYNTHESIS WITHIN THE NEPHRON

The initial studies on the localization of prostaglandins in the nephron was based on immunofluorescence identification of COX, which was localized to arterial and arteriolar endothelial cells and cortical collecting tubules in each of five species studied: cow, guinea pig, rabbit, rat, and sheep (197, 200). COX antigenicity was not detected in the TAL and proximal tubules, indicating that COX is scattered within the nephron. In the renal medulla, collecting tubules showed the highest concentrations of COX antigenicity; medullary interstitial cells exhibited lower concentrations.

Bonvalet, Pradelles, and Farman (13) conducted a segmental analysis of prostaglandin synthesis in the nephron using direct quantitative measurements by either radio or enzyme immunoassay. They concluded, as did Smith and Wilkins (200), that the medullary collecting tubules, the thin limbs of Henle's loop, and, to a lesser extent, the cortical collecting tubules possessed the capacity to synthesize prostaglandins whereas the proximal convoluted tubules and TAL were either devoid of COX activity or exhibited "weak" activity. PGE_2 was the predominant prostaglandin synthesized by the nephron. Alternative pathways to COX metabolism of AA in these nephron segments were not addressed nor could they be as information on the presence of LOX and CYP was fragmentary (120). The absolute values of PG synthesis by the rabbit nephron and glomerulus were much greater than those of the rat. However, in each species, PGE_2 was the predominant prostanoid, exceeding production of PGI_2 by 20 or more and TxA_2 by 100-fold. Human glomeruli synthesize predominantly PGI_2 (9). The completion of this task, assigning eicosanoids to nephron segments, required discovery of the CYP pathway of AA metabolism that filled in large gaps in those segments of the nephron, mainly the proximal tubules and TAL which demonstrated negligible prostaglandin production. These segments were shown later to generate eicosanoid mediators and modulators of transport synthesized by CYP monooxygenases (28, 49, 160). A general statement on the nephron and its capacity to metabolize AA: "The cellular heterogeneity of the kidney has its equivalent in the distinctive eicosanoid profile for each of the more than 12 tubular segments" (193).

Mapping the distribution of oxygenases within the nephron takes on additional importance in view of the multiple isoforms of the CYP pathway of AA metabolism as their activities are individually regulated (38, 176). Localization of CYP-AA metabolites to key renal structures: PGMVs, the TAL, proximal tubules and collecting tubules, is a necessary preliminary to the designation of the CYP pathway of AA metabolism as an essential component in renal vascular and tubular mechanisms.

PROXIMAL TUBULES

The proximal tubules have the greatest concentration of CYP monooxygenases (44, 82, 148) within the kidney and are endowed with the highest renal activity of ω-hydroxylase, estimated to account for the largest component (> 50%) of renal production of 20-HETE (99). EET synthesis by the proximal tubule is located in proximity to or within the brush border membrane (42, 252) and is stimulated by ANG II (148). The 5,6-EET moderates the antinatriuretic action of ANG II by inhibiting the Na^+–H^+ exchanger (NHE-3) producing natriuresis in response to micromolar ANG II concentrations in tubular fluid (178). The effects of ANG II were related to in-

duction of $[Ca^{2+}]$ transients that resulted from Ca^2 influx through verapamil- and nifedipine-sensitive channels; they were reproduced by 5,6-EET and prevented by inhibition of epoxygenase activity. These findings indicate that 5,6-EET is a prime candidate mediator of the effects of ANG II on $[Ca^{2+}]$ transients and Na^+ transport in proximal tubules, particularly as 8,9-, 11,12- and 14,15-EETs were only weakly active.

19-HETE Antagonizes 20-HETE Inhibition of Transport

In a landmark study, Quigley et al. (160) demonstrated a tonic inhibitory action of exogenous 20-HETE on volume transport in the proximal straight tubule that required inhibition of proximal tubular 20-HETE synthesis for its demonstration. The inhibitory action of 20-HETE on Na^+,K^+-ATPase is mediated by activation of protein kinase C (PKC) (143). This mechanism operating through 20-HETE and PKC also may account for inhibition of proximal tubular transport by parathyroid hormone (170) and dopamine (149) Inhibition of Na^+–H^+ exchange by internalization of the NHE3 from the brush border (6) induced by 20-HETE also participates in pressure natriuresis and, presumably, is involved in adjustments in proximal tubular transport evoked by 20-HETE-dependent mechanisms in response to ET-1 (49, 176, 252). The 19-HETE synthesized by ω/ω-1-hydroxylases can antagonize the actions of 20-HETE by stimulating transport, possibly through its capacity to activate renal Na^+,K^+-ATPase (47). Antagonism by 19-HETE of the effects of 20-HETE on vascular tone and reactivity has also been demonstrated in renal blood vessels (247).

Proximal tubular transport increased by as much as 30% in response to inhibition of 20-HETE synthesis. If sustained, volume overload and hypertension will occur in view of the magnitude of reabsorption of the glomerula ultrafiltrate (60%–70%) by the proximal tubules (160). A parallel situation exists in the mTAL of the DS rat: Deficiency of 20-HETE (46) produced enhanced reabsorption of NaCl with elevation of blood pressure (83). Clofibrate, by stimulating 20-HETE production, thereby restoring its ability to modulate TAL transport of NaCl, reduced blood pressure in the DS rat (177).

20-HETE Mediates ET-1 Inhibition of Transport

ET-1 and 20-HETE share unique renal functional effects; viz., diuresis, despite renal vasoconstriction and depression of GFR (96, 153). As 20-HETE mediated the renal functional effects of ET-1 in the anesthetized rat (152), these findings prompted examining the potential role of 20-HETE as a second messenger for ET-1 in proximal tubules. The proximal tubules are ideal for studying 20-HETE–dependent mechanisms because of (1) high rates of 20-HETE synthesis; (2) negligible COX activity that eliminates the difficulties of interpreting the response to 20-HETE in view of its rapid metabolism by COX; and (3) production of NO, a precondition for studying the modulatory effect of NO on 20-HETE-ET-1 interactions (153).

In a dose-dependent manner, ET-1 reduced ^{86}Rb uptake by rat proximal tubules, an effect abolished by inhibiting 20-HETE synthesis. The restraining action of NO on proximal tubular 20-HETE synthesis, once again was demonstrated by increasing conversion of AA to 20-HETE on inhibiting NOS. ET-1 increased release of 20-HETE from proximal tubules that was prevented by either a selective ET$_A$-receptor antagonist or by inhibition of ω-hydroxylase. It should be noted that ET release of 20-HETE is greatly underestimated "because of the rapid disappearance of free 20-HETE by metabolism, conjugation and incorporation into phospholipids" (122).

THE mTAL: CYP- VERSUS COX-DERIVED ARACHIDONATE PRODUCTS

PGE$_2$ inhibited net Cl$^-$ transport across the rabbit mTAL when applied to the luminal or peritubular surfaces (207). PGE$_2$ was without effect on Cl$^-$ transport by the cortical TAL. The mTAL segment occupies a critical role in the excretion of salt and water as well as Ca^{2+} and Mg^{2++}. The osmolar gradient, expressed as increasing medullary tonicity on approaching the papilla, is essential to the regulation of extracellular fluid volume and is established by NaCl transport by the mTAL. PGE$_2$ decreases medullary tonicity by inhibiting mTAL NaCl transport (207) and by dissipating the osmolar gradient via increased medullary blood flow (84), thereby compromising the conservation of ECFV. These effects of PGE$_2$ can be reversed by treatment with NSAIDs as reflected in a sharp increase in renomedullary NaCl concentration (58).

Although the synthesis of prostaglandins by the TAL is negligible under physiological conditions, the tubular fluid contains prostaglandins secreted by the organic acid secretory pathway situated in the proximal tubules (180) as well as filtered prostaglandins, having been synthesized by preglomerular arteries, the glomerulus itself and by prostaglandins entering tubular fluid from the thin limb of Henle (54). In humans, in contrast to rats, 20-HETE is excreted as the glucuronide conjugate (157), secreted by the proximal tubules after glucuronidation. The proximal tubules are endowed with high specific activity of glucuronyl transferase (244).

The mTAL Generates 20-HETE, a Major Product of AA Metabolism

To assign functional significance to renal CYP–AA metabolism, the first step was to identify renal structures that possessed this capacity. The initial study of freshly isolated outer medullary cells of rabbits derived mainly from the mTAL, disclosed avid metabolism of exogenous AA to oxygenated products by a CYP-dependent mechanism (51). Induction of CYP enzymes by 3-methylcholanthrene and

β-naphthoflavone produced a twofold increase in eicosanoid formation by outer medullary cells. Structural identification of these CYP-derived AA metabolites generated by the mTAL disclosed three products: 19- and 20-HETEs and 20-COOH-AA (28); the latter two inhibited Na$^+$,K$^+$-ATPase whereas 19-HETE stimulated the Na$^+$ pump (47). The most important of these arachidonate metabolites synthesized by the mTAL was 20-HETE, which inhibited the Na$^+$-K$^+$-2Cl$^-$ cotransporter, the target of loop diuretics by (1) a direct effect on the cotransporter (46) and (2) inhibiting the 70 pS K$^+$ channel of the mTAL, thereby, reducing K$^+$ recycling that negatively affects the functional integrity of the cotransporter by diminishing availability of K$^+$ (110).

As the cotransporter is the target of furosemide being directly inhibited by the "loop diuretic" (229), a potential relationship between furosemide-induced natriuresis and 20-HETE excretion in hypertensive patients was examined (101). The natriuretic effect of furosemide was related to hypertensive subjects classified as either salt resistant or salt sensitive. Impairment of the natriuretic response to furosemide occurred only in salt-sensitive hypertensive patients and was related to an altered 20-HETE response to the diuretic agent "linked to salt-sensitivity of blood pressure (101)."

COX-2 Expression by the mTAL: Relationship to Tumor Necrosis Factor α

Short-term exposure (15 minutes) of the mTAL to ANG II increased 20-HETE production (110). However, the dominance of AA metabolism by ω-hydroxylase–dependent synthesis of 20-HETE in the TAL is subject to alteration as prolonged exposure (> 3 hours) of isolated TAL cells to ANG II (μM) acting via AT$_1$ receptors induced production of tumor necrosis factor (TNF), an essential link in ANG II induction of COX-2 expression (222). This study is critical to understanding the expression of tissue/cellular oxygenases; namely experimental conditions and diseases such as diabetes (98) can displace/replace the principle oxygenase of a tissue. Prolonged exposure (> 15 minutes) of rat mTAL tubules to either ANG II (110), Ca^{2+} (222), lipopolysaccharide (112), or bradykinin (174) will "shift" the principle pathway of AA metabolism from CYP (20-HETE) to COX-2 (PGE$_2$), thereby, replacing 20-HETE with PGE$_2$ as the principle eicosanoid produced by the mTAL (Fig. 9). This mechanism requires activating TNF within the TAL segment to cause COX-2 expression (112). Proximal tubules (239) and mesangial cells (7) also produce TNF, which has been implicated in the progression of inflammatory renal disease and may contribute to the tubular injury produced by hypercalcemia (40).

Renal TNF-COX-2-PGE$_2$ Buffers Pressor Hormones

ANG II-induced TNF production by isolated TAL tubules can be reproduced in vivo by intravenous infusion of ANG II resulting in increased excretion of PGE$_2$, reflecting co-

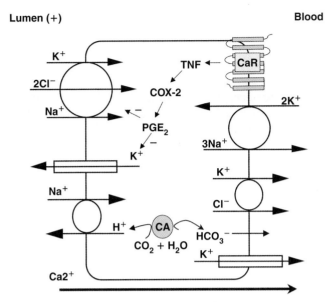

Lumen (+)   **Blood**

FIGURE 9 CaR stimulation of mTAL cells increases tumor necrosis factor production and COX-2–derived prostaglandin E_2 synthesis, which blocks Na^+ entry via inhibitory effects on apical K^+ channels and/or the Na^+-K^+-$2Cl^-$ cotransporter. CA, carbonic anhydrase.

expression of COX-2 and a PGE_2 isomerase in the mTAL and other renal sites (52). Administration of anti-TNF antiserum to rats infused with ANG II intensified the hypertension whereas control rats were unaffected, suggesting a TNF buffer effect that opposed the actions of ANG II and acted through COX-2 and PGE_2 production. This interpretation received support by isolating and incubating TAL tubules from each group of rats. TNF and PGE_2 levels increased three- to fourfold in incubates of TAL tubules obtained from ANG II–infused rats compared with those of vehicle infused rats. Thus, a TNF–COX-2–PGE_2 system that buffers the pressor response to ANG II was demonstrated.

The linkage of COX-2 to antipressor prostanoid production (159) underscores the functional antagonism that exists between the activities of COX-1 and COX-2. The pressor response to ANG II in mice was greatly reduced by either inhibiting COX-1 or COX-1 gene knockout. Inhibition of COX-2 augmented ANG II–induced hypertension and decreased medullary blood flow and urine flow. Several therapeutic strategies are suggested by the study of Qi et al. (159), the most important being the use of COX-1 inhibitors to reduce blood pressure and to inhibit platelet production of TxA_2 while sparing vascular PGI_2 production, which is COX-2–dependent (117). Reduction of thrombotic events and deceleration of atherosclerosis should follow (19).

Calcium Receptors

The Ca^{2+} sensing receptor (CaR) is expressed in abundance on the basolateral surface of the TAL, which reabsorbs divalent minerals in a regulated manner (171). Activation of the

CaR of mTAL cells by elevating extracellular Ca^{2+} for several hours, also increased TNFα production by mTAL cells associated with increased PGE_2 synthesis via a COX-2–dependent mechanism (Fig. 9). Contrastingly, short-term exposure (15 minutes) to elevated Ca^{2+} increased 20-HETE release from the mTAL (110). These temporal-dependent effects of Ca^{2+} on eicosanoid synthesis in the TAL (20-HETE vs. PGE_2) are similar to those effects evoked by ANG II. Ca^{2+}-mediated increase in COX-2 expression and PGE_2 synthesis can be attenuated by anti-TNF antibodies, suggesting that TNF acts in an autocrine fashion in the mTAL (222). Increasing calcium consumption in man produces a small but consistent reduction in blood pressure (118) that may derive from increased TNF production causing COX-2 expression and PGE_2 synthesis by the mTAL that promotes NaCl excretion.

Gain-of-function mutations of CaR have been associated with Bartter syndrome (216, 226), sometimes called hyperprostaglandin E syndrome, and characterized by polyuria, hypokalemia, hypercalciuria, and high levels of PGE_2 in blood and urine (119). NSAID therapy produced reduction of PGE_2 levels, urine volume, and Ca^{2+} excretion (59). The genetic heterogeneity of Bartter syndrome is evident in the mutations expressed in the TAL involving either the apical Na^+-K^+-$2Cl^-$cotransporter (Bartter syndrome, type 1), the ATP-sensitive apical K^+ channel (type 2), or the basolateral Cl^- channel (type 3) (108). High levels of PGE_2 further exacerbate the compromised TAL cell transport function that can be partially rectified by inhibition of COX, thereby diminishing the PGE_2 effect (109).

COLLECTING TUBULES

The renal medullary collecting ducts demonstrate the highest rates of PGE_2 synthesis in the nephron (13). They are invested with both COX-1 and epoxygenase enzymes (148, 186). COX-2 is expressed in collecting ducts as it is in medullary interstitial cells in response to osmotic stress/hypertonicity that stimulates Src kinases acting as osmosensors that transduce the signal to MAPKs with induction of COX-2 expression (236). The chief products are PGE_2, which moderates tonicity of the medulla (13), and 11,12-EET, which inhibits the ENaC in collecting ducts (110). PGE_2 synthesized principally by collecting ducts (13), medullary interstitial cells (128), and mTAL under conditions previously described, reduces medullary tonicity by (1) attenuation of the effects of AVP on the collecting ducts (63, 196) and the TAL (109), which reduces water and NaCl reabsorption, respectively, and (2) enhancement of renomedullary blood flow that dissipates medullary hypertonicity (85). The ability of PGE_2, under physiological conditions, to attenuate the actions of AVP on water permeability of collecting ducts and NaCl reabsorption by the mTAL is mediated by inhibition of vasopressin-induced increase in cAMP through activation

of a PGE$_2$ receptor (EP$_3$) coupled to an inhibitory guanine nucleotide regulatory protein, G$_i$, (201,202). The
hydro-osmotic effect of ADH was potentiated by inhibition of PGE$_2$ synthesis (97) producing (1) "a sharp rise in
medullary NaCl content" (58) and (2) increased urinary
concentration (3).

The first study that addressed the collecting duct response to CYP products demonstrated decreased net Na$^+$
absorption and decreased K$^+$ secretion by microperfused
rabbit cortical collecting ducts in response to micromolar
concentrations of luminal 5,6-EET. As 14,15-EET was
without effect (87), the action of 5,6-EET was considered
to be selective. The 5,6-EET is metabolized by COX (24),
the only EET undergoing extensive transformation by
COX. Of the EETs, only the 5,6-EET inhibited Na$^+$
transport in collecting ducts as measured by changes in
transepithelial voltage (V$_T$), an effect dependent on increased cytosolic Ca^{2+} concentration and mediated by
PGE$_2$. It was abolished by inhibition of COX (183). Further, the action of 5,6-EET was stereoselective; 1 μM
concentration of 5(S), 6(R)-EET was 2.5-fold more potent
than the 5(R), 6(S) enantiomer. This study did not address
the principal CYP-AA metabolite produced by the collecting ducts, the first step in identifying the candidate mediator of the collecting duct mechanism that regulates Na$^+$
reabsorption.

Cortical collecting duct transport was examined with
the patch-clamp technique to determine the effects of AA
and CYP-AA metabolites on the ENaC, the principal
pathway for Na$^+$ reabsorption in the cortical collecting
ducts. These channels are on the luminal surface and respond to aldosterone-regulated Na$^+$ reabsorption. The
11,12-EET was shown to be synthesized by collecting

ducts. Confocal imaging identified the epoxygenase 2C23
isoform as the responsible isoform for 11,12-EET synthesis that maintains normal blood pressure in the face of salt
loading (74). The inhibitory effect of 11,12-EET on
ENaC was activated by an adenosine step that responded
to the stimulus of salt loading (Fig. 10). Activation of
EETs by adenosine, as in the PGMVs (35), was demonstrated by preventing the ability of an adenosine receptor
agonist to inhibit ENaC by blocking either phospholipase
A$_2$ or epoxygenases activity (110). The contribution of
modulating Na$^+$ reabsorption via ENaC to blood pressure
regulation has been emphasized by Lifton (108).

Acknowledgments

This review was made possible by National Institutes of
Health Grants PPG HL-34300 (J.C.M., N.R.F.), RO1-
25394 (J.C.M.), and RO1-56423 (N.R.F.).

The authors wish to thank Melody Steinberg for preparation of the manuscript and editorial assistance and Chiara
Kimmel-Preuss for computer expertise. They also thank
Drs. John Quilley, Mairead A. Carroll, and Wen-Hui Wang
for their help.

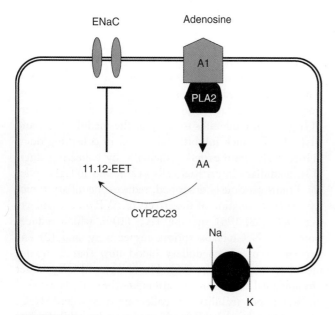

FIGURE 10   A cell schema showing the effect of adenosine on inhibition EnaC via synthesis of 11, 12-EET.

References

1. Abdullah HI, Pedraza PL, Hao S, et al. NFAT regulates calcium sensing receptor-mediated TNF production. *Am J Physiol Renal Physiol* 2005.
2. Alonso Galicia M, Drummond HA, Reddy KK, et al. Inhibition of 20-HETE production contributes to the vascular responses to nitric oxide. *Hypertension* 1997;29:320–325.
3. Anderson RJ, Berl T, McDonald KD, et al. Evidence for an in vivo antagonism between vasopressin and prostaglandin in the mammalian kidney. *J Clin Invest* 1975;56:420–426.
4. Armstrong JM, Blackwell GJ, Flower RJ, et al. Genetic hypertension in rats is accompanied by a defect in renal prostaglandin catabolism. *Nature* 1976;260:582–586.
5. Askari B, Bell-Quilley CP, Fulton D, et al. Analysis of eicosanoid mediation of the renal functional effects of hyperchloremia. *J Pharmacol Exp Ther* 1997;282:101–107.
6. Azuma KK, Balkovetz DF, Magyar CE, et al. Renal Na$^+$/H$^+$ exchanger isoforms and their regulation by thyroid hormone. *Am J Physiol* 1996;270:C585–C592.
7. Baud L, Oudinet JP, Bens M, et al. Production of tumor necrosis factor by rat mesangial cells in response to bacterial lipopolysaccharide. *Kidney Int* 1989;35:1111–1118.
8. Beck LH. Changes in renal function with aging. *Clin Geriatr Med* 1998;14:199–209.
9. Beierwaltes WH, Schryver S, Sanders E, et al. Renin release selectively stimulated by pros-taglandin I2 in isolated rat glomeruli. *Am J Physiol* 1982;243:F276–F283.
10. Bergstrom S. Isolation, structure and action of the prostaglandins. In: Bergstrom S, Samuelsson B (eds.). *Prostaglandins: Proceedings of the Second Nobel Symposium.* New York: John Wiley & Sons;1966:21–30.
11. Bohman SO. Demonstration of prostaglandin synthesis in collecting duct cells and other cell types of the rabbit renal medulla. *Prostaglandins* 1977;14:729–744.
12. Bombardier C, Laine L, Reicin A, et al. Comparison of upper gastrointestinal toxicity of rofe-coxib and naproxen in patients with rheumatoid arthritis. VIGOR Study Group. *N Engl J Med* 2000;343:1520–8, 2.
13. Bonvalet JP, Pradelles P, Farman N. Segmental synthesis and actions of prostaglandins along the nephron. *Am J Physiol* 1987;253:F377–F387.
14. Brater DC. Effects of nonsteroidal anti-inflammatory drugs on renal function: focus on cyclooxygenase-2-selective inhibition. *Am J Med* 1999;107:65S–70S.
15. Bresnahan BA, Wu S, Fenoy FJ, et al. Mesangial cell immune injury. Hemodynamic role of leukocyte- and platelet-derived eicosanoids. *J Clin Invest* 1992;90:2304–2312.
16. Breyer MD, Breyer RM. Prostaglandin E receptors and the kidney. *Am J Physiol Renal Physiol* 2000;279:F12–F23.
17. Briggs JP, Schnermann J. The tubuloglomerular feedback mechanism: functional and bio-chemical aspects. *Annu Rev Physiol* 1987;49:251–273.
18. Bunting S, Gryglewski R, Moncada S, et al. Arterial walls generate from prostaglandin en-doperoxides a substance (prostaglandin X) which relaxes strips of mesenteric and coeliac ateries and inhibits platelet aggregation. *Prostaglandins* 1976;12:897–913.
19. Bunting S, Moncada S, Vane JR. The prostacyclin—thromboxane A2 balance: pathophysi-ological and therapeutic implications. *Br Med Bull* 1983;39:271–276.
20. Burns KD, Capdevila J, Wei S, et al. Role of cytochrome P-450 epoxygenase metabolites in EGF signaling in renal proximal tubule. *Am J Physiol* 1995;269:C831–40.
21. Campbell WB, Gebremedhin D, Pratt PF, et al. Identification of epoxyeicosatrienoic acids as endothelium-derived hyperpolarizing factors. *Circ Res* 1996;78:415–423.

22. Capdevila J, Chacos N, Werringloer J, et al. Liver microsomal cytochrome P-450 and the oxidative metabolism of arachidonic acid. *Proc Natl Acad Sci U S A* 1981;78:5362–5366.
23. Carroll MA, Balazy M, Huang DD, et al. Cytochrome P450-derived renal HETEs: storage and release. *Kidney Int* 1997;51:1696–1702.
24. Carroll MA, Balazy M, Margiotta P, et al. Renal vasodilator activity of 5,6-epoxyeicosatrienoic acid depends upon conversion by cyclooxygenase and release of prostaglandins. *J Biol Chem* 1993;268:12260–12266.
25. Carroll MA, Balazy M, Margiotta P, et al. Cytochrome P-450-dependent HETEs: profile of biological activity and stimulation by vasoactive peptides. *Am J Physiol* 1996;271:R863–R869.
26. Carroll MA, Garcia MP, Falck JR, et al. 5,6-epoxyeicosatrienoic acid, a novel arachidonate metabolite. Mechanism of vasoactivity in the rat. *Circ Res* 1990;67:1082–1088.
27. Carroll MA, Garcia MP, Falck JR, et al. Cyclooxygenase dependency of the renovascular actions of cytochrome P450-derived arachidonate metabolites. *J Pharmacol Exp Ther* 1992; 260:104–109.
28. Carroll MA, Sala A, Dunn CE, et al. Structural identification of cytochrome P450-dependent arachidonate metabolites formed by rabbit medullary thick ascending limb cells. *J Biol Chem* 1991; 266:12306–12312.
29. Carroll MA, Schwartzman M, Capdevila J, et al. Vasoactivity of arachidonic acid epoxides. *Eur J Pharmacol* 1987;138:281–283.
30. Cashman JR, Hanks D, Weiner RI. Epoxy derivatives of arachidonic acid are potent stimulators of prolactin secretion. *Neuroendocrinology* 1987;46:246–251.
31. Castellani S, Paniccia R, Di Serio C, et al. Thromboxane inhibition improves renal perfusion and excretory function in severe congestive heart failure. *J Am Coll Cardiol* 2003;42:133–139.
32. Catella-Lawson F, McAdam B, Morrison BW, et al. Effects of specific inhibition of cyclooxygenase-2 on sodium balance, hemodynamics, and vasoactive eicosanoids. *J Pharmacol Exp Ther* 1999;289:735–741.
33. Chacos N, Capdevila J, Falck JR, et al. The reaction of arachidonic acid epoxides (epoxyeicosatrienoic acids) with a cytosolic epoxide hydrolase. *Arch Biochem Biophys* 1983;223:639–648.
34. Cheng HF, Wang JL, Zhang MZ, et al. Angiotensin II attenuates renal cortical cyclooxygenase-2 expression. *J Clin Invest* 1999;103:953–961.
35. Cheng MK, Doumad AB, Jiang H, et al. Epoxyeicosatrienoic acids mediate adenosine-induced vasodilation in rat preglomerular microvessels (PGMV) via A2A receptors. *Br J Pharmacol* 2004;141:441–448.
36. Cheng MK, McGiff JC, Carroll MA. Renal arterial 20-hydroxyeicosatetraenoic acid levels: regulation by cyclooxygenase. *Am J Physiol Renal Physiol* 2003;284:F474–F479.
37. Ciabattoni G, Pugliese F, Cinotti GA, et al. Characterization of furosemide-induced activation of the renal prostaglandin system. *Eur J Pharmacol* 1979;60:181–187.
38. Cowart LA, Wei S, Hsu MH, et al. The CYP4A isoforms hydroxylate epoxyeicosatrienoic acids to form high affinity peroxisome proliferator-activated receptor ligands. *J Biol Chem* 2002;277:35105–35112.
39. Croft KD, McGiff JC, Sanchez-Mendoza A, et al. Angiotensin II releases 20-HETE from rat renal microvessels. *Am J Physiol Renal Physiol* 2000;279:F544–F551.
40. Cunningham PN, Dyanov HM, Park P, et al. Acute renal failure in endotoxemia is caused by TNF acting directly on TNF receptor-1 in kidney. *J Immunol* 2002;168:5817–5823.
41. Daniels EG, Hinman JW, Leach BE, et al. Identification of prostaglandin E2 as the principal vasodepressor lipid of rabbit renal medulla. *Nature* 1967;215:1298–1299.
42. dos Santos EA, Dahly-Vernon AJ, Hoagland KM, et al. Inhibition of the formation of EETs and 20-HETE with 1-aminobenzotriazole attenuates pressure natriuresis. *Am J Physiol Regul Integr Comp Physiol* 2004;287:R58–R68.
43. Dumoulin M, Salvail D, Gaudreault SB, et al. Epoxyeicosatrienoic acids relax airway smooth muscles and directly activate reconstituted KCa channels. *Am J Physiol* 1998;275:L423–L431.
44. Endou H. Distribution and some characteristics of cytochrome P-450 in the kidney. *J Toxicol Sci* 1983;8:165–176.
45. Epstein M, Berk DP, Hollenberg NK, et al. Renal failure in the patient with cirrhosis. The role of active vasoconstriction. *Am J Med* 1970;49:175–185.
46. Escalante B, Erlij D, Falck JR, et al. Effect of cytochrome P450 arachidonate metabolites on ion transport in rabbit kidney loop of Henle. *Science* 1991;251:799–802.
47. Escalante B, Falck JR, Yadagiri P, et al. 19(S)-hydroxyeicosatetraenoic acid is a potent stimulator of renal Na^+-K^+-ATPase. *Biochem Biophys Res Commun* 1988;152:1269–1274.
48. Escalante B, Sessa WC, Falck JR, et al. Vasoactivity of 20-hydroxyeicosatetraenoic acid is dependent on metabolism by cyclooxygenase. *J Pharmacol Exp Ther* 1989;248:229–232.
49. Escalante BA, McGiff JC, Oyekan AO. Role of cytochrome P-450 arachidonate metabolites in endothelin signaling in rat proximal tubule. *Am J Physiol Renal Physiol* 2002;282: F144–F150.
50. Ferreira SH, Vane JR. Prostaglandins: their disappearance from and release into the circulation. *Nature* 1967;216:868–873.
51. Ferreri NR, Schwartzman M, Ibraham NG, et al. Arachidonic acid metabolism in a cell suspension isolated from rabbit renal outer medulla. *J Pharmacol Exp Ther* 1984;231:441–448.
52. Ferreri NR, Zhao Y, Takizawa H, et al. Tumor necrosis factor-alpha-angiotensin interactions and regulation of blood pressure. *J Hypertens* 1997;15:1481–1484.
53. Fisslthaler B, Popp R, Kiss L, et al. Cytochrome P450 2C is an EDHF synthase in coronary arteries. *Nature* 1999;401:493–497.
54. Frolich JC, Wilson TW, Sweetman BJ, et al. Urinary prostaglandins. Identification and origin. *J Clin Invest* 1975;55:763–770.
55. Fujino T, Nakagawa N, Yuhki K, et al. Decreased susceptibility to renovascular hypertension in mice lacking the prostaglandin I2 receptor IP. *J Clin Invest* 2004;114:805–812.
56. Fulton D, McGiff JC, Quilley J. Pharmacological evaluation of an epoxide as the putative hyperpolarizing factor mediating the nitric oxide-independent vasodilator effect of bradykinin in the rat heart. *J Pharmacol Exp Ther* 1998;287:497–503.
57. Fuson AL, Komlosi P, Unlap TM, et al. Immunolocalization of a microsomal prostaglandin E synthase in rabbit kidney. *Am J Physiol Renal Physiol* 2003;285:F558–F564.
58. Ganguli M, Tobian L, Azar S, et al. Evidence that prostaglandin synthesis inhibitors increase the concentration of sodium and chloride in rat renal medulla. *Circ Res* 1977;40:I135–I139.
59. Gill JR, Jr., Frolich JC, Bowden RE, et al. Bartter's syndrome: a disorder characterized by high urinary prostaglandins and a dependence of hyperreninemia on prostaglandin synthesis. *Am J Med* 1976;61:43–51.
60. Gimbrone MA, Jr., Topper JN, Nagel T, et al. Endothelial dysfunction, hemodynamic forces, and atherogenesis. *Ann N Y Acad Sci* 2000; 902:230–239.
61. Goodwin DC, Landino LM, Marnett LJ. Effects of nitric oxide and nitric oxide-derived species on prostaglandin endoperoxide synthase and prostaglandin biosynthesis. *FASEB J* 1999;13:1121–1136.
62. Granstrom E, Samuelsson B. Quantitative measurement of prostaglandins and thromboxanes: general considerations. In: Samuelsson B, Ramwell PR, Paoletti R (eds). *Advances in Prostaglandin and Thromboxane Research.* New York: Raven Press;1978:1–13.
63. Grantham JJ, Orloff J. Effect of prostaglandin E1 on the permeability response of the isolated collecting tubule to vasopressin, adenosine 3',5'-monophosphate, and theophylline. *J Clin Invest* 1968;47: 1154–1161.
64. Hamberg M, Svensson J, Samuelsson B. Thromboxanes: a new group of biologically active compounds derived from prostaglandin endoperoxides. *Proc Natl Acad Sci U S A* 1975;72: 2994–2998.
65. Harris RC, McKanna JA, Akai Y, et al. Cyclooxygenase-2 is associated with the macula densa of rat kidney and increases with salt restriction. *J Clin Invest* 1994;94:2504–2510.
66. Hasko G, Cronstein BN. Adenosine: an endogenous regulator of innate immunity. *Trends Immunol* 2004;25:33–39.
67. Hassid A, Konieczkowski M, Dunn MJ. Prostaglandin synthesis in isolated rat kidney glomeruli. *Proc Natl Acad Sci U S A* 1979;76:1155–1159.
68. Henning SJ. Plasma concentrations of total and free corticosterone during development in the rat. *Am J Physiol* 1978;235:E451–E456.
69. Hill E, Fitzpatrick F, Murphy RC. Biological activity and metabolism of 20-hydroxyeicosatetraenoic acid in the human platelet. *Br J Pharmacol* 1992;106:267–274.
70. Hiller G, Sundler R. Activation of arachidonate release and cytosolic phospholipase A2 via extracellular signal-regulated kinase and p38 mitogen-activated protein kinase in macrophages stimulated by bacteria or zymosan. *Cell Signal* 1999;11:863–869.
71. Hocherl K, Dreher F, Vitzthum H, et al. Cyclosporine A suppresses cyclooxygenase-2 expression in the rat kidney. *J Am Soc Nephrol* 2002;13:2427–2436.
72. Hockel GM, Cowley AW, Jr. Prostaglandin E2-induced hypertension in conscious dogs. *Am J Physiol* 1979;237:H449–H454.
73. Holla VR, Adas F, Imig JD, et al. Alterations in the regulation of androgen-sensitive CYP 4a monooxygenases cause hypertension. *Proc Natl Acad Sci U S A* 2001;98:5211–5216.
74. Holla VR, Makita K, Zaphiropoulos PG, et al. The kidney cytochrome P-450 2C23 arachidonic acid epoxygenase is upregulated during dietary salt loading. *J Clin Invest* 1999;104:751–760.
75. Imanishi M, Kawamura M, Akabane S, et al. Aspirin lowers blood pressure in patients with renovascular hypertension. *Hypertension* 1989;14:461–468.
76. Imig JD. Eicosanoid regulation of the renal vasculature. *Am J Physiol Renal Physiol* 2000;279: F965–F981.
77. Imig JD. 20-HETE or EETs: which arachidonic acid metabolite regulates proximal tubule transporters and contributes to pressure natriuresis? *Am J Physiol Regul Integr Comp Physiol* 2004;287:R3–R5.
78. Imig JD, Falck JR, Inscho EW. Contribution of cytochrome P450 epoxygenase and hydroxylase pathways to afferent arteriolar autoregulatory responsiveness. *Br J Pharmacol* 1999;127:1399–1405.
79. Imig JD, Navar LG. Afferent arteriolar response to arachidonic acid: involvement of metabolic pathways. *Am J Physiol* 1996;271:F87–93.
80. Imig JD, Navar LG, Roman RJ, et al. Actions of epoxygenase metabolites on the preglomerular vasculature. *J Am Soc Nephrol* 1996; 7:2364–2370.
81. Imig JD, Zou AP, Stec DE, et al. Formation and actions of 20-hydroxyeicosatetraenoic acid in rat renal arterioles. *Am J Physiol* 1996;270:R217–27.
82. Ito O, Alonso GM, Hopp KA, et al. Localization of cytochrome P-450 4A isoforms along the rat nephron. *Am J Physiol* 1998;274:F395–F404.
83. Ito O, Roman RJ. Role of 20-HETE in elevating chloride transport in the thick ascending limb of Dahl SS/Jr rats. *Hypertension* 1999;33:419–423.
84. Itskovitz HD, Stemper J, Pacholczyk D, et al. Renal prostaglandins: determinants of intrarenal distribution of blood flow in the dog. *Clin Sci Mol Med Suppl* 1973;45 Suppl 1:321s–4.
85. Itskovitz HD, Terragno NA, McGiff JC. Effect of a renal prostaglandin on distribution of blood flow in the isolated canine kidney. *Circ Res* 1974;34:770–776.
86. Jackson EK, Oates JA, Branch RA. Indomethacin decreases arterial blood pressure and plasma renin activity in rats with aortic ligation. *Circ Res* 1981;49:180–185.
87. Jacobson HR, Corona S, Capdevila J, et al. Effects of epoxyeicostrienoic acids on ion transport in the rabbit cortical collecting tubule. In: Braquet P, et al. (eds.). *Prostaglandins and Membrane Ion Transport.* New York: Raven Press;1984:311–318.
88. Jensen BL, Schmid C, Kurtz A. Prostaglandins stimulate renin secretion and renin mRNA in mouse renal juxtaglomerular cells. *Am J Physiol* 1996;271:F659–F669.
89. Jiang H, McGiff JC, Quilley J, et al. Identification of 5,6-trans-epoxyeicosatrienoic acid in the phospholipids of red blood cells. *J Biol Chem* 2004;279:36412–36418.
90. Junier MP, Dray F, Blair I, et al. Epoxygenase products of arachidonic acid are endogenous constituents of the hypothalamus involved in D2 receptor-mediated, dopamine-induced release of somatostatin. *Endocrinology* 1990;126:1534–1540.
91. Kennedy CR, Zhang Y, Brandon S, et al. Salt-sensitive hypertension and reduced fertility in mice lacking the prostaglandin EP2 receptor. *Nat Med* 1999;5:217–220.
92. Kieran NE, Maderna P, Godson C. Lipoxins: potential anti-inflammatory, proresolution, and antifibrotic mediators in renal disease. *Kidney Int* 2004;65:1145–1154.
93. Kim SF, Huri DA, Snyder SH. Inducible nitric oxide synthase binds, S-nitrosylates, and activates cyclooxygenase-2. *Science* 2005;310: 1966–1970.
94. Kim YS, Xu ZG, Reddy MA, et al. Novel interactions between TGF-{beta}1 actions and the 12/15-lipoxygenase pathway in mesangial cells. *J Am Soc Nephrol* 2005;16:352–362.
95. Kincaid-Smith P. Effects of non-narcotic analgesics on the kidney. *Drugs* 1986;32 (Suppl 4)109–128.

96. King AJ, Brenner BM, Anderson S. Endothelin: a potent renal and systemic vasoconstrictor peptide. *Am J Physiol* 1989;256:F1051–F1058.

97. Kirschenbaum MA, Lowe AG, Trizna W, et al. Regulation of vasopressin action by prostaglandins. Evidence for prostaglandin synthesis in the rabbit cortical collecting tubule. *J Clin Invest* 1982;70:1193–1204.

98. Komers R, Lindsley JN, Oyama TT, et al. Immunohistochemical and functional correlations of renal cyclooxygenase-2 in experimental diabetes. *J Clin Invest* 2001;107:889–898.

99. Kroetz DL, Huse LM, Thuresson A, et al. Developmentally regulated expression of the CYP4A genes in the spontaneously hypertensive rat kidney. *Mol Pharmacol* 1997;52:362–372.

100. Laethem RM, Balazy M, Falck JR, et al. Formation of 19(S)-, 19(R)-, and 18(R)-hydroxyeicosatetraenoic acids by alcohol-inducible cytochrome P450 2E1. *J Biol Chem* 1993;268:12912–12918.

101. Laffer CL, Laniado-Schwartzman M, Wang MH, et al. 20-HETE and furosemide-induced natriuresis in salt-sensitive essential hypertension. *Hypertension* 2003;41:703–708.

102. Langenbach R, Morham SG, Tiano HF, et al. Prostaglandin synthase 1 gene disruption in mice reduces arachidonic acid-induced inflammation and indomethacin-induced gastric ulceration. *Cell* 1995; 83:483–492.

103. Larsson C, Anggard E. Regional differences in the formation and metabolism of prostaglandins in the rabbit kidney. *Eur J Pharmacol* 1973;21:30–36.

104. Ledent C, Vaugeois JM, Schiffmann SN, et al. Aggressiveness, hypoalgesia and high blood pressure in mice lacking the adenosine A2a receptor. *Nature* 1997;388:674–678.

105. Lee JB. Chemical and physiological properties of renal prostaglandins: the antihypertensive effects of medullin in essential human hypertension. In: Bergstrom S, Samuelsson B (eds.). *Prostaglandins: Proceedings of the Second Nobel Symposium.*. New York: John Wiley & Sons; 1966:197–210.

106. Lee JB, Crowshaw K, Takman BH, et al. Identification of prostaglandins E2, F2a and A2 from rabbit kidney medulla. *Biochem J* 1967;105:1251–1260.

107. Liclican EL, McGiff JC, Pedraza PL, et al. Exaggerated response to adenosine in kidneys from high salt-fed rats: role of epoxyeicosatrienoic acids. *Am J Physiol Renal Physiol* 2005;289:F386–F392.

108. Lifton RP, Gharavi AG, Geller DS. Molecular mechanisms of human hypertension. *Cell* 2001;104:545–556.

109. Liu HJ, Wei Y, Ferreri NR, et al. Vasopressin and PGE(2) regulate activity of apical 70 pS K(+) channel in thick ascending limb of rat kidney. *Am J Physiol Cell Physiol* 2000;278:C905–C913.

110. Lu M, Zhu Y, Balazy M, et al. Effect of angiotensin II on the apical K+ channel in the thick ascending limb of the rat kidney. *J Gen Physiol* 1996;108:537–547.

111. Ma YH, Harder DR, Clark JE, et al. Effects of 12-HETE on isolated dog renal arcuate arteries. *Am J Physiol* 1991;261:H451–6.

112. Macica CM, Escalante BA, Conners MS, et al. TNF production by the medullary thick ascending limb of Henle's loop. *Kidney Int* 1994;46:113–121.

113. Makita K, Takahashi K, Karara A, et al. Experimental and/or genetically controlled alterations of the renal microsomal cytochrome P450 epoxygenase induce hypertension in rats fed a high salt diet. *J Clin Invest* 1994;94:2414–2420.

114. Mangat H, Peterson LN, Burns KD. Hypercalcemia stimulates expression of intrarenal phospholipase A2 and prostaglandin H synthase-2 in rats. Role of angiotensin II AT1 receptors. *J Clin Invest* 1997;100:1941–1950.

115. Mann B, Hartner A, Jensen BL, et al. Furosemide stimulates macula densa cyclooxygenase-2 expression in rats. *Kidney Int* 2001;59:62–68.

116. Martinez-Maldonado M, Gely R, Tapia E, et al. Role of macula densa in diuretics-induced renin release. *Hypertension* 1990;16:261–268.

117. McAdam BF, Catella-Lawson F, Mardini IA, et al. Systemic biosynthesis of prostacyclin by cyclooxygenase (COX)-2: the human pharmacology of a selective inhibitor of COX-2. *Proc Natl Acad Sci U S A* 1999;96:272–277.

118. McCarron DA. Diet and blood pressure—the paradigm shift. *Science* 1998;281:933-934.

119. McGiff JC. Bartter's syndrome results from an imbalance of vasoactive hormones. *Ann Intern Med* 1977;87:369–372.

120. McGiff JC. Cytochrome P-450 metabolism of arachidonic acid. *Annu Rev Pharmacol Toxicol* 1991;31:339–369.

121. McGiff JC, Crowshaw K, Terragno NA, et al. Renal prostaglandins: possible regulators of the renal actions of pressor hormones. *Nature* 1970;227:1255–1257.

122. McGiff JC, Quilley J. 20-HETE and the kidney: resolution of old problems and new beginnings. *Am J Physiol* 1999;277:R607–R623.

123. McGiff JC, Quilley J. 20-hydroxyeicosatetraenoic acid and epoxyeicosatrienoic acids and blood pressure. *Curr Opin Nephrol Hypertens* 2001;10:231–237.

124. McGiff JC, Terragno NA, Malik KU, et al. Release of a prostaglandin E-like substance from canine kidney by bradykinin. *Circ Res* 1972;31:36–43.

125. McGiff JC, Terragno NA, Strand JC, et al. Selective passage of prostaglandins across the lung. *Nature* 1969;223:742–745.

126. McGuire JC, Sun FF. Metabolism of prostacyclin. Oxidation by rhesus monkey lung 15-hydroxyl prostaglandin dehydrogenase. *Arch Biochem Biophys* 1978;189:92–96.

127. Mistry M, Nasjletti A. Prostanoids as mediators of prohypertensive and antihypertensive mechanisms. *Am J Med Sci* 1988;295:263–267.

128. Moeckel GW, Zhang L, Fogo AB, et al. COX2 activity promotes organic osmolyte accumulation and adaptation of renal medullary interstitial cells to hypertonic stress. *J Biol Chem* 2003;278:19352–19357.

129. Moghaddam M, Motoba K, Borhan B, et al. Novel metabolic pathways for linoleic and arachidonic acid metabolism. *Biochim Biophys Acta* 1996;1290:327–339.

130. Morham SG, Langenbach R, Loftin CD, et al. Prostaglandin synthase 2 gene disruption causes severe renal pathology in the mouse. *Cell* 1995;83:473–482.

131. Morrison AR, Pascoe N. Metabolism of arachidonate through NADPH-dependent oxygenase of renal cortex. *Proc Natl Acad Sci U S A* 1981;78:7375–7378.

132. Muirhead EE, Pitcock JA, Nasjletti A, et al. The antihypertensive function of the kidney. Its elucidation by captopril plus unclipping. *Hypertension* 1985;7:I127–I135.

133. Muller DN, Theuer J, Shagdarsuren E, et al. A peroxisome proliferator-activated receptor-alpha activator induces renal CYP2C23 activity and protects from angiotensin II-induced renal injury. *Am J Pathol* 2004;164:521–532.

134. Munger KA, Montero A, Fukunaga M, et al. Transfection of rat kidney with human 15-lipoxygenase suppresses inflammation and preserves function in experimental glomerulonephritis. *Proc Natl Acad Sci U S A* 1999;96:13375–13380.

135. Murakami M, Kuwata H, Amakasu Y, et al. Prostaglandin E2 amplifies cytosolic phospholipase A2- and cyclooxygenase-2-dependent delayed prostaglandin E2 generation in mouse osteoblastic cells: enhancement by secretory phospholipase A2. *J Biol Chem* 1997; 272:19891–19897.

136. Murakami M, Naraba H, Tanioka T, et al. Regulation of prostaglandin E2 biosynthesis by inducible membrane-associated prostaglandin E2 synthase that acts in concert with cyclooxygenase-2. *J Biol Chem* 2000;275:32783–32792.

137. Nakagawa K, Marji JS, Schwartzman ML, et al. Androgen-mediated induction of the kidney arachidonate hydroxylases is associated with the development of hypertension. *Am J Physiol Regul Integr Comp Physiol* 2003;284:R1055–R1062.

138. Natarajan R, Gerrity RG, Gu JL, et al. Role of 12-lipoxygenase and oxidant stress in hyperglycaemia-induced acceleration of atherosclerosis in a diabetic pig model. *Diabetologia* 2002;45:125–133.

139. Navar LG, Inscho EW, Majid SA, et al. Paracrine regulation of the renal microcirculation. *Physiol Rev* 1996;76:425–536.

140. Node K, Huo Y, Ruan X, et al. Anti-inflammatory properties of cytochrome P450 epoxygenase-derived eicosanoids. *Science* 1999;285:1276–1279.

141. Node K, Ruan XL, Dai J, et al. Activation of G alphas mediates induction of tissue-type plasminogen activator gene transcription by epoxyeicosatrienoic acids. *J Biol Chem* 2001; 276:15983–15989.

142. Novy MJ. Effects of indomethacin on labor, fetal oxygenation, and fetal development in rhesus monkeys. *Adv Prostaglandin Thromboxane Res* 1978;4:285–300.

143. Nowicki S, Chen SL, Aizman O, et al. 20-Hydroxyeicosa-tetraenoic acid (20 HETE) activates protein kinase C. Role in regulation of rat renal Na+,K+-ATPase. *J Clin Invest* 1997;99:1224–1230.

144. Ogletree ML, Harris DN, Greenberg R, et al. Pharmacological actions of SQ 29,548, a novel selective thromboxane antagonist. *J Pharmacol Exp Ther* 1985;234:435–441.

145. Oliw EH, Guengerich FP, Oates JA. Oxygenation of arachidonic acid by hepatic monooxygenases: isolation and metabolism of four epoxide intermediates. *J Biol Chem* 1982;257:3771–3781.

146. Olsen UB. Diuretics and kidney prostaglandins. In: *Prostaglandins and the Kidney* Dunn MJ, Patrono C, Cinotti GA (eds). New York and London: Plenum Medical Book Company;1983:205–212.

147. Oltman CL, Weintraub NL, VanRollins M, et al. Epoxyeicosatrienoic acids and dihydroxyeicosatrienoic acids are potent vasodilators in the canine coronary microcirculation. *Circ Res* 1998;83:932–939.

148. Omata K, Abraham NG, Schwartzman ML. Renal cytochrome P-450-arachidonic acid metabolism: localization and hormonal regulation in SHR. *Am J Physiol* 1992;262:F591–599.

149. Ominato M, Satoh T, Katz AI. Regulation of Na-K-ATPase activity in the proximal tubule: role of the protein kinase C pathway and of eicosanoids. *J Membr Biol* 1996;152:235–243.

150. Orloff J, Grantham J. The effect of prostaglandin (PGE1) on the permeability response of rabbit collecting tubules to vasopressin. In: Bergstrom S, Samuelsson B (eds.). *Prostaglandins: Proceedings of the Second Nobel Symposium.* New York: John Wiley & Sons;1966:143–146.

151. Oyekan A, Balazy M, McGiff JC. Renal oxygenases: differential contribution to vasoconstriction induced by ET-1 and ANG II. *Am J Physiol* 1997;273:R293–R300.

152. Oyekan AO, McGiff JC. Cytochrome P-450-derived eicosanoids participate in the renal functional effects of ET-1 in the anesthetized rat. *Am J Physiol* 1998;274:R52–R61.

153. Oyekan AO, McGiff JC. Functional response of the rat kidney to inhibition of nitric oxide synthesis: role of cytochrome p450-derived arachidonate metabolites. *Br J Pharmacol* 1998; 125:1065–1073.

154. Palmer BF. Managing hyperkalemia caused by inhibitors of the renin-angiotensin-aldosterone system. *N Engl J Med* 2004;351:585–592.

155. Piper PJ, Vane JR. Release of additional factors in anaphylaxis and its antagonism by anti-inflammatory drugs. *Nature* 1969;223:29–35.

156. Pomposiello SI, Carroll MA, Falck JR, et al. Epoxyeicosatrienoic acid-mediated renal vasodilation to arachidonic acid is enhanced in SHR. *Hypertension* 2001;37:887–893.

157. Prakash C, Zhang JY, Falck JR, et al. 20-Hydroxyeicosatetraenoic acid is excreted as a glucuronide conjugate in human urine. *Biochem Biophys Res Commun* 1992;185:728–733.

158. Pugliese F, Ciabattoni G. Investigations of renal arachidonic acid metabolites by radioimmunoassay. In: Dunn MJ, Patrono C, Cinotti GA (eds.). *Prostaglandins and the Kidney.* New York: Plenum Medical Books;1983:83–98.

159. Qi Z, Hao CM, Langenbach RI, et al. Opposite effects of cyclooxygenase-1 and -2 activity on the pressor response to angiotensin II. *J Clin Invest* 2002;110:61–69.

160. Quigley R, Baum M, Reddy KM, et al. Effects of 20-HETE and 19(S)-HETE on rabbit proximal straight tubule volume transport. *Am J Physiol Renal Physiol* 2000;278:F949–F953.

161. Quilley J, Fulton D, McGiff JC. Hyperpolarizing factors. *Biochem Pharmacol* 1997;54:1059–1070.

162. Quilley J, McGiff JC. Influence of insulin on urinary eicosanoid excretion in rats with experimental diabetes mellitus. *J Pharmacol Exp Ther* 1986;238:606–611.

163. Quilley J, McGiff JC, Nasjletti A. Role of endoperoxides in arachidonic acid-induced vasoconstriction in the isolated perfused kidney of the rat. *Br J Pharmacol* 1989;96:111–116.

164. Randriamboavonjy V, Kiss L, Falck JR, et al. The synthesis of 20-HETE in small porcine coronary arteries antagonizes EDHF-mediated relaxation. *Cardiovasc Res* 2005;65:487–494.

165. Reckelhoff JF, Granger JP. Role of androgens in mediating hypertension and renal injury. *Clin Exp Pharmacol Physiol* 1999;26:127–131.

166. Reddy MA, Thimmalapura PR, Lanting L, et al. The oxidized lipid and lipoxygenase product 12(S)-hydroxyeicosatetraenoic acid induces hypertrophy and fibronectin transcription in vascular smooth muscle cells via p38 MAPK and cAMP response element-binding protein activation: mediation of angiotensin II effects. *J Biol Chem* 2002;277:9920–9928.

167. Reimann IW, Fischer C, Rosenkranz B, et al. Investigations on renal prostaglandins by gas chromatography-mass spectrometry. In: Dunn MJ (ed.). *Prostaglandins and the Kidney*. New York: Plenum Medical Books;1983:99–107.
168. Reinhold SW, Vitzthum H, Filbeck T, et al. Gene expression of 5-, 12- and 15-lipoxygenases and leukotriene receptors along the rat nephron. *Am J Physiol Renal Physiol* 2006;290:F864–F872.
169. Ren Y, Garvin JL, Carretero OA. Efferent arteriole tubuloglomerular feedback in the renal nephron. *Kidney Int* 2001;59:222–229.
170. Ribeiro CM, Dubay GR, Falck JR, et al. Parathyroid hormone inhibits Na(+)-K(+)-ATPase through a cytochrome P-450 pathway. *Am J Physiol* 1994;266:F497–F505.
171. Riccardi D, Hall AE, Chattopadhyay N, et al. Localization of the extracellular Ca2+/polyvalent cation-sensing protein in rat kidney. *Am J Physiol* 1998;274:F611–F622.
172. Robert A, Nezamis JE, Lancaster C, et al. Cytoprotection by prostaglandins in rats. Prevention of gastric necrosis produced by alcohol, HCl, NaOH, hypertonic NaCl, and thermal injury. *Gastroenterology* 1979;77:433–443.
173. Rodriguez F, Llinas MT, Gonzalez JD, et al. Renal changes induced by a cyclooxygenase-2 inhibitor during normal and low sodium intake. *Hypertension* 2000;36:276–281.
174. Rodriguez JA, Vio CP, Pedraza PL, et al. Bradykinin regulates cyclooxygenase-2 in rat renal thick ascending limb cells. *Hypertension* 2004;44:230–235.
175. Roig F, Llinas MT, Lopez R, et al. Role of cyclooxygenase-2 in the prolonged regulation of renal function. *Hypertension* 2002;40:721–728.
176. Roman RJ. P-450 metabolites of arachidonic acid in the control of cardiovascular function. *Physiol Rev* 2002;82:131–185.
177. Roman RJ, Ma YH, Frohlich B, et al. Clofibrate prevents the development of hypertension in Dahl salt- sensitive rats. *Hypertension* 1993;21:985–988.
178. Romero MF, Hopfer U, Madhun ZT, et al. Angiotensin II actions in the rabbit proximal tubule. Angiotensin II mediated signaling mechanisms and electrolyte transport in the rabbit proximal tubule. *Ren Physiol Biochem* 1991;14:199–207.
179. Romero MF, Madhun ZT, Hopfer U, et al. An epoxygenase metabolite of arachidonic acid 5,6 epoxy- eicosatrienoic acid mediates angiotensin-induced natriuresis in proximal tubular epithelium. *Adv Prostaglandin Thromboxane Leukot Res* 1991;21A:205–208.
180. Rosenblatt SG, Patak RV, Lifschitz MD. Organic acid secretory pathway and urinary excretion of prostaglandin E in the dog. *Am J Physiol* 1978;235:F473–F479.
181. Rzigalinski BA, Willoughby KA, Hoffman SW, et al. Calcium influx factor, further evidence it is 5, 6-epoxyeicosatrienoic acid. *J Biol Chem* 1999;274:175–182.
182. Sacerdoti D, Balazy M, Angeli P, et al. Eicosanoid excretion in hepatic cirrhosis. Predominance of 20-HETE. *J Clin Invest* 1997;100:1264–1270.
183. Sakairi Y, Jacobson HR, Noland TD, et al. 5,6-EET inhibits ion transport in collecting duct by stimulating endogenous prostaglandin synthesis. *Am J Physiol* 1995;268:F931–F933.
184. Salmon JA, Smith DR, Flower RJ, et al. Further studies on the enzymatic conversion of prostaglandin endoperoxide into prostacyclin by porcine aorta microsomes. *Biochim Biophys Acta* 1978; 523:250–262.
185. Samuelsson B. From studies of biochemical mechanism to novel biological mediators: prostaglandin endoperoxides, thromboxanes, and leukotrienes. Nobel Lecture, 8 December 1982. *Biosci Rep* 1983;3:791–813.
186. Schneider A, Zhang Y, Zhang M, et al. Membrane-associated PGE synthase-1 (mPGES-1) is coexpressed with both COX-1 and COX-2 in the kidney. *Kidney Int* 2004;65:1205–1213.
187. Schnermann J. Juxtaglomerular cell complex in the regulation of renal salt excretion. *Am J Physiol* 1998;274:R263–R279.
188. Schnermann J, Schubert G, Hermle M, et al. The effect of inhibition of prostaglandin synthesis on tubuloglomerular feedback in the rat kidney. *Pflugers Arch* 1979;379:269–279.
189. Schreiner GF, Kohan DE. Regulation of renal transport processes and hemodynamics by macrophages and lysmphocytes. *Am J Physiol* 1990;258:F761–F767.
190. Schwartzman M, Carroll MA, Ibraham NG, et al. Renal arachidonic acid metabolism. The third pathway. *Hypertension* 1985;7:I136–44.
191. Schwartzman ML, Abraham NG, Carroll MA, et al. Regulation of arachidonic acid metabolism by cytochrome P-450 in rabbit kidney. *Biochem J* 1986;238:283–290.
192. Schwartzman ML, Falck JR, Yadagiri P, et al. Metabolism of 20-hydroxyeicosatetraenoic acid by cyclooxygenase. Formation and identification of novel endothelium-dependent vasoconstrictor metabolites. *Biol Chem* 1989;264:11658–11662.
193. Schwartzman ML, McGiff JC. Renal cytochrome P450. *J Lipid Mediat Cell Signal* 1995;12:229–242.
194. Sinal CJ, Miyata M, Tohkin M, et al. Targeted disruption of soluble epoxide hydrolase reveals a role in blood pressure regulation. *J Biol Chem* 2000;275:40504–40510.
195. Smith JA, Whitaker EM, Yaktubay N, et al. Regulation of renal adenosine A(1) receptors: effect of dietary sodium chloride. *Eur J Pharmacol* 1999;384:71–79.
196. Smith WL. Prostanoid biosynthesis and mechanisms of action. *Am J Physiol* 1992;263:F181–F191.
197. Smith WL, Bell TG. Immunohistochemical localization of the prostaglandin-forming cyclooxygenase in renal cortex. *Am J Physiol* 1978;235:F451–F457.
198. Smith WL, DeWitt DL. Prostaglandin endoperoxide H synthases-1 and -2. *Adv Immunol* 1996;62:167–215.
199. Smith WL, DeWitt DL, Garavito RM. Cyclooxygenases: structural, cellular, and molecular biology. *Annu Rev Biochem* 2000;69:145–182.
200. Smith WL, Wilkin GP. Immunochemistry of prostaglandin endoperoxide-forming cyclooxygenases: the detection of the cyclooxygenases in rat, rabbit, and guinea pig kidneys by immunofluorescence. *Prostaglandins* 1977;13:873–892.
201. Sonnenburg WK, Smith WL. Regulation of cyclic AMP metabolism in rabbit cortical collecting tubule cells by prostaglandins. *J Biol Chem* 1988;263:6155–6160.
202. Sonnenburg WK, Zhu JH, Smith WL. A prostaglandin E receptor coupled to a pertussis toxin-sensitive guanine nucleotide regulatory protein in rabbit cortical collecting tubule cells. *J Biol Chem* 1990;265:8479–8483.
203. Spector AA, Fang X, Snyder GD, et al. Epoxyeicosatrienoic acids (EETs): metabolism and biochemical function. *Prog Lipid Res* 2004;43:55–90.
204. Spiecker M, Liao JK. Vascular protective effects of cytochrome p450 epoxygenase-derived eicosanoids. *Arch Biochem Biophys* 2005;433:413–420.
205. Sraer J, Foidart J, Chansel D, et al. Prostaglandin synthesis by mesangial and epithelial glomerular cultured cells. *FEBS Lett* 1979;104:420–424.
206. Steinhauslin F, Munafo A, Buclin T, et al. Renal effects of nimesulide in furosemide-treated subjects. *Drugs* 1993;46 (Suppl 1):257–262.
207. Stokes JB. Effect of prostaglandin E2 on chloride transport across the rabbit thick ascending limb of Henle. Selective inhibitions of the medullary portion. *J Clin Invest* 1979;64:495–502.
208. Sun CW, Alonso GM, Taheri MR, et al. Nitric oxide-20-hydroxyeicosatetraenoic acid interaction in the regulation of K+ channel activity and vascular tone in renal arterioles. *Circ Res* 1998;83:1069–1079.
209. Sun FF, Taylor BM, McGuire JC, et al. Metabolic disposition of prostacyclin. In: Vane JRBS (ed.). *Prostacyclin*. New York: Raven Press;1979:119–131.
210. Swan SK, Rudy DW, Lasseter KC, et al. Effect of cyclooxygenase-2 inhibition on renal function in elderly persons receiving a low-salt diet: a randomized, controlled trial. *Ann Intern Med* 2000;133:1–9.
211. Takizawa H, DelliPizzi AM, Nasjletti A. Prostaglandin I2 contributes to the vasodepressor effect of baicalein in hypertensive rats. *Hypertension* 1998;31:866–871.
212. Terragno NA, Terragno DA, McGiff JC. Contribution of prostaglandins to the renal circulation in conscious, anesthetized, and laparotomized dogs. *Circ Res* 1977;40:590–595.
213. Terragno NA, Terragno DA, Pacholczyk D, et al. Prostaglandins and the regulation of uterine blood flow in pregnancy. *Nature* 1974;249:57–58.
214. Thorup C, Persson AE. Inhibition of locally produced nitric oxide resets tubuloglomerular feedback mechanism. *Am J Physiol* 1994;267:F606–F611.
215. van der Heijden BJ, Carlus C, Narcy F, et al. Persistent anuria, neonatal death, and renal microcystic lesions after prenatal exposure to indomethacin. *Am J Obstet Gynecol* 1994;171:617–623.
216. Vargas-Poussou R, Huang C, Hulin P, et al. Functional characterization of a calcium-sensing receptor mutation in severe autosomal dominant hypocalcemia with a Bartter-like syndrome. *J Am Soc Nephrol* 2002;13:2259–2266.
217. Vio CP, An SJ, Cespedes C, et al. Induction of cyclooxygenase-2 in thick ascending limb cells by adrenalectomy. *J Am Soc Nephrol* 2001;12:649–658.
218. Vio CP, Cespedes C, Gallardo P, et al. Renal identification of cyclooxygenase-2 in a subset of thick ascending limb cells. *Hypertension* 1997;30:687–692.
219. von Euler U.S. Welcoming address. In: Bergstrom BS (ed.). *Prostaglandins: Proceedings of the Second Nobel Symposium*. New York: John Wiley & Sons;2006:16–20.
220. Wang D, An SJ, Wang WH, et al. CaR-mediated COX-2 expression in primary cultured mTAL cells. *Am J Physiol Renal Physiol* 2001;281:F658–F664.
221. Wang D, Chabrashvili T, Wilcox CS. Enhanced contractility of renal afferent arterioles from angiotensin-infused rabbits: roles of oxidative stress, thromboxane prostanoid receptors, and endothelium. *Circ Res* 2004;94:1436–1442.
222. Wang D, Pedraza PL, Abdullah HI, et al. Calcium-sensing receptor-mediated TNF production in medullary thick ascending limb cells. *Am J Physiol Renal Physiol* 2002;283:F963–F970.
223. Wang H, Garvin JL, Falck JR, et al. Glomerular cytochrome P-450 and cyclooxygenase metabolites regulate efferent arteriole resistance. *Hypertension* 2005;46:1175–1179.
224. Wang JL, Cheng HF, Harris RC. Cyclooxygenase-2 inhibition decreases renin content and lowers blood pressure in a model of renovascular hypertension. *Hypertension* 1999;34:96–101.
225. Wang W, Lu M. Effect of arachidonic acid on activity of the apical K+ channel in the thick ascending limb of the rat kidney. *J Gen Physiol* 1995;106:727–743.
226. Watanabe S, Fukumoto S, Chang H, et al. Association between activating mutations of calcium-sensing receptor and Bartter's syndrome. *Lancet* 2002;360:692–694.
227. Wei Y, Lin DH, Kemp R, et al. Arachidonic acid inhibits epithelial Na channel via cytochrome P450 (CYP) epoxygenase-dependent metabolic pathways. *J Gen Physiol* 2004; 124:719–727.
228. Welch WJ, Wilcox CS. Potentiation of tubuloglomerular feedback in the rat by thromboxane mimetic. Role of macula densa. *J Clin Invest* 1992;89:1857–1865.
229. Whisenant N, Zhang BX, Khademazad M, et al. Regulation of Na-K-2Cl cotransport in osteoblasts. *Am J Physiol* 1991;261:C433–C440.
230. Wilcox CS, Welch WJ, Murad F, et al. Nitric oxide synthase in macula densa regulates glomerular capillary pressure. *Proc Natl Acad Sci U S A* 1992;89:11993–11997.
231. Wong PY-K, Sun FF, Malik KU, et al. Metabolism of prostacyclin (PGI2) in the isolated kidney and lung of the rabbit. In: Vane JRBS (ed.). *Proceedings of the Workshop on Prostacyclin and Its Analogues*. New York: Raven Press;1979:133–145.
232. Wong PY, McGiff JC, Cagen L, et al. Metabolism of prostacyclin in the rabbit kidney. *J Biol Chem* 1979;254:12–14.
233. Wong PY, McGiff JC, Sun FF, et al. Pulmonary metabolism of prostacyclin (PGI2) in the rabbit. *Biochem Biophys Res Commun* 1978;83:731–738.
234. Wong PY, Sun FF, McGiff JC. Metabolism of prostacyclin in blood vessels. *J Biol Chem* 1978;253:5555–5557.
235. Xie WL, Chipman JG, Robertson DL, et al. Expression of a mitogen-responsive gene encoding prostaglandin synthase is regulated by mRNA splicing. *Proc Natl Acad Sci U S A* 1991; 88:2692–2696.
236. Yang T, Huang Y, Heasley LE, et al. MAPK mediation of hypertonicity-stimulated cyclooxygenase-2 expression in renal medullary collecting duct cells. *J Biol Chem* 2000; 275: 23281–23286.
237. Yang T, Park JM, Arend L, et al. Low chloride stimulation of prostaglandin E2 release and cyclooxygenase-2 expression in a mouse macula densa cell line. *J Biol Chem* 2000;275:37922–37929.
238. Yang T, Singh I, Pham H, et al. Regulation of cyclooxygenase expression in the kidney by dietary salt intake. *Am J Physiol* 1998;274:F481–F489.
239. Yard BA, Daha MR, Kooymans-Couthino M, et al. IL-1 alpha stimulated TNF alpha production by cultured human proximal tubular epithelial cells. *Kidney Int* 1992;42:383–389.

240. Yiu SS, Zhao X, Inscho EW, et al. 12-Hydroxyeicosatetraenoic acid participates in angiotensin II afferent arteriolar vasoconstriction by activating L-type calcium channels. *J Lipid Res* 2003;44:2391–2399.

241. Yu M, Cambj-Sapunar L, Kehl F, et al. Effects of a 20-HETE antagonist and agonists on cerebral vascular tone. *Eur J Pharmacol* 2004;486:297–306.

242. Yu Z, Huse LM, Adler P, et al. Increased CYP2J expression and epoxyeicosatrienoic acid formation in spontaneously hypertensive rat kidney. *Mol Pharmacol* 2000;57:1011–1020.

243. Yu Z, Xu F, Huse LM, et al. Soluble epoxide hydrolase regulates hydrolysis of vasoactive epoxyeicosatrienoic acids. *Circ Res* 2000;87:992–998.

244. Yue QY, Odar-Cederlof I, Svensson JO, et al. Glucuronidation of morphine in human kidney microsomes. *Pharmacol Toxicol* 1988;63:337–341.

245. Zeldin DC. Epoxygenase pathways of arachidonic acid metabolism. *J Biol Chem* 2001; 276:36059–36062.

246. Zewde T, Mattson DL. Inhibition of cyclooxygenase-2 in the rat renal medulla leads to sodium-sensitive hypertension. *Hypertension* 2004;44:424–428.

247. Zhang F, Deng H, Kemp R, et al. Decreased levels of cytochrome P450 2E1-derived eicosanoids sensitize renal arteries to constrictor agonists in spontaneously hypertensive rats. *Hypertension* 2005;45:103–108.

248. Zhang F, Wang MH, Krishna UM, et al. Modulation by 20-HETE of phenylephrine-induced mesenteric artery contraction in spontaneously hypertensive and Wistar-Kyoto rats. *Hypertension* 2001;38:1311–1315.

249. Zhang F, Wang MH, Wang JS, et al. Transfection of CYP4A1 cDNA decreases diameter and increases responsiveness of gracilis muscle arterioles to constrictor stimuli. *Am J Physiol Heart Circ Physiol* 2004;287:H1089–H1095.

250. Zhang JY, Prakash C, Yamashita K, et al. Regiospecific and enantioselective metabolism of 8,9- epoxyeicosatrienoic acid by cyclooxygenase. *Biochem Biophys Res Commun* 1992;183: 138–143.

251. Zhang MZ, Wang JL, Cheng HF, et al. Cyclooxygenase-2 in rat nephron development. *Am J Physiol* 1997;273:F994–1002.

252. Zhang YB, Magyar CE, Holstein-Rathlou NH, et al. The cytochrome P-450 inhibitor cobalt chloride prevents inhibition of renal Na,K-ATPase and redistribution of apical NHE-3 during acute hypertension. *J Am Soc Nephrol* 1998;9:531–537.

253. Zhao X, Inscho EW, Bondlela M, et al. The CYP450 hydroxylase pathway contributes to P2X receptor-mediated afferent arteriolar vasoconstriction. *Am J Physiol Heart Circ Physiol* 2001;281: H2089–H2096.

254. Zhao X, Pollock DM, Inscho EW, et al. Decreased renal cytochrome P450 2C enzymes and impaired vasodilation are associated with angiotensin salt-sensitive hypertension. *Hypertension* 2003;41:709–714.

255. Zhu D, Zhang C, Medhora M, et al. CYP4A mRNA, protein, and product in rat lungs: novel localization in vascular endothelium. *J Appl Physiol* 2002;93:330–337.

256. Zou AP, Fleming JT, Falck JR, et al. 20-HETE is an endogenous inhibitor of the large-conductance Ca(2+)-activated K+ channel in renal arterioles. *Am J Physiol* 1996;270: R228–R237.

257. Zou AP, Fleming JT, Falck JR, et al. Stereospecific effects of epoxyeicosatrienoic acids on renal vascular tone and K(+)-channel activity. *Am J Physiol* 1996;270:F822–832.

258. Zou AP, Imig JD, Kaldunski M, et al. Inhibition of renal vascular 20-HETE production impairs autoregulation of renal blood flow. *Am J Physiol* 1994;266:F275–282.

259. Zou AP, Imig JD, Ortiz de Montellano PR, et al. Effect of P-450 omega-hydroxylase metabolites of arachidonic acid on tubuloglomerular feedback. *Am J Physiol* 1994;266: F934–941.

260. Zusman RM, Caldwell BV, Speroff L, et al. Radioimmunoassay of the A prostaglandins. *Prostaglandins* 1972;2:41–53.

CHAPTER **15**

Kinins and Endothelin

Valentina Kon and Tracy E. Hunley

Vanderbilt University School of Medicine, Memphis, Tennessee, USA
Monroe Carell Jr. Children's Hospital at Vanderbilt, Nashville, Tennessee, USA

KININS

Kinins are bioactive substances with a myriad of functions that encompass regulation of systemic blood pressure and regional blood flow; renal hemodynamic and excretory functions, including vasodilatation and diuresis; modulation of glucose metabolism by enhancing insulin-stimulated glucose uptake and utilization and decreasing gluconeogenesis; and activation of coagulation and fibrinolysis. In addition, kinins have a primary role in inflammation, in which they direct the cardinal features, including pain, through stimulation of sensory C-fiber terminals and substance P; edema, by increasing capillary permeability; and recruitment of leukocytes, through kinin stimulation of other cytokines such interleukin-1 (IL-1) and tumor necrosis factor. With the recent advent of potent antagonists, interest in kinins as pathophysiologic mediators has increased in settings such as inflammatory diseases including asthma, inflammatory bowel disease, arthritis, as well as other disorders such as septic and anaphylactic shock, hypertension, male infertility, and primary and metastatic cancerous proliferation.

History

In 1909, Abelous and Bardier (1) showed that the alcohol-insoluble fraction of human urine caused hypotension when infused into anesthetized dogs. In the 1920s and 1930s, Frey and his colleagues (2, 355) further characterized the substance and demonstrated its existence in blood, salivary glands, and pancreas. The assumption that the hypotensive substance in the urine originates from the pancreas led to the name *kallikrein,* named for the Greek word for pancreas, *kallikreas.* In 1937, the observations that kallikrein itself failed to contract guinea pig ileum or rat uterus but contracted these tissues in the presence of serum suggested an enzyme–substrate relationship and an inactive precursor. In 1948, Werle and Berek (355) named the active substance *kallidin* and the precursor *kallidogen.* In 1949, Rocha e Silva et al. (377) noted that incubation of snake venom with plasma caused a slow contraction of isolated guinea pig ileum and hypotension. Since the response was markedly slower than that of the known vaso-

active substances such as histamine and acetylcholine, the substance was named *bradykinin* (slow movement). In 1960, the nonapeptide bradykinin and the decapeptide kallidin, that is, bradykinin with an additional lysine residue at the amino terminus, were isolated and synthesized (1). In 1980, Regoli et al. (269) separated the kinin receptors into B1 and B2 classes. The period from mid 1985 to 1990 brought kinin receptor antagonists, which increased the physiologic understanding of kinins in physiologic and pathophysiologic settings (32). In the last several years, kinins have come into the limelight as potential mediators of some of the beneficial effects as well as some untoward effects observed with the increased therapeutic use of angiotensin-converting enzyme inhibitors in hypertension, ischemic heart disease, and diabetic and nondiabetic progressive renal damage due to the fact that these inhibitors slow kinin metabolism.

Biochemistry and Pharmacokinetics

The best known of the kinin polypeptides are bradykinin and kallidin (which is also known as *lys-bradykinin*). These peptides are cleaved from precursors, the kininogens. Generation of kinins from kininogens can occur through several different serine proteases; however, the highly specific proteases that release bradykinin and kallidin from kininogens are called *kallikreins* (Fig. 1).

KININOGENS

The kinin precursors, the kininogens (32, 56, 201), are single-chain glycoproteins that are synthesized by the liver. In mammals there are two types of kininogens: high-molecular weight (HMW) and low molecular weight (LMW). In the human, HMW and LMW kininogens are encoded by a single gene located on chromosome 3q26 via alternative splicing at exon 11. They differ in size, structure, and susceptibility to cleavage by plasma and tissue kallikreins. In addition, but exclusively in the rat, a gene duplication exists that produces the gene coding for an acute-phase protein called T-kininogen, the regulation of which is different from the HMW and LMW kininogens.

HMW kininogen is cleaved by both plasma and tissue kallikreins to yield bradykinin and kallidin, respectively.

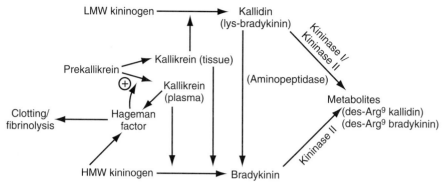

FIGURE 1   Biosynthesis/metabolism of kinins. LMW, low-molecular weight; HMW, high-molecular weight; HF, Hageman factor (factor XII); * kininase II is the identical enzyme as angiotensin-converting enzyme.

LMW kininogen is a substrate only for tissue kallikrein and produces kallidin. Both HMW, and LMW kininogens circulate, and both occupy high-affinity binding sites on platelets, neutrophils, endothelial cells, and vascular smooth muscle cells. This binding has been offered as a mechanism against excessive proteolysis by kallikreins, effectively controlling the availability of kinins. Kininogens are multifunctional glycoproteins that not only serve as precursors for kinins, but are involved in inflammation, protection of cells from damage by inhibition of other proteases, and in the clotting cascade. Thus, together with plasma prekallikrein, Hageman factor (factor XII), and factor XI, kininogens (particularly HMW) trigger contact activation of blood clotting, for which they are essential factors (Fig. 2) (260). Indeed, prekallikrein and factor XI circulate bound to HMW kininogen. A complex of three endothelial surface proteins comprises a binding surface for the circulating HMW kininogen/prekallikrein complex (296, 302). At binding, prekallikrein activation to kallikrein occurs through the serine protease prolylcarboxypeptidase (PRCP), recently shown to colocalize with the kininogen binding complex (303, 304) Activated kallikrein's proximity to HMW kininogen facilitates immediate release of bradykinin at the endothelial cell luminal surface (296, 374).

Factor XII binds to the same endothelial multiprotein receptor complex as HMW kininogen (191, 268). This competitive binding appears to favor HMW kininogen, as factor XII requires a 30-fold higher concentration of zinc (Zn^{2+}) in vitro. Ambient zinc concentration may be augmented by activated platelets and/or other circulating cells and provides a mechanism for activation of the system (191, 304). Underscoring the complex nature of the interaction is the observation that although factor XII is not essential for prekallikrein activation, and in fact competes for the same binding site as PK's carrier (HMW kininogen), factor XII causes dramatic increase in the rate of PK activation, which will tend to foster increased bradykinin synthesis. In addition, factor XII is itself activated by kallikrein and thus serves as a positive feedback for the kinin system.

The physiologic importance of kininogens is underscored by studies in the Brown Norway Katholiek rats, which express kininogen messenger RNA (mRNA) but do not generate the kininogen protein (125). These kininogen-deficient rats are very sensitive to salt loading and sodium retention with resultant systemic hypertension, suggesting that kininogens play a role in normal renal sodium handling and volume homeostasis (125, 193).

KALLIKREINS

Initial understanding of kallikreins derived from their role as kinin-generating enzymes (kininogenases). The two prominent members, plasma and tissue kallikreins, are both serine proteases but differ in several ways: size; substrate specificity, and therefore the specific kinin product that is generated; immunologic characteristics; and susceptibility to inhibitors. These functional differences mirror their origin from two distinct genes on separate chromosomes with little sequence or structural similarity (55). It is important to point out that kinins can be released from kininogens by other systems including mast cell tryptases and microbial gingipains, cysteine proteinases from the major pathogen of periodontal disease. Similarly, neutrophil elastase and cysteine proteinases from *Staphylococcus aureus* may have synergistic kinin generating capabilities (142).

Plasma kallikrein is encoded as a 15-exon single gene on human chromosome 4. It is about 88 kD, is synthesized by the liver in an inactive form (prekallikrein), and circulates as a heterodimer complexed with HMW kininogen (368). This heterodimer docks at the endothelial surface through a multiprotein receptor complex of cytokeratin 1, gC1qR, and urokinase plasminogen activator receptor (uPAR). This complex interaction thus approximates plasma prekallikrein to its activator, the endothelial surface serine protease prolylcarboxypeptidase (PRCP) (see preceding sections). The mature plasma kallikrein then cleaves HMW kininogen to release bradykinin. Functional plasma kallikrein is then rapidly inactivated, primarily by C1 esterase inhibitor, although other proteases may

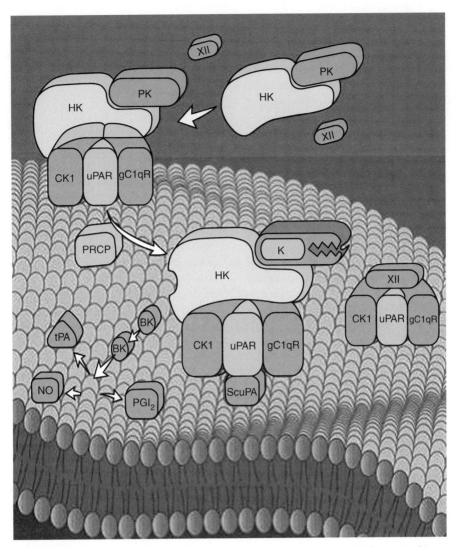

FIGURE 2   Endothelial binding of circulating kininogen (HK)/prekallikrein (PK) complex. Plasma PK circulates in complex with HK which binds to a multiprotein receptor composed of cytokeratin 1 (CK1), urokinase plasminogen activator receptor (uPAR) and gC1qR. After binding, PK is rapidly converted to kallikrein (K) by the enzyme prolylcarboxypeptidase (PRCP), which is constitutively active on endothelial cell membranes. The resulting kallikrein liberates bradykinin (BK), which can liberate nitric oxide (NO), prostacyclin (PGI2), and tissue plasminogen activator (tPA) from endothelial cells. ScuPA, single-chain urokinase plasminogen activator. (From Schmaier AH. The plasma kallikrein-kinin system counterbalances the renin-angiotensin system. *J Clin Invest* 2002;109:1007–1009, with permission)

be inhibitory to lesser degrees. It is noteworthy that patients with hereditary angioneurotic edema (HAE), which is characterized by a decrease in C1 esterase inhibitor, have abdominal pain, laryngeal edema, and local swelling. Fluid in suction-induced blisters obtained from these patients has active plasma kallikrein. Moreover, symptoms of the acute angioneurotic edema attack subside with replacement of C1 inhibition, which is associated with increase in circulating HMW kininogen, suggesting restoration of kallikrein inhibition (60, 161). In C1-inhibitor–deficient mice, the role of kinins in mediating the angioedema of HAE has been further clarified and clearly linked to the kinin system. In these mice, pharmacologic kallikrein inhibition prevented the increase in vascular permeability of the rear footpad assay, as did pharmacologic and mo-

lecular antagonism of the bradykinin type 2 receptor. Angioedema is thus mediated by the kinin kallikrein system through the constitutively present kinin receptor, B2R (see following sections) and does not depend on B1 receptor up-regulation, which concurs with the sudden onset and rapid progression of angioedema symptoms (121).

The tissue kallikrein story has become significantly more complicated in the last decade with the recognition that the human tissue kallikrein locus on chromosome 19 actually encodes 15 different tissue kallikrein genes (*KLK1–KLK15*). Only the product of *KLK1*, hK1, also called pancreatic/renal kallikrein, demonstrates significant kininogenase activity. Current classification as a tissue kallikrein, therefore, is now specifically defined by clustered chromosomal location, and highly conserved genomic and protein organizations rather than biologic function (55, 368). Thus, older discussions of tissue kallikrein in reference to kinin generation refer primarily to hK1. hK1 is smaller than plasma kallikrein at 29 kD, reflecting its smaller gene of five exons. hK1 is synthesized in many organs including the kidney, pancreas, salivary gland, brain, cardiovascular tissue, skeletal muscle, and leukocytes, and its actions are believed to be chiefly local (7, 9, 190). As with plasma kallikrein, hK1 also exists as a precursor in an inactive form which in the circulation is bound to α_1-antitrypsin. hK1 prekallikrein is synthesized as a zymogen from which a 7–amino acid sequence must be cleaved for activation. This activation is known to be affected by several different factors, including aldosterone in the kidney, vagal stimulation in the pancreas, and androgens in other tissues. hK1 activity can be inhibited by aprotinin, the pancreatic trypsin inhibitor, as well as kallistatin, a serine protease inhibitor. Once activated, hK1 cleaves LMW kininogens to release kallidin. Although kallidin has the same structure as bradykinin with an additional lysine residue at the amino terminus (lys-bradykinin), there is only a small amount of conversion from kallidin to bradykinin. This reaction is relatively slow compared with the rate of inactivation by hydrolysis at the carboxy terminal and therefore is not believed to be a physiologically significant pathway for bradykinin synthesis. The decapeptide kallidin and nonapeptide bradykinin have similar biologic activities.

Despite lack of kininogenase activity, other tissue kallikreins warrant mention here due to the extent and potential importance of their biologic actions. Like hK1, all tissue kallikreins are serine proteases encoded in five exons in a small region of chromosome 19. All show strict conservation of the positions of the catalytic triad of histidine, aspartate, and serine and all are synthesized as pre-/propeptides that require activation. Prostate-specific antigen (PSA) is hK3, encoded as KLK3. PSA and hK2 are markers of prostate cancer. Neurosin, hK6, localizes to perivascular and microglial cells in brains affected by Alzheimer disease and has been shown to have amyloidogenic activity. Expression of neuropsin, hK8, mRNA is increased fivefold in the hippocampus of Alzheimer brains. hK5, hK11, and hK14 may have roles in brain physiology including maintenance of plasticity. hK4 through hK9 appear to be important to ovarian cancer whereas hK5, hK10, and hK13 may be particularly relevant to breast cancer. Many of the tissue kallikrein functions can be grouped as growth regulatory, extracellular matrix related, or angiogenic, all of which may be crucial to both neoplastic and central nervous system (CNS) disease (55,368).

Salivary glands are unique in that they show expression for virtually all of the tissue kallikreins, including hK1 (369). Sjögren syndrome is an autoimmune disorder characterized by lymphocytic infiltration of salivary and lacrimal glands, with progression to systemic involvement. A spontaneous model of Sjögren syndrome occurs in IQI/Jic mice after 8 weeks, and antibodies cross-reacting with tissue kallikreins 1 and 13 have recently been identified. By 4 weeks of age,

T-cell autoimmunity against tissue kallikrein 13 is detectable. Cross-reactivity with tissue kallikrein 1 is presumed to develop due to high homology in amino acid sequence and may contribute to the observed systemic progression of Sjögren syndrome (324).

KININASES

Although kinins are formed at various sites, they are rapidly destroyed by the enzymatic actions of peptidases; in plasma the kinin half-life is about 10 to 30 seconds. Moreover, the lungs destroy much of the kinins in a single passage because of their very high concentration of kininases. Thus, the activity of kinins is determined, in large part, by their metabolism. Numerous kininases have been identified that degrade kinins, but none is specific for the peptides. The primary metabolism of kinins is accomplished by the kininase I (KI) family, which removes Arg9 from the kinin molecule, and dipeptidylcarboxypeptide or kininase II (KII), which is more familiar as angiotensin-converting enzyme (ACE) (29), which liberates the terminal Phe8-Arg9. The KII peptidase further degrades the remaining COOH terminus by cleaving the dipeptide SerG-Pr07. The relative importance of each of the peptidase families varies with the species and organ site. For example, in humans, more than 90% of circulating kinins are hydrolyzed by KI, whereas KII/ACE is responsible for tissue metabolism, particularly in the lungs and also in the kidneys. In the rat, KII/ACE is the overwhelmingly important enzyme (7). Distinction between the two kininase families also carries specific clinical implications. Hydrolysis by KI, which includes carboxypeptidase N and carboxypeptidase M, increases levels of des Arg9 metabolite without further degradation of the molecule and may underlie the clinical symptomatology in situations where kinins are increased. Interestingly, systemic hypotension and bronchoconstriction occasionally observed following administration of protamine to reverse the anticoagulant effects of heparin are believed to be due to protamine's inhibition of KI-carboxypeptidase N, which increases kinin levels. In addition, the KI-hydrolyzed metabolite des Arg9-kallidin as well as the KI/KII metabolite des Arg9-bradykinin are potent B1 receptor agonists. This is the receptor that is upregulated in pathophysiologic settings and may even be upregulated by the metabolites themselves (7, 9, 120). Further support for the importance of this pathway comes from observations of a familial KI-carboxypeptidase N deficiency. Affected individuals have low levels of the enzyme, high circulating levels of kinins, and are susceptible to angiodenema, urticaria, dizziness, and hypotension. These findings imply that disruption of this metabolic pathway sufficiently augments kinin activity to produce these symptoms (319).

The KII-ACE family of peptidases includes KII-ACE and KII-neutral endopeptidase (KII-NEP). Both exist as soluble enzymes found in various biologic fluids, but are also present in high concentrations in many different organs including the kidneys, lung, brain, and testis, where they can regulate not only kinin levels but also angiotensin II and atrial natriuretic hormone and thus modulate local vasomotor tone and epithelial cell transport of sodium and water. There has also been keen interest in the finding of KII-NEP in human neutrophils, where it is responsible for chemotaxis. An insertion/deletion (I/D) polymorphism of the ACE gene that affects circulating ACE activity has been shown to modulate bradykinin levels (273). Individuals who are homozygous for the deletion of a 287-base pair (bp) fragment from the ACE gene, that is, the DD genotype, which is associated with the highest circulating levels of ACE, also have the highest levels of BK1-5, the major metabolite of bradykinin. Conversely, individuals homozygous for the presence of the 287-bp fragment, the II genotype, are characterized by the lowest ACE activity and the lowest BK 1-5 levels, indicative of less bradykinin metabolism (224, 225). These observations are intriguing in view of the reports that cough, which is sometimes associated with angiotensin-converting enzyme inhibitor (ACEI) treatment is more frequent in patients with the II genotype (219). This symptom has been linked to accumulation of kinins brought about by inhibition of ACE particularly in the lung. Whether II genotype individuals on ACEI also are at greater risk for other kinin-linked events such as systemic hypotension and fall in glomerular filtration rate (GFR) in response to ACEI is currently under study (292, 207). Not all reports have confirmed the link in ACE II genotype to cough. In Japanese hypertensive patients on ACE inhibitor therapy, cough did not correlate with ACE genotype but rather a B2 receptor polymorphism located in the promoter, the B2 $C^{-58} \rightarrow T$ polymorphism (see subsequent sections). Specifically, cough was associated with the T allele, thought to lead to increased B2 transcriptional rate and possibly increased receptor density (220). Underscoring the role of neutral endopaptidase as a physiologically relevant kininase II, are observations gained from recent clinical trials with a relatively novel class of compounds that inhibits ACE and neutral endopeptidase. One such compound, omapatrilat, recently studied in heart failure and hypertension, was shown to induce angioedema at a threefold higher rate than ACE inhibitors, the symptoms developing hours after the initial dose and ascribed to more pronounced bradykinin effects (15, 329).

Kinin Receptors

Based on the rank order of potency of kinin analogues in isolated tissues, Regoli et al. (6) proposed two kinin receptors, the B1 and B2 receptors. The physiologically prominent B2 receptor binds both bradykinin and kallidin. It is constitutively expressed in normal tissues and is believed to transduce most kinin actions in noninjured tissues. The B1 receptor is less abundant than the B2 receptor and is upregulated under pathophysiologic conditions, in which B1R may actually predominate (198). It is noteworthy that the inducible character of the B1 receptor is unusual among G-protein–coupled receptors (197). The B1 receptor binds the carboxy-

terminal des-Arg metabolites of bradykinin, with a rank order preference for des-Arg kallidin over kallidin, which approximates des-Arg bradykinin and all much higher than bradykinin, indicating a preferential susceptibility to tissue generated kinins over circulating (83). Duration of effect is distinct between the two receptors as well, with B2R usually being transient and B1R eliciting prolonged responses. This underscores differentiation of B2R as functional in physiologic responses and B1R as participating in pathophysiologic and perhaps, at times, maladaptive responses.

Rat and human B2 receptors have been cloned and predict a 366–amino acid, G-protein–coupled, seven-transmembrane receptor. Through G-protein activation of phospholipase C, B2 receptors lead to generation of second messengers inositol triphosphate (IP3), diacylglycerol, and calcium. Through calcium stimulation of cyclic GMP, nitric oxide is generated, which leads to prominent hypotensive effect of kinins in the vasculature. Through B2 coupling to phospholipase A2 and D, kinins can liberate arachidonic acid from membrane-bound phospholipids, which in turn metabolizes a variety of other vasoactive and proinflammatory mediators (34). These observations complement previous studies that show that bradykinin applied to the luminal surfaces of proximal tubules as well as cortical collecting tubular cells or cultured glomerular mesangial cells activates prostaglandin synthesis (92). These findings also dovetail with the well-known observation that infusion of kinins into intact animals produces a prompt increase in prostaglandin excretion. Taken together, these findings reiterate the important role of prostaglandins in mediating kinin actions (see subsequent section). Through diacylglycerol, as well as calcium, B2R can lead to activation of several isoforms of protein kinase C whose functions include regulation of cellular proliferation. Moreover, multiple pathways have been elucidated whereby B2R can activate MAP kinases, which on activation, translocate to the nucleus where they phosphorylate and activate nuclear transcription factors involved in DNA synthesis and cell division. It is important to point out that repeated or continuous stimulation of the B2R will lead to a dampening of its effects, a phenomenon observed for a variety of receptors called desensitization. Recently, the mechanism for desensitization has been assigned to phosphorylation of B2R's intracellular carboxy-terminal tail, which leads to impairment in G-protein activation. In particular, phosphorylation of Ser 346 and Ser348 or Ser349 is sufficient for desensitization of bradykinin-induced phospholipase C activation and phosphorylation of these residues together with threonines 342 and 345 has been shown to trigger internalization of B2R into intracellular compartments, rendering it inaccessible for further bradykinin stimulation (34, 256). That this clustering of residues for B2R desensitization is highly conserved between species attests to the importance of limitation of bradykinin effects through receptor fatigue and sequestration in addition to rapid ligand degradation mentioned previously. Most recent evidence suggests that there may also be novel, direct interaction of the B2 receptor with intracellular signaling proteins phospholipase Cγ1 and tyrosine phosphatase SHP-2 that do not require the interposition of G proteins (69, 70).

The B1 receptor has been cloned from rabbit, mouse, and human. The human receptor sequence predicts a 313–amino acid structure that has about 36% homology with the B2 receptor. B1R was originally isolated in rabbit aortas but is now recognized to be more widely distributed, in a variety of cell types including endothelial cells, smooth muscle cells, mesangial cells, and fibroblasts (120). These receptors are believed to transduce functions that are specific to disease states such as hyperalgesia, increased capillary permeability, and hypotension. Very low-level, constitutive expression in the rat has been documented by Northern blotting in the aorta, uterus, lung, duodenum (slightly higher level), and thymus. Strikingly, after treatment with lipopolysaccharide (LPS), B1R expression is induced in whole-tissue homogenates from the heart, kidney, spleen, and macrophages with further increase in expression in the uterus, lung, duodenum, and thymus (150). Similarly, while B2R is detectable in all segments of the nephron, B1R was detected in the rat nephron only after LPS treatment, where efferent arteriole showed the highest expression, followed by the MTL and distal tubule (203). Similar results have been seen in human kidney where B1R is detectable in the distal tubule and collecting ducts in diseased kidneys but not healthy kidneys being donated for transplantation (228). Substances/mediators known to induce B1R expression include bacterial LPS, endotoxin, Il-1β, EGF, and TNF-α (198, 253). The identity and importance of G-protein subtypes linked to B1R are similar to the ones coupled to B2R, prominent among these being phsopholipase C. However, besides a transient increase in calcium mediated by inositol triphosphate, a sustained or oscillating phase of intracellular calcium increase is seen with B1R activation that is more dependent on extracellular calcium influx and potentially linked to multiple types of calcium channels (198, 206). This sustained calcium signal together with lack of desensitization are thought to mediate the observed longer lasting effects of B1R.

The observation of increased B1R expression in the setting of various perturbations has led to speculation that it may be involved in an appropriate and adaptive response to the injury, or alternatively may be part of these pathological processes per se to which pharmacologic intervention should be directed. In this connection, mice lacking the B2 receptor show increased expression of the B1R in cardiac and renal tissue, an observation thought to reflect B1R assumption of B2R hemodynamic (vasodilating) functions. B1R upregulation, however, appears to be an inadequate response to B2R loss as B2R deficient animals are hypertensive at baseline, despite higher B1R expression, and have more severe hypertension with a variety of hypertensive maneuvers, all of which were accompanied by increased B1R expression (73). In these animals, however, blood pressure remained manipulable as B1R antagonism further increased blood pressure and B1R agonist infusion caused hypotension (72). Among stroke-prone spontaneously hypertensive rats (SHR-SP), B1R mRNA was shown to be dramatically increased at baseline, and immunohistochemistry demonstrated B1R in the renal tubules and glomeruli, neither of which was true for Wistar Kyoto control rats. Administration of B1R agonist increased urinary nitric oxide metabolites fivefold compared to untreated SHR-SP rats. Moreover, B1R antagonism for 4 weeks worsened hypertension and resulted in significant renal pathology with increase in renal TGF-β and collagen III mRNA as well as glomerular and interstitial fibrosis (119). Certainly, hypertension per se, if severe enough, would be sufficient to result in similar renal scarring, but this study raises the possibility that the B1 receptor itself may have renal protective effects which could encompass vasodilatory, antifibrotic, and antiproliferative functions. Indeed, B1R mediates inhibition of neointima formation after angioplasty in rats. Moreover, B1R has recently been shown to mediate some of the beneficial effects of ACE inhibition and AT1 receptor blockade after myocardial infarction or heart failure, other clinical settings characterized by B1R induction (6, 58, 103, 358). Somewhat difficult to reconcile with these apparent beneficial effects of B1R are limited observations of its contribution to proliferation and fibrosis. Immunohistochemistry has shown B1R to be densely expressed in transbronchial lung biopsies from patients with sarcoidosis or progressive systemic sclerosis, but undetectable in control lungs (226). Des-Arg kallidin–induced [³H]thymidine incorporation in rabbit aortic smooth muscle cells pretreated with Il-1β, a system exhibiting the preferred B1R ligand and B1R upregulation (177). Moreover, in human lung embryonic fibroblasts in culture, which constitutively express B1R, des-Arg kallidin aided type I collagen synthesis through stabilization of connective tissue growth factor mRNA (272). Resolution of these apparent contradictory effects of B1R and improved understanding of B1R function in various pathophysiologic settings will no doubt be facilitated by recent synthesis of several selective, nonpeptide B1 receptor antagonists (97, 218, 267).

Kinin Physiology

RENAL REGULATION OF KININ-KALLIKREIN SYSTEM

Although the hypotensive property of human urine was initially thought to originate from the pancreas, in the 1960s, evidence began to accrue that the kidneys are an important source of this hypotensive enzyme. It is now fully established that all of the components of the kinin-kallikrein system are extensively distributed throughout the kidney and exert profound effects on hemodynamic function, tubular reabsorption, and reaction of other vasoactive substances in the kidney. More than 90% of renal kallikrein is found in the cortex with only 1.0% appearing in the medulla and papilla. Immunofluorescence studies localized most of the kallikrein to the distal tubules between the macula densa and cortical duct (7), although glomeruli contained about 15% of the enzyme activity seen in the cortex. Subsequent immunohistochemical studies further localized tissue kallikrein to the connecting tubule in various species including humans (157). Subcellular localization narrowed kallikrein activity to the endoplasmic reticulum, luminal and basolateral cell membranes, Golgi membranes, and secretory-like vesicles in the luminal and basolateral sides of the connecting tubule. Tissue kallikrein is also secreted into the urinary space and the interstitium (Fig. 3).

There are several physiologic regulators of kallikrein activity. Low-sodium diet increases renal levels as well as urinary excretion of tissue kallikrein (7, 9). Whether the converse is true, namely whether high-sodium diet decreases kallikrein activity, remains controversial (157) High-potassium diet also augments renal level and urinary excretion of tissue kallikrein. Notably, high-potassium diets increase tissue kallikrein-containing connecting tubule cells and also the number of immunoreactive secretory vesicles (346). This effect may be mediated by prostaglandins and aldosterone, which are also stimulated by high-potassium diets, which in turn increase the urinary excretion of kallikrein. Indeed, 1% potassium chloride added to the drinking water of spontaneously hypertensive rats decreased systemic blood pressure in association with an increase in urinary excretion of tissue kallikrein. This effect is seen acutely as well, as intravenous infusion of high potassium saline (67.5 mM KCl and 67.5 mM NaCl) in anesthesized rates increased urine volume by nearly 50% and urine Na$^+$ by 32% over 90 minutes, together

with nearly 50% increase in urinary kallikrein. Moreover, K$^+$-induced diuresis and natriuresis appear to be mediated through the B2-receptor, as treatment with B2 receptor antagonist completely eliminated the diuresis and natriuresis (321). Thus, the observed beneficial effect on blood pressure of potassium may be a bradykinin-mediated phenomenon. Hormones also modulate tissue kallikreins. Renal kallikrein mRNA is twice as high in female as in male rats. Chronic deoxycorticosterone acetate (DOCA) treatment increases tissue kallikrein in collecting tubules as well as urinary kallikrein excretion (192). Also, thyroxine, insulin, vasopressin, and oxyt-ocin increase kallikrein synthesis and enzyme activity. Conversely, adrenalin downregulates kallikreins, which is thought to occur via the β-adrenoreceptor since the de novo synthesis of the enzyme can be blocked by β$_1$-adrenergic blockade.

Less is known about the regulation of the kallikrein substrate kininogen. It clearly exists in kidney parenchyma and is found in the urine, where it is present in concentrations of about 1.6 to 6.2 mg/L, which represents about 10% of the total urinary protein normally excreted. According to careful immunocytochemical studies of the distal nephron, kininogen is localized to the collecting duct and especially the luminal sides of principle cells (94). Thus, there is the expectation of significant luminal kinin formation given its close proximity to its enzyme. Taken together, these observations indicate that the terminal segments of the distal nephron and the collecting ducts are rich sources of the substrate as well as the enzyme and are poised to release both into the urinary space as well as abluminally. The regulation of kininogen is akin to kallikrein regulation. Similar to kallikreins, female rat liver kininogen mRNA is found to be some fourfold higher than in male rats. Moreover, estrogen increases liver kininogen expression in ovariectomized rats, whereas progesterone decreases kininogen expression. In the kidney, estradiol and progesterone increase renal kininogen message, indicating tissue-specific regulation of the substrate.

As with the substrate and enzyme, the highest binding activity occurs in the more distal parts of the nephron, particularly in the collecting tubules, although significant binding is also seen in the glomerulus, distal convoluted tubules, proximal collecting tubules, and in the interstitial cells. Indeed, [^{3}H]BK-binding capacity is maximal in the cortical collecting duct and outer medullary collecting duct, with small but significant glomerular and straight proximal tubular binding (332). Moreover, B2 receptors are found in the luminal membranes and colocalize with kallikrein in the connecting tubule and with kininogen in the collecting duct (93). Localization of the B2 receptor thus appears compatible with the observations that bradykinin inhibits the net absorption of sodium in the collecting duct (331). The need for all components of the tubular kinin system to generate functional bradykinin and to effect urinary changes is shown after DOCA treatment in kininogen-deficient Brown Norway Katholiek rats together with controls. While excretion of renal kallikrein increased immediately and equally after

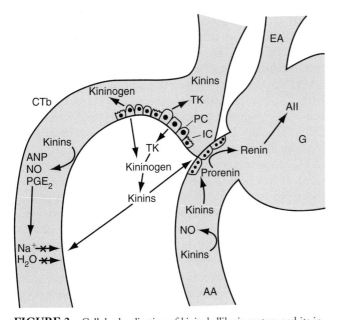

FIGURE 3 Cellular localization of kinin-kallikrein system and its interactions with prostaglandins, renin-angiotensin and nitric oxide (NO). PGE$_2$, prostaglandin E$_2$; AII, angiotensin II; TK, tissue kallikrein; ANP, atrial natriuretic peptide; AA, afferent arteriole; EA, efferent arteriole; G, glomerulus; CTb, connecting tubule; IC, intercalated cell; PC, principle cell; → stimulatory effect; ⇥ inhibitory effect.

the onset of treatment with DOCA in both groups, only the kininogen-replete control animals showed natriuresis/diuresis (192). As noted previously, kinin activity is determined by the rate of its degradation and can occur via both aminopeptidases as well as carboxypeptidases. Both of the enzymes are found prominently in the proximal tubule, with the active site extending to the luminal surface. In fact, ACE is concentrated in the brush border of the proximal tubule and micropuncture studies have demonstrated that [^{3}H]BK injected into the proximal tubule is destroyed there (46, 139). Kininases are also found in the renal vasculature as well as the interstitium, where they are proposed to catalyze the circulating kinins. Importantly, it is now recognized that degradation of tubule bradykinin, especially distal tubule generated bradykinin, is unique. In contrast to plasma, where bradykinin (1–5) is the major metabolite of bradykinin, bradykinin (1–6) predominates in urine (170). Tubular kinin metabolism occurs mainly through carboxypeptidase Y-like exopeptidase (CPY) and neutral endopeptidase (156, 284). Thus, inhibition of CPY with ebelactone increases urinary kinins and results in diuresis and natriuresis without impacting plasma kininases, because of the unique dependence of the tubular kinin system on CPY (194). Kallistatin, a tissue kallikrein inhibitor is synthesized mainly in the liver, but at lower levels in the kidney as well. Renal mRNA expression studies of the analogue of human kallistatin, kallikrein-binding protein (KBP) have shown it to be detected most abundantly in the inner medullary collecting ducts, with only small amounts (<10%) in the cortical collecting duct, proximal tubules, and glomeruli (365). Thus, the nephron location of the kallikrein inhibitor is downstream in the collecting duct from the site of kallikrein and kinogen where it puts an end to the tubule bradykinin signal. It might be predicted therefore, that lessening of kallistatin could augment bradykinin effects or augmenting kallistatin could lessen bradykinin effects. The complexity of the kinin system, as well as the reality of supplementary protein functions beyond their initial characterization, is underscored by the observation that transgenic mice overexpressing kallikrein binding protein have significantly lower blood pressure than wild-type littermates (52). In fact, kallistatin appears to function as a vasodilator and regulator of vascular cell growth independent of its interaction with tissue kallikrein and the kinin system (50, 51)

Kinin Regulation of Renal Function

Clearly a major role of kinins is causing renal vasodilation, diuresis, and natriuresis (7, 9, 27, 48, 57, 301). Even at baseline, it appears that bradykinin is important in maintaining papillary blood flow. Thus, kinin antagonism, which does not affect cortical blood flow or glomerular filtration rate (GFR), decreases papillary blood flow. Moreover, administration of ACEI, which is expected to further elevate bradykinin levels, increases renal papillary blood flow by some 50%. This effect can be abrogated by kinin antagonists.

Vasodilation, systemic as well as renal, is mediated in some part by prostacyclin, but in large part by nitric oxide (NO). The considerable physiologic importance of NO in the kinin effects is underscored by the observation that kinin hydrolysis by both members of kininase I family, carboxypeptidase N and M, releases arginine, which provides the substrate for formation of NO by NO synthase.

Interestingly, in the kidney, kinin-induced vasodilation is not accompanied by an increase in GFR. Baylis et al. (27) showed that increased glomerular plasma flow rate following bradykinin infusion reflected decreases in afferent and efferent arteriolar resistances, particularly in the former. This vasodilation was offset by decrease in the glomerular capillary ultrafiltration coefficient such that the net effect was no change in the GFR. The somewhat surprising finding of a decrease in the glomerular ultrafiltration coefficient response to bradykinin was postulated to be mediated by angiotensin II. Indeed, there are convincing data that kinins as well as kallikreins are powerful stimuli to angiotensin II synthesis; moreover, this stimulation is independent of prostaglandins. Conversely, decreases in kinin synthesis, accomplished by protamine, inhibited basal and diuretic-stimulated renin release in rats, rabbits, and humans. This relationship between the renin-angiotensin system and the kallikrein-kinin system likely forms the basis for an intricate homeostatic mechanism that regulates renal microvasculature.

The kallikrein-kinin system and renin-angiotensin system appear particularly linked in pathophysiologic settings. Indeed, interest in kinins over the last few decades has been propelled by the increased use and observed benefit of ACE inhibition in various settings such as hypertension, ischemic heart disease, and progressive renal damage together with recognition that ACE inhibition augments bradykinin levels. That some of the antihypertensive effects, local vasodilatory effects, vascular remodeling effects, and side effects of ACEI may actually reflect heightened kinin activity has served as an impetus to better delineate the complex interactions of the KKS and RAS. For example, sodium depletion, which activates angiotensin II, also increases bradykinin in the renal interstitium (310). Recently, the angiotensin II stimulation of bradykinin has been found to occur through a non–angiotensin II, type 1 (AT1) receptor, namely the type 2 (AT2) receptor subtype (336). It was postulated that the increased bradykinin levels that typify many pathophysiologic settings such as hypertension, congestive heart failure, and ischemic and toxic renal failure may function to dampen the angiotensin II–induced vasoconstriction. Indeed, therapeutic interventions that target one of the systems can have profound effects on the other, that is, ACE inhibition decreases angiotensin II and increases bradykinin. In this connection, a fall in GFR has been documented in patients treated with ACEI for hypertension or congestive heart failure or to slow progressive renal damage. Importantly, the fall in GFR in response to ACEI in such settings occurs even in the absence of profound systemic hypotensin (205, 63) and likely reflects ACEI's effect to inhibit kininase activity, which leads to accumulation of bradykinin, which in turn has specific effects on the glomerular microcirculation. Bradykinin preferentially decreases efferent arteriolar tone, which has the effect of lowering intraglomerular capillary hydraulic pressure with the net effect of lowering glomerular filtration (165). ACEI-induced hypofiltration in a water-deprived animal model was shown to be ameliorated by treatment with a bradykinin B2-receptor antagonist, Hoe-140. Notably, inhibition of angiotensin without augmenting bradykinin with a specific type I angiotensin II receptor antagonist did not decrease GFR. It is interesting in this connection that the Evaluation of Losartan in the Elderly (ELITE) Trial, which compared safety and efficacy of the ACEI, captopril, and losartan, an angiotensin type 1 receptor antagonist, in elderly patients with heart failure, rather surprisingly found that losartan treatment was associated with less mortality than captopril (255). It was postulated that captopril-induced elevation in bradykinin-stimulated release of norepinephrine contributed to the untoward events.

The KKS and RAS are linked in complex interactions on multiple layers so that the systems appear to counterbalance each other (Fig. 4). There appear to be several links related to concurrent generation and metabolism of effector ligands. Thus, PRCP activates prekallikrein and also converts angiotensin II to angiotensin 1–7, which may have distinct vasodilatory functions (297). Kallikrein can liberate bradykinin from kininogen, but also activates prorenin to renin. As has already been detailed, ACE converts angiotensin I to the prime vasoconstrictor of the RAS, angiotensin II, and at the same time serves as the main degrading enzyme for bradykinin. Through interaction with AT1, Ang II produces vasoconstriction and aldosterone stimulation. Through interaction with AT2, how-

ever, Ang II results in vasodilatation, a response blocked by B2 receptor antagonsism. Thus, through mechanisms not fully understood, AT2 stimulation leads to bradykinin liberation and B2-receptor–mediated vasodilatation. Notably AT2 stimulation did not cause vasodilatation in Brown Norway Katholiek rats deficient in kininogen (155). Importantly, other authors have shown that B2 knockout mice still retain the ability to produce nitric oxide after AT2 stimulation; B1 receptor was not investigated in this model, however, leaving open the possibility that B1R may be stimulated by AT2 as well (1). Receptor interactions have been documented between the KKS and RAS as well. Thus, angiotensin 1-7 may function to resensitize the B2 receptor, a process which has been shown to augment baroreflex sensitivity in conscious Wistar rats (43, 65, 162, 333). ACE inhibitors also appear to participate in resensitizing the B2 receptor through induction of cross talk between ACE and the B2 receptor (202). In addition, recent evidence suggests that chronic ACE inhibitor therapy will induce B1R and that ACE inhibitors can themselves act as B1R agonists, which may have particular relevance for cardiovascular disorders (103, 137). Another important point of interaction of the KKS and RAS involves formation of heterodimers between AT1 and the B2 receptor, a recently recognized phenomenon of G-protein–coupled receptors. AT1/B2 heterodimers enhance AT1 signaling, increasing Ang II–induced inositol phosphatases as well as Ang II–induced increase in intracellular calcium, while lessening bradykinin signaling. One pathophysiologic ramification of AT1/B2 heterodimers is seen in preeclamptic women who have four- to fivefold elevation in levels of B2 on their platelets and omental vessels compared with normotensive pregnant women, with a corresponding increase in AT1/B2 heterodimers and Ang II signaling (2, 3, 107). On balance, the KKS appears to counterbalance the actions of the RAS, although there may be particular settings in which KKS receptor machinery is drafted to serve the purposes of the RAS.

As noted previously, even at baseline, kinins regulate papillary blood flow, which is important in kinin-induced natriuresis and diuresis. Thus, diuresis and natiuresis following ACEI or corticosterone administration are accompanied by increased endogenous bradykinin levels and papillary blood flow. Bradykinin blockers lessened the diuretic/natriuretic response to ACEI or corticosterone (88).The kinin-induced reduction in tubule reabsorption was shown by micropuncture to occur at or beyond the distal nephron, which parallels the availability of the B2 receptors. Conversely, absence of the B2 receptor in mice results in an enhanced urinary oncentrating capacity compared to normal control animals. Kinin modulation of electrogenic ion transport in renal papillary collecting tubule cells may, at least in part, be mediated by prostaglandins, in particular, prostaglandin E_2. Moreover, this effect occurs only on the luminal side of the cortical collecting duct cells, which may enhance the natriuretic actions of kinins since prostaglandin E_2 inhibits reabsorption in isolated perfused rabbit collecting ducts (Fig. 3). Much of the

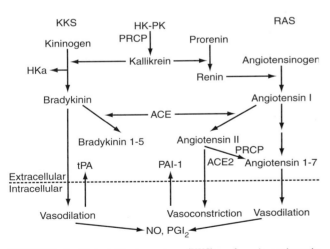

FIGURE 4 Kinin-kalikrein system (KKS) and renin-angiotensin system (RAS) relationships/interactions. HK, high-molecular weight kininogen; PK, prekallikrein; PRCP, prolylcarcoxypeptidase; HKa, plasma kallikrein-cleaved, high-molecular weight kininogen free of bradykinin; ACE, angiotensin-converting enzyme; ACE2, angiotensin converting enzyme 2; tPA, tissue plasminogen activator; PAI-1, plasminogen activator inhibitor-1; NO, nitric oxide; PGI_2, prostaglandin I_2 or prostacyclin. (From Schmaier AH. The kallikrein-kinin and the renin-angiotensin systems have a multilayered interaction. *Am J Physiol Regul Integr Comp Physiol* 2003;285: R1–R13, with permission)

systemic and renal vascular actions of kinins occur through NO and, to a lesser extent, prostaglandins. In addition, kinins have a reciprocal relationship with the renin-angiotensin system in terms of activation and functions. Kinins also interact with other substances. Thus, kallidin inhibits vasopressin-stimulated water permeability, whereas vasopressin stimulates kallikrein excretion. Kallikrein has been shown to stimulate both the production and the metabolism of atrial natriuretic peptide, which is localized in the same nephron segments as the kinin-kallikrein system. Thus, the kinin-kallikrein system may act to regulate the local effect of atrial natriuretic peptide. Taken together these studies indicate that the kinins per se, and through several other cytokines, are important regulators of renal hemodynamics and excretory function (Fig. 3).

Pathophysiologic Implications of the Kinin-Kallikrein System

Infusion of exogenous kinins consistently causes vasodilation, which is in large part dependent on the NO released from endothelial cells. Indeed, bradykinin rather causes vasoconstriction in vessels with damaged endothelium. These observations reiterate the consensus that kinin actions are particularly relevant in pathophysiologic conditions (47, 110, 113, 116, 200). For example, it is widely held that although kinins may not be pivotal in regulating normal blood pressure, they appear particularly important in hypertensive states. This notion is supported by observations in the kininogen-deficient Brown Norway Katholiek rat. At baseline, this strain has normal blood pressure but in response to a saline challenge appears to have impairment in sodium and fluid excretion (125, 157, 193). This impairment is believed to underlie the exaggerated hypertensive response to sodium chloride loading and has been offered as a potential pathophysiologic consequence of impairment in the kinin-kallikrein system. Similar salt sensitivity is seen in B2-receptor knockout mice in which an exaggerated increase in blood pressure is seen with either salt loading or angiotensin II infusion. Moreover, the connection in hypertension and end-organ damage is stronger in B2-receptor knockout mice as they develop heart failure with age, ventricular hypertrophy with loss of myocytes, and myocardial fibrosis, findings, which have subsequently been ascribed to unrestrained angiotensin II effects (80, 189). By contrast, B2R transgenic mice have lower blood pressure than wild-type littermates as well as increased urine production and renal function (351) Taken together, these studies indicate that an impaired kinin system can contribute to pathogenesis of hypertension and end-organ damage particularly in settings of sodium excess. Whether such impairment stems from disturbances in vascular or tubular functions of kinins remains to be clarified, although evidence is accruing that impairment of renal kallikrein may be sufficient for hypertension.

Salt-sensitive hypertension has been observed in settings of renal kallikrein loss produced by renal injury (14)

Thus, three models of renal tubulointerstitial disease, namely chronic N-nitro-L-Arginine Methyl Ester (L-NAME) treatment, 5/6 nephrectomy, and protein overload, have all been shown to result in dramatic reduction in immunohistochemical staining for renal kallikrein. In each model, salt-sensitive hypertension has been observed (9, 10, 143, 290). It appears likely that extensive damage in kallikrein-producing structures of the nephron may disrupt the balance between vasoconstrictors and natriuretic vasodilators, thus setting the stage for hypertension. It is noteworthy that subtle loss of renal tubulointerstitial integrity has recently been implicated as a mechanism in the development of essential hypertension in humans, particularly salt-sensitive hypertension (148, 149). Conversely, augmentation of the kinin system provides protection against hypertensive end-organ damage in experimental animals. Thus, spontaneously hypertensive rats (SHR) underwent tail vein injection of the adenoviral vector containing the human kallikrein (HK) gene. HK-transfected rats indeed showed human kallikrein in urine and kidney as well as heart, liver, and spleen. Blood pressure was reduced, as was urine microalbumin. Renal extracellular matrix was 25% of controls. Similar reduction was seen in cardiac fibrosis and there was amelioration of left ventricular hypertrophy (352). Human kallikrein similarly delivered to Dahl salt-sensitive rats fed a 4% NaCl diet also showed amelioration of renal fibrosis as well as augmentation of urinary nitric oxide and cGMP. In addition, HK transfection induced normalization in renal oxidative stress as assessed by NADH and NADPH activity and superoxide formation, likely a consequence of increased nitric oxide. Reactive oxygen species can contribute to the fibrotic process through TGFβ stimulation. Thus, reduced ROS by increased nitric oxide would be expected to lessen TGFβ. In fact, HK-transfected rats did show reduction in renal TGFβ mRNA and protein, thus, contributing to HK's lessening of renal fibrosis (373).

It has been long observed that humans with hypertension show significantly less urinary excretion of kallikrein than those without hypertension, making the kinin system a recurring target of investigation in search for factors contributing to human essential hypertension (77). Whether the changes in urinary and renal kallikrein levels are causal in the hypertension or simply an epiphenomenon in response to elevated blood pressure remains unclear. In normotensive patients, low-salt diet increases urinary kallikrein but lessens serum bradykinin generation. It appears that with sodium restriction, the renal kinin system is activated and counterbalances the sodium-retaining state induced by activation of the renin-angiotensin-aldosterone axis. Hypertensive patients, particularly African Americans, do not show a comparable increase in urinary kallikrein increase in response to low-salt diet. Importantly, even normotensive African Americans fail to increase urinary kallikrein with low-salt diet, a setting characterized by increased aldosterone, which is known to stimulate urinary kallikrein (223). In another study, normotensive African Americans showed only a 20% increase in urinary kallikrein after fludrocortisone, compared with a 130% increase for whites; note this attenuated increase in kallikrein was superimposed on a marked, baseline disparity, with whites having threefold higher renal kallikrein than African Americans (359). This raises the possibility that diminished capacity to augment renal kallikrein may represent an intermediate phenotype for hypertension and as such may predate the onset of hypertension.

Recently, polymorphisms of the 5′ flanking region of the human tissue kallikrein gene, which could underlie person-to-person differences in renal and urinary kallikrein levels, have been described. Between −133 and −121 upstream from the transcription initiation site, more than 10 haplotype alleles have been defined that encompass both the length and single-nucleotide substitutions found there (KLK1 [−130]G_N). Reporter construct assays have suggested reduced kallikrein promoter activity for alleles D and H. There appear to be wide racial differences with alleles C, D, E, F, I, and P, comprising 40% of the alleles detected in African Americans but only 3% of white alleles (314) Overrepresentation of the K allele was seen in hypertensive end-stage renal disease (ESRD) patients, though no relationship was seen for diabetic ESRD patients (370). Among Taiwanese children developing chronic renal insufficiency (CRI) after vesicoureteral reflux (compared with those who maintained normal renal function), overrepresentation of the K allele was seen again with threefold increase noted. Moreover, among those with CRI, patients with the A allele of KLK1 had significantly higher left ventricular mass index at age 18 years compared with the other alleles (175). This is intriguing as it recalls the finding that B2-receptor knockout mice developed left ventricular hypertrophy and cardiomyopathy.

Interestingly, a polymorphism in the promoter of the human B2-receptor gene has been identified consisting of a C→T transition at −58 bp, the C allele being significantly more frequent in hypertensive African Americans than in normotensive controls. Multivariate analysis revealed an odds ratio of 9 for hypertension for the C allele, even after adjusting for age, weight, and family history of hypertension (100). Some evidence, albeit in reporter constructs in transfected cells, suggests that C^{-58}→T polymorphism may indeed impact B2R transcriptional rate (41). Most recent evidence further indicates an impact of B2 C^{-58}→T polymorphism in baroreflex sensitivity in untreated hypertensive adults. These authors showed a progressive decline in baroreflex sensitivity in relation to number of C alleles; that is, the C allele is associated with less alteration in pulse interval for a given change in blood pressure (209). This is especially interesting considering the dependence of the kinin system on nitric oxide together with recent observations that NO synthetase inhibition induces baroreceptor dysfunction in humans (317).

All components of the kinin system are present in the vasculature. Although vasodilatation is a prime activity of the kinin system, kinin functions are now thought to encompass increased circulation through angiogenesis as well.

Ischemia of the mouse hind limb increases mRNA for tissue kallikrein, B2 receptor, and B1 receptor by 3.3-fold, 3.5-fold, and 7.5–fold, respectively, which reiterates the role of B1 receptor in injurious settings. Interestingly, the native angiogenic response to hind limb ischemia was blunted by chronic infusion of B1 receptor antagonist (but not B2 receptor antagonist). These authors further used an adenoviral vector for gene transfer of the human kallikrein gene (Ad. hTK) into skeletal muscle of mice previously submitted to limb ischemia. The native angiogenic response to ischemia was augmented, and hemodynamic recovery was accelerated. Importantly, histologic analysis of skeletal muscle from Ad.hTK-treated mice showed increased capillary density (79). Diabetes mellitus is characterized by propensity to peripheral vascular disease. In streptozotocin-treated diabetic mice, impaired reparative angiogenesis has been documented as failure to augment skeletal muscle arterioles and capillaries after hind limb ischemia. Prophylactic gene therapy with Ad.hTK in diabetic mice normalized their inadequate ischemia-induced increase in arterioles and capillaries. Further, perfusion of ischemic limbs was increased to the same level as nondiabetic controls (78).

The role of the kinin system in angiogenesis is also seen in pathologic settings in which angiogenesis is not reparative, but rather deleterious. Thus, kininogen-deficient Brown Norway Katholiek rats, when injected with Walker 256 carcinoma cells into dorsal subcutaneous tissues, show less tumor angiogenesis and smaller tumor size than control kininogen-replete rats. In these control animals, treatment with B2-receptor antagonist (but not B1-receptor antagonist) likewise impaired tumor growth and angiogenesis. As expected, B2-receptor knockout mice similarly showed impaired angiogenesis of implanted tumor cells, indicating a dependence on the host kinin system for the angiogenesis necessary for tumor invasion. Notably, host stromal fibroblasts cultured from both Brown Norway Katholiek rats and their kininogen-replete controls both showed an increase in VEGF through the B2 receptor when treated with bradykinin in vitro, indicating intact bradykinin signaling mechanisms in kininogen-deficient animals. Moreover, VEGF is thus, demonstrated to be a prime mediator of kinin-induced angiogenesis (138). Studies with a monoclonal antibody to HMW kininogen (C11C1) have given similar results. Thus, C11C1 significantly inhibited growth of human colon carcinoma cells in a nude mouse xenograft assay and was accompanied by a reduction in mean microvascular density. These observations were not due to a direct tumor effect as in vitro treatment of tumor cells with C11C1 showed no reduction in growth. Interestingly the antibody targets domain 5 of kininogen, one of two domains essential for endothelial cell binding, reiterating the importance of kininogen for initiation of kinin release (313). Bradykinin-increased capillary permeability has recently been used to facilitate delivery of chemotherapy through the blood–brain barrier to central nervous system tumors using the synthetic bradykinin analog lobradimil. In a rodent glioma model, delivery of carboplatin to the tumor was doubled with lobradimil. A phase 2 clinical trial of lobradimil in humans, although potentially limited by inadequate dosing, showed only a trend toward improvement in time to tumor progression. Conversely, bradykinin antagonism shows promise at limiting cerebral tissue edema following ischemia or trauma (81, 259, 372).

Aside from hemodynamic, vascular, and tubular effects, kinins are powerful mediators of inflammation. Increased kinin occurs in many chronic inflammatory diseases including asthma, arthritis, inflammatory bowel disease, rhinitis, and shock associated with sepsis or pancreatitis. In these settings, kinins cause vasodilation, promote pain, and increase capillary permeability and edema. Vasculitis is likewise characterized by abnormal vessel permeability, inflammation, leukocyte influx, and tissue damage. In this connection, serum from children with vasculitis has recently been shown to possess heightened kininogen-degrading capabilities and 30-fold higher bradykinin levels than controls. Moreover, kinins were demonstrated in inflamed skin and kidneys, particularly seen on the luminal side of glomerular capillaries (151). Whether kinin activation in this setting is primary or secondary, pharmacologic manipulation has the potential to lessen inflammatory symptoms.

Exogenous activation of kinins by contact system activation on negatively charged artificial membranes can also trigger these changes (341). Anaphylaxis during hemodialysis was observed in patients dialyzed against a polyacrylonitrile (PAN) membrane (299). Although other hemodialysis membranes have been shown to activate Hageman factor (factor XII), PAN led to earlier and more significant formation of activated Hageman factor and kallikrein after contact with blood than other membranes. PAN thus led to more pronounced generation of bradykinin and likelihood of symptomatic hypotension, especially noted in patients also receiving ACE inhibitors. A related biocompatible membrane, AN69 (acrylonitrile-sodium methallyl sulfonate), used for hemodialysis and hemofiltration, has also been shown to augment bradykinin more than other membranes (while complement activation and histamine release are unaffected) (345). The AN69 reaction may be particularly relevant in pediatric patients in whom small blood volume may necessitate priming of the extracorporeal circuit with blood. Membrane exposure to blood, especially at the relatively acidic pH of banked blood, thus allows for bradykinin formation in the circuit and infusion into the patient at initiation of hemofiltration. Overwhelming hypotension has been noted in critically ill children initiated on hemofiltration with AN69, which was immediately reversed by withdrawal from the hemofiltration circuit. This reaction has been prevented by saline circuit prime and concomitant transfusion of red cells directly to the patient, thus avoiding blood and membrane contact before starting therapy (42).

The pathophysiology of sepsis is also strongly linked to the kinin system. Exposure to both bacterial LPS and inflammatory interleukins upregulate expression of the B1

receptor (198, 253). This may be particularly relevant to the prolonged nature of the hypotensive response in sepsis as B1 receptor (as opposed to the constitutive B2 receptor) does not rapidly desensitize but has more long lasting effects in response to ligand signaling (198, 206) Also, some bacterial components appear to possess requisite protease activity to liberate kinins (127, 142). Evidence also suggests that certain gram negative bacteria possess surface bacterial proteins sufficient for activation of the contact system of kinin generation. Thus, *E. coli* and *Salmonella* strains possessing the proteins curli and thin, respectively (but not mutants lacking these proteins), have been shown to bind radiolabeled factor XI, factor XII (Hageman factor), prekallikrein, and kininogen. Curli/fimbriae-expressing strains are able to hydrolyze factor XII and prekallikrein and to liberate bradykinin when incubated with human plasma. When curli-expressing *E. coli* bacteria were inoculated into mice, clotting was inhibited, which corresponded to an almost complete depletion of fibrinogen. Kinins thus released at the site of infection increase vascular permeability and may facilitate penetration and spreading of bacteria into surrounding tissues, while contributing to reduction in circulating blood volume and hypotension (128, 243).

ENDOTHELINS

In 1985 Hickey et al. detected an endothelium-originating vasoconstrictor (129). In 1988, Yanagisawa et al. (364) generated great excitement with the isolation and cloning of this substance, named, endothelin (ET). In addition to its unprecedented vasoconstrictive potency, ET's effects were found to be exceptionally long-lasting, such that a single bolus produced a pressor response that lasted for hours! An extensive array of actions was soon ascribed to ET. Besides vasoconstriction, ET was found to modulate inotropy and chronotropy, bronchoconstriction, neurotransmission, regulate other hormones and cytokines, act as a mitogen, and stimulate hypertrophy and cellular proliferations—all important processes that are perturbed in a variety of pathophysiologic settings. These characteristics attracted interdisciplinary research interest in both academia and industry.

History

The history of endothelin is explosive and contrasts other vasoactive substances such as bradykinin, whose structural/function characteristics emerged slowly over decades. This striking contrast underscores the tremendous strides made in scientific methodologies and tools in recent years. Endothelin, like many other substances, was first recognized in cell culture supernatant, in this case in the media from porcine endothelial cells. However, Yanagisawa's initial description (364) not only isolated the peptide but cloned the gene and, on the basis of the complement DNA (cDNA) sequencing, predicted the amino acid sequence for preendothelin. They went on to describe the physiologic effects of ET infusion showing it to be some 10 times more potent than angiotensin II (ANG II), vasopressin, or neuropeptide Y. Endothelin was soon renamed endothelin-1 (ET-1), since it was found to belong to a family of functionally and structurally related peptides (ET-1, ET-2, and ET-3) that also included the sarafotoxins (SRTX-a, SRTX-b , SRTX-c, and SRTX-e) from the venom of the Israeli burrowing asp (143). Within a year, much of the structure of the isopeptides, their genes, regulation of gene expression, and signal transduction were defined. In 1990, two simultaneous papers described the cloning of the ETA and ETB receptors (12, 289), and within the next 2 years there was extensive characterization of the synthetic pathway and development of peptide and more recently nonpeptide antagonists. In 1994, genetic engineering produced ET-1– and ET-3–deficient mice and endothelin converting enzyme was cloned (28, 58, 133, 172, 254, 298). These discoveries expanded the biologic importance of endothelins and their role in diseases such as systemic and pulmonary hypertension, heart disease, renal failure, cancer as well as congenital abnormalities of craniofacial development, thoracic blood vessels, enteric neurons and melanocytes. More recent technological advances that permit cell-specific (neurons) and regional (collecting duct, cardiomyocytes) deletions in the ET actions have further defined and expanded the role for ET in systemic hypertension, cardiac hypertrophy, fluid balance, and pain (7, 105, 124, 308). While several studies of the pharmacological antagonism of ET actions are ongoing, in 2001, the orally active ETA/ETB receptor antagonist, bosentan, was approved by the U.S. Food and Drug Administration (FDA) as a therapeutic modality for pulmonary hypertension.

Biochemistry and Pharmacokinetics

The original endothelin, a 21–amino acid peptide discovered in endothelial cells, was soon recognized to be one of at least three isoforms, named ET-1, ET-2, and ET-3. Unless otherwise stated, this chapter describes studies of ET-1 which is the most abundant isoform. ET-2 differs from ET-1 by two amino acids, and ET-3 differs from ET-1 in six of the 21 amino acid residues (115, 143). All three members possess two interachain disulfide bridges and a hydrophobic C-terminal tail. The structure of ET can be regarded in terms of two distinct subdomaines: the N-terminal disulfide loop, which differs among the ET-isoforms, and the conserved C-terminal linear region. The C-terminal Trp21 residue and the two intramolecular disulfide bridges are particularly important for ET-1's effects as removal of the Trp21 residue or cleavage of the disulfide bridges reduces ET-1's vasoconstrictive potency. Deletion of the C-terminal tail causes even further reduction in the constriction. Modification of the N-terminus of ET-1 also lessens its vasoconstriction. These structural domains also dictate, at least in part, interactions of the ET peptide with the ET receptors. The C-terminal portion, particularly the Glu10-Trp21

sequence of the ET molecules, recognizes and interacts with the relatively nonselective ETB receptor. On the other hand, the a-amino group of the Cys1 residue and the N-terminal tertiary (structure including the disulfide bridges) are required for binding to the highly selective ETA receptor. Specific domains within the individual receptors also affect the ligand-receptor interactions (287).

The isoforms of ET are widely distributed among organs in different patterns (68, 115, 164, 204, 279, 354). The most widely distributed, best studied, and the most powerful of the isoforms is the one that was originally isolated from cultured endothelial cells, namely, ET-1. In the kidney, besides endothelial cells, mesangial, glomerular, and tubule epithelial cells all produce ET-l. Circulating cells also secrete ET-1: Macrophages are a source for ET-1, and neutrophils can convert exogenous big ET-1 into the mature form and may, through this mechanism, contribute to pathophysiologic processes. ET-2 has been detected in normal and neoplastic tissue and has recently been linked to macrophage infiltration and neoplastic invasion (117, 118). Finally, ET-3 predominates in the brain and has also been found in various parts of the kidney (190). Each isoform is encoded by a distinct gene: preproendothelin-1 (preproET-l) is on chromosome 6p23-24, preproET-2 on chromosome 1p34, and preproET-3 on chromosome 20q13.2-13.3 (59, 143, 145, 160, 281, 287). The human ET-1 contains five exons and spans 6.8 kilobases (kb) of DNA. Several regulatory elements have been identified: the 5′ flanking region contains consensus-binding sequence motifs for activation protein-1 and nuclear factor-1 through which ANG II and TGF-β, respectively, activate ET-1 expression. There are four copies of the hexanucleotide CTGGGA, the acute-phase reaction regulatory element that induces mRNA under stress conditions and has been postulated to be a mechanism for increased preproET-1 mRNA in disease a states. As described in subsequent sections, a potentially crucial component in fueling ET's effects in pathophysiologic settings is also under transcriptional regulation. Thus, the ET peptide itself is a powerful stimulus for augmenting its own gene expression (146, 282). Whether this autoinduction of ET synthesis is under the control of unique regulatory sites that are distinct from the regulating synthesis following non-ET stimuli (ischemia, thrombin, etc.) remains an unanswered issue. In the 3′ region there is a feature that is conserved among different species, namely a two-AUUUA sequence, which is known to mediate selective mRNA degradation and likely accounts for the short half life of the ET mRNA and the ability of cyclohexamide to cause superinduction.

Figure 5 shows the process by which the mature ET peptide is generated (22, 23, 58, 64, 82, 109, 123, 232, 298, 306). The human prepro-ET-1 gene encodes a 212–amino acid prepropeptide. The prepro-ET-1 is then cleaved by an endopeptidase specific for a pair of furin-like dibasic amino acids, forming a biologically inactive 38–amino acid intermediary structure, big ET-1. Subsequently, the intermediary form is cleaved into the mature ET-1 peptide by freeing the COOH

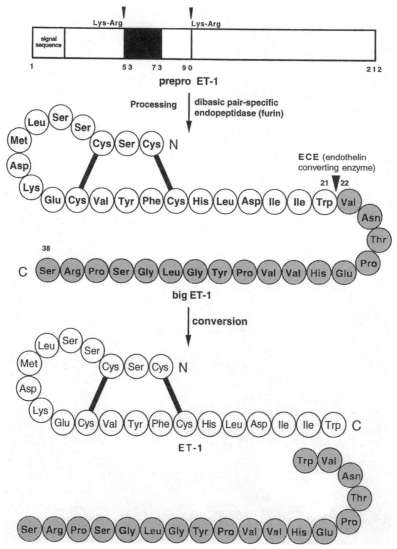

FIGURE 5 Biosynthesis of endothelin-1 (ET-1). The precursor preproET-1 is proteolytically cleaved by dibasic pair-specific endopeptidase to form the intermediary from big ET-1. Big ET-1 is then specifically cleaved by endothelin-converting enzyme (ECE) to form the mature peptide. (From Goto K, Hama H, Kasuya Y. Molecular pharmacology and pathophysiological significance of endothelin. *Jpn J Pharmacol* 1996;72:261–290, with permission)

terminus of the 21-residue. This step requires cleavage between Trp21-Val22 of big ET-1 by endothelin-converting enzyme (ECE). In vivo, big ET has only 1% of the contractile activity of the mature peptide and stresses the importance of ECE which is the rate-limiting enzyme in effecting ET full activity and also provides a potential point for interruption of ET actions. While various peptides were initially considered candidates for ECE, the metallopeptidase inhibitor phosphoramidon was found to inhibit the conversion of big ET-1 to the mature ET-1 peptide. In 1994, three groups simultaneously reported the amino acid sequence of ECE, named ECE-1 (58, 298, 306). ECE-2 was identified in 1995 as having different pH sensitivity from ECE-1. Currently, there are seven isoforms of ECE identified: ECE-1a, ECE-1b, ECE-1c, ECE-1d, ECE-2a, ECE-2b, and

ECE-3. ECE-1 and -2 are membrane metalloproteases that selectively cleave the tryptophan-valine bond in the carboxy terminal of big ET-1. Alternative splice variants of ECE-1 differ in their N-terminus but are similar in their substrate specificity (23, 337, 340). ECE-1 is localized in the plasma cell membrane in various tissues while ECE-2 is localized in the trans-Golgi network most notably in neural tissue (123, 232, 298, 361). ECEs can hydrolyze other peptides including bradykinin, substance P, and insulin. Conversely, big ET-1 can be cleaved by other enzymes. Chymases cleave ET-1 at the tyrosine 31-glycine 32 bond to yield a 31–amino acid peptide that constricts smooth muscle cells of the trachea (232). Matrix metalloprotease 2 cleaves big ET-1 at the glycine 32-leucine 33 peptide to produce a peptide that constricts mesenteric arteries (89). ECE-3 is specific for big

ET-3 and was identified and purified from bovine iris microsomes but its role remains unclear.

Both big ET-1 and the mature ET-1 peptide are present primarily in secretory vesicles indicating that they are released in a constitutive manner and regulated by changes in gene expression through a cyclic-AMP–independent mechanism (37, 122, 280). However, presence of these peptides in Weibel Palade bodies also suggests some regulated secretory pathway that responds to shear stress, TGFβ, interleukin-1 (IL-1), and AII. Innumerable factors have been shown to stimulate ET production including other peptides such as AII, vasopressin, adrenalin, insulin, cortisol, IL-1, TGFβ, thrombin, glucose, low-density lipoprotein, hypoxia, endotoxin, low-shear stress, and endothelin itself (25, 36, 38, 39, 64, 68, 101, 141, 146, 164, 185, 188, 196, 204, 213, 271, 279, 340, 354). ET-1 synthesis can also be downregulated by a number of factors including prostacyclin, NO, atrial natriuretic peptide, heparin, estrogen, and high-shear stress (36, 38, 101, 141). These observations underscore the central role of ET-1 in biology and in disease states.

Endothelin Receptors

The existence of several ET isoforms with varying agonist potencies in different tissues, together with differences in binding characteristics for the individual peptides, suggested that there is more than one receptor. There are two receptors, ETA and ETB (12, 61, 132, 212, 287, 288, 289). Pharmacologic studies imply the existence of other receptor subtypes, however, except for what appears to be an amphibian ETA receptor variant (169), there has been no molecular confirmation for the existence of another mammalian receptor. Indeed, another ET receptor gene is predicted to have little similarity to the two cloned receptors. The known receptors have homology with other heptahelical receptors of the rhodopsin superfamily, with seven transmembrane loops and intracellular actions mediated via signal transducing G proteins. ETA was originally cloned from bovine lung and subsequently from human tissue, contains 427 amino acids, and binds with the rank order of affinities of ET-1 = ET-2 >> ET-3. The human gene for ETA is located on chromosome 4. The ETB receptor was originally cloned in the rat and later in humans, has 442 amino acids, and binds with the order of affinities of ET-1 = ET-2 = ET-3. Sakamoto et al. (28) suggested distinct subdomains of the ET receptors, which determine their relative selectivity for ETA antagonists and ETB agonists. Transmembrane domains (TMDs) I, II, III, and VII, together with the intervening loops of the ETA receptor, were selective for the ETA antagonist (BQ123). TMDs IV, V, and VI, with the adjacent 109ps of the ETB receptor, were selective for the ETB agonist (ET-3). These authors also suggested that the ligand-receptor interaction of the ET system depends on both the ET peptide and receptor, so that the N-terminal loop of the peptide and TMDs IV through VI

with adjacent loops determine isopeptide/subtype selectivity, whereas the C-terminal linear portion of the peptide and TMDs I through III and VII, plus the adjacent loops, determine the binding. The 5′ regulatory regions of the human ETA and ETB receptor genes do not have a canonical TATA or CCAAT box suggesting that transcriptional initiation can originate at many different sites (12, 289). Alternative splicing of the ETB receptor has been noted in brain, placenta, lung, and heart. These ETB receptor isoforms have been postulated to differentiate ETB receptors responsible for release of nitric oxide versus ETB receptors responsible for vasoconstriction (309).

The diversity of ET's effects among a variety of tissues likely reflects differences in the distribution and functions of the receptor subtypes as well as different signal transduction pathways. Endothelins bind very tightly to their receptors and are slow to dissociate. ET-1 has been shown to remain associated with its receptors up to 30 hours after endocytosis (348). Following binding, the ligand-receptor complex is internalized and sequestered into lysosomal compartments. During the endocytosis, sequences in the cytoplasmic domain direct the receptors into different trafficking pathways within the cell. ETA receptor cytoplasmic domain signals trafficking toward recycling endosomes, while ETB receptors are targeted to lysosomes for degradation (4, 246). Such differences in trafficking may underlie differences in duration of actions between the receptors. Interestingly, analysis of intracellular trafficking, while confirming that ETB moves to a lysosomal compartment, also shows that the receptor remains remarkably stable, being held together by disulfide bonding for over 17 hours (96). Whether the ETA receptor is similarly or even more resistant to degradation remains to be clarified. In addition to potential differences in cellular handling of each receptor, the biologic effects of ETs are regulated by the promoter regions of each of the receptors (11, 13, 59, 74, 328). Both ETA and ETB receptors have potential SP-I binding sites, four GATA motifs, are G protein–coupled receptors that result in activation of phospholipase Cβ and induction of the ERK/MAPK signaling cascade. Both receptors regulate adenylyl cyclase through G_s, G_i, and G_{12} subfamilies of G proteins. The most generalized path following ET exposure is activation of phospholipase C and hydrolysis of phosphatidyl inositol to a rapid but transient increase in intracellular calcium. This phase is not dependent on extracellular calcium. By contrast, the later, more sustained increase in calcium is linked to the opening of membrane calcium channels and influx of extracellular calcium. This influx is mediated through pertussis toxin–sensitive guanosine triphosphate (GTP)-binding protein. The phospholipase C activation causes a sustained accumulation of 1,2-diacylglycerol, which activates protein kinase C, which in turn potentiates the calcium-mediated contraction and stimulates the sodium–hydrogen ion exchange pump to alkalinize the intracellular pH. The adenosine triphosphate (ATP)-sensitive potassium channel is also stimulated, further increasing intracellular calcium. ET-1 activates phospholipase A_2 and thus increases arachidonic acid metabolites including prostacyclin and thromboxanes A_2. ET-1's activation of phospholipase D contributes to sustaining diacylglycerol accumulation, which leads to prolonged activation of protein kinase C. Endothelin's mitogenic effects are well recognized and have been confirmed in a variety of different cell lines. The mechanism for this effect includes induction of several proto-oncogenes including c-fos, c-myc, and c-jun. The intracellular pathways have been postulated to include sequential activation of raf-1, mitogen-activated protein kinase (MAPK), and S_6 kinase II. While many of the cellular activities are mediated though ET-1 interactions with specific receptors located on the cell surface, functional ETA and ETB receptors have also been found on nuclei in cardiac ventricular myocytes suggesting "intracrine" regulation of ET-1 actions (36).

Both receptors are extensively distributed throughout all the organ systems of the body. ETA is found in vascular smooth muscle cells and is the predominant subtype in many organs. It is not detected in endothelial cells. In general, the ETA receptor modulates vasoconstriction, cellular proliferation, and matrix deposition (61). The ETB receptor is found primarily in endothelial cells but has also been found in vascular smooth muscle cells (61). ETB receptor mediates release of prostacyclin (PGI_2) and especially NO, which have been viewed as offsetting the vasoconstrictive and mitogenic effects of ET-1 (344). The cellular mechanism for this effect is through ETB-mediated phosphoinositide breakdown via the pertussis toxin–sensitive G protein, which increases intracellular calcium and activates the constitutive Ca^{2+}/calmodulin-dependent NO synthase (180). A critical role for heteromeric G-protein subunit signaling to protein kinaseB/Akt phosphorylation was shown in the activation of NO synthase (181). NO can modulate the actions of ET at several steps. First, NO can suppress production of ET, possibly by blunting the increase in intracellular calcium (38). Further, NO reduces the affinity of the receptor for its ligand (112). Since the unusually strong association of the ET receptor complexes is believed to contribute to the notoriously long-lasting effects of ET, the potential modulation by NO constitutes an important mechanism for termination of ET activity. NO may also interfere with a postreceptor pathway for calcium mobilization, thus providing an additional mechanism by which NO lessens ET's actions. However, ETB also appears to have direct vasoconstrictory actions, including vasoconstriction of pulmonary and renal circulations (215, 309). As noted previously, isoforms of the ETB receptor have been postulated to mediate constrictive effects versus NO and PGI_2 synthesis. Finally, ETB clears circulating ET-1 by internalizing then degrading the peptide (99) and regulates its own gene expression by enhancing prepro-ET-1 synthesis and mRNA stability (146, 282).

The relative number of receptors can be modulated by physiologic and pathophysiologic conditions. For example, increasing passage of aortic vascular smooth muscle cells

decreases ETA receptors, whereas the ETB receptors are upregulated (325). By contrast, renal injury induced by obstruction or cyclosporine that did not to affect the ETA population increased ETB receptors (217, 326), while prostate cancer has been found to have increased ETA receptor and decreased or absent ETB receptor (111, 237). Such modulation in the relative density of each receptor carries great import in the net biologic effect since each receptor has different, and in many cases, diametrically opposing effects. Further, modulation the receptor populations may be of crucial importance in the efficacy of the specific antagonists versus combined antagonism used in clinical diseases (see the following sections).

Additional insights into receptor functions come from studies of genetically mutated mice. Targeted deletion of the ETB receptor causes aganglionic megacolon and abnormal coat pigmentation (28, 133, 261). Notably, the same phenotype was observed in mice whose ET-3 gene was disrupted and reiterates the close relationship of this ligand and receptor (28). Genetic abnormalities in ET-3 or ETB receptor have also been shown in patients with Hirschsprung disease, which is taken to be an abnormality arising from a defect in migration or differentiation of neural crest cells. A frameshift mutation of ET-3 has been reported in congenital central hypoventilation syndrome in humans (37). The mutation consisted of an insertion of a single nucleotide, which caused a premature stop codon and the truncation of the last 41 amino acids of the protein. Further, teratogenicity studies during the preclinical phase of ETA receptor antagonists revealed developmental abnormalities that overlapped with the phenotype in mice with gene knockout for preproendothelin-1, namely, disturbed craniofacial, cardiovascular, and pharyngeal structures (56, 172, 230, 245). Notably, defects in the ETA and ETB receptors have been linked to human Pierre Robin and Treacher Collins syndromes, which are characterized by craniofacial abnormalities (245). These studies reiterate the close relationship between ET-1 and ETA receptors and emphasize their unexpected importance in craniofacial bone development. Notably, ETA receptors are located on osteoblasts, which may be important in adult bone remodeling associated with osteoblastic bone metastases (221, 233).

Overall, the extensive distribution of receptors is paralleled by multiple sources for ET production. The colocalization of peptide and receptors emphasizes the potential importance of paracrine/autocrine mechanisms for ET actions. Indeed, most of the endothelium-derived ET-1 peptide goes in the basolateral, not circulatory direction, where it can interact in a paracrine fashion with receptors on the underlying smooth muscle cells to modulate contractile/proliferating responses to ET-1 (349). Similar observations have been made in tubule epithelial cells where the majority of the ET-1 synthesis is directed to the abluminal (not urinary) side. These observations provide an effective mechanism to localize ET's potent actions to discrete areas. It should be noted that, although epithelial cells and particularly endothelial cells produce a lot of ET, vascular smooth muscles also produce ET-1. Despite lower production, vascular smooth muscles are relatively more abundant than the other types of cells and may contribute substantially to local concentrations of ET-1 in discrete areas. The importance of abluminal secretion was underscored by the findings that more prompt and pronounced vasoconstriction occurred when ET-1 was applied abluminally than when it was applied inside the vessel (240). This type of discrete compartmentalization has several implications. First, this may serve to contain the effects of such a powerful and potentially destructive substance such as ET to damaged areas. In this regard, the concentration of circulating ET-1 in a variety of normal and numerous disease states ranges from 1 to 5 pg/mL, which is below the threshold associated with biologic effects. These findings confirm the consensus that ET functions predominantly as a paracrine/autocrine substance and that its effects are not necessarily dependent on circulating ET levels. Compartmentalization also suggests that susceptibility to ET-1 may vary among tissues and organs, depending on the ability of that tissue to increase or lessen ET production, as well as the distribution and the type of ET receptors prevailing within the tissue. Thus, an autocrine loop may amplify potentially destructive effects of ET-1 via autoinduction of its own synthesis. Conversely, ET-1, through the ETB receptor may promote clearance of the peptide as well as stimulate PGI_2 and NO synthesis that would abrogate its effects.

Renal Physiology

Endothelins affect many aspects of renal function including vasoconstriction, tubule reabsorption, cellular proliferation and matrix deposition. Most conspicuously, endothelins vasoconstrict the renal microcirculation. Although, ET-1 is a powerful vasoconstrictor of all vascular beds, the renal circulation is particularly susceptible to its effects. Pernow et al. (252) measured blood flow in the renal, bronchial, femoral, and coronary vessels and found that the renal vasculature was some 10-fold more sensitive to ET-1 than the other vascular beds. As noted previously, the kidney has several cell types that elaborate ET-1 as well as containing infiltrating inflammatory cells that may further bolster the cumulative production of ET-1 particularly following injury. The cumulative effect of ET-1 activation is vasoconstriction of the microcirculation and glomerular hypofiltration. As in other vascular beds ET-1 mediated vasoconstriction is particularly long lasting. Infusion of ET-1 into one of the branches of the main renal artery in a dose that had no effect on systemic blood pressure or other circulatory parameters caused profound vasoconstriction that lasted for hours (167). The afferent arteriole constricts more in response to ET-1 than the efferent arteriole; however, both contribute to reducing the glomerular plasma flow rate and the rate of filtration. In this study the glomerular capillary ultrafiltration coefficient did not decrease but has been shown in other studies

to fall with higher concentrations of the peptide (17). Recent observations suggest cross-talk between the resident cells of the glomerulus regulates ET-1 activity. Supernatants of cocultured human umbilical vein endothelial cells (HUVECs) together with human mesangial cells contained significantly less ET-1 than HUVEC grown without mesangial cells (184). The study found that the mesangial cells not only increased ET-1 degradation but also had a dramatic effect to lessen mRNA and protein of ECE-1. Interestingly, the AT1 receptor antagonist, losartan, completely abolished the downregulation of ECE-1 in the HUVEC/mesangial cell cultures, while exposure to ANG II alone caused a dose and time/dependent inhibition of ECE-1 expression in these HUVECs. Thus, local ET-1 activity may represent not only cell synthesis but also modulation of this activity by the surrounding cells. Such observations may be important in pathophysiologic settings where damage to one cell type (i.e., mesangial cells) may amplify pro-injurious effects of ET-1 by removing a biologic break on ET-1 activity.

Although the whole kidney is exquisitely sensitive to ET-1 vasoconstriction, intrarenal regional differences exist. The cortical blood flow appears especially sensitive to ET-1 constriction such that most, if not all, of the decrease in total renal blood flow represents reduction in flow to this region. By contrast, the medullary blood flow appears to change very little (66, 86, 168, 242, 265) or even transiently increase following exposure to ET-1 (66, 242, 265). The apparent resistance of the medullary vessels to ET-1 vasoconstriction may reflect the greater expression of the ETB receptor and consequently greater activation of the vasodilatory NO and PGI_2. The importance of intrarenal variation in the activity of the ET system is clearly demonstrated by the recently generated collecting duct-specific knockouts of ET-1 that not only affect tubule reabsorption of sodium and water but also cause systemic hypertension (see following section) (7, 105).

Another aspect of ET-1 actions within the kidney relates to its tubule effects and regulation of salt and water excretion. Tubules elaborate ET-1 and possess ET receptors. Thus, ET-1 can directly regulate tubule function in an autocrine manner. The direct, that is, non-hemodynamic effect of ET-1 on tubule function appears especially relevant in the inner medulla, which contains one of the highest concentrations of ET-1 in the body. The inner medullary collecting duct (IMCD) is the main site for the ET-1 synthesis and has the highest receptor expression within the kidney (158, 262, 339). In vitro, ET-1 inhibits vasopressin-stimulated water flux as well as cyclic-AMP accumulation and osmotic water permeability (195, 162, 227, 327). In IMCDs, ET-1 increases vasopressin V2-receptor expression, an effect that is mediated by the ETB receptor. Although it has long been appreciated that the functional net effect of ET-1 is to reduce fluid reabsorption it was not clear until recently whether this effect was entirely independent of ET-1's hemodynamic effects. Mice expressing Cre recombinase under the control of aquaporin-2 promoter were crossed with mice homozygous for loxP-flanked ET-1 gene to generate collecting duct-specific knockouts for ET-1 (CDET1-KO) (7,105). These CDET1-KO mice were hypertensive and had an impaired ability to excrete a Na load. The authors postulated that the deficiency in collecting duct ET-1 promotes Na and water retention as well as hypertension that reflects impairment in the autocrine activation of ETB receptor and therefore blunts vasopressin-stimulation to accelerate cyclic AMP, decrease Na,K-ATPase, and affect, medullary blood flow (7). These same mice were also shown to have reduced plasma vasopressin levels, enhanced vasopressin responsiveness and reduced acute diuretic response (105). Taken together these observations underscore that ET-1 exerts important nonhemodynamic effects on tubule function that regulate sodium and water excretion. These tubular effects in turn modulate systemic pathophysiologic conditions such as hypertension and may relate to urinary abnormalities observed in other disease states.

Pathophysiologic Implications

The pathophysiologic implications of ET-1 were apparent even from the first report: the powerful and long-lasting vasoconstrictive effects have provided the underpinnings for this idea. These effects initially observed in rats have been reproduced in humans. Infusion of ET-1 into the brachial artery of normal men causes a slowly developing, dose-dependent vasoconstriction and reduction in forearm flow that is sustained for hours after the infusion is stopped (54). Increased ET-1 gene expression and peptide production occur in response to a variety of injurious stimuli. Noteworthy, however, is that this activation can persist for hours, days, and even weeks (95). Since the half-life for prepro-ET-1 mRNA is very short (on the order of minutes), the long-term increase is clearly related to continuous production of new transcripts. Addition of ET-1 peptide caused a dramatic increase in prepro-ET-1 gene expression in mesangial cells (146). The increase was prompt, occurring within 30 minutes, and became maximal at 60 minutes, at which time it was some 450% above baseline levels. The elevation was also persistent such that 24 hours later the signal had not yet returned to prestimulated levels. The increase in gene expression was paralleled by a more than 600% increase in production of the mature peptide. Autoinduction of ET-1 synthesis has been seen in other cell types, including endothelial cells (282). Nuclear transcription runoff analyses revealed that ET-1 significantly increased transcription of the prepro-ET-1 gene. Stabilization of prepro-ET-1 mRNA has also been noted in response to other cytokines. For example, TGF-β increased the half-life of prepro-ET-1 mRNA in Madin-Darby canine kidney cells from 15 to 30 to 45 minutes (131). In bovine aortic endothelial cells, artrial natriuretic peptide increased the half-life of prepro-ET-1 mRNA from 25 minutes to 70 minutes (134).

In addition to vasoconstriction, ET-1 activation stimulates cellular hypertrophy, proliferation and extracellular accumula-tion of matrix which underlies progressive parenchymal destruction in cardiovascular and renal diseases. As noted, the potential importance of ET-1 does not require demonstration of elevated circulating levels of ET, as it is primarily a paracrine system. Moreover, there is ample evidence that even subthreshold concentrations of ET-1 will augment vasoconstriction of other agents such that may as AII, norepinephrine, and serotonin among others. Such cross-talk likely also applies to other potentially important pathophysiologic processes such as enhancement of cellular proliferation and hypertrophy and matrix deposition. Among these, the best studied is the interaction between ANG II and ET-1 (9, 19, 20, 21, 26, 102, 140, 173, 213, 264, 274, 286). Both ANG II and ET-1 have direct effects on all pathophysiologic processes that promote end-organ damage in the heart, blood vessels and kidneys, and each appears to regulate the activity of the other. The AII-ET-1 relationship was first proposed by Lüscher who observed that ANG II increased ET-1 expression in smooth muscle cells from spontaneously hypertensive rates (67). Angiotensin II has been shown to stimulate gene expression and/or ET release by a variety of cultured cells including endothelial, mesangial, and smooth muscle cells (25, 26, 140) as well in kidneys, lungs, and hearts. Systemic hypertension and organ vasoconstriction induced by ANG II has been shown to be attenuated or completely abolished by ETA receptor antagonism suggesting that ET-1 mediates some of the vasoconstriction caused by chronically elevated AII. Notably, the ANG II ET-1 interaction appears sodium dependent because ETA blockade lessens AII-induced hypertension during sodium loading but not during sodium restriction (21). The complexity of interactions between these systems is further underscored by studies that can document the relationship only under specific circumstances. For example, there appears little interaction between ANG II and ET-1 in the two-kidney–one-clip Glodblatt hypertension model or in the renin-dependent hypertensive rat model in which mouse renin is overexpressed TGR (mRen2)27 (29, 154, 179, 277, 293, 322). Neither ETA nor combined ETA/ETB antagonism lessened the systemic blood pressure nor improved structural renal damage in the TGR (mRen2)27 transgenic rat model. By contrast, ANG II receptor blockade dramatically lowered blood pressure, improved renal parenchymal injury, and increased survival of these transgenic mice. Such observations have raised speculations that the ET-ANG II systems interact under specific conditions (277). For example, the magnitude and duration of heightened ANG II may affect stimulation of ET-1 such that persistent and/or exaggerated levels of ANG II are needed to activate the ET system. By contrast, endogenous increase in ANG II may not be sufficient to cause such stimulation of the ET-1 system. The magnitude of blood pressure elevation per se may also modulate ET-1 activation, occurring only with very high systemic blood pressures. Finally, interorgan differences may dictate the sensitivity of the ANG II/ET-1 interactions, being especially sensitive to the relative abundance of ETA vs ETB receptors. This possibility is becoming more widely accepted in view of the increasingly important role ascribed to the ETB receptor in terms of stimulating other cytokines, notably NO. In this connection ACEIs have been shown to increase ETB (but not ETA) gene expression and protein in unilaterally obstructed kidneys (217) as well as in failing hearts (360). The beneficial effects of inhibition of ANG II actions on structural damage were significantly suppressed by concomitant treatment with an ETB receptor antagonist. Similar effect of ACEI was seen in cardiomyopathic hamsters where treatment increased the ETB receptor density (360). These findings would predict that therapy which inhibits ANG II activity would have the additional effect of reducing ET-1 actions and provide synergistic benefit on structural/function abnormalities.

Renal Failure. Activation of ET-1 has been documented in experimental and human acute renal failure (ARF) as well as in chronic renal dysfunction (CRD). ET-1 is elevated in ischemic, cyclosporine, FK-506, myoglobin, contrast media-induced renal damage (95, 114, 154, 184, 278, 325) as well as in acute inflammatory models including immune complex glomerulonephritis, nephrotoxic serum nephritis, and mesangial proliferative glomerulonephritis (68, 126, 186, 279, 375). ET-1 is also elevated in many CRD settings (31, 163, 316) where it is believed to increase cellular hypertrophy, proliferation, and collagen deposition. ET-1 also interacts synergistically with other growth factors, including epidermal growth factor, TGF-α and -β, and platelet-derived growth factor (PDGF) to potentiate cellular proliferation and matrix gene expression, thereby promoting the scarring process. ET-1 increases expression for mRNA for collagen types I, II, and IV and laminin, and, through the ETA receptor, ET-1 induces expression of c-fos and c-myc and fra-1 intermediary genes as well as stimulation of MAPKs, which have been proposed to mediate nuclear signaling and mesangial growth, as well as tyrosine kinases, which are believed to be important regulators of cellular growth and differentiation. In addition to elevating the ET-1 peptide, injurious stimuli can also affect each of the ET receptors (234, 278, 325). Antagonism of ET-1 actions has been seen to lessen functional damage, even in established ARF as well as in renal mass ablation, accelerated passive Heymann nephritis, streptozotocin-induced diabetes, and lupus nephritis (29, 31, 87, 106, 113, 167, 173, 210). Chronic ETA antagonism also lessens renal hypoperfusion and hypofiltration and spares the kidneys from structural damage in the renal ablation model in rats (29). In that study, chronic antagonism of ETA normalized the systemic blood pressure, which may itself have a beneficial effect on progressive functional and structural damage. Even in a nonhypertensive model, that is, chronic cyclosporine nephrotoxicity, glomerular dysfunction can be lessened by ETA or combined ETA/ETB receptor antagonists (136, 166).

These observations have provided the impetus to evaluate antagonism of ET-1 actions in humans. A phase 2 trial of ETA/ETB receptor antagonist, TAK-044, in ischemic ARF was discontinued because of only very limited benefit on renal recovery (182). Another mixed ETA/ETB receptor antagonist, bosentan, showed only limited benefit in protecting against cyclosporine-induce hypoperfusion in normal human volunteers (33). Nonselective ET antagonist, SB209679, given to patients with chronic renal impairment undergoing cardiac angiography also did not protect the kidneys (350). Indeed, treated patients had an increased incidence of contrast media nephrotoxicity. These disappointing results have been interpreted as reflecting differences in magnitude of damage and in receptor distribution between experimental and human renal failure. As in other pathophysiologic settings where ET is predicted to have a central role, the dosing, the choice of specific receptor antagonist and the utility of combining with other therapies offer promise of targeting renal injury. Indeed, the ETA receptor antagonist antisertan is being added to ACEI to evaluate the potential antiproteinuric effect in type II diabetic nephropathy (270).

Systemic Hypertension. The initial observations of ET's remarkable vasoconstrictor effects were complimented by an early report of two patients with malignant hemangioendothelioma who had hypertension and elevated circulating levels of ET-1 (230). Evaluation of the tumor revealed eight times more ET-1 per gram of tissue than in a normal skin. In both cases, excision of the tumor decreased the circulating ET-1 levels and normalized systemic blood pressure. Notably, in one of these patients, recurrence of the tumor was accompanied by increased plasma ET-1 and re-emergence of hypertension. Availability of reliable methodology to measure plasma ET-1 led to many reports of increased circulating ET-1 in patients with secondary hypertension including patients being treated with cyclosporine after transplantation, patients undergoing dialysis and erythropoietin treatment, and patients with sleep-apnea–associated hypertension or preeclampsia (45, 116, 176, 254, 366). Some of these reports describe patients who had already sustained end-organ damage, which raised uncertainty as to whether the hypertension was the cause or the result of elevated levels of circulating ET-1. The relevance of elevated circulating ET-1 in the most common cause of human hypertension remains controversial. Some reports find patients with essential hypertension have increased circulating ET-1 levels (11, 147, 222, 285, 305), whereas others find no correlation between circulating ET-1 and systemic pressure (295, 315, 342). However, findings underscore that circulating ET-1 is affected by several common clinical and biochemical characteristics that may impact interpretation of plasma ET-1 levels in this setting: age (ET-1 increases with age), race (African Americans have higher plasma ET-1 levels), and gender (men have higher levels of ET-1) (85, 211). In addition, low plasma renin activity (PRA), obesity, and insulin resistance have been associated with higher plasma ET levels (11, 147, 176, 250). These characteristics are notable as they overlap with the clinical phenotype of patients with salt-sensitive hypertension.

Salt-sensitivity may identify a subgroup of patients that is especially relevant for ET-1 regulation (76). In this regard, vasoconstrictor and hypertrophic response to ET-1 appears greater in salt-sensitive animal models of hypertension including DOC-salt, aldosterone-induced, Dahl SS, insulin-resistant, and 1K-1C Goldblatt models than salt-independent/renin-dependent models including spontaneously hypertensive rats 2K-1C Goldblatt, L-NAME-induced hypertension, and the (mRen2) 27 transgenic rat (76, 174, 277, 322, 323). Although not uniform (40), there is also accumulating clinical evidence suggesting an important role for ET-1 in salt-sensitive essential hypertension. For example, classification of patients into salt-sensitive and salt resistant groups revealed differences in circulating ET-1 levels, especially during changes in salt balance (75, 90, 91). Classification of hypertensive patients as salt-sensitive, indeterminate, or salt-resistant according to their blood pressure response to salt depletion showed no difference in plasma ET-1 levels. However, acute salt deprivation of these patients caused an 18% increase in plasma ET-1 levels in the salt-sensitive group whereas the salt-resistant group had a 10% reduction in the plasma ET levels from baseline. An indeterminate group did not have a significant change in the plasma ET-1 levels following salt restriction. Notably, the relationship between salt sensitivity of blood pressure and change in plasma ET-1 prevailed across all three groups in this study. It has been postulated that hypertension in the salt-sensitive individuals reflects exaggerated response of the damaged endothelium to salt and or pressure (76, 293). Even as the utility of measuring circulating ET-1 in hypertensive patients remains controversial, it should be underscored that ET-1 elaboration is primarily abluminal, away from the circulation, where its concentration is orders of magnitude higher than plasma. Thus, even a dramatic change in production may only cause a subtle change in ET-1 within the circulation.

As noted previously, ET-1 has major effects on tubule reabsorption of sodium and water that has been recognized as a potentially important mechanism for development and maintenance of systemic hypertension. Urinary ET-1 excretion parallels sodium excretion that is independent of circulating ET-1 and tracks more closely with systemic hypertension circulating ET-1 (30, 195, 283). Renal production of ET-1 is modulated by salt intake and blood pressure (376). Urinary ET-1 decreases with increasing blood pressure in normal as well as hypertensive individuals. This effect is magnified in patients who are salt sensitive (130, 376). The pathophysiologic implications of tubule ET-1 was clarified by the collecting duct-specific knockout of ET-1 (7, 105). The knockout mice had reduced urinary ET-1 excretion. Even on a normal-sodium diet, the animals were hypertensive. On a high-sodium diet, the mice developed worsening hypertension, reduced urinary sodium excretion, and increased weight. Notably, these abnormalities occurred in the absence of changes in aldosterone excretion or changes in PRA. The authors suggest that collecting duct ET-1 may, through the ETB receptor, inhibit vasopressin-stimulated cAMP activation, decrease Na,K-ATPase activity, and inhibit epithelial Na-channel in collecting duct cells. Support for an intermediary role of the ETB receptor comes from several studies that show that chronic pharmacological or genetic disruption of the ETB receptor in mice results in hypertension that is sensitive to sodium (241, 257). Moreover, rats with a natural mutation of the ETB receptor gene (causing toxic megacolon) and rescued with a transgene expressing the ETB receptor under control of a gut-specific promoter (dopamine beta-hydroxylase), developed severe hypertension on a high-salt diet (102, 103). Reduction in medullary ET production may have a dramatic effect on release of NO and/or PGE_2 that may participate in the pathophysiology of hypertension, especially the salt-sensitive variety. Cumulatively, these studies underscore the importance of careful characterization of patients since an ET-1–dependent subset of patients with essential hypertension may be missed.

Only a few clinical studies have evaluated hypertensive patients. An early report examined 293 patients with mild to moderate increase in blood pressure who were treated with a combined ETA/ETB-receptor antagonist, bosentan for 4 weeks (168). The decrease in blood pressure achieved was comparable to that achieved with angiotensin-converting inhibitor. However there were more side effects including headache, flushing, and edema; some patients developed reversible elevations in liver function tests. A multicenter clinical trial of 392 patients with moderate essential hypertension reported treatment with a selective ETA-receptor antagonist, darusenton for 6 weeks (233). This treatment was effective in lowering systolic and diastolic blood pressures. The side effects included headaches, flushing, and edema but there were no instances of liver function abnormalities. These trials were not able to show greater antihypertensive benefit over available therapy and revealed more side effects. It is unclear whether a more narrowly defined population of hypertensive patients (e.g., patients classified as salt-sensitive hypertensives) may reveal a more dramatic benefit to antagonism of ET actions.

Pulmonary Hypertension. Compared with the more extensive repertoire of therapeutic modalities available for systemic hypertension, treatment options for pulmonary hypertension are much more limited and cumbersome. These limitations heightened the anticipation of using ET antagonists in this setting. Animal models of pulmonary hypertension as well as clinical studies show increased activation of ET-1, as well as increased endothelin receptor density, especially the ETA receptor, that correlated with abnormal pulmonary hemodynamics (53, 62, 108, 109, 144, 158, 159, 187, 340). As in other vascular beds, the ETB receptor on endothelial cells was found to counter the pathophysiologic effects via stimulation of NO and prostacyclin although in some instances, the ETB receptor on vascular smooth muscle cells contributed to pulmonary vasoconstriction and cellular proliferation (62). Currently, the only FDA-approved therapy using antagonist of ET actions is the combined ETA-ETB antagonist, bosentan, for patients with pulmonary hypertension who are functional class III or IV.

The first multicentered randomized, placebo-controlled study of chronic oral bosentan studied 32 patients with idiopathic pulmonary hypertension or pulmonary hypertension related to scleroderma (49). Bosentan for 4 weeks significantly improved exercise capacity measured by the 6-minute walk test (6MWT) as well as cardiac output, pulmonary vascular resistance, and mean pulmonary artery pressure. A subsequent larger double-blind, placebo-controlled study of 213 patients also found improvement in the 6MWT after 16 weeks of treatment (101). Longer-term studies also showed sustained improvement in the functional class and pulmonary hemodynamics in patients treated for at least 1 year (312) and improved mortality after 3 years in patients treated with bosentan as first-line therapy (208). One hundred seventy-eight patients with New York Heart Association (NYHA) functional class II, III, or IV were studied using a selective ETA-receptor antagonist sitaxsentan also had improved 6MWT results, although not the maximum oxygen consumption after 12 weeks of treatment (23). These promising results have been clouded by side effects that include headache, flushing, and, in particular, hepatic dysfunction. The combined data of currently available trials reveal a threefold elevation in aminotransferases in 11% of bosentan-treated patients. Although these abnormalities resolved with dose reduction or cessation of treatment, an early pilot study using an ETA receptor antagonist at high doses reported a case of fatal hepatitis (24). Overall, although endothelin antagonism may ultimately find a place in treatment of pulmonary hypertension, issues regarding dose, toxicity, value of selective versus nonselective receptor antagonism, and utility as part of combination therapy remain to be clarified.

Congestive Heart Failure. Patients with ischemic or dilated cardiomyopathy have elevated levels of circulating and intracardiac ET-1 (57, 247). In patients with cardiac failure regardless of the cause, the plasma endothelin is considered to be a good predictor of outcome, with the highest levels of ET-1 portending the worst prognosis (135, 244). Pressure overload or even mechanical stretch induces and stimulates ET-1 mRNA in cardiac myocytes. Coronary artery ligation in rats caused a dramatic increase in cardiac ET-1 and upregulation of ET receptors (271). Continuous infusion of an ETA-receptor antagonist into these rats for 10 days produced improvement in the left ventricular function, lessened ventricular dilatation and hypertrophy, and substantially improved 12-week survival. Circulating ET-1 levels also proved to be an extremely accurate predictor of 1-year survival in this animal model. It was postulated that high ET-1 may be a direct toxin to cardiac tissue, ET-1 may promote cardiac hypertrophy matrix deposition thereby accelerating interstitial fibrosis, and high ET-1 may compound the heart failure by augmenting pulmonary hypertension. Heart failure also appears to affect the absolute density as well as balance of the ET receptors. While not all studies show the same directionality, failing hearts upregulate the ETA receptor and downregulate the ETB receptor (16, 258, 286, 377). The normal ETA:ETB ratio of 60:40 is skewed to 80:20 in the failing heart (16) which may impact the response to therapeutic interventions. ETA-receptor antagonism increases contractility in left ventricular dysfunction while patients with normal ventricular function have reduced contractility following ETA-receptor antagonism. Efficacy of therapeutic interventions will also reflect the function of each receptor. Beneficial effects of antagonism with ETA-receptor blockers may reflect preservation of the vasodilatory effects transduced via the ETB receptor. Indeed, pharmacological blockade or genetic deficiency of the ETB receptor is detrimental in the post ischemic heart model and has been shown to exacerbate cardiac pathology (362). Moreover, antagonism of both ETA/ETB receptors may not only negate potentially beneficial effects of ETB but also remove ETA-mediated inotropy and chronotropy. Clinical heart failure trials have studied mostly the effects of combined ETA/ETB-receptor antagonism; the results of these trials have been disappointing.

Acute and chronic heart failure was studied using intravenous and oral antagonists. Four phase III studies in patients with acute heart failure requiring hospitalizations have been conducted in parallel using the nonselective ET-receptor antagonist tezosentan in the RITZ trials (Randomized Intravenous TeZosentan). RITZ-1 evaluated 669 patients but found no improvement in primary end point of symptoms of dyspnea at 24 hours or secondary end points of time to death or worsening heart failure. Moreover, hypotension, dizziness and renal failure were noted (58). By contrast, RITZ-2 studied 285 patients and found improved cardiac index and decreased pulmonary capillary wedge pressure at 6 hours without serious adverse effects (185). RITZ-4 was a multicenter trial of 193 patients with acute decompensated heart failure with acute coronary syndromes that found no difference in the primary end point of composite of death, worsening heart failure, recurrent ischemia and myocardial infarcts within 72 hours (239). The RITZ-5 trial of 84 patients with acute pulmonary edema also found no difference in the primary end point of improved oxygen saturation or incidence of death, recurrent pulmonary edema, mechanical ventilation and myocardial infarcts at 24 hours (152). REACH-1 (Research on Endothelin Antagonism in Chronic Heart failure) evaluated bosentan in 370 patients with NYHA class III/IV with ejection fraction of less than 35% in patients on diuretics and ACEI. The primary end point was change in the clinical status from baseline after 6 months. The study was prematurely terminated because of concern that liver abnormalities had reached 15.6% in the bosentan group (271). The ENABLE trial (ENdothelin Antagonist Bosentan for Lowering cardiac Events) include NYHA class IIIB and IV congestive heart failure with left ventricular ejection fraction <35% found no improvement in clinical status at the end of 8 months nor improvement in secondary end points. Notably early worsening of congestive heart failure was seen in the bosentan group (248). Selective ETA receptor antagonist, darusentan was evaluated in the HEAT trial (Heart failure ETA receptor blockade trial) in 157 patients with class III heart failure. Cardiac index significantly improved at three weeks. However, there were early exacerbations in heart failure and higher doses of the antagonist were associated with more side effects including death (186). Thus, it has been difficult to support the theoretical benefits of antagonizing ET actions in the clinical heart failure. It is possible that lower doses of ET antagonists, more selective antagonists, perhaps in combination with ANG II antagonism will benefit heart failure patients.

Cancer. An unexpected role for ET-1 has been recognized in cancer pathophysiology. ET-1 and its receptors have been identified in several cancer cell lines as well as tumors including prostate, ovarian, lung, colon, renal, cervical, melanoma and glioma (44, 235). The mechanism for neoplastic effects of ET-1 includes cellular proliferation. In fibroblasts, smooth muscles and epithelial cells, proliferation is mediated through the ETA receptor while in endothelial cells, proliferation is mediated through the ETB receptor (235). Although ET-1 can directly promote cell growth, even more profound proliferative effects occur through its synergism with more powerful growth and survival factors including epidermal growth factor, insulin-like growth factor 1, mitogen-activated protein kinase. ET-1 also inhibits apoptosis of cancer cells and regulates angiogenesis promoting endothelial cell proliferation, invasion, production of proteases and tubule formation. Finally, ET-1 affects development and progression of bone remodeling and metastasis. These novel implications for ET-1 in cancer pathophysiology from in in vitro studies and animals models is being evaluated in a phase II clinical trial in 244 patients with metastatic hormone-refractory prostate cancer treated with an ETA receptor antagonist, atrasentan (44). Available data find delayed time to clinical and PSA progression, and stabilization of biochemical markers of skeletal progression. Although still early, few and only mild side effects have been observed, none of which necessitated discontinuation of therapy.

References

1. Abadir PM, Carey RM, Siragy HM. Angiotensin AT2 receptors directly stimulate renal nitric oxide in bradykinin B2-receptor-null mice. *Hypertension* 2003;42:600–604.
2. AbdAlla S, Lother H, el Massiery A, Quitterer U. Increased AT1 receptor heterodimers in preeclampsia mediate enhanced angiotensin II responsiveness. *Nat Med* 2001;7:1003–1009.
3. AbdAlla S, Lother H, Quitterer U. AT1-receptor heterodimers show enhanced G-protein activation and altered receptor sequestration. *Nature* 2000;407:94–98.
4. Abe Y, Nakayama K, Yamanaka A, et al. Subtype-specific trafficking of endothelin receptors. *J Biol Chem* 2000;275:8664–867.
5. Abelous JE, Bardier E. Les substances hypotensives de l'urine humaine normale. *C R Sac Bioi (Paris)* 1909;66:304.
6. Agata J, Miao RQ, Yayama K, et al. Bradykinin B1 receptor mediates inhibition of neointima formation in rat artery after balloon angioplasty. *Hypertension* 2000;36:364–370.
7. Ahn D, Ge Y, Stricklett PK, et al. Collecting duct-specific knockout of endothelin-1 causes hypertension and sodium retention. *J Clin Invest* 2004;114:504–511.
8. Alanen K, Deng DX, Chakrabarti S. Augmented expression of endothelin-1, endothelin-3 and the endothelin-B receptor in breast carcinoma. *Histopathology* 2000;36:161–167.
9. Alexander BT, Cockrell KL, Rinewalt AN, et al. Enhanced renal expression of preproendothelin mRNA during chronic angiotensin II hypertension. *Am J Physiol Regul Integr Comp Physiol* 2001;280:R1388–R1392.
10. Alvarez V, Quiroz Y, Nava M, Pons H, et al. Overload proteinuria is followed by salt-sensitive hypertension caused by renal infiltration of immune cells. *Am J Physiol Renal Physiol* 2002;283:F1132F1141.
11. Amoroso A, Cossu MF, Mariotti A, et al. Increased plasma levels of endothelin in patients with essential arterial hypertension. *Riv Eur Sci Med Farmacol* 1996;18:33–37.
12. Arai H, Hori S, Aramori I, et al. Cloning and expression of a cDNA encoding an endothelin receptor. *Nature* 1990;348:730–732.
13. Araki S, Haneda M, Togawa M, et al. Endothelin-1 activates c-Jun NH2-terminal kinase in mesangial cells. *Kidney Int* 1997;51:631–639.
14. Ardiles LG, Figueroa CD, Mezzano SA. Renal kallikrein-kinin system damage and salt sensitivity: insights from experimental models. *Kidney Int Suppl* 2003;S2–S8.
15. Armstrong PW, Lorell BH, Nissen S, Borer J. Candesartan. *Circulation* 2002;6:e9011–e9012.
16. Asano K, Bohlmeyer TJ, Westcott JY, et al. Altered expression of endothelin receptors in failing human left ventricles. *J Mol Cell Cardiol* 2002;34:833–846.
17. Badr KF, Murray JJ, Breyer MD, et al. Mesangial cell, glomerular and renal vascular responses to endothelin in the rat kidney. Elucidation of signal transduction pathways. *J Clin Invest* 1989;83:336–342.
18. Bagnato A, Cirilli A, Salani D, et al. Growth inhibition of cervix carcinoma cells in vivo by endothelin A receptor blockade. *Cancer Res* 2002;62:6381–6384.
19. Balakrishnan SM, Wang HD, Gopalakrishnan V, et al. Effect of an endothelin antagonist on hemodynamic responses to angiotensin II. *Hypertension* 1996;28:806–809.
20. Ballew JR, Fink GD. Role of ETA receptors in experimental ANG II-induced hypertension in rats. *Am J Physiol Regul Integr Comp Physiol* 2001;281:R150–R154.
21. Ballew JR, Watts SW, Fink GD. Effects of salt intake and angiotensin II on vascular reactivity to endothelin-1. *J Pharmacol Exp Ther* 2001;296:345–350.
22. Bando K, Vijayaraghavan P, Turrentine MW, et al. Dynamic changes of endothelin-1, nitric oxide, and cyclic GMP in patients with congenital heart disease. *Circulation* 1997;96:II346–II351.
23. Barst RJ, Langleben D, Frost A, et al., Sitaxsentan therapy for pulmonary arterial hypertension. *Am J Respir Crit Care Med* 2004;169:441–447.
24. Barst RJ, Rich S, Widlitz A, et al. Clinical efficacy of sitaxsentan, an endothelin-A receptor antagonist, in patients with pulmonary arterial hypertension: Open-label pilot study. *Chest* 2002;121:1860–1868.
25. Barton M, Shaw S, d"Uscio LV, et al. Angiotensin II increases vascular and renal endothelin-1 and functional endothelin converting enzyme activity in vivo: role of ETA receptors for endothelin regulation. *Biochem Biophys Res Commun* 1997;238:861–865.
26. Barton M, Shaw S, d"Uscio LV, et al. Differential modulation of the renal and myocardial endothelin system by angiotensin II in vivo. *J Cardiovasc Pharmacol* 1998;31:S265–S268.
27. Baylis C, Deen WM, Myers BD, et al. Effects of some vasodilator drugs on transcapillary fluid exchange in renal cortex. *Am J Physiol* 1976;230:1148–1158.
28. Baynash AG, Hosoda K, Giaid A, et al. Interaction of endothelin B receptor is essential for development of epidermal melanocyte and enteric neurons. *Cell* 1994;79:1277.
29. Benigni A, Corna D, Maffi R, et al. Renoprotective effect of contemporary blocking of angiotensin II and endothelin-1 in rats with membranous nephropathy. *Kidney Int* 1998;54:353–359.
30. Benigni A, Perico N, Gaspari F, et al. Increased renal endothelin production in rats with reduced renal mass. *Am J Physiol* 1991;260:F331–339.
31. Benigni A. Endothelin antagonists in renal disease. *Kidney Int* 2000;57:1778–1794.
32. Bhoola KD, Figueroa CD, Worthy K. Bioregulation of kinins: kallikreins, kininogens and kininases. *Pharm Rev* 1992;44:1–80.
33. Binet I, Wallnöfer A, Weber C, et al. Renal hemodynamics and pharmacokinetics of bosentan with and without cyclosporine A. *Kidney Int* 2000;57:224–231.
34. Blaukat A. Structure and signalling pathways of kinin receptors. *Andrologia* 2003;35:17–23.
35. Boissonnas RA, Guitmann S, Jaquenoud PA, et al. Synthesis and biological activity of peptides related to bradykinin. *Experientia* 1960;16:326.
36. Boivin B, Chevalier D, Villeneuve LR, et al. Functional endothelin receptors are present on nuclei in cardiac ventricular myocytes. *J Biol Chem* 2003;278:29153–29163.
37. Bolk S, Angrist M, Xie J, et al. Endothelin-3 frame shift mutation in congenital central hypoventilation syndrome. *Nat Genet* 1996;13:395–396.
38. Boulanger C, Lüscher TF. Release of endothelin from porcine aorta: inhibition by endothelium-derived nitric oxide. *J Clin Invest* 1990;85:587–590.
39. Boulanger CM, Tanner FC, Bea ML, et al. Oxidized low density lipoproteins induced mRNA expression and release of endothelin from human and porane endothelium. *Circ Res* 1992;70:1191–1197.
40. Bragulat E, de la Sierra A, Antonio MT, et al. Endothelial dysfunction in salt-sensitive essential hypertension. *Hypertension* 2001;37:444–448.
41. Braun A, Kammerer S, Maier E, Bohme E, et al. Polymorphisms in the gene for the human B2-bradykinin receptor. New tools in assessing a genetic risk for bradykinin-associated diseases. *Immunopharmacology* 1996;33:32–35.
42. Brophy PD, Mottes TA, Kudelka TL, McBryde KD, et al. AN-69 membrane reactions are pH-dependent and preventable. *Am J Kidney Dis* 2001;381:173–178.
43. Campbell DJ. The renin-angiotensin and the kallikrein-kinin systems. *Int J Biochem Cell Biol* 2003;35:784–791.
44. Carducci MA, Padley RJ, Breul J, et al. Effect of endothelin-A receptor blockade with atrasentan on tumor progression in men with hormone-refractory prostate cancer: a randomized, phase II, placebo-controlled trial. *J Clin Oncol* 2003;21:679–89.
45. Carlini R, Obialo CI, Rothstein M. Intravenous erythropoietin (rHuEPO) administration increases plasma endothelin and blood pressure in hemodialysispatients. *Am J Hypertens* 1993;6:103–107.
46. Carone FA, Pullman TN, Oparil S, Nakamura S. Micropuncture evidence of rapid hydrolysis of bradykinin by rat proximal tubule. *Am J Physiol* 1976;230:1420–1424.
47. Carretero OA, Oza NB, Scicli AG, et al. Renal tissue kallikrein, plasma renin, and plasma aldosterone in renal hypertension. *Acta Physiol Latinoam* 1974;24:448.

48. Carretero OA, Scicli AG. Kinins as regulators of blood flow and blood pressure. In: Laragh JH, Brenner BM, eds. *Hypertension: Pathophysiology, Diagnosis and Management.* New York: Raven Press, 1995:805.
49. Channick RN, Simonneau G, Sitbon O, et al, Effects of the dual endothelin-receptor antagonist bosentan in patients with pulmonary hypertension: A randomized placebo controlled study. *Lancet* 2001;358:1119–1123.
50. Chao J, Miao RQ, Chen V, Chen LM, et. al. Novel roles of kallistatin, a specific tissue kallikrein inhibitor, in vascular remodeling. *Biol Chem* 2001;1:15–21.
51. Chao J, Stallone JN, Liang YM, Chen LM, et. al. Kallistatin is a potent new vasodilator. *J Clin Inves* 1997;1:11–17.
52. Chen LM, Ma J, Liang YM, Chao L, et. al. Tissue kallikrein-binding protein reduces blood pressure in transgenic mice. *J Biol Chem* 1996;44:27590–27594.
53. Chen YF, Oparil S. Endothelin and pulmonary hypertension. *J Cardiovasc Pharmacol* 2000;35:S49–S53.
54. Clarke JG, Benjamin N, Larkin SW, et al. Endothelin is a potent long-lasting vasoconstrictor in men. *Am J Physiol* 1989;257:H2033–2035.
55. Clements JA, Willemsen NM, Myers SA, et al. The tissue kallikrein family of serine proteases: functional roles in human disease and potential as clinical biomarkers. *Crit Rev Clin Lab Sci* 2004;41:265–312.
56. Clouthier DE, Hosoda K, Richardson JA, et al. Cranial and cardiac neural crest defects in endothelin-A receptor-deficient mice. *Development* 1998;125:813–824.
57. Cody RJ, Haas GJ, Binkley PF, et al. Plasma endothelin correlates with the extent of pulmonary hypertension in patients with chronic congestive heart failure. *Circulation* 1992;85: 504–509.
58. Coletta AP, Cleland JG. Clinical trials update: highlights of the Scientific Sessions of the XXIII Congress of the European Society of Cardiology-WARIS II, ESCAMI, PAFAC, RITZ-1 and TIME. *Eur J Heart Fail* 2001;3:747–750.
59. Cramer H, Schmenger K, Heinrich K, et al. Coupling of endothelin receptors to the ERK/MAP kinase pathway. *Eur J Biochem* 2001;268:5449–5459.
60. Curd JG, Prograis LJ, Cochrane CG. Detection of active kallikrein in induced blister fluids of hereditary angioedema patients. *J Exp Med* 1980;152:742–747.
61. Davenport, A. P. International Union of Pharmacology. XXIX. Update on endothelin receptor nomenclature. *Pharmacol Rev* 2002;54:219–226.
62. Davie N, Haleen SJ, Upton PD, et al, ET and ET receptors modulate the proliferation of human pulmonary artery smooth muscle cells. *Am J Respir Crit Care Med* 2002;165:398–405.
63. Deedwania PC. Angiotensin-converting enzyme inhibitors in congestive heart failure. *Arch Intern Med* 1990;150:1798–1805.
64. Denault JB, Claing A, D'Orleans-Juste P, et al. Processing of proendothelin-1 by human furin convertase. *FEBS Lett* 1995;362:276–280.
65. Dendorfer A, Wolfrum S, Dominiak P. Pharmacology and cardiovascular implications of the kinin-kallikrein system. *Jpn J Pharmacol* 1999;79:403–426.
66. Denton KM, Shweta A, Finkelstein L, et al. Effect of endothelin-1 on regional kidney blood flow and renal arteriole caliber in rabbits. *Clin Exp Pharm Physiol* 2004;31:494–501.
67. Dohi Y, Hahn AWA, Boulanger CM, et al. Endothelin stimulated by angiotensin II augments contractility of spontaneously hypertensive rat resistance arteries. *Hypertension* 1992;19:131–137.
68. Duan SB, Liu FY, Luo JA, et al. Assessment of urinary endothelin-1 and nitric oxide levels and their relationship with clinical and pathologic types in primary glomerulonephritis. *Yonsei Med J* 1999;40:425–429.
69. Duchene J, Chauhan SD, Lopez F, Pecher C, Esteve JP, Girolami JP, Bascands JL, Schanstra JP. Direct protein-protein interaction between PLCgamma1 and the bradykinin B2 receptor-importance of growth conditions. *Biochem Biophys Res Commun* 2005;326:894–900.
70. Duchene J, Schanstra JP, Pecher C, Pizard A, et. al. Anovel protein-protein interaction between a G protein-coupled receptor and the phosphatase SHP-2 is involved in bradykinin-induced inhibition of cell proliferation. *J Biol Chem* 2002;277:40375–40383.
71. Duguay D, Der Sarkissian S, Kouz R, et al. Kinin B2 receptor is not involved in enalapril-induced apoptosis and regression of hypertrophy in spontaneously hypertensive rat aorta: possible role of B1 receptor. *Br J Pharmacol* 2004;141:728–736.
72. Duka I, Duka A, Kintsurashvili E, et al. Mechanisms mediating the vasoactive effects of the B1 receptors of bradykinin. *Hypertension* 2003;42:1021–1025.
73. Duka I, Kintsurashvili E, Gavras I, et al. Vasoactive potential of the b(1) bradykinin receptor in normotension and hypertension. *Circ Res* 2001;88:275–281.
74. Egidy G, Juillerat-Jeanneret L, Jeannin JF, et al. Modulation of human colon tumor-stromal interactions by the endothelin system. *Am J Pathol* 2000;157:1863–1874.
75. Elijovich F, Laffer CL, Amador E, et al. Regulation of plasma endothelin by salt in salt-sensitive hypertension. *Circulation* 2001;103:263–268.
76. Elijovich F, Laffer CL. Participation of renal and circulating endothelin in salt-sensitive essential hypertension. *J Hum Hypertens* 2002;16:459–67.
77. Elliot AH, Nuzum FR. The urinary excretion of a depressor substance (kallikrein of Frey and Kraut) in arterial hypertension. *Endocrinology* 1934;18:462–474.
78. Emanueli C, Graiani G, Salis MB, Gadau S, et. al. Prophylactic gene therapy with human tissue kallikrein ameliorates limb ischemia recovery in type 1 diabetic mice. *Diabetes* 2004;4:1096–1103.
79. Emanueli C, Madeddu P. Targeting kinin receptors for the treatment of tissue ischaemia. *Trends Pharmacol Sci* 2001;22:478–484.
80. Emanueli C, Maestri R, Corradi D, Marchione R, et al. Dilated and failing cardiomyopathy in bradykinin B(2) receptor knockout mice. *Circulation* 1999;100:2359–2365.
81. Emerich DF, Snodgrass P, Dean R, Agostino M, Hasler B, Pink M, Xiong H, Kim BS, Bartus RT. Enhanced delivery of carboplatin into brain tumours with intravenous Cereport (RMP-7): dramatic differences and insight gained from dosing parameters. *Br J Cancer* 1999;80:964–970.
82. Emoto N, Yanagisawa M. Endothelin-converting enzyme-2 is a membrane-bound, phosphramidon-sensitive metalloprotease with acidic pH optimum. *J Biol Chem* 1995; 270: 15262–15268.
83. Erdos EG, Deddish PA. The kinin system: suggestions to broaden some prevailing concepts. *Int Immunopharmacol* 2002;2:1741–1746.
84. Erdos EG, Skidgel RA. The angiotensin I-convening enzyme. *Lab Invest* 1987;56:345–348.
85. Ergul S, Parish DC, Puett D, et al. Racial differences in plasma endothelin-1 concentrations in individuals with essential hypertension. *Hypertension* 1996;28:652–655.
86. Evans RG, Madden AC, Denton KM. Diversity of responses of renal cortical and medullary blood flow to vasoconstrictors in conscious rabbits. *Acta Physiol Scan* 2000;169:297–308.
87. Feldman DL, Mogelesky TC, Chou M, et al. Attenuation of puromycin aminonucleoside-induced glomerular lesions in rats by CGS 26303, a dual neutral endopeptidase/endothelin-converting enzyme inhibitor. *J Cardiovasc Pharmacol* 2000;36:S342–S345.
88. Fenoy FJ, Roman RJ. Effect of kinin receptor antagonists on renal hemodynamic and natriuretic responses to volume expansion. *Am J Physiol* 1992;263:R1136.
89. Fernandez-Patron C, Zouki C, Whittal R, et al. Matrix metalloproteinases regulate neutrophil-endothelial cell adhesion through generation of endothelin-1[1-32]. *FASEB J* 2001; 15:2230–2240.
90. Ferri C, Bellini C, Desideri G, et al. Clustering of endothelial markers of vascular damage in human salt-sensitive hypertension: influence of dietary sodium load and depletion. *Hypertension* 1998; 32:862–868.
91. Ferri C, Bellini C, Desideri G, et al. Elevated plasma and urinary endothelin-1 levels in human salt-sensitive hypertension. *Clin Sci* 1997;93:35–41.
92. Figueroa CD, Caorsi I, Subiabre J, et al. Immunoreactive kallikrein localization in the rat kidney: an immunoelectron microscopic Study. *J Histochem Cytochem* 1984;32:117–121.
93. Figueroa CD, Gonzalez CB, Grigoriev S, Abd Alla SA, et. al. Probing for the bradykinin B2 receptor in rat kidney by anti-peptide and anti-ligand antibodies. *J Histochem Cytochem* 1995;43:137–148.
94. Figueroa CD, MacIver AG, Mackenzie JC, Bhoola KD. Localisation of immunoreactive kininogen and tissue kallikrein in the human nephron. *Histochemistry* 1988;89:437–442.
95. Firth JD, Ratcliffe Pl. Organ distribution of the three rat endothelin messenger RNA's and the effects of ischemia on renal gene expression. *J Clin Invest* 1992;90:1023–1031.
96. Foster N, Loi TH, Owe-Young R, et al. Lysosomal traffic of liganded endothelin B receptor. *Biochim Biophys Acta* 2003;1642:45–52.
97. Fox A, Kaur S, Li B, et al. Antihyperalgesic activity of a novel nonpeptide bradykinin B(1) receptor antagonist in transgenic mice expressing the human B(1) receptor. *Br J Pharmacol* 2005;144:889–899.
98. Frey EK, Kraut H. Ein neues Kreislaufhormon und seine Wirkung. *Arch Exp Pathol Pharmkol* 1928;133:1.
99. Fukuroda T, Fujikawa T, Ozaki S, et al. Clearance of circulating endothelin-1 by ETB receptors in rats. *Biochem Biophys Res Commun* 1994;199:1461–1465.
100. Gainer JV, Brown NJ, Bachvarova M, Bastien L, Maltais I, Marceau F, Bachvarov DR. Altered frequency of a promoter polymorphism of the kinin B2 receptor gene in hypertensive African-Americans. *Am J Hyperten* 2000;13:1268–1273.
101. Galie N, Hinderliter AL, Torbicki A, et al, Effects of the oral endothelin-receptor antagonist bosentan on echocardiographic and Doppler measures in patients with pulmonary arterial hypertension. *J Am Coll Cardiol* 2003;41:1380–1386.
102. Gariepy CE, Ohuchi T, Williams SC, et al. Salt-sensitive hypertension in endothelin-B receptor-deficient rats. *J Clin Invest* 2000;105:925–933.
103. Gariepy CE, Williams SC, Richardson JA, et al. Transgenic expression of the endothelin-B receptor prevents congenital intestinal aganglionosis in a rat model of Hirschsprung disease. *J Clin Invest* 1998;102:1092–101.
104. Gavras I. Bradykinin-mediated effects of ACE inhibition. *Kidney Int* 1992;42:1020.
105. Ge Y, Ahn D, Stricklett PK, et al. Collecting duct-specific knockout of endothelin-1 alters vasopressin regulation of urine osmolality. *Am J Physiol Renal Physiol* 2005;288:F912–F920.
106. Gellai M, Jugus M, Fletcher T, et al. Reversal of postischemic acute renal failure with a selective endothelin A receptor antagonist in the rat. *J Clin Invest* 1994;93:900–906.
107. Gerken VMV, Santos RAS. Centrally infused bradykinin increases baroreceptor reflex sensitivity. *Hypertension* 1992;19:II-176–181.
108. Giaid A, Yanagisawa M, Langleben D, et al. Expression of endothelin-1 in the lungs of patients with pulmonary hypertension. *N Engl J Med* 1993;328:1732–1739.
109. Giaid A. Nitric oxide and endothelin-1 in pulmonary hypertension. *Chest* 1998;114: S208–S212.
110. Gilboa N, Rudofsky V; Magro A. Urinary and renal kallikrein in hypertensive Fawn-Hooded (FH/Wjd) rats. *Lab Invest* 1984;50:72.
111. Gohji K, Kitazawa S, Tamada H, et al. Expression of endothelin receptor A associated with prostate cancer progression. *J Urol* 2001;165:1033–1036.
112. Goligorsky MS, Tsukahara H, Magazine H, et al. Termination of endothelin signaling: role of nitric oxide. *J Cell Physiol* 1994;158:485–494.
113. Gomez-Garre D, Largo R, Liu XH, et al. An orally active ETA/ETB receptor antagonist ameliorates proteinuria and glomerular lesions in rats with proliferative nephritis. *Kidney Int* 1996;50:962–972.
114. Goodall T, Kind CN, Hammond TG. FK506-induced endothelin release by cultured rat mesangial cells. *J Card Pharm* 1995;26:S482–S485.
115. Goto K, Hama H, Kasuya Y. Molecular pharmacology and pathophysiological significance of endothelin. *Jpn J Pharmacol* 1996;72:261–290.
116. Greer IA, Leask R, Hodson BA, et al. Endothelin, elastase, and endothelial dysfunction in pre-eclampsia. *Lancet* 1991;337:558.
117. Grimshaw MJ, Hagemann T, Ayhan A, et al. A role for endothelin-2 and its receptors in breast tumor cell invasion. *Cancer Res* 2004;64:2461–2468.
118. Grimshaw MJ, Wilson JL, Balkwill FR. Endothelin-2 is a macrophage chemoattractant: implications for macrophage distribution in tumors. *Eur J Immunol* 2002;32:2393–2400.
119. Hagiwara M, Murakami H, Ura N, et al. Renal protective role of bradykinin B1 receptor in stroke-prone spontaneously hypertensive rats. *Hypertens Res* 2004;27:399–408.
120. Hall JM. Bradykinin receptors. *Gen Pharmacol* 1997;28:1–6.
121. Han ED, MacFarlane RC, Mulligan AN, et al. Increased vascular permeability in C1 inhibitor-deficient mice mediated by the bradykinin type 2 receptor. *J Clin Invest* 2002;109:1057–1063.

122. Harrison VJ, Corder R, Anggard EE, et al. Evidence for vesicles that transport endothelin-1 in bovine aortic endothelial cells. *J Cardiovasc Pharmacol* 1993;22:S57–S60.
123. Hasegawa H, Hiki K, Sawamura T, et al. Purification of a novel endothelin converting enzyme specific for big endothelin-3. *FEBS Lett* 1998;428:304–308.
124. Hasue F, Kuwaki T, Kisanuki YY, et al. Increased sensitivity to acute and persistent pain in neuron-specific endothelin-1 knockout mice. *Neuroscience* 2005;130:349–358.
125. Hayashi I, Maruhashi J, Oh-Ishi S. Functionally active high molecular weight-kininogen was found in the liver but not in the plasma of Brown Norway Katholiek rat. *Thromb Res* 1989;56:179–189.
126. Herman WH, Emancipator SN, Rhoten RL, et al. Vascular and glomerular expression of endothelin-1 in normal human kidney. *Am J Physiol Renal Physiol* 1998;275:F8–F17.
127. Herwald H, Collin M, Muller-Esterl W, Bjorck L. Streptococcal cysteine proteinase releases kinins: a virulence mechanism. *J Exp Med* 1996;184:665–67.
128. Herwald H, Morgelin M, Olsen A, Rhen M, Dahlback B, Muller-Esterl W, Bjorck L. Activation of the contact-phase system on bacterial surfaces—a clue to serious complications in infectious diseases. *Nat Med* 1998;4:298–302.
129. Hickey KA, Rubanyi G, Paul RJ et al., Characterization of coronary vasoconstrictor produced by cultured endothelial cells. *Am J Physiol* 1985;248:C550–C556.
130. Hoffman A, Grossman E, Goldstein DS, et al. Urinary excretion rate of endothelin-1 in patients with essential hypertension and salt sensitivity. *Kidney Int* 1994;45:556–560.
131. Horie M, Uchida S, Yanagisawa M, et al. Mechanisms of endothelin-1 mRNA and peptides induction by TGF-beta and TPA in MDCK cells. *J Cardiovasc Pharmacol* 1991;17:S222–S225.
132. Hosada K, Nakao K, Tamura N, et al. Organization, structure, chromosomal assignment and expression of the gene encoding the human endothelin A receptor. *J Biol Chem* 1992;267:18797–18804.
133. Hosoda K, Hammer RE, Richardson JA, et al. Targeted and natural (piebald-lethal) mutations of endothelin-B receptor gene produce megacolon associated with spotted coat color in mice. *Cell* 1994;79:1267
134. Hu RM, Levin ER, Pedram A, et al. Atrial natriuretic peptide inhibits the production and secretion of endothelin from cultured endothelial cells. Mediation through the C receptor. *J Biol Chem* 1992;267:17384–17389.
135. Hulsmann M, Stanek B, Frey B, et al. Value of cardiopulmonary exercise testing and big endothelin plasma levels to predict short-term prognosis of patients with chronic heart failure. *J Am Coll Cardiol* 1998;32:1695–1700.
136. Hunley TE, Fogo A, Iwasaki S, et al. Endothelin A receptor mediates functional but not structural damage in chronic cyclosporine nephrotoxicity. *J Am Soc Nephrol* 1995;5:1718–1723.
137. Ignjatovic T, Stanisavljevic S, Brovkovych V, Skidgel RA, Erdos EG. Kinin B1 receptors stimulate nitric oxide production in endothelial cells: signaling pathways activated by angiotensin I-converting enzyme inhibitors and peptide ligands. *Mol Pharmacol* 2004;66:1310–1316.
138. Ikeda Y, Hayashi I, Kamoshita E, Yamazaki A, et. al. Host stromal bradykinin B2 receptor signaling facilitates tumor-associated angiogenesis and tumor growth. *Cancer Res* 2004;15:5178–5185.
139. Ikemoto F, Song GB, Tominaga M, Kanayama Y, Yamamoto K. Angiotensin-converting enzyme in the rat kidney. Activity, distribution, and response to angiotensin-converting enzyme inhibitors. *Nephron* 1990;55(Suppl 1):3–9.
140. Imai T, Hirata Y, Emori T, et al. Induction of endothelin-1 gene by angiotensin and vasopressin in endothelial cells. *Hypertension* 1992;19:753–757.
141. Imai T, Hirata Y, Marumo F. Heparin inhibits endothelin-1 and protooncogene c-fos gene expression in cultured bovine endothelial cells. *J Cardiovasc Pharmacol* 1993;22:S49–S52.
142. Imamura T, Potempa J, Travis J. Activation of the kallikrein-kinin system and release of new kinins through alternative cleavage of kininogens by microbial and human cell proteinases. *Biol Chem* 2004;385:989–996.
143. Inoue A, Yanagisawa M, Kimura S, et al. The human endothelin family: three structurally and pharmacologically distinct isopeptides predicted by three separate genes. *Proc Natl Acad Sci U S A* 1989;86:2863–2867.
144. Ishikawa S, Miyauchi T, Sakai S, et al., Elevated levels of plasma endothelin-1 in young patients with pulmonary hypertension caused by congenital heart disease are decreased after successful surgical repair. *J Thorac Cardiovasc Surg* 1995;110:271–273.
145. Itoh Y, Yanagisawa M, Ohkubo S, et al. Cloning and sequence analysis of cDNA encoding the precursor of a human endothelium-derived vasoconstrictor peptide, endothelin: Identity of human and porcine endothelin. *FEBS Lett* 1988;231:440–444.
146. Iwasaki S, Homma T, Matsuda Y, et al. Endothelin receptor subtype B mediates autoinduction of endothelin-1 in rat mesangial cells. *J Biol Chem* 1995;270:6997–7003.
147. Januszewicz A, Lapinski M, Symonides B, et al. Elevated endothelin-1 plasma concentration in patients with essential hypertension. *J Cardiovasc Risk* 1994;1:81–85.
148. Johnson RJ, Herrera-Acosta J, Schreiner GF, Rodriguez-Iturbe B. Subtle acquired renal injury as a mechanism of salt-sensitive hypertension. *N Engl J Med* 2002;346:913–923.
149. Johnson RJ, Rodriguez-Iturbe B, Nakagawa T, Kang DH, et. al. Subtle renal injury is likely a common mechanism for salt-sensitive essential hypertension. *Hypertension* 2005;45:326–330.
150. Jones C, Phillips E, Davis C, et al. Molecular characterisation of cloned bradykinin B1 receptors from rat and human. *Eur J Pharmacol* 1999;374:423–433.
151. Kahn R, Herwald H, Muller-Esterl W, Schmitt R, Sjogren AC, Truedsson L, Karpman D. Contact-system activation in children with vasculitis. *Lancet* 2002 ;360:535–541.
152. Kaluski E, Kobrin I, Zimlichman R, et al. RITZ-5 randomized intravenous tezosentan (an endothelin-A/B antagonist) for the treatment of Pulmonary edema. *J Am Coll Cardiol* 2003;41:204–210.
153. Kanazawa M, Abe K, Yasujima M, Yoshida K, et al: Role of renal kallikrein in the regulation of blood pressure in the rat remnant kidney model of chronic renal failure. *Adv Exp Med Biol* 1989; 247B:121125.
154. Karam H, Bruneval P, Clozel JP, et. al. Role of endothelin in acute renal failure due to rhabdomyolysis in rats. *J Pharm Exp Ther* 1995;274:481–486.
155. Katada J, Majima M. AT(2) receptor-dependent vasodilation is mediated by activation of vascular kinin generation under flow conditions. *Br J Pharmacol* 2002;136:484–491.
156. Katori M, Majima M. Pivotal role of renal kallikrein-kinin system in the development of hypertension and approaches to new drugs based on this relationship. *Jpn J Pharmacol* 1996;70:95–128.
157. Katori M, Majima M. The renal kallikrein-kinin system: its role as a safety valve for excess sodium intake, and its attenuation as a possible etiologic factor in salt-sensitive hypertension. *Crit Rev Clin Lab Sci* 2003;40:43–115.
158. Kim H, Yung GL, Marsh JJ et al. Endothelin mediates pulmonary vascular remodelling in a canine model of chronic embolic pulmonary hypertension. *Eur Respir J* 2000;15:640–648.
159. Kim H, Yung GL, Marsh JJ, et al. Pulmonary vascular remodeling distal to pulmonary artery ligation is accompanied by upregulation of endothelin receptors and nitric oxide synthase. *Exp Lung Res* 2000; 26:287–301.
160. Kimura S, Kasuya Y, Sawamura T, et al. Structure-activity relationships of endothelin: Importance of the C-terminal moiety. *Biochem Biophys Res Commun* 1988;156:1182–1186.
161. Kodama J, Uchida K, Yoshimura S. Studies of four Japanese families with hereditary angioneurotic edema: simultaneous activation of plasma protease systems and exogenous triggering stimuli. *Blut* 1984;49:405–418.
162. Kohan DE, Padilla E, Hughes AK. Endothelin B receptor mediates ET-1 effects on cAMP and PGE2 accumulation in rat IMCD. *Am J Physiol* 1993;265:F670–F676.
163. Kohan DE. Endothelins in the kidney: physiology and pathophysiology. *Am J Kidney Dis* 1993;22:493–510.
164. Kon V, Badr KF. Biological actions and pathophysiologic significance of endothelin in the kidney. *Kidney Int* 1991;40:1–12.
165. Kon V, Fogo A, Ichikawa I. Bradykinin causes selective efferent arteriolar dilation during angiotensin I converting enzyme inhibition. *Kidney Int* 1993;44:545–550.
166. Kon V, Hunley TE, Fogo A. Combined antagonism of endothelin A/B receptors links endothelin to vasoconstriction whereas angiotensin II effects fibrosis. Studies in chronic cyclosporine nephrotoxicity in rats. *Transplantation* 1995;60:89–95.
167. Kon V, Yoshioka T, Fogo A, et al. Glomerular actions of endothelin in vivo. *J Clin Invest* 1989;83:1762–1767.
168. Krum H, Viskoper RJ, Lacourciere Y, et al. The effect of an endothelin-receptor antagonist, Bosentan, on blood pressure in patients with essential hypertension. *N Engl J Med* 1998;338:784–790.
169. Kumar C, Mwangi V, Nuthulaganti P, et al. Cloning and characterization of a novel endothelin receptor from Xenopus heart. *J Biol Chem* 1994;269:13414–13420.
170. Kuribayashi Y, Majima M, Katori M. Major kininases in rat urine are neutral endopeptidase and carboxypeptidase Y-like exopeptidase. *Biomed Res* 1993;14:191–201.
171. Kurihara H et al., Lessons from gene deletion of endothelin systems. In: T.D. Warner (ed.). *Endothelin and its Inhibitors.* Berlin: Springer, 2001;141–154.
172. Kurihara Y, Kurihara H, Oda H, et al. Aortic arch malformations and ventricular septal defect in mice deficient in endothelin-l. *J Clin Invest* 1995;96:293–300.
173. Kusumoto K, Kubo K, Kandori H, et al. Effects of a new endothelin antagonist, TAK 044, on post ischemic acute renal failure in rats. *Life Sci* 1994;55:301–310.
174. Lariviere R, Thibault G, Schiffrin EL. Increased endothelin-1 content in blood vessels of deoxycorticosterone acetate-salt hypertensive but not in spontaneously hypertensive rats. *Hypertension* 1993;21:294–300.
175. Lee-Chen GJ, Liu KP, Lai YC, Juang HS, et. al. Significance of the tissue kallikrein promoter and transforming growth factor-beta1 polymorphisms with renal progression in children with vesicoureteral reflux. *Kidney Int* 2004;65:1467–1472.
176. Letizia C, Cerci S, De Toma G, et al. High plasma endothelin-1 levels in hypertensive patients with low-renin essential hypertension. *J Hum Hypertens* 1997;11:447–451.
177. Levesque L, Larrivee JF, Bachvarov DR, et al. Regulation of kinin-induced contraction and DNA synthesis by inflammatory cytokines in the smooth muscle of the rabbit aorta. *Br J Pharmacol* 1995;116:1673–1679.
178. Levin, ER. Endothelins. *N Engl J Med* 1995;333:356–363.
179. Li JS, Knafo L, Turgeon A, et al. Effect of endothelin antagonism on blood pressure and vascular structure in renovascular hypertensive rats. *Am J Physiol Heart Circ Physiol* 1996;40:H88–H93.
180. Liu B, Wu D. The first inner loop of endothelin receptor type B is necessary for specific coupling to Galpha 13. *J Biol Chem* 2003;278:2384–2387.
181. Liu S, Premont RT, Kontos CD, et al. Endothelin-1 activates endothelial cell nitric-oxide synthase via heterotrimeric G-protein betagamma subunit signaling to protein jinase B/Akt. *J Biol Chem* 2003;278:49929–49935.
182. Lloyd I. Pharma Project Version 2.1 London: PJB Publications, 1999.
183. Lopez-Farre A., Gomez-Garre D, Barnabeu F et al. A role for endothelin in the maintenance of post ischemic renal failure on rats. *J Physiol* 1991;444:513–522.
184. Lopez-Ongil S, Diez-Marques ML, Griera M, et al. Crosstalk between mesangial and endothelial cells: angiotensin II down-regulates endothelin-converting enzyme 1. *Cell Physiol Biochem* 2005;15:135–144.
185. Louis A, Cleland JG, Crabbe S, et al. Clinical trials update: capricorn, copernicus, miracl, staf, ritz-2, recover and renaissance and cachexia and cholesterol in heart failure. highlights of the scientific sessions of the Am College of Cardiology. *Eur J Heart Fail* 2001;3:381–387.
186. Luscher TF, Enseleit F, Pacher R, et al. Hemodynamic and neurohumoral effects of selective endothelin (ET[A]) receptor blockade in chronic heart failure: the Heart Failure ET(A) Receptor Blockade Trial (HEAT). *Circulation* 2002;106:2666–2672.
187. Lutz J, Gorenflo M, Habighorst M, et al. Endothelin-1- and endothelin-receptors in lung biopsies of patients with pulmonary hypertension due to congenital heart disease. *Clin Chem Lab Med* 1999;37:423–428.
188. MacArthur H, Warner TD, Wood EG, et al. Endothelin-1 release from endothelial cells in culture is elevated both acutely and chronically by short periods of mechanical stretch. *Biochem Biophys Res Commun* 1994;200:395–400.
189. Madeddu P, Emanueli C, Maestri R, Salis MB, et. al. Angiotensin II type 1 receptor blockade prevents cardiac remodeling in bradykinin B(2) receptor knockout mice. *Hypertension* 2000;35:391–396.

190. Mahabeer R, Bhoola KD. Kallikrein and kinin receptor genes. *Pharmacol Ther* 2000;88: 77–89.
191. Mahdi F, Madar ZS, Figueroa CD, et al. Factor XII interacts with the multiprotein assembly of urokinase plasminogen activator receptor, gC1qR, and cytokeratin 1 on endothelial cell membranes. *Blood* 2002;99:3585–3596.
192. Majima M, Katori M, Hanazuka M, Mizogami S, et. al. Suppression of rat deoxycorticosterone-salt hypertension by kallikrein-kinin system. *Hypertension* 1991; 17: 806–813.
193. Majima M, Kuribayashi Y, Ikeda Y, Adachi K, Kato H, Katori M, Aoyagi T. Diuretic and natriuretic effect of ebelactone B in anesthetized rats by inhibition of a urinary carboxypeptidase Y-like kininase. *Jpn J Pharmacol* 1994;65:79–82.
194. Majima M, Mizgami S, Kuribayashi Y, et al. Hypertension induced by a nonpressor dose of angiotensin II in kininogen deficient rats. *Hypertension* 1994;24:111–119.
195. Malatino LS, Bellanuova I, Cataliotti A, et al. Renal endothelin-1 is linked to changes in urinary salt and volume in essential hypertension. *J Nephrol* 2000;13:178–184.
196. Malek A, Izumo S. Physiological fluid shear stress causes down regulation of endothelin-1 mRNA in bovine aortic endothelium. *Am J Physiol* 1992;263:C389–C396.
197. Marceau F, Hess JF, Bachvarov DR. The B1 receptors for kinins. *Pharmacol Rev* 1998;50: 357–386.
198. Marceau F, Larrivee JF, Saint-Jacques E, et al. The kinin B1 receptor: an inducible G protein coupled receptor. *Can J Physiol Pharmacol* 1997;75:725–730.
199. Marcic BM, Erdos EG. Protein kinase C and phosphatase inhibitors block the ability of angiotensin I-converting enzyme inhibitors to resensitize the receptor to bradykinin without altering the primary effects of bradykinin. *J Pharmacol Exp Ther* 2000;294:605–612.
200. Margolius HS. Kallikreins and kinins: Some unanswered questions about system characteristics and roles in human disease. *Hypertension* 1995;26:221.
201. Margolius HS. Kallikreins and kinins: molecular characterization and cellular and tissue responses. *Diabetes* 1996:45(Suppl 1):519.
202. Marin-Castano ME, Schanstra JP, Neau E, Praddaude F, Pecher C, Ader JL, Girolami JP, Bascands JL. Induction of functional bradykinin b(1)-receptors in normotensive rats and mice under chronic Angiotensin-converting enzyme inhibitor treatment. *Circulation* 2002;105:627–632.
203. Marin-Castano ME, Schanstra JP, Praddaude F, et al. Differential induction of functional B1-bradykinin receptors along the rat nephron in endotoxin induced inflammation. *Kidney Int* 1998;54:1888–1898.
204. Masaki, T. The endothelin family: an overview. *J Cardiovasc Pharmacol* 2000;35:S3–S5.
205. Maschio G, Alberti D, Janin G, et al. Effect of the angiotensin-enzyme inhibitor benazepril on progression of chronic renal insufficiency. *N Engl J Med* 1996;334:939–945.
206. Mathis SA, Criscimagna NL, Leeb-Lundberg LM. B1 and B2 kinin receptors mediate distinct patterns of intracellular Ca2+ signaling in single cultured vascular smooth muscle cells. *Mol Pharmacol* 1996;50:128–139.
207. Mayer G. ACE genotype and ACE inhibitor response in kidney disease: a perspective. *Am J Kidney Dis* 2002;2:227–235.
208. McLaughlin V, Sitbon O, Badesch DB, et al. Survival with first-line bosentan in patients with primary pulmonary hypertension. *Eur Respir J* 2005;25:244–249.
209. Milan A, Mulatero P, Williams TA, Carra R, Schiavone D, Martuzzi R, Rabbia F, Veglio F. Bradykinin B2 receptor gene (-58T/C) polymorphism influences baroreflex sensitivity in never-treated hypertensive patients. *J Hypertens* 2005;23:63–69.
210. Mino N, Kobayashi M, Nakajima A, et al. Protective effect of selective endothelin receptor antagonist, BQ123, in ischemic acute renal failure in rats. *Eur J Pharmacol* 1992;221:77–83.
211. Miyauchi T, Yanagisawa M, Iida K, et al. Age- and sex-related variation of plasma endothelin-1 concentration in normal and hypertensive subjects. *Am Heart J* 1992;123:1092–1093.
212. Mizono T, Saito Y, Itakura M, et al. Structure of the bovine ETB receptor gene. *Biochem J* 1992;287:305–309.
213. Montanari A, Biggi A, Carra N, et al. Endothelin-A receptors mediate renal hemodynamic effects of exogenous Angiotensin II in humans. *Hypertension* 2003;42:825–30.
214. Morcos SK. Prevention of contrast media nephrotoxicity- the story so far. *Clin Rad* 2004;59:381–389.
215. Moreland S, McMullen DM, Delaney CL, et al. Venous smooth muscle contains vasoconstrictor ETB-like receptors. *Biochem Biophys Res Commun* 1992;184:100–106.
216. Morey AK, Razandi M, Pedram A, et al. Oestrogen and progesterone inhibit the stimulated production of endothelin-1. *Biochem J* 1998;330:1097–1105.
217. Moridaira K, Morrissey J, Fitzgerald M, et al. ACE inhibition increases expression of the ETB receptor in kidneys of mice with unilateral obstruction. *Am J Physiol Renal Physiol* 2003;284:F209–F217.
218. Morissette G, Fortin JP, Otis S, et al. A novel nonpeptide antagonist of the kinin B1 receptor: effects at the rabbit receptor. *J Pharmacol Exp Ther* 2004;311:1121–1130.
219. Mourice AH, Turley AJ, Lintow TK. Human ACE polymorphism and, distilled water induced cough. *Thorax* 1997;52:111–113.
220. Mukae S, Itoh S, Aoki S, Iwata T, Nishio K, Sato R, Katagiri T. Association of polymorphisms of the renin-angiotensin system and bradykinin B2 receptor with ACE-inhibitor-related cough. *J Hum Hypertens* 2002;12:857–863.
221. Mundy GR. Metastasis to bone: causes, consequences and therapeutic opportunities. *Nature Rev Cancer* 2002;2:584–593.
222. Mundy GR. Metastasis to bone: causes, consequences and therapeutic opportunities. *Nature Rev Cancer* 2002;2:584–593.
223. Murphey LJ, Eccles WK, Williams GH, Brown NJ. Loss of sodium modulation of plasma kinins in human hypertension. *J Pharmacol Exp Ther* 2004;308:1046–1052.
224. Murphey LJ, Gainer JV, Vaughan DE, Brown NJ. Angiotensin-converting enzyme insertion/deletion polymorphism modulates the human in vivo metabolism of bradykinin. *Circulation* 2000;102:829–832.
225. Murphey LJ, Hachey DL, Vaughan DE, Brown NJ, et al. Quantification of BK1-5, the stable bradykinin plasma metabolite in humans, by a highly accurate liquid-chromatographic tandem mass spectrometric assay. *Anal Biochem* 2001;292:87–93.
226. Nadar R, Derrick A, Naidoo S, Naidoo Y, Hess F, Bhoola K. Immunoreactive B1 receptors in human transbronchial tissue. *Immunopharmacology* 1996;33:317–320.
227. Nadler SP, Zimplemann JA, Hebert RL. Endothelin inhibits vasopressin-stimulated water permeability in rat terminal inner medullary collecting duct. *J Clin Invest* 1992;90: 1458–1466.
228. Naicker S, Naidoo S, Ramsaroop R, et al. Tissue kallikrein and kinins in renal disease. *Immunopharmacology* 1999;44:183–192.
229. Nakamura S, Naruse M, Naruse K, et al. Immunocytochemical localization of endothelin in cultured bovine endothelial cells. *Histochemistry* 1990;94:475–477.
230. Nakamura T, Ebihara I, Tomino Y et al. Effect of a specific endothelin A receptor antagonist on murine lupus nephritis. *Kidney Int* 1995;47:481–489.
231. Nakanishi S. Substance P precursor and kininogen: their structures, gene organizations, and regulation. *Physiol Rev* 1987;67:1117–1142.
232. Nakano A, Kishi F, Minami K, et al. Selective conversion of big endothelins to tracheal smooth muscle-constricting 31-amino acid-length endothelins by chymase from human mast cells. *J Immunol* 1997;159:1987–1992.
233. Nakov R, Pfarr E, Eberle S. Darusentan: an effective endothelin A receptor antagonist for treatment of hypertension. *Am J Hypertens* 2002;15:583–589.
234. Nambi P, Pullen M, Jugus M, Gellai M. Rat kidney endothelin receptor in ischaemia-induced acute renal failure. *J Pharmacol Exp Ther* 1993;264:345–348.
235. Nelson J, Bagnato A, Battistini B, et al. The endothelin axis: emerging role in cancer. *Nat Rev Cancer* 2003;3:110–116.
236. Nelson JB, Hedican SP, George DJ, et al. Identification of endothelin-1 in the pathophysiology of metastatic adenocarcinoma of the prostate. *Nature Med* 1995;1:944–949.
237. Nelson JB, Lee WH, Nguyen SH, et al. Methylation of the 5′ CpG island of the endothelin B receptor gene is common in human prostate cancer. *Cancer Res* 1997;57:35–37.
238. Nelson JB, Nguyen SH, Wu-Wong JR, et al. New bone formation in an osteoblastic tumor model is increased by endothelin-1 overexpression and decreased by endothelin A receptor blockade. *Urology* 1999;53:1063–1069.
239. O'Connor CM, Gattis WA, Adams KF, et al. Tezosentan in patients with acute heart failure and acute coronary syndromes. *J Am Coll Cardiol* 2003;41:1452–1457.
240. Ogura K, Takayasu M, Dacey RG Jr. Differential effects of intra- and extraluminal endothelin on cerebral arterioles. *Am J Physiol* 1991;261:H531–H537.
241. Ohuchi T, Kuwaki T, Ling G, et al. Elevation of blood pressure by genetic and pharmacological disruption of the ETB receptor in mice. *Am J Physiol Regul Integr Comp Physiol* 1999;276:R1071–R1077.
242. Oliver JJ, Rajapakse NW, Evans RG. Effects of indomethacin on responses of regional kidney perfusion to vasoactive agents in rabbits. *Clin Exp Pharmacol Physiol* 2002;29: 873–879.
243. Olsen A, Herwald H, Wikstrom M, Persson K, Mattsson E, Bjorck L. Identification of two protein-binding and functional regions of curli, a surface organelle and virulence determinant of Escherichia coli. *J Biol Chem* 2002;37:34568–34572.
244. Omland T, Lie RT, Aakvaag A, et al. Plasma endothelin determination as a prognostic indicator of l-year mortality after acute myocardial infarction. *Circulation* 1994;89:1573–1579.
245. Ong ACM. Surprising new roles for endothelins. *Br Med J* 1996;312:195–196.
246. Paasche JD, Attramadal T, Sandberg C, et al. Mechanisms of endothelin receptor sub-type-specific targeting to distinct intracellular trafficking pathways. *J Biol Chem* 2001;276: 34041–34050.
247. Pacher R, Stanek B, Hulsmann M, et al. Prognostic impact of big endothelin-1 plasma concentrations compared with invasive hemodynamic evaluation in severe heart failure. *J Am Coll Cardiol* 1996;27:633–641.
248. Packer M. Effects of the endothelin receptor antagonist bosentan on the morbidity and mortality in patients with chronic heart failure. Results of the ENABLE 1 and 2 trial program. Congress of the American College of Cardiology 2002. Late Breaking Clinical Trials: Special Topic #412.
249. Pagotto U, Arzberger T, Hopfner U, et al. Expression and localization of endothelin-1 and endothelin receptors in human meningiomas. Evidence for a role in tumoral growth. *J Clin Invest* 1995;96:2017–2025.
250. Parrinello G, Scaglione R, Pinto A, et al. Central obesity and hypertension: the role of plasma endothelin. *Am J Hypertens* 1996;9:1186–1191.
251. Paula RD, Lima CV, Khosla MC, et al. Angiotensin-(1-7) potentiates the hypotensive effect of bradykinin in conscious rats. *Hypertension* 1995;26:1154–1159.
252. Pernow J, Boutier J-F, Franco-Cereceda A, et al. Potent selective vasoconstrictor effects of endothelin in the pig kidney in vivo. *Acta Physiol Scand* 1988;134:573–574.
253. Phagoo SB, Poole S, Leeb-Lundberg LM. Autoregulation of bradykinin receptors: agonists in the presence of interleukin-1beta shift the repertoire of receptor subtypes from B2 to B1 in human lung fibroblasts. *Mol Pharmacol* 1999;56:325–333.
254. Phillips BG, Narkiewicz K, Pesek CA, et al. Effects of obstructive sleep apnea on endothelin-1 and blood pressure. *J Hypertens* 1999;17:61–66.
255. Pitt B, Segal R, Martinez FA; et al. Mortality advantage seen with losartan. *Lancet* 1997;349:747–752.
256. Pizard A, Blaukat A, Muller-Esterl W, et al. Bradykinin-induced internalization of the human B2 receptor requires phosphorylation of three serine and two threonine residues at its carboxyl tail. *J Biol Chem* 1999;274:12738–12747.
257. Pollock DM, Pollock JS. Evidence for endothelin involvement in the response to high salt. *Am J Physiol Renal Physiol* 2001;281:F144–F150.
258. Pönicke K, Vogelsang M, Heinroth M, et al. Endothelin receptors in the failing and nonfailing human heart. *Circulation* 1998;97:744–751.
259. Prados MD, Schold SC JR SC, Fine HA, Jaeckle K, Hochberg F, Mechtler L, Fetell MR, Phuphanich S, Feun L, Janus TJ, Ford K, Graney W. A randomized, double-blind, placebo-controlled, phase 2 study of RMP-7 in combination with carboplatin administered intravenously for the treatment of recurrent malignant glioma. *Neuro-oncol* 2003;5:96–103.
260. Proud D, Kaplan AP. Kinin formation mechanisms and role in inflammatory disorders. *Annu Rev Immunol* 1988;6:49–83.

261. Puffenberger EG, Hosoda K, Washington SS, et al. A missense mutation of the endothelin-B receptor gene in multigenic Hirschsprung's disease. *Cell* 1994;79:1257–1266.

262. Pupilli C, Brunori M, Misciglia N, et al. Presence and distribution of endothelin-1 gene expression in human kidney. *Am J Physiol* 1994;267:F679–F687.

263. Quiroz Y, Pons H, Gordon KL, Rincon J et al: Mycophenolate mofetil prevents salt-sensitive hypertension resulting from nitric oxide synthesis inhibition. *Am J Physiol Renal Physiol* 2001;281:F38F47.

264. Rajagopalan S, Laursen JB, Borthayre A, et al. Role for endothelin-1 in angiotensin II–mediated hypertension. *Hypertension* 1997;30:29–34.

265. Rajapakse NW, Oliver JJ, Evans RG. Nitric oxide in responses of regional kidney blood flow to vasoactive agents in anesthetized rabbits. *J Cardiovasc Pharmacol* 2002;40:210–219.

266. Rakugi H, Tabuchi Y, Nakamaru M, et al. Evidence for endothelin-1 release from resistance vessels of rats in response to hypoxia. *Biochem Biophys Res Commun* 1990;169:973–977.

267. Ransom RW, Harrell CM, Reiss DR, et al. Pharmacological characterization and radioligand binding properties of a high-affinity, nonpeptide, bradykinin B1 receptor antagonist. *Eur J Pharmacol* 2004;499:77–84.

268. Reddigari S, Shibayama Y, Brunnee T, et al. Human Hageman factor (factor XII) and high molecular weight kininogen compete for the same binding site on human umbilical vein endothelial cells. *J Biol Chem* 1993;268:11982–11987.

269. Regoli D, Barabe J; Park WK Receptors for bradykinin in rabbit aorta. *Can J Physiol Pharmacol* 1977;55:855.

270. Remuzzi G, Perico N, Benigni A. New therapeutics that antagonize endothelin: promises and frustrations. *Nat Rev Drug Discov* 2002;1:986-1001.

271. Rich S, McLaughlin VV. Endothelin receptor blockers in cardiovascular disease. *Circulation* 2003;108:2184–2190.

272. Ricupero DA, Romero JR, Rishikof DC, et al. Des-Arg(10)-kallidin engagement of the B1 receptor stimulates type I collagen synthesis via stabilization of connective tissue growth factor mRNA. *J Biol Chem* 2000;275:12475–12480.

273. Rigat B, Hubert C, Alhenc-Gelas F, et al. An insertion/deletion polymorphism in the angiotensin I-converting enzyme gene accounting for half the variance of serum enzyme levels. *J Clin Invest* 1990; 86:1343–1346.

274. Riggleman A, Harvey J, Baylis C. Endothelin mediates some of the renal actions of acutely administered angiotensin II. *Hypertension* 2001;38:105–109.

275. Rocha e Silva M, Beraldo WT, Rosenfeld G. Bradykinin hypotensive and smooth muscle stimulating factor released from plasma globulins by snake venoms and by trypsin. *Am J Physiol* 1949;156:261.

276. Rosano L, Salani D, Di Castro V, et al. Endothelin-1 promotes proteolytic activity of ovarian carcinoma. *Clin Sci* 2002;103:306S–309S.

277. Rothermund L, Kossmehl P, Neumayer HH, et al. Renal damage is not improved by blockade of endothelin receptors in primary renin-dependent hypertension. *J Hypertens* 2003;21:2389–2397.

278. Roubert P, Cornet S, Plas P, et al. Upregulation of renal endothelin receptor in glycerol-induced acute renal failure in the rat. *J Cardiovasc Pharmacol* 1993;22:S303–S305.

279. Ruiz-Ortega M, Gomez-Garre D, Liu XH, et al. Quinapril decreases renal endothelin-1 expression and synthesis in a normotensive model of immune-complex nephritis. *J Am Soc Nephrol* 1997;8:756–768.

280. Russell FD, Skepper JN, Davenport AP. Evidence using immunoelectron microscopy for regulated and constitutive pathways in the transport and release of endothelin. *J Cardiovasc Pharmacol* 1998;31:424–430.

281. Saida K, Mitsui Y, Ishida I. A novel peptide, vasoactive intestinal contractor, of a new (endothelin) peptide family. Molecular cloning, expression and biological activity. *J Biol Chem* 1989;264:14613–14616.

282. Saijonmaa O, Nyman T, Fyhrquist F. Endothelin-1 stimulates its own synthesis on human endothelial cells. *Biochem Biophys Res Commun* 1992;188:286–291.

283. Saito I, Mizuno K, Niimura S, et al. Urinary endothelin and sodium excretion in essential hypertension. *Nephron* 1993;65:152–153.

284. Saito M, Majima M, Katori M, Sanjou Y, Suyama I, Shiokawa H, Koshiba K, Aoyagi T. Degradation of bradykinin in human urine by carboxypeptidase Y-like exopeptidase and neutral endopeptidase and their inhibition by ebelactone B and phosphoramidon. *Int J Tissue React* 1995;17:181–190.

285. Saito Y, Nakao K, Mukoyama M et al. Increased plasma endothelin level in patients with essential hypertension. *N Engl J Med* 1990; 322:205.

286. Sakai S, Miyauchi T, Kobayashi M, et al. Inhibition of myocardial endothelin pathway improves long-term survival in heart failure. *Nature* 1996;384:353–355.

287. Sakamoto A, Yanagisawa M, Sakurai T, et al. The ligand-receptor interactions of endothelin systems are mediated by distinct "message" and "address" domains. *J Cardiovasc Pharmacol* 1993;22:S113–S116.

288. Sakurai T, Yanagisawa M, Masaki T. Molecular characterization of endothelin receptors. *Trends Pharmacol Sci* 1992;13:103–108.

289. Sakurai T, Yanagisawa M, Takuwa Y, et al. Cloning of a cDNA encoding a nonisopeptide-selective subtype of the endothelin receptor. *Nature* 1990;348:732–735.

290. Salas SP, Vuletin JF, Giacaman A, Rosso, P et al: Long-term nitric oxide synthase inhibition in rat pregnancy reduces renal kallikrein. *Hypertens* 1999;34:865871.

291. Sasser JM, Pollock JS, Pollock DM. Renal endothelin in chronic angiotensin II hypertension. *Am J Physiol Regul Integr Comp Physiol* 2002;283:R243–R248.

292. Scharplatz M, Puhan MA, Steurer J, Bachmann LM. What is the impact of the ACE gene insertion/deletion (I/D) polymorphism on the clinical effectiveness and adverse events of ACE inhibitors?—Protocol of a systematic review. *BMC Med Genet* 2004;5:23.

293. Schiffrin EL, Thibault G. Plasma endothelin in human essential hypertension. *Am J Hypertens* 1991;4:303–308.

294. Schiffrin EL, Turgeon A, Deng LY. Effect of chronic ET_A-selective endothelin receptor antagonism on blood pressure in experimental and genetic hypertension in rats. *Br J Pharmacol* 1997;121:935–940.

295. Schiffrin EL. The angiotensin-endothelin relationship: does it play a role in cardiovascular and renal pathophysiology? *J Hypertens* 2003;21:2245–2247.

296. Schmaier AH. The kallikrein-kinin and the renin-angiotensin systems have a multilayered interaction. *Am J Physiol Regul Integr Comp Physiol* 2003;285:R1–R13.

297. Schmaier AH. The plasma kallikrein-kinin system counterbalances the renin-angiotensin system. *J Clin Invest* 2002;8:1007–1009.

298. Schmidt M, Kroger B, Jacob E, et al., Molecular characterization of human and bovine endothelin converting enzyme (ECE-1). *FEBS Lett* 1994;356:238–243.

299. Schulman G, Hakim R, Arias R, et al. Bradykinin generation by dialysis membranes: possible role in anaphylactic reaction. *J Am Soc Nephrol* 1993;3:1563.

300. Schweizer A, Valdenaire O, Nelbock P, et al. Human endothelin-converting enzyme (ECE-1): Three isoforms with distinct subcellular localizations. *Biochem J* 1997;328:871–877.

301. Scicli AG, Carretero OA. Renal kallikrein-kinin system. *Kidney Int* 1986;29:120–130.

302. Shariat-Madar Z, Mahdi F, Schmaier AH. Assembly and activation of the plasma kallikrein/kinin system: a new interpretation. *Int Immunopharmacol* 2002;2:1841–1849.

303. Shariat-Madar Z, Mahdi F, Schmaier AH. Identification and characterization of prolylcarboxypeptidase as an endothelial cell prekallikrein activator. *J Biol Chem* 2002;277:17962–17969.

304. Shariat-Madar Z, Mahdi F, Schmaier AH. Recombinant prolylcarboxypeptidase activates plasma prekallikrein. *Blood* 2004;103:4554–4561.

305. Shichiri M, Hirata Y, Ando K, et al. Plasma endothelin levels in hypertension and chronic renal failure. *Hypertension* 1990;15:493–496.

306. Shimada K, Takahashi M, Tanzawa K. Cloning and functional expression of endothelin-converting enzyme from rat endothelial cells. *J Biol Chem* 1994;269:18275–18278.

307. Shimimoto K, Masuda A, Ando T, et al. Mechanisms of suppression of renal kallikrein activity in low renin essential hypertension and renoparenchymal hypertension. *Hypertension* 1989;14:375.

308. Shohet RV, Kisanuki YY, Zhao XS, et al. Mice with cardiomyocyte-specific disruption of the endothelin-1 gene are resistant to hyperthyroid cardiac hypertrophy. *Proc Natl Acad Sci U S A* 2004;101:2088–2093.

309. Shyamala V, Moulthrop THM, Stratton-Thomas J et al. Two distinct endothelin B receptors generated by alternate splicing from a single gene. *Cell Mol Biol Res* 1994;40:285–296.

310. Sigary HM, Ibrahim MM, Jaffa AA, et al. Renal interstitial bradykinin, prostagiandin E2, and cyclic guanosine 3'5'-monophosphate. Effects of altered sodium intake. *Hypertension* 1994;23:1068–1070.

311. Simonson MS, Wann S, Mene P, et al. Endothelin stimulates phospholipase C, Na+/H+ exchange, c-fos expression, and mitogenesis in rat mesangial cells. *J Clin Invest* 1989;83:708–712.

312. Sitbon O, Badesch DB, Channick RN, et al. Effects of the dual endothelin antagonist bosentan in patients with pulmonary arterial hypertension: A 1-year follow-up study. *Chest* 2003;124:247–254.

313. Song JS, Sainz IM, Cosenza SC, Isordia-Salas I, et al. Inhibition of tumor angiogenesis in vivo by a monoclonal antibody targeted to domain 5 of high molecular weight kininogen. *Blood* 2004;7:2065–2072.

314. Song Q, Chao J, Chao L. DNA polymorphisms in the 5'-flanking region of the human tissue kallikrein gene. *Hum Genet* 1997;99:727–734.

315. Sorensen SS, Egeblad M, Eiskjaer H, et al. Endothelin in renovascular and essential hypertension. *Blood Pressure* 1994;3:364–369.

316. Sorokin A, Kohan DE. Physiology and pathology of endothelin-1 in renal mesangium. *Am J Physiol Renal Physiol* 2003;285:F579–F589.

317. Spieker LE, Corti R, Binggeli C, Luscher TF, Noll G. Baroreceptor dysfunction induced by nitric oxide synthase inhibition in humans. *J Am Coll Cardiol* 2000;36:213–218.

318. Stockenhuber F, Gottsauner-Wolf M, Marosi L, et al. Plasma levels of endothelin in chronic renal failure and after renal transplantation: impact on hypertension and cyclosporin A–associated nephrotoxicity. *Clin Sci* 1992;82:255–258.

319. Streeten DH, Kerr CB, Kerr LP, et al. Hyperbradykininism: a new orthostatic syndrome. *Lancet* 1972;2:1048–1053.

320. Sudgen PH. An overview of endothelin signaling in the cardiac myocyte. *J Mol Cell Cardiol* 2003;35:871–886.

321. Suzuki T, Katori M, Fujita T, Kumagai Y, et. al. Involvement of the renal kallikrein-kinin system in K(+)-induced diuresis and natriuresis in anesthetized rats. *Eur J Pharmacol* 2000;399:223–227.

322. Sventek P, Turgeon A, Garcia R, et al. Vascular and cardiac overexpression of endothelin-1 gene in one-kidney one clip Goldblatt hypertensive rats but only in the late phase of two-kidney one clip Goldblatt hypertension. *J Hypertens* 1996;14:57–64.

323. Sventek P, Turgeon A, Schiffrin EL. Vascular endothelin-1 gene expression and effect on blood pressure of chronic ET_A endothelin receptor antagonism after nitric oxide synthase inhibition with L-NAME in normal rats. *Circulation* 1997;95:240–244.

324. Takada K, Takiguchi M, Konno A, Inaba M. Autoimmunity against a Tissue Kallikrein in IQI/Jic Mice: a model for Sjogren's syndrome. *J Biol Chem* 2005;280:3982–3988.

325. Takeda M, Breyer MD, Noland TD, et al. Endothelin-1 receptor antagonist: effects on endothelinand cyclosporine-treated mesangial cells. *Kidney Int* 1992;42:1713–1719.

326. Takeda M, Iwasaki S, Hellings SE, et al. Divergent expression of EtA and EtB receptors in response to cyclosporine in mesangial cells. *Am J Pathol* 1994;144:473–479.

327. Takemoto F, Uchida S, Ogata E, et al. Endothelin-1 and endothelin-3 binding to rat nephrons. *Am J Physiol* 1993;264:F827–F832.

328. Takigawa M, Sakurai T, Kasuya Y, et al. Molecular identification of guanine-nucleotide-binding regulatory proteins which couple to endothelin receptors. *Eur J Biochem* 1995;228:102–108.

329. Tojo A, Fujita T, Wilcox CS. Omapatrilat: still a promise in salt-sensitive hypertension? *J Hypertens* 2003;1:31–32.

330. Tomita K, Nonguchi H, Terada Y, et al. Effects of ET-1 on water and chloride transport in cortical collecting ducts of the rat. *Am J Physiol* 1993;264:F690–F696.

331. Tomita K, Pisano JJ, Knepper MA. Control of sodium and potassium transport in the cortical collecting duct of the rat. Effects of bradykinin, vasopressin, and deoxycorticosterone. *J Clin Invest* 1985;76:132–136.

332. Tomita K, Pisano JJ. Binding of [³H] bradykinin in isolated nephron segments of the rabbit. *Am J Physiol* 1984;246:F732–F737.

333. Tschope C, Schultheiss HP, Walther T. Multiple interactions between the renin-angiotensin and the kallikrein-kinin systems: role of ACE inhibition and AT1 receptor blockade. *J Cardiovasc Pharmacol* 2002;39:478–487.

334. Tschope C, Spillmann F, Altmann C, et al. The bradykinin B1 receptor contributes to the cardioprotective effects of AT1 blockade after experimental myocardial infarction. *Cardiovasc Res* 2004;61:559–569.

335. Tsuchiya K, Naruse M, Sanaka T et al. Effects of endothelin on renal regional blood flow in dogs. *Eur J Pharmacol* 1989;166:541–543.

336. Tsutsumi Y, Matsubara H, Masaki H, et al. Angiotensin II type 2 receptor overexpression activates the vascular kinin system and causes vasodilation. *J Clin Invest* 1999;104:925–935.

337. Turner AJ, Barnes K, Schweizer A, et al. Isoforms of endothelin-converting enzyme: Why and where? *Trends Pharmacol Sci* 1998;19:483–486.

338. Uchida S, Takemoto F, Ogata E, et al. Detection of endothelin-1 mRNA by RT-PCR in isolated rat renal tubules. *Biochem Biophys Res Commun* 1992;188:108–113.

339. Ujiie K, Terada Y, Nonoguchi H, et al. Messenger RNA expression and synthesis of endothelin-1 along rat nephron segments. *J Clin Invest* 1992;90:1043–1048.

340. Valdenaire O, Rohrbacher E, Mattei MG. Organization of the gene encoding the human endothelin-converting enzyme (ECE-1). *J Biol Chem* 1995;270:29794–29798.

341. van der Graaf F, Keus FJ, Vlooswijk RA, Bouma BN. The contact activation mechanism in human plasma: activation induced by dextran sulfate. *Blood* 1982;59:1225–1233.

342. Veglio F, Bertello P, Pinna G, et al. Plasma endothelin in essential hypertension and diabetes mellitus. *J Human Hypertens* 1993;7:321–325.

343. Venuti A, Salani D, Manni V, et al. Expression of endothelin 1 and endothelin A receptor in HPV-associated cervical carcinoma: new potential targets for anticancer therapy. *FASEB J* 2000;14:2277–2283.

344. Verhaar MC, Strachan FE, Newby DE, et al. Endothelin-A receptor antagonist-mediated vasodilatation is attenuated by inhibition of nitric oxide synthesis by endothelin-B receptor blockade. *Circulation* 1998;97:752–756.

345. Verresen L, Fink E, Lemke HD, Vanrenterghem Y. Bradykinin is a mediator of anaphylactoid reactions during hemodialysis with AN69 membranes. *Kidney Int* 1994;45:1497–1503.

346. Vio CP, Figueroa CD. Evidence for a stimulatory effect of high potassium diet on renal kallikrein. *Kidney Int* 1987;31:1327–1334.

347. Wada A, Tsutamato T, Maeda Y, et al. Endogenous atrial natriuretic peptide inhibits endothelin-1 secretion in dogs with severe congestive heart failure. *Am J Physiol* 1996;270: H1819–H1824.

348. Waggoner WG, Genova SL, Rash VA. Kinetic analyses demonstrate that the equilibrium assumption does not apply to [125I]endothelin-1 binding data. *Life Sci* 1992;51:1869–1876.

349. Wagner OF, Christ G, Wojta J, et al. Polar secretion of endothelin-1 by cultured endothelial cells. *J Biol Chem* 1992;267:16066–16068.

350. Wang A, Holcslaw T, Bashmore TM et al. Exacerbation of radiocontrast nephrotoxicity by endothelin receptor antagonism. *Kidney Int* 2000;57:1675–1680.

351. Wang D, Yoshida H, Song Q, Chao L, et. al. Enhanced renal function in bradykinin B(2) receptor transgenic mice. *Am J Physiol Renal Physiol* 2000;278:F484–F491.

352. Wang T, Li H, Zhao C, Chen C, et. al. Recombinant adeno-associated virus-mediated kallikrein gene therapy reduces hypertension and attenuates its cardiovascular injuries. *Gene Ther* 2004;11:1342–1350.

353. Wang Y-X, Gavras I, Lammek B, et al. Effects of bradykinin and prostaglandin inhibition on systemic and regional hemodynamics in conscious normotensive rats. *J Hypertens* 1991;9: 805–812.

354. Webb DJ. Endothelin: from molecule to man. *Br J Clin Pharmacol* 1997;44:9–20.

355. Werle E, Berek U. Zur Kenntnis des Kallikreins. *Angew Chem* 1948;60A:53.

356. Wesson DE, Simoni J, Green DF. Reduced extracellular pH increases endothelin-1 secretion by human renal microvascular endothelial cells. *J Clin Invest* 1998;101:578–583.

357. Wilkins FC Jr, Alberola A, Mizelle HL, et al. Systemic hemodynamics and renal function during long-term pathophysiological increases in circulating endothelin. *Am J Physiol Regul Integr Comp Physiol* 1995;268:R375–R381.

358. Witherow FN, Helmy A, Webb DJ, et al. Bradykinin contributes to the vasodilator effects of chronic angiotensin-converting enzyme inhibition in patients with heart failure. *Circulation* 2001;104:2177–2181.

359. Wong CM, O"Connor DT, Martinez JA, Kailasam MT, et. al. Diminished renal kallikrein responses to mineralocorticoid stimulation in African Americans: determinants of an intermediate phenotype for hypertension. *Am J Hypertens* 2003;16:281–289.

360. Wong WHY, Wong BPH, Wong EFC, et al. Downregulation of endothelin B receptors in cardiomyopathic hamsters. *Cardiology* 1998;89:195–201.

361. Xu D, Emoto N, Giaid A, et al. ECE-1: a membrane-bound metalloprotease that catalyzes the proteolytic activation of big endothelin-1. *Cell* 1994;78:473–485.

362. Yamamoto S, Matsumoto N, Kanazawa M, et al. Different contributions of endothelin-A and endothelin-B receptors in postischemic cardiac dysfunction and norepinephrine overflow in rat hearts. *Circulation* 2005;111:302–309.

363. Yamauchi T, Ohnaka K, Takayanagi R, et al. Enhanced secretion of endothelin-1 by elevated glucose levels from cultured bovine endothelial cells. *FEBS Lett* 1990;267:16–18.

364. Yanagisawa M, Kurihara H, Kimura S, et al, A novel potent vasoconstrictor peptide produced by vascular endothelial cells. *Nature* 1988;332:411–415.

365. Yang T, Terada Y, Nonoguchi H, Tsujino M, Tomita K, Marumo F. Distribution of kallikrein-binding protein mRNA in kidneys and difference between SHR and WKY rats. *Am J Physiol* 1994;267:F325–F330.

366. Yokokawa K, Tahara H, Kohno M, et al. Hypertension associated with endothelin-secreting malignant hemangioendothelioma. *Ann Intern Med* 1991;114:213–215.

367. Yoshimura A, Iwasaki S, Inui K, et al. Endothelin-1 and endothelin B type receptor are induced in mesangial proliferative nephritis in the rat. *Kidney Int* 1995;48:1290–1297.

368. Yousef GM, Diamandis EP. An overview of the kallikrein gene families in humans and other species: emerging candidate tumour markers. *Clin Bioche* 2003;36:443–452.

369. Yousef GM, Diamandis EP. The new human tissue kallikrein gene family: structure, function, and association to disease. *Endocr Rev* 2001;22:184–204.

370. Yu H, Song Q, Freedman BI, Chao J, et. al. Association of the tissue kallikrein gene promoter with ESRD and hypertension. *Kidney Int* 2002;61:1030–1039.

371. Zaporowska-Stachowiak I, Gluszek J, Chodera A. Comparison of the serum insulin and endothelin level in patients with essential and renovascular hyperten- sion. *J Hum Hypertens* 1997;11:795–800.

372. Zausinger S, Lumenta DB, Pruneau D, Schmid-Elsaesser R, Plesnila N, Baethmann A. Therapeutical efficacy of a novel nonpeptide bradykinin B2 receptor antagonist on brain edema formation and ischemic tissue damage in focal cerebral ischemia. *Acta Neurochir Suppl* 2003;86:205–207.

373. Zhang JJ, Bledsoe G, Kato K, Chao L et. al. Tissue kallikrein attenuates salt-induced renal fibrosis by inhibition of oxidative stress. *Kidney Int* 2004;66:722–732.

374. Zhao Y, Qiu Q, Mahdi F, et al. Assembly and activation of HK-PK complex on endothelial cells results in bradykinin liberation and NO formation. *Am J Physiol Heart Circ Physiol* 2001;280:H1821–H1829.

375. Zhou L, Ida T, Marumo F. Role of thromboxane A₂, endothelin-1 and endothelin-3 in rat nephrotoxic serum nephritis. *Tohoku J Exp Med* 1996;178:357–369.

376. Zoccali C, Leonardis D, Parlongo S, et al. Urinary and plasma endothelin-1 in essential hypertension and in hypertension secondary to renoparenchymal disease. *Nephrol Dial Transpl* 1995;10:1320–1323.

377. Zolk O, Quattek J, Sitzler G, et al. Expression of endothelin-1, endothelin-converting enzyme and endothelin receptors in chronic heart failure. *Circulation* 1999;99:2118–2123.

CHAPTER **16**

Adenosine in the Kidney

PHYSIOLOGICAL ROLES AND MECHANISMS OF BIOSYNTHESIS

Edwin K. Jackson* and Raghvendra K. Dubey*†
*University of Pittsburgh School of Medicine, Pittsburgh, Pennsylvania, USA
†University Hospital Zurich, Zurich, Switzerland

RENAL EFFECTS OF ADENOSINE

Introduction

The renal effects of adenosine are mediated by specific adenosine receptors. Adenosine receptors are heptahelical G-protein–coupled receptors and are comprised of four subtypes (A_1, A_{2A}, A_{2B}, and A_3). A_1 receptors exhibit a very high affinity for adenosine (K_D in the low nanomolar range), whereas the affinity of A_{2A} receptors for adenosine is approximately threefold less. Both A_{2B} and A_3 receptors are low-affinity receptors requiring high nanomolar concentrations of adenosine for activation. A_1 and A_{2A} receptors are clearly involved in regulating renal function. Presently there is scant evidence for the involvement of A_{2B} and A_3 receptors in renal physiology.

A_1-Receptor–Mediated Effects

TUBULAR TRANSPORT

A_1 receptors mediate enhancement of renal epithelial transport. In vitro stimulation of A_1 receptors in epithelial cells with a proximal tubular phenotype increases Na^+-glucose and Na^+-phosphate symport (25, 169), and antagonism of A_1 receptors decreases Na^+-dependent phosphate transport in renal proximal tubular cells (19, 20). In vitro stimulation of A_1 receptors in epithelial cells with a proximal tubular phenotype has a bimodal effect on the Na^+-H^+ exchanger 3 (NHE3), stimulating NHE3-mediated transport at low levels of activation and inhibiting NHE3-mediated transport at high levels of stimulation (36, 37). Activation of A_1 receptors in microperfused proximal convoluted tubules enhances basolateral Na^+-$3HCO_3^-$ symport (168).

There is also evidence that A_1 receptors modulate electrolyte reabsorption in the collecting duct: (1) The expression of A_1 receptors is greater in the collecting duct compared with the proximal tubule (159, 184); (2) A_1-receptor antagonists increase sodium excretion, yet have little effect on potassium excretion (89, 92, 150, 172), whereas diuretics that act only proximal to the collecting duct

increase potassium excretion; and (3) A_1-receptor blockade increases the ratio of sodium-to-lithium clearance (5).

RENAL BLOOD FLOW, GLOMERULAR FILTRATION RATE, AND TUBULOGLOMERULAR FEEDBACK

Placement of A_1-receptor agonists into the renal interstitium decreases blood flow to superficial and deep nephrons (1). In the outer cortex, A_1-receptor–mediated vasoconstriction is due to contraction of preglomerular microvessels (66, 71, 81, 117, 118), and thus A_1-receptor agonists decrease glomerular filtration rate (GFR). Stimulation of A_1 receptors may also reduce GFR by causing glomerular contraction (165). Nitric oxide reduces A_1-receptor–mediated preglomerular vasoconstriction (9), and angiotensin II enhances A_1-receptor–induced preglomerular vasoconstriction (34, 65, 67, 116, 127, 162, 174, 180). In juxtaglomerular nephrons, A_1-receptor stimulation causes a more widespread vasoconstriction that includes preglomerular microvessels, efferent arterioles, and outer medullary descending vasa recta (66, 121, 157).

If single-nephron glomerular filtration rate (SNGFR) exceeds the reabsorptive capacity of the proximal tubule, the concentration of NaCl bathing the macula densa increases. In response, the macula densa releases a chemical signal that causes the afferent arteriole servicing that nephron to constrict, thus decreasing glomerular capillary pressure, single nephron blood flow and SNGFR. This negative feedback system is termed "tubuloglomerular feedback" (TGF).

Three mechanisms have been proposed to explain TGF. One mechanism proposes that TGF is mediated by adenosine formed intracellularly and released from macula densa cells (126, 129). In this view, increased NaCl deliver to the macula densa accelerates NaCl reabsorption by the macula densa, which in turn enhances energy utilization and ATP breakdown. Increased utilization of ATP is proposed to increase the production of adenosine within the macula densa, which then exits the macula densa and causes afferent arteriolar vasoconstriction mediated by A_1 receptor activation. A second theory proposes that enhanced transport of NaCl by the macula densa causes depolarization of the basolateral membrane of macula densa cells leading to release of ATP through anion channels (88, 170). ATP is hypothesized to activate P_2 receptors and vasoconstrict preglomerular microvessels. A third theory postulates that the ATP released by the macula densa in response to increased transport of NaCl is metabolized extracellular to adenosine by the sequential actions of ecto-ATPase, ecto-ADPase and ecto-5′-nucleotidase, and it is this extracellularly-derived adenosine that constricts the afferent arteriole via A_1 receptors (24, 143). These three hypotheses to explain TGF are not mutually exclusive.

A role of for adenosine and A_1 receptors in mediating TGF is supported by a large number of observations: (1) Hypertonic saline stimulates adenosine release from mouse thick ascending limbs (10); (2) A high-sodium diet increases renal interstitial levels of adenosine by approximately 18-fold (158) and increases total tissue adenosine levels in the renal cortex and medulla by approximately twofold (190); (3) Nonselective adenosine-receptor antagonists, such as theophylline (126) and DPSPX (55), as well as selective A_1-receptor antagonists, such as DPCPX (151) and FK838 (142), block TGF, as does exogenous adenosine deaminase, the enzyme that metabolizes adenosine to inosine (126); (4) The reduction in renal blood flow induced by intrarenal infusions of hypertonic saline, a model of TGF, is blocked by adenosine receptor antagonists (21, 34, 59); (5) Inhibition of adenosine transport or inhibition of adenosine deaminase augments TGF (125); (6) Intraluminal (55) and peritubular (151) administration of selective A_1-receptor agonists decreases glomerular hydrostatic pressure; (7) TGF responses are completely absent in mice lacking A_1 receptors (16; 163); (8) TGF responses are attenuated in mice deficient in ecto-5′-nucleotidase (24); and (9) TGF in isolated rabbit afferent aterioles with attached macula densas is blocked by inhibition of ecto-5′-nucleotidase (143).

The participation of A_1 receptors in TGF has practical implications. Selective antagonism of A_1 receptors in vivo reproducibly increases sodium excretion (89, 92, 150, 172) without triggering a TGF-induced reduction in GFR (182) and without increasing potassium excretion. Consequently, selective A_1-receptor antagonists are being developed as eukaluretic natriuretics in sodium retaining states such as heart failure (63).

RENIN RELEASE

A_1 receptors may function to restrain renin release responses, a theory known as the *adenosine-brake hypothesis* (76). A_1 receptors are coupled to G_i (98, 183), a G-protein that inhibits adenylyl cyclase. Because most stimuli increase renin release by activating adenylyl cyclase (95), stimulation of juxtaglomerular A_1 receptors attenuates renin release, and antagonism of renal A_1 receptors increases renin release (77). This concept is confirmed by studies in A_1-receptor knockout mice (153).

RENAL INJURY

A_1 receptors appear to mediate in part drug-induced nephrotoxicity. Selective antagonism of A_1 receptors attenuates renal injury caused by several nephrotoxins including cisplatin (87, 119, 164), gentamicin (185), cephaloridine (120), glycerol (84, 131, 156), and radiocontrast media (4, 50). In contrast to nephrotoxins, evidence suggests that A_1 receptors protect the kidney from renal injury caused by renal ischemia followed by reperfusion (100, 102).

A_{2A}-Receptor–Mediated Effects

MEDULLARY BLOOD FLOW AND TUBULAR TRANSPORT

Although there are reports of direct effects of A_{2A} receptors on tubular transport (181), the weight of evidence indicates that A_{2A} receptors importantly modulate tubular transport indirectly via changes in renal medullary blood flow. Selective A_{2A}-receptor agonists increase renal blood flow (104, 105) by dilating the renal medullary microcirculation (1), including afferent and efferent arterioles of juxtaglomerular nephrons (121) and outer medullary descending vasa recta (157). These effects enhance medullary blood flow (189), alter the peritubular forces that modulate sodium reabsorption, and increase NaCl excretion (189).

RENAL INJURY

Activation of A_{2A} receptors engages anti-inflammatory actions that protect the kidneys from injury. Stimulation of A_{2A} receptors inhibits neutrophil–endothelial cell interactions in vitro (27), and in vivo A_{2A} receptor activation decreases ischemia/reperfusion injury–induced neutrophil–endothelial interactions (122). Selective activation of A_{2A} receptors reduces the renal infiltration of neutrophils and decreases renal dysfunction in kidneys subjected to ischemia/reperfusion injury (124). Studies in chimeric mice suggest that A_{2A} receptors residing on bone marrow–derived cells mediate most, if not all, of the renal protective effects of A_{2A}-receptor activation (30).

A_{2B}-Receptor–Mediated Effects

Activation of A_{2B} receptors attenuates proliferation of and extracellular matrix production by vascular smooth muscle cells (41, 43, 46, 47, 48), cardiac fibroblasts (42), and renal mesangial cells (39). Presently, there are insufficient data to judge whether A_{2B} receptors influence renal structure and function in vivo.

A_3-Receptor–Mediated Effects

A_3 receptors do not have an important role with regard to modulating renal excretory function, at least under basal conditions (115). However, mice deficient in A_3 receptors are protected against myoglobinuria-mediated and ischemia-induced acute renal failure (101), and antagonism of A₃ receptors is also renal protective (99, 101).

MECHANISMS OF ADENOSINE PRODUCTION

Introduction

The adenosine that regulates renal function can arise from at least five different biochemical pathways (Fig. 1). Each mechanism of adenosine formation may play a unique role in the regulation of renal function.

Intracellular ATP Pathway

The *intracellular ATP pathway* of adenosine production is due to sequential dephosphorylation of intracellular ATP to adenosine within cells. When cells use ATP more quickly than ATP can be replenished by ADP/AMP rephosphorylation, AMP accumulates and is metabolized to adenosine by cytosolic 5'-nucleotidase (152). Because nucleoside transporters facilitate the movement of adenosine across cell membranes (23), translocation of intracellular adenosine into the extracellular space increases the levels of adenosine at cell surface receptors.

The intracellular ATP pathway is clearly involved in modulating renal function. Increased NaCl transport by the medullary thick ascending limb requires energy and accelerates the breakdown of ATP by basolateral Na⁺, K⁺-ATPase. Because oxygen availability to the renal medulla is marginal (130), increased NaCl transport depletes ATP levels and leads to dephosphorylation of adenine nucleotides to adenosine. That this mechanism exists in the kidney is evidenced by the facts that in vitro a high sodium concentration augments adenosine production by thick ascending limbs (10), and in vivo hypertonic radiocontrast agents (83) and a high NaCl diet (158, 190) increase intrarenal levels of adenosine. Coupling of NaCl concentrations in the lumen of the medullary thick ascending limb to increased renal medullary levels of adenosine importantly regulates sodium excretion (189). In this regard, NaCl-induced increases in medullary adenosine levels activate vasodilatory A₂ₐ receptors in the vasa recta. The resulting decrease in vascular resistance of the vasa recta alters peritubular forces that decrease the rate of NaCl reabsorption. The net result is an enhanced urinary excretion of NaCl (189).

Coupling of NaCl levels at the macula densa to increased adenosine production via the intracellular ATP pathway may participate in TGF and inhibition of renin release by activating vasoconstrictor A₁ receptors in the preglomerular renal microcirculation and juxtaglomerular cells, respectively. However, recent studies suggest that the extracellular ATP pathway is more important in this regard (see following section).

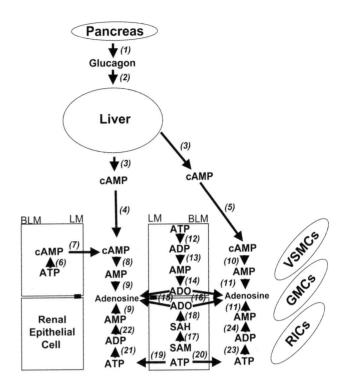

FIGURE 1 Summary of mechanisms mediating adenosine biosynthesis in the kidneys. (*1*) Release of glucagon from the pancreas into the portal circulation; (*2*) Stimulation of hepatocyte adenylyl cyclase by glucagon; (*3*) Efflux of liver-derived cyclic AMP (cAMP) into the systemic circulation; (*4*) Filtration of liver-derived cAMP into the tubular lumen; (*5*) Delivery of liver-derived cAMP into the renal interstitial space via the renal microcirculation; (*6*) Intracellular conversion of ATP to cyclic AMP, mediated by adenylyl cyclase; (*7*) Efflux of cyclic AMP across the luminal membrane (LM) into the tubular lumen, mediated by MRP4 (Note: OAT1 in the basolateral membrane [BLM] transports cAMP into, not out of, cells, so intracellular cyclic AMP would not flux across BLMs into interstitial space.); (*8*) Conversion of cAMP to AMP in the tubular lumen, mediated by ecto-phosphodiesterase in LMs; (*9*) Conversion of AMP to adenosine in the tubular lumen, mediated by ecto-5'-nucleotidase in LMs; (*10*) Conversion of cAMP to AMP in the renal interstitial compartment, mediated by ecto-phosphodiesterase on BLMs; (*11*) Conversion of AMP to adenosine in the renal interstitial compartment, mediated by ecto-5'-nucleotidase on BLMs (Note: Ecto-5'-nucleotidase on VSMCs, GMCs, and RICs may also convert AMP to adenosine); (*12*) and (*13*) Intracellular depletion of high-energy phosphate purine nucleotides to AMP when energy demand exceeds energy supply; (*14*) Intracellular conversion of AMP to adenosine (ADO), mediated by cytosolic 5'-nucleotidase; (*15*) and (*16*) Transport of adenosine into the tubular lumen and renal interstitial space, respectively mediated by adenosine transporters; (*17*) Intracellular methylation reactions convert S-adenosylmethionine (SAM) to S-adenosylhomocysteine (SAH); (*18*) SAH is metabolized to ADO, mediated by SAH hydrolase; (*19*) and (*20*) Transport of ATP across LMs and BLMs, respectively, mediated by anion channels; (*21*) Degradation of ATP to ADP by ecto-ATPases in tubular lumen; (*22*) Degradation of ADP to AMP by ecto-ADPases in tubular lumen; (*23*) Degradation of ATP to ADP by ecto-ATPases in renal interstitial compartment; (*24*) Degradation of ADP to AMP by ecto-ADPases in renal interstitial compartment.

Note that the reactions occurring in the renal interstitial compartment may be mediated in part by enzymes located on the cell surface of renal interstitial cells (RICs), renal vascular smooth muscle cells (VSMCs) and glomerular mesangial cells (GMCs). Also, VSMCs and GMCs may participate in the conversion of systemically derived cyclic AMP to AMP or adenosine before filtration into the tubular lumen or before delivery of these purines to the renal interstitial compartment.

Reactive ischemia is yet another example of the intracellular ATP pathway in the kidney. Because renal ischemia activates the intracellular ATP pathway of adenosine production (112, 128, 140), adenosine causes reactive ischemia via activation of A_1 receptors in the preglomerular microvessels (138, 149). Therefore, a brief period of renal ischemia triggers a short-lived increase in renal vascular resistance.

Studies suggest that brief activation of A_1 receptors preconditions the kidney and protects it from a subsequent prolonged renal ischemia-reperfusion insult (100, 102). Because brief ischemia activates the intracellular ATP pathway, it is likely that this mechanism of adenosine production is involved in renal preconditioning by brief ischemia.

Extracellular ATP Pathway

The *extracellular ATP pathway* of adenosine production is due to sequential dephosphorylation of extracellular adenine nucleotides to adenosine outside cells and is an important mechanism of renal adenosine production (75, 154). Many cell types residing in the kidney, including sympathetic nerve terminals, platelets, endothelial cells, vascular smooth muscle cells, and epithelial cells, can release adenine nucleotides when appropriately stimulated. For example, endothelial cells and vascular smooth muscle cells release adenine nucleotides in response to thrombin (135) and neutrophil-derived proteases (103). Extracellular adenine nucleotides are then metabolized to adenosine by the sequential actions of ecto-ATPases (ATP to ADP), ecto-ADPases (ADP to AMP), and ecto-5'-nucleotidase (AMP to adenosine) (60, 61, 133).

Studies support the view that the extracellular ATP pathway importantly contributes to the TGF mechanism. As mentioned previously, enhanced transport of NaCl by the macula densa depolarizes the macula densa basolateral membrane, thus leading to opening of anion channels that permit the passage of intracellular ATP into the extracellular compartment (88, 170). Studies with inhibitors of ecto-5'-nucleotidase (143) and experiments in ecto-5'-nucleotidase knockout mice (24) strongly support the view that the conversion of ATP to adenosine mediates, at least in part, TGF. This mechanism of adenosine formation may also inhibit renin release in response to high-salt intake.

Transmethylation Pathway

S-adenosyl-L-homocysteine is hydrolyzed to L-homocysteine and adenosine, and this is the *transmethylation pathway* of adenosine biosynthesis (106). Because transfer of a methyl group from *S*-adenosyl-L-methionine to methyl acceptors forms *S*-adenosyl-L-homocysteine, the rate of transmethylation reactions determines the rate of adenosine production by the transmethylation pathway. In cardiomyocytes, approximately one third of the adenosine released to the extracellular space is due to the transmethylation pathway (35); however, the importance of this pathway in the kidney remains to be determined.

Extracellular cAMP-Adenosine Pathway

The *cyclic AMP-adenosine pathway* provides a mechanism for hormonally-mediated adjustments of extracellular adenosine levels in the biophase of adenosine receptors. The cyclic AMP-adenosine pathway has both intracellular and extracellular arms. The *intracellular* cyclic AMP-pathway is mediated by metabolism of intracellular cyclic AMP to AMP by cytosolic phosphodiesterase, followed by metabolism of intracellular AMP by cytosolic 5'-nucleotidase to adenosine. Adenosine formed by the intracellular cyclic AMP-adenosine pathway transverses the cell membrane into the extracellular compartment aided by adenosine transporters.

The intracellular cyclic-AMP-adenosine pathway is most likely less important because of the rapid conversion of intracellular AMP to ADP by AMP kinase. In this regard, at low concentrations, most intracellular AMP is rephosphorylated rather than dephosphorylated (90). In contrast, in the extracellular compartment, dephosphorylation is the predominant fate of extracellular AMP because ecto-5'-nucleotidase, an ubiquitous enzyme attached to the cell membrane by a lipid-sugar linkage, quickly metabolizes AMP to adenosine (113, 134, 187).

Hormonal stimulation of adenylyl cyclase results in efflux of intracellular cyclic AMP into the extracellular compartment, and if ecto-phosphodiesterase is present in the extracellular compartment, hormonal stimulation of adenylyl cyclase would result in extracellular production of adenosine by metabolism of extracellular cyclic AMP to extracellular AMP by ecto-phosphodiesterase, followed by metabolism of extracellular AMP to adenosine by ecto-5'-nucleotidase. This sequence of reactions is called the extracellular cyclic AMP-adenosine pathway.

The extracellular cyclic AMP-adenosine pathway is initiated by efflux of intracellular cyclic AMP. Although cyclic AMP egress was described in pigeon erythrocytes decades ago (29), the mechanism remains insufficiently characterized. The slime mold *Dictyostelium discoideum* evolved the mechanism of cyclic AMP egress several hundred millions years ago as a survival strategy. When nutrients are insufficient for survival, *Dictyostelium discoideum* secretes cyclic AMP, and extracellular cyclic AMP binds to cell-surface receptors on nearby cells to induce chemotaxis. This leads to aggregation of amoebae into a migrating slug (2).

In mammals, cyclic AMP efflux occurs in most cells/tissues including the rat superior cervical ganglia (26), rat glioma cells (38), fibroblasts (85), rat liver (96), rat heart (123), rat adipose tissue (191), and swine adipocytes (53). The speed of cyclic AMP efflux is related to the intracellular levels of cyclic AMP (8, 86), and the process begins within minutes following activation of adenylyl cyclase (52). The mechanism of cyclic AMP efflux is energy-dependent (144) and temperature sensitive (18) and is blocked by probenecid (29), an organic anion transport inhibitor.

Cyclic AMP transport across apical and basolateral membranes of proximal tubular epithelial cells is mediated by multidrug resistance protein type 4 (MRP4; also called ABCC4; 176) and organic acid transporter type 1 (OAT1; 155), respectively. However, it is unknown whether MRP4-like or OAT1-like transporters mediate cyclic AMP efflux in other cell types. Most likely, cyclic AMP egress is mediated by a family of transporters, with the precise transporting proteins depending on the tissue.

The cellular function of the extracellular cyclic AMP pathway is that it provides adenosine to modify the response to hormonal stimulation of adenylyl cyclase. Because adenosine is produced in the unstirred water layer by spatially linked proteins on the cell surface (cyclic AMP transport onto the cell surface, metabolism of cyclic AMP to AMP by ecto-phosphodiesterase and conversion of AMP to adenosine by membrane-bound ecto-5′-nucleotidase), minute increases in cyclic AMP may produce biologically active concentrations of adenosine in the biophase of cell surface adenosine receptors, thus permitting autocrine and paracrine effects of adenosine.

Most components of the extracellular cyclic AMP pathway have been well characterized, and there are molecular descriptions of adenylyl cyclase (91), ecto-5′-nucleotidase (113), and at least some cyclic AMP transporters (155, 176). Moreover, numerous ecto-enyzmes have been cloned that metabolize purine nucleotides, for example, ecto-nucleoside 5′-triphosphate diphosphohydrolases (E-NTPDases 1, 2, 3, 4, 5 and 6), ecto-nucleotide pyrophosphatases (E-NPP 1, 2 and 3), alkaline phosphatases and NAD-glycohydrolases (188).

An increasing amount of information is accumulating to support the existence of ecto-phosphodiesterases that, combined with adenylyl cyclases, cyclic AMP transporters and ecto-5′-nucleotidases, produce an operational cyclic AMP-adenosine pathway. In aortic vascular smooth muscle cells (49) and cardiac fibroblasts (44) in culture, exogenous cyclic AMP is converted to AMP, adenosine and inosine in a concentration- and time-dependent fashion. Significant increases in extracellular adenosine levels occur with concentrations of cyclic AMP in the medium as low as 1 μM, and steady-state levels of adenosine are achieved in the culture medium within 5 minutes of adding exogenous cyclic AMP.

The cyclic AMP-adenosine pathway has been investigated with pharmacological inhibitors. IBMX (3-isobutyl-1-methylxanthine) penetrates cell membranes and is a "broad spectrum" inhibitor of phosphodiesterases that blocks both intracellular and extracellular phosphodiesterases (11). The xanthine DPSPX (1,3-dipropyl-8-p-sulfophenylxanthine) is restricted to the extracellular compartment due to a negative charge at physiological pH (173). At low concentrations, DPSPX blocks adenosine receptors (28), but at high concentrations DPSPX inhibits ecto-phosphodiesterase (109, 186). AMPCP (α,β-methyleneadenosine-5′-diphosphate) is an inhibitor of ecto-5′-nucleotidase, but not cytosolic 5′-nucleotidase (187).

IBMX and DPSPX inhibit the conversion of cyclic AMP to AMP, adenosine and inosine (a metabolite of adenosine) in aortic vascular smooth muscle and cardiac fibroblasts (44, 49). AMPCP blocks the metabolism of cyclic AMP to adenosine and inosine, but not to AMP. In cardiac fibroblasts, stimulation of adenylyl cyclase with norepinephrine, isoproterenol or forskolin raises extracellular levels of endogenous cyclic AMP and adenosine (45), and 2′,5′-dideoxyadenosine, a blocker of adenylyl cyclase, inhibits the increase of extracellular endogenous cyclic AMP and adenosine.

In vascular smooth muscle cells, A$_2$ receptor stimulation increases the first-order rate constant for the efflux of cyclic AMP (52). This implies that in some cell types, the extracellular cyclic AMP-adenosine pathway is involved in a positive-feedback loop in which increases in extracellular adenosine cause activation of the cyclic AMP-adenosine pathway by stimulating adenylyl cyclase and by increasing the rate of cyclic AMP efflux.

In addition to aortic vascular smooth muscle cells and cardiac fibroblasts, the cyclic AMP-adenosine pathway also has been identified in the central nervous system (CNS) (17, 145, 146, 147, 148), in the cerebral vasculature (72), and in adipocytes (82, 186) and hepatocytes (62, 160).

Despite the fact that studies in nonrenal cells/tissues initially provided much of the supporting evidence for the existence of the extracellular cyclic AMP-adenosine pathway, the hypothesis was first explicitly postulated as a "transmembrane negative feedback loop" mechanism in which adenosine formed from cyclic AMP effluxing from juxtaglomerular cells was proposed to inhibit the renin release response to agents that activated renin release by stimulating adenylyl cyclase (76). In support of this view, antagonism of A$_1$ receptors augments renin release responses to agents that release renin by stimulating adenylyl cyclase (137). Studies now provide direct evidence for the extracellular cyclic AMP-adenosine pathway in the kidney.

In the isolated, perfused rat kidney, addition of cyclic AMP to the perfusate augments the renal secretion of AMP, adenosine and inosine (109), and this response is blocked by IBMX and DPSPX. In the perfused kidney, AMPCP blocks the metabolism of cyclic AMP to adenosine and inosine, but does not inhibit the metabolism of cyclic AMP to AMP (109). These data support the existence of a renal cyclic AMP-adenosine pathway. Cyclic AMP is hydrophilic and exogenous cyclic AMP should not penetrate cell membranes, thus the conversion of exogenous cyclic AMP to adenosine in the kidney occurs, for the most part, in the extracellular compartment. This conclusion is supported by the fact that AMPCP inhibits ecto-5′-nucleotidase, not cytosolic 5′-nucleotidase (187). Therefore, the inhibition of cyclic AMP metabolism to adenosine and inosine by AMPCP points to an extracellular site of conversion. DP-SPX is restricted to the extracellular space (173) and blocks the metabolism of cyclic AMP to AMP, adenosine and inosine. This result is also consistent with an extracellular site of cyclic AMP metabolism to AMP and adenosine. However, these data do not rule out the intracellular cyclic AMP-adenosine pathway.

In the isolated perfused rat kidney isoproterenol increases adenosine and inosine secretion (110), an effect that is inhibited by propranolol, a β-adrenoceptor antagonist. These experiments indicate that activation of renal adenylyl cyclase by β-adrenoceptors increases renal adenosine biosynthesis. Inhibition of phosphodiesterase with IBMX and ecto-5'-nucleotidase with AMPCP blocks isoproterenol-induced adenosine production in the isolated, perfused rat kidney, and these results are consistent with endogenous cyclic AMP being converted to adenosine.

The extracellular cyclic AMP-adenosine pathway appears to be present in the renal microcirculation (78). Incubation of preglomerular microvessels with exogenous cyclic AMP increases extracellular adenosine by as much as 60-fold, and this response is blocked by IBMX or DP-SPX. In preglomerular microvessels, isoproterenol plus IBMX increases extracellular cyclic AMP by as much as 30-fold, and there is a linear relationship between intracellular and extracellular cyclic AMP concentrations in preglomerular microvessels. These data demonstrate a robust cyclic AMP efflux following activation of adenylyl cyclase in preglomerular microvessels. In preglomerular microvessels isoproterenol increases extracellular adenosine levels, and this is inhibited by propranolol, IBMX and DPSPX. In cultured rat preglomerular vascular smooth muscle cells, exogenous cyclic AMP stimulates extracellular adenosine concentrations by as much as 40-fold, and this effect is inhibited by IBMX (79). In rat mesangial cells, exogenous cyclic AMP increases extracellular concentrations of adenosine by as much as 25-fold, and this effect is blocked by IBMX, DPSPX and AMPCP (39). Thus the concept that preglomerular microvessels, vascular smooth muscle cells, and mesangial cells transport endogenous cyclic AMP to the extracellular compartment and convert extracellular cyclic AMP to adenosine is supported by a large body of experimental evidence.

Both freshly isolated collecting ducts (CDs) and CD cells in culture convert exogenous cAMP to AMP and adenosine (80), and this conversion of cAMP to AMP and adenosine is affected by IBMX, DPSPX, and AMPCP in a fashion consistent with exogenous cAMP being metabolized by the extracellular cAMP-adenosine pathway. In cultured CD cells, stimulation of adenylyl cyclase augments extracellular concentrations of cAMP, AMP and adenosine, and these changes are also modulated by IBMX, DPSPX, and AMPCP in a manner consistent with the extracellular cAMP-adenosine pathway (80). Similar results have been obtained in freshly isolated proximal tubules and proximal

tubular epithelial cells in culture (80a). Therefore, the extracellular cAMP-adenosine pathway is an important source of adenosine in both the proximal tubule and collecting duct.

Evidence suggests that the extracellular cyclic AMP-adenosine pathway exists *in vivo* in the kidney. Local application of IBMX into the renal cortical interstitial space decreases the renal cortical interstitial levels of adenosine and inosine by approximately 50% (108). Also, intrarenal and intravenous infusions of cyclic AMP and intrarenal infusions of isoproterenol increase urinary excretion rates of both cyclic AMP and adenosine (79a).

The extracellular cyclic AMP-adenosine pathway may contribute to regulation of the function and structure of the renal vasculature. Nitric oxide production importantly contributes to renal vasodilation (107), and in vascular smooth muscle cells the cyclic AMP-adenosine pathway participates in nitric oxide biosynthesis via activation of A_{2B} receptors (40). Therefore, renal vascular tone, in those regions of the kidney microcirculation that express A_{2B} receptors, may be modulated in part by nitric oxide production driven by the extracellular cyclic AMP-adenosine pathway. Moreover, the extracellular cyclic AMP-adenosine pathway, again via A_{2B} receptors, inhibits proliferation of and extracellular matrix production by vascular smooth muscle cells (41, 43, 46, 47, 48), and therefore may influence the structure of those regions of the renal vasculature that express A_{2B} receptors.

The extracellular cyclic AMP-adenosine pathway may also regulate glomerular mesangial cells (GCMs). GMCs express the extracellular cyclic AMP-adenosine pathway (39), and exogenous cyclic AMP reduces proliferation of GMCs and the production of collagen by GMCs (39). As with vascular smooth muscle cells, these effects are mediated by adenosine acting on A_{2B} receptors (39).

The extracellular cyclic AMP-adenosine pathway may regulate noradrenergic neurotransmission in the preglomerular microcirculation, a region of the renal microcirculation that expresses high levels of A_1 receptors. Adenosine potentiates renovascular responses to sympathetic nerve stimulation in the kidney by stimulating postjunctional A_1 receptors (70, 71). Moreover, activation of renal sympathetic nerves releases adenosine and adenosine metabolites by a β-adrenoceptor-mediated mechanism (111). Exocytosis of norepinephrine from renal sympathetic nerve terminals would be expected to activate postjunctional β-adrenoceptors, stimulate adenylyl cyclase and engage the cyclic AMP-adenosine pathway to increase renovascular levels of adenosine. Adenosine formed by this mechanism may enhance renal vascular responses to sympathetic nerve stimulation by sensitizing renal preglomerular vascular smooth muscle cells to norepinephrine.

Juxtaglomerular cells release renin in response to increases in intracellular cyclic AMP (57), and increases in intracellular cyclic AMP cause efflux of cyclic AMP, which activates the extracellular cyclic AMP-adenosine pathway. Because adenosine, via A_1 receptors, blocks renin release

(77), the extracellular cyclic AMP-adenosine pathway may function to provide negative-feedback control of renin release. Several lines of evidence support this concept: (1) Because the extracellular cyclic AMP-adenosine pathway is present in preglomerular microvessels (78), and vascular smooth muscle cells cultured from preglomerular microvessels (79), and because juxtaglomerular cells are derived from preglomerular vascular smooth muscle cells (64), it is likely that the extracellular cyclic AMP-adenosine pathway is present in juxtaglomerular cells; (2) Administration of cyclic AMP (167), AMP (167), and adenosine (31, 33) into the renal artery attenuates renin release; (3) Blockade of A_1 adenosine receptors with nonselective (theophylline, caffeine, and DPSPX) or A_1 selective (DPCPX and FK453) adenosine-receptor antagonists augments renin release (3, 6, 15, 22, 32, 93, 94, 97, 132, 136, 137, 141, 173, 175, 177, 179).

It is likely that the extracellular cyclic AMP-adenosine pathway is involved in the regulation of transport by renal epithelial cells. In cultured opossum kidney cells (a cell model system with a proximal epithelial phenotype), exogenous cyclic AMP is converted rapidly to extracellular adenosine by a mechanism that is blocked by inhibition of ecto-5′-nucleotidase or phosphodiesterase (56). Also, exogenous cyclic AMP is converted to AMP and adenosine in freshly isolated proximal convoluted tubules (80a) and collecting ducts (80) and in proximal (80a) and collecting duct (80) epithelial cells in culture. The conversion of exogenous cyclic AMP to adenosine in these tissues/cell types is blocked by inhibition of ecto-5′-nucleotidase or ecto-phosphodiesterase. Moreover, stimulation of adenylyl cyclase increases adenosine production in proximal (80a) and collecting duct (80) epithelial cells in culture via the cyclic AMP-adenosine pathway. A_1 receptors in cultured epithelial cells that express a proximal tubular phenotype augment both Na^+-glucose symport and Na^+-phosphate symport (25), and activation of A_1 receptors enhances basolateral Na^+-$3HCO_3^-$ symport in microperfused proximal convoluted tubules (168). Thus these data support the existence of a negative feedback mechanism in which stimulation of adenylyl cyclase attenuates epithelial transport, and this effect is moderated by adenosine formation via an epithelial cyclic AMP-adenosine pathway.

Pancreatohepatorenal Cyclic AMP-Adenosine Pathway

The extracellular cyclic AMP-adenosine pathway as described previously is an autocrine/paracrine mechanism of adenosine production. A permutation of this mechanism, the *pancreatohepatorenal cyclic AMP-adenosine pathway*, is an endocrine mechanism of adenosine biosynthesis.

Because the liver is a large organ (approximately 1.5 kg in a healthy adult), activation of hepatic adenylyl cyclase causes release of large quantities of cyclic AMP into the systemic circulation (14, 96). Due to the anatomical relationship between the pancreas and the portal circulation, the pancreas secretes glucagon directly into the portal circulation (139, 166), thereby maximizing the concentration of glucagon delivered to hepatocytes. Because glucagon is a potent and efficacious stimulant of hepatic adenylyl cyclase (13, 73), glucagon release from the pancreas would be expected to cause a substantial increase in plasma levels of cyclic AMP. Once plasma cyclic AMP reaches the kidney, the renal microcirculation would distribute cyclic AMP to the renal interstitial space, and glomerular filtration of cyclic AMP would carry cyclic AMP to the tubular lumen (14). Reabsorption of water by the tubules would further concentrate cyclic AMP in the tubular lumen.

The concept that pancreatic glucagon release may increase delivery of liver-derived cyclic AMP to the kidney was first proposed by Bankir (7), who postulated that liver-derived cyclic AMP may affect tubular transport by binding to cell surface cyclic AMP receptors in the luminal membrane of renal epithelial cells. However, cell surface cyclic AMP receptors have not been identified in mammals. On the other hand, there is increasing evidence that the kidney can convert extracellular cyclic AMP to adenosine. As already mentioned, exogenous cyclic AMP is converted to adenosine by ecto-phosphosphodiesterase and ecto-5′-nucleotidase in freshly isolated proximal convoluted tubules (80a), freshly isolated collecting ducts (80), proximal tubular epithelial cells in culture (80a), collecting duct epithelial cells in culture (80), freshly isolated preglomerular microvessels (78), preglomerular microvascular smooth muscle cells in culture (79), and glomerular mesangial cells in culture (39). It is likely, therefore, that some of the cyclic AMP carried by the circulation to the renal interstitial space and tubular lumen would be converted to adenosine. This adenosine would engage adenosine receptors on the basolateral and luminal membranes of renal epithelial cells and on renal microvascular smooth muscle cells, juxtaglomerular cells and glomerular mesangial cells. Therefore, adenosine formed by this mechanism may regulate epithelial electrolyte transport, renal vascular tone, glomerular filtration rate and renin release.

From the perspective of the pancreatohepatorenal cyclic AMP-adenosine pathway, cyclic AMP is an extracellular pro-hormone. Although cyclic AMP is stable in blood, adenosine has a half-life in human blood of less than one second (114). Clearly, the pancreas and liver could not communicate with the kidneys via the adenosine system by releasing adenosine per se, but could do so by secreting a stable prohormone that can be converted into adenosine at the target tissue.

Does the pancreatohepatorenal cyclic AMP-adenosine system actually exist? We are in the early stages of testing this hypothesis. Thus far our results (79a) demonstrate that (1) intravenous infusions of cyclic AMP increase urinary excretion of both cyclic AMP and adenosine;

(2) intravenous infusions of cyclic AMP increase renal interstitial levels of adenosine and this is blocked by inhibition of ecto-phosphodiesterase and ecto-5'-nucleotidase; (3) intrarenal infusions of cyclic AMP increase urinary excretion of adenosine and this is blocked by inhibition of ecto-phosphodiesterase and ecto-5'-nucleotidase; (4) intraportal infusions of glucagon increase plasma and urinary levels of cyclic AMP and urinary, but not plasma, levels of adenosine; and (5) intraportal, but not intravenous, infusions of glucagon increase renal interstitial levels of cyclic AMP and adenosine.

Does the pancreatohepatorenal cyclic AMP-adenosine system play a role in renal physiology? In normal mammals, exercise and hypoglycemia efficaciously stimulate glucagon secretion (58, 161). Although intrarenal infusions of glucagon do not reduce sodium excretion (12), intraportal infusions of glucagon cause a marked antidiuresis (51). It is possible that activation of the pancreatoheptorenal cyclic AMP-adenosine pathway by exercise enhances sodium transport via A_1 receptors in the renal tubules and thus increases the efficiency of sodium reabsorption. This would provide an adaptive mechanism to avoid volume depletion during sustained physical exertion. Stimulation of the pancreatoheptorenal cyclic AMP-adenosine pathway by hypoglycemia may increase Na^+-glucose symport in proximal tubules and thereby augment the efficiency of glucose transport. This would provide an adaptive mechanism to prevent a further drop in blood glucose levels.

Does the pancreatohepatorenal cyclic AMP-adenosine system play a role in renal pathophysiology? It is conceivable that the pancreatoheptorenal cyclic AMP-adenosine pathway is overly activated in syndrome X (i.e., the metabolic syndrome characterized by obesity, insulin resistance, hyperlipidemia, and hypertension). Normally, oral glucose inhibits glucagon secretion. In contrast, in both animals (178) and people (74) with syndrome X, an oral glucose load augments glucagon secretion by approximately 200%. Therefore, provided the pancreatoheptorenal cyclic AMP-adenosine pathway exists, whenever a syndrome X patient consumes a high-carbohydrate meal, the renal tubules would be exposed to excess adenosine. Because adenosine induces vasoconstriction and sodium reabsorption, the pancreatoheptorenal cyclic AMP-adenosine pathway could contribute to the pathophysiology of hypertension in syndrome X. Moreover, because adenosine receptors also inhibit lipolysis in fat cells (54) and reduce insulin sensitivity in skeletal muscle (171), if adenosine is produced by adipocytes and skeletal muscle from liver-derived cyclic AMP, adenosine may be a common denominator linking obesity, insulin resistance and hypertension. In support of this concept, our studies demonstrate that an oral glucose load in ZSF1 rats (an animal model of syndrome X) increases plasma levels of glucagon and increases urinary levels of cyclic AMP and adenosine (79a).

References

1. Agmon Y, Dinour D, Brezis M. Disparate effects of adenosine A_1- and A_2-receptor agonists on intrarenal blood flow. *Am J Physiol* 1993;26:F802–F806.
2. Albert B, Bray D, Lewis J et al. In: *Molecular biology of the cell.* 2nd ed. New York and London: Garland;1989:825–826.
3. Albinus M, Finkbeiner E, Sosath B, Osswald H. Isolated superfused juxtaglomerular cells from rat kidney: a model for study of renin secretion. *Am J Physiol* 1998;275:F991–F997.
4. Arakawa K, Suzuki H, Naitoh M et al. Role of adenosine in the renal responses to contrast medium. *Kidney Int* 1996;49:1199–1206.
5. Bak M, Thomsen K. Effects of the adenosine A_1 receptor inhibitor FK 838 on proximal tubular fluid output in rats. *Nephrol Dial Transplant* 2004;19:1077–1082.
6. Balakrishnan VS, Coles GA, Williams JD. A potential role for endogenous adenosine in control of human glomerular and tubular function. *Am J Physiol* 1993;265:F504–F510.
7. Bankir L, Ahloulay M, Devreotes PN, Parent CA. Extracellular cAMP inhibits proximal reabsorption: are plasma membrane cAMP receptors involved? *Am J Physiol Renal Physiol* 2002;282:F376–F392.
8. Barber R, Butcher RW. The quantitative relationship between intracellular concentration and egress of cyclic AMP from cultured cells. *Mol Pharmacol* 1981;19:38–43.
9. Barrett RJ, Droppleman DA. Interactions of adenosine A_1 receptor-mediated renal vasoconstriction with endogenous nitric oxide and ANG II. *Am J Physiol* 1993;265:F651–F659.
10. Baudouin-Legros M, Badou A, Paulais M et al. Hypertonic NaCl enhances adenosine release and hormonal cAMP production in mouse thick ascending limb. *Am J Physiol* 1995;269:F103–F109.
11. Beavo JA, Reifsnyder DH. Primary sequence of cyclic nucleotide phosphodiesterase isozymes and the design of selective inhibitors. *Trends Pharmacol Sci* 1990;11:150–155.
12. Briffeuil P, Thu TH, Kolanowski J A lack of direct action of glucagon on kidney metabolism, hemodynamics, and renal sodium handling in the dog. *Metabolism* 1996;45:383–388.
13. Broadus AE, Kaminsky NI, Hardman JG et al. Kinetic parameters and renal clearances of plasma adenosine 3',5'-monophosphate and guanosine 3',5'-monophosphate in man. *J Clin Invest* 1970;49:2222–2236.
14. Broadus AE, Kaminsky NI, Northcutt RC et al. Effects of glucagon on adenosine 3',5'-monophosphate and guanosine 3',5'-monophosphate in human plasma and urine. *J Clin Invest* 1970;49:2237–2245.
15. Brown NJ, Porter J, Ryder D, Branch RA. Caffeine potentiates the renin response to diazoxide in man. Evidence for a regulatory role of endogenous adenosine. *J Pharmacol Exp Ther* 1991;256:56–61.
16. Brown R, Ollerstam A, Johansson B et al. Abolished tubuloglomerular feedback and increased plasma renin in adenosine A_1 receptor-deficient mice. *Am J Physiol Regul Integr Comp Physiol* 2001;281:R1362–R1367.
17. Brundege JM, Diao L, Proctor WR, Dunwiddie TV. The role of cyclic AMP as a precursor of extracellular adenosine in the rat hippocampus. *Neuropharmacology* 1997;36:1201–1210.
18. Brunton LL, Mayer SE. Extrusion of cyclic AMP from pigeon erythrocytes. *J Biol Chem* 1979;254:9714–9720.
19. Cai H, Batuman V, Puschett DB, Puschett JB. Effect of KW-3902, a novel adenosine A_1 receptor antagonist, on sodium-dependent phosphate and glucose transport by the rat renal proximal tubular cell. *Life Sci* 1994;55:839–845.
20. Cai H, Puschett DB, Guan S et al. Phosphate transport inhibition by KW-3902, an adenosine A_1 receptor antagonist, is mediated by cyclic adenosine monophosphate. *Am J Kidney Dis* 1995;26:825–830.
21. Callis JT, Kuan CJ, Branch KR et al. Inhibition of renal vasoconstriction induced by intrarenal hypertonic saline by the nonxanthine adenosine antagonist CGS 15943A. *J Pharmacol Exp Ther* 1989; 248:1123–1129.
22. Cannon ME, Twu BM, Yang CS, Hsu CH. The effect of theophylline and cyclic adenosine 3',5'-monophosphate on renin release by afferent arterioles. *J Hypertens* 1989;7:569–576.
23. Cass CE, Young JD, Baldwin SA. Recent advances in the molecular biology of nucleoside transporters of mammalian cells. *Biochem Cell Biol* 1998;76:761–770.
24. Castrop H, Huang Y, Hashimoto S et al. Impairment of tubuloglomerular feedback regulation of GFR in ecto-5'-nucleotidase/CD73-deficient mice. *J Clin Invest* 2004;114:634–642.
25. Coulson R, Johnson RA, Olsson RA et al. Adenosine stimulates phosphate and glucose transport in opossum kidney epithelial cells. *Am J Physiol* 1991;260:F921–F928.
26. Cramer H, Lindl T. Release of cyclic AMP from rat superior cervical ganglia after stimulation of synthesis in vitro. *Nature* 1974;249:380–382.
27. Cronstein BN. Adenosine, an endogenous anti-inflammatory agent. *J Appl Physiol* 1994;76:5–13.
28. Daly JW, Jacobson KA. Adenosine receptors: Selective agonists and antagonists. In: L Belardinelli, A Pelleg (eds). *Adenosine and Adenine Nucleotides: From Molecular Biology to Intergrative Physiology.* Boston: Kluwer Academic Publishers;1995:157-166.
29. Davorne PR, Sutherland EW. The effect of L-epinephrine and other agents on the synthesis and release of adenosine 3',5'-Phosphate by whole pigeon erythrocytes. *J Biol Chem* 1963; 238:3009–3015.
30. Day YJ, Huang L, McDuffie MJ et al. Renal protection from ischemia mediated by A_{2A} adenosine receptors on bone marrow–derived cells. *J Clin Invest* 2003;112:883–891.
31. Deray G, Branch RA, Herzer WA et al. Adenosine inhibits β-adrenoceptor but not DBcAMP-induced renin release. *Am J Physiol* 1987;252:F46–F52.
32. Deray G, Branch RA, Jackson EK. Methylxanthines augment the renin response to suprarenal-aortic constriction. *Naunyn Schmiedebergs Arch Pharmacol* 1989;339:690–696.
33. Deray G, Branch RA, Ohnishi A, Jackson EK. Adenosine inhibits renin release induced by suprarenal-aortic constriction and prostacyclin. *Naunyn Schmiedebergs Arch Pharmacol* 1989;339:590–595.
34. Deray G, Sabra R, Herzer WA et al. Interaction between angiotensin II and adenosine in mediating the vasoconstrictor response to intrarenal hypertonic saline infusions in the dog. *J Pharmacol Exp Ther* 1990;252:631–635.

35. Deussen A, Lloyd HG, Schrader J Contribution of S-adenosylhomocysteine to cardiac adenosine formation. *J Mol Cell Cardiol* 1989; 21:773–782.

36. Di Sole F, Cerull R, Babich V et al. Acute regulation of Na/H exchanger NHE3 by adenosine A1 receptors is mediated by calcineurin homologous protein. *J Biol Chem* 2004;279:2962–2974.

37. Di Sole F, Cerull R, Petzke S et al. Bimodal acute effects of A1 adenosine receptor activation on Na+/H+ exchanger 3 in opossum kidney cells. *J Am Soc Nephrol* 2003;14:1720–1730.

38. Doore BJ, Bashor MM, Spitzer N et al. Regulation of adenosine 3':5'-monophosphate efflux from rat glioma cells in culture. *J Biol Chem* 1975;250:4371–4372.

39. Dubey RK, Gillespie DG, Mi Z, Jackson EK. Cyclic AMP-adenosine pathway inhibits glomerular mesangial cell growth. *Hypertension* 1997;30:506.

40. Dubey RK, Gillespie DG, Jackson EK. Cyclic AMP-adenosine pathway induces nitric oxide synthesis in aortic smooth muscle cells. *Hypertension* 1998;31:296–302.

41. Dubey RK, Gillespie DG, Jackson EK. Adenosine inhibits collagen and total protein synthesis in vascular smooth muscle cells. *Hypertension* 1999;33:190–194.

42. Dubey RK, Gillespie DG, Mi Z, Jackson EK. Exogenous and endogenous adenosine inhibits fetal calf serum-induced growth of rat cardiac fibroblasts: role of A2B receptors. *Circulation* 1997;96:2656–2666.

43. Dubey RK, Gillespie DG, Mi Z, Jackson EK. Adenosine inhibits growth of human aortic smooth muscle cells via A2B receptors. *Hypertension* 1998;31:516–521.

44. Dubey RK, Gillespie DG, Mi Z, Jackson EK. Cardiac fibroblasts express the cAMP-adenosine pathway. *Hypertension* 2000;36:337–342.

45. Dubey RK, Gillespie DG, Mi Z, Jackson EK. Endogenous cyclic AMP-adenosine pathway regulates cardiac fibroblast growth. *Hypertension* 2001;37:1095–1100.

46. Dubey RK, Gillespie DG, Mi Z et al. Smooth muscle cell-derived adenosine inhibits cell growth. *Hypertension* 1996;27:766–773.

47. Dubey RK, Gillespie DG, Osaka K. et al. Adenosine inhibits fetal calf serum-induced growth of rat aortic smooth muscle cells: Possible role of A2b receptor. *Hypertension* 1996;27:786–793.

48. Dubey RK, Gillespie DG, Shue H, Jackson EK. A2B receptors mediate antimitogenesis in vascular smooth muscle cells. *Hypertension* 2000;35:267–272.

49. Dubey RK, Mi Z, Gillespie DG, Jackson EK. Cyclic AMP-adenosine pathway inhibits vascular smooth muscle cell growth. *Hypertension* 1996;28:765–771.

50. Erley CM, Heyne N, Burgert K et al. Prevention of radiocontrast-induced nephropathy by adenosine antagonists in rats with chronic nitric oxide deficiency. *J Am Soc Nephrol* 1997;8:1125–1132.

51. Faix S, Leng L. The renal response of sheep to intraportal infusion of glucagon. *Exp Physiol* 1997;82:1007–1013.

52. Fehr TF, Dickinson ES, Goldman SJ, Slakey LL. Cyclic AMP efflux is regulated by occupancy of the adenosine receptor in pig aortic smooth muscle cells. *J Biol Chem* 1990;265:10974–10980.

53. Finnegan RB, Carey GB. Characterization of cyclic AMP efflux from swine adipocytes in vitro. *Obes Res* 1998;6:292–298.

54. Foley JE, Anderson RC, Bell PA et al. Pharmacological strategies for reduction of lipid availability. *Ann N Y Acad Sci* 1997;827:231–245.

55. Franco M, Bell PD, Navar LG. Effect of adenosine A1 analogue on tubuloglomerular feedback mechanism. *Am J Physiol* 1989;257:F231–F236.

56. Friedlander G, Couette S, Coureau C, Amiel C. Mechanisms whereby extracellular adenosine 3',5'-monophosphate inhibits phosphate transport in cultured opossum kidney cells and in rat kidney. Physiological implication. *J Clin Invest* 1992;90:848–858.

57. Friis UG, Jensen BL, Hansen PB et al. Exocytosis and endocytosis in juxtaglomerular cells. *Acta Physiol Scand* 2000;168:95–99.

58. Gerich JE, Charles MA, Grodsky GM. Regulation of pancreatic insulin and glucagon secretion. *Annu Rev Physiol* 1976;38:353–388.

59. Gerkens JF, Heidemann HT, Jackson EK, Branch RA. Aminophylline inhibits renal vasoconstriction produced by intrarenal hypertonic saline. *J Pharmacol Exp Ther* 1983;225:611–615.

60. Gordon EL, Pearson JD, Dickinson ES et al. The hydrolysis of extracellular adenine nucleotides by arterial smooth muscle cells. Regulation of adenosine production at the cell surface. *J Biol Chem* 1989;264:18986–18995.

61. Gordon EL, Pearson JD, Slakey LL. The hydrolysis of extracellular adenine nucleotides by cultured endothelial cells from pig aorta. Feed-forward inhibition of adenosine production at the cell surface. *J Biol Chem* 1986;261:15496–15507.

62. Gorin E, Brenner T. Extracellular metabolism of cyclic AMP. *Biochim Biophys Acta* 1976;451:20–28.

63. Gottlieb SS, Skettino SL, Wolff A et al. Effects of BG9719 CVT-124., an A1-adenosine receptor antagonist, and furosemide on glomerular filtration rate and natriuresis in patients with congestive heart failure. *J Am Coll Cardiol* 2000;35:56–59.

64. Hackenthal E, Paul M, Ganten D, Taugner R. Morphology, physiology, and molecular biology of renin secretion. *Physiol Rev* 1990;70:1067–1116.

65. Hall JE, Granger JP. Adenosine alters glomerular filtration control by angiotensin II. *Am J Physiol* 1986;250:F917–F923.

66. Hansen PB, Castrop H, Briggs J, Schnermann J Adenosine induces vasoconstriction through Gi-dependent activation of phospholipase C in isolated perfused afferent arterioles of mice. *J Am Soc Nephrol* 2003;14:2457–2465.

67. Hansen PB, Hashimoto S, Briggs J, Schnermann J Attenuated renovascular constrictor responses to angiotensin II in adenosine 1 receptor knockout mice. *Am J Physiol Regul Integr Comp Physiol* 2003;285:R44–R49.

68. Hansen PB, Schnermann J. Vasoconstrictor and vasodilator effects of adenosine in the kidney. *Am J Physiol Renal Physiol* 2003;285:F590–F599.

69. Hedqvist P, Fredholm BB. Effects of adenosine on adrenergic neurotransmission; prejunctional inhibition and postjunctional enhancement. *Naunyn Schmiedebergs Arch Pharmacol* 1976;293:217–223.

70. Hedqvist P, Fredholm BB, Olundh S. Antagonistic effects of theophylline and adenosine on adrenergic neuroeffector transmission in the rabbit kidney. *Circ Res* 1978;43:592–598.

71. Holz FG, Steinhausen M. Renovascular effects of adenosine receptor agonists. *Ren Physiol* 1987;10:272–282.

72. Hong KW, Shin HK, Kim HH et al. Metabolism of cAMP to adenosine: role in vasodilation of rat pial artery in response to hypotension. *Am J Physiol* 1999;276:H376–H382.

73. Houslay MD. Insulin, glucagon and the receptor-mediated control of cyclic AMP concentrations in liver. Twenty-second Colworth medal lecture. *Biochem Soc Trans* 1986;14:183–193.

74. Iannello S, Campione R, Belfiore F. Response of insulin, glucagon, lactate, and nonesterified fatty acids to glucose in visceral obesity with and without NIDDM: relationship to Hypertension *Mol Genet Metab* 1998;63:214–223.

75. Inscho EW. P2 receptors in regulation of renal microvascular function. *Am J Physiol Renal Physiol* 2001;280:F927–F944.

76. Jackson EK. Adenosine: a physiological brake on renin release. *Annu Rev Pharmacol Toxicol* 1991;31:1–35.

77. Jackson EK. P1 and P2 receptors in the renal system. In: *Handbook of Experimental Pharmacology Volume 151/II: Purinergic and Pryimidinergic Signalling II: Cardiovascular, Respiratory, Immune, Metabolic and Gastrointestinal Tract Function.* MP Abbracchio, M Williams (eds). Berlin: Springer-Verlag;2001:33–71.

78. Jackson EK, Mi Z. Preglomerular microcirculation expresses the cAMP-adenosine pathway. *J Pharmacol Exp Ther* 2000;295:23–28.

79. Jackson EK, Mi Z, Gillespie DG, Dubey RK. Metabolism of cAMP to adenosine in the renal vasculature. *J Pharmacol Exp Ther* 1997; 283:177–182.

79a. Jackson Ek, Mi Z , Zacharia LC, Tofovic SP, Dubey RK. The pancreatoheptorenal cAMP-adenosine mechanism. *J Pharmacol Exp Ther* 2007. Published February 21, 2007; doi:10.1124/jpet.106.119164.

80. Jackson EK, Mi Z, Zhu C, Dubey RK. Adenosine biosynthesis in the collecting duct. *J Pharmacol Exp Ther* 2003;307:888–896.

80a. Jackson EK, Zacharia LC, Zhang M, Gillespie DG, Zhu C, Dubey RK. cAMP-adenosine pathway in the proximal tubule. *J Pharmacol Exp Ther* 2006;317:1219–1229.

81. Joyner WL, Mohama RE, Myers TO, Gilmore JP. The selective response to adenosine of renal microvessels from hamster explants. *Microvasc Res* 1988;35:122–131.

82. Kather H. Beta-adrenergic stimulation of adenine nucleotide catabolism and purine release in human adipocytes. *J Clin Invest* 1990;85:106–114.

83. Katholi RE, Taylor GJ, McCann WP et al. Nephrotoxicity from contrast media: attenuation with theophylline. *Radiology* 1995;195:17–22.

84. Kellett R, Bowmer CJ, Collis MG, Yates MS. Amelioration of glycerol-induced acute renal failure in the rat with 8-cyclopentyl-1,3-dipropylxanthine. *Br J Pharmacol* 1989;98:1066–1074.

85. Kelly LA, Butcher RW. The effects of epinephrine and prostaglandin E-1 on cyclic adenosine 3':5'-monophosphate levels in WI-38 fibroblasts. *J Biol Chem* 1974;249:3098–3102.

86. King CD, Mayer SE. Inhibition of egress of adenosine 3',5'-monophosphate from pigeon erthrocytes. *Mol Pharmacol* 1974;10:941–953.

87. Knight RJ, Collis MG, Yates MS, Bowmer CJ. Amelioration of cisplatin-induced acute renal failure with 8-cyclopentyl-1,3-dipropylxanthine. *Br J Pharmacol* 1991;104:1062–1068.

88. Komlosi P, Peti-Peterdi J, Fuson AL et al. Macula densa basolateral ATP release is regulated by luminal [NaCl] and dietary salt intake. *Am J Physiol Renal Physiol* 2004;286:F1054–F1058.

89. Kost CK, Jr., Herzer WA, Rominski BR et al. Diuretic response to adenosine A1 receptor blockade in normotensive and spontaneously hypertensive rats: role of pertussis toxin-sensitive G-proteins. *J Pharmacol Exp Ther* 2000;292:752–760.

90. Kroll K, Decking UK, Dreikorn K, Schrader J Rapid turnover of the AMP-adenosine metabolic cycle in the guinea pig heart. *Circ Res* 1993;73:846–856.

91. Krupinski J, Coussen F, Bakalyar HA et al. Adenylyl cyclase amino acid sequence: possible channel- or transporter-like structure. *Science* 1989;244:1558–1564.

92. Kuan CJ, Herzer WA, Jackson EK. Cardiovascular and renal effects of blocking A1 adenosine receptors. *J Cardiovasc Pharmacol* 1993; 21:822–828.

93. Kuan CJ, Wells JN, Jackson EK. Endogenous adenosine restrains renin release during sodium restriction. *J Pharmacol Exp Ther* 1989; 249:110–116.

94. Kuan CJ, Wells JN, Jackson EK. Endogenous adenosine restrains renin release in conscious rats. *Circ Res* 1990;66:637–646.

95. Kurtz A, Wagner C. Cellular control of renin secretion. *J Exp Biol* 1999;202:219–225.

96. Kuster J, Zapf J, Jakob A. Effects of hormones on cyclic AMP release in perfused rat livers. *FEBS Lett* 1973;32:73–77.

97. Langard O, Holdaas H, Eide I, Kiil F. Conditions for augmentation of renin release by theophylline. *Scand J Clin Lab Invest* 1983;43:9–14.

98. Leaney JL, Tinker A. The role of members of the pertussis toxin-sensitive family of G proteins in coupling receptors to the activation of the G protein-gated inwardly rectifying potassium channel. *Proc Natl Acad Sci U S A* 2000;97:5651–5656.

99. Lee HT, Emala CW. Protective effects of renal ischemic preconditioning and adenosine pretreatment: role of A1 and A3 receptors. *Am J Physiol Renal Physiol* 2000;278:F380–F387.

100. Lee HT, Gallos G, Nasr SH, Emala CW. A1 adenosine receptor activation inhibits inflammation, necrosis, and apoptosis after renal ischemia-reperfusion injury in mice. *J Am Soc Nephrol* 2004;15:102–111.

101. Lee HT, Ota-Setlik A, Xu H et al. A3 adenosine receptor knockout mice are protected against ischemia- and myoglobinuria-induced renal failure. *Am J Physiol Renal Physiol* 2003;284:F267–F273.

102. Lee HT, Xu H, Nasr SH et al. A1 adenosine receptor knockout mice exhibit increased renal injury following ischemia and reperfusion. *Am J Physiol Renal Physiol* 2004;286:F298–F306.

103. LeRoy EC, Ager A, Gordon JL. Effects of neutrophil elastase and other proteases on porcine aortic endothelial prostaglandin I2 production, adenine nucleotide release, and responses to vasoactive agents. *J Clin Invest* 1984;74:1003–1010.

104. Levens N, Beil M, Jarvis M. Renal actions of a new adenosine agonist, CGS 21680A selective for the A2 receptor. *J Pharmacol Exp Ther* 1991;257:1005–1012.

105. Levens N, Beil M, Schulz R. Intrarenal actions of the new adenosine agonist CGS 21680A, selective for the A2 receptor. *J Pharmacol Exp Ther* 1991;257:1013–1019.

106. Lloyd HG, Deussen A, Wuppermann H, Schrader J The transmethylation pathway as a source for adenosine in the isolated guinea-pig heart. *Biochem J* 1988;252:489–494.
107. Majid DS, Navar LG. Nitric oxide in the control of renal hemodynamics and excretory function. *Am J Hypertens* 2001;14:74S–82S.
108. Mi Z, Herzer WA, Zhang Y, Jackson EK. 3-isobutyl-1-methylxanthine decreases renal cortical interstitial levels of adenosine and inosine. *Life Sci* 1994;54:277–282.
109. Mi Z, Jackson EK. Metabolism of exogenous cyclic AMP to adenosine in the rat kidney. *J Pharmacol Exp Ther* 1995;273:728–733.
110. Mi Z, Jackson EK. Evidence for an endogenous cAMP-adenosine pathway in the rat kidney. *J Pharmacol Exp Ther* 1998;287:926–930.
111. Mi Z, Jackson EK. Effects of α- and β-adrenoceptor blockade on purine secretion induced by sympathetic nerve stimulation in the rat kidney. *J Pharmacol Exp Ther* 1999;288: 295–301.
112. Miller WL, Thomas RA, Berne RM, Rubio R. Adenosine production in the ischemic kidney. *Circ Res* 1978;43:390–397.
113. Misumi Y, Ogata S, Hirose S, Ikehara Y. Primary structure of rat liver 5'-nucleotidase deduced from the cDNA. Presence of the COOH-terminal hydrophobic domain for possible post-translational modification by glycophospholipid. *J Biol Chem* 1990; 265:2178–2183.
114. Moser GH, Schrader J, Deussen A. Turnover of adenosine in plasma of human and dog blood. *Am J Physiol* 1989;256:C799–C806.
115. Mozaffari MS, Abebe W, Warren BK. Renal adenosine A_3 receptors in the rat: assessment of functional role. *Can J Physiol Pharmacol* 2000;78:428–432.
116. Munger KA, Jackson EK. Effects of selective A_1 receptor blockade on glomerular hemodynamics: involvement of renin-angiotensin system. *Am J Physiol* 1994;267:F783–F790.
117. Murray RD, Churchill PC. Effects of adenosine receptor agonists in the isolated, perfused rat kidney. *Am J Physiol* 1984;247:H343–H348.
118. Murray RD, Churchill PC. Concentration dependency of the renal vascular and renin secretory responses to adenosine receptor agonists. *J Pharmacol Exp Ther* 1985;232:189–193.
119. Nagashima K, Kusaka H, Karasawa A. Protective effects of KW-3902, an adenosine A_1-receptor antagonist, against cisplatin-induced acute renal failure in rats. *Jpn J Pharmacol* 1995;67:349–357.
120. Nagashima K, Kusaka H, Sato K, Karasawa A. Effects of KW-3902, a novel adenosine A_1-receptor antagonist, on cephaloridine-induced acute renal failure in rats. *Jpn J Pharmacol* 1994;64:9–17.
121. Nishiyama A, Inscho EW, Navar LG. Interactions of adenosine A_1 and A_{2a} receptors on renal microvascular reactivity. *Am J Physiol Renal Physiol* 2001;280:F406–F414.
122. Nolte D, Lorenzen A, Lehr HA et al. Reduction of postischemic leukocyte-endothelium interaction by adenosine via A_2 receptor. *Naunyn Schmiedebergs Arch Pharmacol* 1992;346: 234–237.
123. O'Brien JA, Strange RC. The release of adenosine 3':5'-cyclic monophosphate from the isolated perfused rat heart. *Biochem J* 1975;152:429–432.
124. Okusa MD, Linden J, Macdonald T, Huang L. Selective A_{2A} adenosine receptor activation reduces ischemia-reperfusion injury in rat kidney. *Am J Physiol* 1999;277:F404–F412.
125. Osswald H, Hermes HH, Nabakowski G. Role of adenosine in signal transmission of tubuloglomerular feedback. *Kidney Int Suppl* 1982;12:S136–S142.
126. Osswald H, Nabakowski G, Hermes H. Adenosine as a possible mediator of metabolic control of glomerular filtration rate. *Int J Biochem* 1980;12:263–267.
127. Osswald H, Schmitz HJ, Heidenreich O. Adenosine response of the rat kidney after saline loading, sodium restriction and hemorrhagia. *Pflugers Arch* 1975;357:323–333.
128. Osswald H, Schmitz HJ, Kemper R. Tissue content of adenosine, inosine and hypoxanthine in the rat kidney after ischemia and postischemic recirculation. *Pflugers Arch* 1977;371:45–49.
129. Osswald H, Vallon V, Muhlbauer B. Role of adenosine in tubuloglomerular feedback and acute renal failure. *J Auton Pharmacol* 1996;16:377–380.
130. Pallone TL, Silldorff EP, Turner MR. Intrarenal blood flow: microvascular anatomy and the regulation of medullary perfusion. *Clin Exp Pharmacol Physiol* 1998;25:383–392.
131. Panjehshahin MR, Munsey TS, Collis MG et al. Further characterization of the protective effect of 8-cyclopentyl-1,3-dipropylxanthine on glycerol-induced acute renal failure in the rat. *J Pharm Pharmacol* 1992;44:109–113.
132. Paul S, Jackson EK, Robertson D et al. Caffeine potentiates the renin response to furosemide in rats. Evidence for a regulatory role of endogenous adenosine. *J Pharmacol Exp Ther* 1989;251:183–187.
133. Pearson JD, Carleton JS, Gordon JL. Metabolism of adenine nucleotides by ectoenzymes of vascular endothelial and smooth-muscle cells in culture. *Biochem J* 1980;190:421–429.
134. Pearson JD, Coade SB, Cusack NJ. Characterization of ectonucleotidases on vascular smooth-muscle cells. *Biochem J* 1985;230:503–507.
135. Pearson JD, Gordon JL. Vascular endothelial and smooth muscle cells in culture selectively release adenine nucleotides. *Nature* 1979;281:384–386.
136. Peart WS, Quesada T, Tenyi I. The effects of cyclic adenosine 3',5'-monophosphate and guanosine 3',5'-monophosphate and theophylline on renin secretion in the isolated perfused kidney of the rat. *Br J Pharmacol* 1975;54:55–60.
137. Pfeifer CA, Suzuki F, Jackson EK. Selective A_1 adenosine receptor antagonism augments β-adrenergic-induced renin release in vivo. *Am J Physiol* 1995;269:F469–F479.
138. Pflueger AC, Schenk F, Osswald H. Increased sensitivity of the renal vasculature to adenosine in streptozotocin-induced diabetes mellitus rats. *Am J Physiol* 1995;269:F529–F535.
139. Radziuk J, Barron P, Najm H, Davies J The effect of systemic venous drainage of the pancreas on insulin sensitivity in dogs. *J Clin Invest* 1993;92:1713–1721.
140. Ramos-Salazar A, Baines AD. Role of 5'-nucleotidase in adenosine-mediated renal vasoconstriction during hypoxia. *J Pharmacol Exp Ther* 1986;236:494–499.
141. Reid IA, Stockigt JR, Goldfien A, Ganong WF. Stimulation of renin secretion in dogs by theophylline. *Eur J Pharmacol* 1972;17:325–332.
142. Ren Y, Arima S, Carretero OA, Ito S. Possible role of adenosine in macula densa control of glomerular hemodynamics. *Kidney Int* 2002;61:169–176.
143. Ren YL, Garvin JL, Liu RS, Carretero OA. Role of macula densa adenosine triphosphate (ATP) in tubuloglomerular feedback. *Kidney Int* 2004;66:1479–1485.
144. Rindler MJ, Bashor MM, Spitzer N, Saier MH, Jr. Regulation of adenosine 3':5'-monophosphate efflux from animal cells. *J Biol Chem* 1978;253:5431–5436.
145. Rosenberg PA, Dichter MA. Extracellular cAMP accumulation and degradation in rat cerebral cortex in dissociated cell culture. *J NeuroSci* 1989;9:2654–2663.
146. Rosenberg PA, Knowles R, Knowles KP, Li Y. Beta-adrenergic receptor-mediated regulation of extracellular adenosine in cerebral cortex in culture. *J NeuroSci* 1994;14: 2953–2965.
147. Rosenberg PA, Li Y. Adenylyl cyclase activation underlies intracellular cyclic AMP accumulation, cyclic AMP transport, and extracellular adenosine accumulation evoked by beta-adrenergic receptor stimulation in mixed cultures of neurons and astrocytes derived from rat cerebral cortex. *Brain Res* 1995;692:227–232.
148. Rosenberg PA, Li Y. Forskolin evokes extracellular adenosine accumulation in rat cortical cultuRes *Neurosci Lett* 1996;211:49–52.
149. Sakai K, Akima M, Nabata H. A possible purinergic mechanism for reactive ischemia in isolated, cross-circulated rat kidney. *Jpn J Pharmacol* 1979;29:235–242.
150. Schnackenberg CG, Merz E, Brooks DP. An orally active adenosine A_1 receptor antagonist, FK838, increases renal excretion and maintains glomerular filtration rate in furosemide-resistant rats. *Br J Pharmacol* 2003;139:1383–1388.
151. Schnermann J, Weihprecht H, Briggs JP. Inhibition of tubuloglomerular feedback during $adenosine_1$ receptor blockade. *Am J Physiol* 1990;258:F553–F561.
152. Schrader J Formation and metabolism of adenosine and adenine nucleotides in cardiac tissue. In *Adenosine and Adenine Nucleotides as Regulators of Cellular Function.* JW Phillis (ed) Boca Raton FL: CRC Press. 1991;55–69.
153. Schweda F, Wagner C, Kramer BK et al. Preserved macula densa-dependent renin secretion in A_1 adenosine receptor knockout mice. *Am J Physiol Renal Physiol* 2003;284:F770–F777.
154. Schwiebert EM, Kishore BK. Extracellular nucleotide signaling along the renal epithelium. *Am J Physiol Renal Physiol* 2001;280:F945–F963.
155. Sekine T, Watanabe N, Hosoyamada M et al. Expression cloning and characterization of a novel multispecific organic anion transporter. *J Biol Chem* 1997;272:18526–18529.
156. Shimada J, Suzuki F, Nonaka H et al. (8-Dicyclopropylmethyl)-1,3-dipropylxanthine: a potent and selective adenosine A_1 antagonist with renal protective and diuretic activities. *J Med Chem* 1991;34:466–469.
157. Silldorff EP, Kreisberg MS, Pallone TL. Adenosine modulates vasomotor tone in outer medullary descending vasa recta of the rat. *J Clin Invest* 1996;98:18–23.
158. Siragy HM, Linden J Sodium intake markedly alters renal interstitial fluid adenosine. *Hypertension* 1996;27:404–407.
159. Smith JA, Sivaprasadarao A, Munsey TS et al. Immunolocalisation of adenosine A_1 receptors in the rat kidney. *Biochem Pharmacol* 2001;61:237–244.
160. Smoake JA, McMahon KL, Wright RK, Solomon SS. Hormonally sensitive cyclic AMP phosphodiesterase in liver cells. An ecto-enzyme. *J Biol Chem* 1981;256:8531–8535.
161. Sperling MA. Glucagon: secretion and actions. *Adv Exp Med Biol* 1979;124:29–61.
162. Spielman WS, Osswald H. Blockade of postocclusive renal vasoconstriction by an angiotensin II antagonists: evidence for an angiotensin-adenosine interaction. *Am J Physiol* 1979;237: F463–F467.
163. Sun D, Samuelson LC, Yang T et al. Mediation of tubuloglomerular feedback by adenosine: evidence from mice lacking adenosine 1 receptors. *Proc Natl Acad Sci U S A.* 2001;98: 9983–9988.
164. Suzuki F, Shimada J, Mizumoto H et al. Adenosine A_1 antagonists. 2. Structure-activity relationships on diuretic activities and protective effects against acute renal failure. *J Med Chem* 1992;35:3066–3075.
165. Szczepanska-Konkel M, Jankowski M, Stiepanow-Trzeciak A et al. Responsiveness of renal glomeruli to adenosine in streptozotocin-induced diabetic rats dependent on hyperglycaemia level. *J Physiol Pharmacol* 2003;54:109–120.
166. Taborsky GJ, Jr., Ahren B, Havel PJ. Autonomic mediation of glucagon secretion during hypoglycemia: implications for impaired alpha-cell responses in type 1 diabetes. *Diabetes* 1998;47:995–1005.
167. Tagawa H, Vander AJ. Effects of adenosine compounds on renal function and renin secretion in dogs. *Circ Res* 1970;26:327–338.
168. Takeda M, Yoshitomi K, Imai M. Regulation of Na^+-$3HCO_3^-$ cotransport in rabbit proximal convoluted tubule via adenosine A_1 receptor. *Am J Physiol* 1993;265:F511–F519.
169. Tang YT, Zhou LB. Characterization of adenosine A_1 receptors in human proximal tubule epithelial (HK-2) cells. *Receptors Channels* 2003;9:67–75.
170. Thomson SC. Adenosine and purinergic mediators of tubuloglomerular feedback. *Curr Opin Nephrol Hypertens* 2002;11:81–86.
171. Thong FS, Graham TE. The putative roles of adenosine in insulin- and exercise-mediated regulation of glucose transport and glycogen metabolism in skeletal muscle. *Can J Appl Physiol* 2002;27:152–178.
172. Ticho B, Whalley E, Gill A et al. Renal effect of BG9928, an A_1 adenosine receptor antagoinist, in rats and nonhuman primates. *Drug Development Rese* 2003;58:486–492.
173. Tofovic SP, Branch KR, Oliver RD et al. Caffeine potentiates vasodilator-induced renin release. *J Pharmacol Exp Ther* 1991; 256:850–860.
174. Traynor T, Yang T, Huang YG et al. Inhibition of adenosine-1 receptor-mediated preglomerular vasoconstriction in AT_{1A} receptor-deficient mice. *Am J Physiol* 1998;275: F922–F927.
175. Tseng CJ, Kuan CJ, Chu H, Tung CS. Effect of caffeine treatment on plasma renin activity and angiotensin I concentrations in rats on a low sodium diet. *Life Sci* 1993;52:883–890.
176. van Aubel RAMH, Smeets PHE, Peters JGP et al. The MRP4/ABCC4 gene encodes a novel apical organic anion transporter in human kidney proximal tubules: Putative efflux pump for urinary cAMP and cGMP. *J Am Soc Nephrol* 2002;13:595–603.
177. van Buren M, Bijlsma JA, Boer P et al. Natriuretic and hypotensive effect of adenosine-1 blockade in essential hypertension. *Hypertension* 1993;22:728–734.
178. Velliquette RA, Koletsky RJ, Ernsberger P. Plasma glucagon and free fatty acid responses to a glucose load in the obese spontaneous hypertensive rat (SHROB) model of metabolic syndrome X. *Exp Biol Med (Maywood)* 2002;227:164–170.

179. Viskoper RJ, Maxwell MH, Lupu AN, Rosenfeld S. Renin stimulation by isoproterenol and theophylline in the isolated perfused kidney. *Am J Physiol* 1977;232:F248–F253.

180. Weihprecht H, Lorenz JN, Briggs JP, Schnermann J Synergistic effects of angiotensin and adenosine in the renal microvasculature. *Am J Physiol* 1994;266:F227–F239.

181. Wengert M, Berto C, Jr., Kaufman J et al. Stimulation of the proximal tubule Na$^+$-ATPase activity by adenosine A$_{2A}$ receptor. *Int J Biochem Cell Biol* 2005;37:155–165.

182. Wilcox CS, Welch WJ, Schreiner GF, Belardinelli L. Natriuretic and diuretic actions of a highly selective adenosine A$_1$ receptor antagonist. *J Am Soc Nephrol* 1999;10:714–720.

183. Wise A, Sheehan M, Rees S et al. Comparative analysis of the efficacy of A$_1$ adenosine receptor activation of Gi/o alpha G proteins following coexpression of receptor and G protein and expression of A$_1$ adenosine receptor-Gi/o alpha fusion proteins. *Biochemistry* 1999;38:2272–2278.

184. Yamaguchi S, Umemura S, Tamura K et al. Adenosine A$_1$ receptor mRNA in microdissected rat nephron segments. *Hypertension* 1995;26:1181–1185.

185. Yao K, Kusaka H, Sato K, Karasawa A. Protective effects of KW-3902, a novel adenosine A$_1$-receptor antagonist, against gentamicin-induced acute renal failure in rats. *Jpn J Pharmacol* 1994;65:167–170.

186. Zacher LA, Carey GB. Cyclic AMP metabolism by swine adipocyte microsomal and plasma membranes. *Comp Biochem Physiol B Biochem Mol Biol* 1999;124:61–71.

187. Zimmermann H. 5′-Nucleotidase: molecular structure and functional aspects. *Biochem J* 1992;285:345–365.

188. Zimmermann H. Ecto-Nucleotidases. In: *MP Abbracchio, M Williams (eds.)*. Handbook of Experimental Pharmacology. Purinergic and pryimidinergic signalling I: molecular, nervous and urogenitary system function. Berlin: Springer-Verlag; 2001:151J: 209-250.

189. Zou AP, Nithipatikom K, Li PL, Cowley AW, Jr. Role of renal medullary adenosine in the control of blood flow and sodium excretion. *Am J Physiol* 1999;276:R790–R798.

190. Zou AP, Wu F, Li PL, Cowley AW, Jr. Effect of chronic salt loading on adenosine metabolism and receptor expression in renal cortex and medulla in rats. *Hypertension* 1999;33: 511–516.

191. Zumstein P, Zapf J, Froesch ER. Effects of hormones on cyclic AMP release from rat adipose tissue in vitro. *FEBS Lett* 1974;49:65–69.

CHAPTER 17

Extracellular Nucleotides and Renal Function

Matthew A. Bailey, David G. Shirley,* Brian F. King,* Geoffrey Burnstock,* and Robert J. Unwin*

University of Edinburgh, Edinburgh, United Kingdom
*University College London, London, United Kingdom

The actions of extracellular adenine nucleotides and nucleosides on physiological functions were first reported as long ago as 1929 (40), but it was not until many years later that ATP was recognized as a transmitter for nonadrenergic, noncholinergic nerves of the autonomic nervous system and the term "purinergic" was coined (20). Early resistance to this concept has since diminished to the extent that purines are now acknowledged not only as neurotransmitters but also as important autocrine/paracrine regulators of diverse cellular processes throughout the body (1, 116).

MOLECULAR PHYSIOLOGY OF PURINOCEPTORS

The purine moiety occurs naturally in the extracellular space in a variety of chemical forms. It can be present as a nucleic acid, nucleoside, nucleotide, and dinucleotide (Fig. 1A) and, as an extracellular signaling molecule, the purine moiety interacts with a large variety of cell surface receptors (Fig. 1B). This array of structurally disparate purinoceptors is highly diverse in its operational properties. Most purinoceptors belong to the Rhodopsin superfamily of heptahelical (seven-transmembrane domains; or serpentine) G-protein–coupled receptors (GPCRs), in the assigned α- and δ-groups of this family (46). The remainder belong to a unique class of ligand-gated ion channels called P2X receptors (110). The actions of extracellularly applied purine-based compounds are highly complex and, as a consequence, often difficult to analyze. Accordingly, it is essential to understand the operational profiles of each class of purinoceptors, before investigating the physiological role of purines in the kidney.

Adenine Receptors

Adenine, the simplest form of the purine moiety (Fig. 1A), specifically activates a GPCR subtype present in modest amounts in rat kidney (14). At present, however, the role of extracellular adenine and its receptors in the control of renal function is unknown.

P1 Receptors

The P1 receptor family consists of four molecularly distinct subtypes: A_1, A_{2a}, A_{2b}, and A_3. Each is a G-protein–coupled receptor and shares structural similarities with other receptors of that class. All four subtypes modulate the activity of adenylate cyclase and thereby affect the cyclic AMP/protein kinase A signaling pathway. A_1 and A_3 receptors inhibit adenylate cyclase while A_{2a} and A_{2b} receptors stimulate it. These receptors are all activated by adenosine. Chapter 16 discusses the renal functions of the P1 receptor family.

P2Y Receptors

When a triphosphate chain is added to the 5′-carbon of the ribose moiety in adenosine (Fig. 1A), the resultant nucleotide (ATP) acts as a ligand for a distinct class of GPCRs called the P2Y receptors. There are eight recognized members of the mammalian P2Y subfamily: $P2Y_1$, $P2Y_2$, $P2Y_4$, $P2Y_6$, $P2Y_{11}$, $P2Y_{12}$, $P2Y_{13}$, and $P2Y_{14}$. These GPCRs were numbered in chronological order, according to their molecular isolation (21). Gaps appear in the sequence because they involve either P2Y receptors with no mammalian equivalent or P2Y-like sequences that were originally misidentified as nucleotide receptors. Thus, several nonmammalian proteins—skate P2Y, turkey P2Y, chick $P2Y_3$ and *Xenopus* $P2Y_8$—are not included in the list of mammalian P2Y receptors; while $P2Y_7$ is a leukotriene B_4 receptor, $P2Y_9$ is a receptor for lysophosphatidic acid, and $P2Y_{15}$ is a receptor for the citric acid cycle intermediates, α-ketoglutarate and succinate. Finally, $P2Y_5$ and $P2Y_{10}$ are orphan receptors with no defined ligand.

The P2Y receptor genes do not normally undergo alternative splicing. However, intergenic splicing occurs for the contiguous $P2Y_{11}$ and SSF1 genes on chromosome 19p31, creating fusion proteins that function in the same way as the wild-type $P2Y_{11}$ receptor (32). Additionally, a functional $P2Y_2$ polymorphism has been reported for a mutation at a single codon (an arginine-cysteine transition) (78). Wild-type P2Y receptor proteins range in length from 328 residues ($P2Y_6$ subtype) to 377 residues ($P2Y_2$ subtype). The amino

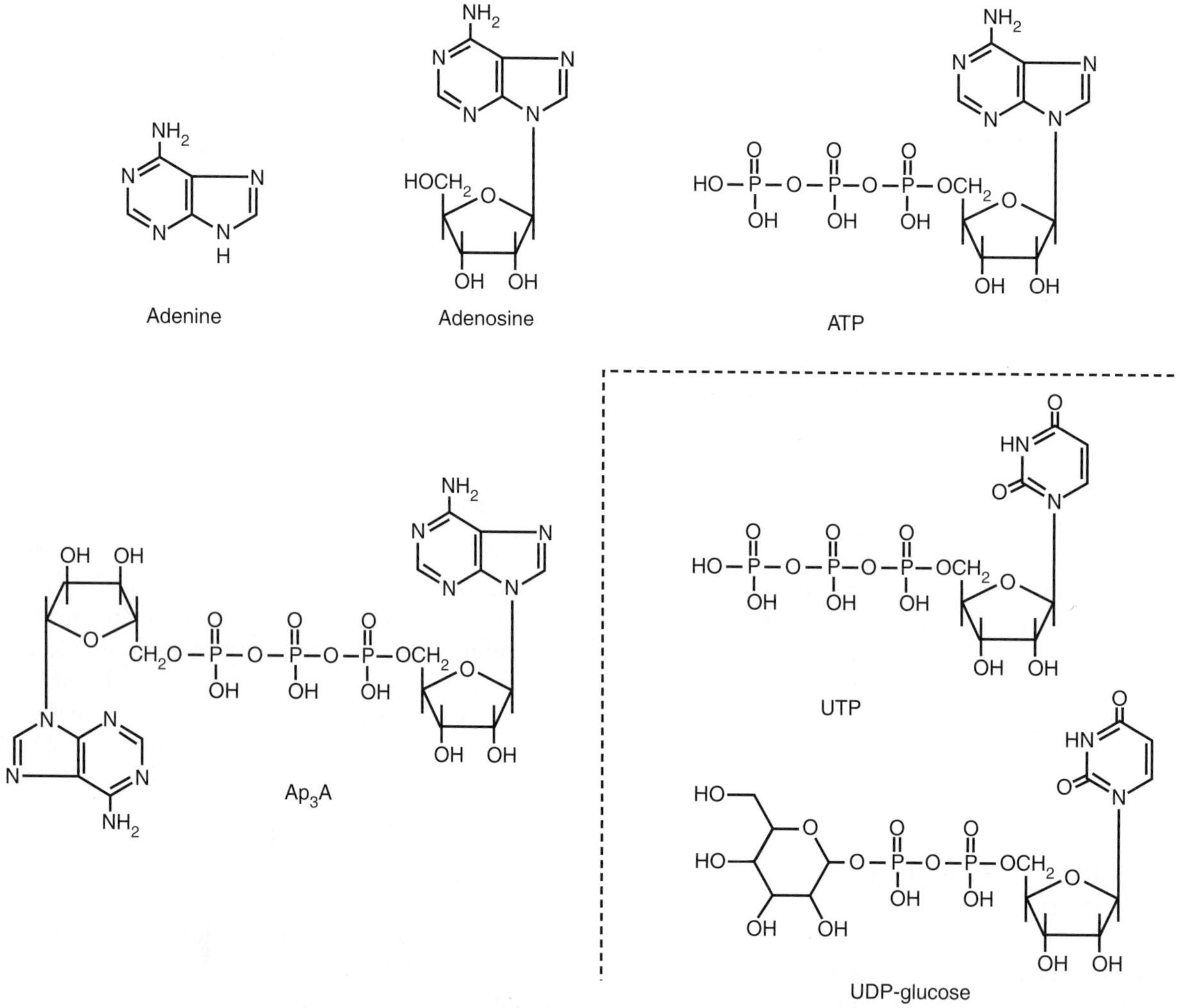

FIGURE 1 A. Molecular structures of selected purines and pyrimidines.

acid sequences of human P2Y receptor proteins are 19% to 55% identical but, where conservative substitutions are considered, these sequences show a 30% to 67% similarity. As noted previously, the P2Y receptor proteins have seven transmembrane spanning regions (TM1-7); the N-terminus projects into the extracellular space and the C-terminus is inside the cell. All the cloned P2Y receptors share the TM6 H-X-X-R/K motif, which is crucial for agonist activity (2). A fuller model of the docking sites for nucleotides—including the involvement of TM2, TM3, TM6, and TM7—has now been defined for the P2Y receptor family (33). Historically, ATP has been viewed as the natural agonist of native P2Y receptors but, from work on recombinant P2Y receptor proteins, it is now known that ATP subserves a range of roles, including agonist, partial agonist, and antagonist, or it may be inert. $P2Y_1$, $P2Y_{12}$, and $P2Y_{13}$ receptors are activated principally by ADP where, in all probability, this nucleoside diphosphate arises from the enzymatic breakdown of extracellular ATP. At very high levels of P2Y receptor expression, ATP can also act as a partial agonist at $P2Y_1$, $P2Y_{12}$, and $P2Y_{13}$ receptors. However, at low levels of P2Y receptor expression, ATP can revert to the role of an antago-

nist at these sites, indicating that its efficacy as an agonist is generally low and highly dependent on receptor reserve (81). The $P2Y_6$ subtype is also activated by ADP, although more potently by UDP and weakly by ATP.

$P2Y_2$ and $P2Y_{11}$ receptors are activated fully by ATP and less potently by ADP. Both these subtypes are also activated by UTP, which, again, is less potent than ATP. In contrast, the human form of $P2Y_4$ is activated primarily by UTP and, surprisingly, antagonized by ATP even at high receptor numbers. The mouse and rat isoforms of $P2Y_4$ are fully activated by both UTP and ATP. Lastly, the $P2Y_{14}$ receptor is potently activated by UDP-glucose (a sugar nucleotide) and completely unaffected by extracellular UTP, ATP, or glycosylated forms of adenine nucleotides. Thus, $P2Y_{14}$ shows the most restricted agonist profile of all the accepted P2Y receptor subtypes.

There are very few ATP analogues that serve as wholly selective agonists for P2Y receptors (Table 1). The *N*-methanocarba-ADP derivative MRS 2365 is a very potent and selective agonist for $P2Y_1$ receptors (29) and the βγ-meATP derivative AR-C67085 is a selective agonist for the $P2Y_{11}$ receptor (32). The remainder of the P2Y subtypes

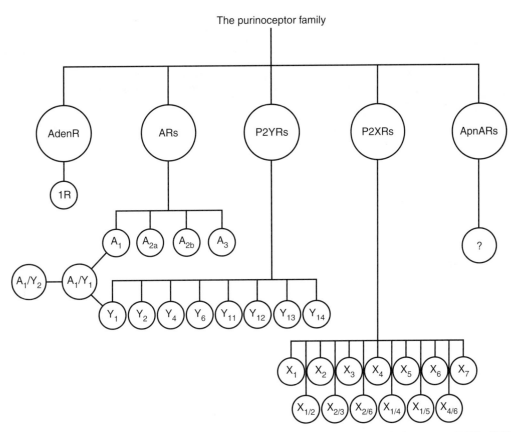

FIGURE 1   B. The purinoceptor family. AdenR, adenine receptor; ARs, adenosine (P1) receptors; P2YRs, P2Y receptors; P2XRs, P2X receptors; ApnARs, dinucleotide receptors.

are stimulated to varying degrees by 2-alkylthio derivatives (e.g. 2meSATP and 2meSADP), phosphorothioate derivatives (ATPγS and ADPβS or, in some cases, UTPγS and UDPβS), or symmetric and asymmetric dinucleotides (e.g., Ap4A, Up4U, and dCp4U). Thus, the pharmacological identification of P2Y receptor subtypes normally requires a cross-comparison of the activity of several nucleotides, to define the relative order of agonist potencies against the reference of ATP.

The concentration range over which P2Y receptor agonists act is neither critically important nor necessarily defining of phenotype, because the absolute number of P2Y receptors in a cell will determine the position of the concentration/response curve. This phenomenon, based on the relationship between the receptor reserve and the G-protein pool in a cell, is a common analytical problem for all types of agonist-activated GPCRs (81).

P2Y receptor–selective antagonists also are few in number. For P2Y₁, the bisphosphate ADP derivatives MRS2179 (2′-deoxy-N^6-methyladenosine-3′,5′-bisphosphate) and MRS2279 (2-Chloro-N^6-methyl-(N)-methanocarba-2′-deoxyadenosine-3′,5′-bisphosphate) are effective and selective antagonists (73); and the P2Y₆ subtype is antagonised by MRS2578 (1,4-di-[phenylthioureido] butane) (101). All members of the P2Y receptor family are nonselectively antagonized by high concentrations of suramin, PPADS (pyridoxal-5-phosphate -6-azophenyl 2′,4′-disulphonic acid), or reactive blue 2 (RB-2).

Heterodimeric P1/P2Y Receptors

The coexpression of A₁ receptors with P2Y₁ or P2Y₂ receptors results in a heterodimeric membrane receptor with mixed pharmacological and signaling properties (162, 163). Heterodimeric complexes may occur constitutively or be promoted by agonist activation of either of the two GPCRs (163). Although dimeric complexes occur naturally in several regions of the rat brain where A₁ and P2Y₁ receptors coexist (164), heterodimeric complexes have not been verified in those regions of the kidney where both A₁ and P2Y receptors are present.

Sugar-Nucleotide Receptor

The addition of a sugar moiety—such as glucose or galactose—to the nucleotide UDP results in an unusual, but potent, signaling molecule called a sugar-nucleotide (Fig. 1A). Cellular release of sugar nucleotides was found to be robust from a series of epithelial cell lines, often exceeding the amounts of ATP released by the same cells (92). The principal sugar nucleotide is UDP-glucose, which potently activates P2Y₁₄ receptor isoforms found in human, rat, and mouse (47). This P2Y subtype is present in rodent kidney, albeit in limited

TABLE 1 Monomeric P2Y Receptor Subtypes

	P2Y$_1$	P2Y$_2$	P2Y$_4$	P2Y$_6$	P2Y$_{11}$	P2Y$_{12}$	P2Y$_{13}$	P2Y$_{14}$
Gene (human)	*3q25.2*	*11q13.5*	*Xq13*	*11q13.5*	*19p13.2*	*3q24-25*	*3q24-25*	*3q24-25*
Protein (human)	372 aa	376 aa	365 aa	328 aa	371 aa	342 aa	333 aa	338 aa
Natural ligands (pEC$_{50}$)	ADP (8.6)	ATP (7.1)	UTP (7.6)	ADP (4.5)	ATP (5.5)	ADP (7.4)	ADP (8.0)	UDP-glucose (7.1)
	ATP (6.5)	UTP (7.7)	ATP (6.0) (r,m*)	UDP (7.0)	UTP (5.2)	ATP (6.2)	ATP (6.6)	
Other agonists (pEC$_{50}$)	Ap$_4$A (6.2)	Up$_4$U (7.0)	GTP (5.2)	IDP (4.5)			IDP (6.3)	
	2MeSATP (8.5)				2MeSATP (4.6)	2MeSATP (10)	2MeSATP (7.9)	
	2MeSADP (8.7)					2MeSADP (10)	2MeSADP (7.1)	
	ATPγS (6.4)	ATPγS (6.2)	UTPγS (5.8)		ATPγS (5.5)			
	ADPβS (6.1)			UDPβS (7.6)		ADPβS (7.0)	ADPβS (7.4)	
	MRS 2365 (9.0)				AR-C67085 (5.8)			
Antagonist: selective (pIC$_{50}$)	MRS 2279 (7.3)			MRS 2578 (7.5)	AMPS (3.5)	2MeSAMP (5.9)	PPADS (4.9)	
						PPADS (3.7)	AR-C69931 (8.3)	
						AR-C69931 (9.0)		
Antagonist: nonselective (pIC$_{50}$)	MRS 2179 (6.5)							
	PPADS (5.4)		PPADS (4.8)					
	suramin (5.8)	suramin (~4.5)			suramin (4.8)	suramin (5.4)	suramin (5.6)	
	RB-2 (6.5) (c*)		RB-2 (4.7) (r,m*)	RB-2 (4.5)		RB-2 (5.9)	RB-2 (5.7)	
Signaling	G$_{q/11}$ PLCβ activation	G$_{q/11}$ PLCβ activation	G$_{q/11}$ PLCβ activation	G$_{q/11}$ PLCβ activation	G$_{q/11}$ and G$_S$ PLCβ and AC activation	G$_{i/o}$ AC inhibition	G$_{i/o}$ AC inhibition	G$_{i/o}$ AC inhibition

Pharmacological and signaling properties of monomeric P2Y receptors, listing the natural and synthetic agonists, and the selective and nonselective antagonists for each subtype. Data are given as $-\log_{10} EC_{50}$ (pEC$_{50}$) and $-\log_{10} IC_{50}$ (pIC$_{50}$). In some cases, data are given for chick (*c**), mouse (*m**) and rat (*r**) isoforms; all other data are for humans. aa, amino acids.

amounts (47). The P2Y$_{14}$ receptor (338 residues) shares 47% to 48% sequence identity with P2Y$_{12}$ and P2Y$_{13}$ receptors, but is only 23% to 27% identical to the remainder of the P2Y receptor family. A striking aspect of the sugar-nucleotide–activated P2Y$_{14}$ receptor is the complete lack of agonist activity by either purine- or pyrimidine-based nucleotides (26). Additionally, no antagonists have been identified.

Dinucleotide Receptors

Where two adenosine molecules are united by a polyphosphate chain by the 5′-carbon of the ribose moieties, the resultant compound creates a purine-based dinucleotide (Fig. 1A). The phosphate chain of these dimeric adenosine molecules can vary in length, from two to seven phosphates (Ap$_n$A; n = 2-7), and all members of this dinucleotide family show biological activity at purinoceptors (62). The diadenosine polyphosphates are examples of symmetrical dinucleotides, but other dimeric species also occur naturally. These include the asymmetrical (Ap$_n$G; n = 3-6) and symmetrical (Gp$_n$G; n = 3-6) dinucleotides, which contain adenosine and guanosine and have been found in human platelets (125). These dinucleotides exert potent vasoconstrictive actions in the renal vasculature (145). Additionally, a newly identified type of vasoconstrictive dinucleotide, Up$_4$A, has been found in vascular endothelial cells and has potent actions in the isolated perfused rat kidney (77).

The molecular targets of symmetrical and asymmetrical dinucleotides are still unresolved. Whereas indirect evidence supports the existence of dinucleotide-specific GPCRs in neuronal and endothelial cells (62), work on recombinant P2Y receptors has revealed many to be sensitive to agonism by various types of dinucleotides (132).

P2X Receptors

P2X receptors are encoded by a family of seven genes (P2X$_1$–P2X$_7$) for human, mouse, or rat (110). Some P2X genes have also been isolated in cDNA libraries of other vertebrates such as chimp, chicken, dog, guinea-pig, frog, and zebrafish and occur in some invertebrates (3). The P2X genes show a complex organization, with the encoding sequences interrupted by up to 14 introns. When transcription proceeds normally, the seven wild-type P2X proteins are 379 residues (P2X$_6$) to 595 residues (P2X$_7$) long and show 30% to 50% identity (19). Hydrophobicity plots of the seven proteins reveal a common pattern of two nonpolar domains that form two transmembrane-spanning α-helices that line and gate the ion-channel pore (134). It is widely accepted that N- and C-termini of P2X proteins are inside the cell. The extracellular loop contains ten conserved cysteine residues, which form five disulphide bridges to give structural complexity and rigidity to the protein.

Three P2X protein subunits come together as a stretched trimer to form a P2X receptor ion channel. The two transmembrane-spanning segments of each subunit line up in a head-to-tail arrangement to form the pore (11). Each of the seven P2X subunits can make homomeric ion channels by assembling three identical subunits, although the efficiency varies from subunit to subunit. Evidence suggests that another 13 combinations of heteromeric assemblies, involving at least two different subunits, can also be made. P2X$_1$ and P2X$_5$ subunits are promiscuous and will form heteromeric ion channels with all other subunits, except for the P2X$_7$ subunit. In contrast, the P2X$_7$ subunit is discerning and only makes homomeric assemblies. In most tissues, the native P2X receptor population is a mixture of homomeric and heteromeric assemblies.

All P2X receptors are activated by ATP, but usually not by ADP, AMP, adenosine, or adenine (Table 2). Some receptors are activated by other naturally occurring agonists. The concentration range of extracellular ATP activating P2X receptors is broadly similar and typically in the low micromolar range. However, the P2X$_1$ receptor stands out as the most sensitive, requiring submicromolar ATP concentrations for activation, whereas P2X$_7$ is the least sensitive and requires near millimolar ATP concentrations for activation. The ATP-binding site involves amino acid residues close to the exofacial ends of the two transmembrane-spanning regions, which interact with the phosphate chain, whereas aromatic residues in the extracellular loop interact with the adenine moiety (119).

P2X receptor ion channels are permeable to Na$^+$ and K$^+$ ions to cause depolarization and to Ca^{2+} ions that interact with intracellular signaling molecules. P2X receptors are sensitized by extracellular pH, the most extreme example being the P2X$_2$ subtype where responses to ATP are potentiated under acidic conditions and inhibited under alkaline conditions; pH changes as small as 0.03 units affect the size of the responses (153). Other P2X receptors are inhibited by H$^+$ ions, so that acidic conditions greatly reduce the potency of extracellular ATP. The precise molecular basis of this inhibitory effect is still unknown. P2X receptors are also sensitive to extracellular metal ions, particularly transition metals such as Zn^{2+} and Cu^{2+}, and to ion species such as Cd^{2+}, Ni^{2+}, Co^{2+}, Gd^{3+}, La^{3+}, and Al^{3+} ions.

Synthetic nucleotides such as methylene phosphonates (αβmeATP and βγmeATP) show a preference for P2X$_1$ and P2X$_3$ receptors, whereas 2-alkylthio derivatives (2meSATP) and phosphorothiates (ATPγS) are nonspecific agonists. A modified ribose derivative, BzATP, is more potent than ATP at P2X$_7$ receptors, but this compound also shows

agonist activity at P2X$_1$, P2X$_3$ and P2X$_5$ receptors and, therefore, is not selective for any particular P2X subtype.

Some modified synthetic nucleotides can act as antagonists at P2X receptors. Ip$_5$I (diinosine pentaphosphate) is highly selective for P2X$_1$ receptors (82); while TNP-ATP (trinitrophenyl-ATP) is a potent antagonist at P2X$_1$ and P2X$_3$ receptors, and less potent at P2X$_2$, P2X$_4$, and P2X$_5$ receptors (150). Several synthetic heterocyclic compounds also act as P2X receptor antagonists. Suramin is a nonselective P2X receptor antagonist, but structurally related derivatives such as NF449 are extremely potent at P2X$_1$ receptors (63). PPADS shows broad antagonist actions at P2X receptors, but some derivatives do show selectivity at P2X$_1$ and P2X$_3$ receptors (18). Reactive blue 2 and brilliant blue 2G (BBG) are active at P2X$_2$ and P2X$_7$ receptors, respectively (Table 2).

NUCLEOTIDE RECEPTORS AND RENAL PHYSIOLOGY

The Renal Vasculature

Immunohistochemical studies in the rat demonstrate a widespread distribution of P2X$_1$ receptors, which are expressed in smooth muscle of the renal artery, arcuate and cortical radial arteries and the afferent, but not the efferent, arteriole (Fig. 2)(28, 142). These studies are supported by functional identification of a P2X$_1$-like receptor in the afferent arteriole (66). P2X$_2$ receptors are the only other member of the P2X family expressed in the vasculature, being limited to the smooth muscle of the larger intrarenal arteries and veins (69, 142). Of the P2Y receptors, P2Y$_1$ has an extensive distribution, being expressed in large arteries and veins as well as in afferent and efferent arterioles (142). A pyrimidine-selective receptor has been functionally identified in the rat afferent arteriole (67), but expression of neither P2Y$_2$ nor P2Y$_4$ could be confirmed immunologically (142).

Infusion of ATP into the renal artery has long been known to alter renal vascular resistance, although the nature and magnitude of the response are species dependent. In the isolated perfused kidney preparation, ATP caused modest vasoconstriction in the rabbit (106), marked and sustained vasoconstriction in the rat (30, 66), and vasodilatation in the dog (100). The net response appears to be determined by the class of the dominant P2 receptor: in the rat, selective agonism of P2Y$_1$ receptors causes nitric oxide–dependent vasodilatation, whereas selective activation of P2X$_1$ receptors evokes constriction (30, 67). Furthermore, the constrictive effects of ATP are augmented by inhibition of nitric oxide synthesis, indicating that the tendency toward vasodilatation, in the rat at least, is masked by the predominant P2X$_1$-mediated vasoconstriction. It is likely that purinergic control of vascular tone (and therefore blood flow) is dependent on the source and local concentration of extracellular nucleotide. ATP released from renal nerve terminals, for example, will act directly on

TABLE 2 Homomeric P2X Receptor Subtypes

	P2X$_1$	P2X$_2$	P2X$_3$	P2X$_4$	P2X$_5$	P2X$_6$	P2X$_7$
Gene (human)	*17p13*	*12q24.33*	*11q12*	*12q24.32*	*17p13*	*22q11.21*	*12q24.31*
Protein (rat)	399 aa	472 aa	397 aa	388 aa	445 aa	379 aa	595 aa
Natural ligands (pEC$_{50}$)	ATP (7.0)	ATP (5.3)	ATP (5.9)	ATP (5.4)	ATP (6.4)	ATP (6.2)	ATP (3.4)
	CTP (4.4)		UTP (4.0)	CTP (3.5)	GTP (4.6)		ADP (2.7) (*m**)
	Ap$_6$A (6.0) Ap$_6$G (5.7)	Ap$_4$A (4.8)	Ap$_6$A (5.9) Ap$_3$A (6.0)	Ap$_4$A (5.5$)	Ap$_4$A (6.6)		
Other agonists (pEC$_{50}$)	2MeSATP (7.0)	2MeSATP (5.1)	2MeSATP (6.7)	2MeSATP (3.6)	2MeSATP (6.4)		2MeSATP (5.0)
	ATPγS (6.2)	ATPγS (5.1)	ATPγS (5.9)	ATPγS (~5.0)	ATPγS (6.5)		
	αβmeATP (5.5)	αβmeATP (3.0)	αβmeATP (5.7)	αβmeATP (4.2$)	αβmeATP (6.0)		
	BzATP (4.6)				BzATP (5.9)		BzATP (5.2)
Antagonist: selective (pIC$_{50}$)	NF449 (9.5)		B^{Z}ATP (7.1) A317491 (7.6)				BBG (8.0)
	Ip$_5$I (8.5)						KN-62 (7.4) (*h**)
Antagonist: nonselective (pIC$_{50}$)	TNP-ATP (9.0)	TNP-ATP (5.9)	TNP-ATP (9.5)	TNP-ATP (4.8)	TNP-ATP (6.3)		TNP-ATP (~4.3)
	PPADS (6.9)	PPADS (5.8)	PPADS (6.7)	PPADS (<4.0)	PPADS (6.7)		PPADS (4.3)
	suramin (5.7)	suramin (5.0)	suramin (5.4)	suramin (<4.0)	suramin (5.8)		
	RB-2 (5.7)	RB-2 (6.4)	RB-2 (4.3)	BBG (3.9)	RB-2 (4.7)		
Signaling	cation channel	cation channel	cation channel	cation channel	cation channel	cation channel	channel/pore pass, <700 Da
	P$_{ca}$/P$_{na}$ ~4	P$_{ca}$/P$_{na}$ ~2	P$_{ca}$/P$_{na}$ ~4	P$_{ca}$/P$_{na}$ ~4	P$_{ca}$/P$_{na}$ ~1.5	nd	

Pharmacological and signaling properties of homomeric P2X receptors, listing the natural and synthetic agonists, and the selective and nonselective antagonists for each subtype. Data are given as $-\log_{10}$ EC$_{50}$ (pEC$_{50}$) and $-\log_{10}$ IC$_{50}$ (pIC$_{50}$). In some cases, data are given for partial agonists ($); in other cases, data are given for human (*h**) and mouse (*m**) isoforms; where not stated, data are rat. aa, amino acids; nd, not determined.

the vascular smooth muscle and thus promote P2X-mediated vasoconstriction (128). Conversely, release of ATP in the vicinity of the endothelial P2Y receptors would be expected to promote nitric oxide synthesis and vasodilatation.

Physiologically, a role for purinergic signaling in the renal vasculature is best illustrated in the myogenic autoregulatory response that, combined with the tubuloglomerular feedback mechanism (vide infra), serves to maintain stable renal blood flow in the face of altered renal perfusion pressure. Using the juxtamedullary nephron preparation, in which the diameter of the afferent arteriole is measured during changes in renal perfusion pressure, Inscho and colleagues have provided compelling pharmacological evidence that P2X$_1$ receptors mediate pressure-induced vasoconstriction (68, 69). More recently, the critical role of this pathway was demonstrated by the ablation of autoregulatory contraction in the afferent arteriole of P2X$_1$ null mice (Fig. 3) (70).

THE GLOMERULUS

The complexity of the glomerular architecture, in which a central tuft of endothelial cells and mesangial cells is encapsulated by a double layer of visceral and parietal epithelial cells,

probably explains why most of the detailed information relating to P2 receptors comes from the study of glomerular cells in culture. These studies, based on mRNA detection and/or agonist profiling, indicate expression of P2Y$_{1, 2, 4, \text{ and } 6}$ and P2X$_{2,3,4,5, \text{ and } 7}$ receptors in glomerular mesangial cells (55, 65, 120, 137), P2Y$_{1,2,6}$ receptors in podocytes (45) and P2Y$_{1, 2}$ receptors in glomerular endothelial cells (17).

Polymerase chain reaction (PCR) studies performed on RNA extracted from the entire glomerulus indicate the expression of P2Y$_{1,2,4,6}$ subtypes (9). Immunohistochemical analysis indicates strong expression of P2Y$_{1,2}$ subtypes in the rat glomerulus (Fig. 2), confirmed functionally by measuring phosphoinositide production in response to receptor-selective agonists (9, 142). Using cell-specific markers, P2Y$_1$ expression was localized to mesangial cells and P2Y$_2$ to podocytes (9, 142). Of all the P2X subtypes, only P2X$_7$ immunoreactivity was found in the rat glomerulus (142), and its expression was very low and highly variable between animals. We were unable to detect expression of P2Y$_4$ and P2Y$_6$ receptor protein either functionally or immunologically, but the high autofluorescence of the rat glomerulus would have made low-level expression difficult to detect.

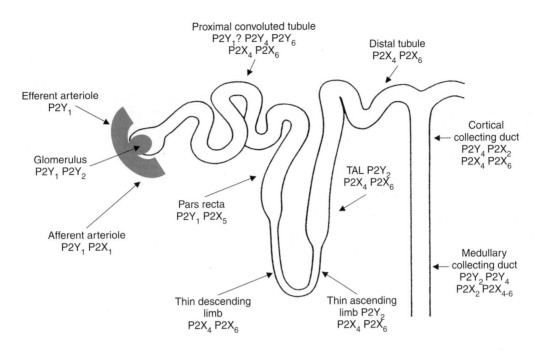

FIGURE 2   P2 receptors in renal vessels and tubule. The figure includes only those receptors in the rat kidney for which firm immunohistochemical evidence has been obtained. Information is from (9, 28, 84, 142, 156). Expression of mRNA has been documented for several additional subtypes (see text for details).

In identifying a functional role for P2 receptors in the control of glomerular filtration rate, it is important to distinguish between those actions mediated by glomerular cells per se and those that occur due to activation of receptors in the afferent or efferent arterioles. The latter events

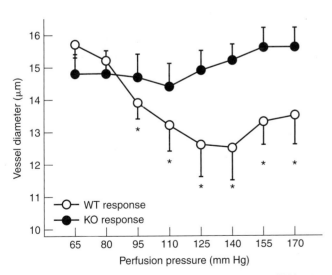

FIGURE 3   Autoregulatory responses in $P2X_1$ knockout (KO) mice versus wild-type (WT) mice. The normal autoregulatory vasoconstrictor response to increases in perfusion pressure is absent in the KO mice. (From EW, Cook AK, Imig JD, et al. Physiological role for $P2X_1$ receptors in renal microvascular autoregulatory behavior. *J Clin Invest* 2003;112:1895-1905, with permission.)

certainly exert a major influence on the formation of the glomerular filtrate. Nevertheless, a growing body of evidence points to purinergic control of nonvascular glomerular cells, which could affect the ultrafiltration coefficient. It is known, for example, that extracellular nucleotides exert bidirectional effects on intracapillary volume in the intact glomerulus devoid of renal arterioles (74). On the one hand, activation of pyrimidine-selective P2Y receptors evokes glomerular contraction consequent upon Rho-kinase−mediated phosphorylation of myosin light chains (76); this is consistent with studies showing P2 receptor-mediated contraction of mesangial cells (114) and of myoepithelial cells in the parietal sheet of Bowman capsule (9). On the other hand, $P2Y_1$ receptor activation relieves angiotensin II−mediated glomerular constriction via activation of endothelial nitric oxide synthase (eNOS) (75). Furthermore, $P2Y_1$ activation underpins the vasodilatory effect on the glomerular capillary bed of third-generation β-adrenoreceptor antagonists such as Nebivolol: β-receptor blockade promotes ATP release through nonselective ion channels in the glomerular endothelial cell that in turn activates eNOS (80).

These studies point to a physiological role for extracellular ATP in the formation of the glomerular filtrate occurring independently of effects mediated by the microvasculature. Such control is likely to be complex, involving both direct action of extracellular nucleotides and modulation of other locally produced vasoactive factors (112).

The Proximal Tubule

The rat proximal tubule expresses mRNA for at least four members of the P2Y receptor family: $P2Y_{1,2,4,6}$ (7, 8). Expression at the mRNA level of other members of the P2Y family or, indeed, of any members of the P2X family has not been investigated in native proximal tubule. However, mRNA for $P2X_1$ (44) and $P2X_4$ (140) has been detected in established proximal tubule cell lines, and quantitative PCR has identified abundant expression of $P2X_4$ and $P2X_5$, and low-level expression of $P2X_7$, in primary cultures of human proximal tubule cells (130).

Like all nephron segments, the proximal tubule is a polarized epithelium and so those P2 receptor subtypes for which mRNA has been identified may be expressed in either membrane domain. To localize specific receptor subtypes to particular membrane domains, both immunohistochemical and functional approaches (the latter using the ubiquitous coupling of P2 receptors to increases in $[Ca^{2+}]_i$) have been used. Most studies have focused on the basolateral membrane, but P2 receptors have also been identified in the apical membrane of rat proximal convoluted and straight tubules.

Basolateral membrane. On the basis of nucleotide-induced increases in $[Ca^{2+}]_i$, the basolateral membrane of the rat proximal tubule appears to contain $P2Y_1$ and $P2Y_6$ receptors (7, 8, 25) and a pyrimidine receptor that has characteristics of $P2Y_2$ and $P2Y_4$ (7). Agonist profiles cannot be used to distinguish between rat $P2Y_2$ and $P2Y_4$ receptors (15, 152), but the use of specific antibodies has shown that the basolateral pyrimidine receptor is $P2Y_4$, there being no expression of $P2Y_2$ in this segment (142). The expression of $P2Y_6$ receptors in the basolateral membrane was confirmed immunologically (9), but this approach failed to detect basolateral $P2Y_1$ receptor expression in the proximal convoluted tubule (142). $P2Y_1$ receptors have been localized basolaterally in the proximal tubule of *Necturus maculosus* (16) and in a variety of proximal cell lines, both primary and immortalized (4, 23, 39, 53, 79). Immunological studies have also identified low-level expression of $P2X_4$ and $P2X_6$ receptors in the rat proximal tubule (142), but $P2X_7$ does not appear to be expressed under normal circumstances.

Apical membrane. Until recently, apical expression of P2 receptors had only been demonstrated in immortalized cell lines with a proximal phenotype. In these, a $P2Y_1$-like receptor was identified on the basis of responses to "selective" agonists (4, 79). Using an in vivo microperfusion approach, pharmacological evidence for expression of $P2Y_1$ receptors in the apical membrane of the rat proximal convoluted tubule has now been obtained (10). This finding appears to be inconsistent with a recent immunohistochemical study in which proximal tubular apical $P2Y_1$ receptor expression was confined to the S3 segment (142). It seems possible, however, that expression was below the limits of detection using this methodology, as Western blot analysis has demonstrated expression of $P2Y_1$ receptors in S2 brush-border membrane vesicles (J. Marks, unpublished observation). Turner and colleagues additionally found expression of apical $P2X_5$ receptors, again in the S3, rather than S1 or S2, segments (142).

In terms of calcium signaling, activation of either $P2Y_1$ or $P2Y_6$ receptors evokes transients equal to those induced by known regulators of proximal function such as norepinephrine and acetylcholine (7, 8). Experimental evidence suggests that these receptors activate the same pool of membrane phosphoinositides (8), raising the question of whether purine and pyrimidine nucleotides induce similar or distinct physiological responses.

There is a growing body of evidence that P2 receptors can influence proximal tubular function. Studies fall into two distinct categories: control of transepithelial electrolyte flux, either directly through actions on membrane transport proteins or indirectly through modulation of hormonal action; and effects on proximal tubular cell metabolism.

TUBULAR TRANSPORT

Direct modulation of proximal tubule transport proteins was initially demonstrated in a rat cell line in which activation of apical $P2Y_1$ receptors induced acute inhibition of basolateral Na,K-ATPase (79), independently of concurrent changes in $[Ca^{2+}]_i$. Separation of calcium signaling from functional consequences was also observed in the amphibian proximal tubule, in which $P2Y_1$ receptors activated basolateral chloride channels (16). More recently, in vivo micropuncture techniques have provided evidence that both apical and basolateral P2 receptors can exert significant (and perhaps coordinated) control of transepithelial bicarbonate reabsorption. Perfusion of the rat proximal tubular lumen with purinoceptor agonists was found to inhibit bicarbonate reabsorption (10). The potency profile of adenine nucleotides/nucleosides implicated $P2Y_1$ receptors, a supposition confirmed by two observations: first, the greatest degree of inhibition was observed using 2meSADP, a potent agonist of $P2Y_1$ receptors; second, 2meSADP did not inhibit bicarbonate flux in the presence of the $P2Y_1$ receptor-specific antagonist MRS2179 (Fig. 4). Maximal inhibition was observed at a lumen 2meSADP concentration of ~100 µmol/l. Although proximal tubular bicarbonate reabsorption was reduced by $\sim50\%$ at this concentration, reported values for proximal tubular endogenous ATP concentrations (vide infra), suggest that submaximal inhibition is the physiological norm.

Further investigation revealed that luminal $P2Y_1$ receptor activation inhibited sodium-hydrogen exchange (in this case mediated by NHE3) by a phospholipase C– and protein kinase A–dependent mechanism (10). Since direct coupling of $P2Y_1$ receptors to Gq or Gs proteins does not occur (122), the $P2Y_1$ receptor-mediated activation of protein kinase A must be indirect, resulting from regulation of adenylate cyclase or phosphodiesterase by $[Ca^{2+}]_i$ (37). Inhibition of NHE3 by a cyclic AMP/protein kinase A–dependent pathway has been observed in A6 cells: mutation of Ser^{552}

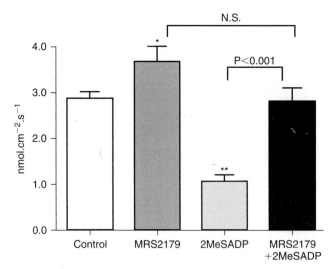

FIGURE 4 Proximal tubule bicarbonate reabsorption: effect of P2Y₁ receptor stimulation and antagonism. Rat proximal convoluted tubules were perfused intraluminally in vivo with the P2Y₁ agonist 2meSADP (100 μmol/l) and/or the P2Y₁ antagonist MRS2179 (1 mmol/l). Note that perfusion with MRS2179 alone caused a significant increase in bicarbonate reabsorption. (From Bailey MA. Inhibition of bicarbonate reabsorption in the rat proximal tubule by activation of luminal P2Y₁ receptors. *Am J Physiol Renal Physiol* 2004;287:F789-F796, with permission.)

and Ser^{605} in the rat NHE3 protein, which prevents phosphorylation of the transporter by protein kinase A (165), eliminates the inhibitory action of P2Y₁ receptor activation (5). Phosphorylation of NHE3 by protein kinase A is facilitated by sodium-hydrogen exchange regulator factor (NHERF). It is not known whether NHERF is a prerequisite for regulation of NHE3 by P2Y₁ receptors as it is for CFTR (52), but P2Y₁ receptors do contain the C-terminal PDZ domain required for such an interaction (54).

In contrast to the effects on the apical domain, in vivo perfusion of the peritubular capillaries with a solution containing ATP caused an *increase* in transepithelial bicarbonate reabsorption (38). Although no attempt was made to identify the receptor subtype, these experiments are of considerable interest. Proximal bicarbonate reabsorption was stimulated by the addition of dextran to the peritubular perfusate, a maneuver that increased fluid viscosity by ~30% yet altered neither osmolality nor charge. This stimulatory action of increased viscosity was abolished by non-selective purinoceptor antagonism or by blockade of nitric oxide synthesis. On the basis of these data, it could be hypothesized that coordinated activation of purinoceptors in apical and basolateral domains might contribute to glomerulotubular balance. In the absence of concomitant changes in renal plasma flow, increased filtration at the glomerulus leads to increases in both peritubular viscosity and luminal flow. zIncreased peritubular fluid viscosity may stimulate ATP release and promote, via a basolateral P2 receptor–dependent release of nitric oxide, transepithelial bicarbonate flux (38), while increased tubular flow may exert a diluting effect on luminal nucleotides (94), thereby attenuating P2Y₁-mediated inhibition of NHE3.

METABOLIC EFFECTS

In the postabsorptive state, the kidney accounts for ~5% of the total body glucose formed by gluconeogenesis (43). There is considerable reserve capacity, however, and the renal contribution to blood glucose rises significantly during fasting. Renal gluconeogenesis is restricted to the proximal tubule (51) and, in the rat at least, has been shown to be stimulated by both adenine and uridine nucleotides (24, 41). These studies were performed on suspensions of proximal tubules isolated from the rat kidney cortex and in most experiments P2 receptor agonists were added to the incubation medium for ~15 minutes. Given the labile nature of extracellular nucleotides and the inherent activity of a variety of degradation products, it is impossible to state with any degree of certainty through which receptor subtypes these effects were mediated. However, UTPγS, which is nonhydrolyzable, has been shown to cause a suramin-sensitive increase in glucose formation, implicating P2 rather than P1 receptors in the response (104). Since agents can access both apical and basolateral membranes under these experimental conditions, the location of the receptor(s) is unknown.

The Loop of Henle

The anatomical loop of Henle consists of the straight portion of the proximal tubule, the thin descending and ascending limbs, and the thick ascending limb of Henle (TAL). The proximal straight tubule has already been discussed. In the descending and ascending thin limbs of Henle, basolateral ATP and UTP were found to be equipotent in terms of increases in [Ca^{2+}]$_i$, suggesting a P2Y₂- or P2Y₄-like receptor in these segments (7). Messenger RNA for P2Y₂ receptors was identified in both segments, whereas P2Y₄ mRNA was expressed only in the ascending thin limb (7). Immunohistochemical analysis, however, suggests that only P2Y₂ receptors are expressed at the protein level (142). P2Y₁ and P2Y₆ receptor mRNAs have also been identified in the descending thin limb; as known agonists for these receptors did not increase [Ca^{2+}]$_i$ when applied to the basolateral membrane, it was concluded that these receptors, if present, are confined to the apical domain (7, 8).

In the rat, the TAL has dense basolateral binding sites for [^{35}S]ATPγS (6). Moreover, the TAL expresses mRNA for four P2Y subtypes (7, 8) and immunohistochemical studies show the presence of P2Y₂, P2X₄ and P2X₆ receptor protein (Fig. 2) (142), although the membrane polarity of expression remains unclear. Rat cortical and medullary TALs are poorly responsive to basolaterally applied ATP, at least in terms of its effect on [Ca^{2+}]$_i$ (7). Interestingly, however, it has been shown recently that the addition of ATP to suspensions of rat TAL stimulates intracellular nitric oxide production, an effect thought to be mediated by P2X receptors (135).

In the mouse TAL, basolateral ATP and UTP consistently evoke large calcium transients (6, 113), indicating important species differences in terms of expression, localization and/or signal transduction of P2Y receptors in the loop. Expression of P2Y$_2$ receptors in both apical and basolateral domains has been reported in isolated perfused mouse TAL (95).

Although the studies described above provide some evidence that P2 receptors have the potential to exert local control over TAL function, this remains circumstantial. It is disappointing that no study has yet addressed the functional consequences of P2 receptor activation in the TAL in terms of transepithelial electrolyte fluxes.

The Macula Densa and Juxtaglomerular Apparatus

The macula densa (MD; a specialized plaque of epithelial cells near the distal end of the TAL), the extraglomerular mesangium (Goormaghtigh cells) and the granular cells of the afferent arteriole comprise the juxtaglomerular apparatus (JGA). The MD functions as an intrarenal sensor, regulating dynamically both the filtration rate at the glomerulus of origin and the synthesis and release of renin in response to altered concentration of NaCl in the tubule lumen. Under sodium replete conditions, an increase in NaCl delivery to the apical membrane of the MD is perceived and transduced to a reduction in single-nephron glomerular filtration rate (tubuloglomerular feedback; TGF) and suppression of renin release.

P2 receptors are expressed throughout the JGA (see Fig. 2). In addition to those in the renal microvasculature and the mesangium (vide supra), calcium-imaging techniques have demonstrated a P2Y$_2$-like receptor in the basolateral membrane of the rabbit MD plaque (97). Microperfusion of the luminal face of the MD with ATP evoked no calcium response, suggesting that P2Y receptor expression is limited to the basolateral membrane. There was no evidence of P1 receptor expression in the basolateral membrane.

In most species, the basolateral membrane of the MD cells is physically separated from the afferent arteriole by the extraglomerular mesangium (EGM). Since there is no evidence of cell-to-cell contact between the MD and EGM, it is hypothesized that communication occurs via paracrine agents released from the basolateral membrane of the MD in response to altered NaCl concentration at the apical membrane. Several putative mediators have been suggested, but recent studies have provided compelling evidence in support of ATP as the initial event in JGA signaling. Bell and colleagues, using the isolated perfused JGA, demonstrated that ATP is released through a maxi-anion channel in the basolateral membrane of the MD plaque in response to increasing the luminal NaCl concentration from 25 to 150 mmol/L (13). Moreover, ATP release correlates strongly with luminal NaCl concentration in the physiological range (88), and the concentration of ATP in the cortical interstitium responds appropriately to inhibition or activation of TGF in vivo (108). On the basis of these experiments, it is estimated that the local concentration of ATP in the cleft

between the MD plaque and the EGM is 10-15 μmol/L. This concentration would be sufficient to activate P2 receptors in the apical membrane of the EGM and is close to the EC$_{50}$ of basolateral P2Y$_2$ receptors of the MD cell (97), suggestive of feedback regulation of MD function. The possible consequences of ATP release on both TGF and renin release are discussed in the following sections.

TUBULOGLOMERULAR FEEDBACK

Gene targeting experiments have provided evidence that P1, rather than P2, receptors mediate TGF. In vivo responses are absent in most tubules from mice lacking A$_1$ receptors (138), and preliminary data suggest that P2X$_1$ receptor knockout mice display normal TGF responses (123), despite impaired pressure-induced autoregulation in the afferent arteriole (71). It has therefore been proposed that hydrolysis of extracellular ATP to adenosine is a prerequisite for TGF, a notion supported by the fact that either pharmacological (118) or genetic ablation (22) of ecto-5'-nucleotidase, an enzyme that catalyses the final stage of the degradation of ATP to adenosine, attenuates the response.

As unequivocal as these data appear to be, the involvement of other receptor systems remains a strong possibility. Schnermann and colleagues have demonstrated impaired TGF responses in mice lacking angiotensin AT$_{1A}$ receptors (124), and desensitization of the P2 receptor system inhibits TGF in rats (109). How is it possible to reconcile these observations? It is noteworthy that ATP released from MD cells in response to increased luminal NaCl cannot impact directly upon the afferent arteriole, being physically separated in most species by the EGM. ATP may be the first cog in the TGF machinery rather than merely the source from which the adenosine required to promote arteriolar vasoconstriction is ultimately generated. Bell and colleagues demonstrated P2Y$_2$-mediated calcium responses in mesangial cells abutting their isolated MD preparation (13), and contraction of the mesangium can reduce the glomerular ultrafiltration coefficient. In this way, the P2 receptor system could be a direct regulator of single-nephron filtration rate. Furthermore, propagation of the nucleotide signal through the mesangial cell syncitium could promote P1-dependent vasoconstriction via the local release (137) and degradation of a second wave of ATP. In support of this hypothesis, an intact mesangium is required for TGF responses (117) and infusion of ATP into the cortical interstitium, a maneuver that would desensitize P2 receptors in the EGM, attenuates this feedback loop (103).

RENIN RELEASE

The renin-angiotensin system is influenced by many factors, the final pathways of which converge at the level of altered [Ca^{2+}]$_i$ in the granular cell; renin secretion is inversely related to [Ca^{2+}]$_i$. The combined use of receptor-specific agonists and antagonists has demonstrated that A$_1$ receptors exert a tonic inhibitory effect on renin secretion at the level of the granular cell (105). However, the P1 receptor system is not vital for the control of renin secretion since A_1 receptor knockout mice are able to raise their secretion appropriately in response to a low salt diet (129), a regimen that increases twofold the sensitivity to luminal NaCl of ATP release by the MD (88).

The role of the P2 receptor system in the regulation of renin release is not entirely clear and to some extent contradictory. Purinergic signaling is a prerequisite for synchronization of the intercellular calcium wave that is required to reduce renin secretion in the JGA (161), and infusion of ATP into the isolated perfused rat kidney causes profound inhibition of renin secretion (161). On the other hand, activation of an ADP-selective receptor, thought to be $P2Y_1$, was shown to *stimulate* renin secretion in rat renal cortical slices via a nitric oxide–dependent mechanism (31). Resolution of this issue awaits further investigation.

Distal Tubule

Current knowledge of the role of P2 receptors in the distal tubule (defined here as that segment of the nephron between the macula densa and the first confluence with another nephron) is confined to findings from in vitro studies, either in primary cultures of native cells or, more commonly, in immortalized distal or "distal-like" cell lines. In native distal tubule, immunohistological techniques have so far identified only $P2X_4$ and $P2X_6$ receptors (142).

There is evidence for a functional role (increased $[Ca^{2+}]_i$ and chloride efflux) for basolateral $P2Y_1$ and apical $P2Y_2$ receptors in *Xenopus* A6 cells (52, 96), commonly used as a model for high-resistance distal epithelia; and the broad-spectrum P2 receptor agonist ATPγS has been shown to reduce the open probability of epithelial sodium channels (ENaC) in cell-attached patches in these cells (99). In contrast, when ATPγS was applied to the basolateral side of A6 monolayers, *stimulation* of amiloride-sensitive sodium transport was observed (50). (Somewhat surprisingly, the P2 receptor antagonist suramin also stimulated sodium conductance.) Another distal-like cell line, Madin-Darby canine kidney (MDCK) cells, also expresses a number of P2Y sub-types, and ATP has long been known to stimulate chloride secretion across MDCK monolayers (136), though the relevance of this observation to native distal tubules is questionable. More recently, it has been demonstrated that (admittedly large) changes in transepithelial pressure can induce transient increases in $[Ca^{2+}]_i$ in MDCK cells, apparently mediated by apical and basolateral nucleotide release (115). In contrast, although flow-induced pressure changes in native rabbit cortical collecting duct (CCD) also caused intracellular calcium transients, a P2-mediated effect here was ruled out (160).

Experiments using an immortalized cell line derived from rabbit distal convoluted tubule (DCT) have indicated that stimulation of apical P2 receptors, pharmacologically characterized as $P2Y_2$, increases apical chloride conductance (144); while Quamme's group, using their immortalized mouse DCT cell line, have provided evidence for P2 receptor-mediated increases in $[Ca^{2+}]_i$, coupled with inhibition of magnesium transport, a physiologically important function of the DCT (35). In the latter instance, pharmacological profiling pointed towards P2X, rather than P2Y, mediation. Given the role of the distal tubule in sodium and calcium transport, it may also be significant that cultured cells from rabbit connecting tubules respond to extracellular ATP with an increased $[Ca^{2+}]_i$, together with inhibition of sodium and calcium absorption [see (130)], probably via $P2Y_2$ receptor stimulation; in this case the functional changes were found not to depend on the calcium transient.

Although these various findings suggest that P2 receptors may have a role to play in distal tubular transport, an appreciation of the full physiological significance of that role awaits a comprehensive in vivo assessment.

Collecting Duct

Multiple P2Y and P2X receptors have been reported in collecting duct cell lines (34, 102, 130); and in native tissue (in the rat), mRNA has been identified for $P2Y_{1, 2, 4 \text{ and } 6}$ receptors in outer medullary collecting duct (7, 8), and for $P2Y_2$ receptors in inner medullary collecting duct (84). However, confirmation of receptor protein using immunohistochemistry has so far been limited to $P2X_{4-6}$ (expressed throughout the collecting duct) and $P2Y_2$ (expressed only in medullary collecting duct) (84, 142). There is some debate over which cell type expresses $P2Y_2$ receptors: in one study, receptor protein was localized to principal cells (84), while in another it was found only in intercalated cells (142).

Despite uncertainties over the precise receptor distribution, a coherent picture is now beginning to emerge concerning the role of P2 receptors in the collecting duct. A combination of approaches has demonstrated that extracellular nucleotides, acting from both apical and basolateral sides, can have significant effects on water and electrolyte handling in this important nephron segment—the final site of regulation of urinary output.

WATER

It is now firmly established that activation of basolateral P2 receptors in the cortical (121) and medullary (83) collecting duct, perfused in vitro, reversibly inhibits vasopressin-stimulated osmotic water permeability. The inhibition is likely to occur at the V_2 receptor level, since by-passing adenylate cyclase activation by administration of forskolin or 8-bromo-cAMP prevented the inhibitory effect of P2 receptor activation (83). In rat inner medullary collecting duct (terminal segment), the inhibitory action was restricted to basolaterally applied nucleotide; luminal application was without effect (42). On the basis that UTP and ATP were equipotent whereas other nucleotides were without effect, the inhibition found in the rat was attributed to basolateral P2Y$_2$ receptors (83). In the rabbit there is additional pharmacological evidence for P2Y$_1$ receptor mediation (121). A recent study in which enhanced expression of P2Y$_2$ mRNA, and of the receptor protein itself, was demonstrated in the inner medulla of hydrated *vs.* dehydrated rats, has provided further evidence for a regulatory role for ATP in modulating collecting duct water reabsorption (85); and this view is supported by the observation that chronic V$_2$ receptor stimulation with dDAVP reduces inner medullary P2Y$_2$ mRNA and protein expression (139).

Interestingly, preliminary data from our laboratory suggest that *apical* P2 receptors may also exert an inhibitory effect on water transport in some parts of the collecting duct, via altered aquaporin-2 trafficking. Immunohistochemical studies identified P2X$_2$ and P2Y$_4$ subtypes in the apical membrane of the rat collecting duct (in addition to basolateral P2Y$_2$ receptors); expression and subsequent activation of these subtypes in *Xenopus* oocytes inhibited aquaporin-2–mediated osmotic water permeability (156).

POTASSIUM

An early study in MDCK cells reported that nucleotides activate K$^+$ channels (48), but more recent evidence in native collecting duct is contradictory. A patch-clamp investigation of split-open mouse native CCDs (allowing access to the apical membrane) has demonstrated that ATP reversibly *inhibits* the activity of the small-conductance K$^+$ channels, which are believed to mediate most potassium secretion in the distal nephron (98). On the basis of equipotency of ATP and UTP and absence of effect of αβmeATP and 2meSATP, it was concluded that apical P2Y$_2$ receptors were responsible. Although this elegant study has not been confirmed or extended to other distal segments, it suggests a potentially important modulatory role for ATP.

SODIUM

Studies in the mouse M-1 cell line have shown that apical application of ATP reduces amiloride-sensitive short-circuit current (SCC; assumed to represent sodium transport) and stimulates chloride secretion (the latter being a characteristic feature of collecting duct cell lines) (34, 141). Pharmacological profiling and reverse transcriptase (RT)-PCR pointed toward P2Y$_2$ receptor mediation (34). Another collecting duct cell model—mIMCD-K2—responds similarly to apical ATP, this time via both P2X and P2Y receptors (102).

Inhibition of sodium reabsorption in the collecting duct has also been reported in native tissue following application of nucleotides. In mouse CCD perfused in vitro, ATP and UTP, applied either luminally or basolaterally, caused an increase in [Ca^{2+}]$_i$ and inhibition of amiloride-sensitive SCC (36, 93), though the apparent reduction in sodium transport did not depend on the calcium transient (93). In CCD isolated from rabbits, however, the picture is not so clear: one group was able to demonstrate an increase in [Ca^{2+}]$_i$ in both principal and intercalated cells following

luminal perfusion with ATPγS or UTP (160), whereas another could not, even though basolateral ATP was effective (36).

Recently, the effect of nucleotides on collecting duct sodium reabsorption in vivo has been investigated in our laboratory, using microperfusion of late distal tubules in rats (133). Addition of ATPγS to the luminal perfusate was found to inhibit ^{22}Na reabsorption (i.e., urinary ^{22}Na recovery was increased), but only when baseline ENaC activity was upregulated by feeding the animals a low sodium diet (Fig. 5). Intriguingly, despite firm evidence from in vitro studies for P2Y$_2$ mediation, "selective" P2Y$_2$/P2Y$_4$ and P2Y$_1$ agonists were ineffective in vivo, and a P2X heteromer-mediated effect was suggested (133). In this connection, another recent study, using the *Xenopus* oocyte expression system, has shown that co-expression of a number of P2X receptors (P2X$_2$, P2X$_{2/6}$, P2X$_4$ or P2X$_{4/6}$) with ENaC leads to its downregulation (155).

In summary, a variety of approaches leave little room for doubt that apical nucleotides, albeit at relatively high concentrations, can inhibit ENaC-mediated sodium reabsorption in the collecting duct. The P2 receptor subtypes responsible remain to be confirmed; species differences seem likely.

Physiological Nucleotide Concentrations in the Kidney

The presence of an array of P2 receptors along the nephron, together with the actions of ATP and its analogs described above, fuels the belief that nucleotides play an autocrine/paracrine role in the kidney. Acceptance of such a role, how-

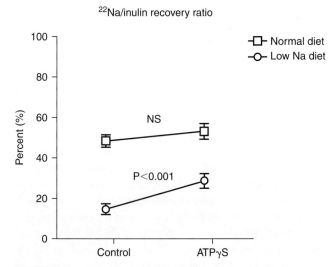

FIGURE 5   Effect of P2 receptor stimulation on collecting duct sodium reabsorption. Late distal tubules were perfused intraluminally in vivo with artificial tubular fluid containing ^{22}Na and inulin ± ATPγS. Urinary ^{22}Na recovery was expressed as a percentage of inulin recovery; the latter averaged 100%, and always exceeded 85% of the delivered dose. Note that ATPγS caused a modest, but reproducible, increase in ^{22}Na recovery in rats on a low sodium diet. (Data from Shirley DG, Bailey MA, Unwin RJ. In vivo stimulation of apical P2 receptors in collecting ducts: evidence for inhibition of sodium reabsorption. *Am J Physiol Renal Physiol* 2005;288: F1243-F1248.)

ever, awaits the demonstration that endogenous nucleotide concentrations in the vicinity of basolateral and apical P2 receptors are adequate for receptor stimulation and that the nucleotides are quickly degraded to terminate their actions.

SECRETION OF NUCLEOTIDES

Evidence for ATP secretion by primary cultures and by cell lines derived from specific nephron segments, grown in vitro, has been obtained by Schwiebert's group (130). These cultures release ATP into both apical and basolateral media, although release across the apical membrane appears to predominate. Cultures derived from proximal tubules produced more ATP than those from more distal segments (130). Recently, using micropuncture, our laboratory has shown that significant concentrations of ATP (100–300 nM) are present in the lumen of the rat proximal tubule in vivo (148). ATP concentrations along the proximal convoluted tubule were markedly higher than those in the distal tubule, echoing the in vitro findings described above. Notably, the ATP concentration of the glomerular filtrate (measured in Munich-Wistar rats) was much lower (four- to fivefold) than that in the proximal convoluted tubule, strongly suggesting secretion of ATP by the proximal tubular cells.

Although any sort of mechanical perturbation can induce cells to release ATP (94), the physiological/pathological stimuli causing ATP secretion within the nephron are unknown (with the exception of MD cells, vide supra). Changes in flow or pressure might be involved, as might osmotically induced cell swelling/shrinkage (at least beyond the proximal tubule). In nonrenal epithelia and cell lines, certain hormones and paracrine factors have been shown to induce ATP secretion, while "constitutive" release of ATP has also been described [see (91)]. The mechanisms of nucleotide exit from cells are also ill understood. Although the concentration gradient is large (intracellular ATP concentration is ~5 mM), simple diffusion is ruled out. With varying degrees of conviction, arguments have been marshalled for ATP making use of stretch-activated channels, ATP binding cassette transporters such as CFTR, or connexin hemichannels; there is also evidence for exocytosis of ATP-loaded vesicles [see (91)]. The latter mechanism is supported by experiments in our laboratory using a proximal tubular S1 cell line, in which quinacrine was used to label ATP-containing vesicles. Exposure of the cells to hypotonic media led to a reduction in intracellular quinacrine fluorescence, coupled with a marked increase in ATP concentration in the medium (146).

ROLE OF ECTONUCLEOTIDASES

Nucleotides secreted/released by cells are rapidly degraded by surface-located enzymes (ectonucleotidases) to other nucleotides/nucleosides that themselves may stimulate P2 or P1 (adenosine) receptors (166). Four families of ectonucleotidases exist: the ectonucleoside triphosphate diphosphohydrolases (NTPDases), the ectonucleotide pyrophosphatase phosphodiesterases (NPPs), ecto-5′-nucleotidase and alkaline phosphatase (Table 3). In addition, the enzyme nucleoside diphosphokinase, which catalyses the reversible interconversion of di- and trinucleosides (e.g., ADP + UTP = ATP + UDP), adds further complexity to the mix.

Although our knowledge of the distribution of these enzymes within the kidney is not yet complete, it is unlikely that any nephron segment is ectonucleotidase-free. It has been known for some time that alkaline phosphatase is expressed in the apical (brush-border) membrane of the proximal tubule (12). Ecto-5′-nucleotidase is also expressed in the proximal tubular brush-border membrane and additionally in the distal tubule and collecting duct, as well as in the peritubular space (49, 147). More recently, immunohistochemical investigations have been extended to the other two families of enzymes. NTPDase 1 was found in the glomerulus, peritubular capillaries and thin ascending limb (86); NTPDase 2 in TAL and distal tubule; and NTPDase 3 in TAL, distal tubule and collecting duct (147). Finally, NPP1 shows strong expression in the distal tubule, and weaker expression in the proximal tubule, of the mouse (56); and prominent staining for NPP3 has been observed in the glomerulus and in the brush-border membrane of the pars recta of the rat (147).

Taking these findings together, it is probable that the hydrolysis of native nucleotides by ectonucleotidases present along the nephron will result in a constantly shifting activation of different purinoreceptor subtypes, and consequent modification of the final physiological response. Moreover, alkaline phosphatase and ecto-5′-nucleotidase are anchored to the cell membrane by glycosyl-phosphatidyl inositol (GPI) linkages that can be cleaved, thereby releasing soluble forms of enzyme.

Potential Role of P2 Receptors in Renal Pathophysiology

The well-documented release of ATP from injured and dying cells, and during thrombosis and platelet aggregation, suggests that the P2 receptor system might be involved in renal pathophysiological processes (27). P2 receptors can mediate changes not only in vascular tone and in fluid and electrolyte reabsorption or secretion (vide supra), but also in renal cell growth (55, 64, 72, 126) and, in the case of the $P2X_7$ receptor, cell death and inflammation (55, 60, 127).

So far, the published work supporting a pathophysiological role for P2 receptors in the kidney is both limited and speculative. Two renal disease models have been the focus of interest: (a) renal cystic disease and (b) glomerular injury and inflammation. The first stems from work on P2 receptors in secretory epithelia (90), in particular the airway epithelium in cystic fibrosis (111), and has been extrapolated to a potential role in renal cyst growth and expansion in polycystic kidney disease (PKD) (131). The second concerns the broadly pro-proliferative effect of stimulating various P2Y receptor subtypes, and the uniquely pro-apoptotic effect of activating the $P2X_7$ receptor, particularly when expressed by mesangial cells and inflammatory macrophages (55, 60, 127).

TABLE 3 Major Hydrolysis Pathways of Ectonucleotidases

Family	Members	Hydrolysis Pathway		
NTPDases	NTPDase 1	$ATP \rightarrow AMP + 2P_i$		
		$ADP \rightarrow AMP + P_i$		
	NTPDase 2	$ATP \rightarrow ADP + P_i$		
		$ADP \rightarrow AMP + P_i$		
	NTPDase 3	$ATP \rightarrow ADP + P_i$		
		$ADP \rightarrow AMP + P_i$		
	NTPDase 4*	$UDP \rightarrow UMP + P_i$		
		$UTP \rightarrow UDP + P_i$		
	NTPDase 5*	$UDP \rightarrow UMP + P_i$		
	NTPDase 6*	$GDP \rightarrow GMP + P_i$		
	NTPDase 7*	$UTP \rightarrow UDP + P_i$		
		$GTP \rightarrow GDP + P_i$		
	NTPDase 8	$ATP \rightarrow ADP + P_i$		
		$ADP \rightarrow AMP + P_i$		
NPPs	NPP1	$ATP \rightarrow AMP + 2P_i$		
		$ADP \rightarrow AMP + P_i$		
		$3',5'\text{-cAMP} \rightarrow AMP$		
	NPP 2	$ATP \rightarrow AMP + 2P_i$	$ATP \rightarrow ADP + P_i$	
		$ADP \rightarrow AMP + P_i$	$GTP \rightarrow GDP + P_i$	
		$3',5'\text{-cAMP} \rightarrow AMP$	$AMP \rightarrow adenosine + P_i$	
	NPP 3	$ATP \rightarrow AMP + 2P_i$		
		$ADP \rightarrow AMP + P_i$		
		$3',5'\text{-cAMP} \rightarrow AMP$		
Ecto-5'-nucleotidase		$AMP \rightarrow adenosine + P_i$		
Alkaline phosphatase		$ATP \rightarrow ADP + P_i$		
		$ADP \rightarrow AMP + P_i$		
		$AMP \rightarrow adenosine + P_i$		

For many of these enzymes, both purine and pyrimidine nucleotides can serve as substrates.

*Intracellular enzymes.

POLYCYSTIC KIDNEY DISEASE

Mutations in polycystin 1, a membrane receptor, or polycystin 2, a putative Ca^{2+} channel, give rise to polycystic kidney disease (PKD), a condition associated with uncontrolled proliferation of renal epithelial cells and disordered fluid transport. This leads to dilatation of tubules and formation of fluid-filled cysts that compress and destroy adjacent normal tissue (159). Cyst-lining cells are thought to exhibit (a) disordered regulation of proliferation and apoptosis; (b) abnormal secretion of fluid and electrolytes; and (c) disturbed polarity of membrane transport proteins and receptors. In culture, these cells have been shown to release more ATP than normal human proximal tubular cells, predominantly from their apical surface (158). The cysts themselves accumulate and concentrate ATP (0.5–10 µM) and their ectonucleotidease activity seems diminished (131). This ATP, acting on P2Y (and possibly P2X) receptors on cyst-lining cells, could not only promote cell growth and fluid secretion, but also, by activating the P2X$_7$ receptor, cell loss and the remodeling necessary for progressive cyst expansion (Fig. 6); and in this context it should be noted that transgenic inactivation of cellular inhibitors of apoptosis causes renal cystic disease in mice (159). However, much of the evidence in support of this attractive hypothesis is indirect and circumstantial. Schwiebert and colleagues performed an in vitro analysis of P2 receptor signaling in cyst-derived epithelial cells. They confirmed ATP release and P2 receptor-mediated stimulation of SCC (Cl$^-$ secretion) and also documented mRNA expression for several P2Y and P2X receptor subtypes (131). At the same time, Hillman and coworkers demonstrated expression of the P2X$_7$ receptor (at mRNA and protein levels) in the cystic epithelium of the *cpk/cpk* mouse model of autosomal recessive PKD (58). Subsequently, a three-dimensional (3D) suspension model of cyst development, using cells isolated from the *cpk/cpk* mouse, was used to study the effects of P2X$_7$ receptor activation on cyst development. Surprisingly, cyst number was *reduced* (59). Furthermore, in a rat model (Han-SPRD) of autosomal dominant PKD, although the P2X$_7$ subtype was again expressed by cyst-lining cells, and its mRNA level increased, other P2X and P2Y receptors were also detected, with particular increases in P2Y$_{2, 4, 6}$ subtypes; thus no clear pattern emerged to provide any functional clues (143).

More mechanistically, expression of a C-terminal polycystin 1 construct, fused to a membrane expression cassette in a mouse collecting duct cell line (M1), upregulates ATP-stimulated Cl$^-$ secretion, associated with a rise in $[Ca^{2+}]_i$ due to an increase in Ca^{2+} entry (61, 154). Tantalizing though these findings are, they unfortunately provide

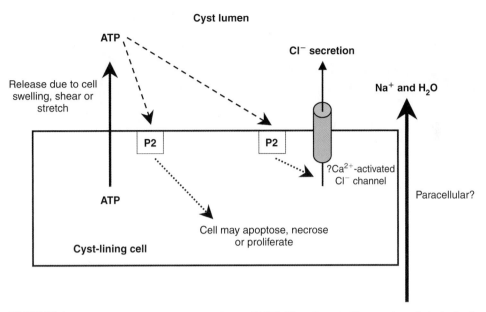

FIGURE 6   P2 receptors in polycystic kidney disease (PKD). The schematic illustrates hypothetical roles for ATP and P2 receptors on cyst-lining cells. See text for details.

more questions than answers, and a role for the purinoceptor system in PKD remains unclear.

The P2X₇ Receptor and Renal Inflammation

As already indicated, P2X$_7$ receptor expression is barely detectable in healthy kidney. However, its renal expression is increased in rodent models of glomerular injury, diabetes mellitus, and renin-dependent hypertension (151). The P2X$_7$ receptor is unique among the P2X receptor family: not only does it form a nonselective ion channel, but it can also initiate cell death by necrosis or apoptosis, and mediate an inflammatory response (Fig. 7) (60). Factors that determine whether P2X$_7$ receptor stimulation will cause cell necrosis or apoptosis, and/or inflammatory cytokine release, will include the cell type, the concentration of nucleotide and duration of exposure, as well as the level of P2X$_7$ receptor surface expression. In cultured human embryonic kidney cells expressing P2X$_7$, membrane blebbing and microvesiculation are seen within seconds to minutes of receptor stimulation, which is associated with cell death by apoptosis (157). More prolonged receptor stimulation leads to formation of a large membrane pore that permits leakage of vital intracellular components (including ATP), and loss of membrane potential, ultimately leading to cell death and necrosis (110).

Activation of the P2X$_7$ receptor promotes release of interleukin (IL)-1β from activated macrophages, and both interferon-γ and tumor necrosis factor-alpha (TNF-α) can increase expression of P2X$_7$ receptors (55, 89, 149), suggesting that this receptor could both regulate, and be regulated by, inflammatory cytokine processing and release. Moreover, we have observed a marked increase in glomerular expression of P2X$_7$ in a rodent model of pro-

liferative glomerulonephritis, reaching a peak that coincides with the onset of proteinuria (143a). Macrophage infiltration and release of inflammatory cytokines are characteristic features of glomerular damage in many forms of glomerulonephritis (87). In the rat diabetic model, both glomerular epithelial (podocytes) and mesangial cells express P2X$_7$ receptors (151): damaged podocytes have been shown to release IL-1β (107); and both IL-1β and TNF-α are increased in diabetic glomeruli (57). Thus, ATP, acting via the P2X$_7$ receptor, could interact with, and control, the inflammatory response, eventually leading to cell death, perhaps as a mechanism for deleting damaged cells without dispersal of their potentially toxic contents.

Clearly, functional studies in these and other models of renal pathophysiology are critical, but still lacking. They await the development of more selective P2 receptor agonists and antagonists suitable for both in vitro and in vivo use, as well as wider availability of the several P2 receptor transgenic mouse models that already exist. Finally, another complexity to consider in any renal disease model is the potential for alterations in the pattern, expression, and activity of nucleotidases (166).

CONCLUDING REMARKS

For extracellular nucleotides to be effective autocrine/paracrine agents, there are three fundamental requirements: release of nucleotides from cells, controlled degradation of the nucleotides once released, and the presence of specific nucleotide receptors that can initiate transduction of the signal to a

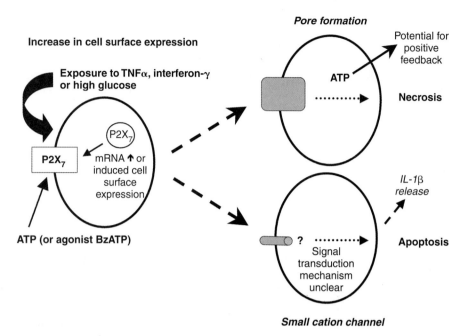

FIGURE 7   P2X$_7$ receptor activation. The schematic illustrates hypothetical roles of P2X$_7$ receptors, whose cell surface expression can be increased by TNF-α, interferon-γ, or exposure to high glucose. Activation of the P2X$_7$ receptors can cause cell necrosis or apoptosis. See text for details.

functional response. The evidence presented here indicates that all three components are present in the kidney, both in the vasculature and the tubule. Thus, it is becoming ever clearer that nucleotides can play important roles in certain key renal functions, but further studies are necessary in order to clarify these roles as well as to assess the potential contribution of the renal purinoceptor system to renal pathology.

Acknowledgments

We thank Dr. C. M. Turner and Dr. R. M. Vekaria for helpful discussion. Work in the authors' laboratories was supported by the Medical Research Council, the Wellcome Trust, Kidney Research UK, and St Peter's Trust for Kidney, Bladder and Prostate Research.

References

1. Abbracchio MP, Burnstock G. Purinergic signalling: pathophysiological roles. *Jpn J Pharmacol* 1998;78:113–145.
2. Abbracchio MP, Boeynaems JM, Barnard EA, et al. Characterization of the UDP-glucose receptor (re-named here the P2Y$_{14}$ receptor) adds diversity to the P2Y receptor family. *Trends Pharmacol Sci* 2003; 24:52–55.
3. Agboh KC, Webb TE, Evans RJ, et al. Functional characterization of a P2X receptor from Schistosoma mansoni. *J Biol Chem* 2004; 279:41650–41657.
4. Anderson RJ, Breckon R, Dixon BS. ATP receptor regulation of adenylate cyclase and protein kinase C activity in cultured renal LLC-PK1 cells. *J Clin Invest* 1991;87:1732–1738.
5. Bagorda A, Guerra L, Di Sole F, et al. Extracellular adenine nucleotides regulate Na$^+$/H$^+$ exchanger NHE3 activity in A6-NHE3 transfectants by a cAMP/PKA-dependent mechanism. *J Membr Biol* 2002;188:249–259.
6. Bailey MA, Hillman KA, Unwin RJ. P2 receptors in the kidney. *J Auton Nerv Syst* 2000;81:264–270.
7. Bailey MA, Imbert-Teboul M, Turner C, et al. Axial distribution and characterization of basolateral P2Y receptors along the rat renal tubule. *Kidney Int* 2000;58:1893–1901.
8. Bailey MA, Imbert-Teboul M, Turner C, et al. Evidence for basolateral P2Y$_6$ receptors along the rat proximal tubule: functional and molecular characterization. *J Am Soc Nephrol* 2001;12:1640–1647.
9. Bailey MA, Turner CM, Hus-Citharel A, et al. P2Y receptors present in the native and isolated rat glomerulus. *Nephron Physiol* 2004;96:p79–90.
10. Bailey MA. Inhibition of bicarbonate reabsorption in the rat proximal tubule by activation of luminal P2Y$_1$ receptors. *Am J Physiol Renal Physiol* 2004;287:F789–F796.
11. Barrera NP, Ormond SJ, Henderson RM, et al. Atomic force microscopy imaging demonstrates that P2X$_2$ receptors are trimers but that P2X$_6$ receptor subunits do not oligomerize. *J Biol Chem* 2005; 280:10759–10765.
12. Beliveau R, Brunette MG, Strevey J. Characterization of phosphate binding by alkaline phosphatase in rat kidney brush border membrane. *Pflügers Arch* 1983;398:227–232.
13. Bell PD, Lapointe JY, Sabirov R, et al. Macula densa cell signaling involves ATP release through a maxi anion channel. *Proc Natl Acad Sci U S A* 2003;100:4322–4327.
14. Bender E, Buist A, Jurzak M, et al. Characterization of an orphan G protein-coupled receptor localized in the dorsal root ganglia reveals adenine as a signaling molecule. *Proc Natl Acad Sci U S A* 2002;99:8573–8578.
15. Bogdanov Y, Rubino A, Burnstock G. Characterisation of subtypes of the P2X and P2Y families of ATP receptors in the foetal human heart. *Life Sci* 1998;62:697–703.
16. Bouyer P, Paulais M, Cougnon M, et al. Extracellular ATP raises cytosolic calcium and activates basolateral chloride conductance in Necturus proximal tubule. *J Physiol* 1998;510:535–548.
17. Briner VA, Kern F. ATP stimulates Ca^{2+} mobilization by a nucleotide receptor in glomerular endothelial cells. *Am J Physiol* 1994;266:F210–F217.
18. Brown SG, Kim YC, Kim SA, et al. Actions of a series of PPADS analogs at P2X$_1$ and P2X$_3$ receptors. *Drug Devel Res* 2001;53:281–291.
19. Buell G, Collo G, Rassendren F. P2X receptors: an emerging channel family. *Eur J Neurosci* 1996;8:2221–2228.
20. Burnstock G. Purinergic nerves. *Pharmacol Rev* 1972;24:509–581.
21. Burnstock G, King BF. Numbering of cloned P2 receptors. *Drug Devel Res* 1996;38:67–71.
22. Castrop H, Huang Y, Hashimoto S, et al. Impairment of tubuloglomerular feedback regulation of GFR in ecto-5'-nucleotidase/CD73-deficient mice. *J Clin Invest* 2004;114:634–642.
23. Cejka JC, Le Maout S, Bidet M, et al. Activation of calcium influx by ATP and store depletion in primary cultures of renal proximal cells. *Pflügers Arch* 1994;427:33–41.
24. Cha SH, Jung KY, Endou H. Effect of P2Y-purinoceptor stimulation on renal gluconeogenesis in rats. *Biochem Biophys Res Commun* 1995; 211:454–461.
25. Cha SH, Sekine T, Endou H. P2 purinoceptor localization along rat nephron and evidence suggesting existence of subtypes P2Y$_1$ and P2Y$_2$. *Am J Physiol* 1998;274:F1006–F1014.
26. Chambers JK, Macdonald LE, Sarau HM, et al. A G protein-coupled receptor for UDP-glucose. *J Biol Chem* 2000;275:10767–10771.
27. Chan CM, Unwin RJ, Burnstock G. Potential functional roles of extracellular ATP in kidney and urinary tract. *Exp Nephrol* 1998;6:200–207.
28. Chan CM, Unwin RJ, Bardini M, et al. Localization of P2X$_1$ purinoceptors by autoradiography and immunohistochemistry in rat kidneys. *Am J Physiol* 1998;274:F799–F804.
29. Chhatriwala M, Ravi RG, Patel RI, et al. Induction of novel agonist selectivity for the ADP-activated P2Y$_1$ receptor versus the ADP-activated P2Y$_{12}$ and P2Y$_{13}$ receptors by conformational constraint of an ADP analog. *J Pharmacol Exp Ther* 2004;311:1038–1043.
30. Churchill PC, Ellis VR. Pharmacological characterization of the renovascular P2 purinergic receptors. *J Pharmacol Exp Ther* 1993; 265:334–338.

31. Churchill PC, Ellis VR. Purinergic P2y receptors stimulate renin secretion by rat renal cortical slices. *J Pharmacol Exp Ther* 1993; 266:160–163.
32. Communi D, Robaye B, Boeynaems JM. Pharmacological characterization of the human $P2Y_{11}$ receptor. *Br J Pharmacol* 1999;128:1199–1206.
33. Costanzi S, Mamedova L, Gao ZG, et al. Architecture of P2Y nucleotide receptors: structural comparison based on sequence analysis, mutagenesis, and homology modeling. *J Med Chem* 2004;47:5393–5404.
34. Cuffe JE, Bielfeld-Ackermann A, Thomas J, et al. ATP stimulates Cl^- secretion and reduces amiloride-sensitive Na^+ absorption in M-1 mouse cortical collecting duct cells. *J Physiol* 2000;524 Pt 1:77–90.
35. Dai LJ, Kang HS, Kerstan D, et al. ATP inhibits Mg^{2+} uptake in MDCT cells via P2X purinoceptors. *Am J Physiol Renal Physiol* 2001;281:F833–840.
36. Deetjen P, Thomas J, Lehrmann H, et al. The luminal P2Y receptor in the isolated perfused mouse cortical collecting duct. *J Am Soc Nephrol* 2000;11:1798–1806.
37. Defer N, Best-Belpomme M, Hanoune J. Tissue specificity and physiological relevance of various isoforms of adenylyl cyclase. *Am J Physiol Renal Physiol* 2000;279:F400–F416.
38. Diaz-Sylvester P, Mac Laughlin M, Amorena C. Peritubular fluid viscosity modulates H^+ flux in proximal tubules through NO release. *Am J Physiol Renal Physiol* 2001;280:F239–F243.
39. Dockrell ME, Noor MI, James AF, et al. Heterogeneous calcium responses to extracellular ATP in cultured rat renal tubule cells. *Clin Chim Acta* 2001;303:133–138.
40. Drury AN, Szent-Gyorgyi A. The physiological activity of adenine compounds with special reference to their action upon the mammalian heart. *J Physiol* 1929;68:213–237.
41. Edgecombe M, Craddock HS, Smith DC, et al. Diadenosine polyphosphate-stimulated gluconeogenesis in isolated rat proximal tubules. *Biochem J* 1997;323:451–456.
42. Edwards RM. Basolateral, but not apical, ATP inhibits vasopressin action in rat inner medullary collecting duct. *Eur J Pharmacol* 2002;438:179–181.
43. Ekberg K, Landau BR, Wajngot A, et al. Contributions by kidney and liver to glucose production in the postabsorptive state and after 60 h of fasting. *Diabetes* 1999;48:292–298.
44. Filipovic DM, Adebanjo OA, Zaidi M, et al. Functional and molecular evidence for P2X receptors in LLC-PK1 cells. *Am J Physiol* 1998;274:F1070–F1077.
45. Fischer KG, Saueressig U, Jacobshagen C, et al. Extracellular nucleotides regulate cellular functions of podocytes in culture. *Am J Physiol Renal Physiol* 2001;281:F1075–F1081.
46. Fredriksson R, Lagerstrom MC, Lundin LG, et al. The G-protein-coupled receptors in the human genome form five main families. Phylogenetic analysis, paralogon groups, and fingerprints. *Mol Pharmacol* 2003;63:1256–1272.
47. Freeman K, Tsui P, Moore D, et al. Cloning, pharmacology, and tissue distribution of G-protein-coupled receptor GPR105 (KIAA0001) rodent orthologs. *Genomics* 2001;78:124–128.
48. Friedrich F, Weiss H, Paulmichl M, et al. Further analysis of ATP-mediated activation of K^+ channels in renal epithelioid Madin Darby canine kidney (MDCK) cells. *Pflügers Arch* 1991;418:551–555.
49. Gandhi R, Le Hir M, Kaissling B. Immunolocalization of ecto-5'-nucleotidase in the kidney by a monoclonal antibody. *Histochemistry* 1990;95:165–174.
50. Gorelik J, Zhang Y, Sanchez D, et al. Aldosterone acts via an ATP autocrine/paracrine system: the Edelman ATP hypothesis revisited. *Proc Natl Acad Sci U S A* 2005;102:15000–15005.
51. Guder WG, Ross BD. Enzyme distribution along the nephron. *Kidney Int* 1984;26:101–111.
52. Guerra L, Favia M, Fanelli T, et al. Stimulation of Xenopus $P2Y_1$ receptor activates CFTR in A6 cells. *Pflügers Arch* 2004;449:66–75.
53. Hafting T, Sand O. Purinergic activation of BK channels in clonal kidney cells (Vero cells). *Acta Physiol Scand* 2000;170:99–109.
54. Hall RA, Ostedgaard LS, Premont RT, et al. A C-terminal motif found in the β2-adrenergic receptor, $P2Y_1$ receptor and cystic fibrosis transmembrane conductance regulator determines binding to the Na^+/H^+ exchanger regulatory factor family of PDZ proteins. *Proc Natl Acad Sci U S A* 1998;95:8496–8501.
55. Harada H, Chan CM, Loesch A, et al. Induction of proliferation and apoptotic cell death via P2Y and P2X receptors, respectively, in rat glomerular mesangial cells. *Kidney Int* 2000;57:949–958.
56. Harahap AR, Goding JW. Distribution of the murine plasma cell antigen PC-1 in non-lymphoid tissues. *J Immunol* 1988;141:2317–2320.
57. Hasegawa G, Nakano K, Sawada M, et al. Possible role of tumor necrosis factor and interleukin-1 in the development of diabetic nephropathy. *Kidney Int* 1991;40:1007–1012.
58. Hillman KA, Johnson TM, Winyard PJ, et al. $P2X_7$ receptors are expressed during mouse nephrogenesis and in collecting duct cysts of the *cpk/cpk* mouse. *Exp Nephrol* 2002;10:34–42.
59. Hillman KA, Woolf AS, Johnson TM, et al. The $P2X_7$ ATP receptor modulates renal cyst development *in vitro*. *Biochem Biophys Res Commun* 2004;322:434–439.
60. Hillman KA, Burnstock G, Unwin RJ. The $P2X_7$ receptor in the kidney: a matter of life of death? *Nephron Exp Nephrol* 2005;101:e24–30.
61. Hooper KM, Unwin RJ, Sutters M. The isolated C-terminus of polycystin-1 promotes increased ATP-stimulated chloride secretion in a collecting duct cell line. *Clin Sci* 2003;104: 217–221.
62. Hoyle CHV, Hilderman R, Pintor J, et al. Diadenosine polyphosphates as extracellular signaling molecules. *Drug Devel Res* 2001; 52:260–273.
63. Hulsmann M, Nickel P, Kassack M, et al. NF449, a novel picomolar potency antagonist at human $P2X_1$ receptors. *Eur J Pharmacol* 2003; 470:1–7.
64. Humes HD, Cieslinski DA. Adenosine triphosphate stimulates thymidine incorporation but does not promote cell growth in primary cultures of renal proximal tubule cells. *Ren Physiol Biochem* 1991; 14:253–258.
65. Huwiler A, Wartmann M, van den Bosch H, et al. Extracellular nucleotides activate the p38-stress-activated protein kinase cascade in glomerular mesangial cells. *Br J Pharmacol* 2000;129:612–618.
66. Inscho EW, Ohishi K, Navar LG. Effects of ATP on pre- and postglomerular juxtamedullary microvasculature. *Am J Physiol Renal Physiol* 1992;263:F886–F893.
67. Inscho EW, Cook AK, Mui V, et al. Direct assesment of renal microvascular responses to P2-purinoceptor agonists. *Am J Physiol Renal Physiol* 1998;274:F718–F727.
68. Inscho EW. P2 receptors in regulation of renal microvascular function. *Am J Physiol Renal Physiol* 2001;280:F927–F944.
69. Inscho EW. Renal microvascular effects of P2 receptor stimulation. *Clin Exp Pharmacol Physiol* 2001;28:332–339.
70. Inscho EW, Cook AK, Imig JD, et al. Physiological role for $P2X_1$ receptors in renal microvascular autoregulatory behavior. *J Clin Invest* 2003;112:1895–1905.
71. Inscho EW, Cook AK, Imig JD, et al. Renal autoregulation in $P2X_1$ knockout mice. *Acta Physiol Scand* 2004;181:445–453.
72. Ishikawa S, Higashiyama M, Kusaka I, et al. Extracellular ATP promotes cellular growth of renal inner medullary collecting duct cells mediated via P2u receptors. *Nephron* 1997;76: 208–214.
73. Jacobson KA, Costanzi S, Ohno M, et al. Molecular recognition at purine and pyrimidine nucleotide (P2) receptors. *Curr Top Med Chem* 2004;4:805–819.
74. Jankowski M, Szczepanska-Konkel M, Kalinowski L, et al. Bidirectional action of extracellular ATP on intracapillary volume of isolated rat renal glomeruli. *J Physiol Pharmacol* 2000;51:491–496.
75. Jankowski M, Szczepanska-Konkel M, Kalinowski L, et al. Cyclic GMP-dependent relaxation of isolated rat renal glomeruli induced by extracellular ATP. *J Physiol* 2001;530:123–130.
76. Jankowski M, Szczepanska-Konkel K, Kalinowski L, et al. Involvement of Rho-kinase in P2Y-receptor-mediated contraction of renal glomeruli. *Biochem Biophys Res Commun* 2003;302:855–859.
77. Jankowski V, Tolle M, Vanholder R, et al. Uridine adenosine tetraphosphate: a novel endothelium-derived vasoconstrictive factor. *Nat Med* 2005;11:223–227.
78. Janssens R, Paindavoine P, Parmentier M, et al. Human $P2Y_2$ receptor polymorphism: identification and pharmacological characterization of two allelic variants. *Br J Pharmacol* 1999;127:709–716.
79. Jin W, Hopfer U. Purinergic-mediated inhibition of Na^+-K^+-ATPase in proximal tubule cells: elevated cytosolic Ca^{2+} is not required. *Am J Physiol* 1997;272:C1169–C1177.
80. Kalinowski L, Dobrucki LW, Szczepanska-Konkel M, et al. Third-generation beta-blockers stimulate nitric oxide release from endothelial cells through ATP efflux: a novel mechanism for antihypertensive action. *Circulation* 2003;107:2747–2752.
81. Kenakin T. Efficacy at G-protein-coupled receptors. *Nat Rev Drug Discov* 2002;1:103–110.
82. King BF, Liu M, Pintor J, et al. Diinosine pentaphosphate (IP5I) is a potent antagonist at recombinant rat $P2X_1$ receptors. *Br J Pharmacol* 1999;128:981–988.
83. Kishore BK, Chou CL, Knepper MA. Extracellular nucleotide receptor inhibits AVP-stimulated water permeability in inner medullary collecting duct. *Am J Physiol* 1995;269: F863–F869.
84. Kishore BK, Ginns SM, Krane CM, et al. Cellular localization of $P2Y_2$ purinoceptor in rat renal inner medulla and lung. *Am J Physiol Renal Physiol* 2000;278:F43–F51.
85. Kishore BK, Krane CM, Miller RL, et al. $P2Y_2$ receptor mRNA and protein expression is altered in inner medullas of hydrated and dehydrated rats: relevance to AVP-independent regulation of IMCD function. *Am J Physiol Renal Physiol* 2005;288:F1164–F1172.
86. Kishore BK, Isaac J, Fausther M, et al. Expression of NTPDase1 and NTPDase2 in murine kidney: relevance to regulation of P2 receptor signaling. *Am J Physiol Renal Physiol* 2005;288: F1032–F1043.
87. Kluth DC, Rees AJ. New approaches to modify glomerular inflammation. *J Nephrol* 1999;12:66–75.
88. Komlosi P, Peti-Peterdi J, Fuson AL, et al. Macula densa basolateral ATP release is regulated by luminal [NaCl] and dietary salt intake. *Am J Physiol Renal Physiol* 2004;286:F1054–F1058.
89. Labasi JM, Petrushova N, Donovan C, et al. Absence of the $P2X_7$ receptor alters leukocyte function and attenuates an inflammatory response. *J Immunol* 2002;168:6436–6445.
90. Lazarowski ER, Boucher RC. UTP as an extracellular signaling molecule. *News Physiol Sci* 2001;16:1–5.
91. Lazarowski ER, Boucher RC, Harden TK. Mechanisms of release of nucleotides and integration of their action as P2X- and P2Y-receptor activating molecules. *Mol Pharmacol* 2003;64:785–795.
92. Lazarowski ER, Shea DA, Boucher RC, et al. Release of cellular UDP-glucose as a potential extracellular signaling molecule. *Mol Pharmacol* 2003;63:1190–1197.
93. Lehrmann H, Thomas J, Kim SJ, et al. Luminal $P2Y_2$ receptor-mediated inhibition of Na^+ absorption in isolated perfused mouse CCD. *J Am Soc Nephrol* 2002;13:10–18.
94. Leipziger J. Control of epithelial transport via luminal P2 receptors. *Am J Physiol Renal Physiol* 2003;284:F419–F432.
95. Leipziger J, Hoeh-Christensen M, Matos JE, et al. The luminal $P2Y_2$ receptor in isolated perfused mouse medullary thick ascending limb. *J Am Soc Nephrol* 2004;15:A42 (Abstract).
96. Leipziger J, Bailey MA, Unwin RJ. Purinergic receptors in the kidney. In Schwiebert, EM ed. *Extracellular Nucleotides and Nucleosides. Release, Receptors, and Physiological and Pathophysiological Effects.* New York Academic Press, 2003:369–394.
97. Liu R, Bell PD, Peti-Peterdi J, et al. Purinergic receptor signaling at the basolateral membrane of macula densa cells. *J Am Soc Nephrol* 2002;13:1145–1151.
98. Lu M, MacGregor GG, Wang W, et al. Extracellular ATP inhibits the small-conductance K channel on the apical membrane of the cortical collecting duct from mouse kidney. *J Gen Physiol* 2000;116:299–310.
99. Ma HP, Li L, Zhou ZH, et al. ATP masks stretch activation of epithelial sodium channels in A6 distal nephron cells. *Am J Physiol Renal Physiol* 2002;282:F501–F505.
100. Majid DS, Navar LG. Suppression of blood flow autoregulation plateau during nitric oxide blockade in canine kidney. *Am J Physiol* 1992;262:F40–F46.
101. Mamedova LK, Joshi BV, Gao ZG, et al. Diisothiocyanate derivatives as potent, insurmountable antagonists of $P2Y_6$ nucleotide receptors. *Biochem Pharmacol* 2004;67:1763–1770.
102. McCoy DE, Taylor AL, Kudlow BA, et al. Nucleotides regulate NaCl transport in mIMCD-K2 cells via P2X and P2Y purinergic receptors. *Am J Physiol* 1999;277:F552–F559.
103. Mitchell KD, Navar LG. Modulation of tubuloglomerular feedback responsiveness by extracellular ATP. *Am J Physiol Renal Physiol* 1993;264:F458–F466.
104. Mo J, Fisher MJ. Uridine nucleotide-induced stimulation of gluconeogenesis in isolated rat proximal tubules. *Naunyn Schmiedebergs Arch Pharmacol* 2002;366:151–157.

105. Modlinger PS, Welch WJ. Adenosine A_1 receptor antagonists and the kidney. *Curr Opin Nephrol Hypertens* 2003;12:497–502.

106. Needleman P, Minkes MS, Douglas JR, Jr. Stimulation of prostaglandin biosynthesis by adenine nucleotides. Profile of prostaglandin release by perfused organs. *Circ Res* 1974;34:455–460.

107. Niemir ZI, Stein H, Dworacki G, et al. Podocytes are the major source of IL-1 alpha and IL-1 beta in human glomerulonephritides. *Kidney Int* 1997;52:393–403.

108. Nishiyama A, Majid DS, Walker M, 3rd, et al. Renal interstitial ATP responses to changes in arterial pressure during alterations in tubuloglomerular feedback activity. *Hypertension* 2001;37:753–759.

109. Nishiyama A, Navar LG. ATP mediates tubuloglomerular feedback. *Am J Physiol Regul Integr Comp Physiol* 2002;283:R273-R275; discussion R278–279.

110. North RA. Molecular physiology of P2X receptors. *Physiol Rev* 2002;82:1013–1067.

111. Novak I. ATP as a signaling molecule: the exocrine focus. *News Physiol Sci* 2003;18:12–17.

112. Oberhauser V, Vonend O, Rump LC. Neuropeptide Y and ATP interact to control renovascular resistance in the rat. *J Am Soc Nephrol* 1999;10:1179–1185.

113. Paulais M, Bandouin-Legros M, Teulon J. Extracellular ATP and UTP trigger calcium entry in mouse cortical thick ascending limb. *Am J Physiol* 1995;268:F496–F502.

114. Pavenstadt H, Gloy J, Leipziger J, et al. Effect of extracellular ATP on contraction, cytosolic calcium activity, membrane voltage and ion currents of rat mesangial cells in primary culture. *Br J Pharmacol* 1993; 109:953–959.

115. Praetorius HA, Frøkiaer J, Leipziger J. Transepithelial pressure pulses induce nucleotide release in polarized MDCK cells. *Am J Physiol Renal Physiol* 2005;288:F133–F141.

116. Ralevic V, Burnstock G. Receptors for purines and pyrimidines. *Pharmacol Rev* 1998;50: 413–492.

117. Ren Y, Carretero OA, Garvin JL. Role of mesangial cells and gap junctions in tubuloglomerular feedback. *Kidney Int* 2002;62:525–531.

118. Ren Y, Garvin JL, Liu R, et al. Role of macula densa adenosine triphosphate (ATP) in tubuloglomerular feedback. *Kidney Int* 2004;66:1479–1485.

119. Roberts JA, Evans RJ. ATP binding at human P2X₁ receptors. Contribution of aromatic and basic amino acids revealed using mutagenesis and partial agonists. *J Biol Chem* 2004;279: 9043–9055.

120. Rost S, Daniel C, Schulze-Lohoff E, et al. P2 receptor antagonist PPADS inhibits mesangial cell proliferation in experimental mesangial proliferative glomerulonephritis. *Kidney Int* 2002;62:1659–1671.

121. Rouse D, Leite M, Suki WN. ATP inhibits the hydrosmotic effect of AVP in rabbit CCT: evidence for a nucleotide P2u receptor. *Am J Physiol* 1994;267:F289–F295.

122. Schachter JB, Boyer JL, Li Q., et al. Fidelity in functional coupling of the rat P2Y₁ receptor to phospholipase C. *Br J Pharmacol* 1997;122:1021–1024.

123. Schnermann J, Castrop H, Hansen P. Adenosine as a paracrine regulator of nephron function. *J Physiol* 2004;560P:SA16 (Abstract).

124. Schnermann JB, Traynor T, Yang T, et al. Absence of tubuloglomerular feedback responses in AT₁A receptor-deficient mice. *Am J Physiol* 1997;273:F315–F320.

125. Schulte EA, Hohendahl A, Stegemann H, et al. Natriuretic peptides and diadenosine polyphosphates modulate pH regulation of rat mesangial cells. *Cell Physiol Biochem* 1999;9: 310–322.

126. Schulze-Lohoff E, Bitzer M, Schagerl S, et al. Regulation of mesangial cell proliferation by purinergic ligands. *Exp Nephrol* 1994;2:136.

127. Schulze-Lohoff E, Hugo C, Rost S, et al. Extracellular ATP causes apoptosis and necrosis of cultured mesangial cells via P2Z/P2X₇ receptors. *Am J Physiol* 1998;275:F962–F971.

128. Schwartz DD, Malik KU. Renal periarterial nerve stimulation-induced vasoconstriction at low frequencies is primarily due to release of a purinergic transmitter in the rat. *J Pharmacol Exp Ther* 1989;250:764–771.

129. Schweda F, Wagner C, Kramer BK, et al. Preserved macula densa-dependent renin secretion in A₁ adenosine receptor knockout mice. *Am J Physiol Renal Physiol* 2003;284:F770–F777.

130. Schwiebert EM, Kishore BK. Extracellular nucleotide signaling along the renal epithelium. *Am J Physiol Renal Physiol* 2001;280:F945–F963.

131. Schwiebert EM, Wallace DP, Braunstein GM, et al. Autocrine extracellular purinergic signaling in epithelial cells derived from polycystic kidneys. *Am J Physiol Renal Physiol* 2002;282: F763–F775.

132. Shaver SR, Rideout JL, Pendergast W, et al. Structure-activity relationships of dinucleotides: potent and selective agonists of P2Y receptors. *Purinergic Signalling* 2005;1:183–191.

133. Shirley DG, Bailey MA, Unwin RJ. In vivo stimulation of apical P2 receptors in collecting ducts: evidence for inhibition of sodium reabsorption. *Am J Physiol Renal Physiol* 2005;288: F1243–F1248.

134. Silberberg SD, Chang TH, Swartz KJ. Secondary structure and gating rearrangements of transmembrane segments in rat P2X₄ receptor channels. *J Gen Physiol* 2005;125:347–359.

135. Silva G, Beierwaltes WH, Garvin JL. Extracellular ATP stimulates NO production in rat thick ascending limb. *Hypertension* 2006;47:563–567.

136. Simmons NL. Identification of a purine (P2) receptor linked to ion transport in a cultured renal (MDCK) epithelium. *Br J Pharmacol* 1981;73:379–384.

137. Solini A, Iacobini C, Ricci C, et al. Purinergic modulation of mesangial extracellular matrix production: role in diabetic and other glomerular diseases. *Kidney Int* 2005;67:875–885.

138. Sun D, Samuelson LC, Yang T, et al. Mediation of tubuloglomerular feedback by adenosine: evidence from mice lacking adenosine 1 receptors. *Proc Natl Acad Sci U S A* 2001;98: 9983–9988.

139. Sun R, Miller RL, Hemmert AC, et al. Chronic dDAVP infusion in rats decreases the expression of P2Y₂ receptor in inner medulla and P2Y₂ receptor-mediated PGE₂ release by IMCD. *Am J Physiol Renal Physiol* 2005;289:F768–F776.

140. Takeda M, Kobayashi M, Endou H. Establishment of a mouse clonal early proximal tubule cell line and outer medullary collecting duct cells expressing P2 purinoceptors. *Biochem Mol Biol Int* 1998;44:657–664.

141. Thomas J, Deetjen P, Ko WH, et al. P2Y₂ receptor-mediated inhibition of amiloride-sensitive short circuit current in M-1 mouse cortical collecting duct cells. *J Membr Biol* 2001;183:115–124.

142. Turner CM, Vonend O, Chan C, et al. The pattern of distribution of selected ATP-sensitive P2 receptor subtypes in normal rat kidney:an immunohistological study. *Cells Tissues Organs* 2003;175:105–117.

143. Turner CM, Ramesh B, Srai SK, et al. Altered ATP-sensitive P2 receptor subtype expression in the Han:SPRD cy/+ rat, a model of autosomal dominant polycystic kidney disease. *Cells Tissues Organs* 2004;178:168–179.

143a. Turner CM, Tam FWT, Lai PC, et al. Increased expression of the proapoptotic ATP-sensitive P2X₇ receptor in experimental and human glomerulonephritis. *Nephrol Dial Transplant* 2007;22:386–395.

144. Unwin RJ, Bailey MA, Burnstock G. Purinergic signaling along the renal tubule: the current state of play. *News Physiol Sci* 2003;18:237–241.

145. van der Giet M, Westhoff T, Cinkilic O, et al. The critical role of adenosine and guanosine in the affinity of dinucleoside polyphosphates to P2X-receptors in the isolated perfused rat kidney. *Br J Pharmacol* 2001;132:467–474.

146. Vekaria RM. Vesicular storage and release of ATP in a rat proximal tubule cell line. *J Physiol* 2004;560P:C17 (Abstract).

147. Vekaria RM, Shirley DG, Sévigny J, et al. Immunolocalization of ectonucleotidases along the rat nephron. *Am J Physiol Renal Physiol* 2006;290:F550–F560.

148. Vekaria RM, Unwin RJ, Shirley DG. Intraluminal ATP concentrations in rat renal tubules. *J Am Soc Nephrol* 2006;17:1841–1847.

149. Verhoef PA, Estacion M, Schilling W, et al. P2X₇ receptor-dependent blebbing and the activation of Rho-effector kinases, caspases, and IL-1 beta release. *J Immunol* 2003;170:5728–5738.

150. Virginio C, Robertson G, Surprenant A, et al. Trinitrophenyl-substituted nucleotides are potent antagonists selective for P2X₁, P2X₃, and heteromeric P2X₂/₃ receptors. *Mol Pharmacol* 1998;53:969–973.

151. Vonend O, Turner CM, Chan CM, et al. Glomerular expression of the ATP-sensitive P2X receptor in diabetic and hypertensive rat models. *Kidney Int* 2004;66:157–166.

152. Webb TE, Henderson DJ, Roberts JA, et al. Molecular cloning and characterization of the rat P2Y₄ receptor. *J Neurochem* 1998;71:1348–1357.

153. Wildman SS, King BF, Burnstock G. Potentiation of ATP-responses at a recombinant P2X₂ receptor by neurotransmitters and related substances. *Br J Pharmacol* 1997;120:221–224.

154. Wildman SS, Hooper KM, Turner CM, et al. The isolated polycystin-1 cytoplasmic COOH terminus prolongs ATP-stimulated Cl⁻ conductance through increased Ca²⁺ entry. *Am J Physiol Renal Physiol* 2003;285:F1168–F1178.

155. Wildman SS, Marks J, Churchill LJ, et al. Regulatory interdependence of cloned epithelial Na⁺ channels and P2X receptors. *J Am Soc Nephrol* 2005;16:2586–2597.

156. Wildman SS, Peppiatt CM, Boone M, et al. Possible role of apical P2 receptors in modulating aquaporin-2-mediated water reabsorption in the collecting duct. *Proc Physiol Soc* 2006;2: PC4 (Abstract).

157. Wilson HL, Wilson SA, Surprenant A, et al. Epithelial membrane proteins induce membrane blebbing and interact with the P2X₇ receptor C terminus. *J Biol Chem* 2002;277:34017–34023.

158. Wilson PD, Hovater JS, Casey CC, et al. ATP release mechanisms in primary cultures of epithelia derived from the cysts of polycystic kidneys. *J Am Soc Nephrol* 1999;10:218–229.

159. Wilson PD. Polycystic kidney disease. *N Engl J Med* 2004;350:151–164.

160. Woda CB, Leite M, Jr., Rohatgi R, et al. Effects of luminal flow and nucleotides on [Ca²⁺]ᵢ in rabbit cortical collecting duct. *Am J Physiol Renal Physiol* 2002;283:F437–F446.

161. Yao J, Suwa M, Li B, et al. ATP-dependent mechanism for coordination of intercellular Ca²⁺ signaling and renin secretion in rat juxtaglomerular cells. *Circ Res* 2003;93:338–345.

162. Yoshioka K, Saitoh O, Nakata H. Heteromeric association creates a P2Y-like adenosine receptor. *Proc Natl Acad Sci U S A* 2001;98:7617–7622.

163. Yoshioka K, Saitoh O, Nakata H. Agonist-promoted heteromeric oligomerization between adenosine A₁ and P2Y₁ receptors in living cells. *FEBS Lett* 2002;523:147–151.

164. Yoshioka K, Hosoda R, Kuroda Y, et al. Hetero-oligomerization of adenosine A₁ receptors with P2Y₁ receptors in rat brains. *FEBS Lett* 2002;531:299–303.

165. Zhao H, Wiederkehr MR, Fan L, et al. Acute inhibition of Na/H exchanger NHE-3 by cAMP. Role of protein kinase A and NHE-3 phosphoserines 552 and 605. *J Biol Chem* 1999;274:3978–3987.

166. Zimmermann H. Extracellular metabolism of ATP and other nucleotides. *Naunyn Schmiedebergs Arch Pharmacol* 2000;362:299–309.

CHAPTER 18

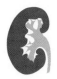

Paracrine Regulation of Renal Function by Dopamine

Ulla Holtbäck and Anita C. Aperia

Astrid Lindgren Children's Hospital, Karolinska University Hospital, Stockholm, Sweden
Astrid Lindgren Children's Hospital, Stockholm, Sweden

DOPAMINE—A NEUROTRANSMITTER

Dopamine was synthesized for the first time in 1910 (23, 143) and its pharmacological effects were at that time thought to mimic those of previously identified sympathomimetic amines. Initially, endogenous dopamine was known only as a precursor to epinephrine and norepinephrine (200); in the late 1950s, Arvid Carlsson demonstrated that dopamine itself had a transmitter role (39). This finding, for which he was awarded the Nobel Prize in Physiology or Medicine 2000, was revolutionary for the understanding of various central functions of the brain, not only to knowledge concerning memory, learning, drug abuse, cognition, and attention, but also to the pathogenesis of various psychiatric and neurological disorders and their treatment.

Dopamine via the basal ganglia controls our movements. Shortage of dopamine, particularly the death of dopamine neurons in the nigrostriatal pathway, causes Parkinson's disease, in which a person loses the ability to execute smooth, controlled movements (22, 218). Increased dopamine on the other hand causes involuntary movements observed in disorders such as Huntington's chorea and Tourette syndrome (3, 145).

Disruption to the dopamine system has been strongly linked to psychosis and schizophrenia (21, 22). The introduction of drugs that modulate effects of dopaminergic neurotransmission, such as haloperidol, dramatically altered the life quality of patients with psychosis. Dopamine neurons in the mesolimbic pathway are particularly associated with psychotic conditions.

Dopamine is commonly associated with the pleasure system of the brain, providing feelings of enjoyment. Dopamine is released (particularly in areas such as the nucleus accumbens and striatum) by naturally rewarding experiences such as food and sex, but also by the use of certain drugs, such as cocaine and amphetamines (205, 229). These drugs can cause psychosis-like behavior.

In the frontal lobes, dopamine controls the flow of information from other areas of the brain. Dopamine disorders in this region of the brain can cause a decline in neurocognitive functions, especially memory, attention, and problem solving (17, 84). Dopamine is not only a neurotransmitter, but also a neuroendocrine hormone and regulates the secretion of prolactin from the anterior pituitary gland (140).

DOPAMINE IN NON-NEURONAL TISSUE

In 1942, Holtz reported that low-dose dopamine in the guinea pig resulted in reducing arterial pressure (105), but the significance of this finding remained unclear for another 20–30 years. Goldberg et al. (82, 83) confirmed the depressor effect of low-dose dopamine in 1959, and in 1962 they demonstrated a direct effect of dopamine on vascular resistance (82, 83). Two years later the same group reported that dopamine increased glomerular filtration rate (GFR) and renal blood flow (RBF), and had a natriuretic effect in humans (148). Early studies from 1963 also demonstrated that the dopamine-producing enzyme, L-aromatic amino acid decarboxylase, was expressed in non-neuronal tissues such the liver, pancreas, intestines, and kidney. Controversial results among the authorities within the field contributed to the fact that it took another 20 years before dopamine was recognized as an endocrine substance with effects outside the neurological system. As recently as 1983, Berkowitz wrote: "It is controversial whether dopamine is a peripheral neurotransmitter in the cardiovascular/renal system" (30). In one sense he was right. Most peripheral effects of dopamine are not mediated via neurons but rather via peripheral production of dopamine.

Since the mid-1980s, the study of dopamine peripheral actions has exploded, and today it is generally recognized that dopamine has various important functions in non-neuronal tissues. Dopamine is an immunomodulatory hormone, produces vasodilatation in various organs, regulates bicarbonate secretion in the duodenum and intestinal motility throughout the intestines, and, as discussed in detail in this chapter, has a key role in renal function.

Dopamine and modulators of dopaminergic activity are today frequently used to treat various conditions of the central nervous system (CNS), such as Parkinson's disease, attention deficit hyperactivity disorder, and psychosis, and in the peripheral system, such as obesity, nausea, shock, renal failure, and hypertension.

DOPAMINE RECEPTORS AND SIGNAL TRANSDUCTION

Receptor Classification

Dopamine (DA) exerts its biological effects via receptors that are categorized as D_1-like and D_2-like based on their ability to stimulate and inhibit adenylate cyclase activity, respectively (119). After the introduction of gene-cloning procedures, three novel DA receptor subtypes have been identified: D_3 and D_4, belonging to the D_2-like group, and D_5 (former D_{1b} in peripheral tissue), which belongs to the D_1 group. Structural, pharmacological, and biochemical studies have demonstrated that all dopamine receptor subtypes fall into one of the initially recognized receptor categories. Thus the pharmacological classification of DA receptors by Kebabian and Calne (119) in 1979 into the D_1- and the D_2-like subtypes is still valid. D_1 and D_5 receptors have a very high homology in transmembrane domains and the first two cytoplasmic loops, whereas the COOH terminus and the third extracellular loop are different. The second extracellular loop is considerably different between D_1 and D_5, being 14 amino acids shorter in the D_1 receptor. In addition, the amino acid sequence of this loop is divergent in rat central and renal D_5 receptors. Similarly, the transmembrane domains are highly conserved among D_2, D_3, and D_4 receptors. The D_2 receptor exists as two alternatively spliced isoforms D_2 long and D_2 short. Both variants share the same distribution pattern and the same pharmacological profile (155).

The general view today is that the interaction between catecholamines and their receptors occurs within the membrane and that transmembrane domains 3, 5, and 6 of the receptor appears to be of particular importance for agonist binding. The C terminal domain of dopamine receptors is known to interact with various proteins including other receptors (see Dopamine Receptor Dimerization section), and the third intracellular loop is another protein interaction domain important for G protein binding (see next section).

Signal Transduction

Dopamine receptors belong to the superfamily of G protein–coupled receptors (GPCR) characterized structurally by an amino-terminal extracellular domain, a carboxyl-terminal intracellular domain, and seven hydrophobic transmembrane domains. To respond to environmental changes, cells must transfer information concerning their environment across their impermeable plasma membranes. One solution to this problem involves three proteins: the GPCR, which detects information outside the cell; an effector molecule that alters the intracellular environment; and a guanine nucleotide regulatory protein (G protein), which couples the receptor to the effector molecule. One characteristic of the entities in this receptor family is that they cycle between the plasma membrane and intracellular compartments. The exposure of GPCR to hormones often results in a rapid attenuation in receptor responsiveness. GPCR desensitization involves the uncoupling of the receptors from its G protein, the internalization of plasma membrane–associated receptors, and an associated downregulation of the total number of receptors at the plasma membrane (208). Today it is well established that receptor desensitization is regulated in a homologous fashion by the cognate agonist and heterologously regulated by protein kinases (123, 240). Resensitization of GPCR was previously believed to be a constitutive process. Recent studies from our laboratory have demonstrated that resensitization and recruitment of GPCR to the plasma membrane is also a regulated process and a crucial step in receptor signaling (35, 103).

In their classical signaling pathways, the D_1-like receptors (D_1 and D_5) couple to the G protein, $G\alpha s$, and in some areas of the brain such as the striatum, $G\alpha olf$ (56, 98) is known to stimulate adenylate cyclase, cAMP formation, and protein kinase A (PKA) activation (Fig. 1). In contrast, the D_2-like receptors (D_2, D_3, and D_4) couple to a $G\alpha i/o$ protein known to inhibit cAMP formation and PKA activation.

In addition to cAMP stimulation, the D_1 receptor also mediates phospholipase C (PLC), (65, 134, 141) and phospholipase A_2 (PLA$_2$) activation in renal tubules (Fig. 1). PLC activation, via a $G\alpha q$ protein, leads to the activation and translocation of several PKC isoforms from the cytoplasm to the plasma membrane (232). The PLC signaling pathway is also associated with Ca^{2+} release from the endoplasmic reticulum (ER) via inositol phosphate-3 receptor (IP$_3$R) activation. PLA$_2$ activation appears to be initiated by D_1 receptor–dependent PKA phosphorylation of PLA$_2$ and subsequent release of arachidonic acid and its metabolites (194). There may be (1) distinct D_1-like receptors utilizing different signaling cascades, which, in this case, demonstrate G protein subunit–coupling specificity with $G\alpha s$ and $G\alpha q$ that is linked to activation of adenylate and phosphoinositol, respectively (170, 183), or (2) protein kinases (53) that, through homologous or heterologous receptor phosphorylation processes, regulate G-protein cross-talk such that individual receptors may shift between different G-proteins.

D_2 receptors also utilize signaling pathways other than $G\alpha i$ inhibition of adenylate cyclase. The G protein is a heterotrimeric protein, which upon receptor binding, dissociates in the α and β/γ units. D_2 receptors alter intracellular signaling through $G\beta/\gamma$ subunits, which can act at a number of intracellular targets (165). D_2 receptors via $G\beta/\gamma$ have been shown to activate the MAP kinase system through several different pathways. Although the effects of D_1-like and D_2-like receptor activation on adenylate cyclase are in opposition, in certain

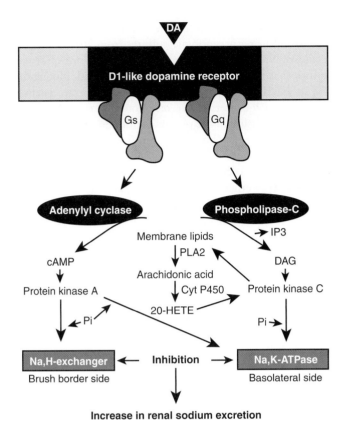

FIGURE 1 D_1-like receptor signaling pathways in the renal tubular cells. Inhibition of sodium-transporting proteins and associated increase in urinary sodium excretion are mediated by activation of D_1-like receptors signaling via PKA- and PKC-dependent pathways. For more detailed information on the PKA signaling pathway, see Fig. 8. DAG, diacylglycerol; P_i inorganic phosphate (phosphorylation). (From Hussain T, Lokhandwala MF. Altered arachidonic acid metabolism contributes to the failure of dopamine to inhibit Na+,K(+)-ATPase in kidney of spontaneously hypertensive rats. *Clin Exp Hypertens* 1996;18:963–974.)

cases it has been demonstrated that D_2-like receptors can activate adenylate cyclase. This activation (by D_2 and D_4, but not by D_3) is mediated by $G\beta/\gamma$ subunits, but occurs only when other activators of adenylate cyclase are present (212, 223). Such synergistic action may underlie the cooperation between D_1 and D_2 receptor activation observed in neurons of the nucleus accumbens (106).

Coactivation of D_1 and D_2 receptors may also activate a novel signaling pathway that involves phospholipase C (PLC)–mediated calcium mobilization. This is distinct from the intracellular responses observed after stimulation of either dopamine receptor alone (185).

Exciting new findings indicate a novel signaling pathway that bypasses the G proteins in dopamine receptor signaling. In response to dopamine receptor activation, a new type of signaling complex involving β-arrestin-2, traditionally associated with receptor desensitization, and two protein kinases, Act and PP2A, is activated. Animals lacking β arrestin-2 show decreases in dopamine-dependent behavior associated with a dissociation of PP2A and Act (25).

Dopamine Signaling and DARPP-32

The dopamine- and cAMP-regulated phosphoprotein, 32 kDa (DARPP-32), was identified initially as a major target for dopamine-activated adenylate cyclase in striatum (88, 217). Since the mid-1980s, DARPP-32 has been acknowledged as a crucial mediator of the biochemical, electrophysiological, transcriptional, and behavioral effects of dopamine (213). The state of DARPP-32 phosphorylation has been shown to provide a mechanism for integrating information arriving at dopaminoceptive neurons, in multiple brain regions, via a variety of neurotransmitters, neuromodulators, neuropeptides, and steroid hormones. Activation of PKA or protein kinase G (PKG) stimulates DARPP-32 phosphorylation at Thr^{34}, and thereby converts DARPP-32 into a potent inhibitor of protein phosphatase-1 (PP1). Protein phosphatase 2-B (PP2B) is the most effective protein phosphatase in dephosphorylating DARPP-32 at Thr^{34}. Thus, DARPP-32 acts as an amplifier of PKA and PKG-mediated signaling when it is phosphorylated on Thr^{34}, which converts it into an inhibitor of PP1. The role of DARPP-32 in signaling has turned out to be very complex. Under basal conditions, DARPP-32 is phosphorylated at Thr^{75} and inhibits PKA. Thus, DARPP-32 has the unique property of acting either as an inhibitor of PP1 or an inhibitor of PKA. However, under hyperdopaminergic conditions, the phosphorylated state of Thr^{75} is reduced allowing increased phosphorylation at Thr^{34}. This positive feedback loop acts as a switch to potentiate dopaminergic signaling. Cdk5, a cyclin-dependent kinase family member, also phosphorylates DARPP-32 at Thr^{75}. Furthermore, protein phosphatase 2 A (PP-2A) dephosphorylates DARPP-32 both at Thr^{34} and Thr^{75} and the state of phosphorylation of DARPP-32 at Thr^{34} depend on the phosphorylation state of two serine residues, Ser^{102} and Ser^{137}.

DARPP-32 has been demonstrated with biochemical, immunohistochemical, and in situ hybridization techniques to have an anatomical distribution similar to that of dopaminoceptive cells possessing D_1 receptors in the CNS (150, 186, 216). DARPP-32 is also expressed in several peripheral tissues, including brown fat cells, parathyroid, retina, and renal tissue (150–154).

Dopamine Receptor Dimerization

Receptor dimerization is a well-known phenomenon, and an obligatory step, in tyrosine kinase–receptor family signaling. An increasing amount of evidence shows that GPCR form receptor dimers as well, or higher-order oligomers, as part of their normal trafficking and function. In fact, certain GPCRs seem to have a strict requirement for heterodimerization to attain proper surface expression and functional activity. Receptor dimerization appears to increase the affinity for the agonist. The idea that GPCRs might also dimerize was first proposed by Fuxe and colleagues (2) in 1982, although the idea did not gain wide acceptance until more than a decade later when Zoli et al. (241) postulated that heterodimerization could explain receptor-receptor interactions between G protein–coupled receptors. Early evidence for GPCR dimerization came from unexplained cooperation observed in ligand-binding assays and unexpectedly large estimates of the size of receptor complexes on gel filtration columns. Even those GPCRs that do not absolutely require heterodimerization may still specifically associate with other GPCR subtypes, sometimes resulting in dramatic effects on receptor pharmacology, signaling, and/or internalization. Understanding the specificity and functional significance of GPCR heterodimerization is of tremendous clinical importance since GPCRs are the molecular targets for numerous therapeutic strategies.

Dopamine D_1, D_2, and D_3 receptors can form homodimers in transfected cell lines and D_2 also in intact human tissue (75, 167, 168). Human and rat D_2 receptors exist either as monomers or as dimers (237). An important feature of normal dopaminergic transmission is that for many behavioral, electrophysiological, and gene-activating effects of dopamine, concomitant stimulation of D_1 and D_2 receptors is required (113, 142, 227), a phenomenon often termed requisite synergism (129). LaHoste et al. (128) have provided further evidence that it is the D_2 receptor itself, not other members of the D_2-like receptor family (D_3 or D_4), that synergizes with the dopamine D_1 receptor. Medium spiny neurons coexpress functional D_1 and D_2 class receptors. It has been shown that concurrent coactivation of D_1 and D_2 receptors within the same cells results in the activation of a novel phospholipase C–dependent calcium signaling pathway (133). Advanced biophysical methods have been used to demonstrate physical interaction of D_1 and D_2 dopamine receptors, which is significantly enhanced upon the concurrent presence of both receptor agonists (59).

Dopamine is a neurotransmitter that can regulate both excitatory and inhibitory fast synaptic transmission. The overlapping dopaminergic, glutamatergic, and GABAergic systems provide a basis for the interaction between these three neurotransmitters (131). A direct interaction has been demonstrated between D_1 receptors and the glutamate NMDA receptor, which is mediated by the binding of various regions of the C-terminal tail of the D1 receptor to either the NR1 or NR2 NMDA receptor subunit (132). Moreover, activation of the one receptor subtype can alter the distribution of other types of receptors. Two studies by Scott et al. (197, 198) are good examples of such receptor interactions. In primary cultures of striatal neurons, activation of NMDA receptors increases the recruitment of D_1 but not D_2 receptors from the interior of the cell to the plasma membrane. This translocation is abolished in the presence of NMDA receptor antagonists or when Ca^{2+} is removed. The newly recruited D_1 receptors are functionally active and stimulate adenylate cyclase activity. In addition, after glutamate treatment, a large increase in the number

of D_1 receptors occurs in the dendritic spines. In the second study, using organotypic cultures from striatum, activation of NMDA causes an increase in D_1 receptor–positive spines that is not depending on Ca^{2+}. Instead, glutamate via its NMDA receptor initiates a diffusion trap mechanism in which subsets of D_1, receptors that typically move by lateral diffusion in the plasma membrane, get trapped in the spines (Fig. 2). Thus, exposure to glutamate reduces the diffusion rate of D_1 receptors and allows the formation of D_1-NMDA receptor dimerization. This phenomenon is highly energy efficient because it depends on D_1 receptor diffusion and NMDA-receptor allosteric regulation, and not the activation of transduction systems or intracellular signaling (197).

Liu et al. (137) found a direct protein–protein interaction between $GABA_A$ and dopamine D_5 receptors in the CNS. One functional meaning of this heterodimerization appears to be to allow mutually inhibitory cross-talk to take place. The formation of the $GABA_A/D_5$ receptor dimer causes a reduction of $GABA_A$-dependent currents and inhibition of D_5, but not D_1, receptor signaling. The latter phenomenon is explained by a reduction in D_5 receptor/$G\alpha s$ coupling. Agonists of either the $GABA_A$ or D_5 receptor induce receptor cotrafficking.

A potential role of this $GABA_A/D_5$ receptor complex in the pathophysiology of schizophrenia has been postulated in view of the fact that alterations in D_1/D_5 and $GABA_{A2}$ containing receptors and their functions may exist in the schizophrenic brain (85, 107, 120, 180).

The D_2 receptor exhibits heterodimerization with the somatostatin receptor 5 ($SSTR_5$). The D_2 receptor/SSTR5 heterodimer displays enhanced signaling and altered pharmacological properties relative to the individually expressed receptors (188), and may help to account for well-known examples of synergistic interactions between somatostatin

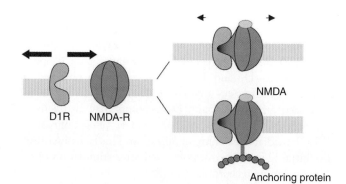

FIGURE 2 D_1R and NMDA receptor dimerization. D_1R randomly diffuses in the plasma membrane and can physically interact with NMDA receptors (NMDA-R), which have undergone an allosteric change, due to ligand occupation of the NMDA/glutamate-binding site. Formation of a D_1R–NMDA receptor complex reduces D_1R mobility. When the NMDA receptor is anchored to postsynaptic density, movement is arrested. (From Scott L, Zelenin S, Malmersjo S, Kowalewski JM, Markus EZ, Nairn AC, Greengard P, Brismar H, Aperia A. Allosteric changes of the NMDA receptor trap diffusible dopamine 1 receptors in spines. *Proc Natl Acad Sci U S A* 2006;103:762–767.)

and dopamine in the CNS (48, 96). The D_2 receptor/SSTR5 heterodimer may have therapeutic implications in the treatment of morbus Parkinson's disease.

Antagonism between adenosine and dopamine at the biochemical and behavioral levels can be explained by heterodimerization of A_1/D_1 receptors (70, 74) as well as A_1/D_2 receptors (73). The A_1/D_1 receptor heterodimerization also appears to have an impact on receptor trafficking (78), whereas A_{2A}/D_2 heterodimeric receptor complexes undergo coaggregation, cointernalization, and codesensitization on D_2 or A_{2A} receptor agonist treatments and especially after combined agonist treatment.

In addition, members within the dopamine subclass families form receptor heterodimers. Scarselli et al. (195) have shown that the two D_2-like receptors D_2 and D_3 receptors can interact with each other to form a functional heterodimer that exhibits unique functional properties, including an increased coupling of D_3 receptor to adenylate cyclase. Again this finding can be used as a therapeutic tool in psychotic patients.

In conclusion, direct intramembrane association among GPCR defines a new level of molecular cross-talk between related G protein–coupled receptor subfamilies.

DOPAMINE: AN INTRARENAL HORMONE

The kidney is an important target for the actions of dopamine (10). Renal effects of dopamine include enhancement of diuresis, regulation of sodium excretion, vasodilatation, and decrease in renal resistance (14, 28, 139, 187). These properties of dopamine are common to all mammalian species investigated including humans (44, 138). Dopamine is a natriuretic and diuretic hormone. These effects involve changes in renal hemodynamics as well as direct tubular actions.

Renal Dopamine Synthesis, Metabolism, and Transport

In the kidney dopamine is primarily synthesized in the proximal tubules and act as an autocrine and paracrine hormone (Fig. 3). The renal precursor to dopamine is filtered L-dopa (40), which enters the tubular cell via a sodium-coupled transporter (87, 104) (Fig. 4). In rats treated with a kidney specific L-dopa analogue, glu-dopa, urinary sodium excretion increases. This effect is abolished by the specific D_1 receptor antagonist, SCH-23390 (62). Intracellularly, L-dopa is converted to dopamine by L-aromatic amino acid decarboxylase (AADC) (18). Immunohistochemistry studies have localized AADC exclusively to the proximal tubules and mainly to proximal convoluted tubules (PCT) (Fig. 5) (19, 33, 97) . The activity of AADC is upregulated by a high-sodium diet and downregulated by a low-salt diet (97). Dopamine is stored in PCT (35), but the mechanisms are unknown. Dopamine is metabolized via methylation by catechol-o-methyl-transferase (COMT) and via deamination by monoamine oxidase A (MAO) and both these enzymes are present in renal tubules (37, 124). In situ hybridization studies have localized COMT to most tubular segments with a particularly strong mRNA signal in PST (149). The enzyme COMT plays an important role for dopamine metabolism and the natriuretic response to dopamine is indeed related to the rate of dopamine metabolism. Nitecapone, an inhibitor of COMT, when given by gavages to rats, induces a dramatic, almost sixfold increase, in urinary sodium excretion associated with an inhibition of Na,K-ATPase activity in both proximal straight tubules and PCT. These effects are completely abolished by the D_1 receptor antagonist, SCH-23390. When rats are treated with both glu-dopa and nitecapone, the effect on natriuresis is additive. COMT in hibition or stimulation of intrarenal dopamine synthesis has no effect on glomerular filtration rate or blood pressure, confirming that tubular effects of dopamine are

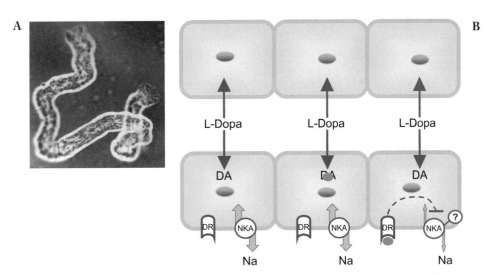

FIGURE 3   Intrarenally produced dopamine inhibits renal tubular Na,K-ATPase activity. (A) Dissected proximal tubule. (B) Intrarenal dopamine, formed from freely filtered L-dopa, decreases the pump activity of Na,K-ATPase in proximal tubules.

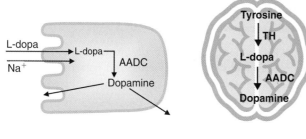

FIGURE 4 Dopamine synthesis in renal proximal tubules and CNS. TH, tyrosine hydroxylase, the rate-limiting enzyme in central dopamine synthesis; AADC, aromatic amino acid decarboxylase, the rate-limiting enzyme in renal dopamine synthesis.

mediated via dopamine produced in proximal tubules (62). The importance of COMT in regulating renal dopamine tonus has been further studied. The natriuretic response to COMT inhibition is highly dependent on D_1 receptor activation, while D_2 receptor activation is not involved. The natriuretic response is a direct tubular effect since regional renal blood flow is unaffected by COMT inhibitors. Furthermore, mice with reduced or absent COMT activity have altered metabolism of catecholamines and the natriuretic response to acute sodium loading is blunted (93, 175–178). Taken together, these findings suggest that manipulations aimed at increasing the intrarenal dopamine tonus result in natriuresis and, ultimately, the renal dopaminergic tonus depends on its capacity to be regulated (Fig. 6). Peripheral inhibitors of dopamine inactivation suggest a new principle in the therapy of salt-sensitive hypertension.

Dopamine can exit the proximal tubular cell at either the apical or basolateral surface via unknown mechanisms. The basolateral outward transporter is dependent on sodium and pH and is developmentally regulated, but little is known about apical dopamine secretion (206). Dopamine-producing areas of CNS express DAT, a dopamine-specific transporter. These transporters uptake released dopamine from the synaptic cleft. This reuptake can be inhibited by certain DAT inhibitors such as cocaine and dopamine transport is reversed by drugs such as amphetamines (117). Caron and colleagues (80) have demonstrated that DAT is an important regulator of the dopaminergic activity in CNS. Ongoing studies demonstrate that mRNA for DAT by RT-PCR amplification and DAT protein by immunohistochemistry and Western blot techniques are present in the kidney. Furthermore, mice lacking the DATz gene develop hypertension and have a blunted renal response to dopamine (101).

Distribution and Signaling Pathways of Renal Dopamine Receptors

Renal dopamine receptor subtypes have been extensively studied in the rat kidney and all of the cloned receptor subtypes have been identified in the kidney (reviewed in Amenta [8] and Jose et al. [116]) (Fig. 7). Peripheral dopamine

receptors were initially named DA_1/DA_2; however, due to extensive similarities between central and peripheral dopamine receptors, today they are also known as D_1/D_2-like receptors. The D_1-like receptors are present in smooth muscles of blood vessels of most major organs, the juxtaglomerular apparatus and in renal tubules along the nephron. The D_2-like receptors are present in the glomeruli, postganglionic sympathetic nerve terminals, and zona glomerulosa cells of the renal cortex and in renal tubules. The D_3 receptor is the predominant member of the D_2-like receptors expressed in the kidney. In situ hybridization studies of renal dopamine receptors mRNA have generally given negative results, but the much more sensitive RT-PCR technique has demonstrated the presence of D_1, D_3, and D_4 in single tubular segments. Immunolabeling techniques have generally given a robust signal of renal dopamine receptors. This apparent discrepancy in the expression between receptor messenger and receptor protein suggest a low turnover of renal dopamine receptors.

VASCULAR RECEPTORS

D_1 receptors have been identified in the renal, mesenteric, and splenic arteries, where they are concentrated in the medial layer. They are mainly located postjunctionally, which has been confirmed by insensitivity to chemical sympathectomy (8). The predominant D_1-like receptor in small renal vessels is the D_5 receptor (7). D_2-like receptors, the D_3 subgroup, are located in the adventitia and intima of renal, mesenteric, and splenic arteries. Chemical denervation reduces the density of D_3 receptors in the adventitia but not in the intima layer, suggesting that both prejunctional and postjunctional D_3 receptors are present in arteries.

GLOMERULAR RECEPTORS

Some controversy exists about whether D_1-like receptors are present in the glomeruli. RT-PCR studies have identified mouse mRNA for both D_1- and D_2-like receptors in glomeruli (27), whereas immunohistochemistry techniques as well as autoradiografic studies have not been able to identify the protein for D_1-like receptors (D_1 and D_5) in the glomeruli (182).

D_2-like receptors, mainly D_2 long and D_3 receptor subtypes, are present in the glomeruli (7, 68). D_3 receptors have been found in the arterioles as well as in podocytes, but not in mesangial cells (157).

RECEPTORS IN JUXTAGLOMERULAR APPARATUS

Immunohistochemistry has revealed the presence of D_1, but not D_3 receptors in juxtaglomerular cells of rat kidney slices and rat juxtaglomerular cells in culture (172, 174). Studies on mRNA expression of dopamine receptors show D_3 and D_4 expression, but not D_5 expression in rat cultured juxtaglomerular cells (192). In humans the predominant D_1-like receptor expressed in the juxtaglomerular apparatus is the D_5 receptor (116).

D_1 receptor stimulates secretion of renin in rat primary cultured cells (92, 233), whereas D_3 activation appears to

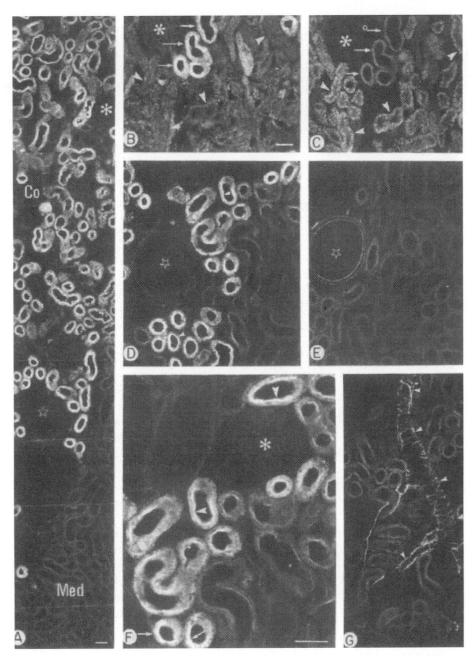

FIGURE 5 Renal tubules express AADC, but not TH. Distribution of AADC along the nephron. Pictures A–D and F show immunoflourescence after incubation with antiserum to AADC. Immunoreactivity is found in numerous tubules in Co, but not in glomeruli (*) blood vessels (☆) or medulla. Figures E and G show the adjacent pictures after incubation with antiserum to TH. No corresponding immunofluorescence of TH can be seen. A distinct TH labeling is found around blood vessels, indicating fiber plexus. Co, cortex; TH, tyrosine hydroxylase. (From Bertorello A, Hokfelt T, Goldstein M, Aperia A. Proximal tubule Na+-K+-ATPase activity is inhibited during high-salt diet: evidence for DA-mediated effect. *Am J Physiol* 1988;254:F795–801.)

have the opposing effect (230). Disruption of the D_3 receptor gene leads to increased renin release and renin-dependent hypertension (16).

TUBULAR RECEPTORS

Both D_1 and D_5 receptors are expressed in almost all tubular segments along the human nephron except the cortical collecting duct (CCD) (116). D_1-like receptors have

not been found in the medullary collecting duct of rat nephrons. Rat PCT (PCT) have the highest expression of D_1-like receptors followed by collecting duct (CD), medullary loop of Henley (mTAL), proximal straight tubules (PST), and distal tubules (DT). Despite the high density of D_1-like receptors in PCT, it is only 25% of the density noted in the brain striatum (234). In PCT, D_1-like receptors are present in luminal (brush border) membrane and basolateral

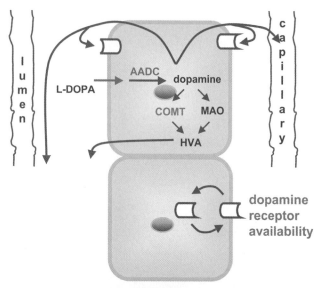

FIGURE 6   Regulation of renal dopamine tonus. The rate of dopamine degradation via COMT and the availability of functionally active dopamine receptors at the plasma membrane are important determinants of renal dopaminergic activity. HVA, homovanillic acid, the end metabolite of dopamine degradation.

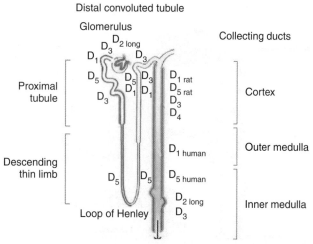

FIGURE 7   Expression of various dopamine receptors along the nephron. D_x human, in humans but not in rats; D_x rat, in rats but not in humans.

membrane. Both subtypes of D_1-like receptors are expressed in PCT, however, the predominant form in human kidney is the D_1 (161, 193). D_5 receptors have been identified in medullary thick ascending loop of Henley (mTAL).

D_2-like receptors are also expressed in PCT at the luminal and basolateral membranes. Although mRNAs for both D_2 long and D_3 have been shown in the rat cortex, only the D_3 protein has been identified in rat PCT. The D_3 receptor is only expressed at the luminal membrane and not the basolateral membrane, at least in rats (172). It is assumed that dopamine receptors have no functions in cTAL (69). D_1-like receptors and D_3 receptors are expressed in human DT.

Hemodynamics and Glomerular Filtration Rate

Selective D_1-like receptor agonists cause hypotension, reduced afterload, and increased blood flow to certain organs. Selective D_2-like receptor agonists produce hypotension, bradycardia, reduced afterload, and vasodilatation in certain organs. D_2 receptor–mediated vasodilatation is explained by the activation of prejunctional receptors on postganglionic sympathetic nerve terminals, causing inhibition of norepinephrine release and an associated inhibition of vasoconstrictor response (8, 47, 81, 139).

In the renal vasculature, D_1-like receptors are linked to vasodilatation. The effect of D_2-like receptors on the renal vasculature is probably dependent on the state of renal nerve activity. Renal vascular effects of dopamine are, in contrast to the tubular effects, elicited by dopamine released from renal nerves and by circulating dopamine. Whereas low-dose dopamine induces vasodilatation, higher doses cause vasoconstriction. This paradoxical effect can be explained by an unselective stimulation of adrenergic receptors (219). Dopamine increases both renal blood flow (RBF) and glomerular filtration rate (GFR). These effects are, however, not consistent, which can partly be explained by the unselective activation of adrenergic receptors, but also by a failure of transglomerular pressure to increase as a consequence of equal vasodilatation of afferent and efferent arterioles.

Studies on a single nephron level have shown that dopamine causes a large increase in single nephron GFR and a more pronounced dilatation in preglomerular than in postglomerular arterioles (15). In humans treated with fenoldopam, a selective D_1-like receptor agonist, RBF increases in a dose-dependent manner with little or no effect on GFR or systemic hemodynamics (146). D_3 receptor activation induces a simultaneous increase in GFR and RBF, suggesting a D_3 receptor–induced vasoconstriction of postglomerular vessels. This effect is at least in part mediated by presynaptical modulation of noradrenalin release (157). D_2 receptor activation reduces GFR and renal plasma flow (RPF), as well as filtration fraction (FF). These results can be explained by a greater afferent than efferent vasoconstriction (201, 202).

Angiotensin II produces mesangial contraction. Dopamine, via activation of D_2-like receptors, attenuates the vasoconstrictor effect of angiotensin II (24).

Tubular Transport

The kidneys respond to high salt intake with increased urinary sodium excretion (99, 209). The finding that dietary sodium could affect urinary dopamine output suggested a role for dopamine in the regulation of urinary sodium excretion (6). When dietary sodium was increased, urine dopamine increased. Administration of carbidopa, an inhibitor of AADC, caused a decrease not only in urinary dopamine but also in urinary sodium excretion (20), and dopamine receptor blockade was found to induce antidiuresis and antinatriuresis (203). The natriuretic effect of dopamine was initially attributed to modulations in renal hemodynamics. However, the natriuretic response to dopamine was still present at dose levels where no effects were observed in renal hemodynamics. The tubular effect of dopamine was established in the 1980s (14, 203). The molecular mechanism of this effect was identified in 1987 when our group demonstrates that dopamine directly inhibits the transport activity of Na,K-ATPase in a preparation of microdissected proximal tubular segments (14) (Fig. 3). Since then numerous of studies have shown that dopamine inhibits the activity of various Na transporters in almost the entire nephron, including PCT, mTAL, DT, and CCD (11).

Importantly, the natriuretic effect of dopamine is prominent during sodium loading and small or negligible during salt depletion (94, 222). Dopamine inhibition of PCT Na,K-ATPase is more pronounced during a high-salt diet than a normal salt diet (33).

Renal nerves have no effect on dopamine-mediated tubular sodium transport. A study by Wang et al. (221) 1999 provided direct evidence for a natriuretic effect of endogenous dopamine. By injecting rats with a D_1-receptor antisense oligodeoxynucleotide into the renal interstitium, the expression of D_1 receptors was reduced, as well as urinary sodium excretion was reduced.

Na,K-ATPase

The Na,K-ATPase, or sodium–potassium pump, is an extensively studied protein in its role as maintainer of electrolyte and fluid balance in all mammals including humans. It is present in the plasma membrane in virtually all eukaryotic cells, where it carries out the coupled active transport of Na ions out of the cell and of K ions into the cell, using the energy of hydrolysis of adenosine triphosphate (ATP) (204). This transport creates the electrochemical gradient across the plasma membrane that in all cells will facilitate the sodium-coupled entry of ions, amino acids, glucose, and many other compounds into the cell. In humans this process accounts for approximately 30% of the energy consumption. Na,K-ATPase consists of an alpha (α) and a beta (β) subunit. The α subunit is the catalytic subunit, where the transport of sodium and potassium occurs, and where the ATP and ouabain-binding sites are located. The β subunit is essential for the assembly of the functional enzyme and its integration into the plasma membrane Na,K-ATPase, present in the basolateral plasma membrane of renal tubular epithelial cells, is an important determinant of tubular sodium reabsorption. Approximately 70% of the oxygen consumed by the kidney is used by Na,K-ATPase to mediate vectorial transport of Na across the tubular cell. This transport generates and maintains low intracellular Na, thereby providing the driving force for Na entry across the apical, brush border membrane. Because of this low intracellular sodium, Na,K-ATPase is generally not saturated with sodium, and any increase in intracellular sodium will lead to an activa-

tion of its transporting activity. In fact, initially the activity of Na,K-ATPase was considered to be regulated only by the concentration of its ligands (Na and K), the availability of ATP, and the presence of Mg. The first demonstration that Na,K-ATPase is a target for hormonal regulation was made in our lab with the use of dissected rat proximal tubules. We showed that activation of dopamine receptors induce an inhibition of Na,K-ATPase activity measured as ATP hydrolysis (14). The method, developed by Doucet et al. (58), has been very useful in studies of the hormonal regulation of Na,K-ATPase activity along the nephron. Today it is well established that renal tubular Na,K-ATPase is bidirectionally regulated by natriuretic and antinatriuretic factors (Fig. 8) (11). These effects are mediated by a reversible phosphorylation on Na,K-ATPase. These findings have contributed to the understanding of regulation of ion transporters in the brain.

Proximal Convoluted Tubule (PCT) Intrarenally formed dopamine causes a dose-dependent decrease in Na,K-ATPase activity (14, 62). Procedures aimed at increasing intrarenal dopamine availability, such as inhibition of the dopamine-metabolizing enzyme COMT or treatment with a specific renal dopamine precursor, causes natriuresis associated with an inhibition of Na,K-ATPase activity (62). Furthermore, high salt intake is associated with a natriuretic response and inhibition of Na,K-ATPase activity. Both of these effects are abolished by an inhibitor of the dopamine synthesizing enzyme, AADC (62). In the PCT, dopamine-induced inhibition of Na,K-ATPase is abolished by a specific D_1 receptor antagonist (SCH-23390), whereas the role of D_2-like receptors is a matter of controversy. In the early 1990s, Bertorello et al. (32, 33) reported that dopamine-induced decrease in Na,K-ATPase activity was abolished by D_2-like receptor antagonists, whereas ongoing studies that use more specific agonists and antagonists, indicate that D_1 receptor activation alone is sufficient for an inhibition of PCT Na,K-ATPase activity. However, D_2-like receptors can act synergistically with D_1-like receptors to increase sodium excretion by inhibition of Na,K-ATPase (32, 86).

In rather recent studies, activation of D_2 receptors has been shown to increase the activity of Na,K-ATPase in a MAPK-tyrosine kinase-dependent manner. This effect is associated with tyrosine phosphorylation of Na,K-ATPase subunits (162, 163).

The classical signaling pathway for D_1-like receptor subtypes is activation of adenylate cyclase which leads to increased cAMP levels and activation of protein kinase A (PKA). The D1-like receptor is also coupled to phospholipase C and protein kinase C (PKC) activation in renal tubular cells. Interestingly, both these signaling pathways need to be activated to obtain an inhibitory effect on PCT Na,K-ATPase (Fig. 1). PKA may stimulate or inhibit Na,K-ATPase activity depending on the concentration of intracellular calcium; low intracellular calcium (<150 nM) is associated with inhibition, whereas high intracellular calcium (>150 nM) is associated with stimulation (43). Studies of

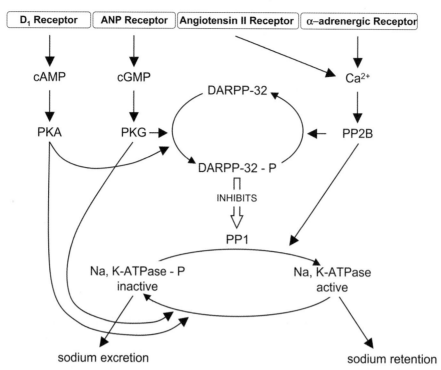

FIGURE 8   Postulated pathways for regulation of sodium metabolism by natriuretic and antinatriuretic factors. Natriuretic substances, such as dopamine and ANP, and antinatriuretic substances, such as norepinephrine via α-adrenergic receptors, and angiotensin II through their respective second messengers and associated protein kinases or phosphatases exert both direct and indirect (via DARRP-32) actions on the phosphorylation state and enzymatic activity of Na,K-ATPase.

dopamine regulation of Na,K-ATPase led to the first demonstration of PKA- and PKC-mediated phosphorylation of the catalytic subunit of Na,K-ATPase (31), and identification of phosphorylation sites for PKA, Ser[943], and PKC, Ser[23]. Site-directed mutagenesis studies have demonstrated that phosphorylation of rat renal Na,K-ATPase catalytic subunits may directly inhibit enzyme activity (71) and cause transient increase in intracellular sodium (29). In addition, PKC may inhibit Na,K-ATPase activity by stimulation of PLA$_2$ activity, and the generation of 20-HETE by cytochrome P-450 (111, 171, 181).

Dopamine-induced regulation of Na,K-ATPase activity involves more steps than phosphorylation of a single amino acid. There is evidence suggesting that dopamine-induced phosphorylation of Na,K-ATPase leads to internalization and subsequent inhibition of the enzyme (45). This process involves a PI$_3$ kinase–induced phosphorylation of Na,K-ATPase (46).

Thick Ascending Limb of Henley (mTAL)   The mTAL segment has the highest concentration of Na,K-ATPase found in any mammalian tissue. The intracellular signaling pathway triggered by dopamine differs between PCT and mTAL. In contrast to PCT, dopamine-induced inhibition of Na,K-ATPase activity is mediated by D$_1$ receptors coupled exclusively to adenylate cyclase (13, 153). In a series of studies, Fryckstedt and colleagues (153) demonstrated the im-

portance of DARPP-32 (see Dopamine Signaling and DARPP-32 section) in dopamine induced inhibition of mTAL Na,K-ATPase. By immunohistochemistry and in situ hybridization techniques, DARPP-32 protein and mRNA have been identified in rat, mouse, and monkey renal slices with the highest abundance in mTAL (153). Activation of D$_1$-like receptors via activation of adenylate cyclase and cAMP leads to activation of PKA and phosphorylation of DARPP-32. Phospho-DARPP-32 inhibits protein phosphatase 1 (PP1) activity, and Na,K-ATPase remains phosphorylated and its activity is decreased (Fig. 8).

Cortical Collecting Duct   In the rat CCD, D$_1$-like receptors inhibit Na,K-ATPase activity via stimulation of AC, PKA, and PLA$_2$ activity (179, 194). The D$_1$-like receptor stimulation of AC activity and inhibition of Na,K-ATPase activity are greater in the rat CCD than in the rat PCT (179).

Na–H Exchanger

The Na–H exchanger (NHE), first analyzed in the kidney (159), mediates approximately 80% of tubular cellular sodium influx and is thereby the quantitatively most important transporter for Na entry. NHE is a secondary active transporter and uses the potential energy of the sodium gradient across the cell membrane, created by Na,K-ATPase, to move Na into the cell in exchange for H ions. In contrast to Na,K-ATPase, NHE activity is not inhibited during a high-salt diet (104), but a small difference is observed between rats on high-salt and low-salt diets (156). Several isoforms of NHE exist with the NHE-3 isoform located at the apical membrane of proximal tubule and thick ascending limb cells. NHE-3 knockouts are hypotonic and cannot survive on a low-salt diet (36). The activity of NHE-3 is under hormonal control. Dopamine, via D_1-like receptor activation, induces a dose-dependent decrease in its activity (Fig. 1) (64). On the other hand, D_2-like receptors stimulate sodium entry via this transporter (166). The inhibitory action of dopamine on NHE-3 is predominantly due to activation of cAMP and PKA (64). NHE-3 is modulated by the NHE regulating factor (NHERF), which interacts with additional proteins, protein kinases, and the cytoskeleton (226). Renal proximal tubule apical NHE-3 activity can also be inhibited by D_1-like receptors via G proteins directly, independently of cAMP and phosphorylation mechanisms (4).

SODIUM-DEPENDENT PHOSPHATE COTRANSPORTER

In 1976, infusion of dopamine as well as the dopamine precursor L-dopa was reported to have a phosphaturic effect in dogs (51). In the early 1990s, several groups observed that dopamine regulates sodium-dependent phosphate (P_i) uptake in renal tubules (54, 55). Intrarenally formed dopamine was found to inhibit P_i uptake via D_1-like receptors. This effect was potentiated by a D_2-like receptor antagonist (184).

The major renal Na^+/phosphate cotransporter, NaP_i-IIa, is regulated by a number of factors including parathyroid hormone (PTH), dopamine, and dietary phosphate intake (158). Currently, it is believed that acute regulation (inhibition) of proximal tubular P_i reabsorption is the result of an increased rate of endocytosis of the NaPi-IIa protein. Like NHE, NaPi-IIa is modulated by NHERF (225).

Dopamine and Water Transport

In the CCD and distal nephron, dopamine inhibits the water permeation effect of vasopressin an effect most probably mediated by the D_4 receptor (57, 160). Vasopressin not only increases osmotic water permeability (P_f) in the rat CCD, but also acts synergistically with aldosterone to augment sodium reabsorption (J_{Na}). These effects are inhibited by catecholamines via a_2-adrenergic receptors and by dopamine via D_4 receptor activation (196, 211).

The water channel, aquaporin-4 (AQP4) plays an important role in the basolateral movement of water in the collecting duct. By confocal microscopy techniques Zelenina et al. (238) showed that AQP4 is a target for dopaminergic regulation. Dopamine decreases the water permeability of AQP4, via a PKC dependent phosphorylation of AQP4 Ser^{180}. AQP2 is mainly located intracellularly in CCD. After exposure to vasopressin, AQP2 is phosphorylated and transported to the apical plasma membrane,

where it forms a pore, allowing water to enter the cell. Dopamine reverses these effects (164).

REGULATION OF RENAL DOPAMINE D_1-RECEPTOR RESPONSIVENESS

GPCR are known to cycle between the plasma membrane and intracellular compartments. Whereas mechanisms of receptor desensitization have been extensively studied, less is known about the reverse pathway, that is, movement of receptors from the cytoplasm to the plasma membrane. Results from our lab show that D_1 receptor recruitment is a regulated phenomenon. The renal D_1 receptor is mainly located intracellularly in the resting cell. After exposure to dopamine, fenoldopam (D_1 receptor agonist), L-dopa, or nitecapone (COMT inhibitor) D_1 receptors are recruited to the plasma membrane, where they become biologically active (Fig. 6) (35, 103). D_1 receptor translocation is prevented by bafilomycin, an inhibitor of vesicular H^+ATPase, indicating that the D_1 receptors are stored, or inserted, in vesicles with an acidic content (35). Using biotinylation procedures to isolate membrane-bound proteins, others have confirmed that recruited D_1 receptors are indeed present within the plasma membrane (60). D_1 receptor recruitment is mediated via cAMP, whereas the PKC signaling pathway is not involved (34). In fact, only newly recruited D_1 receptors are able to activate PKC (128).

DOPAMINE HAS KEY ROLE IN INTERACTIVE REGULATION OF SODIUM

The precision by which sodium balance is regulated suggests an intricate interaction between modulatory factors released from intra- and extra-renal sources. Intrarenally produced dopamine has a central role in this interactive network. Norepinephrine acting via α-adrenoceptors, neuropeptide Y (NPY), and angiotensin II, increase Na,K-ATPase activity and induce antinatriuresis (11, 12), while dopamine, atrial natriuretic peptide (ANP), and norepinephrine acting via β-adrenoceptor decrease the activity of Na,K-ATPase and induce natriuresis. Each of these factors, through their respective second messenger and associated protein kinase or protein phosphatase, exerts both direct and indirect actions on the state of phosphorylation and the enzymatic activity of Na,K-ATPase (11, 12) (Fig. 8). The stimulatory effects of norepinephrine, acting on α-adrenoceptors, and angiotensin II on Na,K-ATPase are opposed by dopamine as well as by ANP (11, 12). The Na–H exchanger is regulated in a similar way; the stimulatory effect of α-adrenoceptor and angiotensin II is blunted by dopamine (76). Conversely, the inhibitory effect of dopamine on Na,K-ATPase activity is opposed by α-adrenoceptor agonists (12). In addition the effects of ANP and isoproterenol on Na,K-ATPase activity are abolished by a D_1 receptor antagonist as well as during inhibition of intrarenal dopamine synthesis (34, 103). DARPP-32 is a phosphoprotein shown to act as a third messenger in the dopamine signaling pathway (see Dopamine Signaling and DARPP-32). Mice, in which the DARPP-32 gene has been inactivated by knockout techniques, develop hypertension and lack the ability to induce ANP-mediated natriuresis (61). Prolactin is a polypeptide involved in various actions in the body including lactation, reproductive and parental behavior, angiogenesis, and osmoregulation (72). It has a crucial role in regulating sodium and water balance in fish that migrate from salt to fresh water. Prolactin is shown to interact with dopamine in several tissues, including CNS, intestines, and lactating breast epithelial cells. In 2005 (112), we reported a novel function of prolactin. Treatment with recombinant prolactin induces a dramatic natriuretic and diuretic response associated with an inhibition of PCT Na,K-ATPase activity. All of these effects are abolished by a D_1 receptor antagonist, whereas D_2 receptor antagonists have no effect. Furthermore, during inhibition of AADC activity prolactin does not inhibit Na,K-ATPase activity (112). The observed effects of prolactin on natriuresis and Na,K-ATPase activity are more pronounced than dopamine alone, suggesting a synergism between dopamine and prolactin (49). Prolactin exerts its effect in renal PCT via its receptor, a tyrosine kinase–coupled receptor identified in PCT, and activation of PKC and PI3 kinase signaling pathways. PKC induces a direct phosphorylation of Na,K-ATPase, a subunit Ser^{23}. New data indicate that prolactin, like dopamine, induces a PI3 kinase–dependent phosphorylation of the α subunit of Na,K-ATPase (49).

In the late 1980s, several laboratories unanimously reported that the natriuretic response to ANP required an intact renal dopamine system. It was observed that the natriuretic effect of ANP is abolished by D_1 receptor antagonists as well as during treatment with carbidopa, an inhibitor of dopamine synthesis (118, 144). Furthermore, a synergistic effect between dopamine and ANP was observed on the Na^+,H^+ exchanger activity (228). The mechanism behind the interaction between ANP and dopamine remained unknown. We examined the effect of ANP on Na,K-ATPase activity and found that threshold doses of ANP and dopamine added together have a synergistic effect on Na,K-ATPase activity, and that ANP-induced decrease in Na,K-ATPase activity is abolished by a D_1 receptor antagonist, SCH-23390 (103). This interaction between ANP and D_1 receptors is explained by the finding that ANP recruits silent D_1 receptors from the interior of renal tubular cells towards the plasma membrane (Fig. 9). The response is mimicked by cGMP, the second messenger for ANP, and requires dopamine binding to the D_1-like receptor (104). This heterologous receptor sensitization of D_1-like receptors by ANP may provide a novel mechanism for synergistic and permissive effects among different factors that modulate sodium balance and blood pressure.

This assumption has been confirmed in the kidney, where the permissive effect of dopamine in the actions of isoproterenol is explained by a heterologous recruitment of D_1 receptors to the plasma membrane (34), as well as in the CNS where insulin is shown to recruit GABA receptors to the plasma membrane (220).

Beside its inhibitory effect on vasopressin induced water permeability, dopamine has additional effects in the CCD; it may exert a modulatory influence on renal aldosterone action. Dopamine, via D_1-like receptors, antagonizes the action of aldosterone in the CCD (160), and the D_1-like action may be enhanced by the ability of D_2-like receptors to inhibit aldosterone release in sodium-*repleted* states (38). In contrast, in rats on a high-K or low-Na diet, D_2-like receptors facilitate aldosterone effects (1).

Dopamine not only opposes the short-term effect of angiotensin II, but has also a more sustained effect on renal angiotensin tonus. Harris and colleagues (41, 42) have demonstrated that dopamine, via D_1 receptors and cAMP, decreases angiotensin-II type 1 (AT_1) mRNA and protein levels in the kidney.

Another dopamine interacting substance is prostaglandin E2. PGE2, produced in the CCD, has a diuretic and natriuretic effect. The diuretic effect is achieved by the ability of PGE2 to counteract the effect of vasopressin. The natriuretic effect may be accomplished by inhibition of several sodium transporters, including Na,K-ATPase. Dopamine has been reported to rapidly stimulate the production of PGE2 in rat medullary collecting-duct cells. This effect is mediated through a D_2-like receptor, possibly a novel type, and PLA_2 activation (108, 109).

Taken together, the observations suggest that dopamine coordinates the effects of antinatriuretic and natriuretic factors and indicate that an intact renal dopamine system is of major importance for the maintenance of sodium homeostasis and, as discussed in the following, normal blood pressure (102).

DOPAMINE AND HYPERTENSION

Hypertension is the single leading risk factor predisposing to stroke, myocardial infarction, heart failure, and renal failure. Essential hypertension affects approximately 30% of the adult population, and of these patients 50%–70% have a salt-sensitive form (224).

The main long-term regulator of blood pressure is the sodium transport system in the kidney. Most cases of hypertension are attributable to minor alterations in the regulation of sodium metabolism (135). A sudden increase in blood pressure greatly increases the rate of sodium and water excretion; these effects are known as pressure natriuresis/diuresis. In all forms of hypertension, including human essential hypertension, pressure natriuresis is abnormal because sodium excretion is the same as in normotension despite increased arterial pressure. Considerable evidence

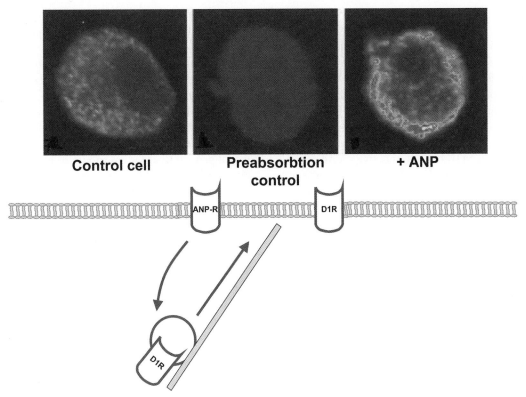

Control cell   **Preabsorbtion control**   **+ ANP**

FIGURE 9   ANP recruits D_1 receptors to the plasma membrane. Confocal micrographs of D_1-like receptors in LLC-PK cells, an immortalized renal tubular cell line. Renal D_1-like receptors are mainly located intracellularly in tubular cells. After exposure to ANP, D_1-like receptors are recruited to the plasma membrane, where they become physiologically active. Many studies have shown that the natriuretic effects of ANP are, to a large extent, mediated by dopamine. The present findings, that ANP recruits silent D_1 receptors to the plasma membrane, provide a plausible explanation for this phenomenon. See color insert.

indicates that this resetting of pressure natriuresis plays a key role in causing hypertension (91). Thus, the basic cause of essential hypertension is the inability to excrete an adequate volume at normal blood pressure (90).

The traditional view has been that hypertension is caused by an excess of factors that produce vasoconstriction and sodium retention. The two most obvious candidates have been norepinephrine and angiotensin II. This hypothesis has been modified after reports showing that a low availability of vasodilative natriuretic factors also predisposes to hypertension. A more likely hypothesis, therefore, is that hypertension is caused by an altered balance between vasoactive, antinatriuretic factors, and vasodilative natriuretic factors.

Several lines of evidence suggest that dopamine has a role in the pathophysiology of hypertension. Two fundamental defects in the renal dopamine system have been described in hypertension: (1) deficient renal dopamine production due to reduced renal uptake and/or decarboxylation of L-dopa (77) and (2) defective D_1-like receptor–G protein coupling, such that renal dopamine is ineffective in transmitting a signal to inhibit sodium excretion (116). Both defects may result in sodium retention and hypertension.

Clinical studies in patients with essential hypertension show that the dopaminuric response to sodium loading, seen in healthy individuals, may be blunted in patients with hypertension (50, 95, 207). Attenuation of the dopaminuric response is also observed in patients with hypertension (114) and in young prehypertensive individuals with a family history of hypertension (189, 190). Patients with β-hydroxylase deficiency (Fig. 1), having low levels of noradrenalin and adrenaline, and high levels of dopamine, suffer from orthostatic hypotension (127).

Infusion with dopamine or D_1 receptor agonists increases urinary sodium excretion in patients with essential hypertension (9, 121), and the natriuretic effect of fenoldopam is increased in young salt-sensitive hypertensive patients (173). The inhibitory effect of dopamine at the proximal tubule, measured as lithium clearance, is impaired in hypertensive individuals. Furthermore, in primary cultured cells isolated from hypertensive patients, dopamine and fenoldopam have an attenuated ability to stimulate adenylate cyclase (193). This impairment is D_1 receptor–specific, since parathyroid hormone–mediated stimulation of adenylate cyclase is similar in cells from both hypertensive and normotensive individuals. Additionally, the blunted effect of D_1 receptors is restricted to the proximal tubules and mTAL and is not present in CCD or CNS (116).

Strong evidence for a role of dopamine in the pathophysiology of hypertension has been provided by experimental studies. A great deal of interest has been focused on abnormalities in D_1 receptor–G protein coupling in two hypertensive strains, the spontaneously hypertensive rats (SHR) and the Dahl salt-sensitive hypertensive rats. The natriuretic effect of D_1 receptor agonist and the antinatriuretic effect of D_1 antagonists are impaired in SHR (117, 122). The first demonstration of a coupling defect between D_1 receptors and G proteins was made in 1989 when Kinoshita et al. (122) found a blunted response to adenylate cyclase activation by D_1 receptor agonist in SHR but not in normotensive control WKY rats. Again this effect is specific for D1 receptors since forskolin and parathyroid hormone activate adenylate cyclase in SHR. Moreover, SHR has a decreased ability to compete for specific 125I–SCH-23982 binding sites. The impaired capacity to increase second messenger response is associated with a blunted response to dopamine in the regulation of PCT and mTAL Na-transporter activity (54, 67, 110, 169). The blunted response to dopamine is not caused by mutations in the coding region or abnormal protein abundance of the D1 receptor (125, 147), defective G proteins (89, 110, 122), defective signaling distal to the G proteins (231), or defective effector proteins (122, 231), and it precedes the onset of hypertension (114).

Studies from 1996 to the present point toward a possible defect in D_1 receptor–G protein complex recycling and recruitment of receptors to the cell membrane. G protein–coupled receptor kinases (GRK) desensitize the D_1 receptor, in part, by serine phosphorylation (214). The D_1 receptor is hyperphosphorylated in renal proximal tubule cells from humans with essential hypertension and from SHR (191, 236). GRK4 desensitizes and phosphorylates D1 receptors. It has been suggested that essential hypertension is caused by constitutively activated polymorphic GRK_4 (66), but this hypothesis needs to be further elucidated. There is also evidence showing that a defect recruitment of D_1 receptors to the plasma membrane is associated with hypertension (116).

Further evidence for an involvement of dopamine as a counter-regulator of hypertension has been obtained from knockout mice lacking the dopamine receptors or dopamine signaling molecules. Jose and collaborators have contributed much of this evidence (116). Disruption of any of the dopamine receptors (D_1, D_2, D_3, D_4, and D_5) results in hypertension (239). Mice lacking one or two alleles of the D_1 receptor gene have a blunted natriuretic response to salt loading and develop hypertension (5). Deletion of the D_2 receptor also leads to hypertension, but the increased blood pressure is related to increased noradrenergic discharge and is not associated with sodium retention (136). D_3 receptor knockout mice develop a renin-dependent form of hypertension and have a blunted natriuretic response to salt loading (16). Disruption of the D_4 receptor gene in mice causes hypertension that is associated with increased expression of AT_1 receptors in the brain and kidney (26). Deletion of the D_5 receptor produces hypertension, which appears to be attributable to increased sympathetic tone with an involvement of adrenal catecholamines (100). DARPP-32 knockout mice as well as DAT knockout mice develop hypertension (61, 101), and have a blunted response to ANP and dopamine, respectively.

The cause(s) of essential hypertension remains elusive, probably because it is a heterogeneous disease in which both genetics and environment contribute to elevate blood pressure. The blood pressure difference between a hypertensive strain of rats and normotensive controls has been attributed to the influence of 2–6 genetic loci (235). Each of the individual genetic loci that contribute to hypertension has specific biochemical or physiological phenotypes. As reviewed previously, there is much evidence of the involvement of dopamine and genes that regulate its function in the pathogenesis of hypertension.

Dopamine coordinates the effects of salt-regulating hormones and peptides. It counteracts the effects of norepinephrine and angiotensin II, and acts permissively for the actions of other natriuretic substances including ANP, prolactin, and isoproterenol. Inability to increase the renal dopamine tonus in situations of sodium retention and/or a defect in the dopamine signaling system would require an extensive adaptation of the other salt-regulating systems to maintain sodium balance and normal blood pressure (Fig. 10).

DOPAMINE AND RENAL FAILURE

Dopamine, in low doses, induces primarily dopaminergic effects, whereas higher doses activate adrenergic receptors. For more than 30 years the so-called "low-dose" dopamine has been used to improve renal perfusion in critically ill adults and children. The rationale for this application of dopamine is based on clinical and experimental studies, where low-dose dopamine is found to cause renal dilatation associated with an increase in RBF, GFR, diuresis, and natriuresis. Additional evidence suggests that dopamine infusion may blunt endogenous norepinephrine-induced vasoconstriction. Higher doses of dopamine augment renal blood flow via activation of adrenergic receptors. However, the use and beneficial effect of low-dose dopamine, particularly during sepsis and acute renal failure (ARF), including ischemic, postischemic, and glycerol-induced ARF, are under debate. Actually in one study (130), low-dose dopamine increased renal vascular resistance in patients with ARF and worsened renal perfusion. There seems to be an association between age and the effects of dopamine on renal perfusion, where vasodilatation is more pronounced in younger than in elderly patients (130). The benefit effect of dopamine in neonates is also controversial. Some studies show no positive correlation between dopamine and renal function (52), whereas others show an improvement in renal perfusion and diuresis (63, 79, 199, 210, 215). Dopamine may also worsen the situation, either by increasing vascular resistance (see previous discussion) or by inducing adverse effects, the most

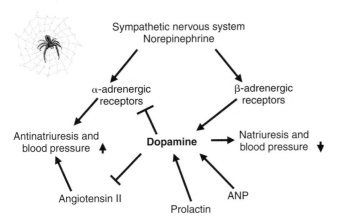

FIGURE 10 Dopamine coordinates the effect of salt-regulating factors. By its capacity to oppose the effect of antinatriuretic substances such as norepinephrine acting on α-adrenergic receptors and angiotensin II, and to act as a permissive factor for other natriuretic substances such as ANP and prolactin, dopamine has a key role in the interactive regulation of sodium balance.

common being gangrene due to peripheral extravasation or, at higher doses, cardiac arrhythmia.

FUTURE PERSPECTIVES

Salt balance is bidirectionally regulated by hormones, which exert an opposing effect on Na,K-ATPase activity. Many of these hormones, including dopamine, exert their effects via GPCR. The principles by which dopamine accomplishes its regulatory function can probably be applied to other hormones acting via GPCR. Clearly, a lot of information on renal dopamine signaling pathways is derived from the CNS, and some findings of dopaminergic principles in the kidney have been adapted to the brain.

It is evident that the biological response to a hormone is dependent not only on the availability of hormone and receptor, but also on the responsiveness of the receptor. Receptor trafficking, including recruitment and endocytosis, is one factor that regulates signaling via GPCR. More research is needed to better elucidate mechanisms involved in GPCR trafficking. Is essential hypertension mediated by defective D_1 receptor trafficking or desensitization? And in that case; by which mechanisms? Receptor dimerization is another important mechanism that alters the responsiveness of a receptor. Dimerization can lead to either a synergistic or an antagonistic effect. Is receptor dimerization a general phenomenon responsible for synergism, antagonism, and permissive effects among various hormones? Can D_1 receptors form dimers with receptors other than GPCR, such as the tyrosine kinase receptor for prolactin? Will this alter the signaling pathway that was heretofore connected to D_1 receptors?

Identification of various steps of importance for the regulation of renal dopamine tonus should provide us with new tools for early genetic diagnosis of hypertension and to new therapeutic strategies in conditions of salt retention and hypertension.

References

1. Adam WR, Adams BA. Production and excretion of dopamine by the isolated perfused rat kidney. *Ren Physiol* 1985;8:150–158.
2. Agnati LF, Fuxe K, Locatelli V, Benfenati F, Zini I, Panerai AE, El Etreby MF, Hokfelt T. Neuroanatomical methods for the quantitative evaluation of coexistence of transmitters in nerve cells. Analysis of the ACTH- and beta-endorphin immunoreactive nerve cell bodies of the mediobasal hypothalamus of the rat. *J Neurosci Methods* 1982; 5:203–214.
3. Albin RL, Mink JW. Recent advances in Tourette syndrome research. *Trends Neurosci* 2006;29:175–182.
4. Albrecht FE, Xu J, Moe OW, Hopfer U, Simonds WF, Orlowski J, Jose PA. Regulation of NHE3 activity by G protein subunits in renal brush-border membranes. *Am J Physiol Regul Integr Comp Physiol* 2000;278:R1064–R1073.
5. Albrecht FE, Drago J, Felder RA, Printz MP, Eisner GM, Robillard JE, Sibley DR, Westphal HJ, Jose PA. Role of the D1A dopamine receptor in the pathogenesis of genetic hypertension. *J Clin Invest* 1996;97:2283–2288.
6. Alexander RW, Gill JR Jr, Yamabe H, Lovenberg W, Keiser HR. Effects of dietary sodium and of acute saline infusion on the interrelationship between dopamine excretion and adrenergic activity in man. *J Clin Invest* 1974;54:194–200.
7. Amenta F. Light microscope autoradiography of peripheral dopamine receptor subtypes. *Clin Exp Hypertens* 1997;19:27–41.
8. Amenta F. Density and distribution of dopamine receptors in the cardiovascular system and in the kidney. *J Auton Pharmacol* 1990; 10(Suppl 1):s11–s18.
9. Andrejak M, Hary L. Enhanced dopamine renal responsiveness in patients with hypertension. *Clin Pharmacol Ther* 1986;40:610–614.
10. Aperia A. Intrarenal dopamine: a key signal in the interactive regulation of sodium metabolism. *Annu Rev Physiol* 2000;62:621–647.
11. Aperia A, Holtback U, Syren ML, Svensson LB, Fryckstedt J, Greengard P. Activation/deactivation of renal Na+,K(+)-ATPase: a final common pathway for regulation of natriuresis. *FASEB J* 1994;8:436–439.
12. Aperia A, Ibarra F, Svensson LB, Klee C, Greengard P. Calcineurin mediates alpha-adrenergic stimulation of Na+,K(+)-ATPase activity in renal tubule cells. *Proc Natl Acad Sci U S A* 1992;89:7394–7397.
13. Aperia A, Fryckstedt J, Svensson L, Hemmings HC Jr, Nairn AC, Greengard P. Phosphorylated Mr 32,000 dopamine- and cAMP-regulated phosphoprotein inhibits Na+,K(+)-ATPase activity in renal tubule cells. *Proc Natl Acad Sci U S A* 1991;88:2798–2801.
14. Aperia A, Bertorello A, Seri I. Dopamine causes inhibition of Na+–K+-ATPase activity in rat proximal convoluted tubule segments. *Am J Physiol* 1987;252:F39–F45.
15. Aperia A, Elinder G. Distal tubular sodium reabsorption in the developing rat kidney. *Am J Physiol* 1981;240:F487–491.
16. Asico LD, Ladines C, Fuchs S, Accili D, Carey RM, Semeraro C, Pocchiari F, Felder RA, Eisner GM, Jose PA. Disruption of the dopamine D3 receptor gene produces renin-dependent hypertension. *J Clin Invest* 1998;102:493–498.
17. Bach MR, Barad M, Son H, Zhuo M, Lu YF, Shih R, Mansuy I, Hawkins RD, Kandel ER. Age-related defects in spatial memory are correlated with defects in the late phase of hippocampal long-term potentiation in vitro and are attenuated by drugs that enhance the cAMP signaling pathway. *Proc Natl Acad Sci U S A* 1999;96:5280–5285.
18. Baines AD, Drangora R, Hatcher C. Dopamine production by isolated glomeruli and tubules from rat kidneys. *Can J Physiol Pharmacol* 1985;63:155–158.
19. Baines AD, Chan W. Production of urine free dopamine from DOPA;a micropuncture study. *Life Sci* 1980;26:253–259.
20. Ball SG, Lee MR. The effect of carbidopa administration on urinary sodium excretion in man. Is dopamine an intrarenal natriuretic hormone? *Br J Clin Pharmacol* 1977;4:115–119.
21. Barbeau A. Dopamine and disease. *CAMJ* 1970;103:824–832.
22. Barbeau A. The "pink spot," 3,4–dimethoxyphenylethylamine and dopamine. Relationship to Parkinson's disease and to schizophrenia. *Rev Can Biol* 1967;26:55–79.
23. Barger G, Dale HH. Chemical structure and sympathomimetic action of amines. *J Physiol* 1910;41:19–59.
24. Barnett R, Singhal PC, Scharschmidt LA, Schlondorff D. Dopamine attenuates the contractile response to angiotensin II in isolated rat glomeruli and cultured mesangial cells. *Circ Res* 1986;59:529–533.
25. Beaulieu JM, Sotnikova TD, Marion S, Lefkowitz RJ, Gainetdinov RR, Caron MG. An Akt/beta-arrestin 2/PP2A signaling complex mediates dopaminergic neurotransmission and behavior. *Cell* 2005; 122:261–273.
26. Bek MJ, Wang X, Asico LD, Jones JE, Zheng S, Li X, Eisner GM, Grandy DK, Carey RM, Soares-da-Silva P, Jose PA. Angiotensin-II type 1 receptor-mediated hypertension in D4 dopamine receptor-deficient mice. *Hypertension* 2006;47:288–295.
27. Bek MJ, Fischer KG, Greiber S, Hupfer C, Mundel P, Pavenstadt H. Dopamine depolarizes podocytes via a D1-like receptor. *Nephrol Dial Transplant* 1999;14:581–587.
28. Bello-Reuss E, Higashi Y, Kaneda Y. Dopamine decreases fluid reabsorption in straight portions of rabbit proximal tubule. *Am J Physiol* 1982;242:F634–F640.
29. Belusa R, Wang Z, Matsubara T, Sahlgren B, Dulubova I, Nairn AC, Ruoslahti E, Greengard P, Aperia A. Mutation of the site of protein kinase C phosphorylation on rat α1 Na+,K+-ATPase alters regulation of intracellular Na+, pH and influences cell shape and adhesiveness. *J Biol Chem* 1997;272:20179–20184.
30. Berkowitz BA. Dopamine and dopamine receptors as target sites for cardiovascular drug action. *Fed Proc* 1983;42:3019–3021.

31. Bertorello AM, Aperia A, Walaas SI, Nairn AC, Greengard P. Phosphorylation of the catalytic subunit of Na+,K(+)-ATPase inhibits the activity of the enzyme. *Proc Natl Acad Sci U S A* 1991; 88:11359–11362.
32. Bertorello A, Aperia A. Inhibition of proximal tubule Na(+)-K(+)-ATPase activity requires simultaneous activation of DA1 and DA2 receptors. *Am J Physiol* 1990;259:F924–928.
33. Bertorello A, Hokfelt T, Goldstein M, Aperia A. Proximal tubule Na+-K+-ATPase activity is inhibited during high-salt diet: evidence for DA-mediated effect. *Am J Physiol* 1988;254: F795–F801.
34. Brismar H, Agren M, Holtback U. beta-Adrenoceptor agonist sensitizes the dopamine-1 receptor in renal tubular cells. *Acta Physiol Scand* 2002;175:333–340.
35. Brismar H, Asghar M, Carey RM, Greengard P, Aperia A. Dopamine-induced recruitment of dopamine D1 receptors to the plasma membrane. *Proc Natl Acad Sci* 1998;95:5573–5578.
36. Burckhardt G, Di Sole F, Helmle-Kolb C. The Na+/H+ exchanger gene family. *J Nephrol* 2002;15(Suppl 5):S3–S21.
37. Caramona MM, Soares-da-Silva P. Evidence for an extraneuronal location of monoamine oxidase in renal tissues. *Naunyn Schmiedebergs Arch Pharmacol* 1990;341:411–413.
38. Carey RM, Sen S. Recent progress in the control of aldosterone secretion. *Recent Prog Horm Res* 1986;42:251–296.
39. Carlsson A, Lindqvist M, Magnusson T, Waldeck B. On the presence of 3-hydroxy-tyramine in brain. *Science* 1958;127:471.
40. Chan YL. Cellular mechanisms of renal tubular transport of L-dopa and its derivates in the rat. *Pharmacol Exp Ther* 1976;199:17–24.
41. Cheng HF, Wang JL, Vinson GP, Harris RC. Young SHR express increased type 1 angiotensin II receptors in renal proximal tubule. *Am J Physiol* 1998;274:F10–F17.
42. Cheng HF, Becker BN, Harris RC. Dopamine decreases expression of type-1 angiotensin II receptors in renal proximal tubule. *J Clin Invest* 1996;97:2745–2752.
43. Cheng Z, Aizman O, Aperia A, Greengard P, Nairn AC. $Ca^{2+}{}_i$ modulates the effects of PKA and PKC activation on renal Na+,K+-ATPase (NKA). *J Am Soc Nephrol* 1997;8:31A.
44. Cheung PY, Barrington KJ. Renal dopamine receptors: mechanisms of action and developmental aspects. *Cardiovasc Res* 1996;31:2–6.
45. Chibalin AV, Pedemonte CH, Katz AI, Feraille E, Berggren PO, Bertorello AM. Phosphorylation of the catalytic alpha-subunit constitutes a triggering signal for Na+,K+-ATPase endocytosis. *J Biol Chem* 1998;273:8814–8819.
46. Chibalin AV, Katz AI, Berggren PO, Bertorello AM. Receptor-mediated inhibition of renal Na(+)-K(+)-ATPase is associated with endocytosis of its alpha- and beta-subunits. *Am J Physiol* 1997;273:C1458–C1465.
47. Clark BJ. 1990. Prejunctional dopamine receptor stimulants. In: Amenta F, ed. *Peripheral Dopamine Pathophysiology*. Boca Raton, FL: CRC Press, 1990:267–306.
48. Chneiweiss H, Glowinski J, Premont J. Modulation by monoamines of somatostatin-sensitive adenylate cyclase on neuronal and glial cells from the mouse brain in primary cultures. *J Neurochem* 1985;44:1825–1831.
49. Crambert S, Sjöberg A, Holtbäck U. Cross talk among prolactin and dopamine in renal tubular cells. In: Proceedings of American Society of Nephrology Annual Meeting 2006 (abstract).
50. Critchley JA, Lee MR. Salt-sensitive hypertension in West Africans: an uncoupling of the renal sodium-dopamine relation. *Lancet* 1986; 2:460.
51. Cuche JL, Marchand GR, Greger RF, Lang RC, Knox FG. Phosphaturic effect of dopamine in dogs. Possible role of intrarenally produced dopamine in phosphate regulation. *J Clin Invest* 1976;58:71–76.
52. Cuevas L, Yeh TF, John EG, Cuevas D, Plides RS. The effect of low-dose dopamine infusion on cardiopulmonary and renal status in premature newborns with respiratory distress syndrome. *Am J Dis Child* 1991;145:799–803.
53. Daaka Y, Luttrell LM, Lefkowitz RJ. Switching of the coupling of the beta2-adrenergic receptor to different G proteins by protein kinase A. *Nature* 1997;390:88–91.
54. Debska-Slizien A, Ho P, Drangova R, Baines AD.Endogenous dopamine regulates phosphate reabsorption but not NaK-ATPase in spontaneously hypertensive rat kidneys. *J Am Soc Nephrol* 1994;5:1125–1132.
55. Debska-Slizien A, Ho P, Drangova R, Baines AD. Endogenous renal dopamine production regulates phosphate excretion. *Am J Physiol* 1994;266:F858–867.
56. De Camilli P, Macconi D, Spada A. Dopamine inhibits adenylate cyclase in human prolactin-secreting pituitary adenomas. *Nature* 1979;278:252–254.
57. Deis RP, Alonso N. Diuretic effect of dopamine in the rat. *J Endocrinol* 1970;47:129–130.
58. Doucet A, Katz AI, Morel F. Determination of Na-K-ATPase activity in single segments of the mammalian nephron. *Am J Physiol* 1979; 237:F105–F113.
59. Dziedzicka-Wasylewska M, Faron-Gorecka A, Andrecka J, Polit A, Kusmider M, Wasylewski Z. Fluorescence studies reveal heterodimerization of dopamine D1 and D2 receptors in the plasma membrane. *Biochemistry* 2006;45:8751–8759.
60. Efendiev R, Budu CE, Cinelli AR, Bertorello AM, Pedemonte CH. Intracellular Na+ regulates dopamine and angiotensin II receptors availability at the plasma membrane and their cellular responses in renal epithelia. *J Biol Chem* 2003;278:28719–28726.
61. Eklof AC, Holtback U, Svennilson J, Fienberg A, Greengard P, Aperia A. Increased blood pressure and loss of anp-induced natriuresis in mice lacking DARPP-32 gene. *Clin Exp Hypertens* 2001;23:449–460.
62. Eklof AC, Holtback U, Sundelof M, Chen S, Aperia A. Inhibition of COMT induces dopamine-dependent natriuresis and inhibition of proximal tubular Na+,K+-ATPase. *Kidney Int* 1997;52:742–747.
63. Emery EF, Greenough A. Efficacy of low-dose dopamine infusion. *Acta Paediatr* 1993;82: 430–432.
64. Felder CC, Campbell T, Albrecht F, Jose PA. Dopamine inhibits Na(+)-H+ exchanger activity in renal BBMV by stimulation of adenylate cyclase. *Am J Physiol* 1990;259:F297–303.
65. Felder CC, Jose PA, Axelrod J. The dopamine-1 agonist, SKF 82526, stimulates phospholipase-C activity independent of adenylate cyclase. *J Pharmacol Exp Ther* 1989;248:171–175.
66. Felder RA, Sanada H, Xu J, Yu PY, Wang Z, Watanabe H, Asico LD, Wang W, Zheng S, Yamaguchi I, Williams SM, Gainer J, Brown NJ, Hazen-Martin D, Wong LJ, Robillard JE, Carey RM, Eisner GM, Jose PA. G protein–coupled receptor kinase 4 gene variants in human essential hypertension. *Proc Natl Acad Sci U S A* 2002;99:3872–3877.
67. Felder RA, Seikaly MG, Eisner GM, Jose PA. Renal dopamine-1 defect in spontaneous hypertension. *Contrib Nephrol* 1988;67:71–74.
68. Felder RA, Blecher M, Eisner GM, Jose PA. Cortical tubular and glomerular dopamine receptors in the rat kidney. *Am J Physiol* 1984; 246:F557–F568.
69. Felder RA, Blecher M, Calcagno PL, Jose PA. Dopamine receptors in the proximal tubule of the rabbit. *Am J Physiol* 1984;247:F499–F505.
70. Ferre S, Fredholm BB, Morelli M, Popoli P, Fuxe K. Adenosine-dopamine receptor-receptor interactions as an integrative mechanism in the basal ganglia. *Trends Neurosci* 1997;20: 482–487.
71. Fisone G, Cheng S X-J, Nairn AC, Czernik AJ, Hemmings HC Jr, Höög J-O, Bertorello AM, Kaiser R, Bergman T, Jörnvall H, Aperia A, Greengard P. Identification of the phosphorylation site for cAMP-dependent protein kinase on Na+,K+ATPase and effects of site-directed mutagenesis *J Biol Chem* 1994;269:9368–9373.
72. Freeman ME, Kanyicska B, Lerant A, Nagy G. Prolactin: Structure, function and regulation of secretion. *Physiol Rev* 2001;80:1523–1631.
73. Fuxe K, Agnati LF, Jacobsen K, Hillion J, Canals M, Torvinen M, Tinner-Staines B, Staines W, Rosin D, Terasmaa A, Popoli P, Leo G, Vergoni V, Lluis C, Ciruela F, Franco R, Ferre S. Receptor heteromerization in adenosine A2A receptor signaling: relevance for striatal function and Parkinson's disease. *Neurology* 2003;61(Suppl 6):S19–S23 (review).
74. Fuxe K, Ferre S, Zoli M, Agnati LF. Integrated events in central dopamine transmission as analyzed at multiple levels. Evidence for intramembrane adenosine A2A/dopamine D2 and adenosine A1/dopamine D1 receptor interactions in the basal ganglia. *Brain Res Rev* 1998; 26:258–273.
75. George SR, Lee SP, Varghese G, Zeman PR, Seeman P, Ng GY, O'Dowd BF. A transmembrane domain-derived peptide inhibits D1 dopamine receptor function without affecting receptor oligomerization. *J Biol Chem* 1998;273:30244–30248.
76. Gesek FA, Schoolwerth AC. Hormonal interactions with the proximal Na, H-exchanger. *Am J Physiol* 2000;258:f514–f521.
77. Gill JR Jr, Gullner G, Lake CR, Lakatua DJ, Lan G. Plasma and urinary catecholamines in salt-sensitive idiopathic hypertension. *Hypertension* 1988;11:312–319.
78. Gines S, Hillion J, Torvinen M, Le Crom S, Casado V, Canela EI, Rondin S, Lew JY, Watson S, Zoli M, Agnati LF, Verniera P, Lluis C, Ferre S, Fuxe K, Franco R. Dopamine D1 and adenosine A1 receptors form functionally interacting heteromeric complexes. *Proc Natl Acad Sci U S A* 2000;97:8606–8611.
79. Girardin E, Berner M, Rouge JC, Rivest RW, Friedli B, Paunier L. Effect of low dose dopamine on hemodynamic and renal function in children. *Pediatr Res* 1989;26:200–203.
80. Giros B, Jaber M, Jones SR, Wightman RM, Caron MG. Hyperlocomotion and indifference to cocaine and amphetamine in mice lacking the dopamine transporter. *Nature* 1996;379: 606–612.
81. Goldberg LI, Kohli JD, Litinsky JJ. Comparison of peripheral pre- and post-synaptic dopamine receptors. In: Langer SZ, Starke K, Dubocovich M, eds. *Presynaptic Receptors*. New York: Pergamon Press, 1979:37–41.
82. Goldberg LI, Horwitz D, Sjoerdsma A. Attenuation of cardiovascular responses to exercise as a possible basis for effectiveness of monoamine oxidase inhibitors in angina pectoris. *J Pharmacol Exp Ther* 1962;137:39–46.
83. Goldberg LI, Sjoerdsma A. Effects of several monoamine oxidase inhibitors on the cardiovascular actions of naturally occurring amines in the dog. *J Pharmacol Exp Ther* 1959;127: 212–218.
84. Goldberg TE, Weinberger DR. The effects of clozapine on neurocognition: an overview. *J Clin Psychiatry* 1994;55(Suppl B):88–90.
85. Goldman-Rakic PS, Selemon LD. Functional and anatomical aspects of prefrontal pathology in schizophrenia. *Schizophr Bull* 1997;23:437–458.
86. Gomes P, Soares-da-Silva T, Katz AI. Apical D1 and D2 dopamine receptor stimulation inhibits Na+,K+-ATPase in OK cells. *J Am Soc Nephrol* 1999;10:454A.
87. Gomes P, Serrao MP, Viera-Coelho MA, Soares-da-Silva P. Opossum kidney cells take up L-DOPA through an organic cation potential–dependent and proton-independent transporter. *Cell Biol Int* 1997; 21:249–255.
88. Greengard P. The neurobiology of slow synaptic transmission. *Science* 2001;294:1024–1030.
89. Gurich RW, Beach RE, Caflish CR. Cloning of the alfa subunit of GS protein from spontaneously hypertensive rats. *Hypertension* 2001;24:R1071–R1078.
90. Guyton AC. Blood pressure control-special role of the kidneys and body fluids. *Science* 1991;252:1813–1816.
91. Hall JE, Guyton AC, Brands MW. Pressure-volume regulation in hypertension. *Kidney Int Suppl* 1996;55:S35–S41.
92. Hano T, Shiotani M, Baba A, Nishio I, Masuyama Y. DA1 receptor-mediated renin release from isolated rat glomeruli. *Hypertens Res* 1995;18(Suppl 1):S141–S143.
93. Hansell P, Odlind C, Mannisto PT. Different renal effects of two inhibitors of catechol-O-methylation in the rat: entacapone and CGP 28014. *Acta Physiol Scand* 1998;162:489–494.
94. Hansell P, Fasching A. The effect of dopamine receptor blockade on natriuresis is dependent on the degree of hypervolemia. *Kidney Int* 1991;39:253–258.
95. Harvey JN, Casson IF, Clayden AD, Cope GF, Perkins CM, Lee MR. A paradoxical fall in urine dopamine output when patients with essential hypertension are given added dietary salt. *Clin Sci (Lond)* 1984;67:83–88.
96. Havlicek V, Rezek M, Friesen H. Somatostatin and thyrotropin releasing hormone: central effect on sleep and motor system. *Pharmacol Biochem Behav* 1976;4:455–459.
97. Hayashi M, Yamaji Y, Kitajima W and saruta T. Aromatic L-amino acid decarboxylase acticity along the rat nephron. *Am J Physiol* 1990; 258:F28–F33.
98. Herve D, Levi-Strauss M, Marey-Semper I, Verney C, Tassin JPJ, Glowinski J. G(olf) and Gs in rat basal ganglia: possible involvement of G(olf) in the coupling of dopamine d1 receptors. *Mol Pharmacol* 1992;40:8–15.
99. Hollenberg NK. Set point for sodium homeostasis: surfeit, deficit, and their implications. *Kidney Int* 1980;17:423–429.

100. Hollon TR, Bek MJ, Lachowicz JE, Ariano MA, Mezey E, Ramachandran R, Wersinger SR, Soares-da-Silva P, Liu ZF, Grinberg A, Drago J, Young WS 3rd, Westphal H, Jose PA, Sibley DR. Mice lacking D5 dopamine receptors have increased sympathetic tone and are hypertensive. *J Neurosci* 2002;22:10801–10810.
101. Holtbäck U, Xiang H, Svensson L-B, Eklöf A-C. The dopamine transporter, DAT, is an important regulator of the renal dopaminergic tone. In: Proceedings of American Society of Nephrology Annual Meeting 2002.
102. Holtback U, Kruse MS, Brismar H, Aperia A. Intrarenal dopamine coordinates the effect of antinatriuretic and natriuretic factors. *Acta Physiol Scand* 2000;168:215–218.
103. Holtbäck U, Brismar H, DiBona GF, Fu M, Greengard P, Aperia A. Receptor recruitment: a mechanism for interactions between G protein-coupled receptors. *Proc Natl Acad Sci U S A* 1999;96:7271–7275.
104. Holtback U, Aperia A, Celsi G. High salt alone does not influence the kinetics of the Na(+)-H+ antiporter. *Acta Physiol Scand* 1993;148:55–61.
105. Holtz P, Credner K. Die enzymatische Entstehung von Oxytyramin im Organismus und die physiologische Bedeutung der Dopadecarboxylase. *Arch Pharmacol Exp Pathol* 1942;200: 356–388.
106. Hopf FW, Cascini MG, Gordon AS, Diamond I, Bonci A. Cooperative activation of dopamine D1 and D2 receptors increases spike firing of nucleus accumbens neurons via G-protein betagamma subunits. *J Neurosci* 2003;23:5079–5087.
107. Huntsman MM, Jones EG. Expression of alpha3, beta3 and gamma1 GABA(A) receptor subunit messenger RNAs in visual cortex and lateral geniculate nucleus of normal and monocularly deprived monkeys. *Neuroscience* 1998;87:385–400.
108. Huo TL, Grenader A, Blandina P, Healy DP. Prostaglandin E2 production in rat IMCD cells. II. Possible role for locally formed dopamine. *Am J Physiol* 1991;261:F655–F662.
109. Huo TL, Healy DP. Prostaglandin E2 production in rat IMCD cells. I. Stimulation by dopamine. *Am J Physiol* 1991;261:F647–F654.
110. Hussain T, Lokhandwala MF. Renal dopamine DA1 receptor coupling with G(S) and G(q/11) proteins in spontaneously hypertensive rats. *Am J Physiol* 1997;272:F339–F346.
111. Hussain T, Lokhandwala MF. Altered arachidonic acid metabolism contributes to the failure of dopamine to inhibit Na+,K(+)-ATPase in kidney of spontaneously hypertensive rats. *Clin Exp Hypertens* 1996;18:963–974.
112. Ibarra F, Crambert S, Eklof AC, Lundquist A, Hansell P, Holtback U. Prolactin, a natriuretic hormone, interacting with the renal dopamine system. *Kidney Int* 2005;68:1700–1707.
113. Ikemoto S, Glazier BS, Murphy JM, McBride WJ. Role of dopamine D1 and D2 receptors in the nucleus accumbens in mediating reward. *J Neurosci* 1997;17:8580–8587.
114. Iimura O, Shimamoto K. Suppressed dopaminergic activity and water–sodium handling in the kidneys at the prehypertensive stage of essential hypertension. *J Auton Pharmacol* 1990;10(Suppl 1):s73–s77.
115. Jones SR, Joseph JD, Barak LS, Caron MG, Wightman RM. Dopamine neuronal transport kinetics and effects of amphetamine. *J Neurochem* 1999;73:2406–2414.
116. Jose PA, Eisner GM, Felder RA. Renal dopamine receptors in health and hypertension. *Pharmacol Ther* 1998;80:149–182.
117. Jose PA, Cody P, Eisner GM. Endogenous dopamine (DA) regulates renal sodium transport in normotensive but not hypertensive rat. *Kidney Int* 1989;35:328.
118. Katoh T, Sophasan S, Kurokawa K. Permissive role of dopamine in renal action of ANP in volume-expanded rats. *Am J Physiol Renal Physiol* 1989;257:F300–F309.
119. Kebabian JW, Calne DB. Multiple receptors for dopamine. *Nature* 1979;277:93–96.
120. Keverne EB. GABA-ergic neurons and the neurobiology of schizophrenia and other psychoses. *Brain Res Bull* 1999;48:467–473.
121. Kikuchi K, Miyama A, Nakao T, Takigami Y, Kondo A, Mito T, Ura N, Tsuzuki M, Imura O. Hemodynamic and natriuretic responses to intravenous infusion of dopamine in patients with essential hypertension. *Jpn Circ J* 1982;46:486–493.
122. Kinoshita S, Sidhu A, Felder RA. Defective dopamine-1 receptor adenylate cyclase coupling in the proximal convoluted tubule from the spontaneously hypertensive rat. *J Clin Invest* 1989;84:1849–1856.
123. Kohout TA, Lefkowitz RJ. Regulation of G protein–coupled receptor kinases and arrestins during receptor desensitization. *Mol Pharmacol* 2003;63:9–18.
124. Kopin IJ. Catecholamine metabolism: basic aspects and clinical significance. *Pharmacol Rev* 1985;37:333–364.
125. Kren V, Pravenec M, Lu S, Krenova D, Wang JM, Wang N, Merriouns T, Wong A, St Lezin E, Lau D, Szpirer C, Szpirer J, Kurtz TW. Genetic isolation of a region of chromosome 8 that exerts major effects on blood pressure and cardiac mass in the spontaneously hypertensive rat. *J Clin Invest* 1997;99:577–581.
126. Kruse MS, Adachi S, Scott L, Holtbäck U, Greengard P, Aperia A, Brismar H. Recruitment of renal dopamine 1 receptors requires an intact microtubulin network. *Pflügers Arch Eur J Physiol* 2003;445:534–539.
127. Kuchel O. Genetic determinants of dopaminergic activity: potential role in blood pressure regulation. *Hypertens Res* 1995;18(Suppl)1:S1–S10.
128. LaHoste GJ, Henry BL, Marshall JF. Dopamine D1 receptors synergize with D2, but not D3 or D4, receptors in the striatum without the involvement of action potentials. *J Neurosci* 2000;20:6666–6671.
129. LaHoste GJ, Yu J, Marshall JF. Striatal Fos expression is indicative of dopamine D1/D2 synergism and receptor supersensitivity. *Proc Natl Acad Sci U S A* 1993;90:7451–7455.
130. Lauschke A, Teichgraber UK, Frei U, Eckardt KU. "Low-dose" dopamine worsens renal perfusion in patients with acute renal failure. *Kidney Int* 2006;69:1669–1674.
131. Lee FJ, Wang YT, Liu F. Direct receptor cross-talk can mediate the modulation of excitatory and inhibitory neurotransmission by dopamine. *J Mol Neurosci* 2005;26:245–252.
132. Lee FJ, Xue S, Pei L, Vukusic B, Chery N, Wang Y, Wang YT, Niznik HB, Yu XM, Liu F. Dual regulation of NMDA receptor functions by direct protein-protein interactions with the dopamine D1 receptor. *Cell* 2002;111:219–230.
133. Lee SP, So CH, Rashid AJ, Varghese G, Cheng R, Lanca AJ, O'Dowd BF, George SR. Dopamine D1 and D2 receptor Co-activation generates a novel phospholipase C-mediated calcium signal. *J Biol Chem* 2004; 279:35671–3578.
134. Lezcano N, Mrzljak L, Eubanks S, Levenson R, Goldman-Rakic P, Bergson C. Dual signaling regulated by calcyon, a D1 dopamine receptor interacting protein. *Science* 2000;287:1660–1664.
135. Lifton RP, Gharavi AG, Geller DS. Molecular mechanisms of human hypertension. *Cell* 2001;104:545–556.
136. Li XX, Bek M, Asico LD, Yang Z, Grandy DK, Goldstein DS, Rubinstein M, Eisner GM, Jose PA. Adrenergic and endothelin B receptor-dependent hypertension in dopamine receptor type-2 knockout mice. *Hypertension* 2001;38:303–308.
137. Liu F, Wan Q, Pristupa ZB, Yu XM, Wang YT, Niznik HB. Direct protein-protein coupling enables cross-talk between dopamine D5 and gamma-aminobutyric acid A receptors. *Nature* 2000;20;403:274–280.
138. Lokhandwala MF, Amenta F. Anatomical distribution and function of dopamine receptors in the kidney. *FASEB J* 1991;5:3023–3030.
139. Lokhandwala MF, Hedge SS. Cardiovascular dopamine receptors: role of renal dopamine and dopamine receptors in sodium excretion. *Pharmacol Toxicol* 1990;66:237–243.
140. MacLeod RM, Login IS. Regulation of prolactin secretion through dopamine, serotonin, and the cerebrospinal fluid. *Adv Biochem Psychopharmacol* 1977;16:147–157.
141. Mahan LC, Burch RM, Monsma FJ Jr, Sibley DR. Expression of striatal D1 dopamine receptors coupled to inositol phosphate production and Ca2+ mobilization in Xenopus oocytes. *Proc Natl Acad Sci U S A* 1990;87:2196–2200.
142. Mailman RB, Schulz DW, Lewis MH, Staples L, Rollema H, Dehaven DL. SCH-23390: a selective D1 dopamine antagonist with potent D2 behavioral actions. *Eur J Pharmacol* 1984;101:159–160.
143. Mannich C, Jacobsohn W. Uber oxyphenyl-alkylamine und dioxyphenyl-alkamine. *Der Deutschen Chem Gesellschaft* 1910;43:189–193.
144. Marin-Grez M, Briggs JP, Schubert G, Schnermann J. Dopamine receptor antagonists inhibit the natriuretic response to atrial natriuretic factor (ANF). *Life Sci* 1985;36:2171–2176.
145. Marsden CD. The neuropharmacology of abnormal involuntary movement disorders (the dyskinesias). *Mod Trends Neurol* 1975;6:141–166.
146. Mathur VS, Swan SK, Lambrecht LJ, Anjum S, Fellmann J, McGuire D, Epstein M, Luther RR. The effects of fenoldopam, a selective dopamine receptor agonist, on systemic and renal hemodynamics in normotensive subjects. *Crit Care Med* 1999;27:1832–1837.
147. Matsumoto T, Ozono R, Sasaki N, Oshima T, Matsuura H, Kajiyama G, Carey RM, Kambe M. Type 1A dopamine receptor expression in the heart is not altered in spontaneously hypertensive rats. *Am J Hypertens* 2000;13:673–677.
148. McDonald RH Jr, Goldberg LI, Mac Navy JL, Tuttle EP. Effects of dopamine in man: augmentation of sodium excretion, glomerular filtration rate and renal plasma flow. *J Clin Invest* 1964;43:1116–1124.
149. Meister B, Bean AJ, Aperia A. Catechol-O-methyltransferase mRNA in the kidney and its appearance during ontogeny. *Kidney Int* 1993; 44:726–733.
150. Meister B, Arvidsson U, Hemmings HC Jr, Greengard P, Hökfelt T. Dopamine- and adenosine-3':5'-monophosphate (cAMP)-regulated phospho-protein of M_r 32,000 (DARPP-32) in the retina of cat, monkey and human. *Neurosci Lett* 1991;131:66–70.
151. Meister B, Askergren J, Tunevall G, Hemmings HC Jr, Greengard P. Identification of a dopamine- and 3'5'-cyclic adenosine monophosphate-regulated phosphoprotein of 32 kD (DARPP-32) in the parathyroid hormone-producing cells of the human parathyroid gland. *J Endocrinol Invest* 1991;14:655–661.
152. Meister B, Schultzberg M, Hemmings HC Jr, Greengard P, Goldtein M, Hökfelt T. Dopamine- and adenosine-3′,5′-monophosphate (cAMP)-regulated phosphoprotein of 32 kDa (DARPP-32) in the adrenal gland: immunohistochemical localization. *J Auton Nerv Syst* 1991;36:75–84.
153. Meister B, Fryckstedt J, Schalling M, Cortes R, Hokfelt T, Aperia A, Hemmings HC Jr, Nairn AC, Ehrlich M, Greengard P. Dopamine- and cAMP-regulated phosphoprotein (DARPP-32) and dopamine DA1 agonist-sensitive Na+,K+-ATPase in renal tubule cells. *Proc Natl Acad Sci U S A* 1989;86:8068–8072.
154. Meister B, Fried G, Hökfelt T, Hemmings HC Jr, Greengard P. Immunohistochemical evidence for the existence of a dopamine- and cyclic AMP–regulated phosphoprotein (DARPP-32) in brown adipose tissue of pigs. *Proc Natl Acad Sci U S A* 1988;85:8713–8716.
155. Missale C, Nash SR, Robinson SW, Jaber M, Caron MG. Dopamine receptors: from structure to function. *Physiol Rev* 1998;78:189–225.
156. Moe OW, Tejedor A, Levi M, Seldin DW, Preisig PA, Alpern RJ. Dietary NaCl modulates Na(+)-H+ antiporter activity in renal cortical apical membrane vesicles. *Am J Physiol* 1991;260:F130–F137.
157. Muhlbauer B, Kuster E, Luippold G. Dopamine D(3) receptors in the rat kidney: role in physiology and pathophysiology. *Acta Physiol Scand* 2000;168:219–223.
158. Murer H, Hernando N, Forster I, Biber J. Proximal tubular phosphate reabsorption: molecular mechanisms. *Physiol Rev* 2000;80:1373–1409.
159. Murer H, Hopfer U, Kinne R. Sodium/proton antiport in brush border membranes vesicles isolated from small intestine and kidney. *Biochem J* 1976;155:597–604.
160. Muto S, Tabei K, Asano Y, Imai M. 1985. Dopaminergic inhibition of the action of vasopressin on the cortical collecting tubule. *Eur J Pharmacol* 1985;114:393–397.
161. Nash SR, Godinot N, Caron MG. Cloning and characterization of the opossum kidney cell D1 dopamine receptor: expression of identical D1A and D1B dopamine receptor mRNAs in opossum kidney and brain. *Mol Pharmacol* 1993;44:918–925.
162. Narkar VA, Hussain T, Lokhandwala MF. Activation of D2-like receptors causes recruitment of tyrosine-phosphorylated NKA alpha 1–subunits in kidney. *Am J Physiol Renal Physiol* 2002;283:F1290–F1295.
163. Narkar VA, Hussain T, Lokhandwala MF. Role of tyrosine kinase and p44/42 MAPK in D-like receptor-mediated stimulation of Na(+), K(+)-ATPase in kidney. *Am J Physiol Renal Physiol* 2002;282:F697–F702.
164. Nejsum LN, Zelenina M, Aperia A, Frokiaer J, Nielsen S. Bidirectional regulation of AQP2 trafficking and recycling: involvement of AQP2–S256 phosphorylation. *Am J Physiol Renal Physiol* 2005;288:F930–F938.
165. Neve KA, Seamans JK, Trantham-Davidson H. Dopamine receptor signaling. *J Recept Signal Transduct Res* 2004;24:165–205.

166. Neve KA, Kozlowski MR, Rosser MP. Dopamine D2 receptor stimulation of Na+/H+ exchange assessed by quantification of extracellular acidification. *J Biol Chem* 1992;267:25748–25753.

167. Ng GY, O'Dowd BF, Lee SP, Chung HT, Brann MR, Seeman P, George SR. Dopamine D2 receptor dimers and receptor-blocking peptides. *Biochem Biophys Res Commun* 1996;227:200–204.

168. Nimchinsky EA, Hof PR, Janssen WG, Morrison JH, Schmauss C. Expression of dopamine D3 receptor dimers and tetramers in brain and in transfected cells. *J Biol Chem* 1997;272:29229–29237.

169. Nishi A, Bertorello AM, Aperia A. Renal Na+,K(+)-ATPase in Dahl salt-sensitive rats: K+ dependence, effect of cell environment and protein kinases. *Acta Physiol Scand* 1993;149:377–384.

170. Niznik HB, Sugamori KS, Clifford JJ, Waddington JL. D1 like dopamine receptors: molecular biology and pharmacology. In: Di Chiara G, ed. *Handbook of Experimental Pharmacology: Dopamine in the CNS 1*. Berlin, Heidelberg, New York: Springer, 2002:121–158.

171. Nowicki S, Chen SL, Aizman O, Cheng XJ, Li D, Nowicki C, Nairn A, Greengard P, Aperia A. 0-Hydroxyeicosa-tetraenoic acid (20 HETE) activates protein kinase C. Role in regulation of rat renal Na+,K+-ATPase. *J Clin Invest* 1997;99:1224–1230.

172. O'Connell DP, Vaughan CJ, Aherne AM, Botkin SJ, Wang ZQ, Felder RA, Carey RM. Expression of the dopamine D3 receptor protein in the rat kidney. *Hypertension* 1998;32:886–895.

173. O'Connell DP, Ragsdale NV, Boyd DG, Felder RA, Carey RM. Differential human renal tubular responses to dopamine type 1 receptor stimulation are determined by blood pressure status. *Hypertension* 1997;29:115–122.

174. O'Connell DP, Botkin SJ, Ramos SI, Sibley DR, Ariano MA, Felder RA, Carey RM. Localization of dopamine D1A receptor protein in rat kidneys. *Am J Physiol* 1995;268: F1185–F1197.

175. Odlind C, Reenila I, Mannisto PT, Juvonen R, Uhlen S, Gogos JA, Karayiorgou M, Hansell P. Reduced natriuretic response to acute sodium loading in COMT gene deleted mice. *BMC Physiol* 2002;2:14.

176. Odlind C, Reenila I, Mannisto PT, Ekblom J, Hansell P. The role of dopamine-metabolizing enzymes in the regulation of renal sodium excretion in the rat. *Pflügers Arch* 2001;442:505–510.

177. Odlind C, Fasching A, Liss P, Palm F, Hansell P. Changing dopaminergic activity through different pathways: consequences for renal sodium excretion, regional blood flow and oxygen tension in the rat. *Acta Physiol Scand* 2001;172:219–226.

178. Odlind C, Goransson V, Reenila I, Hansell P. Regulation of dopamine-induced natriuresis by the dopamine-metabolizing enzyme catechol-O-methyltransferase. *Exp Nephrol* 1999;7:314–322.

179. Ohbu K, Felder RA. DA1 dopamine receptors in renal cortical collecting duct. *Am J Physiol* 1991;261:F890–F895.

180. Okubo Y, Suhara T, Suzuki K, Kobayashi K, Inoue O, Terasaki O, Someya Y, Sassa T, Sudo Y, Matsushima E, Iyo M, Tateno Y, Toru M. Decreased prefrontal dopamine D1 receptors in schizophrenia revealed by PET. *Nature (Lond)* 1997;385:634–636.

181. Ominato M, Satoh T, Katz AI. Regulation of Na-K-ATPase activity in the proximal tubule: role of the protein kinase C pathway and of eicosanoids. *J Membr Biol* 1996;152:235–243.

182. Ozono R, O'Connell DP, Wang ZO, Moore AF, Sanada H, Felder RA, Carey RM. Localization of the dopamine D1 receptor protein in the human heart and kidney. *Hypertension* 1997;30:725–729.

183. Panchalingam S, Undie AS. Optimized binding of [35S]GTPgammaS to Gq-like proteins stimulated with dopamine D1-like receptor agonists. *Neurochem Res* 2000;25:759–767.

184. Perrichot R, Garcia-Ocaña A, Couette S, Comoy E, Amiel C, Friedlander G. Locally formed dopamine modulates renal Na-P$_i$ co-transport through DA1 and DA2 receptors. *Biochem J* 1995;312:433–437.

185. Pollack A. Coactivation of D1 and D2 dopamine receptors: in marriage, a case of his, hers, and theirs. *Sci STKE* 2004;(255):pe50.

186. Quimet CC, Miller PE, Hemmings HC Jr, Walaas SI, Greengard P. DARPP-32, a dopamine- and adenosine 3':5'-monophosphate-regulated phosphoprotein enriched in dopamine-innervated brain regions. III. Immunocytochemical localization. *J Neurosci* 1984;4:111–124.

187. Ricci A, Escaf S, Vega JA, Amenta F. Autoradiographic localization of dopamine D1 receptors in the human kidney. *J Pharmacol Exp Ther* 1993;264:431–437.

188. Rocheville M, Lange DC, Kumar U, Patel SC, Patel RC, Patel YC. Receptors for dopamine and somatostatin: formation of hetero-oligomers with enhanced functional activity. *Science* 2000;288:154–157.

189. Rudberg S, Lemne C, Persson B, Krekula A, de Faire U, Aperia A. The dopaminuric response to high salt diet in insulin-dependent diabetes mellitus and in family history of hypertension. *Pediatr Nephrol* 1997;11:169–173.

190. Saito I, Takeshita E, Saruta T, Nagano S, Sekihara T. Urinary dopamine excretion in normotensive subjects with or without family history of hypertension. *J Hypertens* 1986;4:57–60.

191. Sanada H, Jose PA, Hazen-Martin D, Yu PY, Xu J, Bruns DE, Phipps J, Carey RM, Felder RA. Dopamine-1 receptor coupling defect in renal proximal tubule cells in hypertension. *Hypertension* 1999;33:1036–1042.

192. Sanada H, Yao L, Jose PA, Carey RM, Felder RA. Dopamine D3 receptors in rat juxtaglomerular cells. *Clin Exp Hypertens* 1997;19:93–105.

193. Sanada H, Jose PA, Yu P-Y, Hazen-Martin D, Carey RM, Bruns D, Felder RA. Human hypertensives have a renal proximal tubular defect in dopamine-1 receptor/adenylyl cyclase coupling. *J Am Soc Nephrol* 1997;8:307A.

194. Satoh T, Cohen HT, Katz AI. Intracellular signaling in the regulation of renal Na-K-ATPase. II. Role of eicosanoids. *J Clin Invest* 1993;91:409–415.

195. Scarselli M, Novi F, Schallmach E, Lin R, Baragli A, Colzi A, Griffon N, Corsini GU, Sokoloff P, Levenson R, Vo=gel Z, Maggio R. D2/D3 dopamine receptor heterodimers exhibit unique functional properties. *J Biol Chem* 2001;276:30308–30314.

196. Schafer JA, Li L, Sun D. The collecting duct, dopamine and vasopressin-dependent hypertension. *Acta Physiol Scand* 2000;168:239–244.

197. Scott L, Zelenin S, Malmersjo S, Kowalewski JM, Markus EZ, Nairn AC, Greengard P, Brismar H, Aperia A. Allosteric changes of the NMDA receptor trap diffusible dopamine 1 receptors in spines. *Proc Natl Acad Sci U S A* 2006;103:762–767.

198. Scott L, Kruse MS, Forssberg H, Brismar H, Greengard P, Aperia A. Selective up-regulation of dopamine D1 receptors in dendritic spines by NMDA receptor activation. *Proc Natl Acad Sci U S A* 2002; 99:1661–1664.

199. Seri I, Rudas G, Bors Z, Kanyicska B, Tulassay T. Effects of low-dose dopamine infusion on cardiovascular and renal functions, cerebral blood flow, and plasma catecholamine levels in sick preterm neonates. *Pediatr Res* 1993;34:742–749.

200. Shepherd DM, West GB. Hydroxytyramine and the adrenal medulla. *J Physiol* 1953;120: 15–19.

201. Siragy HM, Felder RA, Peach MJ, Carey RM. Intrarenal DA2 dopamine receptor stimulation in the conscious dog. *Am J Physiol* 1992;262:F932–F938.

202. Siragy HM, Felder RA, Howell NL, Chevalier RL, Peach MJ, Carey RM. Evidence that dopamine-2 mechanisms control renal function. *Am J Physiol* 1990;259:F793–F800.

203. Siragy HM, Felder RA, Howell NL, Chevalier RL, Peach MJ, Carey RM. Evidence that intrarenal dopamine acts as a paracrine substance at the renal tubule. *Am J Physiol* 1989;257: F469–F477.

204. Skou JC. The influence of some cations on an adenosine triphosphatase from peripheral nerves. *Biochim Biophys Acta* 1957;23:394–401.

205. Snyder SH. Catecholamines in the brain as mediators of amphetamine psychosis. *Arch Gen Psychiatry* 1972;27:169–179.

206. Soares-Da-Silva P, Serrao MP, Vieira-Coelho MA. Apical and basolateral uptake and intracellular fate of dopamine precursor L-dopa in LLC-PK1 cells. *Am J Physiol* 1998;274: F243–F251.

207. Sowers JR, Zemel MB, Zemel P, Beck FW, Walsh MF, Zawada ET. Salt sensitivity in blacks. Salt intake and natriuretic substances. *Hypertension* 1988;2:485–490.

208. Stadel JM, Strulovici B, Nambi P, Lavin TN, Briggs MM, Caron MG, Lefkowitz RJ. Desensitization of the beta-adrenergic receptor of frog erythrocytes. Recovery and characterization of the down-regulated receptors in sequestered vesicles. *J Biol Chem* 1983;258:3032–3038.

209. Strauss MB, Lamdin E, Smith WP, Bleifer DJ. Surfeit and deficit of sodium. A kinetic concept of sodium excretion. *Arch Intern Med* 1958;102:527–536.

210. Sulyok E, Seri I, Tulassay T, Kiszel J, Ertl T. The effect of dopamine administration on the activity of the renin-angiotensin-aldosterone system in sick preterm infants. *Eur J Pediatr* 1985;143:191–193.

211. Sun D, Schafer JA. 1996. Dopamine inhibits AVP-dependent Na$^+$ transport and water permeability in rat CCD via a D$_4$-like receptor. *Am J Physiol* 1996;271:F391–F400.

212. Sunahara RK, Taussig R. Isoforms of mammalian adenylyl cyclase: multiplicities of signaling. *Mol Interv* 2002;2:168–184.

213. Svenningsson P, Nishi A, Fisone G, Girault JA, Nairn AC, Greengard P. DARPP-32: an integrator of neurotransmission. *Annu Rev Pharmacol Toxicol* 2004;44:269–296.

214. Tiberi M, Nash SR, Bertrand L, Lefkowitz RJ, Caron MG. Differential regulation of dopamine D1A receptor responsiveness by various G protein-coupled receptor kinases. *J Biol Chem* 1996; 271:3771–3778.

215. Tulassay T, Seri I, Machay T, Kiszel J, Varga J, Csomor S. Effects of dopamine on renal functions in premature neonates with respiratory distress syndrome. *Int J Pediatr Nephrol* 1983;4:19–23.

216. Walaas SI, Greengard P. DARPP-32, a dopamine- and adenosine 3':5'-monophosphate-reglated phosphoprotein enriched in dopamine-innervated brain regions. I. Regional and cellular distribution in the brain. *J Neurosci* 1984;4:84–98.

217. Walaas SI, Aswad DW, Greengard P. A dopamine- and cyclic AMP-regulated phosphoprotein enriched in dopamine-innervated brain regions. *Nature* 1983;301:69–71.

218. van Praag HM. The possible significance of cerebral dopamine for neurology and psychiatry. *Psychiatr Neurol Neurochir* 1967;70:361–379.

219. van Veldhuisen DJ, Girbes AR, de Graeff PA, Lie KI. Effects of dopaminergic agents on cardiac and renal function in normal man and in patients with congestive heart failure. *Int J Cardiol* 1992;37:293–300.

220. Wan Q, Xiong ZG, Man HY, Ackerley CA, Braunton J, Lu WY, Becker LE, MacDonald JF, Wang YT. Recruitment of functional GABA(A) receptors to postsynaptic domains by insulin. *Nature* 1997;388:686–690.

221. Wang ZQ, Felder RA, Carey RM. Selective inhibition of the renal dopamine subtype D1A receptor induces antinatriuresis in conscious rats. *Hypertension* 1999;33:504–510.

222. Wang ZQ, Siragy HM, Felder RA, Carey RM. Intrarenal dopamine production and distribution in the rat. Physiological control of sodium excretion. *Hypertension* 1997;29:228–234.

223. Watts VJ, Neve KA. Activation of type II adenylate cyclase by D2 and D4 but not D3 dopamine receptors. *Mol Pharmacol* 1997;52:181–186.

224. Weinberger MH. Salt sensitivity of blood pressure in humans. *Hypertension* 1996;27:481–490.

225. Weinman EJ, Cunningham R, Wade JB, Shenolikar S. The role of NHERF-1 in the regulation of renal proximal tubule sodium-hydrogen exchanger 3 and sodium-dependent phosphate cotransporter 2a. *J Physiol* 2005;567:27–32.

226. Weinman EJ, Wang Y, Wang F, Greer C, Steplock D, Shenolikar S. A C-terminal PDZ motif in NHE3 binds NHERF-1 and enhances cAMP inhibition of sodium-hydrogen exchange. *Biochemistry* 2003;42:12662–12668.

227. White FJ, Bednarz LM, Wachtel SR, Hjorth S, Brooderson RJ. Is stimulation of both D1 and D2 receptors necessary for the expression of dopamine-mediated behaviors? *Pharmacol Biochem Behav* 1988;30:189–193.

228. Winaver J, Burnett JC, Tyce GM, Dousa TP. ANP inhibits Na(+)-H+ antiport in proximal tubular brush border membrane: role of dopamine. *Kidney Int* 1990;38:1133–1140.

229. Wise RA, Bozarth MA. Brain mechanisms of drug reward and euphoria. *Psychiatr Med* 1985;3:445–460.

230. Worth DP, Harvey JN, Brown J, Worral A, Lee MR. Domperidone treatment in man inhibits the fall in plasma renin activity induced by intravenous gamma-L-glutamyl-L-dopa. *Br J Clin Pharmacol* 1986;21:497–502.

231. Xu J, Li XX, Albrecht FE, Hopfer U, Carey RM, Jose PA. Dopamine receptor, G(salpha), and Na(+)-H(+) exchanger interactions in the kidney in hypertension. *Hypertension* 2000;36:395–399.

232. Yao LP, Li XX, Yu PY, Xu J, Asico LD, Jose PA. Dopamine D1 receptor and protein kinase C isoforms in spontaneously hypertensive rats. *Hypertension* 1998;32:1049–1053.

233. Yamaguchi I, Yao L, Sanada H, Ozono R, Mouradian MM, Jose PA, Carey RM, Felder RA. Dopamine D1A receptors and renin release in rat juxtaglomerular cells. *Hypertension* 1997;29:962–968.

234. Yamaguchi I, Walk SF, Felder RA. Studying the dopaminergic system with transfected receptors. *Hypertens Res* 1995;18 (Suppl 1):S19–S22.

235. Yen TT, Yu P, Roeder H, Willard PW. A genetic study of hypertension in Okamoto-Aoki spontaneously hypertensive rats. *Heredity* 1974;33:309–316.

236. Yu P, Asico LD, Luo Y, Andrews P, Eisner GM, Hopfer U, Felder RA, Jose PA. D1 dopamine receptor hyperphosphorylation in renal proximal tubules in hypertension. *Kidney Int* 2006;70:1072–1079.

237. Zawarynski P, Tallerico T, Seeman P, Lee SP, O'Dowd BF, George SR. Dopamine D2 receptor dimers in human and rat brain. *FEBS Lett* 1998;441:383–386.

238. Zelenina M, Zelenin S, Bondar AA, Brismar H, Aperia A. Water permeability of aquaporin-4 is decreased by protein kinase C and dopamine. *Am J Physiol* 2002;283:F309–F318.

239. Zeng C, Eisner GM, Felder RA, Jose PA. Dopamine receptor and hypertension. *Curr Med Chem Cardiovasc Hematol Agents* 2005;3:69–77.

240. Zhang J, Ferguson SS, Barak LS, Aber MJ, Giros B, Lefkowitz RJ, Caron MG. Molecular mechanisms of G protein-coupled receptor signaling: role of G protein–coupled receptor kinases and arrestins in receptor desensitization and resensitization. *Receptors Channels* 1997;5:193–199.

241. Zoli M, Agnati LF, Hedlund PB, Li XM, Ferre S, Fuxe K. Receptor-receptor interactions as an integrative mechanism in nerve cells. *Mol Neurobiol* 1993;7:293–334.

CHAPTER **19**

Uroguanylin and Guanylin

ENDOCRINE LINK CONNECTING THE INTESTINE AND KIDNEY FOR REGULATION OF SODIUM BALANCE

Leonard Ralph Forte, Jr. and Manasses Claudino Fonteles
University of Missouri School of Medicine, Missouri; The Harry S Truman Memorial Veterans' Hospital, Columbia, Missouri, USA
Universidade Presbiteriana Mackenzie, São Paulo, Brazil

ABSTRACT

Guanylin and uroguanylin are small peptides that are produced in the intestinal mucosa and regulate cellular function through activation of receptor-guanylate cyclase signaling molecules locally in target cells of intestine and at a distance in the body via endocrine pathways. Their discovery stems from studies of bacterial toxins implicated in mechanisms underlying a disorder given the trivial name, traveler's diarrhea. This cholera-like disease is associated with intense diarrhea with marked loss of fluid and electrolytes induced by bacterial peptides that pathologically mimic the actions of guanylin and uroguanylin. However, physiological roles of the natural peptide hormones involve regulation of body sodium balance in times when animals are exposed to excess levels of sodium chloride in the environment or in the diet. Discovery of an orphan receptor-guanylate cyclase for microbial toxins and demonstration that toxin peptides elicit strong natriuretic responses in the isolated perfused kidney opened up a new area of endocrinology involving the peptide hormones, uroguanylin and guanylin. These intestinal natriuretic hormones may act physiologically in the body by a novel endocrine axis linking the intestine and kidney for regulation of body sodium homeostasis. Administration of oral salt loads in vivo elicit marked increases in urinary salt excretion that are uroguanylin-dependent because transgenic uroguanylin$^{-/-}$ mice exhibit impaired natriuretic responses to oral salt loads and have elevated blood pressure. High-salt diets in mammals or adaptation to seawater in the eel stimulate uroguanylin and guanylin mRNA expression in the intestine. The intestine responds to salt with increased secretion of both peptides. High salt also increases uroguanylin mRNA levels in the kidney. Therefore, uroguanylin is likely to serve in an endocrine link between the intestine and kidney, whereas this peptide could also act locally within the kidney as a physiological means of regulating body sodium balance. Additional evidence for uroguanylin's influence on sodium balance is derived from experiments of nature where it has been shown that sodium retention secondary to either heart failure or the nephrotic syndrome is associated with marked increases in uroguanylin levels in vivo. These findings reveal that uroguanylin functions as a counterregulatory hormone in physiological states associated with excess body sodium levels. Finally, we propose that uroguanylin and guanylin may also act to regulate salt excretion by the intestine in times when animals are exposed to high levels of salt in their environment. The physiological actions that regulate body sodium balance may have been important selective pressures guiding the evolution of uroguanylin and guanylin, thus maintaining their distinctive structures and activities for about 400 million years that separate fish and man.

BACKGROUND

Without water there is no life and sodium chloride (NaCl, salt) is essential for life as we know it. Salt and water are inseparable components of what Claude Bernard called the *milieu intérieur* or the internal environment of cells. Sodium, with its attendant anions, contributes greatly to maintaining the osmotic pressure of the fluid bathing all cells of the body. Salt and water go hand in hand in such way that increases in sodium absorption by the gastrointestinal (GI) organ system could ultimately expand the body fluid volume. If this were to occur together with a low of rate of sodium and water excretion by the kidney, it would generate fluid retention and cause edema (91). Naturally, the opposite can occur as well, because loss of salt and water during diarrhea leads to dehydration and electrolyte imbalances, which is one of the leading causes of infant death in developing countries. Management of salt and water links all living vertebrate species to their ancestors and their origins in a seawater environment (92).

Research in the 20th century contributed greatly to understanding how body fluid volume is maintained through mechanisms involving the pituitary gland and one of its peptide hormones, antidiuretic hormone (ADH, vasopressin). Moreover, discovery that the adrenal gland contains hormonelike substances that influence both carbohydrate and salt balance have provided wonderful insights into how body fluid and electrolytes are regulated. ADH secretion is regulated by plasma osmolality and water deprivation leads to the increase of ADH secretion to act on the kidney for water conservation. The mineral-influencing components of adrenal cortex are steroid hormones, such as aldosterone. Production of aldosterone is regulated by the renin–angiotensin axis leading to increased aldosterone secretion, which regulates sodium, chloride, and potassium excretion by the kidney. A contribution of this endocrine system to the regulation of blood pressure has been known for some time and angiotensin II, of course, directly influences blood pressure through its actions to constrict blood vessels. This physiological mechanism involves a regulatory axis that links adrenal glands with juxtaglomerular cells of renal tubules in the kidney. Thus, two factors were recognized as major regulators of body fluid volume and sodium balance and these endocrine mechanisms helped regulate salt and water during times of deprivation. Physiological regulation often works on the principle of counterregulatory forces—a "push-pull" sort of phenomenon. This concept raises a fundamental question concerning the maintenance of sodium balance when the body is flooded with excess salt from the environment. Major physiological forces must exist to deal with this circumstance because simply turning off the hormones that conserve salt and water is not an intellectually satisfying rationale. One or more physiological means to stimulate the excretion of salt from the body should exist to deal with circumstances when excess salt enters the body. One of the concepts, initially proposed more than four decades ago, was the existence of a "third factor," in addition to ADH and aldosterone, which could promote the loss of salt and water by the kidney.

Contemporary thoughts concerning mechanisms for control of body sodium balance assumes that several natriuretic/diuretic substances may exist in the body for regulation of salt and fluid homeostasis in vertebrates. The biological concept of third factor was primarily due to the extensive research by Professor H. E. DeWardener and his colleagues in England. Investigations into the underlying cause of a remarkably robust natriuresis and diuresis caused by blood volume expansion with saline solutions led to their hypothesis that natriuresis and diuresis under these conditions could not be explained by the existing knowledge (14). Therefore, a third factor was postulated to exist for control of salt and fluid volume homeostasis. A search for blood-borne substances with powerful natriuretic and diuretic activities ensued with limited success, including a proposal by originators of the third factor hypothesis concerning putative central nervous system (CNS)–derived factors with such an activity (15). A truly seminal discovery was made in 1981 by Professor Adolfo de Bold and his colleagues in Toronto, Canada who isolated a powerful natriuretic and diuretic factor from atrial muscle of rat hearts that was named atrial natriuretic factor (ANF) (13). We know recognize that ANF represents three small peptide hormones derived from three related, but different genes encoding precursor polypeptides, which have at their C-termini the active peptide domains for atriopeptin-A (ANP), BNP, and CNP. Physiological roles for these hormones are complex, but one fundamental biological activity is germane to this topic. ANP is produced by the myocardium and released into the circulation when the blood volume is increased by saline infusion (80). An endocrine axis between the heart and kidney via ANP appears to be responsible for the saliuresis and diuresis that occurs under this condition of body fluid expansion. This notion is supported by recent gene knock-out (KO) experiments for the ANP receptor, GC-A, which showed that GC-A–deficient mice do not respond appropriately to saline infusion (51). Thus, one of the third factors proposed to exist by DeWardener is likely to be ANP. Atriopeptins, however, do not appear to have major actions in the control of body sodium balance during postprandial states when dietary salt enters the body. Another factor or factors is likely to be the major player for control of sodium balance during times when excess salt is either consumed in the diet or derived from the environment. Therefore, it is likely that third factor is not one, but several endogenous regulatory mechanisms that govern sodium balance. This makes sense because the control of sodium balance is an exceedingly important physiological process that is necessary for life.

One of the sodium-regulating hormones was discovered through investigations focused on the underlying cellular mechanisms associated with a disorder given the trivial name of traveler's diarrhea. An important, but at the time unrecognized, connection between this disease and regulation of postprandial sodium balance was discovered in the mid-1970s. Dr. Robert Carey and his colleagues at the University of Virginia demonstrated initially in sodium-depleted rabbits, and later in human subjects, that oral salt loads cause a sustained natriuresis, which greatly exceeds the increase in urinary sodium excretion produced by intravenous (IV) infusion of the same amount of NaCl (2, 62). It was important to use hypertonic solutions of salt administered IV so that blood volumes were not expanded. Expansion of blood volume would cause a marked natriuresis and diuresis by a different mechanism, thus obscuring the natriuretic effects elicited by oral salt. An intriguing hypothesis was invoked to explain this simple finding. They proposed that oral salt loads are detected by some sensory mechanism within the GI organ system, which causes the release of one or more substances from the GI tract that, in turn, stimulates the urinary excretion of salt. Such a factor could be an "intestinal natriuretic hormone" (e.g., INF) that links together the GI system and kidney for regulation of sodium balance in the postprandial state. It may be accidental that studies leading to Carey's INF hypothesis and investigations of guanosine cyclic 3′,5′-monophosphate (cGMP)–dependent mechanisms underlying traveler's diarrhea both occurred at the University of Virginia in the 1970s. Dr. Richard Guerrant and his collaborators were the first to report that heat-stable enterotoxin (stable toxin, ST) peptides activate guanylate cyclase (GC) in the intestine as a means of stimulating intestinal fluid secretion (46). This finding was extended by an elegant analysis of the biological activity of ST peptides by

Dr. Michael Field and his coworkers (18). Discovery that *Escherichia coli* ST stimulates intestinal secretion via the intracellular second messenger, cGMP, stimulated interest in this area and led to further investigations into the mechanism (35, 39, 83). *E. coli* ST was actually the first agonist molecule that was shown to selectively stimulate cGMP production in any vertebrate tissue. Moreover, this finding would eventually lead to the discovery of two candidate hormones for the INF postulated by Carey for the control of sodium balance (2, 62). This did not occur in a timely fashion, however, because other developments in the field of cGMP signaling would intervene.

DISCOVERY OF GUANYLIN AND UROGUANYLIN

It has been generally forgotten that the first activator of cGMP signal transduction pathways that was discovered in vertebrates is a pharmacological mimic of the native peptide hormones of intestine. ST peptides secreted by enterotoxigenic bacteria that cause a cholera-like form of diarrhea were the first agonists discovered that selectively activate receptor–GC signal transduction. The novel GC molecules targeted by *E. coli* ST are located at their highest densities in the body on the apical surfaces of epithelial cells comprising the intestinal mucosa (reviewed in 30). Activation of this cell-surface GC leads to rapid and large increases in cGMP. In turn, cGMP elicits complex changes in cellular function, which are best described in the intestine for the action to stimulate transepithelial secretion of chloride, bicarbonate, sodium, and water into the intestinal lumen. *E. coli* ST also inhibits sodium absorption by the intestine. Pharmacological actions of ST peptides elicited during an intestinal infection with enterotoxigenic bacteria result in large increases in fecal excretion of salt and water. Discovery that *E. coli* ST activates cGMP production was first reported in 1978 leading to a series of investigations into the basic actions of ST peptides in the intestine (18, 46). This story is a fascinating body of evidence that would, in time, lead to isolation of the endogenous ST-like peptide hormones (10, 40). The path to discovery of guanylin and uroguanylin could have been short and direct so that these cGMP-regulating hormones would be remembered as prototypical for the three types of cGMP-regulating molecules that are known to activate specific types of receptor–GC molecules. However, the cGMP-signaling stage was soon to be dominated by the discovery of another cGMP-regulating substance. Professor Robert Furchgott and his coworker, John Zawadzki, discovered a substance derived from the vascular endothelium that relaxes smooth muscle and lowers blood pressure (33). They named this substance endothelium-derived relaxing factor (EDRF), which was subsequently shown to be nitric oxide. This seminal discovery was soon followed by isolation of ANF from myocardium by de Bold et al. (13). These two major discoveries at the beginning of the 1980s quickly eclipsed previous

reports describing the ST-dependent cGMP pathway of intestine associated with traveler's diarrhea (18, 46). Research leading to the isolation of ST/INF-like peptides would have to wait while the attention of investigators in the cGMP-signaling arena turned to EDRF and ANF.

Diarrhea is one of the main causes of child morbidity and mortality in the developing world. While many different microbes cause diarrhea, the cholera-like disorders produced by enteric infections with bacteria that secrete ST peptides into the intestinal lumen are of major clinical significance (19, 36). One of the main pathogens involved are strains of *E. coli*. However other enteric bacteria carry genes for the inactive pro-ST peptides, which must be cleaved to liberate bioactive ST peptides that stimulate cGMP production in the intestine causing diarrhea (30). During the 1980s when the cGMP world centered its attention on EDRF and ANF, two laboratories, one in the northern and the other in the southern part of the American continent, conducted studies that would ultimately foreshadow the isolation of endogenous ST/INF-like peptides. When ST is injected into ligated loops of rabbit intestine, this toxin promotes intense fluid secretion that imitates clinical diarrhea (64). Considering the intestine as another form of nephron, Lima and Fonteles investigated the renal actions of *E. coli* ST using the isolated perfused rat kidney (65). Using partially purified extract of *E. coli* ST in this preparation, one of the authors (MCF) observed in 1983 that ST has potent natriuretic, kaliuretic, and diuretic actions in the kidney. These data were presented in a symposium at the annual meeting of the Brazilian Society of Physiology (65). Unbeknown to the southerners, investigations in a laboratory in the north also found evidence for actions of ST in the kidney. One of the authors (LRF) and his friend and colleague, the late Professor Arnold A. White, discovered a kidney cell line that exhibits robust cGMP accumulation responses to *E. coli* ST (24, 99). It is quite interesting to reconsider this finding now, with the clear vision of hindsight, because the cells that were used for these studies were the proximal tubular-like, OK cell line. OK is short for opossum kidney and this cell line was originally isolated from the kidney of a North American opossum. OK and PtK-2 cells are the only two kidney cell lines that have been found that have such a robust cGMP response to ST. It is of some interest that both cell lines were derived from marsupial mammals. The PtK-2 cell line was derived from a potaroo, which is a very small kangaroo. Potaroos were not readily available in America, but the opossum is abundant in Missouri and this mammalian species proved to be a valuable animal model. The first report in 1988 derived from this line of inquiry characterized the ST-dependent cGMP signaling mechanism in OK and PtK-2 cells and in opossum kidney cortex (24). Marked increases in cGMP accumulation occurred when OK cells or kidney cortex slices were exposed to *E. coli* ST. Quantitative responses of cGMP to ST are similar in both renal cortex and small intestine (Fig. 1). A series of investigations revealed that bacterial ST peptides activate an orphan receptor

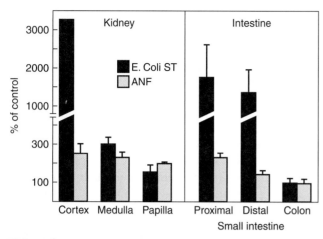

FIGURE 1 Stimulation of guanosine cyclic 3′,5′-monophosphate (cGMP) production by *Escherichia coli* ST and atrial natriuretic factor (ANF) in opossum kidney and intestine. Data are means ± standard error of six animals for kidney cortex and medulla slices, two for papilla, and five animals for intestinal mucosa suspensions. (See Forte, LR, WJ Krause, and RH Freeman. Receptors and cGMP signaling mechanism for *E. coli* enterotoxin in opossum kidney. *Am J Physiol* 1988;255:F1040–F1046, for details.).

found in the kidney, as well as in other organs of the opossum (24, 25, 54, 99). To pharmacologists, orphan receptors provide a clear signal that receptors exist for regulation by one or more endogenous peptide hormones, neurotransmitters, etc. This basic concept must have been overlooked when the ST-dependent GC activities of intestine were first reported (18, 46). Experiments with more highly purified preparations of *E. coli* ST in the isolated perfused kidney model confirmed previous results, which were reported at the USA-Japan Cholera Symposium in 1991 (20). The first published reports demonstrating the natriuretic activity of ST in the perfused kidney by Lima et al. (66, 67) appeared in 1992, shortly before the discovery of guanylin was reported by Currie et al. (10).

Guanylin was initially isolated from rat intestine by Dr. Mark Currie in his laboratory at the Medical University of South Carolina with the final purification steps and sequence analyses accomplished later during his tenure at Monsanto Co (10). The cDNAs encoding rat and human forms of preproguanylin were then isolated by molecular cloning (100, 101). In a collaborative effort between one of the author's (L.R.F.) and Dr. Currie, a second ST-like peptide was purified from opossum urine and named uroguanylin (40). Opossum guanylin was also isolated from opossum intestine, which revealed that at least two different peptides exist to regulate receptor-GC activity in target cells. Prouroguanylin and proguanylin were then isolated from opossum intestine, which defined the primary structures of the precursor polypeptides and demonstrated that the prohormones were inactive in cGMP bioassays (41, 42). Although *E. coli* ST was the first molecule to be recognized as a cGMP-regulating peptide in vertebrates, guanylin and uroguanylin were the third and last of three independent families of cGMP-regulating agonists to be identified at the

molecular level. This delay in identifying the natural ST-like hormones, taken together with the pathway of discovery that meandered through an obscure field of tropical medicine, has led to basic misunderstandings of the possible role(s) for guanylin peptides in the body. We will return to this point later. In analogy to the current view that atriopeptins act locally on the myocardium and serve as endocrine hormones for the kidney and blood vessels, guanylin and uroguanylin, act both locally on the intestine and at distant sites such as renal tubules and other epithelia. Information gathered in the early years of research defining the pathological actions of ST peptides has provided little insight to guide research defining the major physiological roles for the guanylin family of peptide hormones. However, enteric bacteria have performed a useful service by producing potent analogues of guanylin peptides with interesting pharmacological as well as potentially useful therapeutic properties [reviewed in (30)].

Considerable research has revealed that, for most vertebrate species, two genes exist that encode preproguanylin and preprouroguanylin precursor molecules. The primary structures of active guanylin and uroguanylin peptides that are produced in representative vertebrate species compared to selected ST peptides are shown in Fig. 2. Most guanylin and uroguanylin peptides have some similarity, although the shared cysteine residues account for much of the identity between peptides. Disulfide bonds occur between first to third and second to fourth cysteines in guanylin and urogua-

GUANYLIN

Mammalian
Opossum   S H T C E I C A F A A C A G C
Human   P G T C E I C A Y A A C T G C

Teleost
Zebrafish V D V C E I C A F A A C T G C
Fugu   L D L C E I C A F A A C T G C
Eel   Y D E C E I C M F A A C T G C

UROGUANYLIN

Mammalian
Opossum   Q E D C E L C I N V A C T G C
Human   N D D C E L C V N V A C T G C L

Teleost
Zebrafish I D P C E I C A N V A C T G C
Fugu   L D P C E I C A N P S C F G C L N
Eel   P D P C E I C A N A A C T G C L

BACTERIAL ST PEPTIDES

V. cholerae ST   I D C C E I C C N P A C F G C L N
E. coli ST   N Y C C E L C C N P A C T G C Y

FIGURE 2 Primary structures of guanylin, uroguanylin, and bacterial ST peptides. Single-letter abbreviations for the amino acids are used. The peptides are aligned using the conserved cysteine residues found in the three classes of peptides. Sequences for zebrafish and fugu peptides were derived from their respective genome sequencing projects and the eel peptides were taken from Yuge S, Inoue K, Hyodo S, Takei Y. A novel guanylin family (guanylin, uroguanylin, and renoguanylin) in eels. Possible osmoregulatory hormones in intestine and kidney. *J Biol Chem* 2003;278: 22726–22733.

nylin. The disulfides influence conformation, and thus, biological activities of the peptides. ST peptides also exhibit the same cysteine disulfide linkages, but ST peptides have another pair of cysteines and a third disulfide bond that contributes to their biological activities (34). Two vertebrate species have also been identified thus far that produce three different guanylin-like peptides. A novel uroguanylin-related peptide was identified in the opossum by molecular cloning of cDNAs encoding its precursor polypeptide (23, 29). This peptide was named lymphoguanylin because it was first identified as an expressed mRNA in lymphoid tissues of opossums. The euryhaline teleosts, *Anguilla anguilla* and *Anguilla japonica*, also produce a third peptide, which was identified by cloning cDNAs encoding the precursors of guanylin, uroguanylin, and renaguanylin of eels (102). The biological significance of this form of guanylin gene expansion in the opossum and eel is presently unclear. However, it is likely that other examples will be identified when the relatively numerous genome projects are completed in the next few years. It would not be surprising to discover vertebrate species that must rely on a single guanylin/uroguanylin-like gene as well as other species that exhibit three or more genes.

The biological activities of uroguanylin, guanylin and two different *E. coli* ST peptides were compared in kidney and intestinal cell models. Stimulation of cGMP accumulation by agonists in kidney (OK) and intestinal (T84) cell lines are depicted in Figs. 3 and 4. It can be seen that activation of OK-GC in OK cells (68) by the agonists reveals a distinct order of potency with full-length ST being more potent than the N-terminal truncated ST peptide (Fig. 3). Both STs are substantially more potent than uroguanylin, which is more potent than guanylin. This bioassay clearly demonstrates the significant increase in potency that has been achieved by enteric bacteria through microbial evolution of

the active ST peptide domains [reviewed in (30)]. Activation of GC-C in T84 cells demonstrates that human GC-C does not discriminate between full-length and truncated ST peptides, although both ST peptides are more potent than uroguanylin and guanylin (Fig. 4) (43). In T84 cells, similar to findings in the OK cell cGMP bioassay, uroguanylin is more potent than guanylin for activation of the human GC-C receptor. Thus, *E. coli* ST is a superagonist at cognate receptors for guanylin and uroguanylin. Because of this pharmacological property, the microbial ST peptides may turn out to be the most useful peptide agonists for future therapeutic applications (30).

A PHYSIOLOGICAL ROLE FOR UROGUANYLIN AND GUANYLIN IN THE KIDNEY

In the initial studies defining the basic biological properties of guanylin and uroguanylin, it was postulated that the hormones are novel candidates for INF (e.g., intestinal natriuretic factor) that was postulated to exist in the GI system by Professor Carey and his coworkers (2, 62). INF was conceived to be one or more enteric "hormones" that serve in a novel endocrine axis connecting the GI system with the kidney as a means of regulating renal sodium excretion in the postprandial state. The seeds for this concept were initially derived from discovery of an orphan receptor-GC for ST in OK cells and in renal proximal tubules of the opossum (24, 25, 99). The renal responses to *E. coli* ST were measured in the opossum demonstrating that ST elicited marked increases in urinary cGMP without affecting cAMP excretion (24, 25). In the initial experiments, ST did not significantly increase the urinary excretion of NaCl, whereas ANP elicited

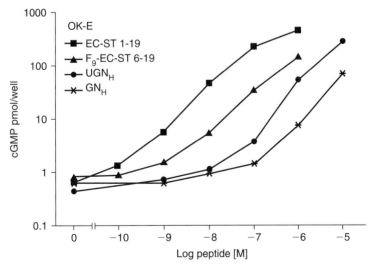

FIGURE 3 Stimulation of guanosine cyclic 3′,5′-monophosphate (cGMP) production in OK cells by uroguanylin, guanylin and *Escherichia coli* ST peptides. Synthetic peptides for human uroguanylin (UGN$_H$), human guanylin (GN$_H$), full-length *E. coli* ST (EC-ST 1-19), and N-terminal truncated *E. coli* ST (F$_9$-EC-ST 6-19). See references 24 and 25 for bioassay description.

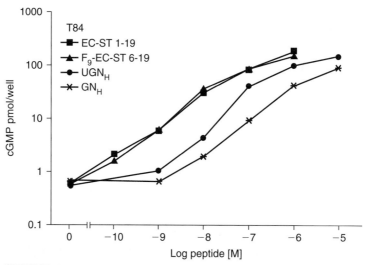

FIGURE 4   Stimulation of guanosine cyclic 3′,5′-monophosphate (cGMP) production in T84 cells by uroguanylin, guanylin, and *Escherichia coli* ST peptides. Synthetic peptides for human uroguanylin (UGN_H), human guanylin (GN_H), full-length *E. coli* ST (EC-ST 1-19) and N-terminal truncated *E. coli* ST (F_9-EC-ST 6-19). See references 24 and 25 for bioassay description.

a characteristic saliuresis (Fig. 5). However, another study was carried out using a larger dose of ST and significant increases in urinary sodium, chloride and cGMP excretion were observed (26). A substantial body of experimental evidence has subsequently accumulated, which clearly demonstrates the natriuretic, chloriuretic, and kaliuretic activities of guanylin, uroguanylin, and ST peptides (3, 7, 20–23, 65–67, 84, 85). Treatment with *E. coli* ST elicits a rapid and sustained increase in the urinary excretion of sodium, chloride and potassium (65–67). Thus, it was clear that activation of receptor-GCs in the kidney resulted in robust natriuretic responses even before guanylin and uroguanylin were identified. However, discovery of receptors for *E. coli* ST in the kidney and defining a natriuretic response of the kidney to this peptide in vivo and ex vivo was insufficient to formulate a clear and distinct working hypothesis to explain the experimental results. The isolation of biologically active ST-like peptides from rat intestine and opossum urine provided a key piece of information to help solve the puzzle (10, 40). Uroguanylin is more closely related to the ST peptides with respect to their primary structures and biological activities than are guanylin peptides (reviewed in 30). Also, urine contains little or no active guanylin (17, 40, 52) and receptors for *E. coli* ST are localized to brush border membranes of opossum kidney proximal tubular cells (24, 25, 54). Studies defining the circulating forms of uroguanylin and guanylin indicate that both peptides circulate in plasma, but only proguanylin, and not active guanylin, circulates in the blood stream (11, 58, 60, 74). Both uroguanylin and prouroguanylin circulate in the plasma (16, 44, 50, 75, 76). Taken together, these findings suggest that uroguanylin and prouroguanylin can be delivered to renal tubules by glomerular filtration. Prouroguanylin appearing in the tubular filtrate, which has

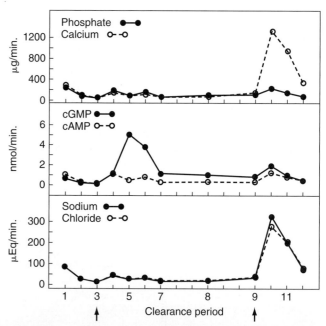

FIGURE 5   Comparison of effects of *Escherichia coli* enterotoxin with atrial natriuretic factor (ANF) on renal excretion of guanosine cyclic 3′,5′-monophosphate (cGMP), cAMP, NaCl, phosphate and calcium in opossums. Each clearance period is 10 minutes long except for periods 7 and 8, which are 30 minutes long. The first arrow denotes intravenous injection of 10 μg ST and the second arrow denotes intravenous injection of 10 μg ANF. (See Forte, LR, WJ Krause, and RH Freeman. Receptors and cGMP signaling mechanism for *E. coli* enterotoxin in opossum kidney. *Am J Physiol* 1988;255:F1040–F1046.)

no biological activity per se, must then be converted into bioactive uroguanylin within renal tubules because prouroguanylin is not detected in urine (40, 75). This finding indicates that uroguanylin-converting enzymes are probably localized to the brush border membranes of renal proximal tubular cells for proteolytic conversion of inactive prouroguanylin to active uroguanylin peptides, which are found in urine at relatively high concentrations. A key structural property, which is uniquely conserved in the uroguanylin and ST peptides, but is not found in guanylin peptides, is the asn residues that make uroguanylin and ST peptides highly resistant to attack by endoproteases like chymotrypsin (41, 42). In contrast, guanylin is readily degraded by chymotrypsin, which attacks the peptide C-terminal to the aromatic amino acids (e.g., tyr or phe) that are uniquely found in guanylin (10, 40). This sensitivity to hydrolysis and inactivation by proteases within renal tubules is likely to account for the relative absence of bioactive guanylin in urine (17, 40, 52). Moreover, hydrolysis and inactivation of filtered proguanylin can be predicted to serve as a physiological mechanism that limits the kidney's response to circulating forms of proguanylin. Experimental support for this concept has been provided by studies using the isolated perfused kidney where it has been clearly demonstrated that renal actions of guanylin ex vivo are greatly enhanced by the administration of protease inhibitors (21, 85). In another experimental approach, the oral administration of protease inhibitors together with guanylin to the suckling mouse model also enhances the action of guanylin to stimulate intestinal secretion. Guanylin administered alone has little effect on the suckling mouse intestine. In contrast, uroguanylin or ST peptides exert potent stimulation of intestinal secretion in the mouse bioassay in vivo even in the absence of treatment with protease inhibitors (37). Thus, guanylin and uroguanylin are quite different peptides with respect to their sensitivity or resistance, respectively, to proteolytic degradation. It is likely that this contrasting property of guanylin versus uroguanylin contributes to the apparent physiological selectivity of target cells in the nephron. It can be postulated that proteases located in proximal tubules cleaves the guanylin peptides within the proguanylin molecules that enter renal tubules via filtration at glomeruli. Alternatively, guanylin peptides could be degraded following the liberation of active guanylin from proguanylin in the filtrate. This type of proteolytic enzyme mechanism could prevent activation of receptors located on the apical side of renal tubular cells by guanylin, thus permitting uroguanylin peptides in the tubular filtrate to selectively activate receptors in the nephron. By this sort of mechanism, kidney function could be regulated by uroguanylin peptides that are secreted by the GI organ system into the circulation to communicate with the kidney in a novel endocrine axis. It was this sort of information that led to the postulate that uroguanylin may act physiologically in the body much like the hypothetical INF postulated by Carey as a physiological means for maintaining body sodium balance in the postprandial state (28). The molecular identity of proteases that act to either degrade guanylin to inactive forms or serve as converting enzymes to release active guanylin and uroguanylin peptides from their prohormone polypeptides are important, but unanswered questions.

Several other features of uroguanylin are consistent with the proposition of uroguanylin as a potential INF that is released from the GI system into the circulation when excess salt is consumed in the diet. Relatively high concentrations of uroguanylin are found in the proximal small intestine and the gastric mucosa produces uroguanylin, and not guanylin (7, 12, 17, 72, 76, 79, 82). The location of uroguanylin-secreting cells in the proximal GI tract seems to be a physiologically appropriate site where uroguanylin could be released into the circulation upon consumption of dietary NaCl (72, 76, 79, 82). A sodium sensor in the GI system has been considered as a physiological mechanism for some time, although no specific cellular machinery for detecting sodium has been revealed in studies thus far. It seems reasonable to consider that a sodium detection mechanism in the GI system exists, which is connected by some other means to physiological processes that regulate secretion of natriuretic hormones, such as uroguanylin, from the stomach and/or intestine into the circulation. This conceptual framework helps explain how uroguanylin (or guanylin) could act in the body to modulate urinary salt excretion in the postprandial state. Moreover, a novel endocrine link between the intestine and kidney is a physiologically sensible as well as an elegant mechanism for maintaining body sodium homeostasis.

EVOLUTION OF TWO GUANYLIN GENES

A key question pertaining to the physiological roles of guanylin and uroguanylin in the body is: Why have the genes encoding guanylin and uroguanylin been so highly conserved throughout vertebrate evolution so that two, apparently similar peptide hormones, exist in vertebrates from fish to mammals? These two genes were derived from duplication (98) of an ancestral gene that occurred at some point quite early during the evolution of vertebrates [reviewed in (30)]. While some differences in primary structures of the active peptide domains have occurred over the course of ~400 million years of time, as revealed in the uroguanylin and guanylin peptides of extant teleosts and mammals, the two cGMP-regulating peptides remain separate and distinct structures (Fig. 2). There must be one or more compelling reasons of substantial physiological significance that have contributed to maintaining the structurally distinct natures of guanylin and uroguanylin hormones over this long period of evolutionary time. We propose the hypothesis that duplication of an ancestral gene encoding a single prototypic guanylin/uroguanylin-like peptide resulted in two genes, which then could evolve separately to produce two distinctly different regulatory hormones with each peptide satisfying different physiological purposes in the body. Furthermore, the evolution of uroguanylin and its companion signaling pathways in target cells is likely to control a particularly important biological activity in vertebrates: the maintenance of body sodium balance. Uroguanylin may, in fact, be a major regulatory factor for maintenance of sodium homeostasis when animals are exposed to excess salt. Emerging information consistent with this concept for uroguanylin as a sodium-regulating hormone is found in recent studies of euryhaline teleosts, such as *Anguilla anguilla* and *Anguilla japonica*. The eel, like some other ocean-dwelling creatures, has the fascinating physiological capability of being able to adapt for life in either fresh water or seawater. This is an extraordinary capability for living exposed to either very low or extremely high concentrations of NaCl in the environment. Following duplication of an ancestral form of guanylin/uroguanylin-like gene, a nascent proto-uroguanylin gene could evolve independently into the genes found in vertebrates today. As the NaCl concentrations of seawater increased over time, ocean-living vertebrates evolved distinct physiological processes for living in a very salty world. The eel has been extensively used as an experimental model for euryhaline fish that live in both fresh water and seawater environments. Experiments with this teleost species have provided key evidence of a biological mechanism involving uroguanylin and sodium homeostasis. Professor Gordon Cramb and his colleagues at St. Andrews University in Scotland have identified and reported a primary structure for the first teleost "guanylin" peptides of fish, which actually turned out to be the eel form of uroguanylin (8). These investigators also cloned partial cDNAs encoding two different forms of GC-C in the eel that are derived from different genes (9). GC-C was first identified as a receptor-GC expressed in rat intestine that binds selectively to and is activated by *E. coli* ST (86, 96). Thus, GC-C was the first cognate receptor identified at the molecular level for the endogenous peptide hormones, uroguanylin and guanylin. Genome projects reveal that only one GC-C gene occurs in Eutherian mammals, indicating that a single cGMP-signaling molecule exists to serve as a cell-surface receptor for the guanylin hormones in placental mammals. However, the eel, living as a mobile fresh to seawater traveler, has evolved two distinct receptor GC-C proteins, and also, has developed a third and structurally unique form of guanylin-like peptide named renoguanylin (102). So, the eel has two different GC-C-like receptors that can bind to and be activated by eel guanylin, uroguanylin, and renoguanylin peptides. Both forms of GC-C receptors in the eel respond to these peptides with increases in cGMP production (personal communication from Professor Y. Takei). Exposure of freshwater–adapted eels to seawater results in the upregulation of one form of GC-C mRNA in the intestinal mucosa (9, 102). Moreover, uroguanylin and guanylin mRNA levels of intestinal mucosa are also increased when fresh-water–adapted eels are exposed to a seawater environment (8, 102). Thus, uroguanylin, guanylin, and GC-C gene expression are upregulated in the intestine when fresh-water–adapted eels are exposed to seawater. The temptation is quite strong to predict that amplification of genes encoding both the first messenger molecules and receptor-GC proteins is linked to the euryhaline nature of eels. This important finding suggests that uroguanylin and guanylin, together with one of their cognate receptors, are upregulated in the intestine as part of a physiological mechanism for adaptation of eels to high salt in the ocean. Although it is clear that eels can adapt to seawater, there are major questions yet to be posed concerning a physiological role for uroguanylin and guanylin in this intriguing form of biological adaptation to salt. It is quite conceivable that uroguanylin and guanylin serve in a novel endocrine axis, perhaps between the GI system and the kidney or other organs involved in body sodium homeostasis such as the gills. Local actions of uroguanylin and guanylin within the intestine per se should also be considered as viable possibilities for controlling body sodium levels. Uroguanylin-regulated cGMP signaling mechanisms connected to body sodium homeostasis may be especially needed by the eel because of the animal's exposure to high levels of salt in seawater. Salt in the ocean inescapably enters their GI system, thus eels are continually ingesting high levels of NaCl. Sodium absorbed by the GI tract must then be excreted to maintain plasma sodium levels within the narrow limits required for normal cellular functions. It is likely that a physiological role for the uroguanylin/guanylin-GC-C–cGMP signaling mechanism appeared early in vertebrate evolution, and such a fundamental role for uroguanylin continues today as an important mechanism for regulating sodium balance. The physiological actions of uroguanylin in the eel may reveal novel biological roles for this peptide hormone that are retained by all vertebrates. In addition, the 400+ million years of time since the last common ancestor of eels and mammals lived is sufficient for the evolution of additional physiological roles for uroguanylin and guanylin. Novel biological actions for both peptide hormones may have arisen during evolution of the "higher" orders of warm-blooded vertebrates, the mammals and birds.

UROGUANYLIN AND BODY SODIUM BALANCE IN MAMMALS

Soon after an orphan receptor-GC was discovered in opossum kidney, a method for in situ labeling of this cell-surface receptor was developed using ^{125}I-ST as a radioligand (25, 54). This receptor assay provided a means to assess both the relative densities and cellular locations of receptor-GC molecules on apical surfaces of epithelial cells within renal tubules, intestinal mucosa, testis, liver, airways, and other epithelial-rich organs of the opossum. Two observations were made that now seem to be of fundamental importance to understanding the biology of uroguanylin-cGMP signaling pathways. Initial observations revealed the location by in situ receptor autoradiography of target epithelial cells bearing this form of receptor-GC in proximal tubules of opossum kidney. Fig. 6 shows the location of target cells for uroguanylin (e.g., ^{125}I-ST) in both the convoluted and straight segments of proximal tubules. It can be

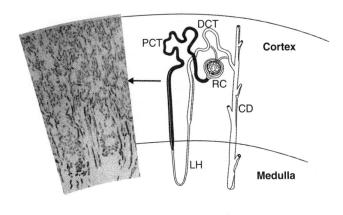

OK-GC receptors

FIGURE 6 Renal tubular cells labeled with ^{125}I-ST to localize uroguanylin/guanylin receptors in opossum kidney. See reference 25 for details of methods. Proximal convoluted tubule (PCT), loop of Henle (LH), distal convoluted tubule (DCT), and collecting duct (CD) describe major portions of the nephron in the diagram adjacent to the autoradiogram depicting silver grains overlying cells that bind to ^{125}I-ST.

seen that glomeruli are not labeled with ^{125}I-ST and these structures appear as holes in this field of view. The relative abundance of receptors in kidney cortex is similar to the densities of receptors on epithelial cells comprising the intestinal mucosa. Thus, opossum kidney produces a remarkably high level of receptor-GCs for uroguanylin, guanylin, and ST peptide agonists that are only matched by receptor densities in the intestinal epithelium. It was fortunate indeed to use OK cells as a model for renal proximal tubules for pilot studies begun in 1987 to see if a ST-stimulated GC activity occurred in the kidney (24, 99). Discovery of receptors for uroguanylin in opossum kidney reinforces the concept that experiments are best carried out where the light shines brightest.

A second basic finding that was made using ^{125}I-ST receptor autoradiography assays with intestinal tissues from vertebrates, including different species of fish, amphibians, reptiles, mammals, and birds, is that virtually all of the epithelial cells comprising the intestinal mucosa exhibit high densities of GC-C-like receptors for guanylin peptides (48, 54–57). Unlike the nephron of opossums, receptors for guanylin peptides are uniformly distributed in epithelial cells lining the intestine. This plain and simple fact was overlooked for some time as investigations described the basic biology of guanylin, uroguanylin, and their cognate receptor-GC signaling molecules. After thinking a bit longer about this fundamental finding in the intestine, it became clear that investigators in this field had been blinded by dogma in the older literature derived from studies of ST-mediated diarrhea. Investigations into the pathological actions of bacterial ST peptides had occurred for many years prior to discovery of guanylin and uroguanylin [reviewed in (19, 36)]. When dogma from the ST years of the 1970s and 1980s was viewed in a different light, a basic concept came to mind. The naturally occurring peptide hormones co-

evolved with GC-C, and thus, guanylin and uroguanylin act specifically for physiological regulation of GC-C receptor activity in the body. Moreover, guanylin and uroguanylin exert their actions on the intestine in a distinctly different way than the pathological actions elicited by toxins secreted by bacteria in an unregulated fashion into the intestinal lumen. Soon after guanylin and uroguanylin were discovered, it was assumed that a prime physiological role for these enteric hormones must be for control of intestinal chloride, bicarbonate and fluid secretion and a number of studies have demonstrated this action (38, 47, 59). Premature assumptions were made that guanylin and uroguanylin act in the body similar to the ST peptides, a view that was extraordinarily short-sighted. One reason for rethinking this concept is that intestinal fluid secretion is carried out by a relatively small fraction of highly specialized cells within the intestinal mucosa. The fact that virtually all epithelial cells comprising the intestinal mucosa express GC-C is inconsistent with a postulate that guanylin and uroguanylin evolved simply to regulate intestinal fluid secretion via cGMP. The remarkably abundant level of GC-C protein in enterocytes, together with a widespread expression of GC-C, in most, if not all epithelial cells comprising the intestinal epithelium, indicates that the guanylin-uroguanylin-dependent GC-C signaling pathway operates at a more fundamental level than merely for regulation of intestinal secretion. In this case, an experiment of nature associated with a common intestinal disorder, traveler's diarrhea, provided insights into and a pathway to discover the natural peptide agonists that regulate cGMP-production in the intestine, but this line of investigation may have obscured the primary physiological roles for guanylin and uroguanylin in the body.

The dogma that guanylin and uroguanylin have physiological actions much like the pathological actions of ST peptides has persisted. The first publication stemming from studies of GC-C KO mice was titled "Disruption of the guanylyl cyclase-C gene leads to a paradoxical phenotype of viable but heat-stable enterotoxin-resistant mice" (87). This title suggests that it was "paradoxical" that mice lacking GC-C were viable. It was certainly not unexpected that GC-C$^{-/-}$ animals failed to respond to the diarrhea-inducing actions of ST peptides. The apparently normal intestinal functions of GC-C KO mice revealed that guanylin peptides regulate some other, heretofore unknown, physiological function(s). Results of experiments in mice with inactivated guanylin genes also revealed animals with an essentially normal phenotype, much like the GC-C KO animals (94). A small difference was observed with respect to the length of intestinal crypts of large intestine in guanylin$^{-/-}$ animals, which was attributed to a potential regulatory action of guanylin on the turnover of epithelial cells in the intestine. Such a potential action of guanylin and/or uroguanylin had been proposed (27). Moreover, additional evidence consistent with physiological regulation of enterocyte turnover by the GC-C signaling pathway was reported following the discovery of potent antitumor actions of uroguanylin. Shailubhai et al. demonstrated that human uroguanylin administered orally to the Min mouse model of colon cancer resulted in a dramatic reduction in the appearance and growth of intestinal tumors (88). Such a biological role for guanylin may be a primary physiological action of this peptide hormone in the colon of mice, where little uroguanylin is produced, but the phenotype of guanylin$^{-/-}$ mice remains essentially that of a normal animal (94). In striking contrast, the physiological characteristics of uroguanylin deficient mice revealed something quite different and these experiments established that uroguanylin has substantial regulatory actions in the body. Professor Mitchell Cohen and his colleagues at the University of Cincinnati demonstrated that uroguanylin$^{-/-}$ animals respond abnormally to oral administration of NaCl loads and also exhibit significant increases in blood pressure (69). When oral salt loads were given to uroguanylin$^{-/-}$ mice, the animals had significantly diminished natriuretic responses compared to the renal responses of wild-type animals. However, natriuretic responses to IV administration of NaCl were similar in uroguanylin$^{-/-}$ and control animals. Elevated blood pressure in uroguanylin deficient mice is also consistent with a defective natriuretic response of uroguanylin$^{-/-}$ animals to oral sodium loads. Both findings provide additional evidence for the hypothesis formulated thirty years earlier that an INF (i.e., natriuretic hormone) may exist in the GI system, which is released into the bloodstream when excess dietary salt is ingested (2, 62). A role for uroguanylin in the control of body sodium balance in postprandial states is strengthened by these novel findings.

Other studies provided additional evidence consistent with this concept. For example, guanylin and uroguanylin are secreted by intestinal cells (71, 73). The intraluminal perfusion of small intestine in vivo with high concentrations of NaCl in the perfusate stimulates the secretion of guanylin, proguanylin, and uroguanylin into the intestinal lumen (53). High NaCl in the perfusate stimulates guanylin secretion greater than the quantitative increase observed for uroguanylin release into the intestinal lumen. Secretion of guanylin and uroguanylin into the circulation was not measured in these experiments. Thus, uroguanylin and/or guanylin peptides may be secreted from small intestine into the circulation when high-salt loads reach the GI tract. In another study with rats fed high-salt diets, it was shown that chronic oral sodium loads causes substantial increases in the urinary excretion of uroguanylin (31). In this study with chronic exposure to high salt in the diet, the plasma levels of uroguanylin were not increased. No reports have been made of studies attempting to define the acute effects of oral sodium loads on plasma levels of either uroguanylin or proguanylin. This type of "Carey" experiment is needed to better define the endocrine nature of intestine in vivo and its response to oral salt loads.

High-salt diets elicit long-lived effects on the intestine in addition to the acute effects on secretion of the enteric peptide hormones. Dietary salt regulates uroguanylin and guanylin gene expression in the intestinal mucosa. Acute treatment of rats with oral sodium loads increases both guanylin and uroguanylin mRNA levels of intestine as early as four hours after salt administration (6). Chronic exposure of rats to high-salt diets also increases guanylin and uroguanylin mRNA levels in the intestine. While increases in the mRNA levels are influenced by intestinal location, the major finding is that guanylin and uroguanylin gene expression appear to be regulated by dietary salt. It is interesting that guanylin mRNA expression in the colon of rats is downregulated by low-salt diets (63). Treatment of rats with low-sodium diets also reduces uroguanylin and guanylin mRNA levels in the intestine (6), thus confirming the earlier finding by Li et al. in rat colon 63). Therefore, demonstrations that dietary sodium influences both the production of guanylin and uroguanylin by intestinal mucosa and the release of bioactive peptides from intestine, coupled together with the phenotype of uroguanylin deficient mice, provides evidence that uroguanylin and/or guanylin may act as "intestinal natriuretic hormones" to help maintain body sodium balance. Two diseases associated with sodium retention and edema may also lend support to a role for uroguanylin as a regulator of sodium balance. In both heart failure and the nephrotic syndrome, marked elevations of uroguanylin have been documented in an apparent connection to sodium retention found in both disorders (4, 49, 50). It may be postulated that uroguanylin acts as a counterregulatory hormone in the body in the physiological states or diseases associated with increased body levels of sodium. Thus, it can be predicted that uroguanylin levels increase under such circumstances to help maintain sodium homeostasis. While uroguanylin and guanylin are only two of several factors that could influence renal sodium excretion in times of sodium excess, it is likely that this particular biological action of uroguanylin per se has served as a selective force for maintaining uroguanylin gene structures during vertebrate evolution. Taken together with observations made in the seawater-adapted eel, and the impaired natriuretic responses of uroguanylin$^{-/-}$ mice to oral sodium loads, it can be concluded that solid experimental substance is emerging for the basic concept that uroguanylin plays a key physiological role for maintenance of body sodium balance.

LOCAL ACTIONS OF UROGUANYLIN AND GUANYLIN IN THE KIDNEY

Initial studies of physiological changes in the uroguanylin$^{-/-}$ mouse reveals an impaired renal response to oral sodium loads and hypertension, but these experiments do not address the in vivo mechanism(s) that may exist for regulation of urinary sodium excretion by uroguanylin (69). Moreover, uroguanylin$^{-/-}$ animals have impaired expression of guanylin mRNA in the intestine, which complicates the interpretation of a phenotype for uroguanylin-deficient animals. This finding may reflect either a technical difficulty in generating the transgenic animal model or uroguanylin could influence the intestinal expression of guanylin. However, uroguanylin KO animals did not exhibit reduced expression of guanylin mRNA in the kidney suggesting that a technical problem may not be the answer. Also, guanylin$^{-/-}$ mice have not been reported thus far with phenotypes exhibiting either impaired renal responses to oral salt loads or the associated elevation of blood pressure (94). However, studies with guanylin KO mice have been limited in scope, and more in depth investigations are needed before definitive conclusions can be made regarding a putative role for guanylin in the regulation of body sodium balance. The quantitative contribution of an endocrine link for uroguanylin between the intestine and/or stomach and the kidney via the blood stream is uncertain because the kidney produces guanylin and uroguanylin (16, 31, 32, 76, 81). Moreover, high-salt diets fed to mice or rats elicit an increase in uroguanylin mRNAs in kidney as well as the intestine (31, 81). High-salt diets exert selective increases in uroguanylin mRNA levels in the kidney without influencing mRNA levels for guanylin. Similar findings have been made in seawater-adapted eels where kidney mRNA levels for uroguanylin, but not guanylin, are increased relative to renal uroguanylin mRNA of eels adapted to fresh water (102). High concentrations of NaCl also appear to influence the expression of uroguanylin in cultured kidney and intestinal cells suggesting that a local mechanism exists for regulation of kidney uroguanylin mRNA expression by salt (81, 93). Therefore, interpretations of the in vivo mechanism of action for uroguanylin-mediated regulation of renal tubular function must consider the possibility that both endocrine and paracrine links involving this natriuretic hormone operate physiologically and that both pathways are influenced by high levels of sodium in the diet. Whether loss of uroguanylin production in both the kidney and intestine contributes to the phenotypic disorders observed in uroguanylin$^{-/-}$ mice, is a fundamental question of substantial significance. At the present time, both endocrine-mediated and local actions of uroguanylin in the kidney should be considered as potential biological mechan-isms for regulation of sodium balance in the postprandial state.

A NOVEL MECHANISM OF ACTION FOR UROGUANYLIN IN THE KIDNEY

Something is peculiarly inconsistent about the phenotype of impaired natriuretic responses of animals to oral salt loads and the associated hypertension found in the uroguanylin$^{-/-}$ mouse model compared to the apparently normal phenotype of GC-C$^{-/-}$ mice (70, 87). Why does the GC-C KO mouse have apparently normal blood pressure? If uroguanylin regulates kidney function through activation of GC-C receptors in renal tubules, then GC-C deficient animals should resemble uroguanylin$^{-/-}$ mice in this regard (5). The mild

phenotype of GC-C$^{-/-}$ animals is consistent with the possibility that one or more additional receptors for uroguanylin may exist and these putative receptors specifically mediate some or all of the renal responses to uroguanylin. Such a phenomenon is likely to be the case because intravenous administration of uroguanylin, guanylin, or *E. coli* ST peptides to GC-C$^{-/-}$ mice results in quantitatively normal increases in the urinary excretion of sodium, chloride, potassium and water (3, 7). Moreover, GC-C$^{-/-}$ animals retain a small number of specific binding sites for the uroguanylin-like agonist, ^{125}I-ST, in plasma membranes isolated from the intestine (70). This biochemical finding is also consistent with the presence of a receptor for guanylin peptides that is not derived from GC-C genes. A recent study using cultured kidney cells has also provided new information consistent with the possibility that one or more additional receptors exist that are activated by uroguanylin, guanylin and ST peptides. The cGMP-regulating peptides elicit changes in potential differences across kidney cell plasma membranes, which resulted in either depolarization or hyperpolarization of the cells (90). Treatment with uroguanylin produces either of the cellular responses, but hyperpolarization responses caused by uroguanylin were selectively blocked by pretreatment of kidney cells with pertussis toxin. It was concluded that hyperpolarization responses to uroguanylin are mediated by a novel receptor located on the surface of kidney cells, which signals via a G-protein that is a substrate for pertussis toxin. These findings provide additional evidence suggesting that another receptor exists for the guanylin peptides in addition to GC-C.

A finding consistent with such a notion may occur in the eel, which has two distinctly different GC-C-like proteins that are derived from two different genes (9). If the eel has evolved two GC-C-like receptors for guanylin peptides by gene duplication, then perhaps other examples of GC-C gene duplication occurred during vertebrate evolution. Such a phenomenon could produce a second cell-surface receptor for guanylin peptides. Results of genome projects in representative mammalian species, such as mouse and man, indicate that a second GC-C-like gene does not exist in Eutherian mammals. One possibility that could explain why a gene duplicated from the GC-C gene is not found when mammalian genomes are interrogated in silico is that a duplicated GC-C gene might change sufficiently over time so that its ancestral relationship to GC-C is difficult to recognize. For example, it is possible that an ancient form of duplicated GC-C could lose most, if not all, of its cytoplasmic domains during evolution, including the C-terminal catalytic domain. Loss of this key domain, together with either a substantial loss and/or otherwise drastic modification of the kinase-homology domain of a duplicated GC-C gene could result in a gene that encodes a cell-surface receptor for guanylin peptides, which has little or no structural similarity to GC-C. It is difficult to recognize membrane GC proteins by their N-terminal domains alone, which are the most variable regions found in GC signaling molecules. Precedence for such a pathway for receptor evolution may be found within the family of atriopeptin receptors (61, 89, 95). One of three established receptors for atriopeptins, that is classified as a "clearance" receptor may have originated by a similar evolutionary pathway. The clearance receptor binds relatively non-selectively to atriopeptins and this receptor has neither a GC catalytic domain nor a kinase-homology domain. However, the residual cytoplasmic tail of the clearance receptor interacts with G-proteins, thus conducting signals into cells (1). A similar pathway to form a second cell-surface receptor for guanylin and uroguanylin can be invoked. Duplication of a GC-C gene with subsequent deletion of the cytosolic GC and kinase-homology domains coupled to the presumptive acquisition of a novel cytosolic domain containing a site for interaction with G-proteins could form another receptor for guanylin and uroguanylin. An illustration of the domain model for OK-GC and GC-C is provided in Fig. 7, which may be useful for visualizing the proposed mechanism for conversion of GC-C into a quite different flavor of receptor that could still bind selectively to guanylin, uroguanylin and ST peptides. It is possible that the N-terminal, ligand-binding domain of such a receptor, could change sufficiently during evolution, yet retain the relatively small site that interacts with guanylin, uroguanylin and ST peptides. Experiments have narrowed the region of GC-C that binds ST peptides to a site close to the transmembrane domain of this protein (45, 97). Thus, a duplicated GC-C gene could evolve into a very different structure given sufficient evolutionary time. Positive selection processes would be required, which could involve participation of this receptor in key regulatory mechanisms

governing body sodium balance. A new receptor for the guanylin family of peptide hormones such as this could be easily missed when gene annotation methods are applied to mammalian genomes to search for membrane receptor-GCs. Classical biochemical means for identification of this postulated receptor might be successful, although such experimental approaches are not ones to be undertaken lightly. If a novel receptor for uroguanylin is derived from GC-C, and it still retains sufficient similarity to GC-C in the ST-binding domain, perhaps interrogation of genomes databases using a strategy to reveal ST binding sites could find a novel receptor for these peptides. Identification of another receptor is clearly one of the important questions in this field of research. A novel receptor for uroguanylin such as this may be involved in the regulation of sodium excretion by the kidney as a physiological means of regulating sodium balance.

TWO DIFFERENT FAMILIES OF NATRIURETIC PEPTIDES: POTENTIAL INTERACTIONS

Two general notions can be proposed concerning the guanylin and atriopeptin families of peptide hormones. Atriopeptins regulate excretion of salt and water by the kidney when the blood (e.g. extracellular fluid) volume is increased and this physiological mechanism acts mainly via receptor-GC-cGMP signaling mechanisms in renal tubules. Second, uroguanylin regulates urinary sodium excretion during postprandial states when excess salt is ingested. It is not clear yet whether cGMP is an important signaling molecule for the mechanism of action of uroguanylin as a natriuretic hormone. However, some evidence exists for possible interactions between atriopeptin and guanylin peptides at the level of renal tubular function. For example, Santos-Neto et al. (84) demonstrated an interesting interaction between guanylin and ANP in the isolated perfused kidney. Experiments were performed using this model system to search for possible synergistic interactions between ANP and guanylin on salt excretion by the kidney. Pretreatment with 0.03 nM ANP, which had no effect when administered alone, markedly enhanced the natriuretic, chloriuretic and kaliuretic responses to 0.19 μM guanylin (Fig. 8). This concentration of guanylin administered alone had no effect on sodium, chloride and potassium excretion in the urine. Furthermore, pretreatment with ANP increased the natriuretic and kaliuretic responses of perfused kidneys to 0.6 μM concentrations of uroguanylin (84). This concentration of uroguanylin elicited submaximal responses in the perfused kidney model. While these novel findings have been published, more research efforts need to be made to further investigate the underlying mechanism(s) that could explain such an interaction between the two different classes of cGMP-regulating agonists. One possibility that comes to mind is derived from the tubular nature of the nephron because inhibition of

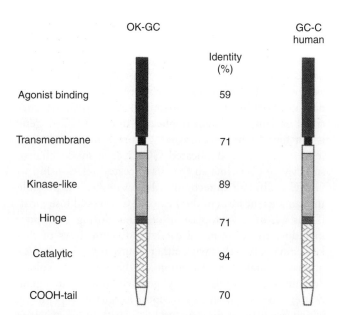

FIGURE 7 Comparison of the primary domains between opossum OK-GC and human GC-C (68). Percentage values refer to the identity comparison of the depicted domains of the two proteins.

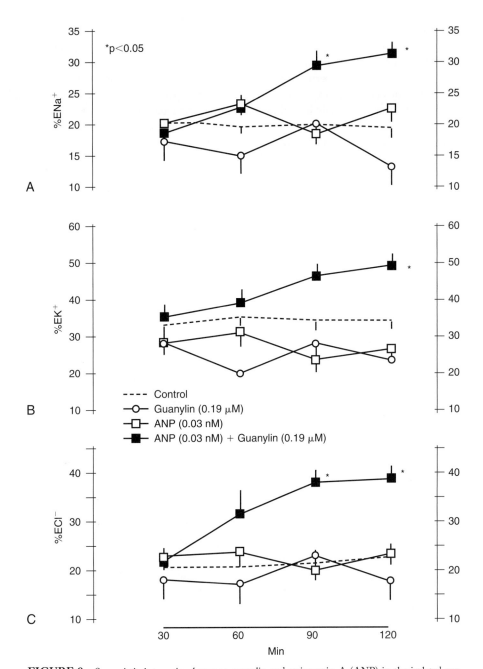

FIGURE 8   Synergistic interaction between guanylin and atriopeptin-A (ANP) in the isolated perfused kidney from rats. Values are given as the percentage of filtered Na+, K+, and Cl⁻ that is excreted in the urine at each time point in the experiment. Inset describes the experimental treatments for each group. Data are the mean ± SE.

sodium reabsorption by an agonist at one site can greatly influence sodium reabsorption downstream in tubules where a second natriuretic agent influences sodium transport. This hypothesis is speculative at the present time, but precedence exists for this type of interaction to occur resulting in greatly enhanced actions of two natriuretic agonists that act at different sites within the nephron. The synergism between guanylin and ANP may also point to a possible interaction at post receptor levels where cGMP derived from both GC-C and GC-A in target cells that express both receptors could stimulate pathways common to both hormones, thus inter-

acting to amplify the natriuretic responses to combinations of guanylin or uroguanylin with ANP. The nephron, of course, is always exposed to both classes of natriuretic hormones in vivo, which is the natural physiological condition.

Coordinated regulation of renal sodium excretion by atriopeptin and guanylin peptides may make considerable physiological sense at this point. Moreover, it is conceivable that coordinate regulation of gene expression for these two families of natriuretic hormones may occur as well. Indeed, the loci of genes encoding atriopeptins are physically close to genes encoding uroguanylin and guanylin on the same chromosomes in mouse and man, and this phenomenon could very well be biologically meaningful. It is unlikely that the location of genes encoding both families of natriuretic hormones occurring close together is merely a fortuitous result of chromosomal evolution. The coordinate expression of atriopeptin and guanylin genes that are physically linked together might occur as part of the physiological mechanisms that have evolved in vertebrates for maintenance of body salt and water balance and for control of blood pressure.

A ROLE FOR THE INTESTINE IN SODIUM BALANCE

Sodium balance has long been the protected turf of those with specialized interests in the kidney and other organs connected with the cardiovascular system. Dogma in the literature clearly indicates that the kidney is a major player for excreting excess salt that is derived from our diets. The intestine has largely been assumed to be an organ that merely absorbs salt into the body so that the kidney can then regulate how much is retained versus the quantity that will be excreted in the urine. However, the enormous concentrations of uroguanylin and guanylin produced in the intestinal mucosa, taken together with a remarkably high density of GC-C receptors in this epithelium, should be viewed as a potential means for regulating sodium absorption, and thus, sodium excretion by the intestine. Perhaps a physiological contribution to sodium balance of the intestine has been overlooked for a very long time. Activation of GC-C by uroguanylin and guanylin can produce actions on the intestinal transport of salt and water like those elicited by the uroguanylin-mimic, *E. coli* ST (30). Stimulation of cGMP production in the intestinal epithelium by these enteric peptide hormones can increase salt and water secretion into the intestinal lumen as well as inhibit sodium absorption (38, 47, 59). Secretion and absorption of NaCl probably resides in two different types of epithelial cells in the intestine. The net effects of cGMP-mediated control of ion transport pathways may culminate in large increases in the excretion of salt and water from the intestine. Indeed, stimulation of salt and water excretion via the intestinal tract is a main action of the uroguanylin-like ST peptides secreted by enteric bacteria that cause traveler's diarrhea. It should be pointed out that activation of the cGMP signaling pathway of intestine has been clearly shown to inhibit sodium absorption in other vertebrate species. In the flounder, stimulation of cGMP production in the intestine by atriopeptins inhibits sodium absorption (77). The possibility should be considered that both the atriopeptins and guanylins, which regulate cGMP signaling pathways through different membrane receptor-GC molecules, may contribute to sodium balance through actions on the intestine as well as the kidney. This type of physiological mechanism in the intestine for excretion of sodium may be more difficult to assess experimentally than are the actions of

these hormones on urinary sodium excretion. This difficulty may have contributed to the general assumption that the kidney, but not the intestine, excretes excess salt derived from the diet. The potential contribution to regulation of urinary sodium excretion through an endocrine axis using enteric uroguanylin for the fine-tuning of sodium reabsorption by renal tubules coupled with local actions of uroguanylin and/or guanylin on the intestinal epithelium to stimulate salt excretion by the GI system makes physiological sense. A similar situation exists for both endocrine and local actions of the atriopeptins. ANP and BNP appear to function in an endocrine pathway between the heart and the kidney, but these peptide hormones also elicit important actions on the myocardium per se. This has been shown in a dramatic fashion by disabling the gene encoding GC-A, which leads to a truly remarkable hypertrophy and deterioration of the heart (78). Thus, atriopeptins work in both endocrine loops and as local regulators of myocardial cell function similar to endocrine and paracrine actions of uroguanylin in the kidney and the intestinal mucosa. Finally, either dietary or environmental exposure to high salt increases the expression of GC-C receptor mRNAs as defined in mammalian species fed high-salt diets and in the eel adapted to life in seawater. Upregulation of a cognate receptor, GC-C, together with the findings that high salt upregulates guanylin and uroguanylin expression in the intestine provides a novel means for regulation of intestinal salt absorption that may contribute to the maintenance of body sodium balance. Conservation of this signal transduction pathway and its physiological responses to high-salt loads in vertebrates from euryhaline teleosts to Eutherian mammals indicates that this physiological mechanism for regulation of sodium balance has been maintained from fish to man. This finding emphasizes the biological significance of uroguanylin, guanylin and the signal transduction pathways that help control body sodium balance.

References

1. Anand-Srivastava MB, Sehl PD, Lowe DG. Cytoplasmic domain of natriuretic peptide receptor-C inhibits adenylyl cyclase. Involvement of a pertussis toxin-sensitive G protein. *J Biol Chem* 1996;271:19324–19329.
2. Carey RM. Evidence for a splanchnic sodium input monitor regulating renal sodium excretion in man: lack of dependence upon aldosterone. *Circul Res* 1978;43:19–23.
3. Carrithers SL, Hill MJ, Johnson BJ, O'Hara SM, Jackson BA, Ott CE, Lorenz J, Mann EA, Giannella RA, Forte LR, Greenberg RN. Renal effects of uroguanylin and guanylin in vivo. *Braz J Med Biol Res* 1999;32:1337–1344.
4. Carrithers SL, Eber SL, Forte LR, Greenberg RN. Increased urinary excretion of uroguanylin in patients with congestive heart failure. *Am J Physiol* 2000;278:H538-H547.
5. Carrithers SL, Taylor B, Cai WY, Johnson BR, Ott BR, Greenberg RN, Jackson BA. Guanylyl cyclase-C receptor mRNA distribution along the rat nephron. *Reg Peptides* 2000;95:65–74.
6. Carrithers SL, Jackson BA, Cai WY, Greenberg RN, Ott CE. Site-specific effects of dietary intake on guanylin and uroguanylin mRNA expression in rat intestine. *Reg Peptides* 2002;107:87–95.
7. Carrithers SL, Ott CE, Hill MJ, Johnson BR, Cai W, Chang JJ, et al. Guanylin and uroguanylin induce natriuresis in mice lacking guanylyl cyclase-C. *Kidney Intl* 2004;65: 40–53.
8. Comrie MM, Cutler CP, Cramb G. Cloning and expression of guanylin from the European eel (*Anguilla anguilla*). *Biochem Biophys Res Commun* 2001;281:1078–1085.
9. Comrie MM, Cutler CP, Cramb G. Cloning and expression of two isoforms of guanylate cyclase C (GC-C) from the European eel (*Anguilla anguilla*). *Comp Biochem Physiol B* 2001;129:575–586.
10. Currie MG, Fok KF, Kato J, Moore RJ, Hamra FK, Duffin KL, Smith CE. Guanylin: an endogenous activator of intestinal guanylate cyclase. *Proc Natl Acad Sci U S A* 1992;89:947–951.

11. Date Y, Nakazato M, Yamaguchi H, Miyazato M, Matsukura S. Tissue distribution and plasma concentration of human guanylin. *Intern Med* 1996;35:171–175.
12. Date Y, Nakazato M, Yamaguchi H, Kangawa K, Kinoshita Y, Chiba T, Ueta Y, Yamashita H, Matsukura S. Enterochromaffin-like cells, a cellular source of uroguanylin in rat stomach. *Endocrinology* 1999;140:2398–2404.
13. de Bold AJ, Borenstein HB, Veress AT, Sonnenberg H. A rapid and potent natriuretic response to intravenous injection of atrial myocardial extract in rats. *Life Sci* 1981;28:89–94.
14. De Wardener HE, Mills IH, Clapham WF, Hayter CJ. Studies on the efferent mechanism of the sodium diuresis which follows the administration of intravenous saline in the dog. *Clin Sci* 1961;21:249–258.
15. De Wardener HE, Clarkson EM. Concept of natriuretic hormone. *Physiol Rev* 1985;65: 658–759.
16. Fan X, Hamra FK, Freeman RH, Eber SL, Krause WJ, et al. Uroguanylin: cloning of preprouroguanylin cDNA, mRNA expression in the intestine and heart and isolation of uroguanylin and prouroguanylin from plasma. *Biochem Biophys Res Commun* 1996;219: 457–462.
17. Fan X, Hamra FK, London RM, Eber SL, Krause WJ, Freeman WH, Smith CE, et al. Structure and activity of uroguanylin isolated from urine and intestine of rats. *Am J Physiol* 1997;273:E957–E964.
18. Field M, Graf, Jr. LH, Laird WJ, Smith PL. Heat-stable enterotoxin of *Escherichia coli*: *in vitro* effects on guanylate cyclase activity, cyclic GMP concentration, and ion transport in small intestine. *Proc Natl Acad Sci U S A* 1978;75:2800–2804.
19. Field M. Intestinal ion transport and the pathophysiology of diarrhea. *J Clin Invest* 2003; 111:931–943.
20. Fonteles MC, Lima AAM, Fang G, Guerrant RL. Effect of STa and cholera toxin on renal eletrolyte transport: possible roles of an endogenous ST-like compound in the isolated kidney. 27th U S Japan Cholera Meeting, Charlottesville, VA 1991;100–105.
21. Fonteles MC, Monteiro HSA, Soares AM, Santos-Neto MS, Greenberg RN, Lima AAM. The lysine-1 analog of guanylin induces intestinal secretion and natriuresis in the isolated perfused kidney. *Braz J Med Biol Res* 1996;29:267–271.
22. Fonteles MC, Greenberg RN, Monteiro HSA, Currie MG, Forte LR. Natriuretic and kaliuretic activities of guanylin and uroguanylin in the isolated perfused rat kidney. *Am J Physiol* 1998;275:F191–F197.
23. Fonteles MC, Carrithers SL, Monteiro HSA, Carvalho AF, Coelho GR, Greenberg RN, et al. Renal effects of serine-7 analog of lymphoguanylin in *ex vivo* rat kidney. *Am J Physiol* 2001;280:F207–F213.
24. Forte LR, Krause WJ, Freeman RH. Receptors and cGMP signaling mechanism for *E. coli* enterotoxin in opossum kidney. *Am J Physiol* 1988;255:F1040–F1046.
25. Forte LR, Krause WJ, Freeman RH. *Escherichia coli* enterotoxin receptors: localization in opossum kidney, intestine and testis. *Am J Physiol* 1989;257:F874–F881.
26. Forte LR, Hamra FK, Fan XH, Krause WJ, Currie MG, Freeman RH. Uroguanylin: an intestinal peptide hormone with natriuretic activity. *Gastroenterology* 1994;106:A808.
27. Forte LR, Currie MG. Guanylin: a peptide regulator of epithelial transport. *FASEB J* 1995;9:643–650.
28. Forte LR, Fan X, Hamra FK. Salt and water homeostasis: uroguanylin is a circulating peptide hormone with natriuretic activity. *Am J Kidney Dis* 1996;28:296–304.
29. Forte LR, Eber SL, Fan X, London RM, Wang Y, Rowland LM, et al. Lymphoguanylin: Cloning and characterization of a unique member of the guanylin peptide family. *Endocrinology* 1999;140:1800–1808.
30. Forte LR. Uroguanylin and guanylin peptides: pharmacology and experimental therapeutics. *Pharmacol Therap* 2004;104:137–162.
31. Fukae H, Kinoshita H, Fujimoto S, Kita T, Nakazato M, Eto T. Changes in urinary levels and renal expression of uroguanylin on low or high salt diets in rats. *Nephron* 2002;92:373–378.
32. Fujimoto S, Kinoshita K, Hara S, Nakazato M, Hisanaga S, Eto T. Immuno-histochemical localization of uroguanylin in the human kidney. *Nephron* 2000;84:88–89.
33. Furchgott RF, Zawadzki JV. The obligatory role of endothelial cells in the relaxation of arterial smooth muscle by acetylcholine. *Nature* 1980;288:373–376.
34. Gariepy J, Judd AK, Schoolnik GK. Importance of disulfide bridges in the structure and activity of *Escherichia coli* enterotoxin ST1b. *Proc Natl Acad Sci U S A* 1987;84:8907–8911.
35. Giannella RA. Suckling mouse model for detection of heat-stable Escherichia coli enterotoxin: characteristics of the model. *Infect Immun* 1976;14:95–99.
36. Giannella RA, Mann EA. *E. coli* heat-stable enterotoxin and guanylyl cyclase C: new functions and unsuspected actions. *Trans Am Clin Climatol Assoc* 2003;114:67–85.
37. Greenberg RN, Hill M, Crytzer J, Krause WJ, Eber SL, Hamra FK, Forte LR. Comparison of effects of uroguanylin, guanylin, *Escherichia coli* heat-stable enterotoxin STa in mouse intestine and kidney: evidence that uroguanylin is an intestinal natriuretic hormone. *J Invest Med* 1997;45:276–282.
38. Guba M, Kuhn M, Forssmann W-G, Classen M, Gregor M, Seidler U. Guanylin strongly stimulates rat duodenal HCO_3^- secretion: proposed mechanism and comparison with other secretagogues. *Gastroenterology* 1996;111:1558–1568.
39. Guerrant RL, Hughes JM, Chang B, Robertson DC, Murad F. Activation of intestinal guanylate cyclase by heat-stable enterotoxin of *Escherichia coli*: studies of tissue specificity, potential receptors, and intermediates. *J Infect Dis* 1980;142:220–228.
40. Hamra FK, Forte LR, Eber SL, Pidhorodeckyj NV, Krause WJ, Freeman RH, et al. Uroguanylin: structure and activity of a second endogenous peptide that stimulates intestinal guanylate cyclase. *Proc Natl Acad Sci U S A* 1993;90:10464–10468.
41. Hamra FK, Fan X, Krause WJ, Freeman RH, Chin DT, Smith CE, et al. Prouroguanylin and proguanylin: purification from colon, structure, and modulation of bioactivity by proteases. *Endocrinology* 1996;137:257–265.
42. Hamra FK, Krause WJ, Smith CE, Freeman RH, Currie MG, Forte LR. Colonic mucosa contains uroguanylin and guanylin peptides. *Am J Physiol* 1996;270:G708–G716.
43. Hamra FK, Eber SL, Chin DT, Currie MG, Forte LR. Regulation of intestinal uroguanylin/guanylin receptor-mediated responses by mucosal acidity. *Proc Natl Acad Sci U S A* 1997, 94:2705–2710.
44. Hess R, Kuhn M, Schulz-Knappe P, Raida M, Fuchs M, Klodt J, et al. Isolation and characterization of the circulating form of human uroguanylin. *FEBS Lett* 1995;374:34–38.
45. Hidaka Y, Matsumoto Y, Shimonishi Y. The micro domain responsible for ligand-binding of guanylyl cyclase C. *FEBS Lett* 2002;526:58–62.
46. Hughes JM, Murad F, Chang B, Guerrant RL. Role of cyclic GMP in the action of heat-stable enterotoxin of *Escherichia coli*. *Nature Lond* 1978;271:755–756.
47. Joo NS, London RM, Kim HD, Forte LR, Clarke LL. Regulation of intestinal Cl^- and HCO_3^- secretion by uroguanylin. *Am J Physiol* 1998;274:G633–G644.
48. Katwa LC, White AA. Presence of functional receptors for the *Escherichia coli* heat-stable enterotoxin in the gastrointestinal tract of the chicken. *Infect Immun* 1992;60:3546–3551.
49. Kikuchi M, Fujimoto S, Fukae H, Kinoshita H, Kita T, Nakazato M, et al. Role of uroguanylin, a peptide with natriuretic activity, in rats with experimental nephritic syndrome. *J Am Soc Nephrol* 2005;16:392–397.
50. Kinoshita H, Fujimoto S, Fukae H, Yokota N, Hisanaga S, Nakazato M, et al. Plasma and urine levels of uroguanylin, a new natriuretic peptide, in nephrotic syndrome. *Nephron* 1999;8:160–164.
51. Kishimoto I, Dubois SK, Garbers DL. The heart communicates with the kidney exclusively through the guanylyl cyclase-A receptor: acute handling of sodium and water in response to volume expansion. *Proc Natl Acad Sci U S A* 1996;93:6215–6219.
52. Kita T, Smith CE, Fok KF, Duffin KL, Moore WM, Karabatsos PJ, et al. Characterization of human uroguanylin: member of the guanylin peptide family. *Am J Physiol* 1994;266: F342–F348.
53. Kita T, Kitamura K, Sakata J, Eto T. Marked increase of guanylin secretion in response to salt loading in the rat small intestine. *Am J Physiol* 1999;277:G960–G966.
54. Krause WJ, Freeman RH, Forte LR. Autoradiographic demonstration of specific binding sites for *E. coli* enterotoxin in various epithelia of the North American opossum. *Cell Tissue Res* 1990;260:387–394.
55. Krause WJ, Cullingford GL, Freeman RH, Eber SL, Richardson KC, Fok KF, et al. Distribution of heat-stable enterotoxin/guanylin receptors in the intestinal tract of man and other mammals. *J Anat* 1994;184:407–417.
56. Krause WJ, Freeman RH, Eber SL, Hamra, FK, Fok KF, Currie MG, et al. Distribution of *E. coli* heat-stable enterotoxin/guanylin/uroguanylin receptors in the avian intestinal tract. *Acta Anat* 1995;153:210–219.
57. Krause WJ, Freeman RH, Eber SL, Hamra FK, Currie MG, Forte LR. Guanylyl cyclase receptors and guanylin-like peptides in reptilian intestine. *Gen Comp Endocrin* 1997;107: 229–239.
58. Kuhn M, Raida M, Adermann K, Schulz-Knappe P, Gerzer R, Heim J-M, et al. The circulating bioactve form of human guanylin is high molecular weight peptide (10.3 kDa). *FEBS Lett* 1993;318:205–209.
59. Kuhn M, Adermann K, Jahne J, Forssmann W-G, Rechkemmer G. Segmental differences in the effects of guanylin and *Escherichia coli* heat-stable enterotoxin on Cl^- secretion in human gut. *J Physiol* 1994; 479:433–440.
60. Kuhn M, Kulaksiz H, Adermann K, Rechkemmer G, Forssmann W-G. Radioimmunoassay for circulating human guanylin. *FEBS Lett* 1994;341:218–222.
61. Kuhn M. Structure, regulation and function of mammalian membrane guanylyl cyclase receptors, with a focus on guanylyl cyclase-A. *Circ Res* 2003;93:700–709.
62. Lennane RJ, Peart WS, Carey RM, Shaw JA. Comparison of natriuresis after oral and intravenous sodium loading in sodium-depleted rabbits: evidence for a gastrointestinal or portal monitor of sodium intake. *Clin Sci Mol Med* 1975;49:433–436.
63. Li Z, Knowles JW, Goyeau D, Prabhakar S, Short DB, Perkins AG, et al. Low salt intake down-regulates the guanylin signaling pathway in rat distal colon. *Gastroenterology* 1996;111:1714–1721.
64. Lima AAM, Master of Science Thesis: Estudo dos efeitos das toxinas do V. cholerae e E. coli no rim isolado do rato. Dept. Fisiologia e Farmacologia, C.C.S.- 3 de Abril, Fortaleza, Ceará, Brazil, 1983.
65. Lima AAM, Fonteles MC. Efeitos das toxinas do V. Cholerae e da *E. coli* no rim perfundido. XVIII Congresso Brasileiro de Fisiologia 1983;S-31:46. São Lourenço, Minas Gerais, Brazil.
66. Lima AA, Monteiro HSA, Fonteles MC. The effects of *Escherichia coli* heat-stable enterotoxin in renal sodium tubular transport. *Pharmacol Toxicol* 1992,70:163–167.
67. Lima AA, Monteiro HS, Fonteles MC. Effects of thermostable *Escherichia coli* enterotoxin peptide on the isolated rat kidney. *Braz J Med Biol Res* 1992;25:633–636.
68. London RM, Eber SL, Visweswariah SS, Krause WJ, Forte LR. Structure and activity of OK-GC: a kidney receptor guanylate cyclase activated by guanylin peptides. *Am J Physiol* 1999;276:F882–F891.
69. Lorenz JN, Nieman M, Sabo J, Sanford LP, Hawkins JA, Elitsur N, et al. Uroguanylin knockout mice have increased blood pressure and impaired natriuretic response to enteral NaCl load. *J Clin Invest* 2003;112:1244–1254.
70. Mann EA, Jump ML, Wu J, Yee E, Giannella RA. Mice lacking the guanylyl cyclase C receptor are resistant to STa-induced intestinal secretion. *Biochem Biophys Res Commun* 1997;239:463–466.
71. Martin S, Adermann K, Forssmann W-G, Kuhn M. Regulated, side-directed secretion of proguanylin from isolated rat colonic mucosa. *Endocrinology* 1999;140:5022–5029.
72. Miyazato M, Nakazato M, Matsukura S, Kangawa K, Matsuo H. Uroguanylin gene expression in the alimentary tract and extra-gastrointestinal tissues. *FEBS Lett* 1996;398:170–174.
73. Moro F, Levenez F, Nemoz-Gaillard E, Pellissier S, Plaisancie P, Cuber JC. Release of guanylin immunoreactivity from the isolated vascularly perfused rat colon. *Endocrinology* 2000;141:2594–2599.
74. Nakazato M, Yamaguchi H, Shiomi K, Date Y, Fujimoto S, Kangawa K, et al. Identification of 10-kDa proguanylin as a major guanylin molecule in human intestine and plasma and its increase in renal insufficiency. *Biochem Biophys Res Commun* 1994;205:1966–1975.
75. Nakazato M, Yamaguchi H, Kinoshita H, Kangawa K, Matsuo H, Chino N, Matsukura S. Identification of biologically active and inactive human uroguanylins in plasma and urine and their increases in renal insufficiency. *Biochem Biophys Res Commun* 1996;220:586–593.

76. Nakazato M, Yamaguchi H, Date Y, Miyazato M, Kangawa K, Goy MF, et al. Tissue distribution, cellular source, and structural analysis of rat immunoreactive uroguanylin. *Endocrinology* 1998;139:5247–5254.

77. O'Grady SM. Cyclic nucleotide-mediated effects of ANF and VIP on flounder intestinal ion transport. *Am J Physiol* 1989;256:C142–C146.

78. Oliver PM, Fox JE, Kim R, Rockman HA, Kim HS, Reddick RL, et al. Hypertension, cardiac hypertrophy, and sudden death in mice lacking natriuretic peptide receptor A. *Proc Natl Acad Sci U S A* 1997; 94:14730–14735.

79. Perkins A, Goy MF, Li Z. Uroguanylin is expressed by enterochromaffin cells in the rat gastrointestinal tract. *Gastroenterology* 1997; 113:1007–1014.

80. Petterson A, Hedner J, Ericksten S, Towle AC, Hedner T. Acute volume expansion as a physiological stimulus for the release of atrial natriuretic peptides in the rat. *Life Sci* 1986;38:1127–1133.

81. Potthast R, Ehler E, Scheving LA, Sindic A, Schlatter E, Kuhn M. High salt intake increases uroguanylin expression in mouse kidney. *Endocrinology* 2001;142:3087–3097.

82. Qian X, Prabhakar S, Nandi A, Visweswariah SS, Goy MF. Expression of GC-C, a receptor-guanylate cyclase, and its endogenous ligands uroguanylin and guanylin along the rostrocaudal axis of the intestine. *Endocrinology* 2000;141:3210–3224.

83. Rao MC, Guandalini S, Smith PL, Field M. Mode of action of heat-stable *Escherichia coli* enterotoxin tissue and subcellular specificities and role of cyclic GMP. *Biochem Biophys Acta* 632:1980;35–46.

84. Santos-Neto MS, Carvalho AF, Forte LR, Fonteles MC. Relationship between the actions of atrial natriuretic peptide (ANP), guanylin and uroguanylin on the isolated kidney. *Braz J Med Biol Res* 1999;32:1015–1019.

85. Santos-Neto MS, Carrithers SL, Carvalho AF, Monteiro HSA, Greenberg RN, Forte LR, et al. Guanylin and its lysine-containing analogue in the isolated perfused rat kidney: Interaction with chymotrypsin inhibitor. *Pharmacol Toxicol* 2003;92:114–120.

86. Schulz S, Green CK, Yuen PST, Garbers DL. Guanylyl cyclase is a heat-stable enterotoxin receptor. *Cell* 1990;63:941–948.

87. Schulz S, Lopez MJ, Kuhn M, Garbers DL. Disruption of the guanylyl cyclase-C gene leads to a paradoxical phenotype of viable but heat-stable enterotoxin-resistant mice. *J Clin Invest* 1997;100:1590–1595.

88. Shailubhai, K, Yu HH, Karunanandaa K, Wang JY, Eber SL, Wang Y, et al. Uroguanylin suppresses polyp formation in the *APC^{Min}/+* mouse and induces apoptosis in human colon adenocarcinoma cells via cyclic GMP. *Cancer Res* 2000;60:5149–5155.

89. Silberbach M, Roberts Jr. CT. Natriuretic peptide signaling: molecular and cellular pathways to growth regulation. *Cell Signal* 2001;13:221–231.

90. Sindice A, Basoglu C, Cerci A, Hirsch JR, Potthast R, Kuhn M, et al. Guanylin, uroguanylin, and heat-stable enterotoxin activate guanylate cyclase C and/or a pertussis toxin-sensitive G protein. *J Biol Chem* 2002;277:17758–17764.

91. Smith HW. From fish to philosopher: the story of our internal environment. Ed. CIBA. NJ. USA. 1959.

92. Smith HW. *Principles of Renal Physiology.* New York: Oxford University Press, 1962.

93. Steinbrecher KA, Rudolph JA, Luo G, Cohen MB. Coordinate upregulation of guanylin and uroguanylin expression by hypertonicity in HT29-18-N2 cells. *Am J Physiol* 2002;283:C1729–C1737.

94. Steinbrecher KA, Wowk SA, Rudolph JA, Witte DP, Cohen MB. Targeted inactivation of the mouse guanylin gene results in altered dynamics of colonic epithelial proliferation. *Am J Pathol* 2002; 161:2169–2178.

95. Tamura N, Chrisman TD, Garbers DL. The regulation and physiological roles of the guanylyl cyclase receptors. *Endocr J* 2001;48:611–634.

96. Vaandrager AB. Structure and function of the heat-stable entertoxin receptor/guanylyl cyclase C. *Mol Cell Biochem* 2002;230:73–83.

97. Wada A, Hirayama T, Kitaura H, Fujisawa J, Hasegawa M, Hidaka Y, et al. Identification of ligand recognition sites in heat-stable enterotoxin receptor, membrane-associated guanylyl cyclase C by site-directed mutational analysis. *Infect Immun* 1996;64:5144–5150.

98. Whitaker TL, Steinbrecher KA, Copeland NG, Gilbert DJ, Jenkins NA, Cohen MB. The uroguanylin gene (Guca1b) is linked to guanylin (Guca2) on mouse chomosome 4. *Genomics* 1997;45:348–354.

99. White AA, Krause WJ, Turner JT, Forte LR. Opossum kidney contains a functional receptor for the *Escherichia coli* heat-stable enterotoxin. *Biochem Biophys Res Commun* 1989;159:363–367.

100. Wiegand RC, Kato J, Currie MG. Rat guanylin cDNA: Characterization of the precursor of the endogenous activator of intestinal guanylate cyclase. *Biochem Biophys Res Commun* 1992;185:812–817.

101. Wiegand RC, Kato J, Huang MD, Fok KF, Kachur JF, Currie MG. Human guanylin: cDNA isolation, structure and activity. *FEBS Lett* 311:1992;150–154.

102. Yuge S, Inoue K, Hyodo S, Takei Y. A novel guanylin family (guanylin, uroguanylin, and renoguanylin) in eels. Possible osmoregulatory hormones in intestine and kidney. *J Biol Chem* 2003;278:22726–22733.

Structural and Functional Organization of the Kidney

Structural Organization

CHAPTER **20**

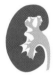

Structural Organization of the Mammalian Kidney

Wilhelm Kriz and Brigitte Kaissling

University of Heidelberg, Heidelberg, Germany
University of Zürich, Zürich, Switzerland

KIDNEY TYPES AND RENAL PELVIS

The mammalian kidney is multiform. The basic architecture is best understood in the unipapillary kidney, which is common in all small species. A coronal section of this kidney shows the main structural parts (Fig. 1A). The renal cortex, as a whole, is cup-shaped, with inverted margins, and surrounds the renal medulla. The medulla can be roughly compared with a pyramid; its top portion, the papilla, projects into the renal pelvis. The pelvis is located within the renal sinus, which opens through the renal hilum to the medial surface of the kidney.

The cortical parenchyma is divided into the cortical labyrinth and the medullary rays. The uppermost part of the cortex, a continuous layer that covers the tops of the medullary rays, is called the cortex corticis. The medulla is divided into an outer medulla (subdivided into outer and inner stripes) and an inner medulla. The innermost part of the inner medulla generally forms the papilla.

The unipapillary kidney is the most simple kidney type; in comparative anatomy, such a kidney as a whole corresponds to

a renculus. All other kidney types may be regarded as adaptations to larger body sizes. The crest kidney and the kidney with tubi maximi are magnifications of a one-renculus unit. The multipapillary kidney (Fig. 2) and the reniculus kidney multiply this unit (234, 256, 585). The human kidney is a multipapillary kidney, however, it is particular because a variable number of papillae are generally fused, forming compound papillae (252).

The renal pelvis (Figs. 1A and 1B) or the renal calyces (Fig. 2) are anchored to the renal parenchyma by connective and smooth muscle tissues that follow the intrarenal arteries. The cavity of the pelvis and calyx surrounds the renal papilla (or its equivalent in other kidney types). In many species the pelvic cavity forms different kinds of pelvic extensions (Fig. 1B) (271, 555, 578). Leaflike extensions called "specialized fornices" accompany the large vessels for some distance along their entry into the renal parenchyma. Secondary pouches protrude toward the hilus, communicating with the primary pelvic cavity only above the free semilunar borders of the pelvic septa. In the sand rat, irregularly shaped extensions penetrate into the outer medullary parenchyma (268). These extensions increase the contact area between

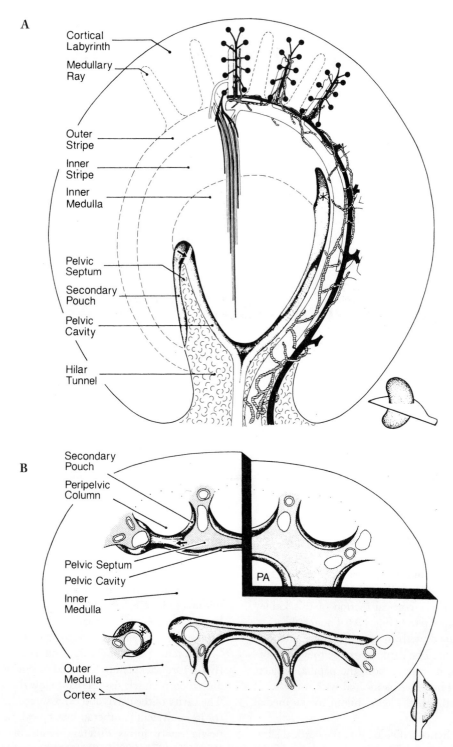

A

Cortical Labyrinth

Medullary Ray

Outer Stripe

Inner Stripe

Inner Medulla

Pelvic Septum

Secondary Pouch

Pelvic Cavity

Hilar Tunnel

B

Secondary Pouch

Peripelvic Column

Pelvic Septum

Pelvic Cavity

Inner Medulla

Outer Medulla

Cortex

PA

FIGURE 1   Schematics of a coronal and two transverse sections through the rabbit kidney. The inset in the right lower corner indicates the section plane. The general architecture of the kidney and the renal pelvis is demonstrated. **A:** Arterial vessels, including glomeruli and descending vasa recta, are shown in black, venous vessels are gray, and lymphatics are hatched. **B:** The section plane of the main drawing runs through the middle part of the inner medulla; a deeper section through the papilla (PA) is shown in the upper right quarter. The cross-sectioned pelvic septa are stippled. The leaflike extensions of the pelvic cavity are marked by a star, the free semilunar edges of the main pelvic septa by an arrow (**A,B**). (From Kaissling B, Kriz W. Structural analysis of the rabbit kidney. *Adv Anat Embryol Cell Biol* 1979;l56:1–123, with permission.)

the pelvic cavity and the renal medulla, especially the outer medulla (339).

RENAL VASCULATURE

Close to the renal hilum and beyond within the renal sinus, the renal artery undergoes several divisions finally establishing the interlobar arteries, which then enter the renal tissue at the border between the cortex and medulla (Figs. 1A and 2). From there they follow an arclike course and are therefore called arcuate arteries. They give rise to the cortical radial arteries, which ascend radially within the cortical labyrinth. The cortex is very densely penetrated by arteries; in contrast, no arteries enter the medulla. The renal veins (cortical radial [interlobular] veins, arcuate veins) accompany the corresponding arteries. In some species (cat, dog, human) the venous blood from the outer cortex drains into veins on the renal surface (in humans called "stellate veins"), which are connected by additional cortical radial veins (interlobular veins) to arcuate veins. Such additional veins are not accompanied by arteries (197).

The microvasculature pattern of the kidney appears to be very similar among mammalian species; a basic pattern can be described (Figs. 3 and 4A) (356, 429, 517). The afferent arterioles arise from the cortical radial arteries (a minor portion from the arcuate arteries) and supply the

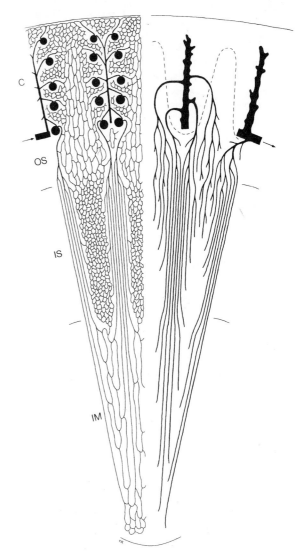

FIGURE 3   Schematic of the microvasculature of the rat kidney. The left panel shows the arterial vessels and capillaries. An arcuate artery (*arrow*) gives rise to a cortical radial (interlobular) artery, from which afferent arterioles originate to supply the glomeruli. The efferent arterioles of the juxtamedullary glomeruli descend into the medulla and divide into the descending vasa recta, which, together with ascending vasa recta, form the vascular bundles of the renal medulla. At intervals, descending vasa recta leave the bundles to feed the adjacent capillaries. The right panel shows the venous vessels. The interlobular veins start in the superficial cortex. In the inner cortex, they, together with the arcuate veins, receive the ascending vasa recta from the medulla. The vasa recta ascending from the inner medulla all traverse the inner stripe within the vascular bundles, whereas most of the vasa recta from the inner stripe ascend outside the bundles. Both of these types of ascending vasa recta traverse the outer stripe as wide, tortuous channels. C, cortex; OS, outer stripe; IS, inner stripe; IM, inner medulla. (Adapted from Kriz W, Lever AF. Renal countercurrent mechanisms: structure and function. *Am Heart J* 1969;78:101–118 and Rollhaeuser H, Kriz W, et al. [The vascular system of the rat kidney.]. *Z Zellforsch Mikrosk Anat* 1964;64:381–403, with permission.)

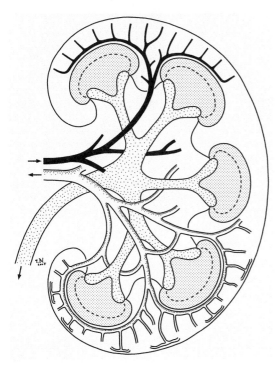

FIGURE 2   Schematic illustration of a compound multipapillary kidney (coronal section) similar to the human kidney. The renal cortex encloses several papillae; fused papillae as typical for the human kidney are not shown. The central region, the renal sinus, contains the calyces and the pelvis (*stippled*), the pattern of branching arteries (*black*), and joining veins (*white*). The arcuate arteries, running at the corticomedullary border, do not form true arches, but rather represent end-arteries. In contrast, the veins form anastomoses at the level of the arcuate and interlobar veins. In the human kidney, there are two types of cortical radial veins (interlobular veins); one group starting as stellate veins drains the most superficial cortex, the second group starts at deeper levels in the cortex; both drain into arcuate veins.

A

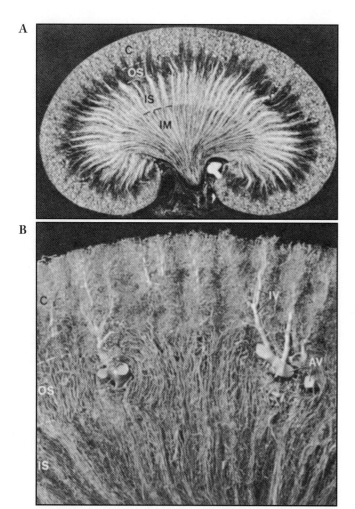

B

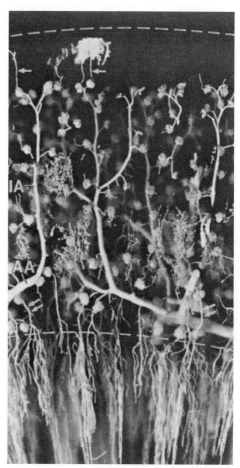

FIGURE 5 Arterial vessels after filling with silicone rubber; rabbit kidney. The broken lines show the renal surface and the corticomedullary border. Arcuate arteries (AA) give rise to cortical radial arteries which split into the afferent arterioles. The efferent arterioles of superficial glomeruli (*arrow*) ascend unbranched to the kidney surface before splitting into capillaries. The efferent arterioles of juxtamedullary nephrons (*arrowheads*) descend into the outer stripe and divide into the descending vasa recta. Magnification × 80. (From Kaissling B, Kriz W. Structural analysis of the rabbit kidney. *Adv Anat Embryol Cell Biol* 1979; 56:1–123, with permission; courtesy of L. Bankir.)

FIGURE 4 Microvasculature. **A**: Rat kidney; silicon rubber (Microfil) filling of the arterial vessels. Cortex (C), outer stripe (OS), inner stripe (IS), and inner medulla (IM) are clearly distinguishable by their vessel patterns. The vascular bundles take shape along the OS and are best developed within the IS. Only a minor part of the descending vasa recta of each bundle enter the IM, where they gradually decrease in number toward the papilla. Note the scantiness of capillaries in the OS. Magnification, ×8. **B**: Rabbit kidney; silicon rubber filling of the venous vessels. The interlobular veins (IV) ac cept the cortical capillaries and a major part of the ascending vasa recta. Note the density of ascending vasa recta within the OS. In the IS, ascending vasa recta are found within the bundles (mostly originating from the IM) and between the vascular bundles (draining the interbundle regions of the IS). AV, arcuate vein. Magnification, × 14. (Courtesy of L. Bankir.)

glomerular tufts of the renal corpuscles. The efferent arterioles drain the glomeruli. Several types of efferent arterioles have been described (58, 192, 517). Basically, a distinction between those of superficial, midcortical and juxtamedullary renal corpuscles is essential (Figs. 3 and 5). The efferent arterioles of juxtamedullary glomeruli turn toward the medulla; they are the supplying vessels of the medulla. Juxtamedullary glomeruli are most exactly defined by this type of an efferent arteriole. The superficial efferent arterioles extend to the kidney surface before dividing. Again, superficial glomeruli are best defined be-

cause of the typical pattern of their efferent arterioles. The efferent arterioles of midcortical nephrons (defined by exclusion) vary in length between those that branch abruptly near the glomerulus and others that extend to a medullary ray before splitting off into capillaries. The efferent arterioles all together (superficial, midcortical, and small branches of the juxtamedullary efferent arterioles) supply the cortical peritubular capillaries. Direct aglomerular arterial supplies to the peritubular capillaries or to the medulla are sparse (105) and have been shown to be frequently the result of degeneration of the corresponding glomeruli (428).

Within the capillary network of the cortex (Figs. 3 and 4), a differentiation between two parts is necessary: namely, the dense, round-meshed capillary plexus of the cortical labyrinth (including the cortex corticis) and the less dense, long-meshed plexus of the medullary rays, both associated with the course of the tubules. Functionally these two plexi are different with respect to their drainage: The blood from the medullary ray plexus has to pass the plexus of the cortical labyrinth to gain access to the interlobular veins. Therefore, the blood that has perfused the straight tubules within the medullary rays mixes with the blood that perfuses the convoluted tubules of the cortical labyrinth.

The medulla (Figs. 3, 4, and 5) is exclusively supplied by the efferent arterioles of the juxtamedullary glomeruli (59, 197, 271, 327, 429, 517). These efferent arterioles descend through the outer stripe and divide into the descending vasa recta. In addition, the efferent arteriole and its first divisions give rise to small side branches that supply the sparse capillary plexus of the outer stripe of the outer medulla. This plexus is continuous with the cortical capillary plexus above and the capillary plexus of the inner stripe below. The descending vasa recta then penetrate the inner stripe of the outer medulla in cone-shaped vascular bundles. At intervals, descending vasa recta leave the bundles to join the capillary plexus at the adjacent medullary level, most leaving the bundle within the inner stripe. Only a small portion of descending vasa recta penetrates the inner medulla, and even fewer reach the tip of the papilla.

The capillary plexuses of the renal medulla (Figs. 3 and 4A) differ in the three regions. The outer stripe is sparse. In contrast, the capillary plexus of the inner stripe is very dense and characteristically round-meshed in appearance. In the inner medulla, the capillary plexus is less dense and long-meshed.

The ascending vasa recta are the draining vessels of the renal medulla (Figs. 3 and 4B). In the inner medulla they arise at every level and ascend as unbranched vessels to the border between the inner medulla and outer medulla. At this point, at the latest, they join the vascular bundles and traverse the inner stripe of the outer medulla within the vascular bundles. The ascending vasa recta, which drain the inner stripe, behave differently. Those of the lowermost part of the inner stripe (and therefore probably a minor portion) join the bundles as they pass through this region. Those from the middle and upper part (and thus probably the majority) do not join the bundles, but ascend directly within the interbundle regions to the outer stripe. There are, however, interspecies differences: In the sand rat (*Psammomys obesus*), all ascending vasa recta that drain the inner stripe ascend directly to the outer stripe without joining the bundles (40).

Within the outer stripe, the vasa recta ascending within the bundles spread out and, together with the directly ascending vasa recta, traverse the outer stripe as individual tortuous channels with wide lumina (Fig. 4B). They contact the tubules like true capillaries, and because the true capillaries, which are derived from direct branches of efferent arterioles, are few in the outer stripe (Fig.3A), they mainly affect the blood supply to the tubules in this

region. At the corticomedullary border, the ascending venous vessels of the medulla empty into the arcuate veins or into the basal parts of interlobular veins. In some species, such as rat, guinea pig, and especially the sand rat (*P. obesus*) some of the venous medullary vessels continue to ascend within the medullary rays of the cortex and finally empty into middle or even upper parts of interlobular veins.

Wall Structure of Intrarenal Vessels

The intrarenal arteries and the proximal portions of the afferent arterioles appear to be similar to arteries and arterioles of the same size elsewhere in the body. The terminal portions of the afferent arterioles are unique because of the occurrence of granular cells (renin-producing cells) which replace ordinary smooth muscle cells in their wall (see following section: Juxtaglomerular Apparatus). It is generally agreed that granular cells are modified smooth muscle cells. Compared with smooth muscle cells proper, granular cells contain fewer myofilaments; thus, the contractile capacity of the very last portion of the afferent arteriole appears to be considerably decreased (601). The endocrine function of granular cells will be considered later in the context of the juxtaglomerular apparatus. The glomerular capillaries will be described together with the glomerulus.

Efferent arterioles are already established inside the glomerular tuft. Thus, in contrast to afferent arterioles, efferent arterioles have an intraglomerular segment that passes through the glomerular stalk (Fig. 6A). The subsequent efferent arterioles have a segment that is narrowly associated with the extraglomerular mesangium (details will be described later in the context of the glomerulus). Thereafter the efferent arterioles are established as arterioles with a proper media made up of smooth muscle cells.

Efferent arterioles from juxtamedullary glomeruli differ considerably from those of cortical (midcortical and superficial) glomeruli (compare Figs. 6B and 6C). Juxtamedullary efferent arterioles are larger in diameter than cortical efferent arterioles; their size even exceeds that of their corresponding afferent arterioles. In the rabbit, the diameters of afferent arterioles throughout the cortex average approximately 20 μm; juxtamedullary efferent arterioles average 28 μm, and cortical efferent arterioles average only 12 μm (38). Similar differences have been found in dog (58), rat (149), and human (182) kidneys.

Cortical efferent arterioles (Fig. 6B) are only sparsely equipped with smooth muscle cells (generally not more than one layer). A striking feature of efferent arterioles (including those from juxtamedullary glomeruli) is the thick, irregular basement membrane. In contrast to the usual appearance of a basement membrane, basement membrane–like material fills the wide and irregular spaces between the endothelium

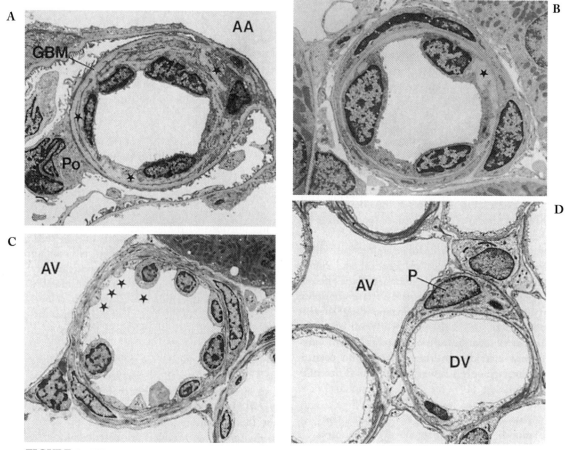

FIGURE 6   Efferent arteriole in rat. **A:** Intraglomerular segment of the efferent arteriole. Between the glomerular basement membrane (GBM) and the endothelium, a mesangial layer is interposed. Note the intimate relationships of the afferent arteriole (AA) to the mesangium. Transmission electron microscopy (TEM) × ~ 4600. **B:** Efferent arteriole of a superficial glomerulus of rat. Note the irregular basement membrane–like material beneath the endothelium (*asterisk*). One to two layers of smooth muscle cells (SM) are encountered. TEM × ~ 3400. **C:** Efferent arteriole of a juxtamedullary glomerulus of rat. Note the many profiles of endothelial cells (*asterisk*); the tight junctions between them are shallow. TEM × ~ 2450. **D:** Descending (DV) and ascending (AV) vasa recta of a vascular bundle in rabbit. The continuous endothelium of the descending vas rectum is surrounded by a pericyte (P). The endothelium of the ascending vas rectum is highly fenestrated (*arrows*). TEM ×~ 2400. PO, podocyte.

and the muscle layer. The juxtamedullary efferent arterioles (Fig. 6C) are surrounded by two to four layers of smooth muscle cells. Their endothelium is composed of a strikingly large number of longitudinally arranged cells: Up to 30 individual cells may be found in cross-sections (149, 319). As in cortical efferent arterioles, the tight junctions between the endothelial cells are shallow (569).

In the descending vasa recta (Fig. 6D) the smooth muscle cells are gradually replaced by pericytes, which form an incomplete layer around the vessel trunk. Pericytes should be regarded as contractile cells. The patterns of these cells, which encircle the endothelial tube–like hoops, and their dense assemblies of microfilaments strongly imply that they have a contractile function. In contrast to smooth muscle cells, they are not contacted by nerve terminals. The descending vasa recta finally lose their pericytes, and the concurrent appearance of endothelial fenestrations marks their gradual transformation into medullary capillaries.

The ultrastructure of the capillaries in the kidney is similar in the cortex and the medulla (with the exception of glomerular capillaries; vide infra). The capillaries of the kidney are of the fenestrated type (Fig. 7). The capillary wall consists of an extremely flat endothelium surrounded by a thin basement membrane. In nonnuclear regions the endothelial cells contain densely and regularly arranged fenestrations that (in contrast to the glomerular capillaries) are bridged by a thin diaphragm. An estimated 50% of the capillary circumference is composed of these fenestration-bearing areas (149). The fenestrations themselves are of rather complex structure. In normal transmission electron microscopy (TEM) sections the diaphragm appears as a very thin (5–6 nm), single-layered membrane provided with a central knob. Deep-etch freezing techniques have revealed a composition of radial fibrils converging to the central knob (56). Recently, a caveolar transmembrane protein, PV-1, has been attributed to the diaphragm (586). The functional significance of this type of capillary has been described in detail elsewhere (580).

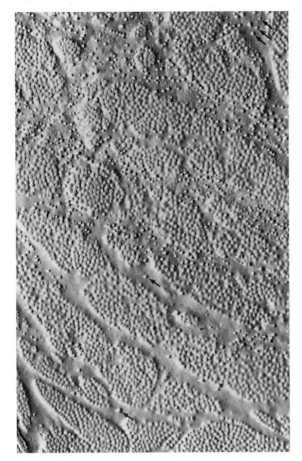

FIGURE 7 Freeze-fracture electron micrograph demonstrating the dense arrangement of fenestrations within the wall of a peritubular capillary; rabbit. Pinocytotic vesicles (*arrows*) are found within areas of thicker cytoplasm, which connects the perikaryon and the more voluminous areas along the cell borders (not shown). Magnification × 7600. (From Schiller A, Taugner R, et al. The thin limbs of Henle's loop in the rabbit. A freeze fracture study. *Cell Tissue Res* 1980;207:249–265, with permission.)

The wall structure of the ascending vasa recta (Fig. 6D) is similar to that of the capillaries. These draining vessels, with wide lumina, are bounded for their entire length by an extremely flat endothelium with extensive fenestrations. The same structure is even found in the large veins of the cortex and at the corticomedullary border (Fig. 8). The interlobular and arcuate veins are not veins in the classic sense, but they have a wall structure fundamentally the same as that of renal capillaries (149, 356). This wall consists solely of an extremely flattened, partly fenestrated endothelium that rests on a basement membrane.

NEPHRONS AND COLLECTING DUCT SYSTEM

The specific structural units of the kidney are the nephrons. In the rat, each kidney contains 30,000 to 35,000 nephrons (32); each human kidney has an estimated 1 million (582) but great interindividual differences exist (8). The nephron

consists of a renal corpuscle connected to a complicated and twisted tube that finally drains into a collecting duct. Based on the location of the renal corpuscles within the cortex, three types of nephrons are distinguished: superficial, midcortical, and juxtamedullary nephrons. Exact definitions of these types, grounded on more than arbitrary decisions, can be based on the different patterns of the efferent arterioles (vide supra).

The tubular part of the nephron consists of a proximal portion and a distal portion connected by a loop of Henle. For details of subdivisions, see Figs. 9 and 10.

According to the lengths of the loops of Henle, two types of nephrons are distinguished (Fig. 9): those with long loops and those with short loops (including those with cortical loops). Short loops turn back in the outer medulla. In many species (rat, rabbit), the bends of the short loops are all located roughly at the same level of the inner stripe, namely, near the junction to the inner medulla. In other species (pig and human), short loops may form their bends at any level of the outer medulla and even in the cortex (cortical loops).

The long loops turn back at successive levels of the inner medulla, many already in its beginning; others reach intermediate levels, and only a few reach the tip of the papilla. Thus, the numbers of loops are successively reduced along the inner medulla toward the papilla. This decrease is paralleled by a decrease in collecting ducts and vasa recta leading to the characteristic form of the inner medulla, which in all species tapers from a broad basis to a papilla (or crest).

The division of nephrons according to the position of their corpuscles in the cortex does not coincide with the division based on the length of their loops. Among species, all three types of renal corpuscles may be attached to both short and long loops. However, within a given species (with short and long loops), the long loops always belong to the deeper renal corpuscles (i.e., juxtamedullary and deep midcortical) and the short loops to the more superficially situated corpuscles.

The numbers of short and long loops vary among species. Some species have only short loops (mountain beaver, muskrat) and consequently lack an inner medulla, which results in a poor ability to concentrate urine (555). Only two species, cat and dog, are known to have only long loops. In comparison with other species, their urine-concentrating ability is considered to be average. In the cat, however, many long loops penetrate into the inner medulla for only a very short distance (less than 0.5 μm (336). If one would define a loop by ultrastructural criteria (vide infra), then a feline kidney does contain many loops resembling the short loops in other species. The formerly held supposition that rodent species with the most powerful ability to concentrate urine, like *Psammomys* or *Meriones*, have only long loops has been proved incorrect (268). Most species have short and long lops, whose ratio varies from species to species. A correlation between the ratio of short and long loops and urine-concentrating ability is not

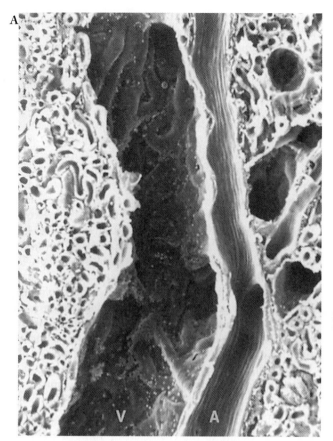
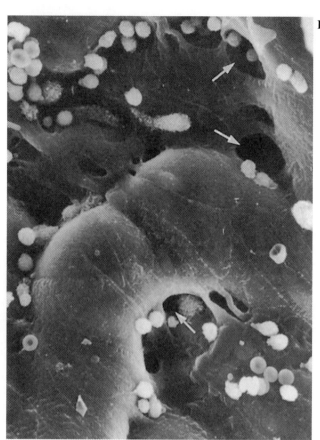

FIGURE 8   Scanning electron micrographs of the inner surface of an arcuate artery and vein; rat. **A:** The tubules underneath the venous wall are clearly discernible through the endothelium, which covers the tubules as a thin coat. Magnification ×~ 120. **B:** Higher magnification of the venous endothelium. The openings in the endothelial wall (*arrows*) mark the positions where venous vasa recta and capillaries empty into the vein. Magnification ×~ 1900. (From Frank M, Kriz W. The luminal aspect of intrarenal arteries and veins in the rat as revealed by scanning electron microscopy. *Anat Embryol (Berl)* 1988;177:371–376, with permission.)

obvious. Most rodent species that have a high urine-concentrating ability (rat, mouse, golden hamster, *Psammomys, Meriones*) have greater numbers of short loops than long loops (268, 315, 699).

The collecting ducts are formed in the renal cortex by the joining of several nephrons (Figs. 9 and 10). The location of the exact border between a nephron and a collecting duct is disputed. According to cytological criteria, a connecting tubule is interposed between a nephron and a cortical collecting duct. Whether this connecting tubule derives from the nephrogenic blastema, and therefore must be considered as a part of the nephron, or from the ureteral bud, and therefore is part of the collecting ducts, remains an open question (271, 465, 471, 482).

Microanatomically, the connecting tubules of deep and superficial nephrons differ (Fig. 9). The connecting tubules of deep nephrons generally join to form an arcade before draining into a collecting duct; superficial nephrons drain via an individual connecting tubule. The numerical ratio between nephrons draining through an arcade and those draining individually varies greatly among species. In rat, rabbit, and pig, most nephrons drain via arcades; as Sperber

(585) observed, some arcades probably exist in all mammalian kidneys.

An arcade ascends within the cortical labyrinth before draining into a cortical collecting duct (Fig. 9). Functionally, an arcade appears to serve as a device that prevents the addition of dilute distal urine to collecting ducts at the corticomedullary junction (266).

The cortical collecting ducts descend within the medullary rays of the cortex and then, as unbranched tubes, traverse the outer medulla (outer medullary collecting ducts). On entering the inner medulla (inner medullary collecting ducts), they fuse successively. In the human kidney, an average of eight fusions has been found (465), a number that may be a good approximation for other species as well (482). Because a cortical collecting duct in the human kidney accepts 11 nephrons on average, it can be calculated that a papillary duct (opening into the renal pelvis) drains a total of 2.750 nephrons. In the rabbit kidney, which has only six nephron tributaries to a cortical collecting duct (271), approximately 1500 nephrons are drained by a terminal collecting duct. It must be emphasized that an inner medullary collecting duct is not a single

lary collecting duct is not a single unbranched tube, but rather is a system of tubules that fuse successively.

INTERSTITIUM AND LYMPHATICS

The interstitial space is bounded by the basement membranes of the renal epithelia and of the blood vessels (Fig. 11), as well as by the renal fibrous capsule. In all renal zones the main cellular constituents of the interstitium are (1) resident fibroblasts and (2) dendritic cells (156, 269). In addition a few lymphocytes and macrophages may be found. The spaces between the cells are filled with extracellular matrix (see following sections).

The peritubular interstitium is involved in virtually all functions of the healthy kidney. A transit across the interstitial extracellular compartment is obligatory for all substances transported from tubules to blood and reciprocally, as well as for many regulatory substances from their site of production to their target site (354). Morphometric measurements have shown that in the cortex only the minor part (about 26% [329] or 42% [480], depending on the definition and used technique of assessment) of the total outer tubular surfaces is directly apposed to capillaries. Thus, it can be concluded that a major part of the reabsorbed tubular fluid has to traverse a true interstitial space before entering the capillaries.

Cellular Constituents

The cells of the interstitium, besides taking part in the modeling of the extracellular matrix, play a role in the production of regulatory substances.

FIBROBLASTS

The peritubular fibroblasts (Fig. 12) establish the scaffolding frame for tubules, renal corpuscles, and blood vessels, and thus maintain the three-dimensional architecture of the tissue. With their filiform and leaflike processes fibroblasts form a continuous network throughout the interstitial space (269, 597), and they are in close touch with all renal structures, including nerve endings. Furthermore, fibroblasts reveal consistent and narrow contacts with all types of migrating interstitial cells (Fig. 12B).

The pericaryon of fibroblasts in healthy interstitium is usually stellate (Fig. 12). The nuclei are surrounded by a strikingly narrow rim of cytoplasm, usually devoid of any cell organelles. In unstimulated fibroblasts the characteristically-prominent apparatus for protein synthesis (i.e., rough endoplasmic reticuli [ERs], ribosomes, Golgi apparatus, and mitochondria) is situated in the large peripheral cell processes. The fibroblast processes are physically connected to the basement membranes of epithelia and vessels and the filiform processes are interconnected by intermediate-like junctions (550) (Fig. 12A). In

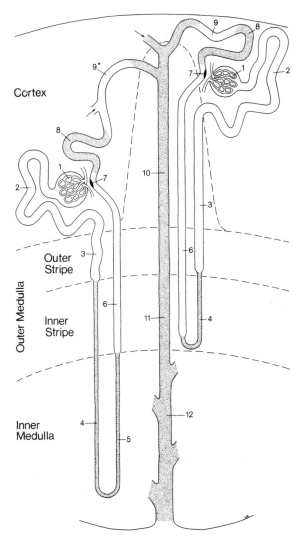

FIGURE 9 Schematic of nephrons and collecting duct. This scheme depicts a short-looped and a long-looped nephron together with the collecting system. Not drawn to scale. Within the cortex a medullary ray is delineated by a dashed line. *1*, Renal corpuscle including Bowman's capsule and the glomerulus (glomerular tuft); *2*, proximal convoluted tubule; *3*, proximal straight tubule; *4*, descending thin limb; *5*, ascending thin limb; *6*, distal straight tubule (thick ascending limb); *7*, macula densa located within the final portion of the thick ascending limb; *8*, distal convoluted tubule; *9*, connecting tubule; *9**, connecting tubule of the juxtamedullary nephron that forms an arcade; *10*, cortical collecting duct; *11*, outer medullary collecting duct; *12*, inner medullary collecting duct. (From Frank M, Kriz W. The luminal aspect of intrarenal arteries and veins in the rat as revealed by scanning electron microscopy. *Anat Embryol (Berl)* 1988;177:371–376, with permission.)

unbranched tube, but rather is a system of tubules that fuse successively. In the human kidney, an average of eight fusions has been found (465), a number that may be a good approximation for other species as well (482). Because a cortical collecting duct in the human kidney accepts 11 nephrons on average, it can be calculated that a papillary duct (opening into the renal pelvis) drains a total of 2.750 nephrons. In the rabbit kidney, which has only six nephron tributaries to a cortical collecting duct (271), approximately 1500 nephrons are drained by a terminal collecting duct. It must be emphasized that an inner medul-

Micro-anatomical terms	Main divisions	Subdivisions	Segmentation	Abbreviation	Cell types	Other frequently used denominations
Proximal convolution	PROXIMAL TUBULE	pars convoluta or convoluted part	Proximal Convoluted Tubule — S1-segment	PCT	S1 cells	P1 segment — PT
			S2-segment		S2 cells	P2 segment
		pars recta or straight part	Proximal Straight Tubule — S3-segment	PST	S3 cells	P3 segment — PR
Loop of HENLE	INTERMEDIATE TUBULE	pars descendens or descending part	Descending Thin Limb — of short loops	DTL	DTL cells Type 1	Short Descending Thin Limb of Henle's loop (SDL)
			of long loops upper part		Type 2	Long Descending Thin Limb, upper part (LDL_u)
			lower part		Type 3	Long Descending Thin Limb, lower part ($LDL_ℓ$)
			pre-bend segment		ATL cells	
		pars ascendens or ascending part	Ascending Thin Limb	ATL	Type 4	TAL Thin Ascending Limb (of long loops only)
Distal convolution	DISTAL TUBULE	pars recta or straight part	Distal Straight Tubule — Medullary straight part	MTAL / DST or TAL	DST or TAL cells	MAL mTALH Thick Ascending Limb of Henle's Loop / Medullary Thick Limb
			or Thick Ascending Limb — Cortical straight part	CTAL		CAL cTALH Cortical Thick Limb (incl. Macula Densa)
			Macula Densa	MD	MD cells	MD
			postmacular segment			DCTa* early distal tubule
		pars convoluta or convoluted part	Distal Convoluted Tubule	DCT	DCT cells (+ IC cells)	DCTb* Distal Tubule
Collecting duct	COLLECTING SYSTEM		CoNnecting Tubule	CNT	CNT cells + IC cells	DCTg* CCTg* late distal tubule Connecting Segment
		COLLECTING DUCT	Cortical Collecting Duct	CCD	CD cells = principal cells = light cells	DCTℓ* CCTℓ* Initial Collecting Tubule / Cortical Collecting Tubule (CCT)
			Outer Medullary Collecting Duct	OMCD	IC cells = intercalated cells = mitochondria-rich cells = carboanhydrase-rich cells = dark cells	Outer Medullary Collecting Tubule (OMCT)
			Inner Medullary Collecting Duct	IMCD	CD cells = principal cells	Inner Medullary Collecting Tubule (IMCT) / Papillary Collecting Duct (PCD) or Ducts of Bellini

FIGURE 10 Segmentation of the renal tubule. This table summarizes the nomenclature of segments and cells of the renal tubule. A continuous serpentine arrow indicates that the transition between the two structures is gradual. An interrupted serpentine arrow indicates that the transition is gradual in some species, abrupt in others. Abbreviations marked by a star were introduced by Morel and coworkers (304). DCTa, distal convoluted tubule, initial portion; DCTb, distal convoluted tubule, bright portion; DCTg, distal convoluted tubule, granular portion; DCTl, distal convoluted tubule, light portion; CCTg, cortical collecting tubule, granular portion; CCTl, cortical collecting tubule, light portion. (From Frank M, Kriz W. The luminal aspect of intrarenal arteries and veins in the rat as revealed by scanning electron microscopy. *Anat Embryol (Berl)* 1988;177:371–376, with permission.)

conventional TEM, peritubular fibroblasts are distinguished from all other cells in the interstitial space (e.g., dendritic cells or lymphocytes) by the conspicuous layers of actin filaments under the plasma membrane of the pericaryons (346), which are concentrated in the thin filiform processes and at the contacts of the processes with the basement membranes of tubules and capillaries (269). The peritubular fibroblasts in the renal cortex have been shown to be the source of renal erythropoietin (24).

DENDRITIC CELLS

Dendritic cells constitute the major antigen-presenting cell (APC) population in the healthy kidney (Fig. 12B) (20). They are distributed in a rather regular pattern throughout the peritubular spaces and are usually found in very close vicinity to fibroblasts (269, 274). Renal dendritic cells are essential immunoregulatory cells. In addition to initiating protective immune responses, they play an active role in maintaining peripheral tolerance (156). In the healthy kidney they are present in their immature phenotype with comparatively low levels of major histocompatibility complex (MHC) class II, CD 11c (333), and costimulatory proteins, but with a high capacity for uptake of antigens (156). They acquire the mature phenotype with high antigen-presenting capacity during their migration to the renal lymph nodes. Dendritic cells possess broad and filiform cell processes that extend into the narrow spaces between tubules and capillaries, in a manner similar to that of fibroblast processes. Unlike fibroblasts, the dendritic cells display mitochondria, ER, and Golgi apparatus in their large pericaryon whereas their processes usually are devoid of cell organelles. Dendritic cells lack the layer of actin filaments beneath the plasma membrane. On this morphological basis distinction between fibroblasts and dendritic is possible by conventional EM in the healthy renal interstitium.

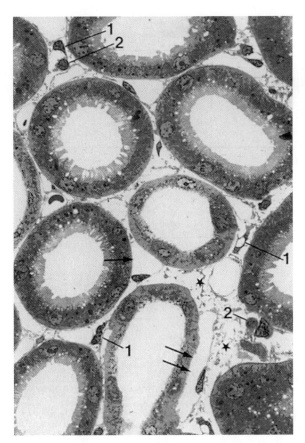

FIGURE 11 Peritubular interstitium of the renal cortex in rat kidney with narrow (*arrows*) and wide (*stars*) portions. Interstitial cells are resident fibroblasts (*1*) and temporarily sojourning dendritic/mononuclear cells (*2*). Transmission electron microscopy (TEM) × ~720.

MACROPHAGES AND LYMPHOCYTES

Macrophages and lymphocytes are rarely found in the healthy renal interstitium but they invade the inters-titial spaces under inflammatory conditions (179). A large proportion of the invading mononuclear cells display besides the established "marker proteins" (CD 45, CD3, CD4, CD 8; ED1, ED2, CD44, etc.) the S100A4 (fibroblast-specific protein, FSP1) protein (346).

Extracellular Matrix

The extracellular matrix of the interstitium is composed of a network of fibers, proteoglycans, glycoproteins, and interstitial fluid (354, 493). Several types of fibers are found, among them typical interstitial collagen fibers (type 1, type 3, and type 6) (282). Type 3 fibers correspond to the reticular fibers that form a network enveloping individual tubules. In addition, microfibrils (collagen type 1) are found throughout the renal interstitium. Proteoglycans are an important component of the interstitial matrix in the kidney, especially in the medulla (vide infra [492]). Elsewhere in the body various glycoproteins (fibronectin, laminin, and others) are found associated with tubular basement membranes as well as to fibrillar structures of the interstitial reticulum. Most of these substances are important substrates for migration of interstitial cells.

Zonal Differences of the Renal Interstitium

CORTICAL INTERSTITIUM AND LYMPHATICS

In the renal cortex, the peritubular interstitium must be distinguished from the periarterial connective tissue.

The *peritubular interstitium* in the cortex of healthy rats (Fig. 11) is scanty, amounting to 7% to 9% by volume (including the interstitial cells; true interstitial spaces approximately 4% (277, 329, 480, 488). In the cortical interstitium of healthy kidneys immunocytochemistry facilitates the discrimination between fibroblasts and dendritic cells. Whereas the plasma membrane of dendritic cells displays, among others, MHC class II, CD11c, and costimulatory proteins (333), that of cortical peritubular fibroblasts is distinguished by the enzyme ecto-5'-nucleotidase (5'NT) (269). In rats this enzyme becomes detectable in renal stromal cells within the second postnatal week, when the expression of the intermediate filament vimentin and α smooth muscle actin (α-SMA) by stromal cells disappears (401). The hydrolysis of 5'-AMP by 5'NT yields (extracellular) adenosine (347). Among others, the glomerular arterioles, the renin-containing granular cells, and the nerve endings along the arterioles (202) in the cortical labyrinth are targets for extracellular adenosine and are found in particularly narrow contact with fibroblasts.

In healthy kidneys the activity of the enzyme is highest in fibroblasts in the deep cortical labyrinth (Fig. 13A) (138). This pattern may change: For instance, under anemia the activity of the enzyme has been found to be strongly upregulated in rat fibroblasts in the superficial cortex and to a lesser extent in the medullary rays (277, 345). Congruent distribution patterns were observed for cells, displaying mRNA for erythropoietin. In normemic rats and mice, mRNA for erythropoietin (EPO) was detected only in peritubular cells in the deep cortical labyrinth, whereas with anemia (313) and hypoxia (177, 178), EPO mRNA was detected in peritubular cells even immediately under the renal capsule (Fig. 13). The striking coincidences in the distribution of 5'NT and EPO mRNA under a variety of functional conditions led to the identification of renal peritubular fibroblasts as source of renal EPO (24, 410).

Extensive phenotypical modulations of cortical peritubular fibroblasts in vivo occur under the concerted action of inflammatory cytokines and growth factors (7, 143, 145). Under these conditions the 5'NT-positive peritubular fibroblasts in the adult kidney seem to transform to *myofibroblasts*, "reexpress" α-SMA and vimentin, and their processes become coupled by gap junctions (535). Myofibroblasts differ from peritubular fibroblasts of the healthy renal interstitium by qualitatively and quantitatively altered extracellular matrix production (7, 143, 145) a reduced potential for erythropoietin gene expression (409), and over time they loose their 5'NT-activity (B. K., unpublished data, July 2002).

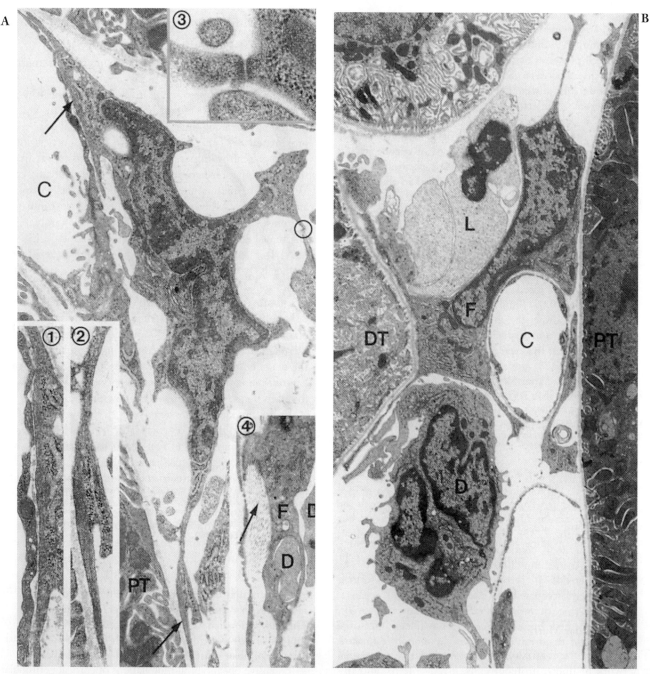

FIGURE 12   **A**: Fibroblast in the cortical peritubular interstitium of a rat kidney; the broad cytoplasmic processes of the sharply outlined pericaryon adhere to the tubular (PT) and capillary (C) basement membranes; the processes show abundant cisterns of rough endoplasmic reticulum and actin filaments (**insets 1 and 2**); filiform fibroblast processes are interconnected by intermediate junctions (*circle*, **inset 3**); collagen fibrils (**inset 4**, *arrow*) closely associated with a fibroblast (F) that encloses part of a dendritic cell (D). Transmission electron microscopy (TEM) ×~ 11,800; inserts 1 and 2, TEM ×~ 23,000; insert 3, TEM ×~ 50,000; insert 4, TEM ×~ 11,800. **B**: Fibroblast (F) in a focal peritubular inflammation, caused by a lesion in a distal tubule; the fibroblast spans the space between a diseased distal (DT) and a healthy proximal tubule (PT) profile, partially encloses a profile of a peritubular capillary (C), and has close contact to migrating cells of the immune system. L, lymphocyte; D, dendritic cell. TEM ×~ 6000.

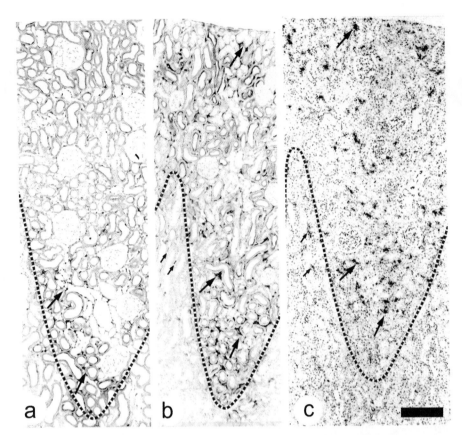

FIGURE 13 Distribution of peritubular ecto-5′nucleotidase activity and erythropoietin mRNA in rat kidney. **A,B:** Enzyme histochemistry; cryostat sections; **(C)** in situ hybridization; paraffin section; the cortical labyrinth is delimited by a *broken line*. **A:** Normemic rat; interstitial enzyme activity (*arrows*) is strongest in the deep cortical labyrinth and decreases toward the superficial cortex; enzyme activity is virtually lacking in the interstitium in the medullary rays and in the outer stripe. **B:** Anemic rat; interstitial enzyme activity is strong (*arrows*) throughout the cortical labyrinth and weakly apparent in the medullary rays. **C:** Same animal as in **B**; signals for erythropoietin mRNA (*arrows*) are detected in the peritubular interstitium throughout the cortex, a few weak signals appear in the medullary rays; in normemic rats (not shown) the signals are found exclusively in the deep cortical labyrinth. Magnification A–C, ×~60; bars, ~ 200 mm. (From Kaissling B, Hegyi I, et al. Morphology of interstitial cells in the healthy kidney. *Anat Embryol* 1996;193:303–318, with permission.)

PERIARTERIAL CONNECTIVE TISSUE

The periarterial tissue is a layer of loose connective tissue surrounding the intrarenal arteries (arcuate arteries, cortical radial arteries) (Fig. 14) and is continuous with the connective tissue underlying the epithelium of the renal pelvis and ureter. The renal veins are apposed to the periarterial sheath (316). At all sites, the periarterial sheath is continuous with the peritubular interstitium and is constituted by large meshes, formed by the extremely attenuated processes of 5′NT-negative, but weakly α-SMA–, and vimentin-positive fibroblasts (269). The meshes are filled with thick bundles of collageneous fibers and interstitial fluid and regularly confine some macrophages. The considerable thickness of the periarterial sheath is apparent in quick-frozen specimens (316) and in perfusion-fixed tissue. It attenuates toward the end of the cortical radial arteries and terminates along the afferent arteriole at the vascular pole of the glomerulus.

The periarterial connective tissue sheath provides the path for renal nerves (see following sections) and for *renal lymphatics* (316). The latter may start in the vicinity of the glomerular vascular pole (320) or at a more proximal level of the afferent arteriole, depending on the species and travel within the periarterial tissue sheath of the branches of the renal arteries toward the renal hilum (Fig. 15). In addition to the lymphatics, the periarterial tissue itself constitutes a pathway for interstitial fluid drainage. Indeed, a tracer, injected under the renal capsule, can be followed within the periarterial interstitium and lymphatics. A pathway toward lymphatics through peritubular and periarterial interstitia may be important for the systemic distribution of regulatory substances that are released into the peritubular interstitium. This suggestion has been made for renin (316) and it may apply for other protein hormones like erythropoietin. The periarterial tissue sheaths have been interpreted as a mixing chamber for a variety of

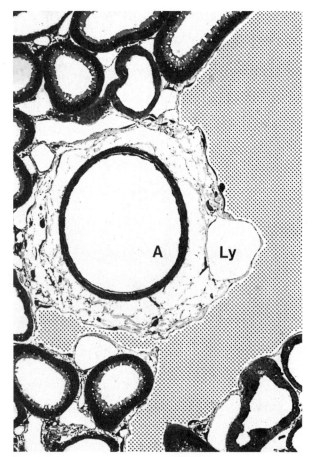

FIGURE 14 Cross-section through the deep cortex in the rat. The cortical radial artery (A) is surrounded by a layer of loose connective tissue that contains the lymphatics (Ly). The cortical radial vein is only partly demonstrated; its lumen and those of direct tributaries have been highlighted by a dotted texture. Note the intimate relationships of the artery, vein, and lymphatic, mediated by the periarterial loose connective tissue. Transmission electron microscopy (TEM) ×~ 360.

vasoactive substances, ultimately determining the contractile status of the renal resistance vessels. While a fraction of cortical interstitial fluid gains access to the periarterial interstitium, and eventually to lymphatics, there is no direct pathway for regulatory substances released in the cortical interstitium to reach medullary targets. It has been proposed that the intimate relationships between cortical radial arteries and veins permit countercurrent exchange of O_2, being responsible—at least in part—for the low partial pressure of O_2 in the superficial cortex (564).

MEDULLARY INTERSTITIUM

The medullary interstitial volume is differently developed in the three medullary zones. In the outer stripe of the outer medulla, the interstitial spaces are extremely sparse (fractional volume ~3%–5%), similar as in the vascular bundle compartment within the inner stripe. In the interbundle compartment of the inner stripe, the fractional volume amounts up to 10% in rat (298, 488). In the inner zone, it continuously increases from the base (10%–15% fractional volume in rat, 20%–25%

in rabbit) to the tip of the papilla (~ 30% in rat; more than 40% in rabbit; (298, 678). The medullary interstitium has no drainage by lymphatics (316, 319).

The phenotype of fibroblasts in the medulla shows progressive transformation from the cortical phenotype to the so-called lipid-laden cell in the inner medulla. The inner medullary fibroblasts are oriented perpendicularly, like "rungs of a ladder," to the longitudinal axis of tubules and vessels (Fig. 16), which in the inner medulla all run in parallel to each other (354, 597).

One striking change in the ultrastructure of medullary fibroblasts is the progressive increase in cytoskeletal elements toward the deep inner zone; actin filaments form a very prominent layer under the plasma membrane of the pericaryon and the processes. The latter may be interconnected by a composite type of intercellular junction (550). Furthermore, the medullary fibroblasts display lipid droplets in their cytoplasm (hence, their designation as lipid-laden cells), the frequency of which usually increases from the inner stripe toward the inner medulla. The capacity for lipid accumulation is, however, not specific for inner medullary interstitial cells but is intrinsic to fibroblasts. Under specific functional conditions (e. g., anemia), lipid droplets are found also in cortical fibroblasts (277) and inner medullary fibroblasts may lack lipid droplets (354). In vitro studies have revealed that the occurrence and amount of lipid droplets in the inner medullary fibroblasts depends on the specific environment of the cells, conditioned by the presence of inner medullary collecting duct cells. Inner medullary fibroblasts can transform to myofibroblasts with upregulation of α-SMA and desmin (219). In medullary fibroblasts, the cisterns of rough endoplasmic reticulum (rER), including the perinuclear cistern, are often strikingly enlarged and they may narrowly enclose mitochondria (Fig. 17). Occasionally the rER membranes are in direct touch with the plasma membrane. The functional interpretation of these particular features, only rarely observed in cortical fibroblasts, is still missing.

The medullary fibroblasts do not display 5′NT or mRNA for EPO. A role of medullary interstitial cells has been proposed in the regulation of urinary osmolality. By their arrangement perpendicular to the longitudinal axis of the papilla they might constitute a barrier against dissipation of the osmotic gradient in the interstitium (354). Glycosaminoglycans are particularly abundant in the inner medullary interstitium (338). Condensed hyaluronate–proteoglycan aggregates are associated with basement membranes, collage fibers, and diffuse reticular structures.

The inner medulla has the greatest capacity for renal prostaglandin (PG) synthesis (434, 641). Cyclooxygenase (COX) isoforms, rate-limiting enzymes in PG biosynthesis, are expressed at substantially higher levels in the inner medulla than in the renal cortex (82, 259, 687, 688). COX-2 is found predominantly in inner medullary interstitial fibroblasts, and its expression increases under chronic salt loading (688).

Dendritic cells are abundant in the inner stripe in the outer medulla and, like in the cortex, are narrowly associated with

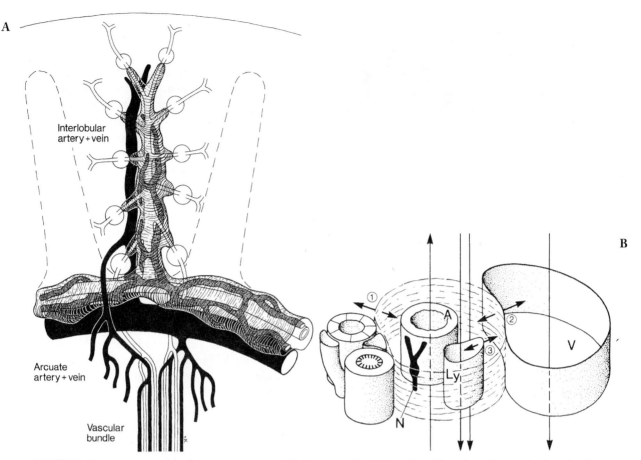

FIGURE 15 Schematics to show **(A)** the distribution and **(B)** the topographical relationships of the periarterial connective tissue sheath. Not drawn to scale. **A:** The periarterial sheath is schematically indicated as a wide "stocking" drawn over the intrarenal arteries and lymphatics. In reality this stocking has no limiting tissue that separates the interior from the surroundings. An arcuate artery transforms into a cortical radial artery, which gives rise to afferent arterioles. These segments are surrounded by the periarterial connective tissue sheath. The efferent arterioles, as well as the veins (*black*), are not included. The lymphatics (*stippled*) originate and travel within the periarterial sheath. Note there are no lymphatics coming up from the medulla. Within the cortex medullary rays are indicated by a broken line. In **B**, a transverse section through an cortical radial artery **(A)** shows the relationships of the periarterial sheath and the possibilities for functional exchanges (*double-headed arrows*) with surrounding structures: (*1*) with the peritubular interstitium; (*2*) with the accompanying vein (V), and (*3*) with lymphatics (Ly). The single-headed arrows indicate the flow of the respective fluid. Note the nerves (N) traveling through the periarterial tissue. In addition, two neighboring tubules, including an arcade and a proximal tubule, together with peritubular capillaries, are drawn. (From Kriz W. A periarterial pathway for intrarenal distribution of renin. *Kidney Int Suppl* 1987;20:S51–S56, with permission.)

fibroblasts. Accumulations of dendritic cells are particularly striking around collecting ducts and thick ascending limbs.

In the inner medulla dendritic cells progressively disappear; in the lower two thirds of the inner medulla bone marrow–derived cells are not detected in the healthy kidney (269, 274).

Nerves

The efferent nerves of the kidney are composed of sympathetic nerves and terminal axons, which accompany the intrarenal arteries and the afferent and efferent arterioles (Fig. 18) (8, 44). The nerve fibers are monoaminergic. Norepinephrine (50, 155, 214) and dopamine have been identified (151). In addition, several neuropeptides are colocalized with norepinephrine in renal nerves (624). The presence of acetylcholinesterase in renal nerves cannot be taken to

indicate cholinergic nerves, but rather that monoaminergic nerves obviously possess acetylcholinesterase activity (48).

The nerve fibers run in the loose connective tissue around the arteries and arterioles. The descending vasa recta within the medulla are innervated by adrenergic nerve terminals as far as they are enveloped by smooth muscle cells (148, 196). A dense assembly of nerves and terminal axons is found around the juxtaglomerular apparatus (JGA) (214) and are described in more detail along with the JGA.

Tubules have direct relationships to terminal axons only when they are located around the arteries or arterioles (44, 214). Tubules adjacent to the JGA (terminal portion of the cortical thick ascending limb) are more frequently touched by terminal axons than at other sites (214). The density of nerve contacts to convoluted proximal tubules (located in the cortical labyrinth) is low (47); nerve contacts to straight proximal tubules (located in the

A

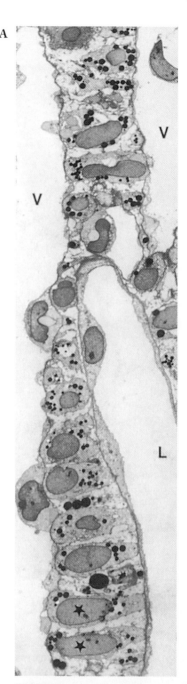

B

certain tubular segments (271). Because nerve fibers pass along the vascular pole of each glomerulus from afferent to efferent arterioles, the distribution of nerves in the renal cortex is dense. Catecholamines (and other transmitters) released from nerve terminals at the vascular poles and at the efferent arterioles may gain access to peritubular capillaries and in this way may perfuse the convoluted tubules of the cortical labyrinth. Tubules arranged around the cortical radial arteries would be reached most easily by transmitters released from periarterially located nerve terminals. This may be of relevance with respect to arcades (connecting tubules), which have been shown to be sensitive to isoproterenol (432). Exposure of the straight tubules within the medullary rays of the cortex to neural transmitters reaching them directly by diffusion from nerve terminal is improbable.

Tubules in the outer medulla may only be reached by neurotransmitters if they are situated adjacent to vascular bundles (a minority of tubules) or, secondarily, by a capillary distribution of the transmitters from nerve terminals accompanying the vascular bundles. The tubules of the inner medulla do not have a chance to be reached by neurotransmitters, directly delivered from nerve terminals in the medulla.

Little is known about the afferent nerves of the kidney; they are commonly believed to be sparse, but the issue remains unresolved (49, 117, 146–148, 189, 195).

TOPOGRAPHICAL RELATIONSHIPS

Cortex

The architectural pattern of the renal cortex is best understood when viewing a cross-section through the midcortex (Figs. 19, 20). Two portions within the cortical parenchyma, the labyrinth and the medullary rays, are distinguished. Within the cortical labyrinth, the vascular axes, which consist of the cortical radial (interlobular) artery, vein, and a lymphatic, are regularly distributed. Around each vascular axis the renal corpuscles and the corresponding convoluted tubules (proximal and distal) are situated. Barriers separating the population of renal corpuscles and convoluted tubules belonging to another vascular axis are not discernible. Thus, the cortical labyrinth is a continuous parenchymal layer that contains the vascular axes of the cortex and the medullary rays in a regular pattern. The straight tubules (proximal and distal), together with the collecting ducts, are located within the medullary rays. Because the number of straight tubules increases toward the corticomedullary border, the medullary rays increase in width toward the outer stripe.

A regular pattern of the convoluted tubules within the labyrinth is not apparent. Proximal and distal convoluted tubules (the latter constitute only a minor portion of profiles in comparison with proximal tubules) are equally embedded in the dense capillary plexus of this region. A strikingly constant position is occupied by the arcades (if they are present). They ascend within the cortical labyrinth and are grouped

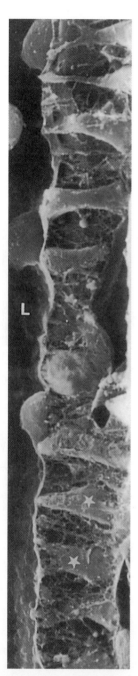

FIGURE 16 Interstitial fibroblasts of the inner medulla, demonstrated in longitudinal sections. The fibroblasts (*asterisks*) are arranged like the rungs of a ladder between parallel running tubules or vessels. The fibroblasts contain numerous lipid granules (*black*) of different sizes (visible in **A**). L, loop limb; V, vessel. **A**: *Psammomys*; transmission electron microscopy (TEM) ×~1350; **B**: Rat; scanning electron microscopy (SEM), ×~ 3400. (Courtesy of J. M. Barrett.)

medullary rays and the outer stripe) have never been encountered. The overwhelming majority of tubular portions have no direct relationships to nerve terminals.

Consequently, morphologists are left with the question of how the neuronal influence on tubular function (147) is mediated. In addition to a systemic distribution of catecholamines, a more specific but indirect mode seems possible for

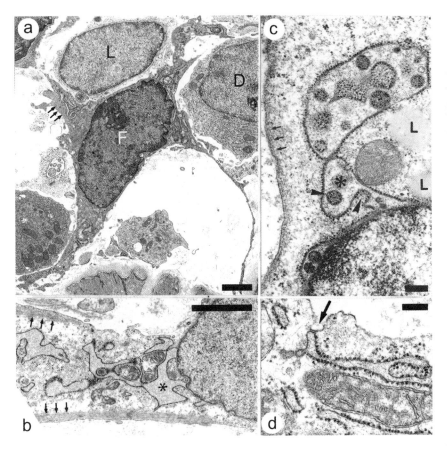

FIGURE 17 Medullary fibroblasts, human fibroblasts from a renal biopsy **(A, B, D)**, and fibroblast from a perfusion-fixed rat kidney **(C)**. **A:** Human fibroblast at the corticomedullary border; stellate pericaryon and microfilament-rich cell processes (*small arrows*), extending between immune cells. **B:** Part of a human fibroblast in the inner stripe of the outer medulla; the cisterns of the rough endoplasmic reticulum are widened and filled with flocculent material (*asterisk*, dilated perinuclear cistern; *small arrows,* accumulations of microfilaments along the plasma membrane). **C:** Rat fibroblast from the inner medulla showing dilated perinuclear and endoplasmic reticulum cisterns (*asterisk*); in-foldings of the endoplasmic reticulum into the cistern (*arrowhead*); L, lipid droplets. **D:** Fibroblast in the outer stripe of the outer medulla; a profile of rough endoplasmic reticulum in direct contact with the plasma membrane (*arrow*). Transmission electron microscopy (TEM): **A,** ×~4760; **B,** × ~8500; **C,** × ~37,400; **D,** ×~33,150; bars: **A,B,** ~ 2 mm; **C,D,** ~0.2 mm. (From Kaissling B, Hegyi I, et al. Morphology of interstitial cells in the healthy kidney. *Anat Embryol* 1996;193:303–318, with permission.)

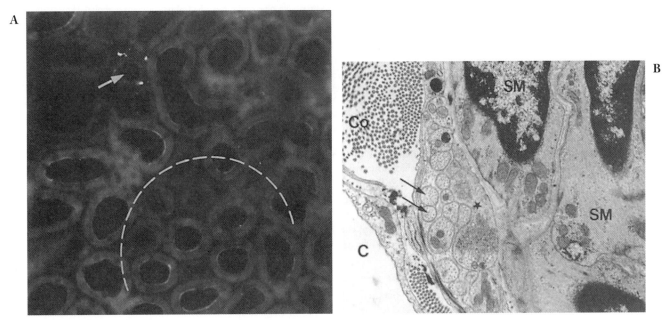

FIGURE 18 The renal nerves accompany **(A)** the intrarenal arteries in the rat. A cortical radial artery (*arrow*) is associated with three nerve bundles, identified by staining with a monoclonal antibody against protein gene product 9.5 (PGP 9.5), which is a universal marker for vertebrate neurons. (From Miner JH. Renal basement membrane components. *Kidney Int* 1999;56:2016–2024.) Among the tubules no nerves are found. A medullary ray is delineated by a hatched line. LM ×~ 240. (Courtesy of M. Siry, W. Kummer, and S. Bachmann). **B:** A large terminal nerve accompanying an afferent arteriole. Several axons (*arrows*) and a varicosity (*star*) with synaptic vesicles are seen. SM, smooth muscle cell; CO, collagen; C, capillary. Rabbit kidney; transmission electron microscopy (TEM) × ~12,000.

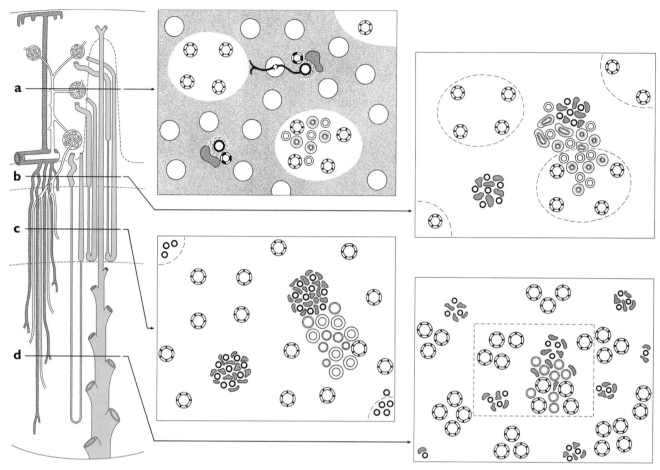

FIGURE 19 Schematics of histotopography. Histotopography of the kidney as revealed by four successive cross-sections through **(A)** cortex, **(B)** outer stripe, **(C)** inner stripe, and **(D)** inner medulla. The simple type of the medulla (rabbit, human) is shown. (From Koushanpour E, Kriz W. *Renal Physiology: Principles, Structure and Function.* New York: Springer-Verlag, 1986, with permission.) **A:** In the cortex the cortical labyrinth (*shaded area*) and the medullary rays (*white*) are shown. The labyrinth contains the cortical radial (interlobular) blood vessels, glomeruli, and the convoluted tubular portions (the latter are not shown). The arcades accompany the interlobular vessels. The medullary rays contain the collecting ducts and the straight proximal and distal tubules. Note the typical grouping of collecting ducts within a medullary ray. **B:** In the outer stripe vascular bundles replace the interlobular vessel axis of the cortex. The continuations of the medullary rays are surrounded by hatched lines. Within these areas the collecting ducts and the loop limbs of superficial and midcortical nephrons are found. The loop limbs of juxtamedullary nephrons are situated around the vascular bundles. **C:** In the inner stripe the vascular bundles are fully developed. Like in the outer stripe, the loop limbs of juxtamedullary nephrons are situated near the bundles, and those from superficial and midcortical nephrons together with the collecting ducts are located distant from the bundles. Note the heterogeneity of the thin limbs: Those of juxtamedullary nephrons lie near the bundles and are thicker in diameter, whereas those of the superficial nephrons lie distant from the bundles. **D:** Inner medulla. The area defined by the dashed rectangle corresponds to the entire area shown in **C.** This reduction in size is because short loops and many vasa recta have turned back in the inner stripe. Note the grouping of collecting ducts reflecting their medullary ray arrangement in the cortex. Thin limbs (both descending and ascending) are associated with vasa recta or collecting ducts.

immediately around the vascular axes. The topographical relationships within the JGA will be described later.

Within the medullary rays, the straight tubules of superficial nephrons (proximal and distal) generally occupy a central position, those of midcortical nephrons a peripheral position. The collecting ducts are situated between the two groups and therefore are situated neither in the center nor at the very border of a medullary ray. Efferent arterioles do not enter the medullary rays but frequently do break off into capillaries just at the border between the labyrinth and the medullary rays. As a result, the blood supply of the medul-

lary ray tubules is as direct as that of the tubules within the cortical labyrinth. However, blood that perfuses the straight tubules of the medullary rays later mixes with the blood that perfuses the convoluted tubules (vide supra).

Medulla

The three regions of the medulla contain different populations of nephron segments. The outer stripe contains straight parts of the proximal tubule (S_3 segments), straight parts of the distal tubule (thick ascending limbs), and collecting

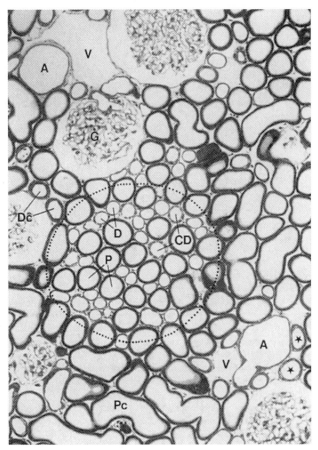

FIGURE 20   Renal cortex of the rat; 1-μm cross-section. The architectural pattern of the cortex is demonstrated. A medullary ray is delineated by a dashed line. It contains the straight proximal (P), the straight distal tubules (thick ascending limb; *asterisks*), and the collecting ducts (C). The cortical radial vessels (A, artery; V, vein), glomeruli (G), and convoluted proximal (Pc) and distal (D) tubules establish the cortical labyrinth. Arcades (*stars*) ascend close to the cortical radial vessels. Magnification, ×~200.

ducts. The inner stripe is composed of descending thin limbs, ascending thick limbs (distal straight tubules), and collecting ducts. The inner medulla contains thin descending and ascending limbs and collecting ducts.

The architectural organization of the medulla can best be described by considering the vascular bundles as central axes and studying how the tubules are arranged around them (315, 646). "Simple" and "complex" types of renal medulla are distinguished (Fig. 21) ; the differences between both are mainly found in the inner stripe.

In the *outer stripe* the vascular bundles develop (Figs. 19, 22). At the beginning of the bundles the straight proximal and distal tubules of juxtamedullary nephrons are grouped immediately around the bundles. In continuation of the medullary rays, the tubules of superficial and midcortical nephrons, together with the collecting ducts, fill the spaces between the bundles and their adjacent juxtamedullary tubules. Although in the outer stripe straight proximal tubules and straight distal tubules (thick ascending limbs) should

theoretically be present in equal numbers, a cross-section through the outer stripe shows that proximal tubular profiles are much more prominent than distal tubules. In the rat, proximal tubules occupy roughly 68% of the space in the outer stripe, in contrast to approximately 13% by the thick ascending limbs and 5% by the collecting ducts (488). The dominance of the proximal tubules is rooted in the fact that the straight proximal tubules of juxtamedullary nephrons are not straight (as their name indicates) but rather take a tortuous course when descending through the outer stripe; this holds true for the mouse kidney (697). In addition, straight proximal tubules are much thicker in diameter than the straight distal tubules, and proximal tubules of juxtamedullary nephrons are even thicker than those of the midcortical and superficial nephrons (271).

The tubules of the outer stripe are perfused by a specific "capillary" plexus. True capillaries, derived from direct branches of efferent arterioles, are few; the dominating capillary vessels in the outer stripe are the ascending vasa recta (Figs. 3 and 4B). They traverse the outer stripe as wide tortuous channels contacting the tubules in a manner similar to the capillaries proper. Because these vessels carry the entire venous blood from the medulla, the outer stripe tubules are mainly supplied by venous blood from deeper parts of the medulla.

It should be mentioned that the outer stripe varies considerably in thickness among species. In the rat (315) and mouse (699), it is very well developed and constitutes approximately one third of the outer medulla. In contrast, in *Psammomys* (268), cat (482), and humans (482) the outer stripe is thin, and in dog (93) it is almost completely absent; thus, a correlation between the elaboration of the outer stripe and the urine-concentrating capacity is absent.

The *inner stripe* of the outer medulla is the most constant part of the renal medulla, consisting of the prominent vascular bundles (VBs), which are regularly distributed within the interbundle region (IBR) (Figs. 19 and 23). Two types of vascular bundles must be distinguished. These differences in bundle structure are the basis for the discrimination of a simple and a complex type of medulla.

In most species (271, 317), vascular bundles of the so-called simple type are present, which exclusively contain descending and ascending vasa recta. The tubules are found in the IBR and are arranged around the bundles in a pattern similar to that found in the outer stripe. The loops of Henle, originating from juxtamedullary nephrons (generally the longest long loops), lie nearest to the bundles, whereas those loops derived from superficial and midcortical nephrons (in most species, short loops) lie distant from the bundles. The collecting ducts are generally arranged in distant rings around the bundles and are intermingled with loops derived from superficial and midcortical nephrons. Altogether, they are perfused by the dense capillary plexus of this region.

The complex type of vascular bundle (Fig. 24) is present in several rodents with a high urine-concentrating ability, including rat (315), mouse (327, 699), *Meriones* (321), and *Psammomys* (268). Its difference from the simple type

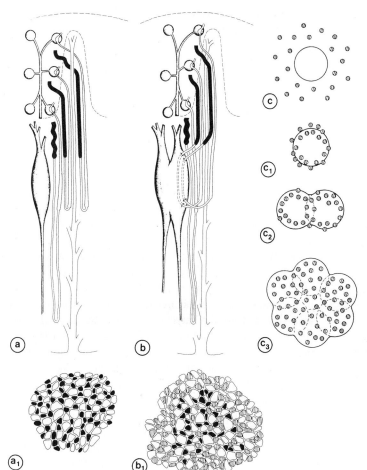

FIGURE 21 Schematic to demonstrate the difference between the simple (**A** and **A₁**) and complex (**B** and **B₁**) types of medulla. In the simple medulla (**A**), loops of Henle surround the vascular bundle according to the pattern established in the cortex. The long loops lie nearest to the bundle, the short loops of superficial nephrons farthest away. The collecting ducts are situated at a distance from the bundle. The bundle itself (**A₁**) contains only descending (*black*) and ascending (*white*) vasa recta. In the complex medulla (**B**), the descending thin limbs of short loops descend within the vascular bundles. The complex bundle (**B₁**) contains, in addition to descending (*black*) and ascending (*white*) vasa recta, the descending thin limbs of short loops (*hatched*). **C₁–C₃**: Schematics of cross-sections through vascular bundles to show different degrees of bundle fusing and loop integration in the complex type of renal medulla (**C₁–C₃**) compared with the simple type (**C**). Large circle, vascular bundle; small hatched circles, descending thin limbs of short loops. In the simple type of medulla (**C**), the descending thin limbs of short loops are all located outside the bundle. Complex bundles (**C₁–C₃**) may be established in different degrees. In rat (**C₁**), descending thin limbs of short loops are arranged in the periphery of the bundles; bundles generally do not fuse. In mouse (**C₂**), bundles frequently fuse; descending thin limbs of short loops have penetrated deeper into the bundle. In *Psammomys* or *Meriones* (**C₃**), bundle fusing has produced giant bundles; descending thin limbs of short loops are distributed over the entire bundle area. (**A,B**: From Jamison R, Kriz W. *Urinary Concentrating Mechanism: Structure and Function*. New York: Oxford University Press, 1982, with permission; **C**: From Kriz W. Structural organization of the renal medulla: comparative and functional aspects. *Am J Physiol* 1981;241:R3–R16, with permission.)

arises from the fact that the descending thin limbs of short loops (SDLTs; only of short loops!) descend within the vascular bundle (Fig. 25). Consequently, the bundles within the inner stripe change from the classic countercurrent arrangement of a rete mirabile, consisting of descending vasa rectas (DVRs) and ascending vasa rectas (AVRs), to a system in which one ascending tube (AVR) is closely packed together with two descending tubes (DVRs and SDTLs). In addition, the vascular bundles in the complex type of medulla tend to fuse and to form larger bundles up to giant bundles (*Psammomys*). These complex bundles are developed at the transition from the outer stripe to the inner stripe and are maintained only throughout the inner stripe. At the border to the inner medulla, the SDTLs leave the bundles, and the fused bundles split into the original number of bundles. The characteristics of the complex type are developed to different degrees in the species so far investigated. A somewhat gradual transition from the rat via the mouse to *Meriones* and *Psammomys* is observed.

The tubular pattern around these complex bundles is different from that of the simple type. At the border between the outer stripe and inner stripe, the SDTLs leave their position distant from the bundles, then turn toward a bundle and descend within the bundle. Their thick ascending limbs

(TALs) maintain a position distant from the bundles and near a collecting duct throughout the outer medulla. As observed in the simple type, the tubules of the interbundle regions are embedded in a dense capillary plexus. In contrast to what is observed in the simple type, it is worthwhile to stress the fact that in the complex type only the LDTLs, scattered among the TALs of short and long loops, traverse this region. Very specific variations in mice (433) and *Psammomys* (40, 268) are described elsewhere.

To understand the possible functional implications of the inner stripe architecture, as well as the differences between the simple type and the complex type, we have to consider precisely the composition of the vascular bundles.

The vascular bundles of the simple type contain all descending and all ascending vasa recta servicing the inner medulla. Furthermore, they contain most of the descending vasa recta, which service the inner stripe, but only few of the ascending vasa recta, which drain the inner stripe. The numerical relationship between descending and ascending vasa recta is about 1 to 1 (at the level of the inner stripe). Thus, in the simple type of vascular bundle, the venous blood from the inner medulla contacts in a countercurrent arrangement the arterial blood that supplies both the inner medulla and the inner stripe of the outer medulla. Therefore, inner

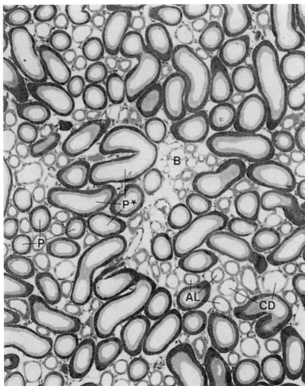

FIGURE 22 Outer stripe of rat kidney; 1-μm cross-section. The vascular bundle (B) is surrounded by the straight proximal tubules of juxtamedullary nephrons (*asterisk*), which are larger in diameter than those of superficial and midcortical nephrons (P), which lie distant from the bundles. Interstitial spaces are sparsely developed. Magnification × ~220. *, thick ascending limb; CD, collecting duct.

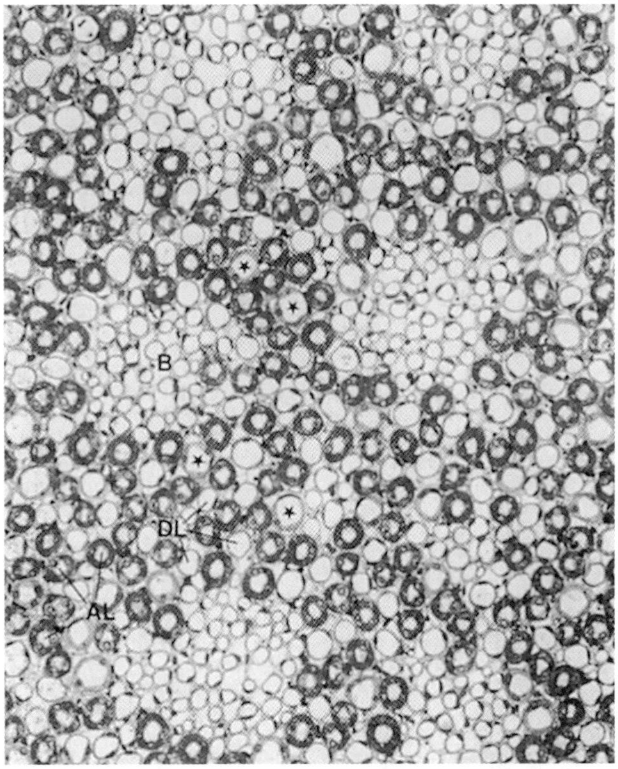

FIGURE 23 Inner stripe of rabbit kidney (simple medulla); 1-μm cross-section. The vascular bundles (B) are regularly distributed. The collecting ducts (CD) lie distant from the bundles. Descending thin limbs (*asterisks*) and thick ascending limbs (*stars*) are situated within the interbundle regions. Magnification × ~ 200.

medullary venous blood may exchange not only with the arterial blood that is predetermined for the inner medulla but also with blood predetermined for the inner stripe. Substances originating form the inner medulla could be trapped by countercurrent exchange to the inner medulla, but could also be shifted to the inner stripe capillary plexus and thereby be offered to inner stripe tubules (see following sections).

In the complex type of medulla, the vascular bundles incorporate the descending thin limbs of short loops In *Psammomys*, at the level of the inner stripe, the bundles consist of approximately 10% descending vasa recta, 45% ascending vasa recta, and 45% descending thin limbs (268). Evaluation of these numerical relationships indicates that the countercurrent arrangement between ascending vasa recta and descending thin limbs seems to be more important than the "classic" arrangement between descending and ascending vasa recta. The difference between the simple and the complex types of bundles is even more pronounced when one observes that the bundles in *Psammomys* no longer contain vasa recta servicing the inner stripe. All vasa recta present in the giant bundles of *Psammomys* either descend to the inner medulla or ascend from the inner medulla. The vasa recta servicing the inner stripe in *Psammomys* descend or ascend, respectively, independent of the bundles. Thus, the giant

bundles of the inner stripe in *Psammomys* appear to form a countercurrent trap for the inner medullary blood, although located in the inner stripe. In other species with complex bundles (rat, mouse), vasa recta servicing the inner stripe are not strictly excluded from the bundles as in *Psammomys*. Rather, even in these species the vascular bundles appear to be a countercurrent trap concerning mainly the inner medullary circulation.

The functionally more important countercurrent exchanges in the complex bundles would seem to occur between the venous blood from the inner medulla and the descending limb fluid within the SDTLs. As will be discussed in some more detail later, countercurrent exchange of urea between the AVRs coming up from the EM and the SDTLs provide the essential step of a recycling route for urea via short nephrons and collecting ducts back to the inner medulla.

The *inner medulla* is very differently developed among species. Species with only short loops of Henle (555) do not have an inner medulla; their urine-concentrating ability is poor. All species with high urine-concentrating ability have a well-developed inner medulla (554, 585). It is characteristic for the inner medulla to taper from a broad basis to a papilla (or a crest). The mass of the inner medulla is therefore unevenly distributed along the longitudinal axis.

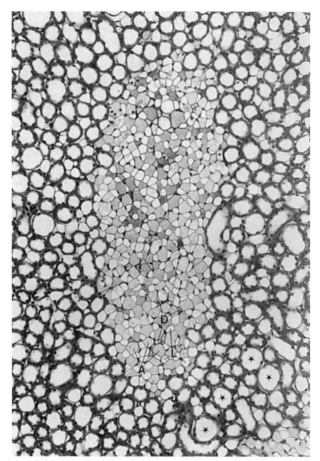

FIGURE 24   Inner stripe of *Meriones shawii* kidney (complex medulla); paraffin cross-section. The large vascular bundle originates by fusing of primary bundles. In addition to descending (D) and ascending (A) vasa recta, complex vascular bundles contain descending thin limbs of short loops (L). Collecting ducts (*asterisks*) are situated distant from the bundles. Magnification × 190.

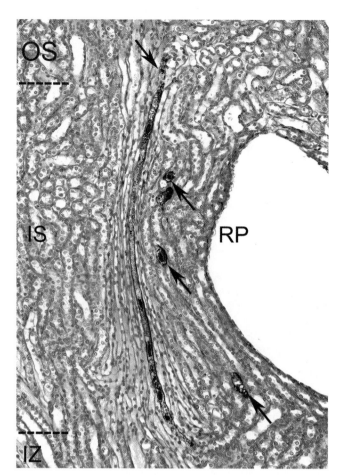

FIGURE 25   Longitudinal section through a vascular bundle in the inner stripe of a gerbil kidney (complex medulla); paraffin section. One superficial nephron has been injected with Microfi; at the transition from the outer (OS) to the inner stripe (IS) the proximal tubule transforms to the intermediate tubule (thin descending limb; *left arrow*), which descends within the vascular bundle; the tubule leaves the bundle at the border between inner stripe and the inner zone (IZ) and ascends as thick ascending limb (*right arrows*) within the interbundle region; RP, extension of the renal pelvis. Magnification ×~200.

A study in the rat (57, 222, 256) has shown that the decrease in the mass of the inner medulla along the longitudinal axis follows an exponential function. The first part of the inner medulla accounts for approximately 80% of the total inner medullary volume, and consequently only 20% is left for the second, the papillary part.

Regarding the ratio between Henle loops and collecting ducts along the inner medulla, considerable differences are found when comparing the base with the tip of the inner medulla, as well as notable interspecies differences (298). In the rat, the ratio is about 2.5 (2.5 loops per collecting duct) at the beginning of the inner medulla; this ratio rapidly decreases to about 1 toward the papilla. In the rabbit, the ratio increases from 3 at the beginning of the inner medulla to 9 within the papilla, then later decreases to 5 in the papillary tip. These data all await functional interpretation, thus indicating the limitation of our knowledge concerning structure-function correlations in the inner medulla.

An architectural pattern within the inner medulla is less apparent than in the outer medulla (271, 332, 699). Constant histotopographical relationships between certain

structures or spatial separations of others do not seem to be as important to the function of the inner medulla compared to the outer medulla. The vascular bundles have already drastically decreased in numbers of vasa recta when entering the inner medulla. Toward the papilla they are further diminished, and finally are totally absent. Descending vasa recta then continue as individual vessels to the tip of the papilla. Ascending vasa recta frequently ascend independent of the bundles, which they finally join at the border to the inner stripe. Thus, in the inner medulla, the vasa recta are never as closely packed to bundles as they are in the inner stripe.

As far as vascular bundles are discernible, the collecting ducts are generally distanced from them. At the beginning of the inner medulla, collecting ducts are still arranged in groups that reflect their grouping within the medullary rays of the cortex (Fig. 26). Joining of collecting ducts first occurs among the ducts of one group. Descending and ascending

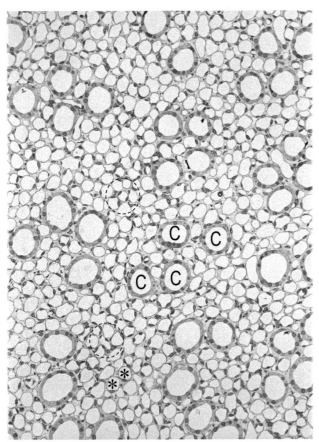

FIGURE 26 Inner medulla of the rabbit kidney; 1-μm cross-section through the upper part of medulla. The collecting ducts are still arranged in groups, reflecting the pattern in the medullary rays of the cortex. Vascular bundles (*dashed circles*) are poorly delineated. Thin loop limbs (*asterisks*) lay near collecting ducts (C) and vasa recta of the vascular bundles. Magnification × ∼ 240.

thin loop limbs, together with individually running vasa recta and capillaries, fill the spaces between the bundle centers and the collecting ducts. Even if the DTLs in general tend to be more distant from CDs, and the ATLs tend to be positioned more closely to CDs (332, 477), a given thin limb, regardless of whether descending or ascending, may be associated with both collecting ducts and vasa recta. Obviously, the wide interstitial spaces mediate the interactions of the structures in the inner medulla.

Regarding the functional connections of the inner medulla with the outer medulla, it is notable that all descending vasa recta servicing the inner medulla have already been established as individual vessels in the outer stripe and traverse the inner stripe within the bundles. All ascending vasa recta from the inner medulla traverse the inner stripe within the bundles without joining with ascending vasa recta from the inner stripe. The blood flow of the inner stripe and that of the inner medulla are apparently distinct from each other. In the outer stripe, however, venous vasa recta coming up from the inner medulla and those from the inner stripe finally take an identical route. Both traverse the outer stripe as wide capillary

channels representing the major capillary supply of the outer stripe tubules.

GLOMERULUS (RENAL CORPUSCLE)

The renal corpuscle consists of a tuft of specialized capillaries that protrudes into Bowman space (urinary space) surrounded by Bowman capsule (BC). The tuft consists of specialized capillaries held together by the mesangium and covered—as a whole—by the glomerular basement membrane (GBM) followed by a layer of unique epithelial cells, the podocytes. Traditionally, this layer is called the visceral epithelium of BC, which—at the vascular pole of the glomerular tuft—reflects into the parietal epithelium of BC. Today, the term Bowman capsule is generally used only for this parietal cell layer which, together with its basement membrane (parietal BM [PBM]), form the outer wall of a glomerulus. At the urinary pole, BC transforms into the proximal tubule epithelium, Bowman's space opens into the tubular lumen (Figs. 27 and 28).

The diameters of the more or less spherical renal corpuscles in different species range from approximately 100 μm (mouse) to up to 300 μm (elephant), in humans they are approximately 200 μm, in rat 120 μm, and in rabbit 150 μm (465, 482, 582). In many species (rodents), the diameter of juxtamedullary renal corpuscles may exceed that of midcortical and superficial nephrons by up to 50% (38, 482, 582, 699); this does not hold true for the human kidney (533).

Architecture of the Glomerulus

The reflection of the parietal epithelium of Bowman's capsule into the visceral epithelium creates an oval opening in the glomerulus, which is called glomerular hilum. Actually, it is the reflection of the GBM into the parietal basal membrane (PBM) (i.e., the basement membrane of the parietal epithelium of Bowman's capsule) that borders the opening. Through it, the glomerular arterioles and glomerular mesangium enter the inner space of the GBM, which forms a complexly folded sack. Inside this sack, the glomerular capillaries pursue a tortuous course around centrally located mesangial axes. Capillaries and mesangium totally fill the labyrinthine spaces inside the GBM. The outer aspect of the GBM is covered by the visceral epithelium (i.e., by the podocytes). The glomerular tuft therefore consists of the glomerular capillaries and the mesangium inside the sack of the GBM and the podocytes covering this sack from outside (7).

The glomerular capillaries are derived from the afferent arteriole (which, strictly at the entrance level, divides into several [two to five] primary capillary branches) (185, 440). Each of these branches gives rise to an anastomosing capillary network that runs toward the urinary pole and then turns back running toward the vascular pole. Thereby the glomerular tuft is subdivided into several (two to five) lobules, each of which contains an afferent and efferent capillary portion. The lobules

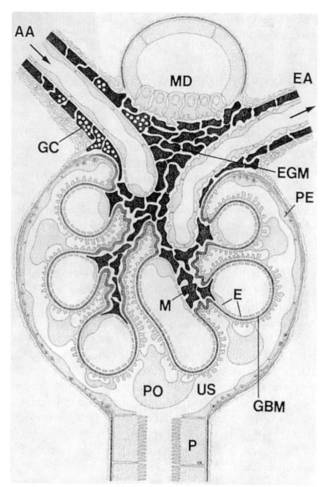

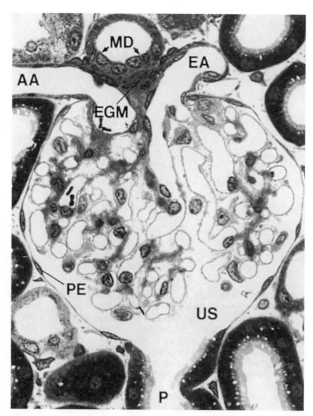

FIGURE 28   Longitudinal section through a glomerulus; rat. At the vascular pole the afferent arteriole (AA), the efferent arteriole (EA), the extraglomerular mesangium (EGM), and the macula densa (MD) are seen. At the urinary pole the beginning of the proximal tubule is seen (P). PE, parietal epithelial of Bowman's capsule; US, urinary space. LM × ∼ 490.

FIGURE 27   Diagram of a longitudinal section through a glomerulus and its juxtaglomerular apparatus (JGA). The capillary tuft consists of a network of specialized capillaries, which are outlined by a fenestrated endothelium (From Cunningham R, et al. Defective PTH regulation of sodium-dependent phosphate transport in NHERF-1⁻/⁻ renal proximal tubule cells and wild-type cells adapted to low-phosphate media. *Am J Physiol Renal Physiol* 2005;289:F933–938, with permission.) At the vascular pole, the afferent arteriole (AA) enters branching into capillaries immediately after its entrance; the efferent arteriole (EA) is established inside the tuft and passes through the glomerular stalk before leaving at the vascular pole. The capillary network and mesangium are enclosed in a common compartment bounded by the glomerular basement membrane (GBM). Note, that there is no basement membrane at the interface between the capillary endothelium and the mesangium. The glomerular visceral epithelium consists of highly branched podocytes (PO), which, in a typical interdigitating pattern, cover the outer aspect of the GBM. At the vascular pole, the visceral epithelium and the GBM are reflected into the parietal epithelium (PE) of Bowman's capsule, which passes over into the epithelium of the proximal tubule (PT) at the urinary pole. At the vascular pole the glomerular mesangium is continuous with the extraglomerular mesangium (EGM) consisting of extraglomerular mesangial cells and an extraglomerular mesangial matrix. The extraglomerular mesangium together with the granular cells (G) of the afferent arteriole and the macula densa (MD) establish the JGA. All cells that are considered to be of smooth muscle origin are shown in black. F, foot processes; N, sympathetic nerve terminals; US, urinary space. (From Kriz W, Sakai T, et al. Morphological aspects of glomerular function. In: Davison AM (ed.). *Nephrology: Proceedings of the X International Congress of Nephrology*, vol. 1. London: Bailliere Tindall, 1988:3–23, with permission.)

are not strictly separated from each other; some anastomoses between lobules occur. The efferent portions of all lobules together establish the efferent domain of the capillary network out of which the efferent arteriole develops.

In contrast to the afferent arteriole, the efferent arteriole is established already inside the glomerular tuft; thus, the efferent arteriole has a significant intraglomerular segment that runs through the glomerular stalk (Figs. 29, 30, 31) (185). At this site, the efferent arteriole has a close spatial relation to the primary branching site of the afferent arteriole. After leaving the tuft, the efferent arteriole has a segment that is narrowly associated with the extraglomerular mesangium (see Juxtaglomerular apparatus). The intraglomerular segment is made up of a continuous endothelium that is fully separated from the GBM by a "mesangial layer" consisting of mesangial cell processes and matrix. Thus, this initial segment of the EA is fully embedded into the mesangium. Along the course through the extraglomerular mesangium, the mesangial and/or extraglomerular mesangial cells in its wall are gradually replaced by smooth muscle cells (185). Thereafter the efferent vessel is established as a proper arteriole.

Glomerular capillaries are a specific type of blood vessel whose wall is made up of an endothelial tube only. A small strip of the outer circumference of this tube is in touch with

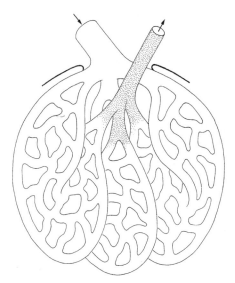

FIGURE 29 Schematic to show the branching pattern of the glomerular tuft. Immediately after its entrance into the tuft, the afferent arteriole splits into large superficial located capillaries which are the supplying vessels of glomerular lobules (three are shown). The capillaries run toward the urinary pole. After turning back they unite to establish the efferent arteriole still inside the glomerular tuft. Thus, in contrast to the afferent arteriole, the efferent arteriole has an intraglomerular segment (*stippled*). Afferent and an efferent capillary domains are distinguished. The efferent capillary domain occupies roughly a quarter sector of the tuft; it is partly covered by the afferent domain. (From Winkler D, Elger M, et al. Branching and confluence pattern of glomerular arterioles in the rat. *Kidney Int Suppl* 1991;32:S2–8, with permission.)

the mesangium, the major part bulges toward the urinary space and is covered by the GBM followed by the layer of podocyte foot processes. These peripheral portions of the capillary wall in total represent the filtration area. The small juxtamesangial portion of the capillary wall is not underlaid by a basement membrane but directly abuts the mesangium (532). The glomerular mesangium constitutes the axis of a glomerular lobule, to which the glomerular capillaries are attached by their juxtamesangial portion. Apart from this attachment site, the mesangium is bounded by the perimesangial part of the GBM. Like the peripheral GBM it is covered at its outer aspect by the layer of podocyte processes.

The Glomerular Basement Membrane

The GBM represents the skeletal backbone of the glomerular tuft. Topographically, the GBM consists of a peripheral (pericapillary) and a perimesangial part. At the border between both parts the GBM changes from a convex pericapillary into a concave perimesangial course; the turning points are called mesangial angles (532).

The GBM originates in development from fusion of a dual basement membrane between endothelial cells and podocytes. After fusion, and thus in the adult, newly synthesized material is primarily derived from podocytes (1, 536). In the adult, podocytes are capable of synthesizing all the components of the GBM (73, 424); glomerular endothelial cells and mesan-

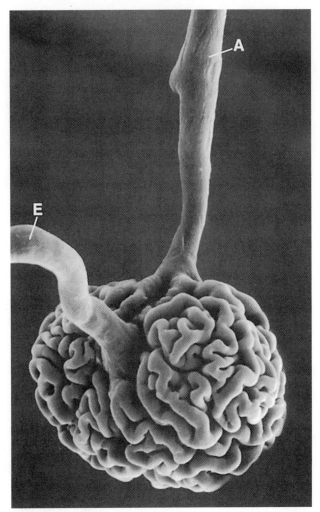

FIGURE 30 Scanning electron micrograph of a vascular cast of a dog glomerulus with afferent (*A*) and efferent (*E*) arterioles. Note the superficially located branching pattern of the afferent arteriole, out of which the afferent capillary domain is supplied. The efferent arteriole emerges from inside of the glomerular tuft.

gial cells may contribute to the formation of the GBM (350). The GBM is subject to a continuous turnover (2, 504), but few details are known where and how new components are added and others removed and degraded. Several extracellular matrix degrading enzymes have been found to be produced by podocytes and mesangial cells (137, 397, 398), however, the relevance of these enzymes for the turnover of the GBM remains to be established.

The GBM varies in width among species. In humans the thickness ranges between 240 and 370 nm (473, 590), in rat and other experimental animals between 110 and 190 nm (620). In electron micrographs of traditionally fixed tissue the GBM appears as a trilaminar structure made up of a lamina densa bounded by two less dense layers: the lamina rara interna and externa. Recent studies using freeze techniques reveal only one dense layer directly attached to the bases of the epithelium and endothelium (253, 503).

The major components of the mature GBM include type IV collagen, type 11 laminin (laminin 521), heparan sulfate

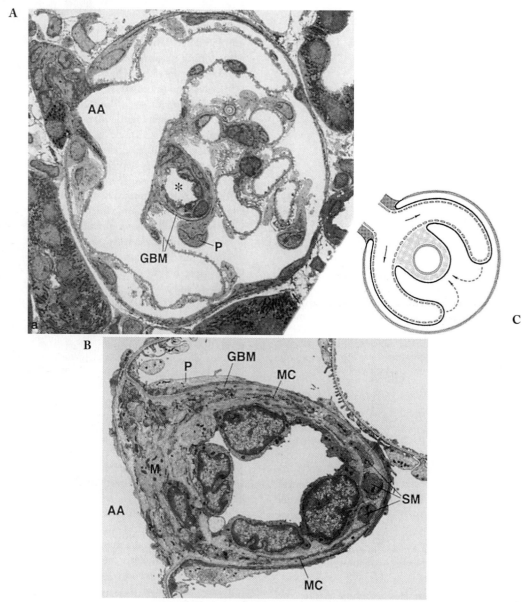

FIGURE 31   A: Narrow association between the afferent arteriole (AA) and the intraglomerular segment of the efferent arteriole (*asterisk*, EA) as seen in a section approximately 15 μm inside a glomerulus. The AA splits into primary branches. The branching point of the AA has a narrow spatial relationship to the intraglomerular segment of the EA (*asterisk*), which is located in the center of the tuft. The intraglomerular segment of the EA is enclosed—together with the AA—in a common compartment bordered by the GBM. **B:** Higher magnification of the intraglomerular segment in a subsequent section with several conspicuous features: the lumen is narrow; the continuous endothelium consists of four cell bodies that bulge into the lumen; the endothelium is surrounded by a mesangial envelope made up of mesangial cells (MC) and matrix; a few smooth muscle cell processes (SM) are interspersed. AA and EA are separated only by mesangial tissue (M); there is no basement membrane separating the AA and EA. *P,* cell body of a podocyte attached to the GBM surrounding the EAs. **C:** Schematic of a cross-section through the glomerular vascular pole, showing the spatial relationships of the AA and EA within the glomerular stalk corresponding to the situation in A. Immediately after its entry into the glomerulus, the AA splits into wide capillary branches with open endothelial pores. The branching point of the AA has a narrow spatial association with the outflow segment of the EA. The outflow segment is enclosed together with the AA in a common compartment bordered by the GBM. The EA is completely surrounded by a layer of mesangial tissue (shown in *gray*) and is separated from the AA only by this layer; there is no basement membrane between AA and EA. Broken arrows represent blood flow from afferent branches through the capillary network to the outflow segment. Transmission electron microscopy (TEM): **A** ×~1500, **B** ×~4300; **C** (From Elger M, Sakai T, et al. The vascular pole of the renal glomerulus of rat. *Adv Anat Embryol Cell Biol* 1998;139:1–98, with permission.)

proteoglycans (perlecan, agrin) and the glycoproteins entactin/nidogen and fibronectin (1, 608, 694); type V and VI collagen have also been demonstrated (400).

The mature GBM is established during the development of a glomerulus from the S-shaped body to the capillary loop stage. During this transition the collagen IV α_1 and α_2 chains are replaced by α_3, α_4, and α_5 chains and the laminin α_1 and β_1 chains are replaced by the α_5 and β_2 chains, the γ_1 chain remains preserved forming together laminin-11, termed laminin-521 (314, 422–425). The components of the mature GBM are all synthesized by the podocytes. The functional importance of this specific composition of the GBM compared with basement membranes elsewhere in the body becomes evident when looking at their involvement in glomerular diseases: the various forms of Alport syndrome are caused by mutations in the genes encoding the α_3, α_4, and α_5 chains of collagen type IV; Goodpasture syndrome is mediated by antibodies against the α_3 collagen IV chain (246).

Current models depict the basic structure of the basement membrane as a three-dimensional network of collagen type IV (245, 334, 607). Monomers of type IV collagen consist of a triple helix of α_3, α_4, and α_5 chains measuring 400 nm in length 400, which, at its carboxy-terminal end, has a large noncollagenous globular domain, called NC1. At the amino-terminus the helix possesses a triple helical rod of length 60 nm, the 7S domain. Interactions between the 7S domains of two triple helices or the NC1 domains of four triple helices allow collagen type IV monomers to form dimers and tetramers. In addition, triple helical strands interconnect by lateral associations via binding of NC1 domains to sites along the collageneous region.

Fibronectin, laminin, and entactin are the glycoproteins of the GBM (399); the major one is laminin-11. Laminin forms a second network that is superimposed to the collageneous network. Laminin is a noncollagenous glycoprotein consisting of three polypeptide chains, two of which are glycolylated and cross-linked by disulfide bridges (123, 425, 607). Laminin, via entactin, binds to specific sites on the polymerized network of type IV collagen as well as to integrin and dystroglycan surface receptors of the podocytes and endothelial cells (see following sections). This combined network of type IV collagen and laminin is considered to provide mechanical strength to the basement membrane and to serve as a scaffold for alignment of other matrix components.

The proteoglycans of the GBM consist of core proteins and covalently bound glycosaminoclycans that are concentrated in the laminae rarae internae and externae. The electronegative charge of the GBM is mainly due to these polyanionic proteoglycans (594). The major proteoglycans of the GBM are heparan sulfate proteoglycans; most prominent is agrin but perlecan is present also (218, 424, 462). Proteoglycan molecules aggregate to form a meshwork that is kept highly hydrated by water molecules trapped in the interstices of the matrix. Within the GBM, heparan sulfate proteoglycans may act as anticlogging agents to prevent hydrogen bonding and adsorption of anionic plasma proteins and maintain an effi-

cient flow of water through the membrane. Digestion of these molecules with heparinase lead to a dramatic increase in the permeability of the GBM to anionic compounds (280).

The Cells of the Glomerular Tuft

Within the glomerular tuft three cell types (Fig. 32) are found, which all are in narrow contact with the GBM: (1) mesangial cells, (2) endothelial cells, and (3) podocytes

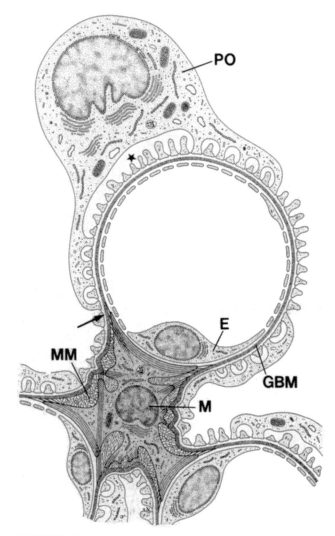

FIGURE 32 Schematic to show the arrangement of the structures in the glomerular tuft; part of a glomerular lobule is shown with three glomerular capillaries (two are only partly shown) attached to a mesangial center. The glomerular capillary is made up of a fenestrated endothelium. The peripheral part of the endothelial tube is surrounded by the GBM which, at the mesangial angles (*arrow*), deviates from a pericapillary course and covers with the mesangium. The interdigitated pattern of the podocyte (PO) foot processes form the external layer of the filtration barrier. Note the sub–cell body space (*star*). Podocyte foot processes are also found covering the paramesangial GBM. In the center a mesangial cell (M) is shown. Its many processes contain microfilament bundles and run toward the GBM to which they are connected. The mesangial matrix (MM) contains an interwoven network of microfilaments (From Venkatachalam MA, Kriz W. Anatomy of the kidney. In: Heptinsall R (ed.). *Pathology of the Kidney.* Boston: Little, Brown and Company, 1992:1–92, with permission).

(visceral epithelial cells). In rats, their numerical ratio has been calculated to amount to 3:2:1, respectively (233).

Mesangial cells together with the mesangial matrix establish the *glomerular mesangium* (Fig. 33). Mesangial cells are irregular in shape with many processes extending from the cell body toward the GBM (193, 701). In these processes (to a lesser extent also in cell bodies) dense assemblies of microfilaments are found, which have been shown to contain actin, myosin, and α-actinin (184).

The processes of mesangial cells run toward the GBM to which they are attached, either directly or mediated by the interposition of microfibrils (see following sections). The GBM represents the effector structure of mesangial contractility (323, 532). Mesangial cell–GBM connections are especially prominent alongside the capillaries. At these sites mesangial cell processes (densely stuffed with microfilament bundles) extend underneath the capillary endothelium toward the mesangial angles

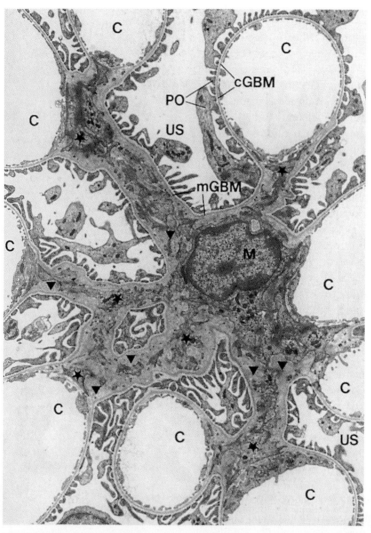

FIGURE 33   Section through a glomerular lobule in the rat. The relationships of glomerular capillaries to the mesangium in the lobule center are seen. Glomerular capillaries (C) and the glomerular mesangium occupy a common compartment enclosed by the glomerular basement membrane (GBM). The mesangial cell body (M) gives rise to several processes (some are marked by *stars*) which extend toward the peripherally located capillaries. Note the abundant mesangial matrix (*triangles*). The layer of podocytes (PO) covers the outer aspect of the GBM. Thus, neither the GBM nor the podocyte layer encircles the capillaries completely; both form a common surface cover around the entire lobule. Therefore, two subdomains of the GBM (as well as of the podocyte layer) can be delineated: the pericapillary (peripheral) GBM (cGBM; faced by podocytes and the endothelium) and the perimesangial GBM (mGBM) bordered by podocytes and the mesangium. The peripheral part of the capillary wall establishes the filtration barrier. Note the mesangial cell body (M) giving rise to many cell processes (some are marked by *stars*) which are embedded in the mesangial matrix (*triangles*). US, urinary space. Transmission electron microscopy (TEM) × ~5500.

of the GBM where they are anchored. Generally, these processes interconnect the GBM from two opposing mesangial angles (Fig. 34B). Functionally, the microfilament bundles bridge the entire distance between both mesangial angles. In the axial mesangial region, numerous microfilament bundles extending through mesangial cell bodies and processes bridge opposing parts of the GBM. The connection of mesangial cell processes to the GBM is mediated by the integrin $\alpha_3\beta_1$ and the Lutheran glycoprotein, which both adhere to the laminin α_5 chain (290).

The *mesangial matrix* fills the highly irregular spaces between the mesangial cells and the perimesangial GBM (for review see [124, 323]). A large number of common extracellular matrix proteins have been demonstrated within the mesangial matrix, including several types of

collagens (III, IV, V, and VI); heparan sulfate proteoglycans (including the small proteoglycans biglycan and decorin) (542); fibronectin, laminin, entactin, fibrillin-1, and other specific elastic fiber proteins (125, 208, 389, 399, 592). Among these components, fibronectin is the most abundant and has been shown to be associated with microfibrils (125, 566).

The basic ultrastructural organization of the matrix is a network of microfibrils. In specimens prepared for TEM by routine methods a fine filamentous network is seen with structures that possibly correspond to collageneous filaments. In specimens prepared by a technique that avoids osmium tetroxide and uses tannic acid for staining, the mesangial matrix is seen to contain abundant elastic microfibrils (436, 532). Microfibrils are unbranched, noncollagenous tubular structures that have an indefinite

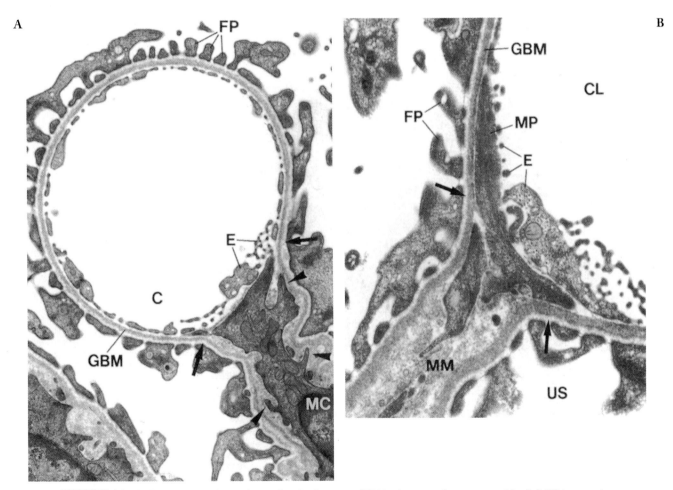

FIGURE 34 **A:** Overview of a glomerular capillary in the mouse. Within the mesangium, a mesangial cell (MC) is seen whose processes extend toward the peripherally located capillary (C). Microprojections (*arrowheads*) originating from the primary process extend toward the glomerular basement membrane (GBM). Note that the GBM (as well as the podocyte layer) deviates from its pericapillary course at the two mesangial angles (*arrows*) continuing as a cover of the mesangium. Thus, the juxtamesangial part of the glomerular capillary lacks a basement membrane; at this site the endothelium is directly exposed to the mesangium. The capillary endothelium is thin and fenestrated. The podocyte layer consists of interdigitating foot processes (FP), which abut the GBM on its outside surface. Transmission electron microscopy (TEM) × ~13,500. **B:** Capillary-mesangium interface in the rat. At this site a basement membrane is not developed. Beneath the endothelium, tonguelike mesangial cell processes (MP) are found which run toward both opposing mesangial angles. They contain microfilament bundles, which interconnect the GBM of both mesangial angles (*arrows*). CL, capillary lumen; US, urinary space; MM, mesangial matrix; FP, foot processes. TEM × ~23,000.

length with a diameter of about 15 nm. They form a dense three-dimensional network establishing a functionally continuous medium anchoring the mesangial cells to the GBM (323, 592). Distinct bundles of microfibrils may be regarded as "microtendons" that allow the transmission of contractile force of mesangial cells to specific sites of the GBM, predominantly to mesangial angles (436, 532). The α_8 integrin serves as a specific matrix receptor in the mesangium (67).

Glomerular endothelial cells (Figs. 32–34) are large flat cells consisting of a cell body (which contains all the usual cell organelles) and extremely attenuated highly "fenestrated" peripheral parts. These peripheral parts are characterized by round to oval pores that are 50 to 100 nm in diameter. The pores of glomerular endothelial cells lack a diaphragm, they are virtually open (56) (Figs. 35B and 36B). Fenestrae bridged by diaphragms in glomerular capillaries are only found along the intraglomerular segment of the efferent arteriole and its tributaries (185). In rat, about 60% of the capillary surface is covered by the porous regions; the total area of pores occupies about 13% of the capillary surface (95). Micropinocytotic vesicles are rare in glomerular endothelial cells, corroborating the fact that the open pores make transcytotic processes unnecessary.

Glomerular endothelial cells contain the usual inventory of cytoplasmic organelles, generally located within the cell body cytoplasm. The endothelial skeleton comprises intermediate filaments and microtubules; individual pores are lined by clusters of microfilaments (633).

The luminal membrane of endothelial cells is highly negatively charged due to a cell coat that also fills the pores like "sieve plugs" (520). It consists of several polyanionic glycoproteins including a sialoprotein called podocalyxin, which is considered as the major surface polyanion of glomerular endothelial as well as epithelial cells (240). Endothelial cells are active participants in the processes controlling coagulation, inflammation, and immune processes (see other chapters in this book). Glomerular endothelial cells synthesize and release endothelin-1, endothelium-derived relaxing factor (EDRF) (540), and platelet-derived growth factor-β (PDGF-β) (62). Glomerular endothelial cells have receptors for VEGF-α and angiopoietin that are produced by podocytes (190, 537). The continuous stimulation of glomerular endothelial cells by VEGF-α has a major relevance for the maintenance of glomerular capillaries (34).

Within the conspicuously narrow portion of the efferent arteriole (outflow segment) the endothelial cells are arranged in an eye-scratching pattern: Their cell bodies bulge

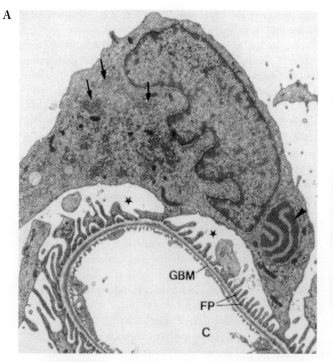

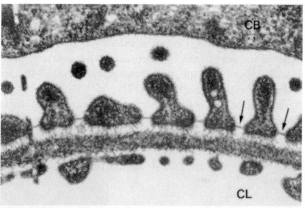

FIGURE 35   **A:** Podocyte in the rat. The cell body contains a large nucleus with indentations. The cytoplasm contains a well developed Golgi apparatus (*arrows*) and a conspicuous lamellated inclusion body (*arrowhead*). The cell processes run toward the glomerular basement membrane (GBM) forming there the interdigitating pattern of foot processes (FP). Note the sub–cell body space (*stars*). C, capillary. Transmission electron microscopy (TEM) × ~7600. **B:** Filtration barrier in the rat. The peripheral part of the glomerular capillary wall comprises three layers: the endothelium with large open pores, the GBM, and the layer of interdigitating podocyte foot processes. The GBM consists of a lamina densa, a lamina rara interna toward the endothelium, and a lamina rara externa toward the epithelium. Note the slit diaphragms bridging the floor of the filtrations slits (*arrows*). CL, capillary lumen; CB, cell body of a podocyte. TEM × ~57,000.

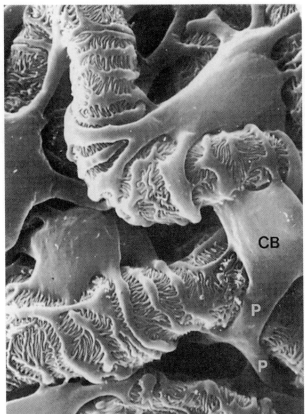

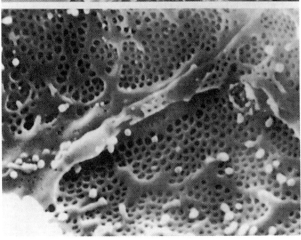

FIGURE 36 **A:** Outer surface of glomerular capillaries in the rat. Processes (P) of podocytes run from the cell body (CB) toward the capillaries where they ultimately split into foot processes. By interdigitation, foot processes from neighboring cells create the filtration slits. Scanning electron microscopy (SEM) × ~3400. **B:** Inner surface of a glomerular capillary in the rat. The open fenestrations (not bridged by a diaphragm) are shown. SEM × ~16,000.

into the lumen by longitudinal stretching suggesting a specific shear stress receptor of glomerular circulation (185, 198).

The mature *podocytes* are highly differentiated cells. In the developing glomerulus at the S-shaped body stage, podocytes have a simple polygonal shape and are connected by apical tight junctions. At the transition to the capillary

loop stage, the mitotic activity of the cells is completed and the final number of podocytes is established. In rats, this point is reached soon after birth; in humans it is reached during prenatal life. Differentiated podocytes are unable to perform regenerative cell replication (438); thus in the adult, lost podocytes cannot be replaced by division of the remaining cells. However, in response to extreme mitogenic stimulation (e.g., by a basic fibroblast growth factor, FGF-2) the cells may undergo mitotic division but are unable to perform cytokinesis, resulting in binucleated or multinucleated cells (325). Under certain conditions (HIV nephropathy), podocytes may dedifferentiate followed by an uncontrolled multiplication leading to the collapse of the glomerular tuft (51).

Podocytes have a voluminous smooth surfaced cell body, which floats within the urinary space; its shape appears to adapt to the surrounding flow conditions created by the filtrate. The cells give rise to long primary processes (frequently branching another time) that extend toward the capillaries, finally splitting apart into terminal processes, called foot processes, which affix to the GBM. The foot processes of neighboring podocytes interdigitate with each other, leaving between them meandering slits (filtration slits), which are bridged by an extracellular structure, the so-called slit diaphragm. Podocytes are polarized epithelial cells with a luminal and a basal cell membrane domain; the latter corresponds to the sole plates of the foot processes, which are embedded into the GBM to a depth of 40 to 60 nm. The border between basal and luminal membrane is represented by the insertion of the slit diaphragm (438).

The cell body contains a prominent nucleus, a well-developed Golgi system (Fig. 35A), abundant rough and smooth endoplasmic reticulum, prominent lysosomes (including abundant multivesicular bodies), and many mitochondria. In contrast to the cell body, the cell processes contain only a few organelles. The density of organelles in the cell body indicates a high level of anabolic and catabolic activity. In addition to the work necessary to sustain structural integrity of these specialized cells, all components of the GBM are synthesized by podocytes (1, 424).

A well-developed cytoskeleton accounts for the complex shape of the cells. In the cell body and the primary processes, microtubules and intermediate filaments (vimentin, desmin) dominate whereas microfilaments are densely accumulated in the foot processes. In addition, in the cell body and the primary processes, microfilaments are seen as a thin layer underlying the cell membrane (165, 248, 633).

The prominent bundles of microtubules in the large processes are associated with microtubule-associated proteins including MAP3/MAP4 and tau (243, 478). Moreover, as in neuronal dendrites the microtubes of the podocyte foot processes are nonuniformly arranged with peripheral plus- and minus-end microtubules associated with the specific protein CHO1/MKLP1 (303). In addition, the large processes contain the intermediate-type filament protein vimentin (165). In the foot processes, a complete microfilament-based contractile apparatus is present. The microfilaments form loop-shaped bundles, with their limbs running in the longitudinal axis of the foot processes. The bends of these loops are located centrally at the transition to the primary processes and are probably connected to the microtubules by "tau," which is concentrated at those sites (534). Tau is known from other places to mediate connections between microtubules and microfilaments (127). The microfilament bundles contain actin, myosin II, α-actinin, and synaptopodin (165, 437, 439); synaptopodin, a novel podocyte–specific, actin-associated protein interacts with α-actinin inducing the formation of long unbranched parallel bundles of microfilaments (19). Peripherally, the actin bundles anchor in the dense cytoplasm associated with the basal cell membrane of podocytes (i.e., the sole plates of foot processes) (438). Anchoring of the sole plates to the GBM is achieved by specific transmembrane receptors; two systems are known (Fig. 37). First, a specific integrin heterodimer, consisting of $\alpha_3\beta_1$ integrins, which bind within the GBM to collagen type IV, fibronectin, and laminin-11 (3, 133, 314). Second, a dystroglycan complex connects the intracellular molecule utrophin to laminin-11, agrin, and perlecan in the GBM (501, 506). Both, integrins and dystroglycans are coupled via adepter molecules (paxillin, vinculin, α-actinin, and others) to the podocyte cytoskeleton, allowing outside-in and inside-out signaling and transmission of mechanical force in both directions. Integrin-linked kinase plays a major role in this issue (70).

A huge body of data has been accumulated in recent years concerning the inventory of receptors and signaling processes starting from them in podocytes. cGMP signaling (stimulated by ANP, BNP, CNP, and NO), cAMP signaling (stimulated by prostaglandin E_2, dopamine, isoproterenol, PTH/PTHrP) and Ca^{++} signaling (stimu-

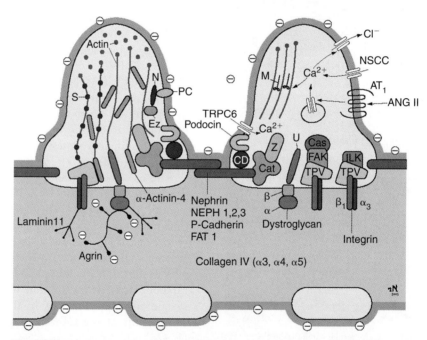

FIGURE 37 Glomerular filtration barrier. Two podocyte foot processes bridged by the slit membrane, the glomerular basement membrane (GBM) and the porous capillary endothelium are shown. The surfaces of podocytes and of the endothelium are covered by a negatively charged glycocalix containing the sialoprotein podocalyxin (PC). The GBM is mainly composed of collagen IV (α_3, α_4, and α_5), of laminin-11 (α_5, β_2, and γ_1 chains) and the heparan sulfate proteoglycan agrin. The slit membrane represents a porous proteinaceous membrane composed of (as far as known) Nephrin; Neph-1, -2, and -3; P-cadherin; and FAT1. The actin-based cytoskeleton of the foot processes connects to both the GBM and the slit membrane. Regards the GBM, β_1/α_3 integrin dimers specifically interconnect the TVP complex (talin, paxillin, vinculin) to laminin-11; the β and a dystroglycans interconnect utrophin to agrin. The slit membrane proteins are joined to the cytoskeleton via various adaptor proteins including podocin, Zonula occludens protein-1 (ZO-1; Z), CD2-associated protein (CD), and catenins (Cat). TRPC6 associates with podocin (and nephrin; not shown) at the slit membrane. Among the many surface receptors only the angiotensin II (ANG II) type 1 receptor (AT1) is shown. Cas, p130Cas; Ez, ezrin; FAK, focal adhesion kinase; ILK, integrin-linked kinase; M, myosin; N, NHERF2 (Na^+-H^+ exchanger regulatory factor); NSCC, nonselelective cation channel; S, synaptopodin. (From Endlich K, Kriz W, Witzgall R. Update in podocyte biology. *Curr Opin Nephrol Hypertens* 2001;10:331–340, with permission.)

lated by a huge number of ligands including angiotensin II, acetylcholine, PGF_2, AVP, ATP, endothelin, histamine, and others) have been identified. Among the cation channels, TRPC6, a nonselective Ca^{2+} channel, has received attention because mutations in the respective gene lead to hereditary FSGS (509, 674). The major target of this signaling orchestra is the cytoskeleton, the concrete effects however are poorly understood. Other receptors, such as those for C3b (287), transforming growth factor β (TGFβ) (546, 677), FGF2 (325), and other cytokines and chemokines have been shown to be involved in the development of podocyte diseases (for details see [479]). Megalin, a multiligand endocytotic receptor is associated with coated bits (288, 289, 469); it represents the major antigen of rat Heymann nephritis (531).

The filtration slits are the site of convective fluid flow through the visceral epithelium. They have a width of 30 to 40 nm and are bridged by the slit membrane. The structure and molecular composition of this proteinaceous membrane are insufficiently understood. Chemically fixed and tannic acid–treated tissue reveals a zipperlike structure with a row of "pores" approximately 4 × 14 nm on either side of a central bar (515). According to its dimension and its components (as far as known) the slit diaphragm may be considered as a specific adherens-like intercellular junction. Intensive research in recent years has uncovered several transmembrane proteins that participate in the formation of the slit membrane, including nephrin (525), Neph1 (157), P-cadherin (508), and FAT (254) (Fig. 37). Other molecules, such as ZO1 (557), podocin (78), CD2AP (360), and catenins mediate the connection to the actin cytoskeleton (see following sections). Nephrin is a member of the immunoglobin superfamily (IgCAM); its gene *NPHS1* has been identified as the gene whose mutations cause congenital nephritic syndrome of the Finnish type (525). In addition to its role as a structural component, nephrin acts as a signaling molecule that can activate MAP kinase cascades (244). Neph1 is considered as a ligand for nephrin. Podocin belongs to the raft associated stomatin family, whose gene *NPHS2* is mutated in a subgroup of patients with autosomal recessive, steroid-resistant nephrotic syndrome (78). These patients show disease onset in early childhood and rapid progression to end-stage renal failure. Podocin interacts with nephrin and CD2AP (571). FAT is a novel member of the cadherin superfamily with 34 tandem cadherin-like extracellular repeats and a molecular weight of 516 kD (172). Because FAT has a huge extracellular domain, it is speculated that it dominates the molecular structure of the slit membrane (254); the FAT mutant mouse fails to develop a slit membrane (116). P-cadherin (508) is thought to mediate with its intracellula r domain the linkage to β- and γ-catenin, a complex that then connects to the actin cytoskeleton via α-catenin and α-actinin. Taken together, many components of the slit membrane are known, but an integrative model of its substructure including all components is so far lacking.

The luminal membrane and the slit diaphragm are covered by a thick surface coat that is rich in sialoglycoproteins (including podocalyxin, podoendin, and others) that are responsible for the high negative surface charge of the podocytes (242, 541). Podocalyxin is anchored to the subplasma membrane actin cytoskeleton via the linker protein NHERF 2 ($Na^+–H^+$ exchanger regulatory factor 2) and ezrin (247, 598). The surface charge of podocytes contributes to the maintenance of the interdigitating pattern of the foot processes. In response to neutralization of the surface charge by cationic substances (e.g., protamine sulfate), the foot processes retract and tight junctions may be formed between adjacent foot processes (206, 573).

Filtration Barrier

The walls of glomerular capillaries represent a specific barrier that is very permeable to water and yet able to prevent all but very minute losses of serum albumin and other major plasma proteins from the circulation. The glomerular capillary wall consists of three distinct layers. Starting at the capillary lumen, there is the porous endothelium, followed by the GBM, and the layer of interdigitating foot processes with the filtration slits in between.

The high hydraulic permeability of this barrier suggests that the filtrate pathway is entirely extracellular, passing through the endothelial fenestrae, across the GBM, and through the slit diaphragms of the filtration slits (169). According to a calculation by Drumond and Deen (169) the hydraulic resistance of the endothelium is negligible. The GBM and the filtration slits each comprise approximately one half of the total hydraulic resistance of the filtration barrier.

Charge, size, and shape determine the specific permeability of a macromolecule. It is now generally accepted that the charge barrier plays an important part in preventing polyanionic macromolecules such as albumin from passing through the glomerular filter. All components of the glomerular filter are heavily laden with negative charges. In vivo studies analyzing the distribution of differently charged electron dense tracers (279) suggested that especially the charges of the GBM are responsible for restricting the passage of polyanionic macromolecules. Research does not support this view (72, 135); it appears that the negative residues of the endothelium play the major role establishing a negative charge field that considerably decreases already the entry of polyanionic macromolecules (i.e., albumin into the filter). However, there is an ongoing debate on this issue.

In terms of the size selectivity, direct experimental findings (167–169, 180, 181) and findings about the molecular composition of the slit membrane and the consequences of genetic mutations in these components suggest that is primarily the slit membrane that is responsible for the size selectivity; it appears to be the main barrier for albumin and larger molecules.

The lack of precise knowledge of slit membrane structure underlies another major problem in glomerular physiology, namely the regulation of the ultrafiltration coefficient K_f. K_f is the product of the local hydraulic permeability and the filtration area. There has been a widespread belief that K_f is regulated through changes in filtration area due to an action of the mesangium (173). However, the structural arrangement of the mesangium (532) and morphometric studies (13, 142) do not support such an assumption. Dimensional changes in just the slit membrane area have also been regarded as a reasonable and, theoretically, very effective site to change K_f (14). In pathological conditions (e.g., in membranous nephropathy) (170), the decrease in K_f correlates with the decrease of total slit length. With respect to acute regulatory mechanisms under physiological conditions, however, no convincing morphometric data have been published showing that changes in K_f are correlated with corresponding dimensional changes of the slit membrane. Thus, the questions as to where and how K_f is regulated remain unanswered.

Stability of the Glomerular Tuft

The glomerular tuft is constantly exposed to comparably high intraglomerular pressures within glomerular capillaries and mesangium. The high intraglomerular pressures challenge not only the glomerular capillaries themselves but also the folding pattern of the glomerular tuft. Increased pressures lead to the loss of the folding pattern and to dilation of the glomerular capillaries. Therefore, we have to ask what are the specific structures and mechanisms that counteract the expansile forces in the glomerular tuft. To answer this question, we must distinguish between the structures and mechanisms maintaining (1) the folding pattern of the glomerular tuft and those maintaining (2) the width of glomerular capillaries (Fig. 38).

The folding pattern of the glomerular tuft is primarily sustained by the mesangium (322, 323, 532). Mesangial cells are connected to the GBM by their contractile processes (see preceding sections); by centripetal contractions they maintain the in-foldings of the GBM, thereby allowing for the capillaries to arrange in the peripheral expansion of the GBM. This supporting role of mesangial cells is best illustrated under circumstances with loss of mesangial cells, such as Thy-1 nephritis (324). Under those circumstances the folding pattern of the GBM is progressively lost, finally resulting in mesangial aneurysms. Podocytes clearly contribute to the maintenance of the folding pattern by specific cell processes that interconnect opposing parts of the GBM from outside (i.e., within the niches of the in-foldings). This function is again clearly illustrated in Thy-1 nephritis under circumstances with loss of mesangial support: Podocytes are capable of maintaining a high degree of the GBM folding pattern for 2 to 4 days, after which they fail and mesangial aneurysms become prominent (324).

The width of glomerular capillaries is probably controlled by growth processes accounting for differently sized capillaries. The width of a given capillary, in an acute situation being exposed to changes in blood pressure, appears to be stabilized by the GBM, which is a strong elastic structure (662) and, together with the mesangial cell bridges (see preceding sections), capable of developing wall

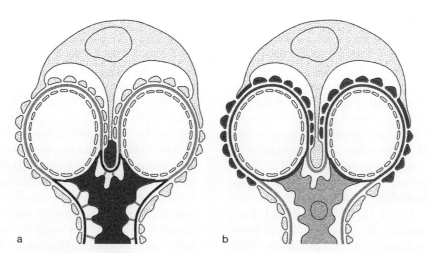

FIGURE 38   Schematic to show the mechanisms that stabilize the glomerular tuft against expansion (relevant structures, *dark gray*). **A:** The folding pattern of the glomerular basement membrane (GBM) is sustained by mesangial cells from inside and by specific podocyte processes located in the depth between two capillaries from outside. **B:** The width of capillaries against transmural pressure gradients is maintained by wall tension, which is generated by the rigidity of the GBM, by the mesangial cell processes that interconnect opposing turning points of the GBM and by the tonus of podocyte foot processes.

tension (323, 328). In addition, the tensile strength of the GBM is reinforced by podocytes. Podocytes are a kind of pericytes; their foot processes represent a unique type of pericyte process, which, like elsewhere in the body, counteract the dilation of the vessel. Podocyte processes are firmly attached to the underlying GBM (see preceding sections); their cytoskeletal tonus counteracts the elastic extension of the GBM. In this function, podocytes cannot be replaced by any other cell; failure in this function will lead to capillary dilation.

Parietal Epithelium of Bowman's Capsule

The parietal layer of Bowman's capsule consists of squamous epithelial cells resting on a basement membrane (8). The polygonal cells contain prominent bundles of actin filaments running in all directions. Microfilament bundles are especially prominent in the parietal cells surrounding the vascular pole, where they are located within cytoplasmic ridges that run in a circular fashion around the glomerular entrance (185).

The basement membrane of the parietal epithelium (PBM) is, at variance to the GBM, composed of several dense layers that are separated by translucent layers and contain bundles of fibrils (microligaments [411]). Some studies suggest a role of type XIV collagen in the organization of the multilayered PBM (357). In contrast to the GBM, the predominant proteoglycan of the PBM is a chondroitin sulfate proteoglycan (124). The transition from the GBM to the PBM borders the glomerular entrance. This transitional region is mechanically connected to the smooth muscle cells of the afferent and efferent arterioles and to extraglomerular mesangial cells.

At the urinary pole, the flat parietal cells transform into proximal tubule cells. In some cases the flat cells may continue for a certain distance as a so-called neck segment of the tubule (rabbit) (562) or the typical proximal tubule epithelium generally starts already within the glomerular capsule. This is the case in the mouse (449, 697), the most pronounced in males.

In rare cases, parietal epithelial cells may be replaced by podocytes ("parietal podocytes"), which display a process pattern identical to that of podocytes proper of the tuft (207). At such sites, the PBM is similar to the GBM and capillaries may attach from outside.

STRUCTURAL ORGANIZATION OF RENAL ELECTROLYTE TRANSPORTING EPITHELIA

General Overview of Renal Epithelial Organization

The renal tubular epithelia function as selective barriers between the tubular fluid in the luminal compartment and the interstitial compartment that communicates with the blood compartment. The epithelium consists of a single

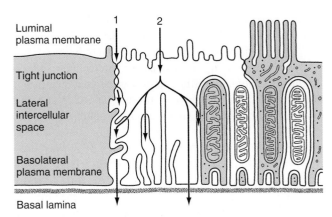

FIGURE 39 Schematic drawing demonstrating the essential structural features of renal transporting epithelia: (1) paracellular route through the tight junction and the lateral intercellular spaces; (2) transcellular route, across the apical plasma membrane, of which the area may be augmented by short microvilli, microfolds (not shown) or long microvilli of uniform length, called "brush border," across the cytoplasm, and across the basolateral plasma membrane; the latter may be augmented by in-foldings of the basal plasma membrane or by basolateral processes of the cells, which narrowly interdigitate with each other: the lateral interdigitating processes contain large mitochondria.

layer of cells, resting on a basement membrane composed of extracellular matrix. The cells are interconnected by *junctional complexes* that encircle each individual cell like a belt. The *tight junction* (zonula occludens) separates the luminal compartment from the lateral intercellular space and is the boundary between the apical plasma membrane domain, facing the tubular fluid, and the basolateral membrane domain, which lines the intercellular compartments and is in contact with the basement membrane. The *intermediate junctions* (zonula adherens) and the patches of *desmosomes* (maculae adherentes) provide mechanical adherence. Gap junctions that provide intercellular communication exist exclusively in the proximal tubule.

This basic organization of the epithelium (Fig. 39) implies two *transepithelial transport pathways* for solutes and macromolecules: (1) the paracellular pathway across the tight junctions and the lateral intercellular spaces; the passage of solutes through the paracellular pathway is driven by the transepithelial electrochemical and oncotic gradients; and (2) the transcellular pathway across the luminal membrane domain, the cellular cytoplasm and the basolateral membrane domain, and vice versa; the passage of solutes via the transcellular pathway occurs mostly against electrochemical gradients and is energy dependent.

PARACELLULAR PATHWAY

As seen in freeze fracture replicas, *tight junctions* are composed of globular particles, arranged in one or several, roughly parallel strands or in a netlike pattern (Fig. 40A) (558). The more or less densely packed particles in the strands presumably represent the transmembrane proteins that participate in the junction formation.

The tight junctions function as barriers between the luminal compartment and the lateral intercellular spaces. At the same time, they allow a selective, regulated paracellular flow of small inorganic cations (426, 622) and the passage of some large organic cations and uncharged molecules (403, 558). The selectivity of tight junctions for different solutes varies among the different tubular epithelia (263, 362, 387, 691, 692). Claudins, a large family of integral membrane proteins make up the bulk of tight junctional strands (362, 691, 692) and play a key role in determining and regulating the paracellular permeability for small inorganic cations (33, 621). They act as size-, charge-, ion concentration–, and pH-dependent channels or pores in the intercellular space (120, 121, 600) and seem to be targets of the serine-threonine kinases WNK1 and WNK4 (119, 239, 263, 683), The dynamic regulation of paracellular flux does not seem to involve structural changes of the tight junctional complexes. Mutations in claudin members (581, 669) or defects in the WNK-signaling cascades may have major implications on volume homeostasis (110, 263, 265, 670, 671, 683).

Occludin, another integral membrane protein is interspersed with claudins in the tight junctional strands. The cytoplasmic domain of occludin is associated with ZO1, thereby providing a linkage of the membrane to its scaffolding actin cytoskeleton (558, 622). The interaction of occludins with the actin skeleton may be important in regulating the paracellular passage for larger molecules and for "macropermeation" across the epithelium as well as in the transduction of signals from apoptotic cells (693). Further, ZO1 seems to be associated with the "fence" function of tight junctions (i.e., the ability of the tight junction to prevent diffusion of lipids from the apical to the basolateral membrane domain) (558).

Cell adhesion proteins at the extracellular face of the basolateral surface of renal tubular cells maintain a basal level of cell–cell adhesion, in addition to strong cellular adhesion provided by the junctional complexes and/or desmosomes. The cell adhesion proteins in the intercellular spaces can be made visible by electron microscopy with specific fixation procedures (Fig. 40B). The "classical" cell adhesion proteins N- and E-cadherin (296a, 488a, 488b, 494a), as well as the "atypical" kidney-specific (ksp) cadherin 16 (527, 605) have been located by immunostainings on the basolateral membranes all along the tubular system. The classical cell adhesion molecules are linked to the scaffolding actin skeleton, as well as to β-catenin, at the cytoplasmic face of the basolateral membranes (447). This connection provides a pathway for coupling extracellular signals (among others, binding of a hormone to its receptor, mechanical stresses) to intracellular signaling cascades that control various cellular responses, such as endocytosis, ubiquitination of proteins, transcription, proliferation, or apoptosis (447).

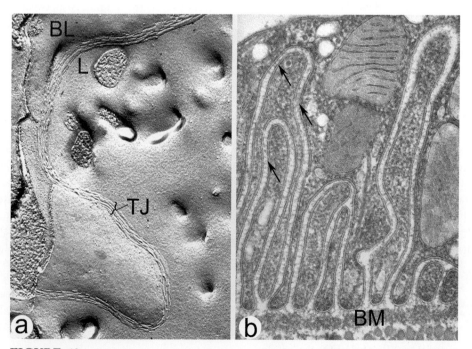

FIGURE 40   Tight junction and intercellular space. Freeze fracture electron micrograph of thick ascending limb cells. **A:** The tight junction (TJ) consists of several densely arranged parallel strands. BL, basolateral membrane. L, luminal membrane. Rabbit; transmission electron microscopy (TEM), × ~45,000. (Cooperation with A. Schiller and R. Taugner). **B:** Thick ascending limb epithelium after tannic acid staining. Cell adhesion molecules are contrasted within the intercellular spaces (*arrows*). BM, basement membrane. Rat; TEM, × ~54,000. (In cooperation with T. Sakai.)

TRANSCELLULAR PATHWAY

The prerequisite for transcellular vectorial transport of solutes across epithelia is the asymmetric or polarized distribution of cotransporters, exchangers, channels, and enzymes in the luminal and basolateral membrane domains.

Basolateral Membrane Domain The Na, K-ATPase, the so-called sodium pump, is present in the basolateral membrane domain of all tubular cells where it is firmly linked to the actin cytoskeleton by interacting proteins, such as ankyrin, spectrin/fodrin, and NHERF (85). The Na, K-ATPase provides the ATP-dependent driving force for all sodium-coupled transcellular solute movements (204). In renal epithelia ATP is mainly made available by mitochondria.

Characteristic differences in Na, K-ATPase activity/protein exist among the different tubular segments (164, 286). They rely on cell-type–specific differences in the density of the enzyme molecules per area basolateral membrane and differences in the surface area of basolateral membranes per unit tubular length (275, 348). Basically two modes of increases of the basolateral membrane surface are distinguished in renal epithelia:

Lateral interdigitating folds (basolateral interdigitations) increase in number and decrease in size with cell depth (Fig. 41) (661). The width of the spaces between the lateral membranes is usually narrow (~ 20 nm) and varies little with function. The characteristic palisade-like arrangement of mitochondria in the basal parts of proximal and distal tubules in histological sections is rooted in the confinement of mitochondria in the lateral folds. By this arrangement the Na, K-ATPase in the lateral plasma membrane is very close to mitochondria. The folds terminate in basal ridges, which contain densely packed actin filaments, arranged in a circular manner (519, 521, 616)

and provide attachment of the cells to the underlying basement membrane. The plasma membrane portions adjacent to the basement membrane are exempt from Na, K-ATPase (283, 312).

The intercellular spaces between the folds converge toward the tight junctional belt, which often has a very tortuous course. The common compartment of para- and transcellular transport routes is extensive. In interdigitated epithelia, the tight junctions are composed of one or several parallel strands with more or less high particle density. The

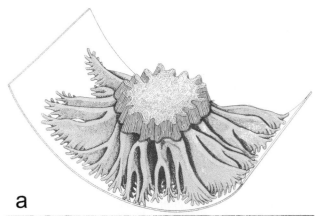

a

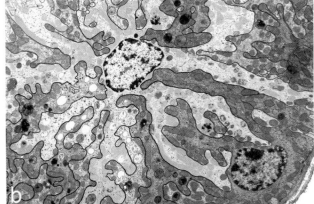

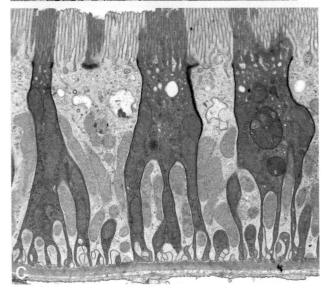

FIGURE 41 Augmentation of apical and basolateral plasma membrane surfaces by microvilli and interdigitating lateral cell processes. **A:** Three-dimensional model of a rabbit proximal tubule cell. The dark line indicates the position of the tight junctional belt between the apical and basolateral membrane domains; the apical membrane domain is amplified by microvilli, which form a *brush border*; the basolateral membrane domain is augmented by interdigitating lateral cell processes, that split in apicobasal direction to primary and secondary processes and basal plicae; the latter are anchored in the basement membrane. **B,C:** Sections through S1 proximal tubule *(Psammomys obesus)*; the dark contrast of the intercellular spaces *(black lines)*, and the differential contrast of adjacent cells result from fixation with reduced osmium. **B:** The section, cut approximately in parallel to the basement membrane through the center of the cell reveals the complex interdigitation of the lateral cell processes. **C:** In the section in apicobasal direction apical interdigitation by lateral processes is revealed by the different contrast in the brush border; the lateral interdigitating processes increasingly split up toward the cell base; the larger ones are filled out with mitochondria. Transmission electron microscopy (TEM) × ~9000. (From Welling LW, Welling DJ. Surface areas of brush border and lateral cell walls in the rabbit proximal nephron. *Kidney Int* 1975;8:343–348, with permission.)

epithelia of the proximal tubule (Fig. 41), Henle's loop, and the distal convoluted tubule are made up by interdigitating cells.

In-foldings of the basal plasma membrane into the cell body. The spaces between the infolded membranes open via so-called basal slits directly toward the underlying basement membrane and are not directly continuous with the lateral intercellular spaces. The luminal outline of the cells is usually polygonal. Therefore the tight junctional belt, constituted by networks of anastomosing strands with high particle density, is short and interference of para- and transcellular pathways is less than that in interdigitated epithelia. The width of the intercellular spaces is variable, depending on the functional conditions. The lateral membranes are interconnected by small desmosomes, present on small *fingerlike villi or folds*, which might enforce the mechanical cohesion of the cells under expansion of the intercellular space. Epithelia with noninterdigitating cells are found in the collecting duct system Increases in membrane area by lateral interdigitating folds and basal in-foldings may well be found in the same cell (e.g., connecting tubule cells; see following sections).

Luminal Membrane Domain The permeation of many small solutes across the luminal membrane occurs via cotransporters, exchangers, and channels and takes advantage of the electrochemical gradient for sodium across the plasma membrane, maintained by the sodium pump in the basolateral membrane. Various enzymes (e.g., phosphatases, peptidases) in the luminal membrane contribute to the reabsorption of organic compounds by hydrolyzing poorly permeable molecules in readily permeable ones. Many of the apical transport proteins are linked to the actin-based cytoskeleton under the plasma membrane via adaptor proteins containing PDZ interactive domains (158, 174, 648, 649, 658, 660) namely NHERF-1, -2, and -3, and are thereby maintained in the specific cell membrane areas (107)

The given assembly of transport proteins in the apical plasma membrane of a segment confers the *specificity* for transported solutes. The *rate* of solute permeation across the membrane critically depends on type (cotransporter, exchanger, channel) and quantity of active transport systems in the apical cell membrane domain. The latter is ultimately related to the available surface area. Thus, in many epithelia with high transport rates the apical membrane area is much larger than the area of a virtual plane at the level of the tight junctional belt.

Interestingly, in the interdigitated type of epithelia, sodium movements across the luminal membrane are mediated mainly via cotransporters and exchangers, whereas in the noninterdigitated epithelia they proceed mainly via the epithelial sodium channel. The striking differences in mitochondrial density between both epithelial types suggest differential energy requirements for transepithelial solute movements.

Three modes of amplification of apical membrane surface are distinguished (Fig. 39): (1) densely arranged fingerlike microvilli, all of similar dimensions, evenly distributed over the entire cell surface, forming the so-called ***brush border*** (Figs. 41–44). The microvilli have an axial cytoskeleton of actin filaments, arranged in a 6 + 1 pattern, associated with villin and fimbrin in the microvillar core (516). The actin filaments extend into the terminal web, located in the subapical cytoplasm immediately beneath the base of the microvilli. Brush border formation characterizes the proximal tubule; (2) short ***microvilli***, found on all other tubular cells; their density and distribution on the cell surface varies considerably; and (3) ***microfolds***, found on cells, in which regulation of the permeation rates for given solutes is associated with rapid transient modulation of the luminal cell surface area (subtypes of intercalated cells and occasionally also in collecting duct cells; see below).

CORRELATION BETWEEN STRUCTURE AND TRANSPORT

Microquantitative analyses of Na, K-ATPase protein (286) or activity (348), combined with morphometric estimations of basolateral membrane areas, mitochondrial volume density (275), and transport studies in defined nephron and collecting duct segments (278, 587, 588, 647) established the consistent quantitative correlation between the "workload" on one side and the surface area of basolateral membrane and the volume density of mitochondria on the other side (589). Prolonged increases or decreases of the workloads in vivo are manifest by respective adaptations of the given parameters.

Transient changes of the permeation rates for a given solute across the luminal cell membrane are brought about by rapidly reversible changes in the availability of active transport systems in the luminal cell surface. Several mechanisms are known, from *gating of transport channels* (e.g., ENaC in collecting duct cells), which are already present at the cell surface (85); *redistribution of a given protein between microdomains* in the apical membrane (e.g., NHE3 in the brush border of proximal tubuli [65, 414]); *cycling of membrane portions* containing the respective transport proteins (e.g., AQP2 in collecting duct cells; H+ATPase in intercalated cells) between the cell surface and intracellular vesicles (84); and *exocytotic insertion* into or *endocytotic retraction* from the membrane, respectively, of specific transport proteins (31, 383).

Prolonged duration of altered workload entails regulation of luminal transport protein quantity at the transcriptional level (175). The resulting sustained changes in luminal solute permeation and transcellular transport rates go along with respective adaptation of the basolateral membrane area, correlated changes in Na, K-ATPase, and of the amount of mitochondria. The persistent adaptation is associated with readily recognizable epithelial hypertro-

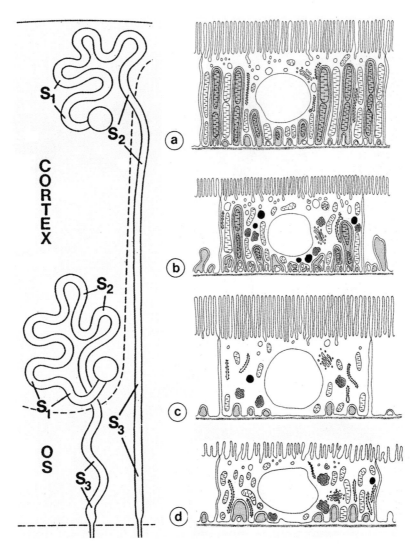

FIGURE 42 Survey on location and ultrastructure of proximal tubule segments. **A:** S1 segments start at the urinary pole of the renal corpuscle in the cortex, transform gradually to S2 segments within the labyrinth, and S2 give way to S3 at different levels (depending on the nephron generation) within the medullary rays; S3 terminates at the border (*dashed line*) of the outer stripe (OS) to the inner stripe. **B:** Salient features of S1, S2, and S3 proximal tubule cells; neighboring cells are shaded to reveal the interdigitation by lateral cell processes; the vacuolar apparatus in the subapical cytoplasm, mitochondria, ER, Golgi apparatus, lysosomes (*black spots*), and peroxisomes (*cross-hatched*) are indicated in rat S3 segments. **C:** The brush border microvilli are the highest in rabbit **(D)** and most other species they are the shortest. (From Kaissling B, Kriz W. Structural analysis of the rabbit kidney. *Adv Anat Embryol Cell Biol* 1979; 56:1–123, with permission.)

phy or hypotrophy, respectively, including changes in cell number by cell proliferation and/or apoptosis (370, 371).

On this background it is tempting to interpret the *inter-nephron heterogeneity* (i.e., the different tubular dimensions between juxtamedullary, intermediate, and superficial nephrons) as reflection of their different workloads. In rats the juxtamedullary nephrons have the largest glomeruli and highest filtration rates (35), thus the heaviest workload, they have the longst nephrons and their epithelia display the largest largest basolateral membrane area, Na, K-ATPase activity and mitochondrial volume density (488). The super-

ficial nephrons have the smallest glomeruli, filtration rates and tubular dimensions.

PRIMARY SINGLE CILIA

All renal cell types, except the intercalated cells, carry a central single primary cilium on their luminal surface. The primary cilia are regarded as mechanosensors that sense changes in luminal flow rate and circumferential stretch (365). The extracellular mechanical stimulus caused by the urinary flow is transduced via the transmembrane proteins polycystin 1 (PC-1) and polycystin 2 (PC-2) (689), located in

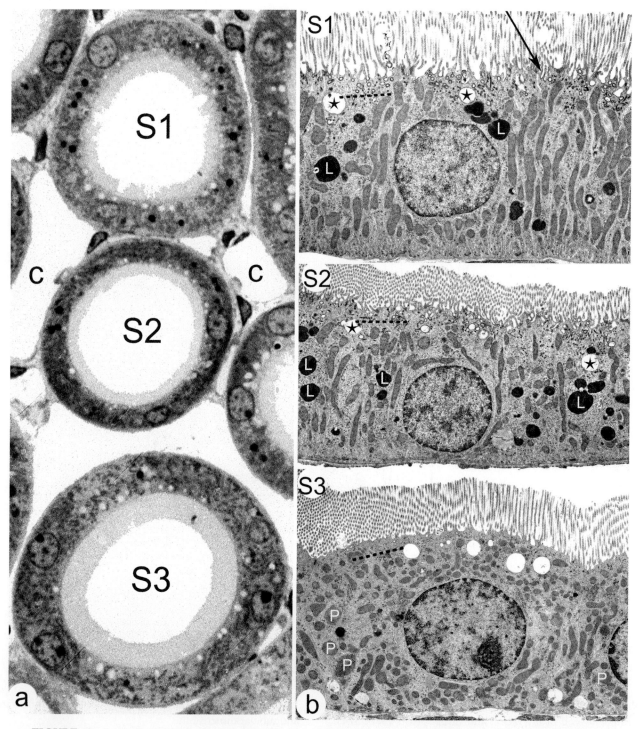

FIGURE 43   Proximal tubule in the rat. **A:** Profiles of S1, S2, and S3 segments of juxtamedullary proximal tubules. Note the differences in brush border length, cell height, cytoplasmic density, and outer diameter. Size, 1-mm Epon section; magnification, × ~1000. **B:** Ultrastructure of S1, S2, and S3 proximal tubule cell in the rat. The mitochondria in S1 and S2 are located in lateral cell processes, in S3 they are mainly scattered throughout the cytoplasm. The endocytotic apparatus in the subapical cytoplasm (roughly delimited by *broken lines*) is most prominent in S1 and S2 early; endosomes (*stars*) and lysosomes (L) are located deeper in the cytoplasm. In S3 the vacuolar apparatus and lysosomes are virtually absent, whereas peroxisomes (P) are more frequent than in S1 and S2; interdigitation by lateral folds is almost lacking. C, peritubular capillaries. Transmission electron microscopy (TEM) × ~ 5400.

the membrane of the cilium (361, 700). Together they form a complex required for the flow-mediated calcium entry in response to the deflection of the axoneme (136). This subsequently results in release of calcium stores from the endoplasmic reticulum, possibly mediated by PC-2 (100, 136, 385). By these pathways, the primary cilia of renal epithelial cells may be involved in the functional differentiation of polarized cells (241), in the maintenance of normal tubular architecture (100), in regulation of tissue morphogenesis (446) and in inducing gene transcription (e.g., in lack of fluid flow or tubular obstruction) (100, 136, 385). Loss-of-function mutations in the genes for PC-1 or PC-2 cause ciliary abnormalities (249) and the autosomal dominant form of polycystic kidney disease (ADPKD) (461, 700).

Proximal Tubule

GENERAL ORGANIZATION

The proximal tubule begins at the urinary pole of the renal corpuscle and ends at the transition to the descending thin limb of Henle's loop, which defines the border between the outer and the inner stripes. It has a convoluted part, situated in the cortical labyrinth, and a straight part (pars recta, the thick descending limb of Henle's loop), located in the cortical medullary rays and in the outer stripe (Fig. 42). The volume fraction of proximal tubules is about 48% in the rat cortex and about 54% in the outer stripe (488). From the collected tubular volume in the cortical labyrinth of an adult rat the convoluted proximal tubule takes a fraction of 80% to 85% (277).

The proximal tubule is subdivided into three segments, S1, S2, and S3 (406, 407). S1 cells line the initial half of the convoluted portion and transform to S2 cells within the second half of the convoluted part. All proximal tubule segments touching the renal capsule are S2 (162), and S2 cells form the beginning of the straight part in the medullary rays. S3 cells supersede S2 cells at various levels (depending on the nephron generation) in the medullary rays (162, 697, 699) and line the terminal portion of the proximal tubule.

MORPHOLOGY OF PROXIMAL TUBULAR EPITHELIUM

The proximal tubule is lined by an *interdigitated epithelium* (see previous section). The cells display a characteristic *brush border* at the apical pole and their basal part is expanded by complex *interdigitating basolateral folds* enclosing large *mitochondria* (Fig. 43). The *tight junctions* are shallow, mostly consisting of a single strand with low particle density (516) in agreement with the low-resistance shunt pathway in parallel with a high-resistance pathway across the limiting cell membranes (215, 386). The proximal tubule cells are electrically coupled by *gap junctions*.

The subapical cytoplasm immediately under the base of the brush border microvilli is a membrane-rich region, called *vacuolar apparatus* (Fig. 44). It contains intermicro-

villar in-foldings (*clefts*), small *clathrin-coated vesicles*, uncoated *dense apical tubules* (*DATs*) 70 to 90 nm in diameter, and *large uncoated vesicles*. The vacuolar apparatus is the structural correlate of the early endocytotic apparatus (see following sections). The *nucleus* is encircled in its equatorial plane by well-developed *Golgi apparatus*, and abundant *lysosomes* are present in the center of the cells. Cisterns of *rough ER* are preferentially found between the lateral cell membranes and the adjacent mitochondrial profiles, *ribosomes* are abundant throughout the cytoplasm. In the terminal portions of the proximal tubule fenestrated cisterns of *smooth ER (sER)*, containing xenobiotic-metabolizing enzymes (367) are particularly abundant. The cisterns of the sER often extend along the lateral membranes and narrowly enwrap mitochondria and *peroxisomes* (60). The latter are generally situated in the basal portions of the cells (695). The amount of lysosomes, peroxisomes, and *lipid droplets* in proximal tubule cells strongly varies with the functional stage of the animal, food intake, and sex hormones (134, 545, 696).

The *subdivision into S1, S2, and S3* is based on gradually occurring changes in ultrastructure along the proximal tubule in rats and rabbits. S2 cells have less basolateral surface area and Na, K-ATPase activity per unit membrane area, as well as a lower mitochondrial density. The microvilli in S2 are markedly shorter than in S1 (in rat S1: ~ 4. 5 to 4.0 μm; S2: ~ 4.0 to 1.5 μm). In rats, the brush border microvilli of S3 are much longer than in S2. In rabbits, dogs, and humans, the height of microvilli

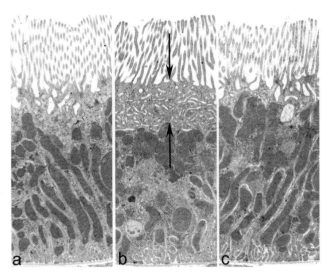

FIGURE 44 S1 cells of the proximal tubule of rats after a single injection of parathyroid hormone (PTH). PTH induces a rapid shift of the sodium phosphate cotransporter NaPi-IIa from the brush border membrane into the subapical compartment, where the tubular and vesicular structures of the endocytotic apparatus (*between arrows*) transiently expand. **A:** Control; **(B)** 15 minutes after PTH-injection; **(C)** 60 minutes after PTH-injection. Transmission electron microscopy (TEM) × ~10,000. (From Lotscher M, Scarpetta Y, et al. Rapid downregulation of rat renal Na/P(i) cotransporter in response to parathyroid hormone involves microtubule rearrangement. *J Clin Invest* 1999;104:483–494, with permission.)

decreases along S3 (93, 271, 407). In mice, differences in the length of the brush border microvilli among the three segments are not very apparent (697, 698). In all species S3 cells have only little membrane in-foldings and, thus, a rather small basolateral surface. The volume density of mitochondria in S3 of rat and mice is rather high. In contrast to S1 and S2 most mitochondria are scattered throughout the cytoplasm. Structural correlates for endocytosis (see following sections), including lysosomes, are abundant in S1 and S2, but are almost absent in S3. The amount and size of peroxisomes increase from S2 toward S3.

FUNCTIONAL ASPECTS

The proximal tubule **reabsorbs** from the tubular fluid the major fraction of *water* and filtered *solutes*, and it **secretes** various *organic compounds* into the tubular lumen (680, 681). In addition, filtered *proteins* are almost completely recovered from the tubular fluid by **endocytosis**.

Luminal and Basal Membrane Domains Transcellular *water reabsorption* in the proximal tubule is mediated by the constitutive water channel, aquaporin-1 (AQP1), located in both membrane domains (408, 452, 455, 530, 560). In mice another water channel, AQP4, is located in the basolateral membranes of S3 segments and associated with orthogonal arrays of intramembrane particles, as revealed by freeze fracture studies (632).

The plasma membrane of the microvilli is covered by a glycocalix containing hydrolases (phosphatases, peptidases, nucleotidases), which cleave their substrates in the tubular fluid (ectoenzymes). The microvillus membrane holds a large variety of transport proteins for uptake of *solutes* from the tubular fluid. Many of the transport proteins are anchored by adaptor proteins, such as PDZ-proteins and NHERF-1/-2, to the underlying apical scaffold (64, 159, 211, 649, 659).

The density of a given sodium cotransport protein in the microvillus membrane can be dissimilar along the segments of the proximal tubule and among nephron generations and can vary with the functional conditions. For instance, the expression of the sodium phosphate cotransporter NaPi-IIa usually decreases in nephron generations from S1 to S3. In the three proximal tubule segments of juxtamedullary nephrons, it is much more abundant than in those of superficial nephrons (388). These patterns may be profoundly modified by the functional conditions (132, 359, 376, 383, 514, 613). Inversely, the sodium glucose cotransporter SGLT1 has its highest expression in the brushborder membrane (BBM) of S3 and is almost undetectable in S1. In females SGLT1 is higher expressed than in males (529).

The *sodium/hydrogen exchanger* NHE3 is responsible for most, if not all, apical membrane Na^+-H^+ exchange in the proximal tubule and the reabsorption of the bulk of filtered sodium (17, 238). The N–H exchanger is enriched in the intermicrovillar microdomain (12), where it interacts with the scavenger receptor megalin (10, 65, 414). Changes in the

NHE3-mediated sodium transport rates might involve rapid and reversible redistribution between the two microdomains (61, 302, 414, 415, 419, 685).

Secretion of organic amphiphilic electrolytes from the blood into the tubular fluid is a pathway for clearance and detoxification of xenobiotics and drugs, including diuretics (305, 351, 502, 680, 681, 690). The uptake into the proximal tubule epithelium proceeds via multispecific organic anion transporters (OATs) and organic cation transporters (OCTs) in the basolateral membrane domain. Most members of the OAT and OCT families have been immunolocalized to the basolateral cell membrane of S3 proximal tubule (281, 626, 627), yet OAT 1 has been detected mainly in S2 (612), a few of them also in S1. The expression of the OATs and OCTs is strongly regulated by sex hormones (97, 284, 285, 366, 625, 628).

The export into the tubular lumen of conjugated and unconjugated lipophilic anionic substrates involves various OATs and primarily active transporters with ATP-binding cassette motifs, belonging to the MRP family (574) and located in the brush border membrane of S1, S2, and S3 proximal tubule segments (544, 574).

Endocytotic Apparatus Tubular reabsorption of filtered proteins results from fluid phase or receptor-mediated endocytosis (69, 113). Receptor-mediated endocytosis is the most efficient. By multiphoton microscopy the passage of proteins across the different endocytotic compartments has been directly observed in vivo (430).

The first requirement for receptor-mediated endocytosis is binding of a ligand to a receptor protein on the surface of the tubular cell. The multireceptors *megalin, cubilin,* and *amnionless* (226, 427), binding to partially differential ligands, have all been located in the proximal tubule, mainly at the base of the microvillus plasma membrane, in the *intermicrovillar membrane invaginations* (clefts), and in subapical *clathrin-coated pits*. Megalin, belonging to the LDL-receptor family, is bound with its cytoplasmic tail to cytoplasmic adaptor proteins (443, 599), forms a tandem with the peripheral protein cubilin (642, 643) and is responsible for the internalization of its own ligands and of cubilin with its ligands (113). Amnionless protein is essential for the membrane association and trafficking of cubilin. The receptor–ligand complexes are gathered in the *clathrin-coated membrane pits* and are directed by *clathrin-coated vesicles* to larger, uncoated *early and late endosomes*, located slightly deeper in the cytoplasm. In the endosomes the receptors are cleaved from the ligands and travel back to the luminal membrane via uncoated DATs (114, 225, 406, 407). The DATs form an elaborate, moving dynamic network of anastomosing tubules (130, 225), which are transiently connected to the larger endosomes and display at their other end small clathrin-coated domains (129-131, 194). From the endosomes the ligands are sorted for degradation to lysosomes or for ubiquitination via the proteasome pathway. The trafficking of internalized material from the vacuolar apparatus to lysosomes critically depends on the *microtubular system* (382). Microtubules normally form a loose network across the proximal tubule cells and become highly oriented in an apicobasal direction during vesicular transport of endocytosed cargo to lysosomes (383).

The dimensions of the vacuolar apparatus (Fig. 44) and the location of megalin in proximal tubule cells are correlated with the rate of endocytosis. If endocytosis does not take place, either due to paucity of ligands in the tubular fluid (e.g., normally in S3) or lack or low levels of the endocytosis receptor (26, 28, 113), the vacuolar apparatus is barely developed.

The processing of material in the vesicular compartments of the endocytotic pathway relies on acidification. NHE3, the proton-ATPase, and the chloride channel ClC-5 are highly expressed and colocalized in the intermicrovillous clefts as well as in the vesicular membranes in the early endocytotic pathway (112, 205, 654). Dysfunction of one or several of these acidifying proteins may cause primary defects in endocytosis. Knockout of the ClC-5 channel, for instance, impairs the clearance of PTH from the tubular fluid, entailing hyperphosphaturia and hypercalciuria (112, 654). This mechanism can explain the high incidence of kidney stones in Dent disease, with functionally impaired ClC-5 channels (144, 260, 261).

Endocytosis contributes also to *acute regulation of transport rates* by selective retraction of transport proteins from the microvillous membrane. For instance, the drastic decrease of the brush border protein NaPi-IIa protein, occurring within minutes after an injection of PTH (383, 441), soon after acute high phosphate intake (359), or following activation of dopamine receptors (27), relies on withdrawal of NaPi-IIa, first, from its anchoring NHERF1/2 and PDZ proteins in the apical scaffold (63, 141) and, second, by subsequent endocytotic uptake of the protein by endocytosis (358, 382, 383). Absence or reduced expression of megalin markedly slows down the endocytosis of NaPi-IIa (26, 28).

The passage of NaPi-IIa across the successive endocytotic compartments, namely, the megalin-containing clefts, the clathrin-coated-vesicle compartment (614), through the early and late endosomal compartment, and finally its disposal in lysosomes, where NaPi-IIa is degraded (29–31) has been tracked by immunofluorescence (29). The shifting of the protein through the early endocytotic compartments goes along with a dramatic, rapidly transient expansion and remodeling of the vacuolar apparatus in the subapical compartment (Fig. 44) (383).

Thin Limbs of Henle's Loop (Intermediate Tubule)

The intermediate tubule comprises the thin tubular portions, interposed between the proximal and the distal tubules (Fig. 45). Ultrastructurally, the intermediate tubule has four structurally different segments: (1) the descending thin limbs of short loops (SDTLs), (2) the upper part, (3) the lower part of descending thin limbs of long loops (LDTLup and LDTL lp), and (4) the ascending thin limbs (ATLs). This pattern has been observed in various species, including rat (331, 570), mouse (150, 699), golden hamster (22), rabbit (271, 548), *Perognathus* (444), *Octodon degus* (46), *Meriones shawii* (321), and *Psammomys obesus* (52, 53, 330). An additional subsegment of thin limbs has been identified in *Chinchilla* (111). The thin limbs in human have so far not been studied in comparable completeness (153, 318, 326).

These thin epithelia are strikingly different from each other with respect to ultrastructure and function, not only the ascending from the descending limbs but, most remarkably, the descending limbs of short from those of long loops. Furthermore, within the descending segments (SDTL, LDTLup, LDTL lp) the proximal portion, though structurally not different from the distal portion, displays considerable functional differences. In the inner medulla (IM) a high percentage of thin limbs was found that consisted of a patchwork of descending and ascending type epithelia (475, 476). Beyond all these heterogeneities, there are prominent differences among species. This complex situation appears to account for the persistent discussion about the integrated function of thin limbs in the urine concentrating process.

The *type 1 epithelium* (Fig. 46), which is characteristic for SDTLs, has a simple and uniform organization. It is composed of flat, noninterdigitating cells reposing on a thin basement membrane. The luminal cell membrane bears only a few short microvilli that are mainly found along the cell borders. The tight junction consists of several anastomosing junctional strands; desmosomes are frequently encountered. The SDTLs in the rat have, among all other thin limb segments, a particularly prominent cytoskeleton with a high content of cytokeratins and desmoplakins (23). Cell organelles, such as mitochondria, profiles of rough and smooth endoplasmic reticulum etc. are exceedingly sparse in type 1 epithelium.

Functionally, this segment contains AQP1 and the urea transporter UT-A2 in its cell membranes (43, 293, 455, 457), thus it is water and urea permeable. However, these properties are unequally distributed; within the proximal part the water permeability, within the distal part the urea permeability is high (43, 293, 459). In species with complex vascular bundles (rat, mouse, and others), the short descending limbs lie within the vascular bundles (317); in these surroundings, the thin limbs are in an ideal position to recycle urea from the ascending vasa recta into the short loop nephrons (see subsequent sections).

This simple type 1 epithelium is found also in many descending loop profiles in the inner stripe of feline and canine kidneys, which by the microanatomical definition possess only "long" loops. Consequently, it may be assumed that these simple profiles belong to those long loops that descend into the inner medulla for only very short distances,

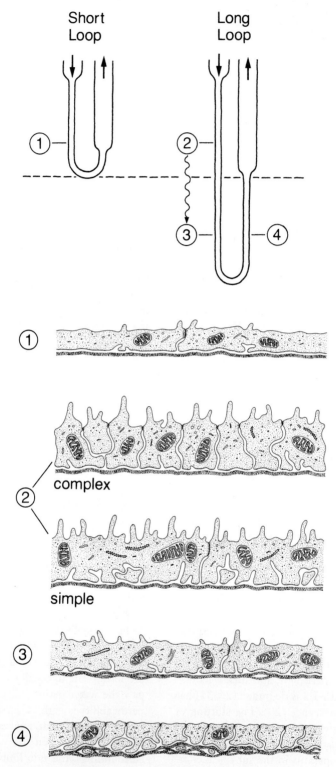

FIGURE 45   Survey of thin limb ultrastructure. Four thin limb segments are discernible: (*1*) Descending thin limb of short loops. (*2*) Descending thin limbs of long loops, upper part. This segment is differently developed among species: A complex type (*upper panel*) found in rat, mouse, and *Psammomys* is distinguished from a simple type (*lower panel*) found in rabbit and guinea pig. (*3*) Descending thin limb of long loops, lower part. The transition between upper and lower parts is gradual. (*4*) Ascending thin limb. (From Kriz W, Schiller A, et al. Comparative and functional aspects of thin loop limb ultrastructure. In: Maunsbach AB (ed.). *Functional Ultrastructure of the Kidney*. London: Academic Press, 1980:239–250 and Kaissling B, Kriz W. Morphology of the loop of Henle, distal tubule and collecting duct. In: Windhager EE (ed.). *Handbook of Physiology: Section on Renal Physiology*. New York: Oxford University Press, 1992:109–167, with permission.)

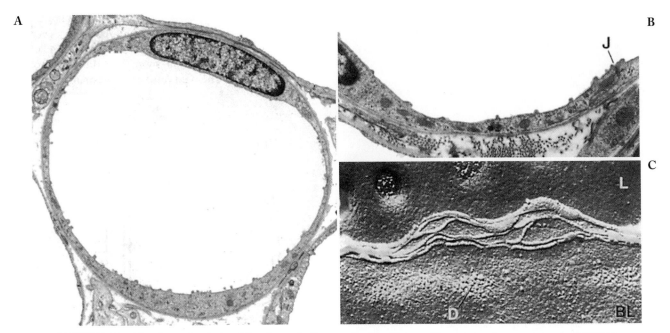

FIGURE 46   Thin descending limbs of short loops. **A:** Cross-sectional profile in rat. Transmission electron microscopy (TEM) × ~4100. **B:** The simplicity of the epithelium is demonstrated in the rat. J, junctional complex. TEM, × ~11,000. **C:** Freeze-fracture electron micrograph of rabbit. The tight junction consists of several anastomosing strands. L, luminal membrane; BL, basolateral membrane; D, desmosome. TEM ×~71,000.

frequently less than 500 μm (336). The epithelial characteristics of these loops may be more important than their short descent into the inner zone for determining their functional role. From this point of view, "short loops" are also present in the cat kidney. The short descending thin limbs of cortical loops—studied in the minipig (152) and guinea pig (unpublished results from our laboratory; Kriz 1974)—are also established by the simple type 1 epithelium.

The **descending thin limbs of long loops** are generally much larger in diameter and have a thicker epithelium than those of short loops. Moreover, the LDTLs are heterogeneous: Obviously, those of the "longest" long loops begin in the inner stripe as a much thicker tubule than those of "shorter" long loops. The character of the epithelium gradually changes as the limbs descend toward and into the inner medulla. The subdivision of these thin limbs into an upper part (*type 2 epithelium*) (Fig. 47A) and a lower part (*type 3 epithelium*) (Fig. 47B) is an approximation and reflects the gradual change to a more structurally simplified epithelium. Moreover, this process of epithelial simplification appears to be individually related to the length of each loop. It occurs earlier and more quickly in "short" long loops and is delayed in the longest of the long loops (270, 330, 569, 570, 699). This explains the heterogeneity among descending thin limb profiles in a given cross-section through the medulla: Profiles lined with the lower part of the epithelium (type 3) may already be found at the end of the inner stripe. Even deep in the inner medulla, profiles with the upper-part epithelium (type 2; in reduced elaboration) are still present.

Furthermore, considerable interspecies differences, concerning in particular the upper parts of LDTLs complicate

the understanding of the long descending thin limbs. Two patterns may be distinguished (270). In one group of species (mouse, rat, golden hamster, *Perognathus*, *Psammomys*, *O. degus*, cat), *the epithelium (type 2)* of the LDTLup is characterized by an extremely high degree of cellular interdigitation. In a single cross-section, more than 100 cell processes may be encountered (Figs. 47A and 48A,B). The tight junctions are extremely shallow, usually consisting of one junctional strand. Thus, the most characteristic features of this epithelium are the prominent paracellular pathways. The junctions are "leaky," and the amount of junctional area available per unit area of epithelial surface is increased several-fold by the tortuosity of the junction due to cellular interdigitation. The lateral cellular spaces form an elaborate "labyrinth," bordered by correspondingly amplified basolateral membranes. Additional structural characteristics of the epithelium are numerous apical microvilli, considerable numbers of mitochondria, and a strikingly high density of uniform intramembranous particles in the luminal and basolateral membrane. In addition, cytochemical and immunohistochemical studies have revealed that the LDTLup exhibits a Na, K-ATPase in both membranes (191, 393), suggesting active salt secretion. Like all descending limb segments, LDTLups are highly permeable to water due to the abundance of the constitutive water channel AQP1 in both membranes (454), probably correlating with the high density of intramembrane particles. Carbonic anhydrase activity was found in both, short and long descending thins limbs (154).

In a second group of species that includes rabbit (548, 551), minipig (152), and guinea pig the upper parts of

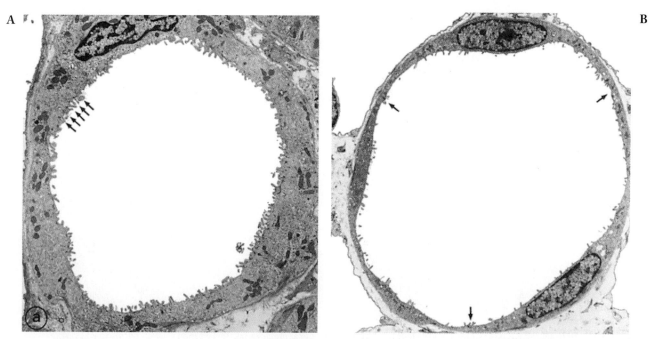

FIGURE 47   Descending thin limb of long loops, upper part. **A:** Complex type in *Psammomys*; note the many tight junctions (*arrows*). Transmission electron microscopy (TEM) × ~3000. **B:** Simple type in rabbit; only three junctions are encountered (*arrows*). TEM × ~3000.

LDTLs are more simply organized. The prominent paracellular pathways typical of the first group are lacking. The epithelial cells in this group do not interdigitate and are joined by much deeper tight junctions, consisting of several anastomosing junctional strands (Figs. 47B and 48C). In other respects, however, the epithelia are similar in the two groups. Numerous luminal microvilli, many mitochondria, and the dense assembly of intramembrane particles in luminal and basolateral membranes are present in type 2 epithelium also in this group. The high density of intramembrane particles may be partially due to the high density of AQP1 channels in both membranes; corresponding to the decrease of particle density along its descending course also the density of AQP1 channels decreases (341, 459, 635).

The epithelium of the lower part of LDTLs (*type 3 epithelium*) is comparably simple (Fig. 49); interspecies differences are no longer prominent. The epithelium consists of relatively flat, noninterdigitating cells bearing some sparse microvilli; in the rat it is covered by an unusually thick surface coat (570). The tight junctions are of an intermediate apicobasal depth, composed of several junctional strand (in rabbit: 138 ± 37 nm and 3.5 ± 0.7 strands; in *Psammomys*, 51 ± 28 nm) (270). The basolateral membrane regularly forms basal in-foldings similar to those found in the simple type of the LDTLup (270). The fluid spaces between the in-foldings are not continuous with the lateral intercellular spaces, and thus they are not part of a paracellular pathway route. The pattern and density of intramembrane particles in the luminal and

basolateral membranes are inconspicuous; the dense packing, typical for the upper parts, has disappeared. This appears to correlate with the decrease in density of AQP1 channels that, in the terminal portions of this segment, may completely disappear. Thus, the water permeability probably decreases toward the loop bend (341, 459); the terminal segment may accordingly be suggested to have low water permeability. Regarding the permeability to urea and the distribution of the urea transporter UT-A, conflicting data are published, especially when comparing data from different species (232, 293, 341, 476, 577, 617).

With respect to the descending thin limbs of the human kidney, the published data do not allow a final conclusion. In an older TEM investigation (96), a thin limb profile is shown with a heavily interdigitated epithelium corresponding to the thin limb epithelium described previously as the complex type in other species. However, in that text the descending thin limbs in the human kidney are described as being outlined by a simply structured epithelium. In 1967, when that paper was published, it was not yet known that there are four different thin limb epithelia.

The axial, the internephron, and interspecies differences in descending thin limb epithelia are surprisingly prominent compared with other nephron segments. Differences among thin limb segments were also found with respect to the cholesterol content of their cell membranes (468). Binding studies with various lectins have revealed distinct labeling patterns in the descending as

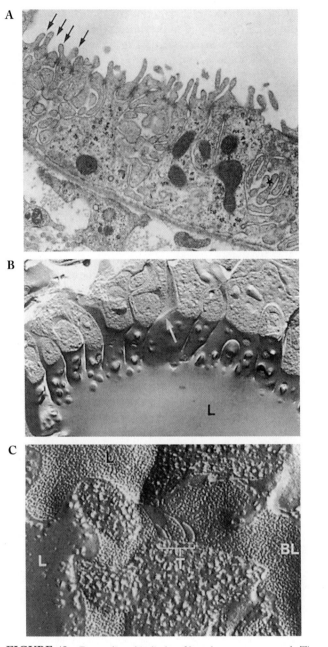

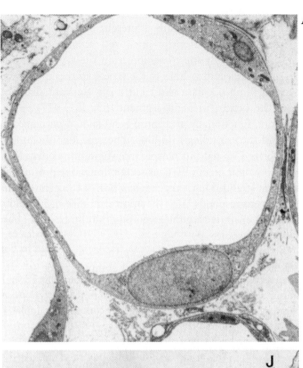

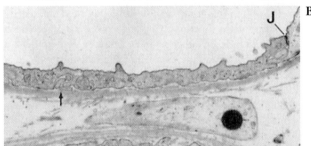

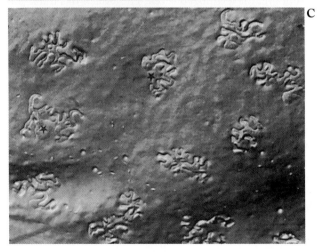

FIGURE 48 Descending thin limbs of long loops, upper part. **A:** The complex epithelium is characterized by numerous tight junctions (*arrows*) indicating the extensive intercellular digitations in rat. The interdigitation of the basolateral membrane forms a "labyrinth" of extracellular spaces within the cell body (*asterisk*). Transmission electron microscopy (TEM) × ~11,000. **B:** Freeze-fracture electron micrograph exhibiting the luminal aspect of the complex epithelium demonstrating the extensive cellular interdigitation. The tight junction consists of one strand only (*arrow*). L, lumen of the tubule. TEM × ~13,000. (From Kriz W, Schiller A, et al. Comparative and functional aspects of thin loop limb ultrastructure. In: Maunsbach AB (ed.). *Functional Ultrastructure of the Kidney*. London: Academic Press, 1980:239–250, with permission.) **C:** Freeze-fracture electron micrograph of the simple type epithelium in rabbit. The tight junction (T) consists of several junctional strands. Note the dense pattern of intramembrane particles on the P face of luminal (L) and basolateral (BL) membranes (an equally dense particle pattern is also found in the complex type). L, tubular lumen. TEM ×~66,000. (From Schiller A, Taugner R, et al. The thin limbs of Henle's loop in the rabbit. A freeze fracture study. *Cell Tissue Res* 1980;207:249–265, with permission.)

FIGURE 49 Descending thin limbs of long loops, lower part. **A:** Cross-sectional profile in rat. Transmission electron microscopy (TEM) ×~3800. **B:** The epithelium is simply organized; basal in-foldings (*arrow*) are regularly encountered in rabbit. TEM ×~10200. **C:** Freeze-fracture electron micrograph of *Psammomys* demonstrating the regular pattern of basal in-foldings within the basal cell membrane (*asterisk*). TEM × ~12800. J, junctional complex. (Cooperation with A. Schiller and R. Taugner.)

well as the ascending thin limbs in rat and rabbit (343, 344, 522).

The ascending thin limb is present only in long-loop nephrons and is uniformly organized among mammals (Fig. 50). Generally the transition from the type 3 epithelium of the descending limb to the type 4 epithelium of the ascending limb occurs a short but fairly constant distance before the bend ("prebend segment"[53, 331, 477, 699]). Therefore, functionally, the entire bend should be regarded as part of the ascending thin limb. The type 4 epithelium is characterized by flat but heavily interdigitating cells joined by shallow tight junctions, consisting of only one prominent junctional strand. This leaky organization of the paracellular pathways corresponds with functional studies (250, 257), which demonstrate that the ascending thin limbs are highly permeable for ions.

The change from the type 3 epithelium to the type 4 epithelium coincides with the full disappearance of the urea transporter UT-A and the abrupt beginning of the expression of the chloride channel ClC-K1 (341, 475); aquaporins are completely lacking. Thus, the ascending thin limb is water and urea impermeable, but highly permeable for Cl^- and Na^+. Surprisingly, in mouse, rat, and rabbit a high fraction of "mixed" thin limbs was found, consisting of alternating stretches of descending- and ascending-type epithelia, thus changing from water permeable, Na^+ and Cl^- impermeable to highly Na^+ and Cl^- permeable but water impermeable along a descending (or an ascending?) thin limb.

In most species, the transition from the ascending thin limb to the thick ascending limb (distal straight tubule) is abrupt over the length of one cell. The level of this transition defines the border between the inner medulla and the inner stripe of the outer medulla. In the canine (92) and human kidney (96), a gradual transition between the thin and thick ascending parts of the limb has been observed.

Thick Ascending Limb of Henle's Loop

The thick ascending limb of Henle's loop (TAL; straight part of the distal tubule) ascends through the outer medulla and the cortical medullary rays, enters the cortical labyrinth for a short distance before its "macula densa" contacts the vascular pole of its parent glomerulus (Fig. 51). After a short "postmacular" segment, the TAL transforms to the distal convoluted tubule (DCT). While the length of the medullary part of the TAL (mTAL) differs little among nephron generations, the length of the cortical part of the TAL (cTAL) depends on the location of the corresponding renal corpuscle in the cortex (36, 272). Juxtamedullary nephrons have the shortest, superficial nephrons the longest cTAL (Fig. 51). The length of the postmacular segment varies not only among species (<500 μm in rabbits) but also among nephrons within the same kidney (270, 272, 482). An association of its length with nephron types has not been established.

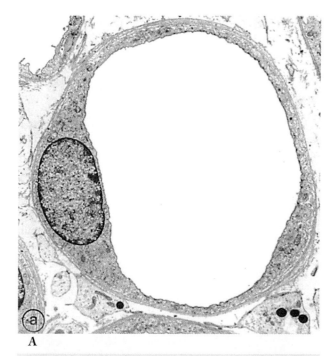

A

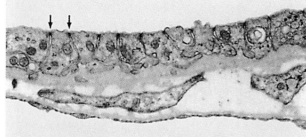

B

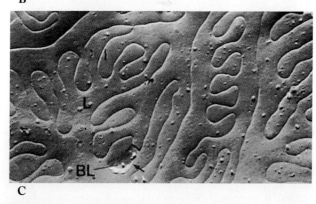

C

FIGURE 50   Ascending thin limbs. **A:** Cross-sectional profile; note the many junctions in *Psammomys* (*arrows*). Transmission electron microscopy (TEM) ×~3500. **B:** Epithelium in golden hamster exhibiting extensive intercellular interdigitation; numerous tight junctions are encountered (*arrows*). TEM ×~13,500. **C:** Freeze-fracture electron micrograph. Luminal aspect of the tubule demonstrating the mode of cellular interdigitation and the shallow tight junction (*arrow*) in *Psammomys*. BL, basolateral membrane; C, capillary; L, luminal membrane. TEM ×~4800. (From Kriz W, Schiller A, et al. Comparative and functional aspects of thin loop limb ultrastructure. In: Maunsbach AB (ed.). *Functional Ultrastructure of the Kidney*. London: Academic Press, 1980:239–250, with permission.)

The virtually water impermeable thick ascending limb reabsorbs actively sodium chloride from the tubular fluid. The apical transport system, which functionally characterizes the TAL, is the *Na+,K+,2 Cl− (NKCC2) symporter* (229). It is located exclusively in the TAL cells (including the macula densa cells) (176, 458, 464). The NKCC2 is specifically inhibitable by loop diuretics, such as bumetanide and furosemide (217).

The salt subtraction along the segment progressively dilutes the salt concentration in the tubular fluid. Such a "diluting segment" exists also in lower species (e.g., amphibians), which lack formation of loops (505, 553). Salt reabsorption by the TAL epithelium is crucial for the urinary concentrating mechanism (see subsequent sections).

The *TAL-epithelium* is typically interdigitated (Fig. 51). The interdigitating *lateral cell processes* (665) are the most conspicuous, each of them is usually completely filled by a single *large mitochondrial profile* (Fig. 52) and occasionally a few cisterns of rough endoplasmic reticulum (rER). The large nucleus is located between the in-foldings and usually (except in the deep inner stripe) spans the entire cell height. The cytoplasm in the nuclear region displays small, round mitochondrial profiles, a particularly *extensive Golgi apparatus* (36), polyribosomes, and some short cisternae of rER. The subapical cytoplasm displays varying amounts of narrow tubular profiles and smooth *vesicles* that might indicate trafficking of apical transport proteins (see following section). The *apical membrane* of the cells carries short stubby microvilli (93, 94), which border the tight junctional belt (309). Variations in the amount of microvilli on the luminal surface of the TAL have been found among species and even among nephrons of the same animal. Scanning electron microscopy revealed that "rough" cells with numerous microvilli may be present side by side with rather smooth cells with only a few microvilli (5). In rat

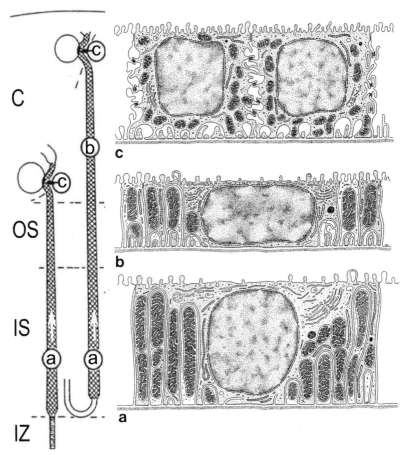

FIGURE 51 Survey on location and ultrastructure of the thick ascending limb of Henle s loop (TAL, distal straight tubule, including macula densa); the direction of the urinary flow is indicated by white arrows, interdigitated cells with large mitochondria, enclosed in the lateral processes. **A:** Medullary part, **(B)** cortical part, **(C)** macula densa. Note the difference in the organization of the lateral intercellular spaces between macula densa cells other TAL cells. C, cortex; IS, inner stripe; OS, outer stripe; IZ, inner zone. (From Kaissling B, Kriz W. Structural analysis of the rabbit kidney. *Adv Anat Embryol Cell Biol* 1979;56:1–123 and Kaissling B, Kriz W. Morphology of the loop of Henle, distal tubule and collecting duct. In: Windhager EE (ed.). *Handbook of Physiology: Section on Renal Physiology*. New York: Oxford University Press, 1992:109–167, with permission.)

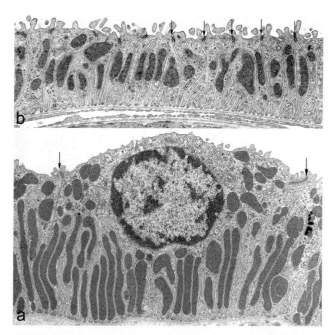

FIGURE 52 Thick ascending limb cells in rat. **A:** Deep level of the inner stripe; the lateral interdigitated foldings contain large mitochondria and do not reach up to the lumen. **B:** Cortical part; in the much lower cells the lateral interdigitated foldings reach up to the lumen, causing a folded course of the tight junctions (*arrows*). Transmission electron microscopy (TEM) × ~14,500. (From Kaissling B, Kriz W. Morphology of the loop of Henle, distal tubule and collecting duct. In: Windhager EE (ed.). *Handbook of Physiology: Section on Renal Physiology.* New York: Oxford University Press, 1992:109–167, with permission.)

TAL the latter cells display strong immunoreactivity for EGF, which seems to play a role in the regulation of growth and differentiation of cells in the loop of Henle (262).

The epithelium gradually changes from the inner stripe toward the cortex (Figs. 51 and 52) (36, 272). The most obvious is a continuous decrease in epithelial height, which goes along with a reduction and finally a lack of the apical cytoplasm, covering the interdigitating processes (Fig. 52A). This results in heavy interdigitation of the apical cell portion and a considerable increase in the *length* of the tight junctional belt (309), evident by the frequent hits of the junction in sections across the cortical TAL epithelium (Fig. 52B) and a marked increase in the density of microvilli on the luminal surface, since they border the junctions.

The *tight junctions* in the TAL are of low to intermediate apicobasal depth (Fig. 40A). The construction of the tight junction with strands arranged in parallel with high particle density might contribute to the *low water permeability* of the paracellular pathway in the TAL. At the same time the junctions in the TAL display a selective permeability for Mg^{2+} and Ca^{2+}, due to the presence of the tight junction protein claudin 16 (paracellin-1) (310). The much greater length of the tight junctional belt in the cTAL than in the mTAL might explain the higher paracellular move-

ment of Mg^{2+} and Ca^{2+} in the cTAL than in the mTAL (310, 311). Impaired function of paracellin-1 leads to urinary losses specifically of magnesium and calcium (186, 301, 496, 623).

The activity/density of the Na-K-ATPase in basolateral plasma membrane, which drives the entry of Na^+, K^+, and $2Cl^-$ into the cell, exceeds by far that of more proximal tubular sites (164, 286). The K ions entering the cell at the luminal side via NKCC2 recycle over the apical membrane by the inwardly rectifying *renal outer medullary K channel, ROMK*, which is particularly abundant in the apical plasma membrane of TAL cells (209, 227, 261, 364).

Regulation of salt transport rates in the TAL involves peptide hormones that increase cAMP in the TAL, among them vasopressin and glucagon (140, 176, 228, 230, 231, 251, 299, 416, 431, 433, 676). *Cyclooxygenase-2* (COX2), which has been located in the TAL cells including the macula densa cells (74), contributes to the handling of ions by the TAL through local production of prostaglandins (224, 227, 258, 644).

The *acute response* to decreases or increases in cAMP seems to consist of endocytotic and exocytotic, respectively, membrane translocation (416, 470). The various amounts of vesicular and tubular structures in the apical cytoplasm of TAL cells, which display NKCC2 (174, 291, 299) might be related with trafficking of the transport proteins. Similar as in the proximal tubule, endocytosis relies on *NHE3*-mediated acidification and presence of the chloride channel *CLC5*. NHE3 and ClC5 are located in the apical cytoplasm of TAL cells (364, 489).

The basolateral extrusion of Cl occurs passively through *ClC-K* and *ClC-Kb* channels (227). The trafficking of ClC-K to the basolateral membrane requires the protein barttin (227). Impaired function of one or several of the genes for these proteins and/or channels, or of the respective signaling cascade, causes severe renal salt wasting associated with lowered blood pressure, hypokalemic metabolic alkalosis, and hypercalciuria, and variable risk of kidney stones, symptoms characterizing Bartter syndrome (83, 227, 384, 559, 651, 652).

Prolonged changes in salt reabsorption rates induce structural adaptation (hypertrophy or hypotrophy) of the TAL epithelium. The heterogeneity of cell height, mitochondrial density, and basolateral plasma membrane surface (i.e., Na, K-ATPase) along the TAL might reflect adaptation of the cortical portions to the physiologically lower tubular salt load at this site and ensuing lower transport rates (229). Under physiological conditions the overall reduction of the cell height, membrane area, and mitochondrial volume (per unit tubular length) along the TAL is much more pronounced in rabbits than in rats and mice.

The plasticity of the TAL epithelium in response to variations in plasma levels of vasopressin (ADH) or cAMP had been revealed by studies on Brattleboro rats, which genetically lack ADH and suffer from diabetes insipidus (DI) (629). In these rats the medullary and cortical portion of the TAL are equally thin (618). In healthy rats with chronic *low* plasma levels of ADH due to chronic high water intake, the structural appearance of the TAL resembles that seen in DI rats (39). Several weeks of substitution of ADH in DI rats or of endogenously increased ADH levels, associated with chronic water restriction, restore the normal axial heterogeneity (76, 77).

The transport rates by the TAL epithelium seem to be positively correlated with the *DNA synthesis rate* of TAL cells. Specific inhibition of NaCl reabsorption in the TAL of rats by furosemide reduces transiently the incidence of TAL cells showing DNA synthesis (assessed by nuclear detection of the proliferating cell nuclear antigen [PCNA] and incorporation of the thymidine analogue bromodesoxyuridine) from about 1%, the basal rate in the rat TAL epithelium, to zero (370).

The function of the TAL plays also an important role in maintaining *acid-base homeostasis.* The TAL reabsorbs about 15% to 20% of the filtered bicarbonate (98, 99, 103, 104). Bicarbonate reabsorption involves the activity of the sodium/hydrogen exchangers *NHE3* and *NHE2* in the luminal plasma membrane of the TAL cells (10, 66, 381, 596) and the NEM-sensitive *vacuolar H^+-ATPase* (650). The apical N–H exchange is tightly coupled with the basolateral Cl^-–$HCO3^-$ exchange that proceeds by the Cl^-–$HCO3^-$ exchanger *AE2* (495, 500). The abundance of the NHE3 protein in the apical plasma membrane of the TAL has been shown to increase with functional adaptation to reduced renal mass (103), under metabolic acidosis (9), and with high levels of glucocorticoids (376).

The *Tamm-Horsfall glycoprotein* (THP) the most abundant urinary protein in mammals, relevant, among others, in the pathogenesis of cast nephropathy and urolithiasis (575), is synthesized in the kidney exclusively by the TAL epithelium. THP has been located in high density on the apical plasma membrane and in low density also on the basolateral plasma membrane (21, 25).

SEGMENTS DOWNSTREAM THE TAL: DISTAL CONVOLUTED TUBULE, CONNECTING TUBULE, AND COLLECTING DUCT

The electrolyte and water reabsorption by the tubular portions downstream of the TAL determines the final renal electrolyte and acid/base excretion.

Detailed electron microscopic studies on renal distal tubules in the 1970s and 1980s (reviewed in [369]) resulted in the *morphological segmentation* of the distal convolution, (DC), located in the cortical labyrinth, in the *distal convoluted tubule* (**DCT**) and the *connecting tubule* (**CNT**). The CNT opens into a short branch ("initial collecting tubule") of the *cortical collecting duct* (**CCD**) located the in

the medullary rays (Fig. 53). The successive CD portions traverse the outer medulla as *outer medullary* CD (OMCD) and the inner medulla as *inner medullary* CD (IMCD) (Fig. 53).

In the DCT, CNT, and CCD of rabbits (272), rats (126, 392, 556), *P. obesus* (266), and mice (375), four cell types have been described (Fig. 53). Three are segment-specific cell types: the DCT cells in the DCT, the CNT cells in the CNT, and the CD cells (formerly called "principle cells") in the CCD and OMCD (Fig. 53). The fourth cell type, the intercalated cells (IC cells), are interspersed among the segment-specific cells of all these segments (Fig. 53) (161, 270, 272, 352, 369). The few studies on the human nephron (68, 442, 609) agree with the data obtained from experimental animals. The IMCD is lined by cells, which are distinguished from those in the OMCD as "IMCD cells" (Fig. 53).

The *functional segmentation* (Fig. 54) of the tubular portions downstream of the TAL is based on the distribution of the major apical sodium, calcium, magnesium and water transport proteins (see following sections). The transcellular transports, initiated by the solute entry via the apical transporters, rely on functionally correlated cytoplasmic and/or basolateral membrane proteins, taking part in the movement of the solute trough the cells, and in its extrusion through the basolateral plasma membrane (see following sections). The distribution of some of these latter proteins is congruent with that of the given apical transporter.

Because each change in the apical transport proteins is translated by distinct, though often subtle, changes in cellular organization, the subdivisions of the tubular system on account of structure and function are necessarily congruent. The criteria for the delineation of the segments are a matter of definition (369).

Distal Convoluted Tubule

The transition from the TAL to the DCT is marked in all species by an abrupt rise in epithelial height (Fig. 55) (369, 372). This structural change coincides with the replacement of the NKCC2, characterizing the TAL cells, by the thiazide-inhibitable sodium chloride cotransporter, NCC, characterizing the DCT cells (507).

DCT cells are typically interdigitated (Figs. 56A and 57A). The surface area of the basolateral membranes, the amount of Na, K-ATPase (163, 275, 286), and the volume density of mitochondria in the DCT cells are the highest from all tubular cells (275, 488). The prominent equipment for active transport, characterizing the DCT, might be related to the fact that the NCC-mediated NaCl reabsorption occurs at the nephron site with the steepest transepithelial concentration gradients for sodium in the kidney. The large *lamella-like mitochondria* are narrowly enclosed by the plasma membrane of the *lateral interdigitating processes,* all other cell organelles are situated in the apical cytoplasm: the *nucleus,* the distinct *Golgi apparatus,* numerous *small mitochondrial profiles,* short cisterns of *rough endoplasmic reticulum,* and

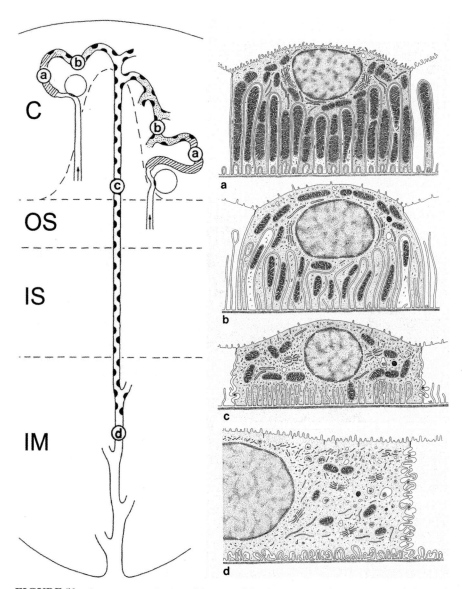

FIGURE 53 Survey on organization of the cortical distal segments and collecting ducts (left panel) and on ultrastructure of the segment-specific cells (right panel). Dashed line delimits the medullary ray; **(A)** distal convoluted tubule (DCT) and DCT cell; **(B)** connecting tubule (CNT) and CNT cell; **(C)** CCD and CCD cell; **(D)** inner medulla (IM) and IMCD cell; the black semicircles indicate the occurrence of intercalated (IC) cells; each DCT opens into one CNT. In superficial nephrons the CNT opens directly into a CCD; connecting tubules of deeper nephrons join to form an arcades which ascend in the cortical labyrinth, before they open into a CCD; the collecting ducts descends in the medullary rays and through the outer and inner stripes of the outer medulla; the lower two thirds of the collecting duct are lined by IMCD cells, exclusively; the IMCD open as papillary ducts on the renal papilla. C, cortex; OS, outer stripe; IS, inner stripe of the outer medulla; IM, inner medulla. (From Kaissling B, Kriz W. Morphology of the loop of Henle, distal tubule and collecting duct. In: Windhager EE (ed.). *Handbook of Physiology: Section on Renal Physiology.* New York: Oxford University Press, 1992:109–167, with permission.)

abundant *smooth small, invaginated vesicles* closely beneath the apical plasma membrane (270, 272, 391). The microtubular system in DCT cells is much more prominent than in proximal tubule cells. The *tight junctional belt* has a similar organization as in the TAL, but is shorter since the apical portions of the DCT cells are not interdigitated and, thus, have a polygonal outline. The apical plasma membrane carries numerous *stubby microvilli*.

The recent detection of *TRPM6* in the apical membrane of the DCT, so far shown only in mice (552, 645), in addition to NCC, substantiates former suggestions on the role of the DCT in determining the final urinary excretion of magnesium (496, 539, 645). Transcellular magnesium reabsorption via *TRPM6* seems to critically depend on the presence of the *gamma subunit of the renal Na, K-APTase* (204) in the basolateral membrane of the DCT cells (417) and on low

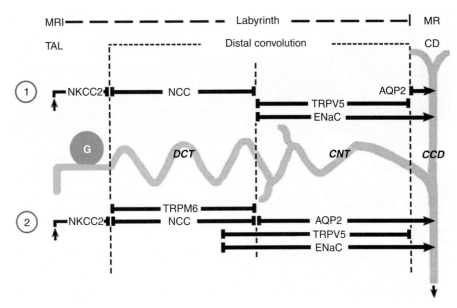

FIGURE 54 Schematic distribution of the major apical transport proteins (NKCC2, NCC, TRPM6, TRPV5, ENaC, and AQP2) along the cortical distal segments (*1*) in rabbit and (*2*) in rat, mouse and human. Sharp beginning and stop of a transporter along the cortical nephron is indicated by vertical bars, the continuation along the CD by arrows. MR, medullary ray; TAL, thick ascending limb; G, renal corpuscle; DCT, distal convoluted tubule; CNT, connecting tubule; CCD, cortical collecting duct.

levels of free intracellular magnesium, putatively kept low by the cytoplasmic *calcium-binding protein parvalbumin (PV)*. PV has a several-fold higher binding capacity for magnesium than the calcium-binding protein calbindinD28k and is seen in the early part of the DCT of mice (375). The key player for paracellular Mg^{2+} transport *Claudin 16* (paracellin-1) is present in the DCT tight junction (310) and enables paracellular Mg movement across the DCT epithelium.

The *regulation of NCC expression* in the apical plasma membrane, and thus of the NaCl-transport rates by the DCT epithelium, is controlled by the luminal *NaCl-load, mineralocorticoids* (186), and *sex hormones*. In female rats the expression of NCC in the DCT is higher than that in males (640).

Chronic increases in the NaCl-transport rates in the DCT, induced in *rabbits* by high dietary Na intake combined with low K intake (275, 348) or in *rats* by raises in NaCl delivery due to impaired NaCl reabsorption in the preceding TAL (187, 267, 304), provoke extensive structural hypertrophy in the DCT (278, 588) (187, 267), including substantial increases in the DNA synthesis rate in DCT cells (370, 589). These changes occur in the presence and absence of increased plasma levels of mineralocorticoids (589).

On the other hand, the renal abundance and the NCC labeling in DCT was found to be profoundly and selectively decreased in aldosterone-escape rats (653). In rabbits on a chronic low-sodium diet, combined with high potassium intake and associated endogenous high plasma levels of aldosterone, from all distal segments only the DCT epithelium was markedly atrophied. The structural atrophy revealed that under these conditions the Na-transport rates by

the DCT epithelium were chronically low (275, 348). Some data suggest that the thiazide-sensitive NaCl cotransporter may be the chief molecular target for regulatory processes responsible for mineralocorticoid escape via a posttranscriptional mechanism (653).

The *downregulation of NCC activity* in the apical plasma membrane involves "with-no-lysine" (WNK) kinases (201, 595) and WNK signaling is implicated in the coordination of transcellular and paracellular flux to achieve NaCl and K^+ homeostasis (264). Mutations in the WNK 4 cause pseudo-hypoaldosteronism type II (PHAII) (264, 683).

NCC-mediated NaCl transport activity in the DCT is specifically inhibited by thiazide diuretics, which are frequently used in treatment of hypertension (507). In rats, treatment with thiazide diuretics induces massive rates of cell death by apoptosis of DCT cells in the early part of the DCT (371). The late part of the segment in which the cells express in addition to NCC other apical sodium entry pathways (see following sections) remains intact. If the transport activity of the early DCT cells is inhibited only for a few days, the epithelium rapidly and fully recovers within a few days after removal of the drug. By contrast, in loss-of-function mutations of the NCC gene in mice (563) permanent, dramatic atrophy of the early DCT portion is seen (379). These data highlight the importance of the transport activity in maintaining and modeling the tubular epithelium. Loss-of-function mutations in the NCC gene in humans cause Gitelman syndrome, which is characterized by mild renal sodium wasting, hypocalciuria, hypomagnesiuria, hypokalemic alkalosis, and reduced blood pressure in humans (128, 139, 418, 510). Loss-of-function mutations of one or several of the genes involved

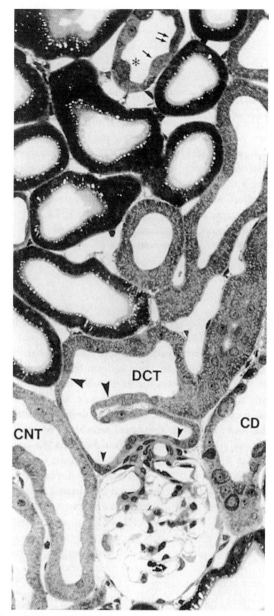

FIGURE 55   Distal tubular segments in rat beyond the macula densa; small arrowheads delimit the macula densa, large arrowheads point to the transition from the epithelium of the thick ascending limb to the distal convoluted tubule (DCT). The tubule profile in the upper portion of the micrograph has a mixed cell population, composed of connecting tubule (CNT) cells (*arrow*), cortical collecting duct (CD) cells (*double arrow*) and IC cells (*asterisk*) and represents the transition from a CNT to a cortical CD. Transmission electron microscopy (TEM) × ~500.

in Mg²⁺ reabsorption are associated with hypomagnesaemia, characteristic of Gordon syndrome (340).

TRANSITION TO CNT

In rat, mice, *Psammomys*, and human the DCT cells in the second half of the DCT, the *late part of the DCT* (designated also as "transitional" segment [369, 375], or DCT2 [102]), display less lateral interdigitating cell processes but more basal plasma membrane in-foldings, and

less mitochondria (Fig. 57B) (126). Furthermore, Intercalated cells (IC cells) make their most upstream appearances in the "late" DCT (Fig. 57B) (126). The subtle structural change in the late DCT cells goes along with the most upstream appearance of the *epithelial sodium channel*, ENaC, as well as the *epithelial calcium channel*, TRPV5 (formerly called ECaC) (Fig. 54). The *cessation of NCC* defines the beginning of the *connecting tubule* (CNT) (Fig. 54) (372).

In *rabbits*, the transition from the DCT to the CNT, is sharp and marked by an abrupt change in cell structure (272, 275), coinciding with the abrupt onset of *ENaC* (372) in the apical membrane, as well as the onset of the *TRPV5* (630) (Fig. 54) and also the appearance of IC cells.

CONNECTING TUBULE

In all species the epithelium of the CNT is lined by two distinct cell types: the segment-specific CNT cells and the IC cells (Fig. 58).

The organization of *CNT cells* (Figs. 53B, 56B, and 58B) is intermediate between the interdigitated DCT cells and the noninterdigitating epithelia (CD cells). The organization of the *tight junction* changes along the CNT from parallel strands to a complex network of anastomosing strands (548). Irregular deep in-foldings of the basal plasma membrane supersede interdigitation by lateral processes. The *intercellular spaces* and the spaces between the basal infolded plasma membrane are narrow. The basolateral plasma membrane is frequently adorned by *caveolae* (81, 270) (Fig. 58 inset). The *nucleus* with the *Golgi apparatus* and *large mitochondria* are usually situated between the in-folded membranes, whereas *small mitochondrial profiles* and *smooth vesicles* are often found on top of the nucleus. *Polyribosomes* and very short profiles of *rER* are particularly abundant in the apical half of CNT cells. In contrast to the DCT cells small *lysosomes* are frequent. The apical membrane of CNT cells is adorned with short slender *microvilli*.

From the beginning to the end of the segment the height of the CNT cells, their extent of basal plasma membrane and their volume density of mitochondria decrease. The steepness of the *axial changes* is more pronounced in rabbits (275) and mice than in rats and varies with the functional conditions (372, 377).

In *rats, mice, and humans* the connecting tubule cells express *ENaC and TRPV5*, similar as the cells in the late DCT, and in addition, the *vasopressin-regulated water channel, aquaporin-2* (AQP2). In *rabbits*, however, the CNT cells do **not** express AQP2 (Fig. 54).

The *amiloride-sensitive sodium channel, ENaC*, is the key player in the final sodium recovery by the kidney (518, 656). The activity of amiloride-sensitive transport is under the tight control of aldosterone (402). Whereas *mineralocorticoid receptors* (MR) seem to be present all along the rat distal nephron, the enzyme 11-β-hydroxy steroid dehydrogenase (11-βHSD2), which confers mineralocorticoid specificity to

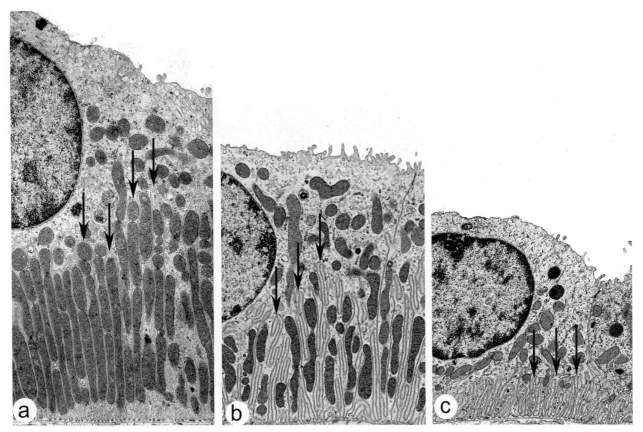

FIGURE 56   Organization of distal and collecting duct cells in the renal cortex. **A,B:** *Psammomys obesus*; **(C)** rat; fixation by reduced osmium. **A:** Distal convoluted tubule (DCT) cell, interdigitating, lateral cell processes (*arrows*) narrowly enclose large mitochondria. **B:** Connecting tubule (CNT) cell, displaying a few interdigitating lateral cell processes and abundant in-foldings of the basal plasma membrane (*arrows*), extending up into the apical cell half; most mitochondria are aligned between the infolded membranes. **C:** Noninterdigitating CCD cell; all in-foldings of the basal plasma membrane are restricted to the basal cell portion; the location of mitochondria above the basal rim of in-folded membranes is characteristic for CD cells. Transmission electron microscopy (TEM) × ~10,000.

the MR (75, 91, 337) is detected only in the *aldosterone-sensitive distal nephron (ASDN),* the *late DCT,* the *CNT,* and the *CD* in the cortex and medulla of rats, mice, and humans, in rabbits, only in the CNT and collecting ducts (372, 378, 380). The extensions of the ASDN and of ENaC-expression are congruent.

ENaC is composed of three different *subunits,* α, β, and γ, which are all needed to form the functional Na-channel in the apical plasma membrane (171). The insertion of the three subunits into the apical plasma membrane, and thus the abundance of functional channels, is differentially regulated. The abundance of functional channels, detectable by immunostainings for the subunits in the apical plasma membrane, decreases from the late DCT along the CNT toward the CD. The decrease of immunostaining in the apical plasma membrane goes along with accumulation of immunostaining (with the available antibodies evident in particular for β-ENaC) in the cytoplasm (377, 380). The decline in available channels in the luminal membrane is paralleled by structural changes in the CNT epithelium (see preceding sections), which suggests progressively lower transport rates

along the segment. The steepness of these changes is modulated by dietary salt intake and aldosterone plasma levels (275, 348, 377, 380).

Convincing evidence for the predominant functional importance of the more proximal portions of the ASDN (i.e., the late DCT and the CNT) to achieve sodium and potassium balance has been provided by collecting-duct–specific gene inactivation of the αsubunit of ENaC in mouse kidney (524). Functional ENaC (all three subunits) was present only in the late DCT and in the CNT, whereas in the CD no ENaC activity was measurable. Nevertheless, the animals were able to maintain sodium and potassium balance, even when challenged by salt restriction, water deprivation, or potassium loading (524). In fact, recent data on the three-dimensional reconstruction of the mouse nephron show that five to seven nephrons are connected via a CNT to one CCD (699). Thus, the available luminal surface for ENaC-mediated sodium reabsorption in the late DCTs and the CNT, (482, 122), is several-fold greater than that available in the CCD itself. Under conditions of low sodium availability or high levels of plasma aldosterone, the more

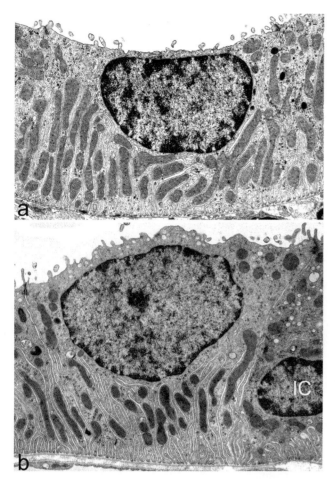

FIGURE 57   Ultrastructure of distal convoluted tubule (DCT) cells, rat kidney. **A:** Cell in the early and **(B)** late portion of the DCT. In **(A)** characteristic apical position of the nucleus and location of the mitochondria in basolateral interdigitating cell processes, the volume density of mitochondria is high. In **(B)** the amount of basal plasma membrane in-foldings is higher than in **(A),** the amount of mitochondria is lower; the most upstream appearance of intercalated cells (IC) is in the late DCT. Transmission electron microscopy (TEM) × ~5400.

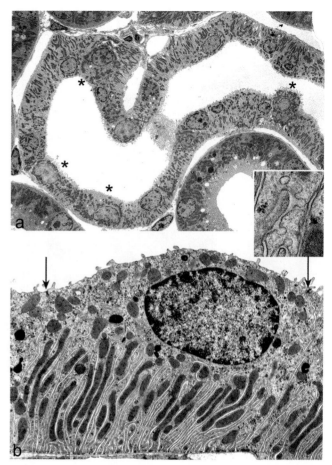

FIGURE 58   Connecting tubule in rat kidney. **A:** The epithelium is composed of CNT cells and intercalated cells (*asterisks*). **B:** Characteristic CNT cell with abundant in-foldings of the basal cell membrane; the arrows point to the tight junction. **Inset:** The infolded plasma membranes reveal numerous caveolae. **A:** Transmission electron microscopy (TEM) × ~1400; **B:** × ~6100.

distal portions of the ASDN in the CD can be recruited for salt reabsorption by insertion of the ENaC-subunits into the apical plasma membrane (377, 420).

Mutations in the genes coding for ENaC subunits and for proteins involved in the correct targeting into or removal from the membrane (e.g., SGK1, Nedd4-2) are associated with severe disturbances of blood pressure regulation (363, 494, 518, 543, 547, 655, 656).

The sodium reabsorption via ENaC is tightly coupled with *K secretion via ROMK* in the apical membrane in the segment-specific cells along the ASDN. ROMK interacts with PDZ proteins (NHERF2) in the apical membrane of collecting duct cells (649). By which mechanisms the strict quantitative association of Na-reabsorption via ENaC and K secretion via ROMK in ENaC-positive cells can be mitigated is not precisely known. Other potassium pathways, such as BK channels, might play a role. Putatively, *intercalated cells* (IC cells; see following sections) might be involved therein. IC cells are consistently found

among the ENaC-displaying cells and only there. Whereas in ENaC-positive cells the electrochemical gradient created by sodium reabsorption via ENaC drives K secretion via ROMK, in intercalated cells the proton secretion via H, K-ATPase (673) can be apparently coupled with K reabsorption.

The discovery of the *epithelial calcium channel* (235, 236), *TRPV5,* in the late DCT and in the CNT confirmed the role of these tubular portions in *transcellular calcium transport.* Immunostainings revealed in these tubular portions the consistent association of TRPV5 with high abundance of *calbindin D28k (CB)* in the cytoplasm, and in the basolateral plasma membrane with the *sodium-calcium exchanger, NCX,* and with $Ca2^+$-$Mg2^+$-*ATPase.* Interestingly, TRPV5 progressively shifts in tubular flow direction from the apical plasma membrane into the cytoplasm (375). The simultaneous decrease of TRPV5 channel abundance in the apical plasma membrane, of CB abundance in the cytoplasm, and of Ca^{2+}-Mg^{2+}-ATPase and NCX abundance in the basolateral plasma membrane indicate a parallel decrease of the transcellular calcium transport rates.

Recent data suggest that regulation of both the renal Mg^{2+}(TRPM6) and the renal Ca^{2+}(TRPV5) transport proteins is involved in the effects of acid-base status on renal divalent cation handling (460).

The *PTH/PTHrP*- and the extracellular Ca^{2+}-sensing receptor have been located in the distal tubule (511, 512, 686). Although the authors of the respective studies did not distinguish between the DCT and CNT cells, it is probable that these proteins are present in the cells of the late DCT and possibly in the CNT.

The sites of tissue *kallikrein* synthesis in the kidney are approximately congruent with the sites of calcium reabsorption (i.e., the late DCT and CNT) (466). Tissue kallikrein deficiency impairs renal tubular calcium absorption but has no effect on the renal abundance of distal Ca-transporter mRNA (490). These findings suggest that tissue kallikrein may be a physiologic regulator of renal tubular calcium transport, acting through a nonkinin mechanism (16, 466, 490, 630, 631).

In rodents and humans AQP2 is expressed along the CNT. Thus, in contrast to rabbits, in rodents and humans (68) vasopressin-regulated water subtraction is possible in the CNTs, located in cortical labyrinth (122, 372). This suggests the possibility of delivery of less-diluted tubular fluid to the cortical collecting duct.

TRANSITION TO THE CCD

In *rabbits* the transition from the CNT to the CCD is marked by a distinct change in the morphology of the segment-specific cells. At the site of the morphological change TRPV5 and Ca^{2+}-transport related proteins (calbindin D28k, NCX, Ca-Mg-ATPase) stop, and the *vasopressin-regulated water channel AQP2* appears in the CCD cells (Fig. 54) (372). In rabbits the abrupt appearance of dilated intercellular spaces indicates the change from the water-impermeable CNT epithelium to the water-permeable CCD epithelium (272, 275).

In *rodents and humans*, where AQP2 begins further upstream in the CNT, no sharp morphological transition from the CNT to the CCD is detectable. In rats and mice the transition from the CNT to the CCD is marked by the stop of TRPV5 (Fig. 54) and related proteins (369, 375), in humans NCX and calbindin D28k have been detected also in the CCD (68). Decisive for the diagnosis of the CCD is the location in the medullary ray.

Collecting Ducts

The CCD, the OMCD, and the upper part of the IMCD are composed of the segment-specific cells (CD cells) and intercalated cells (IC cells; see subsequent sections) (Fig. 53). Functionally, the collecting duct cells are characterized by expression of the vasopressin (V)–regulated AQP2 (Fig. 54).

The *CD cells* (Figs. 53, 56, 59 and 60) belong to the noninterdigitated cell type and have simple polygonal basal and apical outlines (663, 664). The *tight junctional belt* is deep and consists of anastomosing strands with high particle density (549). The apical plasma membrane generally bears only a few short *microvilli or microfolds* and a prominent central single cilium (Fig. 61A). The *subapical zone* often reveals small round or elongated vesicles, oriented perpendicularly or in an oblique angle to the luminal membrane (Fig. 60C). These vesicles contain aggregates of the AQP2 and are called *aggrephores*. AQP2 is colocalized with dynein and dynactin (396, 453). Many of the aggrephores carry spherical clathrin-coated heads. *Laterally* the CD cells are connected by numerous, small *desmosomes*, located on the abundant short villi or folds of the lateral plasma membrane (Fig. 61B) (23). In the *basal cell portion*, abundant, narrowly arranged in-foldings of the basal plasma membrane form a rim of uniform height (Figs. 53, 56, and 59). The *nucleus*, mitochondria, numerous small *Golgi fields*, abundant profiles of *smooth ER*, a few *r ERs* (60), *lysosomes, multivesicular bodies*, and occasional glycogen accumulations are located in the zone above the in-folded membranes.

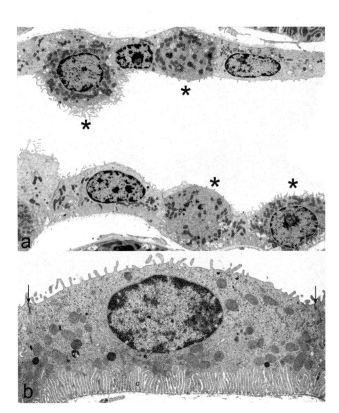

FIGURE 59 Cortical collecting duct in rat kidney. **A:** The epithelium is composed of CD and IC cells. **B:** CCD cell; in-foldings of the basal plasma membrane are restricted to the basal cell portion; all mitochondria and cell organelles are located above the infolded membranes. Arrows represent tight junctions. **A:** Transmission electron microscopy (TEM), $\times \sim$ 2700; **B:** $\times \sim$ 8500. (From Kaissling B, Kriz W. Morphology of the loop of Henle, distal tubule and collecting duct. In: Windhager EE (ed.). *Handbook of Physiology: Section on Renal Physiology.* New York: Oxford University Press, 1992:109–167, with permission.)

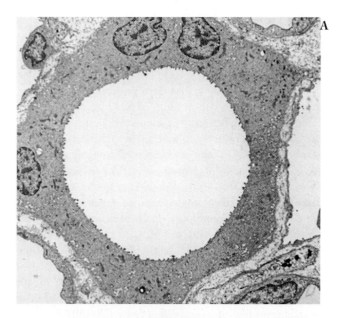

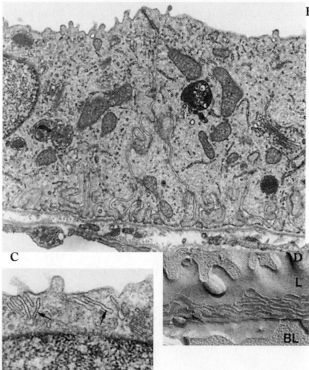

FIGURE 60 Inner medullary collecting duct in rat. **A:** Tubular profile showing the homogenous epithelium in rat. Transmission electron microscopy (TEM) × ~3400. **B:** Epithelium of the middle portion of an IMCD. Within the epithelium three zones are seen: a basal zone with basal in-foldings; a middle zone containing Golgi fields, mitochondria, and lysosomal elements; and a thin apical zone with tubular and vesicular profiles. Note the deep tight junction in the rat. TEM × ~17,000. **C:** Apical zone of a CD cell with many elongated tubular profiles (*arrows*), which represent aggrephores. TEM × ~38,000. **D:** Freeze-fracture electron micrograph to show the multistranded tight junction of the collecting duct epithelium in rabbit. L, luminal membrane; BL, basolateral membrane. TEM × ~34,000.

Because all cell organelles are usually located in the cytoplasm above this rim, CD cells of all species are recognizable in light and electron microscopy by their *light basal boundary* (Figs. 53, 56, and 59).

Receptors for vasopressin (V_1 and V_2) have been found in the collecting ducts (629) and, in rodents, also in the arcades (CNT) (18, 212, 251, 300). Binding of vasopressin (ADH) to the V_2-receptor at the basolateral membrane of CD cells triggers the signal transduction cascade leading to exocytotic insertion of AQP2 from stores in the subapical cytoplasm into the apical cell membrane, thereby conferring water permeability to the luminal membrane. The vasopressin-induced water flow across the epithelium is manifested by the dilated *intercellular spaces* (Fig. 61B) (203, 216, 610). With low levels of vasopressin the AQP2-containing membrane portions recycle back into the subapical cytoplasm (84, 530, 637).The movement of aggrephores critically depends on microtubules and actin filaments in the apical cytoplasm.

The water channel AQP3 and AQP4 are both located in the basolateral membrane of CD cells. AQP4 is associated with orthogonal arrays of intramembrane particles, as revealed by freeze fracture studies in the outer medullary collecting duct (603, 636).

The *cytoskeleton* is particularly prominent in CD cells and increases in CD cells from the CCD toward the tip of the papilla. Actin filaments and microtubules form a dense meshwork along the apical and lateral plasma membrane. The prominent cytoskeleton may be one mean, among others, to withstand the varying osmotic pressure in the collecting ducts.

The CD cells (and CNT cells in rodents) consistently coexpress the amiloride-sensitive Na-channel ENaC (see preceding sections) and AQP2 (Fig. 54) (455). The coexistence of the differentially regulated pathways for Na and water reabsorption in the same cell suggests the possibility for mutual interactions (448, 451).

The CD cell undergoes gradual, though considerable changes from the deep cortex (CCD) downstream to the upper third of the inner zone (IMCD) (Fig. 60). The extents of basal in-foldings and the volume density of mitochondria decrease, whereas the volume density of lysosomes and the density of cytoskeletal proteins increase. The degree of changes along the CD differs among species (270, 272, 442).

The CD cells in the lower two thirds of the *inner medulla* (in the papilla) are distinguished as *IMCD cells* (390). In rabbit (272) and guinea pig IMCD cells increase in height toward the papilla up to the 20-fold. A substantial, albeit less drastic increase occurs in rhesus monkey (15) and in human kidney (442). In other species (e.g., rat, mouse, *Psammomys*, and dog) (270), the epithelium near the tip of the papilla is cuboidal or low columnar. The luminal membrane of IMCD cells is covered by numerous *stubby microvilli* and generally lacks the central cilium (118). The lateral intercellular spaces are conspicuous by their dense assembly of *microvilli and microfolds*, projecting from the lateral cell membranes.

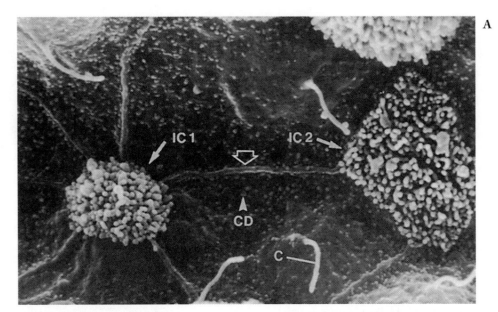

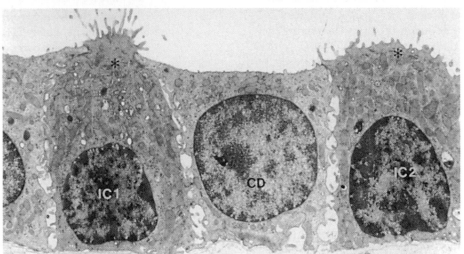

FIGURE 61 Intercalated cells from the rabbit. **A:** Scanning electron micrograph of a cortical collecting duct with collecting duct–specific CD cells (CD) and intercalated cells (IC). The CD cells carry single cilia (C) and short microvilli (*arrowhead*). The straight ridges (*open arrow*) represent the cell borders between CD cells. From the IC cells one (IC1) has a narrow, constricted apical cell pole, the other one (IC2) a large apical cell pole, both adorned with numerous long microvilli. Transmission electron microscopy (TEM) ×~13,000. **B:** Section across corresponding cells. Note the position and accumulation of flat vesicles (*asterisk*) in the apical cell pole of the IC cells. TEM × ~7500.

In the beginning of the inner medulla the *tight junctions* of the IMCD are complex, consisting of several anastomosing strands (270). Toward the papillary tip in rat and rabbit, there is a considerable decrease in the number of strands and in the apicobasal depth of the junction (270).

The IMCD cells coexpress with the amiloride-sensitive sodium channel (ENaC) and the *vasopressin-regulated AQP2*, the *vasopressin-regulated urea transporters UT-A1/3*, and possibly *UT-A4* (for review see [682]). The abundance of UT-A1/3 in the apical membrane is rate-limiting for transepithelial, vasopressin-dependent urea reabsorption (456, 682). In the basolateral membranes of the IMCD cells the water channels AQP3 (300), permeability to glyc-erol, urea and water (255), and AQP4 (199, 603) with an apparently low urea permeability have been demonstrated.

The genes coding for proteins, which are involved in cellular accumulation of organic osmolytes, such as the vasopressin-regulated urea transporter UT-A and heat shock protein 70 (223) are target genes of the tonicity-response enhancer binding protein (TonEBP), a transcriptional activator of the REL-family. During kidney development expression of TonEBP precedes that of the urea transporter. It is first detected in the renal medulla of mice at the fetal age of 16 days and increases up to postnatal day 21, when the medulla is fully developed and the urinary concentrating ability is achieved (335).

INTERCALATED CELLS

Intercalated cells (IC cells) are interspersed as single cells in the ENaC-displaying epithelium of the DCT, the CNT, and the CD (Fig. 53) (390). In rabbits the DCT lacks IC cells (272). IC cells are involved in the final regulation of acid-base excretion. This function of IC cells is achieved by the presence of an electrogenic V-type proton-ATPase in one membrane domain and a bicarbonate/chloride exchanger (HCO_3^-/Cl^-) in the other membrane domain, and it is facilitated by a high level of carbonic anhydrase II (CAII) in the cytoplasm.

The *proportion of IC cells* varies slightly among species and between the nephron segments. In the CNT IC cells amount between 25% to 40%, in the CCD up to about 40%, in the outer stripe of the OMCD they may constitute up to 50% of the tubular cell population (272), and their frequency decreases along the OMCD in the inner stripe (88, 89) to about 10% in the upper part of the IMCDs (390). In the papillary CD IC cells are usually absent. In kidneys of *juvenile rodents* IC cells may be found deep in the papilla and in the epithelium lining the renal papilla (445).

The luminal outline of IC cells appears usually more rounded than that of the surrounding polygonal CD cells (160, 352) and the pattern of elaborate *microfolds or microprojections* on the apical cell pole differs from that of the neighboring segment-specific cells (Figs. 58, 59, and 61A) (160, 352, 392, 442, 611). IC cells usually lack the single cilium (Fig. 61A) (392, 611). By light and electron microscopy IC cells usually appear darker than the neighboring cells and display a higher mitochondrial density (Figs. 61B, 62, and 63). Therefore they have been called *dark cells* (221) and *mitochondria-rich cells*, respectively (86), in analogy to similar cells in the amphibian bladder. The dark appearance as well as the high density of mitochondria are, however, no "safe" criteria for recognizing IC cells (270). Because of their high level of CAII (80, 94, 154, 292, 513, 568) they have been called also "carboanhydrase-rich" cells. Interestingly, it had been reported that IC cells lack significant levels of Na, K-ATPase in the basolateral membranes (283). However, more recently, weak to moderate Na, K-ATPase was revealed in cortical and outer medullary IC cells, whereas IC cells in the upper part of the inner medullary collecting duct showed a staining intensity that was similar or even stronger than that in adjacent IMCD cells (528).

On at least one membrane domain (more often on the luminal and vesicular than on the basolateral), most IC cells display the AMP-degrading phosphatidyl-inositol-anchored *ecto-enzyme 5′nucleotidase (5′NT)* (90, 138, 202) and the protein *Connexin 30*, which might function as plasma membrane ATP channel (412). Both might play a role in the purinergic autocrine and/or paracrine regulation of salt and water reabsorption (353, 413, 634). The integral membrane proteins *syntaxin-3* (395) and *synaptotagmin-VIII*, demonstrated in the basolateral membrane of IC cells

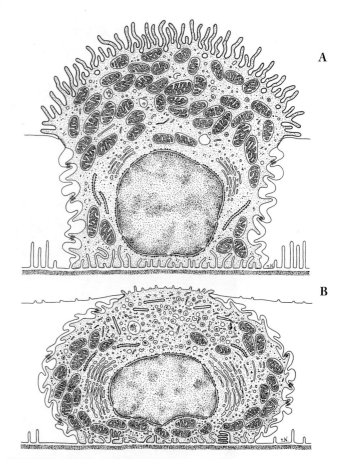

FIGURE 62 Survey of ultrastructure of intercalated cells. **A:** A-type intercalated (IC) cell; **(B)** B-type IC cell. (From Kaissling B, Kriz W. Morphology of the loop of Henle, distal tubule and collecting duct. In: Windhager EE (ed.). *Handbook of Physiology: Section on Renal Physiology.* New York: Oxford University Press, 1992:109–167, with permission.)

(297), are possibly involved in the targeting of acid-base transporters and may participate in the basolateral membrane remodeling of IC cells in response to systemic acid-base perturbations.

To date, two well-defined forms, type A IC cells and type B IC cells, with opposite structural and functional features, are distinguished among the IC cell population. IC cells that do not fit in either group are classified as "non A–non B" cells.

TYPE A IC CELLS

Type A IC cells are considered the *proton-secreting cells.* They are found in the late DCT, the CNT, and they represent a small minority among the IC cell population in the CCD and constitute the entire IC cell population in the medullary CD portions.

Morphologically, the type A IC cell has a broad *apical cell pole*, which is covered with elaborate *microfolds* (Figs. 62A and 63A) (392, 638) and contains numerous characteristic *tubulo-vesicular profiles* (diameter 80–200 nm) (160). The cytoplasmic faces of the apical plasma membrane and tubulovesicular profiles carry an IC-cell–specific

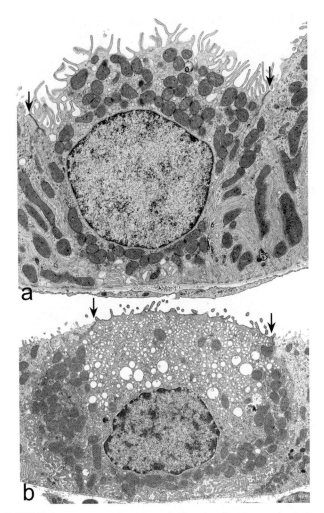

FIGURE 63 Intercalated cells; rat. **A:** Type A cell with many luminal microfolds and abundant mitochondria in the apical cell pole. **B:** Type B cell with a rather narrow apical cell pole, a narrow rim of dense cytoplasm exempt of vesicles under the apical plasma membrane, abundant smooth-surfaced vesicles in the apical cytoplasm, a huge Golgi complex (G), and abundant mitochondria along the basolateral plasma membrane (*arrows*, tight junction). Transmission electron microscopy (TEM) × ~7000.

coat of electron-dense "*studs*" (Figs. 64A) 10 nm in diameter, arranged in paracrystalline hexagonal arrays (86, 87). These studs represent one subunit of the *electrogenic V-type proton pump*, detectable by immunostainings (for review see [54, 87, 650]). To mediate net H$^+$ secretion the proton ATPase functions in series with a *bicarbonate/Cl* (HCO$_3^-$/ Cl$^-$) *exchanger* located in the *basolateral membrane* domain (for review see [650]). In type A-IC cells the HCO$_3^-$/Cl$^-$ exchanger is the anion exchanger *AE1* (6) (encodrd by Slc4a1), a splice variant product of the erythrocyte band 3 gene (166). The presence of AE1 in the basolateral membrane is decisive for diagnosis of type A-IC cells.

The membrane surface areas of the microfolds and tubular–vesicular profiles seem to be inversely related and vary with the functional conditions. For instance, under acute metabolic and respiratory acidosis and/or potassium

depletion H$^+$-ATPase subunits are translocated from the vesicular pool into the apical membrane, thereby the proton extrusion increases. *Mitochondria* with rather short profiles and narrowly arranged cristae are amassed in the apical cell pole. Under acidotic conditions the mitochondria lie in particularly close vicinity to the apical cell membrane. Many *microtubules* and *clathrin-coated vesicles* are apparent between the tubulovesicular profiles and the mitochondria. The *nucleus* is shifted to the basal cell portion (Figs. 62A and 63A).

In addition to the V-type proton ATPase type A IC cells—at least in the outer stripe—display a *P-type (gastric-type) K, H-ATPase*, shown in rats and rabbits (188, 579, 587, 672, 673). This K-reabsorbing ATPase seems to be associated with clusters of *rod-shaped particles*, revealed by freeze fracture studies on the P-face of cell membranes (Fig. 64B) in rabbit IC cells (593). Thus, the type A IC cells could be involved in recovering potassium, secreted via ROMK, in association with ENaC-mediated Na-reabsorption by the segment-specific cells.

Type A cells express also the chloride channel *ClC 5* (463). The secretory isoform of the Na, K-Cl-cotransporter, *NKCC-1*, has been detected in the basolateral membrane of type A cells in the outer stripe (210).

The type A IC cells express the nonerythroid Rh-associated glycoproteins *RhBG* in the basolateral membrane and *RhCG* in the apical plasma membrane (109, 498, 639, 650, 657), which mediate transport of ammonia/ammonium (*NH4$^+$/NH3*) (183, 498), when expressed in *Xenopus laevis* oocytes (394).

In chronic metabolic acidosis and prolonged high-proton secretion the type A IC cells hypertrophy (for review see [650]) and IC cells in the OMCD and IMCD show increased RhCG expression (576). However, genetic ablation of the *RhBG* gene is not a critical determinant of NH4$^+$ excretion by the kidney under acidic or control conditions (109). Furthermore, under chronic acidosis, the type A IC cells proliferate, evident by upregulation of cell cycle proteins, by incorporation of the thymidine analogue bromodeoxyuridine (BrdU) and mitotic ures (D. Bacic and C. Wagner, personal communication; November 2005).

TYPE B IC CELLS

Type B IC cells are considered as the bicarbonate-secreting cells. They occur exclusively in the renal cortex. In the CNT they constitute the minority, whereas in the CCD they are the large majority of the IC cell population.

The type B-IC cells (Figs. 61B, 62B, and 63B) seem to be in many respects a "mirror" image of type A. The *apical cell pole* is narrow, and is covered with rather few and short *microvilli*. Below the luminal membrane, at the level of the tight junctional belt, the cells reveal a type B–characteristic *band of dense cytoplasm*, consistently devoid of any vesicles, and containing filamentous material (160, 270, 272, 602). The profiles of type B cells are typically

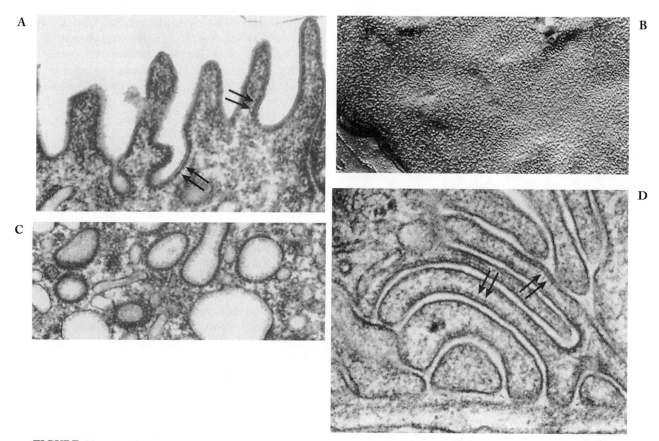

FIGURE 64   Intercalated cells in rat. **A:** Luminal membrane; its cytoplasmic face is coated with studs (*arrows*). Transmission electron microscopy (TEM) × ~61,000. **B:** Freeze-fracture electron micrograph showing the rod-shaped intramembrane particles (*stars*) of a luminal membrane. TEM × ~32,000. **C:** Apical cytoplasm of a type A cell. The specific vesicles are coated with studs. TEM × ~64,000. **D:** Membrane of basal in-foldings of type B cell; its cytoplasmic face is covered with studs (*arrows*). TEM × ~61,000.

oval (Figs. 62B and 63B), the lateral faces bulging into the adjacent cells, and have often a large *basal cell pole*. The latter usually reveals abundant, narrowly arranged plasma membrane in-foldings, which frequently display the *proton pump*, apparent in the cytoplasmic coat of densely arranged studs (Fig. 64D). The *mitochondria* are preferentially aligned along the basolateral plasma membranes (Figs. 62B and 63B). Polyribosomes and microtubules are apparent. The *nucleus* has an exocentric position, leaving place for a huge *Golgi complex*, with the *trans* side pointing toward the base of the cell (160). Small vesicles of *smooth endoplasmic reticulum*, often with *clathrin-coated heads*, are abundant. Type B cells reveal less carbonic anhydric activity than type A cells (292), and they express the chloride channel ClC 3 (463) in the apical cell pole.

Type B IC cells mediate secretion of HCO_3^- through *apical Cl^-/HCO_3^- exchange*, which functions in series with H^+-ATPase-mediated H^+ *efflux* across the *basolateral plasma membrane* (421). In distinction to type A IC cells the *HCO_3^-/Cl^- exchange* in type B IC cells is mediated by *pendrin*, encoded by the PDS/pds gene (*Slc26a4*) (523). Detection of pendrin in the apical plasma membrane of IC cells allows the unequivocal diagnosis of type B IC cells (294, 497).

Metabolic alkalosis is compensated by the kidney by reducing bicarbonate reabsorption and increased bicarbonate secretion by type B IC cells. Type B IC cells adapt under chronic metabolic alcalosis with cellular hypertrophy (486). DNA synthesis and mitoses of type B cells have been recorded under this condition (660a). Adaptive downregulation of pendrin in metabolic acidosis indicates the important role of this exchanger in acid-base regulation in the CCD (486).

NON A–NON B CELLS

A third type of IC cells without evident polarity with respect to proton APTase and so far undefined function are called "non A–non B" cells (294). In mice this latter population of intercalated cells is more frequent than in rats (602). It decreases in pronounced chronic metabolic acidosis or pronounced chronic metabolic alkalosis.

The observations on non A–non B cells, the striking structural diversity (54, 55), and the apparent plasticity of IC cells raised the question whether one, two, or more distinct cell types are subsumed in the IC cell population.

Based on studies in adult rabbit collecting ducts in vitro and IC cells cultured in vitro (404, 405, 565, 567), where IC cells with the morphology of type B were identified by apical binding to peanut lectin (349), it was speculated that the

IC cells might reverse their polarity in response to the specific functional environmental conditions. The type A would present the terminal differentiation of IC cells. This hypothesis received support from studies in vitro showing that the *matrix protein hensin* could reverse the functional phenotype of cultured intercalated cells (for review see [650]) and induce the A type of IC cells. The non A–non B cells might represent intermediate stages. The diminution of this latter population under chronic acidotic or alkalotic conditions would support with this hypothesis.

Another view was that the non A–non B cells could be precursors for either A or B cells, or only of B cells (for review see [650]). Also this hypothesis would be supported by the finding of a diminution of non A–non B cells under chronic acidosis or alkalosis. However, in the studies on isolated rabbit collecting ducts the coexistence of the two different bicarbonate/chloride exchangers, AE1 and pendrin, in rabbit IC cells has not been investigated nor been observed in non A–non B IC cells of other species. This and the observations on mitosis in fully differentiated type A, as well as in type B IC cells (Wehrli et al. 2007) do not agree with hypothesis on reversal of polarity nor with the hypothesis, claiming a common precursor cell of type A and B.

Inheritable forms of distal renal tubular acidosis (dRTA) most often affect the physiology of type A IC cells (450). Disruption of one of the IC cell characteristic genes leads to profound structural alterations of IC cell types. In mice with functional deletion of carbonic anhydrase II the frequency of IC cells is drastically reduced (79). The genetic disruption of pendrin (Slc26a4) leads to marked reduction of type B cell size with reduced H^+/OH^- transporters expressions (294). In mice with disruption of the *Foxi1* gene, which is upstream of several anion transporters, proton pumps, and anion exchange proteins expressed by intercalated cells, the normal collecting duct epithelium with its two major cell populations—collecting ducts cells (principle) and intercalated cells—has been replaced by a single cell type positive for markers for both cell types (71).

ARCHITECTURAL–FUNCTIONAL RELATIONSHIPS

So far we have emphasized the relationships between structure and function. However, we have neglected the important relationships between architecture and function (i.e., arrangements through which the close relationships between certain nephron and vascular portions permit the carrying out and coordination of complex regulatory functions). The two most obvious examples in this respect are the juxtaglomerular apparatus (JGA) regulating glomerular perfusion and renin secretion, and the renal medulla permitting the production of urine, varying from dilution to concentration.

Juxtaglomerular Apparatus

The JGA is a composite assembly of specialized structures at the vascular pole of the glomerulus The thick ascending limb of Henle's loop (TAL) returns to its parent glomerulus and extends through the angle between afferent and efferent arterioles (Fig. 65A) where it is firmly attached to the extraglomerular mesangium. At the attachment point, the TAL changes its character: a plaque of specialized cells, known as the macula densa (MD), represents the contact site of the tubule. Around this attachment, other specialized structures are developed, which together with the MD, comprise the JGA. These are the terminal portion of the afferent arteriole housing the renin-producing granular cells, the initial portion of the efferent arteriole, and the extraglomerular mesangium (EGM). The latter is in continuity with the intraglomerular mesangium and has intimate relationships to the parietal epithelium of Bowman's capsule (185). The JGA, more precisely the granular cells and the smooth muscle cells of afferent and efferent arterioles, are richly innervated by sympathetic nerves.

The MD comprises some 20 to 30 specialized epithelial cells within the end portion of the cortical thick ascending limb. Shortly after the macula densa the TAL transforms into the distal convoluted tubule (271, 276). The basal surface of the MD attaches to the extraglomerular mesangium, which fills the angle between the two glomerular arterioles. In addition, the MD contacts variable portions of the afferent and/or efferent arterioles (46). However, the only consistent histotopographical relationships of the MD are those established with the extraglomerular mesangium (115). Discrepancies in the literature concerning the histotopographical relationships of the MD appear to be due to the fact that the MD frequently has not been clearly distinguished from adjacent portions of the distal tubule. Considering the relationships of the outer surface of only the MD, the latter always covers the base of the extraglomerular mesangium; it appears, that for guaranteeing a total cover, it overlaps and contacts other neighboring structures (i.e., portions of the afferent and efferent arterioles).

The cells of the MD (Figs. 65 and 51C) are clearly different from the surrounding cells of the TAL (46, 271, 273). Although cell size is variable among species, MD cells are generally taller than the surrounding cells of the TAL so that the entire plaque of the MD protrudes into the tubule lumen. In contrast to the cells of the TAL, MD cells do not interdigitate with each other by large lateral processes; rather, the lateral cell membranes of MD cells run in a fairly straight fashion from the tight junction toward the base of the epithelium. They possess slender microplicae or microvilli that protrude into the lateral intercellular spaces, contacting (frequently by desmosomes) corresponding protrusions from opposite cells. At the very base, the cells ramify into slender processes. MD cells contain conspicuously large cell nuclei, accounting for the appearance of narrowly packed nuclei, the feature from which the entire cell plaque derives the name macula densa. Otherwise, the cells contain the usual cytoplasmic organelles: some small mitochondria, a Golgi apparatus, and smooth endoplasmic reticulum; free ribosomes are abundant, but rough endoplasmic reticulum is infrequent.

Functionally, the cells of the MD are similar to those of the TAL in many respects. Notably, they possess the same

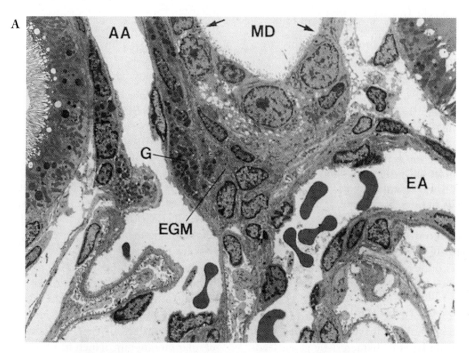

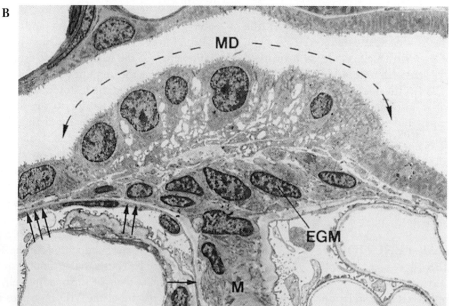

FIGURE 65   Juxtaglomerular apparatus. **A:** Meridional section through a glomerulus which runs through both glomerular arterioles; rat. The macula densa (MD) is attached to the extraglomerular mesangium (EGM), which fills the angle between the afferent (AA) and the efferent (EA) arteriole. Within the wall of the afferent arteriole granular cells (G) are seen. Note the intraglomerular segment of the efferent arteriole. Transmission electron microscopy (TEM) × ~1850. **B:** Meridional section through a glomerulus running in between both arterioles; rabbit. The macula densa (MD) is a prominent cell plaque within the thick ascending limb. It covers the extraglomerular mesangium (EGM). Within the glomerular stalk the EGM continues into the mesangium (M). The EGM interconnects opposing parts of the GBM (*one arrow*), of the reflection of the GBM to the basement membrane of Bowman's capsule (BCBM) (*two arrows*) as well as the beginning parts of the BCBM (*three arrows*). Note the dilated intercellular spaces between macula densa cells.

salt reabsorption machinery (i.e., the bumetanide-sensitive $Na^+,K^+, -2Cl^-$ cotransporter NKCC2 in the apical membrane). In contrast to the TAL, MD cells lack the Tamm-Horsfall protein (21), quite specifically they express nitric oxide synthase I (435, 667) and cyclooxygenase-2 (224).

The lateral intercellular spaces are a prominent feature of the MD (Fig. 65B). Electron microscopic studies (273) and studies on isolated MD segments in vitro (296) have shown that the width of the lateral interspaces varies under different functional conditions. In agreement with the suggestion that water flow through the MD epithelium is secondary to active sodium reabsorption, compounds such as furosemide that block sodium transport by MD cells as well as high osmolalities of impermeable solutes in the tubular fluid, such as Mannitol, are associated with narrow intercellular spaces (4, 273). The spaces are apparently dilated under most physiological conditions, usual regarded as normal conditions. Previously it had been suggested that the MD epithelium is water permeable (273), but so far no aquaporins have been found at this site.

The *granular cells* (often termed "juxtaglomerular cells") (Fig. 66) (45) are assembled in clusters (up to 15 cells, but generally not more than four or five) within the wall of the terminal portion of the afferent arteriole replacing ordinary smooth muscle cells. Occasionally, they are also found within the wall of the efferent arteriole, again occupying the space where one would otherwise expect to find an ordinary smooth muscle cell. In rare cases, extraglomerular mesangial cells may be replaced by granular cells. The name "granular" cell points to the specific cytoplasmic granules that may densely fill the cell body cytoplasm. They are electron-dense, membrane-bound, and irregular in size and shape. Small granules with crystalline substructure represent protogranules, which are developed within the prominent Golgi apparatus and are then transformed into the major amorphous granules. Immunocytochemical studies with two antibodies against the renin prosegment and against mature renin have shown that only protogranules are prosegment positive whereas a signal of mature renin was found in mature as well as protogranules. These findings show that the cleavage of the prosegment (i.e., the maturation of renin) takes place in the juvenile granules. Details of this process together with the molecular biology of renin synthesis are found in former reviews (220, 601).

Renin release occurs by exocytosis into the surrounding interstitium (601) and may then be taken up by peritubular capillaries or be distributed within the periarterial connective tissue sheaths, in a retrograde manner along the outside of intrarenal arterioles and arteries (316). From a structural point of view, renin release directly into the arterial lumen would appear improbable.

Granular cells are modified smooth muscle cells. Within the peripheral parts of the cytoplasm, especially within the many cell processes, granular cells contain myofibrils. In situations that require enhanced renin synthesis

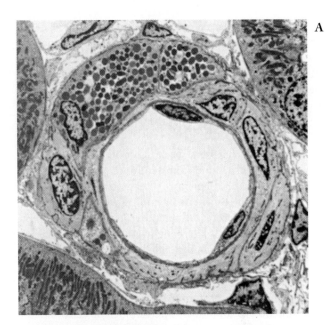

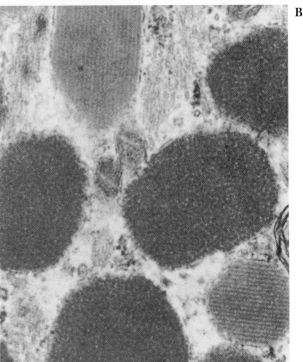

FIGURE 66   **A:** Juxtaglomerular portion of an afferent arteriole in rabbit. Smooth muscle cells are replaced by two granular cells. Transmission electron microscopy (TEM) × ~2700. **B:** Granular cell in rat. Renin granules are membrane-bound. Granules with a crystalline substructure are considered as "protogranule," which will develop into mature amorphous granules. TEM ×~48,000.

(e.g., volume depletion or stenosis of the renal artery) additional smooth muscle cells located upstream in the wall of the afferent arteriole transform into granular cells (601).

Granular cells have processes of manifold shape (214). Because of them, granular cells have extensive membrane contacts to all surrounding cells (e.g., other granular cells, smooth muscle cells, and extraglomerular mesangial cells). At these contacts, gap junctions are frequently encountered (601). Like ordinary smooth muscle cells, granular cells have membrane contacts also to endothelial cells, in the manner that footlike processes of endothelial cells penetrate the basement membrane and come into contact with granular cells; gap junctions are found at these contact sites (214).

Peripolar cells have first been described in sheep where they are routinely found (526); in most other species, including man, they are rare (200). Peripolar cells are parietal cells of Bowman's capsule, which are located around the glomerular hilum (i.e., at the vascular pole, therefore "peripolar") and contain numerous cytoplasmic membrane–bound granules filled homogeneously with electron-dense fibrillogranular material (526). Subsequent studies have shown that these granules contain a neuron-specific enolaselike protein (615) and transthyretin (237); their function is unknown. The number of cells and the number of granules per cell vary greatly among species and, furthermore, are dependent on age (200). In the rat kidney, granulated peripolar cells have only been found very rarely (200).

Extraglomerular mesangial cells (EGM cells, Goormaghtigh cells, lacis cells) together with the surrounding matrix establish the extraglomerular mesangium (polar cushion). The EGM represents a solid cell complex that is not penetrated by blood vessels or lymphatic capillaries. Nerves pass on both sides of it from the afferent to the efferent arteriole but do not enter the cell complex (214).

The EGM is located within the triangular space bordered by the two glomerular arterioles and the macula densa (45) (Figs. 65, 67). Reconstruction studies have shown that EGM cells are flat and elongated, separating into two bunches of long cell processes at their poles (584). They are arranged in several layers parallel to the base of the macula densa. The cells nearest to the glomerular stalk, thus filling the deepest portion of the triangle, loose this parallel grouping, but extend into the stalk of the glomerular tuft mixing with mesangial cells proper. The cells are separated by a conspicuous matrix that appears to be different from the intraglomerular mesangial matrix by the fact that microfibrils are rarely found in the EGM (185); details are largely unknown.

EGM cells are characterized by the scantiness of their cytoplasm and their extensive ramifications (Fig. 68) (45, 538). A Golgi apparatus and some profiles of granulated endoplasmic reticulum are regularly encountered. Although direct evidence is lacking, EGM cells can be expected to be contractile for several reasons. First, they contain a good amount of microfilaments, mainly in their processes and peripherally within cell bodies. Second, intimate structural similarities are found among arteriolar smooth muscle cells, granular cells, and intra- and EGM cells suggesting that they have the same origin. Third, they are extensively coupled by gap junctions). Gap junc-

tions not only bridge different cells, but also regularly bridge individual processes of the same cell (583). Moreover, gap junction contacts consistently occur to all other cells of the JGA (except the macula densa!), i.e., to granular cells, to ordinary smooth muscle cells of both arterioles, and to the mesangial cells proper (601).

From a biomechanical point of view the contractile apparatus of EGM cells is conspicuous. Microfilament bundles are contained within the periphery of cell bodies and within the cell processes which are connected to the walls of both glomerular arterioles and to the basement membrane of the parietal layer of Bowman's capsule (PBM) surrounding the glomerular hilum (Figs. 67 and 68). As a

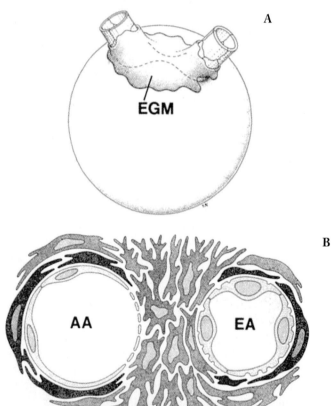

FIGURE 67   A: Schematic of the extraglomerular mesangium (EGM). The glomerulus is shown as a globe. Its outer aspect is represented by the parietal basement membrane of Bowman's capsule (PBM). The EGM lies between the two arterioles above the opening of Bowman's capsule (*broken line*). It is attached to the PBM and has extensive contacts with the two arterioles. The macula densa and the smooth muscle layers of the arterioles are not shown. **B:** Schematic cross-section through the vascular pole just above Bowman's capsule. Afferent (AA) and efferent arterioles (EA) are cut traversely. EGM cells are shown in moderate gray, smooth muscle cells in dark gray, and endothelial cells in light gray. Note differences in the wall of AA and EA: The AA already displays endothelial fenestration on the side facing the EGM. Conversely, the EA has a continuous endothelium with many cell bodies. In both AA and EA the smooth muscle layer (SM) is not complete: toward the center of the EGM the SM cells are replaced by EGM cells (From Elger M, Sakai T, et al. The vascular pole of the renal glomerulus of rat. *Adv Anat Embryol Cell Biol* 1998;139:1–98, with permission.)

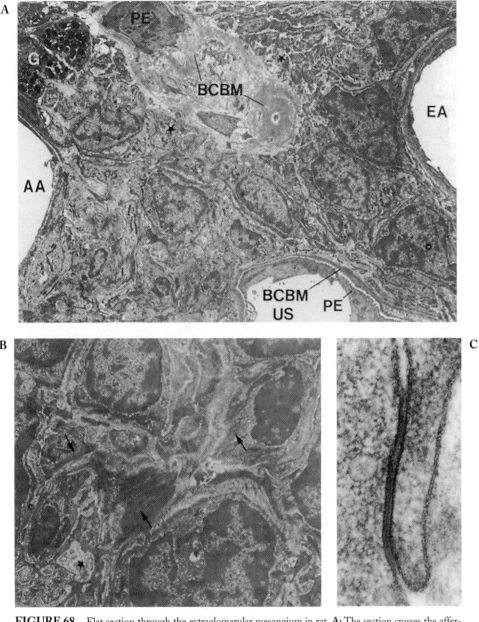

FIGURE 68 Flat section through the extraglomerular mesangium in rat. **A:** The section crosses the afferent (AA) and efferent (EA) arterioles; it grazes through the top of Bowman's capsule, showing the basement membrane of Bowman's capsule (BCBM), the parietal epithelium (PE), and the urinary space (US). The extraglomerular mesangium forms a complicated texture by which the structures of the vascular pole are interconnected. Note that toward their insertion in the BCBM the extraglomerular mesangial cells fall apart into many processes (*stars*). G, granular cells. Transmission electron microscopy (TEM) × ~2650. **B:** Higher magnification of extraglomerular mesangial cells. Note the microfilament bundles within the periphery of cell bodies as well as within cell processes (*arrows*). Note the irregular extracellular spaces filled with a matrix of varying appearance (*star*). TEM × ~6000. **C:** Gap junction between two mesangial cells. TEM ×~147,000.

whole, the EGM can be considered as a spider-like contractile clamp sitting above the glomerular entrance interconnecting all structures at this site (185). The EGM probably represents some sort of a closure device of the glomerular entrance, maintaining the structural integrity of the entrance against the distending forces exerted to it by the high intraglomerular pressure. Moreover, from the view point that the glomerular mesangium represents a high pressure compartment (mesangial interstitial pressures are expected to range in the same magnitude as glomerular capillary pressures; [323]), the EGM would seem to be the structure which mediates a gradual pressure drop toward the cortical interstitium and toward the base of the macula densa (185).

The function of the EGM cells is obscure. Because of their central position within the JGA, their constant relationships to the macula densa and their gap junction coupling to all smooth muscle–derived cells of the JGA, the EGM cells have repeatedly been considered as the necessary functional link between the macula densa and any possible effector cell within the regulatory mechanisms of the JGA (185, 214). Thus, they are widely considered as an integrating system of signals derived from the reabsorptive function of the MD and the function of the EGM as a pressure sentinel mirroring the blood pressure in the afferent–efferent arteriolar system, but details are unknown.

The intimate and systematic juxtaposition of tubular and vascular cells within the JGA has given rise to early speculations about a feed back system between tubular and glomerular function (213). It has now become clear that the JGA serves two different functions: It regulates the flow resistance of afferent arterioles in the so-called tubuloglomerular feedback mechanism, and it participates in the control of renin synthesis and release from granular cells in the afferent arteriole (561). Researchers originally assumed that the two responses might be related to each other in that renin released from the granular cells not only has systematic relevance, but locally triggers the formation of angiotensin II and thus is responsible for the afferent vasoconstriction as well; however, it now appears that the final activation of smooth muscle and granular effector cells occurs through largely independent pathways. Renin release from granular cells is the major source of systemic angiotensin II and thus plays an essential role in controlling extracellular volume and blood pressure, whereas the vasoconstriction of the afferent arteriole locally serves to modulate the filtration of this nephron.

For both mechanisms it is well established that a change in NaCl concentration in the tubular fluid at the MD initiate the appropriate signal. Thus the MD, situated at the very end of the TAL, controls the work of the TAL; the short postmacular segment of the TAL may be interpreted as to guarantee that the composition of the tubular fluid at the MD might not be influenced by the function of the subsequent DCT. Expressed in general terms, the MD translates changes in the tubular fluid NaCl concentration into a graded release of mediators that reach their target by diffusion, thus acting in a paracrine fashion. Note that the extraglomerular mesangium that mediates the contact between the MD and the effector cells is not vascularized, so that the build up of any paracrine agent would not be perturbed by blood flow.

With respect to renin release, the most likely paracrine mediators of this process are prostaglandin E_2 and nitric oxide (485, 572, 668). With respect to the vasoconstrictor response purinergic mediators, ATP or adenosine, as first suggested by Oswald and colleagues (472), appear to play the major role (106, 561, 606). For an up-to-date discussion of the function of the JGA see the reviews by Schnermann und Levine (561), Persson and colleagues (481), and Komlosi and colleagues (308).

The Renal Medulla

During phylogeny the renal medulla (Fig. 69) has developed in response to the necessity to conserve water by excreting a concentrated urine (582). Loops of Henle, collecting ducts, and a specific blood supply through vascular bundles have developed into a complex structural system that accounts for this function. However, the details are insufficiently understood.

The overall mechanism (Fig. 69) is clear: Reabsorption of NaCl from the MTALs in the outer medulla represents the driving force to produce an interstitial corticomedullary osmotic gradient that provokes the osmotic water withdrawal from the collecting duct when the latter descend toward the papillary tip. The reabsorbed water is brought back into the systemic circulation by venous vasa recta (256, 474).

The unresolved problem is the generation of a cortico-papillary solute gradient, notably in the inner medulla. In the discussions concerning the formation of a medullary solute gradient "countercurrent multiplication" has occupied a center stage as the decisive mechanism. This mechanism has been experimentally established in artificial tubes (675) and has been imposed on the renal medulla, conceding immense deviations from the original conditions. From a structural point of view, the preconditions for countercurrent multiplication in the renal medulla would appear to be quite incompletely developed: The limbs of Henle's loop are not juxtaposed to each other at any site. Even when allowing a mediating interstitial space between both loop limbs, the DTLs in no case behave homogenously in an adequate way but change their function gradually on their descent, they even change their transport characteristics to the ascending limb type a considerable distance before the bend; most relevant in the present context: The terminal third of the SDTLs in the mouse kidney are equipped with the TAL epithelium (327, 699). Without going in more details, everyone who has been engaged in this problem knows that the principle of countercurrent multiplication has been extensively bent to make it fitting with the structural organization of the renal medulla, in our view, with little benefit in facilitating the understanding of the function of the renal medulla. If at all, this principle can only be applied to describe the mechanism in the outer medulla. In the inner medulla, a process that could be regarded as a "single concentrating effect" is not apparent. Several "passive models" (307, 341, 591, 604, 666) attempting to explain the concentrating mechanism in the inner medulla have greatly refined our understanding of the problem but have not reached the level of general acceptance.

In this situation, it might be worth an attempt to start with the available functional data—including the recent data on the distribution of transporters—confronting them with the structure (i.e., the architecture of the renal medulla as well as the cellular organization of the individual compo-

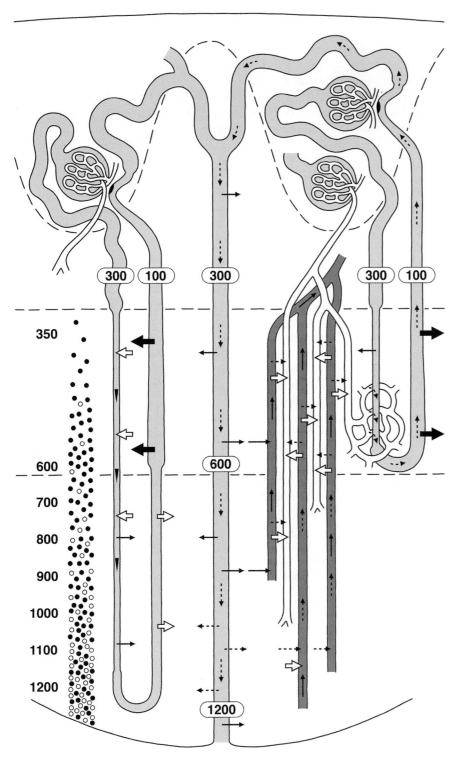

FIGURE 69 Schematic to show the functional interactions in the medulla as they are derived from the histotopography of the structures, the distribution of channels and transporters and direct measurements of transport characteristics in the various tubular and vessel segments. A long looped nephron, a short looped nephrons and a collecting duct are shown in light gray. Descending vasa rectas (DVRs) derived from the efferent arteriole of a juxtamedullary glomerulus are shown in white (including the capillaries), ascending vasa rectas (AVRs) in dark gray: both together establish a vascular bundle. The osmolar concentration in the medulla rises from the corticomedullary border to the papillary tip from 300 to 1200 mOsm/L, mainly established by the increase in the concentration of salt (*dark dots*) and urea (*open circles*). The driving force of the concentrating mechanism is the dumping of salt into the medullary interstitium from thick ascending limbs (TALs; *thick black arrows*), leaving behind a diluted fluid (indicated by an osmolar concentration of 100 mOsm/L at the re-entry into the cortex). Osmotic water withdrawal from CCDs (*thin arrows*) into the cortical circulation again elevates the tubular urine to 300 mOsm/L when re-entering into the medulla. Continuous water reabsorption along the MCDs (*thin arrows*) will produce a final urine concentration of about 1200 mOsm/L (in humans). The source for the inner medullary solute gradient is shown to consist of (*i*) dragging of salt from the IS into the IM by LDTLs (*arrowheads*) and (*ii*) re-entry of urea from the IMCDs into the terminal portion of the IM (*hatched arrows*). The gain in osmotic energy by urea re-entry originates from urea recycling, which starts with a shift of urea from the AVRs into the SDTLs in the IS (follow the *hatched arrows*) and concentration of this urea by water reabsorption in the CCDs, OMCDs and beginning portions of IMCDs (see text for further explanation). The removal of the water from the medulla regained from the CDs (thus the final step in urine concentration) is effected by AVRs (follow the *thin arrows*). These vessels are the core structures in the complex countercurrent exchange system of the medulla equilibrating at any level with the local concentrations of salt and urea. Open thick arrows show passive movements of salt. See text for further explanation.

nents) to arrive at a novel view of "function–structure correlation."

Let us first regard the three regions of the medulla with such an approach. The most constant region is the IS; there is no renal medulla known without an IS. In contrast, an OS is frequently quite incompletely developed and an IM may be fully absent.

THE INNER STRIPE OF THE OUTER MEDULLA

The IS (Figs. 19 and 23) is made up of two portions: the vascular bundles (VBs) and the interbundle region (IBR). The IBR contains the tubules (DTLs, TALs, CDs) supplied by a dense capillary plexus that is drained upward by the gradual transition of capillaries into AVRs that directly ascend into the OS. Since all the salt reabsorbed by MTALs accumulates in this area, the interstitium of the IBR is rich in salt (355).

The VBs, structurally, are part of the IS but, functionally, they belong to the IM. They represent a perfectly developed countercurrent exchange system primarily handling the blood descending to and ascending from the IM by respective DVRs and AVRs. However, since the DVRs supplying the capillary plexus of the IBR of the IS are contained within the VBs (not the respective AVRs), the VBs provide the possibility to shift solutes coming up from the IM into the IBR of the IS. Since the dominating solute of the IM is urea (355), the VBs are rich in urea. The handling of urea as a main function of the VBs becomes most obvious in the complex bundles (see following sections).

THE INNER MEDULLA

The IM (Figs. 19 and 26) including the papilla, at the transverse level, is homogenously organized; a separation into VBs and an IBR is no longer possible. Even if there may be a prevalence that the ATLs are more frequently gathered around CDs than DTLs (306, 699), it appears doubtful that this is of any functional relevance. The AVRs (including the capillaries) are homogenously distributed among all other components and, most important, a wide homogenous interstitial space permits the interaction of every descending tube with every ascending tube. The IM provides strict countercurrent arrangements of all involved structures but without giving prevalence to any specific lateral interaction. Thus, the IM may be considered as a countercurrent system that allows countercurrent exchange—mediated by the interstitium—between all descending (DVRs, DTLs, CDs) and all ascending tubes (AVRs, ATLs) according to the transport characteristics of the individual tubes.

A most important feature of the IM is its particular shape reflecting its longitudinal organization. The inner medulla tapers from a broad basis to a tiny papilla ([256]; see also preceding section). This shape perfectly reflects what happens with the structures within the inner medulla: loops of Henle, vasa recta, and collecting ducts (by fusing together) all decrease rapidly in number from the base to the tip of the papilla (57, 222). It has been calculated that of an estimated 10,000 long loops entering the inner medulla at its base, only about 1500 reach the papillary half of the inner medulla and only a few of them the papillary tip (256). Most long loops, the "short" long loops, turn back shortly after entering the inner medulla, a smaller but still substantial number of long loops reach the middle part of the inner medulla and only a small population of "long" long loops really reach the papilla.

THE OUTER STRIPE OF THE OUTER MEDULLA

The OS (Figs. 19 and 22) is a transitional region that separates the medulla from the cortex mediating the transition between an hyperosmotic and an iso-osmotic environment. The OS does not seem to make any particular contribution to the creation of the corticomedullary solute gradient but it greatly helps to maintain it. The OS contains the nascent (or dissolving) VBs (performing the same function as in the IS but quantitatively of minor importance) and the AVRs, which are directly coming up form the IBR of the IS (Fig. 70). Together with the AVRs spreading out from the dissolving VBs, the AVRs transverse the OS as individual vessels intimately associated with the tubules of this region; they represent the major "capillary" supply of the OS (see preceding section). In addition, among all regions of the kidney, the OS exhibits the smallest fraction of interstitial space, thus the vessels are most closely juxtaposed to the tubules (lymphatics are absent [320]). Since the PSTs of juxtamedullary nephrons, in contrast to their name, take a tortuous course when descending through the OS, most tubular profiles in the OS consists of PSTs (S3 segments). This arrangement—AVRs closely associated with descending PTs (and, to some extent, CDs)—represent an ultimate countercurrent trap to prevent the loss of osmotic energy into the systemic circulation (Fig. 70C). Since reabsorption from PTs is iso-osmotic, the hypertonic environment created by AVRs will allow water withdrawal not only from CDs (starting the concentrating process) but also from the PTs increasing their osmolality already at the level of the OS—with a clear prevalence of the PTs of juxtamedullary nephrons (tortuous course!) that give rise to the "long long loops." The TALs of the OS are already of the cortical type (equipped with a comparably flat epithelium; see preceding section) capable of maintaining and even increasing large salt gradient but incapable of transporting large quantities (36).

So far, a summary of the essential architectural features of the three medullary regions; let us now talk about the functional connections between them. This needs, first, to talk about the overall mechanism underlying urine concentration in some more detail, followed by discussion about the individual mechanisms.

THE BASIC MECHANISM

The renal medulla contains the phylogenetically ancient "diluting segments" of the nephrons (i.e., the TALs that separate salt from water; Fig. 69). The salt is dumped into the medullary interstitium, the water is carried up into the cortex, and—if ADH is available—recovered by the systemic circulation through osmotic withdrawal from the CCDs. Thus, the tubular urine that re-enters the renal medulla in the collecting duct is iso-osmotic with respect to plasma concentration and considerably reduced in quantity compared with the amount that originally entered the renal medulla in descending limbs after filtration. Thus, the salt that is available to drive the concentrating mechanism has emerged from a much larger quantity of iso-osmotic fluid than the quantity of iso-osmotic fluid that is subject to concentration. Moreover,

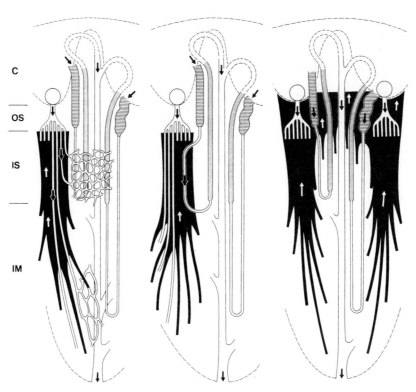

FIGURE 70 Schematics to demonstrate the possible recycling routes within the medulla. A short loop and a long loop of Henle and a collecting duct are shown. The straight proximal tubules are hatched; the thin limbs, collecting ducts, and capillaries are white; the thick ascending limbs are gray. Ascending vasa recta are drawn black en bloc. **A:** Simple type of medulla: recycling route from the ascending vasa recta in the inner stripe, via descending vasa recta, to inner stripe tubules. **B:** Complex type of medulla: recycling route from ascending vasa recta in the inner stripe to descending thin limbs of short loops. **C.** Recycling route from the ascending vasa recta in the outer stripe to descending tubules (proximal tubules and collecting ducts); valid for both the simple type and the complex type of medulla. C, cortex OS, outer stripe; IS, inner stripe; IM, inner medulla. (From Kaissling B, Kriz W. Morphology of the loop of Henle, distal tubule and collecting duct. In: Windhager EE (ed.). *Handbook of Physiology: Section on Renal Physiology.* New York: Oxford University Press, 1992:109–167, with permission.)

along with the progressing concentration of the CD urine, less water has to be reclaimed to achieve the same increment in concentration; the work that is necessary to account for a progressively increasing urine concentration decreases steeply toward the tip of the papilla.

In the IM, in addition to salt, urea is a major solute accounting for the solute gradient toward the tip of the papilla. Since in the IM no up hill transport of salt or of urea is known, the crucial problem consists of how explaining the increasing concentration of salt (flat increase) and of urea (steep increase) toward the papillary tip. If both depend on the work of the TALs in the OM, how can part of the osmotic energy be carried down from the OM into the IM and piled up there to a steep solute gradient toward the tip of the papilla?

In our view, it is apparent that three major mechanisms are responsible for the distribution of salt and urea into a corticopapillary gradient (Fig. 69). They all depend on salt reabsorption by TALs in the OM; they all fit with the morphology. Specific structural elaborations in highly concentrating species appear to lay stress on them. These

are (1) salt dragging by flow to deeper medullary levels, (2) countercurrent exchange of solutes and water to maintain the corticopapillary gradient, and (3) urea recycling by short loops of Henle as a major mechanism to create the inner medullary solute gradient toward the papilla.

Dragging of Solutes by Flow to Deeper Medullary Levels In all descending tubes of the renal medulla (DVRs, DTLs, CDs) solutes are dragged by flow to deeper medullary levels. This appears to be relevant for salt in the DTLs and for urea in the CDs (see urea recycling).

Continuous uptake and dragging of salt by SDTLs down to their bends at the end of the IS has been considered as an essential mechanism in the original countercurrent multiplication concept. Actually, compared to water withdrawal and addition of urea recycling (see following sections), such a mechanism does not seem to be of crucial importance. However, the salt that enters the SDTLs in the OS, left from filtration, will be dragged down by flow until the loop bends and will return in the TALs allowing for the active salt reabsorption to start at higher than systemic concentration levels (this is the only essential step that is left from the countercurrent multiplication principle). Part of the reabsorbed salt may—via the interstitium—re-enter the descending limb, thus being trapped within the SDTLs.

Continuous uptake of salt by LDTLs in the OM and dragging it by flow down into the IM appears to be the essential mechanism for salt accumulation in the IM; no other source of salt (apart from a small quantity reabsorbed by IMCDs) for the IM is obvious. Available models of the inner medullary concentrating process do not put so much emphasis on this mechanism but the structural data strongly do suggest it. Layton and colleagues (341) were the first to include this idea into a model. The structural arguments are the following:

1. The upper portions of the LDTLs, most obvious in the IS, have an epithelial organization that suggest ion transport through extensively developed tight junctions (Fig. 47A). Since the salt concentration is higher outside the LDTLs (see following sections), salt can readily be expected to diffuse into the lumen. This process may become reinforced by active salt-secretion into the lumen based on the abundant occurrence of Na^+, K^+-ATPase in the upper portions of LDTLs (191, 393). Water removal may occur in parallel through AQP1 channels (see following sections). Both processes will lead to high salt concentrations within LDTLs at the transition from the OM to the IM. Measured data are not available, but it seems reasonable to suggest considerably higher salt concentrations inside than outside.

2. The LDTLs on their descent through the inner stripe always pass through the sodium richest area (i.e., distant from the vascular bundles among the TALs of short loops) (355) (Fig. 21). In the mouse kidney, two modifications in this system appear to reinforce the ability of LDTLs to participate in salt uptake. First, the LDTLs take a tortuous course when descending through the IS (increasing their lengths by 27%) (699), and, second, at the end of the IS before entering the IM, they traverse the so-called innermost stripe, which has a thickness of about half of the IS proper and in which the SDTLs are already equipped with the TAL epithelium (327, 699). Thus, the density of TALs dumping salt into the interstitium is extremely high at this level (three times higher than any other lever of the OM). Consequently, the interstitial salt concentration (even after continuous dilution due to water withdrawal from the CDs) should be very high. The LDTLs transverses this region and may readily be expected to take up some of the accumulated salt.

3. After challenging urine concentration in rats by water deprivation (or treatment with ADH) the TALs hypertrophy with the most prominent increase in epithelial salt transport capacity of the initial portions in the deep IS (41, 618). Thus again, a prominent "surplus" in

salt accumulation occurs just at the border to the inner medulla.

4. As described previously, the LDTLs are heterogeneous with respect to their length and epithelial differentiation of their upper parts (318, 355). Most important, the actual length of a LDTL strictly correlates with the degree of epithelial elaboration of its upper part in the IS. The small fraction of longest long loops extending down into the papilla clearly have the most prominent upper parts in the IS: They are thicker with larger lumina and with more elaborate epithelia composed of heavily interdigitating cells; their abundance in Na,K-ATPase is spectacular (191). Comparing these longest long loops with those extending down into the IM for only short or intermediate distances, there is a continuous spectrum also with respect to the epithelial elaboration in the IS. Thus, the idea is plausible that salt is taken up by the upper portions of LDTLs and subsequently carried down through the salt impermeable lower portions to the bend region. Beginning abruptly with a prebend segment, the loop becomes ion permeable, allowing the salt to be dumped into the interstitium. In the mouse the prebend segments are quite prominent, with lengths up to 700 μm (699). Thus, the entire loop bend appears to represent a loop segment that delivers salt into the interstitium.

Since the lower portions of LDTLS are water permeable (the extent to which is the case is unclear [341, 459]), water withdrawal may further increase the salt concentration in these segments. The problem consists of the driving force for such a process. A possibility offered from a structural view is that the heterogeneous longitudinal distribution of loops within the inner medulla (as described previously) might account for a cascadelike transport of salt toward the papilla. The large fraction of "short" long loops carries salt into the first third of the IM. Together with some urea (emerging from recycling; see subsequent sections) the total interstitial osmolality will be elevated above DTL fluid osmolality at the respective level allowing them to reclaim water from DTLs, elevating the total osmolality and salt concentration in all the DTLs underway to deeper medullary levels. A major fraction of those will reach an intermediate level of the IM before bending, dumping some of the salt at this level into the interstitium. Again together with some urea a driving force will be established accounting for some water withdrawal from the small fraction of "long" long loops that will carry their salt into the papillary tip. No question, this is a hypothetical idea but from a structural point of view would be worth of modeling. Ideas in this direction have been published previously (318), and mathematical models for some features of such a mechanism have been presented (341, 342).

Countercurrent Exchange of Solutes and Water Countercurrent exchange in an U-type countercurrent exchanger may have two functions: (1) trapping of solutes within the system by transfer of solutes from the ascending to the descending limb and (2) preventing water from entering the system by short circuiting from the descending to the ascending limb. Both mechanisms per se do not build up any solute gradient, they are only capable of maintaining a gradient (with little loss). However, incorporated into the complex countercurrent arrangement of the renal medulla they decisively participate in the creation of the corticopapillary gradient. In agreement with others (474), in our view, the relevance of countercurrent exchange has always been underestimated compared with countercurrent multiplication in the urine concentrating mechanism. From a structural point of view, the renal medulla should be considered as an extremely complex countercurrent exchange system that is fuelled by two mechanisms at two sites: by salt reabsorption through TALs in the OS and by urea addition through terminal CDs in the IM. These solutes are distributed by countercurrent exchange into a corticomedullary gradient that—due to continuous fueling—allows water withdrawal from CDs and the transport of this water into the systemic circulation in the cortex.

As discussed previously, a direct countercurrent exchange between juxtaposed countercurrent tubes may only occur within the VBs of the IS. In contrast, in the IBR of the IS and within the entire IM the countercurrent tubes are consistently separated from each other by comparably wide interstitial spaces, thus any exchange at a traverse level is mediated by the interstitium. No doubt, this decreases the effectiveness of the exchanges but allows countercurrent exchanges between more than two structures Any solute dumped into the inner medullary interstitium (i.e., predominantly salt from LDTLs [at their bends] and urea from CDs [at their terminal portion]) or left in ATL and AVRs at their beginning in the IM, will be subject to countercurrent trapping (or used to drive countercurrent short circuiting of water; see following sections), between AVRs and ATLs on one site and DVRs and DTLs on the other.

In addition to solute trapping, countercurrent exchange of water preventing the flow of water to deeper levels by short circuiting seems of major relevance. The recent elucidation of the distribution of aquaporins in medullary structures has shed considerable light on the handling of water in the urine concentrating process. All descending structures (DTLs, DVRs, CDs) are equipped with aquaporins, thus they are water permeable (in the CDs the permeability is ADH dependent). The only ascending structures that are water permeable are the AVRs (based on the hydrophilic fenestrae providing a direct route of water flow than through the cells). Thus, any water withdrawn from any descending structure finally enters an AVR by which it is brought back to the cortex. This cardinal function of AVRs has been analyzed in detail by Pallone and colleagues (474).

The ability of AVRs to take up water appears to be based on an elevated oncotic pressure (resulting from short circuiting of water between DVRs and AVRs within the VBs) and on the reasonable assumption that the blood in capillaries at any level of the medulla is in osmotic equilibrium with the interstitial fluid (due to the hydrophilic fenestrae in capillary and AVR endothelia). Thus, when capillary blood at any level of the medulla starts to gather (to assemble) in AVRs and to ascend, it will—after any small ascent—become hyperosmotic compared with the surrounding interstitium. Due to the abundant hydrophilic fenestrae of the AVR endothelium osmotic equilibrium will most easily be achieved by water uptake.

The water to be taken up originates mainly from the CDs, but water may also originate from DTLs. In SDTLs only the upper portions are stuffed with aquaporins suggesting that in this subsegment osmotic equilibration is predominantly achieved by water removal leading to an increase in salt concentration. The lower portions of SDTLs are instead equipped with the urea transporter UTA1, favoring equilibration by urea entry (see subsequent sections).

In LTDLs, the upper parts have abundant aquaporins (type 1) in both membranes surprisingly contained in an epithelium that exhibits the features of an ion permeable epithelium (i.e., an extremely lengthened leaky tight junction due to extensive cellular interdigitation). Thus, this epithelium, in addition to being water permeable, allows the transport of large amounts of ions. From what we have reported previously, salt dragging by flow in LDTLs appears to be the only mechanism to bring down the salt into the IM; large volumes of a salt-enriched urine would be the best precondition for this goal. It appears that the transport capabilities of the upper portions of LDTLs have not been completely elucidated. Along the lower portions of LDTLs in the IM, the water permeability progressively decreases but appears to fully cease only at the transition to the prebend segment (475, 476). This offers the possibility (described previously) that water withdrawal from the LDTLs by an osmotic driving force established at each medullary level by salt and urea might lead to a cascadelike transport of salt toward the tip of the papilla.

Urea Recycling Solute recycling is a different mechanism compared with solute trapping by countercurrent exchange; this difference is rarely appreciated. Urea appears to be the only solute, recycling of which plays an essential role in the urine concentrating process. Recycling of urea defines a process that starts with a molecule of urea in the inner medullary interstitium and brings this molecule back into the IM via the normal tubular route, finally re-entering the inner medullary interstitium via exit from the terminal IMCD (Fig. 69). As described previously, the terminal portion of the IMCDs contains the urea transporters UTA1 and UTA3 that allow the facilitated diffusion of urea from the CD into the surrounding interstitium (43). A precondition for this reuptake of urea is that the concentration of urea in the tubular urine of IMCDs has reached a higher level than in the medullary interstitium at the same level. This is achieved by water removal through urea-impermeable tubular segments (i.e., CNTs and CCDs in the cortex, OMCDs and upper IMCDs in the medulla). The reabsorption of urea through IMCDs compromises the reclaiming of water through IMCDs, decreasing urine concentration instead of increasing. Thus, urea does both: Reabsorption of urea increases the inner medullary solute gradient thereby decreasing urine osmolality and the increased solute gradient increases the driving force for water reabsorption thereby increasing urine osmolality. This sounds like a story from Baron Münchhausen who was able to help himself getting out of a swamp by pulling on his own hairs. However, the two opposing functions of urea have a solid base: A given molecule of urea may become active a second (or a third) time. This is what urea recycling means. After entering the inner medullary interstitium from an IMCD, a given molecule of urea will travel toward the cortex within an AVR, thereby balancing (together with other molecules and other solutes) a certain amount of water that enters the AVR along its ascent and that finally has to be delivered into the systemic circulation at the corticomedullary border. However, this specific molecule of urea participates in water balancing on its way from a hyperosmotic to an iso-osmotic environment only up to an intermediate level (i.e., up to the IS). Here it re-enters the nephron; its relevance in balancing water that continuously enters the AVR and needs to be transported further up into the cortex is taken over by salt, which, due to the active Na^+ reabsorption by TALs, is available in abundance at this level. Thus, the urea molecule has spent only part of its osmotic energy for the transport of water before it re-enters the nephron, precisely the SDTL, and becomes again the subject of a concentrating process in subsequent urea-impermeable, but water–permeable, tubular segments. This urea molecule started the intratubular concentrating process at a higher energy level than a urea molecule that entered the tubule by filtration. In our view, this difference in osmotic energy between a recycling and a freshly filtered urea molecule, entering the nephron in the IS versus in the cortex and becoming subject to a concentrating process by water removal along the DCT, CNT, CCD, OMCD, and upper IMCD represents a gain in osmotic energy that is finally available for water reabsorption in the inner medulla. Entry of urea to the LTDLs somewhere in the IM (i.e., recycling of urea via long loops) would not have a similar effect, simply because at this site there is no surplus salt available to replace urea in its role of water balancing.

At the present stage of knowledge, urea recycling via short loops appears to be an essential process in urine concentration and represents the most obvious evidence for the numerical dominance of short loops of Henle in every highly concentrating species. Note, that also species that by definition are commonly reported to have 100% long loops (e.g., *P. obesus*) actually have a majority of short loops.

Moreover, as described previously, the SDTLs in such highly concentrating rodent species are directly incorporated into the vascular bundles and thus provide a more direct route for urea recycling than the simple bundles (Figs. 21, 24, 25, and 70) (268, 317, 318, 327). Within the VBs of such species, AVRs coming up from the IM are arranged in a countercurrent fashion not only with DVRs but also with the SDTLs. Thus urea, by countercurrent exchange, may directly enter the SDTLs through the urea transporter UT-A2 (42, 43) (the hydrophilic fenestrae of the endothelium of the AVRs may readily be expected to be highly permeable for urea). In a renal medulla with "simple" vascular bundles (as they are found in most species) countercurrent exchange of urea first occurs from AVRs to DVRs (which contain the urea transporter UT-B1) (37, 619), which later will deliver their blood to the capillary plexus of the IBR in the IS, which perfuses the SDTLs on their descending way. Thus, even if probably much less effective, urea from the inner medulla has access to the SDTLs (43, 318, 355) and may start its recycling route to the terminal CD in the papilla (43, 318, 619).

The locus of urea redelivery (i.e., in the papilla, thus at the "ultimate bend" of the complex) countercurrent exchange system in the papilla, is optimal, since by countercurrent exchange in vasa recta and thin limbs, urea is largely trapped and distributed in a longitudinal gradient within the inner medulla. The fraction of urea that escapes this process in the inner medulla is subject to recycling via short loops (starting in the IS) back into the inner medulla and is thus available another time within the papillary interstitium ready to withdraw and/or to balance water reabsorption from the collecting duct.

CONCLUSION

The urine-concentrating mechanism certainly does not belong to the most urgent problems in medicine but it represents a highly challenging biological enigma. We are aware that several aspects of our view are hypothetical but they are based on particular structural features (the ultrastructural organization and particular histotopographical relationships of LDTLs, the incorporation of SDTLs into the VBs in highly concentrating rodent species) for which no better functional relevance is available. Whether the proposed mechanisms are sufficient to build an effective solute gradient in the IM (in rodents up to several osmoles) or whether there are additional sources complementing the solute gradients (i.e., continuous production of osmotic active substances) is presently unknown.

References

1. Abrahamson D. Structure and development of the glomerular capillary wall and basement membrane. *Am J Physiol* 1987;253:F783–F794.
2. Abrahamson DR. Origin of the glomerular basement membrane visualized after in vivo labeling of laminin in newborn rat kidneys. *J Cell Biol* 1985;100:1988–2000.
3. Adler S. Integrin receptors in the glomerulus: potential role in glomerular injury. *Am J Physiol* 1992;262:F697–F704.
4. Alcorn D, Anderson W, Ryan G. Morphological changes in the renal macula densa during natriuresis and diuresis. *Renal Physiol* 1986; 9:335–347.
5. Allen F, Tisher CC. Morphology of the ascending thick limb of Henle. *Kidney Int* 1976;9:8–22.
6. Alper SL. The band 3-related anion exchanger (AE) gene family. *Annu Rev Physiol* 1991;53:549–564.
7. Alpers CE, Hudkins KL, Floege J, Johnson RJ. Human renal cortical interstitial cells with some features of smooth muscle cells participate in tubulointerstitial and crescentic glomerular injury. *J Am Soc Nephrol* 1994;5:201–209.
8. Amann K, Plank C, Dotsch J. Low nephron number—a new cardiovascular risk factor in children? *Pediatr Nephrol* 2004;19:1319–1323.
9. Ambühl P, Amemiya M, Danzkay M, Lötscher M, Kaissling B, Moe O, Preisig P, Alpern R. Chronic metabolic acidosis increases NHE-3 protein abundance in rat kidney. *Am J Physiol* 1996;271:F917–F925.
10. Amemiya M, Loffing J, Lötscher M, Kaissling B, Alpern R, Moe O. Expression of NHE-3 in the apical membrane of rat renal proximal tubule and thick ascending limb. *Kidney Int* 1995;48:1206–1215.
11. Deleted in proof.
12. Amemiya M, Loffing J, Lotscher M, Kaissling B, Alpern RJ, Moe OW. Expression of NHE-3 in the apical membrane of rat renal proximal tubule and thick ascending limb. *Kidney Int* 1995;48:1206–1215.
13. Anderson W, Alcorn D, Gilchrist A, Whiting J, Ryan G. Glomerular actions of ANG II during reduction of renal artery pressure: a morphometric analysis. *Am J Physiol* 1989;256: F1021–F1026.
14. Andrews PM. Morphological alterations of the glomerular (visceral)epithelium in response to pathological and experimental situations. *J Electron Microsc Tech* 1988;9:115–144.
15. Andrews PM. Scanning electron microscopy of the nephrotic kidney. *Virchows Arch B Cell Pathol* 1975;17:195–211.
16. Ardiles LG, Loyola F, Ehrenfeld P, Burgos ME, Flores CA, Valderrama G, Caorsi I, Egido J, Mezzano SA, Figueroa CD. Modulation of renal kallikrein by a high potassium diet in rats with intense proteinuria. *Kidney Int* 2006;69:53–59.
17. Aronson PS. Ion exchangers mediating NaCl transport in the renal proximal tubule. *Cell Biochem Biophys* 2002;36:147–153.
18. Arpin-Bott MP, Kaissling B, Waltisperger E, Rabhi M, Saussine P, Freund-Mercier MJ, Stoeckel ME. Historadioautographic localization of oxytocin and V1a vasopressin binding sites in the kidney of developing and adult rabbit, mouse and merione and of adult human. *Exp Nephrol* 2002;10:196–208.
19. Asanuma K, Kim K, Oh J, Giardino L, Chabanis S, Faul C, Reiser J, Mundel P. Synaptopodin regulates the actin-bundling activity of alpha-actinin in an isoform-specific manner. *J Clin Invest* 2005; 115:1188–1198.
20. Austyn JM, Hankins DF, Larsen CP, Morris PJ, Rao AS, Roake JA. Isolation and characterization of dendritic cells from mouse heart and kidney. *J Immunol* 1994;152:2401–2410.
21. Bachmann S, Koeppen-Hagemann I, Kriz W. Ultrastructural localization of Tamm-Horsfall glycoprotein (THP) in rat kidney as revealed by protein A-gold immunocytochemistry. *Hystochemistry* 1985; 83:531–538.
22. Bachmann S, Kriz W. Histotopography and ultrastructure of the thin limbs of the loop of Henle in the hamster. *Cell Tissue Res* 1982;225:111–127.
23. Bachmann S, Kriz W, Kuhn C, Franke WW. Differentiation of cell types in the mammalian kidney by immunofluorescence microscopy using antibodies to intermediate filament proteins and desmoplakins. *Histochemistry* 1983;77:365–394.
24. Bachmann S, Le Hir M, Eckardt KU. Co-localization of erythropoietin mRNA and ecto-5'-nucleotidase immunoreactivity in peritubular cells of rat renal cortex indicates that fibroblasts produce erythropoietin. *J Histochem Cytochem* 1993;41:335–341.
25. Bachmann S, Metzger R, Bunnemann B. Tamm-Horsfall protein-mRNA synthesis is localized to the thick ascending limb of Henle's loop in rat kidney. *Histochem Cell Biol* 1990;94:517–523.
26. Bachmann S, Schlichting U, Geist B, Mutig K, Petsch T, Bacic D, Wagner CA, Kaissling B, Biber J, Murer H, Willnow TE. Kidney-specific inactivation of the megalin gene impairs trafficking of renal inorganic sodium phosphate cotransporter (NaPi-IIa). *J Am Soc Nephrol* 2004;15:892–900.
27. Bacic D, Capuano P, Baum M, Zhang J, Stange G, Biber J, Kaissling B, Moe OW, Wagner CA, Murer H. Activation of dopamine D1-like receptors induces acute internalization of the renal Na+/phosphate cotransporter NaPi-IIa in mouse kidney and OK cells. *Am J Physiol Renal Physiol* 2005;288:F740–747.
28. Bacic D, Capuano P, Gisler SM, Pribanic S, Christensen EI, Biber J, Loffing J, Kaissling B, Wagner CA, Murer H. Impaired PTH-induced endocytotic down-regulation of the renal type IIa Na+/Pi-cotransporter in RAP-deficient mice with reduced megalin expression. *Pflugers Arch* 2003;446:475–484.
29. Bacic D, Lehir M, Biber J, Kaissling B, Murer H, Wagner CA. The renal Na(+)/phosphate cotransporter NaPi-IIa is internalized via the receptor-mediated endocytic route in response to parathyroid hormone. *Kidney Int* 2006;69:495–503.
30. Bacic D, M. Le Hir, J. Biber, B. Kaissling, CA. Wagner, H. Murer. The renal Na+/Phosphate cotransporter NaPI-IIa is internalized via receptor-mediated endocytotic route in response to parathyroid hormone. *Kidney Int* 2006. in press.
31. Bacic D, Wagner CA, Hernando N, Kaissling B, Biber J, Murer H. Novel aspects in regulated expression of the renal type IIa Na/Pi-cotransporter. *Kidney Int Suppl* 2004;S5–S12.
32. Baines AD, de Rouffignac C. Functional heterogeneity of nephrons. II. Filtration rates, intraluminal flow velocities and fractional water reabsorption. *Pflugers Arch* 1969;308: 260–276.
33. Balkovetz DF. Claudins at the gate: determinants of renal epithelial tight junction paracellular permeability. *Am J Physiol Renal Physiol* 2006;290:F572–579.
34. Ballermann BJ. Glomerular endothelial cell differentiation. *Kidney Int* 2005;67:1668–1671.
35. Bankir L, Bouby N, Trinh-Trang-Tan MM. Heterogeneity of nephron anatomy. *Kidney Int Suppl* 1987;20:S25–39.
36. Bankir L, Bouby N, Trinh-Trang-Tan MM, Kaissling B. Thick ascending limb—anatomy and function: role in urine concentrating mechanisms. Advances in Nephrology from the Necker Hospital 1987;16:69–102.
37. Bankir L, Chen K, Yang B. Lack of UT-B in vasa recta and red blood cells prevents urea-induced improvement of urinary concentrating ability. *Am J Physiol Renal Physiol* 1984;286: F144–F151.
38. Bankir L, Farman N. [Heterogeneity of the glomeruli in the rabbit]. *Arch Anat Microsc Morphol Exp* 1973;62:281–291.
39. Bankir L, Fischer C, Fischer S, Jukkala K, Specht HC, Kriz W. Adaptation of the rat kidney to altered water intake and urine concentration. *Pflugers Arch* 1988;412:42–53.
40. Bankir L, Kaissling B, de Rouffignac C, Kriz W. The vascular organization of the kidney of Psammomys obesus. *Anat Embryol (Berl)* 1979;155:149–160.
41. Bankir L, Kriz W. Adaptation of the kidney to protein intake and to urine concentrating activity: similar consequences in health and CRF. *Kidney Int* 1995;47:7–24.
42. Bankir L, Trinh-Trang-Tan MM. Urea and the kidney. In: Brenner B (ed.). *The Kidney*. Philadelphia: Saunders, 2000:637–679.
43. Bankir LT, Trinh-Trang-Tan MM. Renal urea transporters. Direct and indirect regulation by vasopressin. *Exp Physiol* 2000;85:243S–252S.
44. Barajas L. Innervation of the renal cortex. *Fed Proc* 1978;37:1192–1201.
45. Barajas L. The juxtaglomerular apparatus: anatomical considerations in feedback control of glomerular filtration rate. *Fed Proc* 1981;40:78–86.
46. Barajas L. The ultrastructure of the juxtaglomerular apparatus as disclosed by three-dimensional reconstructions from serial sections. The anatomical relationship between the tubular and vascular components. *J Ultrastruct Res* 1970;33:116–147.
47. Barajas L, Powers K. Innervation of the renal proximal convoluted tubule of the rat. *Am J Anat* 1989;186:378–388.
48. Barajas L, Wang P. Demonstration of acetylcholinesterase in the adrenergic nerves of the renal glomerular arterioles. *J Ultrastruct Res* 1975;53:244–253.
49. Barajas L, Wang P. Myelinated nerves of the rat kidney. A light and electron microscopic autoradiographic study. *J Ultrastruct Res* 1978; 65:148–162.
50. Barajas L, Wang P. Simultaneous ultrastructural visualization of acetylcholinesterase activity and tritiated norepinephrine uptake in renal nerves. *Anat Rec* 1983;205:185–195.
51. Barisoni L, Kriz W, Mundel P, D'Agati V. The dysregulated podocyte phenotype: a novel concept in the pathogenesis of collapsing idiopathic focal segmental glomerulosclerosis and HIV-associated nephropathy. *J Am Soc Nephrol* 1999;10:51–61.
52. Barrett JM, Kriz W, Kaissling B, de Rouffignac C. The ultrastructure of the nephrons of the desert rodent (Psammomys obesus) kidney, I: thin limb of Henle of short-looped nephrons. *Am J Anat* 1978; 151:487–497.
53. Barrett JM, Kriz W, Kaissling B, de Rouffignac C. The ultrastructure of the nephrons of the desert rodent (Psammomys obesus) kidney, II: thin limbs of Henle of long-looped nephrons. *Am J Anat* 1978; 151:499–514.
54. Bastani B. Immunocytochemical localization of the vacuolar H(+)-ATPase pump in the kidney. *Histol Histopathol* 1997;12:769–779.
55. Bastani B, Haragsim L. Immunocytochemistry of renal H-ATPase. *Miner Electrolyte Metab* 1996;22:382–395.
56. Bearer EL, Orci L. Endothelial fenestral diaphragms: a quick-freeze, deep-etch study. *J Cell Biol* 1985;100:418–428.
57. Becker B. *Quantitative Beschreibung der Innenzone der Rattenniere*. Medical Dissertation, University Muenster, Münster, Germany 1978.
58. Beeuwkes R, 3rd. Efferent vascular patterns and early vascular-tubular relations in the dog kidney. *Am J Physiol* 1971;221:1361–1374.
59. Beeuwkes R, III, Bonventre JV. Tubular organization and vascular-tubular relations in the dog kidney. *Am J Physiol* 1975;229:695–713.
60. Bergeron M, Gaffiero P, Thiery G. Segmental variations in the organization of the endoplasmic reticulum of the rat nephron. A stereomicroscopic study. *Cell Tissue Res* 1987;247: 215–225.
61. Besse-Eschmann V, Klisic J, Nief V, Le Hir M, Kaissling B, Ambuhl PM. Regulation of the proximal tubular sodium/proton exchanger NHE3 in rats with puromycin aminonucleoside (PAN)-induced nephrotic syndrome. *J Am Soc Nephrol* 2002;13:2199–2206.
62. Betsholtz C, Lindblom P, Bjarnegard M, Enge M, Gerhardt H, Lindahl P. Role of platelet-derived growth factor in mesangium development and vasculopathies: lessons from platelet-derived growth factor and platelet-derived growth factor receptor mutations in mice. *Curr Opin Nephrol Hypertens* 2004;13:45–52.
63. Biber J, Gisler SM, Hernando N, Murer H. Protein/protein interactions (PDZ) in proximal tubules. *J Membr Biol* 2005;203:111–118.
64. Biber J, Gisler SM, Hernando N, Wagner CA, Murer H. PDZ interactions and proximal tubular phosphate reabsorption. *Am J Physiol Renal Physiol* 2004;287:F871–875.
65. Biemesderfer D, DeGray B, Aronson PS. Active (9.6 s) and inactive (21 s) oligomers of NHE3 in microdomains of the renal brush border. *J Biol Chem* 2001;276:10161–10167.
66. Biemesderfer D, Rutherford PA, Nagy T, Pizzonia JH, Abu-Alfa AK, Aronson PS. Monoclonal antibodies for high-resolution localization of NHE3 in adult and neonatal rat kidney. *Am J Physiol* 1997;273:F289–F299.
67. Bieritz B, Spessotto P, Colombatti A, Jahn A, Prols F, Hartner A. Role of alpha8 integrin in mesangial cell adhesion, migration, and proliferation. *Kidney Int* 2003;64:119–127.

68. Biner HL, Arpin-Bott MP, Loffing J, Wang X, Knepper M, Hebert SC, Kaissling B. Human cortical distal nephron: distribution of electrolyte and water transport pathways. *J Am Soc Nephrol* 2002;13:836–847.
69. Birn H, Willnow TE, Nielsen R, Norden AG, Bonsch C, Moestrup SK, Nexo E, Christensen EI. Megalin is essential for renal proximal tubule reabsorption and accumulation of transcobalamin-B(12). *Am J Physiol Renal Physiol* 2002;282:F408–416.
70. Blattner SM, Kretzler M. Integrin-linked kinase in renal disease: connecting cell-matrix interaction to the cytoskeleton. *Curr Opin Nephrol Hypertens* 2005;14:404–410.
71. Blomqvist SR, Vidarsson H, Fitzgerald S, Johansson BR, Ollerstam A, Brown R, Persson AE, Bergstrom GG, Enerback S. Distal renal tubular acidosis in mice that lack the forkhead transcription factor Foxi1. *J Clin Invest* 2004;113:1560–1570.
72. Bolton GR, Deen WM, Daniels BS. Assessment of the charge selectivity of glomerular basement membrane using Ficoll sulfate. *Am J Physiol* 1998;274:F889–F896.
73. Bonadio JF, Sage H, Cheng F, Bernstein J, Striker GE. Localization of collagen types IV and V, laminin, and heparan sulfate proteoglycan to the basal lamina of kidney epithelial cells in transfilter metanephric culture. *Am J Pathol* 1984;116:289–296.
74. Bostanjoglo M, Reeves W, Reilly R, Velazquez H, Robertson N, Litwack G, Morsing P, Dorup J, Bachmann S, Ellison D, Bostonjoglo M$[corrected to Bostanjoglo M, eds. 11Beta-hydroxysteroid dehydrogenase, mineralocorticoid receptor, and thiazide-sensitive Na-Cl cotransporter expression by distal tubules [published erratum appears in *J Am Soc Nephrol* 1998;9:2179]. 1998;9:1347–1358.
75. Bostanjoglo M, Reeves WB, Reilly RF, Velazquez H, Robertson N, Litwack G, Morsing P, Dorup J, Bachmann S, Ellison DH. 11Beta-hydroxysteroid dehydrogenase, mineralocorticoid receptor, and thiazide-sensitive Na-Cl cotransporter expression by distal tubules. *J Am Soc Nephrol* 1998;9:1347–1358.
76. Bouby N, Bankir L. Effect of high protein intake on sodium, potassium-dependent adenosine triphosphatase activity in the thick ascending limb of Henle's loop in the rat. *Clin Sci (Lond)* 1988; 74: 319–329.
77. Bouby N, Trinh-Trang-Tan MM, Coutaud C, Bankir L. Vasopressin is involved in renal effects of high-protein diet: study in homozygous Brattleboro rats. *Am J Physiol Renal Physiol* 1991;260:F96–100.
78. Boute N, Gribouval O, Roselli S, Benessy F, Lee H, Fuchshuber A, Dahan K, Gubler MC, Niaudet P, Antignac C. NPHS2, encoding the glomerular protein podocin, is mutated in autosomal recessive steroid-resistant nephrotic syndrome. *Nat Genet* 2000;24: 349–354.
79. Breton S, Alper SL, Gluck SL, Sly WS, Barker JE, Brown D. Depletion of intercalated cells from collecting ducts of carbonic anhydrase II-deficient (CAR2 null) mice. *Am J Physiol* 1995;269:F761–F774.
81. Breton S, Lisanti MP, Tyszkowski R, McLaughlin M, Brown D. Basolateral distribution of caveolin-1 in the kidney. Absence from H+-atpase-coated endocytic vesicles in intercalated cells. *J Histochem Cytochem* 1998;46:205–214.
82. Breyer MD, Harris RC. Cyclooxygenase 2 and the kidney. *Curr Opin Nephrol Hyperten* 2001;10:89–98.
83. Brooks HL, Sorensen A-M, Terris J, Schultheis PJ, Lorenz JN, Shull GE, Knepper MA. Profiling of renal tubule Na+ transporter abundances in NHE3 and NCC null mice using targeted proteomics. *J Physiol (Lond)* 2001;530:359–366.
84. Brown D. The ins and outs of aquaporin-2 trafficking. *Am J Physiol Renal Physiol* 2003;284: F893–901.
85. Brown D. Targeting of membrane transporters in renal epithelia: when cell biology meets physiology. *Am J Physiol Renal Physiol* 2000; 278:F192–201.
86. Brown D, Breton S. Mitochondria-rich, proton-secreting epithelial cells. *J Exp Biol* 1996;199:2345--2358.
87. Brown D, Gluck S, Hartwig J. Structure of the novel membrane-coating material in proton-secreting epithelial cells and identification as an H+ATPase. *J Cell Biol* 1987;105:1637–1648.
88. Brown D, Hirsch S, Gluck S. An H+-ATPase in opposite plasma membrane domains in kidney epithelial cell subpopulations. *Nature* 1988;331:622–624.
89. Brown D, Hirsch S, Gluck S. Localization of a proton-pumping ATPase in rat kidney. *J Clin Invest* 1988;82:2114–2126.
90. Brown D, Waneck GL. Glycosyl-phosphatidylinositol-anchored membrane proteins. *J Am Soc Nephrol* 1992;3:895–906.
91. Brown RW, Diaz R, Robson AC, Kotelevtsev YV, Mullins JJ, Kaufman MH, Seckl JR. The ontogeny of 11 beta-hydroxysteroid dehydrogenase type 2 and mineralocorticoid receptor gene expression reveal intricate control of glucocorticoid action in development. Endocrinology 1996;137:794–797.
92. Bulger RE. The shape of rat kidney tubular cells. *Am J Anat* 1965; 116:237–255.
93. Bulger RE, Cronin RE, Dobyan DC. Survey of the morphology of the dog kidney. *Anat Rec* 1979;194:41–65.
94. Bulger RE, Dobyan DC. Recent structure-function relationships in normal and injured mammalian kidneys. *Anat Rec* 1983;205:1–11.
95. Bulger RE, Eknoyan G, Purcell DJ, 2nd, Dobyan DC. Endothelial characteristics of glomerular capillaries in normal, mercuric chloride-induced, and gentamicin-induced acute renal failure in the rat. *J Clin Invest* 1983;72:128–141.
96. Bulger RE, Tisher CC, Myers CH, Trump BF. Human renal ultrastructure, II: the thin limb of Henle's loop and the interstitium in healthy individuals. *Lab Invest* 1967;16: 124–141.
97. Burckhardt BC, Burckhardt G. Transport of organic anions across the basolateral membrane of proximal tubule cells. *Rev Physiol Biochem Pharmacol* 2003;146:95–158.
98. Burckhardt G, Di Sole F, Helmle-Kolb C. The Na+/H+ exchanger gene family. *J Nephrol* 2002;15(Suppl 5):S3–21.
99. Burckhardt G, Wolff NA, Bahn A. Molecular characterization of the renal organic anion transporter 1. *Cell Biochem Biophys* 2002;36:169–174.
100. Calvert JP. New insights into ciliary fundtion: Kidney cysts and photoreceptors. *Proc Natl Acad Sci U S A* 2003;100:5583–5585.
101. Deleted in proof.
102. Campean V, Kricke J, Ellison D, Luft FC, Bachmann S. Localization of thiazide-sensitive Na(+)-Cl(-) cotransport and associated gene products in mouse DCT. *Am J Physiol Renal Physiol* 2001;281:F1028–1035.
103. Capasso G, Rizzo M, Pica A, Di Maio FS, Moe OW, Alpern RJ, De Santo NG. Bicarbonate reabsorption and NHE-3 expression: abundance and activity are increased in Henle's loop of remnant rats. *Kidney Int* 2002;62:2126–2135.
104. Capasso G, Unwin R, Rizzo M, Pica A, Giebisch G. Bicarbonate transport along the loop of Henle: molecular mechanisms and regulation. *J Nephrol* 2002;15(Suppl 5):S88–96.
105. Casellas D, Mimran A. Shunting in renal microvasculature of the rat: a scanning electron microscopic study of corrosion casts. *Anat Rec* 1981;201:237–248.
106. Castrop H, Huang Y, Hashimoto S, Mizel D, Hansen P, Theilig F, Bachmann S, Deng C, Briggs J, Schnermann J. Impairment of tubuloglomerular feedback regulation of GFR in ecto-5'-nucleotidase/CD73-deficient mice. *J Clin Invest* 2004;114:634–642.
107. Cha B, Kenworthy A, Murtazina R, Donowitz M. The lateral mobility of NHE3 on the apical membrane of renal epithelial OK cells is limited by the PDZ domain proteins NHERF1/2, but is dependent on an intact actin cytoskeleton as determined by FRAP. *J Cell Sci* 2004;117:3353–3365.
108. Deleted in proof.
109. Chambrey R, Goossens D, Bourgeois S, Picard N, Bloch-Faure M, Leviel F, Geoffroy V, Cambillau M, Colin Y, Paillard M, Houillier P, Cartron JP, Eladari D. Genetic ablation of Rhbg in the mouse does not impair renal ammonium excretion. *Am J Physiol Renal Physiol* 2005;289:F1281–1290.
110. Choate KA, Kahle KT, Wilson FH, Nelson-Williams C, Lifton RP. WNK1, a kinase mutated in inherited hypertension with hyperkalemia, localizes to diverse Cl- -transporting epithelia. *Proc Natl Acad Sci U S A* 2003;100:663–668.
111. Chou CL, Nielsen S, Knepper MA. Structural-functional correlation in chinchilla long loop of Henle thin limbs: a novel papillary subsegment. *Am J Physiol* 1993;265:F863–F874.
112. Christensen EI, Devuyst O, Dom G, Nielsen R, Van der Smissen P, Verroust P, Leruth M, Guggino WB, Courtoy PJ. Loss of chloride channel ClC-5 impairs endocytosis by defective trafficking of megalin and cubilin in kidney proximal tubules. *Proc Natl Acad Sci U S A* 2003; 100:8472–8477.
113. Christensen EI, Gburek J. Protein reabsorption in renal proximal tubule-function and dysfunction in kidney pathophysiology. *Pediatr Nephrol* 2004;19:714–721.
114. Christensen EI, Nielsen S, Moestrup SK, Borre C, Maunsbach AB, de Heer E, Ronco P, Hammond TG, Verroust P. Segmental distribution of the endocytosis receptor gp330 in renal proximal tubules. *Eur J Cell Biol* 1995;66:349–364.
115. Christensen JA, Bjaerke HA, Meyer DS, Bohle A. The normal juxtaglomerular apparatus in the human kidney. A morphological study. *Acta Anat* 1979;103:374–383.
116. Ciani L, Patel A, Allen ND, ffrench-Constant C. Mice lacking the giant protocadherin mFAT1 exhibit renal slit junction abnormalities and a partially penetrant cyclopia and anophthalmia phenotype. *Mol Cell Biol* 2003;23:3575–3582.
117. Ciriello J, de Oliveira CV. Renal afferents and hypertension. *Curr Hypertens Rep* 2002; 4:136–142.
118. Clapp WL, Madsen KM, Verlander JW, Tisher CC. Intercalated cells of the rat inner medullary collecting duct. *Kidney Int* 1987;31:1080–1087.
119. Clarke H, Marano CW, Peralta Soler A, Mullin JM. Modification of tight junction function by protein kinase C isoforms. *Adv Drug Deliv Rev* 2000;41:283–301.
120. Colegio OR, Van Itallie C, Rahner C, Anderson JM. Claudin extracellular domains determine paracellular charge selectivity and resistance but not tight junction fibril architecture. *Am J Physiol Cell Physiol* 2003;284:C1346–1354.
121. Colegio OR, Van Itallie CM, McCrea HJ, Rahner C, Anderson JM, eds. Claudins create charge-selective channels in the paracellular pathway between epithelial cells. *Am J Physiol Cell Physiol* 2002;283:C142–C147.
122. Coleman RA, Wu DC, Liu J, Wade JB. Expression of aquaporins in the renal connecting tubule. *Am J Physiol Renal Physiol* 2000;279:F874–883.
123. Colognato H, Yurchenco PD. Form and function: the laminin family of heterotrimers. *Dev Dyn* 2000;218:213–234.
124. Couchman JR, Beavan LA, McCarthy KJ. Glomerular matrix: synthesis, turnover and role in mesangial expansion. *Kidney Int* 1994; 45:328–335.
125. Courtoy PJ, Timpl R, Farquhar MG. Comparative distribution of laminin, type IV collagen, and fibronectin in the rat glomerulus. *J Histochem Cytochem* 1982;30:874–886.
126. Crayen ML, Thoenes W. Architecture and cell structures in the distal nephron of the rat kidney. *Cytobiologie* 1978;17:197–211.
127. Cross D, Vial C, Maccioni RB. A tau-like protein interacts with stress fibers and microtubules in human and rodent cultured cell lines. *J Cell Sci* 1993;105(Pt 1):51–60.
128. Cruz DN, Shaer AJ, Bia MJ, Lifton RP, Simon DB. Gitelman's syndrome revisited: an evaluation of symptoms and health-related quality of life. *Kidney Int* 2001;59: 710–717.
129. Cui S, Christensen EI. Three-dimensional organization of the vacuolar apparatus involved in endocytosis and membrane recycling of rat kidney proximal tubule cells: an electron-microscopic study of serial sections. *Exp Nephrol* 1993;1:175–184.
130. Cui S, Mata L, Maunsbach AB, Christensen EI. Ultrastructure of the vacuolar apparatus in the renal proximal tubule microinfused in vivo with the cytological stain light green. *Exp Nephrol* 1998; 6:359–367.
131. Cui S, Verroust PJ, Moestrup SK, Christensen EI. Megalin/gp330 mediates uptake of albumin in renal proximal tubule. *Am J Physiol* 1996;271:F900–F907.
132. Custer M, Lotscher M, Biber J, Murer H, Kaissling B. Expression of Na-P(i) cotransport in rat kidney: localization by RT-PCR and immunohistochemistry. *Am J Physiol* 1994;266: 767–774.
133. Cybulsky AV, Carbonetto S, Huang Q, McTavish AJ, Cyr MD. Adhesion of rat glomerular epithelial cells to extracellular matrices: role of beta 1 integrins. *Kidney Int* 1992;42: 1099–1106.
134. Daigeler R. Sex-dependent changes in the rat kidney after hypophysectomy. *Cell Tissue Res* 1981;216:423–443.

135. Daniels BS. Increased albumin permeability in vitro following alterations of glomerular charge is mediated by the cells of the filtration barrier. *J Lab Clin Med* 1994;124: 224–230.
136. Davenport JR, Yoder BK. An incredible decade for the primary cilium: a look at a once-forgotten organelle. *Am J Physiol Renal Physiol* 2005;289:F1159–1169.
137. Davies M, Thomas GJ, Shewring LD, Mason RM. Mesangial cell proteoglycans: synthesis and metabolism. *J Am Soc Nephrol* 1992;2:S88–S94.
138. Dawson TP, Gandhi R, Le Hir M, Kaissling B. Ecto-5'-nucleotidase: localization in rat kidney by light microscopic histochemical and immunohistochemical methods. *J Histochem Cytochem* 1989;37:39–47.
139. De Jong JC, Van Der Vliet WA, Van Den Heuvel LP, Willems PH, Knoers NV, Bindels RJ. Functional expression of mutations in the human NaCl cotransporter: evidence for impaired routing mechanisms in Gitelman's syndrome. *J Am Soc Nephrol* 2002;13: 1442–1448.
140. De Rouffignac C, Di Stefano A, Wittner M, Roinel N, Elalouf JM. Consequences of differential effects of ADH and other peptide hormones on thick ascending limb of mammalian kidney. *Am J Physiol* 1991;260:R1023–1035.
141. Deliot N, Hernando N, Horst-Liu Z, Gisler SM, Capuano P, Wagner CA, Bacic D, O'Brien S, Biber J, Murer H. Parathyroid hormone treatment induces dissociation of type IIa Na+-P(i) cotransporter-Na+/H+ exchanger regulatory factor-1 complexes. *Am J Physiol Cell Physiol* 2005;289:C159–167.
142. Denton KM, Fennessy PA, Alcorn D, Anderson WP. Morphometric analysis of the actions of angiotensin II on renal arterioles and glomeruli. *Am J Physiol* 1992;262:F367–F372.
143. Desmouliere A, Gabbiani G. Myofibroblast differentiation during fibrosis. *Exp Nephrol* 1995;3:134–139.
144. Devuyst O. Chloride channels and endocytosis: new insights from Dent's disease and CLC-5 knockout mice. *Bull Mem Acad R Med Belg* 2004;159:212–217.
145. Diamond JR, van Goor H, Ding G, Engelmyer E. Myofibroblasts in experimental hydronephrosis. *Am J Pathol* 1995;146:121–129.
146. DiBona GF. Differentiation of vasoactive renal sympathetic nerve fibers. *Acta Physiol* Scand 2000;168:195–200.
147. DiBona GF, Kopp UC. Neural control of renal function. *Physiol Rev* 1997;77:75–197.
148. Dieterich HJ. Electron microscopic studies of the innervation of the rat kidney. *Z Anat Entwicklungsgesch* 1974;145:169–186.
149. Dieterich HJ. [Structure of blood vessels in the kidney]. *Norm Pathol Anat (Stuttg)* 1978;35:1–108.
150. Dieterich HJ, Barrett JM, Kriz W, Bulhoff JP. The ultrastructure of the thin loop limbs of the mouse kidney. *Anat Embryol (Berl)* 1975;147:1–18.
151. Dinerstein RJ, Vannice J, Henderson RC, Roth LJ, Goldberg LI, Hoffmann PC. Histofluorescence techniques provide evidence for dopamine-containing neuronal elements in canine kidney. *Science* 1979;205:497–499.
152. Dobyan DC, Bulger RE. Morphology of the minipig kidney. *J Electron Microsc Tech* 1988;9:213–234.
153. Dobyan DC, Jamison R. Structure and function of the renal papilla. *Semin Nephrol* 1984;4:5.
154. Dobyan DC, Magill LS, Friedman PA, Hebert SC, Bulger RE. Carbonic anhydrase histochemistry in rabbit and mouse kidneys. *Anat Rec* 1982;204:185–197.
155. Dolezel S, Edvinsson L, Owman C, Owman T. Fluorescence histochemistry and autoradiography of adrenergic nerves in the renal juxtaglomerular complex of mammals and man, with special regard to the efferent arteriole. *Cell Tissue Res* 1976;169:211–220.
156. Dong X, Swaminathan S, Bachman LA, Croatt AJ, Nath KA, Griffin MD. Antigen presentation by dendritic cells in renal lymph nodes is linked to systemic and local injury to the kidney. *Kidney Int* 2005; 68:1096–1108.
157. Donoviel DB, Freed DD, Vogel H, Potter DG, Hawkins E, Barrish JP, Mathur BN, Turner CA, Geske R, Montgomery CA, Starbuck M, Brandt M, Gupta A, Ramirez-Solis R, Zambrowicz BP, Powell DR. Proteinuria and perinatal lethality in mice lacking NEPH1, a novel protein with homology to NEPHRIN. *Mol Cell Biol* 2001;21:4829–4836.
158. Donowitz M, Cha B, Zachos NC, Brett CL, Sharma A, Tse CM, Li X. NHERF family and NHE3regulation. *J Physiol* 2005;567:3–11.
159. Donowitz M, Milgram S, Murer H, Kurachi Y, Yun C, Weinman E. Coming out of the NHERF family. *J Physiol* 2005;567:1.
160. Dorup J. Structural adaptation of intercalated cells in rat renal cortex to acute metabolic acidosis and alkalosis. *J Ultrastruct Res* 1985;92:119–131.
161. Dorup J. Ultrastructure of distal nephron cells in rat renal cortex. *J Ultrastruct Res* 1985;2:101–118.
162. Dorup J, Maunsbach AB. Three-dimensional organization and segmental ultrastructure of rat proximal tubules. *Exp Nephrol* 1997; 5:305–317.
163. Doucet A. H+, K(+)-ATPASE in the kidney: localization and function in the nephron. *Exp Nephrol* 1997;5:271–276.
164. Doucet A, Katz AI, Morel F. Determination of Na-K-ATPase activity in single segments of the mammalian nephron. *Am J Physiol* 1979; 237:F105–113.
165. Drenckhahn D, Franke RP. Ultrastructural organization of contractile and cytoskeletal proteins in glomerular podocytes of chicken, rat, and man. *Lab Invest* 1988;59:673–682.
166. Drenckhahn D, Schluter K, Allen DP, Bennett V. Colocalization of band 3 with ankyrin and spectrin at the basal membrane of intercalated cells in the rat kidney. *Science* 1985;230:1287–1289.
167. Drumond MC, Deen WM. Hindered transport of macromolecules through a single row of cylinders: application to glomerular filtration. *J Biomech Eng* 1995;117:414–422.
168. Drumond MC, Deen WM. Stokes flow through a row of cylinders between parallel walls: model for the glomerular slit diaphragm. *J Biomech Eng* 1994;116:184–189.
169. Drumond MC, Deen WM. Structural determinants of glomerular hydraulic permeability. *Am J Physiol* 1994;266:F1–F12.
170. Drumond MC, Kristal B, Myers BD, Deen WM. Structural basis for reduced glomerular filtration capacity in nephrotic humans. *J Clin Invest* 1994;94:1187–1195.
171. Duc C, Farman N, Canessa CM, Bonvalet JP, Rossier BC. Cell-specific expression of epithelial sodium channel alpha, beta, and gamma subunits in aldosterone-responsive epithelia from the rat: localization by in situ hybridization and immunocytochemistry. *J Cell Biol* 1994; 127:1907–1921.
172. Dunne J, Hanby AM, Poulsom R, Jones TA, Sheer D, Chin WG, Da SM, Zhao Q, Beverley PC, Owen MJ. Molecular cloning and tissue expression of FAT, the human homologue of the Drosophila fat gene that is located on chromosome 4q34-q35 and encodes a putative adhesion molecule. *Genomics* 1995;30:207–223.
173. Dworkin L, Brenner B. Biophysical basis of glomerular filtration. In: Seldin D (ed.). *The Kidney: Physiology and Pathophysiology*. New York: Raven Press, 1992:979–1016.
174. Ecelbarger CA, Kim GH, Wade JB, Knepper MA. Regulation of the abundance of renal sodium transporters and channels by vasopressin. *Exp Neurol* 2001;171:227–234.
175. Ecelbarger CA, Knepper MA, Verbalis JG. Increased abundance of distal sodium transporters in rat kidney during vasopressin escape. *J Am Soc Nephrol* 2001;12:207–217.
176. Ecelbarger CA, Terris J, Hoyer JR, Nielsen S, Wade JB, Knepper MA. Localization and regulation of the rat renal Na(+)-K(+)-2Cl- cotransporter, BSC-1. *Am J Physiol* 1996;271: F619–F628.
177. Eckardt KU, Koury ST, Tan CC, Schuster SJ, Kaissling B, Ratcliffe PJ, Kurtz A. Distribution of erythropoietin producing cells in rat kidneys during hypoxic hypoxia. *Kidney Int* 1993; 43:815–823.
178. Eckardt KU, LeHir M, Tan CC, Ratcliffe PJ, Kaissling B, Kurtz A. Renal innervation plays no role in oxygen-dependent control of erythropoietin mRNA levels. *Am J Physiol* 1992;263:925–930.
179. Eddy AA. Interstitial nephritis induced by protein-overload proteinuria. *Am J Pathol* 1989;135:719–733.
180. Edwards A, Daniels BS, Deen WM. Hindered transport of macromolecules in isolated glomeruli. II. Convection and pressure effects in basement membrane. *Biophys J* 1997;72: 214–222.
181. Edwards A, Deen WM, Daniels BS. Hindered transport of macromolecules in isolated glomeruli, I: diffusion across intact and cell-free capillaries. *Biophys J* 1997;72:204–213.
182. Edwards JG. Efferent arterioles of glomeruli in the juxtamedullary zone of the human kidney. *Anat Rec* 1956;125:521–529.
183. Eladari D, Cheval L, Quentin F, Bertrand O, Mouro I, Cherif-Zahar B, Cartron JP, Paillard M, Doucet A, Chambrey R. Expression of RhCG, a new putative NH(3)/NH(4)(+) transporter, along the rat nephron. *J Am Soc Nephrol* 2002;13:1999–2008.
184. Elger M, Drenckhahn D, Nobiling R, Mundel P, Kriz W. Cultured rat mesangial cells contain smooth muscle alpha-actin not found in vivo. *Am J Pathol* 1993;142:497–509.
185. Elger M, Sakai T, Kriz W. The vascular pole of the renal glomerulus of rat. *Adv Anat Embryol Cell Biol* 1998;139:1–98.
186. Ellison DH. Divalent cation transport by the distal nephron: insights from Bartter's and Gitelman's syndromes. *Am J Physiol Renal Physiol* 2000;279:F616–625.
187. Ellison DH, Velazquez H, Wright FS. Thiazide-sensitive sodium chloride cotransport in early distal tubule. *Am J Physiol* 1987;253:546–554.
188. Emmons C, Kurtz I. H+/base transport pathways in the cortical collecting duct. *Exp Nephrol* 1993;1:325–333.
189. Eppel GA, Luff SE, Denton KM, Evans RG. Type 1 neuropeptide Y receptors and {alpha}1-adrenoceptors in the neural control of regional renal perfusion. *Am J Physiol Regul Integr Comp Physiol* 2006;290:R331–R340.
190. Eremina V, Quaggin SE. The role of VEGF-A in glomerular development and function. *Curr Opin Nephrol Hypertens* 2004;13:9–15.
191. Ernst SA, Schreiber JH. Ultrastructural localization of Na+,K+-ATPase in rat and rabbit kidney medulla. *J Cell Biol* 1981;91:803–813.
192. Evan AP, Dail WG, Jr. Efferent arterioles in the cortex of the rat kidney. *Anat Rec* 1977;187:135–145.
193. Farquhar MG, Palade G. Functional evidence for the existence of a third cell type in the renal glomerulus. Phagocytosis of filtration residues by a distinctive "third" cell. *J Cell Biol* 1962;13:55–87.
194. Farquhar MG, Saito A, Kerjaschki D, Orlando RA. The Heymann nephritis antigenic complex: megalin (gp330) and RAP. *J Am Soc Nephrol* 1995;6:35–47.
195. Ferguson M, Bell C. Ultrastructural localization and characterization of sensory nerves in the rat kidney. *J Comp Neurol* 1988;274:9–16.
196. Fourman J. The adrenergic innervation of the efferent arterioles and the vasa recta in the mammalian kidney. *Experientia* 1970;26:293–294.
197. Fourman J, Moffat D. *The Blood Vessels of the Kidney*. Oxford: Blackwell Scientific, 1971.
198. Fretschner M, Endlich K, Fester C, Parekh N, Steinhausen M. A narrow segment of the efferent arteriole controls efferent resistance in the hydronephrotic rat kidney. *Kidney Int* 1990;37:1227–1239.
199. Frigeri A, Gropper MA, Turck CW, Verkman AS. Immunolocalization of the mercurial-insensitive water channel and glycerol intrinsic protein in epithelial cell plasma membranes. *Proc Natl Acad Sci U S A* 1995;92:4328–4331.
200. Gall JA, Alcorn D, Butkus A, Coghlan JP, Ryan GB. Distribution of glomerular peripolar cells in different mammalian species. *Cell Tissue Res* 1986;244:203–208.
201. Gamba G. Role of WNK kinases in regulating tubular salt and potassium transport and in the development of hypertension. *Am J Physiol Renal Physiol* 2005;288:F245–252.
202. Gandhi R, Le Hir M, Kaissling B. Immunolocalization of ecto-5'-nucleotidase in the kidney by a monoclonal antibody. *Histochemistry* 1990;95:165–174.
203. Ganote CE, Grantham JJ, Moses HL, Burg MB, Orloff J. Ultrastructural studies of vasopressin effect on isolated perfused renal collecting tubules of the rabbit. *J Cell Biol* 1968;36: 355–367.
204. Geering K. FXYD proteins: new regulators of Na-K-ATPase. *Am J Physiol Renal Physiol* 2006;290:F241–250.
205. Gekle M, Volker K, Mildenberger S, Freudinger R, Shull GE, Wiemann M. NHE3 Na+/H+ exchanger supports proximal tubular protein reabsorption in vivo. *Am J Physiol Renal Physiol* 2004;287:F469–473.

206. Gelberg H, Healy L, Whiteley H, Miller LA, Vimr E. In vivo enzymatic removal of alpha 2->6-linked sialic acid from the glomerular filtration barrier results in podocyte charge alteration and glomerular injury. *Lab Invest* 1996;74:907–920.

207. Gibson IW, Downie I, Downie TT, Han SW, More IA, Lindop GB. The parietal podocyte: a study of the vascular pole of the human glomerulus. *Kidney Int* 1992;41:211–214.

208. Gibson MA, Kumaratilake JS, Cleary EG. The protein components of the 12-nanometer microfibrils of elastic and nonelastic tissues. *J Biol Chem* 1989;264:4590–4598.

209. Giebisch G. Renal potassium channels: function, regulation, and structure. *Kidney Int* 2001;60:436–445.

210. Ginns SM, Knepper MA, Ecelbarger CA, Terris J, He X, Coleman RA, Wade JB. Immunolocalization of the secretory isoform of Na-K-Cl cotransporter in rat renal intercalated cells. *J Am Soc Nephrol* 1996;7:2533–2542.

211. Gisler SM, Pribanic S, Bacic D, Forrer P, Gantenbein A, Sabourin LA, Tsuji A, Zhao ZS, Manser E, Biber J, Murer H. PDZK1, I: a major scaffolder in brush borders of proximal tubular cells. *Kidney Int* 2003;64:1733–1745.

212. Gonzalez CB, Figueroa CD, Reyes CE, Caorsi CE, Troncoso S, Menzel D. Immunolocalization of V1 vasopressin receptors in the rat kidney using anti-receptor antibodies. *Kidney Int* 1997;52:1206–1215.

213. Goormaghtigh N. Facts in favour of an endocrine function of the renal arterioles. *J Pathol Bacteriol* 1945;57:392.

214. Gorgas K. [Structure and innervation of the juxtaglomerular apparatus of the rat (author's transl)]. *Adv Anat Embryol Cell Biol* 1978;54:3–83.

215. Grandchamp A, Boulpaep EL. Pressure control of sodium reabsorption and intercellular backflux across proximal kidney tubule. *J Clin Invest* 1974;54:69–82.

216. Grantham JJ. Mode of water transport in mammalian renal collecting tubules. *Fed Proc* 1971;30:14–21.

217. Greger R, Schlatter E, Lang F. Evidence for electroneutral sodium chloride cotransport in the cortical thick ascending limb of Henle's loop of rabbit kidney. *Pflugers Arch* 1983;396:308–314.

218. Groffen AJ, Buskens CA, van Kuppevelt TH, Veerkamp JH, Monnens LA, van den Heuvel LP. Primary structure and high expression of human agrin in basement membranes of adult lung and kidney. *Eur J Biochem* 1998;254:123–128.

219. Grupp C, Lottermoser J, Cohen DI, Begher M, Franz HE, Muller GA. Transformation of rat inner medullary fibroblasts to myofibroblasts in vitro. *Kidney Int* 1997;52:1279–1290.

220. Hackenthal E, Paul M, Ganten D, Taugner R. Morphology, physiology, and molecular biology of renin secretion. *Physiol Rev* 1990;70:1067–1116.

221. Hagege J, Richet G. Dark cells of the distal convoluted tubules and collecting ducts, I: morphological data. *Fortschr Zool* 1975;23:288–298.

222. Han JS, Thompson KA, Chou CL, Knepper MA. Experimental tests of three-dimensional model of urinary concentrating mechanism. *J Am Soc Nephrol* 1992;2:1677–1688.

223. Han KH, Woo SK, Kim WY, Park SH, Cha JH, Kim J, Kwon HM. Maturation of TonEBP expression in developing rat kidney. *Am J Physiol Renal Physiol* 2004;287:F878–885.

224. Harris RC, McKanna JA, Akai Y, Jacobson HR, Dubois RN, Breyer MD. Cyclooxygenase-2 is associated with the macula densa of rat kidney and increases with salt restriction. *J Clin Invest* 1994;94:2504–2510.

225. Hatae T, Ichimura T, Ishida T, Sakurai T. Apical tubular network in the rat kidney proximal tubule cells studied by thick-section and scanning electron microscopy. *Cell Tissue Res* 1997;288:317–325.

226. He Q, Madsen M, Kilkenney A, Gregory B, Christensen EI, Vorum H, Hojrup P, Schaffer AA, Kirkness EF, Tanner SM, de la Chapelle A, Giger U, Moestrup SK, Fyfe JC. Amnionless function is required for cubilin brush-border expression and intrinsic factor-cobalamin (vitamin B12) absorption in vivo. *Blood* 2005;106:1447–1453.

227. Hebert SC. Bartter syndrome. *Curr Opin Nephrol Hypertens* 2003;12:527–532.

228. Hebert SC, Andreoli TE. Control of NaCl transport in the thick ascending limb. *Am J Physiol* 1984;246:F745–F756.

229. Hebert SC, Culpepper RM, Andreoli TE. NaCl transport in mouse medullary thick ascending limbs. I. Functional nephron heterogeneity and ADH-stimulated NaCl cotransport. *Am J Physiol* 1981;241: F412–431.

230. Hebert SC, Culpepper RM, Andreoli TE. NaCl transport in mouse medullary thick ascending limbs. II. ADH enhancement of transcellular NaCl cotransport; origin of transepithelial voltage. *Am J Physiol* 1981;241:F432–442.

231. Hebert SC, Culpepper RM, Andreoli TE. NaCl transport in mouse medullary thick ascending limbs, III: modulation of the ADH effect by peritubular osmolality. *Am J Physiol* 1981;241: F443–451.

232. Hediger MA, Knepper MA. Introduction: recent insights into the urinary concentrating mechanism: from cDNA cloning to dodelin renal function. *Am J Physiol* 1998;275:F317.

233. Helmchen U. Die Zahl der Mesangiumzellen in einem normalen Glomerulum der Rattenniere. Eine dreidimensionale elektronenoptische Analyse. Tübingen, 1980.

234. Hodson J. The lobar structure of the kidney. *Br J Urol* 1972;44:246–261.

235. Hoenderop JG, Nilius B, Bindels RJ. ECaC: the gatekeeper of transepithelial Ca2+ transport. *Biochim Biophys Acta* 2002;1600:6–11.

236. Hoenderop JG, Nilius B, Bindels RJ. Epithelial calcium channels: from identification to function and regulation. *Pflugers Arch* 2003; 446:304–308.

237. Hollywell CA, Jaworowski A, Thumwood C, Alcorn D, Ryan GB. Immunohistochemical localization of transthyretin in glomerular peripolar cells of newborn sheep. *Cell Tissue Res* 1992;267:193–197.

238. Honegger KJ, Capuano P, Winter C, Bacic D, Stange G, Wagner CA, Biber J, Murer H, Hernando N. Regulation of sodium-proton exchanger isoform 3 (NHE3) by PKA and exchange protein directly activated by cAMP (EPAC). *PNAS* 2006;103:803–808.

239. Hopkins AM, Li D, Mrsny RJ, Walsh SV, Nusrat A. Modulation of tight junction function by G protein-coupled events. *Adv Drug Deliv Rev* 2000;41:329–340.

240. Horvat R, Hovorka A, Dekan G, Poczewski H, Kerjaschki D. Endothelial cell membranes contain podocalyxin—the major sialoprotein of visceral glomerular epithelial cells. *J Cell Biol* 1986;102: 484–491.

241. Hou X, Mrug M, Yoder BK, Lefkowitz EJ, Kremmidiotis G, D'Eustachio P, Beier DR, Guay-Woodford LM. Cystin, a novel cilia-associated protein, is disrupted in the cpk mouse model of polycystic kidney disease. *J Clin Invest* 2002;109:533–540.

242. Huang TW, Langlois JC. Podoendin. A new cell surface protein of the podocyte and endothelium. *J Exp Med* 1985;162:245–267.

243. Huber G, Matus A. Microtubule-associated protein 3 (MAP3) expression in non-neuronal tissues. *J Cell Sci* 1990;95(Pt 2):237–246.

244. Huber TB, Kottgen M, Schilling B, Walz G, Benzing T. Interaction with podocin facilitates nephrin signaling. *J Biol Chem* 2001;276:41543–41546.

245. Hudson BG, Reeders ST, Tryggvason K. Type IV collagen: structure, gene organization, and role in human diseases. Molecular basis of Goodpasture and Alport syndromes and diffuse leiomyomatosis. *J Biol Chem* 1993;268:26033–26036.

246. Hudson BG, Tryggvason K, Sundaramoorthy M, Neilson EG. Alport's syndrome, Goodpasture's syndrome, and type IV collagen. *N Engl J Med* 2003;348:2543–25563.

247. Hugo C, Nangaku M, Shankland SJ, Pichler R, Gordon K, Amieva MR, Couser WG, Furthmayr H, Johnson RJ. The plasma membrane-actin linking protein, ezrin, is a glomerular epithelial cell marker in glomerulogenesis, in the adult kidney and in glomerular injury. *Kidney Int* 1998;54:1934–1944.

248. Ichimura K, Kurihara H, Sakai T. Actin filament organization of foot processes in rat podocytes. *J Histochem Cytochem* 2003;51:1589–1600.

249. Igarashi P, Somlo S. Genetics and pathogenesis of polycystic kidney disease. *J Am Soc Nephrol* 2002;13:2384–2398.

250. Imai M. Function of the thin ascending limb of Henle of rats and hamsters perfused in vitro. *Am J Physiol* 1977;232:F201–F209.

251. Imbert-Teboul M, Charbardes D, Morel F. Vasopressin and catecholamines sites of action along rabbit, mouse and rat nephron. *Contrib Nephrol* 1980;21:41–47.

252. Inke G. *The Protolobar Structure of the Human Kidney*. New York: Alan R. Liss, Inc., 1988.

253. Inoue S. Ultrastructural architecture of basement membranes. *Contrib Nephrol* 1994;107:21–28.

254. Inoue T, Yaoita E, Kurihara H, Shimizu F, Sakai T, Kobayashi T, Ohshiro K, Kawachi H, Okada H, Suzuki H, Kihara I, Yamamoto T. FAT is a component of glomerular slit diaphragms. *Kidney Int* 2001; 59:1003 –1012.

255. Ishibashi K, Sasaki S, Fushimi K, Yamamoto T, Kuwahara M, Marumo F. Immunolocalization and effect of dehydration on AQP3, a basolateral water channel of kidney collecting ducts. *Am J Physiol* 1997;272:F235–F241.

256. Jamison R, Kriz W. Urinary Concentrating Mechanism: Structure and Function. New York, Oxford University Press, 1982.

257. Jamison RL. Micropuncture study of segments of thin loop of Henle in the rat. *Am J Physiol* 1968;215:236–242.

258. Jeck N, Schlingmann KP, Reinalter SC, Komhoff M, Peters M, Waldegger S, Seyberth HW. Salt handling in the distal nephron: lessons learned from inherited human disorders. *Am J Physiol Regul Integr Comp Physiol* 2005;288:R782–795.

259. Jensen BL, Kurtz A. Differential regulation of renal cyclooxygenase mRNA by dietary salt intake. *Kidney Int* 1997;52:1242–1249.

260. Jentsch TJ. Chloride transport in the kidney: lessons from human disease and knockout mice. *J Am Soc Nephrol* 2005;16:1549–1561.

261. Jentsch TJ, Hubner CA, Fuhrmann JC. Ion channels: function unravelled by dysfunction. *Nat Cell Biol* 2004;6:1039–1047.

262. Jung J-Y, Song J-H, Li C, Yang C-W, Kang T-C, Won M-H, Jeong Y-G, Han K-H, Choi K-B, Lee S-H, Kim J. Expression of epidermal growth factor in the developing rat kidney. *Am J Physiol Renal Physiol* 2005;288:F227–235.

263. Kahle KT, Gimenez I, Hassan H, Wilson FH, Wong RD, Forbush B, Aronson PS, Lifton RP. WNK4 regulates apical and basolateral Cl- flux in extrarenal epithelia. *Proc Natl Acad Sci U S A* 2004;101:2064–2069.

264. Kahle KT, Gimenez I, Hassan H, Wilson FH, Wong RD, Forbush B, Aronson PS, Lifton RP. WNK4 regulates apical and basolateral Cl- flux in extrarenal epithelia. *Proc Natl Acad Sci U S A* 2004;101:2064–2069.

265. Kahle KT, Wilson FH, Leng Q, Lalioti MD, O'Connell AD, Dong K, Rapson AK, MacGregor GG, Giebisch G, Hebert SC, Lifton RP. WNK4 regulates the balance between renal NaCl reabsorption and K+ secretion. *Nat Genet* 2003;35:372–376.

266. Kaissling B. Ultrastructural organization of the transition from the distal nephron to the collecting duct in the desert rodent *Psammomys obesus*. *Cell Tissue Res* 1980;212:475–495.

267. Kaissling B, Bachmann S, Kriz W. Structural adaptation of the distal convoluted tubule to prolonged furosemide treatment. *Am J Physiol* 1985;248:F374–381.

268. Kaissling B, de Rouffignac C, Barrett JM, Kriz W. The structural organization of the kidney of the desert rodent Psammomys obesus. *Anat Embryol (Berl)* 1975;148:121–143.

269. Kaissling B, Hegyi I, Loffing J, Le Hir M. Morphology of interstitial cells in the healthy kidney. *Anat Embryol (Berl)* 1996;193:303–318.

270. Kaissling B, Kriz W. Morphology of the loop of Henle, distal tubule and collecting duct. In: Windhager EE (ed.). *Handbook of Physiology: Section on Renal Physiology*. New York: Oxford University Press, 1992:109–167.

271. Kaissling B, Kriz W. Structural analysis of the rabbit kidney. *Adv Anat Embryol Cell Biol* 1979;56:1–123.

272. Deleted in proof.

273. Kaissling B, Kriz W. Variability of intercellular spaces between macula densa cells: a transmission electron microscopic study in rabbits and rats. *Kidney Int Suppl* 1982;12: S9–S17.

274. Kaissling B, Le Hir M. Characterization and distribution of interstitial cell types in the renal cortex of rats. *Kidney Int* 1994;45:709–720.

275. Kaissling B, Le Hir M. Distal tubular segments of the rabbit kidney after adaptation to altered Na- and K-intake, I: structural changes. *Cell Tissue Res* 1982;224:469–492.

276. Kaissling B, Peter S, Kriz W. The transition of the thick ascending limb of Henle's loop into the distal convoluted tubule in the nephron of the rat kidney. *Cell Tissue Res* 1977;182: 111–118.
277. Kaissling B, Spiess S, Rinne B, Le Hir M. Effects of anemia on morphology of rat renal cortex. *Am J Physiol* 1993;264:F608–F617.
278. Kaissling B, Stanton BA. Adaptation of distal tubule and collecting duct to increased sodium delivery, I: ultrastructure. *Am J Physiol Renal Physiol* 1988;255:F1256–1268.
279. Kanwar Y, Venkatachalam M. Renal Physiology. In: Windhager EE, ed. *Handbook of Physiology*. New York: Oxford University Press, 1992:3–40.
280. Kanwar YS, Linker A, Farquhar MG. Increased permeability of the glomerular basement membrane to ferritin after removal of glycosaminoglycans (heparan sulfate) by enzyme digestion. *J Cell Biol* 1980; 86:688–693.
281. Karbach U, Kricke J, Meyer-Wentrup F, Gorboulev V, Volk C, Loffing-Cueni D, Kaissling B, Bachmann S, Koepsell H. Localization of organic cation transporters OCT1 and OCT2 in rat kidney. *Am J Physiol Renal Physiol* 2000;279:F679–687.
282. Karkavelas G, Kefalides NA, Amenta PS, Martinez-Hernandez A. Comparative ultrastructural localization of collagen types III, IV, VI and laminin in rat uterus and kidney. *J Ultrastruct Mol Struct Res* 1988;100:137–155.
283. Kashgarian M, Biemesderfer D, Caplan M, Forbush B, 3rd. Monoclonal antibody to Na,K-ATPase: immunocytochemical localization along nephron segments. *Kidney Int* 1985;28:899–913.
284. Kato Y, Kuge K, Kusuhara H, Meier PJ, Sugiyama Y. Gender difference in the urinary excretion of organic anions in rats. *J Pharmacol Exp Ther* 2002;302:483–489.
285. Kato Y, Sai Y, Yoshida K, Watanabe C, Hirata T, Tsuji A. PDZK1 directly regulates the function of organic cation/carnitine transporter OCTN2. *Mol Pharmacol* 2005;67:734–743.
286. Katz AI, Doucet A, Morel F. Na-K-ATPase activity along the rabbit, rat, and mouse nephron. *Am J Physiol* 1979;237:F114–120.
287. Kazatchkine MD, Fearon DT, Appay MD, Mandet C, Bariety J. Immunohistochemical study of the human glomerular C3b receptor in normal kidney and in seventy-five cases of renal diseases: loss of C3b receptor antigen in focal hyalinosis and in proliferative nephritis of systemic lupus erythematosus. *J Clin Invest* 1982; 69:900–912.
288. Kerjaschki D, Exner M, Ullrich R, Susani M, Curtiss LK, Witztum JL, Farquhar MG, Orlando RA. Pathogenic antibodies inhibit the binding of apolipoproteins to megalin/gp330 in passive Heymann nephritis. *J Clin Invest* 1997;100:2303–2309.
289. Kerjaschki D, Farquhar MG. Immunocytochemical localization of the Heymann nephritis antigen (GP330) in glomerular epithelial cells of normal Lewis rats. *J Exp Med* 1983;157:66–686.
290. Kikkawa Y, Virtanen I, Miner JH. Mesangial cells organize the glomerular capillaries by adhering to the G domain of laminin alpha5 in the glomerular basement membrane. *J Cell Biol* 2003;161:187–196.
291. Kim GH, Ecelbarger CA, Mitchell C, Packer RK, Wade JB, Knepper MA. Vasopressin increases Na-K-2Cl cotransporter expression in thick ascending limb of Henle's loop. *Am J Physiol* 1999;276:F96–F103.
292. Kim J, Tisher CC, Linser PJ, Madsen KM. Ultrastructural localization of carbonic anhydrase II in subpopulations of intercalated cells of the rat kidney. *J Am Soc Nephrol* 1990;1: 245–256.
293. Kim YH, Kim DU, Han KH, Jung JY, Sands JM, Knepper MA, Madsen KM, Kim J. Expression of urea transporters in the developing rat kidney. *Am J Physiol Renal Physiol* 2002;282: F530–F540.
294. Kim Y-H, Verlander JW, Matthews SW, Kurtz I, Shin W, Weiner ID, Everett LA, Green ED, Nielsen S, Wall SM. Intercalated cell H+/OH- transporter expression is reduced in Slc26a4 null mice. *Am J Physiol Renal Physiol* 2005;289:F1262–1272.
295. Deleted in proof.
296. Kirk KL, Bell PD, Barfuss DW, Ribadeneira M. Direct visualization of the isolated and perfused macula densa. *Am J Physiol* 1985;248:F890–F894.
296a. Kiuchi-Saishin Y, Gotoh S, Furuse M, Takasuga A, Tano Y, and Tsukita S. Differential expression patterns of claudins, tight junction membrane proteins, in mouse nephron segments. *J Am Soc Nephrol* 2002;13:875-886.
297. Kishore BK, Wade JB, Schorr K, Inoue T, Mandon B, Knepper MA. Expression of synaptotagmin VIII in rat kidney. *Am J Physiol* 1998;275:F131–F142.
298. Knepper MA, Danielson RA, Saidel GM, Post RS. Quantitative analysis of renal medullary anatomy in rats and rabbits. *Kidney Int* 1977;12:313–323.
299. Knepper MA, Kim GH, Fernandez-Llama P, Ecelbarger CA. Regulation of thick ascending limb transport by vasopressin. *J Am Soc Nephrol* 1999;10:628–634.
300. Knepper MA, Wade JB, Terris J, Ecelbarger CA, Marples D, Mandon B, Chou CL, Kishore BK, Nielsen S. Renal aquaporins. *Kidney Int* 1996;49:1712–1717.
301. Knohl SJ, Scheinman SJ. Inherited hypercalciuric syndromes: Dent's disease (CLC-5) and familial hypomagnesemia with hypercalciuria (paracellin-1). *Semin Nephrol* 2004;24: 55–60.
302. Kobayashi K, Monkawa T, Hayashi M, Saruta T. Expression of the Na+/H+ exchanger regulatory protein family in genetically hypertensive rats. *J Hypertens* 2004;22:1723–1730.
303. Kobayashi N, Reiser J, Kriz W, Kuriyama R, Mundel P. Nonuniform microtubular polarity established by CHO1/MKLP1 motor protein is necessary for process formation of podocytes. *J Cell Biol* 1998; 143:1961–1970.
304. Koechlin N, Elalouf JM, Kaissling B, Roinel N, de Rouffignac C. A structural study of the rat proximal and distal nephron: effect of peptide and thyroid hormones. *Am J Physiol* 1989;256:814–822.
305. Koepsell H. Polyspecific organic cation transporters: their functions and interactions with drugs. *Trends Pharmacol Sci* 2004;25:375–381.
306. Koepsell H, Kriz W, Schnermann J. Pattern of luminal diameter changes along the descending and ascending thin limbs of the loop of Henle in the inner medullary zone of the rat kidney. *Z Anat Entwicklungsgesch* 1972;138:321–328.
307. Kokko JP, Rector FC, Jr. Countercurrent multiplication system without active transport in inner medulla. *Kidney Int* 1972;2:214–223.
308. Komlosi P, Fintha A, Bell PD. Current mechanisms of macula densa cell signalling. *Acta Physiol Scand* 2004;181:463–469.
309. Kone BC, Madsen KM, Tisher CC. Ultrastructure of the thick ascending limb of Henle in the rat kidney. *Am J Anat* 1984;171:217–226.
310. Konrad M, Schlingmann KP, Gudermann T. Insights into the molecular nature of magnesium homeostasis. *Am J Physiol Renal Physiol* 2004;286:F599–605.
311. Konrad M, Weber S. Recent advances in molecular genetics of hereditary magnesium-losing disorders. *J Am Soc Nephrol* 2003;14:249–260.
312. Koob R, Zimmermann M, Schoner W, Drenckhahn D. Colocalization and coprecipitation of ankyrin and Na+,K+-ATPase in kidney epithelial cells. *Eur J Cell Biol* 1988;45:230–237.
313. Koury ST, Bondurant MC, Koury MJ. Localization of erythropoietin synthesizing cells in murine kidneys by in situ hybridization. *Blood* 1988;71:524–527.
314. Kreidberg JA, Symons JM. Integrins in kidney development, function, and disease. *Am J Physiol Renal Physiol* 2000;279:F233–F242.
315. Kriz W. [The architectonic and functional structure of the rat kidney]. *Z Zellforsch Mikrosk Anat* 1967;82:495–535.
316. Kriz W. A periarterial pathway for intrarenal distribution of renin. *Kidney Int Suppl* 1987;20: S51–S56.
317. Kriz W. Structural organization of the renal medulla: comparative and functional aspects. *Am J Physiol* 1981;241:R3–R16.
318. Kriz W. Structural organization of the renal medullary counterflow system. *Fed Proc* 1983;42:2379–2385.
319. Kriz W, Dieterich H. *The Supplying and Draining vessels of the Renal Medulla in Mammals. Proceedings of the 4th International Congress of Nephrology*. Basel: Karger, 1970:138–144.
320. Kriz W, Dieterich HJ. [The lymphatic system of the kidney in some mammals. Light and electron microscopic investigations]. *Z Anat Entwicklungsgesch* 1970;131:111–147.
321. Kriz W, Dieterich HJ, Hoffmann S. [Construction of vascular bundles in the renal medulla of desert mice]. *Naturwissenschaften* 1968; 55:40.
322. Kriz W, Elger M, Lemley K, Sakai T. Structure of the glomerular mesangium: a biomechanical interpretation. *Kidney Int Suppl* 1990;30:S2–S9.
323. Kriz W, Elger M, Mundel P, Lemley KV. Structure-stabilizing forces in the glomerular tuft. *J Am Soc Nephrol* 1995;5:1731–1739.
324. Kriz W, Hahnel B, Hosser H, Ostendorf T, Gaertner S, Kranzlin B, Gretz N, Shimizu F, Floege J. Pathways to recovery and loss of nephrons in anti-Thy-1 nephritis. *J Am Soc Nephrol* 2003;14:1904–1926.
325. Kriz W, Hahnel B, Rosener S, Elger M. Long-term treatment of rats with FGF-2 results in focal segmental glomerulosclerosis. *Kidney Int* 1995;48:1435–1450.
326. Kriz W, Kaissling B. Structural organization of the mammalian kidney. In: Seldin D (ed.). *The Kidney: Physiology and Pathophysiology*, vol. 1, 3rd ed. New York: Raven Press, 2000:586–654.
327. Kriz W, Koepsell H. The structural organization of the mouse kidney. *Z Anat Entwicklungsgesch* 1974;144:137–163.
328. Kriz W, Mundel P, Elger M. The contractile apparatus of podocytes is arranged to counteract GBM expansion. *Contrib Nephrol* 1994; 107:1–9.
329. Kriz W, Napiwotzky P. Structural and functional aspects of the renal interstitium. *Contrib Nephrol* 1979;16:104–108.
330. Kriz W, Schiller A, Taugner R. Freeze-fracture studies on the thin limbs of Henle's loop in Psammomys obesus. *Am J Anat* 1981;162:23–33.
331. Kriz W, Schnermann J, Dieterich H. Differences in the morphology of descending limbs of short and long loops of Henle in the rat kidney. In: Wirz H (ed.). *Recent Advances in Renal Physiology*. Basel: Karger, 1972:140–144.
332. Kriz W, Schnermann J, Koepsell H. The position of short and long loops of Henle in the rat kidney. *Z Anat Entwicklungsgesch* 1972; 138: 301–319.
333. Kruger T, Benke D, Eitner F, Lang A, Wirtz M, Hamilton-Williams EE, Engel D, Giese B, Muller-Newen G, Floege J, Kurts C. Identification and functional characterization of dendritic cells in the healthy murine kidney and in experimental glomerulonephritis. *J Am Soc Nephrol* 2004;15:613–621.
334. Kühn K. Basement membrane (type IV) collagen. *Matrix Biol* 1994;14:439–445.
335. Kultz D. Hypertonicity and TonEBP promote development of the renal concentrating system. *Am J Physiol Renal Physiol* 2004;287:F876–877.
336. Küttler T. *Verlauf und histotopographische Beziehungen oberflächlich gelegener Nephrone der Katzenniere*. Heidelberg, 1980.
337. Kyossev Z, Walker PD, Reeves WB. Immunolocalization of NAD-dependent 11 beta-hydroxysteroid dehydrogenase in human kidney and colon. *Kidney Int* 1996;49:271–281.
338. LÃ1/4llmann-Rauch R. Lysosomal storage of sulfated glycosaminoglycans in renal interstitial cells of rats treated with tilorone. *Cell Tissue Res* 1987;250:641–648.
339. Lacy ER, ed. The mammalian renal pelvis: physiological implications from morphometric analyses. *Anat Embryol (Berl)* 1980;160:131–144.
340. Lang F, Capasso G, Schwab M, Waldegger S. Renal tubular transport and the genetic basis of hypertensive disease. *Clin Exp Nephrol* 2005;9:91–99.
341. Layton AT, Pannabecker TL, Dantzler WH, Layton HE. Two modes for concentrating urine in rat inner medulla. *Am J Physiol Renal Physiol* 2004;287:F816–F839.
342. Layton HE. Distribution of Henle's loops may enhance urine concentrating capability. *Biophys J* 1986;49:1033–1040.
343. Le Hir M, Dubach UC. The cellular specificity of lectin binding in the kidney, I: a light microscopical study in the rat. *Histochemistry* 1982;74:521–530.
344. Le Hir M, Dubach UC. The cellular specificity of lectin binding in the kidney, II, a light microscopical study in the rabbit. *Histochemistry* 1982;74:531–540.
345. Le Hir M, Eckardt KU, Kaissling B, Koury ST, Kurtz A. Structure-function correlations in erythropoietin formation and oxygen sensing in the kidney. *Klin Wochensch* 1991;69:567–575.
346. Le Hir M, Hegyi I, Cueni-Loffing D, Loffing J, Kaissling B. Characterization of renal interstitial fibroblast-specific protein 1/S100A4-positive cells in healthy and inflamed rodent kidneys. *Histochem Cell Biol* 2005;123:335–346.
347. Le Hir M, Kaissling B. Distribution and regulation of renal ecto-5'-nucleotidase: implications for physiological functions of adenosine. *Am J Physiol* 1993;264:377–387.

348. Le Hir M, Kaissling B, Dubach UC. Distal tubular segments of the rabbit kidney after adaptation to altered Na- and K-intake. II. Changes in Na-K-ATPase activity. *Cell Tissue Res* 1982;224:493–504.
349. Le Hir M, Kaissling B, Koeppen BM, Wade JB. Binding of peanut lectin to specific epithelial cell types in kidney. *Am J Physiol* 1982;242:F521–530.
350. Lee LK, Pollock AS, Lovett DH. Asymmetric origins of the mature glomerular basement membrane. *J Cell Physiol* 1993;157:169–177.
351. Lee W, Kim RB. Transporters and renal drug elimination. *Ann Rev Pharmacol Toxicol* 2004;44:137–166.
352. LeFurgey A, Tisher CC. Morphology of rabbit collecting duct. *Am J Anat* 1979;155:111–124.
353. Leipziger J. Control of epithelial transport via luminal P2 receptors. *Am J Physiol Renal Physiol* 2003;284:F419–432.
354. Lemley KV, Kriz W. Anatomy of the renal interstitium. *Kidney Int* 1991;39:370–381.
355. Lemley KV, Kriz W. Cycles and separations: the histotopography of the urinary concentrating process. *Kidney Int* 1987:31:538–548.
356. Lemley KV, Kriz W. *Structure and Function of the Renal Vasculature.* Philadelphia: JB Lippincott, 1989.
357. Lethias C, Aubert-Foucher E, Dublet B, Eichenberger D, Font B, Goldschmidt D, Labourdette L, Mazzorana M, van der Rest M. Structure, molecular assembly and tissue distribution of FACIT collagen molecules. *Contrib Nephrol* 1994;107:57–63.
358. Levi M, Arar M, Kaissling B, Murer H, Biber J. Low-Pi diet increases the abundance of an apical protein in rat proximal-tubular S3 segments. *Pflugers Arch Eur J Physio*l 1994;426:5–11, 1994.
359. Levi M, Lotscher M, Sorribas V, Custer M, Arar M, Kaissling B, Murer H, Biber J. Cellular mechanisms of acute and chronic adaptation of rat renal P(i) transporter to alterations in dietary P(i). *Am J Physiol* 1994;267:F900–908.
360. Li C, Ruotsalainen V, Tryggvason K, Shaw AS, Miner JH. CD2AP is expressed with nephrin in developing podocytes and is found widely in mature kidney and elsewhere. *Am J Physiol Renal Physiol* 2000;279:F785–F792.
361. Li Q, Montalbetti N, Shen PY, Dai XQ, Cheeseman CI, Karpinski E, Wu G, Cantiello HF, Chen XZ. Alpha-actinin associates with polycystin-2 and regulates its channel activity. *Hum Mol Genet* 2005;14:1587–1603.
362. Li WY, Huey CL, Yu AS. Expression of claudin-7 and -8 along the mouse nephron. *Am J Physiol Renal Physiol* 2004;286:F1063–1071.
363. Lifton RP, Gharavi AG, Geller DS. Molecular mechanisms of human hypertension. *Cell* 2001;104:545–556.
364. Lin D-H, Sterling H, Wang W-H. The Protein Tyrosone Kinase-Dependent Pathway Mediates the Effect of K Intake on Renal K Secretion. *Physiology* 2005;20:140–146.
365. Liu W, Xu S, Woda C, Kim P, Weinbaum S, Satlin LM. Effect of flow and stretch on the [Ca2+]i response of principal and intercalated cells in cortical collecting duct. *Am J Physiol Renal Physiol* 2003;285:F998–F1012.
366. Ljubojevic M, Herak-Kramberger CM, Hagos Y, Bahn A, Endou H, Burckhardt G, Sabolic I. Rat renal cortical OAT1 and OAT3 exhibit gender differences determined by both androgen stimulation and estrogen inhibition. *Am J Physiol Renal Physiol* 2004;287:F124–138.
367. Lock EA, Reed CJ. Xenobiotic metabolizing enzymes of the kidney. *Toxicol Pathol* 1998;26:18–25.
368. Deleted in proof.
369. Loffing J, Kaissling B. Sodium and calcium transport pathways along the mammalian distal nephron: from rabbit to human. *Am J Physiol Renal Physiol* 2003;284:F628–43.
370. Loffing J, Le Hir M, Kaissling B. Modulation of salt transport rate affects DNA synthesis in vivo in rat renal tubules. *Kidney Int* 1995;47:1615–1623.
371. Loffing J, Loffing-Cueni D, Hegyi I, Kaplan MR, Hebert SC, Le Hir M, Kaissling B. Thaizide treatment of rats provokes apoptosis in distal tubule cells. *Kidney Int* 1996;50:1180–1190.
372. Loffing J, Loffing-Cueni D, Macher A, Hebert SC, Olson B, Knepper MA, Rossier BC, Kaissling B. Localization of epithelial sodium channel and aquaporin-2 in rabbit kidney cortex. *Am J Physiol Renal Physiol* 2000;278:F530–539.
373. Deleted in proof.
374. Deleted in proof.
375. Loffing J, Loffing-Cueni D, Valderrabano V, Klausli L, Hebert SC, Rossier BC, Hoenderop JG, Bindels RJ, Kaissling B, Distribution of transcellular calcium and sodium transport pathways along mouse distal nephron. *Am J Physiol Renal Physiol* 2001;281: F1021–1027.
376. Loffing J, Lotscher M, Kaissling B, Biber J, Murer H, Seikaly M, Alpern RJ, Levi M, Baum M, Moe OW, Renal Na/H exchanger NHE-3 and Na-PO4 cotransporter NaPi-2 protein expression in glucocorticoid excess and deficient states. *J Am Soc Nephrol* 1998;9:1560–1567.
377. Loffing J, Pietri L, Aregger F, Bloch-Faure M, Ziegler U, Meneton P, Rossier BC, Kaissling B. Differential subcellular localization of ENaC subunits in mouse kidney in response to high- and low-Na diets. *Am J Physiol Renal Physiol* 2000;279:F252–258.
378. Loffing J, Summa V, Zecevic M, Verrey F. Mediators of aldosterone action in the renal tubule. *Curr Opin Nephrol Hypertens* 2001;10:667–675.
379. Loffing J, Vallon V, Loffing-Cueni D, Aregger F, Richter K, Pietri L, Bloch-Faure M, Hoenderop JG, Shull GE, Meneton P, Kaissling B. Altered renal distal tubule structure and renal Na(+) and Ca(2+) handling in a mouse model for Gitelman's syndrome. *J Am Soc Nephrol* 2004; 15:2276–2288.
380. Loffing J, Zecevic M, Feraille E, Kaissling B, Asher C, Rossier BC, Firestone GL, Pearce D, Verrey F. Aldosterone induces rapid apical translocation of ENaC in early portion of renal collecting system: possible role of SGK. *Am J Physiol Renal Physiol* 2001:280:F675–682.
381. Lorenz JN, Schultheis PJ, Traynor T, Shull GE, Schnermann J, Micropuncture analysis of single-nephron function in NHE3-deficient mice. *Am J Physiol Renal Physiol* 1999;277: F447–453.
382. Lotscher M, Kaissling B, Biber J, Murer H, Levi M. Role of microtubules in the rapid regulation of renal phosphate transport in response to acute alterations in dietary phosphate content. *J Clin Invest* 1997;99:1302–1312.
383. Lotscher M, Scarpetta Y, Levi M, Halaihel N, Wang H, Zajicek HK, Biber J, Murer H, Kaissling B. Rapid downregulation of rat renal Na/P(i) cotransporter in response to parathyroid hormone involves microtubule rearrangement. *J Clin Invest* 1999;104:483–494.
384. Lu M, Wang T, Yan Q, Wang W, Giebisch G, Hebert SC. ROMK is required for expression of the 70-pS K channel in the thick ascending limb. *Am J Physiol Renal Physiol* 2004;286: F490–495.
385. Luo Y, Vassilev PM, Li X, Kawanabe Y, Zhou J. Native polycystin 2 functions as a plasma membrane Ca2+-permeable cation channel in renal epithelia. *Mol Cell Biol* 2003;23:2600–2607.
386. Lutz MD, Cardinal J, Burg MB. Electrical resistance of renal proximal tubule perfused in vitro. *Am J Physiol* 1973;225:729–734.
387. Madara JL. Regulation of the movement of solutes across tight junctions. In: *Annu Rev Physiol,* 1998.
388. Madjdpour C, Bacic D, Kaissling B, Murer H, Biber J. Segment-specific expression of sodium-phosphate cotransporters NaPi-IIa and -IIc and interacting proteins in mouse renal proximal tubules. *Pflugers Arch* 2004:448:402–410.
389. Madri JA, Roll FJ, Furthmayr H, Foidart JM. Ultrastructural localization of fibronectin and laminin in the basement membranes of the murine kidney, *J Cell Biol* 1980;86: 682–687.
390. Madsen KM, WL, Verlander JW. Structure and function of the inner medullary collecting duct. *Kidney Clapp Int* 1988;34:441–454.
391. Madsen KM, Harris RH, Tisher CC. Uptake and intracellular distribution of ferritin in the rat distal convoluted tubule. *Kidney Int* 1982;21:354–3-61.
392. Madsen KM, Verlander JW, Tisher CC. Relationship between structure and function in distal tubule and collecting duct. *J Electron Microsc Tech* 1988;9:187–208.
393. Majack RA, Paull WK, Barrett JM. The ultrastructural localization of membrane ATPase in rat thin limbs of the loop of Henle. *Histochemistry* 1979;63:23–33.
394. Mak D-OD, Dang B, Weiner ID, Foskett JK, Westhoff CM. Characterization of ammonia transport by the kidney Rh glycoproteins RhBG and RhCG. *Am J Physiol Renal Physiol* 2006;290:F297–305.
395. Mandon B, Nielsen S, Kishore BK, Knepper MA. Expression of syntaxins in rat kidney. *Am J Physiol* 1997;273:F718–F730.
396. Marples D, Schroer TA, Ahrens N, Taylor A, Knepper MA, Nielsen S. Dynein and dynactin colocalize with AQP2 water channels in intracellular vesicles from kidney collecting duct. *Am J Physiol* 1998;274:F384–394.
397. Martin J, Eynstone L, Davies M, Steadman R. Induction of metalloproteinases by glomerular mesangial cells stimulated by proteins of the extracellular matrix. *J Am Soc Nephrol* 2001;12:88–96.
398. Martin J, Steadman R, Knowlden J, Williams J, Davies M. Differential regulation of matrix metalloproteinases and their inhibitors in human glomerular epithelial cells in vitro. *J Am Soc Nephrol* 1998; 9:1629–1637.
399. Martinez-Hernandez A, Chung AE. The ultrastructural localization of two basement membrane components: entactin and laminin in rat tissues. *J Histochem Cytochem* 1984;32:289–298.
400. Martinez-Hernandez A, Gay S, Miller EJ. Ultrastructural localization of type V collagen in rat kidney. *J Cell Biol* 1982;92:343–349.
401. Marxer-Meier A, Hegyi I, Loffing J, Kaissling B. Postnatal maturation of renal cortical peritubular fibroblasts in the rat. *Anat Embryol (Berl)* 1998;197:143–153.
402. Masilamani S, Kim GH, Mitchell C, Wade JB, Knepper MA. Aldosterone-mediated regulation of ENaC alpha, beta, and gamma subunit proteins in rat kidney. *J Clin Invest* 1999;104: R19–23.
403. Matlin KS. Clues to occluding: focus on "knockdown of occludin expression leads to diverse phenotypic alterations in epithelial cells." *Am J Physiol Cell Physiol* 2005;288: C1191–1192.
404. Matsumoto T, Fejes-Toth G, Schwartz GJ. Postnatal differentiation of rabbit collecting duct intercalated cells. *Pediatr Res* 1996;39:1–12.
405. Matsumoto T, Fejes-Toth G, Schweartz GJ. Developmental expression of acid-base-related proteins in the rabbit kidney. *Pediatric Nephrol* 1993;7:792–799.
406. Maunsbach AB. Functional ultrastructure of the proximal tubule. In: Windhager E (ed.). *Handbook of Physiology: Section on Renal Physiology.* New York: Oxford University, 1992: 41–108.
407. Maunsbach AB. Observations on the segmentation of the proximal tubule in the rat kidney. Comparison of results from phase contrast, fluorescence and electron microscopy. *J Ultrastruct Res* 1966;16:239–258.
408. Maunsbach AB, Marples D, Chin E, Ning G, Bondy C, Agre P, Nielsen S. Aquaporin-1 water channel expression in human kidney. *J Am Soc Nephrol* 1997;8:1–14.
409. Maxwell PH, Ferguson DJ, Nicholls LG, Johnson MH, Ratcliffe PJ. The interstitial response to renal injury: fibroblast-like cells show phenotypic changes and have reduced potential for erythropoietin gene expression. *Kidney Int* 1997;52:715–724.
410. Maxwell PH, Osmond MK, Pugh CW, Heryet A, Nicholls LG, Tan CC, Doe BG, Ferguson DJ, Johnson MH, Ratcliffe PJ. Identification of the renal erythropoietin-producing cells using transgenic mice. *Kidney Int* 1993;44:1149 –1162.
411. Mbassa G, Elger M, Kriz W. The ultrastructural organization of the basement membrane of Bowman's capsule in the rat renal corpuscle. *Cell Tissue Res* 1988;253:151–163.
412. McCulloch F, Chambrey R, Eladari D, Peti-Peterdi J. Localization of connexin 30 in the luminal membrane of cells in the distal nephron. *Am J Physiol Renal Physiol* 2005;289: F1304–1312.
413. McCulloch F, Chambrey R, Eladari D, Peti-Peterdi J. Localization of connexin 30 in the luminal membrane of cells in the distal nephron. *Am J Physiol Renal Physiol* 2005;89: F1304–1312.
414. McDonough AA, Biemesderfer D. Does membrane trafficking play a role in regulating the sodium/hydrogen exchanger isoform 3 in the proximal tubule? *Curr Opin Nephrol Hypertens* 2003;12:533–541.
415. McDonough AA, Leong PK, Yang LE. Mechanisms of pressure natriuresis: how blood pressure regulates renal sodium transport. *Ann N Y Acad Sci* 2003;986:669–677.

416. Meade P, Hoover RS, Plata C, Vazquez N, Bobadilla NA, Gamba G, Hebert SC. cAMP-dependent activation of the renal-specific Na+-K+-2Cl- cotransporter is mediated by regulation of cotransporter trafficking. *Am J Physiol Renal Physiol* 2003;284:F1145–1154.

417. Meij IC, Koenderink JB, De Jong JC, De Pont JJ, Monnens LA, Van Den Heuvel LP, Knoers NV. Dominant isolated renal magnesium loss is caused by misrouting of the Na+,K+-ATPase gamma-subunit. *Ann N Y Acad Sci* 2003;986:437–443.

418. Melander O, Orho-Melander M, Bengtsson K, Lindblad U, Rastam L, Groop L, Hulthen UL. Genetic variants of thiazide-sensitive NaCl-cotransporter in Gitelman's syndrome and primary hypertension. *Hypertension* 2000;36:389–394.

419. Meneton P. Comparative roles of the renal apical sodium transport systems in blood pressure control. *J Am Soc Nephrol* 2000;11(Suppl 16):S135–139.

420. Meneton P, Loffing J, Warnock DG. Sodium and potassium handling by the aldosterone-sensitive distal nephron: the pivotal role of the distal and connecting tubule. *Am J Physiol Renal Fl Electrol Physiol* 2004;287:F593–601.

421. Milton AE, Weiner ID. Regulation of B-type intercalated cell apical anion exchange activity by CO2/HCO3. *Am J Physiol* 1998;274:F1086–F1094.

422. Miner JH. Building the glomerulus: a matricentric view. *J Am Soc Nephrol* 2005;16:857–861.

423. Miner JH. Developmental biology of glomerular basement membrane components. *Curr Opin Nephrol Hypertens* 1998;7:13–19.

424. Miner JH. Renal basement membrane components. *Kidney Int* 1999; 56:2016–2024.

425. Miner JH, Yurchenco PD. Laminin functions in tissue morphogenesis. *Annu Rev Cell Dev Biol* 2004;20:255–284.

426. Mitic LL, Anderson JM. Molecular architecture of tight junctions. *Annu Rev Physiol* 1998; 121–142.

427. Moestrup SK, Nielsen LB. The role of the kidney in lipid metabolism. *Curr Opin Lipidol* 2005;16:301–306.

428. Moffat D. *The Mammalian Kidney*. London: Cambridge University, 1975.

429. Moffat DB, Fourman J. The vascular pattern of the rat kidney. *J Anat* 1963;97:543-553.

430. Molitoris BA, Sandoval RM. Intravital multiphoton microscopy of dynamic renal processes. *Am J Physiol Renal Physiol* 2005;288:F1084–1089.

431. Molony DA, Reeves WB, Hebert SC, Andreoli TE. ADH increases apical Na+, K+, 2Cl- entry in mouse medullary thick ascending limbs of Henle. *Am J Physiol* 1987;252:F177–187.

432. Morel F, Chabardes D, Imbert-Teboul M. Heterogeneity of hormonal control in the distal nephron. In: Barcelo R (ed.). *Proceedings of the VII International Congress of Nephrology*. Basel: Karger, 1978; 209–216.

433. Morel F, Imbert-Teboul M, Chabardes D. Receptors to vasopressin and other hormones in the mammalian kidney. *Kidney Int* 1987; 31:512–520.

434. Muirhead EE. Discovery of the renomedullary system of blood pressure control and its hormones. *Hypertension* 1990;15:114–116.

435. Mundel P, Bachmann S, Bader M, Fischer A, Kummer W, Mayer B, Kriz W. Expression of nitric oxide synthase in kidney macula densa cells. *Kidney Int* 1992;42:1017–1019.

436. Mundel P, Elger M, Sakai T, Kriz W. Microfibrils are a major component of the mesangial matrix in the glomerulus of the rat kidney. *Cell Tissue Res* 1988;254:183–187.

437. Mundel P, Heid HW, Mundel TM, Kruger M, Reiser J, Kriz W. Synaptopodin: an actin-associated protein in telencephalic dendrites and renal podocytes. *J Cell Biol* 1997;139: 193–204.

438. Mundel P, Kriz W. Structure and function of podocytes: an update. *Anat Embryol (Berl)* 1995;192:385–397.

439. Mundel P, Reiser J, Zuniga Mejia Borja A, Pavenstadt H, Davidson GR, Kriz W, Zeller R. Rearrangements of the cytoskeleton and cell contacts induce process formation during differentiation of conditionally immortalized mouse podocyte cell lines. *Exp Cell Res* 1997; 236: 248–258.

440. Murakami T, Miyoshi M, Fujita T. Glomerular vessels of the rat kidney with special reference to double efferent arterioles. A scanning electron microscope study of corrosion casts. *Arch Histol Jpn* 1971;33:179–198.

441. Murer H, Hernando N, Forster I, Biber J. Regulation of Na/Pi transporter in the proximal tubule. *Annu Rev Physiol* 2003;65:531–542.

442. Myers CE, Bulger RE, Tisher CC, Trump BF. Human ultrastructure, IV: collecting duct of healthy individuals. *Lab Invest* 1966;15:1921–1950.

443. Nagai J, Christensen EI, Morris SM, Willnow TE, Cooper JA, Nielsen R. Mutually dependent localization of megalin and Dab2 in the renal proximal tubule. *Am J Physiol Renal Physiol* 2005;289:F569–576.

444. Nagle RB, Altschuler EM, Dobyan DC, Dong S, Bulger RE. The ultrastructure of the thin limbs of Henle in kidneys of the desert heteromyid (*Perognathus penicillatus*). *Am J Anat* 1981;161:33–47.

445. Narbaitz R, Vandorpe D, Levine DZ. Differentiation of renal intercalated cells in fetal and postnatal rats. *Anat Embryol (Berl)* 1991;183:353–361

446. Nauli SM, Alenghat FJ, Luo Y, Williams E, Vassilev P, Li X, Elia AE, Lu W, Brown EM, Quinn SJ, Ingber DE, Zhou J. Polycystins 1 and 2 mediate mechanosensation in the primary cilium of kidney cells. *Nat Genet* 2003;33:129–137.

447. Nelson WJ, Nusse R. Convergence of Wnt, beta-catenin, and cadherin pathways. *Science* 2004;303:1483–1487.

448. Nicco C, Wittner M, DiStefano A, Jounier S, Bankir L, Bouby N. Chronic exposure to vasopressin upregulates ENaC and sodium transport in the rat renal collecting duct and lung. *Hypertension* 2001;38:1143–1149.

449. Nicholes BK, Krakower CA, Greenspon SA. The chemically isolated lamina densa of the renal glomerulus. *Proc Soc Exp Biol Med* 1973;142:1316–1321.

450. Nicoletta JA, Schwartz GJ. Distal renal tubular acidosis. *Curr Opin Pediatr* 2004;16:194–198.

451. Nielsen J, Kwon T-H, Praetorius J, Frokiaer J, Knepper MA, Nielsen S. Aldosterone increases urine production and decreases apical AQP2 expression in rats with diabetes insipidus. *Am J Physiol Renal Physiol* 2006;290: F438–449.

452. Nielsen S. Renal aquaporins: an overview. *Br J Urol Int* 2002;90(Suppl 3)1–6.

453. Nielsen S, Chou CL, Marples D, Christensen EI, Kishore BK, Knepper MA. Vasopressin increases water permeability of kidney collecting duct by inducing translocation of aquaporin-CD water channels to plasma membrane. *Proc Natl Acad Sci U S A* 1995;92: 1013–1017.

454. Nielsen S, DiGiovanni SR, Christensen EI, Knepper MA, Harris HW. Cellular and subcellular immunolocalization of vasopressin-regulated water channel in rat kidney. *Proc Natl Acad Sci U S A* 1993; 90:11663–11667.

455. Nielsen S, Frokiaer J, Marples D, Kwon TH, Agre P, Knepper MA. Aquaporins in the kidney: from molecules to medicine. *Physiol Rev* 2002;82:205–244.

456. Nielsen S, Knepper MA. Vasopressin activates collecting duct urea transporters and water channels by distinct physical processes. *Am J Physiol* 1993;265:F204-213.

457. Nielsen S, Kwon TH, Christensen BM, Promeneur D, Frokiaer J, Marples D. Physiology and pathophysiology of renal aquaporins. *J Am Soc Nephrol* 1999;10:647–663.

458. Nielsen S, Maunsbach AB, Ecelbarger CA, Knepper MA. Ultrastructural localization of Na-K-2Cl cotransporter in thick ascending limb and macula densa of rat kidney. *Am J Physiol* 1998;275:F885–893.

459. Nielsen S, Pallone T, Smith BL, Christensen EI, Agre P, Maunsbach AB. Aquaporin-1 water channels in short and long loop descending thin limbs and in descending vasa recta in rat kidney. *Am J Physiol* 1995;268:F1023–F1037.

460. Nijenhuis T, Renkema KY, Hoenderop JGJ, Bindels RJM. Acid-base status determines the renal expression of Ca2+ and Mg2+ transport proteins. *J Am Soc Nephrol* 2006;17: 617–626.

461. Nishio S, Hatano M, Nagata M, Horie S, Koike T, Tokuhisa T, Mochizuki T. Pkd1 regulates immortalized proliferation of renal tubular epithelial cells through p53 induction and JNK activation. *J Clin Invest* 2005;115:910–918.

462. Noonan DM, Fulle A, Valente P, Cai S, Horigan E, Sasaki M, Yamada Y, Hassell JR. The complete sequence of perlecan, a basement membrane heparan sulfate proteoglycan, reveals extensive similarity with laminin A chain, low density lipoprotein-receptor, and the neural cell adhesion molecule. *J Biol Chem* 1991;266:22939–22947.

463. Obermuller N, Gretz N, Kriz W, Reilly RF, Witzgall R. The swelling-activated chloride channel ClC-2, the chloride channel ClC-3, and ClC-5, a chloride channel mutated in kidney stone disease, are expressed in distinct subpopulations of renal epithelial cells. *J Clin Invest* 1998;101:635–642.

464. Obermuller N, Kunchaparty S, Ellison DH, Bachmann S. Expression of the Na-K-2Cl cotransporter by macula densa and thick ascending limb cells of rat and rabbit nephron. *J Clin Invest* 1996; 98:635–640.

465. Oliver J. *Nephrons and Kidneys*. New York: Harper & Row, Hoeber Medical, 1968.

466. Omata K, Carretero OA, Scicli AG, Jackson BA. Localization of active and inactive kallikrein (kininogenase activity) in the microdissected rabbit nephron. *Kidney Int* 1982;22: 602–607.

467. Deleted in proof.

468. Orci L, Brown D. Distribution of filipin-sterol complexes in plasma membranes of the kidney, II: the thin limbs of Henle's loop. *Lab Invest* 1983;48:80–89.

469. Orlando RA, Rader K, Authier F, Yamazaki H, Posner BI, Bergeron JJ, Farquhar MG. Megalin is an endocytic receptor for insulin. *J Am Soc Nephrol* 1998;9:1759–1766.

470. Ortiz PA. cAMP increases surface expression of NKCC2 in rat thick ascending limbs: role of VAMP. *Am J Physiol Renal Physiol* 2006;290: F608–616

471. Osathanondh V, Potter EL. Development of human kidney as shown by microdissection, III: formation and interrelationship of collecting tubules and nephrons. *Arch Pathol* 1963;76:290–302.

472. Osswald H, Nabakowski G, Hermes H. Adenosine as a possible mediator of metabolic control of glomerular filtration rate. *Int J Biochem* 1980;12:263–267.

473. Osterby R. Morphometric studies of the peripheral glomerular basement membrane in early juvenile diabetes, I: development of initial basement membrane thickening. *Diabetologia* 1972;8:84–92.

474. Pallone TL, Turner MR, Edwards A, Jamison RL. Countercurrent exchange in the renal medulla. *Am J Physiol Regul Integr Comp Physiol* 2003;284:R1153–R1175.

475. Pannabecker TL, Abbott DE, Dantzler WH. Three-dimensional functional reconstruction of inner medullary thin limbs of Henle's loop. *Am J Physiol Renal Physiol* 2004;286:F38–F45.

476. Pannabecker TL, Dahlmann A, Brokl OH, Dantzler WH. Mixed descending- and ascending-type thin limbs of Henle's loop in mammalian renal inner medulla. *Am J Physiol Renal Physiol* 2000;278:F202–F208.

477. Pannabecker TL, Dantzler WH. Three-dimensional lateral and vertical relationships of inner medullary loops of Henle and collecting ducts. *Am J Physiol Renal Physiol* 2004;287:F767–F774.

478. Parysek LM, Wolosewick JJ, Olmsted JB. MAP 4: a microtubule-associated protein specific for a subset of tissue microtubules. *J Cell Biol* 1984;99:2287–2296.

479. Pavenstadt H, Kriz W, Kretzler M. Cell biology of the glomerular podocyte. *Physiol Rev* 2003;83:253–307.

480. Pedersen J, Persson A, Maunsbach AB. Ultrastructure and quantitative characterization of the cortical interstitium in the rat kidney. In: Maunsbach AB (ed.). *Functional Ultrastructure of the Kidney*. London: Academic Press, 1980:443–457.

481. Persson AE, Ollerstam A, Liu R, Brown R. Mechanisms for macula densa cell release of renin. *Acta Physiol Scand* 2004;181:471–474.

482. Peter K. *Untersuchungen über Bau und Entwicklung der Niere*. Jena: Gustav Fischer, 1909.

483. Deleted in proof.

484. Deleted in proof.

485. Peti-Peterdi J, Komlosi P, Fuson AL, Guan Y, Schneider A, Qi Z, Redha R, Rosivall L, Breyer MD, Bell PD. Luminal NaCl delivery regulates basolateral PGE2 release from macula densa cells. *J Clin Invest* 2003;112:76–82.

486. Petrovic S, Wang Z, Ma L, Soleimani M. Regulation of the apical Cl-/HCO-3 exchanger pendrin in rat cortical collecting duct in metabolic acidosis. *Am J Physiol Renal Physiol* 2003;284:F103–112.

487. Deleted in proof.

488. Pfaller W. Structure function correlation on rat kidney. Quantitative correlation of structure and function in the normal and injured rat kidney. *Adv Anat Embryol Cell Biol* 1982;70:1–106.

488a. Piepenhagen PA and Nelson WJ. Differential expression of cell-cell and cell-substratum adhesion proteins along the kidney nephron. *Am J Physiol* 1995;269:C1433–1449.

488b. Piepenhagen PA, Peters LL, Lux SE, and Nelson WJ. Differential expression of Na(+)-K(+)-ATPase, ankyrin, fodrin, and E-cadherin along the kidney nephron. *Am J Physiol* 1995;269:C1417–1432.

489. Pham PC, Devuyst O, Pham PT, Matsumoto N, Shih RN, Jo OD, Yanagawa N, Sun AM. Hypertonicity increases CLC-5 expression in mouse medullary thick ascending limb cells. *Am J Physiol Renal Fuidl Electr Physiol* 2004;287:F747–752.

490. Picard N, Van Abel M, Campone C, Seiler M, Bloch-Faure M, Hoenderop JG, Loffing J, Meneton P, Bindels RJ, Paillard M, Alhenc-Gelas F, Houillier P. Tissue kallikrein-deficient mice display a defect in renal tubular calcium absorption. *J Am Soc Nephrol* 2005; 16: 3602–3610.

491. Deleted in proof.

492. Pitcock JA, Lyons H, Brown PS, Rightsel WA, Muirhead EE. Glycosaminoglycans of the rat renomedullary interstitium: ultrastructural and biochemical observations. *Exp Mol Pathol* 1988;49:373–387.

493. Postlethwaite A, Kang A. Fibroblasts and matrix proteins. In: Gallin J (ed.). *Inflammation: Basic Principles and Clinical Correlates.* New York: Raven Press, 1992;747–773.

494. Pradervand S, Vandewalle A, Bens M, Gautschi I, Loffing J, Hummler E, Schild L, Rossier BC. Dysfunction of the epithelial sodium channel expressed in the kidney of a mouse model for Liddle syndrome. *J Am Soc Nephrol* 2003;14: 2219–2228.

494a. Prozialeck WC, Lamar PC, and Appelt DM. Differential expression of E-cadherin, N-cadherin and beta-catenin in proximal and distal segments of the rat nephron. *BMC Physiol* 2004;4:10.

495. Pushkin A, Kurtz I. SLC4 base (HCO_3^-, CO32-) transporters: classification, function, structure, genetic diseases, and knockout models. *Am J Physiol Renal Physiol* 2006;290: F580–599.

496. Quamme GA, de Rouffignac C. Epithelial magnesium transport and regulation by the kidney. *Front Biosci* 2000;5:D694–711.

497. Quentin F, Chambrey R, Trinh-Trang-Tan MM, Fysekidis M, Cambillau M, Paillard M, Aronson PS, Eladari D. The Cl−/HCO3− exchanger pendrin in the rat kidney is regulated in response to chronic alterations in chloride balance. *Am J Physiol Renal Physiol* 2004;287: F1179–1188.

498. Quentin F, Eladari D, Cheval L, Lopez C, Goossens D, Colin Y, Cartron J-P, Paillard M, Chambrey R. RhBG and RhCG, the putative ammonia transporters, are expressed in the same cells in the distal nephron. *J Am Soc Nephrol* 2003;14:545–554.

500. Quentin F, Eladari D, Frische S, Cambillau M, Nielsen S, Alper SL, Paillard M, Chambrey R. Regulation of the Cl-/HCO_3^- Exchanger AE2 in rat thick ascending limb of Henle's loop in response to changes in acid-base and sodium balance. *J Am Soc Nephrol* 2004; 15:2988–2997.

501. Raats CJ, van den Born J, Bakker MA, Oppers-Walgreen B, Pisa BJ, Dijkman HB, Assmann KJ, Berden JH. Expression of agrin, dystroglycan, and utrophin in normal renal tissue and in experimental glomerulopathies. *Am J Pathol* 2000;156:1749–1765.

502. Rafey MA, Lipkowitz MS, Leal-Pinto E, Abramson RG. Uric acid transport. *Curr Opin Nephrol Hypertens* 2003;12:511–516.

503. Reale E, Luciano L. The laminae rarae of the glomerular basement membrane. Their manifestation depends on the histochemical and histological techniques. *Contrib Nephrol* 1990;80:32–40.

504. Reddi AS. Metabolism of glomerular basement membrane in normal, hypophysectomized, and growth-hormone-treated diabetic rats. *Exp Mol Pathol* 1985;43:196–208.

505. Regel J. *Comparative Physiology of Renal Excretion.* New York: Hafner, 1972.

506. Regele HM, Fillipovic E, Langer B, Poczewki H, Kraxberger I, Bittner RE, Kerjaschki D. Glomerular expression of dystroglycans is reduced in minimal change nephrosis but not in focal segmental glomerulosclerosis. *J Am Soc Nephrol* 2000;11:403–412.

507. Reilly RF, Ellison DH. Mammalian distal tubule: physiology, pathophysiology, and molecular anatomy. *Physiol Rev* 2000;80:277–313.

508. Reiser J, Kriz W, Kretzler M, Mundel P. The glomerular slit diaphragm is a modified adherens junction. *J Am Soc Nephrol* 2000; 11:1–8.

509. Reiser J, Polu KR, Moller CC, Kenlan P, Altintas MM, Wei C, Faul C, Herbert S, Villegas I, Avila-Casado C, McGee M, Sugimoto H, Brown D, Kalluri R, Mundel P, Smith PL, Clapham DE, Pollak MR. TRPC6 is a glomerular slit diaphragm-associated channel required for normal renal function. *Nat Genet* 2005;37:739 –744.

510. Reissinger A, Ludwig M, Utsch B, Promse A, Baulmann J, Weisser B, Vetter H, Kramer HJ, Bokemeyer D. Novel NCCT gene mutations as a cause of Gitelman's syndrome and a systematic review of mutant and polymorphic NCCT alleles. *Kidney Blood Press Res* 2002;25:354–362.

511. Riccardi D, Hall AE, Chattopadhyay N, Xu JZ, Brown EM, Hebert SC. Localization of the extracellular Ca2+/polyvalent cation-sensing protein in rat kidney. *Am J Physiol* 1998;274: F611–622.

512. Riccardi D, Lee WS, Lee K, Segre GV, Brown EM, Hebert SC. Localization of the extracellular Ca(2+)-sensing receptor and PTH/PTHrP receptor in rat kidney. *Am J Physiol* 1996;271:F951–956.

513. Ridderstrale Y, Wistrand PJ, Tashian RE. Membrane-associated carbonic anhydrase activity in the kidney of CA II-deficient mice. *J Histochem Cytochem* 1992;40:1665–1673.

514. Ritthaler T, Traebert M, Lotscher M, Biber J, Murer H, Kaissling B. Effects of phosphate intake on distribution of type II Na/Pi cotransporter mRNA in rat kidney. *Kidney Int* 1999;55:976–983.

515. Rodewald R, Karnovsky MJ. Porous substructure of the glomerular slit diaphragm in the rat and mouse. *J Cell Biol* 1974;60:423–433.

516. Rodman JS, Mooseker M, Farquhar MG. Cytoskeletal proteins of the rat kidney proximal tubule brush border. *Eur J Cell Biol* 1986;42:319–327.

517. Rollhaeuser H, Kriz W, Heinke W. [the Vascular System of the Rat Kidney.]. *Z Zellforsch Mikrosk Anat* 1964;64:381–403.

518. Rossier BC, Pradervand S, Schild L, Hummler E. Epithelial sodium channel and the control of sodium balance: interaction between genetic and environmental factors. *Annu Rev Physiol* 2002;64:877–897.

519. Rostgaard J. Electron microscopy of filaments in the basal part of rat kidney tubule cells, and their in situ interaction with heavy meromyosin. *Z Zellforsch Mikrosk Anat* 1972;132:497–521.

520. Rostgaard J, Qvortrup K. Sieve plugs in fenestrae of glomerular capillaries—site of the filtration barrier? *Cells Tissues Organs* 2002; 170:132–138.

521. Rostgaard J, Thuneberg L. Electron microscopic evidence suggesting a contractile system in the base of tubular cells of rat kidney. *J Ultrastruct Res* 1969;29:570.

522. Roth J, Taatjes DJ. Glycocalix heterogeneity of rat kidney urinary tubule: Demonstration with lecitin-gold technique specific for sialic acid. *Eur J Cell Biol* 1985;39:449–457.

523. Royaux IE, Wall SM, Karniski LP, Everett LA, Suzuki K, Knepper MA, Green ED. Pendrin, encoded by the Pendred syndrome gene, resides in the apical region of renal intercalated cells and mediates bicarbonate secretion. *Proc Natl Acad Sci U S A* 2001;98: 4221–4226.

524. Rubera I, Loffing J, Palmer LG, Frindt G, Fowler-Jaeger N, Sauter D, Carroll T, McMahon A, Hummler E, Rossier BC. Collecting duct-specific gene inactivation of alphaENaC in the mouse kidney does not impair sodium and potassium balance. *J Clin Invest* 2002;112:554–565.

525. Ruotsalainen V, Ljungberg P, Wartiovaara J, Lenkkeri U, Kestila M, Jalanko H, Holmberg C, Tryggvason K. Nephrin is specifically located at the slit diaphragm of glomerular podocytes. *Proc Natl Acad Sci U S A* 1999;96:7962–7967.

526. Ryan GB, Coghlan JP, Scoggins BA. The granulated peripolar epithelial cell: a potential secretory component of the renal juxtaglomerular complex. *Nature* 1979;277:655–656.

527. Rybak JN, Ettorre A, Kaissling B, Giavazzi R, Neri D, Elia G. In vivo protein biotinylation for identification of organ-specific antigens accessible from the vasculature. *Nat Methods* 2005;2:291–298.

528. Sabolic I, Herak-Kramberger CM, Breton S, Brown D. Na/K-ATPase in intercalated cells along the rat nephron revealed by antigen retrieval. *J Am Soc Nephrol* 1999;10:913–922.

529. Sabolic I, Skarica M, Gorboulev V, Ljubojevic M, Balen D, Herak-Kramberger CM, Koepsell H. Rat renal glucose transporter SGLT1 exhibits zonal distribution and androgen-dependent gender differences. *Am J Physiol Renal Physiol* 2005;270:.

530. Sabolic I, Valenti G, Verbavatz JM, Van Hoek AN, Verkman AS, Ausiello DA, Brown D. Localization of the CHIP28 water channel in rat kidney. *Am J Physiol* 1992;263:C1225–C1233.

531. Saito A, Pietromonaco S, Loo AK, Farquhar MG. Complete cloning and sequencing of rat gp330/"megalin," a distinctive member of the low density lipoprotein receptor gene family. *Proc Natl Acad Sci U S A* 1994;91:9725–9729.

532. Sakai T, Kriz W. The structural relationship between mesangial cells and basement membrane of the renal glomerulus. *Anat Embryol (Berl)* 1987;176:373–386.

533. Samuel T, Hoy WE, Douglas-Denton R, Hughson MD, Bertram JF. Determinants of glomerular volume in different cortical zones of the human kidney. *J Am Soc Nephrol* 2005;16:3102 –3109.

534. Sanden W, Elger M, Mundel P, Kriz W. The architecture of podocyte cytoskeleton suggests a role in glomerular filtration dynamics. *Ann Anat* 1995;177:44–45.

535. Sappino AP, Schurch W, Gabbiani G. Differentiation repertoire of fibroblastic cells: expression of cytoskeletal proteins as marker of phenotypic modulations. *Lab Invest* 1990;63:144–161.

536. Sariola H, Timpl R, von der Mark K, Mayne R, Fitch JM, Linsenmayer TF, Ekblom P. Dual origin of glomerular basement membrane. *Dev Biol* 1984;101:86–96.

537. Satchell SC, Anderson KL, Mathieson PW. Angiopoietin 1 and vascular endothelial growth factor modulate human glomerular endothelial cell barrier properties. *J Am Soc Nephrol* 2004;15:566–574.

538. Satlin LM, Schwartz GJ. Cellular remodeling of HCO3(−)-secreting cells in rabbit renal collecting duct in response to an acidic environment. *J Cell Biol* 1989;109:1279–1288.

539. Satoh J, Romero MF. Mg2+ transport in the kidney. Biometals. Vol. 15, pp. 285-95, 2002.

540. Savage CO. The biology of the glomerulus: endothelial cells. *Kidney Int* 1994;45:314–319.

541. Sawada H, Stukenbrok H, Kerjaschki D, Farquhar MG. Epithelial polyanion (podocalyxin) is found on the sides but not the soles of the foot processes of the glomerular epithelium. *Am J Pathol* 1986;125:309–318.

542. Schaefer L, Grone HJ, Raslik I, Robenek H, Ugorcakova J, Budny S, Schaefer RM, Kresse H. Small proteoglycans of normal adult human kidney: distinct expression patterns of decorin, biglycan, fibromodulin, and lumican. *Kidney Int* 2000;58:1557–1568.

543. Schafer JA. Abnormal regulation of ENaC: syndromes of salt retention and salt wasting by the collecting duct. *Am J Physiol Renal Physiol* 2002;283:F221–235.

544. Schaub TP, Kartenbeck J, Konig J, Vogel O, Witzgall R, Kriz W, Keppler D. Expression of the conjugate export pump encoded by the mrp2 gene in the apical membrane of kidney proximal tubules. *J Am Soc Nephrol* 1997;8:1213–1221.

545. Schiebler TH, Danner KG. The effect of sex hormones on the proximal tubules in the rat kidney. *Cell Tissue Res* 1978;192:527–549.

546. Schiffer M, Schiffer LE, Gupta A, Shaw AS, Roberts IS, Mundel P, Bottinger EP. Inhibitory smads and tgf-Beta signaling in glomerular cells. *J Am Soc Nephrol* 2002;13:2657–2666.

547. Schild L. The epithelial sodium channel: from molecule to disease. *Rev Physiol Biochem Pharmacol* 2004;151:92–106.

548. Schiller A, Forssmann WG, Taugner R. The tight junctions of renal tubules in the cortex and outer medulla. A quantitative study of the kidneys of six species. *Cell Tissue Res* 1980;12:395–413.

549. Schiller A, Taugner R. Heterogeneity of tight junctions along the collecting duct in the renal medulla. A freeze-fracture study in rat and rabbit. *Cell Tissue Res* 1982;223:603–614.

550. Schiller A, Taugner R. Junctions between interstitial cells of the renal medulla: a freeze-fracture study. *Cell Tissue Res* 1979;203:231–240.

551. Schiller A, Taugner R, Kriz W. The thin limbs of Henle's loop in the rabbit: a freeze fracture study. *Cell Tissue Res* 1980;207:249–265.

552. Schlingmann KP, Gudermann T. A critical role of TRPM channel-kinase for human magnesium transport. *J Physiol* 2005;566:301–308.

553. Schmidt-Nielsen B. Organ *Systems in Adaption: The Excretory System—Handbook of Physiology.* Washington, D.C.: American Physiological Society, 1964:215–243.

554. Schmidt-Nielsen B, O'Dell R. Structure and concentrating mechanism in the mammalian kidney. *Am J Physiol* 1961;200:1119–1124.

555. Schmidt-Nielsen B, Pfeiffer EW. Urea and urinary concentrating ability in the mountain beaver *Aplodontia rufa*. *Am J Physiol* 1970; 218:1370–1375.

556. Schmitt R, Ellison DH, Farman N, Rossier BC, Reilly RF, Reeves WB, Oberbaumer I, Tapp R, Bachmann S. Developmental expression of sodium entry pathways in rat nephron. *Am J Physiol* 1999;276:F367–F381.

557. Schnabel E, Anderson JM, Farquhar MG. The tight junction protein ZO-1 is concentrated along slit diaphragms of the glomerular epithelium. *J Cell Biol* 1990;111:1255–1263.

558. Schneeberger EE, Lynch RD. The tight junction: a multifunctional complex. *Am J Physiol Cell Physiol* 2004;286:C1213–C1228.

559. Schnermann J. Sodium transport deficiency and sodium balance in gene-targeted mice. *Acta Physiol Scand* 2001;173:59–66.

560. Schnermann J, Chou CL, Ma T, Traynor T, Knepper MA, Verkman AS. Defective proximal tubular fluid reabsorption in transgenic aquaporin-1 null mice. *Proc Natl Acad Sci U S A* 1998;95:9660–9664.

561. Schnermann J, Levine DZ. Paracrine factors in tubuloglomerular feedback: adenosine, ATP, and nitric oxide. *Annu Rev Physiol* 2003;65:501–529.

562. Schonheyder H, Maunsbach AB. Ultrastructure of a specialized neck region in the rabbit nephron. *Kidney Int* 1975;7:145–153.

563. Schultheis PJ, Lorenz JN, Meneton P, Nieman ML, Riddle TM, Flagella M, Duffy JJ, Doetschman T, Miller ML, Shull GE. Phenotype resembling Gitelman's syndrome in mice lacking the apical Na+−Cl− cotransporter of the distal convoluted tubule. *J Biol Chem* 1998;273:29150–29155.

564. Schurek HJ, Jost U, Baumgartl H, Bertram H, Heckmann U. Evidence for a preglomerular oxygen diffusion shunt in rat renal cortex. *Am J Physiol* 1990;259:F910–F915.

565. Schwaderer AL, Vijayakumar S, Al-Awqati Q, Schwartz GJ. Galectin-3 expression is induced in renal beta-intercalated cells during metabolic acidosis. *Am J Physiol Renal Physiol* 2006;290:F148–158.

566. Schwartz E, Goldfischer S, Coltoff-Schiller B, Blumenfeld OO. Extracellular matrix microfibrils are composed of core proteins coated with fibronectin. *J Histochem Cyto Chem* 1985; 33:268–274.

567. Schwartz GJ, Satlin LM. Fluorescent characterization of intercalated cells in the rabbit renal cortical collecting duct. *Semin Nephrol* 1989;9:79–82.

568. Schwartz GJ, Winkler CA, Zavilowitz BJ, Bargiello T. Carbonic anhydrase II mRNA is induced in rabbit kidney cortex during chronic metabolic acidosis. *Am J Physiol* 1993;265:F764–F772.

569. Schwartz MM, Karnovsky MJ, Vehkatachalam MA. Ultrastructural differences between rat inner medullary descending and ascending vasa recta. *Lab Invest* 1976;35:161–170.

570. Schwartz MM, Vehkatachalam MA. Structural differences in thin limbs of Henle: physiological implications. *Kidney Int* 1974;6:193–208.

571. Schwarz K, Simons M, Reiser J, Saleem MA, Faul C, Kriz W, Shaw AS, Holzman LB, Mundel P. Podocin, a raft-associated component of the glomerular slit diaphragm, interacts with CD2AP and nephrin. *J Clin Invest* 2001;108:1621–1629.

572. Schweda F, Kurtz A. Cellular mechanism of renin release. *Acta Physiol Scand* 2004;181: 383–390.

573. Seiler MW, Rennke HG, Venkatachalam MA, Cotran RS. Pathogenesis of polycation-induced alterations ("fusion") of glomerular epithelium. *Lab Invest* 1977;36:48–61.

574. Sekine T, Miyazaki H, Endou H. Molecular physiology of renal organic anion transporters. *Am J Physiol Renal Physiol* 2006;297:F251–261.

575. Serafini-Cessi F, Malagolini N, Cavallone D. Tamm-Horsfall glycoprotein: biology and clinical relevance. *Am J Kidney Dis* 2003;42:658–676.

576. Seshadri RM, Klein JD, Kozlowski S, Sands JM, Kim Y-H, Han K-H, Handlogten ME, Verlander JW, Weiner ID. Renal expression of the ammonia transporters, Rhbg and Rhcg, in response to chronic metabolic acidosis. *Am J Physiol Renal Physiol* 2006;290:F397–408.

577. Shayakul C, Knepper MA, Smith CP, DiGiovanni SR, Hediger MA. Segmental localization of urea transporter mRNAs in rat kidney. *Am J Physiol* 1997;272:F654–F660.

578. Sheehan HL, Davis JC. Anatomy of the pelvis in the rabbit kidney. *J Anat* 1959;93:499–502.

579. Silver RB, Frindt G, Mennitt P, Satlin LM. Characterization and regulation of H-K-ATPase in intercalated cells of rabbit cortical collecting duct. *J Exp Zool* 1997;279:443–455.

580. Simionescu N. Cellular aspects of transcapillary exchange. *Physiol Rev* 1983;63: 1536–1579.

581. Simon DB, Lu Y, Choate KA, Velazquez H, Al-Sabban E, Praga M, Casari G, Bettinelli A, Colussi G, Rodriguez-Soriano J, McCredie D, Milford D, Sanjad S, Lifton RP. Paracellin-1, a renal tight junction protein required for paracellular Mg2+ resorption. *Science* 1999; 285:103–106.

582. Smith H. *The Kidney: Structure and Function in Health and Disease*. New York: Oxford University Press, 1951.

583. Spanidis A, Wunsch H. *Rekonstruktion einer Goormaghtigh'schen und einer Epitheloiden Zelle der Kaninchenniere*. Heidelberg, 1979.

584. Spanidis A, Wunsch H, Kaissling B, Kriz W. Three-dimensional shape of a Goormaghtigh cell and its contact with a granular cell in the rabbit kidney. *Anat Embryol (Berl)* 1982;165:239–252.

585. *Studies of the Mammalian Kidney* [program]. Uppsala: Almqvist & Wiksells Boktryckeri AB, 1944.

586. Stan RV, Kubitza M, Palade GE. PV-1 is a component of the fenestral and stomatal diaphragms in fenestrated endothelia. *Proc Natl Acad Sci U S A* 1999;96:13203–13207.

587. Stanton BA. Renal potassium transport: morphological and functional adaptations. *Am J Physiol* 1989;257:R989–R997.

588. Stanton BA, Kaissling B. Adaptation of distal tubule and collecting duct to increased Na delivery. II. Na+ and K+ transport. *Am J Physiol* 1988;255:F1269–1275.

589. Stanton BA, Kaissling B. Regulation of renal ion transport and cell growth by sodium. *Am J Physiol Renal Physiol* 1989;257:F1–10.

590. Steffes MW, Barbosa J, Basgen JM, Sutherland DE, Najarian JS, Mauer SM. Quantitative glomerular morphology of the normal human kidney. *Lab Invest* 1983;49:82–86.

591. Stephenson JL. Concentration of urine in a central core model of the renal counterflow system. *Kidney Int* 1972;2:85–94.

592. Sterzel RB, Hartner A, Schlotzer-Schrehardt U, Voit S, Hausknecht B, Doliana R, Colombatti A, Gibson MA, Braghetta P, Bressan GM. Elastic fiber proteins in the glomerular mesangium in vivo and in cell culture. *Kidney Int* 2000;58:1588–1602.

593. Stetson DL, Wade JB, Giebisch G. Morphologic alterations in the rat medullary collecting duct following potassium depletion. *Kidney Int* 1980;17:45–56.

594. Stow JL, Sawada H, Farquhar MG. Basement membrane heparan sulfate proteoglycans are concentrated in the laminae rarae and in podocytes of the rat renal glomerulus. *Proc Natl Acad Sci U S A* 1985; 82:3296–3300.

595. Subramanya AR, Yang C-L, Zhu X, Ellison DH. Dominant-negative regulation of WNK1 by its kidney-specific kinase-defective isoform. *Am J Physiol Renal Physiol* 2006;290: F619–624.

596. Sun AM, Liu Y, Dworkin LD, Tse CM, Donowitz M, Yip KP. Na+/H+ exchanger isoform 2 (NHE2) is expressed in the apical membrane of the medullary thick ascending limb. *J Membr Biol* 1997; 160:85–90.

597. Takahashi-Iwanaga H. The three-dimensional cytoarchitecture of the interstitial tissue in the rat kidney. *Cell Tissue Res* 1991;264:269–281.

598. Takeda T, McQuistan T, Orlando RA, Farquhar MG. Loss of glomerular foot processes is associated with uncoupling of podocalyxin from the actin cytoskeleton. *J Clin Invest* 2001;108:289–301.

599. Takeda T, Yamazaki H, Farquhar MG. Identification of an apical sorting determinant in the cytoplasmic tail of megalin. *Am J Physiol Cell Physiol* 2003;284:C1105–1113.

600. Tang VW, Goodenough DA. Paracellular ion channel at the tight junction. *Biophys J* 2003;84:1660–1673.

601. Taugner R, Hackenthal E. *The Juxtaglomerular Apparatus*. Berlin: Springer, 1989.

602. Teng-Umnuay P, Verlander JW, Yuan W, Tisher CC, Madsen KM. Identification of distinct subpopulations of intercalated cells in the mouse collecting duct. *J Am Soc Nephrol* 1996; 7:260–274.

603. Terris J, Ecelbarger CA, Marples D, Knepper MA, Nielsen S. Distribution of aquaporin-4 water channel expression within rat kidney. *Am J Physiol* 1995;269:F775–F785.

604. Thomas SR. Cycles and separations in a model of the renal medulla. *Am J Physiol* 1998;275: F671–F690.

605. Thomson RB, Aronson PS. Immunolocalization of Ksp-cadherin in the adult and developing rabbit kidney. *Am J Physiol Renal Physiol* 1999;277: F146–156.

606. Thomson S, Bao D, Deng A, Vallon V. Adenosine formed by 5'-nucleotidase mediates tubuloglomerular feedback. *J Clin Invest* 2000; 106:289–298.

607. Timpl R, Brown JC. Supramolecular assembly of basement membranes. *Bioessays* 1996;18:123–132.

608. Timpl R, Dziadek M. Structure, development, and molecular pathology of basement membranes. *Int Rev Exp Pathol* 1986;29:1–112.

609. Tisher CC, Bulger RE, Trump BF. Human renal ultrastructure, 3: the distal tubule in healthy individuals. *Lab Invest* 1968;18:655–668.

610. Tisher CC, Bulger RE, Valtin H. Morphology of renal medulla in water diuresis and vasopressin-induced antidiuresis. *Am J Physiol* 1971;220:87–94.

611. Tisher CC, Madsen KM. Anatomy of the kidney. In: Brenner B (ed.). *The Kidney*. Philadelphia: Saunders, 1996:3–71.

612. Tojo A, Sekine T, Nakajima N, Hosoyamada M, Kanai Y, Kimura K, Endou H. Immunohistochemical localization of multispecific renal organic anion transporter 1 in rat kidney. *J Am Soc Nephrol* 1999; 10:464–471.

613. Traebert M, Lotscher M, Aschwanden R, Ritthaler T, Biber J, Murer H, Kaissling B. Distribution of the sodium/phosphate transporter during postnatal ontogeny of the rat kidney. *J Am Soc Nephrol* 1999; 10:1407–1415.

614. Traebert M, Roth J, Biber J, Murer H, Kaissling B. Internalization of proximal tubular type II Na-P(i) cotransporter by PTH: immunogold electron microscopy. *Am J Physiol Renal Physiol* 2000;278:F148–154.

615. Trahair JF, Ryan GB. Co-localization of neuron-specific enolase-like and kallikrein-like immunoreactivity in ductal and tubular epithelium of sheep salivary gland and kidney. *J Histochem Cyto Chem* 1989;37:309–314.

616. Trenchev P, Dorling J, Webb J, Holborow EJ. Localization of smooth muscle-like contractile proteins in kidney by immunoelectron microscopy. *J Anat* 1976;121:85–95.

617. Trinh-Trang-Tan MM, Bankir L. Integrated function of urea transporters in the mammalian kidney. *Exp Nephrol* 1998;6:471–479.

618. Trinh-Trang-Tan MM, Bouby N, Kriz W, Bankir L. Functional adaptation of thick ascending limb and internephron heterogeneity to urine concentration. *Kidney Int* 1987; 31:549–555.

619. Trinh-Trang-Tan MM, Lasbennes F, Gane P, Roudier N, Ripoche P, Cartron JP, Bailly P. UT-B1 proteins in rat: tissue distribution and regulation by antidiuretic hormone in kidney. *Am J Physiol Renal Physiol* 2002;283:F912–F922.

620. Trump BF, Bulger RE. Morphology of the kidney. In: Becker B (ed.). *Structural Basis of Renal Disease*. New York: Harper & Row, 1968:1–92.

621. Tsukita S, Furuse M. Claudin-based barrier in simple and stratified cellular sheets. *Curr Opin Cell Biol* 2002;14:531–536.

622. Tsukita S, Furuse M, Itoh M. Multifunctional strands in tight junctions. *Nat Rev Mol Cell Biol* 2001;2:285–293.

623. Unwin RJ, Capasso G, Shirley DG. An overview of divalent cation and citrate handling by the kidney. *Nephron Physiol* 2004;98:15–20.

624. Unwin RJ, Ganz MD, Sterzel RB. Brain-gut peptides, renal function and cell growth. *Kidney Int* 1990;37:1031–1047.

625. Urakami Y, Nakamura N, Takahashi K, Okuda M, Saito H, Hashimoto Y, Inui K-i. Gender differences in expression of organic cation transporter OCT2 in rat kidney. *FEBS Letters* 1999;461:339–342.

626. Urakami Y, Okuda M, Masuda S, Akazawa M, Saito H, Inui K-i. Distinct characteristics of organic cation transporters, OCT1 and OCT2, in the basolateral membrane of renal tubules. *Pharmaceut Res* 2001;18:1528–1534.

627. Urakami Y, Okuda M, Masuda S, Saito H, Inui K-I. Functional characteristics and membrane localization of rat multispecific organic cation transporters, OCT1 and OCT2, mediating tubular secretion of cationic drugs. *J Pharmacol Exp Ther* 1998;287: 800–805.

628. Urakami Y, Okuda M, Saito H, Inui K-i. Hormonal regulation of organic cation transporter OCT2 expression in rat kidney. *FEBS Letters* 2000;473:173–176.

629. Valtin H. Physiological effects of vasopressin on the kidney. In: Gash D (ed.). *Vasopressin.* New York: Plenum, 1987:369–387.

630. van Abel M, Hoenderop JG, Bindels RJ. The epithelial calcium channels TRPV5 and TRPV6: regulation and implications for disease. *Naunyn Schmiedebergs Arch Pharmacol* 2005;371:295–306.

631. van Abel M, Hoenderop JG, van der Kemp AW, Friedlaender MM, van Leeuwen JP, Bindels RJ. Coordinated control of renal Ca(2+) transport proteins by parathyroid hormone. *Kidney Int* 2005;68:1708–1721.

632. van Hoek AN, Ma T, Yang B, Verkman AS, Brown D. Aquaporin-4 is expressed in basolateral membranes of proximal tubule S3 segments in mouse kidney. *Am J Physiol Renal Physiol* 2000;278: F310–316.

633. Vasmant D, Maurice M, Feldmann G. Cytoskeleton ultrastructure of podocytes and glomerular endothelial cells in man and in the rat. *Anat Rec* 1984;210:17–24.

634. Vekaria RM, Shirley DG, Sevigny J, Unwin RJ. Immunolocalization of ectonucleotidases along the rat nephrons. *Am J Physiol Renal Physiol* 2006;290:F550–560.

635. Verbavatz JM, Brown D, Sabolic I, Valenti G, Ausiello DA, Van Hoek AN, Ma T, Verkman AS. Tetrameric assembly of CHIP28 water channels in liposomes and cell membranes: a freeze-fracture study. *J Cell Biol* 1993;123:605–618.

636. Verkman AS. Lessons on renal physiology from transgenic mice lacking aquaporin water channels. *J Am Soc Nephrol* 1999;10:1126–1135.

637. Verkman AS, Shi LB, Frigeri A, Hasegawa H, Farinas J, Mitra A, Skach W, Brown D, Van Hoek AN, Ma T. Structure and function of kidney water channels. *Kidney Int* 1995;48:1069–1081.

638. Verlander JW, Madsen KM, Tisher CC. Effect of acute respiratory acidosis on two populations of intercalated cells in rat cortical collecting duct. *Am J Physiol* 1987;253:F1142–F1156.

639. Verlander JW, Miller RT, Frank AE, Royaux IE, Kim YH, Weiner ID. Localization of the ammonium transporter proteins RhBG and RhCG in mouse kidney. *Am J Physiol* 2003;284: F323–337.

640. Verlander JW, Tran TM, Zhang L, Kaplan MR, Hebert SC. Estradiol enhances thiazide-sensitive NaCl cotransporter density in the apical plasma membrane of the distal convoluted tubule in ovariectomized rats. *J Clin Invest* 1998;101:1661–1669.

641. Vernace MA, Mento PF, Maita ME, Girardi EP, Chang MD, Nord EP, Wilkes BM. Osmolar regulation of endothelin signaling in rat renal medullary interstitial cells. *J Clin Invest* 1995;96:183–191.

642. Verrout PJ, Birn H, Nielsen R, Kozyraki R, Christensen EI. The tandem endocytic receptors megalin and cubilin are important proteins in renal pathology. *Kidney Int* 2002;62: m745–756.

643. Verrout PJ, Christensen EI. Megalin and cubilin—the story of two multipurpose receptors unfolds. *Nephrol Dial Transplant* 2002;17:1867–1871.

644. Vio CP, Cespedes C, Gallardo P, Masferrer JL. Renal identification of cyclooxygenase-2 in a subset of thick ascending limb cells. Hypertension 1997;30:687–692.

645. Voets T, Nilius B, Hoefs S, van der Kemp AW, Droogmans G, Bindels RJ, Hoenderop JG. TRPM6 forms the Mg2+ influx channel involved in intestinal and renal Mg2+ absorption. *J Biol Chem* 2004;279:19–25.

646. von Möllendorff W. Exkretionsapparat und weibliche Genitalorgane. In: von Möllendorff WH (ed.). *Handbuch der mikroskopischen Anatomie des Menschen.* vol. 7. Berlin: Julius Springer Verlag, 1930:1–328.

647. Wade JB, O'Neil RG, Pryor JL, Boulpaep EL. Modulation of cell membrane area in renal collecting tubules by corticosteroid hormones. *J Cell Biol* 1979;81:439–445.

648. Wade JB, Stanton BA, Brown D. Structural correlates of transport in distal tubule and collecting duct segments. In: Windhager EE (ed.). *Handbook of Physiology: Renal.* New York: Oxford University Press, 1992:1–10.

649. Wade JB, Welling PA, Donowitz M, Shenolikar S, Weinman EJ. Differential renal distribution of NHERF isoforms and their colocalization with NHE3, ezrin, and ROMK. *Am J Physiol Cell Physiol* 2001; 280:C192–198.

650. Wagner CA, Finberg KE, Breton S, Marshansky V, Brown D, Geibel JP. Renal vacuolar H+-ATPase. *Physiol Rev* 2004;84:1263–1314.

651. Wang W. Renal potassium channels: recent developments. *Curr Opin Nephrol Hypertens* 2004;13:549–555.

652. Wang W-H. Regulation of ROMK (Kir1.1) channels: new mechanisms and aspects. *Am J Physiol Renal Physiol* 2006;290:F14–19.

653. Wang XY, Masilamani S, Nielsen J, Kwon TH, Brooks HL, Nielsen S, Knepper MA. The renal thiazide-sensitive Na-Cl cotransporter as mediator of the aldosterone-escape phenomenon. *J Clin Invest* 2001; 108:215–222.

654. Wang Y, Cai H, Cebotaru L, Hryciw DH, Weinman EJ, Donowitz M, Guggino SE, Guggino WB. ClC-5: role in endocytosis in the proximal tubule. *Am J Physiol Renal Physiol* 2005;289:F850–862.

655. Warnock DG. Liddle syndrome: genetics and mechanisms of Na+ channel defects. *Am J Med Sci* 2001;322:302–307.

656. Warnock DG, Rossier BC. Renal sodium handling: the role of the epithelial sodium channel. *J Am Soc Nephrol* 2005;16:3151–3153.

657. Weiner ID, Miller RT, Verlander JW. Localization of the ammonium transporters, Rh B glycoprotein and Rh C glycoprotein, in the mouse liver. *Gastroenterology* 2003;5:1432–1440.

658. Weinman EJ, Cunningham R, Shenolikar S. NHERF and regulation of the renal sodium-hydrogen exchanger NHE3. *Pflugers Arch* 2005;450:137–144.

659. Weinman EJ, Cunningham R, Wade JB, Shenolikar S. The role of NHERF-1 in the regulation of renal proximal tubule sodium-hydrogen exchanger 3 and sodium-dependent phosphate cotransporter 2a. *J Physiol* 2005;567:27–32.

660. Weinman EJ, Cunningham R, Wade JB, Shenolikar S. The role of NHERF-1 in the regulation of renal proximal tubule sodium-hydrogen exchanger 3 and sodium-dependent phosphate co-transporter 2a. *J Physiol* 2005;567:27–32.

660a. Wehrli Ph, Loffing.Cueni D, Kaissling B, Loffing J. Replication of segment-specific and intercalated cells in mouse renal collecting system. Histochem Cell Biol 2006;

661. Welling D, Urani J, Welling L, Wagner E. Fractal analysis and imaging of the proximal nephron cell. *Am J Physiol* 1996;270:C953–963.

662. Welling L, Zupka M, Welling D. Mechanical properties of basement membrane. *News Physiol Sci* 1995;10:30–35.

663. Welling LW, Evan AP, Welling DJ. Shape of cells and extracellular channels in rabbit cortical collecting ducts. *Kidney Int* 1981;20:211–222.

664. Welling LW, Evan AP, Welling DJ, Gattone VH, 3rd. Morphometric comparison of rabbit cortical connecting tubules and collecting ducts. *Kidney Int* 1983;23:358–367.

665. Welling LW, Welling DJ, Hill JJ. Shape of cells and intercellular channels in rabbit thick ascending limb of Henle. *Kidney Int* 1978;13:144–151.

666. Wexler AS, Kalaba RE, Marsh DJ. Three-dimensional anatomy and renal concentrating mechanism, I: modeling results. *Am J Physiol* 1991;260:F368–F383.

667. Wilcox CS, Welch WJ. Macula densa nitric oxide synthase: expression, regulation, and function. *Kidney Int* 1998;67(Suppl):S53–S57.

668. Wilcox CS, Welch WJ, Murad F, Gross SS, Taylor G, Levi R, Schmidt HH. Nitric oxide synthase in macula densa regulates glomerular capillary pressure. *Proc Natl Acad Sci U S A* 1992;89:11993–11997.

669. Wilcox ER, Burton QL, Naz S, Riazuddin S, Smith TN, Ploplis B, Belyantseva I, Ben-Yosef T, Liburd NA, Morell RJ, Kachar B, Wu DK, Griffith AJ, Riazuddin S, Friedman TB. Mutations in the gene encoding tight junction claudin-14 cause autosomal recessive deafness DFNB29. *Cell* 2001;104:165–172.

670. Wilson FH, Disse-Nicodeme S, Choate KA, Ishikawa K, Nelson-Williams C, Desitter I, Gunel M, Milford DV, Lipkin GW, Achard JM, Feely MP, Dussol B, Berland Y, Unwin RJ, Mayan H, Simon DB, Farfel Z, Jeunemaitre X, Lifton RP. Human hypertension caused by mutations in WNK kinases. *Science* 2001;293:1107–1112.

671. Wilson FH, Kahle KT, Sabath E, Lalioti MD, Rapson AK, Hoover RS, Hebert SC, Gamba G, Lifton RP. Molecular pathogenesis of inherited hypertension with hyperkalemia: the Na-Cl cotransporter is inhibited by wild-type but not mutant WNK4. *Proc Natl Acad Sci U S A* 2003;100:680–684.

672. Wingo CS, Cain BD. The renal H-K-ATPase: physiological significance and role in potassium homeostasis. *Annu Rev Physiol* 1993; 55:323–347.

673. Wingo CS, Smolka AJ. Function and structure of H-K-ATPase in the kidney. *Am J Physiol* 1995;269:F1–F16.

674. Winn MP, Conlon PJ, Lynn KL, Farrington MK, Creazzo T, Hawkins AF, Daskalakis N, Kwan SY, Ebersviller S, Burchette JL, Pericak-Vance MA, Howell DN, Vance JM, Rosenberg PB. A mutation in the TRPC6 cation channel causes familial focal segmental glomerulosclerosis. *Science* 2005;308:1801–1814.

675. Wirz H. Countercurrent principle. *Protoplasma* 1967;63:322–327.

676. Wittner M, Di Stefano A, Mandon B, Roinel N, de Rouffignac C. Stimulation of NaCl reabsorption by antidiuretic hormone in the cortical thick ascending limb of Henle's loop of the mouse. *Pflugers Arch* 1991;419:212–214.

677. Wogensen L, Nielsen CB, Hjorth P, Rasmussen LM, Nielsen AH, Gross K, Sarvetnick N, Ledet T. Under control of the Ren-1c promoter, locally produced transforming growth factor-beta1 induces accumulation of glomerular extracellular matrix in transgenic mice. *Diabetes* 1999;48:182–192.

678. Wolgast M, Larson M, Nygren K. Functional characteristics of the renal interstitium. *Am J Physiol* 1981;241:F105–F111.

679. Deleted in proof.

680. Wright SH. Role of organic cation transporters in the renal handling of therapeutic agents and xenobiotics. *Toxicol Appl Pharmacol* 2005;204:309–319.

681. Wright SH, Dantzler WH. Molecular and cellular physiology of renal organic cation and anion transport. *Physiol Rev* 2004;84:987–1049.

682. Yang B, Bankir L. Urea and urine concentrating ability: new insights from studies in mice. *Am J Physiol Renal Physiol* 2005;288:F881–896.

683. Yang CL, Angell J, Mitchell R, Ellison DH. WNK kinases regulate thiazide-sensitive Na-Cl cotransport. *J Clin Invest* 2003;111:1039–1045.

684. Deleted in proof.

685. Yang LE, Maunsbach AB, Leong PK, McDonough AA. Differential traffic of proximal tubule Na+ transporters during hypertension or PTH: NHE3 to base of microvilli vs. NaPi2 to endosomes. *Am J Physiol Renal Physiol* 2004;287:F896–906.

686. Yang T, Hassan S, Huang YG, Smart AM, Briggs JP, Schnermann JB. Expression of PTHrP, PTH/PTHrP receptor, and Ca(2+)-sensing receptor mRNAs along the rat nephron. *Am J Physiol* 1997;272:F751–758.

687. Yang T, Singh I, Pham H, Sun D, Smart A, Schnermann JB, Briggs JP. Regulation of cyclooxygenase expression in the kidney by dietary salt intake. *Am J Physiol* 1998;274:F481–489.

688. Ye W, Zhang H, Hillas E, Kohan DE, Miller RL, Nelson RD, Honeggar M, Yang T. Expression and function of COX isoforms in renal medulla: evidence for regulation of salt sensitivity and blood pressure. *Am J Physiol Renal Physiol* 2006;290:F542–549.

689. Yoder BK, Hou X, Guay-Woodford LM. The polycystic kidney disease proteins, polycystin-1, polycystin-2, polaris, and cystin, are co-localized in renal cilia. *J Am Soc Nephrol* 2002; 13:2508–2516.

690. You C. Structure, function, and regulation of renal organic anion transporters. *Med Res Rev* 2002;22:602–616.

691. Yu AS. Claudins and epithelial paracellular transport: the end of the beginning. *Curr Opin Nephrol Hypertens* 2002;12:503–509.

692. Yu AS, Enck AH, Lencer WI, Schneeberger EE. Claudin-8 expression in Madin-Darby canine kidney cells augments the paracellular barrier to cation permeation. *J Biol Chem* 2002; 278:17350–17359.

693. Yu ASL, McCarthy KM, Francis SA, McCormack JM, Lai J, Rogers RA, Lynch RD, Schneeberger EE. Knockdown of occludin expression leads to diverse phenotypic alterations in epithelial cells. *Am J Physiol Cell Physiol* 2005;288:C1231–1241.

694. Yurchenco P. Assembly of laminin and type IV collagen into basement membrane networks. In: Yurchenco P, (ed.) *Extracellular Matrix Assembly and Structure*. San Diego: Academic Press, 1994:351–388.

695. Zaar K. Structure and function of peroxisomes in the mammalian kidney. *Eur J Cell Biol* 1992;59:233–254.

696. Zabel M, Schiebler TH. Histochemical, autoradiographic and electron microscopic investigations of the renal proximal tubule of male and female rats after castration. *Histochemistry* 1980;69:255–276.

697. Zhai XY, Birn H, Jensen KB, Thomsen JS, Andreasen A, Christensen EI. Digital three-dimensional reconstruction and ultrastructure of the mouse proximal tubule. *J Am Soc Nephrol* 2003;14:611–619.

698. Zhai XY, Birn H, Jensen KB, Thomsen JS, Andreasen A, Christensen EI. Digital three-dimensional reconstruction and ultrastructure of the mouse proximal tubule. *J Am Soc Nephrol* 2003;14:611–619.

699. Zhai XY, Thomsen JS, Birn H, Kristoffersen IB, Andreasen A, Christensen EI. Three-dimensional reconstruction of the mouse nephron. *J Am Soc Nephrol* 2006;17:77-88.

700. Zhang Q, Taulman PD, Yoder BK. Cystic kidney diseases: all roads lead to the cilium. *Physiology (Bethesda)* 2004;19:225–230.

701. Zimmermann KW. Ueber den Bau des Glomerulus der Saeugerniere. Z Mikrosk Anat Forsch 1933;32:176-278.

Functional Organization

CHAPTER **21**

Biophysical Basis of Glomerular Filtration

Scott C. Thomson and Roland C. Blantz

University of California and VA San Diego Healthcare System, San Diego, California, USA

INTRODUCTION

Aristotle (384–322 BC) surmised that surplus liquid becomes separated from the blood within the renal meat (77). In 1666, Marcello Malpighi discovered the glomerulus with aid of a microscope (76). After two centuries of failed attempts by others, William Bowman finally established the anatomic relation between the glomerular capillary tuft and the uriniferous tubule in 1842 (15). One year later, Carl Ludwig proffered the notion of the glomerulus as a simple filter in which, under the pressure of the blood in the glomerular capillaries, the watery and crystalloid constituents of the plasma become separated from the "proteid" constituents (73). Ludwig's theory was not universally accepted until several years later. The most forceful objection came from Heidenhain who favored the secretory formation of glomerular urine based on studies on the passage of indigo carmine from blood to urine. Heidenhain was able to find this dye in tubular structures, but not in the glomerulus (51).

The physical process known as osmosis was discovered by Dutrochet, who was studying plants in the early 19th century (34). Ludwig was aware of this and even postulated that the hyperproteinaemia brought about by glomerular filtration causes concentration of the urine by endosmosis into the peritubular capillaries (74). However, it was only after van't Hoff and others had applied thermodynamic principles to explain osmosis in terms of pressure (130) that Ernest Henry Starling contemplated a role for the osmotic pressure of the plasma colloids in glomerular filtration. Starling had noted that the minimal blood pressure compatible with urine formation was about 40 mm Hg and he wondered

whether 40 mm Hg might also equal the osmotic pressure of the plasma colloids that oppose filtration. In 1897, he set out to determine "more exactly the probability of the filtration hypothesis"(121). First, using a colloid osmometer of his own design, he found the osmotic pressure of the blood plasma colloids to be 25 to 30 mm Hg or about 0.4 mm Hg-gram^{-1}-liter^{-1}. Then, he observed that raising the ureteral pressure to within 30 to 45 mm Hg of the arterial blood pressure would stop the flow of urine in a dog undergoing diuresis. Thus, the hydraulic pressure across the glomerular epithelium must exceed the plasma colloid osmotic pressure by some small amount in order for urine to form. On this basis, Ludwig's filtration hypothesis was deemed credible. Starling's paper does not contain any equation for transcapillary flux or for the "force" that bears his name. Further evidence for glomerular filtration was published in 1924 by Wearn and Richards, who performed the first renal micropuncture experiments and succeeded in collecting fluid from Bowman's space in frogs (Fig. 1). From these collections, they verified the presence of sugar and chloride in glomerular fluid when there was none in the urine, thereby proving that the tubule reabsorbs these substances. They also directly visualized the passage of indigo carmine into Bowman's space from the blood, thus refuting Heidenhain's objection to the filtration theory. Wearn and Richards interpreted their own findings as "indirect evidence that the process in the glomerulus is physical" (135).

Glomerular filtration eventually received theoretical consideration as a case of coupled transport subject to the fundamental rules of nonequilibrium thermodynamics. The cardinal theory for this was articulated by Onsager in

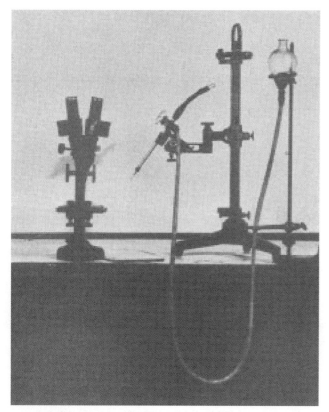

FIGURE 1   Micropuncture apparatus used by Wearn and Richards to sample fluid from Bowman's space in the frog. (From Wearn JT, Richards AN. *Am J Physiol* 1924; 71:209–227.)

1931 (89) and became the basis for his Nobel Prize in 1968. Applying Onsager's theory to the movement of sub-stances across a membrane, the behavior of a membrane system containing n components is fully characterized by ($\frac{1}{2}$ $n(n+1)$) "phenomenological constants." For the case of a two-component system consisting of a solvent and a nonelectrolyte solute, one can describe the transcapillary flux of water J_w and the solute J_s. Each of the components is driven by a conjugate force equivalent to its difference in free energy across the membrane. The conjugate forces for water and nonelectrolyte solute are

$$\Delta\mu_w = V_w \Delta P + RT\Delta \ln \gamma_w X_w \qquad (1)$$
$$\Delta\mu_s = V_s \Delta P + RT\Delta \ln \gamma_s X_s$$

where V is a partial molar volume, ΔP is the pressure difference, X is the mole fraction, and γ is an activity function, empirically derived as a function of X. Since water flux affects X_s and solute flux affects X_w, the two conjugate forces and fluxes are coupled. For a small deviation from equilibrium this coupling can be taken into account by the following linear flux equations:

$$J_w = L_{11}\Delta\mu_w + L_{12}\Delta\mu_s \qquad (2)$$
$$J_s = L_{21}\Delta\mu_w + L_{22}\Delta\mu_s$$

where Lxy are the, so-called phenomenological constants. A central principle of nonequilibrium thermodynamics, the Onsager reciprocity principle, says that $L_{21} = L_{12}$. Therefore, if the three coefficients, L_{11}, L_{22}, and $L_{21} = L_{12}$, are known along with baseline values of Jw and Js, then one can predict the changes in Jw and Js that will arise from any alteration in $\Delta\mu_w$ or $\Delta\mu_s$. However, the physical meanings of the phenomenological constants are difficult to appreciate and a more familiar form of the Onsager equations was provided in 1958 by Kedem and Katchalsky to describe transport across biological membranes (64).

$$J_v = L_p \cdot \left(\Delta P - \sigma_s \Delta\Pi\right) \qquad (3a,b)$$
$$J_s = P_s \cdot \Delta C_s + J_V \left(1 - \sigma_s\right) \cdot \overline{C}_s$$

When applied to movement across a capillary wall, the effluxes per unit area of volume v (which is mostly water) and solute s are given by J_v and J_s, respectively; ΔP, $\Delta\Pi$, and ΔC are opposites of the gradients for hydrostatic pressure, osmotic pressure, and concentration integrated across the membrane; σ_s is the reflection coefficient of the membrane for s; L_p is the hydraulic permeability per unit area of membrane; and P_s is the diffusive permeability of the membrane to s; $\overline{c}_s$ is the mean concentration of s within the membrane. Π is a function of C. σ_s assumes a value between 0 and 1. Three of these parameters, L_p, P_s, and σ_s are characteristics of the membrane, in keeping with the Onsager theory, which requires exactly three coefficients to describe the coupled transport of the two entities, v and s. Equation 3a, though developed from Onsager's theory and articulated by Kedem and Katchalsky, is often referred to as the "Starling equation." Equation 3b expresses J_s as the sum of diffusive and convective components. Equations 3a and 3b are coupled. J_s explicitly depends on J_v. J_v depends on J_s because J_s affects $\Delta\Pi$.

There are limitations to irreversible thermodynamics and to the simplified equations, beginning with the assumption of a linear relationship between fluxes and forces. For example, one can imagine how increasing ΔP might cause a capillary wall to stretch, thereby changing the geometry of its pores and altering L_p. Also, $\overline{c}_s$ can take a variety of forms depending on whether σ is taken to be active throughout the membrane or to be a membrane entrance phenomenon and this will affect how J_s is parsed into its diffusive and convective components (62). Finally, as water efflux causes protein to accumulate near the capillary wall, this could raise the local colloid osmotic pressure at the wall and cause L_p to be underestimated when calculated on the basis of $\Delta\Pi$ for the bulk plasma. Nonetheless, these equations remain the basis for all current understanding of the physical factors that determine transport of water and solutes between the glomerular capillary plasma and the urinary space.

Depending on the context, different simplifying assumptions are made that streamline the description of capillary flux in the glomerulus. For example, when considering J_v (i.e., glomerular filtration), the solutes are divided into two groups, large and small. Large solutes are the colloids and it is assumed that P_s for these is zero and σ_s is unity. All other solutes are assumed to be small and it is assumed that σ_s (and ΔC) for these is zero. Solutes with intermediate permeability are ignored. Therefore, $\Delta\Pi$ can be substituted by the colloid osmotic pressure of the glomerular plasma and a full description of J_v is provided by Eq. 3a. This obviates the need to consider coupled transport. Although the contribution of filtered macromolecules to the transcapillary oncotic pressure may be negligible, there are times when it is critical to understand the sieving properties of the glomerulus for large molecules. In such cases, simplifying assumptions are made regarding the geometry of the filtration barrier and the shape of the solute molecules so that the process can be conveniently described using hydrodynamic theory.

THE MAGNITUDE OF RENAL BLOOD FLOW AND GLOMERULAR FILTRATION

In humans, the kidneys constitute 0.5% of the body weight but receive 20% of the cardiac output. The caliber of the resistance vessels (15–25 μm) is similar to that in other organs and the low resistance to renal blood flow owes to the large number of parallel conductances, with each human kidney containing about 1 million glomeruli (116). The cardiac ouptut in a human is about 8000 L per day. Approximately 20 L of this is filtered through systemic capillaries into the interstitium to give a filtration fraction of 0.25% for organs other than the kidney (66). In contrast, the glomerular capillaries filter 180 L per day into Bowman's space, for a filtration fraction of ~20%. The Starling force for filtration at the upstream end of the glomerular capillary has been measured in several species of mammal and is 15 to 20 mm Hg. This is comparable to other, nonrenal, capillaries (41, 93, 136). Hence, the high rate of filtration by the kidney relative to other organs must be due to a greater surface area for filtration or to a greater hydraulic permeability. The surface area available for filtration in the human kidney is on the order of 1.2 m² overall, or 0.6 mm² per glomerulus. A meaningful number is difficult to assign to the capillary surface area in other major organs where the number of capillaries perfused at any given moment is highly variable. The hydraulic permeability L_p of fenestrated glomerular capillaries has been estimated from 2.5 to 4.0 μl/min/mm Hg/cm² in rats and humans (30, 106, 107), which is 50-fold higher than L_p for nonfenestrated skeletal muscle (115). Another unique feature of the glomerular circulation is the low-resistance pathway provided by the tubule, which enables 180 L per day to pass through Bowman's space at a pressure of only 10 to 15 mm Hg. In other organs, where filtrate must be cleared by lymphatics or reverse filtration,

filtration is limited by the resistance encountered by fluid leaving the interstitium.

GLOMERULAR HEMODYNAMICS BY INFERENCE

Homer W. Smith, who also deserves credit for identifying inulin as a marker of glomerular filtration rate (GFR)(113) and para amino hippuric acid (PAH) as a marker of renal plasma flow (RPF) (118), conjectured as to the microvascular control of glomerular filtration. Smith injected humans with pyrogens or adrenaline to manipulate the renal blood flow and observed a marked reciprocal relation between RPF and filtration fraction (21). He realized that this reciprocal relation is contrary to what should occur if the changes in RPF were mediated by a preglomerular resistance and he presented a series of equations to argue that the renal resistance changed in these experiments due to dilation and constriction of the efferent arteriole. His formulation required a strong inverse effect of efferent resistance on filtration fraction, which could be achieved by assuming that the net ultrafiltration pressure vanishes at some point along the capillary as hydrostatic pressure declines and plasma oncotic pressure increases. Based on knowledge that this occurs in the mesenteric circulation, Smith was willing to assume that this also happens in the kidney and coined the term *filtration pressure equilibrium* in reference to it the phenomenon (Fig. 2) (117). Smith later recanted his notion of filtration pressure equilibrium in the glomerular capillary, arguing, on teleologic grounds, that the hydrostatic null point should occur in the proximal portion of the efferent arteriole in order to promote maximal GFR and maximal reabsorption in the peritubular capillary (116). His revised thinking was likely influenced by the theoretical contemplations of Gomez (44).

GLOMERULAR HEMODYNAMICS AND MICROPUNCTURE

A full and direct assessment of the filtration forces and hydraulic permeability in a mammalian glomerulus was first published by Brenner et al. in 1971(18). Three developments made this possible. First, a mutant rat strain (Munich Wistar) was discovered with glomeruli on the kidney surface making them accessible for glomerular micropuncture. Second, a servo-null device was invented that enabled accurate and rapid pressure measurements in capillaries and tubules (39). Third, a microadaptation of the Lowry method (72) was developed for measuring the protein concentration in a few nanoliters of plasma, which could be obtained by micropuncture from a postglomerular arteriole (16).

   Given values for the pressure in the glomerular capillary P_{GC} and Bowman's space P_{BS}, pre- and postglomerular plasma protein concentrations c_0 and c_1, single-nephron ³H-inulin

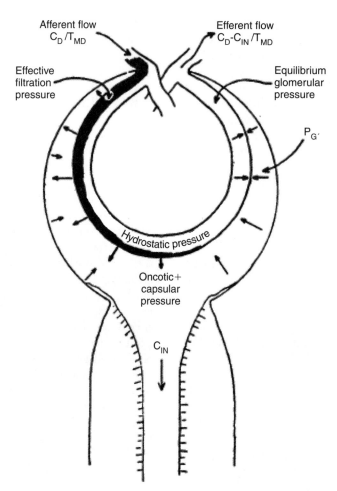

FIGURE 2   Supposition of filtration equilibrium illustreated in the glomerulus. (From HW Smith et al. *J Clin Invest* 1940.)

clearance, or single nephron GFR, *SNGFR*, and a simple mathematical model for computing changes in the ultrafiltration pressure P_{UF} along the glomerular capillary, it is possible to obtain values for the glomerular plasma flow Q_0 and ultrafiltration coefficient LpA. LpA is the product of the hydraulic permeability Lp (see Eq. 3a) and the filtration surface area A.

The mathematical model for computing the physical determinants of *SNGFR* from micropuncture data was developed by Deen, Robertson, and Brenner in 1972 (28). This model treats the glomerular capillary as a circular cylinder of unit length and surface area, uniform permeability to water and small solutes, and zero permeability to protein (Fig. 3). As in Eq. 3a, the filtration flux at any point along the capillary is equal to the product of the Starling force, $\Delta P - \Delta \Pi$, and the hydraulic permeability, L_p. *SNGFR* is obtained by integrating the flux along the capillary length

$$SNGFR = \int_0^1 Jv \cdot dx$$
$$= LpA \int_0^1 (\Delta P - \Delta \Pi)dx \qquad (4)$$
$$= LpA \langle P_{UF} \rangle$$

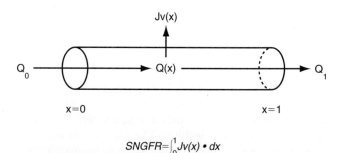

$$SNGFR = \int_0^1 Jv(x) \cdot dx$$

FIGURE 3   Glomerular capillary represented by a homogenous circular circular cylinder with unit length and surface area. Q-plasma flow. Jv, filtration water flux. X, axial position along the capillary.

Where $\Delta P = P_{GC} - P_{BS}$, $\Delta \Pi + \Pi_{GC} - \Pi_{BS}$, and $\langle P_{UF} \rangle$ is the mean ultrafiltration pressure. The term LpA represents the product of the hydraulic permeability Lp and filtration surface area A. For the nondimensionalized capillary A equals unity. For the real capillary, micropuncture data do not distinguish between changes in Lp and changes in A.

To perform the integration in Eq. 4 it is necessary to know how the integrand varies along the capillary. In theory, both ΔP and $\Delta \Pi$ should change along the capillary since P_{GC} must decline due to axial flow resistance and Π_{GC} must rise as water moves from the plasma into Bowman's space. It has always been assumed that the decline in P_{GC} along the capillary is small relative to the increase in Π_{GC}. This assumption was eventually justified by a three-dimensional reconstruction of the rat glomerulus submitted to computational analysis (97). It is our custom to ignore the small axial pressure drop and represent ΔP as a constant, since including a 1– to 2–mm Hg axial pressure drop in the model has a minimal effect on $\langle P_{UF} \rangle$. However, to better illustrate certain principles in this chapter, we have incorporated a 1–mm Hg decline in P_{GC} from the beginning to the end of the glomerular capillary.

For purposes of determining $\Delta \Pi$ it is assumed that all solutes in the system are completely impermeant plasma proteins that exert their full osmotic potential ($\sigma = 1$, $Ps = 0$) and reside solely in the plasma or small molecules that are freely filtered ($\sigma = 0$) and contribute nothing to $\Delta \Pi$. Thus $\Delta \Pi$ is reduced to the plasma oncotic pressure, Π_{GC}. The oncotic pressure in a plasma sample is determined from the protein concentration c, according to an empiric relationship developed by Landis and Pappenheimer

$$\Pi = \alpha_1 c + \alpha_2 c^2 \qquad (5)$$

The values of α_1 and α_2 in Eq. 5 vary according to the ratio of albumin to globulin in the plasma. When Π is expressed in mm Hg and c in g/100 ml, for rat plasma, α_1 and α_2 are 1.73 and 0.28, respectively (66). According to Eq. 5, Π_{GC} will increase from 18 to 35 mm Hg along the length of a glomerular capillary if the systemic plasma contains 6 g/dl of protein and the nephron filtration fraction is 0.29. Such values are typical of the rat.

LpA is computed from $SNGFR$ and $\langle P_{UF} \rangle$, according to Eq. 4. To obtain $\langle P_{UF} \rangle$ it is necessary to know the profile for Π_{GC} along the capillary. This profile is computed from the following mass balance considerations for protein and water. First are three conservation of mass equations

$$Q_0 = SNGFR \left(\frac{c_1}{c_1 - c_0} \right) \qquad (6a\text{-}c)$$

$$cQ = c_0 Q_0$$

$$J_v = \frac{dQ}{dx}$$

where Q_0 is the nephron plasma flow and c_0 and c_1 are the pre- and postcapillary plasma protein concentrations. Differentiating Eq. 6b and substituting Eqs. 6c, 5, and 3a:

$$\begin{aligned} \frac{dc}{dx} &= \frac{c^2}{c_0 Q_0} J_v \\ &= \frac{Lp \cdot c^2}{c_0 Q_0} \left(\Delta P - \left(\alpha_1 c + \alpha_2 c^2 \right) \right) \end{aligned} \qquad (7)$$

A standard root-finding algorithm is used to obtain a value for LpA by numerical integration of Eq. (7) along the entire capillary to obtain an estimate for the plasma protein concentration at the end of the capillary (c_1^*) and adjusting the value of LpA until c_1^* is arbitrarily close to the measured value of c_1.

$$c_1^* = c_0 + \frac{LpA}{c_0 Q_0} \int_0^1 c^2 \left(\Delta P - \left(\alpha_1 c + \alpha_2 c^2 \right) \right) \cdot dx \qquad (8)$$

In a typical experiment, $SNGFR$, ΔP, and c_1 are measured in several nephrons. Most often, these parameters are not obtained from the same nephrons. The mean values for an experiment are inserted into the model to calculate the determinants of $SNGFR$ for an idealized nephron.

From the foregoing description, we see that $SNGFR$ is fully determined by ΔP, Q_0, c_0, and LpA. Typical values for these parameters are shown in Table 1 for Munich Wistar rats from two different breeding colonies under different volume states. In concept, $SNGFR$ can be made to increase by raising ΔP, Q_0, or LpA, or by reducing c_0. But the magnitude of the dependence on each of the four determinants depends on the values of the other three. Some of these interactions are shown in Figs. 4 through 7 and discussed in subsequent sections.

Ultrafiltration Coefficient, LpA, and Filtration Pressure Equilibrium

If the ratio of LpA to Q_0 is great enough, then Π_{GC} will rise to become arbitrarily near to ΔP at some point along the glomerular capillary, resulting in filtration pressure equilibrium. The remaining capillary surface downstream from the equilibration point will not contribute to the flux. It is possible to infer the presence of filtration equilibrium from micropuncture data, but it is not possible to know at what point along the length of the capillary equilibrium occurs. Therefore, it is not possible to compute actual values for $\langle P_{UF} \rangle$ or LpA for nephrons in filtration equilibrium. When Eqs. 4 through 8 are applied to data from a nephron in filtration pressure equilibrium, the values generated for LpA and $\langle P_{UF} \rangle$ are respective minimum and maximum estimates for the actual LpA and $\langle P_{UF} \rangle$. If a change in LpA occurs while a nephron remains in filtration pressure equilibrium, the equilibrium point will shift along the capillary, but $SNGFR$ will not be affected. For $SNGFR$ to be affected by a change in LpA, the nephron must not be in filtration equilibrium.

A debate over whether filtration pressure equilibrium occurs dates back to Homer Smith who used conjecture and teleology to argue both sides of the issue at different points in his career (vide supra). Brenner and colleagues found filtration equilibrium in each of 12 consecutive published series, suggesting that filtration equilibrium is universal for hydropenic or euvolemic Munich Wistar rats. However, contrary data were generated by other micropuncture laboratories. At one point, this led to consternation (86). The issue was resolved after experiments done with rats exchanged between different

TABLE 1   Representative Micropuncture Data in Munich Wistar Rats from the Blantz Laboratory in San Diego and Brenner Laboratory in Boston

Laboratory	State of hydration	SNGFR (nl/min)	ΔP (mm Hg)	Π_0 (mm Hg)	Q_0 (nl/min)	LpA (nl/s/mm Hg)	Filtration pressure equilibrium	Reference no.
Blantz	Hydropenia	30	30.5	18.3	86	0.08*	Yes	8
	Euvolemia	31	37.2	19.7	121	0.06	No	125
	Acute 2.5% plasma volume expansion	45	42.2	18.2	177	0.05	No	125
Brenner	Hydropenia	21	35.3	19.4	65	0.08*	Yes	18
	Euvolemia	32	33.4	19.4	114	0.08*	Yes	55
	Acute 5% plasma volume expansion	50	41.2	22.9	201	0.08	No	30

SNGFR, single-nephron glomerular filtration rate.

*Minimum estimate due to filtration pressure equilibrium. *LpA* values that show differently from the original papers were originally calculated based on a linear estimate of the oncotic pressure profile and are recalculated here using the nonlinear model.

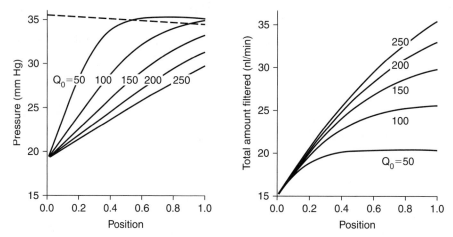

FIGURE 4   Pressure (left) and total flux (right) along the length of the glomerular capillary. In left panel solid curves represent Π_{GC} which rises due to removal of water while dashed line represents ΔP, which declines by 1 mm Hg along the capillary due to flow resistance. SNGFR is the total amount filtered at position =1. Other inputs include systemic plasma protein concentration 5.8 g/dl and LpA=0.08 nl/s/mm Hg. Filtration ceases where $\Delta P - \Pi_{GC} =0$ as occurs when Q_0 is low.

laboratories led to the conclusion that filtration equilibrium prevails in some rat strains or breeding colonies, but not in others and that the difference is attributable to differences in *LpA* (4). This finding detracts some-what from teleologic arguments for or against filtration pressure equilibrium.

Nephron Plasma Flow, Q_0

Q_0 does not appear in the Starling equation for water flux (Eq. 3a) or in the flux integral that defines *SNGFR* (Eq. 4). Nonetheless, Q_0 is an important determinant of *SNGFR*. In fact, increased renal plasma flow underlies many of the physiologic increases in GFR that occur in the normal course of life, such as during pregnancy (6) or after protein feeding (53, 95, 112). According to Eq. 4, *SNGFR* is equal to the product of

LpA and $\langle P_{UF} \rangle$. Q_0 influences $\langle P_{UF} \rangle$ by affecting the rate of rise in the plasma oncotic pressure along the capillary. Removing a given amount of water from the plasma will cause a lesser increase in the plasma oncotic pressure if that water is subtracted from a larger initial plasma volume. Hence increasing Q_0 will cause Π_{GC} to rise more slowly all along the capillary. Therefore, $\langle P_{UF} \rangle$ will increase along with Q_0. The precise effect of Q_0 on the rate of rise in plasma protein concentration along the nephron is described mathematically in Eq. 7. *SNGFR* will be most sensitive to changes in Q_0 under conditions of filtration pressure equilibrium where the filtration fraction remains constant as Q_0 increases. In filtration disequilibrium, c_1, ergo filtration fraction, will decline with increasing Q_0 to reduce the impact of Q_0 on *SNGFR*. Homer Smith recognized that renal plasma flow should affect GFR by this mechanism, and that his experiments (vide supra) failed to confirm a plasma flow dependence of *GFR* only because the particular tools that he used to manipulate the renal blood flow were confounded by offsetting effects on P_{GC} (117).

Systemic Plasma Protein Concentration, C_0

In the idealized glomerulus, an isolated change in c_0 will cause opposite changes in $\langle P_{UF} \rangle$ and, therefore, *SNGFR*. However, it is difficult to demonstrate this experimentally because it is nearly impossible to manipulate oncotic pressure of the arterial plasma without affecting the neurohumoral milieu of the entire body, thereby altering other determinants of *SNGFR*. In fact, the circumstances associated with low oncotic pressure in real life (e.g., generalized capillary leak, sepsis, malnutrition, or nephrosis) are generally associated with a low GFR. When c_0 is manipulated by whatever means, changes in other determinants occur to offset the impact on *SNGFR*. These changes are discussed under Interactions Among the Determinants of SNGFR.

Hydrostatic Pressure, P_{GC} and ΔP

Whereas *SNGFR* is insensitive to *LpA* when Q_0 is low and insensitive to Q_0 when *LpA* is low, *SNGFR* will always be sensitive to an isolated change in ΔP unless ΔP is so low as to be exceeded by the incoming plasma oncotic pressure, in which case *SNGFR* will be zero. This is true because the proportional increase in $\langle P_{UF} \rangle$ brought about by any increment in $\Delta P - \Pi_0$ is relatively insensitive to the other determinants of SNGFR. This is illustrated in Fig. 5 and in the lower half of Fig. 6.

The interposition of the efferent arteriole between the glomerulus and peritubular capillary provides a simple mechanism for regulating ΔP independently of Q_0. Furthermore, this arrangement provides an opportunity to elicit reciprocal changes in P_{GC} and pressure in the downstream peritubular capillary P_{PTC}. Tying an increase in P_{GC} to a decrease in P_{PTC} has teleologic appeal as this will facilitate homeostasis of the effective circulating blood volume while stabilizing GFR. If the efferent arteriole reacts to sustain P_{GC} and reduce P_{PTC} during a decline in renal perfusion pressure or effective circulating blood volume, then GFR will be relatively spared from declining while filtration fraction will increase, thus affecting both the hydraulic and oncotic components of the Starling force that drives reabsorption by the peritubular capillary.

Regulating the efferent arteriole in this way is largely the purview of the renin-angiotensin system, which figures prominently among the myriad neurohumoral mechanisms contained in models of blood pressure and salt homeostasis. Angiotensin II is antinatriuretic and constricts arterioles throughout the body but, in balance, its effect on the glomerulus is always to elevate ΔP (49, 52, 111, 129). Thus, in spite of being a renal vasoconstrictor, angiotensin II protects GFR from total decline while contributing to antinatriuresis when the arterial blood pressure is low or when the preglomerular resistance is high.

Although unduly low P_{GC} must impair glomerular filtration, P_{GC} and *SNGFR* are poorly correlated under normal circumstances, as are P_{GC} and arterial blood pressure. This implies that the kidney generally protects P_{GC} against the influence of arterial blood pressure and uses determinants other than ΔP to effect those physiological changes in *SNGFR* that normally occur throughout life. Furthermore, it has recently been demonstrated that the preglomerular myogenic elements, long associated with static renal blood flow autoregulation, efficiently buffer the glomerular capillary against systolic pressure pulses delivered at the heart-rate frequency (71). Teleologic reasoning behind sheltering the glomerular capillary from high pressure is that high P_{GC} augments wall stress in the glomerular capillary, which elicits a trophic

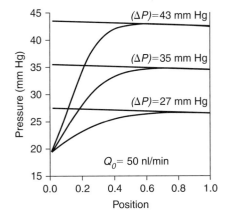
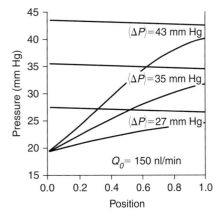

FIGURE 5 ΔP (lines) and Π_{GC} (curves) along the length of a glomerular capillary for three different values of ΔP and allowing for 1 mm Hg decline in ΔP along the capillary. Left panel: $Q_0 = 50$ nl/min. Right panel: $Q_0 = 150$ nl/min. Other inputs include systemic plasma protein concentration 5.8 g/dl and $LpA = 0.06$ nl/s/mm Hg. ΔP has little effect on whether or not filtration pressure equilibrium is achieved over a 3-fold range of afferent PUF (8-24 mm Hg). In contrast, increasing Q_0 from 50 (left) to 150 nl/min (right) eliminates filtration equilibrium regardless of ΔP.

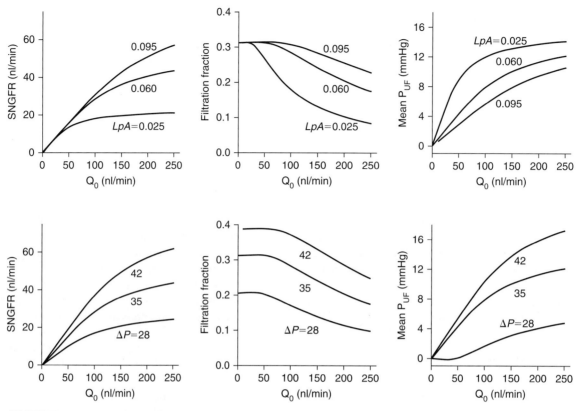

FIGURE 6   SNGFR, filtration fraction, or mean P_{UF} vs Q_0. Curves in the top panels were generated for 3 different values of *LpA*. Curves in the bottom panel were generated for 3 values of ΔP. Unless otherwise stated, $LpA=0.06$ nl/s/mm Hg, $\Delta P=35$ mm Hg, systemic plasma oncotic pressure $=19.5$ mm Hg. Values over this range are seen in the rat at varying levels of volume expansion. P_{GC} is assumed to decline by 1 mm Hg along the length of the capillary.

response. If unchecked, this response will ultimately sclerose and destroy the glomerulus. Therefore, high P_{GC} is always pathologic, and treating glomerular capillary hypertension has been a cornerstone of nephrology practice for more than two decades. Some examples of glomerular capillary hypertension include angiotensin II–mediated hypertension (43), experimental glomerulonephritis (9, 42), and residual nephrons after subtotal nephrectomy (3). It has been asserted, and commonly accepted, that glomerular capillary hypertension also underlies glomerular hyperfiltration in early diabetes mellitus (54, 137). However, there are more than 10 published micropuncture studies in which diabetic hyperfiltration occurred in the absence of glomerular capillary hypertension or in which glomerular capillary hypertension was treated with no mitigating effect on diabetic hyperfiltration (25, 57, 79, 80, 83, 84, 99, 110, 114, 128, 138). This does not detract from the salutary effect of therapy to reduce P_{GC}, which applies to all glomerular diseases (5, 68, 78, 124).

Interactions Among the Determinants of SNGFR

According to the standard model of Deen and Brenner (18), *SNGFR* is completely determined by a set of four parameters, which includes ΔP, Q_0, *LpA*, and c_0 (or Π_0). To state that *SNGFR* can be calculated from these four deter-

minants is a mathematical truism which requires no consideration of how the four determinants might correlate in actual physiology. In fact, the individual components of the glomerular microvasculature that influence determinants of *SNGFR* generally affect more than one of them at a time. For example, an isolated increase in resistance of the preglomerular arteriole will directly reduce both ΔP and Q_0 and will reliably reduce *SNGFR*. In contrast, an isolated increase in resistance of the efferent arteriole will directly augment ΔP and reduce Q_0. Since these two effects exert opposing influences on *SNGFR*, increasing efferent arteriolar resistance might cause SNGFR to increase, decrease, or remain the same depending on other circumstances. For example if P_{GC} is low enough to be at or below Π_{GC}, then raising the efferent resistance can only cause *SNGFR* to increase, whereas if efferent resistance increases toward infinity, Q_0 must tend toward zero while P_{GC} cannot exceed the arterial blood pressure and, therefore, *SNGFR* must decline. The point where the impact of increasing the efferent resistance switches from positive to negative is within the domain of values that occur in vivo. Much of the acute renal failure encountered in contemporary medical practice occurs when drugs that reduce the ratio of efferent: afferent resistance are taken by patients who operate to the left of that point (Fig. 7).

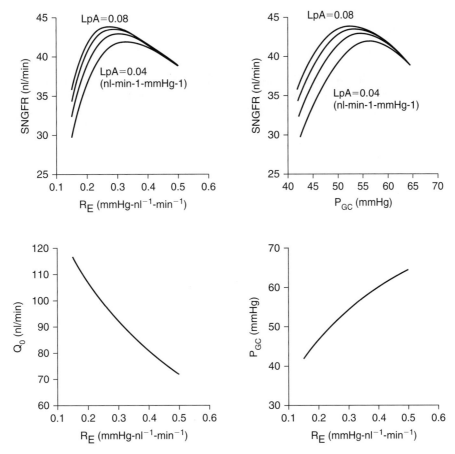

FIGURE 7 Effects of efferent arteriolar resistance (RE) on SNGFR, nephron plasma flow (Q_0), and glomerular capillary pressure (P_{GC}). In top right panel, P_{GC} is made an independent variable by manipulating RE. Effects on Q_0, and P_{GC} are nonlinear because the filtration fraction rises along with RE such that that a lesser fraction of the blood flow transits the efferent arteriole. The Q_0 and P_{GC} curves (bottom) are insensitive to *LpA*. The apex of the SNGFR curve occurs within the physiological range of P_{GC} (48-52 mm Hg). Medical treatments of glomerular capillary hypertension that reduce RE until P_{GC} is normal will not reduce SNGFR. However, for $P_{GC} < 48$ mm Hg, reducing RE causes a precipitous decline in SNGFR.

There are other correlations between determinants of *SNGFR* that are more difficult to explain. For example, since *LpA* is computed as the ratio of *SNGFR* to $\langle P_{UF} \rangle$, random uncorrelated errors in ΔP and SNGFR will cause an inverse correlation to appear between ΔP and *LpA*. Also, an isolated reduction in *LpA*, if sufficient to reduce *SNGFR*, will remove a shunt pathway for fluid to bypass the efferent arteriole, thereby increasing ΔP. Furthermore, the physical orientation of the glomerular mesangium relative to the intraglomerular portion of the efferent arteriole allows activation of the same contractile elements to simultaneously reduce *LpA* and constrict the efferent arteriole (38). This appears to explain why, angiotensin II, the prototype effector of glomerular hemodynamics, simultaneously increases ΔP and reduces *LpA* (11) and why lysing mesangial cells with an antibody negate the effects of angiotensin II on ΔP and *LpA* (10).

Another interesting interaction among two determinants of *SNGFR* involves ΔP and the systemic plasma oncotic pressure Π_0. As mentioned previously, experiments targeted at confirm-

ing the role of Π_0 as a determinant of *SNGFR* are encumbered by the difficulty of manipulating the plasma protein concentration independent of the neurohumoral environment. To get around this, Brenner (7) and Blantz (8, 12, 127) drew on a wide variety of infusion and exchange protocols to alter the systemic plasma protein concentration in multiple ways that were likely to yield contrary effects on the effective circulating volume and hematocrit. These differences were roughly intended to cancel each other and reveal the underlying impact of Π_0 on *SNGFR*, ΔP, Q_0, and *LpA*. Both groups of investigators confirmed that the four determinants of *SNGFR* are not independent of one another. In particular, they discovered that, regardless of the experimental means for invoking a change in Π_0, a change in Π_0 causes a parallel change in ΔP, and reciprocal change in *LpA*. In contrast, neither *SNGFR* nor Q_0 are predictably tied to Π_0. Most remarkably, ΔP is so strongly dependent on Π_0 that the afferent effective filtration pressure, $\Delta P - \Pi_0$, is independent of Π_0. A biophysical or anatomic explanation for this interaction between Π_0 and ΔP has not been forthcoming. It seems, instead, that a physiological mechanism is involved in autoregulating the afferent effective filtration pressure (Table 2).

Brenner and Blantz also observed an inverse correlation between Π_0 and LpA (7, 8, 12, 127). It is possible that this is an artifact of concentration polarization that causes plasma proteins to accumulate near the capillary wall. Concentration polarization will lead to an overestimate of P_{UF} because the calculation of P_{UF} will be based on a lower value of Π than is present at the plasma interface with the capillary wall. Using an overestimate of $\langle P_{UF} \rangle$ in Eq. 4 will lead to an underestimate for LpA. If concentration polarization occurs in the glomerular capillary, the effect will be greatest when c_0 is least. Hence, the appearance could arise of an inverse dependence of LpA on c_0 even though c_0 has no actual effect on the capillary wall. However, there is likely to be enough scrubbing by red blood cells to prevent concentration polarization. Furthermore, concentration polarization cannot explain the correlation between Π_0 and ΔP. Finally, we have already discussed a mechanism for the inverse relation between ΔP and LpA. Therefore, the inverse correlation of between LpA and Π_0 might arise because LpA is affected, as an innocent bystander, by a mechanism that is postulated to autoregulate afferent P_{UF}.

THE FILTRATION BARRIER AND FILTRATION OF MACROMOLECULES

A striking feature of glomerular filtration is the ability of the capillary wall to discriminate among molecules of varying size. Solutes up to the size of inulin pass freely from the plasma to Bowman's space while passage becomes progressively difficult for substances that are larger such that all but the smallest plasma proteins are screened almost entirely. Hence, when describing the determinants of SNGFR, the concentration of macromolecules in the filtrate is low enough that these contribute negligibly to the Starling forces. However, the filtration of small amounts of macromolecules is important for other reasons. For example, the plasma transiting a normal pair of human kidneys in 1 day contains 50,000 g of protein, while the appearance of 1 g/day of protein in the urine is sufficient to establish the presence of glomerular disease. Discerning how this small amount of

protein winds up in Bowman's space is key to explaining how the filtration barrier operates normally and to understanding the physical aspects of glomerular disease.

The filtration of a macromolecule is most often quantified in terms of its sieving coefficient, Θ, which is the ratio of solute concentration in the filtrate relative to filtrand. The earliest direct test for protein in mammalian glomerular filtrate was performed by Walker in 1941 who reported that micropuncture fluid obtained from Bowman's space in rat, guinea pig, or opossum contained "either no protein or, at most, very small amounts." The assay in use at the time would have detected an overall sieving coefficient for protein of 0.4%, which made it insensitive by later standards (133). Several subsequent micropuncture studies during the 1970s yielded widely varying amounts of albumin in proximal tubular fluid, even within an experiment. This variability was reasonably ascribed to contamination of samples by extratubular proteins since only 1% contamination of a tubular fluid sample with plasma from the peritubular capillary would markedly alter the apparent result (87). Performing micropuncture with a system of concentric pipettes to reduce contamination, Tojo and Endou (126) succeeded in confirming a strong inverse relationship between TF/P inulin and albumin concentration in fluid collected from rat proximal tubules due to removal of filtered albumin along the proximal tubule. By linear extrapolation to TF/P inulin of unity, which represents Bowman's space, the sieving coefficient for albumin was estimated at 0.062%. Meanwhile the sieving coefficient of low-molecular-weight proteins was almost 99%, confirming the size-selective nature of protein sieving (Fig. 8) (126). But micropuncture remains an unwieldy technique for studying glomerular sieving of macromolecules and most of what is known about glomerular sieving has been learned by other means (vide infra).

Pore Theory

The glomerular capillary wall clearly screens solutes according to size, and it is usually taught that the glomerulus also screens macromolecules according to charge. The physical basis of molecular sieving is often modeled using pore theory. In pore theory, the coupled flux Eq. 3ab are modified to fit an idealized model of the glomerular capillary wall. The usual model con-

---

TABLE 2   Multivariate regression applied to combined micropuncture data to test for interactions between ΔP and the other determinants of SNGFR

Dependent variable	Independent terms in multivariate regression		
ΔP (mm Hg)	Π_0 (mm Hg)	LpA (nl/sec/mm Hg)	Q_0 (nl/min)
Regression coefficient	0.84 ± 0.09	-72 ± 10	~ 0
P value associated with regression coefficient	2×10^{-10}	1×10^{-10}	0.750

The original regression model included the protocol for manipulating the systemic plasma protein and the laboratory where the work was performed, neither of which influenced the result.

From Brenner [7] and Blantz [127]

sists of a solid barrier perforated by cylindrical pores. In some models, the pores form a homogenous population whereas other models use a mixture of pores of different sizes. This paradigm for describing the flow of material through porous membranes was applied to diffusion and filtration of solutes by capillaries and an early review of the subject was published by Pappenheimer in 1953 (92). Mathematical descriptions were developed for pores shaped like circular cylinders or rectangular slits. At about the same time, theories were developed by others to explain the migration of large solutes through fibrous gels (85). Given what is now known about the physical structure of the glomerular capillary wall, pores, slits, and fibrous gels are all relevant to glomerular sieving. Hence, descriptions based solely on cylindrical pores have become more obviously phenomenological. Nonetheless, pore theory remains the most popular paradigm for describing nuances of glomerular sieving in humans (12, 26, 67, 82).

Pore theory builds on the Kedem-Katchalsky flux Eq. 3ab by associating the three membrane parameters, Lp, Ps, and σ_s with an idealized physical structure. This structure incorporates the membrane geometry, the Stokes-Einstein radius of the solute molecules, temperature, viscosity, and the Boltzman constant. The solutes are represented by rigid spheres that interact with the solvent medium and with the pores, but not with each other. This makes the problem mathematically tractable. The filtration properties of a membrane with circular pores turns out to depend on two things, (1) the ratio of pore diameter to membrane thickness and (2) the overall fraction of the membrane area covered by pores.

An explanation begins with Fick's first law of diffusion for a solute s

$$J_s^{diffusion} = -D_s \frac{dC_s}{dx} \tag{9}$$

Where

$$D_s = \frac{RT}{fN} \tag{10}$$

is the diffusion coefficient, N is Avogadro's number, and f is the frictional force that opposes diffusion of s. Stokes' law states that a sphere of radius a falling at unit velocity in a medium of viscosity η faces a frictional force given by

$$f = 6\pi\eta a \tag{11}$$

Einstein (37) combined Fick's law of diffusion and Stokes law to describe the diffusion coefficient for a spherical molecule in free solution D_0 in terms of its molecular radius a

$$D_0 = \frac{RT}{6\pi\eta aN} \tag{12}$$

Since molecules are rarely spherical, the Stokes-Einstein radius, a, of a molecule, as determined by its diffusibility, is

a virtual quantity represented by a sphere of equivalent radius. Determining the radius of a solute in this way, then using the solute as a marker for pore radius will lead to an overestimate of the pore radius if the marker solute is not rigid and can squeeze through a smaller pore than a rigid sphere with the same Stokes-Einstein radius.

For the diffusion of small molecules through a membrane that contains large pores, Fick's first law is rewritten

$$J_s^{diffusion} = D_0 \frac{A_p}{\delta} \Delta C_s \tag{13}$$

where A_p is the fraction of the membrane surface covered by pores and δ is the membrane thickness. Therefore, the diffusion through a membrane of a small solute with known D_0 is a convenient method to determine the ratio of pore area to thickness for the membrane.

However, when the molecular radius of the solute molecule is on the same scale as the pore size, diffusion through the membrane is less than predicted from Eq. 13. In other words, mobility of the solute is restricted. There are two factors that contribute to restricted mobility. First, there is steric hindrance to the solute entering or residing within the pore. Second, solute molecules within the pore experience greater friction than predicted by Stokes' law for solute molecules in free solution. Although it makes sense to us to represent the steric hindrance by a reduced effective pore area and the increased friction as a reduced effective diffusion coefficient, most of the literature rolls both effects into an expression for the effective pore area. This is described in the following section.

DIFFUSION THROUGH A POROUS MEMBRANE: STERIC HINDRANCE AND ALTERED FRICTION

Restricted passage of solutes of increasing molecular radius is a basic property of membrane structures made of impermeable matrix with pores or of fibrous gels. The basis for molecular sieving in all cases is the exclusion of large solute molecules from a portion of the membrane that is otherwise available to be occupied by water and other small molecules. The formulae for describing steric hindrance are different for pores than for gels. Here we will describe the phenomenon for cylindrical pores.

The center of a spherical molecule cannot approach any closer than its own radius to the edge of any pore. Hence, the fraction of a cylindrical pore, area V_p and radius r, that is available to be occupied by a solute with molecular radius a, is

$$\frac{V}{V_p} = \frac{\pi(r-a)^2}{\pi r^2} = \left(1 - \frac{a}{r}\right)^2 \tag{14}$$

When solvent flow is added due to Starling forces, the steric hindrance is more complex as shown by Ferry (40)

$$\frac{V}{Vp} = \left(1 - \frac{a}{r}\right)^2 \cdot \left(2 - \left(1 - \frac{a}{r}\right)^2\right) \tag{15}$$

The frictional drag on a solute molecule moving through a pore is also different from that described by Stokes' law for a solute in an unbounded free solution. The drag according to Stokes' law for the unbounded condition and the drag encountered in a pore are given by Eq. (16a,b) for a solute moving with velocity μ in a fluid with velocity v; k_1 and k_2 are component drag coefficients that weight the contributions of the particle and fluid velocities; k_1 and k_2 are functions of a/r.

$$f_{unbounded} = 6\pi\eta a(u-v)$$
$$f_{pore} = 6\pi\eta a(u \cdot k_1 - v \cdot k_2) \qquad (16a, b)$$

Theoretical treatments have provided approximate solutions for k_1 and k_2 for particles in cylindrical tubes (48). The actual values of k_1 and k_2 depend on an infinite set of infinite linear equations and approximations are made by laborious computation. For this reason k_1 and k_2 were originally provided for only a few values of a/r and a polynomial equation was fit to these points to allow interpolation. This approximation expression was in-accurate for a/r greater than 0.6, but this was the only method available until better computers were built in the 1970s (91).

Accounting for steric hindrance and dividing Eq. 16b by Eq. 16a to correct for the departure from Stokes' law, the diffusive flux is rewritten from Eq. 13 to become

$$J_s^{diffusion} = D_0 \frac{A_p}{\delta}\left(\left(1-\frac{a}{r}\right)^2\left(2-\left(1-\frac{a}{r}\right)^2\right)\right)\cdot\left(\frac{u-v}{uk_1-vk_2}\right)\Delta C_s$$
$$= D_0 \frac{A_{eff}}{\delta}\Delta C_s \qquad (17)$$

where A_{eff} represents the "effective" pore area and depends on a/r as well as the solute and bulk flow velocities. The com-

bined effects of steric hindrance and friction on A_{eff} are illustrated in Fig. 9 using published values or k_1 and k_2 (91). The approximation equation used by Landis and Pappenheimer (66) in 1963 is also shown where

$$\frac{f_{unbounded}}{f_{pore}} = 1 - 2.104\cdot\left(\frac{a}{r}\right) + 2.09\left(\frac{a}{r}\right)^3 - 0.95\left(\frac{a}{r}\right)^5 + \cdots \quad (18)$$

From Fig. 9 it is clear that restricted diffusion will cause a membrane to discriminate between two solute molecules of different radii even when the radii of both are considerably less than the radius of the pore. Also, note that Eq. 17 reduces to Eq. 13 in the absence of bulk flow and as a/r approaches zero.

PORE THEORY AND HYDRODYNAMIC FLOW

It is statistically valid to describe bulk flow within a cylindrical pore using Poiseulle's law even when the pore radius is only several-fold the radius of a water molecule. Accordingly,

$$q = \frac{-\pi r^4}{8\eta}\frac{dP}{dy} \qquad (19)$$

where q represents bulk flow within a single pore and dP/dy is the axial pressure gradient along the pore. For flow per unit area across a membrane, pressure is replaced by the Starling forces (96, 109) such that

$$J_v = \frac{n\pi r^4}{8\eta\delta}(\Delta P - \Delta\Pi) = \frac{A_w r^2}{8\eta\delta}(\Delta P - \Delta\Pi) \qquad (20)$$

where n is the number of pores per unit area and A_w is the restricted pore area available to water. Comparing Eq. 20 to

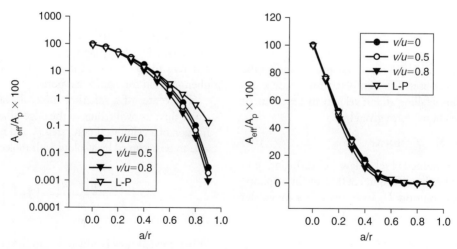

FIGURE 9   Ratio of effective pore area A_{eff} to true pore area A_p that applies to diffusion of solute with radius a through circular pore with radius r. The model accounts for both steric hindrance and friction. u and v refer to solute and bulk flow velocities. Friction is calculated based on published coefficients (Paine 1975). L-P was generated from an approximating equation used by Landis and Pappenheimer in 1963, which works well only for $a/r < 0.6$. Semilog (left) and linear (right) representations are included.

Eq. 3a, the hydraulic permeability L_p for an isoporous membrane is given in terms of the pore radius r and the ratio of total pore area to membrane thickness A_w/δ.

$$L_p = \frac{A_w r^2}{8\eta\delta} \qquad (21)$$

COMBINING BULK FLOW AND RESTRICTED DIFFUSION

The solute flux equation (Eq. 3b) includes terms for diffusion and convection. Convective transport and restricted diffusion occur simultaneously in the glomerulus and each contributes to the presence of large molecules in the filtrate. Furthermore, convection and diffusion are coupled, and a theory that unravels this coupling is necessary for a full understanding of glomerular sieving. We will present two approaches to this that are both based on pore theory and rely on the sieving coefficient, Θ to draw inferences regarding the filtration barrier. The first approach is early work of Pappenheimer and the second approach is that of Chang and Deen who based their method on the prior work of Patlak. It is the latter approach to interpreting sieving data that is used in by most authors who publish in the physiology or clinical literature nowadays.

There are some intuitive features of glomerular sieving and some that are not so intuitive. First, it is intuitive that Θ cannot be a negative number, nor can it exceed unity. If Θ exceeds unity, a model other than pore theory is required to explain the flux. It is also intuitive that Θ will approach unity for small solutes and that Θ will equal zero for any solute that is larger than the largest pore. A feature that is not so intuitive is how intermediate Θ can arise from an isoporous membrane, although we have shown

intermediate A_{eff} for an isoporous membrane in Fig. 8. Intermediate Θ also owes to the effect of filtration rate on molecular sieving, which appears as the second term in Eq. 3b. If the passage of a solute is restricted relative to the passage of water, the filtrate will become diluted during filtration. This will give rise to a concentration gradient for diffusion. Thus, the overall sieving coefficient is determined by competition between the filtration rate, which tends to dilute the filtrate, and the restricted diffusion, which fights to reduce the concentration difference that arises from molecular sieving.

It is intuitive that, if A_{eff} is nonzero and J_v is low enough, then solute will eventually equilibrate between the plasma and Bowman's space ($\Theta = 1$). It is also intuitive that, at high rates of J_v, Θ will approach the ratio of restricted pore area for solute relative to water. Pappenheimer (66) provided a quantitative expression for Θ that satisfies these two conditions. This derivation begins with a bulk-flow sieving step to create an initial filtrate to plasma concentration ratio

$$\frac{C_{filtrate}}{C_{plasma}} = \left(1 - \sigma_s\right) = \frac{A_s}{A_w} \qquad (22)$$

where C is the concentration of the solute in question, A_w and A_s are the effective pore areas for water and solute, and s_s is the sieving coefficient from Eq. 3. Next, diffusion is superimposed according to Fick's law. Assuming that the concentration gradient is constant within the membrane

$$J_s^{diffusion} = D_0 \frac{A_s}{\delta}\left(C_{plasma} - C_{filtrate}\right) \qquad (23)$$

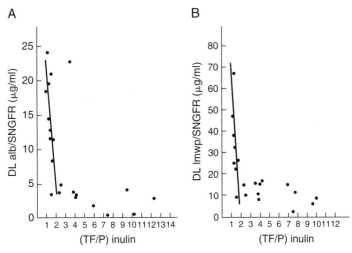

FIGURE 8   Albumin (A) and low-molecular-weight protein (LMWP) delivery (B) along the nephron. Linear regression over the domain of TF/Pinulin from 1 to 2 was used to calculate the protein concentration in Bowman's space. (From Tojo et al. *Am J Physiol* 1992;263(4 Pt 2):F601–606.)

where D_0 is the free solute diffusion coefficient and δ is the membrane thickness. Summing the effects of bulk-flow sieving and diffusion

$$C_{filtrate} = \left(\frac{A_s}{A_w}\right) C_{plasma} + \frac{J_s^{diffusion}}{J_v} \qquad (24)$$

Inserting Eq. 23 into Eq. 24 and rearranging yields

$$\Theta = \frac{C_{filtrate}}{C_{plasma}} = \frac{\left(1 + \dfrac{D_0 Aw}{J_v \delta}\right)}{\left(\dfrac{A_w}{A_s} + \dfrac{D_0 Aw}{J_v \delta}\right)} \qquad (25)$$

The assumption of a constant solute gradient within the membrane is a serious shortcoming of Pappenheimer's approach. This shortcoming was later overcome, based on the work of Patlak (94) who developed a more rigorous approach for quantifying filtration-diffusion interactions in isoporous membranes. Variations on the Patlak approach form the basis for the pore models that are applied to animal and clinical investigations of glomerular sieving nowadays (2). A modified Patlak equation for solute flux begins again with the Kedem-Katchalsky solute flux equation (Eq. 3b). Diffusion-convection coupling in Eq. 3b is contained in the parameter, $\overline{C_s}$ which is the average value of C_s within the membrane. However, $\overline{C_s}$ can't be measured or derived without prior knowledge of the coupled flux that we are trying to determine. Therefore, the challenge is to come up with a form of Eq. 3b that doesn't contain $\overline{C_s}$. The first step toward accomplishing this is to divide the capillary wall of thickness δ into a series of infinitesimally thin laminae. The Kedem-Katchalsky equation for a thin lamina is

$$J_s = -D_s \frac{dC_s}{dy} + J_v (1 - \sigma_s) C_s \qquad (26)$$

where y is the position along the length of the pore, which runs perpendicular to the membrane surface. Next, separating variables and integrating across the membrane yields

$$\int_{plasma}^{filtrate} \frac{dy}{-D_s} = \int_{plasma}^{filtrate} \frac{dC_s}{J_s - J_v(1-\sigma_s)C_s}$$

$$\frac{\delta}{-D_s} = \frac{1}{-P_s} = \frac{1}{-J_v(1-\sigma_s)} \left[ln\left(J_s - J_v(1-\sigma_s)C_s\right)\right]_{plasma}^{filtrate}$$

$$exp\left(\frac{J_v(1-\sigma_s)}{P_s}\right) = \left[\frac{J_s - J_v(1-\sigma_s)C_{filtrate}}{J_s - J_v(1-\sigma_s)C_{plasma}}\right] \qquad (27a\text{-}c)$$

Making the substitutions,

$$P_e = \frac{J_v(1-\sigma_s)}{P_s} \text{ and } C_{filtrate} = \frac{J_s}{J_v} \qquad (28a,b)$$

and rearranging Eq. 27c to solve for J_s yields

$$J_s = \frac{C_{plasma} J_v (1-\sigma_s)}{1 - \sigma_s \exp(-P_e)} \qquad (29)$$

Equation 29 expresses the solute flux as a function of plasma solute concentration, filtration rate, and the membrane characteristics s_s and P_s without referring to C_s anywhere inside the membrane. P_e is the Peclet number, which represents the ratio of convective to diffusive solute flux.

The remaining steps involve relating P_s and s_s to the idealized membrane geometry using the equations for the hydrodynamics of cylindrical pores developed above.

$$P_s = \frac{D_0 A_s}{\delta A_p} \text{ and } \sigma_s = 1 - \frac{A_s}{A_w} \qquad (30)$$

Pore Theory and Experiments in the Glomerulus. To characterize the filtration properties of a particular membrane by applying pore theory as described above, one begins with tracer solute(s) of known concentration(s) and Stokes-Einstein radii and a membrane of unknown microscopic dimensions. The water flux and sieving coefficient of the tracer solute(s) are measured along with the filtrand tracer concentration(s) and transmembrane pressure. A best fit of these data is made to the theoretical model to determine the size and density of idealized pore(s). A better fit can always be achieved by allowing subpopulations of pores with various sizes. This is often justifiable on grounds of common sense. For example, in glomerular disease there is increased permeability to macromolecules, but not to water. This is easily explained by the appearance of a small population of large pores (sometimes called shunts) that allow for the passage of macromolecules that are excluded from the main population of small pores. A scant population of shunt pores could account for most of the macromolecular sieving but contribute negligibly to the ultrafiltration coefficient, LpA, because the pore area available to water is much larger.

To convert solute flux to overall sieving for the glomerulus, flux must be integrated over the entire capillary surface. Using c_{plasma} to represent the plasma concentration of s and x as the position along the capillary

$$\Theta_s = \frac{1}{C_{plasma}(0)} \cdot \frac{\int_0^1 J_s dx}{\int_0^1 J_v dx} \qquad (31)$$

But the forces driving J_v and J_s change along the length of the capillary since C_{plasma}, rises as filtration occurs and J_v declines as oncotic pressure in the capillary pressure rises. For the idealized cylindrical capillary of unit length

$$C_{plasma}(x) = \frac{C_{plasma}(0)Q_0 - \int_0^x J_s(z)dz}{Q_0 - \int_0^x J_v(z)dz} \qquad (32a, b)$$

$$J_v(x) = Lp(\Delta P - \Pi(x))$$

where Q_0 is the incident plasma flow, and the oncotic pressure Π is given by Eq. 5.

To solve for the total sieving of solute by a glomerular capillary, Eq. 32 is iterated to provide the inputs for Eq. 29, which is then integrated along the capillary according to Eq. 31. Although the actual glomerular capillary bed is a complex and heterogeneous network of branching blood vessels, the sieving coefficients predicted for the idealized homogeneous circular cylinder differ negligibly from those predicted from a reconstruction that incorporates the complex anatomy (98).

Sieving Curves To compute the size-selective properties of the glomerular barrier it is necessary to know the sieving coefficient Θ for multiple tracer solutes with different radii. Therefore, tracer solutes are required whose concentration in Bowman's space can be measured or inferred. Direct sampling from Bowman's space is inconvenient or impossible in most circumstances, so it is usually necessary to infer sieving coefficient(s) from urinary clearance(s). The sieving coefficient of a tracer solute is equal to its urinary clearance divided by the GFR, as long as the test solute is not secreted, reabsorbed, or metabolized by the tubule. Polysaccharides fulfill this criterion of being impervious to processing by the tubule. Also, it is possible to generate mixtures of polysaccharides with a range of Stokes-Einstein radii. These mixtures can be used to plot Θ as a function of Stokes-Einstein radius with many data points in a single experiment. These sieving curves can be used to determine pore size and relative abundance of different pores in heteroporous models.

The most commonly used tracer polysaccharide is dextran, an inert polymer of glucopyranose. There are more than 50 published human and animal studies in which the size-selective characteristics of the glomerular barrier have been analyzed from dextran sieving curves. As a rule, dextran sieving data are consistent with a two-pore model (102) of the glomerular capillary wall where the vast majority are small pores with radius of 48 to 60 Å and the remainder are shunt pores with radius exceeding 100 Å [reviewed in (131)]. However, this use of dextran is seriously encumbered because the equations of pore theory were developed for rigid spheres whereas dextran exists as a flexible random coil (45). Due to its flexibility, a dextran molecule is far less hindered at crossing the filtration barrier than is a rigid spherical molecule of equivalent Stokes-Einstein radius (101). Based on pore sizes computed from dextran sieving data, Θ for albumin (Stokes-Einstein radius 36 Å) should exceed the experimental value by roughly 500-fold. The realization that this discrepancy in Θ between albumin and 36 Å neutral dextran owes mainly to the flexibility of the dextran molecule has reduced the need explain the low sieving coefficient for albumin based on something other than size. Hence, less emphasis is now placed on the charge selectivity of the glomerular capillary wall than there was during the 1970s. Clearly, one must be cautious when using dextran sieving data to predict the sieving of nondextrans. Nonetheless, dextran sieving is reproduc-

ible and precise and predicts the structural changes that befall diseased glomeruli even though they give a biased estimate of pore size.

Ficoll is an inert spherical sucrose polymer with internal cross-linking that confers some rigidity (14). Ficoll has been tested against dextran in rats and found to have sieving coefficient substantially less than size-matched dextran for Stokes-Einstein radii greater than 30 Å (88). Lower sieving coefficients for Ficoll relative to size-matched dextran have also been confirmed in healthy and nephrotic humans (1, 12). However, Ficoll is less convenient to use than dextran in humans because potential toxicity limits the amount that can be given. Also, Ficoll molecules are more compressible than globular proteins such that pore sizes estimated from Ficoll sieving data will overestimate the sieving coefficients of like-sized globular proteins, albeit to a lesser degree than dextran (131).

The glomerular sieving of polysaccharides is useful to the extent that it helps explain the permselectivity for endogenous proteins. Ultimately, however, the predictions based on polysaccharide sieving must be verified for proteins. As already discussed, the direct approach of measuring protein sieving by micropuncture is difficult. Other strategies have been used to estimate sieving coefficients for proteins without requiring micropuncture. We will mention two of these. One alternative to micropuncture is to reduce the tubular processing of proteins by cooling the isolated perfused rat kidney to 8°C (cold IPK) to stop the tubule from degrading or transporting filtered proteins, then assuming that the filtered protein equals the protein excretion. Adding furosemide and nitroprusside to the cold IPK eliminates water reabsorption almost completely and reportedly yields stable values for albumin fractional clearance. However, GFR is low in the cold IPK and perfusate flow is high, which means that the determinants of glomerular filtration are quite different than in vivo. This should pose a problem for the cold IPK because fractional solute clearance must depend on the determinants of glomerular filtration rate given that convection and diffusion both contribute to solute transport (20). Nonetheless, cooling seems to have minimal effect on the urine to plasma ratio for Ficoll, and the cold IPK has been used to address a variety of issues related to glomerular protein sieving (50, 59–61, 69, 70, 119).

Tenstad et al. (123) have made direct estimates of glomerular sieving coefficents for proteins based on tracer radioactivity retained in the kidney 6 minutes after administering radiolabeled proteins to rats. The rationale behind this approach is that there is a several-minute window of opportunity when a tracer protein will remain in the kidney after being filtered and taken up by the proximal tubule and before being degraded or reabsorbed back to the body. An estimate of this time window was first made using cystatin C, which is a freely filtered protein that is completely degraded by the tubule. As such, the rate at which cystatin C enters the urinary space is equal to its plasma concentration × GFR. Administering a bolus of labeled cystatin C along with a GFR marker, then stopping the experiment at various time points and counting tracer activity in the kidney revealed that cystatin C remains in the kidney for at least 6 minutes after undergoing filtration (123). In tracer uptake experiments using neutral horseradish peroxidase, myoglobin, and charge-neutralized albumin, the sieving coefficients for each of these proteins was significantly less than for Ficoll or dextran of equal hydrodynamic radius (75). The principle pore radius computed by pore theory is 37.5, 46, and 55 Å for protein, Ficoll, and dextran, respectively (Fig. 10) (131).

Charge Selectivity of the Filtration Barrier

Since the 1970s it has been generally accepted that the glomerular capillary wall is less permeable to proteins that are negatively charged. In addition to the low Θ for albumin compared to neutral dextran of equivalent Stokes-Einstein radius, the impression of charge selectivity was supported by experiments that compared sieving of anionic, neutral, and cationic dextrans (17, 19). It has since been learned that anionic dextran-sulfate can be taken up by glomerular cells, desulfated, then secreted to appear in the urine as neutral dextran (122, 132). In addition, sieving of dextran sulfate is reduced through binding to plasma proteins (46). These effects could create the appearance of charge selectivity of the filtration barrier where none exists. Furthermore, other experiments using Ficoll or hydroxyethyl starch failed to show a charge-selective barrier to either of these alternative polysaccharide molecules (47, 108).

Although the notion of charge selectivity for polysaccharides has lost some of its currency, the bulk of evidence still

favors the notion that charge selectivity applies to the filtration of globular proteins. Rennke showed a lesser sieving coefficient for anionic horseradish peroxidase (HRP) than neutral HRP in rats (100), allowing that part of the effect may have been due to degradation of anionic HRP during filtration (90). Lindström showed charge selectivity for the somewhat larger protein, lactate dehydrogenase (70). Using the tissue tracer uptake technique described previously, Lund (75) calculated sieving coefficients and reflection coefficients for several proteins, including charge-neutralized and native anionic human serum albumin. Θ for anionic albumin was remarkably similar to the micropuncture result of Tojo (vide supra) while Θ for neutral albumin was 10-fold higher (Table 3).

THEORETICAL BASIS OF CHARGE SELECTIVE SIEVING

Deen et al. (29) presented a theory for glomerular filtration of charged solutes based on a homogeneous distribution of fixed negative charges within the glomerular capillary wall (29) as idealized in Fig. 11. The mathematical description of this model begins with an equation for flux through an imaginary thin surface within a membrane. This is the same as Eq. 26, except that the full electrochemical potential is included in the diffusion force to yield

$$J_s = -D_s \left(\frac{dC_s}{dx} + z_s C_s \frac{d\Psi}{dx} \right) + J_v \left(1 - \sigma_s \right) C_s \qquad (33)$$

where $D_s = D_0 \times A_{eff}$, Z_s is the valence of s and ψ is a dimensionless electrical potential. Next, it is assumed that there is electrochemical equilibrium at both membrane-solution interfaces. This allows the step change in Cs at each interface

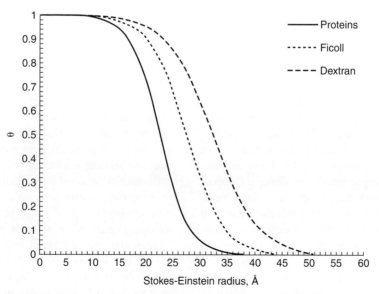

FIGURE 10   Sieving curves for dextran, Ficoll, and neutral proteins constructed from the literature. (From Venturoli D, Rippe B. Ficoll and dextran vs. globular proteins as probes for testing glomerular permselectivity: effects of molecular size, shape, charge, and deformability. *Am J Physiol Renal Physiol* 2005; 288(4):F605–613.)

TABLE 3 Charge Permselectivity of the Glomerulus in Rats Confirmed by the Tracer Uptake Method Using Neutralized or Native Anionic Human Serum Albumin

	Stokes-Einstein radius (Å)	Isoelectric pH	Θ	σ
Neutral albumin	35.0	7.4	0.0055	0.996
Anionic albumin	35.5	4.9	0.0006	0.9997

Since these experiments were performed in vivo, they reflect the normal contributions of diffusion and convection to albumin flux.

Θ, glomerular sieving coefficient. σ, Staverman reflection coefficient.

Source: Adapted from Lund U, Rippe A, Venturoli D, Tenstad O, Grubb A, and Rippe B. Glomerular filtration rate dependence of sieving of albumin and some neutral proteins in rat kidneys. *Am J Physiol Renal Physiol* 2003;284: F1226–F1234.

to be calculated from the Nernst equation and the steric hindrance

$$C_s'(0)=C_{plasma}\left(1-\sigma_s\right)\exp\left(z_s\left(\psi_{plasma}-\psi'(0)\right)\right)$$
$$C_s'(\delta)=C_{filtrate}\left(1-\sigma_s\right)\exp\left(z_s\left(\psi_{B.S.}-\psi'(\delta)\right)\right) \quad (34)$$

where (') refers to values within the membrane just inside its interface with the plasma or Bowman's space dψ/dx, and *B.S.* refers to Bowman's space. Within the membrane, is small so that the same integration can be done as was done to Eq. 27. Integrating from 0 to δ within the membrane and substituting and rearranging yields the following charged-solute flux equation which is analogous to Eq. 29

$$J_s=\frac{C_{plasma}J_v\left(1-\sigma\right)\exp\left(z_s\left(\psi_{plasma}-\psi'(0)\right)\right)}{1-\exp\left(-P_e\right)\left(1-\left(1-\sigma\right)\exp\left(z_s\left(\psi_{B.S.}-\psi'(\delta)\right)\right)\right)} \quad (35)$$

The two electrical potential differences in Eq. 35 are next to be determined. These cannot be measured, but are given by the Donnan potentials for Na^+

$$\psi-\psi'=\ln\left(\frac{C_{Na^+}'}{C_{Na^+}}\right) \quad (36)$$

Since there must be zero net charge in each compartment

$$C_{Na}=C_{An} \text{ and } C_{Na}'=C_{An}'+C_m \quad (37)$$

where *An* refers to mobile anions and *Cm* is the density of negative charges in the membrane. At Donnan equilibrium

$$\frac{C_{An}'}{C_{An}}=\frac{C_{Na}}{C_{Na}'} \quad (38)$$

Combining Eqs. 37 and 38 yields a quadratic equation for C_{Na}' with the positive root

$$C_{Na^+}'=\frac{C_m+\sqrt{C_m^2+4C_{Na^+}C_{An^-}}}{2} \quad (39)$$

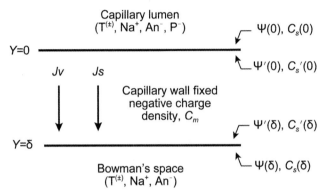

FIGURE 11 Idealized capillary wall with fixed negative charge density C_m that causes Donnan potentials (ψ-ψ') to form at interfaces of the membrane with the capillary lumen and Bowman's space. These Donnan potentials retard the flux of anionic tracer T^- and accelerate the flux of cationic tracer T^+ according to equations shown in the text. An, mobile anions. Panionic proteins. (Adapted from Deen et al. *Am J Physiol* 238:F126, 1980.)

Inserting Eq. 39 into the numerator of Eq. 36 gives the Donnan potentials. Inserting these into Eq. 35 gives an expression for solute flux that incorporates the effect of C_m. If C_m or z_s is zero, this reduces to Eq. 29, as it should. Θ_s for the glomerulus is obtained by integrating J_s along the capillary surface as per Eq. 31.

Deen's model predicts that a single parameter, C_m, can account for charge selective sieving. This is shown in Fig. 12 where the theory was applied to anionic dextran sulfate on the basis of other model inputs from the normal rat in which neutral dextran was used to determine a pore radius.

This theory of charge-selective filtration has been criticized because isolated GBM was found to have too low a density of anionic charge to satisfy model predictions for what is required of the GBM to operate as barrier to albumin (22). However, the inflated 50-Å pore radius calculated from neutral dextran sieving may account for the discrepancy. It should also be noted that this model explains charge-related sieving entirely on the basis of Donnan potentials at the two membrane interfaces. It makes no allowance for any effect that the fixed membrane charges might have on the steric hindrance

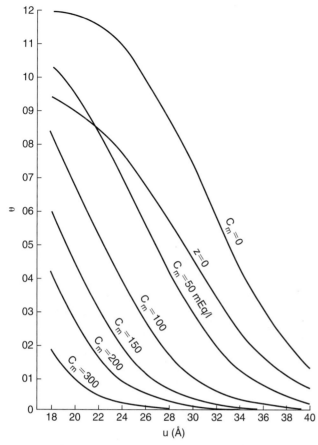

FIGURE 12 Sieving coeffcient (Θ) for dextran sulfate as function of Stokes-Einstein radius, a. C_m-membrane fixed negative charge density in mEq/liter. Valence, z, of dextran $= -0.245xa$. z=0 is curve for neutral dextran. (From Deen et al. *Am J Physiol* 238:F126, 1980.)

relative to free solution (D_{eff}) can be expressed as the product of its diffusion coefficient in the gel relative to free solution (D_{gel}/D_0)and the fraction of the gel volume available to be occupied by the protein (e.g. its partition coefficient, Φ).

$$D_{eff} = \frac{D_{gel}}{D_0}\Phi \qquad (40)$$

Therefore, it is conceivable that electrostatic interactions with a negatively charged gel might impede the transit of like-charged molecules by reducing D_{gel} or Φ.

One way to study the role of electrostatic interactions between proteins and gels is to inhibit these interactions by increasing the ionic strength of the solvent. Ions in the solvent have the effect of screening the charged solute protein from the coulomb forces that would otherwise be exerted on it by the fixed charges on the gel fibers. (This phenomenon, which is known as field screening, also explains why a submarine cannot receive radio communications while submerged under the ocean.)

Adding a point charge at a fixed position in any medium generates an electric field that attracts mobile ions of opposite charge. An electric field formed by those charges will offset the field associated with the fixed charge so that at some distance from the fixed charge, one can no longer "sense" its presence. If a fixed charge is added, causing mobile charges to reposition in response, it can be shown from the density of repositioned charges that the influence of the fixed charge decays exponentially with distance. The reciprocal of the decay constant is known as the Debye length. The Debye length can be derived by rearranging the equation for electrochemical potential into a Boltzman distribution for the concentration of redistributed charges, using the first term of the Taylor series expansion for this Boltzmann distribution to approximate concentration as a linear function of voltage, then plugging the result into the Poisson equation from classical electrical theory, which expresses the second derivative of voltage as a function of charge density. This yields

$$C(r) = \frac{l}{d}\exp\left(\frac{-r}{d}\right)\text{ where }d = \sqrt{\frac{k_B T \epsilon}{q^2 C_0}} \qquad (41)$$

$C(r)$ is the probability density of relocated charges at distance r from the fixed charge, d is the Debye length, k_B is Boltzmann's constant, ϵ is the permitivity, q is the elementary charge, and C_0 is the baseline concentration of mobile charges, e.g. the ionic strength of the buffer. Accordingly, increasing the salinity of the buffer will shorten the Debye length and the influence of the fixed charge wanes almost completely beyond two or three Debye lengths. For a material with a typical dielectric constant and 0.15 molar mobile charges, the Debye length is about 2 Å, which is similar to the difference between the main pore radius estimated from sieving of neutral proteins (37.5 Å, vide supra) and the molecular radius of albumin (36 Å).

or friction within the pore. Such effects are likely and would further reduce the amount of fixed negative membrane charge required to account for any degree of charge selectivity. To date, there is no theory for quantifying this, although it has been argued that a phenomenon known as "charge screening" can be used to show reduced partitioning of anionic proteins in the glomerular capillary wall (vide infra). Furthermore, the relevant Donnan potential may arise at the plasma interface with the negatively charged endothelial glycocalyx rather than the basement membrane, in which case the charge density of the GBM is not the appropriate straw man for arguments against charge-based sieving.

ENDOTHELIAL GLYCOCALYX AS A POSSIBLE CHARGE BARRIER

Although the lack of detailed information about the dimensions and electrical properties of the glycocalyx forestalls a definitive analysis, arguments have been made for the glycocalyx as a principal charge barrier. The endothelial glycocalyx forms a hydrated gel within the fenestrae and contains fixed negative charges on its gel fibers. As for a pore, the effective permeability of a solute in a gel

Johnson et al. (58) made use of charge screening to examine the role of electrostatic interactions on diffusion and partitioning of bovine serum albumin in 6% sulfated agarose gels by varying the ionic strength of the buffer from 0.01 to 1.0 M. Increasing the ionic strength to shorten the Debye length and reduce the distance over which repulsive coulomb forces from gel anions can be "felt" had minimal effect on the diffusion coefficient for albumin, but caused a major increase in its partitioning coefficient, Φ. Therefore, the anionic gel poses a selective barrier to sieving of anionic proteins not because it restricts the diffusive mobility of albumin within the gel, but because electrostatic forces reduce the amount of space available within the gel to be occupied by albumin (58).

The notion of altering buffer strength to manipulate the Debye length has also been applied to study the filtration of charged proteins in the cold IPK (120). Perfusion with physiologic concentration of buffer salts (152 mM) yielded respective sieving coefficients of 0.11 and 0.045 for neutral and anionic horseradish peroxidase (HRP). Reducing the total salts in the buffer to from 152 to 34 mM did not affect the sieving of neutral HRP, but reduced the sieving coefficient for anionic HRP by about half. Thus, there appears to be selective screening out of anionic HRP by the glomerulus that increases along with the distance over which coulomb forces between the barrier and albumin are able to act. A note of caution is warranted when ascribing the effect of buffer salinity to charge screening within the membrane, since increasing the buffer salinity will also reduce the Donnan potential at the membrane-solution interface, according to Eqs. 35–39.

Glomerular sieving properties have also been examined in the cold isolated perfused kidney of mice treated with glycosaminoglycan-degrading enzymes intended to disrupt the endothelial glycocalyx. This treatment was estimated to reduce the fiber charge density by 10% and increased the sieving coefficient for albumin by fivefold but only increased sieving of Ficoll by 1.5-fold, thus demonstrating that hyaluronic acid, chondroitin sulfate, and heparan sulfate are important for glomerular charge selectivity (56). If the endothelial glycocalyx contributes to the screening of albumin, this removes some of the burden of showing how the GBM can do this when it appears that the GBM contains too few fixed charges. Screening by the glycocalyx at the interface with the well-stirred plasma also reduces the burden on the epithelial slit diaphragm which might otherwise clog.

Combining Fiber Matrix Theory with the Pore Model

Using a wider range of dextran radii than previously used by others, Katz et al. (63) generated dextran sieving curves that were not uniformly convex upward, but flattened out slightly above 40 Å. This nuance could be explained by a two-pore model in which the pores were filled with a fiber matrix, but it could not be explained by any open-pore model of equal

complexity. Citing the location of albumin molecules found in glomerular sections (105) and confocal tracking of dextran in isolated glomeruli (23), it was hypothesized that the albumin barrier does not reside in the GBM anyway and that the endothelial fenestrae, filled with fibrous glycocalyx, justify the mathematical model. The pore–matrix model has features corresponding to the pore theory model described. For example, steric hindrance occurs due to the presence of the gel fibers. There is also reduced solute mobility due to the gel fibers. The specific formulae for these were developed from the theoretical groundwork for gel permeation by solutes provided by Ogston (85) and combined with pore theory by Katz et al. (63).

Structure-Based Models of the Filtration Barrier

Since the 1990s there has been progress toward relating the filtration properties of the glomerulus to its actual physical structure. This is mainly the work of Deen and colleagues who apply modern numerical methods in fluid mechanics to a specific structural model that is based on morphometry (27, 32). The defined structural elements of the model include the endothelial cells and fenestrae, the GBM represented as homogeneous porous material, and the epithelial cell foot processes with filtration slits bridged by slit diaphragms. These elements form a filtering subunit that is repeated many times to form the glomerular capillary. Each filtration subunit consists of one filtration slit, several fenestrae, and the GBM in between (Fig. 13). Water movement is assumed to be paracellular. In some instances consideration is given to the endothelial glycocalyx, although untestable assumptions are required for this, since the permeability characteristics of the glycocalyx are not known.

The hydraulic conductances of the endothelium, GBM and filtration slits are treated as separate conductances arranged in series such that the overall conductance is given by a reciprocal of summed resistance

$$\frac{P_{UF}}{J_v} = \frac{1}{k} = \frac{1}{k_{endo}} + \frac{1}{k_{GBM}} + \frac{1}{k_{epi}} \tag{42}$$

where P_{UF} is the ultrafiltration pressure and k is the hydraulic permeability.

By analogy to the first term in Eq. 3a, the hydraulic permeability for a single endothelial fenestra is equal to

$$k_{endo} = \frac{\epsilon_F \overline{v}_Z}{\left(P_G - \overline{P}_0\right)} \tag{43}$$

where z is the direction perpendicular to the membrane, v_Z is the average z-component of the flow velocity within the fenestra, $\overline{P}_0$ is the average pressure at the outflow, P_G is the capillary pressure, and ϵ_F is the fraction of the endothelial surface covered by fenestrae. $\overline{P}_0$ and $\overline{v}_{0\,Z}$ are determined from pressure and velocity fields calculated by finite element analysis applied to a

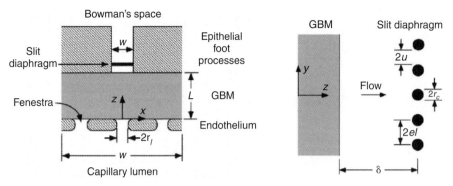

FIGURE 13   Left: Idealized structural unit of glomerular capillary wall corresponding to one filtration slit. Right: Idealized structure of slit diaphragm in relation to GBM. Dimensions in nm: W 360, L 200, w 39, rf 30, rc 2, 2u 20±15, δ 500, fractional area of fenestrae 0.2, fractional area of filtration slits 0.11. (From Edwards et al. *Am J Physiol* 1999;276:F892–902.)

simplified Navier-Stokes' equation, which relates fluid flow to pressure and external forces acting on a fluid.

Hydraulic permeability of the basement membrane is estimated from Darcy's law, which describes the flow of water through porous media when the structural details of the media are unknown

$$v = -\nabla P \frac{k_D}{\mu} \qquad (44)$$

where v is the velocity vector, μ is the viscosity, and k_D is the so-called Darcy permeability of the medium. The Darcy permeability is related to L_p in Eq. 3a and must be determined empirically. Values for k_D/μ are available from measurements made on isolated glomerular basement membrane (24, 35, 103). It is a complicated problem to solve for the pressures and flows within the GBM due to streaming and bulging of the velocity and pressure fields that arise because fluid must enter only through fenestrae and leave only through epithelial slits that cover only part of the basement membrane. These pressure and flow fields are determined numerically after setting the appropriate conditions for zero flow in the z-direction at boundary areas covered by cells and setting the divergence of flow equal to zero to satisfy conservation of mass for a noncompressible fluid. Calculating k_{GBM} in this way is somewhat artificial inasmuch as the apparent conductance of the GBM will increase along with the fraction of its surface that is covered by fenestrae and filtration slits. Therefore, as the number of fenestrae and filtration slits declines the apparent hydraulic resistance of the GBM will increase even though there has been no actual change to the GBM.

Hydraulic permeability of the epithelial layer is calculated, again by applying the simplified Navier-Stokes' equation, this time to an ultrastructural model of the filtration slit as a rectangular channel bridged by fibers (31). This particular geometry for the slit diaphragm is based on microscopy of Rodewald and Karnovsky (104), who suggested that the filtration slit consists of a central fiber

connected by bridging fibers to the cell membranes on either side (Fig. 14). Solving the model reveals that the slit diaphragm is the main site of resistance to flow through the filtration slit and there is little resistance to flow along the remainder of the filtration slit, which is a channel whose walls are formed by two adjacent foot processes. One caveat to these predictions has arisen from molecular sieving data, which suggest that the true pore dimensions provided by the Rodewald-Karnovsky model are too small and are better explained if the slit diaphragm is represented by a single row of parallel cylindrical fibers rather than two rows of pores separated by a central fiber (36). However, a more detailed image of the slit diaphragm has now been obtained by electron tomography, which vali-

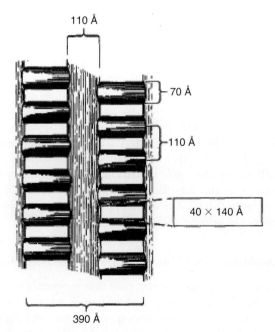

FIGURE 14   Schematic drawing of the epithelial slit diaphragm. Typical cross-sectional dimensions of pores between cross-bridges are 40 x 140 D. (From Rodewald R, Karnovsky MJ. *J Cell Biol* 1974;60:432–433.)

dates the basic zipperlike configuration with pores on each side that approximate the dimension of albumin. As depicted by electron tomography, these pores appear more irregular and tortuous than previously imagined (134).

The morphometric parameters and hydraulic permeabilities calculated from the ultrastructural model of Deen et al. (32) are shown in Table 4, which also shows that the hydraulic permeability predicted by the model is consistent with values obtained by micropuncture in normal rats. Some other predictions of the model cannot be tested by micropuncture. For example, a main prediction of the model is that the GBM and epithelial layers contribute equally and, together, account for most of the resistance to glomerular filtration. The endothelial fenestrae pose little resistance to bulk flow except that reducing their fractional area reduces the apparent permeability of the GBM. Furthermore, as already mentioned, most resistance of the filtration slit is due to the slit diaphragm rather than to drag along the length of the slit.

An important test of the model is that it predicts changes in the ultrafiltration coefficient that occur when the glomerular structure is altered. The model has successfully forecasted changes in ultrafiltration coefficient brought about by manipulating dietary protein and/or renal mass to alter glomerular morphology in rats with adriamycin nephrosis (81).

Computation based on morphometry has also been used to estimate glomerular ultrafiltration coefficient from renal biopsies in patients with reduced GFR due to membranous or minimal change nephropathies (33) and preeclampsia (65). In each of these conditions, GFR was reduced in spite of normal PAH clearance. For GFR to decline while nephron plasma flow remains constant there must be a decrease in either glomerular ultrafiltration pressure or ultrafiltration coefficient. While it is not possible to measure ultrafiltration pressure in humans, the determinants of *SNGFR* have been extensively evaluated in a wide range of animal models of glomerular disease. With the single exception of cyclosporine toxicity (125), low pressure in the glomerular capillary does not provide the basis for low *SNGFR* in any of these models. Therefore, it is reasonable to assume that ultrafiltration pressure is not reduced in humans with idiopathic nephrotic syndrome or preeclampsia, and that the low filtration fraction in these patients is likely to be the consequence of a decline in ultrafiltration coefficient. Once this premise is accepted, there are several potential explanations for an apparent decline in ultrafiltration coefficient in a glomerulus. First, this could be due to a loss of capillary surface area. Second, it could result from mismatched blood flow among capillary loops within the glomerulus such that those loops with low flow manifest filtration equilibrium early in their course, which eliminates their latter portions from contributing to the working area. A third mechanism for reducing ultrafiltration coefficient could be to alter in the chemical composition of the GBM or slit diaphragm to make them less permeable to water. Finally, ultrafiltration coefficient could decline due to changes in geometry of the individual filtration unit. The latter of these possibilities is amenable to testing by applying computational fluid dynamics to morphometry. Based on this approach, changes in geometry of the filtration unit predict that ultrafiltration coefficient will be different between normal subjects and those with minimal change disease, membranous nephropthy, and preeclampsia. Although each disease has its own morphology, reduced frequency of filtration slits, increased basement membrane thickness, loss of fenestral area, or loss of capillary surface area predicted changes in the ultrafiltration coefficient consistent with what would be necessary to explain the associated declines in GFR, given the reasonable assumption that glomerular capillary pressure was not profoundly reduced and a less-certain assumption that the Darcy permeability for the GBM is unaffected. One interesting prediction of the model is that, while the GBM is thickened in membranous nephropathy, this has little importance to the GFR because an even greater augmentation of the average distance traveled from fenestra to slit diaphragm results from the lower filtration slit density which requires much of the filtrate to stream obliquely through the GBM rather than crossing it directly.

TABLE 4 Microstructural Parameters and Ultrafiltration Coefficient in the Rat used by Drumond et al.

Width of filtration unit	360 nm
Thickness of glomerular basement membrane (GBM)	200 nm
Width of filtration slit	39 nm
Fractional area of fenestrae	0.2
Number of fenestrae per unit	3
Fractional area of slits	0.11
Darcy permeability of GBM	2.7 nm^2
k_{endo}	$2.0 \times 10^{-7} \text{ m-s}^{-1}\text{-Pa}^{-1}$
k_{GBM}	$8.3 \times 10^{-9} \text{ m-s}^{-1}\text{-Pa}^{-1}$
k_{epi}	$8.6 \times 10^{-9} \text{ m-s}^{-1}\text{-Pa}^{-1}$
k	$4.1 \times 10^{-9} \text{ m-s}^{-1}\text{-Pa}^{-1}$
k estimated from micropuncture and morphometry	$3 \times 10^{-9} - 5 \times 10^{-9} \text{ m-s}^{-1}\text{-Pa}^{-1}$

Drumond MC, Deen WH. Structural determinants of glomerular hydraulic permeability. *Am J Physiol Renal Fluid Electrolyte Physiol* 1994;266: F1–F12.

See also Figure 13.

SUMMARY

Details about the physics of glomerular filtration have become known over the past century. Different approaches to describing glomerular filtration use different admixtures of phenomenology and structural detail. The spectrum of useful models extends from the glomerular capillary as an idealized circular cylinder with homogenous permeability to water and small solutes and zero permeability to macromolecules, to a tube perforated by discreet cylindrical pores with differential permeability to solutes based on size and electrical charge, to a representation that incorporates actual physical dimensions to determine the contributions of endothelial, basement membrane and epithelial layers to the filtration barrier. In the final analysis, each of these paradigms begins with Kedem and Katchalsky's application of nonequilibrium thermodynamics to the coupled transport of solute and solvent across membranes.

Acknowledgment

This work was performed with grant support from NIH, NIDDK, DK28602 and the Department of Veterans Affairs Research Service.

References

1. Andersen S, Blouch K, Bialek J, Deckert M, Parving HH, and Myers BD. Glomerular permselectivity in early stages of overt diabetic nephropathy. *Kidney Int* 2000;58:2129–2137.
2. Anderson JL, Quinn JA. Restricted transport in small pores A model for steric exclusion and hindered particle motion. *Biophys J* 1974; 14:130–150.
3. Anderson S, Meyer TW, Rennke HG, Brenner BM. Control of glomerular hypertension limits glomerular injury in rats with reduced renal mass. *J Clin Invest* 1985;76(2):612–619.
4. Arendshorst WJ, Gottschalk CW. Glomerular ultrafiltration dynamics: historical perspective. *Am J Physiol* 1985;248(2 Pt 2):F163–174.
5. Bakris GL, Weir MR. Angiotensin-converting enzyme inhibitor-associated elevations in serum creatinine: is this a cause for concern? *Arch Intern Med* 2000;160(5):685–693.
6. Baylis C. The mechanism of the increase in glomerular filtration rate in the twelve-day pregnant rat. *J Physiol* 1980;305:405–414.
7. Baylis C, Ichikawa I, Willis WT, Wilson CB, Brenner BM. Dynamics of glomerular ultrafiltration. IX. Effects of plasma protein concentration. *Am J Physiol* 1977;232(1):F58–71.
8. Blantz RC. Effect of mannitol on glomerular ultrafiltration in the hydropenic rat. *J Clin Invest* 1974;54(5):1135–1143.
9. Blantz RC, Gabbai F, Gushwa LC, Wilson CB. The influence of concomitant experimental hypertension and glomerulonephritis. *Kidney Int* 1987;32(5):652–663
10. Blantz RC, Gabbai FB, Gushwa LC, Peterson OW, Wilson CB. Role of mesangial cell in glomerular response to volume and angiotensin II. *Am J Physiol* 1993;264(1 Pt 2):F158–165.
11. Blantz RC, Konnen KS, Tucker BJ. Angiotensin II effects upon the glomerular microcirculation and ultrafiltration coefficient of the rat. *J Clin Invest* 1976;57(2):419–434.
12. Blantz RC, Rector FC Jr, Seldin DW. Effect of hyperoncotic albumin expansion upon glomerular ultrafiltration in the rat. *Kidney Int* 1974;6(4):209–221.
13. Blouch K, Deen WM, Fauvel JP, Bialek J, Derby G, Myers BD: Molecular configuration and glomerular size selectivity in healthy and nephrotic humans. *Am J Physiol* 1997;273: F430–F437.
14. Bohrer MP, Deen WM, Robertson CR, Troy JL, Brenner BM. Influence of molecular configuration on the passage of macromolecules across the glomerular capillary wall. *J Gen Physiol* 1979;74(5):583–593.
15. Bowman W. *On the Structure and Use of the Malpighian Bodies of the Kidney, with Observations on the Circulation.* London: Printed by R. and J. E. Taylor, 1842. Offprint from *Philosophical Transactions of the Royal Society, Part I for 1842.*
16. Brenner BM, Falchuk KH, Keimowitz RI, Berliner RW. The relationship between peritubular capillary protein concentration and fluid reabsorption by the renal proximal tubule. *J Clin Invest* 1969;48(8):1519–1531.
17. Brenner BM, Hostetter TH, and Humes HD. Glomerular permselectivity: barrier function based on discrimination of molecular size and charge. *Am J Physiol Renal Fluid Electrolyte Physiol* 1978;234:F455–F460.
18. Brenner BM, Troy JL, Daugharty TM. The dynamics of glomerular ultrafiltration in the rat. *J Clin Invest* 1971;50(8):1776–1780.
19. Chang RL, Deen WM, Robertson CR, and Brenner BM. Permselectivity of the glomerular capillary wall. III. Restricted transport of polyanions. *Kidney Int* 1975;8:212–218.
20. Chang RL, Robertson CR, Deen WM, Brenner BM. Permselectivity of the glomerular capillary wall to macromolecules, I: Theoretical considerations. *Biophys J* 1975;15(9):861–886.
21. Chasis H, Ranges HA, Goldring W, Smith HW. The control of renal blood flow and glomerular filtration in normal man. *J Clin Invest* 1938;17:683–697.
22. Comper WD, Lee AS, Tay M, Adal Y. Anionic charge concentration of rat kidney glomeruli and glomerular basement membrane. *Biochem J* 1993;289 :647–652.
23. Daniels BS, Deen WM, Mayer G, Meyer T, Hostetter TH. Glomerular permeability barrier in the rat. Functional assessment by in vitro methods. *J Clin Invest* 1993;92(2):929–936.
24. Daniels BS, Hauser EH, Deen WM, Hostetter TH. Glomerular basement membrane: in vitro studies of water and protein permeability. *Am J Physiol Renal Fluid Electrolyte Physiol* 1992;262:F919–F926.

25. De Nicola L, Blantz RC, Gabbai FB. Renal functional reserve in the early stage of experimental diabetes. *Diabetes* 1992;41(3):267–273.
26. Deen WM, Bridges CR, Brenner BM, Myers BD: Heteroporous model of glomerular size selectivity: Application to normal and nephrotic humans. *Am J Physiol* 1985;249:F374–F389.
27. Deen WM, Lazzara MJ, Myers BD. Structurual determinants of glomerular permeability. *Am J Physiol Renal Physiol* 2001;281:F579–F596.
28. Deen WM, Robertson CR, Brenner BM. A model of glomerular ultrafiltration in the rat. *Am J Physiol* 1971;223:1178–1183.
29. Deen WM, Satvat B, Jamieson JM. Theoretical model for glomerular filtration of charged solutes. *Am J Physiol* 1980;238(2):F126–139.
30. Deen WM, Troy JL, Robertson CR, Brenner BM. Dynamics of glomerular ultrafiltration in the rat. IV. Determination of the ultrafiltration coefficient. *J Clin Invest* 1973;52(6):1500–1508.
31. Drumond MC, Deen WM. Stokes flow through a row of cylinders between parallel walls: model for the glomerular slit diaphragm. *J Biomech Eng* 1994;116(2):184–189.
32. Drumond MC, Deen WH. Structural determinants of glomerular hydraulic permeability. *Am J Physiol Renal Fluid Electrolyte Physiol* 1994;266:F1–F12.
33. Drumond MC, Kristal B, Myers BD, Deen WM. Structural basis for reduced glomerular filtration capacity in nephrotic humans. *J Clin Invest* 1994;94(3):1187–1195.
34. Dutrochet H. *L'agent immédiat du mouvement vital dévoilé dans la nature et dans son mode d'action chez les végétaux et les animaux.* Paris: JB Ballière, 1826. See also: Nouvelles recherches sur l'endosmose et l'exosmose. Paris: JB Ballière, 1828.
35. Edwards A, Daniels BS, Deen WM. Hindered transport of macromolecules in isolated glomeruli II. Convection and pressure effects in basememt membrane. *Biophys J* 1997;72:214–222.
36. Edwards A, Daniels BS, Deen WM. Ultrastructural model for size selectivity in glomerular filtration. *Am J Physiol* 1999;276(6 Pt 2):F892–902.
37. Einstein A. Uber die von der molekularkinetistchen Theorie der Waerme geforderte Bewegung von in ruhenden Fluessigkeiten suspendierten Teilchen. *Ann Physik* 1905;17:549–560.
38. Elger M, Sakai T, Kriz W. The vascular pole of the renal glomerulus of rat. *Adv Anat Embryol Cell Biol* 1998;139:1–98.
39. Falchuk HK Berliner RW. Hydrostatic pressures in peritubular capillaries and tubules in the rat kidney *Am J Physiol* 1971;220:1422–1426.
40. Ferry JD. Ultrafilter membranes and ultrafiltration. *Chem Rev* 1936;18:373.
41. Fronek K, Zweifach BW. Microvascular pressure distribution in skeletal muscle and the effect of vasodilation. *Am J Physiol* 1975; 228(3):791–796.
42. Gabbai FB, Gushwa LC, Wilson CB, Blantz RC. An evaluation of the development of experimental membranous nephropathy. *Kidney Int* 1987;31(6):1267–1278.
43. Gabbai FB, Gushwa LC, Peterson OW, Wilson CB, Blantz RC. Analysis of renal function in the two-kidney Goldblatt model. *Am J Physiol* 1987;252(1 Pt 2):F131–137.
44. Gomez DM. Evaluation of renal resistances, with special reference to changes in essential hypertension. *J Clin Invest* 1951;30:1143–1155.
45. Granath KA. Solution properties of branched dextrans. *J Colloid Sci* 1958;13:308–328.
46. Guasch A, Deen WM, and Myers BD. Charge selectivity of the glomerular filtration barrier in healthy and nephrotic humans. *J Clin Invest* 1993;92:2274–2282.
47. Guimarãães MA, Nikolovski J, Pratt LM, Greive K, and Comper WD. Anomalous fractional clearance of negatively charged Ficoll relative to uncharged Ficoll. *Am J Physiol Renal Physiol* 2003;285:F1118–F1124.
48. Haberman WL, Sayre RM. Motion of rigid and fluid spheres in stationary and moving liquids inside cylindrical tubes. David Taylor Model Basin. Report No. 1143, Washington, DC: US Navy, 1958.
49. Hall JE, Guyton AC, Smith MJ Jr, Coleman TG. Blood pressure and renal function during chronic changes in sodium intake: role of angiotensin. *Am J Physiol* 1980;239:F271–280.
50. Haraldsson BS, Johnsson EK, Rippe B. Glomerular permselectivity is dependent on adequate serum concentrations of orosomucoid. *Kidney Int* 1992;41:310–316.
51. Heidenhain, RP. Absonderungsvorgaenge. Sechster Abschnitt. Die Harnabsonderung (Viertes Capitel. Die Absonderung der festen Harnbestandteile). In: Leipzig HL (ed.). *Handbuch d. Physiol Fuenfter Teil.* Germany: Vogel, 1883. 341–343.
52. Heller J, Horacek V. Angiotensin II: preferential efferent constriction? *Ren Physiol* 1986;9:357–365.
53. Hostetter TH. Human renal response to a meat meal. *Am J Physiol* 1986;250(Pt 2):F613–618.
54. Hostetter TH, Troy JL, Brenner BM. Glomerular hemodynamics in experimental diabetes mellitus. *Kidney Int* 1981;19:410–415.
55. Ichikawa I, Brenner BM. Local intrarenal vasoconstrictor-vasodilator interactions in mild partial ureteral obstruction. *Am J Physiol* 1979;236:F131–140.
56. Jeansson M, Haraldsson B. Glomerular size and charge selectivity in the mouse after exposure to glucosaminoglycan-degrading enzymes. *J Am Soc Nephrol* 2003;14:1756–1765.
57. Jensen PK, Christiansen JS, Steven K, Parving HH. Renal function in streptozotocin-diabetic rats. *Diabetologia* 1981;21(4):409–414.
58. Johnson EM, Berk DA, Jain RK, Deen WM. Diffusion and partitioning of proteins in charged agarose gels. *Biophys J* 1995;68(4):1561–1568.
59. Johnsson E, Haraldsson B. An isolated perfused rat kidney preparation designed for assessment of glomerular permeability characteristics. *Acta Physiol Scand* 1992;144(1):65–73.
60. Johnsson E, Rippe B, Haraldsson B. Analysis of the pressure-flow characteristics of isolated perfused rat kidneys with inhibited tubular reabsorption. *Acta Physiol Scand* 1994;150(2):189–199.
61. Johnsson E, Rippe B, Haraldsson B. Reduced permselectivity in isolated perfused rat kidneys following small elevations of glomerular capillary pressure. *Acta Physiol Scand* 1994;150(2):201–209.
62. Katz MA, Bressler EH. Osmosis. In: Staub N, Taylor A (eds.). *Edema: Basic Science and Clinical Manifestations.* New York: Raven Press, 1984:39–60.
63. Katz MA, Schaeffer RC Jr, Gratrix M, Mucha D, Carbajal J. The glomerular barrier fits a two-pore-and-fiber-matrix model: derivation and physiologic test. *Microvasc Res* 1999;57(3):227–243.
64. Kedem O, Katchalsky A. Thermodynamic analysis of the permeability of biological membranes to non-electrolytes. *Biochim Biophys Acta* 1958;27:229–246.

65. Lafayette RA, Druzin M, Sibley R, Derby G, Malik T, Huie P, Polhemus C, Deen WM, Myers BD. Nature of glomerular dysfunction in pre-eclampsia. *Kidney Int* 1998;54(4):1240–1249.

66. Landis EM, Pappenheimer JR. Exchange of substances through the capillary walls. In: Hamilton WF, Dow, P (eds.). *Handbook of Physiology. Circulation.* Washington, DC: American Physiological Society, 963:961 –1034.

67. Lemley KV, Blouch K, Abdullah I, Boothroyd DB, Bennett PH, Myers BD, Nelson RG. Glomerular permselectivity at the onset of nephropathy in type 2 diabetes mellitus. *J Am Soc Nephrol* 2000;11:2095–2105.

68. Lewis EJ, Hunsicker LG, Bain RP, Rohde RD for the Collaborative Study Group. The effect of angiotensin-converting-enzyme inhibition on diabetic nephropathy. *N Engl J Med* 1993;329:1456–1462.

69. Lindström KE, Blom A, Johnsson E, Haraldsson B, Fries E. High glomerular permeability of bikunin despite similarity in charge and hydrodynamic size to serum albumin. *Kidney Int* 1997;51(4):1053–1058.

70. Lindström KE, Johnsson E, Haraldsson B. Glomerular charge selectivity for proteins larger than serum albumin as revealed by lactate dehydrogenase isoforms. *Acta Physiol Scand* 1998;162(4):481–488.

71. Loutzenhiser R, Bidani A, Chilton L. Renal myogenic response: kinetic attributes and physiological role. *Circ Res* 2002;90(12):1316–1324.

72. Lowry OH, Rosebrough NJ, Farr AL, randall RJ. Protein measurement with the Folin phenol reagent. *J Biol Chem* 1951;193:265–275.

73. Ludwig, CFW, Beitraege zur Lehre vom Mechanismus der Harnsekretion. Marburg: N.G. Elwert 1843.

74. Ludwig C. *De viribus physicis secretionem urinae adjuvantibus.* Thesis, Marburg 1842. Reprinted with a translation into English in *Kidney Int* 1994;Suppl 46:1–23.

75. Lund U, Rippe A, Venturoli D, Tenstad O, Grubb A, and Rippe B. Glomerular filtration rate dependence of sieving of albumin and some neutral proteins in rat kidneys. *Am J Physiol Renal Physiol* 2003;284:F1226–F1234.

76. Malpighi, M. *De viscerum structura exercitatio anatomica Bononias.* Iacoi Montiz, 1666. For English translation see: JM Hayman Jr. Maipighi's "Concerning the structure of the kidney." *Ann Med Hist.* 1925;7:242–263.

77. Marandola P, Musitelli S, Jallous H, et al. The aristotelian kidney. *Am J Nephrol* 1994;14: 302–306.

78. Maschio G, Alberti D, Janin G, et al. Effect of the angiotensin-converting-enzyme inhibitor benazepril on the progression of chronic renal insufficiency: the Angiotensin-Converting Enzyme Inhibition in Progressive Renal Disease Trial. *N Engl J Med* 1996;334:939–945.

79. Michels LD, Davidman M, Keane WF. Determinants of glomerular filtration and plasma flow in experimental diabetic rats. *J Lab Clin Med* 1981;8(6):869–885.

80. Michels LD, O'Donnell MP, Keane WF. Glomerular hemodynamic and structural correlations in long-term experimental diabetic rats. *J Lab Clin Med* 1984;103(6):840–847.

81. Miller PL, Scholey JW, Rennke HG, Meyer TW. Glomerular hypertrophy aggravates epithelial cell injury in nephrotic rats. *J Clin Invest* 1990;85(4):1119–1126.

82. Myers BD, Nelson RG, Williams GW, Bennett PH, Hardy SA, Berg RL, Loon N, Knowler WC, Mitch WE. Glomerular function in Pima Indians with noninsulin-dependent diabetes mellitus of recent onset. *J Clin Invest* 1991;88(2):524–530.

83. O'Donnell MP, Kasiske BL, Daniels FX, Keane WF. Effects of nephron loss on glomerular hemodynamics and morphology in diabetic rats. *Diabetes* 1986;35(9):1011–1015.

84. O'Donnell MP, Kasiske BL, Keane WF. Glomerular hemodynamic and structural alterations in experimental diabetes mellitus. *FASEB J* 1988;(8):2339–2347.

85. Ogston, A. G. The spaces in a uniform random suspension of fibRes *Trans Faraday Soc* 1958;54;1754 –1757.

86. Oken DE, Choi SC. Filtration pressure equilibrium: a statistical analysis. *Am J Physiol* 1981;241(2):F196–200.

87. Oken DE, Flamenbaum W. Micropuncture studies of proximal tubule albumin concentrations in normal and nephrotic rats. *J Clin Invest* 1971;50(7):1498–1505.

88. Oliver JD, Anderson S, Troy JL, Brenner BM, Deen WH. Determination of glomerular size-selectivity in the normal rat with Ficoll. *J Am Soc Nephrol* 1992;3:214–218.

89. Onsager, L. Reciprocal relations in irreversible processes. *Int Phys Rev* 1931;37:405–491.

90. Osicka TM and Comper WD. Glomerular charge selectivity for anionic and neutral horseradish peroxidase. *Kidney Int* 1995;47:1630–1637.

91. Paine PL, Scherr P. Drag coefficients for the movement of rigid spheres through liquid-filled cylindrical pores. *Biophys J* 1975;15:1087–1091.

92. Pappenheimer JR. Passage of molecules through capillary walls. *Physiol Rev* 1953;33: 387–423.

93. Parazynski SE, Tucker BJ, Aratow M, Crenshaw A, Hargens AR. Direct measurement of capillary blood pressure in the human lip. *J Appl Physiol* 1993;74(2):946–950.

94. Patlak C S, Goldstein DA, Hoffman JF. The flow of solute and solvent across a two-membrane system. *J Theoret Biol* 1963;5:426–442.

95. Pullman TN, Alving AS, Dern RJ, Landowne M. The influence of dietary protein intake on specific renal functions in normal man. *J Lab Clin Med* 1954;44:320–332.

96. Ray PM. On the theory of osmotic water movement. *Plant Physiol* 1960;35:783–795.

97. Remuzzi A, Brenner BM, Pata V, Tebaldi G, Mariano R, Belloro A, Remuzzi G. Three-dimensional reconstructed glomerular capillary network: blood flow distribution and local filtration. *Am J Physiol* 1992;263(Pt 2):F562–F572.

98. Remuzzi A, Ene-Iordache B. Capillary network structure does not affect theoretical analysis of glomerular size selectivity. *Am J Physiol* 1995;268(Pt 2):F972–979.

99. Remuzzi A, Fassi A, Sangalli F, Malanchini B, Mohamed EI, Bertani T, Remuzzi G. Prevention of renal injury in diabetic MWF rats by angiotensin II antagonism. *Exp Nephrol* 1998;6:28–38.

100. Rennke HG, Patel Y, and Venkatachalam MA. Glomerular filtration of proteins: clearance of anionic, neutral, and cationic horseradish peroxidase in the rat. *Kidney Int* 1978;13:278–288.

101. Rennke HG, Venkatachalam MA. Glomerular permeability of macromolecules: effect of molecular configuration on the fractional clearance of uncharged dextran and neutral horseradish peroxidase in the rat. *J Clin Invest* 1979;63(4):713–717.

102. Rippe B and Haraldsson B. Transport of macromolecules across microvascular walls: the two-pore theory. *Physiol Rev* 1994;74:163–219.

103. Robinson GB, Walton HA. Glomerular basement membrane as a compressible ultrafilter. *Microvasc Res* 1989;38:36–48.

104. Rodewald R, Karnovsky MJ. Porous substructure of the glomerular slit diaphragm in the rat and mouse. *J Cell Biol* 1974;60:423–433.

105. Russo PA, Bendayan M. Distribution of endogenous albumin in the glomerular wall of proteinuric patients. *Am J Pathol* 1990;137:1481–1490.

106. Savin VJ. Ultrafiltration in single isolated human glomeruli. *Kidney Int* 1983;24:748–753.

107. Savin VJ, Terreros DA. Filtration in single isolated mammalian glomeruli. *Kidney Int* 1981;20:188–197.

108. Schaeffer RC Jr, Gratrix ML, Mucha DR, and Carbajal JM. The rat glomerular filtration barrier does not show negative charge selectivity. *Microcirculation* 2002;9:329–342.

109. Schlogl R. Zurtheorie der anomalen osmose. *Z Physik Chem* 1955;3:73–102.

110. Scholey JW, Meyer TW. Control of glomerular hypertension by insulin administration in diabetic rats. *J Clin Invest* 1989;83:1384–1389.

111. Schor N, Ichikawa I, Brenner BM. Glomerular adaptations to chronic dietary salt restriction or excess. *Am J Physiol* 1980;238(5):F428–436.

112. Shannon JA, Jolliffe N, and. Smith HW. The excretion of urine in the dog IV. The effect of maintenance diet, feeding, etc., upon the quantity of the glomerular filtrate. *Am J Physiol* 1932;101:625–638.

113. Shannon JA, Smith HW. The excretion of inulin, xylose and urea by normal and phlorinized man. *J Clin Invest* 1935;112:405–413.

114. Slomowitz LA, Peterson OW, Thomson SC. Converting enzyme inhibition and the glomerular hemodynamic response to glycine in diabetic rats. *J Am Soc Nephrol* 1999;10:1447–1454.

115. Smaje L, Zweifach BW, Intaglietta M. Micropressures and capillary filtration coefficients in single vessels of the cremaster muscle of the rat. *Microvasc Res* 1970;2:96–110.

116. Smith HW. *The Kidney: Structure and Function in Health and Disease.* New York: Oxford Univ. Press, 1951.

117. Smith HW, Chasis H, Goldring W, Ranges HA. Glomerular dynamics in the normal human kidney. *J Clin Invest* 1940;19:751–764.

118. Smith HW, Finkelstein N, Aliminosa L, et al. The renal clearance of substituted hippuric acid derivatives and other aromatic acids in dog and man *J Clin Invest* 1945;24:388–404.

119. Sorensson J, Ohlson M, Lindström K, Haraldsson B. Glomerular charge selectivity for horseradish peroxidase and albumin at low and normal ionic strengths. *Acta Physiol Scand* 1998;163:83–91.

120. Sorensson J, Ohlson M, Lindström K, Haraldsson B. Glomerular charge selectivity for horseradish peroxidase and albumin at low and normal ionic strengths. *Acta Physiol Scand* 1998;163:83–91.

121. Starling EH. The glomerular functions of the kidney. *J Physiol London* 1899;24:317–330.

122. Tay M, Comper WD, and Singh AK. Charge selectivity in kidney ultrafiltration is associated with glomerular uptake of transport probes. *Am J Physiol Renal Fluid Electrolyte Physiol* 1991;260:F549–F554.

123. Tenstad, O, Roald AB, Grubb A, and Aukland K. Renal handling of radiolabelled human cystatin C in the rat. *Scand J Clin Lab Invest* 1996;56:409–414.

124. The Sixth Report of the Joint National Committee on Prevention, Detection, Evaluation and Treatment of High Blood Pressure. *Arch Intern Med* 1997;157:2413–2446.

125. Thomson SC, Tucker BJ, Gabbai FB, Blantz RC. Functional effects on glomerular hemodynamics of short-term chronic cyclosporine in male rats. *J Clin Invest* 1989;83:960–969.

126. Tojo A, Endou H. Intrarenal handling of proteins in rats using fractional micropuncture technique. *Am J Physiol* 1992;263(Pt 2):F601–606.

127. Tucker BJ, Blantz RC. Effects of glomerular filtration dynamics on the glomerular permeability coefficient. *Am J Physiol* 1981;240:F245–254.

128. Tucker BJ, Anderson CM, Thies RS, Collins RC, Blantz RC. Glomerular hemodynamic alterations during acute hyperinsulinemia in normal and diabetic rats. *Kidney Int* 1992;42:1160–1168.

129. Tucker BJ, Mundy CA, Blantz RC. Adrenergic and angiotensin II influences on renal vascular tone in chronic sodium depletion. *Am J Physiol* 1987;252(Pt 2):F811–817.

130. van't Hoff J. *L'Équilibre chimique dans les Systèmes gazeux ou dissous à l'État dilué.* (Chemical equilibria in gaseous systems or strongly diluted solutions), 1885. From *Nobel Lectures, Chemistry 1901-1921.* Amsterdam: Elsevier, 1966.

131. Venturoli D, Rippe B. Ficoll and dextran vs. globular proteins as probes for testing glomerular permselectivity: effects of molecular size, shape, charge, and deformability. *Am J Physiol Renal Physiol* 2005;288(4):F605–613.

132. Vyas SV and Comper WD. Dextran sulfate binding to isolated rat glomeruli and glomerular basement membrane. *Biochim Biophys Acta* 1994;1201:367–372.

133. Walker AM, Bott PA, Oliver J, MacDowell M. The collection and analysis of fluid from single nephrons of the mammalian kidney. *Am J Physiol* 1941;134:580–585.

134. Wartiovaara J, Ofverstedt LG, Khoshnoodi J, Zhang J, Makela E, Sandin S, Ruotsalainen V, Cheng RH, Jalanko H, Skoglund U, Tryggvason K. Nephrin strands contribute to a porous slit diaphragm scaffold as revealed by electron tomography. *J Clin Invest* 2004;114:1475–1483.

135. Wearn JT, Richards AN. From: Observations on the composition of glomerular urine, with particular reference to the problem of reabsorption in the renal tubules. *Am J Physiol* 1924;71:209–227.

136. Wiederhielm CA, Weston BV. Microvascular, lymphatic, and tissue pressures in the unanesthetized mammal. *Am J Physiol* 1973;225:992–996.

137. Zatz R, Dunn BR, Meyer TW, Anderson S, Rennke HG, Brenner BM. Prevention of diabetic glomerulopathy by pharmacological amelioration of glomerular capillary hypertension. *J Clin Invest* 1986;77: 1925–1930.

138. Zatz R, Meyer TW, Rennke HG, Brenner BM. Predominance of hemodynamic rather than metabolic factors in the pathogenesis of diabetic glomerulopathy. *Proc Natl Acad Sci U S A* 1985;82:5963–5967.

CHAPTER **22**

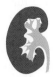

Function of the Juxtaglomerular Apparatus:

CONTROL OF GLOMERULAR HEMODYNAMICS AND RENIN SECRETION

Jürgen B. Schnermann and Josephine P. Briggs

National Institute of Diabetes, and Digestive and Kidney Diseases, National Institutes of Health, Bethesda, Maryland, USA
Howard Hughes Medical Institute, Chevy Chase, Maryland, USA

Description of the function of a complex organ like the kidney requires consideration not only of the properties of the individual cells, but also of the structural connections between them. A striking example in which anatomical relationships between epithelial cells, interstitial cells, and vascular smooth muscle cells must be considered to understand function is furnished by the juxtaglomerular apparatus (JGA). More than a century ago, Golgi observed that "the ascending limb of the loop of Henle returns with invariable constancy to its capsule of origin" (122), creating a structural connection between tubules and vessels that has at least two distinct functions. Changes in fluid composition in the tubular segment at the contact point produce changes in vascular tone of the associated glomerular arterioles and alterations in the rate of renin secretion from the granular cells at the vascular hilum. Full comprehension of the mechanisms of these two responses requires knowledge of both the properties of the individual juxtaglomerular cell types and of their interactions. In this chapter, we will discuss the structural and functional characteristics of the JGA cells, the evidence for the existence of macula densa control of filtration rate and renin secretion, and the available information about the cellular mechanisms by which changes in tubular fluid composition produce changes in filtration rate and renin release.

CELLULAR ELEMENTS OF THE JGA

The afferent and efferent arterioles at the glomerular hilum, together with the adherent distal tubule, form a wedge-shaped compartment that contains the three cell types of the JGA (Fig. 1). The *macula densa* (MD) cells in the wall of the tubule abut on a cushion of closely packed specialized interstitial cells called *Goormaghtigh* or lacis cells. Since these cells are indistinguishable in their fine structure from mesangial cells (205) and actually extend into the stalk of the mesangium, they are often referred to as extraglomerular mesangial (EGM) cells. The third JGA cell type refers to the *juxtaglomerular granular* (JG) cells located in the media of the arteriolar wall.

Serial reconstructions of the JGA have established an extensive and regular contact of the MD cells with the extraglomerular mesangium. In fact, the MD area often extends beyond the borders of the EM cell field (77) so that the only tubular epithelium with regular access to this compartment is the MD. Contacts between the MD and afferent and efferent arterioles are seen, but they are less extensive and less consistent than the apposition to the extraglomerular mesangium. In the rabbit a regular area of contact exists between the efferent arteriole and the thick ascending limb, either immediately before or immediately after the MD (205). Furthermore, a region of tubulovascular contact has been noted in the distal tubule where afferent arterioles make contact with the connecting tubule (78, 95, 473).

Macula Densa Cells

MORPHOLOGY

The MD cells consist of a plaque of epithelial cells located at the distal end of the thick ascending limb, approximately 100 to 200 μm upstream from the transition to the distal convoluted tubule (204, 205). An unusually high nucleus-to-cytoplasm ratio causes the dense appearance of this cell group that was the distinguishing feature noted by early anatomists (569). MD cells do not have the extensive basal infoldings, and elongated mitochondria found in many transporting epithelia; mitochondria, although numerous, are not in contact with the basal membrane, but rather scattered throughout the cytosol (205). The basement membrane is thinner than found in other areas of the tubule and shows discontinuities in scanning electron micrographs (33). The difference in basement membrane appearance is paralleled by a macromolecular composition that differs from that of adjacent thick ascending limb (TAL) cells (326).

NaCl AND WATER MOVEMENT

Although morphologically distinct, MD cells and neighboring TAL cells share similar NaCl transport mechanisms (Fig. 2). Like in TAL cells, NaCl uptake is mostly through the apical Na,K,2Cl-cotransporter (NKCC₂/

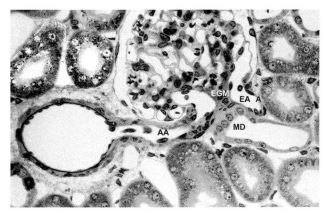

FIGURE 1   Low-power electron micrograph of the juxtaglomerular apparatus and surrounding cortical tissue (magnification, ×320). AA, afferent arteriole; EA, efferent arteriole; MD, macula densa; EGM, extraglomerular mesangium. (Courtesy of Brigitte Kaissling and Wilhelm Kriz, University of Heidelberg, Germany.)

BSC_1). Conventional electrophysiology and patch clamp evidence has established its presence functionally (249, 401, 402). Presence of the $NKCC_2$ cotransporter has also been shown at the mRNA expression level by in situ hybridization and RT-PCR (324, 555), and at the protein

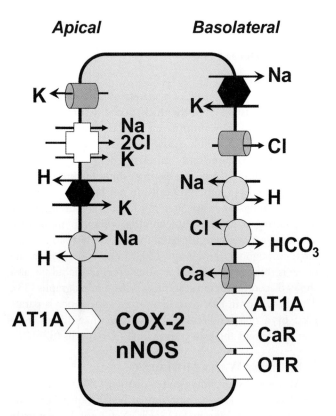

FIGURE 2   Representation of transport proteins and receptors in apical and basolateral membranes of macula densa cells. Experimental evidence comes from work in rats and rabbits.

level by immunocytochemistry (319). Of the three full—length isoforms of the cotransporter, both the A and the B types are expressed in the MD (121, 332, 341, 555). From the rates of MD cell acidification by luminal ammonium, it has been concluded that apical $NKCC_2$-mediated flux rates are not markedly different from those in TAL cells (246). Apical membranes of MD cells are rich in low-conductance K channels of the ROMK type that are required for K recycling (180, 323, 401, 402, 552). Na/H exchange activity, probably representing the presence of NHE2 rather than NHE3, provides a second pathway for a smaller fraction of Na uptake by MD cells (4, 102, 245, 355). In the rabbit, the apical membrane may also be the site of active Na extrusion since the luminal presence of ouabain has been found to elevate basal intracellular Na concentration in MD and TAL cells; in addition, luminal ouabain prevented the recovery of intracellular Na from the elevated levels resulting from increased luminal NaCl (356). The presence of a luminal H/K-ATPase in MD cells is indicated by immunocytochemical evidence and by the finding that an increase of luminal K in a NaCl-free environment caused the cytosolic pH to recover from the acidification caused by increased luminal NaCl in an ouabain-inhibitable fashion (356, 511). Since the colonic H/K-ATPase has been shown previously to mediate active Na efflux, it is possible that apical Na extrusion through an ouabain-sensitive H/K-ATPase contributes to the regulation of intracellular Na in MD cells (374).

Immunocytochemical and microenzymatic evidence agrees that Na,K-ATPase abundance and activity in the basolateral membrane of MD cells in rabbit kidneys is low compared to neighboring cells (213, 356, 417). In the rat, however, detailed immunocytochemical studies have discovered that the basolateral membrane of MD cells (identified by nNOS counterstaining) expresses the Na,K-ATPase $\alpha 1$ subunit together with the β_1 subunit, and a γ subunit that may be either γ_a, or both γ_a and γ_b (9, 97, 373, 462, 538, 539). Cl exit across the basolateral membrane occurs through abundant Cl channels (250, 402). Immunocytochemical evidence indicates the presence of the AE2 anion exchanger in basolateral membranes of MD cells in both the rat and the mouse, and Cl/HCO_3 exchange activity has been observed in the isolated rabbit JGA preparation (3, 230). Together with the apical Na/H exchanger basolateral AE2 may play a role in the absorption of HCO_3 or it may act as a pHi-controlling housekeeping gene.

The effect of changes in luminal fluid composition on the volume of macula densa cells has remained a controversial issue. At constant luminal osmolarity of around 300 mOsm, changes in luminal NaCl concentration caused parallel changes in the volume of MD cells (231, 267, 270). Changes in volume were to some extent transient, indicating some ability of MD cells for volume regulation (270). Both increases and decreases in MD cell volume have been observed with concomitant increments in Na (25–135 mM) and osmolarity (210–300 mOsm; 231,

357). When NaCl concentration was kept constant, MD cells behaved like osmometers, swelling with a reduction and shrinking with an increase in osmolarity (270). Transcellular osmotic water permeability of MD cells, assessed from the initial cell volume change in response to an osmotic step change, was estimated to be similar to that of cortical collecting tubules in the absence of ADH (124, 125). The main restriction to water movement resides in the apical membrane (125). Transmembrane pathways for water movement have not been identified; apical membranes of MD cells lack aquaporin-1 (428), and the presence of other aquaporins has not been established. TRPV4, a nonselective cation channel thought to be involved in cell volume regulation, has been found in TALs and distal convoluted tubules, but it was conspicuously absent in MD cells (488).

OTHER CELLULAR CHARACTERISTICS

Nitric oxide synthase type I (NOS I or nNOS), a constitutive and Ca-dependent NOS isoform, is highly and selectively expressed in MD cells and has become a useful marker of this cell type (309, 541). Catalysis of the conversion of L-arginine to NO and L-citrulline by NOS requires the participation of a number of cofactors. One of these cofactors is NADPH, and it is possible that the relatively high activity of glucose-6-phosphate dehydrogenase (G6PDH) in MD cells is related to the NADPH requirement of NOS (321). A functional connection between nNOS and G6PDH is suggested by the parallel upregulation of the expression of both enzymes during NaCl restriction (321, 436, 447). Alternatively, the high pentose shunt activity suggested by the abundance of G6PDH may serve to provide ribose-5-phosphate for nucleic acid synthesis. Avid uptake of labeled uridine has been shown to occur in MD cells, a process inhibited by actinomycin D and therefore indicative of incorporation of the pyrimidine precursor into the RNA pool (510).

Cyclo-oxygenase-2 (COX-2), typically induced by lipopolysaccharide (LPS) and cytokines in the inflammatory process, is constitutively expressed in the renal medulla and to a lesser extent in the cortex (152, 556). Cortical expression of COX-2 in the mature rat and rabbit kidney is restricted to a subgroup of MD and perimacular cells of the TAL (131, 152, 156, 280). Species differences have been described with MD expression of COX-2 being a characteristic of rodents and dogs, but not of primates or humans. Nevertheless, MD expression of COX-2 has been observed in humans older than 60 years and in patients with Bartter syndrome (227, 312), suggesting that the difference between species may be merely quantitative and that its assessment is limited by the sensitivity of the detection system. Condensation of COX-2 expression is the remnant of a more intense expression in early postnatal kidneys where the enzyme can be found in a more contiguous pattern in TAL cells proximal and distal of the MD. At this early stage COX-2 appears to be specifically excluded from MD cells (567). Conversion of PGH_2 into the bioactive prostaglandin E_2 (PGE_2) is catalyzed by PGE_2 synthases of which both a microsomal and cytosolic isoform have been described (311). Immunocytochemical evidence has demonstrated the presence of a membrane-associated PGE_2 synthase in MD cells of both rats and rabbits (51, 112). Colocalization of COX-2 with phospholipase A2 has been described in the MD at the level of single cells (280). Table 1 lists a number of other differences in the expression pattern of MD compared to surrounding TAL cells where the function has remained unclear.

Extraglomerular Mesangial Cells

MORPHOLOGY

The extraglomerular mesangial (EGM) cells (Goormaghtigh or lacis cells are synonyms) are the cells of the JGA that have the most intimate and regular contact with the

TABLE 1 Proteins With Expression Pattern That Differs Between Macula Densa and Surrounding Tubular Cells

Macula densa	Comments	Reference
Tamm–Horsfall protein	Neg, ideal negative selection marker	176
Epidermal growth factor	Neg, present in TAL and DCT	393
Hepcidin	Neg, present in TAL, apical	237
PKD2	Neg, present in TAL, mostly basolateral	325
Oxytocin receptors	Pos, not in TAL, mostly basolateral	459
Angiotensin II receptors	Pos, apical and basolateral	154
Benzodiazepine receptors	Pos, peripheral type receptors	13
Ca-sensing receptor	Pos, basolateral	388
PTHrP	Pos, microvessels, PCT and DCT	285
Stanniocalcin	Pos, also in TAL, DCT, and CD	142
Integrin-β6	Pos, fibronectin receptor	39
P2Y receptors	Pos, basolateral	266
WNK3	Pos, cytosolic	339

CD, collecting duct; DCT, distal collecting tubule; TAL, thick ascending limb; PCT, proximal collecting tubule.

MD (77). MD cells and EGM cells are separated by an interstitial cleft of variable width that does not appear to be bridged by gap junctional connections. In three-dimensional reconstructions, EGM cells are elongated cells with long cytoplasmic processes that in general run parallel to the base of the MD cells (454). EGM cells are extensively coupled by gap junctions with each other as well as with mesangial cells and granular cells (371, 470). The gap junctional connexins 37 and 40 are abundantly expressed in extra- and intraglomerular mesangial cells, and together with connexin 43 in endothelial cells of the renal vasculature (8, 566). The presence of myofilaments in EM cells suggests that EGM cells, like mesangial cells, have contractile potential (254).

The extraglomerular mesangial cell field is free of capillaries, lymph terminals, or nerve fibers. The absence of blood capillaries may cause a retardation of fluid entry and fluid removal from this compartment. Electron microscopical assessment has shown that the interstitial volume density of the EGM cell field increased from 17% during volume depletion to 29% during volume expansion while no changes were noted in the peritubular interstitium (403).

BIOCHEMICAL AND FUNCTIONAL ASPECTS

Localization studies using histochemical, autoradiographic, or immunological methods usually do not distinguish between intra- and extraglomerular mesangial expression patterns. Nevertheless, in some cases it seems justified to assume parallel expression in both cell types. For example, autoradiographic localization of angiotensin II and atrial natriuretic factor binding suggests the presence of receptors on both intra- and extraglomerular mesangial cells (10, 336). Relative predominance of AT_1 receptor mRNA in EGM cells has been observed by in situ hybridization (206). While EGM cells normally do not synthesize renin, they can be recruited to form renin with long-standing stimulation such as chronic diuretic abuse (79, 473).

Differential expression patterns in intra- and extraglomerular mesangium are relatively discrete. EGM cells do not stain with antibodies against Thy-1 while the glomerular mesangium does (340). Conversely, decay-accelerating factor (DAF), a glycoprotein that limits complement activation on cell surfaces, is restricted to the EGM cells, at least in the human kidney (82). Heat shock protein (HSP)–25 expression has also been reported to be expressed in extraglomerular, but not intraglomerular mesangium (308). Of particular interest may be the demonstration that two Na,K-ATPase-associated proteins, the FXYD protein phospholemman (FXYD1) and the $\beta2$ subunit, are expressed in the extraglomerular mesangium while being excluded from both MD cells and intraglomerular mesangial cells (539). Although a specific Na,K-ATPase α not been identified thus far, a relation to EGM transport function is conceivable.

Cultures of mesangial cells have in some instances been used as a model to study properties of specific significance for the function of the extraglomerular mesangium. Exis-

tence of functional gap junctions is suggested by lucifer yellow transfer between cells and by the propagation of a calcium wave in response to KCl depolarization of single cells (183). Syncytial organization of mesangial cells may play a role in MD to afferent arteriole signal transmission. Cultured mesangial cells possess Ca-activated Cl channels that mediate the cell depolarization caused by agonists such as angiotensin II (236, 327). A reduction in extracellular Cl concentration attenuated the rise in cytosolic Ca elicited by angiotensin II as well as its contractile effect, and this result may be the consequence of a concomitant increase in PGE_2 production (327). A decrease in NaCl has also been shown to stimulate the production of nitric oxide through a Ca-dependent NO synthase (494). Cl-dependent changes in mesangial cell activity, PGE_2, and NO production may be of functional importance in the context of the anion specificity of JGA-mediated responses addressed in the following sections. Whether these studies permit inferences about the JGA signaling mechanisms in vivo is not clear.

Granular Cells

MORPHOLOGY

It is well established that the granular cells in the arteriolar walls are the main renin-producing cells of the kidney. With a rough endoplasmic reticulum, a well-developed Golgi apparatus, and numerous cytoplasmic granules, they have the fine structure of protein-secreting cells (205, 254). The renin-containing granules are membrane bound. Some granules, believed to be the more newly formed, have a crystalline lattice appearance and may mainly contain prorenin; others, with an amorphous electron-dense content, are believed to represent the mature form (12, 473). Myofibrils and smooth muscle myosin are sparse and may be even absent in granular cells at the vascular pole (472). In the mature rat kidney under control conditions, granular cells are clustered at the vascular pole over a length of about 30 μm or about 20% of the afferent arteriole, but single, ringlike renin-positive regions in more proximal locations are sometimes seen (57). In the developing kidney as well as during stimulation of renin synthesis, for example with converting enzyme blockade, renin-positive cells can be found all along the afferent arteriole and in larger vessels as well (123).

Coexistence of renin and angiotensin II in granules of rat and human epithelioid cells has been shown by light and electron microscopy (62, 471). Granular angiotensin II appears to increase in parallel to renin following adrenalectomy and renal artery stenosis (53, 471). Granular angiotensin II may reflect uptake through either nonspecific endocytosis or receptor internalization, or intracellular de novo generation (286, 313). Not unexpectedly, granular cells contain AT1 receptor mRNA with rats expressing both AT1A and AT1B receptor mRNA and mice expressing only AT1A receptor mRNA (50, 115). Granular cells express the mRNA for D1- and D2-like dopamine receptors mediating stimulation and inhibition of renin secretion (396, 553). The gap-junctional protein connexin 40 has been shown to colocalize with renin demonstrating linkage between granular and endothelial cells of the glomerular arterioles (143). Other proteins found in JG cells include cyclic guanylate kinase II (113), the ubiquitous basolateral form of the Na/2Cl/K-cotransporter NKCC1/BSC2 (210), and GLUT4 (5).

FUNCTIONAL ASPECTS

In isolated afferent arterioles, the release of renin is quantal with about one release episode per 5 minutes under basal conditions (449). The episodic nature of renin release is most consistent with granule exocytosis, although EM studies rarely document the classic omega configuration with an open pore to the cell exterior, probably because of the low frequency of the exocytotic event (473). Exocytosis has been studied in dissected glomerulus/vessel preparations using optical labeling of renin granules with quinacrine and LysoTracker-Red, fluorophores that are taken up into acidic organelles. When stimulated by isoproterenol or a low arteriolar pressure, labeled granules were noted to disappear at a rate of about five to 10 granules per minute (359). In renin-releasing As4.1 cells, the extinction of individual granules was followed by the appearance of an extracellular quinacrine cloud presumably representing the released granule contents (359). Electrophysiological evidence for renin exocytosis has also been obtained in single isolated granular cells in which isoproterenol and cAMP caused an increase in membrane capacitance, a proven method to detect membrane fusion events (107).

Studies of the membrane characteristics of JG cells in the hydronephrotic mouse kidney by the whole-cell, patch-clamp technique have identified an inward rectifying K current whose inhibition was shown to be partly responsible for the depolarizing effect of angiotensin II (240). In addition, JG cells expressed Ca-activated Cl channels in high density (240). In contrast, inwardly rectifying K channels were not detected in isolated JG cells from rat kidneys (109). Instead, Ca-dependent and voltage-gated large conductance K channels (BK_{Ca}) were identified that largely determined the resting potential of -32 mV (109). Presence of BK_{Ca} channels was verified at the mRNA level by reverse-transcriptase–polymerase chain reaction (RT-PCR) and at the protein level by immunocytochemistry. The increased outward current caused by cAMP was also due to activation of BK_{Ca} channels suggesting that they were of the cAMP-stimulated ZERO splice variant (109). There is also evidence for the presence of K_{ATP} channels in JG cells, but their functional role is not clear (391). While earlier studies failed to obtain functional evidence for the presence of voltage-dependent Ca channels (241), the presence of L-type Ca channels and their activation by strong depolarizations has been established in isolated JG cells (110).

MACULA DENSA CONTROL OF VASCULAR TONE

The Tubuloglomerular Feedback Loop

EFFECT OF DISTAL TUBULE FLOW PERTURBATIONS ON SINGLE-NEPHRON GLOMERULAR FILTRATION RATE

Changes in flow rate past the MD, induced in single nephrons with the aid of a microperfusion pipette in the late proximal tubule, are followed by inverse changes in glomerular filtration rate of the same nephron (404). This flow-induced change of glomerular filtration rate (GFR) is called the tubuloglomerular feedback (TGF) response. The average maximum reduction of single-nephron GFR (SNGFR) in superficial nephrons in 15 independent studies in the rat was 13 ± 1 nl/min or $40 \pm 3\%$ (refs. in [428]). Repeated measurements of SNGFR in the same superficial rat nephron at eight loop perfusion rates (Fig. 3) revealed that TGF responses occur over a defined flow range and show nonlinear saturation kinetics (47). Data can be fitted to a four-parameter logistic equation (Fig. 4) by an iterative method that minimizes the sum of squares of deviations of measured from computed values (40) or by linear regression of log-transformed data (442). From the results shown in Fig. 3, $V_{1/2}$, the flow resulting in the half-maximum response, was

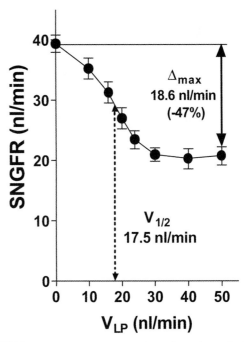

FIGURE 3 Relationship between single-nephron glomerular filtration rate (SNGFR) and loop of Henle perfusion rate (V_{LP}). The diagram shows mean values from nine tubules in which single-nephron glomerular filtration rate (SNGFR) was determined at eight different flow rates. Δ_{max}, maximum reduction of SNGFR; $V_{1/2}$, perfusion rate causing half maximal reduction of SNGFR. (From Briggs JP, Schubert G, Schnermann J. Quantitative characterization of the tubuloglomerular feedback response: effect of growth. *Am J Physiol Renal Physiol* 1984;247:F808–F815, with permission.)

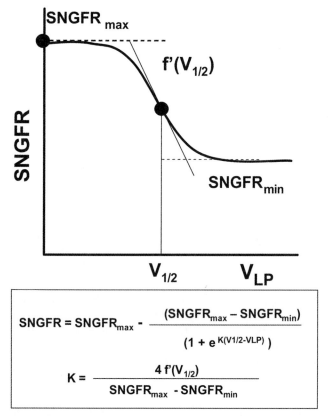

FIGURE 4 Four-parameter equation (logistic equation) used to describe the sigmoidal relationship between single-nephron glomerular filtration rate (SNGFR) and late proximal flow rate (V_{LP}). Parameters are $SNGFR_{max}$, $SNGFR_{min}$, $V_{1/2}$, the flow rate at which the response is half-maximum, and f' $V_{1/2}$, the slope at the midpoint. (From Briggs J. A simple steady-state model for feedback control of glomerular filtration rate. *Kidney Int* 1982;22[Suppl 12]:S143–S150, with permission.)

calculated to be 17.5 nl/min, a value that is close to the ambient end-proximal flow rate determined in separate experiments. Feedback functions established for animals of different size and GFR showed that maximum responses, $V_{1/2}$, and the slope of the function at the midpoint were directly dependent on body weight (47).

TGF responses are not confined to superficial nephrons of rats in which they have been studied most intensely. In juxtamedullary nephrons of both rats and hamsters, increased flow past the MD by perfusion of thin ascending limbs produced a reduction in SNGFR by about 25 nl/min or approximately 50% (306, 307). In addition to the rat, TGF responses have been observed in all mammalian species tested thus far (dog, hamster, mouse, humans) as well as in two nonmammalian species (*Amphiuma means* and *Necturus maculosus*) (refs. in [428]).

TONIC SUPPRESSION OF GFR BY TGF

TGF is a homeostatic control mechanism that is active under basal conditions and suppresses SNGFR to a level that is lower than it would be without TGF. One piece of evidence is provided by the position of steady-state values of end-proximal flow and SNGFR at the midpoint of the

independently determined feedback relationship (47). The precise location of the TGF operating point has been determined directly by adding or withdrawing small volumes of fluid from the proximal tubule and determining the resulting changes in proximal fluid flow rate by quasicontinuous videometric flow velocimetry (476). In these studies, small increases and decreases in loop flow rate were equally and maximally effective in altering SNGFR, an observation that directly demonstrates position of the operating point at the midpoint of the feedback function curve (474, 476). Finally, since fluid collections in the proximal tubule eliminate the TGF signal, while the signal is undisturbed during fluid sampling in the distal tubule, the proximal–distal SNGFR difference is a measure of the GFR-reducing effect of ambient distal flow (Fig. 5). A summary of 39 experimental series is shown in Fig. 6 (refs. in [428]). Proximal SNGFR exceeded distal SNGFR by an average of 6.0 ± 0.54 nl/min, suggesting that under normal free-flow conditions GFR of superficial nephrons is suppressed by about 16% through the operation of the TGF mechanism. Systematically higher values of SNGFR of superficial nephrons determined in proximal compared to distal tubule segments have also been observed in the dog and mouse (316, 504). Measurements of juxtamedullary SNGFR by micropuncture cannot be made without interrupting distal flow. However, another technique not requiring interruption of distal delivery, the ferrocyanide

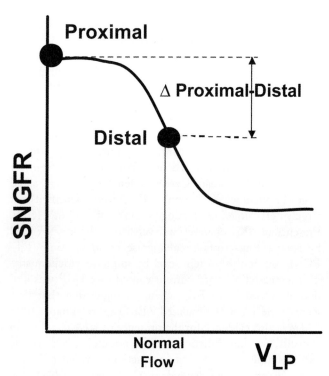

FIGURE 5 Difference between single-nephron glomerular filtration rate (SNGFR) measured in the distal and in the proximal tubule (ΔProximal-Distal); its magnitude is an index of the SNGFR-reducing effect of ambient flow rates past the macula densa.

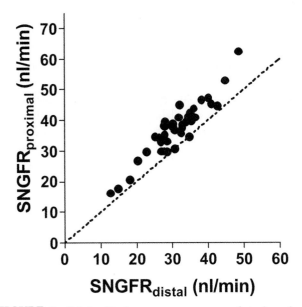

FIGURE 6 Relationship between measurements of single-nephron glomerular filtration rate (SNGFR) in proximal and distal segments of the same nephron. Each point is the mean of an experimental series taken from the literature. (See Schnermann J, Briggs JP. Function of the juxtaglomerular apparatus: control of glomerular hemodynamics and renin secretion. In: Seldin DW, Giebisch G (eds.). *The Kidney: Physiology and Pathophysiology.* Philadelphia: Lippincott Williams & Wilkins, 2000:945–980.)

technique, has been shown to yield values of SNGFR consistently lower than found by micropuncture measurements (90, 193) suggesting that, as in superficial nephrons, filtration rate is suppressed by the TGF mechanism.

TGF OSCILLATIONS

The operation of the TGF system in the closed-loop mode can result in stable oscillations of filtration pressure and filtration rate. Studies in halothane-anesthetized rats have shown that proximal tubular pressure can oscillate with a periodicity of two to three cycles/min (35–50 mHz) and an amplitude of up to 8 mm Hg (168, 259, 260). Similar oscillations were recorded in chloralose/ketamine anesthetized mice (504). Synchronous pressure oscillations were seen in efferent arteriolar blood flow with blood flow leading tubular pressure by an about 1-second lag. This phase shift suggests that oscillations in blood flow were the cause for the changes in tubular pressure (563). Pressure fluctuations were sometimes seen spontaneously, but were more commonly induced by small elevations in tubular flow rate (259, 260). Oscillations were unrelated to circulatory or respiratory rhythms, suggesting that they are of intrarenal and probably of single-nephron origin since oscillations in random adjacent nephrons were not in phase (259). However, synchronized pressures can occasionally be observed in adjacent nephrons whose afferent arterioles originate from the same interlobular artery (169, 562). Pressure oscillations were abolished by loop diuretics, and they were absent in mice that lack TGF responses, suggesting that they were generated by the TGF system (262, 504). This contention

was further supported by the finding that distal flow rate and Cl concentration oscillate with the same frequency, but with a fixed phase shift (170). These results show that the TGF system has temporal characteristics that can cause stable oscillations of intratubular pressure and proximal flow rate. Mathematical modeling of the TGF system indicates that oscillations are the result of a relatively high feedback gain in combination with delays in the transmission of the signal across the JGA and along the nephron (171, 256). The physiological significance of these oscillations remains to be established.

Spontaneously hypertensive rats (SHR) as well as Goldblatt hypertensive rats, but not salt-sensitive Dahl rats with hypertension, display irregular fluctuations of proximal tubular pressure that have been characterized as deterministic chaos (68, 168, 212, 561). Since most of the power spectrum remains concentrated around the same frequency as the regular oscillations it is likely that a change in TGF parameters is the cause for the chaotic dynamics (561). In fact, the complexity in the power spectra observed in SHR has also been interpreted as the result of known interactions and parameter variations of the TGF system (255).

In addition to the slow TGF-induced oscillations, laser-Doppler velocimetry identified an oscillation in star vessel blood flow with a frequency of about 100 to 200 Hz, probably reflecting myogenic vessel activity (563). Oxygen tension on the renal surface has also been found to oscillate at the same 30-mHz frequency, and it has been speculated that a switch of TAL cell energy production from aerobic to anaerobic metabolism may cause the instability in MD NaCl concentration that activates TGF oscillations (437).

The Tubular Signal and Sensing Mechanism

EFFECT OF LOOP OF HENLE FLOW ON MD NaCl CONCENTRATION

Experimental evidence favors the notion that the MD cells respond to changes in luminal NaCl concentration and that the flow dependency of TGF responses described previously reflects flow dependence of luminal [NaCl] in the MD region of the nephron (487). In situ microperfusion of loops of Henle has revealed a biphasic relationship between flow rate and distal [NaCl] measured 300 to 600 μm downstream from the MD, the earliest accessible site along the distal convoluted tubule (136, 297, 404). The increase of distal solute concentrations at subnormal flow rates is the result of modifications of tubular fluid between the MD region and the distal tubule. NaCl influx along the early post-MD epithelium causes NaCl to increase over the levels existing at the MD, and the effect of this addition of NaCl is particularly evident at low flow rates (136, 411). Although mechanical perturbations through activation of mechanosensors, for example central cilia, can be important factors in initiating flow-dependent events (370), considerable experimental evidence has indicated that the effects elicited by MD cells in situ are not in any discernible way related to the mechanical effects of flow rate per se. Nevertheless, in the isolated perfused JGA preparation, changes in flow at constant NaCl of 10 mM were even more efficient than NaCl concentration changes in eliciting vasoconstriction and increases of cytosolic calcium in vascular cells at the glomerular pole (360). The reasons for this major discrepancy between the in vivo and in vitro effects of flow are unclear.

Effect of MD NaCl Concentration on SNGFR

The relationship between MD NaCl concentration and SNGFR was established by perfusing loops of Henle from their distal ends in a retrograde direction (407). In this approach the distance between perfusion and sensing sites is shortened and changes in perfusate composition by tubular transport activities are minimized. Furthermore, this technique permits an assessment of the effects of perfusate composition on SNGFR at constant flow rate and pressure. At a flow rate of 20 nl/min, SNGFR varied inversely with changes in perfusate NaCl concentration between 15 and 60 mM (or 30 and 120 mOsm), values that extend over the hypotonic range normally occurring at the end of the TAL (20, 407, 441). Increments in NaCl concentration above 60 mM did not further suppress filtration rate. Maximum changes of SNGFR caused by saturating flow rates during orthograde perfusion and during saturating NaCl concentrations during retrograde perfusion were identical. Fitting the equation of a hyperbolic tangent to these results (Fig. 7) indicates that the half-maximum decrease in SNGFR is caused by a NaCl concentration of 33.5 mM, and that the maximum slope is about 0.5 nl/min mM.

No attempt was made in these studies to discriminate between ionic or osmotic effects of the perfusion fluid. Substantial additional evidence, however, suggests that total

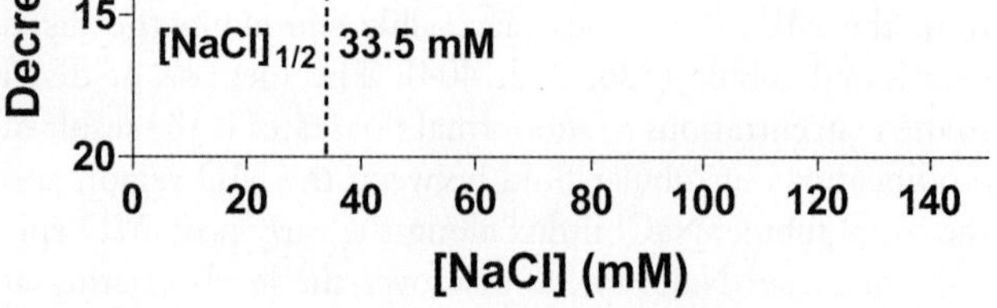

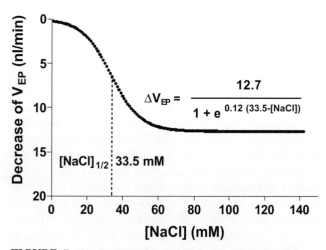

FIGURE 7 Logistic equation describing the relationship between NaCl at the macula densa and early proximal flow rate (V_{EP}), a close correlate of single-nephron glomerular filtration rate (SNGFR). Changes in NaCl concentration at the macula densa were produced by retrograde microperfusion. $[NaCl]_{1/2}$, NaCl concentration causing half-maximum reduction of V_{EP}. (From Schnermann J, Ploth DW, Hermle M. Activation of tubulo-glomerular feedback by chloride transport. *Pfluegers Arch.* 1976;362: 229–240, with permission.)

solute concentration at the MD does not seem to measurably participate in TGF-mediated reductions of SNGFR. Orthograde perfusion with isotonic mannitol solutions in the rat is usually not associated with sustained reductions in SNGFR even though distal tubular fluid osmolality is greatly increased (41, 404, 548). TGF responses correlating with alterations in osmolality have been observed during orthograde perfusion with various perfusion solutions, but the variations in distal osmolality were outside the critical osmolality range of 30 to 120 mOsm observed in retrograde perfusion studies (18). In retrograde perfusion experiments in which fluid osmolality and NaCl concentration were varied independently, TGF responses were exclusively determined by NaCl concentration and not by osmolality in a range between 130 and 400 mOsm (43). Finally, the pattern of SNGFR responses during retrograde perfusion with isotonic solutions in which either Na or Cl was replaced, but in which osmolality was kept constant, indicates dependence on the ionic composition and independence of osmolality (407, 441). Thus, the cells initiating the vascular TGF response are activated by changes in luminal NaCl concentration while changes in osmolality do not appear to play a major role.

TGF Response and NaCl Transport

Transport Inhibitor Studies The observation that inhibition of NaCl transport along the loop of Henle is associated with blockade of the TGF mechanism has been of fundamental importance in understanding the initiation of the TGF signaling pathway (547). Transport inhibition elevates distal Na and Cl concentration, which would normally be expected to activate the TGF response. The dissociation between changes in distal NaCl concentration and feedback responses caused by transport inhibitors indicates that the MD cells do not possess receptors sensitive to changes in luminal NaCl concentration, but that a change in cellular NaCl uptake is the necessary initiating event that leads to the vascular response. The concentration dependence of feedback responses is probably the result of concentration dependence of NaCl uptake.

TGF inhibition has been reported to be rather uniformly observed in the presence of loop diuretics such as furosemide, bumetanide, piretanide, ethacrynic acid, triflocin, or L-ozolinone (refs. in [428]). Concentrations causing half maximal inhibition of transport and feedback appear to be similar, about 5×10^{-5} M for furosemide and about 10^{-6} M for bumetanide ([284) and own unpublished data). Furosemide also blocked TGF responses during retrograde perfusion suggesting that metabolic consequences of TAL inhibition are not transmitted by convective transport to the MD cells. Studies in mice with selective deletions of the A or B isoform of $NKCC_2$ indicate that $NKCC_2B$ mediates TGF in the low NaCl concentration range while $NKCC_2A$ is required for responsiveness to higher NaCl concentrations (332). Thus, the presence of two isoforms of $NKCC_2$ in the macula densa extends the NaCl range over which TGF op-

erates. The concept that TGF responses are generated by the successive activation of NKCC$_2$B and NKCC$_2$A is supported by expression studies in *Xenopus* oocytes that have shown a higher Cl affinity of NKCC$_2$B than NKCC$_2$A, 9 mM versus 45 mM (121). Other aspects, such as the dependence of the inhibitory potency of furosemide on Cl concentration, have also been found to hold true for the TGF response (223, 412). Diuretic agents with primary actions outside the loop of Henle such as acetazolamide, chlorothiazide and amiloride do not possess TGF-inhibitory properties (329, 547). Transport inhibition caused by metabolic inhibitors such as cyanide, antimycin A, or uncouplers of oxidative phosphorylation has also been found to reduce TGF responsiveness (44, 547). TGF responses are not affected by peritubular application of ouabain, and this is probably related to the fact that due to the presence of an arginine in position 111 and an aspartate in position 122, the α1 Na,K-ATPase in rodents is very insensitive to cardiac glycoside inhibition (372). In fact, when α1 Na,K-ATPase was genetically engineered to become ouabain-sensitive, intravenous or luminal administration of the glycoside caused marked reductions of TGF responses (276). The effect of luminal ouabain may not be related to H,K-ATPase inhibition since TGF responses were unaltered in H,K-ATPase deficient mice (276). The striking effect of loop transport blockade suggests that NaCl uptake through the furosemide sensitive Na,K,2Cl-cotransporter and Na extrusion through an energy-dependent pathway are critical steps in generating feedback responses.

Whereas the inhibitory effect of luminal Ba on TGF responses was diminished by a pronounced direct vascular constrictor action (425), retrograde application of the K channel blocker U37883A caused an almost complete inhibition of TGF responsiveness (500). This effect is mediated by ROMK type K channels since TGF responses were largely absent in mice with targeted ROMK deletion (275), a finding that has been confirmed in mice in which selective breeding of surviving animals has generated ROMK-deficient mice with less compromised kidney function and well maintained blood pressure (Fig. 8; 279). The observation that inhibition of NKCC$_2$ and ROMK has similar effects on TGF responses argues against a specific "sensor" function of these transport proteins and for a critical role of some consequence of MD NaCl transport. Since ambient distal K concentrations near the MD are close to the K affinity of the cotransporter it is possible that variations in luminal K may in part regulate TGF response magnitude (500). Nevertheless, the increase in distal K concentration accompanying acute hyperkalemia was associated with attenuation, not enhancement of TGF responses (36).

Ion-Substitution Studies That NaCl transport is the initial step in the feedback transmission pathway is further supported by parallelisms in the ionic requirements for both TGF responses and NKCC$_2$-mediated NaCl transport across thin ascending loop of Henle (TALH). During retrograde perfusion of the MD segment (Fig. 9B), TGF re-

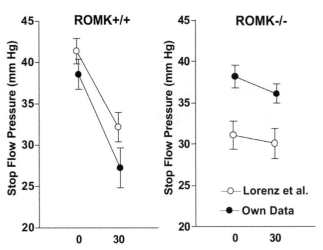

FIGURE 8   Mean responses of stop flow pressure to an increase in loop of Henle perfusion rate from 0 to 30 nl/min in wildtype (ROMK$^{+/+}$) and ROMK-deficient mice (ROMK$^{-/-}$). Open symbols, data taken from Lorenz JN, Baird NR, Judd LM, Noonan WT, Andringa A, Doetschman T, Manning PA, Liu LH, Miller ML, Shull GE. Impaired renal NaCl absorption in mice lacking the ROMK potassium channel, a model for type II Bartter's syndrome. *J Biol Chem* 2002;277:37871–37880; own data, data obtained in our laboratory using mice in which selective breeding had increased survival and reduced arterial hypotension (generated and donated to us by S. C. Hebert and T. Wang, Yale University).

sponses were not seen during perfusion with isotonic or hypotonic solutions of Na salts such as NaHCO$_3$, NaNO$_3$, NaI, NaSCN, Na acetate, Na gluconate, or Na isethionate (407, 441). In contrast, isotonic solutions of Cl salts (Fig. 9A) accompanied by small monovalent cations such as K, Rb, Cs, or NH$_4$ elicited full TGF responses, as did the Br salts of Na and K (407). It is to be noted that some of these small cations have been found to be substrates for the Na or K site on the cotransporter (223, 224).

The requirement for sizable Cl or Br concentrations and the apparent lack of dependence on Na concentration are consistent with an involvement of Na,K,2Cl-cotransport since the apparent overall affinity of NKCC$_2$ for Cl in both TAL and MD cells is much lower than that for Na or K (129, 251). Thus, the relatively low Cl affinity would predictably create an apparent Cl dependency of transport while the small amounts of Na or K entering initially Na- or K-free solutions are sufficient to sustain near-normal NKCC$_2$ activity. When Na was replaced with large cations such as choline or tetramethylammonium (TMA), TGF responses of normal magnitude were not seen even though Cl was present in sufficiently high concentrations (407, 441). Considering the cationic selectivity of the paracellular shunt, replacing luminal Na for choline will result in a sizable lumen positive Na diffusion potential (129) that is predicted to reduce NaCl absorption by increasing Cl backflux. This explanation is consistent with the observation that NaCl transport rates of isolated TAL were found unaltered when studied under symmetric conditions with high choline Cl on both sides of the epithelium (129). In this case, Na back-diffusion and

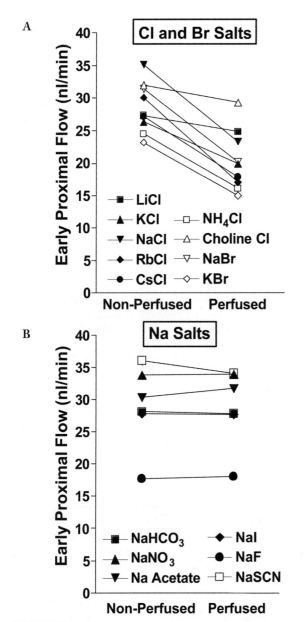

FIGURE 9   A: Effect of Cl and Br salts with various cationic substitutions on the response of early proximal flow rate (V_{EP}) to retrograde perfusion of the macula densa segment. **B:** Effect of Na salts with various anionic substitutions on the response of V_{EP} to retrograde perfusion of the macula densa segment. (From Schnermann J, Ploth DW, Hermle M. Activation of tubulo-glomerular feedback by chloride transport. *Pfluegers Arch.* 1976;362: 229–240, with permission.)

voltage-dependent inhibition of NaCl absorption is not to be expected as long as low concentrations of Na and K are present.

Stimulation of NaCl transport by a rise in luminal NaCl concentration is associated with profound changes in composition and membrane polarity of MD cells. These changes include increases in cytosolic Na and Cl concentrations, increases in cytosolic pH, and membrane depolarization (102, 251, 356, 395, 401). Increasing luminal NaCl to 150 mM causes depolarization of MD cells by about 30 mV due to

increased Cl efflux across the basolateral Cl channels. Most of this change in membrane potential occurs over the 20- to 60-mM range, and it therefore parallels the TGF response curve (24). MD depolarization may be directly involved in TGF responses since the cation ionophore nystatin elicited afferent arteriolar vasoconstriction in the presence of low luminal NaCl and furosemide (378). TGF responses were also seen when MD cells were depolarized by luminal application of the K ionophore valinomycin together with 50 mM KCl. The valinomycin-induced vascular response was not affected by the Cl channel inhibitor NPPB (5-nitro-2-(3-phenylpropylamino) benzoic acid), whereas the normal NaCl-induced response was fully blocked by NPPB (378). Although the magnitude of the membrane potential changes was not directly measured in these studies, it appears that TGF responses depend on MD cell depolarization independent of the specific mechanism underlying the PD change.

MD cell depolarization may be linked to TGF responsiveness through its effect on MD cytosolic calcium [Ca]i. Transport-induced changes in MD [Ca]i have been suggested to play a specific role in coupling the luminal electrolyte signal to the vascular response (19). In support of this proposal, it was shown that the small response of stop-flow pressure (P_{SF}) to a hypotonic NaCl solution was restored to the full response by adding 5 μM of the Ca ionophore A 23187 to the retrograde perfusate, whereas the response to an isotonic NaCl solution was only marginally affected (19, 21). To demonstrate the effect of the Ca ionophore, the presence of Ca in the perfusate was required (19). Adding 8–(*N,N*-diethyl-amino)-octyl-3,4,5-trimethoxybenzoate (TMB-8), a blocker of Ca release from intracellular stores, induced a dose-dependent reduction in the TGF response produced by an isotonic electrolyte solution (21). In the perfused JGA preparation, the Ca chelator BAPTA-AM has been found to prevent TGF responses (382). The mechanism of the Ca increase is unclear. Some evidence supports the presence of a nifedipine-sensitive, voltage-dependent Ca channel in the basolateral membrane, and thereby a direct link to the cell depolarization discussed previously (354). Patch-clamp studies of the basolateral membrane have discovered the presence of a 20-pS nonselective cation channel with finite Ca permeability, perhaps representing a member of the TRP channel family (252). In contrast, TGF responses in the perfused JGA preparation were blocked by inhibitors of Na/Ca exchange activity suggesting that the TGF-relevant [Ca]i change was secondary to reduced Ca extrusion (382). Finally, a reduction of luminal calcium to zero caused afferent vasodilatation, and this effect was accompanied by MD cell hyperpolarization, compatible with the presence of a conductive Ca entry pathway across the apical cell membrane (314). Taken together, these experiments have identified an important role of [Ca]i on TGF responses under certain experimental conditions. It is questionable, however, whether the [Ca]i changes occurring in response to fluctuations of luminal NaCl between 20 and 60 mM in vivo are large and consistent enough to establish a systematic and causal association between MD [Ca]i and the TGF response. In fact, the relationship between luminal NaCl and MD cytosolic calcium has been described as positive (354), negative (270), or entirely absent (360). Since the dissection strategies appear to be identical and the use of the fluorescent Ca indicators similar in principle, one must conclude that the changes of [Ca]i in MD cells may be too small to be safely distinguishable from experimental noise in this technically demanding approach.

The Vascular Effector Mechanism

The vascular response to a change in perfusion of single loops of Henle occurs without alterations in systemic arterial pressure, renal sympathetic tone, or in the resistance of larger renal vessels such as the cortical radial arteries (interlobular arteries). Therefore, the alteration in the hemodynamic determinants of filtration must be caused by a change in the contractile state of glomerular vascular elements. To determine the effect of TGF on glomerular arteriolar resistance, both the pressure fall and the rate of arteriolar blood flow have to be assessed while the perfusion in the loop of Henle of the same nephron is altered.

PRESSURE GRADIENTS

Stop-flow Pressure Measurement of stop-flow pressure (P_{SF}) in single nephrons was introduced as a method to estimate glomerular capillary pressure (P_{GC}) in nephrons that do not possess superficial glomeruli (118). P_{SF} can be measured reliably over extended periods of time, and it has therefore been used extensively as an index of TGF-dependent hemodynamic effects. In response to a saturating increase in loop flow mean P_{SF} of 23 studies fell by 22%, from 39.0 ± 0.8 to 30.3 ± 0.8 mm Hg (for refs. [428]). A reduction in P_{SF} was also observed in the dog when loop flow was increased from zero to normal and supranormal values (17, 317). In the mouse, TGF responses of P_{SF} are similar in magnitude as seen in rats, but the sensitivity range is shifted to lower flows (431). Since multiple determinations of P_{SF} can be made in the same nephron with small perfusion flow increments, the nonlinear relationship between loop of Henle flow and P_{SF} was apparent long before a similar feedback function for SNGFR was defined (405). In 15 experimental series, the maximum P_{SF} decrease averaged 7.9 ± 0.6 mm Hg with a mean $V_{\{1/2\}}$ of 20.1 ± 1.1 nl/min. The maximum sensitivity varied substantially between different studies, but in general was between 1 and 2 mm Hg min/nl (for refs. [428]).

Direct Glomerular Capillary Pressure Measurements Direct measurements of P_{GC} in superficial glomeruli of Munich-Wistar rats during changes in loop perfusion have confirmed that saturating flow increments cause a significant fall in P_{GC} with fractional decreases ranging between 15 and 22% (22, 46, 353, 474). The slope of the P_{GC} change in the most sensitive flow range was 1.3 mm Hg min/nl (474). P_{GC} measured directly in an in vitro preparation of juxta-

medullary nephrons also fell during TGF activation (56). Two laboratories have reported that the TGF-induced change in P_{SF} was identical to the TGF-induced change in P_{GC} (46, 346).

The main uncertainty in the determination of feedback-induced changes in the glomerular arteriolar pressure drop results from the evidence that at least in the rat a portion of the preglomerular resistance resides in the cortical radial arteries rather than in the afferent arterioles (32, 166). As a consequence, afferent arteriolar resistance, calculated from the artery to glomerulus pressure difference, overestimates true afferent resistance, while the relative change caused by the TGF mechanism is underestimated. If preglomerular resistance is equally apportioned between interlobular artery and afferent arteriole, the TGF-induced resistance change along the afferent arteriole would be about 15% greater.

GLOMERULAR PLASMA FLOW

Estimation of glomerular plasma flow (GPF) by micropuncture requires measurements of SNGFR and single-nephron filtration fraction (SNFF), with SNFF being derived from the increase in protein concentration or hematocrit in collected samples of early postglomerular blood. Increasing loop perfusion rate has been found to reduce plasma flow entering the glomerulus by about 20%, a change accompanied by a fall in SNFF (42, 182). Laser-Doppler shift analysis showed that saturation of the TGF mechanism caused an about 40% reduction in efferent arteriolar blood flow while TGF inhibition with furosemide increased blood flow by about 25% (563). Supportive evidence for TGF-induced reductions in GPF came from the observation that glomerular blood flow, estimated from the change in the arrival of fluorescent particles in a single glomerular capillary (457), fell by about 25% to 30% when loop flow was increased (M. Steinhausen and J. Schnermann, 1980, unpublished data). A 30% reduction in afferent arteriolar blood flow was also seen in *Amphiuma* and *Necturus* kidneys when distal flow rate was increased (350, 351).

EFFECTOR SITE

Preglomerular Resistance The micropuncture studies agree that increasing loop of Henle flow produces a 30% to 40% increase of preglomerular resistance (42, 182). Direct observations of TGF-induced changes in afferent arteriolar diameter in the blood-perfused juxtamedullary nephron preparation and in an isolated perfused tubule/vessel preparation showed that increases in MD NaCl concentration were followed by reductions in afferent arteriolar diameters that were most pronounced close to the glomerular entry site of the arteriole and near the MD cells (56, 190, 295). TGF-induced resistance changes estimated from diameter observations are consistently much larger than measured with the micropuncture approach. As suggested previously, the location of a sizable resistance along large intrarenal arteries would lead to an underestimation of the TGF-induced resistance change. It is also possible that in the small preglomerular arterioles resistance estimates may deviate from Poiseuille law. Finally, withdrawal of distal tubular fluid downstream from the MD caused an increase in maximum TGF responses, suggesting that the connecting tubule-arteriolar contact point may mediate vasorelaxation when exposed to increased NaCl concentrations (302). Preliminary results support this finding by showing in an isolated connecting tubule/arteriolar preparation that perfusion of the connecting tubule with increasing NaCl concentrations induced a marked relaxation of preconstricted afferent arterioles (384). Thus, the composite TGF response in vivo would be less than the in vitro response since it would include the late nephron dilator component.

The ultimate cause for TGF-induced vasoconstriction is a rise in intracellular calcium that at least to a large extent is mediated by activation of voltage-dependent calcium channels. The presence of L-type Ca channels in afferent arterioles has been amply documented, and intravenous or peritubular application of Ca channel blockers virtually completely inhibits TGF responses (55, 99, 140, 288, 304). A decrease in protein kinase A (PKA) activation may be an additional component of TGF-mediated vasoconstriction of afferent arterioles. When Db-cAMP was administered in the presence of 50 μM IBMX (3-isobutyl-1-methylxanthine), an inhibitor of cyclic nucleotide phosphodiesterase, TGF responses were reduced to a larger extent than seen with IBMX alone (23). Furthermore, luminal application of forskolin, a stimulator of adenyl cyclase, significantly reduced the TGF response to an isotonic solution (23, 426).

Observation of the TGF response indicates that the afferent arteriole immediately adjacent to the glomerulum is the main direct target of the TGF mediator (56). The glomerular entrance segment of the vessel is the part of the afferent arteriole in which agents affecting TGF response magnitude like adenosine and angiotensin II exert their largest constrictor action (147, 525). If only the segments of the arteriole that are in physical contact with the juxtaglomerular apparatus are directly affected by the tubular signal, TGF-induced local constriction may elicit a vascular-conducted response that spreads to proximal portions of the arteriole by electrotonic coupling or myogenic excitation (134, 296). Spreading of contractile responses during local application of KCl has been observed in juxtamedullary nephrons indicating electrotonic coupling of afferent arteriolar smooth muscle cells (513). Expression of connexin 40 has been observed in the media of afferent arterioles (8). Upstream propagation of TGF-induced vasoconstriction is also responsible for the functional coupling of nephrons that are supplied by a common interlobular artery (68, 169, 207). In view of the functional connection between afferent arteriolar smooth muscle cells, one may conclude that the total vasoconstrictor response to a NaCl step change is composed of a local MD-generated effect and an upstream myogenic constrictor component.

Postglomerular Resistance Evidence for a concomitant constriction of efferent arterioles during TGF activation has been obtained by micropuncture studies showing a reduc-

tion of GFR with unaltered glomerular capillary pressure, suggesting proportional increases in the tone of afferent and efferent vessels (182, 346, 495). Furthermore, an increase of flow within the low-to–ambient flow range is associated with a greater change of SNGFR than of P_{SF} suggesting that there was balanced afferent and efferent vasoconstriction with the SNGFR fall being a consequence of the reduced plasma flow or that total resistance did not change and the SNGFR change was a consequence of a reduced K_f (421, 474). Direct observations of juxtamedullary efferent arterioles during TGF activation did not reveal any vasoactivity of efferent arterioles (56). In contrast to these observations, a direct dilator effect of luminal NaCl was observed during retrograde perfusion of the efferent vessel in the double-perfused nephron preparation of the rabbit (377). This effect was prevented by antagonists of adenosine A2 receptors, and it may have been precipitated by the high norepinephrine-induced baseline tone. There is some experimental evidence in support of the possibility that a reduction in the filtration coefficient may contribute to the TGF-induced reduction of GFR (182).

PURINERGIC MEDIATION OF THE VASCULAR RESPONSE

As discussed in the previous sections, an increase in loop of Henle flow rate produces increases in NaCl concentration and NaCl transport at the MD, and this functional alteration elicits a vasoconstrictor response of the glomerular microvasculature as well as a reduction in the rate of renin secretion. Propagation of the signal across the JGA interstitium and subsequent changes in vasomotor tone occurs through the transport-dependent generation and action of purinergic mediators (Fig. 10).

Adenosine Adenosine was originally proposed as a mediator of the TGF response since it provided a conceptual link between the energy expended for NaCl transport and the generation of a vasoactive ATP metabolite (337, 455). Stimulation of Na transport in the proximal tubule is in fact associated with a decrease in cellular ATP, and increased NaCl secretion in the shark rectal gland causes a decrease in ATP as well as an increase in adenosine release (14, 217).

The vasomotor action of adenosine in most organs and vascular beds consists of vasorelaxation that reflects the wide distribution of the two types of A2 adenosine receptors, A2aAR and A2bAR. Although the kidney is usually considered an exception to this rule (505), several studies have shown that the steady-state response to an intravenous administration of adenosine is a clear reduction of renal vascular resistance whereas the initial constrictor response is only short-lasting (145, 149, 463). In contrast, persistent vasoconstriction of afferent arterioles by adenosine and A1 adenosine (A₁)-analogues was observed in the hydronephrotic kidney and in isolated perfused afferent arterioles when adenosine receptors were activated from the interstitial aspect of the vessel (147, 175, 526). The constrictor effect was absent in arterioles from A1 adenosine receptor (A1AR)–deficient

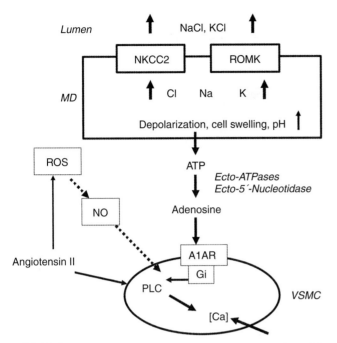

FIGURE 10 Schematic summary of our current understanding of the pathway by which an increase in luminal NaCl at the macula densa causes activation of vascular smooth muscle cells (VSMCs) in the afferent arteriole. Some consequence of NaCl uptake is linked to the release of ATP, subsequent generation of adenosine, interaction with adenosine 1 receptors (A1AR), Gi-dependent activation of PLC, and increases in Ca by release from stores and opening of Ca channels. Angiotensin II is an important cofactor that augments the impact of A1AR activation. NO is a response-attenuating factor whose levels are to some extent modulated by reactive oxygen species (ROS).

mice (147, 248). Thus, adenosine causes vasoconstriction only when the nucleoside is generated in a restricted interstitial region so that A1AR can be accessed without general activation of the more dominant A2 receptors. Expression data as well as functional observations indicate that the terminal afferent arteriole is a vessel with high representation of A1AR (523, 526). A1AR-mediated vasoconstriction of afferent arterioles is initiated by Gi-dependent activation of phospholipase C, release of Ca from intracellular stores, and subsequent Ca entry through L-type Ca channels (147, 148). The A1AR-mediated vasoconstrictor effect of adenosine in afferent arterioles was stable for extended periods of time indicating absence of rapid receptor desensitization (147, 148). Tubular administration of A1AR agonists augments the vasoconstrictor response to increased loop flow rates (105, 419). This effect does not appear to be mediated through apical A1AR, but rather reflects a direct interaction with A1AR on afferent arterioles, and thereby demonstrates the vasoconstrictor potency of A1AR activation and its effect on glomerular capillary pressure in vivo (424).

Two laboratories have independently generated mouse strains with targeted deletion of A1AR, and both groups observed a complete absence of TGF responses in A1AR$^{-/-}$ animals using micropuncture measurements of stop-flow pressure or single-nephron GFR (Fig. 11) (48, 461). Fur-

thermore, specific A1AR antagonists such as 8–cyclopentyl-1,3-dipropylxanthine (DPCPX) inhibit TGF responses when added to the tubular lumen or the peritubular blood (424). A similar effect has been seen earlier with nonspecific blockers such as theophylline or IBMX (23, 105, 337, 408). Addition of the nonxanthine A$_1$ receptor antagonist FK838 to the perfusate or the bath also eliminated TGF responses in an isolated tubule preparation (379).

Interference with adenosine transport or metabolism has been used as a tool to test the effect of predicted changes in interstitial adenosine levels on TGF responsiveness. Dipyridamole, an inhibitor of equilibrative nucleoside transporters (ENTs), has been reported to increase TGF responses (337, 496), but a more recent study with the water-soluble ENT inhibitor dilazep failed to show TGF enhancement during intravenous administration: The authors reported blunting of TGF with high luminal concentrations (215). ENT inhibition would be expected to change baseline interstitial adenosine levels in the vicinity of cells that express the transporters without altering adenosine formation or A1AR signaling. It is unclear how the acute adenosine formation postulated to occur during TGF activation would be affected by such a baseline change.

A 5'-nucleotidase ectoenzyme (e-5'NT) is present on glomerular mesangial cells as well as on interstitial fibrocytes surrounding the arterioles at the glomerular vascular pole in a cufflike fashion (257, 456). Evidence has been obtained suggesting that adenosine formation by e-5'NT may be critical in the generation of adenosine during the TGF response. Blocking adenosine formation with the e-5'NT-inhibitor α,β-methylene adenosine 5'-diphosphate (MADP) significantly reduced the compensatory TGF efficiency and the slope of the TGF relationship (475). When the level of TGF activation was fixed by saturating concentrations of cyclohexyl adenosine (CHA), TGF efficiency was further reduced, and retrograde administration of MADP in combination with CHA caused vasoconstriction and abolition of TGF responsiveness (475). Consistent with these data are observations in mice with targeted deletion of e-5'NT in which TGF responses were found to be markedly compromised (59, 178). Finally, in the double-perfused JGA preparation, bath addition of the ecto-ATPase apyrase enhanced, and MADP abolished, TGF responses suggesting that extracellular generation of adenosine from ATP is critical for JGA signaling (383). Exogenous e-5'NT was also found to improve the defective TGF-component of renal autoregulation in Thy-1 nephritic rats (466).

ATP ATP is another purinergic agent that has been proposed to participate in MD regulation of vascular tone (320). ATP causes rapid and reversible constriction of afferent arterioles, an effect that may be more pronounced in juxtamedullary than superficial nephrons (187, 526). A similar effect is seen with the P2X receptor-specific ligand α,β-methylene ATP, suggesting mediation of vasoconstriction by P2X purinoceptors (187). The presence of P2X$_1$ receptors on afferent arterioles as well as larger intrarenal arteries has been demonstrated

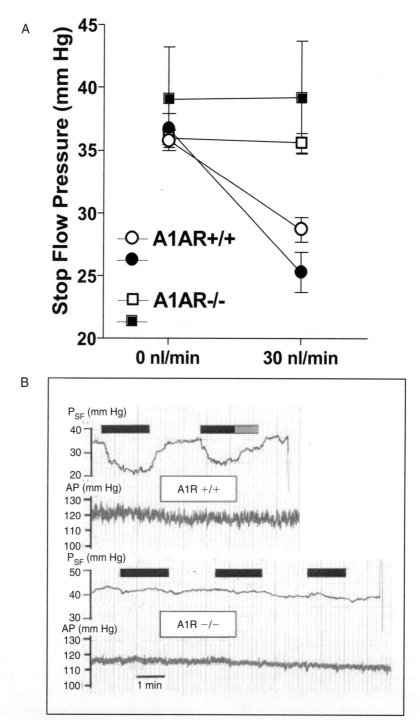

FIGURE 11 **A:** Mean responses of stop-flow pressure to an increase in loop of Henle perfusion rate from 0 to 30 nl/min in wildtype (A1AR[+/+]) and in adenosine-1 receptor–deficient mice (A1AR[−/−]). Gene targeting and phenotypic studies were performed by two independent groups of investigators. Closed symbols, data from Brown R, Ollerstam A, Johansson B, Skott O, Gebre-Medhin S, Fredholm B, Persson AE. Abolished tubuloglomerular feedback and increased plasma renin in adenosine A1 receptor-deficient mice. *Am J Physiol Regul Integr Comp Physiol* 2001;281:R1362–1367, with permission; open symbols, data from Sun D, Samuelson LC, Yang T, Huang Y, Paliege A, Saunders T, Briggs J, Schnermann J. Mediation of tubuloglomerular feedback by adenosine: Evidence from mice lacking adenosine 1 receptors. *Proc Natl Acad Sci U S A* 2001;98:9983–9988, with permission. **B:** Recordings of stop-flow pressure (PSF) and arterial blood pressure (AP) in a wild-type mouse (A1R[+/+]) and in an adenosine 1 receptor-deficient mouse (A1R[−/−]). During periods indicated by black bars, loop of Henle perfusion rate was increased to activate the TGF mechanism. Note absence of perfusion-related changes of PSF in the nephron of the A1 receptor–deficient animal.

by immunohistochemistry and ligand binding (64). Infusion of ATP or the ATP analogue β,γ-methylene ATP into peritubular capillaries revealed marked blunting of TGF responses when the TGF test was performed after the direct constrictor effect of ATP had waned (289). Maintaining saturating concentrations of ATP may have rendered P2X receptors inaccessible to endogenous ATP or it may have caused desensitization of P2 receptors. Suramin, a nonspecific P2 receptor antagonist, did not alter TGF responses in the double-perfused JGA preparation suggesting that P2 receptors do not contribute importantly to the TGF response (383). In the perfused juxtamedullary nephron preparation, suramin and pyridoxalphosphate-6-azophenyl-2′,4′-disulfonic acid (PPADS) prevented autoregulatory adjustments of afferent arteriolar tone (186), and the same observation was made in a similar preparation from $P2X_1$-deficient mice (188). Additional experiments support the notion that autoregulation was incomplete because of a deficiency in the TGF component of autoregulation (186, 188). However, TGF responses in superficial nephrons of $P2X_1$ knockout mice were not statistically distinguishable from wildtype animals so that the autoregulatory and possibly TGF deficit may be restricted to juxtamedullary nephrons.

Nevertheless, a role for ATP in JGA signaling is strongly supported by the observation that the basolateral membranes of MD cells appear to have an ATP release pathway that is modulated by changes in luminal NaCl (25, 229). Patch-clamp studies in cell-attached and -excised patches of the basolateral membrane of MD cells showed the presence of an anion channel of 380 pS whose activity was dependent on the presence of extracellular NaCl and that was active in the presence of ATP as the only anion (25, 229). Channel activity was blocked by gadolinium, but not by the Cl channel inhibitors DPC or NPPB (25). The molecular nature of this large-conductance anion channel has not been identified, but it may be identical to that functionally described in a mouse mammary gland cell line (392). In vivo release of ATP was suggested by the observation that PC12 or mesangial cells placed near the basolateral MD cell membrane responded to changes in luminal NaCl over the 20- to 60-mM range with an increase in cytosolic calcium (25, 229). This Ca response reflects P2 receptor activation since it was inhibited by suramin (25, 229). It is conceivable that ATP released into the JGA interstitium serves as substrate for membrane-bound ecto-ATPases and nucleotidases resulting in the formation of the final mediator adenosine as outlined in prior sections. Alternatively, it is possible that ATP activates P2 receptors (other than $P2X_1$) on mesangial cells to elicit TGF responses. Mesangial cells in culture respond to nucleotides including UTP and ATP-γ-S with an increase in cytosolic calcium suggesting the presence of the P2Y type of nucleotide receptor (25, 135). Activation of mesangial cells and signal transmission through gap junctions may be an intermediate step in the TGF pathway since mesangial destruction with a Thy-1 antibody abolished TGF responses in the double-perfused JGA preparation (381). Alternatively, mesangial cell lysis may disrupt the

ATP degradation pathway since ecto-5′-nucleotidase is expressed on the surface of mesangial cells.

Integrated Function of the TGF Mechanism

The JGA control system is constructed as a negative, homeostatic feedback loop. The physiological purpose of this regulatory loop has been the subject of a substantial body of investigation using both experimental approaches and mathematical modeling. One potential effect of the operation of the TGF feedback loop is to reduce fluctuations of NaCl concentration at the MD, thus reducing the variability in the delivery of NaCl into the relatively low-capacity transport system of the distal nephron. Another role hypothesized for the TGF loop is in the autoregulatory adjustments in vascular resistance that promote constancy of GFR when arterial pressure changes.

The two hypothesized roles, regulation of distal salt delivery and control of GFR, are functionally interrelated; the feedback loop may contribute to stabilization of NaCl excretion, rendering it relatively independent of fast and irregular fluctuations in perturbing forces that are not the expression of an adaptation to a change in body Na balance. Such variations are represented, for example, by the marked fluctuations in blood pressure that have been observed to occur in conscious dogs throughout the day and with changing body activities (282). In the absence of tight control of vascular resistance, glomerular capillary pressure and hence GFR would be expected to fluctuate in parallel with blood pressure, causing changes in Na excretion unrelated to the NaCl status of the organism. Since, however, changes in GFR will in general be followed by changes in distal NaCl concentration in the same direction, the TGF system can dampen the amplitude of the predicted GFR changes. Similar rapid hemodynamic adjustments will occur with other acute perturbations of MD NaCl concentration resulting from variations in cardiac output, renal blood flow or proximal tubular transport. As discussed in the following sections, the TGF mechanism changes its response characteristics when perturbations of MD NaCl concentration are sustained for extended periods of time (477).

FEEDBACK LOOP EFFICIENCY

Mathematical approaches have been applied to assess the homeostatic effectiveness of the TGF mechanism as a negative-feedback controller. In analogy to technical control systems, the TGF mechanism can be modeled as a negative-feedback loop in which the NaCl concentration at the sensing site is the controlled variable, the juxtaglomerular apparatus the controller, and the blood vessels the effector. The output determined by the effector is SNGFR, which is fed back to the controlled variable after being modified by proximal absorption. Estimates of the homeostatic efficiency with which distal salt delivery is controlled need to consider both the TGF response of SNGFR and the response of absorption to a change in GFR. Thus, the error compensation following a perturbation of SNGFR is composed of two parts: an adjustment of transport and an adjustment of SNGFR.

The homeostatic efficiency of the intact loop can be expressed as the magnification (M) or open loop gain (OLG) of distal salt delivery or of SNGFR; these indices of control need not be identical. M and OLG are technical indices of control efficiency with M being defined as the ratio of the perturbation-induced change of the regulated variable in the presence of control and its change in the absence of control. OLG is an inverse function of M and is defined as $1/M-1$. In studies where early proximal flow was elevated by microperfusion, OLG of SNGFR was about 1.5 (292, 294), a value similar to that estimated by using data from open-feedback loop experiments (40, 138). Because OLG of distal delivery was about the same, fractional error compensation in this experimental setting was about 0.5 and almost entirely due to TGF (292). When proximal absorption rate was increased by hemorrhage, OLG for distal delivery was higher than OLG for SNGFR, indicating that modifications in proximal transport contributed to compensating for the induced perturbation (292). Closed-loop studies designed to assess fractional compensation in the vicinity of the operating point have reported higher values, between 0.6 and 0.75, and higher OLG, around 3 (172, 476).

PARTICIPATION OF THE TGF MECHANISM IN AUTOREGULATION

Acute changes in mean arterial pressure induce adjustments in renal vascular resistance that stabilizes renal blood flow and glomerular filtration rate over a wide range of pressures. Pressure-induced resistance changes in the kidney have been proposed to be TGF-mediated (137, 485). A role of TGF in steady-state autoregulation was first supported by the observation in both dogs and rats that interruption of the TGF loop in single nephrons causes SNGFR and P_{SF} to vary directly with arterial pressure (290, 293, 316, 317, 361, 362, 415, 448). Pressure dependency of SNGFR was noted regardless of whether the TGF loop was physically disrupted by injecting an oil block, blocked acutely by adding furosemide to the perfusate (290), or inhibited by chronic treatment with DOCA and a high-salt diet (290). In contrast, arterial pressure had little effect on GFR when the TGF loop was intact (290, 293, 316, 361, 362, 415). In the in vitro perfused juxtamedullary nephron preparation, interference with the TGF mechanism by furosemide or physical interruption of the feedback loop markedly diminished autoregulatory diameter alterations of afferent arterioles (295, 397, 465), and constancy of afferent arteriolar blood flow was no longer maintained (465).

There is equally solid evidence for the existence of TGF-independent autoregulatory resistance changes. Glomerular arterioles in kidney tissue transplanted to the cheek pouch of the hamster showed marked autoregulation of vessel diameters (120). In the hydronephrotic kidney model, which does not possess an operating TGF system, a decrease in arterial pressure increased vessel diameters along the entire preglomerular vasculature except for the portion of the afferent arteriole near the glomerulus (458). Isolated afferent arterioles and interlobular arteries maintained their diameter when luminal pressure increased, although they did not significantly constrict (96, 150). The nature of the TGF-independent regulator is unclear, but an intrinsic myogenic mechanism responding to wall tension or mechanical stress is the most likely possibility.

Existence of at least two regulators is further supported by studies in which the dynamic response of renal blood flow to random fluctuations of blood pressure has been analyzed. Frequency domain analysis of renal blood flow using linear techniques revealed the presence of a regulator with a frequency response compatible with the TGF mechanism, about 0.01 Hz, and a faster mechanism with a frequency characteristics consistent with myogenic vasomotion, about 0.1 Hz (86, 173, 565). Since the TGF system is nonlinear, it is important that a similar conclusion has been reached from the more recent application of nonlinear system analysis (74, 75, 174). The existence of two regulators with similar frequencies has also been established in spontaneously hypertensive and Dahl rats (67, 87, 211). There is some evidence for the operation of two regulating mechanisms in conscious dogs (544). Interference with the slow component was observed during ureteral obstruction, converting enzyme inhibition and in the perfused hydronephrotic kidney, experimental models of TGF interruption (83, 87, 161). Temporal resolution of the adjustment of renal vascular resistance to step changes in renal arterial pressure is consistent with the sequential operation of several mechanisms with different response times (200, 202, 549). In addition to the TGF and myogenic components, this approach has yielded evidence for the presence of a third mechanism with a slow response time that may by of particular importance at low perfusion pressures (202, 549). Furthermore, an afferent arteriolar constrictor mechanism has been identified that responds to the systolic pressure peaks rather than to mean arterial pressure and therefore must possess a response time in the frequency of the heart rate (277, 278). This mechanism is thought to protect the glomerular vasculature against the high pressures exerted during systole.

The evidence of a functional role for both TGF and TGF-independent mechanisms in autoregulation raises the question of the quantitative contribution of each component to the total regulatory response. In early studies in rats, the experimentally determined pressure dependence of SNGFR in the absence of TGF was compared to the passive pressure–SNGFR relationship (290). The passive slope was estimated from model predictions or from the change of SNGFR in the subautoregulatory pressure range (290, 415). The deviation from the predicted passive slope after eliminating a TGF contribution indicated residual autoregulatory capacity, with a relative contribution of about 50% of the total resistance change. This conclusion was confirmed in studies in which the fractional change in stop-flow pressure was found to be clearly smaller than the fractional change in arterial pressure (293). A more direct demonstration of two mechanisms and their approximate relative contributions is the demonstration in the blood-perfused juxtaglomerular nephron preparation that selective TGF blockade by furosemide or an oil block caused a smaller reduction of pressure-induced vasoconstriction of afferent arterioles than a Ca channel blocker that presumably blocked both TGF and myogenic mechanisms (56, 465). Similarly, the rise of afferent blood flow following TGF inhibition was less than that caused by Ca channel blockade (465). Consistent with earlier conclusions TGF inhibition was estimated to cause a 60% loss of autoregulation (465).

Interaction between the two autoregulatory mechanisms may lead to amplification of vascular responses. Models of autoregulation suggest that a TGF-dependent vasoconstriction can induce a myogenic response in upstream vascular regions and amplify the resistance increase (88, 141, 296). In fact, mathematical modeling suggests that a myogenic contribution from proximal vascular segments is necessary for distal mechanisms such as TGF to contribute to resistance regulation (98). Spatial separation between the two regulatory mechanisms along the afferent arteriole has been noted, with TGF being most effective in the region of the afferent arteriole close to the glomerulus and the myogenic component being more pronounced in more proximal portions of the afferent arteriole (295). Interactions between the myogenic response and TGF have been demonstrated at the single-nephron and whole-kidney levels (74, 420), and they have been the subject of extensive mathematical modeling (76, 174, 283). One of the conclusions is that elimination of a variable TGF signal enhances myogenic responsiveness (76, 200, 420, 516). Evidence indicates that the restraining effect of TGF on the myogenic mechanism is mediated by nitric oxide (203, 445). Functional coupling of small ensembles of nephrons by ascending myogenic or conducted vascular responses adds to the complexity of regulation of preglomerular vascular tone (169, 207). Enhanced nephron-to-nephron coupling has been suggested to be responsible for the more efficient dynamic autoregulation in spontaneously hypertensive rats (67, 513, 562).

ROLE OF TGF IN RESPONSE TO TRANSPORT ALTERATIONS

Hypertonic NaCl Administration of hypertonic NaCl causes vasodilatation in most vascular beds, but in the kidney it results in an anomalous vasoconstriction (315). This response may be a whole-kidney equivalent of the response of SNGFR to increased loop flow rate. Both TGF- and NaCl-induced vasoconstriction are enhanced by salt depletion (92, 540), and inhibited by furosemide, theophylline or DOCA-salt treatment (116, 117, 406, 408, 547). Furthermore, hypertonic non–chloride-containing solutions usually do not produce vasoconstriction (540). A micropuncture study in the rat revealed that an infusion of hypertonic NaCl reduced proximal tubular fluid absorption from 16 to 11 nl/min with a concomitant increase in loop flow rate from 13.7 to

17.0 nl/min (410). As a consequence of this increase in flow, SNGFR fell from 31.4 to 27.9 nl/min (410). When the increased flow was prevented from reaching the MD area by a tubular block, SNGFR rose instead of falling, supporting the conclusion that the GFR fall was TGF-mediated. In these studies, an increase of loop flow of 3.3 nl/min resulted in a fall in SNGFR of 3.5 nl/min. This response is in reasonable agreement with the sensitivity predicted from microperfusion studies.

Protein Feeding The vasodilatation caused by acute and chronic protein feeding may include a TGF-dependent component. In conscious dogs, furosemide and ethacrynic acid blocked the acute rise in GFR following a meat meal, suggesting that the postprandial vasodilatation may be TGF dependent (546). It has been proposed that the rise in filtered amino acids causes an increase in proximal Na and fluid absorption and a decrease in MD Na delivery (546).

Chronic consumption of a high-protein diet induced a rightward resetting in the feedback curve of normal and Goldblatt hypertensive rats so that higher flows were necessary to suppress GFR than in control or low-protein fed animals (416, 442). In normotensive animals, the response amplitude and the slope of the feedback function were unaltered (442). These effects appear to be due to alterations in transport along the loop of Henle (443). NaCl concentrations in distal tubular fluid during loop perfusion were 30% lower in rats on a high-protein diet than in rats on a low-protein diet, and this reduction is responsible for the rise in SNGFR produced by a high-protein diet (443). Consistent with this notion is the observation that TGF responses were the same in the two groups of rats when loops of Henle were perfused in a retrograde fashion, indicating that functional changes in the loop of Henle rather than at the level of the JGA were responsible for the protein-induced changes in TGF characteristics. The increased rate of NaCl transport along the loop of Henle caused by high-protein feeding may result from structural adaptations (35).

Inhibition of Proximal Transport Diuretics that inhibit predominantly proximal tubular fluid absorption may cause a TGF-dependent decrease in GFR as a result of increased distal NaCl delivery. In support of this hypothesis, several studies using carbonic anhydrase inhibitors as well as chlorothiazide suggest that these agents cause SNGFR to fall more with the TGF loop intact than with the TGF loop interrupted (329, 349, 495). In view of the Cl dependency of TGF, however, the acute TGF activation by carbonic anhydrase inhibition is unexpected since these drugs, while causing an increase of early distal Na, do not elevate distal Cl concentrations (329, 349). There is no evidence to show that HCO_3 can substitute for Cl in initiating TGF responses. In fact, studies have shown that the effect of benzolamide to reduce GFR and RBF was maintained in $A1AR^{-/-}$ mice, which are unable to generate a TGF response (160). Thus, the mechanism of the renal vasoconstriction caused by CA inhibitors is not entirely clear, but it appears that a rise in tubular pressure may be an important contributor (263, 264). In addition, studies in rats and mice indicate that major increases in urine flow including those caused by furosemide may lead to increases in total renal vascular resistance even when a participation of TGF is a priori unlikely (194, 331).

Aquaporin-1 and NHE3 Knockout Mice SNGFR of mice with targeted deletion of AQP1 was found to be significantly reduced compared with wildtype when it was determined in distal nephron segments with the TGF pathway intact (427). The fall in GFR was dependent upon distal fluid delivery since it was not observed when SNGFR was measured in the proximal tubule with the TGF loop interrupted (427). Mice deficient in both AQP1 and A1AR, which combine a proximal transport defect with absent TGF responsiveness, have been found to have a normal distal SNGFR, supporting the notion that the fall of GFR in AQP1$^{-/-}$ mice is TGF-mediated (159).

Very similar results were obtained in mice with a knockout mutation in the apical Na/H exchanger NHE3, another model of established proximal tubular NaCl and fluid malabsorption (274). Considering that distal flow rates were not different between wildtype and AQP1 or NHE3 knockout mice it seems unlikely that TGF activation is due to an increased NaCl concentration at the MD. Resetting of the TGF function curve (discussed in subsequent sections) subsequent to extracellular volume depletion seems to be more likely as causation for enhanced TGF engagement.

Adaptation of TGF Response Characteristics

Adaptations in the TGF function occur whenever MD NaCl concentrations deviate from normal for an extended period of time. Typically such deviations result from alterations in body Na content, with volume expansion associated with persistently increased, and volume depletion associated with decreased MD NaCl concentrations. Formally, two types of adaptation in the TGF relationship can be distinguished. TGF *resetting* refers to a shift in the range over which the system is operating, either a shift to the right, to higher flows or concentrations, or a shift to the left, to lower flows or concentrations. A change in TGF response *sensitivity* refers to an altered response either altered slope and/or maximum response magnitude. By and large, volume depletion is associated with a left shift and an increase in response magnitude, and volume expansion with the opposite, but the actual adaptation observed has varied with the protocol used.

A number of studies have established that acute expansion of the extracellular space by infusion of isotonic saline or plasma reduces the TGF response magnitude and slope and increases $V_{1/2}$ in superficial and juxtamedullary nephrons (30, 31, 307, 344, 348, 363, 422). Similar changes are observed with chronic volume expansion; administration of DOCA together with isotonic saline as drinking fluid virtually abolishes TGF responses (290, 291, 406). The combination of a right shift and a reduced response magnitude is not invariant. Short-term volume expansion by a bolus injection

of dilute rat plasma shifted the responsive range to higher flows although this protocol produced an increase rather than a decrease in the maximum response magnitude (89); SNGFR at zero loop flow rose 60%, whereas kidney GFR and free-flow SNGFR rose only moderately, with the position of the operating point and a large proximal–distal SNGFR difference indicating that the suppressing effect of the TGF mechanism was greater than normal. Thus, in these studies, the TGF mechanism appeared to counteract TGF-independent vasodilator influences on the renal vasculature. These data are consistent with closed-loop studies in which acute volume expansion with plasma did not reduce the maximum homeostatic efficiency, but shifted it away from ambient flows to lower flows, enhancing its dilatory and reducing its constrictor potency (476).

The effects of an acute decrease of extracellular volume (ECV) have been studied in rats after acute hypotensive hemorrhage (292, 294) and in dehydrated rats (439). In general, these interventions are accompanied by an increase in TGF response magnitude. Hypotensive hemorrhage induced a shift of the feedback curve to the left (214, 292, 294). Since proximal absorption increased at the same time, the operating point tended to move toward the shoulder of the reset feedback function (292). Thus, in this circumstance the resetting results in reduced dilatory and enhanced constrictor capacity.

Studies have been performed to determine the time course of TGF adaptation. When single nephrons were perfused for extended periods of time, resetting developed over the initial 30 to 40 minutes of hyperperfusion, whereas changes in response magnitude were slower, requiring 40 to 60 minutes (477). Similarly, acute volume depletion by furosemide restored TGF responses in chronically volume-expanded rats within 60 to 120 minutes (291).

OTHER CONDITIONS ASSOCIATED WITH TGF ADAPTATION

Ureteral and Nephron Obstruction In the first few hours following complete unilateral ureteral obstruction (UUO) TGF reactivity appears to be completely abolished (300, 347, 515). Elimination of the restraining effect of TGF is reflected by increased renal and glomerular plasma flows and elevated glomerular capillary pressures (84). After persistence of ureteral obstruction for 24 hours, TGF activity is restored and possibly slightly enhanced as indicated by a reduced $V_{1/2}$ (469, 515). The dominant effect of prolonged ureteral obstruction is a marked reduction of glomerular capillary pressure and glomerular plasma flow, changes that result in a dramatic reduction of GFR (85, 347). The apparent absence of a luminal signal suggests that vasoconstriction is not equivalent to the standard TGF response discussed so far. On the other hand, obstruction of a single nephron for 4 hours also causes marked vasoconstriction, indicating that persistent interruption of distal delivery produces a local constrictor signal of unknown nature (7, 467, 468).

Following release of short-lasting ureteral obstruction TGF reactivity is increased (347), and it is maintained in its somewhat activated state after release of an obstruction of 24–hour duration (469, 515). It is possible that the activated TGF mechanism is in part responsible for the continued vasoconstriction following release of both ureteral and single-nephron obstruction (469). However, additional mechanisms appear to contribute to the reduction in filtration after release of obstruction since SNGFR at zero flow increased only slightly above distal values (469). Furthermore, nephron and kidney filtration rates were also markedly suppressed after release of bilateral ureteral obstruction even though in this experimental condition TGF responses were blunted rather than enhanced (469, 515).

During partial unilateral ureteral obstruction for 3 to 6 weeks, TGF reactivity appears to be in the normal range (298, 299). During volume expansion, on the other hand, TGF reactivity increased in the hydronephrotic kidney whereas it was strongly inhibited in the nonobstructed contralateral kidney (298). The enhanced TGF reactivity seen in hydronephrotic kidneys during volume expansion could be prevented by thromboxane synthase inhibition (299). A similar paradoxical enhancement of TGF reactivity by volume expansion was less pronounced during chronic bilateral ureteral obstruction (303).

Loss of Renal Mass In the first hours following unilateral nephrectomy, TGF responses in the residual kidney may be enhanced, and ambient distal flows may exert a GFR-depressing effect as judged from an increase in the proximal-distal SNGFR difference without a change in the proximal value (28). However, at later time points uninephrectomy or 5/6 ablation has been shown to shift the TGF function to the right with (305) or without increasing the maximum response (322, 394). A similar response to nephrectomy was noted in transplanted kidneys (322). To the extent that the most striking change is a TGF-independent increase in GFR (Y-intercept of the TGF function or proximal SNGFR), these results are reminiscent of the findings during growth-related increases in renal weight and suggest an adaptation of the TGF function curve to a primary increase in GFR (47, 368).

Hyperglycemia Moderate hyperglycemia produced by either acute glucose infusion (27) or streptozotocin-induced diabetes mellitus (199) reduced the amplitude of the TGF response and shifted $V_{1/2}$ to higher flow rates (27). This reduced capacity to compensate for experimentally induced perturbations was also demonstrable under closed-loop conditions (497). The reduction in the TGF response magnitude may in part be caused by a reduction in NaCl concentration and the presence of glucose in tubular perfusion fluid (26, 27, 502).

One hypothesis under active investigation is the possibility that the hyperfiltration of early diabetes may be caused by excessive salt reabsorption in the nephron segments upstream from the MD and the resulting reduction in MD NaCl concentration (480, 503). In support of this

hypothesis, it has been demonstrated by micropuncture that tubular transport proximal to the macula densa is in fact enhanced in diabetic animals (478, 502). On the other hand, it has been argued that TGF may be fully active and may actually prevent excessive hyperfiltration in diabetes (367). Structural adaptations may participate in tubular hyperreabsorption: Inhibition of the enzyme ornithine decarboxylase blocked the renal hypertrophy in a rat model of diabetes mellitus (342), and attenuated both the enhanced proximal reabsorption and the increase in GFR (478). In streptozotocin-treated rats and in diabetic humans, a paradoxical relationship between salt intake and GFR or renal plasma flow has been observed, with high salt intake producing a decrease instead of the expected rise of GFR (499, 502). These observations are consistent with the notion that the TGF adaptation during changes in extracellular fluid volume may be defective in diabetic animals. Whereas TGF desensitization normally prevents a nonhomeostatic reduction of GFR during volume expansion, absent or incomplete resetting of TGF in diabetes appears to permit persistent GFR deviations. Altered resetting in diabetic animals could be a consequence of abnormal RAS activation or dysregulation of NO generation, factors thought to be involved in TGF adaptation. Nevertheless, the paradoxical low-salt–induced increase and high-salt–induced decrease of GFR has not been found in all studies of diabetic patients and animals (2, 11, 52).

Renal Sympathetic Nerve Activity Whereas some experiments did not detect an effect of acute denervation or renal nerve stimulation on the TGF function curve in normotensive animals (165, 464), other studies have reported that denervation causes a time-dependent resetting of TGF to higher values of $V_{1/2}$ without changes in the maximum response (482). Changes in TGF function persisted for at least 1 week and were associated with increased GFR and Na excretion (483).

MECHANISMS OF TGF ADAPTATION

Renin-Angiotensin System The local activity of the renin-angiotensin system appears to be the most consistent determinant of TGF sensitivity. Converting enzyme inhibitors or angiotensin-receptor blockers in relatively high doses cause a reduction of the TGF response magnitude by about 50% to 60% (364, 366, 414, 460, 530). An essentially complete inhibition of TGF responsiveness was seen in mice with a null mutation in the AT1A receptor, the major renal receptor for angiotensin I (431). Similarly, TGF responses were essentially absent in angiotensin-converting enzyme (ACE) knockout mice, an effect that was in part reversible with infusion of subpressor doses of angiotensin II (492). Studies in mice with deletion of tissue ACE or with selective expression of ACE in blood vessels or proximal tubules suggest that the angiotensin II that is required for full TGF responsiveness is derived from the action of membrane-associated ACE in endothelial cells and from systemic ACE (158) while exclusive expression of ACE in proximal tubules is unable to sustain normal TGF responses (218). This conclusion is consistent with earlier observations that angiotensin infusion partly restored feedback responsiveness during captopril-induced TGF inhibition (179, 365). Intravenous or peritubular infusion of angiotensin II enhanced TGF responses in untreated control rats, a property not shared by other vasoconstrictors such as vasopressin and norepinephrine (287, 421). Conversely, the arteriolar constrictor response to angiotensin II was greater during simultaneous TGF activation in both the afferent arteriole/MD double-perfused preparation and in the blood-perfused juxtamedullary nephron technique (184, 385). Since local adenosine levels are thought to increase during TGF activation, this augmentation is possibly due to the effect of adenosine in preventing angiotensin II desensitization (247). In accordance with the role of TGF in autoregulation, angiotensin II has been noted to enhance the TGF component of dynamic autoregulation (94, 133, 201). The suppression of TGF responsiveness caused by acute volume expansion could be fully overcome by the infusion of angiotensin II at doses that restored normal plasma angiotensin II levels (422). Taken together, these results indicate that an AT1A receptor–mediated effect of angiotensin II is a required constituent of the TGF pathway. It is likely that the requirement for angiotensin II results from the well-described synergistic interaction between the vascular effects of angiotensin II and of the TGF mediator, adenosine (430, 491, 527). Another possibility may be an upregulation of MD NaCl transport by angiotensin II (234).

The TGF modifying effect of angiotensin II gains special importance in view of the fact that changes in NaCl in the tubular fluid in the MD region not only affect vascular tone, but also regulate renin secretion (see subsequent sections). This dual effect of MD NaCl has the potential of automatically adjusting TGF sensitivity to the NaCl status of the organism. When the combined external forces determining GFR and proximal and loop of Henle absorption cause deflections in MD NaCl concentration that exceed the range over which TGF operates effectively, persistent changes in MD NaCl occur that will cause an inverse change in renin secretion. The change in angiotensin II concentration resulting from the altered rate of renin secretion in turn is predicted to alter TGF sensitivity. For example, an increase in MD NaCl resulting from extracellular volume expansion will decrease renin secretion, and the decrease of angiotensin II concentration expected to gradually develop is then predicted to uncouple GFR from MD control.

Eicosanoids The presence of both isoforms of cyclo-oxygenase (COX) in the juxtaglomerular region raises the possibility of a participation of prostaglandins in JGA cell-to-cell signaling. COX-1 is expressed in mesangial cells and in endothelial cells of afferent arterioles (453), whereas COX-2 activity has been demonstrated in epithelial cells of thick ascending limb and MD (153). Maximum TGF responses have been found to be inhibited by the intravenous or luminal application of high concentrations of nonspecific

COX inhibitors suggesting that the net effect of any MD-dependent PG production is vasoconstriction (301, 409, 413, 529). The juxtaglomerular operation of a potential eicosanoid-dependent constrictor pathway is supported by the finding that arachidonic acid elicits a constrictor rather than a dilator response when administered by retrograde luminal infusion (104). Thromboxane (TP) is a vasoconstrictor prostaglandin that has been implicated in TGF on the basis of the finding that the intravenous administration of inhibitors of TP receptors or of TP synthesis reduced the magnitude of the TGF-induced vasoconstrictor response (299, 529, 530). Furthermore, activation of TP-receptors by U-46,619 or by the isoprostane 8–isoprostaglandin F2α enhanced TGF responses (537). However, low levels of glomerular thromboxane synthase may limit thromboxane formation under basal and low-salt conditions (531, 554); in fact, attenuation of TGF responses by systemic or luminal application of blockers of TP receptors or of TP synthesis has not been found in all laboratories (104, 299, 529, 530), and normal TGF responses have been observed in TP receptor knockout mice (429). Administration of a high-salt diet, on the other hand, caused a 20fold increase of thromboxane synthase expression as well as a stimulation of TP receptor levels (531, 543). These observations provide an explanation for the finding that the TGF response in the presence of the TP mimetic U 46,619 is augmented in high-salt fed animals (531). TP receptor activation may also contribute to the exaggerated TGF responses observed in young SHR (38). In contrast to these conclusions, studies in the blood-perfused juxtamedullary nephron preparation indicate that TGF activation is accompanied by nNOS-dependent enhancement of COX-2 activity and subsequent generation of vasodilatory PG metabolites that counteract TGF-mediated vasoconstriction (181).

Whether the clear inhibitory effect of nonsteroidal COX blockers is consistent with a role of constrictor prostanoids in TGF is unclear because of the very high doses needed to see this effect. For example, a dose of 5 mg/kg indomethacin was required to obtain more than 50% inhibition of either the SNGFR (409) or the P_{SF} response (529) despite the fact that maximum inhibition of PG synthesis as judged from urinary excretion of PGE_2 or PGF_2 was achieved with a lower dose of indomethacin (409). Similarly, inhibition of TGF responses by luminal administration of indomethacin required concentrations in the millimolar range (104, 409). There is some reason to suspect that the attenuation of TGF responses by indomethacin may not be specifically related to COX inhibition. Intravenous administration of indomethacin did not reduce the maximum TGF response of SNGFR in animals kept on a low-salt diet even though PG synthesis was inhibited to a similar extent (409). Normal TGF responses returned about 80 minutes after the intravenous administration of either indomethacin or carprofen whereas PG production continued to be depressed (409). Similarly, the inhibition of the TGF response achieved by retrograde administration of indomethacin was acutely reversible (104,

409). With high doses of indomethacin applied by retrograde perfusion a marked increase in SNGFR rather than the normal decrease was observed (409) indicating that indomethacin in this study acted by producing active vasodilatation rather than by blocking the generation of a PG mediator with direct or indirect vasoconstrictor properties. Thus, the effect of indomethacin may reflect an interference with cAMP degradation, cellular Ca metabolism, or cytochrome P-450 function (54, 100). Inhibition of the lipoxygenase pathway by nordihydroguaiaretic acid did not alter TGF responsiveness (104).

There is some evidence that 20-hydroxyeicosatetraenoic acid (20-HETE), an arachidonic acid metabolite endogenously generated in afferent arterioles by the 4A family of cytochrome P-450 enzymes, may be involved in the TGF response (568). Two inhibitors of cytochrome P-450 enzymes, 17-octadecynoic acid (ODYA) and clotrimazole, caused a marked attenuation of the TGF response when added to the luminal perfusate for an extended period of time, and this inhibition could be overcome by the administration of exogenous 20-HETE (570). The presence of the mRNAs for cytochrome P-450 4A2, 4A3, and 4A8 has been demonstrated by RT-PCR in glomeruli and most segments of the tubule while preglomerular arterioles appear to express only the 4A2 isoform (189). Immunocytochemistry with a polyclonal nonspecific P-450 4A antibody showed cortical presence of P-450 4A protein in proximal tubules, thick ascending limbs, glomeruli, and preglomerular arterioles (189). Exactly how locally formed 20-HETE affects the TGF pathway is unclear. In addition to its vasoconstrictor properties, 20-HETE has been shown to inhibit TAL NaCl transport by blocking Na,K/2Cl cotransport, Na,K-ATPase, and by closing K channels (398). This combination of effects should result in a powerful inhibition of NaCl transport in thick ascending limb and presumably MD cells so that increments in 20-HETE production would be expected to attenuate, not enhance TGF responses. It is conceivable therefore that ODYA and clotrimazole inhibit the TGF response in a nonspecific way by causing a reduction in baseline afferent arteriolar tone (418). It is also possible that 20-HETE acts as an intracellular second messenger for the TGF mediating agent (151, 568).

Nitric Oxide The addition of nonspecific and nNOS-selective inhibitors of NO synthases to the luminal fluid has been shown to enhance MD-mediated vasoconstrictor responses both in vivo and in vitro (37, 191, 484, 498, 541). These findings demonstrate tonic attenuation of TGF responsiveness by NO generated by nNOS in MD cells, an effect that is cyclic guanosine monophosphate (cGMP) dependent (479). TGF responses of stop-flow pressure in situ and afferent arteriolar diameter reductions in vitro in response to elevated MD [NaCl] were similar in nNOS-deficient and wildtype mice indicating compensatory events during chronic absence of MD NO formation (387, 501). Nevertheless, the proximal-distal SNGFR difference was significantly higher in the $nNOS^{-/-}$ animals, and lu-

minal administration of a nonspecific NOS inhibitor (NLA 10^{-3} M) caused an augmentation of TGF responses only in wildtype, but not in nNOS knockout mice (501). Luminal and systemic administration of NOS inhibitors reversed the attenuation of TGF responses caused by an acute saline infusion suggesting that NO contributes to the TGF resetting caused by volume expansion (49). While there is convincing evidence that NO generated and released by MD cells tonically suppresses the full effect of the vasoconstrictor TGF mediator, the mechanism of TGF modulation by NO is not entirely clear.

In the absence of hemoglobin, the biological half-life of NO in relation to the diffusion distance across the JGA would seem long enough to permit a direct interaction of NO released by MD cells with smooth muscle cells of the afferent arterioles. Nevertheless, NO inactivation may be an important modulator of the effect of NO on TGF. Reactive oxygen species have been identified as a factor that can markedly reduce bioactive NO levels. Immunohistochemical evidence has been obtained for the presence of several components of NADPH oxidase in the JGA (p47phox, p67phox, p22phox) implicating this enzyme in juxtaglomerular formation of superoxide (63). The membrane-permeant superoxide dismutase mimetic tempol diminished TGF responses in vivo and in the perfused JGA preparation (268, 380, 535). Since tempol had no effect in the presence of a NOS inhibitor, it appears that this effect was due to an increase in NO bioavailability (268, 380). In spontaneously hypertensive rats (SHRs), the expression of NADPH oxidase subunits was increased, and the TGF-inhibiting effect of tempol was enhanced compared to normotensive controls suggesting increased oxidative stress in SHR and reduced bioavailability of NO (63, 535). This observation is concordant with the earlier finding that inhibition of nNOS did not enhance TGF responses in SHR (534). Angiotensin II may be in part responsible for the activation of NADPH oxidase in SHR since candesartan restored normal TGF responses to NOS inhibition (536). A high salt intake may be another situation in which the generation of superoxide is increased as indicated by increased expression of NADPHase subunits, and increased excretion of isoprostanes (226). However, the TGF-enhancing effect of NOS inhibition was augmented rather than reduced in rats on a high-salt diet (532, 542). Another mechanism by which NO may reduce TGF responses is inhibition of ecto-5'-nucleotidase, an intervention that would be predicted to reduce extracellular adenosine levels (399, 446).

Further evidence indicates that NO may affect TGF by altering the function of MD cells. In the isolated double-perfused JGA preparation, inhibition of soluble guanylate cyclase or cGMP-dependent protein kinase mimicked the TGF-potentiating effect of a nNOS inhibitor when administered from the tubular side, whereas there was no effect when inhibitors were added to the vascular perfusate (386). The cGMP-dependent mechanism may be inhibition of NaCl uptake since inhibition of Cl fluxes by NO is mediated by soluble guanylate cyclase in TAL cells (334). Formation of NO may occur in MD cells, but a contribution of NO produced by eNOS in TAL cells appears to also affect MD cell function (517).

The relationship between luminal NaCl concentration and NO formation in MD cells has been addressed by using the NO-binding agents DAF-AM DA and DAF-AM. Two independent studies agree that an increase of luminal NaCl causes an increase in fluorescence in MD cells as well as in their surroundings, and that this increase was prevented by an inhibitor of nNOS (235, 267, 269). Since the concentration steps causing increased NO formation were between 35 and 135 mM in one study and between 60 and 150 mM in the other, it has been concluded that supraphysiological NaCl changes are necessary to stimulate NOS (235). Whether the stimulation of nNOS activity by high luminal NaCl is Ca dependent is unclear since NaCl does not consistently elevate [Ca]I and an activation of NOS was seen in Ca-free medium (267). Another explanation for the increased formation of NO is based on the fact that the pH optimum of NOS is in the slightly alkaline range (560). Since an increase in luminal NaCl caused cell alkalinization, it is conceivable that pH-dependent disinhibition of nNOS is responsible for the enhanced NO generation (102). This notion is supported by the observation that dimethyl amiloride increased TGF responses and an nNOS-specific inhibitor in the presence of the NHE blocker did not further enhance the TGF reaction (269, 518). Furthermore, amiloride as well as 7-nitroindazole blunted the increase in NO formation caused by elevated luminal NaCl (269). Stimulation of NO formation by high luminal NaCl is consistent with the earlier observations that the effect of NOS blockade on TGF-dependent vasoconstriction is greater at high than at low flows (533). On the background of this evidence it is remarkable that direct NO measurements performed with carbon fiber electrodes in the distal tubule have shown an increase in the amount of NO and in NO concentration during perfusion of loops of Henle with furosemide suggesting that transport inhibition along the entire loop of Henle stimulates emission and downstream convection of NO (258). While this study did not specifically identify flow as a factor controlling NO emission, NO formation along isolated perfused TAL segments was stimulated by increases in luminal flow rate (335).

Other Vasoactive Factors A reduction in TGF reactivity has been observed subsequent to the systemic administration of renal vasodilators such as atrial natriuretic factor (45, 177), histamine (418), dopamine (423), high concentrations of PGI_2 (29), bradykinin (300), uroguanylin (521), and a number of vasodilating drugs (288, 304, 418, 522). Furthermore, TGF reactivity is decreased by an acute reduction of arterial blood pressure (420), probably as a consequence of non–TGF-mediated autoregulatory vasodilatation. It seems unlikely that all these agents specifically interact with the TGF mechanism at the JGA level to cause a reduction of renal vascular resistance. Rather, the adjustment of TGF

responsiveness may be the nonspecific consequence of vasodilatation reflecting a dependency of vascular resistance changes on the initial wall thickness/radius ratio (101). Since the predominant effector of the TGF response is the afferent arteriole, a resistance change at this site would appear to be most likely to modulate TGF sensitivity.

Interstitial Pressure TGF reactivity has been shown to increase during peritubular capillary perfusion with a hyperoncotic solution, whereas perfusion with protein free solutions reduced TGF responses (343). Changes in response were seen after a time delay of about 20 minutes (343). Based on these observations, the concept was developed that net interstitial pressure (the difference between interstitial hydrostatic pressure and interstitial oncotic pressure) may be an important determinant of TGF reactivity in general. It was subsequently shown that TGF reactivity correlated inversely with net interstitial pressure during acute NaCl infusion (30, 31, 348, 440), during short-lasting ureteral obstruction (347), and after contralateral nephrectomy (144, 305). In all these conditions, $V_{1/2}$ increased and the TGF response amplitude decreased. Conversely, net interstitial pressure was found to be reduced by 24 hours of dehydration (439, 440) and before and after release of 24-hour unilateral ureteral occlusion (515). TGF reactivity was increased in these experimental situations. Exactly how net interstitial pressure affects TGF reactivity is unclear.

Ionic and Osmotic Effects Because of the absence of blood capillaries and lymphatics in the juxtaglomerular interstitium, changes in local interstitial NaCl concentration may result from changes in NaCl transport and may play a role in mediating MD-dependent responses. In fact, NaCl concentrations in the periglomerular interstitium of *Amphiuma* kidneys have been found to increase with increasing flow rates to values much higher than plasma (350). There is no experimental evidence for the occurrence of similar concentration changes in the mammalian JGA. Nevertheless, mathematical modeling has shown that juxtaglomerular interstitial NaCl concentration may vary with changes in NaCl transport although the determining parameters, transport rate, epithelial water permeability, and interstitial space volume, are not known with the degree of certainty necessary to safely predict interstitial ion concentrations (389). In cultured mesangial cells, decrements in extracellular Cl concentration can inhibit the contractile response to agonists such as angiotensin II (238, 328), an effect that is accompanied by a reduction in the rise of intracellular Ca and IP3, and by an increase in PGE_2 formation (328). Furthermore, a decrease in NaCl has been shown to stimulate NO release by mesangial cells in a calcium-dependent manner, and this inverse relationship between NaCl and NO formation has been suggested to mediate TGF responses (494). In the intact JGA, however, neither luminal nor systemic administration of PGE_2 causes inhibition of TGF responses (345, 413), and neither NOS I nor NOS III mRNA is found in freshly dissected glomeruli by in situ hybridization or the highly sensitive RT-PCR method (309, 447, 541). Furthermore, NO is unlikely to be a vasodilator mediator of the TGF response since inhibition of NO synthesis has been reported to augment vasoconstriction, not to abolish vasodilatation (481, 541). Changes in osmolarity, if they occur, are unlikely to be directly involved in TGF mediation since the effect of an increase in tonicity on glomerular afferent tone appears to be vasodilatation, not vasoconstriction (318).

Resetting by Luminal Factors There are a number of circumstances in which unidentified factors in tubular fluid have been shown to modify responses. During chronic dietary salt loading TGF control was inhibited when native tubular fluid was used as perfusate, whereas responses were only slightly blunted during perfusion with an artificial fluid (139). A luminal factor has also been reported to modify TGF during the infusion of atrial natriuretic peptide (369), but this factor appears to enhance TGF responses compared to the blunting observed with artificial solutions. Loop of Henle perfusion with electrolyte-free plasma dialysates from patients with acute renal failure and liver dysfunction produced exaggerated TGF responses that could not be blocked by furosemide (550), suggesting that the plasma in certain disease states contains a factor that can elicit NaCl-independent vasoconstriction when present in the tubular lumen.

MACULA DENSA CONTROL OF RENIN SECRETION

Following Goormaghtigh's early speculation (126), Vander suggested that renin release might be influenced by tubular fluid composition at the macula densa (507). With a variety of manipulations he and his colleagues observed an inverse correlation between plasma renin activity and sodium excretion, but no correlation between renin and mean arterial pressure or renal blood flow (506, 508). The overall conclusion from these studies was that an increased delivery of NaCl to the MD cells inhibits renin secretion. Studies using micropuncture techniques to manipulate MD NaCl appeared to suggest a different relationship, however. Two groups of investigators observed that injection of fluid with a high NaCl concentration into the distal nephron stimulated the activity of renin in the associated glomerulus, which was isolated by microdissection after completion of micropuncture (119, 486). Since renin secretion was not measured in these studies, these observations were not in direct conflict with those of Vander. Nonetheless, the two data sets were considered discrepant leading to a vigorous debate as to whether renin secretion was stimulated or inhibited by a high MD NaCl concentration. The significance of the NaCl dependency of intracellular renin activity has not been pursued further. Nevertheless, granular cells in culture have been found to contain both angiotensin I and angiotensin II as well as all other components of the RAS suggesting intracellular synthesis of angiotensin peptides (185). Furthermore, angiotensin II microinjected into vascular smooth muscle cells can elicit calcium responses suggest-

ing intracellular angiotensin binding sites and transduction pathways (146). If similar mechanisms for an intracellular action of angiotensin II exist in JG cells, it is possible that the increased renin activity caused by increased luminal NaCl is followed by increased angiotensin II formation and JG cell activation. While this aspect of MD-dependent regulation of JG renin remains speculative, substantial additional evidence from whole-animal studies and from isolated in vitro systems has established the concept that a high NaCl concentration at the macula densa inhibits renin secretion (450, 507).

Evidence for MD Control of Renin Secretion

STUDIES IN INTACT ANIMALS

Vander's proposal that renin secretion depends on MD NaCl concentration was studied more directly by comparing renin secretion from normal or nonfiltering kidneys. In dogs in which basal levels of renin were elevated by thoracic caval constriction, intrarenal infusion of NaCl or KCl inhibited renin secretion, but such a response was not seen in similarly treated animals in which the infused kidney had been rendered nonfiltering by ureteral occlusion (444).

Attempts have been made to evaluate the effect of changes in MD NaCl concentration at the single-nephron level in vivo. In these studies in rats, renin concentration in proximal tubular fluid and in postglomerular blood collected by micropuncture was found to vary inversely with changes in distal NaCl (261).

STUDIES IN THE ISOLATED PERFUSED TAL/ GLOMERULUS PREPARATION

With the isolated perfused tubule technique it has been possible to study MD-dependent renin secretion in the absence of baroreceptor and regulated adrenergic inputs and during precise control of tubular fluid composition (450, 452). Another important aspect of the isolated JGA preparation is that it limits the possible sites of tubulovascular information transfer to MD cells and possibly a small number of surrounding TAL cells as the only cells present in the area of contact. In this preparation, there is unequivocal evidence that increasing NaCl concentration in the tubular perfusate suppresses renin secretion and reducing NaCl concentration stimulates it (127, 271, 272, 524). As can be seen in Fig. 12, these results yield clear evidence for an inverse relationship between renin secretion and MD NaCl concentration. MD-dependent renin secretion is characterized by a rapid onset and offset following step changes in NaCl concentration and by reversibility of the induced changes (271, 524). Renin responses were independent of whether the tubule was perfused in an orthograde fashion from the TALH or in a retrograde fashion from the distal convoluted tubule (271). Similar to the TGF response, MD-dependent renin secretion was not altered when NaCl concentration was reduced from isotonicity to about 80 mM, but the full renin response was seen when NaCl concentrations were varied between 7 and 61 mM of Cl

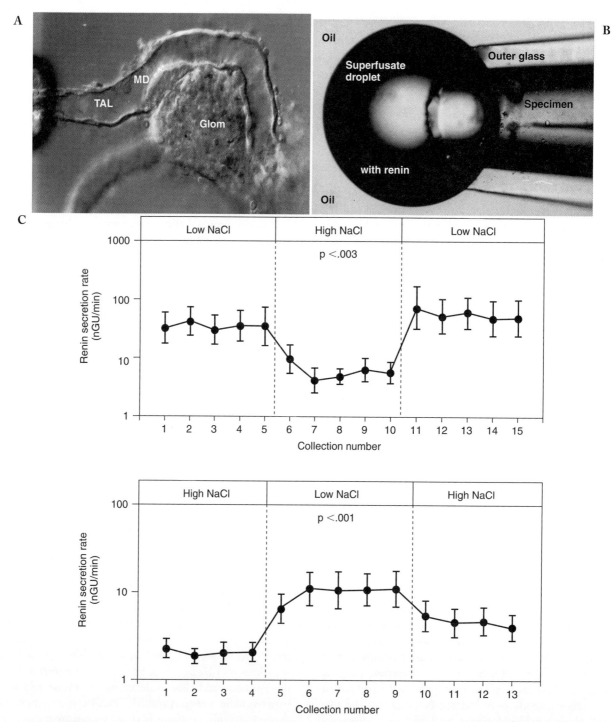

FIGURE 12   A: Isolated perfused thick ascending limb (TAL) with attached glomerulus (glom); macula densa (MD) cells can be seen to protrude into the luminal space. **B:** The perfused specimen is superfused through an outer glass pipette; emerging superfusate containing the secreted renin is collected under oil in defined time intervals. (From Skott O, Briggs JP. A method for superfusion of the isolated perfused tubule. *Kidney Int* 1988;33:1009–1012, with permission.) **C:** Macula densa–mediated changes in renin secretion showing the time course of changes in renin release to an increase (*top*) and to a decrease (*bottom*) in perfusate NaCl concentration. (From Lorenz JN, Weihprecht H, Schnermann J, Skott O, Briggs JP. Characterization of the macula densa stimulus for renin secretion. *Am J Physiol Renal Physiol* 1990;259:F186–193; and Lorenz JN, Weihprecht H, Schnermann J, Skott O, Briggs JP. Renin release from isolated juxtaglomerular apparatus depends on macula densa chloride transport. *Am J Physiol Renal Physiol* 1991;260:F486–493, with permission.) See color insert.

and between 26 and 80 mM of Na, which is within the range that is physiologically relevant (162).

These studies yield a quantitative estimate of the effect of MD NaCl concentration on renin secretion (162). In the most sensitive concentration range between 7 and 47 of Cl, renin secretion increased by about 2 nanoGoldblatt/min per mM decrease in NaCl concentration whereas it fell by 0.4 nGU/min per mM when NaCl concentration was raised from 47 to 87 mM (162). The NaCl concentration causing a half-maximum renin response is estimated to be between 25 and 30 mM, values close to the estimated ambient NaCl concentration and close to the NaCl concentration causing a half-maximum TGF response. Thus, both decreases and increases of NaCl concentration are predicted to affect renin secretion. Quantitative extrapolation from this in vitro system to the in vivo response must be made with caution. In vitro renin secretory responses are assessed in the absence of stabilizing feedback loops that may be important in vivo. For example, stimulation of renin secretion in vivo will increase angiotensin II levels and thereby depress steady-state renin secretion below that predicted for the prevailing MD NaCl concentration. Since renin is effectively removed in the in vitro preparation this negative feedback is eliminated. The TGF mechanism is another feedback system that would tend to minimize deviations in NaCl concentration at the MD and thereby dampen the signal for renin release.

Sensing Mechanism for MD-Mediated Renin Secretion

RENIN SECRETORY RESPONSE AND NaCl TRANSPORT

Early studies in intact animals suggested that in certain conditions renin secretion correlates more closely with distal tubular NaCl load than NaCl concentration, for example, during the infusion of hypertonic mannitol (80, 93, 508). However, a re-investigation of early distal NaCl concentration during mannitol diuresis showed a clear concentration decrease, in agreement with the stimulation of renin release typically seen in this condition (265). In the isolated JGA preparation, an 80% reduction in luminal NaCl load by decreasing perfusate flow at constant NaCl concentration caused only a small, approximately twofold increase in the rate of renin secretion. In contrast, when NaCl load was reduced to a similar degree by decreasing perfusate NaCl concentration, renin secretion increased nearly eightfold (271). These studies show clearly that, at least in the isolated perfused JGA, NaCl concentration is a more important determinant of renin release than NaCl delivery.

Based on the stimulatory effect of loop diuretics in intact animals it was concluded that MD NaCl transport plays a critical role as an early step in NaCl-dependent control of renin secretion (16, 60, 216, 507-509). The first direct evidence for a MD-mediated effect of transport inhibition on renin secretion was obtained in nonperfused afferent arterioles in which furosemide stimulated renin release only when the MD segment was included in the dissected specimen, but

not in its absence (192). In the isolated perfused JGA preparation, luminal application of bumetanide at 10^{-6} M increased renin secretion during perfusion with high NaCl solutions (272). Furthermore, the presence of furosemide at 5×10^{-5} M essentially abolished the dependence of renin secretion on luminal NaCl concentration (162). Studies have shown that plasma renin concentration is significantly elevated in $NKCC_1$-deficient compared to wildtype mice (61). Studies in isolated JG cells indicate that $NKCC_1$ exerts a direct inhibitory effect on basal renin release (61). This effect appears to be independent of the $NKCC_2$-dependent inhibitory pathway through the macula densa since the stimulatory effect of furosemide on renin release was essentially normal in $NKCC_1^{-/-}$ mice.

Ion Specificity of Renin Secretory Responses

MD control of renin secretion shows an apparent Cl dependency that is reminiscent of that described for TGF responses. Whereas the acute or chronic administration of various Cl or Br salts without Na inhibited renin secretion, Na salts without Cl as the accompanying anion had no effect (225, 233). Furthermore, changes in renin secretion under these conditions correlated with loop of Henle Cl absorption (528). Conversely, an acute selective depletion of Cl by peritoneal dialysis increased plasma renin activity (1), and substitution of Cl by nitrate or thiocyanate in the perfusate of isolated kidneys stimulated renin secretion (390). In the isolated perfused JGA, ion selectivity has been examined by measuring the inhibitory effect of adding various Na and Cl salts to a low NaCl perfusate. The inhibitory response was unchanged when most of luminal Na was replaced by choline or rubidium (272). On the other hand, substituting Cl by isethionate or acetate virtually eliminated the response to increased Na concentration (272). These results support the hypothesis that the initiating signal for MD control of renin secretion is a change in the rate of NaCl uptake via a luminal Na,K,2Cl-cotransporter whose physiological activity is determined by a change in luminal Cl concentration.

The Stimulus-Response Coupling Mechanism

NITRIC OXIDE

The presence of NOS I in MD cells raises the possibility that NO may act as an epithelium-derived factor that participates in MD control of renin secretion. This notion is supported by observations showing that the expression of MD nNOS changes in parallel with renin expression in a number of circumstances. MD cells of rats on a low-salt diet have increased levels of nNOS mRNA and protein expression (34, 310, 436, 447, 489). Furthermore, the administration of furosemide also causes a marked increase in MD nNOS expression (34, 436), as does renal artery constriction (34, 436). The mechanism responsible for the upregulation of nNOS expression in these states is unclear, but a reduced

NaCl transport at the MD is a common feature. Since the expression and secretion of renin is known to be elevated in these conditions, it is possible that NO generation is an upstream signal in the control of the RAS. The suggestion that a chronically reduced NaCl transport may stimulate MD nNOS expression is not immediately reconcilable with the evidence discussed earlier that acute changes in NaCl concentration appear to increase nNOS activity and NO formation. The expression of nNOS in MD cells is stabilized by negative feedback influences exerted by angiotensin II and PGE_2 since nNOS expression was markedly upregulated in mice with AT1 receptor or angiotensinogen deficiencies as well as in COX-$2^{-/-}$ mice (219, 220, 338).

Understanding of the role of NO in renin secretion is complicated by the fact that NO can elicit both stimulatory and inhibitory effects. While both pathways are relatively well defined, the factors causing predominance of one or the other are not entirely clear. Isolated JG cells in short-term culture respond to brief exposure of nitroprusside with a dose-dependent inhibition of renin secretion that is accompanied by a prompt rise of cyclic GMP (cGMP) levels (128, 433). Inhibition of renin secretion by cGMP was prevented by methylene blue, suggesting that it was mediated by activation of cGMP-dependent protein kinases (128, 433). Inhibition of renin release in JG cell cultures and kidney slices by ANP, which causes increases in cellular cGMP through activation of particulate guanylate cyclase, supports this notion (164, 239). NO has also been found to exert inhibitory effects on renin secretion in kidney slices (15, 512). Furthermore, 8–bromo-cGMP reduced isoproterenol- and bumetanide-stimulated renin secretion in isolated perfused rat kidneys (242, 514).

The inhibitory effect is likely to be the direct result of activation of cGMP-dependent protein kinases (cGK). Two isoforms of cGK have been identified, cGK I and cGK II, and both isoforms have been found in granular cells (113). A direct activator of cGK, 8–para-chlorophenylthio-cGMP, has been shown to inhibit isoproterenol- or forskolin-stimulated renin secretion in isolated perfused rat kidneys and microdissected afferent arterioles, and this stimulation could be reversed by an inhibitor of cGK (114). A role for cGKII is suggested by the finding that 8–bromo-cGMP reduced basal and forskolin-stimulated stimulated renin secretion in JG cells isolated from wildtype and cGK $I^{-/-}$ mice, but that it had no effect in cultures from cGK $II^{-/-}$ mice (514). Furthermore, adenovirus-mediated transfection of JG cells with either cGK I or cGK II enhanced the inhibitory effect of a cGK activator on forskolin-stimulated renin release (114).

While the immediate effect of NO on renin secretion in JG cells is inhibition, incubation for longer than 5 hours caused a marked increase in renin release as well as an increase in renin mRNA expression (91, 433). In the isolated perfused JGA preparation, the addition of L-arginine during perfusion with low NaCl further enhanced renin release, and this effect was blocked in the presence of a NOS blocker (163). The mechanism of the stimulatory effect of NO on renin secretion

is related to an activation of the cAMP/protein kinase A pathway, and this activation results from an inhibition of PDEIII, a cAMP-degrading phosphodiesterase that is inhibited by cGMP (155). An early report showing that the PDEIII inhibitor milrinone increased basal and isoproterenol-stimulated renin release in conscious rabbits has now been corroborated by substantial additional evidence (73). In the isolated perfused rat kidney, Na nitroprusside increased renin secretion, and this increase was attenuated by the PKA inhibitor Rp-8–CPT-cAMPS. Since membrane-permeable cGMP analogues also reduced the stimulatory effect of sodium nitroprusside (SNP), stimulation of renin secretion by NO was clearly related to the A kinase, not G kinase pathway (242). PDEIII inhibition by cGMP as the cause for the increase in cAMP is suggested by the observation that two inhibitors of this enzyme, milrinone and trequinsin, markedly elevated renin secretion, and that a specific guanylate cyclase inhibitor abolished the stimulatory effect of SNP (243). Furthermore, trequinsin elevated cellular cAMP content in JG cells, and enhanced renin secretion, an effect that was abolished by PKA inhibition (108). Inhibition of PDE IV, a phosphodiesterase with predominant effects on cGMP degradation, also increased renin secretion (400). This effect was blunted by nNOS inhibition, suggesting that nNOS contributed to cGMP formation. Thus, the stimulatory pathway of NO is initiated by guanylate cyclase-dependent generation of cGMP, inhibition of PDEIII-dependent degradation of cAMP, and activation of the PKA pathway. The major open question is to evaluate the nature of the mechanism that determines whether activation of cGK or PKA predominates.

NO in MD-Dependent Renin Release In view of the dual effects of NO on renin secretion and the ambiguity about the directional changes of juxtaglomerular NO with changes in loop of Henle flow rates, it is not surprising that the precise role of NO in MD control of renin release has remained equivocal. In the isolated perfused JGA preparation during perfusion with a low NaCl concentration, the luminal addition of L-arginine stimulated renin secretion and this stimulation was abolished by NOS blockade, suggesting that in this setting NO is renin-stimulatory (163). Consistent with this conclusion is our observation that the NaCl dependency of renin secretion was essentially abolished in the presence of a NOS blocker in the tubular lumen, a change that was due entirely to prevention of the rise of renin secretion caused by a low luminal NaCl (Fig. 13A; 163). The conclusion that a low NaCl concentration at the MD stimulates renin secretion in an NO-dependent fashion is also supported by findings showing that the increased renin secretion caused by a reduction in arterial or perfusion pressure in kidneys of conscious dogs and in isolated rat kidneys was markedly and consistently blunted by NOS inhibition (352, 432). In other studies, the administration of a loop diuretic has been used to simulate a reduction in MD NaCl concentration. In dissected rat renal microvessels, NOS inhibition abolished the increase in renin release caused by furosemide pretreatment (65). Similarly, the stim-

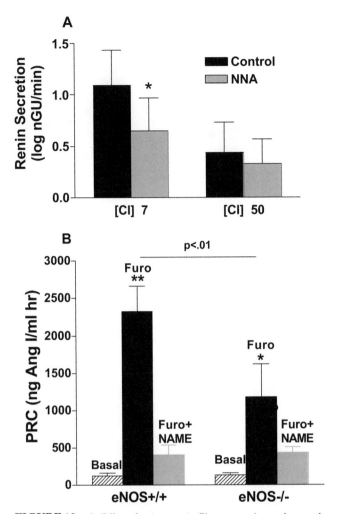

FIGURE 13 **A:** Effect of an increase in Cl concentration at the macula densa on renin secretion during control and during NOS inhibition with nitro-L-arginine (NNA). Studies were performed in the isolated perfused thick ascending limb/glomerulus preparation of the rabbit. (From He XR, Greenberg SG, Briggs JP, Schnermann JB. Effect of nitric oxide on renin secretion, II: studies in the perfused juxtaglomerular apparatus. *Am J Physiol Renal Physiol* 1995;268:F953–959, with permission.) **B:** Plasma renin concentrations (PRC) under basal conditions and following the injection of furosemide in the absence and presence of the NOS inhibitor L-NAME in conscious wildtype (eNOS$^{+/+}$) and eNOS-deficient mice (eNOS$^{-/-}$). (From Castrop H, Schweda F, Mizel D, Huang Y, Briggs J, Kurtz A, Schnermann J. Permissive role of nitric oxide in macula densa control of renin secretion. *Am J Physiol Renal Physiol* 2004;286:F848–857, with permission.)

ulation of renin secretion by furosemide in vivo was inhibited by the administration of NOS inhibitors (16, 375, 434). Plasma renin activity in nNOS knockout mice and basal renin secretion in isolated perfused kidneys from nNOS$^{-/-}$ or eNOS$^{-/-}$ mice were found to be consistently lower than in wildtype animals suggesting that tonic release of NO enhances renin release in mice (60, 338). The relative increases of renin secretion by furosemide were essentially normal in nNOS$^{-/-}$ or eNOS$^{-/-}$ mice, but were markedly reduced by general NOS inhibition (Fig. 13B; 60). Furthermore, the administration of the NO donor SNAP in kidneys in which endogenous NO production was blocked by

L-NAME completely restored the stimulatory effect of loop diuretics. According to this evidence it would appear that exposition of JG cells to NO regardless of its exact cellular source is necessary for the MD pathway to operate normally. The nature of this permissive effect of NO may be to inhibit PDEIII, and thereby to sensitize the renin secretory mechanism to the renin mediator that we assume to act through activation of the cAMP/PKA pathway (Fig. 14).

PROSTAGLANDINS

Starting with the early observations by Larsson et al. (253) that arachidonic acid increases and indomethacin reduces plasma renin activity, various metabolites of arachidonic acid, most notably prostaglandins, have been established as potent regulators of renin secretion in a variety of experimental conditions (216). Stimulation of renin secretion is most consistently seen with administration of prostaglandins of the E and I series (196). The effect of PGs on renin secretion is mediated by G-protein–coupled receptors, IP receptors in the case of PGI$_2$ and EP$_2$/EP$_4$ receptors in the case of PGE$_2$ (198). Selective deletion of floxed Gsα in JG cells by cre recombinase driven by the endogenous renin promoter was associated with marked reductions of plasma renin concentration (66).

Relation between MD COX-2 and Renin Cyclooxygenases catalyze the hydroxylation and oxygenation of arachidonic acid that leads to the generation of endoperoxides (or PGH$_2$). Subsequent processing by a number of enzymes converts PGH$_2$ into the biologically active spectrum of prostaglandins. The potential of prostaglandins to regulate renin secretion became highly relevant for the MD-dependent pathway by the demonstration that one of the cyclo-oxygenases, the inducible isoform COX-2, was constitutively expressed in MD cells (152). The abundance of COX-2 in the MD and adjacent TAL cells is highly regulated, and the pattern of COX-2 regulation parallels that of nNOS in the macula densa and of renin in JG cells.

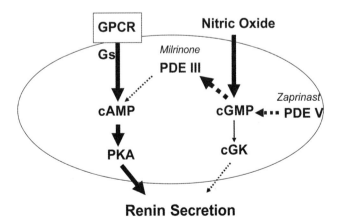

FIGURE 14 Schematic representation of the pathways by which nitric oxide can inhibit or stimulate renin secretion. Inhibition of phosphodiesterase by cyclic guanosine monophosphate (cGMP) and subsequent reduced degradation of cAMP appears to be the dominant pathway under many conditions. Milrinone, an inhibitor of PDEIII, consistently stimulates renin secretion.

Parallel increases in COX-2 and renin have been observed in rats treated chronically with furosemide and in patients with Bartter syndrome, suggesting that, COX-2 expression, like nNOS may be in some way linked to NaCl uptake by MD cells (58, 208, 228, 281, 376). An increase of MD COX-2 expression and of JG cell renin is induced by administration of a low-sodium diet or by renal artery stenosis (152, 157, 197, 520, 556). Stimulation of COX-2 expression has also been found following partial renal ablation and in active lupus nephritis (490, 519). A low-sodium diet also caused a two- to threefold increase in the expression of PGE_2 synthase in MD cells (51). Conversely, mice with genetic COX-2 deficiency have a marked reduction of renin expression and of plasma renin concentration (221, 557). On the other hand, angiotensin II appears to play the role of a negative-feedback regulator of COX-2 synthesis: a strong and consistent stimulation of COX-2 expression is induced by ACE inhibition or AT1 receptor blockade, and COX-2 expression is increased in AT1 receptor knockout mice (58, 69, 545) as well as in other states of low angiotensin action (66).

Regulation of PGE_2 Production   The application of a biosensor technique has provided a missing piece of evidence linking MD NaCl delivery to local PGE_2 release (358). In this approach, HEK293 cells were stably transfected with the mouse PGE_2 receptor EP_1, a receptor subtype that is coupled to the IP_3 pathway and whose activation therefore causes an increase in cytosolic Ca. Transfected HEK cells responded to PGE_2 with a dose-dependent increase in [Ca]i, and this effect was blocked by the EP_1 inhibitor SC51322. In perfused TAL/MD preparations dissected from kidneys of salt-restricted rabbits, a transfected and fura-2–loaded sensor cell was then positioned at the basolateral aspect of MD cells, and changes in [Ca]i were used as an index of PGE_2 release. In preparations obtained from rabbits fed a low-salt diet, removal of luminal NaCl caused a significant increase in sensor cell [Ca]I, while no effect was seen when NaCl was reduced to zero in the presence of luminal furosemide. This effect appeared to be cell-specific since the positioning of the sensor cell close to a TAL cell had no affect on [Ca]i. Of major importance is the observation that most of the change in [Ca]i occurred in a NaCl concentration range of between 20 and 40 mM, exactly the concentration range in which NaCl concentration affects renin secretion in a similar preparation (Fig. 15) .

The mechanisms by which a reduction in luminal NaCl may cause stimulation of PGE_2 release and COX-2 expression have been studied in cell lines derived from the MD and from TAL cells (70, 559). In both lines of cells, a reduction in medium NaCl caused a prompt and dose-dependent increase in PGE_2 release that was essentially completely inhibited by NS-398 and was therefore largely mediated by COX-2. The onset of this response preceded any increase in COX-2 expression, suggesting that it was the result of an increase in COX-2 activity and/or of an activation of PLA2 followed by increased availability of arachidonic acid. Pres-

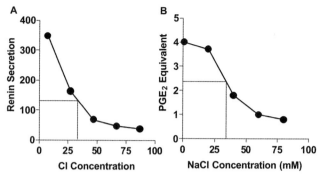

FIGURE 15   **A:** Relationship between perfusate Cl concentration and renin release in the isolated perfused JGA preparation; data from He XR, Greenberg SG, Briggs JP, Schnermann J. Effects of furosemide and verapamil on the NaCl dependency of macula densa-mediated renin secretion. *Hypertension* 1995;26:137–142, with permission. **B:** Relationship between perfusate NaCl concentration and prostaglandin E_2 (PGE_2) release by macula densa cells. The PGE_2 equivalent corresponds to the EP1-mediated increase in cytosolic Ca in HEK cells transfected with EP1 receptor cDNA, and placed at the basolateral aspect of macula densa cells. (From Peti-Peterdi J, Komlosi P, Fuson AL, Guan Y, Schneider A, Qi Z, Redha R, Rosivall L, Breyer MD, Bell PD. Luminal NaCl delivery regulates basolateral PGE_2 release from macula densa cells. *J Clin Invest* 2003;112:76–82, with permission.)

ence of PLA2 in macula densa cells and regulation of PLA2 in parallel to that of COX-2 have been demonstrated (280). In TAL and MD cells in culture, a reduction in medium NaCl also augmented the expression of the mRNA and protein expression of COX-2 (70, 559). Ion-substitution studies indicate that the extracellular signal for COX-2 stimulation appears to be a reduction in Cl rather than in Na concentration, a finding that is remarkably concordant with the Cl dependency of renin secretion shown earlier in an entirely different preparation. The intracellular signaling events leading to the stimulation of COX-2 activity and expression are initiated by rapid phosphorylation of p38 and Erk1/2 kinases (559). Participation of MAP kinases in COX-2 expression is supported by the inhibitory effects of SB 203580 and PD 98059, inhibitors of p38 and Erk1/2-mediated signaling events (70, 559). The increased expression of COX-2 through the MAP kinase pathway appears to reflect both a transcriptional activation and an increased stability of the mRNA (72). These observations are in agreement with findings in other cell types in which MAP kinases are critically involved in regulating COX-2 expression in response to cytokines, growth factors, and hypertonicity (132, 551, 558)

PGs in MD-Dependent Renin Release   Studies in the isolated rabbit JGA have shown that acute, nonspecific COX inhibition with flufenamic acid or flurbiprofen virtually completely abolished the increase in renin secretion caused by a decrease in MD NaCl concentration (127). Since the concentration change from minimal to maximal was done in a single step, it is not clear whether the effect of these agents was symmetrical around the midpoint or whether it mainly affected the stimulation in the subnormal concentration range. Direct evidence for a role of COX-2 has been obtained in an extension of these studies in which the specific COX-2 inhibitor NS-398 was also found to prevent the stimulation of renin secretion by low NaCl while the putative COX-1 blocker valerylsalicylate did not have this effect (Fig. 16) (493). The significance of these findings is substantial since as pointed out earlier, the isolated perfused rabbit JGA preparation is the only available technique capable of assessing MD-dependent renin release unencumbered by simultaneous sympathetic and baroreceptor input. Earlier support for a role of PGs in MD-mediated renin release came from studies examining the response to supraaortic constriction in denervated kidneys of dogs treated with papaverine; in this model, designed to isolate MD-dependent responses, stimulation of renin secretion was blocked by indomethacin and meclofenamate (330). Furthermore, indomethacin prevented the increase of plasma renin that accompanied the reduction of distal NaCl caused by dietary salt restriction (103).

In addition to the attenuation of MD-mediated renin release by acute COX-2 inhibition, chronic interference with COX-2 signaling is associated with a reduction of renin expression that has secondary consequences for acute renin secretory responses. Thus, COX-2–deficient mice have been shown to have a markedly reduced renin mRNA expression and plasma renin, and this effect was greater on a 129J or C57Bl/6 than mixed genetic background (71, 221, 557). Chronic administration of COX-2 blockers, on the other hand, did not consistently reduce renin expression (111, 167, 209). Acute stimulation of renin release by furosemide, hydralazine, or isoproterenol was markedly reduced in COX-2–deficient compared to wildtype mice, suggesting that the acute release response was dependent upon basal

renin expression levels (221). Furthermore, stimulation of renin release by angiotensin-converting enzyme or AT1 blockers was also markedly reduced in animals with genetic or pharmacologic COX-2 deficiency (69, 71, 221). Overall these studies reveal that the level of renin expression is an important and nonspecific determinant of the acute secretory response independent of whether the stimulus acts through the MD, baroreceptor, sympathetic, or any other pathway. The strong relationship between basal levels of renin release or its surrogate, plasma renin, and the acute release response suggests the existence of an acutely releasable renin pool in JG cells whose magnitude depends on renin synthesis (221, 244). Figure 17 provides a schematic summary of the pathways causing stimulation of renin secretion during reduction of MD NaCl concentration.

Adenosine

In general, exogenous adenosine inhibits renin release in intact rats or dogs (6, 81, 463), an effect that is produced by activation of A1AR (81). Nevertheless, it is unclear to what extent adenosine participates in the renin inhibition caused by high luminal NaCl concentrations. In the isolated perfused JGA, the selective adenosine$_1$-receptor blocker 8–cyclopentyl-1,3-dipropylxanthine (CPX) blunted the fall in

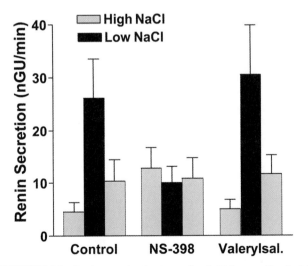

FIGURE 16 Renin secretion in the perfused thick ascending limb/glomerulus preparation of the rabbit in response to perfusion with solutions containing high and low NaCl concentrations during control conditions, during inhibition of COX-2 with NS-398, and during inhibition of COX-1 with valerylsalicylate. (From Traynor TR, Smart A, Briggs JP, Schnermann J. Inhibition of macula densa-stimulated renin secretion by pharmacological blockade of cyclooxygenase-2. *Am J Physiol Renal Physiol* 1999;277:F706–F710, with permission.)

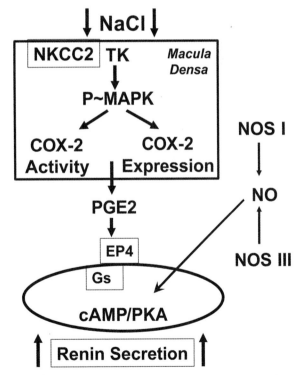

FIGURE 17 Schematic summary of the pathway by which a decrease in luminal NaCl concentration causes stimulation of renin secretion. Activation of several MAP kinases causes activation of COX-2 as well as transcriptional upregulation of COX-2 synthesis, augmented release of prostaglandin E$_2$, and stimulation of the cAMP/PKA pathway through EP4 receptors. Nitric oxide, derived from both NOS I and NOC III, supports renin secretion by stabilizing cAMP.

renin secretion caused by an elevation in luminal NaCl, but did not abolish it (524). Adenosine itself was found to be only a weak inhibitor of MD-stimulated renin secretion when added to the bathing fluid (273). This may reflect effective degradation of exogenous adenosine since the addition of the adenosine deaminase inhibitor pentostatin (deoxycoformycin) augmented the renin inhibitory effect of adenosine somewhat (273). Additional studies may have clarified the role of adenosine in MD-dependent renin release. In isolated perfused kidneys, it was found that the stimulation of renin release by bumetanide was not measurably different between wildtype and A1AR-deficient mice (438). This observation argues against a role of A1AR and adenosine in the stimulation of renin secretion during inhibition of NaCl transport below ambient levels without excluding a role in the inhibitory pathway activated by increases in MD NaCl. The injection of a bolus of NaCl has been used previously as a method to acutely expose the MD segment to an increased NaCl load. The resulting decrease of renin secretion appears to be MD-mediated since it requires the presence of Cl ions (232). In agreement with earlier results in rats, we have found in mice that the injection of NaCl reduced PRC, whereas the injection of $NaHCO_3$ did not (222). However, this effect was not seen in A1AR-deficient mice, suggesting that the renin-inhibitory effect of increased NaCl concentrations is mediated by adenosine whereas the renin-stimulatory effect is not (Fig. 18).

The cellular mechanisms of inhibition of renin release by adenosine are not clear, but it is likely that an increase in [Ca]i may play a role. Considerable progress has been made in understanding the paradoxical inhibition of renin release by elevated [Ca]i. In primary cultures of JG cells it has been observed that an increase of [Ca]i by thapsigargin, angiotensin II, or endothelin was associated with a marked decrease in isoproterenol or forskolin-stimulated cellular cAMP and a

decrease of renin release (130). Conversely, a decrease of [Ca]i by the Ca chelator BAPTA-AM caused an increase in cellular cAMP accompanied by an increase in renin release (333). The inverse relation between [Ca]i and cAMP was suggested to reflect regulation of adenylyl cyclase (AC) by [Ca]i. In fact, the Ca-inhibitable AC5 and AC6 isoforms were shown to be expressed in JG cells (130, 333), and siRNAs directed against AC5 and AC6 were able to prevent cAMP stimulation by forskolin or isoproterenol as well as renin secretion in As4.1 cells (130).

Ionic and Osmotic Effects

Changes in external juxtaglomerular osmolarity, such as those observed in *Amphiuma*, may mediate the renin secretory response to a change of luminal NaCl. In a number of different preparations hypoosmolarity stimulates and hyperosmolarity inhibits renin secretion, and such changes would seem to be directionally plausible in mediating MD-dependent renin release (106, 195, 435, 451). However, a study in isolated perfused rat or mouse kidneys established a direct rather than an inverse relationship between renin release and external osmolarity (244), a finding that confirms an earlier in vivo observation (564). Osmotic stimulation of renin release was not prevented by L-NAME, indomethacin, or bumetanide and was therefore suggested to reflect a direct effect on JG cells (244).

Acknowledgment

Research from the laboratory of the authors was supported by intramural funds of the National Institute of Diabetes, and Digestive and Kidney Diseases, National Institutes of Health.

References

1. Abboud HE, Luke RG, Galla JH, Kotchen TA. Stimulation of renin by acute selective chloride depletion in the rat. *Circ Res* 1979;44:815–821.
2. Allen TJ, Waldron MJ, Casley D, Jerums G, Cooper ME. Salt restriction reduces hyperfiltration, renal enlargement, and albuminuria in experimental diabetes. *Diabetes* 1997;46:19–24.
3. Alper SL, Stuart-Tilley AK, Biemesderfer D, Shmukler BE, Brown D. Immunolocalization of AE2 anion exchanger in rat kidney. *Am J Physiol Renal Physiol* 1997;273:F601–614.
4. Amemiya M, Loffing J, Lotscher M, Kaissling B, Alpern RJ, Moe OW. Expression of NHE-3 in the apical membrane of rat renal proximal tubule and thick ascending limb. *Kidney Int* 1995;48:1206–1215.
5. Anderson TJ, Martin S, Berka JL, James DE, Slot JW, Stow JL. Distinct localization of renin and GLUT-4 in juxtaglomerular cells of mouse kidney. *Am J Physiol* 1998;274:F26–33.
6. Arend LJ, Haramati A, Thompson CI, Spielman WS. Adenosine-induced decrease in renin release: dissociation from hemodynamic effects. *Am J Physiol Renal Physiol* 1984;247:F447–452.
7. Arendshorst WJ, Finn WF, Gottschalk CW. Nephron stop-flow pressure response to obstruction for 24 hours in the rat kidney. *J Clin Invest* 1974;53:1497–1500.
8. Arensbak B, Mikkelsen HB, Gustafsson F, Christensen T, Holstein-Rathlou NH. Expression of connexin 37, 40, and 43 mRNA and protein in renal preglomerular arterioles. *Histochem Cell Biol* 2001;115:479–487.
9. Arystarkhova E, Wetzel RK, Sweadner KJ. Distribution and oligomeric association of splice forms of Na(+)-K(+)-ATPase regulatory gamma-subunit in rat kidney. *Am J Physiol Renal Physiol* 2002;282:F393–407.
10. Bacay AC, Mantyh CR, Cohen AH, Mantyh PW, Fine LG. Glomerular atrial natriuretic factor receptors in primary glomerulopathies: studies on human renal biopsies. *Am J Kidney Dis* 1989;14:386–395.
11. Bank N, Lahorra G, Aynedjian HS, Wilkes BM. Sodium restriction corrects hyperfiltration of diabetes. *Am J Physiol* 1988;254:F668–676.
12. Barajas L. The development and ultrastructure of the juxtaglomerular cell granule. *J Ultrastruct Res* 1966;15:400–413.

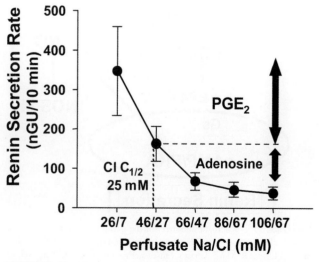

FIGURE 18 Control of macula densa–dependent renin secretion by prostaglandin E_2 (PGE_2) and adenosine with PGE_2 being responsible for the larger stimulatory effect during reduced luminal NaCl, and adenosine causing a smaller inhibitory effect during increases in macula densa NaCl.

13. Beaumont K, Healy DP, Fanestil DD. Autoradiographic localization of benzodiazepine receptors in the rat kidney. *Am J Physiol* 1984;247:F718–724.
14. Beck JS, Breton S, Mairbaurl H, Laprade R, Giebisch G. Relationship between sodium transport and intracellular ATP in isolated perfused rabbit proximal convoluted tubule. *Am J Physiol* 1991;261:F634–639.
15. Beierwaltes WH, Carretero OA. Nonprostanoid endothelium-derived factors inhibit renin release. *Hypertension* 1992;19:II68–73.
16. Beierwaltes WH. Selective neuronal nitric oxide synthase inhibition blocks furosemide-stimulated renin secretion in vivo. *Am J Physiol Renal Physiol* 1995;269:F134–139.
17. Bell PD, Thomas C, Williams RH, Navar LG. Filtration rate and stop-flow pressure feedback responses to nephron perfusion in the dog. *Am J Physiol* 1978;234:F154–165.
18. Bell PD, McLean CB, Navar LG. Dissociation of tubuloglomerular feedback responses from distal tubular chloride concentration in the rat. *Am J Physiol Renal Physiol* 1981;240:F111–119.
19. Bell PD, Navar LG. Cytoplasmic calcium in the mediation of macula densa tubuloglomerular feedback responses. *Science* 1982;215:670–673.
20. Bell PD, Navar LG. Relationship between tubulo-glomerular feedback responses and perfusate hypotonicity. *Kidney Int* 1982;22:234–239.
21. Bell PD,Reddington M. Intracellular calcium in the transmission of tubuloglomerular feedback signals. *Am J Physiol Renal Physiol* 1983;245:F295–302.
22. Bell PD, Reddington M, Ploth D, Navar LG. Tubuloglomerular feedback-mediated decreases in glomerular pressure in Munich-Wistar rats. *Am J Physiol Renal Physiol* 1984;247:F877–880.
23. Bell PD. Cyclic AMP-calcium interaction in the transmission of tubuloglomerular feedback signals. *Kidney Int* 1985;28:728–732.
24. Bell PD, Lapointe JY, Cardinal J. Direct measurement of basolateral membrane potentials from cells of the macula densa. *Am J Physiol Renal Physiol* 1989;257:F463–468.
25. Bell PD, Lapointe JY, Sabirov R, Hayashi S, Peti-Peterdi J, Manabe K, Kovacs G, Okada Y. Macula densa cell signaling involves ATP release through a maxi anion channel. *Proc Natl Acad Sci U S A* 2003;100:4322–4327.
26. Blantz RC, Konnen KS. Relation of distal tubular delivery and reabsorptive rate to nephron filtration. *Am J Physiol Renal Physiol* 1977;233:F315–324.
27. Blantz RC, Peterson OW, Gushwa L, Tucker BJ. Effect of modest hyperglycemia on tubuloglomerular feedback activity. *Kidney Int Suppl* 1982;12:S206–212.
28. Blantz RC, Peterson OW, Thomson SC. Tubuloglomerular feedback responses to acute contralateral nephrectomy. *Am J Physiol Renal Physiol* 1991;260:F749–756.
29. Boberg U, Hahne B, Persson AE. The effect of intraarterial infusion of prostacyclin on the tubuloglomerular feedback control in the rat. *Acta Physiol Scand* 1984;121:65–72.
30. Boberg U, Persson AE. Tubuloglomerular feedback during elevated renal venous pressure. *Am J Physiol Renal Physiol* 1985;249:F524–531.
31. Boberg U, Persson AE. Increased tubuloglomerular feedback activity in Milan hypertensive rats. *Am J Physiol Renal Physiol* 1986;250:F967–974.
32. Boknam L, Ericson AC, Aberg B, Ulfendahl HR. Flow resistance of the interlobular artery in the rat kidney. *Acta Physiol Scand* 1981;111:159–163.
33. Bonsib SM. The macula densa tubular basement membrane: a unique plaque of basement membrane specialization. *J Ultrastruct Mol Struct Res* 1986;97:103–108.
34. Bosse HM, Bohm R, Resch S, Bachmann S. Parallel regulation of constitutive NO synthase and renin at JGA of rat kidney under various stimuli. *Am J Physiol Renal Physiol* 1995;269:F793–805.
35. Bouby N, Trinh-Trang-Tan MM, Kriz W, Bankir L. Possible role of the thick ascending limb and of the urine concentrating mechanism in the protein-induced increase in GFR and kidney mass. *Kidney Int Suppl* 1987;22:S57–61.
36. Braam B, Boer P, Koomans HA. Tubuloglomerular feedback and tubular reabsorption during acute potassium loading in rats. *Am J Physiol Renal Physiol* 1994;267:F223–230.
37. Braam BKoomans HA. Reabsorption of nitro-L-arginine infused into the late proximal tubule participates in modulation of TGF responsiveness. *Kidney Int* 1995;47:1252–1257.
38. Brannstrom KArendshorst WJ. Thromboxane A2 contributes to the enhanced tubuloglomerular feedback activity in young SHR. *Am J Physiol Renal Physiol* 1999;276:F758–F766.
39. Breuss JM, Gillett N, Lu L, Sheppard D, Pytela R. Restricted distribution of integrin beta 6 mRNA in primate epithelial tissues. *J Histochem Cytochem* 1993;41:1521–1527.
40. Briggs J. A simple steady-state model for feedback control of glomerular filtration rate. *Kidney Int* 1982;22[Suppl 12]:S143–S150.
41. Briggs J, Schubert G, Schnermann J. Further evidence for an inverse relationship between macula densa NaCl concentration and filtration rate. *Pflugers Arch* 1982;392:372–378.
42. Briggs JP, Wright FS. Feedback control of glomerular filtration rate: site of the effector mechanism. *Am J Physiol* 1979;236:F40–47.
43. Briggs JP, Schnermann J, Wright FS. Failure of tubule fluid osmolarity to affect feedback regulation of glomerular filtration. *Am J Physiol Renal Physiol* 1980;239:F427–432.
44. Briggs JP, Schnermann J. The effect of metabolic inhibitors on feedback response of nephron filtration rate. *Pflugers Arch* 1981;389[Suppl]:R40.
45. Briggs JP, Steipe B, Schubert G, Schnermann J. Micropuncture studies of the renal effects of atrial natriuretic substance. *Pflugers Arch* 1982;395:271–6.
46. Briggs JP. Effect of loop of Henle flow rate on glomerular capillary pressure. *Ren Physiol* 1984;7:311–320.
47. Briggs JP, Schubert G, Schnermann J. Quantitative characterization of the tubuloglomerular feedback response: effect of growth. *Am J Physiol Renal Physiol* 1984;247:F808–F815.
48. Brown R, Ollerstam A, Johansson B, Skott O, Gebre-Medhin S, Fredholm B, Persson AE. Abolished tubuloglomerular feedback and increased plasma renin in adenosine A1 receptor-deficient mice. *Am J Physiol Regul Integr Comp Physiol* 2001;281:R1362–1367.
49. Brown R, Ollerstam A, Persson AE. Neuronal nitric oxide synthase inhibition sensitizes the tubuloglomerular feedback mechanism after volume expansion. *Kidney Int* 2004;65:1349–1356.
50. Burson JM, Aguilera G, Gross KW, Sigmund CD. Differential expression of angiotensin receptor 1A and 1B in mouse. *Am J Physiol* 1994;267:E260–267.
51. Campean V, Theilig F, Paliege A, Breyer M, Bachmann S. Key enzymes for renal prostaglandin synthesis: site-specific expression in rodent kidney (rat, mouse). *Am J Physiol Renal Physiol* 2003;285:F19–32.
52. Campese VM, Wurgaft A, Safa M, Bianchi S. Dietary salt intake, blood pressure and the kidney in hypertensive patients with non-insulin dependent diabetes mellitus. *J Nephrol* 1998;11:289–295.
53. Cantin M, Gutkowska J, Lacasse J, Ballak M, Ledoux S, Inagami T, Beuzeron J, Genest J. Ultrastructural immunocytochemical localization of renin and angiotensin II in the juxtaglomerular cells of the ischemic kidney in experimental renal hypertension. *Am J Pathol* 1984;115:212–224.
54. Capdevila J, Gil L, Orellana M, Marnett LJ, Mason JI, Yadagiri P, Falck JR. Inhibitors of cytochrome P-450–dependent arachidonic acid metabolism. *Arch Biochem Biophys* 1988;261:257–263.
55. Carmines PK, Navar LG. Disparate effects of Ca channel blockade on afferent and efferent arteriolar responses to ANG II. *Am J Physiol* 1989;256:F1015–120.
56. Casellas DMoore LC. Autoregulation and tubuloglomerular feedback in juxtamedullary glomerular arterioles. *Am J Physiol Renal Physiol* 1990;258:F660–669.
57. Casellas D, Dupont M, Kaskel FJ, Inagami T, Moore LC. Direct visualization of renin-cell distribution in preglomerular vascular trees dissected from rat kidney. *Am J Physiol Renal Physiol* 1993;265:F151–156.
58. Castrop H, Schweda F, Schumacher K, Wolf K, Kurtz A. Role of renocortical cyclooxygenase-2 for renal vascular resistance and macula densa control of renin secretion. *J Am Soc Nephrol* 2001;12:867–874.
59. Castrop H, Huang Y, Hashimoto S, Mizel D, Hansen P, Theilig F, Bachmann S, Deng C, Briggs J, Schnermann J. Impairment of tubuloglomerular feedback regulation of GFR in ecto-5'-nucleotidase/CD73–deficient mice. *J Clin Invest* 2004;114:634–642.
60. Castrop H, Schweda F, Mizel D, Huang Y, Briggs J, Kurtz A, Schnermann J. Permissive role of nitric oxide in macula densa control of renin secretion. *Am J Physiol Renal Physiol* 2004;286:F848–857.
61. Castrop H, Lorenz JN, Hansen PB, Friis U, Mizel D, Oppermann M, Jensen BL, Briggs J, Skott O, Schnermann J. Contribution of the basolateral isoform of the Na-K-2Cl⁻ cotransporter (NKCC1/BSC2) to renin secretion. *Am J Physiol Ren Physiol* 2005; 289:F1185–1192.
62. Celio MR, Inagami T. Angiotensin II immunoreactivity coexists with renin in the juxtaglomerular granular cells of the kidney. *Proc Natl Acad Sci U S A* 1981;78:3897–3900.
63. Chabrashvili T, Tojo A, Onozato ML, Kitiyakara C, Quinn MT, Fujita T, Welch WJ, Wilcox CS. Expression and cellular localization of classic NADPH oxidase subunits in the spontaneously hypertensive rat kidney. *Hypertension* 2002;39:269–274.
64. Chan CM, Unwin RJ, Bardini M, Oglesby IB, Ford AP, Townsend-Nicholson A, Burnstock G. Localization of P2X1 purinoceptors by autoradiography and immunohistochemistry in rat kidneys. *Am J Physiol* 1998;274:F799–804.
65. Chatziantoniou C, Pauti MD, Pinet F, Promeneur D, Dussaule JC, Ardaillou R. Regulation of renin release is impaired after nitric oxide inhibition. *Kidney Int* 1996;49:626–633.
66. Chen L, Kim SM, Oppermann M, Faulhaber-Walter R, Huang YG, Mizel D, Chen M, Sequeira Lopez ML, Weinstein LS, Gomez RA, Briggs JP, Schnermann JB. Regulation of renin in mice with cre recombinase-mediated deletion of G protein Gsα in juxtaglomerular cells. *Am J Physiol Renal Physiol* 2006;292:F27–31.
67. Chen YM, Holstein-Rathlou NH. Differences in dynamic autoregulation of renal blood flow between SHR and WKY rats. *Am J Physiol Renal Physiol* 1993;264:F166–174.
68. Chen YM, Yip KP, Marsh DJ, Holstein-Rathlou NH. Magnitude of TGF-initiated nephron-nephron interactions is increased in SHR. *Am J Physiol Renal Physiol* 1995;269:F198–204.
69. Cheng HF, Wang JL, Zhang MZ, Miyazaki Y, Ichikawa I, McKanna JA, Harris RC. Angiotensin II attenuates renal cortical cyclooxygenase-2 expression. *J Clin Invest* 1999;103:953–961.
70. Cheng HF, Wang JL, Zhang MZ, McKanna JA, Harris RC. Role of p38 in the regulation of renal cortical cyclooxygenase-2 expression by extracellular chloride. *J Clin Invest* 2000;106:681–688.
71. Cheng HF, Wang JL, Zhang MZ, Wang SW, McKanna JA, Harris RC. Genetic deletion of COX-2 prevents increased renin expression in response to ACE inhibition. *Am J Physiol Renal Physiol* 2001;280:F449–456.
72. Cheng HF, Harris RC. Cyclooxygenase-2 expression in cultured cortical thick ascending limb of Henle increases in response to decreased extracellular ionic content by both transcriptional and post-transcriptional mechanisms. Role of p38–mediated pathways. *J Biol Chem* 2002;277:45638–45643.
73. Chiu T, Reid IA. Role of cyclic GMP-inhibitable phosphodiesterase and nitric oxide in the beta adrenoceptor control of renin secretion. *J Pharmacol Exp Ther* 1996;278:793–799.
74. Chon KH, Chen YM, Marmarelis VZ, Marsh DJ, Holstein-Rathlou NH. Detection of interactions between myogenic and TGF mechanisms using nonlinear analysis [published erratum appears in *Am J Physiol Renal Physiol* 1994 Dec;267(6 Pt 3):section F following table of contents]. *Am J Physiol Renal Physiol* 1994;267:F160–173.
75. Chon KH, Chen YM, Holstein-Rathlou NH, Marmarelis VZ. Nonlinear system analysis of renal autoregulation in normotensive and hypertensive rats. *IEEE Trans Biomed Eng* 1998;45:342–353.
76. Chon KH, Raghavan R, Chen YM, Marsh DJ, Yip KP. Interactions of TGF-dependent and myogenic oscillations in tubular pressure. *Am J Physiol Renal Physiol* 2005;288:F298–307.
77. Christensen JA, Meyer DS, Bohle A. The structure of the human juxtaglomerular apparatus. A morphometric, lightmicroscopic study on serial sections. *Virchows Arch A Pathol Anat Histol* 1975;367:83–92.
78. Christensen JA, Bohle A. The juxtaglomerular apparatus in the normal rat kidney. *Virchows Arch A Pathol Anat Histol* 1978;379:143–150.
79. Christensen JA, Bohle A, Mikeler E, Taugner R. Renin-positive granulated Goormaghtigh cells. Immunohistochemical and electron-microscopic studies on biopsies from patients with pseudo-Bartter syndrome. *Cell Tissue Res* 1989;255:149–153.
80. Churchill PC, Churchill MC, McDonald FD. Effects of saline and mannitol on renin and distal tubule Na in rats. *Circ Res* 1979;45:786–792.
81. Churchill PC, Churchill MC. A1 and A2 adenosine receptor activation inhibits and stimulates renin secretion of rat renal cortical slices. *J Pharmacol Exp Ther* 1985;232:589–594.

82. Cosio FG, Sedmak DD, Mahan JD, Nahman NS, Jr. Localization of decay accelerating factor in normal and diseased kidneys. *Kidney Int* 1989;36:100–107.
83. Cupples WA, Loutzenhiser RD. Dynamic autoregulation in the in vitro perfused hydronephrotic rat kidney. *Am J Physiol Renal Physiol* 1998;275:F126–130.
84. Dal Canton A, Stanziale R, Corradi A, Andreucci VE, Migone L. Effects of acute ureteral obstruction on glomerular hemodynamics in rat kidney. *Kidney Int* 1977;12:403–411.
85. Dal Canton A, Corradi A, Stanziale R, Maruccio G, Migone L. Effects of 24-hour ureteral obstruction on glomerular hemodynamics in rat kidney. *Kidney Int* 1979;15:457–462.
86. Daniels FH, Arendshorst WJ. Tubuloglomerular feedback kinetics in spontaneously hypertensive and Wistar-Kyoto rats. *Am J Physiol Renal Physiol* 1990;259:F529–534.
87. Daniels FH, Arendshorst WJ, Roberds RG. Tubuloglomerular feedback and autoregulation in spontaneously hypertensive rats. *Am J Physiol Renal Physiol* 1990;258:F1479–1489.
88. Davis JM, Haberle DA, Kawata T. The control of glomerular filtration rate and renal blood flow in chronically volume-expanded rats. *J Physiol (Lond)* 1988;402:473–495.
89. Davis JM, Takabatake T, Kawata T, Haberle DA. Resetting of tubuloglomerular feedback in acute volume expansion in rats. *Pflugers Arch* 1988;411:322–327.
90. de Rouffignac C, Bonvalet JP. Use of sodium ferrocyanide as glomerular indicator to study the functional heterogeneity of nephrons. *Yale J Biol Med* 1972;45:243–253.
91. Della Bruna R, Pinet F, Corvol P, Kurtz A. Opposite regulation of renin gene expression by cyclic AMP and calcium in isolated mouse juxtaglomerular cells. *Kidney Int* 1995;47:1266–1273.
92. Dev B, Drescher C, Schnermann J. Resetting of tubulo-glomerular feedback sensitivity by dietary salt intake. *Pflugers Arch* 1974;346:263–277.
93. DiBona GF. Effect of mannitol diuresis and ureteral occlusion on distal tubular reabsorption. *Am J Physiol* 1971;221:511–514.
94. DiBona GF, Sawin LL. Effect of endogenous angiotensin II on the frequency response of the renal vasculature. *Am J Physiol Renal Physiol* 2004;287:F1171–1178.
95. Dorup J, Morsing P, Rasch R. Tubule-tubule and tubule-arteriole contacts in rat kidney distal nephrons. A morphologic study based on computer-assisted three-dimensional reconstructions. *Lab Invest* 1992;67:761–769.
96. Edwards RM. Segmental effects of norepinephrine and angiotensin II on isolated renal microvessels. *Am J Physiol* 1983;244:F526–534.
97. Farman N, Fay M, Cluzeaud F. Cell-specific expression of three members of the FXYD family along the renal tubule. *Ann N Y Acad Sci* 2003;986:428–436.
98. Feldberg R, Colding-Jorgensen M, Holstein-Rathlou NH. Analysis of interaction between TGF and the myogenic response in renal blood flow autoregulation. *Am J Physiol Renal Physiol* 1995;269:F581–593.
99. Fleming JT, Parekh N, Steinhausen M. Calcium antagonists preferentially dilate preglomerular vessels of hydronephrotic kidney. *Am J Physiol* 1987;253:F1157–1163.
100. Flower RJ. Drugs which inhibit prostaglandin biosynthesis. *Pharmacol Rev* 1974;26:33–67.
101. Folkow B. Physiological aspects of primary hypertension. *Physiol Rev* 1982;62:347–504.
102. Fowler BC, Chang YS, Laamarti A, Higdon M, Lapointe JY, Bell PD. Evidence for apical sodium proton exchange in macula densa cells. *Kidney Int* 1995;47:746–751.
103. Francisco LL, Osborn JL, DiBona GF. Prostaglandins in renin release during sodium deprivation. *Am J Physiol Renal Physiol* 1982;243:F537–F542.
104. Franco M, Bell PD, Navar LG. Evaluation of prostaglandins as mediators of tubuloglomerular feedback. *Am J Physiol Renal Physiol* 1988;254:F642–649.
105. Franco M, Bell PD, Navar LG. Effect of adenosine A1 analogue on tubuloglomerular feedback mechanism. *Am J Physiol Renal Physiol* 1989;257:F231–236.
106. Frederiksen O, Leyssac PP, Skinner SL. Sensitive osmometer function of juxtaglomerular cells in vitro. *J Physiol* 1975;252:669–679.
107. Friis UG, Jensen BL, Aas JK, Skott O. Direct demonstration of exocytosis and endocytosis in single mouse juxtaglomerular cells. *Circ Res* 1999;84:929–936.
108. Friis UG, Jensen BL, Sethi S, Andreasen D, Hansen PB, Skott O. Control of renin secretion from rat juxtaglomerular cells by cAMP-specific phosphodiesterases. *Circ Res* 2002;90:996–1003.
109. Friis UG, Jorgensen F, Andreasen D, Jensen BL, Skott O. Molecular and functional identification of cyclic AMP-sensitive BKCa potassium channels (ZERO variant) and L-type voltage-dependent calcium channels in single rat juxtaglomerular cells. *Circ Res* 2003;93:213–220.
110. Friis UG, Jorgensen F, Andreasen D, Jensen BL, Skott O. Membrane potential and cation channels in rat juxtaglomerular cells. *Acta Physiol Scand* 2004;181:391–396.
111. Fujino T, Nakagawa N, Yuhki K, Hara A, Yamada T, Takayama K, Kuriyama S, Hosoki Y, Takahata O, Taniguchi T, Fukuzawa J, Hasebe N, Kikuchi K, Narumiya S, Ushikubi F. Decreased susceptibility to renovascular hypertension in mice lacking the prostaglandin I2 receptor IP. *J Clin Invest* 2004;114:805–82.
112. Fuson AL, Komlosi P, Unlap TM, Bell PD, Peti-Peterdi J. Immunolocalization of a microsomal prostaglandin E synthase in rabbit kidney. *Am J Physiol Renal Physiol* 2003;285:F558–64.
113. Gambaryan S, Hausler C, Markert T, Pohler D, Jarchau T, Walter U, Haase W, Kurtz A, Lohmann SM. Expression of type II cGMP-dependent protein kinase in rat kidney is regulated by dehydration and correlated with renin gene expression. *J Clin Invest* 1996;98:662–670.
114. Gambaryan S, Wagner C, Smolenski A, Walter U, Poller W, Haase W, Kurtz A, Lohmann SM. Endogenous or overexpressed cGMP-dependent protein kinases inhibit cAMP-dependent renin release from rat isolated perfused kidney, microdissected glomeruli, and isolated juxtaglomerular cells. *Proc Natl Acad Sci U S A* 1998;95:9003–9008.
115. Gasc JM, Shanmugam S, Sibony M, Corvol P. Tissue-specific expression of type 1 angiotensin II receptor subtypes: an in situ hybridization study. *Hypertension* 1994;24:531–537.
116. Gerber JG, Branch RA, Nies AS, Hollifield JW, Gerkens JF. Influence of hypertonic saline on canine renal blood flow and renin release. *Am J Physiol* 1979;237:F441–446.
117. Gerkens JF, Heidemann HT, Jackson EK, Branch RA. Aminophylline inhibits renal vasoconstriction produced by intrarenal hypertonic saline. *J Pharmacol Exp Ther* 1983;225:611–615.
118. Gertz KH, Mangos JA, Braun G, Pagel HD. Pressure in the glomerular capillaries of the rat kidney and its relation to arterial blood pressure. *Pflugers Arch Gesamte Physiol Menschen Tiere* 1966;288:369–374.
119. Gillies A, Morgan T. Renin content of individual juxtaglomerular apparatuses and the effect of diet, changes in nephron flow rate and in vitro acidification on the renin content. *Pflugers Arch* 1978;375:105–110.
120. Gilmore JP, Cornish KG, Rogers SD, Joyner WL. Direct evidence for myogenic autoregulation of the renal microcirculation in the hamster. *Circ Res* 1980;47:226–230.
121. Gimenez I, Isenring P, Forbush B. Spatially distributed alternative splice variants of the renal Na-K-Cl cotransporter exhibit dramatically different affinities for the transported ions. *J Biol Chem* 2002;277:8767–8770.
122. Golgi C. Annotazioni intorno all'istologia dei reni dell'uomo e di altri mammiferi e sull'istogenesi dei canalicoli oriniferi. *Atti della Reale Accademia dei Lincei* 1889;5:334–342.
123. Gomez RA, Chevalier RL, Everett AD, Elwood JP, Peach MJ, Lynch KR, Carey RM. Recruitment of renin gene-expressing cells in adult rat kidneys. *Am J Physiol* 1990;259:F660–665.
124. Gonzalez E, Salomonsson M, Muller-Suur C, Persson AE. Measurements of macula densa cell volume changes in isolated and perfused rabbit cortical thick ascending limb, I: isosmotic and anisosmotic cell volume changes. *Acta Physiol Scand* 1988;133:149–157.
125. Gonzalez E, Salomonsson M, Muller-Suur C, Persson AE. Measurements of macula densa cell volume changes in isolated and perfused rabbit cortical thick ascending limb, II: apical and basolateral cell osmotic water permeabilities. *Acta Physiol Scand* 1988;133:159–166.
126. Goormaghtigh N. Une glande endocrine dans la paroi des arterioles renales. *Bruxelles Med* 1939;19:1541–1549.
127. Greenberg SG, Lorenz JN, He XR, Schnermann JB, Briggs JP. Effect of prostaglandin synthesis inhibition on macula densa-stimulated renin secretion. *Am J Physiol Renal Physiol* 1993;265:F578–583.
128. Greenberg SG, He XR, Schnermann JB, Briggs JP. Effect of nitric oxide on renin secretion. I. Studies in isolated juxtaglomerular granular cells. *Am J Physiol* 1995;268:F948–952.
129. Greger R. Ion transport mechanism in thick ascending limb of Henle's loop of mammalian nephron. *Physiol Rev* 1985;65:760–797.
130. Grunberger C, Obermayer B, Klar J, Kurtz A, Schweda F. The calcium paradoxon of renin release: calcium suppresses renin exocytosis by inhibition of calcium-dependent adenylate cyclases AC5 and AC6. *Circ Res* 2006;99:1197–1206.
131. Guan Y, Chang M, Cho W, Zhang Y, Redha R, Davis L, Chang S, DuBois RN, Hao CM, Breyer M. Cloning, expression, and regulation of rabbit cyclooxygenase-2 in renal medullary interstitial cells. *Am J Physiol Renal Physiol* 1997;273:F18–26.
132. Guan Z, Buckman SY, Miller BW, Springer LD, Morrison AR. Interleukin-1beta-induced cyclooxygenase-2 expression requires activation of both c-Jun NH2-terminal kinase and p38 MAPK signal pathways in rat renal mesangial cells. *J Biol Chem* 1998;273:28670–28676.
133. Guan Z, Willgoss DA, Matthias A, Manley SW, Crozier S, Gobe G, Endre ZH. Facilitation of renal autoregulation by angiotensin II is mediated through modulation of nitric oxide. *Acta Physiol Scand* 2003;179:189–201.
134. Gustafsson F, Holstein-Rathlou N. Conducted vasomotor responses in arterioles: characteristics, mechanisms and physiological significance. *Acta Physiol Scand* 1999;167:11–21.
135. Gutierrez AM, Lou X, Erik A, Persson G, Ring A. Ca2+ response of rat mesangial cells to ATP analogues. *Eur J Pharmacol* 1999;369:107–112.
136. Gutsche HU, Muller-Suur R, Hegel U, Hierholzer K. Electrical conductivity of tubular fluid of the rat nephron: micropuncture study of the diluting segment in situ. *Pflugers Arch* 1980;383:113–121.
137. Guyton AC, Langston JB, Navar G. Theory for renal autoregulation by feedback at the juxtaglomerular apparatus. *Circ Res* 1964;15[Suppl]:187–197.
138. Haberle DA, Davis JM. Interrelationship between proximal tubular hydrodynamics and tubuloglomerular feedback in the rat kidney. *Kidney Int* 1982;12[Suppl]:S193–197.
139. Haberle DA, Davis JM. Resetting of tubuloglomerular feedback: evidence for a humoral factor in tubular fluid. *Am J Physiol Renal Physiol* 1984;246:F495–500.
140. Haberle DA, Kawata T, Davis JM. The site of action of nitrendipine in the rat kidney. *J Cardiovasc Pharmacol* 1987;9[Suppl 1]:S17–23.
141. Haberle DA. Hemodynamic interactions between intrinsic blood flow control mechanisms in the rat kidney. *Ren Physiol Biochem* 1988;11:289–315.
142. Haddad M, Roder S, Olsen HS, Wagner GF. Immunocytochemical localization of stanniocalcin cells in the rat kidney. *Endocrinology* 1996;137:2113–2117.
143. Haefliger JA, Demotz S, Braissant O, Suter E, Waeber B, Nicod P, Meda P. Connexins 40 and 43 are differentially regulated within the kidneys of rats with renovascular hypertension. *Kidney Int* 2001;60:190–201.
144. Hahne B, Persson AEG. Prevention of interstitial pressure change at unilateral nephrectomy by prostaglandin synthesis inhibition. *Kidney Int* 1984;25:42–46.
145. Hall JE, Granger JP, Hester RL. Interactions between adenosine and angiotensin II in controlling glomerular filtration. *Amer J Physiol Renal Physiol* 1985;248:F340–F346.
146. Haller H, Luft FC. Angiotensin II acts intracellularly in vascular smooth muscle cells. *Basic Res Cardiol* 1998;93[Suppl 2]:30–36.
147. Hansen PB, Castrop H, Briggs J, Schnermann J. Adenosine induces vasoconstriction through Gi-dependent activation of phospholipase c in isolated perfused afferent arterioles of mice. *J Am Soc Nephrol* 2003;14:2457–2465.
148. Hansen PB, Schnermann J. Vasoconstrictor and vasodilator effects of adenosine in the kidney. *Am J Physiol Renal Physiol* 2003;285:F590–599.
149. Hansen PB, Hashimoto S, Oppermann M, Huang Y, Briggs JP, Schnermann J. Vasoconstrictor and vasodilator effects of adenosine in the mouse kidney due to preferential activation of A1 or A2 adenosine receptors. *J Pharmacol Exp Ther* 2005;315:1150–1157.
150. Harder DR, Gilbert R, Lombard JH. Vascular muscle cell depolarization and activation in renal arteries on elevation of transmural pressure. *Am J Physiol* 1987;253:F778–781.
151. Harder DR, Lange AR, Gebremedhin D, Birks EK, Roman RJ. Cytochrome P450 metabolites of arachidonic acid as intracellular signaling molecules in vascular tissue. *J Vasc Res* 1997;34:237–243.

152. Harris RC, McKanna JA, Akai Y, Jacobson HR, Dubois RN, Breyer MD. Cyclooxygenase-2 is associated with the macula densa of rat kidney and increases with salt restriction. *J Clin Invest* 1994;94:2504–2510.

153. Harris RCBreyer MD. Physiological regulation of cyclooxygenase-2 in the kidney. *Am J Physiol Renal Physiol* 2001;281:F1–11.

154. Harrison-Bernard LM, Navar LG, Ho MM, Vinson GP, el-Dahr SS. Immunohistochemical localization of ANG II AT1 receptor in adult rat kidney using a monoclonal antibody. *Am J Physiol* 1997;273:F170–177.

155. Harrison SA, Reifsnyder DH, Gallis B, Cadd GG, Beavo JA. Isolation and characterization of bovine cardiac muscle cGMP-inhibited phosphodiesterase: a receptor for new cardiotonic drugs. *Mol Pharmacol* 1986;29:506–514.

156. Hartner A, Goppelt-Struebe M, Hilgers KF. Coordinate expression of cyclooxygenase-2 and renin in the rat kidney in renovascular hypertension. *Hypertension* 1998;31:201–205.

157. Hartner A, Cordasic N, Goppelt-Struebe M, Veelken R, Hilgers KF. Role of macula densa cyclooxygenase-2 in renovascular hypertension. *Am J Physiol Renal Physiol* 2003;284:F498–502.

158. Hashimoto S, Adams JW, Bernstein KE, Schnermann J. Micropuncture determination of nephron function in mice without tissue angiotensin converting enzyme. *Am J Physiol Renal Physiol* 2005;288:F445–452.

159. Hashimoto S, Huang Y, Mizel D, Briggs J, Schnermann J. Compensation of proximal tubule malabsorption in AQP1-deficient mice without TGF-mediated reduction of GFR. *Acta Physiol Scand* 2004;181:455–462.

160. Hashimoto S, Huang YG, Castrop H, Hansen PB, Mizel D, Briggs J, Schnermann J. Effect of carbonic anhydrase inhibition on GFR and renal hemodynamics in adenosine-1 receptor-deficient mice. *Pflugers Arch* 2004;448:621–628.

161. He J, Marsh DJ. Effect of captopril on fluctuations of blood pressure and renal blood flow in rats. *Am J Physiol Renal Physiol* 1993;264:F37–44.

162. He XR, Greenberg SG, Briggs JP, Schnermann J. Effects of furosemide and verapamil on the NaCl dependency of macula densa-mediated renin secretion. *Hypertension* 1995;26:137–142.

163. He XR, Greenberg SG, Briggs JP, Schnermann JB. Effect of nitric oxide on renin secretion. II. Studies in the perfused juxtaglomerular apparatus. *Am J Physiol Renal Physiol* 1995;268:F953–959.

164. Henrich WL, McAllister EA, Smith PB, Campbell WB. Guanosine 3′,5′-cyclic monophosphate as a mediator of inhibition of renin release. *Am J Physiol* 1988;255:F474–478.

165. Hermansson K, Kallskog O, Wolgast M. Effect of renal nerve stimulation on the activity of the tubuloglomerular feedback mechanism. *Acta Physiol Scand* 1984;120:381–385.

166. Heyeraas Tonder KJ, Aukland K. Interlobular arterial pressure in the rat kidney. *Renal Physiol.* 1979/80;2:214–221.

167. Hocherl K, Kammerl MC, Schumacher K, Endemann D, Grobecker HF, Kurtz A. Role of prostanoids in regulation of the renin-angiotensin-aldosterone system by salt intake. *Am J Physiol Renal Physiol* 2002;283:F294–301.

168. Holstein-Rathlou NH, Leyssac PP. TGF-mediated oscillations in the proximal intratubular pressure: differences between spontaneously hypertensive rats and Wistar-Kyoto rats. *Acta Physiol Scand* 1986;126:333–339.

169. Holstein-Rathlou NH. Synchronization of proximal intratubular pressure oscillations: evidence for interaction between nephrons. *Pflugers Arch* 1987;408:438–443.

170. Holstein-Rathlou NH, Marsh DJ. Oscillations of tubular pressure, flow, and distal chloride concentration in rats. *Am J Physiol Renal Physiol* 1989;256:F1007–1014.

171. Holstein-Rathlou NH, Marsh DJ. A dynamic model of the tubuloglomerular feedback mechanism. *Am J Physiol Renal Physiol* 1990;258:F1448–1459.

172. Holstein-Rathlou NH. A closed-loop analysis of the tubuloglomerular feedback mechanism. *Am J Physiol Renal Physiol* 1991;261:F880–889.

173. Holstein-Rathlou NH, Wagner AJ, Marsh DJ. Tubuloglomerular feedback dynamics and renal blood flow autoregulation in rats. *Am J Physiol Renal Physiol* 1991;260:F53–68.

174. Holstein-Rathlou NH, Marsh DJ. Renal blood flow regulation and arterial pressure fluctuations: a case study in nonlinear dynamics. *Physiol Rev* 1994;74:637–681.

175. Holz FG, Steinhausen M. Renovascular effects of adenosine receptor agonists. *Renal Physiol.* 1987;10:272–282.

176. Hoyer JR, Sisson SP, Vernier RL. Tamm-Horsfall glycoprotein: ultrastructural immunoperoxidase localization in rat kidney. *Lab Invest* 1979;41:168–173.

177. Huang CL, Cogan MG. Atrial natriuretic factor inhibits maximal tubuloglomerular feedback response. *Am J Physiol Renal Physiol* 1987;252:F825–828.

178. Huang DY, Vallon V, Zimmermann H, Koszalka P, Schrader J, Osswald H. Ecto-5′-nucleotidase (cd73)-dependent and -independent generation of adenosine participates in the mediation of tubuloglomerular feedback in vivo. *Am J Physiol Renal Physiol* 2006;291:F282–288.

179. Huang WC, Bell PD, Harvey D, Mitchell KD, Navar LG. Angiotensin influences on tubuloglomerular feedback mechanism in hypertensive rats. *Kidney Int* 1988;34:631–637.

180. Hurst AM, Lapointe JY, Laamarti A, Bell PD. Basic properties and potential regulators of the apical K+ channel in macula densa cells. *J Gen Physiol* 1994;103:1055–1070.

181. Ichihara A, Imig JD, Inscho EW, Navar LG. Cyclooxygenase-2 participates in tubular flow-dependent afferent arteriolar tone: interaction with neuronal NOS. *Am J Physiol Renal Physiol* 1998;275:F605–612.

182. Ichikawa I. Direct analysis of the effector mechanism of the tubuloglomerular feedback system. *Am J Physiol Renal Physiol* 1982;243:F447–455.

183. Iijima K, Moore LC, Goligorsky MS. Syncytial organization of cultured rat mesangial cells. *Am J Physiol* 1991;260:F848–855.

184. Ikenaga H, Fallet RW, Carmines PK. Contribution of tubuloglomerular feedback to renal arteriolar angiotensin II responsiveness. *Kidney Int* 1996;49:34–39.

185. Inagami T, Mizuno K, Higashimori K. Juxtaglomerular cells as a source of intrarenal angiotensin II production. *Kidney Int* 1991;32[Suppl]:S20–22.

186. Inscho EW, Cook AK, Navar LG. Pressure-mediated vasoconstriction of juxtamedullary afferent arterioles involves P2-purinoceptor activation. *Am J Physiol* 1996;271:F1077–1085.

187. Inscho EW. P2 receptors in regulation of renal microvascular function. *Am J Physiol Renal Physiol* 2001;280:F927–944.

188. Inscho EW, Cook AK, Imig JD, Vial C, Evans RJ. Physiological role for P2X1 receptors in renal microvascular autoregulatory behavior. *J Clin Invest* 2003;112:1895–1905.

189. Ito O, Alonso-Galicia M, Hopp KA, Roman RJ. Localization of cytochrome P-450 4A isoforms along the rat nephron. *Am J Physiol* 1998;274:F395–404.

190. Ito S, Carretero OA. An in vitro approach to the study of macula densa-mediated glomerular hemodynamics. *Kidney Int* 1990;38:1206–1210.

191. Ito S, Ren YL. Evidence for the role of nitric oxide in macula densa control of glomerular hemodynamics. *J Clin Invest* 1993;92:1093–1098.

192. Itoh S, Carretero OA. Role of the macula densa in renin release. *Hypertension* 1985;7:I49–154.

193. Jamison RL, Lacy FB. Effect of saline infusion on superficial and juxtamedullary nephrons in the rat. *Am J Physiol* 1971;221:690–697.

194. Janssen BJ, Eerdmans PH, Smits JF. Mechanisms of renal vasoconstriction following furosemide in conscious rats. *Naunyn Schmiedebergs Arch Pharmacol* 1994;349:528–537.

195. Jensen BL, Skott O. Osmotically sensitive renin release from permeabilized juxtaglomerular cells. *Am J Physiol* 1993;265:F87–95.

196. Jensen BL, Schmid C, Kurtz A. Prostaglandins stimulate renin secretion and renin mRNA in mouse renal juxtaglomerular cells. *Am J Physiol Renal Physiol* 1996;271:F659–F669.

197. Jensen BL, Kurtz A. Differential regulation of renal cyclooxygenase mRNA by dietary salt intake. *Kidney Int* 1997;52:1242–1249.

198. Jensen BL, Mann B, Skott O, Kurtz A. Differential regulation of renal prostaglandin receptor mRNAs by dietary salt intake in the rat. *Kidney Int* 1999;56:528–537.

199. Jensen PK, Kristensen KS, Rasch R, Persson AEG. Decreased sensitivity of the tubuloglomerular feedback mechanism in experimental diabetic rats. In: Persson AEG, Boberg U (eds.). *The Juxtaglomerular Apparatus.* Amsterdam: Elsevier, 1988:333–338.

200. Just A, Ehmke H, Toktomambetova L, Kirchheim HR. Dynamic characteristics and underlying mechanisms of renal blood flow autoregulation in the conscious dog. *Am J Physiol Renal Physiol* 2001;280:F1062–1071.

201. Just A, Ehmke H, Wittmann U, Kirchheim HR. Role of angiotensin II in dynamic renal blood flow autoregulation of the conscious dog. *J Physiol* 2002;538:167–177.

202. Just A, Arendshorst WJ. Dynamics and contribution of mechanisms mediating renal blood flow autoregulation. *Am J Physiol Regul Integr Comp Physiol* 2003;285:R619–631.

203. Just A, Arendshorst WJ. Nitric oxide blunts myogenic autoregulation in rat renal but not skeletal muscle circulation via tubuloglomerular feedback. *J Physiol* 2005;569:959–974.

204. Kaissling B, Peter S, Kriz W. The transition of the thick ascending limb of Henle's loop into the distal convoluted tubule in the nephron of the rat kidney. *Cell Tissue Res* 1977;182:111–118.

205. Kaissling B, Kriz W. Structural analysis of the rabbit kidney. *Adv Anat Embryol Cell Biol* 1979;56:1–123.

206. Kakinuma Y, Fogo A, Inagami T, Ichikawa I. Intrarenal localization of angiotensin II type 1 receptor mRNA in the rat. *Kidney Int* 1993;43:1229–1235.

207. Kallskog O, Marsh DJ. TGF-initiated vascular interactions between adjacent nephrons in the rat kidney. *Am J Physiol Renal Physiol* 1990;259:F60–64.

208. Kammerl MC, Nusing RM, Richthammer W, Kramer BK, Kurtz A. Inhibition of COX-2 counteracts the effects of diuretics in rats. *Kidney Int* 2001;60:1684–1691.

209. Kammerl MC, Nusing RM, Seyberth HW, Riegger GA, Kurtz A, Kramer BK. Inhibition of cyclooxygenase-2 attenuates urinary prostanoid excretion without affecting renal renin expression. *Pflugers Arch* 2001;442:842–847.

210. Kaplan MR, Plotkin MD, Brown D, Hebert SC, Delpire E. Expression of the mouse Na-K-2Cl cotransporter, mBSC2, in the terminal inner medullary collecting duct, the glomerular and extraglomerular mesangium, and the glomerular afferent arteriole. *J Clin Invest* 1996;98:723–730.

211. Karlsen FM, Andersen CB, Leyssac PP, Holstein-Rathlou NH. Dynamic autoregulation and renal injury in Dahl rats. *Hypertension* 1997;30:975–983.

212. Karlsen FM, Leyssac PP, Holstein-Rathlou NH. Tubuloglomerular feedback in Dahl rats. *Am J Physiol Renal Physiol* 1998;274:R1561–1569.

213. Kashgarian M, Biemesderfer D, Caplan M, Forbush B, 3rd. Monoclonal antibody to Na,K-ATPase: immunocytochemical localization along nephron segments. *Kidney Int* 1985;28:899–913.

214. Kaufman JS, Hamburger RJ, Flamenbaum W. Tubuloglomerular feedback response after hypotensive hemorrhage. *Ren Physiol* 1982;5:173–181.

215. Kawabata M, Haneda M, Wang T, Imai M, Takabatake T. Effects of a nucleoside transporter inhibitor, dilazep, on renal microcirculation in rats. *Hypertens Res* 2002;25:615–621.

216. Keeton TK, Campbell WB. The pharmacologic alteration of renin release. *Pharmacol Rev* 1980;32:81–227.

217. Kelley GG, Aassar OS, Forrest JN, Jr. Endogenous adenosine is an autacoid feedback inhibitor of chloride transport in the shark rectal gland. *J Clin Invest* 1991;88:1933–1939.

218. Kessler SP, Hashimoto S, Senanayake PS, Gaughan C, Sen GC, Schnermann J. Nephron function in transgenic mice with selective vascular or tubular expression of angiotensin-converting enzyme. *J Am Soc Nephrol* 2005;16:3535–3542.

219. Kihara M, Umemura S, Kadota T, Yabana M, Tamura K, Nyuui N, Ogawa N, Murakami K, Fukamizu A, Ishii M. The neuronal isoform of constitutive nitric oxide synthase is up- regulated in the macula densa of angiotensinogen gene-knockout mice. *Lab Invest* 1997;76:285–294.

220. Kihara M, Umemura S, Sugaya T, Toya Y, Yabana M, Kobayashi S, Tamura K, Kadota T, Kishida R, Murakami K, Fukamizu A, Ishii M. Expression of neuronal type nitric oxide synthase and renin in the juxtaglomerular apparatus of angiotensin type-1a receptor gene-knockout mice. *Kidney Int* 1998;53:1585–1593.

221. Kim SM, Chen L, Mizel D, Huang YG, Briggs JP, Schnermann JB. Low plasma renin and reduced renin secretory responses to acute stimuli in conscious COX-2-deficient mice. *Am J Physiol Renal Physiol* 2006;292:415–422.

222. Kim SM, Mizel D, Huang YG, Briggs JP, Schnermann J. Adenosine as a mediator of macula densa-dependent inhibition of renin secretion. *Am J Physiol Renal Physiol* 2006;290:F1016–1023.

223. Kinne R, Koenig B, Hannafin J, Kinne-Saffran E, Scott DM, Zierold K. The use of membrane vesicles to study the NaCl/KCl cotransporter involved in active transepithelial chloride transport. *Pflugers Arch* 1985;405[Suppl 1]:S101–105.
224. Kinne R, Kinne-Saffran E, Schutz H, Scholermann B. Ammonium transport of medullary thick ascending limb of rabbit kidney: involvement of the Na+,K+,Cl-cotransporter. *J Membr Biol* 1986;94:279–284.
225. Kirchner KA, Kotchen TA, Galla JH, Luke RG. Importance of chloride for acute inhibition of renin by sodium chloride. *Am J Physiol* 1978;235:F444–450.
226. Kitiyakara C, Chabrashvili T, Chen Y, Blau J, Karber A, Aslam S, Welch WJ, Wilcox CS. Salt intake, oxidative stress, and renal expression of NADPH oxidase and superoxide dismutase. *J Am Soc Nephrol* 2003;14:2775–2782.
227. Komhoff M, Seyberth HW, Nusing RM, Breyer MD. Cyclooxygenase-2 expression is associated with the macula densa in kidneys from patients with Bartter like syndrome. *J Am Soc Nephrol* 1999;10:437A.
228. Komhoff M, Jeck ND, Seyberth HW, Grone HJ, Nusing RM, Breyer MD. Cyclooxygenase-2 expression is associated with the renal macula densa of patients with Bartter-like syndrome. *Kidney Int* 2000;58:2420–2424.
229. Komlosi P, Peti-Peterdi J, Fuson AL, Fintha A, Rosivall L, Bell PD. Macula densa basolateral ATP release is regulated by luminal [NaCl] and dietary salt intake. *Am J Physiol Renal Physiol* 2004;286:F1054–1058.
230. Komlosi P, Frische S, Fuson AL, Fintha A, Zsembery A, Peti-Peterdi J, Bell PD. Characterization of basolateral chloride/bicarbonate exchange in macula densa cells. *Am J Physiol Renal Physiol* 2005;288:F380–386.
231. Komlosi P, Fintha A, Bell PD. Unraveling the relationship between macula densa cell volume and luminal solute concentration/osmolality. *Kidney Int* 2006;70:865–871.
232. Kotchen TA, Galla JH, Luke RG. Contribution of chloride to the inhibition of plasma renin by sodium chloride in the rat. *Kidney Int* 1978;13:201–207.
233. Kotchen TA, Luke RG, Ott CE, Galla JH, Whitescarver S. Effect of chloride on renin and blood pressure responses to sodium chloride. *Ann Intern Med* 1983;98:817–822.
234. Kovacs G, Peti-Peterdi J, Rosivall L, Bell PD. Angiotensin II directly stimulates macula densa Na-2Cl-K cotransport via apical AT(1) receptors. *Am J Physiol Renal Physiol* 2002;282: F301–306.
235. Kovacs G, Komlosi P, Fuson A, Peti-Peterdi J, Rosivall L, Bell PD. Neuronal nitric oxide synthase: its role and regulation in macula densa cells. *J Am Soc Nephrol* 2003;14:2475–2483.
236. Kremer SG, Breuer WV, Skorecki KL. Vasoconstrictor hormones depolarize renal glomerular mesangial cells by activating chloride channels. *J Cell Physiol* 1989;138:97–105.
237. Kulaksiz H, Theilig F, Bachmann S, Gehrke SG, Rost D, Janetzko A, Cetin Y, Stremmel W. The iron-regulatory peptide hormone hepcidin: expression and cellular localization in the mammalian kidney. *J Endocrinol* 2005;184:361–370.
238. Kurokawa K, Okuda T. Chloride conductance of mesangial cells: insight into the transcellular signaling of tubuloglomerular feedback. *Contrib Nephrol* 1991;95:76–81.
239. Kurtz A, Della Bruna R, Pfeilschifter J, Taugner R, Bauer C. Atrial natriuretic peptide inhibits renin release from juxtaglomerular cells by a cGMP-mediated process. *Proc Natl Acad Sci U S A* 1986;83:4769–4773.
240. Kurtz A, Penner R. Angiotensin II induces oscillations of intracellular calcium and blocks anomalous inward rectifying potassium current in mouse renal juxtaglomerular cells. *Proc Natl Acad Sci U S A* 1989;86:3423–3427.
241. Kurtz A, Skott O, Chegini S, Penner R. Lack of direct evidence for a functional role of voltage-operated calcium channels in juxtaglomerular cells. *Pflugers Arch* 1990;416:281–287.
242. Kurtz A, Gotz KH, Hamann M, Kieninger M, Wagner C. Stimulation of renin secretion by NO donors is related to the cAMP pathway. *Am J Physiol Renal Physiol* 1998;274: F709–717.
243. Kurtz A, Gotz KH, Hamann M, Wagner C. Stimulation of renin secretion by nitric oxide is mediated by phosphodiesterase 3. *Proc Natl Acad Sci U S A* 1998;95:4743–4747.
244. Kurtz A, Schweda F. Osmolarity-induced renin secretion from kidneys: evidence for readily releasable renin pools. *Am J Physiol Renal Physiol* 2006;290:F797–805.
245. Kwon TH, Nielsen J, Kim YH, Knepper MA, Frokiaer J, Nielsen S. Regulation of sodium transporters in the thick ascending limb of rat kidney: response to angiotensin II. *Am J Physiol Renal Physiol* 2003;285:F152–165.
246. Laamarti MA, Lapointe JY. Determination of NH4+/NH3 fluxes across apical membrane of macula densa cells: a quantitative analysis. *Am J Physiol Renal Physiol* 1997;273: F817–824.
247. Lai EY, Martinka P, Fahling M, Mrowka R, Steege A, Gericke A, Sendeski M, Persson PB, Persson AE, Patzak A. Adenosine restores angiotensin II-induced contractions by receptor-independent enhancement of calcium sensitivity in renal arterioles. *Circ Res* 2006;99:1117–1124.
248. Lai EY, Patzak A, Steege A, Mrowka R, Brown R, Spielmann N, Persson PB, Fredholm BB, Persson AE. Contribution of adenosine receptors in the control of arteriolar tone and adenosine-angiotensin II interaction. *Kidney Int* 2006;70:690–698.
249. Lapointe JY, Bell PD, Cardinal J. Direct evidence for apical Na+:2Cl-:K+ cotransport in macula densa cells. *Am J Physiol Renal Physiol* 1990;258:F1466–1469.
250. Lapointe JY, Bell PD, Hurst AM, Cardinal J. Basolateral ionic permeabilities of macula densa cells. *Am J Physiol Renal Physiol* 1991;260:F856–860.
251. Lapointe JY, Laamarti A, Hurst AM, Fowler BC, Bell PD. Activation of Na:2Cl:K cotransport by luminal chloride in macula densa cells. *Kidney Int* 1995;47:752–757.
252. Lapointe JY, Bell PD, Sabirov RZ, Okada Y. Calcium-activated nonselective cationic channel in macula densa cells. *Am J Physiol Renal Physiol* 2003;285:F275–280.
253. Larsson C, Weber P, Anggard E. Arachidonic acid increases and indomethacin decreases plasma renin activity in the rabbit. *Eur. J. Pharmacol.* 1974;28:391–394.
254. Latta HMaunsbach AB. The juxtaglomerular apparatus as studied electron microscopically. *J Ultrastruct Res* 1962;6:547–561.
255. Layton AT, Moore LC, Layton HE. Multistability in tubuloglomerular feedback and spectral complexity in spontaneously hypertensive rats. *Am J Physiol Renal Physiol* 2006;291:F79–97.
256. Layton HE, Pitman EB, Moore LC. Bifurcation analysis of TGF-mediated oscillations in SNGFR. *Am J Physiol Renal Physiol* 1991;261:F904–919.
257. Le Hir M, Kaissling B. Distribution and regulation of renal ecto-5'-nucleotidase: implications for physiological functions of adenosine. *Am J Physiol* 1993;264:F377–387.
258. Levine DZ, Burns KD, Jaffey J, Iacovitti M. Short-term modulation of distal tubule fluid nitric oxide in vivo by loop NaCl reabsorption. *Kidney Int* 2004;65:184–189.
259. Leyssac PP, Baumbach L. An oscillating intratubular pressure response to alterations in Henle loop flow in the rat kidney. *Acta Physiol Scand* 1983;117:415–419.
260. Leyssac PP. Further studies on oscillating tubulo-glomerular feedback responses in the rat kidney. *Acta Physiol Scand* 1986;126:271–277.
261. Leyssac PP. Changes in single nephron renin release are mediated by tubular fluid flow rate. *Kidney Int* 1986;30:332–339.
262. Leyssac PP, Holstein-Rathlou NH. Effects of various transport inhibitors on oscillating TGF pressure responses in the rat. *Pflugers Arch* 1986;407:285–291.
263. Leyssac PP, Karlsen FM, Skott O. Dynamics of intrarenal pressures and glomerular filtration rate after acetazolamide. *Am J Physiol Renal Physiol* 1991;261:F169–178.
264. Leyssac PP, Karlsen FM, Holstein-Rathlou NH, Skott O. On determinants of glomerular filtration rate after inhibition of proximal tubular reabsorption. *Am J Physiol Renal Physiol* 1994;266:R1544–1550.
265. Leyssac PP, Holstein-Rathlou NH, Skott O. Renal blood flow, early distal sodium, and plasma renin concentrations during osmotic diuresis. *Am J Physiol Regul Integr Comp Physiol* 2000;279:R1268–1276.
266. Liu R, Bell PD, Peti-Peterdi J, Kovacs G, Johansson A, Persson AE. Purinergic receptor signaling at the basolateral membrane of macula densa cells. *J Am Soc Nephrol* 2002;13: 1145–1151.
267. Liu R, Pittner J, Persson AE. Changes of cell volume and nitric oxide concentration in macula densa cells caused by changes in luminal NaCl concentration. *J Am Soc Nephrol* 2002;13:2688–2696.
268. Liu R, Ren Y, Garvin JL, Carretero OA. Superoxide enhances tubuloglomerular feedback by constricting the afferent arteriole. *Kidney Int* 2004;66:268–274.
269. Liu R, Carretero OA, Ren Y, Garvin JL. Increased intracellular pH at the macula densa activates nNOS during tubuloglomerular feedback. *Kidney Int* 2005;67:1837–1843.
270. Liu R, Persson AE. Simultaneous changes of cell volume and cytosolic calcium concentration in macula densa cells caused by alterations of luminal NaCl concentration. *J Physiol* 2005;205:895–901.
271. Lorenz JN, Weihprecht H, Schnermann J, Skott O, Briggs JP. Characterization of the macula densa stimulus for renin secretion. *Am J Physiol Renal Physiol* 1990;259:F186–193.
272. Lorenz JN, Weihprecht H, Schnermann J, Skott O, Briggs JP. Renin release from isolated juxtaglomerular apparatus depends on macula densa chloride transport. *Am J Physiol Renal Physiol* 1991;260:F486–493.
273. Lorenz JN, Weihprecht H, He XR, Skott O, Briggs JP, Schnermann J. Effects of adenosine and angiotensin on macula densa-stimulated renin secretion. *Am J Physiol Renal Physiol* 1993;265:F187–194.
274. Lorenz JN, Schultheis PJ, Traynor T, Shull GE, Schnermann J. Micropuncture analysis of single-nephron function in NHE3–deficient mice. *Am J Physiol Renal Physiol* 1999;277: F447–F453.
275. Lorenz JN, Baird NR, Judd LM, Noonan WT, Andringa A, Doetschman T, Manning PA, Liu LH, Miller ML, Shull GE. Impaired renal NaCl absorption in mice lacking the ROMK potassium channel, a model for type II Bartter's syndrome. *J Biol Chem* 2002;277:37871–37880.
276. Lorenz JN, Dostanic-Larson I, Shull GE, Lingrel JB. Ouabain inhibits tubuloglomerular feedback in mutant mice with ouabain-sensitive alpha1 Na,K-ATPase. *J Am Soc Nephrol* 2006;17:2457–2463.
277. Loutzenhiser R, Bidani A, Chilton L. Renal myogenic response: kinetic attributes and physiological role. *Circ Res* 2002;90:1316–1324.
278. Loutzenhiser R, Bidani AK, Wang X. Systolic pressure and the myogenic response of the renal afferent arteriole. *Acta Physiol Scand* 2004;181:407–413.
279. Lu M, Wang T, Yan Q, Yang X, Dong K, Knepper MA, Wang W, Giebisch G, Shull GE, Hebert SC. Absence of small conductance K+ channel (SK) activity in apical membranes of thick ascending limb and cortical collecting duct in ROMK (Bartter's) knockout mice. *J Biol Chem* 2002;277:37881–37887.
280. Mangat H, Peterson LN, Burns KD. Hypercalcemia stimulates expression of intrarenal phospholipase A_2 and prostaglandin H synthase-2 in rats. *J Clin Invest* 1997;100: 1941–1950.
281. Mann B, Hartner A, Jensen BL, Kammerl M, Kramer BK, Kurtz A. Furosemide stimulates macula densa cyclooxygenase-2 expression in rats. *Kidney Int* 2001;59:62–68.
282. Marsh DJ, Osborn JL, Cowley AW, Jr. 1/f fluctuations in arterial pressure and regulation of renal blood flow in dogs. *Am J Physiol* 1990;258:F1394–1400.
283. Marsh DJ, Sosnovtseva OV, Chon KH, Holstein-Rathlou NH. Nonlinear interactions in renal blood flow regulation. *Am J Physiol Regul Integr Comp Physiol* 2005;288:R1143–1159.
284. Mason J, Takabatake T, Olbricht C, Thurau K. The early phase of experimental acute renal failure. III. Tubologlomerular feedback. *Pflugers Arch* 1978;373:69–76.
285. Massfelder T, Stewart AF, Endlich K, Soifer N, Judes C, Helwig JJ. Parathyroid hormone-related protein detection and interaction with NO and cyclic AMP in the renovascular system. *Kidney Int* 1996;50:1591–1603.
286. Mercure C, Ramla D, Garcia R, Thibault G, Deschepper CF, Reudelhuber TL. Evidence for intracellular generation of angiotensin II in rat juxtaglomerular cells. *FEBS Lett* 1998;422: 395–399.
287. Mitchell KD, Navar LG. Enhanced tubuloglomerular feedback during peritubular infusions of angiotensins I and II. *Am J Physiol Renal Physiol* 1988;255:F383–390.
288. Mitchell KD, Navar LG. Tubuloglomerular feedback responses during peritubular infusions of calcium channel blockers. *Am J Physiol Renal Physiol* 1990;258:F537–544.
289. Mitchell KD, Navar LG. Modulation of tubuloglomerular feedback responsiveness by extracellular ATP. *Am J Physiol Renal Physiol* 1993;264:F458–466.

290. Moore LC, Schnermann J, Yarimizu S. Feedback mediation of SNGFR autoregulation in hydropenic and DOCA- and salt-loaded rats. *Am J Physiol Renal Physiol* 1979;237:F63–74.
291. Moore LC, Yarimizu S, Schubert G, Weber PC, Schnermann J. Dynamics of tubuloglomerular feedback adaptation to acute and chronic changes in body fluid volume. *Pflugers Arch* 1980;387:39–45.
292. Moore LC, Mason J. Perturbation analysis of tubuloglomerular feedback in hydropenic and hemorrhaged rats. *Am J Physiol Renal Physiol* 1983;245:F554–563.
293. Moore LC. Tubuloglomerular feedback and SNGFR autoregulation in the rat. *Am J Physiol Renal Physiol* 1984;247:F267–276.
294. Moore LC, Mason J. Tubuloglomerular feedback control of distal fluid delivery: effect of extracellular volume. *Am J Physiol Renal Physiol* 1986;250:F1024–1032.
295. Moore LC, Casellas D. Tubuloglomerular feedback dependence of autoregulation in rat juxtamedullary afferent arterioles. *Kidney Int* 1990;37:1402–1408.
296. Moore LC, Rich A, Casellas D. Ascending myogenic autoregulation: interactions between tubuloglomerular feedback and myogenic mechanisms. *Bull Math Biol* 1994;56:391–410.
297. Morgan T, Berliner RW. A study by continuous microperfusion of water and electrolyte movements in the loop of Henle and distal tubule of the rat. *Nephron* 1969;6:388–405.
298. Morsing P, Stenberg A, Muller-Suur C, Persson AE. Tubuloglomerular feedback in animals with unilateral, partial ureteral occlusion. *Kidney Int* 1987;32:212–218.
299. Morsing P, Stenberg A, Persson AE. Effect of thromboxane inhibition on tubuloglomerular feedback in hydronephrotic kidneys. *Kidney Int* 1989;36:447–452
300. Morsing P, Persson AE. Kinin and tubuloglomerular feedback in normal and hydronephrotic rats. *Am J Physiol Renal Physiol* 1991;260:F868–873.
301. Morsing P, Persson AE. Effect of prostaglandin synthesis inhibition on the tubuloglomerular feedback control in the rat kidney. *Ren Physiol Biochem* 1992;15:66–72.
302. Morsing P, Velazquez H, Ellison D, Wright FS. Resetting of tubuloglomerular feedback by interrupting early distal flow. *Acta Physiol Scand* 1993;148:63–68.
303. Morsing P, Stenberg A, Wahlin N, Persson AE. Tubuloglomerular feedback in rats with chronic partial bilateral ureteral obstruction. *Ren Physiol Biochem* 1995;18:27–34.
304. Muller-Suur R, Gutsche HU, Schurek HJ. Acute and reversible inhibition of tubuloglomerular feedback mediated afferent vasoconstriction by the calcium-antagonist verapamil. *Curr Probl Clin Biochem* 1976;6:291–298.
305. Muller-Suur R, Norlen BJ, Persson AE. Resetting of tubuloglomerular feedback in rat kidneys after unilateral nephrectomy. *Kidney Int* 1980;18:48–57.
306. Muller-Suur R, Ulfendahl HR, Persson AE. Evidence for tubuloglomerular feedback in juxtamedullary nephrons of young rats. *Am J Physiol Renal Physiol* 1983;244:F425–431.
307. Muller-Suur R, Persson AE. Influence of water-diuresis or saline volume expansion on deep nephron tubuloglomerular feedback. *Acta Physiol Scand* 1986;126:139–146.
308. Muller E, Neuhofer W, Ohno A, Rucker S, Thurau K, Beck FX. Heat shock proteins HSP25, HSP60, HSP72, HSP73 in isoosmotic cortex and hyperosmotic medulla of rat kidney. *Pflugers Arch* 1996;431:608–617.
309. Mundel P, Bachmann S, Bader M, Fischer A, Kummer W, Mayer B, Kriz W. Expression of nitric oxide synthase in kidney macula densa cells. *Kidney Int* 1992;42:1017–1019.
310. Murakami K, Tsuchiya K, Naruse M, Naruse K, Demura H, Arai J, Nihei H. Nitric oxide synthase I immunoreactivity in the macula densa of the kidney is angiotensin II dependent. *Kidney Int Suppl* 1997;63:S208–210.
311. Murakami M, Nakatani Y, Tanioka T, Kudo I. Prostaglandin E synthase. *Prostaglandins Other Lipid Mediat* 2002;68–69:383–399.
312. Nantel F, Meadows E, Denis D, Connolly B, Metters KM, Giaid A. Immunolocalization of cyclooxygenase-2 in the macula densa of human elderly. *FEBS Lett* 1999;457:475–477.
313. Naruse K, Inagami T, Celio MR, Workman RJ, Takii Y. Immunohistochemical evidence that angiotensins I and II are formed by intracellular mechanism in juxtaglomerular cells. *Hypertension* 1982;4:70–74.
314. Naruse M, Inoue T, Nakayama M, Sato T, Kurokawa K. Effect of luminal Cl- and Ca2+ on tubuloglomerular feedback mechanism. *Jpn J Physiol* 1994;44:S269–272.
315. Nashat FS, Tappin JW, Wilcox CS. The renal blood flow and the glomerular filtration rate of anaesthetized dogs during acute changes in plasma sodium concentration. *J Physiol* 1976;256:731–745.
316. Navar LG, Burke TJ, Robinson RR, Clapp JR. Distal tubular feedback in the autoregulation of single nephron glomerular filtration rate. *J Clin Invest* 1974;53:516–525.
317. Navar LG, Chomdej B, Bell PD. Absence of estimated glomerular pressure autoregulation during interrupted distal delivery. *Am J Physiol* 1975;229:1596–1603.
318. Navar LG, Inscho EW, Majid SA, Imig JD, Harrison-Bernard LM, Mitchell KD. Paracrine regulation of the renal microcirculation. *Physiol Rev* 1996;76:425–536.
319. Nielsen S, Maunsbach AB, Ecelbarger CA, Knepper MA. Ultrastructural localization of Na-K-2Cl cotransporter in thick ascending limb and macula densa of rat kidney. *Am J Physiol Renal Physiol* 1998;275:F885–893.
320. Nishiyama A, Navar LG. ATP mediates tubuloglomerular feedback. *Am J Physiol Regul Integr Comp Physiol* 2002;283:R273–275; discussion R278–279.
321. Norgaard T. Quantitation of glucose-6-phosphate dehydrogenase activity in cortical fractions of the nephron in sodium-depleted and sodium-loaded rabbits. *Histochemistry* 1980; 69:49–59.
322. Norlen BJ, Muller-Suur R, Persson AE. Tubulo-glomerular feedback response and excretory characteristics of the transplanted rat kidney. *Scand J Urol Nephrol* 1978;12:27–33.
323. Nusing RM, Pantalone F, Grone HJ, Seyberth HW, Wegmann M. Expression of the potassium channel ROMK in adult and fetal human kidney. *Histochem Cell Biol* 2005;123: 553–559.
324. Obermuller N, Kunchaparty S, Ellison DH, Bachmann S. Expression of the Na-K-2Cl cotransporter by macula densa and thick ascending limb cells of rat and rabbit nephron. *J Clin Invest* 1996;98:635–640.
325. Obermuller N, Gallagher AR, Cai Y, Gassler N, Gretz N, Somlo S, Witzgall R. The rat pkd2 protein assumes distinct subcellular distributions in different organs. *Am J Physiol* 1999;277: F914–925.
326. Ojeda J, LPiedra S. Lectin-binding sites and silver affinity of the macula densa basement membranes in the rabbit kidney. *J Anat* 1994;185:529–35.
327. Okuda T, Yamashita N, Kurokawa K. Angiotensin II and vasopressin stimulate calcium-activated chloride conductance in rat mesangial cells. *J Clin Invest* 1986;78:1443–1448.
328. Okuda T, Kojima I, Ogata E, Kurokawa K. Ambient Cl^- ions modify rat mesangial cell contraction by modulating cell inositol trisphosphate and Ca2+ via enhanced prostaglandin E2. *J Clin Invest* 1989;84:1866–1872.
329. Okusa MD, Persson AE, Wright FS. Chlorothiazide effect on feedback-mediated control of glomerular filtration rate. *Am J Physiol Renal Physiol* 1989;257:F137–144.
330. Olson RD, Skoglund ML, Nies AS, Gerber JG. Prostaglandins mediate the macula densa stimulated renin release. *Adv Prostaglandin Thromboxane Res* 1980;7:1135–1137.
331. Oppermann M, Castrop H, Briggs J, Schnermann J. Influence of furosemide on renal hemodynamics in mice. *J Am Soc Nephrol* 2005;16:393A.
332. Oppermann M, Castrop H, Huang Y, Mizel D, Deng C, Briggs JP, Schnermann J. Macula densa regulation in mice lacking the B-isoform of the renal Na/K/2Cl cotransporter $NKCC_2$. *FASEB J.* 2005;19:A151.
333. Ortiz-Capisano MC, Ortiz PA, Harding P, Garvin JL, Beierwaltes WH. Decreased intracellular calcium stimulates renin release via calcium-inhibitable adenylyl cyclase. *Hypertension* 2007;49:162–169.
334. Ortiz PAGarvin JL. NO Inhibits NaCl absorption by rat thick ascending limb through activation of cGMP-stimulated phosphodiesterase. *Hypertension* 2001;37:467–471.
335. Ortiz PA, Hong NJ, Garvin JL. Luminal flow induces eNOS activation and translocation in the rat thick ascending limb. *Am J Physiol Renal Physiol* 2004;287:F274–280.
336. Osborne MJ, Droz B, Meyer P, Morel F. Angiotensin II: renal localization in glomerular mesangial cells by autoradiography. *Kidney Int* 1975;8:245–254.
337. Osswald H, Nabakowski G, Hermes H. Adenosine as a possible mediator of metabolic control of glomerular filtration rate. *Int J Biochem* 1980;12:263–267.
338. Paliege A, Mizel D, Medina C, Pasumarthy A, Huang YG, Bachmann S, Briggs JP, Schnermann JB, Yang T. Inhibition of nNOS expression in the macula densa by COX-2–derived prostaglandin E(2). *Am J Physiol Renal Physiol* 2004;287:F152–159.
339. Paliege A, Yang C-L, Theilig F, Ellison D, Bachmann S. Expression and regulation of WNK3 in the macula densa. *J Am Soc Nephrol* 2006;17:475A (abstract).
340. Paul LC, Rennke HG, Milford EL, Carpenter CB. Thy-1.1 in glomeruli of rat kidneys. *Kidney Int* 1984;25:771–777.
341. Payne JA, Forbush B. Alternatively spliced isoforms of the putative renal Na-K-Cl cotransporter are differently distributed within the rabbit kidney. *Proc Natl Acad Sci U S A* 1994; 91: 4544–4548.
342. Pedersen SB, Flyvbjerg A, Richelsen B. Inhibition of renal ornithine decarboxylase activity prevents kidney hypertrophy in experimental diabetes. *Am J Physiol* 1993;264:C453–456.
343. Persson AE, Muller-Suur R, Selen G. Capillary oncotic pressure as a modifier for tubuloglomerular feedback. *Am J Physiol Renal Physiol* 1979;236:F97–102.
344. Persson AE, Schnermann J, Wright FS. Modification of feedback influence on glomerular filtration rate by acute isotonic extracellular volume expansion. *Pflugers Arch* 1979;381: 99–105.
345. Persson AE, Hahne B, Selen G. The effect of tubular perfusion with PGE2, PGF2 alpha, and PGI2 on the tubuloglomerular feedback control in the rat. *Can J Physiol Pharmacol* 1983;61:1317–1323.
346. Persson AE, Gushwa LC, Blantz RC. Feedback pressure-flow responses in normal and angiotensin-prostaglandin-blocked rats. *Am J Physiol Renal Physiol* 1984;247:F925–931.
347. Persson AE, Wahlberg J, Safirstein R, Wright FS. The effect of 2 hours of complete unilateral ureteral obstruction on tubuloglomerular feedback control. *Acta Physiol Scand* 1984;122: 35–43.
348. Persson AE, Bianchi G, Boberg U. Tubuloglomerular feedback in hypertensive rats of the Milan strain. *Acta Physiol Scand* 1985;123:139–146.
349. Persson AEG, Wright FS. Evidence for feedback mediated reduction of glomerular filtration rate during infusion of acetazolamide. *Acta Physiol. Scand.* 1982;114:1–7.
350. Persson BE, Sakai T, Marsh DJ. Juxtaglomerular interstitial hypertonicity in *Amphiuma*: tubular origin-TGF signal. *Am J Physiol* 1988;254:F445–449.
351. Persson BE, Sakai T, Ekblom M, Marsh DJ. Effect of bumetanide on tubuloglomerular feedback in *Necturus maculosus*. *Acta Physiol Scand* 1989;137:93–99.
352. Persson PB, Baumann JE, Ehmke H, Hackenthal E, Kirchheim HR, Nafz B. Endothelium-derived NO stimulates pressure-dependent renin release in conscious dogs. *Am J Physiol* 1993;264:F943–947.
353. Peterson OW, Gushwa LC, Wilson CB, Blantz RC. Tubuloglomerular feedback activity after glomerular immune injury. *Am J Physiol Renal Physiol* 1989;257:F67–71.
354. Peti-Peterdi J, Bell PD. Cytosolic [Ca2+] signaling pathway in macula densa cells. *Am J Physiol Renal Physiol* 1999;277:F472–476.
355. Peti-Peterdi J, Chambrey R, Bebok Z, Biemesderfer D, St John PL, Abrahamson DR, Warnock DG, Bell PD. Macula densa Na(+)/H(+) exchange activities mediated by apical NHE2 and basolateral NHE4 isoforms. *Am J Physiol Renal Physiol* 2000;278:F452–463.
356. Peti-Peterdi J, Bebok Z, Lapointe JY, Bell PD. Novel regulation of cell [Na(+)] in macula densa cells: apical Na(+) recycling by H-K-ATPase. *Am J Physiol Renal Physiol* 2002;282: F324–329.
357. Peti-Peterdi J, Morishima S, Bell PD, Okada Y. Two-photon excitation fluorescence imaging of the living juxtaglomerular apparatus. *Am J Physiol Renal Physiol* 2002;283:F197–201.
358. Peti-Peterdi J, Komlosi P, Fuson AL, Guan Y, Schneider A, Qi Z, Redha R, Rosivall L, Breyer MD, Bell PD. Luminal NaCl delivery regulates basolateral PGE2 release from macula densa cells. *J Clin Invest* 2003;112:76–82.
359. Peti-Peterdi J, Fintha A, Fuson AL, Tousson A, Chow RH. Real-time imaging of renin release in vitro. *Am J Physiol Renal Physiol* 2004;287:F329–35.
360. Peti-Peterdi J. Calcium wave of tubuloglomerular feedback. *Am J Physiol Renal Physiol* 2006;291:F473–480.
361. Ploth DW, Schnermann J, Dahlheim H, Hermle M, Schmidmeier E. Autoregulation and tubuloglomerular feedback in normotensive and hypertensive rats. *Kidney Int* 1977;12:253–267.

362. Ploth DW, Dahlheim H, Schmidmeier E, Hermle M, Schnermann J. Tubuloglomerular feedback and autoregulation of glomerular filtration rate in Wistar-Kyoto spontaneously hypertensive rats. *Pflugers Arch* 1978;375:261–267.
363. Ploth DW, Rudulph J, Thomas C, Navar LG. Renal and tubuloglomerular feedback responses to plasma expansion in the rat. *Am J Physiol Renal Physiol* 1978;235:F156–162.
364. Ploth DW, Rudulph J, LaGrange R, Navar LG. Tubuloglomerular feedback and single nephron function after converting enzyme inhibition in the rat. *J Clin Invest* 1979;64:1325–1335.
365. Ploth DW, Roy RN. Renin-angiotensin influences on tubuloglomerular feedback activity in the rat. *Kidney Int Suppl* 1982;12:S114–121.
366. Ploth DW, Roy RN. Renal and tubuloglomerular feedback effects of [Sar1,Ala8]angiotensin II in the rat. *Am J Physiol Renal Physiol* 1982;242:F149–157.
367. Pollock CA, Lawrence JR, Field MJ. Tubular sodium handling and tubuloglomerular feedback in experimental diabetes mellitus. *Am J Physiol Renal Physiol* 1991;260:F946–952.
368. Pollock CA, Bostrom TE, Dyne M, Gyory AZ, Field MJ. Tubular sodium handling and tubuloglomerular feedback in compensatory renal hypertrophy. *Pflugers Arch* 1992;420:159–166.
369. Pollock DM, Arendshorst WJ. Native tubular fluid attenuates ANF-induced inhibition of tubuloglomerular feedback. *Am J Physiol Renal Physiol* 1990;258:F189–198.
370. Praetorius HA, Spring KR. The renal cell primary cilium functions as a flow sensor. *Curr Opin Nephrol Hypertens* 2003;12:517–520.
371. Pricam C, Humbert F, Perrelet A, Orci L. Gap junctions in mesangial and lacis cells. *J Cell Biol* 1974;63:349–354.
372. Price EM, Lingrel JB. Structure-function relationships in the Na,K-ATPase alpha subunit: site-directed mutagenesis of glutamine-111 to arginine and asparagine-122 to aspartic acid generates a ouabain-resistant enzyme. *Biochemistry* 1988;27:8400–8408.
373. Pu HX, Cluzeaud F, Goldshleger R, Karlish SJ, Farman N, Blostein R. Functional role and immunocytochemical localization of the gamma a and gamma b forms of the Na,K-ATPase gamma subunit. *J Biol Chem* 2001;276:20370–20378.
374. Rajendran VM, Sangan P, Geibel J, Binder HJ. Ouabain-sensitive H,K-ATPase functions as Na,K-ATPase in apical membranes of rat distal colon. *J Biol Chem* 2000;275:13035–13040.
375. Reid IA, Chou L. Effect of blockade of nitric oxide synthesis on the renin secretory response to frusemide in conscious rabbits. *Clin Sci (Colch)* 1995;88:657–663.
376. Reinalter SC, Jeck N, Brochhausen C, Watzer B, Nusing RM, Seyberth HW, Komhoff M. Role of cyclooxygenase-2 in hyperprostaglandin E syndrome/antenatal Bartter syndrome. *Kidney Int* 2002;62:253–260.
377. Ren Y, Garvin JL, Carretero OA. Efferent arteriole tubuloglomerular feedback in the renal nephron. *Kidney Int* 2001;59:222–229.
378. Ren Y, Yu H, Wang H, Carretero OA, Garvin JL. Nystatin and valinomycin induce tubuloglomerular feedback. *Am J Physiol Renal Physiol* 2001;281:F1102–1108.
379. Ren Y, Arima S, Carretero OA, Ito S. Possible role of adenosine in macula densa control of glomerular hemodynamics. *Kidney Int* 2002;61:169–176.
380. Ren Y, Carretero OA, Garvin JL. Mechanism by which superoxide potentiates tubuloglomerular feedback. *Hypertension* 2002;39:624–628.
381. Ren Y, Carretero OA, Garvin JL. Role of mesangial cells and gap junctions in tubuloglomerular feedback. *Kidney Int* 2002;62:525–531.
382. Ren Y, Liu R, Carretero OA, Garvin JL. Increased intracellular Ca++ in the macula densa regulates tubuloglomerular feedback. *Kidney Int* 2003;64:1348–1355.
383. Ren Y, Garvin JL, Liu R, Carretero OA. Role of macula densa adenosine triphosphate (ATP) in tubuloglomerular feedback. *Kidney Int* 2004;66:1479–1485.
384. Ren Y, Garvin JL, Liu R, Carretero OA. A novel mechanism of afferent arteriole regulation: a cross-talk between the connecting tubule and afferent arteriole. *J Am Soc Nephrol* 2006;17:715A (abstract).
385. Ren YL, Carretero OA, Ito S. Influence of NaCl concentration at the macula densa on angiotensin II-induced constriction of the afferent arteriole. *Hypertension* 1996;27:649–652.
386. Ren YL, Garvin JL, Carretero OA. Role of macula densa nitric oxide and cGMP in the regulation of tubuloglomerular feedback. *Kidney Int* 2000;58:2053–2060.
387. Ren YL, Garvin JL, Ito S, Carretero OA. Role of neuronal nitric oxide synthase in the macula densa. *Kidney Int* 2001;60:1676–1683.
388. Riccardi D, Hall AE, Chattopadhyay N, Xu JZ, Brown EM, Hebert SC. Localization of the extracellular Ca2+/polyvalent cation-sensing protein in rat kidney. *Am J Physiol* 1998;274:F611–622.
389. Rich A, Moore LC. Transport-coupling hypothesis of tubuloglomerular feedback signal transmission. *Am J Physiol Renal Physiol* 1989;257:F882–892.
390. Rostand SG, Work J, Luke RG. Effect of reduced chloride reabsorption on renin release in the isolated rat kidney. *Pflugers Arch* 1985;405:46–51.
391. Russ U, Rauch U, Quast U. Pharmacological evidence for a KATP channel in renin-secreting cells from rat kidney. *J Physiol* 1999;517[Pt 3]:781–790.
392. Sabirov RZ, Dutta AK, Okada Y. Volume-dependent ATP-conductive large-conductance anion channel as a pathway for swelling-induced ATP release. *J Gen Physiol* 2001;118:251–266.
393. Salido EC, Yen PH, Shapiro LJ, Fisher DA, Barajas L. In situ hybridization of prepro-epidermal growth factor mRNA in the mouse kidney. *Am J Physiol* 1989;256:F632–638.
394. Salmond R, Seney FJ. Reset tubuloglomerular feedback permits and sustains glomerular hyperfunction after extensive renal ablation. *Am J Physiol Renal Physiol* 1991;260:F395–401.
395. Salomonsson M, Gonzalez E, Westerlund P, Persson AE. Chloride concentration in macula densa and cortical thick ascending limb cells. *Kidney Int Suppl* 1991;32:S51–54.
396. Sanada H, Yao L, Jose PA, Carey RM, Felder RA. Dopamine D3 receptors in rat juxtaglomerular cells. *Clin Exp Hypertens* 1997;19:93–105.
397. Sanchez-Ferrer CF, Roman RJ, Harder DR. Pressure-dependent contraction of rat juxtamedullary afferent arterioles. *Circ Res* 1989;64:790–798.
398. Sarkis A, Roman RJ. Role of cytochrome P450 metabolites of arachidonic acid in hypertension. *Curr Drug Metab* 2004;5:245–256.
399. Satriano J, Wead L, Cardus A, Deng A, Boss GR, Thomson SC, Blantz RC. Regulation of ecto-5'-nucleotidase by NaCl and nitric oxide: potential roles in tubuloglomerular feedback and adaptation. *Am J Physiol Renal Physiol* 2006;291:F1078–1082.
400. Sayago CM, Beierwaltes WH. Nitric oxide synthase and cGMP-mediated stimulation of renin secretion. *Am J Physiol Regul Integr Comp Physiol* 2001;281:R1146–1151.
401. Schlatter E, Salomonsson M, Persson AE, Greger R. Macula densa cells sense luminal NaCl concentration via furosemide sensitive Na+2Cl-K+ cotransport. *Pflugers Arch* 1989;414:286–290.
402. Schlatter E. Effect of various diuretics on membrane voltage of macula densa cells: whole-cell patch-clamp experiments. *Pflugers Arch* 1993;423:74–77.
403. Schnabel E, Kriz W. Morphometric studies of the extraglomerular mesangial cell field in volume expanded and volume depleted rats. *Anat Embryol (Berl)* 1984;170:217–222.
404. Schnermann J, Wright FS, Davis JM, Stackelberg Wv, Grill G. Regulation of superficial nephron filtration rate by tubulo-glomerular feedback. *Pflugers Arch* 1970;318:147–175.
405. Schnermann J, Persson AE, Agerup B. Tubuloglomerular feedback. Nonlinear relation between glomerular hydrostatic pressure and loop of henle perfusion rate. *J Clin Invest* 1973;52:862–869.
406. Schnermann J, Hermle M, Schmidmeier E, Dahlheim H. Impaired potency for feedback regulation of glomerular filtration rate in DOCA escaped rats. *Pflugers Arch* 1975;358:325–338.
407. Schnermann J, Ploth DW, Hermle M. Activation of tubulo-glomerular feedback by chloride transport. *Pfluegers Arch.* 1976;362:229–240.
408. Schnermann J, Osswald H, Hermle M. Inhibitory effect of methylxanthines on feedback control of glomerular filtration rate in the rat. *Pflugers Arch.* 1977;369:39–48.
409. Schnermann J, Schubert G, Hermle M, Herbst R, Stowe NT, Yarimizu S, Weber PC. The effect of inhibition of prostaglandin synthesis on tubuloglomerular feedback in the rat kidney. *Pflugers Arch* 1979;379:269–279.
410. Schnermann J, Briggs J, Wright FS. Feedback-mediated reduction of glomerular filtration rate during infusion of hypertonic saline. *Kidney Int* 1981;20:462–468.
411. Schnermann J, Briggs J, Schubert G. In situ studies of the distal convoluted tubule in the rat. I. Evidence for NaCl secretion. *Am J Physiol* 1982;243:F160–166.
412. Schnermann J, Briggs JP. Concentration-dependent sodium chloride transport as the signal in feedback control of glomerular filtration rate. *Kidney Int* 1982;22[Suppl 12]:S82–S89.
413. Schnermann J, Weber PC. Reversal of indomethacin-induced inhibition of tubuloglomerular feedback by prostaglandin infusion. *Prostaglandins* 1982;24:351–361.
414. Schnermann J, Briggs JP, Schubert G, Marin-Grez M. Opposing effects of captopril and aprotinin on tubuloglomerular feedback responses. *Am J Physiol Renal Physiol* 1984;247:F912–918.
415. Schnermann J, Briggs JP, Weber PC. Tubuloglomerular feedback, prostaglandins, and angiotensin in the autoregulation of glomerular filtration rate. *Kidney Int* 1984;25:53–64.
416. Schnermann J, Gokel M, Weber PC, Schubert G, Briggs JP. Tubuloglomerular feedback and glomerular morphology in Goldblatt hypertensive rats on varying protein diets. *Kidney Int* 1986;29:520–529.
417. Schnermann J, Marver D. ATPase activity in macula densa cells of the rabbit kidney. *Pflugers Arch* 1986;407:82–86.
418. Schnermann J, Vascular tone as a determinant of tubuloglomerular feedback responsiveness. In: Persson AEG, Boberg U (eds.). *The Juxtaglomerular Apparatus.* Amsterdam: Elsevier, 1988:167–176.
419. Schnermann J. Effect of adenosine analogues on tubuloglomerular feedback responses. *Am J Physiol Renal Physiol* 1988;255:F33–42.
420. Schnermann J, Briggs JP. Interaction between loop of Henle flow and arterial pressure as determinants of glomerular pressure. *Am J Physiol Renal Physiol* 1989;256:F421–F429.
421. Schnermann J, Briggs JP. Single nephron comparison of the effect of loop of Henle flow on filtration rate and pressure in control and angiotensin II-infused rats. *Miner Electrolyte Metab* 1989;15:103–107.
422. Schnermann J, Briggs JP. Restoration of tubuloglomerular feedback in volume-expanded rats by angiotensin II. *Am J Physiol Renal Physiol* 1990;259:F565–572.
423. Schnermann J, Todd KM, Briggs JP. Effect of dopamine on the tubuloglomerular feedback mechanism. *Am J Physiol Renal Physiol* 1990;258:F790–798.
424. Schnermann J, Weihprecht H, Briggs JP. Inhibition of tubuloglomerular feedback during adenosine1 receptor blockade. *Am J Physiol Renal Physiol* 1990;258:F553–561.
425. Schnermann J. Effects of barium ions on tubuloglomerular feedback. *Am J Physiol Renal Physiol* 1995;268:F960–966.
426. Schnermann J. Juxtaglomerular cell complex in the regulation of renal salt excretion. *Am J Physiol Renal Physiol* 1998;274:R263–279.
427. Schnermann J, Chou C-L, Ma T, Traynor T, Knepper MA, Verkman AS. Defective proximal tubular fluid reabsorption in transgenic aquaporin-1 null mice. *Proc Natl Acad Sci U S A* 1998;95:9660–9664.
428. Schnermann J, Briggs JP. Function of the juxtaglomerular apparatus: control of glomerular hemodynamics and renin secretion. In: Seldin DW, Giebisch G (eds.). *The Kidney Physiology and Pathophysiology*. Philadelphia: Lippincott Williams &Wilkins, 2000:945–980.
429. Schnermann J, Traynor T, Pohl H, Thomas DW, Coffman TM, Briggs JP. Vasoconstrictor responses in thromboxane receptor knockout mice: tubuloglomerular feedback and ureteral obstruction. *Acta Physiol Scand* 2000;168:201–207.
430. Schnermann J, Levine DZ. paracrine factors in tubuloglomerular feedback: adenosine, ATP, and nitric oxide. *Annu Rev Physiol* 2003;65:501–529.
431. Schnermann JB, Traynor T, Yang T, Huang YG, Oliverio MI, Coffman T, Briggs JP. Absence of tubuloglomerular feedback responses in AT1A receptor- deficient mice. *Am J Physiol Renal Physiol* 1997;273:F315–320.
432. Scholz H, Kurtz A. Involvement of endothelium-derived relaxing factor in the pressure control of renin secretion from isolated perfused kidney. *J Clin Invest* 1993;91:1088–1094.
433. Schricker K, Kurtz A. Liberators of NO exert a dual effect on renin secretion from isolated mouse renal juxtaglomerular cells. *Am J Physiol* 1993;265:F180–186.
434. Schricker K, Hamann M, Kurtz A. Nitric oxide and prostaglandins are involved in the macula densa control of the renin system. *Am J Physiol Renal Physiol* 1995;269:F825–830.
435. Schricker K, Kurtz A. Role of membrane-permeable ions in renin secretion by renal juxtaglomerular cells. *Am J Physiol* 1995;269:F64–69.

436. Schricker K, Potzl B, Hamann M, Kurtz A. Coordinate changes of renin and brain-type nitric-oxide-synthase (b- NOS) mRNA levels in rat kidneys. *Pflugers Arch* 1996;432: 394–400.

437. Schurek HJ, Johns O. Is tubuloglomerular feedback a tool to prevent nephron oxygen deficiency? *Kidney Int* 1997;51:386–392.

438. Schweda F, Wagner C, Kramer BK, Schnermann J, Kurtz A. Preserved macula densa-dependent renin secretion in A1 adenosine receptor knockout mice. *Am J Physiol Renal Physiol* 2003;284:F770–777.

439. Selen G, Muller-Suur R, Persson AE. Activation of the tubuloglomerular feedback mechanism in dehydrated rats. *Acta Physiol Scand* 1983;117:83–89.

440. Selen G, Persson AE. Hydrostatic and oncotic pressures in the interstitium of dehydrated and volume expanded rats. *Acta Physiol Scand* 1983;117:75–81.

441. Seney FD, Wright FS. Signal for tubuloglomerular feedback control of GFR: separate changes of sodium and chloride at constant osmolality. *Kidney Int* 1986;29:388.

442. Seney FD, Jr.Wright FS. Dietary protein suppresses feedback control of glomerular filtration in rats. *J Clin Invest* 1985;75:558–568.

443. Seney FD, Jr., Persson EG, Wright FS. Modification of tubuloglomerular feedback signal by dietary protein. *Am J Physiol Renal Physiol* 1987;252:F83–90.

444. Shade RE, Davis JO, Johnson JA, Witty RT. Effects of renal arterial infusion of sodium and potassium on renin secretion in the dog. *Circ Res* 1972;31:719–727.

445. Shi Y, Wang X, Chon KH, Cupples WA. Tubuloglomerular feedback-dependent modulation of renal myogenic autoregulation by nitric oxide. *Am J Physiol Regul Integr Comp Physiol* 2006;290:R982–991.

446. Siegfried G, Amiel C, Friedlander G. Inhibition of ecto-5'-nucleotidase by nitric oxide donors. Implications in renal epithelial cells. *J Biol Chem* 1996;271:4659–4664.

447. Singh I, Grams M, Wang WH, Yang T, Killen P, Smart A, Schnermann J, Briggs JP. Coordinate regulation of renal expression of nitric oxide synthase, renin, and angiotensinogen mRNA by dietary salt. *Am J Physiol Renal Physiol* 1996;270:F1027–1037.

448. Sjoquist M, Goransson A, Kallskog O, Ulfendahl HR. The influence of tubulo-glomerular feedback on the autoregulation of filtration rate in superficial and deep glomeruli. *Acta Physiol Scand* 1984;122:235–242.

449. Skott O. Episodic release of renin from single isolated superfused rat afferent arterioles. *Pflugers Arch* 1986;407:41–45.

450. Skott O, Briggs JP. Direct demonstration of macula densa-mediated renin secretion. *Science* 1987;237:1618–1620.

451. Skott O. Do osmotic forces play a role in renin secretion? *Am J Physiol* 1988;255:F1–10

452. Skott O, Briggs JP. A method for superfusion of the isolated perfused tubule. *Kidney Int* 1988;33:1009–1012.

453. Smith WL, Bell TG. Immunohistochemical localization of the prostaglandin-forming cyclooxygenase in renal cortex. *Am J Physiol Renal Physiol* 1978;235:F451–F457.

454. Spanidis A, Wunsch H, Kaissling B, Kriz W. Three-dimensional shape of a Goormaghtigh cell and its contact with a granular cell in the rabbit kidney. *Anat Embryol (Berl)* 1982;165:239–52.

455. Spielman WS, Thompson CI. A proposed role for adenosine in the regulation of renal hemodynamics and renin release. *Am J Physiol* 1982;242:F423–435.

456. Stefanovic V, Savic V, Vlahovic P, Ardaillou N, Ardaillou R. Ecto-5'-nucleotidase of cultured rat mesangial cells. *Ren Physiol Biochem* 1988;11:89–102.

457. Steinhausen M, Zimmerhackl B, Thederan H, Dussel R, Parekh N, Esslinger HU, von Hagens G, Komitowski D, Dallenbach FD. Intraglomerular microcirculation: measurements of single glomerular loop flow in rats. *Kidney Int* 1981;20:230–9.

458. Steinhausen M, Blum M, Fleming JT, Holz FG, Parekh N, Wiegman DL. Visualization of renal autoregulation in the split hydronephrotic kidney of rats. *Kidney Int* 1989;35: 1151–1160.

459. Stoeckel ME, Freund-Mercier MJ. Autoradiographic demonstration of oxytocin-binding sites in the macula densa [published erratum appears in *Am J Physiol Renal Physiol* 1990 Jan;258(1 Pt 2):preceding F1]. *Am J Physiol Renal Physiol* 1989;257:F310–314.

460. Stowe N, Schnermann J, Hermle M. Feedback regulation of nephron filtration rate during pharmacologic interference with the renin-angiotensin and adrenergic systems in rats. *Kidney Int* 1979;15:473–486.

461. Sun D, Samuelson LC, Yang T, Huang Y, Paliege A, Saunders T, Briggs J, Schnermann J. Mediation of tubuloglomerular feedback by adenosine: Evidence from mice lacking adenosine 1 receptors. *Proc Natl Acad Sci U S A* 2001;98:9983–9988.

462. Sweadner KJ, Arystarkhova E, Donnet C, Wetzel RK. FXYD proteins as regulators of the Na,K-ATPase in the kidney. *Ann N Y Acad Sci* 2003;986:382–387.

463. Tagawa H, Vander AJ. Effects of adenosine compounds on renal function and renin secretion in dogs. *Circ Res* 1970;26:327–338.

464. Takabatake T, Ushiogi Y, Ohta K, Hattori N. Attenuation of enhanced tubuloglomerular feedback activity in SHR by renal denervation. *Am J Physiol Renal Physiol* 1990;258:F980–985.

465. Takenaka T, Harrison-Bernard LM, Inscho EW, Carmines PK, Navar LG. Autoregulation of afferent arteriolar blood flow in juxtamedullary nephrons. *Am J Physiol Renal Physiol* 1994;267:F879–887.

466. Takenaka T, Okada H, Kanno Y, Inoue T, Ryuzaki M, Nakamoto H, Kawachi H, Shimizu F, Suzuki H. Exogenous 5'-nucleotidase improves glomerular autoregulation in Thy-1 nephritic rats. *Am J Physiol Renal Physiol* 2006;290:F844–853.

467. Tanner GA. Effects of kidney tubule obstruction on glomerular function in rats. *Am J Physiol* 1979;237:F379–385.

468. Tanner GA. Nephron obstruction and tubuloglomerular feedback. *Kidney Int Suppl* 1982;12: S213–218.

469. Tanner GA. Tubuloglomerular feedback after nephron or ureteral obstruction. *Am J Physiol Renal Physiol* 1985;248:F688–697.

470. Taugner R, Schiller A, Kaissling B, Kriz W. Gap junctional coupling between the JGA and the glomerular tuft. *Cell Tissue Res* 1978;186:279–285.

471. Taugner R, Mannek E, Nobiling R, Buhrle CP, Hackenthal E, Ganten D, Inagami T, Schroder H. Coexistence of renin and angiotensin II in epitheloid cell secretory granules of rat kidney. *Histochemistry* 1984;81:39–45.

472. Taugner R, Rosivall L, Buhrle CP, Groschel-Stewart U. Myosin content and vasoconstrictive ability of the proximal and distal (renin-positive) segments of the preglomerular arteriole. *Cell Tissue Res* 1987;248:579–588.

473. Taugner R, Hackenthal E. *The Juxtaglomerular Apparatus*. Springer-Verlag, Berlin Heidelberg, 1989.

474. Thomson S, Vallon V, Blantz RC. Asymmetry of tubuloglomerular feedback effector mechanism with respect to ambient tubular flow. *Am J Physiol Renal Physiol* 1996;271:F1123–F1130.

475. Thomson S, Bao D, Deng A, Vallon V. Adenosine formed by 5'-nucleotidase mediates tubuloglomerular feedback. *J Clin Invest* 2000;106:289–298.

476. Thomson SC, Blantz RC. Homeostatic efficiency of tubuloglomerular feedback in hydropenia, euvolemia, and acute volume expansion. *Am J Physiol Renal Physiol* 1993;264:F930–936.

477. Thomson SC, Blantz RC, Vallon V. Increased tubular flow induces resetting of tubuloglomerular feedback in euvolemic rats. *Am J Physiol Renal Physiol* 1996;270:F461–468.

478. Thomson SC, Deng A, Bao D, Satriano J, Blantz RC, Vallon V. Ornithine decarboxylase, kidney size, and the tubular hypothesis of glomerular hyperfiltration in experimental diabetes. *J Clin Invest* 2001;107:217–224.

479. Thomson SC, Deng A. Cyclic GMP Mediates Influence of Macula densa Nitric Oxide over Tubuloglomerular Feedback. *Kidney Blood Press Res* 2003;26:10–18.

480. Thomson SC, Vallon V, Blantz RC. Kidney function in early diabetes: the tubular hypothesis of glomerular filtration. *Am J Physiol Renal Physiol* 2004;286:F8–15.

481. Thorup C, Persson AE. Inhibition of locally produced nitric oxide resets tubuloglomerular feedback mechanism. *Am J Physiol Renal Physiol* 1994;267:F606–611.

482. Thorup C, Kurkus J, Morsing P, Persson AE. Acute renal denervation causes time-dependent resetting of the tubuloglomerular feedback mechanism. *Acta Physiol Scand* 1995;153:43–49.

483. Thorup C, Kurkus J, Ollerstam A, Persson AE. Effects of acute and chronic unilateral renal denervation on the tubuloglomerular feedback mechanism. *Acta Physiol Scand* 1996;156: 139–145.

484. Thorup C, Persson AEG. Macula densa derived nitric oxide in regulation of glomerular capillary pressure. *Kidney Int* 1996;49:430–436.

485. Thurau K. Renal hemodynamics. *Am. J. Med.* 1964;36:850–860.

486. Thurau K, Gruner A, Mason J, Dahlheim H. Tubular signal for the renin activity in the juxtaglomerular apparatus. *Kidney Int Suppl* 1982;12:S55–62.

487. Thurau K, Schnermann J. The Na concentration at the macula densa cells as a factor regulating glomerular filtration rate (micropuncture studies). 1965 [classical article]. *J Am Soc Nephrol* 1998;9:925–934.

488. Tian W, Salanova M, Xu H, Lindsley JN, Oyama TT, Anderson S, Bachmann S, Cohen DM. Renal expression of osmotically responsive cation channel TRPV4 is restricted to water-impermeant nephron segments. *Am J Physiol Renal Physiol* 2004;287:F17–24.

489. Tojo A, Madsen KM, Wilcox CS. Expression of immunoreactive nitric oxide synthase isoforms in rat kidney. Effects of dietary salt and losartan. *Jpn Heart J* 1995;36:389–398.

490. Tomasoni S, Noris M, Zappella S, Gotti E, Casiraghi F, Bonazzola S, Benigni A, Remuzzi G. Upregulation of renal and systemic cyclooxygenase-2 in patients with active lupus nephritis. *J Am Soc Nephrol* 1998;9:1202–1212.

491. Traynor T, Yang T, Huang YG, Arend L, Oliverio MI, Coffman T, Briggs JP, Schnermann J. Inhibition of adenosine-1 receptor-mediated preglomerular vasoconstriction in AT1A receptor-deficient mice. *Am J Physiol Renal Physiol* 1998;275:F922–927.

492. Traynor T, Yang T, Huang YG, Krege JH, Briggs JP, Smithies O, Schnermann J. Tubuloglomerular feedback in ACE-deficient mice. *Am J Physiol Renal Physiol* 1999;276:F751–757.

493. Traynor TR, Smart A, Briggs JP, Schnermann J. Inhibition of macula densa-stimulated renin secretion by pharmacological blockade of cyclooxygenase-2. *Am J Physiol Renal Physiol* 1999;277:F706–F710.

494. Tsukahara H, Krivenko Y, Moore LC, Goligorsky MS. Decrease in ambient [Cl-] stimulates nitric oxide release from cultured rat mesangial cells. *Am J Physiol Renal Physiol* 1994;267: F190–195.

495. Tucker BJ, Steiner RW, Gushwa LC, Blantz RC. Studies on the tubulo-glomerular feedback system in the rat. The mechanism of reduction in filtration rate with benzolamide. *J Clin Invest* 1978;62:993–1004.

496. Vallon V, Osswald H. Dipyridamole prevents diabetes-induced alterations of kidney function in rats. *Naunyn Schmiedebergs Arch Pharmacol* 1994;349:217–222.

497. Vallon V, Blantz RC, Thomson S. Homeostatic efficiency of tubuloglomerular feedback is reduced in established diabetes mellitus in rats. *Am J Physiol Renal Physiol* 1995;269:F876–883.

498. Vallon V, Thomson S. Inhibition of local nitric oxide synthase increases homeostatic efficiency of tubuloglomerular feedback. *Am J Physiol Renal Physiol* 1995;269:F892–F899.

499. Vallon V, Kirschenmann D, Wead LM, Lortie MJ, Satriano J, Blantz RC, Thomson SC. Effect of chronic salt loading on kidney function in early and established diabetes mellitus in rats. *J Lab Clin Med* 1997;130:76–82.

500. Vallon V, Osswald H, Blantz RC, Thomson S. Potential role of luminal potassium in tubuloglomerular feedback. *J Am Soc Nephrol* 1997;8:1831–1837.

501. Vallon V, Traynor T, Barajas L, Huang YG, Briggs JP, Schnermann J. Feedback control of glomerular vascular tone in neuronal nitric oxide synthase knockout mice. *J Am Soc Nephrol* 2001;12:1599–1606.

502. Vallon V, Huang DY, Deng A, Richter K, Blantz RC, Thomson S. Salt-sensitivity of proximal reabsorption alters macula densa salt and explains the paradoxical effect of dietary salt on glomerular filtration rate in diabetes mellitus. *J Am Soc Nephrol* 2002;13:1865–1871.

503. Vallon V, Blantz RC, Thomson S. Glomerular hyperfiltration and the salt paradox in early [corrected] type 1 diabetes mellitus: a tubulo-centric view. *J Am Soc Nephrol* 2003;14: 530–537.

504. Vallon V, Richter K, Huang DY, Rieg T, Schnermann J. Functional consequences at the single-nephron level of the lack of adenosine A1 receptors and tubuloglomerular feedback in mice. *Pflugers Arch* 2004;448:214–221.

505. Vallon V, Muhlbauer B, Osswald H. Adenosine and kidney function. *Physiol Rev* 2006;86:901–40.

506. Vander AJ, Miller R. Control of renin secretion in the anesthetized dog. *Am. J Physiol* 1964;207:537–546.

507. Vander AJ. Control of renin release. *Physiol Rev* 1967;47:359–382.

508. Vander AJ. Renin secretion during mannitol diuresis and ureteral occlusion. *Proc Soc Exp Biol Med* 1968;128:518–520.

509. Vander AJ, Carlson J. Mechanism of the effects of furosemide on renin secretion in anesthetized dogs. *Circ Res* 1969;25:145–152.

510. Vandewalle A, Farman N, Cluzeaud F, Bonvalet JP. Heterogeneity of uridine incorporation along the rabbit nephron. I. Autoradiographic study. *Am J Physiol* 1984;246:F417–426.

511. Verlander JW, Moudy RM, Campbell WG, Cain BD, Wingo CS. Immunohistochemical localization of H-K-ATPase alpha(2c)-subunit in rabbit kidney. *Am J Physiol Renal Physiol* 2001;281:F357–365.

512. Vidal MJ, Romero JC, Vanhoutte PM. Endothelium-derived relaxing factor inhibits renin release. *Eur J Pharmacol* 1988;149:401–402.

513. Wagner AJ, Holstein-Rathlou NH, Marsh DJ. Internephron coupling by conducted vasomotor responses in normotensive and spontaneously hypertensive rats. *Am J Physiol* 1997;272:F372–379.

514. Wagner C, Pfeifer A, Ruth P, Hofmann F, Kurtz A. Role of cGMP-kinase II in the control of renin secretion and renin expression. *J Clin Invest* 1998;102:1576–1582.

515. Wahlberg J, Stenberg A, Wilson DR, Persson AE. Tubuloglomerular feedback and interstitial pressure in obstructive nephropathy. *Kidney Int* 1984;26:294–301.

516. Walker M, 3rd, Harrison-Bernard LM, Cook AK, Navar LG. Dynamic interaction between myogenic and TGF mechanisms in afferent arteriolar blood flow autoregulation. *Am J Physiol Renal Physiol* 2000;279:F858–865.

517. Wang H, Carretero OA, Garvin JL. Nitric oxide produced by THAL nitric oxide synthase inhibits TGF. *Hypertension* 2002;39:662–666.

518. Wang H, Carretero OA, Garvin JL. Inhibition of apical Na+/H+ exchangers on the macula densa cells augments tubuloglomerular feedback. *Hypertension* 2003;41:688–691.

519. Wang JL, Cheng HF, Zhang MZ, McKanna JA, Harris RC. Selective increase of cyclooxygenase-2 expression in a model of renal ablation. *Am J Physiol Renal Physiol* 1998;275:F613–622.

520. Wang JL, Cheng HF, Harris RC. Cyclooxygenase-2 inhibition decreases renin content and lowers blood pressure in a model of renovascular hypertension. *Hypertension* 1999;34:96–101.

521. Wang T, Kawabata M, Haneda M, Takabatake T. Effects of uroguanylin, an intestinal natriuretic peptide, on tubuloglomerular feedback. *Hypertens Res* 2003;26:577–582.

522. Wang T, Takabatake T. Effects of vasopeptidase inhibition on renal function and tubuloglomerular feedback in spontaneously hypertensive rats. *Hypertens Res* 2005;28:611–618.

523. Weaver DR, Reppert SM. Adenosine receptor gene expression in rat kidney. *Am J Physiol Renal Physiol* 1992;263:F991–995.

524. Weihprecht H, Lorenz JN, Schnermann J, Skott O, Briggs JP. Effect of adenosine1-receptor blockade on renin release from rabbit isolated perfused juxtaglomerular apparatus. *J Clin Invest* 1990;85:1622–1628.

525. Weihprecht H, Lorenz JN, Briggs JP, Schnermann J. Vasoconstrictor effect of angiotensin and vasopressin in isolated rabbit afferent arterioles. *Am J Physiol Renal Physiol* 1991;261:F273–282.

526. Weihprecht H, Lorenz JN, Briggs JP, Schnermann J. Vasomotor effects of purinergic agonists in isolated rabbit afferent arterioles. *Am J Physiol Renal Physiol* 1992;263:F1026–1033.

527. Weihprecht H, Lorenz JN, Briggs JP, Schnermann J. Synergistic effects of angiotensin and adenosine in the renal microvasculature. *Am J Physiol Renal Physiol* 1994;266:F227–239.

528. Welch WJ, Ott CE, Lorenz JN, Kotchen TA. Effects of chlorpropamide on loop of Henle function and plasma renin. *Kidney Int* 1986;30:712–6.

529. Welch WJ, Wilcox CS. Modulating role for thromboxane in the tubuloglomerular feedback response in the rat. *J Clin Invest* 1988;81:1843–1849.

530. Welch WJ, Wilcox CS. Feedback responses during sequential inhibition of angiotensin and thromboxane. *Am J Physiol Renal Physiol* 1990;258:F457–466.

531. Welch WJ, Peng B, Takeuchi K, Abe K, Wilcox CS. Salt loading enhances rat renal TxA2/PGH2 receptor expression and TGF response to U-46,619. *Am J Physiol Renal Physiol* 1997;273:F976–983.

532. Welch WJ, Wilcox CS. Role of nitric oxide in tubuloglomerular feedback: effects of dietary salt. *Clin Exp Pharmacol Physiol* 1997;24:582–586.

533. Welch WJ, Wilcox CS. Tubuloglomerular feedback and macula densa-derived NO, In: Goligorsky MS, Gross SS (eds.). *Nitric Oxide and the Kidney*. New York: Chapman & Hall, 1997:216–232.

534. Welch WJ, Tojo A, Lee JU, Kang DG, Schnackenberg CG, Wilcox CS. Nitric oxide synthase in the JGA of the SHR: expression and role in tubuloglomerular feedback. *Am J Physiol Renal Physiol* 1999;277:F130–138.

535. Welch WJ, Tojo A, Wilcox CS. Roles of NO and oxygen radicals in tubuloglomerular feedback in SHR. *Am J Physiol Renal Physiol* 2000;278:F769–776.

536. Welch WJ, Wilcox CS. AT1 receptor antagonist combats oxidative stress and restores nitric oxide signaling in the SHR. *Kidney Int* 2001;59:1257–1263.

537. Welch WJ. Effects of isoprostane on tubuloglomerular feedback: roles of TP receptors, NOS, and salt intake. *Am J Physiol Renal Physiol* 2005;288:F757–762.

538. Wetzel RK, Sweadner KJ. Immunocytochemical localization of Na-K-ATPase alpha- and gamma-subunits in rat kidney. *Am J Physiol Renal Physiol* 2001;281:F531–545.

539. Wetzel RK, Sweadner KJ. Phospholemman expression in extraglomerular mesangium and afferent arteriole of the juxtaglomerular apparatus. *Am J Physiol Renal Physiol* 2003;285:F121–129.

540. Wilcox CS. Regulation of renal blood flow by plasma chloride. *J Clin Invest* 1983;71:726–735.

541. Wilcox CS, Welch WJ, Murad F, Gross SS, Taylor G, Levi R, Schmidt HH. Nitric oxide synthase in macula densa regulates glomerular capillary pressure. *Proc Natl Acad Sci U S A* 1992;89:11993–11997.

542. Wilcox CS, Deng X, Welch WJ. NO generation and action during changes in salt intake: roles of nNOS and macula densa. *Am J Physiol* 1998;274:R1588–1593.

543. Wilcox CS, Welch WJ. Thromboxane synthase and TP receptor mRNA in rat kidney and brain: effects of salt intake and ANG II. *Am J Physiol Renal Physiol* 2003;284:F525–531.

544. Wittmann U, Nafz B, Ehmke H, Kirchheim HR, Persson PB. Frequency domain of renal autoregulation in the conscious dog. *Am J Physiol* 1995;269:F317–322.

545. Wolf K, Castrop H, Hartner A, Goppelt-Strube M, Hilgers KF, Kurtz A. Inhibition of the renin-angiotensin system upregulates cyclooxygenase-2 expression in the macula densa. *Hypertension* 1999;34:503–507.

546. Woods LL, DeYoung DR, Smith BE. Regulation of renal hemodynamics after protein feeding: effects of loop diuretics. *Am J Physiol Renal Physiol* 1991;261:F815–823.

547. Wright FS, Schnermann J. Interference with feedback control of glomerular filtration rate by furosemide, triflocin, and cyanide. *J Clin Invest* 1974;53:1695–1708.

548. Wright FS, Mandin H, Persson AE. Studies of the sensing mechanism in the tubuloglomerular feedback pathway. *Kidney Int Suppl* 1982;12:S90–96.

549. Wronski T, Seeliger E, Persson PB, Forner C, Fichtner C, Scheller J, Flemming B. The step response: a method to characterize mechanisms of renal blood flow autoregulation. *Am J Physiol Renal Physiol* 2003;285:F758–764.

550. Wunderlich PF, Brunner FP, Davis JM, Haberle DA, Tholen H, Thiel G. Feedback activation in rat nephrons by sera from patients with acute renal failure. *Kidney Int* 1980;17:497–506.

551. Xie W, Herschman HR. Transcriptional regulation of prostaglandin synthase 2 gene expression by platelet-derived growth factor and serum. *J Biol Chem* 1996;271:31742–31748.

552. Xu JZ, Hall AE, Peterson LN, Bienkowski MJ, Eessalu TE, Hebert SC. Localization of the ROMK protein on apical membranes of rat kidney nephron segments. *Am J Physiol Renal Physiol* 1997;273:F739–F748.

553. Yamaguchi I, Yao L, Sanada H, Ozono R, Mouradian MM, Jose PA, Carey RM, Felder RA. Dopamine D1A receptors and renin release in rat juxtaglomerular cells. *Hypertension* 1997;29:962–968.

554. Yanagisawa H, Jin Z, Kurihara N, Klahr S, Morrissey J, Wada O. Increases in glomerular eicosanoid production in rats with bilateral ureteral obstruction are mediated by enhanced enzyme activities of both the cyclooxygenase and 5–lipoxygenase pathways. *Proc Soc Exp Biol Med* 1993;203:291–296.

555. Yang T, Huang YG, Singh I, Schnermann J, Briggs JP. Localization of bumetanide- and thiazide-sensitive Na-K-Cl cotransporters along the rat nephron. *Am J Physiol* 1996;271:F931–939.

556. Yang T, Singh I, Pham H, Sun D, Smart A, Schnermann JB, Briggs JP. Regulation of cyclooxygenase expression in the kidney by dietary salt intake. *Am J Physiol Renal Physiol* 1998;274:F481–F489.

557. Yang T, Endo Y, Huang YG, Smart A, Briggs JP, Schnermann J. Renin expression in COX-2–knockout mice on normal or low-salt diets. *Am J Physiol Renal Physiol* 2000;279:F819–825.

558. Yang T, Huang Y, Heasley LE, Berl T, Schnermann JB, Briggs JP. MAPK mediation of hypertonicity-stimulated cyclooxygenase-2 expression in renal medullary collecting duct cells. *J Biol Chem* 2000;275:23281–23286.

559. Yang T, Park JM, Arend L, Huang Y, Topaloglu R, Pasumarthy A, Praetorius H, Spring K, Briggs JP, Schnermann J. Low chloride stimulation of prostaglandin E2 release and cyclooxygenase-2 expression in a mouse macula densa cell line. *J Biol Chem* 2000;275:37922–37929.

560. Yaqoob M, Edelstein CL, Wieder ED, Alkhunaizi AM, Gengaro PE, Nemenoff RA, Schrier RW. Nitric oxide kinetics during hypoxia in proximal tubules: effects of acidosis and glycine. *Kidney Int* 1996;49:1314–1319.

561. Yip KP, Holstein-Rathlou NH, Marsh DJ. Chaos in blood flow control in genetic and renovascular hypertensive rats. *Am J Physiol Renal Physiol* 1991;261:F400–408.

562. Yip KP, Holstein-Rathlou NH, Marsh DJ. Dynamics of TGF-initiated nephron-nephron interactions in normotensive rats and SHR. *Am J Physiol Renal Physiol* 1992;262:F980–988.

563. Yip KP, Holstein-Rathlou NH, Marsh DJ. Mechanisms of temporal variation in single-nephron blood flow in rats. *Am J Physiol Renal Physiol* 1993;264:F427–434.

564. Young DB, Rostorfer HH. Renin release responses to acute alterations in renal arterial osmolarity. *Am J Physiol* 1973;225:1009–1014.

565. Young DK, Marsh DJ. Pulse wave propagation in rat renal tubules: implications for GFR autoregulation. *Am J Physiol* 1981;240:F446–458.

566. Zhang J, Hill CE. Differential connexin expression in preglomerular and postglomerular vasculature: accentuation during diabetes. *Kidney Int* 2005;68:1171–1185.

567. Zhang MZ, Wang JL, Cheng HF, Harris RC, McKanna JA. Cyclooxygenase-2 in rat nephron development. *Am J Physiol Renal Physiol* 1997;273:F994–1002.

568. Zhao X, Imig JD. Kidney CYP450 enzymes: biological actions beyond drug metabolism. *Curr Drug Metab* 2003;4:73–84.

569. Zimmermann KW. Ueber den Bau des Glomerulus der Saeugeniere. *Z. Mikr. Anat. Forsch.* 1933;32:176–278.

570. Zou AP, Imig JD, Ortiz de Montellano PR, Sui Z, Falck JR, Roman RJ. Effect of P-450 omega-hydroxylase metabolites of arachidonic acid on tubuloglomerular feedback. *Am J Physiol Renal Physiol* 1994;266:F934–941.

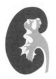

CHAPTER 23

Renal Cortical and Medullary Microcirculations

STRUCTURE AND FUNCTION

Thomas L. Pallone and Chunhua Cao
University of Maryland at Baltimore, Baltimore, Maryland, USA

INTRODUCTION

Approximately 170 L/day of glomerular filtrate is formed in the human renal cortex. Nephrons and collecting ducts perform the enormous task of reabsorbing ~99% of the filtrate while regulating the small quantity excreted. The renal microcirculation returns the reabsorbed fluid to the systemic circulation. Highly specific tubular–vascular relationships in the cortex and medulla accommodate that task. Anatomically, postglomerular capillaries in the cortex form a dense plexus that surrounds proximal and distal tubules while, in contrast, the medullary microcirculation is organized as a countercurrent exchanger that traps and recycles NaCl and urea. Tubular–vascular relationships are well maintained across mammalian species and the capacity for regional control of perfusion within the kidney is highly developed. A growing body of literature supports the hypothesis that differential regulation of blood flow to the cortex and medulla plays a mechanistic role in the regulation of salt and water excretion.

In this chapter, we first focus on microanatomy and tubular–vascular relationships. Subsequently, transport properties of cortical capillaries and medullary vasa recta are reviewed. Finally, topics relevant to control of vasoactivity and the modulation of intrarenal blood flow are covered. Important related topics, treated in depth in other chapters of this text, include glomerular hemodynamics and filtration, the juxtaglomerular apparatus, macula densa signaling, and tubuloglomerular feedback.

ANATOMY OF THE RENAL CIRCULATION

Cortical Microcirculation

The basic vascular pattern of the kidney is preserved across mammalian species (24, 26, 28, 265, 266, 301) (Fig. 1). The renal artery branches into interlobar arteries that ascend within the renal pelvis to enter the parenchyma. In multipapillate organisms, the interlobar arteries travel to-ward the cortex along the columns of Bertin. These vessels change direction and follow an arc-like course near the corticomedullary border to become arcuate arteries. The arcuate artery gives rise to the interlobular arteries that ascend, in radial fashion, toward the cortical surface. Afferent arterioles arise from interlobular arteries at angles that vary with their cortical depth. Afferents that supply deep glomeruli near the corticomedullary junction (juxtamedullary glomeruli) leave the interlobular artery at a recurrent angle. In contrast, superficial afferent arterioles that supply glomeruli near the surface of the kidney line up with the interlobular artery as its termination.

In some species (rat, cat, dog, and *Meriones*) a pair of intra-arterial "cushions" exist as parallel ridges that project from the origin of the juxtamedullary afferent arteriole into the lumen of the parent intralobular artery (Fig. 2A) (152, 153). The cushions are 18 to 30 μm in length, composed of a ground substance in which smooth muscle cells are embedded and covered by a layer of continuous endothelium (Fig. 2B) (392). The cushions are ideally placed to regulate blood flow distribution within the cortex. Given that blood flow to the renal medulla arises largely from the efferent flow of juxtamedullary glomeruli, it is also plausible that the cushions play a role in the regulation of blood flow to the medulla. The cushions have been hypothesized to separate plasma and red blood cells and alter medullary hematocrit by "skimming" plasma from a red cell–free layer near the vessel wall (152, 459).

The structure of afferent and efferent arterioles varies with cortical location. Afferent arterioles are composed of one to three layers of smooth muscle cells. Muscle and elastic tissue diminish near the glomerulus and the media is replaced by granular cells of the juxtaglomerular apparatus. The diameters of efferent arterioles vary from as small as 12 μm in the superficial cortex to 28 μm for juxtamedullary glomeruli. Efferent arterioles in the superficial cortex branch to form a dense peritubular capillary plexus. Ten different branching patterns have been described (37). In contrast to the efferent arterioles of superficial glomeruli, those of juxtamedullary glomeruli most frequently cross the corticomedullary junction to enter the outer stripe of the outer medulla where they give rise to descending vasa recta (DVR). DVR are transitional vessels along which smooth muscle is replaced by contractile pericytes (256, 301). A small fraction of blood flow to the renal medulla may bypass juxtamedullary glomeruli in "shunt" vessels

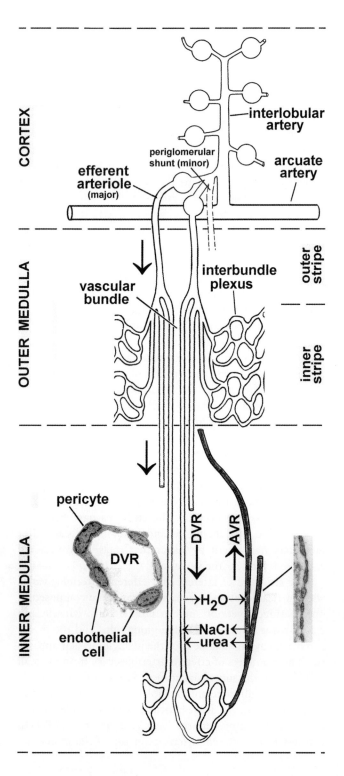

(*dashed line*, Fig. 1). Casellas and Mimran have described variations of those shunts as (1) branches of afferent arterioles, (2) continuous vessels from which afferent arterioles arise as side branches, (3) short vascular connections between afferent and efferent arterioles, and (4) pelvic arterioles derived from afferent arterioles near the renal hilus (Fig. 3) (69). Several reviews of arteriolar patterns in the renal cortex have been written (26, 153, 448).

The bulk of glomerular filtrate is reabsorbed by the proximal convoluted tubule (PCT). That reabsorbate is conducted through the cortical interstitium and taken up by peritubular capillaries. The peritubular interstitium of the cortex has been divided into "narrow" and "wide" portions comprising 0.6% and 3.4% of tissue volume (17, 467). The narrow interstitium is flanked by highly fenestrated capillary wall on one side and the basolateral membrane of the PCT on the other (Fig. 4) (303, 317). Since only 26% of the tubular surface faces the narrow interstitium if follows that substantial quantities of fluid must flow from the wide to the narrow portion, implying that some spatial hydrostatic pressure gradients must exist within the cortical interstitium (17, 617).

Medullary Microcirculation

Blood flow to the renal medulla is supplied by DVR. In the rat, DVR are generally about one half the diameter of the parent efferent arteriole; however, a few are larger, in the range of 20 μm. The larger DVR lie in the center of vascular bundles and penetrate to the deepest regions of

FIGURE 1 Microcirculation of the renal cortex and medulla. Within the renal cortex, interlobular arteries, derived from the arcuate artery, ascend toward the cortical surface. Superficial and midcortical glomeruli arise at obtuse and right angles while juxtamedullary glomeruli arise at an acute, recurrent angle from the interlobular artery. Most blood flow to the medulla arises from juxtamedullary efferent arterioles. A minor fraction might also be derived from periglomerular shunt pathways (*dashed lines*). In the outer stripe of the outer medulla, juxtamedullary efferent arterioles give rise to descending vasa recta (DVR) that combine with ascending vasa recta (AVR), and sometimes, thin descending limbs of Henle, to form vascular bundles. Vascular bundles are the prominent feature of the inner stripe of the outer medulla. DVR on the periphery of vascular bundles perfuse the interbundle capillary plexus that supplies nephrons (thick ascending limb, collecting duct, long looped thin descending limbs, not shown). DVR in the center of the bundles continue across the inner-outer medullary junction to perfuse the inner medulla. In some species, thin descending limbs of short looped nephrons migrate toward or become associated with vascular bundles. In the inner medulla, vascular bundles disappear and vasa recta become dispersed with thin loops of Henle and collecting ducts. Blood from the interbundle capillary plexus is returned without rejoining vascular bundles. DVR have a continuous endothelium (*inset*) and are surrounded by contractile pericytes. Like cortical peritubular capillaries, the AVR endothelium is highly fenestrated. As blood flows toward the papillary tip, NaCl and urea diffuse into DVR and out of AVR. Transmural gradients of NaCl and urea drive water efflux across the DVR wall via aquaporin-1 water channels. The increasing size of the circled "P" is to represent the rise in DVR plasma protein concentration with medullary depth. (From Pallone TL, Turner MR, Edwards A, Jamison RL. Countercurrent exchange in the renal medulla. *Am J Physiol Regul Integr Comp Physiol* 2003;284:R1153–R1175, with permission.)

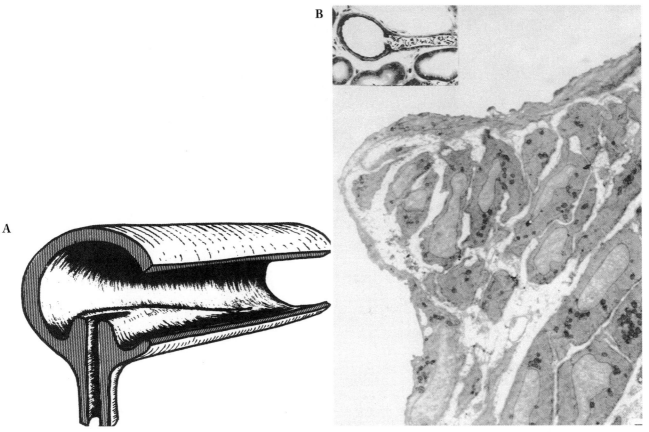

FIGURE 2   The intra-arterial cushion. **A:** In some species intra-arterial cushions are present where juxtamedullary afferent arterioles arise from interlobular arterioles. **B:** A longitudinal section through an afferent arteriole shows an intra-arterial cushion at its origin from the interlobular artery (inset, × 160). The cushion protrudes into the lumen of the parent vessel. Smooth muscle cells of the cushion are embedded in a copious matrix (×4000). Intra-arterial cushions might affect the relative volume fraction of red blood cells versus plasma (hematocrit) that is directed from intralobular arterioles to juxtamedullary glomeruli and renal medulla. It is also conceivable that they regulate the relative distribution of blood flow between the superficial and juxtamedullary cortex (see text). (From Fourman J, Moffat DB. *The Blood Vessels of the Kidney.* Oxford: Osney Mead, 1971; Moffat DB, Creasey M. The fine structure of the intra-arterial cushions at the origins of the juxtamedullary afferent arterioles in the rat kidney. *J Anat* 1971;110:409–419, with permission.)

the inner medulla (256, 301, 448). The smooth muscle of the efferent arteriole is gradually replaced by pericytes (Fig. 5). Pericytes are smooth muscle–like cells that surround DVR and continuous capillaries of other organ beds (538). Pericytes may become more sparce with medullary depth but are retained well into the inner medulla (Fig 6.) (462). DVR have a continuous endothelium with tight junctions, whereas the ascending vasa recta (AVR) that arises from them has a highly fenestrated endothelium (Figs. 5 and 7) (386, 534).

The most striking characteristic of the outer medullary circulation is its separation into vascular bundles and the dense capillary plexus in the interbundle region of the inner stripe (Fig. 8). Vascular–tubular relationships in the inner stripe separate blood flow destined to perfuse the outer and inner medulla. In addition, certain peribundle nephron segments lie within diffusion distance of vascular bundles. The "simple" vascular bundle of the rabbit, guinea pig, dog, cat, monkey, and human comprises only DVR and AVR but no nephrons (26, 301, 448). DVR that supply blood flow to the interbundle capillary plexus peel off

from the periphery of the vascular bundles as they pass through the inner stripe (316). AVR within vascular bundles are only those that originate from inner medullary DVR. In contrast, blood leaving the outer medullary interbundle plexus ascends directly to the cortex without rejoining vascular bundles. Thus countercurrent exchange in the inner stripe involves all DVR and those AVR that drain the inner medulla (simple bundles). The "complex" vascular bundle of some rodent species incorporates the descending thin limbs of short-looped nephrons (nephrons that turn at the inner–outer medullary junction). That pattern varies with species; the degree to which thin, descending limbs are incorporated into vascular bundles is greatest in the mouse (Fig. 9) (26, 256, 301, 448). The parallel arrangement of DVR in the vascular bundles of all species strongly suggests that they play a role to modulate regional blood flow. It is logical to assume that constriction of vessels on the bundle periphery would favor perfusion of the inner medulla. Conversely, preferential constriction of DVR in the bundle center should favor perfusion of the outer medullary interbundle region. As

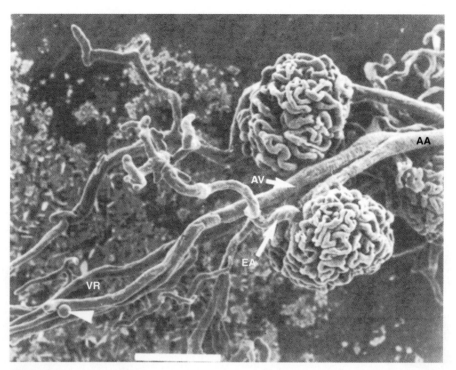

FIGURE 3   Corrosion cast showing a periglomerular shunt vessel at the corticomedullary junction. The afferent arteriole (AA) of a juxtamedullary glomerulus gives rise to a side branch (AV), which forms descending vasa recta (VR). The efferent arteriole (EA) of the juxtamedullary glomerulus is visible; *arrowhead*, 16 μm sphere; *bar*, 100 μm. It is probable that some blood flow that reaches the renal medulla bypasses juxtamedullary glomeruli by shunts such as the one illustrated, but the overall fraction of medullary blood flow derived from shunts is probably small (i.e., < 10%). (From Casellas D, Mimran A. Shunting in renal microvasculature of the rat: a scanning electron microscopic study of corrosion casts. *Anat Rec* 1981;201:237–248, with permission.)

illustrated in Fig. 8A, individual vascular bundles combine in the outer stripe to form "giant" vascular bundles in *Psammomys* but not other species such as the rat (Figs. 8B and 8C).

Below the inner–outer medullary junction, vascular bundles disappear and individual DVR and AVR become dispersed among thin limbs of Henle and collecting ducts. Throughout the medulla, AVR are larger and more numerous than DVR. As a consequence, during passage of blood from the juxtamedullary efferent arteriole to DVR and then AVR, single-vessel flow rate successively falls as the sum of overall microvessel circumference increases (219, 362, 448). Interstitial space in the outer medullary vascular bundles is sparse, but in the inner medulla the fraction of attributable to interstitium rises substantially (256, 285, 448). In some species, renal medullary interstitial cells (RMICs) of the inner medulla appear to be tethered between thin limbs of Henle and vasa recta (Fig. 10) (317). Their horizontal arrangement might help to preserve corticomedullary solute gradients by limiting diffusion along the corticomedullary axis (378, 400, 570). RMICs have receptors for angiotensin II (ANG II), bradykinin and endothelin, and release vasoactive agents (prostaglandin E$_2$ [PGE$_2$], medullipin). RMICs are contractile (220, 580, 644, 658).

TRANSPORT FUNCTIONS AND PROPERTIES

The Renal Cortex and Capillary Uptake of Tubular Reabsorbate

Cortical peritubular capillaries are fenestrated, with large surface areas and high hydraulic conductivity. It is generally accepted that fluid is driven into the cortical interstitium from the PCT due to the generation of a locally hypertonic fluid within the lateral intercellular space between PCT epithelial cells. The local hypertonicity results from the secretion of small hydrophilic solutes by proximal tubular cells. Dilution of the interstitium in the vicinity of the capillary wall with protein-free fluid both lowers interstitial oncotic pressure and raises interstitial hydraulic pressure. These effects generate Starling forces that favor capillary reabsorption.

A substantial body of evidence has demonstrated that modulation of cortical peritubular capillary oncotic pressure alters PCT reabsorption. Intra-aortic injection or peritubular perfusion of colloid-free or hyperoncotic fluid leads to decreases or increases proximal reabsorption, respectively (47, 48, 550). Although it seems inviting to surmise that protein oncotic pressure acts directly to enhance fluid movement out of the PCT, several lines of evi-

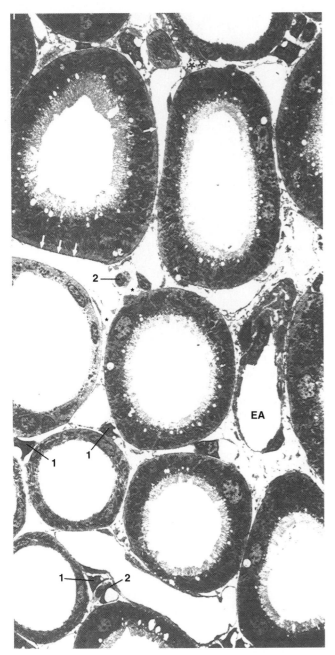

FIGURE 4 Peritubular interstitium of the renal cortex. The narrow portion of the cortical interstitium *(arrows)* lies immediately adjacent to the basement membrane of the proximal tubule. The wide portion *(stars)* lies between peritubular capillaries and cortical nephrons. Interstitial cells are fibroblast-like (1) or rounded (2) (× 1000). EA, efferent arteriole. (From Lemley KV, Kriz W. Anatomy of the renal interstitium. *Kidney Int* 1991;39:370–381, with permission.)

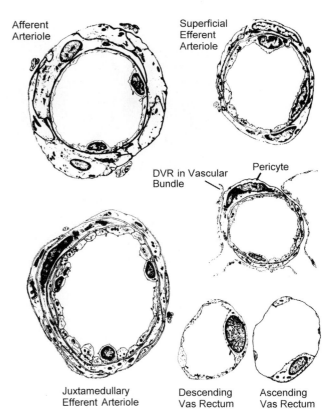

FIGURE 5 Structure and transition of cortical and medullary vessels. The proximal afferent arteriole is composed of at least two layers of smooth muscle cells. The muscularity and size of cortical efferent arterioles differ with location. Note the difference between the superficial and juxtamedullary efferent arterioles. The juxtamedullary efferent arteriole is larger, has a thicker, multilayered media, and its endothelium is composed of more numerous endothelial cells. In the illustration, a descending vas rectum (DVR) in a vascular bundle is adjacent to three fenestrated ascending vasa recta (AVR). The DVR wall is surrounded by a contractile pericyte. At the bottom right, DVR and AVR from the inner medulla are shown. Inner medullary DVR have a continuous endothelium through most of their length as pericytes become more scarce with medullary depth. Terminal DVR and the entire AVR wall is fenestrated. (From Jamison RL, Kriz W. *Urinary Concentrating Mechanism: Structure and Function.* Oxford: Oxford University Press, 1982, with permission.)

dence suggest otherwise. Oncotic pressure changes fail to modulate reabsorption when active transport by PCT epithelia is inhibited (520), PCT reabsorption rates correlate with glomerular filtration rates (GFRs) but not with interstitial Starling forces (589), hydropenia blunts the capacity of hyperoncotic albumin to enhance PCT reabsorption (427), and elevation of luminal pressure in the PCT fails to enhance reabsorption (179). The osmotic water permea-

bility of the proximal convoluted tubule ($P_f = 0.1 - 0.4$ cm/s) is probably too low for small oncotic pressure changes to substantially affect transmembrane water flux (9, 180). It has been suggested that peritubular oncotic pressure might modulate PCT volume reabsorption by affecting solute reabsorption rate (33, 181) or by enhancing paracellular backleak into the PCT lumen (223).

Whatever the mechanisms that influence PCT reabsorption, an immense peritubular volume reabsorption from the cortical interstitium must be accommodated by the cortical microcirculation. Since lymphatics remove less than 1% of the reabsorbate (469), the route for return to the systemic circulation must be via peritubular capillaries. As reviewed by Aukland et al. (17), the high oncotic pressure of postglomerular plasma cannot be invoked as the primary driving force for capillary uptake in all cases. Older rats in which renal lymphatic (and therefore

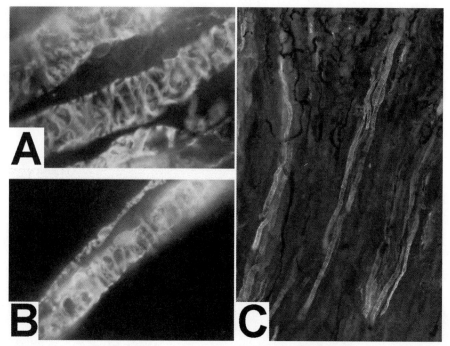

FIGURE 6   Distribution of descending vasa recta pericytes. **A,B:** Immunofluorescent staining of descending vas rectum (DVR) pericytes using anti–α-smooth muscle actin as primary antibody. The pericytes are present on DVR from outer medullary vascular bundles (**A**) and those from the inner medulla (**B**) (× 1000). **C:** Low-power image of immunofluorescent staining of DVR pericytes using anti–α-smooth muscle actin antibody. Some vessels show pericytes throughout their length to the papillary tip. Black vessels are filled with India ink (× 100). (From Park F, Mattson DL, Roberts LA, Cowley AW, Jr. Evidence for the presence of smooth muscle alpha-actin within pericytes of the renal medulla. *Am J Physiol* 1997;273:R1742–R1748, with permission.)

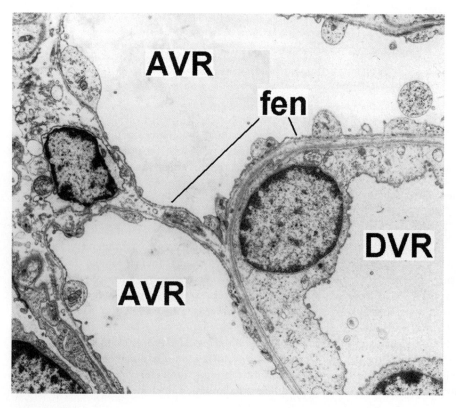

FIGURE 7   Electron micrograph of descending vas rectum (DVR) and ascending vas rectum (AVR). Electron micrograph of DVR and AVR in rat vascular bundles. DVR have a continuous endothelium and AVR are fenestrated. Note the minimal interstitium that exists between vessels in this region (× 12,400). (From Pallone TL, Work J, Myers RL, Jamison RL. Transport of sodium and urea in outer medullary descending vasa recta. *J Clin Invest* 1994;93:212–222, with permission.)

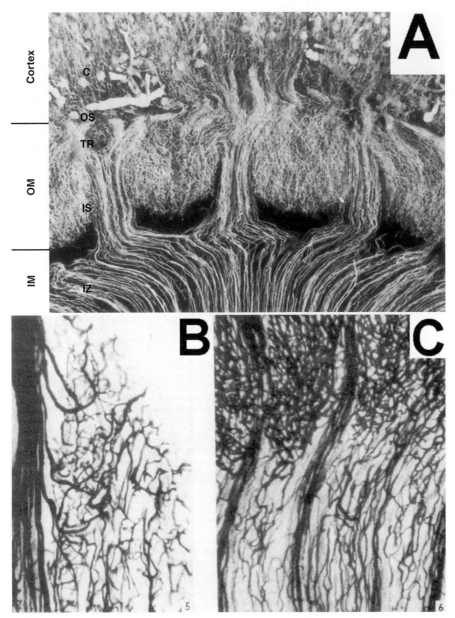

FIGURE 8   Arterial injection of *Psammomys obesus*. **A:** Photograph of the microvasculature of the desert rodent *Psammomys obesus* obtained by injecting the arteries of the kidney with Microfil and digesting the tissue. The distinct arteriolar patterns of the cortex and outer and inner medulla are apparent. In *Psammomys*, the separation of the outer medulla into vascular bundles and the dense capillary plexus of the interbundle region (*) is striking because vasa recta coalesce into giant vascular bundles. OM, outer medulla; IM, inner medulla. Designations on the original figure are c, cortex; TR, transitional region (outer stripe of the outer medulla); IS, inner stripe of the outer medulla; IZ, inner zone (inner medulla). (From Bankir L, Kaissling B, de Rouffignac C, Kriz W. The vascular organization of the kidney of *Psammomys obesus*. *Anat Embryol (Berl)* 1979;155:149–160, with permission.). **B,C:** India ink injection study of vascular bundles in the outer medulla of the rat. In contrast to *Psammomys*, individual vascular bundles do not coalesce into giant bundles. The bundles are more evenly dispersed throughout the inner stripe of the outer medulla. This pattern is typical of many mammalian species including the rat, mouse and human. (From Moffat DB, Fourman J. The vascular pattern of the rat kidney. *J Anat* 1963;97:543–553, with permission.)

presumably interstitial) protein concentration is equal to that of plasma continue to reabsorb tubular fluid (469). Furthermore, PCT reabsorption occurs even in kidneys perfused with colloid-free solutions (533). Particularly in the latter case, it is apparent that interstitial pressure must exceed intracapillary luminal pressure to provide the driving force for transcapillary volume flux. It also follows that the peritubular capillaries must be tethered to the interstitium in a way that prevents an inwardly directed transmural pressure from collapsing the lumen.

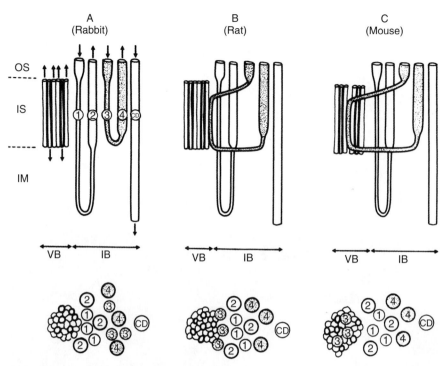

FIGURE 9   Tubular–vascular relationships in the outer medulla. Organization of the inner stripe of the outer medulla. Top and bottom panels show longitudinal and cross-sectional views, respectively. The extent to which the thin descending limbs (tDLH) of short-looped nephrons associate with vascular bundles varies between species. In the rabbit, no association exists whereas in the rat and mouse, the tDLH migrates to the periphery or becomes incorporated within vascular bundles, respectively. VB, vascular bundle; IB, interbundle region; 1 and 2, thin descending and thick ascending limbs of long looped nephrons; 3 and 4, thin descending and thick ascending limbs of short looped nephrons. (From Bankir L, de Rouffignac C. Urinary concentrating ability: insights from comparative anatomy. *Am J Physiol* 1985;249:R643–R666, with permission.)

The Renal Medulla and Countercurrent Exchange

Like the capillary bed of other organs, the renal medullary microcirculation supplies oxygen and nutrients to the surrounding tissue. Additionally, however, corticomedullary gradients of NaCl and urea must be preserved to enable urinary concentration. This task is accommodated by countercurrent exchange between DVR and AVR (307, 384, 448, 453). Countercurrent exchange is an adaptation found throughout nature. The maintenance of high gas tensions in swim bladders of deep sea fish and the minimization of heat loss from the extremities of aquatic and arctic animals relies on this strategy (453, 530).

The microcirculation of the renal medulla traps NaCl and urea deposited to the interstitium by the loops of Henle and collecting ducts. Countercurrent exchange provides the means by which blood flow through the medulla is concentrated and then diluted to preserve corticomedullary solute gradients established by countercurrent multiplication. The hypothesis that vasa recta are a purely "U-tube" diffusive countercurrent exchanger implies the following function. NaCl and urea diffuse from interstitium into DVR plasma enroute from the corticomedullary

junction toward the papillary tip. The solutes diffuse out from AVR plasma to be returned to the interstitium as blood returns to the cortex. That theory predicts that countercurrent exchanger efficiency will be favored if permeability to solute is high.

In fact, vasa recta probably do not function as a purely diffusive countercurrent exchanger. Several features point to greater complexity. Tubular–vascular relationships in the outer and inner medulla differ markedly (Figs. 1 and 9) and the endotheliums of DVR and AVR are continuous and fenestrated, respectively (Fig. 5). The discoveries of aquaporin-1 (AQP1) water channels and the facilitated urea carrier, urea transporter type B (UTB), in DVR endothelia (see following section) shows that transcellular and paracellular pathways involving water and urea are involved in equilibration of DVR plasma with the interstitium. Efflux of water across the DVR wall to the medullary interstitium occurs across AQP1 water channels and AQP1 excludes NaCl and urea, implying that both water removal and diffusive influx of solute contribute to transmural equilibration (442, 444, 452, 453).

Transport of Small Solutes and Water by Vasa Recta and Red Blood Cells

TRANSPORT OF WATER ACROSS THE DVR WALL: SMALL SOLUTES, OSMOTIC PRESSURE, AND STARLING FORCES

Mass balance dictates that water, NaCl, and urea must be remhoved from the medullary interstitium at a rate that equals deposition by the loops of Henle and collecting tubules (302, 448). Papillary micropuncture studies in the hydropenic rat (260) and hamster (176, 361) have shown that DVR and AVR plasma osmolality rises in parallel with tubular fluid from the loops of Henle and collecting ducts. DVR plasma protein also becomes concentrated along the direction of flow, implying that water is lost from DVR lumen to the interstitium (Table 1, Fig. 1) (514, 515). Uptake of fluid into AVR exceeds that lost from DVR, accounting for mass balance in the medulla (118, 256, 456, 585, 647). Volume efflux from the DVR occurs despite an intracapillary oncotic pressure that exceeds hydraulic pressure so that "Starling forces" cannot fully explain transmural volume efflux. According to Starling, volume flux (J_v) across a capillary wall is a function of capillary (P_c) and interstitial hydraulic pressure (P_i) and luminal (π_c) and interstitial (π_i) oncotic pressure (308).

$$J_V = L_P[(P_c - P_i) - (\pi_c - \pi_i)] \qquad \text{(Eq. 1)}$$

where L_p is the hydraulic conductivity. To explain volume efflux from the DVR in a manner compatible with Eq. 1, a negative interstitial hydraulic pressure or very high interstitial oncotic pressure has to be postulated. In either of those cases, however, interstitial driving forces would prevent volume uptake by AVR violating mass balance. Neither possibility can be the explanation (446, 448, 515).

Due to the lag in equilibration of DVR plasma with the interstitium, NaCl and urea concentrations in the interstitium exceed those in DVR so that a transendothelial osmotic gradient favors water efflux across the DVR wall. That driving force could account for water efflux only if there is a transendothelial pathway across which small solutes are effective to drive water movement (515). Volume flux across a membrane can be simulated by Eq. 2 that accounts for osmotic reflection coefficients (σ) to individual solutes. In the current context, small solutes (σ_{ss}) and proteins (σ_{pr}) are of importance, leading to (274)

$$J_V = L_P[\Delta P - \sigma_{pr}\Delta\pi_{pr} - \sigma_{ss}\Delta\pi_s] \qquad \text{(Eq. 2)}$$

where ΔP is transmembrane hydraulic pressure, $\Delta\pi_{pr}$ and $\Delta\pi_{SS}$ are the transmembrane osmotic pressure due to protein and small solutes, respectively (515). The hypothesis that small solutes act to promote volume movement across the DVR is equivalent to postulating that $\sigma_{ss} > 0$. Support for this was readily obtained. Volume efflux from DVR was prevented by elimination of corticomedullary (and therefore transendothelial) NaCl and urea gradients by furosemide (456) and in vivo microperfusion of DVR with buffers made

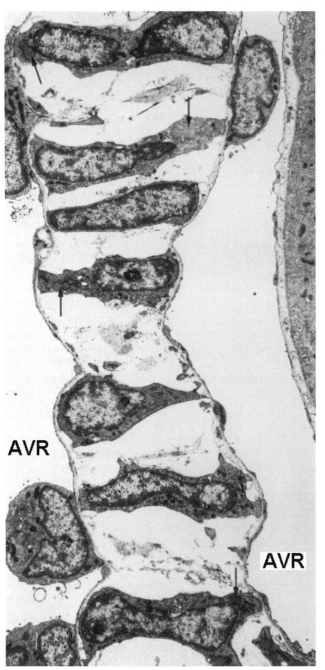

FIGURE 10 Renal medullary interstitial cells (RMICs). RMIC from the rat kidney appear to be tethered between thin limbs and vasa recta in the inner medulla. Interstitial spaces lie between the cells and the cells are stacked like rungs of a ladder. RMIC are contractile and secrete vasoactive paracrine agents (see text). The stacked arrangement or RMICs in some species has been suggested to help retard axial diffusion that would otherwise tend to dissipate corticomedullary gradients of NaCl and urea. V, venous or ascending vasa recta. Arrows point to lipid droplets within RMIC. (From Lemley KV, Kriz W. Anatomy of the renal interstitium. *Kidney Int* 1991;39:370–381, with permission.)

TABLE 1 Vasa Recta Plasma Protein Concentration, Hydraulic and Oncotic Pressures Measured in Rats and Hamsters

Location	VR/P	Cp (g/dl)	Oncotic Pressure (mm Hg)	Hydraulic Pressure (mm Hg)	Osmolality (mOsm)	Condition (reference)
DVR-base	1.76	7.1	26.0	9.2	—	Hydropenia
DVR-tip	—	—	—	—	—	(514)
AVR-base	1.38	5.6	18.1	7.8	—	
DVR-base	1.43	7.1	26.0	6.6	688	Hydropenia
DVR-tip	1.66	6.4	21.8	7.4	759	(515)
AVR-base	—	—	—	—	—	
DVR-base	1.0–1.8[a]	—	—	—	—	Hydropenia
DVR-tip	2.1–2.9	—	—	—	—	(585)
DVR-base	1.42	5.1	16.0	—	—	Hydropenia
DVR-tip	—	—	—	—	—	(647)
AVR-base	1.11	4.0	11.2	—	—	
DVR-base	—	—	—	15.7	—	Hydropenia
DVR-tip	—	—	—	11.4	—	(173)
AVR-base	—	—	—	10.2	—	
DVR-base	1.08	5.2	16.7	9.5	573	Hydropenia
DVR-tip	1.42	6.8	18.2	9.1	1011	(456)
AVR-base	—	—	—	—	—	
DVR-base	1.10	5.4	17.6	12.2	356	Furosemide
DVR-tip	1.12	5.5	18.2	11.2	377	(456)
AVR-base	—	—	—	—	—	
DVR-base	1.19	5.7	18.6	11.7	380	Furosemide
DVR-tip	—	—	—	11.2	386	(454)
AVR-base	1.17	5.6	18.4	9.6	—	
AVR-mid	—	5.2	16.7	8.0	—	Hydropenia
AVR-mid	—	5.2	16.7	16.0	—	Furosemide (437)
DVR-mid	—	—	—	9.1–15.5[b]	—	Plasma/ANP[c]
AVR-mid	—	—	—	7.8–14.3	—	Plasma/ANP
DVR-mid	—	—	—	8.4–10.8	—	Plasma/furosemide
AVR-mid	—	—	—	7.8–10.0	—	Plasma/furosemide (381)

—, Not measured as part of the study.

VR/P, vasa recta to plasma ratio; Cp, plasma protein concentration; DVR, descending vasa recta; AVR, ascending vasa recta; base, mid, tip, micropuncture site along exposed papilla (inner one third of the inner medulla, blood flows from base to tip in DVR and tip to base in AVR); ANP, atrial natriuretic peptide.

[a]Ratio measured from ^{131}I-albumin activity.

[b]Values refer to changes before and after administration of either ANP or furosemide.

[c]Measured after replacement of surgical fluid losses with plasma.

hypertonic or hypotonic to the papillary interstitium generated volume uptake or efflux, respectively ($\sigma_{NaCl} > 0$) (432).

DVR HYDRAULIC CONDUCTIVITY AND OSMOTIC WATER PERMEABILITY

The predominant pathway that conducts water efflux across the DVR is the AQP1 water channel. AQP1 but not other aquaporins are expressed by DVR endothelia (414, 415).

Diffusional water permeability (P_D) of isolated, microperfused DVR, measured by efflux of ^3H_2O was reduced by the AQP1-blocking mercurial agent p-chloromercuribenzenesulfonate (pCMBS). Dramatic confirmation was provided by the demonstration that *osmotic* water permeability (P_f) of microperfused DVR, measured by driving water flux with transmural gradients of NaCl, was driven from ~1100 μm/s to nearly 0 by pCMBS (Fig. 11A). In contrast, when albumin rather than

NaCl was used to drive water flux, P_f was much higher, ~16,700 μm/s and insensitive to pCMBS, implying that a different pathway conducts transmural volume flux driven by oncotic pressure (444, 452). The results support the notion that NaCl and urea drive water flux across the DVR wall exclusively through AQP1 (contribution to total transmural water conductivity is $P_f \sim 1100$ μm/s), while hydraulic pressure and oncotic pressure drive most water flux through a high conductivity parallel pathway (paracellular or other). Mathematically the AQP1 and parallel pathways are best stimulated as (117, 118),

$$J_{V,P} = L_{P,P}[\Delta P - \sigma_{pr}\Delta\pi_{pr}] \text{ and, } J_{V,C} = L_{P,C}[\Delta P - \sum_i \Delta\pi_i]$$

(Eq. 3A,B)

where the additional subscript "P" (probably pericellular) refers to the high conductivity pathway for which $\sigma_{NaCl} = \sigma_{urea} = 0$ (590) and the subscript "C" refers to the transcellular AQP1 pathway for which $\sigma_{NaCl} = \sigma_{urea} = 1$. Hydraulic conductivity (L_p) and osmotic water permeability (P_f) are related according to $L_p = (P_f \times V_w)/(RT)$, where V_W is the partial molar volume of water. Existing measurements of DVR osmotic water permeability are summarized in Table 2. A rigorous discussion of the measurement of and relationships between these transport parameters has been provided (452, 590).

The AQP1 knockout mouse provided additional confirmation of the role of AQP1 in DVR water transport. P_f of DVR in AQP1 knockout mice, driven by NaCl, was indeed very low (Fig. 11B). An intriguing finding was that urea and larger solutes (raffinose, molecular weight [MW] 594; glucose, MW 180) drive significant water flux despite AQP1 deletion, a finding that implies the existence of a non-AQP1 route across which those solutes are osmotically active. A potential candidate for the non-AQP1, pCMBS-insensitive pathway is the UTB urea trans-porter (see following section), which is expressed by the DVR endothelium and can function as a water channel (480, 621, 623).

INSIGHTS FROM MODELING: AQP1 AND THE ENHANCEMENT OF EXCHANGER EFFICIENCY

Mathematical models of the urinary concentration have played an important role in the evolution of our understanding. Simulation of nephrons and the microcirculation is difficult so that investigators prefer to account for one while neglecting the other. Vasa recta models typically assume

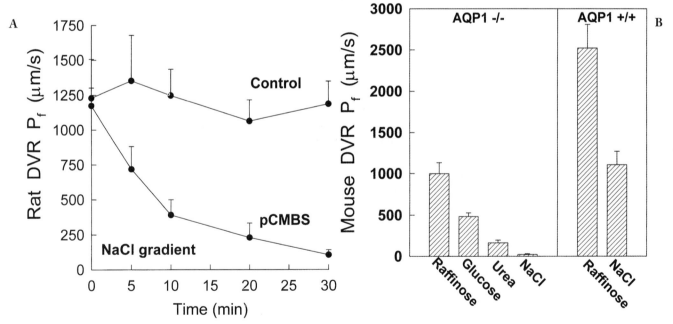

FIGURE 11 Osmotic water permeability (P_f) of outer medullary DVR. **A:** P_f was measured in glutaraldehyde-fixed rat descending vas rectum (DVR) by measuring the rate of transmural water flux generated by a bath greater than lumen NaCl gradient. Sequential measurements in controls were stable. In contrast, exposure to p-chloromercuribenzene sulfonate (pCMBS, 2 mM), an agent that covalently binds to cysteine residues on aquaporin-1, reduced P_f to nearly zero. In these experiments, glutaraldehyde fixation was necessary to prevent deterioration of the vessel caused by pCMBS and other harsh conditions of the experiment. **B:** P_f was measured in AQP1 null ($^{-/-}$) or replete ($^{+/+}$) murine DVR by transmural gradients of NaCl, urea, glucose, or raffinose. When NaCl was the solute used to drive water flux, deletion of AQP1 reduced P_f from ~1100 μm/s to nearly zero. Water flux driven by raffinose (molecular weight [MW], 564) was markedly reduced by AQP1deletion (compare AQP1 $^{-/-}$ to $^{+/+}$), but remained unexpectedly high. Similarly, glucose (MW, 180) and urea (MW, 60) gradients drove measurable water flux across AQP1 ($^{-/-}$) DVR. (From Pallone TL, Edwards A, Ma T, Silldorff EP, Verkman AS. Requirement of aquaporin-1 for NaCl-driven water transport across descending vasa recta. *J Clin Invest* 2000;105:215–222 and Pallone TL, Kishore BK, Nielsen S, Agre P, Knepper MA. Evidence that aquaporin-1 mediates NaCl-induced water flux across descending vasa recta. *Am J Physiol* 1997;272:F587–F59, with permission.)

TABLE 2 Hydraulic Conductivity, Osmotic Water Permeability, and Solute Reflection Coefficients of Vasa Recta

Parameter	Driving Force	OMDVR	IMDVR	IMAVR	Reference
$L_p \times 10^{-6}$ (cm $\times$ s^{-1} $\times$ mm Hg^{-1})	Albumin gradient	—	1.4[a]	—	454
$L_p \times 10^{-6}$ (cm $\times$ s^{-1} $\times$ mm Hg^{-1})	Albumin gradient	1.6	—	—	590
$L_p \times 10^{-6}$ (cm $\times$ s^{-1} $\times$ mm Hg^{-1})	NaCl gradient	0.12[b]	—	—	442, 444
$L_p \times 10^{-6}$ (cm $\times$ s^{-1} $\times$ mm Hg^{-1})	Hydraulic pressure	—	—	12.5	347, 432

Parameter	Method	OMDVR	IMDVR	IMAVR	Reference
$\sigma_{Albumin}$	Sieving	0.89[c]	—	—	590
$\sigma_{Albumin}$	Sieving	—	—	0.78	435
$\sigma_{Albumin}$	Osmotic	—	—	0.70	347
σ_{Na}	Osmotic	—	< 0.05[d]	0.00[d]	432, 434
σ_{Na}	Osmotic	~ 0.03[d]	—	—	452
σ_{Na}	Sieving	~ 1.0[e]	—	—	452
$\sigma_{Raffinose}$	Sieving	~ 1.0[e]	—	—	452

—, Not measured as part of the study.

OMDVR, outer medullary descending vasa recta; IMAVR, inner medullary ascending vasa recta; IMDVR, inner medullary descending vasa recta.

[a] Assumes a reflection coefficient to albumin of 1.0.

[b] Evidence shows that transmural NaCl gradients drive water flux exclusively through water channels, whereas albumin drives water flux predominantly through water channels along with a small component via other pathway(s); see text and references 444, 452, and 590.

[c] Not significantly different from 1.0.

[d] Measurement of σ_{Na} for the vessel wall as a whole.

[e] σ_{Na}, $\sigma_{Raffinose}$ for the putative aquaporin-1 water channel pathway through which NaCl gradients drive water flux, see text and references 444, and 452.

specified corticomedullary solute concentrations and simulate transport properties of the vessel wall. Wang and Michel revised this approach by specifying the rate of deposition of NaCl, urea and water to the medullary interstitium as though they are generated within the interstitium. In agreement with electron probe measurements, they predicted an exponential increase in corticomedullary solute concentration in the medulla (286, 604, 605). A weakness of models that neglect simulation of loops of Henle and collecting ducts is that solute generation rates in the interstitium are assigned as inputs and interstitial solute concentrations calculated as predictions. Variations of blood flow and transport properties cannot affect the interstitial appearance of NaCl, urea and water from nephrons as would occur in vivo. Convincing evidence has been provided that structure and properties of nephrons can abruptly vary with medullary depth (81, 82, 458, 462, 580).

Many key parameters needed to simulate microvascular exchange in the renal medulla (solute permeabilities, reflection coefficients, hydraulic conductivities) have been measured. Those data have been combined with more complete simulations of transcellular pathways for urea and water transport to perform additional simulations. The models predict that AQP1 might play an important role in raising medullary interstitial osmolality by driving water

efflux from DVR to the medullary interstitium across AQP1 water channels (see previous sections). That water movement effectively shunts DVR plasma volume to the AVR, reducing blood flow to the deep medulla. This favors high diffusive exchanger efficiency in the deep inner medulla where urea is added to the interstitium from the collecting duct. Stated another way, it reduces the lag in equilibration that leads to solute "washout" from the deep medulla (116, 442, 442, 581). The net effect is to enhance interstitial osmolality (Fig. 12). Interest in this intriguing prediction is heightened by the observation that transmural water flux can be driven across the wall of AQP1 null mice by solutes other than NaCl (Fig. 11B). If the non-AQP1 pathway is important in vivo, it might also enhance shunting of water from DVR to AVR (116, 442, 453).

TRANSPORT OF SMALL HYDROPHILIC SOLUTES ACROSS THE DVR WALL

It is likely that most NaCl and urea equilibration across the DVR wall occurs by diffusive influx. AQP1 contributes to the process of equilibration through molecular sieving. Evidence supports the notion that small hydrophilic solutes (NaCl, urea) diffuse through the same "shared" pathway that conducts the component of water flux driven by Starling forces because

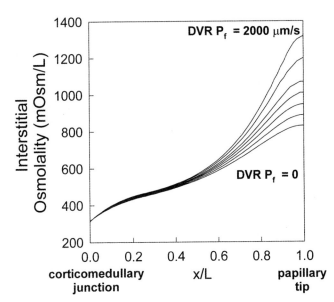

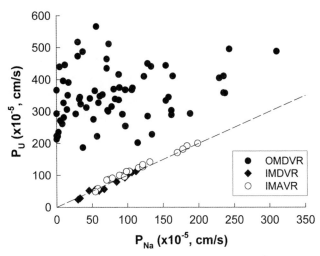

FIGURE 12 Effect of AQP1 deletion on predictions of renal medullary interstitial osmolality. A mathematical simulation of the renal medulla was solved to predict interstitial osmolality. Interstitial osmolality is shown as a function of corticomedullary axis (x/L = 0 is the corticomedullary junction, x/L = 1 is the papillary tip). Various curves denote predictions for different values of P_f (descending vas rectum [DVR] osmotic water permeability). P_f was varied between 0 (equivalent to AQP1 deletion) and 2000 μm/s. AQP1 expression in DVR is predicted to enhance concentrating ability by conducting water flux from DVR to interstitium where after it is taken up by AVR. The net result is a secondary reduction of blood flow in the deepest regions of the inner medulla (papillary tip). (From Pallone TL, Edwards A, Ma T, Silldorff EP, Verkman AS. Requirement of aquaporin-1 for NaCl-driven water transport across descending vasa recta. *J Clin Invest* 2000;105:215–222, with permission.)

FIGURE 13 Vasa recta solute permeabilities. [^{14}C]urea permeability (P_U, ordinate) versus ^{22}Na permeability (P_{Na}, abscissa) is shown for outer medullary descending vas rectum (OMDVR) isolated from Sprague-Dawley rats and perfused in vitro. Results are also shown for inner medullary DVR and ascending vas rectum (AVR) (IMDVR, IMAVR, respectively) perfused on the surface of the exposed papilla of Munich-Wistar rats in vivo. The dashed line is identity. P_U and P_{Na} are highly correlated and nearly equal in inner medullary vasa recta. In contrast, P_U of outer medullary DVR is always very high and is not correlated with P_{Na}. The dissociation of P_{Na} and P_U in OMDVR results (at least in part) from the expression of the urea transporter type B (UTB)–facilitated urea carrier. In separate experiments (not shown), P_U of OMDVR was inhibited by exposure to urea analogues or phloretin. (From Pallone TL, Work J, Myers RL, Jamison RL. Transport of sodium and urea in outer medullary descending vasa recta. *J Clin Invest* 1994;93:212–222, with permission.)

DVR permeability to tracers (^{22}Na, ^{36}Cl, ^{3}HRaffinose, ^{14}Cinulin) correlate with each other and hydraulic conductivity (447, 453, 455, 590). Urea transport across the DVR wall is more complicated because it diffuses both via paracellular and transcellular routes. A summary of available solute diffusive permeability measurements is provided in Table 3.

FACILITATED TRANSPORT OF UREA ACROSS DVR AND RBCs

Transmural flux of urea across the DVR wall is complicated because DVR endothelia express a facilitated urea carrier (436, 481). Sodium and urea have similar free-water diffusivity and are therefore expected to have the same transvessel permeability if they diffuse, sterically unrestricted, through a large pore. In contrast to this, some outer medullary DVR have low or moderate P_{Na} but high P_U (Fig. 13). DVR permeability to ^{14}Curea can be partially inhibited by phloretin, pCMBS, and structural analogs of urea, verifying the presence of an endothelial carrier (436, 455). Histochemical evidence and in situ hybridization studies have shown that the DVR urea carrier is the same as that in the RBC (UTB) and distinct from the urea carrier in the thin limbs of Henle (UTA2) and collecting duct (UTA1, UTA3, UTA4) (25, 536, 537, 619, 621, 622).

Rat UTB carries the Kidd blood group antigen, has 62% identity to UTA2, and is expressed in RBCs, DVR endothelium, papillary surfaces, and pelvic epithelium of the kidney (513, 621). The presence of UTB in the DVR endothelium and RBCs facilitates medullary urea recycling. Urea tends to exit the renal medulla in AVR plasma and RBCs. To prevent associated dissipation of corticomedullary urea gradients, urea recycles from AVR into DVR plasma and RBCs via UTB, and into thin limbs of Henle via UTA2 (Fig. 14). Those processes are highly evolved in the outer medullary inner stripe where DVR and AVR are closely positioned in vascular bundles. Many water-conserving species also incorporate UTA2 expressing thin limbs of Henle within or on the periphery of vascular bundles (Fig. 9) (28, 256, 265, 301, 316). Interesting insights into function have been obtained from the study of UTB null mice. UTB deficiency results in reduced urinary concentrating ability, reduced urea clearance, and increased plasma urea concentration (25, 621, 622). In contrast to wild-type mice, infusion of urea into UTB null animals fails to enhance urinary concentrating ability (25). Acute regulation of UTB by vasopressin or other factors has not been demonstrated. In contrast to upregulation of UTA transporters (513), chronic vasopressin treatment may reduce UTB expression (480, 587). UTB expression in the renal medulla increases during osmotic diuresis induced by urea but not NaCl or glucose infusion

TABLE 3 Diffusional Permeability of Vasa Recta to Hydrophilic Solutes

*Permeability × 10^{-5}cm/s	Species	OMDVR[a]	IMDVR[b]	IMAVR[b]	Reference
P_{Na}	Hamster	—	28	51	362
P_{Na}	Rat	76	75	115	455
P_{Na}	Rat	—	67	116	432, 434
P_{Na}	Mouse	207–314	—	—	442
P_{Urea}	Rat	—	47	—	395
P_{Urea}	Rat	360	76	121	455
P_{Urea}	Rat	$343 \rightarrow 191$[c]	—	—	436
P_{Urea}	Mouse	661[d]	—	—	442
P_D	Rat	476[e]	—	—	414, 447
$P_{Raffinose}$	Rat	40	—	—	447, 590
$P_{Raffinose}$	Mouse	80, 111[d]	—	—	442

Permeability Ratio	Species	OMDVR[a]	IMDVR[b]	IMAVR[b]	Reference
P_{Urea}/P_{Na}	Rat	4.7	1.1	0.98	442, 447
	Mouse[D]	3.2			455
P_{Cl}/P_{Na}	Rat	1.3	—	—	
$P_{Raffinose}/P_{Na}$	Rat	0.35	—	—	
	Mouse	0.35, 0.39[d]			
P_{Inulin}/P_{Na}	Rat	0.22	—	—	
	Mouse	0.31[d]			

—, Not measured as part of the study.

OMDVR, outer medullary descending vasa recta; IMDVR, inner medullary descending vasa recta; IMAVR, inner medullary ascending vasa recta.

[a] Values obtained with in vitro microperfusion are highly dependent upon perfusion rate; see text and references (444, 447, 590).

[b] Values obtained with in vivo microperfusion in the exposed papilla, probably underestimated due to boundary layer effects; see text.

[c] Values are before and after inhibition with 50 mM thiourea.

[d] Value from DVR of AQP1 null mice (442).

[e] Diffusional water permeability measured with ^{3}H$_2$O efflux.

(279). In contrast, UTB expression is depressed by ureteral obstruction, lithium treatment, potassium deficiency and cyclosporine toxicity (262, 284, 322, 330).

UTB expression in RBCs should limit AQP1-mediated water transport and the associated osmotic shrinking and swelling that would otherwise accompany RBC transit through the medulla. Macey and Yousef proposed that this might prevent osmotic lysis (346). Against this hypothesis is the finding that humans devoid of Kidd antigen have mildly depressed urinary concentrating ability but no hemolytic anemia. It seems most likely that RBC expression of UTB serves to increase the overall mass of urea that is efficiently recycled from the AVR and DVR lumens (621).

TRANSPORT OF SOLUTES AND WATER ACROSS THE AVR WALL

Transport of solutes and water in AVR has not been as thoroughly evaluated as that in DVR because AVR cannot be isolated for in vitro microperfusion. Measurements of

AVR transport properties have been performed by in vivo micropuncture and microperfusion of vessels on the surface of the exposed papilla (inner one third of the inner medulla) of rats. Some reliable measurements of AVR hydraulic conductivity (L_p) have been obtained. Consistent with the highly fenestrated endothelium, L_p is high, about 12.5×10^{-6} cm/(s×mm Hg) ($P_f = 13.4$ cm/s) (347, 433). The reflection coefficient of the AVR wall to albumin has been measured by molecular sieving (435) and by osmosis (347). Mean values of 0.78 and 0.70 were obtained, respectively. A summary of AVR hydraulic conductivity and reflection coefficient measurements is provided in Table 2.

When blood ascends toward the cortex in AVR, it encounters decreasing NaCl and urea concentrations so that luminal osmolality exceeds that of the adjacent interstitium. Perfusing AVR in vivo with buffers made hypertonic or hypotonic to the papillary interstitium with NaCl generated no measurable water flux, suggesting that, for the AVR wall, $\sigma_{SS} = 0$ (Eq. 2) (434). Transmural AVR NaCl and

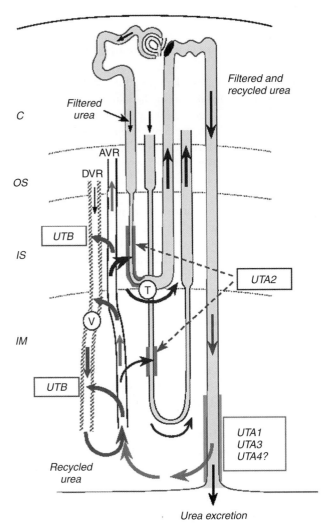

Vasa recta diffusional solute permeabilities, measured in the rat (395, 434) and hamster (362), are higher than those in DVR (Table 3). Even so, AVR permeabilities have probably been underestimated because all measurements relied upon ^{22}Na and ^{14}Curea efflux during microperfusion in vivo. That method probably underestimates permeability because accumulation of tracers near the abluminal surface during microperfusion violates the assumption that abluminal tracer concentrations are zero (432, 434).

Transport of Macromolecules in the Cortex and Medulla

It is generally accepted that lymphatics are sparse in the outer medulla and absent from the inner medulla (41, 302). It has long been recognized that proteins permeate the walls of capillaries (308, 313, 491) to be drained by lymphatics and returned to the systemic circulation. Given the absence of lymphatics in the inner medulla, the mechanisms that regulate interstitial oncotic pressure and protein trafficking through the interstitium have been enigmatic. Early studies led to the conclusion that a large extravascular pool of albumin is present within the medulla (312, 328, 546). Leakage of fluorescent albumin (68, 474) and Evans blue dye–labeled albumin (391, 615) into the medullary interstitium were observed. Ultrastructural studies with horse radish peroxidase (molecular radius, 50 Å), catalase (elliptical molecule, 240,000 D; major axis, 240 Å), and ferritin (spherical molecule, 500,000 D; 110 Å) demonstrated that these markers can cross the fenestrations of cortical peritubular cortical capillaries (596) and medullary AVR (539).

Measurements of albumin transport rates across the DVR and AVR walls have been technically limited. Using molecular sieving of Texas red–labeled albumin, Turner estimated the reflection coefficient of the DVR wall to albumin to be 0.89 (not significantly different from unity) (590). In separate studies with different methods, the reflection coefficient of the AVR wall to albumin was estimated to be 0.7 and 0.78 (347, 435). No reliable measurements of the diffusional permeability of either the DVR or AVR wall to albumin exist. Attempts have been made to determine Starling forces within the medullary interstitium through direct measurement of interstitial protein concentration. Using a differential centrifugation technique, MacPhee and Michel obtained a mean value of 0.9 g/dl (347). By an alternative approach interstitial protein concentrations of 4 to 6 g/dl were predicted and interstitial hydraulic pressures in the range of 5 to 10 mm Hg were found (437).

Whatever the concentration of albumin in the medullary interstitium, the fundamental question remains, in the absence of lymphatics, how is medullary interstitial protein deposited and cleared by the microcirculation? Protein transport into the AVR lumen by convective influx is the most likely answer (347, 384, 437). Michel pointed out that molecular sieving at the AVR wall would prevent convective movement of protein into the AVR lumen were it not for continuous deposition of

FIGURE 14 Urea transporter type B (UTB) and urea recycling in the medulla. Schematic of vascular and tubular urea recycling in the kidney. Short and long loops of Henle and vasa recta are shown. The UTA2 urea transporter is expressed in the thin descending limbs of Henle. The UTB urea transporter is expressed in DVR endothelium and red blood cells (not shown). Thin descending limbs of short looped nephrons become associated with vascular bundles (see Figure 9) so that urea recycling from thin limbs to descending vas rectum (DVR) via UTA2 and UTB is accommodated. UTB is not expressed by the ascending vas rectum (AVR) endothelium but AVR are fenestrated and urea permeability is high. Thus urea in AVR plasma and red blood cells (RBCs) can readily recycle back to DVR in vascular bundles using UTB in the RBC membrane and DVR endothelium. The UTA1, A3, and A4 collecting duct conduct urea transporters conduct urea from the lumen to the inner medullary interstitium. C, cortex; OS, outer stripe of outer medulla; IS, inner stripe of outer medulla; IM, inner medulla. (From Yang B, Bankir L. Urea and urine concentrating ability: new insights from studies in mice. *Am J Physiol Renal Physiol* 2005;288: F881–F896, with permission.)

urea gradients in vivo are likely to be smaller than those in DVR because AVR blood flow rates are lower. AVR are larger in diameter and more numerous than DVR (219, 362, 647). Consequently, high permeability, high surface area and an increased transit time of blood all favor a high degree of equilibration between AVR plasma and interstitium (117, 446).

protein free fluid by medullary nephrons (384). The plausibility of convective protein uptake is also supported by the finding that papillary AVR withstand an inwardly directed hydraulic pressure without collapsing (348).

INTRARENAL HEMATOCRIT

When the volumes of distribution of plasma and red blood cells within the kidney were examined by injecting labeled albumin and red blood cells (RBCs), intrarenal hematocrit was found to be less than systemic hematocrit. Given the observation of Fahreaus that red cells migrate to the center of small vessels, Pappenheimer and Kinter proposed that cell free blood is "skimmed" from the periphery of the interlobular arteries to enter the afferent arterioles of deep glomeruli (134, 459), an effect that might be facilitated by intra-arterial cushions (Fig. 2) (152, 153, 392). This possibility was tested by Lilienfield et al. (329) who found that RBC transit time was shorter than plasma transit time and that tissue hematocrit varies with medullary axis. Rasmussen performed a technically superior examination using ^{131}I-IgM, a larger and therefore more reliable plasma marker. Simultaneous injection with ^{51}Cr-RBCs led to the estimates of tissue hematocrit shown in Fig. 15 (489). Using videomicroscopic techniques, Zimmerhackl estimated the "dynamic" or "tube" hematocrit of the papillary

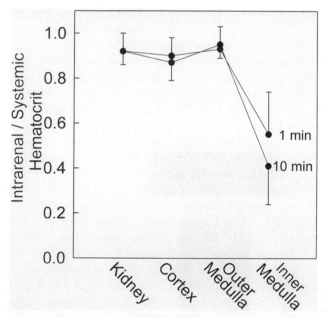

FIGURE 15 Distribution of hematocrit in the kidney. ^{51}Cr-RBCs and ^{131}I-IgM (plasma volume marker) were simultaneously infused into the kidney. An equilibration period of either 1 or 10 minutes followed before ligation of the renal artery and vein. The distribution of red blood cells and plasma were inferred by measuring activity of the isotopes in tissue and dividing their ratio by the systemic ratio. Results show that the hematocrit of inner medullary blood is lower than than whole kidney, cortex, or outer medulla. (From Rasmussen SN. Red cell and plasma volume flows to the inner medulla of the rat kidney: determinations by means of a step function input indicator technique. *Pflugers Arch* 1978;373:153–159, with permission.)

DVR and AVR to be 26% and 25%, respectively (645). Direct measurements with micropuncture gave similar results. A low microvessel hematocrit in the renal medulla has been consistently found.

In addition to plasma skimming (152, 459), other mechanisms could reduce medullary hematocrit. Fahreaus demonstrated that the hematocrit of a microvessel is reduced by migration of RBCs to the centerline where the velocity of flow is highest (134). Based on this alone, vasa recta (10–20 µm diameter) are expected to have hematocrits reduced by 40% to 50% of that in a large vessel (158). Pries et al. (477) have shown that a "network" Fahreaus effect can further reduce microvessel hematocrit by as much as 20%. When a vessel bifurcates, the higher flow branch receives blood of higher hematocrit. Conservation of RBC and plasma dictates that the increase of hematocrit in one branch must be less than the reduction in the other branch, tending to reduce average capillary hematocrit. Shrinkage of RBCs in the hypertonic medulla must also tend to lower medullary microvessel hematocrit (448).

METHODS FOR MEASUREMENT OF REGIONAL BLOOD FLOW TO THE CORTEX AND MEDULLA

The relative contribution of various renal microvessels to renal vascular resistance can be inferred from the luminal hydrostatic pressure profile. As shown in Fig. 16, the largest pressure drop, and therefore the dominant resistance, is the afferent arteriole. Glomerular capillaries offer little resistance to flow. Efferent arterioles and DVR (Fig. 5) contribute significantly to renal vascular resistance, but less than that attributed to afferent arterioles. The vasomotor tone of the afferent arteriole is governed by myogenic autoregulation and tubuloglomerular feedback, important topics covered by other chapters of this text. Measurement of regional blood flows in the kidney that result from the actions and distributions of resistance arterioles has been the frequently pursued. Early approaches to the measurement of regional blood flow within the kidney relied upon tracers, gave widely varying estimates of tissue blood flow and have fallen into disfavor. Results from those methods are summarized in Table 4, from which one can conclude that inner medullary tissue blood flow rate is much lower than that in the cortex (18, 22, 34, 83, 84, 87, 137, 161, 162, 204, 219, 272, 299, 327, 489, 505, 547, 554, 583, 584, 616, 626). The associated details have been reviewed in prior versions of this text and other sources (439, 448). Videomicroscopic measurement of RBC velocity is a more reliable means for calculating single-vessel blood flow rates, but it is limited to surface microvessels in the cortex or exposed papilla (645, 648). Use of a pencil lens camera for measurement of glomerular and cortical peritubular RBC velocities has been described by Goligorsky and colleagues (620). Laser-Doppler flowmetry is the dominant method for examining

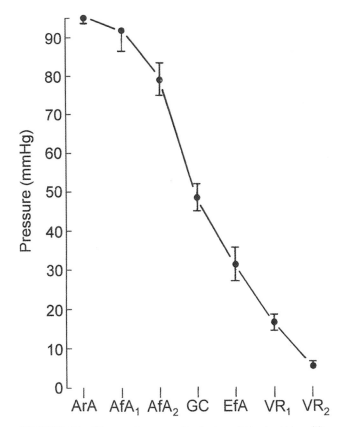

FIGURE 16 Microvessel pressure distribution within the kidney. The values on the ordinate were obtained by micropuncture and servo-nulling pressure measurements using the juxtamedullary nephron preparation. Pressure falls successively from the arcuate artery to vasa recta. ArA, arcuate artery; AfA_1 and AfA_2, early and late afferent arteriole; GC, glomerular capillaries; EfA, efferent arterioles; VR_1, descending vasa recta; VR_2, ascending vasa recta. (From Casellas D, Navar LG. In vitro perfusion of juxtamedullary nephrons in rats. *Am J Physiol* 1984;246:F349–F358, with permission.)

regional blood flow due to the ease of applying optical fibers to the kidney surface or inserting them into otherwise inaccessible regions within the parenchyma (505).

Videomicroscopy

Measurement of microvessel diameter and RBC velocity (V_{RBC}) can be combined to calculate single vessel blood flow rates (362). Gussis and colleagues measured V_{RBC} in vasa recta on the surface of the exposed renal papilla following which Holliger and coworkers coupled V_{RBC} with diameter measurement to calculate single-vessel blood flow rates (185, 219). In later refinements, contrast between red cells, plasma, and the capillary wall was enhanced by injection of fluorescein isothiocyanate–labeled gamma globulin and V_{RBC} was determined from the video images captured with a silicon intensified target camera. Additionally, the Fahraeus effect (134) was accounted for by calibrating RBC streaming effects in quartz capillaries (648). Application of videomicroscopy to measurement of renal blood flow is limited by regional accessibility. Observation of the medulla for videomicroscopy is limited to the

papilla (distal one third of the inner medulla) because only that part of the medulla can be exposed for visualization by excising the ureter of young rodents.

Laser-Doppler

The laser-Doppler method for measuring tissue blood flow rates relies upon the frequency shift of light emitted from a laser due to scattering by flowing RBCs (557). Among other advantages, sequential measurements in the same region are possible and signals can be obtained on the renal surface or from optical fibers implanted into the parenchyma. The counterflow arrangement of vasa recta within the medulla would appear to violate the requirement that the laser-Doppler receive *random* back-scattered light. Despite this concern, agreement between laser-Doppler and videomicroscopy (144) or ^{51}Cr-RBC accumulation (505) has been demonstrated. The laser-Doppler device provides a voltage proportional to tissue perfusion in the immediate vicinity of the fiber-optic probe. Calibration to convert the signal to absolute units that quantitatively describe local perfusion is generally not possible. This limits absolute comparisons of measurements between regions of the kidney of the same or different animals.

METHODS FOR DIRECT MEASUREMENTS OF MICROVESSEL REACTIVITY

Another category of important methods for investigation of the regulation of regional blood flow involves direct examination of the effects of vasoactive agents on pressurized microvessels. Important information on the sites of action, the concentrations at which specific hormones modulate reactivity and receptor subtypes responsible for mediating vasoactivity can be obtained. Extrapolation of results to arrive at conclusions concerning the effects of hormones and autocoids on regional blood flow within the kidney is fraught with uncertainty. This topic has been frequently reviewed (16, 63, 256, 410, 454, 500).

In Vitro Microperfusion

The in vitro microperfusion method commonly used for study of transport processes in renal tubules has also been applied to microvessels (Fig. 17) (54, 440). The first applications of this method were in canine glomeruli (425). Subsequent adaptations in rabbits permitted examination of vasomotor tone in afferent and efferent arterioles (119, 246–249). Using this approach, it has been possible to measure effects of vasoactive agents on afferent arterioles (Fig. 18A) and vasa recta (Figs. 18B and 18C) (192, 438, 455). As with all methods, limitations exist. Hormones that cause vasoconstriction often activate compensatory mechanisms that inhibit their actions. Endothelium-dependent vasodilators such as nitric oxide, prostacyclin, and hyperpolarizing factors (413) might be

TABLE 4   Regional Tissue Plasma Inflow Rates Measured in the Kidney

Method	Species	Cortex	Outermedulla	Innermedulla	Reference
Dye transit	Dog	—	1.3	0.2–0.7	584
	Dog	5.35	3.22	0.38	299
^{32}P transit	Dog	—	1.8	0.5–0.7	616
^{85}Kr washout	Dog	4.72	1.32	0.17	583
H_2 washout	Dog	2.6–5.0	—	—	18
^{86}Rb uptake	Dog	4.4–7.4	1.2–2.3	1.1	554
	Dog	4.84	2.81	0.8	22
	Rat	4.76	1.35	0.66	204
	Rat	—	0.60–0.88[a]	0.2–0.3[a]	87
	Rat	5.2	1.5–2.2	0.69	272
	Rat	4.7–7.3	2.4	2.4	626
Albumin accumulation	Dog	—	—	0.25	327
	Dog	—	—	0.22	137
	Dog	—	—	0.23	83
	Rat	—	—	0.38–0.42	161, 162
	Rat	—	—	0.32	547
	Rat	—	—	0.27	34
	Rat	—	—	0.36	84
	Rat	—	—	0.38–0.64	489
	Rat	—	—	0.06–0.08[b]	489
	Rat	—	—	0.18[c,d]	505
	Rat	—	—	0.31[c,e]	505
RBC velocity	Rat	—	—	1.3–5.9[c,f]	219

—, Not measured as part of the study.

RBC, red blood cell.

Note: Inflow Rate, ml × min × g^{-1}.

[a] Probably underestimated.

[b] RBC inflow rate.

[c] Total blood (RBC and plasma) inflow rate.

[d] Young rats.

[e] Old rats.

[f] Probably overestimated.

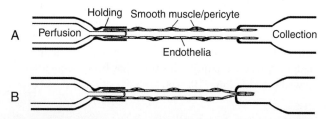

FIGURE 17 In vitro microperfusion. **A:** An isolated microvessel is cannulated on concentric pipettes by drawing the vessel into an outer holding pipette and cannulating its orifice with a perfusion pipette. By pressurizing the perfusion pipette, fluid is forced to flow through the vessel lumen into a collection pipette. **B:** The collection end can be crimped to create a "stop flow" condition in which the lumen is pressurized to that of the holding pipette in the absence of flow. (From Zhang Z, Pallone TL. Response of descending vasa recta to luminal pressure. *Am J Physiol Renal Physiol* 2004;287:F535–F542, with permission.)

blunted, substrate limited (52), or simply diluted into the bathing buffer. The actions of nitric oxide (NO) might be enhanced in vitro due to the absence of hemoglobin, an NO scavenger (365), or reduced by endothelial damage during vessel isolation.

Juxtamedullary Nephron Preparation

The ingenious blood-perfused juxtamedullary nephron preparation was devised by Casellas and Navar (Fig. 19, *top panel*). The surgically isolated kidney, perfused with artificial buffers or blood is hemisected. Dissection of perihilar fat and reflection of the papilla exposes the juxtamedullary circulation to enable observation of RBC flow and microvessel diameters. Advantages of the method are many, including relative preservation of tubular–vascular relationships, continuous oxygenation of the tissue under study, the ability to measure pressures by servo-nulling, and the ability to control hormone concentrations in the perfusate and superfusate (70).

The Split Hydronephrotic Kidney

Steinhausen et al. (555, 556) developed a method for reducing the kidney to a transparent layer of tissue within which transilluminated microvessels are readily visualized. After transient ischemia to the kidney, ureteral ligation is performed, inducing hydronephrosis. Weeks later, the hydronephrotic kidney,

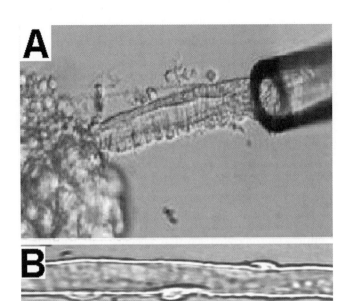

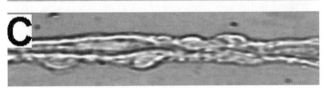

FIGURE 18 In vitro microperfusion. **A:** An afferent arteriole is cannulated with concentric pipettes and perfused toward the glomerulus. Perfusion of an isolated descending vas rectum (DVR). Images obtained before **(B)** and after **(C)** exposure to angiotensin II. Compare the thick smooth muscle layer of the afferent arteriole to the sporadically distributed pericyte cell bodies of DVR. (From Hansen PB, Hashimoto S, Briggs J, Schnermann J. Attenuated renovascular constrictor responses to angiotensin II in adenosine 1 receptor knockout mice. *Am J Physiol Regul Integr Comp Physiol* 2003;285:R44–R49, with permission.)

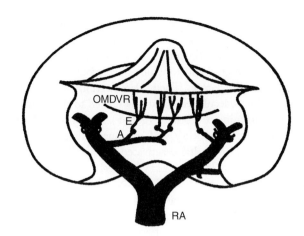

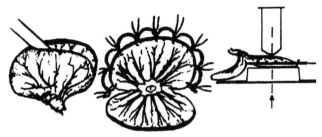

FIGURE 19 Juxtamedullary nephron and split hydronephrotic kidney preparations. **Top panel:** The juxtamedullary nephron preparation is created by perfusing the kidney, sectioning it longitudinally and reflecting the papilla to expose the underlying microvasculature. **Bottom panel:** The split hydronephrotic kidney preparation is created by ligating the ureter for 3 to 10 weeks prior to isolation of the kidney. Ureteral ligation eventually reduces the kidney to a thin sheet of tissue in which tubules have atrophied but the vasculature remains. The kidney is exposed, split along the greater curvature and sutured onto a chamber for observation and experimentation. RA, renal artery; A and E, afferent and efferent arterioles; OMDVR, outer medullary descending vasa recta. (From Navar LG, Inscho EW, Majid SA, Imig JD, Harrison-Bernard LM, Mitchell KD. Paracrine regulation of the renal microcirculation. *Physiol Rev* 1996;76:425–536, with permission.)

reduced to a thin layer, can be split along its curvature and suspended on a microscope stage for study (Fig. 19, *bottom panel*). The actions of vasoactive agents can be studied by infusing them into the rat or by applying them directly onto the preparation. Changes in blood flow rate can be measured by videomicroscopy and the reactivity of microvessels quantitated as changes in luminal diameter. The possibility of phenotypic drift in the altered tissue has to be considered.

VASOACTIVITY OF THE RENAL MICROCIRCULATION: ION CHANNEL ARCHITECTURE

Voltage-Gated Ca^{2+} Channels

Contraction of microvessels is generally tied to elevation of cytoplasmic calcium ($[Ca^{2+}]_{CYT}$) of smooth muscle cells (SMCs). The increase of $[Ca^{2+}]_{CYT}$ is often mediated by influx through voltage-gated channels that are activated by membrane depolarization. This is observed experimentally; exposing SMC to high extracellular KCl induces depolariza-

tion by raising the K$^+$ equilibrium potential (Keq), activating voltage-gated Ca^{2+} entry and inducing vasoconstriction. Studies have shown that KCl depolarization constricts afferent arterioles more than efferent arterioles (65, 194, 194, 338). A role for high voltage–gated, L-type channels to mediate afferent SMC contraction is supported by the observation that both $[Ca^{2+}]_{CYT}$ elevation and vasoconstriction are blocked by diltiazem (89, 242). In the split hydronephrotic kidney preparation, ANG II constricts afferent and efferent arterioles but depolarizes only the former (335). Application of agonists such as ANG II, endothelin, and ATP to preglomerular smooth muscle preparations consistently elicits $[Ca^{2+}]_{CYT}$ and current responses that are sensitive to L-type antagonists (10, 209, 245, 251, 333). Taken together, sensitivity of the preglomerular microcirculation to L-type calcium channel blockade has been a very consistent finding (66, 151, 337, 339, 409, 572). Reduction of afferent vasoconstriction due to impairment of L-channel function could conceivably lead to transmission of elevated pressures to the glomerulus, resulting in injury. Such a mechanism has been invoked in rodent models of diabetes and hypertension (67, 139, 252).

Voltage-gated Ca^{2+} channels (CaVs) exist as a variety of subtypes, the designations of which have evolved through a confusing nomenclature. Their classification is currently dominated by molecular designations related to the identity of the pore forming α subunit (Table 5). Isoforms of classic high-voltage–activated (HVA), L-channels are CaV 1.1 to 1.3 and those of low-voltage–activated (LVA), T-type channels are CaV 3.1 to 3.3. Other HVA types, originally identified in neurons, are the P/Q, R and N, which are CaV 2.1 to 2.3. Reverse transcriptase–polymerase chain reaction (RT-PCR) and immunochemistry have been effectively used to examine the distribution of voltage-gated Ca^{2+} channel α subunits in the kidney. In addition to the anticipated expression of L-type (CaV1.x, where x is either 1,2,3, or 4; see Table 5) in the afferent circulation, T-type as well as unexpected P/Q-type Ca^{2+} channels were found (193, 194, 259, 428, 429, 511). Of great interest, CaVs are not just confined to the preglomerular circulation, juxtamedullary efferent arterioles and DVR express them. In a manner consistent with the earlier literature (see prior sections), superficial efferent arterioles do not (194). Functional confirmation CaV expression in the afferent and efferent circulation has been obtained. The CaV 1.x, L-type blocker diltiazem, partially reversed ANG II vasoconstriction and $[Ca^{2+}]_{CYT}$ elevation in DVR pericytes (495, 637). Similarly, the L-type blocker calciseptine and nonselective T-type blockers nilvadipine, mibefradil, pimozide, and Ni^{2+} reversed KCl and ANG II–induced constriction of afferent and efferent arterioles (142, 194, 207, 428, 429). Elegant patch clamp recordings by Gordienko et al. (174) demonstrated signature currents consistent with both high- and low-voltage–gated Ca^{2+} entry into isolated preglomerular smooth muscle (174). Glomerular mesangial cells have a smooth muscle phenotype and express L-type dihydropyridine–sensitive voltage-gated Ca^{2+} channels (189).

Nonselective Cation Channels, Store-Operated Channels, Trp Channels

Early study of store-operated Ca^{2+} entry (SOC) in mast cells pointed to a highly Ca^{2+} selective pathway of immeasurably low single channel conductance that was referred to as a "calcium release activated current" (CRAC or I_{CRAC}) (460). It now is clear that many other pathways partici-pate in cellular Ca^{2+} entry in response to receptor activation and intracellular Ca^{2+} store depletion. The routes involved are not always highly selective for Ca^{2+}, but instead also conduct other cations including Na^+. Their promiscuous transport of cations led to the designation "nonselective cation channels" (NSCCs). Both receptor-operated and store-operated Ca^{2+} entry into cells can occur via NSCC, and channels of the transient receptor potential (TRP) families are now recognized as the major participants (86). Fellner and Arendshorst (138, 139) showed that SOC entry into renal SMCs occurs and may be increased in the spontaneously hypertensive rat. Using SKF-96365 as a NSCC blocker, it has been shown that ANG II induced Ca^{2+} responses (333) and vasoconstriction (573) of the efferent arteriole involves NSCC. There is currently little information concerning the molecular identity of store-operated and receptor-operated cation channels in the renal microcirculation. Assigning subtype-specific functional roles to the ubiquitously expressed TRP channel family members has proven generally difficult (86). Takenaka and colleagues demonstrated that TRPC1 is expressed in glomerular arterioles and might conduct store- or receptor-operated Ca^{2+} entry (86, 573). The presence and activation of SOC have been most thoroughly examined in glomerular mesangial cells. Sansom and colleagues identified a small, 2.1 pS cation channel that is activated by thapsigargin-induced store depletion (86, 344). In whole-cell patch-clamp experiments, identical currents were elicited by either thapsigargin or epidermal growth factor activation (324, 343). Activation of the pathway requires signaling through $PKC\alpha$ (341, 342). TRPC1 and

TABLE 5   Expression of Voltage-Activated Ca2+ Channels in the Renal Microcirculation (193, 194, 259, 428, 429, 510, 561)

		CaV	α Subunit	Renal SMC[a]	Locations
HVA	L	1.1	1S	−	Preglomerular SMC
	L	1.2	1C	+	Afferent arteriole
	L	1.3	1D	−	Mesangial cells
	L	1.4	1F	−	JM efferent arteriole DVR
HVA	P/Q	2.1	1A	+	Afferent arteriole
	N	2.2	1B	−	Mesangial cells
	R	2.3	1E	−	DVR
LVA	T	3.1	1G	+	Afferent arteriole
	T	3.2	1H	+	Efferent arteriole
	T	3.3	1I	−	DVR

DVR, descending vasa recta; HVA, high voltage activated by depolarization to greater than − 40 mV; JM, juxtamedullary; LVA, low voltage activated by depolarization to greater than − 55 mV; SMC, smooth muscle cell.

[a]Detection by immunochemistry, polymerase chain reaction.

TRPC4 are expressed in the murine mesangium whereas antisense-induced suppression of TRPC4 was accompanied by inhibition of SOCs (606). TRPC4 has also been identified in DVR pericytes and endothelium where it is in physical association with isoform 2 of the Na^+/H^+ exchange regulatory factor (NHERF-2), a scaffolding protein that facilitates protein–protein interactions (314). The function of the NHERF-TRPC4 association is unknown.

Chloride Channels

For CaVs to mediate Ca^{2+} entry into smooth muscle, they must depolarize the cell membrane to potentials greater than the CaV activation threshold. The equilibrium potential for K^+ ion is about -90 mV, and SMC membrane potential is held at negative values because overall conductance of the cell membrane is dominated by permeability to K^+. In many SMCs, depolarization that presages CaV-mediated Ca^{2+} entry is achieved by increasing the conductance to Cl^- ion, the equilibrium potential of which is generally -35 to -20 mV. This is accomplished through activation of Ca^{2+}-dependent Cl^- channels (ClCa) (282, 309). In the kidney, activation of ClCa channels appears to be necessary for ANG II and endothelin induced constriction of afferent but not efferent arterioles (62, 195, 258, 571). Presumably, based on the juxtamedullary efferent expression of CaV (194), ClCa plays a similar role in that location, but this has not been demonstrated. DVR pericyte depolarization and constriction is dependent on ClCa activation (443, 457, 634). It has also been shown that high concentrations of ANG II also depolarize DVR pericytes by inhibiting K^+ channels (441). The extent to which Cl^- channel activity regulates overall renal vascular resistance is uncertain (511, 552).

Potassium Channels

Most SMCs express an array of K^+ channels. These include inward rectifier (K_{IR}), calcium-dependent (K_{Ca}), voltage-dependent (K_V), and ATP-dependent (K_{ATP}) varieties (412).

SMCs of renal vessels are no exception, and many studies have been dedicated to the determination of their distribution and function (Table 6).

K_{Ca} channels are activated by depolarization and elevation of $[Ca^{2+}]_{CYT}$. They can be further subdivided into larger conductance (maxiK_{Ca} or BK_{Ca}) channels sensitive to charybdotoxin and iberotoxin and medium- and low-conductance channels blocked by apamin. K_{Ca} channels are ubiquitous in smooth muscle. When stimulated by Ca^{2+} entry, they may provide a "breaking" function that opposes depolarization and deactivates CaV.

K_V channels, also referred to as delayed rectifiers, activate with depolarization, are insensitive to $[Ca^{2+}]_{CYT}$, and are specifically blocked by 4-aminopyridine. K_V can contribute to resting potential and their voltage-dependent activation probably limits membrane depolarization.

K_{IR}S are named for their avid permeation of K^+ at membrane potentials that lie below Keq. Above Keq, where the physiological function of K_{IR} occurs, K_{IR}S conduct K^+ efflux from cells in a complex manner. Conductance, at membrane potentials greater than Keq, declines as the difference between membrane potential and Keq increases. The latter property imparts a very important characteristic. Small elevations of extracellular K^+ (e.g., 5–20 mM) raise Keq to a level that enhances K_{IR} conductance but still lies below the resting membrane potential. The result is hyperpolarization of the membrane that favors inhibition of Ca^{2+} entry and vasodilation (483). That mechanism may enable extracellular K^+ ion to function as an endothelium-dependent hyperpolarizing factor (EDHF). The increase in extracellular K^+ needed for the EDHF process to occur is thought to arise from endothelial K^+ secretion. Vasodilators such as bradykinin and acetylcholine increase $[Ca^{2+}]_{CYT}$ and stimulate endothelial K_{Ca} channels so that they secrete K^+ ion into the extracellular space of adjacent SMCs (55, 150, 476, 484). Stated another way, K^+ may be an EDHF the function of which depends upon endothelial K^+ secretion and SMC K_{IR} expression. Extracellular K^+ can also activate electrogenic Na^+,K^+-ATPase activity in SMC, which, by exchanging

TABLE 6 Potassium Channel Expression in the Renal Microcirculation

Site	K_{Ca}	K_V	K_{IR}	K_{ATP}	Reference
Main renal artery	+	+	ND	ND	42, 169, 170
Preglomerular SMCs	+	+	+	+	168, 315, 323, 349, 565, 652, 653
Interlobar artery	+	+	ND	ND	8, 145, 174, 264
Arcuate artery	+	+	+	ND	145, 174, 345, 478, 479
Interlobular arteriole	+	+	ND	ND	363, 364, 563, 564
Afferent arteriole	+	+	+	+	80, 115, 135, 280, 340, 383, 492, 493, 509, 577, 600, 607
Mesangial cells	+	+	ND	+	30, 73, 305, 367, 516-518, 558-561, 566
Efferent arteriole	+	ND	+	+	359, 492
DVR	+	ND	ND	+	441, 637

Table entries are + for existence of functional evidence based on electrophysiology, vasoactivity, and use of specific channel blockers.

DVR, descending vasa recta; KCa, small, medium, or large/maxi calcium-dependent potassium channel; K_v, voltage-gated (delayed rectifier) potassium channel; K_{IR}, inward rectifier potassium channel; K_{ATP}, ATP-dependent potassium channel; ND, no data; SMC, smooth muscle cell.

$3Na^+$ for $2K^+$, favors hyperpolarization. Participation of Na^+ pumps versus K_{IR} in SMC hyperpolarization must be experimentally distinguished, generally by examining the sensitivity to ouabain.

SMC K_{ATP} channels are generally composed of four KIR 6.1 α subunits combined with four type 2B sulfonurea receptors (SUR2Bs). Despite the participation of K_{IR} 6.1, K_{ATP} channels lack the strongly inward rectifying characteristics of other K_{IR} isoforms. K_{ATP} channels are widely expressed in SMC and, with high specificity, are inhibited by antagonists such as glybenclamide that bind to the SUR subunits. K_{ATP} channels are named for their inhibition by intracellular ATP. In addition to ATP, nucleotide diphosphates (NDPs) regulate most K_{ATP} channels. It was initially considered that reduction of ATP during metabolic stress might serve to activate K_{ATP} channels leading to hyperpolarization, microvessel dilation, and enhanced perfusion. It is now recognized that this is an oversimplification because K_{ATP} channels can contribute to resting potential and are sensitive to a variety of regulatory influences (483).

SMCs of the main renal, interlobar, and arcuate arteries have been shown to express both BK_{Ca} and K_V channels that exhibit slow inactivation after depolarization (42, 145, 168–170, 174, 478). Preglomerular renal microvessels of varying caliber are often obtained by hand dissection or by filling them with iron oxide particles and isolating them from collagenase-digested tissue with a magnet. SK_{Ca}, BK_{Ca}, and K_V channels have been observed in afferent SMCs (363, 364, 479). Synthesis of the P450 cyclooxygenase constrictor, 20-hydroxyeicosatetraenoic acid (20-HETE), inhibits preglomerular K_{Ca} channel activity (345, 349, 652) probably through activation of MAP kinase (564) without affecting K_V. Preg lomerular K_{Ca} channels can be activated through NO (563) and CO generated by hemoxygenase (264). The cytochrome P450 synthesis of epoxyeicosatrienoic acids (EETs) has been shown to activate BK_{Ca} and may participate in the function of EETs as an EDHF (224, 600, 653). Inhibition of 20-HETE synthesis by NO may dominate over cyclic GMP generation as the signaling pathway that activates BK_{Ca} in preglomerular SMC (8, 349). Preglomerular expression of K_{ATP} component subunits has been variably observed (323, 565).

Afferent arterioles are the dominant resistance of the renal microcirculation and play vital roles in autoregulation through myogenic constriction and tubuloglomerular feedback. The K^+ channel architecture of afferent arterioles has been intensely studied and evidence for expression of K_{Ca}, K_{IR}, K_V, and K_{ATP} channels has been obtained. Afferent dilation by acetylcholine during inhibition of NO and prostaglandin synthesis has been traced to the participation of K_{IR} and K_{Ca} channels because it is blocked by the combined K_{Ca} inhibitors, charybdotoxin and apamin (600, 607). As described previously, the EDHF response may be related to local elevations of K^+ outside the SMC membrane. Direct participation of K_{IR} has been demonstrated by Chilton and Loutzenhiser (80), who found that small elevations of K^+ dilate afferent arterioles. The dilation is sensitive to low concentrations of Ba^{2+} (<100 μM), that selectively blocks K_{IR} channels (80, 115). Juxtaglomerular cells express the strong inward rectifier, K_{IR} 2.1, where it plays a role in setting membrane potential (315). Vasodilation of afferent arterioles by the K^+ channel activator, NS-1619, supports a role for K_{Ca} channels in that structure (135, 315). Myogenic constriction appears to be modulated through PKC that acts, at least in part, by inhibiting 4-aminopyridine–sensitive K_V channels (280). A role for K_{ATP} channel activity to affect afferent arterioles has been repeatedly verified. K_{ATP} channels activated by hypoxia, pinacidil, calcitonin gene-related peptide (CGRP), or adenosine modulate constriction (340, 492, 493, 577) and levakromlin hyperpolarizes renin secreting cells of the afferent arteriole (509). K_{ATP} expression in afferent arterioles is supported by the observation of [^{3}H]P-1075 binding to membranes (383).

The role of K^+ channels in the activity of the efferent circulation has not been as thoroughly explored as that of afferent smooth muscle. The K_{ATP} opener, pinacidil, dilates the efferent arteriole (492) . Pinacidil dilates DVR and hyperpolarizes DVR smooth muscle/pericytes (637). High concentrations of ANG II inhibit DVR K^+ channel activity (441). A modulatory role for K_{IR} and K_{Ca} channels to affect [Ca^{2+}]$_{CYT}$ signaling by ANG II in efferent arteriolar smooth muscle has been described (359).

Mesangial cells are smooth muscle/pericytes that contract to modulate filtration by glomerular capillaries (561). The ability to study mesangial cells in culture has permitted study of their channel architecture. Molecular evidence exists for expression of K_V, K_{ATP}, and K_{Ca} channels in rat primary and immortalized murine mesangial cells (30, 566). Both medium- and large-conductance K_{Ca} channels are present (367, 479, 517, 558–560). The BK_{Ca} channel in mesangial cells is activated by arachidonic acid (562) and Ca^{2+}/calmodulin-dependent protein kinase (516). Atrial natriuretic peptide (73) or NO, acting through cGMP-dependent protein kinase, also activates K_{Ca} channels through phosphorylation of the hβ1 subunit (305). Mesangial BK_{Ca} activation leads to a transient increase in open probability that is prolonged when protein phosphatase 2A is inhibited (518).

Connexins

In addition to permitting exchange of ions with the extracellular space, specialized channel proteins, the connexins, electrically couple smooth muscle and endothelia in the vascular wall. Of more than 20 connexins, Cx37, Cx40, Cx43, and Cx45 have been found in the vasculature where they form endothelial and myoendothelial gap junctions. Connexins are four-transmembrane–spanning proteins with two extracellular loops that combine as homomeric or heteromeric hexamers. Docking of the extracellular loops combines two hexameric hemichannels from adjacent cells into the transcellular "connexon" conduit that mediates cell–cell communication. Mimetic peptides have been designed that interfere with binding of the extracellular loops (100). Connexons are true channels that generally have high conductivity (15–300 pS), high open probability, and can occupy multiple subconductance states. They are highly regulated by pH, Ca^{2+}, signaling molecules and phosphorylation events. Their pores are sufficiently large to pass signaling molecules as well as anions and cations; communication between cells is often documented by cell to cell spreading of high-molecular-weight fluorescent molecules (e.g., Lucifer yellow, 457 D) (95, 133, 147). The physiological roles of vascular gap junctions are under study. A role for endothelial to smooth muscle transfer of vasodilators has been postulated (55, 150). This has received support from the observation that Cx40-deficient mice are hypertensive, have abnormal vasomotion, and exhibit deficient spreading of vasodilation (95–97). Endothelial deficiency of Cx43 also leads to abnormal spreading of vasodilation (148, 325) and targeting of Cx43 and Cx37 with the extracellular peptide mimetic, Gap27, inhibits myogenic responses (114). Like other vascular beds, the renal microcirculation expresses gap junctions (221, 386, 545). Their role is less well explored than that in other organs. NO- and COX-independent (EDHF mediated) dilation of the main renal artery with carbachol were shown to be sensitive to Gap27 (271). Similarly, arachidonic acid– and bradykinin-mediated, NO- and COX-independent dilation of arcuate and interlobar arterioles was inhibited by the gap junction blocker, 18-α glycyrrhetinic acid (592). Salmonsson and colleagues have documented Ca^{2+} spreading along interlobular arterioles that is likely to be mediated by gap junctions (510).

REGULATION OF BLOOD FLOW AND MICROVESSEL CONTRACTION

The most effective locations at which regional perfusion of cortex and medulla can be controlled are readily inferred from renal microanatomy (Fig. 1). For example, constriction of intralobular arterioles should favor redistribution of blood flow toward the medulla via the juxtamedullary glomeruli. Similarly, closure of juxtamedullary intra-arterial cushions (Fig. 2) or constriction of juxtamedullary afferent or efferent arterioles should favor perfusion of the superficial cortex. DVR are the final resistance vessels involved in the control of medullary perfusion. The fraction of the total resistance to blood flow into the renal medulla accounted for by DVR versus juxtamedullary afferent and efferent arterioles is uncertain. The parallel arrangement of DVR within vascular bundles does, however, imply a probable role for them to modulate regional perfusion to the outer versus inner medulla. For example, contraction of DVR that are destined to perfuse the inner medulla should favor redirection of blood flow toward the outer medullary interbundle capillary plexus.

Factors that control regional perfusion within the kidney are the subject of intense investigation.

Autoregulation and Pressure Natriuresis

Blood flow to the kidney remains relatively constant despite physiological variation of renal perfusion pressure (RPP), a phenomenon called autoregulation. Two major mechanisms account for renal autoregulation. The first is "myogenic," whereby stretch of the afferent arteriole leads to reflex vasoconstriction (334). The second component, that reacts more slowly than the myogenic reflex, is tubuloglomerular feedback (TGF). TGF occurs when an increase in RPP, transiently transmitted to glomerular capillaries, results in rise in glomerular filtration rate. After a delay traversing the nephron, the increased tubular fluid delivery is sensed at the macula densa where a signaling cascade leads to release of ATP and adenosine formation via 5′-ecto-nucleotidase. The adenosine so formed constricts the afferent arteriole thereby reducing filtration pressure and returning glomerular filtration rate to its set point (39, 40, 71, 290, 490, 529).

The phenomenon of "pressure natriuresis" may be tied to variation of medullary autoregulation. Pressure natriuresis refers to the observation that elevation of RPP causes natriuresis even in isolated, denervated kidneys (177, 270). Increased RPP leads to increased sodium delivery to papillary thin descending limbs of Henle, implying that a mechanism exists to inhibit reabsorption by the proximal tubule of deep nephrons (187, 498). Internalization of proximal Na^+/H^+ exchanger from the apical membrane might participate. Pressure natriuresis has been traced to alteration of renal interstitial hydrostatic pressure (RIHP). An increase in RIHP occurs when RPP is elevated (275) and both the increase in RIHP and natriuresis can be blunted through renal decapsulation (276). Garcia-Estan and Roman have suggested that residual effects after decapsulation might be traced to the inability of decapsulation to modulate interstitial pressure in the renal medulla (163). A role for RIHP in the phenomenon of pressure natriuresis is supported by experiments in which it has been altered without changing RPP. Infusion of 2.5% albumin into the renal interstitium increases RIHP and causes natriuresis through inhibition of sodium reabsorption by superficial and deep nephrons (178, 188).

It is accepted that renal cortical blood flow is autoregulated over a physiological range of RPP. In contrast, the extent to which medullary blood flow is autoregulated is controversial. It has been proposed that lack of medullary autoregulation is essential to pressure natriuresis and the control of salt and water excretion (91, 93, 143, 144, 368, 374, 442). The renal medulla is largely perfused by postglomerular blood. Flow through a small population of shunt vessels that bypass glomeruli has been invoked to explain the escape of the medulla from tubuloglomerular feedback–mediated autoregulation (Figs. 1 and 3) (69, 91).

Nearly 50 years of investigation have failed to completely support or refute the hypothesis that blood flow to the renal medulla lacks autoregulation. Work with microvascular transit time indicators favored lack of autoregulation (584) but several early studies favored its presence (88, 160, 557). Studies performed in the rat suggest that the efficiency of medullary autoregulation is a function of volume status. Measurement of blood flow to the cortex and medulla using videomicroscopy or laser-Doppler probes placed on the renal surface (501) or within the parenchyma (372) showed that medullary blood flow of volume expanded rats does not autoregulate but instead increases with perfusion pressure (Fig. 20). Both an increase in single-vessel blood flow rate and recruitment of flow through previously unperfused vasa recta may contribute to the process (501). In contrast to volume-expanded animals, hydropenic rats autoregulate medullary blood flow and minimal pressure natriuresis (Fig. 21) (91–93, 368). Studies of regional blood flow in the sodium-replete dogs by Majid and in rabbits by Eppel et al. support intact medullary autoregulation (129, 350). Zhang and colleagues recently demonstrated that pressurizing the DVR lumen leads to endothelial $[Ca^{2+}]_{CYT}$ elevation and generation of NO (635). If transmission of pressure to the medulla is a key event in pressure natriuresis, release of NO could conceivably inhibit salt reabsorp-

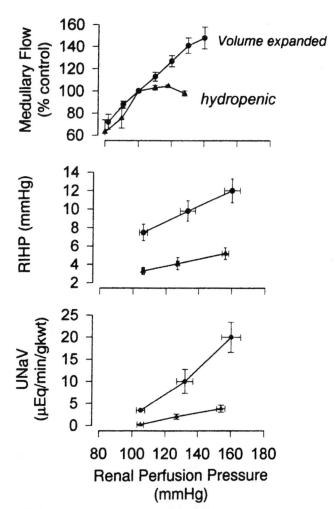

FIGURE 21 Pressure natriuresis. **A:** Medullary blood flow is autoregulated in hydropenic but not volume-expanded rats. **B:** Renal interstitial hydrostatic pressure (RIHP) is higher and increases to a greater degree with renal perfusion pressure in volume expanded animals. **C:** When renal perfusion pressure is increased, urinary sodium excretion (UNaV) increases much more markedly in volume expanded than in hydropenic animals. (From Cowley AW, Jr. Role of the renal medulla in volume and arterial pressure regulation. *Am J Physiol* 1997;273:R1–15, with permission.)

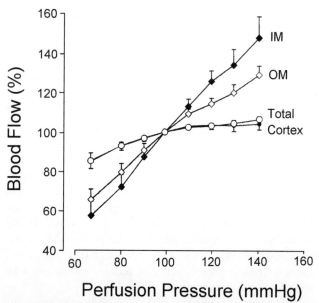

FIGURE 20 Autoregulation in different regions of the kidney. An electromagnetic flow device on the renal artery was used to measure total renal blood flow. Laser-Doppler flow probes were inserted into the renal parenchyma at various depths to measure regional blood flow in the outer and inner medulla. Total renal blood flow and cortical tissue blood flow shows intact autoregulation (stability of blood flow over a range of perfusion pressure). In contrast, in these volume-expanded rats (see text), the small fraction of blood flow that reaches the outer or inner medulla is not autoregulated. (From Mattson DL, Lu S, Roman RJ, Cowley AW, Jr. Relationship between renal perfusion pressure and blood flow in different regions of the kidney. *Am J Physiol* 1993;264:R578–R583, with permission.)

tion by adjacent nephrons generating pressure natriuresis. Such a paracrine role for NO to signal between the vasculature and nephrons is frequently postulated (93, 109, 451, 542, 544).

Blood flow to the renal medulla is particularly dependent on generation of NO (93, 368). This is particularly true in the spontaneously hypertensive rat (SHR) (485). Roald and colleagues observed poor autoregulation of juxtamedullary blood flow in the SHR. They proposed that the tendency toward early tissue damage in the juxtaglomerular cortex is due to poor autoregulation (497). The superoxide dismutase mimetic, tempol, enhances tissue NO levels by eliminating its reaction with superoxide (578). Feng and colleagues found that tempol reduced blood pressure and enhanced medullary blood flow in the SHR (141).

Vasopressin, Sodium, and Water Excretion

Changes in medullary blood flow might have diuretic effects by reducing the efficiency of countercurrent exchange, leading to "solute washout" and loss of corticomedullary axial gradients of NaCl and urea (448). The role of vasopressin to modulate medullary blood flow during antidiuresis has been the focus of much investigation (23, 91, 92, 410). Early studies, based on indicator transit times, showed that vasopressin reduces medullary blood flow (584). Homozygous Brattleboro rats that lack vasopressin secretion have elevated papillary plasma flow (34). The effect of vasopressin and specific V_1 (vasoconstrictor) and V_2 (antidiuretic) receptor subtype inhibitors on vasa recta blood flow was studied with videomicroscopy. Vasopressin reduces vasa recta blood flow in a manner that was partially blocked with either vasopressin V_1 or V_2 receptor subtype inhibitors (186, 277, 646).

Laser-Doppler flowmetry confirmed that intrarenal infusion of a selective V_1 receptor agonist reduces *inner* medullary blood flow to a greater extent than *outer* medullary blood flow without affecting the cortex (405). Elevation of plasma vasopressin within the physiological range, stimulated by depriving conscious rats of water, led to selective reduction of inner medullary but not cortical or outer medullary blood flow. The reduction of inner medullary blood flow correlated inversely with urine osmolality. Intramedullary infusion of a V_1 antagonist through implanted capsules blocked the decline in inner medullary perfusion and interfered with urinary concentration (154). When vasopressin was infused into decerebrate rats to maintain plasma levels within a physiological range of 2.9 to 11.2 pg/ml (about 10^{-12} to 10^{-11} M), inner medullary blood flow fell to an extent that correlated with urinary osmolality (Fig. 22) (155). Taken together, these studies provide important support for the vascular effects of vasopressin, mediated via the V_1 receptor, to modulate inner medullary blood flow and favor antidiuresis. The renal cortex might be spared from V_1 receptor–mediated vasoconstriction by reflex generation of vasodilator epoxyeicosatrienoic acids (486).

Vasopressin could reduce inner medullary perfusion by acting at various sites. It constricts juxtamedullary afferent (10^{-12} to 10^{-9} M) and efferent (10^{-9} M) arterioles in isolated, blood-perfused rat kidneys (201). Afferent AVP constriction is dependent on voltage-gated Ca^{2+} entry whereas efferent constriction may be related to Ca^{2+} mobilization from stores (136). Vasopressin also constricts rabbit afferent arterioles (608), efferent arterioles (10^{-13} to 10^{-7} M), and rat outer medullary DVR (10^{-10} to 10^{-6} M) in vitro (121, 591). Correia and colleagues showed that vasopressin V_1 agonist reduced medullary blood flow in rabbits but did not constrict either juxtamedullary afferent and efferent arterioles. They concluded that DVR might be the primarily site at which vasopressin acts to regulate inner medullary blood flow (90).

In addition to the constrictor effects of vasopressin, mediated by the V_1 receptor, it has been demonstrated that vasodilation of some vessels can be mediated through vascular V_2 receptors leading to elevation of NO (5, 326, 403, 507). Selective V_2 agonists have been shown to dilate preconstricted afferent arterioles (575) and outer medullary DVR (591) in vitro. In contrast, however, efforts to date have failed to show V_2 receptor mRNA in dissected renal microvessels by RT-PCR (463). Chronic infusion of the V_2 agonist dDAVP was shown to elevate renal medullary NO and increase medullary blood flow (464). Blockade of NO production during vasopressin elevation leads to hypertension: This finding suggests that V_2-mediated NO production in the medulla serves as a buffer to protect the outer medulla from ischemia as well as prevent salt retention and hypertension (132, 567). The probable source of V_2-mediated NO production is the inner medullary collecting duct (397).

Angiotensins

Using isolated microvessel perfusion (246, 247, 438, 542, 608, 630), the juxtamedullary nephron preparation (62, 65, 202), or the split hydronephrotic kidney (335, 556), studies have shown that ANG II constricts afferent arterioles, efferent arterioles, and DVR. Cultured mesangial cells also contract in response to ANG II (561). ANG II tonically constricts the juxtamedullary microcirculation in vivo (94, 137, 173, 502). Several vasodilators modulate ANG II–induced vasoconstriction. Blockade of NOS induces basal constriction of afferent arterioles and DVR and intensifies constriction by ANG II stimulation (246, 247, 287, 288, 624). Paracrine agents such as prostaglandin E_2 (PGE_2) and adenosine counteract ANG II constriction of glomerular arterioles and DVR (366, 438, 543, 576). Blockade of prostaglandin production may have a greater effect to augment constriction of juxtamedullary than superficial glomerular arterioles (366).

ANG II exerts its effects through type 1 ($AT1_A$ and $AT1_B$) and type 2 (AT2) receptors. $AT1_A$ and $AT1_B$ receptors are

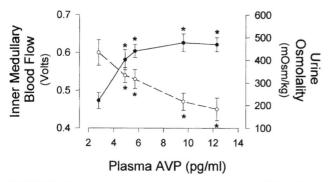

FIGURE 22 Effect of arginine vasopressin on inner medullary blood flow and urine osmolality. To control plasma vasopressin concentrations, decerebrate rats were infused with vasopressin. Increasing vasopressin concentration within the physiological range caused a reduction of inner medullary blood flow and an improvement in urinary concentration. (From Franchini KG, Cowley AW, Jr. Sensitivity of the renal medullary circulation to plasma vasopressin. *Am J Physiol* 1996;271:R647–R653, with permission.)

seven-membrane–spanning G-protein–coupled receptors with 95% amino acid sequence homology. AT1 stimulation activates phospholipase C (PLC) to generate inositol trisphosphate (IP_3) and elevate $[Ca^{2+}]_{CYT}$ (10, 333). $AT1_A$ receptor null mice have blunted afferent and absent efferent arteriolar responses to ANG II (203). Study of the distribution of receptors on juxtamedullary efferent arterioles revealed expression of $AT1_A$, $AT1_B$, and AT2 on muscular efferents destined to perfuse the medulla. In contrast, the $AT1_B$ subtype was absent in efferent arterioles that give rise to juxtamedullary capillary plexus in the cortex (208). AT2 receptor activation has been reported to favor vasodilation via generation of NO (60, 61). In the afferent arteriole, however, AT2 stimulation favors synthesis of vasodilatory CYP450 epoxygenase products (EETs) (11, 287, 288) rather than NO. Thus, evidence favors compensatory NO generation due to AT1 stimulation (465, 466). AT2 activation also vasodilates efferent arterioles (127) and DVR where it both inhibits reactive oxygen species formation and facilitates endothelium-dependent $[Ca^{2+}]_{CYT}$ signaling in response to vasodilators (451, 494, 636). The vasodilatory response to AT2 receptors may be impaired in forms of hypertension (128, 175). AT1 and AT2 receptors are widely expressed in vascular and tubular elements of in the kidney (389).

The role of ANG II AT1 and AT2 receptors in modulating regional perfusion in the kidney has been investigated. ANG II constricts DVR that supply the medulla (438, 451), but ANG II infusion reduces blood flow only to the renal cortex. Interestingly, reports of ANG II–induced enhancement of medullary perfusion have been provided (19, 113). The resistance of the renal medulla to ANG II–induced vasoconstriction has been traced to reflex generation of compensatory vasodilators, particularly NO (19, 109, 408, 451, 569, 656). Pressure natriuresis has been tied to renal medullary perfusion (see previous sections). Possibly related to this, AT2 receptor null mice are hypertensive and lack the pressure natriuretic response (182).

ANG II constricts renal microvessels over a broad range of concentrations with efferent arterioles and DVR showing the greatest sensitivity (EC_{50}, ∼ 0.5 nM). Although circulating plasma ANG II concentrations are in the range of 100 pM, renal interstitial and intratubular concentrations approach 1 to 10 nM, implying an intrarenal mechanism for generation and sequestration (Fig. 23). Interstitial concentrations are greatest in the renal medulla where ANG II receptor density is high (407, 411, 419, 420, 535).

ANG II is derived from angiotensin I through the actions of angiotensin-converting enzyme (ACE). ANG II has a short half-life and is itself degraded by angiotensinases to form several fragments including ANG[1–7] and ANG [3–8]. Angiotensin-converting enzyme type 2 (ACE2) is a metalloprotease that hydrolyzes ANG I and ANG II to form the heptapeptide, ANG[1–7]. ACE2 is not blocked by conventional converting enzyme inhibitors. ACE2 reduces formation of ANG II by degrading ANG I to other fragments (60, 146, 419). ANG[1–7] is a dilator of the renal and other capillary beds (512) and accumulates during ACE inhibition,

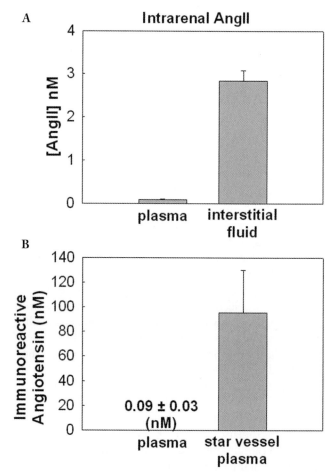

FIGURE 23 Intrarenal angiotensin II concentrations. **A:** Graph shows a comparison of angiotensin II (ANG II) concentration in plasma and renal interstitial fluid obtained by microdialysis. Cortical interstitial ANG II concentrations are markedly higher than plasma values. **B:** Comparison of immunoreactive angiotensins in systemic plasma and star vessel plasma (efferent arteriolar, precapillary blood) by micropuncture of the rat kidney. ANG II concentration is estimated to be ∼10% to 25% of the immunoreactive angiotensins in various compartments. (From Nishiyama A, Seth DM, Navar LG. Angiotensin II type 1 receptor-mediated augmentation of renal interstitial fluid angiotensin II in angiotensin II-induced hypertension. *J Hypertens* 2003;21:1897–1903; and Seikaly MG, Arant BS, Jr., Seney FD, Jr. Endogenous angiotensin concentrations in specific intrarenal fluid compartments of the rat. *J Clin Invest* 1990;86:1352–1357, with permission.)

potentially contributing to antihypertensive actions of those pharmaceuticals (553). In the kidney, ANG [1–7] specifically binds to the Mas receptor. Mas null mice lack binding, aortic relaxation and antidiuretic response to ANG[1–7] (519).

Aldosterone

Aldosterone increases transcription of molecular machinery dedicated to salt reabsorption in the distal nephron. It has been shown to increase mRNA for renin in juxtaglomerular cells in manner that is blocked by the mineralocorticoid receptor antagonist, spironoloactone (283). Research has shown that aldosterone acts as a paracrine agent in the vasculature to have acute "nongenomic" effects on vasoactivity (593) as evidenced by the work of Schmidt and colleagues who showed that aldosterone increased human forearm blood flow. With NOS inhibition, aldosterone enhanced blood flow reduction mediated by phenyephrine. The data were interpreted to show that aldosterone causes vasoconstriction via smooth muscle activation and compensatory vasodilation via release of NO (523). Similarly, Arima et al. (12, 13) showed that aldosterone caused concentration-dependent constriction of afferent and efferent arterioles, an effect that was insensitive to spironoloactone. The constriction was prevented by PLC inhibition and involved voltage-gated Ca^{2+} entry into myocytes. In other studies, aldosterone was found to blunt afferent arteriolar constriction by enhancing NO production (12, 13).

Adrenomedullin

Adrenomedullin is a 53–amino acid peptide (human) with homology to CGRP. It circulates in picomolar concentrations and is widely synthesized by tissues including vascular smooth muscle and endothelium. It has potent vasodilatory and hypotensive effects at least partially mediated by NO (46, 53, 214). Deletion of the gene for adrenomedullin is lethal in utero. Heterozygotes live to adulthood but are hypertensive, have defective synthesis of NO, and are vulnerable to renal ischemia (417, 540). Renal synthesis of adrenomedullin is enhanced by hypoxia (401). Intrarenal infusion induces vasodilation that is attenuated by NO synthase inhibition (164, 352, 385). Effects of adrenomedullin on renal arteriolar segments have not been extensively studied. However, studies have shown that adrenomedullin dilates afferent and efferent arterioles of the hydronephrotic kidney preparation (215) and increases canine cortical and medullary blood flow (352). Chronic infusion of adrenomedullin was found to limit hypertensive injury in deoxycorticosterone (DOCA) salt hypertensive rats (398, 416).

Nitric Oxide

Endothelia secrete paracrine modulators of vascular tone, including NO, prostacyclin (prostaglandin I_2, PGI_2), and endothelium-derived hyperpolarizing factors (EDHFs). NO regulates vessel tone, regional distribution of blood flow, autoregulation, pressure natriuresis, TGF, and salt reabsorption. Its effects on the microcirculation of the kidney have been frequently reviewed (93, 171, 172, 291–293, 354, 368, 370, 374, 408, 445, 651).

Infusions of the NO synthase inhibitor N^w-nitro-L-arginine methyl ester (L-NAME) into the renal artery of rats and dogs increase renal vascular resistance and blunt the pressure natriuretic response (38, 355). Imig and colleagues showed that NOS inhibition constricts the preglomerular microcirculation of the juxtamedullary nephron preparation and that effects are enhanced when RBCs, which trap NO, are included in the perfusate (226, 230). The ability of NO to modulate

afferent arteriolar tone results from its synthesis by the endothelium (246-248, 261) and signaling in the macula densa (249). Study of the effects of NO on renal resistance vessels showed that NOS inhibition interferes with the modulation of medullary autoregulation that accompanies pressure natriuresis (see previous sections) (217, 230). Infusion of an NO synthase inhibitor into rats restored medullary autoregulation and blunted pressure natriuresis (143). Similarly, Larson and Lockhart found that infusion of L-arginine altered medullary autoregulation and normalized pressure natriuresis in the SHR (310). The endothelium-dependent vasodilators, acetylcholine and bradykinin, enhance NO production and dilate preconstricted DVR (450, 494, 496, 624).

Chronic intravenous or intrarenal infusion of L-NAME into rats causes hypertension and selective reduction of renal medullary blood flow (371, 404). NO production in the renal medulla exceeds that in the cortex (43, 374, 379, 399, 649). L-Arginine supplementation enhances NO levels in the renal medullary interstitium (649) and abrogates hypertension in the Dahl rat and SHR (310, 388, 390). Selective nitric oxide synthase type 1 (nNOS or NOS1) or type 2 (iNOS or NOS2) isoform inhibition in the medulla of rats by antisense infusion or pharmacological blockade, leads to salt-sensitive hypertension that, unlike L-NAME infusion, does not reduce medullary perfusion (269, 369, 373). The data may indicate that eNOS- or NOS3-derived NO is responsible for the effects on vascular resistance while NO derived from all NOS isoforms favors saliuresis (167, 423, 424).

NO is released in response to administration of the vasoconstrictor agents norepinephrine, ANG II, and vasopressin (464, 567–569, 650, 656). Evidence also favors an important role for NO to abrogate tissue hypoxia that would otherwise arise from the action of vasoconstrictors. Low-dose, subpressor infusion of L-NAME into the renal interstitium does not affect MBF or PO_2 but enables otherwise ineffective doses of ANG II (656), norepinephrine (568, 650), or vasopressin (567, 629) to reduce those parameters. Reduced expression of NOS isoforms and NO generation in the Dahl rat may contribute to it sensitivity to ANG II and hypertension (569). In the absence of NOS blockade, constrictors enhance medullary NO levels, implying that a reflex increase in medullary NO probably serves to protect the hypoxic medulla from ischemia. NO generation has also been found to protect the medulla from the blood flow redistribution induced by endotoxemic hypotension (213, 255).

NOS isoforms are expressed by nephrons and vessels throughout the kidney (292, 368, 370, 374) but expression is greatest in the inner medullary collecting duct and vasa recta (375). It has also been shown that NO generation by collecting duct is regulated by uptake of L-arginine via the CAT1 cationic amino acid transporter (267, 268, 618, 632). Infusion of competing cationic amino acids reduced medullary NO, reduced medullary blood flow and induced hypertension (267).

Given that NO has vasodilatory and saliuretic effects and is widely synthesized by nephrons and endothelium, attention has been drawn to possible tubular–vascular interactions.

Hypothetically, NO generated by the medullary thick ascending limb could influence DVR tone (93, 109, 396, 451, 457, 494, 496) and be subject to regulation by reaction with superoxide to form peroxynitrite (396). Conversely, NO generated by DVR might influence salt reabsorption by adjacent nephrons (451, 635). The latter might explain the association of medullary perfusion with pressure natriuresis because pressurization of the DVR lumen leads to endothelial $[Ca^{2+}]_{CYT}$ responses and NO generation (635). If hemoglobin in vascular bundles is the major sink for NO, then net diffusion should be directed toward the vasa recta lumen. Local NO concentration should, however, be influenced by the slope of the NO gradient and the rate of its generation by both nephrons and vessels. NOS expression and NO generation by the collecting duct is also modulated by shear (56). Contractile smooth muscle pericytes surround DVR in the inner medulla (462) so that similar concepts potentially apply along the entire corticomedullary axis.

Reactive Oxygen Species

Oxygen-free radicals are generated by one and two electron reductions of O_2 that generate superoxide (O_2^-) and hydrogen peroxide (H_2O_2). In turn, reactions of those species yield hypochlorous acid and hydroxyl radical (OH). Reaction of NO with O_2^- forms peroxynitrite ($ONOO^-$), reducing the availability of NO to act as a vasodilator. Oxygen-derived radicals are collectively referred to as "reactive oxygen species" (ROS). ROS can be generated through many pathways. Auto-oxidation of cysteine can generate O_2^- and H_2O_2. Oxygen-using enzymes such as cyclooxygenase, lipoxygenase, epoxygenase, and xanthine oxidase can generate ROS. When oxidative stress reduces the ratio of the NOS cofactor tetrahydrobiopterin (BH_4) relative to di hydrobiopterin (BH_2) NOS produces O_2^- rather than NO. It is generally accepted that the dominant source of ROS for bacterocidal activity in leukocytes and signaling in other cells is NADPH oxidase. NADPH oxidase consists of cytosolic components (p47phox, p67phox), a G-protein– (Rac1 or Rac2) and membrane-associated cytochrome b_{558} composed of p22phox and gp91phox. In nonphagocytic cells, the gp91phox subunit may be substituted by another isoform such as RENOX/NOX4 (578). Antioxidant systems exist within all cells. Superoxide dismutase (SOD) catalyzes the conversion of O_2^- to H_2O_2, which is then converted to water by catalase. Extracellular, cytoplasmic (Cu/ZnSOD), and mitochondrial (MnSOD) forms of SOD participate in the control of oxidative stress. Endogenous free radical scavengers also serve to limit the potential for oxidative damage to cellular macromolecules (112).

ROS generation plays a role in the agonist-induced constriction of renal microvessels (524). Schnackenberg et al. (526) found that elimination of O_2^- with the cell permeant superoxide dismutase mimetic, tempol, largely abrogated afferent constriction by the TxA2/prostaglandin H_2 (TP) receptor agonist U46619 (526). Tempol also enhanced bio-

available NO in bradykinin-stimulated DVR and vasodilated ANG II–constricted vessels (496). Zhang et al. found that ROS are generated upon stimulation of DVR with ANG II and PKC agonists. Interestingly, the ANG II–mediated generation of ROS was pronounced when ANG II AT2 receptors were blocked with PD123, 319 (636). The role of ROS in the mediation of vasoconstriction probably varies with the vasoactive stimulus (430).

Intrarenal generation of ROS plays a role in vasoactivity and generation of hypertension. Blood pressure elevation in the SHR is associated with enhanced urinary excretion of the ROS marker, 8-iso prostaglandin F2α. Both hypertension and 8-Iso PGF2α excretion are blunted by treatment of the SHR with the superoxide dismutase (SOD) mimetic, tempol. Infusion of L-NAME eliminates the antihypertensive effect of tempol, implying that reduction of NO availability through reaction with O_2^- partially underlies the genesis of SHR hypertension (525, 527). Slow-pressor hypertension due to chronic infusion of ANG II is also associated with an increase in cortical ROS generation (74) but the medulla may be spared in that model (638). Intrarenal oxygen tension and the efficiency of renal oxygen utilization are low in rodent models of hypertension (611, 612).

Enhancement of renal medullary ROS generation occurs in hypertensive models and intramedullary infusion of the SOD inhibitor, diethylthiocarbamate, reduces medullary blood flow and raises arterial blood pressure (77, 356, 357). Conversely, infusion of the SOD mimetic, tempol, increases medullary blood flow and sodium excretion, an effect that is enhanced when H_2O_2 is eliminated with catalase (77, 356, 655). A role for renal medullary generation of ROS was reinforced by Meng et al. (382) who showed that hypertension of Dahl salt sensitive rats is accompanied by reduced expression of Cu/Zn SOD and Mn SOD in the medulla. In contrast to those findings, slow-pressor hypertension generated by chronic ANG II infusion failed to increase ROS generation by isolated DVR (638). Instead, ANG II hypertension was accompanied by increased DVR generation of NO, a finding that agrees with earlier reports by Zou and Cowley (93, 656). It is possible that ROS production by medullary nephrons contributes to ANG II–induced slow-pressor hypertension. NO is an endogenous diuretic and its consumption by ROS could favor hypertension (167, 423). Enhanced generation of ROS may also play a role to enhance arteriolar constriction in diabetes (531).

Adenosine and P1 Purinoceptors

Adenosine acts via A1, A2$_A$, A2$_B$, and A3 receptors (P_1 purinoceptors). In the kidney, A1 and A2 receptors predominate, A2$_A$ are primarily vascular, and A3 may be absent (254, 598). Through their actions, adenosine modulates vasoactivity and epithelial transport (196, 253, 254). The microvascular effects of adenosine vary with intrarenal location

(376). Adenosine A1 receptor activation transiently reduces cortical and medullary blood flow and constricts afferent arterioles (3, 64, 609). When afferent A1 receptors are blocked, however, A2-mediated vasodilation can be elicited (418). Afferent constriction by adenosine is of particular importance because data support it as the primary mediator of TGF (51, 528, 582). Macula densa release of ATP via maxi-anion channels followed by ecto-5′-nucleotidase–mediated ATP hydrolysis to form adenosine are intrinsic steps (39, 39, 40, 71, 239, 490). Adenosine constriction of the afferent arteriole is complex because proximal portions away from the glomerulus may be regulated by A2 dilatory and A1 constrictor interactions. In contrast, the afferent arteriole near the glomerular hilus may lack A2 vasodilatory receptors so that it undergoes monotonic constriction as adenosine concentration is increased (196).

Adenosine A2 receptor stimulation leads to preferential vasodilation, saliuresis, and enhanced perfusion of the medulla (Fig. 24) (3, 376, 387). A1 and A2 receptors are expressed by DVR (300) and their respective stimulation induces constriction or dilation (542). Interstitial adenosine concentrations are near the affinity for the A2 receptor so that changes should modulate vasodilatory and saliuretic

effects (29). In preglomerular vessels, A1-induced constriction is mediated by pertussis toxin–sensitive Gi protein and phospholipase C activation (191). A2-mediated dilation has been traced to activation of K_{ATP} channels (577), probably activated through 11,12-epoxyeicosatrienoic acid (79).

Evidence for and against synergism between ANG II and adenosine exists (192, 239). Several studies have favored the interdependence of adenosine A1 receptor and ANG II AT1 receptor–mediated constriction (110, 190, 426, 549, 610), while others have not (32, 64, 236). The availability of adenosine A1 and ANG II $AT1_A$ receptor–deficient mice have permitted re-examination of the issue. Infusion of NG II led to less reduction of renal blood flow and less constriction of afferent arterioles in A1 knockout mice (192). Similarly, favoring synergism, intranephron infusion of an adenosine A1 agonist induced greater reduction of stop-flow pressure (reflecting afferent constriction) in wild-type than in ANG II $AT1_A$ receptor–deficient mice (586).

A consequence of countercurrent exchange is that renal medullary oxygen tensions (PO_2) are low (Fig. 25) (111). During hypoxia, the medullary thick ascending limb of Henle (mTAL) synthesizes adenosine (36). That finding, coupled with the close proximity of the mTAL to outer medullary

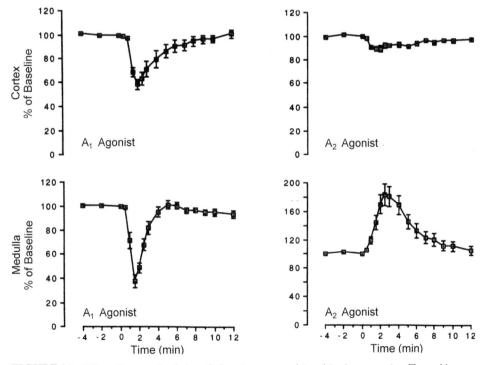

FIGURE 24 Effect of intrarenal infusion of adenosine receptor A1 or A2 subtype agonists. Top and bottom panels show the effect of adenosine agonist infusions on intrarenal blood flow. Cortical and medullary measurements were obtained using laser-Doppler flowmetry with optical fibers placed on the kidney surface or inserted into the renal parenchyma, respectively. Left and right panels show the respective effects of either A1 or A2 receptor stimulation with subtype specific agonists. At time = 0, the A1 agonist N^6-cyclopentyladenosine (*left panels*) or the A2 agonist CGS-21680C (*right panels*) were transiently infused (1 minute) into the renal parenchyma. The A1 agonist transiently reduced both cortical and medullary blood flow while the A2 agonist caused a preferential increase in blood flow to the medulla. From Agmon Y, Dinour D, Brezis M. Disparate effects of adenosine A1- and A2-receptor agonists on intrarenal blood flow. *Am J Physiol* 1993;265:F802–F806 and Nishiyama A, Seth DM, Navar LG. Angiotensin II type 1 receptor-mediated augmentation of renal interstitial fluid angiotensin II in angiotensin II-induced hypertension. *J Hypertens* 2003;21:1897–1903, with permission.)

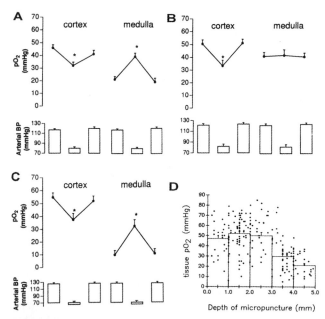

FIGURE 25 Hemodynamic effects on intrarenal oxygenation. Intrarenal oxygen tension (PO₂) was measured in the cortex and medulla with a microelectrode. Cortical PO₂ falls and medullary PO₂ increases during an episode of hypotension induced by hemorrhage, aortic ligation, or nitroprusside infusion **(A)**. Inhibition of transport in the thick ascending limb of Henle with a loop diuretic **(B)**. increases basal PO₂ in the medulla (compare to **A**) and eliminates the effect of hypotension to raise medullary PO₂. Inhibition of vasodilatory prostaglandins and nitric oxide, or blockade of adenosine receptors reduces basal PO₂ in the medulla and accentuates the increase in PO₂ caused by hypotension **(C)**. Intrarenal tissue PO₂ decreases with medullary depth **(D)**. (From Brezis M, Agmon Y, Epstein FH. Determinants of intrarenal oxygenation, I: effects of diuretics. *Am J Physiol* 1994;267:F1059–F1062; and Brezis M, Heyman SN, Dinour D, Epstein FH, Rosen S. Role of nitric oxide in renal medullary oxygenation: studies in isolated and intact rat kidneys. *J Clin Invest* 1991;88:390–395, with permission.)

vascular bundles, led to the hypothesis that adenosine, like NO and prostaglandins (see previous sections), acts as a paracrine vasodilator to preserve medullary perfusion, raising medullary PO₂ (35). Inhibition of mTAL transport by adenosine A2 receptor activation, like the effects of furosemide, probably raises medullary PO₂ by reducing O₂ consumption (35, 49). Rats fed high salt diet increase tissue adenosine levels and downregulate A1 receptor expression, the activation of which encourages sodium reabsorption (657).

Extracellular ATP and Renal P₂ Purinoceptors

In addition to the actions of adenosine mediated by P1 purinoceptors (A1, A2 adenosine receptors), micromolar concentrations of ATP modulate vasoactivity through P2 purinoceptors (235, 236, 239). P2 receptors are subdivided into P2X and P2Y families, encoded by separate genes, that yield ligand-gated nonselective cation channels or seven transmembrane–spanning, G-protein–coupled receptors, respectively. Unlike adenosine receptors, P2 receptors seem confined to the preglomerular microcirculation (21, 75, 321).

P2 antagonists such as suramin are somewhat nonselective, however α,β-methylene-ATP and β,γ-methylene-ATP are relatively selective agonists for P2X receptors. UTP largely stimulates P2Y (21, 234, 236, 487). The experimental effects of ATP on the vasculature are variable depending on luminal versus abluminal application, the preparation, and species (234). Both constrictor and dilator effects can be observed. Intrarenal infusion of α,β-methylene-ATP leads to constriction, but ATP (mixed P2X, P2Y agonist) and UTP (selective P2Y agonist) yield NO-dependent dilation at low concentrations or constriction at high concentrations (85). Exposure of preconstricted afferent arterioles of rabbit and human kidneys to ATP leads to dilation via NO generation (234, 235, 508). In the juxtamedullary nephron preparation of the rat, activation of P2X leads to afferent but not efferent constriction that is dependent on generation of 20-HETE and Ca²⁺ influx involving L-type Ca²⁺ channel blockade (243, 244, 639, 640). Stimulation of P2Y receptors yields sustained constriction that is independent of 20-HETE and dependent on Ca²⁺ release from cellular stores (241, 245, 613).

Of great importance, myogenic autoregulatory constriction of afferent arterioles has been traced to activation of P2 receptors (Fig. 26). In the juxtamedullary nephron preparation, prior desensitization or nonspecific blockade of P2 receptors attenuated pressure-induced afferent constriction (240). Similarly, infusion of excess ATP into the dog kidney during NO synthase blockade eliminated autoregulatory constriction (351, 353). Finally, P2X1 receptor–deficient mice were shown to retain TGF responses but to lack autoregulatory adjustments to changes in perfusion pressure (238).

Arachidonic Acid Metabolites

Once liberated from the membrane by phospholipases, arachidonic acid undergoes metabolism to a large array of metabolites that function as paracrine, autocrine, and intracellular signaling molecules. These metabolites have profound effects on vascular tone and solute and water excretion (Fig. 27). Three generalized pathways are recognized, cyclooxygenases (COXs) that generate prostaglandins (PGs) and thromboxanes (TBXs), lipoxygenases that generate leukotrienes (LTs) and hydroxyeicosatetraenoic acids (HETEs), and cytochrome P450 pathways that synthesize HETEs and epoxyeicosatrienoic acids (EETs).

PROSTAGLANDINS
Prostaglandins (PGs) are generated from arachidonic acid by COX (Fig. 27A) and exert wide effects on solute reabsorption, TGF, and intrarenal hemodynamics. When injected into the renal artery, PGE₂ and PGI₂ enhance renal blood flow (76). Early efforts showed that stimulation of PG synthesis redistributes blood flow toward the juxtamedullary cortex (250, 311). A consistent finding has been that renal medullary perfusion is protected from vasoconstrictors by NO (see previous sections) and PGs. Nonselective COX blockade decreased vasa recta blood flow (318) and augmented the ability of ANG

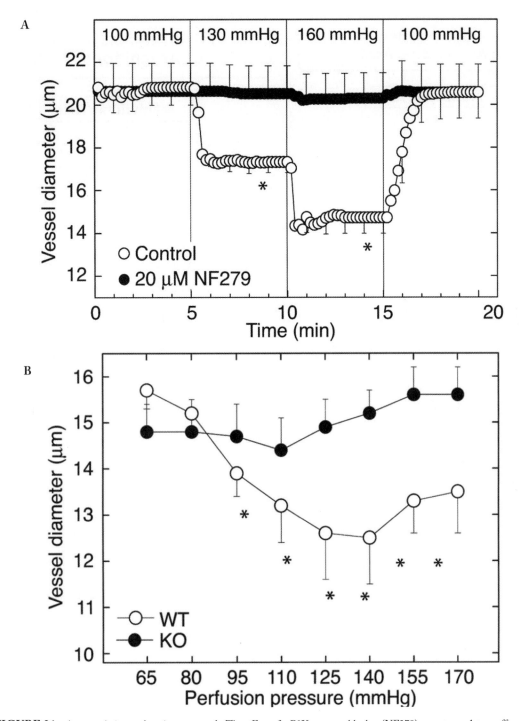

FIGURE 26 Autoregulation and purinoceptors. **A:** The effect of a P2X receptor blocker (NF279) on autoregulatory afferent arteriolar constriction resulting from step changes in perfusion pressure from 100 to 120 and 160 mm Hg. P2X blockade eliminates the afferent myogenic response associated with autoregulation. **B:** Summary of the changes in murine afferent arteriolar diameter elicited by graded change of perfusion pressure. Autoregulatory vasoconstriction occurs in wild-type (WT) but not P2X1 receptor null mice. Data obtained using the juxtamedullary nephron preparation. (From Inscho EW, Cook AK, Imig JD, Vial C, Evans RJ. Physiological role for P2X1 receptors in renal microvascular autoregulatory behavior. *J Clin Invest* 2003;112:1895–1905, with permission.)

II infusion to decrease single-vessel blood flow in the exposed papilla (94). Laser-Doppler studies indicate that COX blockade reduces medullary blood flow with relative sparing of cortical perfusion (20, 421, 461, 503). Radiocontrast agents can lower cortical and medullary oxygen content predisposing

to hypoxic insult. Indomethacin potentiates medullary hypoxia and the parenchymal damage induced by radiocontrast agents or ureteral excision (4, 211, 212).

COX-1 and COX-2 isoforms contribute to renal PG synthesis. Of the two, COX-1 is expressed to a greater extent

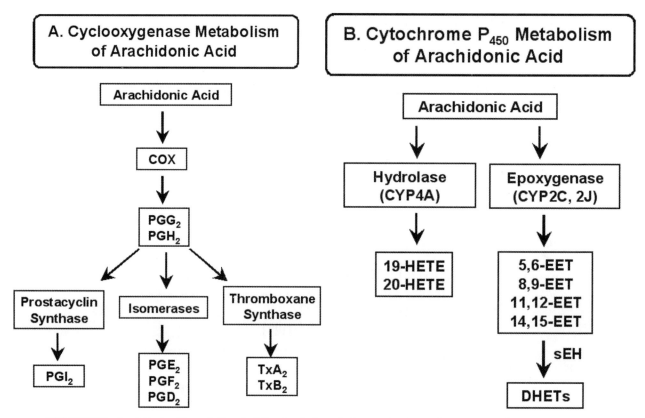

FIGURE 27   Arachidonic acid metabolites. **A:** Abbreviated schematic showing signaling molecules generated from arachadonic acid by cyclooxygenase (COX). Prostaglandins (PGs) and thromboxanes (Tx's) are vasoactive end products. **B:** Abbreviated schematic showing signaling molecules generated cytochrome P450 metabolism of arachidonic acid (COX). Hydrolases generate the potent constrictor 20-hydroxyeicosatetraenoic acid (20-HETE) and epoxygenases generate the epoxyeicosatrienoic acids (EETs) that most often function as vasodilators. The lipoxygenase pathway of arachidonic acid metabolism is not shown.

while COX-2 is more highly regulated (57, 78, 199, 200, 625). In a manner that predicts the effects of its inhibition, COX-2 expression is pronounced in macula densa (57). Release of renin by juxtaglomerular cells and release of PGE$_2$ by the macula densa is COX-2–dependent (156, 431, 468). In the macula densa, COX-2 is coexpressed with NOS1. Simultaneous inhibition of COX-2 and NOS in the dog markedly enhances sensitivity to vasoconstriction. Norepinephrine infusion, which otherwise has minor effects, induces a remarkable rise in renal vascular resistance and sharp reduction of GFR (331). COX-2 blockade blunts adaptation of TGF (98) and augments afferent constriction associated with benzolamide inhibition of proximal transport (222). Renomedullary interstitial cells express receptors for vasoconstrictors, release paracrine substances such as PGE$_2$ and medullipin, and express COX-1 and COX-2 (57, 644). Zhang et al. (633) showed that COX-2 expression is stimulated by medullary tonicity. Genetic deficiency of COX-2 or its inhibition leads to reduction of medullary perfusion and salt-sensitive hypertension and enhanced response to infusion of ANG II (44, 482, 631, 642).

In isolated vessels, Edwards (120) first showed that prostaglandins dilate in vitro–perfused rabbit afferent (PGE$_2$ and PGI$_2$) and efferent (PGI$_2$) arterioles. In contrast, Inscho et al.

(237) found that PGE$_2$ enhanced ANG II and norepinephrine constriction of the afferent arteriole while PGI$_2$ counteracted their effects. In rabbit afferent arterioles, indomethacin enhanced vasoconstriction when perfusate passed through the glomerulus but not during retrograde perfusion, implying that glomerular PGs influence efferent vasoactivity (14). Abluminal PGE$_2$ blunts ANG II–induced constriction of DVR (438, 544). Few studies of the effects of selective COX-2 inhibition in isolated vessel preparations are available. Wang et al. (602) determined that augmented constriction of afferent arterioles during slow-pressor ANG II hypertension is partially mediated by a COX-2 product from the endothelium. PGE$_2$ is abundant in the kidney, and its local actions are governed by the receptor subtype activated. For example, stimulation of the EP3 receptor inhibits cAMP formation, favoring vasoconstriction, while stimulation of EP2 and EP4 receptors increases cAMP, favoring vasodilation (224). The ability of PGE$_2$ to act as a vasoconstrictor has also been observed (237), and EP3 receptor deficiency leads to reduction of renal vascular resistance (15, 224).

COX products can be metabolized by thromboxane synthase to stimulate the thromboxane/PGH$_2$ receptor and induce vasoconstriction. In the afferent arteriole and DVR, ANG II–induced constriction is reduced by TP receptor blockade, inhibition of COX with indomethacin, or inhibition of thromboxane synthesis (206, 541, 543, 614). Thromboxane-mediated constriction may be exaggerated during ANG II slow-pressor hypertension due to enhanced synthesis of reactive oxygen species (273, 601),

CYTOCHROME P450 METABOLITES OF ARACHIDONIC ACID

Vasoactive products of arachidonic acid are generated by cytochrome P450 (CYP) isoforms (Fig. 27B) in the form of EETs, the HETEs, and their products, dihydroxyeicosatetraneoic acids (DHETs) (197). More than 400 CYP isoforms are recognized in various species. Those that have more than 40% homology are classified by an Arabic numeral and those with more than 55% homology by a capital letter. CYP monooxygenases metabolize arachidonic acid to 19- and 20-HETE (ω/ω-1 hydroxylase) and to 5,6-; 8,9-; 11,12-; and 14,15-EETs (epoxygenases). For the purposes of focusing on the microvasculature of the kidney, it is important to recognize that CYP2C and CYC2J isoforms are largely responsible for synthesis of EETs, and CYP4A isoforms for synthesis of the HETEs. This topic has been frequently reviewed (149, 197, 229, 349, 377, 422, 484, 499, 504, 521).

The 20 ω-hydroxylation product, 20-HETE, is a potent vasoconstrictor the synthesis of which is rate limited by O_2 (198, 233). The 20-HETE depolarizes and increases $[Ca^{2+}]_{CYT}$ in smooth muscle (345) and mediates constriction by ANG II (7, 287), endothelin-1 (210, 229), and ATP via P2X stimulation (640). The 20-HETE plays an important role in blood flow autoregulation of the cerebral and renal microcirculations (197, 654) and inhibits K_{Ca} channel activity (233, 504, 563, 564, 652, 653) through the actions of tyrosine and MAP kinases (564). It is generally recognized that NO inhibits vascular smooth muscle contraction through cGMP formation. Roman and colleagues have shown that most NO effects in the kidney involve inhibition of CYP4A and reduction of 20-HETE synthesis (6, 8). The 20 ω-hydroxylation products play a role in blood pressure regulation. Chronic inhibition of 20-HETE synthesis induces salt-sensitive hypertension in the rat (216, 551). Similarly, disruption of murine CYP4A14 leads to hypertension, and a variant of the CYP4A11 homologue in humans has been associated with essential hypertension (58, 59, 159).

The EET epoxygenase metabolites, arachidonic acids, have several important roles in the renal microcirculation. In addition, EETs have been broadly identified as EDHFs (55, 150). The EETs are largely vasodilatory but some of their metabolites can induce COX-dependent vasoconstriction (224, 228, 548). Simulation of preglomerular arteriolar A2A adenosine receptors leads to enhanced synthesis of EETs and vasodilation (79). Similarly, ANG II dilation via AT2 receptor stimulation has been traced to these epoxygenase products (11, 287). Afferent vasodilation by 11,12-EET is partially mediated by PKA (227). In contrast to inhibition by 20-HETE, 11,12-EET and 5,6-EET are associated with K_{Ca} channel activation (157, 475, 504, 653).

The ability to activate large conductance K_{Ca} channels may be tied to the role of 11,12-EET as an EDHF. Putative EDHFs are agents that elevate endothelial $[Ca^{2+}]_{CYT}$, hyperpolarize endothelium and smooth muscle, and vasodilate, independent of NO and COX. Work in this area has failed to identify a single EDHF, but much evidence points to a role for EET formation and K_{Ca} channel activation in the endothelium. Adjacent smooth muscle hyperpolarization may be tied to diffusion of secondary signaling molecules or electrogenic spread of current from the endothelium via myoendothelial gap junctions (476, 484). It might also be tied to release of K^+ ion into the myoendothelial intercellular space via EET-stimulated endothelial K_{Ca} channels, resulting in hyperpolarization via activation of smooth muscle K_{IR} or Na,K-ATPase (55, 150). In the kidney, evidence points to a role for afferent arteriolar EET formation in the EDHF-related actions of bradykinin (225) and acetylcholine (600). Evidence for K_{IR} expression in afferent smooth muscle has been provided (80).

Reduction of vasodilatory EET formation may accompany hypertension. Imig et al. (231, 232) showed that enhanced afferent constriction during slow-pressor ANG II hypertension is reversed by an 11,12-EET analogue and that reduction of EET degradation through soluble epoxide hydrolase inhibition reverses ANG II hypertension. Lack of ability to upregulate CYP2C and CYP2J isoforms of P450 might underlie the abnormality (641). Similarly, it has been found that enhancement of EET through inhibition of soluble epoxide hydrolase reverses hypertension and protects the kidney from damage (627, 628, 642).

Endothelins

Endothelins are 21–amino acid vasoactive peptides synthesized by a variety of cell types in the kidney. Three ETs have been identified (ET1, ET2, ET3). These agents are autocrine/paracrine hormones derived from ~200–amino acid preproendothelins that undergo successive proteolytic cleavage to form large (Big ET) intermediates that are processed by endothelin-converting enzymes. ETs stimulate ETA and ETB receptors on smooth muscle to induce potent vasoconstriction. Endothelia express ETB receptors, stimulation of which leads to synthesis of NO. In addition to their vascular actions, ETs have an important role to inhibit sodium reabsorption through inhibition of transport by NO and downregulation of the epithelial Na^+ of the collecting duct (298, 304, 402, 470). Renal ET receptors have been identified on collecting ducts, vascular bundles and RMIC (579, 643).

The highest concentrations of ET1 occur in the renal medulla where it is synthesized by collecting duct and other cells (2, 289). ET1 is a potent vasoconstrictor and reduces overall renal blood flow via combined ETA and ETB stimulation.

Isolated ETB receptor stimulation, however, can have net vasodilatory effects (263). In the renal cortex, ET1 constricts afferent and efferent arterioles and arcuate and interlobular arteries (45, 72, 125, 281, 294, 336, 410). Afferent constriction by ET1 partially depends on voltage-gated Ca^{2+} entry, is modulated by endothelial generation of NO (122, 248), and is mediated by 20-HETE and COX products (210, 229). Preglomerular smooth muscle cells show biphasic $[Ca^{2+}]_{CYT}$ responses to ETA agonists but small or absent responses to ETB agonists (140, 473, 532). Isolated DVR from the outer medulla are intensely constricted by low concentrations of endothelins (449, 457, 544).

The actions of ETB stimulation in the medulla favor natriuresis and vasodilation. Bolus injection of ET1 (a mixed ETA and ETB receptor agonist) selectively reduced cortical blood flow while transiently increasing medullary blood flow. Medullary vasodilation and saliuresis are abrogated by blocking ETB receptors or synthesis of NO (132, 184, 218, 281, 294). The effects on medullary blood flow may vary with dietary salt intake (594). ETB receptor–deficient "spotted lethal" rats have been identified that have been rescued from lethal abnormalities by selective ETB gene replacement into ganglionic cells of the intestine. Those rats have salt-sensitive hypertension (165, 166). Injection of Big ET1 into ETB receptor–deficient rats or wild-type rats in which ETB receptor have been blocked, fails to elicit saliuresis (294, 472). Chronic ANG II infusion, combined with salt loading, increases cortical and medullary immunoreactive ET (471, 522). Reduction of endothelin induced saliuresis may play a role in human and rodent models of hypertension (304, 304, 394, 471). ETs might play significant roles in other pathological states, for example, renal hypoxia stimulates ET production and ET receptor antagonists attenuate ischemic injury and hyperfiltration in remnant kidneys created by surgical ablation (289).

Natriuretic Peptides

The diuretic effect of injection of extracts of atrial tissue extracts into rats led to the discovery of atrial (ANP), brain (BNP), and C- (CNP) natriuretic peptides. Each is derived by proteolytic cleavage of different gene products. They act through stimulation of guanylyl cyclase A (GC-A) (ANP, BNP ligands), GC-B type (CNP ligand), and GC-C receptors. GC-C may play a role in peptide clearance and inhibition. Deletion of ANP or its receptor leads to hypertension whereas overexpression results in hypotension (306). In the kidney, expression and alternate processing of ANP prohormone yield urodilatin (320, 597). Studies showed that that ANP infusions increased renal blood flow, GFR, papillary plasma flow, and sodium excretion. Diuresis and natriuresis, however, begin before the increase in medullary blood flow so that medullary dilation is not required for the natriuretic effect (257, 278, 574, 588). Examination of the vasoactive effects of natriuretic peptides revealed dilation of preglomerular vasculature (1, 205, 360, 595). Edwards and

Weidley found no effect of ANP on in vitro–perfused rabbit afferent or efferent arterioles (123). In the efferent arteriole, a lack of effect (123, 595) or constriction (126) was reported while urodilatin mediated vasodilation (124). Vasodilatory effects of ANP may be mediated through cGMP formation, activation of smooth muscle K_{Ca} channels, hyperpolarization, and inhibition of Ca^{2+} signaling (305, 561). Natriuresis from an oral salt load is more brisk than that from an intravenous route, a finding that may be related to intestinal release of guanylin and uroguanylin, peptide hormones that activate ANP receptors. Like ANP, these agents inhibit TGF, but their specific effects on renal arterioles have not been reported (332, 603).

Renal Innervation

Type 1 sympathetic nerves supply glomerular afferent and efferent arterioles and type 2 supply efferent arterioles alone with neuropeptide Y immunoreactive fibers (99). Sympathetic innervation includes juxtamedullary arterioles and DVR in the renal outer medulla. Renal sympathetic nerve stimulation enhances salt reabsorption, renin release, vascular tone, and TGF. Recruitment of these effects increases with the frequency of nerve stimulation. Renin release without effects on vascular resistance or sodium excretion occurs at low frequencies. Progressive enhancement of sodium uptake, accompanied by decrease in blood flow and GFR, occurs at high frequencies (102, 104). High-frequency stimulation may set average vascular tone, whereas low-frequency stimulation yields superimposed low-frequency oscillations of renal blood flow (358). Tubular and vascular effects of sympathetic activation are also dependent on the pattern of stimulation (105, 106). Barret and colleagues concluded that basal sympathetic nerve activity does not set renal vascular resistance in conscious rabbits but that vascular tone responds to episodic changes in sympathetic input to the kidney (31). Activation of the renin-angiotensin axis through salt deprivation reduces vascular frequency responsiveness to renal nerve stimulation while selectively increasing the slow TGF-mediated component of autoregulation (107). Sympathetic nerve activity is augmented by volume contraction, hypoxia, and hemorrhage, and renal hypoperfusion is accompanied by a redistribution of blood flow from the outer to the juxtamedullary cortex and renal medulla (27, 380, 448). Similarly, renal sympathetic nerve stimulation reduces cortical blood flow more than medullary blood flow (130, 131, 183, 406, 506). Medullary perfusion is more responsive to nerve stimulation occurring at high frequency (319) or when NO synthesis is inhibited (130, 599).

A role for modulation of renal sympathetic nerve activity in hypertension has been established (101, 103, 104). An increase in renal sympathetic nerve activity arising from the central nervous system accompanies some forms of hypertension. This is accompanied by an increase in renal vascular resistance and inhibition of the capacity for pressure natriuresis (488). Denervation enhanced renal blood flow in spontaneously hypertensive rats and improved autoregulation (108). Furthermore, denervation can significantly improve hypertension (103, 104).

Renal sympathetic nerve activity can also be modulated through a reflex arc involving sensory innervation of the renal pelvic wall. Sensory nerves containing substance P are activated by pelvic pressure (297). The associated sensory output leads to a reflex decrease in sympathetic nerve activity to the kidney, favoring saliuresis through inhibition of sodium reabsorption. The associated sensory output is inhibited by ANG II and augmented by high-salt diet. Denervation reduces the reflex, resulting in the need for higher blood pressure and extracellular fluid volume to facilitate natriuresis. Reduced effectiveness of this renorenal reflex occurs in hypertension (295, 296)

Acknowledgments

Our efforts are supported by NIH R37 DK42495, P01 HL 78870, and R01 DK67621. We are grateful to Professor Lise Bankir for helpful discussions.

References

1. Aalkjaer C, Mulvany MJ, Nyborg NC. Atrial natriuretic factor causes specific relaxation of rat renal arcuate arteries. *Br J Pharmacol* 1985;86:447–453.

2. Abassi ZA, Ellahham S, Winaver J, Hoffman A. The intrarenal endothelin system and hypertension. *News Physiol Sci* 2001;16:152–156.

3. Agmon Y, Dinour D, Brezis M. Disparate effects of adenosine A1- and A2-receptor agonists on intrarenal blood flow. *Am J Physiol* 1993;265:F802–F806.

4. Agmon Y, Peleg H, Greenfeld Z, Rosen S, Brezis M. Nitric oxide and prostanoids protect the renal outer medulla from radiocontrast toxicity in the rat. *J Clin Invest* 1994;94:1069–1075.

5. Aki Y, Tamaki T, Kiyomoto H, He H, Yoshida H, Iwao H, Abe Y. Nitric oxide may participate in V2 vasopressin-receptor-mediated renal vasodilation. *J Cardiovasc Pharmacol* 1994;23: 331–336.

6. Alonso-Galicia M, Drummond HA, Reddy KK, Falck JR, Roman RJ. Inhibition of 20-HETE production contributes to the vascular responses to nitric oxide. *Hypertension* 1997;29:320–325.

7. Alonso-Galicia M, Maier KG, Greene AS, Cowley AW, Jr., Roman RJ. Role of 20-hydroxyeicosatetraenoic acid in the renal and vasoconstrictor actions of angiotensin II. *Am J Physiol Regul Integr Comp Physiol* 2002;283:R60–R68.

8. Alonso-Galicia M, Sun CW, Falck JR, Harder DR, Roman RJ. Contribution of 20-HETE to the vasodilator actions of nitric oxide in renal arteries. *Am J Physiol* 1998;275:F370–F378.

9. Andreoli TE, Schafer JA, Troutman SL. Perfusion rate-dependence of transepithelial osmosis in isolated proximal convoluted tubules: estimation of the hydraulic conductance. *Kidney Int* 1978;14:263–269.

10. Arendshorst WJ, Brannstrom K, Ruan X. Actions of angiotensin II on the renal microvasculature. *J Am Soc Nephrol* 1999;10 (Suppl 11):S149–S161.

11. Arima S, Endo Y, Yaoita H, Omata K, Ogawa S, Tsunoda K, Abe M, Takeuchi K, Abe K, Ito S. Possible role of P-450 metabolite of arachidonic acid in vasodilator mechanism of angiotensin II type 2 receptor in the isolated microperfused rabbit afferent arteriole. *J Clin Invest* 1997;100:2816–2823.

12. Arima S, Kohagura K, Xu HL, Sugawara A, Abe T, Satoh F, Takeuchi K, Ito S. Nongenomic vascular action of aldosterone in the glomerular microcirculation. *J Am Soc Nephrol* 2003;14: 2255–2263.

13. Arima S, Kohagura K, Xu HL, Sugawara A, Uruno A, Satoh F, Takeuchi K, Ito S. Endothelium-derived nitric oxide modulates vascular action of aldosterone in renal arteriole. *Hypertension* 2004;43:352–357.

14. Arima S, Ren Y, Juncos LA, Carretero OA, Ito S. Glomerular prostaglandins modulate vascular reactivity of the downstream efferent arterioles. *Kidney Int* 1994;45:650–658.

15. Audoly LP, Ruan X, Wagner VA, Goulet JL, Tilley SL, Koller BH, Coffman TM, Arendshorst WJ. Role of EP(2) and EP(3) PGE(2) receptors in control of murine renal hemodynamics. *Am J Physiol Heart Circ Physiol* 2001;280:H327–H333.

16. Aukland K. Methods for measuring renal blood flow: total flow and regional distribution. *Annu Rev Physiol* 1980;42:543–555.

17. Aukland K, Bogusky RT, Renkin EM. Renal cortical interstitium and fluid absorption by peritubular capillaries. *Am J Physiol* 1994;266:F175–F184.

18. Aukland K, Bower BF, Berliner RW. Measurement of local blood flow with hydrogen gas. *Circ Res* 1964;14:164–187.

19. Badzynska B, Grzelec-Mojzesowicz M, Dobrowolski L, Sadowski J. Differential effect of angiotensin II on blood circulation in the renal medulla and cortex of anaesthetised rats. *J Physiol* 2002;538:159–166.

20. Badzynska B, Grzelec-Mojzesowicz M, Sadowski J. Prostaglandins but not nitric oxide protect renal medullary perfusion in anaesthetised rats receiving angiotensin II. *J Physiol* 2003;548:875–880.

21. Bailey MA, Hillman KA, Unwin RJ. P2 receptors in the kidney. *J Auton Nerv Syst* 2000;81:264–270.

22. Balint P, Bartha J, Fekete A. Intrarenal distribution of blood flow in the dog. *Acta Physiol Acad Sci Hung* 1969;36:1–11.

23. Bankir L. Antidiuretic action of vasopressin: quantitative aspects and interaction between V1a and V2 receptor-mediated effects. *Cardiovasc Res* 2001;51:372–390.

24. Bankir L, Bouby N, Trinh-Trang-Tan MM. Heterogeneity of nephron anatomy. *Kidney Int Suppl* 1987;20:S25–S39.

25. Bankir L, Chen K, Yang B. Lack of UT-B in vasa recta and red blood cells prevents urea-induced improvement of urinary concentrating ability. *Am J Physiol Renal Physiol* 2004;286: F144–F151.

26. Bankir L, de Rouffignac C. Urinary concentrating ability: insights from comparative anatomy. *Am J Physiol* 1985;249:R643–R666.

27. Bankir L, Farman N, Grunfeld JP, De la Tour EH, Funck-Brentano JL. Radioactive microsphere distribution and single glome-rular blood flow in the normal rabbit kidney. *Pflugers Arch* 1973;342:111–123.

28. Bankir L, Kaissling B, de Rouffignac C, Kriz W. The vascular organization of the kidney of *Psammomys obesus. Anat Embryol (Berl)* 1979;155:149–160.

29. Baranowski RL, Westenfelder C. Estimation of renal interstitial adenosine and purine metabolites by microdialysis. *Am J Physiol* 1994;267:F174–F182.

30. Barber RD, Woolf AS, Henderson RM. Potassium conductances and proliferation in conditionally immortalized renal glomerular mesangial cells from the H-2Kb-tsA58 transgenic mouse. *Biochim Biophys Acta* 1997;1355:191–203.

31. Barrett CJ, Navakatikyan MA, Malpas SC. Long-term control of renal blood flow: what is the role of the renal nerves? *Am J Physiol Regul Integr Comp Physiol* 2001;280:R1534–R1545.

32. Barrett RJ, Droppleman DA. Interactions of adenosine A1 receptor-mediated renal vasoconstriction with endogenous nitric oxide and ANG II. *Am J Physiol* 1993;265:F651–F659.

33. Baum M, Berry CA. Peritubular protein modulates neutral active NaCl absorption in rabbit proximal convoluted tubule. *Am J Physiol* 1985;248:F790–F795.

34. Bayle F, Eloy L, Trinh-Trang-Tan MM, Grunfeld JP, Bankir L. Papillary plasma flow in rats. I. Relation to urine osmolality in normal and Brattleboro rats with hereditary diabetes insipidus. *Pflugers Arch* 1982;394:211–216.

35. Beach RE, Good DW. Effects of adenosine on ion transport in rat medullary thick ascending limb. *Am J Physiol* 1992;263:F482–F487.

36. Beach RE, Watts BA, III, Good DW, Benedict CR, DuBose TD, Jr. Effects of graded oxygen tension on adenosine release by renal medullary and thick ascending limb suspensions. *Kidney Int* 1991;39:836–842.

37. Beeuwkes R, III. The vascular organization of the kidney. *Annu Rev Physiol* 1980;42:531–542.

38. Beierwaltes WH, Sigmon DH, Carretero OA. Endothelium modulates renal blood flow but not autoregulation. *Am J Physiol* 1992;262:F943–F949.

39. Bell PD, Lapointe JY, Peti-Peterdi J. Macula densa cell signaling. *Annu Rev Physiol* 2003;65:481–500.

40. Bell PD, Lapointe JY, Sabirov R, Hayashi S, Peti-Peterdi J, Manabe K, Kovacs G, Okada Y. Macula densa cell signaling involves ATP release through a maxi anion channel. *Proc Natl Acad Sci U S A* 2003; 100:4322–4327.

41. Bell RD, Keyl MJ, Shrader FR, Jones EW, Henry LP. Renal lymphatics: the internal distribution. *Nephron* 1968;5:454–463.

42. Betts LC, Kozlowski RZ. Electrophysiological effects of endothelin-1 and their relationship to contraction in rat renal arterial smooth muscle. *Br J Pharmacol* 2000;130:787–796.

43. Biondi ML, Dousa T, Vanhoutte P, Romero JC. Evidences for the existence of endothelium-derived relaxing factor in the renal medulla. *Am J Hypertens* 1990;3:876–878.

44. Birck R, Krzossok S, Knoll T, Braun C, Der Woude FJ, Rohmeiss P. Preferential COX-2 inhibitor, meloxicam, compromises renal perfusion in euvolemic and hypovolemic rats. *Exp Nephrol* 2000;8:173–180.

45. Bloom IT, Bentley FR, Wilson MA, Garrison RN. In vivo effects of endothelin on the renal microcirculation. *J Surg Res* 1993;54:274–280.

46. Brain SD, Grant AD. Vascular actions of calcitonin gene-related peptide and adrenomedullin. *Physiol Rev* 2004;84:903–934.

47. Brenner BM, Falchuk KH, Keimowitz RI, Berliner RW. The relationship between peritubular capillary protein concentration and fluid reabsorption by the renal proximal tubule. *J Clin Invest* 1969;48:1519–1531.

48. Brenner BM, Troy JL. Postglomerular vascular protein concentration: evidence for a causal role in governing fluid reabsorption and glomerulotubular balance by the renal proximal tubule. *J Clin Invest* 1971;50:336–349.

49. Brezis M, Agmon Y, Epstein FH. Determinants of intrarenal oxygenation, I: effects of diuretics. *Am J Physiol* 1994;267:F1059–F1062.

50. Brezis M, Heyman SN, Dinour D, Epstein FH, Rosen S. Role of nitric oxide in renal medullary oxygenation: studies in isolated and intact rat kidneys. *J Clin Invest* 1991;88:390–395.

51. Brown R, Ollerstam A, Johansson B, Skott O, Gebre-Medhin S, Fredholm B, Persson AE. Abolished tubuloglomerular feedback and increased plasma renin in adenosine A1 receptor-deficient mice. *Am J Physiol Regul Integr Comp Physiol* 2001;281:R1362–R1367.

52. Buckley BJ, Mirza Z, Whorton AR. Regulation of Ca(2+)-dependent nitric oxide synthase in bovine aortic endothelial cells. *Am J Physiol* 1995;269:C757–C765.

53. Bunton DC, Petrie MC, Hillier C, Johnston F, McMurray JJ. The clinical relevance of adrenomedullin: a promising profile? *Pharmacol Ther* 2004;103:179–201.

54. Burg M, Grantham J, Abramow M, Orloff J. Preparation and study of fragments of single rabbit nephrons. *Am J Physiol* 1966;210:1293–1298.

55. Busse R, Edwards G, Feletou M, Fleming I, Vanhoutte PM, Weston AH. EDHF: bringing the concepts together. *Trends Pharmacol Sci* 2002;23:374–380.

56. Cai Z, Xin J, Pollock DM, Pollock JS. Shear stress-mediated NO production in inner medullary collecting duct cells. *Am J Physiol Renal Physiol* 2000;279:F270–F274.

57. Campean V, Theilig F, Paliege A, Breyer M, Bachmann S. Key enzymes for renal prostaglandin synthesis: site-specific expression in rodent kidney (rat, mouse). *Am J Physiol Renal Physiol* 2003;285:F19–F32.
58. Capdevila JH, Falck JR. The CYP P450 arachidonic acid monooxygenases: from cell signaling to blood pressure regulation. *Biochem Biophys Res Commun* 2001;285:571–576.
59. Capdevila JH, Nakagawa K, Holla V. The CYP P450 arachidonate monooxygenases: enzymatic relays for the control of kidney function and blood pressure. *Adv Exp Med Biol* 2003;525:39–46.
60. Carey RM. Update on the role of the AT2 receptor. *Curr Opin Nephrol Hypertens* 2005;14: 67–71.
61. Carey RM, Jin X, Wang Z, Siragy HM. Nitric oxide: a physiological mediator of the type 2 (AT2) angiotensin receptor. *Acta Physiol Scand* 2000;168:65–71.
62. Carmines PK. Segment-specific effect of chloride channel blockade on rat renal arteriolar contractile responses to angiotensin II. *Am J Hypertens* 1995;8:90–94.
63. Carmines PK, Fleming JT. Control of the renal microvasculature by vasoactive peptides. *FASEB J* 1990;4:3300–3309.
64. Carmines PK, Inscho EW. Renal arteriolar angiotensin responses during varied adenosine receptor activation. *Hypertension* 1994;23:I114–I119.
65. Carmines PK, Morrison TK, Navar LG. Angiotensin II effects on microvascular diameters of in vitro blood-perfused juxtamedullary nephrons. *Am J Physiol* 1986;251:F610–F618.
66. Carmines PK, Navar LG. Disparate effects of Ca channel blockade on afferent and efferent arteriolar responses to ANG II. *Am J Physiol* 1989;256:F1015–F1020.
67. Carmines PK, Ohishi K, Ikenaga H. Functional impairment of renal afferent arteriolar voltage-gated calcium channels in rats with diabetes mellitus. *J Clin Invest* 1996;98:2564–2571.
68. Carone FA, Everett BA, Blondeel NJ, Stolarczyk J. Renal localization of albumin and its function in the concentrating mechanism. *Am J Physiol* 1967;212:387–393.
69. Casellas D, Mimran A. Shunting in renal microvasculature of the rat: a scanning electron microscopic study of corrosion casts. *Anat Rec* 1981;201:237–248.
70. Casellas D, Navar LG. In vitro perfusion of juxtamedullary nephrons in rats. *Am J Physiol* 1984;246:F349–F358.
71. Castrop H, Huang Y, Hashimoto S, Mizel D, Hansen P, Theilig F, Bachmann S, Deng C, Briggs J, Schnermann J. Impairment of tubuloglomerular feedback regulation of GFR in ecto-5'-nucleotidase/CD73-deficient mice. *J Clin Invest* 2004;114:634–642.
72. Cavarape A, Bartoli E. Effects of BQ-123 on systemic and renal hemodynamic responses to endothelin-1 in the rat split hydronephrotic kidney. *J Hypertens* 1998;16:1449–1458.
73. Cermak R, Kleta R, Forssmann WG, Schlatter E. Natriuretic peptides increase a K+ conductance in rat mesangial cells. *Pflugers Arch* 1996;431:571–577.
74. Chabrashvili T, Kitiyakara C, Blau J, Karber A, Aslam S, Welch WJ, Wilcox CS. Effects of ANG II type 1 and 2 receptors on oxidative stress, renal NADPH oxidase, and SOD expression. *Am J Physiol Regul Integr Comp Physiol* 2003;285:R117–R124.
75. Chan CM, Unwin RJ, Bardini M, Oglesby IB, Ford AP, Townsend-Nicholson A, Burnstock G. Localization of P2X1 purinoceptors by autoradiography and immunohistochemistry in rat kidneys. *Am J Physiol* 1998;274:F799–F804.
76. Chatziantoniou C, Arendshorst WJ. Prostaglandin interactions with angiotensin, norepinephrine, and thromboxane in rat renal vasculature. *Am J Physiol* 1992;262:F68–F76.
77. Chen YF, Cowley AW, Jr., Zou AP. Increased H(2)O(2) counteracts the vasodilator and natriuretic effects of superoxide dismutation by tempol in renal medulla. *Am J Physiol Regul Integr Comp Physiol* 2003;285:R827–R833.
78. Cheng HF, Harris RC. Cyclooxygenases, the kidney, and hypertension. *Hypertension* 2004;43:525–530.
79. Cheng MK, Doumad AB, Jiang H, Falck JR, McGiff JC, Carroll MA. Epoxyeicosatrienoic acids mediate adenosine-induced vasodilation in rat preglomerular microvessels (PGMV) via A2A receptors. *Br J Pharmacol* 2004;141:441–448.
80. Chilton L, Loutzenhiser R. Functional evidence for an inward rectifier potassium current in rat renal afferent arterioles. *Circ Res* 2001;88:152–158.
81. Chou CL, Knepper MA. In vitro perfusion of chinchilla thin limb segments: segmentation and osmotic water permeability. *Am J Physiol* 1992;263:F417–F426.
82. Chou CL, Nielsen S, Knepper MA. Structural-functional correlation in chinchilla long loop of Henle thin limbs: a novel papillary subsegment. *Am J Physiol* 1993;265:F863–F874.
83. Chou SY, Spitalewitz S, Faubert PF, Park IY, Porush JG. Inner medullary hemodynamics in chronic salt-depleted dogs. *Am J Physiol* 1984;246:F146–F154.
84. Chuang EL, Reineck HJ, Osgood RW, Kunau RT, Jr., Stein JH. Studies on the mechanism of reduced urinary osmolality after exposure of renal papilla. *J Clin Invest* 1978;61:633–639.
85. Churchill PC, Ellis VR. Pharmacological characterization of the re-novascular P2 purinergic receptors. *J Pharmacol Exp Ther* 1993;265: 334–338.
86. Clapham DE. TRP channels as cellular sensors. *Nature* 2003;426:517–524.
87. Coelho JB. Heterogeneity of intracortical peritubular plasma flow in the rat kidney. *Am J Physiol* 1977;233:F333–F341.
88. Cohen HJ, Marsh DJ, Kayser B. Autoregulation in vasa recta of the rat kidney. *Am J Physiol* 1983;245:F32–F40.
89. Conger JD, Falk SA. KCl and angiotensin responses in isolated rat renal arterioles: effects of diltiazem and low-calcium medium. *Am J Physiol* 1993;264:F134–F140.
90. Correia AG, Denton KM, Evans RG. Effects of activation of vasopressin-V1-receptors on regional kidney blood flow and glomerular arteriole diameters. *J Hypertens* 2001;19:649–657.
91. Cowley AW, Jr. Role of the renal medulla in volume and arterial pressure regulation. *Am J Physiol* 1997;273:R1–15.
92. Cowley AW, Jr. Control of the renal medullary circulation by vasopressin V1 and V2 receptors in the rat. *Exp Physiol* 2000;85 Spec No:223S–231S.
93. Cowley AW, Jr., Mori T, Mattson D, Zou AP. Role of renal NO production in the regulation of medullary blood flow. *Am J Physiol Regul Integr Comp Physiol* 2003;284:R1355–R1369.
94. Cupples WA, Sakai T, Marsh DJ. Angiotensin II and prostaglan-dins in control of vasa recta blood flow. *Am J Physiol* 1988;254:F417–F424.
95. De Wit C. Connexins pave the way for vascular communication. *News Physiol Sci* 2004;19: 148–153.
96. De Wit C, Roos F, Bolz SS, Kirchhoff S, Kruger O, Willecke K, Pohl U. Impaired conduction of vasodilation along arterioles in connexin40-deficient mice. *Circ Res* 2000;86:649–655.
97. De Wit C, Roos F, Bolz SS, Pohl U. Lack of vascular connexin 40 is associated with hypertension and irregular arteriolar vasomotion. *Physiol Genomics* 2003;13:169–177.
98. Deng A, Wead LM, Blantz RC. Temporal adaptation of tubuloglomerular feedback: effects of COX-2. *Kidney Int* 2004;66:2348–2353.
99. Denton KM, Luff SE, Shweta A, Anderson WP. Differential neural control of glomerular ultrafiltration. *Clin Exp Pharmacol Physiol* 2004;31:380–386.
100. Dhein S. Peptides acting at gap junctions. *Peptides* 2002;23:1701–1709.
101. DiBona GF. Sympathetic nervous system and the kidney in hypertension. *Curr Opin Nephrol Hypertens* 2002;11:197–200.
102. DiBona GF. Neural control of the kidney: past, present, and future. *Hypertension* 2003;41: 621–624.
103. DiBona GF. The sympathetic nervous system and hypertension: recent developments. *Hypertension* 2004;43:147–150.
104. DiBona GF, Kopp UC. Neural control of renal function. *Physiol Rev* 1997;77:75–197.
105. Dibona GF, Sawin LL. Functional significance of the pattern of renal sympathetic nerve activation. *Am J Physiol* 1999;277:R346–R353.
106. Dibona GF, Sawin LL. Effect of renal nerve stimulation on responsiveness of the rat renal vasculature. *Am J Physiol Renal Physiol* 2002;283:F1056–F1065.
107. DiBona GF, Sawin LL. Effect of endogenous angiotensin II on the frequency response of the renal vasculature. *Am J Physiol Renal Physiol* 2004;287:F1171–F1178.
108. DiBona GF, Sawin LL. Effect of renal denervation on dynamic autoregulation of renal blood flow. *Am J Physiol Renal Physiol* 2004;286:F1209–F1218.
109. Dickhout JG, Mori T, Cowley AW, Jr. Tubulovascular nitric oxide crosstalk: buffering of angiotensin II-induced medullary vasoconstriction. *Circ Res* 2002;91:487–493.
110. Dietrich MS, Endlich K, Parekh N, Steinhausen M. Interaction between adenosine and angiotensin II in renal microcirculation. *Microvasc Res* 1991;41:275–288.
111. Dinour D, Brezis M. Effects of adenosine on intrarenal oxygenation. *Am J Physiol* 1991;261: F787–F791.
112. Droge W. Free radicals in the physiological control of cell function. *Physiol Rev* 2002;82: 47–95.
113. Duke LM, Eppel GA, Widdop RE, Evans RG. Disparate roles of AT2 receptors in the renal cortical and medullary circulations of anesthetized rabbits. *Hypertension* 2003;42:200–205.
114. Earley S, Resta TC, Walker BR. Disruption of smooth muscle gap junctions attenuates myogenic vasoconstriction of mesenteric resistance arteries. *Am J Physiol Heart Circ Physiol* 2004;287:H2677–H2686.
115. Eckman DM, Nelson MT. Potassium ions as vasodilators: role of inward rectifier potassium channels. *Circ Res* 2001;88:132–133.
116. Edwards A, Delong MJ, Pallone TL. Interstitial water and solute recovery by inner medullary vasa recta. *Am J Physiol Renal Physiol* 2000;278:F257–F269.
117. Edwards A, Pallone TL. Facilitated transport in vasa recta: theoretical effects on solute exchange in the medullary microcirculation. *Am J Physiol* 1997;272:F505–F514.
118. Edwards A, Pallone TL. A multiunit model of solute and water removal by inner medullary vasa recta. *Am J Physiol* 1998;274:H1202–H1210.
119. Edwards RM. Segmental effects of norepinephrine and angiotensin II on isolated renal microvessels. *Am J Physiol* 1983;244:F526–F534.
120. Edwards RM. Effects of prostaglandins on vasoconstrictor action in isolated renal arterioles. *Am J Physiol* 1985;248:F779–F784.
121. Edwards RM, Trizna W, Kinter LB. Renal microvascular effects of vasopressin and vasopressin antagonists. *Am J Physiol* 1989;256:F274–F278.
122. Edwards RM, Trizna W, Ohlstein EH. Renal microvascular effects of endothelin. *Am J Physiol* 1990;259:F217–F221.
123. Edwards RM, Weidley EF. Lack of effect of atriopeptin II on rabbit glomerular arterioles in vitro. *Am J Physiol* 1987;252:F317–F321.
124. Endlich K, Forssmann WG, Steinhausen M. Effects of urodilatin in the rat kidney: comparison with ANF and interaction with vasoactive substances. *Kidney Int* 1995;47:1558–1568.
125. Endlich K, Hoffend J, Steinhausen M. Localization of endothelin ETA and ETB receptor-mediated constriction in the renal microcirculation of rats. *J Physiol* 1996;497(Pt 1):211–218.
126. Endlich K, Steinhausen M. Natriuretic peptide receptors mediate different responses in rat renal microvessels. *Kidney Int* 1997;52:202–207.
127. Endo Y, Arima S, Yaoita H, Omata K, Tsunoda K, Takeuchi K, Abe K, Ito S. Function of angiotensin II type 2 receptor in the postglomerular efferent arteriole. *Kidney Int Suppl* 1997;63:S205–S207.
128. Endo Y, Arima S, Yaoita H, Tsunoda K, Omata K, Ito S. Vasodilation mediated by angiotensin II type 2 receptor is impaired in afferent arterioles of young spontaneously hypertensive rats. *J Vasc Res* 1998; 35:421–427.
129. Eppel GA, Bergstrom G, Anderson WP, Evans RG. Autoregulation of renal medullary blood flow in rabbits. *Am J Physiol Regul Integr Comp Physiol* 2003;284:R233–R244.
130. Eppel GA, Denton KM, Malpas SC, Evans RG. Nitric oxide in responses of regional kidney perfusion to renal nerve stimulation and renal ischaemia. *Pflugers Arch* 2003;447:205–213.
131. Eppel GA, Malpas SC, Denton KM, Evans RG. Neural control of renal medullary perfusion. *Clin Exp Pharmacol Physiol* 2004;31:387–396.
132. Evans RG, Madden AC, Denton KM. Diversity of responses of renal cortical and medullary blood flow to vasoconstrictors in conscious rabbits. *Acta Physiol Scand* 2000;169:297–308.
133. Evans WH, Martin PE. Gap junctions: structure and function (Review). *Mol Membr Biol* 2002;19:121–136.
134. Fahraeus R. The suspension stability of blood. *Physiol Rev* 1929;9:241–274.
135. Fallet RW, Bast JP, Fujiwara K, Ishii N, Sansom SC, Carmines PK. Influence of Ca(2+)-activated K(+) channels on rat renal arteriolar responses to depolarizing agonists. *Am J Physiol Renal Physiol* 2001;280:F583–F591.
136. Fallet RW, Ikenaga H, Bast JP, Carmines PK. Relative contributions of Ca2+ mobilization and influx in renal arteriolar contractile responses to arginine vasopressin. *AJP - Renal Physiology* 2005;288:F545–F551.

137. Faubert PF, Chou SY, Porush JG. Regulation of papillary plasma flow by angiotensin II. *Kidney Int* 1987;32:472–478.
138. Fellner SK, Arendshorst WJ. Capacitative calcium entry in smooth muscle cells from preglomerular vessels. *Am J Physiol* 1999;277:F533–F542.
139. Fellner SK, Arendshorst WJ. Store-operated Ca2+ entry is exaggerated in fresh preglomerular vascular smooth muscle cells of SHR. *Kidney Int* 2002;61:2132–2141.
140. Fellner SK, Arendshorst WJ. Endothelin A and B receptors of preglomerular vascular smooth muscle cells. *Kidney Int* 2004;65:1810–1817.
141. Feng MG, Dukacz SA, Kline RL. Selective effect of tempol on renal medullary hemodynamics in spontaneously hypertensive rats. *Am J Physiol Regul Integr Comp Physiol* 2001;281: R1420–R1425.
142. Feng MG, Navar LG. Angiotensin II-Mediated Constriction of Afferent and Efferent Arterioles Involves T-Type Ca Channel Activation. *Am J Nephrol* 2004;24:641–648.
143. Fenoy FJ, Ferrer P, Carbonell L, Garcia-Salom M. Role of nitric oxide on papillary blood flow and pressure natriuresis. *Hypertension* 1995;25:408–414.
144. Fenoy FJ, Roman RJ. Effect of volume expansion on papillary blood flow and sodium excretion. *Am J Physiol* 1991;260:F813–F822.
145. Fergus DJ, Martens JR, England SK. Kv channel subunits that contribute to voltage-gated K+ current in renal vascular smooth muscle. *Pflugers Arch* 2003;445:697–704.
146. Ferrario CM, Chappell MC. Novel angiotensin peptides. *Cell Mol Life Sci* 2004;61:2720–2727.
147. Figueroa XF, Isakson BE, Duling BR. Connexins: gaps in our knowledge of vascular function. *Physiology (Bethesda)* 2004;19:277–284.
148. Figueroa XF, Paul DL, Simon AM, Goodenough DA, Day KH, Damon DN, Duling BR. Central role of connexin40 in the propagation of electrically activated vasodilation in mouse cremasteric arterioles in vivo. *Circ Res* 2003;92:793–800.
149. Fleming I. Cytochrome p450 and vascular homeostasis. *Circ Res* 2001;89:753–762.
150. Fleming I. Cytochrome P450 epoxygenases as EDHF synthase(s). *Pharmacol Res* 2004;49: 525–533.
151. Fleming JT, Parekh N, Steinhausen M. Calcium antagonists preferentially dilate preglomerular vessels of hydronephrotic kidney. *Am J Physiol* 1987;253:F1157–F1163.
152. Fourman J, Moffat DB. The effect of intra-arterial cushions on plasma skimming in small arteries. *J Physiol* 1961;158:374–380.
153. Fourman J, Moffat DB. *The Blood Vessels of the Kidney.* Oxford: Osney Mead, 1971.
154. Franchini KG, Cowley AW, Jr. Renal cortical and medullary blood flow responses during water restriction: role of vasopressin. *Am J Physiol* 1996;270:R1257–R1264.
155. Franchini KG, Cowley AW, Jr. Sensitivity of the renal medullary circulation to plasma vasopressin. *Am J Physiol* 1996;271:R647–R653.
156. Fujino T, Nakagawa N, Yuhki K, Hara A, Yamada T, Takayama K, Kuriyama S, Hosoki Y, Takahata O, Taniguchi T, Fukuzawa J, Hasebe N, Kikuchi K, Narumiya S, Ushikubi F. Decreased susceptibility to renovascular hypertension in mice lacking the prostaglandin I2 receptor IP. *J Clin Invest* 2004;114:805–812.
157. Fukao M, Mason HS, Kenyon JL, Horowitz B, Keef KD. Regulation of BK(Ca) channels expressed in human embryonic kidney 293 cells by epoxyeicosatrienoic acid. *Mol Pharmacol* 2001;59:16–23.
158. Gaehtgens P. Flow of blood through narrow capillaries: rheological mechanisms determining capillary hematocrit and apparent viscosity. *Biorheology* 1980;17:183–189.
159. Gainer JV, Bellamine A, Dawson EP, Womble KE, Grant SW, Wang Y, Cupples LA, Guo CY, Demissie S, O'Donnell CJ, Brown NJ, Waterman MR, Capdevila JH. Functional variant of CYP4A11 20-hydroxyeicosatetraenoic acid synthase is associated with essential hypertension. *Circulation* 2005;111:63–69.
160. Galskov A, Nissen OI. Autoregulation of directly measured blood flows in the superficial and deep venous drainage areas of the cat kidney. *Circ Res* 1972;30:97–103.
161. Ganguli M, Tobian L, Azar S, O'Donnell M. Evidence that prostaglandin synthesis inhibitors increase the concentration of sodium and chloride in rat renal medulla. *Circ Res* 1977;40: I135–I139.
162. Ganguli M, Tobian L, Dahl L. Low renal papillary plasma flow in both Dahl and Kyoto rats with spontaneous hypertension. *Circ Res* 1976;39:337–341.
163. Garcia-Estan J, Roman RJ. Role of renal interstitial hydrostatic pressure in the pressure diuresis response. *Am J Physiol* 1989;256:F63–F70.
164. Gardiner SM, Kemp PA, March JE, Bennett T. Regional haemodynamic effects of human and rat adrenomedullin in conscious rats. *Br J Pharmacol* 1995;114:584–591.
165. Gariepy CE, Ohuchi T, Williams SC, Richardson JA, Yanagisawa M. Salt-sensitive hypertension in endothelin-B receptor-deficient rats. *J Clin Invest* 2000;105:925–933.
166. Gariepy CE, Williams SC, Richardson JA, Hammer RE, Yanagisawa M. Transgenic expression of the endothelin-B receptor prevents congenital intestinal aganglionosis in a rat model of Hirschsprung disease. *J Clin Invest* 1998;102:1092–1101.
167. Garvin JL, Ortiz PA. The role of reactive oxygen species in the regulation of tubular function. *Acta Physiol Scand* 2003;179:225–232.
168. Gebremedhin D, Kaldunski M, Jacobs ER, Harder DR, Roman RJ. Coexistence of two types of Ca(2+)-activated K+ channels in rat renal arterioles. *Am J Physiol* 1996;270: F69–F81.
169. Gelband CH, Hume JR. Ionic currents in single smooth muscle cells of the canine renal artery. *Circ Res* 1992;71:745–758.
170. Gelband CH, Ishikawa T, Post JM, Keef KD, Hume JR. Intracellular divalent cations block smooth muscle K+ channels. *Circ Res* 1993;73:24–34.
171. Goligorsky MS, Brodsky SV, Noiri E. NO bioavailability, endothelial dysfunction, and acute renal failure: new insights into pathophysiology. *Semin Nephrol* 2004;24:316–323.
172. Goligorsky MS, Li H, Brodsky S, Chen J. Relationships between caveolae and eNOS: everything in proximity and the proximity of everything. *Am J Physiol Renal Physiol* 2002;283: F1–10.
173. Goransson A, Sjoquist M, Ulfendahl HR. Superficial and juxtamedullary nephron function during converting enzyme inhibition. *Am J Physiol* 1986;251:F25–F33.
174. Gordienko DV, Clausen C, Goligorsky MS. Ionic currents and endothelin signaling in smooth muscle cells from rat renal resistance arteries. *Am J Physiol* 1994;266:F325–F341.
175. Goto M, Mukoyama M, Sugawara A, Suganami T, Kasahara M, Yahata K, Makino H, Suga S, Tanaka I, Nakao K. Expression and role of angiotensin II type 2 receptor in the kidney and mesangial cells of spontaneously hypertensive rats. *Hypertens Res* 2002;25:125–133.
176. Gottschalk CW, Mylle M. Micropuncture study of the mammalian urinary concentrating mechanism: evidence for the countercurrent hypothesis. *Am J Physiol* 1959;196:927–936.
177. Granger JP, Alexander BT, Llinas M. Mechanisms of pressure natriuresis. *Curr Hypertens Rep* 2002;4:152–159.
178. Granger JP, Haas JA, Pawlowska D, Knox FG. Effect of direct increases in renal interstitial hydrostatic pressure on sodium excretion. *Am J Physiol* 1988;254:F527–F532.
179. Grantham JJ, Qualizza PB, Welling LW. Influence of serum proteins on net fluid reabsorption of isolated proximal tubules. *Kidney Int* 1972;2:66–75.
180. Green R, Giebisch G. Luminal hypotonicity: a driving force for fluid absorption from the proximal tubule. *Am J Physiol* 1984;246:F167–F174.
181. Green R, Giebisch G, Unwin R, Weinstein AM. Coupled water transport by rat proximal tubule. *Am J Physiol* 1991;261:F1046–F1054.
182. Gross V, Schunck WH, Honeck H, Milia AF, Kargel E, Walther T, Bader M, Inagami T, Schneider W, Luft FC. Inhibition of pressure natriuresis in mice lacking the AT2 receptor. *Kidney Int* 2000;57:191–202.
183. Guild SJ, Eppel GA, Malpas SC, Rajapakse NW, Stewart A, Evans RG. Regional responsiveness of renal perfusion to activation of the renal nerves. *Am J Physiol Regul Integr Comp Physiol* 2002;283:R1177–R1186.
184. Gurbanov K, Rubinstein I, Hoffman A, Abassi Z, Better OS, Winaver J. Differential regulation of renal regional blood flow by endothelin-1. *Am J Physiol* 1996;271:F1166–F1172.
185. Gussis GL, Jamison RL, Robertson CR. Determination of erythrocyte velocities in the mammalian inner renal medulla by a video velocity-tracking system. *Microvasc Res* 1979;18: 370–383.
186. Gussis GL, Robertson CR, Jamison RL. Erythrocyte velocity in vasa recta: effect of antidiuretic hormone and saline loading. *Am J Physiol* 1979;237:F326–F332.
187. Haas JA, Granger JP, Knox FG. Effect of renal perfusion pressure on sodium reabsorption from proximal tubules of superficial and deep nephrons. *Am J Physiol* 1986;250:F425–F429.
188. Haas JA, Granger JP, Knox FG. Effect of intrarenal volume expansion on proximal sodium reabsorption. *Am J Physiol* 1988;255:F1178–F1182.
189. Hall DA, Carmines PK, Sansom SC. Dihydropyridine-sensitive Ca(2+) channels in human glomerular mesangial cells. *Am J Physiol Renal Physiol* 2000;278:F97–F103.
190. Hall JE, Granger JP. Adenosine alters glomerular filtration control by angiotensin II. *Am J Physiol* 1986;250:F917–F923.
191. Hansen PB, Castrop H, Briggs J, Schnermann J. Adenosine induces vasoconstriction through Gi-dependent activation of phospholipase C in isolated perfused afferent arterioles of mice. *J Am Soc Nephrol* 2003;14:2457–2465.
192. Hansen PB, Hashimoto S, Briggs J, Schnermann J. Attenuated renovascular constrictor responses to angiotensin II in adenosine 1 receptor knockout mice. *Am J Physiol Regul Integr Comp Physiol* 2003;285:R44–R49.
193. Hansen PB, Jensen BL, Andreasen D, Friis UG, Skott O. Vascular smooth muscle cells express the alpha(1A) subunit of a P-/Q-type voltage-dependent Ca(2+) channel, and it is functionally important in renal afferent arterioles. *Circ Res* 2000;87:896–902.
194. Hansen PB, Jensen BL, Andreasen D, Skott O. Differential expression of T- and L-type voltage-dependent calcium channels in renal resistance vessels. *Circ Res* 2001;89:630–638.
195. Hansen PB, Jensen BL, Skott O. Chloride regulates afferent arteriolar contraction in response to depolarization. *Hypertension* 1998;32:1066–1070.
196. Hansen PB, Schnermann J. Vasoconstrictor and vasodilator effects of adenosine in the kidney. *Am J Physiol Renal Physiol* 2003;285:F590–F599.
197. Harder DR, Campbell WB, Roman RJ. Role of cytochrome P-450 enzymes and metabolites of arachidonic acid in the control of vascular tone. *J Vasc Res* 1995;32:79–92.
198. Harder DR, Narayanan J, Birks EK, Liard JF, Imig JD, Lombard JH, Lange AR, Roman RJ. Identification of a putative microvascular oxygen sensor. *Circ Res* 1996;79:54–61.
199. Harris RC, Breyer MD. Physiological regulation of cyclooxygenase-2 in the kidney. *Am J Physiol Renal Physiol* 2001;281:F1–11.
200. Harris RC, Zhang MZ, Cheng HF. Cyclooxygenase-2 and the renal renin-angiotensin system. *Acta Physiol Scand* 2004;181:543–547.
201. Harrison-Bernard LM, Carmines PK. Juxtamedullary microvascular responses to arginine vasopressin in rat kidney. *Am J Physiol* 1994;267:F249–F256.
202. Harrison-Bernard LM, Carmines PK. Impact of cyclo-oxygenase blockade on juxtamedullary microvascular responses to angiotensin II in rat kidney. *Clin Exp Pharmacol Physiol* 1995;22:732–738.
203. Harrison-Bernard LM, Cook AK, Oliverio MI, Coffman TM. Renal segmental microvascular responses to ANG II in AT1A receptor null mice. *Am J Physiol Renal Physiol* 2003;284: F538–F545.
204. Harsing L, Pelley K. [The determination of renal medullary blood flow based on Rb-86 deposit and distribution]. *Pflugers Arch Gesamte Physiol Menschen Tiere* 1965;285:302–312.
205. Hayashi K, Epstein M, Loutzenhiser R. Determinants of renal actions of atrial natriuretic peptide. Lack of effect of atrial natriuretic peptide on pressure-induced vasoconstriction. *Circ Res* 1990;67:1–10.
206. Hayashi K, Loutzenhiser R, Epstein M. Direct evidence that thromboxane mimetic U44069 preferentially constricts the afferent arteriole. *J Am Soc Nephrol* 1997;8:25–31.
207. Hayashi K, Ozawa Y, Wakino S, Kanda T, Homma K, Takamatsu I, Tatematsu S, Saruta T. Cellular mechanism for mibefradil-induced vasodilation of renal microcirculation: studies in the isolated perfused hydronephrotic kidney. *J Cardiovasc Pharmacol* 2003;42:697–702.
208. Helou CM, Imbert-Teboul M, Doucet A, Rajerison R, Chollet C, Alhenc-Gelas F, Marchetti J. Angiotensin receptor subtypes in thin and muscular juxtamedullary efferent arterioles of rat kidney. *Am J Physiol Renal Physiol* 2003;285:F507–F514.
209. Helou CM, Marchetti J. Morphological heterogeneity of renal glomerular arterioles and distinct [Ca2+]i responses to ANG II. *Am J Physiol* 1997;273:F84–F96.
210. Hercule HC, Oyekan AO. Cytochrome P450 omega/omega-1 hydroxylase-derived eicosanoids contribute to endothelin(A) and endothelin(B) receptor-mediated vasoconstriction

to endothelin-1 in the rat preglomerular arteriole. *J Pharmacol Exp Ther* 2000;292: 1153–1160.
211. Heyman SN, Brezis M, Epstein FH, Spokes K, Silva P, Rosen S. Early renal medullary hypoxic injury from radiocontrast and indomethacin. *Kidney Int* 1991;40:632–642.
212. Heyman SN, Fuchs S, Jaffe R, Shina A, Ellezian L, Brezis M, Rosen S. Renal microcirculation and tissue damage during acute ureteral obstruction in the rat: effect of saline infusion, indomethacin and radiocontrast. *Kidney Int* 1997;51:653–663.
213. Heyman SN, Rosen S, Darmon D, Goldfarb M, Bitz H, Shina A, Brezis M. Endotoxin-induced renal failure. II. A role for tubular hypoxic damage. *Exp Nephrol* 2000;8:275–282.
214. Hinson JP, Kapas S, Smith DM. Adrenomedullin, a multifunctional regulatory peptide. *Endocr Rev* 2000;21:138–167.
215. Hirata Y, Hayakawa H, Suzuki Y, Suzuki E, Ikenouchi H, Kohmoto O, Kimura K, Kitamura K, Eto T, Kangawa K. Mechanisms of adrenomedullin-induced vasodilation in the rat kidney. *Hypertension* 1995;25:790–795.
216. Hoagland KM, Flasch AK, Roman RJ. Inhibitors of 20-HETE formation promote salt-sensitive hypertension in rats. *Hypertension* 2003;42:669–673.
217. Hoffend J, Cavarape A, Endlich K, Steinhausen M. Influence of endothelium-derived relaxing factor on renal microvessels and pressure-dependent vasodilation. *Am J Physiol* 1993;265: F285–F292.
218. Hoffman A, Abassi ZA, Brodsky S, Ramadan R, Winaver J. Mechanisms of big endothelin-1-induced diuresis and natriuresis : role of ET(B) receptors. *Hypertension* 2000;35:732–739.
219. Holliger C, Lemley KV, Schmitt SL, Thomas FC, Robertson CR, Jamison RL. Direct determination of vasa recta blood flow in the rat renal papilla. *Circ Res* 1983;53:401–413.
220. Hughes AK, Barry WH, Kohan DE. Identification of a contractile function for renal medullary interstitial cells. *J Clin Invest* 1995;96:411–416.
221. Hwan SK, Beyer EC. Heterogeneous localization of connexin40 in the renal vasculature. *Microvasc Res* 2000;59:140–148.
222. Ichihara A, Imig JD, Inscho EW, Navar LG. Cyclooxygenase-2 participates in tubular flow-dependent afferent arteriolar tone: interaction with neuronal NOS. *Am J Physiol* 1998;275: F605–F612.
223. Imai M, Kokko JP. Effect of peritubular protein concentration on reabsorption of sodium and water in isolated perfused proxmal tubules. *J Clin Invest* 1972;51:314–325.
224. Imig JD. Eicosanoid regulation of the renal vasculature. *Am J Physiol Renal Physiol* 2000;279: F965–F981.
225. Imig JD, Falck JR, Wei S, Capdevila JH. Epoxygenase metabolites contribute to nitric oxide-independent afferent arteriolar vasodilation in response to bradykinin. *J Vasc Res* 2001;38: 247–255.
226. Imig JD, Gebremedhin D, Harder DR, Roman RJ. Modulation of vascular tone in renal microcirculation by erythrocytes: role of EDRF. *Am J Physiol* 1993;264:H190–H195.
227. Imig JD, Inscho EW, Deichmann PC, Reddy KM, Falck JR. Afferent arteriolar vasodilation to the sulfonimide analog of 11, 12-epoxyeicosatrienoic acid involves protein kinase A. *Hypertension* 1999; 33:408–413.
228. Imig JD, Navar LG, Roman RJ, Reddy KK, Falck JR. Actions of epoxygenase metabolites on the preglomerular vasculature. *J Am Soc Nephrol* 1996;7:2364–2370.
229. Imig JD, Pham BT, LeBlanc EA, Reddy KM, Falck JR, Inscho EW. Cytochrome P450 and cyclooxygenase metabolites contribute to the endothelin-1 afferent arteriolar vasoconstrictor and calcium responses. *Hypertension* 2000;35:307–312.
230. Imig JD, Roman RJ. Nitric oxide modulates vascular tone in preglomerular arterioles. *Hypertension* 1992;19:770–774.
231. Imig JD, Zhao X, Capdevila JH, Morisseau C, Hammock BD. Soluble epoxide hydrolase inhibition lowers arterial blood pressure in angiotensin II hypertension. *Hypertension* 2002;39: 690–694.
232. Imig JD, Zhao X, Falck JR, Wei S, Capdevila JH. Enhanced renal microvascular reactivity to angiotensin II in hypertension is ameliorated by the sulfonimide analog of 11, 12-epoxyeicosatrienoic acid. *J Hypertens* 2001;19:983–992.
233. Imig JD, Zou AP, Stec DE, Harder DR, Falck JR, Roman RJ. Formation and actions of 20-hydroxyeicosatetraenoic acid in rat renal arterioles. *Am J Physiol* 1996;270: R217–R227.
234. Inscho EW. P2 receptors in regulation of renal microvascular function. *Am J Physiol Renal Physiol* 2001;280:F927–F944.
235. Inscho EW. Renal microvascular effects of P2 receptor stimulation. *Clin Exp Pharmacol Physiol* 2001;28:332-339.
236. Inscho EW. Modulation of renal microvascular function by adenosine. *Am J Physiol Regul Integr Comp Physiol* 2003;285:R23–R25.
237. Inscho EW, Carmines PK, Navar LG. Prostaglandin influences on afferent arteriolar responses to vasoconstrictor agonists. *Am J Physiol* 1990;259:F157–F163.
238. Inscho EW, Cook AK, Imig JD, Vial C, Evans RJ. Physiological role for P2X1 receptors in renal microvascular autoregulatory behavior. *J Clin Invest* 2003;112:1895–1905.
239. Inscho EW, Cook AK, Imig JD, Vial C, Evans RJ. Renal autoregulation in P2X1 knockout mice. *Acta Physiol Scand* 2004;181:445–453.
240. Inscho EW, Cook AK, Navar LG. Pressure-mediated vasoconstriction of juxtamedullary afferent arterioles involves P2-purinoceptor activation. *Am J Physiol* 1996;271:F1077–F1085.
241. Inscho EW, LeBlanc EA, Pham BT, White SM, Imig JD. Purinoceptor-mediated calcium signaling in preglomerular smooth muscle cells. *Hypertension* 1999;33:195–200.
242. Inscho EW, Mason MJ, Schroeder AC, Deichmann PC, Stiegler KD, Imig JD. Agonist-induced calcium regulation in freshly isolated renal microvascular smooth muscle cells. *J Am Soc Nephrol* 1997;8:569–579.
243. Inscho EW, Ohishi K, Cook AK, Belott TP, Navar LG. Calcium activation mechanisms in the renal microvascular response to extracellular ATP. *Am J Physiol* 1995;268:F876–F884.
244. Inscho EW, Ohishi K, Navar LG. Effects of ATP on pre- and postglomerular juxtamedullary microvasculature. *Am J Physiol* 1992;263:F886–F893.
245. Inscho EW, Schroeder AC, Deichmann PC, Imig JD. ATP-mediated Ca2+ signaling in preglomerular smooth muscle cells. *Am J Physiol* 1999;276:F450-F456.
246. Ito S, Arima S, Ren YL, Juncos LA, Carretero OA. Endothelium-derived relaxing factor/nitric oxide modulates angiotensin II action in the isolated microperfused rabbit afferent but not efferent arteriole. *J Clin Invest* 1993;91:2012–2019.
247. Ito S, Johnson CS, Carretero OA. Modulation of angiotensin II-induced vasoconstriction by endothelium-derived relaxing factor in the isolated microperfused rabbit afferent arteriole. *J Clin Invest* 1991;87:1656–1663.
248. Ito S, Juncos LA, Nushiro N, Johnson CS, Carretero OA. Endothelium-derived relaxing factor modulates endothelin action in afferent arterioles. *Hypertension* 1991;17:105 2–1056.
249. Ito S, Ren Y. Evidence for the role of nitric oxide in macula densa control of glomerular hemodynamics. *J Clin Invest* 1993;92:1093–1098.
250. Itskovitz HD, Stemper J, Pacholczyk D, McGiff JC. Renal prostaglandins: determinants of intrarenal distribution of blood flow in the dog. *Clin Sci Mol Med Suppl* 1973;45 (Suppl 1): 321s–4.
251. Iversen BM, Arendshorst WJ. ANG II and vasopressin stimulate calcium entry in dispersed smooth muscle cells of preglomerular arterioles. *Am J Physiol* 1998;274:F498–F508.
252. Iversen BM, Arendshorst WJ. Exaggerated Ca2+ signaling in preglomerular arteriolar smooth muscle cells of genetically hypertensive rats. *Am J Physiol* 1999;276:F260–F270.
253. Jackson EK, Dubey RK. Role of the extracellular cAMP-adenosine pathway in renal physiology. *Am J Physiol Renal Physiol* 2001;281:F597–F612.
254. Jackson EK, Zhu C, Tofovic SP. Expression of adenosine receptors in the preglomerular microcirculation. *Am J Physiol Renal Physiol* 2002;283:F41–F51.
255. James PE, Bacic G, Grinberg OY, Goda F, Dunn JF, Jackson SK, Swartz HM. Endotoxin-induced changes in intrarenal pO2, measured by in vivo electron paramagnetic resonance oximetry and magnetic resonance imaging. *Free Radic Biol Med* 1996;21:25–34.
256. Jamison RL, Kriz W. *Urinary Concentrating Mechanism: Structure and Function.* Oxford: Oxford University Press, 1982.
257. Janssen WM, Beekhuis H, de Bruin R, de Jong PE, de Zeeuw D. Noninvasive measurement of intrarenal blood flow distribution: kinetic model of renal 123I-hippuran handling. *Am J Physiol* 1995;269:F571–F580.
258. Jensen BL, Ellekvist P, Skott O. Chloride is essential for contraction of afferent arterioles after agonists and potassium. *Am J Physiol* 1997;272:F389–F396.
259. Jensen BL, Friis UG, Hansen PB, Andreasen D, Uhrenholt T, Schjerning J, Skott O. Voltage-dependent calcium channels in the renal microcirculation. *Nephrol Dial Transplant* 2004;19:1368–1373.
260. Johnston PA, Battilana CA, Lacy FB, Jamison RL. Evidence for a concentration gradient favoring outward movement of sodium from the thin loop of Henle. *J Clin Invest* 1977;59: 234–240.
261. Juncos LA, Ito S, Carretero OA, Garvin JL. Removal of endothelium-dependent relaxation by antibody and complement in afferent arterioles. *Hypertension* 1994;23:I54–I59.
262. Jung JY, Madsen KM, Han KH, Yang CW, Knepper MA, Sands JM, Kim J. Expression of urea transporters in potassium-depleted mouse kidney. *Am J Physiol Renal Physiol* 2003;285: F1210–F1224.
263. Just A, Olson AJ, Arendshorst WJ. Dual constrictor and dilator actions of ET(B) receptors in the rat renal microcirculation: interactions with ET(A) receptors. *Am J Physiol Renal Physiol* 2004;286:F660–F668.
264. Kaide JI, Zhang F, Wei Y, Jiang H, Yu C, Wang WH, Balazy M, Abraham NG, Nasjletti A. Carbon monoxide of vascular origin attenuates the sensitivity of renal arterial vessels to vasoconstrictors. *J Clin Invest* 2001;107:1163–1171.
265. Kaissling B, de Rouffignac C, Barrett JM, Kriz W. The structural organization of the kidney of the desert rodent Psammomys obesus. *Anat Embryol (Berl)* 1975;148:121–143.
266. Kaissling B, Kriz W. Structural analysis of the rabbit kidney. *Adv Anat Embryol Cell Biol* 1979;56:1–123.
267. Kakoki M, Kim HS, Arendshorst WJ, Mattson DL. L-Arginine uptake affects nitric oxide production and blood flow in the renal medulla. *Am J Physiol Regul Integr Comp Physiol* 2004;287:R1478–R1485.
268. Kakoki M, Wang W, Mattson DL. Cationic amino acid transport in the renal medulla and blood pressure regulation. *Hypertension* 2002;39:287–292.
269. Kakoki M, Zou AP, Mattson DL. The influence of nitric oxide synthase 1 on blood flow and interstitial nitric oxide in the kidney. *Am J Physiol Regul Integr Comp Physiol* 2001;281: R91–R97.
270. Kaloyanides GJ, DiBona GF, Raskin P. Pressure natriuresis in the isolated kidney. *Am J Physiol* 1971;220:1660–1666.
271. Karagiannis J, Rand M, Li CG. Role of gap junctions in endothelium-derived hyperpolarizing factor-mediated vasodilatation in rat renal artery. *Acta Pharmacol Sin* 2004;25:1031–1037.
272. Karlberg L, Kallskog O, Ojteg G, Wolgast M. Renal medullary blood flow studied with the 86-Rb extraction method. Methodological considerations. *Acta Physiol Scand* 1982;115:11–18.
273. Kawada N, Dennehy K, Solis G, Modlinger P, Hamel R, Kawada JT, Aslam S, Moriyama T, Imai E, Welch WJ, Wilcox CS. TP receptors regulate renal hemodynamics during angiotensin II slow pressor response. *Am J Physiol Renal Physiol* 2004;287:F753–F759.
274. Kedem O, Katchalsky A. Thermodynamic analysis of the permeability of biological membranes to non-electrolytes. *Biochim Biophys Acta* 1958;27:229–246.
275. Khraibi AA, Haas JA, Knox FG. Effect of renal perfusion pressure on renal interstitial hydrostatic pressure in rats. *Am J Physiol* 1989;256:F165–F170.
276. Khraibi AA, Knox FG. Effect of renal decapsulation on renal interstitial hydrostatic pressure and natriuresis. *Am J Physiol* 1989;257:R44–R48.
277. Kiberd B, Robertson CR, Larson T, Jamison RL. Effect of V2-receptor-mediated changes on inner medullary blood flow induced by AVP. *Am J Physiol* 1987;253:F576–F581.
278. Kiberd BA, Larson TS, Robertson CR, Jamison RL. Effect of atrial natriuretic peptide on vasa recta blood flow in the rat. *Am J Physiol* 1987;252:F1112–F1117.
279. Kim D, Klein JD, Racine S, Murrell BP, Sands JM. Urea may regulate urea transporter protein abundance during osmotic diuresis. *Am J Physiol Renal Physiol* 2005;288:F188–F197.
280. Kirton CA, Loutzenhiser R. Alterations in basal protein kinase C activity modulate renal afferent arteriolar myogenic reactivity. *Am J Physiol* 1998;275:H467–H475.

281. Kitamura K, Tanaka T, Kato J, Eto T, Tanaka K. Regional distribution of immunoreactive endothelin in porcine tissue: abundance in inner medulla of kidney. *Biochem Biophys Res Commun* 1989;161:348–352.
282. Kitamura K, Yamazaki J. Chloride channels and their functional roles in smooth muscle tone in the vasculature. *Jpn J Pharmacol* 2001;85:351–357.
283. Klar J, Vitzthum H, Kurtz A. Aldosterone enhances renin gene expression in juxtaglomerular cells. *Am J Physiol Renal Physiol* 2004;286:F349–F355.
284. Klein JD, Gunn RB, Roberts BR, Sands JM. Down-regulation of urea transporters in the renal inner medulla of lithium-fed rats. *Kidney Int* 2002;61:995–1002.
285. Knepper MA, Danielson RA, Saidel GM, Post RS. Quantitative analysis of renal medullary anatomy in rats and rabbits. *Kidney Int* 1977;12:313–323.
286. Koepsell H, Nicholson WA, Kriz W, Hohling HJ. Measurements of exponential gradients of sodium and chlorine in the rat kidney medulla using the electron microprobe. *Pflugers Arch* 1974;350:167–184.
287. Kohagura K, Arima S, Endo Y, Chiba Y, Ito O, Abe M, Omata K, Ito S. Involvement of cytochrome P450 metabolites in the vascular action of angiotensin II on the afferent arterioles. *Hypertens Res* 2001;24:551–557.
288. Kohagura K, Endo Y, Ito O, Arima S, Omata K, Ito S. Endogenous nitric oxide and epoxyeicosatrienoic acids modulate angiotensin II-induced constriction in the rabbit afferent arteriole. *Acta Physiol Scand* 2000;168:107–112.
289. Kohan DE. Endothelins in the normal and diseased kidney. *Am J Kidney Dis* 1997;29:2–26.
290. Komlosi P, Fintha A, Bell PD. Current mechanisms of macula densa cell signalling. *Acta Physiol Scand* 2004;181:463–469.
291. Kone BC. Nitric oxide synthesis in the kidney: isoforms, biosynthesis, and functions in health. *Semin Nephrol* 2004;24:299–315.
292. Kone BC, Baylis C. Biosynthesis and homeostatic roles of nitric oxide in the normal kidney. *Am J Physiol* 1997;272:F561–F578.
293. Kone BC, Kuncewicz T, Zhang W, Yu ZY. Protein interactions with nitric oxide synthases: controlling the right time, the right place, and the right amount of nitric oxide. *Am J Physiol Renal Physiol* 2003;285:F178–F190.
294. Konishi F, Okada Y, Takaoka M, Gariepy CE, Yanagisawa M, Matsumura Y. Role of endothelin ET(B) receptors in the renal hemodynamic and excretory responses to big endothelin-1. *Eur J Pharmacol* 2002;451:177–184.
295. Kopp UC, Cicha MZ, Farley DM, Smith LA, Dixon BS. Renal substance P-containing neurons and substance P receptors impaired in hypertension. *Hypertension* 1998;31:815–822.
296. Kopp UC, Cicha MZ, Smith LA. Dietary sodium loading increases arterial pressure in afferent renal-denervated rats. *Hypertension* 2003;42:968–973.
297. Kopp UC, Farley DM, Cicha MZ, Smith LA. Activation of renal mechanosensitive neurons involves bradykinin, protein kinase C, PGE(2), and substance P. *Am J Physiol Regul Integr Comp Physiol* 2000;278:R937–R946.
298. Kotelevtsev Y, Webb DJ. Endothelin as a natriuretic hormone: the case for a paracrine action mediated by nitric oxide. *Cardiovasc Res* 2001;51:481–488.
299. Kramer K, Thurau K, Deetjen P. [Hemodynamics of kidney medullary substance. Part I. Capillary passage time, blood volume, circulation, tissue hematocrit and oxygen consumption of kidney medullary substance in situ]. *Pflugers Arch Gesamte Physiol Menschen Tiere* 1960; 270:251–269.
300. Kreisberg MS, Silldorff EP, Pallone TL. Localization of adenosine-receptor subtype mRNA in rat outer medullary descending vasa recta by RT-PCR. *Am J Physiol* 1997;272:H1231–H1238.
301. Kriz W. Structural organization of the renal medulla: comparative and functional aspects. *Am J Physiol* 1981;241:R3–16.
302. Kriz W, Dieterich HJ. [The lymphatic system of the kidney in some mammals. Light and electron microscopic investigations]. *Z Anat Entwicklungsgesch* 1970;131:111–147.
303. Kriz W, Napiwotzky P. Structural and functional aspects of the renal interstitium. *Contrib Nephrol* 1979;16:104–108.
304. Krum H, Viskoper RJ, Lacourciere Y, Budde M, Charlon V. The effect of an endothelin-receptor antagonist, bosentan, on blood pressure in patients with essential hypertension. Bosentan Hypertension Investigators. *N Engl J Med* 1998;338:784–790.
305. Kudlacek PE, Pluznick JL, Ma R, Padanilam B, Sansom SC. Role of hbeta1 in activation of human mesangial BK channels by cGMP kinase. *Am J Physiol Renal Physiol* 2003;285: F289–F294.
306. Kuhn M. Molecular physiology of natriuretic peptide signalling. *Basic Res Cardiol* 2004;99: 76–82.
307. Kuhn W, Ryffel R. Herstellung konzentrierter Losungen aus verdunnten durch blosse Membranwirkung. (Ein Modellversuch zur Function der Niere). *Hoppe-Seylers Z Physiol Chem* 1942;276:145–178.
308. Landis EM, Pappenheimer JR. Exchange of substances through the capillary wall. In: *Handbook of Physiology. Circulation,* edited by W.F. Hamilton. Washington, DC: American Physiological Society, 1963:962–1034.
309. Large WA, Wang Q. Characteristics and physiological role of the Ca(2+)-activated Cl-conductance in smooth muscle. *Am J Physiol* 1996;271:C435–C454.
310. Larson TS, Lockhart JC. Restoration of vasa recta hemodynamics and pressure natriuresis in SHR by L-arginine. *Am J Physiol* 1995;268:F907–F912.
311. Larsson C, Anggard E. Increased juxtamedullary blood flow on stimulation of intrarenal prostaglandin biosynthesis. *Eur J Pharmacol* 1974;25:326–334.
312. Lassen NA, Longley JB, Lilienfield LS. Concentration of albumin in renal papilla. *Science* 1958;128:720–721.
313. LeBrie SJ. Renal peritubular capillary permeability to macromolecules. *Am J Physiol* 1967;213:1225–1232.
314. Lee-Kwon W, Wade JB, Zhang Z, Pallone TL, Weinman E. Expression of TRPC 4 channel protein that interacts with NHERF-2 in rat descending vasa recta. *Am J Physiol Cell Physiol* 2005288(4):C942–949.
315. Leichtle A, Rauch U, Albinus M, Benohr P, Kalbacher H, Mack AF, Veh RW, Quast U, Russ U. Electrophysiological and molecular characterization of the inward rectifier in juxtaglomerular cells from rat kidney. *J Physiol* 2004;560:365–376.
316. Lemley KV, Kriz W. Cycles and separations: the histotopography of the urinary concentrating process. *Kidney Int* 1987;31:538–548.
317. Lemley KV, Kriz W. Anatomy of the renal interstitium. *Kidney Int* 1991;39:370–381.
318. Lemley KV, Schmitt SL, Holliger C, Dunn MJ, Robertson CR, Jamison RL. Prostaglandin synthesis inhibitors and vasa recta erythrocyte velocities in the rat. *Am J Physiol* 1984;247: F562–F567.
319. Leonard BL, Evans RG, Navakatikyan MA, Malpas SC. Differential neural control of intrarenal blood flow. *Am J Physiol Regul Integr Comp Physiol* 2000;279:R907–R916.
320. Levin ER, Gardner DG, Samson WK. Natriuretic peptides. *N Engl J Med* 1998;339:321–328.
321. Lewis CJ, Evans RJ. P2X receptor immunoreactivity in different arteries from the femoral, pulmonary, cerebral, coronary and renal circulations. *J Vasc Res* 2001;38:332–340.
322. Li C, Klein JD, Wang W, Knepper MA, Nielsen S, Sands JM, Frokiaer J. Altered expression of urea transporters in response to ureteral obstruction. *Am J Physiol Renal Physiol* 2004;286: F1154–F1162.
323. Li L, Wu J, Jiang C. Differential expression of Kir6.1 and SUR2B mRNAs in the vasculature of various tissues in rats. *J Membr Biol* 2003;196:61–69.
324. Li WP, Tsiokas L, Sansom SC, Ma R. Epidermal growth factor activates store-operated Ca2+ channels through an inositol 1, 4, 5-trisphosphate-independent pathway in human glomerular mesangial cells. *J Biol Chem* 2004;279:4570–4577.
325. Liao Y, Day KH, Damon DN, Duling BR. Endothelial cell-specific knockout of connexin 43 causes hypotension and bradycardia in mice. *Proc Natl Acad Sci U S A* 2001;98:9989–9994.
326. Liard JF. L-NAME antagonizes vasopressin V2-induced vasodilatation in dogs. *Am J Physiol* 1994;266:H99–106.
327. Lilienfield LS, Maganzini HC, Bauer MH. Renal medullary blood flow. *Fed Proc* 1960;19:363–265.
328. Lilienfield LS, Maganzini HC, Bauer MH. Blood flow in the renal medulla. *Circ Res* 1961;9:614–617.
329. Lilienfield LS, Rose JC, Lassen NA. Diverse distribution of red cells and albumin in the dog kidney. *Circ Res* 1958;6:810–815.
330. Lim SW, Li C, Sun BK, Han KH, Kim WY, Oh YW, Lee JU, Kador PF, Knepper MA, Sands JM, Kim J, Yang CW. Long-term treatment with cyclosporine decreases aquaporins and urea transporters in the rat kidney. *Am J Physiol Renal Physiol* 2004;287: F139–F151.
331. Lopez R, Llinas MT, Roig F, Salazar FJ. Role of nitric oxide and cyclooxygenase-2 in regulating the renal hemodynamic response to norepinephrine. *Am J Physiol Regul Integr Comp Physiol* 2003;284:R488–R493.
332. Lorenz JN, Nieman M, Sabo J, Sanford LP, Hawkins JA, Elitsur N, Gawenis LR, Clarke LL, Cohen MB. Uroguanylin knockout mice have increased blood pressure and impaired natriuretic response to enteral NaCl load. *J Clin Invest* 2003;112:1244–1254.
333. Loutzenhiser K, Loutzenhiser R. Angiotensin II-induced Ca(2+) influx in renal afferent and efferent arterioles: differing roles of voltage-gated and store-operated Ca(2+) entry. *Circ Res* 2000;87:551–557.
334. Loutzenhiser R, Bidani AK, Wang X. Systolic pressure and the myogenic response of the renal afferent arteriole. *Acta Physiol Scand* 2004;181:407–413.
335. Loutzenhiser R, Chilton L, Trottier G. Membrane potential measurements in renal afferent and efferent arterioles: actions of angiotensin II. *Am J Physiol* 1997;273:F307–F314.
336. Loutzenhiser R, Epstein M, Hayashi K, Horton C. Direct visualization of effects of endothelin on the renal microvasculature. *Am J Physiol* 1990;258:F61–F68.
337. Loutzenhiser R, Epstein M, Horton C. Inhibition by diltiazem of pressure-induced afferent vasoconstriction in the isolated perfused rat kidney. *Am J Cardiol* 1987;59:72A–75A.
338. Loutzenhiser R, Hayashi K, Epstein M. Divergent effects of KCl-induced depolarization on afferent and efferent arterioles. *Am J Physiol* 1989;257:F561–F564.
339. Loutzenhiser RD, Epstein M, Fischetti F, Horton C. Effects of amlodipine on renal hemodynamics. *Am J Cardiol* 1989;64:122I–127I.
340. Loutzenhiser RD, Parker MJ. Hypoxia inhibits myogenic reactivity of renal afferent arterioles by activating ATP-sensitive K+ channels. *Circ Res* 1994;74:861–869.
341. Ma R, Kudlacek PE, Sansom SC. Protein kinase Calpha participates in activation of store-operated Ca2+ channels in human glomerular mesangial cells. *Am J Physiol Cell Physiol* 2002;283:C1390–C1398.
342. Ma R, Pluznick J, Kudlacek P, Sansom SC. Protein kinase C activates store-operated Ca(2+) channels in human glomerular mesangial cells. *J Biol Chem* 2001;276:25759–25765.
343. Ma R, Sansom SC. Epidermal growth factor activates store-operated calcium channels in human glomerular mesangial cells. *J Am Soc Nephrol* 2001;12:47–53.
344. Ma R, Smith S, Child A, Carmines PK, Sansom SC. Store-operated Ca(2+) channels in human glomerular mesangial cells. *Am J Physiol Renal Physiol* 2000;278:F954–F961.
345. Ma YH, Gebremedhin D, Schwartzman ML, Falck JR, Clark JE, Masters BS, Harder DR, Roman RJ. 20-Hydroxyeicosatetraenoic acid is an endogenous vasoconstrictor of canine renal arcuate arteries. *Circ Res* 1993;72:126–136.
346. Macey RI, Yousef LW. Osmotic stability of red cells in renal circulation requires rapid urea transport. *Am J Physiol* 1988;254:C669–C674.
347. MacPhee PJ, Michel CC. Fluid uptake from the renal medulla into the ascending vasa recta in anaesthetized rats. *J Physiol* 1995;487(Pt 1):169–183.
348. MacPhee PJ, Michel CC. Subatmospheric closing pressures in individual microvessels of rats and frogs. *J Physiol* 1995;484(Pt 1):183–187.
349. Maier KG, Roman RJ. Cytochrome P450 metabolites of arachidonic acid in the control of renal function. *Curr Opin Nephrol Hypertens* 2001;10:81–87.
350. Majid DS, Godfrey M, Omoro SA. Pressure natriuresis and autoregulation of inner medullary blood flow in canine kidney. *Hypertension* 1997;29:210–215.
351. Majid DS, Inscho EW, Navar LG. P2 purinoceptor saturation by adenosine triphosphate impairs renal autoregulation in dogs. *J Am Soc Nephrol* 1999;10:492–498.
352. Majid DS, Kadowitz PJ, Coy DH, Navar LG. Renal responses to intra-arterial administration of adrenomedullin in dogs. *Am J Physiol* 1996;270:F200–F205.
353. Majid DS, Navar LG. Suppression of blood flow autoregulation plateau during nitric oxide blockade in canine kidney. *Am J Physiol* 1992;262:F40–F46.

354. Majid DS, Navar LG. Nitric oxide in the control of renal hemodynamics and excretory function. *Am J Hypertens* 2001;14:74S–82S.

355. Majid DS, Williams A, Navar LG. Inhibition of nitric oxide synthesis attenuates pressure-induced natriuretic responses in anesthetized dogs. *Am J Physiol* 1993;264:F79–F87.

356. Makino A, Skelton MM, Zou AP, Cowley AW, Jr. Increased renal medullary H2O2 leads to hypertension. *Hypertension* 2003;42:25–30.

357. Makino A, Skelton MM, Zou AP, Roman RJ, Cowley AW, Jr. Increased renal medullary oxidative stress produces hypertension. *Hypertension* 2002;39:667–672.

358. Malpas SC, Leonard BL. Neural regulation of renal blood flow: a re-examination. *Clin Exp Pharmacol Physiol* 2000;27:956–964.

359. Marchetti J, Praddaude F, Rajerison R, Ader JL, Alhenc-Gelas F. Bradykinin attenuates the [Ca(2+)](i) response to angiotensin II of renal juxtamedullary efferent arterioles via an EDHF. *Br J Pharmacol* 2001;132:749–759.

360. Marin-Grez M, Fleming JT, Steinhausen M. Atrial natriuretic peptide causes pre-glomerular vasodilatation and post-glomerular vasoconstriction in rat kidney. *Nature* 1986;324:473–476.

361. Marsh DJ, Azen SP. Mechanism of NaCl reabsorption by hamster thin ascending limbs of Henle's loop. *Am J Physiol* 1975;228:71–79.

362. Marsh DJ, Segel LA. Analysis of countercurrent diffusion exchange in blood vessels of the renal medulla. *Am J Physiol* 1971;221:817–828.

363. Martens JR, Gelband CH. Alterations in rat interlobar artery membrane potential and K+ channels in genetic and nongenetic hypertension. *Circ Res* 1996;79:295–301.

364. Martens JR, Gelband CH. Ion channels in vascular smooth mus-cle: alterations in essential hypertension. *Proc Soc Exp Biol Med* 1998;218:192–203.

365. Martin W, Villani GM, Jothianandan D, Furchgott RF. Selective blockade of endothelium-dependent and glyceryl trinitrate-induced relaxation by hemoglobin and by methylene blue in the rabbit aorta. *J Pharmacol Exp Ther* 1985;232:708–716.

366. Matsuda H, Hayashi K, Arakawa K, Kubota E, Honda M, Tokuyama H, Suzuki H, Yamamoto T, Kajiya F, Saruta T. Distinct modulation of superficial and juxtamedullary arterioles by prostaglandin in vivo. *Hypertens Res* 2002;25:901–910.

367. Matsunaga H, Yamashita N, Miyajima Y, Okuda T, Chang H, Ogata E, Kurokawa K. Ion channel activities of cultured rat mesangial cells. *Am J Physiol* 1991;261:F808–F814.

368. Mattson DL. Importance of the renal medullary circulation in the control of sodium excretion and blood pressure. *Am J Physiol Regul Integr Comp Physiol* 2003;284:R13–R27.

369. Mattson DL, Bellehumeur TG. Neural nitric oxide synthase in the renal medulla and blood pressure regulation. *Hypertension* 1996;28:297–303.

370. Mattson DL, Lu S, Cowley AW, Jr. Role of nitric oxide in the control of the renal medullary circulation. *Clin Exp Pharmacol Physiol* 1997;24:587–590.

371. Mattson DL, Lu S, Nakanishi K, Papanek PE, Cowley AW, Jr. Effect of chronic renal medullary nitric oxide inhibition on blood pressure. *Am J Physiol* 1994;266:H1918–H1926.

372. Mattson DL, Lu S, Roman RJ, Cowley AW, Jr. Relationship between renal perfusion pressure and blood flow in different regions of the kidney. *Am J Physiol* 1993;264:R578–R583.

373. Mattson DL, Maeda CY, Bachman TD, Cowley AW, Jr. Inducible nitric oxide synthase and blood pressure. *Hypertension* 1998;31:15–20.

374. Mattson DL, Wu F. Control of arterial blood pressure and renal sodium excretion by nitric oxide synthase in the renal medulla. *Acta Physiol Scand* 2000;168:149–154.

375. Mattson DL, Wu F. Nitric oxide synthase activity and isoforms in rat renal vasculature. *Hypertension* 2000;35:337–341.

376. McCoy DE, Bhattacharya S, Olson BA, Levier DG, Arend LJ, Spielman WS. The renal adenosine system: structure, function, and regulation. *Semin Nephrol* 1993;13:31–40.

377. McGiff JC, Quilley J. 20-HETE and the kidney: resolution of old problems and new beginnings. *Am J Physiol* 1999;277:R607–R623.

378. McGowan HM, Vandongen R, Codde JP, Croft KD. Increased aortic PGI2 and plasma lyso-PAF in the unclipped one-kidney hypertensive rat. *Am J Physiol* 1986;251:H1361–H1364.

379. McKee M, Scavone C, Nathanson JA. Nitric oxide, cGMP, and hormone regulation of active sodium transport. *Proc Natl Acad Sci U S A* 1994;91:12056–12060.

380. McNay JL, Abe Y. Pressure-dependent heterogeneity of renal cortical blood flow in dogs. *Circ Res* 1970;27:571–587.

381. Mendez RE, Dunn BR, Troy JL, Brenner BM. Atrial natriuretic peptide and furosemide effects on hydraulic pressure in the renal papilla. *Kidney Int* 1988;34:36–42.

382. Meng S, Roberts LJ, Cason GW, Curry TS, Manning RD, Jr. Superoxide dismutase and oxidative stress in Dahl salt-sensitive and -resistant rats. *Am J Physiol Regul Integr Comp Physiol* 2002;283:R732–R738.

383. Metzger F, Quast U. Binding of [3H]-P1075, an opener of ATP-sensitive K+ channels, to rat glomerular preparations. *Naunyn Schmiedebergs Arch Pharmacol* 1996;354:452–459.

384. Michel CC. Renal medullary microcirculation: architecture and exchange. *Microcirculation* 1995;2:125–139.

385. Minami K, Segawa K, Uezono Y, Shiga Y, Shiraishi M, Ogata J, Shigematsu A. Adrenomedullin inhibits the pressor effects and decrease in renal blood flow induced by norepinephrine or angiotensin II in anesthetized rats. *Jpn J Pharmacol* 2001;86:159–164.

386. Mink D, Schiller A, Kriz W, Taugner R. Interendothelial junctions in kidney vessels. *Cell Tissue Res* 1984;236:567–576.

387. Miyamoto M, Yagil Y, Larson T, Robertson C, Jamison RL. Effects of intrarenal adenosine on renal function and medullary blood flow in the rat. *Am J Physiol* 1988;255:F1230–F1234.

388. Miyata N, Cowley AW, Jr. Renal intramedullary infusion of L-arginine prevents reduction of medullary blood flow and hypertension in Dahl salt-sensitive rats. *Hypertension* 1999;33:446–450.

389. Miyata N, Park F, Li XF, Cowley AW, Jr. Distribution of angiotensin AT1 and AT2 receptor subtypes in the rat kidney. *Am J Physiol* 1999;277:F437–F446.

390. Miyata N, Zou AP, Mattson DL, Cowley AW, Jr. Renal medullary interstitial infusion of L-arginine prevents hypertension in Dahl salt-sensitive rats. *Am J Physiol* 1998;275:R1667–R1673.

391. Moffat DB. Extravascular protein in the renal medulla. *Q J Exp Physiol Cogn Med Sci* 1969;54:60–67.

392. Moffat DB, Creasey M. The fine structure of the intra-arterial cushions at the origins of the juxtamedullary afferent arterioles in the rat kidney. *J Anat* 1971;110:409–419.

393. Moffat DB, Fourman J. The vascular pattern of the rat kidney. *J Anat* 1963;97:543–553.

394. Molero MM, Giulumian AD, Reddy VB, Ludwig LM, Pollock JS, Pollock DM, Rusch NJ, Fuchs LC. Decreased endothelin binding and [Ca2+]i signaling in microvessels of DOCA-salt hypertensive rats. *J Hypertens* 2002;20:1799–1805.

395. Morgan T, Berliner RW. Permeability of the loop of Henle, vasa recta, and collecting duct to water, urea, and sodium. *Am J Physiol* 1968;215:108–115.

396. Mori T, Cowley AW, Jr. Angiotensin II-NAD(P)H oxidase-stimulated superoxide modifies tubulovascular nitric oxide cross-talk in renal outer medulla. *Hypertension* 2003;42:588–593.

397. Mori T, Dickhout JG, Cowley AW, Jr. Vasopressin increases intracellular NO concentration via Ca2(+) signaling in inner medullary collecting duct. *Hypertension* 2002;39:465–469.

398. Mori Y, Nishikimi T, Kobayashi N, Ono H, Kangawa K, Matsuoka H. Long-term adrenomedullin infusion improves survival in malignant hypertensive rats. *Hypertension* 2002;40:107–113.

399. Moridani BA, Kline RL. Effect of endogenous L-arginine on the measurement of nitric oxide synthase activity in the rat kidney. *Can J Physiol Pharmacol* 1996;74:1210–1214.

400. Muirhead EE, Germain G, Leach BE, Pitcock JA, Stephenson P, Brooks B, Brosius WL, Daniels EG, Hinman JW. Production of renomedullary prostaglandins by renomedullary interstitial cells grown in tissue culture. *Circ Res* 1972;31(Suppl2):161–172.

401. Nagata D, Hirata Y, Suzuki E, Kakoki M, Hayakawa H, Goto A, Ishimitsu T, Minamino N, Ono Y, Kangawa K, Matsuo H, Omata M. Hypoxia-induced adrenomedullin production in the kidney. *Kidney Int* 1999;55:1259–1267.

402. Naicker S, Bhoola KD. Endothelins: vasoactive modulators of renal function in health and disease. *Pharmacol Ther* 2001;90:61–88.

403. Naitoh M, Suzuki H, Murakami M, Matsumoto A, Ichihara A, Nakamoto H, Yamamura Y, Saruta T. Arginine vasopressin produces renal vasodilation via V2 receptors in conscious dogs. *Am J Physiol* 1993;265:R934–R942.

404. Nakanishi K, Mattson DL, Cowley AW, Jr. Role of renal medullary blood flow in the development of L-NAME hypertension in rats. *Am J Physiol* 1995;268:R317–R323.

405. Nakanishi K, Mattson DL, Gross V, Roman RJ, Cowley AW, Jr. Control of renal medullary blood flow by vasopressin V1 and V2 receptors. *Am J Physiol* 1995;269:R193–R200.

406. Navakatikyan MA, Leonard BL, Evans RG, Malpas SC. Modelling the neural control of intrarenal blood flow. *Clin Exp Pharmacol Physiol* 2000;27:650–652.

407. Navar LG. The intrarenal renin-angiotensin system in hypertension. *Kidney Int* 2004;65:1522–1532.

408. Navar LG, Ichihara A, Chin SY, Imig JD. Nitric oxide-angiotensin II interactions in angiotensin II-dependent hypertension. *Acta Physiol Scand* 2000;168:139–147.

409. Navar LG, Inscho EW, Imig JD, Mitchell KD. Heterogeneous activation mechanisms in the renal microvasculature. *Kidney Int Suppl* 1998;67:S17–S21.

410. Navar LG, Inscho EW, Majid SA, Imig JD, Harrison-Bernard LM, Mitchell KD. Paracrine regulation of the renal microcirculation. *Physiol Rev* 1996;76:425–536.

411. Navar LG, Nishiyama A. Why are angiotensin concentrations so high in the kidney? *Curr Opin Nephrol Hypertens* 2004;13:107–115.

412. Nelson MT, Quayle JM. Physiological roles and properties of potassium channels in arterial smooth muscle. *Am J Physiol* 1995;268:C799–C822.

413. Newby AC, Henderson AH. Stimulus-secretion coupling in vascular endothelial cells. *Annu Rev Physiol* 1990;52:661–674.

414. Nielsen S, Pallone T, Smith BL, Christensen EI, Agre P, Maunsbach AB. Aquaporin-1 water channels in short and long loop descending thin limbs and in descending vasa recta in rat kidney. *Am J Physiol* 1995;268:F1023–F1037.

415. Nielsen S, Smith BL, Christensen EI, Agre P. Distribution of the aquaporin CHIP in secretory and resorptive epithelia and capillary endothelia. *Proc Natl Acad Sci U S A* 1993;90:7275–7279.

416. Nishikimi T, Mori Y, Kobayashi N, Tadokoro K, Wang X, Akimoto K, Yoshihara F, Kangawa K, Matsuoka H. Renoprotective effect of chronic adrenomedullin infusion in Dahl salt-sensitive rats. *Hypertension* 2002;39:1077–1082.

417. Nishimatsu H, Hirata Y, Shindo T, Kurihara H, Kakoki M, Nagata D, Hayakawa H, Satonaka H, Sata M, Tojo A, Suzuki E, Kangawa K, Matsuo H, Kitamura T, Nagai R. Role of endogenous adrenomedullin in the regulation of vascular tone and ischemic renal injury: studies on transgenic/knockout mice of adrenomedullin gene. *Circ Res* 2002;90:657–663.

418. Nishiyama A, Inscho EW, Navar LG. Interactions of adenosine A1 and A2a receptors on renal microvascular reactivity. *Am J Physiol Renal Physiol* 2001;280:F406–F414.

419. Nishiyama A, Seth DM, Navar LG. Renal interstitial fluid angiotensin I and angiotensin II concentrations during local angiotensin-converting enzyme inhibition. *J Am Soc Nephrol* 2002;13:2207–2212.

420. Nishiyama A, Seth DM, Navar LG. Angiotensin II type 1 receptor-mediated augmentation of renal interstitial fluid angiotensin II in angiotensin II-induced hypertension. *J Hypertens* 2003;21:1897–1903.

421. Oliver JJ, Eppel GA, Rajapakse NW, Evans RG. Lipoxygenase and cyclo-oxygenase products in the control of regional kidney blood flow in rabbits. *Clin Exp Pharmacol Physiol* 2003;30:812–819.

422. Ortiz PA, Garvin JL. Intrarenal transport and vasoactive substances in hypertension. *Hypertension* 2001;38:621–624.

423. Ortiz PA, Garvin JL. Role of nitric oxide in the regulation of nephron transport. *Am J Physiol Renal Physiol* 2002;282:F777–F784.

424. Ortiz PA, Garvin JL. Superoxide stimulates NaCl absorption by the thick ascending limb. *Am J Physiol Renal Physiol* 2002;283:F957–F962.

425. Osgood RW, Patton M, Hanley MJ, Venkatachalam M, Reineck HJ, Stein JH. In vitro perfusion of the isolated dog glomerulus. *Am J Physiol* 1983;244:F349–F354.

426. Osswald H, Schmitz HJ, Heidenreich O. Adenosine response of the rat kidney after saline loading, sodium restriction and hemorrhagia. *Pflugers Arch* 1975;357:323–333.

427. Ott CE, Haas JA, Cuche JL, Knox FG. Effect of increased peritubule protein concentration on proximal tubule reabsorption in the presence and absence of extracellular volume expansion. *J Clin Invest* 1975;55:612–620.

428. Ozawa Y, Hayashi K, Nagahama T, Fujiwara K, Saruta T. Effect of T-type selective calcium antagonist on renal microcirculation: stu-dies in the isolated perfused hydronephrotic kidney. *Hypertension* 2001;38:343–347.
429. Ozawa Y, Hayashi K, Nagahama T, Fujiwara K, Wakino S, Saruta T. Renal afferent and efferent arteriolar dilation by nilvadipine: studies in the isolated perfused hydronephrotic kidney. *J Cardiovasc Pharmacol* 1999;33:243–247.
430. Ozawa Y, Hayashi K, Wakino S, Kanda T, Homma K, Takamatsu I, Tatematsu S, Yoshioka K, Saruta T. Free radical activity depends on underlying vasoconstrictors in renal microcirculation. *Clin Exp Hypertens* 2004;26:219–229.
431. Paliege A, Mizel D, Medina C, Pasumarthy A, Huang YG, Bachmann S, Briggs JP, Schnermann JB, Yang T. Inhibition of nNOS expression in the macula densa by COX-2-derived prostaglandin E(2). *Am J Physiol Renal Physiol* 2004;287:F152–F159.
432. Pallone TL. Effect of sodium chloride gradients on water flux in rat descending vasa recta. *J Clin Invest* 1991;87:12–19.
433. Pallone TL. Resistance of ascending vasa recta to transport of water. *Am J Physiol* 1991;260: F303–F310.
434. Pallone TL. Transport of sodium chloride and water in rat ascending vasa recta. *Am J Physiol* 1991;261:F519–F525.
435. Pallone TL. Molecular sieving of albumin by the ascending vasa recta wall. *J Clin Invest* 1992;90:30–34.
436. Pallone TL. Characterization of the urea transporter in outer medullary descending vasa recta. *Am J Physiol* 1994;267:R260–R267.
437. Pallone TL. Extravascular protein in the renal medulla: analysis by two methods. *Am J Physiol* 1994;266:R1429–R1436.
438. Pallone TL. Vasoconstriction of outer medullary vasa recta by angiotensin II is modulated by prostaglandin E2. *Am J Physiol* 1994;266:F850–F857.
439. Pallone TL. The extraglomerular circulation of the kidney. In: Seldin DW, Giebisch G, eds. *The Kidney: Physiology and Pathophysiology*. Philadelphia, PA: Lippincott Williams & Wilkins; 2000:791–822.
440. Pallone TL. Microdissected perfused vessels. *Methods Mol Med* 2003;86:443–456.
441. Pallone TL, Cao C, Zhang Z. Inhibition of K+ conductance in descending vasa recta pericytes by ANG II. *Am J Physiol Renal Physiol* 2004;287:F1213–F1222.
442. Pallone TL, Edwards A, Ma T, Silldorff EP, Verkman AS. Requirement of aquaporin-1 for NaCl-driven water transport across descending vasa recta. *J Clin Invest* 2000;105:215–222.
443. Pallone TL, Huang JM. Control of descending vasa recta pericyte membrane potential by angiotensin II. *Am J Physiol Renal Physiol* 2002;282:F1064–F1074.
444. Pallone TL, Kishore BK, Nielsen S, Agre P, Knepper MA. Evidence that aquaporin-1 mediates NaCl-induced water flux across descending vasa recta. *Am J Physiol* 1997;272:F587–F596.
445. Pallone TL, Mattson DL. Role of nitric oxide in regulation of the renal medulla in normal and hypertensive kidneys. *Curr Opin Nephrol Hypertens* 2002;11:93–98.
446. Pallone TL, Morgenthaler TI, Deen WM. Analysis of microvascular water and solute exchanges in the renal medulla. *Am J Physiol* 1984;247:F303–F315.
447. Pallone TL, Nielsen S, Silldorff EP, Yang S. Diffusive transport of solute in the rat medullary microcirculation. *Am J Physiol* 1995;269:F55–F63.
448. Pallone TL, Robertson CR, Jamison RL. Renal medullary microcirculation. *Physiol Rev* 1990;70:885–920.
449. Pallone TL, Silldorff EP. Pericyte regulation of renal medullary blood flow. *Exp Nephrol* 2001;9:165–170.
450. Pallone TL, Silldorff EP, Cheung JY. Response of isolated rat descending vasa recta to bradykinin. *Am J Physiol* 1998;274:H752–H759.
451. Pallone TL, Silldorff EP, Zhang Z. Inhibition of calcium signaling in descending vasa recta endothelia by ANG II. *Am J Physiol Heart Circ Physiol* 2000;278:H1248–H1255.
452. Pallone TL, Turner MR. Molecular sieving of small solutes by outer medullary descending vasa recta. *Am J Physiol* 1997;272:F579–F586.
453. Pallone TL, Turner MR, Edwards A, Jamison RL. Countercurrent exchange in the renal medulla. *Am J Physiol Regul Integr Comp Physiol* 2003;284:R1153–R1175.
454. Pallone TL, Work J, Jamison RL. Resistance of descending vasa recta to the transport of water. *Am J Physiol* 1990;259:F688–F697.
455. Pallone TL, Work J, Myers RL, Jamison RL. Transport of sodium and urea in outer medullary descending vasa recta. *J Clin Invest* 1994;93:212–222.
456. Pallone TL, Yagil Y, Jamison RL. Effect of small-solute gradients on transcapillary fluid movement in renal inner medulla. *Am J Physiol* 1989;257:F547–F553.
457. Pallone TL, Zhang Z, Rhinehart K. Physiology of the renal medullary microcirculation. *Am J Physiol Renal Physiol* 2003;284:F253–F266.
458. Pannabecker TL, Dahlmann A, Brokl OH, Dantzler WH. Mixed descending- and ascending-type thin limbs of Henle's loop in mammalian renal inner medulla. *Am J Physiol Renal Physiol* 2000;278:F202–F208.
459. Pappenheimer JR, Kinter WB. Hematocrit ratio of blood within mammalian kidney and its significance for renal hemodynamics. *Am J Physiol* 1956;185:377–390.
460. Parekh AB. Store-operated Ca2+ entry: dynamic interplay between endoplasmic reticulum, mitochondria and plasma membrane. *J Physiol* 2003;547:333–348.
461. Parekh N, Zou AP. Role of prostaglandins in renal medullary circulation: response to different vasoconstrictors. *Am J Physiol* 1996;271:F653–F658.
462. Park F, Mattson DL, Roberts LA, Cowley AW, Jr. Evidence for the presence of smooth muscle alpha-actin within pericytes of the renal medulla. *Am J Physiol* 1997;273:R1742–R1748.
463. Park F, Mattson DL, Skelton MM, Cowley AW, Jr. Localization of the vasopressin V1a and V2 receptors within the renal cortical and medullary circulation. *Am J Physiol* 1997;273: R243–R251.
464. Park F, Zou AP, Cowley AW, Jr. Arginine vasopressin-mediated stimulation of nitric oxide within the rat renal medulla. *Hypertension* 1998;32:896–901.
465. Patzak A, Kleinmann F, Lai EY, Kupsch E, Skelweit A, Mrowka R. Nitric oxide counteracts angiotensin II induced contraction in efferent arterioles in mice. *Acta Physiol Scand* 2004;181: 439–444.
466. Patzak A, Lai EY, Mrowka R, Steege A, Persson PB, Persson AE. AT1 receptors mediate angiotensin II-induced release of nitric oxide in afferent arterioles. *Kidney Int* 2004;66:1949–1958.
467. Pedersen JC, Persson AEG, Maunsbach AB. Ultrastructure and quantitative characterization of the cortical interstitium in the rat kidney. In: *Functional Ultrastructure of the Kidney*. London: Academic Press; 1980:443–457.
468. Peti-Peterdi J, Komlosi P, Fuson AL, Guan Y, Schneider A, Qi Z, Redha R, Rosivall L, Breyer MD, Bell PD. Luminal NaCl delivery regulates basolateral PGE2 release from macula densa cells. *J Clin Invest* 2003;112:76–82.
469. Pinter GG, Gartner K. Peritubular capillary, interstitium, and lymph of the renal cortex. *Rev Physiol Biochem Pharmacol* 1984;99:184–202.
470. Plato CF, Garvin JL. Nitric oxide, endothelin and nephron transport: potential interactions. *Clin Exp Pharmacol Physiol* 1999;26:262–268.
471. Pollock DM. Renal endothelin in hypertension. *Curr Opin Nephrol Hypertens* 2000;9:157–164.
472. Pollock DM. Contrasting pharmacological ETB receptor blockade with genetic ETB deficiency in renal responses to big ET-1. *Physiol Genomics* 2001;6:39–43.
473. Pollock DM, Jenkins JM, Cook AK, Imig JD, Inscho EW. L-type calcium channels in the renal microcirculatory response to endothelin. *Am J Physiol Renal Physiol* 2005. 288(4):F771–777.
474. Pomerantz RM, Slotkoff LM, Lilienfield LS. Histochemical and microanatomical differences between renal cortical and medullary interstitium. In: Kass EH (ed.). *Progress in Pyelonephritis*. Philadelphia: F.A. Davis Co., 1965:434.
475. Pomposiello SI, Quilley J, Carroll MA, Falck JR, McGiff JC. 5, 6-epoxyeicosatrienoic acid mediates the enhanced renal vasodilation to arachidonic acid in the SHR. *Hypertension* 2003;42:548–554.
476. Popp R, Brandes RP, Ott G, Busse R, Fleming I. Dynamic modulation of interendothelial gap junctional communication by 11, 12-epoxyeicosatrienoic acid. *Circ Res* 2002;90:800–806.
477. Pries AR, Ley K, Gaehtgens P. Generalization of the Fahraeus principle for microvessel networks. *Am J Physiol* 1986;251:H1324–H1332.
478. Prior HM, Yates MS, Beech DJ. Functions of large conductance Ca2+-activated (BKCa), delayed rectifier (KV) and background K+ channels in the control of membrane potential in rabbit renal arcuate artery. *J Physiol* 1998;511(Pt 1):159–169.
479. Prior HM, Yates MS, Beech DJ. Role of K+ channels in A2A adenosine receptor-mediated dilation of the pressurized renal arcuate artery. *Br J Pharmacol* 1999;126:494–500.
480. Promeneur D, Bankir L, Hu MC, Trinh-Trang-Tan MM. Renal tubular and vascular urea transporters: influence of antidiuretic hormone on messenger RNA expression in Brattleboro rats. *J Am Soc Nephrol* 1998;9:1359–1366.
481. Promeneur D, Rousselet G, Bankir L, Bailly P, Cartron JP, Ripoche P, Trinh-Trang-Tan MM. Evidence for distinct vascular and tubular urea transporters in the rat kidney. *J Am Soc Nephrol* 1996;7:852–860.
482. Qi Z, Hao CM, Langenbach RI, Breyer RM, Redha R, Morrow JD, Breyer MD. Opposite effects of cyclooxygenase-1 and -2 activity on the pressor response to angiotensin II. *J Clin Invest* 2002;110:61–69.
483. Quayle JM, Nelson MT, Standen NB. ATP-sensitive and inwardly rectifying potassium channels in smooth muscle. *Physiol Rev* 1997;77:1165–1232.
484. Quilley J, Fulton D, McGiff JC. Hyperpolarizing factors. *Biochem Pharmacol* 1997;54: 1059–1070.
485. Racasan S, Joles JA, Boer P, Koomans HA, Braam B. NO dependency of RBF and autoregulation in the spontaneously hypertensive rat. *Am J Physiol Renal Physiol* 2003;285:F105–F112.
486. Rajapakse NW, Roman RJ, Falck JR, Oliver JJ, Evans RG. Modulation of V1-receptor-mediated renal vasoconstriction by epoxyeicosatrienoic acids. *Am J Physiol Regul Integr Comp Physiol* 2004;287:R181–R187.
487. Ralevic V, Burnstock G. Receptors for purines and pyrimidines. *Pharmacol Rev* 1998;50: 413–492.
488. Ramchandra R, Barrett CJ, Guild SJ, Malpas SC. Neural control of the renal vasculature in angiotensin II-induced hypertension. *Clin Exp Pharmacol Physiol* 2002;29:867–872.
489. Rasmussen SN. Red cell and plasma volume flows to the inner medulla of the rat kidney: determinations by means of a step function input indicator technique. *Pflugers Arch* 1978;373:153–159.
490. Ren Y, Garvin JL, Liu R, Carretero OA. Role of macula densa adenosine triphosphate (ATP) in tubuloglomerular feedback. *Kidney Int* 2004;66:1479–1485.
491. Renkin EM. Capillary transport of macromolecules: pores and other endothelial pathways. *J Appl Physiol* 1985;58:315–325.
492. Reslerova M, Loutzenhiser R. Divergent mechanisms of ATP-sensitive K+ channel-induced vasodilation in renal afferent and efferent arterioles. Evidence of L-type Ca2+ channel-dependent and -independent actions of pinacidil. *Circ Res* 1995;77:1114–1120.
493. Reslerova M, Loutzenhiser R. Renal microvascular actions of calcitonin gene-related peptide. *Am J Physiol* 1998;274:F1078–F1085.
494. Rhinehart K, Handelsman CA, Silldorff EP, Pallone TL. ANG II AT2 receptor modulates AT1 receptor-mediated descending vasa recta endothelial Ca2+ signaling. *Am J Physiol Heart Circ Physiol* 2003;284:H779–H789.
495. Rhinehart K, Zhang Z, Pallone TL. Ca(2+) signaling and membrane potential in descending vasa recta pericytes and endothelia. *Am J Physiol Renal Physiol* 2002;283:F852–F860.
496. Rhinehart KL, Pallone TL. Nitric oxide generation by isolated descending vasa recta. *Am J Physiol Heart Circ Physiol* 2001;281:H316–H324.
497. Roald AB, Ofstad J, Iversen BM. Attenuated buffering of renal perfusion pressure variation in juxtamedullary cortex in SHR. *Am J Physiol Renal Physiol* 2002;282:F506–F511.
498. Roman RJ. Pressure-diuresis in volume-expanded rats. Tubular reabsorption in superficial and deep nephrons. *Hypertension* 1988;12:177–183.
499. Roman RJ. P-450 metabolites of arachidonic acid in the control of cardiovascular function. *Physiol Rev* 2002;82:131–185.
500. Roman RJ, Carmines PK, Loutzenhiser R, Conger JD. Direct studies on the control of the renal microcirculation. *J Am Soc Nephrol* 1991;2:136–149.
501. Roman RJ, Cowley AW, Jr., Garcia-Estan J, Lombard JH. Pressure-diuresis in volume-expanded rats. Cortical and medullary hemodynamics. *Hypertension* 1988;12:168–176.

502. Roman RJ, Kaldunski ML, Scicli AG, Carretero OA. Influence of kinins and angiotensin II on the regulation of papillary blood flow. *Am J Physiol* 1988;255:F690–F698.

503. Roman RJ, Lianos E. Influence of prostaglandins on papillary blood flow and pressure-natriuretic response. *Hypertension* 1990;15:29–35.

504. Roman RJ, Maier KG, Sun CW, Harder DR, Alonso-Galicia M. Renal and cardiovascular actions of 20-hydroxyeicosatetraenoic acid and epoxyeicosatrienoic acids. *Clin Exp Pharmacol Physiol* 2000;27:855–865.

505. Roman RJ, Smits C. Laser-Doppler determination of papillary blood flow in young and adult rats. *Am J Physiol* 1986;251:F115–F124.

506. Rudenstam J, Bergstrom G, Taghipour K, Gothberg G, Karlstrom G. Efferent renal sympathetic nerve stimulation in vivo. Effects on regional renal haemodynamics in the Wistar rat, studied by laser-Doppler technique. *Acta Physiol Scand* 1995;154:387–394.

507. Rudichenko VM, Beierwaltes WH. Arginine vasopressin-induced renal vasodilation mediated by nitric oxide. *J Vasc Res* 1995;32:100–105.

508. Rump LC, Oberhauser V, von K, I. Purinoceptors mediate renal vasodilation by nitric oxide dependent and independent mechanisms. *Kidney Int* 1998;54:473–481.

509. Russ U, Rauch U, Quast U. Pharmacological evidence for a KATP channel in renin-secreting cells from rat kidney. *J Physiol* 1999;517(Pt 3):781–790.

510. Salomonsson M, Gustafsson F, Andreasen D, Jensen BL, Holstein-Rathlou NH. Local electric stimulation causes conducted calcium response in rat interlobular arteries. *Am J Physiol Renal Physiol* 2002;283:F473–F480.

511. Salomonsson M, Sorensen CM, Arendshorst WJ, Steendahl J, Holstein-Rathlou NH. Calcium handling in afferent arterioles. *Acta Physiol Scand* 2004;181:421–429.

512. Sampaio WO, Nascimento AA, Santos RA. Systemic and regional hemodynamic effects of angiotensin-(1-7) in rats. *Am J Physiol Heart Circ Physiol* 2003;284:H1985–H1994.

513. Sands JM. Renal urea transporters. *Curr Opin Nephrol Hypertens* 2004;13:525–532.

514. Sanjana VM, Johnston PA, Deen WM, Robertson CR, Brenner BM, Jamison RL. Hydraulic and oncotic pressure measurements in inner medulla of mammalian kidney. *Am J Physiol* 1975;228:1921–1926.

515. Sanjana VM, Johnston PA, Robertson CR, Jamison RL. An examination of transcapillary water flux in renal inner medulla. *Am J Physiol* 1976;231:313–318.

516. Sansom SC, Ma R, Carmines PK, Hall DA. Regulation of Ca(2+)-activated K(+) channels by multifunctional Ca(2+)/calmodulin-dependent protein kinase. *Am J Physiol Renal Physiol* 2000;279:F283–F288.

517. Sansom SC, Stockand JD. Physiological role of large, Ca2+-activated K+ channels in human glomerular mesangial cells. *Clin Exp Pharmacol Physiol* 1996;23:76–82.

518. Sansom SC, Stockand JD, Hall D, Williams B. Regulation of large calcium-activated potassium channels by protein phosphatase 2A. *J Biol Chem* 1997;272:9902–9906.

519. Santos RA, Simoes e Silva AC, Maric C, Silva DM, Machado RP, de B, I, Heringer-Walther S, Pinheiro SV, Lopes MT, Bader M, Mendes EP, Lemos VS, Campagnole-Santos MJ, Schultheiss HP, Speth R, Walther T. Angiotensin-(1-7) is an endogenous ligand for the G protein-coupled receptor Mas. *Proc Natl Acad Sci U S A* 2003;100:8258–8263.

520. Sapirstein LA. Regional blood flow by fractional distribution of indicators. *Am J Physiol* 1958;193:161–168.

521. Sarkis A, Lopez B, Roman RJ. Role of 20-hydroxyeicosatetraenoic acid and epoxyeicosatrienoic acids in hypertension. *Curr Opin Nephrol Hypertens* 2004;13:205–214.

522. Sasser JM, Pollock JS, Pollock DM. Renal endothelin in chronic angiotensin II hypertension. *Am J Physiol Regul Integr Comp Physiol* 2002;283:R243–R248.

523. Schmidt BM, Oehmer S, Delles C, Bratke R, Schneider MP, Klingbeil A, Fleischmann EH, Schmieder RE. Rapid nongenomic effects of aldosterone on human forearm vasculature. *Hypertension* 2003;42:156–160.

524. Schnackenberg CG. Physiological and pathophysiological roles of oxygen radicals in the renal microvasculature. *Am J Physiol Regul Integr Comp Physiol* 2002;282:R335–R342.

525. Schnackenberg CG, Welch WJ, Wilcox CS. Normalization of blood pressure and renal vascular resistance in SHR with a membrane-permeable superoxide dismutase mimetic: role of nitric oxide. *Hypertension* 1998;32:59–64.

526. Schnackenberg CG, Welch WJ, Wilcox CS. TP receptor-mediated vasoconstriction in microperfused afferent arterioles: roles of O(2)(-) and NO. *Am J Physiol Renal Physiol* 2000;279:F302–F308.

527. Schnackenberg CG, Wilcox CS. Two-week administration of tempol attenuates both hypertension and renal excretion of 8-Iso prostaglandin f2alpha. *Hypertension* 1999;33:424–428.

528. Schnermann J. Adenosine mediates tubuloglomerular feedback. *Am J Physiol Regul Integr Comp Physiol* 2002;283:R276–R277.

529. Schnermann J. Homer W. Smith Award lecture. The juxtaglomerular apparatus: from anatomical peculiarity to physiological relevance. *J Am Soc Nephrol* 2003;14:1681–1694.

530. Scholander PF. The wonderful net. *Scient Am* 1957;196:96–107.

531. Schoonmaker GC, Fallet RW, Carmines PK. Superoxide anion curbs nitric oxide modulation of afferent arteriolar ANG II responsiveness in diabetes mellitus. *Am J Physiol Renal Physiol* 2000;278:F302–F309.

532. Schroeder AC, Imig JD, LeBlanc EA, Pham BT, Pollock DM, Inscho EW. Endothelin-mediated calcium signaling in preglomerular smooth muscle cells. *Hypertension* 2000;35:280–286.

533. Schurek HJ, Alt JM. Effect of albumin on the function of perfused rat kidney. *Am J Physiol* 1981;240:F569–F576.

534. Schwartz MM, Karnovsky MJ, Vehkatachalam MA. Ultrastructural differences between rat inner medullary descending and ascending vasa recta. *Lab Invest* 1976;35:161–170.

535. Seikaly MG, Arant BS, Jr., Seney FD, Jr. Endogenous angiotensin concentrations in specific intrarenal fluid compartments of the rat. *J Clin Invest* 1990;86:1352–1357.

536. Shayakul C, Knepper MA, Smith CP, DiGiovanni SR, Hediger MA. Segmental localization of urea transporter mRNAs in rat kidney. *Am J Physiol* 1997;272:F654–F660.

537. Shayakul C, Steel A, Hediger MA. Molecular cloning and characterization of the vasopressin-regulated urea transporter of rat kidney collecting ducts. *J Clin Invest* 1996;98:2580–2587.

538. Shepro D, Morel NM. Pericyte physiology. *FASEB J* 1993;7:1031–1038.

539. Shimamura T, Morrison AB. Vascular permeability of the renal medullary vessels in the mouse and rat. *Am J Pathol* 1973;71:155–163.

540. Shindo T, Kurihara Y, Nishimatsu H, Moriyama N, Kakoki M, Wang Y, Imai Y, Ebihara A, Kuwaki T, Ju KH, Minamino N, Kangawa K, Ishikawa T, Fukuda M, Akimoto Y, Kawakami H, Imai T, Morita H, Yazaki Y, Nagai R, Hirata Y, Kurihara H. Vascular abnormalities and elevated blood pressure in mice lacking adrenomedullin gene. *Circulation* 2001;104:1964–1971.

541. Silldorff EP, Hilbun LR, Pallone TL. Angiotensin II constriction of rat vasa recta is partially thromboxane dependent. *Hypertension* 2002;40:541–546.

542. Silldorff EP, Kreisberg MS, Pallone TL. Adenosine modulates vasomotor tone in outer medullary descending vasa recta of the rat. *J Clin Invest* 1996;98:18–23.

543. Silldorff EP, Pallone TL. Adenosine signaling in outer medullary descending vasa recta. *Am J Physiol Regul Integr Comp Physiol* 2001;280:R854–R861.

544. Silldorff EP, Yang S, Pallone TL. Prostaglandin E2 abrogates endothelin-induced vasoconstriction in renal outer medullary descending vasa recta of the rat. *J Clin Invest* 1995;95:2734–2740.

545. Silverstein DM, Thornhill BA, Leung JC, Vehaskari VM, Craver RD, Trachtman HA, Chevalier RL. Expression of connexins in the normal and obstructed developing kidney. *Pediatr Nephrol* 2003;18:216–224.

546. Slotkoff LM, Lilienfield LS. Extravascular renal albumin. *Am J Physiol* 1967;212:400–406.

547. Solez K, Kramer EC, Fox JA, Heptinstall RH. Medullary plasma flow and intravascular leukocyte accumulation in acute renal failure. *Kidney Int* 1974;6:24–37.

548. Spiecker M, Liao JK. Vascular protective effects of cytochrome p450 epoxygenase-derived eicosanoids. *Arch Biochem Biophys* 2005;433:413–420.

549. Spielman WS, Osswald H. Blockade of postocclusive renal vasoconstriction by an angiotensin II antagonists: evidence for an angiotensin-adenosine interaction. *Am J Physiol* 1979;237:F463–F467.

550. Spitzer A, Windhager EE. Effect of peritubular oncotic pressure changes on proximal tubular fluid reabsorption. *Am J Physiol* 1970;218:1188–1193.

551. Stec DE, Mattson DL, Roman RJ. Inhibition of renal outer medullary 20-HETE production produces hypertension in Lewis rats. *Hypertension* 1997;29:315–319.

552. Steendahl J, Holstein-Rathlou NH, Sorensen CM, Salomonsson M. Effects of chloride channel blockers on rat renal vascular responses to angiotensin II and norepinephrine. *Am J Physiol Renal Physiol* 2004;286:F323–F330.

553. Stegbauer J, Oberhauser V, Vonend O, Rump LC. Angiotensin-(1-7) modulates vascular resistance and sympathetic neurotransmission in kidneys of spontaneously hypertensive rats. *Cardiovasc Res* 2004;61:352–359.

554. Steiner SH, King RD. Nutrient renal blood flow and its distribution in the unanesthetized dog. *J Surg Res* 1970;10:133–146.

555. Steinhausen M, Ballantyne D, Fretschner M, Parekh N. Sex differences in autoregulation of juxtamedullary glomerular blood flow in hydronephrotic rats. *Am J Physiol* 1990;258:F863–F869.

556. Steinhausen M, Kucherer H, Parekh N, Weis S, Wiegman DL, Wilhelm KR. Angiotensin II control of the renal microcirculation: effect of blockade by saralasin. *Kidney Int* 1986;30:56–61.

557. Stern MD, Bowen PD, Parma R, Osgood RW, Bowman RL, Stein JH. Measurement of renal cortical and medullary blood flow by laser-Doppler spectroscopy in the rat. *Am J Physiol* 1979;236:F80–F87.

558. Stockand JD, Sansom SC. Large Ca(2+)-activated K+ channels responsive to angiotensin II in cultured human mesangial cells. *Am J Physiol* 1994;267:C1080–C1086.

559. Stockand JD, Sansom SC. Activation by methylene blue of large Ca(2+)-activated K+ channels. *Biochim Biophys Acta* 1996;1285:123–126.

560. Stockand JD, Sansom SC. Role of large Ca(2+)-activated K+ channels in regulation of mesangial contraction by nitroprusside and ANP. *Am J Physiol* 1996;270:C1773–C1779.

561. Stockand JD, Sansom SC. Glomerular mesangial cells: electrophysiology and regulation of contraction. *Physiol Rev* 1998;78:723–744.

562. Stockand JD, Silverman M, Hall D, Derr T, Kubacak B, Sansom SC. Arachidonic acid potentiates the feedback response of mesangial BKCa channels to angiotensin II. *Am J Physiol* 1998;274:F658–F664.

563. Sun CW, Alonso-Galicia M, Taheri MR, Falck JR, Harder DR, Roman RJ. Nitric oxide-20-hydroxyeicosatetraenoic acid interaction in the regulation of K+ channel activity and vascular tone in renal arterioles. *Circ Res* 1998;83:1069–1079.

564. Sun CW, Falck JR, Harder DR, Roman RJ. Role of tyrosine kinase and PKC in the vasoconstrictor response to 20-HETE in renal arterioles. *Hypertension* 1999;33:414–418.

565. Sun X, Cao K, Yang G, Huang Y, Hanna ST, Wang R. Selective expression of Kir6.1 protein in different vascular and non-vascular tissues. *Biochem Pharmacol* 2004;67:147–156.

566. Szamosfalvi B, Cortes P, Alviani R, Asano K, Riser BL, Zasuwa G, Yee J. Putative subunits of the rat mesangial KATP: a type 2B sulfonylurea receptor and an inwardly rectifying K+ channel. *Kidney Int* 2002;61:1739–1749.

567. Szentivanyi M, Jr., Park F, Maeda CY, Cowley AW, Jr. Nitric oxide in the renal medulla protects from vasopressin-induced hypertension. *Hypertension* 2000;35:740–745.

568. Szentivanyi M, Jr., Zou AP, Maeda CY, Mattson DL, Cowley AW, Jr. Increase in renal medullary nitric oxide synthase activity protects from norepinephrine-induced hypertension. *Hypertension* 2000;35:418–423.

569. Szentivanyi M, Jr., Zou AP, Mattson DL, Soares P, Moreno C, Roman RJ, Cowley AW, Jr. Renal medullary nitric oxide deficit of Dahl S rats enhances hypertensive actions of angiotensin II. *Am J Physiol Regul Integr Comp Physiol* 2002;283:R266–R272.

570. Takahashi-Iwanaga H. The three-dimensional cytoarchitecture of the interstitial tissue in the rat kidney. *Cell Tissue Res* 1991;264:269–281.

571. Takenaka T, Kanno Y, Kitamura Y, Hayashi K, Suzuki H, Saruta T. Role of chloride channels in afferent arteriolar constriction. *Kidney Int* 1996;50:864–872.

572. Takenaka T, Ohno Y, Hayashi K, Saruta T, Suzuki H. Governance of arteriolar oscillation by ryanodine receptors. *Am J Physiol Regul Integr Comp Physiol* 2003;285:R125–R131.

573. Takenaka T, Suzuki H, Okada H, Inoue T, Kanno Y, Ozawa Y, Hayashi K, Saruta T. Transient receptor potential channels in rat renal microcirculation: actions of angiotensin II. *Kidney Int* 2002;62:558–565.

574. Takezawa K, Cowley AW, Jr., Skelton M, Roman RJ. Atriopeptin III alters renal medullary hemodynamics and the pressure-diuresis response in rats. *Am J Physiol* 1987;252:F992–1002.
575. Tamaki T, Kiyomoto K, He H, Tomohiro A, Nishiyama A, Aki Y, Kimura S, Abe Y. Vasodilation induced by vasopressin V2 receptor stimulation in afferent arterioles. *Kidney Int* 1996;49:722–729.
576. Tang L, Loutzenhiser K, Loutzenhiser R. Biphasic actions of prostaglandin E(2) on the renal afferent arteriole : role of EP(3) and EP(4) receptors. *Circ Res* 2000;86:663–670.
577. Tang L, Parker M, Fei Q, Loutzenhiser R. Afferent arteriolar adenosine A2a receptors are coupled to KATP in in vitro perfused hydronephrotic rat kidney. *Am J Physiol* 1999;277: F926–F933.
578. Taniyama Y, Griendling KK. Reactive oxygen species in the vasculature: molecular and cellular mechanisms. *Hypertension* 2003;42:1075–1081.
579. Terada Y, Tomita K, Nonoguchi H, Marumo F. Different localization of two types of endothelin receptor mRNA in microdissected rat nephron segments using reverse transcription and polymerase chain reaction assay. *J Clin Invest* 1992;90:107–112.
580. Thomas CJ, Woods RL, Evans RG, Alcorn D, Christy IJ, Anderson WP. Evidence for a renomedullary vasodepressor hormone. *Clin Exp Pharmacol Physiol* 1996;23:777–785.
581. Thomas SR. Cycles and separations in a model of the renal medulla. *Am J Physiol* 1998;275: F671–F690.
582. Thomson S, Bao D, Deng A, Vallon V. Adenosine formed by 5'-nucleotidase mediates tubuloglomerular feedback. *J Clin Invest* 2000;106:289–298.
583. Thorburn GD, Kopald HH, Herd JA, Hollenberg M, O'morchoe CC, Barger AC. Intrarenal distribution of nutrient blood flow determined with krypton 85 in the unanesthetized dog. *Circ Res* 1963;13:290–307.
584. Thurau K. Renal hemodynamics. *Am J Med* 1964;36:698–719.
585. Thurau K, Sugiura T, Lilienfield LS. Micropuncture of renal vasa recta in hydropenic hamsters. *Circ Res* 1960;8:383–383.
586. Traynor T, Yang T, Huang YG, Arend L, Oliverio MI, Coffman T, Briggs JP, Schnermann J. Inhibition of adenosine-1 receptor-mediated preglomerular vasoconstriction in AT1A receptor-deficient mice. *Am J Physiol* 1998;275:F922–F927.
587. Trinh-Trang-Tan MM, Lasbennes F, Gane P, Roudier N, Ripoche P, Cartron JP, Bailly P. UT-B1 proteins in rat: tissue distribution and regulation by antidiuretic hormone in kidney. *Am J Physiol Renal Physiol* 2002;283:F912–F922.
588. Tsuchiya K, Sanaka T, Nitta K, Ando A, Sugino N. Effects of atrial natriuretic peptide on regional renal blood flow measured by a thermal diffusion technique. *Jpn J Exp Med* 1989;59:27–35.
589. Tucker BJ, Blantz RC. Determinants of proximal tubular reabsorption as mechanisms of glomerulotubular balance. *Am J Physiol* 1978;235:F142–F150.
590. Turner MR, Pallone TL. Hydraulic and diffusional permeabilities of isolated outer medullary descending vasa recta from the rat. *Am J Physiol* 1997;272:H392–H400.
591. Turner MR, Pallone TL. Vasopressin constricts outer medullary descending vasa recta isolated from rat kidneys. *Am J Physiol* 1997;272:F147–F151.
592. Udosen IT, Jiang H, Hercule HC, Oyekan AO. Nitric oxide-epoxygenase interactions and arachidonate-induced dilation of rat renal microvessels. *Am J Physiol Heart Circ Physiol* 2003;285: H2054–H2063.
593. Uhrenholt TR, Jensen BL, Skott O. Rapid nongenomic effect of aldosterone on vasoconstriction. *Hypertension* 2004;43:415–419.
594. Vassileva I, Mountain C, Pollock DM. Functional role of ETB receptors in the renal medulla. *Hypertension* 2003;41:1359–1363.
595. Veldkamp PJ, Carmines PK, Inscho EW, Navar LG. Direct evaluation of the microvascular actions of ANP in juxtamedullary nephrons. *Am J Physiol* 1988;254:F440–F444.
596. Venkatachalam MA, Karnovsky MJ. Extravascular protein in the kidney. An ultrastructural study of its relation to renal peritubular capillary permeability using protein tracers. *Lab Invest* 1972;27:435–444.
597. Vesely DL. Atrial natriuretic peptides in pathophysiological diseases. *Cardiovasc Res* 2001;51:647–658.
598. Vitzthum H, Weiss B, Bachleitner W, Kramer BK, Kurtz A. Gene expression of adenosine receptors along the nephron. *Kidney Int* 2004;65:1180–1190.
599. Walkowska A, Badzynska B, Kompanowska-Jezierska E, Johns EJ, Sadowski J. Effects of renal nerve stimulation on intrarenal blood flow in rats with intact or inactivated NO synthases. *Acta Physiol Scand* 2005;183:99–105.
600. Wang D, Borrego-Conde LJ, Falck JR, Sharma KK, Wilcox CS, Umans JG. Contributions of nitric oxide, EDHF, and EETs to endothelium-dependent relaxation in renal afferent arterioles. *Kidney Int* 2003;63:2187–2193.
601. Wang D, Chabrashvili T, Wilcox CS. Enhanced contractility of renal afferent arterioles from angiotensin-infused rabbits: roles of oxidative stress, thromboxane prostanoid receptors, and endothelium. *Circ Res* 2004;94:1436–1442.
602. Wang D, Chabrashvili T, Wilcox CS. Enhanced contractility of renal afferent arterioles from angiotensin-infused rabbits: roles of oxidative stress, thromboxane prostanoid receptors, and endothelium. *Circ Res* 2004;94:1436–1442.
603. Wang T, Kawabata M, Haneda M, Takabatake T. Effects of uroguanylin, an intestinal natriuretic peptide, on tubuloglomerular feedback. *Hypertens Res* 2003;26:577–582.
604. Wang W, Michel CC. Effects of anastomoses on solute transcapillary exchange in countercurrent systems. *Microcirculation* 1997;4:381–390.
605. Wang W, Parker KH, Michel CC. Theoretical studies of steady-state transcapillary exchange in countercurrent systems. *Microcirculation* 1996;3:301–311.
606. Wang X, Pluznick JL, Wei P, Padanilam BJ, Sansom SC. TRPC4 forms store-operated Ca2+ channels in mouse mesangial cells. *Am J Physiol Cell Physiol* 2004;287:C357–C364.
607. Wang X, Trottier G, Loutzenhiser R. Determinants of renal afferent arteriolar actions of bradykinin: evidence that multiple pathways mediate responses attributed to EDHF. *Am J Physiol Renal Physiol* 2003;285:F540–F549.
608. Weihprecht H, Lorenz JN, Briggs JP, Schnermann J. Vasoconstrictor effect of angiotensin and vasopressin in isolated rabbit afferent arterioles. *Am J Physiol* 1991;261:F273–F282.
609. Weihprecht H, Lorenz JN, Briggs JP, Schnermann J. Vasomotor effects of purinergic agonists in isolated rabbit afferent arterioles. *Am J Physiol* 1992;263:F1026–F1033.
610. Weihprecht H, Lorenz JN, Briggs JP, Schnermann J. Synergistic effects of angiotensin and adenosine in the renal microvasculature. *Am J Physiol* 1994;266:F227–F239.
611. Welch WJ, Baumgartl H, Lubbers D, Wilcox CS. Renal oxygenation defects in the spontaneously hypertensive rat: role of AT1 receptors. *Kidney Int* 2003;63:202–208.
612. Welch WJ, Blau J, Xie H, Chabrashvili T, Wilcox CS. Angiotensin-induced defects in renal oxygenation: role of oxidative stress. *Am J Physiol Heart Circ Physiol* 2005;288: H22–H28.
613. White SM, Imig JD, Kim TT, Hauschild BC, Inscho EW. Calcium signaling pathways utilized by P2X receptors in freshly isolated preglomerular MVSMC. *Am J Physiol Renal Physiol* 2001;280:F1054–F1061.
614. Wilcox CS, Welch WJ, Snellen H. Thromboxane mediates renal hemodynamic response to infused angiotensin II. *Kidney Int* 1991;40:1090–1097.
615. Wilde WS, Vorburger C. Albumin multiplier in kidney vasa recta analyzed by microspectrophotometry of T-1824. *Am J Physiol* 1967;213:1233–1243.
616. Wolgast M. Studies on the regional renal blood flow with p32-labelled red cells and small beta-sensitive semiconductor detectors. *Acta Physiol Scand Suppl* 1968;313:1–109.
617. Wolgast M, Larson M, Nygren K. Functional characteristics of the renal interstitium. *Am J Physiol* 1981;241:F105–F111.
618. Wu F, Cholewa B, Mattson DL. Characterization of L-arginine transporters in rat renal inner medullary collecting duct. *Am J Physiol Regul Integr Comp Physiol* 2000;278:R1506–R1512.
619. Xu Y, Olives B, Bailly P, Fischer E, Ripoche P, Ronco P, Cartron JP, Rondeau E. Endothelial cells of the kidney vasa recta express the urea transporter HUT11. *Kidney Int* 1997;51: 138–146.
620. Yamamoto T, Tada T, Brodsky SV, Tanaka H, Noiri E, Kajiya F, Goligorsky MS. Intravital videomicroscopy of peritubular capillaries in renal ischemia. *Am J Physiol Renal Physiol* 2002;282:F1150–F1155.
621. Yang B, Bankir L. Urea and urine concentrating ability: new insights from studies in mice. *Am J Physiol Renal Physiol* 2005;288:F881–F896.
622. Yang B, Bankir L, Gillespie A, Epstein CJ, Verkman AS. Urea-selective concentrating defect in transgenic mice lacking urea transporter UT-B. *J Biol Chem* 2002;277:10633–10637.
623. Yang B, Verkman AS. Urea transporter UT3 functions as an efficient water channel. Direct evidence for a common water/urea pathway. *J Biol Chem* 1998;273:9369–9372.
624. Yang S, Silldorff EP, Pallone TL. Effect of norepinephrine and acetylcholine on outer medullary descending vasa recta. *Am J Physiol* 1995;269:H710–H716.
625. Yang T. Regulation of cyclooxygenase-2 in renal medulla. *Acta Physiol Scand* 2003;177: 417–421.
626. Yarger WE, Boyd MA, Schrader NW. Evaluation of methods of measuring glomerular and nutrient blood flow in rat kidneys. *Am J Physiol* 1978;235:H592–H600.
627. Yu Z, Huse LM, Adler P, Graham L, Ma J, Zeldin DC, Kroetz DL. Increased CYP2J expression and epoxyeicosatrienoic acid formation in spontaneously hypertensive rat kidney. *Mol Pharmacol* 2000;57:1011–1020.
628. Yu Z, Xu F, Huse LM, Morisseau C, Draper AJ, Newman JW, Parker C, Graham L, Engler MM, Hammock BD, Zeldin DC, Kroetz DL. Soluble epoxide hydrolase regulates hydrolysis of vasoactive epoxyeicosatrienoic acids. *Circ Res* 2000;87:992–998.
629. Yuan B, Cowley AW, Jr. Evidence that reduced renal medullary nitric oxide synthase activity of dahl s rats enables small elevations of arginine vasopressin to produce sustained hypertension. *Hypertension* 2001;37:524–528.
630. Yuan BH, Robinette JB, Conger JD. Effect of angiotensin II and norepinephrine on isolated rat afferent and efferent arterioles. *Am J Physiol* 1990;258:F741–F750.
631. Zewde T, Mattson DL. Inhibition of cyclooxygenase-2 in the rat renal medulla leads to sodium-sensitive hypertension. *Hypertension* 2004;44:424–428.
632. Zewde T, Wu F, Mattson DL. Influence of dietary NaCl on L-arginine transport in the renal medulla. *Am J Physiol Regul Integr Comp Physiol* 2004;286:R89–R93.
633. Zhang MZ, Sanchez LP, McKanna JA, Harris RC. Regulation of cyclooxygenase expression by vasopressin in rat renal medulla. *Endocrinology* 2004;145:1402–1409.
634. Zhang Z, Huang JM, Turner MR, Rhinehart KL, Pallone TL. Role of chloride in constriction of descending vasa recta by angiotensin II. *Am J Physiol Regul Integr Comp Physiol* 2001;280:R1878–R1886.
635. Zhang Z, Pallone TL. Response of descending vasa recta to luminal pressure. *Am J Physiol Renal Physiol* 2004;287:F535–F542.
636. Zhang Z, Rhinehart K, Kwon W, Weinman E, Pallone TL. ANG II signaling in vasa recta pericytes by PKC and reactive oxygen species. *Am J Physiol Heart Circ Physiol* 2004;287: H773–H781.
637. Zhang Z, Rhinehart K, Pallone TL. Membrane potential controls calcium entry into descending vasa recta pericytes. *Am J Physiol Regul Integr Comp Physiol* 2002;283: R949–R957.
638. Zhang Z, Rhinehart K, Solis G, Pittner J, Lee-Kwon W, Welch WJ, Wilcox CS, Pallone TL. Chronic ANG II infusion increases NO generation by rat descending vasa recta. *Am J Physiol Heart Circ Physiol* 2005;288:H29–H36.
639. Zhao X, Falck JR, Gopal VR, Inscho EW, Imig JD. P2X receptor-stimulated calcium responses in preglomerular vascular smooth muscle cells involves 20-hydroxyeicosatetraenoic acid. *J Pharmacol Exp Ther* 2004;311:1211–1217.
640. Zhao X, Inscho EW, Bondlela M, Falck JR, Imig JD. The CYP450 hydroxylase pathway contributes to P2X receptor-mediated afferent arteriolar vasoconstriction. *Am J Physiol Heart Circ Physiol* 2001;281:H2089–H2096.
641. Zhao X, Pollock DM, Inscho EW, Zeldin DC, Imig JD. Decreased renal cytochrome P450 2C enzymes and impaired vasodilation are associated with angiotensin salt-sensitive hypertension. *Hypertension* 2003;41:709–714.
642. Zhao X, Yamamoto T, Newman JW, Kim IH, Watanabe T, Hammock BD, Stewart J, Pollock JS, Pollock DM, Imig JD. Soluble epoxide hydrolase inhibition protects the kidney from hypertension-induced damage. *J Am Soc Nephrol* 2004;15:1244–1253.

643. Zhuo J, Dean R, Maric C, Aldred PG, Harris P, Alcorn D, Mendelsohn FA. Localization and interactions of vasoactive peptide receptors in renomedullary interstitial cells of the kidney. *Kidney Int Suppl* 1998;67:S22–S28.

644. Zhuo JL. Renomedullary interstitial cells: a target for endocrine and paracrine actions of vasoactive peptides in the renal medulla. *Clin Exp Pharmacol Physiol* 2000;27:465–473.

645. Zimmerhackl B, Dussel R, Steinhausen M. Erythrocyte flow and dynamic hematocrit in the renal papilla of the rat. *Am J Physiol* 1985;249:F898–F902.

646. Zimmerhackl B, Robertson CR, Jamison RL. Effect of arginine vasopressin on renal medullary blood flow. A videomicroscopic study in the rat. *J Clin Invest* 1985;76:770–778.

647. Zimmerhackl B, Robertson CR, Jamison RL. Fluid uptake in the renal papilla by vasa recta estimated by two methods simultaneously. *Am J Physiol* 1985;248:F347–F353.

648. Zimmerhackl B, Tinsman J, Jamison RL, Robertson CR. Use of digital cross-correlation for on-line determination of single-vessel blood flow in the mammalian kidney. *Microvasc Res* 1985;30:63–74.

649. Zou AP, Cowley AW, Jr. Nitric oxide in renal cortex and medulla. An in vivo microdialysis study. *Hypertension* 1997;29:194–198.

650. Zou AP, Cowley AW, Jr. alpha(2)-adrenergic receptor-mediated increase in NO production buffers renal medullary vasoconstriction. *Am J Physiol Regul Integr Comp Physiol* 2000;279:R769–R777.

651. Zou AP, Cowley AW, Jr. Reactive oxygen species and molecular regulation of renal oxygenation. *Acta Physiol Scand* 2003;179:233–241.

652. Zou AP, Fleming JT, Falck JR, Jacobs ER, Gebremedhin D, Harder DR, Roman RJ. 20-HETE is an endogenous inhibitor of the large-conductance Ca(2+)-activated K+ channel in renal arterioles. *Am J Physiol* 1996;270:R228–R237.

653. Zou AP, Fleming JT, Falck JR, Jacobs ER, Gebremedhin D, Harder DR, Roman RJ. Stereospecific effects of epoxyeicosatrienoic acids on renal vascular tone and K(+)-channel activity. *Am J Physiol* 1996;270:F822–F832.

654. Zou AP, Imig JD, Kaldunski M, Ortiz de Montellano PR, Sui Z, Roman RJ. Inhibition of renal vascular 20-HETE production impairs autoregulation of renal blood flow. *Am J Physiol* 1994;266:F275–F282.

655. Zou AP, Li N, Cowley AW, Jr. Production and actions of superoxide in the renal medulla. *Hypertension* 2001;37:547–553.

656. Zou AP, Wu F, Cowley AW, Jr. Protective effect of angiotensin II-induced increase in nitric oxide in the renal medullary circulation. *Hypertension* 1998;31:271–276.

657. Zou AP, Wu F, Li PL, Cowley AW, Jr. Effect of chronic salt loading on adenosine metabolism and receptor expression in renal cortex and medulla in rats. *Hypertension* 1999;33:511–516.

658. Zusman RM, Keiser HR. Prostaglandin biosynthesis by rabbit renomedullary interstitial cells in tissue culture. Stimulation by angiotensin II, bradykinin, and arginine vasopressin. *J Clin Invest* 1977;60:215–223.

Renal Differentiation and Growth

CHAPTER **24**

Molecular and Cellular Mechanisms of Kidney Development

Hiroyuki Sakurai and Sanjay K. Nigam
University of California, San Diego, La Jolla, California, USA

OVERVIEW

In the course of its development, the mammalian kidney goes through three distinct forms: the pronephros, the mesonephros, and the metanephros, ultimately leading to the formation of the mature kidney (Fig. 1). At day 22 of gestation in humans, or at day 8 in mice, an epithelial streak called the pronephric duct arises in the cervical region of the developing embryo. The pronephric duct then extends caudally to form the nephric duct or Wolffian duct. The most primitive kidney, the pronephros, is formed as the pronephric duct induces surrounding mesenchyme to form the pronephric tubules. The pronephros is functional only in fish and amphibians; it is thought to be rudimentary and nonfunctional in higher vertebrates.

Next, a more complex "protokidney," the mesonephros, arises just caudal to the pronephros at day 24 in humans or day 9.5 in mice. As with the pronephros, mesonephric development starts with induction of the surrounding mesenchyme by the Wolffian duct. Unlike the pronephros, however, the mesonephros glomeruli are linked to the Wolffian duct via mesonephric tubules. In humans, about 30 nephrons are observed in the mesonephros; their function is unclear. The mesonephric duct and some tubules persist and are ultimately integrated into the male genital system. In females, the mesonephros degenerates and disappears.

The permanent kidney of amniotes, the metanephros, starts to form at day 28 in humans or day 11 in mice. Unlike the pronephros and mesonephros, which are induced by the Wolffian duct, metanephric tubules are induced by an epithelial structure derived from the Wolffian duct: the ureteric bud. As the ureteric bud invades the surrounding mesen-

chyme, it induces the mesenchymal cells to form metanephric tubules that eventually differentiate into the proximal through distal portions of the nephron. The ureteric bud, reciprocally induced by the metanephric mesenchyme, undergoes branching morphogenesis, eventually giving rise to the collecting system. Morphologically, nephron formation is completed by birth in humans, although only after birth does the nephron become fully functional (154).

DEVELOPMENT OF THE METANEPHROS

Here, the development of the metanephros is described in more detail (Fig. 2), since it becomes the final kidney in mammals. As discussed in the previous section, the ureteric bud, the inducer of metanephric development, is formed from the Wolffian duct. This structure invades the metanephric mesenchyme, whereupon mesenchymal cells condense at the tip of the ureteric bud. The condensed mesenchymal cells then differentiate into epithelial cells: the so-called mesenchymal-epithelial transformation. The newly formed epithelial cells gradually develop into distinct structures called "comma-shaped bodies," which subsequently become "S-shaped bodies." The S-shaped bodies, which begin to exhibit tubular morphology, continue to elongate; the end closest to the ureteric bud connects to it, while the opposite end forms podocytes and Bowman's capsule. The middle part ultimately differentiates into the proximal through distal tubules of the nephron. At the same time, the tips of the ureteric bud, induced by the metanephric mesenchyme, continue to branch to ultimately form the collecting ducts, renal pelvis, calyces, and papillae.

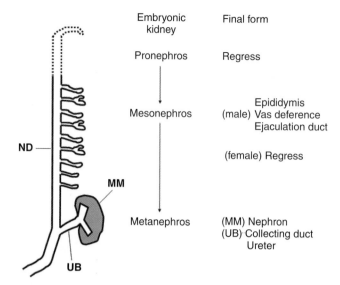

FIGURE 1 Schematic drawings of mammalian kidney development. The pronephros appears at a relatively higher position in the embryo. Then the mesonephros forms caudally around the nephric duct (ND) or Wolffian duct. In the male, the mesonephric tubules become a part of the genital system. The permanent kidney, the metanephros, forms caudally to the mesonephros. The ureteric bud (UB) derives from the Wolffian duct, ultimately becoming the collecting system. The metanephric mesenchyme, induced by the ureteric bud, forms nephron tubules and glomeruli.

The process of collecting system development has been studied in detail by microdissection of the human kidney (116, 117). Initial ureteric bud branching is dichotomous and symmetric; the ureteric bud takes on a T shape in this early stage of metanephrogenesis. Subsequently, the ureteric bud elongates, and eventually branches again dichotomously. At later branching events, the angle between

branches lessens and branching may not be completely symmetrical so that somehow ureteric tree structure "fits" into the final shape of the kidney. The initial branches become dilated to form the renal pelvis, while terminal branches become collecting ducts. As the ureteric bud undergoes branching morphogenesis, its tips continue to induce more nephrons from the metanephric mesenchyme.

Vascular development occurs along with nephron development. Dissection of the developing kidney reveals that large vessels branch off from the dorsal aorta invading into the kidneys (118). As will be discussed later, the extent to which the microvasculature of the kidney derives from the metanephric mesenchyme versus derived from outside the kidney is still unclear. The origin of the mesangial cells, which are in close association with the endothelial cells in the glomerulus, is also uncertain.

Thus, the key event in metanephric epithelial tissue development is mutual induction between the ureteric bud and the metanephric mesenchyme. This leads to branching morphogenesis of the ureteric bud together with epithelialization and tubulogenesis of the metanephric mesenchyme (Fig. 3). To better understand the mechanisms underlying induction, it is necessary to identify and analyze the key molecules that mediate signals between the metanephric mesenchyme and the ureteric bud.

EXPERIMENTAL APPROACHES TO KIDNEY DEVELOPMENT

Over the years, a variety of experimental approaches have been used for evaluation of the mechanistic details of the induction process between the ureteric bud and meta-

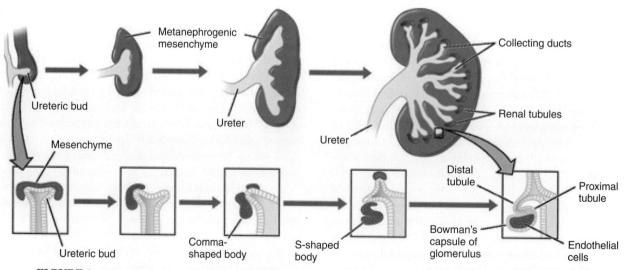

FIGURE 2 Schematic drawings of metanephros development. Top panel shows macroscopic view of kidney collecting system development through ureteric bud branching morphogenesis. Bottom panel shows nephron development from metanephric mesenchyme. (Adapted from Sampogna RV, Nigam SK. Implications of gene networks for understanding resilience and vulnerability in the kidney branching program. *Physiology (Bethesda)* 2004;19:339–347, with permission.)

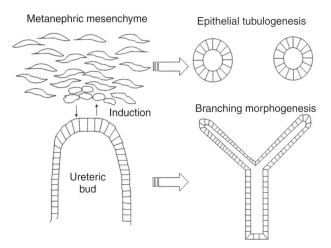

FIGURE 3 Schematic drawings of mutual induction. The metanephric mesenchyme cells become epithelial nephron tubules (induced by the ureteric bud), while the ureteric bud undergoes branching morphogenesis to form the collecting system (induced by the metanephric mesenchyme).

nephric mesenchyme. For example, the developing kidney has been found to be amenable to extensive in vitro analysis. In addition to this "whole embryonic kidney organ culture," it has been demonstrated that progenitor tissues (i.e., Wolffian duct, ureteric bud, and metanephric mesenchyme) can be isolated and cultured individually. Advances in genetic manipulation have allowed the analysis of kidney development in vivo in genetically engineered mice. As in vitro culture techniques and in vivo genetic manipulation become increasingly sophisticated, it is becoming clear that these approaches should be viewed as complementary.

Organ Culture

WHOLE EMBRYONIC KIDNEY ORGAN CULTURE

The transfilter culture system, used by Grobstein and coworkers in the 1950s (49–51) has been the mainstay of in vitro organ culture work in the developing kidney. In this system, microdissected kidneys, from as early as the beginning of metanephrogenesis (gestational day 11.5 in mice or day 13.5 in rats), are cultured on top of filters for several days. In the presence of appropriate defined serum-free medium, kidney rudiments grow and differentiate (41). It is possible to observe branching morphogenesis of the ureteric bud, induction of the metanephric mesenchyme, and formation of nephrons by microscopy as the cultured embryonic kidneys develop (Fig. 4A). Only vascular development does not occur to an appreciable extent. Thus, not only does the whole embryonic kidney culture resemble in vivo developmental processes but it also appears to retain the inherent spatiotemporal complexity.

In this whole embryonic kidney culture, it is possible to manipulate humoral factors that play a role in nephrogenesis. The effects of growth factors or their inhibitors on kidney development can be evaluated in vitro by analysis of total kidney size, ureteric bud branching events, and metanephric mesenchyme tubulogenesis. For example, ureteric bud branching can be assayed by staining with a fluorescently labeled lectin from *Dolichos biflorus*, which has been shown to bind specifically to the cells derived from the ureteric bud (74) (Fig. 4B). However, the organ culture method is not without its limitations. For example, when antibodies and antisense oligonucleotides are used to perturb in vitro nephrogenesis, care must be taken to ensure that the agent is delivered to the sites of interest, since antisense

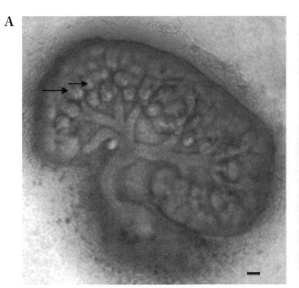

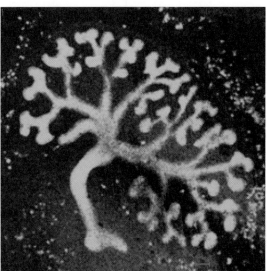

FIGURE 4   **A:** A rat embryonic kidney isolated at embryonic day 13 and cultured for 3 days on Transwell filter. Ureteric bud branch and epithelial nephron formation (*arrows*) are visible. **B:** The same specimen was stained with fluorescent-labeled lectin from *Dolichos biflorus* to visualize ureteric bud-derived structures. Bars, = 100 μm. See color insert.

oligonucleotides do not seem to penetrate the ureteric bud as well as the metanephric mesenchyme (37). In addition, oligonucleotide toxicity may, in some instances, nonspecifically inhibit kidney growth (37). However, recent development of RNAi technology to perturb specific gene function may prove useful in this setting (27, 141).

WOLFFIAN DUCT CULTURE

It is possible to culture the entire mesonephros-metanephros area on top of transfilters. Addition of humoral factors can induce outgrowth of ureteric bud–like structures from the Wolffian duct (12, 167). This system may prove useful in the elucidation of the mechanism of ureteric bud budding (91a).

ISOLATED URETERIC BUD CULTURE

Since the 1950s, in vitro culture of the two individual components of metanephros, the ureteric bud and the metanephric mesenchyme, has been attempted. Of the two progenitor tissues, in vitro growth of the isolated ureteric bud proved to be more difficult, and it was argued that cell–cell contact between the ureteric bud and metanephric mesenchyme was an important component in the process of ureteric bud branching. However, the isolated ureteric bud has since been shown to grow and branch extensively in the presence of appropriate extracellular matrix and soluble factors in the absence of direct contact with the metanephric mesenchyme (Fig. 5) (129). The epithelial cells of the ureteric bud in this culture system appear to retain similar morphological characteristics to those of the ureteric bud in the whole embryonic kidney culture (100). This system has allowed for the isolation and identification of soluble factors that modulate ureteric bud branching morphogenesis (14, 128, 143).

ISOLATED METANEPHRIC MESENCHYME CULTURE AND HETEROLOGOUS RECOMBINATION OF METANEPHRIC MESENCHMYE AND INDUCTIVE TISSUES

Another setting in which organ culture has been used focuses on metanephric mesenchyme induction and transformation to an epithelial phenotype. In this system, the isolated mesenchyme is cultured on one side of a filter, while, on the other side of the filter, heterologous inducing tissues are placed. Various stages of metanephric mesenchyme induction (i.e., condensation, epithelialization, and tubulogenesis) can be observed depending on the inductive capacity of the tissue. Using this method, it has been shown that embryonic spinal cord, salivary gland, and other tissues can induce the metanephric mesenchyme (52, 155). As is the case for isolated ureteric bud branching described previously, a key question here is the relative contribution of humoral factor(s) or cell–cell contact in this process. Electron microscopic examination revealed that the inducing tissue can contact the metanephric mesenchyme via cellular processes extending through the filter (77). In fact, filters with pore sizes greater than 0.1 μm are unable to block cell-to-cell contact completely (154), favoring the importance of cell–cell contact. However, complete mesenchymal induction has been demonstrated in the presence of soluble factors without cell–cell contact with inductive tissue (6, 121).

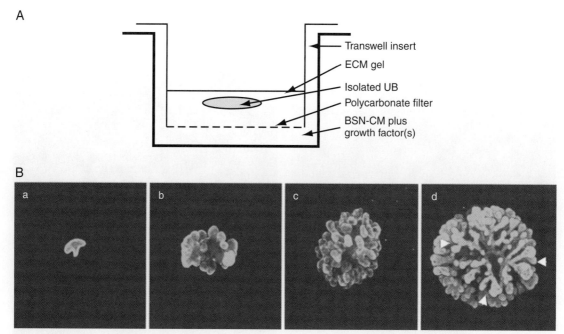

FIGURE 5   A: Schematic drawing of isolated ureteric bud culture system. **B:** Cultured ureteric buds were stained with fluorescein-conjugated lectin from Dolichos biflorus at (a) 0 day (freshly isolated ureteric bud), (b) 3 days, (c) 6 days, and (d) 12 days. Arrows indicate branch points. (Adapted from Qiao J, Sakurai H, Nigam SK. Branching morphogenesis independent of mesenchymal-epithelial contact in the developing kidney. *Proc Natl Acad Sci U S A* 1999;96:7330–7335.). See color insert.

ISOLATED URETERIC BUD AND METANEPHRIC MESENCHYME RECOMBINATION CULTURE

It has been shown that when cocultured with freshly isolated metanephric mesenchyme, the isolated ureteric bud in culture (as described previously) is capable of inducing nephron tubules from the metanephric mesenchyme (129). At the same time, the pattern of ureteric bud growth is altered by the presence of the metanephric mesenchyme; the ureteric bud tubules become slender as they elongate into the metanephric mesenchyme. This "mesenchyme effect" may be mediated by cell–cell contact.

Another potential application of this "recombination" system is to pinpoint the defective tissue in knockout mice with a kidney phenotype. Through recombination of wild-type and gene knockout tissues (e.g., wild-type ureteric bud with knockout metanephric mesenchyme), it may be possible to determine the source of the kidney defect.

The aforementioned tissue culture systems allow one to observe certain key phenomenon in metanephric kidney development in vitro. The analysis of genetically engineered kidneys (and/or their component tissues) in these in vitro systems in combination with an advanced method of gene perturbation (e.g., RNAi) will undoubtedly provide a more mechanistic picture of kidney development.

Genetically Engineered Mice

Genetically engineered mice allow one to manipulate the process of kidney development in vivo. Introducing null mutations of the gene of interest into mouse embryonic stem cells can be used to generate gene knockout mice (17, 18, 45). Generally speaking, knockout mice grow from conception without normal expression of the gene product. If the mice develop beyond the stage of kidney development, the effect of the gene disruption on nephrogenesis can be observed in vivo by direct examination of the tissue histology. In such cases, the abnormal kidney phenotype can be directly or indirectly ascribed to disruption of the gene. In fact, many important molecules involved in kidney development have been identified by gene knockout technology (75, 187). In particular, the contribution of many transcription factors, molecules acting in the nucleus to regulate gene expression in the cell, has been demonstrated by this technique. However, knockout technology has its limitations. For example, although gene knockout mice can demonstrate the indispensability of a particular gene, how the gene product acts in the complex process of kidney development often remains unclear owing to the spatiotemporal complexity of the developing organ. Thus, if one observes defective ureteric bud branching in knockout mice, the deleted/disrupted gene product could be affecting the ureteric bud directly or it could be affecting the metanephric mesenchyme, resulting in incompetent induction of the ureteric bud. To resolve this problem, some have used organ culture type approaches ("recombination") (103). Another limitation of gene knockouts is that the mice may not have an apparent phenotype due to redundancy. In other words, the expression of other molecules with features or functions that overlap with the targeted gene could compensate for the defect from the gene knockout. In other cases, the function of the targeted gene is critical for early embryonic survival, rendering the analysis of kidney development impossible as the embryo dies before organogenesis. Some of these issues may be overcome by the gene disruption in a time and organ specific manner. This conditional gene targeting is performed by crossing two transgenic mouse lines: "floxed" mice that carry loxP sites franking the gene of interest and Cre-recombinase transgenic mice under the control of a tissue-specific promoter (46).

Cell Culture

Cell culture models have the advantage of simplicity. Since they use homogenous cell populations grown under controlled conditions, it is possible to perform biochemical analysis in great detail. Moreover, gene introduction by plasmid transfection and gene knockdown by RNAi is simpler in comparison to the organ culture system. Here, the most relevant system for branching morphogenesis of the ureteric bud, the three-dimensional cell culture system, is discussed.

When certain kidney-derived epithelial cells are suspended in an extracellular matrix gel (type I collagen or a collagen–Matrigel mixture) in the presence of morphogenetic humoral factors, they form tubules and undergo branching morphogenesis in vitro. The tubules in the three-dimensional culture have lumens and retain apical-basolateral polarity (149). The effect of humoral factors in epithelial tube and/or branch formation can be studied here. In addition to the humoral factors, the effect of extracellular matrix composition on morphogenesis and the cellular details of morphogenesis can be examined in this system. MDCK cells and murine inner medullary collecting duct (mIMCD3) cells have been used in the past (7, 16, 144, 145), but these have the limitation of being derived from mature renal epithelial cells. To address this issue, an in vitro cell culture system using ureteric bud (UB) cells directly derived from embryonic day (E) 11.5 mouse ureteric bud has also been established (142). Although there is some difference in the responsiveness of the different cell lines to growth factors, all three cell lines respond to soluble factors produced by the metanephric mesenchyme by forming branching tubules.

A detailed mechanism of hepatocyte growth factor (HGF)–induced MDCK cell tubulogenesis model has been described (188). There appear to be two steps involved in this process of invasion: epithelial–mesenchymal transition and the reestablishment of epithelial intercellular junctions. However, it has also been shown that ureteric buds in in vitro culture undergo branching morphogenesis through budding, a process in which epithelial cells never lose their junctions (100). It remains to be seen where and when these two morphogenetic processes, branching through invasion ("invadopodic") and branching through budding, are utilized in vivo (165).

MOLECULAR MECHANISMS OF KIDNEY DEVELOPMENT

Development of high-density DNA microarray technology allows one to analyze changes in gene expression profiles during kidney development (166). In this study, mRNA encoding transcription factors and growth factors were found to be upregulated early in organogenesis (group 1). Among the genes whose expression level peaked in the middle of kidney organogenesis (group 2), many extracellular matrix related genes were found (Fig. 6). As described in the following section, some of these molecules have been shown to be involved in kidney development. Ultimately, high-throughput gene profiling may provide mechanistic insight into this very complex system. This may enable the development of a systems perspective on nephrogenesis. Attempts at creation of "coarse granuled" models of kidney development has clearly begun (14, 104a, 111a, 146).

TRANSCRIPTION FACTORS IN METANEPHROGENESIS

Transcription factors bind to DNA and regulate the expression of other genes that are involved in, among other things, morphogenesis and differentiation. As a result of many gene disruption studies, several important transcrip-

tion factors in kidney development have been demonstrated. With careful molecular marker analysis, it will soon be possible to draw a whole network of these molecules in this process.

Glial Cell Line–Derived Neurotrophic Growth Factor Regulating Transcription Factors

As will be described later, a key molecule in the process of the initial stage of metanephros development, ureteric bud formation from the Wolffian duct, is glial cell line–derived neurotrophic growth factor (GDNF). Many transcription factors regulating expression of this growth factor affect ureteric bud development.

Hox GENES

Hox genes, mammalian homologues of *Drosophilia* homeotic genes, have been shown to be critically important for early nephrogenesis. While null mutants for *Hoxa11* or *Hoxd11* mice do not have a kidney phenotype, double knockouts of *Hoxa11* and *Hoxd11* show kidney agenesis or hypogenesis (29). Moreover, complete elimination of *Hox11* paralogs (*Hoxa11, Hoxc11,* and *Hoxd11*) results in a lack of ureteric bud outgrowth from the Wolffian duct (177). In this mutant, expression of another transcription factor, *Six2* as well as *Gdnf* is lacking, suggesting that *Hox11* paralogs regulate *Gdnf* expression.

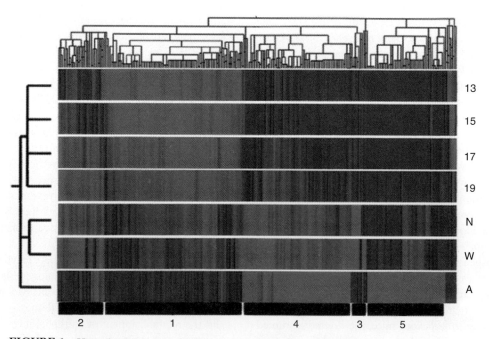

FIGURE 6 Hierarchical clustering of 873 genes identified as changing significantly at some point in kidney development (out of 8740 genes examined). Numbers at the bottom indicate group numbers derived from k-means clustering. Group 1 genes are upregulated (red) in the early embryonic period and decrease thereafter. Group 2 genes rise to a mid-late embryonic peak. Group 3 genes peak in the neonatal period. Group 4 genes rise somewhat linearly throughout development. Group 5 genes display a distinct peak in the adult versus all earlier times. 13, 15, 17, 19, embryonic days; N, newborn; W, 1 week old; A, adult. (From Stuart RO, Bush KT, Nigam SK. Changes in global gene expression patterns during development and maturation of the rat kidney. *Proc Natl Acad Sci U S A* 2001;98:5649–5654.) See color insert.

PAX GENES

Additional members of the homeotic gene family, the *Pax* genes, have been implicated in nephrogenesis. Compared with *Hox* genes, *Pax* genes appear to be restricted to certain tissues or organs. *Pax2* and *Pax8* have been shown to be expressed in the kidney. These *Pax* genes can be considered as early nephric lineage specification genes as it is first expressed in pronephric duct and their simultaneous disruption causes failure in the formation of the epithelial pronephric duct from the intermediate mesoderm (11). After the pronephric duct, *Pax2* expression is sequentially found in its extension, the Wolffian duct, the ureteric bud, as well as the condensed metanephric mesenchyme and the newly formed nephron tubules. As the kidney tubules mature, *Pax2* expression decreases (31, 32). The expression pattern suggests a role for *Pax2* in mesenchymal–epithelial transformation. Homozygous null mutant mice lacking *Pax2* show only a partially developed Wolffian duct, leading to kidney agenesis (169). It has also been shown that the mutant Wolffian duct does not respond to GDNF to form the ureteric bud. Furthermore, the mutant metanephric mesenchyme not only lacks *Gdnf* expression, it is not competent to form nephron tubules in response to wild-type spinal cord (12). Heterozygous *Pax2* mutant mice have hypoplastic kidneys (169). In fact, there are PAX2 binding sites in the promoter region of *Gdnf*, and PAX2 can promote *Gdnf* expression in vitro (12).

Pax8 has a similar tissue expression pattern to *Pax2*; however, *Pax8* expression peaks later than *Pax2* (120). Although kidney development is apparently normal in *Pax8* knockout mice (94), double knockouts of *Pax2* and *Pax8* show a complete absence of urogenital system due to failure in the formation of the pronephric duct from the intermediate mesoderm (11), suggesting some overlap in the roles of these two *Pax* genes in pronephric duct induction.

EYA1, SIX1, AND SIX2 GENES

These genes have been implicated in *Drosophila* eye development together with *Pax6* (175) and are expressed in the metanephric mesenchyme in the kidney. Homozygous null mutants for *Eya1* show kidney agenesis with loss of *Gdnf* and *Six* expression (183), suggesting that EYA1 acts upstream of SIX and together, they regulate *Gdnf* expression. In fact, EYA1 is shown to act as a co-activator (183) of the genes regulated by SIX (83). In *Six1* knockouts, which show various kidney phenotypes ranging from hypogenesis to agenesis, *Gdnf* expression is reduced but *Eya1* expression is preserved (83, 184). Interestingly, metanephric mesenchyme derived from *Six1* knockout mice is not competent in nephron tubule formation when it is cultured with spinal cord, a potent inducer of nephron tubulogenesis, suggesting that these factors not only control *Gdnf* expression but also have a role in maintaining certain characteristics of metanephric mesenchyme (184). As described previously, another member of the *Six* family, *Six2* appears to regulate *Gdnf* expression downstream of *Hox11* paralogs (177). Although *Six1* and *Six2* show overlapping areas of expression, the fact that *Six2* expression is reduced in

Six1 knockouts (83, 184) suggests a close relationship between these 2 molecules.

SALL1 GENE

Sall1 is a transcription related protein expressed in the metanephric mesenchyme of the developing kidney (112). It is also expressed in extrarenal tissues such as the limb buds and central nervous systems. Knockout of this gene results in failure of the ureteric bud to invade the metanephric mesenchyme. Although *Gdnf* expression just before ureteric bud formation is reported to be normal, its expression in the metanephric mesenchyme subsequently decreases (112). It is unclear whether this reduction of *Gdnf* expression is due to a direct effect of the *Sall1* mutation or if it is secondary to a loss of a ureteric bud derived signal. *Sall1* null metanephric mesenchyme is still able to respond to spinal cord to form nephron tubules.

FOXC1 GENE

Although some of the aforementioned genes affect a number of other genes, they all normally stimulate *Gdnf* expression. However, it is also important to restrict the area of *Gdnf* expression to avoid multiple kidneys arising from a single Wolffian duct. In this regard, a member of the forkhead transcription factor superfamily, *Foxc1*, appears to restrict *Gdnf* expression to the intermediate mesoderm around the Wolffian duct (i.e., metanephric mesenchyme). *Foxc1* homozygous null mutants display ectopic ureteric bud outgrowth resulting in duplex kidneys (73). In this mutant, the restrictive expression pattern of *Gdnf* as well as *Eya1* is perturbed and is abnormally extended along the Wolffian duct.

Other Transcription Factors Regulating Ureteric Bud Formation (or Early Kidney Development)

LIM1 GENE

Lim1 is a homeotic gene expressed in both the central nervous system and kidneys. By whole-mount in situ hybridization, its transcript is detected from the pronephric stage to the metanephros (44). In the metanephros, its expression is detected in the renal vesicles, S-shaped bodies, and ureteric bud branches (44). Knockout of *Lim1* leads to kidney agenesis, suggesting its distinct role in early nephrogenesis (161). Since *Pax2* expression in the mesonephros is detected in *Lim1* knockouts (170), and the ectopic expression of *Pax2* was found to induce *Lim1* in the intermediate mesoderm (11), it is likely that *Lim1* acts downstream of *Pax2* in pronephros development. However, the exact role of *Lim1* in metanephrogenesis remains to be determined.

WT1 GENE

One of the Wilms tumor suppressor genes, *Wt1*, a zinc-finger transcription factor, is required for kidney development. *Wt1* generally acts as a transcriptional repressor and has been shown to repress *Igf2* (33), *Igf1* receptor (178), *Pax2* (139), *Myc* (55), and *Bcl2* (55) expression. Most of these genes are related to cell proliferation, supporting the notion that loss of *Wt1*-mediated repression could lead to disregulated proliferation (i.e., cancer). It seems paradoxical that the *Wt1* knockout suffers from kidney agenesis, not tumors (72). In the homozygous deletion mutant of *Wt1*, the ureteric bud fails to form despite relatively normal development of the mesonephros and in the presence of *Gdnf* expression (30), suggesting that factor(s) other than GDNF might be required for the ureteric bud initiation. In normal embryonic kidneys, *Wt1* is expressed in uninduced mesenchyme, renal vesicles, and glomerular podocytes (110). *Wt1* mutant mesenchyme is not responsive to the inductive signal from wild-type spinal cord, while the mutant Wolffian duct can induce wild-type metanephric mesenchyme, suggesting that the primary defect is in the mesenchyme (30).

LIMB DEFORMITY GENE/*FMN1*

Kidney agenesis is observed in mice homozygous for the *limb deformity (ld)* gene, *Fmn1*, mutation. The initial outgrowth of the ureteric bud is not observed in mutant mice. The metanephric mesenchyme from *Fmn1* mutant mice is induced by embryonic spinal cord, suggesting that the defect is in the ureteric bud (91). The *Fmn* gene encodes formin, a gene product, which is present in both the ureteric bud and the metanephric mesenchyme (20, 95). While knockouts of certain formin isoforms display limb deformity and kidney defects, specific elimination of isoform 4 results in a pure kidney phenotype (182).

MYC GENES

The *Myc* family members were first recognized as proto-oncogenes that function as transcription factors. While *Myc* is expressed in the uninduced metanephric mesenchyme and newly formed epithelium, *Nmyc1* is transiently expressed in the area of mesenchymal-epithelial transformation (108). Another *Myc* family member, *Lmyc1*, is expressed in ureteric bud derived structures and its expression increases as these structures mature (108). Both *Myc* and *Nmyc1* gene knockouts are lethal at E9.5–10.5 and E10.5–12.5, respectively (21, 28, 163). *Myc* mutants apparently have no specific kidney phenotype. In *Nmyc1* mutants, mesonephric development is affected. In both cases, mice die before metanephric development, which therefore cannot be assessed. The distinct pattern of expression of the various *Myc* genes makes them useful as markers: Mesenchymal stromal cells are negative for *Myc*; *Nmyc1* is a marker for induced mesenchyme or early mesenchymal epithelialization; *Lmyc1* is a marker for the collecting duct.

Transcription Factors Regulating Ureteric Bud Survival/Branching

EMX2 GENE

Disruption of a homeotic gene, *Emx2* results in urogenital defects in mice (103). In mutant mice, the initial formation of the Wolffian duct and ureteric bud is normal as is the initial induction of the metanephric mesenchyme. Normal *Pax2* expression is observed in these structures. However,

the ureteric bud starts to degenerate around E12.5. At the same time, the expression of *Pax2* and *Ret*, a receptor tyrosine kinase normally expressed at the tip of growing ureteric bud, is greatly reduced. Recombinant organ culture between wild type and mutant ureteric bud and metanephric mesenchyme indicates a defect in the ureteric bud. *Emx2* expression is observed at a later stage of epithelialization than is *Pax2* in normal mice. The expression pattern suggests that *Emx2* regulates maturation and/or survival of epithelial cells rather than formation of epithelial cells.

TIMELESS GENE

By differential gene expression screening in the epithelial cell three-dimensional culture system for branching tubulogenesis, the mammalian ortholog of *Timeless* gene was identified as a candidate for regulation of epithelial branching morphogenesis. Its expression is detected in the active region of ureteric bud branching in the developing kidney. Selective inhibition of this gene in various in vitro culture models resulted in inhibition of ureteric bud branching (85). Deletion of this gene is embryonic lethal prior to the onset of kidney development (46a). The kidney (or ureteric bud)–specific knockout data are needed to provide a definitive role of this molecule in kidney development.

Transcription Factors Regulating Stroma Development

FOXD1 GENE

Study of one of the forkhead box transcription factor superfamily members, *Foxd1 (Bf2),* shed light on the role of the third cellular component of the developing kidney, the stroma. In developing kidneys, *Foxd1* is expressed by the cortical stromal mesenchyme. Homozygous null mutants for *Foxd1* die soon after birth due to renal failure. Mutant kidneys are small, fused, and located in the pelvis (53). Both ureteric bud branching morphogenesis and kidney tubulogenesis in the metanephric mesenchyme–derived segments are perturbed. Further analysis of this knockout mouse reveals that the mutant kidney capsule abnormally contains cells expressing bone morphogenetic protein (BMP) 4 or PECAM (endothelial marker). Abnormal signals from these cells are likely to cause disruption of normal ureteric bud branching and nephrogenesis (82). One of the target genes for this transcription factor is placental growth factor, a family member of vascular endothelial growth factor (190).

POD1 GENE

The *Pod1* gene, a transcription factor expressed in mesenchymal cells surrounding the ureteric bud and visceral glomerular podocytes in the developing kidney (132), also plays a role in regulating ureteric bud branching and nephron formation. Null mutants for this gene exhibit a phenotype similar to that seen in *Foxd1* knockouts; initial ureteric budding and mesenchymal condensation occurs, but the process appears to slow down beyond this point (131). By chimeric mouse analysis, *Pod1* expression was shown to be critical for the medullary stroma (25).

Pbx1 Gene

Pbx1 gene encodes a homeodomain containing transcription factor expressed in metanephric mesenchyme and both cortical and medullary stroma in the developing kidney. The kidney phenotype of *Pbx1* knockouts is similar to that of *Pod1*/*Foxd1* knockouts (157). It appears that expression of these genes is not dependent upon the others and all three genes are required for the functioning stroma capable of supporting ureteric bud branching and nephron differentiation. Identifying the molecular nature of this "stromal effect" will provide considerable insight into kidney development.

Retinoic Acid Receptor Genes

One possible mechanism for control of ureteric bud branching morphogenesis by the stromal cells is through vitamin A/retinoic acid pathway. Vitamin A deficiency has been known to result in small kidneys (180). Dietary vitamin A is converted to its active form, retinoic acid, and its signal is mediated through the retinoic acid receptor, which acts as a transcription factor. Retinoic acid synthesizing enzyme localizes to the cortical stromal cells (9) and double knockout of retinoic acid receptor *Rara* and *Rarb2* results in *Ret* downregulation and impaired ureteric branching (99).

Transcription Factors Regulating Functional Maturation of Nephron Tubules

Hnf1 Gene

Hepatocyte nuclear factor (Hnf)–1 is a homeotic gene mainly expressed in liver and kidney. *Hnf1* knockout mice have an enlarged liver and Fanconi syndrome, resulting in urinary wasting of sugars, amino acids, and electrolytes that normally are reabsorbed in the renal proximal tubules (125), suggesting an important role for *Hnf1* in regulating the expression of proximal tubule transporters.

Brn1 Gene

Maturation of Henle's loop and distal tubule is controlled by *Brn1*, a POU transcription factor. *Brn1* is expressed only in part of the mesenchymal condensate, then the prospective Henle's loop and distal tubule in the maturing kidney. There is no expression in the glomerulus, proximal tubule, or collecting duct. Knockout of this transcription factor results in an elongation and maturation defect of the Henle's loop, macula densa, and distal tubule (111).

URETERIC BUD BRANCHING MORPHOGENESIS

As discussed previously, ureteric bud branching morphogenesis is induced by signals from the metanephric mesenchyme. Soluble growth factors, direct cell-to-cell contact,

and cell–matrix contact play key roles in the process. The molecules likely to be involved in ureteric bud branching morphogenesis are summarized in Table 1.

Growth Factors

The embryonic kidney or isolated metanephric mesenchyme can induce branching morphogenesis of MDCK, mIMCD3 or UB cells grown in type I collagen gels in the absence of apparent cell contact (7, 142, 148). Moreover, isolated ureteric buds from E13 rats have been shown to undergo branching morphogenesis in the presence of soluble factors (129). This suggests that the metanephric mesenchyme elaborates soluble growth factors capable of inducing branching morphogenesis in the ureteric bud. A number of key growth factors have been identified.

GLIAL CELL LINE–DERIVED NEUROTROPHIC FACTOR

The importance of GDNF and its receptors GFRa1 and RET in kidney development is strongly supported by gene knockout data. Kidney agenesis or severe kidney hypogenesis is found in *Gdnf* (107, 119, 147), *Gfra1* (41a), or *Ret* knockout mice (35, 158). GDNF is expressed in the

TABLE 1 Molecules Likely to Be Involved in Ureteric Bud Branching Morphogenesis

	Soluble Factors	Transcription Factors	ECM/ Protease/ Integrin
Initiation	GDNF WNT2b	*Pax2* *Lim1* *Six1, 2* *Eya1* *Wt1* *Hox11 paralog* *Formin* *Foxc1*	
Branching morphogenesis	GDNF Pleiotrophin Wnt11 Gremlin TGFβ superfamily Slit/Robo HGF IGF	*Sall1* *Timeless*	Proteoglycans MMP9 Integrin $\alpha_3\beta_1$
Maintenance/ maturation of collecting system	EGFR ligands	*Emx2* *Foxd1* *Pbx1* *Pod1*	

ECM, extracellular matrix; EGFR, epidermal growth factor receptor; GDNF, glial cell line–derived neurotrophic growth factor; HGF, hepatocyte growth factor; IGF, insulin-like growth factor; TGF, transforming growth factor.

prospective metanephric mesenchyme area, while GFRa1 and RET are expressed in the Wolffian duct at the time of the ureteric bud induction. As discussed previously, a wide variety of genetic manipulations affecting the transcription of the GDNF/GFRα1/RET axis lead to disruption of kidney development. Moreover, in vitro application of GDNF-soaked beads to the whole genitourinary tract culture induces ectopic budding from the Wolffian duct (140). GDNF is also important in subsequent branching morphogenesis of the ureteric bud, as inhibition of this factor perturbs further branching of the isolated ureteric bud in vitro (129). Gene dosage of *Gdnf* is important as heterozygous null mutants of this gene have smaller kidneys (26). However, unlike ureteric budding from the Wolffian duct, where GDNF appears necessary and sufficient, GDNF is necessary but not sufficient to support ureteric bud branching morphogenesis, at least in the isolated ureteric bud culture system (129).

FIBROBLAST GROWTH FACTORS

Many fibroblast growth factors (FGFs) and their receptors are expressed in the developing kidney (15). Initial demonstration of the importance of this signaling pathway came from an analysis of transgenic mice that overexpress a soluble chimera of FGFR 2IIIb and human IgG Fc. In these animals, where FGF signaling is broadly inhibited, kidney agenesis or severe hypogenesis ensue (19). In addition, minor kidney defects are reported in *Fgf7* (130), *Fgf10* (115), and *Fgfr2IIIb* (134) knockout mice. In the isolated ureteric bud culture system, FGF2 and FGF7 induce a less branched globular ureteric bud growth, while FGF1 and FGF10 support branching growth (128), suggesting that FGFs may play a role in ureteric bud morphogenesis. In addition, a recent ureteric bud specific knockout of *Fgfr2*, (but not *Fgfr1*) was found to result in abnormal ureteric bud growth as well as abnormally thickened cortical stroma (191).

PLEIOTROPHIN

This heparin-binding growth factor has been implicated in neurite outgrowth (84) and mesenchymal-epithelial interaction during organogenesis (102). In the context of kidney development, pleiotrophin (isolated from the conditioned medium made by metanephric mesenchyme-derived cells) was found to induce ureteric bud branching morphogenesis in the presence of GDNF in the in vitro culture system (143). It is present in the developing kidney at the basement membrane of the ureteric bud. Although pleiotrophin may act as a mitogen for the ureteric bud after its budding through GDNF action, knockout of this gene does not appear to have a major affect in kidney development (1).

WNTS AND RELATED MOLECULES (FRIZZLED-RELATED PROTEINS)

A member of WNT family of secreted glycoprotein, WNT2b is expressed in the stroma and its presence promotes ureteric bud branching in vitro (86). Null mutants of the gene encoding another member of WNT family, *Wnt11* results in decreased ureteric bud branching with reduced *Gdnf* expression in the mesenchyme (92). *Ret* knockout mice also show reduced expression of *Wnt11* (92).

Secreted frizzled-related proteins (sFRPs) are secreted proteins that function as WNT modulators. sFRP1 is expressed in the stroma and periureter area, and sFRP2 is expressed in early mesenchymal condensates and also in the periureter area in the developing kidney (80, 186). Exogenous administration of sFRP1 to embryonic kidney organ culture leads to decreased ureteric bud branching and nephron induction. While exogenous sFRP2 alone does not have a major effect, its administration to the organ culture treated with sFRP1 partially reverses the inhibitory effect of sFRP1 (186).

TRANSFORMING GROWTH FACTOR β SUPERFAMILY

Most of the soluble factors discussed thus far facilitate ureteric bud branching and growth. However, unopposed proliferation and branching is not desirable for normal kidney development. Potential candidates for these "negative regulators" include members of the transforming growth factor (TGF) β superfamily. Generally, TGFβ inhibits epithelial cell growth. In organ culture, exogenous TGFβ1 or another member of the TGFβ superfamily, activin, inhibits ureteric bud development and/or disrupts the branching pattern (135), suggesting their role not only in regulating proliferation but also in correct patterning. In this regard, it is interesting that TGFβ selectively inhibits HGF-induced mIMCD3 branching events with little effect on tubule formation (144); HGF plus TGFβ induces long, straight tubules, whereas HGF alone induces branching tubules. Furthermore, detailed image analysis reveals alteration in the ureteric bud branching pattern in embryonic kidneys treated with TGFβ superfamily members (14). In isolated ureteric bud culture, administration of TGFβ superfamily members causes growth inhibition as well as morphological changes similar (though not so striking) to that observed in mIMCD cell culture (14).

Heterozygous mutation of another family member, bone morphogenetic protein (*Bmp*) 4 reveals loss of ureteric bud elongation together with ectopic budding from Wolffian duct (104). Its expression is detected at the intermediate mesoderm surrounding the Wolffian duct and metanephric mesenchyme surrounding the stalk of the ureteric bud

(104, 133). Taken together, these data suggest that TGFβ superfamily members inhibit branching events but have somewhat less effect on ureteric bud elongation (and may even facilitate it in the presence of stimulatory growth factors) and play a role in regulating the pattern of ureteric bud branching.

Another member of this family, growth/differentiation factor (*Gdf*)11 is expressed in the Wolffian duct and the metanephric mesenchyme. Knockouts of this gene result in kidney hypoplasia to agenesis, thought to be caused by downregulation of *Gdnf* in the mesenchyme (42, 98). In these mice, molecules known to regulate *Gdnf* expression such as *Eya1*, *Six2*, *Pax2*, and *Wt1* are expressed in the metanephric mesenchyme region, and the metanephric mesenchyme from this mutant undergoes nephron tubule formation when it is cultured with embryonic spinal cord. Molecular markers for Wolffian duct such as *Ret*, *Pax2*, *Emx2*, and *Lim1* were expressed in the right place, and "mutant Wolffian duct responds to exogenous GDNF (42). Thus, GDF11 is likely to be indispensable for *Gdnf* expression.

Outside the kidney, this mutant mouse shows deranged anterior/posterior patterning with alteration of *Hox* gene expression pattern (98). Given the fact that *Hox11* paralogs control *Gdnf* expression (177), downregulation of *Gdnf* in *Gdf11* mutants may be mediated through *Hox11* expression. GDF11 acts through the activin receptor (ACVR) IIA and IIB (114) and knockouts of *Acvr2b* results in similar though milder phenotype than that of *Gdf11* knockouts (113).

GREMLIN

Gremlin is a secreted BMP antagonist (56) expressed initially in the Wolffian duct, followed by induced mesenchyme in metanephros development (101). Knockout of this gene results in kidney agenesis. The ureteric bud forms but fails to invade the metanephric mesenchyme (101). Subsequently the metanephric mesenchyme undergoes apoptosis. Gremlin might antagonize BMP at the tip of the ureteric bud thereby allowing its branching growth. Although the kidney phenotype of *Gremlin1* knockouts resembles that of *Sall1* knockouts, *Sall1* expression is unchanged in *Gremlin1* knockouts (101).

SLIT-ROBO AND SPROUTY (INTRACELLULAR PROTEIN)

We have discussed a transcription factor, *Foxc1*, as a regulator to restrict *Gdnf* spatial expression. The secreted protein *Slit2* and its receptor *Robo2*, previously reported as a chemo-repellant factor for axon guidance (181), also functions to restrict *Gdnf* expression. Null mutations of either *Slit2* or *Robo2* result in supernumerary ureteric buds, caused by an abnormally extended *Gdnf* expression area

(47). In these mutants, however, *Foxc1* expression is normal, suggesting that the Slit/Robo pathway lies downstream of *Foxc1*, or the existence of multiple parallel pathways for regulating *Gdnf* expression.

Sprouty (Spry) is a intercellular protein that acts as a negative feedback regulator for FGF and other receptor tyrosine kinase mediated signaling (70). Knockouts of *Spry1* display multiple ureters and multiplex kidneys (8). It appears that mutant Wolffian ducts are abnormally more sensitive to GDNF as reduction of *Gdnf* expression rescues the phenotype (8).

HEPATOCYTE GROWTH FACTOR

Embryonic kidneys express HGF and its receptor Met (148). Neutralizing anti-HGF antibodies inhibit the growth of the embryonic kidney and disrupt ureteric bud branching morphogenesis in serum-free organ culture (148). These results support the notion that HGF is an important morphogen for the ureteric bud that is secreted from metanephric mesenchyme. However, kidney development appears to be unaffected up to embryonic day 14 in *Hgf* or *Met* knockout mice, which die around this time from liver failure (10, 156). Although HGF may act at later stages of ureteric bud branching morphogenesis, it is probably not critically important in the initial stages.

EPIDERMAL GROWTH FACTOR RECEPTOR LIGANDS

Epidermal growth factor (EGF), transforming growth factor α (TGFα), heparin-binding epidermal growth factor like growth factor (HBEGF), amphiregulin, and betacellulin all bind and activate the EGF receptor (96). TGFα is present in the embryonic kidney, and disruption of TGFα signaling by neutralizing antibodies results in a small, less well-developed kidney in organ culture (138). As mentioned above, when mIMCD3 cells grown in collagen gels are co-cultured with embryonic kidney, the cells undergo branching morphogenesis. Unlike MDCK cells, which only undergo branching morphogenesis in the presence of HGF (105, 148), mI MCD3 cells respond to EGF receptor ligands as well (7, 145). Similar results are obtained with the UB cell three-dimensional culture system (142). Moreover, *Met* (HGF receptor) knockout kidney epith-elial cells grown in three-dimensional extracellular matrix (ECM) gels undergo in vitro tubulogenesis in response to EGF or TGFα (65). Although *Tgfα* knockout mice do not have a kidney phenotype (89, 93), knockout of the *EGF receptor* in mice with a certain genetic background leads to dilated collecting ducts and renal dysfunction (168). These results suggest an important role for EGF receptor ligands in later collecting duct development.

INSULIN-LIKE GROWTH FACTORS

In serum-free organ culture, the embryonic kidney produces insulin-like growth factors (IGFs) 1 and 2 (137). When neutralizing antibodies against IGFs are added to the culture, kidney growth is suppressed (137). The ureteric bud expresses IGF1 receptor (173). Addition of antisense oligonucleotides against IGF1 receptor to the embryonic kidney in organ culture leads to a small kidney with disrupted ureteric bud branching morphogenesis (173). However, knockout mice for either *Igf1* or *Igf2* do not display a kidney phenotype (3, 126). Molecular redundancy may be part of the explanation; however, as with HGF, the apparent discrepancies between the in vitro and in vivo data need to be addressed experimentally.

Extracellular Matrix

Soluble growth factors are not the only molecules involved in ureteric bud branching morphogenesis. Cells of the ureteric bud are surrounded by ECM proteins, and to form branching tubules, the cells must digest the ECM. Cells have receptors for ECM proteins, such as integrins as well as other specific receptors. Integrins can transmit signals to cytosolic and intranuclear proteins in a fashion similar to growth factor receptors. The cell modifies its behavior in response to the combined signals from growth factors and ECM proteins (60).

The importance of the specific composition of the ECM in kidney epithelial cell branching morphogenesis has been shown using the three-dimensional cell culture model. When MDCK cells are cultured in type I collagen gels in the presence of HGF, the cells undergo branching morphogenesis. When MDCK cells are suspended in growth factor–reduced Matrigel, a basement membrane protein mixture secreted by EHS sarcoma cells, HGF-induced tubulogenesis is inhibited (150). By mixing individual Matrigel component proteins into type I collagen gels, it was found that collagen I, laminin, fibronectin, and entactin facilitate MDCK cell tubulogenesis, whereas collagen IV, vitronectin, and heparan sulfate proteoglycan inhibit it (150). However, a mixture of type I collagen and Matrigel, not pure type I collagen, is the optimum ECM for UB cell (a cell line derived from embryonic kidney tissue) tubulogenesis. Interestingly, when these cells are cultured in growth factor–reduced Matrigel alone, UB cells develop into cystic structures (Fig. 7) (142). Together with the fact that isolated ureteric buds can be cultured in an ECM containing Matrigel but not in pure type 1 collagen gels (129). This indicates that ECM composition modulates tubulogenesis and branching morphogenesis.

LAMININ

Laminins are the major component of the mature basement membrane. The role of laminin in epithelial branching morphogenesis has been shown in lung organ culture in vitro. Antilaminin antibodies perturb branching morphogenesis of embryonic lung in culture (159). In the kidney, studies have shown a role for laminin in epithelial cell formation from the induced metanephric mesenchyme. It is known that antibodies against nidogen, a basement membrane protein secreted by mesenchymal cells, perturb epithelial morphogenesis in lung and kidney (39). Nidogen binds to the γ1 chain of laminin. Thus, it is conceivable that the mesenchyme regulates epithelial branching morphogenesis through nidogen-laminin interaction. Moreover, knockouts of one of the laminin receptors, $\alpha_3\beta_1$ integrin, result in decreased ureteric bud branching morphogenesis (71). In in vitro whole organ culture and isolated ureteric bud culture, branching is inhibited in the presence of blocking antibodies against integrins α_3, α_6, β_1, or β_4. Interestingly, a common ligand for $\alpha_3\beta_1$ and $\alpha_6\beta_4$, laminin-5 is present in the developing ureteric bud and its inhibition results in decreased branching in both whole embryonic kidney culture and isolated ureteric bud culture (189).

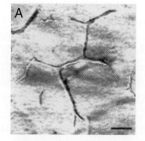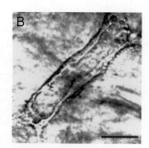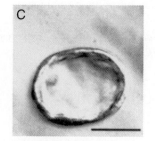

FIGURE 7 Photomicrograph of ureteric bud (UB) cells cultured in three-dimensional extracellular matrix (ECM) gels. In the presence of conditioned medium from BSN cells, which derive from the metanephric mesenchyme, the UB cells form branching cordlike structures in 3 to 5 days **(A)**. In 10 to 15 days tubules with clear lumens can be observed **(B)**. Even in the presence of BSN-conditioned medium, the UB cells form multicellular cysts when cultured in pure Matrigel **(C)** instead of collagen I/Matrigel mixture **(A** and **B)**. Bars, 50 μm. (From Sakurai H, Barros EJ, Tsukamoto T, Barasch J, Nigam SK. An in vitro tubulogenesis system using cell lines derived from the embryonic kidney shows dependence on multiple soluble growth factors. *Proc Natl Acad Sci U S A* 1997;94;6279–6284, with permission.)

PROTEOGLYCANS

Proteoglycans are protein molecules containing many bound glycosaminoglycan (GAG) chains (64). The common GAG chains include chondroitin sulfate, dermatan sulfate, heparan sulphate, heparin, and keratan sulfate. Proteoglycans are mostly found at the cell surface or in the extracellular matrix. In embryonic kidneys, sulfated proteoglycans are concentrated around the tip of the ureteric bud and perturbation of their synthesis by β-xyloside results in the inhibition of ureteric bud branching morphogenesis (66, 78). This perturbation also abolishes the expression of *Wnt11* at the tip of the ureteric bud (63). As described previously, loss of *Wnt11* expression at the tip of the ureteric bud can lead to loss of *Gdnf* expression in the metanephric mesenchyme. However, the linking mechanism between inhibition of sulfated proteoglycan and the loss of *Wnt11* expression is unclear. Along the same lines, genetic inactivation of an enzyme, heparan sulfate 2-o-sulfotransferase, involved in heparan sulfate proteoglycan synthesis results in kidney agenesis (13). In this case, the ureteric bud forms from the Wolffian duct, but subsequent invasion of the metanephric mesenchyme is perturbed. As for the mesenchyme, initial specification of the metanephric mesenchyme appears intact, but subsequent mesenchymal condensation is affected. Consistent with the in vitro result described above, heparan sulfate biosynthesis perturbation results in loss of *Wnt11* expression and reduced *Gdnf* expression. Given the fact that many growth factors that regulate branching morphogenesis of the ureteric bud are heparin (a heavily sulfated form of GAG chain) binding, it is likely that global inhibition of GAG chain synthesis or its sulfation could compromise actions of these heparin binding growth factors.

In contrast, inhibition of specific heparan sulfate proteoglycans results in less clear effects. One exception is *glypican* (*Gpc*) 3, a gene encoding a heparan sulfate proteoglycan linked to the cell surface via a glycosyl-phosphatidylinositol anchor. *Gpc3* knockout mice display enhanced ureteric branching and dysplastic kidneys (48). *Gpc3* is expressed in the ureteric bud cells and modulates BMP and FGF action on the ureteric bud (48). A potent angiogenesis inhibitor, endostatin, a breakdown product of extracellular proteoglycan, collagen XVIII, inhibits ureteric bud branching morphogenesis (62). Interestingly, this action is likely to be mediated through its binding to glypicans (62).

Although it is not a proteoglycan in the strict sense, because it lacks a protein core, hyaluronic acid (HA) also plays a role in branching morphogenesis. Synthetic enzymes for this GAG are expressed in the developing kidney and the addition of HA to three-dimensional culture of UB cells promotes tubulogenesis and survival of cells. Blocking antibodies against its receptor CD44 abolishes this effect (123).

FIBRILLIN1

Fibrillin1 is made in the metanephric mesenchyme and it binds to integrin $\alpha_v\beta_3$, which is expressed in the ureteric bud. Antisense oligonucleotides directed against this extracellular matrix molecule induces dysmorphogenesis of cultured metanephros (58), suggesting a role for this protein in kidney development.

EXTRACELLULAR PROTEINASES AND THEIR INHIBITORS

The idea that ECM-degrading proteases are involved in branching morphogenesis is supported by work from in vitro three-dimensional culture and organ culture. Two classes of proteases appear to be involved: metalloproteases (MMPs) and serine proteases. In HGF-induced MDCK cell tubulogenesis, inhibitors of collagenase (MMP1) perturb the morphogenetic events when the cells are suspended in type I collagen gels (106). The broadly active MMP inhibitor, 1,10-phenanthroline, inhibits TGFα- or HGF-induced mIMCD3 cell tubulogenesis in collagen gels (145). Furthermore, tubulogenic growth factors such as HGF or EGF receptor ligands upregulate the expression of MMPs and urokinase in the epithelial cells as they undergo tubulogenesis (145, 165). Interestingly, in the case of long, nonbranching mIMCD3 cell tubules induced by HGF plus TGFβ, the balance between proteases (MMP1 and urokinase) and their inhibitors (TIMP1 and PAI1) expressed by mIMCD3 cells changes in parallel with tubular morphology (144). In embryonic ureteric bud derived UB cells, expression of MMPs and TIMPs changes in response to surrounding ECM and soluble factors (122). These results suggest that tubulogenic growth factors act, at least in part, through changing the expression patterns of extracellular proteases and their inhibitors in in vitro tubulogenesis. It has also been shown that "tubulogenic ECM" and highly tubulogenic conditioned medium secreted by metanephric mesenchyme-derived cells contain MMP activity, and that the expression level of regulators for these MMPs in UB cells alters as branching morphogenesis progresses (122), suggesting local control of proteolytic activity is important in the morphogenetic process. In the embryonic kidney in organ culture, antibodies against MMP9, but not MMP2, inhibit the branching morphogenesis of the ureteric bud (79). Furthermore, *Mmp9* knockout mice do not show a kidney phenotype (2). Both of these enzymes act as a gelatinase, which is required to digest ECMs in basement membranes. In another study, however, antisense oligonucleotides against mesenchymal MMP2 or epithelial cell surface–expressed membrane type (MT)1–MMP inhibit metanephrogenesis in organ culture (59).

In summary, ureteric bud branching outgrowth and morphogenesis is modulated in large part by a combination of positive and negative soluble growth factors secreted by the metanephric mesenchyme that act synergistically. In many cases, these pathways are more parallel than interdependent. These growth factors subsequently regulate downstream effector molecules such as ECM or ECM-degrading proteinases (Fig. 8).

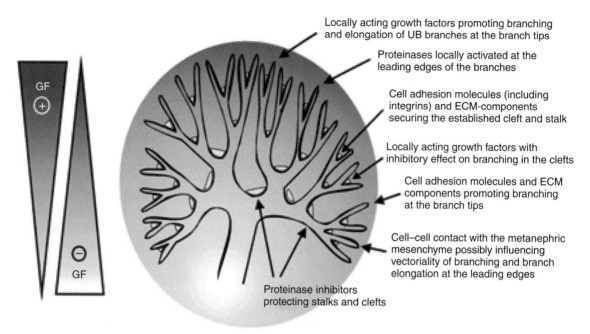

FIGURE 8   Model for ureteric bud branching morphogenesis. After induction of the ureteric bud (UB), in which the GDNF appears to play a critical role, UB branching may be guided by gradients of branching promoting (GF+) and inhibiting growth factors (GF−). Promoting factors might include GDNF, pleiotrophin, FGFs, EGFs, whereas TGFβ superfamily members may inhibit branching. Distal effector molecules probably include facilitating and inhibiting extracellular matrix (ECM) components together with signal transducing–cell adhesion molecules such as integrins, CD44, membrane-bound proteinase activators such as MT1-MMP, and active proteinases (e.g., MMP9), as well as proteinase inhibitors such as TIMP3, which binds to the ECM and could protect the matrix around the stalks from degradation. Reprinted with permission from the *Annual Review of Physiology*, Volume 62 © 2000 by Annual Reviews www.annualreviews.org.

TUBULOGENESIS AFTER INDUCTION OF THE METANEPHRIC MESENCHYME

Early mesenchymally derived nephrons, which will go on to form Bowman's capsule, as well as the proximal and distal tubules, are induced in the metanephric mesenchyme by the ureteric bud. In the process, mesenchymal cells transform into epithelial cells. The induced epithelial cells differentiate into kidney tubules. This transformation can be induced by a number of inducer tissues other than the ureteric bud, including embryonic spinal cord, embryonic salivary mesenchyme, and embryonic bone (52, 155, 171). Many embryonic epithelial, neural, or mesenchymal tissues can thus induce the metanephric mesenchyme, though various tissues have different potency. For example, brain can only induce metanephric mesenchyme to the condensation stage, while spinal cord can induce tubule formation (87). Thus, it is conceivable that there are several steps in the induction process: (1) rescue of metanephric mesenchyme and/or later tubular structures from apoptosis; (2) mesenchymal cell condensation; (3) epithelial polarization and junction formation; (4) tubule formation. The molecules likely involved in the process are summarized in Table 2.

Prevention of Apoptosis

During kidney tubule development, apoptosis is observed among cells surrounding newly formed epithelial tubules (69). In fact, significant amounts of apoptosis appear to be occurring in many parts of the kidney during development (24). When the metanephric mesenchyme is cultured with inducer tissues or EGF, apoptosis becomes less prominent (24, 69). These results suggest that an important early signal from the inducer tissue prevents metanephric mesenchyme cell apoptosis. In in vitro culture of metanephric mesenchyme, conditioned medium from UB cells also exhibits an anti-apoptotic effect (4). One of the anti-apoptotic molecules in UB conditioned medium is FGF2 (5). Consistent with these findings, RUB cell (derived from rat ureteric bud)–conditioned medium requires supplementation of FGF2 and TGFα to induce kidney tubule formation in the absence of inductive tissues (61).

In addition, analysis of bone morphogenetic protein (*Bmp*)7–deficient mice suggests that BMP7 may act as an anti-apoptotic factor (34, 90). BMP7 belongs to the TGFβ superfamily and is expressed in the Wolffian duct, ureteric bud, and nephron structures after induction (34). *Bmp7* knockout mice exhibit defects in eye and kidney development. Although there is a difference in the early kidney phenotype between knockout mice created by different groups, ureteric bud formation and initial induction appears unaffected; at least a few comma- and S-shaped bodies are observed at E12.5 (34, 90). However, soon after this, both the ureteric bud and the metanephric mesenchyme start to degenerate, ultimately resulting in nonfunctioning disorganized kidneys. This raises the possibility that BMP7 maintains induced tubules, preventing

TABLE 2 Molecules Likely to Be Involved in Metanephric Mesenchyme Induction

	Transcription Factors	Soluble Factors	ECM/Other Molecules
Define nephrogenic mesenchyme	*Wt1* *Pax2* *Six1* *Myc* (uninduced MM)		
Rescue from apoptosis		FGF2 EGFR ligands BMP7	
Condensation/epithelialization	*Pax2* *Pax8* *Nmyc* *Foxd1* *Pod1* *Pbx1*	LIF TGFβ2 Lipocalin Wnt4	Laminin (βγ chain)/laminin receptor (α$_6$β$_1$ integrin, nonmuscle dystroglycan) α$_8$β$_1$ integrin
Tubule formation	*Hnf1* (proximal tubule) *Brn1* (Henle, distal)		Laminin (α chain)/laminin receptor

ECM, extracellular matrix; LIF, leukemia inhibiting factor; TGF, transforming growth factor.

them from apoptosis rather than directly inducing the metanephric mesenchyme (34). On the other hand, in vitro application of BMP7 has been reported to induce E11.5 mouse metanephric mesenchyme to form epithelial glomeruli without inductive tissues (172). Whether BMP7 directly induces the metanephric mesenchyme remains to be determined.

Molecules Involved in Metanephric Mesenchyme Induction and Nephron Tubule Formation

As discussed in the transcription factor section, certain transcription factors such as *Pax2*, *Wt1*, or *Six1* are necessary to retain competency of the metanephric mesenchyme to the signals from the ureteric bud.

Early experiments using transfilter coculture of the metanephric mesenchyme with various inductive tissues defined several expected characteristics of "inductive molecules" (154). Experiments using different pore-size filters and multiple filters to separate the metanephric mesenchyme and inducer suggest that inductive molecules do not simply diffuse, rather, they seem to require close association of cells. In other words, direct cell-to-cell contact and/or soluble molecules associated with the cell surface are likely to be required for induction. In fact, direct interaction between the inductive tissue and the metanephric mesenchyme cells have been observed through the filter pores by electron microscopy (76).

However, in vitro work indicates that combinations of soluble factors are sufficient to induce tubulogenesis of the metanephric mesenchyme. Leukemia inhibitory factor (LIF), FGF2, and TGFα (6) or this combination plus TGFβ2 (121) can induce nephron tubules in metanephric mesenchyme cultured in the absence of inductive tissues. The 24p3, a member of the lipocalin superfamily, also has been shown to induce epithelialization of metanephric mes-

enchyme in the presence of FGFs (185) and delivers iron to the cell and iron is required for mesenchymal induction by this molecule (185).

Cell surface glycoproteins of the Wnt family are candidate molecules for coordinating morphogenesis at the interface of metanephric mesenchyme and inductive tissues, as WNT1 expressing fibroblasts induce the metanephric mesenchyme to form glomeruli (54). Although the *Wnt1* gene is not expressed in embryonic kidneys (179), this result raises the possibility of an important role for other Wnt family members in nephrogenesis. Another Wnt family member, *Wnt4* is expressed in the embryonic kidneys; it first appears in condensed metanephric mesenchyme, and its expression continues in comma- and S-shaped bodies, finally becoming restricted to the area where newly formed epithelial tubules are connected to collecting ducts (164). Based on its expression pattern, WNT4 may not be mediating the inductive signal from the ureteric bud. Nevertheless, WNT4 plays an important role in metanephric mesenchyme induction perhaps as an autocrine or paracrine factor for metanephric mesenchymal cells. The metanephric mesenchyme of mutant mice lacking the *Wnt4* gene is able to condense around the branching ureteric bud but fails to form peritubular aggregates (164). There is no apparent kidney tubule development in these knockout animals. The expression of markers for early mesenchymal induction, *Pax2* and *Nmyc*, does not seem to be affected in *Wnt4* mutant mice, suggesting that *Wnt4* acts at a later stage than *Pax2* or *Nmyc*. However, *Pax8* expression by metanephric mesenchyme-derived structures cannot be detected in the mutant mice.

The cell-surface–signaling molecule Notch has also been implicated in tubulogenesis. *Notch 1, 2,* and *3* have been shown to be expressed in the developing kidney (22, 176). *Notch2* mutation leads to hypoplastic kidneys with glomerular defects (97). Proteolytic cleavage of Notch1 by γ-secretase is required for the Notch activation and this inhibition in kidney organ culture results in decreased S-shaped bodies despite having normal condensation (23). Knockout and partial rescue of *Presenilin1 and 2* that are required for γ-secretase activity lead to the similar phenotype (174).

Extracellular matrix proteins are important for maintaining epithelial tubular structures. Much work has been done on the basement membrane glycoprotein laminin and the integrins that bind laminin. Laminin1 is composed of three chains: α1, β1, γ1. Of these, β1 and γ1 expression increases early (day 1) when the metanephric mesenchyme is induced, while the α1 chain is expressed after epithelial cell polarization begins (38, 67). The laminin α1 chain is exclusively expressed by the epithelial cells (38), and perturbation of this chain by antibodies inhibits kidney tubulogenesis in vitro (68). The kidney epithelial cell has at least two laminin receptors: $\alpha_6\beta_1$ integrin and nonmuscle dystroglycan. Perturbation of these receptors inhibits kidney tubulogenesis in vitro (36, 43). Moreover, in in vitro culture of embryonic lung, it has been demonstrated that heterotypic cell-to-cell contact between epithelial cells and mesenchymal cells is required to synthesize the laminin α_1 chain (160). If this result is applicable to embryonic kidney, further differentiation after cell-to-cell contact may be a function of expression of the laminin α_1 chain.

In addition to laminin binding integrins, knockouts of integrin a8 have been shown to have severe defects in kidney development (109). The ureteric bud initiation and initial mesenchymal induction appear unaffected; the metanephric mesenchyme cells condense around the ureteric bud and start to express *Pax2* and p75 NGFR. However, further steps toward epithelialization and tubule formation are not observed. In normal mice, $\alpha8\beta1$ integrin is transiently expressed in the condensing mesenchymal cells. Both spatiotemporal localization and knockout phenotype suggest that $\alpha_8\beta_1$ integrin plays an important role after the initial induction step of mesenchymal-epithelial transformation.

Evidence is beginning to accumulate on the functional maturation of the kidney tubules. Kidney tubules further differentiate into several segments. In each segment the tubular cells express different sets of transporters. For example, northern blot analysis shows that the organic anion transporter Oat1 begins to be expressed at around E16 kidney (88). It is likely that expression of many transporters, characteristic of mature tubules, is tightly regulated. In this regard, elucidation of the roles of transcription factors *Hnf1* (proximal tubules) and *Brn1* (Henle's loop and distal tubule) is important and other unknown factors may be involved in this process.

VASCULAR AND GLOMERULAR DEVELOPMENT

The origin of glomerular endothelial cells and mesangial cells, and how the vascular system is integrated in the developing kidney, has been an area of controversy for years. Vascular development occurs by (1) angiogenesis, in which new vessels arise from existing vasculature; and/or (2) vasculogenesis, in which de novo endothelial cells are formed. As mentioned previously, in vitro kidney organ culture gives rise to epithelial glomerular structures, not mesangial cells nor endothelial cells, suggesting that either the culture conditions are not suitable for endothelial cell growth or there are no angioblasts in the metanephric mesenchyme. To study kidney vascular development, interspecies grafting techniques have been used in which E11 murine embryonic kidneys are transplanted into the chick chorioallantoic-membranes (CAM) (127). When E11 mouse kidneys, which have no apparent vascular development, are grown in chick CAM, the kidneys form glomeruli containing blood vessels from the chick as determined by staining with species specific antibodies against basement membranes (40, 151). However, when E11 mouse kidneys are grafted into the rat anterior eye chamber, newly formed glomerular endothelial cells appear to be derived from the graft (57). Moreover, the same group has demonstrated that vascular endothelial cell growth factor receptor FLK1 positive cells are found in the E12 mouse kidney, and that these cells are likely to be angioblasts, which differentiate into blood vessels in the glomeruli (136). Thus, depending on the culture and grafting conditions, glomerular capillaries can be derived by an angiogenic process (i.e., outside of the metanephric mesenchyme or a vasculogenic process; inside of the metanephric mesenchyme). Which of these processes is more important in vivo remains uncertain, and it is of course possible that both are important.

The origin of mesangial cells also remains uncertain. In the aforementioned different kidney graft systems, mesangial cells appear to behave similarly to glomerular endothelial cells; in CAM grafts, the mesangial cells are derived from the hosts; (152, 153) while in the anterior eye chamber grafts, they are derived from the grafts (57). *Platelet-derived growth factor (Pdgf)-B receptor* knockout mice do not have mesangial cells and exhibited dilated capillary loops resulting in defective glomeruli (81, 162).

Acknowledgments

The authors thank Dr. Kevin Bush for providing valuable comments on this manuscript. S. K. Nigam is funded by the National Institutes of Health and Established Investigator Awards from American Heart Association. H. Sakurai is supported by a Scientist Development Grant from American Heart Association.

References

1. Amet LE, Lauri SE, Hienola A, et al. Enhanced hippocampal long-term potentiation in mice lacking heparin-binding growth-associated molecule. *Mol Cell Neurosci* 2001;17:1014–1024.

2. Andrews KL, Betsuyaku T, Rogers S, Shipley JM, Senior RM, Miner JH. Gelatinase B (MMP-9) is not essential in the normal kidney and does not influence progression of renal disease in a mouse model of Alport syndrome. *Am J Pathol* 2000;157:303–311.

3. Baker J, Liu JP, Robertson EJ, Efstratiadis A. Role of insulin-like growth factors in embryonic and postnatal growth. *Cell* 1993;75:73–82.
4. Barasch J, Pressler L, Connor J, Malik A. A ureteric bud cell line induces nephrogenesis in two steps by two distinct signals. *Am J Physiol* 1996;271:F50–F61.
5. Barasch J, Qiao J, McWilliams G, Chen D, Oliver JA, Herzlinger D. Ureteric bud cells secrete multiple factors, including bFGF, which rescue renal progenitors from apoptosis. *Am J Physiol* 1997;273:F757–767.
6. Barasch J, Yang J, Ware CB, et al. Mesenchymal to epithelial conversion in rat metanephros is induced by LIF. *Cell* 1999;99:377–386.
7. Barros EJ, Santos OF, Matsumoto K, Nakamura T, Nigam SK. Differential tubulogenic and branching morphogenetic activities of growth factors: implications for epithelial tissue development. *Proc Natl Acad Sci U S A* 1995;92:4412–4416.
8. Basson MA, Akbulut S, Watson-Johnson J, et al. Sprouty1 is a critical regulator of GDNF/RET-mediated kidney induction. *Dev Cell* 2005;8:229–239.
9. Batourina E, Gim S, Bello N, et al. Vitamin A controls epithelial/mesenchymal interactions through Ret expression. *Nat Genet* 2001; 27:74–78.
10. Bladt F, Riethmacher D, Isenmann S, Aguzzi A, Birchmeier C. Essential role for c-met receptor in the migration of myogenic precursor cells into the limb bud. *Nature (Lond)* 1995;376: 768–771.
11. Bouchard M, Souabni A, Mandler M, Neubuser A, Busslinger M. Nephric lineage specification by Pax2 and Pax8. *Genes Dev* 2002; 16:2958–2970.
12. Brophy PD, Ostrom L, Lang KM, Dressler GR. Regulation of ureteric bud outgrowth by Pax2-dependent activation of the glial derived neurotrophic factor gene. *Development* 2001;128:4747–4756.
13. Bullock SL, Fletcher JM, Beddington RS, Wilson VA. Renal agenesis in mice homozygous for a gene trap mutation in the gene encoding heparan sulfate 2-sulfotransferase. *Genes Dev* 1998;12:1894–1906.
14. Bush KT, Sakurai H, Steer DL, et al. TGF-beta superfamily members modulate growth, branching, shaping, and patterning of the ureteric bud. *Dev Biol* 2004;266:285–298.
15. Cancilla B, Davies A, Cauchi JA, Risbridger GP, Bertram JF. Fibroblast growth factor receptors and their ligands in the adult rat kidney. *Kidney Int* 2001;60:147–155.
16. Cantley LG, Barros EJ, Gandhi M, Rauchman M, Nigam SK. Regulation of mitogenesis, motogenesis, and tubulogenesis by hepatocyte growth factor in renal collecting duct cells. *Am J Physiol* 1994;267:F271–F280.
17. Capecchi MR. Altering the genome by homologous recombination. *Science* 1989;244: 1288–1292.
18. Capecchi MR. Targeted gene replacement. *Sci Am* 1994;270:52–59.
19. Celli G, LaRochelle WJ, Mackem S, Sharp R, Merlino G. Soluble dominant-negative receptor uncovers essential roles for fibroblast growth factors in multi-organ induction and patterning. *EMBO J* 1998;17:1642–1655.
20. Chan DC, Wynshaw-Boris A, Leder P. Formin isoforms are differentially expressed in the mouse embryo and are required for normal expression of fgf-4 and shh in the limb bud. *Development* 1995;121:3151–3162.
21. Charron J, Malynn BA, Fisher P, et al. Embryonic lethality in mice homozygous for a targeted disruption of the N-myc gene. *Genes Dev* 1992;6:2248–2257.
22. Chen L, Al-Awqati Q. Segmental expression of Notch and Hairy genes in nephrogenesis. *Am J Physiol Renal Physiol* 2005;288:F939–952.
23. Cheng HT, Miner JH, Lin M, Tansey MG, Roth K, Kopan R. Gamma-secretase activity is dispensable for mesenchyme-to-epithelium transition but required for podocyte and proximal tubule formation in developing mouse kidney. *Development* 2003;130: 5031–5042.
24. Coles HS, Burne JF, Raff MC. Large-scale normal cell death in the developing rat kidney and its reduction by epidermal growth factor. *Development* 1993;118:777–784.
25. Cui S, Schwartz L, Quaggin SE. Pod1 is required in stromal cells for glomerulogenesis. *Dev Dyn* 2003;226:512–522.
26. Cullen-McEwen LA, Drago J, Bertram JF. Nephron endowment in glial cell line-derived neurotrophic factor (GDNF) heterozygous mice. *Kidney Int* 2001;60:31–36.
27. Davies JA, Ladomery M, Hohenstein P, et al. Development of an siRNA-based method for repressing specific genes in renal organ culture and its use to show that the Wt1 tumour suppressor is required for nephron differentiation. *Hum Mol Genet* 2004;13:235–246.
28. Davis AC, Wims M, Spotts GD, Hann SR, Bradley A. A null c-myc mutation causes lethality before 10.5 days of gestation in homozygotes and reduced fertility in heterozygous female mice. *Genes Dev* 1993;7:671–682.
29. Davis AP, Witte DP, Hsieh-Li HM, Potter SS, Capecchi MR. Absence of radius and ulna in mice lacking hoxa-11 and hoxd-11. *Nature* 1995;375:791–795.
30. Donovan MJ, Natoli TA, Sainio K, et al. Initial differentiation of the metanephric mesenchyme is independent of WT1 and the ureteric bud. *Dev Genet* 1999;24:252–262.
31. Dressler GR, Deutsch U, Chowdhury K, Nornes HO, Gruss P. Pax2, a new murine paired-box-containing gene and its expression in the developing excretory system. *Development* 1990;109:787–795.
32. Dressler GR, Douglass EC. Pax-2 is a DNA-binding protein expressed in embryonic kidney and Wilms tumor. *Proc Natl Acad Sci U S A* 1992;89:1179–1183.
33. Drummond IA, Madden SL, Rohwer-Nutter P, Bell GI, Sukhatme VP, Rauscher FJd. Repression of the insulin-like growth factor II gene by the Wilms tumor suppressor WT1. *Science* 1992;257:674–678.
34. Dudley AT, Lyons KM, Robertson EJ. A requirement for bone morphogenetic protein-7 during development of the mammalian kidney and eye. *Genes Dev* 1995;9:2795–2807.
35. Durbec P, Marcos-Gutierrez CV, Kilkenny C, et al. GDNF signalling through the Ret receptor tyrosine kinase (see comments). *Nature* 1996:381:789–793.
36. Durbeej M, Larsson E, Ibraghimov-Beskrovnaya O, Roberds SL, Campbell KP, Ekblom P. Non-muscle alpha-dystroglycan is involved in epithelial development. *J Cell Biol* 1995;130: 79–91.
37. Durbeej M, Soderstrom S, Ebendal T, Birchmeier C, Ekblom P. Differential expression of neurotrophin receptors during renal development. *Development* 1993;119:977–989.
38. Ekblom M, Klein G, Mugrauer G, et al. Transient and locally restricted expression of laminin A chain mRNA by developing epithelial cells during kidney organogenesis. *Cell* 1990;60: 337–346.
39. Ekblom P, Ekblom M, Fecker L, et al. Role of mesenchymal nidogen for epithelial morphogenesis in vitro. *Development* 1994;120:2003–2014.
40. Ekblom P, Sariola H, Karkinen-Jaaskelainen M, Saxen L. The origin of the glomerular endothelium. *Cell Differ* 1982;11:35–39.
41. Ekblom P, Thesleff I, Miettinen A, Saxen L. Organogenesis in a defined medium supplemented with transferrin. *Cell Differ* 1981;10:281–288.
41a. Enomoto H, Araki T, Jackman A, et al. GFR alpha1-deficient mice have deficits in the enteric nervous system and kidneys. *Neuron* 1998; 21:317–324.
42. Esquela AF, Lee SJ. Regulation of metanephric kidney development by growth/differentiation factor 11. *Dev Biol* 2003;257:356–370.
43. Falk M, Salmivirta K, Durbeej M, et al. Integrin alpha 6B beta 1 is involved in kidney tubulogenesis in vitro. *J Cell Sci* 1996:109:2801–2810.
44. Fujii T, Pichel JG, Taira M, Toyama R, Dawid IB, Westphal H. Expression patterns of the murine LIM class homeobox gene lim1 in the developing brain and excretory system. *Dev Dyn* 1994;199:73–83.
45. Galli-Taliadoros LA, Sedgwick JD, Wood SA, Korner H. Gene knock-out technology: a methodological overview for the interested novice. *J Immunol Meth* 1995;181:1–15.
46. Gawlik A, Quaggin SE. Deciphering the renal code: advances in conditional gene targeting. *Physiology (Bethesda)* 2004;19:245–252.
46a. Gotter AL, Manganaro T, Weaver DR, et al. A time-less function for mouse timeless. *Nat Neurosci* 2000;3:755–756.
47. Grieshammer U, Le M, Plump AS, Wang F, Tessier-Lavigne M, Martin GR. SLIT2-mediated ROBO2 signaling restricts kidney induction to a single site. *Dev Cell* 2004;6:709–717.
48. Grisaru S, Cano-Gauci D, Tee J, Filmus J, Rosenblum ND. Glypican-3 modulates BMP- and FGF-mediated effects during renal branching morphogenesis. *Dev Biol* 2001;231:31–46.
49. Grobstein C. Inductive epithelio-mesenchymal interaction in cultured organ rudiments of the mouse. *Science (Wash, DC)* 1953;118:52–55.
50. Grobstein C. Inductive interaction in the development of the mouse metanephros. *J. Exp. Zool.* 1955;130:319–340.
51. Grobstein C. Morphogenetic interaction between embryonic mouse tissues separated by a membrane filter. *Nature (Lond)* 1953;172:869–871.
52. Grobstein C. Trans-filter induction of tubules in mouse metanephrogenic mesenchyme. *Exp Cell Res* 1956;10:424–440.
53. Hatini V, Huh SO, Herzlinger D, Soares VC, Lai E. Essential role of stromal mesenchyme in kidney morphogenesis revealed by targeted disruption of Winged Helix transcription factor BF-2. *Genes Dev* 96;10:1467–1478.
54. Herzlinger D, Qiao J, Cohen D, Ramakrishna N, Brown AM. Induction of kidney epithelial morphogenesis by cells expressing Wnt-1. *Develop Biol* 1994;166:815–818.
55. Hewitt SM, Hamada S, McDonnell TJ, Rauscher FJ, 3rd, Saunders GF. Regulation of the proto-oncogenes bcl-2 and c-myc by the Wilms' tumor suppressor gene WT1. *Cancer Res* 1995;55:5386–5389.
56. Hsu DR, Economides AN, Wang X, Eimon PM, Harland RM. The Xenopus dorsalizing factor Gremlin identifies a novel family of secreted proteins that antagonize BMP activities. *Mol Cell* 1998;1:673–683.
57. Hyink DP, Abrahamson DR. Origin of the glomerular vasculature in the developing kidney. *Seminars in Nephrology* 1995;15:300–314.
58. Kanwar YS, Ota K, Yang Q, et al. Isolation of rat fibrillin-1 cDNA and its relevance in metanephric development. *Am J Physiol* 1998;275:F710–723.
59. Kanwar YS, Ota K, Yang Q, et al. Role of membrane-type matrix metalloproteinase 1 (MT-1-MMP), MMP-2, and its inhibitor in nephrogenesis. *Am J Physiol* 1999;277:F934–947.
60. Kanwar YS, Wada J, Lin S, et al. Update of extracellular matrix, its receptors, and cell adhesion molecules in mammalian nephrogenesis. *Am J Physiol Renal Physiol* 2004;286:F202–215.
61. Karavanova ID, Dove LF, Resau JH, Perantoni AO. Conditioned medium from a rat ureteric bud cell line in combination with bFGF induces complete differentiation of isolated metanephric mesenchyme. *Development* 1996:122:4159–4167.
62. Karihaloo A, Karumanchi SA, Barasch J, et al. Endostatin regulates branching morphogenesis of renal epithelial cells and ureteric bud. *Proc Natl Acad Sci U S A* 2001;98:12509–12514.
63. Kispert A, Vainio S, Shen L, Rowitch DH, McMahon AP. Proteoglycans are required for maintenance of Wnt-11 expression in the ureter tips. *Development* 1996:122:3627–3637.
64. Kjellen L, Lindahl U. Proteoglycans: structures and interactions (published erratum appears in *Annu Rev Biochem* 1992;61:following viii). *Annu Rev Biochem* 1991;60:443–475.
65. Kjelsberg C, Sakurai H, Spokes K, et al. Met -/- kidneys express epithelial cells that chemotax and form tubules in response to EGF receptor ligands. *Am J Physiol* 1997;272:F222–228.
66. Klein DJ, Brown DM, Moran A, Oegema TR, Jr., Platt JL. Chondroitin sulfate proteoglycan synthesis and reutilization of beta-D- xyloside-initiated chondroitin/dermatan sulfate glycosaminoglycans in fetal kidney branching morphogenesis. *Dev Biol* 1989:133:515–528.
67. Klein G, Ekblom M, Fecker L, Timpl R, Ekblom P. Differential expression of laminin A and B chains during development of embryonic mouse organs. *Development* 1990;110:823–837.
68. Klein G, Langegger M, Timpl R, Ekblom P. Role of laminin A chain in the development of epithelial cell polarity. *Cell* 1988:55:331–341.
69. Koseki C, Herzlinger D, al-Awqati Q. Apoptosis in metanephric development. *J Cell Biol* 1992;119:1327–1333.
70. Kramer S, Okabe M, Hacohen N, Krasnow MA, Hiromi Y. Sprouty: a common antagonist of FGF and EGF signaling pathways in Drosophila. *Development* 1999;126:2515–2525.
71. Kreidberg JA, Donovan MJ, Goldstein SL, et al. Alpha 3 beta 1 integrin has a crucial role in kidney and lung organogenesis. *Development* 1996:122:3537–3547.
72. Kreidberg JA, Sariola H, Loring JM, et al. WT-1 is required for early kidney development. *Cell* 1993;74:679–691.
73. Kume T, Deng K, Hogan BL. Murine forkhead/winged helix genes Foxc1 (Mf1) and Foxc2 (Mfh1) are required for the early organogenesis of the kidney and urinary tract. *Development* 2000;127:1387–1395.

74. Laitinen L, Virtanen I, Saxen L. Changes in the glycosylation pattern during embryonic development of mouse kidney as revealed with lectin conjugates. *J Histochem Cytochem* 1987:35:55–65.
75. Lechner MS, Dressler GR. The molecular basis of embryonic kidney development. *Mech Dev* 1997;62:105–120.
76. Lehtonen E. Epithelio-mesenchymal interface during mouse kidney tubule induction in vivo. *J Embryol Exp Morphol* 1975:34:695–705.
77. Lehtonen E, Wartiovaara J, Nordling S, Saxen L. Demonstration of cytoplasmic processes in Millipore filters permitting kidney tubule induction. *J Embryol Exp Morphol* 1975:33:187–203.
78. Lelongt B, Makino H, Dalecki TM, Kanwar YS. Role of proteoglycans in renal development. *Dev Biol* 1988:128:256–276.
79. Lelongt B, Trugnan G, Murphy G, Ronco PM. Matrix metalloproteinases MMP2 and MMP9 are produced in early stages of kidney morphogenesis but only MMP9 is required for renal organogenesis in vitro. *J Cell Biol* 1997;36:1363–1373.
80. Lescher B, Haenig B, Kispert A. sFRP-2 is a target of the Wnt-4 signaling pathway in the developing metanephric kidney. *Dev Dyn* 1998;213:440–451.
81. Leveen P, Pekny M, Gebre-Medhin S, Swolin B, Larsson E, Betsholtz C. Mice deficient for PDGF B show renal, cardiovascular, and hematological abnormalities. *Genes Dev* 1994;8: 1875–1887.
82. Levinson RS, Batourina E, Choi C, Vorontchikhina M, Kitajewski J, Mendelsohn CL. Foxd1-dependent signals control cellularity in the renal capsule, a structure required for normal renal development. *Development* 2005;132:529–539.
83. Li X, Oghi KA, Zhang J, et al. Eya protein phosphatase activity regulates Six1-Dach-Eya transcriptional effects in mammalian organogenesis. *Nature* 2003;426:247–254.
84. Li YS, Milner PG, Chauhan AK, et al. Cloning and expression of a developmentally regulated protein that induces mitogenic and neurite outgrowth activity. *Science* 1990;250: 1690–1694.
85. Li Z, Stuart RO, Qiao J, et al. A role for Timeless in epithelial morphogenesis during kidney development. *Proc Natl Acad Sci U S A* 2000;97:10038–10043.
86. Lin Y, Liu A, Zhang S, et al. Induction of ureter branching as a response to Wnt-2b signaling during early kidney organogenesis. *Dev Dyn* 2001;222:26–39.
87. Lombard MN, Grobstein C. Activity in various embryonic and postembryonic sources for induction of kidney tubules. *Dev Biol* 1969:19:41–51.
88. Lopez-Nieto CE, You G, Bush KT, Barros EJ, Beier DR, Nigam SK. Molecular cloning and characterization of NKT, a gene product related to the organic cation transporter family that is almost exclusively expressed in the kidney. *J Biol Chem* 1997;272:6471–6478.
89. Luetteke NC, Qui TH, Peiffer RL, Oliver P, Smithies O, Lee DC. TGF-a deficiency results in hair follicle and eye abnormalities in targeted and waved-1 mice. *Cell* 1993;73:263–278.
90. Luo G, Hofmann C, Bronckers AL, Sohocki M, Bradley A, Karsenty G. BMP-7 is an inducer of nephrogenesis, and is also required for eye development and skeletal patterning. *Genes Dev* 1995;9:2808–2820.
91. Maas R, Elfering S, Glaser T, Jepeal L. Deficient outgrowth of the ureteric bud underlies the renal agenesis phenotype in mice manifesting the limb deformity (ld) mutation. *Dev Dyn* 1994;199:214–228.
91a. Maeshima A, Vaughn DA, Choi Y, Nigam SK. Activin A is an endogenous inhibitor of ureteric bud outgrowth from the Wolffian duct. *Dev Biol* 2006;295:473–485.
92. Majumdar A, Vainio S, Kispert A, McMahon J, McMahon AP. Wnt11 and Ret/Gdnf pathways cooperate in regulating ureteric branching during metanephric kidney development. *Development* 2003;130:3175–3185.
93. Mann GB, Fowler KJ, Gabriel A, Nice EC, Williams RL, Dunn AR. Mice with a null mutation of TGFa gene have abnormal skin architecture, wavy hair, and curly whiskers and often develop corneal inflammation. *Cell* 1993;73:249–261.
94. Mansouri A, Chowdhury K, Gruss P. Follicular cells of the thyroid gland require Pax8 gene function. *Nat Genet* 1998;19:87–90.
95. Mass RL, Zeller R, Woychik RP, Vogt TF, Leder P. Disruption of formin-encoding transcripts in two mutant limb deformity alleles. *Nature* 1990;346:853–855.
96. Massague J, Pandiella A. Membrane-anchored growth factors. *Annu Rev Biochem* 1993;62: 515–541.
97. McCright B, Gao X, Shen L, et al. Defects in development of the kidney, heart and eye vasculature in mice homozygous for a hypomorphic Notch2 mutation. *Development* 2001;128:491–502.
98. McPherron AC, Lawler AM, Lee SJ. Regulation of anterior/posterior patterning of the axial skeleton by growth/differentiation factor 11. *Nat Genet* 1999;22:260–264.
99. Mendelsohn C, Batourina E, Fung S, Gilbert T, Dodd J. Stromal cells mediate retinoid-dependent functions essential for renal development. *Development* 1999;126:1139–1148.
100. Meyer TN, Schwesinger C, Bush KT, et al. Spatiotemporal regulation of morphogenetic molecules during in vitro branching of the isolated ureteric bud: toward a model of branching through budding in the developing kidney. *Dev Biol* 2004;275:44–67.
101. Michos O, Panman L, Vintersten K, Beier K, Zeller R, Zuniga A. Gremlin-mediated BMP antagonism induces the epithelial-mesenchymal feedback signaling controlling metanephric kidney and limb organogenesis. *Development* 2004;131:3401–3410.
102. Mitsiadis TA, Salmivirta M, Muramatsu T, et al. Expression of the heparin-binding cytokines, midkine (MK) and HB-GAM (pleiotrophin) is associated with epithelial-mesenchymal interactions during fetal development and organogenesis. *Development* 1995;121:37–51.
103. Miyamoto N, Yoshida M, Kuratani S, Matsuo I, Aizawa S. Defects of urogenital development in mice lacking Emx2. *Development* 1997;124:1653–1664.
104. Miyazaki Y, Oshima K, Fogo A, Hogan BL, Ichikawa I. Bone morphogenetic protein 4 regulates the budding site and elongation of the mouse ureter. *J Clin Invest* 2000;105:863–873.
104a. Monte JC, Sakurai H, Bush KT, Nigam SK. The developmental nephrome: systems biology in the developing kidney. *Curr Opin Nephrol Hypertens* 2007;16:3–9.
105. Montesano R, Matsumoto K, Nakamura T, Orci L. Identification of a fibroblast-derived epithelial morphogen as hepatocyte growth factor. *Cell* 1991;67:901–908.
106. Montesano R, Schaller G, Orci L. Induction of epithelial tubular morphogenesis in vitro by fibroblast-derived soluble factors. *Cell* 1991;66:697–711.
107. Moore MW, Klein RD, Farinas I, et al. Renal and neuronal abnormalities in mice lacking GDNF. *Nature* 1996:382:76–79.
108. Mugrauer G, Ekblom P. Contrasting expression patterns of three members of the myc family of protooncogenes in the developing and adult mouse kidney. *J Cell Biol* 1991;112:13–25.
109. Muller U, Wang D, Denda S, Meneses JJ, Pedersen RA, Reichardt LF. Integrin alpha8beta1 is critically important for epithelial-mesenchymal interactions during kidney morphogenesis. *Cell* 1997; 88:603–613.
110. Mundlos S, Pelletier J, Darveau A, Bachmann M, Winterpacht A, Zabel B. Nuclear localization of the protein encoded by the Wilms' tumor gene WT1 in embryonic and adult tissues. *Development* 1993;119:1329–1341.
111. Nakai S, Sugitani Y, Sato H, et al. Crucial roles of Brn1 in distal tubule formation and function in mouse kidney. *Development* 2003;130:4751–4759.
111a. Nigam SK. From the ureteric bud to the penome. *Kidney Int* 2003;64:2320–2322.
112. Nishinakamura R, Matsumoto Y, Nakao K, et al. Murine homolog of SALL1 is essential for ureteric bud invasion in kidney development. *Development* 2001;128:3105–3115.
113. Oh SP, Li E. The signaling pathway mediated by the type IIB activin receptor controls axial patterning and lateral asymmetry in the mouse. *Genes Dev* 1997;11:1812–1826.
114. Oh SP, Yeo CY, Lee Y, Schrewe H, Whitman M, Li E. Activin type IIA and IIB receptors mediate Gdf11 signaling in axial vertebral patterning. *Genes Dev* 2002;16:2749–2754.
115. Ohuchi H, Hori Y, Yamasaki M, et al. FGF10 acts as a major ligand for FGF receptor 2 IIIb in mouse multi-organ development. *Biochem Biophys Res Commun* 2000;277:643–649.
116. Osathanondh V, Potter E. Development of human kidney as shown by microdissection, II: renal pelvis, calyses, and papillae. *Arch Pathol* 1963;76:277–289.
117. Osathanondh V, Potter E. Development of human kidney as shown by microdissection, III: Formation and interrelationships of collecting tubules and nephrons. *Arch Pathol* 1963;76:290–302.
118. Osathanondh V, Potter EL. Development of human kidney as shown by microdissection, V: development of vascular pattern of glomerulus. *Arch Pathol* 1966:82:403–411.
119. Pichel JG, Shen L, Sheng HZ, et al. Defects in enteric innervation and kidney development in mice lacking GDNF. *Nature* 1996:382:73–76.
120. Plachov D, Chowdhury K, Walther C, Simon D, Guenet JL, Gruss P. Pax8, a murine paired box gene expressed in the developing excretory system and thyroid gland. *Development* 1990;110:643–651.
121. Plisov SY, Yoshino K, Dove LF, Higinbotham KG, Rubin JS, Perantoni AO. TGF beta 2, LIF and FGF2 cooperate to induce nephrogenesis. *Development* 2001;128:1045–1057.
122. Pohl M, Sakurai H, Bush KT, Nigam SK. Matrix metalloproteinases and their inhibitors regulate in vitro ureteric bud branching morphogenesis. *Am J Physiol Renal Physiol* 2000;279: F891–900.
123. Pohl M, Sakurai H, Stuart RO, Nigam SK. Role of hyaluronan and CD44 in in vitro branching morphogenesis of ureteric bud cells. *Dev Biol* 2000;224:312–325.
124. Pohl M, Stuart RO, Sakurai H, Nigam SK. Branching morphogenesis during kidney development. *Annu Rev Physiol* 2000;62:595–620.
125. Pontoglio M, Barra J, Hadchouel M, et al. Hepatocyte nuclear factor 1 inactivation results in hepatic dysfunction, phenylketonuria, and renal Fanconi syndrome. *Cell* 1996:84:575–585.
126. Powell-Braxton L, Hollingshead P, Warburton C, et al. IGF-I is required for normal embryonic growth in mice. *Genes Dev* 1993;7:2609–2617.
127. Preminger GM, Koch WE, Fried FA, Mandell J. Utilization of the chick chorioallantoic membrane for in vitro growth of the embryonic murine kidney. *Am J Anat* 1980:159:17–24.
128. Qiao J, Bush KT, Steer DL, et al. Multiple fibroblast growth factors support growth of the ureteric bud but have different effects on branching morphogenesis. *Mech Dev* 2001;109:123–135.
129. Qiao J, Sakurai H, Nigam SK. Branching morphogenesis independent of mesenchymal-epithelial contact in the developing kidney. *Proc Natl Acad Sci U S A* 1999;96:7330–7335.
130. Qiao J, Uzzo R, Obara-Ishihara T, Degenstein L, Fuchs E, Herzlinger D. FGF-7 modulates ureteric bud growth and nephron number in the developing kidney. *Development* 1999;126: 547–554.
131. Quaggin SE, Schwartz L, Cui S, et al. The basic-helix-loop-helix protein pod1 is critically important for kidney and lung organogenesis. *Development* 1999;126:5771–5783.
132. Quaggin SE, Vanden Heuvel GB, Igarashi P. Pod-1, a mesoderm-specific basic-helix-loop-helix protein expressed in mesenchymal and glomerular epithelial cells in the developing kidney. *Mech Dev* 1998;71:37–48.
133. Raatikainen-Ahokas A, Hytonen M, Tenhunen A, Sainio K, Sariola H. BMP-4 affects the differentiation of metanephric mesenchyme and reveals an early anterior-posterior axis of the embryonic kidney. *Dev Dyn* 2000;217:146–158.
134. Revest JM, Spencer-Dene B, Kerr K, De Moerlooze L, Rosewell I, Dickson C. Fibroblast growth factor receptor 2-IIIb acts upstream of Shh and Fgf4 and is required for limb bud maintenance but not for the induction of Fgf8, Fgf10, Msx1, or Bmp4. *Dev Biol* 2001;231:47–62.
135. Ritvos O, Tuuri T, Eramaa M, et al. Activin disrupts epithelial branching morphogenesis in developing glandular organs of the mouse. *Mech Dev* 1995;50:229–245.
136. Robert B, St. John PL, Hyink DP, Abrahamson DR. Evidence that embryonic kidney cells expressing flk-1 are intrinsic, vasculogenic angioblasts. *Am J Physiol* 1996:271:F744–753.
137. Rogers SA, Ryan G, Hammerman MR. Insulin-like growth fact-ors I and II are produced in the metanephros and are requi-red for growth and development in vitro. *J Cell Biol* 1991;113:1447–1453.
138. Rogers SA, Ryan G, Hammerman MR. Metanephric transforming growth factor-alpha is required for renal organogenesis in vitro. *Am J Physiol* 1992;262:F533–539.
139. Ryan G, Steele-Perkins V, Morris JF, Rauscher FJ, 3rd, Dressler GR. Repression of Pax-2 by WT1 during normal kidney development. *Development* 1995;121:867–875.
140. Sainio K, Suvanto P, Wartiovaara J, et al. Glial-cell-line-derived neurotrophic factor is required for bud initiation from ureteric epithelium. *Dev Suppl* 1997;124:4077–4087.
141. Sakai T, Larsen M, Yamada KM. Fibronectin requirement in branching morphogenesis. *Nature* 2003;423:876–881.
142. Sakurai H, Barros EJ, Tsukamoto T, Barasch J, Nigam SK. An in vitro tubulogenesis system using cell lines derived from the embryonic kidney shows dependence on multiple soluble growth factors. *Proc Natl Acad Sci U S A* 1997;94:6279–6284.

143. Sakurai H, Bush KT, Nigam SK. Identification of pleiotrophin as a mesenchymal factor involved in ureteric bud branching morphogenesis. *Development* 2001;128:3283–3293.

144. Sakurai H, Nigam SK. Transforming growth factor-beta selectively inhibits branching morphogenesis but not tubulogenesis. *Am J Physiol* 1997;272:F139–146.

145. Sakurai H, Tsukamoto T, Kjelsberg CA, Cantley LG, Nigam SK. EGF receptor ligands are a large fraction of in vitro branching morphogens secreted by embryonic kidney. *Am J Physiol* 1997;273:F463–472.

146. Sampogna RV, Nigam SK. Implications of gene networks for understanding resilience and vulnerability in the kidney branching program. *Physiology (Bethesda)* 2004;19:339–347.

147. Sanchez MP, Silos-Santiago I, Frisen J, He B, Lira SA, Barbacid M. Renal agenesis and the absence of enteric neurons in mice lacking GDNF. *Nature* 1996:382:70–73.

148. Santos OF, Barros EJ, Yang XM, et al. Involvement of hepatocyte growth factor in kidney development. *Dev Biol* 1994;163:525–529.

149. Santos OF, Moura LA, Rosen EM, Nigam SK. Modulation of HGF-induced tubulogenesis and branching by multiple phosphorylation mechanisms. *Dev Biol* 1993;159:535–548.

150. Santos OF, Nigam SK. HGF-induced tubulogenesis and branching of epithelial cells is modulated by extracellular matrix and TGF-beta. *Dev Biol* 1993;160:293–302.

151. Sariola H, Ekblom P, Lehtonen E, Saxen L. Differentiation and vascularization of the metanephric kidney grafted on the chorioallantoic membrane. *Dev Biol* 1983;96:427–435.

152. Sariola H, Kuusela P, Ekblom P. Cellular origin of fibronectin in interspecies hybrid kidneys. *J Cell Biol* 1984;99:2099–2107.

153. Sariola H, Timpl R, von der Mark K, et al. Dual origin of glomerular basement membrane. *Dev Biol* 1984;101:86–96.

154. Saxen L. *Organogenesis of the Kidney*. Cambridge UK: Cambridge University Press; 1987.

155. Saxen L, Lehtonen E. Embryonic kidney in organ culture. *Differentiation* 1987:36:2–11.

156. Schmidt C, Bladt F, Goedecke S, et al. Scatter factor/hepatocyte growth factor is essential for liver development. *Nature (Lond)* 1995;373:699–702.

157. Schnabel CA, Godin RE, Cleary ML. Pbx1 regulates nephrogenesis and ureteric branching in the developing kidney. *Dev Biol* 2003;254:262–276.

158. Schuchardt A, D'Agati VD, Pachnis V, Costantini F. Renal agenesis and hypodysplasia in ret-k- mutant mice result from defects in ureteric bud development. *Development* 1996:122:1919–1929.

159. Schuger L, S OS, Rheinheimer J, Varani J. Laminin in lung development:effects of anti-laminin antibody in murine lung morphogenesis. *Dev Biol* 1990;137:26–32.

160. Schuger L, Skubitz AP, Zhang J, Sorokin L, He L. Laminin alpha1 chain synthesis in the mouse developing lung: requirement for epithelial-mesenchymal contact and possible role in bronchial smooth muscle development. *J Cell Biol* 1997;139:553–562.

161. Shawlot W, Behringer RR. Requirement for Lim1 in head-organizer function (see comments). *Nature* 1995;374:425–430.

162. Soriano P. Abnormal kidney development and hematological disorders in PDGF beta-receptor mutant mice. *Genes Dev* 1994;8:1888–1896.

163. Stanton BR, Perkins AS, Tessarollo L, Sassoon DA, Parada LF. Loss of N-myc function results in embryonic lethality and failure of the epithelial component of the embryo to develop. *Genes Dev* 1992;6:2235–2247.

164. Stark K, Vainio S, Vassileva G, McMahon AP. Epithelial transformation of metanephric mesenchyme in the developing kidney regulated by Wnt-4. *Nature (Lond)* 1994;372:679–683.

165. Stuart RO, Barros EJ, Ribeiro E, Nigam SK. Epithelial tubulogenesis through branching morphogenesis: relevance to collecting system development (editorial). *J Am Soc Nephrol* 1995;6:1151–1159.

166. Stuart RO, Bush KT, Nigam SK. Changes in global gene expression patterns during development and maturation of the rat kidney. *Proc Natl Acad Sci U S A* 2001;98:5649–5654.

167. Tang MJ, Cai Y, Tsai SJ, Wang YK, Dressler GR. Ureteric bud outgrowth in response to RET activation is mediated by phosphatidylinositol 3-kinase. *Dev Biol* 2002;243:128–136.

168. Threadgill DW, Dlugosz AA, Hansen LA, et al. Targeted disruption of mouse EGF receptor: effect of genetic background on mutant phenotype. *Science (Wash, DC)* 1995;269:230–234.

169. Torres M, Gomez-Pardo E, Dressler GR, Gruss P. Pax-2 controls multiple steps of urogenital development. *Development* 1995;121:4057–4065.

170. Tsang TE, Shawlot W, Kinder SJ, et al. Lim1 activity is required for intermediate mesoderm differentiation in the mouse embryo. *Dev Biol* 2000;223:77–90.

171. Unsworth B, Grobstein C. Induction of kidney tubules in mouse metanephrogenic mesenchyme by various embryonic mesenchymal tissues. *Dev Biol* 1970:21:547–556.

172. Vukicevic S, Kopp JB, Luyten FP, Sampath TK. Induction of nephrogenic mesenchyme by osteogenic protein 1 (bone morphogenetic protein 7). *Proc Natl Acad Sci U S A* 1996:93:9021–9026.

173. Wada J, Liu ZZ, Alvares K, et al. Cloning of cDNA for the alpha subunit of mouse insulin-like growth factor I receptor and the role of the receptor in metanephric development. *Proc Natl Acad Sci U S A* 1993;90:10360–10364.

174. Wang P, Pereira FA, Beasley D, Zheng H. Presenilins are required for the formation of comma- and S-shaped bodies during nephrogenesis. *Development* 2003;130:5019–5029.

175. Wawersik S, Maas RL. Vertebrate eye development as modeled in Drosophila. *Hum Mol Genet* 2000;9:917–925.

177. Wellik DM, Hawkes PJ, Capecchi MR. Hox11 paralogous genes are essential for metanephric kidney induction. *Genes Dev* 2002;16:1423–1432.

178. Werner H, Re GG, Drummond IA, et al. Increased expression of the insulin-like growth factor I receptor gene, IGF1R, in Wilms tumor is correlated with modulation of IGF1R promoter activity by the WT1 Wilms tumor gene product. *Proc Natl Acad Sci U S A* 1993;90:5828–5832.

179. Wilkinson DG, Bailes JA, McMahon AP. Expression of the proto-oncogene int-1 is restricted to specific neural cells in the developing mouse embryo. *Cell* 1987:50:79–88.

180. Wilson JG, Roth CB, Warkany J. An analysis of the syndrome of malformations induced by maternal vitamin A deficiency. Effects of restoration of vitamin A at various times during gestation. *Am J Anat* 1953;92:189–217.

181. Wong K, Park HT, Wu JY, Rao Y. Slit proteins: molecular guidance cues for cells ranging from neurons to leukocytes. *Curr Opin Genet Dev* 2002;12:583–591.

182. Wynshaw-Boris A, Ryan G, Deng CX, et al. The role of a single formin isoform in the limb and renal phenotypes of limb deformity. *Mol Med* 1997;3:372–384.

183. Xu PX, Adams J, Peters H, Brown MC, Heaney S, Maas R. Eya1-deficient mice lack ears and kidneys and show abnormal apoptosis of organ primordia. *Nat Genet* 1999;23:113–117.

184. Xu PX, Zheng W, Huang L, Maire P, Laclef C, Silvius D. Six1 is required for the early organogenesis of mammalian kidney. *Development* 2003;130:3085–3094.

185. Yang J, Blum A, Novak T, Levinson R, Lai E, Barasch J. An epithelial precursor is regulated by the ureteric bud and by the renal stroma. *Dev Biol* 2002;246:296–310.

186. Yoshino K, Rubin JS, Higinbotham KG, et al. Secreted Frizzled-related proteins can regulate metanephric development. *Mech Dev* 2001;102:45–55.

187. Yu J, McMahon AP, Valerius MT. Recent genetic studies of mouse kidney development. *Curr Opin Genet Dev* 2004;14:550–557.

188. Zegers MM, O'Brien LE, Yu W, Datta A, Mostov KE. Epithelial polarity and tubulogenesis in vitro. *Trends Cell Biol* 2003;13:169–176.

189. Zent R, Bush KT, Pohl ML, et al. Involvement of laminin binding integrins and laminin-5 in branching morphogenesis of the ureteric bud during kidney development. *Dev Biol* 2001;238:289–302.

190. Zhang H, Palmer R, Gao X, et al. Transcriptional activation of placental growth factor by the forkhead/winged helix transcription factor FoxD1. *Curr Biol* 2003;13:1625–1629.

191. Zhao H, Kegg H, Grady S, et al. Role of fibroblast growth factor receptors 1 and 2 in the ureteric bud. *Dev Biol* 2004;276:403–415.

CHAPTER 25

Molecular and Cellular Mechanisms of Glomerular Capillary Development

Jeffrey H. Miner and Dale R. Abrahamson

Washington University School of Medicine, St. Louis, Missouri, USA
University of Kansas Medical Center, Kansas City, Kansas, USA

Among all of the capillaries in the body, the glomerulus is arguably the most unusual and important, if not the most aesthetically interesting. In this chapter, we review the morphogenesis of this unique capillary, discuss the origins of its cells and extracellular matrices, and describe some of the primary regulatory events that occur during glomerular development.

GLOMERULAR MORPHOGENESIS

Formation of the permanent, metanephric kidney begins at embryonic day 11 in mice, day 12 in rats, and during the fourth to fifth weeks of gestation in humans (135). As the ureteric bud projects from the mesonephric duct and enters the metanephric anlage, mesenchymal cells begin condensing around the bud's advancing tip. Soon thereafter, the condensed mesenchyme converts to an epithelial phenotype and proceeds through a developmental sequence of nephric structures, which are termed *vesicle, comma- and S-shaped, developing capillary loop*, and *maturing glomerulus stages* (4, 135). These processes of mesenchymal cell induction and aggregation, conversion to epithelium, and glomerular and tubule differentiation occur repeatedly until the full complement of nephrons has developed. Nephrogenesis concludes ~1 week after birth in rodents (135), and during the 34th gestational week in humans (162).

Vesicle Stage

At the inception of the vesicle stage of nephron development, the aggregated mesenchymal cells near the ureteric bud tips convert to a cluster of epithelial cells (vesicle) and begin assembling a basement membrane matrix containing collagen type IV, laminin, and basement membrane proteoglycans around the basal surface of the vesicle (3, 28, 86). As development progresses through the comma- and then S-shaped stages, a groove (vascular cleft) forms in the lower aspect of the vesicle, into which migrate endothelial precursor cells (angioblasts) (Fig. 1). Two epithelial layers can be distinguished beneath the vascular cleft: visceral epithelial cells of Bowman's capsule (which ultimately differentiate into podocytes) and

parietal epithelial cells (which will become the thin epithelium lining Bowman's capsule of the mature nephron). Epithelial cells above the vascular cleft ultimately develop into proximal, Henle's loop, and distal tubule epithelium. During the S-shaped phase of nephron development, the distal segment fuses with the same ureteric bud branch tip that initially induced the nephric structure, so that the lumen of the forming nephron is now continuous with that of the developing collecting system. Continued growth and branching of the ureteric bud leads to the induction of new mesenchymal aggregates, and glomerulo- and tubulogenesis continue until the full complement of nephrons is achieved (135).

Vascular Clefts of Comma- and S-Shaped Stage

With the progressive invasion and differentiation of endothelial cells, the developing capillary endothelium assembles a subendothelial basement membrane matrix. Similarly, the developing podocyte cell layer assembles a subepithelial basement membrane, so that two distinct basal laminae can be seen between the endothelial and epithelial cells (Fig. 2). As nephrons develop further, these two basement membranes layers merge to form the glomerular basement membrane (GBM), with endothelial cells lining its inner surface and podocytes adherent to its outer surface (6).

Capillary Loop

As glomerular capillary loops begin to form, the endothelial cells gradually flatten and become extensively fenestrated (Figs. 3 and 4). Initially, the fenestrations are spanned by diaphragms but these structures soon disappear. The epithelial podocytes, which originally were columnar with apical junctional complexes, also begin to flatten and begin sending out basolateral cytoplasmic projections that interdigitate with similar projections from neighboring cells (Fig. 3). As glomeruli mature, these projections go on to develop into the podocyte pedicels or foot processes (Figs. 3 and 4). The apical junctional complexes migrate basolaterally between these cellular projections, and, although the mechanism is not fully understood (see

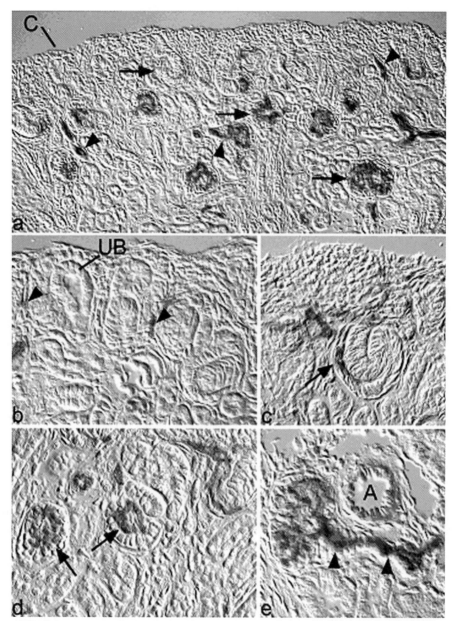

FIGURE 1   Sections of developing kidney from a heterozygous Flk1/LacZ transgenic mouse. Blue reaction product reflects cellular sites of Flk1 (VEGFR2) gene transcription. **A:** Kidney cortex contains a range of glomeruli at different stages of development (*arrows*) that are lined by endothelial cells expressing Flk1. Vascular endothelium throughout the cortex also express Flk1 (*arrowheads*). **B:** Higher magnification view of outer cortex. Note blue cells scattered in mesenchyme (*arrowheads*). **C:** Nephric figure at S-shaped stage. Endothelial cells expressing Flk1 can be seen migrating into the vascular cleft (*arrow*), which is the initial site of glomerlar formation. **D:** Two capillary loop–stage glomeruli can be seen (*arrows*). **E:** Maturing stage glomerulus with attached arteriole (*arrowheads*). A, small artery; C, capsule; UB, branch of ureteric bud. (Reprinted from Robert B, Abrahamson DR. Control of glomerular capillary development by growth factor/receptor kinases. *Pediatr Nephrol* 2001;16:294–301, with permission). See color insert.

following section), seem to convert into the slit diaphragm complex between foot processes (117) (Fig. 4). Metabolic labeling studies, histochemical and immunohistochemical techniques, and interspecies transplantation experiments (2, 74, 86, 118, 134) have all shown that both the endothelium and epithelium are actively synthesizing GBM proteins at this time (3).

Maturing Glomeruli

Here, capillary loop diameters expand, and endothelial and podocyte cell layers differentiate further until the fully mature glomerular morphology is achieved. Unfused basement membranes are rarely seen in maturing glomeruli. On the other hand, complex, irregular projections of basement membrane

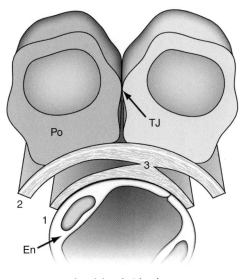

Laminin α1, β1, γ1
α4, β1, γ1
Collagen α1, α2(IV)

FIGURE 2 Diagram showing spatial relationships during development of glomerular capillary wall. During initial glomerular development, endothelial cells (En) migrate into vascular clefts of comma- and S-shaped nephrons. Dual sheets of subendothelial (1) and subepithelial (2) basement membranes separate the endothelium from the developing podocyte (Po) cell layers. Areas of basement membrane fusion can be seen (3). The immature glomerular basement membrane contains laminin α1, β1, γ1; laminin α4, β1, and γ1; and collagen α1 and α2(IV) at this time. Apical tight junctional complexes (*TJ*) exist between immature podocytes.

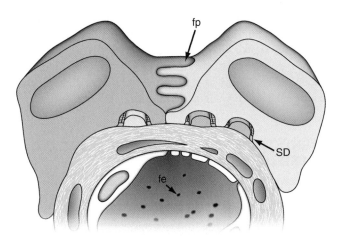

Laminin α5, β1, γ1
α5, β2, γ1
Collagen α1, α2(IV)
α3, α4, α5 (IV)

FIGURE 3 During intermediate, capillary loop and maturing stages of glomerular development, fenestrae (*fe*) form in the endothelial cells. Foot process (*fp*) extension occurs between podocytes and epithelial slit diaphragms (*SD*) first appear. Remodeling and splicing of newly synthesized glomerular capillary membrane (GBM) into existing, fused, GBM takes place, and new isoforms of GBM laminin and type IV collagen are seen.

are commonly found beneath podocytes at this stage, particularly in areas where foot process formation is still incomplete. In vivo labeling studies have shown that these subepithelial basement membrane segments are somehow spliced or inserted into the existing fused GBM, possibly to provide the additional GBM material necessary for the inflating capillaries (5, 23). Shortly after the initial, vascular cleft stage, and continuing into maturing glomeruli, modification and remodeling of the GBM occurs with the appearance of new basement membrane protein isoforms and disappearance of earlier species. As discussed in subsequent sections, however, we do not understand how these events are regulated at either the gene or protein level. Additionally, once the glomerulus is fully mature (Fig. 4), matrix synthesis and cell morphogenesis virtually halt (except for some poorly understood activities responsible for GBM "maintenance" or "turnover") and how these processes are downregulated are also not known.

ORIGIN OF THE GLOMERULAR ENDOTHELIUM

Extrarenal Origins

Although compelling evidence has accumulated showing that nephron epithelial cells, including the visceral and parietal epithelium of Bowman's capsule, all derive originally from the metanephric mesenchyme, the origin of vascular endothelial cells during kidney organogenesis has been more difficult to understand (69). Studies conducted nearly 25 years ago convincingly showed that cells of extrarenal origin grew into the metanephros and established the microvasculature, including the glomerular capillary tufts. These studies involved the grafting of embryonic, avascular mouse or quail kidney rudiments onto avian chorioallantoic membranes. After culturing in ovo, the kidney grafts contained glomerular endothelial and mesangial cells stemming from host chorioallantoic tissues, therefore signifying the ingress of vessel progenitors from sites outside the kidney (133, 134).

Intrarenal Origins

Contrary to the view discussed previously, several lines of evidence from a number of more recent experiments have shown that the metanephros contains its own pool of endothelial progenitors (angioblasts) capable of vascularizing nephrons in vivo. The first clues about the existence of these intrinsic metanephric angioblasts came from transplantation studies between mice and rats. For example, when embryonic day (E)–12 mouse kidneys are grafted into anterior eye chambers of rats, the vascular and glomerular basement membranes that develop within the grafts after transplantation are almost entirely of mouse (graft) origin (70). Similarly, when E12 kidneys are transplanted under kidney capsules of adult ROSA26 mice (which bear a ubiquitously expressed LacZ reporter gene useful as a lineage marker) all

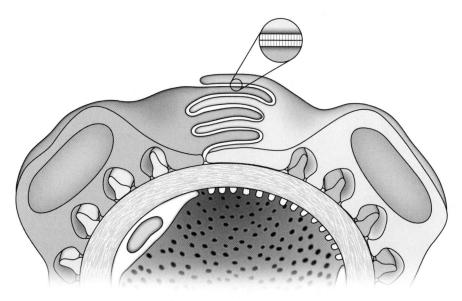

Laminin α**5**, β**2**, γ**1**
Collagen α3, α4, α5 (IV)

FIGURE 4   As glomeruli approach full maturation, the endothelium becomes extensively fenestrated, and the mature glomerular basement membrane (GBM) laminin and collagen type IV isoforms are now in place. In the podocyte layer, foot process extension and interdigitation finalizes, and epithelial slit diaphragms completely span the filtration slits. Inset shows structure of SD viewed en face.

of the microvascular and glomerular endothelial *cells* within grafts are derived from the engrafted kidney, not from the host (125). Furthermore, when kidneys from E12 ROSA26 mice are grafted into the nephrogenic renal cortices of newborn wild-type hosts, endothelial cells stemming from the grafts can be seen integrating into host vasculature (125). In additional experiments, when embryonic kidneys from Flk1 (VEGF receptor-2)–LacZ heterozygous mice are grown under routine organ culture conditions, Flk1-LacZ–positive microvessels do not develop in vitro, despite the extensive formation of metanephric tubules and avascular glomerular epithelial tufts (124). When these same cultured kidneys are then transplanted into anterior eye chambers of wild-type host mice, the grafts develop microvessels and vascularized glomeruli lined by Flk1-LacZ–expressing cells, indicating again that the endothelium originates from the engrafted kidney itself and not from the host (124). Several other research groups have reached similar conclusions independently. For example, when avascular metanephroi from E11 Tie1/LacZ transgenic mice are transplanted into newborn wild-type hosts, widespread expression of Tie1/LacZ is found within glomeruli developing within grafts (90). Others have immunolocalized putative angioblasts in the metanephric mesenchyme of prevascular embryonic rat kidney (151).

Although current evidence shows that the embryonic kidney contains a pool of angioblasts capable of establishing the glomerular endothelium, whether these progenitors originate initially from outside the metanephric blastema or instead stem directly from metanephric mesenchyme is not yet clear. Nevertheless, immunolabeling experiments in developing rat kidney shows that endothelial as well as mesangial cell precursors share common markers during glomerulogenesis (RECA-1 and Thy1.1, respectively), suggesting that they may indeed derive from metanephric mesenchyme (122). Other immunolocalization and transplantation experiments have also shown that juxtaglomerular cells in developing kidney also originate from metanephric mesenchyme, although they appear to stem from a different lineage than endothelial and mesangial cells (138).

ENDOTHELIAL CELL RECRUITMENT AND DIFFERENTIATION

Mechanisms controlling vascular development are highly complex and involve several different transcription factors, cell–cell and cell–matrix interactions, and many membrane receptor–ligand signaling cascades. Although our knowledge of these systems in a variety of vascular beds has improved dramatically during the past several years, many key questions regarding temporal and spatial controls still persist. With respect to the formation of glomerular capillaries, the process can be considered to progress through four interrelated events: (1) angioblast survival, proliferation, and differentiation into endothelium; (2) endothelial cell recruitment; (3) initial assembly of the glomerular capillary tuft and associated mesangium; and (4) glomerular capillary stabilization and maturation (21, 123).

VEGF Signaling

Among all of the mechanisms involved with development of the systemic vasculature, signals evoked by binding of VEGF to its cellular receptors, VEGFR1 and VEGFR2 (or in mice, Flt1 and Flk1, respectively) are singularly critical. Mice with homozygous *VEGF* gene deletions die by E9.5 with severe vascular deficits. Remarkably, *VEGF* heterozygote mutants also succumb by E12 with vascular phenotypes, indicating that a single *VEGF* allele is insufficient to direct normal vascular development (15, 33). Homozygous (but not heterozygous) *Flk1* and *Flt1* mutants die at mid-gestation due to failure of endothelial differentiation (139) and vessel integrity (34), respectively.

Developing podocytes are key sources of VEGF (142), and its secretion and binding to angioblasts bearing VEGF receptors may initiate their recruitment into the vascular cleft of comma- and S-shaped nephrons (150), which is the initial site of glomerulogenesis. Because *VEGF* and *VEGFR2* knockout mice die with vascular phenotypes before glomerulogenesis commences, the precise role of this ligand/receptor pair in mediating glomerular endothelial development has been difficult to analyze fully. Nevertheless, and underscoring the importance of the VEGF signaling system, injection of VEGF blocking antibodies into developing mouse kidney cortex inhibits glomerular capillary formation in vivo (80). With the advent of cell-selective and/or inducible gene-deletion technologies, additional evidence for the importance of podocyte-derived VEGF has been obtained. For example, homozygous deletion of VEGF selectively in podocytes (obtained in bitransgenic mice carrying nephrin-cre recombinase and floxed VEGF-A alleles) results in animals that die perinatally with nonvascularized glomeruli (30). Heterozygous deletion of VEGF causes no evident phenotype initially. By 2.5 weeks of age, however, mice become proteinuric, and glomeruli contain swollen endothelial cells and hyaline deposits similar to those seen in patients with preeclampsia. By contrast, overexpression of the VEGF$_{164}$ isoform specifically in podocytes leads to collapsing glomerulopathy and death at ~5 days of age (31). Clearly, the cellular controls for maintaining VEGF protein expression within an optimal range are critically important for the appropriate establishment and maintenance of the glomerular capillary.

Regulation of Endothelial Development

HYPOXIA-INDUCIBLE TRANSCRIPTION FACTORS

Transcription of *VEGF* and *VEGFR* genes is activated by hypoxia-inducible transcription factors (HIFs), which consist of heterodimers of HIF α and β subunits (159). Under normal oxygen concentrations, the HIFα subunit undergoes prolyl hydroxylation, binding to von Hippel Lindau (VHL) protein, polyubiquitination, and proteasomal degradation. In hypoxia, the prolyl hydroxylase enzyme is inhibited, and HIFα chain degradation is avoided. Hypoxia-stabilized HIFαβ heterodimers bind to hypoxia-responsive elements (HREs) located in promoter/enhancer regions of inducible genes (92), many of which are proteins expressed in response to hypoxic stress. For example, erythropoietin, transferrin, *VEGF*, *VEGFR1*, and *VEGFR2* are among the more than 70 distinct genes known to be transcriptionally activated by HIFs (159).

There are at least three distinct HIFα and two β subunits known at present, making a variety of different HIF isoforms possible. Because HIF stabilization is enhanced in cells experiencing subnormal oxygen tensions, such as those in rapidly growing tissues, robust VEGF and VEGFR synthesis commonly occurs during organogenesis. Increased VEGF/VEGFR signaling stimulates mitosis in endothelial progenitor cells, phosphorylation of the anti-apoptotic kinases Akt/PKB (41) and focal adhesion kinase (FAK) (1), and upregulation of the survival factors Bcl2 and A1 (40). In time, these events can lead to the creation of new blood vessels, which can then provide appropriate levels of oxygen specifically to the formerly hypoxic tissue sites.

RENAL HIF EXPRESSION

The expression patterns for several of the different HIF α and β subunits have been documented in developing human, rat, and mouse kidney using in situ hybridization and immunohistochemistry. In general, both HIF-1 and -2α are found in glomeruli, with specific immunolocalization of -2α protein to immature podocytes (which are rich sources of VEGF) (13, 37). HIF-2α is also expressed by developing vascular endothelial cells in the kidney (most of which express VEGFR-2), whereas HIF-1α is found in cortical and medullary collecting duct epithelium. HIF-1α and -2α protein are undetectable in fully mature glomeruli. Interestingly, HIF-1β is apparently ubiquitously expressed by all cells in kidney, but HIF-2β distribution is greatly restricted during development, and, in mice, becomes confined to nuclei in cells of the thick ascending limb of Henle's loop (36).

The selective expression of certain HIF isoforms in different tissue compartments of developing kidney may reflect the coordinated regulation of different sets of HIF target genes (35). Importantly, individuals with mutations in VHL, a key protein in mediating HIFα chain degradation and thereby reducing expression of HIF target genes, are prone to developing hemangioblastomas and clear cell–renal cell carcinomas (49, 50, 72). A recent study showed that HIF-1α and -2α had differential and sometimes antagonistic effects on the growth of clear cell–renal cell carcinomas, with HIF-1α retarding and HIF-2α promoting tumor growth (116). These new findings provide further evidence for differential effects of different HIF isoforms and call for more studies examining the expression of HIF and HIF gene targets in developing kidney.

Once glomeruli are vascularized and fully mature, podocytes still continue VEGF synthesis. Likewise, expression of Flk1 is also maintained by glomerular endothelial cells of mature kidneys. VEGF-Flk1 signaling in glomeruli therefore probably exerts functions extending well beyond those needed for mobilization of angioblasts and initial formation of the capillary tuft. For example, in co-cultures of epithelial cells with endothelium, epithelial-derived VEGF has been shown to induce fenestrae formation in the endothelium (32). Perhaps the continued expression of VEGF by podocytes and Flk1 by glomerular endothelial cells in vivo is therefore necessary for maintenance of the highly fenestrated state seen in the endothelium.

OTHER GROWTH FACTOR/RECEPTORS

Beyond VEGF and VEGFR, several other growth factor–receptor signaling systems important for vessel development systemically are also crucial for glomerular capillary formation, including the Tie/angiopoietin, and PDGFR/PDGF families (21, 123). Developing glomerular endothelial cells express Tie-2, and one of its ligands, angiopoietin-1, is important for vascular organization and remodeling. Another Tie-2 ligand, angiopoietin-2, may mediate vascular integrity and permeability. The coordinated expression of these two angiopoietins may therefore regulate the maturation and stabilization phases of glomerular development (reviewed in 163). Additionally, Tie-2 and at least some members of the angiopoietins contain defined HREs in their promoters, making their transcriptional regulation by hypoxia/HIFs seem likely (159). Similarly, an HRE is found in the *PDGFB* gene promoter, although this may not necessarily be responsive to hypoxia (152). During early glomerular development, PDGFB protein is expressed by podocytes. This may be important for the glomerular recruitment of immature mesangial cells, which express the PDGFB receptor, PDGFRβ (7). In later developmental stages, both PDGF and PDGFRβ expression becomes confined to the mesangium, which may provide autocrine signals required for mesangial cell proliferation and/or maturation (7) (see following sections).

Like other developing vessels, at least some neuronal axon guidance receptors and ligands are also found in developing glomeruli (27, 81, 126). For example, neuropilin-1 (Np1), which is a coreceptor with VEGFR2 for VEGF$_{164}$ (but lacks a cytoplasmic signaling domain), immunolocalizes to glomerular endothelial cells. Semaphorins-3A and -3F, which are ligands for Np1, have been found on podocytes, suggesting that semaphorin-Np1 signaling between podocytes and endothelium may help pattern glomerular morphogenesis (155). One study, however, has also reported that Np1 is expressed by podocytes in vivo (53). Experiments also showed that podocyte-derived VEGF may act as an autocrine survival factor for cultured podocytes in vitro (46). Additionally, these same studies found an upregulation of VEGFR2 in cultured podocytes, suggesting that VEGF/VEGFR2 signaling is important not only for glomerular capillary formation and maintenance but also for podocyte differentiation (46).

Other receptor–ligand signaling systems probably crucial for glomerular capillary formation include members of the Eph/ephrin receptor/counterreceptor families (21, 124). Specifically, the receptor tyrosine kinase EphB1 and its ligand, ephrin-B1, which itself is also a transmembrane protein receptor, are both expressed in similar distribution patterns in developing kidney microvasculature (22). Although the precise roles for Eph/ephrin signaling in the glomerulus are still uncertain, knockout mice display lethal vascular phenotypes including defects in vessel patterning, sprouting and remodeling (reviewed in 21). Reciprocal gradients of Eph and ephrin protein concentrations have been identified in the developing brain, where they appear to direct accurate neuronal patterning in the visual system. Perhaps analogous events take place in the developing glomerulus, where spatial signals conveyed between endothelial cells help target them to correct microanatomical domains (21).

DEVELOPMENT OF THE MESANGIUM

Fundamentals regarding the development of the intercapillary mesangium, as well as the origin and recruitment of mesangial cell progenitors, are still largely unresolved issues in glomerular biology. Nevertheless, we have known for some time that PDGFB and its receptor, PDGFR, are both expressed by mesangial cells of mature glomeruli (7). Additionally, studies in developing kidney have shown that immature podocytes produce PDGFB, which may help recruit mesangial cell progenitors expressing PDGFR into glomeruli. Later, podocyte expression of PDGF declines and the synthesis of both PDGF and PDGFR becomes confined to the mesangial cells, perhaps to promote their proliferation or maturation (7). Gene-deletion studies in mice have conclusively shown an absolute requirement for PDGFB/PDGFRB signaling. Null mutants for either gene die perinatally with massive hemorrhaging systemically (87, 143). Importantly, glomeruli in these mutants entirely lack mesangial cells and consist of one or only a few large, swollen capillary loops (87, 143).

Interestingly, once the glomerulus has fully matured, there appears to be a small population of extraglomerular mesangial cells capable of completely repopulating the glomerulus if the intraglomerular mesangium becomes severely injured. These mesangial reserve cells reside in the juxtaglomerular apparatus and are distinct from renin-secreting cells, macrophages, vascular smooth muscle cells, and endothelial cells (68). In an anti-Thy 1 model of proliferative glomerulonephritis in rats, these extraglomerular mesangial reserve cells migrate into the glomerulus and entirely restore the depleted intraglomerular mesangium (68). Alternatively, some studies suggest that bone marrow hematopoietic stem cells can be a source of mesangial cells (91). Perhaps additional studies based on these fascinating observations can shed more light on the origin and development of mesangial cells during glomerulogenesis. Similarly, much more work needs to be done on the assembly and maintenance of the mesangial matrix. Although this matrix undergoes morphologic and compositional changes throughout glomerulogenesis, it has not yet been the topic of thorough study. Whether the mesangial matrix is produced exclusively by mesangial cells, or whether glomerular endothelial cells and podocytes also contribute components, are also not understood. On the other hand, and as discussed later, considerable progress has been made in understanding assembly of the GBM.

FACTORS REGULATING PODOCYTE DIFFERENTIATION

Determination of podocyte identity and regulation of podocyte differentiation are fundamental aspects of glomerulogenesis about which little is known. Although the podocyte transcription factors described in the following sections have been shown to be crucial for proper differentiation, how these regulators interact to orchestrate the complex acquisition of the podocyte phenotype remains a mystery. Recent studies aimed at defining the entire glomerular transcriptome (148) will hopefully lead to a better understanding of exactly how the podocyte achieves its unique and important properties.

WT1

The protein that likely has one of the earliest roles in podocyte differentiation is Wilms tumor 1 (WT1), a zinc finger protein that is involved in transcription and RNA processing (56). WT1 is expressed at the initial stages of nephrogenesis, but once glomerulogenesis begins, there is a dramatic increase in the level of WT1 in podocyte precursors, and podocytes continue to express WT1 throughout life (reviewed in 82). One potentially important function of WT1 is to downregulate expression of Pax2 in the immature podocytes of S-shaped–stage nephrons (130). Indeed, transgene-driven overexpression of Pax2 widely, including in podocytes, causes severe nephrotic syndrome (25). In addition, WT1 has been shown to regulate a number of genes, and two reports suggest direct regulation of *NPHS1* (47, 156), the gene encoding nephrin, which is a component of the epithelial slit diaphragm protein complex, and required for filtration barrier function. This provides a clear mechanism whereby alteration in WT1 function directly affects glomerular function.

Several lines of investigation reveal important roles for WT1 in promoting proper podocyte differentiation (reviewed in 56, 82, 113). Most notable is that heterozygous mutations that affect the zinc finger structure of WT1 cause Denys-Drash syndrome in human. This rare disease is characterized by proteinuria, nephrotic syndrome, diffuse mesangial sclerosis, and end-stage renal disease (ESRD). Expression of mutant WT1 forms associated with Denys-Drash syndrome in transgenic mice, either globally or specifically in podocytes, causes various glomerular and podocyte defects that are consistent with the human pathology (56, 109). Moreover, heterozygous mutations in *WT1* that affect the normal pattern of WT1 RNA alternative splicing to generate the so-called $^+$KTS

and $^-$KTS isoforms of WT1 cause Frasier syndrome (132). The renal component of this disease includes proteinuria that begins in early childhood and progresses to focal segmental glomerulosclerosis (FSGS), but the course to ESRD is slower than observed in Denys-Drash syndrome. Mice engineered to express only the $^+$KTS or only the $^-$KTS isoforms develop severe podocyte and glomerular defects, further emphasizing the important role that WT1 and these specific splice variants play in glomerular development and function (52).

LMX1B

LMX1B, a LIM-homeodomain protein, is another transcription factor expressed in podocytes that is affected in human disease. Heterozygous mutations in *LMX1B* cause nail-patella syndrome (26), an autosomal dominant disease with skeletal abnormalities, nail hypoplasia, and variably penetrant nephropathy associated with accumulation of fibrillar material in the GBM that appears to be collagen type III (57). Although *LMX1B*$^{+/-}$ mice do not exhibit a phenotype, *LMX1B*$^{-/-}$ mice die shortly after birth with abnormalities in dorsal limb structures, including absence of nails and patellae, abnormal glomeruli, attenuated podocyte maturation with lack of normal slit diaphragms, and tubular protein casts (16). Analysis of gene expression in *LMX1B*$^{-/-}$ podocytes has revealed decreases in collagen α3 and α4(IV), podocin, and CD2AP (100, 106, 128), which are all known to be important for proper glomerular filtration. The reduced expression in *LMX1B*$^{-/-}$ mice suggests a basis for the partially penetrant nephropathy in *LMX1B*$^{+/-}$ humans, but gene expression studies in affected individuals do not support this hypothesis (57). Thus, exactly how LMX1B haploinsufficiency causes nephropathy in humans remains a mystery. If there really is not a reduction in the expression of relevant podocyte genes, then perhaps there is a lack of repression, either direct or indirect, of genes injurious to glomerular function, as previously proposed (108).

Pod1/Tcf21

Pod1, a basic helix-loop-helix transcription factor also known as epicardin, capsulin, and Tcf21, is highly expressed early during kidney development in condensing metanephric mesenchyme and in stromal cells. In the developing nephron, Pod1 is expressed in podocyte precursors at the S-shaped stage and persists in adult podocytes (113, 115). The kidney phenotype in *Pod1*$^{-/-}$ mice, which die at birth due to heart and lung defects, is complex, but it is clear that there are fewer glomeruli associated with defects in ureteric bud branching. In addition, there is a striking arrest of glomerular development at the capillary loop stage, and podocytes fail to mature properly, elaborating only rudimentary foot processes (114). Interestingly, studies in chimeric mice demonstrate that the presence of wild-type stromal cells can rescue the glomerulogenesis defects, suggesting a non–cell-autonomous role for Pod1 in these cells (20). Gene expression profiling studies of *Pod1*$^{-/-}$ glomeruli revealed 3986 genes expressed differently than in wild-type glomeruli, demonstrating that Pod1 has profound effects on gene expression (19).

Kreisler/Mafb

Kreisler/Mafb is a basic domain leucine zipper transcription factor expressed in podocytes from the capillary loop stage onward (131). Mice that are homozygous for a point mutation affecting the kreisler DNA binding domain die within 24 hours of birth. The podocytes of these mice fail to extend foot processes or establish slit diaphragms, and there is a slight reduction in expression of nephrin and podocin (another slit diaphragm component discussed in more detail below). Interestingly, whereas *Pod1* is expressed in *kreisler*$^{-/-}$ podocytes, *kreisler* is not expressed in *Pod1*$^{-/-}$ podocytes. This suggests the existence of a transcriptional hierarchy in which Pod1 may activate expression of kreisler (131), but this remains to be formally proven.

Foxc2

Foxc2 is a member of the forkhead/winged-helix family of transcription factors. During nephrogenesis, Foxc2 is first expressed in a subset of cells in the comma-shaped body and then is expressed in developing podocytes at the S-shaped and capillary loop stages and more weakly at maturity (147). *Foxc2*$^{-/-}$ mice exhibit small kidneys and reduced numbers of glomeruli with ballooned capillaries, suggesting a defect in adhesion of mesangial cells (which are present) to the GBM. Ultrastructural analyses revealed that podocytes fail to extend processes or assemble slit diaphragms, and endothelial cells fail to become fenestrated, suggesting an arrest of differentiation of these two cell types. Gene expression profiling studies of *Foxc2*$^{-/-}$ glomeruli showed reductions in a number of known podocyte genes, such as *kreisler/Mafb*, *Nphs2* (podocin) and *Podxl1* (podocalyxin), though others, such as *Nphs1*, *Wt1*, and *Cd2ap*, were not affected (147).

Notch2

Notch2 is expressed in developing podocytes from as early as the comma-shaped stage (96). Although the total absence of Notch2 in mice results in embryonic lethality at E11.5, before glomerulogenesis begins, homozygosity for a hypomorphic *Notch2* allele allows survival until 24 hours after birth. These latter *Notch2*$^{-/-}$ mice exhibit small kidneys with cortical vascular lesions. Some glomeruli arrested before the capillary loop stage and were not vascularized, whereas others became vascularized but had ballooned capillaries due to an absence of mesangial cells. In addition, genetic interaction studies demonstrated that Jagged1, a Notch ligand, is required for proper Notch2 signaling during glomerulogenesis (96).

FORMATION OF THE SLIT DIAPHRAGM COMPLEX

In mature glomeruli, the slit diaphragm (SD) represents the only known connection between adjacent podocyte foot processes. The SD spans the space between the interdigitated podocyte foot processes (Fig. 4) and has been proposed to play a crucial role in glomerular filtration by serving as the major barrier to albumin (157). More recently, the SD has been shown to mediate important signaling events that are responsible for maintaining podocyte health (59). Thus, it plays dual roles in ensuring proper glomerular function.

Slit Diaphragm Components

NEPHRIN AND THE NEPH FAMILY

The relatively recent explosion of information on the SD began with the identification of the protein, nephrin, as an integral component of the SD (Fig. 5) (58). The nephrin gene (*NPHS1*) is mutated in congenital nephrotic syndrome of the Finnish type (77). Nephrin is an immunoglobulin (Ig) superfamily member containing extracellular Ig-like domains, a transmembrane domain, and a cytoplasmic tail. Humans and mice lacking nephrin never establish SDs, demonstrating the importance of nephrin for SD formation. A group of three related Ig superfamily molecules that interact with nephrin, Neph1, Neph2, and Neph3, are also found at the SD, and it is clear that at least Neph1 is required for maintenance of the filtration barrier (24). Interestingly, nephrin interacts directly with the Neph proteins (Fig. 5) (12, 42, 43), and disturbing their association in vivo causes proteinuria (89).

ZO-1 AND PODOCIN

Before the identification of nephrin, zonula occludens-1 (ZO-1), an epithelial tight junction protein, was shown to be localized to the cytoplasmic face of the SD (136). ZO-1 has been shown to interact with Neph1-3, which may serve to anchor it to the SD. In turn, podocin, whose encoding gene (*NPHS2*) is mutated in familial steroid resistant nephrotic syndrome, appears important for anchoring nephrin and the Neph family to the SD (Fig. 5). Podocin is a hairpin-shaped integral membrane protein that interacts with the cytoplasmic tails of nephrin and Neph family members (137) and is required to target nephrin to lipid raft microdomains, which are proposed to be crucial for SD organization and function (64).

CADHERINS

Consistent with the notion that the SD is a modified adherens junction (119), two cadherins, P-cadherin and the FAT1 protocadherin, have been localized to the SD. P-cadherin was found to associate with ZO-1 and the catenins at the SD, but the functional importance of P-cadherin at the SD has yet to be demonstrated. FAT1, an extremely large member of the cadherin family, is involved in regulating actin cytoskeleton dynamics and cell polarization (105).

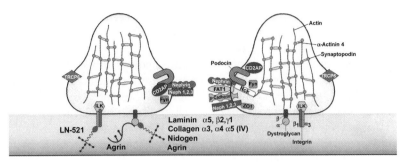

FIGURE 5 Diagram showing clustering of the slit diaphragm complex proteins at the basolateral surfaces of podocyte foot processes, which are attached to the underlying glomerular basement membrane (GBM) (shown as the gray ribbon beneath the foot processes). Molecules are not drawn to scale, but many known extracellular and intracellular protein–protein interactions are represented. Exactly how the several protein ectodomains interact to form the characteristic slit diaphragm ultrastructure is not yet fully defined. See Formation of the Slit Diaphragm Complex, pp. 698–700, for details.

Mice lacking FAT1 die within 2 days of birth, and their podocytes lack SDs and significant foot process formation. This underscores the importance of FAT1 in establishment or maintenance of SDs. A model of the SD that can accommodate the very large extracellular domain of FAT1 has not yet been presented, but FAT1 may somehow contribute to the central density of the SD that is apparent in ultrastructural analyses (127, 157).

CD2AP

CD2-associated protein (CD2AP) is a modular cytoplasmic docking protein that interacts with multiple slit diaphragm components, including nephrin and podocin, as well as with the actin cytoskeleton (Fig. 5) (158, 164). Mice lacking CD2AP exhibit congenital nephrotic syndrome with progressive loss of SDs and foot processes, and they die at 6 to 7 weeks of age (141). In addition, CD2AP haploinsufficiency has been associated with renal disease in mice and humans (62, 79). CD2AP is thought to be an adaptor that forms a bridge between the SD and the cytoskeleton (140), but it also appears to play a role in the trafficking of endocytic vesicles (79, 158).

NCK

That mice lacking CD2AP are able to form normal foot processes and SDs initially suggested the existence of other adaptor proteins in podocytes that might play an earlier role in organizing SDs and linking them to the cytoskeleton. Indeed, the Nck adaptor proteins (Nck1 and Nck2), which contain three Src homology 3 (SH3) domains and one SH2 domain, bind to phosphotyrosine-containing motifs in the cytoplasmic tail of nephrin via their SH2 domains. In addition, clustering of nephrin/Nck complexes reorganized the actin cytoskeleton in transfected cells (71, 153). Importantly, genetically engineered mice lacking Nck1 and Nck2 in podocytes failed to elaborate foot processes or assemble SDs (71). These exciting findings establish a potentially pivotal role for the Nck adaptor proteins in organizing SDs and

suggest one mechanism whereby the Fin minor mutation in *NPHS1*, which results in a nephrin protein lacking most of its cytoplasmic tail and all of the intracellular tyrosines (77), causes congenital nephrotic syndrome.

TRPC6

TRPC6 is a member of the transient receptor potential family of cation channel proteins and is associated with the SD. Mutations in *TRPC6* have been shown to cause autosomal dominant FSGS in several different families, and this was associated with increased calcium current amplitude in some cases (121, 161). Calcium flux mediated by TRPC6 could have an important role in regulating podocyte and SD homeostasis.

Slit Diaphragm Assembly Mechanisms

As mentioned previously, the slit diaphragm bears some relationship to adherens junctions, and ZO-1 immunolocalizes to the cytoplasmic domains on the lateral surfaces of podocytes adjacent to the extracellular diaphragm spanning the slit pore. The synthetic patterns of all of the SD components during glomerular development have not yet been studied in detail. However, nephrin and podocin first appear during the late S-shaped and early capillary loop stages of nephron development, which is when foot process interdigitation first occurs and simultaneous with the first ultrastructural appearance of SDs (58, 104). The precise sequence of SD assembly, including how the linkages between the ectodomains of SD proteins are made, as well as connections with the internal cytoskeleton and associated elements, are not known. Similarly, the extent that the SD may be dynamic and undergo modification with age is poorly understood. Nevertheless, an increasing number of studies have shown that the SD does not merely represent a static component of the glomerular filtration barrier, but it also functions to influence podocyte behavior (59).

Signaling at the Slit Diaphragm

The first evidence that the SD complex may have a signaling role came from studies of nephrin activity in cultured cells. Transfection of cells with nephrin increased activator protein-1 (AP1)–mediated transcriptional activation, and this effect on intracellular signaling was augmented by co-transfection with podocin, to which nephrin binds (61). These authors later showed that podocin recruits nephrin to lipid rafts (64), which are cholesterol-enriched plasma membrane microdomains associated with high concentrations of signaling proteins and high levels of signaling activity. Furthermore, as alluded to previously, nephrin contains multiple tyrosines in its cytoplasmic tail. Some of these can be phosphorylated by the Src-family tyrosine kinase, Fyn (154); and clustering of nephrin by Fyn increases phosphorylation (85). Phosphorylation of nephrin augments its interaction with podocin (88) and allows Nck adaptor proteins to bind its tail and influence the organization of the adjacent actin cytoskeleton (71, 153). Consistent with this, $Fyn^{-/-}$ mice have variably coarsened or effaced foot processes (154). In addition, trans-heterozygous $Fyn^{+/-}$; $Cd2ap^{+/-}$ mice exhibit marked proteinuria and FSGS, and CD2AP can be immunoprecipitated with Fyn from glomerular lysates. These findings demonstrate that Fyn-mediated signaling likely depends on interactions with CD2AP (62).

Nephrin-mediated signaling has also been shown to involve stimulation of phosphoinositide 3-OH kinase (PI3K). Nephrin and CD2AP interact with the p85 regulatory subunit of PI3K, recruit PI3K to the plasma membrane, and, with podocin, stimulate PI3K activation of AKT signaling in podocytes (60). This is proposed to regulate the behavior of podocytes and protect them from detachment-induced apoptosis (anoikis), which suggests that proper signaling at the SD is important for maintaining podocyte health.

Neph family proteins, like nephrin, have cytoplasmic tails containing tyrosines that can be phosphorylated. Also like nephrin, Neph1 can induce AP-1–mediated transcriptional activation (137). ZO-1, which binds to the cytoplasmic tail of Neph proteins, enhances tyrosine phosphorylation of Neph1 and augments AP-1 activation (63). As ZO-1 can also interact with the actin cytoskeleton, one can envision how the podocin/CD2AP/nephrin/Neph/ZO-1 complex can activate signaling in podocytes and provide stability to the SD via linkage to actin (Fig. 5). Interfering with any of these interactions likely leads to abnormal podocyte behavior and proteinuria. In this regard, the actin cytoskeleton in podocyte foot processes also has specialized components. These include α-actinin-4, which is mutated in autosomal dominant FSGS (75), and synaptopodin, which regulates α-actinin's actin bundling activity (9) and binds to CD2AP (62). That trans-heterozygous $Synpo^{+/-}/Cd2ap^{+/-}$ mice develop proteinuria and FSGS-like lesions (62) provides further support for the importance of the SD/actin cytoskeleton linkage in maintaining podocyte health, structure, and function.

DEVELOPMENTAL/ORGANIZATIONAL ROLE OF THE GLOMERULAR BASEMENT MEMBRANE

An important extracellular matrix component of developing and mature glomeruli is the GBM. Basement membranes are the thin sheets of specialized extracellular matrix that underlie all epithelial cells, including the vascular endothelium. The GBM is somewhat unique in that it is an unusually thick basement membrane that forms by fusion of two independent basement membranes, one secreted by podocytes and one by endothelial cells. Thus, both cell types contribute components to the GBM. Like all basement membranes, the GBM contains laminin, type IV collagen, nidogen/entactin, and sulfated proteoglycans (149). These are all relatively large glycoproteins of which there are multiple isoforms, but only specific ones are found in the GBM (98). These isoforms are thought to impart properties to the GBM that are important for maintaining glomerular structure and function.

Laminin

Most laminins are cruciform heterotrimers consisting of evolutionarily related α, β, and γ chains (10). There are five α, four β, and three γ chains that associate nonrandomly and become disulfide bonded to each other to form at least 15 different heterotrimers, most of which are ~800 kD (101). Assembly of trimers occurs intracellularly within the endoplasmic reticulum, and then trimers are secreted into the extracellular space where they interact with cellular receptors, such as integrins and dystroglycan, and polymerize with each other to form laminin networks (17). This network provides the foundation of the basement membrane; as shown in knockout mice, basement membranes do not form without laminin (101).

Only a subset of the known laminin heterotrimers is expressed in glomeruli, and only a single heterotrimer, laminin α5β2γ1 (designated LM-521 in a recently developed nomenclature [10]), is found in the mature GBM (98) (Fig. 4). The mesangial matrix, on the other hand, which is structurally and compositionally similar, but distinct from, basement membranes, contains an assortment of laminins, including LM-111, LM-211, LM-411, and LM-511 (98). Whether these mesangial laminins have any specific functions in glomerular biology is not yet clear, but they could certainly influence the behavior of mesangial cells and interact with laminins or other components of the GBM to strengthen the adhesion of the mesangium to GBM segments at the bases of the glomerular capillary loops. In contrast, as discussed below, the laminin content of the GBM is well known to be extremely important for both glomerular development and function.

DEVELOPMENTAL TRANSITIONS IN GBM LAMININ COMPOSITION

During glomerulogenesis there are well-characterized developmental transitions in the deposition of laminin isoforms in the GBM and its precursor (97). From the comma-shaped through the S-shaped stage, LM-111 and LM-411 are present, but they are eliminated from the GBM during the transition to the capillary loop stage (Figs. 2 and 3). At the S-shaped stage, LM-511 is first deposited in the nascent GBM by the presumptive podocytes and the invading endothelial cells. At the capillary loop stage, both LM-511 and LM-521 are present in the maturing GBM, but LM-511 is gradually eliminated as the glomerulus begins functioning as a filter. LM-521 is from then on the major GBM laminin (97). Although little is known about the transcriptional control of these isoform transitions during glomerular development, it is clear that the in vivo setting is important, as metanephroi grown ex vivo do not deposit LM-521. This deficiency is rescued upon reimplantation and subsequent glomerular vascularization in vivo, suggesting that glomerular endothelial cells are required for proper laminin isoform substitution (145).

Laminin α-Chain Transitions. Experiments primarily in knockout mice have revealed the importance of some of these developmental transitions for successful glomerulogenesis and proper glomerular function. A targeted mutation in *Lama5*, the gene encoding laminin α5, results in breakdown of the GBM at the stage when LM-511 should begin to replace LM-111 (late S-shaped stage) (99). In the absence of LM-511, LM-111 is still eliminated from the nascent GBM, and without a full-sized laminin trimer, GBM architecture cannot be maintained. The loss of the GBM at this critical stage of glomerulogenesis has severe consequences, as podocytes lose their cup-shaped arrangement and instead contract into a ball of cells, leaving no place for the endothelial and mesangial cells to form capillaries. Thus, glomerular vascularization completely fails (99). Additional studies aimed at defining the function of the laminin α5 COOH-terminal globular (α5LG) domain in glomerulogenesis showed that this domain is not important for maintenance of GBM integrity, but rather serves as a ligand for mesangial cells to adhere to the GBM at the bases of the glomerular capillary loops so that they can maintain and perhaps modulate capillary loop structure and diameter, as previously proposed (84). When this ligand is missing, the capillaries balloon in a fashion similar to that observed in the absence of mesangial cells (discussed previously), yet here mesangial cells are clearly present but apparently unable to adhere to the GBM under the stress of capillary blood flow (78). These studies show that the GBM and the laminin that it contains serve important organizational roles both during and after glomerulogenesis.

Laminin β-Chain Transitions. In contrast to the requirement for laminin α5 for successful glomerulogenesis, laminin β2 is dispensable. This is best demonstrated by the structurally normal glomeruli that form in *LAMB2⁻/⁻* mice, which correlates with maintenance of GBM integrity during glomerulogenesis (111). The GBM is able to remain intact without LM-521, the only isoform normally found in mature GBM, because of persistence or continued expression of laminin β1, resulting in a GBM containing LM-511 instead of LM-521. However, despite normal glomerulogenesis, *LAMB2⁻/⁻* mice exhibit congenital nephrotic syndrome and are proteinuric (111). Similarly, humans with mutations in *LAMB2* exhibit congenital nephrotic syndrome and diffuse mesangial sclerosis that is sometimes associated with distinct ocular and other abnormalities, a disease entity called Pierson syndrome (165–167). Together these results show that laminin β2 in the GBM (as part of LM-521) is uniquely qualified to ensure that the glomerular barrier to protein is intact. This could be due to either direct effects on GBM porosity or indirect effects on behavior of the attached endothelium and overlying podocytes as well as assembly and function of the slit diaphragm complex.

Collagen Type IV

There are six genetically distinct collagen IV chains, called α chains, that assemble in a defined fashion to form three different triple helical protomers (65, 67). These are designated $(\alpha1)_2\alpha2$, $\alpha3\alpha4\alpha5$, and $(\alpha5)_2\alpha6$. Like all collagen chains, collagen IV chains contain long stretches of Gly-X-Y amino-acid triplet repeats that favor formation of a triple helix. However, unlike most other collagens, type IV contains interspersed interruptions of the triplet repeats that provide flexibility both to the protomers and to the collagen IV network. This is in turn thought to impart needed flexibility to basement membranes (66).

Collagen IV protomers interact with each other via covalent and noncovalent interactions to form a chicken wire–like network, and a substantial amount of cross-linking stabilizes the network. Surprisingly, knockout mice demonstrate that collagen IV is not absolutely required for basement membrane formation, but it is crucial for basement membrane maintenance and stability (112).

Most basement membranes in the body contain the $(\alpha1)_2\alpha2$ protomer, and this is also true of the early nephrogenic epithelial structures (Fig. 2). However, at the capillary loop stage, the α3, α4, and α5 chains become detectable in the GBM (97) (Fig. 3). At maturity the α3α4αa5 protomer represents the major collagen IV component of the GBM (Fig. 4), though apparently small amounts of presumably residual $(\alpha1)_2\alpha2$ can also be detected, more so in human than in mouse GBM. On the other hand, the α1 and α2(IV) chains are abundant in the mesangial matrix, whereas the α3, α4, and α5 chains are absent (98). Interestingly, the basement membrane of Bowman's capsule contains $(\alpha1)_2\alpha2$ and $(\alpha5)_2\alpha6$ protomers (110).

As implied by the existence of only three different collagen IV protomers in vivo, the α3 and α4(IV) chains exist exclusively in combination with α5(IV) to make the α3α4α5 protomer (65, 67). Thus, if any one of the three genes encoding these chains is altered by genetic mutation, this protomer is affected. Mutations that prevent proper assembly of this protomer cause Alport syndrome, or hereditary glomerulonephritis, in humans, dogs, and mice (65, 67), as discussed in detail in Chapter 93. In the absence of the α3α4α5 protomer, there are no defects in glomerulogenesis, primarily due to compensation by the collagen IV network containing the $(\alpha1)_2\alpha2$ protomer. However, as affected individuals age, the abnormal GBM develops characteristic lesions, including thickening and splitting, that eventually leads to renal failure in most cases (76).

Nidogen/Entactin

Nidogens are dumbbell-shaped molecules (149). There are two isoforms of nidogen, nidogen-1 and -2, and both have been reported to be present in the GBM (102). Nidogen-1 was previously considered to be an obligatory link between the laminin and collagen IV networks because it binds well to each of them (149). However, mutant mice lacking both nidogens-1 and -2 survive to birth with most basement membranes intact, demonstrating that nidogen is not required for the integrity of all basement membranes (11). Although the double knockouts died on the day of birth, urine removed from their bladders showed only a marginal increase in low-molecular-weight proteins (11), suggesting that the glomerular barrier to albumin was intact and therefore not dependent on the presence of nidogen in the GBM.

Nidogen-1 binds to laminin trimers via a high-affinity interaction with a specific domain of the laminin γ1 chain (93). To determine the biological importance of this interaction, 56 amino acids encompassing this domain of γ1 were deleted in mice such that nidogen-1 could no longer bind laminin (160). Interestingly, the result was a phenotype that is in many ways more severe than the total absence of both nidogen-1 and -2. For example, homozygotes died immediately after birth rather than surviving for many hours. Renal agenesis was very common, and glomerular capillary aneurisms and hydronephrosis occurred in those few kidneys that did form (160). Together, the results of these two studies (11, 160) suggest that the alteration to laminin γ1 affects more than just its ability to bind nidogens, but the phenotype of the *Lamc1* mutant also underscores the importance of laminin for proper glomerulogenesis.

Sulfated Proteoglycans

Proteoglycans consist of a core protein with covalently attached glycosaminoglycan side chains (GAGs). Those proteoglycans present in basement membranes are usually modified further on their GAGs by addition of heparan sulfate and/or chondroitin sulfate. The anionic character of these sulfate-containing adducts provides much of the basement membrane's net negative charge. A large number of experiments performed in animals suggest that the glomerular filtration barrier possesses charge selectivity, and the sulfated proteoglycans that are present in the GBM are attractive candidates to provide the basis for at least part of

this selectivity against the passage of negatively charged molecules into the urine. However, studies suggest that anionic charges within the GBM may not be involved in establishment of the glomerular filtration barrier under normal circumstances (52).

PERLECAN

There are four major sulfated proteoglycans with relevance to the glomerulus and the best studied biochemically is perlecan. Perlecan consists of a 400-kD core protein with three heparan sulfate chains linked to residues near the NH2-terminus. It is widely found in basement membranes and is abundant in the mesangial matrix, but perlecan is only weakly detected in the GBM (45). Cleavage of the COOH-terminus of perlecan produces a fragment with antiangiogenic activity called endorepellin (14).

Knockout mice lacking perlecan die during embryogenesis or in the neonatal period with multiple developmental defects. Most basement membranes form normally, but mechanical stress causes disruptions in meningeal and cardiomyocyte basement membranes. Perlecan is also normally found in cartilage extracellular matrix, and this matrix is severely disrupted in perlecan mutants (8, 18). No defects in kidneys were noted in these mice.

To investigate further the function of perlecan as a heparan sulfate proteoglycan, a deletion was made that affects only the small part of the protein to which the GAGs are normally attached. Mice carrying this mutation are viable, but they have defects in the lens capsule (129). Neither functional nor structural defects were noted in kidney glomeruli under normal circumstances, but these mice exhibit elevated levels of urinary protein after bovine serum albumin overload (107). Because little perlecan is detectable in the GBM, it is somewhat surprising that removal of its GAGs can have an effect on the filtration barrier.

AGRIN

Agrin is a widely expressed modular proteoglycan that consists of a core protein of ~220 kD with two glycosaminoglycan side chains that carry heparan sulfate and/or chondroitin sulfate. These increase the molecular weight of agrin to greater than 400 kD. Agrin exhibits robust binding to the coiled-coil domain of the laminin γ1 chain in vitro (73), and this might indicate that agrin is involved in organization of basement membrane architecture.

Agrin has been intensively studied by the neuroscience community because a specific splice form of agrin is deposited by motor neurons on developing skeletal muscle fibers, where it serves as a signal that is in part responsible for maintaining the aggregation of acetylcholine receptors to ensure the proper assembly of the neuromuscular junction (39, 103). In kidney, agrin is highly concentrated in the GBM (44), significantly more so than perlecan, but there is as yet no evidence that it serves any signaling functions. Agrin has, however, been proposed to be responsible for the anionic charge that is present in the GBM and that is presumed to be involved in establishing the charge-selective aspect of the glomerular barrier to protein.

Several different mutations have been made in the mouse agrin gene. Whereas all but the most subtle of these have dramatic effects on the differentiation of the neuromuscular junction, no defects in the kidney have been found. Because agrin-mutant mice die at birth due to an inability to breathe, agrin-null kidneys beyond the neonatal period have not been studied. Nevertheless, no defects in glomerulogenesis were noted in agrin-deficient kidneys at perinatal stages (55). In addition, a conditional knockout of agrin in podocytes using the Cre/loxP system was successful at removing both agrin and fixed anionic sites from the GBM, yet there were no detectable defects in glomerular filtration (54). These results show that agrin likely plays no role in glomerulogenesis or establishment of the glomerular barrier to protein. Further, these findings suggest that glomerular charge selectivity may be contributed by podocyte and endothelial cell surface molecules rather than by GBM proteoglycans.

OTHER PROTEOGLYCANS

Although perlecan and agrin are the best studied GBM proteoglycans, two others have been shown to be present. Collagen XVIII, whose COOH-terminus is cleaved to form the antiangiogenic molecule endostatin (14), is unique in that it is a basement membrane collagen with heparan sulfate glycosaminoglycan side chains (51). It is present in the GBM, but its function there, if any, is unknown. Mutant mice lacking collagen XVIII have no reported glomerular defects but do exhibit abnormal blood vessel formation in the eye and retinal defects (38). Consistent with this, Knobloch syndrome in humans is caused by mutations in *COL18A1* (146).

A basement membrane chondroitin sulfate proteoglycan that exhibits transient deposition in postnatal rat GBM has been described (95). Although nothing is known about the function of this protein, of potential interest is the fact that increased levels of this proteoglycan were detected in the GBM of diabetic rats, compared to the normal situation where it is not detected in mature GBM (94).

RECEPTORS AND RECEPTOR-ASSOCIATED PROTEINS MEDIATING GLOMERULAR CELL INTERACTIONS WITH THE GBM

To interact appropriately with the GBM, glomerular cells must express the required matrix receptors and the associated cytoplasmic proteins that mediate responses to the engagement of ligand. Although there are a plethora of these molecules, only a limited set have been studied in the context of glomerulogenesis and glomerular function.

The best-characterized matrix receptors are the integrins. Integrins are a large family of transmembrane αβ heterodimers that bind to extracellular matrix proteins, mediate adhesion, and transduce signals that govern cell prolifera-

tion, survival, and migration. The most studied integrin in the glomerulus is $\alpha_3\beta_1$. This is primarily a laminin binding integrin, though it has also been shown to bind collagen IV. Biochemical studies suggest that $\alpha_3\beta_1$ preferentially binds laminins containing the α_3 and α_5 chains. This would include the LM-511 and LM-521 heterotrimers that, as discussed previously, are so important for glomerular development and function.

The first indication that integrin $\alpha_3\beta_1$ is important for glomerulogenesis came from studies of *Itga3* mutant mice, which lack integrin α_3 (83). These mice die in the neonatal period due to defects in both kidney and lung. Glomerulogenesis occurs in a mostly normal fashion, but ultrastructural analysis reveals that formation of podocyte foot processes is defective, and the GBM appears highly disorganized (83). These data are consistent with the fact that podocytes express integrin $\alpha_3\beta_1$ at a high level and suggest that $\alpha_3\beta_1$ is involved in organizing GBM architecture, perhaps by modulating polymerization of secreted laminins, and in regulating foot process extension. In vitro studies of injured podocytes show that integrin $\alpha_3\beta_1$ is anti-adhesive and involved in localizing cathepsin L, a protease associated with migratory podocytes (120). In functioning glomeruli, $\alpha_3\beta_1$ serves as a mesangial cell receptor for the COOH-terminal LG domain of laminin α_5 in the GBM. Their interaction at the base of the glomerular capillary loops allows mesangial cells to maintain loop structure. If this interaction is impaired, either by alteration of the composition of the LG domain or by deletion of integrin α_3, capillary ballooning occurs (78, 83). Ballooning is more severe in the former case, indicating that there is likely a receptor on mesangial cells besides integrin $\alpha_3\beta_1$ that mediates binding to the GBM. One possibility is integrin $\alpha_8\beta_1$, as older *Itga8*$^{-/-}$ mice exhibit widening of the glomerular capillaries, although the effect is mild (48).

Integrin $\alpha_3\beta_1$ is one of many integrins that use the integrin-linked kinase (ILK) as an intermediate in signal transduction. ILK binds to integrins and to various actin-binding proteins and therefore serves to bridge the actin cytoskeleton with the cell's major linkage to the extracellular matrix. Whereas mice lacking ILK die as very early peri-implantation embryos, mice with a podocyte-specific deletion of ILK survive for a few months, but they eventually succumb to an ESRD that begins with thickening and broadening of the GBM, followed by focal segmental glomerulosclerosis (29). These data further underscore the importance of the podocyte in organizing GBM architecture.

CONCLUDING REMARKS

Although much progress has been made in understanding certain aspects of glomerular development, many important questions remain. First and foremost, the fundamental morphogenic events that initiate, propel, and conclude glomerulogenesis are still poorly defined. In this chapter, we discussed a series of different transcription factors, intracellular and transmembrane proteins, growth factors, and signaling mechanisms associated with glomerular endothelial cell and podocyte biology. With only a few exceptions, however, most of these proteins and processes are expressed by many other cells and tissues throughout the body, and therefore are not likely to be solely or directly responsible for development of the glomerulus. On the other hand, there are a few features of the glomerulus that are both compositionally and structurally distinct, and these include the GBM and epithelial slit diaphragm. Similarly, the intercapillary mesangial cell and its matrix are also unusual structures not found in other vascular beds. We believe that more research aimed at investigating the regulation of the synthesis, assembly, and maintenance of the GBM, SD, and mesangium specifically may yield detailed new insights on how the glomerulus develops and is maintained normally. Perhaps new therapies that retrace parts of the normal developmental pathway could then be designed and used successfully to repair glomerular injury.

Acknowledgments

We thank Erin Cambron and Eileen Roach for help with the illustrations. Funds came from the National Institutes of Health and the American Heart Association.

References

1. Abedi H, Zachary, I. Vascular endothelial growth factor stimulates tyrosine phosphorylation and recruitment to new focal adhesions of focal adhesion kinase and paxillin in endothelial cells. *J Biol Chem* 1997;272:15442–15451.
2. Abrahamson DR. Origin of the glomerular basement membrane visualized after in vivo labeling of laminin in newborn rat kidneys. *J Cell Biol* 1985;100:1988–2000.
3. Abrahamson DR. Structure and development of the glomerular capillary wall and basement membrane. *Am J Physiol* 1987;253:F783–794.
4. Abrahamson DR. Glomerulogenesis in the developing kidney. *Semin Nephrol* 1991;11:375–389.
5. Abrahamson DR, Perry EW. Evidence for splicing new basement membrane into old during glomerular development in newborn rat kidneys. *J Cell Biol* 1986;103:2489–2498.
6. Abrahamson DR, Wang R. Development of the glomerular capillary and its basement membrane. In: Vize PD, Woolf AS, Bard JBL, eds. *The Kidney: From Normal Development to Congenital Disease.* London: Academic Press, 2003:221–249.
7. Alpers CE, Seifert RA, Hedkins KL, Johnson RJ, Bowen-Pope DR. Developmental patterns of PDGF B-chain, PDGF-receptor, and ∀-actin expression in human glomerulogenesis. *Kidney Int* 1992;42:390–399.
8. Arikawa-Hirasawa E, Watanabe H, Takami H, Hassell JR, Yamada Y. Perlecan is essential for cartilage and cephalic development. *Nat Genet* 1999;23:354–358.
9. Asanuma K, Kim K, Oh J, et al. Synaptopodin regulates the actin-bundling activity of alpha-actinin in an isoform-specific manner. *J Clin Invest* 2005;115:1188–1198.
10. Aumailley M, Bruckner-Tuderman L, Carter WG, et al. A simplified laminin nomenclature. *Matrix Biol* 2005;24:326–332.
11. Bader BL, Smyth N, Nedbal S, et al. Compound genetic ablation of nidogen 1 and 2 causes basement membrane defects and perinatal lethality in mice. *Mol Cell Biol* 2005;25:6846–6856.
12. Barletta GM, Kovari IA, Verma RK, Kerjaschki D, Holzman LB. Nephrin and Neph1 co-localize at the podocyte foot process intercell-ular junction and form cis hetero-oligomers. *J Biol Chem* 2003;278:19266–19271.
13. Bernhardt WM, Schmitt R, Rosenberger C, et al. Expression of hypoxia-inducible transcription factors in developing human and rat kidneys. *Kidney Int* 2006;69:114–122.
14. Bix G, Iozzo RV. Matrix revolutions: "tails" of basement-membrane components with angiostatic functions. *Trends Cell Biol* 2005;15:52–60.
15. Carmeliet P, Ferreira V, Breier G, et al. Abnormal blood vessel development and lethality in embryos lacking a single VEGF allele. *Nature* 1996;380:435–439.
16. Chen H, Lun Y, Ovchinnikov D, et al. Limb and kidney defects in Lmx1b mutant mice suggest an involvement of LMX1B in human nail patella syndrome. *Nat Genet* 1998;19:51–55.
17. Colognato H, Yurchenco PD. Form and function: the laminin family of heterotrimers. *Dev Dyn* 2000;218:213–234.
18. Costell M, Gustafsson E, Aszodi A, et al. Perlecan maintains the integrity of cartilage and some basement membranes. *J Cell Biol* 1999;147:1109–1122.
19. Cui S, Li C, Ema M, Weinstein J, Quaggin SE. Rapid isolation of glomeruli coupled with gene expression profiling identifies downstream targets in Pod1 knockout mice. *J Am Soc Nephrol* 2005;16:3247–3255.
20. Cui S, Schwartz L, Quaggin SE. Pod1 is required in stromal cells for glomerulogenesis. *Dev Dyn* 2003;226:512–522.
21. Daniel TO, Abrahamson DR. Endothelial signal integration in vascular assembly. *Ann Rev Physiol* 2000;62:649–671.
22. Daniel TO, Stein E, Cerretti DP, St John PL, Robert B, Abrahamson DR. ELK and LERK-2 in developing kidney and microvascular endothelial assembly. *Kidney Int* 1996;50(Suppl):73–81.
23. Desjardins M, Bendayan M. Ontogenesis of glomerular base-ment membrane: structural and functional properties. *J Cell Biol* 1991;113:689–700.
24. Donoviel DB, Freed DD, Vogel H, et al. Proteinuria and perinatal lethality in mice lacking neph1, a novel protein with homology to nephrin. *Mol Cell Biol* 2001;21:4829–4836.
25. Dressler GR, Wilkinson JE, Rothenpieler UW, Patterson LT, Williams-Simons L, Westphal H. Deregulation of Pax-2 expression in transgenic mice generates severe kidney abnormalities. *Nature* 1993;362:65–67.
26. Dreyer SD, Zhou G, Baldini A, et al. Mutations in LMX1B cause abnormal skeletal patterning and renal dysplasia in nail patella syndrome. *Nat Genet* 1998;19:47–50.
27. Eichmann A, Makinen T, Alitalo K. Neural guidance molecules regulate vascular remodeling and vessel navigation. *Genes Dev* 2005;19:1013–1021.
28. Ekblom P. Formation of basement membranes in the embryonic kidney: an immunohistological study. *J Cell Biol* 1981;91:1–10.
29. El-Aouni C, Herbach N, Blattner SM, et al. Podocyte specific deletion of integrin-linked kinase results in severe glomerular basement membrane alterations and progressive glomerulosclerosis. *J Am Soc Nephrol* 2006;17:1334–1344.
30. Eremina V, Cui S, Gerber H, et al. Vascular endothelial growth factor-A signaling in the podocyte-endothelial compartment is required for mesangial cell migration and survival. *J Am Soc Nephrol* 2006;17:724–735.
31. Eremina V, Sood M, Haigh J, et al. Glomerular-specific alterations of VEGF-A expression lead to distinct congenital and acquired renal diseases. *J Clin Invest* 2003;111:701–716.
32. Esser S, Wolburg K, Wolburg H, Breier G, Kurzchalia T, Risau W. Vascular endothelial growth factor induces endothelial fenestrations in vitro. *J Cell Biol* 1998;140:947–959.
33. Ferrara N, Carver-Moore K, Chen H, et al. Heterozygous embryonic lethality induced by targeted inactivation of the VEGF gene. *Nature* 1996;380:439–442.
34. Fong G-H, Rossant J, Gertsenstein M, Breitman ML. Role of the Flt-1 receptor kinase in regulating the assembly of vascular endothelium. *Nature* 1995;376:66–70.
35. Freeburg PB, Abrahamson DR. Hypoxia-inducible factors and kidney vascular development. *J Am Soc Nephrol* 2003;14:2723–2730.
36. Freeburg PB, Abrahamson DR. Divergent expression patterns for hypoxia-inducible factor-1beta and aryl hydrocarbon receptor nuclear transporter-2 in developing kidney. *J Am Soc Nephrol* 2004;15:2569–2578.
37. Freeburg PB, Robert B, St John PL, Abrahamson DR. Podocyte expression of hypoxia-inducible factor (HIF)-1 and HIF-2 during glomerular development. *J Am Soc Nephrol* 2003;14:927–938.
38. Fukai N, Eklund L, Marneros AG, et al. Lack of collagen XVIII/endostatin results in eye abnormalities. *EMBO J* 2002;21:1535–1544.
39. Gautam M, Noakes PG, Moscoso L, et al. Defective neuromuscular synaptogenesis in agrin-deficient mutant mice. *Cell* 1996;85:525–535.
40. Gerber HP, Dixit V, Ferrara N. Vascular endothelial growth factor induces expression of the anti-apoptotic proteins Bcl-2 and A1 in vascular endothelial cells. *J Biol Chem* 1998;273:13313–13316.
41. Gerber HP, Hillan KJ, Ryan AM, Kowalski J, Keller GA, Rangell L, Wright BD, Radtke F, Aguet M, Ferrara N. VEGF is required for growth and survival in neonatal mice. *Development* 1999;126:149–1159.
42. Gerke P, Huber TB, Sellin L, Benzing T, Walz G. Homodimerization and heterodimerization of the glomerular podocyte proteins nephrin and NEPH1. *J Am Soc Nephrol* 2003;14:918–926.
43. Gerke P, Sellin L, Kretz O, et al. NEPH2 is located at the glomerular slit diaphragm, interacts with nephrin and is cleaved from podocytes by metalloproteinases. *J Am Soc Nephrol* 2005;16:1693–1702.
44. Groffen AJ, Ruegg MA, Dijkman H, et al. Agrin is a major heparan sulfate proteoglycan in the human glomerular basement membrane. *J Histochem Cytochem* 1998;46:19–27.
45. Groffen AJA, Hop FWH, Tryggvason K, et al. Evidence for the existence of multiple heparan sulfate proteoglycans in the human glomerular basement membrane and mesangial matrix. *Eur J Biochem* 1997;247:175–182.
46. Guan F, Villegas G, Teichman J, et al. Autocrine VEGF system in podocytes regulates podocin and its interaction with CD2AP. *Am J Physiol Renal Physiol* 2006;291:F422–428.
47. Guo G, Morrison DJ, Licht JD, Quaggin SE. WT1 activates a glomerular-specific enhancer identified from the human nephrin gene. *J Am Soc Nephrol* 2004;15:2851–2856.
48. Haas CS, Amann K, Schittny J, Blaser B, Muller U, Hartner A. Glomerular and renal vascular structural changes in alpha8 integrin-deficient mice. *J Am Soc Nephrol* 2003;14:2288–2296.
49. Haase VH. The VHL/HIF oxygen sensing pathway and its relevance to kidney disease. *Kidney Int* 2006;69:1302–1307.
50. Haase VH. Hypoxia-inducible factors in the kidney. *Am J Physiol Renal Physiol* 2006;291:F271–281.
51. Halfter W, Dong S, Schurer B, Cole GJ. Collagen XVIII is a basement membrane heparan sulfate proteoglycan. *J Biol Chem* 1998;273:25404–25412.
52. Hammes A, Guo JK, Lutsch G, et al. Two splice variants of the Wilms' tumor 1 gene have distinct functions during sex determination and nephron formation. *Cell* 2001;106:319–329.
53. Harper SJ, Xing CY, Whittle C, et al. Expression of neuropilin-1 by human glomerular epithelial cells in vitro and in vivo. *Clin Sci* 2001;101:439–446.

54. Harvey SJ, Burgess R, Miner JH. Podocyte-derived agrin is responsible for glomerular basement membrane anionic charge. *J Am Soc Nephrol* 2005;16:1A.
55. Harvey SJ, Miner JH. Renal phenotype of agrin-deficient mice: agrin contributes to the fixed negative charge of the glomerular basement membrane. *J Am Soc Nephrol* 2004;15:37A.
56. Hastie ND. Life, sex, and WT1 isoforms: three amino acids can make all the difference. *Cell* 2001;106:391–394.
57. Heidet L, Bongers EM, Sich M, et al. In vivo expression of puta-tive LMX1B targets in nail-patella syndrome kidneys. *Am J Pathol* 2003;163:145–155.
58. Holzman LB, John PL, Kovari IA, Verma R, Holthofer H, Abrahamson DR. Nephrin localizes to the slit pore of the glomerular epithelial cell. *Kidney Int* 1999;56:1481–1491.
59. Huber TB, Benzing T. The slit diaphragm: a signaling platform to regulate podocyte function. *Curr Opin Nephrol Hypertens* 2005;14:211–216.
60. Huber TB, Hartleben B, Kim J, et al. Nephrin and CD2AP associate with phosphoinositide 3-OH kinase and stimulate AKT-dependent signaling. *Mol Cell Biol* 2003;23:4917–4928.
61. Huber TB, Kottgen M, Schilling B, Walz G, Benzing T. Interaction with podocin facilitates nephrin signaling. *J Biol Chem* 2001;276:41543–41546.
62. Huber TB, Kwoh C, Wu H, et al. A bigenic mouse model of focal segmental glomerulosclerosis involving pairwise interaction of CD2AP, Fyn and synaptopodin. *J Clin Invest* 2006;116:1337–1345.
63. Huber TB, Schmidts M, Gerke P, et al. The carboxy terminus of Neph family members binds to the PDZ domain protein Zonula occludens-1. *J Biol Chem* 2003;278:13417–13421.
64. Huber TB, Simons M, Hartleben B, et al. Molecular basis of the functional podocin-nephrin complex: mutations in the NPHS2 gene disrupt nephrin targeting to lipid raft microdomains. *Hum Mol Genet* 2003;12:3397–3405.
65. Hudson BG. The molecular basis of Goodpasture and Alport syndromes: beacons for the discovery of the collagen IV family. *J Am Soc Nephrol* 2004;15:2514–2527.
66. Hudson BG, Reeders ST, Tryggvason K. Type IV collagen: structure, gene organization, and role in human diseases. *J Biol Chem* 1993;268:26033–26036.
67. Hudson BG, Tryggvason K, Sundaramoorthy M, Neilson EG. Alport's syndrome, Goodpasture's syndrome, and type IV collagen. *N Engl J Med* 2003;348:2543–2556.
68. Hugo C, Shankland SJ, Bowen-Pope DF, Couser WG, Johnson RJ. Extraglomerular origin of the mesangial cell after injury. A new role of the juxtaglomerular apparatus. *J Clin Invest* 1997;100:786–794.
69. Hyink DP, Abrahamson DR. Origin of the glomerular vasculature in the developing kidney. *Semin Nephrol* 1995;15:300–314.
70. Hyink DP, Tucker DC, St John PL, et al. Endogenous origin of glomerular endothelial and mesangial cells in grafts of embryonic kidneys. *Am J Physiol* 1996;270:F886–899.
71. Jones N, Blasutig IM, Eremina V, et al. Nck adaptor proteins link nephrin to the actin cytoskeleton of kidney podocytes. *Nature* 2006;440:818–823.
72. Kaelin WG. The von Hippel-Lindau tumor suppressor gene and kidney cancer. *Clin Can Res* 2004;10:6290s–6295s.
73. Kammerer RA, Schulthess T, Landwehr R, et al. Interaction of agrin with laminin requires a coiled-coil conformation of the agrin-binding site within the laminin gamma1 chain. *EMBO J* 1999;18:6762–6770.
74. Kanwar YS, Jakubowski ML, Rosenzweig LJ, Gibbons JT. De novo cellular synthesis of sulfated proteoglycans of the developing renal glomerulus in vivo. *Proc Natl Acad Sci U S A* 1984;81:7108–7111.
75. Kaplan JM, Kim SH, North KN, et al. Mutations in ACTN4, encoding alpha-actinin-4, cause familial focal segmental glomerulosclerosis. *Nat Genet* 2000;24:251–256.
76. Kashtan CE. Alport syndrome. *Kidney Int* 1997;51(Suppl):S69–S71.
77. Kestila M, Lenkkeri U, Mannikko M, et al. Positionally cloned gene for a novel glomerular protein—nephrin—is mutated in congenital nephrotic syndrome. *Mol Cell* 1998;1:575–582.
78. Kikkawa Y, Virtanen I, Miner JH. Mesangial cells organize the glomerular capillaries by adhering to the G domain of laminin alpha5 in the glomerular basement membrane. *J Cell Biol* 2003;161:187–196.
79. Kim JM, Wu H, Green G, et al. CD2-associated protein haplo-insufficiency is linked to glomerular disease susceptibility. *Science* 2003;300:1298–1300.
80. Kitamoto Y, Tokunaga H, Tomita K. Vascular endothelial growth factor is an essential molecule for mouse kidney development: glomerulogenesis and nephrogenesis. *J Clin Invest* 1997;99:2351–2357.
81. Klagsbrun M, Eichmann A. A role for axon guidance receptors and ligands in blood vessel development and tumor angiogenesis. *Cytokine Growth Fact Rev* 2005;16:535–548.
82. Kreidberg JA. Podocyte differentiation and glomerulogenesis. *J Am Soc Nephrol* 2003;14:806–814.
83. Kreidberg JA, Donovan MJ, Goldstein SL, et al. Alpha 3 beta 1 integrin has a crucial role in kidney and lung organogenesis. *Development* 1996;122:3537–3547.
84. Kriz W, Elger M, Mundel P, Lemley KV. Structure-stabilizing forces in the glomerular tuft. *J Am Soc Nephrol* 1995;5:1731–1739.
85. Lahdenpera J, Kilpelainen P, Liu XL, et al. Clustering-induced tyrosine phosphorylation of nephrin by Src family kinases. *Kidney Int* 2003;64:404–413.
86. Lelongt B, Makino H, Kanwar YS. Maturation of the developing renal glomerulus with respect to basement membrane proteoglycans. *Kidney Int* 1987;32:498–506.
87. Leveen P, Pekny M, Gebre-Medhin S, Swolin B, Larsson E, Betsholtz C. Mice deficient for PDGF B show renal, cardiovascular, and hematological abnormalities. *Genes Dev* 1994;8:1875–1887.
88. Li H, Lemay S, Aoudjit L, Kawachi H, Takano T. SRC-family kinase Fyn phosphorylates the cytoplasmic domain of nephrin and modulates its interaction with podocin. *J Am Soc Nephrol* 2004;15:3006–3015.
89. Liu G, Kaw B, Kurfis J, Rahmanuddin S, Kanwar YS, Chugh SS. Neph1 and nephrin interaction in the slit diaphragm is an important determinant of glomerular permeability. *J Clin Invest* 2003;112:209–221.
90. Loughna S, Hardman P, Landels E, et al. A molecular and genetic analysis of renal glomerular capillary development. *Angiogenesis* 1997;1:84–101.
91. Masuya M, Drake CJ, Fleming PA, et al. Hematopoietic origin of glomerular mesangial cells. *Blood* 2003;101:2215–2218.
92. Maxwell PH, Ratcliffe PJ. Oxygen sensors and angiogenesis. *Semin Cell Dev Biol* 2002;13:29–37.
93. Mayer U, Nischt R, Poschl E, et al. A single EGF-like motif of laminin is responsible for high affinity nidogen binding. *EMBO J* 1993;12:1879–1885.
94. McCarthy KJ, Abrahamson DR, Bynum KR, St John PL, Couchman JR. Basement membrane-specific chondroitin sulfate proteoglycan is abnormally associated with the glomerular capillary basement membrane of diabetic rats. *J Histochem Cytochem* 1994;42:473–484.
95. McCarthy KJ, Bynum K, St. John PL, Abrahamson DR, Couchman JR. Basement membrane proteoglycans in glomerular morphogenesis: chondroitin sulfate proteoglycan is temporally and spatially restricted during development. *J Histochem Cytochem* 1993;41:401–414.
96. McCright B, Gao X, Shen L, et al. Defects in development of the kidney, heart and eye vasculature in mice homozygous for a hypomorphic Notch2 mutation. *Development* 2001;128:491–502.
97. Miner JH. Developmental biology of glomerular basement membrane components. *Curr Opin Nephrol Hypertens* 1998;7:13–19.
98. Miner JH. Renal basement membrane components. *Kidney Int* 1999;56:2016–2024.
99. Miner JH, Li C. Defective glomerulogenesis in the absence of laminin a5 demonstrates a developmental role for the kidney glomerular basement membrane. *Dev Biol* 2000;217:278–289.
100. Miner JH, Morello R, Andrews KL, et al. Transcriptional induction of slit diaphragm genes by Lmx1b is required in podocyte differentiation. *J Clin Invest* 2002;109:1065–1072.
101. Miner JH, Yurchenco PD. Laminin functions in tissue morphogenesis. *Annu Rev Cell Dev Biol* 2004;20:255–284.
102. Miosge N, Kother F, Heinemann S, Kohfeldt E, Herken R, Timpl R. Ultrastructural colocalization of nidogen-1 and nidogen-2 with laminin-1 in murine kidney basement membranes. *Histochem Cell Biol* 2000;113:115–124.
103. Misgeld T, Kummer TT, Lichtman JW, Sanes JR. Agrin promotes synaptic differentiation by counteracting an inhibitory effect of neurotransmitter. *Proc Natl Acad Sci U S A* 2005;102:11088–11093.
104. Moeller MJ, Sanden SK, Soofi A, Wiggins RC, Holzman LB. Podocyte-specific expression of cre recombinase in transgenic mice. *Genesis* 2003;35:39–42.
105. Moeller MJ, Soofi A, Braun GS, et al. Protocadherin FAT1 binds Ena/VASP proteins and is necessary for actin dynamics and cell polarization. *EMBO J* 2004;23:3769–3779.
106. Morello R, Zhou G, Dreyer SD, et al. Regulation of glomerular basement membrane collagen expression by LMX1B contributes to renal disease in nail patella syndrome. *Nat Genet* 2001;27:205–208.
107. Morita H, Yoshimura A, Inui K, et al. Heparan sulfate of perlecan is involved in glomerular filtration. *J Am Soc Nephrol* 2005;16:1703–1710.
108. Mutter WP, Peng H, Goldring MB, Knebelmann B, Karumanchi A. Role of LMX1B in proteinuria. *J Am Soc Nephrol* 2005;16:670A.
109. Natoli TA, Liu J, Eremina V, et al. A mutant form of the Wilms' tumor suppressor gene WT1 observed in Denys-Drash syndrome interferes with glomerular capillary development. *J Am Soc Nephrol* 2002;13:2058–2067.
110. Ninomiya Y, Kagawa M, Iyama K, et al. Differential expression of two basement membrane collagen genes, COL4A6 and COL4A5, demonstrated by immunofluorescence staining using peptide-specific monoclonal antibodies. *J Cell Biol* 1995;130:1219–1229.
111. Noakes PG, Miner JH, Gautam M, Cunningham JM, Sanes JR, Merlie JP. The renal glomerulus of mice lacking s-laminin/laminin b2: nephrosis despite molecular compensation by laminin b1. *Nat Genet* 1995;10:400–406.
112. Poschl E, Schlotzer-Schrehardt U, Brachvogel B, Saito K, Ninomiya Y, Mayer U. Collagen IV is essential for basement membrane stability but dispensable for initiation of its assembly during early development. *Development* 2004;131:1619–1628.
113. Quaggin SE. Transcriptional regulation of podocyte specification and differentiation. *Microsc Res Tech* 2002;57:208–211.
114. Quaggin SE, Schwartz L, Cui S, et al. The basic-helix-loop-helix protein pod1 is critically important for kidney and lung organogenesis. *Development* 1999;126:5771–5783.
115. Quaggin SE, Vanden Heuvel GB, Igarashi P. Pod-1, a mesoderm-specific basic-helix-loop-helix protein expressed in mesenchymal and glomerular epithelial cells in the developing kidney. *Mech Dev* 1998;71:37–48.
116. Raval RR, Lau KW, Tran MGB, et al. Contrasting properties of hypoxia-inducible factor 1 (HIF-1) and HIF-2 in von hippel-lindau-associated renal cell carcinoma. *Molec Cell Biol* 2005;25:5675–5686.
117. Reeves W, Caulfield JP, Farquhar MG. Differentiation of epithelial foot processes and filtration slits. Sequential appearance of occluding junctions, epithelial polyanion, and slit membranes in developing glomeruli. *Lab Invest* 1978;39:90–100.
118. Reeves WH, Kanwar YS, Farquhar MG. Assembly of the glomerular filtration surface. Differentiation of anionic sites in glomerular capillaries of newborn rat kidney. *J Cell Biol* 1980;85:735–753.
119. Reiser J, Kriz W, Kretzler M, Mundel P. The glomerular slit diaphragm is a modified adherens junction. *J Am Soc Nephrol* 2000;11:1–8.
120. Reiser J, Oh J, Shirato I, et al. Podocyte migration during nephrotic syndrome requires a coordinated interplay between cathepsin L and alpha3 integrin. *J Biol Chem* 2004;279:34827–34832.
121. Reiser J, Polu KR, Moller CC, et al. TRPC6 is a glomerular slit diaphragm-associated channel required for normal renal function. *Nat Genet* 2005;37:739–744.
122. Ricono JM, Xu YC, Arar M, et al. Morphological insights into the origin of glomerular endothelial and mesangial cells and their precursors. *J Histochem Cytochem* 2003;51:141–150.
123. Robert B, Abrahamson DR. Control of glomerular capillary development by growth factor/receptor kinases. *Pediatr Nephrol* 2001;16:294–301.
124. Robert B, St John PL, Abrahamson DR. Direct visualization of renal vascular morphogenesis in Flk1 heterozygous mutant mice. *Am J Physiol* 1998;275:F164–F172.
125. Robert B, St John PL, Hyink DP, Abrahamson DR. Evidence that embryonic kidney cells expressing flk-1 are intrinsic, vasculogenic angioblasts. *Am J Physiol* 1996;271:F744–F753.

126. Robert B, Zhao X, Abrahamson DR. Coexpression of neuropilin-1, Flk1, and VEGF(164) in developing and mature mouse kidney glomeruli. *Am J Physiol Renal Physiol* 2000;279: F275–F282.

127. Rodewald R, Karnovsky MJ. Porous substructure of the glomerular slit diaphragm in the rat and mouse. *J Cell Biol* 1974;60:423–433.

128. Rohr C, Prestel J, Heidet L, et al. The LIM-homeodomain transcription factor Lmx1b plays a crucial role in podocytes. *J Clin Invest* 2002;109:1073–1082.

129. Rossi M, Morita H, Sormunen R, et al. Heparan sulfate chains of perlecan are indispensable in the lens capsule but not in the kidney. *EMBO J* 2003;22:236–245.

130. Ryan G, Steele-Perkins V, Morris JF, Rauscher FJ, 3rd, Dressler GR. Repression of Pax-2 by WT1 during normal kidney development. *Development* 1995;121:867–875.

131. Sadl V, Jin F, Yu J, et al. The mouse Kreisler (Krml1/MafB) segmentation gene is required for differentiation of glomerular visceral epithelial cells. *Dev Biol* 2002;249:16–29.

132. Salomon R, Gubler MC, Niaudet P. Genetics of the nephrotic syndrome. *Curr Opin Pediatr* 2000;12:129–134.

133. Sariola H, Ekblom P, Lehtonen E, Saxen L. Differentiation and vascularization of the metanephric kidney grafted on the chorioallantoic membrane. *Dev Biol* 1983;96:427–435.

134. Sariola H, Timpl R, von der Mark K, Mayne R, Fitch JM, Linsenmayer TF, Ekblom P. Dual origin of the glomerular basement membrane. *Dev Biol* 1984;101:86–96.

135. Saxen, L. *Organogenesis of Kidney.* Cambridge, UK: Cambridge University Press; 1987:1–173.

136. Schnabel E, Anderson JM, Farquhar MG. The tight junction protein ZO-1 is concentrated along slit diaphragms of the glomerular epithelium. *J Cell Biol* 1990;111:1255–1263.

137. Sellin L, Huber TB, Gerke P, Quack I, Pavenstadt H, Walz G. NEPH1 defines a novel family of podocin interacting proteins. *FASEB J* 2003;17:115–117.

138. Sequeira Lopez ML, Pentz ES, Robert B, et al. Embryonic origin and lineage of juxtaglomerular cells. *Am J Physiol Renal Physiol* 2001;281:F345–F356.

139. Shalaby F, Rossant J, Yamaguchi TP, Gertsenestein M, Wu XF, Breitman ML, Schuh, AC. Failure of blod-island formation and vasculogenesis in Flk-1-deficient mice. *Nature* 1995;376:62–66.

140. Shih N-Y, Li J, Cotran R, Mundel P, Miner JH, Shaw AS. CD2AP localizes to the slit diaphragm and binds to nephrin via a novel C-terminal domain. *Am J Pathol* 2001;159: 2303–2308.

141. Shih N-Y, Li J, Karpitskii V, et al. Congenital nephrotic syndrome in mice lacking CD2-associated protein. *Science* 1999;286:312–315..

142. Simon M, Grone HJ, Johren O, et al. Expression of vascular endothelial growth factor and its receptors in human renal ontogenesis and in adult kidney. *Am J Physiol* 1995;268:F240–F250.

143. Soriano P. Abnormal kidney development and hematological disorders in platelet-derived growth factor Ǝ receptor knock out mice. *Genes Dev* 1994;8:1888–1896.

144. St John PL, Abrahamson DR. Glomerular endothelial cells and podocytes jointly synthesize laminin-1 and -11 chains. *Kidney Int* 2001;60:1037–1046.

145. St. John PL, Wang R, Yin Y, Miner JH, Robert B, Abrahamson DR. Glomerular laminin isoform transitions: errors in metanephric culture are corrected by grafting. *Am J Physiol Renal Physiol* 2001;280:F695–705.

146. Suzuki OT, Sertie AL, Der Kaloustian VM, et al. Molecular analysis of collagen XVIII reveals novel mutations, presence of a third isoform, and possible genetic heterogeneity in Knobloch syndrome. *Am J Hum Genet* 2002;71:1320–1329.

147. Takemoto M, Asker N, Gerhardt H, et al. A new method for large scale isolation of kidney glomeruli from mice. *Am J Pathol* 2002;161:799–805.

148. Takemoto M, He L, Norlin J, et al. Large-scale identification of genes implicated in kidney glomerulus development and function. *EMBO J* 2006;25:1160–1174.

149. Timpl R. Structure and biological activity of basement membrane proteins. *Eur J Biochem* 1989;180:487–502.

150. Tufro A. VEGF spatially directs angiogenesis during metanephric development in vitro. *Dev Biol* 2000;227:558–566.

151. Tufro A, Norwood VF, Carey RM, Gomez RA. Vascular endothelial growth factor induces nephrogenesis and vasculogenesis. *J Am Soc Nephrol* 1999;10:2125–2134.

152. Ulleras E, Wilcock A, Miller SJ, Franklin GC. The sequential activation and repression of the human PDGF-B gene during chronic hypoxia reveals antagonistic roles for the depletion of oxygen and glucose. *Growth Factors* 2001;19:233–245.

153. Verma R, Kovari I, Soofi A, Nihalani D, Patrie K, Holzman LB. Nephrin ectodomain engagement results in Src kinase activation, nephrin phosphorylation, Nck recruitment, and actin polymerization. *J Clin Invest* 2006;116:1346–1349.

154. Verma R, Wharram B, Kovari I, et al. Fyn binds to and phosphorylates the kidney slit diaphragm component Nephrin. *J Biol Chem* 2003;278:20716–20723.

155. Villegas G, Tufro A. Ontogeny of semaphorins 3A and 3F and their receptors neuropilins 1 and 2 in the kidney. *Mech Dev* 2002;119:S149—S53.

156. Wagner N, Wagner KD, Xing Y, Scholz H, Schedl A. The major podocyte protein nephrin is transcriptionally activated by the Wilms' tumor suppressor WT1. *J Am Soc Nephrol* 2004;15:3044–3051.

157. Wartiovaara J, Ofverstedt LG, Khoshnoodi J, et al. Nephrin strands contribute to a porous slit diaphragm scaffold as revealed by electron tomography. *J Clin Invest* 2004;114:1475–1483.

158. Welsch T, Endlich N, Gokce G, et al. Association of CD2AP with dynamic actin on vesicles in podocytes. *Am J Physiol Renal Physiol* 2005;289:F1134–1143.

159. Wenger RH, Stiehl DP, Camenisch G. Integration of oxygen signaling at the consensus HRE. *Sci STKE* 2005;(306): re12.

160. Willem M, Miosge N, Halfter W, et al. Specific ablation of the nidogen-binding site in the laminin gamma1 chain interferes with kidney and lung development. *Development* 2002;129:2711–2722.

161. Winn MP, Conlon PJ, Lynn KL, et al. A mutation in the TRPC6 cation channel causes familial focal segmental glomerulosclerosis. *Science* 2005;308:1801–1804.

162. Woolf AS. The life of the human kidney before birth: its secrets unfold. *Pediatr Res* 2001;49:8–10.

163. Woolf AS, Yuan HT. Angiopoietin growth factors and Tie receptor tyrosine kinases in renal vascular development. *Pediatr Nephrol* 2001;16:177–184.

164. Yuan H, Takeuchi E, Salant DJ. Podocyte slit-diaphragm protein nephrin is linked to the actin cytoskeleton. *Am J Physiol Renal Physiol* 2002;282:F585–591.

165. Zenker M, Aigner T, Wendler O, et al. Human laminin beta2 deficiency causes congenital nephrosis with mesangial sclerosis and distinct eye abnormalities. *Hum Mol Genet* 2004;13: 2625–2632.

166. Zenker M, Pierson M, Jonveaux P, Reis A. Demonstration of two novel LAMB2 mutations in the original Pierson syndrome family reported 42 years ago. *Am J Med Genet A* 2005;138: 73–74.

167. Zenker M, Tralau T, Lennert T, et al. Congenital nephrosis, mesangial sclerosis, and distinct eye abnormalities with microcoria: an autosomal recessive syndrome. *Am J Med Genet A* 2004;130:138–145.

CHAPTER **26**

Postnatal Renal Development

Michel Baum, Raymond Quigley, and Lisa M. Satlin*

University of Texas Southwestern Medical Center, Dallas, Texas, USA
*Mount Sinai School of Medicine, New York, New York, USA

INTRODUCTION

The adult kidney functions to keep the organism in a steady state and protect against changes in the volume and composition of the extracellular fluid. Unlike the adult, the neonate must maintain a positive balance for many solutes to promote growth. This chapter focuses on maturational changes in kidney function that occur during postnatal renal development with a focus on the differences between the mature and neonatal kidney.

RENAL BLOOD FLOW AND GLOMERULAR FILTRATION RATE

Renal Blood Flow

Renal blood flow in the adult human is 660 ml/min, which is 20%–25% of the cardiac output. In contrast, the fetal kidney receives only 2% of the cardiac output from mid-gestation to term (173, 174). The developmental increase in renal blood flow is due in part to an increase in cardiac output, but predominantly due to a decrease in renal vascular resistance (76, 105, 209). When corrected for a body surface area of 1.73 m^2, the human neonate has a renal blood flow of only 15%–20% of that measured in adults (40,172). Renal blood flow doubles in the first month of life and is comparable to adults by 1 to 2 years of age (172). The maturational changes in renal vascular resistance are due to anatomical changes in the renal vasculature as well as changes in the balance between vasoconstrictors such as catecholamines and angiotensin II and vasodilators such as nitric oxide.

The kidney develops in a centrifugal fashion. Juxtamedullary nephrons are formed before those in the superficial cortex. Renal blood flow distribution measured by both xenon washout and injection of microspheres is characterized by a paucity of blood flow to the outer cortex compared to the deep cortex in neonates (16, 105, 142). With renal maturation there is a redistribution of blood flow with enhanced perfusion of the outer cortex (16, 105, 142), which is due to a decrease in renal vascular resistance.

Autoregulation

Renal blood flow (RBF) and glomerular filtration rate (GFR) remain stable over a wide range of perfusion pressures (240). As perfusion pressure falls there is vasodilatation of the afferent arteriole and vasoconstriction of the efferent arteriole which maintains RBF and GFR. As blood pressure increases during development, the range in pressure where autoregulation of renal blood flow and GFR occurs shifts accordingly (106). While neonates can autoregulate GFR in response to changes in blood pressure, this protective mechanism is far less than the autoregulatory capability of adults (240), an observation attributed to, at least in part, to an attenuated release and efferent arteriolar response to angiotensin II in neonates (240).

Glomerular Filtration Rate

Initiation of glomerular filtration, as evidenced by the flow of urine, begins between 9 and 12 weeks gestation in the human (69). The GFR is lower in neonates than adults even when corrected for body surface area (13, 172). In premature human infants, creatinine clearance increases as a function of postconceptual age (the sum of gestational age and postnatal age) (13). GFR is constant at ~0.5 ml/min in infants with a postconceptional age of 28–34 weeks despite the increase in renal size (12). GFR increases to 1.0 ml/min at 34–37 weeks and to 2 ml/min at a postconceptional age of 40 weeks (12). In absolute terms, the GFR increases 25-fold from birth to adulthood. Corrected for a surface area of 1.73 m^2, the GFR in the human term neonate is 30 ml/min/1.73 m^2 in the first week of life (13, 53). GFR continues to increase during the first ~1–2 years of life to reach adult levels when factored for body surface area (172) (Fig. 1).

At birth, juxtamedullary glomeruli have a larger volume and greater single-nephron GFR than superficial nephrons (208). In the guinea pig there is a seven-fold increase in GFR from 1 day to 38 days of age (208). The increase in total kidney GFR during the first week of life, a time when superficial nephron GFR is relatively constant, was predominantly due to an increase in juxtamedullary nephron GFR (208). After 2 weeks of age, however, the rise in total

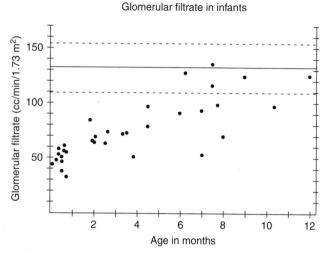

FIGURE 1 Glomerular filtration rate (GFR) in infants in the first year of life (values are corrected for a surface area of 1.73 m²). The *horizontal line* is the mean adult value and the *broken line* represents one standard deviation. (With permission, from Rubin MI, Bruck E, Rapoport M. Maturation of renal function in childhood: clearance studies. *J Clin Invest* 1949;28:1144–1162.)

kidney GFR was predominantly due to an increase in GFR in superficial nephrons, which increases ,20-fold in the guinea pig during the next 2 weeks (Fig. 2) (208).

The increase in single-nephron GFR with postnatal maturation is due to a number of factors. Single-nephron GFR is the product of the net ultrafiltration pressure and the glomerular ultrafiltration coefficient, K_f. The effective ultrafiltration pressure is the difference between the hydrostatic and oncotic pressures across the glomerular capillary bed. Studies comparing newborn rats and guinea pigs to adults have shown a maturational increase in effective ultrafiltration pressure (2, 209). However, these changes contribute at most 10% to the 20-fold increase in single-nephron GFR (101, 209, 220). The maturational increase in GFR is predominantly the result of the increase in K_f, which is the product of the hydraulic permeability of the glomerular capillary and the glomerular capillary surface

area (72, 103, 116, 220). Studies using neutral dextrans have found that the permeability characteristics change only slightly with maturation (72). The increase in K_f, and thus single-nephron GFR, is predominately due to the 7.5-fold increase in glomerular capillary surface area during renal maturation (103, 116).

SODIUM CHLORIDE TRANSPORT

The transition from fetal to neonatal life is characterized by a dramatic decrease in urinary sodium excretion despite an increase in GFR. The early fetus excretes ~20% of the filtered sodium while the late-gestation fetus excretes only ~0.2% (166, 201). Term neonates are able to maintain a positive sodium balance over a wide range of sodium intake, which is essential for growth (5, 207). Compared to adults, neonates have a limited capacity to excrete an acute sodium load and will develop volume expansion and hypernatremia with a sodium load (5, 51). This phenomenon was exemplified in a study where adult and neonatal dogs were given an isotonic saline infusion equal in volume to 10% of the animal's weight (71). The results of the cumulative excretion of sodium with time are shown in Fig. 3. Adult dogs had a brisk natriuresis and diuresis excreting 50% of the sodium within 2 hours of the infusion. Dogs

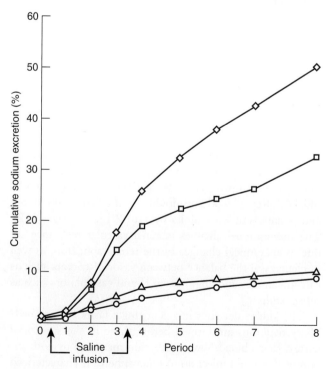

FIGURE 3 Cumulative sodium excretion in dogs of various ages after infusion of isotonic saline equal to 10% of body weight over 30 minutes. Period 8 is approximately 120 minutes after initiation of saline infusion. (With permission, from Goldsmith DI, Drukker A, Blaufox MD, et al. Hemodynamic and excretory response of the neonatal canine kidney to acute volume expansion. *Am J Physiol Renal Fluid Electrolyte Physiol* 1979;237:F392–F397.)

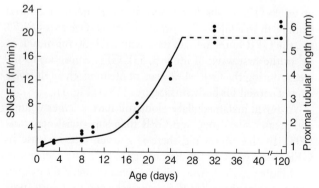

FIGURE 2 Single nephron GFR (SNGFR) in guinea pigs with age. Each point represents two to six determinations of SNGFR in an animal. (With permission, from Spitzer A, Brandis M. Functional and morphologic maturation of the superficial nephrons. *J Clin Invest* 1974;53:279–287.)

less than 1 week of age excreted less than 10% of the sodium infused by 2 hours. The limited ability to excrete a sodium load in neonates was not explained by a low GFR since there was a comparable change with volume expansion in neonates and adults. Unlike term infants, premature neonates have high urinary sodium losses and fractional excretion of sodium and are unable to conserve sodium efficiently (1, 4, 5, 60). The following section discusses the maturation of tubular transport, which maintains the positive sodium balance in growing neonates.

Glomerulotubular Balance

In the adult, glomerulotubular balance, defined as the ratio of absolute reabsorptive rate to single-nephron GFR, remains fairly constant under a number of conditions that alter the GFR. During postnatal development, the maturational increase in the GFR is paralleled by a concomitant increase in the rate of tubule solute absorption (97, 208). If this did not occur, there would be loss of essential solutes that would jeopardize the life of the developing organism.

Several studies have examined whether there is a parallel increase in GFR to proximal tubular reabsorption capacity during renal maturation. The fraction of fluid reabsorbed by the proximal convoluted tubule remained constant in dogs between the ages of 3 and 11 weeks despite a seven-fold increase in GFR (97). Similar findings were also found in rat and guinea pig micropuncture studies (208).

In the fetus, however, the GFR and delivery of solutes and water to the tubules can surpass the reabsorptive capacity of the tubules. In a clearance study examining the fractional reabsorption of volume and sodium after salt loading in fetal, young, and adult guinea pigs, the fractional reabsorption of volume and sodium were lower in the fetus and 1-day-old animals. By 2–5 days of age, the fractional reabsorption of sodium and water were at the adult level (136). The glomerular-tubular imbalance is not only present in the fetus but can also be manifested in the premature neonate. This is exemplified by the fact that glucosuria is frequently present in premature human neonates born before 30 weeks of gestation (12, 89, 223). In human neonates born before 34 weeks gestation, 93% of the filtered glucose is reabsorbed (12), which is comparable to the fractional reabsorption in the guinea pig fetus (136). By 34 weeks of gestation, the human neonate can reabsorb over 99% of the filtered glucose load (12).

Maturation of Proximal Tubule Volume Reabsorption

The developing kidney exhibits a centrifugal pattern of nephron maturation with juxtamedullary nephrons being formed before superficial nephrons (61). The glomerular and tubular morphology of juxtamedullary nephrons are more mature than those in the superficial cortex (61). In many species, including the rat and rabbit, nephrogenesis continues after birth in the superficial cortex. Nephrogenesis

also continues postnatally in humans born before 36 weeks gestation.

The reabsorptive capacity of neonatal superficial and juxtamedullary proximal tubules is less than that in adults. The rate of volume absorption in superficial proximal convoluted tubules increases twofold between the 22–24-day-old weanling to 40–45-day-old adult rat (9). In rabbit superficial proximal tubules, the rate of volume absorption increased fourfold between 1 week and 1 month of age (117), while the rate of volume absorption in rabbit juxtamedullary proximal convoluted tubules did not change appreciably during that time (186). There is a twofold increase in volume absorption in juxtamedullary nephrons between 4 and 6 weeks of age in the rabbit (186).

Proximal tubule transport for each solute is the sum of transport mediated by passive diffusion, solvent drag, and active transport. Active transport of many solutes by the proximal tubule is sodium dependent where the low intracellular sodium concentration generated by the basolateral Na,K-ATPase provides the driving force for apical solute entry. The maturational changes in proximal tubule transporter activities mediating active solute transport are discussed in detail below.

There is evidence that a greater fraction of solute transport by the neonatal proximal tubule may be due to passive diffusion than by the adult segment (18, 112). Urinary recovery of mannitol microinjected into an early proximal tubule loop increased from 92% in neonates to 100% in adult guinea pigs (111). Since mannitol is only transported passively across the paracellular pathway, these data are consistent with greater paracellular permeability of this and likely other solutes. Histologic studies have demonstrated an almost twofold maturational increase in the length of the proximal tubule intercellular channels; however, there was no difference in length of the zonulae occludens or the width of the intercellular channels (111).

Direct measurements of chloride and bicarbonate permeability of the rabbit proximal convoluted tubule demonstrate that neonatal segments have a lower permeability to both solutes than observed in the adult (151, 154, 198). In addition, the resistance of the proximal tubule is higher in the neonatal rabbit proximal tubule than in the adult, providing further evidence that there are developmental changes in the paracellular pathway in neonates (154). Finally, studies have demonstrated that solvent drag does not contribute significantly to volume absorption in the neonatal tubule, since the reflection coefficients for both NaCl and $NaHCO_3$ were not different than 1 (153).

The vast majority of water transport in the proximal tubule is transcellular and not across the paracellular pathway. Water movement in this segment is through a 28-Kd membrane protein designated aquaporin-1 (203). Aquaporin-1 is present in equal abundance in the apical and basolateral membranes of the proximal tubule (203). The fetal proximal tubule has a paucity of detectable aquaporin-1; however, at the time of birth there is substantial increase in aquaporin-1 expression on the apical and basolateral membrane in juxta-medullary proximal tubules (203).

Adult proximal tubule water reabsorption is characterized by a higher osmotic than diffusional water permeability, low activation energy, and sensitivity to mercurial compounds (30, 158, 227). In vitro microperfusion of rabbit neonatal proximal tubules have similar characteristics (153). Interestingly, while the diffusional water permeability was the same in neonatal and adult proximal tubules, the osmotic water permeability was greater in the neonatal segment (153). We have examined the reason for the high osmotic water permeability in the neonatal proximal tubule and found that the proximal tubule osmotic permeability of both the apical and basolateral membranes could not explain the higher osmotic permeability of the intact tubule and that the expression of aquaporin-1 was actually far less in neonatal apical and basolateral membranes than in the mature segment (139, 155, 157, 158). The cytoplasm accounts for over half the resistance to transcellular water movement (30), and this resistance is much lower in neonates, which explains the high osmotic permeability in the intact neonatal tubule (155).

Maturation of Proximal Tubule NaCl Transport

In the early proximal tubule there is preferential reabsorption of bicarbonate over chloride ions. This leaves the proximal tubule with a higher luminal chloride concentration and a lower bicarbonate concentration than the peritubular fluid. Chloride transport is the sum of active transcellular reabsorption and chloride diffusion across the paracellular pathway down its concentration gradient. In the adult rabbit proximal convoluted tubule two thirds of NaCl transport is active and transcellular and one-third is passive and paracellular (22). In the adult rat proximal convoluted tubule one-third of NaCl transport is active and two thirds is mediated by passive diffusion (3).

Active chloride transport by the proximal convoluted tubule is mediated by the parallel operation of the Na–H antiporter and Cl–base exchangers (15, 196, 199). Cl–OH, Cl–oxalate, and Cl–formate exchange have all been found to mediate chloride uptake into the proximal tubule (15); however, the relative importance of these transporters remains controversial. In the rabbit superficial convoluted tubule, there is evidence for both Cl–OH and Cl–formate exchangers (199). However, in juxtamedullary proximal convoluted tubules, only Cl–OH exchange is present (199). In the guinea pig there is a large increase in Na^+–H^+ antiporter activity and Cl–formate exchange in brush-border membrane vesicles during the transition from fetus to newborn (77). In isolated perfused rabbit proximal straight tubules, we found that the rate of active NaCl transport was twofold greater in adult proximal straight tubules compared to neonatal tubules (195). Both Cl–OH and Na–H exchange activities were fivefold less in neonatal tubules compared to that in adult tubules (195).

The relative contribution of passive chloride transport to total NaCl transport may be species specific. In the adult rat

the late proximal tubular chloride concentration is significantly higher than that in the glomerular ultrafiltrate (122). However, in the neonatal rat, the proximal tubule luminal chloride concentration remained the same as that in the glomerular ultrafiltrate. The constant luminal chloride concentration could be due to equal rates of chloride and bicarbonate reabsorption by the immature segment or to a higher chloride permeability in the neonate, which mediates higher rates of passive chloride transport than in adults (122). Direct measurements of chloride permeability and the relative contributions of passive chloride transport have not been examined in vivo. Thus, the reason for the lack of the chloride gradient in neonatal rat proximal tubules is unknown.

Passive chloride transport has been characterized in the rabbit using in vitro microperfusion (154, 195, 198). The chloride permeability of rabbit superficial and juxtamedullary proximal convoluted tubule was directly measured. There was no difference in the chloride permeability in neonatal and adult superficial proximal convoluted tubules. In both neonates and adults, the chloride permeability was extremely low, indicating that passive chloride transport does not contribute significantly to chloride absorption in this nephron segment (198). The permeability of chloride in neonatal juxtamedullary proximal convoluted tubules was more than 10-fold lower than that of the adult segment (198). In adult rabbit proximal straight tubules, there is a substantive rate of passive chloride transport (154, 195). However, the neonatal rabbit proximal tubule is impermeable to chloride ions, and thus there is no passive chloride transport in the neonatal proximal straight tubule (154, 195). The rate of passive NaCl transport in neonatal rabbit proximal straight tubules perfused in vitro was half that of the mature segment. Compared to the mature segment, the neonatal proximal tubule has a higher transepithelial resistance and higher sodium-to-chloride and bicarbonate-to-chloride permeability ratios (154). These maturational changes indicated that there must be a developmental change in the composition of tight junction proteins. We have shown that there is a maturational decrease in claudin-2 and increase in occludin in the rat which may explain these permeability differences (80).

Na,K-ATPase Activity

The Na,K-ATPase provides the driving force for all sodium-dependent transport along the nephron by generating and maintaining a low intracellular sodium concentration. Inhibition of Na,K-ATPase activity with ouabain causes a reduction in the rate of volume absorption to a level not different from zero in neonatal and adult isolated rabbit proximal convoluted tubules perfused with an ultrafiltrate-like solution (186). Thus, maturation of Na,K-ATPase activity plays a key role in the maturation of solute transport along the nephron.

The Na,K-ATPase is made up of an α subunit and a regulatory β subunit. There are four α isoforms and three β isoforms (34). The α subunit is the catalytic subunit and has an ATP binding site as well as the binding site for cardiac glycosides. The adult kidney predominantly expresses the α1 and β1 isoforms (63, 143). There is a postnatal increase in renal Na,K-ATPase activity (10, 11, 67, 184, 187). In dissected rabbit tubules, the neonatal Na,K-ATPase activity is lower than the adult level in each nephron segment examined (184) (Fig. 4). The V_{max} Na,K-ATPase activity increases fivefold during renal maturation with no change in the K_m for sodium, potassium, or ATP.

The increase in Na,K-ATPase activity in rabbit juxtamedullary proximal convoluted tubule lags behind by 1 week the maturational increase in bicarbonate and volume absorption (184). This suggests that the maturational increase in apical membrane transport is the driving force for the increase in Na,K-ATPase on the basolateral membrane. Several studies have supported this hypothesis. An increase in intracellular sodium stimulates Na,K-ATPase activity (48, 86, 119). In rat proximal tubule cells in culture, stimulation of the Na^+–H^+ antiporter increases intracellular sodium and leads to an increase in Na,K-ATPase activity (86). An increase in intracellular sodium not only increases pump activity, but also increases α and β Na,K-ATPase subunit mRNA and protein abundance (48). Chronic increases in Na^+–H^+ antiporter activity in rats in vivo induced by metabolic acidosis result in an increase in Na,K-ATPase activity in growing but not adult rats, an effect not seen when the rats were administered amiloride, an inhibitor of the Na^+–H^+ antiporter (66). Thus, the maturational increase in Na^+–H^+ antiporter activity may be responsible for the increase in Na,K-ATPase activity.

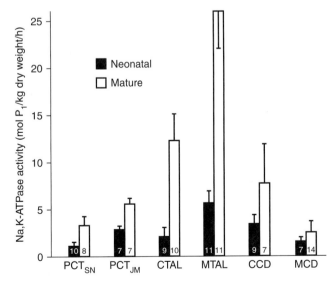

FIGURE 4 Na,K-ATPase activity in neonatal and adult rabbit nephron segments. PCT_{SN}, superficial proximal convoluted tubule; PCT_{JM}, juxtamedullary proximal convoluted tubule; CTAL and MTAL, cortical and medullary thick ascending limbs; CCD and MCD, cortical and medullary collecting ducts. (With permission, from Schmidt U, Horster M. NA-K–activated ATPase: activity maturation in rabbit nephron segments dissected in vitro. *Am J Physiol Renal Fluid Electrolyte Physiol* 1977;233:F55–F60.)

Distal Tubule NaCl Transport

The thick ascending limb and distal convoluted tubule reabsorb NaCl and are impermeable to water, processes (or transport pathways) that are essential for the generation of concentrated and dilute urine. The osmolality of the luminal fluid collected by micropuncture of rat early distal tubules was 40% lower in adults compared to neonates (242), and the fraction of filtered sodium remaining in the early distal tubule was higher in neonatal than adult rats (6) consistent with a maturational increase in the rate of sodium transport in the thick ascending limb. In vivo micropuncture of 13- to 39-day-old rats showed an increase in loop NaCl reabsorption during postnatal maturation (122), and in vitro microperfusion of the rabbit cortical thick ascending limb demonstrated that the rate of sodium transport in the adult segment was fivefold greater than that of the neonate (95). Both rat and rabbit cortical and medullary thick ascending limb Na,K-ATPase activity increase approximately fourfold during postnatal maturation consistent with a large developmental increase in sodium reabsorption by both segments (160, 184). The maturational increase in Na,K-ATPase activity in the rat is mediated by glucocorticoids (160).

A direct comparison of NaCl transport in neonatal and adult medullary thick ascending limb has not been performed; however, there is a maturational increase in Na,K-ATPase activity in this segment (54, 184). In the adult medullary thick ascending limb vasopressin increases the rate of NaCl reabsorption and in rats there is a fourfold increase in cAMP formation in the medullary thick ascending limb in response to vasopressin during postnatal maturation (102). Whether vasopressin directly stimulates sodium transport in neonatal segments is unknown.

As noted earlier, one of the most striking differences in sodium transport is the fact that compared to adults, neonates have a limited capacity to excrete a sodium load that is not due solely to a lower GFR (5, 51, 71). None of the nephron segments thus far discussed is responsible for this phenomenon, as this requires a segment where the relative transport rates are higher in neonates than in adults. The adult distal convoluted tubule reabsorbs only 5% of the filtered sodium but sodium transport rates are higher in neonates (6). In an in vivo micropuncture study distal tubule transport was assayed during hydropenia and during volume expansion in 24- and 40-day-old rats. While 24-day-old hydropenic rats had a higher fraction of filtered sodium remaining in the early distal tubule than 40-day-old animals, this difference had disappeared by the late distal tubule puncture site. With volume expansion there was a comparable fraction of filtered sodium remaining in the early distal tubule in the two age groups, but there was enhanced late distal tubule sodium reabsorption in the younger rats (6). Thus, this segment is, at least in part, responsible for the blunted natriuresis with salt loading in neonates.

The cortical collecting duct is the nephron segment responsible for the final modulation of sodium transport under the control of aldosterone. In the isolated perfused cortical collecting tubule, there is a three- to fivefold increase in sodium transport between 1 week and adult rabbits (175, 224, 226, 284). Most of the maturational increase occurs between the first and second weeks of life. Sodium enters in neonatal and adult cortical collecting tubule via an apical sodium channel termed ENaC. ENaC is the rate-limiting step in collecting tubule sodium transport, and neonatal cortical collecting ducts have fewer apical conducting sodium channels adult segments (Fig. 5) (100, 179). ENaC is composed of α, β, and γ subunits, and the mRNA and protein abundance of each increases during postnatal life (100, 226, 230, 243). The driving force for conductive sodium entry across the apical conductance is the basolateral Na,K-ATPase, which increases in activity twofold during maturation in this segment (184). Interestingly, the fetal collecting duct expresses α and $β_2$ Na,K-ATPase on the apical membrane (39, 96).

REGULATION OF SODIUM TRANSPORT

Renin-Angiotensin-Aldosterone Axis

The plasma concentrations of both renin and aldosterone are higher in the neonate than in the adult and contribute to the regulation of sodium transport by the neonatal nephron (70, 213). Plasma renin activity responds appropriately to changes in extracellular fluid volume in the fetus, premature infant, and neonate (56, 70, 104, 269, 270). In human neonates the plasma renin activity varies inversely with alterations in dietary sodium intake, demonstrating that this limb of the renin-angiotensin-aldosterone axis is intact (70). Premature neonates also respond to the negative salt balance of prematurity with appropriate increases in plasma renin activity (213).

Plasma aldosterone levels are also significantly higher in preterm and term neonates than in adults (7, 29, 200, 213). Cord blood from term infants born to mothers who ingested a normal salt diet had significantly lower plasma aldosterone levels than those whose mothers who ingested a low-salt diet or who were taking diuretics (29). These data imply that the human fetus can also respond to volume contraction with an increase in serum aldosterone. The plasma aldosterone level has also been shown to vary inversely with sodium intake in preterm infants with respiratory distress syndrome (200). Although the newborn can increase aldosterone secretion, the effect of aldosterone to increase distal tubule sodium reabsorption and potassium secretion is blunted (7, 213). For example, in adult rats adrenalectomy produces a 40-fold increase in urinary Na/K ratio, but in neonatal rats adrenalectomy has no effect on urinary electrolyte excretion (211). Administration of exogenous aldosterone to adult adrenalectomized rats

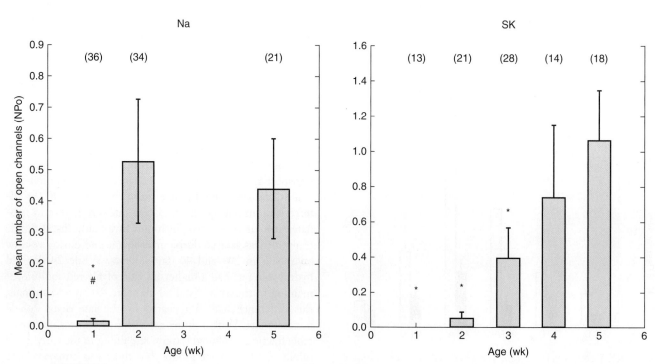

FIGURE 5 Postnatal changes in number of conducting Na (ENaC) and secretory potassium (SK) channels per cell-attached patch of apical membrane of rabbit principal cells. The number of functional Na channels increased ~30-fold between the first and second weeks of life, whereas the number of SK channels increased gradually after the second postnatal week. (With permission, from Satlin LM, Palmer LG. Apical Na+ conductance in maturing rabbit principal cell. *Am J Physiol Renal Fluid Electrolyte Physiol* 1996;270: F391–F397; and Satlin LM, Palmer LG. Apical Na+ conductance in maturing rabbit principal cell. *Am J Physiol Renal Fluid Electrolyte Physiol* 1997;272:F397–F404).)

decreases the urinary Na/K ratio profoundly, but administration of aldosterone had no effect on these urinary electrolytes in adrenalectomized neonatal rats (211). Isolated perfused cortical collecting tubules from adult rabbits treated with mineralocorticoid had a significant increase in sodium absorption compared to control rabbits, but neonatal cortical collecting tubules were unaffected by prior mineralocorticoid treatment (224). This resistance to aldosterone in neonates is not due to a paucity of mineralocorticoid receptors but to a postreceptor phenomenon (211).

Angiotensin II augments proximal tubule sodium reabsorption by binding to both basolateral and luminal receptors. Recent studies have demonstrated that endogenously produced angiotensin II can modulate proximal tubule transport in the adult rat and rabbit (150). While neonatal rats have a blunted diuresis and natriuresis in response to volume expansion, this was not the case in neonates that received Losartan, an AT_I receptor blocker, consistent with an augmented effect of angiotensin II in the neonate (44).

Atrial Natriuretic Peptide

Atrial natriuretic peptide (ANP) is normally released under conditions of volume expansion and produces natriuresis and an increase in the GFR. ANP levels are higher in the fetus than in the maternal plasma (171, 232). While adult ANP production is solely from the atria, fetal ANP is produced by both the atria and ventricles (232). Shortly after birth, ANP declines to a level close to the adult, and atrial production of atriopeptins increases concomitantly with a fall in ventricular production (232).

The fetus and neonate respond to alterations in extracellular fluid volume with appropriate changes in plasma ANP levels (168, 171). ANP levels are elevated in the perinatal period, which contributes to the diuresis as well as the maintenance of volume homeostasis in the neonate (33, 222). Compared to adults, however, the human fetus and neonate have a less sustained rise in ANP plasma levels in response to volume expansion, which may be a factor in the attenuated natriuresis with volume expansion in the neonate (38).

Prostaglandins

PGE2 has a direct inhibitory action on sodium transport in the cortical and outer medullary collecting tubule and promotes a natriuresis and diuresis in adults (144, 212). This is not the case in neonates or the fetus where indomethacin does not affect salt and water excretion (129, 144). Indomethacin has no effect on sodium transport in neonatal tubules suggesting that endogenous production of prostaglandin does not modulate transport by the neonatal segment (163). These data are consistent with studies demonstrating a low synthetic rate of prostaglandins by neonatal cortical and medullary collecting tubules (182).

Renal Nerves and Catecholamines

Renal nerve stimulation produces an increase in renal vascular resistance and reduction in renal blood flow in the fetus and newborn as it does in the adult, although the effect is lower in immature animals (167). Renal denervation of the fetus and neonatal lamb does not significantly alter renal blood flow, with GFR or renal sodium handling indicating that basal renal function is not significantly affected by renal nerves (165, 204, 205). However, in the transition from fetal to neonatal life, renal nerves may play a role in the decrease in sodium excretion that occurs during this period (206). Sheep with denervated kidneys had a greater urine volume and sodium excretion in the first 24 hours after birth as well as lower plasma ANP and renin levels (206). There was no difference in urinary sodium or volume excretion after the first day of life, indicating that other unknown variables play an important role in mediating the profound decrease in urinary sodium and volume excretion after birth (206).

Dopamine is a natriuretic hormone that is increased with volume expansion. Dopamine increases renal blood flow and GFR and inhibits sodium transport in the proximal tubules, thick ascending limb, and collecting duct (8). The concentration of dopamine is higher in fetal rat plasma and amniotic fluid than the maternal blood (39). Administration of exogenous dopamine to human premature neonates with respiratory distress syndrome increases GFR, and produces a natriuresis and diuresis (221). However, comparative studies have demonstrated that the inhibitory effect of dopamine on sodium transport is attenuated in neonates compared to adults. The inhibitory effect of dopamine on the $Na^+–H^+$ antiporter and Na,K-ATPase is less in neonatal than in adult tubules (8, 67, 107, 125).

RENAL ACIDIFICATION

The serum bicarbonate concentration in human infants in the first year of life averages 22 mEq/L, a value significantly less than that of adults (59). Premature human neonates can have serum bicarbonate levels as low as 14.5 mEq/L (189). The lower serum bicarbonate concentration in neonates and infants is due to a lower threshold for bicarbonate by the immature kidney (59). This section will discuss the salient differences between the neonatal and adult kidney with regard to renal acidification.

Proximal Tubules

The adult proximal tubule reabsorbs 80% of the filtered bicarbonate. The lower bicarbonate threshold in neonates is, in large part, due to a lower bicarbonate reabsorptive capacity of the neonatal proximal tubule. In juxtamedullary proximal convoluted tubules perfused in vitro, the rate of bicarbonate reabsorption in proximal tubules from 1-week-old rabbits was one third that of the adult proximal tubule (186). The rate of bicarbonate absorption did not vary significantly until the time of weaning at 4 weeks of age. Adult rates of bicarbonate absorption were attained at 6 weeks of age. The maturational pattern of glucose and total volume reabsorption was quite similar to that for bicarbonate absorption (186). The rate of bicarbonate absorption has not been directly measured in superficial nephrons. However, micropuncture studies in rats and in vitro microperfusion studies in rabbits have demonstrated a similar maturational increase in the rate of volume absorption in these segments (9, 117, 122). Since a substantial fraction of volume absorption reflects bicarbonate absorption, a similar maturational pattern for bicarbonate is assumed to occur.

There are several potential explanations for the lower rate of bicarbonate transport in neonatal proximal tubules. In the adult proximal tubule, there is a preferential reabsorption of bicarbonate over chloride ions. This leaves the luminal fluid with a higher chloride concentration and a lower bicarbonate concentration than that in the peritubular capillaries. This bicarbonate concentration difference could potentially allow bicarbonate to diffuse from the peritubular capillaries back to the luminal fluid. The amount of bicarbonate passive backflux is dependent on the permeability of the paracellular pathway of the neonatal proximal tubule to bicarbonate.

As discussed previously, there is evidence for a maturational change in paracellular pathway permeability (111, 151, 154, 195, 197, 198). Direct measurements of bicarbonate permeability in juxtamedullary rabbit proximal convoluted tubules demonstrate that bicarbonate permeability was actually significantly lower in neonatal juxtamedullary proximal tubules perfused in vitro than that of the adult segment (151). Thus, the lower rate of bicarbonate transport in neonatal juxtamedullary proximal tubules is not explained by enhanced back diffusion, but is entirely due to a lower rate of active transcellular bicarbonate transport.

In the adult proximal tubule, two thirds of apical proton secretion is mediated by an apical Na^+-H^+ antiporter and one-third is via a H^+-ATPase (20, 149). The driving force for the Na^+-H^+ antiporter is the low intracellular sodium concentration generated by the Na,K-ATPase. In the adult proximal tubule, bicarbonate exit occurs through the $Na(HCO_3)_3$ symporter. A lower rate of bicarbonate reabsorption by the neonatal proximal tubule could be due to lower activity of any of these transport processes.

Studies using a variety of different techniques have demonstrated a maturational increase in Na^+-H^+ antiporter activity in the proximal tubule apical membrane (19, 20, 28, 194). In isolated, perfused, rabbit juxtamedullary proximal convoluted tubules, the rate of Na^+-H^+ antiporter activity was approximately one-third that of the adult rate, and adult values were measured at 6 weeks of age (19). These results compare well to the maturational changes in bicarbonate absorption measured in isolated perfused rabbit convoluted

tubules (186). While this study solely examined juxtamedullary proximal tubules, similar findings have been demonstrated in brush-border membrane vesicles from renal-cortex (28). Na^+-H^+ antiporter activity in late rabbit fetal kidney cortex was found to be one fourth that of the adult cortex. This difference was entirely due to a lower V_{max} with no change in the K_M for sodium (28).

The H^+-ATPase present on the apical membrane of the adult proximal tubules does not contribute significantly to bicarbonate absorption in the neonatal proximal tubule. To study the relative contribution of the Na^+-H^+ antiporter and the H^+-ATPase to proximal tubule acidification, the rates of these two transporters were assayed by measuring proton secretory rates in adult and neonatal proximal convoluted tubules in response to an intracellular acid load (20). As has previously been demonstrated, the rate of neonatal Na^+-H^+ antiporter activity was less than that in the adult. In the adult rabbit proximal tubule, two-thirds of the pH recovery from an acid load was due to the Na^+-H^+ antiporter and one third was due to a sodium-independent mechanism, likely the H^+-ATPase. In the neonate, 95% of pH recovery was due to the Na^+-H^+ antiporter, and only 5% was due to a sodium-independent mechanism. Thus, both the Na^+-H^+ antiporter and the H^+-ATPase undergo a significant increase in activity during maturation and presumably limit bicarbonate absorption by the neonatal proximal tubule.

Three isoforms of the Na^+-H^+ antiporter, NHE-1, NHE-3, and NHE-8 have been localized to the proximal tubule (31, 32, 75, 244). NHE-1 has a ubiquitous distribution in tissues and is found on the basolateral membrane of the proximal tubule (32). NHE-3 is the apical membrane Na^+-H^+ antiporter that mediates most luminal proton secretion by the adult proximal tubule (31, 239). There is a substantive postnatal maturational increase in NHE-3 mRNA and protein abundance (23). Interestingly, neonates have Na^+-H^+ antiporter activity at a time when NHE-3 protein abundance is barely detectable. This Na^+-H^+ antiporter activity is likely mediated by NHE-8, a recently cloned proximal tubule isoform that is more highly expressed in the neonatal proximal tubule than in the adult. NHE-1 protein abundance does not vary significantly with postnatal maturation (23).

The $Na(HCO_3)_3$ symporter, which is located on the basolateral membrane, facilitates bicarbonate exit from the proximal tubule. $Na(HCO_3)_3$ symporter activity in neonates is only slightly less than such activity in adults (19). This transporter not only plays a role in bicarbonate exit, but is the predominant mechanism for the defense against changes in intracellular pH by the proximal tubule (19).

Distal Tubule Acidification

The adult cortical collecting duct can absorb or secrete bicarbonate depending on the acid-base status of the animal (134). Proton and bicarbonate secretion are mediated by α- and β-intercalated cells, respectively, which are far fewer in number than principal cells, the predominant cells in the cortical collecting duct. The number of α- and β-intercalated cells per millimeter of tubular length increases several fold during maturation of the rabbit cortical collecting duct (62, 178).

Isolated perfused cortical collecting tubules from neonatal rabbits exhibit no net bicarbonate transport, whereas adult cortical collecting ducts secrete bicarbonate (135). Bicarbonate secretion by the β-intercalated cell occurs via an apical chloride-bicarbonate exchanger that functions at a reduced rate in the neonatal segment (178). Removal of bath chloride inhibits basolateral membrane chloride-base exchanger on α-intercalated cells and inhibits luminal proton secretion. Removal of bath chloride had no effect on the rate of bicarbonate transport in cortical collecting tubules from neonatal rabbits, but increased net bicarbonate secretion in adult segments (135). There is also evidence for reduced activity of the α-intercalated cell in the cortical collecting duct (178, 181). The number of acidic vesicles and the intracellular pH is lower in neonatal cells consistent with reduced proton pump activity compared to the adult (178).

The outer medullary collecting duct is an important segment for urinary acidification. Unlike the cortical collecting tubule, the number of intercalated cells per millimeter tubular length does not change significantly with postnatal development (62, 181). The rate of bicarbonate absorption is only slightly less in the neonatal outer medullary collecting ducts compared to the adult rabbit segment (135). Thus, there is a significant difference in the relative maturity of the cortical and medullary segments in neonates.

Titratable Acid and Ammonia Excretion

In addition to reclaiming the filtered load of bicarbonate, the kidney must excrete an amount of acid equivalent to the acid generated from metabolism. The growing animal must also excrete protons liberated during the formation of bone (114, 115). This is in part compensated for by the gastrointestinal absorption of alkali (114, 115, 229), but as in the adult, the neonatal kidney plays a major role in acid excretion. Thus, the kidney of the growing neonate must excrete 50%–100% more acid per kilogram than in the adult.

To excrete the quantity of acid generated from metabolism of proteins and growing bones, there must be urinary buffers to accept the secreted protons. If there were not titratable acids and ammonia in our urine, the secretion of a few protons would decrease the urine pH to levels that would inhibit further proton secretion. Net acid excretion, the sum of ammonium and titratable acid excretion, per kilogram of body weight is significantly less in neonates than adults (132). However, by 7 days of age cow's milk formula fed infants had comparable rates of ammonium and titratable acid excretion as that of adults when normalized per kilogram of body weight (131, 132). Breast milk–fed infants, however, had significantly less phosphate intake than infants

fed cow's milk formula and have been shown to have lower rates of titratable acid excretion (52, 65, 88, 132). Thus, the rate of renal maturation of net acid excretion is quite brisk. However, neonates, unlike adults, function at near maximal capacity of net acid excretion to eliminate metabolically generated acid (131), and have a limited ability to respond to an exogenous acid load by increasing titratable acid and ammonia excretion. In comparison to adults, neonates given an acid load had a smaller increase of both titratable acid and ammonium excretion, making them more prone to develop acidosis when so challenged (47, 88). By 1 month of age, the rate of net acid excretion in response to acid load was comparable to that of adults (59, 74, 138, 147, 216). However, young infants responded to an acid load with higher rates of titratable acid excretion to compensate for the lower rates of ammonium excretion (59, 138). In vitro studies have shown that the rate of renal ammonia production in kidney slices is lower in neonates compared to adults (93). The low rate of ammonia production in neonates is due predominantly to lower rates of renal glutaminase activity (73, 228) and, to a lesser extent, a lower concentration of glutamine, the substrate for ammonia production, secondary to lower glutamine synthetase activity (73, 228).

Premature neonates have significantly lower rates of titratable acid and ammonia excretion than do term infants (113, 214, 217). Preterm infants are thus less tolerant of high-protein formulas than term infants because sulfur-containing amino acids generate an acid load that cannot be eliminated due to low rates of net acid excretion (49, 216). Administration of NH_4Cl to premature infants resulted in an increase in net acid excretion, but premature infants had lower rates of ammonium and titratable acid excretion and a higher urine pH than did term neonates (74, 113, 214–217). As with term infants, there is a rapid maturation of the ability of premature infants to excrete an exogenous acid load (113, 214, 217).

Carbonic Anhydrase Activity

Carbonic anhydrase facilitates the conversion of CO_2 and H_2O to H_2CO_3 (188). Carbonic anhydrase II is located in the cytosol of all acidifying renal tubules and comprises 95% of carbonic anhydrase activity in the kidney (108). Carbonic anhydrase IV comprises approximately 5% of total renal carbonic anhydrase activity, and is located on the apical and basolateral membrane of the proximal tubule and on the apical membrane of acid-secreting cells in the distal nephron (188, 190, 191, 235). Carbonic anhydrase XII is also present on the basolateral membrane of acidifying segments, but its role in renal acidification is unclear at present (145). Carbonic anhydrase plays an important role in proximal tubule bicarbonate reabsorption, as evidenced by the fact that there is a 90% inhibition of bicarbonate reabsorption when this enzyme is inhibited (128). Thus, a lower rate of carbonic anhydrase activity by acidifying proximal and distal nephron segments may be a factor that limits the rate of bicarbonate absorption. Carbonic anhydrase II protein abundance, normalized per millimeter of tubular length, increases approximately 10-fold in rat proximal convoluted tubules, cortical collecting tubules, and outer medullary collecting tubules between 1 and 12 weeks of age (108). In the rabbit, carbonic anhydrase II increases only twofold during postnatal maturation compared to carbonic anhydrase IV, which undergoes a 10-fold increase in mRNA and protein abundance with cortical maturation (235).

INDUCTION OF NEPHRON MATURATION

There are substantive changes in nephron maturation during postnatal development. Most of our knowledge of postnatal maturation comes from work examining changes that occur with the proximal tubule, which will be the focus here. There are a number of potential factors that may be responsible for the postnatal maturational changes in proximal tubule transport. The maturational increase in GFR may induce the maturation of transporters on the apical membrane by increasing solute delivery. As previously discussed, an increase in apical membrane sodium transport could increase intracellular sodium and play a potential role in the maturational increase in Na,K-ATPase activity (48, 87, 119). There are also significant postnatal maturational changes in several hormones that affect proximal tubular transport, including thyroid hormone and glucocorticoids, which increase 3-fold and 20-fold, respectively, in the postnatal period (92).

Glucocorticoids increase renal cortical Na^+–H^+ antiporter activity. This effect can, in part, be mediated by an increase in GFR, which will increase sodium delivery to the proximal tubule. However, glucocorticoids and thyroid hormone have direct epithelial action on the proximal tubule to increase the rate of bicarbonate absorption and Na^+–H^+ antiporter activity (21, 24). This effect of glucocorticoids and thyroid hormone is due to a direct action to increase NHE-3 transcription (21, 41). Administration of glucocorticoids to pregnant rabbits 2 days prior to the delivery increases the V_{max} of the Na^+–H^+ antiporter to levels seen in adults (28). The K_m for sodium was unaffected. Similarly, proximal convoluted tubules from neonatal rabbits whose mothers received dexamethasone before delivery had infants with an almost twofold increase in the rate of bicarbonate absorption to levels comparable to that measured in adult animals (26). In addition, the rate of Na^+–H^+ antiporter and $Na(HCO_3)_3$ activity in proximal tubules increased twofold in dexamethasone treated neonates (26). The effect of dexamethasone was specific for the NHE-3 isoform, the isoform present on the apical membrane of the proximal tubule and responsible for the majority of Na^+–H^+ antiporter activity in adults (23). Prevention of the maturational increase of glucocorticoids or thyroid hormone limits the maturational increase in Na^+–H^+ antiporter activity and NHE-3 protein abundance to adult levels (25, 79). While glucocorticoids are the most important factor in the matu-

rational increase in NHE-3, adrenalectomy in the neonatal period did not prevent an increase in both in Na^+–H^+ antiporter activity and NHE-3 protein and mRNA abundance, suggesting that thyroid hormone can compensate, to some extent, in the absence of glucocorticoids (79). This was definitively demonstrated in studies using the hypothyroid-glucocorticoid–deficient rats where the maturational increase in both hormones was prevented and where Na^+–H^+ antiporter activity and NHE-3 protein and mRNA abundance remained at neonatal levels into adulthood (78).

As will be discussed, there is a maturational decrease in the rate of phosphate transport during postnatal maturation (45, 52, 94, 164). This is observed at a time when there is an increase in serum glucocorticoid levels (91). Administration of glucocorticoids to neonatal rats produced a significant inhibition in the rate of sodium-dependent phosphate uptake. This was due to a reduction in the V_{max} with no change in the K_M for phosphate (14). This glucocorticoid-induced decrease in phosphate uptake was not accompanied by a change in NaP_i mRNA abundance; however, there was a threefold decrease in NaP_i transporter protein abundance (14). Thus, glucocorticoids appear to stimulate most apical and basolateral transporters which increase with maturation and also may play a role in the maturational decrease in phosphate transport.

Thyroid hormone appears to play an important role in postnatal development of mitochondrial enzymes in the rat proximal convoluted tubule. The normal maturational increase in the proximal tubule mitochondrial enzymes 3-keto acid-CoA transferase, an enzyme involved in ketone body oxidation, citrate synthase and carnitine acetyltransferase, were impaired in hypothyroid rats (233). The enzyme activities were restored with thyroid replacement. Acetoacetyl-CoA thiolase, however, was not decreased in 21-day-old hypothyroid rats (233). Finally, thyroid hormone may play a role in the maturational changes that occur in the permeability properties of the paracellular pathway (27, 197). As noted above, the adult rabbit proximal straight tubule has a high chloride permeability that results in high rates of passive chloride transport (197). The neonatal rabbit proximal straight tubule is impermeable to chloride (154). Neonatal proximal straight tubules have higher P_{Na}/P_{Cl} (sodium-to-chloride permeability ratio) and P_{HCO3}/P_{Cl} ratios than adult segments. Many, but not all, of the maturational changes in paracellular permeability properties of the proximal tubule can be accelerated by administration of thyroid hormone to neonates (197), or prevented if the neonates are made hypothyroid (197).

PHOSPHATE TRANSPORT

Phosphate is essential for the growing animal, and unlike adults who are in phosphate balance, only 60% of absorbed phosphate is excreted in the urine of neonates. Human neonates and infants have a higher serum phosphate concentration than that of adults. While the high serum phosphate in neonates could be due to the lower GFR in neonates compared to adults, this is not the case. Studies have demonstrated that increasing the GFR by arginine infusion in young rats does not increase phosphate excretion and lowering the GFR in adult rats by constricting the abdominal aorta does not increase the rate of phosphate absorption to that seen in the neonate (84). The tubular reabsorptive capacity for phosphate is higher in neonates and infants than in adults (45, 52, 94, 164). Approximately 90% of the filtered phosphate is reabsorbed in human neonates during the first week of life, and growing children continue to maintain a higher maximal tubular reabsorption of phosphate than adults (45, 94).

A number of variables such as parathyroid hormone, dietary phosphate content and growth factors can modulate phosphate transport and could potentially explain the higher rate of phosphate transport by the neonatal kidney. However, a higher intrinsic rate of renal phosphate transport has been demonstrated in the isolated perfused guinea pig kidney where these factors were eliminated (104). The maximal tubular reabsorption of phosphate per volume of glomerular filtrate in 3- to 7-day-old neonatal kidneys was 40% greater than that measured in adult animals. A higher intrinsic rate of proximal tubular phosphate reabsorption was also directly demonstrated in micropuncture studies where neonatal guinea pigs reabsorbed a higher fraction of filtered phosphate than adults (110). The maximal rate of phosphate uptake in brush-border membrane vesicles is fivefold higher in neonates than in adults, in the absence of a maturational change in the K_M for phosphate in growing animals (141).

In addition to the difference in the rate of sodium-dependent phosphate cotransport with maturation, other factors may play a role in the higher rates of phosphate transport in growing animals. The intracellular phosphate concentration measured in isolated perfused kidneys using nuclear magnetic resonance was significantly lower in growing animals than adults (17). This provides a greater driving force for phosphate transport in growing animals. The lower intracellular phosphate concentration in the presence of a higher rate of apical phosphate transport implies that the rate of basolateral phosphate exit is also higher in growing animals, although this has not been directly examined.

Membrane fluidity also has been shown to affect phosphate transport (123, 124, 137). The brush-border membrane content of cholesterol, sphingomyelin, and phosphatidylinositol increases with age (124). This change in lipid composition decreases membrane fluidity (124, 137), which directly decreases the rate of phosphate transport (123, 137). Thus, the lipid composition and high membrane fluidity of the neonate and growing animal provides an environment that increases the V_{max} of the NaPi cotransporter. Glucocorticoids, which increase during the time of weaning, decrease membrane fluidity and likely play a role in the postnatal decrease in phosphate transport (14).

The predominant brush-border membrane NaPi cotransporter has been designated NaPi-2A. NaPi-2A mRNA is first detected in early proximal convolutions in the post–S-shaped body segment of the developing nephron (185). However, NaPi-2A protein is not detected until the proximal tubules have a distinct brush-border membrane (219). Brush-border membrane NaPi-2A expression is twofold higher in 4-week-old juvenile rats than in adult rats consistent with the higher rate of phosphate transport in growing animals (236).

While there is increased expression of NaPi-2A in growing animals, it does not fully explain the disparity in the rate of NaPi cotransport between growing animals and adults. There is evidence that the higher rate of phosphate transport in growing animals is due to a growth-related, sodium-dependent phosphate transporter other than NaPi-2A (236). Recently, a growth-related NaPi cotransporter has been cloned and designated NaPi-2C (193). Unlike NaPi-2A, NaPi-2C is electroneutral. It is highly expressed in weanling animals and, like NaPi-2A, regulated by dietary phosphate intake (193).

Dietary phosphate content regulates renal phosphate transport in adult and in growing animals (42, 109, 140, 236). Thyroparathyroidectomized growing rats had a greater increase in their maximal tubular capacity of phosphate reabsorption in response to a low-phosphate diet and a blunted decrease in phosphate reabsorption on a high-phosphate diet compared to adult thyroparathyroidectomized rats (42, 140). In addition, the adaptive increase in maximal tubular capacity of phosphate reabsorption in response to phosphate deprivation took longer to occur in adult animals than in growing animals (42). A low-phosphate diet increases the rate of sodium-dependent phosphate uptake by brush-border membrane vesicles in growing rats (43). In addition, ingestion of a low-phosphate diet increases the abundance of Na-Pi transporters on the apical membrane of the proximal tubule, whereas a high-phosphate diet produces the opposite effect (236). In each of these phosphate diets, the expression of NaPi-2A was higher in growing rats than in adult rats (236).

The plasma concentration of PTH is lower in human neonates than in adults (50). Fetal and neonatal rats can respond to changes in serum calcium with appropriate changes in PTH levels (218), but there is a blunted response to PTH (231). However, infusion of PTH in 1-day-old human neonates produces no increase in urinary phosphate excretion (45, 126). By 3 days of age, infusion of parathyroid hormone results in an increase in phosphate excretion and increase in urinary cAMP (45, 126, 133). However, the phosphaturic response to PTH is markedly lower in neonates than adults (126). Furthermore, in micropuncture studies, the proximal tubule response to infusion of pharmacologic doses of PTH is attenuated in young rats compared to adults (236). Despite the fact that PTH did not significantly increase phosphate excretion in young animals, the urinary cAMP per milliliter GFR in response to PTH infusion was similar in all ages (231). Thus, there is clearly a disassociation between the PTH-induced increase in cAMP production in neonates and the effect on phosphate excretion.

Growth hormone administration can result in an increase in serum phosphate (90). Brush-border–membrane vesicle phosphate transport is increased in dogs that received growth hormone compared to controls (82). The effect of growth hormone on phosphate transport is mediated by IGF-1 (152). While growth hormone is not a significant regulator of phosphate transport in the adult, this may not be the case in the growing animal. Administration of growth hormone–releasing factor antagonist, which suppresses growth hormone secretion, has no effect on the maximal rate of phosphate absorption in adult rats but significantly reduces phosphate absorption in growing rats (85).

POTASSIUM TRANSPORT

The placenta is responsible for the maintenance of a potassium gradient that ensures adequate delivery of potassium to the growing fetus. Both premature and term neonates have very low rates of renal potassium excretion, which maintains a positive potassium balance necessary for growth (213). The low rate of renal potassium excretion is also responsible for the higher serum potassium concentration in neonates than in adults (213). Renal potassium clearance in infants less than 1 year of age is lower than that of older children even if corrected for GFR (176, 213). Neonates can respond to potassium loading with net tubular secretion but this response is lower than that of adults (127).

The proximal tubule of neonatal and adult rats reabsorbs approximately 50% of the filtered potassium (122). There is a maturational increase in potassium reabsorption by the loop of Henle (55, 122). The loop of Henle of adult rats has been shown to reabsorb 79% of the delivered load while only 56% was reabsorbed by 13- to 15-day-old neonates (122). The limited capability of the thick ascending limb of the neonate to reabsorb potassium will increase distal delivery of potassium. Thus, neither the proximal tubule nor the loop of Henle is responsible for the limited capability of the neonate to excrete potassium.

The connecting tubule and cortical collecting duct ultimately regulate potassium excretion in adults and neonates. Clearance studies in dogs have demonstrated that the amiloride-sensitive component of potassium secretion was substantially less in neonates than adults, providing indirect evidence for a limited distal nephron potassium-secretory capacity (127). A low rate of potassium excretion early in life could be due to the low rate of conductive apical sodium transport, reflecting the low number of apical conducting sodium channels (179), which in turn, limits the electrochemical driving force for conductive potassium secretion. Low rates of sodium absorption and potassium secretion could also be explained by the low rate of Na,K-ATPase activity in this segment in neonates (184). While low rates of luminal flow and distal sodium delivery can limit potassium secretion in adults, these are unlikely to be significant variables in neonates, which have high rates of distal nephron flow and sodium delivery (6, 122).

The maturation of cortical collecting tubule potassium transport has been directly examined in the rabbit using in vitro microperfusion (175). Potassium secretory rates were not different from zero during the first 3 weeks of life, and did not reach mature rates until 6 weeks of age (175). Maturation of sodium transport by this segment and the concomitant generation of a lumen negative potential difference occurred at an earlier age than potassium secretion first became detectable. The absence of potassium secretion in neonates was not due to the inability of Na,K-ATPase to increase intracellular potassium and create the chemical driving force for luminal secretion, as intracellular potassium levels in cortical collecting tubules were the same as that in adults (177). The limitation in potassium secretion is likely due to a paucity of apical potassium-secretory channels, since the driving force for potassium secretion exists in the neonate (Figure 5).

There are two distinct potassium channels in the collecting duct principal cell. The secretory K (SK) channel, encoded by ROMK, is a small conductance channel with a high open probability. The SK/ROMK channel is considered to mediate baseline potassium secretion (180), while the high conductance maxi-K channel mediates flow-dependent potassium secretion (237, 238). Both potassium channels increase in abundance during postnatal maturation (180, 238, 243). The H,K-ATPase is a third potassium transporter, which is present in intercalated cells in the distal nephron. The H,K-ATPase has little functional role except under conditions of potassium deficiency and metabolic acidosis, when it mediates potassium absorption and proton secretion. The activity of this transporter is comparable in neonates and adult collecting tubules (46).

URINARY CONCENTRATING AND DILUTING ABILITY

Deprived of water for sufficient time, an adult human can concentrate the urine to 1200 mOsm/kg of water; the term and premature neonatal kidney can achieve urine osmolalities of only 400–600 mOsm/kg of water (64, 83, 146, 148). By 6 months of age, the infant can increase the urine osmolality to 600 mOsm/kg of water (148), and by 12 to 18 months, the human infant can concentrate the urine to levels comparable to that of the adult (148, 234). The neonate also has a limited capacity to excrete free water compared to that of adults (121, 130). However, both term and premature infants can excrete diluted urine with an osmolality approaching 50 mOsm/kg of water (170). Thus, the primary limiting factor in the ability of the neonate to excrete free water is the low GFR that limits the distal delivery of fluid.

The ability to maximally concentrate the urine in the human requires that the hypothalamus and pituitary can synthesize and secret vasopressin, that the renal medulla can form and maintain an adequate osmotic gradient, and that the renal collecting duct can respond to vasopressin by increasing its water permeability. In the developing human, there are a number of factors in the concentrating mechanism that limit the ability to maximally concentrate urine. The neonate and late-gestation fetus respond to changes in plasma osmolality and volume with appropriate changes in plasma vasopressin (81, 120, 161, 162). These changes in plasma vasopressin are comparable in magnitude to that measured under similar conditions in the adult (120, 161). Perinatal stress also results in the secretion of vasopressin (81, 162). However, infusion of vasopressin in late-gestation fetal sheep resulted in a smaller increase in urinary osmolality than that measured in adult animals (169). Thus, while the fetus and neonate can secrete vasopressin at concentrations comparable to the adult, they are less responsive to its action.

The osmotic gradient in the renal medulla is composed of urea and sodium chloride. The urea concentration in the neonatal renal medulla is limited in part by the low dietary protein intake and the high volume of fluids normally ingested (57, 58). Augmentation of protein or addition of urea to the diet of neonates increases their maximal concentrating ability, albeit not to the levels measured in adults (57, 58). The capacity of the thick ascending limb to reabsorb sodium chloride is significantly less in neonates than in adult animals, and thus plays a significant role in the inability of the neonate to concentrate urine to the same extent as that of adults (6, 95, 98, 160, 184, 242). Furthermore, the vasopressin-mediated increase in medullary thick ascending limb, adenylate-cyclase activity is lower in the neonate than in the adult, which would attenuate the vasopressin-mediated increase in sodium chloride transport in this segment (102). The developmental changes that occur in transport with age in the thick ascending limb are paralleled by an increase in the concentration of sodium and urea in the medulla and papilla (161, 210). The urinary concentrating ability of neonatal rats can be induced by the administration of betamethasone (161). Adrenalectomy in rats prevents the maturational increase in papillary sodium and urea concentration, but not the growth of the papilla consistent with a role for glucocorticoids in the maturation of the tubular transport processes responsible for development of maximally concentrated urine (161). Sorbitol, a major intracellular osmolite in the inner medulla, is formed by aldose reductase. Aldose reductase mRNA and activity in rat neonatal inner medulla are significantly less than that in the adult (192). Fluid restriction increases aldose reductase activity in the adult medulla, but not in the neonate (192).

In addition to the limited osmotic gradient in the neonatal kidney, the neonatal collecting duct does not respond to vasopressin to the same extent as the adult tubule. The basal osmotic water permeability of the adult and neonatal inner medullary collecting duct is very low (202). In both the outer medullary collecting tubule and inner medullary collecting duct, vasopressin results in an increase in osmotic permeability, yet the response is far less than that measured in the adult segment (99, 202).

The limited response to vasopressin by the neonatal collecting tubule is due to several factors. There are fewer vasopressin-binding sites in medullopapillary membranes from neonatal rats compared to adults (159). The vasopressin-mediated increase in adenylate cyclase activity is also lower in the neonatal collecting tubule (68, 102, 159, 183). Recent studies have demonstrated that mRNA and protein abundance of the apical collecting tubule water channel, aquaporin-2, is less in the renal medulla of neonatal rats than that of adult animals (241). Both aquaporin-2 mRNA and protein abundance are increased by betamethasone (241), providing further evidence that glucocorticoids are important in the maturation of the urinary concentrating mechanism.

Prostaglandins also play a role in the limited response of the neonatal collecting duct to vasopressin. When exposed to vasopressin, cAMP generation by neonatal tubules was less than that measured in adult tubules (35). However, in the presence of indomethacin, the cAMP production of the neonatal collecting ducts increased to the level detected in the adult (36). In addition, it has been shown that the neonatal kidney has a higher level of expression of prostaglandin receptors when compared to the adult kidney (35). However, when neonatal collecting ducts were perfused in the presence of indomethacin to inhibit the production of prostaglandins, there was no improvement in the response to vasopressin (37). Thus, the role of prostaglandins in the limited response to vasopressin in the neonatal collecting duct remains unclear.

Recently, the role of phosphodiesterase was examined (156). Neonatal collecting ducts were shown to have an elevated phosphodiesterase activity (which degrades cAMP) when compared to adult tubules, which could limit the response to vasopressin (156). In the presence of inhibitors of phosphodiesterase, response of the neonatal collecting duct to vasopression was not different from the adult tubules (156). Thus, developmental changes in phosphodiesterase could play an important role in the development of the concentrating ability.

References

1. Al-Dahhan J, Haycock GB, Chantler C, Stimmler L. Sodium homeostasis in term and preterm neonates. *Arch Dis Child* 1983;58:335–342.
2. Allison ME, Lipham EM, Gottschalk CW. Hydrostatic pressure in the rat kidney. *Am J Physiol* 1972;223:975–983.
3. Alpern RJ, Howlin KJ, Preisig PA. Active and passive components of chloride transport in the rat proximal convoluted tubule. *J Clin Invest* 1985;76:1360–1366.
4. Aperia A, Broberger O, Elinder G, Herin P, Zetterstrom R. Postnatal development of renal function in pre-term and full-term infants. *Acta Paediatr Scand* 1981;70:183–187.
5. Aperia A, Broberger O, Thodenius K, Zetterstrom R. Renal response to an oral sodium load in newborn full-term infants. *Acta Paediatr Scand* 1972;61:670–676.
6. Aperia A, Elinder G. Distal tubular sodium reabsorption in the developing rat kidney. *Am J Physiol* 1981;240:F487–F491.
7. Aperia A, Broberger O, Herin P, Zetterstrom R. Sodium excretion in relation to sodium intake and aldosterone excretion in newborn preterm and fulterm infants. *Acta Paediatr Scand* 1979;68:813–817.
8. Aperia AC. Intrarenal dopamine: a key signal in the interactive regulation of sodium metabolism. *Annu Rev Physiol* 2000;62:621–647.
9. Aperia A, Larsson L. Corrrelation between fluid reabsorption and proimal tubule ultrastructure during development of the rat kidney. *Acta Physiol Scand* 1979;105:11–22.
10. Aperia A, Larsson L. Induced development of proximal tublar NaKATPase, basolateral cell membranes and fluid reabsorption. *Acta Physiol Scand* 1984;121:133–141.
11. Aperia A, Larsson L, Zetterstrom R. Hormonal induction of Na-K-ATPase in developing proximal tubular cells. *Am J Physiol* 1981;241:F356–F360.
12. Arant BS Jr. Developmental patterns of renal functional maturation compared in the human neonate. *J Pediatr* 1978;92:705–712.
13. Arant BS, Edelmann CM, Nash MA. The renal reabsorption of glucose in the developing canine kidney: a study of glomerulotubular balance. *Pediatr Res* 1974;8:638–646.

14. Arar M, Levi M, Baum M. Maturational effects of glucocorticoids on neonatal brush-border membrane phosphate transport. *Pediatr Res* 1994;35:474–478.
15. Aronson PS. Role of ion exchangers in mediating NaCl transport in the proximal tubule. *Kidney Int* 1996;49:1665–1670.
16. Aschinberg LC, Goldsmith DI, Olbing H, Spitzer A, Edelmann CM Jr, Blaufox MD. Neonatal changes in renal blood flow distribution in puppies. *Am J Physiol* 1975;228:1453–1461.
17. Barac-Nieto M, Dowd TL, Gupta RK, Spitzer A. Changes in NMR-visible kidney cell phosphate with age and diet: relationship to phosphate transport. *Am J Physiol* 1991;261: F153–F162.
18. Barac-Nieto M, Spitzer A. The relationship between renal metabolism and proximal tubule transport during ontogeny. *Pediatr Nephrol* 1988;2:356–367.
19. Baum M. Neonatal rabbit juxtamedullary proximal convoluted tubule acidification. *J Clin Invest* 1990;85:499–506.
20. Baum M. Developmental changes in rabbit juxtamedullary proximal convoluted tubule acidification. *Pediatr Res* 1992;31:411–414.
21. Baum M, Amemiya M, Dwarakanath V, Alpern RJ, Moe OW. Glucocorticoids regulate NHE-3 transcription in OKP cells. *Am J Physiol* 1996;270:F164–F169.
22. Baum M, Berry CA. Evidence for neutral transcellular NaCl transport and neutral basolateral chloride exit in the rabbit convoluted tubule. *J Clin Invest* 1984;74:205–211.
23. Baum M, Biemesderfer D, Gentry D, Aronson PS. Ontogeny of rabbit renal cortical NHE3 and NHE1: effect of glucocorticoids. *Am J Physiol* 1995;268:F815–F820.
24. Baum M, Cano A, Alpern RJ. Glucocorticoids stimulate Na+/H+ antiporter in OKP cells. *Am J Physiol* 1993;264:F1027–F1031.
25. Baum M, Dwarakanath V, Alpern RJ, Moe OW. Effects of thyroid hormone on the neonatal renal cortical Na+/H+ antiporter. *Kidney Int* 1998;53:1254–1258.
26. Baum M, Quigley R. Prenatal glucocorticoids stimulate neonatal juxtamedullary proximal convoluted tubule acidification. *Am J Physiol* 1991;261:F746–F752.
27. Baum M, Quigley R. Thyroid hormone modulates rabbit proximal straight tubule paracellular permeability. *Am J Physiol Ren Physiol* 2004;286:F477–F482.
28. Beck JC, Lipkowitz MS, Abramson RG. Ontogeny of Na/H antiporter activity in rabbit renal brush border membrane vesicles. *J Clin Invest* 1991;87:2067–2076.
29. Beitins IZ, Bayard F, Levitsky L, Ances IG, Kowarski A, Migeon CJ. Plasma aldosterone concentration at delivery and during the newborn period *J Clin Invest* 1972;51:386–394.
30. Berry CA. Characteristics of water diffusion in the rabbit proximal convoluted tubule. *Am J Physiol* 1985;249:F729–F738.
31. Biemesderfer D, Pizzonia J, Abu-Alfa A, Exner M, Reilly R, Igarashi P, Aronson PS. NHE3: a Na+/H+ exchanger isoform of renal brush border. *Am J Physiol* 1993;265:F736–F742.
32. Biemesderfer D, Reilly RF, Exner M, Igarashi P, Aronson PS. Immunocytochemical characterization of Na(+)-H+ exchanger isoform NHE-1 in rabbit kidney. *Am J Physiol* 1992;263: F833–F840.
33. Bierd TM, Kattwinkel J, Chevalier RL, Rheuban KS, Smith DJ, Teague WG, Carey RM, Linden J. Interrelationship of atrial natriuretic peptide, atrial volume, and renal function in premature infants *J Pediatr* 1990;116:753–759.
34. Blanco G, Mercer RW. Isozymes of the Na-K-ATPase: heterogeneity in structure, diversity in function. *Am J Physiol* 1998;275:F633–F650.
35. Bonilla-Felix M, Jiang W. Expression and localization of prostaglandin EP3 receptor mRNA in the immature rabbit kidney. *Am J Physiol* 1996;271:F30–F36.
36. Bonilla-Felix M, John-Phillip C. Prostaglandins mediate the defect in AVP-stimulated cAMP generation in immature collecting duct. *Am J Physiol* 1994;267:F44–F48.
37. Bonilla-Felix M, Vehaskari VM, Hamm LL. Water transport in the immature rabbit collecting duct. *Pediatr Nephrol* 1999;13:103–107.
38. Brace RA, Miner LK, Siderowf AD, Cheung CY. Fetal and adult urine flow and ANF responses to vascular volume expansion. *Am J Physiol* 1988;255:R846–R850.
39. Burrow CR, Devuyst O, Li X, Gatti L, Wilson PD. Expression of the beta2-subunit and apical localization of Na+-K+-ATPase in metanephric kidney *Am J Physiol* 1999;277: F391–F403.
40. Calcagno PL, Rubin MI. Renal extraction of paraaminohippurate in infants and children. *J Clin Invest* 1963;42:1632–1639.
41. Cano A, Baum M, Moe OW. Thyroid hormone stimulates the renal Na/H exchanger NHE3 by transcriptional activation. *Am J Physiol* 1999;276:C102–C108.
42. Caverzasio J, Bonjour JP, Fleisch H. Tubular handling of Pi in young growing and adult rats. *Am J Physiol* 1982;242:F705–F710.
43. Caverzasio J, Murer H, Fleisch H, Bonjour JP. Phosphate transport in brush border membrane vesicles isolated from renal cortex of young growing and adult rats. Comparison with whole kidney data. *Pflugers Arch* 1982;394:217–221.
44. Chevalier RL, Thornhill BA, Belmonte DC, Baertschi AJ. Endogenous angiotensin II inhibits natriuresis after acute volume expansion in the neonatal rat. *Am J Physiol* 1996;270: R393–R397.
45. Connelly JP, Crawford JD, Watson J. Studies of neonatal hyperphosphatemia. *Pediatrics* 1962;30:425–432.
46. Constantinescu A, Silver RB, Satlin LM. H-K-ATPase activity in PNA-binding intercalated cells of newborn rabbit cortical collecting duct. *Am J Physiol* 1997;272:F167–F177.
47. Cort JPMRA. The renal response of puppies to an acidosis. *J Physiol (London)* 1954;124: 358–369.
48. Cramb G, Cutler CP, Lamb JF, McDevitt T, Ogden PH, Owler D, Voy C. The effects of monensin on the abundance of mRNA(alpha) and sodium pumps in human cultured cells. *Q J Exp Physiol* 1989;74:53–63.
49. Darrow DC, DaSilva MM, Stevenson SS. Production of acidosis in premature infants by protein milk. *J Pediatr* 1945;27:43–58.
50. David L, Anast CS. Calcium metabolism in newborn infants. The interrelationship of parathyroid function and calcium, magnesium, and phosphorus metabolism in normal, "sick," and hypocalcemic newborns. *J Clin Invest* 1974;54:287–296.
51. Dean RF, McCance RA. The renal response of infants and adults to the administration of hypertonic solutions of sodium chloride and urea. *J Physiol (London)* 2004;109:81–87.
52. Dean RFA, McCance RA. Phosphate clearance in infants and adults. *J Physiol (London)* 1948;107:182–186.
53. Dean RFAMRA. Inulin, diodone, creatinine and urea clearance in newborn infants. *J Physiol (London)* 1947;106:431–439.
54. Djouadi F, Wijkhuisen A, Bastin J. Coordinate development of oxidative enzymes and Na-K-ATPase in thick ascending limb: role of corticosteroids. *Am J Physiol* 1992;263:F237–F242.
55. Dlouha H. A micropuncture study of the development of renal function in the young rat. *Biol Neonate* 1976;29:117–128.
56. Drukker A, Goldsmith DI, Spitzer A, Edelmann CM Jr, Blaufox MD. The renin angiotensin system in newborn dogs: developmental patterns and response to acute saline loading. *Pediatr Res* 1980;14:304–307.
57. Edelmann CM Jr, Barnett HL, Stark H. Effect of urea on concentration of urinary nonurea solute in premature infants. *J Appl Physiol* 1966;21:1021–1025.
58. Edelmann CM Jr, Barnett HL, Troupkou V. Renal concentrating mechanisms in newborn infants. Effect of dietary protein and water content, role of urea, and responsiveness to antidiuretic hormone. *J Anat* 1960;1062–1069.
59. Edelmann CMJ, Soriano JR, Boichis H, Gruskin AB, Acosta M. Renal bicarbonate reabsorption and hydrogen ion excretion in normal infants. *J Clin Invest* 1967;46:1309–1317.
60. Engelke CS, Shah LB, Vasan U, Raye RJ. Sodium balance in very-low-birth-weight infants. *J Pediatr* 1978;93:837–841.
61. Evan AP, Gattone IJ, Schwartz GJ. Development of solute transport in rabbit proximal tubule. II. Morphologic segmentation. *Am J Physiol* 1983;245:F391–F407.
62. Evan AP, Satlin LM, Gattone VH, Connors B, Schwartz GJ. Postnatal maturation of rabbit renal collecting duct. II. Morphological observations. *Am J Physiol* 1991;261: F91–F107.
63. Farman N. Na,K-pump expression and distribution in the nephron. *Miner Electrolyte Metab* 1996;22:272–278.
64. Fisher DA, Pyle HR Jr, Porter JC, Beard AG, Panos TC. Control of water balance in the newborn. *Am J Dis Child* 1963;106:137–146.
65. Fomon SJHDMJRL. Acidification of the urine by infants fed human milk and whole cow's milk. *Pediatrics* 1959;23:113–120.
66. Fukuda Y, Aperia A. Differentiation of Na+-K+ pump in rat proximal tubule is modulated by Na+-H+ exchanger. *Am J Physiol* 1988;255:F552–F557.
67. Fukuda Y, Bertorello A, Aperia A. Ontogeny of the regulation of Na+,K(+)-ATPase activity in the renal proximal tubule cell. *Pediatr Res* 1991;30:131–134.
68. Gengler WR, Forte LR. Neonatal development of rat kidney adenyl cyclase and phosphodiesterase. *Biochim Biophys Acta* 1972;279:367–372.
69. Gersh I. The correlation of structure and function in the developing mesonephros and metanephros. *Contrib Embryol* 1937;153:35–58.
70. Godard C, Geering JM, Geering K, Vallotton MB. Plasma renin activity related to sodium balance, renal function and urinary vasopressin in the newborn infant. *Pediatr Res* 1979;13: 742–745.
71. Goldsmith DI, Drukker A, Blaufox MD, Edelmann CM Jr, Spitzer A. Hemodynamic and excretory response of the neonatal canine kidney to acute volume expansion. *Am J Physiol* 1979;237:F392–F397.
72. Goldsmith DI, Jodorkovsky RA, Sherwinter J, Kleeman SR, Spitzer A. Glomerular capillary permeability in developing canines. *Am J Physiol* 1986;251:F528–F531.
73. Goldstein L. Ammonia metabolism in kidneys of suckling rats. *Am J Physiol* 1971;220: 213–217.
74. Gordon HHMHBHR. The response of young infants to ingestion of ammonium chloride. *Pediatrics* 1948;2:290–302.
75. Goyal S, Vanden Heuvel G, Aronson PS. Renal expression of novel Na+/H+ exchanger isoform NHE8. *Am J Physiol Renal Physiol* 2003;284:F467–F473.
76. Gruskin AB, Edelmann CM Jr, Yuan S. Maturational changes in renal blood flow in piglets. *Pediatr Res* 1970;4:7–13.
77. Guillery EN, Huss DJ. Developmental regulation of chloride/formate exchange in guinea pig proximal tubules. *Am J Physiol* 1995;269:F686–F695.
78. Gupta N, Dwarakanath V, Baum M. Maturation of the Na+/H+ antiporter (NHE3) in the proximal tubule of the hypothyroid adrenalectomized rat. *Am J Physiol Renal Physiol* 2004;287: F521–F527.
79. Gupta N, Tarif SR, Seikaly M, Baum M. Role of glucocorticoids in the maturation of the rat renal Na+/H+ antiporter (NHE3). *Kidney Int* 2001;60:173–181.
80. Haddad M, Lin F, Dwarakanath V, Cordes K, Baum M. Developmental changes in proximal tubule tight junction proteins. *Pediatr Res* 2005;57:453–457.
81. Hadeed AJ, Leake RD, Weitzman RE, Fisher DA. Possible mechanisms of high blood levels of vasopressin during the neonatal period. *J Pediatr* 1979;94:805–808.
82. Hammerman MR, Karl IE, Hruska KA. Regulation of canine renal vesicle Pi transport by growth hormone and parathyroid hormone. *Biochim Biophys Acta* 1980;603:322–335.
83. Hansen JOL, SmithC.A. Effects of withholding fluid in the immediate post-natal period. *Pediatrics* 1953;12:99–113.
84. Haramati A, Mulroney SE. Enhanced tubular capacity for phosphate reabsorption in immature rats—role of glomerular-filtration rate (GFR). *Fed Proc* 1987;46:1288.
85. Haramati A, Mulroney SE, Lumpkin MD. Regulation of renal phosphate reabsorption during development: implications from a new model of growth hormone deficiency. *Pediatr Nephrol* 1990;4:387–391.
86. Harris RC, Seifter JL, Lechene C. Coupling of Na-H exchange and Na-K pump activity in cultured rat proximal tubule cells. *Am J Physiol* 1986;251:C815–C824.
87. Harris RC, Seifter JL, Lechene C. Coupling of Na-H exchange and Na-K pump activity in cultured rat proximal tubule cells. *Am J Physiol* 1986;251:C815–C824.
88. Hatemi N, McCance RA. Response to acidifying drugs. *Acta Paediatr Scand* 1961;50:603–616.
89. Haworth J, MacDonald MS. Reducing sugars in the urine and blood of premature babies. *Arch Dis Child* 1957;32:417–421.
90. Henneman PH, Forbes AP, Moldawer M, Dempsey EF, Carroll EL. Effects of human growth hormone in man. *J Clin Invest* 1960;39:1223–1238.

91. Henning SJ. Plasma concentrations of total and free corticosterone during development in the rat. *Am J Physiol* 1978;235:E451–E456.

92. Henning SJ. Plasma concentrations of total and free corticosterone during development in the rat. *Am J Physiol* 1978;235:E451–E456.

93. Hines BK, McCance RA. Ammonia formation from glutamine by kidney slices from adult and newborn animals. *J Physiol (London)* 1954;124:8–16.

94. Hohenauer L, Rosenberg TF, Oh W. Calcium and phosphorus homeostasis on the first day of life. *Biol Neonate* 1970;15:49–56.

95. Horster M. Loop of Henle functional differentiation: in vitro perfusion of the isolated thick ascending segment. *Pflugers Arch* 1978;378: 15–24.

96. Horster M, Huber S, Tschop J, Dittrich G, Braun G. Epithelial nephrogenesis. *Pflugers Arch* 1997;434:647–660.

97. Horster M, Valtin H. Postnatal development of renal function: micropuncture and clearance studies in the dog. *J Clin Invest* 1971;50:779–795.

98. Horster MF, Gilg A, Lory P. Determinants of axial osmotic gradients in the differentiating countercurrent system. *Am J Physiol* 1984;246:F124–F132.

99. Horster MF, Zink H. Functional differentiation of the medullary collecting tubule: influence of vasopressin. *Kidney Int* 1982;22:360–365.

100. Huber SM, Braun GS, Horster MF. Expression of the epithelial sodium channel (ENaC) during ontogenic differentiation of the renal cortical collecting duct epithelium. *Pflugers Arch* 1999;437:491–497.

101. Ichikawa I, Maddox DA, Brenner BM. Maturational development of glomerular ultrafiltration in the rat. *Am J Physiol* 1979;236:F465–F471.

102. Imbert-Teboul M, Chabardes D, Clique A, Montegut M, Morel F. Ontogenesis of hormone-dependent adenylate cyclase in isolated rat nephron segments. *Am J Physiol* 1984;247:F316–F325.

103. John E, Goldsmith DJ, Spitzer A. Quantitative changes in the canine glomerular vasculature during development: physiologic implications. *Kidney Int* 1981;20:223–229.

104. Johnson V, Spitzer A. Renal reabsorption of phosphate during development: whole-kidney events. *Am J Physiol* 1986;251:F251–F256.

105. Jose PA, Slotkoff LM, Lilienfield LS, Calcagno PL, Eisner GM. Sensitivity of neonatal renal vasculature to epinephrine. *Am J Physiol* 1974;226:796–799.

106. Jose PA, Slotkoff LM, Montgomery S, Calcagno PL, Eisner G. Autoregulation of renal blood flow in the puppy. *Am J Physiol* 1975;229:983–988.

107. Kaneko S, Albrecht F, Asico LD, Eisner GM, Robillard JE, Jose PA. Ontogeny of DA1 receptor-mediated natriuresis in the rat: in vivo and in vitro correlations. *Am J Physiol* 1992;263:R631–R638.

108. Karashima S, Hattori S, Ushijima T, Furuse A, Nakazato H, Matsuda I. Developmental changes in carbonic anhydrase II in the rat kidney. *Pediatr Nephrol* 1998;12:263–268.

109. Karlen J. Renal response to low and high phosphate intake in weanling, adolescent and adult rats. *Acta Physiol Scand* 1989;135:317–322.

110. Kaskel FJ, Kumar AM, Feld LG, Spitzer A. Renal reabsorption of phosphate during development: tubular events. *Pediatr Nephrol* 1988;2:129–134.

111. Kaskel FJ, Kumar AM, Lockhart EA, Evan A, Spitzer A. Factors affecting proximal tubular reabsorption during development. *Am J Physiol* 1987;252:F188–F197.

112. Deleted in proof.

113. Kerpel-Fronius E, Heim T, Solyuk E. The development of the renal acidifying processes and their relation to acidosis in low-birth-weight infants. *Biol Neonate* 1979;15:156–168.

114. Kildeberg P, Engel K, Winters RW. Balance of net acid in growing infants. Endogenous and transintestinal aspects. *Acta Paediatr Scand* 1969;58:321–329.

115. Kildeberg P, Winters R. Infant feeding and blood acid–base status. *Pediatrics* 1972;49:801–802.

116. Knutson DW, Chieu F, Bennett CM, Glassock RJ. Estimation of relative glomerular capillary surface area in normal and hypertrophic rat kidneys. *Kidney Int* 1978;14:437–443.

117. Larsson L, Horster M. Ultrastructure and net fluid transport in isolated perfused developing proximal tubules. *J Ultrastruc Res* 1976;54:276–285.

118. Deleted in proof.

119. Larsson SH, Rane S, Fukuda Y, Aperia A, Lechene C. Changes in Na influx precede postnatal increase in Na, K-ATPase activity in rat renal proximal tubular cells. *Acta Physiol Scand* 1990;138:99–100.

120. Leake RD, Weitzman RE, Weinberg JA, Fisher DA. Control of vasopressin secretion in the newborn lamb. *Pediatr Res* 1979;13:257–260.

121. Leake RD, Zakauddin S, Trygstad CW, Fu P, Oh W. The effects of large volume intravenous fluid infusion on neonatal renal function. *J Pediatr* 1976;89:968–972.

122. Lelievre-Pegorier M, Merlet-Benichou C, Roinel N, de Rouffignac C. Developmental pattern of water and electrolyte transport in rat superficial nephrons. *Am J Physiol* 1983;245:F15–F21.

123. Levi M, Baird BM, Wilson PV. Cholesterol modulates rat renal brush border membrane phosphate transport. *J Clin Invest* 1990;85:231–237.

124. Levi M, Jameson DM, van der Meer BW. Role of BBM lipid composition and fluidity in impaired renal Pi transport in aged rat. *Am J Physiol* 1989;256:F85–F94.

125. Li XX, Albrecht FE, Robillard JE, Eisner GM, Jose PA. Gbeta regulation of Na/H exchanger-3 activity in rat renal proximal tubules during development. *Am J Physiol Regul Integr Comp Physiol* 2000;278:R931–R936.

126. Linarelli LG. Nephron urinary cyclic AMP and developmental renal responsiveness to parathyroid hormone. *Pediatrics* 1972;50:14–23.

127. Lorenz JM, Kleinman LJ, Disney TA. Renal response of newborn dog to potassium loading. *Am J Physiol* 1986;251:F513–F519.

128. Lucci MS, Pucacco LR, DuBose TD Jr, Kokko JP, Carter NW. Direct evaluation of acidification by rat proximal tubule: role of carbonic anhydrase. *Am J Physiol* 1980;238:F372–F379.

129. Matson JR, Stokes JB, Robillard JE. Effects of inhibition of prostaglandin synthesis on fetal renal function. *Kidney Int* 1981;20:621–627.

130. McCance RA, Naylor NJ, Widdowson EM. The response of infants to a large dose of water. *Arch Dis Child* 1954;29:104–109.

131. McCance RA, HN. Control of acid–base stability in the newly born. *Lancet* 1961;1:293–297.

132. McCance RA, Widdowson EM. Renal aspects of acid–base control in the newly born. *Acta Paediatr Scand* 1960;49:409–414.

133. McCrory WW, Forman CW, McNamara H, Barnett HL. Renal excretion of inorganic phosphate in newborn infants. *J Clin Invest* 1952;31:357–366.

134. McKinney TD, Burg MB. Bicarbonate transport by rabbit cortical collecting tubules. Effect of acid and alkali loads in vivo on transport in vitro. *J Clin Invest* 1977;60:766–768.

135. Mehrgut FM, Satlin LM, Schwartz GJ. Maturation of HCO_3^- transport in rabbit collecting duct. *Am J Physiol* 1990;259:F801–F808.

136. Merlet-Benichou C, Pegorier M, Muffat-Joly M, Augeron C. Functional and morphologic patterns of renal maturation in the developing guinea pig. *Am J Physiol* 1981;36:H1467–H1475.

137. Molitoris BA, Simon FR. Renal cortical brush-border and basolateral membranes: cholesterol and phospholipid composition and relative turnover. *J Membr Biol* 1985;83:207–215.

138. Monnens L, Schretlen E, van Munster P. The renal excretion of hydrogen ions in infants and children. *Nephron* 1974;12:29–43.

139. Mulder J, Baum M, Quigley R. Diffusional water permeability (PDW) of adult and neonatal rabbit renal brush border membrane vesicles. *J Membr Biol* 2002;187:167–174.

140. Mulroney SE, Haramati A. Renal adaptation to changes in dietary phosphate during development. *Am J Physiol* 1990;258:F1650–F1656.

141. Neiberger RE, Barac-Nieto M, Spitzer A. Renal reabsorption of phosphate during development: transport kinetics in BBMV. *Am J Physiol* 1989;257:F268–F274.

142. Olbing H, Blaufox MD, Aschinberg LC, Silkalns GI, Bernstein J, Spitzer A, Edelmann CM Jr. Postnatal changes in renal glomerular blood flow distribution in puppies. *J Clin Invest* 1973;52:2885–2895.

143. Orlowski J, Lingrel JB. Tissue-specific and developmental regulation of rat Na,K-ATPase catalytic alpha isoform and beta subunit mRNAs. *J Biol Chem* 1988;263:10436–10442.

144. Osborn JL, Hook JB, Bailie MD. Effect of saralasin and indomethacin on renal function in developing piglets. *Am J Physiol* 1980;238:R438–R442.

145. Parkkila S, Parkkila AK, Saarnio J, Kivela J, Karttunen TJ, Kaunisto K, Waheed A, Sly WS, Tureci O, Virtanen J, Rajaniemi H. Expression of the membrane-associated carbonic anhydrase isozyme XII in the human kidney and renal tumors. *J Histochem C ytochem* 2000;48: 1601–1608.

146. Pellegrini L, Burke DF, von Delft F, Mulloy B, Blundell TL. Crystal structure of fibroblast growth factor receptor ectodomain bound to ligand and heparin. *Nature* 2000;407:1029–1034.

147. Peonides A, Levin B, Young WF. The renal excretion of hydrogen ions in infants and children. *Arch Dis Child* 1965;40:33–39.

148. Polacek E, Vocel J, Neugebaurova L, Sebkova M, Vechetova E. The osmotic concentrating ability in healthy infants and children. *Arch Dis Child* 1965;40:291–295.

149. Preisig PA, Ives HE, Cragoe EJ Jr, Alpern RJ, Rector FC Jr. Role of the Na+/H+ antiporter in rat proximal tubule bicarbonate absorption. *J Clin Invest* 1987;80:970–978.

150. Quan A, Baum M. Regulation of proximal tubule transport by angiotensin II. *Semin Nephrol* 1997;17:423–430.

151. Quigley R, Baum M. Developmental changes in rabbit juxtamedullary proximal convoluted tubule bicarbonate permeability. *Pediatr Res* 1990;28:663–666.

152. Quigley R, Baum M. Effects of growth hormone and insulin-like growth factor I on rabbit proximal convoluted tubule transport. *J Clin Invest* 1991;88:368–374.

153. Quigley R, Baum M. Developmental changes in rabbit juxtamedullary proximal convoluted tubule water permeability. *Am J Physiol* 1996;271:F871–F876.

154. Quigley R, Baum M. Developmental changes in rabbit proximal straight tubule paracellular permeability. *Am J Physiol Renal Physiol* 2002;283:F525–F531.

155. Quigley R, Baum M. Water transport in neonatal and adult rabbit proximal tubules. *Am J Physiol Renal Physiol* 2002;283:F280–F285.

156. Quigley R, Chakravarty S, Baum M. Antidiuretic hormone resistance in the neonatal cortical collecting tubule is mediated in part by elevated phosphodiesterase activity. *Am J Physiol Renal Physiol* 2004;286:F317–F322.

157. Quigley R, Gupta N, Lisec A, Baum M. Maturational changes in rabbit renal basolateral membrane vesicle osmotic water permeability. *J Membr Biol* 2000;174:53–58.

158. Quigley R, Mulder J, Baum M. Ontogeny of water transport in the rabbit proximal tubule. *Pediatr Nephrol* 2003;18:1089–1094.

159. Rajerison RM, Butlen D, Jard S. Ontogenic development of antidiuretic hormone receptors in rat kidney: comparison of hormonal binding and adenylate cyclase activation. *Mol Cell Endocrinol* 1976;4:271–285.

160. Rane S, Aperia A. Ontogeny of Na-K-ATPase activity in thick ascending limb and of concentrating capacity. *Am J Physiol* 1985;249:F723–F728.

161. Rane S, Aperia A, Eneroth P, Lundin S. Development of urinary concentrating capacity in weaning rats. *Pediatr Res* 1985;19:472–475.

162. Rees L, Forsling ML, Brook CG. Vasopressin concentrations in the neonatal period. *Clin Endocrinol (Oxf)* 1980;12:357–362.

163. Reyes JL, Roch-Ramel F, Besseghir K. Net sodium and water movements in the newborn rabbit collecting tubule: lack of modifications by indomethacin. *Biol Neonate* 1987;51: 212–216.

164. Richmond JB, Kravitz H, Segar W, Waisman HA. Renal clearance of endogenous phosphate in infants and children. *Proc Soc Exp Biol Med* 1951;77:83–87.

165. Robillard JE, Nakamura KT, DiBona GF. Effects of renal denervation on renal responses to hypoxemia in fetal lambs. *Am J Physiol* 1986;250:F294–F301.

166. Robillard JE, Sessions C, Kennedey RL, Hamel-Robillard L, Smith FG Jr. Interrelationship between glomerular filtration rate and renal transport of sodium and chloride during fetal life. *Am J Obstet Gynecol* 1977;128:727–734.

167. Robillard JE, Smith FG, Nakamura KT, Sato T, Segar J, Jose PA. Neural control of renal hemodynamics and function during development. *Pediatr Nephrol* 1990;4:436–441.

168. Robillard JE, Weiner C. Atrial natriuretic factor in the human fetus: effect of volume expansion. *J Pediatr* 1988;113:552–555.

169. Robillard JE, Weitzman RE. Developmental aspects of the fetal renal response to exogenous arginine vasopressin. *Am J Physiol* 1980;238:F407–F414.

170. Rodriguez-Soriano J, Vallo A, Oliveros R, Castillo G. Renal handling of sodium in premature and full-term neonates: a study using clearance methods during water diuresis. *Pediatr Res* 1983;17:1013–1016.
171. Ross MG, Ervin MG, Lam RW, Castro L, Leake RD, Fisher DA. Plasma atrial natriuretic peptide response to volume expansion in the ovine fetus. *Am J Obstet Gynecol* 1987;157:1292–1297.
172. Rubin MI, Bruck E, Rapoport M, Snively M, McKay H, Baumler A. Maturation of renal function in childhood: clearance studies. *J Clin Invest* 1949;28:1144–1162.
173. Rudolph AM, Heymann MA. The circulation of the fetus in utero. Methods for studying distribution of blood flow, cardiac output and organ blood flow. *Circ Res* 1967;21:163–184.
174. Rudolph AM, Heymann MA. Circulatory changes during growth in the fetal lamb. *Circ Res* 1970;26:289–299.
175. Satlin LM. Postnatal maturation of potassium transport in rabbit cortical collecting duct. *Am J Physiol* 1994;266:F57–F65.
176. Satlin LM. Regulation of potassium transport in the maturing kidney. *Semin Nephrol* 1999;19:155–165.
177. Satlin LM, Evan AP, Gattone VH, IIJ, Schwartz GJ. Postnatal maturation of the rabbit cortical collecting duct. *Pediatr Nephrol* 1988;2:135–145.
178. Satlin LM, Matsumoto T, Schwartz GJ. Postnatal maturation of rabbit renal collecting duct. III. Peanut lectin-binding intercalated cells. *Am J Physiol* 1992;262:F199–F208.
179. Satlin LM, Palmer LG. Apical Na+ conductance in maturing rabbit principal cell. *Am J Physiol* 1996;270:F391–F397.
180. Satlin LM, Palmer LG. Apical K+ conductance in maturing rabbit principal cell. *Am J Physiol* 1997;272:F397–F404.
181. Satlin LM, Schwartz GJ. Postnatal maturation of rabbit renal collecting duct: intercalated cell function. *Am J Physiol* 1987;253:F622–F635.
182. Schlondorff D, Satriano JA, Schwartz GJ. Synthesis of prostaglandin E2 in different segments of isolated collecting tubules from adult and neonatal rabbits. *Am J Physiol* 1985;248: F134–F144.
183. Schlondorff D, Weber H, Trizna W, Fine LG. Vasopressin responsiveness of renal adenylate cyclase in newborn rats and rabbits. *Am J Physiol* 1978;234:F16–F21.
184. Schmidt U, Horster M. Na-K-activated ATPase: activity maturation in rabbit nephron segments dissected in vitro. *Am J Physiol* 1977;233:F55–F60.
185. Schmitt R, Ellison DH, Farman N, Rossier BC, Reilly RF, Reeves WB, Oberbaumer I, Tapp R, Bachmann S. Developmental expression of sodium entry pathways in rat nephron. *Am J Physiol* 1999;276:F367–F381.
186. Schwartz GH, Evan AP. Development of solute transport in rabbit proximal tubule. I. HCO_3 and glucose absorption. *Am J Physiol* 1983;245:F382–F390.
187. Schwartz GH, Evan AP. Development of solute transport in rabbit proximal tubule. III. Na-K-ATPase activity. *Am J Physiol* 1984;246:F845–F852.
188. Schwartz GJ. Physiology and molecular biology of renal carbonic anhydrase. *J Nephrol* 2002;15(Suppl 5):S61–S74.
189. Schwartz GJ, Haycock GB, Edelmann CM Jr, Spitzer A. Late metabolic acidosis: a reassessment of the definition. *J Pediatr* 1979;95:102–107.
190. Schwartz GJ, Kittelberger AM, Barnhart DA, Vijayakumar S. Carbonic anhydrase IV is expressed in H(+)-secreting cells of rabbit kidney. *Am J Physiol Renal Physiol* 2000;278: F894–F904.
191. Schwartz GJ, Olson J, Kittelberger AM, Matsumoto T, Waheed A, Sly WS. Postnatal development of carbonic anhydrase IV expression in rabbit kidney. *Am J Physiol* 1999;276: F510–F520.
192. Schwartz GJ, Zavilowitz BJ, Radice AD, Garcia-Perez A, Sands JM. Maturation of aldose reductase expression in the neonatal rat inner medulla. *J Clin Invest* 1992;90:1275–1283.
193. Segawa H, Kaneko I, Takahashi A, Kuwahata M, Ito M, Ohkido I, Tatsumi S, Miyamoto K. Growth-related renal type II Na/Pi cotransporter. *J Biol Chem* 2002;277:19665–19672.
194. Shah M, Gupta N, Dwarakanath V, Moe OW, Baum M. Ontogeny of Na+/H+ antiporter activity in rat proximal convoluted tubules. *Pediatr Res* 2000;48:206–210.
195. Shah M, Quigley R, Baum M. Maturation of rabbit proximal straight tubule chloride/base exchange. *Am J Physiol* 1998;274:F883–F888.
196. Shah M, Quigley R, Baum M. Neonatal rabbit proximal tubule basolateral membrane Na+/H+ antiporter and Cl-/base exchange. *Am J Physiol* 1999;276:R1792–R1797.
197. Shah M, Quigley R, Baum M. Maturation of proximal straight tubule NaCl transport: role of thyroid hormone. *Am J Physiol Renal Physiol* 2000;278:F596–F602.
198. Sheu JN, Baum M, Bajaj G, Quigley R. Maturation of rabbit proximal convoluted tubule chloride permeability. *Pediatr Res* 1996;39:308–312.
199. Sheu JN, Quigley R, Baum M. Heterogeneity of chloride/base exchange in rabbit superficial and juxtamedullary proximal convoluted tubules. *Am J Physiol* 1995;268:F847–F853.
200. Siegel SR, Fisher DA, Oh W. Serum aldosterone concentrations related to sodium balance in the newborn infant. *Pediatrics* 1974;53:410–413.
201. Siegel SR, Oh W. Renal function as a marker of human fetal maturation. *Acta Paediatr Scand* 1976;65:481–485.
202. Siga E, Horster MF. Regulation of osmotic water permeability during differentiation of inner medullary collecting duct. *Am J Physiol* 1991; 260:F710–F716.
203. Smith B, Baumgarten R, Nielsen S, Raben D, Zeidel ML, Agre P. Concurrent expression of erythroid and renal aquaporin CHIP, appearance of water channel activity in perinatal rats. *J Clin Invest* 1993;92:2035–2041.
204. Smith FG, Sato T, McWeeny OJ, Klinkefus JM, Robillard JE. Role of renal sympathetic nerves in response of the ovine fetus to volume expansion. *Am J Physiol* 1990;259:R1050–R1055.
205. Smith FG, Sato T, McWeeny OJ, Torres L, Robillard JE. Role of renal nerves in response to volume expansion in conscious newborn lambs. *Am J Physiol* 1989;257:R1519–R1525.
206. Smith FG, Smith BA, Guillery EN, Robillard JE. Role of renal sympathetic nerves in lambs during the transition from fetal to newborn life. *J Clin Invest* 1991;88:1988–1994.
207. Spitzer A. The role of the kidney in sodium homeostasis during maturation. *Kidney Int* 1982;21:539–545.
208. Spitzer A, Brandis M. Functional and morphologic maturation of the superficial nephrons. Relationship to total kidney function. *J Clin Invest* 1974;53:279–287.
209. Spitzer A, Edelmann CM Jr. Maturational changes in pressure gradients for glomerular filtration. *Am J Physiol* 1971;221:1431–1435.
210. Stanier MW. Development of intra-renal solute gradients in foetal and post-natal life. *Pflugers Arch* 1972;336:263–270.
211. Stephenson G, Hammet M, Hadaway G, Funder JW. Ontogeny of renal mineralocorticoid receptors and urinary electrolyte responses in the rat. *Am J Physiol* 1984;247:F665–F671.
212. Stokes JB, Kokko JP. Inhibition of sodium transport by prostaglandin E2 across the isolated, perfused rabbit collecting tubule. *J Clin Invest* 1977;59:1099–1104.
213. Sulyok E, Nemeth M, Tenyi I, Csaba IF, Varga F, Gyory E, Thurzo V. Relationship between maturity, electrolyte balance and the function of the renin-angiotensin-aldosterone system in newborn infants. *Biol Neonate* 1979;35:60–65.
214. Sulyok EHT. Assessment of maximal urinary acidification in prematuare infants. *Biol Neonate* 1971;19:200–210.
215. Sulyok EHT. The influence of matauarity on renal control of acidosis in newborn infants. *Biol Neonate* 1972;21:418–435.
216. Svenningsen NW. Renal acid–base titration studies in infants with and without metabolic acidosis in the postneonatal period. *Pediatr Res* 1973;8:659–672.
217. Svenningsen NWLB. Postnatal development of renal hydrogen ion excretion capacity in relation to age and protein intake. *Acta Paediatr Scand* 1974;63:721–731.
218. Thomas ML, Anast CS, Forte LR. Regulation of calcium homeostasis in the fetal and neonatal rat. *Am J Physiol* 1981;240:E367–E372.
219. Traebert M, Lotscher M, Aschwanden R, Ritthaler T, Biber J, Murer H, Kaissling B. Distribution of the sodium/phosphate transporter during postnatal ontogeny of the rat kidney. *J Am Soc Nephrol* 1999;10:1407–1415.
220. Tucker BJ, Blantz RC. Factors determining superficial nephron filtration in the mature, growing rat. *Am J Physiol* 1977;232:F97–104.
221. Tulassay T, Rascher W, Hajdu J, Lang RE, Toth M, Seri I. Influence of dopamine on atrial natriuretic peptide level in premature infants. *Acta Paediatr Scand* 1987;76:42–46.
222. Tulassay T, Rascher W, Seyberth HW, Lang RE, Toth M, Sulyok E. Role of atrial natriuretic peptide in sodium homeostasis in premature infants. *J Pediatr* 1986;109:1023–1027.
223. Tuvad FVJ. The maximal tubular transfer of glucose and para-aminohippurate in premature infants. *Acta Paediatr Scand* 1953;42:337–345.
224. Vehaskari VM. Ontogeny of cortical collecting duct sodium transport. *Am J Physiol* 1994;267: F49–F54.
225. Deleted in proof.
226. Vehaskari VM, Hempe JM, Manning J, Aviles DH, Carmichael MC. Developmental regulation of ENaC subunit mRNA levels in rat kidney. *Am J Physiol* 1998;274:C1661–C1666.
227. Verkman AS. Mechanisms and regulation of water permeability in renal epithelia. *Am J Physiol* 1989;257:C837–C850.
228. Wacker GR, Zarkowsky HS, Bruch HB. Changes in kidney enzymes of rats after birth. *Am J Physiol* 1961;200:367–369.
229. Wamberg S, . Balance of net base in the rat. II. Reference values in relation to growth rate. *Biol Neonate* 1976;28:171–190.
230. Watanabe S, Matsushita K, McCray PB Jr, Stokes JB. Developmental expression of the epithelial Na+ channel in kidney and uroepithelia. *Am J Physiol* 1999;276:F304–F314.
231. Webster SK, Haramati A. Developmental changes in the phosphaturic response to parathyroid hormone in the rat. *Am J Physiol* 1985;249:F251–F255.
232. Wei YF, Rodi CP, Day ML, Wiegand RC, Needleman LD, Cole BR, Needleman P. Developmental changes in the rat atriopeptin hormonal system. *J Clin Invest* 1987;79:1325–1329.
233. Wijkhuisen A, Djouadi F, Vilar J, Merlet-Benichou C, Bastin J. Thyroid hormones regulate development of energy metabolism enzymes in rat proximal convoluted tubule. *Am J Physiol* 1995;268:F634–F642.
234. Winberg J. Determination of renal concentrating capacity in infants and children without renal disease. *Acta Paediatr Scand* 1959;48:318–328.
235. Winkler CA, Kittelberger AM, Watkins RH, Maniscalco WM, Schwartz GJ. Maturation of carbonic anhydrase IV expression in rabbit kidney. *Am J Physiol Renal Physiol* 2001;280: F895–F903.
236. Woda C, Mulroney SE, Halaihel N, Sun L, Wilson PV, Levi M, Haramati A. Renal tubular sites of increased phosphate transport and NaPi-2 expression in the juvenile rat. *Am J Physiol Regul Integr Comp Physiol* 2001;280:R1524–R1533.
237. Woda CB, Bragin A, Kleyman TR, Satlin LM. Flow-dependent K+ secretion in the cortical collecting duct is mediated by a maxi-K channel. *Am J Physiol Renal Physiol* 2001;280: F786–F793.
238. Woda CB, Miyawaki N, Ramalakshmi S, Ramkumar M, Rojas R, Zavilowitz B, Kleyman TR, Satlin LM. Ontogeny of flow-stimulated potassium secretion in rabbit cortical collecting duct: functional and molecular aspects. *Am J Physiol Renal Physiol* 2003;285:F629–F639.
239. Wu MS, Biemesderfer D, Giebisch G, Aronson PS. Role of NHE3 in mediating renal brush border Na+-H+ exchange. Adaptation to metabolic acidosis. *J Biol Chem* 1996;271:32749–32752.
240. Yared A, Yoshioka T. Autoregulation of glomerular filtration in the young. *Semin Nephrol* 1989;9:94–97.
241. Yasui M, Marples D, Belusa R, Eklof AC, Celsi G, Nielsen S, Aperia A. Development of urinary concentrating capacity: role of aquaporin-2. *Am J Physiol* 1996;271:F461–F468.
242. Zink H, Horster M. Maturation of diluting capacity in loop of Henle of rat superficial nephrons. *Am J Physiol* 1977;233:F519–F524.
243. Zolotnitskaya A, Satlin LM. Developmental expression of ROMK in rat kidney. *Am J Physiol* 1999;276:F825–F836.
244. Zweifach A, Desir GV, Aronson PS, Giebisch G. Inhibition of Ca-activated K+ channels from renal microvillus membrane vesicles by amiloride analogs. *J Membr Biol* 1992;128:115–122.

CHAPTER 27

Renal Hyperplasia and Hypertrophy

ROLE OF CELL CYCLE REGULATORY PROTEINS

Sian V. Griffin and Stuart J. Shankland

University Hospital Wales, Health Park, Cardiff, Wales
University of Washington, Seattle, Washington, USA

INTRODUCTION

The tight regulation of cell growth and division within an organ is essential for the development and maintenance of correct structure and function. Perturbations of renal growth occurring either developmentally (such as agenesis), or following injury to mature renal cells (such as occurs in glomerulonephritis or acute tubular necrosis) contribute to the abnormalities observed in a wide range of diseases. The changes in growth are increasingly recognized to influence progression of the initial disease process and the ultimate clinical outcome. Abnormal cell growth is classified according to the presence of an increase in cell number or cell size. Hyperplasia refers to abnormal growth resulting in an increased absolute number of cells (i.e., proliferation), whereas hypertrophy refers to an increase in individual cell size. Both processes may be present in a given cell population and contribute to the increase in overall kidney size.

Of particular interest to clinical nephrologists and renal pathologists is that the kidney has several different resident cell types. Within the glomerulus, the growth responses of the mesangial cell, podocyte, parietal epithelial cell, and endothelial cell differ. The tubulointerstitial cells and vascular smooth muscle cells also vary in their growth responses following injury. Thus, characterizing the mechanisms that regulate each cell's growth response enables the potential development of specific therapies that will modify these to injury. We recognize that renal cell hyperplasia and hypertrophy are regulated by numerous pathways, involving growth factors, signaling pathways, and transcription factors. However, the focus of this review is to update the reader on recent advances in the regulation of these growth processes at the level of the cell cycle. We will first describe cell cycle regulation by specific cell cycle proteins, and then discuss hyperplasia and hypertrophy for individual glomerular and tubular cell types.

Although highly metabolically active, under normal conditions the cells of the mature kidney are relatively quiescent with respect to cell cycle entry. Following injury to either the glomerulus or the tubules, cell cycle progression with proliferation is often an essential part of the reparative process.

However, if unchecked, proliferation can lead to compromise of renal function. Similarly, renal hypertrophy may occur as a compensatory physiological response, but unregulated hypertrophy is maladaptive, and is one of the hallmarks of diabetic nephropathy.

Cell proliferation is ultimately regulated at the level of the cell cycle, which occurs within the nucleus. Within the kidney, the control of the cell cycle is particularly intriguing given the contrasting responses of the various resident cell types to injury. For example, the mesangial cell is capable of marked proliferation, often accompanied by the deposition of extracellular matrix. In contrast, the podocyte has been considered a relatively inert cell, although this view has recently been challenged, and the reparative proliferation of glomerular endothelial cells following injury has also been described. Renal tubular cells readily undergo both proliferative and hypertrophic responses following injury. The last decade has seen a rapid expansion in our understanding of the molecular mechanisms underlying the cell cycle, and therapeutic options for its manipulation are becoming available. There is currently increasing awareness of the need to reduce the progression of renal diseases. Knowledge of the cell cycle and an understanding of how this can be influenced may be crucial to the prevention, control, and amelioration of a wide range of renal diseases.

MEASUREMENT OF CELL GROWTH

Hyperplasia

During a hyperplastic response, the number of proliferating cells is increased. A number of methods are available for measuring this increase, both in vivo and in cell culture. The majority of these have as their basis the detection of increased DNA synthesis. This may be done by determining the presence of proteins known to be associated with DNA synthesis, such as proliferating cell nuclear antigen (PCNA) or Ki-67, or by exogenously labeling cells with a compound known to be incorporated into newly synthesized DNA, such as ^3H thymidine or bromodeoxyuridine

(BrdU). In cell culture, a convenient and high-throughput method for determining cell number is the MTT assay, in which the yellow tetrazolium salt is reduced in metabolically active cells to form insoluble formazan crystals, which are solubilized by the addition of detergent. The color intensity may then be quantified spectrophotometrically, allowing quantification of changes in proliferation. A caveat for this method is that a decrease in cell viability will mimic a decrease in proliferation, and concomitant apoptosis should be excluded. Analysis by fluorescent activated cell sorting (FACS) is a valuable tool for the assessment of hyperplasia, because it also allows quantification of the number of cells in each phase of the cell cycle.

Hypertrophy

Cellular hypertrophy may be defined as an increase in cell size due to an increase in protein and RNA content without DNA replication (52, 53), and this forms the basis for the majority of methods for detection of hypertrophy. Upon entry into G1, cells undergo a physiologic increase in protein synthesis prior to the DNA synthesis of S phase. Thus, one mechanism underlying hypertrophy is cell cycle arrest at the G1/S checkpoint, so that while protein synthesis, and hence content increase, there is no subsequent increase in DNA. Hypertrophy may also result independently of the cell cycle due to an inhibition of protein synthesis, and this mechanism is considered

to contribute to tubular cell hypertrophy (59, 181). Measurement of leucine or proline incorporation and comparison to ^{3}H thymidine incorporation allow determination of cell protein/DNA content and hence assessment of hypertrophy. FACS analysis is also useful and enables direct measurement of cell size. Defining the growth response to a given stimulus as either hyperplastic or hypertrophic is important, as each will result from different alterations in cell signaling pathways, with implications for possible interventions.

CELL CYCLE AND CELL CYCLE REGULATORY PROTEINS

Cell Cycle

The cell cycle is divided into distinct phases, each representing a different function, and each being regulated by specific proteins (Fig. 1) (155). Quiescent cells are termed as in G0, and upon mitogenic stimuli enter the cell cycle at early G1. Cells pass through the restriction point in late G1, beyond which they are typically unresponsive to extracellular cues, and are committed to complete the cell cycle despite the withdrawal of mitogenic stimuli. DNA synthesis occurs in S phase. Cells then progress through G2, in preparation for mitosis (M phase). Ultimately, cell division follows during cytokinesis. Our current understanding

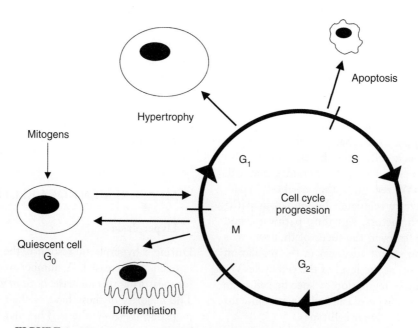

FIGURE 1   The cell cycle and possible consequences of cell cycle exit. Mitogens stimulate quiescent cells to engage the cell cycle at G1 phase. Hyperplasia then requires a coordinated and sequential series of events, including DNA synthesis at S phase, followed by a resting G2 phase and mitosis in M phase. This is followed by cell division. Cells that then exit the cell cycle and are quiescent again are in many cases differentiated. Of note is that if cells arrest at the G1/S phase, they can develop a hypertrophic phenotype. Cell cycle exit with apoptosis may also occur.

suggests there are at least two checkpoints to ensure fidelity of DNA duplication, at G1/S and G2/M, where cell cycle progression may be arrested. The length of the cell cycle is cell-type specific, but this variability is largely due to differences in the duration of G1. For mammalian cells, the typical duration of G1 is approximately 12 hours, S and G2 phases 6 hours, and mitosis 30 minutes.

Cyclins and Cyclin-Dependent Kinases: Positive Regulators of the Cell Cycle

OVERVIEW

The progress of a somatic cell through the cell cycle is dependent on the sequential and coordinated activation of the cyclin-dependent kinases (Cdks), a family of serine/threonine kinases, by their specific partners, called cyclins (Fig. 2). Once active, Cdks phosphorylate downstream targets, ultimately to induce DNA synthesis (81). While the levels of the Cdk catalytic subunits remain constant throughout the cell cycle, they are only functional following the binding of their specific cyclin partners. In contrast, cyclins are unstable proteins that are sequentially expressed and subsequently degraded by ubiquitination throughout the cell cycle (104), which activate their partner Cdks by inducing conformational changes. Originally described for their fluctuation during the cell cycle (46), members of the cyclin family are now defined by the presence of a conserved 100–amino-acid cyclin box, which binds their complementary Cdk. In addition, the binding of inhibitors and accessory proteins, subcellular localization and both inhibitory and activating phosphorylations influence the functional activity of the Cdk-cyclin complex (175).

JUMPSTARTING THE CYCLE

The cell cycle is initiated by the mitogen-driven induction of cyclin D (2, 51, 233). Depending on the cell type, three forms of cyclin D have been described (D1, D2, and D3), which interact allosterically with Cdk4 and Cdk6. Receptor-activated Ras signaling pathways lead to accu-

mulation of cyclin D by three mechanisms: gene transcription, assembly, and stabilization of the cyclin D-Cdk complex (70). The Ras-Raf-1-mitogen-activated, protein kinase kinase (MEK), extracellular signal-related protein kinase (ERK) pathway both induces cyclin D transcription and promotes assembly of cyclin D-Cdk (24, 169). The rate of degradation of cyclin D is controlled by a separate Ras signaling pathway involving phosphatidylinositol 3-kinase (PI3K) and protein kinase B (PKB/Akt), which inhibits the phosphorylation of cyclin D on threonine-286 (Thr-286) by glycogen synthase kinase 3β (GSKβ) (38). Thr-286 phosphorylated cyclin D would otherwise be exported to the cytoplasm for ubiquitination and degradation (39). This requirement for mitogen signaling prevents the cell from autonomous cycling. Although ectopic expression of cyclin D is insufficient to drive cell cycle progression, constitutive activation of the cyclin D pathway can reduce the reliance of the cell on mitogenic stimulation and lower the threshold for oncogenic transformation (208). The cyclin D-Cdk4/6 complex enters the cell nucleus and is phosphorylated by Cdk-activating kinase (CAK) (97).

Once DNA replication begins, active cyclin D–dependent kinase activity is not required until mitosis is complete and the cell re-enters the next G1 phase (131). In continuously dividing cells, cyclin D1 is exported to the cytoplasm during S phase, and its turnover is accelerated (7, 38). However, cyclin D1 synthesis stimulated by Ras is stabilized in G2 as described above, allowing reaccumulation before cells divide (74). Hence, in the presence of continuous mitogen stimulation, the second and subsequent cell cycles are shorter than the first. Withdrawal of mitogens results in a rapid decline in cyclin D kinase activity, and cell cycle exit.

Active cyclin D–dependent kinases phosphorylate the retinoblastoma protein (pRb), which in quiescent cells has a growth-inhibitory effect (130, 227). In its hypophosphorylated state, pRb suppresses the transcription of several genes whose proteins are required for DNA synthesis, including the E2F transcription factors. Upon phosphorylation of pRb, the E2Fs are released from inhibition, leading to the

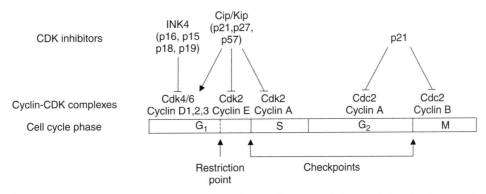

FIGURE 2 Cell cycle progression: timing of activation of cyclins and Cdks, and site of action of Cdk inhibitors. Each Cdk is activated by a partner cyclin in each phase of the cell cycle, and the resulting cyclin–Cdk complex can be inhibited by specific Cdk inhibitors.

transcription of cyclins E and A and many genes whose products are required for DNA replication (223). Furthermore, cyclin D-Cdk4 complexes also phosphorylate Smad3, negatively regulating the functions of transcriptional proteins responsible for mediating the growth inhibitory effects of transforming growth factor β (TGFβ) (132). Cyclin D–dependent kinases therefore affect the activity of at least two pathways that independently inhibit the expression of cell cycle promoting genes.

The activity of cyclin E-Cdk2 is maximal at the G1- to S-phase transition (42, 105), when its function to further phosphorylate pRb releases the cell from mitogen dependency (102, 124). In addition to preferentially phosphorylating pRb on different sites to the cyclin D–dependent kinases, which may modify the interaction with E2Fs (79), cyclin E-Cdk2 phosphorylates a second set of substrates involved in cell replication, thus affecting histone gene expression, centrosome duplication (261). The timing of expression and wider range of substrates suggest a role for cyclin E-Cdk2 in coordinating G1 regulation and the core cell cycle machinery.

The abrupt decline in cyclin E-Cdk2 activity in early S phase results from cyclin E degradation. Phosphorylation by GSK-3β and Cdk2 itself target cyclin E for ubiquitination by the SCF^{Fbw7} E3 ligase, leading to proteasomal destruction (26, 229, 251).

Low levels of cyclin A-Cdk2 activity are first detected in late G1 phase, increase as cells begin to replicate their DNA, and decline as cyclin A is degraded in early mitosis. The substrate specificity of cyclin A-Cdk2 is different from that of cyclin E-Cdk2. In S phase, cyclin A-Cdk2 is thought to phosphorylate substrates that control the start of DNA replication from preassembled replication initiation complexes (29, 91, 111), and control the integration of the end of S phase with the activation of the mitotic Cdks (140). The apparently central role of Cdk2 in coordinating cell cycle progression through S phase and entry into mitosis has been challenged by the surprising observation that Cdk2 null mice are viable (11, 160). The possibility that other Cdks compensate for loss of Cdk2 is currently a focus of intense research.

The entry to mitosis is controlled by cyclin B–Cdc2 (4, 213). Cell cycle–regulated transcription of cyclin B begins at the end of S phase. Phosphorylation on Thr161 by CAK parallels cyclin B binding to Cdc2 (107). During G2, cyclin B–Cdc2 complexes are maintained in an inactive state by phosphorylation on two inhibitory sites, Thr14 and tyrosine 15 (Tyr15) (Fig. 3). Phosphorylation on Tyr15 is mediated by the nuclear Wee1 kinases (166), and that on Thr14 by the membrane-bound Myt1 (118). In late G2 phase, both Thr14 and Tyr15 are dephosphorylated by Cdc25, thus activating cyclin B–Cdc2, and initiating mitosis (153). Inappropriate triggering of mitosis is also prevented by the translocation of cyclin B to the cytoplasm by the nuclear export factor CRM1 (exportin 1) during S and G2 phases (259). Phosphorylation of cyclin B is thought to promote nuclear import at the G2/M transition (75). Cyclin B–Cdc2 phosphorylates numerous downstream targets responsible for the structural reorganization of the cell to enable mitosis.

Although what is described above represents the basic paradigm of the control of cell cycle progression in mammalian cells, recent studies of knockout mice have demonstrated that much of fetal development can occur normally despite the absence of cyclins and Cdks formerly considered to be vital (210). Clearly, individual cyclins and Cdks are able to act more promiscuously than previously appreciated to enable compensation for the lack of a specific cell cycle protein.

Stopping the Cell Cycle: Cdk Inhibitors Act as Negative Regulators

In essence, Cdk inhibitors bind and inhibit target cyclin–Cdk complexes. Two classes of Cdk inhibitors have been described, the *INK4 proteins* and the *Cip/Kip family* (149, 211). Within each family, individual proteins are named according to their molecular weight. INK4 proteins were originally named for their ability to *in*hibit Cd*k4*. This family comprises four proteins, namely p16^{INK4a}, p15^{INK4b}, p18^{INK4c}, and p19^{INK4d}. Structurally these proteins are made up of multiple ankyrin repeats and bind only to the catalytic subunits Cdk4 and Cdk6, thus inhibiting G1 progression. An alternate reading

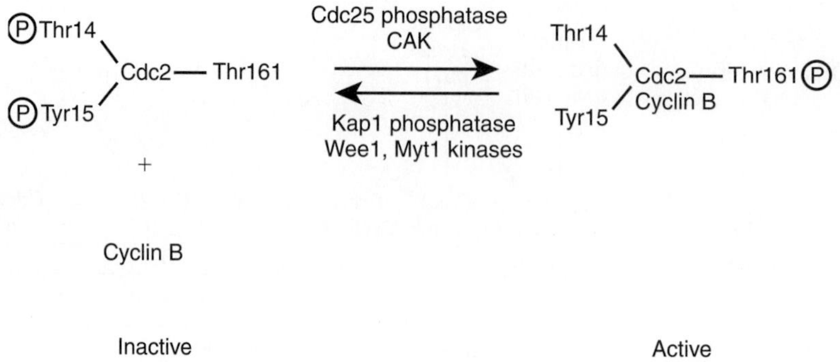

FIGURE 3 Regulation of the phosphorylation status of Cdc2. Wee1 and Myt1 kinases phosphorylate Cdc2 on Thr14 and Tyr15, inhibiting activity. Phosphorylation by CAK on Thr161 results in a 200-fold increase in kinase activity. Cdk2 is similarly phosphorylated on Thr160.

frame of the genetic locus encoding p16^{INK4a} also encodes a second structurally and functionally unrelated protein named p19^{ARF} in the mouse (p14^{ARF} in the human) (182). Whereas p16^{INK4a} acts to stabilize Rb by inhibition of Cdk4/6, p19^{ARF} stabilizes p53 by binding its negative regulator, Mdm2 (207). Data from knockout mice suggest that p19^{ARF}, rather than p16^{INK4a}, is responsible for the tumor suppressor function of this locus (209).

The second class of Cdk inhibitors is the Cip/Kip family and includes p21^{Cip1}, p27^{Kip1}, and p57^{Kip2}, which share a conserved N-terminal Cdk-binding domain (149). They are capable of binding a wider range of targets and can variably affect the activities of cyclin D–, E–, A–, and B–dependent kinases (19, 211, 212). Although potent inhibitors of cyclin E– and A–dependent CDK2, and to a lesser extent Cdc2, the Cip/Kip proteins have recently also been characterized, paradoxically, as positive regulators of the cyclin D–dependent kinases (23).

p21^{Cip1} was the first member of the family to be identified (44, 80, 252), and is usually present at a low level in quiescent cells. As the cell enters the replicative cycle, p21^{Cip1} levels rise, displace INK4 proteins from binding to Cdk 4/6, and promote the assembly of cyclin D-Cdk complexes (114, 168). This stabilizes the active complex and additionally provides a nuclear localization signal (NLS). The transcription of p21^{Cip1} is increased by both p53-dependent (41) and independent (167) pathways, such as those mediated by TGFβ (248). The inhibitory role of p21^{Cip1} becomes dominant later in the cell cycle, and levels are also increased in senescent cells (154).

In contrast to p21^{Cip1}, the level of p27^{Kip1} is usually high in quiescent cells, where its primary role is as an inhibitor of cell division (179, 222). Whereas p21^{Cip1} is a principal mediator of the p53-dependent G1 arrest that occurs following DNA damage (91), p27^{Kip1} appears to be primarily responsible for mediating extracellular anti-proliferative signals (179, 222). The levels and activity of p27^{Kip1} are post-transcriptionally regulated by changes in the rates of translation, ubiquitination, and phosphorylation (83, 161). As cyclin D levels rise in response to mitogens, both p21^{Cip1} and p27^{Kip1} are sequestered by cyclin D–Cdk complexes, and therefore are unable to inhibit Cdk2 (211). Cyclin E-Cdk2 phosphorylates p27^{Kip1} on Thr 187 (204, 225), proving a recognition motif for an E3 ligase that targets p27^{Kip1} for ubiquitination and proteasomal degradation (13, 45).

The most recently identified member of the family, p57^{Kip2}, was cloned in 1995 (115, 128). While tissue expression of p21^{Cip1} and p27^{Kip1} is widespread, that of p57^{Kip2} is restricted to placenta, muscle, heart, brain, lung, and kidney. In addition to the Cdk inhibitory domain and putative C terminal NLS, p57^{Kip2} also has a proline-rich domain containing a consensus ERK phosphorylation site, and an acidic domain, the functions of which are not known (115, 128). A role for p57^{Kip2} in the cell cycle exit that accompanies terminal differentiation has been suggested.

Despite their structural similarities, knockout studies have demonstrated divergent roles for the three Cip/Kip Cdk inhibitors. While p21^{Cip1} and p27^{Kip1} are not essential for normal embryogenesis (50, 148, 235), lack of p57^{Kip2} results in profound developmental abnormalities (217, 257, 263). Most p57^{Kip2} null mice die shortly after birth and have severe cleft palates, abdominal wall and gastrointestinal tract defects, and abnormal skeletal ossification. Unlike adult p21^{Cip1}−/− mice (35, 235), p27^{Kip1}−/− mice are larger than wildtype animals and have hyperplasia of organs that usually express high levels of p27^{Kip1}, such as the thymus, spleen, adrenal and pituitary glands, testes, and ovaries (50, 148). In contrast, only 10% of p57^{Kip2}−/− mice survive the weaning period and are much smaller than wildtype (217). The kidneys of p57^{Kip2}−/− mice have medullary dysplasia, although glomerular development appears normal.

HYPERPLASIA: AN INCREASE IN CELL NUMBER DUE TO PROLIFERATION

Glomerular Hyperplasia

MESANGIAL CELL PROLIFERATION

Mesangial cell proliferation characterizes many forms of both experimental and human glomerular disease, including IgA nephropathy, lupus nephritis, diabetic nephropathy, and other forms of membranoproliferative glomerulonephritis (Fig. 4). It is frequently associated with, and likely underlies, matrix expansion and subsequent glomerulosclerosis, the significance of which has been shown in a range of experimental models (28, 58, 94, 103, 170, 215). This simple observation provides the impetus for understanding what switches mesangial proliferation on and what switches it off. Several growth factors and cytokines are mitogens for mesangial cells, including platelet-derived growth factor (PDGF) (92, 95), basic fibroblast growth factor (bFGF) (54), interleukin 6 (187, 189), and the product of growth arrest–specific gene 6 (Gas6) (258). Intervention to reduce mesangial proliferation also reduces matrix expansion, confirming the tight link between these two processes. This has been achieved in experimental models using complement depletion (15, 56), heparin infusion (55), blocking the action PDGF (67, 96) and bFGF (28), and inhibiting their specific intracellular signaling pathways with phosphodiesterase inhibitors (224). Warfarin has been used with mixed results in the treatment of glomerular diseases since the 1970s, and was originally hypothesized to reduce fibrin deposition. However, low-dose warfarin may also be effective, suggesting a mechanism of action not directly related to anticoagulation. Gas6 is a vitamin K–dependent growth factor for mesangial cells, and its inhibition by warfarin is likely to underlie the reported benefits of this treatment in human disease (258). Careful research since the

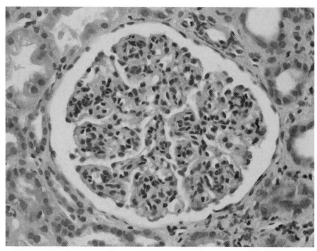

FIGURE 4   Global mesangial cell proliferation occurring in the context of membranoproliferative glomerulonephritis. (Haematoxylin and eosin, × 400). Histology courtesy of Dr Meryl Griffiths, Addenbrooke's Hospital, Cambridge.

mid-1990s has delineated the role of individual cell cycle proteins in both mesangial cell proliferation, and also its resolution by apoptosis (Fig. 5).

Role of Cdk2 in Mesangial Cell Proliferation   Cdk2 protein and kinase activity increase in cultured mesangial cells in response to mitogenic growth factors (21, 193). The Thy1 model of experimental mesangial proliferative glomerulonephritis, induced in rats by an antibody directed against the mesangial Thy1 antigen, has provided an opportunity to study the regulation and consequences of mesangial cell proliferation in vivo (255, 256). The initial complement-dependent mesangiolysis is followed by a phase of marked mesangial proliferation, paralleled by an increase in extracellular matrix accumulation and a decline in renal function. This model is useful as not only may the fluctuations of cell cycle proteins during proliferation be defined, but also the effect of their manipulation. Mesangial cell proliferation is associated with an increase in cyclin D1 and A, and their partners Cdk4 and Cdk2 (200). Cdk2 expression is absent in the normal rat glomerulus. Proliferation is associated with increased Cdk2 activity, measured by the histone H1 kinase assay on protein extracted from isolated glomeruli. Cdk2 protein levels are also increased in the remnant kidney model, a nonimmune glomerular disease associated with mesangial proliferation (199). Taken together, these studies show that in contrast to most nonrenal cells (200), Cdk2 protein is at low levels in quiescent mesangial cells, and its levels and activity increase following injury.

Cdk Inhibitors and Mesangial Cell Proliferation

The Cdk inhibitor $p27^{Kip1}$ is constitutively expressed in quiescent mesangial cells both in vitro (202) and in vivo (200), whereas $p21^{Cip1}$ and $p57^{Kip2}$ are essentially absent (84, 200). In cultured mesangial cells, proliferation induced

Mesangial cell

Baseline expression	$p21-$, $p27+$, $p57-$

Injury

Change in expression of cell cycle proteins	• ↑ Cyclin D1/Cdk4
	• ↑ Cyclin A/Cdk2
	• ↓ p27

Response to injury	Proliferation

	Resolution
	• ↑ p21, ↑ p27

FIGURE 5   Changes in cell cycle protein activity following injury to glomerular mesangial cells. At baseline, quiescent mesangial cells express $p27^{Kip1}$, but not $p21^{Cip1}$ or $p57^{Kip2}$. Following injury, there is an increase in the positive cell cycle regulators cyclin D1/Cdk4 and cyclin A/Cdk2, with a decline in $p27^{Kip1}$, resulting in promotion of cell cycle progression and proliferation. During the resolution phase, there is an increase in the Cdk-inhibitors $p21^{Cip1}$ and $p27^{Kip1}$, with cessation of proliferation.

by mitogenic growth factors reduces $p27^{Kip1}$ levels (202). Mesangial cells derived from $p27^{Kip1}-/-$ mice have augmented proliferation in response to mitogens (86), and lowering $p27^{Kip1}$ levels with antisense oligonucleotides has a similar effect in rat mesangial cells (202).

Complement (C5b-9)-induced injury in the Thy1 model is associated with a marked decrease in $p27^{Kip1}$ levels (200). However, there is de novo synthesis of $p21^{Cip1}$ in the resolution phase of the disease, coincident with a decrease in proliferation. To further explore the role of $p27^{Kip1}$ in inflammatory disease, we induced experimental glomerulonephritis in $p27^{Kip1}-/-$ mice (158). Our results showed a marked increase in the onset and magnitude of glomerular cell proliferation and cellularity in nephritic $p27^{Kip1}-/-$ mice compared to control nephritic $p27^{Kip1}+/+$ mice. Moreover, this was associated with increased extracellular matrix proteins and a decline in renal function. To demonstrate that this result was not specific to glomerular cells or immune-mediated injury, we also obstructed a ureter by ligation to induce nonimmune injury to tubuloepithelial cells (158). Our results showed that tubuloepithelial proliferation was increased in obstructed

$p27^{Kip1}-/-$ mice compared to obstructed $p27^{Kip1}+/+$ mice. Taken together, these studies were the first to show that in inflammatory diseases, renal cell proliferation is regulated by the CKI $p27^{Kip1}$, supporting a role for $p27^{Kip1}$ in controlling the threshold at which proliferation occurs.

ROLE OF CELL CYCLE PROTEINS IN RESOLUTION OF MESANGIAL HYPERPLASIA: APOPTOSIS

Although a characteristic response to mesangial cell injury is proliferation, apoptosis is often simultaneously increased (6). Studies have shown that apoptosis is a vital mechanism required to normalize cell number in the reparative phase of injury (191). However, the cellular pathways linking these opposing responses remain unclear. Many cells undergoing apoptosis have entered the cell cycle, but rather than completing their replication, they are destined to leave by programmed cell death. This suggests a role for the cell cycle proteins in directing these alternative outcomes.

Evidence to support this hypothesis was the observation that the resolution phase of Thy1 mesangial proliferation in the rat is characterized by mesangial cell apoptosis, a process that peaks when the levels of $p27^{Kip1}$ are at their lowest (200). Considering glomerulonephritis or unilateral ureteric obstruction in $p27^{Kip1}-/-$ mice as described above, in addition to the increase in either glomerular or tubuloepithelial cell proliferation following injury, there was a marked increase in apoptosis in the $p27^{Kip1}-/-$ mice compared to wildtype disease controls (158). Moreover, apoptosis was also increased in $p27^{Kip1}-/-$ mesangial cells in culture following growth factor deprivation or cycloheximide, and reconstituting $p27^{Kip1}$ levels by transfection-rescued cells from apoptosis (86). In wildtype rat mesangial cells, apoptosis was increased following treatment with anti-$p27^{Kip1}$ antisense oligonucleotides (86). These results showed for the first time that $p27^{Kip1}$ has a role beyond the regulation of proliferation, in that it also protects cells from apoptosis. This dual role of regulating the proliferative threshold and governing apoptosis makes $p27^{Kip1}$ a potent regulator of overall mesangial cell number.

How does $p27^{Kip1}$ Protect Cells from Apoptosis? A clue to a possible mechanism was the increase in Cdk2 activity in $p27^{Kip1}-/-$ mesangial cells when deprived of growth factors (86). The increase was due specifically to cyclin A-Cdk2, and not cyclin E-Cdk2. Moreover, inhibition of cyclin A-Cdk2 activity by roscovitine or a dominant negative mutant reduced apoptosis in mesangial cells and fibroblasts. In apoptotic $p27^{Kip1}-/-$ mesangial cells, Cdk2 was bound to cyclin A, without a preceding increase in cyclin E-Cdk2 activity. We suggest that in the absence of $p27^{Kip1}$, uncoupling of Cdk2 activity from the scheduled sequence of cell cycle protein expression may lead to an inappropriate and premature initiation of G_1/S phase transition, causing the cell to respond by undergoing apoptosis, rather than inappropriately progressing through an unscheduled cell cycle.

How Might Cdk2 Control Growth and Apoptotic Fate of Cells? Apoptosis typically begins in the cytoplasm, whereas DNA synthesis and mitosis are nuclear events.

Accordingly, we tested the hypothesis that the subcellular localization of Cdk2 determines if cells undergo apoptosis or proliferation (85). As expected, Cdk2 protein was cytoplasmic in quiescent, and nuclear in proliferating, mesangial cells. However, in proliferating cells injured by an apoptotic stimulus, Cdk2 localized to the cytoplasm, was no longer nuclear, and importantly, remained active. Our results also showed that cyclin A, and not cyclin E, colocalized to the cytoplasm with Cdk2 in apoptotic cells, to form an active cytoplasmic cyclin A–Cdk2 complex. The translocation of Cdk2 is not p53 dependent, and inhibiting the nuclear localization signal has no effect. That inhibiting Cdk2 decreased apoptosis provides further support for a critical role for cytoplasmic Cdk2 in triggering programmed cell death. Thus, the subcellular localization of active Cdk2 determines the fate of a cell: when nuclear, cells proliferate; when cytoplasmic, cells die by apoptosis. The mechanism by which nuclear Cdk2 is translocated to the cytoplasm remains to be elucidated. These studies provide the novel paradigm that specific cell cycle regulatory proteins have a role in glomerular disease beyond the regulation of proliferation.

THERAPEUTIC INHIBITION OF MESANGIAL PROLIFERATION AT CELL CYCLE LEVEL

In vitro and animal studies have recently revealed the potential of three novel therapies to modulate glomerular cell proliferation: the purine analog roscovitine, which inhibits Cdk2 activity; retinoids, derived from vitamin A; and lipoxins, endogenously produced eicosanoids. Roscovitine and retinoids have also been used to beneficial effect in the treatment of podocyte diseases, discussed in the next sections.

Roscovitine The significance of increased Cdk2 activity in mesangial proliferation was demonstrated by Pippin et al. (177), using roscovitine to inhibit Cdk2 in rats with Thy1 mesangioproliferative gomerulonephritis. Given immediately after disease induction, roscovitine significantly reduced mesangial cell proliferation. Moreover, administering roscovitine to rats once mesangial proliferation was already established also reduced proliferation. This inhibition of Cdk2 activity was accompanied by a marked reduction in the accumulation of glomerular extracellular matrix proteins (collagen IV, laminin, and fibronectin) and an improvement in renal function compared to controls. These results suggest that inhibiting Cdk2 may be a potential therapeutic target in glomerular diseases characterized by proliferation.

Retinoids Retinoic acid (RA) has an established role in kidney development (69, 253). RA binds to specific nuclear receptors, and the RA receptor complex then binds to DNA–RA response elements to cause the transcription of target genes (126). RA is used therapeutically in acute promyelocytic leukemia to slow proliferation and promote differentiation. RA-induced cell cycle arrest in nonrenal cells has been reported to involve reduction in c-Myc, cyclin D1, and cyclin E levels, with upregulation of $p21^{Cip1}$ and $p27^{Kip1}$ (40, 90, 196). The treatment of rats with experimental Thy1

glomerulonephritis with RA reduced mesangial cell proliferation, glomerular lesions, and albuminuria (33). In addition to a direct antiproliferative action, RA has also been reported to modulate both the renin-angiotensin system (34) and TGFβ signaling (143), in addition to anti-inflammatory and immune modulatory effects (253). The efficacy of RA in the treatment of glomerulonephritis is likely due to its pleiotropic effects on these numerous pathways.

Lipoxins Lipoxins are endogenously produced eicosanoids with potent anti-inflammatory actions (134), and are generated during the resolution phase of an acute inflammatory insult (117). Lipoxin A_4 biosynthesis has been demonstrated in glomerulonephritis (163), and its effects include modulation of leukocyte trafficking and phagocytic clearance of apoptotic cells (117, 134). In vitro, lipoxin A4 inhibits PDGF-induced activation of Akt/PKB in human mesangial cells and modulates PDGF-induced decrements of $p21^{Cip1}$ and $p27^{Kip1}$ (139). PDGF-induced increases in Cdk2–cyclin E complex formation are also inhibited by lipoxin A_4. Prolonged exposure of mesangial cells to PDGF is associated with autocrine TGFβ production, and this is ameliorated by lipoxin A_4.

In vivo, lipoxins are rapidly metabolized. To enable study of these compounds in disease models, stable synthetic analogs have been developed that are modified at C-15, C-16, and/or C20 (25). These compounds retain the biological activity and receptor-binding affinity of the native lipoxin. The effect of a lipoxin A_4 analog, 15-epi-16-(FPho)-LXA-Me, has been studied in the immediate phase of experimental anti-GBM nephritis in mice, and found to inhibit neutrophil infiltration and glomerular nitrotyrosine staining (156). Although animal studies with lipoxins are at an earlier stage than those with roscovitine or retinoids, their potential to augment the resolution phase of glomerulonephritis suggests that they may in the future have an important therapeutic role.

THE PODOCYTE AND CELL CYCLE: WHY IS LACK OF PODOCYTE PROLIFERATION IMPORTANT?

The podocyte, or visceral glomerular epithelial cell, is a highly specialized, terminally differentiated cell overlying the outer aspect of the glomerular basement membrane. In contrast to the mesangial cell, numerous studies of both animal models and human disease have shown that aside from a few specific conditions, podocytes do not typically proliferate in vivo (Fig. 6). Indeed, following injury, podocyte numbers may become depleted, because following cell loss by detachment or apoptosis, the lack of proliferation prevents normalization of podocyte number. Although initially the remaining podocytes may undergo a degree of compensatory hypertrophy, the decrease in podocyte number will eventually result in areas of "denuded" basement membrane, which is thought to predispose to the formation of synechiae between the GBM and Bowman's capsule, leading to the development of secondary focal glomerulosclerosis and subsequent decline in renal function (65, 108–110, 184). Podocytes provide a size- and charge-dependent barrier to protein leakage into the urine,

and are therefore a critical component of the glomerular filtration apparatus. Several studies in diverse renal diseases have shown a close correlation between the onset and progression of proteinuria and reduced podocyte number (32, 87, 116, 138, 147, 231, 232). These events provide a compelling rationale to define the mechanisms underlying the lack of podocyte proliferation.

Mature Podocyte Has Exited Cell Cycle and Is Postmitotic During glomerulogenesis, immature podocytes are capable of proliferation (84, 145). However, during the critical S-shaped body stage of glomerular development, podocytes exit the cell cycle in order to become terminally differentiated and quiescent, which are necessary requirements for normal function. Thus, in podocytes, proliferation and differentiation are closely linked, akin to neurons and cardiac myocytes. In both mouse and human glomerulogenesis, immunostaining for $p27^{Kip1}$ and $p57^{Kip2}$

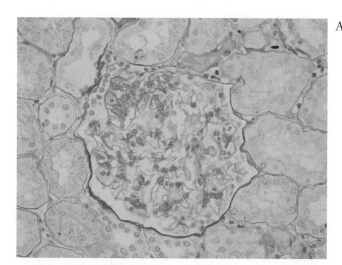

A

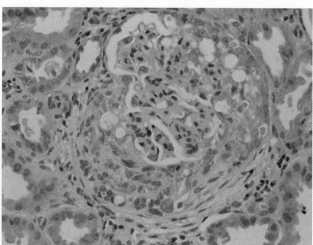

B

FIGURE 6 The podocyte response to injury in human glomerulonephritis – to proliferate or not to proliferate? **A:** No proliferation, with development of segmental sclerosis, as occurs in idiopathic focal and segmental glomerulosclerosis (Periodic Acid Schiff, × 400). **B:** Proliferation, with the development of a cellular crescent in a patient with vasculitis (Haematoxylin and eosin, × 400). Histology courtesy of Dr Meryl Griffiths, Addenbrooke's Hospital, Cambridge.

is absent in proliferating podocytes during the S-shaped body stage (84, 145). On cessation of proliferation, there is strong expression of both Cdk inhibitors, so that p27^{Kip1} and p57^{Kip2} are constitutively expressed in mature podocytes. The Cdk inhibitors p21^{Cip1}, p27^{Kip1}, and p57^{Kip2} alone are not required for normal glomerular development, because as described previously the glomeruli from null mice are histologically normal. However, functional redundancy of p27^{Kip1} and p57^{Kip2}, at least within the podocyte, has been suggested by studies of E13.5 embryonic metanephroi from double p27^{Kip1}/p57^{Kip2}−/− mice. Glomeruli from these mice have been reported to be significantly larger than those from wildtype or single mutants, due to an increase in podocyte number. Differentiation of podocytes was judged to be normal by electron microscopy and immunostaining for WT-1, suggesting a synergistic role for p27^{Kip1} and p57^{Kip2} in determining the final complement of podocytes.

Resistance of Podocytes to Proliferation: Role of Cell Cycle Regulatory Proteins Studies have shown that the frequently observed lack of podocyte proliferation may be due to abnormalities in DNA synthesis or mitosis and cytokinesis (Fig. 7).

The passive Heymann nephritis (PHN) model, induced by the administration of an antibody reactive against the Fx1A antigen on the rat podocyte, has many similarities to human membranous nephropathy (31, 190). In common with the Thy1 model of mesangial proliferative glomerulonephritis, PHN is complement (C5b-9) dependent. However, in contrast to the observed mesangial cell proliferation in response to complement-mediated injury, there is no increase in podocyte number. Mitotic figures and an increase in ploidy are seen in the acute phase of disease, but over time the number of podocytes decreases. The comparison of patterns of expression of cell cycle proteins between the PHN and Thy-1 disease models has provided an opportunity to elucidate the role of cell cycle proteins in experimental podocyte disease.

Following C5b-9 induced injury in PHN rats, protein levels for cyclin A and Cdk2 rise (198), indicating engagement of the cell cycle. However, only a limited increase in DNA synthesis occurs, suggesting the presence of an inhibitor to cell cycle progression. Indeed, the levels of the Cdk inhibitors p21^{Cip1} and p27^{Kip1} increase specifically in podocytes following the induction of PHN (198). The increase in p21^{Cip1} is attenuated by administering the mitogen bFGF to PHN rats, and this augments the increase in podocyte DNA synthesis and ploidy. Furthermore, upregulation of M phase cell cycle proteins Cdc2 and cyclin B is also observed in PHN podocytes, suggesting that a disturbance in cytokinesis is ultimately responsible for the development of polynucleated cells and lack of podocyte proliferation in this experimental glomerular disease (173).

Cell culture studies have further explored the inability of podocytes to proliferate following C5b-9-induced injury, and support the hypothesis of a defect in completing mitosis. When cultured podocytes are exposed to sublytic C5b-9 attack, the cells engage the cell cycle. However, there is a delay or inhibition in entering mitosis, suggesting a block in the G$_2$/M transition and involvement of mechanisms that regulate this checkpoint. The delay in entering mitosis was associated with a marked increase in p53 levels, which was accompanied by an increase in p21^{Cip1} (43), observations that were confirmed in PHN in vivo (178). This response is typical of that following DNA damage, to which podocytes appear to be particularly susceptible. The occurrence of DNA damage following exposure to sublytic C5b-9 has subsequently been confirmed (176), together with increased checkpoint kinase-1 and -2 protein levels, thus arresting cells at G$_2$/M. The mechanism by which DNA damage occurs in podocytes is not currently well understood, but is thought to involve the generation of reactive oxygen radicals. Further studies are needed to explore the role of DNA damage in podocyte disease.

A key role for p21^{Cip1} in limiting the proliferative response of podocytes has been demonstrated in studies using p21^{Cip1} knockout mice (100, 203). The administration of an antiglomerular antibody to induce experimental podocyte injury caused podocyte dedifferentiation and proliferation in p21^{Cip1}−/− mice compared to control mice receiving the same antibody. Glomerular extracellular

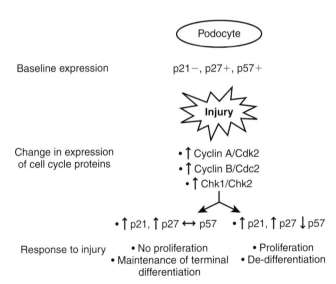

FIGURE 7 Changes in cell cycle protein activity following injury to glomerular podocytes: the critical role of Cdk inhibitors in determining podocyte fate. In contrast to mesangial cells, at baseline quiescent podocytes express both p27^{Kip1} and p57^{Kip2}. Following injury, there is an increase in the positive cell cycle regulators cyclin A/Cdk2 and cyclin B/Cdc2; however, this is accompanied by an increase in checkpoint kinases 1 and 2. The subsequent podocyte response depends on changes in the Cdk inhibitors. If p21^{Cip1} and p27^{Kip1} increase, cell cycle entry remains inhibited, there is no proliferation, and terminal differentiation is maintained. However, if there is a decline in the levels of p21^{Cip1}, p27^{Kip1}, and p57^{Kip2}, then the cell cycle is engaged and proliferation and dedifferentiation occur.

matrix accumulation was also increased in p21^{Cip1}−/− mice, and was associated with a significant decrease in renal function.

The resistance of podocytes to proliferation in the majority of animal models has been confirmed in human diseases, and similar underlying mechanisms have been observed. Normal quiescent podocytes express p27^{Kip1} and p57^{Kip2}, and immunostaining for these proteins is maintained in conditions without proliferation, namely minimal change diseases and membranous glomerulopathy (197). In contrast, expression of both these proteins is uniformly decreased in diseases characterized by podocyte proliferation, that is, cellular FSGS, collapsing glomerulopathy and HIV-associated nephropathy. This is accompanied by the de novo expression of p21^{Cip1}. The mechanisms by which the podocyte eludes the usual constraints on proliferation are discussed below.

Resistance of Podocytes to Proliferation: Role of Mechanical Stretch An additional factor reported to influence the proliferative capacity of the podocyte is the presence of mechanical stress (171). Independent of the site of initial injury, a common pathway to progressive glomerulosclerosis is an increase in intraglomerular pressure, also known as glomerular hypertension (16, 65, 109). Lowering intraglomerular pressure reduces progression in a number of glomerular diseases, including diabetic nephropathy (228). Glomerular hypertension is associated with glomerular hypertrophy (see below), and the resultant mechanical stretch causes injury to all three glomerular cell types. Whereas applying mechanical stretch to cultured mesangial cells increases proliferation (82), the opposite response is seen in cultured podocytes (171). Stretching mouse podocytes in culture decreased the levels of cyclins D1, A, and B1 and Cdc2, in association with an increase in the Cdk inhibitors. Stretch caused an early increase in p21^{Cip1}, followed by an increase in p27^{Kip1} at 24 hours and p57^{Kip2} at 72 hours. In contrast to the growth arrest seen in wildtype cells exposed to stretch, p21^{Cip1}−/− podocytes exposed to stretch continued to proliferate, suggesting a role for p21^{Cip1} in the inability of the podocyte to progress through the cell cycle in response to stretch. These studies show that in addition to being injurious to mesangial cells, mechanical stretch affects podocytes and reduces their proliferative potential by altering specific cell cycle proteins.

Podocyte Proliferation Although the majority of both experimental animal models of podocyte injury and human podocyte diseases are not associated with proliferation, this has been reported to occur in a limited number of settings. The true ability of the mature podocyte to proliferate remains controversial, principally because glomerular cells believed to be proliferating podocytes frequently lack defining cell-type–specific markers (146). However, the use of transgenic animals has been invaluable in resolving the debate. A well-studied animal model of podocyte proliferation is crescentic glomerulonephritis in the mouse, which has been examined in detail by several groups. In this model, predictable proliferation of glomerular cells occurs, and early in the course of the disease, this is not associated with rup-

ture of Bowman's capsule, nor with the presence of infiltrating cells (159). It is therefore a useful model for studying the contribution of intrinsic glomerular cells to crescent formation. Using Cre/loxP recombination, Moeller et al. generated a mouse with constitutive expression of β galactosidase specifically in podocytes in vivo (141). Experimental crescentic nephritis was induced by injecting rabbit IgG IP, followed 6 days later by an intravenous injection of rabbit antimouse GBM antibody (141). The crescents contained numerous β-galactosidase–expressing cells, confirming their podocyte origin. Furthermore, expression of the nuclear proliferation marker Ki-67 by these cells demonstrated the capability of these podocyte-derived cells to undergo proliferation. An alternative approach was taken by Matsusaka et al. (129). They generated a transgenic mouse with podocyte-specific expression of human CD25. Injury was then induced using an immunotoxin, resulting in a proliferative glomerular lesion. However, immunohistochemistry indicated that the proliferating cells were of parietal epithelial origin, not podocytes. The disparity between these two results likely results from the different initiating injuries used, but illustrates the ongoing debate. As described above, once podocytes proliferate they lose several of their defining characteristic proteins, such as WT-1, making identification difficult. However, there is broad agreement that the proliferating resident glomerular cells making up crescents are of epithelial origin, although the relative contributions of parietal cells and podocytes remain disputed.

In human disease, podocyte proliferation is considered to occur in collapsing glomerulopathy, cellular focal segmental glomerulosclerosis, and HIV-associated nephropathy (9, 10). In these diseases, there is increased expression of cyclin A and the proliferation marker Ki-67, with a marked reduction in p27^{Kip1} and p57^{Kip2} (10, 197). In contrast, all other diseases of podocytes in humans, including membranous nephropathy, minimal change disease, and focal segmental glomerulosclerosis, are not associated with a decrease in Cdk inhibitor levels, and typical markers of proliferation are absent. Interestingly, the rate of progression to end-stage renal failure is increased in glomerular diseases characterized by podocyte proliferation (36, 195). The pathogenesis of HIV-associated nephropathy has been further detailed using transgenic mice expressing HIV-1 genes (8, 18, 37). The Tg26 mouse model develops murine HIVAN secondary o renal expression of HIV-1 mRNAs from the HIV-1 NL4-3 gag-pol proviral transgene (37). This model has enabled characterization of the cellular effects of HIV-1 using both the intact animal and conditionally immortalized podocytes in culture. HIV-1 induces loss of contact inhibition in podocytes (194), and expression of cyclin D1 and phosphorylation of pRb (151). The cells become dedifferentiated, with loss of specific podocyte-expressed proteins (8, 27). Interestingly, there have been reports of reversibility of HIV nephropathy in both mice (discussed below) and human disease (192) following treatment with highly active antiretroviral therapy, suggesting that once the virus is cleared, the podocyte is capable of exiting the cell cycle and redifferentiating to its mature phenotype.

Therapeutic Inhibition of Podocyte Proliferation at Cell Cycle Level As with glomerular diseases principally affecting the mesangial cell, both roscovitine and retinoids have shown promise as therapeutic agents in modulating the podocyte response to injury.

Roscovitine We hypothesized that inhibition of podocyte proliferation with the Cdk2 inhibitor roscovitine in a mouse model of crescentic glomerulonephritis would improve renal outcome (71), similarly to that observed following inhibition of mesangial cell proliferation in Thy 1 nephritis (177) described previously. Inhibition of Cdk2 activity was confirmed by a histone kinase assay, and podocyte DNA synthesis measured by incorporation of BrdU. Compared to control nephritic animals receiving the vehicle, in mice treated with roscovitine there was a significant decrease in BrdU at day 5 of nephritis. This was accompanied by less accumulation of laminin at day 14, and significantly improved renal function, suggesting a similar intervention may be beneficial in human diseases. Roscovitine has also been demonstrated to be beneficial in the treatment of Tg26 mice at doses that did not decrease HIV-1 transgene expression, suggesting an effect mediated by inhibition of cell cycle progression (68).

Retinoids Retinoids are particularly attractive agents for the treatment of podocyte disease, as it has been demonstrated that following podocyte injury, both decrease podocyte proliferation and maintain the expression of markers of differentiation (216, 221). The promoter region of the human nephrin gene (NPHS1) contains three putative retinoic acid–response elements and shows enhancer activity in response to all-trans-retinoic acid (ATRA) in a dose-dependent manner. We have recently demonstrated that ATRA in vitro significantly retards podocyte proliferation as measured by the MTT assay, while inducing process formation and increasing the expression of both nephrin and podocin (221). Similarly, in mice with anti-glomerular antibody nephritis, treatment with ATRA both reduces podocyte proliferation, and prevents the decreases in nephrin, podocin, and synaptopodin in experimental animals. This was accompanied by a reduction in proteinuria. The dual roles of retinoids to both inhibit proliferation while promoting differentiation underscore their potential value as therapeutic agents for human podocyte diseases.

GLOMERULAR ENDOTHELIAL CELL PROLIFERATION

The endothelial cells of mature glomeruli are quiescent but retain the capacity to proliferate and form new capillaries following injury (99). The degree of proliferation appears to be dependent on the local balance of proangiogenic factors, such as vascular endothelial growth factor (VEGF), and antiangiogenic factors, such as thrombospondin-1. An inadequate proliferative response may lead to loss of the glomerular microvasculature and contribute to glomerulosclerosis and progressive renal impairment. The beneficial effects of VEGF administration have been demonstrated in animal models of acute glo-merulonephritis (98, 101, 127), suggesting that amelioration of human diseases may be achieved by augmenting the reparative potential of the glomerular endothelial cells. However, the underlying role of individual cyclins, Cdk, and Cdk inhibitors in these cells remains unknown.

Tubular Cell Hyperplasia

Renal tubular hyperplasia is most frequently encountered during the reparative phase following an acute injury, such as ischemia or toxin exposure (14). Tubular injury results in cell loss by either necrosis or apoptosis, and therefore there is a requirement for the remaining cells to spread and migrate to cover the exposed basement membrane. These cells then dedifferentiate and proliferate to restore cell number, and finally differentiate again to restore the functional integrity of the nephron. Interestingly, the tubular repair recapitulates organogenesis in patterns of gene expression, including vimentin; neural cell adhesion molecule; growth factors such as IGF-1, fibroblast growth factor, and hepatocyte growth factor; and matrix molecules such as osteopontin (14). This dedifferentiated phenotype is likely to be important for the spreading and proliferative properties of the viable tubular epithelial cells as they cover the denuded basement membrane to replace lost cells. However, the factors controlling the reversion to a less differentiated phenotype, and the subsequent re-establishment of the mature phenotype, remain poorly understood.

As might be expected, the proliferation observed following a transient ischemic injury is associated with an increase in the mRNA and protein expression of cyclins D1, D3, and B, mRNA expression of cyclin A, and protein expression of Cdks 2 and 4 (164). Both cyclin-D and -E kinase activities are increased (122, 164). Thus, the proliferative response is due to increased expression of both the regulatory and catalytic subunits of the G1 kinases, and an increase in their activity.

The Cdk inhibitors appear to have a critical role in limiting the proliferative response. Following acute renal injury induced by ischemia, ureteral obstruction, or cisplatin, p21[Cip1] protein expression is increased in the thick ascending limb of the loop of Henle and in the distal convoluted tubule (137). Induction of the same injury in p21[Cip1]−/− mice was associated with increased proliferation, as assessed by BrdU incorporation and PCNA staining (136). The p21[Cip]−/− mice had a more rapid onset of acute renal failure, developed more severe morphological damage, and had a higher mortality, emphasizing the requirement for proliferation following injury to be at a controlled and appropriate level.

HYPERTROPHY

Hypertrophy has been described in most segments of the nephron, but proximal tubular hypertrophy is observed most frequently. Hypertrophy of the proximal tubule has been described in compensatory renal growth, chronic metabolic acidosis and chronic hypokalemia, diabetes mellitus, and during protein loading (113). In compensatory renal growth, there is also hypertrophy of the glomerulus and collecting tubules; in diabetes, hypertrophy of glomerular cells is well described, and with prolonged protein-loading hypertrophy of the initial segments of the thick ascending limb occurs.

As mentioned previously, cellular hypertrophy may result from either cell cycle–dependent or –independent mechanisms. Within the glomerulus, an increase in cell size is predominantly due to cell cycle re-entry without progression, whereas in the tubules there appears to be a more significant contribution from the inhibition of protein synthesis.

Glomerular Hypertrophy

Glomerular cell hypertrophy occurs during many forms of chronic renal disease, and may herald the development of glomerulosclerosis (65, 89, 262). Glomerular diseases associated with glomerular hypertrophy include diabetic nephropathy (264), minimal change nephropathy (220), focal segmental glomerulosclerosis (57, 144), and a reduction in renal mass (218). However, there are clear differences in the prognosis of glomerular hypertrophy, depending on the underlying disease. Following uninephrectomy, the hypertrophy is compensatory and is not typically associated with the development of glomerulosclerosis. In contrast, the hypertrophy of diabetic nephropathy antecedes and probably underlies the development of glomerulosclerosis (37). Diabetic nephropathy is the leading cause of end-stage renal disease in Western countries, and is discussed further below. Pathological glomerular hypertrophy leads to progressive glomerulosclerosis and scarring by a number of different mechanisms (89). The increased metabolic rate of cells undergoing hypertrophy results in enhanced mitochondrial oxygen consumption, which may lead to tissue injury due to the generation of reactive oxygen radicals and the subsequent peroxidation of proteins and lipids. The hypertrophy is often initiated by growth factors that also stimulate the cells to increase production of extracellular matrix components, such as type IV collagen.

DIABETIC NEPHROPATHY

Diabetes mellitus is now the most frequent cause of end-stage renal failure in Western countries (152), and the pathogenesis of diabetic nephropathy is discussed in detail elsewhere in this book. The focus of this chapter is on the disordered cell growth seen in association with diabetic renal involvement. The hallmarks of human diabetic nephropathy are similar in both type I and type II diabetes, and consist of mesangial cell hypertrophy and podocyte loss, with accumulation of extracellular matrix in the mesangium and tubulointerstitium, resulting in glomerulosclerosis and tubulointerstitial fibrosis (133, 162, 185). Research has concentrated principally on the ability of hyperglycemia and TGF-β to induce mesangial cell hypertrophy, and more recently the roles of RAGE (17) and hyperinsulinemia (30) have also been studied.

Diabetes and Mesangial Cells

Hyperglycemia In vitro culture of mesangial cells in high glucose media causes cell cycle entry and a biphasic growth response (260). Following initial proliferation, the cells arrest in G1 phase and there is progressive hypertrophy. Both kidney and glomerular hypertrophy induced by hyperglycemia are associated with an early and sustained increase in expression of cyclin D1 and activation of Cdk4 (49). An arrested cell cycle suggests a role for the Cdk inhibitors in mediating hypertrophy, and indeed high glucose increases the levels of both $p21^{Cip1}$ (112) and $p27^{Kip1}$ (245) in cultured mesangial cells. This is mediated by a number of factors including glucose itself; TGF-β, which then acts in an autocrine fashion (246, 265, 265); and CTGF (1). High glucose directly stimulates the transcription of $p21^{Cip1}$ (243), and activates MAP kinases, which prolong the half-life of $p27^{Kip1}$ by phosphorylation on serine residues (242). Lowering $p21^{Cip1}$ (47) or $p27^{Kip1}$ (245) levels with antisense oligonucleotides reduces the hypertrophic effects of high glucose. Moreover, hypertrophy is not induced by high glucose in $p21^{Cip1}-/-$ (unpublished observations) and $p27^{Kip1}-/-$ (244) mesangial cells in vitro. Indeed, high glucose increases proliferation in $p27^{Kip1}-/-$ mesangial cells, whereas it arrests cell cycle progression in $p27^{Kip1}+/+$ mesangial cells (244). Reconstituting $p27^{Kip1}$ levels in $p27^{Kip1}-/-$ mesangial cells by transfection restores the hypertrophic phenotype (244). These studies show a compelling role for the Cdk inhibitors $p21^{Cip1}$ and $p27^{Kip1}$ in mediating the hypertrophy induced by high glucose.

These in vitro findings have been confirmed in experimental models of both type I and type II diabetic nephropathy. Considering type I diabetes, the glomerular protein levels of $p21^{Cip1}$ are increased in the streptozotocin (STZ)-induced model in the mouse (112), and both $p21^{Cip1}$ and $p27^{Kip1}$ levels are increased in the glomeruli of diabetic BBdp rats (248). A similar increase was noted in glomeruli of *db/db* mice (243) and the Zucker diabetic fatty rat (88), models of type II diabetic nephropathy. Diabetic $p21^{Cip1}-/-$ mice are protected from glomerular hypertrophy (3). Diabetic $p27^{Kip1}-/-$ mice have only mild mesangial expansion and no glomerular or renal hypertrophy compared to control diabetic $p27^{Kip1}+/+$ mice despite upregulation of glomerular TGF-β (5). These results support a critical role for the Cdk inhibitors $p21^{Cip1}$ and $p27^{Kip1}$ in mediating the glomerular hypertrophy seen not only in association with diabetes, but also as described in the following, a reduction in nephron number.

Transforming Growth Factor β The cytokine TGF-β has been shown in numerous settings to be a key mediator of progressive fibrosis in renal disease (106, 186, 201). TGF-β also decreases proliferation in mesangial cells, an effect that appears to be independent of $p21^{Cip1}$ and $p27^{Kip1}$, and induces cell hypertrophy (125, 142, 250). To determine the role of Cdk inhibitors in mediating the hypertrophic effects of TGF-β, mesangial cells derived from single and double null mice were studied (142). Compared to wildtype mice, hypertrophy was significantly reduced in double p21^{Cip1}/p27^{Kip1}−/− mesangial cells. A less marked reduction in hypertrophy was seen in the single p21^{Cip1}−/− and p27^{Kip1}−/− cells. These results show that although p21^{Cip1} and p27^{Kip1} each contribute to the hypertrophic action of TGFβ, the presence of both is required for maximal effect.

The expression of Cdk inhibitors has also been explored in response to CTGF, considered to be a principle mediator of the downstream effects of TGFβ. Abdel Wahab et al. (1) demonstrated that CTGF is a hypertrophic factor for human mesangial cells, and that this hypertrophy is associated with the induction of p15^{INK4b}, p21^{Cip1}, and p27^{Kip1}, with the maintenance of pRb in a hypophosphorylated state.

DIABETES AND PODOCYTES

Compared to the accumulated depth of knowledge concerning the effect of the diabetic milieu on the mesangial cell, studies of the podocyte remain in their infancy. Recent morphometric analyses have demonstrated that the podocyte undergoes hypertrophy early in the course of both animal models of diabetic nephropathy (72, 73, 88, 254) and in human disease (230, 231). This hypertrophy may be in direct response to the metabolic changes associated with diabetes, or compensatory, consequent to the loss of podocytes that is known to occur (12, 174).

At the level of the cell cycle, mRNA and protein expression of p27^{Kip1} is increased in both cultured podocytes exposed to high glucose and in glomeruli isolated from streptozotocin-induced diabetic rats (254). High glucose also significantly increased angiotensin II levels both in cell lysates and media compared with normal glucose, and exogenous angiotensin II increased p27^{Kip1} mRNA and protein expression. Exposure of cultured cells and treatment of diabetic rats with an angiotensin II receptor antagonist (ARB) inhibited the increase in p27^{Kip1}. Glomerular hypertrophy was also significantly prevented by ARB treatment. Although the data are currently limited, it appears likely that similar cell cycle mechanisms drive both mesangial cell and podocyte hypertrophy in diabetic nephropathy, suggesting that podocytes in this setting are also capable of engaging the cell cycle.

COMPENSATORY GLOMERULAR HYPERTROPHY

A reduction in nephron number results in compensatory hypertrophy in the remaining viable nephron (234). Uninephrectomy does not alter the protein expression of cyclins D1 or D2, nor of Cdk2 or Cdk4, when total renal lysates are studied at day 7 (165). However, there may be a differential effect in specific renal compartments (121), and an increase in tubular cyclin E-Cdk2 activity was demonstrated during compensatory hypertrophy following uninephrectomy. Prior to hypertrophy, severe renal ablation produced by 5/6 nephrectomy resulted in an early proliferative glomerular response, associated with an increase in cyclin E expression and phosphorylation of pRb (199).

A role for the Cdk inhibitors is now emerging in the pathogenesis of glomerular hypertrophy. Following partial renal ablation, p21^{Cip1}−/− mice develop glomerular hyperplasia rather than hypertrophy and increased intraglomerular pressure, with protection from the development of progressive renal failure (135). Increased intraglomerular pressure is a final pathway toward glomerulosclerosis in systemic hypertension, diabetes, and focal segmental glomerulosclerosis (FSGS). This glomerular hypertension causes stress-tension, or stretch, on resident glomerular cells, with differing consequences for the different cell types. Exposure of mesangial cells to cyclical mechanical stretch results in cell cycle entry and proliferation (93). In contrast, mechanical stretch reduces cell cycle progression and induces podocyte hypertrophy in vitro (172). This is unchanged in p27^{Kip1}−/− cells, but hypertrophy was not induced in p21^{Cip1} and double p21^{Cip1}/p27^{Kip1}−/− podocytes, indicating a requirement for p21^{Cip1}. Stretch-induced hypertrophy required cell cycle entry, and was prevented by specifically blocking Erk1/2 or Akt. However, it is not clear whether podocyte hypertrophy represents a beneficial adaptive response to raised intraglomerular pressure, or whether this change in podocyte phenotype is accompanied by a disturbance in function that is detrimental to the glomerulus.

TUBULAR HYPERTROPHY

The compensatory growth capacity of the kidney was known to the ancient Greeks: Aristotle (384–322 BC) described that animals born with a single kidney have a larger organ compared to those born with two. More contemporary studies have documented that the increase in renal size following nephron reduction by disease or surgical resection is due primarily to proximal tubular epithelial hypertrophy (183). The initial hypertrophic response is considered adaptive (234, 236, 240); however, with time persistent hypertrophy is associated with the infiltration of macrophages, T cells, and fibroblasts into the tubulointerstitial space (89, 103). This hypertrophy is no longer beneficial to organ function, and the cellular infiltrate results in tubular atrophy and tubulointerstitial fibrosis, the final convergent pathway of many renal diseases of diverse etiologies.

CELL CYCLE–DEPENDENT TUBULAR CELL HYPERTROPHY

Transforming Growth Factor β As in the glomerulus, TGFβ is an important mediator of tubular cell hypertrophy. The hypertrophy induced by both angiotensin II and high glucose (22) is also dependent on TGFβ. TGFβ converts a mitogen-induced proliferative response to cellular hypertrophy, and this has been studied in detail in cultures of proximal tubule cells by examining the effects of epidermal growth factor (EGF) plus TGFβ. TGFβ alone has an antiproliferative effect on tubular cell growth, but does not induce hypertrophy (62). EGF-induced hyperplasia is associated with cell cycle entry, hyperphosphorylation of pRb, and an increase in thymidine incorporation, but no change in cell size or protein/DNA ratio (62). In the presence of additional TGFβ cell cycle entry is not impaired and cyclin-E protein levels increase, but there is no increase in DNA synthesis and pRb remains hypophosphorylated, with arrest of the cells in mid to late G1. Inactivation of pRb by expression of either SV40 large-T antigen (inactivates both pRb and p53) or HPV E7 (inactivates pRb alone) prevents TGFβ from converting EGF-induced hyperplasia to hypertrophy. In contrast, inactivation of p53 alone with HPV E6 has no effect on the induction of hypertrophy, confirming the importance of pRb in the cell cycle arrest of tubular cells resulting from TGFβ.

The maintenance of pRb in its hypophosphorylated state suggests TGFβ modifies the activity of G1 kinases. Consistent with the observation that cell cycle entry is not impaired in the presence of TGFβ, TGFβ has no effect on EGF-induced increase in Cdk4/6–cyclin D kinase activity (120, 180). However, there is no increase in cyclin E kinase activity, with a decrease number of Cdk2–cyclin E complexes and retention of p57, but not p27 or p21, in those complexes that do form.

In summary, the proposed paradigm for the development of hypertrophy in response to TGFβ in renal tubular cells is as follows. After a proliferative stimulus, there is cell cycle entry and activation of cyclin D kinase. This is associated with an increase in protein synthesis, and hence cell size. As the cell reaches mid to late G1, if cyclin E kinase is sufficiently activated, pRb is further phosphorylated and becomes inactivated, allowing the cell to progress to S phase and hyperplasia to occur. However, in the presence of TGFβ, cyclin E kinase is not sufficiently activated, pRb remains hypophosphorylated, the cell is arrested, and hypertrophy results.

Angiotensin II Angiotensin II has an established role in stimulating hypertrophy of proximal tubular cells, mediated by the high-affinity AT_1 receptor (241). Both angiotensin II and EGF induce the expression of early immediate genes in tubule cells, suggesting that angiotensin II–mediated hypertrophy is also dependent on cell cycle entry (238). Indeed, angiotensin II–treated cells are arrested in G1 and do not progress to S phase (20, 241), reminiscent of cells exposed to TGFβ. It has subsequently been shown that angiotensin II stimulates the transcription and protein synthesis of TGFβ in proximal tubule cells (239). Exposure of cells to a neutralizing antibody to TGFβ abrogated the ability of angiotensin II to induce hypertrophy, demonstrating its dependency on the induction and autocrine activity of TGFβ (239). In contrast to proximal tubules cells exposed to EGF and TGFβ, angiotensin II increases protein (but not mRNA) levels for $p27^{Kip1}$ (247). To characterize the functional role of $p27^{Kip1}$ in angiotensin II–mediated hypertrophy, proximal tubule cells were cultured from $p27^{Kip1}$ null mice (237), which responded to angiotensin II with cell cycle progression but no hypertrophy. Cdk4/6–cyclin D kinase activity was stimulated in both wildtype and null cells, but Cdk2–cyclin E kinase activity only increased in the null cells, indicating that $p27^{Kip1}$ inhibits this

complex, and is required for angiotensin II–mediated hypertrophy of proximal tubular cells.

The mechanism by which angiotensin II increases $p27^{Kip1}$ expression has been studied in detail (77). Angiotensin II upregulates p22phox, a subunit of membrane-bound NADPH oxidase, and hence increases the concentration of intracellular reactive oxygen species. This results in phosphorylation and activation of the mitogen-activated protein kinases Erk 1,2 that in turn leads to serine phosphorylation of $p27^{Kip1}$ (78, 242). Serine phosphorylated $p27^{Kip1}$ has increased stability and decreased degradation by the ubiquitin pathway (242). Atrial natriuretic peptide attenuates angiotensin II–mediated $p27^{Kip1}$ expression and proximal tubule cell hypertrophy, by a mechanism that appears to involve activation of the phosphatase MKP-1, which dephosphorylates Erk1,2 (76). The importance of this pathway has also been shown in vivo (249). Infusion of angiotensin II into normal rats for 7 days increased the formation of reactive oxygen species in tubular cells and augmented $p27^{Kip1}$ expression. Immunostaining for PCNA decreased, indicating G1 cell cycle arrest, although hypertrophy was not observed.

As with mesangial cells, a role for CTGF has been described in mediating tubular cell hypertrophy in response to angiotensin II. Systemic infusion of angiotensin II into normal rats induced overexpression of CTGF in glomeruli, tubules, and renal arteries, with associated tubular injury and increase in fibronectin expression (188). A similar effect was demonstrated in cultured tubular cells, with angiotensin II acting through the AT_1 receptor. The importance of CTGF in angiotensin II–mediated hypertrophy was explored in detail by another group using HK2 cells (123). Angiotensin II induced CTGF expression, G1 cell cycle arrest, and cell hypertrophy, which were reversed by treatment with an anti-CTGF antibody. In addition to the well-described roles in apoptosis and fibrosis, further detrimental renal effects of angiotensin II are likely to be secondary to its recently described effects of cell cycle arrest and hypertrophy.

A summary of the changes in cell cycle proteins occurring in glomerular and tubular hyperplasia, and in cell cycle–dependent hypertrophy, is shown in Table 1. Data from knockout mice are shown in Table 2.

CELL CYCLE–INDEPENDENT TUBULAR CELL HYPERTROPHY

In addition to increased new protein synthesis, a decrease in the rate of protein breakdown may contribute to cell hypertrophy (59). Within the kidney, this is best characterized for tubular cells. Although diabetes and acidosis are catabolic states, both are associated with decreases in renal proteolysis, which makes a significant contribution to the associated growth of the kidney (157, 205, 206).

An estimated 60% of total intracellular proteolysis in renal tubular cells occurs by the ubiquitin–proteasome pathway (60); however, this does not appear to be a major factor in the regulation of proteolysis during the hypertrophic response of renal tubular cells. Two lines of evidence support an alteration

TABLE 1 Summary of Cell Cycle Proteins in Hyperplasia and Hypertrophy of Renal Cells

Experiment	Cyclin CDK			CDK Inhibitor			Reference
	Increased	Decreased	No Change	Increased	Decreased	No Change	
Mesangial Cell							
Proliferation							
In vitro exposure to mitogens (PDGF, bFGF)	D1, E, A			p21	p27	p57	176,193,99
Animal models							
Thy1	D1, E	Cdk4,2		p15, p21	p27		200
Remnant kidney	E, Cdk2		Cdk4				199
Suppression of proliferation							
In vitro exposure to antimitogens (TGFβ, SPARC, heparin)		D1, E, A Cdk4, 2		p15, p21, p27			193,203,246
Hypertrophy							
In vitro exposure							
Glucose			Cdk2	p21, p27			112,245
TGFβ				p16, p21, p27			201,248
CTGF				p15, p21, p27			1
Animal models							
Type I diabetes (STZ mouse, BBdp rat)			E, A	p21, p27			112,248
Type II diabetes (db/db mouse, Zucker rat)			Cdk2	p27			88,243
Apoptosis							
Cytoplasmic location of Cdk2							85
Podocyte							
Immune injury							
In vitro exposure to C5b9				p21			43
Animals models							
PHN	A, Cdk2			p21	p57		176,98
Antiglomerular antibody	A, Cdk2			p21, p27	p57		203
Proliferation							
In vitro exposure to HIV-1	D1						151
Human disease							
Collapsing GN	A						10,202
Response to stretch							
In vitro		D, A, B		D, A p21, p27, p57	p27, p57		171
Tubular epithelial cell							
Proliferation							
Animal models							
Uninephroctomy	E, Cdk2						122
Ischemic injury	D1, D3, A, B Cdk2, 4						137,164
UUO, cisplatin		E					164
Hypertrophy							
In vitro exposure EGF + TGFβ	D, Cdk4			p21			62,120

TABLE 2   Data from Knockout Mice

	Experiment	Outcome	Reference
p21−/−	Mesangial cells exposed to high glucose in vitro	Resistant to hypertrophy	—[a]
	Animal models		
	STZ diabetes	Reduced glomerular hypertrophy	3
	Antiglomerular antibody	Increased podocyte proliferation	100
	Remnant kidney	Glomerular hyperplasia, not hypertrophy	135
	Acute tubular injury (ischemia, UUO, cisplatin)	Increased proliferation, worse renal function, increased mortality	136
p27−/−	Mesangial cells exposed to high glucose in vitro	Resistant to hypertrophy	244
	Mesangial cells deprived of growth factors	Increased apoptosis	84
	Animal models		
	STZ diabetes	Reduced glomerular hypertrophy	5
	Antiglomerular antibody	Increased mesangial cell proliferation and apoptosis	158
	UUO	Increased tubular apoptosis	158
p57−/−	Unmanipulated animal	Normal glomerulogenesis in embryonic mice	217, 257, 263

[a]Unpublished.

UUO, Unilateral ureteral obstruction.

in lysosomal function as underlying the reduced proteolysis observed in certain cases of tubular hypertrophy, and a possible mechanism by which this occurs has recently begun to be clarified (63). First, in addition to stimulating cell cycle entry, EGF increases protein half-life by approximately 30% in cultured primary proximal tubular cells, primarily by affecting lysosomal proteolysis (60). Second, exposure of tubular cells to ammonia leads to alkalinization of acidic intracellular compartments, including lysosomes, thus modifying their function, and stimulates hypertrophy that is independent of cell cycle entry (61).

Several studies have demonstrated proximal tubule cell hypertrophy in response to ammonia in vitro (61, 66, 119), and renal ammonia synthesis is increased in several apparently diverse clinical conditions associated with hypertrophy (113, 150). In chronic metabolic acidosis and chronic hypokalemia, mitochondrial ammoniagenesis is directly stimulated. In contrast, the increase in ammonia in diabetes mellitus, following uninephrectomy and during protein loading, is thought to be stimulated by an increase in single-nephron glomerular filtration rate (SNGFR). Cell culture studies involving either reducing the media pH (221) or lowering potassium concentration (226) do not induce hypertrophy, indicating that it is not changes in the extracellular milieu per se that initiate the hypertrophic growth response. The results from direct application of ammonium chloride suggest that the accumulation of this molecule, in response to acidosis or hypokalemia, drives the development of hypertrophy. This hypothesis is supported by studies of hypertrophy in the setting of chronic hypokalemia in the rat (219). In this model, renal ammonia production is significantly increased. Administration of bicarbonate both decreases the rate of ammonia synthesis and the hypertrophy.

Renal generation of ammonia has recently been studied in patients with metabolic acidosis and normal renal function (66). Compared to individuals with normal acid–base balance, kidney protein degradation was significantly lower and urinary ammonia excretion significantly higher. As with cell and animal studies, it was suggested that in human metabolic acidosis the increase ammonia synthesis drives the decrease in protein degradation, and is potentially responsible for kidney hypertrophy.

What is the mechanism by which altered lysosomal function affects protein degradation? Chaperone-mediated autophagy allows lysosomal import of proteins containing a specific consensus sequence, KFERQ, by the binding of heat-shock cognate protein 73 (Hsc73) to lysosomal membrane protein 2a (LAMP2a). In cultured NRK-52E cells (a rat kidney epithelial cell line) exposed to EGF or ammonia (but not TGFβ alone), there was an increase in the half-life of KFERQ-containing proteins (63) associated with a decrease in total cellular and lysosomal LAMP2a. Furthermore, declines in LAMP2a and Hsc73 have also been demonstrated in lysosomes isolated from the hypertrophied cortex of acutely diabetic rats, and was accompanied by an increase in KFERQ-containing proteins (214). Other lysosomal pathways may also be affected during renal hypertrophy (59). EGF-induced suppression of proteolysis in NRK-52E cells was prevented by inhibitors of Ras and PI-3 kinase, but not by inhibitors of MAP kinase or Src (64). PI-3 kinase and Akt activities are increased in the renal cortex of diabetic *db/db* mice and correlate with hypertrophy (48). Products of the PI-3 kinase pathway control membrane and protein trafficking, and the suppression of chaperone-mediated autophagy may be part of a generalized abnormality in trafficking to and from lysosomes.

CONCLUSIONS

The last 16 years has seen an explosion in our understanding of the underlying mechanisms governing renal hyperplasia and hypertrophy has literally burgeoned since 1991. The goal for the next 15 years will be to identify specific modifiable targets to alter or even reverse these pathological processes. Numerous agents have been demonstrated to be beneficial in ameliorating the course of animal models of disease, and the hope is that certain of these will transfer to be of use in human disease. Indeed, Cdk2 inhibitors are now in human trials for treatment of proliferative glomerulonephritis. With the discovery of drugs that target either the network of mitogens responsible for stimulating abnormal cell growth or specific cell cycle–regulatory proteins, potential therapies may be on the horizon for patients with renal diseases in which hyperplasia or hypertrophy is a dominant feature. Much has been learned, but in addition to characterizing the role of conventional cyclins, Cdks and Cdk inhibitors, the challenge remains to identify novel cell cycle proteins, determine their role in renal disease, and the consequences of their manipulation.

References

1. Abdel Wahab N, Weston BS, Roberts T, Mason RM. Connective tissue growth factor and regulation of the mesangial cell cycle: role in cellular hypertrophy. *J Am Soc Nephrol* 2002;13:2437–2445.
2. Aktas H, Cai H, Cooper GM. Ras links growth factor signalling to the cell cycle machinery via regulation of cyclin D1 and the cdk inhibitor p27kip1. *Mol Cell Biol* 1997;17:3850–3857.
3. Al-Douahji M, Brugarolas J, Brown PAJ, et al. The cyclin kinase inhibitor p21Waf1/Cip1 is required for glomerular hypertrophy in experimental diabetic nephropathy. *Kidney Int* 1999;56:1691–1699.
4. Atherton-Fessler S, Parker LL GR, Piwnica-Worms H. Mechanisms of p34cdc2 regulation. *Mol Cell Biol* 1993;13:1675–1685.
5. Awazu M, Omori S, Ishikura K, Hida M, Fujita H. The lack of cyclin kinase p27Kip1 ameliorates progression of diabetic nephropathy. *J Am Soc Nephrol* 2003;14:699–708.
6. Baker AJ, Mooney A, Lombardi D, Johnson RJ, Savill J. Mesangial cell apoptosis: the major mechanism for resolution of glomerular hypercellularity in experimental mesangial proliferative nephritis. *J Clin Invest* 1994;94:2105–2116.
7. Baldin V, Lukas J, Marcote MJ, Pagano M, Draetta GF. Cyclin D1 is a nuclear protein required for cell cycle progression in G1 cells. *Genes Dev* 1993;7:812–821.
8. Barisoni L, Bruggeman LA, Mundel P, D'Agati V, Klotman PE. HIV-1 induces renal epithelial dedifferentiation in a transgenic model of HIV-associated nephropathy. *Kidney Int* 2000;58:173–181.
9. Barisoni L, Kriz W, Mundel P, D'Agati V. The dysregulated podocyte phenotype: a novel concept in the pathogenesis of collapsing idiopathic focal segmental glomerulosclerosis and HIV associated nephropathy. *J Am Soc Nephrol* 1999;10:51–61.
10. Barisoni L, Mokrzycki M, Sablay L, et al. Podocyte cell cycle regulation and proliferation in collapsing glomerulonephropathies. *Kidney Int* 2000;58:137–143.
11. Berthet C, Aleem E, Coppola V, Tessarollo L, Kaldis P. Cdk2 knockout mice are viable. *Curr Biol* 2003;13:1775–1785.
12. Bhathena DB. Glomerular basement membrane length to podocyte ratio in human nephropenia: implications for focal segmental glomerulosclerosis. *Am J Kidney Dis* 2003;41:1179–1188.
13. Bloom J, Pagano G. Deregulated degradation of the cdk inhibitor p27 and malignant transformation. *Semin Cancer Biol* 2003;13:41–47.
14. Bonventre JV. Dedifferentiation and proliferation of surviving epithelial cells in acute renal failure. *J Am Soc Nephrol* 2003;14:555–561.
15. Brandt J, Pippin J, Schulze M, et al. Role of complement membrane attack complex (C5b-9) in mediating experimental mesangioproliferative glomerulonephritis. *Kidney Int* 1996;49:335–343.
16. Brenner BM. Nephron adaptation to renal injury or ablation. *Am J Physiol* 1985;249:F324–F337.
17. Brizzi MF, Dentelli P, Rosso A, et al. RAGE- and TGF-beta receptor-mediated signals converge on STAT5 and p21waf to control cell-cycle progression of mesangial cells: a possible role in the developement and progression of diabetic nephropathy. *FASEB J* 2004;18:1249–1251.
18. Bruggeman LA, Dikman S, Meng C, et al. Nephropathy in human immunodeficiency virus-1 transgenic mice is due to renal transgene expression. *J Clin Invest* 1997;100:84–92.
19. Bunz F, Dutriaux A, Lengauer C, et al. Requirement for p53 and p21 to sustain G2 arrest after DNA damage. *Science* 1998;282:1497–1501.
20. Burns KD, Harris RC. Signalling and growth responses of LLC-PK1/CI4 cells transfected with the rabbit AT1 ang II receptor. *Am J Physiol* 1995;268:C925–C935.
21. Caspary T, Cleary MA, Perlman EJ, et al. Oppositely imprinted genes p57Kip2 and Igf2 interact in a mouse model for Beckwith–Wiedemann syndrome. *Genes Dev* 1999;13:3115–3124.
22. Chen S, Hoffman BB, Lee JS, et al. Cultured tubule cells from TGF b1 null mice exhibit impaired hypertrophy and fibronectin expression in high glucose. *Kidney Int* 2004;65:1191–1204.
23. Cheng M, Olivier P, Diehl JA, et al. The p21cip1 and p27kip1 cdk "inhibitors" are essential activators of cyclin D–dependent kinases in murine fibroblasts. *EMBO J* 1999;18:1571–1583.
24. Cheng M, Sexl V, Sherr CJ, Roussel M. Assembly of cyclin D dependent kinase and titration of p27Kip1 regulated by mitogen-activated protein kinase kinase (MEK1). *PNAS* 1998;95:1091–1096.
25. Clish CB, O'Brien JA, Gronert K, et al. Local and systemic delivery of an aspirin-triggered lipoxin prevents neutrophil recruitment in vivo. *Proc Natl Acad Sci U S A* 1999;96:8247–8252.
26. Clurman BE, Sheaff RJ, Thress K, Groudine M, Roberts JM. Turnover of cyclin E by the ubiquitin-proteasome pathway is regulated by cdk2 binding and cyclin phosphorylation. *Genes Dev* 1996;10:1979–1990.
27. Conaldi PG, Bottelli A, Baj A, et al. Human immunodeficiency virus-1 tat induces hyperproliferation and dysregulation of renal glomerular epithelial cells. *Am J Pathol* 2002;161:53–61.
28. Couser WG, Johnson RJ. Mechanisms of progressive renal disease in glomerulonephritis. *Am J Kidney Dis* 1994;23:193–198.
29. Coverley D, Laman H, Laskey RA. Distinct roles for cyclins E and A during DNA replication complex assembly and activation. *Nat Cell Biol* 2002;4:523–528.
30. Cusumano AM, Bodkin NL, Hansen BC, et al. Glomerular hypertrophy is associated with hyperinsulinaemia and precedes overt diabetes in aging rhesus monkeys. *Am J Kidney Dis* 2002;40:1075–1085.
31. Cybulsky AV, Rennke HG, Feintzeig ID, Salant DJ. Complement-induced glomerular epithelial cell injury: role of membrane attack complex in rat membranous nephropathy. *J Clin Invest* 1986;77:1096–1107.
32. Dalla Vestra M, Masiero A, Roiter AM, et al. Is podocyte injury relevant in diabetic nephropathy? Studies in patients with type II diabetes mellitus. *Diabetes* 2003;52:1031–1035.
33. Dechow C, Morath C, Lehrke I, et al. Retinoic acid reduces glomerular injury in a rat model of glomerular damage. *J Am Soc Nephrol* 2000;11:1479–1487.
34. Dechow C, Morath C, Peters J, et al. Effects of all-trans retinoic acid on the renin angiotensin system in rats with experimental nephritis. *Am J Physiol Renal Physiol* 2001.
35. Deng C, Zhang P, Harper JW, Elledge SJ, Leder S. Mice lacking p21Cip1/Waf1 undergo normal development but are defective in G1 checkpoint control. *Cell* 1995;82:675–684.
36. Detwiler RK, Falk RJ, Hogan SL, Jenette JC. Collapsing glomerulopathy: a clinically and pathologically distinct variant of focal segmental glomerulosclerosis. *Kidney Int* 1994;45:1416–1424.
37. Dickie P, Felser J, Eckhaus M, et al. HIV-associated nephropathy in transgenic mice expressing HIV-1 genes. *Virology* 1991;185:109–119.
38. Diehl JA, Cheng M, Roussel M, Sherr CJ. Glycogen synthase kinase-3b regulates cyclin D1 proteolysis and subcellular localisation. *Genes Dev* 1998;12:3499–3511.
39. Diehl JA, Zindy F, Sherr CJ. Inhibition of cyclin D1 phosphorylation on threonine-286 prevents its rapid degradation via the ubiquitin-proteasome pathway. *Genes Dev* 1997;11:957–972.
40. Dimberg A, Bahram F, Karlberg I, et al. Retinoic acid induced cell cycle arrest of human myeloid cell lines is associated with sequential down-regulation of cMyc and cyclin E and posttranscriptional upregulation of p27Kip1. *Blood* 2002;99:2199–2206.
41. Dulic V, Kaufmn W, Wilson S, et al. p53-dependent inhibition of cyclin-dependent kinase activities in human fibroblasts during radiation-induced G1 arrest. *Cell* 1994;76:1013–1023.
42. Dulic V, Lees E, Reed SI. Association of human cyclin E with a periodic G1-S phase protein kinase. *Science* 1992;257:1958–1961.
43. Durvasula RV, Pippin J, Petermann AT, et al. Sublytic C5b-9 induces DNA damage in podocytes in vitro: a novel response to injury which prevents proliferation. *J Am Soc Nephrol* 2001;12:609A.
44. El-Deiry WS, Tokino Y, Velculescu VE, et al. WAF1, a potential mediator of p53 tumour suppression. *Cell* 1993;75:817–825.
45. Elledge SJ, Harper JW. The role of protein stability in the cell cycle and cancer. *Biochim Biophys Acta* 1998;1377:M61–M70.
46. Evans T, Rosenthal TE, Youngblom J, Distel D, Hunt T. Cyclin: a protein specified by maternal mRNA in seas urchin eggs that is destroyed at each cleavage division. *Cell* 1983;33:389–396.
47. Fan Y-P, Weiss RH. Exogenous attenuation of p21Waf1/Cip1 decreases mesangial hypertrophy as a result of hyperglycemia and IGF-1. *J Am Soc Nephrol* 2004;15:575–584.
48. Feliers D, Duraisamy S, Faulkner JL, et al. Activation of renal signalling pathways in db/db mice with type 2 diabetes. *Kidney Int* 2001;60:495–504.
49. Feliers D, Frank MA, Riley DJ. Activation of cyclin D1-CDK4 and CDK4-directed phosphorylation of RB protein in diabetic mesangial hypertrophy. *Diabetes* 2002;51:3290–3299.
50. Fero ML, Rivkin M, Tasch M, et al. A syndrome of multiorgan hyperplasia with features of gigantism, tumorigenesis and female sterility in p27kip1–deficient mice. *Cell* 1996;85:733–744.
51. Filmus J, Robles AI, Shi W, et al. Induction of cyclin D1 overexpression by activated ras. *Oncogene* 1994;9:3627–3633 (abstract).
52. Fine LG. The biology of renal hypertrophy. *Kidney Int* 1986;29:619–634.
53. Fine LG, Norman J. Cellular events in renal hypertrophy. *Annu Rev Physiol* 1989;51:19–32.
54. Floege J, Eng E, Lindner V, et al. Rat glomerular mesangial cells synthesize basic fibroblast growth factor. Release, upregulated synthesis and mitogenecity in mesangial proliferative glomerulonephritis. *J Clin Invest* 1992;90:2362–2369.
55. Floege J, Eng E, Young BA, Couser WG, Johnson RJ. Heparin suppresses mesangial cell proliferation and matrix expansion in experimental mesangioproliferative glomerulonephritis. *Kidney Int* 1993;43: 369–380.

56. Floege J, Johnson RJ, Gordon KL, et al. Increased synthesis of extracellular matrix in mesangial proliferative nephritis. *Kidney Int* 1991;40:477–488.

57. Fogo A, Hawkins EP, Berry PL, et al. Glomerular hypertrophy in minimal change disease predicts subsequent progression to focal glomerular sclerosis. *Kidney Int* 1990;38:123.

58. Fogo A, Ichikawa I. Evidence for the central role of glomerular growth promoters in the developement of sclerosis. *Semin Nephrol* 1989;9:329–342.

59. Franch HA. Pathways of proteolysis affecting renal cell growth. *Curr Opin Nephrol Hypertens* 2002;11:445–450.

60. Franch HA, Curtis PV, Mitch WE. Mechanisms of renal tubular cell hypertrophy: mitogen-induced suppression of proteolysis. *Am J Physiol* 1997;273:C843–C851.

61. Franch HA, Prei. NH4Cl-induced hypertrophy is mediated by weak base effects and is independent of cell cycle processes. *Am J Physiol* 1996;270:C932–C938.

62. Franch HA, Shay JW, Alpern RJ, Preiseig P. Involvement of pRB family in TGFb-dependent epithelial cell hypertrophy. *J Cell Biol* 1995;129:245–254.

63. Franch HA, Sooparb S, Du J. A mechanism regulating proteolysis of specific proteins during renal tubular cell growth. *J Biol Chem* 2001;276:19126–19131.

64. Franch HA, Wang X, Sooparb S, Brown NS, Du J. Phosphatidylinositol 3-kinase activity is required for epidermal growth factor to suppress proteolysis. *J Am Soc Nephrol* 2002;13:903–908.

65. Fries JW, Sandstrom DJ, Meyer TW, Rennke HG. Glomerular hypertrophy and epithelial cell injury modulate progressive glomerulosclerosis in the rat. *Lab Invest* 1989;60:205–218.

66. Garibotto G, Sofia A, Robaudo C, et al. Kidney protein dynamics and ammoniagenesis in humans with chronic metabolic acidosis. *J Am Soc Nephrol* 2004;15:1606–1615.

67. Gesualdo L, Di Paolo S, Ranieri E, Schena FP. Trapidil inhibits human mesangial cell proliferation: effect on PDGF B-receptor binding and expression. *Kidney Int* 1994;46:1002–1009.

68. Gheradi D, D'Agati V, Tearina Chu T-H, et al. Reversal of collapsing glomerulopathy in mice with the cyclin-dependent kinase inhibitor CYC202. *J Am Soc Nephrol* 2004;15:1212–1222.

69. Gilbert T, Merlet-Benichon C. Retinoids and nephron mass control. *Pediatr Nephrol* 2000;14:1137–1144.

70. Gille H, Downward J. Multiple Ras effector pathways contribute to G1 cell cycle progression. *J Biol Chem* 1999;274:22033–22040.

71. Griffin SV, Krofft R, Pippin J, Shankland SJ. Limitation of podocyte proliferation improves renal function in experimental crescentic glomerulonephritis. *Kidney Int* 2005;67:977–986.

72. Gross ML, El-Shakmak A, Szabo A, et al. ACE inhibitors but not endothelin receptor blockers prevent podocyte loss in early diabetic nephropathy. *Diabetologia* 2003;46:856–868.

73. Gross ML, Ritz E, Schoof A, et al. Comparison of renal morphology in the streptozotocin and the SHR/N-cp models of diabetic nephropathy. *Lab Invest* 2004;84:452–464.

74. Guo Y, Stacey DW, Hitomi M. Post-transcriptional regulation of cyclin D1 expression during G2 phase. *Oncogene* 2002;21:7545–7556.

75. Hagting A, Jackman M, Simpson K, Pines J. Translocation of cyclin B1 to the nucleus at prophase requires a phosphorylation-dependent nuclear import signal. *Curr Biol* 1999;9:680–689.

76. Hannken T, Schroeder R, Stahl RAK, Wolf G. Atrial natriuretic peptide attenuates Ang II-induced hypertrophy of renal tubular cells. *Am J Physiol* 2001;281:F81–F90.

77. Hannken T, Schroeder R, Stahl RAK, Wolf G. Angiotensin II-mediated expression of p27 (kip1) and induction of cellular hypertrophy in renal tubular cells depend on the generation of oxygen radicals. *Kidney Int* 1998;54:1923–1933.

78. Hannken T, Schroeder R, Zahner G, Stahl RAK, Wolf G. Reactive oxygen species stimulate p44/42 mitogen-activated protein kinase and induce p27Kip1: role in angiotensin II–mediated hypertrophy of proximal tubular cells. *J Am Soc Nephrol* 2000;11:1387–1397.

79. Harbour JW, Dean DC. The Rb/E2F pathway: Expanding roles and emerging paradigms. *Genes Dev* 2000;14:2393–2409.

80. Harper JW, Adami GR, Wei N, Keyomarsi K, Elledge SJ. The p21 CDK-interacting protein Cip1 is a potent inhibitor of G1 cyclin-dependent kinases. *Cell* 1993;75:805–816.

81. Harper JW, Adams PD. Cyclin dependent kinases. *Chem Rev* 2001;101:2511–2526.

82. Harris RC, Haralson MA, Badr KF. Continuous stretch-relaxation in culture alters rat mesangial cell morphology, growth characteristics, and metabolic activity. *Biochem J* 1992;313:697–710.

83. Hengst L, Reed SI. Translational control of p27Kip1 accumulation during the cell cycle. *Science* 1996;271:1861–1864.

84. Hiromura K, Haseley LA, Zhang P, et al. Podocyte expression of the CDK-inhibitor p57 during development and disease. *Kidney Int* 2001;60:2235–2246.

85. Hiromura K, Pippin J, Blonski MJ, Roberts JM, Shankland SJ. The subcellular localisation of cyclin dependent kinase 2 determines the fate of mesangial cells: role in apoptosis and proliferation. *Oncogene* 2002;21:1750–1758.

86. Hiromura K, Pippin J, Fero ML, Roberts JM, Shankland SJ. Modulation of apoptosis by the cyclin-dependent kinase inhibitor p27kip1. *J Clin Invest* 1999;103:597–604.

87. Hishiki T, Shirato I, Takahashi Y, et al. Podocyte injury predicts prognosis in patients with IgA nephropathy using a small amount of renal biopsy tissue. *Kidney Blood Press Res* 2001;24:99–104.

88. Hoshi S, Shu Y, Yoshida F, et al. Podocyte injury promotes progressive nephropathy in Zucker diabetic fatty rats. *Lab Invest* 2002;82:25–35.

89. Hostetter TH. Progression of renal disease and renal hypertrophy. *Annu Rev Physiol* 1995;57:263–278.

90. Hsu SL, Hsu JW, Liu MC, Chen LY, Chang CD. Retinoic acid-mediated G1 arrest is associated with induciotn of p27Kip1 and inhibition of cyclin dependent kinase 3 in human lung squamous carcinoma CH27 cells. *Exp Cell Res* 2000;258:322–331.

91. Hua XH, Newport J. Identification of a preinitiation step in DNA replication that is independent of origin recognition complex and cdc6, but dependent on Cdk2. *J Cell Biol* 1998;140:271–281.

92. Hudkins KL, Gilbertson DG, Carling M, et al. Exogenous PDGF-D is a potent mesangial cell mitogen and causes a severe mesangial proliferative glomerulopathy. *J Am Soc Nephrol* 2004;15:286–298.

93. Ingram AJ, Ly H, Thai K, Kang M, Scholey JW. Activation of mesangial cell signaling cascades in response to mechanical strain. *Kidney Int* 1999;55:476–485.

94. Johnson RJ. The glomerular response to injury: progression or resolution? *Kidney Int* 1994;45:1769–1782.

95. Johnson RJ, Floege J, Couser WG, Alpers CE. Role of platelet-derived growth factor in glomerular disease. *J Am Soc Nephrol* 1993;4:119–128.

96. Johnson RJ, Raines EW, Floege J, et al. Inhibition of mesangial cell proliferation and matrix expansion in glomerulonephritis in the rat by antibody to platelet derived growth factor. *J Exp Med* 1993;175:1413–1416.

97. Kaldis P. The cdk-activating kinase (CAK): from yeast to mammals. *Cell Mol Life Sci* 1999;55:284–296.

98. Kang D-H, Hughes J, Mazzali M, Schreiner GF, Johnson RJ. Impaired angiogenesis in the remnant kidney model. II. Vascular endothelial growth factor administration reduces renal fibrosis and stabilises renal function. *J Am Soc Nephrol* 2001;12:1448–1457.

99. Kang D-H, Kanellis J, Hugo C, et al. Role of the microvascular endothelium in progressive renal disease. *J Am Soc Nephrol* 2002;13:806–816.

100. Kim Y-G, Alpers CE, Brugarolas J, et al. The cyclin kinase inhibitor p21Cip1/Waf1 limits glomerular epithelial cell proliferation in experimental glomerulonephritis. *Kidney Int* 1999;55:2349–2361.

101. Kim Y-G, Suga S-I, Kang D-H, et al. Vascular endothelial growth factor accelerates renal recovery in experimental thrombotic microangiopathy. *Kidney Int* 2000;58:2390–2399.

102. Kitagawa M, Higashi H, Jung HK, et al. The consensus motif for phosphorylation by cyclin D1-Cdk4 is different from that for phosphorylation by cyclin A/E-Cdk2. *EMBO J* 1996;15:7060–7069.

103. Klahr S, Schreiner G, Ichikawa I. Progression in renal disease. *N Engl J Med* 1988;318:1666.

104. Koepp DM, Harper JW, Elledge SJ. How the cyclin became a cyclin: regulated proteolysis in the cell cycle. *Cell* 1999;97:431–434.

105. Koff A, Giordano A, Desai D, et al. Formation and activation of a cyclin E-cdk2 complex during the G1 phase of the human cell cycle. *Science* 1992;257:1689–1694.

106. Kopp JB, Factor VM, Mozes M, et al. Transgenic mice with increased plasma levels of TGF-beta 1 develop progressive renal disease. *Lab Invest* 1996;74:991–1003.

107. Krek W, Nigg EA. Differential phosphorylation of vertebrate p34cdc2 kinase at the G1/S nd G2/M transitions of the cell cycle: identification of major phosphorylation sites. *EMBO J* 1991;10:305–316.

108. Kriz W. Podocyte is the major culprit accounting for the progression of chronic renal disease. *Microsc Res Tech* 2002;57:189–195.

109. Kriz W, Gretz N, Lemley KV. Progression of glomerular diseases: is the podocyte the culprit? *Kidney Int* 1998;54:687–697.

110. Kriz W, Lemley KV. The role of the podocyte in glomerulosclerosis. *Curr Opin Nephrol Hypertens* 1999;8:489–497.

111. Krude T, Jackman M, Pines J, Laskey RA. Cyclin/cdk-dependent initiation of DNA replication in a human cell–free system. *Cell* 1997;88:109–119.

112. Kuan C-J, Al-Douahji M, Shankland SJ. The cyclin kinase inhibitor p21waf1,cip1 is increased in experimental diabetic nephropathy: potential role in glomerular hypertrophy. *J Am Soc Nephrol* 1998;9:986–993.

113. Kurtz I. Role of ammonia in the induction of renal hypertrophy. *Am J Kidney Dis* 1991;17:650–653.

114. LaBaer J, Garrett M, Stevenson L, et al. New functional activities for the p21 family of CDK inhibitors. *Genes Dev* 1997;11:847–862.

115. Lee M-H, Reynisdottir I, Massague J. Cloning of p57Kip2, a cyclin dependent kinase inhibitor with unique domain structure and tissue distribution. *Genes Dev* 1995;9:639–649.

116. Lemley KV, Lafayette RA, Safai M, et al. Podocytopenia and disease severity in IgA nephropathy. *Kidney Int* 2002;61:1475–1485.

117. Levy BD, Clish CB, Schmidt B, Gronert K, Serhan CN. Lipid mediator class switching during acute inflammation: signals in resolution. *Nat Med* 2001;2:612–619.

118. Li J, Meyer AN, Donoghue DJ. Requirement for phosphorylation of cyclin B1 for *Xenopus* oocyte maturation. *Mol Cell Biol* 1995;6:1111–1124.

119. Ling H, Vamvakas S, Gekle M, et al. Role of lysosomal cathepsin activities in cell hypertrophy induced by NH4Cl in cultured renal proximal tubule cells. *J Am Soc Nephrol* 1996;7:73–80.

120. Liu B, Preiseig P. TGFb-mediated hypertrophy in rat renal epithelial cells involves inhibiting pRb phosphorylation by preventing activation of cdk2/cyclin E kinase. *Am J Physiol* 1999;277:F186–F194.

121. Liu B, Preisig P. Compensatory renal hypertrophy is mediated by a cell cycle–dependent mechanism. *Kidney Int* 2002;62:1650–1658.

122. Liu B, Preisig P. Renal hypertrophy following uninephrectomy is associated with the activation of Cdk2/cyclin E, but not Cdk4/cyclin D1 kinase. *J Am Soc Nephrol* 1997;8:424A.

123. Liu BC, Sun J, Chen Q, et al. Role of connective tissue growth factor in mediating hypertrophy of human proximal tubular cells induced by angiotensin II. *Am J Nephrol* 2003;23:429–437.

124. Lundberg AS, Weinberg RA. Functional inactivation of the retinoblastoma protein requires sequential modification by at least two distinct cyclin-CDK complexes. *Mol Biol Cell* 1998;18:753–761.

125. Mackay K, Striker LJ, Stauffer JW, et al. Transforming growth factor beta. Murine glomerular receptors and responses of isolated glomerular cells. *J Clin Invest* 1989;83:1160–1167.

126. Marill J, Idres N, Capron CE, Nguyen E, Chabot GG. Retinoic acid metabolism and mechanism of action. *Curr Drug Metab* 2003;4:1–10.

127. Masuda Y, Shimizu A, Mori T, et al. Vascular endothelial growth factor enhances glomerular capillary repair and accelerates resolution of experimentally induced glomerulonephritis. *Am J Path* 2001;159:599–608.

128. Matsuoka S, Edwards MC, Bai C, et al. p57Kip2, a structurally distinct member of the p21Cip1 CDK inhbitor family, is a candidate tumour suppressor gene. *Genes Dev* 1995;9:650–662.

129. Matsusaka T, Xin J, Niwa S, et al. Genetic engineering of glomerular sclerosis in the mouse via onset and severity controlled podocyte-specific injury. *J Am Soc Nephrol* 2005;16:1013–1023.

130. Matsushime H, Quelle DE, Shurtleff SA, et al. D-type cyclin-dependent kinase activity in mammalian cells. *Mol Cell Biol* 1994;14:2066–2076.

131. Matsushime H, Roussel MF, Ashmun RA, Sherr CJ. Colony-stimulating factor-1 regulates novel cyclins during the G1 phase of the cell cycle. *Cell* 1991;65:701–705.

132. Matsuura I, Denissova NG, Wang G, et al. Cyclin-dependent kinases regulate the anti-proliferative effects of Smads. *Nature* 2004;430:226–231.
133. McGowan TA, McCue P, Sharma K. Diabetic nephropathy. *Clin Lab Med* 2001;21:111–146.
134. McMahon BM, Mitchell S, Brady HR, Godson C. Lipoxins: revelations on resolution. *Trends Pharmacol Sci* 2001;22:391–395.
135. Megyesi J, Price P, Tamayo E, Safirstein RL. The lack of a functional p21Waf1/Cip1 gene ameliorates progression to chronic renal failure. *Proc Natl Acad Sci U S A* 1999;96:10830–10835.
136. Megyesi J, Safirstein R, Price PM. Induction of p21Waf1/Cip1/Sdi1 in kidney tubule cells affects the course of cisplatin-induced acute renal failure. *J Clin Invest* 1998;101:777–782.
137. Megyesi J, Udvarhelyi N, Safirstein R, Price PM. The p53-independent activation of transcription of p21Waf1/Cip1/Sdi1 after acute renal failure. *Am J Physiol* 1996;271:F1211–F1216.
138. Meyer TW, Bennett PH, Nelson RG. Podocyte number predicts long term urinary albumin excretion in Pima Indians with type II diabetes and microalbuminuria. *Diabetologia* 1999;42:1341–1344.
139. Mitchell D, Rodgers K, Hanly J, et al. Lipoxins inhibit Akt/PKB activation and cell cycle progression in human mesangial cells. *Am J Pathol* 2004;164:937–946.
140. Mitra J, Enders GH. Cyclin A/Cdk2 complexes regulate activation of Cdk1 and Cdc2 phosphatases in human cells. *Oncogene* 2004;23:3361–3367.
141. Moeller MJ, Soofi A, Hartmann I, et al. Podocytes populate cellular crescents in a murine model of inflammatory glomerulonephritis. *J Am Soc Nephrol* 2004;15:61–67.
142. Monkawa T, Hiromura K, Wolf G, Shankland SJ. The hypertrophic effect of TGF beta is reduced in the absence of the cyclin dependent kinase inhibitors p21 and p27. *J Am Soc Nephrol* 2002;13:1172–1178.
143. Morath C, Dechow C, Lehrke I, et al. Effects of retinoids on the TGFb system and extracellular matrix in experimental glomerulonephritis. *J Am Soc Nephrol* 2001;12:2300–2309.
144. Muda AO, Feriozzi S, Cinotti GA, Faraggiana T. Glomerular hypertrophy and chronic renal failure in focal segmental glomerulosclerosis. *Am J Kidney Dis* 1994;23:237–241.
145. Nagata M, Nakayama K, Terada Y, Hoshi S, Watanabe N. Cell cycle regulation and differentiation in the human podocyte lineage. *Am J Kidney Dis* 1998;153:1511–1520.
146. Nagata M, Tomari S, Kanemoto K, Usui J, Lemley KV. Podocytes, parietal cells and glomerular pathology: the role of cell cycle proteins. *Pediatr Nephrol* 2003;18:3–8.
147. Nakamura T, Ushiyama C, Hara M, et al. Comparative effects of plasma exchange and intravenous cyclophosphamide on urinary podocyte excretion in patients with proliferative lupus nephritis. *Clin Nephrol* 2002;57:108–113.
148. Nakayama K, Ishida N, Shirane M, et al. Mice lacking p27kip1 display increased body size, multiple organ hyperplasia, retinal dysplasia and pituitary tumours. *Cell* 1996;85:707–720.
149. Nakayama K-I, Nakayama K. Cip/Kip cyclin-dependent kinase inhibitors: brakes of the cell cycle engine during development. *Bioessays* 1998;20:1020–1029.
150. Nath KA, Hostetter MK, Hostetter TH. Increased ammoniagenesis as a determinant of progressive renal injury. *Am J Kidney Dis* 1991;17: 654–657.
151. Nelson PJ, Sunamoto M, Husain M, Gelman IH. HIV-1 expression induces cyclin D1 expression and pRb phosphorylation in infected podocytes: cell-cycle mechanisms contributing to the proliferative phenotype in HIV-associated nephropathy. *BMC Microbiology* 2002;2:26.
152. National Institute of Diabetic and Digestive and Kidney Disease. U.S. Renal Data System, USRDS 2001 annual data report. In: *Atlas of End-Stage Renal Diseases in the United States.* Bethesda, MD: National Institutes of Health, 2002.
153. Nilsson I, Hoffmann I. Cell cycle regulation by the Cdc25 phosphatase family. *Prog Cell Cycle Res* 2000;4:107–114.
154. Noda A, Ning Y, Venable SF, Pereira-Smith OM, Smith JR. Cloning of senescent cell-derived inhibitors of DNA synthesis using an expression screen. *Exp Cell Res* 1994;211:90–98.
155. Nurse P. A long twentieth century of the cell cycle and beyond. *Cell* 2000;100:71–78.
156. Ohse T, Ota T, Kieran N, et al. Modulation of interferon-induced genes by lipoxin analogue in anti-GBM nephritis. *J Am Soc Nephrol* 2004;15:919–927.
157. Olbricht CJ, Geissinger E. Renal hypertrophy in streptozotocin diabetic rats: role of proteolytic lysosomal enzymes. *Kidney Int* 1992;41:966–972.
158. Ophascharoensuk V, Fero ML, Hughes J, Roberts JM, Shankland SJ. The cyclin-dependent kinase inhbitor p27kip1 safeguards against inflammatory injury. *Nat Med* 1998;4:575–580.
159. Ophascharoensuk V, Pippin J, Gordon KL, et al. Role of intrinsic renal cells versus infiltrating cells in glomerular crescent formation. *Kidney Int* 1998;54:416–425.
160. Ortega S, Prieto I, Odajima J, et al. Cyclin dependent kinase 2 is essential for meiosis but not for mitotic cell division in mice. *Nat Genet* 2003;35:25–31.
161. Pagano M, Tam SW, Theodoras AM, et al. Role of the ubiquitin-proteasome pathway in regulating abundance of the cyclin dependent kinase inhibitor p27. *Science* 1995;269:682–685.
162. Pagtalunan ME, Miller PL, Jumping-Eagle S, et al. Podocyte loss and progressive glomerular injury in type II diabetes. *J Clin Invest* 1997;99:342–348.
163. Papayianni A, Serhan CN, Phillips ML, Rennke HG, Brady HR. Transcellular biosynthesis of lipoxin A4 during adhesion of platelets and neutrophils in experimental immune complex glomerulonephritis. *Kidney Int* 1995;47:1295–1302.
164. Park SK, Kang MJ, Kim W, Koh GY. Renal tubule regeneration after ischaemic injury is coupled to the up-regulation and activation of cyclins and cyclin dependent kinases. *Kidney Int* 1997;52:706–714.
165. Park SK, Kang SK, Lee DY, et al. Temporal expressions of cyclins and cyclin dependent kinases during renal development and compensatory growth. *Kidney Int* 1997;51:762–769.
166. Parker LL, Piwnica-Worms H. Inactivation of the p34cdc2–cyclin B complex by the human WEE1 tyrosine kinase. *Science* 1992;257:1955–1957.
167. Parker S, Eichele G, Zhang P, et al. p53-independent expression of p21Cip1 in muscle and other terminal differentiating cells. *Science* 1995;267:1024–1027.
168. Parry D, Mahony D, Wills K, Lees E. Cyclin D-CDK subunit arrangement is dependent on the availability of competing INK4 and p21 class inhibitors. *Mol Cell Biol* 1999;19:1775–1783.
169. Peeper DS, Upton TM, Ladha MH, et al. Ras signalling linked to the cell cycle machinery by the retinoblastoma protein. *Nature* 1997;386:177–181.
170. Pesce CM, Striker LJ, Peten E, Elliott SJ, Striker GE. Glomerulosclerosis at both early and late stages is associated with increased cell turnover in mice transgenic for growth hormone. *Lab Invest* 1991;65:601–605.
171. Petermann AT, Hiromura K, Blonski MJ, et al. Mechanical stress reduces podocyte proliferation in vitro. *Kidney Int* 2002;61:40–50.
172. Petermann AT, Pippin J, Durvasula R, et al. Mechanical stretch induces podocyte hypertrophy in vitro. *Kidney Int* 2005;67:157–166.
173. Petermann AT, Pippin J, Hiromura K, et al. Mitotic cell cycle proteins increase in podocytes despite lack of proliferation. *Kidney Int* 2003;63:113–122.
174. Petermann AT, Pippin J, Krofft R, et al. Viable podocytes detach in experimental diabetic nephropathy: potential mechanism underlying glomerulsclerosis. *Nephron Exp Nephrol* 2004;98:e114–e123.
175. Pines J. Cyclins and cyclin dependent kinases: a biochemical view. *Biochem J* 1995;308:697–711.
176. Pippin J, Durvasula R, Petermann AT, et al. DNA damage is a novel response to sublytic complement C5b-9–induced injury in pododcytes. *J Clin Invest* 2003;111:877–885.
177. Pippin J, Qu Q, Meijer L, Shankland SJ. Direct in vivo inhibition of the nuclear cell cycle cascade in experimental mesangial proliferative glomerulonephritis with roscovitine, a novel cyclin-dependent kinase antagonist. *J Clin Invest* 1997;100:2512–2520.
178. Pippin JW, Durvasula RV, Petermann AT, et al. Podocytes exhibit DNA damage in vivo in experimental membranous nephropathy. *J Am Soc Nephrol* 2001;12:638A.
179. Polyak K, Lee M-H, Erdjument-Bromage H, et al. Cloning of p27kip1, a cyclin-dependent kinase inhibitor and a potent mediator of extracellular antimitogenic signals. *Cell* 1994;78:59–66.
180. Preiseig P. What makes cells grow larger and how do they do it: hypertrophy revisited. *Exp Nephrol* 1999;7:273–283.
181. Preiseig P. A cell cycle–dependent mechanism of renal tubule epithelial cell hypertrophy. *Kidney Int* 1999;56:1193–1198.
182. Quelle DE, Zindy F, Ashman RA, Sherr CJ. Alternative reading frames of the INK4a tumor suppressor gene encode two unrelated proteins capable of inducing cell cycle arrest. *Cell* 1995;83:993–1000.
183. Rabkin R, Fervenza FC. Renal hypertrophy and kidney disease in diabetes. *Diabetes Metab Rev* 1996;12:217–241.
184. Rennke HG. How does glomerular epithelial cell injury contribute to glomerular damage? *Kidney Int* 1994;S45:S58–S63.
185. Ritz E, Keller C, Bergis K, Strojek K. Pathogenesis and course of renal disease in IDDM/NIDDM: differences and similarities. *Am J Hypertens* 1997;10:202S–207S.
186. Roberts AB, McCune BK, Sporn MB. TGF beta: regulation of extracellular matrix. *Kidney Int* 1992;41:557–559.
187. Ruef C, Budde K'Lacy J, Nothemann W, et al. Interleukin 6 is an autocrine growth factor for mesangial cells. *Kidney Int* 1990;38:249–257.
188. Ruperez MR, Ruiz-Ortega M, Esteban V, et al. Angiotensin II increases connective tissue growth factor in the kidney. *Am J Pathol* 2003;163:1937–1947.
189. Ryffel B, Car BD, Gunn H, et al. Interleukin 6 exacerbates glomerulonephritis in (NZB x NZW)F1 mice. *Am J Path* 1994;144:927–937.
190. Salant DJ, Darby C, Couser WG. Experimental membranous glomerulonephritis in rats. *J Clin Invest* 1980;66:71–81.
191. Savill J. Regulation of glomerular cell number by apoptosis. *Kidney Int* 1999;56:1216–1222.
192. Scheurer D. Rapid reversal of renal failure after intiation of HAART: a case report. *AIDS Read* 2004;14:443–447.
193. Schoecklmann HO, Rupprecht HD, Zauner I, Sterzel RB. TGF-beta1 induced cell cycle arrest in renal mesangial cells involves inhibition of cyclin E–CDK2 activation and retinoblastoma protein phosphorylation. *Kidney Int* 1996;51:1228–1236.
194. Schwartz EJ, Cara A, Snoeck H, et al. HIV-1 induces loss of contact inhibition in podocytes. *J Am Soc Nephrol* 2001;12:1677–1684.
195. Schwartz MM, Evans J, Bain R, Korbet SM. Focal segmental glomerulosclerosis: prognostic implications of the cellular lesion. *J Am Soc Nephrol* 1999;10:1900–1907.
196. Seewaldt VL, Dietze EC, Johnson BS, Collins SJ, Parker MB. Retinoic acid mediated G1-S phase arrest of normal human mammary epithelial cells is independent of the level of p53 protein expression. *Cell Growth Differ* 1999;10:49–59.
197. Shankland SJ, Eitner F, Hudkins KL, et al. Differential expression of cyclin-dependent kinase inhibitors in human glomerular disease: role in podocyte proliferation and maturation. *Kidney Int* 2000;58:674–683.
198. Shankland SJ, Floege J, Thomas SE, et al. Cyclin kinase inhibitors are increased during experimental membranous nephropathy: potential role in limiting glomerular epithelial proliferation in vivo. *Kidney Int* 1997;522:404–413.
199. Shankland SJ, Hamel P, Scholey JW. Cyclin and cyclin-dependent kinase expression in the remnant glomerulus. *J Am Soc Nephrol* 1997;8:368–375.
200. Shankland SJ, Hugo C, Coats SR, et al. Changes in cell-cycle protein expression during experimental mesangial proliferative nephritis. *Kidney Int* 1996;50:1230–1239.
201. Shankland SJ, Johnson RJ. TGF beta in glomerular disease. *Miner Electrolyte Metab* 1998;24:168–173.
202. Shankland SJ, Pippin J, Flanagan M, et al. Mesangial cell proliferation mediated by PDGF and bFGF is determined by levels of the cyclin kinase inhibitor p27kip1. *Kidney Int* 1997;51:1088–1099.
203. Shankland SJ, Wolf G. Cell cycle regulatory proteins in renal disease: role in hypertrophy, proliferation and apoptosis. *Am J Physiol* 2000;278:F515–F529.
204. Sheaff RJ, Groudine M, Gordon M, Roberts JM, Clurman BE. Cyclin E–cdk2 is a regulator of p27kip1. *Genes Dev* 1997;11:1464–1478.
205. Shecter P, Boner G, Rabkin R. Tubular cell protein degradation in early diabetic renal hypertrophy. *J Am Soc Nephrol* 1994;4:1582–1587.

206. Shecter P, Shi JD, Rabkin R. Renal tubular cell protein breakdown in uninephrectomized and ammonium chloride-loaded rats. *J Am Soc Nephrol* 1994;5:1201–1207.
207. Sherr CJ. The INK4a/ARF network in tumour suppression. *Nat Rev Mol Cell Biol* 2001;2:731–737.
208. Sherr CJ. Mammalian G1 cyclins. *Cell* 1993;73:1065.
209. Sherr CJ. Parsing Ink4a/Arf: "pure" p16-null mice. *Cell* 2001;106:531–534.
210. Sherr CJ, Roberts JM. Living with or without cyclins and cyclin dependent kinases. *Genes Dev* 2005;18:2699–2711.
211. Sherr CJ, Roberts JM. CDK inhibitors: positive and negative regulators of G1 phase progression. *Genes Dev* 1999;13:1501–1512.
212. Smits VAJ, Klompmaker R, Vallenius T, Rijksen G, Makela TP. p21 inhibits Thr161 phosphorylation of Cdc2 to enforce the G2 DNA damage checkpoint. *J Biol Chem* 2000;275:30638–30643.
213. Smits VAJ, Medema RH. Checking out the G2/M transition. *Biochim Biophys Acta* 2001;1519:1–12.
214. Sooparb S, Price SR, Shaoguang J, Franch HA. Suppression of chaperone-mediated autophagy in the renal cortex during acute diabetes mellitus. *Kidney Int* 2004;65:2135–2144.
215. Striker LJ, Doi T, Elliott SJ, Striker GE. The contribution of glomerular mesangial cells to progressive glomerulosclerosis. *Semin Nephrol* 1989;9:318–328.
216. Suzuki A, Ito T, Imai E, et al. Retinoids regulate the repairing process of the podocytes in puromycin aminonucleoside-induced nephrotic rats. *J Am Soc Nephrol* 2003;14:981–991.
217. Takahashi K, Nakayama K-I, Nakayama K. Mice lacking a CDK inhibitor, p57Kip2, exhibit skeletal abnormalities and growth retardation. *J Biochem* 2000;127:73–83.
218. Tenschert S, Elger M, Lemley KV. Glomerular hypertrophy after subtotal nephrectomy: relationship to early glomerular injury. *Virchows Arch* 1995;426:517.
219. Tollins JP, Hostetter MK, Hostetter TH. Hypokalemic nephropathy in the rat: role of ammonia in chronic tubular injury. *J Clin Invest* 1987;79:1447–1458.
220. Toth T, Takebayashi S. Glomerular hypertrophy in relapsing minimal change nephropathy. *Nephron* 1996;74:64–71.
221. Tovbin D, Franch HA, Alpern RJ, Preisig PA. Media acidification inibits TGFb-mediated growth suppression in cultured rabbit proximal tubule cells. *Proc Assoc Am Physicians* 1997;109:572–579.
222. Toyoshima H, Hunter T. p27, a novel inhibitor of G1 cyclin–cdk protein kinase activity, is related to p21. *Cell* 1994;78:67–74.
223. Trimarchi JM, Lees JA. Sibling rivalry in the E2F family. *Nat Rev Mol Cell Biol* 2002;3:11–20.
224. Tsuboi Y, Shankland SJ, Grande JP, et al. Suppression of mesangial proliferative glomerulonephritis development in rats by inhibition of cAMP phosphodiesterase isoenzymes types III and IV. *J Clin Invest* 1996;98:262–270.
225. Vlach J, Hennecke S, Amati B. Phosphorylation-dependent degradation of the cyclin-dependent kinase inhibitor p27Kip1. *EMBO J* 1997;16:5334–5344.
226. Walsh-Reitz MM, Toback FG. Kidney epithelial cell growth is stimulated by lowering extracellular potassium concentration. *Am J Physiol* 1983;244:C429–C432.
227. Weinberg RA. The retinoblastoma protein and cell cycle control. *Cell* 1995;81:323–330.
228. Weir MR. Diabetes and hypertension: blood pressure control and consequences. *Am J Hypertens* 1999;12:170S–178S.
229. Welcker M, Singer JD, Loeb KR, et al. Multisite phosphorylation by Cdk2 and GSK3 controls cyclin E degradation. *Mol Cell* 2003;12:381–392.
230. White KE, Bilous RW. Estimation of podocyte number: a comparison of methods. *Kidney Int* 2004;66:663–667.
231. White KE, Bilous RW. Structural alterations to the podocyte are related to proteinuria in type 2 diabetic patients. *Nephrol Dial Transplant* 2004;19:1437–1440.
232. White KE, Bilous RW, Marshall SM, et al. Podocyte number in normotensive type I diabetic patients with albuminuria. *Diabetes* 2002;51:3083–3089.
233. Winston JT, Coats SR, Wang Y-Z, Pledger WJ. Regulation of the cell cycle machinery by oncogenic Ras. *Oncogene* 1996;12:127–134.
234. Wolf G. Changing concepts of compensatory renal growth: from humoral pathology to molecular biology. *Am J Nephrol* 1992;12:369–373.
235. Wolf G. Molecular mechanisms of renal hypertrophy: role of p27Kip1. *Kidney Int* 1999;56:1262–1265.
236. Wolf G. Cellular mechanisms of tubule hypertrophy and hyperplasia in renal injury. *Miner Electrolyte Metab* 1995;21:303–316.
237. Wolf G, Jablonski K, Schroeder R, et al. Angiotensin II–induced hypertrophy of proximal tubular cells requires p27Kip1. *Kidney Int* 2003;64:71–81.
238. Wolf G, Kuncio GS, Sun MJ, Neilson EG. Expression of homeobox genes in a proximal tubule cell line derived from adult mice. *Kidney Int* 1991;39:1027–1033.
239. Wolf G, Mueller E, Stahl RAK, Ziyadeh FN. Angiotensin II–induced hypertrophy of cultured murine proximal tubular cells is mediated by endogenous transforming growth factor beta. *J Clin Invest* 1993;92:1366–1372.
240. Wolf G, Neilson EG. Molecular mechanisms of tubulointerstitial hypertrophy and hyperplasia. *Kidney Int* 1991;39:401–420.
241. Wolf G, Neilson EG. Angiotensin II induces cellular hypertrophy in cultured murine proximal tubular cells. *Am J Physiol Renal Fluid Electrolyte Physiol* 1990;259:F768–F777.
242. Wolf G, Reinking R, Zahner G, Stahl RAK, Shankland SJ. Erk 1,2 phosphorylates p27Kip1: functional evidence for a role in high glucose-induced hypertrophy of mesangial cells. *Diabetologica* 2003;46:1090–1099.
243. Wolf G, Schroeder R, Thaiss F, et al. Glomerular expression of p27Kip1 in diabetic db/db mouse: role of hyperglycaemia. *Kidney Int* 1998;53:869–879.
244. Wolf G, Schroeder R, Zahner G, Stahl RAK, Shankland SJ. High glucose-induced hypertrophy of mesangial cells requires p27Kip1, an inhibitor of cyclin dependent kinases. *Am J Path* 2001;158:1091–1100.
245. Wolf G, Schroeder R, Ziyadeh FN, et al. High glucose stimulates expression of p27Kip1 in cultured mouse mesangial cells. *Am J Physiol* 1997;42:F348–F356.
246. Wolf G, Sharma K, Chen Y, Ericksen M, Ziyadeh FN. High glucose-induced proliferation in mesangial cells is reversed by autocrine TGF beta. *Kidney Int* 1992;42:647–656.
247. Wolf G, Stahl RAK. Angiotensin II–stimulated hypertrophy of LLC-PK1 cells depends on the induction of the cyclin dependent kinase inhibitor p27Kip1. *Kidney Int* 1996;50:2112–2119.
248. Wolf G, Wengel U, Ziyadeh FN, Stahl RAK. Angiotensin converting enzyme inhibitor treatment reduces glomeular p16INK4a and p27Kip1 expression in diabetic BBdp rats. *Diabetologica* 1999;42:1425–1432.
249. Wolf G, Wenzel U, Hannken T, Stahl RAK. Angiotensin II induces p27Kip1 expression in renal tubules in vivo: role of reactive oxygen species. *J Mol Med* 2001;79:383–389.
250. Wolf G, Ziyadeh FN. Molecular mechanisms of diabetic renal hypertrophy. *Kidney Int* 1999;56:393–405.
251. Won K-A, Reed SI. Activation of cyclin E/CDK2 is coupled to site-specific autophosphorylation and ubiquitin-dependent degradation of cyclin E. *EMBO J* 1996;15:4182–4193.
252. Xiong Y, Hannon GJ, Zhang H, et al. p21 is a universal inhibitor of cyclin kinases. *Nature* 1993;366:701–704.
253. Xu Q, Lucio-Cazana FJ, Kitamura M, et al. Retinoids in nephrology: promises and pitfalls. *Kidney Int* 2004;66:2119–2131.
254. Xu ZG, Yoo TH, Ryu DR, et al. Angiotensin II receptor blocker inhibits p27Kip1 expression in glucose stimulated podocytes and in diabetic glomeruli. *Kidney Int* 2005;67:944–952.
255. Yamamoto T, Wilson CB. Complement dependence of antibody-induced mesangial cell injury in the rat. *J Immunol* 1987;138:3758–3765.
256. Yamamoto T, Wilson CB. Quantitative and qualitative studies of antibody-induced mesangial cell damage in the rat. *Kidney Int* 1987;32:514–525.
257. Yan Y, Frisen J, Lee M-H, Massaque J, Barbacid M. Ablation of the CDK inhibitor p57Kip2 results in increased apoptosis and delayed differentiation during mouse development. *Genes Dev* 1997;11:973–983.
258. Yanagita M. The role of the vitamin K–dependent growth factor Gas6 in glomerular pathophysiology. *Curr Opin Nephrol Hypertens* 2004;13:465–470.
259. Yang J, Bardes ESG, Moore JD, et al. Control of cyclin B1 localisation through regulated binding of the nuclear export factor CRM1. *Genes Dev* 2002;12:2131–2143.
260. Young BA, Johnson RJ, Alpers CE, et al. Cellular events in the evolution of experimental diabetic nephropathy. *Kidney Int* 1995;47:935–944.
261. Yu Q, Sicinski P. Mammalian cell cycles without cyclin E-CDK2. *Cell Cycle* 2004;3:292–295.
262. Zatz R, Fujihara CK. Glomerular hypertrophy and progressive glomerulopathy: is there a definitive pathogenetic correlation? *Kidney Int* 1994;45:S27–S29.
263. Zhang P, Liegeois NJ, Wong C, et al. Altered cell differentiation and proliferation in mice lacking p57Kip2 indicates a role in Beckwith–Wiedemann syndrome. *Nature* 1997;387:151–158.
264. Ziyadeh FN, Sharma K. Role of transforming growth factor b in diabetic glomerulosclerosis and renal hypertrophy. *Kidney Int* 1995;48:S34–S36.
265. Ziyadeh FN, Sharma K, Wolf G. Stimulation of collagen gene expression and protein synthesis in murine mesangial cells by high glucose is mediated by autocrine activation of transforming growth factor beta. *J Clin Invest* 1994;93:536–542.

Fluid and Electrolyte Regulation and Dysregulation

Regulation and Disorders of Sodium Chloride Homeostasis

CHAPTER **28**

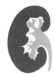

Epithelial Na$^+$ Channels

Shaohu Sheng, John P. Johnson, and Thomas R. Kleyman
University of Pittsburgh, Pittsburgh, Pennsylvania, USA

INTRODUCTION

From the late distal convoluted tubule and connecting tubule and throughout the collecting duct, Na$^+$ exits the urinary space by passive diffusion through an apical membrane epithelial Na$^+$ channel, referred to as ENaC. The Na$^+$,K$^+$-ATPase mediates active Na$^+$ exit from cells across basolateral membranes. This model of electrogenic transepithelial Na$^+$ transport, with diffusion of Na$^+$ across an apical membrane conductance pathway, was initially proposed by Koefoed-Johnson and Ussing in 1958 (192). Subsequent studies using both noise analysis and single-channel recordings demonstrated the presence of apical membrane Na$^+$-selective ion channels (127, 249, 252, 336).

Electrophysiologic Characteristics

The basic electrophysiologic characteristics of epithelial Na$^+$ channels have been defined using both macroscopic and single-channel studies, and are presented in Fig. 1. ENaCs are Na$^+$ and Li$^+$ permeable channels that exhibit negligible K$^+$ conductance, with a single-channel conduc-

tance of 4 to 5 pS at room temperature with Na$^+$ as the charge carrier (48, 128, 252). These channels exhibit a slight increase in open probability under hyperpolarizing membrane potentials (250, 253). ENaCs characteristically exhibit long open and closed times, on the order of seconds to tens of seconds, although a population of ENaCs has been described that has brief open times and long closed times (45, 183, 253). Channels are blocked by submicromolar concentrations of amiloride, a pyrazinoyl-guanidine derivative (24, 186). Amiloride is a weak base, with a pK$_a$ of 8.8 in water. It is the charged, or protonated, form of amiloride that blocks ENaC (186). Other organic weak bases, including triamterene, trimethoprim, and pentamidine also inhibit ENaC (59, 189, 275, 282).

Biochemical and Molecular Characteristics of ENaC

Amiloride was first demonstrated to inhibit electrogenic transepithelial Na$^+$ transport in 1968 (24). With an IC$_{50}$ of ~100 nM, amiloride and several related compounds proved to be highly selective Na$^+$ channel inhibitors (186). Prior to the cloning of ENaC subunits, these compounds provided

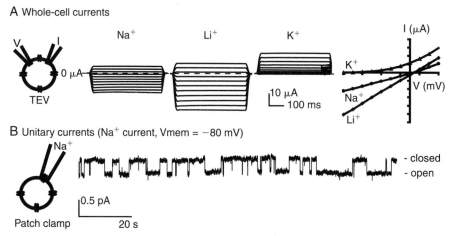

FIGURE 1 Biophysical properties of epithelial Na$^+$ channels. **A:** Whole-cell currents were recorded in *Xenopus* oocytes expressing αβγ ENaC that were bathed with NaCl, LiCl, or KCl solutions. Current-voltage curves are shown on the right. **B:** Single-channel recording was performed with cell-attached patch and NaCl in the pipette. (Recordings in part A are reprinted with permission from Sheng S, McNulty KA, Harvey JM, Kleyman TR. Second transmembrane domains of ENaC subunits contribute to ion permeation and selectivity. *J Biol Chem* 2001;276:44091–44098.)

investigators with tools to purify Na$^+$ channels using standard biochemical techniques. Sariban-Sohraby and coworkers (22, 23, 245) isolated a complex of polypeptides from bovine kidney that, when reconstituted in lipid bilayers, exhibited characteristics of an amiloride-blockable cation channel. However, the single-channel conductance, Na$^+$/K$^+$ selectivity ratio, and gating properties of the purified channel differed from the properties of Na$^+$ channels in epithelia. The relationship of this purified channel complex to ENaC is still unclear, although antibodies raised against a subunit of the cloned Na$^+$ channel have been observed to recognize a polypeptide within the purified channel complex (156, 268). Kleyman and coworkers used an anti-idiotypic approach to generate monoclonal antibodies directed against the amiloride-binding domain of the Na$^+$ channel (188). These antibodies were shown to inhibit Na$^+$ transport across an epithelial monolayer, and recognized one of the cloned subunits of ENaC (185, 188).

The molecular characteristics of this channel were elucidated in elegant studies by Canessa and coworkers and Lingueglia and coworkers in 1993 and 1994 (46, 48, 208, 209). An expression cloning technique led to the identification of a cDNA, termed alpha ENaC, whose cRNA-induced expression of amiloride-sensitive Na$^+$ currents when injected into *Xenopus* oocytes (46, 209). However, Na$^+$ current levels were considerably smaller than expected. Two subsequent cDNA clones were isolated based on their ability to complement alpha ENaC cRNA in the expression of amiloride-sensitive Na$^+$ currents in *Xenopus* oocytes, and were termed beta and gamma ENaC (48). *Xenopus* oocytes coinjected with the three cRNA species expressed amiloride-sensitive Na$^+$ channels with characteristics nearly identical to those of Na$^+$ channels expressed in renal cortical collecting tubules and in cultured cell lines derived from the distal nephron. Na$^+$ currents were not observed when the beta or gamma subunits were expressed alone.

The three subunits share limited (~30%–40%) sequence identity, suggesting that they are derived from a common ancestral gene. ENaC cRNAs have been cloned from a variety of species, including rat, human, mouse, rabbit, guinea pig, chicken, cattle, clawed African frog (*Xenopus laevis*), and bullfrog (5, 46, 48, 106, 117, 162, 208, 209, 233, 234, 264, 283). The human alpha subunit gene *Scnn1a* spans 17 kb on chromosome 12p13. The beta and gamma subunit *Scnn1b* and *Scnn1g* are closely linked on human chromosome 16p12-p13 (37, 338). The genes encoding the three ENaC subunits have a conserved exon–intron architecture, with up to 13 exons (217, 328). Splice variants have been described that alter the cytoplasmic N-termini or alter the extracellular domains (63, 327, 332). Variants that result in a premature truncation of the extracellular domain of the alpha subunit have also been reported (57, 332). Some of these variants are associated with a reduction or loss of channel activity when expressed in heterologous systems, and with an autosomal recessive loss of function phenotype (pseudohypoaldosteronism) in humans (57).

ENaC/Degenerin Gene Family

Canessa and coworkers noted that ENaC subunits were related to genes identified in *Caenorhabditis elegans* that participate in mechanosensation in which specific mutations result in degeneration of selected neurons (67, 118, 146). The three ENaC subunits are members of the ENaC/DEG gene family (Fig. 2). There are two additional ENaC subunits, referred to as delta and epsilon, that appear to be functionally related to the alpha subunit. Delta ENaC is a proton-activated channel, although its physiologic role has not been elucidated (345, 361). The epsilon subunit was identified in *Xenopus* and has an

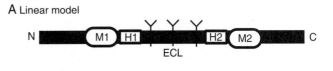

A Linear model

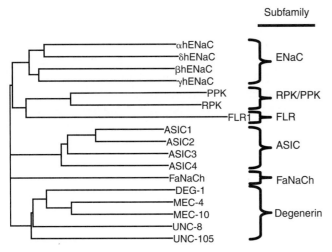

FIGURE 2 Phylogenetic tree of the ENaC/DEG superfamily. Gene products are grouped into six subfamilies: ENaCs; RPK (ripped pocket)/PPK (pickpocket), expressed in *Drosophila*; FLR, expressed in *Caenorhabditis elegans*; ASICs, or acid-sensing ion channels; FaNaCh, a peptide-gated channel expressed in marine snails; and degenerins, expressed in *C. elegans*.

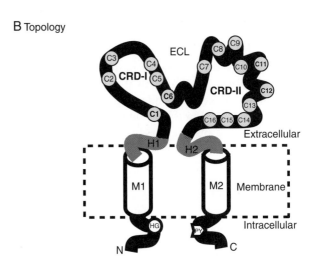

B Topology

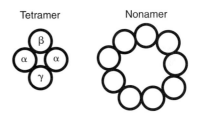

C Subunit stoichiometry

FIGURE 3 Structural features of ENaC subunits. **A:** Linear model of an ENaC subunit. M1, M2, the first and second membrane-spanning domains; H1 and H2 (or pre-M2), the hydrophobic segments following M1 or preceding M2; ECL, extracellular loop connecting M1/H1 and H2/M2; N, amino-terminus and C, carboxyl-terminus. Several of the glycosylation sites are shown as branched lines. **B:** Topology model of an ENaC subunit. Conserved extracellular Cys residues are within two cysteine rich domains (CDRs). HG is a gating domain with key His and Gly residues within the amino-terminus. The PY motif mediates ENaC interactions with Nedd4-2. **C:** Two models of ENaC subunit stoichiometry.

altered Na⁺ self-inhibition response suggesting altered gating properties (14). Members of this family also include genes identified in *Caenorhabditis elegans* that are involved in mechanosensation (*mecs* and *degs*) or control of defecation rhythm (*flrs*); H⁺-gated channels (referred to as acid-sensing ion channels [ASICs]) that are expressed in mammalian central and peripheral nervous systems and have a role in nociception and mechanosensation (197, 261, 343, 344); a family of 16 genes expressed in *Drosophila*, referred to as pickpocket, that may have roles in airway fluid clearance, mechanosensation, salt sensation, and detection of pheromones (2, 75, 204, 211, 212, 323); and peptide-gated channels expressed in marine snails (70, 163, 207).

Overview of Structural Features of ENaC Subunits

Each ENaC subunit has only two predicted membrane-spanning domains, similar to the topology of members of the Kir family of K⁺ channels and members of the P2X family of purinergic receptors that are ligand-gated ion channels (141, 334) (Fig. 3). Topologic analyses of ENaC subunits were published by three independent groups (47, 267). Each subunit has two membrane-spanning domains and intracellular amino- and carboxyl-termini. The cytoplasmic domains have sites that are phosphorylated by specific kinases, have specific motifs that direct protein–protein and protein–lipid interactions that affect channel gating or trafficking, and sites that may directly influence channel gating or trafficking. The membrane-spanning domains are presumably alpha helical. Short hydrophobic regions immediately follow the first membrane-spanning domain and precede the second membrane-spanning domain (48). Amino acid residues from the three subunits that are within and preceding the second membrane-spanning domain line

the channel's pore. The hydrophobic region immediately preceding the second membrane-spanning domain, referred to as H2, pre-M2, or pore region, contains the channel's main selectivity filter and amiloride-binding site (179, 180, 281, 288–291, 306). Linking these hydrophobic regions within each subunit is a large extracellular domain, comprised of ~450 residues. Recent studies, outlined below, have begun to elucidate the roles of these extracellular domains in the regulation of channel gating (148, 287, 292, 293). These largely hydrophilic extracellular domains have 16 cysteine resides whose locations are conserved among the three subunits and are grouped within two cysteine-rich domains. The functional roles of these cysteine residues remain to be defined, although mutagenesis of several specific cysteine residues results in a loss of channel activity associated with a decrease in surface expression (100). At present, it is unclear whether these cysteine residues form inter- or intra-subunit disulfide bonds that could have a role in stabilizing the heteroligomeric structure of the mature channel.

Subunit Stoichiometry

Investigators have used a number of approaches to assess the number of each ENaC subunit that assembles to form a Na$^+$ channel complex. Biophysical approaches, similar to that initially described by McKinnon in 1991 (220), have been used by several investigators to determine the subunit stoichiometry of αβγ Na$^+$ channels. Firsov and coworkers and Kosari and coworkers independently suggested a stoichiometry of two alpha subunits, one beta subunit, and one gamma subunit (99, 195). This quaternary structure is similar to that reported for voltage-gated and inwardly rectifying K$^+$ channels, as well as voltage-gated Na$^+$ and Ca^{2+} channels that have fourfold internal symmetry. Consistent with a proposed tetrameric organization of this family of channels, Na$^+$ channels composed solely of alpha subunits as well as homomeric peptide-activated Na$^+$ channels were reported to have a tetrameric organization (26, 69). Studies using concatameric ENaC constructs suggested the alpha subunits are on opposite sides of the pore, separated by beta and gamma subunits (99) (Fig. 3). Snyder and coworkers, using a similar biophysical approach, suggested a subunit stoichiometry of three alpha, three beta, and three gamma subunits (Fig. 3) (305). This higher-ordered organization has been supported by studies estimating the number of transmembrane alpha helices within a putative channel complex by freeze-fracture electron microscopy (95), and recently by studies using fluorescence resonance energy transfer (311, 312). Future studies using structural approaches will likely resolve this dispute.

ENaC Biogenesis

Na$^+$ channel subunits likely undergo assembly in the endoplasmic reticulum (ER), where core, high-mannose asparagine (or N)-linked glycans are added at specific sites (4, 58, 76, 131, 150, 231, 262, 272, 333, 350). Within each subunit there are multiple sites that undergo N-linked glycosylation. For example, rat alpha, beta, and gamma subunits have 6, 12, and 5 consensus sites (Asn-X-Ser/Thr) for N-linked oligosaccharide addition, respectively. Exit of assembled channels from the ER appears to be inefficient in *Xenopus* oocytes (333). In epithelial cells, exit of assembled channels from the ER may also be inefficient, but the evidence is somewhat controversial. Weisz and coworkers reported that ~20% of the total pool of channels (detected by immunoblots of whole-cell lysates) was expressed at the plasma membrane (350). Channel subunits that do not exit the ER are likely degraded via proteosome-mediated ER-associated degradation (ERAD). While specific signals have been identified within other ion channels that either facilitate retention within the ER, or facilitate ER exit (218, 365), similar signals have not yet been identified within ENaC subunits. Integral membrane proteins are cotranslationally inserted into the ER membrane. The proper folding and assembly of polypeptides synthesized in the ER involves interactions with a variety of chaperone proteins, including heat shock/stress proteins, lectin-like proteins such as calnexin and calreticulin, and protein disulfide isomerase (92, 98, 194). Specific chaperones that participate in ENaC folding and assembly are starting to be defined.

The half-life of newly synthesized subunits, determined by metabolic labeling/pulse-chase experiments, is approximately an hour (76, 131, 221, 231, 333, 350), consistent with the notion that the majority of ENaC subunits synthesized within the ER are targeted for degradation via ERAD. Conflicting reports have been published regarding the half-life of channels that have reached the surface. Several groups have suggested that the rate of degradation of channels that have reached the surface may be on the order of many hours to days (42, 191, 239, 350). Other investigators have reported a short half-life for channels that have reached the cell surface of A6 cells and MDCK cells expressing exogenous ENaCs (76, 131).

ENaC PROCESSING IN BIOSYNTHETIC PATHWAY

As assembled ENaCs exit the ER, it is has been thought that channels follow the route used by other proteins in the secretory pathway. This involves trafficking through the Golgi where most N-glycans are processed, and the trans-Golgi network where channels are sorted into endosomes that are delivered to the apical membrane. N-glycan processing is often monitored by the enzyme endoglycosidase H, an enzyme that removes high-mannose N-linked glycans prior to processing events that occur in the medial Golgi complex. A number of investigators have reported that ENaC subunits do not undergo modification of N-linked sugars to an endoglycosidase H-resistant form (131, 262, 333, 350). One group suggested that N-linked glycans are removed from subunits expressed at the plasma membrane (262).

Recent studies have shown that N-glycans on all three subunits of assembled channels are modified to complex-type Endo H-resistant forms (76, 150). Surprisingly, endoglycosidase H-resistant N-glycans were observed only on forms of the alpha and gamma subunits that had also undergone proteolytic processing (150). Hughey and coworkers reported that two distinct pools of ENaC subunits were expressed at the plasma membrane: subunits with processed N-glycans and cleaved alpha and gamma subunits; and full-length subunits that have nonprocessed N-glycans (150). Furthermore, they observed that individual channel complexes with processed subunits lacked nonprocessed subunits. Processing of subunits within a channel complex is an all-or-none event (149). These findings suggest that a population of channel complexes exiting the ER transits through Golgi and post-Golgi compartments where subunits are processed. This likely represents the pool of active, functional channels. A distinct population of channels exiting the ER appears to bypass Golgi and post-Golgi processing (Fig. 4). This distinct pool of nonprocessed channels is likely a functionally inactive pool, as proteolysis of ENaC subunits appears to have a dramatic effect on increasing channel open probability (44, 45, 62, 148). Proteolytic cleavage of these inactive channels provides a potential mechanism to increase rates of Na⁺ transport in the distal nephron. The role of proteolysis of ENaC subunits in regulating channel gating is discussed in detail later in this chapter.

Intracellular Trafficking of ENaC

Functional channels are delivered to the apical plasma membrane via the traditional secretory pathway (Fig. 4) (149). The exocytic insertion of channels into the apical plasma membrane occurs as a regulated process that is increased in response to a variety of hormones, including vasopressin, aldosterone, and insulin. Vesicle and target soluble N-ethylmaleimide sensitive factor attachment protein receptors (SNAREs) participate in this process, as overexpression of

specific SNARE proteins disrupts the intracellular trafficking of ENaC subunits (25, 64, 65, 279). Specific SNARE proteins may interact directly with ENaC subunits and affect its gating (65). Once channels reach the plasma membrane, they appear to reside within specific compartments. Several groups have reported that a population of channels resides within lipid-rich microdomains, referred to as lipid rafts (139, 300), although other groups have not confirmed this finding (131). Lipid rafts facilitate the localization of integral membrane proteins and signaling molecules within the plasma membrane. However, the functional consequence of localization of ENaC within lipid rafts remains to be determined. ENaCs interact with cytoskeletal elements including actin and alpha-spectrin, which may have a role in localizing the channel to the plasma membrane and in modulating ENaC activity (27, 66, 271, 374). The residency time of channels at the plasma membrane has been examined by several groups, with reported half-lives on the order of minutes to hours (42, 50, 76, 131, 239, 297). Mutations within a carboxyl-terminal PY motif within the beta and gamma subunits are associated with increases in the half-life of the channel at the plasma membrane via mechanisms that are

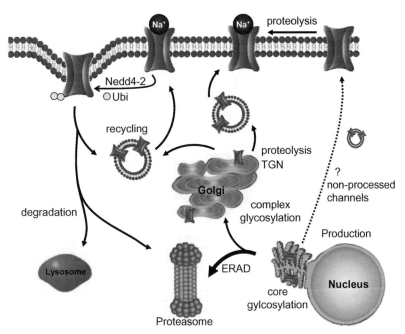

FIGURE 4 Model of ENaC biogenesis and intracellular trafficking. ENaC subunits are assembled and undergo addition of high-mannose asparagine (N)–linked glycans within the endoplasmic reticulum (ER). The majority of newly synthesized subunits are targeted for ER associated degradation (ERAD) that occurs within proteasomes. Assembled ENaCs that exit the ER transit to the apical plasma membrane via distinct routes. ENaCs traffic through the Golgi where most N-glycans are processed, the trans-Golgi network (TGN) where channels are processed by the protease furin before delivery to apical membrane. Alternatively, ENaCs exiting the ER may be delivered directly to the apical plasma membrane, bypassing processing steps that occur in the Golgi and TGN. These nonprocessed channels are functionally inactive, but are potentially activated by proteases present at the plasma membrane or within the urinary space. ENaCs at the plasma membrane pool are targeted for internalization following Nedd4-2–dependent ubiquitination (Ubi). Internalized channels are degraded within lysosomes or proteasomes. Alternatively, internalized channels are likely deubiquitinated and recycled to the plasma membrane in a regulated manner. See color insert.

discussed later in this chapter (280, 297). Internalization of channels from the plasma membrane has been proposed to occur via a dynamin-dependent process (297). Dynamin is required for clatherin-dependent endocytosis, as well as for caveolae-dependent endocytosis (137, 244, 324). Ubiquitin conjugation of defined lysine residues within ENaC subunits at the plasma membrane targets the channels for endocytosis (316), presumably via a clatherin-dependent mechanism (Fig. 4). Once internalized, some channels are targeted for degradation via proteosomes or possibly lysosomes (76, 221, 316). A significant fraction of the pool of endocytosed channels may undergo recycling to the plasma membrane in a regulated manner (Fig. 4) (42). The fate of individual subunits following internalization may differ, as rates of degradation of beta subunits have been reported to be more rapid than rates of alpha and gamma subunit degradation (350).

Localization Within the Nephron

The aldosterone-sensitive distal nephron represents the final site within the nephron where filtered Na^+ is reabsorbed. ENaCs are expressed in principal cells in the late distal convoluted tubule, connecting tubule and through the collecting duct, and are the major pathway for Na^+ entry across the apical plasma membrane. In the more proximal segments of the aldosterone-sensitive distal nephron, Na^+ reabsorption via ENaC is coupled to K^+ secretion mediated by apical membrane K^+ channels, including Kir1.1 (or ROMK) and the large conductance Ca^{2+}-activated K^+ channel (maxi-K) (354, 355, 360). The regulated reabsorption of Na^+ via ENaC in the distal nephron has a key role in the control of extracellular fluid volume, blood pressure, and renal K^+ secretion.

Within the nephron, the cellular localization of individual ENaC subunits may differ. When rats were maintained on a normal laboratory diet, beta and gamma subunits were localized within an intracellular compartment in principal cells within the cortical and outer medullary segments of the aldosterone-sensitive distal nephron (126). One group reported that the alpha subunit was localized primarily to apical part of principal cells (126), whereas other groups have observed either modest cytoplasmic localization or have failed to detect the alpha subunit (213, 227). Within the inner medullary collecting duct, all three ENaC subunits were localized primarily within an intracellular compartment (126). When placed on a low Na^+ diet or following administration of aldosterone, all three subunits were expressed at the apical membrane of principal cells (213, 214).

Mice lacking expression of the beta or gamma subunits, or that have reduced expression of the alpha subunit, exhibit renal Na^+ wasting (18, 152, 235, 260). Mice that lack expression of the alpha subunit are unable to clear airway fluids at birth, leading to death in the early postnatal period (151). Recent work suggests that the density of ENaC expression may be greatest in the connecting tubule, an early segment within the aldosterone-sensitive distal nephron that connects the distal convoluted tubule to the collecting tubule (104).

Mice that lack expression of alpha ENaC beyond the connecting tubule are able to maintain Na^+ and K^+ balance, even in the setting of dietary Na^+ restriction or K^+ loading (274).

In addition to its expression in the nephron, ENaCs are expressed within numerous other organs. They are expressed throughout the airways, as well as in both type I and type II alveolar cells (34, 41, 161, 229, 325). ENaC has a key role in the reabsorption of airway fluids (151, 223). Maintaining an appropriate volume of airway surface liquids has an important role in facilitating mucociliary clearance (35, 223). ENaCs are also expressed in the distal colon, sweat ducts, salivary ducts, inner ear, lingular epithelium, keritinocytes, lymphocytes, and vascular smooth muscle. ENaC expression has also been reported in endothelium and in various sites within the eye (epithelia within retina, lens, and pigmented ciliary body and iris (38, 40, 48, 71, 85, 88, 122, 196, 237)). The functional role of ENaC within many of these tissues is, at present, unclear.

STRUCTURAL FEATURES OF ENaC SUBUNITS

The biophysical properties of ENaC are determined by key structural domains within the channel subunits. All three ENaC subunits contribute to the formation of the conduction pore, as pore properties are altered by mutations within each of the three subunits (281). It is likely that the ENaC pore is primarily formed by the second membrane-spanning (M2) domains (200, 290) and the regions (referred to as pore, H2, or pre-M2) immediately preceding the M2 domains (Fig. 5) (179, 288, 306). Other sites within the extracellular domains and cytoplasmic amino- and carboxyl-termini also have roles in modulating channel gating and trafficking. The functional roles of individual domains within ENaC subunits, and potential mechanisms of ion permeation, ion selectivity, channel gating, and amiloride block are reviewed.

Functional Domains Within ENaC Subunits

AMINO TERMINUS
The cytoplasmic amino-termini have regions that affect channel gating, trafficking, and regulation by intracellular factors. Chalfant and coworkers identified a Lys-Gly-Asp-Lys tract within the rat alpha subunit, corresponding to residues 47–50, which may function as an endocytic signal that regulates the number of channels in the plasma membrane (55). A domain that affects channel gating has been characterized within the distal portion of the amino-terminus of the alpha subunit, which includes a highly conserved His-Gly tract (Fig. 5) (120, 121). A mutation in the corresponding Gly in the beta subunit was described in a patient with pseudohypoaldosteronism. Reduced channel activity attributed to a decreased open probability was observed with a mutation of the conserved Gly in each subunit, suggesting that the His-Gly tract within the amino-termini of all three subunits influences channel gating (57, 120, 121).

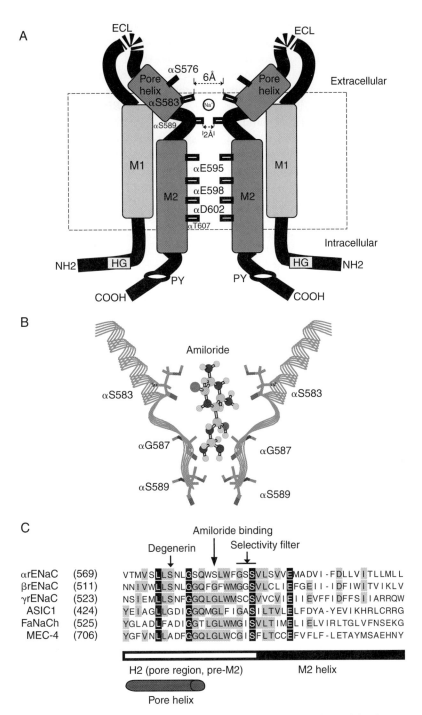

FIGURE 5 ENaC pore models. **A:** Only two subunits are shown in this model with putative helices as rectangles and non-helices as curved thick lines. The open bars attached to the various domains identify key residues within the alpha subunit of mouse ENaC. These include the degenerin site (αS576), amiloride-binding site (αS583), a key selectivity filter residue (αS589), polar residues within the second membrane-spanning domain (αE595, αE598, αD602, and αT607). Space dimensions at the amiloride-binding site and selectivity filter are in angstroms. The majority of the extracellular domain is omitted for clarity. **B:** Structural model of amiloride binding to the ENaC pore. The amino and carboxyl-terminal portions of the pore region are modeled as helical and nonhelical, respectively, with αS583 at the transition point. Amiloride interacts with both αS583 and selectivity filter residue αG587. **C:** Sequence alignments of pore-forming regions. Identical residues are shown on black background and conserved residues are shadowed with grey background. Key sites are labeled with arrows. (Part B is reprinted with permission from Sheng S, Perry CJ, Kashlan OB, Kleyman TR. Side chain orientation of residues lining the selectivity filter of epithelial Na⁺ channels. *J Biol Chem* 2005;280:8513–8522.)

Phosphatidylinositol 4,5-bisphosphate (PIP2) activates ENaCs (219, 367), an effect that reflects an increase in channel open probability as a result of direct interactions between PIP2 and ENaC. Several groups have proposed that the amino-termini of the beta and gamma subunits of ENaC harbor putative PIP2-binding domains containing basic amino acid residues (198, 367). The ENaC amino-termini also contain Cys residues that are required for the channel to respond to intracellular metals (Cd^{2+} and Zn^{2+}) and thiol-reactive chemicals with a reduction in open probability (175). Mutations within a region (pre-M1) in the amino-terminus near the first membrane-spanning domain of ASIC2 and ASIC3, members in the ENaC/DEG family, altered ion selectivity and pH dependence, suggesting a participation of the region in the ion pore (68). Whether the homologous regions in ENaC subunits contribute to the channel pore is not known.

First Membrane-Spanning Domain (M1)

Structures of K^+ channels that are composed of subunits with two membrane-spanning domains have been resolved (84, 199). If the membrane-spanning domains of ENaC subunits are arranged in a manner similar to that of the K^+ channels, the M1 domains of ENaC would be located at the interface between the pore-lining second membrane-spanning domains and the membrane lipids (Fig. 5). However, Poet and coworkers suggested that M1 domains of a peptide-gated channel and of an acid-sensing ion channel, members of the ENaC/DEG family, contribute to the pore based on the response of channels with introduced Cys residues to sulfhydryl-reactive reagents (259). The functional roles of the M1 domains of ENaC subunits are being explored.

Extracellular Domains

Each ENaC subunit has a large, ~450-residue extracellular domain with 16 conserved Cys residues clustered within two cysteine-rich domains (CRD I and II) (Fig. 3) (100). Other members of the ENaC/DEG family also possess extracellular cysteine-rich domains (225). The size and apparently conserved structural organization of the extracellular domain suggest that this region has important functional roles. Recent studies have examined the role of the extracellular domain in modulating channel gating in response to proteases, external Na^+, metals, and amiloride (100, 150, 157, 182, 292). It is likely that these domains facilitate the assembly of the heteroligomeric channel complex within the ER or delivery to the plasma membrane (39, 100).

Proteolytic Cleavage Several serine proteases, including prostasin and related channel-activating proteases, furin, trypsin, chymotrypsin, and elastase, have been shown to activate ENaC (1, 44, 62, 125, 148, 335, 342). Activation of ENaC by proteases appears to be a result of proteolytic cleavage of ENaC extracellular domains at defined sites (149, 150). Proteolytic activation of ENaC by furin is dependent on cleavage of the alpha and gamma subunits at

distinct sites between the first and second conserved Cys residues (148). Prostasin cleavage occurs at polybasic tracts, and potential prostasin cleavage sites are present within ENaC extracellular domains (299). Mechanisms by which proteases activate ENaCs are discussed below.

Amiloride Binding A six-residue tract (Trp-Tyr-Arg-Phe-His-Tyr) within the extracellular domain of the alpha subunit was identified as a putative amiloride-binding site based on its homology with the antigen-binding domain of an anti-amiloride antibody (157, 185). Specific mutations within this tract alter the amiloride sensitivity of channels composed solely of alpha subunits that were reconstituted in lipid bilayers or expressed in CHO cells (157, 182). However, these mutations were not associated with a significant change in the apparent amiloride affinity when all three ENaC subunits were expressed (180). Residues in the pre-M2 regions of the alpha, beta, and gamma subunits have been identified as a putative amiloride-binding site (281), as discussed below.

Na^+ Self-Inhibition and Gating Na^+ self-inhibition represents the decline from a peak ENaC current that occurs following a rapid increase in the extracellular Na^+ concentration (105, 203). It is considered an intrinsic response of the Na^+ channels to extracellular Na^+, as the self-inhibition response has been observed in both model epithelia expressing native channels and *Xenopus* oocytes expressing cloned human, rat, *Xenopus*, and mouse ENaCs (14, 61, 254, 287, 337). Several lines of evidence suggest that a reduction of open probability underscores the mechanism of channel inhibition by extracellular Na^+ (61, 110, 287, 336). Therefore, Na^+ self-inhibition is a gating event and may be a target process for various extracellular factors that regulate ENaC gating. The structural basis of Na^+ self-inhibition has begun to emerge from mutagenesis studies. *Xenopus* $\alpha\beta\gamma$ and $\epsilon\beta\gamma$ channels exhibit different Na^+ self-inhibition responses, and analyses of *Xenopus* α/ϵ ENaC chimeras suggested that a region in the proximal portion of the extracellular domain was responsible for the difference in Na^+ self-inhibition responses (14). Sheng and coworkers concluded that a His residue (γH239) within the extracellular domain has a critical role in the Na^+ self-inhibition response, based on the observation that mutations of γH239 resulted in a complete loss of the response (287). Interestingly, mutations of mouse αH282, the site analogous to mouse γH239, led to an enhanced Na^+ self-inhibition. At present, mechanisms by which the binding of Na^+ to sites within the extracellular domains of ENaC leads to a reduction in channel open probability have not been defined.

The extracellular domains either directly participate in or regulate ENaC gating. Consistent with this notion, mutations of αH282 affect gating kinetics of channels composed solely of alpha subunits (182). Furthermore, the extracellular domains of other members of the ENaC/DEG family have been implicated in the regulation of channel gating (225). We have proposed that αHis282 and γH239 are present within a region that functions as an extracellular allosteric regulator of ENaC gating (287).

Transition Metal-Binding Site External Ni^{2+} is an inhibitor of rat and mouse αβγ ENaC (42, 286, 292). Ni^{2+} block was diminished by mutations at either mouse αH282 or its corresponding site in the gamma subunit (mouse γH239), and was not observed when both His residues were mutated. Sheng and coworkers proposed that these two His residues within the extracellular domains of the alpha and gamma subunits form a Ni^{2+}-binding site (292). The inhibitory effect of external Ni^{2+} reflects a reduction of ENaC open probability (286, 292). Ni^{2+} block and Na⁺ self-inhibition may share a common mechanism, as Ni^{2+} pretreatment prevents further inhibition by extracellular Na⁺ (293). In contrast, external Ni^{2+} stimulates Na⁺ channels present in A6 cells, derived from the *Xenopus laevis* kidney (72). These seemingly conflicting results may reflect structural or functional differences among ENaC species (e.g., rat, mouse, and *Xenopus*) and warrant further investigation.

External Zn^{2+} also affects ENaC activity in a species-specific manner. Amuzescu and coworkers reported that external Zn^{2+} is a voltage-dependent blocker of *Xenopus* ENaC. High (100 μM) concentrations of Zn^{2+} stimulated rat ENaC, although lower concentrations were inhibitory (8). Sheng and coworkers also observed that extracellular Zn^{2+} at concentrations of less than 1 mM activated mouse and human ENaC by increasing channel open probabilityy, due to a loss of Na⁺ self-inhibition (293), although an inhibitory effect at higher concentrations of Zn^{2+} was not observed. These opposing effects of external Ni^{2+} and Zn^{2+} on ENaCs derived from different species suggest the presence of species-dependent differences in the structural organization of the extracellular domain.

Role of Extracellular Cysteine Residues in ENaC Expression The roles of the conserved cysteine residues within the extracellular domains were investigated by systematic mutagenesis of these cysteine residues. Firsov and colleagues proposed that specific cysteines (the 1st and 6th cysteines in alpha, beta, and gamma ENaC as well as the 11th and 12th cysteine in the alpha and beta subunits) have an essential role in the efficient transport of assembled channels to the plasma membrane (100).

PRE-M2 (PORE) REGION

The region preceding M2 within each subunit contains both hydrophobic and hydrophilic residues, and is highly conserved among members of the ENaC/DEG family (Fig. 5). The pre-M2 regions harbor important functional domains that affect channel gating, cation selectivity, and amiloride binding.

Amiloride Binding Schild and coworkers identified a ring of residues at homologous positions within each of the three subunits (αS583, βG525, and γG537 in rat ENaC) as a putative amiloride-binding site (Fig. 5) (281). The substitution of βG525 or γG537 with any residue weakened

amiloride IC_{50} by about three orders of magnitude, suggesting that the loss of backbone torsion angles unique to Gly were responsible for the reduction in amiloride affinity. In contrast, amino acids bearing side chains with different functional groups (e.g., Gly, Leu, Asn, Gln) had only a slight effect on amiloride block, suggesting that the side chain of αS583 does not participate in amiloride binding (173). However, amino acids with aromatic side chains introduced at αS583 led to a large reduction in amiloride affinity, suggesting that large side chains at position α583 protrude into the pore and limit access of amiloride to this site (173). The effects of Cys mutations at the amiloride-binding ring on the inhibitory constant largely reflected an increase in the microscopic k_{off} rate, consistent with an effect on the bound complex (178). An adjacent three-residue Gly/Ser-X-Ser tract that forms the primary selectivity filter may also have an important role in amiloride binding (Fig. 5B). Mutations introduced in the first position of this tract in the alpha or beta subunit were associated with a large reduction in amiloride affinity (180, 202, 291), suggesting that amiloride interacts with this site (Fig. 5).

The introduction of Cys residues at the amiloride-binding ring rendered channels sensitive to block by external Zn^{2+}, Cd^{2+}, and sulfhydryl-reactive methanthiosulfonate (MTS) derivatives (195, 202, 281, 289, 306). Moreover, mutations of these residues reduced single-channel conductance (173, 281). This site was also shown to be located within the membrane electrical field (173, 281, 289). These observations suggest that this ring of residues lines the conducting pore.

Selectivity Filter A three-residue tract (Gly/Ser-X-Ser), starting four residues distal to the amiloride-binding site, has a key role in conferring cation selectivity (Fig. 5). Systematic examination of the pre-M2 region of ENaC subunits by several groups found that the introduction of Cys residues within the amino-terminal portion of this region did not affect cation selectivity. However, mutations of either the first and/or third residue within the Gly/Ser-X-Ser tract in the carboxyl-terminal part of the pre-M2 region of the alpha, beta, and gamma subunits resulted in significant K⁺ permeation (174, 179, 180, 202, 288, 306). Certain substitutions of the third residue in this tract in the alpha subunit also increase permeability to Ca^{2+} and other divalent cations that do not permeate wildtype ENaCs (179). Alterations of the Li⁺/Na⁺ selectivity ratio were observed with mutants at multiple sites within the pre-M2 region, as well as within the M2 region. The three-residue Gly/Ser-X-Ser tract has been proposed to function as the channel's primary selectivity filter (174, 179, 180, 202, 288, 306).

Channel Gating In addition to a role in amiloride binding and conferring cation selectivity, the pore region (pre-M2) also has a role in channel gating. A key residue that affects channel gating is amino-terminal to the amiloride-binding ring. Members of the ENaC/DEG family have a residue present at this site that has a small or negligible side chain, e.g., Ser (ENaCs), Ala (DEGs and MECs) or Gly

(ASICs). This site is often referred to as the degeneration site, as a substitution at this site in a MEC subunit with a bulky residue results in degeneration of specific neurons in *Caenorhabditis elegans* (143) and activation of ASICs and ENaCs (3, 177, 289, 304). External sulfhydryl reagents activate ENaCs with a Cys substitution at the degenerin site by increasing channel open probability (177, 289, 304). Modification of ENaCs with Cys substitutions at the degenerin site is dependent on channels being in an open state, suggesting that (i) there is an extracellular gate controlling access to the degenerin site or (ii) that this site undergoes a conformational change in association with channel gating that alters its accessibility to chemical reagents (304). In addition to the degenerin site, external sulfhydryl reagents activate channels with Cys substitutions at nearby sites with a periodicity suggestive of an alpha-helical structure (289). Secondary structure prediction algorithms have also suggested that the amino-terminal part of the pore region (pre-M2) has an alpha-helical structure, which may be similar to the pore helix of KcsA and Kir channels (Fig. 5) (84, 199). These results suggest that the helical region as a whole, rather than a single degeneration residue (mouse αS576) (Fig. 5), may function as a gating domain (289), which may be involved in the regulation of ENaC gating by various external and internal factors. Consistent with this idea, Na^+ self-inhibition and channel activation by laminar shear stress are eliminated in αS580Cβγ mouse ENaC upon external application of the sulfhydryl reagent MTSET, which locks the channels in a fully open state (51, 287). Carattino and coworkers recently reported that mutations at multiple sites within the pore region of the alpha subunit altered the magnitude and time course of ENaC activation by laminar shear stress, suggesting a role of the region in channel mechanoregulation (52).

Several amiloride-binding site mutants exhibited an altered single-channel conductance, although cation selectivity was preserved (173, 195, 281). Moreover, the channels with a Cys residue at the gamma site exhibited a high open probability, failed to respond to shear stress stimulus, and lacked a Na^+ self-inhibition response (52). These results suggest that the αS583-βG525-γG537 ring participates, either directly or indirectly, in ion permeation and channel gating in addition to its role in amiloride binding.

SECOND MEMBRANE-SPANNING DOMAIN (M2)

The M2 domains of ENaC subunits may be equivalent to the second transmembrane domains (inner helices) of K^+ channels that have subunits with two membrane-spanning domains (e.g., members of the Kir family), or the sixth membrane-spanning domain (S6) in voltage-gated channels that are thought to line the channel's inner pore (84, 140, 168). M2 residues are predicted to be alpha helical and their primary sequence is highly conserved among the three ENaC subunits, including three negatively charged residues that likely line one face of an alpha helix (Fig. 5). These negatively charged residues are not present in other highly selective cation channels,

and may play structural or functional roles in channel permeation, selectivity, or gating. The introduction of mutations at specific sites containing acidic residues has been reported to reduce channel activity without altering surface expression (200) and results in K^+ permeation, suggesting that these residues have a direct or indirect role in conferring cation selectivity (290). The carboxyl-terminal portion of M2 may also have a role in the regulation of gating (108, 368).

CYTOPLASMIC CARBOXYL TERMINUS

The region immediately following M2 contains clusters of basic residues that affect cation selectivity, as well as channel gating through interactions with acidic phospholipids, such as PIP3. (33, 166, 258). The major function of the carboxyl-termini appears to be related to the internalization of the channel complex, through a well-characterized Pro-Tyr (PY) motif (PPPXYXXL) that interacts with the ubiquitin ligase Nedd4-2 (170, 280, 309, 316). ENaC subunit ubiquitination likely serves as a signal for channel internalization from the plasma membrane (316). It is unclear whether the YXXL sequence within this motif serves as an independent signal for channel internalization. Other sites within the carboxyl-termini may influence rates of channel endocytosis. For example, an A663T polymorphism in the alpha subunit of the human hENaC affects rates of channel internalization from the plasma membrane (276, 362).

The carboxyl-termini have sites that are targeted by specific protein kinases that modulate ENaC activity via phosphorylation. These kinases include an extracellular regulated kinase (ERK), casein kinase 2, a glucocorticoid, and serum-regulated kinase (Sgk), a G protein–coupled receptor kinase (Grk2), and IkappaB kinase-beta (IKKβ) kinase (79, 81, 201, 294, 295). EKR1/2-dependent phosphorylation of the carboxyl-termini of the beta and gamma subunits enhances ENaC interactions with Nedd4 (294). Both forskolin and phorbol 12-myristate 13-acetate (PMA) have been reported to enhance phosphorylation of the beta and gamma subunits, although the target residues that are phosphorylated have not been identified (296). A region in the proximal part of the carboxyl-terminus of the alpha subunit has a role in conferring sensitivity to a staurosporine-sensitive kinase that has not been identified (340). The carboxyl-termini also bind alpha spectrin and possibly actin, linking the channel to the cytoskeleton (66, 271). Grk2 activates ENaC by phosphorylating the carboxyl-terminus of the beta subunit and preventing Nedd4-2–dependent inhibition of ENaC (81). Cys residues in the amino and carboxyl-termini of ENaC subunits may participate in the inhibition of ENaC that is observed with intracellular thiol-reactive reagents (175).

PORE STRUCTURE

Elegant structural studies of bacterial K^+ channels have provided a three-dimensional view of the conduction pore. The pore is lined by the distal part of the pore region (or P loop) that contains the selectivity filter, and by the most distal membrane-spanning domain (84, 140, 199). The pore regions of K⁺ channels are structured as reentry loops with an amino-terminal alpha helix that enters the membrane, followed by a hairpin turn and an extended region that contains the selectivity filter. A distinct model of the ENaC pore has been proposed by several groups. This model has a gradually narrowing outer pore extending from the alpha-helical proximal part of the pre-M2 domain and the amiloride-binding ring (αS583-βG525-γG537) to the three-residue tract (Gly/Ser-X-Ser) that forms the selectivity filter (Fig. 5) (173, 179, 180, 281, 291, 306). The M2 region follows the selectivity filter, the narrowest part of the pore (Fig. 5). M2 segments may reside at an angle relative to the membrane normal (i.e., a tepee-like structure), with charged and polar residues facing an aqueous pore (200, 290). This model is in agreement with a growing body of observations derived from mutagenesis studies, suggesting that (i) the amiloride-binding ring is external to the selectivity filter, and (ii) the first residue in the selectivity filter (Gly/Ser-X-Ser) is external to the third residue (281, 291, 306).

Cation Permeation and Selectivity

While a detailed understanding of the molecular mechanisms underlying permeation and selectivity awaits a high-resolution structure of ENaC, recent studies have yielded important clues regarding ion permeation and selectivity (181, 247). Organic or inorganic cations larger than Na⁺ are unable to pass through the channel, in contrast to voltage-gated Na⁺ channels, suggesting that permeant cations must dehydrate to cross the narrowest part of the channel pore (i.e., the selectivity filter) (21, 248). Within the Gly/Ser-X-Ser tract that comprises the ENaC selectivity filter (174, 180, 288), backbone carbonyl oxygens and hydroxyl oxygens present on the side chains of Ser residues may coordinate permeating Na⁺ or Li⁺ ions (174, 291).

The selectivity sequence of ENaC (Li⁺ > Na⁺ >>> K⁺, organic cations) suggests that the relative permeability of an ion is inversely related to its ionic size, a relationship consistent with a mechanism in which ENaC discriminates cations through molecular sieving (174, 179). Alternatively, cation selectivity could be achieved by placing a negatively (or partially negatively) charged site with strong field strength that preferentially binds small cations within the channel pore (21, 248). In this regard, the selectivity sequence for ENaC corresponds to the Eisenman sequence XI. This sequence was determined based on the presence of strong electrostatic interactions between ions and the selectivity site that overrides differences in dehydration energies for ions (91).

Selectivity filters appear to be flexible and are not static structures (28, 184, 273). A potentially flexible selectivity filter provides another variable that will need to be taken into account when developing models of the ENaC selectivity filter. Clearly, additional studies are needed to enhance

our understanding of the molecular mechanisms by which ENaC achieves ion selectivity.

Mechanisms of ENaC Gating

ENaC gating is characterized by unusually long open and close times (up to seconds or even tens of seconds) compared to other channels such as voltage-gated channels (Fig. 1) (111). This gating pattern seems appropriate for this channel, given its major physiologic role of mediating bulk Na⁺ transport across the apical membrane of epithelial cells and for which slow transitions between open and close states may be beneficial in the terms of transport efficiency. Transitions between open and closed states appear to occur spontaneously. Another feature of ENaC gating is the high variability in open probability observed by patch clamp (56, 111, 253). Subunit composition and regulatory factors that affect gating may account for this variability (107, 111). As discussed above, proteolytic cleavage of ENaC subunits converts channels that have a low open probability to channels that exhibit "normal" gating behavior (44, 45, 148, 150). Mechanical forces, external metals, and temperature have also been shown to affect channel gating (51, 52, 61, 287, 292, 293). Studies on Na⁺ self-inhibition and effects of metals on ENaC gating have raised the question of whether ENaCs should be considered a ligand-gated channel, similar to FaNaCh and ASIC (145, 293).

A detailed understanding of ENaC gating mechanisms is lacking, despite the identification of several sites within ENaC where the introduction of mutations affected ENaC gating kinetics. These sites are present within the amino-terminal domain (120, 121), the extracellular domain (44, 45, 148, 182, 287, 292, 293), the pore region (pre-M2) (52, 177, 289, 304), the M2 domain (108), and the intracellular carboxyl-terminal domain (33, 164, 258). However, it is unclear whether these various regions control channel gating in an independent or collaborative manner, nor is it known whether there is a single gate or multiple gates. The location of the channel gate is another open question, although the pore region seems to be an attractive candidate.

Several recent studies have suggested that the pore helix of cation channels may be a central gating structure (6, 52, 116, 210, 285, 363). Yeh and coworkers have suggested that the regulation of TRPV5 (a member of transient receptor potential channel subfamily) gating by extracellular and intracellular protons is mediated by a rotational movement of the pore helix and the subsequent closing of a gate within the selectivity filter (363). As the amino-terminal helical portion of the pore region of ENaC participates in channel gating (177, 289, 304), it is possible that rotation of this helix that is initiated by conformational changes at other sites within the channels alters ENaC gating kinetics.

Permeation and gating of ion channels were proposed to be two independent processes nearly 50 years ago (142). While previous studies have supported this concept, recent studies suggest that connections exist between permeation and gating (370, 371). For example, channel gating is often modulated by permeant or blocking ions (78, 322). Mutations within selectivity filters are associated with changes in gating kinetics in K^+ channels, voltage-gated Na^+ channels, and ENaC (52, 180, 346). Lu and coworkers recently provided evidence suggesting conformational changes of the selectivity filter contribute directly to the spontaneous gating of an inward rectifier K^+ channel (Kir2.1) (216). Significant differences in the selectivity filter structure of KcsA K^+ channel were observed when the crystals were soaked in low-K^+ and high-K^+ solutions (372), suggesting that the selectivity filter of this channel is flexible. Molecular simulations using the high-resolution structures of bacterial K^+ channels have confirmed the idea (82, 83). Conformational changes in the selectivity filter have been proposed to occur in the ligand-initiated gating of cyclic nucleotide-gated ion channels (230). A similar notion has been proposed for inward rectifier K^+ channels (263, 357). We anticipate that future studies will examine whether ENaC's selectivity filter serves as its gate.

Amiloride Interaction with ENaC

Although amiloride is generally accepted as a pore blocker of ENaC and other members of the ENaC/DEG family, published observations support a more complex interaction between amiloride and ion channels (110). For example, some amiloride analogues stimulate activity of epithelial Na^+ channels (337). Current models of amiloride binding to ENaC, based on analyses of ENaC mutants, must take into account interactions that are occurring at the amiloride-binding ring (αS583-βG525-γG537), as well as interactions at the start of the selectivity filter. It was proposed that the positively charged guanidine moiety of amiloride interacts with the first residue within the Gly/Ser-X-Ser tract of the selectivity filter, whereas that the pyrazine ring interacts with a more external stretch of residues, including the amiloride-binding ring (αS583-βG525-γG537) (Fig. 5) (173, 291). Residues within the extracellular domains, including αHis282, might help stabilize the binding of amiloride to the channel (190).

ENaC REGULATION

ENaC is subject to a wide variety of regulatory influences that alter channel activity over long or short time periods in order to respond to the physiologic needs of the organism. In the kidney, these regulatory influences determine the final Na^+ concentration of the urine, which may vary from virtually Na^+ free to more than 100 mM. Abnormalities in these regulatory mechanisms in the cortical collecting duct have been convincingly linked to excess Na^+ reabsorption and hypertension when disordered regulation leads to gain of function, and salt wasting and hypotension when abnormal regulation leads to loss of function (270). Altered or

abnormal regulation of ENaC in the lung has been linked to abnormal alveolar fluid clearance in disease states such as cystic fibrosis, high-altitude pulmonary edema, and acute lung injury (35, 223, 228). In many cases, studies of abnormal ENaC function in disease states have complemented basic observations concerning channel function made in experimental settings and led to remarkable insights concerning molecular mechanisms of regulating channel activity.

Until quite recently, it has been accepted that ENaC present in the apical membrane of Na^+ reabsorbing epithelia is constitutively active. Channel activity could therefore be subject to regulation through alteration of one of its intrinsic kinetic properties: its number (N), open probability (P_o), or single-channel conductance (i). Since significant changes in single-channel conductance are not found under physiologic conditions, channel regulation may be considered primarily as a matter of alterations in either channel number or open probability. Thinking about channel regulation from this perspective would seem to simplify the subject, and certainly provides a framework within which regulation may be considered; however, the subject remains enormously complex because of the number of regulatory influences that may modify either channel number or open probability. There is a significant paradigm shift in that we now recognize that "near silent" channels are present in the membrane, in addition to constitutively active channels (45, 183, 253). These "near silent" channels are capable of activation and may be viewed as the extreme case of open probability regulation, where channels move from very low to a measurable open probability given the appearance of increased numbers of channels (45). Levels of expression of "near silent" channels in the distal nephron under varying physiologic states remains to been determined. Channel regulation serves to either enhance or diminish Na^+ reabsorption from luminal fluids of distal nephron, lung, or colon in accord with the needs of the organism. Given the wide variations in rates of Na^+ reabsorption and luminal Na^+ gradients that this involves, other intrinsic regulatory influences are required to maintain constant cell volume and ion gradients. In order to respond to these needs under normal physiologic conditions, channel activity is regulated by a number of hormones, including steroids, vasopressin, and insulin; by a variety of accessory proteins; by kinases, proteases, and methyltransferases; by other channels such as cystic fibrosis transmembrane regulator (CFTR); and by ion concentrations and pH.

Cellular Regulation

NEDD4

Liddle's syndrome is a hereditary form of salt-sensitive hypertension associated with increased ENaC activity (270, 298, 347). The most common defects in ENaC primary structure leading to this disorder involve the proline-rich regions of carboxyl-termini of the beta or gamma subunit (129, 130, 298, 326). Rotin and colleagues used this region of the ENaC beta subunit as bait in a yeast two-hybrid screen to identify proteins that interact with ENaC and might regulate ENaC expression. They isolated the protein Nedd4 (neuronal precursor cells expressed developmentally downregulated) using this technique, and in a series of elegant studies, examined the role of this protein in regulating ENaC expression (314–316). Nedd4 is an E3 ubiquitin ligase composed of a C2 domain, three or four WW domains that are protein interaction modules, and a ubiquitin-ligase Hect domain. The WW domains serve to mediate the interaction between Nedd4 and ENaC with the strongest interaction being between the carboxyl-terminus of beta ENaC and the third WW domain. The Hect domain is an E3 ligase that receives ubiquitin from an E2 protein and transfers ubiquitin to lysines in target proteins. The C2 region is a Ca^{2+}- and phospholipid-binding domain. It is not present on all Nedd4 isoforms and, based on oocyte studies, does not appear to be essential for inhibition of ENaC expression (158, 159, 170). This domain does, however, serve to localize Nedd4 to plasma membrane in response to an increase in cytosolic $[Ca^{2+}]$ (257), and mediates association with annexin XIIIb, which may be involved in apical membrane targeting in epithelia (256).

Nedd4-2, the isoform most active in binding ENaC, is detected in tissues that express ENaC. The Nedd4-2 WW domains interact in vitro with the proline-rich region of carboxyl terminus of the beta subunit (102, 171, 215). Considerable evidence indicates that the interaction between Nedd4 and ENaC results in ubiquitination of the channel (Fig. 6). ENaC has been shown to be ubiquitinated in endogenously expressing A6 cells and when overexpressed along with Nedd4-2 in HEK-293 cells (221, 316). Coexpression studies with Nedd4 and ENaC in oocytes demonstrated that Nedd4 decreases ENaC surface expression, and that this is dependent both on the E3 ligase domain of Nedd4 and on the presence of lysine residues on the amino-

termini of the target subunits (316). Taken together, these studies strongly support the model that surface expression of ENaC is regulated by ubiquitination, which serves as a signal for retrieval from the plasma membrane. It is likely that ENaC is ubiquitinated at other cellular sites, including the ER. Unassembled subunits are likely degraded by the proteosome by a process involving polyubiquitination, while fully assembled trimeric channels are degraded by either the proteasome or lysosomal-endosomal pathway following ubiquitination at the cell surface (76, 221, 272, 316). At present, it is unclear whether monoubiquitination of ENaC occurs at the cell surface, nor is it known by what mechanism ubiquitinated ENaC at the cell surface is internalized. As discussed above, channel internalization from the plasma membrane is a dynamin-dependent process (297). Whatever the mechanism, it seems clear that the bulk of available evidence indicate that surface expression of ENaC is negatively regulated by ubiquitination mediated by Nedd4-2. The interaction between Nedd4-2 and ENaC is itself subject to regulation by specific hormones and kinases (81, 232, 294, 301, 303), and is involved as the final common pathway of several regulatory influences affecting ENaC surface expression, providing further evidence for the importance of this interaction in ENaC regulation (see below).

KINASES

Protein phosphatase inhibitors, such as okadaic acid, result in activation of ENaC (19), while nonspecific kinase inhibitors, such as staurosporine, inhibit basal channel activity (339, 340); both observations are consistent with kinase regulation of the channel. In many cases, the regulation of ENaC by a protein kinase is indirect, with kinase activation occurring within a pathway of hormonal regulation. Examples of this follow:

1. Activation of SGK1 by steroid hormones that phosphorylates the Nedd4-2. A 14-3-3 protein binds to phosphorylated Nedd4-2 and inhibits the interaction

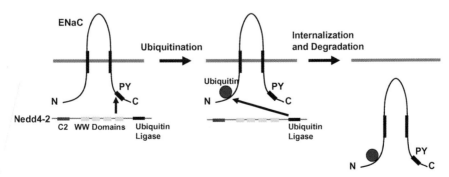

FIGURE 6 Nedd4-2–dependent regulation of ENaC surface expression. Nedd4-2 binding to ENaC subunits is facilitated through interactions between WW domains on Nedd4-2 and the PY motif on ENaC beta and gamma subunits. Nedd4-2–dependent ubiquitination of ENaC subunits targets the channel for internalization and degradation. (Adapted with permission from Snyder PM. The epithelial Na+ channel: cell surface insertion and retrieval in Na+ homeostasis and hypertension. *Endocrinol Rev* 2002;23:258–275.)

between ENaC subunits and Nedd4-2, thereby increasing surface expression of channels through inhibition of ubiquitin-based retrieval (Fig. 7) (29, 77, 101, 153, 308).

2. Activation of phosphatidyl-insoitol 3 kinase by insulin, which in turn leads to phosphorylation and activation of SGK1 by 3-phosphoinositide-dependent kinase 1, and activation of ENaC by the same distal cascade (30, 101).

3. Protein kinase A, which is activated by adenylate cyclase and cAMP in response to vasopressin or beta-adrenergic stimulation and leads to exocytotic insertion of channels into the membrane (42, 240, 302), as well as phosphorylation and activation of SGK1 (307).

4. Src kinase, which is activated by endothelin and mediates inactivation of ENaC by decreasing open probability without directly phosphorylating the channel (115).

5. Protein kinase C, which inactivates ENaC by decreasing open probability possibly through a Ca^{2+}-dependent mechanism and decreasing expression of beta and gamma ENaC by activating ERK kinase (32, 205, 366).

6. IKKβ, the kinase regulating NfκB activation, directly interacts with beta ENaC and enhances channel surface expression through an unknown mechanism, suggesting an interaction between the inflammatory cascade and ENaC activation (201).

7. AMP-activated kinase, a ubiquitous metabolic sensor, has been shown to inhibit ENaC in oocytes and cultured cells, although it does not directly phosphorylate the channel (49).

ENaC is also a substrate for kinases that are involved in its regulation. Studies of ENaC expressed in MDCK cells have demonstrated increased phosphorylation of the beta and gamma subunits in response to stimulation by aldosterone and insulin (296). Phosphopeptide mapping indicated that the sites phosphorylated were carboxyl-terminal serine and threonine residues (296). Shi and colleagues described phosphorylation of βS631 by casein kinase-2, but it is unclear whether casein kinase-2 regulates ENaC activity (295). The same

group described phosphorylation of βThr613 and γThr623 by the extracellular regulated kinase (ERK) (294). ERK-dependent phosphorylation of ENaC facilitates interactions between the channel and Nedd4, thereby inhibiting ENaC activity. Recent work suggests that Sgk increases channel open probability by directly phosphorylating the carboxyl-terminus of the alpha subunit (79). Finally, insulin has been described to increase phosphorylation of a fully mature 65-kDa form of alpha ENaC in cultured epithelial cells, which correlated with an increase in channel activity (369). The kinase mediating this effect was not directly identified, but the protein kinase C inhibitor chelerythrine blocked the insulin stimulation of transport and subunit phosphorylation.

Of considerable interest is the report that the G protein–coupled receptor kinase, Grk2, phosphorylates S633 in carboxyl-terminus of beta ENaC (81). Phosphorylation at this site renders the channel insensitive to regulation by Nedd4-2, resulting in increased surface expression and channel activity. This finding is particularly important, as (1) it is the first report of a G-protein receptor kinase directly regulating an ion channel, and (2) increased Grk2 activity has been associated with hypertension (97). Such observations add to a growing body of literature that associates abnormalities of ENaC activity, whether due to trafficking defects as in Liddle's syndrome or polymorphisms resulting in increased activity, with low-renin hypertension in humans (270).

Another family of kinases linked to human hypertension is the WNK (with no lysine) family of serine-threonine kinases (169). These kinases are prominently expressed in the distal tubule and collecting ducts of the kidney and mutations lead to hypertension and hyperkalemia typical of psuedohypoaldosteronism type II (PHA II) (353). WNK4 has been shown to inhibit the renal Na–Cl cotransporter and ROMK, and mutations associated with hypertension relieve Na–Cl cotransporter inhibition, but enhance inhibition of ROMK (169). These observations suggested that under normal physiologic conditions, WNK4 regulates the balance between renal Na^+ reabsorption and K^+ excretion, but mutations would lead to exaggerated Na^+ reabsorption and hypertension with hyperkalemia

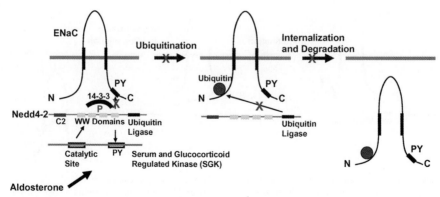

FIGURE 7   Aldosterone modulation of the interaction of Nedd4-2 and ENaC. Sgk is targeted to Nedd4-2 through interactions between a PY motif on Sgk and WW domains on Nedd4-2. Sgk-dependent phosphorylation of Nedd4-2 results in the recruitment of a 14-3-3 protein that prevents Nedd4-2 binding to ENaC.

due to impaired K⁺ excretion. Recently another member of this family, WNK1, has been implicated in regulation of ENaC. Interestingly, intronic deletions that could lead to hypertension and hyperkalemia result in overexpression of WNK1 (358). Aldosterone has also been shown to stimulate expression of a kidney-specific isoform of WNK1, and overexpression of this kinase stimulates Na⁺ reabsorption in cultured collecting duct cells and in overexpression systems (242). Cobb and colleagues have shown that WNK1 expression leads to activation of SGK1 in a PI-3 kinase–dependent manner, indicating that the kinase activates ENaC by increasing its expression at the apical membrane of collecting duct cells, contributing to the human hypertension seen in association with PHA II (359).

Proteases A growing body of evidence suggests that proteolysis of ENaC subunits has an important role in regulating ENaC activity. Vallet and coworkers in 1997 used a functional complementation assay in *Xenopus* oocytes expressing ENaC to clone a channel-activating protease (CAP) (335). Chraibi and coworkers reported in 1998 that extracellular trypsin activated ENaCs due to an increase in channel open probability (62). These observations provided the first hints that proteases may have a role in the regulation of ENaC. Since that time, a growing number of proteases have been identified that, when coexpressed with ENaC or added to a solution bathing cells expressing ENaCs, result in channel activation. Several channel-activating serine proteases have been identified, based on their ability to activate ENaC when coexpressed in oocytes. These include prostasin (also referred to as CAP1) and two additional proteases, CAP2 and CAP3 (335, 341). These CAPs are primarily expressed at the plasma membrane and exhibit parallel patterns of tissue expression with alpha ENaC, except that CAP2 is poorly expressed in the kidney (341). CAPs 1 and 2 are inhibited by the bovine serine protease inhibitor aprotinin, a prototypical Kunitz type protease inhibitor (341). Extracellular elastase and chymotrypsin also activate ENaC (44, 62).

As discussed above, proteolytic processing of ENaC subunits occurs within the biosynthetic pathway. This is likely mediated by a furin, a member of the proprotein convertase family of serine proteases that is expressed primarily in the trans-Golgi network (148, 329). There are three putative furin cleavage sites within the extracellular domain of the alpha subunit, and a single site within the extracellular domain of the gamma subunit. Hughey and coworkers demonstrated that furin-dependent cleavage occurs at the proximal and distal furin cleavage sites within the alpha subunit, excising a 26-mer peptide fragment, and at the furin cleavage site within the gamma subunit (148). Channel activation in CHO cells and *Xenopus* oocytes appears to be dependent on cleavage by furin at these sites (148).

How does proteolysis affect ENaC activity? At a single-channel level, ENaCs exhibit open and closed times on the order of seconds to tens of seconds. Several groups have identified a distinct population of ENaCs that have brief open times and long closed times, referred to as near-silent channels (45, 183, 253). Caldwell and coworkers have shown that it is this latter population of channels that responds to external trypsin with a dramatic increase in channel open probability (45). These observations suggest that proteases convert channels which are near silent to channels that have the characteristically long open and closed times. Both processed (i.e., cleaved) and unprocessed subunits are expressed at the cell surface (76, 149). These nonprocessed channels provide a pool of ENaCs that could be activated by proteases in a regulated manner. In this regard, recent studies suggest that rats placed on a low-Na⁺ diet or receiving exogenous aldosterone have increased levels of whole kidney expression of the processed form of the gamma subunit (103, 227, 243). When *Xenopus* A6 cells deprived of serum were treated with aldosterone, a conversion of near silent channels to channels that exhibited normal gating behavior was observed (183).

The extracellular domains of ENaC subunits are ~450 residues in length, and have multiple sites that might be targets for cleavage by specific proteases. Which are the key proteases that modulate ENaC activity in epithelia? Both furin and prostasin regulate ENaC activity in epithelial cells. Hughey and coworkers have shown that the recombinant furin inhibitor α₁-antitrypsin Portland inhibits ENaC activity in a mouse cortical connecting duct cell line, suggesting that furin has an important role in the processing and activation of ENaC in the nephron (148). Both Kunitz-type inhibitors, as well as inhibition of prostasin expression by a small interfering RNA, were particularly effective in inhibiting ENaC activity in airway epithelial cells (36, 331).

SYNTAXIN 1A

The factors regulating ENaC delivery to the apical membrane in epithelial cells have not been fully defined. The SNARE proteins have been linked to directed exocytosis and intracellular trafficking in a number of tissues (114). A typical interaction involves binding of vesicle-associated v-SNARES to target membrane–associated t-SNARES. These interactions may be regulated by accessory proteins such as Munc 18 (310). The t-SNARE syntaxin-1A has been demonstrated to interact directly with ENaC in coimmunoprecipitation experiments, and overexpression of this protein inhibited ENaC expression in oocytes (265, 279). This effect was blocked by coexpression of Munc 18. These findings are interesting in that they implicate the SNARE proteins in the process of exocytosis of ENaC, but are somewhat counterintuitive in that overexpression of the trafficking partners results in downregulation of the channel. The results suggest that the balance of t- and v-SNAREs may regulate this process, and that overexpression alters this interaction in a negative fashion.

The direct interaction of syntaxin-1A and ENaC is also of interest in that it suggests there are cargo-specific interactions between SNARE proteins and apical-membrane resident proteins such as ENaC. In a series of studies, Condliffe and colleagues identified domain-specific interactions between carboxyl-termini of ENaC subunits and the H3 domain of syntaxin-1A. Interestingly, H3 was observed to decrease ENaC open probability, suggesting that SNARE proteins may regulate both channel exocytosis and gating (64, 65). If SNAREs are involved in the rapid activation of channels following exocytosis, a decrease in open probability would tend to counterregulate Na^+ entry.

CFTR

Patients with cystic fibrosis (CF) have been shown to have increased amiloride-sensitive transport in airway epithelia, suggesting increased ENaC activity (222). Indeed, increased activity of ENaC in airway epithelia has been proposed as one mechanism for the drying of airway fluids that promotes progression of airway disease. Lung-specific overexpression of beta ENaC results in a phenotype similar to CF airway disease in humans (223). CF is caused by function-impairing mutations in the CFTR (CF transmembrane conductance regulator), an ATP-dependent Cl^- channel (74). On the basis of studies comparing ENaC activity in the presence and absence of CFTR expressed in MDCK cells, Stutts and colleagues proposed that CFTR functions as a cAMP-dependent regulator of ENaC, and the absence of this function in CF airways explained the increased ENaC activity in CF patients (320, 321). Ling and coworkers demonstrated that inhibiting CFTR expression in a renal distal nephron cell line (A6) led to an increase in ENaC open probability (206). A number of studies in *Xenopus* oocytes or other overexpression systems have demonstrated that CFTR inhibits ENaC activity (53, 193, 320), although this has recently been disputed (144, 241). Studies have also shown that ENaC enhances the activity of CFTR due to an increase in the number of channels expressed at the plasma membrane as well as an increase in CFTR open probability (167).

It is unclear if the interaction between CFTR and ENaC is indirect or results from a direct physical interaction. Changes in the intracellular $[Cl^-]$, as well as electrochemical coupling have been proposed as potential mechanisms by which CFTR regulates ENaC (15, 144). One group has proposed that there are interactions between the regulatory domain of CFTR and ENaC (284), although the manner in which this interaction results in ENaC regulation is not clear. Moreover, ENaC-CFTR interactions appear to vary depending on tissue of expression. For example, in sweat ducts, CFTR enhances ENaC activity (266). Although both CFTR and ENaC are expressed in collecting duct principal cells, there have been no abnormalities of renal Na^+ handling described in CF patients. Overexpression of an alternative Cl^- channel, CLC-0, has also been shown to inhibit ENaC activity in response to cAMP in oocytes (15). Interestingly, coexpression of CLC-5, the endosomal channel linked to Dent's disease, results in decreased expression of ENaC, apparently through a trafficking defect (238). In summary, with current data it is difficult to explain the regu-

latory interactions between CFTR and ENaC solely on the basis of physical interactions or alterations in electrochemical driving forces or the intracellular Cl^- concentration. These regulatory interactions may reflect changes in ENaC open probability and surface expression and vary among differing tissues, which has led to the speculation that other proteins or factors may be critical for expression of functional CFTR–ENaC interactions (147).

METHYLTRANSFERASES

Methylation reactions have been implicated in the activation of ENaC by aldosterone (277, 318). Aldosterone stimulates carboxylmethylation of proteins and phospholipids, and inhibition of these reactions blunts the ENaC response to steroid stimulation (351). Two potential target proteins of methyltransferases have been identified, k-ras and the beta subunit of ENaC. Aldosterone induces k-ras in a *Xenopus* distal nephron cell line (A6) cells and this small G-protein is methylated by isoprenylcysteine carboxylmethyltransferase (PCMTase). PCMTase is not induced by aldosterone, but is regulated by the enzyme s-adenosyl-homocysteine hydrolase that is stimulated by aldosterone and results in increased activity of PCMTase (317). The enzyme (PCMTase) itself does not appear to stimulate ENaC, so it is unlikely to directly methylate the channel. Induction and processing of k-ras appear to be important for regulating ENaC in A6 cells, but it is not clear that this occurs in mammalian tissues (319). Direct methylation of beta ENaC has been demonstrated using a partially purified membrane preparation as a source of enzyme, but the enzyme itself has not been identified. Methylation of ENaC in planar lipid bilayers has been shown to lead to an increase in open probability of the channel (268). Methylation does not appear to play a role in basal channel activity.

CALCIUM

Increases in intracellular calcium have been shown to inhibit ENaC activity by several groups (109, 111, 155, 251). This appears to happen as a biphasic process with a very quick early response and a slower downregulation after 5 minutes (155). This is likely an indirect effect on the channel, as the activity of channels from cortical collecting ducts in excised patches exposed to increased cytosolic $[Ca^{2+}]$ was not altered (251). Activation of protein kinase C has been suggested to mediate the Ca^{2+}-dependent inhibition of ENaC, since this is known to decrease channel activity (205). A second intriguing possibility, related to the delayed effect of Ca^{2+} on ENaC activity, is Ca^{2+}-dependent recruitment of Nedd4-2 isoforms that possess a C2 domain to the plasma membrane mediated by the domain (158, 159), with a subsequent increase in channel retrieval from the apical membrane.

pH AND OXIDATIVE STRESS

Acidic intracellular pH, below 7.2, has been shown to decrease amiloride-sensitive Na^+ transport in isolated epithelial tissues, suggesting that intracellular pH may act as an intrinsic regulator of ENaC activity (54, 133, 251). In conditions of ischemia or hypoxia where intracellular pH might fall, activation of AMPK might act to decrease channel activity as noted previously (49). Hypoxia is known to decrease activity of ENaC through a decrease in channel expression in cultured type II alveolar cells, but the mechanism of this response is unknown. The effect of pH on channel activity appears to be direct. In excised, inside-out patches from apical membrane of rat cortical collecting tubule, a fall in pH from 7.4 to 6.4 resulted in a progressive and dramatic fall in channel open probability. The mechanism of this regulation is unknown. However, ENaC activity is clearly downregulated under cellular conditions where ATP is limiting (154). It has been proposed that ENaC may be sensitive to changes in intracellular redox potential through oxidation of intracellular cysteine residues (175).

NITRIC OXIDE

Several studies have shown that nitric oxide (NO) inhibits ENaC activity in both alveolar type II (AT II) cells and in cultured renal epithelial cells (80, 132, 160). This effect may be important in inflammatory conditions, such as acute respiratory distress syndrome, where NO levels may be elevated due to increased expression of inducible nitric oxide synthase (iNOS) (80). NO appears to inhibit channel open probability in a cGMP-dependent manner (160). Interestingly, aldosterone has also been shown to inhibit NO production from ATII cells, and this appears to be related to an effect of SGK1 (136). These results suggest a second, novel mechanism by which SGK1 could enhance ENaC activity through downregulation of iNOS activity and a decrease in NO inhibition of ENaC open probability.

LIPIDS

A number of membrane lipids and lipid intermediates have been shown to modify ENaC activity, often in complex ways. Inhibition of phospholipase A2 (PLA2) by the agent aristolochic acid reduced arachidonic acid (AA) levels and increased ENaC activity in both *Xenopus* oocytes and A6 cells in culture (50, 356). Direct application of arachidonic acid to rat cortical collecting duct markedly reduced ENaC activity (number of channels × open probability, NPo) in a dose-dependent manner. While this effect was not reproduced by application of a nonmetabolized analogue of AA, 5,8,11,14-eicosatetraynoic acid (ETYA), it was reproduced by the CYP-epoxygenase metabolite 11,12-epoxyeicosatrienoic acid (EET) (348). These results suggest that the AA effect is mediated by a CYP epoxygenase metabolite. In contrast, in A6 cells, current stimulation by PLA2 inhibition was blocked by ETYA, suggesting a direct effect of AA on the channel, rather than the effect of a metabolite. The effect of ETYA on ENaC was to reduce open probability (356). In oocytes, however, both AA and ETYA inhibited ENaC and this was due to an alteration in the number of surface channels. Analysis of ENaC surface expression showed downregulation of channels consistent with a trafficking effect mediated by both increased endocytosis and decreased exocytosis (50). All these experimental observations

indicate that PLA2 activity leads to increased AA levels that inhibit ENaC activity, but the precise molecular mechanisms remain in dispute.

Cellular phosphoinositides also affect ENaC function. Phosphatidylinositol-4,5-bisphosphate (PIP2) is a signaling molecule associated with a number of intracellular processes, including endocytosis (246) and exocytosis (138). It has also been implicated in activation of a number of ion channels, although the exact mechanisms are often not clear (138). Patch clamp studies have shown that anionic phospholipids, including PIP2 and PI-3,4,5-P3 can directly alter channel activity, presumably by binding to cationic sequences of beta and gamma ENaC (219, 367). A distinct PIP3-binding site has been identified in the initial part of the carboxyl-terminus of the gamma subunit (258). Phosphoinositides directly interact with the channel and alter its gating. Interestingly, increases in cellular PIP2 levels have been shown to increase surface expression of ENaC presumably by stimulating exocytosis (313). Kunzelmann and colleagues demonstrated that purinergic inhibition of ENaC by extracellular ATP in tracheal epithelia resulted in depletion of PIP2 from cells and appeared to require a PIP2-binding region of amino-terminus of the beta subunit (198). There are three isoforms of phosphoinositide-5-kinase, which produces PI-4,5-P2 from PI4P. These kinases have differing effects on cellular processes such as endocytosis (246). PIP2 may induce varying effects on ENaC function depending on the PI5K isoform that is activated or the spatial localization of kinases and phosphatases that regulate PIP2 activity within the cellular microenvironment. In summary, phosphoinositides functioning as signaling agents or by directly binding to ENaC affect channel activity.

INTRACELLULAR Na$^+$

Since ENaC is present in epithelia that generate a steep lumen-to-bath Na$^+$ gradient, it is potentially exposed to significant variations in both internal and external [Na$^+$]. ENaC has been shown to be modulated by both. Low levels of extracellular [Na$^+$] increase ENaC activity while elevated levels decrease activity, a process known as Na$^+$ self-inhibition (337). Cytoplasmic [Na$^+$] is usually maintained quite low through the action of the Na$^+$,K$^+$-ATPase on the basolateral surface of epithelial cells. Since the pump is normally functioning well below its maximum capacity, Na$^+$ entry into cells is the rate-limiting step for Na$^+$ reabsorption. Under conditions of rapid increases in ENaC activity, regulation may also be achieved through increases in the intracellular [Na$^+$], a process referred to as feedback inhibition. This phenomenon has been observed in epithelial cells and *Xenopus* oocytes (11, 155). Feedback inhibition in response to increased intracellular [Na$^+$] is a slow process that occurs over a period of minutes, in contrast to Na$^+$ self-inhibition, which occurs over seconds (111). Studies in oocytes indicated that this feedback inhibition was not readily seen in cells expressing ENaC with the Liddle's mutations that inhibit Nedd4-2 binding and ubiquitin-dependent internalization (176). This finding focused attention on

Nedd4-2 as the potential mediator of Na^+ feedback inhibition. In a series of studies in mouse mandibular duct cells, it was demonstrated that Na^+ feedback inhibition was dependent on Nedd4-2 and required binding of the second and third WW domains to carboxyl-termini of beta and gamma ENaC (134, 135). The mechanism by which increased intracellular Na^+ leads to altered interaction between Nedd4-2 and ENaC is not known.

EXTRACELLULAR Na^+

Rapid increases in the extracellular $[Na^+]$ inhibit ENaC activity, a process referred to as Na^+ self-inhibition. This phenomenon was originally observed in studies of native epithelial tissues in the setting of a rapid increase in extracellular Na^+ concentration (105). This process reflects a decrease in channel open probability and is not dependent on Na^+ influx (61, 110, 287, 336). Chaibi and Horisberger demonstrated that Na^+ self-inhibition is an intrinsic property of ENaC and can be abolished by treatment with extracellular proteases (61). Na^+ self-inhibition is a temperature-dependent phenomenon with a large activation energy, suggesting that a conformational change occurs in association with the inhibition of channel activity by extracellular Na^+ that is presumably initiated by Na^+ binding to an extracellular site (60, 61). Two His residues that have important roles in Na^+ self-inhibition have been identified within the amino-terminal part of the extracellular domain of the alpha and gamma subunits (287). A number of important questions remain to be addressed regarding the Na^+ self inhibition response, including the following:

1. Where are the external Na^+-binding site(s)?
2. What are the conformation changes that occur in response to Na^+ binding that result in a reduction in channel open probability?
3. How do external proteases, presumably by cleaving ENaC subunits, diminish Na^+ self-inhibition response?

PPARs

The peroxisome proliferator-activated receptors (PPARs) have been implicated in regulation of a wide variety of cellular processes. PPARγ is the pharmacologic target of thiazolidinediones (TZDs), which are used in management of hyperglycemia associated with type II diabetes mellitus (364). PPARγ is localized along the collecting duct in kidney (124), and it is known that a side effect of PPAR stimulation by TZDs is fluid retention (123). Recently, it has been shown that TZD-induced weight gain was prevented in mice by amiloride, or by deletion of the gene encoding PPARγ from collecting duct (123) tissue. In these studies, TZDs increased ENaC activity in collecting duct cells, and increased mRNA for gamma ENaC. These interesting results implicate PPARs in the regulation of transcription of at least one ENaC subunit transcription that apparently leads to increased ENaC activity.

Hormonal Regulation

ALDOSTERONE

The major hormones regulating ENaC activity in a broad variety of tissues are corticosteroids. ENaC regulation by steroids is the subject of Chapter 32, and will not be discussed in detail here. Although nongenomic actions of aldosterone have been described in vascular and nonabsorptive tissues (373), the bulk of the available evidence supports the notion that steroid regulation of ENaC in Na^+-absorptive organs including kidney, lung, and colon, is mediated by processes dependent on the transcription and translation of new proteins. This transcriptional activity is driven by translocation of the steroid receptor to the nucleus following binding to its cognate ligand, and binding to specific domains within the genome. Interestingly, ENaC regulation varies somewhat by tissue. Steroid regulation of ENaC activity is largely due to an increase in the number of active channels in the apical membrane, although there is evidence for an early effect on open probability as well (183). Increase in the number of active channels is not apparently a simple one-step procedure. An early increase in channels appears to be a trafficking event, with altered insertion or retrieval of already synthesized subunits (214, 227). A large part, but not all, of this effect is regulated by the aldosterone-induced protein SGK1 altering Nedd4-2–ENaC interactions and leading to increased membrane expression of the channel (Fig. 7) (101). Synthesis and delivery of new channel subunits can be detected somewhat later in the course of steroid action in responsive tissues, and, interestingly, also varies somewhat by tissue. In the kidney, the predominant induced subunit is alpha ENaC, while in the colon, the beta and gamma subunits are primarily induced (9). This is true at both the mRNA and protein levels. This phenomenon has been referred to as noncoordinate regulation, and suggests a degree of complexity of ENaC trafficking still not fully understood (349, 350).

VASOPRESSIN

Vasopressin has been shown to lead to stimulation of ENaC activity in kidney and a number of epithelial cell lines derived from the kidney (10, 111, 240). The response is relatively rapid, with a time course of minutes, and does not appear to depend on transcription or translation of new proteins, at least in its initial phase (111). Vasopressin binds to V_2 receptors on the basolateral surface of responsive epithelia, and activates adenylate cyclase. In almost all tissues studied, the action of vasopressin on Na^+ transport is fully reproduced by exogenous cAMP and is felt to be secondary to activation of protein kinase-A (PKA) (20, 90, 111). PKA has not been shown to phosphorylate any subunit of the channel, so its actions are thought to be indirect (20). There has been no consistent demonstration of an effect of PKA on ENaC open probability; thus it is likely that the primary effect of PKA on ENaC is to increase the number of channels at the plasma membrane. Indeed, there are now numerous demonstrations that PKA stimulation leads to an increase in surface expression of ENaC by biochemical, immunohistochemical, and electrophysiologic techniques (42, 43, 94, 187, 240). By analogy to its well-described effects on insertion of aquaporins in kidney cortex and medulla, it seems reasonable to expect that the primary event in PKA stimulation of ENaC is therefore exocytosis of channels into the apical membrane from some preexisting cytoplasmic pool. Strong evidence supports this likelihood. Studies by patch clamp indicate a rapid increase in the number of surface channels in response to cAMP stimulation (226). Stimulation of adenylate cyclase by forskolin or addition or cAMP analogs leads to an increase in biochemical and immunohistochemically measured apical channel number (187, 240), and this increase is temporally associated with an increase in apical membrane capacitance typical of exocytic events (42, 43). Butterworth and colleagues proposed in 2005 that cAMP stimulation leads to exocytic insertion of channels from a subapical recycling pool of channels that is distinct from constitutive turnover of the channel, exactly analogous to vasopressin regulation of water channels (Fig. 4) (42).

It is also possible that vasopressin, acting through cAMP, alters channel retrieval. In 2004, Snyder and colleagues described Nedd4-2 as a substrate for phosphorylation by PKA, and related cAMP regulation of ENaC to inhibition of Nedd4–ENaC interactions (307). These observations suggest also that basal SGK activation may be to some degree regulated by PKA activity. There is an obvious interplay between the hormonal regulation of ENaC by aldosterone and vasopressin, and it is possible that it occurs at the point of kinase regulation. However, the fact that aldosterone and vasopressin are synergistic and that epithelial Na$^+$ channels with Liddle's mutations, which should be unresponsive to Nedd4-2 inhibition, are still responsive to vasopressin stimulation (10), suggests that, at a minimum, different afferent pathways of ENaC regulation are involved in the actions of these two hormones. It is also interesting to note that a long-term (days) effect of vasopressin to stimulate transcription of ENaC subunits would clearly complement and be synergistic with aldosterone effects in situations of significant Na$^+$ avidity (89).

INSULIN

Insulin stimulates ENaC activity in renal epithelia (111, 352). The exact mechanism(s) of this effect are a subject of considerable controversy. This would seem odd, as it is clear that insulin stimulates phosphoinositide 3-kinase (PI3K), which in turn regulates the activity of 3-phosphoinositide–dependent kinase 1. The latter kinase phosphorylates SGK1 and converts it to an active form (255). This represents an obvious convergence point for the effects of aldosterone and insulin, which have been shown to be synergistic, on the stimulation of ENaC activ-

ity (31, 96, 255). Indeed, noise analysis indicates that the primary effect of insulin is to increase the number of active apical membrane channels with little effect on open probability (31). All these observations are consistent with insulin increasing ENaC activity via decreasing Nedd4-2–dependent retrieval.

It is possible, however, that the action of insulin is more complex. Stimulation of ENaC activity by insulin is quite rapid (minutes), and has been associated with exocytosis and delivery of preformed channels to the apical membrane in a PI3K-dependent manner (30). Additionally, it has been proposed that insulin may directly activate channels by phosphorylation that is dependent on protein kinase C (369), or by interaction with active metabolites of PI3K, phosphoinositol 3,4 phosphate and phosphoinositol 3,4,5 phosphate, both of which activate ENaC in excised patches (330). As with aldosterone and vasopressin, although a great deal has been learned about the regulation and trafficking of ENaC, the final control mechanisms by which hormones regulate the channel are complex and only partially understood.

Regulation by Mechanical Forces

Members of the ENaC/DEG family expressed in *C. elegans* are mechanosensitive ion channels. Early studies directed at examining the mechanosensitivity of ENaC produced conflicting results that have led to lively debates (269). Different responses of ENaC expressed in *Xenopus* oocytes to cell swelling or shrinking have been reported (13, 165). Application of a negative hydrostatic pressure to rat CCD cells by patch pipettes led to a variable increase in the open probability of Na$^+$ channels (253). An increase in hydrostatic pressure across planar lipid bilayers containing ENaC led to an increase in channel open probability with a decrease in amiloride sensitivity (12).

The distal nephron is subject to varying flow rates and volumes, dependent in part on extracellular volume status and use of pharmacologic agents, such as loop and thiazide diuretics. Changes in flow rates within the distal nephron affects ENaC activity. Micropuncture and microperfusion studies of distal nephron segments have demonstrated that increases in flow rates within the physiologic range led to increases in rates of net transepithelial Na$^+$ flux (93, 224, 278). Increases in tubular flow rates will expose channels to a variety of mechanical forces including hydrostatic pressure and shear stress. Carattino and coworkers demonstrated that ENaCs expressed in oocytes are activated when exposed to laminar shear stress at levels that are likely to be present at the surface of principal cells within collecting ducts exposed to flow rates within a physiologic range (51, 52). The increase in ENaC activity is due to an increase in channel open probability, as channels expressed in oocytes that have a high intrinsic open probability do not respond to shear stress. ENaCs are also expressed in vascular smooth muscle where they are also exposed to mechanical forces. Recent studies suggest that the channel functions as an arterial baroreceptor (85–87).

ENaC AND HUMAN DISORDERS

Liddle's syndrome is a rare, autosomal dominant disorder characterized by extracellular fluid volume expansion, hypertension, and hypokalemia. Mutations have been described in patients with this disorder in genes encoding the beta or gamma subunits of ENaC that result in either a truncation or frame shift within the intracellular carboxyl-termini, or amino acid substitutions within the PY motifs (129, 130, 298, 326). These mutations disrupt the binding of Nedd4-2 to ENaC, prevent Nedd4-2–dependent ubiquitination of ENaC subunits, and significantly retard rates of channel internalization from the plasma membrane and degradation (119, 172, 280, 297, 315). Liddle's mutations are also associated with an increase in channel open probability by mechanisms that are being defined. Given the increased half-life of channels at the plasma membrane, it is possible that the increase in open probability reflects a conversion of nonprocessed (i.e., noncleaved) channels to processed channels by proteases expressed at the plasma membrane, such as prostasin, or by proteases secreted into the urinary space.

It is likely that rare mutations that result in a Liddle's syndrome phenotype that are not associated with the PY motif will be identified. These mutations would result in either an increase in channel open probability or an increase in surface expression. For example, a beta-subunit N530K mutation has been described in a patient with diabetic nephropathy (236). This mutation is within a region where mutations, or chemical modification of substituted cysteine residues, lead to an increase in channel open probability (177, 289, 304). Common human epithelial Na^+-channel polymorphisms segregate with blood pressure, including βT594M and αA663T (7, 16), and are associated with altered channel activity (17, 73, 276). A mutation in the gene encoding the mineralocortoid receptor has been described as resulting in receptor activation by progesterone and early onset hypertension (112). Specific disorders of mineralocorticoid and glucocorticoid metabolism are also associated with increases in ENaC activity and hypertension.

A decrease in airway fluid volume has been observed in patients with CF. ENaCs are expressed throughout the airway. It has been suggested that the CFTR , a cAMP regulated Cl^- channel, inhibits ENaC activity in airway epithelia. In the absence of functional CFTR, ENaC activity is increased, although mechanisms by which this occurs are unclear, as discussed previously (206, 222, 320). The increase in ENaC activity in CF is thought to contribute to a reduced airway surface–liquid volume and associated increases in the viscosity of airway fluids and reduction in mucociliary clearance (35). A mouse model with overexpression of the ENaC beta subunit in the lung, leading to an increase in ENaC activity in the lung, exhibits a lung phenotype with characteristics that are remarkably similar to the CF lung phenotype (223).

ENaC loss-of-function mutations have been described in the autosomal recessive variant of type I pseudohypoaldosteronism. This disorder is characterized by volume depletion, hypotension, and hyperkalemia. Many of the mutations described to date are due to a frame shift or premature stop codon (57). A missense mutation within the beta subunit G37S led to the identification of an N-terminal domain that affects channel gating (120, 121). Mutations in the mineralocorticoid receptor have been described in the autosomal dominant variant of type I pseudohypoaldosteronism (113).

CONCLUSIONS

ENaCs have a key role in the regulation of extracellular fluid volume and blood pressure. Since the initial characterization in 1993 of ENaCs at a molecular level, investigators have identified key structural features within channel subunits and have defined mechanisms by which hormones and other factors regulate ENaC activity. Investigators have identified mutations within ENaC subunits that result in a gain or loss of function, which have profound effects on blood pressure. The identification of Liddle's syndrome mutations led to the elucidation of a network of proteins, including Sgk and Nedd4-2, which have important roles in the regulation of ENaC activity. Numerous groups have examined the contributions of polymorphisms within ENaC subunits in the development of salt-sensitive hypertension. However, the role of polymorphisms within proteins that regulate ENaC activity in salt-sensitive hypertension has received limited attention. The lack of even a low-resolution structure has limited our ability to advance our understanding of the mechanisms of ENaC selectivity and gating. Clearly, important questions regarding ENaC remain to be addressed.

References

1. Adachi M, Kitamura K, Miyoshi T, Narikiyo T, Iwashita K, Shiraishi N, Nonoguchi H, Tomita K. Activation of epithelial sodium channels by prostasin in *Xenopus* oocytes. *J Am Soc Nephrol* 2001;12:1114–1121.
2. Adams CM, Anderson MG, Motto DG, Price MP, Johnson WA, Welsh MJ. Ripped pocket and pickpocket, novel *Drosophila* DEG/ENaC subunits expressed in early development and in mechanosensory neurons. *J Cell Biol* 1998;140:143–152.
3. Adams CM, Snyder PM, Price MP, Welsh MJ. Protons activate brain Na+ channel 1 by inducing a conformational change that exposes a residue associated with neurodegeneration. *J Biol Chem* 1998;273:30204–30207.
4. Adams CM, Snyder PM, Welsh MJ. Interactions between subunits of the human epithelial sodium channel. *J Biol Chem* 1997;272:27295–27300.
5. Ahn YJ, Brooker DR, Kosari F, Harte BJ, Li J, Mackler SA, Kleyman TR. Cloning and functional expression of the mouse epithelial sodium channel. *Am J Physiol* 1999;277:F121–F129.
6. Alagem N, Yesylevskyy S, Reuveny E. The pore helix is involved in stabilizing the open state of inwardly rectifying K+ channels. *Biophys J* 2003;85:300–312.
7. Ambrosius WT, Bloem LJ, Zhou L, Rebhun JF, Snyder PM, Wagner MA, Guo C, Pratt JH. Genetic variants in the epithelial sodium channel in relation to aldosterone and potassium excretion and risk for hypertension. *Hypertension* 1999;34:631–637.
8. Amuzescu B, Segal A, Flonta ML, Simaels J, Van Driessche W. Zinc is a voltage-dependent blocker of native and heterologously expressed epithelial Na+ channels. *Pflugers Arch* 2003;446:69–77.

9. Asher C, Wald H, Rossier BC, Garty H. Aldosterone-induced increase in the abundance of Na+ channel subunits. *Am J Physiol* 1996;271:C605–C611.
10. Auberson M, Hoffmann-Pochon N, Vandewalle A, Kellenberger S, Schild L. Epithelial Na+ channel mutants causing Liddle's syndrome retain ability to respond to aldosterone and vasopressin. *Am J Physiol Renal Physiol* 2003;285:F459–F471.
11. Awayda MS. Regulation of the epithelial Na(+) channel by intracellular Na(1). *Am J Physiol* 1999;277:C216–C224.
12. Awayda MS, Ismailov II, Berdiev BK, Benos DJ. A cloned renal epithelial Na+ channel protein displays stretch activation in planar lipid bilayers. *Am J Physiol* 1995;268:C1450–C1459.
13. Awayda MS, Subramanyam M. Regulation of the epithelial Na+ channel by membrane tension. *J Gen Physiol* 1998;112:97–111.
14. Babini E, Geisler HS, Siba M, Grunder S. A new subunit of the epithelial Na+ channel identifies regions involved in Na+ self-inhibition. *J Biol Chem* 2003;278:28418–28426.
15. Bachhuber T, Konig J, Voelcker T, Murle B, Schreiber R, Kunzelmann K. Cl2 interference with the epithelial Na+ channel ENaC. *J Biol Chem* 2005;280:31587–31594.
16. Baker EH, Dong YB, Sagnella GA, Rothwell M, Onipinla AK, Markandu ND, Cappuccio FP, Cook DG, Persu A, Corvol P, Jeunemaitre X, Carter ND, MacGregor GA. Association of hypertension with T594M mutation in beta subunit of epithelial sodium channels in black people resident in London. *Lancet* 1998;351:1388–1392.
17. Baker EH, Duggal A, Dong Y, Ireson NJ, Wood M, Markandu ND, MacGregor GA. Amiloride, a specific drug for hypertension in black people with T594M variant? *Hypertension* 2002;40:13–17.
18. Barker PM, Nguyen MS, Gatzy JT, Grubb B, Norman H, Hummler E, Rossier B, Boucher RC, Koller B. Role of gammaENaC subunit in lung liquid clearance and electrolyte balance in newborn mice. Insights into perinatal adaptation and pseudohypoaldosteronism. *J Clin Invest* 1998;102:1634–1640.
19. Becchetti A, Malik B, Yue G, Duchatelle P, Al-Khalili O, Kleyman TR, Eaton DC. Phosphatase inhibitors increase the open probability of ENaC in A6 cells. *Am J Physiol Renal Physiol* 2002;283:F1030–F1045.
20. Benos DJ, Awayda MS, Ismailov II, Johnson JP. Structure and function of amiloride-sensitive Na+ channels. *J Membr Biol* 1995;143:1–18.
21. Benos DJ, Mandel LJ, Simon SA. Cationic selectivity and competition at the sodium entry site in frog skin. *J Gen Physiol* 1980;76:233–247.
22. Benos DJ, Saccomani G, Brenner BM, Sariban-Sohraby S. Purification and characterization of the amiloride-sensitive sodium channel from A6 cultured cells and bovine renal papilla. *Proc Natl Acad Sci U S A* 1986;83:8525–8529.
23. Benos DJ, Saccomani G, Sariban-Sohraby S. The epithelial sodium channel. Subunit number and location of the amiloride binding site. *J Biol Chem* 1987;262:10613–10618.
24. Bentley PJ. Amiloride: a potent inhibitor of sodium transport across the toad bladder. *J Physiol* 1968;195:317–330.
25. Berdiev BK, Jovov B, Tucker WC, Naren AP, Fuller CM, Chapman ER, Benos DJ. ENaC subunit–subunit interactions and inhibition by syntaxin 1A. *Am J Physiol Renal Physiol* 2004;286:F1100–F1106.
26. Berdiev BK, Karlson KH, Jovov B, Ripoll PJ, Morris R, Loffing-Cueni D, Halpin P, Stanton BA, Kleyman TR, Ismailov II. Subunit stoichiometry of a core conduction element in a cloned epithelial amiloride-sensitive Na+ channel. *Biophys J* 1998;75:2292–2301.
27. Berdiev BK, Latorre R, Benos DJ, Ismailov II. Actin modifies Ca2+ block of epithelial Na+ channels in planar lipid bilayers. *Biophys J* 2001;80:2176–2186.
28. Berneche S, Roux B. A gate in the selectivity filter of potassium channels. *Structure* 2005;13:591–600.
29. Bhalla V, Daidie D, Li H, Pao AC, LaGrange LP, Wang J, Vandewalle A, Stockand JD, Staub O, Pearce D. SGK1 regulates ubiquitin ligase Nedd4-2 by inducing interaction with 14-3-3. *Mol Endocrinol* 2005;19:3073–3084.
30. Blazer-Yost BL, Esterman MA, Vlahos CJ. Insulin-stimulated trafficking of ENaC in renal cells requires PI 3-kinase activity. *Am J Physiol Cell Physiol* 2003;284:C1645–C1653.
31. Blazer-Yost BL, Liu X, Helman SI. Hormonal regulation of ENaCs: insulin and aldosterone. *Am J Physiol* 1998;274:C1373–C1379.
32. Booth RE, Stockand JD. Targeted degradation of ENaC in response to PKC activation of the ERK1/2 cascade. *Am J Physiol Renal Physiol* 2003;284:F938–F947.
33. Booth RE, Tong Q, Medina J, Snyder PM, Patel P, Stockand JD. A region directly following the second transmembrane domain in gamma ENaC is required for normal channel gating. *J Biol Chem* 2003;278:41367–41379.
34. Borok Z, Liebler JM, Lubman RL, Foster MJ, Zhou B, Li X, Zabski SM, Kim KJ, Crandall ED. Na transport proteins are expressed by rat alveolar epithelial type I cells. *Am J Physiol Lung Cell Mol Physiol* 2002;282:L599–L608.
35. Boucher RC. Regulation of airway surface liquid volume by human airway epithelia. *Pflugers Arch* 2003;445:495–498.
36. Bridges RJ, Newton BB, Pilewski JM, Devor DC, Poll CT, Hall RL. Na+ transport in normal and CF human bronchial epithelial cells is inhibited by BAY 39-9437. *Am J Physiol Lung Cell Mol Physiol* 2001;281:L16–L23.
37. Brooker DR, Kozak CA, Kleyman TR. Epithelial sodium channel genes Scnn1b and Scnn1g are closely linked on distal mouse chromosome 7. *Genomics* 1995;29:784–786.
38. Brouard M, Casado M, Djelidi S, Barrandon Y, Farman N. Epithelial sodium channel in human epidermal keratinocytes: expression of its subunits and relation to sodium transport and differentiation. *J Cell Sci* 1999;112:3343–3352.
39. Bruns JB, Hu B, Ahn YJ, Sheng S, Hughey RP, Kleyman TR. Multiple epithelial Na+ channel domains participate in subunit assembly. *Am J Physiol Renal Physiol* 2003;285: F600–F609.
40. Bubien JK, Watson B, Khan MA, Langloh AL, Fuller CM, Berdiev B, Tousson A, Benos DJ. Expression and regulation of normal and polymorphic epithelial sodium channel by human lymphocytes. *J Biol Chem* 2001;276:8557–8566.
41. Burch LH, Talbot CR, Knowles MR, Canessa CM, Rossier BC, Boucher RC. Relative expression of the human epithelial Na+ channel subunits in normal and cystic fibrosis airways. *Am J Physiol* 1995;269:C511–C518.
42. Butterworth MB, Edinger RS, Johnson JP, Frizzell RA. Acute ENaC stimulation by cAMP in a kidney cell line is mediated by exocytic insertion from a recycling channel pool. *J Gen Physiol* 2005;125:81–101.
43. Butterworth MB, Helman SI, Els WJ. cAMP-sensitive endocytic trafficking in A6 epithelia. *Am J Physiol Cell Physiol* 2001;280:C752–C762.
44. Caldwell RA, Boucher RC, Stutts MJ. Neutrophil elastase activates near-silent epithelial Na+-channels and increases airway epithelial Na+ transport. *Am J Physiol Lung Cell Mol Physiol* 2005;288:L813–L819.
45. Caldwell RA, Boucher RC, Stutts MJ. Serine protease activation of near-silent epithelial Na+ channels. *Am J Physiol Cell Physiol* 2004;286:C190–C194.
46. Canessa CM, Horisberger JD, Rossier BC. Epithelial sodium channel related to proteins involved in neurodegeneration. *Nature* 1993;361:467–470.
47. Canessa CM, Merillat AM, Rossier BC. Membrane topology of the epithelial sodium channel in intact cells. *Am J Physiol* 1994;267:C1682–C1690.
48. Canessa CM, Schild L, Buell G, Thorens B, Gautschi I, Horisberger JD, Rossier BC. Amiloride-sensitive epithelial Na+ channel is made of three homologous subunits. *Nature* 1994;367:463–467.
49. Carattino MD, Edinger RS, Grieser HJ, Wise R, Neumann D, Schlattner U, Johnson JP, Kleyman TR, Hallows KR. Epithelial sodium channel inhibition by AMP-activated protein kinase in oocytes and polarized renal epithelial cells. *J Biol Chem* 2005;280:17608–17616.
50. Carattino MD, Hill WG, Kleyman TR. Arachidonic acid regulates surface expression of epithelial sodium channels. *J Biol Chem* 2003;278:36202–36213.
51. Carattino MD, Sheng S, Kleyman TR. Epithelial Na+ channels are activated by laminar shear stress. *J Biol Chem* 2004;279:4120–4126.
52. Carattino MD, Sheng S, Kleyman TR. Mutations in the pore region modify epithelial sodium channel gating by shear stress. *J Biol Chem* 2004;280:4393–4401.
53. Chabot H, Vives MF, Dagenais A, Grygorczyk C, Berthiaume Y, Grygorczyk R. Downregulation of epithelial sodium channel (ENaC) by CFTR co-expressed in *Xenopus* oocytes is independent of Cl^- conductance. *J Membr Biol* 1999;169:175–188.
54. Chalfant ML, Denton JS, Berdiev BK, Ismailov II, Benos DJ, Stanton BA. Intracellular H+ regulates the alpha-subunit of ENaC, the epithelial Na+ channel. *Am J Physiol* 1999;276: C477–C486.
55. Chalfant ML, Denton JS, Langloh AL, Karlson KH, Loffing J, Benos DJ, Stanton BA. The NH(2) terminus of the epithelial sodium channel contains an endocytic motif. *J Biol Chem* 1999;274:32889–32896.
56. Chalfant ML, Peterson-Yantorno K, O'Brien TG, Civan MM. Regulation of epithelial Na+ channels from M-1 cortical collecting duct cells. *Am J Physiol* 1996;271:F861–F870.
57. Chang SS, Grunder S, Hanukoglu A, Rosler A, Mathew PM, Hanukoglu I, Schild L, Lu Y, Shimkets RA, Nelson-Williams C, Rossier BC, Lifton RP. Mutations in subunits of the epithelial sodium channel cause salt wasting with hyperkalaemic acidosis, pseudohypoaldosteronism type 1. *Nat Genet* 1996;12:248–253.
58. Cheng C, Prince LS, Snyder PM, Welsh MJ. Assembly of the epithelial Na+ channel evaluated using sucrose gradient sedimentation analysis. *J Biol Chem* 1998;273:22693–22700.
59. Choi MJ, Fernandez PC, Patnaik A, Coupaye-Gerard B, D'Andrea D, Szerlip H, Kleyman TR. Brief report: trimethoprim-induced hyperkalemia in a patient with AIDS. *N Engl J Med* 1993;328:703–706.
60. Chraibi A, Horisberger JD. Dual effect of temperature on the human epithelial Na+ channel. *Pflugers Arch* 2003;447:316–320.
61. Chraibi A, Horisberger JD. Na self-inhibition of human epithelial Na channel: temperature dependence and effect of extracellular proteases. *J Gen Physiol* 2002;120:133–145.
62. Chraibi A, Vallet V, Firsov D, Hess SK, Horisberger JD. Protease modulation of the activity of the epithelial sodium channel expressed in *Xenopus* oocytes. *J Gen Physiol* 1998;111:127–138.
63. Chraibi A, Verdumo C, Merillat AM, Rossier BC, Horisberger JD, Hummler E. Functional analyses of a N-terminal splice variant of the alpha subunit of the epithelial sodium channel. *Cell Physiol Biochem* 2001;11:115–122.
64. Condliffe SB, Carattino MD, Frizzell RA, Zhang H. Syntaxin 1A regulates ENaC via domain-specific interactions. *J Biol Chem* 2003;278:12796–12804.
65. Condliffe SB, Zhang H, Frizzell RA. Syntaxin 1A regulates ENaC channel activity. *J Biol Chem* 2004;279:10085–10092.
66. Copeland SJ, Berdiev BK, Ji HL, Lockhart J, Parker S, Fuller CM, Benos DJ. Regions in the carboxy terminus of alpha-bENaC involved in gating and functional effects of actin. *Am J Physiol Cell Physiol* 2001;281:C231–C240.
67. Corey DP, Garcia-Anoveros J. Mechanosensation and the DEG/ENaC ion channels. *Science* 1996;273:323–324.
68. Coscoy S, de Weille JR, Lingueglia E, Lazdunski M. The pre-transmembrane 1 domain of acid-sensing ion channels participates in the ion pore. *J Biol Chem* 1999;274:10129–10132.
69. Coscoy S, Lingueglia E, Lazdunski M, Barbry P. The Phe-Met-Arg-Phe-amide-activated sodium channel is a tetramer. *J Biol Chem* 1998;273:8317–8322.
70. Cottrell GA. The first peptide-gated ion channel. *J Exp Biol* 1997;200:2377–2386.
71. Couloigner V, Fay M, Djelidi S, Farman N, Escoubet B, Runembert I, Sterkers O, Friedlander G, Ferrary E. Location and function of the epithelial Na channel in the cochlea. *Am J Physiol Renal Physiol* 2001;280:F214–F222.
72. Cucu D, Simaels J, Van Driessche W, Zeiske W. External Ni2 + and ENaC in A6 cells: Na+ current stimulation by competition at a binding site for amiloride and Na+. *J Membr Biol* 2003;194:33–45.
73. Cui Y, Su YR, Rutkowski M, Reif M, Menon AG, Pun RY. Loss of protein kinase C inhibition in the beta-T594M variant of the amiloride-sensitive Na+ channel. *Proc Natl Acad Sci U S A* 1997;94:9962–9966.
74. Dalemans W, Barbry P, Champigny G, Jallat S, Dott K, Dreyer D, Crystal RG, Pavirani A, Lecocq JP, Lazdunski M. Altered chloride ion channel kinetics associated with the delta F508 cystic fibrosis mutation. *Nature* 1991;354:526–528.
75. Darboux I, Lingueglia E, Pauron D, Barbry P, Lazdunski M. A new member of the amiloride-sensitive sodium channel family in *Drosophila melanogaster* peripheral nervous system. *Biochem Biophys Res Commun* 1998;246:210–216.

76. De La Rosa DA, Li H, Canessa CM. Effects of aldosterone on biosynthesis, traffic, functional expression of epithelial sodium channels in a6 cells. *J Gen Physiol* 2002;119:427–442.
77. Debonneville C, Flores SY, Kamynina E, Plant PJ, Tauxe C, Thomas MA, Munster C, Chraibi A, Pratt JH, Horisberger JD, Pearce D, Loffing J, Staub O. Phosphorylation of Nedd4-2 by Sgk1 regu-lates epithelial Na(+) channel cell surface expression. *EMBO J* 2001;20:7052–7059.
78. Demo SD, Yellen G. Ion effects on gating of the Ca(2+)-activated K+ channel correlate with occupancy of the pore. *Biophys J* 1992;61:639–648.
79. Diakov A, Korbmacher C. A novel pathway of epithelial sodium channel activation involves a serum- and glucocorticoid-inducible kinase consensus motif in the C terminus of the channel's alpha-subunit. *J Biol Chem* 2004;279:38134–38142.
80. Ding JW, Dickie J, O'Brodovich H, Shintani Y, Rafii B, Hackam D, Marunaka Y, Rotstein OD. Inhibition of amiloride-sensitive sodium-channel activity in distal lung epithelial cells by nitric oxide. *Am J Physiol* 1998;274:L378–L387.
81. Dinudom A, Fotia AB, Lefkowitz RJ, Young JA, Kumar S, Cook DI. The kinase Grk2 regulates Nedd4/Nedd4-2–dependent control of epithelial Na+ channels. *Proc Natl Acad Sci U S A* 2004;101:11886–11890.
82. Domene C, Grottesi A, Sansom MS. Filter flexibility and distortion in a bacterial inward rectifier K+ channel: simulation studies of KirBac1.1. *Biophys J* 2004;87:256–267.
83. Domene C, Sansom MS. Potassium channel, ions, water: simulation studies based on the high resolution x-ray structure of KcsA. *Biophys J* 2003;85:2787–2800.
84. Doyle DA, Morais Cabral J, Pfuetzner RA, Kuo A, Gulbis JM, Cohen SL, Chait BT, MacKinnon R. The structure of the potassium channel: molecular basis of K+ conduction and selectivity. *Science* 1998;280:69–77.
85. Drummond HA, Gebremedhin D, Harder DR. Degenerin/epithelial Na+ channel proteins: components of a vascular mechanosensor. *Hypertension* 2004;44:643–648.
86. Drummond HA, Price MP, Welsh MJ, Abboud FM. A molecular component of the arterial baroreceptor mechanotransducer. *Neuron* 1998;21:1435–1441.
87. Drummond HA, Welsh MJ, Abboud FM. ENaC subunits are molecular components of the arterial baroreceptor complex. *Ann N Y Acad Sci* 2001;940:42–47.
88. Duc C, Farman N, Canessa CM, Bonvalet JP, Rossier BC. Cell-specific expression of epithelial sodium channel alpha, beta, and gamma subunits in aldosterone-responsive epithelia from the rat: localization by in situ hybridization and immunocytochemistry. *J Cell Biol* 1994;127:1907–1921.
89. Ecelbarger CA, Kim GH, Terris J, Masilamani S, Mitchell C, Reyes I, Verbalis JG, Knepper MA. Vasopressin-mediated regulation of epithelial sodium channel abundance in rat kidney. *Am J Physiol Renal Physiol* 2000;279:F46–F53.
90. Ecelbarger CA, Kim GH, Wade JB, Knepper MA. Regulation of the abundance of renal sodium transporters and channels by vasopressin. *Exp Neurol* 2001;171:227–234.
91. Eisenman G. Cation selective glass electrodes and their mode of operation. *Biophys J* 1962;2:259–323.
92. Ellgaard L, Molinari M, Helenius A. Setting the standards: quality control in the secretory pathway. *Science* 1999;286:1882–1888.
93. Engbretson BG, Stoner LC. Flow-dependent potassium secretion by rabbit cortical collecting tubule in vitro. *Am J Physiol* 1987;253:F896–F903.
94. Erlij D, De Smet P, Mesotten D, Van Driessche W. Forskolin increases apical sodium conductance in cultured toad kidney cells (A6) by stimulating membrane insertion. *Pflugers Arch* 1999;438:195–204.
95. Eskandari S, Snyder PM, Kreman M, Zampighi GA, Welsh MJ, Wright EM. Number of subunits comprising the epithelial sodium channel. *J Biol Chem* 1999;274:27281–27286.
96. Faletti CJ, Perrotti N, Taylor SI, Blazer-Yost BL. sgk: an essential convergence point for peptide and steroid hormone regulation of ENaC-mediated Na+ transport. *Am J Physiol Cell Physiol* 2002;282:C494–C500.
97. Feldman RD. Deactivation of vasodilator responses by GRK2 overexpression: a mechanism or the mechanism for hypertension? *Mol Pharmacol* 2002;61:707–709.
98. Fewell SW, Travers KJ, Weissman JS, Brodsky JL. The action of molecular chaperones in the early secretory pathway. *Annu Rev Genet* 2001;35:149–191.
99. Firsov D, Gautschi I, Merillat AM, Rossier BC, Schild L. The heterotetrameric architecture of the epithelial sodium channel (ENaC). *EMBO J* 1998;17:344–352.
100. Firsov D, Robert-Nicoud M, Gruender S, Schild L, Rossier BC. Mutational analysis of cysteine-rich domains of the epithelium sodium channel (ENaC). Identification of cysteines essential for channel expression at the cell surface. *J Biol Chem* 1999;274:2743–2749.
101. Flores SY, Loffing-Cueni D, Kamynina E, Daidie D, Gerbex C, Chabanel S, Dudler J, Loffing J, Staub O. Aldosterone-induced serum and glucocorticoid-induced kinase 1 expression is accompanied by Nedd4-2 phosphorylation and increased Na+ transport in cortical collecting duct cells. *J Am Soc Nephrol* 2005;16:2279–2287.
102. Fotia AB, Dinudom A, Shearwin KE, Koch JP, Korbmacher C, Cook DI, Kumar S. The role of individual Nedd4-2 (KIAA0439) WW domains in binding and regulating epithelial sodium channels. *FASEB J* 2003;17:70–72.
103. Frindt G, Masilamani S, Knepper MA, Palmer LG. Activation of epithelial Na channels during short-term Na deprivation. *Am J Physiol Renal Physiol* 2001;280:F112–F118.
104. Frindt G, Palmer LG. Na channels in the rat connecting tubule. *Am J Physiol Renal Physiol* 2004;286:F669–F674.
105. Fuchs W, Larsen EH, Lindemann B. Current-voltage curve of sodium channels and concentration dependence of sodium permeability in frog skin. *J Physiol* 1977;267:137–166.
106. Fuller CM, Awayda MS, Arrate MP, Bradford AL, Morris RG, Canessa CM, Rossier BC, Benos DJ. Cloning of a bovine renal epithelial Na+ channel subunit. *Am J Physiol* 1995;269: C641–C654.
107. Fyfe GK, Canessa CM. Subunit composition determines the single channel kinetics of the epithelial sodium channel. *J Gen Physiol* 1998;112:423–432.
108. Fyfe GK, Zhang P, Canessa CM. The second hydrophobic domain contributes to the kinetic properties of epithelial sodium channels. *J Biol Chem* 1999;274:36415–36421.
109. Garty H, Asher C, Yeger O. Direct inhibition of epithelial Na+ channels by a pH-dependent interaction with calcium, and by other divalent ions. *J Membr Biol* 1987;95:151–162.
110. Garty H, Benos DJ. Characteristics and regulatory mechanisms of the amiloride-blockable Na+ channel. *Physiol Rev* 1988;68:309–373.
111. Garty H, Palmer LG. Epithelial sodium channels: function, structure, and regulation. *Physiol Rev* 1997;77:359–396.
112. Geller DS, Farhi A, Pinkerton N, Fradley M, Moritz M, Spitzer A, Meinke G, Tsai FT, Sigler PB, Lifton RP. Activating mineralocorticoid receptor mutation in hypertension exacerbated by pregnancy. *Science* 2000;289:119–123.
113. Geller DS, Rodriguez-Soriano J, Vallo Boado A, Schifter S, Bayer M, Chang SS, Lifton RP. Mutations in the mineralocorticoid receptor gene cause autosomal dominant pseudohypoaldosteronism type I. *Nat Genet* 1998;19:279–281.
114. Gerst JE. SNAREs and SNARE regulators in membrane fusion and exocytosis. *Cell Mol Life Sci* 1999;55:707–734.
115. Gilmore ES, Stutts MJ, Milgram SL. SRC family kinases mediate epithelial Na+ channel inhibition by endothelin. *J Biol Chem* 2001;276:42610–42617.
116. Giorgetti A, Nair AV, Codega P, Torre V, Carloni P. Structural basis of gating of CNG channels. *FEBS Lett* 2005;579:1968–1972.
117. Goldstein O, Asher C, Garty H. Cloning and induction by low NaCl intake of avian intestine Na+ channel subunits. *Am J Physiol* 1997;272:C270–C277.
118. Goodman MB, Ernstrom GG, Chelur DS, O'Hagan R, Yao CA, Chalfie M. MEC-2 regulates *C. elegans* DEG/ENaC channels needed for mechanosensation. *Nature* 2002;415:1039–1042.
119. Goulet CC, Volk KA, Adams CM, Prince LS, Stokes JB, Snyder PM. Inhibition of the epithelial Na+ channel by interaction of Nedd4 with a PY motif deleted in Liddle's syndrome. *J Biol Chem* 1998;273:30012–30017.
120. Grunder S, Firsov D, Chang SS, Jaeger NF, Gautschi I, Schild L, Lifton RP, Rossier BC. A mutation causing pseudohypoaldosteronism type 1 identifies a conserved glycine that is involved in the gating of the epithelial sodium channel. *EMBO J* 1997;16:899–907.
121. Grunder S, Jaeger NF, Gautschi I, Schild L, Rossier BC. Identification of a highly conserved sequence at the N-terminus of the epithelial Na+ channel alpha subunit involved in gating. *Pflugers Arch* 1999;438:709–715.
122. Grunder S, Muller A, Ruppersberg JP. Developmental and cellular expression pattern of epithelial sodium channel alpha, beta and gamma subunits in the inner ear of the rat. *Eur J Neurosci* 2001;13:641–648.
123. Guan Y, Hao C, Cha DR, Rao R, Lu W, Kohan DE, Magnuson MA, Redha R, Zhang Y, Breyer MD. Thiazolidinediones expand body fluid volume through PPARgamma stimulation of ENaC-mediated renal salt absorption. *Nat Med* 2005;11:861–866.
124. Guan Y, Zhang Y, Davis L, Breyer MD. Expression of peroxisome proliferator-activated receptors in urinary tract of rabbits and humans. *Am J Physiol* 1997;273:F1013–F1022.
125. Guipponi M, Vuagniaux G, Wattenhofer M, Shibuya K, Vazquez M, Dougherty L, Scamuffa N, Guida E, Okui M, Rossier C, Hancock M, Buchet K, Reymond A, Hummler E, Marzella PL, Kudoh J, Shimizu N, Scott HS, Antonarakis SE, Rossier BC. The transmembrane serine protease (TMPRSS3) mutated in deafness DFNB8/10 activates the epithelial sodium channel (ENaC) in vitro. *Hum Mol Genet* 2002;11:2829–2836.
126. Hager H, Kwon TH, Vinnikova AK, Masilamani S, Brooks HL, Frokiaer J, Knepper MA, Nielsen S. Immunocytochemical and immunoelectron microscopic localization of alpha-, beta-, and gamma-ENaC in rat kidney. *Am J Physiol Renal Physiol* 2001;280:F1093–F1106.
127. Hamilton KL, Eaton DC. Single-channel recordings from amiloride-sensitive epithelial sodium channel. *Am J Physiol* 1985;249:C200–C207.
128. Hamilton KL, Eaton DC. Single-channel recordings from two types of amiloride-sensitive epithelial Na+ channels. *Membr Biochem* 1986;6:149–171.
129. Hansson JH, Nelson-Williams C, Suzuki H, Schild L, Shimkets R, Lu Y, Canessa C, Iwasaki T, Rossier B, Lifton RP. Hypertension caused by a truncated epithelial sodium channel gamma subunit: genetic heterogeneity of Liddle syndrome. *Nat Genet* 1995;11:76–82.
130. Hansson JH, Schild L, Lu Y, Wilson TA, Gautschi I, Shimkets R, Nelson-Williams C, Rossier BC, Lifton RP. A de novo missense mutation of the beta subunit of the epithelial sodium channel causes hypertension and Liddle syndrome, identifying a proline-rich segment critical for regulation of channel activity. *Proc Natl Acad Sci U S A* 1995;92:11495–11499.
131. Hanwell D, Ishikawa T, Saleki R, Rotin D. Trafficking and cell surface stability of the epithelial Na+ channel expressed in epithelial Madin–Darby canine kidney cells. *J Biol Chem* 2002;277:9772–9779.
132. Hardiman KM, McNicholas-Bevensee CM, Fortenberry J, Myles CT, Malik B, Eaton DC, Matalon S. Regulation of amiloride-sensitive Na(+) transport by basal nitric oxide. *Am J Respir Cell Mol Biol* 2004;30:720–728.
133. Harvey BJ, Thomas SR, Ehrenfeld J. Intracellular pH controls cell membrane Na+ and K+ conductances and transport in frog skin epithelium. *J Gen Physiol* 1988;92:767–791.
134. Harvey KF, Dinudom A, Cook DI, Kumar S. The Nedd4-like protein KIAA0439 is a potential regulator of the epithelial sodium channel. *J Biol Chem* 2001;276:8597–8601.
135. Harvey KF, Dinudom A, Komwatana P, Jolliffe CN, Day ML, Parasivam G, Cook DI, Kumar S. All three WW domains of murine Nedd4 are involved in the regulation of epithelial sodium channels by intracellular Na+. *J Biol Chem* 1999;274:12525–12530.
136. Helms MN, Yu L, Malik B, Kleinhenz DJ, Hart CM, Eaton DC. Role of SGK1 in nitric oxide inhibition of ENaC in Na+-transporting epithelia. *Am J Physiol Cell Physiol* 2005;289: C717–C726.
137. Henley JR, Krueger EW, Oswald BJ, McNiven MA. Dynamin-mediated internalization of caveolae. *J Cell Biol* 1998;141:85–99.
138. Hilgemann DW, Feng S, Nasuhoglu C. The complex and intriguing lives of PIP2 with ion channels and transporters. *Sci STKE* 2001;2001:RE19.
139. Hill WG, An B, Johnson JP. Endogenously expressed epithelial sodium channel is present in lipid rafts in A6 cells. *J Biol Chem* 2002;277:33541–33544.
140. Hille B. *Ion Channels of Excitable Membranes*. Sunderland, MA: Sinauer Associates, 2001.
141. Ho K, Nichols CG, Lederer WJ, Lytton J, Vassilev PM, Kanazirska MV, Hebert SC. Cloning and expression of an inwardly rectifying ATP-regulated potassium channel. *Nature* 1993;362: 31–38.
142. Hodgkin AL, Huxley AF. A quantitative description of membrane current and its application to conduction and excitability in nerve. *J Physiol* 1952;117:500–544.

143. Hong K, Driscoll M. A transmembrane domain of the putative channel subunit MEC-4 influences mechanotransduction and neurodegeneration in *C. elegans*. *Nature* 1994;367: 470–473.
144. Horisberger JD. ENaC-CFTR interactions: the role of electrical coupling of ion fluxes explored in an epithelial cell model. *Pflugers Arch* 2003;445:522–528.
145. Horisberger JD, Chraibi A. Epithelial sodium channel: a ligand-gated channel? *Nephron Physiol* 2004;96:37–41.
146. Huang M, Chalfie M. Gene interactions affecting mechanosensory transduction in *Caenorhabditis elegans*. *Nature* 1994;367:467–470.
147. Huang P, Gilmore E, Kultgen P, Barnes P, Milgram S, Stutts MJ. Local regulation of cystic fibrosis transmembrane regulator and epithelial sodium channel in airway epithelium. *Proc Am Thorac Soc* 2004;1:33–37.
148. Hughey RP, Bruns JB, Kinlough CL, Harkleroad KL, Tong Q, Carattino MD, Johnson JP, Stockand JD, Kleyman TR. Epithelial sodium channels are activated by furin-dependent proteolysis. *J Biol Chem* 2004;279:18111–18114.
149. Hughey RP, Bruns JB, Kinlough CL, Kleyman TR. Distinct pools of epithelial sodium channels are expressed at the plasma membrane. *J Biol Chem* 2004;279:48491–48494.
150. Hughey RP, Mueller GM, Bruns JB, Kinlough CL, Poland PA, Harkleroad KL, Carattino MD, Kleyman TR. Maturation of the epithelial Na+ channel involves proteolytic processing of the alpha- and gamma-subunits. *J Biol Chem* 2003;278:37073–37082.
151. Hummler E, Barker P, Gatzy J, Beermann F, Verdumo C, Schmidt A, Boucher R, Rossier BC. Early death due to defective neonatal lung liquid clearance in alpha-ENaC–deficient mice. *Nat Genet* 1996;12:325–328.
152. Hummler E, Barker P, Talbot C, Wang Q, Verdumo C, Grubb B, Gatzy J, Burnier M, Horisberger JD, Beermann F, Boucher R, Rossier BC. A mouse model for the renal salt-wasting syndrome pseudohypoaldosteronism. *Proc Natl Acad Sci U S A* 1997;94: 11710–11715.
153. Ichimura T, Yamamura H, Sasamoto K, Tominaga Y, Taoka M, Kakiuchi K, Shinkawa T, Takahashi N, Shimada S, Isobe T. 14-3-3 proteins modulate the expression of epithelial Na+ channels by phosphorylation-dependent interaction with Nedd4-2 ubiquitin ligase. *J Biol Chem* 2005;280:13187–13194.
154. Ishikawa T, Jiang C, Stutts MJ, Marunaka Y, Rotin D. Regulation of the epithelial Na+ channel by cytosolic ATP. *J Biol Chem* 2003;278:38276–38286.
155. Ishikawa T, Marunaka Y, Rotin D. Electrophysiological characterization of the rat epithelial Na+ channel (rENaC) expressed in MDCK cells. Effects of Na+ and Ca2+. *J Gen Physiol* 1998;111:825–846.
156. Ismailov II, Berdiev BK, Bradford AL, Awayda MS, Fuller CM, Benos DJ. Associated proteins and renal epithelial Na+ channel function. *J Membr Biol* 1996;149:123–132.
157. Ismailov II, Kieber-Emmons T, Lin C, Berdiev BK, Shlyonsky VG, Patton HK, Fuller CM, Worrell R, Zuckerman JB, Sun W, Eaton DC, Benos DJ, Kleyman TR. Identification of an amiloride binding domain within the alpha-subunit of the epithelial Na+ channel. *J Biol Chem* 1997;272:21075–21083.
158. Itani OA, Campbell JR, Herrero J, Snyder PM, Thomas CP. Alternate promoters and variable splicing lead to hNedd4-2 isoforms with a C2 domain and varying number of WW domains. *Am J Physiol Renal Physiol* 2003;285:F916–F929.
159. Itani OA, Stokes JB, Thomas CP. Nedd4-2 isoforms differentially associate with ENaC and regulate its activity. *Am J Physiol Renal Physiol* 2005;289:F334–F346.
160. Jain L, Chen XJ, Brown LA, Eaton DC. Nitric oxide inhibits lung sodium transport through a cGMP-mediated inhibition of epithelial cation channels. *Am J Physiol* 1998;274:L475–L484.
161. Jain L, Chen XJ, Malik B, Al-Khalili O, Eaton DC. Antisense oligonucleotides against the alpha-subunit of ENaC decrease lung epithelial cation-channel activity. *Am J Physiol* 1999;276:L1046–L1051.
162. Jensik P, Holbird D, Cox T. Cloned bullfrog skin sodium (fENaC) and xENaC subunits hybridize to form functional sodium channels. *J Comp Physiol [B]* 2002;172:569–576.
163. Jeziorski MC, Green KA, Sommerville J, Cottrell GA. Cloning and expression of a FM-RFamide-gated Na(+) channel from *Helisoma trivolvis* and comparison with the native neuronal channel. *J Physiol* 2000;526 Pt 1:13–25.
164. Ji HL, Fuller CM, Benos DJ. Intrinsic gating mechanisms of epithelial sodium channels. *Am J Physiol Cell Physiol* 2002;283:C646–C650.
165. Ji HL, Fuller CM, Benos DJ. Osmotic pressure regulates alpha beta gamma-rENaC expressed in *Xenopus* oocytes. *Am J Physiol* 1998;275:C1182–C1190.
166. Ji HL, Parker S, Langloh AL, Fuller CM, Benos DJ. Point mutations in the post-M2 region of human alpha-ENaC regulate cation selectivity. *Am J Physiol Cell Physiol* 2001;281:C64–C74.
167. Jiang Q, Li J, Dubroff R, Ahn YJ, Foskett JK, Engelhardt J, Kleyman TR. Epithelial sodium channels regulate cystic fibrosis transmembrane conductance regulator chloride channels in *Xenopus* oocytes. *J Biol Chem* 2000;275:13266–13274.
168. Jiang Y, Lee A, Chen J, Ruta V, Cadene M, Chait BT, MacKinnon R. X-ray structure of a voltage-dependent K+ channel. *Nature* 2003;423:33–41.
169. Kahle KT, Wilson FH, Leng Q, Lalioti MD, O'Connell AD, Dong K, Rapson AK, MacGregor GG, Giebisch G, Hebert SC, Lifton RP. WNK4 regulates the balance between renal NaCl reabsorption and K+ secretion. *Nat Genet* 2003;35:372–376.
170. Kamynina E, Debonneville C, Bens M, Vandewalle A, Staub O. A novel mouse Nedd4 protein suppresses the activity of the epithelial Na+ channel. *FASEB J* 2001;15:204–214.
171. Kamynina E, Staub O. Concerted action of ENaC, Nedd4-2, and Sgk1 in transepithelial Na(+) transport. *Am J Physiol Renal Physiol* 2002;283:F377–F387.
172. Kamynina E, Tauxe C, Staub O. Distinct characteristics of two human Nedd4 proteins with respect to epithelial Na(+) channel regulation. *Am J Physiol Renal Physiol* 2001;281: F469–F477.
173. Kashlan OB, Sheng S, Kleyman TR. On the interaction between amiloride and its putative alpha-subunit epithelial Na+ channel binding site. *J Biol Chem* 2005;280:26206–26215.
174. Kellenberger S, Auberson M, Gautschi I, Schneeberger E, Schild L. Permeability properties of ENaC selectivity filter mutants. *J Gen Physiol* 2001;118:679–692.
175. Kellenberger S, Gautschi I, Pfister Y, Schild L. Intracellular thiol-mediated modulation of epithelial sodium channel activity. *J Biol Chem* 2005;280:7739–7747.
176. Kellenberger S, Gautschi I, Rossier BC, Schild L. Mutations causing Liddle syndrome reduce sodium-dependent downregulation of the epithelial sodium channel in the *Xenopus* oocyte expression system. *J Clin Invest* 1998;101:2741–2750.
177. Kellenberger S, Gautschi I, Schild L. An external site controls closing of the epithelial Na+ channel ENaC. *J Physiol* 2002;543:413–424.
178. Kellenberger S, Gautschi I, Schild L. Mutations in the epithelial Na+ channel ENaC outer pore disrupt amiloride block by increasing its dissociation rate. *Mol Pharmacol* 2003;64:848–856.
179. Kellenberger S, Gautschi I, Schild L. A single point mutation in the pore region of the epithelial Na+ channel changes ion selectivity by modifying molecular sieving. *Proc Natl Acad Sci U S A* 1999;96:4170–4175.
180. Kellenberger S, Hoffmann-Pochon N, Gautschi I, Schneeberger E, Schild L. On the molecular basis of ion permeation in the epithelial Na+ channel. *J Gen Physiol* 1999;114: 13–30.
181. Kellenberger S, Schild L. Epithelial sodium channel/degenerin family of ion channels: a variety of functions for a shared structure. *Physiol Rev* 2002;82:735–767.
182. Kelly O, Lin C, Ramkumar M, Saxena NC, Kleyman TR, Eaton DC. Characterization of an amiloride binding region in the alpha-subunit of ENaC. *Am J Physiol Renal Physiol* 2003;285: F1279–F1290.
183. Kemendy AE, Kleyman TR, Eaton DC. Aldosterone alters the open probability of amiloride-blockable sodium channels in A6 epithelia. *Am J Physiol* 1992;263:C825–C837.
184. Khakh BS, Lester HA. Dynamic selectivity filters in ion channels. *Neuron* 1999;23:653–658.
185. Kieber-Emmons T, Lin C, Foster MH, Kleyman TR. Antiidiotypic antibody recognizes an amiloride binding domain within the alpha subunit of the epithelial Na+ channel. *J Biol Chem* 1999;274:9648–9655.
186. Kleyman TR, Cragoe EJ Jr. Cation transport probes: the amiloride series. *Methods Enzymol* 1990;191:739–755.
187. Kleyman TR, Ernst SA, Coupaye-Gerard B. Arginine vasopressin and forskolin regulate apical cell surface expression of epithelial Na+ channels in A6 cells. *Am J Physiol* 1994;266: F506–F511.
188. Kleyman TR, Kraehenbuhl JP, Ernst SA. Characterization and cellular localization of the epithelial Na1 channel. Studies using an anti-Na+ channel antibody raised by an antiidiotypic route. *J Biol Chem* 1991;266:3907–3915.
189. Kleyman TR, Roberts C, Ling BN. A mechanism for pentamidine-induced hyperkalemia: inhibition of distal nephron sodium transport. *Ann Intern Med* 1995;122:103–106.
190. Kleyman TR, Sheng S, Kosari F, Kieber-Emmons T. Mechanism of action of amiloride: a molecular prospective. *Semin Nephrol* 1999;19:524–532.
191. Kleyman TR, Zuckerman JB, Middleton P, McNulty KA, Hu B, Su X, An B, Eaton DC, Smith PR. Cell surface expression and turnover of the alpha-subunit of the epithelial sodium channel. *Am J Physiol Renal Physiol* 2001;281:F213–F221.
192. Koefoed-Johnson V, Ussing HH. The nature of frog skin potential. *Acta Physiol Scand* 1958;42:298–308.
193. Konstas AA, Koch JP, Korbmacher C. cAMP-dependent activation of CFTR inhibits the epithelial sodium channel (ENaC) without affecting its surface expression. *Pflugers Arch* 2003;445:513–521.
194. Kopito RR. ER quality control: the cytoplasmic connection. *Cell* 1997;88:427–430.
195. Kosari F, Sheng S, Li J, Mak DO, Foskett JK, Kleyman TR. Subunit stoichiometry of the epithelial sodium channel. *J Biol Chem* 1998;273:13469–13474.
196. Kretz O, Barbry P, Bock R, Lindemann B. Differential expression of RNA and protein of the three pore-forming subunits of the amiloride-sensitive epithelial sodium channel in taste buds of the rat. *J Histochem Cytochem* 1999;47:51–64.
197. Krishtal O. The ASICs: signaling molecules? Modulators? *Trends Neurosci* 2003;26:477–483.
198. Kunzelmann K, Bachhuber T, Regeer R, Markovich D, Sun J, Schreiber R. Purinergic inhibition of the epithelial Na+ transport via hydrolysis of PIP2. *FASEB J* 2005;19: 142–143.
199. Kuo A, Gulbis JM, Antcliff JF, Rahman T, Lowe ED, Zimmer J, Cuthbertson J, Ashcroft FM, Ezaki T, Doyle DA. Crystal structure of the potassium channel KirBac1.1 in the closed state. *Science* 2003;300:1922–1926.
200. Langloh AL, Berdiev B, Ji HL, Keyser K, Stanton BA, Benos DJ. Charged residues in the M2 region of alpha-hENaC play a role in channel conductance. *Am J Physiol Cell Physiol* 2000;278: C277–C291.
201. Lebowitz J, Edinger RS, An B, Perry CJ, Onate S, Kleyman TR, Johnson JP. Ikappab kinase-beta (ikkbeta) modulation of epithelial sodium channel activity. *J Biol Chem* 2004;279:41985–41990.
202. Li J, Sheng S, Perry CJ, Kleyman TR. Asymmetric organization of the pore region of the epithelial sodium channel. *J Biol Chem* 2003;278:13867–13874.
203. Li JH, Lindemann B. Competitive blocking of epithelial sodium channels by organic cations: the relationship between macroscopic and microscopic inhibition constants. *J Membr Biol* 1983;76:235–251.
204. Lin H, Mann KJ, Starostina E, Kinser RD, Pikielny CW. A *Drosophila* DEG/ENaC channel subunit is required for male response to female pheromones. *Proc Natl Acad Sci U S A* 2005; 102:12831–12836.
205. Ling BN, Eaton DC. Effects of luminal Na+ on single Na+ channels in A6 cells, a regulatory role for protein kinase C. *Am J Physiol* 1989;256:F1094–F1103.
206. Ling BN, Zuckerman JB, Lin C, Harte BJ, McNulty KA, Smith PR, Gomez LM, Worrell RT, Eaton DC, Kleyman TR. Expression of the cystic fibrosis phenotype in a renal amphibian epithelial cell line. *J Biol Chem* 1997;272:594–600.
207. Lingueglia E, Champigny G, Lazdunski M, Barbry P. Cloning of the amiloride-sensitive FMRFamide peptide-gated sodium channel. *Nature* 1995;378:730–733.
208. Lingueglia E, Renard S, Waldmann R, Voilley N, Champigny G, Plass H, Lazdunski M, Barbry P. Different homologous subunits of the amiloride-sensitive Na+ channel are differently regulated by aldosterone. *J Biol Chem* 1994;269:13736–13739.
209. Lingueglia E, Voilley N, Waldmann R, Lazdunski M, Barbry P. Expression cloning of an epithelial amiloride-sensitive Na+ channel. A new channel type with homologies to *Caenorhabditis elegans* degenerins. *FEBS Lett* 1993;318:95–99.

210. Liu J, Siegelbaum SA. Change of pore helix conformational state upon opening of cyclic nucleotide-gated channels. *Neuron* 2000;28:899–909.

211. Liu L, Johnson WA, Welsh MJ. *Drosophila* DEG/ENaC pickpocket genes are expressed in the tracheal system, where they may be involved in liquid clearance. *Proc Natl Acad Sci U S A* 2003; 100:2128–2133.

212. Liu L, Leonard AS, Motto DG, Feller MA, Price MP, Johnson WA, Welsh MJ. Contribution of *Drosophila* DEG/ENaC genes to salt taste. *Neuron* 2003;39:133–146.

213. Loffing J, Pietri L, Aregger F, Bloch-Faure M, Ziegler U, Meneton P, Rossier BC, Kaissling B. Differential subcellular localization of ENaC subunits in mouse kidney in response to high- and low-Na diets. *Am J Physiol Renal Physiol* 2000;279:F252–F258.

214. Loffing J, Zecevic M, Feraille E, Kaissling B, Asher C, Rossier BC, Firestone GL, Pearce D, Verrey F. Aldosterone induces rapid apical translocation of ENaC in early portion of renal collecting system: possible role of SGK. *Am J Physiol Renal Physiol* 2001;280: F675–F682.

215. Lott JS, Coddington-Lawson SJ, Teesdale-Spittle PH, McDonald FJ. A single WW domain is the predominant mediator of the interaction between the human ubiquitin-protein ligase Nedd4 and the human epithelial sodium channel. *Biochem J* 2002;361:481–488.

216. Lu T, Ting AY, Mainland J, Jan LY, Schultz PG, Yang J. Probing ion permeation and gating in a K+ channel with backbone mutations in the selectivity filter. *Nat Neurosci* 2001;4:239–246.

217. Ludwig M, Bolkenius U, Wickert L, Marynen P, Bidlingmaier F. Structural organisation of the gene encoding the alpha-subunit of the human amiloride-sensitive epithelial sodium channel. *Hum Genet* 1998;102:576–581.

218. Ma D, Zerangue N, Lin YF, Collins A, Yu M, Jan YN, Jan LY. Role of ER export signals in controlling surface potassium channel numbers. *Science* 2001;291:316–319.

219. Ma HP, Saxena S, Warnock DG. Anionic phospholipids regulate native and expressed epithelial sodium channel (ENaC). *J Biol Chem* 2002;277:7641–7644.

220. MacKinnon R. Determination of the subunit stoichiometry of a voltage-activated potassium channel. *Nature* 1991;350:232–235.

221. Malik B, Schlanger L, Al-Khalili O, Bao HF, Yue G, Price SR, Mitch WE, Eaton DC. ENaC degradation in A6 cells by the ubiquitin-proteosome proteolytic pathway. *J Biol Chem* 2001;276:12903–12910.

222. Mall M, Bleich M, Greger R, Schreiber R, Kunzelmann K. The amiloride-inhibitable Na+ conductance is reduced by the cystic fibrosis transmembrane conductance regulator in normal but not in cystic fibrosis airways. *J Clin Invest* 1998;102:15–21.

223. Mall M, Grubb BR, Harkema JR, O'Neal WK, Boucher RC. Increased airway epithelial Na+ absorption produces cystic fibrosis-like lung disease in mice. *Nat Med* 2004;10:487–493.

224. Malnic G, Berliner RW, Giebisch G. Flow dependence of K+ secretion in cortical distal tubules of the rat. *Am J Physiol* 1989;256:F932–F941.

225. Mano I, Driscoll M. DEG/ENaC channels: a touchy superfamily that watches its salt. *Bioessays* 1999;21:568–578.

226. Marunaka Y, Eaton DC. Effects of vasopressin and cAMP on single amiloride-blockable Na channels. *Am J Physiol* 1991;260:C1071–C1084.

227. Masilamani S, Kim GH, Mitchell C, Wade JB, Knepper MA. Aldosterone-mediated regulation of ENaC alpha, beta, and gamma subunit proteins in rat kidney. *J Clin Invest* 1999;104: R19–23.

228. Matalon S, Lazrak A, Jain L, Eaton DC. Invited review: biophysical properties of sodium channels in lung alveolar epithelial cells. *J Appl Physiol* 2002;93:1852–1859.

229. Matsushita K, McCray PB Jr, Sigmund RD, Welsh MJ, Stokes JB. Localization of epithelial sodium channel subunit mRNAs in adult rat lung by in situ hybridization. *Am J Physiol* 1996;271:L332–L339.

230. Matulef K, Zagotta WN. Cyclic nucleotide-gated ion channels. *Annu Rev Cell Dev Biol* 2003;19:23–44.

231. May A, Puoti A, Gaeggeler HP, Horisberger JD, Rossier BC. Early effect of aldosterone on the rate of synthesis of the epithelial sodium channel alpha subunit in A6 renal cells. *J Am Soc Nephrol* 1997;8:1813–1822.

232. McCormick JA, Bhalla V, Pao AC, Pearce D. SGK1: a rapid aldosterone-induced regulator of renal sodium reabsorption. *Physiology (Bethesda)* 2005;20:134–139.

233. McDonald FJ, Price MP, Snyder PM, Welsh MJ. Cloning and expression of the beta- and gamma-subunits of the human epithelial sodium channel. *Am J Physiol* 1995;268:C1157–C1163.

234. McDonald FJ, Snyder PM, McCray PB Jr, Welsh MJ. Cloning, expression, and tissue distribution of a human amiloride-sensitive Na+ channel. *Am J Physiol* 1994;266:L728–L734.

235. McDonald FJ, Yang B, Hrstka RF, Drummond HA, Tarr DE, McCray PB Jr, Stokes JB, Welsh MJ, Williamson RA. Disruption of the beta subunit of the epithelial Na+ channel in mice: hyperkalemia and neonatal death associated with a pseudohypoaldosteronism phenotype. *Proc Natl Acad Sci U S A* 1999;96:1727–1731.

236. Melander O, Orho M, Fagerudd J, Bengtsson K, Groop PH, Mattiasson I, Groop L, Hulthen UL. Mutations and variants of the epithelial sodium channel gene in Liddle's syndrome and primary hypertension. *Hypertension* 1998;31:1118–1124.

237. Mirshahi M, Nicolas C, Mirshahi S, Golestaneh N, d'Hermies F, Agarwal MK. Immunochemical analysis of the sodium channel in rodent and human eye. *Exp Eye Res* 1999;69:21–32.

238. Mo L, Wills NK. ClC-5 chloride channel alters expression of the epithelial sodium channel (ENaC). *J Membr Biol* 2004;202:21–37.

239. Mohan S, Bruns JR, Weixel KM, Edinger RS, Bruns JB, Kleyman TR, Johnson JP, Weisz OA. Differential current decay profiles of epithelial sodium channel subunit combinations in polarized renal epithelial cells. *J Biol Chem* 2004;279:32071–32078.

240. Morris RG, Schafer JA. cAMP increases density of ENaC subunits in the apical membrane of MDCK cells in direct proportion to amiloride-sensitive Na(+) transport. *J Gen Physiol* 2002;120:71–85.

241. Nagel G, Barbry P, Chabot H, Brochiero E, Hartung K, Grygorczyk R. CFTR fails to inhibit the epithelial sodium channel ENaC, when expressed in *Xenopus laevis* oocytes. *J Physiol* 2005;5643:671–682.

242. Naray-Fejes-Toth A, Snyder PM, Fejes-Toth G. The kidney-specific WNK1 isoform is induced by aldosterone and stimulates epithelial sodium channel-mediated Na+ transport. *Proc Natl Acad Sci U S A* 2004;101:17434–17439.

243. Nielsen J, Kwon TH, Masilamani S, Beutler K, Hager H, Nielsen S, Knepper MA. Sodium transporter abundance profiling in kidney: effect of spironolactone. *Am J Physiol Renal Physiol* 2002;283:F923–F933.

244. Oh P, McIntosh DP, Schnitzer JE. Dynamin at the neck of caveolae mediates their budding to form transport vesicles by GTP-driven fission from the plasma membrane of endothelium. *J Cell Biol* 1998;141:101–114.

245. Oh Y, Benos DJ. Single-channel characteristics of a purified bovine renal amiloride-sensitive Na+ channel in planar lipid bilayers. *Am J Physiol* 1993;264:C1489–C1499.

246. Padron D, Wang YJ, Yamamoto M, Yin H, Roth MG. Phosphatidylinositol phosphate 5-kinase Ibeta recruits AP-2 to the plasma membrane and regulates rates of constitutive endocytosis. *J Cell Biol* 2003;162:693–701.

247. Palmer LG. Epithelial Na channels: the nature of the conducting pore. *Ren Physiol Biochem* 1990;13:51–58.

248. Palmer LG. Ion selectivity of the apical membrane Na channel in the toad urinary bladder. *J Membr Biol* 1982;67:91–98.

249. Palmer LG, Edelman IS, Lindemann B. Current-voltage analysis of apical sodium transport in toad urinary bladder: effects of inhibitors of transport and metabolism. *J Membr Biol* 1980;57:59–71.

250. Palmer LG, Frindt G. Conductance and gating of epithelial Na channels from rat cortical collecting tubule. Effects of luminal Na and Li. *J Gen Physiol* 1988;92:121–138.

251. Palmer LG, Frindt G. Effects of cell Ca and pH on Na channels from rat cortical collecting tubule. *Am J Physiol* 1987;253:F333–F339.

252. Palmer LG, Frindt G. Epithelial sodium channels: characterization by using the patch-clamp technique. *Fed Proc* 1986;45:2708–2712.

253. Palmer LG, Frindt G. Gating of Na channels in the rat cortical collecting tubule: effects of voltage and membrane stretch. *J Gen Physiol* 1996;107:35–45.

254. Palmer LG, Sackin H, Frindt G. Regulation of Na1 channels by luminal Na+ in rat cortical collecting tubule. *J Physiol* 1998;509 (Pt 1):151–162.

255. Pearce D. The role of SGK1 in hormone-regulated sodium transport. *Trends Endocrinol Metab* 2001;12:341–347.

256. Plant PJ, Lafont F, Lecat S, Verkade P, Simons K, Rotin D. Apical membrane targeting of Nedd4 is mediated by an association of its C2 domain with annexin XIIIb. *J Cell Biol* 2000;149:1473–1484.

257. Plant PJ, Yeger H, Staub O, Howard P, Rotin D. The C2 domain of the ubiquitin protein ligase Nedd4 mediates Ca2+-dependent plasma membrane localization. *J Biol Chem* 1997;272:32329–32336.

258. Pochynyuk O, Staruschenko A, Tong Q, Medina J, Stockand JD. Identification of a functional phosphatidylinositol 3,4,5-trisphosphate binding site in the epithelial Na+ channel. *J Biol Chem* 2005;280:37565–37571.

259. Poet M, Tauc M, Lingueglia E, Cance P, Poujeol P, Lazdunski M, Counillon L. Exploration of the pore structure of a peptide-gated Na+ channel. *EMBO J* 2001;20:5595–5602.

260. Pradervand S, Barker PM, Wang Q, Ernst SA, Beermann F, Grubb BR, Burnier M, Schmidt A, Bindels RJ, Gatzy JT, Rossier BC, Hummler E. Salt restriction induces pseudohypoaldosteronism type 1 in mice expressing low levels of the beta-subunit of the amiloride-sensitive epithelial sodium channel. *Proc Natl Acad Sci U S A* 1999; 96:1732–1737.

261. Price MP, Snyder PM, Welsh MJ. Cloning and expression of a novel human brain Na+ channel. *J Biol Chem* 1996;271:7879–7882.

262. Prince LS, Welsh MJ. Cell surface expression and biosynthesis of epithelial Na+ channels. *Biochem J* 1998;336:705–710.

263. Proks P, Antcliff JF, Ashcroft FM. The ligand-sensitive gate of a potassium channel lies close to the selectivity filter. *EMBO Rep* 2003;4:70–75.

264. Puoti A, May A, Canessa CM, Horisberger JD, Schild L, Rossier BC. The highly selective low-conductance epithelial Na channel of *Xenopus laevis* A6 kidney cells. *Am J Physiol* 1995;269:C188–C197.

265. Qi J, Peters KW, Liu C, Wang JM, Edinger RS, Johnson JP, Watkins SC, Frizzell RA. Regulation of the amiloride-sensitive epithelial sodium channel by syntaxin 1A. *J Biol Chem* 1999;274:30345–30348.

266. Reddy MM, Quinton PM. Functional interaction of CFTR and ENaC in sweat glands. *Pflugers Arch* 2003;445:499–503.

267. Renard S, Lingueglia E, Voilley N, Lazdunski M, Barbry P. Biochemical analysis of the membrane topology of the amiloride-sensitive Na+ channel. *J Biol Chem* 1994;269: 12981–12986.

268. Rokaw MD, Wang JM, Edinger RS, Weisz OA, Hui D, Middleton P, Shlyonsky V, Berdiev BK, Ismailov I, Eaton DC, Benos DJ, Johnson JP. Carboxylmethylation of the beta subunit of xENaC regulates channel activity. *J Biol Chem* 1998;273:28746–28751.

269. Rossier BC. Mechanosensitivity of the epithelial sodium channel (ENaC): controversy or pseudocontroversy? *J Gen Physiol* 1998;112:95–96.

270. Rossier BC, Pradervand S, Schild L, Hummler E. Epithelial sodium channel and the control of sodium balance: interaction between genetic and environmental factors. *Annu Rev Physiol* 2002;64:877–897.

271. Rotin D, Bar-Sagi D, O'Brodovich H, Merilainen J, Lehto VP, Canessa CM, Rossier BC, Downey GP. An SH3 binding region in the epithelial Na+ channel (alpha rENaC) mediates its localization at the apical membrane. *EMBO J* 1994;13:4440–4450.

272. Rotin D, Kanelis V, Schild L. Trafficking and cell surface stability of ENaC. *Am J Physiol Renal Physiol* 2001;281:F391–F399.

273. Roux B. Ion conduction and selectivity in K(+) channels. *Annu Rev Biophys Biomol Struct* 2005;34:153–171.

274. Rubera I, Loffing J, Palmer LG, Frindt G, Fowler-Jaeger N, Sauter D, Carroll T, McMahon A, Hummler E, Rossier BC. Collecting duct-specific gene inactivation of alphaENaC in the mouse kidney does not impair sodium and potassium balance. *J Clin Invest* 2003;112: 554–565.

275. Salako LA, Smith AJ. Effects of the diuretics, triamterene and mersalyl on active sodium transport mechanisms in isolated frog skin. *Br J Pharmacol* 1971;41:552–557.

276. Samaha FF, Rubenstein RC, Yan W, Ramkumar M, Levy DI, Ahn YJ, Sheng S, Kleyman TR. Functional polymorphism in the carboxyl terminus of the alpha-subunit of the human epithelial sodium channel. *J Biol Chem* 2004;279:23900–23907.

277. Sariban-Sohraby S, Burg M, Wiesmann WP, Chiang PK, Johnson JP. Methylation increases sodium transport into A6 apical membrane vesicles: possible mode of aldosterone action. *Science* 1984;225:745–746.

278. Satlin LM, Sheng S, Woda CB, Kleyman TR. Epithelial Na(+) channels are regulated by flow. *Am J Physiol Renal Physiol* 2001;280:F1010–F1018.

279. Saxena S, Quick MW, Tousson A, Oh Y, Warnock DG. Interaction of syntaxins with the amiloride-sensitive epithelial sodium channel. *J Biol Chem* 1999;274:20812–20817.

280. Schild L, Lu Y, Gautschi I, Schneeberger E, Lifton RP, Rossier BC. Identification of a PY motif in the epithelial Na channel subunits as a target sequence for mutations causing channel activation found in Liddle syndrome. *EMBO J* 1996;15:2381–2387.

281. Schild L, Schneeberger E, Gautschi I, Firsov D. Identification of amino acid residues in the alpha, beta, and gamma subunits of the epithelial sodium channel (ENaC) involved in amiloride block and ion permeation. *J Gen Physiol* 1997;109:15–26.

282. Schlanger LE, Kleyman TR, Ling BN. K(+)-sparing diuretic actions of trimethoprim: inhibition of Na+ channels in A6 distal nephron cells. *Kidney Int* 1994;45:1070–1076.

283. Schnizler M, Mastroberardino L, Reifarth F, Weber WM, Verrey F, Clauss W. cAMP sensitivity conferred to the epithelial Na+ channel by alpha-subunit cloned from guinea-pig colon. *Pflugers Arch* 2000;439:579–587.

284. Schreiber R, Hopf A, Mall M, Greger R, Kunzelmann K. The first-nucleotide binding domain of the cystic-fibrosis transmembrane conductance regulator is important for inhibition of the epithelial Na+ channel. *Proc Natl Acad Sci U S A* 1999;96:5310–5315.

285. Seebohm G, Westenskow P, Lang F, Sanguinetti MC. Mutation of colocalized residues of the pore helix and transmembrane segments S5 and S6 disrupt deactivation and modify inactivation of KCNQ1 K+ channels. *J Physiol* 2005;563:359–368.

286. Segal A, Cucu D, Van Driessche W, Weber WM. Rat ENaC expressed in *Xenopus laevis* oocytes is activated by cAMP and blocked by Ni(2+). *FEBS Lett* 2002;515:177–183.

287. Sheng S, Bruns JB, Kleyman TR. Extracellular histidine residues crucial for Na+ self-inhibition of epithelial Na+ channels. *J Biol Chem* 2004;279:9743–9749.

288. Sheng S, Li J, McNulty KA, Avery D, Kleyman TR. Characterization of the selectivity filter of the epithelial sodium channel. *J Biol Chem* 2000;275:8572–8581.

289. Sheng S, Li J, McNulty KA, Kieber-Emmons T, Kleyman TR. Epithelial sodium channel pore region: structure and role in gating. *J Biol Chem* 2001;276:1326–1334.

290. Sheng S, McNulty KA, Harvey JM, Kleyman TR. Second transmembrane domains of ENaC subunits contribute to ion permeation and selectivity. *J Biol Chem* 2001;276:44091–44098.

291. Sheng S, Perry CJ, Kashlan OB, Kleyman TR. Side chain orientation of residues lining the selectivity filter of epithelial Na+ channels. *J Biol Chem* 2005;280:8513–8522.

292. Sheng S, Perry CJ, Kleyman TR. External nickel inhibits epithelial sodium channel by binding to histidine residues within the extracellular domains of alpha and gamma subunits and reducing channel open probability. *J Biol Chem* 2002;277:50098–50111.

293. Sheng S, Perry CJ, Kleyman TR. Extracellular Zn2+ activates epithelial Na+ channels by eliminating Na+ self-inhibition. *J Biol Chem* 2004;279:31687–31696.

294. Shi H, Asher C, Chigaev A, Yung Y, Reuveny E, Seger R, Garty H. Interactions of beta and gamma ENaC with Nedd4 can be facilitated by an ERK-mediated phosphorylation. *J Biol Chem* 2002;277:13539–13547.

295. Shi H, Asher C, Yung Y, Kligman L, Reuveny E, Seger R, Garty H. Casein kinase 2 specifically binds to and phosphorylates the carboxy termini of ENaC subunits. *Eur J Biochem* 2002;269:4551–4558.

296. Shimkets RA, Lifton R, Canessa CM. In vivo phosphorylation of the epithelial sodium channel. *Proc Natl Acad Sci U S A* 1998;95:3301–3305.

297. Shimkets RA, Lifton RP, Canessa CM. The activity of the epithelial sodium channel is regulated by clathrin-mediated endocytosis. *J Biol Chem* 1997;272:25537–25541.

298. Shimkets RA, Warnock DG, Bositis CM, Nelson-Williams C, Hansson JH, Schambelan M, Gill JR Jr, Ulick S, Milora RV, Findling JW, et al. Liddle's syndrome: heritable human hypertension caused by mutations in the beta subunit of the epithelial sodium channel. *Cell* 1994;79:407–414.

299. Shipway A, Danahay H, Williams JA, Tully DC, Backes BJ, Harris JL. Biochemical characterization of prostasin, a channel activating protease. *Biochem Biophys Res Commun* 2004;324:953–963.

300. Shlyonsky VG, Mies F, Sariban-Sohraby S. Epithelial sodium channel activity in detergent-resistant membrane microdomains. *Am J Physiol Renal Physiol* 2003;284:F182–F188.

301. Snyder PM. The epithelial Na+ channel: cell surface insertion and retrieval in Na+ homeostasis and hypertension. *Endocrinol Rev* 2002;23:258–275.

302. Snyder PM. Liddle's syndrome mutations disrupt cAMP-mediated translocation of the epithelial Na(+) channel to the cell surface. *J Clin Invest* 2000;105:45–53.

303. Snyder PM. Regulation of epithelial Na+ channel trafficking. *Endocrinology* 2005;146:5079–5085.

304. Snyder PM, Bucher DB, Olson DR. Gating induces a conformational change in the outer vestibule of ENaC. *J Gen Physiol* 2000;116:781–790.

305. Snyder PM, Cheng C, Prince LS, Rogers JC, Welsh MJ. Electrophysiological and biochemical evidence that DEG/ENaC cation channels are composed of nine subunits. *J Biol Chem* 1998;273:681–684.

306. Snyder PM, Olson DR, Bucher DB. A pore segment in DEG/ENaC Na(+) channels. *J Biol Chem* 1999;274:28484–28490.

307. Snyder PM, Olson DR, Kabra R, Zhou R, Steines JC. cAMP and serum and glucocorticoid-inducible kinase (SGK) regulate the epithelial Na(+) channel through convergent phosphorylation of Nedd4-2. *J Biol Chem* 2004;279:45753–45758.

308. Snyder PM, Olson DR, Thomas BC. Serum and glucocorticoid-regulated kinase modulates Nedd4-2-mediated inhibition of the epithelial Na+ channel. *J Biol Chem* 2002;277:5–8.

309. Snyder PM, Price MP, McDonald FJ, Adams CM, Volk KA, Zeiher BG, Stokes JB, Welsh MJ. Mechanism by which Liddle's syndrome mutations increase activity of a human epithelial Na+ channel. *Cell* 1995;83:969–978.

310. Sollner TH. Regulated exocytosis and SNARE function. *Mol Membr Biol* 2003;20:209–220 (review).

311. Staruschenko A, Adams E, Booth RE, Stockand JD. Epithelial Na+ channel subunit stoichiometry. *Biophys J* 2005;88:3966–3975.

312. Staruschenko A, Medina JL, Patel P, Shapiro MS, Booth RE, Stockand JD. Fluorescence resonance energy transfer analysis of subunit stoichiometry of the epithelial Na+ channel. *J Biol Chem* 2004;279:27729–27734.

313. Staruschenko A, Nichols A, Medina JL, Camacho P, Zheleznova NN, Stockand JD. Rho small GTPases activate the epithelial Na(+) channel. *J Biol Chem* 2004;279:49989–49994.

314. Staub O, Abriel H, Plant P, Ishikawa T, Kanelis V, Saleki R, Horisberger JD, Schild L, Rotin D. Regulation of the epithelial Na1 channel by Nedd4 and ubiquitination. *Kidney Int* 2000;57:809–815.

315. Staub O, Dho S, Henry P, Correa J, Ishikawa T, McGlade J, Rotin D. WW domains of Nedd4 bind to the proline-rich PY motifs in the epithelial Na+ channel deleted in Liddle's syndrome. *EMBO J* 1996;15:2371–2380.

316. Staub O, Gautschi I, Ishikawa T, Breitschopf K, Ciechanover A, Schild L, Rotin D. Regulation of stability and function of the epithelial Na+ channel (ENaC) by ubiquitination. *EMBO J* 1997;16:6325–6336.

317. Stockand JD, Edinger RS, Al-Baldawi N, Sariban-Sohraby S, Al-Khalili O, Eaton DC, Johnson JP. Isoprenylcysteine-O-carboxyl methyltransferase regulates aldosterone-sensitive Na(+) reabsorption. *J Biol Chem* 1999;274:26912–26916.

318. Stockand JD, Edinger RS, Eaton DC, Johnson JP. Toward understanding the role of methylation in aldosterone-sensitive Na(+) transport. *News Physiol Sci* 2000;15:161–165.

319. Stockand JD, Spier BJ, Worrell RT, Yue G, Al-Baldawi N, Eaton DC. Regulation of Na(+) reabsorption by the aldosterone-induced small G protein K-Ras2A. *J Biol Chem* 1999;274:35449–35454.

320. Stutts MJ, Canessa CM, Olsen JC, Hamrick M, Cohn JA, Rossier BC, Boucher RC. CFTR as a cAMP-dependent regulator of sodium channels. *Science* 1995;269:847–850.

321. Stutts MJ, Rossier BC, Boucher RC. Cystic fibrosis transmembrane conductance regulator inverts protein kinase A–mediated regulation of epithelial sodium channel single channel kinetics. *J Biol Chem* 1997;272:14037–14040.

322. Swenson RP Jr, Armstrong CM. K+ channels close more slowly in the presence of external K+ and Rb+. *Nature* 1981;291:427–429.

323. Take-Uchi M, Kawakami M, Ishihara T, Amano T, Kondo K, Katsura I. An ion channel of the degenerin/epithelial sodium channel superfamily controls the defecation rhythm in *Caenorhabditis elegans*. *Proc Natl Acad Sci U S A* 1998;95:11775–11780.

324. Takei K, McPherson PS, Schmid SL, De Camilli P. Tubular membrane invaginations coated by dynamin rings are induced by GTP-gamma S in nerve terminals. *Nature* 1995;374:186–190.

325. Talbot CL, Bosworth DG, Briley EL, Fenstermacher DA, Boucher RC, Gabriel SE, Barker PM. Quantitation and localization of ENaC subunit expression in fetal, newborn, and adult mouse lung. *Am J Respir Cell Mol Biol* 1999;20:398–406.

326. Tamura H, Schild L, Enomoto N, Matsui N, Marumo F, Rossier BC. Liddle disease caused by a missense mutation of beta subunit of the epithelial sodium channel gene. *J Clin Invest* 1996;97:1780–1784.

327. Thomas CP, Auerbach S, Stokes JB, Volk KA. 5' heterogeneity in epithelial sodium channel alpha-subunit mRNA leads to distinct NH2-terminal variant proteins. *Am J Physiol* 1998;274:C1312–C1323.

328. Thomas CP, Auerbach SD, Zhang C, Stokes JB. The structure of the rat amiloride-sensitive epithelial sodium channel gamma subunit gene and functional analysis of its promoter. *Gene* 1999;228:111–122.

329. Thomas G. Furin at the cutting edge: from protein traffic to embryogenesis and disease. *Nat Rev Mol Cell Biol* 2002;3:753–766.

330. Tong Q, Gamper N, Medina JL, Shapiro MS, Stockand JD. Direct activation of the epithelial Na(+) channel by phosphatidylinositol 3,4,5-trisphosphate and phosphatidylinositol 3,4-bisphosphate produced by phosphoinositide 3-OH kinase. *J Biol Chem* 2004;279:22654–22663.

331. Tong Z, Illek B, Bhagwandin VJ, Verghese GM, Caughey GH. Prostasin, a membrane-anchored serine peptidase, regulates sodium currents in JME/CF15 cells, a cystic fibrosis airway epithelial cell line. *Am J Physiol Lung Cell Mol Physiol* 2004;287:L928–L935.

332. Tucker JK, Tamba K, Lee YJ, Shen LL, Warnock DG, Oh Y. Cloning and functional studies of splice variants of the alpha-subunit of the amiloride-sensitive Na+ channel. *Am J Physiol* 1998;274:C1081–C1089.

333. Valentijn JA, Fyfe GK, Canessa CM. Biosynthesis and processing of epithelial sodium channels in *Xenopus* oocytes. *J Biol Chem* 1998;273:30344–30351.

334. Valera S, Hussy N, Evans RJ, Adami N, North RA, Surprenant A, Buell G. A new class of ligand-gated ion channel defined by P2x receptor for extracellular ATP. *Nature* 1994;371:516–519.

335. Vallet V, Chraibi A, Gaeggeler HP, Horisberger JD, Rossier BC. An epithelial serine protease activates the amiloride-sensitive sodium channel. *Nature* 1997;389:607–610.

336. Van Driessche W, Lindemann B. Concentration dependence of currents through single sodium-selective pores in frog skin. *Nature* 1979;282:519–520.

337. Van Driessche W, Zeiske W. Ionic channels in epithelial cell membranes. *Physiol Rev* 1985;65:833–903.

338. Voilley N, Bassilana F, Mignon C, Merscher S, Mattei MG, Carle GF, Lazdunski M, Barbry P. Cloning, chromosomal localization, and physical linkage of the beta and gamma subunits (SCNN1B and SCNN1G) of the human epithelial amiloride-sensitive sodium channel. *Genomics* 1995;28:560–565.

339. Volk KA, Husted RF, Snyder PM, Stokes JB. Kinase regulation of hENaC mediated through a region in the COOH-terminal portion of the alpha-subunit. *Am J Physiol Cell Physiol* 2000;278:C1047–C1054.

340. Volk KA, Snyder PM, Stokes JB. Regulation of epithelial sodium channel activity through a region of the carboxyl terminus of the alpha-subunit. Evidence for intracellular kinase-mediated reactions. *J Biol Chem* 2001;276:43887–43893.

341. Vuagniaux G, Vallet V, Jaeger NF, Hummler E, Rossier BC. Synergistic activation of ENaC by three membrane-bound channel-activating serine proteases (mCAP1, mCAP2, and mCAP3) and serum- and glucocorticoid-regulated kinase (Sgk1) in *Xenopus* oocytes. *J Gen Physiol* 2002;120:191–201.

342. Vuagniaux G, Vallet V, Jaeger NF, Pfister C, Bens M, Farman N, Courtois-Coutry N, Vandewalle A, Rossier BC, Hummler E. Activation of the amiloride-sensitive epithelial sodium channel by the serine protease mCAP1 expressed in a mouse cortical collecting duct cell line. *J Am Soc Nephrol* 2000;11:828–834.

343. Waldmann R. Proton-gated cation channels—neuronal acid sensors in the central and peripheral nervous system. *Adv Exp Med Biol* 2001;502:293–304.

344. Waldmann R, Champigny G, Bassilana F, Heurteaux C, Lazdunski M. A proton-gated cation channel involved in acid-sensing. *Nature* 1997;386:173–177.

345. Waldmann R, Champigny G, Bassilana F, Voilley N, Lazdunski M. Molecular cloning and functional expression of a novel amiloride-sensitive Na+ channel. *J Biol Chem* 1995;270:27411–27414.

346. Waldmann R, Champigny G, Lazdunski M. Functional degenerin-containing chimeras identify residues essential for amiloride-sensitive Na+ channel function. *J Biol Chem* 1995;270:11735–11737.

347. Warnock DG. Liddle syndrome: genetics and mechanisms of Na+ channel defects. *Am J Med Sci* 2001;322:302–307.

348. Wei Y, Lin DH, Kemp R, Yaddanapudi GS, Nasjletti A, Falck JR, Wang WH. Arachidonic acid inhibits epithelial Na channel via cytochrome P450 (CYP) epoxygenase-dependent metabolic pathways. *J Gen Physiol* 2004;124:719–727.

349. Weisz OA, Johnson JP. Noncoordinate regulation of ENaC: paradigm lost? *Am J Physiol Renal Physiol* 2003;285:F833–F842.

350. Weisz OA, Wang JM, Edinger RS, Johnson JP. Non-coordinate regulation of endogenous epithelial sodium channel (ENaC) subunit expression at the apical membrane of A6 cells in response to various transporting conditions. *J Biol Chem* 2000;275:39886–39893.

351. Wiesmann WP, Johnson JP, Miura GA, Chaing PK. Aldosterone-stimulated transmethylations are linked to sodium transport. *Am J Physiol* 1985;248:F43–F47.

352. Wiesmann WP, Sinha S, Klahr S. Insulin stimulates active sodium transport in toad bladder by two mechanisms. *Nature* 1976;260:546–547.

353. Wilson FH, Disse-Nicodeme S, Choate KA, Ishikawa K, Nelson-Williams C, Desitter I, Gunel M, Milford DV, Lipkin GW, Achard JM, Feely MP, Dussol B, Berland Y, Unwin RJ, Mayan H, Simon DB, Farfel Z, Jeunemaitre X, Lifton RP. Human hypertension caused by mutations in WNK kinases. *Science* 2001;293:1107–1112.

354. Woda CB, Bragin A, Kleyman TR, Satlin LM. Flow-dependent K+ secretion in the cortical collecting duct is mediated by a maxi-K channel. *Am J Physiol Renal Physiol* 2001;280:F786–F793.

355. Woda CB, Miyawaki N, Ramalakshmi S, Ramkumar M, Rojas R, Zavilowitz B, Kleyman TR, Satlin LM. Ontogeny of flow-stimulated potassium secretion in rabbit cortical collecting duct: functional and molecular aspects. *Am J Physiol Renal Physiol* 2003;285:F629–F639.

356. Worrell RT, Bao HF, Denson DD, Eaton DC. Contrasting effects of cPLA2 on epithelial Na+ transport. *Am J Physiol Cell Physiol* 2001;281:C147–C156.

357. Xiao J, Zhen XG, Yang J. Localization of PIP2 activation gate in inward rectifier K+ channels. *Nat Neurosci* 2003;6:811–818.

358. Xu BE, Stippec S, Chu PY, Lazrak A, Li XJ, Lee BH, English JM, Ortega B, Huang CL, Cobb MH. WNK1 activates SGK1 to regulate the epithelial sodium channel. *Proc Natl Acad Sci U S A* 2005;102:10315–10320.

359. Xu BE, Stippec S, Lazrak A, Huang CL, Cobb MH. WNK1 activates SGK1 by a PI-3 kinase-dependent and non-catalytic mechanism. *J Biol Chem* 2005;280:34218–34223.

360. Xu JZ, Hall AE, Peterson LN, Bienkowski MJ, Eessalu TE, Hebert SC. Localization of the ROMK protein on apical membranes of rat kidney nephron segments. *Am J Physiol* 1997;273:F739–F748.

361. Yamamura H, Ugawa S, Ueda T, Nagao M, Shimada S. Protons activate the delta-subunit of the epithelial Na+ channel in humans. *J Biol Chem* 2004;279:12529–12534.

362. Yan W, Suaud L, Kleyman TR, Rubenstein RC. Differential modulation of a polymorphism in the COOH terminus of the {alpha}-subunit of the human epithelial sodium channel by protein kinase C[delta]. *Am J Physiol Renal Physiol* 2006;290:F279–F288.

363. Yeh BI, Kim YK, Jabbar W, Huang CL. Conformational changes of pore helix coupled to gating of TRPV5 by protons. *EMBO J* 2005;24:3224–3234.

364. Yki-Jarvinen H. Thiazolidinediones. *N Engl J Med* 2004;351:1106–1118.

365. Yoo D, Fang L, Mason A, Kim BY, Welling PA. A phosphorylation-dependent export structure in ROMK (KIR 1.1) channel overrides an ER-localization signal. *J Biol Chem* 2005;280:35281–35289.

366. Yue G, Edinger RS, Bao HF, Johnson JP, Eaton DC. The effect of rapamycin on single ENaC channel activity and phosphorylation in A6 cells. *Am J Physiol Cell Physiol* 2000;279:C81–C88.

367. Yue G, Malik B, Yue G, Eaton DC. Phosphatidylinositol 4,5–bisphosphate (PIP2) stimulates epithelial sodium channel activity in A6 cells. *J Biol Chem* 2002;277:11965–11969.

368. Zhang P, Fyfe GK, Grichtchenko II, Canessa CM. Inhibition of alphabeta epithelial sodium channels by external protons indicates that the second hydrophobic domain contains structural elements for closing the pore. *Biophys J* 1999;77:3043–3051.

369. Zhang YH, Alvarez de la Rosa D, Canessa CM, Hayslett JP. Insulin-induced phosphorylation of ENaC correlates with increased sodium channel function in A6 cells. *Am J Physiol Cell Physiol* 2005;288:C141–C147.

370. Zhang ZR, McDonough SI, McCarty NA. Interaction between permeation and gating in a putative pore domain mutant in the cystic fibrosis transmembrane conductance regulator. *Biophys J* 2000;79:298–313.

371. Zheng J, Sigworth FJ. Selectivity changes during activation of mutant Shaker potassium channels. *J Gen Physiol* 1997;110:101–117.

372. Zhou Y, Morais-Cabral JH, Kaufman A, MacKinnon R. Chemistry of ion coordination and hydration revealed by a K+ channel-Fab complex at 2.0 A resolution. *Nature* 2001;414:43–48.

373. Zhou ZH, Bubien JK. Nongenomic regulation of ENaC by aldosterone. *Am J Physiol Cell Physiol* 2001;281:C1118–C1130.

374. Zuckerman JB, Chen X, Jacobs JD, Hu B, Kleyman TR, Smith PR. Association of the epithelial sodium channel with Apx and alpha-spectrin in A6 renal epithelial cells. *J Biol Chem* 1999;274:23286–23295.

CHAPTER **29**

Anion Channels

Yinghong Wang, William B. Guggino, and Peying Fong

Albany Medical Center, Albany, New York, USA
The Johns Hopkins University School of Medicine, Baltimore, Maryland, USA
Kansas State University, Manhattan, Kansas, USA

INTRODUCTION

Transporting epithelial cells such as those of the kidney utilize the energy expended in generating ionic gradients to sustain anion fluxes by either secondary active or passive mechanisms. These movements are critical to housekeeping functions, such as volume regulation and acid–base homeostasis, as well as to the specialized task that characterizes epithelial tissue, vector ial transport. In the case of the kidney, the goal is to defend total body ionic homeostasis by regulating the composition of the extracellular milieu. Because chloride is the most abundant anion in the body, these fluxes often involve at least one chloride-transporting pathway. This pathway could be a transporter, such as a cation-coupled chloride transporter, or it could be any of an expanding array of chloride channels that belong to one of several well-studied families. The classic example of the concerted action of these pathways is the thick ascending limb, the site of NaCl absorption. Here, the intracellular accumulation of chloride above electrochemical equilibrium, via an apical $Na^+/K^+/2Cl^-$ cotransporter, NKCC, is coupled to the sodium gradient. That gradient is generated and maintained by the expenditure of ATP by the Na^+/K^+-ATPase. The accumulated chloride then passively exits through a basolateral chloride channel complex, ClC-Kb/Barttin.

The mammalian kidney evolved highly specialized cellular mechanisms as well as an intricate structural organization to permit the efficient recovery of essential solutes and water, as well as the concomitant excretion of metabolic waste. This also means that kidney epithelial cells must have a robust means of generating a high extracellular osmolality, an enormous capacity to recover sodium, low-molecular-weight proteins, glucose and bicarbonate, and an exquisite sensitivity to hormones secreted in response to either loading or deprivation of salt and water. Moreover, in the face of these extreme osmotic and metabolic challenges, kidney cells still must maintain volume and pH homeostasis. Practically all of these functions involve anion transport.

This chapter will examine the anion channels that contribute to these aspects of kidney function. We will start with an overview of physiological methods used to classify renal anion channels into functional classes. A discussion of the known, as well as putative, molecular correlates of these channels follows. Lastly, we will consider the disease phenotypes resulting from disrupting these channels or their regulation, evaluate what these phenotypes tell us about the normal physiological roles of these channels, and explore the avenues that have been opened by current knowledge.

METHODS COMMONLY USED TO STUDY RENAL ANION CHANNEL FUNCTION

Anion conductances had long been postulated to exist in most segments of the nephron, largely on the basis of microelectrode and transepithelial potential difference measurements of isolated, perfused tubules. Polarized renal epithelial cell lines, such as those from opossum (OK, [276]), pig (LLCPK-1 [207]), and dog (MDCK [188]) kidney; mouse medullary thick ascending limb (mTAL [178]), and mouse inner medullary collecting duct (IMCD-3 [221]) lines, as well as the development of differentiated primary renal cell cultures, have also proven useful (52). Both primary cell cultures, as well as cell lines, may be grown on permeable supports and their function assessed using Ussing's short-circuit current method (286). Recently, short-circuit current measurements of polarized primary renal cultures has enjoyed a renaissance. This method has proven critical in analyses of function in collecting ducts of knockout and transgenic mice (37, 195) as well as in diseased human tissue with limited availability (90).

The advent of tight-seal recording techniques (101) represented a major breakthrough in functional analysis of the ionic channels in a wide variety of cells, and this proved no exception in investigations of renal anion channels. Tight seal, or "patch clamp," methods allow the recording of membrane currents conducted by small numbers of channels, or even a single channel, in isolated patches of cell membrane. The formation of a highly resistive ("gigaohm") seal between the tip of a recording electrode and the cell membrane permits the resolution of extremely small currents on the order of picoamperes (pA) that flow during the fleeting (submillisecond) openings and closings of the channel(s). The membrane patch can be held at different command potentials and so facilitate the evaluation of the resultant currents as a function of the applied voltages.

Patch clamp recording methods have proven extremely versatile, and have become the standard for the classification of ion channels on the basis of their single-channel conductance, gating kinetics, current–voltage (I–V or i–V, with uppercase designating macroscopic currents and lowercase designating single-channel currents) relationship/rectification properties, selectivity, regulation, and pharmacology. In particular, the range of recording configurations permits excellent control of both intra- and extra-cellular sides of the membrane. This affords extreme versatility in detailed studies of selectivity and pharmacology that are necessary for the proper distinction between anion channels. Tight-seal recording also can be applied to studies of channels in their native context as well as channels that are expressed heterologously. With the identification of many putative chloride channels by molecular cloning, the functional verification of channel activity in expression systems has become essential. Patch clamp measurements of transiently or stably transfected mammalian cell lines, such as HEK293, COS-7, and CHO, thus also occupy another important niche as a critical assay for molecular predictions. Conversely, molecular methods such as site-directed mutagenesis and reverse transcription polymerase chain reaction (RT-PCR) continue to complement and enhance functional studies. Most recently, the availability of high-resolution crystal structures have extended the collective understanding of CLC protein function (64, 65).

Another electrophysiological assay uses oocytes of the South African clawed toad, *Xenopus laevis*, which readily express cRNA encoding exogenous proteins. These large (~1-mm diameter) cells are easily manipulated and measured using two microelectrode voltage clamp methods. Removal of the vitelline membrane permits patch recording as well. Oocytes have become an essential tool for characterizing cloned ion channels, including those of the kidney. One caveat does exist: oocytes express background calcium-activated chloride channels, as well as native volume-sensitive and hyperpolarization-activated anion channels (6, 15, 184). Thus, endogenous channel currents have the potential to obscure measurements of heterologously expressed chloride channels. Although oocytes provide a well-studied example of this confounding factor, mammalian cells also endogenously express background chloride currents.

Channels also can be distinguished on the basis of their drug sensitivities. Until recently, highly specific and potent inhibitors of anion channels were rare (76, 253). Widely used, but also notably nonspecific and weak, inhibitors include (1) stilbenes such as DIDS and DNDS; (2) anthranilic acid derivatives such as 9-anthracene carboxylate (9-AC), diphenylamine-2-carboxylic acid (DPC) and 5-nitro-2-(3-phenylpropylamino)-benzoate (NPPB); (3) nonsteroidal anti-inflammatory agents (niflumic acid and flufenamic acid); and (4) the sulfonylurea receptor antagonist, glibenclamide. In addition, heavy metals such as cadmium, zinc, and nickel have been used to inhibit CLC chloride channels (126). Marginal distinctions can be drawn from criteria such as sidedness and voltage dependence of block. The inhibitor sensitivities of members of the CLC family are summarized in Table 1.

TABLE 1   Properties of CLC Proteins

	Distribution	I-V	Anionic Selectivity	Inhibition by[a]	Activation by	Human Disease	Knockout Phenotype
ClC-1	Skeletal muscle	Inward	$Cl^- > Br^- > I^-$	9-AC, clofibrate, CPP, DPC, nifumic acid, Zn^{2+}	Depolarization	Myotonia congenita	Myotonic (*Adr*) mouse
ClC-2	Broad	Inward	$Cl^- > Br^- > I^-$	Zn^{2+}, Cd^{2+}, NPPB, DPC, 9-AC, DIDS	Hyperpolarization, hypotonicity, $\downarrow pH_o$		Retinal and testicular degeneration
ClC-Ka[b]	Kidney, inner ear	linear	$Br^- > Cl^- > I^-$	DIDS, CPP, $\downarrow pH_o$	Ca^{2+}_o		Nephrogenic diabetes insipidus
ClC-Kb[b]	Kidney, inner ear	Outward	$Cl^- > Br^- > I^-$	$\downarrow pH_o$, CPP, DIDS	Ca^{2+}_o	Bartter's syndrome	
ClC-3	Broad; high in brain	Outward	$Cl^- > Br^- > I^-$				Hippocampal and retinal degeneration
ClC-4	Broad	Outward	$Cl^- > Br^- > I^-$				
ClC-5	Broad; high in kidney	Outward	$Cl^- > Br^- > I^-$	$\downarrow pH_o$		Dent's disease	Endocytosis defect, nephrocalcinosis, hypercalciuria
ClC-6	Broad						
ClC-7	Broad					Osteopetrosis	Osteopetrosis

[a] Inhibitors are listed in the order of their relative efficacy.

[b] Stated functional properties for ClC-Ka and -Kb channels are those obtained with barttin coexpression.

Recently, high-throughput screening efforts yielded CFTR$_{inh}$-172 and GlyH-101, two highly specific, small-molecule inhibitors of cystic fibrosis transmembrane conductance regulator (CFTR), a cAMP-regulated chloride channel (171, 193). On the other hand, targeted drug design based on the crystal structure of a bacterial CLC protein has led to the generation of 2-(p-chlorophenoxy) propionic acid (CPP) derivatives that are not only potent but very selective between highly homologous CLC channels (211).

BIOPHYSICAL AND OTHER FUNCTIONAL CHARACTERISTICS OF RENAL ANION CHANNELS STUDIED IN SITU

Anion channels that display the gamut of conductance, rectification properties, selectivity, and pharmacological profile have been measured in epithelial cells derived from every segment of the nephron. Brief descriptions of notable examples follow.

Anion Channels Measured in Isolated Tubules and Primary Cultures

Patch clamp measurements in intact cells of isolated renal tubules pose a challenge. Access to the basolateral membrane can be gained only with collagenase treatment or physical disruption of the basement membrane. Moreover, apical access is limited by the tubular geometry. Hence, the study of apical channels necessitates either splitting the tubules open or acute isolation and subsequent primary culture. Despite these limitations, tight seal recording of intact tubules is a powerful tool for the analysis of channel function in nephronal segments isolated from transgenic animals.

Chloride handling by the proximal tubule largely occurs via electroneutral processes, and the presence of low-conductance chloride channels in this nephronal segment is consistent with this observation (97). That stated, this does not exclude a role for anion channels in either transepithelial transport or volume regulation. Gogelein and Greger (86) identified a low-conductance (28.0 ± 1.2 pS), basolaterally localized channel in cells of rabbit single-cannulated proximal tubules. This channel conducted chloride and was reversibly blocked by DPC. Because this channel also passed sodium and potassium indiscriminately, a role in cell volume regulation was proposed. Apical, cAMP-activated chloride channels were also described in primary cultures of rabbit proximal tubule cells, and in vivo microperfusion studies support a role for these in transcellular transport (54, 271, 292).

Small- and intermediate-conductance (7–9 and 45 pS, respectively), linear chloride channels have been measured from basolateral membrane patches of the mouse cortical thick ascending limb (98). Forskolin and cAMP agonists activated both channels. In addition, cytosolic ATP stimulated the small conductance channel in a Mg^{2+}-dependent fashion. The two channels differed in their anion selectivity. The small conductance channel had a selectivity sequence of $NO_3^- > Br^- > Cl^- > F^- >$ gluconate, whereas selectivity of the intermediate conductance channel was $Cl^- > Br^- > NO_3^- > F^-$. Furthermore, the small conductance channel could be inhibited by application of NPPB, glibenclamide, DIDS, and DPC to the intracellular side. At the time, the anionic selectivity and inhibition by intracellular DIDS seemed at odds with the idea that the small-conductance chloride channel was CFTR. In hindsight, the findings of later studies on the biophysical properties and pharmacology of CFTR support this notion. Similarly, the anion selectivity of the 45-pS channel suggests that this is a member of the CLC family.

More recently, the cell-attached and inside-out patch clamp studies of isolated mouse distal convoluted tubules, together with single-cell RT-PCR analysis, yielded informative findings about both functional and molecular heterogeneity of basolateral chloride channels in this nephronal segment (199). Nissan and colleagues found evidence for small (9 pS) channels that likely represent ClC-K2 homodimers in one cell population, as well as other channels (also 9 pS) in another group that may be a mixture of ClC-K1 and/or -K2 homo- and/or heterodimers. These channels were inhibited by acidic intracellular pH, and their anionic selectivity was $Cl^- > NO_3^- = Br^-$. Another anion channel, also with 9 pS conductance, showed $I^- > NO_3^- > Br^- > Cl^-$ selectivity. The molecular identity of this channel remains unknown, although its anion selectivity overlaps with those previously reported for volume- and calcium-sensitive chloride channels.

Sansom and coworkers (234) patched principal cells from the isolated rabbit cortical collecting duct and recorded single chloride channel currents. This basolaterally localized channel gated swiftly between three substates of 0, 23, and 46 pS, and slowly between the closed state and the first open substate (0 pS). The two conductive states had a linear I–V relationship and the currents reversed at a potential that was consistent with a chloride to potassium selectivity ratio of ~15:1. Thus, this suggested the presence, in mammalian collecting duct cells, of a "double-barreled" CLC chloride channel similar to that previously observed in reconstituted *Torpedo californicus* electroplax membranes (18, 186, 187).

Primary cultures of rat inner medullary collecting duct show an outwardly rectifying, intermediate conductance anion conductance when measured using both outside-out and excised patch configurations (27). In chloride-rich recording solutions, this channel has chord conductances of ~34 pS between −100 and −50 mV and ~77 pS between +50 and +120 mV. These channels resemble the volume-sensitive, outwardly rectifying anion channels described in a number of systems, including glioma (C6 [121]) and human colonic epithelial (T84 [203, 301]) cell lines, as well as primary cell cultures of human tracheal epithelia and eccrine sweat duct (260). This suggests a role in cell volume regulation. Importantly, these channels conduct taurine, an organic osmolyte that is abundant in the kidney (28). Thus, in the inner medulla, it is a likely solute for maintaining intracellular osmolality.

Anion Channels in Renal Cell Lines

The availability of several cell lines derived from renal epithelia greatly extends the range of functional experimentation. Not only do they facilitate functional analysis, but cell lines open the possibility of molecular identification using biochemical, molecular, and cell biological tools.

Electrophysiological studies of chloride channels using proximal tubule lines such as OK and LLC-PK1 have been limited. However, aspects of chloride channel function, such as their role in endosomal acidification and endocytosis, have been addressed using these lines in studies that primarily utilize biochemical and cell biological methods (105, 106, 116). The mouse mTAL line recently has been used in evaluations of the stimulatory effect of hypertonicity on ClC-5 expression, a process that may be necessary for the proper expression and turnover of Tamm–Horsfall protein (210). Tamm–Horsfall protein in turn may be protective against nephrolithiasis and/or inflammation.

In contrast, the electrophysiological properties of anion channels from cell lines derived from the distal nephron have been studied more extensively. Intermediate-conductance outwardly rectifying chloride channels, as well as large conductance ("maxi") anion channels, have been measured in the RCCT-28A rabbit, cortical collecting duct cell line (9, 61, 246, 247). The former, which appeared exclusively in basolateral membrane patches, had a 96-pS conductance at a holding potential of $+80$ mV and a conductance of 13 pS when measured at a holding potential of -80 mV. These channels appeared heterogeneous in their activation properties, with a PKA-activated subset and another PKA-indifferent subset. In contrast, the "maxi" chloride channel was found exclusively in the apical patches. This channel had a linear I–V relationship, a single channel conductance of 305 pS, and a Cl^- to Na^- permeability ratio of 9:1 (247). Furthermore, the "maxi" chloride channel can be activated by cell swelling, as well as short actin filaments (248). Thus, the actin polymerization state may mediate regulatory volume decrease by influencing the activity of the 305-pS chloride channel. A similar, large conductance channel has been described in MDCK cells (141), rat cortical astrocytes (122), and neuroblastoma cells (75).

The mouse inner medullary collecting duct line, IMCD-K2, has proven extremely versatile (24–26, 135, 136, 288). In addition to volume-sensitive, outwardly rectifying chloride currents similar to those found in the RCCT-28 cells and inner medullary collecting duct primary cultures, calcium-activated chloride channels, and CFTR have been identified in IMCD-K2 cells. In addition to patch clamp measurements, IMCD-K2 cells form confluent, electrically tight epithelial monolayers. Thus, the contributions of these chlo-

ride channels to transepithelial transport can be assessed directly by measuring the short-circuit current (25, 26, 135, 136). Boese et al. (26) offered pharmacological and RT-PCR evidence that ClC-3 underlies the volume-sensitive current. The debate over the molecular identity of volume-sensitive chloride channels persists and will be discussed further in the following sections.

MOLECULAR IDENTITIES OF RENAL ANION CHANNELS

CLC Channels/Transporters

ClC-0, the chloride channel of the *Torpedo* electric organ, represents the prototypic CLC protein (126, 127). Jentsch and coworkers (127) first elucidated the primary structure of this protein and studied the chloride currents resulting from heterologous expression in the *Xenopus* oocyte system. Subsequent single-channel analysis showed that expression of this single cRNA recapitulated all properties of the bilayer-reconstituted channel studied by Miller (18, 186, 187), who dubbed it "double-barreled" because of its unusual, voltage-dependent gating between two equal protochannel conductive states. Thus, no accessory subunit was required. The molecular cloning of ClC-0 paved the way for a plethora of related mammalian, plant, and prokaryotic family members (124, 126). The *Torpedo* electroplax derives from muscle, so it stands to reason that ClC-0 shares significant 54% amino acid identity with ClC-1, the major skeletal muscle chloride conductance. Figure 1 depicts relatedness between mammalian CLC proteins.

The bacterial CLCs likely act as Cl^-/H^+ exchangers, but chloride channel function has been confirmed or at least remains highly likely for most CLC proteins to date (4, 5, 12). The first crystal structure of the *Salmonella typhimurium* CLC protein (StClC), at 3 Å resolution, revealed a structure that was both predictable and surprising (64, 125). Two monomers, each consisting of 18 intramembrane α-helices that form a self-contained unit, interact at a plane perpendicular to the membrane to form a two-pore, homodimeric assembly. The amino and carboxyl halves of each monomer show structural similarity, and span the membrane in an antiparallel fashion, reminiscent of the structure of aquaporins (Fig. 2). The subsequent cocrystallization of the *Escherichia coli* CLC protein, ClC-ecl, with Fab fragments yielded a higher resolution (2.5 Å) structure that permitted analysis of its pore region and selectivity filter (65). Importantly, information extracted from these findings has led to the identification of potentially useful pharmacological probes for renal CLCs (211). Early structure–function studies suggested that CLCs exist as functional dimers, so this aspect of the structure is not altogether unexpected (168, 169, 183, 235, 295). On the other hand, the complex, antiparallel membrane topology deviates considerably from the original models formed largely on the basis of hydrophobicity analysis (237). Importantly, the availability of

Mammalian CLC proteins

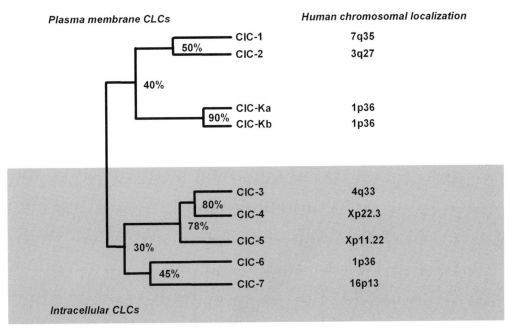

FIGURE 1 A dendrogram that depicts the relationship between the nine mammalian CLC proteins appears at left. On the right side, the corresponding human chromosomal localizations are provided.

the structure provides a context for reevaluating many of the data from early mutagenesis studies that could not be reconciled on the basis of the former topological model.

The bacterial CLC proteins lack the extended carboxyl terminus of mammalian CLCs. Thus, this important structural feature was not provided by the StClC and CLC-ecl crystal structures (64, 65). Mammalian CLC carboxyl termini contain two copies of a highly conserved structural motif, called CBS domains (for cystathionine β-synthase, a protein in which the motif was originally described [17, 213]). Another protein in which two CBS domain copies exist is inosine monophosphate dehydrogenase (IMPDH), and the structure of this protein is known (258). An interesting recent finding demonstrated that tandem pairs of CBS domains bind AMP, ATP, and S-adenosyl methionine, thus suggesting a role in sensing the cellular metabolic status (250). Thus, these findings are provocative because they may provide a link between the activity of mammalian CLCs and cellular metabolism.

INFERENCES FROM LOCALIZATION STUDIES, FUNCTIONAL EXPRESSION, AND ANALYSIS OF KNOCKOUT MICE

Several members of the CLC family play critical roles in kidney function. The nephron expresses eight of the nine identified mammalian CLCs. To begin with, it is useful to consider these on the basis of their cellular localization (see Fig. 1 for a broad breakdown). Those that can be expressed in heterologous systems can also be assessed according to their biophysical and pharmacological properties. The avail-

ability of mouse models has enhanced the overall mechanistic understanding of CLC channels, and has also proven particularly invaluable for garnering information about those for which functional expression has been problematic. Table 1 summarizes the properties of human CLC proteins.

Of those CLCs that reside in the plasma membrane, ClC-2 is expressed in most cells of the body (47, 277). Analysis of ClC-2–expressing oocytes suggests that this channel likely plays a role in volume regulation, as well as in neuronal excitability (48). A specific role in kidney function is obscure, as the ClCn-2$^{-/-}$ mouse does not show a renal phenotype. Rather, these animals have severe retinal and testicular degeneration. However, single-cell RT-PCR and whole-cell measurements of embryonic rat uretic bud cells imply that ClC-2 participates in early nephrogenesis (118).

Sharing about 43% amino acid homology with ClC-2, and occupying a separate division of the plasma membrane branch of CLC channels, are ClC-Ka and -Kb (133, 285). Human ClC-Ks are about 90% related to each other. The rodent orthologues, ClC-K1 and -K2, share ~80% relatedness with each other and with both human ClC-Ks. This, and the discrepancy in the conclusions of early expression attempts (133, 285), precluded a straightforward assignment of which human ClC-K corresponded to a given rodent ClC-K. Genetic analysis did link mutations in CLCNKB to the salt-wasting disease, Bartter's syndrome type III (255). Thus, ClC-Kb probably functions in the mechanism of salt absorption by the thick ascending limb.

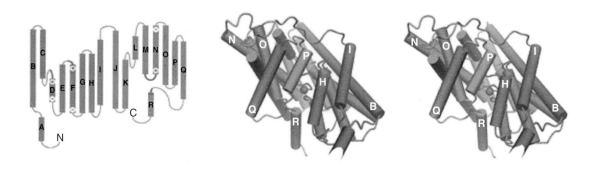

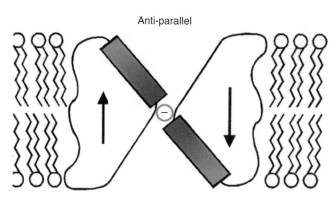

FIGURE 2   The top panel (left) shows the helical structure of the StClC monomer. The extracellular loop between helices I and J rests between the two halves of the molecule; α-helical regions appear as rectangles. Note that helices A-I and J-R are organized in an antiparallel manner. The loop regions immediately 5' to helices D and F, the loop between helices M and N, and a short stretch before and including part of helix R form the selectivity filter. The helix dipoles are indicated by the "+" and "−" signs. Two monomers form a functional StClC protein. The top panel (right) shows a stereoview of the monomer viewed from within the plane of the membrane, from the perspective of the dimer interface. The selectivity filter surrounds the permeating chloride ion, represented by the ball. Bottom panel shows the antiparallel architecture of CLCs that permits similar dipole charges of the α-helices to organize from opposing sides of the membrane, hence contributing to the selectivity filter. (From Dutzler R, Campbell EB, Cadene M, Chait BT, MacKinnon R. X-ray structure of a ClC chloride channel at 3.0 Å reveals the molecular basis of anion selectivity, *Nature* 2002;415:287-294.)

Furthermore, Clcnk1$^{-/-}$ mice display nephrogenic diabetes insipidus, a phenotype that suggests a role for ClC-K1 in the concentrating mechanism, with an appropriate localization to the thin ascending limb (177). Together with the immunolocalization data of Kobayashi and colleagues (139), it can be surmised that ClC-Ka and -Kb represent the human forms of rodent ClC-K1 and -K2, respectively.

Another major advance came with the discovery that ClC-Ks require an accessory protein, barttin, for their plasma membrane expression in the distal nephron, including the thin ascending limb and thick ascending limb of Henle's loop (72). Notably, ClC-K/barttin channel assemblies are also present in the stria vascularis of the inner ear. There, they contribute to the secretion of high potassium endolymph. As a result, mutation of the BSND gene results in type IV Bartter's, which is characterized by deafness (22). Thus, in summary, ClC-K/barttin complexes contribute to transepithelial Cl transport that is critical to the renal concentrating mechanism and the absorption of salt (138, 139, 177, 284) as well as proper function of the auditory system (see Fig. 5).

The two branches of the intracellular CLCs share about 30% homology on the amino acid level. Members of the first branch are ClC-3, -4, and -5, and these proteins share ~80% identity. ClC-3 and -4 are more broadly distributed than ClC-5, which is found prevalently in the kidney. All three show outwardly rectifying currents when expressed in heterologous systems. Their likely function rests in facilitating the acidification of intracellular compartments by shunting the lumen-positive potential difference generated by the proton-ATPase (105, 106). Dent's disease, an X-linked nephrolithiasis resulting from mutations sin the CLCN5 gene, illustrates the consequences of limited acidification capacity. Affected individuals have low-molecular-weight proteinuria that has been attributed to a defect in endocytosis. Indeed, primary proximal tubule cell cultures from the ClC-5 knockout mouse also show attenuated uptake of fluorescently labeled albumin, and impairment of early endosomal acidification (105).

Based on early heterologous expression data in transfected mammalian (NIH/3T3) cells, Duan and colleagues (62) raised the possibility that ClC-3 mediates volume-sensitive currents, $I_{Clswell}$. However, the biophysical properties of the reported currents differed substantially from those of the highly related ClC-4 and -5, thus raising a red flag. The hypothesis rapidly fell into disfavor with the demonstration that $I_{Clswell}$ persists in Clcn3 knockout mice (266). Recently, the possibility that ClC-3 mediates the CaMKII-modulated chloride currents of T84 and HT-29 cells, as well as aortic smooth cells, has emerged (117, 229).

ClC-6 and -7 are broadly expressed members of the second branch of the intracellular CLCs. Despite the lack of verifiable functional expression, these likely also act to modify the pH of intracellular compartments. Northern blot analysis indicates that they are distributed broadly in many tissues, including kidney (29). To date, attempts at heterologous expression have not produced functional currents. ClC-6 functionally complements the gef1 yeast phenotype (132). When overexpressed in COS cells, the c-myc–tagged splice variants ClC-6a and -6c colocalize with the sarco/endoplasmic reticulum calcium pump, SER-CA2b (34). The ClC-7 knockout mouse ($Clcn7^{-/-}$) has osteopetrosis, thus revealing the importance of this protein in the acidification of the resorptive lacunae (142). More recent work shows that the loss of ClC-7 function results in lysosomal storage abnormalities, even in the absence of gross lysosomal pH changes. $Clcn7^{-/-}$ mice also show severe degeneration of the central nervous system (130). Taken together, these studies suggest a role for ClC-6 and -7 in modulating the composition of intracellular compartments. Their possible roles in the physiology of the kidney remain obscure and likely are minimal, based on their apparent failure to compensate for ClC-5 in Dent's patients and the ClC-5 knockout mouse.

SIGNATURE BIOPHYSICAL PROPERTIES OF CLC CHANNEL PROTEINS

At steady state, the current–voltage relationships exhibited by CLC channels range from the inwardly rectifying (ClC-2) to the strongly outwardly rectifying (ClC-3, -4, and -5). The inward rectification of ClC-2 makes it well suited to promoting chloride exit during volume load. On the other hand, at first glance the marked outward rectification of ClC-3, -4, and -5 seems poorly suited to shunting the proton pump efficiently. This can be explained by recalling that the turnover rates of channels can exceed those of carriers and pumps by a thousand-fold. Thus, however small, the inward currents carried by the intracellular CLCs may be sufficient to match the turnover rate of the pump.

With the exception of ClC-K1 and -Ka, the anionic selectivity of CLC channels favors chloride over other halides (126). This characteristic has proved useful in distinguishing the contributions of CLC channels from those of other chloride channels. Similarly, CLCs exhibit pH-sensitive gating that may represent a vestige of the bacterial ClC-ecl's function as a H^+/Cl^- antiporter (5). Extracellular acidification apparently activates ClC-2, whereas it inhibits both

ClC-4 and ClC-5 (79, 128, 189). At steady state, ClC-2 shows inward rectification, whereas ClC-3, -4, and -5 currents rectify in the outward direction.

Because CLCs often are expressed in the same cells, the potential exists for the formation of heterodimeric channels. Coexpression studies of CLC channels using the *Xenopus oocyte* system support this concept (166, 295). Co-immunoprecipitation experiments using rat kidney suggest that ClC-4 and -5 form heterodimers (190). In principle, the presence of heteromeric assemblies would lead to a variety of dimeric configurations, thus accounting for the diverse spectrum of characteristics exhibited by CLC-like channels in native cell systems. This could explain the range of acidification capacities characteristic of various intracellular, organellar compartments. Because ClC-3, -4, and -5 all localize intracellularly in vesicular and tubulovesicular structures, their heterodimerization conceivably could generate novel assemblies that promote acidification to different degrees. Thus, whether heterodimers indeed assemble and function in native tissues poses a provocative question for future studies.

PHARMACOLOGY

In general, the traditional chloride channel blockers such as anthracene derivatives, stilbenes, and heavy metal ions block CLC channels with variable, but overall weak, sensitivities. At best, DPC and DIDS almost uniformly require concentrations in excess of 1 mM. In the case of ClC-3, neither DIDS nor NPPB inhibit (154, 190), whereas DPC, DIDS, NPPB, and 9-AC do not block ClC-5 at all (264). An indanyloxyacetic acid (IAA-94) has been used to isolate, as well as block, the p64 channel of bovine kidney cortex; it inhibits these channels with an IC_{50} of 2 µM (147). Only a few compounds block CLC channels at micromolar concentrations. For instance, 9-anthracene-carboxylate at 100 µM inhibits ClC-1, but the block of other CLC channels requires substantially higher levels, with ClC-0 and ClC-2 only modestly inhibited by 1 mM (263, 277). Clofibrates, long known to induce myotonia (148), inhibit the muscle chloride conductance, ClC-1 (56). Zinc inhibits ClC-0 potently ($IC_{50} \sim 1$–3 µM), whereas cadmium block is weaker (38). Both zinc and cadmium efficiently block ClC-2 at submillimolar concentrations (48, 243).

The availability of the bacterial crystal structure catalyzed a series of experiments that explored the inhibition of the muscle CLC, ClC-1, by 9-AC and clofibrates, specifically the clofibric acid derivative, p-chloro-phenoxy-acetic acid (CPA [73]). These compounds block ClC-1 from the intracellular side. Information provided by the crystal structure of bacterial CLCs (64, 65) formed the basis of extensive mutagenesis studies of ClC-1 that provided further clues to the structure of the inhibitor-binding site. Resting close to the chloride-binding site is a partially hydrophobic pocket that is accessible from the cytoplasm, consistent with the observed intracellular block by 9-AC and CPA.

Until recently, the pharmacology of ClC-K/barttin channels has been hampered by their strong molecular similarity. Structure–activity screening studies by Liantonio et al. (155, 156) led to the fortuitous finding that clofibrates, which incorporate a phenoxy and a phenoxy-alkyl group on the chiral center (bis-phenoxy derivatives), also block ClC-K1/barttin when applied to the extracellular bath solution. Specifically, 2-(p-chlorophenoxy) propionic acid (CPP), blocks ClC-K1 channels from the extracellular side, with an affinity on the order of 150 μM. Furthermore, this compound had negligible effects on ClC-2 and ClC-5 (155, 156). Recently, Picollo et al. (211) showed that 3-phenyl-CPP, as well as the unrelated stilbene blocker, DIDS, inhibit the human ClC-Ka and -Kb channels with differential sensitivities. Guided by the bacterial crystal structure (64), residues that were likely to confer the fivefold higher extracellular sensitivity of ClC-Ka to these drugs were identified. Mutagenesis and subsequent functional expression pinpointed the neutral amino acids N68 and G72 as crucial for the better block by 3-phenyl-CPP and DIDS, respectively. Replacement with the negatively charged D68 and E72 that are found in ClC-Kb diminished the block. The side groups of these amino acids project into the external mouth of the channel pore. One model postulates that electrostatic interactions at these points permit (as in the case of ClC-Ka) or impede (in ClC-Kb) the interaction of the negatively charged groups of either drug with other binding sites deeper within the pore. If this proves to be the case, a basis for designing specific inhibitors of other CLC channels may be at hand.

CYSTIC FIBROSIS TRANSMEMBRANE CONDUCTANCE REGULATOR

Cystic fibrosis is a life-limiting, autosomal recessive human disease that results from mutations in CFTR and causes impaired ion transport in the airways, pancreas, and other tissues. CFTR, a member of the ATP–binding cassette (ABC) transporter family, mediates the vectorial transport of chloride by a variety of epithelia (242), including kidney. It is found in full-length and truncated forms in the kidney (191). The CFTR gene encodes a 160-kD protein, comprising two regions of six transmembrane-spanning domains (TMD1 and TMD2), two cytoplasmic nucleotide-binding domains (NBD1 and NBD2), and a regulatory (R) domain (Fig. 3, top). CFTR is a small (5–8 pS), linear channel that has a relative halide selectivity of $Br^- \geq Cl^- > I^-$ (8). Gating of CFTR requires (1) phosphorylation at the R domain by protein kinase A, and (2) the binding and hydrolysis of ATP (NBDs). The recent solution of the crystal structures of NBD1 in unbound as well as both ATP- and ADP-bound states (152) provides insight into the role of NBD1 in the gating cycle and bodes well for attempts to crystallize CFTR en toto.

In addition to the abovementioned functional domains, the CFTR carboxyl terminus ends with four amino acids,

DTRL, which interact with PDZ domains. PDZ domain regions consist of approximately 80–90 amino acids organized as six antiparallel β-strands and two α-helices. The term "PDZ" originates from the names of proteins in which these domains were initially described: postsynaptic density (PSD-95 [42, 152]), the septate junctions linking *Drosophila* epithelia (discs-large [dlg] protein, the product of the dlg tumor suppressor gene [300]), and the tight junctions of mammalian epithelia (ZO-1 [120, 297]). PDZ domain-containing proteins act as molecular linkers and as such provide exceptionally dynamic and plastic scaffolds upon which complex regulatory systems can be built. Thus, CFTR's PDZ protein interactions have profound implications for its role as a regulator, as well as for its own biosynthesis and regulation (39, 40, 185, 273).

Classification of CFTR Mutations

To date, more than a 1000 mutations in CFTR have been identified (www.genet.sickkids.on.ca). The most common mutation is a deletion of phenylalanine at position 508 (ΔF508) that leads to misprocessing in the synthetic pathway. CFTR mutations range in severity and can be categorized roughly into five classes (43). On the severe end of the spectrum are the Class I–III mutations, which are associated with lung disease and pancreatic insufficiency. Class I comprises null mutations, in which no CFTR at all is made. Folding and trafficking mutants such as ΔF508 fall into Class II; these are targeted for degradation by the endoplasmic reticulum quality control machinery. The Class III mutations result in channels that are trafficked to the membrane, but are gated and regulated improperly. On the other end of the spectrum are the Class IV (altered conductance) and V (reduced synthesis) mutations; these patients are pancreatic sufficient. Individuals affected with Class V mutations are often asymptomatic, but are identified when presenting with idiopathic pancreatitis or congenital bilateral absence of the vas deferens (41, 44).

CFTR Pharmacology

CFTR can be inhibited in two distinct ways: allosterically or by open channel block (253). Allosteric block involves intervention at the level of the ATP-dependent gating by the NBDs. On the other hand, open channel blockers exert their effects in a voltage-dependent manner and in addition are affected by the external chloride concentration (316). Most basic characterizations of CFTR channel behavior in renal systems have used open channel blockers as structurally diverse as the sulfonylurea receptor antagonist, glibenclamide, and classical anthracene derivatives such as DPC. When applied to the cytosolic side in excised, inside-out patches, these compounds block CFTR, but only at high concentrations. Using patch recording in conjunction with site-directed mutagenesis, Linsdell (157) recently identified K95 as a critical residue that functions in CFTR inhibition by these anionic compounds by attracting them into an accommodating inner vestibule.

A. Full-length CFTR

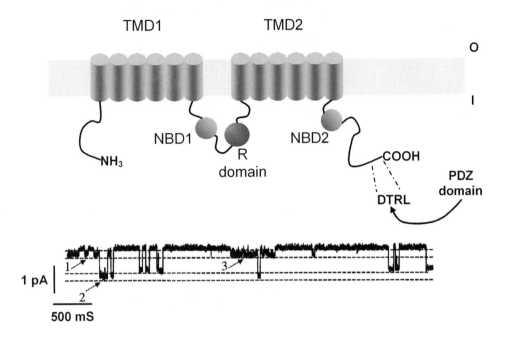

B. TNR CFTR

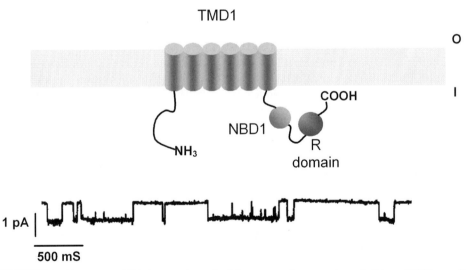

FIGURE 3 The top panel (A) shows a schematic of the transmembrane topology of wildtype CFTR, as well as a representative trace depicting the typical chloride channel activity that arises upon activation of full-length CFTR with 75-nM PKA and 0.5-mM ATP. The patch was held at a membrane potential of −85 mV. Note the presence of a low conductance state, which can gate either directly from the closed state (labeled 1 or together with the large conductance state (labeled 2 or 3). The bottom panel (B) shows a schematic of the kidney-specific, truncated variant of CFTR, TNR. Also shown is a representative recording of a patch containing a single TNR channel, which opens only to the larger conductance level when stimulated with PKA and ATP. This recording was obtained on a patch held at a membrane potential of −75 mV. (Current traces from Yue H, Devidas S, Guggino WB. The two halves of CFTR form a dual-pore ion channel. *J Biol Chem* 2000;275:10030–10034.)

High throughput screening efforts to identify CFTR activators, and inhibitors have yielded small molecule activators (307), as well as two novel chemical classes of high-affinity (K_i on the order of micromolar) CFTR inhibitors, thiazolidinones (CFTR$_{inh}$-172 [171]) as well as glycine hydrazides (GlyH-101 [193]). Li et al. (153) showed inhibition of MDCK cyst expansion by CFTR$_{inh}$-172, a finding that has implications for the management of polycystic kidney disease. Although GlyH-101 has been evaluated thoroughly for its effects on cholera toxin-challenged, CFTR-mediated, murine small intestinal fluid secretion (193), to date it has not been used on kidney-derived systems.

CFTR in Kidney

RT-PCR STUDIES

Numerous studies have identified CFTR in the mammalian kidney (261). Although its function there is not completely understood, its relative abundance in both fetal and adult kidney suggests a role in renal epithelial chloride transport. CFTR mRNA is expressed in all segments of the nephron, albeit in varying degrees. For instance, fluorescence-activated cell sorting of rabbit CCD cells enabled RT-PCR studies that demonstrate expression of mRNA encoding CFTR in principal cells, as well as both α- and β-intercalated cells (279). In tubule segments dissected from rat kidney, RT-PCR showed very low amounts in the thin limbs, as well as the outer and inner medullary collecting ducts. Interestingly, a short form (TNR) consisting of TMD1, NBD1, and R domain, which was not detected in the more proximal nephron, was found in those segments (191). TNR lacks 145 base pairs of exons 13 and 14, resulting in a frameshift that leads to a premature termination stop codon. Figure 3 schematizes the difference between the full-length CFTR and TNR proteins. Heterologous expression in both *Xenopus* oocytes and mammalian epithelial cells and subsequent electrophysiological analysis indicated that, despite an overall lower expression level, TNR encodes a cAMP-activated chloride channel with most the biophysical and pharmacological properties of wildtype CFTR (312). Interestingly, however, a smaller subconductance state that is seen in wildtype CFTR did not appear in TNR single-channel traces. To date, the physiological role of TNR remains enigmatic.

DETECTION OF CFTR PROTEIN IN KIDNEY

Devuyst and colleagues (60) used a panel of six different CFTR antibodies in immunohistochemical localization studies. In 12-week human fetal kidneys, CFTR is expressed primarily in the apical membrane region of the ureteric bud epithelial cells. The cells of the proximal tubules and loops of Henle show diffuse cytoplasmic staining for CFTR by 15 weeks. No glomerular staining was seen at any gestational state. From 15 to 24 weeks of gestation this staining pattern remains constant. Using the rabbit polyclonal antibody 169, directed against the R-domain of CFTR and also used in the human studies mentioned previously, Murray and coworkers (191, 194) showed that the newborn rat kidney mirrors this same general pattern of CFTR protein expression.

Functional Measurements of CFTR in Renal Epithelia

Early studies using light-scattering measurements detected PKA-activated chloride conductance in vesicles derived from rat kidney cortical brush-border membrane and outer medulla (19). The pharmacological properties of this conductance included glibenclamide sensitivity. Whole-cell patch measurements of cultured rabbit distal convoluted tubule cells (275), as well as cultured mouse cortical collecting duct cells (151), also indicated the presence of cAMP-activated chloride channel activity. The presence of CFTR in proximal nephronal segments suggests a role in chloride absorption. There is some evidence that more distal segments such as the medullary collecting duct can also secrete chloride. The presence of chloride channels with properties identical to CFTR in both mouse (288) and rat (119) medullary collecting duct suggests a role in chloride secretion by this segment.

Although life-threatening renal disease does not occur in cystic fibrosis (CT), some aspects of renal function do arise. In CF, the excretion of drugs is altered, and in some cases the renal concentrating mechanism and the ability to excrete a salt load are compromised. Moreover, CF patients have an increased risk of kidney stones that may result from hyperoxaluria and hypocitraturia (100, 131). The lack of severe, overt kidney disease may reflect sufficient redundancy in the renal chloride channel pool to compensate for the lack of functional CFTR. Precedence for similar compensation by another channel has been established as the result of studies on the CFTR knockout mouse (259, 259). Unlike humans with CF, the CF mouse does not have significant lung disease. Apparently, Ca^{2+}-activated chloride conductance adequately compensates for the lack of CFTR in the airways and rescues lung function (49). In addition, it remains possible that chloride transport per se constitutes a minor role of renal CFTR; indeed, its primary function may be as a regulator of other renal channels and transporters.

CFTR as Regulator

CFTR is known to regulate other processes. For example, cAMP-dependent protein kinase A activates outwardly rectifying Cl⁻ channels (ORCC) (83). The effect of CFTR activation on that of epithelial sodium channels (ENaC) differs, depending on the tissue studied (59, 223, 242). Both ORCC and ENaC lose their pattern(s) of protein kinase sensitivity when the function of CFTR is severely compromised in CF. In addition, sulfonylurea sensitivity of the renal outer medullary potassium channel, ROMK, appears to be modulated by CFTR (36, 180, 181).

ACTIVATED CFTR ACTIVATES ORCC

A clear functional relationship between CFTR and the ORCC has been established (68, 83, 96, 129, 244, 245). ORCC's persistence, but lower overall frequency of detection, in CFTR (-/-) mice led to the conclusion that it represents a molecular entity distinct from CFTR (83). Schwiebert and colleagues (244) proposed that protein kinase A-mediated stimulation of CFTR leads to ATP release, with subsequent paracrine activation of purinergic receptors then leading to ORCC activation. Alternatively, released ATP could directly activate ORCC. A minimalistic model, based on the findings of bilayer reconstitution experiments, is illustrated in Fig. 4 (top) (241).

Despite the amassment of substantial knowledge concerning the functional relationship between CFTR and the ORCC, the lack of a molecular identity for ORCC has hampered further progress. Recently, Ogura et al. (202) put forth the hypothesis that a long splice form of ClC-3 (ClC-3b), which contains a PDZ protein-binding motif, may encode the ORCC. These workers presented evidence that PDZ protein interactions linking ClC-3b to EBP-50 lead to protein kinase A-regulated, outwardly rectifying chloride currents. In this scenario, CFTR regulates ORCC via its PDZ interaction with EBP-50 (see Fig. 4, bottom). However, the subcellular localization studies of Gentzsch and coworkers (85) argue to the contrary. Thus, at present, the molecular identity of the ORCC remains a topic of intense scrutiny and awaits conclusive resolution.

CFTR AND ENaC

This inhibitory function of CFTR on ENaC requires functionally active NBD1 and R domains (144), and moreover, depends on the ability to conduct chloride. CFTR inhibition of ENaC in airway cells has been suggested to be defective in CF individuals (137, 172). Heterologous expression experiments using *Xenopus* oocytes show inhibition of ENaC consequent to IBMX activation of wildtype CFTR. Similar treatment of ΔF508-CFTR and ENaC coexpressing oocytes did not influence ENaC activity (144, 173). Thus, these data are consistent with the notion that CFTR normally inhibits Na+ reabsorption (30, 144, 151, 269). Studies conducted on M-1 mouse cortical collecting duct cells showed that activation of protein kinase A reduced amiloride-sensitive Na+ currents in a manner similar to the previously observed effects on airway epithelia (151). These data support the notion that, in the kidney as in the airways, CFTR normally inhibits Na+ reabsorption (30, 144, 151, 269). In contrast, recent work using an MDCK cell line that stably expresses rat ENaC subunits provides evidence suggesting otherwise (303). Increased levels of intracellular chloride inhibit amiloride-sensitive sodium currents. By extension, decreased levels, such as those expected when chloride secretion is engaged by cAMP stimulation, would promote ENaC-mediated currents. Similarly, primary cultures of collecting duct cells derived from a Liddle's syndrome mouse model that carries the activating β-ENaC

stop codon mutation, display a greater AVP-stimulated, CFTR-mediated chloride current (37). These data are consistent with the scenario that previously has been described in studies on the sweat duct, with concomitant activation of both CFTR and ENaC by cAMP stimulation (223).

CFTR: A COMPONENT OF K_{ATP}?

Renal ATP-sensitive, inward rectifier potassium channels (K_{ATP}) modulate Na+, K+ and Cl− reabsorption in the thick ascending limb of the loop of Henle, as well as K+ secretion in the cortical collecting tubule (293). The molecular biology of a class of inwardly rectifying potassium channels (KIR; also known as ROMK for renal outer medullary K+) has

CFTR regulation of ORCC: 2 proposed models

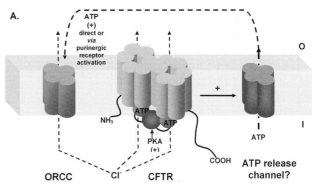

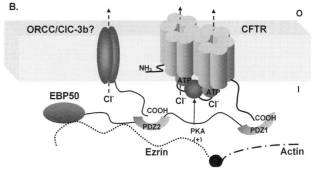

FIGURE 4 Two proposed models for regulation of ORCC by CFTR. The top panel (A) summarizes a minimalistic model derived from reconstitution studies discussed in Schwiebert et al. (241). ATP binding at the NBDs of CFTR, together with PKA-mediated phosphorylation of the R domain, not only leads to CFTR gating and conduction of chloride, but also elicits the release of ATP. This release hypothetically occurs through a closely associated, ATP release pathway. Subsequently, ATP either activates ORCC directly or indirectly by stimulating a purinergic receptor, resulting in further chloride exit from the cell. Note that the molecular identity of both the ORCC and the ATP release channel are not specified in this model. The lower panel (B) illustrates the model. In this scenario, the longer splice form of ClC-3, ClC-3b, encodes the ORCC, and its regulation by CFTR is mediated by their mutual interactions with the PDZ domains of EBP50, which by virtue of its interaction with ezrin, connects to the actin cytoskeleton. Note that the two models do not necessarily conflict. (Model in lower panel from Ogura T, Furukawa T, Toyozaki T, Yamada K, Zheng YJ, Katayama Y, Nakaya H, Inagaki N. ClC-3B, a novel ClC-3 splicing variant that interacts with EBP50 and facilitates expression of CFTR-regulated ORCC. *FASEB J* 2002;16:863–865.)

been studied extensively (113). These channels are expressed in distal nephron segments of the mammalian kidney and display many of the characteristics of low conductance, ATP-sensitive K^+ currents previously described in the apical membranes of thick ascending limb, macula densa, and principal cells. One such trait is sensitivity (with micromolar affinity) to the sulfonylurea compound, glibenclamide.

One conundrum encountered in early studies was that, although expression of Kir 1.1a (ROMK2) in *Xenopus* oocytes yielded secretory K_{ATP} currents, these had negligible sensitivity to glibenclamide. Coexpression studies with CFTR, however, conferred sensitivity (180). Mutagenesis studies point to a role for the first nucleotide-binding fold (NBF1) motif of CFTR in this effect (181). Interestingly, although truncated, the kidney-specific splice form, TNR CFTR, does contain NBD1 (191). Phosphorylation of the R domain attenuates the interaction between CFTR and ROMK2 (36).

Interestingly, the relationship between ROMK2 and CFTR mirrors that between the KIR6.x and the sulfonylurea receptor (SUR) proteins underlying the K_{ATP} of pancreatic β cells (reviewed recently by Neagoe and Schwappach [196]). KIR6.x and KIR1.1a are members of a transmembrane-spanning domain potassium-channel family; SUR and CFTR are members of the ABC transporter superfamily. Further evidence to support the notion that native K_{ATP} channels are composed of KIR 1.1a and CFTR comes from experiments showing that KIR 1.1a and CFTR have overlapping distribution with low sulfonylurea affinity K_{ATP} in the kidney tubules TAL and CCD (232). Important recent studies that elucidate the mechanism by which coassembly with SUR facilitates the trafficking of KIR6.x/SUR complexes thus are likely to bear relevance to that of renal KIR1.1a/CFTR (239, 313).

DOES CFTR PARTICIPATE IN INTRAORGANELLAR ACIDIFICATION?

Rabbit kidney endosomes have protein kinase A–mediated chloride permeability, and CFTR has been identified in these endosomes (13, 51). Thus, CFTR may play a role in regulating and maintaining an acidic pH in intracellular compartments. Indeed, a significant acidification defect exists in the trans-Golgi and prelysosomal compartments in respiratory epithelial cells and nasal polyps from CF patients (14). However, cellubrevin-labeled endosomes in CF lung epithelial cells hyperacidify; these observations therefore are at odds with the notion that CFTR is needed to acidify intracellular compartments (214). Experiments showing that the presence or absence of CFTR did not alter endosomal pH further challenge this hypothesis (251). However, the advent of more sensitive reagents and morphological methods has revealed the existence of distinct endosomal subpopulations. Thus, it remains possible that the lack of unambiguous identification between heterogeneous intracellular compartments in the previously mentioned studies may account for the reported discrepancies.

AQUAPORIN-6

Yasui and coworkers (309) identified aquaporin-6 (AQP6), an intracellular member of the AQP family of water-permeant membrane channels, which they subsequently determined to function as an anion channel. Immunohistochemical microscopy and immunogold electron microscopy localized AQP6 to vesicles in glomerular podocytes, cells of the proximal tubular S2 and S3 segments, and α intercalated cells of the inner medullary collecting duct. The proximal tubule cells showed AQP6 in the subapical vesicles, whereas the staining of α intercalated cells appeared in vesicles in all cellular regions. AQP6 localizes to neither the apical nor basolateral membranes, thus suggesting a role other than transepithelial water movement. Subsequent functional analysis revealed external acidity-activated, linear anion currents, but little water permeability, in AQP6-expressing *Xenopus* oocytes (308). Curiously, Hg^{+2}, an inhibitor of other aquaporins, augmented both the ionic current and the osmotic water permeability. β-mercaptoethanol partially reversed the effect, but classical chloride channel inhibitors such as DPC, DIDS, NPPB and niflumic acid, as well as the heavy metal inhibitors of ClC-2, zinc, and cadmium, did not block AQP6.

The K72E charge mutation alters ionic selectivity. Wild-type AQP6 selects for chloride approximately fourfold over sodium, whereas the substitution of glutamate for lysine normalizes the permeability ratio. Thus, AQP6 likely functions as an anion channel (308). Alignment of the amino acid sequence of AQP6 with other mammalian aquaporins shows a single asparagine residue (N60) in place of a conserved glycine residue (G57). Interestingly, AQP6 can be converted into a channel that discriminates against anions and exhibits higher osmotic water permeability by mutation of this residue back to glycine (158).

Together with activation of anion currents at low pH, the colocalization of AQP6 with the V-type H^+-ATPase suggests a role in vesicular acidification. Like ClC-5, AQP6 might promote acidification by the H^+-ATPase by shunting the development of the vesicular lumen-positive potential difference. Interestingly, ClC-5 itself is inhibited at a pH that is lower than 6.5, precisely the range at which AQP-6 anion permeability becomes activated (79).

CALCIUM-ACTIVATED CHLORIDE CHANNELS: CLCAS, BESTROPHIN

Other anion transporting proteins, particularly those underlying calcium-activated chloride currents (CaCCs), have resisted straightforward molecular identification until recently. The heterogeneity of CaCCs further complicates the matter; roughly, they can be categorized on the basis of their requirements for activation (215). Thus, they can be (1) strictly and exclusively dependent on intracellular calcium levels, (2) regulated by the calcium/calmodulin-dependent protein kinase II (CAMKII), or (3) regulated by cGMP.

Despite these hurdles, the last several years have witnessed steps toward realizing this goal.

CaCCs have been implicated in the pathogenesis of polycystic kidney disease (114, 296). They have been measured in a range of renal epithelial cells, including those acutely isolated from the proximal and distal convoluted tubules (16, 21, 231) as well as in collecting duct primary cultures (24) or lines (24, 25, 182, 217). In particular, studies using the mouse IMCD-K2 cell line (24, 217), as well as the IMCD-3 line (221), have proven exceptionally informative. The current studied in IMCD-K2 cells strongly resembles the well-studied, endogenous, calcium-activated chloride current of Xenopus oocytes (15, 108), with outward rectification at stimulated physiological (submillimolar) calcium levels, rapid closure at excessive intracellular calcium levels, voltage-dependent calcium affinity and block by niflumic acid at micromolar concentrations. On the other hand, the CaCCs observed in IMCD-3 cells appear open at resting intracellular calcium activities. Moreover, although outwardly rectifying, these currents showed neither the time-dependent kinetics nor the voltage-dependence described for the currents in IMCD-K2 cells (265).

Two families of putative calcium-activated chloride channels, the CLCAs and the bestrophins are summarized in the next sections. For in-depth treatments of CaCCs, see the excellent reviews by Eggermont (69), Hartzell et al. (108), and Jentsch et al. (126).

CLCAs

As early as 1991, a 38-kD protein had been purified from bovine tracheal epithelium and, subsequent to successful functional reconstitution in liposomes and bilayers, identified as a calcium-activated chloride channel (218–220). Cloning of the cDNA for this bovine channel followed (53). Now known as bCLCA1, this cDNA encodes a 100–140-kD membrane protein of 903 amino acids that initially was predicted to span four transmembrane domains and contain two sites for N-linked glycosylation, as well as several consensus sites for phosphorylation. Post-translational cleavage may underlie the discrepancy between the size of this product and the purified 38-kD protein, but to date this has not yet been addressed rigorously. The expression of the bCLCA1 cRNA in Xenopus oocytes yielded channels with similar functional properties (53). Biophysical traits include a single-channel conductance between 25 and 30 pS, linear I–V relationship, and a halide selectivity sequence of $I^- > Br^- > Cl^-$. Importantly, like the reconstituted protein (80), the expressed bCLCA1 currents showed modulation by CaMKII that increased the sensitivity to intracellular calcium levels (53). DIDS and DTT both inhibited the expressed channel currents. Bovine CLCA1 currents proved relatively insensitive to niflumic acid, a compound known to block the endogenous oocyte CaCC, as well as those previously characterized in epithelial cells (53).

It soon became clear that bCLCA1 represented the founding member of a diverse molecular family (71, 74, 84, 91, 230). A plethora of roles has been attributed to bovine, human, porcine, and mouse members of the CLCA family. These include (1) regulation of ionic channels (162–165), (2) action as extracellular matrix proteins (1–3) and tumor suppressors (33, 70, 92), (3) functioning as targets for cytokine signaling (11, 115, 278, 315), and (4) upregulation of mucin secretion by induction of MUC2 (179).

Overall, agreement on CLCA topology is lacking, with predictions ranging between one and five membrane-spanning domains (94, 230). More perplexing is the paucity of structure-function information pinpointing which of several proteolytic fragments forms the anion-conducting domain. Moreover, hCLCA3 encodes a truncated protein that lacks transmembrane domains and is secreted, further complicating the picture (93).

Even among the CLCA isoforms that express functional chloride currents, considerable heterogeneity in biophysical and pharmacological properties exist. Moreover, several of these characteristics are at odds with those documented for the endogenous CaCCs in renal epithelial cells, and may even depend on the choice of expression system. These include calcium (and CaMKII) dependence and rectification properties, as well as sensitivity to inhibitors such as niflumic acid and DTT (discussed in Eggermont [69]). Moreover, CLCA expression is undetectable in some cell types that clearly show CaCC activity (77, 205), although they have been detected in the mouse kidney. Therefore, at this time, whether CLCAs encode the channels comprising CaCCs or regulators of yet-to-be-identified native proteins remains controversial and will require continued careful scrutiny.

Bestrophins

The first member of the bestrophin family was identified by positional cloning as the product of VMD2, the gene that is disrupted in the autosomal dominant retinopathy, Best (or, alternatively, vitelloform) macular dystrophy (175, 209, 268). The 585-amino-acid bestrophin protein was predicted to have multiple transmembrane-spanning regions, and many disease-associated bestrophin mutations fall in highly conserved regions in the vicinity of predicted transmembrane domains. Best's disease–affected individuals accumulate fluid in the subretinal space and show an attenuated, slow light peak of the electro-oculogram (58, 78), a feature attributed to the activity of chloride conductance in the basolateral membrane of retinal pigment epithelial (RPE) cells (262). These points led Sun et al. (270) to hypothesize that VMD2 encodes a chloride channel, and thus undertake functional analysis by heterologous expression in HEK 293 cells (270). Biophysical properties of the expressed whole-cell currents of the two human homologues, hBest1 and hBest2, include an anion permeability sequence of $NO_3^- > I^- > Br^- > Cl^-$, a linear I–V relationship, and inhibition by 500-μM DIDS, DTT, and the sulfhydryl-reactive agents, MTSEA and MT-SET. The expression of cysteine-less hBest1 mutants resulted in currents that resisted block by MTSEA and MTSET. Photorelease of calcium augmented the current, thus further characterizing bestrophin as a calcium-activated channel. The expression of Best's disease–associated mutants reduced the whole-cell current. The successful expression of bestrophin permitted a detailed topographical mapping of hBest1 that predicted three extracellular loops, four transmembrane domains, and both the amino and carboxyl termini on the cytosolic side (282).

To date, four human and four mouse bestrophin family members have been identified (267, 282). A recent in-depth functional analysis further identifies mouse bestrophin-2 (mBest2) as a time-independent, calcium-activated chloride channel, with an EC_{50} for calcium of 230 nM as well as block of chloride conductance by external SCN^- and a permeability sequence of $SCN^- > I^- > Br^- > Cl^- > F^-$ (216). Structure–function analysis of residues in the second putative transmembrane domain, together with sulfhydryl modification studies, identified S79 as a pore-lining residue that acts as an anion-binding site and determines anion selectivity by a mechanism independent from electrostatic interaction. Thus, these findings confirm that bestrophin family members do indeed function as chloride channels.

Northern analysis revealed strong expression of VMD2 in the retina (209) and RPE (175). Prolonged exposure also resulted in signals in the brain and spinal cord, and RT-PCR also produced a band of the correct size in the kidney (209). Do renal CaCCs reflect bestrophin channel activity? RT-PCR data indicate that bestrophins are expressed in IMCD-K2 cells (217). However, the biophysical properties of CaCCs measured in IMCD-K2 cells differ substantially from those of bestrophins. Thus, an involvement of bestrophins in mediating the CaCCs in IMCD-K2 cells is highly unlikely.

Certainly, the advent of siRNA technology will enable attempts to knock down CaCC. This will permit identification of the responsible molecular species as well as exclusion of those that are irrelevant.

I_{CLN}: CHANNEL OR CHANNEL MODULATOR?

Using expression cloning methods, Paulmichl et al. (206) isolated a unique cDNA, pI_{Cln}, from the MDCK cell line. pI_{Cln} encodes a 235-amino-acid, 26-kD protein that, by initial hydrophobicity analysis, has no α-helical transmembrane domains. This led these authors to propose that pI_{Cln} organizes as a unique structure consisting of a dimer of four β sheets each (206). Expression of the cDNA in *Xenopus* oocytes resulted in the appearance of a chloride-selective, outwardly rectifying current. pI_{Cln}-associated currents displayed slow inactivation at depolarized holding potentials and calcium insensitivity. DIDS and NPPB, as well as extra-

cellular nucleotides (cAMP, cGMP, and ITP), block these currents in a dose-dependent fashion. The mutation of a putative nucleotide-binding site at the predicted external mouth of the pore not only abolished sensitivity to cAMP, but also rendered the currents sensitive to the depletion of extracellular calcium (206). However, several lines of evidence rapidly emerged that suggest pI_{Cln} encodes a mediator of endogenous chloride channels, rather a bona fide chloride channel. Among these points were the observations that its expression was almost entirely restricted to the cytosol and furthermore its overexpression in the Sf9 (*Spodoptera frugiperda* pupal ovary) cell line did not produce detectable channel activity (143). The peculiar structural features of pI_{Cln}, such as the lack of hydrophobic regions, also raised concerns. Moreover, the expression of a structurally unrelated protein, ClC-6, elicited I_{Cln}-like currents in *Xenopus* oocytes (35). In contrast, a polyclonal antibody raised against a synthetic peptide from the C-terminus of I_{Cln} detected expression of I_{Cln} protein at equivalent levels in the cortex, outer and inner medullae, and papilla of rat kidney (145). Western blotting of isolated membrane vesicles indicated expression in the apical, but not basolateral, membrane (145). Biochemical evidence exists for association of pI_{Cln} with β-actin in reticulocytes, and laser confocal microscopy localized it to the reticulocyte membrane (240). An association with soluble actin was previously reported by Krapivinsky et al. (143), who also postulated a role for pI_{Cln} in linking the cytoskeleton with an unidentified, volume-sensitive chloride channel. Recent fluorescence-resonance energy-transfer experiments demonstrated that pI_{Cln} redistributes from the cytosol to the plasma membrane in response to cell swelling, with kinetics that correlate with those measured for regulatory volume decrease (228).

Thus, the possibility that pI_{Cln} functions as an accessory chloride-channel regulator could account for the observations to date. Certainly, its high expression in the kidney speaks to an important role in normal renal physiology in general and perhaps specifically to the process of volume regulation.

CLIC/p64: PUTATIVE INTRACELLULAR CHLORIDE CHANNELS

In recent years, information about how proteins of the CLIC/p64 family contribute to the physiology of intracellular compartments has increased at an astonishing rate. For further details, see Ashley's (10) excellent and concise review. Initial studies utilizing IAA-affinity chromatography resulted in the partial isolation of chloride channels from the bovine kidney cortex, as well as bovine tracheal epithelium (147). Reconstitution of this protein into planar bilayers and liposomes resulted in, respectively, chloride channel activity and potential-driven ^{36}Cl uptake. Subsequently, a 64-kD protein, dubbed p64, was purified and determined to be the component that supported ^{36}Cl

uptake (225). This same study localized p64 to intracellular organellar membranes as well as the apical membrane of CFPAC cells, a CF pancreatic ductal line. In the T84 colonic epithelial cell line, p64 was detected in perinuclear dense core vesicles (224). Screening of a bovine renal cortex cDNA expression library led to the isolation of a 6160 nucleotide, full-length clone encoding a novel protein of 437 amino acids (146). Like the CLCAs and pI$_{Cln}$, the initial predicted structures bore no resemblance to then-perceived notions of channel structure. Among recognizable features, however, are between two and four transmembrane-spanning regions, as well as consensus sites for phosphorylation by protein kinase C, tyrosine kinase, and casein kinase II within the cytoplasmic amino terminus. The expression of p64 in *Xenopus* oocytes did not produce apparent currents, nor did surface biotinylation experiments reveal its presence in the plasma membrane, but isolated intracellular microsomes did show the insertion of the 64-kD protein (146). Edwards et al. (67) determined the channel properties of p64 by bilayer reconstitution of membranes isolated from expressing HeLa cells. They found p64 to be outwardly rectifying, with a single-channel conductance of 42 pS, and Cl$^-$ to K$^+$ selectivity of 20:1, as well as activated by dephosphorylation. Curiously, p64 primarily associated with the soluble fraction of these preparations, a finding belying its apparent ability to function as a membrane channel.

The identification of p64 set the stage for the cloning of broadly distributed, homologous proteins, and hence also for the birth of the intracellular chloride channel (CLIC) family (Table 2). Of these, CLIC1, a human homologue, perhaps has been studied to a similar level of detail as p64. CLIC1 was predicted to assume an even more minimal structure than p64, with fewer amino acids (241) and only one transmembrane domain (112). CLIC1 is expressed in the glomeruli and the proximal tubular brush border. Like p64, CLIC predominantly is found in soluble protein fractions (283).

When overexpressed, intracellular channels often traffic to the plasma membrane. Single-channel recordings of over-expressing, transfected CHO-K1 cells showed activity with a single-channel conductance of 22 pS in 140-mM symmetrical chloride, a relative permeability of SCN$^-$ > F$^-$ > Cl$^-$ > NO$_3^-$ ~ I$^-$ = HCO$_3^-$ > acetate, and a linear i–V relationship (280, 287). FLAG tagging of either the amino or carboxyl terminus of CLIC1 (FLAG-CLIC1 and CLIC1-FLAG, respectively) enabled Tonini et al. (280) to probe transmembrane topology. In excised, outside-out patch recordings of CHO-K1 cells transfected with FLAG-CLIC1, the bath application of anti-FLAG M2 antibody–silenced chloride channel activity. On the other hand, bath application of M2 blocked channel currents measured on inside-out patches from cells transfected with CLIC1-FLAG. Thus, the amino terminus of CLIC1 must project outward, whereas the carboxyl terminus must project inward. One peculiarity, however, is that the biophysical traits of bilayer-reconstituted CLIC1 channels differ from those acquired from measurements on overexpressing cells, with a single-channel conductance of 70 pS in 150-mM chloride and an outwardly rectifying i–V. These discrepancies may arise from the loss of a regulatory protein, and hence disrupted channel modulation in the

TABLE 2   Summary of CLIC/p64 Family Members

	Predicted Molecular Mass	Functional Expression	Localization	Initial Identification	Other Distribution	Other [a]
p64	49 kD	+[a]	Cytosol/intracellular membranes	Bovine renal cortex	CF-PAC1	Electrophysiological (bilayer recording) and chloride flux
Parchorin	65 kD	+[a]	Cytosol/translocates to plasma membrane with stimulation[a]	Rabbit gastric parietal cell	Rabbit airway epithelia; rabbit choroid plexus; porcine (LLCPK-1) cells	Dye assay for chloride flux; cAMP stimulation causes membrane association
CLIC1	26.9 kD	+[a]		Human myelomonocytes		Electrophysiological (patch clamp⁻ excised patches)
CLIC2	27 kD			Skeletal muscle		
CLIC3	23.6 kD	+[a]	Nuclear	Human fetal brain	Human heart, placenta, lung	Whole-cell recordings; nuclear localization argues instead for a role as a regulator
CLIC4	28.6 kD[a]	+[a]	Cytosol/intracellular membranes	Rat brain neurons	Human pancreatic (Panc-1) line; human kidney proximal tubule	Sites for PKA, PKC phosphorylation; molecular mass ~43 kD with PKC
CLIC5	28 kD			Human placenta		

bilayer system. However, until mutagenesis of CLIC1 itself reveals a change in pore properties, the issue awaits resolution. Similar reservations apply to parchorin, a family member that has been found to associate with the cell membrane on cAMP stimulation and mediate chloride fluxes in LLCPK-1 cells (198), as well as to CLIC4, a family member that has been detected in human kidney proximal tubule (66).

More recent work utilizing database searches has revealed a likeness of the soluble form of CLIC1 to omega-class glutathione S-transferases (GSTs), sharing the glutaredoxin fold that is characteristic of these enzymes (63). Omega-class GSTs modulate ryanodine receptors, potentiating skeletal muscle ryanodine receptors, and inhibiting those of cardiac muscle (63). Interestingly, IAA-94, used to purify p64 and also known to inhibit CLIC currents, is structurally related to ethacrynic acid, an inhibitor of GSTs (107). However, to date, GSTs have not been observed to form ion channels under any circumstances. Together, these observations have led to the elucidation of the CLIC1 structure at 1.4 Å resolution (protein database file 1K0O) (107, 107). Without a doubt, the quest to obtain the structure of the membrane-inserted species has commenced. The availability of both structures will provide insights into the dramatic structural rearrangements that are necessary for CLICs to convert among a compact, globular, and soluble species and assume the conformation of a membrane protein.

BACK TO FUNCTION: LESSONS FROM DISEASE MODELS

The central role of chloride channels to renal function is highlighted by the insights gained from recent studies of diseases that result from their genetic disruption. Bartter's syndrome types III and IV, Dent's disease, and polycystic kidney disease all attest to the central role of chloride channels in renal physiology.

Bartter's Syndrome

Bartter's syndrome is an autosomal recessive renal tubular disorder characterized by renal salt wasting, hypokalemic metabolic alkalosis, elevated renin and aldosterone levels, normal or low blood pressure, hypercalciuria, and normal serum magnesium levels (20). Mutations in five different genes account for the five Bartter's variants. Figure 5 summarizes the transport processes that are pertinent to Bartter's. Types I to III are caused by loss-of-function mutations in the genes encoding transport proteins that directly mediate NaCl reabsorption by the thick ascending limb: NKCC2, ROMK, and ClC-Kb, respectively (20, 255–257). The ClC-K channel accessory protein, barttin, enhances membrane expression of both ClC-Ka and -Kb (72). Barttin is a two-transmembrane domain, integral membrane protein present

A. TALH Cell

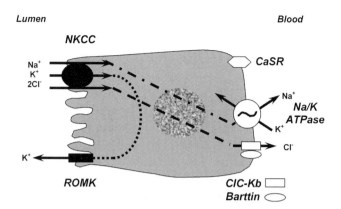

B. Cell of Stria Vascularis

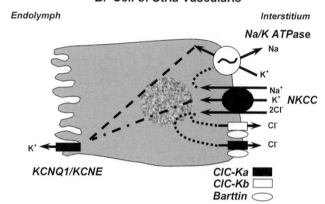

FIGURE 5 These schema illustrate the basic transport processes in the kidney and inner ear that can explain the differences between type III and type IV Bartter's syndrome. Mutations in CLCNKB disrupt chloride absorption by the thick ascending limb (TALH cell; top panel, A) by creating the loss of basolaterally located, heteromeric ClC-Kb/barttin channel function. Thus, the uptake of chloride from the lumen cannot proceed, leading to the salt wasting that is characteristic of type III Bartter's syndrome. Type IV Bartter's presents with not only renal salt wasting, but also congenital deafness, due to mutations in barttin. This is because the cells of the inner ear (cell of stria vascularis; bottom panel, B) require basolateral chloride conductance to secrete a high-potassium endolymph that is essential to the excitability of the cochlear hair cells. Both ClC-Ka/barttin and ClC-Kb/barttin channel complexes subserve this chloride conductance. Type III Bartter's patients escape the deafness phenotype because ClC-Ka/barttin complexes presumably sufficiently compensate for the defect in ClC-Kb.

in all nephron segments that express either of the ClC-Ks, as well as the stria vascularis of the inner ear, which also expresses ClC-K channels. Its mutation accounts for the more severe salt wasting, as well as the additional consequence of sensorineural deafness, that characterizes type IV Bartter's syndrome (22, 72, 123, 140, 290). Type V results from gain-of-function mutations in the calcium-sensing receptor (CaSR) (109, 111, 252). The CaSR is a G protein–coupled surface receptor that belongs to family C of the G-protein receptor superfamily. It resides at the basolateral membranes of the thick ascending limb, and its normal activation by high extracellular calcium inhibits salt transport (32, 110, 227). Thus, Bartter's type V mutations inappropriately attenuate salt absorption. Here, we focus on the molecular basis of type III and type IV Bartter's syndrome, which result from disruption of the basolateral chloride channel complex, ClC-Kb/barttin.

The rodent orthologue of ClC-Ka, ClC-K1, localizes to the apical and basolateral membrane of thin ascending limbs and inner medullary collecting ducts (138, 284, 289, 310). In contrast, ClC-K2, the orthologue of human ClC-Kb, is broadly expressed in the basolateral membrane of the cells that make up the distal nephron, including the thick ascending limb, distal convoluted tubule, connecting tubule, and α-intercalated cells of the collecting duct (289, 310). Thus, the lack of overlap in the kidney contrasts with the distribution in the inner ear, where both ClC-K1 and -K2 likely are present in the stria vascularis.

The renal distribution pattern predicts that loss-of-function mutations in the human orthologue of ClC-K2, ClC-Kb, cause impairment in salt absorption. Note that, compared to Bartter's type III, patients with type IV Bartter's syndrome have more severe salt wasting. This suggests that, at least in humans, salt absorption by the distal nephron might also rely on the presence of ClC-Ka, as well as ClC-Kb. Although the immunolocalization studies in mice suggest that the distributions of the rodent orthologues do not overlap, a recent electrophysiological and single-cell RT-PCR study does suggest that both ClC-K1 and -K2 are present in mouse distal convoluted tubule cells (199).

Mouse knockout models have been produced for type I and type II Bartter's syndrome, but so far not for type III or IV (167, 274). It is anticipated that the creation of these models will further extend the collective understanding of these diseases.

Dent's Disease

Dent's disease, X-linked recessive nephrolithiasis (XRN), X-linked recessive hypophosphatemic rickets (XLRH), and idiopathic low-molecular-weight proteinuria of Japanese children are now considered the same genetic disorder. All of these exhibit loss-of-function mutations in the CLCN5 gene identified on chromosome Xp11.22 by linkage analysis and positional cloning (126, 160). Various mutations have been identified in families from Britain, Japan, and North America, including nonsense, missense, donor splice site mutations, deletions, frameshifts, and insertions in CLCN5 (159–161). These mutations either abolish or reduce ClC-5 channel activity (126). The common disease symptoms in human patients include low-molecular-weight (LMW) proteinuria, hypercalciuria, aminoaciduria, phosphaturia, nephrocalcinosis, nephrolithiasis, and renal failure (7, 160). Among these, LMW proteinuria is the most consistent manifestation and is almost always present in female carriers (161, 226). However, there is variability in other manifestations, such as hypercalciuria, proximal tubule solute wasting,

distal tubule disorders, and rickets (236, 302, 311). The independent generation of two Clcn5 knockout mouse models enabled more extensive studies directed at exploring the disease mechanisms (212, 291). Both knockout mouse models exhibit the LMW proteinuria phenotype. Both show evidence that knockout of Clcn5 disrupts both receptor-mediated and fluid-phase endocytosis (212, 291). Moreover, the internalization of the transporters, NaP_i-2 and NHE3, appears inhibited (212). Hyperphosphaturia and hypercalciuria are variable in these models.

Further studies have been carried out to study the role of ClC-5 in facilitating endosomal acidification, ostensibly by shunting the lumen-positive transvacuolar potential difference generated by activity of the H^+-ATPase. The acidification rate of cortical endosomes purified from ClC-5 knockout mice was reduced, compared to that measured for endosomes isolated from wildtype mice (99, 176). However, the biophysical properties of expressed ClC-5—specifically, outward rectification and inhibition by external acidic pH—do not support this proposed role ideally (79, 159).

Moulin and coworkers (192) conducted an immunohistochemical study using renal biopsies from Dent's patients and demonstrated a consistent and specific inversion of H^+-ATPase polarity to the basolateral membrane of proximal tubule cells. No other ultrastructural differences appeared. The inversion of polarity contrasts sharply with the apical localization seen in proximal tubule cells from control kidney biopsies. These workers also noted the absence of apical H^+-ATPase expression in the α-intercalated cells of the collecting duct (192). These data suggest that coordination and cooperativity between ClC-5 and the proton pump are critical for the function of both proteins in the renal proximal tubules.

Megalin, a 600-kD member of the low-density lipoprotein receptor family, and cubulin, also known as the intrinsic-factor cobalamin receptor, are multiligand receptors that reside at the proximal tubular brush border membrane. Together, they scavenge LMW proteins that enter the proximal tubule through the glomerular filtrate. Megalin knockout mice and cubulin-deficient dogs and humans all have LMW proteinuria (23, 45, 81, 150, 314). Subcellular fractionation experiments, as well as ultrastructural immunogold analysis, indicated that megalin and cubulin expression are reduced in cells from ClC-5 knockout animals. These findings led Christensen et al. (46) to hypothesize that loss of ClC-5 causes defective recycling of endosomes back to the plasma membrane, hence bringing about this reduction in megalin and cubulin expression at the brush border. Given the role that megalin plays in binding low-molecular-weight proteins for uptake into the cells, its reduced expression would also contribute to the formation of LMW proteinuria (46, 212).

The reason that Dent's patients and ClC-5 knockout mice have hypercalciuria remains unresolved. Luyckx et al. (170) attributed the hypercalciuria in their knockdown mouse model to increased intestinal Ca^{2+} absorption. Alternatively, the loss of vitamin D–binding protein could underlie the hypercalciuria seen in two murine ClC-5 knockout models (212, 291). A marked increase in the urinary excretion of the 50-kD vitamin D–binding protein is expected to reduce the 25-hydroxyvitamin D substrate delivered to the 1-hydroxylase localized in proximal tubule cells. With less 25-hydroxyvitamin D to be converted to the active form, 1,25-dihydroxyvitamin D, intestinal Ca^{2+} absorption is predicted to fall. However, compared to normal individuals, ClC-5 knockout mice and Dent's patients (236, 254) show an increase in the ratio of serum 1,25-dihydroxyvitamin D to 25-hydroxyvitamin D. How can this be explained? Two models have been proposed.

One model proposes that an increase in proximal tubule luminal fluid PTH, resulting from defective endocytosis in proximal tubules, may cause this apparent paradox by elevating the level of 1-hydroxylase (99). Elevated luminal fluid PTH also is hypothesized to reduce the expression of the sodium-phosphate transporter, NaP_i-2, as well as enhance its internalization in the proximal tubule. This may explain the hyperphosphaturia exhibited by ClC-5 knockout mice (212). Alternatively, another investigation of the Ca^{2+} handling in ClC-5 knockout mice suggests that hypercalciuria is of bone and renal origin and is not caused by increased intestinal calcium absorption under the effect of elevated serum 1,25-dihydroxyvitamin D (254, 291).

Polycystic Kidney Disease

Polycystic kidney disease (PKD) is an inheritable systemic disorder that primarily affects the kidneys. Its symptoms include hypertension, cardiovascular abnormalities, and cysts in other organs (liver and pancreas). PKD is characterized by progressively enlarging cysts derived from the massive enlargement of fluid-filled renal tubules and/or collecting ducts. This, together with interstitial fibrosis, severely compromises the normal kidney architecture and eventually leads to renal failure (82, 222).

To date, two polycystic kidney diseases have been identified: autosomal dominant PKD (ADPKD) and autosomal recessive PKD (ARPKD). ADPKD is the most common monogenic cause of kidney failure, and occurs with an incidence of 1:1000 in Caucasians. It is caused by mutations in either PKD1 (chromosome 16) or PKD2 (chromosome 4), which encode, respectively, the integral membrane proteins polycystin 1 and polycystin 2. Polycystin 1 is a large (4302 amino acid) protein with a long amino terminus, and extracellular domain containing a multitude of motifs that suggest a role in protein interactions. Following a region of homology to the sea urchin receptor for egg jelly and a proteolytic cleavage site are 11 transmembrane domains and a cytoplasmic carboxyl terminus with a coiled-coil domain and a variety of potential phosphorylation sites. Polycystin 1 may have one important role as a G protein coupled receptor (57). Polycystin 2, a member of the Trp family of ion channels, contains six transmembrane domains, consists of 968 amino acids and shares modest homology with the transmembrane-spanning regions of polycystin 1. These proteins likely associate and form a receptor–cation channel complex (87, 104, 197, 281, 305). Mutations in PKD1 account for ~85% of ADPKD cases and ~15% of PKD2 cases. Mutations in a yet-to-be unidentified gene account for the remaining, very small number of ADPKD patients (134, 208, 233, 238). On the other hand, mutations in the PKHD1 (for polycystic kidney and hepatic disease) gene, located on chromosome 6, underlie ARPKD (204, 294, 304). It encodes a novel protein dubbed polyductin (204) or, alternatively, fibrocystin (294). The structure of fibrocystin suggests that it functions as a cell surface receptor. Truncated transcripts that are predicted to encode a secreted protein also exist.

Two key features associated with cyst formation in AD-PKD are fluid secretion and cell proliferation, both of which are stimulated by cAMP (95, 103, 306). These form the basis of two models by which cyst growth can be explained. In addition, ADPKD cells change their EGF receptor distribution and response to signals (89). The effects of EGF and cAMP on cell proliferation are additive. Thus, EGF-activated cell proliferation in ADPKD proceeds via a separate signal transduction cascade that is distinct from that initiated by cAMP (103).

Transepithelial potential difference measurements of forskolin-stimulated fluid secretion using excised, intact ADPKD cysts, as well as polarized monolayers grown from cysts, indicate that fluid secretion is driven by that of anions, predominantly chloride (90). CFTR likely mediates chloride secretion into cysts (88, 90). Similar to other chloride-secreting epithelia, chloride enters cystic epithelial cells through a bumetanide-sensitive, basolateral NKCC1, and then exits across the apical membrane into the luminal cavity via CFTR (174).

Immunolocalization studies using antibodies directed against CFTR, as well as NKCC1, support the fluid secretion model (149). CFTR was detected in the apical membrane of primary cultures of ADPKD cells and the luminal membrane of ADPKD cyst sections (31, 102, 149, 298). Patch-clamp studies in primary cultures of ADPKD cells identified linear, cAMP-activated chloride currents. These currents were sensitive to glibenclamide and DPC, but not DIDS, and displayed an anion selectivity sequence of $Br^- > Cl^- > I^- >$ glutamate, properties consistent with those of CFTR (102). Furthermore, antisense oligonucleotide disruption of CFTR function in ADPKD cells dramatically reduced fluid secretion (55). Interestingly, patients affected with both ADPKD and CF have less severe renal disease compared to non-CF, ADPKD patients (50, 200). With the EGF and forskolin stimulation, cells isolated from wildtype mice form cysts readily but those derived from CF mice form cysts poorly (272). These data further support a role for CFTR in the formation of cysts, and that modulating its function could be a target for treatment of ADPKD.

Notably, a study in 2004 by Li et al. (153) tested the effects of a dozen classical and novel inhibitors of CFTR and overall transepithelial secretion on cAMP-activated chloride current, cell proliferation, and cyst growth in MDCK cells grown as electrically tight monolayers and as cysts in collagen gels. The data show strong correlation between inhibition of transepithelial chloride current and suppression of cyst growth, yet at best only a marginal correlation between decreased cell proliferation and diminishment of cyst growth.

ATP-activated chloride currents may also contribute to cyst expansion via autocrine and/or paracrine purinergic receptor–mediated mechanisms (249). Wilson and colleagues (299) measured ATP levels as high as 10 μM in cyst fluid, which is enough to activate purinoceptors. Overall, their findings support a scenario whereby ATP is released into the cyst lumen, activates either or both ionotropic P2X or metabotropic P2Y receptors, elevates intracellular calcium, and activates calcium-activated chloride channels, thus driving fluid secretion. Stable transfection of the polycystin-1 carboxyl terminus in the M-1 mouse collecting duct line produces a dominant negative effect, and recapitulates the ATP-stimulated ADPKD chloride and fluid transport phenotype (114). Detailed analysis indicates that the purinergic response in these M-1 transfectants involves a prolongation of both the ATP-stimulated calcium transient and the whole cell chloride current, in a manner dependent on extracellular calcium (296).

In the (cy/+) rat model of ADPKD, the loss of ClC-5 and megalin in cysts correlates well with an inability of cyst-lining cells to internalize FITC-dextran (201). Hence, the ensuing entrapment of hormones and growth factors, as well as purines, in cyst fluid could exacerbate matters by promoting cyst expansion.

In contrast to ADPKD, no extensive studies specifically testing the involvement of chloride channels in ARPKD are presently available. However, cyst growth and renal dysfunction persist in double mutant mice derived from crossing the BPK mouse model for ARPKD (bpk -/-) and the CFTR knockout (cftr -/-) mouse (195). These findings clearly indicate that aberrant CFTR activity does not underlie the development of ARPKD. Some evidence for a role of purinergic mechanisms does exist, as an elevated basal release of ATP has been determined for collecting duct primary cultures from the cpk mouse model for ARPKD. Whether this ultimately alters chloride secretion and contributes to cyst formation and growth in ARPKD awaits further elucidation.

SUMMARY

With the merging of highly sophisticated physiological, cell biological, molecular biological, genetic, and structural approaches, the cumulative knowledge of anion channel and transport protein families has grown explosively. We can determine with some degree of confidence where these important proteins localize in the nephron, and just now are beginning to understand what they do once they find their way to those places. The contributions of CFTR, calcium-activated chloride channels, pI_{Cln}, and the CLICs to renal function are less straightforward than those of some CLC proteins. Thus, these issues will require further work directed at understanding their biophysical potential and their roles in generic cells before their function in the kidney can be explored fully. How do these proteins look on the atomic level and how do submolecular movements contribute to normal function and regulation? Certainly, the recent elucidation of the crystal structure of bacterial CLC proteins represents a landmark achievement. Insights offered by these structures, and that of the soluble form of CLIC1, have catapulted the field of anion channel and transporter research onto another level, and have opened up many more exciting questions. The availability of knockout and transgenic animals now permits direct physiological measurements determining the consequences of genetic ablation of these channels and transporters, and has already unearthed critical insights. All of the open questions funnel into three: How do these proteins work? What happens when they go awry? How can we manipulate them pharmacologically? Increasingly more refined answers to these deceptively plain questions surely will deepen the collective understanding of renal function, as well as the physiological chaos that ensues when these proteins become dysfunctional.

References

1. Abdel-Ghany M, Cheng HC, Elble RC, Lin H, DiBiasio J, Pauli BU. The interacting binding domains of the beta (4) integrin and calcium-activated chloride channels (CLCAs) in metastasis. *J Biol Chem* 2003;278:49406–49416.
2. Abdel-Ghany M, Cheng HC, Elble RC, Pauli BU. The breast cancer beta 4 integrin and endothelial human CLCA2 mediate lung metastasis. *J Biol Chem* 2001;276:25438–25446.
3. Abdel-Ghany M, Cheng HC, Elble RC, Pauli BU. Focal adhesion kinase activated by beta(4) integrin ligation to mCLCA1 mediates early metastatic growth. *J Biol Chem* 2002;277:34391–34400.
4. Accardi A, Kolmakova-Partensky L, Williams C, Miller C. Ionic currents mediated by a prokaryotic homologue of CLC Cl- channels. *J Gen Physiol* 2004;123:109–119.
5. Accardi A, Miller C. Secondary active transport mediated by a prokaryotic homologue of ClC Cl- channels. *Nature* 2004;427:803–807.
6. Ackerman MJ, Wickman KD, Clapham DE. Hypotonicity activates a native chloride current in *Xenopus* oocytes. *J Gen Physiol* 1994;103:153–179.
7. Akuta N, Lloyd SE, Igarashi T, Shiraga H, Matsuyama T, Yokoro S, Cox JP, Thakker RV. Mutations of CLCN5 in Japanese children with idiopathic low molecular weight proteinuria, hypercalciuria and nephrocalcinosis. *Kidney Int* 1997;52:911–916.
8. Anderson MP, Gregory RJ, Thompson S, Souza DW, Paul S, Mulligan RC, Smith AE, Welsh MJ. Demonstration that CFTR is a chloride channel by alteration of its anion selectivity. *Science* 1991;253:202–205.
9. Arend LJ, Handler JS, Rhim JS, Gusovsky F, Spielman WS. Adenosine-sensitive phosphoinositide turnover in a newly established renal cell line. *Am J Physiol* 1989;256:F1067–F1074.
10. Ashley RH. Challenging accepted ion channel biology: p64 and the CLIC family of putative intracellular anion channel proteins. *Mol Membr Biol* 2003;20:1–11 (review).
11. Atherton H, Mesher J, Poll CT, Danahay H. Preliminary pharmacological characterisation of an interleukin-13–enhanced calcium-activated chloride conductance in the human airway epithelium. *Naunyn Schmiedebergs Arch Pharmacol* 2003;367:214–217.
12. Babini E, Pusch M. A two-holed story: structural secrets about ClC proteins become unraveled. *Physiology (Bethesda)* 2004;19:293–299.
13. Bae HR, Verkman AS. Protein kinase A regulates chloride conductance in endocytic vesicles from proximal tubule. *Nature* 1990;348:637–639.
14. Barasch J, Kiss B, Prince A, Saiman L, Gruenert D, Al Awqati Q. Defective acidification of intracellular organelles in cystic fibrosis. *Nature* 1991;352:70–73.
15. Barish ME. A transient calcium-dependent chloride current in the immature *Xenopus* oocyte. *J Physiol* 1983;342:309–325.
16. Barriere H, Belfodil R, Rubera I, Tauc M, Poujeol C, Bidet M, Poujeol P. CFTR null mutation altered cAMP-sensitive and swelling-activated Cl- currents in primary cultures of mouse nephron. *Am J Physiol Renal Physiol* 2003;284:F796–F811.
17. Bateman A. The structure of a domain common to archaebacteria and the homocystinuria disease protein. *Trends Biochem Sci* 1997;22:12–13.

18. Bauer CK, Steinmeyer K. Schwarz JR, Jentsch TJ. Completely functional double-barreled chloride channel expressed from a single Torpedo cDNA. *Proc Natl Acad Sci U S A* 1991;88: 11052–11056.

19. Benharouga M, Fritsch J, Banting G, Edelman A. Properties of chloride-conductive pathways in rat kidney cortical and outer-medulla brush-border membranes—inhibition by anti-(cystic fibrosis transmembrane regulator) mAbs. *Eur J Biochem* 1997;246:367–372.

20. Bettinelli A, Bianchetti MG, Girardin E, Caringella A, Cecconi M, Appiani AC, Pavanello L, Gastaldi R, Isimbaldi C, Lama G. Use of calcium excretion values to distinguish two forms of primary renal tubular hypokalemic alkalosis: Bartter and Gitelman syndromes. *J Pediatr* 1992;120:38–43.

21. Bidet M, Tauc M, Rubera I, De RG, Poujeol C, Bohn MT, Poujeol P. Calcium-activated chloride currents in primary cultures of rabbit distal convoluted tubule. *Am J Physiol* 1996; 271:F940–F950.

22. Birkenhager R, Otto E, Schurmann MJ, Vollmer M, Ruf EM, Maier-Lutz I, Beekmann F, Fekete A, Omran H, Feldmann D, Milford DV, Jeck N, Konrad M, Landau D, Knoers NV, Antignac C, Sudbrak R, Kispert A, Hildebrandt F. Mutation of BSND causes Bartter syndrome with sensorineural deafness and kidney failure. *Nat Genet* 2001;29:310–314.

23. Birn H, Fyfe JC, Jacobsen C, Mounier F, Verroust PJ, Orskov H, Willnow TE, Moestrup SK, Christensen EI. Cubilin is an albumin binding protein important for renal tubular albumin reabsorption. *J Clin Invest* 2000;105:353–1361.

24. Boese SH, Aziz O, Simmons NL, Gray MA. Kinetics and regulation of a Ca2+-activated Cl- conductance in mouse renal inner medullary collecting duct cells. *Am J Physiol Renal Physiol* 2004;286:F682–F692.

25. Boese SH, Glanville M, Aziz O, Gray MA, Simmons NL. Ca2+ and cAMP-activated Cl- conductances mediate Cl- secretion in a mouse renal inner medullary collecting duct cell line. *J Physiol* 2000;5232:325–338.

26. Boese SH, Glanville M, Gray MA, Simmons NL. The swelling-activated anion conductance in the mouse renal inner medullary collecting duct cell line mIMCD-K2. *J Membr Biol* 2000;177:51–64.

27. Boese SH, Kinne RK, Wehner F. Single-channel properties of swelling-activated anion conductance in rat inner medullary collecting duct cells. *Am J Physiol* 1996;271:F1224–F1233.

28. Boese SH, Wehner F, Kinne RK. Taurine permeation through swelling-activated anion conductance in rat IMCD cells in primary culture. *Am J Physiol* 1996;271:F498–F507.

29. Brandt S, Jentsch TJ. ClC-6 and ClC-7 are two novel broadly expressed members of the CLC chloride channel family. *FEBS Lett* 1995;377:15–20.

30. Briel M, Greger R, Kunzelmann K. Cl- transport by cystic fibrosis transmembrane conductance regulator (CFTR) contributes to the inhibition of epithelial Na+ channels (ENaCs) in *Xenopus* oocytes co-expressing CFTR and ENaC. *J Physiol* 1998;508:825–836.

31. Brill SR, Ross KE, Davidow CJ, Ye M, Grantham JJ, Caplan MJ. Immunolocalization of ion transport proteins in human autosomal dominant polycystic kidney epithelial cells. *Proc Natl Acad Sci U S A* 1996;93:10206–10211.

32. Brown EM, Chattopadhyay N, Vassilev PM, Hebert SC. The calcium-sensing receptor (CaR) permits Ca2+ to function as a versatile extracellular first messenger. *Recent Prog Horm Res* 1998;53:257–280.

33. Bustin SA, Li SR, Dorudi S. Expression of the Ca2+-activated chloride channel genes CLCA1 and CLCA2 is downregulated in human colorectal cancer. *DNA Cell Biol* 2001;20:331–338.

34. Buyse G, Trouet D, Voets T, Missiaen L, Droogmans G, Nilius B, Eggermont J. Evidence for the intracellular location of chloride channel (ClC)-type proteins: co-localization of ClC-6a and ClC-6c with the sarco/endoplasmic-reticulum Ca2+ pump SERCA2b. *Biochem J* 1998;330:1015–1021.

35. Buyse G, Voets T, Tytgat J, De Greef C, Droogmans G, Nilius B, Eggermont J. Expression of human pICln and ClC-6 in *Xenopus* oocytes induces an identical endogenous chloride conductance. *J Biol Chem* 1997;272:3615–3621.

36. Cahill P, Nason MW, Jr, Ambrose C, Yao TY, Thomas P, Egan ME. Identification of the cystic fibrosis transmembrane conductance regulator domains that are important for interactions with ROMK2. *J Biol Chem* 2000;275:16697–16701.

37. Chang CT, Bens M, Hummler E, Boulkroun S, Schild L, Teulon J, Rossier BC, Vandewalle A. Vasopressin-stimulated CFTR Cl- currents are increased in the renal collecting duct cells of a mouse model of Liddle's syndrome. *J Physiol* 2005;562:271–284.

38. Chen TY. Extracellular zinc ion inhibits ClC-0 chloride channels by facilitating slow gating. *J Gen Physiol* 1998;112:715–726.

39. Cheng J, Moyer BD, Milewski M, Loffing J, Ikeda M, Mickle JE. Cutting GR, Li M, Stanton BA, Guggino WB. A Golgi-associated PDZ domain protein modulates cystic fibrosis transmembrane regulator plasma membrane expression. *J Biol Chem* 2002;277: 3520–3529.

40. Cheng J, Wang H, Guggino WB. Modulation of mature cystic fibrosis transmembrane regulator protein by the PDZ domain protein CAL. *J Biol Chem* 2004;279:1892–1898.

41. Chillon M, Casals T, Mercier B, Bassas L, Lissens W, Silber S, Romey MC, Ruiz-Romero J, Verlingue C, Claustres M. Mutations in the cystic fibrosis gene in patients with congenital absence of the vas deferens. *N Engl J Med* 1995;332:1475–1480.

42. Cho KO, Hunt CA, Kennedy MB. The rat brain postsynaptic density fraction contains a homolog of the Drosophila discs-large tumor suppressor protein. *Neuron* 1992;9: 929–942.

43. Choo-Kang LR, Zeitlin PL. Type I, II, III, IV, and V cystic fibrosis transmembrane conductance regulator defects and opportunities for therapy. *Curr Opin Pulm Med* 2000;6:521–529.

44. Choudari CP, Lehman GA, Sherman S. Pancreatitis and cystic fibrosis gene mutations. *Gastroenterol Clin North Am* 1999;28:543–549, vii–viii.

45. Christensen EI, Birn H. Megalin and cubilin: synergistic endocytic receptors in renal proximal tubule. *Am J Physiol Renal Physiol* 2001;280:F562–F573.

46. Christensen EI, Devuyst O, Dom G, Nielsen R, Van der Smissen P, Verroust P, Leruth M, Guggino WB, Courtoy PJ. Loss of chloride channel ClC-5 impairs endocytosis by defective trafficking of megalin and cubilin in kidney proximal tubules. *Proc Natl Acad Sci U S A* 2003;100:8472–8477.

47. Cid LP, Montrose-Rafizadeh C, Smith DI, Guggino WB, Cutting GR. Cloning of a putative human voltage-gated chloride channel (ClC-2) cDNA widely expressed in human tissues. *Hum Mol Genet* 1995;4:407–413.

48. Clark S, Jordt SE, Jentsch TJ, Mathie A. Characterization of the hyperpolarization-activated chloride current in dissociated rat sympathetic neurons. *J Physiol* 1998;506:665–678.

49. Clarke LL, Grubb BR, Yankaskas JR, Cotton CU, McKenzie A, Boucher RC. Relationship of a non-cystic fibrosis transmembrane conductance regulator-mediated chloride conductance to organ-level disease in Cftr(-/-) mice. *Proc Natl Acad Sci U S A* 1994;91: 479–483.

50. Cotton CU, Avner ED. PKD and CF: an interesting family provides insight into the molecular pathophysiology of polycystic kidney disease. *Am J Kidney Dis* 1998;32:1081–1083.

51. Crawford IT, Maloney PC. Identification of cystic fibrosis transmembrane conductance regulator in renal endosomes. *Methods Enzymol* 1998;292:652–663.

52. Cunningham R, Steplock D, Wang F, Huang H, E X Shenolikar S, Weinman EJ. Defective parathyroid hormone regulation of NHE3 activity and phosphate adaptation in cultured NHERF-1-/- renal proximal tubule cells. *J Biol Chem* 2004;279:37815–37821.

53. Cunningham SA, Awayda MS, Bubien JK, Ismailov II, Arrate MP, Berdiev BK, Benos DJ, Fuller CM. Cloning of an epithelial chloride channel from bovine trachea. *J Biol Chem* 1995;270:31016–31026.

54. Darvish N, Winaver J, Dagan D. Diverse modulations of chloride channels in renal proximal tubules. *Am J Physiol* 1994;267:F716–F724.

55. Davidow CJ, Maser RL, Rome LA, Calvet JP, Grantham JJ. The cystic fibrosis transmembrane conductance regulator mediates transepithelial fluid secretion by human autosomal dominant polycystic kidney disease epithelium in vitro. *Kidney Int* 1996;50:208–218.

56. De Luca A, Tricarico D, Wagner R, Bryant SH, Tortorella V, Conte-Camerino D. Opposite effects of enantiomers of clofibric acid derivative on rat skeletal muscle chloride conductance: antagonism studies and theoretical modeling of two different receptor site interactions. *J Pharmacol Exp Ther* 1992;260:364–368.

57. Delmas P, Nomura H, Li X, Lakkis M, Luo Y, Segal Y, Fernandez-Fernandez JM, Harris P, Frischauf AM, Brown DA, Zhou J. Constitutive activation of G-proteins by polycystin-1 is antagonized by polycystin-2. *J Biol Chem* 2002;277:11276–11283.

58. Deutman AF. Electro-oculography in families with vitelliform dystrophy of the fovea. Detection of the carrier state. *Arch Ophthalmol* 1969;81:305–316.

59. Devidas S, Guggino WB. The cystic fibrosis transmembrane conductance regulator and ATP. *Curr Opin Cell Biol* 1997;9:547–552.

60. Devuyst O, Burrow CR, Schwiebert EM, Guggino WB, Wilson PD. Developmental regulation of CFTR expression during human nephrogenesis. *Am J Physiol* 1996;271: F723–F735.

61. Dietl P, Stanton BA. Chloride channels in apical and basolateral membranes of CCD cells (RCCT-28A) in culture. *Am J Physiol* 1992;263:F243–F250.

62. Duan D, Winter C, Cowley S, Hume JR, Horowitz B. Molecular identification of a volume-regulated chloride channel. *Nature* 1997;390:417–421.

63. Dulhunty A, Gage P, Curtis S, Chelvanayagam G, Board P. The glutathione transferase structural family includes a nuclear chloride channel and a ryanodine receptor calcium release channel modulator. *J Biol Chem* 2001;276:3319–3323.

64. Dutzler R, Campbell EB, Cadene M, Chait BT, MacKinnon R. X-ray structure of a ClC chloride channel at 3.0 A reveals the molecular basis of anion selectivity. *Nature* 2002; 415:287–294.

65. Dutzler R, Campbell EB, MacKinnon R. Gating the selectivity filter in ClC chloride channels. *Science* 2003;300:108–112.

66. Edwards JC. A novel p64-related Cl- channel: subcellular distribution and nephron segment-specific expression. *Am J Physiol* 1999;276:F398–F408.

67. Edwards JC, Tulk B, Schlesinger PH. Functional expression of p64, an intracellular chloride channel protein. *J Membr Biol* 1998;163:119–127.

68. Egan ME, Schwiebert EM, Guggino WB. Differential expression of ORCC and CFTR induced by low temperature in CF airway epithelial cells. *Am J Physiol* 1995;268:C243–C251.

69. Eggermont J. Calcium-activated chloride channels (un)known, (un)loved? *Proc Am Thorac Soc* 2004;1:22–27.

70. Elble RC, Pauli BU. Tumor suppression by a proapoptotic calcium-activated chloride channel in mammary epithelium. *J Biol Chem* 2001;276:40510–40517.

71. Elble RC, Widom J, Gruber AD, Abdel-Ghany M, Levine R, Goodwin A, Cheng HC, Pauli BU. Cloning and characterization of lung-endothelial cell adhesion molecule-1 suggest it is an endothelial chloride channel. *J Biol Chem* 1997;272:27853–27861.

72. Estevez R, Boettger T, Stein V, Birkenhager R, Otto E, Hildebrandt F, Jentsch TJ. Barttin is a Cl- channel beta-subunit crucial for renal Cl- reabsorption and inner ear K+ secretion. *Nature* 2001;414:558–561.

73. Estevez R, Schroeder BC, Accardi A, Jentsch TJ, Pusch M. Conservation of chloride channel structure revealed by an inhibitor binding site in ClC-1. *Neuron* 2003;38:47–59.

74. Evans SR, Thoreson WB, Beck CL. Molecular and functional analyses of two new calcium-activated chloride channel family members from mouse eye and intestine. *J Biol Chem* 2004;279:41792–41800.

75. Falke LC, Misler S. Activity of ion channels during volume regulation by clonal N1E115 neuroblastoma cells. *Proc Natl Acad Sci U S A* 1989;86:3919–3923.

76. Fong P. CLC-K channels: if the drug fits, use it. *EMBO Rep* 2004;5:565–566.

77. Fong P, Argent BE, Guggino WB, Gray MA. Characterization of vectorial chloride transport pathways in the human pancreatic duct adenocarcinoma cell line HPAF. *Am J Physiol Cell Physiol* 2003;285:C433–C445.

78. Francois J, De RA, Fernandez-Sasso D. Electro-oculography in vitelliform degeneration of the macula. *Arch Ophthalmol* 1967;77:726–733.

79. Friedrich T, Breiderhoff T, Jentsch TJ. Mutational analysis demonstrates that ClC-4 and ClC-5 directly mediate plasma membrane currents. *J Biol Chem* 1999;274:896–902.

80. Fuller CM, Ismailov II, Keeton DA, Benos DJ. Phosphorylation and activation of a bovine tracheal anion channel by Ca2+/calmodulin-dependent protein kinase II. *J Biol Chem* 1994;269:26642–26650.

81. Fyfe JC, Ramanujam KS, Ramaswamy K, Patterson DF, Seetharam B. Defective brush-border expression of intrinsic factor-cobalamin receptor in canine inherited intestinal cobalamin malabsorption. *J Biol Chem* 1991;266:4489–4494.
82. Gabow PA. Autosomal dominant polycystic kidney disease—more than a renal disease. *Am J Kidney Dis* 1990;16:403–413.
83. Gabriel SE, Clarke LL, Boucher RC, Stutts MJ. CFTR and outward rectifying chloride channels are distinct proteins with a regulatory relationship. *Nature* 1993;363:263–268.
84. Gandhi R, Elble RC, Gruber AD, Schreur KD, Ji HL, Fuller CM, Pauli BU. Molecular and functional characterization of a calcium-sensitive chloride channel from mouse lung. *J Biol Chem* 1998; 273: 32096–32101.
85. Gentzsch M, Cui L, Mengos A, Chang XB, Chen JH, Riordan JR. The PDZ-binding chloride channel ClC-3B localizes to the Golgi and associates with cystic fibrosis transmembrane conductance regulator-interacting PDZ proteins. *J Biol Chem* 2003;278:6440–6449.
86. Gogelein H, Greger R. A voltage-dependent ionic channel in the basolateral membrane of late proximal tubules of the rabbit kidney. *Pflugers Arch* 1986; 407(Suppl2):S142–S148.
87. Gonzalez-Perrett S, Kim K, Ibarra C, Damiano AE, Zotta E, Batelli M, Harris PC, Reisin IL, Arnaout MA, Cantiello HF. Polycystin-2, the protein mutated in autosomal dominant polycystic kidney disease (ADPKD), is a Ca2+-permeable nonselective cation channel. *Proc Natl Acad Sci U S A* 2001;98:1182–1187.
88. Grantham JJ. Pathogenesis of renal cyst expansion: opportunities for therapy. *Am J Kidney Dis* 1994;23:210–218.
89. Grantham JJ. Mechanisms of progression in autosomal dominant polycystic kidney disease. *Kidney Int* 1997; 63(Suppl): S93–S97.
90. Grantham JJ, Ye M, Gattone VH, Sullivan LP. In vitro fluid secretion by epithelium from polycystic kidneys. *J Clin Invest* 1995;95:195–202.
91. Gruber AD, Elble RC, Ji HL, Schreur KD, Fuller CM, Pauli BU. Genomic cloning, molecular characterization, and functional analysis of human CLCA1, the first human member of the family of Ca2+-activated Cl- channel proteins. *Genomics* 1998;54:200–214.
92. Gruber AD, Pauli BU. Tumorigenicity of human breast cancer is associated with loss of the Ca2+-activated chloride channel CLCA2. *Cancer Res* 1999;59:5488–5491.
93. Gruber AD, Pauli BU. Molecular cloning and biochemical characterization of a truncated, secreted member of the human family of Ca2+-activated Cl- channels. *Biochim Biophys Acta* 1999;1444:418–423.
94. Gruber AD, Schreur KD, Ji HL, Fuller CM, Pauli BU. Molecular cloning and transmembrane structure of hCLCA2 from human lung, trachea, and mammary gland. *Am J Physiol* 1999;276:C1261–C1270.
95. Guggino WB. Cystic fibrosis and the salt controversy. *Cell* 1999;96:607–610.
96. Guggino WB. Outwardly rectifying chloride channels and CF: a divorce and remarriage. *J Bioenerg Biomembr* 1993;25:27–35.
97. Guggino WB, Boulpaep EL, Giebisch G. Electrical properties of chloride transport across the necturus proximal tubule. *J Membr Biol* 1982;65:185–196.
98. Guinamard R, Chraibi A, Teulon J. A small-conductance Cl- channel in the mouse thick ascending limb that is activated by ATP and protein kinase A. *J Physiol* 1995;485:97–112.
99. Gunther W, Piwon N, Jentsch TJ. The ClC-5 chloride channel knock-out mouse—an animal model for Dent's disease. *Pflugers Arch* 2003;445:456–462.
100. Gutknecht DR. Kidney stones and cystic fibrosis. *Am J Med* 2001;111:83.
101. Hamill OP, Marty A, Neher E, Sakmann B, Sigworth FJ. Improved patch-clamp techniques for high-resolution current recording from cells and cell-free membrane patches. *Pflugers Arch* 1981;391:85–100.
102. Hanaoka K, Devuyst O, Schwiebert EM, Wilson PD, Guggino WB A role for CFTR in human autosomal dominant polycystic kidney disease. *Am J Physiol* 1996;270:C389–C399.
103. Hanaoka K, Guggino WB cAMP regulates cell proliferation and cyst formation in autosomal polycystic kidney disease cells. *J Am Soc Nephrol* 2000;11:1179–1187.
104. Hanaoka K, Qian F, Boletta A, Bhunia AK, Piontek K, Tsiokas L, Sukhatme VP, Guggino WB, Germino GG. Co-assembly of polycystin-1 and -2 produces unique cation-permeable currents. *Nature* 2000;408:990–994.
105. Hara-Chikuma M, Wang Y, Guggino SE, Guggino WB, Verkman AS. Impaired acidification in early endosomes of ClC-5 deficient proximal tubule. *Biochem Biophys Res Commun* 2005;329:941–946.
106. Hara-Chikuma M, Yang B, Sonawane ND, Sasaki S, Uchida S, Verkman AS. ClC-3 chloride channels facilitate endosomal acidification and chloride accumulation. *J Biol Chem* 2005;280:1241–1247.
107. Harrop SJ, DeMaere MZ, Fairlie WD, Reztsova T, Valenzuela SM, Mazzanti M, Tonini R, Qiu MR, Jankova L, Warton K, Bauskin AR, Wu WM, Pankhurst S, Campbell TJ, Breit SN, Curmi PM. Crystal structure of a soluble form of the intracellular chloride ion channel CLIC1 (NCC27) at 1.4-A resolution. *J Biol Chem* 2001;276:44993–45000.
108. Hartzell C, Putzier I, Arreola J. Calcium-activated chloride channels. *Annu Rev Physiol* 2005;67:719–758.
109. Hatta S, Sakamoto J, Horio Y. Ion channels and diseases. *Med Electron Microsc* 2002;35: 117–126.
110. Hebert SC. Extracellular calcium-sensing receptor: implications for calcium and magnesium handling in the kidney. *Kidney Int* 1996; 50:2129–2139.
111. Hebert SC. Bartter syndrome. *Curr Opin Nephrol Hypertens* 2003;12:527–532.
112. Heiss NS, Poustka A. Genomic structure of a novel chloride channel gene, CLIC2 in Xq28. *Genomics* 1997;45:224–228.
113. Ho K, Nichols CG, Lederer WJ, Lytton J, Vassilev PM, Kanazirska MV, Hebert SC. Cloning and expression of an inwardly rectifying ATP-regulated potassium channel. *Nature* 1993;362:31–38.
114. Hooper KM, Unwin RJ, Sutters M. The isolated C-terminus of polycystin-1 promotes increased ATP-stimulated chloride secretion in a collecting duct cell line. *Clin Sci (Lond)* 2003;104:217–221.
115. Hoshino M, Morita S, Iwashita H, Sagiya Y, Nagi T, Nakanishi A, Ashida Y, Nishimura O, Fujisawa Y, Fujino M. Increased expression of the human Ca2+-activated Cl- channel 1 (CaCC1) gene in the asthmatic airway. *Am J Respir Crit Care Med* 2002;165:1132–1136.
116. Hryciw DH, Wang Y, Devuyst O, Pollock CA, Poronnik P, Guggino WB. Cofilin interacts with ClC-5 and regulates albumin uptake in proximal tubule cell lines. *J Biol Chem* 2003;278:40169–40176.
117. Huang P, Liu J, Di A, Robinson NC, Musch MW, Kaetzel MA, Nelson DJ. Regulation of human CLC-3 channels by multifunctional Ca2+/calmodulin-dependent protein kinase. *J Biol Chem* 2001; 276: 20093–20100.
118. Huber S, Schroppel B, Kretzler M, Schlondorff D, Horster M. Single cell RT-PCR analysis of ClC-2 mRNA expression in ureteric bud tip. *Am J Physiol* 1998;274:F951–F957.
119. Husted RF, Volk KA, Sigmund RD, Stokes JB. Anion secretion by the inner medullary collecting duct. Evidence for involvement of the cystic fibrosis transmembrane conductance regulator. *J Clin Invest* 1995;95:644–650.
120. Itoh M, Furuse M, Morita K, Kubota K, Saitou M, Tsukita S. Direct binding of three tight junction-associated MAGUKs, ZO-1, ZO-2, and ZO-3, with the COOH termini of claudins. *J Cell Biol* 1999; 147:1351–1363.
121. Jackson PS, Strange K. Single-channel properties of a volume-sensitive anion conductance. Current activation occurs by abrupt switching of closed channels to an open state. *J Gen Physiol* 1995;105:643–660.
122. Jalonen T. Single-channel characteristics of the large-conductance anion channel in rat cortical astrocytes in primary culture. *Glia* 1993;9:227–237.
123. Jeck N, Reinalter SC, Henne T, Marg W, Mallmann R, Pasel K, Vollmer M, Klaus G, Leonhardt A, Seyberth HW, Konrad M. Hypokalemic salt-losing tubulopathy with chronic renal failure and sensorineural deafness. *Pediatrics* 2001;108:E5.
124. Jentsch TJ. Chloride channels: a molecular perspective. *Curr Opin Neurobiol* 1996;6:303–310.
125. Jentsch TJ. Chloride channels are different. *Nature* 2002;415:276–277.
126. Jentsch TJ, Stein V, Weinreich F, Zdebik AA. Molecular structure and physiological function of chloride channels. *Physiol Rev* 2002;82:503–568.
127. Jentsch TJ, Steinmeyer K, Schwarz G. Primary structure of Torpedo marmorata chloride channel isolated by expression cloning in *Xenopus* oocytes. *Nature* 1990;348:510–514.
128. Jordt SE, Jentsch TJ. Molecular dissection of gating in the ClC-2 chloride channel. *EMBO J* 1997;16:1582–1592.
129. Jovov B, Ismailov II, Berdiev BK, Fuller CM, Sorscher EJ, Dedman JR, Kaetzel MA, Benos DJ. Interaction between cystic fibrosis transmembrane conductance regulator and outwardly rectified chloride channels. *J Biol Chem* 1995;270:29194–29200.
130. Kasper D, Planells-Cases R, Fuhrmann JC, Scheel O, Zeitz O, Ruether K, Schmitt A, Poet M, Steinfeld R, Schweizer M, Kornak U, Jentsch TJ. Loss of the chloride channel ClC-7 leads to lysosomal storage disease and neurodegeneration. *EMBO J* 2005;24:1079–1091.
131. Katz SM, Krueger LJ, Falkner B. Microscopic nephrocalcinosis in cystic fibrosis. *N Engl J Med* 1988;319:263–266.
132. Kida Y, Uchida S, Miyazaki H, Sasaki S, Marumo F. Localization of mouse CLC-6 and CLC-7 mRNA and their functional complementation of yeast CLC gene mutant. *Histochem Cell Biol* 2001;115:189–194.
133. Kieferle S, Fong P, Bens M, Vandewalle A, Jentsch TJ. Two highly homologous members of the ClC chloride channel family in both rat and human kidney. *Proc Natl Acad Sci U S A* 1994;91:6943–6947.
134. Kimberling WJ, Kumar S, Gabow PA, Kenyon JB, Connolly CJ, Somlo S. Autosomal dominant polycystic kidney disease: localization of the second gene to chromosome 4q13–q23. *Genomics* 1993;18:467–472.
135. Kizer NL, Lewis B, Stanton BA. Electrogenic sodium absorption and chloride secretion by an inner medullary collecting duct cell line (mIMCD-K2). *Am J Physiol* 1995;268:F347–F355.
136. Kizer NL, Vandorpe D, Lewis B, Bunting B, Russell J, Stanton BA. Vasopressin and cAMP stimulate electrogenic chloride secretion in an IMCD cell line. *Am J Physiol* 1995;268: F854–F861.
137. Knowles M, Gatzy J, Boucher R. Increased bioelectric potential difference across respiratory epithelia in cystic fibrosis. *N Engl J Med* 1981;305:1489–1495.
138. Kobayashi K, Uchida S, Mizutani S, Sasaki S, Marumo F. Developmental expression of CLC-K1 in the postnatal rat kidney. *Histochem Cell Biol* 2001;116:49–56.
139. Kobayashi K, Uchida S, Mizutani S, Sasaki S, Marumo F. Intrarenal and cellular localization of CLC-K2 protein in the mouse kidney. *J Am Soc Nephrol* 2001;12:1327–1334.
140. Kobayashi K, Uchida S, Okamura HO, Marumo F, Sasaki S. Human CLC-KB gene promoter drives the EGFP expression in the specific distal nephron segments and inner ear. *J Am Soc Nephrol* 2002;13:1992–1998.
141. Kolb HA, Brown CD, Murer H. Identification of a voltage-dependent anion channel in the apical membrane of a Cl(-)-secretory epithelium (MDCK). *Pflugers Arch* 1985;403: 262–265.
142. Kornak U, Kasper D, Bosl MR, Kaiser E, Schweizer M, Schulz A, Friedrich W, Delling G, Jentsch TJ. Loss of the ClC-7 chloride channel leads to osteopetrosis in mice and man. *Cell* 2001;104:205–215.
143. Krapivinsky GB, Ackerman MJ, Gordon EA, Krapivinsky LD, Clapham DE. Molecular characterization of a swelling-induced chloride conductance regulatory protein, pICln. *Cell* 1994;76:439–448.
144. Kunzelmann K, Kiser GL, Schreiber R, Riordan JR. Inhibition of epithelial Na+ currents by intracellular domains of the cystic fibrosis transmembrane conductance regulator. *FEBS Lett* 1997;400:341–344.
145. Laich A, Gschwentner M, Krick W, Nagl UO, Furst J, Hofer S, Susanna A, Schmarda A, Deetjen P, Burckhardt G, Paulmichl M. ICln, a chloride channel cloned from kidney cells, is activated during regulatory volume decrease. *Kidney Int* 1997;51:477–478.
146. Landry D, Sullivan S, Nicolaides M, Redhead C, Edelman A, Field M, Al Awqati Q, Edwards J. Molecular cloning and characterization of p64, a chloride channel protein from kidney microsomes. *J Biol Chem* 1993;268:14948–14955.
147. Landry DW, Akabas MH, Redhead C, Edelman A, Cragoe EJ, Jr, Al Awqati Q. Purification and reconstitution of chloride channels from kidney and trachea. *Science* 1989;244:1469–1472.
148. Langer T, Levy RI. Acute muscular syndrome associated with administration of clofibrate. *N Engl J Med* 1968;279:856–858.

149. Lebeau C, Hanaoka K, Moore-Hoon ML, Guggino WB, Beauwens R, Devuyst O. Basolateral chloride transporters in autosomal dominant polycystic kidney disease. *Pflugers Arch* 2002;444:722–731.

150. Leheste JR, Rolinski B, Vorum H, Hilpert J, Nykjaer A, Jacobsen C, Aucouturier P, Moskaug JO, Otto A, Christensen EI, Willnow TE. Megalin knockout mice as an animal model of low molecular weight proteinuria. *Am J Pathol* 1999;155:1361–1370.

151. Letz B, Korbmacher C. cAMP stimulates CFTR-like Cl- channels and inhibits amiloride-sensitive Na+ channels in mouse CCD cells. *Am J Physiol* 1997;272:C657–C666.

152. Lewis HA, Buchanan SG, Burley SK, Conners K, Dickey M, Dorwart M, Fowler R, Gao X, Guggino WB, Hendrickson WA, Hunt JF, Kearins MC, Lorimer D, Maloney PC, Post KW, Rajashankar KR, Rutter ME, Sauder JM, Shriver S, Thibodeau PH, Thomas PJ, Zhang M, Zhao X, Emtage S. Structure of nucleotide-binding domain 1 of the cystic fibrosis transmembrane conductance regulator. *EMBO J* 2004;23: 282–293.

153. Li H, Findlay IA, Sheppard DN. The relationship between cell proliferation, Cl- secretion, and renal cyst growth: a study using CFTR inhibitors. *Kidney Int* 2004;66:1926–1938.

154. Li X, Shimada K, Showalter LA, Weinman SA. Biophysical properties of ClC-3 differentiate it from swelling-activated chloride channels in Chinese hamster ovary-K1 cells. *J Biol Chem* 2000;275: 35994–35998.

155. Liantonio A, Accardi A, Carbonara G, Fracchiolla G, Loiodice F, Tortorella P, Traverso S, Guida P, Pierno S, De LA, Camerino DC, Pusch M. Molecular requisites for drug binding to muscle CLC-1 and renal CLC-K channel revealed by the use of phenoxy-alkyl derivatives of 2-(p-chlorophenoxy)propionic acid. *Mol Pharmacol* 2002;62:265–271.

156. Liantonio A, Pusch M, Picollo A, Guida P, De LA, Pierno S, Fracchiolla G, Loiodice F, Tortorella P, Conte CD. Investigations of pharmacologic properties of the renal CLC-K1 chloride channel co-expressed with barttin by the use of 2-(p-chlorophenoxy)propionic acid derivatives and other structurally unrelated chloride channels blockers. *J Am Soc Nephrol* 2004;15:13–20.

157. Linsdell P. Location of a common inhibitor binding site in the cytoplasmic vestibule of the cystic fibrosis transmembrane conductance regulator chloride channel pore. *J Biol Chem* 2005;280:8945–8950.

158. Liu K, Kozono D, Kato Y, Agre P, Hazama A, Yasui M. Conversion of aquaporin 6 from an anion channel to a water-selective channel by a single amino acid substitution. *Proc Natl Acad Sci U S A* 2005;102: 2192–2197.

159. Lloyd SE, Gunther W, Pearce SH, Thomson A, Bianchi ML, Bosio M, Craig IW, Fisher SE, Scheinman SJ, Wrong O, Jentsch TJ, Thakker RV. Characterisation of renal chloride channel, CLCN5, mutations in hypercalciuric nephrolithiasis (kidney stones) disorders. *Hum Mol Genet* 1997;6:1233–1239.

160. Lloyd SE, Pearce SH, Fisher SE, Steinmeyer K, Schwappach B, Scheinman SJ, Harding B, Bolino A, Devoto M, Goodyer P, Rigden SP, Wrong O, Jentsch TJ, Craig IW, Thakker RV. A common molecular basis for three inherited kidney stone diseases. *Nature* 1996;379:445–449.

161. Lloyd SE, Pearce SH, Gunther W, Kawaguchi H, Igarashi T, Jentsch TJ, Thakker RV. Idiopathic low molecular weight proteinuria associated with hypercalciuric nephrocalcinosis in Japanese children is due to mutations of the renal chloride channel (CLCN5). *J Clin Invest* 1997;99:967–974.

162. Loewen ME, Bekar LK, Gabriel SE, Walz W, Forsyth GW. pCLCA1 becomes a cAMP-dependent chloride conductance mediator in Caco-2 cells. *Biochem Biophys Res Commun* 2002;298:531–536.

163. Loewen ME, Gabriel SE, Forsyth GW. The calcium-dependent chloride conductance mediator pCLCA1. *Am J Physiol Cell Physiol* 2002;283:C412–C421.

164. Loewen ME, MacDonald DW, Gaspar KJ, Forsyth GW. Isoform-specific exon skipping in a variant form of ClC-2. *Biochim Biophys Acta* 2000;1493:284–288.

165. Loewen ME, Smith NK, Hamilton DL, Grahn BH, Forsyth GW. CLCA protein and chloride transport in canine retinal pigment epithelium. *J Physiol Cell Physiol* 2003;285: C1314–C1321.

166. Lorenz C, Pusch M, Jentsch TJ. Heteromultimeric CLC chloride channels with novel properties. *Proc Natl Acad Sci U S A* 1996;93:13362–13366.

167. Lorenz JN, Baird NR, Judd LM, Noonan WT, Andringa A, Doetschman T, Manning PA, Liu LH, Miller ML, Shull GE. Impaired renal NaCl absorption in mice lacking the ROMK potassium channel, a model for type II Bartter's syndrome. *J Biol Chem* 2002;277:37871–37880.

168. Ludewig U, Pusch M, Jentsch TJ. Independent gating of single pores in CLC-0 chloride channels. *Biophys J* 1997;73:789–797.

169. Ludewig U, Pusch M, Jentsch TJ. Two physically distinct pores in the dimeric ClC-0 chloride channel. *Nature* 1996;383:340–343.

170. Luyckx VA, Leclercq B, Dowland LK, Yu AS. Diet-dependent hypercalciuria in transgenic mice with reduced CLC5 chloride channel expression. *Proc Natl Acad Sci U S A* 1999;96:12174–12179.

171. Ma T, Thiagarajah JR, Yang H, Sonawane ND, Folli C, Galietta LJ, Verkman AS. Thiazolidinone CFTR inhibitor identified by high-throughput screening blocks cholera toxin-induced intestinal fluid secretion. *J Clin Invest* 2002;110:1651–1658.

172. Mall M, Grubb BR, Harkema JR, O'Neal WK, Boucher RC. Increased airway epithelial Na+ absorption produces cystic fibrosis-like lung disease in mice. *Nat Med* 2004;10: 487–493.

173. Mall M, Hipper A, Greger R, Kunzelmann K. Wild type but not deltaF508 CFTR inhibits Na+ conductance when coexpressed in *Xenopus* oocytes. *FEBS Lett* 1996;381: 47–52.

174. Mangoo-Karim R, Ye M, Wallace DP, Grantham JJ, Sullivan LP. Anion secretion drives fluid secretion by monolayers of cultured human polycystic cells. *Am J Physiol* 1995;269: F381–F388.

175. Marquardt A, Stohr H, Passmore LA, Kramer F, Rivera A, Weber BH. Mutations in a novel gene, VMD2, encoding a protein of unknown properties cause juvenile-onset vitelliform macular dystrophy (Best's disease). *Hum Mol Genet* 1998;7:1517–1525.

176. Marshansky V, Ausiello DA, Brown D. Physiological importance of endosomal acidification: potential role in proximal tubulopathies. *Curr Opin Nephrol Hypertens* 2002;11:527–537.

177. Matsumura Y, Uchida S, Kondo Y, Miyazaki H, Ko SB, Hayama A, Morimoto T, Liu W, Arisawa M, Sasaki S, Marumo F. Overt nephrogenic diabetes insipidus in mice lacking the CLC-K1 chloride channel. *Nat Genet* 1999;21:95–98.

178. McManus M, Fischbarg J, Sun A, Hebert S, Strange K. Laser light-scattering system for studying cell volume regulation and membrane transport processes. *Am J Physiol* 1993;265: C562–C570.

179. McNamara N, Gallup M, Khong A, Sucher A, Maltseva I, Fahy J, Basbaum C. Adenosine up-regulation of the mucin gene, MUC2, in asthma. *FASEB J* 2004;18:1770–1772.

180. McNicholas CM, Guggino WB, Schwiebert EM, Hebert SC, Giebisch G, Egan ME. Sensitivity of a renal K+ channel (ROMK2) to the inhibitory sulfonylurea compound glibenclamide is enhanced by coexpression with the ATP-binding cassette transporter cystic fibrosis transmembrane regulator. *Proc Natl Acad Sci U S A* 1996;93: 8083–8088.

181. McNicholas CM, Nason MW, Jr, Guggino WB, Schwiebert EM, Hebert SC, Giebisch G, Egan ME. A functional CFTR-NBF1 is required for ROMK2-CRTR interaction. *Am J Physiol* 1997;273:F843–F848.

182. Meyer K, Korbmacher C. Cell swelling activates ATP-dependent voltage-gated chloride channels in M-1 mouse cortical collecting duct cells. *J Gen Physiol* 1996;108:177–193.

183. Middleton RE, Pheasant DJ, Miller C. Homodimeric architecture of a ClC-type chloride ion channel. *Nature* 1996;383:337–340.

184. Miledi R, Parker I. Chloride current induced by injection of calcium into *Xenopus* oocytes. *J Physiol* 1984;357:173–183.

185. Milewski MI, Mickle JE, Forrest JK, Stafford DM, Moyer BD, Cheng J, Guggino WB, Stanton BA, Cutting GR. A PDZ-binding motif is essential but not sufficient to localize the C terminus of CFTR to the apical membrane. *J Cell Sci* 2001;114:719–726.

186. Miller C, White MM. A voltage-dependent chloride conductance channel from *Torpedo electroplax* membrane. *Ann N Y Acad Sci* 1980; 341:534–551.

187. Miller C, White MM. Dimeric structure of single chloride channels from *Torpedo electroplax*. *Proc Natl Acad Sci U S A* 1984;81:2772–2775.

188. Misfeldt DS, Hamamoto ST, Pitelka DR. Transepithelial transport in cell culture. *Proc Natl Acad Sci U S A* 1976;73:1212–1216.

189. Mo L, Hellmich HL, Fong P, Wood T, Embesi J, Wills NK. Comparison of amphibian and human ClC-5: similarity of functional properties and inhibition by external pH. *J Membr Biol* 1999;168:253–264.

190. Mohammad-Panah R, Harrison R, Dhani S, Ackerley C, Huan LJ, Wang Y, Bear CE. The chloride channel ClC-4 contributes to endosomal acidification and trafficking. *J Biol Chem* 2003;278:29267–29277.

191. Morales MM, Carroll TP, Morita T, Schwiebert EM, Devuyst O, Wilson PD, Lopes AG, Stanton BA, Dietz HC, Cutting GR, Guggino WB. Both the wild type and a functional isoform of CFTR are expressed in kidney. *Am J Physiol* 1996;270:F1038–F1048.

192. Moulin P, Igarashi T, Van der SP, Cosyns JP, Verroust P, Thakker RV, Scheinman SJ, Courtoy PJ, Devuyst O. Altered polarity and expression of H+-ATPase without ultrastructural changes in kidneys of Dent's disease patients. *Kidney Int* 2003;63:1285–1295.

193. Muanprasat C, Sonawane ND, Salinas D, Taddei A, Galietta LJ, Verkman AS. Discovery of glycine hydrazide pore-occluding CFTR inhibitors: mechanism, structure-activity analysis, and in vivo efficacy. *J Gen Physiol* 2004;124:125–137.

194. Murray CB, Chu S, Zeitlin PL. Gestational and tissue-specific regulation of C1C-2 chloride channel expression. *Am J Physiol* 1996;271:L829–L837.

195. Nakanishi K, Sweeney WE, Jr, Macrae DK, Cotton CU, Avner ED. Role of CFTR in autosomal recessive polycystic kidney disease. *J Am Soc Nephrol* 2001;12:719–725.

196. Neagoe I, Schwappach B. Pas de deux in groups of four-the biogenesis of K(ATP) channels. *J Mol Cell Cardiol* 2005;38:887–894.

197. Newby LJ, Streets AJ, Zhao Y, Harris PC, Ward CJ, Ong AC. Identification, characterization, and localization of a novel kidney polycystin-1-polycystin-2 complex. *J Biol Chem* 2002;277:20763–20773.

198. Nishizawa T, Nagao T, Iwatsubo T, Forte JG, Urushidani T. Molecular cloning and characterization of a novel chloride intracellular channel-related protein, parchorin, expressed in water-secreting cells. *J Biol Chem* 2000;275:11164–11173.

199. Nissant A, Lourdel S, Baillet S, Paulais M, Marvao P, Teulon J, Imbert-Teboul M. Heterogeneous distribution of chloride channels along the distal convoluted tubule probed by single-cell RT-PCR and patch clamp. *Am J Physiol Renal Physiol* 2004;287:F1233–F1243.

200. O'Sullivan DA, Torres VE, Gabow PA, Thibodeau SN, King BF, Bergstralh EJ. Cystic fibrosis and the phenotypic expression of autosomal dominant polycystic kidney disease. *Am J Kidney Dis* 1998;32: 976–983.

201. Obermuller N, Kranzlin B, Blum WF, Gretz N, Witzgall R. An endocytosis defect as a possible cause of proteinuria in polycystic kidney disease. *Am J Physiol Renal Physiol* 2001;280: F244–F253.

202. Ogura T, Furukawa T, Toyozaki T, Yamada K, Zheng YJ, Katayama Y, Nakaya H, Inagaki N. ClC-3B, a novel ClC-3 splicing variant that interacts with EBP50 and facilitates expression of CFTR-regulated ORCC. *FASEB J* 2002;16:863–865.

203. Okada Y, Petersen CC, Kubo M, Morishima S, Tominaga M. Osmotic swelling activates intermediate-conductance Cl- channels in human intestinal epithelial cells. *Jpn J Physiol* 1994;44:403–409.

204. Onuchic LF, Furu L, Nagasawa Y, Hou X, Eggermann T, Ren Z, Bergmann C, Senderek J, Esquivel E, Zeltner R, Rudnik-Schoneborn S, Mrug M, Sweeney W, Avner ED, Zerres K, Guay-Woodford LM, Somlo S, Germino GG. PKHD1, the polycystic kidney and hepatic disease 1 gene, encodes a novel large protein containing multiple immunoglobulin-like plexin-transcription-factor domains and parallel beta-helix 1 repeats. *Am J Hum Genet* 2002;70:1305–1317.

205. Papassotiriou J, Eggermont J, Droogmans G, Nilius B. Ca(2+)-activated Cl- channels in Ehrlich ascites tumor cells are distinct from mClCA1, 2 and 3. *Pflugers Arch* 2001;442:273–279.

206. Paulmichl M, Li Y, Wickman K, Ackerman M, Peralta E, Clapham D. New mammalian chloride channel identified by expression cloning. *Nature* 1992;356:238–241.

207. Perantoni A, Berman JJ. Properties of Wilms' tumor line (TuWi) and pig kidney line (LLC-PK1) typical of normal kidney tubular epithelium. *In Vitro* 1979;15:446–454.

208. Peters DJ, Spruit L, Saris JJ, Ravine D, Sandkuijl LA, Fossdal R, Boersma J, van Eijk R, Norby S, Constantinou-Deltas CD. Chromosome 4 localization of a second gene for autosomal dominant polycystic kidney disease. *Nat Genet* 1993;5:359–362.
209. Petrukhin K, Koisti MJ, Bakall B, Li W, Xie G, Marknell T, Sandgren O, Forsman K, Holmgren G, Andreasson S, Vujic M, Bergen AA, Garty-Dugan V, Figueroa D, Austin CP, Metzker ML, Caskey CT, Wadelius C. Identification of the gene responsible for Best macular dystrophy. *Nat Genet* 1998;19:241–247.
210. Pham PC, Devuyst O, Pham PT, Matsumoto N, Shih RN, Jo OD, Yanagawa N, Sun AM. Hypertonicity increases CLC-5 expression in mouse medullary thick ascending limb cells. *Am J Physiol Renal Physiol* 2004;287:F747–F752.
211. Picollo A, Liantonio A, Didonna MP, Elia L, Camerino DC, Pusch M. Molecular determinants of differential pore blocking of kidney CLC-K chloride channels. *EMBO Rep* 2004;5:584–589.
212. Piwon N, Gunther W, Schwake M, Bosl MR, Jentsch TJ. ClC-5 Cl-channel disruption impairs endocytosis in a mouse model for Dent's disease. *Nature* 2000;408:369–373.
213. Ponting CP. CBS domains in CIC chloride channels implicated in myotonia and nephrolithiasis (kidney stones). *J Mol Med* 1997;75:160–163.
214. Poschet JF, Skidmore J, Boucher JC, Firoved AM, Van Dyke RW, Deretic V. Hyperacidification of cellubrevin endocytic compartments and defective endosomal recycling in cystic fibrosis respiratory epithelial cells. *J Biol Chem* 2002;277:13959–13965.
215. Pusch M. Ca(2+)-activated chloride channels go molecular. *J Gen Physiol* 2004;123:323–325.
216. Qu Z, Fischmeister R, Hartzell C. Mouse bestrophin-2 is a bona fide Cl(-) channel: identification of a residue important in anion binding and conduction. *J Gen Physiol* 2004;123:327–340.
217. Qu Z, Wei RW, Hartzell HC. Characterization of Ca2+-activated Cl- currents in mouse kidney inner medullary collecting duct cells. *Am J Physiol Renal Physiol* 2005;285:F326–F335.
218. Ran S, Benos DJ. Isolation and functional reconstitution of a 38-kDa chloride channel protein from bovine tracheal membranes. *J Biol Chem* 1991;266:4782–4788.
219. Ran S, Benos DJ. Immunopurification and structural analysis of a putative epithelial Cl-channel protein isolated from bovine trachea. *J Biol Chem* 1992;267:3618–3625.
220. Ran S, Fuller CM, Arrate MP, Latorre R, Benos DJ. Functional reconstitution of a chloride channel protein from bovine trachea. *J Biol Chem* 1992;267:20630–20637.
221. Rauchman MI, Nigam SK, Delpire E, Gullans SR. An osmotically tolerant inner medullary collecting duct cell line from an SV40 transgenic mouse. *Am J Physiol* 1993;265:F416–F424.
222. Ravine D, Walker RG, Gibson RN, Forrest SM, Richards RI, Friend K, Sheffield LJ, Kincaid-Smith P, Danks DM. Phenotype and genotype heterogeneity in autosomal dominant polycystic kidney disease. *Lancet* 1992;340:1330–1333.
223. Reddy MM, Quinton PM. Functional interaction of CFTR and ENaC in sweat glands. *Pflugers Arch* 2003;445:499–503.
224. Redhead C, Sullivan SK, Koseki C, Fujiwara K, Edwards JC. Subcellular distribution and targeting of the intracellular chloride channel p64. *Mol Biol Cell* 1997;8:691–704.
225. Redhead CR, Edelman AE, Brown D, Landry DW, Al Awqati Q. A ubiquitous 64-kDa protein is a component of a chloride channel of plasma and intracellular membranes. *Proc Natl Acad Sci U S A* 1992;89:3716–3720.
226. Reinhart SC, Norden AG, Lapsley M, Thakker RV, Pang J, Moses AM, Frymoyer PA, Favus MJ, Hoepner JA, Scheinman SJ. Characterization of carrier females and affected males with X-linked recessive nephrolithiasis. *J Am Soc Nephrol* 1995;5:1451–1461.
227. Riccardi D, Hall AE, Chattopadhyay N, Xu JZ, Brown EM, Hebert SC. Localization of the extracellular Ca2+/polyvalent cation-sensing protein in rat kidney. *Am J Physiol* 1998;274: F611–F622.
228. Ritter M, Ravasio A, Jakab M, Chwatal S, Furst J, Laich A, Gschwentner M, Signorelli S, Burtscher C, Eichmuller S, Paulmichl M. Cell swelling stimulates cytosol to membrane transposition of ICln. *J Biol Chem* 2003;278:50163–50174.
229. Robinson NC, Huang P, Kaetzel MA, Lamb FS, Nelson DJ. Identification of an N-terminal amino acid of the CLC-3 chloride channel critical in phosphorylation-dependent activation of a CaMKII-activated chloride current. *J Physiol* 2004;556:353–368.
230. Romio L, Musante L, Cinti R, Seri M, Moran O, Zegarra-Moran O, Galietta LJ. Characterization of a murine gene homologous to the bovine CaCC chloride channel. *Gene* 1999;228:181–188.
231. Rubera I, Tauc M, Bidet M, Verheecke-Mauze C, De RG, Poujeol C, Cuiller B, Poujeol P. Extracellular ATP increases (Ca(2+))(i) in distal tubule cells. II. Activation of a Ca(2+)-dependent Cl(-) conductance. *Am J Physiol Renal Physiol* 2000;279:F102–F111.
232. Ruknudin A, Schulze DH, Sullivan SK, Lederer WJ, Welling PA. Novel subunit composition of a renal epithelial KATP channel. *J Biol Chem* 1998;273:14165–14171.
233. San Millan JL, Viribay M, Peral B, Martinez I, Weissenbach J, Moreno F. Refining the localization of the PKD2 locus on chromosome 4q by linkage analysis in Spanish families with autosomal dominant polycystic kidney disease type 2. *Am J Hum Genet* 1995;56:248–253.
234. Sansom SC, La BQ, Carosi SL. Double-barreled chloride channels of collecting duct basolateral membrane. *Am J Physiol* 1990;259:F46–F52.
235. Saviane C, Conti F, Pusch M. The muscle chloride channel ClC-1 has a double-barreled appearance that is differentially affected in dominant and recessive myotonia. *J Gen Physiol* 1999;113:457–468.
236. Scheinman SJ. X-linked hypercalciuric nephrolithiasis: clinical syndromes and chloride channel mutations. *Kidney Int* 1998;53:3–17.
237. Schmidt-Rose T, Jentsch TJ. Transmembrane topology of a CLC chloride channel. *Proc Natl Acad Sci U S A* 1997;94:7633–7638.
238. Schneider MC, Rodriguez AM, Nomura H, Zhou J, Morton CC, Reeders ST, Weremowicz S. A gene similar to PKD1 maps to chromosome 4q22: a candidate gene for PKD2. *Genomics* 1996;38:1–4.
239. Schwappach B, Zerangue N, Jan YN, Jan LY. Molecular basis for K(ATP) assembly: transmembrane interactions mediate association of a K+ channel with an ABC transporter. *Neuron* 2000;26:155–167.
240. Schwartz RS, Rybicki AC, Nagel RL. Molecular cloning and expression of a chloride channel-associated protein pICln in human young red blood cells: association with actin. *Biochem J* 1997;327:609–616.
241. Schwiebert EM, Benos DJ, Egan ME, Stutts MJ, Guggino WB. CFTR is a conductance regulator as well as a chloride channel. *Physiol Rev* 1999;79:S145–S166.
242. Schwiebert EM, Benos DJ, Fuller CM. Cystic fibrosis: a multiple exocrinopathy caused by dysfunctions in a multifunctional transport protein. *Am J Med* 1998;104:576–590.
243. Schwiebert EM, Cid-Soto LP, Stafford D, Carter M, Blaisdell CJ, Zeitlin PL, Guggino WB, Cutting GR. Analysis of ClC-2 channels as an alternative pathway for chloride conduction in cystic fibrosis airway cells. *Proc Natl Acad Sci U S A* 1998;95:3879–3884.
244. Schwiebert EM, Egan ME, Hwang TH, Fulmer SB, Allen SS, Cutting GR, Guggino WB. CFTR regulates outwardly rectifying chloride channels through an autocrine mechanism involving ATP. *Cell* 1995;81:1063–1073.
245. Schwiebert EM, Flotte T, Cutting GR, Guggino WB. Both CFTR and outwardly rectifying chloride channels contribute to cAMP-stimulated whole cell chloride currents. *Am J Physiol* 1994;266:C1464–C1477.
246. Schwiebert EM, Karlson KH, Friedman PA, Dietl P, Spielman WS, Stanton BA. Adenosine regulates a chloride channel via protein kinase C and a G protein in a rabbit cortical collecting duct cell line. *J Clin Invest* 1992;89:834–841.
247. Schwiebert EM, Light DB, Fejes-Toth G, Naray-Fejes-Toth A, Stanton BA. A GTP-binding protein activates chloride channels in a renal epithelium. *J Biol Chem* 1990;265: 7725–7728.
248. Schwiebert EM, Mills JW, Stanton BA. Actin-based cytoskeleton regulates a chloride channel and cell volume in a renal cortical collecting duct cell line. *J Biol Chem* 1994;269:7081–7089.
249. Schwiebert EM, Wallace DP, Braunstein GM, King SR, Peti-Peterdi J, Hanaoka K, Guggino WB, Guay-Woodford LM, Bell PD, Sullivan LP, Grantham JJ, Taylor AL. Autocrine extracellular purinergic signaling in epithelial cells derived from polycystic kidneys. *Am J Physiol Renal Physiol* 2002;282:F763–F775.
250. Scott JW, Hawley SA, Green KA, Anis M, Stewart G, Scullion GA, Norman DG, Hardie DG. CBS domains form energy-sensing modules whose binding of adenosine ligands is disrupted by disease mutations. *J Clin Invest* 2004;113:274–284.
251. Seksek O, Biwersi J, Verkman AS. Evidence against defective trans-Golgi acidification in cystic fibrosis. *J Biol Chem* 1996;271:15542–15548.
252. Shaer AJ. Inherited primary renal tubular hypokalemic alkalosis: a review of Gitelman and Bartter syndromes. *Am J Med Sci* 2001;322: 316–332.
253. Sheppard DN. CFTR channel pharmacology: novel pore blockers identified by high-throughput screening. *J Gen Physiol* 2004;124:109–113.
254. Silva IV, Cebotaru V, Wang H, Wang XT, Wang SS, Guo G, Devuyst O, Thakker RV, Guggino WB, Guggino SE. The ClC-5 knockout mouse model of Dent's disease has renal hypercalciuria and increased bone turnover. *J Bone Miner Res* 2003;18:615–623.
255. Simon DB, Bindra RS, Mansfield TA, Nelson-Williams C, Mendonca E, Stone R, Schurman S, Nayir A, Alpay H, Bakkaloglu A, Rodriguez-Soriano J, Morales JM, Sanjad SA, Taylor CM, Pilz D, Brem A, Trachtman H, Griswold W, Richard GA, John E, Lifton RP. Mutations in the chloride channel gene, CLCNKB, cause Bartter's syndrome type III. *Nat Genet* 1997;17:171–178.
256. Simon DB, Karet FE, Hamdan JM, DiPietro A, Sanjad SA, Lifton RP. Bartter's syndrome, hypokalaemic alkalosis with hypercalciuria, is caused by mutations in the Na-K-2Cl cotransporter NKCC2. *Nat Genet* 1996;13:183–188.
257. Simon DB, Karet FE, Rodriguez-Soriano J, Hamdan JH, DiPietro A, Trachtman H, Sanjad SA, Lifton RP. Genetic heterogeneity of Bartter's syndrome revealed by mutations in the K+ channel, ROMK. *Nat Genet* 1996;14:152–156.
258. Sintchak MD, Fleming MA, Futer O, Raybuck SA, Chambers SP, Caron PR, Murcko MA, Wilson KP. Structure and mechanism of inosine monophosphate dehydrogenase in complex with the immunosuppressant mycophenolic acid. *Cell* 1996;85:921–930.
259. Snouwaert JN, Brigman KK, Latour AM, Malouf NN, Boucher RC, Smithies O, Koller BH. An animal model for cystic fibrosis made by gene targeting. *Science* 1992;257:1083–1088.
260. Solc CK, Wine JJ. Swelling-induced and depolarization-induced C1-channels in normal and cystic fibrosis epithelial cells. *Am J Physiol* 1991; 261:C658–C674.
261. Stanton BA. Cystic fibrosis transmembrane conductance regulator (CFTR) and renal function. *Wien Klin Wochenschr* 1997;109:457–464.
262. Steinberg RH. Interactions between the retinal pigment epithelium and the neural retina. *Doc Ophthalmol* 1985;60:327–346.
263. Steinmeyer K, Ortland C, Jentsch TJ. Primary structure and functional expression of a developmentally regulated skeletal muscle chloride channel. *Nature* 1991;354:301–304.
264. Steinmeyer K, Schwappach B, Bens M, Vandewalle A, Jentsch TJ. Cloning and functional expression of rat CLC-5, a chloride channel related to kidney disease. *J Biol Chem* 1995;270:31172–31177.
265. Stewart GS, Glanville M, Aziz O, Simmons NL, Gray MA. Regulation of an outwardly rectifying chloride conductance in renal epithelial cells by external and internal calcium. *J Membr Biol* 2001;180:49–64.
266. Stobrawa SM, Breiderhoff T, Takamori S, Engel D, Schweizer M, Zdebik AA, Bosl MR, Ruether K, Jahn H, Draguhn A, Jahn R, Jentsch TJ. Disruption of ClC-3, a chloride channel expressed on synaptic vesicles, leads to a loss of the hippocampus. *Neuron* 2001;29:185–196.
267. Stohr H, Marquardt A, Nanda I, Schmid M, Weber BH. Three novel human VMD2-like genes are members of the evolutionary highly conserved RFP-TM family. *Eur J Hum Genet* 2002;10:281–284.
268. Stohr H, Milenkowic V, Weber BH. (VMD2 and its role in Best's disease and other retinopathies.) *Ophthalmologe* 2005;102:116–121.
269. Stutts MJ, Canessa CM, Olsen JC, Hamrick M, Cohn JA, Rossier BC, Boucher RC. CFTR as a cAMP-dependent regulator of sodium channels. *Science* 1995;269:847–850.
270. Sun H, Tsunenari T, Yau KW, Nathans J. The vitelliform macular dystrophy protein defines a new family of chloride channels. *Proc Natl Acad Sci U S A* 2002;99:4008–4013.
271. Suzuki M, Morita T, Hanaoka K, Kawaguchi Y, Sakai O. A Cl- channel activated by parathyroid hormone in rabbit renal proximal tubule cells. *J Clin Invest* 1991;88:735–742.
272. Sweeney WE, Avner ED, Elmer H, Cotton CU. CFTR is required for cAMP-dependent in vivo renal cyst formation. *J Am Soc Nephrol* 1998;9:38A.

273. Swiatecka-Urban A, Duhaime M, Coutermarsh B, Karlson KH, Collawn J, Milewski M, Cutting GR, Guggino WB, Langford G, Stanton BA. PDZ domain interaction controls the endocytic recycling of the cystic fibrosis transmembrane conductance regulator. *J Biol Chem* 2002;277:40099–40105.

274. Takahashi N, Chernavvsky DR, Gomez RA, Igarashi P, Gitelman HJ, Smithies O. Uncompensated polyuria in a mouse model of Bartter's syndrome. *Proc Natl Acad Sci U S A* 2000;97:5434–5439.

275. Tauc M, Bidet M, Poujeol P. Chloride currents activated by calcitonin and cAMP in primary cultures of rabbit distal convoluted tubule. *J Membr Biol* 1996;150:255–273.

276. Teitelbaum AP, Strewler GJ. Parathyroid hormone receptors coupled to cyclic adenosine monophosphate formation in an established renal cell line. *Endocrinology* 1984;114:980–985.

277. Thiemann A, Grunder S, Pusch M, Jentsch TJ. A chloride channel widely expressed in epithelial and non-epithelial cells. *Nature* 1992;356:57–60.

278. Toda M, Tulic MK, Levitt RC, Hamid Q. A calcium-activated chloride channel (HCLCA1) is strongly related to IL-9 expression and mucus production in bronchial epithelium of patients with asthma. *J Allergy Clin Immunol* 2002;109:246–250.

279. Todd-Turla KM, Rusvai E, Naray-Fejes-Toth A, Fejes-Toth G. CFTR expression in cortical collecting duct cells. *Am J Physiol* 1996;270:F237–F244.

280. Tonini R, Ferroni A, Valenzuela SM, Warton K, Campbell TJ, Breit SN, Mazzanti M. Functional characterization of the NCC27 nuclear protein in stable transfected CHO-K1 cells. *FASEB J* 2000;14:1171–1178.

281. Tsiokas L, Kim E, Arnould T, Sukhatme VP, Walz G. Homo- and heterodimeric interactions between the gene products of PKD1 and PKD2. *Proc Natl Acad Sci U S A* 1997;94:6965–6970.

282. Tsunenari T, Sun H, Williams J, Cahill H, Smallwood P, Yau KW, Nathans J. Structure–function analysis of the bestrophin family of anion channels. *J Biol Chem* 2003;278:41114–41125.

283. Tulk BM, Edwards JC. NCC27, a homolog of intracellular Cl- channel p64, is expressed in brush border of renal proximal tubule. *Am J Physiol* 1998;274:F1140–F1149.

284. Uchida S. In vivo role of CLC chloride channels in the kidney. *Am J Physiol Renal Physiol* 2000;279:F802–F808.

285. Uchida S, Sasaki S, Furukawa T, Hiraoka M, Imai T, Hirata Y, Marumo F. Molecular cloning of a chloride channel that is regulated by dehydration and expressed predominantly in kidney medulla. *J Biol Chem* 1993;268:3821–3824.

286. Ussing HH, Zerahn K. Active transport of sodium as the source of electric current in the short-circuited isolated frog skin. *Acta Physiol Scand* 1951;23:110–127.

287. Valenzuela SM, Martin DK, Por SB, Robbins JM, Warton K, Bootcov MR, Schofield PR, Campbell TJ, Breit SN. Molecular cloning and expression of a chloride ion channel of cell nuclei. *J Biol Chem* 1997;272:12575–12582.

288. Vandorpe D, Kizer N, Ciampollilo F, Moyer B, Karlson K, Guggino WB, Stanton BA. CFTR mediates electrogenic chloride secretion in mouse inner medullary collecting duct (mIMCD-K2) cells. *Am J Physiol* 1995;269:C683–C689.

289. Vitzthum H, Castrop H, Meier-Meitinger M, Riegger GA, Kurtz A, Kramer BK, Wolf K. Nephron specific regulation of chloride channel CLC-K2 mRNA in the rat. *Kidney Int* 2002;61:547–554.

290. Waldegger S, Jeck N, Barth P, Peters M, Vitzthum H, Wolf K, Kurtz A, Konrad M, Seyberth HW. Barttin increases surface expression and changes current properties of ClC-K channels. *Pflugers Arch* 2002;444:411–418.

291. Wang SS, Devuyst O, Courtoy PJ, Wang XT, Wang H, Wang Y, Thakker RV, Guggino S, Guggino WB. Mice lacking renal chloride channel, CLC-5, are a model for Dent's disease, a nephrolithiasis disorder associated with defective receptor-mediated endocytosis. *Hum Mol Genet* 2000;9:2937–2945.

292. Wang T, Segal AS, Giebisch G, Aronson PS. Stimulation of chloride transport by cAMP in rat proximal tubules. *Am J Physiol* 1995;268:F204–F210.

293. Wang T, Wang WH, Klein-Robbenhaar G, Giebisch G. Effects of a novel KATP channel blocker on renal tubule function and K channel activity. *J Pharmacol Exp Ther* 1995;273:1382–1389.

294. Ward CJ, Hogan MC, Rossetti S, Walker D, Sneddon T, Wang X, Kubly V, Cunningham JM, Bacallao R, Ishibashi M, Milliner DS, Torres VE, Harris PC. The gene mutated in autosomal recessive polycystic kidney disease encodes a large, receptor-like protein. *Nat Genet* 2002;30:259–269.

295. Weinreich F, Jentsch TJ. Pores formed by single subunits in mixed dimers of different CLC chloride channels. *J Biol Chem* 2001;276:2347–2353.

296. Wildman SS, Hooper KM, Turner CM, Sham JS, Lakatta EG, King BF, Unwin RJ, Sutters M. The isolated polycystin-1 cytoplasmic COOH terminus prolongs ATP-stimulated Cl- conductance through increased Ca2+ entry. *Am J Physiol Renal Physiol* 2003;285:F1168–F1178.

297. Willott E, Balda MS, Fanning AS, Jameson B, Van Itallie C, Anderson JM. The tight junction protein ZO-1 is homologous to the Drosophila discs-large tumor suppressor protein of septate junctions. *Proc Natl Acad Sci U S A* 1993;90:7834–7838.

298. Wilson PD. Cystic fibrosis transmembrane conductance regulator in the kidney: clues to its role? *Exp Nephrol* 1999;7:284–289.

299. Wilson PD, Hovater JS, Casey CC, Fortenberry JA, Schwiebert EM. ATP release mechanisms in primary cultures of epithelia derived from the cysts of polycystic kidneys. *J Am Soc Nephrol* 1999;10:218–229.

300. Woods DF, Bryant PJ. The discs-large tumor suppressor gene of Drosophila encodes a guanylate kinase homolog localized at septate junctions. *Cell* 1991;66:451–464.

301. Worrell RT, Butt AG, Cliff WH, Frizzell RA. A volume-sensitive chloride conductance in human colonic cell line T84. *Am J Physiol* 1989; 256:C1111–C1119.

302. Wrong OM, Norden AG, Feest TG. Dent's disease; a familial proximal renal tubular syndrome with low-molecular-weight proteinuria, hypercalciuria, nephrocalcinosis, metabolic bone disease, progressive renal failure and a marked male predominance. *Q J Med* 1994;87:473–493.

303. Xie Y, Schafer JA. Inhibition of ENaC by intracellular Cl- in an MDCK clone with high ENaC expression. *Am J Physiol Renal Physiol* 2004;287:F722–F731.

304. Xiong H, Chen Y, Yi Y, Tsuchiya K, Moeckel G, Cheung J, Liang D, Tham K, Xu X, Chen XZ, Pei Y, Zhao ZJ, Wu G. A novel gene encoding a TIG multiple domain protein is a positional candidate for autosomal recessive polycystic kidney disease. *Genomics* 2002;80:96–104.

305. Xu GM, Gonzalez-Perrett S, Essafi M, Timpanaro GA, Montalbetti N, Arnaout MA, Cantiello HF. Polycystin-1 activates and stabilizes the polycystin-2 channel. *J Biol Chem* 2003;278:1457–1462.

306. Yamaguchi T, Nagao S, Takahashi H, Ye M, Grantham JJ. Cyst fluid from a murine model of polycystic kidney disease stimulates fluid secretion, cyclic adenosine monophosphate accumulation, and cell proliferation by Madin–Darby canine kidney cells in vitro. *Am J Kidney Dis* 1995;25:471–477.

307. Yang H, Shelat AA, Guy RK, Gopinath VS, Ma T, Du K, Lukacs GL, Taddei A, Folli C, Pedemonte N, Galietta LJ, Verkman AS. Nanomolar affinity small molecule correctors of defective delta F508-CFTR chloride channel gating. *J Biol Chem* 2003;278:35079–35085.

308. Yasui M, Hazama A, Kwon TH, Nielsen S, Guggino WB, Agre P. Rapid gating and anion permeability of an intracellular aquaporin. *Nature* 1999;402:184–187.

309. Yasui M, Kwon TH, Knepper MA, Nielsen S, Agre P. Aquaporin-6: an intracellular vesicle water channel protein in renal epithelia. *Proc Natl Acad Sci U S A* 1999;96:5808–5813.

310. Yoshikawa M, Uchida S, Yamauchi A, Miyai A, Tanaka Y, Sasaki S, Marumo F. Localization of rat CLC-K2 chloride channel mRNA in the kidney. *Am J Physiol* 1999;276:F552–F558.

311. Yu AS. Role of ClC-5 in the pathogenesis of hypercalciuria: recent insights from transgenic mouse models. *Curr Opin Nephrol Hypertens* 2001;10:415–420.

312. Yue H, Devidas S, Guggino WB. The two halves of CFTR form a dual-pore ion channel. *J Biol Chem* 2000;275:10030–10034.

313. Zerangue N, Schwappach B, Jan YN, Jan LY. A new ER trafficking signal regulates the subunit stoichiometry of plasma membrane K(ATP) channels. *Neuron* 1999;22:537–548.

314. Zhai XY, Nielsen S, Birn H, Drumm K, Mildenberger S, Freudinger R, Moestrup SK, Verroust PJ, Christensen EI, Gekle M. Cubilin- and megalin-mediated uptake of albumin in cultured proximal tubule cells of opossum kidney. *Kidney Int* 2000;58:1523–1533.

315. Zhou Y, Dong Q, Louahed J, Dragwa C, Savio D, Huang M, Weiss C, Tomer Y, McLane MP, Nicolaides NC, Levitt RC. Characterization of a calcium-activated chloride channel as a shared target of Th2 cytokine pathways and its potential involvement in asthma. *Am J Respir Cell Mol Biol* 2001;25:486–491.

316. Zhou Z, Hu S, Hwang TC. Probing an open CFTR pore with organic anion blockers. *J Gen Physiol* 2002;120:647–662.

CHAPTER 30

Sodium and Chloride Transport

PROXIMAL NEPHRON

Alan M. Weinstein

Cornell University Weill Medical College, New York, New York, USA

INTRODUCTION

The main function of the proximal tubule is the nearly isosmotic reabsorption of some two-thirds to three-fourths of the glomerular filtrate. This means, primarily, the reabsorption of Na^+, Cl^-, HCO_3, and in smaller quantities, potassium, phosphate, and various filtered organic compounds. In view of the large quantities of solutes and water filtered by the glomeruli, proximal tubular reabsorption plays a crucial role in maintaining the body's fluid and electrolyte balance. In particular, modern hypertension research has considered it essential to identify the proximal tubule Na^+ transporters and understand the signals and second messengers that regulate these transporters. Proximal tubular transport is energized by the metabolic reactions within the proximal tubular epithelium, either directly by ATP-driven "ion pumps" (primary active transport), or indirectly by the coupling of solute fluxes to Na transport (secondary active transport). The workload to this epithelium is prescribed by the glomerular filtration rate (GFR), which can vary severalfold in the course of a day, so that the ensemble of epithelial transport systems are also asked to modulate their function responsively, and in a coordinated manner.

All segments of isolated proximal tubules are capable of reabsorbing the same solutes when perfused with bicarbonate-containing Ringer's solution to which glucose and other organic solutes have been added. Quantitatively, however, marked differences exist along the tubule: reabsorption of sodium, water, glucose, and bicarbonate in the early proximal tubule is about threefold greater than that in the mid-portion of the convoluted proximal tubule and nearly ten times that of the straight segment of the tubule. Furthermore, in vivo, the transtubular concentration gradients of the luminal solutes, as well as the electrical potential of the lumen, change as one moves from early to late proximal tubule. In the earliest part of the proximal tubule, preferential reabsorption of organic solutes (glucose and amino acids, etc.) and of sodium bicarbonate, lactate, acetate, phosphate, and citrate occurs. Consequently, the luminal concentration of these solutes is reduced in the remaining portion of the proximal tubule. As a consequence of the preferential bicarbonate reabsorption, the luminal chloride concentration in all but the first 1–2 mm of proximal tubule is increased above that of the peritubular plasma. Since convoluted tubules, and to an even greater extent, straight proximal tubules, are more permeable to Cl^- ions than to bicarbonate, chloride ions diffuse out of the tubule, rendering the lumen electrically positive with respect to the peritubular capillary.

Following the delineation of whole tubule transport properties, transepithelial fluxes and tubular permeabilities, the major experimental focus was to decipher the array of transporters within luminal and peritubular cell membranes. The experimental techniques brought to bear have been diverse. Assessment of the cellular compartment was first done electrophysiologically, using both conventional and ion-selective microelectrodes. In addition, a great deal of important information has derived from studies using pH- or cation-sensitive fluorescent dyes. From knowledge of whole epithelial fluxes and the concurrent change in cytosolic solute activity, luminal and peritubular transport mechanisms could often be inferred. More direct information about the membrane transporters derived from vesicle preparations enriched in fractions from luminal (brush border) or peritubular cell membranes. Despite the inaccuracies associated with inhomogeneous preparations, the inferences derived from this approach have generally been reliable. The patch clamp techniques (whole-cell or excised patch) also provide for study of a single membrane, with the advantage of a more precise focus on the transporter of interest, but with the limitation to ion channels. A major boost in our understanding of proximal tubule function has come over the last decade, with the capability of molecular definition of the transporters, of expressing these transporters in cells that are convenient for study, of developing antibodies for precise location (and quantification) within tubular cell membranes, and of examination of tubules from mice in which the transporter has been knocked out. Basically, molecular techniques have complemented earlier work, with the provision of considerable precision in the quantification of transporter density and kinetics.

Central to its role in body fluid homeostasis is the responsiveness of proximal tubule sodium transport to changes in GFR, as well as to direct neural and hormonal signals. In large measure, changes in sodium reabsorption that accompany changes in GFR may be understood in terms of transepithelial oncotic and hydrodynamic forces which impact on the tubule cells. In some circumstances, peritubular pressures may directly alter the structure of the paracellular pathway, by changing tight junctional transport properties. The neurohumoral regulation of proximal tubule transport must begin with a cellular signal, followed by transduction of the signal to impact the membrane transporters, ultimately producing a change in solute affinity or in transporter density within the cell membrane. The signaling pathways for the important neurohumoral regulators have been an object of intense investigation over the past decade. Nevertheless, the effort to understand the regulation of proximal tubule transporters has gone slowly, having to deal with a number of second messenger molecules, with a number of kinases and phosphatases, with identification of anchoring proteins that secure the local action of a signal, and with the cytoskeletal elements responsible for transporter traffic. At times the same second messenger has been found to be stimulatory and at times inhibitory, depending upon the "state" of the tubule. Although much information is available, a facile description of the path from neurohumoral signal to transporter flux is not yet at hand.

The organization of this chapter starts with the description of whole tubule function, fluxes and the associated driving forces, and tubule permeabilities. Historically, this is the section with the oldest data, and the section that has undergone the least revision from earlier chapter versions. The second section is devoted to the description of the epithelial components: luminal and peritubular cell membranes, the tight junction, and modulation of tubule transport by the lateral intercellular space. With respect to the membrane components, the focus is on identifying what is there and the nature of its kinetics. In this section, there is a mix of data, with substantial molecular input, but not to the exclusion of its precedents. The last section describes the regulation of proximal transport, and is very much a new chapter component. In this section, a number of uncertainties are presented, in the spirit of acknowledging conflicts within the literature, but without forcing a judgment or guessing at an ultimate resolution.

EPITHELIAL FUNCTION

Net Fluxes

The filtered load of a solute to the proximal tubule is, by definition, the product of the single nephron glomerular filtration rate (SNGFR) and the ultrafilterable concentration of the solute. For small nonelectrolyte species the ultrafilterable concentration is that in plasma water. For electrolytes, negatively charged serum proteins produce a Donnan potential, which acts to decrease ultrafilterable Na^+ and increase Cl^- concentration with respect to that of plasma water (577). In amphibian and mammalian proximal tubules, the net effect of proximal

tubule transport is the reabsorption of the luminal solution, resulting in a diminished axial flow rate as one proceeds along the tubules. The systemic infusion of a substance, such as inulin, which is filtered at the glomerulus, not reabsorbed (or secreted) by the proximal tubule, and which may be assayed in aliquots of tubular fluid, permits the calculation of the net volume reabsorption by the tubule from the glomerulus to the point of sampling. Thus, for example, in the rat superficial cortical nephrons, the tubular fluid (TF) inulin concentration at the end of the convoluted proximal tubules is twice that of plasma (P), indicating that one-half of the filtrate is reabsorbed proximally (241). In *Necturus*, the TF/P ratio suggests that about one-third of the filtrate is reabsorbed by the proximal tubule (629). In certain species of fish the net effect of proximal tubule transport is secretion of fluid into the lumen (85). Nevertheless, in view of the considerably greater experimental effort to understand proximal transport by the mammalian kidney, only reabsorption will be considered in this chapter.

When micropuncture techniques are used to sample fluid from the proximal tubule, the fractional reabsorption of the glomerular filtrate is ascertained directly in the TF/P inulin ratio. If a complete collection of tubule fluid is made, then the absolute transport rate of the nephron segment is known and can be expressed as a flux per unit area of epithelium. This was the approach used to obtain the transport data for *Necturus* proximal tubule and rat proximal convoluted tubule shown in Table 1. Alternatively, one may perfuse dissected segments of tubule to directly establish the epithelial fluxes under well defined luminal and peritubular conditions. One must then obtain an independent measure of SNGFR to estimate the fractional reabsorption. The advantage of this approach is that proximal nephron segments not accessible to micropuncture may be examined. For the data from the perfused proximal convoluted tubule of the rabbit shown in Table 1, the measured sodium flux, referred to a 5.4 mm segment of tubule, implies sodium reabsorption of 1.2 nEq/min. With a SNGFR of 20 nl/min, the filtered load of sodium is 2.9 nEq/min, so that the fractional reabsorption is predicted to be about 40%. In the instances of successful micropuncture of rabbit proximal tubule, the observed fractional reabsorption of sodium has been 50% (156) and 45% (806). This type of comparison is particularly important in that it suggests a reasonably well maintained transport capacity for the tubule examined in vitro. When examined carefully, however, conditions in vitro can produce subtle differences from the tubule in vivo. As might be expected, dissection conditions of isolated rabbit proximal tubules can decrease the peritubular membrane electrical potential and increase cytosolic Na^+ concentration, however, they can also engender a peritubular membrane K^+ channel, not seen in vivo, and change the Na^+:HCO_3^- stoichiometry of the peritubular membrane Na–HCO_3 cotransporter from 3:1 to 2:1 (516, 518).

Unfortunately, any attempt to present a concise tabulation of proximal transport (Table 1) must be tempered by an appreciation of inter-nephron heterogeneity and the structural

TABLE 1 Net Fluxes Across Proximal Tubules

	Necturus PT	Rat PCT	Rabbit PCT	Rabbit PST
SNGFR (nl/s)	0.23[h]	0.50[f]	0.33[d]	
PT diameter (μm)	140[k]	20[f]	26[a]	22[j]
Length (cm)	1.4[k]	0.55[f]	0.54[d]	0.33[b]
J_v (nl/s • cm^2)	1.0[k]	65[l]	30[i]	9.76[j]
J_{Na} (nEq/s • cm^2)	0.097[k]	9.4[l]	4.5[i]	1.52[j]
J_{Cl}	0.047[g]	5.1[l]		1.29[j]
J_{HCO_3}		2.65[l]	1.7[c]	0.23[j]
J_{Ca}			0.18[e]	

Sources: [a]Andreoli TE, Schafer JA, Troutman SL. Perfusion rate-dependence of transepithelial osmosis in isolated proximal convoluted tubules: estimation of the hydraulic conductance. *Kidney Int* 1978;14:263–269.

[b]Bankir L, de Rouffignac C (1976). Anatomical and functional heterogeneity of nephrons in the rabbit: microdissection studies and SNGFR measurements. *Pflugers Arch* 1976;366:89–93.

[c]Burg MB, Green N. Bicarbonate transport by isolated perfused rabbit proximal convoluted tubules. *Am J Physiol* 1977;233:F307–F314.

[d]Chonko AM, Osgood RW, Nickel AE, Ferris TF, Stein JH. The measurement of nephron filtration rate and absolute reabsorption in the proximal tubule of the rat kidney. *J Clin Invest* 1975;56:232–235.

[e]Friedman PA, Figueiredo JF, Maack T, Windhager EE. Sodium-calcium interactions in the renal proximal convoluted tubule of the rabbit. *Am J Physiol* 1981;240:F558–F568.

[f]Gertz KH, Boylan JW. Glomerular-tubular balance. In: Orloff J, Berliner RW, eds. *Handbook of Physiology*. Section 8: Renal Physiology. Washington, DC: American Physiological Society; 1973:783–790.

[g]Giebisch G, Windhager EE. Measurement of chloride movement across single proximal tubules of *Necturus* kidney. *Am J Physiol* 1963;204:387–391.

[h]Giebisch G. Measurements of pH, chloride and inulin concentrations in proximal tubule fluid of *Necturus*. *Am J Physiol* 1956;1985:171–174.

[i]Kokko JP, Burg MB, Orloff J. Characteristics of NaCl and water transport in the renal proximal tubule. *J Clin Invest* 1971;50:69–76.

[j]Schafer JA, Patlak CS, Andreoli TE. Fluid absorption and active and passive ion flows in the rabbit superficial pars recta. *Am J Physiol* 1977;233:F154–F167.

[k]Windhager EE, Whittembury G, Oken DE, Schatzmann HJ, Solomon AK. Single proximal tubules of the *Necturus* kidney. III Dependence of H2O movement on NaCl concentration. *Am J Physiol* 1959;197:313–318.

[l]Windhager EE. Sodium chloride transport. Giebisch G, ed. *Transport Organs*. Vol. IV, *Membrane Transport in Biology*. Berlin: Springer-Verlag; 1979:145–214.

changes along the individual tubule. In many mammalian species, the juxtamedullary glomeruli are larger and have a greater SNGFR than the mid cortical or superficial cortical nephrons (577). Thus, in the rat, for example, single nephron inulin clearance obtained by micropuncture of a superficial cortical nephron is only 40% of what must be an average SNGFR, based on whole kidney GFR and nephron number (241). In the rabbit, an indirect technique has given estimates for both superficial and juxtamedullary nephrons at 23 and 29 nl/min (38). An extensive comparison of the transport properties of the superficial cortical and juxtamedullary proximal tubules is

available (76). Corresponding to the greater SNGFR of the juxtamedullary nephrons, there is a greater overall rate of volume and sodium reabsorption, although beyond this quantitative distinction, the relative importance of specific transport mechanisms may also differ between the two nephron populations (350, 492, 666).

The capacity for volume transport is thought to gradually diminish as one proceeds along the mammalian proximal nephron (358). This occurs in association with morphologic changes at the electron-microscopic level that have prompted the division of mammalian proximal tubule into three segments (Fig. 1) (479). The early proximal convoluted tubule, S1, is characterized by tall, densely packed apical microvilli, numerous mitochondria, and an intricate pattern of folding

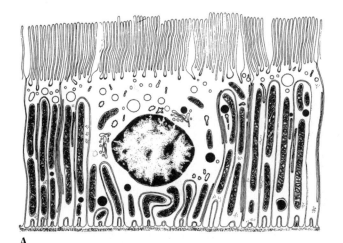

A

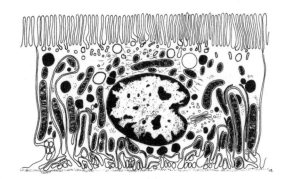

B

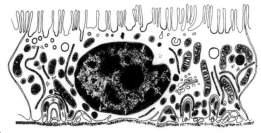

C

FIGURE 1 Proximal tubule cells within the (**A**) S1, (**B**) S2, and (**C**) S3 segments of the rabbit nephron. (With permission, from Kaissling B, Kriz W. *Structural Analysis of the Rabbit Kidney*. Berlin: Springer-Verlag, 1979.)

and interdigitation of the lateral cell membranes (778). There is a gradual transition to the S2 segment which comprises the remainder of the proximal convoluted tubule and the very beginning of the proximal straight tubule. Here there are fewer mitochondria and less amplification of membrane area. Finally, the proximal straight tubule, S3, shows a more cuboidal cell with fewer mitochondria and rare inter-digitations. Welling and Welling (777) compared the cell membrane areas in the S1 and S3 segments of rabbit proximal tubule and found that for each segment, the apical and basolateral areas are nearly equal. In S1, however, the absorptive area of the cell is increased by membrane folding to 36 cm^2/cm^2 of epithelium, whereas in S3 this value is 15 cm^2/cm^2 of epithelium. The spontaneous transport of solutes and water has been measured in segments of the rabbit proximal tubule that had been dissected free and perfused with a solution analogous to an ultrafiltrate of plasma. It is clear that the spontaneous transport rate is substantially less in the proximal straight tubule than in the convoluted segments (125, 396) (Table 1). In the rat, microperfusion of proximal tubule segments in vivo (with comparable flow rates and luminal fluid composition) has demonstrated a lower volume reabsorption rate for segments more than 1–2 mm from the glomerulus (168). Serial micropuncture along a single proximal tubule with filtered fluid flowing freely confirmed the sharp decline in reabsorptive flux of volume (sodium) and anions after the first 1–2 mm of tubule (Fig. 2) (445, 446).

The proximal tubule of the amphibian salamander, *Necturus*, shows fewer mitochondria and little of the membrane amplification found in the mammalian kidney (479). Morphometric analysis of tubules taken from free flow conditions shows an apical area of only 1.5 cm^2/cm^2 of epithelium and basolateral cell membrane area of 11.6 cm^2/cm^2 (480). The rate of volume transport per square centimeter of tubule is correspondingly low, roughly 1 to 2 orders of magnitude less than in mammalian nephron (803) (Table 1). Nevertheless, there is some differentiation of the tubule along its length with shorter cells in the latter, straight portion (479). Corresponding to morphologic differences along the proximal tubule of the amphibian, *Amphiuma*, are substantial changes in the conductance properties of the cell membranes (420). For any of the luminal solutes, if the concentration in the reabsorbed fluid is the same as that in the lumen, then the luminal concentration of the solute will remain unchanged along the proximal tubule. This is the case for sodium, chloride and bicarbonate in the kidneys of *Necturus* (243, 377, 629) and another amphibian, *Ambystoma* (829). In rat and rabbit kidneys, the sodium concentration and hence the total osmolality also remain relatively constant along the proximal tubule (259, 396). This constancy of tubule fluid osmolality has been termed "isotonic transport" and poses a special problem for understanding the forces at work in water reabsorption (vide infra). The fate of chloride and bicarbonate in the mammalian proximal tubule differs, however, from that in *Necturus*. Here the chloride rapidly rises to a level above that of the glomerular filtrate and the bicarbonate falls (125, 221, 259, 727). This shift in anion composi-

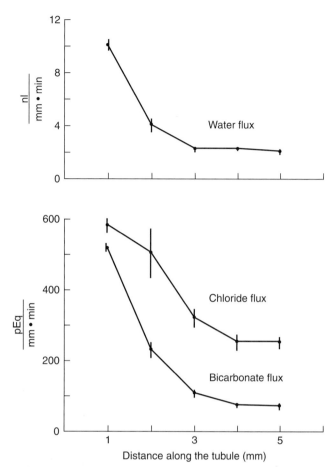

FIGURE 2 Reabsorption of water, bicarbonate, and chloride along the rat proximal convoluted tubule. (From Liu F-Y, Cogan MG. Axial heterogeneity of bicarbonate chloride and water transport in the rat proximal convoluted tubule. *J Clin Invest* 1986;78:1547–1557.)

tion occurs early in the proximal tubule, that is to say, within the S1 segment. This is referred to as "preferential bicarbonate reabsorption" and received much attention as a clue to transport activity at the cellular level. The transepithelial ionic differences have been tabulated for *Necturus* and for the rat (Table 2).

The key features of the compositional changes in tubular fluid during its passage through the mammalian proximal tubule are illustrated in Fig. 3 (572). The tubular fluid/plasma (TF/P) concentration ratio of several solutes is plotted as a function of proximal tubular length. TF/P inulin rises to approximately 2.0, indicating water reabsorption. Glucose and amino acids are rapidly reabsorbed so that at 25% proximal tubular length their concentrations decline to some 10% of the filtrate concentration. Preferential bicarbonate reabsorption lowers the bicarbonate concentration of tubular fluid to approximately 5–8 mM. Along the initial portion of the proximal tubule, the chloride concentration is increased by reabsorption of water (27). In the initial segment, the transepithelial voltage is lumen negative (41, 226), due to the electrogenic nature of co-transport of sodium with glucose or amino acids (227, 395). As the concentration of these solutes

TABLE 2   Composition Differences Between Luminal and Peritubular Solutions

Concentrations (mmol/liter)	*Necturus* PT		Rat PCT	
	Lumen	Capillary	Lumen	Capillary
Na⁺	97.5[k]	97.5[l]	14[c]	144[c]
K⁺	5/8[k]	3.2[l]	3.2–4.6[c, i]	4.0[c]
Cl⁻	76.0[e]	76.0[e]	135[c]	115[c]
HCO₃⁻	7.9[e]	7.9[e]	5–10[c]	30[c]
Ca²⁺	1.4[a, j]	1.8[a, j]	1.8[h]	2.6[h]
Pressure (mm Hg)	3.2[f]	2.9[f]	10.9[b]	6.5[b]
Oncotic pressure (mm Hg)	—	12.1[f]	—	60[g]
Transepithelial PD (mV)	−10 to −15[a]		+1.0[d]	

[a]Free [Ca²⁺] in perfused kidney.

Sources: [a]Boulpaep EL. Electrophysiology of the kidney. In: Giebisch G, ed. *Transport Organs*. Vol. IV, *Membrane Transport in Biology*. Berlin: Springer-Verlag; 1979:97–144.

[b]Falchuk KH, Berliner RW. Hydrostatic pressures in peritubular capillaries and tubules in the rat kidney. *Am J Physiol* 1971;220:1422–1426.

[c]Fromter E. Electrophysiology and isotonic fluid absorption of proximal tubules of mammalian kidney. In: Thurau KT, ed. *Kidney and Urinary Tract Physiology*. MTP International Reviews of Science Physiology Series I, Vol. 6. Baltimore: University Park Press, 1974:1–38.

[d]Fromter E. Solute transport across epithelia: What can we learn from micropuncture studies on kidney tubules? *J PhysiolJ Physiol (Lond)* 1979;288:1–31.

[e]Giebisch G. Measurements of pH, chloride and inulin concentrations in proximal tubule fluid of *Necturus*. *Am J Physiol* 1956;1985:171–174.

[f]Grandchamp A, Boulpaep EL. Pressure control of sodium reabsorption and intercellular backflux across proximal kidney tubule. *J Clin Invest* 1974;54:69–82.

[g]Green R, Windhager EE, Giebisch G. Protein oncotic pressure effects on proximal tubular fluid movement in the rat. *Am J Physiol* 1974;226:265–276.

[h]Harris CA, Baer PG, Chirito E, Dirks JH. Composition of mammalian glomerular filtrate. *Am J Physiol* 1974;227:972–976.

[i]Le Grimellec C. Micropuncture study along the proximal convoluted tubule. *Pflugers Arch* 1975;354:133–150.

[j]Lee CO, Taylor A, Windhager EE. Cytosolic calcium ion activity in epithelial cells of *Necturus* kidney. *Nature* 1980;287:859–861.

[k]Oken DE, Solomon AK. Single proximal tubules of *Necturus* kidney. VI: Nature of potassium transport. *Am J Physiol* 1963;204:377–380.

[l]Shipp JC, Hanenson IB, Windhager EE, Schatzmann HJ, Whittembury G, Yoshimura H, Solomon AK. Single proximal tubules of the *Necturus* kidney. Methods for micropuncture and microperfusion. *Am J Physiol* 1958;195:563–569.

declines and that of chloride rises, the polarity of the transepithelial electrical potential difference changes to lumen positive values (41, 226). This voltage is, at least in part, a diffusion potential, generated by the chloride and bicarbonate concentration gradients and the greater permeability of the tubular wall to chloride than to bicarbonate.

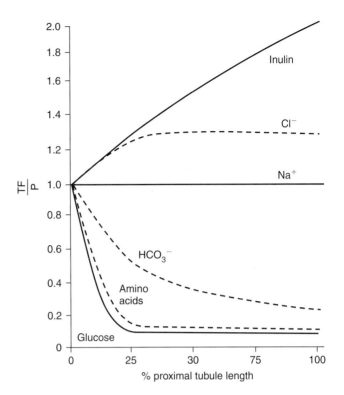

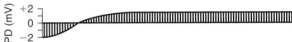

FIGURE 3   Compositional changes in proximal tubule fluid along the mammalian nephron (With permission, from Rector FC Jr. Sodium bicarbonate and chloride absorption by the proximal tubule. *Am J Physiol* 1983;244:F461–F471.)

Transport Forces

In order to evaluate the mechanisms of transport, the observed fluxes across the proximal tubule must be resolved as a function of the responsible driving forces. Experience with non-living membranes had suggested to early authors that a certain fraction of transport might be driven by differences in ion concentration or electrical potential differences across the epithelium. This "passive transport" was to be distinguished from the remaining "active transport" driven by the metabolism of the living epithelium. Early attempts, however, to quantify these notions and to precisely define active transport were confounded by the observations that the flux of one species across the epithelium may affect the transport of another. Thus, for example, a flow of water from lumen to blood, driven by peritubular oncotic pressure, may drag with it a certain amount of sodium. This transepithelial sodium flux cannot be attributed to a difference in sodium concentration across the epithelium, nor to direct metabolic energy input, but is an example of coupled transport.

The equations of epithelial transport are usually written in a form in which all terms containing a volume are consolidated to express the transepithelial volume flow, J_v (ml/sec • cm² of epithelium), as a function of hydrostatic and osmotic driving forces:

$$J_v = L_p \left[\Delta p - RT \sum_{i=1}^{n} \sigma_i \Delta C_i \right] \qquad (1)$$

or

$$\frac{J_v}{V_w} = P_f \left[\frac{\Delta p}{RT} - \sum_{i=i}^{n} \sigma_i \Delta C_i \right] \qquad (1a)$$

Here the "water permeability" of the epithelium is represented either by the coefficient L_p (ml/sec • cm^2 • mm Hg) or by P_f (cm/sec). Both coefficients are commonly used and related according to the formula

$$P_f = \frac{RTL_p}{V_w}$$

where V_w is the partial molar volume of water (0.018 ml/mmol). In Eqs. 1 and 1a the osmotic effect of any species is incorporated in the "reflection coefficient," σ_i, ($0 \le \sigma_i \le 1$). For $\sigma_i = 1$, the species exerts a full osmotic effect and the epithelium is an ideal semipermeable membrane. When $\sigma_i = 0$, the species exerts no osmotic force. To determine the reflection coefficient for a specific solute, the change in the transepithelial volume flow produced by a transepithelial concentration gradient, Δc_i, is compared to the volume flow produced by an equal concentration gradient of an impermeant species. The ratio of these two volume flows is just the reflection coefficient, σ_i.

The representation of solute transport, J_i (mmol/sec • cm^2), the flux equation takes on the form

$$J_i = J_v \left(1 - \sigma_i \right) \bar{c}_i + \sum_{j=1}^{n} L_{ij} \Delta \bar{\mu}_j^c \qquad (2)$$

where

$$\Delta \bar{\mu}_j^c = RT \Delta \ln c_j + z_j F \Delta \psi$$

contains only the concentration and electrical terms of the potential and

$$\bar{c}_i = \frac{\Delta c_i}{\Delta \ln c_i} \approx \frac{1}{2} \left[c_i(1) + c_i(p) \right]$$

is a mean epithelial solute concentration, generally expressed as a logarithmic mean. When the luminal and peritubular concentrations ($c_i(1)$, $c_i(p)$) are not too different, their mean, $\bar{c}_i$, may be approximated by their average value. It is a consequence of thermodynamic theory (Onsager symmetry) that σ_i also appears in the Eq. 2 for solute flux in the term for convective solute drag. This formalizes the intuitive notion that the smaller solutes, which are least osmotically effective, are more likely to be entrained in the volume flow. It is also a consequence of Onsager symmetry that $L_{ij} = L_{ji}$. When the coefficient L_{ij} is positive (for $i \ne j$), then a reabsorptive driving force on solute i will also promote reabsorption of

solute j, so that this coefficient may be considered to represent cotransport of the two solutes. Such cotransport obviously arises when a common carrier transports the two species, but may also occur as a result of intraepithelial convective flows (769).

Some of the most precise experimental measurements that can be made are those of electrical potentials and currents. In the absence of solute–solute interaction, the transepithelial solute flux is the sum of convective and electrodiffusive components and may be written

$$J_i = J_v \left(1 - \sigma_i \right) \bar{c}_i + P_i \left[\Delta c_i + \left(\frac{z_i F}{RT} \right) \bar{c}_i \Delta \psi \right] \qquad (3)$$

where P_i (cm/sec) is the conventional solute permeability and is related to L_{ii} by

$$P_i = \frac{RTL_{ii}}{\bar{c}_i}$$

Equation 3 has generally been the starting point for the application of electrophysiology to characterize proximal tubule. For example, if luminal and peritubular solutions were to have equal ionic concentrations ($\Delta c_i = 0$), the application of an electrical potential difference ($\Delta \psi$) would result in the change in ionic flux

$$J_i = P_i \left(\frac{z_i F}{RT} \right) \bar{c}_i \Delta \psi$$

This can be translated into an ionic current, I_i, and written

$$I_i = z_i F J_i = g_i \Delta \psi \qquad (4)$$

where

$$g_i = P_i \left(\frac{z_i^2 F^2}{RT} \right) \bar{c}_i = z_i^2 F^2 L_{ii} \qquad (5)$$

is the partial conductance of the species i. The total change in current through the epithelium, I, is

$$I = \sum_{i=1}^{n} I_i = \left(\sum_{i=1}^{n} g_i \right) \Delta \psi = g \Delta \psi \qquad (6)$$

Thus, from the electrical resistance, $R = 1/g$, one obtains a measure of the sum of the ionic permeabilities.

When the luminal and peritubular solutions are unequal, the open-circuit potential in the absence of net transepithelial volume flow ($J_v = 0$), gives useful information about the relative ionic permeabilities. In this case, $I = 0$, so that

$$0 = \sum_{i=1}^{n} g_i \left(\frac{RT}{z_i F} \right) \Delta \ln c_i + g \Delta \psi$$

and the open-circuit potential is

$$\Delta\psi = -\sum_{i=1}^{n}\frac{g_i}{g}\frac{RT}{z_iF}\Delta\ln c_i \qquad (7)$$

If, for example, the only concentration differences across the epithelium are equal and opposite anion gradients (such as chloride and bicarbonate), Eq. 7 shows that the difference in ionic conductances determines the magnitude of the transepithelial potential, namely, a "diffusion potential."

Table 3 is a compilation of the permeability properties of the proximal tubules of several species. Again, the inclination to present such tabulation must be tempered by the acknowledgment of permeability variation along the nephron and of differences between superficial and juxtamedullary nephrons. With respect to water permeability, it has been suggested that there is a decline in L_p from the S1 to the S2 segment of the rat tubule (452). Nevertheless, the water permeability remains at least as large in the straight segment as in the convoluted segment (625). With respect to solute permeabilities, an increase in the electrical conductance of the rat proximal tubule has been observed upon moving from the earliest to the latest accessible segments (652). Experiments in perfused rabbit tubules suggest that the increase in total conductance is due to an increase in the chloride permeability (351). Furthermore, these segmental changes appear to be absent in juxtamedullary nephrons.

There is no doubt that proximal tubule metabolism is required for transport to proceed at its normal rate. In the absence of ionic concentration gradients across the epithelium, reabsorption still proceeds and cooling or poisoning with metabolic inhibitors abolishes transport. A generally accepted treatment of active transport by the proximal tubule has been that of Frömter (221), in which Eq. 2 is extended by the simple inclusion of a term for metabolically driven transport, J_i^a:

$$J_i = J_v(1-\sigma_i)\overline{c}_i + \sum_{j=1}^{n}L_{ij}\Delta\overline{\mu}_j^c + J_i^a \qquad (8)$$

or in the absence of coupled fluxes

$$J_i = J_v(1-\sigma_i)\overline{c}_i + P_i\left[\Delta c_i + \left(\frac{z_iF}{RT}\right)\overline{c}_i\Delta\psi\right] + J_i^a \qquad (8a)$$

It may also occur that water flux is linked to metabolic reactions in a way that reabsorption proceeds in the absence of transepithelial driving forces. This flux, J_v^a has been termed "active water transport," and, by analogy with Eq. 8, the transepithelial volume flow has been written as follows (273, 770):

$$J_v = L_p\left[\Delta p - RT\sum_{i=1}^{n}\sigma_i\Delta C_i\right] + J_v^a \qquad (9)$$

A derivation of J_v^a from considerations of the internal structure of the tubule epithelium will be indicated below.

TRANSCELLULAR PATHWAY

Cytosolic Concentrations

In the foregoing, the transport properties of the proximal tubule have been treated from the perspective of the epithelium as a homogeneous entity. The reabsorptive properties of the tubule have been inferred from the transepithelial fluxes resulting from changes in luminal and peritubular solutions. Over the last decades, however, a more microscopic view of proximal tubule transport has come into focus. Crucial to this perspective were the observations that the intercellular tight junctions could serve as a low resistance route for transepithelial ion permeation (229, 800). This defines a "paracellular pathway" for fluxes, across the tight junction, into the lateral intercellular space, and out across the basement membrane to the peritubular capillaries. The "transcellular pathway" enters the cell cytosol via the luminal membrane and exits across the basal cell surface, or across the lateral cell membrane into the lateral intercellular space. The final transepithelial transport is the sum of the fluxes via each pathway.

To discern solute transport across individual cell membranes, one must be able to monitor changes in intracellular concentrations (106). Historically, the first estimates of cell ion content derived from chemical analysis of tissue. Difficulties with this method include the inaccuracy associated with the subtraction of the extracellular contribution to the total, as well as the limitation of examining the concentration at only a single point in time. An additional concern arises when one tries to estimate transmembrane chemical potential differences, if some of the cell ion content is bound or sequestered, and thus not available to the "transport pool." Application of the electron probe to determine cell solutes is somewhat akin to the chemical assay. With the small beam of this technique, true intracellular sampling can be assured. Nevertheless, the estimate of cell water remains indirect and is an important source of uncertainty. Nuclear magnetic resonance (NMR) spectroscopy has been used as a non-destructive method for measuring intracellular sodium of proximal tubules in suspension (284, 409). Unfortunately, only a portion of the cell sodium is "visible" by NMR and additional steps must be taken to estimate the total pool (107). Perhaps the most fruitful technique for probing the cell interior has been the use of microelectrodes capable of penetrating the cell membrane, presumably without destroying the functional integrity of the cell. The electrodes may record the electrical potential of the cytosol or, when fashioned with a substance that reacts selectively with an ion, the cytosolic electrochemical potential of the selected ion species. Though technically challenging, these measurements provide precisely the information necessary for establishing the driving forces for ionic fluxes (225, 375). More recently, ion-sensitive fluorescent dyes have become an important tool for the study of proximal tubule function. When loaded intracellularly, they can be used to monitor continuous changes in pH (8), calcium (178), or chloride (339, 407).

The large cells of the *Necturus* proximal tubule have been most accessible to micropuncture and their intracellular electrical potential has been known for some time (244). More recently, the activities of the various ionic species have been determined and these are indicated in Table 3, along with the electrochemical potential differences between cytosol and peritubular capillary. It should be noted that the low concentration of cell sodium and extremely low concentration of cell calcium, along with the cell electronegativity place these species within a potential well inside the cell. The cytosolic activity of Na^+, is kept low by the Na-K activated ATPase; that of Ca^{++} by Na^+/Ca^{++} exchange and an ATP-driven Ca^{++} pump in the contraluminal cell membrane. Permeability of either luminal or basolateral cell membranes to these species permits influx while metabolic energy is required for their extrusion from the cell. It has been known from chemical data that the tubule cell concentration of potassium is high and of

chloride, low, consistent with the negative electrical potential (789). The data of Table 3 indicate, however, a potential hill for both these species within the cell. For potassium this is due to active inward transport by the Na^+,K^+-ATPase located within the basolateral cell membrane (408). The elevation of cell chloride above what would be found with a purely passive distribution is an observation of several investigators (192, 281, 375, 685). The case for coupled Na-Cl entry across the luminal membrane will be considered in the following section. Finally, the elevation of cell bicarbonate to achieve a neutral cell pH (376) is compatible with either active or coupled bicarbonate entry or active or coupled proton extrusion (598).

Despite the difficulties associated with study of the smaller mammalian proximal tubules, a reasonably complete picture of the intracellular milieu is now available (Table 3B and C). In the rat, the intracellular potential has been found to be slightly more negative than in *Necturus*, −76 mV (193). As in *Necturus*,

TABLE 3 Ion Activities in Proximal Tubule of Three Species

	Cell Concentration (mM)	Cell Activity (mM)	Capillary Concentration (mM)	Electrochemical Potential Difference (Cell–Capillary)[a] (J/mmol)
(A) Necturus				
Na^+	9.6	7.4[a]	100	−11.8
K^+	79	61[a]	2.5	2.7
Cl^-	27	20[c]	98	2.7
HCO_3^-	11[b]	8.3	10	6.2
Ca^{2+}	232×10^{-6}	82×10^{-6d}	1.8	−34.3
PD		−62 mV[c]		
(B) Rat				
Na^+	17.5	13[i]	145	−12.8
K^+	113	82[h]	4	1.3
Cl^-	18	13[f]	118	2.5
HCO_3^-	17[e]	12	25	6.3
Ca^{2+}	250×10^{-6}	87×10^{-6g}	2.3	−38.1
PD		−76 mV[h]		
(C) Rabbit				
Na^+	44[m]	32	145	−9.0
K^+	68	49[k]	5	0.8
Cl^-	25	18[n]	118	1.9
HCO_3^-	16[o]	12	25	4.7
Ca^{2+}	450×10^{-6}	160×10^{-6l}	2.3	−33.7
PD		−61 mV[j]		

[a]For *Necturus*, RT = 2.49 J/mmol and F = 96.5 coul/mmol; for rat and rabbit, RT = 2.57 J/mmol.

Sources: **(A)** [a]Cemerikic D, Giebisch G. Intracellular sodium activity in *Necturus* kidney proximal tubule. *Fed Proc* 1980;39:1080 (abstract); [b]Khuri RN, Agulian SK, Bogharian K, Nassar R, Wise W. Intracellular bicarbonate in single cells of *Necturus* kidney proximal tubule. *Pflugers Arch* 1974;349:295–299; [c]Spring KR, Kimura G. Chloride reabsorption by renal proximal tubules of *Necturus*. *J Membr Biol* 1978;38:233–254; [d]Yang JM, Lee CO, Windhager EE. Regulation of cytosolic free calcium in isolated perfused proximal tubules of *Necturus*. *Am J Physiol* 1988;255:F787–F799. **(B)** [e]Alpern RJ. Mechanism of basolateral membrane $H^+/OH^-/HCO_3^-$ transport in the rat proximal convoluted tubule. A sodium-coupled electrogenic process. *J Gen Physiol* 1985;86: 613–636; [f]Cassola AC, Mollehauer M, Fromter E. The intracellular chloride activity of rat kidney proximal tubular cells. *Pflugers Arch* 1983;399:259–265; [g]Dominguez JH, Rothrock JK, Macias WL, Price J. Na^+ electrochemical gradient and Na^+–Ca^{++} exchange in rat proximal tubule. *Am J Physiol* 1989;257: F531–F538; [h]Edelman A, Curci S, Samarzija I, Fromter E. Determination of intracellular K^+ activity in rat kidney proximal tubular cells. *Pflugers Arch* 1978;378:37–45; [i]Yoshitomi K, Fromter E. How big is the electrochemical potential difference of Na^+ across rat renal proximal tubular cell membranes in vivo. *Pflugers Arch* 1985;405(Suppl 1):S121–S126. **(C)** [j]Bello-Reuss E. Electrical properties of the basolateral membrane of the straight portion of the rabbit proximal renal tubule. *J Physiol (Lond)* 1982;326:49–63; [k]Biagi B, Sohtell M, Giebisch G. Intracellular potassium activity in the rabbit proximal straight tubule. *Am J Physiol* 1981;241:F677–F686; [l]Dolson GM, Hise MK, Weinman EJ. Relationship among parathyroid hormone cAMP, and calcium on proximal tubule sodium transport. *Am J Physiol* 1985;249:F409–F416; [m]Gullans SR, Avison MJ, Ogino T, Giebisch G, Shulman RG. NMR measurements of intracellular sodium in the rabbit proximal tubule. *Am J Physiol* 1985;249:F160–F168; [n]Ishibashi K, Sasaki S, Yoshiyama N. Intracellular chloride activity of rabbit proximal straight tubule perfused in vitro. *Am J Physiol* 1988;255:F49–F56; [o]Sasaki S, Shiigai T, Takeuchi J. Intracellular pH in the isolated perfused rabbit proximal straight tubule. *Am J Physiol* 1985;249:F417–F423.

however, potassium is actively accumulated (145, 193). Good agreement has been reported for the cell sodium concentration estimated electrophysiologically (17.5 mmol/liter) (826) and with the electron probe (20.3 mmol/liter) (56). Although an early investigation suggested passive distribution of chloride across the proximal tubule (672), subsequent work established cellular chloride uptake against a potential gradient (140). The mechanism underlying this elevation of cytosolic chloride will be considered below. At this point, it suffices to acknowledge that the potential hill for chloride is linked via several anion exchangers to the bicarbonate potential. In turn, the elevation of cytosolic bicarbonate is regulated and maintained well above the equilibrium value (1.4 mmol/liter) by a number of transport processes, including Na^+/H^+ exchange and metabolically driven proton extrusion from the cell (H^+ ATPase) (10, 598).

It has also been possible to impale the cells of the isolated perfused rabbit proximal tubule. The intracellular potentials of the proximal convoluted and proximal straight tubules were first found to be -51 and -47 mV, respectively (88), and subsequent determinations have been confirmatory (-50 mV [616]; -61 mV [65]). In the proximal straight tubule, the cell potassium activity is higher than its electrical equilibrium. Both the cell potassium activity and the cell potential fall (depolarize) with the peritubular application of ouabain (89). As in the rat, the chloride activity is elevated above equilibrium, and there is good agreement between the electrophysiologic determination (18 mmol/liter) (345) and that found using a fluorescent dye (21 mmol/liter) (407).

The intracellular pH of rabbit proximal tubules in suspension was first investigated using a radio-labeled weak organic acid. Under control conditions, the cells were found to be alkaline at 7.51, becoming acid with the application of ouabain at 7.42 (91). Subsequent determinations have revealed the pH to be lower (7.22 [616]), and thus more akin to that found in the rat proximal tubule.

Luminal Membrane

GENERAL PROPERTIES

Important information about membrane solute permeabilities and species-species interactions has been obtained from studies in vesicle suspensions prepared from proximal tubule brush border. One result of such studies has been the determination of the water permeability of the luminal membrane, as assessed by the response of vesicle volume (light scattering) to an osmotic shock (723, 725, 730). Corresponding to the approximate doubling of transepithelial water permeability from proximal convoluted tubule to proximal straight tubule of the rabbit (Table 4), is the observation of a comparable increase in water permeability of luminal membranes from these two segments (721). Critical insight into the mechanism of water transport came with the discovery of a specific integral membrane protein (designated AQP-1), which serves as a water channel, or aquaporin, and is the principal water pathway for luminal and peritubular membranes of proximal tubule (reviewed by

Agre et al. [4]). Consistent with the membrane water permeability measurements, the abundance of AQP-1 along the proximal tubule has been found to double as from S2 to S3 segments (470). In mice, the importance of AQP-1 for proximal tubule water flux was demonstrated with the study of S2 segments from AQP-1 knockout mice, whose water permeability (P_f) was about 20% that of wildtype mice (639). Additional vesicle studies indicated that across the luminal membrane, solute–water interaction appears to be minimal, with a reflection coefficient for NaCl of 1.0 (546, 722, 723). This is consistent with absence of solute permeability of AQP-1, when expressed and studied in oocytes (4). Thus, in the application of Eq. 8 to the luminal membrane, the terms for convective solute flux may be ignored.

Early electrophysiologic investigation of the proximal tubule revealed that luminal membrane electrical resistance was between one and two orders of magnitude greater than total epithelial resistance (Table 4). For the *Necturus* proximal tubule, this resistance is 7200 ohm•cm^2 (110, 283), and for the rat, 260 ohm•cm^2 (223, 224). In both species, the effects of altering luminal ionic composition on intracellular potential suggested that the potassium permeability of the luminal cell membrane was much greater than the sodium permeability, and that the chloride permeability was negligible (222, 244). For the *Necturus* proximal tubule, the driving force for sodium across the luminal membrane is about 7.3 J/mmol, or 76 mV (143). If all of the membrane conductance were attributed to a passive sodium pathway, then (combining Eqs. 4 and 5) the sodium flux would be 110 pEq/sec • cm^2, or just about the observed rate of net sodium reabsorption. Yet the estimate of the sodium permeability, determined from purely electrical measurements, placed it at only one-tenth of the total membrane conductance (244). These observations provided strong evidence that sodium entry was coupled to the entry or exit of other solute species.

Direct examination of the conductive channels within this membrane using the patch clamp technique has been possible only to a limited extent. In the first successful attempt, Gogelein and Greger (252) identified a channel in the luminal membrane of rabbit proximal convoluted tubule, which showed a greater conductance to K^+ than to Na^+. In *Necturus* proximal tubule, a luminal channel was identified that was activated by cytosolic calcium and had K^+ permeability 32-fold greater than that of Na^+ (369). Luminal K^+ channels have also been identified in patch clamp studies of primary culture of rabbit S1 proximal tubule (495). Additional K^+ channels have been identified immunohistochemically in the luminal cell membrane of mammalian proximal tubule, including the voltage-gated channel KCNA10 (820), and the voltage-dependent K^+ channel complex, KCNE1/KCNQ1 (717). Both are thought to play a role in stabilizing the membrane potential against the depolarizing effect of Na^+-dependent uptake of glucose and amino acids. Luminal membrane sodium channels ($P_{Na}/P_K \geq 19$ and blocked by amiloride) have been found in a patch clamp study of the rabbit proximal straight tubule (253). Confirming this result,

TABLE 4 Permeabilities of Proximal Tubules

	Necturus	**Rat PCT**	**Rabbit PCT**	**Rabbit PST**
$L_p (\times 10^8$ ml/s $\cdot$ cm$^2 \cdot$ mm Hg)	0.44[a]	22.6[g]	32.6	48.5[f]
P_f (cm/s)	0.46×10^{-2}	0.24	0.35[e]	0.52[e]
σ(Na)		0.7[g]		0.9–1.0[e]
σ(Cl)		0.43[g]		0.78–0.95[e]
σ(HCO$_3$)		1.0[g]		0.97[e]
P(Na) ($\times 10^5$ cm/s)	0.14[j]	24.7[g]	4.0–11.9[e]	2.3–2.6[e]
P(K)	1.56[j]	27.1[g]		
P(Cl)	0.53[j]	21.2[g]	1.9–6.5[e]	5.6–7.3[e]
P(HCO$_3$)	0.13[c]	6.7[g]	1.3–2.3[d,i]	0.4–2.0[e]
P(Ca)		23[h]		
R($\Omega \cdot$ cm^2)	102[b]	5[a]	7.0[f]	8.2[e]

Sources: [a]Bentzel CJ, Davies M, Scott WN, Zatzman M, Solomon AK. Osmotic volume flow in the proximal tubule of *Necturus* kidney. *J Gen Physiol* 1968;51:517–533.

[b]Boulpaep EL. Electrophysiology of the kidney. In: Giebisch G, ed. *Transport Organs*. Vol. IV, *Membrane Transport in Biology*. Berlin: Springer-Verlag; 1979:97–144.

[c]Edelman A, Anagnostopoulos T. Further studies on ion permeation in proximal tubule of *Necturus* kidney. *Am J Physiol* 1978;235:F89–F95.

[d]Holmberg C, Kokko JP, Jacobson HR. Determination of chloride bicarbonate permeabilities in proximal convoluted tubules. *Am J Physiol* 1981;241:F386–F394.

[e]Schafer JA, Andreoli TE. Perfusion of isolated mammalian renal tubules. Giebisch G, ed. *Transport Organs*. Vol. IV, *Membrane Transport in Biology*. Berlin: Springer-Verlag; 1979:473–528.

[f]Schafer JA, Troutman SL, Watkins ML, Andreoli TE. Volume absorption in the pars recta. I "Simple" active Na$^+$ transport. *Am J Physiol* 1978;234:F332–F339.

[g]Ullrich KJ. Permeability characteristics of the mammalian nephron. In: Orloff J, Berliner RW, eds. *Handbook of Physiology*. Section 8: Renal Physiology. Washington, DC: American Physiological Society; 1973:377–398.

[h]Ullrich KJ, Rumrich G, Kloss S. Active Ca^{++} reabsorption in the proximal tubule of the rat kidney. *Pflugers Arch* 1976;364:223–228.

[i]Warnock DG, Yee VJ. Anion permeabilities of the isolated perfused rabbit proximal tubule. *Am J Physiol* 1982;242:F395–F405.

[j]Whittembury G, Sugino N, Solomon AK. Ionic permeability and electrical potential differences in *Necturus* kidney cells. *J Gen Physiol* 1961;44:689–712.

is the finding of voltage-sensitive, amiloride-blockable sodium entry across luminal membrane vesicles of this tubule segment (349), and across the luminal membrane of cultured LLC-PK1 cells (133). The LLC-PK1 cell line is derived from pig kidney and is thought to resemble S3 proximal tubule. A later study of the S3 segment of rat proximal tubule demonstrated a luminal membrane conductance, which could be inhibited by micromolar concentrations of amiloride, and which could be enhanced by a low-sodium diet or mineralocorticoid injection (797). Under conditions of enhanced channel expression, the mRNA which encodes for the ENaC sodium channel could be detected in these proximal tubule cells. It is natural to surmise that the capacity of the proximal straight tubule of the rabbit to reabsorb sodium in the absence of a cotransported solute (626) might be a consequence of such channels.

Chloride channels have also been identified within proximal tubule cell membranes. A careful electrophysiologic study of *Ambystoma* proximal tubule, measuring cytosolic Cl$^-$ activity and membrane potentials, has identified Cl$^-$ conductances in both luminal and peritubular cell membranes. The elevation in cytosolic Cl$^-$ potential was referable solely to a peritubular Cl$^-$/HCO$_3^-$ exchanger (1). In the mammalian kidney, an interesting finding has been the appearance of a chloride conductance after addition of cyclic AMP (443) or by modulating cytosolic production of cyclic AMP (444). These observations, made in a preparation of brush border membrane vesicles, were confirmed in a patch clamp study of the luminal membrane of proximal tubule cells in primary culture (171, 599, 688), and parallels observations in other epithelia. Under the cellular conditions of Table 3B, one would expect such a channel to be a pathway for Cl$^-$ secretion, however, in the presence of a lumen to blood chloride gradient, application of cyclic AMP induces a reabsorptive transcellular chloride flux, which can be inhibited by luminal application of a chloride channel blocker (745). The physiologic role of this chloride channel in proximal tubule function remains to be delineated.

SODIUM–GLUCOSE AND SODIUM–AMINO ACID COTRANSPORT

Perhaps the first sodium entry pathway to receive intensive study was its coupled transport with glucose. Considerable insight had been derived from intestinal and renal preparations, and the description of cotransport that emerged received confirmation as molecular biology provided expression and study of these transporters in other cells (312, 808–810). The cotransport of glucose with sodium was clearly demonstrated in vesicles prepared from the luminal membranes of rabbit (25) and rat (381) proximal tubules. In the presence of a sodium gradient (medium to vesicle), vesicle glucose concentration rises to levels above that in the medium, and then slowly equilibrates with the ambient concentration. This glucose uptake, which carries a net positive current, can be enhanced by short-circuiting the vesicle membrane (57). Conversely, glucose gradients (medium to vesicles) may be used to drive vesicle sodium concentrations transiently well above those of the bathing solution (317). In the intact epithelium, the presence of glucose and sodium in the luminal perfusate depolarizes the luminal cell membrane (223, 474, 614). In a study on the rat proximal tubule in vivo, Samarzija et al. (614) observed that the magnitude of this luminal membrane depolarization is diminished by lowering either the luminal glucose or sodium concentration, by depolarizing the luminal membrane, or by elevating the cell glucose concentration. In *Necturus* proximal tubule, a rise in the intracellular sodium activity accompanies the reabsorptive flux of glucose (375). In *Ambystoma*, this glucose-mediated increase in cell sodium is blunted both by elevations in cell sodium concentration, or by luminal membrane depolarization (511). In sum, the reabsorptive flux of the Na^+–glucose pair has been shown to be dependent upon the electrochemical potentials for each species across the luminal membrane. These qualitative features of Na^+-dependent glucose flux could be captured using a linear nonequilibrium thermodynamic model of the cotransporter (768).

Studies of the kinetics of glucose uptake across the luminal membrane have been presented within the framework of carrier mediated transport, characterized by a maximal transport rate and a luminal glucose concentration for which transport is half-maximal (K_m). When Turner and Silverman (709) examined the sodium-dependent uptake of glucose into vesicles prepared from dog renal cortex their data suggested the presence of two such carrier sites. In their preparation, a high-velocity, low-affinity site had a $K_m = 4.5$ mmol/liter, while the second site had a low velocity and high affinity ($K_m = 0.2$ mmol/liter). The possibility was suggested that these two carriers might correspond to different sites of glucose uptake along the nephron. In pursuit of this issue, Turner and Moran (671, 706) prepared vesicles from both the outer cortex and outer medulla of rabbit kidney. Here, the low affinity carrier localized to the outer cortical region (presumably containing S1 and S2 segments of the proximal tubule) and the high-affinity carrier localized to the outer medullary vesicles (presumably containing S3 segments). Corresponding to the affinity difference, is the determination of a 1:1 (glucose:Na^+) stoichiometry of the cortical cotransporter (324, 707), and a 1:2 stoichiometry of the high-affinity carrier (708). More direct studies localizing glucose uptake

were performed in isolated segments of rabbit proximal tubule by Barfuss and Schafer (40). Their data were compatible with a single high capacity carrier in the proximal convoluted tubule ($J_{max} = 1800$ pmol/sec • cm^2 and $K_m = 1.7$ mmol/liter) and low capacity, high-affinity transporters in the proximal straight tubule ($J_{max} = 170–270$ pmol/sec • cm^2 and $K_m = 0.35–0.70$). Thus these experiments presented a coherent picture of a system of proximal glucose transport which would, under normal conditions, deliver only negligible quantities of glucose to the distal nephron. It should be noted that Na^+–glucose cotransport appears in cultured cell systems and its identification was useful in establishing the similarity of the LLC-PK1 cell line to proximal tubule (568). As in the straight tubule, the stoichiometry of glucose:Na^+ is 1:2 (433, 500). Cotransport was also identified in primary cultures of proximal tubule cells (157, 821), again as high affinity with 1:2 stoichiometry (6, 609), although electrophysiologic study of one preparation suggested a lower-affinity transporter (69).

An important step in the study of Na^+–glucose cotransport came with the cloning of the gene for the intestinal cotransporter, SGLT1 (or, using the Human Genome Organization nomenclature, SoLute Carrier SLC5A1) (311). When this cotransporter was expressed in amphibian oocytes (338) or in mammalian cells (96), it had high glucose affinity and kinetics indicating 1:2 stoichiometry. Early on, the availability of the intestinal transporter allowed identification of antigenic similarity with renal brush border proteins (320). Subsequent in-situ hybridization studies localized SGLT1 to the S3 segment of proximal tubule, precisely the site suggested by the kinetic data (429). Prior to the cloning of this transporter, a number of detailed mathematical representations of Na^+-cotransport had been developed (313, 373, 578, 704). In each of these models, the cotransport of glucose and sodium was represented as a series of reactions: substrate binding to carrier, translocation of loaded carrier, unbinding at the opposite membrane face, and cycle completion by translocation of empty carrier. The expression of SGLT1 in an oocyte enabled more extensive electrophysiologic investigation and reformulation of a more secure model. Steady-state experiments revealed several salient features of the transporter: solute binding affinity is asymmetric, comparing inside and outside of the carrier; translocation of empty carrier is an important rate limiting step and sensitive to the transmembrane PD; and solute binding is not sufficiently rapid as to be considered at equilibrium with respect to translocation (150, 544, 545). This expression system also enabled time-dependent studies to directly examine individual potential-dependent steps within the transport cycle. These have been useful in confirming charge of the unloaded carrier and identifying similarity in kinetics of SGLT1 from human, rat, and rabbit (309, 457, 543).

The cloning of SGLT1 also yielded insights not suspected from earlier studies, namely that protons could substitute for sodium in the transport of glucose (318) and that in the translocation of 2 Na^+ and 1 glucose, SGLT1 also transports over

200 water molecules (458, 493). This degree of water transport is certainly important with respect to intestinal function, although in the kidney, these fluxes through SGLT1 will be tiny. The discrepancy between the limited abundance of SGLT1 and the high capacity for glucose transport of cortical brush border membrane vesicles was readily apparent (542). Homology screening revealed a gene which encoded for a second Na^+–glucose cotransport, termed SGLT2 (SLC5A2), expressed in kidney, for which the stoichiometry is 1:1 and which, by in situ hybridization localizes to the S1 segment of proximal tubule (359). More detailed kinetic studies indicated that SGLT2 is the low affinity, high capacity system identified in kinetic studies (828). When SGLT2 is expressed in oocytes and studied electrophysiologically, a kinetic scheme similar to that for SGLT1 could be developed to represent this transporter (466). While still other sodium–glucose cotransporters have been identified, any significance with respect to renal transport remains to be established.

Owing to the diversity of amino acid transport systems, their description is considerably more complex than that for glucose, and these transporters span several solute carrier families within the SLC-taxonomy (141, 256, 491, 732). Nevertheless, it has been established that with respect to the quantitative reabsorption of amino acids, the most important pathways across the luminal membrane of proximal tubule all exhibit sodium-dependent uptake (628, 712, 831, 830). A series of electrophysiologic investigations in the rat by Samarzija and Frömter (611–613) documented several luminal membrane carriers for neutral amino acids as well as separate carriers for basic and acidic amino acids. In those studies, all of the amino acid uptake occurred in association with Na^+ and in all cases was associated with depolarization of the luminal cell membrane. Among these systems, perhaps the most carefully examined was that for alanine. Electrophysiologically, it showed an apparent K_m for alanine of about 6 mmol/liter (328, 611) and a Hill coefficient suggesting 1:1 Na^+:alanine stoichiometry. Studies in renal brush border membrane vesicles confirmed the K_m (465). This carrier purified as a single protein band and its activity could be recovered following reconstitution into phospholipid vesicles (183). The relatively low affinity of this carrier was of obvious concern when trying to rationalize the ability of proximal tubule to clear the urine of filtered amino acids. In this regard, another sodium-dependent neutral amino acid transporter, SAAT1, was obtained from a proximal tubule cell line (LLCPK1), with amino acid sequence 89% identical to SGLT1, and with amino acid K_m less than 1 mmol/liter (403). Some of the complexity of amino acid transport is indicated with acknowledgment of other ions that can be involved in cotransport. Turner (705) demonstrated that a lumen-to-cell chloride gradient enhanced the sodium-dependent transport of alanine, and chloride has been found to be required for the transport of glycine (621), as well as taurine and proline (832). A cell-to-lumen K^+ gradient enhances glutamate uptake (638) and a lumen-to-cell proton gradient enhances the uptake of glutamate (527), proline (589), and glycine (569).

SODIUM/PROTON EXCHANGE

Of greatest quantitative importance for sodium flux across the luminal cell membrane is the Na^+/H^+ counter transport system (654). The Na^+/H^+ exchanger was securely established by Murer et al. (520), using a suspension of vesicles composed predominately of luminal membrane. Their basic observation was that a sodium concentration gradient from suspension medium to vesicle interior resulted in acidification of the medium. This effect required the presence of intact vesicles but was undisturbed when electrical potential differences between the vesicle interior and the medium were eliminated. Further, a suspension medium alkaline with respect to vesicle interior stimulated sodium uptake by the vesicles. These results were confirmed in rabbit proximal tubule vesicles by Kinsella and Aronson (Fig. 4) (383), who further demonstrated alkalinization of the vesicle interior by the inwardly directed sodium gradient. This counter transport is reversibly inhibited by amiloride (384), and proceeds with a Na^+:H^+ stoichiometry of 1:1 (385). Following those early observations, kinetics of the proximal tubule luminal membrane Na^+/H^+ antiporter were studied intensively (22, 276, 504). Vesicle preparations revealed a transport site that bound a single Na^+ (753) with an affinity roughly one tenth that of the external Na^+ concentration and with competitive binding by H^+ or NH^+_4 (26, 384). Studies of the antiporter at lower temperatures indicated that Na^+ uptake and H^+ extrusion occurred in a sequential ("ping-pong") fashion with H^+ transport likely to be the rate-limiting step (538, 539). The effect of intracellular pH is more complex, with cytosolic

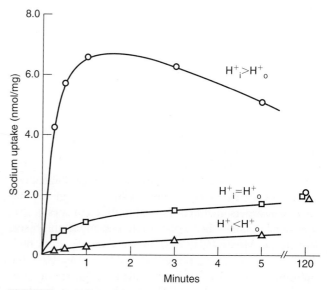

FIGURE 4 Effect of proton gradients on sodium uptake by luminal membrane vesicles prepared from rabbit renal cortex. Low internal pH $(H^+_i>H^+_o)$ enhances and elevated internal pH $(H^+_i<H^+_o)$ retards sodium entry relative to the rate of entry in the absence of pH gradients. The vesicles were prepared in sodium-free medium, and uptake was measured in solutions containing 1 mM Na^+. (With permission, from Kinsella JL, Aronson PS. Properties of the Na^+–H^+ exchanger in renal microvillus membrane vesicles. *Am J Physiol* 1980;238:F461–F469.)

alkalosis shutting off Na^+/H^+ exchange more sharply than a simple substrate depletion effect (24). Cytosolic pH appears to have little impact on the Na^+ affinity of the antiporter (386), but rather modifies the turnover rate (539). With respect to the kinetic properties of this transporter, the information gained from renal brush border membrane vesicles has generally received confirmation in studies of isolated proximal tubule cell suspensions (92, 529), and in vesicles prepared from established cell lines (507), or from primary culture of proximal tubule cells (213, 686).

The function of the Na^+/H^+ exchanger in the maintenance of cytosolic pH was studied extensively by Boron and Boulpaep (102) in the isolated perfused tubule of the salamander, *Ambystoma tigrinum*. This preparation, which permits both intracellular recordings, as well as rapid change of the perfusion solutions, had been developed by Sackin and Boulpaep (607) and shown to be comparable to the proximal tubule of *Necturus* in terms of sodium transport rate and electrical resistances. Bathed in Ringers media, the cell cytosol is -57 mV with respect to the peritubular solution, at pH $= 7.43$, and with sodium and chloride activities 27 and 18 mmol/liter, respectively (compare *Necturus*; see Table 3) (102). The prototype experiment of Boron and Boulpaep was the equilibration of the tubule with an NH_4Cl-containing solution followed by the instantaneous removal of this solution. This left the cell cytosol with an abundance of the acid species NH^+_4 and electrically depolarized. Over a period of several minutes the cytosolic pH returned toward normal. This recovery was accompanied by an overshoot of the cell sodium activity above control and recovery was substantially impaired in the absence of external sodium or in the presence of amiloride. During recovery there was no change in cytosolic chloride, nor any effect of anion transport inhibition. This work demonstrated the presence of the Na^+/H^+ exchanger in both luminal and basolateral membranes of this epithelium as well as its function in the recovery from an intracellular acid load.

In the mammalian proximal tubule, examination of brush border and basolateral membrane vesicles showed that the Na^+/H^+ exchanger is primarily within the luminal cell membrane (347, 647). Schwartz (647) presented evidence for the direct coupling of Na^+ and H^+ fluxes in the intact proximal convoluted tubule perfused with an acidic solution. He found that ouabain inhibition of sodium reabsorption, presumably raising cell sodium concentration, could run the luminal Na^+/H^+ exchanger in reverse, increasing proton exit from the lumen into the cell. Examination of vesicles from cortical and outer medullary regions of the kidney indicated that the Na^+/H^+ exchanger is present along both convoluted and straight segments of proximal tubule (348, 508). More direct evidence for the presence of the luminal membrane Na^+/H^+ exchanger in the S3 segment was offered by Kurtz (412). Using tubules whose cells had been loaded with the pH-sensitive fluorescent dye, BCECF, he found acidification of the cell interior with removal of luminal sodium. Nevertheless, the vesicle studies indicated that

the maximal Na^+/H^+ exchange rate was lower in the outer medullary population, suggesting a lower density of the transporter in straight proximal tubules (348). This also received confirmation by Baum (47), who perfused both convoluted and straight proximal tubules with cells containing BCECF. By studying the impact of changes in luminal sodium on intracellular pH, he was able to conclude that in comparison to the convoluted segment, the straight tubule had a 30% capacity for Na^+/H^+ exchange.

In the molecular era, the Na^+/H^+ exchangers came to be recognized as a family of transport proteins, NHE^-, with the luminal membrane exchanger of proximal tubule identified as NHE3 (SLC9A3). The gene for NHE3 was cloned and sequenced (537, 699) and the product identified immunocytochemically in the brush border membrane (94). Kinetic studies of the NHE3 in expression systems generally confirmed the properties noted a decade earlier in the membrane preparations (536, 700). With respect to the Na^+/H^+ exchange activity of the peritubular membrane, the NHE1 isoform was identified in both basolateral membrane vesicles and in immunohistochemical staining of rabbit proximal tubule (95). Failure to detect NHE3 protein in proximal straight tubule prompted speculation that another NHE isoform may be operative in this segment (14). More generally, even in tubule segments in which NHE3 was abundant, the magnitude of the Na^+/H^+ flux that traversed this isoform was of interest. Based on the observation that the inhibitor profile of rat brush border vesicle Na^+/H^+ exchange was identical to the inhibitor profile of NHE3 in expression systems, it was concluded that NHE3 was the sole exchanger within the luminal cell membrane (743). That view was quickly amended with the development of the NHE3 knockout mouse, in which proximal microperfusion revealed rates for Na^+ and HCO_3^- reabsorption of 25% and 40%, respectively, compared with wildtype (641). In subsequent in vivo microperfusion studies, residual Na^+ reabsorption was found to be slightly greater, 60% (462) and 45% (746). When the proximal tubules from knockout mice were dissected, loaded with BCECF, and perfused in vitro, the magnitude of luminal Na^+/H^+ exchange could be assessed as the change in intracellular pH in response to restoration of luminal Na^+ (155). In those experiments, the Na^+-dependent proton secretion in knockout tubules was about 50% of the wildtype, and completely inhibitable by amiloride. The magnitude of NHE3 flux was also assessed in rat proximal tubules perfused in vivo, in which a specific NHE3 inhibitor reduced Na^+ reabsorption by 30% (718) and 40% (743). These values are likely to be underestimates of the NHE3 flux, in view of the fact that amiloride inhibition was only 50% (743). In sum, it seems safe to attribute about half of the luminal membrane Na^+/H^+ exchange to NHE3. With respect to the molecular identity of the residual transport, both NHE2 knockout (155) and specific inhibitor studies (743) have eliminated NHE2 as a candidate. Recently, Goyal and coworkers identified a new NHE^- isoform, NHE8, within kidney cortex (262) and expressed on proximal tubule brush border (261). Its quantitative role in luminal Na^+/H^+ exchange remains to be defined.

Regarding the functional importance of the luminal membrane Na^+/H^+ exchanger in the proximal nephron, two caveats are in order. It is important to distinguish total HCO_3^- reabsorption from the Na^+-dependent portion of HCO_3^- reabsorption. The luminal membrane contains a H^+-ATPase (120), and amiloride block of the Na^+/H^+ transporter has been used to identify a significant component of proton secretion via the H^+-ATPase (36, 327, 412, 558). The second caveat is that total Na^+-dependent proton secretion may be considerably greater than tubular HCO_3^- reabsorption. Preisig and Rector (559) microperfused rat proximal convoluted tubules with a late proximal solution, low in bicarbonate and high in chloride. In this situation, where net bicarbonate absorption was virtually absent, amiloride still inhibited 44% of NaCl reabsorption. These findings were taken as evidence for the importance of parallel pathways through the luminal membrane for Na^+ (via the Na^+/H^+ exchanger) and for Cl^- (via a Cl^-/base exchanger) in the net reabsorption of NaCl. The implication of such a scheme is that the net flux of Na^+ across the Na^+/H^+ transporter can well exceed the total reabsorptive bicarbonate flux. To date, only one mathematical model of NHE3 has been developed, based on a scheme of Na^+ binding, translocation, and release, H^+ binding, translocation, and release, and which also includes competing NH_4^+ binding, translocation, and release (773). In this model, all binding was assumed to be rapid (equilibrium) and affinity coefficients were assumed to be symmetric with respect to internal and external faces of the transporter. With one additional assumption, namely the inclusion of an internal modifier site, which enhances translocation in response to cytosolic acidification, most of the kinetic behavior described in vesicle studies could be represented. When this simulation of NHE3 was incorporated into a mathematical model of rat proximal tubule, Na^+/H^+ exchange functioned directly to reabsorb luminal $NaHCO_3$, and in parallel with a luminal membrane Cl^-/base exchanger, effected net NaCl reabsorption. An additional prediction of this kinetic model was that Na^+/NH_4^+ exchange via luminal NHE3 is the most important mechanism for ammonia secretion by proximal tubule. This strengthened earlier conclusions, drawn from observation of tubules in vitro, that luminal ammonia entry from cellular ammonia genesis could be blocked by inhibition of NHE3 (521).

CHLORIDE/BASE EXCHANGE

To gain entry to the cell across the luminal membrane, chloride must be transported up an electrochemical potential gradient (Table 3); either cotransport with luminal Na^+ or exchange for cytosolic base is energetically feasible. In *Necturus* proximal tubule, Spring and Kimura used both Cl^-- (685) and Na^+-selective (379) microelectrodes, as well as tracer fluxes (378), to look for NaCl cotransport. Their

data indicated that intracellular chloride activity was depressed when either chloride or sodium is omitted from the bathing solution, and paralleled the cotransport of sodium and chloride in gallbladder epithelium (220). The dependence of cell chloride concentration on luminal sodium received confirmation in the electrophysiologic study of Guggino et al. (282), who in addition, showed a lack of effect of luminal bicarbonate on cell chloride. The results obtained with the Cl^--selective electrode, however, could not be reproduced by Edelman et al. (192). Furthermore, Na^+-dependent Cl^- uptake is difficult to rationalize with experiments using luminal membrane vesicles from *Necturus*, which revealed no direct coupling of Na^+ and Cl^- fluxes, but did indicate the presence of both Na^+/H^+ and Cl^-/HCO_3^- exchangers (653). The absence of Na^+-Cl^- cotransport had been a consistent finding in vesicles prepared from brush border membranes of the mammalian kidney (519, 655). In the straight proximal tubule of rabbit, a Cl^- microelectrode study has failed to detect Na^+-dependent luminal chloride entry (345).

In the rat, Lucci and Warnock (464) found that furosemide inhibited two-thirds of the fluid transport, when the luminal perfusion was a high chloride, low bicarbonate solution. Since the transported solute was sodium chloride and since furosemide does not effect the tight junction permeability, their observations were interpreted as indicating a predominantly transcellular route of sodium and chloride transport. (The absence of a furosemide effect on junctional permeability is suggested by finding no change in transepithelial resistance in rabbit proximal tubule [127] nor a change in glucose-induced transepithelial potential [228].) In view of the ability of a known inhibitor of erythrocyte anion exchange (SITS) to also inhibit proximal volume reabsorption in their preparation, Lucci and Warnock (464) suggested that NaCl transport occurred via parallel luminal Na^+/H^+ and Cl^-/OH^- (or Cl^-/HCO_3^-) exchangers.

Warnock and colleagues supported this hypothesis with the demonstration of pH-gradient driven, electroneutral Cl^- fluxes across brush border membrane vesicles (751, 754, 755). Similar conclusions were drawn by Liedtke and Hopfer (440) whose investigation of luminal membrane vesicles from rat small intestine indicated that coupled NaCl cotransport was unlikely. Their work also indicated an inhibitory effect of furosemide on the Cl^-/OH^- exchanger (441). Although a number of reports confirmed the presence of a Cl^-/OH^- exchanger in renal brush border membrane vesicles (130, 148, 670), the absence of quantitatively significant flux through such an exchanger was indicated by others (139, 346, 602, 655). Methodologic concerns relating to vesicle experiments were raised on both sides of this issue. Chen et al. (148) indicated that proton permeation of the luminal membrane could limit the ability to detect a Cl^--driven pH gradient. Seifter et al. (655) also suggested that Cl^-/OH^- exchange in a brush border vesicle preparation could arise from basolateral membrane contamination. Schwartz (648) examined intact rabbit convoluted proximal tubules, looking for evidence of luminal Cl$^-$/OH$^-$ exchange. When perfused with a sodium-free acidic fluid, there was no significant effect of luminal Cl$^-$ on the appearance of bicarbonate within the tubule fluid.

Critical insight into the process of luminal membrane chloride transport came with the work of Karniski and Aronson (361), who demonstrated the presence of a chloride-formate (Cl$^-$/HCO$_2^-$) exchanger in brush border membrane vesicles from the rabbit. In their experiments they found that a formate gradient could drive transmembrane chloride flux and that a chloride gradient could drive formate flux. This process was electroneutral and could be blocked by the anion exchange inhibitor, DIDS. Most significantly, they found (Fig. 5) that while a pH gradient only slightly enhanced chloride uptake, this same gradient in the presence of a physiologic concentration of formate could drive substantial chloride flux. To account for this formate effect, they indicated that a backflux of formic acid, down its concentration gradient, from the acidic bath to the alkaline vesicle interior, would serve to constantly resupply the Cl$^-$/HCO$_2^-$ exchanger. Karniski and Aronson (361) proposed that in the intact tubule, the concurrent operation of Cl$^-$/HCO$_2^-$ and Na$^+$/H$^+$ exchangers, along with back diffusion of formic acid, would yield a net flux of NaCl across the luminal cell membrane.

Subsequently, this mechanism was refined with the identification of a luminal membrane HCO$_2^-$/OH$^-$ exchanger (equivalently HCO$_2^-$-H$^+$ cotransport) which could act to recycle secreted formate back into the cell (610). (By virtue of its inhibitor profile, this anion exchanger is distinct from the Cl$^-$/HCO$_2^-$ antiporter.) One point of difficulty with this proposal was the subsequent finding that the diffusional permeability of the luminal membrane to formic acid was far too low to sustain a flux comparable to the estimated chloride flux (556). An effort was made to rationalize this discrepancy mathematically, by considering the possibility of formic acid accumulation within an unstirred layer defined by the brush border. It was found, however, that with realistic diffusion coefficients, the microvilli were sufficiently short that no significant differences of formic acid concentration could develop between the bulk luminal solution and that near the cell membrane (405, 406). At this time, the possibility of a microdomain of low pH adjacent to the luminal membrane in which the formic acid to formate concentration ratio is enhanced, remains the least secure element of this proposed mechanism.

Acknowledging points of uncertainty, a scheme emerged in which Cl$^-$/base exchange in the proximal tubule is effected by two or more anion exchangers functioning in parallel (Fig. 6) (23). To pursue this scheme further, a candidate protein for the Cl$^-$-HCO$_2^-$ antiporter was sought and purified from brush border membrane vesicles (675). Of uncertain significance was the observation that when reconstituted into phospholipid vesicles, this protein could also mediate direct Cl$^-$/HCO$_3^-$ exchange (674). The effect of formate has been examined in intact tubules, with cells containing BCECF, in which luminal chloride is able to acidify the cell in the presence (but not the absence) of formate (9, 46). It must also be acknowledged that one protocol which could detect formate stimulation of Cl$^-$/base exchange in superficial proximal convoluted tubules, failed to detect it in tubules from juxtamedullary nephrons (666). There has also been the observation of a negative formate effect in a study of proximal straight tubule (414), again raising the possibility of nephron heterogeneity with respect to the mechanism of chloride entry. In their search for chloride entry mechanisms, Karniski and Aronson (362) also demonstrated a Cl$^-$/oxalate exchanger within brush border vesicles, on a carrier distinct from that for Cl$^-$/HCO$_2^-$. The subsequent finding of luminal membrane pathways for oxalate recycling, either in exchange for SO$_4$ or OH$^-$ (410), supported the possibility that the Cl$^-$/oxalate exchanger may also be an important route for luminal membrane Cl$^-$ entry (Fig. 6). Aronson and colleagues (410, 741) envisioned the possibility that three carriers in parallel, Cl$^-$/oxalate and oxalate/SO$_4^=$ antiporters plus the 2 Na$^+$-SO$_4^=$ cotransporter, would effect luminal entry of NaCl.

Confirmation of the importance of luminal chloride/base exchangers came with measurements of fluxes in intact proximal tubules. When any segment of rabbit proximal tubule (S1–S3) was perfused with an acidic (high Cl$^-$,

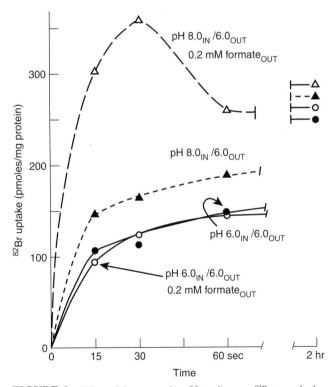

FIGURE 5 Effect of formate and a pH gradient on ^{82}Br$^-$ uptake by luminal membrane vesicles prepared from rabbit renal cortex. While a pH gradient (8.0$_{in}$/6.0$_{out}$) only slightly enhances ^{82}Br$^-$ transport, this same gradient in the presence of 0.2-mM formate produces a substantial increase in uptake, with an overshoot above the equilibrium concentration. (From Karniski LP, Aronson PS. Chloride/formate exchange with formic acid recycling: a mechanism of active chloride transport across epithelial membranes. *Proc Natl Acad Sci U S A* 1985;82:6362–6365.)

LUMEN   **CELL**

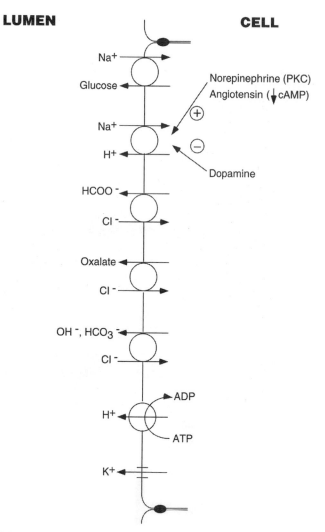

FIGURE 6   Transport pathways across the luminal cell membrane of the mammalian proximal tubule.

low HCO_3^-) solution, there was a substantial impact of formate to stimulate volume (NaCl) reabsorption (632, 633). In perfusions with a relatively alkaline solution (such as an ultrafiltrate of plasma) there was no such enhancement, presumably due to the limited recycling of formate. In reviewing these observations, Berry and Rector (81) pointed out that the pH-dependence of formic acid permeation effectively prioritizes proximal anion reabsorption along the tubule, HCO_3^- taking precedence over Cl^-. The increased volume reabsorption observed with formate was subsequently found to occur in association with an increase in cell volume, thus supporting the transcellular route for the increment in chloride flux (630). With perfusion of proximal tubules of the intact rat kidney, both luminal formate and oxalate enhance NaCl reabsorption from an acidic, high-chloride, luminal solution (741, 742, 749). The ability of a chloride channel blocker, DPC, within the peritubular perfusate to block the formate and oxalate effects, is additional evidence that the increment in NaCl flux is transcellular.

The effort to delineate the luminal membrane anion transporters received a major boost with their molecular identification and examination in expression systems. In particular, attention has focused on the SLC26 family of anion exchangers (515). Of the members in this family, the SLC26A4 transporter (pendrin) was demonstrated to be a Cl^-/formate exchanger when expressed in Xenopus oocytes (650), and its mRNA was identified in rat kidney cortex (678). The protein however, was not detected immunohistochemically in mouse proximal tubule brush border (390). Furthermore, in pendrin knockout mice Cl^-/formate exchange in brush border membrane vesicles was normal, and microperfusion of proximal tubules showed normal formate stimulation of volume reabsorption (363). The transporter SLC26A6 (CFEX, PAT1) could also mediate Cl^-/formate exchange in oocytes, and the protein was expressed in brush border of mouse proximal tubules (390). Further study of SCL26A6 revealed that it had a broad transport capacity, which included Cl^-/oxalate, Cl^-/HCO_3^-, and Cl^-/OH^- (152, 816). The observation that low concentrations of oxalate could inhibit Cl^-/HCO_3^- exchange led Jiang et al. (352) to surmise that the primary function of SLC26A6 in proximal tubule was as the luminal Cl^-/oxalate exchanger. This prediction was borne out in study of mice deficient in SLC26A6 (748). The mice had normal serum electrolytes and normal proximal tubule volume reabsorption under control conditions; oxalate stimulation of proximal volume flux was absent. These knockout mice showed only a tendency toward deficient formate stimulation of volume reabsorption, so that at this time, the identity of the Cl^-/formate exchanger(s) remains uncertain.

Suspicion that formate may have other effects on proximal transport, beyond luminal anion exchange, was raised in a mathematical model of rat proximal convoluted tubule which included representation of luminal membrane Cl^-/HCO_2^- exchange (772). Simulation of formate addition reproduced the observed cell swelling and increase in cytosolic chloride concentration, however, the density of the chloride/formate exchanger had virtually no effect on overall NaCl reabsorption along the tubule. In similar simulations, the density of the Na^+/H^+ exchanger had a powerful impact on NaCl reabsorption, indicating that for the model tubule, sodium reabsorption was rate limiting for NaCl flux. Subsequent experimental examination of mice deficient in NHE3 found that formate stimulation of proximal sodium (volume) and chloride reabsorption was absent, although oxalate stimulation was entirely preserved (743). These authors surmised that in the normal tubule, there might be a functional coupling between NHE3 and the Cl^-/formate exchanger. A direct study of the impact of formate on NHE3 function was undertaken by Petrovic et al. (550). In the absence of CO_2/HCO_3, addition of formate to the bath and lumen of mouse microperfused kidney proximal tubule caused intracellular alkalinization, with cell pH increasing from baseline level 7.17 to 7.55. Removal of sodium from the lumen or addition of EIPA completely prevented the alkalinization. It was concluded that formate stimulates the apical Na^+/H^+ exchanger NHE3 in kidney proximal tubule, and that formate stimulation of chloride reabsorption could be indirect and secondary to activation of NHE3. An intriguing possibility is that the Cl^-/formate exchanger may be acting as a formate receptor to modulate NHE3 (550).

Peritubular Membrane

GENERAL PROPERTIES

The cell sodium content reflects the balance among conductive, coupled, and metabolically driven fluxes across both luminal and peritubular cell membranes. The Na^+ conductance of the peritubular membrane appears to be small. In *Necturus*, the ratio of potassium to sodium permeabilities has been estimated at 30:1 (108). The total electrical resistance of this membrane is 2550 ohm•cm^2, roughly one-third that of the luminal membrane (110, 283). In the rat the potassium to sodium permeability ratio is about 20:1 (221), and the electrical resistance of this membrane is 90 ohm•cm^2, again roughly a third of the luminal membrane (223). A similar apportionment of electrical resistance appears in the proximal convoluted tubule of the rabbit, where the peritubular and luminal resistances are, respectively, 39 and 118 ohm•cm^2 (425). In the straight proximal tubule of the rabbit, Bello-Reuss (65) has found the peritubular sodium conductance undetectable. In the first successful application of a patch pipette to the peritubular membrane of rabbit proximal tubule, only a potassium channel was clearly identified (252). With respect to convective sodium fluxes across this membrane, all the data are negative with one exception. Welling et al. (779, 781), applied an osmotic shock to the peritubular surface of isolated rabbit tubules and recorded the change in cell volume. A comparison of the effect of raffinose and NaCl indicated a reflection coefficient, σ_{NaCl}, of 0.5, suggesting that water flow across this membrane would carry significant quantities of NaCl. This surprising result did not receive confirmation however, in two subsequent studies of basolateral membrane vesicles. Using either light scattering (723) or a fluorescent indicator (546) to assess vesicle volume, salt reflection coefficients of 1.0 were obtained. Subsequent experiments in whole tubule preparations, with optical measurement of cell volume (289) or using a fluorescent indicator (667) indicated $\sigma_{NaCl} = 1.0$, implying that no NaCl flowed convectively across the peritubular membrane.

SODIUM BICARBONATE COTRANSPORT

The cotransport of sodium with bicarbonate is an important pathway for sodium and the principal pathway for bicarbonate exit across the peritubular membrane in both amphibian and mammalian proximal nephron (10, 104, 556). The delineation of this coupled transport followed from the careful examination of bicarbonate exit from the salamander proximal tubule by Boron and Boulpaep (103). Using pH- and Na^+-sensitive microelectrodes, they observed that a reduction in peritubular bicarbonate concentration led to a

decline in cytosolic pH, a peritubular depolarization, and a decline in cell sodium activity. Further, a reduction in peritubular sodium also led to a decline in cytosolic pH and, in contrast to the expectation from a conductive Na^+ pathway, peritubular depolarization.

All of these effects could be blocked by the anion transport inhibitor, SITS. These results suggested the operation of a coupled Na^+ and HCO_3^- cotransporter with the exit of at least two bicarbonate ions for each sodium ion. In the salamander, the electrochemical gradient of bicarbonate across the peritubular membrane was sufficient to drive sodium exit from the cell, if the stoichiometry were 2:1 or greater (HCO_3^-:Na^+). Subsequent study of the *Necturus* proximal tubule confirmed the presence of substantial voltage-sensitive HCO_3^- exit across the peritubular membrane (476), which was later shown to be coupled Na^+ and HCO_3^- transport (460). Here it was suggested that the stoichiometry might well be 3:1. With regard to the issue of HCO_3^-:Na^+ stoichiometry, one interesting set of observations in *Necturus* was the finding that when functioning in the normal reabsorptive direction, this ratio was 3:1, but when bath conditions were changed to reverse the flux direction, the ratio changed to 2:1 (553). This suggested an asymmetry with respect to the affinities of the substrates, perhaps secondary to the conformational changes of the transporter during the translocation step.

In the rat proximal tubule, experiments using conventional microelectrodes indicated that elimination of bicarbonate from the perfused peritubular capillaries produced a large instantaneous depolarization (231). In this early work, the investigators attributed the depolarization to a conductive bicarbonate pathway and estimated (Eq. 7) that nearly half the conductance of the peritubular membrane might be mediated by bicarbonate. Electrophysiologic study of the perfused straight proximal tubule of the rabbit also disclosed a steady-state depolarization with removal of peritubular bicarbonate (65, 88). In that work, however, the depolarization was attributed to a pH-dependent decrease in peritubular membrane K^+ conductance, and thus a decreased contribution of the K^+ potential to the overall membrane potential. The rat proximal tubule was then reexamined, and still the results indicated that the immediate depolarization produced by peritubular bicarbonate removal did not depend upon changes in membrane K^+ conductance (123, 124). This depolarization was inhibited by SITS, but a clear implication of Na^+ in the bicarbonate exit step was not confirmed. Within a short period of time, a number of investigators securely established the presence of Na^+–HCO_3^- cotransport in the peritubular membrane of the mammalian kidney. Sasaki et al. (616) using pH-sensitive microelectrodes demonstrated that in the straight proximal tubule of rabbit, elimination of bath sodium resulted in cellular acidification and peritubular depolarization, an effect that was partially blocked by SITS. Biagi and Sohtell (86, 87) used conventional microelectrodes to document a peritubular depolarization with sodium removal in both convoluted and straight proximal segments. The effect was substantially blocked by SITS and attributed to coupled HCO_3^- transport. Yoshitomi et al. (825) reexamined the rat proximal tubule, now using both Na^+-sensitive and pH-sensitive microelectrodes. The removal of peritubular sodium or bicarbonate led to the expected depolarization, acidification and decrease in cell sodium activity. When these investigators compared the (SITS-inhibitable) depolarization with either 10-fold reductions of peritubular Na^+ or HCO_3^- (equal changes in chemical potential) they found that the impact of the bicarbonate removal was 3.0 fold greater. They concluded that the HCO_3^-:Na^+ stoichiometry was 3:1. In an independent set of experiments, the sudden reduction in peritubular bicarbonate resulted in peritubular HCO_3^- and Na^+ fluxes (estimated from cell size and buffering power), which confirmed a 3:1 coupling ratio (825).

The peritubular bicarbonate pathway in the rat proximal tubule was also investigated using the fluorescence of intracellular BCECF to monitor changes in cytosolic pH (8). In this first use of BCECF in the rat, Alpern was able to document SITS-inhibitable acidification of the cell with reduction of peritubular sodium. When BCECF was used to detect pH changes along the nephron, the transporter was identified in the S3 segment, but in clearly reduced capacity compared with S2 (47, 239). Abuladze et al. (3) used BCECF to quantify Na^+-HCO_3^- transport capacity in all three proximal tubule segments from both cortical and juxtamedullary rabbit kidneys. They reported S1 fluxes three- to five-fold greater than those of S2, and S2 fluxes eight-fold greater than those of S3. Examination of isolated basolateral membrane vesicles prepared from rabbit (5, 267) and rat kidney (268) permitted the kinetics of the transporter to be studied in relative isolation. By analysis of driving forces that would just transport through this pathway, Soleimani et al. (677) confirmed that three negative charges were transported for each sodium. Subsequently, the cotransported species were identified as one HCO_3^- plus one $CO_3^=$ (673). Identification of the transported species was also pursued electrophysiologically. In rabbit proximal tubules in vitro, under "standard" conditions, the stoichiometry of peritubular HCO_3^-:Na^+ flux through this cotransporter was 2:1 and insensitive to carbonic anhydrase inhibition. However, with perfusion conditions more closely approximating those in vivo, the stoichiometry shifted to 3:1 and sensitive to carbonic anhydrase inhibition. This change in transport was interpreted as a shift of the transported species from 2 HCO_3^-–HCO_3^-–Na^+ to $CO_3^=$–HCO_3^-–Na^+, as in vivo (518, 657). Gross and Hopfer (1998) studied the Na^+–HCO_3^- cotransporter in a cell line derived from the S1 segment of rat proximal tubule, grown to confluence on filters. When the luminal cell membrane of this artificial epithelium was permeabilized with amphotericin, cytosolic solute concentrations were identified with those of the luminal solution, and the stilbene-sensitive transepithelial current with current through the Na^+–HCO_3^- cotransporter. Data from this preparation indicated a 3:1 flux stoichiometry

(280), and provided information with which to construct a detailed kinetic model for this transporter (279, 280).

Major advances in the study of the Na^+–HCO_3^- cotransporter came with its cloning, first from *Ambystoma* kidney (595), and then from the human (128) and rat kidneys (129, 594). Denoted akNBC, hkNBC, and rkNBC, respectively, all three cotransporters are comprised of 1035 amino acids, and structural comparisons have been presented (593, 676). Using antibody developed against rNBC, the protein was demonstrated in rat proximal tubule in an exclusively basolateral pattern, with intense staining in S1, rapid decline in S2, and no detectable staining in S3 (636). Staining in *Ambystoma* proximal tubule was also basolateral, but considerably weaker. Immunohistochemistry at the electron microscopic level confirmed these findings (484). When rkNBC was expressed in Xenopus oocytes, transporter function could be studied electrophysiologically, and the stoichiometry of HCO_3^- to Na^+ fluxes was found to be 2:1 (187, 649). It was concluded that the function of this transporter in mammalian cells in vivo was clearly different from its function in an amphibian cell. The conundrum was sharpened with experiments in artificial epithelia derived from mouse proximal tubule or collecting duct, each deficient in NBC. In these two mammalian cells, transfected kNBC showed 3:1 or 2:1 stoichiometry for proximal and collecting duct cells, respectively (277). Important insight came from Müller-Berger et al. (517) who examined rkNBC in oocytes electrophysiologically, and found that with elevation of cytosolic calcium concentration, there was a relatively slow (30 seconds) activation of the NBC conductance plus a shift in stoichiometry from 2:1 to 3:1. They understood that such events in the proximal tubule in vivo would constitute a switch from zero (or secretory) peritubular HCO_3 flux to brisk HCO_3 reabsorption. This switch was deciphered by Gross et al. (277), working with the artificial mouse proximal tubule epithelium, transfected with kNBC. They found that addition of cAMP caused a shift in stoichiometry from the basal 3:1 to 2:1, and this was PKA-dependent. Replacing the single PKA phosphorylation site of the transfected transporter eliminated the stoichiometry shift.

CHLORIDE TRANSPORTERS

In early electrophysiologic investigation of both amphibian (281, 668) and mammalian (65, 123, 134) proximal tubules, peritubular membrane chloride conductance appeared to be virtually absent, or at least negligible. In proximal convoluted tubules of the rabbit, perfused in vitro, peritubular application of a chloride channel blocker had no effect on NaCl reabsorption (48). Subsequently, Welling and O'Neil (783) found that in rabbit proximal straight tubule the conductive chloride pathway in peritubular membrane could account for about 6% of the total membrane conductance. However, after cell swelling induced by a 150 mOsmol hypotonic osmotic shock, the chloride conductance increased to 20% of the total peritubular membrane conductance. In proximal convoluted tubule of the rabbit, using quantitative video microscopy, the volume of control tubules was unaffected by changes in peritubular chloride concentration. However, prior hypotonic cell swelling rendered the cell volume sensitive to peritubular chloride concentration, and this effect was eliminated by application of a chloride channel blocker (631). Peritubular chloride channel blockers have also been effective at blunting the changes in the membrane electrical potential following a change in peritubular chloride concentration (658). Further electrophysiologic study of rabbit convoluted tubule during osmotic shock estimated the fractional chloride conductance to increase from 3% to a maximum of 16%, with relaxation to 8%. During these same experiments, the fractional conductance of the Na^+–$3HCO_3^-$ pathway declined from 41%–16%, with little change in the absolute conductance through this pathway.

The data from this type of experiment give enough information to estimate the reabsorptive flux of chloride through the peritubular channels. If one assumes that the peritubular membrane under control conditions has an electrical resistance of 100 $\Omega \cdot cm^2$ (425), equivalently a conductance of 10 mS/cm^2, then the conductance of the Na^+–$3HCO^-$ pathway is about 5 mS/cm^2, as is the maximal chloride conductance after the osmotic shock. With reference to Table 3C, the cytosolic chloride electrochemical potential across this channel is about 2 J/mmol, or 20 mV. Multiplication by the steady-state chloride conductance of the swollen cell, 2.5 mS/cm^2, yields a chloride current of 50 nA, or 0.5 $nmol/sec \cdot cm^2$. This estimate may be compared with the overall transepithelial sodium flux of late proximal convoluted tubule 4.5 $nmol/sec \cdot cm^2$. Thus the conductive chloride flux is not insignificant, and yet it cannot be the whole story. Further, concern over the magnitude of the osmotic shocks used in these experiments prompted reexamination with smaller perturbations by Breton et al. (117). When the cell volumes increased by only 20%–25%, the peritubular chloride conductance increased only three- to four-fold from control. Another important observation from the study of Breton et al. (117) was that the time course of chloride channel activation was delayed with respect to the time course of cell swelling, suggesting perhaps a chemical modification of the channel, rather than an immediate stretch-activated response. As in the luminal membrane, increases in cytosolic cAMP also activate a chloride channel within the peritubular membrane of rabbit (659, 660) and rat (745).

From the considerations above, chloride fluxes across the peritubular membrane must also occur as electroneutral coupled transport process with other ions. Guggino and associates (282, 456) examined the mechanism of chloride transport across the peritubular membrane of *Necturus* proximal tubule, using Cl^- and pH-sensitive microelectrodes. They found that following either the removal of peritubular Cl^- or the increase of cytosolic Cl^-, the exit of chloride from the cell was substantially blunted by the removal of either peritubular Na^+ or HCO_3^-. This chloride exit was inhibited by SITS. In view of the electroneutral nature of the process,

they proposed a coupled transport mechanism in which intracellular Cl^- was exchanged for Na^+ and $2HCO_3^-$ from the peritubular side (Fig. 7). Such coupled transport systems had been established previously in invertebrate neurons (598). Examination of the free energy change of such a transporter (Table 3A) reveals that it is favorable for reabsorptive chloride flux. Other studies of chloride permeation of the peritubular membrane of amphibian proximal tubule have suggested the presence of a Cl^-/HCO_3^- exchanger that was independent of sodium (192, 827). It is clear from the energy balance, however, that such a transporter would mediate chloride uptake by the cell. Its contribution to the overall chloride economy of the proximal tubule remains uncertain.

In the mammalian proximal tubule, peritubular $Cl^-/$$HCO_3^-$ exchange had been suspected from peritubular capillary perfusion studies in the rat (119, 713). More convincing evidence for the presence of Na^+-dependent Cl^-/HCO^- exchange in the peritubular membrane of rat proximal tubule came with the experiments of Alpern and Chambers (11). In these tubules loaded with BCECF, restoration of peritubular capillary chloride produced cellular acidification. This acidification did not occur in the absence of ambient (luminal and peritubular) Na^+ and was blocked by SITS. Consistent with these findings was the observation of Grassl et al. (268), that in basolateral membrane vesicles from rat renal cortex, an

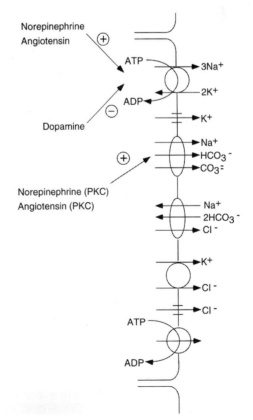

FIGURE 7   Transport pathways across the basolateral cell membrane of the mammalian proximal tubule.

oppositely directed Cl^- gradient (inside to outside) stimulated Na^+ uptake, driven by an (outside to inside) HCO_3^- gradient. In vesicles from the rabbit, in which Cl^- uptake was assayed, it was found to be enhanced by an outwardly directed HCO_3^- gradient and further stimulated by the addition of a Na^+ gradient (149). In a Cl^- microelectrode study of rabbit proximal convoluted tubule, Ishibashi et al. (343) found that removal of either HCO_3^- or Na^+ from the peritubular bath increased cytosolic Cl^-, an effect which could be inhibited by SITS, and which was interpreted as confirmation of Na^+-dependent Cl^-/HCO_3^- exchange. In subsequent examination of the rate of decline of cell Cl^- following perturbations of the peritubular bath, these authors concluded that this transporter was the dominant pathway for Cl^- exit across the peritubular membrane (344).

Examination of the straight proximal tubule of the rabbit has not yielded consistent findings regarding the Na^+ dependence of Cl^-/HCO_3^- exchange. Sasaki and associates (617), using pH-sensitive microelectrodes first found a small cellular alkalinization with the removal of peritubular chloride. Subsequent study with a Cl^--sensitive electrode demonstrated a substantial increase in intracellular chloride with reduction of peritubular bicarbonate, an effect that was blunted by the complete removal of sodium and blocked by SITS (619). Using straight proximal tubules containing BCECF, Kurtz (413) found a peritubular Cl^-/HCO_3^- exchanger that could function in the absence of Na^+. A basolateral Cl^-/HCO_3^- exchanger in this segment was also identified by Nakhoul et al. (525), but its Na^+ dependence could not be defined. A careful microelectrode study of the S3 segment of the rabbit was performed by Kondo and Frömter (400) who found that removal of bath Cl^- decreased intracellular Cl^-, alkalinized the cell, and produced no change in cytosolic Na^+. This effect was blocked by peritubular SITS. Further, reduction of peritubular HCO_3^- increased cell Cl^-, so that a strong case was advanced for the presence of a Na^+-independent Cl^-/HCO_3^- exchanger in the peritubular membrane. With reference to Table 3C, this exchanger must mediate chloride uptake by the cell. A cycle of this exchanger in association with a cycle of the luminal Na^+/H^+ transporter would yield net cellular uptake of NaCl and could increase the volume of the tubule cell. Indeed, the peritubular Cl^-/HCO_3^- exchanger has been implicated in the recovery of cell volume after shrinkage in a hyperosmolar medium (454, 455, 592).

Electrically silent chloride exit across the peritubular membrane may also occur as cotransport of KCl (752). In consideration of their data on the conductive properties of the basolateral membrane of *Necturus* gallbladder, Reuss and associates (579, 581) proposed KCl cotransport as a means of rationalizing the necessary Cl^- exit with the low membrane chloride conductance. This proposal was subsequently confirmed with the demonstration that intracellular chloride activity could be made to vary with variation in the basolateral potassium concentration (166, 580). Such a mechanism was proposed for the *Necturus* proximal tubule by Shindo and Spring (668),

based on their concern for a chloride exit pathway. With respect to the mammalian proximal tubule, beyond the need for Cl^- exit, the brisk influx of K^+ via the Na-K-ATPase mandates substantial peritubular K^+ exit. For the rat proximal tubule, it was estimated that the conductive pathway was inadequate to account completely for this exit, so that in construction of a mathematical model of this epithelium a peritubular KCl cotransporter was incorporated (766). The first evidence for the proximal tubule KCl cotransporter came with the experiments of Eveloff and Warnock (203) on rabbit renal basolateral membrane vesicles. Here K^+ or Cl^- gradients drove uptake of the other species in a voltage-independent manner. These findings received support with observations of furosemide-sensitive cell volume decrease in rabbit proximal straight tubule (782) and furosemide-sensitive K^+ exit in proximal tubule suspensions (29, 402). In the proximal straight tubule, Sasaki et al. (615) used both K^+-and Cl^--sensitive microelectrodes to demonstrate the mutual interaction of K^+ and Cl^- across the peritubular membrane. This interaction was independent of membrane electrical potential and independent of Na^+. These findings received confirmation in the proximal convoluted tubule, examined with Cl^--sensitive microelectrodes by Ishibashi et al. (343), although in this work, coupled K–Cl exit appeared to be insensitive to furosemide. A subsequent electrophysiologic investigation also failed to detect furosemide-sensitive coupled K^+ and Cl^- fluxes (658). At the molecular level, at least four K^+–Cl^- cotransporters have been identified within the SLC12 family (SLC12A4–7), also known as KCC1–4, respectively (310, 514). KCC3 is limited to nerve, but the isoform within the proximal tubule has not yet been established.

NA,K-ATPASE

Metabolically driven sodium extrusion from the cell and potassium uptake are affected by the Na,K-ATPase situated exclusively within the peritubular cell membrane (364, 415). The biochemical properties of the pump have been intensively investigated and extensively reviewed (249, 354–356). The functional transport unit of the Na,K-ATPase consists of an alpha subunit bound to cytoplasmic structural proteins (512) and an externally protruding beta subunit. Although there are three isoforms for the alpha subunit, only a single isoform (α1) appears to be expressed in proximal tubule (490, 703). Together the alpha-beta unit spans the peritubular membrane and contains within its interior, cation binding sites. The most widely held scheme (356) for the operation of the pump envisions a cycle which begins with an E1 state, in which ATP is bound to the alpha subunit and the cation binding sites are open to the cytoplasmic surface for the binding of three Na^+ ions. With the binding of Na^+, ADP is released, leaving a phosphorylated unit in which the cations are initially inaccessible to either membrane face (occluded). A conformational change in the transport unit brings it to the E2 state in which the cationic binding sites are open to the external surface. At this point the release of the Na^+ is followed by the binding of $2K^+$ ions, and with hydrolysis of the phosphate bond, these K^+ ions are occluded. Binding of ATP is associated with the conformational transition back to the E1 state and release of K^+ into the cytoplasm.

The stoichiometry of the Na,K-ATPase was first established in nonrenal systems (249, 388, 528). In the kidney, Kinne (380) interpreted whole organ oxygen uptake data, in light of an "active" fraction of tubular sodium transport, to obtain approximately three sodium transported per ATP hydrolyzed. Harris and associates (305) approached this problem by examining potassium uptake and oxygen consumption in a suspension of rabbit renal cortical tubules. Their data confirmed the uptake of two potassium ions per ATP hydrolyzed (306). A suspension of rabbit renal cortical tubules has been examined, where NMR was used to monitor Na^+ transport from the cell and a K^+ electrode in the suspending medium determined K^+ uptake (28). Over nearly an order of magnitude of transport rates of the Na,K-ATPase, the Na:K stoichiometry remained 3:2. By virtue of this stoichiometry, the Na,K-ATPase generates a net outward current across the peritubular membrane. Pump inhibition with ouabain induces prompt depolarization of the peritubular membrane in the rat proximal tubule (228). In the perfused *Ambystoma* proximal tubule held in K^+-free bathing solution, the restoration of bath potassium induces a peritubular hyperpolarization directly attributable to the Na,K-ATPase (608).

The development of a microassay system for Na,K-ATPase by Schmidt and Dubach (634, 635) permitted the first estimate of enzyme activity within individual tubule segments. Subsequently, Morel and colleagues developed a technically simpler assay and studied the distribution of Na,K-ATPase along the nephron (181, 366). They found comparable distribution in rat, rabbit, and mouse, with substantially greater concentration of ATPase in proximal convoluted tubule than in the straight segment. In the study of Garg et al. (236), the Na,K-ATPase activities of the S1, S2, and S3 segments of the rabbit proximal tubule were determined to be 17.5, 6.7 and 3.8 pmol ATP/sec • cm of tubule. Under conditions of the assay, maximal hydrolytic activity of the enzyme is determined, so that maximal Na^+ transport will be three times these values. Corresponding to the transport activity of the Na,K-ATPase, there is a free energy change of 28.6 J/mmol (Table 3C) or 6.8 cal/mmol. The energy change is certainly compatible with the free energy of hydrolysis of ATP of 13–14 cal/mmol, which has been determined in several tissues (728). El Mernissi and Doucet (199) quantified ouabain binding sites of rabbit PCT and found 0.109 pmol/cm or 25×10^6 sites/cell. Thus the ATPase activity of 10 pmol/sec • cm would correspond to about 100 cycles/sec of a single Na,K-ATPase unit.

The actual rate of sodium transport by the Na,K-ATPase is usually less than maximal enzyme activity, and is dependent on the levels of intracellular Na^+, peritubular K^+, and intracellular ATP. Of these three factors, in the proximal tubule in vivo, cytosolic Na^+ concentration is the most important regu-

lator of pump activity (354, 365). The half-maximal enzyme activation occurs at 31 mmol/liter (249, 680), a level comparable to normal intracellular chemical concentrations. The physiologic correlate to this biochemical data is the observation in *Necturus* proximal tubule that the rate of sodium transport responds to variations in the cytosolic sodium concentrations (684). It had been a previous observation in *Necturus* that the increase in luminal membrane sodium permeability achieved by the luminal addition of amphotericin B produced an increase in proximal tubule volume reabsorption (687). Spring and Giebisch (684) measured both reabsorptive rates of luminal droplets as well as cell sodium content by chemical analysis. It was found that isotonic water transport increased linearly, and steeply, in response to increased cytosolic sodium (Fig. 8). This suggested that under normal conditions the luminal cell membrane is the rate limiting step for sodium transport. With respect to peritubular K^+,-half maximal ATPase activation occurs at concentrations under 1.0 mmol/liter (249, 306, 680). In lysed membrane preparations the-half maximal saturation of ATPase activity, with respect to ATP, occurs at 0.4 mmol/liter (354, 681). Thus, at

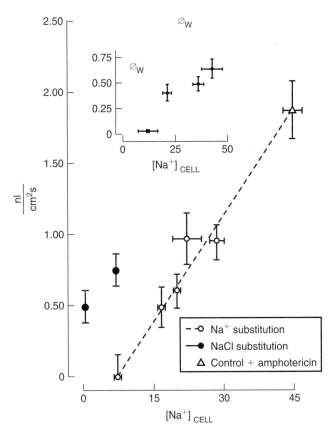

FIGURE 8 Transepithelial water flow, Φ_w, (or, equivalently, transepithelial sodium flux) is plotted as a function of intracellular sodium concentration in *Necturus* proximal tubules. Intracellular sodium is decreased from the control value (30 mM) by substitution of luminal Na+ with tetramethylammonium (or substitution of luminal NaCl with mannitol; see inset); sodium is increased above the control level by the luminal application of amphotericin. (With permission, from Spring KR, Giebisch G. Kinetics of Na^+ transport in *Necturus* proximal tubule. *J Gen Physiol* 1977;70: 307–328.)

normal levels of intracellular ATP (1–3 mmol/liter) there should be little change in the rate of hydrolysis with variation of the ATP concentration. Nevertheless in the intact tubule, partial inhibition of mitochondrial respiration produced proportional declines in cellular ATP and transport (285). In a more extensive study, Soltoff and Mandel (679, 681) found a linear correlation between cellular respiration and ion transport spanning a range of cellular ATP concentrations of 0–4 mmol/liter. Thus in the intact cell, it appears that ATP concentration can serve as an intermediary between transport and metabolism.

CALCIUM EXIT

The peritubular membrane contains both a Ca^{++}-dependent ATPase and a Na^+/Ca^{++} exchanger (251). Either transporter, in association with a luminal entry step, could provide the mechanism for the active reabsorption of calcium by proximal tubule. The Na^+/Ca^{++} exchanger would also provide a mechanism for the blunting of calcium transport by removal of peritubular sodium (711). Studies of transport across membrane vesicles have suggested that the Ca^{++}-ATPase mediates the bulk of the peritubular calcium flux. Both transporters have comparable affinities for cytosolic calcium, but the maximal transport rate of the ATPase may be fivefold greater than that of the Na^+/Ca^{++} exchanger (250, 724). Further, under normal conditions the Na^+/Ca^{++} exchanger appears to be poised near its equilibrium. The $Na^+:Ca^{++}$ stoichiometry of the exchanger, whether in heart (575) or kidney (690) appears to be 3:1. Thus, with reference to Table 3, the large free energy changes associated with Ca^{++} entry and Na^+ exit appear to almost balance (180, 250). Studies in the intact tubule, however, have revealed circumstances in which peritubular Na^+/Ca^{++} exchange is manifest. The first demonstration was in *Necturus* proximal tubule, where Ca^{++}-sensitive microelectrodes indicated a sustained increase in intracellular Ca^{++} following removal of peritubular Na^+ (428). A subsequent experiment in rat proximal tubule examined isotopic calcium fluxes and found that low peritubular Na^+ enhanced Ca^{++} influx across this membrane (180). If peritubular Na^+ were lowered first, the enhanced Ca^{++} efflux induced by lowering peritubular Ca^{++} was eliminated; this effect could be reproduced by peritubular application of a blocker of Na^+/Ca^{++} exchange (179). In *Necturus* it has also been shown that elevation of cell Na^+ concentration, whether by blunting Na-K ATPase activity with ouabain (463) or removal of peritubular K^+ (818), or by increasing luminal Na^+ entry with gramicidin channels (219), increase cytosolic Ca^{++}. Conversely, decreasing cell Na^+ concentration with either low Na^+ luminal perfusate (219) or removal of luminal organics (818) decreased cytosolic Ca^{++}.

Coordination of Entry and Exit

Under normal circumstances, there may be several-fold variations in glomerular filtration rate, to which the proximal tubule responds with nearly proportional changes in sodium reabsorption (vide infra). Although the mechanism underlying this glomerulotubular balance is not completely understood, the wide swings in the transcellular fluxes of sodium and bicarbonate pose a definite threat to the proximal tubule cell, with respect to maintaining a viable cell volume and pH. Such challenges are not unique to proximal tubule, but threaten all transporting cells, particularly the gastrointestinal epithelia, which experience swings in sodium-dependent glucose and amino acid uptake. In part, enhanced exit will be affected by the kinetic response of the Na,K-ATPase to increases in cell Na^+ concentration (Fig. 8), but this is generally not sufficient to account for cellular homeostasis. Schultz and associates have emphasized the need for peritubular exit pathways to keep pace with luminal entry in order to preserve the integrity of cell composition and cell volume (642–644). Beyond this, considerable attention has focused on the positive correlation between the potassium permeability of the peritubular membrane and the rate of epithelial sodium transport (61, 172). Increasing peritubular potassium conductance, beyond enhancing potassium exit, should be expected to hyperpolarize the membrane, thus enhancing chloride and bicarbonate exit as well. The critical experimental observations were made in the epithelium of the small intestine of *Necturus*, from recordings with conventional and K^+-selective microelectrodes (266, 286). It was found that with the addition of alanine to the luminal solution there was a prompt depolarization of the cell interior in association with a doubling of sodium reabsorption. Over a period of several minutes the K^+ conductance of the basolateral membrane increased, producing a repolarization of the cell and a further enhancement of sodium transport. The parallel response of peritubular K^+-conductance with reabsorptive Na^+ flux was subsequently documented in frog proximal tubule, following the application of phenylalanine to the tubule lumen (497, 498), and in the mammalian proximal tubule with luminal application of glucose and alanine (62, 423, 424). Direct examination of the K^+ channel of the peritubular membrane via patch clamp has shown that the increase in K^+-conductance with luminal application of organics is the result of an increase in the open probability of this channel (60). Thus attention was focused on identifying the signal by which luminal solute entry could activate these channels. The two principal candidates for the modulators of peritubular exit have been (1) cell volume and (2) coupling of the Na,K-ATPase activity with K^+-channel open probability (pump-leak parallelism) via cytosolic ATP concentration. The signaling and transport effectors for cell volume regulation have been extensively reviewed (418, 419).

Examination of *Necturus* small intestine indicated that both increased sodium transport and hypotonic cell swelling had similar impact on the basolateral membrane. These observations led to the proposal that a transport-associated increase in cell volume might mediate the enhanced K^+-conductance found with increased Na^+ reabsorption (427). It had been known since the experiments of MacRobbie and Ussing (467) that frog skin epithelium could volume regulate. When the skin was placed in a hypotonic bathing solution, the initial swelling of the epithelial cells was followed by a gradual restoration of cell volume, presumably with the loss of cell solute. A critical observation was that hypotonic swelling of the toad urinary bladder was associated with increased basolateral membrane conductance (214). In his analysis of cell volume regulation, Ussing (716) articulated the hypothesis that cell swelling was associated with the appearance or activation of both K^+ and Cl^- channels within the basolateral cell membrane, and loss of KCl via these pathways. With respect to proximal tubule, there has been considerable attention focused on the response of the peritubular membrane to increases in cell volume (202, 505, 735). It was first noted in proximal tubules from the rabbit that exposure to a hypotonic solution was followed by a "volume regulatory decrease" (173). This VRD was associated with a loss of cytosolic potassium (265). In both *Necturus* (459) and rabbit tubules (387) cell swelling enhances peritubular K^+-conductance. Further, Kirk et al. (389) made the important observation that proximal tubule VRD occurred during isotonic swelling, where cell volume increased as a result of enhanced luminal Na^+ entry (rather than a hypotonic shock).

Proposed mechanisms of volume-induced K^+-conductance have included the direct effect of stretch on the K^+ channel, or a volume-driven increase in cytosolic Ca^{++}, with secondary channel activation. Patch clamp studies have demonstrated stretch activated K^+ channels within the peritubular membrane of amphibian proximal tubule (368, 605), as well as stretch-activated, nonselective cation channels which are permeable to Ca^{++} (211, 212). In frog proximal tubule cells, subjected to Na^+-alanine uptake, there is also evidence for stretch-activated anion channels (499, 587). In the mammalian tubule stretch-activated K^+ channels have not been identified, however it was observed that hypotonic cell swelling resulted in a rise in cytosolic calcium concentration (486–488). This finding, in association with the appearance of Ca^{++}-activated K^+ channels during hypotonic shock (370) supplied a plausible mechanism for the increase in peritubular membrane K^+ permeability. In part the rise in cytosolic calcium is derived from internal stores, and in part from volume-activated peritubular entry. In these studies (proximal straight tubules of the rabbit), blocking the rise in cytosolic calcium eliminated the hypotonic VRD. Questions were raised, however, by experiments in proximal convoluted tubule (116), which indicated that VRD persists despite elimination of the rise in cell calcium. Most germane to the problem of coordinating entry and exit is the observation that when proximal convoluted tubules are exposed to luminal glucose and alanine, there is no significant increase in cytosolic calcium (59). The importance of this result is the demonstration of differences in the cellular response to hypotonic swelling and that due to enhanced luminal entry. Indeed, even in amphibian tubules, differences between hypotonic and isotonic VRD have been discerned, with Na^+-coupled alanine uptake, the VRD is independent of external Ca^{++} (513).

Critical insight into the coupling of transport to peritubular K^+ permeability came with the discovery that the peritubular K^+ channel open probability was decreased by increases in cytosolic ATP concentration in the physiologic range (701). With application of luminal glucose and alanine to rabbit proximal convoluted tubule, sodium transport increased, cytosolic ATP decreased, and peritubular K^+ conductance increased in proportion to the decrease in ATP (59, 701). When ATP was applied exogenously, this effect of luminal organics to increase peritubular K^+ conductance was eliminated (701). Conversely, application of an inhibitor of the Na,K-ATPase increased cytosolic ATP concentration, and thus decreased the open probability of the peritubular K^+ channel (332). In the proximal tubule of the amphibian, the situation is less clear. In *Ambystoma*, ATP-sensitive peritubular K^+ channels have been identified, and as in the mammalian tubules, open probability increases with application of alanine, an effect that is eliminated by application of ATP (477, 478). In the frog proximal tubule, phenylalanine application activated a volume-sensitive channel, and this effect was not reduced by ATP (144).

One question that has received relatively little attention in these investigations, is whether the observed changes in peritubular membrane K^+ permeability are sufficient to rationalize the observed volume homeostasis. Contributing to this homeostatic effect is the impact of increased K^+ permeability to hyperpolarize the peritubular membrane, and thus augment chloride and bicarbonate exit. These events are complicated by the fact that peritubular hyperpolarization will also enhance luminal entry via the Na^+-glucose cotransporter, and cytosolic acidification (increased peritubular HCO_3^- exit) will enhance luminal entry via the Na^+/H^+ exchanger. The quantitative issue of the sufficiency of the documented pump-leak parallelism to maintain cell volume was examined in a mathematical model of proximal tubule (774). In those calculations, it was found that with realistic bounds on the electrical conductance of the peritubular membrane, variation of K^+-permeability by itself does not provide adequate homeostasis for proximal tubule. Satisfactory volume regulation was achieved, however, when the activity of the peritubular Na^+–$3HCO_3^-$ cotransporter was allowed to vary directly in response to changes in the rate of luminal Na^+/H^+ exchange. Evidence for the coordination of these two transporters will be considered below. There are data regarding the anion lost in association with K^+ during cell swelling, and it appears to show some variability among species. In *Necturus* (459) and mouse tubules (734) omission of bicarbonate impairs VRD and cell swelling is associated with enhanced peritubular HCO_3^- conductance (733). In the straight proximal tubule of rabbit, however, removal of chloride impaired VRD, while omission of bicarbonate or the application of SITS had no inhibitory effect (782). In the proximal convoluted tubule of the rabbit, hypotonic swelling increases both K^+-conductance and Cl^--conductance of the peritubular cell membrane (117, 783, 784). An intriguing examination of cell volume was undertaken in primary culture of mouse proximal tubule cells, comparing wildtype with knockouts of the peritubular K^+ channel, KCNE1 (42). The wildtype cells showed VRD with the appearance of swelling-induced K^+-and Cl^- channels; the knockouts showed neither K^+ nor Cl^- currents during swelling. When knockout cells were transfected with KCNE1, both swelling-activated K^+ and Cl^- currents were restored. These experiments demonstrated a close functional linkage between the two channels allowing a coordinated response to a volume challenge.

There is one additional paradigm for cellular homeostasis, in which increases in cell volume or cytosolic Na^+, rather than enhancing a peritubular exit step, exert negative feedback on luminal entry. A possible role for the peritubular Na^+/Ca^{++} exchanger in the regulation of transepithelial Na^+ reabsorption was indicated by the experiments of Friedman et al. (218). These investigators found that in perfused rabbit proximal convoluted tubules removal of peritubular sodium inhibited sodium efflux from the tubule lumen. Decreasing the ambient calcium concentration protected against this inhibition. Thus it was proposed (218, 801, 802) that decreases in peritubular Na^+/Ca^{++} exchange would elevate cytosolic calcium, and then via calcium-mediated decrease in luminal sodium entry, inhibit sodium reabsorption. In particular, this would provide a mechanism in which increases in cell sodium concentration would blunt sodium entry. At this time, however, the putative calcium effects on the luminal entry pathways remain to be documented. Toward this end, Lang and associates (421, 422) have examined glucose-induced depolarization in frog proximal tubules treated with ouabain. (Ouabain clamps intracellular Ca^{++} concentration at abnormally high levels.) In these experiments, the apparent entry of glucose (glucose-induced depolarization) remained a linear function of the cytosolic sodium potential, so that no clear down regulation of this entry step could be discerned. In rat S1 proximal convoluted tubule, maneuvers designed to increase cytosolic Ca^{++} enhanced $NaHCO_3$ reabsorptive flux (450).

PARACELLULAR PATHWAY

Lateral Intercellular Space

It had long been recognized that certain epithelia, such as gallbladder or small intestine, could transport water from lumen to blood against an adverse osmotic gradient. Curran (170) and Durbin (188), hypothesized that metabolically driven salt transport into an intraepithelial compartment could drive transepithelial water flow, if the membranes bounding this compartment had suitable permeability properties. Subsequently, several groups of investigators (246, 714, 785) proposed that the space between the basolateral cell membrane and the basement membrane qualifies as the "middle compartment" within the epithelium. Salt transport into the interspace across the lateral cell membrane would

induce an osmotic water flow across this membrane. The accumulation of salt and water within the interspace would then create a sufficient hydrostatic pressure to drive this solution out across the permeable basement membrane and connective tissue. This proposal identifies the lateral intercellular space as part of the pathway for the bulk of transepithelial water flow. Morphologic observations on gall bladder (372, 697), intestine (794), *Necturus* proximal tubule (74, 480, 481), and the isolated perfused rabbit proximal tubule (695) have all been confirmatory, showing interspace dilatation with reabsorptive flow and interspace collapse with cessation or reversal of flow.

It is also a secure finding that along the length of the proximal tubule the luminal sodium concentration differs little, if at all, from that in peritubular blood. This means that water reabsorption must occur in a constant proportion to sodium reabsorption. Windhager et. al. (803) demonstrated that in the *Necturus* proximal tubule the sodium flux drives the net water reabsorption. These investigators introduced into the tubule lumen solutions isosmotic with plasma but with varying sodium concentration, in order to obtain a wide range of values for the sodium flux. Over the course of the experiment, the luminal osmolality did not change, indicating a negligible external driving force in the passive movement of water. Nevertheless, a plot of the net water flux as a function of the net sodium flux shows a line, the slope of which indicates that transport occurred isotonically (Fig. 9A). A similar series of experiments was performed in the rat proximal convoluted tubule by Morel and Murayama (506). They again verified over a wide range of luminal sodium concentrations (and sodium fluxes) that the flux of sodium determined the flow of water. Further, the water flow occurred so as to maintain the lumen isotonic to plasma (Fig. 9B).

The apparent dependence of isotonic water reabsorption on sodium reabsorption has been referred to as "coupled water transport" to distinguish it from water flux referable to a demonstrable transepithelial osmotic gradient. One useful approach to rationalize this coupled water transport has been an approximate analysis of the lateral intercellular space as an intraepithelial middle compartment (770, 775, 776). As in Fig. 10, the lateral interspace is represented with a tight junction (A), basement membrane (B) and lateral cell membranes (L). A reference osmolality, c_0, is assumed (such as that of the blood) and the osmolality of the interspace, $c_0 + c_E$, of the lumen and cell interior, $c_0 + c_M$, and of the peritubular solution, $c_0 + c_S$, are written in terms of increments above or below the reference. Each membrane, α (α = A, B, L), has water and solute permeabilities $L_{p\alpha}$ and H_α and a reflection coefficient σ_α. The transmembrane fluxes for volume and solute are denoted by $J_{v\alpha}$ and $J_{s\alpha}$. Several assumptions may be made, which simplify the analysis considerably, but which maintain most of the important features of the lateral interspace model: (1) the tight junction is relatively impermeable, $L_{pA} = H_A = 0$; (2) the lateral cell membrane is relatively solute impermeable, $H_L = 0$, and $\sigma_L = 1$; but (3) there is fixed solute transport

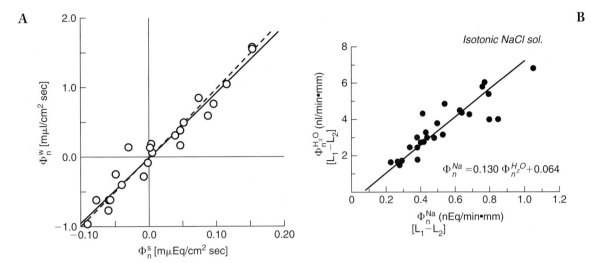

FIGURE 9   **A:** Correlation of net solute flux, Φ_n^s, and net water flux, Φ_n^w, across the perfused proximal tubule of *Necturus*. The least-squares line of regression for the data points (*solid line*) is not statistically different from the line through the origin (*dashed line*), whose slope is that for isotonic water reabsorption. (With permission, from Windhager EE, Whittembury G, Oken DE, Schatzmann HJ, Solomon AK. Single proximal tubules of the *Necturus* kidney. III. Dependence of H2O movement on NaCl concentration. *Am J Physiol* 1959;197:313–318.) **B:** Correlation of net sodium flux, Φ_n^{Na}, and net water flux, $\Phi_n^{H_2O}$, occurring between two collection sites (L1 and L2) of a perfused rat proximal tubule. The line of regression for the data points (*solid line*) indicates isotonic transport of sodium. (With permission, from Morel F, Murayama Y. Simultaneous measurement of unidirectional and net sodium fluxes in microperfused rat proximal tubules. *Pflugers Arch* 1970;320:1–23.)

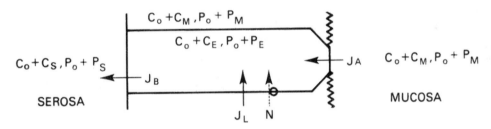

FIGURE 10   Schematic representation of the lateral intercellular space. The cell and mucosal medium are assumed to be at the same osmolality and pressure. (With permission, from Weinstein AM, Stephenson JL. Models of coupled salt and water transport across leaky epithelial. *J Membr Biol* 1981;60:1–20.)

across the lateral membrane at a rate, N; and (4) the reflection coefficient for the interspace basement membrane and underlying tissue is zero, $\sigma_B = 0$. With these assumptions the transport equations for each membrane may be written, for volume flow

$$J_{vL} = L_{pL}\left[\left(p_M - p_E\right) + RT\left(c_E - c_M\right)\right]$$
$$J_{vB} = L_{pB}\left(p_E - p_s\right) \tag{10}$$

and solute flux

$$J_{sL} = N$$
$$J_{sB} = J_{vB}c_0 + H_B\left(c_E - c_s\right) \tag{11}$$

where p_M, p_E, and p_S are the hydrostatic pressures in the respective compartments. It may be noted that an additional

approximation has been introduced into Eq. 11, in which the reference concentration, c_0, has replaced the mean basement membrane concentration.

In the steady state, the mass entry across the lateral membrane must be equal to that leaving the channel mouth

$$J_v = J_{vL} = J_{vB}$$
$$J_s = J_{sL} = J_{sB} \tag{12}$$

These mass balance relations (Eq. 12) can be used to eliminate the unknowns p_E and c_E from Eqs. 10 and 11 to arrive at the following expressions for transepithelial volume and solute flow:

$$J_v = L_p\left(p_M - p_s\right) + RTL_p\left(c_s - c_M + \frac{N}{H_B}\right)$$
$$J_s = N \tag{13}$$

where

$$L_p = \frac{L_{pLB}H_B}{H_B + RTL_{pLB}c_0} \tag{14}$$

and

$$L_{pLB} = \frac{L_{pL}L_{pB}}{L_{pL} + L_{pB}}$$

Equation 13 describes the volume flow of the whole epithelial model in terms of the permeability parameters of the component membranes. It shows the volume flow to be a linear function of the pressure and osmolality of the bathing solutions. When there are exactly equal bathing media ($c_M = c_S = p_M = p_S = 0$) there is still transepithelial volume flow,

$$J_v^a = RTL_p\frac{N}{H_B} = RTL_p\hat{c} \tag{15}$$

This "active water transport," referenced in Eq. 9, thus arises naturally as a component of volume flow driven by intraepithelial solute-solvent coupling, that is, the empirically described "coupled water transport." It increases with larger rates of solute transport and decreases when there is little solute trapping by the basement membrane (large H_B). The virtual concentration $\hat{c} = N/H_B$, represents the strength of transport of the epithelium, in that volume flow just ceases when the osmolality of the luminal solution is raised by this amount. For a proximal tubule model one must also verify isotonic transport. In approximate terms, this means that only a small decrement in luminal osmolality is required for the reabsorbate tonicity to be equal to that of the peritubular fluid. Formally, one seeks the osmotic deviation, c^*, such that if $c_S = c_0$, and $c_M = c_0 - c^*$, then $J_s/J_v = c_0$. This corresponds to solving the equation

$$c_0 = \frac{J_s}{J_v} = \frac{N}{RTL_p(\hat{c}+c_S-c_M)} = \frac{N}{RTL_p(\hat{c}+c^*)} \tag{16}$$

which has the solution

$$c^* = \frac{N}{RTL_{pLB}c_0} \tag{17}$$

When the luminal osmolality is decreased by the amount, c^*, transport is isotonic to plasma. Provided that c^* is at most a few mOsmol per liter, there will be no experimentally detectable difference between lumen and blood. Transport is generally considered isotonic if c^* is within 2% of c_0. It should also be noted that isotonic transport depends only upon the water permeabilities of the epithelial membranes. The notion of solute trapping within the interspace, which was crucial to uphill water transport, is really unimportant in the dynamics of isotonic transport.

Perhaps one of the confusing features of transport isotonicity is that the membrane permeabilities relevant here, may be quite different from the whole epithelial water permeability that is actually measured. The expression for L_p (Eq. 14) shows that both water permeabilities and solute trapping effects are involved. Intuitively, this corresponds to the fact that water flow across the lateral membrane, driven by a hypotonic lumen, will tend to dilute the interspace, and hence, negate some of the osmotic flow. The interspace dilution will be smaller for larger basement membrane permeabilities. This "intraepithelial solute polarization" effect is an inescapable feature of the lateral interspace. The expression for L_p may be rewritten

$$\frac{L_p}{L_{pLB}} = \frac{1}{1+\hat{c}/c^*} \tag{18}$$

which shows that to the extent that an epithelium can transport against a gradient (large $\hat{c}$) and yet reabsorb water isotonically (small c^*), the observed epithelial L_p must be substantially smaller than the cell membrane water permeabilities. In this regard, Persson and Spring (547) have been able to estimate the apical and basolateral membrane water permeabilities of *Necturus* gallbladder cells by recording the time course of cell volume changes after a unilateral change in bath osmolality. They found the permeability of the apical and basolateral membranes in series to be more than four times the transepithelial water permeability.

In Table 5, this model is applied to the data of Tables 1 and 4 for proximal tubules of rat, rabbit, and *Necturus*. The top rows are rates of isotonic reabsorption, along with the measured water permeabilities. For the rat, two values for L_p are given, corresponding to the older (710) and more recent determinations (557). A value for the equilibrium deviation from isotonicity (c^*) has been assumed to be at most 2% of the ambient osmolality. At least in the rat, this is comparable to experimental determinations (271, 452). The quantities in the lower portion of the table are derived from the experimental data using the model equations. The estimate of cell membrane water permeability required for isotonic transport, RTL_{pLB}, is just J_v/c^*. If the value of RTL_{pLB} computed for the rabbit tubule, is referred to the luminal and lateral cell membranes in series, each of 36 cm²/cm² (777), then one obtains a unit membrane water permeability, consistent with direct estimates, using rapid video techniques (137, 780). In theory, the AQP1 knock-out mouse, deficient in water channels from both luminal and peritubular cell membranes, provides a pure decrease in the parameter RTL_{pLB}. The experimental observations in this knockout were an overall epithelial water permeability (L_p) about 22% that of wildtype (639), and luminal hypotonicity (c^*) about fourfold greater than wildtype (719). In terms of the model developed here, and with the assumption that active Na⁺ transport is little changed in the knockout mouse, the change in c^* should reflect a 78% reduction in L_{pLB}. The fact that the fractional change in overall L_p is comparable indicates that in the mouse, one would expect little intraepithelial solute polarization, and

TABLE 5 Application of Interspace Model to Proximal Tubule

	Rat PCT	Rat PCT	Rabbit PCT	*Necturus*
J_s (nOsm/s • cm^2)	19	19	9.0	0.2
J_v (nl/s • cm^2)	65	65	30	1.0
RTL_p (cm/s • Osm × 10^4)	44	22	63	0.82
P_f (cm/s)	0.24	0.12	0.35	0.0046
c^* (mOsm/liter)	6	6	6	4
RTL_{pLB} (cm/s • Osm × 10^4)	105	105	50	2.5
$\hat{c}$ (mOsm/liter)	8	23	—	8
J_v^a (nl/s • cm^2)	35	51	—	0.66
H_B (cm/s × 10^4)	24	8.3	—	0.25
$c_E - c_0$ (mOsm/liter)	3.4	4.8	—	2.7

thus little capacity for water reabsorption against an adverse osmotic gradient.

The discrepancy between the overall epithelial water permeability and that of the cell membranes in series, allows the calculation of the strength of transport, $\hat{c}$ in Eq. 18. Williams and Schafer (796) have emphasized that the middle compartment need not be the true lateral interspace, but could actually be the cortical interstitial space. In their model of rat proximal tubule, the salt permeability of the peritubular capillary corresponds to the term H_B used here. With estimates of cell membrane water permeability and capillary solute permeability comparable to those of the first column in Table 5, they also predicted that solute polarization would reduce the epithelial L_p to about 50% of that of the cell membranes. For the rat (and for *Necturus*), the discrepancy between L_p and L_{pLB} require that active water transport be substantial, i.e., from 55%–80% of the isotonic flux (Table 5). In the more detailed models of proximal tubule epithelium that have been developed, there is considerable disagreement in the estimates of coupled water flux, ranging from predominant (333, 334, 606, 693) to negligible (16, 622, 750, 796). In a simulation of the rat proximal tubule, in which both isotonic transport and the whole epithelial L_p were reproduced faithfully, coupled water flux was estimated to be about two-thirds of the isotonic transport rate (766). This corresponded to a transport strength of 23 mOsm/liter of NaCl.

There are few experimental studies examining uphill water transport by the proximal tubule. Bomsztyk and Wright (99) reported that in rat tubules, microperfused with a low bicarbonate (10 mEq/liter) luminal solution, an additional 30 mmol/liter of mannitol was required within the lumen to nullify volume reabsorption. Although the interpretation of this experiment was complicated by the presence of several forces favoring water reabsorption (anion gradients and protein oncotic forces), the findings suggested a substantial component of solute-linked water reabsorption by the rat proximal tubule. Green et al. (273) examined the doubly perfused rat proximal tubule, specifically with the aim of determining the presence of active water transport. Using low bicarbonate solutions in both tubule and capillary perfusions, an isotonic luminal solution yielded reabsorptive

water flux of 1 nl/mm • min. Varying only the luminal NaCl concentration allowed the determination of volume flux as a linear function of the transepithelial salt gradient (Fig. 11). Regression analysis indicated that a luminal osmolality ($\hat{c}$) between 13 and 29 mOsm/liter (depending on peritubular protein concentration) greater than in peritubular blood would be required to null volume reabsorption. These experiments document active water transport by rat proximal tubule, quantitatively close to model predictions, and thus provide support for solute–solvent coupling within the lateral intercellular space.

The interspace outlet permeability, H_B, is a parameter of critical importance. It directly determines the strength of transport (Eq. 15), and when this solute permeability is sufficiently small ($H_B < RTL_{pLB}c_0$), it is dominant in determining the epithelial L_p (Eq. 14). Persson and Spring (548) examined the subepithelial tissue of *Necturus* gallbladder and found that it has only about twice the resistivity of free solution. They argue, therefore, that any important limitation to solute exit from the interspace must derive from the small area of the lateral interspace as it abuts the basement membrane. More recent experiments using photo activation of caged fluorescent dyes have indicated that solute diffusion within the lateral interspace is comparable to that in free solution (814). Such had been the assumption in analytical estimates of the electrical resistance of the interspace fluid of proximal tubule from ultrastructural data. Mathias (475), using data from the rabbit (778) estimated interspace resistance about 4% that of tight junction, and Maunsbach and Boulpaep (482) calculated 4%–21% of epithelial resistance may be attributed to the interspace. Welling et al. (779) have indicated that beyond the limitations of interspace width, interdigitating cellular elements at the base of the interspace may provide the most important barrier to mass exit. With reference to Table 5, Eq. 15 defines the outlet permeability required by the model ($H_B = N/\hat{c} = J_S/\hat{c}$). For the rat, H_B is predicted to be 8.3–24 × 10^{-4} cm/sec. When interpreted as an electrical resistance (Eq. 5), this is 0.4–1.1 ohm • cm^2, and is not incompatible with the whole epithelial resistance of 5–10 ohm • cm^2.

The idea of interspace hypertonicity has often been paramount in discussions of active water transport. The estimate

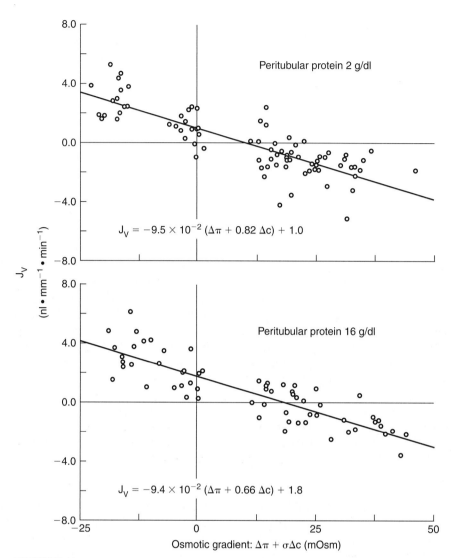

FIGURE 11   Volume flux as a function of transepithelial osmotic driving force in rat proximal tubules, in which both lumen and peritubular capillaries have been perfused. Each point corresponds to a single tubule perfusion. The abscissa is the transepithelial osmotic driving force, $\Delta\pi + \sigma\Delta C$; the ordinate is the measured volume flux, Jv. For each protein concentration, the line shown is the graph of Eq. 11, so that the ordinate intercept, J_v^a, is the coupled water transport (water flux in the absence of a transepithelial driving force). The abscissa intercept is the concentration of the luminal impermeant required to null volume reabsorption. (With permission, from Green R, Giebisch G, Unwin R, Weinstein AM. Coupled water transport by rat proximal tubule. *Am J Physiol* 1991;261:F1046–F1054.

for the osmolality of the interspace, c_E, when both bathing media are at the reference, c_0, is

$$c_E = c_0 + \frac{\hat{c}\, c^*}{\hat{c} + c^*} \qquad (19)$$

The significance of this formula is that it displays the interspace osmolality as a function of the two measurable whole epithelial quantities, the strength of transport ($\hat{c}$) and the deviation from isotonicity (c^*). Furthermore, it shows that the interspace hypertonicity must be smaller than either $\hat{c}$ or c^*. Of note, careful electrophysiologic studies by Sackin

(604) in *Ambystoma* proximal tubule have found interspace hypertonicity ($c_E - c_0$) to be some 8 mOsm/liter.

Tight Junction

The tight junction of the proximal tubule provides a low resistance pathway between the luminal solution and the lateral intercellular space. Morphologically, the tight junctions have been identified with the "zonula occludentes," visualized in electron microscopy, in which there is no detectable space between the epithelial cells. Freeze-fracture techniques indicated the fibrillar structure of these junctions, with relatively few fibrils present in the junctions of the proximal tubule (159, 560). In epithelia with greater electrical resistance, there are, correspondingly, a greater number of fibrils (158, 159). The TJ strands may be viewed as chains of particles, with typical spacing of these particles, as seen in freeze-fracture electron micrographs, being on the order of 20 nm (535). The structural composition of these strands has been deciphered slowly (501, 637). Occludin was the first of the transmembrane proteins to be associated with the tight junction (234) and to be implicated in a functional role in junctional permeability (485). An important advance came with the identification of claudin-1 and claudin-2 within the junctional strands (232, 235). When claudin-2 was introduced into the Madin–Darby canine kidney (MDCK) cells, a conversion from a very "tight" junction to a leaky junction was observed (233). This suggested that claudin-2 could be responsible for the leakiness of the MDCK epithelium and the formation of pores between apposing TJ strands. Indeed, when the claudins expressed in MDCK cells are selectively modified, the paracellular conductance of small electrolytes can be modulated, including the anion/cation selectivity preference (162). Claudin-2 exists throughout the proximal tubule and in a contiguous early segment of the thin descending limb of long-looped nephrons in mouse kidney (200).

The low electrical resistance of proximal tubule also correlates with the permeation of lanthanum, a heavy cation that does not penetrate cell membranes. After placement within the lumen, lanthanum may be found within the tight junctions and lateral intercellular spaces of the rat proximal tubule, but not in those of high resistance epithelia (472, 696, 788). These junctional properties qualify the proximal tubule as a typical leaky epithelium. Like the proximal tubule, other leaky epithelia (gallbladder, small intestine) also transport large volumes of salt solutions isotonically and this has encouraged speculation as to the function of the tight junction in isotonic water transport. Several mathematical simulations of proximal tubule, incorporating a permeable tight junction, have been fashioned to try to reveal some role for the paracellular pathway in solute–solvent coupling (333, 334, 606, 683, 693). These theoretical investigations have simply not provided an answer as to why electrical leakiness should correlate with the ability to transport isotonically. Further, an approximate mathematical analysis of the lateral interspace with a permeable tight junction was developed, similar to that of the previous section (775, 776). With respect to water reabsorption, this model functioned qualitatively like its simpler version and has failed to reveal a special role for the tight junction.

The fraction of reabsorptive water flow which actually traverses the tight junction is also unknown. Arguments in favor of transjunctional water flow in proximal tubules have included: substantial solvent drag of ionic species (18, 100, 230, 272, 315, 367, 623); the appearance of streaming potentials with the application of an impermeant osmotic agent (167, 227, 698); and ionic permeabilities roughly in proportion to their mobility in free solution (404). None of these findings, however, provides proof of tight junctional water flow. Either streaming potentials or solvent drag can come as the result of a solute polarization effect within the interspace. With solute polarization, water flux across the cell and through the lateral interspace alters interspace ion concentrations, thus promoting either a diffusion potential or diffusive flux across the tight junction. For a true streaming potential, water flux across the tight junction must be present and carry either an anion or cation preferentially. This issue was addressed by Tripathi and Boulpaep (698) in their measurements of streaming potentials across the proximal tubule of *Ambystoma*. With the application of peritubular sucrose, a lumen-positive potential appeared, consistent with either a streaming potential or interspace NaCl depletion (and an anion-selective junction). When ambient chloride was replaced by cyclamate, the junction became cation-selective and its total conductance substantially decreased. Repeat application of peritubular sucrose produced the same lumen-positive potential, now inconsistent with a diffusion potential. With respect to the solvent drag measurements, it is undisputed that intraepithelial solute polarization may produce an overall reflection coefficient that is substantially less than that of the cell and tight junction, taken in parallel. The question is thus a quantitative one, as to whether one could construct a model of proximal tubule with just the right solute polarization to yield realistic reflection coefficients as well as a proper L_p. So far, this does not appear possible. For the rat, the data of Frömter et al. (230) were used to determine composite interspace models for this epithelium (769). It was found that all of the acceptable interspace models required substantial tight junction convective chloride flux.

An apparently direct argument for tight junctional flux in rabbit tubules came from Whittembury and associates (136, 257, 787), whose estimate of the water permeability of the peritubular cell membrane indicated transcellular water permeability less than the overall epithelial L_p. The unit membrane water permeability obtained with this technique was confirmed in a vesicle preparation (729, 731), although higher values have also been obtained (725). Strong evidence for tight junction water flow was also obtained in the rat, with observation of substantial convective entrainment of sucrose, despite relatively small diffusional flux (786). The small diffusive component effectively rules out interspace solute polarization as a confounding factor. Nevertheless, an objection had been raised by Rector and Berry (77, 573) who presented calculations based on pore theory, which indicated that the tight junctions were not large enough to allow passage of a significant fraction of transepithelial water flow. Subsequently, Preisig and Berry (557) measured the permeation of sucrose and mannitol across the rat proximal tubule. Applying the Renkin equations to their data, they computed the dimensions of the "sucrose pore," and indicated that it could be responsible for at most 2% of the tubule water permeability. It was acknowledged, however, that a smaller paracellular pore that did not admit the sucrose molecule could account for up to one-third of the water permeability. An important contribution to this discussion came with the suggestion of Fraser and Baines (217) that the tight junction might be more realistically represented as a fiber matrix, rather than as a collection of pores. The critical feature of the fiber matrix equations is that for a given solute permeability, the water permeability can be substantially greater than that predicted from the Renkin equations. It was demonstrated that this formulation was compatible with the known permeabilities of rat proximal tubule (217). Alternatively, Guo et al. (287) reproduced a pore-theoretic representation of the tight junction, utilizing two pores to fit the mannitol and sucrose data of Preisig and Berry (557). In this model, the two pores were given anatomic correlates: the small pore was referred to gaps in the apposition of claudins molecules, while the large pore corresponded to breaks within a strand, occupying about 2% of its length. With these dimensions, tight junction water permeability was predicted to be about 21% of transepithelial water permeability.

Once the tight junction had been established as a route for reabsorptive solute flux, a hypothesis was advanced that the junction might be an important site for the regulation of proximal sodium reabsorption. Lewy and Windhager found that in rats, both with and without acutely elevated renal venous pressure, there was a direct correlation between single nephron filtration fraction and proximal tubule sodium reabsorption (434). Given that lower filtration fractions would result in reduced protein oncotic pressure within the peritubular capillaries, they surmised that this would lead to reduced capillary uptake of fluid from the renal interstitium and lateral intercellular space, and, hence, elevated interspace pressure. This, in turn, would result in increased backflux of the sodium, already transported into the interspace, that is, backflux across the tight junction into the lumen. At the time of this proposal, considerable attention had focused on the intrarenal mechanisms responsible for the natriuresis of extracellular fluid volume expansion with saline (190, 392, 393). Dirks et al. (177) had shown that proximal tubule sodium reabsorption was depressed following saline expansion. In the intact dog, the ability to reverse the natriuresis with infusion of hyperoncotic albumin provided a strong indication that peritubular oncotic pressure could influence sodium reabsorption and Earley and associates (189, 473) had proposed that renal interstitial pressure might be an intermediate variable. Subsequent micropuncture experiments in the rat documented the enhancement of proximal sodium reabsorption by peritubular protein (112, 113, 394). In particular, the depression of proximal tubule sodium reabsorption which occurs with saline infusion could be reversed by perfusion of the efferent arteriole with a solution whose protein concentration is comparable to that under control conditions (114, 682). Normally aortic constriction is associated with decreased glomerular capillary pressure and plasma flow, decreased

filtration fraction, decreased peritubular capillary oncotic pressure, and decreased proximal tubule sodium reabsorption (205). When, under conditions of plasma expansion, aortic constriction produced decreased GFR but little change in peritubular protein, there was also little change in proximal sodium reabsorption (115).

It has been well documented that changes in the ambient protein concentration alter sodium reabsorption by the perfused proximal tubule. In *Necturus*, the elimination of peritubular colloid caused sodium reabsorption to fall by 40% (263). This occurred in association with a 60% increase in the electrical conductivity of the epithelium but no perceptible change in the cell membrane conductance. Similarly, the elimination of colloid from the bath surrounding a perfused salamander proximal tubule has been shown to produce a 15% fall in reabsorptive volume flux (607). In the isolated perfused rabbit proximal tubule Imai and Kokko (340) also found an enhancement of sodium reabsorption with increasing concentrations of protein in the bathing solution. In the absence of peritubular colloid, the permeability of the tubule to sucrose was increased. In the rat kidney, Green et al. (275) studied proximal tubule volume reabsorption when albumin was present in varying concentrations in luminal or peritubular capillary perfusates. Figure 12 shows the asymmetry (luminal vs peritubular protein) and the nonlinearity of the reabsorptive enhancement by peritubular colloid. This implies that the colloid effect is not a simple oncotic force, such as might be reckoned using Eq. 1 and a known water permeability. It does suggest that the increase in peritubular capillary albumin changes the "state" of the epithelium to make active sodium transport more efficient at driving volume reabsorption. A comparable asymmetric effect of protein on salt reabsorption was also documented in the rabbit proximal convoluted tubule in vitro (341).

It is a tenet of the backflux hypothesis that the action of peritubular protein is mediated through an effect on renal interstitial pressure and hence, pressures within the lateral intercellular spaces. In substantiation of this point, it has been shown that decreases in peritubular capillary oncotic pressure, which occur with saline volume expansion, result in increases in renal interstitial pressure (as least as assessed by renal subcapsular pressures) (540, 541, 567, 661). Prevention of this rise in interstitial pressure by applying a renal artery clamp also prevents the fall in absolute proximal reabsorption associated with saline expansion (216, 337). Further, the deliberate increase of renal interstitial pressure by the instillation of fluid decreases proximal sodium reabsorption and produces a natriuresis (264, 292). Morphologic examination of the proximal tubule of *Necturus* (72, 480) and of the rat (70, 142) has shown progressive dilation of the lateral intercellular space, as well as opening of the interspace at the tubule basement membrane, with increments of saline volume expansion. Indeed, some widening of the tight junction (72) or disruption of junctional strands (331) has been reported in proximal tubules of *Necturus* undergoing saline expansion, although no discernible changes occurred in the rat (201).

The precise mechanism of the "backflux" of sodium across the tight junction remains to be delineated. One possibility is that with increased interstitial pressure there is junctional widening and back-diffusion of sodium from interspace to lumen. Evidence from several sources has documented increased junctional permeability with volume expansion. Boulpaep (109) found in the *Necturus* kidney that volume expansion produced a fall in sodium reabsorption to about half of control levels in association with an increase in junctional electrical conductivity by a factor of three. A decrease in epithelial electrical resistance, albeit considerably smaller, has also been documented with saline loading in the rat (651). In the rat, mannitol injected into the proximal tubule does not permeate and is completely recovered in the urine. However, with massive saline diuresis, as with renal venous constriction or elevated ureteral pressure, a significant fraction of the mannitol traversed the tubular epithelium into the systemic circulation (461). Similarly, sucrose infused into the systemic circulation may permeate the proximal tubule epithelium during periods of renal vein constriction (37). Perhaps the strongest objection to the view that sodium diffuses back across widened junctions is that, at least in the rat proximal tubule, the electrodiffusive force on sodium is likely to be in the reabsorptive direction. Given a 1 mV lumen positive potential (Table 2), Eq. 2 (with electrical constants from Table 3) shows that an interspace sodium concentration greater than 4% of the luminal concentration would be required to produce back-diffusion. This corresponds to an interspace osmolality some 11 mOsm/liter hypertonic to the lumen. From the considerations of the previous section (and Table 5) this degree of interspace hypertonicity is unlikely to be achieved in rat proximal tubule.

A second possibility is that backflux of sodium across the tight junction occurs by convective flow. The tight junctions of the leaky epithelia are very sensitive to hydrostatic pressures applied from the contraluminal side. In the rabbit gallbladder (726) and the *Necturus* proximal tubule (263, 308) contraluminal pressures drive substantially greater volume flow across the epithelium than an equal luminal pressure. In *Necturus*, volume expansion was found to decrease the proximal tubule NaCl reflection coefficient (75). In these experiments, it is likely that the junctional structure is distorted, forming relatively large pores with negligible sieving of solute, as both salt and water return to the lumen. Indeed, in the meticulous study of van Os et al. (726) on the rabbit gallbladder, it was found that serosal pressures drove water back into the lumen at a rate 30-fold greater than would have been predicted from the osmotic water permeability of this epithelium. This occurred with little change in diffusional solute permeability. These investigators suggested that their results were most compatible with a serosal pressure effect of opening up relatively large water channels at a small number of junctional loci. Convective backflux across the tight junction of rat proximal tubule has been invoked by Ramsey et al. (570) to explain their observation that the luminal appearance of lanthanum deposited within the renal interstitium is enhanced during saline volume expansion.

The mathematical model of the lateral interspace, set out in the previous section, cannot represent the peritubular oncotic effects on sodium reabsorption considered above. Even when this model is extended with the inclusion of a permeable tight junction and a compliant lateral intercellular space, the impact of peritubular protein is negligible (767). However, when this model is extended by the inclusion of a compliant tight junction, the regulatory effect of peritubular Starling forces can be simulated (771). In this case, "compliance" of the tight junction signifies that both the junctional salt and water permeability increase and the salt reflection coefficient decreases in response to small pressure differences from lateral interspace to tubule lumen. Although these compliance properties were completely empirical, they provided a model in which decreases in peritubular protein (which increased interspace hydrostatic pressure) opened the tight junction, and produced a secretory salt flux. This backflux was a combination of both diffusive and convective terms and did not specifically require either component to dominate. When this model was used to simulate the experiments of Green et al. (275), the model predictions were consistent with the observed reabsorption. The predicted fluxes appear as the dashed curve in Fig. 12.

In this model of the tight junction, once the interspace pressure falls below that of the lumen, the junction is closed and junctional properties are fixed. The consequence of junction closure in the simulation of Fig. 12 is that beyond a certain value of peritubular protein, one may expect little influence of peritubular Starling forces on volume reabsorption. In this light, it is not surprising that a number of investigators found no significant influence of peritubular protein on proximal reabsorption (35, 164, 323) and even interstitial Starling forces could correlate poorly with sodium transport (97, 496, 702). Consistent with this view are the observations by Ott et al. (541) that in the dog, hyperoncotic albumin infusion increased proximal reabsorption only in the previously volume expanded group. In the isolated perfused proximal tubule of the rabbit, several reports have indicated a lack of effect of peritubular bath protein on paracellular permeability (77, 80, 425). Pirie and Potts (551) explored the influence of pressure gradients in this preparation. They found that elevations in intraluminal hydrostatic pressures abolished the effect of peritubular protein to enhance sodium reabsorption. Although they did not offer a specific explanation for their data, the present considerations might suggest that with higher luminal pressures, the tight junction always stayed closed.

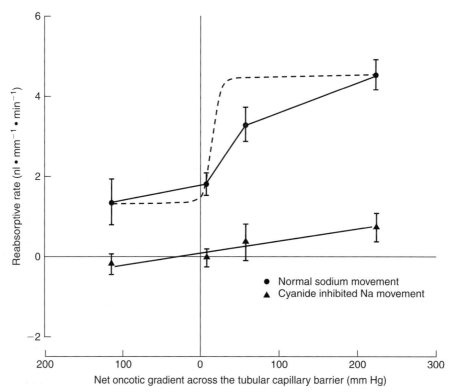

FIGURE 12   Effects of transtubular oncotic pressure gradients on volume reabsorption by rat proximal tubule. Both tubule lumen and peritubular capillaries are perfused with identical Ringer's solutions to which variable amounts of albumin have been added. In the tubules perfused with cyanide (lower curve), spontaneous sodium reabsorption has ceased and the effect of oncotic pressure is blunted. (With permission, from Green R, Windhager EE, Giebisch G. Protein oncotic pressure effects on proximal tubular fluid movement in the rat. *Am J Physiol* 1974;226:265–276.) The dashed curve represents the prediction of an interspace model in which the tight junction is compliant. (From Weinstein AM. Glomerulotubular balance in a mathematical model of the proximal nephron. *Am J Physiol* 1990;258:F612–F626.)

REGULATION OF PROXIMAL NACL TRANSPORT

Convergence on NHE3

To this point, the proximal tubule has been treated much as an isolated epithelium in which sodium transport has been examined as a function of luminal and peritubular solutions. Considerable attention has been given to understanding proximal sodium reabsorption in relation to neural and hormonal signals (209), and to changes in glomerular filtration rate. The luminal membrane Na^+/H^+ exchanger is responsible for both $NaHCO_3$ reabsorption and a substantial component of NaCl reabsorption. This, along with the fact that luminal entry is rate-limiting for transcellular sodium flux, renders the antiporter ideally suited as a regulatory site for proximal reabsorption. Indeed, a coherent picture has emerged in which every signal that regulates proximal Na^+ reabsorption converges on NHE3. A remarkable diversity of pathways have been identified as proximate modifiers of the antiporter (242, 276, 307, 502, 757). Of these, perhaps the most the most important is inhibition by cAMP-dependent phosphorylation of the

antiporter by protein kinase A (PKA) (357, 503, 762). Liu and Cogan (449) examined bicarbonate reabsorption by the S1 segment of rat proximal tubule following a variety of maneuvers designed to affect cellular cAMP concentration. When luminal appearance of cAMP is used as a measure of cytosolic concentration, the correlation with bicarbonate transport, over nearly a 10-fold range is striking (Fig. 13). The acute nature of these experimental maneuvers must be emphasized, since the impact of chronic stimulation by cAMP is different (132). Beyond cAMP effects, NHE3 activity is also regulated acutely via phosphorylation by the calcium-phospholipid-dependent protein kinase, PKC (360, 494, 760, 761, 792), by direct signals from G-proteins (7), and perhaps by a tyrosine kinase (247). Beyond transporter phosphorylation, rapid regulation of sodium reabsorption via NHE3 is achieved through cellular machinery that makes NHE3 physically available within the brush border membrane, including insertion and retrieval of transporter from cytosolic pools (98, 206, 314, 835). Ultimately, chronic NHE3 regulation must be referable to the protein synthetic machinery (131, 248, 325).

Of the signals that impact NHE3 flux, perhaps the most intensively and most fruitfully studied has been the

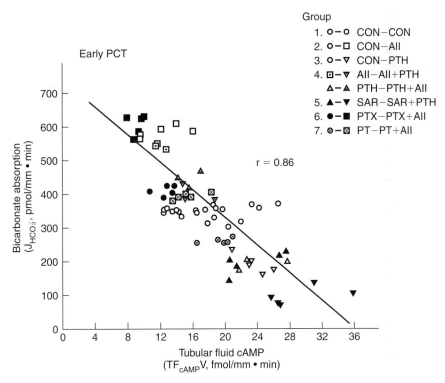

FIGURE 13 Relationship of bicarbonate absorption to tubular fluid cAMP delivery in the early S1 segment of PCT. A variety of maneuvers have been used to alter cellular content of cAMP, including parathyroidectomy (PTX) or infusion of angiotensin II (AII), parathyroid hormone (PTH), saralasin (SAR), or pertussis toxin (PT). (From Liu F-Y, Cogan MG. Angiotensin II stimulates early proximal bicarbonate absorption in the rat by decreasing cyclic adenosine monophosphate. *J Clin Invest* 1989;84:83–91.)

effect of parathyroid hormone (PTH) and cAMP to decrease Na^+/H^+ exchange. The PTH effect was documented in isolated perfused proximal tubules (175, 298), and paralleled the effect of cAMP when examined in tubule suspension (178), or brush border membrane vesicles (357). A major advance came with the identification of a protein cofactor, since termed NHERF (NHE regulatory factor), which is required for the cAMP effect (763, 765). The OK cell is a proximal tubule line from opossum kidney that expresses NHE3 and NHERF, and which displays cAMP-dependent inhibition of NHE3. This cell served as a preparation in which to demonstrate a physical link between NHE3 and NHERF, as well as a link between NHERF and ezrin (417). Ezrin is a protein kinase A (PKA) anchoring protein, as well as a linking molecule to the actin cytoskeleton. The hypothesis that emerged was that of a multiprotein signal complex, in which NHERF and ezrin brought PKA and NHE3 into proximity (Fig. 14) (758, 764). Supporting this picture in the intact kidney was immunocytochemical colocalization of NHE3, NHERF, and ezrin within the brush border of rat proximal tubule (736). Although mice with homozygous deficiency of NHERF show normal electrolytes (664), cultured proximal tubule cells from these mice display absent regulation of NHE3 by PTH, which could be

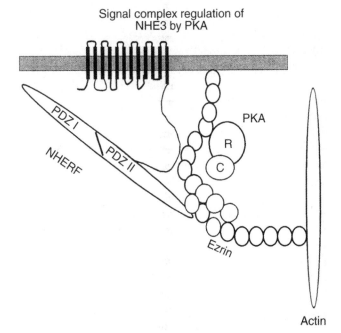

FIGURE 14 Proposed signal complex regulation of NHE3 by cAMP. NHERF links NHE3 to the actin cytoskeleton through the scaffolding protein, ezrin. In this scheme ezrin also functions as a PKA anchoring protein, enabling cAMP-dependent phosphorylation of NHE3. (From Weinman EJ, Steplock D, Shenolikar S. Acute regulation of NHE3 by protein kinase A requires a multiprotein signal complex. *Kidney Int* 2001;60:450–454.)

restored via transfection with adenovirus containing the gene for NHERF (169).

Beyond chemical modification of a fixed contingent of microvillous Na^+/H^+ exchangers, there is regulation of the NHE3 density within the luminal membrane (489, 665). An early observation in cultured proximal tubule cells was that PTH perturbed actin filament structure and caused microvillous shortening, events not replicated with application of cAMP alone (254). Subsequently, density-gradient centrifugation of cell homogenates permitted examination of distinct membrane vesicle populations from rat proximal tubule suspension. It was found that PTH treatment resulted in migration of Na^+/H^+-exchange activity from one fraction to another, and then disappeared (314). With the availability of NHE3 specific antibody, the distinction between Na^+/H^+ activity and NHE3 abundance could be made. Using vesicles prepared from the kidneys of parathyroidectomized rats treated acutely with PTH, it was found that within minutes of treatment, Na^+/H^+ activity decreased and phosphorylated NHE3 appeared. Over the course of hours, brush border NHE3 antigen declined, and this could be blocked by pretreating the animals with colchicine (206). The ability of PTH to couple to adenylate cyclase appears to be critical to its ability to provoke NHE3 redistribution (835). Events in vivo were mimicked in OK cells in which PTH induced a rapid phosphorylation of membrane-bound NHE3 and a parallel decrease in function, and then a slower retrieval of the cell surface transporter into an endocytic pathway (163). Disruption of the actin cytoskeleton in proximal tubule suspension produced an increase in NHE3 abundance in luminal membrane vesicles prepared from these tubules (146). A precise role, however, for the actin cytoskeleton in the regulation of NHE3 function has been elusive. Beyond transporter retrieval, the state of cellular actin fibers has been implicated in modulation of PKA phosphorylation of NHE3, consistent with its physical association with the NHERF-ezrin complex (411, 689). An additional complication is that the retrieval destination of apical transporters may be transporter dependent. Whereas PTH in vivo produces transfer to endosomes of the luminal membrane sodium-phosphate transporter, the destination of NHE3 appears to be to a reserve compartment at the base of the microvilli (819), perhaps in association with megalin (93). Possible differences between the membrane retrieval machinery between proximal tubules in vivo and stable cell lines in culture limit the ability to extrapolate in vitro observations to the intact kidney, at least with respect to regulation of microvillous NHE3 density.

Modulation of Na,K-ATPase

All of the regulatory signals that impact on the luminal Na^+/H^+ exchanger also modulate the Na,K-ATPase (209). Nevertheless, this aspect of the coordinate control of transcellular Na^+ flux has been much more difficult to decipher. This may be due to the multiplicity of cellular signals that impact on the Na,K-ATPase, as well as from the distortion of the cellular milieu required for experimental determination of its activity. Early study of the action of PTH in OK cells identified the release of inositol triphosphate (IP3) and diacyl glycerol, along with an increase in cytosolic Ca^{++}. In intact proximal tubule cells and basolateral membrane vesicles, it was possible to confirm the IP3 release (329). With this information, it was natural to focus on the role of protein kinase C (PKC) in mediating the PTH-induced decrease in proximal Na^+ reabsorption. Baum and Hays (50) were first to examine the effect of PKC activation on PCT transport, and demonstrated inhibition of bicarbonate, chloride, and glucose transport by rabbit tubules in vitro. This global effect on multiple solutes was certainly consistent with inhibition of the Na,K-ATPase, and this was the finding of Bertorello and Aperia (82) who determined maximal Na,K-ATPase activity in rat proximal tubules preincubated with a PKC activator. The logical connection of these portions of the story was the demonstration that PTH inhibited maximal Na,K-ATPase activity in tubules in which cytosolic Na^+ was elevated by the ionophore, monensin (583). This stimulation also occurred when a truncated PTH analog was used, which had no PKA activity, so that the Na,K-ATPase inhibition was dissociated from cAMP generation. These observations were supported by the finding in intact tubules that the PTH effect on Na,K-ATPase is eliminated by inhibition of PKC with staurosporine (620) or with calphostin (534).

Considerable interest has focused on the structural correlates of Na,K-ATPase regulation, and these have been depicted by Feraille and Doucet (Fig. 15) (209). The first observation is that regulatory phosphorylation occurs on the alpha subunit, and this catalytic unit can be phosphorylated by both PKA and PKC (83). There is a single PKA phosphorylation site at a serine within the last cytoplasmic loop, while PKC phosphorylation occurs on the N-terminal cytoplasmic tail (63, 210). The rate of alpha-chain phosphorylation by PKC was influenced by the ionic environment, enhancing with K^+ and diminishing with Na^+, suggesting preference for the E2 over the E1 conformation (210). The converse of this observation has also been reported, namely that PKC phosphorylation impacts on the conformational equilibrium of the enzyme, favoring the E1-Na state (453). Although an inhibitory effect of PKC phosphorylation had been reported (83), Feschenko and Sweadner (210) found no effect of alpha subunit phosphorylation on Na,K-ATPase kinetics, neither on maximal velocity or Na^+ affinity. They concluded that the regulatory impact of PKC must derive from the cellular environment, and other signals. This view echoed the observation of Satoh et al. (620), that along the nephron, the effect of phosphorylation on Na,K-ATPase activity differed between proximal and distal nephron cells.

One complicating aspect of the PTH effect on proximal tubule Na,K-ATPase is the interaction with the cytochrome P450 pathway. Ribeiro et al. (582) demonstrated that PTH released arachidonic acid in proximal tubule suspension, that

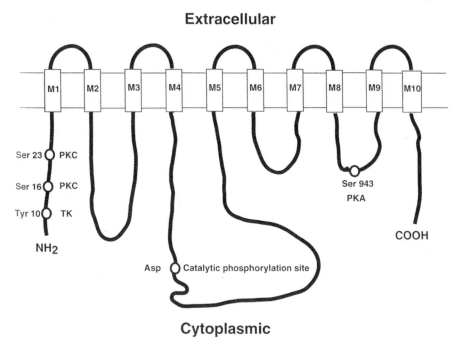

FIGURE 15 Transmembrane looping of the alpha subunit of Na,K-ATPase, with localization of phosphorylated amino acids. The PKA site is located at serine-943; PKC sites are on the NH2 cytoplasmic tail. The aspartate residue within the M4–M5 loop is phosphorylated during the catalytic cycle of the pump. (From Feraille E, Doucet A. Sodium-potassium-adenosine triphosphatase-dependent sodium transport in the kidney: hormonal control. *Physiol Rev* 2001;81:345–418.)

a specific inhibitor of P450 prevented the inhibitory effect of PTH on the Na,K-ATPase, and that the effects of 20-hydroxyeicosate-traenoic acid (20-HETE) and PTH on the Na,K-ATPase were not additive. These observations were extended by Ominato et al. (534) working with rat proximal tubules, who showed that inhibition of cytochrome P450 not only blocked the PTH effect, but also Na,K-ATPase inhibition by activators of PKC as well as inhibition by a PKC catalytic fragment. These authors drew the conclusion that the P450 product was an effector for PKC on the Na,K-ATPase. A slightly different conclusion was reached by Nowicki et al. (531) working in a cultured cell line (COS cells), who observed that 20-HETE had no effect on Na,K-ATPase in the absence of PKC, and that inhibitors of PKC (or mutation of the PKC catalytic site) eliminated the 20-HETE effect. These authors drew the conclusion that the P450 product was an effector for PKC on the Na,K-ATPase. A second complicating aspect of the regulation of Na,K-ATPase is the interaction with the cell's endocytic machinery. In proximal tubule cells in suspension, dopamine treatment caused phosphorylation of the alpha subunit of Na,K-ATPase, decreasing its activity, and resulting in its appearance in endosomes (154). Dopamine-induced phosphorylation was blocked by PKC inhibition. In OK cells, phosphorylation of the alpha subunit and its uptake into endosomes could be prevented with either PKC inhibition or by transfection with an alpha subunit lacking the PKC phosphorylation site (154).

The undercutting of this picture of PKC modulation of the Na,K-ATPase began with the microperfusion of rat proximal tubules by Liu and Cogan (450), and their observation that Na$^+$ and HCO$_3$ reabsorption was stimulated by PKC activation and depressed by PKC inhibition. Wang and Chan (740) sharpened this picture with their report of a time-dependent effect of PKC activation on microperfused rat proximal tubules, with early stimulation (0 to 10 minutes), yielding to late inhibition after 25 to 35 minutes of perfusion. In rat proximal tubule cells in suspension, Feraille et al. (208) examined the effect of PKC activation on Na,K-ATPase activity, and reproduced prior observations that with standard incubation conditions PKC activation inhibited Na,K-ATPase activity. However, the thrust of their report was that in a well oxygenated preparation, PKC was stimulatory, due to an increase in the Na$^+$ affinity. Enhancement of the transport activity occurred in parallel with phosphorylation of the alpha subunit of the Na,K-ATPase (138). In contrast to the findings of Chibalin et al. (154), Efendiev et al. (195) reported that in OK cells, PKC activation increased Na,K-ATPase activity by recruiting new transporters to the cell membrane. With regard to the inhibitory or stimulatory effect of PKC on the Na,K-ATPase, Efendiev et al. (196) have focused attention on cytosolic Na$^+$ concentration to act as a switch. Working in OK cells, they manipulated cell Na$^+$ using the ionophore monensin, and used rubidium uptake to assay Na$^+$,K$^+$-ATPase activity in intact tubules. They found that PKC activation stimulated the pump at low cell [Na$^+$], had no effect at estimated [Na$^+$] around

12 mM, and was inhibitory at cell [Na⁺] greater than 16 mM. The inhibition, but not the stimulation, was abrogated with P450 inhibition. This work was extended by experiments in rat proximal tubules in which the phosphorylation of the PKC site of the alpha subunit was measured (336). It was found that at the normally low cell Na⁺, the sites were largely phosphorylated, and only at abnormally high cell Na⁺ were they dephosphorylated and susceptible to the action of PKC.

Neural and Humoral Factors

RENAL NERVES

Renal sympathetic nerves have long been known to modulate proximal tubule sodium transport and are perhaps the most important regulator (176, 260). Denervation of the rat kidney reduced proximal reabsorption by 40% in the absence of any change in single nephron glomerular filtration (66). Stimulation of the sympathetic nerves can increase reabsorption by 30%, again without change in filtration (68). In the isolated perfused convoluted proximal tubule of the rabbit (but not the straight portion) both alpha and beta catecholamines enhance sodium transport (64). Similar stimulation by both adrenergic agonists is observed in the doubly microperfused rat tubule (759). In *Ambystoma*, application of the beta adrenergic agonist, isoproterenol, depolarized the cell and decreased the apical to basolateral membrane resistance ratio (510). In the perfused mammalian tubule, norepinephrine increases both bicarbonate and chloride transport (55). Nord and associates (530) found that in a suspension of tubule cells from the rabbit, sodium uptake was enhanced by alpha agonists. The elimination of this effect by ethylisopropylamiloride implicated alpha stimulation of brush border Na⁺/H⁺ exchange as the underlying mechanism.

Subsequently, Wong et al. (805) demonstrated that in the microperfused S1 segment of rat proximal tubule, both acute renal denervation or acute alpha-1 blockade reduce chloride reabsorption by 40%, while manipulation of alpha-2 activity had little impact. The effect of alpha-1 blockade could be eliminated by pre-activation of PKC, suggesting that the calcium-phospholipid-dependent kinase was the important signaling pathway for renal sympathetic activity. In view of the increase in cellular cAMP with beta-adrenergic agonists, the mechanism by which beta agonists enhance proximal sodium reabsorption must be indirect, and the evidence implicates NHERF: the activated beta-2 receptor binds NHERF, and thus eliminates cAMP-dependent downregulation of NHE3. When binding was prevented with a mutated beta receptor, the PKA-dependent decrease in NHE3 flux was also prevented (297).

A coordinated effect of sympathetic activity on luminal and peritubular cell membranes was suggested by the observation that PKC activation also enhanced activity of the peritubular Na⁺−3 HCO₃⁻ cotransporter (600). Of greater significance with respect to luminal-peritubular coordination, is the observation that norepinephrine also increases the activity of the Na,K-ATPase (55, 84). The effect on the

sodium pump, however, is more likely mediated by a phosphatase, since PKC is inhibitory here (21, 322, 435). In *Ambystoma*, norepinephrine application also produces activation of the Na,K-ATPase, and a decrease in cytosolic sodium concentration (2).

ANGIOTENSIN

Angiotensin II has been intensely studied as a regulator of proximal sodium transport (161, 301, 302, 562, 645). In the intact animal, selective blockade of angiotensin II is diuretic, so that it appears that under normal conditions, there is tonic stimulation of the proximal tubule (815). In physiologic doses, it enhances reabsorption in rat (304) or rabbit tubules (646), and the stimulatory effect appears to be more pronounced in the S1 segment (447). Specific receptors for angiotensin exist on both luminal (121) and peritubular membranes (122), and the hormone effect may be achieved from either side of the cell (448). Distinguished on the basis of inhibitor binding, several distinct receptor types have been identified on proximal tubule, each with affinity for angiotensin in the nanomolar range (182, 194). In intact rat tubules, the most prominent effect of angiotensin, in picomolar concentrations, is the stimulation of NaHCO₃ reabsorption via Na⁺/H⁺ exchange (448), and this is mediated by binding to AT1 receptors (564, 807). In a suspension of proximal tubule cells, angiotensin II enhances both Na⁺ uptake and cell pH recovery after an acid load (603). The increase in tubular reabsorption due to angiotensin is correlated with the inhibition of cAMP generation (449), and these findings are reproduced in cultured proximal tubule cells transfected with the AT1 angiotensin receptor (692).

While systemic angiotensin concentrations may be in the 0.01–0.1 nM range, luminal concentrations are 100-fold higher (656), due to tubular synthesis and secretion of angiotensin (111). Microperfusion studies, combining luminal perfusion of angiotensin with simultaneous inhibition of local synthesis, have confirmed the stimulation of transport starting in the picomolar range (52, 561). However, over a broad range of luminal concentrations (0.01–10.0 nM) these authors found the stimulatory effect of luminal angiotensin to be relatively flat. With respect to the peritubular action of angiotensin, inhibition of Na⁺ transport becomes apparent at concentrations above 0.1 nM as an attenuation of the stimulation seen at lower doses. Inhibition may dominate at concentrations greater than 100 nM (302), and may involve binding to an AT2 receptor (296). Pursuit of the signaling pathway underlying the inhibitory effect of angiotensin has indicated formation (via phospholipase-A2) of an epoxygenase metabolite of arachidonic acid (182, 299, 326, 469, 597).

Microperfusion experiments have also revealed a coordinated action of luminal angiotensin and renal nerve activity. In volume contracted animals, proximal reabsorption is brisk, additional luminal angiotensin adds little, and luminal AT1 antagonism has a dramatic inhibitory effect on reabsorption; in volume expanded animals, there is only small impact of luminal AT1 inhibition, while luminal angiotensin sharply increases volume reabsorption (563). Quan and Baum (566) made the observation that when renal nerves were cut, luminal perfusion of an angiotensin-converting enzyme inhibitor (enalaprilat) failed to decrease proximal volume reabsorption, although the tubule remained sensitive to the stimulatory effect of directly applied luminal angiotensin. Conversely, stimulation of renal nerves conferred enalaprilat-sensitivity to proximal reabsorption (565). These studies suggested that renal nerves amplified their signal to enhance proximal sodium reabsorption by switching on the local angiotensin synthetic machinery. A mysterious aspect of luminal angiotensin signaling is the luminal angiotensin concentration maintained well above that needed for maximal stimulation. One explanation that has been advanced is that in such a system, regulation of transport might then be determined by the AT1 receptor density (398).

With respect to specific proximal tubule transporters, angiotensin is pleiotropic. Beyond the effect of decreasing cAMP to increase NHE3 flux, there is evidence that angiotensin can act to increase NHE3 membrane density in both intact tubules (431) and in proximal tubule cells in culture (186). It is likely that the increase in NHE3 activity contributes to the observed increase in NH_4^+ secretion by perfused mouse proximal tubule (523), although the finding of increased NH_4^+ production in perfused S3 segments is evidence for a more global angiotensin action (522). Within the proximal tubules of rats with renovascular hypertension, there is increased expression of the Na^+–glucose cotransporter (SGLT2) that is blunted by AT1 inhibition (54). Additionally, angiotensin augments proximal acidification by the luminal membrane H^+-ATPase, at least in part through transporter insertion (737). In the picomolar to nanomolar concentration range, angiotensin stimulates HCO_3 exit via the peritubular Na^+–3 HCO_3^- cotransporter (165, 197, 240), perhaps via a pathway which activates PKC (601), and perhaps by increasing the membrane content of this transporter (585). Within the concentration range of angiotensin that stimulates proximal reabsorption, there is increased peritubular Na,K-ATPase (237); this occurs promptly and with changes in the phosphorylation of the Na,K-ATPase (822). There is also increased peritubular K^+ conductance (165). Despite enhancement of peritubular exit pathways, the net effect of angiotensin on cytosolic Na^+ concentration is an increase (576).

DOPAMINE

The proximal tubule is also the target of natriuretic signals, and dopamine has emerged as the most important (19, 135). Among the key early observations were the findings that urinary dopamine could derive from circulating L-DOPA (32), that on balance, the whole kidney synthesized dopamine (consuming DOPA), with tubular secretion providing the bulk of urinary dopamine (34), and that proximal tubules could be a source for this excreted dopamine (33).

Within proximal tubule, conversion from DOPA to dopamine is due to the enzyme L-amino acid decarboxylase (L-AADC), and the importance of the local generation of dopamine was underscored by the demonstration that maximal L-AADC activity was modulated by dietary salt intake (663). Proximal tubules are also a target for the locally generated dopamine. Dopamine inhibits sodium reabsorption in the isolated perfused straight tubule (65) and in tubule suspensions (426). In proximal convoluted tubules (in vitro), however, dopamine decreased sodium reabsorption only in tubules in which transport had been stimulated by norepinephrine (53), consistent with the observation in vivo that a DA-1 agonist is not natriuretic in a denervated kidney (335). RNA message for the DA-1 dopamine receptor was demonstrated in proximal tubule (817), and subsequently the protein was identified on both luminal and peritubular cell membranes (532). In cell culture (LLCPK) dopamine can act to recruit its own DA-1 receptor to the cell membrane (118); in rats, an additional dopamine effect is the down regulation of the AT1 angiotensin receptor (151). Studies of dopamine action via the DA-1 receptor have implicated a number of second messenger systems (reviewed by Aperia [19]).

As with angiotensin, dopamine impacts on transporters of both luminal and peritubular cell membranes, most notably but not exclusively NHE3 and the Na,K-ATPase. When renal cortical tissue is incubated with dopamine or DA-1 agonists, Na^+/H^+ exchange in brush border membrane vesicles is diminished; and this effect is blocked by inhibitors of either adenylate cyclase or PKA (207). Use of OK cells permitted the direct demonstration that dopamine (via DA-1) and PKA phosphorylated NHE3 on identical sites (791). In large measure, the decrease in Na^+/H^+ exchange reflects a dopamine-mediated decrease in NHE3 within the luminal cell membrane (30). This conclusion is based on experiments in which mouse cortical slices were treated with dopamine, and brush border membrane vesicles assayed for NHE3 activity and antigen. A prior observation had been made in OK cells that dopamine produced endocytosis of NHE3 in a PKA-dependent manner (330). With respect to other luminal transporters, dopamine also induces internalization of the Na^+-phosphate cotransporter (30). The impact of dopamine on the Na,K-AT-Pase is demonstrable as a decrease of enzyme activity in microdissected tubules (20) or as a decrease in oxygen consumption by proximal tubules in suspension in which cell Na^+ is kept high by nystatin permeabilization (662). The dopamine-mediated decrease in proximal tubule cellular Na,K-ATPase activity has been shown to occur in association with endocytosis of the enzyme, and blocking the endocytosis with an actin stabilizer, phallaciclin, eliminated the decrease in enzyme activity (153). An early event in the endocytic process is PKC-dependent phosphorylation of the alpha subunit of the Na,K-ATPase (154). An early observation in rat proximal tubule was that like ouabain, dopamine produced an increase in tubule diameter (20). More recent study of rabbit PST with Na^+-sensitive microelectrodes has demonstrated a prompt rise in cell Na^+ in response to dopamine (Kunimi et al., 2000). This indicates that with inhibition of both Na^+ entry and exit pathways, on balance, the effect of dopamine on the Na,K-ATPase dominates. In an electro-physiologic study, it was also found that dopamine blunted peritubular HCO_3 exit via the Na^+–$3HCO_3^-$ cotransporter (Kunimi et al., 2000).

NITRIC OXIDE

Nitric oxide provides a paracrine signal from renal nerves or renal endothelial cells to affect proximal tubule Na^+ transport (439). Due to its short half-life and difficulty in measurement, the impact of NO has been assessed indirectly, in experiments in which NO synthase (NOS) has been inhibited or NO donors have been infused, so that renal tubular dose-response for NO is not available. In whole animals, infusion of a NOS inhibitor at a dose which does not increase arterial blood pressure or glomerular filtration leads to a reduction in sodium excretion (416). Majid et al. (1993) found that with NOS inhibition, urinary Na^+ excretion failed to increase as a function of renal perfusion pressure, and this prompted them to propose that NO may be a mediator of the pressure-natriuresis response (see below). At apparent odds with the natriuretic effect of NO was the micropuncture observation that systemic NOS inhibition decreased proximal tubule Na^+ reabsorption (174). These findings received support from a study in which rat peritubular capillaries were perfused with agents promoting NO release and the effect was an increase in Na^+-dependent luminal proton secretion (15). However, other microperfusion studies arrived at an opposite conclusion. When the NO donor, sodium nitroprusside (SNP), was added to tubule lumen or to peritubular capillaries, it decreased proximal Na^+ reabsorption (198). In another study, proximal fluid reabsorption was increased by a NOS inhibitor added to the tubule lumen, and it was decreased by perfusion with SNP; this effect was dependent on the presence of intact renal nerves (812). Wang (738) observed a dose-dependent effect of tubule perfusion with SNP, in which low dose increased and high dose decreased proximal Na^+ and HCO_3 reabsorption; perfusion with a NOS inhibitor decreased reabsorption, consistent with the enhancing effect of low-dose SNP. A cautionary observation came from Liang et al. (436) who sampled renal interstitial fluid during systemic infusion with a low dose of a NOS inhibitor, and found that contrary to the expected decrease in NO, both nitrate/nitrite and cyclic GMP (cGMP) concentrations increased. With these increases, however, there was no change in proximal tubule fluid reabsorption, but an increase in distal delivery and natriuresis.

With respect to identifying the transporters affected by NO, treatment with cGMP of brush border membrane vesicles from rabbit kidney produced a relatively minor increase (22%) in Na^+/H^+ exchange (273). In primary culture of rabbit proximal tubule cells, the effect was opposite: SNP stimulated cGMP in a dose-dependent fashion, but only at the very highest dose was there a modest (35%) inhibition of Na^+/H^+ exchange (588). In a primary culture of mouse proximal tubule cells, SNP produced a modest decrease in Na,K-ATPase activity, and this effect was not reproduced by application of cGMP (290). In OK cells, SNP-induced inhibition of Na,K-ATPase was reproduced, and cGMP was equally effective (437); the downstream signal of cGMP was later identified as a PKC isoform (438). In human proximal tubule cells in primary culture, application of an NO donor resulted in accumulation of cGMP and a decrease in cell Na^+ content, consistent with a dominance of an inhibitory effect on Na^+ entry pathways (618). Of interest, these authors also observed that prevention of cGMP exit from the cell diminished the impact on cell Na^+, suggesting an autocrine role for cGMP. The proximal tubule epithelial cells do not contain RNA message for constitutive nitric oxide synthases (endothelial or neuronal NOS), but have abundant message for guanylate cyclase (691). In primary culture, rat proximal tubule cells showed little cGMP production in response to NO inducers, but coincubation with bovine pulmonary endothelial cells rendered the cells sensitive and resulted in a sharp increase in cGMP, a decrease in Na,K-ATPase activity, and a decrease in vectorial Na^+ transport from apical to basal surfaces (442). Of note, when mice lacking endothelial NOS were studied by micropuncture, there was no abnormality of proximal tubule transport, although maneuvers to elicit pressure natriuresis were not performed (739). A relationship between renal NO generation and the proximal tubule response to adrenergic stimulation has also been identified. In a rat micropuncture study, Thomson and Vallon (694) observed: (1) NOS inhibition decreased proximal sodium reabsorption, but the effect was absent when either renal nerves were cut or an alpha-2 adrenergic blocker was infused, and (2) in the denervated kidney, decrease in proximal reabsorption could be restored by systemic infusion of an alpha-2 adrenergic agonist. The observation of Wang et al. (744) that mice with deficient neuronal NOS had defective proximal $NaHCO_3$ reabsorption is consistent with these findings. Although Wu et al. (812) observed that NOS inhibition increased proximal sodium reabsorption, they also found that transection of renal nerves abrogated this effect; and the NOS inhibition effect was reproduced with specific inhibition of neuronal NOS. With renal nerve stimulation, proximal Na^+ reabsorption increased, but not in the presence of neuronal NOS inhibition (813). One possible reconciliation of these divergent findings is that NO may either stimulate or inhibit proximal Na^+ transport, depending on the concurrent neurohumoral signals, but the modulation of those signals requires an intact NOS system.

VOLUME EXPANSION AND PRESSURE NATRIURESIS

The influence of physical factors on the paracellular pathway does not preclude important effects of volume expansion on the cell itself. This was the supposition of Robson et al. (586) who reported the depression of glucose reabsorption in the kidney of the volume expanded rat. This view found support in a whole organ tracer study which failed to discern a pattern of increased glucose backflux during volume expansion (316). Micropuncture of the proximal tubule documented the decreased capacity for glucose reabsorption during volume expansion (31) and the correlation of proximal sodium and glucose reabsorption under the influence of albumin infusion (371). The microperfusion study of Boonjarern et al. (101) demonstrated decreased reabsorptive flux of labeled glucose in the presence of volume expansion. The case for a cellular effect of peritubular protein has also been presented by Berry and associates (79), who first noted in the isolated tubule a specific depression of chloride reabsorption with the removal of protein bath. The evidence was strengthened considerably in subsequent experiments in which transepithelial concentration gradients were adjusted to virtually eliminate electrodiffusive forces across the epithelium. In that study, the increase of peritubular protein from 6 to 10 g/dl still produced a 42% increase in NaCl reabsorption (49). Consistent with these findings, micropuncture of volume expanded rats has also indicated a greater depression of proximal reabsorption of NaCl than $NaHCO_3$ (90, 160). Pursuing this issue in another coupled transport system, Pitts et al. found that prior volume expansion of the rabbit depressed phosphate transport in straight proximal tubule removed and perfused over 90 minutes (552). In the same study, prior volume expansion also depressed Na^+-coupled phosphate transport in brush border membrane vesicles.

At this time, the cellular effects of volume expansion are not well characterized. Electron probe analysis of rat kidney has suggested that cell Na^+ concentration increases following saline infusion (291). When the kidney from the volume expanded rat is protected from physical factors using an arterial snare, the increase in cell Na^+ is eliminated (574). These findings were interpreted as most consistent with a decrease in Na,K-ATPase activity during volume expansion. "Pressure natriuresis," in which systemic arterial pressure is increased, has been another acute model in which the impact of physical factors on proximal sodium reabsorption has been examined (526, 596). In these animals, renal autoregulation maintains a relatively constant renal blood flow and glomerular filtration rate, but renal sodium excretion increases in association with an increase in renal interstitial hydrostatic pressure (374). In previous studies, Kinoshita and Knox (382) had shown that the decrease of proximal sodium reabsorption that normally follows increased renal interstitial pressure could be eliminated by blocking prostaglandin synthesis. In pressure natriuresis during block of prostaglandin synthesis with indomethacin, renal interstitial hydrostatic pressure still increases, but sodium and lithium reabsorption are no longer decreased (258). Complementing this observation is the finding that with directly applied increase in interstitial hydrostatic pressure, treatment with indomethacin eliminated the increase in tight junctional

lanthanum permeability (571). Although physical factors are involved, these results are best rationalized by an impact on the cell, rather than a direct tight-junction effect.

To pursue this issue, membrane fractions were obtained from kidneys undergoing pressure natriuresis, and examined for content of NHE3 and Na,K-ATPase (834). This study revealed that acute hypertension prompted the retrieval of luminal membrane transporters (change in membrane fraction in which transport activity appeared), and a sharp reduction in the activity of Na,K-ATPase. Extending this approach, it was found that the retrieval of NHE3 was prompt (within 5 minutes of acute hypertension), reversible (within 20 minutes), and concurrent with the acute changes in lithium clearance (833). With respect to the Na,K-ATPase, the decrease in activity was not accompanied by any loss of immunoreactivity of its subunits within the membrane fractions. Intact tubules were examined during acute hypertension, using immunohistochemical staining of NHE3 plus confocal microscopy to localize the transporter. In this way, there was direct observation that with acute hypertension, NHE3 redistributed from the brush border into the base of the microvilli, confirming the inference from the membrane fraction analysis (Fig. 16). Complementing these structural changes, functional changes in luminal membrane Na^+/H^+ exchange could be identified in vivo. When proximal tubule cells were loaded with BCECF, cytosolic pH could be monitored continuously during luminal microperfusion, and in particular, the time course of cellular acidification following luminal Na^+ removal could be determined. It was found that within 20 minutes of acute hypertension, the Na^+-dependent change in cytosolic pH was reduced 52% from control (824). When brush border membrane vesicles were examined both for NHE3 protein and for Na^+/H^+ exchange activity, it was found that despite retrieval (change in membrane fraction), the activity per transporter remained constant (819). Thus, in contrast to the changes in Na,K-ATPase activity, the reduction in Na^+/H^+ activity could not be attributed to kinetic modification of the NHE3 transporter. With acute volume contraction, however, transporter kinetics do appear to change, since the increase in lithium reabsorption is not accompanied by the appearance of new NHE3 (432). Over time, however, chronic volume depletion does increase NHE3 message in proximal tubule (215).

The signals from interstitium to tubule have also been pursued in more detail, and there is evidence from several authors that arachidonic acid metabolites of cytochrome P-450 are implicated. Acknowledging the prior identification of eicosanoids (specifically 20-hydroxyeicosate-traenoic acid, 20-HETE) as inhibitors of Na,K-ATPase, Zhang et al. (833) sought evidence for their role as mediators of pressure natriuresis. They examined pressure natriuresis in rats pretreated with cobalt chloride to blunt cytochrome P-450 metabolism, and found that this treatment blocked the pressure-associated increase in lithium clearance. This occurred in association with failure of NHE3 retrieval from

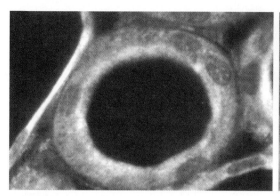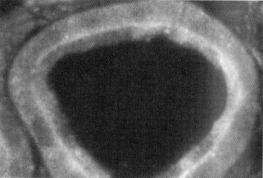

FIGURE 16   Effect of acute hypertension on NHE3 distribution in rat proximal tubules. Panels show NHE3 immunoflourescence under control conditions (left) and after 20 minutes of acute hypertension. Under control conditions, NHE3 appears along microvilli; with pressure natriuresis, there is redistribution of the exchanger to the base of the brush border. (From Yip KP, Tse CM, McDonough AA, Marsh DJ. Redistribution of Na+/H+ exchanger isoform NHE3 in proximal tubules induced by acute and chronic hypertension. *Am J Physiol* 1998;275:F565–F575.)

brush border vesicles, and failure of Na,K-ATPase activity to decrease within its membrane fraction (833). These findings received support with the observation that proximal convoluted tubule contains abundant cytochrome P-450 4A isoforms (345a). Furthermore, rabbit proximal straight tubules in suspension produce 20-HETE, and when 20-HETE production is inhibited in an isolated perfused tubule, volume reabsorption is enhanced (566a). With the availability of a specific inhibitor of eicosanoid formation, Dos Santos et al. (180a) reexamined pressure natriuresis in pretreated rats. In these animals, 20-HETE excretion was nearly eliminated, and the pressure-induced increase in sodium excretion and lithium clearance was substantially blunted. This occurred in association with blunted retrieval of NHE3 from brush border and blunted decrease in Na,K-ATPase activity (180a). It must be acknowledged, however, that this work leaves unanswered the identity of the signal from interstitial hydrostatic pressure to cell. A role for nitric oxide was examined in the rat, but NOS inhibition blunted transmission of renal perfusion pressure to the interstitium, so that the failure to observe pressure natriuresis may simply have been a consequence of low interstitial pressure (524). More recently, renal interstitial cyclic GMP concentration was found to increase with renal perfusion pressure, and guanylyl cyclase inhibition blunted the pressure-associated decrease in proximal Na+ reabsorption (353).

GLOMERULOTUBULAR BALANCE

In response to spontaneous variations in glomerular filtration rate, the rate of proximal tubule reabsorption is found to vary proportionally. This "glomerulotubular balance" is demonstrated by the study of Schnermann et al. (640) in the rat, where, despite fourfold variation in GFR, the proximal tubule continued to reabsorb roughly 40% of the filtered load (Fig. 17). Although glomerulotubular balance may obviously prevent loss of solute following increases in GFR, perhaps its most important effect is the preservation of adequate distal

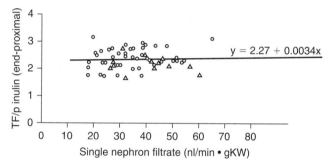

FIGURE 17   End-proximal tubular fluid was sampled from rat nephrons and plotted as a function of SNGFR. With spontaneous variation in SNGFR over a fourfold range, there is virtually no change in the fractional water reabsorption. (With permission, from Schnermann J, Wahl M, Liebau G, Fischbach H. Balance between tubular flowrate and net fluid reabsorption in the proximal convolution of the rat kidney. *Pflugers Arch* 1968;304:90–103.)

delivery of sodium (permitting distal regulation of acid and potassium excretion) in times of low GFR. The mechanisms for balanced tubular reabsorption include both peritubular capillary effects and luminal factors (241, 295, 793). Peritubular oncotic forces are generally recognized as a major force in the maintenance of balanced tubular reabsorption (190). Any increase in filtration fraction must result in an increased peritubular protein concentration, and thus, enhanced proximal reabsorption. Experimental maneuvers which distort this oncotic force (such as saline infusion or albumin administration) disrupt glomerulotubular balance. Nevertheless, in a mathematical model comprised of glomerulus, proximal tubule, peritubular capillary, and interstitium, simulation of only the filtration fraction effect on tubular transport failed to reproduce glomerulotubular balance (771). In simulations of glomerular arteriolar resistance changes, it was found that fractional changes in proximal sodium reabsorption were smaller than the fractional changes in GFR. This derived from the fact that the variation in GFR came as a result of changes in glomerular plasma flow, as well as in filtration fraction. In order to achieve glomerulotubular balance, there must be a mechanism by which alterations in plasma flow, independent of peritubular Starling forces, can influence proximal reabsorption.

The impact of isolated changes in glomerular plasma flow has been approached by examination of the effect of luminal flow rate on tubular reabsorption, that is, "perfusion-absorption balance" (793). One mechanism which may contribute to flow-dependent reabsorption is what may be referred to as "substrate utilization." In this case, the perfusion solution contains a substance which enhances sodium reabsorption and which may be depleted at slower perfusion rates. Thus, starting at the slower rates, more rapid perfusion will, up to a point, increase fluid transport. Kokko and Rector (397) had suggested that substrate utilization might be important in interpreting their observations of the transepithelial potential of the perfused rabbit proximal convoluted tubule. It was found that when the perfusate was an ultrafiltrate of rabbit serum, there was a clear decline in voltage at perfusion rates less than 10 nl/min. In view of the complete abolition of the transepithelial electrical potential difference in the absence of tubular glucose and amino acids, this depletion with the slower perfusion rate was expected. This study was invoked several years later to understand the observations of Imai et al. on water reabsorption in the perfused rabbit proximal convoluted tubule (342). Again when perfusion was with an ultrafiltrate of serum, there was a clear decline in sodium reabsorption at initial flow rates less than 11 nl/min. The earlier result of Burg and Orloff (126) showing no effect of flow on reabsorptive rate was attributed to the higher flow rates used by these investigators (9–18 nl/mm[1]min). The relevance of the substrate utilization model to glomerulotubular balance, however, remains to be demonstrated. In the rat, there is no enhancement of reabsorption in the presence of luminal glucose (270). Further, theoretical calculations by Marsh (471) suggest at most a small role for Na^+–glucose cotransport in the maintenance of glomerulotubular balance. Nevertheless, using a more detailed model of proximal tubule and invoking preferential reabsorption of all luminal organics, Barfuss and Schafer (39) have estimated that up to 30% of glomerulotubular balance might be attributed to a substrate utilization mechanism.

Perhaps the most important factor underlying perfusion-absorption balance is a direct effect of axial flow velocity on reabsorption. Such an effect has been found to influence the transport of glucose (391), bicarbonate (13, 147, 447), and chloride (274, 804). One of the best illustrations of this phenomenon is the micropuncture data of Chan et al. (147) shown in Fig. 18, in which a threefold increase in luminal perfusion rate (with trivial changes in luminal HCO_3^- concentration) produced a doubling of the rate of bicarbonate reabsorption. More pronounced effects have been reported with "native" tubular fluid, in comparison with artificial microperfusion solutions, suggesting the presence of a filtered, transport-promoting factor (44, 293). It may also be the case

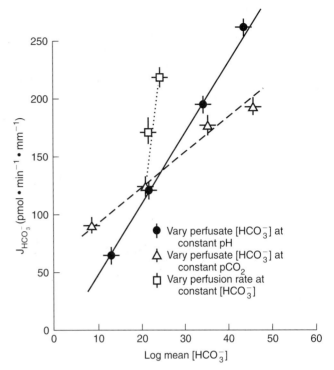

FIGURE 18 Net bicarbonate reabsorption, J_{HCO3}, by perfused rat proximal tubule as a function of mean luminal bicarbonate concentration. At a constant pCO_2, bicarbonate transport varies linearly with the transepithelial concentration gradient (dashed line). Elevation of pCO_2 enhances, and depression of pCO_2 diminishes, bicarbonate reabsorption (solid line). There is a steep dependence of J_{HCO3} on luminal flow rate. (With permission, from Chan YL, Biagi B, Giebisch G. Control mechanisms of bicarbonate transport across the rat proximal convoluted tubule. *Am J Physiol* 1982;242:F532–F543.)

that reductions (rather than increases) in luminal flow, are more faithfully followed by proportional changes in transport (43, 294, 549, 591). Nevertheless, the range over which modulation of luminal flow produces proportional changes in proximal reabsorption is broad (590). The underlying mechanism for flow-dependent changes in reabsorption has not been established. One perennial consideration is that of an unstirred layer effect within the brush border (584). The morphologic observations of Maunsbach et al. (483) demonstrate that lower tubule flow rates are associated with diminished tubule distention and a compaction of the brush border microvilli. Nevertheless, model calculations indicate it unlikely that there is any appreciable convective stirring within this pile (45), nor should the diffusion barrier between the bulk luminal fluid and the cell membrane pose any significant hindrance to Na^+/H^+ exchange (406). An intriguing mechanism for flow-dependent transport gained support from two studies, using very different methodology, which both suggested that increases in axial flow velocity recruit new transporters into the luminal membrane. Preisig (554) loaded rat proximal tubule cells with the pH indicator BCECF and examined recovery from an acute acid load in vivo (ammonium pulse). With increases in luminal flow rate, the pH recovery mediated by Na$^+$/H$^+$ exchange was enhanced. Maddox et al. (468) subjected rats to acute changes in vascular volume in order to obtain hydropenic, euvolemic, and volume expanded groups, with respective grouping according to decreased, normal, and increased GFR. When brush border membrane vesicles were prepared from each of these groups, and Na$^+$/H$^+$ kinetic parameters assessed, it was found that the V$_{max}$ determinations stratified in parallel with GFR.

Guo et al. (288) have proposed that the brush border microvilli serve as the sensor for axial flow along the proximal tubule. In that hypothesis, the drag force on each microvillus produced torque on an actin filament core that was transmitted to the underlying cytoskeleton. The close spacing and uniform height of the microvilli allowed a precise calculation of that torque, and using the known bending moment for an actin filament, the Young's modulus for a microvillus was estimated. This yielded the prediction that for microvilli 2.5 μm in height, the tip deflection under axial flows of 30 nl/min would be about 4 nm, in effect depicting the microvilli as a set of stiff bristles that would retain their configuration through the physiologic range of flows (288). In a subsequent analysis, a simplified equation for microvillous torque was derived which has been useful for assessment of experimental data (185). The essence of that derivation was identifying the microvillous drag with the force on the axial tubular flow

$$D \cdot N = \frac{dp}{dz} \cdot \pi \cdot R^2 \qquad (20)$$

where D is the drag per microvillus, N is the number of microvilli per unit length of tubule, p is luminal hydrostatic pressure, z is axial length, and R is the tubule radius from center-line to microvillus tip. Assuming Poiseuille flow,

$$\frac{dp}{dz} = 8\mu Q / \pi R^4 \qquad (21)$$

where Q is luminal flow rate and μ is the tubule fluid viscosity. This provides the estimate of microvillous drag

$$D \cdot N = 8\mu Q / R^2 \qquad (22)$$

and for a microvillus of height, L, the torque, T, is

$$T \cdot N = 8\mu Q / R^2 \qquad (23)$$

Since the number of microvilli, N, is not easily obtained, Eq. 23 is most useful in comparison of two experimental trials in which flow is varied and the assumption is made that neither N nor L change with the experimental conditions:

$$\frac{T}{T_r} = \left[\frac{\mu\ Q}{\mu_r\ Q_r} \right] \cdot \left[\frac{R_r^2}{R^2} \right] \qquad (24)$$

in which the subscript *r* denotes a reference flow. This equation reveals the microvillous torque to vary directly with lu-

minal flow and fluid viscosity, and inversely as the square of the luminal radius.

Du et al. (185) applied a slightly more detailed version of Eq. 24 to analyze the first experimental study of flow-dependent volume reabsorption, J$_v$, in isolated perfused mouse proximal tubules. The key finding of that work was that fractional changes in perfusion were greater than the fractional changes in J$_v$, but when changes in luminal diameter were included in the calculation, the fractional change in microvillous torque and J$_v$ were identical. Furthermore, luminal fluid viscosity increased J$_v$ at a constant perfusion rate. And finally, disruption of the cytoskeleton with cytochalasin D eliminated the perfusion-dependent increase in J$_v$. More recently, Du et al. (184) reexamined flow-dependent transport in mouse proximal tubule, with measurement of HCO$_3$ reabsorption, J$_{HCO3}$. Over a five-fold variation of luminal perfusion rate, there was a predicted twofold variation in microvillous torque, which scaled identically with the reabsorption (Fig. 19). Du et al. (185) also reconsidered the data of Burg and Orloff (126), widely cited as a negative effect of flow on proximal sodium reabsorption in isolated perfused rabbit proximal convoluted tubule. Burg and Orloff had observed that a threefold increase in tubule perfusion rate produced a 37% increase in volume reabsorption, a value that did not achieve statistical significance. However, they also noted that with the highest flow, there was a 41% increase in tubule diameter. Du et al. (185) estimated that these changes of flow and diameter would yield a 43% increase in microvillous torque, certainly compatible with the observed impact on J$_v$. In sum, it appears that the rabbit proximal tubules were more distensible than mouse tubules, so that perfusion-dependent changes in luminal diameter precluded large deviations in microvillous torque. At present, the cellular signals from torque to Na$^+$/H$^+$ exchange remain to be delineated.

PERSPECTIVE

Sodium reabsorption along the proximal tubule, rather than a specific transport process, refers to a multiplicity of processes, occurring in series and in parallel along a heterogeneous epithelium. Sodium transport cannot be considered out of context of the secretion of protons, or the reabsorption of chloride, bicarbonate, potassium, calcium, and organic solutes. Furthermore, the precise interrelationship of these coupled transport processes, depends upon the location along the proximal tubule, as well as upon physiologic parameters external to the nephron (such as the plasma electrolyte composition, or the extracellular volume status of the organism).

The focus of this chapter has been on the dynamics of transport, namely the delineation of the responsible driving forces for each of the intraepithelial transport steps. The feasibility of such an approach was due entirely to the development of experimental technology which permits the study

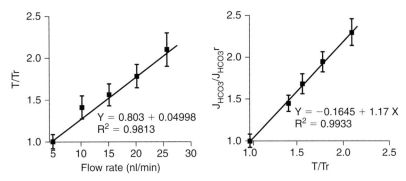

FIGURE 19   Impact of luminal flow rate on bicarbonate (J_{HCO3}) reabsorption in mouse proximal tubules perfused in vitro. The panel on the left shows the computed microvillous torque, T, at each flow, relative to the torque when perfusion is at 5 nl/min (T_r). In the right panel, the observed J_{HCO3} is plotted as a function of the relative torque. (Du Z, Yan Q, Duan Y, Weinbaum S, Weinstein AM, Wang T. Axial flow modulates proximal tubule NHE3 and H-ATPase activities by changing microvillous bending moments. *Am J Physiol* 2006;290: F289–F296.)

of cellular membranes and the recording of intracellular composition. With this technology, the first order of business had been the definition and localization of the coupled transport processes. More recent molecular methods have enhanced this aspect of tubule physiology by providing a means of securely identifying a transporter within proximal tubule, and of distinguishing distinct isoforms, which may have different membrane locations and subserve different functions. The ability to clone and express transporters in high density in otherwise quiet systems (in which flux through the pathway of interest dominates) has yielded advances in the definition of transport kinetics.

The second order of business has been identification of the important regulatory factors. This means an understanding of how changes in cell volume or ionic composition translate into alterations of proximal tubular sodium reabsorption, of the intraepithelial effects of alterations in luminal and peritubular composition, and of the biochemical signals operative in the modulation of transport. The complexity of this task derives from the observations that single hormones may activate more than one second messenger system, with possibly opposing effects, and that the overall effect on sodium transport by one hormone may depend upon the state of activation of the other systems. Nevertheless, one recurring theme in descriptions of transport regulation has been the targeting of luminal and peritubular membranes in a coordinated fashion.

Enrichment of our perspective of proximal tubule function must ultimately confer a quantitative understanding of its roles in pathologic states of the organism. Traditionally, this has focused on the secondary renal response to disorders of extracellular volume homeostasis, such as the edema forming states (i.e., heart failure, cirrhosis, and nephrotic syndrome). It is entirely likely, however, that a role for proximal tubule may come to be identified in primary pathogenesis, as perhaps in volume-dependent hypertension. One anticipates, as a consequence of such information,

that therapeutic intervention which seeks to alter renal sodium transport will be achieved with greater accuracy and greater safety.

Acknowledgment

This work was supported by National Institute of Diabetes and Digestive and Kidney Disease (grant 1-RO1-DK-29857).

References

1. Abdulnour-Nakhoul S, Boulpaep EL. Transcellular chloride pathways in *Ambystoma* proximal tubule. *J Membr Biol* 1998;166:15–35.
2. Abdulnour-Nakhoul S, Khuri RN, Nakhoul NL. Effect of norepinephrine on cellular sodium transport in Ambystoma kidney proximal tubule. *Am J Physiol* 1994;267:F725–36.
3. Abuladze N, Lee I, Newman D, Hwang J, Pushkin A, Kurtz I. Axial heterogeneity of sodium-bicarbonate cotransporter expression in the rabbit proximal tubule. *Am J Physiol* 1998;274: F628–F633.
4. Agre P, Preston GM, Smith BL, Jung JS, Raina S, Moon C, Guggino WB, Nielsen S. Aquaporin CHIP: the archetypal molecular water channel. *Am J Physiol* 1993;265:F463–F476.
5. Akiba T, Alpern RJ, Eveloff J, Calamina J, Warnock DG. Electrogenic sodium/bicarbonate cotransport in rabbit renal cortical basolateral membrane vesicles. *J Clin Invest* 1986;78:1472–1478.
6. Alavi N, Spangler RA, Jung CY. Sodium-dependent glucose transport by cultured proximal tubule cells. *Biochim Biophys Acta* 1987;899:916.
7. Albrecht FE, Xu J, Moe OW, Hopfer U, Simonds WF, Orlowski J, Jose PA. Regulation of NHE3 activity by Gprotein subunits in renal brush-border membranes. *Am J Physiol* 2000;278: R1064–R1073.
8. Alpern RJ. Mechanism of basolateral membrane H⁺/OH⁻/HCO₃ transport in the rat proximal convoluted tubule. A sodium-coupled electrogenic process. *J Gen Physiol* 1985;86: 613–636.
9. Alpern RJ. Apical membrane chloride/base exchange in the rat proximal convoluted tubule. *J Clin Invest* 1987;79:1026–30.
10. Alpern RJ. Cell mechanisms of proximal tubule acidification. *Physiol Rev* 1990;70:79–114.
11. Alpern RJ, Chambers M. Basolateral membrane Cl/HCO₃ exchange in the rat proximal convoluted tubule. Na-dependent and-independent modes. *J Gen Physiol* 1987;89:581–98.
12. Alpern RJ, Howlin KJ, Preisig PA. Active and passive components of chloride transport in the rat proximal convoluted tubule. *J Clin Invest* 1985;76:1360–1366.
13. Alpern RJ, Cogan MG, Rector FC Jr. Flow dependence of proximal tubular bicarbonate absorption. *Am J Physiol* 1983;245:F478–F484.
14. Amemiya M, Loffing Lotscher M, Kaissling B, Alpern RJ, Moe OW. Expression of NHE-3 in the apical membrane of rat renal proximal tubule and thick ascending limb. *Kidney Int* 1995;48:1206–1215.
15. Amorena C, Castro AF. Control of proximal tubule acidification by the endothelium of the peritubular capillaries. *Am J Physiol* 1997;272: R691–R694.
16. Andreoli TE, Schafer JA. Volume absorption in the pars recta. III. Luminal hypotonicity as a driving force for isotonic volume absorption. *Am J Physiol* 1978;234:F349–F355.

17. Andreoli TE, Schafer JA, Troutman SL. Perfusion rate–dependence of transepithelial osmosis in isolated proximal convoluted tubules: estimation of the hydraulic conductance. *Kidney Int* 1978;14:263–269.
18. Andreoli TE, Schafer JA, Troutman SL, Watkins ML. Solvent drag component of Cl^- flux in superficial proximal straight tubules: evidence for a paracellular component of isotonic fluid absorption. *Am J Physiol* 1979;237:F455–F462.
19. Aperia AC. Intrarenal dopamine: a key signal in the interactive regulation of sodium metabolism. *Ann Rev Physiol* 2000;62:621–647.
20. Aperia A, Bertorello A, Seri I. Dopamine causes inhibition of Na^+-K^+-ATPase activity in rat proximal convoluted tubule segments. *Am J Physiol* 1987;252:F39–F45.
21. Aperia A, Ibarra F, Svensson L-B, Klee C, Greengard P. Calcineurin mediates alpha-adrenergic stimulation of Na^+-K^+-ATPase activity in renal tubule cells. *Proc Natl Acad Sci U S A* 1992;89:7394–7397.
22. Aronson PS. Kinetic properties of the plasma membrane Na^+–H^+ exchanger. *Ann Rev Physiol* 1985;47:545–560.
23. Aronson PS, Giebisch G. Mechanisms of chloride transport in the proximal tubule. *Am J Physiol* 1997;273:F179–F192.
24. Aronson PS, Nee J, Suhm MA. Modifier role of internal H in activating the Na^+–H^+ exchanger in renal microvillus membrane vesicles. *Nature* 1982;299:161–163.
25. Aronson PS, Sacktor B. The Na^+ gradient-dependent transport of D-glucose in renal brush border membranes. *J Biol Chem* 1975;250:6032–6039.
26. Aronson PS, Suhm MA, NeeJ. Interaction of external H^+ with the Na^+–H^+ exchanger in renal microvillus membrane vesicles. *J Biol Chem* 1983;258:6767–6771.
27. Atherton JC. Comparison of chloride concentration and osmolality in proximal tubular fluid peritubular capillary plasma and systemic plasma in the rat. *J Physiol (Lond)* 1977;273: 765–773.
28. Avison MJ, Gullans SR, Ogino T, Giebisch G, Shulman RG. Measurement of Na^+–K^+ coupling ratio of Na^+-K^+-ATPase in rabbit proximal tubules. *Am J Physiol* 1987;253:C126–C136.
29. Avison MJ, Gullans SR, Ogino T, Giebisch G. Na^+ and K^+ fluxes stimulated by Na^+-coupled glucose transport: evidence for a Ba2$^+$-insensitive K^+ efflux pathway in rabbit proximal tubules. *J Membr Biol* 1988;105:197–205.
30. Bacic D, Kaissling B, McLeroyP, Zou L, Baum M, Moe OW. Dopamine acutely decreases apical membrane Na/H exchanger NHE3 protein in mouse renal proximal tubule. *Kidney Int* 2003;64:2133–2141.
31. Baines AD. Effect of extracellular fluid volume expansion on maximum glucose reabsorption rate and glomerular tubular balance in single rat nephrons. *J Clin Invest* 1971;50:2414–2425.
32. Baines AD, Chan W. Production of urine free dopamine from DOPA: a micropuncture study. *Life Sci* 1980;26:253–259.
33. Baines AD, Drangova R, Hatcher C. Dopamine production by isolated glomeruli and tubules from rat kidneys. *Can J Physiol Pharmacol* 1985;63:155–158.
34. Ball SG, Gunn IG, Douglas IHS. Renal handling of dopa, dopamine norepinephrine and epinephrine in the dog. *Am J Physiol* 1982;242:F56–F62.
35. Bank N, Aynedjian HS. Failure of changes in intracapillary pressures to alter proximal fluid reabsorption. *Kidney Int* 1984;26:275–282.
36. Bank N, Aynedjian HS, Mutz BF. Proximal bicarbonate absorption independent of Na^+–H^+ exchange: effect of bicarbonate load. *Am J Physiol* 1989;256:F577–F582.
37. Bank N, Yarger WE, Aynedjian HS. A microperfusion study of sucrose movement across the rat proximal tubule during renal vein constriction. *J Clin Invest* 1971;50:294–302.
38. Bankir L, de Rouffignac C. Anatomical and functional heterogeneity of nephrons in the rabbit: microdissection studies and SNGFR measurements. *Pflugers Arch* 1976;366:89–93.
39. Barfuss DW, Schafer JA. Flow dependence of nonelectrolyte absorption in the nephron. *Am J Physiol* 1979;236:F163–F174.
40. Barfuss DW, Schafer JA. Differences in active and passive glucose transport along the proximal nephron. *Am J Physiol* 1981;240:F322–332.
41. Barratt LJ, Rector FC Jr, Kokko JP, Seldin DW. Factors governing the transepithelial potential difference across the proximal tubule of the rat kidney. *J Clin Invest* 1974;53:454–464.
42. Barriere H, Rubera I, Belfodil R, Tauc M, Tonnerieux N, Poujeol C, Barhanin J, Poujeol P. Swelling-activated chloride and potassium conductance in primary cultures of mouse proximal tubules. Implication of KCNE1 protein. *J Membr Biol* 2003;193:153–170.
43. Bartoli E, Conger JD, Earley LE. Effect of intraluminal flow on proximal tubular reabsorption. *J Clin Invest* 1973;52:843–849.
44. Bartoli E, Earley LE. Importance of ultrafilterable plasma factors in maintaining tubular reabsorption. *Kidney Int* 1973;3:142–150.
45. Basmadjian D, Dykes DS, Baines AD. Flow through brush borders and similar protuberant wall structures. *J Membr Biol* 1980;56:183–190.
46. Baum M. Effect of luminal chloride on cell pH in rabbit proximal tubule. *Am J Physiol* 1988;254:F677–F683.
47. Baum M. Axial heterogeneity of rabbit proximal tubule luminal H^+ and basolateral HCO_3^- transport. *Am J Physiol* 1989;256:F335–F341.
48. Baum M, Berry CA. Evidence for neutral transcellular NaCl transport and neutral basolateral chloride exit in the rabbit proximal convoluted tubule. *J Clin Invest* 1984;74: 205–211.
49. Baum M, Berry CA. Peritubular protein modulates neutral active NaCl absorption in rabbit proximal convoluted tubule. *Am J Physiol* 1985;248:F790–F795.
50. Baum M, Hays SR. Phorbol myristate acetate and dioctanoylglycerol inhibit transport in rabbit proximal convoluted tubule. *Am J Physiol* 1988;254:F9–F14.
51. Baum M, Quigley R. Inhibition of proximal convoluted tubule transport by dopamine. *Kidney Int* 1998;54:1593–1600.
52. Baum M, Quigley R, Quan A. Effect of luminal angiotensin II on rabbit proximal convoluted tubule bicarbonate absorption. *Am J Physiol* 1997;273:F595–F600.
53. Deleted in proof.
54. Bautista R, Manning R, Martinez F, Avila-Casado M, Soto V, Medina A, Escalante B. Angiotensin II–dependent increased expression of Na^+-glucose cotransporter in hypertension. *Am J Physiol* 2004;286:F127–F133.
55. Beach RE, Schwab SJ, Brazy PC, Dennis VW. Norepinephrine increases Na^+-K^+-ATPase and solute transport in rabbit proximal tubules. *Am J Physiol* 1987;252:F215–F220.
56. Beck FX, Dorge A, Rick R, Schramm M, Thurau K. Effect of potassium adaptation on the distribution of potassium sodium and chloride across the apical membrane of renal tubular cells. *Pflugers Arch* 1987;409:477–485.
57. Beck JC, Sacktor B. Energetics of the Na^+-dependent transport of D-glucose in renal brush border membrane vesicles. *J Biol Chem* 1975;250:8674–8680.
58. Beck JS, Breton S, Laprade R, Giebisch G. Volume regulation and intracellular calcium in the rabbit proximal convoluted tubule. *Am J Physiol* 1991;60:F861–F867.
59. Beck JS, Breton S, Mairbaurl H, Laprade R, Giebisch G. Relationship between sodium transport and intracellular ATP in isolated perfused rabbit proximal convoluted tubule. *Am J Physiol* 1991;261:F634–F639.
60. Beck JS, Hurst AM, Lapointe J-Y, Laprade R. Regulation of basolateral K channels in proximal tubule studied during continuous microperfusion. *Am J Physiol* 1993;264:F496–F501.
61. Beck JS, Laprade R, Lapointe J-Y. Coupling between transepithelial Na transport and basolateral K conductance in renal proximal tubule. *Am J Physiol* 1994;266:F517–F527.
62. Beck JS, Potts DJ. Cell swelling co-transport activation and potassium conductance in isolated perfused rabbit kidney proximal tubules. *J Physiol* 1990;425:369–378.
63. Beguin P, Beggah AT, Chibalin AV, Burgener-Kairuz P, Jaisser F, Mathews PM, Rossier BC, Cotecchia S, Geering K. Phosphorylation of the Na K-ATPase alpha-subunit by protein kinase A and C in vitro and in intact cells. *J Biol Chem* 1994;269:24437–24445.
64. Bello-Reuss E. Effect of catecholamines on fluid reabsorption by the isolated proximal convoluted tubule. *Am J Physiol* 1980;238:F347–F352.
65. Bello-Reuss E. Electrical properties of the basolateral membrane of the straight portion of the rabbit proximal renal tubule. *J Physiol (Lond)* 1982;326:49–63.
66. Bello-Reuss E, Colindres RE, Pastoriza-Munoz E, Mueller RA, Gottschalk CW. Effects of acute unilateral renal denervation in the rat. *J Clin Invest* 1975;56:208–217.
67. Bello-Reuss E, Higashi Y, Kaneda Y. Dopamine decreases fluid reabsorption in straight portions of rabbit proximal tubule. *Am J Physiol* 1982;242:F634–F640.
68. Bello-Reuss E, Trevino DL, Gottschalk CW. Effect of renal sympathetic nerve stimulation on proximal water and sodium reabsorption. *J Clin Invest* 1976;57:1104–1107.
69. Bello-Reuss E, Weber MR. Electrophysiological studies on primary cultures of proximal tubule cells. *Am J Physiol* 1986;251:F490–F498.
70. Bengele HH, Evan AP. The effects of Ringer-Locke or blood infusions on the lateral intercellular spaces of the rat proximal tubule. *Anat Rec* 1975;182:201–214.
71. Bennett E, Kimmich GA. The molecular mechanism and potential dependence of the Na^+/glucose cotransporter. *Biophys J* 1996;70:1676–1688.
72. Bentzel CJ. Proximal tubule structure–function relationships during volume expansion in *Necturus*. *Kidney Int* 1972;2:324–335.
73. Bentzel CJ, Davies M, Scott WN, Zatzman M, Solomon AK. Osmotic volume flow in the proximal tubule of *Necturus* kidney. *J Gen Physiol* 1968;51:517–533.
74. Bentzel CJ, Parsa B, Hare DK. Osmotic flow across proximal tubule of *Necturus*: correlation of physiologic and anatomic studies. *Am J Physiol* 1969;217:570–580.
75. Bentzel CJ, Reczek PR. Permeability changes in *Necturus* proximal tubule during volume expansion. *Am J Physiol* 1978;234:F225–F234.
76. Berry CA. Heterogeneity of tubular transport processes in nephron. *Ann Rev Physiol* 1982;44:181–201.
77. Berry CA. Lack of effect of peritubular protein on passive NaCl transport in the rabbit proximal tubule. *J Clin Invest* 1983;71:268–281.
78. Berry CA. Water permeability and pathways in the proximal tubule. *Am J Physiol* 1983;245: F279–F294.
79. Berry CA, Cogan MG. Influence of peritubular protein on solute absorption in the rabbit proximal tubule. A specific effect on NaCl transport. *J Clin Invest* 1981;68:506–516.
80. Berry CA, Rector FC Jr. Relative sodium-to-chloride permeability in the proximal convoluted tubule. *Am J Physiol* 1978;235:F592–F604.
81. Berry CA, Rector FC Jr.. Electroneutral NaCl absorption in the proximal tubule: mechanisms of apical Na-coupled transport. *Kidney Int* 1989;36:403–411.
82. Bertorello A, Aperia A. Na^+-K^+-ATPase is an effector protein for protein kinase C in renal proximal tubule cells. *Am J Physiol* 1989;256:F370–F373.
83. Bertorello A, Aperia A, Walaas SI, Nairn AC, Greengard P. Phosphorylation of the catalytic subunit of Na^+, K^+-ATPase inhibits the activity of the enzyme. *Proc Natl Acad Sci U S A* 1991;88:11359–11362.
84. Bertorello AM, Katz AI. Short-term regulation of renal Na-K-ATPase activity: physiological relevance and cellular mechanisms. *Am J Physiol* 1993;265:F743–F755.
85. Beyenbach KW. Secretory NaCl and volume flow in renal tubules. *Am J Physiol* 1986;250: R753–R763.
86. Biagi BA, Sohtell M. pH sensitivity of the basolateral membrane of the rabbit proximal tubule. *Am J Physiol* 1986;250:F261–F266.
87. Biagi BA, Sohtell M. Electrophysiology of basolateral bicarbonate transport in the rabbit proximal tubule. *Am J Physiol* 1986;250:F267–F272.
88. Biagi B, Kubota T, Sohtell M, Giebisch G. Intracellular potentials in rabbit proximal tubules perfused in vitro. *Am J Physiol* 1981;240:F200–F210.
89. Biagi B, Sohtell M, Giebisch G. Intracellular potassium activity in the rabbit proximal straight tubule. *Am J Physiol* 1981;241:F677–F686.
90. Bichara M, Paillard M, Corman B, de-Rouffignac C, Leviel F. Volume expansion modulates $NaHCO_3$ and NaCl transport in the proximal tubule and Henle'sloop. *Am J Physiol* 1984;247: F140–F150.
91. Bichara M, Paillard M, Leviel F, Gardin J-P. Hydrogen transport in rabbit kidney proximal tubules—Na:H exchange. *Am J Physiol* 1980;238:F445–F451.
92. Bidet M, Tauc M, Merot J, Vandewalle A, Poujeol P. Na^+–H^+ exchanger in proximal cells isolated from rabbit kidney. I. Functional characteristics. *Am J Physiol* 1987;253:F935–F944.
93. Biemesderfer D, Nagy T, DeGray B, Aronson PS. Specific association of megalin and the Na^+/H^+ exchanger isoform NHE3 in the proximal tubule. *J Biol Chem* 1999;274: 17518–17524.

94. Biemesderfer D, Pizzonia J, Abu-AlfaA, Exner M, Reilly R, Igarashi P, Aronson PS. NHE3: a Na^+/H^+ exchanger isoform of renal brush border. *Am J Physiol* 1993;265:F736–F742.
95. Biemesderfer D, Reilly RF, Exner M, Igarashi P, Aronson PS. Immunocytochemical characterization of Na^+–H^+ exchanger isoform NHE-1 in rabbit kidney. *Am J Physiol* 1992;263: F833–F840.
96. Birnir B, Lee H-S, Hediger MA, Wright EM. Expression and characterization of the intestinal Na^+/glucose cotransporter in COS-7 cells. *Biochim Biophys Acta* 1990;1048:100–104.
97. Blantz RC, Tucker BJ. Determinants of peritubular capillary fluid uptake in hydropenia and saline and plasma expansion. *Am J Physiol* 1975;228:1927–1935.
98. Bloch RD, Zikos D, Fisher KA, Schleicher L, Oyama M, Cheng J-C, Skopicki HA, Sukowski EJ, Cragoe EJ Jr, Peterson DR. Activation of proximal tubular Na^+–H^+ exchange by angiotensin II *Am J Physiol* 1992;263:F135–F143.
99. Bomsztyk K, Wright FS. Effects of transepithelial fluid flux on transepithelial voltage and transport of calcium sodium chloride and potassium by renal proximal tubule. *Kidney Int* 1982;21:269 (abstract).
100. Bomsztyk K, Wright FS. Dependence of ion fluxes on fluid transport by rat proximal tubule. *Am J Physiol* 1986;250:F680–F689.
101. Boonjarern S, Leski ME, Kurtzman NA. Effects of extracellular volume expansion on the tubular reabsorption of glucose. *Pflugers Arch* 1976;366:67–71.
102. Boron WF, Boulpaep EL. Intracellular pH regulation in the renal proximal tubule of the salamander: Na–H exchange. *J Gen Physiol* 1983;81:29–52.
103. Boron WF, Boulpaep EL. Intracellular pH regulation in the renal proximal tubule of the salamander: basolateral HCO_3^- transport. *J Gen Physiol* 1983;81:53–94.
104. Boron WF, Boulpaep EL. The electrogenic Na/HCO_3 cotransporter. *Kidney Int* 1989;36: 392–402.
105. Boron WF, Hediger MA, Boulpaep EL, Romero MF. The renal electrogenic $Na^+:HCO_3^-$ cotransporter. *J Exp Biol* 1997;200:263–268.
106. Boron WF, Sackin H. Measurement of intracellular ionic composition and activities in renal tubules. *Ann Rev Physiol* 1983;45:483–496.
107. Boulanger Y, Vinay P, Boulanger M. NMR monitoring of intracellular sodium in dog and rabbit kidney tubules. *Am J Physiol* 1987;253:F904–F911.
108. Boulpaep EL. Electrophysiological properties of the proximal tubule: importance of cellular and intercellular transport pathways. In: Giebisch G, ed. *Electrophysiology of Epithelial Cells*. Stuttgart: Schattauer Verlag; 1971:91–118.
109. Boulpaep EL. Permeability changes of the proximal tubule of *Necturus* during saline loading. *Am J Physiol* 1972;222:517–531.
110. Boulpaep EL. Electrophysiology of the kidney. In: Giebisch G, ed. *Transport Organs*. Vol. IV. *Membrane Transport in Biology*. Berlin: Springer-Verlag; 1979:97–144.
111. Braam B, Mitchell KD, Fox J, Navar LG. Proximal tubular secretion of angiotensin II in rats. *Am J Physiol* 1993;264:F891–F898.
112. Brenner BM, Falchuk KH, Keimowitz RI, Berliner RW. The relationship between peritubular capillary protein concentration and fluid reabsorption by the renal proximal tubule. *J Clin Invest* 1969;48:1519–1531.
113. Brenner BM, Troy JL. Postglomerular vascular protein concentration: evidence for a causal role in governing fluid reabsorption and glomerulotubular balance by the renal proximal tubule. *J Clin Invest* 1971;50:336–349.
114. Brenner BM, Troy JL, Daugharty TM. On the mechanism of inhibition in fluid reabsorption by the renal proximal tubule of the volume-expanded rat. *J Clin Invest* 1971;50: 1596–1602.
115. Brenner BM, Troy JL, Daugharty TM, MacInnes RM. Quantitative importance of changes in postglomerular colloid osmotic pressure in mediating glomerulotubular balance in the rat. *J Clin Invest* 1973;52:190–197.
116. Breton S, Beck JS, Cardinal J, Giebisch G, Laprade R. Involvement and source of calcium in volume regulatory decrease of collapsed proximal convoluted tubule. *Am J Physiol* 1992;263: F656–F664.
117. Breton S, Marsolais M, Lapointe JY, Laprade R. Cell volume increases of physiologic amplitude activate basolateral K and CI conductances in the rabbit proximal convoluted tubule. *J Am Soc Nephrol* 1996;7:2072–2087.
118. Brismar H, Asghar M, Carey RM, Greengard P, Aperia A. Dopamine-induced recruitment of dopamine D1 receptors to the plasma membrane. *Proc Natl Acad Sci U S A* 1998;95: 5573–5578.
119. Brisolla-Diuana A, Amorena C, Malnic G. Transfer of base across the basolateral membrane of cortical tubules of rat kidney. *Pflugers Arch* 1985;405:209–215.
120. Brown D, Hirsch S, Gluck S. Localization of proton-pumping ATPase in rat kidney. *J Clin Invest* 1988;82:2114–2126.
121. Brown GP, Douglas JG. Angiotensin II binding sites on isolated rat renal brush border membranes. *Endocrinology* 1982;111:1830–1836.
122. Brown GP, Douglas JG. Angiotensin II binding sites in rat and primate isolated renal tubular basolateral membranes. *Endocrinology* 1983;112:2007–2014.
123. Burckhardt B-Ch, Cassola AC, Frömter E. Electrophysiological analysis of bicarbonate permeation across the peritubular cell membrane of rat kidney proximal tubule. II. Exclusion of HCO_3^- effects on other ion permeabilities and of coupled electroneutral HCO_3^- transport. *Pflugers Arch* 1984;401:43–51.
124. Burckhardt B-Ch, Sato K, Frömter E. Electrophysiological analysis of bicarbonate permeation across the peritubular cell membrane of rat kidney proximal tubule. I. Basic observations. *Pflugers Arch* 1984;401:34–42.
125. Burg MB, Green N. Bicarbonate transport by isolated perfused rabbit proximal convoluted tubules. *Am J Physiol* 1977;233:F307–F314.
126. Burg MB, Orloff J. Control of fluid absorption in the renal proximal tubule. *J Clin Invest* 1968;47:2016–2024.
127. Burg MB, Stoner L, Cardinal J, Green N. Furosemide effect on isolated perfused tubules. *Am J Physiol* 1973;225:119–124.
128. Burnham CE, Amlal H, Wang Z, Shull GE, Soleimani M. Cloning and functional expression of a human kidney $Na^+:HCO_3^-$ cotransporter. *J Biol Chem* 1997;272:19111–19114.
129. Burnham CE, Flagella M, Wang Z, Amlal H, Shull GE, Soleimani M. Cloning renal distribution and regulation of the rat $Na^+:HCO_3^-$ cotransporter. *Am J Physiol* 1998;274:F1119–F1126.
130. Burnham C, Munzesheimer C, Rabon E, Sachs G. Ion pathways in renal brush border membranes. *Biochim Biophys Acta* 1982;685:260–272.
131. Cano A, Baum M, Moe OW. Thyroid hormone stimulates the renal Na/H exchanger NHE3 by transcriptional activation. *Am J Physiol* 1999;276:C102–C108.
132. Cano A, Preisig P, Alpern RJ. Cyclic adenosine monophosphate acutely inhibits and chronically stimulates Na/H antiporter in OKP cells. *J Clin Invest* 1993;92:1632–1638.
133. Cantiello HF, Scott JA, Rabito CA. Conductive Na^+ transport in an epithelial cell line (LLC-PK1) with characteristics of proximal tubular cells. *Am J Physiol* 1987;252:F590–F597.
134. Cardinal J, Lapointe J-Y, Laprade R. Luminal and peritubular ionic substitutions and intracellular potential of the rabbit proximal convoluted tubule. *Am J Physiol* 1984;247:F352–F364.
135. Carey RM. Theodore Cooper Lecture. Renal dopamine system: paracrine regulator of sodium homeostasis and blood pressure. *Hypertension* 2001;38:297–302.
136. Carpi-Medina P, Gonzalez E, Whittembury G. Cell osmotic water permeability of isolated rabbit proximal convoluted tubules. *Am J Physiol* 1983;244:F554–F563.
137. Carpi-Medina P, Lindemann B, Gonzalez E, Whittembury G. The continuous measurement of tubular volume changes in response to step changes in contraluminal osmolality. *Pflugers Arch* 1984;400:343–348.
138. Carranza ML, Feraille E, Favre H. Protein kinase C-dependent phosphorylation of Na^+-K^+-ATPase alpha-subunit in rat kidney cortical tubules. *Am J Physiol* 1996;271:C136–C143.
139. Cassano G, Stieger B, Murer H. Na/H and Cl/OH exchange in rat jejunal and rat proximal tubular brush border membrane vesicles. *Pflugers Arch* 1984;400:309–317.
140. Cassola AC, Mollehauer M, Frömter E. The intracellular chloride activity of rat kidney proximal tubular cells. *Pflugers Arch* 1983;399:259–265.
141. Castagna M, Shayakul C, Trotti D, Sacchi VF, Harvey WR, Hediger MA. Molecular characteristics of mammalian and insect amino acid transporters: implications for amino acid homeostasis. *J Exp Biol* 1997;200:269–286.
142. Caulfield JB, Trump BF. Correlation of ultrastructure with function in the rat kidney. *Am J Pathol* 1962;40:199–218.
143. Cemerikic D, Giebisch G. Intracellular sodium activity in *Necturus* kidney proximal tubule. *Fed Proc* 1980;39:1080 (abstract).
144. Cemerikic D, Sackin H. Substrate activation of mechanosensitive whole cell currents in renal proximal tubule. *Am J Physiol* 1993;264:F697–F714.
145. Cemerikic D, Wilcox CS, Giebisch G. Intracellular potential and K^+ activity in rat kidney proximal tubular cells in acidosis and K^+ depletion. *J Membr Biol* 1982;69:159–165.
146. Chalumeau C, du Cheyron D, Defontaine N, Kellermann O, Paillard M, Poggioli J. NHE3 activity and trafficking depend on the state of actin organization in proximal tubule. *Am J Physiol* 2001;280:F283–F290.
147. Chan YL, Biagi B, Giebisch G. Control mechanisms of bicarbonate transport across the rat proximal convoluted tubule. *Am J Physiol* 1982;242:F532–F543.
148. Chen P-Y, Illsley NP, Verkman AS. Renal brush-border chloride transport mechanisms characterized using a fluorescent indicator. *Am J Physiol* 1988;254:F114–F120.
149. Chen P-Y, Verkman AS. Sodium-dependent chloride transport in basolateral membrane vesicles isolated from rabbit proximal tubule. *Biochemistry* 1988;27:655–660.
150. Chen XZ, Coady MJ, Jackson F, Berteloot A, Lapointe JY. Thermodynamic determination of the Na^+:glucose coupling ratio for the human SGLT1 cotransporter. *Biophys J* 1995;69:2405–2414.
151. Cheng H, Becker BN, Harris RC. Dopamine decreases expression of type-1 angiotensin II receptors in renal proximal tubule. *J Clin Invest* 1996;97:2745–2752.
152. Chernova MN, Jiang L, Friedman DJ, Darman RB, Lohi H, Kere J, Vandorpe DH, Alper SL. Functional comparison of mouse slc26a6 anion exchanger with human SLC26A6 polypeptide variants. *J Biol Chem* 2005;280:8564–8580.
153. Chibalin AV, Katz AI, Berggren PO, Bertorello AM. Receptor-mediated inhibition of renal Na^+-K^+-ATPase is associated with endocytosis of its alpha and beta subunits. *Am J Physiol* 1997;273:C1458–C1465.
154. Chibalin AV, Pedemonte CH, Katz AI, Feraille E, Berggren PO, Bertorello AM. Phosphorylation of the catalytic alpha-subunit constitutes a triggering signal for Na^+, K^+-ATPase endocytosis. *J Biol Chem* 1998;273:8814–8819.
155. Choi JY, Shah M, Lee MG, Schultheis PJ, Shull GE, Muallem S, Baum M. Novel amiloride-sensitive sodium-dependent proton secretion in the mouse proximal convoluted tubule. *J Clin Invest* 2000;105:1141–1146.
156. Chonko AM, Osgood RW, Nickel AE, Ferris TF, Stein JH. The measurement of nephron filtration rate and absolute reabsorption in the proximal tubule of the rat kidney. *J Clin Invest* 1975;56:232–235.
157. Chung SD, Alavi N, Livingston D, Hiller S, TaubM. Characterization of primary rabbit kidney cultures that express proximal tubule functions in a hormonally defined medium. *J Cell Biol* 1982;95:118–126.
158. Claude P. Morphological factors influencing transepithelial permeability: a model for the resistance of the zonula occludens. *J Membr Biol* 1978;39:219–232.
159. Claude P, Goodenough DA. Fracture faces of zonulae occludentes from "tight" and "leaky" epithelia. *J Cell Biol* 1973;58:390–400.
160. Cogan MG. Volume expansion predominantly inhibits proximal reabsorption of NaCl rather than $NaHCO_3$. *Am J Physiol* 1983;245:F272–F275.
161. Cogan MG. Angiotensin II: a powerful controller of sodium transport in the early proximal tubule. *Hypertension* 1990;15:451–458.
162. Colegio OR, van Itallie CM, McCrea HJ, Rahner C, Anderson JM. Claudins create charge-selective channels in the paracellular pathway between epithelial cells. *Am J Physiol* 2002;283: C142–C147.
163. Collazo R, Fan L, Hu MC, Zhao H, Wiederkehr MR, Moe OW. Acute regulation of Na^+/H^+ exchanger NHE3 by parathyroid hormone via NHE3 phosphorylation and dynamin-dependent endocytosis. *J Biol Chem* 2000;275:31601–31608.

164. Conger JD, Bartoli E, Earley LE. A study in vivo of peritubular oncotic pressure and proximal tubular reabsorption in the rat. *Clin Sci Mol Med* 1976;51:379–392.
165. Coppola S, Frömter E. An electrophysiological study of angiotensin II regulation of Na-HCO_3 cotransport and K conductance in renal proximal tubules. I. Effect of picomolar concentrations. *Pflugers Arch* 1994;427:143–150.
166. Corcia A, Armstrong WM. KCl cotransport: a mechanism for basolateral chloride exit in *Necturus* gallbladder. *J Membr Biol* 1983;76:173–182.
167. Corman B. Streaming potentials and diffusion potentials across rabbit proximal convoluted tubule. *Pflugers Arch* 1985;403:156–163.
168. Corman B, Roinel N, de Rouffignac C. Water reabsorption capacity of the proximal convoluted tubule: a microperfusion study on rat kidney. *J Physiol* 1981;316:379–392.
169. Cunningham R, Steplock D, Wang F, Huang H, Xiaofei E, Shenolikar S, Weinman EJ. Defective parathyroid hormone regulation of NHE3 activity and phosphate adaptation in cultured NHERF-1-/- renal proximal tubule cells. *J Biol Chem* 2004;279:37815–37821.
170. Curran PF. Na Cl and water transport by rat ileum in vitro. *J Gen Physiol* 1960;43: 1137–1148.
171. Darvish N, Winaver J, Dagan D. Diverse modulations of chloride channels in renal proximal tubules. *Am J Physiol* 1994;267:F716–F724.
172. Dawson DC, Richards NW. Basolateral K conductance: role in regulation of NaCl absorption and secretion. *Am J Physiol* 1990;259:C181–C195.
173. Dellasega M, Grantham JJ. Regulation of renal tubule cell volume in hypotonic media. *Am J Physiol* 1973;224:1288–1294.
174. DeNicola L, Blantz RC, Gabbai FB. Nitric oxide and angiotensin II: Glomerular and tubular interactions in the rat. *J Clin Invest* 1992;89:1248–1256.
175. Dennis VW. Influence of bicarbonate on parathyroid hormone-induced changes in fluid absorption by the proximal tubule. *Kidney Int* 1976;10:373–380.
176. DiBona GF. Neural regulation of renal tubular sodium reabsorption and renin secretion. *Fed Proc* 1985;44:2816–2822.
177. Dirks JH, Cirksena WJ, Berliner RW. The effect of saline infusion on sodium reabsorption by the proximal tubule of the dog. *J Clin Invest* 1965;44:1160–1170.
178. Dolson GM, Hise MK, Weinman EJ. Relationship among parathyroid hormone cAMP, and calcium on proximal tubule sodium transport. *Am J Physiol* 1985;249:F409–F416.
179. Dominguez JH, Mann R, Rothrock JK, Bhati V. Na^+-Ca^{++} exchange and Ca^{++} depletion in rat proximal tubules. *Am J Physiol* 1991;261:F328–F335.
180. Dominguez JH, Rothrock JK, Macias WL, Price J. Na^+ electrochemical gradient and Na^+–Ca^{++} exchange in rat proximal tubule. *Am J Physiol* 1989;257:F531–F538.
180a. Dos Santos EA, Dahly-Vernon AJ, Hoagland KM, and Roman RJ (2004). Inhibition of the formation of EETs and 20-HETE with 1-aminobenzotriazole attenuates pressure natriuresis. *Am J Physiol* 287:R58–R68.
181. Doucet A, Katz AI, Morel F. Determination of Na-K-ATPase activity in single segments of the mammalian nephron. *Am J Physiol* 1979;237:F105–F113.
182. Douglas JG, Hopfer U. Novel aspect of angiotensin receptors and signal transduction in the kidney. *Ann Rev Physiol* 1994;56:649–669.
183. Doyle FA, McGivan JD. Reconstitution and identification of the major Na (+)-dependent neutral amino acid-transport protein from bovine renal brush-border membrane vesicles. *Biochem J* 1992;281:95–102.
184. Du Z, Yan Q, Duan Y, Weinbaum S, Weinstein AM, Wang T. Axial flow modulates proximal tubule NHE3 and H-ATPase activities by changing microvillous bending moments. *Am J Physiol* 2006;290:F289–F296.
185. Du Z, Duan Y, Yan Q, Weinstein AM, Weinbaum S, Wang T. Mechanosensory function of microvilli of the kidney proximal tubule. *Proc Natl Acad Sci U S A* 2004;101:13068–13073.
186. du Cheyron D, Chalumeau C, Defontaine N, Klein C, Kellermann O, Paillard M, Poggioli J. Angiotensin II stimulates NHE3 activity by exocytic insertion of the transporter:role of PI 3-kinase. *Kidney Int* 2003;64:939–949.
187. Ducoudret O, Diakov A, Muller-Berger S, Romero MF, Frömter E. The renal Na-HCO_3^- cotransporter expressed in Xenopus laevis oocytes: inhibition by tenidap and benzamil and effect of temperature on transport rate and stoichiometry. *Pflugers Arch* 2001;442:709–717.
188. Durbin RP. Osmotic flow of water across permeable cellulose membranes. *J Gen Physiol* 1960;44:315–326.
189. Earley LE, Martino JA, Friedler RM. Factors affecting sodium reabsorption by the proximal tubule as determined during blockade of distal sodium reabsorption. *J Clin Invest* 1966;45:1668–1684.
190. Earley LE, Schrier RW. Intrarenal control of sodium excretion by hemodynamic and physical factors. In: Orloff J, Berliner RW, eds. *Handbook of Physiology*. Section 8: Renal Physiology. Washington, DC: American Physiological Society; 1973:721–762.
191. Edelman A, Anagnostopoulos T. Further studies on ion permeation in proximal tubule of *Necturus* kidney. *Am J Physiol* 1978;235:F89–F95.
192. Edelman A, Bouthier M, Anagnostopoulos T. Chloride distribution in the proximal convoluted tubule of *Necturus* kidney. *J Membr Biol* 1981;62:7–17.
193. Edelman A, Curci S, Samarzija I, Frömter E. Determination of intracellular K^+ activity in rat kidney proximal tubular cells. *Pflugers Arch* 1978;378:37–45.
194. Edwards RM, Alyar N. Angiotensin II receptor subtypes in the kidney. *J Am Soc Nephrol* 1993;3:1643–1652.
195. Efendiev R, Bertorello AM, PressleyTA, Rousselot M, Feraille E, Pedemonte CH. Simultaneous phosphorylation of Ser11 and Ser18 in the alpha-subunit promotes the recruitment of Na (+), K (+)-ATPase molecules to the plasma membrane. *Biochemistry* 2000;39:9884–9892.
196. Efendiev R, Bertorello AM, Zandomeni R, Cinelli AR, Pedemonte CH. Agonist-dependent regulation of renal Na^+, K^+-ATPase activity is modulated by intracellular sodium concentration. *J Biol Chem* 2002;277:11489–11496.
197. Eiam-Ong S, Hilden SA, Johns CA, Madias NE. Stimulation of basolateral Na^+–HCO_3^- cotransporter by angiotensin II in rabbit renal cortex. *Am J Physiol* 1993;265:F195–F203.
198. Eitle E, Hiranyachattada S, Wang H, Harris PJ. Inhibition of proximal tubular fluid absorption by nitric oxide and atrial natriuretic peptide in rat kidney. *Am J Physiol* 1998;274: C1075–C1080.
199. El Mernissi G, Doucet A. Quantitation of [3H]ouabain binding and turnover of Na-K-ATPase along the rabbit nephron. *Am J Physiol* 1984;247:F158–F167.
200. Enck AH, Berger UV, YuAS. Claudin-2 is selectively expressed in proximal nephron in mouse kidney. *Am J Physiol* 2001;281:F966–F974.
201. Evan AP, Baker JT, Bengele HH. Zonulae occludentes of the rat nephron under conditions of experimental expansion of blood and/or fluid volume. *Anat Res* 1976;186:139–150.
202. Eveloff JL, Warnock DG. Activation of ion transport systems during cell volume regulation. *Am J Physiol* 1987;252:F1–F10.
203. Eveloff J, Warnock DG. K-Cl transport systems in rabbit renal basolateral membrane vesicles. *Am J Physiol* 1987;252:F883–F889.
204. Falchuk KH, Berliner RW. Hydrostatic pressures in peritubular capillaries and tubules in the rat kidney. *Am J Physiol* 1971;220:1422–1426.
205. Falchuk KH, Brenner BM, Tadokoro M, Berliner RW. Oncotic and hydrostatic pressures in peritubular capillaries and fluid reabsorption by proximal tubule. *Am J Physiol* 1971;220:1427–1433.
206. Fan L, Wiederkehr MR, CollazoR, Wang H, Crowder LA, Moe OW. Dual mechanisms of regulation of Na/H exchanger NHE-3 by parathyroid hormone in rat kidney. *J Biol Chem* 1999;274:11289–11295.
207. Felder CC, Campbell T, Albrecht F, Jose PA. Dopamine inhibits Na^+–H^+ exchanger activity in renal BBMV by stimulation of adenylate cyclase. *Am J Physiol* 1990;259:F297–F303.
208. Feraille E, Carranza ML, Buffin-Meyer B, Rousselot M, Doucet A, Favre H. Protein kinase C-dependent stimulation of Na^+-K^+-ATPase in rat proximal convoluted tubule. *Am J Physiol* 1995;268:C1277–C1283.
209. Feraille E, Doucet A. Sodium-potassium-adenosine triphosphatase-dependent sodium transport in the kidney: hormonal control. *Physiol Rev* 2001;81:345–418.
210. Feschenko MS, Sweadner KJ. Conformation-dependent phosphorylation of Na K-ATPase by protein kinase A and protein kinase C *J Biol Chem* 1994;269:30436–30444.
211. Filipovic D, Sackin H. A calcium-permeable stretch-activated cation channel in renal proximal tubule. *Am J Physiol* 1991;260:F119–F129.
212. Filipovic D, Sackin H. Stretch-and volume-activated channels in isolated proximal tubule cells. *Am J Physiol* 1992;262:F857–F870.
213. Fine LG, Sakhrani LM. Proximal tubular cells in primary culture. *Miner Electrolyte Metab* 1986;12:51–57.
214. Finn AL, Reuss L. Effects of changes in the composition of the serosal solution on the electrical properties of the toad urinary bladder epithelium. *J Physiol* 1975;250:541–558.
215. Fisher KA, Lee SH, Walker J, Dileto-Fang C, Ginsberg L, Stapleton SR. Regulation of proximal tubule sodium/hydrogen antiporter with chronic volume contraction. *Am J Physiol* 2001;280:F922–F926.
216. Fitzgibbons JP, Gennari FJ, Garfinkel HB, Cortell S. Dependence of saline-induced natriuresis upon exposure of the kidney to the physical effects of extracellular fluid volume expansion. *J Clin Invest* 1974;54:1428–1436.
217. Fraser WD, Baines AD. Application of a fiber-matrix model to transport in renal tubules. *J Gen Physiol* 1989;94:863–879.
218. Friedman PA, Figueiredo JF, Maack T, Windhager EE. Sodium-calcium interactions in the renal proximal convoluted tubule of the rabbit. *Am J Physiol* 1981;240:F558–F568.
219. Frindt G, Lee CO, Yang JM, Windhager EE. Potential role of cytoplasmic calcium ions in the regulation of sodium transport in renal tubules. *Miner Electrolyte Metab* 1988;14:40–47.
220. Frizzell RA, Dugas MC, Schultz SG. Sodium chloride transport by rabbit gallbladder. *J Gen Physiol* 1975;65:769–795.
221. Frömter E. Electrophysiology and isotonic fluid absorption of proximal tubules of mammalian kidney. In: Thurau KT, ed. *Kidney and Urinary Tract Physiology*. MTP International Reviews of Science Physiology Series I, Vol. 6. Baltimore: University Park Press; 1974:1–38.
222. Frömter E. Magnitude and significance of the paracellular shunt path in rat kidney proximal tubule. In: Kramer M, Lauterbach F, eds. *Intestinal Permeation*. Vol. 4. Amsterdam: Excerpta Medica; 1977:393–405.
223. Frömter E. Solute transport across epithelia: what can we learn from micropuncture studies on kidney tubules? *J Physiol (Lond)* 1979;288:1–31.
224. Frömter E. Electrophysiological analysis of rat renal sugar and amino acid transport. *Pflugers Arch* 1982;393:179–189.
225. Frömter E. Viewing the kidney through microelectrodes. *Am J Physiol* 1984;247:F695–F705.
226. Frömter E, Gessner K. Free-flow potential profile along rat kidney proximal tubule. *Pflugers Arch* 1974;351:69–83.
227. Frömter E, Gessner K. Active transport potentials membrane diffusion potentials and streaming potentials across rat kidney proximal tubule. *Pflugers Arch* 1974;351:85–98.
228. Frömter E, Gessner K. Effect of inhibitors and diuretics on electrical potential differences in rat kidney proximal tubule. *Pflugers Arch* 1975;357:209–224.
229. Frömter E, Muller CW, Wick T. Permeability properties of the proximal tubular epithelium of the rat kidney studied with electrophysiological methods. In: Giebisch G, ed. *Electrophysiology of Epithelial Cells*. Stuttgart: Schattauer Verlag; 1971:119–148.
230. Frömter E, Rumrich G, Ullrich KJ. Phenomenologic description of Na^+ Cl^- and HCO_3^- absorption from proximal tubules. *Pflugers Arch* 1973;343:189–220.
231. Frömter E, Sato K. Electrical events in active H^+/HCO_3^- transport across rat kidney proximal tubular epithelium. In: Kasbeker DK, Sachs G, Rehm WS, eds. *Gastric Hydrogen Ion Secretion*. New York: Marcel Dekker; 1976:382–403.
232. Furuse M, Fujita K, Hiiragi T, Fujimoto K, Tsukita S. Claudin-1 and -2: novel integral membrane proteins localizing at tight junctions with no sequence similarity to occludin. *J Cell Biol* 1998;141:1539–1550.
233. Furuse M, Furuse K, Sasaki H, Tsukita S. Conversion of zonulae occludentes from tight to leaky strand type by introducing claudin-2 into Madin–Darby canine kidney I cells. *J Cell Biol* 2001;153:263–272.
234. Furuse M, Hirase T, Itoh M, Nagafuchi A, Yonemura S, Tsukita S, Tsukita S. Occludin: a novel integral membrane protein localizing at tight junctions. *J Cell Biol* 1993;123:1777–1788.
235. Furuse M, Sasaki H, Fujimoto K, Tsukita S. A single gene product claudin-1 or -2, reconstitutes tight junction strands and recruits occludin in fibroblasts. *J Cell Biol* 1998;43:391–401.

236. Garg LC, Knepper MA, Burg MB. Mineralocorticoid effects on Na-K-ATPase in individual nephron segments. *Am J Physiol* 1981;240:F536–F544.
237. Garvin JL. Angiotensin stimulates bicarbonate transport and Na^+/K^+ ATPase in rat proximal straight tubules. *J Am Soc Nephrol* 1991;1:1146–1152.
238. Garvin JL. ANF inhibits norepinephrine-stimulated fluid absorption in rat proximal straight tubules. *Am J Physiol* 1992;263:F581–F585.
239. Geibel J, Giebisch G, Boron WF. Basolateral sodium-coupled acid–base transport mechanisms of the rabbit proximal tubule. *Am J Physiol* 1989;257:F790–F797.
240. Geibel J, Giebisch G, Boron WF. Angiotensin II stimulates both Na^+/H^+ exchange and Na^+/HCO_3^- cotransport in the rabbit proximal tubule. *Proc Natl Acad Sci U S A* 1990;87: 7917–7920.
241. Gertz KH, Boylan JW. Glomerular-tubular balance. In: Orloff J, Berliner RW, eds. *Handbook of Physiology*. Section 8: Renal Physiology. Washington, DC: American Physiological Society; 1973:763–790.
242. Gesek FA, Schoolwerth AC. Hormonal interactions with the proximal Na^+–H^+ exchanger. *Am J Physiol* 1990;258:F514–F521.
243. Giebisch G. Measurements of pH, chloride and inulin concentrations in proximal tubule fluid of *Necturus*. *Am J Physiol* 1956;1985:171–174.
244. Giebisch G. Measurements of electrical potential differences on single nephrons of the perfused *Necturus* kidney. *J Gen Physiol* 1961;44:659–678.
245. Giebisch G, Windhager EE. Measurement of chloride movement across single proximal tubules of *Necturus* kidney. *Am J Physiol* 1963;204:387–391.
246. Giebisch G, Windhager EE. Renal tubular transfer of sodium chloride and potassium. *Am J Med* 1964;36:643–669.
247. Girardi AC, Knauf F, Demuth HU, Aronson PS. Role of dipeptidyl peptidase IV in regulating activity of Na^+/H^+ exchanger isoform NHE3 in proximal tubule cells. *Am J Physiol* 2004;287: C1238–C1245.
248. Girardi AC, Titan SMO, Malnic G, Reboucas NA. Chronic effect of parathyroid hormone on NHE3 expression in rat renal proximal tubules. *Kidney Int* 2000;58:1623–1631.
249. Glynn IM, Karlish SJD. The sodium pump. *Annu Rev Physiol* 1975;37:13–55.
250. Gmaj P, Murer H. Calcium transport mechanisms in epithelial cell membranes. *Miner Electrolyte Metab* 1988;14:22–30.
251. Gmaj P, Murer H, Kinne R. Calcium ion transport across plasma membranes isolated from rat kidney cortex. *Biochem J* 1979;178:549–557.
252. Gogelein H, Greger R. Single channel recordings from basolateral and apical membranes of renal proximal tubules. *Pflugers Arch* 1984;401:424–426.
253. Gogelein H, Greger R. Na^+ selective channels in the apical membrane of rabbit late proximal tubules (pars recta). *Pflugers Arch* 1986;406:198–203.
254. Goligorsky MS, Menton DN, Hruska KA. Parathyroid hormone-induced changes of the brush border topography and cytoskeleton in cultured renal proximal tubular cells. *J Membr Biol* 1986;92:151–162.
255. Gomes GN, Aires MM. Interaction of atrial natriuretic factor and angiotensin II in proximal HCO_3^- reabsorption. *Am J Physiol* 1992;262:F303–F308.
256. Gonska T, Hirsch JR, Schlatter E. Amino acid transport in the renal proximal tubule. *Amino Acids* 2000;19:395–407.
257. Gonzalez E, Carpi-Medina P, Whittembury G. Cell osmotic water permeability of isolated rabbit proximal straight tubules. *Am J Physiol* 1982;242:F321–F330.
258. Gonzalez-Campoy JM, Long C, Roberts D, Berndt TJ, Romero JC, Knox FG. Renal interstitial hydrostatic pressure and PGE2 in pressure natriuresis. *Am J Physiol* 1991;260: F643–F649.
259. Gottschalk CW. Renal tubular function: lessons from micropuncture. In: *The Harvey Lectures*, series 58. New York and London: Academic Press; 1963:99–124.
260. Gottschalk CW. Renal nerves and sodium excretion. *Ann Rev Physiol* 1979;41:229–240.
261. Goyal S, Mentone S, Aronson PS. Immunolocalization of NHE8 in rat kidney. *Am J Physiol* 2005;288:F530–F538.
262. Goyal S, Vanden Heuvel G, Aronson PS. Renal expression of novel Na^+/H^+ exchanger isoform NHE8. *Am J Physiol* 2003;284:F467–F473.
263. Grandchamp A, Boulpaep EL. Pressure control of sodium reabsorption and intercellular backflux across proximal kidney tubule. *J Clin Invest* 1974;54:69–82.
264. Granger JP, Haas JA, Pawlowska D, Knox FG. Effect of direct increases in renal interstitial hydrostatic pressure on sodium excretion. *Am J Physiol* 1988;254:F527–F532.
265. Grantham JJ, Lowe CM, Dellasega M, Cole BR. Effect of hypotonic medium on K and Na content of proximal renal tubules. *Am J Physiol* 1977;232:F42–F49.
266. Grasset E, Gunter-Smith P, Schultz SG. Effects of Na-coupled alanine transport on intracellular K activities and the K conductance of the basolateral membranes of *Necturus* small intestine. *J Membr Biol* 1983;71:89–94.
267. Grassl SM, Aronson PS. Na^+/HCO_3^- co-transport in basolateral membrane vesicles isolated from rabbit renal cortex. *J Biol Chem* 1986;261:8778–8783.
268. Grassl SM, Holohan PD, Ross CR. HCO_3^- transport in basolateral membrane vesicles isolated from rat renal cortex. *J Biol Chem* 1987;262:2682–2687.
269. Green M, Ruiz OS, Kear F, Arruda JAL. Dual effect of cyclic GMP on renal brush border Na–H antiporter. *Proc Soc Exp Biol Med* 1991;198:846–851.
270. Green R, Giebisch G. Ionic requirements of proximal tubular sodium transport. I. Bicarbonate and chloride. *Am J Physiol* 1975;229:1205–1215.
271. Green R, Giebisch G. Luminal hypotonicity: a driving force for fluid absorption from the proximal tubule. *Am J Physiol* 1984;246:F167–F174.
272. Green R, Giebisch G. Reflection coefficients and water permeability in rat proximal tubule. *Am J Physiol* 1989;257:F658–F668.
273. Green R, Giebisch G, Unwin R, Weinstein AM. Coupled water transport by rat proximal tubule. *Am J Physiol* 1991;261:F1046–F1054.
274. Green R, Moriarty RJ, Giebisch G. Ionic requirements of proximal tubular fluid reabsorption: flow dependence of fluid transport. *Kidney Int* 1981;20:580–587.
275. Green R, Windhager EE, Giebisch G. Protein oncotic pressure effects on proximal tubular fluid movement in the rat. *Am J Physiol* 1974;226:265–276.
276. Grinstein S, Rothstein A. Mechanisms of regulation of the Na^+/H^+ exchanger. *J Membr Biol* 1986;90:1–12.
277. Gross E, Hawkins K, Abuladze N, Pushkin A, Cotton CU, Hopfer U, Kurtz I. The stoichiometry of the electrogenic sodium bicarbonate cotransporter NBC1 is cell-type dependent. *J Physiol* 2001;531:597–603.
278. Gross E, Hawkins K, Pushkin A, Sassani P, Dukkipati R, Abuladze N, Hopfer U, Kurtz I. Phosphorylation of Ser(982) in the sodium bicarbonate cotransporter kNBC1 shifts the HCO_3^-:Na^+ stoichiometry from 3:1 to 2:1 in murine proximal tubule cells. *J Physiol* 2001;537:659–665.
279. Gross E, Hopfer U. Effects of pH on kinetic parameters of the Na–HCO_3 cotransporter in renal proximal tubule. *Biophys J* 1999;76:3066–3075.
280. Gross E, Hopfer U. Voltage and cosubstrate dependence of the Na–HCO_3 cotransporter kinetics in renal proximal tubule cells. *Biophys J* 1998;75:810–824.
281. Guggino WB, Boulpaep EL, Giebisch G. Electrical properties of chloride transport across the *Necturus* proximal tubule. *J Membr Biol* 1982;65:185–196.
282. Guggino WB, London R, Boulpaep EL, Giebisch G. Chloride transport across the basolateral cell membrane of the *Necturus* proximal tubule: dependence on bicarbonate and sodium. *J Membr Biol* 1983;71:227–240.
283. Guggino WB, Windhager EE, Boulpaep EL, Giebisch G. Cellular and paracellular resistances of the *Necturus* proximal tubule. *J Membr Biol* 1982;67:143–154.
284. Gullans SR, Avison MJ, Ogino T, Giebisch G, Shulman RG. NMR measurements of intracellular sodium in the rabbit proximal tubule. *Am J Physiol* 1985;249:F160–F168.
285. Gullans SR, Brazy PC, Soltoff SP, Dennis VW, Mandel LJ. Metabolic inhibitors: effects on metabolism and transport in the proximal tubule. *Am J Physiol* 1982;243: F133–F140.
286. Gunter-Smith PJ, Grasset E, Schultz SG. Sodium-coupled amino acid and sugar transport by *Necturus* small intestine. An equivalent electrical circuit analysis of a rheogenic cotransport system. *J Membr Biol* 1982;66:25–39.
287. Guo P, Weinstein AM, Weinbaum S. A dual-pathway ultrastructural model for the tight junction of rat proximal tubule epithelium. *Am J Physiol* 2003;285:F241–F257.
288. Guo P, Weinstein AM, Weinbaum S. A hydrodynamic mechanosensory hypothesis for brush border microvilli. *Am J Physiol* 2000;279:F698–F712.
289. Gutierrez AM, Gonzalez E, Echevarria M, Hernandez CS, Whittembury G. The proximal straight tubule (PST) basolateral cell membrane water channel: selectivity characteristics. *J Membr Biol* 1995;143:189–197.
290. Guzman NJ, Fang M-Z, Tang S-S, Ingelfinger JR, Garg LC. Autocrine inhibition of Na^+/K^+-ATPase by nitric oxide in mouse proximal tubule epithelial cells. *J Clin Invest* 1995;95: 2083–2088.
291. Gyory AZ, Beck F, Rick R, Thurau K. Electron microprobe analysis of proximal tubule cellular Na Cl and K element concentrations during acute mannitol-saline volume expansion in rats: evidence for inhibition of the Na pump. *Pflugers Arch* 1985;403:205–209.
292. Haas JA, Granger JP, Knox FG. Effect of intrarenal volume expansion on proximal sodium reabsorption. *Am J Physiol* 1988;255:F1178–F1182.
293. Haberle DA, Shiigai T. Flow-dependent volume reabsorption in the proximal convolution of the rat kidney-the role of glomerular-born tubular fluid for the maintenance of glomerulotubular balance. In: Vogel HGV, Ullrich KJ, eds. *New Aspects of Renal Function*. Amsterdam: Excerpta Medica; 1978:198–206.
294. Haberle DA, Shiigai TT, Maier G, Schiffl H, Davis JM. Dependency of proximal tubular fluid transport on the load of glomerular filtrate. *Kidney Int* 1981;20:18–28.
295. Haberle DA, von Baeyer H. Characteristics of glomerulotubular balance. *Am J Physiol* 1983;244:F355–F366.
296. Haithcock D, Jiao H, Cui XL, Hopfer U, Douglas JG. Renal proximal tubular AT2 receptor: signaling and transport. *J Am Soc Nephrol* 1999;10(Suppl 11):S69–S74.
297. Hall RA, Premont RT, ChowCW, Blitzer JT, Pitcher JA, Claing A, Stoffel RH, Barak LS, Shenolikar S, Weinman EJ, Grinstein S, Lefkowitz RJ. The beta2-adrenergic receptor interacts with the Na^+/H^+-exchanger regulatory factor to control Na^+/H^+ exchange. *Nature* 1998;392:626–630.
298. Hamburger RJ, Lawson NL, Schwartz JH. Response to parathyroid hormone in defined segments of proximal tubule. *Am J Physiol* 1976;230:286–290.
299. Han HJ, Park SH, Koh HJ, TaubM. Mechanism of regulation of Na^+ transport by angiotensin II in primary renal cells. *Kidney Int* 2000;57:2457–2467.
300. Harris CA, Baer PG, Chirito E, Dirks JH. Composition of mammalian glomerular filtrate. *Am J Physiol* 1974;227:972–976.
301. Harris PJ. Regulation of proximal tubule function by angiotensin. *Clin Exp Pharmacol Physiol* 1992;19:213–222.
302. Harris PJ, Navar LG. Tubular transport responses to angiotensin. *Am J Physiol* 1985;248: F621–F630.
303. Harris PJ, Thomas D, Morgan TO. Atrial natriuretic peptide inhibits angiotensin-stimulated proximal tubular sodium and water reabsorption. *Nature* 1987;326:697–698.
304. Harris PJ, Young JA. Dose-dependent stimulation and inhibition of proximal tubular sodium reabsorption by angiotensin II in the rat kidney. *Pflugers Arch* 1977;367:295–297.
305. Harris SI, Balaban RS, Mandel LJ. Oxygen consumption and cellular ion transport: evidence for adenosine triphosphate to O2 ratio near 6 in intact cell. *Science* 1980;208: 1148–1150.
306. Harris SI, Patton L, Barrett L, Mandel LJ. (Na^+K^+)-ATPase kinetics within the intact renal cell. *J Biol Chem* 1982;257:6996–7002.
307. Hayashi H, Szaszi K, Grinstein S. Multiple modes of regulation of Na^+/H^+ exchangers. *Ann N Y Acad Sci* 2002;976:248–258.
308. Hayslett JP. Effect of changes in hydrostatic pressure in peritubular capillaries on the permeability of the proximal tubule. *J Clin Invest* 1973;52:1314–1319.
309. Hazama A, Loo DD, Wright EM. Pre-steady-state currents of the rabbit Na^+/glucose cotransporter (SGLT1). *J Membr Biol* 1997;155:175–186.
310. Hebert SC, Mount DB, Gamba G. Molecular physiology of cation-coupled Cl^- cotransport: the SCL12 family. *Pflugers Arch* 2004;447:580–593.

311. Hediger MA, Coady MJ, Ikeda TS, Wright EM. Expression cloning and cDNA sequencing of the Na^+/glucose co-transporter. *Nature* 1987;330:379–381.
312. Hediger MA, Rhoads DB. Molecular physiology of sodium-glucose cotransporters. *Physiol Rev* 1994;74:993–1026.
313. Heinz E, Weinstein AM. The overshoot phenomenon in cotransport. *Biochim Biophys Acta* 1984;776:83–91.
314. Hensley CB, Bradley ME, Mircheff AK. Parathyroid hormone-induced translocation of Na–H antiporters in rat proximal tubules. *Am J Physiol* 1989;257:C637–C645.
315. Hierholzer K, Kawamura S, Seldin DW, Kokko JP, Jacobson HR. Reflection coefficients of various substrates across superficial and juxtamedullary proximal convoluted segments of rabbit nephrons. *Miner Electrolyte Metab* 1980;3:172–180.
316. Higgins JT Jr, Meinders AE. Quantitative relationship of renal glucose and sodium reabsorption during ECF expansion. *Am J Physiol* 1975;229:66–71.
317. Hilden SA, Sacktor B. D-glucose–dependent sodium transport in renal brush border membrane vesicles. *J Biol Chem* 1979;254:7090–7096.
318. Hirayama BA, Loo DD, Wright EM. Protons drive sugar transport through the Na^+/glucose cotransporter (SGLT1). *J Biol Chem* 1994;269:21407–21410.
319. Hirayama BA, Lostao MP, Panayotova-Heiermann M, Loo DD, Turk E, Wright EM. Kinetic and specificity differences between rat human and rabbit Na^+-glucose c transporters (SGLT-1). *Am J Physiol* 1996;270:G919–C926.
320. Hirayama BA, Wong HC, Smith CD, Hagenbuch BA, Hediger MA, Wright EM. Intestinal and renal Na^+/glucose c transporters share common structures. *Am J Physiol* 1991;261:C296–C304.
321. Holmberg C, Kokko JP, Jacobson HR. Determination of chloride bicarbonate permeabilities in proximal convoluted tubules. *Am J Physiol* 1981;241:F386–F394.
322. Holtback U, Eklof AC. Mechanism of FK 506/520 action on rat renal proximal tubular Na^+, K^+-ATPase activity. *Kidney Int* 1999;56:1014–1021.
323. Holzgreve H, Schrier RW. Variation of proximal tubular reabsorptive capacity by volume expansion and aortic constriction during constancy of peritubular capillary protein concentration in rat kidney. *Pflugers Arch* 1975;356:73–86.
324. Hopfer J, Groseclose R. The mechanism of Na^+-dependent D-glucose transport. *J Biol Chem* 1980;255:4453–4462.
325. Horie S, Moe O, Tejedor A, Alpern RJ. Preincubation in acid medium increases Na/H antiporter activity in cultured renal proximal tubule cells. *Proc Natl Acad Sci U S A* 1990;87:4742–4745.
326. Houillier P, Chambrey R, Achard JM, Froissart M, Poggioli J, Paillard M. Signaling pathways in the biphasic effect of angiotensin II on apical Na/H antiport activity in proximal tubule. *Kidney Int* 1996;50:1496–1505.
327. Howlin KJ, Alpern RJ, Rector FC Jr. Amiloride inhibition of proximal tubular acidification. *Am J Physiol* 1985;248:F773–F778.
328. Hoyer J, Gogelein H. Sodium-alanine cotransport in renal proximal tubule cells investigated by whole-cell recording. *J Gen Physiol* 1991;97:1073–1094.
329. Hruska KA, Moskowitz D, Esbrit P, Civitelli R, Westbrook S, Huskey M. Stimulation of inositol trisphosphate and diacylglycerol production in renal tubular cells by parathyroid hormone. *J Clin Invest* 1987;79:230–239.
330. Hu MC, Fan L, Crowder LA, Karim-Jimenez Z, Murer H, Moe OW. Dopamine acutely stimulates Na^+/H^+ exchanger (NHE3) endocytosis via clathrin-coated vesicles: dependence on protein kinase A–mediated NHE3 phosphorylation. *J Biol Chem* 2001;276: 26906–26915.
331. Humbert F, Grandchamp A, Pricam C, Perrelet A, Orci L. Morphological changes in tight junctions of *Necturus* maculosus proximal tubules undergoing saline diuresis. *J Cell Biol* 1976;69:90–96.
332. Hurst AM, Beck JS, Laprade R, Lapointe J-Y. Na^+ pump inhibition downregulates an ATP-sensitive K^+ channel in rabbit proximal convoluted tubule. *Am J Physiol* 1993;264: F760–F764.
333. Huss RE, Marsh DJ. A model of NaCl and water flow through paracellular pathways of renal proximal tubules. *J Membr Biol* 1975;23:305–347.
334. Huss RE, Stephenson JL. A mathematical model of proximal tubule absorption. *J Membr Biol* 1979;47:377–399.
335. Ibarra F, Aperia A, Svensson L-B, Eklof A-C, Greengard P. Bidirectional regulation of Na^+K^+-ATPase activity by dopamine and an alpha-adrenergic agonist. *Proc Natl Acad Sci U S A* 1993;90:21–24.
336. Ibarra FR, Cheng SX, Agren M, Svensson LB, Aizman O, Aperia A. Intracellular sodium modulates the state of protein kinase C phosphorylation of rat proximal tubule Na^+, K^+-ATPase. *Acta Physiol Scand* 2002;175:165–171.
337. Ichikawa I, Brenner BM. Mechanism of inhibition of proximal tubule fluid reabsorption after exposure of the rat kidney to the physical effects of expansion of extracellular fluid volume. *J Clin Invest* 1979;64:1466–1474.
338. Ikeda TS, Hwang E-S, Coady MJ, Hirayama BA, Hediger MA, Wright EM. Characterization of a Na^+/glucose cotransporter cloned from rabbit small intestine. *J Membr Biol* 1989;110:87–95.
339. Illsley NP, Verkman AS. Membrane chloride transport measured using a chloride sensitive fluorescent probe. *Biochemistry* 1987;26:1215–1219.
340. Imai M, Kokko JP. Effect of peritubular protein concentration on reabsorption of sodium and water in isolated perfused proximal tubules. *J Clin Invest* 1972;51:314–325.
341. Imai M, Kokko JP. Transtubular oncotic pressure gradients and net fluid transport in isolated proximal tubules. *Kidney Int* 1974;6:138–145.
342. Imai M, Seldin DW, Kokko JP. Effect of perfusion rate on the fluxes of water sodium chloride and urea across the proximal convoluted tubule. *Kidney Int* 1977;11:18–27.
343. Ishibashi K, Rector FC Jr, Berry CA. Chloride transport across the basolateral membrane of rabbit proximal convoluted tubules. *Am J Physiol* 1990;258:F1569–F1578.
344. Ishibashi K, Rector FC Jr, Berry CA. Role of Na-dependent Cl/HCO_3 exchange in basolateral Cl transport of rabbit proximal tubules. *Am J Physiol* 1993;264:F251–F258.
345. Ishibashi K, Sasaki S, Yoshiyama N. Intracellular chloride activity of rabbit proximal straight tubule perfused in vitro. *Am J Physiol* 1988;255:F49–F56.
345a. Ito O, Alonso-Galicia M, Hopp KA, and Roman RJ (1998). Localization of cytochrome P-450 4A isoforms along the rat nephron. *Am J Physiol* 274:F395–F404.
346. Ives HE, Chen P-Y, Verkman AS. Mechanism of coupling between Cl^- and OH^- transport in renal brush-border membranes. *Biochim Biophys Acta* 1986;863:91–100.
347. Ives HE, Yee VJ, Warnock DG. Asymmetric distribution of the Na^+/H^+ antiporter in the renal proximal tubule epithelial cell. *J Biol Chem* 1983;258:13513–13516.
348. Jacobsen C, Kragh-Hansen U, Sheikh MI. Na^+–H^+ exchange in luminal-membrane vesicles from rabbit proximal convoluted and straight tubules in response to metabolic acidosis. *Biochem J* 1986;239:411–416.
349. Jacobsen C, Rigaard-Petersen H, Sheikh MI. Demonstration of Na^+-selective channels in the luminal-membrane vesicles isolated from pars recta of rabbit proximal tubule. *FEBS Lett* 1988;236:95–99.
350. Jacobson HR. Effects of CO2 and acetazolamide on bicarbonate and fluid transport in rabbit proximal tubules. *Am J Physiol* 1981;240:F54–F62.
351. Jacobson HR, Kokko JP. Intrinsic differences in various segments of the proximal convoluted tubule. *J Clin Invest* 1976;57:818–825.
352. Jiang Z, Grichtchenko II, Boron WF, Aronson PS. Specificity of anion exchange mediated by mouse slc26a6. *J Biol Chem* 2002;277:33963–33967.
353. Jin XH, McGrath HE, Gildea JJ, Siragy HM, Felder RA, Carey RM. Renal interstitial guanosine cyclic 3', 5'-monophosphate mediates pressure-natriuresis via protein kinase G. *Hypertension* 2004;43:1133–1139.
354. Jorgensen PL. Sodium and potassium ion pump in kidney tubules. *Physiol Rev* 1980;60: 864–917.
355. Jorgensen PL. Structure, function and regulation of Na K-ATPase in the kidney. *Kidney Int* 1986;29:10–20.
356. Jorgensen PL, Andersen JP. Structural basis for E1–E2 conformational transitions in Na K-pump and Ca-pump proteins. *J Membr Biol* 1988;103:95–120.
357. Kahn AM, Dolson GM, Hise MK, Bennett SC, Weinman EJ. Parathyroid hormone and dibutyryl cAMP inhibit Na^+–H^+ exchange in renal brush border vesicles. *Am J Physiol* 1985;248:F212–F218.
358. Kaissling B, Kriz W. *Structural Analysis of the Rabbit Kidney*. Berlin: Springer-Verlag; 1979.
359. Kanai Y, Lee W, You G, Brown D, Hediger MA. The human kidney low affinity Na^+/ glucose cotransporter SGLT2. Delineation of the major renal reabsorptive mechanism for D-glucose. *J Clin Invest* 1994;93:397–404.
360. Karim ZG, Chambrey R, Chalumeau C, Defontaine N, Warnock DG, Paillard M, Poggioli J. Regulation by PKC isoforms of Na $(^+)$/H $(^+)$ exchanger in luminal membrane vesicles isolated from cortical tubules. *Am J Physiol* 1999;277:F773–F778.
361. Karniski LP, Aronson PS. Chloride/formate exchange with formic acid recycling: a mechanism of active chloride transport across epithelial membranes. *Proc Natl Acad Sci U S A* 1985;82:6362–6365.
362. Karniski LP, Aronson PS. Anion exchange pathways for Cl^- transport in rabbit renal microvillus membranes. *Am J Physiol* 1987;253:F513–F521.
363. Karniski LP, Wang T, Everett LA, Green ED, Giebisch G, Aronson PS. Formate-stimulated NaCl absorption in the proximal tubule is independent of the pendrin protein. *Am J Physiol* 2002;283:F952–F956.
364. Kashgarian M, Biemesderfer D, Caplan M, Forbush B III. Monoclonal antibody to Na K-ATPase: immunocytochemical localization along nephron segments. *Kidney Int* 1985;28: 899–913.
365. Katz AI. Renal Na-K-ATPase: its role in tubular sodium and potassium transport. *Am J Physiol* 1982;242:F207–F219.
366. Katz AI, Doucet A, Morel F. Na-K-ATPase activity along the rabbit rat and mouse nephron. *Am J Physiol* 1979;237:F114–F120.
367. Kaufman JS, Hamburger RJ. Passive potassium transport in the proximal convoluted tubule. *Am J Physiol* 1985;248:F228–F232.
368. Kawahara K. A stretch-activated K^+ channel in the basolateral membrane of Xenopus kidney proximal tubule cells. *Pflugers Arch* 1990;415:624–629.
369. Kawahara K, Hunter M, Giebisch G. Potassium channels in *Necturus* proximal tubule. *Am J Physiol* 1987;253:F488–F494.
370. Kawahara K, Ogawa A, Suzuki M. Hyposmotic activation of Ca-activated K channels in cultured rabbit kidney proximal tubule cells. *Am J Physiol* 1991;260:F27–F33.
371. Kawamura J, Mazumdar DC, Lubowitz H. Effect of albumin infusion on renal glucose reabsorption in the rat. *Am J Physiol* 1977;232:F286–F290.
372. Kaye GI, Wheeler HO, Whitlock RT, Lane N. Fluid transport in the rabbit gallbladder. *J Cell Biol* 1966;30:237–268.
373. Kessler M, Semenza G. The small intestinal Na^+ D-glucose cotransporter: an asymmetric gated channel (or pore) responsive to $\Delta\psi$. *J Membr Biol* 1983;76:27–56.
374. Khraibi AA, Haas JA, Knox FG. Effect of renal perfusion pressure on renal interstitial hydrostatic pressure in rats. *Am J Physiol* 1989;256:F165–F170.
375. Khuri RN. Electrochemistry of the nephron. In: Giebisch G, ed. *Membrane Transport in Biology*. Vol. IV. *Transport Organs*. Berlin: Springer-Verlag; 1979:47–96.
376. Khuri RN, Agulian SK, Bogharian K, Nassar R, Wise W. Intracellular bicarbonate in single cells of *Necturus* kidney proximal tubule. *Pflugers Arch* 1974;349:295–299.
377. Khuri RN, Goldstein DA, Maude DL, Edmonds C, Solomon AK. Single proximal tubules of *Necturus* kidney. VIII. Na^+ and K^+ determinations by glass electrodes. *Am J Physiol* 1963;204:743–748.
378. Kimura G, Spring KR. Transcellular and paracellular tracer chloride fluxes in *Necturus* proximal tubule. *Am J Physiol* 1978;235:F617–F625.
379. Kimura G, Spring KR. Luminal Na^+ entry into *Necturus* proximal tubule cells. *Am J Physiol* 1979;236:F295–F301.
380. Kinne R. Metabolic correlates of tubular transport. In: Giebisch G, ed. *Transport Organs*. Vol. IV. *Membrane Transport in Biology*. Berlin: Springer-Verlag; 1979:529–562.
381. Kinne R, Murer H, Kinne-Saffran E, Thees M, Sachs G. Sugar transport by renal plasma membrane vesicles. *J Membr Biol* 1975;21:375–395.

382. Kinoshita Y, Knox FG. Role of prostaglandins in proximal tubule sodium reabsorption: response to elevated renal interstitial hydrostatic pressure. *Circ Res* 1989;64:1013–1018.

383. Kinsella JL, Aronson PS. Properties of the Na⁺–H⁺ exchanger in renal microvillus membrane vesicles. *Am J Physiol* 1980;238:F461–F469.

384. Kinsella JL, Aronson PS. Amiloride inhibition of the Na⁺–H⁺ exchanger in renal microvillus membrane vesicles. *Am J Physiol* 1981;241:F374–F379.

385. Kinsella JL, Aronson PS. Determination of the coupling ratio for Na⁺–H⁺ exchange in renal microvillus membrane vesicles. *Biochim Biophys Acta* 1982;689:161–164.

386. Kinsella JL, Cujdik T, Sacktor B. Kinetic studies on the stimulation of Na⁺–H⁺ exchange activity in renal brush border membranes isolated from thyroid hormone-treated rats. *J Membr Biol* 1986;91:183–191.

387. Kirk KL, DiBona DR, Schafer JA. Regulatory volume decrease in perfused proximal nephron: evidence for a dumping of cell K⁺. *Am J Physiol* 1987;252:F933–F942.

388. Kirk KL, Halm DR, Dawson DC. Active sodium transport by turtle colon via an electrogenic Na-K exchange pump. *Nature* 1980;287:237–239.

389. Kirk KL, Schafer JA, DiBona DR. Cell volume regulation in rabbit proximal straight tubule perfused in vitro. *Am J Physiol* 1987;252:F922–F932.

390. Knauf F, Yang CL, Thomson RB, Mentone SA, Giebisch G, Aronson PS. Identification of a chloride–formate exchanger expressed on the brush border membrane of renal proximal tubule cells. *Proc Natl Acad Sci U S A* 2001;98:9425–9430.

391. Knight TF, Senekjian HO, Sansom SC, Weinman EJ. Proximal tubule glucose efflux in the rat as a function of delivered load. *Am J Physiol* 1980;238:F499–F503.

392. Knox FG, Haas JA. Factors influencing renal sodium reabsorption in volume expansion. *Rev Physiol Biochem Pharmacol* 1982;92:75–113.

393. Knox FG, Mertz JI, Burnett JC Jr, Haramati A. Role of hydrostatic and oncotic pressures in renal sodium reabsorption. *Circ Res* 1983;52:491–500.

394. Knox FG, Schneider EG, Willis LR, Strandhoy JW, Ott CE. Effect of volume expansion on sodium excretion in the presence and absence of increased delivery from superficial proximal tubules. *J Clin Invest* 1973;52:1642–1646.

395. Kokko JP. Proximal tubule potential difference: dependence on glucose HCO₃ and amino acids. *J Clin Invest* 1973;52:1362–1367.

396. Kokko JP, Burg MB, Orloff J. Characteristics of NaCl and water transport in the renal proximal tubule. *J Clin Invest* 1971;50:69–76.

397. Kokko JP, Rector FC. Flow dependence of transtubular potential difference in isolated perfused segments of rabbit proximal convoluted tubule. *J Clin Invest* 1971;50:2745–2750.

398. Kolb RJ, Woost PG, Hopfer U. Membrane trafficking of angiotensin receptor type-1 and mechanochemical signal transduction in proximal tubule cells. *Hypertension* 2004;44:352–359.

399. Kondo Y, Frömter E. Axial heterogeneity of sodium-bicarbonate cotransport in proximal straight tubule of rabbit kidney. *Pflugers Arch* 1987;410:481–486.

400. Kondo Y, Frömter E. Evidence of chloride/bicarbonate exchange mediating bicarbonate efflux from S3 segments of rabbit renal proximal tubule. *Pflugers Arch* 1990;415:726–733.

401. Kondo Y, Kudo K, Abe K, Hoshi S, Igarashi Y. Na⁺/HCO₃ cotransporter in basolateral membrane of proximal tubule. *Lancet* 1991;337:1355.

402. Kone BC, Brady HR, Gullans SR. Coordinated regulation of intracellular K⁺ in the proximal tubule: Ba²⁺ blockade down-regulates the Na⁺, K⁺-ATPase and up-regulates two K⁺ permeability pathways. *Proc Natl Acad Sci U S A* 1989;86:6431–6435.

403. Kong C-T, Yet S-F, Lever J E. Cloning and expression of a mammalian Na⁺/amino acid cotransporter with sequence similarity to Na⁺/glucose cotransporters. *J Biol Chem* 1993;268:1509–1512.

404. Kottra G, Frömter E. Functional properties of the paracellular pathway in some leaky epithelia. *J Exp Biol* 1983;106:217–229.

405. Krahn TA, Aronson PS, Weinstein AM. Weak acid permeability of a villous membrane: formic acid transport across rat proximal tubule. *Bull Math Biol* 1994;56:459–490.

406. Krahn TA, Weinstein AM. Acid/base transport in a model of the proximal tubule brush border: impact of carbonic anhydrase. *Am J Physiol* 1996;270:F344–F355.

407. Krapf R, Berry CA, Verkman AS. Estimation of intracellular chloride activity in isolated perfused rabbit proximal convoluted tubules using a fluorescent indicator. *Biophys J* 1988;53:955–962.

408. Kubota T, Biagi BA, Giebisch G. Intracellular potassium activity measurements in single proximal tubules of *Necturus* kidney. *J Membr Biol* 1983;73:51–60.

409. Kumar AM, Spitzer A, Gupta RK. ²³Na NMR spectroscopy of proximal tubule suspensions. *Kidney Int* 1986;29:747–751.

409a. Kumini M, Muller-Berger S, Hara C, Samarzija I, Seki G, and Fromter E (2000). Incubation in tissue culture media allows isolated rabbit proximal tubules to regain in-vivo-like transport function: response of HCO₃ absorption to norepinephrine. *Pflugers Arch* 440:908–917.

410. Kuo S-M, Aronson PS. Pathways for oxalate transport in rabbit renal microvillus membrane vesicles. *J Biol Chem* 1996;271:15491–15497.

411. Kurashima K, D'Souza S, Szaszi K, Ramjeesingh R, Orlowski J, Grinstein S. The apical Na⁺/H⁺ exchanger isoform NHE3 is regulated by the actin cytoskeleton. *J Biol Chem* 1999;274:29843–29849.

412. Kurtz I. Apical Na⁺/H⁺ antiporter and glycolysis-dependent H⁺-ATPase regulate intracellular pH in the rabbit S3 proximal tubule. *J Clin Invest* 1987;80:928–935.

413. Kurtz I. Basolateral membrane Na⁺/H⁺ antiport Na⁺/base cotransport and Na⁺-independent Cl⁻/base exchange in the rabbit S3 proximal tubule. *J Clin Invest* 1989;83:616–622.

414. Kurtz I, Nagami G, Yanagawa N, Li L, Emmons C, Lee I. Mechanism of apical and basolateral Na⁺-independent Cl⁻/base exchange in the rabbit superficial proximal straight tubule. *J Clin Invest* 1994;94:173–183.

415. Kyte J. Immunoferritin determination of the distribution of (Na⁺ K⁺)ATPase over the plasma membranes of renal convoluted tubules. II. Proximal segment. *J Cell Biol* 1976;68:304–318.

416. Lahera V, Salom MG, Miranda-Guardiola F, Moncada S, Romero JC. Effects of NG-nitro-L-arginine methyl ester on renal function and blood pressure. *Am J Physiol* 1991;261:F1033–F1037.

417. Lamprecht G, Weinman EJ, Yun CH. The role of NHERF and E3KARP in the cAMP mediated inhibition of NHE3. *J Biol Chem* 1998;273:29972–29978.

418. Lang F, Busch GL, Ritter M, Volkl H, Waldegger S, Gulbins E, Haussinger D. Functional significance of cell volume regulatory mechanisms. *Physiol Rev* 1998;78:247–306.

419. Lang F, Busch GL, Volkl H. The diversity of volume regulatory mechanisms. *Cell Physiol Biochem* 1998;8:1–45.

420. Lang F, Messner G, Rehwald W. Electrophysiology of sodium-coupled transport in proximal renal tubules. *Am J Physiol* 1986;250:F953–F962.

421. Lang F, Messner G, Wang W, Paulmichl M, Oberleithner H, Deetjen P. The influence of intracellular sodium activity on the transport of glucose in proximal tubule of frog kidney. *Pflugers Arch* 1984;401:14–21.

422. Lang F, Oberleithner H, Giebisch G. Electrophysiological heterogeneity of proximal convoluted tubules in *Amphiuma* kidney. *Am J Physiol* 1986;251:F1063–F1072.

423. Lapointe J-Y, Duplain M. Regulation of basolateral membrane potential after stimulation of Na⁺ transport in proximal tubules. *J Membr Biol* 1991;120:165–172.

424. Lapointe J-Y, Garneau L, Bell PD, Cardinal J. Membrane crosstalk in the mammalian proximal tubule during alterations in transepithelial sodium transport. *Am J Physiol* 1990;258:F339–F345.

425. Lapointe J-Y, Laprade R, Cardinal J. Transepithelial and cell membrane electrical resistances of the rabbit proximal convoluted tubule. *Am J Physiol* 1984;247:F637–F649.

426. Laradi A, Sakhrani LM, Massry SG. Effect of dopamine on sodium uptake by renal proximal tubule cells of rabbit. *Miner Electrolyte Metab* 1986;12:303–307.

427. Lau KR, Hudson RL, Schultz SG. Cell swelling increases a barium-inhibitable potassium conductance in the basolateral membrane of *Necturus* small intestine. *Proc Natl Acad Sci U S A* 1984;81:3591–3594.

428. Lee CO, Taylor A, Windhager EE. Cytosolic calcium ion activity in epithelial cells of *Necturus* kidney. *Nature* 1980;287:859–861.

429. Lee WS, Kanai Y, Wells RG, Hediger MA. The high affinity Na⁺/glucose cotransporter. Reevaluation of function and distribution of expression. *J Biol Chem* 1994;269:12032–12039.

430. Le Grimellec C. Micropuncture study along the proximal convoluted tubule. *Pflugers Arch* 1975;354:133–150.

431. Leong PK, Yang LE, Holstein-Rathlou NH, McDonough AA. Angiotensin II clamp prevents the second step in renal apical NHE3 internalization during acute hypertension. *Am J Physiol* 2002;283:F1142–F1150.

432. Leong PK, Yang LE, Lin HW, Holstein-Rathlou NH, McDonough AA. Acute hypotension induced by aortic clamp vs. PTH provokes distinct proximal tubule Na⁺ transporter redistribution patterns. *Am J Physiol* 2004;287: R878–R885.

433. Lever JE. A two sodium ion/D-glucose symport mechanism: membrane potential effect on phlorizin binding. *Biochemistry* 1984;23:4697–4702.

434. Lewy JE, Windhager EE. Peritubular control of proximal tubular fluid reabsorption in the rat kidney. *Am J Physiol* 1968;214:943–954.

435. Li D, Xian S, Cheng J, Fisone G, Caplan MJ, Ohtomo Y, Aperia A. Effects of okadaic acid calyculin A, and PDBu on state of phosphorylation of rat renal Na⁺–K⁺-ATPase. *Am J Physiol* 1998;275:F863–F869.

436. Liang M, Berndt TJ, Knox FG. Mechanism underlying diuretic effect of L-NAME at a subpressor dose. *Am J Physiol* 2001;281:F414–F419.

437. Liang M, Knox FG. Nitric oxide activates PKC alpha and inhibits Na⁺-K⁺-ATPase in opossum kidney cells. *Am J Physiol* 1999;277:F859–F865.

438. Liang M, Knox FG. Nitric oxide reduces the molecular activity of Na⁺, K⁺-ATPase in opossum kidney cells. *Kidney Int* 1999;56:627–634.

439. Liang M, Knox FG. Production and functional roles of nitric oxide in the proximal tubule. *Am J Physiol* 2000;278: R1117–R1124.

440. Liedtke CM, Hopfer U. Mechanism of Cl⁻ translocation across small intestinal brush-border membrane. I. Absence of Na⁺-Cl⁻ cotransport. *Am J Physiol* 1982;242:G263–G271.

441. Liedtke CM, Hopfer U. Mechanism of Cl⁻ translocation across small intestinal brush-border membrane. II. Demonstration of Cl⁻–OH⁻ exchange and Cl⁻ conductance. *Am J Physiol* 1982;242:G272–G280.

442. Linas SL, Repine JE. Endothelial cells regulate proximal tubule epithelial cell sodium transport. *Kidney Int* 1999;55:1251–1258.

443. Lipkowitz MS, Abramson RG. Modulation of the ionic permeability of renal cortical brush-border membranes by cAMP. *Am J Physiol* 1989;257:F769–F776.

444. Lipkowitz MS, London RD, Beck JC, Abramson RG. Hormonal regulation of rat renal proximal tubule brush-border membrane ionic permeability. *Am J Physiol* 1992;263:F144–F151.

445. Liu F-Y, Cogan MG. Axial heterogeneity in the rat proximal convoluted tubule. I. Bicarbonate chloride and water transport. *Am J Physiol* 1984;247:F816–F821.

446. Liu F-Y, Cogan MG. Axial heterogeneity of bicarbonate chloride and water transport in the rat proximal convoluted tubule. *J Clin Invest* 1986;78:1547–1557.

447. Liu F-Y, Cogan MG. Flow dependence of bicarbonate transport in the early (S1) proximal convoluted tubule. *Am J Physiol* 1988;254:F851–F855.

448. Liu F-Y, Cogan MG. Angiotensin II stimulation of hydrogen ion secretion in the rat early proximal tubule. Modes of action mechanism and kinetics. *J Clin Invest* 1988;82:601–607.

449. Liu F-Y, Cogan MG. Angiotensin II stimulates early proximal bicarbonate absorption in the rat by decreasing cyclic adenosine monophosphate. *J Clin Invest* 1989;84:83–91.

450. Liu F, Cogan MG. Role of protein kinase C in proximal bicarbonate absorption and angiotensin signaling. *Am J Physiol* 1990;258:F927–F933.

451. Liu F-Y, Cogan MG. Effects of intracellular calcium on proximal bicarbonate absorption. *Am J Physiol* 1990;259:F451–F457.

452. Liu F-Y, Cogan MG, Rector FC Jr. Axial heterogeneity in the rat proximal convoluted tubule. II. Osmolality and osmotic water permeability. *Am J Physiol* 1984;247:F822–F826.

453. Logvinenko NS, Dulubova I, Fedosova N, Larsson SH, Nairn AC, Esmann M, Greengard P, Aperia A. Phosphorylation by protein kinase C of serine-23 of the alpha-1 subunit of rat Na⁺, K⁺-ATPase affects its conformational equilibrium. *Proc Natl Acad Sci U S A* 1996;93:9132–9137.

454. Lohr JW, Grantham JJ. Isovolumetric regulation of isolated S2 proximal tubules in anisotonic media. *J Clin Invest* 1986;78:1165–1172.

455. Lohr JW, Sullivan LP, Cragoe EJ Jr, Grantham JJ. Volume regulation determinants in isolated proximal tubules in hypertonic medium. *Am J Physiol* 1989;256:F622–F631.

456. London R, Cohen B, Guggino WB, Giebisch G. Regulation of intracellular chloride activity during perfusion with hypertonic solutions in the *Necturus* proximal tubule. *J Membr Biol* 1983;75:253–258.

457. Loo DD, Hazama A, Supplisson S, Turk E, Wright EM. Relaxation kinetics of the Na+/glucose cotransporter. *Proc Natl Acad Sci U S A* 1993;90:5767–5771.

458. Loo DD, Zeuthen T, Chandy G, Wright EM. Cotransport of water by the Na+/glucose cotransporter. *Proc Natl Acad Sci U S A* 1996;93:13367–13370.

459. Lopes AG, Guggino WB. Volume regulation in the early proximal tubule of the *Necturus* kidney. *J Membr Biol* 1987;97:117–125.

460. Lopes AG, Siebens AW, Giebisch G, Boron WF. Electrogenic Na/HCO₃ cotransport across basolateral membrane of isolated perfused *Necturus* proximal tubule. *Am J Physiol* 1987;253:F340–F350.

461. Lorentz WB Jr, Lassiter WE, Gottschalk CW. Renal tubular permeability during increased intrarenal pressure. *J Clin Invest* 1972;51:484–492.

462. Lorenz JN, Schultheis PJ, Traynor T, Shull GE, Schnermann J. Micropuncture analysis of single-nephron function in NHE3-deficient mice. *Am J Physiol* 1999;277:F447–F453.

463. Lorenzen M, Lee CO, Windhager EE. Cytosolic Ca++ and Na+ activities in perfused proximal tubules of *Necturus* kidney. *Am J Physiol* 1984;247:F93–F102.

464. Lucci MS, Warnock DG. Effects of anion-transport inhibitors on NaCl reabsorption in the rat superficial proximal convoluted tubule. *J Clin Invest* 1979;64:570–579.

465. Lynch AM, McGivan JD. Evidence for a single common Na+-dependent transport system for alanine glutamine leucine and phenylalanine in brush-border membrane vesicles from bovine kidney. *Biochim Biophys Acta* 1987;899:176–184.

466. Mackenzie B, Loo DDF, Panayotova-Heiermann M, Wright EM. Biophysical characteristics of the pig kidney Na+/glucose cotransporter SGLT2 reveal a common mechanism for SGLT1 and SGLT2. *J Biol Chem* 1996;271:32678–32683.

467. MacRobbie EAC, Ussing HH. Osmotic behavior of the epithelial cells of frog skin. *Acta Physiol Scand* 1961;53:348–365.

468. Maddox DA, Fortin SM, Tartini A, Barnes WD, Gennari FJ. Effect of acute changes in glomerular filtration rate on Na+/H+ exchange in rat renal cortex. *J Clin Invest* 1992;89:1296–1303.

469. Madhun ZT, Goldthwait DA, McKay D, Hopfer U, Douglas JG. An epoxygenase metabolite of arachidonic acid mediates angiotensin II–induced rises in cytosolic calcium in rabbit proximal tubule epithelial cells. *J Clin Invest* 1991;88:456–461.

470. Maeda Y, Smith BL, Agre P, Knepper MA. Quantification of aquaporin-CHIP water channel protein in microdissected renal tubules by fluorescence-based ELISA *J Clin Invest* 1995;95:422–428.

470a. Majid DSA, Williams A, and Navar LG (1993). Inhibition of nitric oxide synthesis attenuates pressure-induced natriuretic responses in anesthetized dogs. *Am J Physiol* 264:F79–F87.

471. Marsh DJ. Models of flow and pressure modulated isoosmotic reabsorption in mammalian proximal tubules. In: Salanki J, ed. *Advances in Physiological Science*. Vol. 3. *Physiology of Non-excitable Cells*. London: Pergamon Press; 1981:47–55.

472. Martinez-Palomo A, Erlij D. The distribution of lanthanum in tight junctions of the kidney tubule. *Pflugers Arch* 1973;343:267–272.

473. Martino JA, Earley LE. Demonstration of a role of physical factors as determinants of the natriuretic response to volume expansion. *J Clin Invest* 1967;46:1963–1978.

474. Maruyama T, Hoshi T. The effect of D-glucose on the electrical potential profile across the proximal tubule of newt kidney. *Biochim Biophys Acta* 1972;282:214–225.

475. Mathias RT. Epithelial water transport in a balanced gradient system. *Biophys J* 1985;47:823–836.

476. Matsumura Y, Cohen B, Guggino WB, Giebisch G. Electrical effects of potassium and bicarbonate on proximal tubule cells of *Necturus*. *J Membr Biol* 1984;79:145–152.

477. Mauerer UR, Boulpaep EL, Segal AS. Properties of an inwardly rectifying ATP-sensitive K+ channel in the basolateral membrane of renal proximal tubule. *J Gen Physiol* 1998;111:139–160.

478. Mauerer UR, Boulpaep EL, Segal AS. Regulation of an inwardly rectifying ATP-sensitive K+ channel in the basolateral membrane of renal proximal tubule. *J Gen Physiol* 1998;111:161–180.

479. Maunsbach AB. Ultrastructure of the proximal tubule. In: Orloff J, Berliner RW, eds. *Handbook of Physiology*. Section 8: Renal Physiology. Washington, DC: American Physiological Society; 1973:31–80

480. Maunsbach AB, Boulpaep EL. Hydrostatic pressure changes related to paracellular shunt ultrastructure in proximal tubule. *Kidney Int* 1980;17:732–748.

481. Maunsbach AB, Boulpaep EL. Paracellular shunt ultrastructure and changes in fluid transport in *Necturus* proximal tubule. *Kidney Int* 1983;24:610–619.

482. Maunsbach AB, Boulpaep EL. Quantitative ultrastructure and functional correlates in proximal tubule of *Ambystoma* and *Necturus*. *Am J Physiol* 1984;246:F710–F724.

483. Maunsbach AB, Giebisch GH, Stanton BA. Effects of flow rate on proximal tubule ultrastructure. *Am J Physiol* 1987;253:F582–F587.

484. Maunsbach AB, Vorum H, Kwon TH, Nielsen S, Simonsen B, Choi I, Schmitt BM, Boron WF, Aalkjaer C. Immunoelectron microscopic localization of the electrogenic Na/HCO₃ cotransporter in rat and Ambystoma kidney. *J Am Soc Nephrol* 2000;11:2179–2189.

485. McCarthy KM, Skare IB, Stankewich MC, Furuse M, Tsukita S, Rogers RA, Lynch RD, Schneeberger EE. Occludin is a functional component of the tight junction. *J Cell Sci* 1996;109:2287–2298.

486. McCarty NA, O'Neil RG. Dihydropyridine-sensitive cell volume regulation in proximal tubule: the calcium window. *Am J Physiol* 1990;259:F950–F960.

487. McCarty NA, O'Neil RG. Calcium-dependent control of volume regulation in renal proximal tubule cells: I. Swelling-activated Ca2+ entry and release. *J Membr Biol* 1991;123:149–160.

488. McCarty NA, O'Neil RG. Calcium-dependent control of volume regulation in renal proximal tubule cells: II Roles of dihydropyridine-sensitive and-insensitiveCa2+ entry pathways. *J Membr Biol* 1991;123:161–170.

489. McDonough AA, Biemesderfer D. Does membrane trafficking play a role in regulating the sodium/hydrogen exchanger isoform 3 in the proximal tubule? *Curr Opin Nephrol Hypertens* 2003;12:533–541.

490. McDonough AA, Magyar CE, Komatsu Y. Expression of Na+-K+-ATPase alpha-and beta-subunits along rat nephron: isoform specificity and response to hypokalemia. *Am J Physiol* 1994;267:C901–C908.

491. McGivan JD, Pastor-Anglada M. Regulatory and molecular aspects of mammalian amino acid transport. *Biochem J* 1994;299:321–334.

492. McKeown J, Brazy PC, Dennis VW. Intrarenal heterogeneity for fluid phosphate and glucose absorption in the rabbit. *Am J Physiol* 1979;234:F312–F318.

493. Meinild AK, Klaerke DA, Loo DDF, Wright EM, Zeuthen T. The human Na+-glucose cotransporter is a molecular water pump. *J Physiol* 1998;508:15–21.

494. Mellas J, Hammerman MR. Phorbol ester-induced alkalinization of canine renal proximal tubular cells. *Am J Physiol* 1986;250:F451–F459.

495. Merot J, Bidet M, Le Maout S, Tauc M, Poujeol P. Two types of K+ channels in the apical membrane of rabbit proximal tubule in primary culture. *Biochim Biophys Acta* 1989;978:134–144.

496. Mertz JJ, Haas JA, Berndt TJ, Burnett JC Jr, Knox FG. Effects of bradykinin on renal interstitial pressures and proximal tubule reabsorption. *Am J Physiol* 1984;247:F82–F85.

497. Messner G, Koller A, Lang F. The effect of phenylalanine on intracellular pH and sodium activity in proximal convoluted tubule cells of the frog kidney. *Pflugers Arch* 1985;404:145–149.

498. Messner G, Oberleithner H, Lang F. The effect of phenylalanine on the electrical properties of proximal tubule cells in the frog kidney. *Pflugers Arch* 1985;404:138–144.

499. Millar ID, Robson L. Na+-alanine uptake activates a Cl− conductance in frog renal proximal tubule cells via nonconventional PKC. *Am J Physiol* 2001;280:F758–F767.

500. Misfeldt DS, Sanders MJ. Transepithelial transport in cell culture: stoichiometry of Na/phlorizin binding and Na/D-glucose cotransport. A two-step two-sodium model of binding and translocation. *J Membr Biol* 1982;70:191–198.

501. Mitic LL, Anderson JM. Molecular architecture of tight junctions. *Annu Rev Physiol* 1998;60:121–142.

502. Moe OW. Acute regulation of proximal tubule apical membrane Na/H exchanger NHE-3: role of phosphorylation protein trafficking and regulatory factors. *J Am Soc Nephrol* 1999;10:2412–2425.

503. Moe OW, Amemiya M, Yamaji Y. Activation of protein kinase A acutely inhibits and phosphorylates Na/H exchanger NHE-3. *J Clin Invest* 1995;96:2187–2194.

504. Montrose MH, Murer H. Kinetics of Na+/H+ exchange. In: Grinstein S, ed. *Na+–H+ Exchange*. Boca Raton, FL: CRC Press; 1988:57–75.

505. Montrose-Rafizadeh C, Guggino WB. Cell volume regulation in the nephron. *Ann Rev Physiol* 1990;52:761–772.

506. Morel F, Murayama Y. Simultaneous measurement of unidirectional and net sodium fluxes in microperfused rat proximal tubules. *Pflugers Arch* 1970;320:1–23.

507. Moran A, Biber J, Murer H. A sodium–hydrogen exchange system in isolated apical membrane from LLC-PK1 epithelia. *Am J Physiol* 1986;251:F1003–F1008.

508. Moran A, Stange G, Murer H. Sodium-hydrogen exchange system in brush border membranes from cortical and medullary regions of the proximal tubule. *Biochem Biophys Res Commun* 1989;163:269–275.

509. Morgan T, Berliner RW. In vivo perfusion of proximal tubules of the rat: glomerulotubular balance. *Am J Physiol* 1969;217:992–997.

510. Morgunov NS. Electrophysiological analysis of beta-receptor stimulation in salamander proximal tubules. *Am J Physiol* 1987;253:F636–F641.

511. Morgunov N, Boulpaep EL. Electrochemical analysis of renal Na+-glucose cotransport in salamander proximal tubules. *Am J Physiol* 1987;252:F154–F169.

512. Morrow JS, Cianci CD, Ardito T, Mann AS, Kashgarian M. Ankyrin links fodrin to the alpha subunit of Na K-ATPase in Madin–Darby canine kidney cells and in intact renal tubule cells. *J Cell Biol* 1989;108:455–465.

513. Mounfield PR, Robson L. The role of Ca2+ in volume regulation induced by Na+-coupled alanine uptake in single proximal tubule cells isolated from frog kidney. *J Physiol* 1998;510:145–153.

514. Mount DB, Gamba G. Renal potassium–chloride cotransporters. *Curr Opin Nephrol Hypertens* 2001;10:685–691.

515. Mount DB, Romero MF. The SLC26 gene family of multifunctional anion exchangers. *Pflugers Arch* 2004;447:710–721.

516. Müller-Berger S, Coppola S, Samarzija I, Seki G, Frömter E. Partial recovery of in vivo function by improved incubation conditions of isolated renal proximal tubule. I. Change of amiloride-inhibitable K+ conductance. *Pflugers Arch* 1997;434:373–382.

517. Müller-Berger S, Ducoudret O, Diakov A, Frömter E. The renal Na–HCO₃ cotransporter expressed in Xenopus laevis oocytes: change in stoichiometry in response to elevation of cytosolic Ca2+ concentration. *Pflugers Arch* 2001;442:718–728.

518. Müller-Berger S, Nesterov VV, Frömter E. Partial recovery of in vivo function by improved incubation conditions of isolated renal proximal tubule. II. Change of Na–HCO₃ cotransport stoichiometry and of response to acetazolamide. *Pflugers Arch* 1997;434:383–391.

519. Murer H, Burckhardt G. Membrane transport of anions across epithelia of mammalian small intestine and kidney proximal tubule. *Rev Physiol Biochem Pharmacol* 1983;96:1–51.

520. Murer H, Hopfer U, Kinne R. Sodium/proton antiportin brush-border–membrane vesicles isolated from rat small intestine and kidney. *Biochem J* 1976;154:597–604.

521. Nagami GT. Luminal secretion of ammonia in the mouse proximal tubule perfused in vitro. *J Clin Invest* 1988;81:159–164.

522. Nagami GT. Enhanced ammonia secretion by proximal tubules from mice receiving NH4Cl: role of angiotensin II. *Am J Physiol* 2002;282:F472–F477.

523. Nagami GT. Ammonia production and secretion by S3 proximal tubule segments from acidotic mice: role of ANG II. *Am J Physiol* 2004;287:F707–F712.
524. NakamuraT, Alberola AM, Salazar FJ, Saito Y, Kurashina T, Granger JP, Nagai R. Effects of renal perfusion pressure on renal interstitial hydrostatic pressure and Na^+ excretion: role of endothelium-derived nitric oxide. *Nephron* 1998;78:104–111.
525. Nakhoul NL, Chen LK, Boron WF. Intracellular pH regulation in rabbit S3 proximal tubule: basolateral Cl^- HCO_3^- exchange and Na–HCO_3^- cotransport. *Am J Physiol* 1990;258:F371–F381.
526. Navar LG, Majid DSA. Interactions between arterial pressure and sodium excretion. *Curr Opin Nephrol Hypertens* 1996;5:64–71.
527. Nelson PJ, Dean GE, Aronson PS, Rudnick G. Hydrogen ion cotransport by the renal brush border glutamate transporter. *Biochemistry* 1983;22:5459–5463.
528. Nielsen R. A 3 to 2 coupling of the Na-K pump responsible for the transepithelial Na transport in frog skin disclosed by the effect of Ba. *Acta Physiol Scand* 1979;107:189–191.
529. Nord EP, Goldfarb D, Mikhail N, Moradeshagi P, Hafezi A, Vaystub S, Cragoe EJ Jr, Fine LG. Characteristics of the Na^+–H^+ antiporter in the intact renal proximal tubular cell. *Am J Physiol* 1986;250:F539–F550.
530. Nord EP, Howard MJ, Hafezi A, Moradeshagi P, Vaystub S, Insel PA. Alpha 2 adrenergic agonists stimulate Na^+–H+ antiport activity in the rabbit renal proximal tubule. *J Clin Invest* 1987;80:1755–1762.
531. Nowicki S, Chen SL, Aizman O, Cheng XJ, Li D, Nowicki C, Nairn A, Greengard P, Aperia A. 20-Hydroxyeicosa-tetraenoic acid (20-HETE) activates protein kinase C Role in regulation of rat renal Na^+, K^+-ATPase. *J Clin Invest* 1997;99:1224–1230.
532. O'Connell DP, Botkin SJ, Ramos SI, Sibley DR, Ariano MA, Felder RA, Carey RM. Localization of dopamine D1A receptor protein in rat kidneys. *Am J Physiol* 1995;268:F1185–F1197.
533. Oken DE, Solomon AK. Single proximal tubules of *Necturus* kidney. VI. Nature of potassium transport. *Am J Physiol* 1963;204:377–380.
534. Ominato M, Satoh T, Katz AI. Regulation of Na-K-ATPase activity in the proximal tubule: role of the protein kinase C pathway and of eicosanoids. *J Membr Biol* 1996;152:235–243.
535. Orci L, Humbert F, Brown D, Perrelet A. Membrane ultrastructure in urinary tubules. *Int Rev Cytol* 1981;73:183–242.
536. Orlowski J. Heterologous expression and functional properties of amiloride high affinity (NHE-1) and low affinity (NHE-3) isoforms of the rat Na/H exchanger. *J Biol Chem* 1993;268:16369–16377.
537. Orlowski J, Kandasamy RA, Shull GE. Molecular cloning of putative members of the Na/H exchanger gene family. cDNA cloning deduced amino acid sequence and mRNA tissue expression of the rat Na/H exchanger NHE-1 and two structurally related proteins. *J Biol Chem* 1992;267:9331–9339.
538. Otsu K, Kinsella JL, Koh E, Froehlich JP. Proton dependence of the partial reactions of the sodium–proton exchanger in renal brush border membranes. *J Biol Chem* 1992;267: 8089–8096.
539. Otsu K, Kinsella JL, Sacktor B, Froehlich JP. Transient state kinetic evidence for an oligomer in the mechanism of Na^+–H+ exchange. *Proc Natl Acad Sci U S A* 1989;86:4818–4822.
540. Ott CE. Effect of saline expansion on peritubule capillary pressures and reabsorption. *Am J Physiol* 1981;240:F106–F110.
541. Ott CE, Haas JA, Cuche J-L, Knox FG. Effect of increased peritubule protein concentration on proximal tubule reabsorption in the presence and absence of extracellular volume expansion. *J Clin Invest* 1975;55:612–620.
542. Pajor AM, Hirayama BA, Wright EM. Molecular evidence for two renal Na^+/glucose cotransporters. *Biochim Biophys Acta* 1992;1106:216–220.
543. Panayotova-Heiermann M, Loo DD, Wright EM. Kinetics of steady-state currents and charge movements associated with the rat Na^+/glucose cotransporter. *J Biol Chem* 1995;270:27099–27105.
544. Parent L, Supplisson S, Loo DDF, Wright EM. Electrogenic properties of the cloned Na^+/ glucose cotransporter: I Voltage-clamp studies. *J Membr Biol* 1992;125:49–62.
545. Parent L, Supplisson S, Loo DDF, Wright EM. Electrogenic properties of the cloned Na^+/ glucose cotransporter: II A transport model under nonrapid equilibrium conditions. *J Membr Biol* 1992;125:63–79.
546. Pearce D, Verkman AS. NaCl reflection coefficients in proximal tubule apical and basolateral membrane vesicles. Measurement by induced osmosis and solvent drag. *Biophys J* 1989;55:1251–1259.
547. Persson B, Spring KR. Gallbladder epithelial cell hydraulic water permeability and volume regulation. *J Gen Physiol* 1982;79:481–505.
548. Persson B, Spring KR. Permeability properties of the subepithelial tissues of *Necturus* gallbladder. *Biochim Biophys Acta* 1984;772:135–139.
549. Peterson OW, Gushwa LC, Blantz RC. An analysis of glomerular-tubular balance in the rat proximal tubule. *Pflugers Arch* 1986;407:221–227.
550. Petrovic S, Barone S, Weinstein AM, Soleimani M. Activation of the apical Na^+/H^+ exchanger NHE3 by formate: a basis of enhanced fluid and electrolyte reabsorption by formate in the kidney. *Am J Physiol* 2004;287:F336–F346.
551. Pirie SC, Potts DJ. The effect of peritubular protein upon fluid reabsorption in rabbit proximal convoluted tubules perfused in vitro. *J Physiol* 1983;337:429–440.
552. Pitts TO, McGowan JA, Chen TC, Silverman M, Rose ME, Puschett JB. Inhibitory effects of volume expansion performed in vivo on transport in the isolated rabbit proximal tubule perfused in vitro. *J Clin Invest* 1988;81:997–1003.
553. Planelles G, Thomas SR, Anagnostopoulos T. Change of apparent stoichiometryof proximal-tubule Na(+)-HCO_3 cotransport upon experimental reversal of its orientation. *Proc Natl Acad Sci U S A* 1993;90:7406–7410.
554. Preisig PA. Luminal flow rate regulates proximal tubule H-HCO_3 transporters. *Am J Physiol* 1992;262:F47–F54.
555. Preisig PA, Alpern RJ. Basolateral membrane H-OH-HCO_3 transport in the proximal tubule. *Am J Physiol* 1989;256:F751–F765.
556. Preisig PA, Alpern RJ. Contributions of cellular leak pathways to net $NaHCO_3$ and NaCl absorption. *J Clin Invest* 1989;83:1859–1867.
557. Preisig PA, Berry CA. Evidence for transcellular osmotic water flow in rat proximal tubules. *Am J Physiol* 1985;249:F124–F131.
558. Preisig PA, Ives HE, Cragoe EJ Jr, Alpern RJ, Rector FC Jr. Role of the Na^+/H^+ antiporter in rat proximal tubule bicarbonate absorption. *J Clin Invest* 1987;80:970–978.
559. Preisig PA, Rector FC Jr. Role of Na^+–H+ antiport in rat proximal tubule NaCl absorption. *Am J Physiol* 1988;255:F461–F465.
560. Pricam C, Humbert F, Perrelet A, Orci L. A freeze-etch study of the tight junctions of the rat kidney tubules. *Lab Invest* 1974;30:286–291.
561. Quan A, Baum M. Endogenous production of angiotensin II modulates rat proximal tubule transport. *J Clin Invest* 1996;97:2878–2882.
562. Quan A, Baum M. Regulation of proximal tubule transport by angiotensin II. *Semin Nephrol* 1997;17:423–430.
563. Quan A, Baum M. Endogenous angiotensin II modulates rat proximal tubule transport with acute changes in extracellular volume. *Am J Physiol* 1998;275:F74–F78.
564. Quan A, Baum M. Effect of luminal angiotensin II receptor antagonists on proximal tubule transport. *Am J Hypertens* 1999;12:499–503.
565. Quan A, Baum M. Renal nerve stimulation augments effect of intraluminal angiotensin II on proximal tubule transport. *Am J Physiol* 2002;282:F1043–F1048.
566. Quan A, Baum M. The renal nerve is required for regulation of proximal tubule transport by intraluminally produced ANG II. *Am J Physiol* 2001;280:F524–F529.
566a. Quigley R, Baum M, Reddy KM, Griener JC, and Falck JR (2000). Effects of 20-HETE and 19(S)-HETE on rabbit proximal straight tubule volume transport. *Am J Physiol* 278: F949–F953.
567. Quinn MD, Marsh DJ. Peritubular capillary control of proximal tubule reabsorption in the rat. *Am J Physiol* 1979;236:F478–F487.
568. Rabito CA, Ausiello DA. Na^+-dependent sugar transport in a cultured epithelial cell line from pig kidney. *J Membr Biol* 1980;54:31–38.
569. Rajendran VM, Barry JA, Kleinman JG, Ramaswamy K. Proton gradient-dependent transport of glycine in rabbit renal brush border membrane vesicles. *J Biol Chem* 1987;262:14974–14977.
570. Ramsey CR, Berndt T, Knox FG. Effect of volume expansion on the paracellular flux of lanthanum in the proximal tubule. *J Am Soc Nephrol* 1998;9:1147–1152.
571. Ramsey CR, Berndt TJ, Knox FG. Indomethacin blocks enhanced paracellular backflux in proximal tubules. *J Am Soc Nephrol* 2002;13:1449–1454.
572. Rector FC Jr. Sodium bicarbonate and chloride absorption by the proximal tubule. *Am J Physiol* 1983;244:F461–F471.
573. Rector FC Jr, Berry CA. Role of the paracellular pathway in reabsorption of solutes and water by proximal convoluted tubule of the mammalian kidney. In: Bradley SE, Purcell EF, eds. *The Paracellular Pathway*. New York: Josiah Macy Jr. Foundation; 1982:135–157.
574. Reddy S, Gyory AZ, Bostrom T, Dyne M, Salipan-Moore N, Field MJ, Pollock CA, Cockayne DJ. Proximal tubular cell electrolytes during volume expansion in the rat. *J Physiol* 1994;481: 217–222.
575. Reeves JP, Hale CC. The stoichiometry of the cardiac sodium-calcium exchange system. *J Biol Chem* 1984;259:7733–7739.
576. Reilly AM, Harris PJ, Williams DA. Biphasic effect of angiotensin II on intracellular sodium concentration in rat proximal tubules. *Am J Physiol* 1995;269:F374–F380.
577. Renkin EM, Gilmore JP. Glomerular filtration. In: Orloff J, Berliner RW, eds. *Handbook of Physiology*. Washington, DC: American Physiological Society; 1973:185–248.
578. Restrepo D, Kimmich GA. Kinetic analysis of mechanism of intestinal Na^+-dependent sugar transport. *Am J Physiol* 1985;248:C498–C509.
579. Reuss L. Electrical properties of the cellular transepithelial pathway in *Necturus* gallbladder. III. Ionic permeability of the basolateral cell membrane. *J Membr Biol* 1979;47:239–259.
580. Reuss L. Basolateral KCl co-transport in a NaCl-absorbing epithelium. *Nature* 1983;305: 723–726.
581. Reuss L, Weinman SA, Grady TP. Intracellular K^+ activity and its relation to basolateral membrane ion transport in *Necturus* gallbladder epithelium. *J Gen Physiol* 1980;76: 33–52.
582. Ribeiro CMP, Dubay GR, Falck JR, Mandel LJ. Parathyroid hormone inhibits Na^+-K^+-ATPase through a cytochrome P-450 pathway. *Am J Physiol* 1994;266:F497–F505.
583. Ribeiro CP, Mandel LJ. Parathyroid hormone inhibits proximal tubule Na^+-K^+-AT-Pase activity. *Am J Physiol* 1992;262:F209–F216.
584. Richardson IW, Licko V, Bartoli E. The nature of passive flows through tightly folded membranes. *J Membr Biol* 1973;11:293–308.
585. Robey RB, Ruiz OS, Espiritu DJ, Ibanez VC, Kear FT, Noboa OA, Bernardo AA, Arruda JA. Angiotensin II stimulation of renal epithelial cell Na/HCO_3 cotransport activity: a central role for Src family kinase/classic MAPK pathway coupling. *J Membr Biol* 2002;187:135–145.
586. Robson AM, Srivastava PL, Bricker NS. The influence of saline loading on renal glucose reabsorption in the rat. *J Clin Invest* 1968;47:329–335.
587. Robson L, Hunter M. Stimulation of Na^+-alanine cotransport activatesa voltage-dependent conductance in single proximal tubule cells isolated from frog kidney. *J Physiol* 1999;517: 193–200.
588. Roczniak A, Burns KD. Nitric oxide stimulates guanylate cyclase and regulates sodium transport in rabbit proximal tubule. *Am J Physiol* 1996;270:F109–F115.
589. Roigaard-Petersen H, Jacobsen H, Sheikh MI. H^+-L-proline cotransport by vesicles from pars convoluta of rabbit proximal tubule. *Am J Physiol* 1987;253:F15–F20.
590. Romano G, Favret G, Damato R, Bartoli E. Proximal reabsorption with changing tubular fluid inflow in rat nephrons. *Exp Physiol* 1998;83:35–48.
591. Romano G, Favret G, Federico E, Bartoli E. The effect of intraluminal flowrate on glomerulotubular balance in the proximal tubule of the rat kidney. *Exp Physiol* 1996;81: 95–105.
592. Rome L, Grantham J, Savin V, Lohr J, Lechene C. Proximal tubule volume regulation in hyperosmotic media: intracellular K^+ Na^+ and Cl^-. *Am J Physiol* 1989;257:C1093–C1100.
593. Romero MF, Boron WF. Electrogenic Na^+/HCO_3^- cotransporters: cloning and physiology. *Ann Rev Physiol* 1999;61:699–723.

594. Romero MF, Fong P, Berger UV, Hediger MA, Boron WF. Cloning and functional expression of rNBC, an electrogenic Na (+)-HCO₃ (-) cotransporter from rat kidney. *Am J Physiol* 1998;274:F425–F432.

595. Romero MF, Hediger MA, Boulpaep EL, Boron WF. Expression cloning and characterization of a renal electrogenic Na⁺/HCO₃ cotransporter. *Nature* 1997;387:409–413.

596. Romero JC, Knox FG. Mechanisms underlying pressure-related natriuresis: the role of the renin-angiotensin and prostaglandin systems. *Hypertension* 1988;11:724–738.

597. Romero MF, Hopfer U, Madhun ZT, Zhou J, Douglas JG. Angiotensin II mediated signaling mechanisms and electrolyte transport in the rabbit proximal tubule. *Renal Physiol Biochem* 1991;14:199–207.

598. Roos A, Boron WF. Intracellular pH. *Physiol Rev* 1981;61:296–434.

599. Rubera I, Tauc M, Bidet M, Poujeol C, Cuiller B, Watrin A, Touret N, Poujeol P. Chloride currents in primary cultures of rabbit proximal and distal convoluted tubules. *Am J Physiol* 1998;275:F651–F663.

600. Ruiz OS, Arruda JAL. Regulation of the renal Na-HCO₃ cotransporter by cAMP and Ca-dependent protein kinases. *Am J Physiol* 1992;262:F560–F565.

601. Ruiz OS, Qiu Y-Y, Wang L-J, Arruda JAL. Regulation of the renal Na-HCO₃ cotransporter: IV Mechanisms of the stimulatory effect of angiotensin II. *J Am Soc Nephrol* 1995;6:1202–1208.

602. Sabolic J, Burckhardt G. Proton pathways in rat renal brush border and basolateral membranes. *Biochim Biophys Acta* 1983;734:210–220.

603. Saccomani G, Mitchell KD, Navar LG. Angiotensin II stimulation of Na⁺–H+ exchange in proximal tubule cells. *Am J Physiol* 1990;258:F1188–F1195.

604. Sackin H. Electrophysiology of salamander proximal tubule. II. Interspace NaCl concentrations and solute-coupled water transport. *Am J Physiol* 1986;251:F334–F347.

605. Sackin H. Stretch-activated potassium channels in renal proximal tubule. *Am J Physiol* 1987;253:F1253–F1262.

606. Sackin H, Boulpaep EL. Models for coupling of salt and water transport. *J Gen Physiol* 1975;66:671–733.

607. Sackin H, Boulpaep EL. Isolated perfused salamander proximal tubule: methods, electrophysiology, and transport. *Am J Physiol* 1981;241:F39–F52.

608. Sackin H, Boulpaep EL. Rheogenic transport in the renal proximal tubule. *J Gen Physiol* 1983;82:819–851.

609. Sakhrani LM, Badie-Dezfooly B, Trizna W, Mikhail N, Lowe AG, Taub M, Fine LG. Transport and metabolism of glucose by renal proximal tubular cells in primary culture. *Am J Physiol* 1984;246:F757–F764.

610. Saleh AM, Rudnick H, Aronson PS. Mechanism of H⁺-coupled formate transport in rabbit renal microvillus membranes. *Am J Physiol* 1996;271:F401–F407.

611. Samarzija I, Frömter E. Electrophysiological analysis of rat renal sugar and amino acid transport. III. Neutral amino acids. *Pflugers Arch* 1982;393:199–209.

612. Samarzija I, Frömter E. Electrophysiological analysis of rat renal sugar and amino acid transport. IV. Basic amino acids. *Pflugers Arch* 1982;393:210–214.

613. Samarzija I, Frömter E. Electrophysiological analysis of rat renal sugar and amino acid transport. V Acidic amino acids. *Pflugers Arch* 1982;393:215–221.

614. Samarzija I, Hinton BT, Frömter E. Electrophysiological analysis of rat renal sugar and amino acid transport. II. Dependence on various transport parameters and inhibitors. *Pflugers Arch* 1982;393:190–197.

615. Sasaki S, Ishibashi K, Yoshiyama N, Shiigai T. KCl co-transport across the basolateral membrane of rabbit renal proximal straight tubules. *J Clin Invest* 1988;81:194–199.

616. Sasaki S, Shiigai T, Takeuchi J. Intracellular pH in the isolated perfused rabbit proximal straight tubule. *Am J Physiol* 1985;249:F417–F423.

617. Sasaki S, Shiigai T, Yoshiyama N, Takeuchi J. Mechanism of bicarbonate exit across basolateral membrane of rabbit proximal straight tubule. *Am J Physiol* 1987;252:F11–F18.

618. Sasaki S, Siragy HM, Gildea JJ, Felder RA, Carey RM. Production and role of extracellular guanosine cyclic 3', 5' monophosphate in sodium uptake in human proximal tubule cells. *Hypertension* 2004;43:286–291.

619. Sasaki S, Yoshiyama N. Interaction of chloride and bicarbonate transport across the basolateral membrane of rabbit proximal straight tubule. Evidence for sodium coupled chloride/bicarbonate exchange. *J Clin Invest* 1988;81:1004–1011.

620. Satoh T, Cohen HT, Katz AI. Different mechanisms of renal Na-K-ATPase regulation by protein kinases in proximal and distal nephron. *Am J Physiol* 1993;265:F399–F405.

621. Scalera V, Corcelli A, Frassanito A, Carlo S. Chloride dependence of the sodium-dependent glycine transport in pig kidney cortex brush-border membrane vesicles. *Biochim Biophys Acta* 1987;903:1–10.

622. Schafer JA, Andreoli TE. Perfusion of isolated mammalian renal tubules. In: Giebisch G, ed. *Transport Organs*. Vol. IV. *Membrane Transport in Biology*. Berlin: Springer-Verlag; 1979:473–528.

623. Schafer JA, Patlak CS, Andreoli TE. A component of fluid absorption linked to passive ion flows in the superficial pars recta. *J Gen Physiol* 1975;66:445–471.

624. Schafer JA, Patlak CS, Andreoli TE. Fluid absorption and active and passive ion flows in the rabbit superficial pars recta. *Am J Physiol* 1977;233:F154–F167.

625. Schafer JA, Patlak CS, Troutman SL, Andreoli TE. Volume absorption in the pars recta. II. Hydraulic conductivity coefficient. *Am J Physiol* 1978;234:F340–F348.

626. Schafer JA, Troutman SL, Watkins ML, Andreoli TE. Volume absorption in the pars recta. I. "Simple" active Na⁺ transport. *Am J Physiol* 1978;234:F332–F339.

627. Schafer JA, Troutman SL, Watkins ML, Andreoli TE. Flow dependence of fluid transport in the isolated superficial pars recta: Evidence that osmotic disequilibrium between external solutions drives isotonic fluid absorption. *Kidney Int* 1981;20:588–597.

628. Schafer JA, Williams JC. Transport of metabolic substrates by the proximal nephron. *Ann Rev Physiol* 1985;47:103–125.

629. Schatzmann HJ, Windhager EE, Solomon AK. Single proximal tubules of the *Necturus* kidney. II. Effect of 2, 4-dinitrophenol and ouabain on water reabsorption. *Am J Physiol* 1958;195:570–574.

630. Schild L, Aronson PS, Giebisch G. Effects of apical membrane Cl-formate exchange on cell volume in rabbit proximal tubule. *Am J Physiol* 1990;258:F530–F536.

631. Schild L, Aronson PS, Giebisch G. Basolateral transport pathways for K⁺ and Cl⁻ in rabbit proximal tubule: effects on cell volume. *Am J Physiol* 1991;260:F101–F109.

632. Schild L, Giebisch G, Karniski L, Aronson PS. Chloride transport in the mammalian proximal tubule. *Pflugers Arch* 1986;407(Suppl 2):S156–S159.

633. Schild L, Giebisch G, Karniski LP, Aronson PS. Effect of formate on volume reabsorption in the rabbit proximal tubule. *J Clin Invest* 1987;79:32–38.

634. Schmidt U, Dubach UC. Activity of (Na⁺, K⁺)-stimulated adenosinetriphosphatase in the rat nephron. *Pflugers Arch* 1969;306:219–226.

635. Schmidt U, Schmid H, Funk B, Dubach UC. The function of Na K-ATPase in single portions of the rat nephron. *Ann N Y Acad Sci* 1974;242:489–500.

636. Schmitt BM, Biemesderfer D, Romero MF, Boulpaep EL, Boron WF. Immunolocalization of the electrogenic Na⁺-HCO₃ cotransporter in mammalian and amphibian kidney. *Am J Physiol* 1999;276:F27–F38.

637. Schneeberger EE, Lynch RD. Structure function and regulation of cellular tight junctions. *Am J Physiol* 1992;262:L647–L661.

638. Schneider EG, Sacktor B. Sodium gradient-dependent L-glutamate transport in renal brush border membrane vesicles. Effect of an intravesicular > extravesicular potassium gradient. *J Biol Chem* 1980;255:7645–7649.

639. Schnermann J, Chou CL, Ma T, Traynor T, Knepper MA, Verkman AS. Defective proximal tubular fluid reabsorption in transgenic aquaporin-1 null mice. *Proc Natl Acad Sci U S A* 1998;95:9660–9664.

640. Schnermann J, Wahl M, Liebau G, FischbachH. Balance between tubular flow rate and net fluid reabsorption in the proximal convolution of the rat kidney. *Pflugers Arch* 1968;304:90–103.

641. Schultheis PJ, Clarke LL, Meneton P, Miller ML, Soleimani M, Gawenis LR, Riddle TM, Duffy JJ, Doetschman T, Wang T, Giebisch G, Aronson PS, Lorenz JN, Shull GE. Renal and intestinal absorptive defects in mice lacking the NHE3 Na⁺/H⁺ exchanger. *Nature Genet* 1998;19:2282–2285.

642. Schultz SG. Homocellular regulatory mechanisms in sodium-transporting epithelia: Avoidance of extinction by "flush-through." *Am J Physiol* 1981;241:F579–F590.

643. Schultz SG. Membrane cross-talk in sodium-absorbing epithelial cells. In: Seldin DW, Giebisch G, eds. *The Kidney: Physiology and Pathophysiology*. New York: Raven Press; 1992:287–299.

644. Schultz SG, Hudson RL, Lapointe JY. Electrophysiological studies of sodium cotransport in epithelia: toward a cellular model. *Ann N Y Acad Sci* 1985;456:127–135.

645. Schuster VL. Effects of angiotensin on proximal tubular reabsorption. *Fed Proc* 1986;45:1444–1447.

646. Schuster VL, Kokko JP, Jacobson HR. Angiotensin II directly stimulates sodium transport in rabbit proximal convoluted tubules. *J Clin Invest* 1984;73:507–515.

647. Schwartz GJ. Na⁺-dependent H⁺ efflux from proximal tubule: evidence for reversible Na⁺–H+ exchange. *Am J Physiol* 1981;241:F380–F385.

648. Schwartz GJ. Absence of Cl⁻-OH⁻ or Cl⁻-HCO⁻ exchange in the rabbit renal proximal tubule. *Am J Physiol* 1983;245:F462–F469.

649. Sciortino CM, Romero MF. Cation and voltage dependence of rat kidney electrogenic Na (+)-HCO₃ (-) cotransporter rkNBC, expressed in oocytes. *Am J Physiol* 1999;277:F611–F623.

650. Scott DA, Karniski LP. Human pendrin expressed in Xenopus laevis oocytes mediates chloride/formate exchange. *Am J Physiol* 2000;278:C207–C211.

651. Seely JF. Effects of peritubular oncotic pressure on rat proximal tubule electrical resistance. *Kidney Int* 1973;4:28–35.

652. Seely JF. Variation in electrical resistance along length of rat proximal convoluted tubule. *Am J Physiol* 1973;225:48–57.

653. Seifter JL, Aronson PS. Cl⁻ transport via anion exchange in *Necturus* renal microvillus membranes. *Am J Physiol* 1984;247:F888–F895.

654. Seifter JL, Aronson PS. Properties and physiologic roles of the plasma membrane sodium-hydrogen exchanger. *J Clin Invest* 1986;78:859–864.

655. Seifter JL, Knickelbein R, Aronson PS. Absence of Cl⁻OH exchange and NaCl transport in rabbit renal microvillus membrane vesicles. *Am J Physiol* 1984;247:F753–F759.

656. Seikaly MG, Arant BS Jr, Seney FD Jr. Endogenous angiotensin concentrations in specific intrarenal fluid compartments of the rat. *J Clin Invest* 1990;86:1352–1357.

657. Seki G, Coppola S, Yoshitomi K, Burckhardt BC, Samarzija I, Muller-Berger S, Frömter E. On the mechanism of bicarbonate exit from renal proximal tubular cells. *Kidney Int* 1996;49:1671–1677.

658. Seki G, Taniguchi S, Uwatoko S, Suzuki K, Kurokawa K. Evidence for conductive Cl⁻ pathway in the basolateral membrane of rabbit renal proximal tubule S3 segment. *J Clin Invest* 1993;92:1229–1235.

659. Seki G, Taniguchi S, Uwatoko S, Suzuki K, Kurokawa K. Activation of the basolateral Cl⁻ conductance by cAMP in rabbit renal proximal tubule S3 segments. *Pflugers Arch* 1995;430:88–95.

660. Seki G, Yamada H, Taniguchi S, Uwatoko S, Suzuki K, Kurokawa K. Mechanism of anion permeation in the basolateral membrane of isolated rabbit renal proximal tubule S3 segment. *Am J Physiol* 1997;272:C837–C846.

661. Selen G, Persson AEG. Hydrostatic and oncotic pressures in the interstitium of dehydrated and volume expanded rats. *Acta Physiol Scand* 1983;117:75–81.

662. Seri I, Kone BC, Gullans SR, Aperia A, Brenner BM, Ballerman BJ. Locally formed dopamine inhibits Na⁺-K⁺-ATPase activity in rat renal cortical tubule cells. *Am J Physiol* 1988;255:F666–F673.

663. Seri I, Kone BC, Gullans SR, Aperia A, Brenner BM, Ballerman BJ. Influence of Na⁺ intake on dopamine-induced inhibition of renal cortical Na⁺-K⁺-ATPase. *Am J Physiol* 1990;258:F52–F60.

664. Shenolikar S, Voltz JW, Minkoff CM, Wade JB, Weinman EJ. Targeted disruption of the mouse NHERF-1 gene promotes internalization of proximal tubule sodium-phosphate cotransporter type IIa and renal phosphate wasting. *Proc Natl Acad Sci U S A* 2002;99:11470–11475.

665. Shenolikar S, Weinman EJ. NHERF: targeting and trafficking membrane proteins. *Am J Physiol* 2001;280:F389–F395.
666. Sheu J-N, Quigley R, Baum M. Heterogeneity of chloride/base exchange in rabbit superficial and juxtamedullary proximal convoluted tubules. *Am J Physiol* 1995;268:F847–F853.
667. Shi L-B, Fushimi K, Verkman AS. Solvent drag measurement of transcellular and basolateral membrane NaCl reflection coefficient in kidney proximal tubule. *J Gen Physiol* 1991;98: 379–398.
668. Shindo T, Spring KR. Chloride movement across the basolateral membrane of proximal tubule cells. *J Membr Biol* 1981;58:35–42.
669. Shipp JC, Hanenson IB, Windhager EE, Schatzmann HJ, Whittembury G, Yoshimura H, Solomon AK. Single proximal tubules of the *Necturus* kidney. Methods for micropuncture and microperfusion. *Am J Physiol* 1958;195:563–569.
670. Shiuan D, Weinstein SW. Evidence for electroneutral chloride transport in rabbit renal cortical brush border membrane vesicles. *Am J Physiol* 1984;247:F837–F847.
671. Silverman M. Glucose reabsorption in the kidney. *Can J Physiol Pharmacol* 1981;59: 209–224.
672. Sohtell M. Electrochemical forces for chloride transport in the proximal tubules of the rat kidney. *Acta Physiol Scand* 1978;103:363–369.
673. Soleimani M, Aronson PS. Ionic mechanism of Na^+-HCO_3^- cotransport in rabbit renal basolateral membrane vesicles. *J Biol Chem* 1989;264 (31):18302–18308.
674. Soleimani M, Bizal GL. Functional indentity of a purified proximal tubule anion exchange protein: mediation of chloride/formate and chloride/bicarbonate exchange. *Kidney Int* 1996;50:1914–1921.
675. Soleimani M, Bizal GL, Anderson CC. Aprotein with anion exchange properties found in the kidney proximal tubule. *Kidney Int* 1993;44:565–573.
676. Soleimani M, Burnham CE. Na^+:HCO_3^- cotransporters (NBC): cloning and characterization. *J Membr Biol* 2001;183:71–84.
677. Soleimani M, Grassi SM, Aronson PS. Stoichiometry of Na^+-HCO_3^- cotransport in basolateral membrane vesicles isolated from rabbit renal cortex. *J Clin Invest* 1987;79:1276–1280.
678. Soleimani M, Greeley T, Petrovic S, Wang Z, Amlal H, Kopp P, Burnham CE. Pendrin: an apical Cl^-/OH^-/HCO_3^- exchanger in the kidney cortex. *Am J Physiol* 2001;280:F356–F364.
679. Soltoff SP, Mandel LJ. Active ion transport in the renal proximal tubule. I. Transport and metabolic studies. *J Gen Physiol* 1984;84:601–622.
680. Soltoff SP, Mandel LJ. Active ion transport in the renal proximal tubule. II. Ionic dependence of the Na pump. *J Gen Physiol* 1984;84:623–642.
681. Soltoff SP, Mandel LJ. Active ion transport in the renal proximal tubule. III. The ATP dependence of the Na pump. *J Gen Physiol* 1984;84:643–662.
682. Spitzer A, Windhager EE. Effect of peritubular oncotic pressure changes on proximal tubular fluid reabsorption. *Am J Physiol* 1970;218:1188–1193.
683. Spring KR. A parallel path model for *Necturus* proximal tubule. *J Membr Biol* 1973;13: 323–352.
684. Spring KR, Giebisch G. Kinetics of Na^+ transport in *Necturus* proximal tubule. *J Gen Physiol* 1977;70:307–328.
685. Spring KR, Kimura G. Chloride reabsorption by renal proximal tubules of *Necturus*. *J Membr Biol* 1978;38:233–254.
686. Stanton RC, Mendrick DL, RennkeHG, Seifter JL. Use of monoclonal antibodies to culture rat proximal tubule cells. *Am J Physiol* 1986;251:C780–C786.
687. Stroup RF, Weinman E, Hayslett JP, Kashgarian M. Effect of luminal permeability on net transport across the amphibian proximal tubule. *Am J Physiol* 1974;226:1110–1116.
688. Suzuki M, Morita T, Hanaoka K, Kawaguchi Y, Sakai O. A Cl^- channel activated by parathyroid hormone in rabbit renal proximal tubule cells. *J Clin Invest* 1991;88:735–742.
689. Szaszi K, Kurashima K, Kaibuchi K, Grinstein S, Orlowski J. Role of the cytoskeleton in mediating cAMP-dependent protein kinase inhibition of the epithelial Na^+/H^+ exchanger NHE3. *J Biol Chem* 2001;276:40761–40768.
690. Talor Z, Arruda JAL. Partial purification and reconstitution of renal basolateral Na^+-Ca^{++} exchanger into liposomes. *J Biol Chem* 1985;260:15473–15476.
691. Terada Y, Tomita K, Nonoguchi H, Marumo F. Polymerase chain reaction localization of constitutive nitric oxide synthase and soluble guanylate cyclase messenger RNAs in microdissected rat nephron segments. *J Clin Invest* 1992;90:659–665.
692. Thekkumkara TJ, Cookson R, Linas SL. Angiotensin (AT1A) receptor-mediated increases in transcellular sodium transport in proximal tubule cells. *Am J Physiol* 1998;274:F897–905.
693. Thomas SR, Mikulecky DC. A network thermodynamic model of salt and water flow across the kidney proximal tubule. *Am J Physiol* 1978;235:F638–F648.
694. Thomson SC, Vallon V. Alpha-2–adrenoceptors determine the response to nitric oxide inhibition in the rat glomerulus and proximal tubule. *J Am Soc Nephrol* 1995;6:1482–1490.
695. Tisher CC, Kokko JP. Relationship between peritubular oncotic pressure gradients and morphology in isolated proximal tubules. *Kidney Int* 1974;6:146–156.
696. Tisher CC, Yarger WE. Lanthanum permeability of the tight junction (zonula occludens) in the renal tubule of the rat. *Kidney Int* 1973;3:238–250.
697. Tormey JM, Diamond JM. The ultrastructural route of fluid transport in rabbit gall bladder. *J Gen Physiol* 1967;50:2031–2060.
698. Tripathi S, Boulpaep EL. Cell membrane water permeabilities and streaming currents in Ambystoma proximal tubule. *Am J Physiol* 1988;255:F188–203.
699. Tse C-M, Brant SR, Walker MS, Pouyssegur J, Donowitz M. Cloning and sequencing of a rabbit cDNA encoding an intestinal and kidney-specific Na^+/H^+ exchanger isoform (NHE-3). *J Biol Chem* 1992;267:9340–9346.
700. Tse C-M, Levine SA, Yun CHC, Brant SR, Pouyssegur J, Montrose MH, Donowitz M. Functional characteristics of a cloned epithelial Na^+/H^+ exchanger (NHE3): resistance to amiloride and inhibition by protein kinase C. *Proc Natl Acad Sci U S A* 1993;90:9110–9114.
701. Tsuchiya K, Wang W, Giebisch G, Welling PA. ATP is a coupling modulator of parallel Na K-ATPase-K-channel activity in the renal proximal tubule. *Proc Natl Acad Sci U S A* 1992;89:6418–6422.
702. Tucker BJ, Blantz RC. Determinants of proximal tubular reabsorption as mechanisms of glomerulotubular balance. *Am J Physiol* 1978;235:F142–F150.
703. Tumlin JA, Hoban CA, Medford RM, Sands JM. Expression of Na-K-ATPase alpha- and beta-subunit mRNA and protein isoforms in the rat nephron. *Am J Physiol* 1994;266:F240–F245.
704. Turner RJ. Quantitative studies of cotransport systems: models and vesicles. *J Membr Biol* 1983;76:1–15.
705. Turner RJ. βamino acid transport across the renal brush border membrane is coupled to both Na and Cl. *J Biol Chem* 1986;261:16060–16066.
706. Turner RJ, Moran A. Further studies of proximal tubular brush border membrane D-glucose transport heterogeneity. *J Membr Biol* 1982;70:37–45.
707. Turner RJ, Moran A. Heterogeneity of sodium-dependent D-glucose transport sites along the proximal tubule: Evidence from vesicle studies. *Am J Physiol* 1982;242:F406–F414.
708. Turner RJ, Moran A. Stoichiometric studies of the renal outer cortical brush border membrane D-glucose transporter. *J Membr Biol* 1982;67:73–80.
709. Turner RJ, Silverman M. Sugar uptake into brush border vesicles from dog kidney. II. Kinetics. *Biochim Biophys Acta* 1978;511:470–486.
710. Ullrich KJ. Permeability characteristics of the mammalian nephron. In: Orloff J, Berliner RW, eds. *Handbook of Physiology*. Section 8: Renal Physiology. Washington, DC: American Physiological Society; 1973:377–398.
711. Ullrich KJ. Renal tubular mechanisms of organic solute transport. *Kidney Int* 1976;9: 134–148.
712. Ullrich KJ. Sugar amino acid and Na^+ cotransport in the proximal tubule. *Annu Rev Physiol* 1979;41:181–195.
713. Ullrich KJ, Papavassiliou F. Contraluminal bicarbonate transport in the proximal tubule of the rat kidney. *Pflugers Arch* 1987;410:501–504.
714. Ullrich KJ, Rumrich G. Direkte Messung der Waser permabilitat corticaler Nephronabschnitte bei Verschiedenen Diuresezustanden. *Pflugers Arch* 1963;351:35–48.
715. Ullrich KJ, Rumrich G, Kloss S. Active Ca^{++} reabsorption in the proximal tubule of the rat kidney. *Pflugers Arch* 1976;364:223–228.
716. Ussing HH. Volume regulation of frog skin epithelium. *Acta Physiol Scand* 1982;114: 363–369.
717. Vallon V, Grahammer F, Richter K, Bleich M, Lang F, Barhanin J, Volkl H, Warth R. Role of KCNE1–dependent K^+ fluxes in mouse proximal tubule. *J Am Soc Nephrol* 2001;12:2003–2011.
718. Vallon V, Schwark JR, Richter K, Hropot M. Role of Na (+)/H (+) exchanger NHE3 in nephron function: micropuncture studies with S3226, an inhibitor of NHE3. *Am J Physiol* 2000;278:F375–F379.
719. Vallon V, Verkman AS, Schnermann J. Luminal hypotonicity in proximal tubules of aquaporin-1–knockout mice. *Am J Physiol* 2000;278:F1030–F1033.
720. Vance BA, Biagi BA. Microelectrode characterization of the basolateral membrane of rabbit S3 proximal tubule. *J Membr Biol* 1989;108:53–60.
721. Van der Goot F, Corman B. Axial heterogeneity of apical water permeability along rabbit kidney proximal tubule. *Am J Physiol* 1991;260: R186–R191.
722. Van der Goot FG, Podevin RA, Corman BJ. Water permeabilities and salt reflection coefficients of luminal basolateral and intracellular membrane vesicles isolated from rabbit kidney proximal tubule. *Biochim Biophys Acta* 1989;986:332–340.
723. Van der Goot F, Ripoche P, Corman B. Determination of solute reflection coefficients in kidney brush-border membrane vesicles by light scattering: influence of the refractive index. *Biochim Biophys Acta* 1989;979:272–274.
724. van Heeswijk MPE, Geertsen JAM, van Os CH. Kinetic properties of the ATP-dependent Ca^{++} pump and the Na^+/Ca^{++} exchange system in basolateral membranes from rat kidney cortex. *J Membr Biol* 1984;79:19–31.
725. van Heeswijk MPE, van Os CH. Osmotic water permeabilities of brush border and basolateral membrane vesicles from rat renal cortex and small intestine. *J Membr Biol* 1986;92:183–193.
726. van Os CH, Wiedner G, Wright EM. Volume flows across gallbladder epithelium induced by small hydrostatic and osmotic gradients. *J Membr Biol* 1979;49:1–20.
727. Vari RC, Ott CE. In vivo proximal tubular fluid-to-plasma chloride concentration gradient in the rabbit. *Am J Physiol* 1982;242:F575–F579.
728. Veech RL, Lawson JWR, Cornell NW, Krebs HA. Cytosolic phosphorylation potential. *J Biol Chem* 1979;254:6538–6547.
729. Verkman AS. Mechanisms of regulation of water permeability in renal epithelia. *Am J Physiol* 1989;257:C837–C850.
730. Verkman AS, Dix JA, Seifter JL. Water and urea transport in renal microvillus membrane vesicles. *Am J Physiol* 1985;248:F650–F655.
731. Verkman AS, Ives HE. Water permeability and fluidity of renal basolateral membranes. *Am J Physiol* 1986;250:F633–F643.
732. Verrey F, Ristic Z, Romeo E, Ramadan T, Makrides V, DaveMH, Wagner CA, Camargo SMR. Novel renal amino acid transporters. *Annu Rev Physiol* 2005;67:557–572.
733. Volkl H, Lang F. Electrophysiology of cell volume regulation in proximal tubules of the mouse kidney. *Pflugers Arch* 1988;411:514–519.
734. Volkl H, Lang F. Ionic requirement for regulatory cell volume decrease in renal straight proximal tubules. *Pflugers Arch* 1988;412:1–6.
735. Volkl H, Paulmichl M, Lang F. Cell volume regulation in renal cortical cells. *Renal Physiol Biochem* 1988;11:158–173.
736. Wade JB, Welling PA, Donowitz M, Shenolikar S, Weinman EJ. Differential renal distribution of NHERF isoforms and their colocalization with NHE3, ezrin and ROMK. *Am J Physiol* 2001;280:C192–C198.
737. Wagner CA, Giebisch G, Lang F, Geibel JP. Angiotensin II stimulates vesicular H^+-ATPase in rat proximal tubular cells. *Proc Natl Acad Sci U S A* 1998;95:9665–9668.
738. Wang T. Nitric oxide regulates HCO_3^- and Na^+ transport by a cGMP-mediated mechanism in the kidney proximal tubule. *Am J Physiol* 1997;272:F242–F248.
739. Wang T. Role of iNOS and eNOS in modulating proximal tubule transport and acid–base balance. *Am J Physiol* 2002;283:F658–F662.
740. Wang T, Chan YL. Time and dose-dependent effects of protein kinase C on proximal bicarbonate transport. *J Membr Biol* 1990;117:131–139.

741. Wang T, Egbert AL Jr, Abbiati T, Aronson PS, Giebisch G. Mechanisms of stimulation of proximal tubule chloride transport by formate and oxalate. *Am J Physiol* 1996;271:F446–F450.
742. Wang T, Giebisch G, Aronson PS. Effects of formate and oxalate on volume absorption in rat proximal tubule. *Am J Physiol* 1992;263:F37–F42.
743. Wang T, Hropot M, Aronson PS, Giebisch G. Role of NHE isoforms in mediating bicarbonate reabsorption along the nephron. *Am J Physiol* 2001;281:F1117–F1122.
744. Wang T, Inglis FM, Kalb RG. Defective fluid and HCO_3^- absorption in proximal tubule of neuronal nitric oxide synthase-knockout mice. *Am J Physiol* 2000;279:F518–F524.
745. Wang T, Segal AS, Giebisch G, Aronson PS. Stimulation of chloride transport by cAMP in rat proximal tubules. *Am J Physiol* 1995;268:F204–F210.
746. Wang T, Yang CL, Abbiati T, Schultheis PJ, Shull GE, Giebisch G, Aronson PS. Mechanism of proximal tubule bicarbonate absorption in NHE3 null mice. *Am J Physiol* 1999;277: F298–302.
747. Wang T, Yang CL, Abbiati T, Shull GE, Giebisch G, Aronson PS. Essential role of NHE3 in facilitating formate-dependent NaCl absorption in the proximal tubule. *Am J Physiol* 2001;281:F288–F292.
748. Wang Z, Wang T, Petrovic S, Tuo B, Riederer B, Barone S, Lorenz JN, Seidler U, Aronson PS, Soleimani M. Renal and intestinal transport defects in Slc26a6-null mice. *Am J Physiol* 2005;288:C957–C965.
749. Wareing M, Green R. Effect of formate and oxalate on fluid reabsorption from the proximal convoluted tubule of the anaesthetized rat. *J Physiol* 1994;477:347–354.
750. Warner RR, Lechene C. Isosmotic volume reabsorption in rat proximal tubule. *J Gen Physiol* 1980;76:559–586.
751. Warnock DG, Eveloff J. NaCl entry mechanisms in the luminal membrane of the renal tubule. *Am J Physiol* 1982;42:F561–F574.
752. Warnock DG, Eveloff J. K-Cl cotransport systems. *Kidney Int* 1989;36:412–417.
753. Warnock DG, Reenstra WW, Yee VJ. Na^+/H^+ antiporter of brush border vesicles: studies with acridine orange uptake. *Am J Physiol* 1982;242:F733–F739.
754. Warnock DG, Yee VJ. Neutral NaCl cotransport in the proximal tubule: Evidence for the parallel exchanger model. *Clin Res* 1981;29:479A (abstract).
755. Warnock DG, Yee VJ. Chloride uptake by brush border membrane vesicles isolated from rabbit renal cortex. *J Clin Invest* 1981;67:103–115.
756. Warnock DG, Yee VJ. Anion permeabilities of the isolated perfused rabbit proximal tubule. *Am J Physiol* 1982;242:F395–F405.
757. Weinman EJ, Dubinsky W, Shenolikar S. Regulation of the renal Na^+–H+ exchanger by protein phosphorylation. *Kidney Int* 1989;36:519–525.
758. Weinman EJ, Minkoff C, Shenolikar S. Signal complex regulation of renal transport proteins: NHERF and regulation of NHE3 by PKA. *Am J Physiol* 2000;279:F393–F399.
759. Weinman EJ, Sansom SC, Knight TF, Senekjian HO. Alpha and beta adrenergic agonists stimulate water absorption in the rat proximal tubule. *J Membr Biol* 1982;69:107–111.
760. Weinman EJ, Shenolikar S. Protein kinase C activates the renal apical membrane Na^+/H^+ exchanger. *J Membr Biol* 1986;93:133–139.
761. Weinman EJ, Shenolikar S. Regulation of the renal brush border membrane Na^+/H^+ exchanger. *Ann Rev Physiol* 1993;55:289–304.
762. Weinman EJ, Shenolikar S, Kahn AM. cAMP-associated inhibition of Na^+–H+ exchanger in rabbit kidney brush-border membranes. *Am J Physiol* 1987;252:F19–F25.
763. Weinman EJ, Steplock D, Shenolikar S. cAMP-mediated inhibition of the renal brush border membrane Na^+–H+ exchanger requiresa dissociable phosphoprotein cofactor. *J Clin Invest* 1993;92:1781–1786.
764. Weinman EJ, Steplock D, Shenolikar S. Acute regulation of NHE3 by protein kinase A requires a multiprotein signal complex. *Kidney Int* 2001;60:450–454.
765. Weinman EJ, Steplock D, Wang Y, Shenolikar S. Characterization of a protein cofactor that mediates protein kinase A regulation of the renal brush border membrane Na^+–H+ exchanger. *J Clin Invest* 1995;95:2143–2149.
766. Weinstein AM. A nonequilibrium thermodynamic model of the rat proximal tubule epithelium. *Biophys J* 1983;44:153–170.
767. Weinstein AM. Transport by epithelia with compliant lateral intercellular spaces: asymmetric oncotic effects across the rat proximal tubule. *Am J Physiol* 1984;247:F848–F862.
768. Weinstein AM. Glucose transport in a model of the rat proximal tubule epithelium. *Math Biosci* 1985;76:87–115.
769. Weinstein AM. Convective paracellular solute flux: a source of ion–ion interaction in the epithelial transport equations. *J Gen Physiol* 1987;89:501–518.
770. Weinstein AM. Modeling the proximal tubule: complications of the paracellular pathway. *Am J Physiol* 1988;254:F297–F305.
771. Weinstein AM. Glomerulotubular balance in a mathematical model of the proximal nephron. *Am J Physiol* 1990;258:F612–F626.
772. Weinstein AM. Chloride transport in mathematical model of the rat proximal tubule. *Am J Physiol* 1992;263:F784–F798.
773. Weinstein AM. Performance of a kinetically defined Na^+/H^+ antiporter within a mathematical model of the rat proximal tubule. *J Gen Physiol* 1995;105:617–641.
774. Weinstein AM. Coupling of entry to exit by Peritubular K^+-permeability in a mathematical model of the rat proximal tubule. *Am J Physiol* 1996;271:F158–F168.
775. Weinstein AM, Stephenson JL. Models of coupled salt and water transport across leaky epithelia. *J Membr Biol* 1981;60:1–20.
776. Weinstein AM, Stephenson JL, Spring KR. The coupled transport of water. In: Bonting SL, de Pont JJHHM, eds. Amsterdam: Elsevier/North-Holland Biomedical Press; 1981:311–351.
777. Welling LW, Welling DJ. Surface areas of brush border and lateral cell walls in the rabbit proximal nephron. *Kidney Int* 1975;8:343–348.
778. Welling LW, Welling DJ. Shape of epithelial cells and intracellular channels in the rabbit proximal nephron. *Kidney Int* 1976;9:385–394.
779. Welling LW, Welling DJ, Holsapple JW, Evan AP. Morphometric analysis of distinct microanatomy near the base of proximal tubule cells. *Am J Physiol* 1987;22:F126–F140.
780. Welling LW, Welling DJ, Ochs TJ. Video measurement of basolateral membrane hydraulic conductivity in the proximal tubule. *Am J Physiol* 1983;245:F123–F129.
781. Welling LW, Welling DJ, Ochs TJ. Relative osmotic effects of raffinose KCl and NaCl across basolateral cell membrane. *Am J Physiol* 1990;259:F594–F597.
782. Welling PA, Linshaw MA. Importance of anion in hypotonic volume regulation of rabbit proximal straight tubule. *Am J Physiol* 1988;255:F853–F860.
783. Welling PA, O'Neil RG. Ionic conductive properties of rabbit proximal straight tubule basolateral membrane. *Am J Physiol* 1990;258:F940–F950.
784. Welling PA, O'Neil RG. Cell swelling activates basolateral membrane Cl and K conductances in rabbit proximal tubule. *Am J Physiol* 1990;258:F951–F962.
785. Whitlock RT, Wheeler HO. Coupled transport of solute and water across rabbit gallbladder epithelium. *J Clin Invest* 1964;48:2249–2265.
786. Whittembury G, Malnic G, Mello-Aires M, Amorena C. Solvent drag of sucrose during absorption indicates paracellular water flow in the rat kidney proximal tubule. *Pflugers Arch* 1988;412:541–547.
787. Whittembury G, Pas-Aliaga A, Biondi A, Carpi-Medina P, Gonzalez E, Linares H. Pathways for volume flow and volume regulation in leaky epithelia. *Pflugers Arch* 1985;405:S17–S22.
788. Whittembury G, Rawlins FA. Visualization of tubular interspaces in the kidney with the aid of lanthanum. *Yale J Biol Med* 1972;45:446–450.
789. Whittembury G, Sugino N, Solomon AK. Ionic permeability and electrical potential differences in *Necturus* kidney cells. *J Gen Physiol* 1961;44:689–712.
790. Wiederholt M, Hierholzer K, Windhager EE, Giebisch G. Microperfusion study of fluid reabsorption in proximal tubules of rat kidneys. *Am J Physiol* 1967;213:809–818.
791. Wiederkehr MR, Di Sole F, Collazo R, Quinones H, Fan L, Murer H, Helmle-Kolb C, Moe OW. Characterization of acute inhibition of Na/H exchanger NHE-3 by dopamine in opossum kidney cells. *Kidney Int* 2001;59:197–209.
792. Wiederkehr MR, Zhao H, Moe OW. Acute regulation of Na/H exchanger NHE3 activity by protein kinase C: role of NHE3 phosphorylation. *Am J Physiol* 1999;276:C1205–C1217.
793. Wilcox CS, Baylis C. Glomerular-tubular balance and proximal regulation. In: Seldin DW, Giebisch G, eds. *The Kidney. Physiology and Pathophysiology*. New York: Raven Press; 1985:985–1012.
794. Williams AW. Electron microscopic changes associated with water absorption in the jejunum. *Gut* 1963;4:1–7.
795. Williams JC Jr, Schafer JA. A model of osmotic and hydrostatic pressure effects on volume absorption in the proximal tubule. *Am J Physiol* 1987;253:F563–F575.
796. Williams JC, Schafer JA. Cortical interstitium as a site for solute polarization during tubular absorption. *Am J Physiol* 1988;254:F813–F823.
797. Willmann JK, Bleich M, Rizzo M, Schmidt-Hieber M, Ullrich KJ, Greger R. Amiloride-inhibitable Na^+ conductance in rat proximal tubule. *Pflugers Arch* 1997;434:173–178.
798. Winaver J, Burnett JC, Tyce GM, Dousa TP. ANP inhibits Na^+–H+ antiport in proximal tubular brush border membrane: role of dopamine. *Kidney Int* 1990;38:1133–1140.
799. Windhager EE. Sodium chloride transport. In: Giebisch G, ed. *Transport Organs*. Vol. IV. *Membrane Transport in Biology*. Berlin: Springer-Verlag; 1979:145–214.
800. Windhager EE, Boulpaep EL, Giebisch G. Electrophysiological studies on single nephrons. In: *Proceedings of the 3rd International Congress of Nephrology*. Washington, DC: Karger Basel; 1967:35–47.
801. Windhager EE, Taylor A. Regulatory role of intracellular calcium ions in epithelial Na transport. *Ann Rev Physiol* 1983;45:519–532.
802. Windhager EE, Taylor A, Maack T, Lee CO, LorenzenM. Studies on renal tubular function. In: Corradino RA, ed. *Functional Regulation at the Cellular and Molecular Levels*. Amsterdam: Elsevier/North Holland; 1982:299–319.
803. Windhager EE, Whittembury G, Oken DE, Schatzmann HJ, Solomon AK. Single proximal tubules of the *Necturus* kidney. III. Dependence of H2O movement on NaCl concentration. *Am J Physiol* 1959;197:313–318.
804. Wong KR, Berry CA, Cogan MG. Flow dependence of chloride transport in rat S1 proximal tubules. *Am J Physiol* 1995;269:F870–F875.
805. Wong KR, Berry CA, Cogan MG. Alpha-1 adrenergic control of chloride transport in the rat S1 proximal tubule. *Am J Physiol* 1996;270:F1049–F1056.
806. Wong NL, Whiting SJ, Mizgala CL, Quamme GA. Electrolyte handling by the superficial nephron of the rabbit. *Am J Physiol* 1986;250:F590–F595.
807. Wong PS, Johns EJ. The receptor subtype mediating the action of angiotensin II on intracellular sodium in rat proximal tubules. *Br J Pharmacol* 1998;124:41–46.
808. Wright EM. The intestinal Na^+/glucose cotransporter. *Ann Rev Physiol* 1993;55:575–589.
809. Wright EM. Renal Na ($^+$)-glucose cotransporters. *Am J Physiol* 2001;280:F10–F18.
810. Wright EM, Loo DDF, Panayotova-Heiermann M, Lostao MP, Hirayama BH, Mackenzie B, Boorer K, Zampighi G. "Active" sugar transport in eukaryotes. *J Exp Biol* 1994;196:197–212.
811. Wu M, Biemesderfer D, Giebisch G, Aronson PS. Role of NHE3 in mediating renal brush border Na^+/H^+ exchange. *J Biol Chem* 1996;271(51):32749–32752.
812. Wu XC, Harris PJ, Johns EJ. Nitric oxide and renal nerve-mediated proximal tubular reabsorption in normotensive and hypertensive rats. *Am J Physiol* 1999;277:F560–F566.
813. Wu XC, Johns EJ. Nitric oxide modulation of neurally induced proximal tubular fluid reabsorption in the rat. *Hypertension* 2002;39:790–793.
814. Xia P, Bungay PM, Gibson CC, Kovbasnjuk ON, Spring KR. Diffusion coefficients in the lateral intercellular spaces of Madin–Darby canine kidney cell epithelium determined with caged compounds. *Biophys J* 1998;74:3302–3312.
815. Xie M-H, Liu F-Y, Wong PC, Timmermans PBMWM, Cogan MG. Proximal nephron and renal effects of DuP 753, a nonpeptide angiotensin II receptor antagonist. *Kidney Int* 1990;38:473–479.
816. Xie Q, Welch R, Mercado A, Romero MF, Mount DB. Molecular characterization of the murine Slc26a6 anion exchanger: functional comparison with Slc26a1. *Am J Physiol* 2002;283: F826–F838.
817. Yamaguchi I, Jose PA, Mouradian MM, Canessa LM, Monsma FJ Jr, Sibley DR, Takeyasu K, Felder RA. Expression of dopamine D1A receptor gene in proximal tubule of rat kidneys. *Am J Physiol* 1993;264:F280–F285.
818. Yang JM, Lee CO, Windhager EE. Regulation of cytosolic free calcium in isolated perfused proximal tubules of *Necturus*. *Am J Physiol* 1988;255:F787–F799.

819. Yang LE, Maunsbach AB, Leong PK, McDonough AA. Differential traffic of proximal tubule Na$^+$ transporters during hypertension or PTH: NHE3 to base of microvilli vs. NaPi2 to endosomes. *Am J Physiol* 2004;287:F896–F906.

820. Yao X, Tian S, Chan HY, Biemesderfer D, Desir GV. Expression of KCNA10, a voltage-gated K channel in glomerular endothelium and at the apical membrane of the renal proximal tubule. *J Am Soc Nephrol* 2002;13:2831–2839.

821. Yau C, Rao L, Silverman M. Sugar uptake into a primary culture of dog kidney proximal tubular cells. *Can J Physiol Pharmacol* 1985;63:417–426.

822. Yingst DR, Massey KJ, Rossi NF, Mohanty MJ, Mattingly RR. Angiotensin II directly stimulates activity and alters the phosphorylation of Na-K-ATPase in rat proximal tubule with a rapid time course. *Am J Physiol* 2004;287:F713–F721.

823. Yip KP, Tse CM, McDonough AA, Marsh DJ. Redistribution of Na$^+$/H$^+$ exchanger isoform NHE3 in proximal tubules induced by acute and chronic hypertension. *Am J Physiol* 1998;275:F565–F575.

824. Yip KP, Wagner AJ, Marsh DJ. Detection of apical Na$^{(+)}$/H$^{(+)}$ exchanger activity inhibition in proximal tubules induced by acute hypertension. *Am J Physiol* 2000;279:R1412–R1418.

825. Yoshitomi K, Burckhardt BC, Frömter E. Rheogenic sodium-bicarbonate cotransport in the peritubular cell membrane of rat renal proximal tubule. *Pflugers Arch* 1985;405:360–366.

826. Yoshitomi K, Frömter E. How big is the electrochemical potential difference of Na$^+$ across rat renal proximal tubular cell membranes in vivo. *Pflugers Arch* 1985;405(Suppl 1):S121–S126.

827. Yoshitomi K, Hoshi T. Intracellular Cl$^-$ activity of the proximal tubule of *Triturus* kidney: dependence on extracellular ionic composition and transmembrane potential. *Am J Physiol* 1983;245:F359–F366.

828. You G, Lee W, Barros EJG, Kanai Y, Huo T, Khawaja S, Wells RG, Nigam SK, Hediger MA. Molecular characterization of Na$^+$-coupled glucose transporters in adult and embryonic rat kidney. *J Biol Chem* 1995;270:29365–29371.

829. Yucha CB, Stoner LC. Bicarbonate transport by amphibian nephron. *Am J Physiol* 1986;251:F865–F872.

830. Zelikovic I, Budreau-Patters A. Cl$^-$ and membrane potential dependence of amino acid transport across the rat renal brush border membrane. *Mol Gen Metab* 1999;67:236–247.

831. Zelikovic I, Chesney RW. Sodium-coupled amino acid transport in renal tubule. *Kidney Int* 1989;36:351–359.

832. Zelikovic I, Stejskal-Lorenz E, Lohstroh P, Budreau A, Chesney RW. Anion dependence of taurine transport by rat renal brush border membrane vesicles. *Am J Physiol* 1989;256:F646–F655.

833. Zhang Y, Magyar CE, Norian JM, Holstein-Rathlou NH, Mircheff AK, McDonough AA. Reversible effects of acute hypertension on proximal tubule sodium transporters. *Am J Physiol* 1998;274:C1090–C1100.

834. Zhang Y, Mircheff AK, Hensley CB, Magyar CE, Warnock DG, Chambrey R, Yip KP, Marsh DJ, Holstein-Rathlou NH, McDonough AA. Rapid redistribution and inhibition of renal sodium transporters during acute pressure natriuresis *Am J Physiol* 1996;270:F1004–F1014.

835. Zhang Y, Norian JM, Magyar CE, Holstein-Rathlou NH, Mircheff AK, McDonough AA. In vivo PTH provokes apical NHE3 and NaPi2 redistribution and Na-K-ATPase inhibition. *Am J Physiol* 1999;276:F711–F719.

CHAPTER **31**

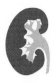

Sodium Chloride Transport in the Loop of Henle, Distal Convoluted Tubule, and Collecting Duct

W. Brian Reeves and Thomas E. Andreoli

Penn State College of Medicine, Milton S. Hershey Medical Center, Hershey, Pennsylvania, USA
University of Arkansas College of Medicine, Little Rock, Arkansas, USA

INTRODUCTION

In this chapter we review the transport of Na^+ by the loop of Henle, distal convoluted tubule, and collecting ducts. We will place special emphasis on the cellular and molecular mechanisms responsible for Na^+ transport in these regions as well as the factors that regulate Na^+ transport.

ANATOMIC CONSIDERATIONS

The mammalian loop of Henle contains the descending thin limb, the ascending thin limb and the thick ascending limb. The thin descending segment begins in the outer medulla after a gradual transition from the pars recta and ends at the hairpin turn at the tip of Henle's loop. The thin ascending limb begins at the tip of Henle's loop and ends with its abrupt transition to the thick ascending limb. Loops of Henle that arise from superficial or midcortical nephrons may lack a thin ascending limb. In these short loops, thick limbs generally begin at, or slightly before, the hairpin turn.

The thick ascending limbs of Henle (TAL) of long-looped nephrons begin at the boundary between the inner and outer medulla. The TAL of short-looped nephrons does not extend as far into the medulla, and may, in fact, be entirely cortical (246). The TAL extends up into the cortex where it abuts the glomerulus of origin for that nephron and forms the macula densa part of the juxtaglomerular apparatus. The TAL is composed of two parts: a medullary portion and a cortical portion. The ratio of medullary to cortical TAL for a given nephron is a function of the depth of the glomerulus of the nephron such that superficial nephrons have primarily cortical thick limbs, while juxtamedullary nephrons possess primarily medullary thick limbs.

The distal nephron may be divided into three segments: the distal convoluted tubule (DCT), the connecting tubule (CNT), and the collecting duct. While these segments are clearly delineated in the rabbit (245), in many species the

transition between contiguous segments is gradual (282). Therefore, distal tubule segments are most accurately defined by their respective cell types: the DCT cell, found only in the DCT; the CNT cell, found only in the CNT; and the principal cell, found in cortical collecting tubules and in medullary collecting tubules.

The distal convoluted tubule (DCT) begins about 50–100 μm beyond the macula densa, and in the rabbit has an average length of about 0.5 mm (335). The DCT is lined by a single type of cell: the DCT cell (245, 282). (Na^+, K^+)-ATPase activity is particularly high in the basolateral membrane of this segment.

The connecting tubule (CNT) forms a transition zone between the DCT and the cortical collecting duct (CCD). This segment is sometimes referred to as the "late distal tubule" or "initial collecting duct." In superficial nephrons, a single connecting tubule drains the DCT into the collecting duct. The connecting tubules of deep nephrons, however, form arcades that ascend through the cortex draining several DCTs into a cortical collecting duct (282). The CNT is lined by two types of cells: the CNT cell, exclusive to the CNT, and the intercalated cell, also found in the collecting duct (245).

The collecting duct begins at, or slightly before the confluence of two or more connecting tubules, and may be divided into three main parts: the cortical collecting duct (CCD), the outer medullary collecting duct (OMCD), and the inner medullary collecting duct (IMCD) (336). The CCD consists of at least three cell types: principal cells, responsible for Na^+ and K^+ transport, and two types of intercalated cells, responsible for H^+ and HCO_3^- transport. In the rabbit, principal cells account for 65%–75% of cells in the CCD (293). The OMCD can be divided into two regions based on location: the outer stripe and the inner stripe. Approximately 80%–90% of cells within the OMCD are principal cells (293). However, as will be discussed later, the functional properties of principal cells in the OMCD differ from those of the CCD. The IMCD extends from the junction between the inner and outer medulla to the tip of the papilla. The IMCD has been divided into three subsegments based on functional differences, including Na$^+$ transport. Intercalated cells account for about 10% of all cells in the initial portion of the IMCD, but are absent from the terminal IMCD (293).

NA$^+$ TRANSPORT IN LOOP OF HENLE

The loop of Henle is responsible for absorbing 25% to 40% of the filtered sodium load (28, 146, 291). Moreover, the dissociation of salt and water absorption by the loop of Henle is ultimately responsible for the capacity of the kidney either to concentrate or to dilute the urine. The active absorption of NaCl in the water-impermeable TAL serves both to dilute the urine and supply the energy for the single effect of countercurrent multiplication.

Salt Transport by Thin Descending and Thin Ascending Segments

There is morphologic and functional evidence of interspecies and both inter- and intra-nephron heterogeneity in the thin loop segments. The morphologic characteristics of the loop of Henle are covered in detail in Chapter 20 of this volume. Generally, loops of Henle can be divided into two groups: long loops and short loops (227). The thin descending limb of short-loop nephrons is a simple, flat epithelium with few organelles and deep junctional complexes (245, 246). The thin descending limbs of long-loop nephrons are

heterogeneous. The upper segment of these thin limbs has a larger diameter and thicker epithelium than short loops. The cells in this region have complicated basolateral interdigitations and apical microvilli, but shallow junctional complexes consist of a single junctional strand. These characteristics are most pronounced in rodents, while in rabbits and humans the upper portion of the thin descending limb has a simpler organization with less extensive interdigitation and deeper junctional complexes (245).

The lower portion of the thin descending limb consists of flat, noninterdigitating cells with a few apical microvilli and with junctional complexes of intermediate depth. There is little interspecies variability in this portion of the descending limb. The thin ascending limb, present only in long-loop nephrons, consists of very flat cells connected by very shallow junctional complexes (507).

According to the passive models for urinary concentration (see Chapter 40, and [276,479]), the thin descending limb should have very high water permeability such that the tubular fluid is concentrated by water abstraction rather than solute entry. In vitro microperfusion studies, with one exception (491), have confirmed that both the upper and lower portions of mammalian descending limbs are very permeable to water (222, 227, 275, 326, 338) (Table 1). In contrast, the descending limbs of birds (355) are rather impermeable to water. The passive models also require that the thin ascending limb be rather impermeable to water, highly permeable to sodium chloride, and only modestly permeable to urea. As indicated in Table 1, in vitro microperfusion studies of thin ascending limb seg-

TABLE 1   Permeability Properties of Thin Limb of Henle Segments

	P_f (10^{-3}cm/sec)	P_{Na} (10^{-5}cm/sec)	P_{Cl} (10^{-5}cm/sec)	P_{Na}/P_{Cl}		P_{urea} (10^{-5}cm/sec)
				SDL	LDLu	
Descending Limb						
Rabbit	240–250	1.61	—	0.75	0.76	1.5
Rat	227	34–47	—	0.61	5.0	
Hamster SDL	285	4.2	1.3	0.68	—	7.4
Hamster LDL$_u$	403	45.6	4.2	—	4–6	1.5
Ascending Limb						
Rabbit	0	25.5	117	0.29		6.7
Rat	2.5	67.9	183.7	0.43		23.0
Hamster	3	87.6	196	0.47		18.5

Note: P_{Na} and P_{Cl} determined from isotope flux measurements. P_{Na}/P_{Cl} determined from salt dilution voltages.

LDLu, upper portion of long-loop descending limb; P_f, osmotic water permeability; SDL, short-loop descending limb.

Data from Imai M. Function of the thin ascending limb of Henle of rats and hamsters perfused in vitro. *Am J Physiol* 1977;232:F201–F209; Imai M. Functional heterogeneity of the descending limbs of Henle's loop. II. Interspecies defferences among rabbits, rats, and hamsters. *Pflugers Arch* 1984;402:393–401; Imai M, Kokko JP. NaCl, urea, and water transport in the thin ascending limb of Henle: generation of osmotic gradients by passive diffusion of solutes. *J Clin Invest* 1974;53:393–402; Imai M, Taniguchi J, Tabei K. Function of thin loops of Henle. *Kidney Int* 1987;31:565–57; Isozaki T, Yoshitomi K, Imai M. Effects of Cl$^-$ transport inhibitors on Cl$^-$ permeability across hamster ascending thin limb. *Am J Physiol* 1989;257:F92–F98; Kokko JP. Sodium chloride and water transport in the descending limb of Henle. *J Clin Invest* 1970;49:1838–1846; Miwa T, Imai M. Flow-dependent water permeability of the rabbit descending limb of Henle's loop. *Am J Physiol* 1983;245:F743–F754; Morgan T, Berliner RW. Permeability of loop of Henle, vasa recta, and collecting duct to water, urea, and sodium. *Am J Physiol* 1968;215:108–115.

ments have demonstrated that these requirements are, in fact, satisfied.

The permeability of thin descending limb segments to sodium and chloride has been measured in hamster, rats, and rabbits. In hamsters and rats, the upper portion of long-looped descending limbs have a higher sodium permeability and higher P_{Na}/P_{Cl} ratio than do descending limbs of short-looped nephrons (222, 227). In contrast, there is little difference in P_{Na}/P_{Cl} between long- and short-loop nephrons in rabbits (221). These results are consistent with the morphologic evidence of greater heterogeneity in rats and hamsters than in rabbits. The pathways for transepithelial movement of sodium and chloride in the descending limb are not defined. Lopes et al. (302) studied the mechanism of cell volume regulation in rabbit descending limb cells and concluded that the basolateral membrane contains Cl^- and K^+ channels and a KCl cotransport process.

The formation of dilute urine begins in the thin ascending limb of Henle. Fluid from the thin ascending limb is more dilute than fluid obtained from the descending limb at the same level (237, 238). The decrease in osmolality is due primarily to a fall in the NaCl content of the luminal fluid. The mechanism for NaCl transport across the thin ascending limb epithelium is incompletely understood. Measurements of salt dilution potentials in microperfused thin ascending limb segments reveal them to be chloride selective with P_{Cl}/P_{Na} ratios of 2.2 to 3.5 in rats and hamsters (220). Segments perfused and bathed with symmetric solutions do not generate a spontaneous transepithelial voltage (220, 223, 225, 226) and do not show net transport of solute (225). These observations, together with the very low activity of (Na^+, K^+)-ATPase in this segment (252), have been interpreted to indicate that salt transport in vivo results from passive electrodiffusion rather than active transport. Although driven by passive electrochemical gradients, Cl^- movement across the TAL proceeds through a transcellular, and regulated, pathway. $^{36}Cl^-$ flux ratios and salt dilution voltages indicate that the Cl^- pathway discriminates among anions and is saturable (220, 223). Reduction of the Cl^- concentration of the basolateral solution causes a spike-like depolarization of the basolateral cell membrane (570). Likewise, reductions of the luminal perfusate Cl^- concentration caused a depolarization of the apical membrane. These results are consistent with the presence of conductive pathways for Cl^- in both the apical and basolateral membranes of TAL cells (570). The basolateral Cl^- conductance is inhibited at low pH (570), by low intracellular Ca^{2+} concentrations (279) and by compounds known to block Cl^- channels in other tissues (278).

A chloride channel cloned from the renal medulla, ClC-Ka, may represent the major Cl^- channel in the thin ascending limb (515). This channel, which belongs to the ClC family of Cl channels, is expressed exclusively within the kidney and has been localized by immunohistochemistry to both the apical and basolateral membranes of the thin ascending limb of Henle (516). The expression of ClC-Ka is increased by dehydration (515, 519). The initial reports of

the functional characteristics of ClC-Ka showed some similarities with the Cl conductance observed in isolated thin ascending limb segments, suggesting that this channel formed the primary Cl conductance in this segment (515). Genetic knockout of the ClC-Ka gene in mice produced a urinary concentrating defect confirming the role of passive NaCl transport in the thin ascending limb in the urinary concentrating mechanism (314).

NaCl Absorption in Thick Ascending Limb

GENERAL FEATURES

Rocha and Kokko (412) and Burg and Green (56) first demonstrated the salient characteristics of salt absorption in rabbit medullary and cortical TAL segments, respectively. First, net salt absorption resulted in a lumen-positive transepithelial voltage (Ve, mV), which could be abolished by furosemide, and in dilution of the luminal fluid. Second, the transport of Cl^- under these circumstances occurred against both electrical and chemical gradients and hence involved an active transport process; however, the nature of the active process was not specified at that time. Third, both net chloride absorption and the transepithelial voltage depended on (Na^+, K^+)-ATPase activity, present in large amounts along the basolateral membrane of this segment (252). A final curious feature of the TAL is that this segment is a "hybrid epithelium" possessing a very low permeability to water, yet a high ionic conductance (Table 2). The ionic conductance determined from the fluxes of $^{22}Na^+$ and $^{36}Cl^-$ is approximately 20–50 mS/cm^2 and is cation selective (P_{Na}/P_{Cl} = 2–6). This high electrical conductance is unusual among epithelia with low water permeabilities.

Table 2 presents a summary of the important transport properties of the rabbit, mouse, and rat TAL that are relevant to the concentrating and diluting functions of this nephron segment. A low permeability to water is required for the TAL to function as a diluting segment. Hebert et al. (198, 200), and subsequently Hebert (195) demonstrated that the apical cell membrane constitutes the major barrier to transcellular water flow in this segment. A similar conclusion was reached by Guggino et al. (177) regarding the water permeability of the *Amphiuma* diluting segment. Note that the water permeability of the paracellular pathway must also be low in order to achieve dilution of the luminal fluid.

Studies of the electrophysiologic (Table 3) and biochemical properties of intact, isolated, perfused thick limb segments, and of apical and basolateral membranes of thick limb cells have provided insights into the specific transport mechanisms involved in salt absorption, and the origin of the lumen-positive transepithelial voltage in this nephron segment (158–160, 162–165, 198–200, 203). A model for salt absorption by the TAL, which integrates the results of these studies is shown in Fig. 1. A similar model has been proposed for amphibian (176), avian (327, 354), and marine elasmobranch (127, 202) diluting segments.

TABLE 2 Transport Properties of Cortical and Medullary Thick Ascending Limb of Henle

	V_{Te} (mV)	P_f (μm/sec)	P_{Na} (μm/sec)	P_{Cl} (μm/sec)	J_{Cl} (pEq/cm²/sec)
Rabbit					
cTAL	3–10	11	0.28	0.14	2500
mTAL	3–7	0	0.63	0.11	5600
Mouse					
cTAL	8–12		0.63	0.51	5200
mTAL					
−ADH	5	6–23	0.23	0.10	3000
+ADH	10	6–23	0.25	0.12	10,900
Rat					
cTAL	7–8	0			8405
mTAL	5–6	0			9300

Note: Values of J_{Cl} for rat were calculated assuming an inner tubule diameter of 20 μm.

J_{Cl}, chemically determined net rate of Cl⁻ absorption; P_f, osmotic water permeability; P_{Na}, P_{Cl}, isotopically determined Na+ and Cl⁻ permeabilities; V_{Te}, transepithelial voltage (lumen positive).

Data from Burg MB, Green N. Function of the thick ascending limb of Henle's loop. *Am J Physiol* 1973;224:659–668; Friedman PA, Andreoli TE. CO₂-stimulated NaCl absorption in the mouse renal cortical thick ascending limb of Henle. *J Gen Physiol* 1982;80:683–711; Friedman PA, Andreoli TE. CO₂-stimulated NaCl absorption in the mouse renal cortical thick ascending limb of Henle. *J Gen Physiol* 1982;80:683–711; Good DW, Knepper MA, Burg MB. Ammonia and bicarbonate transport by thick ascending limb of rat kidney. *Am J Physiol* 1984;247:F35–F44; Hebert SC, Friedman PA, Andreoli TE. Effects of antidiuretic hormone on cellular conductive pathways in mouse medullary thick ascending limbs of Henle. I. ADH increases transcellular conductance pathways. *J Membr Biol* 1984;80:201–219; Molony DA, Reeves WB, Hebert SC, Andreoli TE. ADH increases apical Na⁺-K⁺-2Cl⁻ entry in mouse medullary thick ascending limbs of Henle. *Am J Physiol* 1987;252:F177–F187; Rocha AS, Kokko JP. Sodium chloride and water transport in the medullary thick ascending limb of Henle. *J Clin Invest* 1973;52:612–623; Schlatter E, Greger R. cAMP increases the basolateral Cl⁻ conductance in the isolated perfused medullary thick ascending limb of Henle's loop of the mouse. *Pflugers Arch* 1985;405:367–376; Wittner M, Di Stefano A, Wangemann P, Nitschke R, Greger R, Bailly C, Amiel C, Roinel N, deRouffignac C. Differential effects of ADH on sodium, chloride, potassium, calcium, and magnesium transport in cortical and medullary thick ascending limbs of mouse nephron. *Pflugers Arch* 1988;412:516–523.

TABLE 3 Basal Electrophysiologic Parameters of Thick Ascending Limb Segments

	V_e (mV)	G_e	G_c (mS/cm²)	G_s	V_a (mV)	V_{bl}	R_a/R_b	Reference
Rabbit cTAL	4–8	33	12	21	76	−69	2.0	165
Mouse mTAL	3–7	70–100	45–50	40–60	55.4	−50.7	1.2	196, 329, 331
Mouse cTAL	7–14	88	39	49				126
Hamster mTAL	4.0	934				−72		571

G_c, transcellular conductance; G_e, transepithelial conductance; G_s, paracellular conductance; V_a, apical membrane voltage; V_{bl}, basolateral membrane voltage; V_e, transepithelial voltage; R_a/R_b, apical to basolateral membrane resistance.

According to the model shown in Fig. 1, net Cl⁻ absorption by the TAL is a secondary active transport process. Luminal Cl⁻ entry into the cell is mediated by an electroneutral Na⁺-K⁺-2Cl⁻ cotransport process driven by the favorable electrochemical gradient for sodium entry. More specifically, the net driving force for the entry of Cl⁻ into the cell is determined by the sum of the chemical gradients for Na⁺, K⁺, and Cl⁻. Unfortunately, the intracellular activities of all three of these ions have not been determined in the mammalian TAL (Table 4). However, in the diluting segment of *Amphiuma*, these measurements (359–361) confirm that there is a favorable gradient for Na⁺-K⁺-2Cl⁻ entry into cells and that the gradient for Na⁺ accounts for the majority of this favorable integrated chemical gradient (360). Since the Na⁺ gradient is maintained by the continuous operation of the basolateral membrane (Na⁺, K⁺)-ATPase pump, apical entry of Cl⁻ via the cotransporter ultimately depends on the operation of the basolateral (Na⁺, K⁺)-ATPase. Accordingly, maneuvers that inhibit ATPase activity, such as removal of K⁺ from, or addition of ouabain to, peritubular solutions leads to dissipation of the Na⁺ gradient and subsequent inhibition of apical membrane Cl⁻ entry (198, 412).

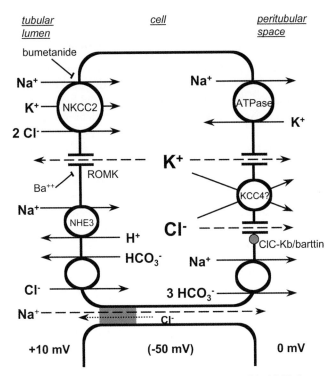

FIGURE 1 A model depicting the major elements of the NaCl absorption mechanism by the thick ascending limb. Dashed lines indicate passive ion movements down electrochemical gradients.

tially above the equilibrium value (5 mM) predicted from the intracellular voltage. Intracellular Cl⁻ is maintained at concentrations above electrochemical equilibrium by the continued entry of Cl⁻ via the apical Na⁺-K⁺-2Cl⁻ cotransporter. Blocking Cl⁻ entry through this pathway with furosemide, or substitution of extracellular Cl⁻ by gluconate, caused the intracellular Cl⁻ activity to fall to a value close to its equilibrium (162). Measurements of intracellular Cl⁻ activity in *Amphiuma* diluting segments using double-barreled microelectrodes have also documented a favorable electrochemical gradient for basolateral Cl⁻ efflux under transporting conditions (360).

In addition to electrodiffusive efflux of Cl⁻ across the basolateral membrane, a component of electroneutral KCl cotransport has been proposed in some species (164). As will be discussed below, the evidence for KCl cotransport is strongest in the low basolateral conductance cells of the *Amphiuma* diluting segment (175, 177).

In addition, according to the model in Fig. 1, the potassium that enters TAL cells via the Na⁺-K⁺-Cl⁻ cotransporter recycles does so, to a large extent, across the apical membrane by way of a K⁺ conductive pathway. This apical K⁺ recycling serves several purposes. First, it ensures a continued supply of luminal potassium in order to sustain Na⁺-K⁺-Cl⁻ cotransport. Without recycling, the luminal K⁺ concentration would fall rapidly as a consequence of K⁺ entry via Na⁺-K⁺-Cl⁻ cotransport and would limit net NaCl absorption. Second, the apical membrane potassium current provides a pathway for net potassium secretion by the TAL. In mouse mTAL, for example, the rate of K⁺ secretion amounts to about 10% of the rate of net Cl⁻ absorption (203). K⁺ secretion in this segment is an active process, ultimately driven by the (Na⁺, K⁺)-ATPase, proceeding in the face of a lumen-positive transepithelial potential. Third, under open circuit conditions, the transcellular and paracellular pathways form a cur-

In contrast to the electroneutral entry of Cl⁻ across the apical membrane, the majority of Cl⁻ efflux across the basolateral membrane proceeds through conductive pathways (196, 203, 445). A favorable electrochemical gradient for Cl⁻ efflux through dissipative pathways has been demonstrated by Greger et al. (162) in the rabbit cTAL. In this study, an intracellular Cl⁻ activity of 22 mM, measured using single barreled Cl⁻-selective microelectrodes, was substan-

TABLE 4 Intracellular Ion Activities and Electrochemical Potentials in Diluting Segments

	Rabbit cTAL			**Amphiuma Diluting Segments**				
	V_e (mV)	G_e	G_c(mS/cm²)	G_s	V_a (mV)	V_{bl}	R_a/R_b	Reference
Rabbit cTAL	4–8	33	12	21	76	−69	2.0	165
Mouse mTAL	3–7	70–100	45–50	40–60	55.4	−50.7	1.2	196, 329, 331
Mouse cTAL	7–14	88	39	49				126
Hamster mTAL	4.0	934				−72		571

Ion	PD$_x$(mV)	Cell Activity (mM)	Reference	PD$_x$(mV)	Cell Activity (mM)	Reference
Na⁺				129	12	360
K⁺	−15	113	167	−16	76	359
Cl⁻	−33	22	162	−40	64	361

Note: Negative values favor movement of ions out of cells.

PD$_x$, electrochemical potential of the respective ion.

rent loop in which the currents traversing the two pathways are of equal size but opposite direction. The potassium current from cell to lumen polarizes the lumen and causes an equivalent current to flow from lumen to bath through the paracellular pathway (165, 330). Since the paracellular pathway is cation-selective ($P_{Na}/P_{Cl} = 2$–6), the majority of the current through the paracellular pathway is carried by sodium moving from the lumen to the interstitium. This paracellular absorption of sodium increases the efficiency of sodium transport by the TAL (204). With reference to Fig. 1, for each Na^+ transported through the cell—and requiring utilization of ATP—one Na^+ is transported through the paracellular pathway without any additional expenditure of energy. Finally, the apical K^+ current satisfies the continuity requirement imposed by a high degree of conductive Cl^- efflux across basolateral membranes (196, 331).

A small component of sodium transport by the TAL is accounted for by sodium bicarbonate absorption (148). In the rat TAL, the rate of sodium bicarbonate absorption is roughly 5%–10% of that for sodium chloride absorption. Sodium bicarbonate absorption is thought to be mediated by an apical membrane amiloride-sensitive Na^+/H^+ exchanger and a basolateral membrane electrogenic $3Na^+/(HCO_3^-)$ cotransporter (148, 281).

The following sections will describe the individual components of the mechanism for TAL salt transport (Fig. 1) in greater detail.

APICAL Na^+-K^+-Cl^- COTRANSPORT

Studies of Cl^- transport across apical membranes of intact TAL segments (158, 198, 203) and in isolated membrane vesicle preparations (268) established that the predominant mode for Cl^- entry into the TAL cell is via a Na^+-K^+-$2Cl^-$ cotransporter. A characteristic feature of this transporter is its sensitivity to inhibition by furosemide, bumetanide and other 5-sulfamoylbenzoic acid derivatives (405).

The first demonstration of dependence on luminal sodium for Cl^- absorption was reported by Greger in isolated perfused rabbit cortical TAL segments (158). In these studies, extreme care was taken to remove all sodium from the luminal perfusate, including the use of perfusion pipettes constructed of sodium-free glass. Under these conditions, the removal of sodium from the luminal perfusate resulted in a prompt and reversible decline in both the transepithelial voltage and short-circuit current. The relation of luminal sodium concentration to the magnitude of the equivalent short-circuit current followed typical saturation kinetics with a $K_{0.5}$ for sodium of 2–4 mM (158). Comparable replacement experiments, except for the use of sodium free glass, in mouse medullary TAL segments showed that luminal sodium deletion reduced the transepithelial voltage by 70% (198). A similar sodium requirement for Cl^- absorption has been documented in amphibian (176) and avian (354) diluting segments. Moreover, a requirement for luminal potassium has been demonstrated for sodium and chloride

absorption in both mouse medullary (203) and rabbit (163) cortical thick ascending segments perfused in vitro. As a result of these studies, it is now recognized that Cl^- absorption in the TAL generally depends on the simultaneous presence of Na^+ and K^+ (or NH_4^+) in the lumen. Under certain circumstances, which will be discussed below, apical membrane NaCl entry may be independent of luminal potassium.

Measurement of isotope flux into TAL cells or membrane vesicles prepared from the inner stripe of outer medulla have delineated further the ionic requirements and stoichiometry of Na^+-K^+-$2Cl^-$ cotransport (58, 260, 268). Koenig et al. (268) demonstrated Cl^- dependence of $^{22}Na^+$ accumulation and Na^+ dependence of $^{86}Rb^+$ accumulation into membrane vesicles prepared from rabbit outer renal medulla. Elimination of either Na^+ or Cl^- from the external solutions inhibited the rate of $^{86}Rb^+$ uptake by 31%–44%. Likewise, the initial rate of $^{22}Na^+$ accumulation was inhibited 37%–54% with Cl^-- or K^+- removal from the extravesicular solution. Furthermore, this Cl^-- and K^+- dependent component of sodium uptake could be completely inhibited by loop diuretics. Analysis of the Hill coefficients for the concentration effects of each ion on sodium uptake yielded a stoichiometry of $1Na:1K:2Cl$ (268). A stoichiometry of $1Na:1K:2Cl$ has also been demonstrated for the Na^+-K^+-$2Cl^-$ cotransporter in the shark rectal gland (460), MDCK cell (321), Ehrlich ascites cell (141), duck red cell (182), and flounder intestine (366). Although there is general agreement that the cotransporter in the thick ascending limb conforms to the $1Na^+:1K^+:2Cl^-$ stoichiometry under most experimental conditions, there remains some disagreement with regard to (1) the kinetics of the cotransport process, and (2) whether under certain conditions the cotransporter might operate as a simple NaCl symporter.

From the dependence of the equivalent short-circuit current on luminal Cl^- concentration in perfused rabbit cortical TAL segments, Greger (160) determined an apparent affinity constant for chloride of 50 mM. That is, chloride had a much lower affinity for the cotransporter than did sodium ($K_a \sim 3$ mM). Likewise, from an examination of the coupling of ion transport to metabolic CO_2 production in rat cortical TAL segments, Hus-Citharel and Morel (216) determined an apparent affinity for Cl^- of 41 mM. In that study, CO_2 production from ^{14}C-labeled lactate by microdissected TAL segments was increased in a sigmoidal fashion as a function of the extracellular Cl^- concentration. A relatively low affinity for Cl^- was also observed by Eveloff et al. (113) in isolated rabbit mTAL cells. In that study, reduction of either the Na^+ or Cl^- concentration of the incubation solution reduced the rate of O_2 consumption by TAL cells. The concentration of Cl^- that supported half-maximal O_2 consumption was 79 mM. However, the concentration of sodium that supported half-maximal O_2 consumption was also quite high, 66 mM. The latter finding illustrates the hazards of performing kinetic analysis using indirect measures, such as O_2 consumption or CO_2 production, in intact cells.

Koenig et al. (268), studying $Na^+/K^+/Cl^-$ transport directly in isolated plasma membrane vesicles, demonstrated a significantly higher Cl^- affinity for the cotransporter, 15 mM, than did Greger. The findings of Burnham et al. (58) that maximal bumetanide-sensitive Rb^+ accumulation into rabbit renal outer medullary membrane vesicles was supported by Cl^- concentrations of less than 50 mM are in accord with the results of Koenig et al. (268). The relevance of this issue derives from the fact that the luminal Cl^- concentration in the early distal convoluted tubule is in the range of 50 mM. Thus, from the results of Greger, Cl^- absorption may be significantly substrate limited at low luminal Cl^- concentration. In contrast, Koenig's results indicate that substrate, that is, Cl^-, availability is not a significant limit to Cl^- transport at physiologic lumenal Cl^- concentrations. The differences in these data may reflect axial heterogeneity in the properties of the Na^+-K^+-$2Cl^-$ cotransporter. Greger (160) and Hus-Citharel and Morel (216) examined the cortical TAL, while Koenig et al. (268) and Burnham et al. (58) prepared membranes from the medulla. An axial heterogeneity in the regulation of cotransporter activity as the thick limb ascends from the medulla into the cortex might be anticipated.

Evidence for a model of two distinct binding sites for Cl^- with differing affinities follows from studies of Forbush and Palfrey (123) on ^3H-bumetanide binding to renal medullary membranes. In these studies, Na^+, K^+, and Cl^- were all required for bumetanide to bind to canine renal medullary membranes. The K_a values for sodium and potassium were 2 mM and 1 mM, respectively. The effect of Cl^- concentration on bumetanide binding was biphasic. At low concentrations (<5 mM), Cl^- enhanced ^3H-bumetanide binding. Higher Cl^- concentrations, however, inhibited bumetanide binding. Kinetic studies of ion fluxes in LLC-PK (54) cells and HeLa cells (328) also indicate the presence of two Cl^--binding sites with differing affinities. Further, in red blood cells, bumetanide and Cl^- were shown to compete for a common binding site (181). Taken together, these data are consistent with a model in which the binding of Cl^- to a high-affinity site exposes a second lower-affinity site that may be occupied either by bumetanide or by the second Cl^-.

The binding of ions to the cotransporter is thought to be ordered and cooperative (292). Thus, sodium binds to the cotransporter first, and promotes binding of a Cl^- and then K^+. Binding of K^+ to its site, in turn, promotes binding of the second Cl^- to the cotransporter. Once fully occupied, the cotransporter–ion complex translocates to the internal surface of the cell membrane where debinding occurs in the same order. The full reaction sequence of binding and debinding results in inward $Na^+/K^+/2Cl^-$ transport. Partial reactions permit K^+/K^+ and Na^+/Na^+ exchange.

A second area of controversy centers on the possibility that the cotransporter might operate as a simple NaCl symporter under certain conditions. Eveloff and coworkers have reported potassium-independent, furosemide-sensitive NaCl transport in isolated rabbit TAL cells and membrane vesicles prepared from TAL cells (115). Potassium dependence of the cotransporter might be subject to physiologic regulation. Eveloff and Calamia (114) have shown that under isotonic conditions the chloride dependent, furosemide-sensitive component of sodium uptake is independent of potassium, but that under hypertonic conditions the sodium uptake becomes K^+ dependent. Sun et al. (494) have also reported that, in perfused mouse medullary TAL segments, basal sodium chloride transport was K^+ independent, but that upon stimulation of salt transport by ADH NaCl transport became dependent on luminal K^+.

Proteins that mediate Na^+-K^+-$2Cl^-$ cotransport have now been cloned. An absorptive form of Na:K:2Cl cotransporter, referred to as BSC1 or NKCC2, was initially cloned by Gamba et al. (134) based on sequence homology to the thiazide-sensitive Na:Cl cotransporter (see subsequent discussion). A second Na^+-K^+-$2Cl^-$ cotransporter, NKCC1, was cloned by Payne et al. (386). Several lines of evidence indicate that NKCC2 (BSC1) is the protein that mediates apical salt entry in the thick ascending limb. First, in situ hybridization and single nephron RT-PCR studies demonstrated expression of NKCC2 primarily in the MTAL and CTAL (134, 250, 567). Moreover, immunohistochemical studies using antibodies to NKCC2 indicate that the protein is localized to the apical membrane of the MTAL and CTAL (250). The most compelling evidence, however, is the identification of inactivating mutations in the NKCC2 gene in some patients with Bartter syndrome. This syndrome, characterized by hypokalemia, metabolic alkalosis, hyperaldosteronism, and normal blood pressure, results from a defect in salt absorption by the TAL. Simon et al. (463) first reported the linkage of Bartter syndrome to mutations in the NKCC2 (BSC1) gene. Subsequently, a large number of different NKCC2 mutations have been found in families with Bartter syndrome (465, 521). These results provide strong support for the conclusion that NKCC2 is responsible for apical Na^+-K^+-$2Cl^-$ cotransport in the thick ascending limb.

The NKCC2 cDNA encodes a protein containing ~1100 amino acids and having a predicted molecular weight of 115–120 kDa (134). The observed molecular weight, however, is approximately 150 kDa due to extensive glycosylation. Hydropathy analysis of the amino acid sequence predicts a protein having 12 putative transmembrane spanning domains. Six isoforms of NKCC2 have been identified that are results of alternative splicing in the 5′ and 3′ regions of the NKCC2 gene. Three 5′ splice products, termed A, B, and F, were reported by Payne and Forbush (385). These variants differ only in a 96-bp region, which encodes the amino acids forming the second transmembrane domain. The isoforms show differential expression within the thick ascending limb. Using RT-PCR, Yang et al. (567) examined the distribution of NKCC2 isoforms in single nephron segments. The A isoform was found in both the cortical and medullary TAL, the B isoform was restricted to the cortical TAL, while the F isoform was present in the medullary, but not cortical, TAL and, to a lesser extent, in the outer medullary collecting duct. All three products are capable of mediating Na^+-K^+-$2Cl^-$ cotransport. However, the isoforms have different transport properties that may have physiologic relevance. Specifically, the A and B isoforms have higher affinities for Na^+, K^+ and Cl^- than the F isoform. The F isoform appears to have a greater transport capacity than the other isoforms (392). Thus, the presence of the F isoform in the medullary thick ascending limb could account for the observed high rates of NaCl transport relative to the cortical segment (Table 2) while the expression of the A and B isoforms in the cortical thick ascending limb may subserve the ability to achieve lower luminal NaCl concentrations in that segment. Alternative splicing at the 3' end of NKCC2 produces additional isoforms with either long (C9) or short (C4) carboxy termini (339). Under isotonic conditions, the truncated (C4) isoforms do not mediate Na:K:2Cl cotransport and inhibit the transport activity of the full-length (C9) isoforms when the two are coexpressed (393). This inhibition is relieved by cAMP (393). Under hypotonic conditions, however, the C4 isoforms mediate K^+-independent NaCl cotransport, which is stimulated by cAMP (391) and may account for the K^+-independent NaCl transport noted in earlier studies (115, 494).

The inhibition of C9 NKCC2 isoforms by C4 isoforms suggests a physical interaction between these proteins. Biochemical studies have recently established that NKCC2 exists as a dimer (478). Thus, it is possible that different combinations of NKCC2 isoforms within the dimer could produce transporters with a wide variety of functional properties. Moreover, the subunit composition of the dimers may be a point of physiologic regulation. Alternatively, the C4 isoform could alter membrane trafficking or stability of the C9 isoform. The C4 isoform resides predominantly in subapical vesicles rather than the cell membrane (339). Meade et al. (321a) found that coexpression of the C4 isoform reduced the abundance of C9 isoform in *Xenopus* oocyte membranes. The reduction in cell surface C9 isoform was reflected by a commensurate reduction in bumetanide-sensitive Rb uptake. The inhibitory effect of C4 on C9 cell surface localization could be prevented by cAMP or by disruption of microtubules, suggesting that C4 alters the trafficking of C9 in or out of the apical membrane.

APICAL K^+ CONDUCTANCE

As described in a previous section, an important feature of the luminal membrane of the TAL and nonmammalian diluting segments is a barium-inhibitable potassium conductance (165, 176, 203). Studies of isolated, perfused, thick limb segments have established that the predominant, and perhaps only, conductance across the apical membrane is to potassium (165, 197). Blockade of the apical potassium conductance by luminal barium in mouse mTAL decreases the transepithelial electrical conductance (G_e) by roughly 50%, while increasing the apical to basolateral membrane resistance ratio (Ra/Rb) from 1.9 to 12.9 (196). Moreover, changes in the luminal K^+ concentration produce essentially Nernstian changes in the apical membrane electrical potential (196). Virtually identical results have been obtained for the rabbit cTAL (165) and the *Amphiuma* diluting segments (360).

The apical K^+ conductance in all of these tissues can be inhibited by the luminal application of millimolar concentrations of barium. Electrophysiologic studies using cable analysis and the ability to block completely the apical membrane conductance with Ba^{2+} have allowed quantitation of the apical membrane conductances in the mouse mTAL (197, 331), rabbit cTAL (165) and *Amphiuma* diluting segments (176). In each segment, using measured values of intracellular potassium activity (rabbit cTAL [167] and *Amphiuma* [359]), apical membrane conductance, and intracellular voltage, it can be shown that the measured apical membrane conductance is sufficient to provide for the recycling of all of the potassium uptake via the Na^+-K^+-$2Cl^-$ cotransporter.

The properties of the apical membrane K^+ conductance have been studied in plasma membrane vesicles prepared from outer renal medulla (58, 404). Conductive potassium fluxes in these vesicles can be measured by loading the vesicles with a high concentration of potassium and then removing the potassium from the external solutions, usually by passing the vesicles through an ion exchange column. Tracer amounts of ^{86}Rb are then added to the extravesicular solutions to begin uptake. Under these conditions, the outwardly directed K^+ gradient creates an inside-negative diffusion potential that drives ^{86}Rb uptake into the vesicles. The advantages of this method are that only vesicles which contain a K^+ conductance will generate a diffusion potential for $^{86}Rb^+$ uptake and the rate of uptake is prolonged, thereby facilitating measurement of initial rates of uptake (147). Burnham et al. (58) and Reeves et al. (404) were thus able to demonstrate barium-sensitive $^{86}Rb^+$ flux in membranes from rabbit outer medulla. The Rb^+ flux was conductive as judged by its inhibition by collapse of the intravesicular voltage or by measurement of intravesicular voltage using voltage-sensitive dyes. The $K_{0.5}$ value for barium inhibition of Rb^+ flux was 50–100 μM (58). The barium-sensitive Rb flux was also dependent on the calcium activity within the vesicles (58). Moreover, in reconstituted proteoliposomes prepared from porcine outer medulla, the calcium dependence of the K^+ conductance was modulated by a high-affinity ($K_{0.5} = 0.1$ nM) calmodulin-binding site (261). Klaerke et al. (261) applied solubilized membrane proteins from the pig outer medulla to a calmodulin-sepharose affinity column. After extensive washing, specifically bound proteins were eluted by a calcium-free buffer. When reconstituted into liposomes, the eluted proteins, primarily peptides of 86 and 51 kD, exhibited calcium but not barium-sensitive conductive $^{86}Rb^+$ flux. Because these vesicle preparations are admixtures of both apical and basolateral membranes from several cell types, it is impossible to state with certainty that the conductive pathways demonstrated in these studies do, in fact, represent the apical potassium conductance of the TAL.

The patch clamp technique has identified three types of apical potassium channels in intact TAL segments or cultured TAL cells. In cultured TAL cells, Guggino et al. (174) identified a 140–150-pS calcium-activated "maxi" potassium channel that can be blocked by barium, TEA, quinidine, and charybdotoxin (173). The open probability of this channel at physiologic apical membrane voltage and intracellular calcium concentration is too low to account for the observed K$^+$ conductance of the TAL (174); rather, it may play a role in cell volume regulation (503). Wang and coworkers described a low-conductance (35 pS) potassium channel in the apical membrane of rabbit (537) and rat (533) cortical TAL segments. The channel was insensitive to changes in membrane voltage or cytoplasmic calcium concentration. However, exposure of the cytoplasmic surface of the patch to ATP inhibited channel activity. The inhibition of activity to ATP was reversible and was dependent on the ratio of ATP to ADP in solution. These properties would render the channels sensitive to changes in cell metabolism. For example, during an increase in transcellular salt absorption ATP would be consumed and ADP produced. The fall in the ATP/ADP ratio, then, might activate apical K$^+$ channels providing more K$^+$ recycling to support further salt absorption.

Bleich et al. (34) and Wang (533) described an intermediate conductance (60–70 pS) K$^+$ channel in rat TAL segments. Like the low conductance channel described by Wang et al. (537), this channel was inhibited by ATP and by barium. In addition, the channel activity was voltage dependent with depolarization increasing activity; could be blocked by quinine, verapamil, and diltiazem; and was inhibited at low cytosolic pH. The activities of both the intermediate and low conductance channels are increased by high dietary potassium (303). The general features of K$^+$ transport across the apical membrane of TAL cells are summarized in Fig. 2.

An ATP-dependent potassium channel was cloned from rat kidney by Ho et al. (212). This channel, termed ROMK, is the prototype for a large family of inward rectifying K channels (K$_{IR}$ channels). K$_{IR}$ channels have two transmembrane spanning domains, intracellular N and C-termini, and an extracellular helical domain between the two transmembrane domains (Fig. 3). Structural studies of other K$_{IR}$ channels have established that the channels exist as heteromers of four K$_{IR}$ subunits (231, 286, 353). The extracellular helical domain appears to form the outer vestibule and selectivity filter of the channel, while the second transmembrane domain lines the pore cavity.

Alternative splicing of 5′ exons of ROMK produces four isoforms (ROMK1–3 and 6) that differ at the N-terminus (37, 277, 580). These isoforms are differentially expressed along the distal tubule. Single-nephron PCR analysis indicated that ROMK1 is expressed in the collecting duct, while

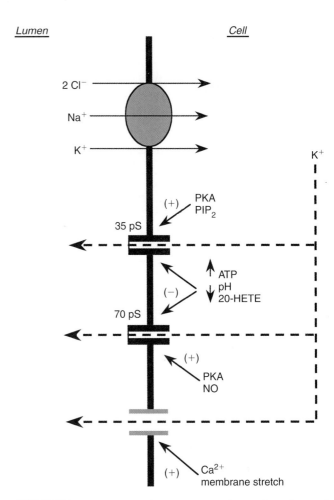

FIGURE 2 Pathways for K$^+$ transport across the apical membrane of TAL cells. K$^+$ entry occurs via the Na$^+$-K$^+$-2Cl$^-$ cotransporter. The majority of K$^+$ recycling to the lumen occurs through ATP-sensitive channels. Two such channels, having conductances of 35 and 70 pS, respectively, have been described. A large (150 pS) calcium-activated channel may contribute to K$^+$ efflux during cell volume regulation (lower channel). The minus (−) and plus (+) signs refer to agents that inhibit or stimulate channel activity, respectively. See text for more details.

both ROMK2 and ROMK3 are expressed in the medullary and cortical thick ascending limb (36). Immunolocalization of ROMK proteins, using antibodies that recognized all three isoforms, revealed apical membrane localization in the medullary and cortical thick ascending limb, the connecting tubule, and the cortical collecting duct (322, 564). Oddly, the expression of ROMK in the thick limb was heterogeneous, with some cells lacking demonstrable staining. In contrast, the expression of the Na$^+$-K$^+$-2Cl$^-$ cotransporter was uniform within the TAL (251, 564). This implies that either the ROMK-negative cells express a different apical K$^+$ channel or that apical K$^+$ recycling by the ROMK-positive cells is sufficient to supply K$^+$ for Na$^+$-K$^+$-2Cl$^-$ transport in the ROMK-negative cells. In this regard, it is possible that the 60–70 pS K$^+$ channel described in the rat thick limb (34, 533) constitutes the apical membrane K$^+$ conductance in the ROMK-negative cells.

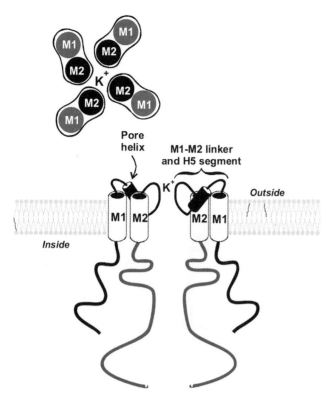

FIGURE 3 A schematic representation of ROMK (Kir 1.1) potassium-channel structure. **A:** Tetrameric structure of the channel, with the second transmembrane domains (M2) lining the pore. **B:** The pore-forming region, H5, is flanked by two transmembrane domains. The H5 region is highly conserved within the Kir family. (With permission, from Hebert SC, Desir G, Giebisch G, Wang W. Molecular diversity and regulation of renal potassium channels. *Physiol Rev* 2005;85:319–371.)

The properties of K_{IR} channels are the subject of an extensive recent review (201) and are discussed in Chapter 44. The single-channel conductance of ROMK, 35 pS, corresponds to the low conductance channel described by Wang et al. (533, 537). The current–voltage relations exhibit weak inward rectification, which is due to blocking of the channel by intracellular Mg^{2+} or polyamines. The activity of this channel is modulated by intracellular pH and by intracellular ATP through both phosphorylation-dependent and phosphorylation-independent pathways (320). The maintenance of ROMK channel activity requires protein kinase A (PKA)–mediated phosphorylation (320). ROMK contains three PKA phosphorylation sites, each of which contributes about 30%–40% to total channel activity (307). Phosphorylation of ROMK affects both channel activity (P_o) and the number of functional channels in the plasma membrane (201). ROMK activity is increased by phosphatidylinositol phosphates (PIP_2), at least in part through competition for nucleotide binding (306).

Nucleotides have both inhibitory and stimulatory effects on ROMK activity. At micromolar concentrations, ATP stimulates ROMK activity via PKA-mediated phosphorylation and production of PIP_2 (see previous discussion). Mil-

limolar concentrations of ATP inhibit ROMK activity (534). The inhibition by ATP can be relieved by increasing concentrations of ADP or by PIP_2. Certain other members of the K_{IR} family are also inhibited by ATP. The ATP sensitivity of these channels—for example, $K_{IR}6.2$—is endowed by the association of regulatory subunits (76). These regulatory subunits, such as the sulfonylurea receptor (SUR) and CFTR (4, 229, 230), belong to the ABC gene family, which are characterized by nucleotide-binding domains. The sulfonylurea receptor together with $K_{IR}6.2$ forms the glibenclamide-sensitive, ATP-sensitive K channel that controls insulin secretion by pancreatic β-cells (230). The K_{IR}/SUR channels are much more sensitive to inhibition by ATP than are heterologously expressed ROMK channels. In addition, the native 35-pS K^+ channel, but not the heterologously expressed ROMK channel, is inhibited by glibenclamide (325). These observations have prompted the search for regulatory subunits for the ROMK channel. Both SUR2B (26) and CFTR (333) are expressed in the thick ascending limb and collecting duct, making them candidates for ROMK regulation. In transfection studies, coexpression of ROMK with either SUR2B (13) or CFTR (318, 319, 420, 502) dramatically increases both the nucleotide dependence and glibenclamide sensitivity of ROMK. Immunoprecipitation studies confirmed that one of the ROMK isoforms, ROMK2, physically interacts with SUR2B (502). The interaction between CFTR and ROMK may be mediated by a bridging protein, NHERF-2 (568). However, the identities of the regulatory proteins that may be associated with native ROMK channels have not been established.

The electrophysiologic properties of the ROMK channels, their regulation by intracellular pH (74), ATP, phosphorylation (320) and dietary K^+ and their localization (36, 322, 564) all suggest that ROMK is the low conductance K^+ channel of the thick ascending limb (145). Further support for this view comes from studies of ROMK knockout mice. Specifically, no low conductance K^+ channels were detected by patch clamp analysis in ROMK(-/-), mice while channels in heterozygous ROMK(+/-) mice were detected at a rate approximately half that of wildtype ROMK(+/+) mice (304). Complicating this interpretation is the observation that ROMK(-/-) mice also lack intermediate conductance K^+ channels in the thick ascending limb (303). It has been proposed that the intermediate conductance channel may be a heteromeric protein containing ROMK and other, as yet, unidentified subunits.

The notion that one of the ROMK channels is the predominant channel responsible for apical K^+ recycling in the thick ascending limb is strongly supported by the finding of mutations in the ROMK gene in some families with Bartter syndrome (15, 88, 464, 465, 530). At least some of these mutations have been confirmed to result in defective K^+ channel function (452). As noted above, Bartter syndrome results from a defect in thick ascending limb salt transport. Thus, the presence of ROMK mutations as a cause of Bartter syndrome indicates the important role of ROMK in net salt absorption by the thick ascending limb.

Basolateral Membrane Cl⁻ Transport

Cl⁻ exit across the basolateral membrane of TAL cells is largely conductive, proceeding down its electrochemical gradient through Cl⁻-selective channels in the basolateral membrane. The notion that basolateral Cl⁻ transport is electrogenic first derived from observations that, in the mouse medullary TAL (198) and rabbit cTAL, net Cl⁻ absorption accounts for about 90% of the equivalent short-circuit current. Measurements of the basolateral membrane voltage by Greger and Schlatter (164) confirmed that reductions in bath chloride concentration depolarized the basolateral membrane while reductions in intracellular chloride concentration produced by blocking Cl⁻ entry with furosemide, hyperpolarized the basolateral membrane. Both sets of observations are consistent with the presence of a Cl⁻ conductance in the basolateral membrane. Yoshitomi et al. (571) also identified a large chloride conductance in the basolateral membrane of hamster TAL cells. In their study, two populations of TAL cell were identified, one having a high basolateral membrane conductance (fractional resistance of the basolateral membrane, $FR_b = 0.05$) and one with a low basolateral conductance ($FR_b = 0.8$). Both cell types contained a basolateral Cl⁻ conductance with the high conductance cells also possessing a basolateral barium-sensitive potassium conductance. Similar cell heterogeneity has been noted in the *Amphiuma* diluting segments (175). Electrophysiologic studies of the mouse (203, 329, 445) and rabbit TAL (164) have not disclosed two populations of cells, although in the rabbit, there was considerable variability in the responses of V_{bl} to changes in bath Cl⁻ concentration.

Consistent with the view that basolateral Cl⁻ transport is via chloride channels, a variety of compounds known to block Cl⁻ channels also inhibit salt absorption in TAL segments. Wangemann et al. (538) have catalogued the electrophysiologic effects, relative potencies, and structure-function relations of over 200 such compounds. The major effects of these agents, when present in the peritubular bathing solutions, are inhibition of transepithelial voltage, inhibition of the equivalent short-circuit current, and hyperpolarization of the basolateral membrane.

Application of the patch clamp technique to the TAL has established that Cl⁻ channels are present in the basolateral membrane of TAL cells. Paulais and Teulon (384) detected a 40-pS anion selective channel ($P_{Cl}/P_{Na} = 20$) in the basolateral membrane of collagenase treated mouse cortical TAL segments. The I–V relations of the channel were linear in both the cell-attached and excised configurations. The open probability of the channel in the cell attached state was voltage dependent, increasing as the membrane was depolarized. In the excised patch configuration, the open probability was no longer voltage dependent. Greger et al. (161) described a Cl⁻ channel in the basolateral membrane of rat TAL segments. This channel also has a conductance of about 40 pS, but rather than having a linear I–V relation, this channel exhibits outward rectification. The open probability increases with depolarization in both the cell attached and excised patch configuration. A low conductance Cl⁻ channel (8–10 pS) having linear I–V relations has also been detected in the basolateral membrane of TAL cells (178, 179). The activity of this channel is increased following incubation with cAMP-dependent protein kinase and ATP (178).

Evidence for TAL Cl⁻ channels also comes from studies of Cl⁻ flux in renal medullary membrane vesicles. Since TALs comprise approximately 70% of the volume in the inner stripe of outer medulla, vesicles prepared from this region should be predominantly derived from this segment. ³⁶Cl⁻ flux into vesicles from porcine (46) and rabbit outer medulla (24) is electrogenic, cation independent, inhibitable by chloride channel blockers, and has a low activation energy ($E_a = 6.4$ kcal/mole), characteristic of transport through a channel. Moreover, when vesicles from rabbit outer medulla were incorporated into planar lipid bilayers, chloride channel activity was demonstrated (401). These channels were anion selective ($P_{Cl}/P_K = 10$) and had a single-channel conductance of 80–90 pS in 320-mM KCl solution. The I–V relations in symmetric solution were linear, and in asymmetric solutions the I–V relations conformed to the Goldman–Hodgkin–Katz equation. The open probability of this channel was voltage dependent, increasing activity with depolarizing voltages. These channels are also seen in vesicles made from highly purified suspensions of mouse thick ascending limb (554) and from cultured mouse medullary thick limb cells (406), which confirms their origin as the thick ascending limb.

A unique feature of these medullary chloride channels is the asymmetric dependence of channel activity on the chloride activity of the solutions bathing the lipid bilayer (406, 553). Increases in the Cl⁻ concentration of the cis, or extracellular, solution over the range 50–300 mM produced almost linear increases in channel open probability. In contrast, the Cl⁻ concentration dependence of the trans, or intracellular surface of the channel, was most pronounced in the range of 0–50 mM Cl⁻ and was almost saturated at 50 mM Cl⁻. Similar Cl⁻ dependence was observed in channels studied in excised patches of cultured TAL cells indicating that the effect is not an artifact of the lipid bilayer reconstitution technique (406). Dependence of channel activity on extracellular Cl⁻ has also been shown for certain members of the ClC family of Cl⁻ channels (399). As will be discussed, it is believed that the basolateral Cl⁻ channel of the TAL is a member of this family of channels.

A chloride channel, termed ClC-0, was cloned from the electric organ of the *Torpedo* ray by Jentsch et al. (242) using an expression cloning strategy. This work led to the identification of a large number of related chloride channels that form the ClC family of channels (241). Based on homology to the ClC-0 channel, Uchida et al. (515), Adachi et al. (2), and Kieferle et al. (256) reported the cloning of two chloride channels, ClC-K1 and ClC-K2, that are expressed exclusively within the rat kidney. In the human, the two corresponding channels are denoted hCLC-Ka and hCLC-Kb and are located contiguously on chromosome 1 (424). Due to the high degree of sequence similarity between hCLC-Ka and hCLC-Kb, it is not certain which of the human channels correspond to CLC-K1 versus CLC-K2, although the distribution of ClC-K2 along the nephron most closely matches that of hClC-Kb (500). Zimniak and colleagues (582) have cloned cDNA from rabbit renal outer medulla, named rbClC-Ka, which shares 80% homology to the rat CLC-K1 and CLC-K2. The distribution of rbClC-Ka along the nephron resembles that of CLC-K2 rather than ClC-K1 (581, 582). Several lines of evidence support the view that CLC-K2 (or the probable human homologue hCLC-Kb) is the channel that mediates chloride efflux across the basolateral membrane of the thick ascending limb. First, using polymerase chain reaction amplification of single tubule segments, the ClC-K2 and rbClC-Ka channels were shown to be expressed primarily in the thick ascending limb and the collecting duct (2, 582). Second, immunohistochemical studies using an antibody against the rbClC-Ka channel revealed predominantly basolateral staining in the medullary and cortical thick ascending limb (556). Similar results were obtained by Vandewalle and colleagues using an antibody that recognized both CLC-K1 and CLC-K2 (519). Third, treatment of cultured thick ascending limb cells with an antisense oligonucleotide to rbClC-Ka reduced the expression of chloride channels (581). Fourth, an antibody against rbClC-Ka that inhibited chloride channel activity in lipid bilayers (581) also reduced chloride efflux in intact thick ascending limb segments (556). Finally, and most compelling, is the identification of mutations in hCLC-Kb in patients with neonatal Bartter syndrome (462). Thus, as was the case for the NKCC2 and ROMK proteins, linkage of ClC-Kb to Bartter syndrome establishes the importance of its gene product in transepithelial NaCl transport. Activating mutations of CLC-Kb have also been reported (239). Specifically, substitution of threonine by serine at position 481 of CLC-Kb results in a dramatic increase in Cl^- currents without a change in channel selectivity or cell surface expression. The T481S polymorphism is relatively common in the general population, particularly in African populations. Among Caucasians, the presence of the T481S polymorphism was associated with higher systolic and diastolic blood pressures and a higher prevalence of hypertension (240). Thus, ClC-Kb is an attractive candidate gene for certain forms of essential hypertension, particularly salt-sensitive hypertension. Additional studies in different populations will be required to determine the significance of these ClC-Kb polymorphisms.

Some of the difficulty in assigning a role for CLC-K2/hCLC-Kb in thick ascending limb Cl^- transport was the inability to achieve functional expression in heterologous systems. This was recently shown to be due to the requirement of an additional subunit for channel activity. This subunit, named barttin, was originally identified by positional cloning of the BSND gene, which is responsible for a form of Bartter syndrome accompanied by sensorineural deafness (32). By in situ hybridization (32) and immunohistochemistry (112), barttin is located in the basolateral membranes of the thin and thick ascending limb and also in the stria vascularis of the inner ear, where it is believed to play a role in K^+ secretion into endolymph. Although expression of ClC-Kb or barttin alone in *Xenopus* oocytes produces no significant conductance, their coexpression results in a large Cl^- conductance (112, 531). Barttin is believed to act, at least in part, by increasing the cell surface expression of ClC-Kb (112, 531). The mutations of barttin identified in Bartter patients generally, though not always, impair the ability of barttin to produce a Cl^- conductance when expressed with ClC-Kb (112, 531).

Some uncertainty remains regarding the role of basolateral electrochemical KCl symport in net Cl^- efflux across that membrane. In the rabbit cortical TAL, Greger and Schlatter (164) concluded that KCl symport accounted for about one-third of basolateral Cl^- efflux. This conclusion is based on the following observations: an increase in the K^+ concentration or decrease in the Cl^- concentration of the basolateral solution depolarized the basolateral membrane, bath barium depolarized the basolateral membrane and abolished the K^+-induced changes in V_{bl}, and barium had no discernible effect on the transepithelial resistance or fractional resistance of the basolateral membrane. The lack of an effect of barium on resistance persuaded the investigators to propose that a barium-sensitive KCl cotransporter was present (164). Alternatively, these data are compatible with parallel conductive pathways for K^+ and Cl^-. The absence of a barium effect on transepithelial resistance could be due to an offsetting increase in basolateral Cl^- conductance or to changes in basolateral membrane resistance below the experimental limits of detection. In the *Amphiuma* diluting segment, the low basolateral conductance cells transport both K^+ and Cl^- across the basolateral membrane via an electroneutral cotransporter (175). In the high basolateral conductance cells, Cl^- efflux is via basolateral membrane channels (175). A cloned KCl cotransporter, KCC4, is present in the basolateral membrane of the thick ascending limb (527). However, its physiologic role in thick ascending limb function is not known.

SYNCHRONOUS Na^+/H^+:Cl^-/HCO_3^- EXCHANGE

An additional form of apical membrane NaCl entry has been observed in the mouse cTAL. Friedman and Andreoli (125) found that net Cl^- absorption and the transepithelial voltage were doubled when CO_2 and HCO_3^- were added to the external solutions bathing cTAL segments. Since the $(CO_2 + HCO_3^-)$ stimulated rate of NaCl absorption did not result in net CO_2 transport and could be abolished by the lipophilic carbonic anhydrase inhibitor ethoxyzolamide or by the luminal addition of the anion exchange inhibitor SITS or DIDS, it was proposed that the apical membrane of the mouse cTAL contains parallel, near-synchronous Na^+/H^+:Cl^-/HCO_3^- exchangers in addition to a Na^+-K^+-Cl^- cotransporter. Subsequent studies have shown that, like the mouse mTAL, the apical membrane of the mouse cTAL contains a potassium conductance and that both the (CO_2 + HCO_3^-)-dependent and (CO_2 + HCO_3^-)-independent components of NaCl absorption require luminal potassium (126). Thus, the cation exchange process may proceed as (Na^+, K^+)/$2H^+$. Both the (CO_2 + HCO_3^-)-dependent and -independent components of NaCl absorption in mouse cTAL segments were equally susceptible to inhibition by luminal bumetanide (K_i = 5–8 × 10–7 M) (124). Addition of CO_2 and HCO_3^- to the bathing solutions has no effect on net NaCl transport in either the rabbit cTAL or the mouse mTAL. Both the rat and mouse mTAL do contain Na^+/H^+ exchangers in their apical membranes. However in these segments, Na^+/H^+ exchange plays a role in net HCO_3^- transport and cell pH regulation rather than transcellular NaCl absorption (148, 257). The NHE-3 isoform of the Na^+/H^+ exchanger is the major isoform expressed in the apical membrane of the thick ascending limb (11).

Bicarbonate and Ammonium Transport

Medullary and cortical TAL segments from the rat absorb bicarbonate and acidify the luminal fluid (148, 149). The rates of bicarbonate absorption measured in vitro perfused TAL segments account for most of the filtered bicarbonate that is reabsorbed by the loop of Henle in vivo (148, 153). The rate of sodium bicarbonate absorption in the rat TAL is, however, only a small fraction (5%–10%) of total sodium absorption by this segment (148). Thus, while bicarbonate transport by the TAL may play an important role in urinary acidification in some species, bicarbonate transport has little impact on net salt balance or free water excretion. There is considerable species variation in the rates of bicarbonate absorption by the TAL. No significant bicarbonate transport was detected in mouse (125) and rabbit TAL (232). In the rabbit, this correlates with the absence of carbonic anhydrase activity in the TAL (95). In the mouse cTAL, which possesses considerable type IV carbonic anhydrase activity (55), the lack of net bicarbonate transport is due to the synchronous operation of luminal Cl^-/HCO_3^- and Na^+/H^+ exchangers (125) such that no net acid or base transport occurs.

The mechanism of bicarbonate absorption by the rat TAL has been reviewed by Good (150). Transcellular bicarbonate absorption results from proton secretion across the apical membrane and bicarbonate reabsorption across the basolateral membrane. The apical proton secretion occurs primarily by Na^+/H^+ exchange. Evidence for functional apical Na^+/H^+ exchange has been presented for the rat (149, 152, 155, 281, 540) and mouse TAL (125, 257) and the *Amphiuma* diluting segment (362, 363). In these segments, acidification of luminal fluid is sodium dependent and amiloride-sensitive (149, 362). Moreover, removal of luminal sodium or luminal amiloride results in cytoplasmic acidification (155, 257, 362). As noted above, the NHE3 isoform of the Na^+/H^+ exchanger is expressed in the apical membrane of the thick ascending limb (11). NHE3 expression in the TAL is in-

creased by chronic metabolic acidosis (289), providing a mechanism for enhanced HCO_3^- absorption in this setting. An apical membrane H^+-ATPase may also contribute to bicarbonate absorption in the TAL (148).

Inhibition of the Na^+-K^+-Cl^- cotransporter by furosemide stimulates bicarbonate absorption in the rat TAL (150). Thus, this transporter is not directly involved in bicarbonate absorption. Rather, the reduction in cell Na^+ activity that attends inhibition of Na^+-K^+-Cl^- cotransport provides a greater driving force for apical Na^+/H^+ exchange.

Krapf (281) has demonstrated that base efflux across the basolateral membrane of perfused rat TAL segments occurs as $Na^+(HCO_3^-)$ cotransport. This process is electrogenic (probable stoichiometry 1Na:3HCO3), sodium dependent, Cl^- independent and SITS-sensitive. $Na^+(HCO_3^-)$ cotransport has been demonstrated in mouse medullary TAL as well (257). In the mouse, the apical Na^+/H^+ exchanger and basolateral $Na^+(HCO_3^-)$ cotransporter play a role in cell pH regulation rather than transcellular bicarbonate transport. An electroneutral $Na^+:HCO_3^-$ cotransporter has also been localized in the basolateral membrane of the medullary TAL. This transporter mediates net HCO_3^- influx into the cell rather than efflux (365). Accordingly, the role of this transporter in net HCO_3^- absorption in unclear.

Origin of Transepithelial Voltage

The spontaneous, lumen-positive transepithelial potential that accompanies net NaCl absorption is, in principle, the sum of at least two terms: an electrogenic voltage arising from rheogenic cellular pathways, and a zero-current dilution voltage referable to salt accumulation in intercellular spaces during salt absorption. Given the cation selectivity of the paracellular pathway (P_{Na}/P_{Cl} ~2–6), an accumulation of Na^+ in the lateral intracellular space mediated by the (Na^+, K^+)-ATPase could create a lumen-positive diffusion potential across the junctional complex. As discussed earlier, the lumen-positive potential arising from rheogenic cellular transport serves to drive a proportion of net sodium reabsorption through the paracellular pathway. However, this paracellular sodium absorption will be diminished by the extent to which paracellular diffusion potential accounts for the spontaneous transepithelial voltage, V_e. Thus, it is pertinent to consider the relative contributions of both electrogenic and diffusion potentials to the total transepithelial voltage.

Hebert and Andreoli (197) assessed the possible contributions of a paracellular diffusion potential to V_e in the mouse TAL. The conductance of the paracellular pathway, G_s, was measured by blocking the transcellular conductance with 20-mM Ba^{2+} in the lumen. The junctional complexes were then disrupted by the imposition of large osmotic gradients produced by the addition of urea to the luminal perfusate. Using the value of G_s in the presence of 800-mM luminal urea as an estimate of the ionic conductance of the lateral interspace, exclusive of the junctional complex,

Hebert and Andreoli (197) calculated that, during net NaCl transport, the maximal rise in NaCl concentration in the lateral interspace was 10 mEq/liter and that the resulting dilution potential was less than 1 mV. These results are consistent with the notion that virtually all of the transepithelial voltage is the result of rheogenic transcellular processes.

Specifically, because the apical membrane is exclusively conductive to potassium and because the Na^+-K^+-$2Cl^-$ cotransporter is electroneutral, the apical membrane voltage, V_a, will approximate the K^+ equilibrium voltage, E_K. The basolateral membrane voltage, V_{bl}, in contrast, is a function of several conductive pathways; examples include K^+ and Cl^- channels, $Na^+HCO_3^-$ symport, (Na^+, K^+)-ATPase. Of these, Cl^- is likely the most important conductive species across the basolateral membrane. V_{bl}, therefore, will be greater than E_{Cl}, but less that E_K and hence less than V_a (Table 3). The lumen-positive V_e then is the result of differing conductance characteristics of the apical and basolateral membranes. The exact value of V_e will be determined by the relative magnitude of the basolateral K^+ and Cl^- conductances and on the currents passing through the apical and basolateral membranes.

According to these arguments, the electrogenic nature of V_e should allow for a significant fraction of net sodium absorption to proceed via the paracellular pathway. Indeed, for a constant stoichiometry of the Na^+-K^+-$2Cl^-$ entry, the ratio of net Cl^- absorption to paracellular sodium absorption should have a value of 2. The rate of net paracellular Na^+ absorption depends on a variety of factors, such as V_e, G_s, and P_{Na}/P_{Cl}, which vary considerably from tubule to tubule. When each of these variables was measured in the same tubule, however, the ratio of net Cl^- absorption to paracellular Na^+ absorption was reasonably constant at 2.4 ± 0.3 (197). Thus, the stoichiometry of Na^+-K^+-$2Cl^-$ entry may be constant under those experimental conditions, that is, ADH stimulated mTAL segments, and the variables G_e, G_s, and P_{Na}/P_{Cl} are related in a given tubule in such a way as to maintain the net Cl^- to paracellular Na^+ ratio at 2.

Coupling of Substrate Utilization to Ion Transport

Several studies have examined the utilization of metabolic substrates by the TAL and the coupling of substrate utilization to transepithelial salt absorption. The rates of active salt absorption and the activity of (Na^+, K^+)-ATPase in the TAL are among the highest of any nephron segment (180). Indeed, transepithelial NaCl absorption accounts for the single largest expenditure of energy by TAL cells. Inhibition of the (Na^+, K^+)-ATPase by ouabain reduces O_2 consumption by rabbit (64, 113), rat (512) and mouse (257) TAL segments by 50%. The majority of the ouabain-sensitive components of O_2 consumption can be abolished by furosemide. Furosemide, however, has no effect on O_2 consumption in the presence of the sodium ionophore nystatin. Likewise, as shown in Fig. 4, the deletion of either Na^+ or Cl^- from the incubation solutions reduces O_2 consumption

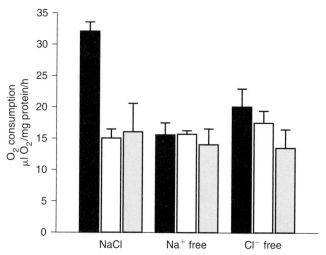

FIGURE 4   Oxygen consumption by isolated rabbit mTAL cells in suspension. O_2 consumption was measured in the presence of NaCl (left three bars), and in the absence of either Na^+ (middle bars) or Cl^- (right three bars). In each case, the black bar represents the control condition, white bars 0.1 mM ouabain, and gray bars 1 mM furosemide. (Data from Eveloff J, Bayerdorffer E, Silva P, Kinne R. Sodium-chloride transport in the thick ascending limb of Henle's loop. Oxygen consumption studies in isolated cells. *Pflugers Arch* 1981;389:263–270.)

by 50% and virtually eliminates any further response to either furosemide or ouabain (64, 113). Taken together, these data indicate that about one-half of the total cellular ATP supply is consumed by the basolateral membrane (Na^+, K^+)-ATPase pump and that this pump operates almost exclusively for the purpose of transepithelial NaCl transport.

TAL segments utilize a variety of metabolic substrates to support the high ATP requirement imposed by salt transport. Wittner et al. (559) examined the ability of various substrates to support NaCl transport in perfused rabbit cTAL segments. In the absence of exogenous substrate, NaCl transport fell by 73% in 10 minutes. When substrates were present only in the luminal perfusate, butyrate was the only substrate capable of supporting NaCl transport. In contrast, several substrates were capable of supporting transport when added to the basolateral solutions: D-glucose, D-mannose, butyrate, β-OH-butyrate, acetoacetate, lactate, acetate, and pyruvate (559). TCA cycle intermediates such as citrate, α-keto-glutarate and succinate, as well as glutamine, glutamate, proprionate, caprylate, and oleate did not sustain transport.

Substrate utilization by rat medullary and cortical TAL segments has been examined by measuring $^{14}CO_2$ release from ^{14}C-labeled substrates (216, 262). In the mTAL, $^{14}CO_2$ was produced from labeled glucose, lactate, 2-oxyglutarate, glutamate, glutamine, and palmitate. Little succinate, citrate or malate were oxidized in this segment. A similar pattern of substrate utilization was seen with cortical TAL segments (262). As noted with O_2 consumption, $^{14}CO_2$ production from ^{14}C-lactate or ^{14}C-glucose was coupled to ion transport. In both cTAL and mTAL segments, furosemide or ouabain reduced $^{14}CO_2$ production by 50%–60% (216). $^{14}CO_2$ production was also dependent on extracellular ions. Analysis of the relation between extracellular Cl⁻ concentrations and $^{14}CO_2$ production revealed an apparent K_m for Cl⁻ of 41 mM and a Hill coefficient for Cl⁻ of 2.1 (216). These results are consistent with the view that Cl⁻ entry via the Na^+-K^+-$2Cl^-$ cotransporter is a prime determinant of the rate of oxidative metabolism in TAL cells.

Chamberlin and Mandel (65) assessed the ability of various endogenous and exogenous substrates to support oxidative metabolism in suspensions of rabbit mTAL segments. Unlike the findings of Wittner et al. (559) in rabbit cTAL, where depletion of exogenous substrates reduced transport by 73%, these mTAL suspensions maintained 85% of their basal O_2 consumption in the absence of exogenous substrates. Inhibitors of glycolysis, fatty acid oxidation and amino acid oxidation reduced O_2 consumption indicating that glucose, fatty acids, and amino acids all serve as endogenous substrates capable of supporting oxidative metabolism when the availability of exogenous substrate is limited (65).

Uchida and Endou (514) determined the ability of various substrates to maintain cellular ATP concentrations in microdissected mouse TAL segments. In mTAL segments, glucose, lactate, and β-hydroxybutyrate all conserved cellular ATP content equally well. In cTAL, lactate and β-hydroxybutyrate increased cellular ATP more than did glucose. Glutamine was not a good substrate for ATP production in either segment (514).

Several studies have addressed the relative contributions of anaerobic and oxidative metabolism in supporting cellular energy needs. This issue is particularly important and may have clinical implications for the medullary TAL. In perfused cTAL segments, Wittner et al. (559) demonstrated that salt transport was preserved even at very low ambient oxygen tensions. However, inhibition of oxidative metabolism with cyanide markedly reduced transport. Moreover, in the presence of cyanide, glucose, and lactate were almost equal in their ability to support transport (559). They concluded that oxidative metabolism mainly supported salt absorption in the cTAL even at very low oxygen tension. Glycolysis made only a minor contribution to ATP production, even when oxidative metabolism was inhibited by cyanide.

In renal tubule segments, glycolysis is the sole source of lactate production (20). Hence, the production of lactate provides a measure of the rate of the glycolytic production of ATP. Cortical and medullary rat TAL segments produce small, but detectable amounts of lactate under basal conditions. When oxidative phosphorylation was inhibited with antimycin A, lactate production increased by 98% in the cTAL and by 1400% in the mTAL (20). However, even at these enhanced rates, anaerobic metabolism was unable to maintain cellular ATP levels in these segments (514).

The above data indicate that the TAL, particularly the medullary portion with its high rate of salt transport, relies almost exclusively on oxidative metabolism as its source of energy. Somewhat paradoxically, the mTAL resides in an oxygen poor environment. The oxygen tension in the outer medulla is about 10 mm Hg (294). Apparently, like the cTAL (559), the O_2 affinity of the mTAL is sufficiently high that oxidative metabolism is maintained even at low oxygen pressures. Nonetheless, the high oxygen requirement in an oxygen poor environment might predispose the mTAL to injury if oxygen delivery falls or salt transport requirements increase. Brezis and coworkers have shown that the medullary TAL is, in fact, exquisitely susceptible to hypoxic injury (51). Moreover, the metabolic work load of TAL cells seems to correlate with the susceptibility to hypoxic injury. Maneuvers that increase TAL salt transport, such as feeding rats a high protein diet, exacerbate hypoxic injury (109) while agents that diminish TAL salt transport, such as furosemide, exert a marked protective effect against hypoxic injury (52). Apparently, the susceptibility to hypoxic injury is not related to depletion of cellular ATP stores since inhibition of oxidative metabolism also protects TAL cells from hypoxic injury (53). Likewise, acidosis protects TAL cells from hypoxic injury without altering medullary ATP content (454).

Regulation of Salt Absorption in TAL

The rate of salt absorption by the thick ascending limb is modulated by at least two general classes of factors: physical factors, such as luminal flow rate and the composition and osmolality of luminal and peritubular fluids; and hormones, such as vasopressin and glucagon, which exert their effects through interactions with specific cellular receptor proteins. The regulation of TAL salt transport is characterized by considerable interspecies variation as well as intranephron heterogeneity. It is worth noting, again, that the cortical and medullary portions of the TAL have different transport properties (Table 2) and subserve different functions. Salt absorption in both segments creates luminal fluid dilution and the potential for free water excretion; however, only salt absorption by the medullary TAL enriches the medullary interstitial osmolality and enhances urinary concentrating power. Given these differences, it is not surprising that the rates of transport in the medullary and cortical TAL are modulated quite differently. A good example of both species and intranephronal heterogeneity is the effect of antidiuretic hormone on TAL transport.

ANTIDIURETIC HORMONE
The notion that ADH might affect NaCl absorption in the ascending limb of Henle and thereby regulate the countercurrent multiplication process was first suggested by Wirz (557). Support for this contention was provided by the demonstration, in some species, of an ADH-induced increase in adenylate cyclase activity (62, 87) and protein kinase activity (101) in the medullary, but not cortical, portions of the TAL.

Table 5 summarizes the effects of ADH on salt transport in vitro microperfused medullary TAL segments of mouse, rat, and rabbit. Hall and Varney (183) established that ADH

TABLE 5   Effects of ADH on NaCl Transport by Thick Ascending Limb Segments

Species	ADH	V_e (mV)	J_{NaCl} (pmol/sec/cm^2)	Reference
Mouse	−	5	2600	183, 198, 203, 437
	+	11	10,800	183, 198, 203, 437
Rat	−	2.4–3.3	4825	29, 437, 560
	+	3.6–4.7	7770	29, 437, 560
Rabbit	−	3–7	6400	412, 437
	+	3–7	Unchanged	412, 437

increased the lumen-positive transepithelial voltage and the net rate of tracer Cl⁻ absorption in the mouse medullary TAL. Several laboratories have confirmed these effects of ADH on the transepithelial voltage and unidirectional Cl⁻ flux in the mouse and demonstrated that the effect of ADH on NaCl transport was restricted to the medullary portion of this segment (198, 437, 445, 558). Moreover, the maximal stimulation of the transepithelial voltage in the mouse medullary TAL occurred at hormone concentrations, approximately 10–11 M (20 pg/ml or 10 μU/ml), found during states of antidiuresis (198). A similar increase in transepithelial voltage can be obtained in the mouse medullary TAL, but not the cortical TAL, by the addition of cAMP analogs, or forskolin, a nonhormonal activator of adenylate cyclase to the peritubular media (80, 198). In contrast, ADH, even at peritubular concentrations of 250 μU/ml, has no effect on V_e in the mouse cortical TAL (198). Taken together, these results indicate that the mouse medullary TAL and cortical TAL are functionally heterogeneous with respect to the effect of ADH on net NaCl absorption and that stimulation of net NaCl absorption in the mouse medullary TAL by ADH is mediated by cAMP. In contrast, while ADH causes a variable increase in cyclic AMP production in the rabbit TAL, pharmacologic concentrations of ADH had no effects on either the transepithelial voltage or tracer Cl⁻ efflux in this species (437).

Observations on the homozygous Brattleboro (central diabetes insipidus) rat indicated that ADH or the V_2 selective analog dDAVP increased NaCl absorption from the TAL of this species, when assessed either by in vitro perfusion of the loop of Henle or by in vitro microperfusion of medullary TAL segments (560).

Given this species variability, it is reasonable to ask whether ADH influences salt absorption in the human medullary TAL. Chabardés and coworkers (62) did not detect an effect of ADH on cAMP production in human medullary TAL segments obtained from pump-perfused kidneys rejected for transplantation, while cortical collecting tubules from the same kidneys responded to the hormone with a large increase in cAMP production. Similarly, Ruggles et al. (419) demonstrated ADH-sensitive adenylate cyclase activity in collecting ducts but not in TAL segments obtained from human kidneys immediately after surgical removal. This lack of response of human TAL segments to ADH may reflect an inherent in vivo unresponsiveness, an artifact resulting from pump-perfusion injury or ischemia (6), or a combination of both factors. Since the ability of humans to elaborate concentrated urine is limited compared to the mouse, the failure of ADH to increase cAMP in the human TAL is consistent with Morel's suggestion that the response of medullary TAL segments to ADH correlates directly with urinary concentrating ability (337).

MECHANISMS OF ADH EFFECT ON TAL

The mechanism whereby ADH stimulates salt transport in the medullary TAL has been studied most extensively in the mouse. It appears that the effects of ADH in this segment are mediated predominantly through interaction of the hormone with the vasopressin V_2 receptor coupled to adenylate cyclase. Thus, ADH stimulates adenylate cyclase activity in the TAL (334, 337) and cAMP analogues (198) and forskolin (80) mimic the effects of ADH on transport in this segment. Cholera toxin stimulates salt transport in the TAL indicating that the V_2 receptor is coupled to the catalytic subunit of adenylate cyclase by a stimulatory guanine nucleotide-binding protein, G_s (45). cAMP subsequently binds to the regulatory subunit of cAMP-dependent protein kinase and both the RI and RII isozymes are present in the TAL (136). The catalytic subunit of adenylate cyclase may, in turn, be influenced by calmodulin. Takaichi and Kurokawa (496) have shown that calmodulin inhibitors inhibited ADH-sensitive cAMP production in isolated mouse medullary TAL segments. Likewise, Ausiello and Hall (17) showed that the addition of exogenous calmodulin stimulated ADH-sensitive cAMP production by LLC PK$_1$ cells.

Table 6 lists the effects of ADH on several electrophysiologic parameters of mouse medullary TAL segments perfused in vitro. The approximate doubling of the equivalent short-circuit current results from an increase in the transepithelial voltage (198, 203, 331) and an increase of roughly 20% in the transepithelial conductance (203, 331, 445). Moreover, the ADH-induced increase in transepithelial conductance, G_e, is referable to an increase in the barium-sensitive, or transcellular conductance, Gc (196, 203, 331). ADH has no effect on the magnitude or permselectivity of the paracellular conductance, G_s (Table 6) (203).

ADH increases both the apical and basolateral membrane conductance (203, 331). The apical membrane of

TABLE 6 Effects of ADH on Electrophysiologic Parameters in Mouse Medullary TAL Segments

ADH (μU/ml)	V_e (mV)	G_e (mS/cm²)	G_c (mS/cm²)	G_s (mS/cm²)	V_a (mV)	V_{bl} (mV)	R_a/R_b
0	5.6	103.7	45.1	58.6	54.4	−50.7	1.2
250	10.3	121.3	60.2	61.0	47.3	−38.9	2.2

Data from Guggino WB. Functional heterogeneity in the early distal tubule of the *Amphiuma* kidney: evidence for two modes of Cl⁻ and K⁺ transport across the basolateral cell membrane. *Am J Physiol* 1986;250:F430–F440; Guggino WB, Oberleithner H, Giebisch G. The amphibian diluting segment. *Am J Physiol* 1988;254:F615–F627; Molony DA, Reeves WB, Hebert SC, Andreoli TE. ADH increases apical Na-:K-:2Cl⁻ entry in mouse medullary thick ascending limbs of Henle. *Am J Physiol* 1987;252:F177–F187.

TAL cells is, as noted previously, predominantly K⁺ conductive. In the presence of luminal furosemide to block K⁺ uptake via the Na⁺-K⁺-2Cl⁻ cotransporter, mouse TAL segments exhibit net K⁺ secretion that is increased by ADH (203). Because the electrochemical driving force for K⁺ secretion is presumably constant in the presence of furosemide, it was suggested that the increase in K⁺ secretion was due to an increase in apical membrane K⁺ conductance (203). In support of this notion, using membrane vesicles prepared from rabbit outer medulla, Reeves et al. (404) demonstrated that in vitro exposure to cAMP-dependent protein kinase and ATP specifically enhanced barium-sensitive rates of ⁸⁶Rb⁺ uptake. As noted above, this finding has been confirmed in subsequent work that examined the effects of phosphorylation on the activity of ROMK channels. As discussed above, the ROMK channels are believed to comprise a major component of the apical membrane K⁺ conductance in the thick ascending limb. ROMK is phosphorylated by cAMP-dependent protein kinase at a number of sites (565), and this phosphorylation increases the activity of the channel (320).

The ADH-induced increase in transepithelial NaCl absorption can be blocked by luminal furosemide and therefore represents an increase in apical Na⁺-K⁺-2Cl⁻ cotransport activity. The mechanism whereby ADH increases apical cotransport activity is unclear. Sun et al. (494) demonstrated that in isolated perfused mouse TAL segments, ADH changed the stoichiometry of NaCl entry from 1Na⁺:1Cl⁻ to 1Na⁺:1K⁺:2Cl⁻. This change in stoichiometry, accompanied by apical K⁺ recycling, could create a lumen-positive potential to drive Na⁺ reabsorption via the paracellular pathway. Phosphorylation of the cloned Na⁺-K⁺-2Cl⁻ cotransporter NKCC2 by cAMP-dependent protein kinase does not appear to directly increase cotransporter activity. However, phosphorylation may influence cotransporter activity by modulating the interactions between NKCC2 isoforms. As noted above, an isoform with a truncated C terminus, denoted C4, is itself nonfunctional but can inhibit the activity of the full-length NKCC2 (393). However, the inhibition by the C4 isoform can be relieved by phosphorylation by cAMP-dependent protein kinase (393). Thus, ADH may increase apical Na:K2Cl entry by releasing NKCC2 from tonic inhibition by truncated isoforms. Chronic exposure to ADH may increase apical Na:K:2Cl entry by increasing the abundance of NCKK2 (100).

The predominant portion of the ADH-induced increase in cellular conductance is accounted for by an increase in the basolateral membrane Cl⁻ conductance (196, 331). Two mechanisms have been suggested for the hormone-dependent increase in basolateral Cl⁻ conductance. Schlatter and Greger (445) have proposed that the ADH-induced increase in intracellular cAMP results in a direct increase in chloride channel activity. Such a mechanism has been amply demonstrated in Cl⁻ secreting epithelial such as the trachea and intestine. In support of their proposal, Schlatter and Greger demonstrated that cAMP and ADH elicited a fall in the fractional resistance of the basolateral membrane in mouse medullary TAL segments even when cell Cl⁻ activity was kept at low levels by blocking apical Cl⁻ entry with furosemide (445). Likewise, using patch clamp analysis, Paulais and Teulon (384) found that preincubation of mouse cortical TAL segments with forskolin or cAMP analogues increased the number of Cl⁻ channels observed in basolateral membrane patches.

Alternatively, ADH might enhance Cl⁻ conductance indirectly by increasing apical membrane Cl⁻ entry (196, 331). According to this proposal, an ADH-dependent activation of apical membrane Na⁺-K⁺-2Cl⁻ cotransporter and K⁺ channels leads to an increase in intracellular Cl⁻ activity and subsequent increase in basolateral Cl⁻ conductance. In support of this view, Molony et al. (331) found, also in mouse medullary TAL, that the ADH-dependent rise in cellular and basolateral conductance were much lower when Cl⁻ entry was inhibited by furosemide than in control conditions.

Studies of Cl⁻ channels incorporated from basolaterally enriched renal medullary membrane vesicles into planar lipid bilayers have demonstrated several properties of these channels that may account for an intracellular Cl⁻ concentration-dependent rise in basolateral Cl⁻ conductance (401, 407, 553). First, the activity of the Cl⁻ channels is increased with membrane depolarization evident to the basolateral membrane depolarization that follows ADH stimulation of TAL segments (401). Second, Cl⁻ channels in the vesicles behave like Goldman rectifiers so that increases in intracellular Cl⁻ cause an increase in the outward single-channel conductance (401). Third, channel activity is dependent on the intracellular Cl⁻ concentration such that increases in Cl⁻ over the range of 2–50 mM results in large increases in the open time probability of these Cl⁻ channels (406, 553). In this respect, it should be recognized that the time-averaged conductance of a basolateral Cl⁻ channel is given by the product $g_{Cl}P_o$, where g_{Cl} is unit channel conductance and P_o is open time probability.

Thus, an ADH-dependent increase in apical Cl⁻ entry could stimulate basolateral Cl⁻ conductance to a far greater extent than expected from simple Goldman rectification. In that connection, at least two laboratories have found, in mTAL segments, that reducing intracellular Cl⁻ with luminal furosemide produced a three-fold reduction in basolateral Cl⁻ conductance (331, 445).

Winters et al. (552, 554) have examined the possible interactions between direct protein kinase activation of Cl⁻ channels and Cl⁻-dependent activation of Cl⁻ channels. At low intracellular Cl⁻ concentrations (≤ 2 mM), exposure of the intracellular face of the channel to ATP and purified cAMP-dependent protein kinase resulted in an increase in channel open probability from 0.31 to 0.50. However, at higher intracellular Cl⁻ concentration (50 mM), the channel open probability was higher (0.52) under control conditions and did not increase further upon addition of ATP and protein kinase (406, 552). Thus, both cAMP-dependent protein kinase and increases in cell Cl⁻ activity can, independently, increase basolateral membrane Cl⁻ conductance. However, these two effects may not be additive. The relative importance of these two mechanisms depends on the transporting state of the cell and on the relative rates of apical Cl⁻ entry and basolateral Cl⁻ efflux. Of interest, Cl⁻ channels in the basolateral membrane of cortical TAL cells share a similar single-channel conductance and voltage dependence to channels from medullary TAL cells. However, the cortical TAL channels differ in one key respect, namely, that open probability of the cortical channels is not dependent on intracellular Cl⁻ activity (555). This lack of response to intracellular Cl⁻ may be one factor that accounts for the failure of ADH to increase net NaCl absorption in the cortical TAL (198).

MODULATION OF ADH EFFECT ON TAL SEGMENTS

The actions of ADH on NaCl absorption in the thick ascending limb can be modulated by a number of factors. Three of these, increases in peritubular osmolality, prostaglandins, and increases in peritubular calcium concentration, will be considered briefly.

In isolated mouse and rabbit TAL segments, increases in peritubular osmolality, produced either with permeant solutes such as urea or with impermeant solutes such as mannitol, rapidly and reversibly inhibit the ADH-stimulated rate of net Cl⁻ absorption (200, 329). Peritubular hypertonicity results in a prompt reduction in the transepithelial voltage and in the cellular conductance (329). Molony and Andreoli (329) determined that hypertonicity inhibits the basolateral membrane chloride conductance. This inhibition of transcellular salt absorption occurs at a locus beyond the generation of cAMP, since supramaximal concentrations of either ADH or cAMP are unable to reverse the hypertonicity-mediated effect (200).

Thus, increasing the absolute magnitude of interstitial osmolality provides a negative feedback signal that can reduce ADH-dependent salt absorption by the mTAL. Hypertonicity increases the expression of ROMK in the mTAL (133). Since an increase in ROMK activity would tend to increase NaCl absorption and transepithelial voltage, it is not clear how this finding relates to the observed inhibition of transport by hypertonicity.

PGE₂ also participates in a local negative feedback system in the renal medulla that modulates the rate of net NaCl absorption by the mTAL (210, 482). In the in vitro mouse mTAL (79, 80), PGE₂ has no effect on NaCl salt absorption when ADH is absent. In the presence of ADH, PGE₂ reduces the ADH-dependent values for transepithelial voltage and net NaCl absorption to ADH-independent values. Likewise, reported biochemical studies in the mTAL (348, 511) indicate that PGE₂ has no effect on cellular cAMP concentrations in the absence of ADH, and that PGE₂ markedly inhibits the ADH-dependent stimulation of cytosolic cAMP concentrations.

PGE₂ does not inhibit the component of NaCl transport in the mouse mTAL stimulated by the nonhormonal catalytic subunit activator forskolin, but PGE₂ does inhibit transport stimulation by cholera toxin, which activates adenylate cyclase specifically and irreversibly at G_s (80). Thus, it is likely that PGE₂ inhibits ADH-stimulated generation of cAMP in the mTAL by activating G_i (80, 348).

Although interstitial cells are a major source of PGE2 production in the renal medulla, thick ascending limb cells can metabolize arachidonic acid through at least two pathways (see Chapter 14). McGiff and coworkers (110) demonstrated that purified medullary thick ascending limb cells produce 20-hydroxyeicosatetraenoic acid (20-HETE) via the cytochrome P450 enzyme, ω-hydroxylase. 20-HETE was subsequently shown to inhibit NaCl transport in the thick ascending limb at steps that include the apical K⁺ channel (305) and the Na⁺-K⁺-2Cl⁻ cotransporter (12, 110). Thick ascending limb cells, particularly in the macula densa, also express COX-2 (188). COX-2 expression in these cells may be coupled to renin secretion. Thus, COX-2 expression is increased by salt restriction, diuretics and in Bartter syndrome, all conditions characterized by hyperreninemia (73). Moreover, COX-2 inhibitors reduce renin secretion in these settings (187, 388).

Hypercalcemia often results in an ADH-resistant urinary concentrating defect, that is, nephrogenic diabetes insipidus (402). At least part of this concentrating defect results from the inhibition of ADH-stimulated cAMP production in the TAL by calcium. Takaichi and Kurokawa demonstrated that cAMP production in response to ADH or glucogen was significantly blunted when the calcium concentration of the incubation medium was raised from 1 mM (497). High ambient calcium also inhibited cAMP production stimulated by forskolin indicating that the inhibition probably involved the catalytic subunit of adenylate cyclase. Preincubation of tubule segments with pertussis toxin abolishes the effect of hypercalcemia on cAMP generation, indicating that the inhibition of cAMP generation is mediated through activation of G_i (498). The effects of hypercalcemia on cAMP production are mediated by a G-protein coupled calcium-sensing receptor (CaSR) present on the basolateral membrane of TAL cells (410, 411). Activation of this receptor also inhibits the activity of the 70-pS apical K channel via the production of 20-HETE, a P450 metabolite of arachidonic acid (535, 536). Even changes in serum calcium within the physiologic range can alter NaCl absorption via the CaSR (131). This may help to explain the hypotensive effect of high calcium intake in salt-sensitive hypertensive individuals (316).

In addition to ADH, a number of other peptide hormones stimulate adenylate cyclase activity in the TAL. The effects of these hormones on sodium transport are discussed in Chapters 34 and 35.

ADRENERGIC AGENTS

β agonist-sensitive adenylate cyclase activity is present in the rat, but not rabbit TAL (63, 334). Likewise, β-adrenoceptors have been detected along the rat TAL by autoradiographic localization (342, 493). The physiologic effects of adrenergic agents have been tested in micropunctures and in vitro microperfusion studies. DiBona and Sawin (89) demonstrated an enhancement of loop NaCl absorption during low-frequency renal nerve stimulation. Acute renal denervation, on the other hand, depressed NaCl absorption by the loop of Henle (27).

Micromolar concentrations of isoproterenol stimulate net Cl^- absorption by the in vitro perfused mouse medullary and cortical TAL (21). The effects of isoproterenol on NaCl absorption in these segments can be blocked by propranolol.

MINERALOCORTICOIDS

Several lines of evidence suggest that mineralocorticoids influence NaCl transport in the TAL (90). First, clearance studies indicate that aldosterone increases free water clearance in adrenalectomized animals (416), consistent with an increase in NaCl absorption by the TAL. Second, nuclear mineralocorticoid receptors are present in both the medullary and cortical portions of the TAL of rat and rabbit (117, 311). The mere presence of mineralocorticoid receptors, however, is no guarantee that the TAL is a specific target site of aldosterone. In vitro, mineralocorticoid receptors bind aldosterone, cortisol and corticosterone with equal affinity. The specificity of the receptor is conferred, in vivo, by the enzyme 11β-hydroxysteroid dehydrogenase type 2, which metabolizes cortisol and corticosterone so that they do not bind to the mineralocorticoid receptor (132). 11β-hydroxysteroid dehydrogenase has been detected in the TAL using enzymatic assays (38) and by immunohistochemistry (288). Third, aldosterone appears to modulate the activity of certain transport related enzymes in the TAL. Specifically, adrenalectomy reduces the activity of (Na^+, K^+)-ATPase (213, 312) and citrate

synthase (312) in the rabbit TAL. The activity of these enzymes can be restored almost to normal by aldosterone but not by dexamethasone (213, 312). In the adrenal-intact mouse, pharmacologic doses of mineralocorticoid increased (Na^+, K^+)-ATPase activity of mTAL segments by 25% (170). Other studies, however, have failed to show an effect of mineralocorticoids on (Na^+, K^+)-ATPase activity in the TAL (103, 137, 400).

Finally, in vivo and in vitro microperfusion studies have demonstrated effects of aldosterone on TAL sodium transport. In an in vivo microperfusion study of superficial loop segments, Stanton (477) showed that adrenalectomy inhibited loop of Henle sodium absorption by 33%. Aldosterone, but not dexamethasone, increased sodium transport to control levels. Work and Jamison (561) demonstrated, using in vitro perfusion, that the rate of salt absorption and the transepithelial voltage in TAL segments dissected from adrenalectomized rats were reduced by 50% compared to tubules from adrenal intact rats. Moreover, administration of aldosterone to the adrenalectomized rats returned salt absorption and transepithelial voltage back to control values. Also in the rat medullary TAL, adrenalectomy decreases $NaHCO_3$ absorption by 33% (154). Taken together, these data indicate that aldosterone stimulates sodium absorption by the mammalian TAL. The mechanisms of aldosterone actions are discussed in Chapter 32.

NITRIC OXIDE

Acute administration of nitric oxide donors or L-arginine, the substrate for NOS, decreases NaCl absorption in isolated perfused thick ascending limb segments (374, 395). The effect of L-arginine on NaCl transport can be blocked by L-NAME, and inhibitor of NOS, indicating that endogenous production of NO mediates the effect of L-arginine. The inhibitory effect of NO on net NaCl absorption appears to involve, at least in part, inhibition of NKCC2 activity (375). The thick ascending limb expresses all three isoforms of nitric oxide synthase (373). Plato et al. (394) used mice deficient in the various NOS isoforms in determining that the effect of L-arginine is mediated by e-NOS rather than i-NOS or n-NOS. In contrast to its effect on NaCl absorption, NO stimulates $NaHCO_3^-$ absorption in the thick ascending limb (151). Finally, although short-term exposure to NO inhibits NaCl absorption, chronic exposure increases NKCC2 expression (513), which could translate into increased NaCl absorption.

SODIUM BALANCE

Dietary sodium restriction in rats results in a transient decrease in NKCC2 expression (313) while high-sodium intake has no major effect on NKCC2 expression (471). Chronic treatment with furosemide in conjunction with a high-sodium diet increases NKCC2 expression (346). The latter phenomenon may account for the development of diuretic resistance and the inter-dose rebound in sodium absorption in patients treated chronically with loop diuretics.

TROPHIC EFFECTS OF PROTEIN INTAKE AND ADH

Selective hypertrophy of the medullary TAL can be induced by chronic administration of ADH to ADH deficient (Brattleboro) rats (41). The hypertrophy is most pronounced in the inner stripe of outer medulla. High protein intake also causes an increase in the thickness of the inner stripe of outer medulla and an increase in the epithelial volume of TAL segments in that region (42). Concomitantly, there occurs an increase in urinary concentrating ability and of (Na$^+$, K$^+$)-ATPase activity in TAL segments (42). The high protein diet did not induce hypertrophy in Brattleboro rats suggesting that ADH may be necessary for this effect (43).

NA$^+$ TRANSPORT IN DISTAL CONVOLUTED TUBULE AND CONNECTING SEGMENT

General Characteristics

Much of the information regarding salt transport in the distal tubule has derived from micropuncture studies that did not distinguish between the early and late distal tubule. For this reason, the distal convoluted tubule and the connecting segment will be discussed together. The DCT absorbs roughly 10% of the filtered sodium load (105, 208, 255). Fluid enters the DCT with a sodium concentration of 25–30 mM, but salt is added along the initial 20% of the DCT, so that the sodium concentration averages 50 mM at a point 200–300 μm from the macula densa (449). From there, tubular sodium concentration decreases along the DCT to a value of approximately 30 mM at the end (209, 255). Tubular fluid to plasma sodium ratios as low as 0.10 have been observed during stationary microperfusion (209, 291, 309). This finding, together with the presence of the lumen-negative potential difference (see subsequent discussion), establishes clearly the active nature of sodium absorption in this segment.

Sodium absorption by the DCT is load dependent. That is, over a wide range of delivery rates, the proportion of sodium absorbed by the DCT remains constant at 80% (255).

At high tubular fluid flow rates, the fall in luminal sodium concentration along the tubule is attenuated; thus, more sodium is available to distal sodium absorptive sites at high flow rates than at low flow rates.

Sodium absorption in the rat DCT has been reported to be 25–30 pEq/mm^2/sec, that is, about one-third of the rate occurring in the PCT (549). However, rates comparable to those in the PCT have been reported in isolated perfused DCT (77, 78, 107).

Electrophysiologic Considerations

The electrophysiologic and transport properties of the DCT and CNT are summarized in Table 7. The transepithelial voltage in the earliest loops of the DCT, measured with fine tip electrodes, ranges from −9 to −19 mV, lumen-negative (192, 562). Small lumen-positive voltages, +3.7 to 5.7 mV, have been measured both in micropuncture experiments, by using low resistance micropuncture electrodes (9, 23), and in isolated, perfused early DCT segments (455). The variation in lumen voltages may reflect differences in the experimental conditions under which the measurements were made. When the composition of the luminal perfusate resembled distal tubular fluid, that is, having a low NaCl concentration (see earlier discussion), the lumen voltage tended to be slightly positive whereas when tubules were perfused with solutions resembling plasma, that is, high NaCl concentration, the lumen voltage was negative (9). The lumen-negative potential measured with high NaCl solutions was abolished by luminal amiloride, an inhibitor of epithelial sodium channels. The positive voltage under "in vivo" conditions is a salt dilution potential arising from the differential permeability of the DCT to Na and Cl, while the lumen-negative potential under symmetric solutions reflects active Na$^+$ reabsorption via amiloride-sensitive sodium channels (see subsequent discussion).

The transepithelial electrical potential in the late DCT of rats measured in vivo ranges from −37 to −60 mV (44). Values in isolated rabbit DCT and CNT segments perfused with symmetric solutions are less negative, −5 to −30 mV (166, 219, 455, 457, 574). The voltage can be inhibited by

TABLE 7   Electrophysiologic and Transport Properties of DCT

	V_t (mV) (References)	R_t (Ω-cm^2) (References)	V_{bl} (mV) (References)	fRa (References)	J_{Na} (pmol/mm/min) (References)	J_{Cl} (pmol/mm/min) (References)
Rat DCT	+8 to −19 (7–9, 192, 308, 562)	81–382 (81, 308, 562)	−57 to −65 (308, 562)		128–258 (77, 78, 107)	285 (107)
Rabbit DCT	−2 to −40 (168, 169, 219, 457, 458, 525, 526, 572)	22–116 (525, 526, 574)	−78 to −84 (525, 526, 574)	0.78–0.99 (525, 526, 574)	82 (458)	
Rabbit CNT	−4 to −27 (10, 219, 456–458)	29–31 (10)	−71 to −83 (456, 572, 573)		62–121 (10, 455)	405 (457)

Table from Koeppen BM, Stanton BA. Sodium chloride transport—distal nephron. In: Seldin DW, Giebisch G, eds. *The Kidney: Physiology and Pathophysiology*, 2nd ed. New York: Raven Press; 1992:2003–2039.

peritubular ouabain or luminal amiloride (168, 574), and is quite sensitive to changes in perfusion pressure and flow rate, decreasing with high pressures or flow rates (219).

The transepithelial resistance of the rat DCT decreases from 337 Ω-cm^2 in the early DCT to 135 Ω-cm^2 in the late DCT (81, 308). Hypotonic luminal fluids increase and hypertonic perfusates decrease the transepithelial resistance with respect to isotonic luminal fluid (81). Somewhat lower electrical resistances have been found in isolated perfused rabbit DCT (166, 574) and CNT (10). The passive ionic permeability determined by single ion dilution voltages (191) reveals the following sequence: $K^+ > Na^+ > Cl^-$.

Intracellular microelectrode analysis of rabbit DCT cells has yielded conflicting results. Yoshitomi et al. (574) found evidence for both K^+ and Na^+ conductive pathways in the apical membrane and K^+ and Cl^- conductive pathways in the basolateral membrane. The apical membrane accounted for 80% of the total cellular resistance. In contrast, Velazquez et al. (524, 526) found the apical membrane to comprise over 99% of the cellular resistance and could not detect any Na^+ or K^+ conductances in that membrane. Perhaps some of this discrepancy could have arisen from the examination of different portions of the DCT in the two laboratories. Ellison et al. have demonstrated that sodium reabsorption in the early DCT is largely mediated by a thiazide-sensitive, neutral NaCl cotransporter, while sodium absorption in the late DCT involves an amiloride-sensitive electrogenic pathway (107). Thus, Yoshitomi et al. (574) may have described the late DCT and Velazquez et al. (524, 526) the early DCT.

MECHANISM OF NA$^+$ ABSORPTION

The available evidence permits the delineation of certain facets of Na$^+$ absorption in the DCT. A general model for these mechanisms is presented in Fig. 5. Cardinal among these are the characteristics discussed in the following subsections.

Apical NaCl Cotransport The absorption of sodium and chloride in the early DCT is mutually dependent on each other (524). Sodium absorption is a function of the luminal chloride concentration, and chloride absorption is a function of the luminal sodium concentration. The half-maximal concentrations of both sodium and chloride are 10 mM (524). Furthermore, the intracellular Cl$^-$ activity is above its electrochemical equilibrium (39) such that Cl$^-$ entry into the cell must involve active transport. The early distal tubule is the site of action of thiazide diuretics (78, 107, 457). Autoradiographic studies (25) and immunocytochemical studies (104) have demonstrated thiazide-binding sites in the apical membranes of DCT and connecting tubule cells.

A thiazide-sensitive neutral NaCl cotransporter (TSC) was cloned from the flounder urinary bladder using an expression cloning strategy (135). A homologous transporter, NCC (SLC12A3) was subsequently cloned from the mammalian kidney (134). The transporter shares considerable sequence homology to the bumetanide-sensitive

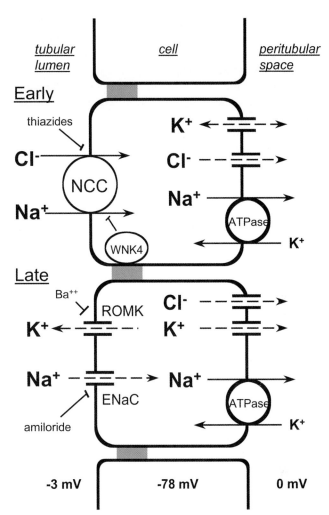

FIGURE 5   Model of NaCl absorption by cells of the early (top) and late DCT/CNT (bottom). See text for details. (Modified from Reeves WB, Andreoli TE. Tubular sodium transport. In: Schrier RW, ed. *Diseases of the Kidney and Urinary Tract*, 7th ed. Philadelphia: Lippincott Williams & Wilkins; 2001:135–176.)

Na$^+$-K$^+$-Cl$^-$ cotransporter (NKCC2) present in the TAL (134, 385), yet exhibits markedly different inhibitor sensitivity and ionic requirements compared to the latter transporter. NCC transports NaCl with a 1:1 stoichiometry, is K independent, and is inhibited by thiazide diuretics (332). The expression of NCC within the kidney has been determined by in situ hybridization (19, 364), RT-PCR of single nephron segments (567), and by immunohistochemistry (19, 31, 104, 396, 528). The results indicate that NCC is expressed in the apical membrane of DCT cells and extends, in most species, into the connecting segment. In addition, mutations in the NCC gene have been linked to the pathogenesis of Gitelman syndrome (1, 397, 465, 466, 499). This syndrome resembles Bartter syndrome (hypokalemia, alkalosis, sodium wasting), except that urinary calcium excretion is reduced in Gitelman syndrome but is elevated in most cases of Bartter syndrome. Thus, physiologically, Gitelman syndrome mimics the effects of thiazide diuretics. The Gitelman mutations have little effect on the functional and biochemical properties of NCC protein, but markedly reduce its cell surface expression (285, 423). That mutations in the NCC gene are seen in Gitelman syndrome provides further support for the view that the NCC gene product is the thiazide-sensitive cotransporter of the DCT.

In addition to thiazide-sensitive NaCl cotransport, a component of electroneutral NaCl absorption may be mediated by parallel actions of Na^+/H^+ and Cl^-/organic anion exchangers. The net effect of synchronous Na^+/H^+ and Cl^-/base exchange is the reabsorption of NaCl with recycling of the organic anion. In this regard, the addition of either formate or oxalate to the perfusate of microperfused rat distal tubules stimulated chloride transport (532). Moreover, the formate or oxalate stimulated component of Cl^- transport was not inhibited by thiazide diuretics. The protein(s) that mediate the Cl^-/anion exchange is not known. CFEX, which may mediate proximal tubule Cl^-/anion exchange, is not expressed in the distal tubule (265).

Apical Conductive Sodium Channels The entry of sodium into the *Amphiuma* distal tubular cell (543) and late rat DCT cell (77) is inhibited by amiloride, a sodium channel blocker. A sodium channel in the apical membrane would serve to depolarize the membrane and create the observed lumen-negative transepithelial potential. This transepithelial voltage, in turn, is a driving force for passive chloride reabsorption. Sodium channel subunits have been found by immunolocalization in the late DCT in mouse and rat kidney (301, 448) but not human kidney (31).

Basolateral Electrogenic Na^+ Pump The voltage (V_{bl}) across the basolateral membrane of the *Amphiuma* (542) and rabbit (166, 526, 574) DCT is −60 to −90 mV. A reduction in the luminal sodium concentration causes V_{bl} to depolarize, while increases in the sodium concentration hyperpolarize V_{bl} (542, 543). In addition, V_{bl} depolarizes after ouabain treatment (525). These observations are consistent with the notion that apical sodium entry stimulates the electrogenic (Na^+, K^+)-ATPase system in the basolateral membrane.

Basolateral Potassium Channels The basolateral membrane of DCT cells contains a large, barium-sensitive potassium conductance (166). Patch clamp studies of the basolateral membrane of DCT cells have identified three different potassium channels. Two of the channels have similar conductances (50–60 pS) and kinetics, and both are blocked by barium (504). The third channel is seen less frequently, has a conductance of 80 pS, and is not blocked by barium.

Basolateral Chloride Channels Microelectrode studies by Yoshitomi et al. (574) provided evidence for a chloride conductive pathway in the basolateral membrane of rabbit DCT cells. Likewise, Gesek and Friedman (143, 144) found evidence for basolateral membrane Cl^- channels in cultured mouse DCT cells. Specifically, inhibition of apical Cl^- entry with thiazide diuretics resulted in a fall in intracellular Cl^- activity and a hyperpolarization of the membrane voltage (143). The thiazide-induced hyperpolarization could be abolished by either a reduction in the extracellular Cl^- concentration or by NPPB, a Cl^- channel blocker (143, 144), suggesting that a Cl^- channel accounts for the basolateral Cl^- conductance. The single-channel properties of Cl^- channels in DCT cells have not been reported. The basolateral Cl^- conductance was increased by parathyroid hormone, presumably acting via cAMP (144). A cAMP-activated Cl^- conductance regulator having 30% homology to CFTR has been cloned from rabbit ileum (518). The protein is expressed in the basolateral membranes of the thick ascending limb and the DCT. The possible relation of this protein to the basolateral membrane Cl^- conductance in the DCT remains to be determined.

REGULATION OF NaCl TRANSPORT IN DCT

Na^+ Delivery As noted earlier, NaCl reabsorption in the DCT is dependent on the delivered load of NaCl (255). Chronic increases in the delivery of NaCl to the DCT can be achieved using furosemide to inhibit NaCl reabsorption in the thick ascending limb. The DCT responds to such a maneuver with an increase in the capacity for NaCl transport (97, 98, 105) as well as marked ultrastructural changes in the DCT cell. These morphologic changes include an increase in the size of the DCT cell, an increase in the basolateral membrane surface area, and in increase in the size of mitochondria (105, 248). Accompanying the functional and morphologic changes are an increase in (Na^+, K^+)-ATPase activity and an increase in thiazide-binding sites (70, 106). These effects appear to result from an increase in sodium entry into the DCT cell rather than the increase in distal NaCl delivery or changes in plasma aldosterone or ADH levels that occur with chronic furosemide treatment. Thus, the same structural and functional changes are observed in adrenalectomized animals receiving physiologic steroid hormone replacement (249). In addition, an increase in dietary sodium alone, which increases distal NaCl delivery but not distal Na^+ absorption (105), does not, in the rat, result in an increase in cell height (105) or an increase in thiazide-binding sites (70, 116). Moreover, inhibition of NaCl entry into DCT cells with chronic thiazide treatment resulted in a loss of cell height, loss of normal polarity, and apoptosis of the DCT cells (300). The cellular mechanisms whereby NaCl entry affects transport function and morphology are not known.

Dietary Na^+ Studies in rats and rabbits have yielded conflicting results regarding the effects of increased dietary sodium on DCT morphology and sodium transport. In rats, no consistent effect of a high-sodium diet on cell morphology, transport rates, or thiazide receptor density could be demonstrated (70, 105, 116). In contrast, rabbits fed a high-sodium diet developed hypertrophy of DCT cells, an increased rate of DCT sodium reabsorption, and an increase in (Na^+, K^+)-ATPase activity (247, 458).

Steroid Hormones Currently available evidence suggests that adrenal steroid hormones regulate sodium transport in the DCT. The presence of both mineralocorticoid and glucocorticoid receptors in the DCT has been demonstrated by immunohistochemistry and by hormone binding (40, 96, 117–119, 421). In addition, adrenalectomy resulted in a decrease in (Na^+, K^+)-ATPase activity in the DCT (103). The (Na^+, K^+)-ATPase activity could be restored by replacement doses of glucocorticoids (102, 103, 138) but not by mineralocorticoids (102, 103, 137). Microperfusion studies of superficial distal tubules (containing both DCT and CNT), however, demonstrated an increase in sodium transport in animals receiving aldosterone infusions (477, 523). Both the thiazide-sensitive and thiazide-insensitive components of sodium transport were increased by aldosterone (523). The former may reflect neutral NaCl cotransport in the DCT while the latter reflects electrogenic sodium absorption in the late DCT or CNT. Aldosterone infusion also resulted in an increase in thiazide-binding sites in the renal cortex, as determined by [³H]metolazone binding, and an increase in the natriuretic response to thiazide diuretics, and a large increase in NCC protein (71, 258, 523). These findings establish NCC as an aldosterone regulated transporter. By combining immunohistochemical and in situ hybridization techniques, Bostonjoglo et al. (40) determined that DCT cells coexpress NCC, mineralocorticoid receptors, and 11β-hydroxysteroid dehydrogenase type 2, an enzyme typically found in mineralocorticoid target sites. Thus, DCT cells, particularly those in the late portions of the DCT, express the key elements required for selective mineralocorticoid actions.

As just mentioned, glucocorticoids increase (Na^+, K^+)-ATPase activity following adrenalectomy in the DCT (102, 103, 138). This effect was not blocked by spironolactone, a mineralocorticoid receptor antagonist, suggesting that glucocorticoids were acting via glucocorticoid receptors rather than mineralocorticoid receptors (102). In addition, dexamethasone infusions increased thiazide-sensitive NaCl transport and [³H]metolazone-binding sites in adrenalectomized rats (71, 523). Nonetheless, the role of glucocorticoids in the physiologic regulation of sodium transport in the DCT remains unclear.

Gonadal steroid hormones may also influence NaCl transport in the DCT. Chen et al. (72) first reported gender differences in the density of thiazide receptors and in the natriuretic response to thiazides in rats. Female rats had higher levels of thiazide-binding sites in the renal cortex than males. The levels in females fell following ovariectomy while levels rose in males following orchiectomy. Moreover, the increase in urinary sodium excretion caused by thiazides was greater in females than in males suggesting that the differences in thiazide-binding sites were reflective of differences in thiazide-sensitive salt transport in vivo. Likewise, using antibodies against the cloned thiazide-sensitive NaCl cotransporter (NCC), Verlander et al. (528) found that estrogen treatment increased NCC expression in the DCT. These results are consistent with the view that male sex hormones (e.g., testosterone) may downregulate NCC expression and salt transport while estrogens increase NCC expression and salt transport in the DCT. These authors are not aware of gender differences in the response of humans to thiazide diuretics.

Protein Kinases Studies of an inherited disorder of distal sodium transport, Gordon's syndrome, have yielded additional insights into the regulation of NCC function. Gordon's syndrome, or pseudohypoaldosteronism type II (PHAII) is the phenotypic opposite of Gitelman syndrome and is characterized by hypertension, hyperkalemia and metabolic acidosis. The disorder is largely corrected by thiazide diuretics. These features suggested that an increase in NCC activity may be involved in the pathogenesis of PHAII. Positional cloning demonstrated that PHAII is caused by mutations in either of two serine-threonine kinases, WNK1 and WNK4 (546). Subsequent studies have shown that WNK4 normally acts to inhibit NCC-mediated NaCl transport, likely by reducing cell surface expression of NCC (547, 566). Mutant WNK4, in contrast, is unable to inhibit NCC activity and results in higher rates of NaCl transport (547, 566). WNK4 also affects the activity of apical ROMK channels (243) and the Cl^- permeability of the paracellular pathway (244). The mechanism whereby WNK1 produces PHAII is less well defined. Yang et al. (566) found that WNK1 does not directly affect NCC activity, but modulates the inhibition of NCC by WNK4. They propose that mutations which increase the activity of WNK1 prevent WNK4 from inhibiting NCC-mediated transport. It is interesting that WNK4 also inhibits CFEX activity (243). Although CFEX is not expressed in the distal tubule, perhaps a homologous distal tubule Cl^-/anion exchanger is also regulated by WNK4.

The factors that regulate WNK activity and the role of WNK kinases in the regulation of DCT NaCl absorption in response to physiologic and pathophysiologic stimuli remain to be determined.

NA⁺ TRANSPORT IN COLLECTING DUCT

General Considerations

The transport processes in the collecting duct are responsible for the final adjustments in urinary composition. The collecting duct is a major locus of action of mineralocorticoid hormones, and plays a major role in potassium homeostasis and acid–base balance. Quantitatively, it is a minor site of sodium absorption, reclaiming only about 2% of the filtered sodium load (550).

ELECTROPHYSIOLOGIC ASPECTS

The electrophysiologic and transport properties of the CCD are summarized in Table 8. The transepithelial voltage in the cortical collecting duct (CCD) varies widely, but generally in a range from +10 to −100 mV (44, 78, 156, 184, 433). This variability is largely the result of differences in the mineralocorticoid status of animals. The voltages in isolated human CCD segments averaged +6.8 mV, lumen-positive

TABLE 8   Electrophysiologic and Transport Properties of CCD

	V_t (mV) (References)	R_t (Ω-cm^2) (References)	V_{bl} (mV) (References)	fRa (References)	J_{na} (pmol/mm/min) (References)	J_{cl} (pmol/mm/min) (References)
Rabbit CCD	−2 to −27 (273, 287, 343, 344, 372, 432-434, 453, 456, 487, 510)	86–133 (273, 343, 344, 372, 432–434)	−73 to −85 (273, 343, 344, 372, 432–434)	0.31–0.53 (273, 343, 344, 372, 432–434)	5.7–24.3 (453, 486, 487, 551)	−3.4 to 4.0 (483, 484)
Rat CCD	−1 to −5 (67, 189, 408, 418, 439)	51–64 (440, 447)	−77 to −83 (440, 446, 447)	0.76–0.84 (440, 447)	−2.3 to 0.2 (408, 510)	

Note: Intracellular data from principal cells only.

Table modified from Koeppen BM, Stanton BA. Sodium chloride transport—distal nephron. In: Seldin DW, Giebisch G, eds. *The Kidney: Physiology and Pathophysiology*, 2nd ed. New York: Raven Press; 1992:2003–2039.

(236). The lumen-negative voltage in other mammalian CCD segments is abolished by ouabain (156, 185), luminal amiloride (371, 485, 490), and luminal sodium deletion (185, 486, 490). The lumen-negative voltage is increased by a high-K$^+$, low-Na$^+$ diet, and mineralocorticoid treatment (184, 219, 371, 453, 486).

The reported values for transepithelial resistance vary from 30 Ω-cm^2 to 2700 Ω-cm^2 (57, 205, 206, 434). The apical membrane contains a sodium conductance and a potassium conductance, as shown by the effects of luminal amiloride and luminal barium, respectively, on transepithelial resistance (273, 372, 433, 434). The basolateral membrane is conductive to K$^+$ and, at least in rabbits, Cl$^-$ (431, 432, 434, 447).

MECHANISMS OF SALT ABSORPTION IN COLLECTING DUCTS

A proposed model for sodium absorption and potassium secretion in the CCD is presented in Fig. 6. As indicated above, apical membranes of principal cells of the CCD possess conductive pathways for sodium and for potassium (215, 273, 372, 486). Sodium enters principal cells through sodium channels in the apical membrane, along its electrochemical gradient. In the rabbit CCD, these sodium channels mediate virtually all of Na$^+$ reabsorption. Sodium is then pumped across the basolateral membrane by (Na$^+$, K$^+$)-ATPase in exchange for potassium. The sodium current across the apical membrane depolarizes the latter, so that the cellular potassium is above its equilibrium concentration, and hence leaves the cell through the conductive pathway in the apical membrane (430).

Mechanisms of Salt Absorption in Collecting Ducts The conductive entry of sodium depolarizes the apical cell membrane relative to the basolateral membrane resulting in a lumen-negative transepithelial voltage. This lumen-negative voltage, in turn, provides the driving force for Cl$^-$ reabsorption through the paracellular pathway.

Patch clamp studies of collecting duct cells and A6 cells, from amphibian urinary bladder, have provided some details regarding the electrophysiologic properties and regulation of

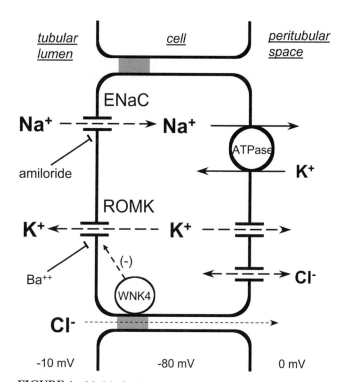

FIGURE 6   Model of salt transport by the principal cell of the cortical collecting duct. Apical Na$^+$ entry proceeds via amiloride-sensitive Na$^+$ channels (ENaC). Apical K$^+$ channels mediate K$^+$ secretion by this segment. Cl$^-$ absorption is driven by the lumen-negative voltage through the paracellular pathway. (Modified from Reeves WB, Andreoli TE. Tubular sodium transport. In: Schrier RW, ed. *Diseases of the Kidney and Urinary Tract*, 7th ed. Philadelphia: Lippincott Williams & Wilkins; 2001:135–176.).

the apical membrane sodium channels (99, 130, 140, 298, 299, 377, 380, 382, 461). The amiloride-sensitive sodium channel in these cells has a single-channel conductance of 4–5 pS, and is highly selective for sodium over potassium ($P_{Na}/P_K > 20$). A somewhat larger (8 pS) and less sodium-selective ($P_{Na}/P_K < 10$) channel has been observed under certain conditions (298). However, it appears that the 4–5 pS, highly selective channel accounts for the sodium permeability of the apical membrane of the CCD (99, 140). This channel exhibits rather slow gating, with openings and closings that last several seconds (298, 380). Amiloride causes a flickering block of the channel at submicromolar concentrations (298, 378, 380), that is, much lower than required to inhibit Na^+/H^+ exchange.

An amiloride-sensitive sodium channel has been cloned (59, 61). The channel, termed ENaC, consists of three homologous subunits (α, β, and γ) (61). The subunits share a common structure consisting of two transmembrane domains, intracellular N- and C-termini, and a large extracellular loop (60, 467). While the α subunit of ENaC can form sodium channels on its own (59), the coexpression of all three subunits dramatically increases the membrane sodium conductance (61). The native channel appears to be a heterotetramer consisting of two α, one β, and one γ subunit (91, 121, 280). The single-channel properties of the expressed channel, that is, single-channel conductance, voltage dependence, gating kinetics, and inhibitor sensitivity, all closely resemble those of the 4–5 pS highly selective channel studied in native tissues (61, 121). That ENaC actually is the sodium channel responsible for Na^+ reabsorption in the collecting duct has been confirmed by two experiments of nature. Specifically, mutations in the ENaC gene are responsible for Liddle syndrome, an autosomal dominant form of hypertension, and pseudohypoaldosteronism type 1, an autosomal recessive form of salt wasting. In Liddle syndrome, mutations in either the β or γ subunit result in an increase in amiloride-sensitive Na^+ channel activity with a consequent increase in sodium reabsorption and volume-mediated hypertension (186, 459, 501). The increase in sodium absorption in Liddle syndrome is due to both an increase in the cell surface expression of ENaC as well as an increase in the open probability of individual ENaC channels (122, 186, 253, 442, 443, 459, 469, 501). Most Liddle mutations occur in the cytoplasmic C-termini of the γ (SCNN1G) and β (SCNN1B) subunits (376, 459). These mutations affect a conserved PY motif in the C-terminus that is necessary for interaction with Nedd4-2 and subsequent internalization and degradation of ENaC (470). As a result of the mutation, excessive ENaC accumulates in the cell membrane leading to increased sodium absorption. A mutation in the extracellular domain of the γ subunit was found in one family with Liddle syndrome (211). This mutation increased the activity of ENaC channels without affecting cell surface expression. Pseudohypoaldosteronism type I (PHAI), the clinical opposite of Liddle syndrome, is caused by homozygous inactivating mutations in the ENaC channel resulting in a syndrome of sodium-wasting, hypotension, and hyperkalemia (66, 214). The majority of mutations causing PHA-1 are frameshift or nonsense mutations that result in truncated, nonfunctional ENaC proteins (441). Additional details concerning the electrophysiologic and molecular properties of the amiloride-sensitive sodium channels are available in Chapter 28.

Apical Electroneutral NaCl Transport In the rat, a portion of Na^+ entry across the apical membrane of principal cells may be mediated by a neutral, thiazide-sensitive NaCl cotransporter (506). Specifically, in perfused rat CCD segments, luminal hydrochlorothiazide inhibited Na^+ and Cl^- absorption without changing the transepithelial voltage (506). Similarly, amiloride, which completely blocks Na^+ transport in the rabbit CCD, inhibited Na^+ transport in the rat by only 50%. Finally, the effects of amiloride and hydrochlorothiazide were additive. Thus, the rat CCD may possess two parallel transport pathways for Na^+: an electrogenic pathway involving amiloride-sensitive Na^+ channels, and a thiazide-sensitive neutral NaCl cotransport pathway. However, these results contrast with the studies of Schafer and colleagues in rat CCD, which provided no evidence for thiazide-sensitive NaCl cotransport (408, 418, 440, 446). Likewise, the cloned thiazide-sensitive cotransporter (NCC) has not been detected in the collecting duct using either RT-PCR, in situ hybridization, or immunohistochemistry (19, 40, 396, 567). The reasons for these contradictory findings are not known.

Basolateral Cl^- Conductance The basolateral membrane of the principal cell of the rabbit is highly conductive to Cl^- (270, 432, 434). A "double-barrel" Cl^- channel with two conductance states, 23 and 46 pS, was described by Sansom et al. (431) in a patch clamp study of the basolateral membrane of rabbit principal cells. Some Cl^- channels in the ClC family display such a double-barrel conductance, with two independently gating pores (323, 324). Several members of the ClC family are expressed in the kidney, including the collecting duct. However, it is not known if any of these channels correspond to the basolateral channel studied by Sansom. The function of this Cl^- conductance is not known. Unlike the rabbit, the basolateral membrane of the rat principal cell is dominated by a K^+ conductance; the Cl^- conductance is negligible under most conditions (440, 446, 447).

CONTROL OF Na^+ ABSORPTION IN CCD

Aldosterone Aldosterone is one of the most important regulators of Na^+ transport in the collecting duct, where it increases the rates of Na^+ absorption and K^+ secretion (369, 371, 432, 433, 440, 453). The actions of aldosterone are reviewed in detail in Chapter 32, and are discussed here briefly. The major target site for mineralocorticoid effects is the principal cell of the CCD (369). Mineralocorticoid effects are produced by the binding of either mineralocorticoids or glucocorticoids (351) to type I steroid receptors found predominantly in the CCD (96, 117, 118, 438). In addition, the binding of glucocorticoids to type II receptors can also produce mineralocorticoid responses (351). This lack of specificity is due to two factors. First, type I (mineralocorticoid) receptors do not discriminate between aldosterone and glucocorticoids (132) so that either class of steroids can bind to, and activate, the receptor. Second, the DNA-binding domains of type I and type II receptors are highly conserved such that both receptors can activate many of the same genes (387). The specificity for mineralocorticoids in vivo is provided by the selective degradation of glucocorticoids, but not mineralocorticoids, by the enzyme 11β-

steroid dehydrogenase (132). 11β-steroid dehydrogenase activity is high in CCD segments (38, 352, 363, 422). The type 2 isoform of 11β-hydroxysteroid dehydrogenase (3, 5, 350), specifically, is expressed almost exclusively by aldosterone target cells including the principal cell of the cortical collecting duct (283, 288, 541). Illustrating the important role of this enzyme in regulating access of hormones to the mineralocorticoid receptor, genetic deficiency of this enzyme produces a syndrome, apparent mineralocorticoid excess, which resembles hyperaldosteronism (hypertension, hypokalemia, metabolic alkalosis) except that aldosterone levels are low (340, 341, 548). The clinical manifestations result from the stimulation of mineralocorticoid (type I) receptors by circulating glucocorticoids.

In isolated perfused CCDs from mineralocorticoid treated rabbits, there is an increase in both the Na^+ and K^+ conductance of the apical membrane and an increase in basolateral (Na^+, K^+)-ATPase activity (370, 390, 433). The functional changes after aldosterone treatment are accompanied by morphologic changes in principal cells. The basolateral membrane length of principal cells falls by 35% after adrenalectomy, and administration of aldosterone, but not dexamethasene, restores the membrane length to control levels (475).

Table 9 summarizes the mineralocorticoid-induced changes in the specific ionic conductances of the rabbit CCD principal cell. With respect to sodium transport, an early effect of aldosterone, occurring within a few hours of exposure, is an increase in the sodium permeability of the apical membrane. Results from electrophysiologic (139, 254, 381) and immunologic (263, 264) studies support the view that the early aldosterone-induced increase in apical sodium permeability is due to the activation of quiescent Na^+ channels rather than the synthesis and/or insertion of new Na^+ channels into the membrane. Several pathways have been implicated in the aldosterone-mediated increase in Na^+ channel activity. An important downstream mediator of aldosterone is Sgk, serum, and glucocorticoid-regulated kinase (69, 349). Sgk, a serine and threonine kinase, is expressed in the thick ascending limb, DCT, connecting segment, and cortical collecting tubules

(82). Aldosterone increases the transcription of Sgk in vitro (69, 349), although the effects of aldosterone on Sgk protein expression in vivo are minor (82). Coexpression of Sgk with ENaC results in markedly greater sodium currents than seen with ENaC alone (69, 207, 349). Sgk is required for the stimulation of sodium transport by aldosterone both in vitro (207) and in vivo (563). Sgk increases sodium currents by increasing cell surface expression of ENaC (83) and also increasing the open probability of individual ENaC channels (84). The effect of Sgk on cell surface expression of ENaC may be mediated via Nedd4-2. Specifically, Nedd4-2 is a substrate for Sgk. Upon phosphorylation by Sgk, the affinity of Nedd4-2 for the PY domains of ENaC is diminished (468). In addition, Sgk itself contains a PY motif and might compete with ENaC for Nedd4-2 binding. As discussed earlier, binding of Nedd4-2 leads to the internalization and degradation of ENaC channels. Accordingly, Sgk may increase cell surface ENaC by decreasing Nedd4-2 binding and/or availability. In parallel, Sgk also phosphorylates ROMK on serine 44 and increases the cell surface expression of that channel (569). The effect of sgk on ROMK cell surface expression appears to involve the scaffolding protein NHERF2 (575). Methylation of proteins and lipids is increased by aldosterone. It has been suspected for almost two decades that methylation may mediate the effects of aldosterone on Na^+ transport (435). Recent work supports this view. As reviewed recently (480), aldosterone increases the activity of a number of cellular methyltransferase enzymes. Moreover, the β subunit of ENaC itself is a substrate for methylation, and, when methylated, exhibits increased Na^+ transport activity (417, 436). The effects of aldosterone on Na^+ channel activity may also involve small GTP-binding proteins, such as Ras (481) and phosphatidylinositol 3-kinase (33). Sgk may be a downstream mediator of phosphoinositide-3-kinase (383).

Somewhat after the increase in apical membrane Na^+ conductance occurs, the basolateral membrane (Na^+, K^+)-ATPase activity and pump current increase (432). This increase is due initially to an effect of increased cell sodium activity on existing pump units (22, 35). Later, aldosterone induces synthesis

TABLE 9 Effects of Mineralocorticoids on Electrophysiologic Characteristics of Rabbit CCD

| | V_T (mV) | V_T (mV) | G_a (mS/cm²) | | G_b (mS/cm²) | | Ipump (mS/cm²) |
			Na	K	K	Cl	
Low ALDO	−2	−64	0.2	1.4	3.4 (total)	9	
Control	−7	−80	0.7	5	1.0	4.2	40
High ALDO	−34	−100	1.7	7.6	3.7	10.5	195

Studies performed using in vitro perfused CCD segments were obtained from adrenalectomized rabbits (low ALDO), adrenal intact rabbits (control), and rabbits treated with mineralocorticoid (DOCA) for 9–16 days (high ALDO).

V_T, V_b-transepithelial and basolateral membrane voltage; G_a Na, G_a K, G_bNa, G_bK, conductances of the apical and basolateral membranes to the indicated ions; Ipump, current generated by (Na^+, K^+)-ATPase.

Data from Muto S, Giebisch G, Sansom S. Effects of adrenalectomy on CCD: evidence for differential response of two cell types. *Am J Physiol* 1987;253: F742–F752; Sansom S, Muto S, Giebisch G. Na-dependent effects of DOCA on cellular transport properties of CCDs from ADX rabbits. *Am J Physiol* 1987;253:F753–F759; Sansom SC, O'Neil RG. Effects of mineralocorticoids on transport properties of cortical collecting duct basolateral membrane. *Am J Physiol* 1986;251:F743–F757; Sansom SC, O'Neil RG. Mineralocorticoid regulation of apical cell membrane Na^+ and K^+ transport of the cortical collecting duct. *Am J Physiol* 1985;248:F858–F868.

of additional (Na^+, K^+)-ATPase pump units (529). There is evidence that increased apical membrane Na^+ entry may modulate the late synthesis of (Na^+,K^+)-ATPase. Inhibition of sodium entry by amiloride markedly reduced the aldosterone-induced increase in (Na^+,K^+)-ATPase activity (370, 379, 390, 429). Aldosterone also exerts an additional, late effect on the amiloride-sensitive Na^+ conductance. Patch clamp studies in rats exposed to high levels of aldosterone for several days demonstrated a large increase in the amiloride-sensitive whole cell Na^+ conductance (129). The increase in whole cell conductance correlated with an increase in the number of active Na^+ channels in the apical membrane (377). In contrast, the single-channel conductance and open probability of individual Na^+ channels was not affected by aldosterone (377). Northern blot (16, 108, 111, 315) and Western blot analysis (266) has shown an increase in ENaC mRNA and protein levels in aldosterone-treated tissues suggesting that the synthesis of new ENaC channels may contribute to the late aldosterone-induced increase in Na^+ conductance. Sgk, in addition to increasing cell surface expression of ENaC, also regulates the transcription of ENaC subunits (45).

The pump current associated with the increased rate of (Na^+, K^+)-ATPase activity in aldosterone treated tubules hyperpolarizes the basolateral membrane to the degree that potassium entry, rather than efflux, occurs through basolateral membrane potassium channels (430, 432). The basolateral K^+ influx provides K^+ for secretion into the tubular lumen.

ADH Exposure of rat CCD segments in vitro to antidiuretic hormone results in a sustained stimulation of Na^+ absorption (408). ADH increases the transepithelial potential, depolarizes the apical membrane, and increases the conductance of the tubule and, more specifically, of the apical membrane of principal cells (447). These changes are entirely reversed by luminal amiloride, indicating that ADH increases the apical membrane sodium conductance of the principal cell. These effects of ADH are mediated intracellularly by cAMP (439). Moreover, the effects of ADH on Na^+ transport in the rat CCD are enhanced by prior treatment of the animals with mineralocorticoids (189, 408). In contrast, in rabbit CCD, ADH produces only a transient stimulation, or even inhibition, of Na^+ transport and this effect is lost after treatment with mineralocorticoids (68, 128, 450). The transient response to ADH in the rabbit is not due to downregulation of ADH-stimulated cAMP generation as the response to cAMP analogues is also transient (49). Rather, the transient response may be due to a protein kinase C (PKC)–mediated inhibition of Na^+ transport. According to this view, the initial increase in apical Na^+ entry induced by ADH leads to an increased intracellular $[Na^+]$ with a consequent rise in intracellular $[Ca^{2+}]$ via basolateral Na^+/Ca^{2+} exchange (47). The increase in $[Ca^{2+}]$ then activates PKC with the subsequent inhibition of further apical Na^+ entry. Supporting this notion are studies that show a transient increase in intracellular $[Na^+]$ following ADH exposure (49), and that the stimulation of Na^+ transport by

ADH in CCD cells is sustained, rather than transient, in the presence of a low calcium bath (47) or after downregulation of PKC (85). As will be discussed in the following, PGE2 inhibits Na^+ transport in the rabbit CCD. Since ADH stimulates prostaglandin synthesis in renal tissue, it has been suggested that PGE2 may be responsible for the eventual decline in transport after the transient stimulation by ADH observed in the rabbit. In this regard, pretreatment of CCD segments with indomethacin to inhibit PG synthesis prevented the late inhibition of Na^+ transport following ADH exposure (193). PGE2 also inhibits ADH-mediated water transport in the CCD (157, 347). However, the effects of PGE2 on ADH-induced Na^+ transport and water transport appear to be mediated via different pathways (194). The inhibition of water transport by PGE2 can be traced to a pertussin-toxin–sensitive inhibition of ADH-stimulated cAMP production (347, 356). The effects of PGE2 on ADH modulation of Na^+ transport, however, are not mediated via changes in cAMP but rather via an increase in intracellular $[Ca^{2+}]$ (193). In the rat, which has a sustained response to ADH (409), PGE2 does not inhibit sodium transport by the CCD (67).

While both ADH and aldosterone increase the apical membrane sodium conductance, their mechanisms of action are different. In contrast to aldosterone, which activates quiescent channels, ADH, via cAMP, leads to the insertion of additional Na^+ channels into the apical membrane (99, 310). In addition, cAMP, via protein kinase A-mediated phosphorylation also directly stimulates the activity of sodium channels already present in the apical membrane (18, 233, 367). Long-term exposure to ADH may also increase the capacity of the collecting duct for Na^+ transport by increasing the expression of both Na^+, K^+-ATPase and amiloride-sensitive Na^+ channels (94, 100). ADH also increases the apical membrane K^+ conductance. As noted previously, ROMK contains three sites for protein kinase A–mediated phosphorylation. Phosphorylation of these sites affects both channel activity (P_o), by increasing the affinity of the channel for PIP2, and, at serine 44, the number of functional channels in the plasma membrane (201).

Other Agents Bradykinin is produced in the connecting duct (368, 398) and binds to specific receptors in the CCD (120, 508). Intrarenal infusion of bradykinin produces a diuresis. However, the evidence that bradykinin affects Na^+ transport in the CCD is equivocal. Bradykinin has been reported to reduce Na^+ absorption in rat CCD segments (509, 510). Since sodium transport fell in the absence of any change in transepithelial voltage, it was proposed that this agent inhibits neutral NaCl cotransport. However, other laboratories have found no effect of bradykinin on Na^+ transport in rat CCD (418, 444). There is no obvious explanation for these discrepancies. In the rabbit, bradykinin had no effect on basal Na^+ transport, and only slightly reduced the effect of ADH on Na^+ reabsorption (450). Bradykinin did significantly reduce the hydroosmotic response of rabbit CCD to ADH (451). The effect of bradykinin on ADH-induced water permeability appears to involve prostaglandins and protein kinase C (93, 290, 450).

As will be discussed below, the major site of action of atrial natriuretic peptide (ANP) is the inner medullary collecting duct. ANP stimulates cGMP production in the CCD (357), and inhibits the hydroosmotic actions of ADH in the CCD (92, 358). In addition, Nonoguchi et al. (358) reported that ANP reduced Na^+ transport in the rat CCD by 90%. The inhibition of Na^+ transport occurred without a change in the transepithelial voltage (358), suggesting that ANP inhibited electroneutral NaCl cotransport. However, Rouch et al. (418) and Schlatter et al. (444) found no effect of either ANP or cGMP analogues on Na^+ transport in the rat CCD. Again, there is no obvious explanation for these discrepancies.

α2-adrenergic agonists inhibit sodium reabsorption in the rat CCD (418). This inhibition is associated with an increase in the apical membrane resistance reflecting a decrease in sodium movement through amiloride-sensitive sodium channels (418). These changes appear to result from an inhibition of adenylate cyclase by α2-agonists (142). In the rabbit CCD, clonidine, an α2 adrenergic agonist, does not inhibit sodium transport (67) or adenylate cyclase activity (142).

β-*Adrenergic Agonists* β-adrenergic agonists reduce the transepithelial voltage in the CCD (218, 259). However, in spite of their effects on transepithelial voltage, these agents produce no change in net Na^+ transport. Rather, the effects of β-adrenergic agents on transepithelial voltage may be due to stimulation of electrogenic H^+ secretion by α-intercalated cells (274).

Prostaglandin E_2 exerts diuretic and natriuretic effects on the kidney. Part of this action is mediated by an inhibition of Na^+ absorption in the CCD (488). Application of PGE2 to the basolateral surface of perfused rabbit CCD segments reversibly inhibits the negative transepithelial voltage and net sodium absorption (193, 456, 488). The effect of PGE2 on sodium transport is pertussis toxin-insensitive, is coupled to a rise in intracellular $[Ca^{2+}]$, and is dependent on activation of PKC (193, 194). Four PGE2 receptor subtypes, designated EP1, EP2, EP3, and EP4, have been characterized. EP1 and EP3 were identified in the CCD of human kidney by in situ hybridization (48). Recent studies using receptor subtype-specific agonists and antagonists suggest that the EP1 receptor mediates PGE2-dependent inhibition of Na^+ transport in the CCD (172). In contrast to the inhibitory effect of basolateral PGE2 on Na^+ transport, luminal PGE2 increases transepithelial voltage (and presumably Na^+ absorption) (14, 425). The effects of luminal PGE2 may be mediated via the EP4 receptor (425).

Epidermal growth factor (EGF) reduces Na^+ absorption in rabbit CCD by about 50% (50, 522). The electrophysiologic effects of EGF have been examined in isolated perfused CCD segments (343) and in cultured CCD cells (539). In both cases, EGF reduces the transepithelial volt-

age, hyperpolarizes the apical cell membrane, increases the transepithelial resistance, and increases the resistance of the apical membrane (343, 539). These effects are consistent with an inhibition of apical electrogenic Na^+ entry via the amiloride-sensitive Na^+ channel.

Nitric oxide decreases Na^+ transport in rat CCD segments by 40%–80% (492). The addition of nitric oxide to tubules decreased the intracellular $[Na^+]$ but did not affect the activity of basolateral (Na^+, K^+)-ATPase, suggesting that the primary effect of nitric oxide was to inhibit apical Na^+ entry.

Dopamine inhibits ADH-dependent Na^+ transport and transepithelial voltage in rat CCD segments (495). The actions of dopamine are believed to be mediated via the D4 receptor subtype.

Angiotensin II (AII) stimulates sodium channel activity in rabbit and mouse cortical collecting ducts (389). Chronic AII infusion also increases the abundance of the α subunit of ENaC, the rate-limiting subunit for ENaC assembly (30). Both the acute effects of AII on ENaC activity and the chronic effects on ENaC abundance are mediated by the AT1 receptor (30, 389).

NA$^+$ TRANSPORT IN OUTER MEDULLARY COLLECTING DUCT

The transport properties of the outer medullary collecting duct (OMCD) have been studied by in vitro perfusion of isolated tubule segments (Table 10). The functional properties of the OMCD differ depending on the location of the segment within the outer medulla. Segments within the outer stripe of the outer medulla (OMCD$_o$) exhibit electrophysiologic properties resembling the cortical collecting duct, that is, a lumen-negative transepithelial voltage and electrogenic apical Na^+ entry (270). Compared to the CCD, the OMCD$_o$ displays a less-negative transepithelial voltage, much lower ionic permeabilities and a lower rate of active reabsorption of Na^+ (484). Electrophysiologic studies have shown that as the collecting duct descends into the medulla, principal cells, which mediate Na^+ and K^+ transport in the CCD (see previous discussion), are replaced by cells whose electrical properties are similar to intercalated cells of the CCD, that is, the apical membrane lacks a demonstrable Na^+ or K^+ conductance (269). Within the inner stripe of outer medulla (OMCD$_i$), principal cells are virtually absent and no net Na^+ absorption occurs (483, 484, 487).

NA$^+$ TRANSPORT IN INNER MEDULLARY COLLECTING DUCT

Mechanism of Na$^+$ Transport

The analysis of salt transport by the IMCD has been confounded by problems of axial tubule heterogeneity, species variability, and differences in experimental approach. Based on

TABLE 10   Electrophysiologic and Transport Properties of Rabbit OMCD

	V_t (mV) (References)	R_t (Ω-cm^2) (References)	Vbl (mV) (References)	fRa (References)	J_{Na} (pmol/mm/min) (References)	J_{Cl} (pmol/mm/min) (References)
Outer OMCD	−2 to −11 (270, 317, 483, 484)	233–272 (270, 271)	−65 (270, 271)	0.81 (270, 271)	7.9 (483, 484)	−1.4 (483, 484)
Inner OMCD	+2 to +48 (269, 272, 345, 483, 484, 487, 489)	294–534 (269, 272, 345)	−24 to −36 (235, 269, 272, 345)	0.96–0.99 (269, 272, 345)	1.5 (483, 484)	−9.8 (235, 483, 484)

Table from Koeppen BM, Stanton BA. Sodium chloride transport—distal nephron. In: Seldin DW, Giebisch G, eds. *The Kidney: Physiology and Pathophysiology*, 2nd ed. New York: Raven Press; 1992:2003–2039.

morphologic factors, the IMCD has been divided into three subsegments: IMCD1, IMCD2, and IMCD3 (75). This morphologic heterogeneity is paralleled, to some extent, by functional heterogeneity. For example, the urea permeability of IMCD1 is low, and not affected by ADH, while IMCD2 and IMCD3 segments have a higher basal urea permeability that is increased further by ADH (428). Further complicating the analysis is the observation that similar subsegments from different species exhibit different properties relating to salt transport (228, 476). Finally, for unknown reasons, studies examining IMCD function in vivo—for instance, by microcatheterization or micropuncture—have yielded markedly different results than have in vitro studies of isolated perfused tubules. For example, in vivo microcatheterization studies and microperfusion studies have demonstrated that the IMCD reabsorbs about 80% of the sodium delivered to it (473, 474) while, with one exception (284), little sodium transport occurs in in vitro perfused IMCD tubules (427, 476).

Electrophysiologic studies of the IMCD (Table 11) have found that the transepithelial voltage is generally in the range of 0 to −5 mV (lumen-negative) and that the transepithelial resistance is in the range of 40 to 100 ohm cm^2 (228, 284, 427, 476). Limited data regarding the conductive properties of IMCD cells are available. Stanton performed microelectrode impalements of IMCD segments from rat (476). The apical membrane constituted the major cellular resistance (FRa = 0.92). Luminal application of amiloride resulted in an increase in the apical membrane voltage and apical membrane resistance and a fall in the transepithelial voltage. These results and others (296, 472, 473) are consistent with the presence of an amiloride-sensitive sodium conductance in the apical membrane of IMCD cells. Patch

clamp studies of cultured rat IMCD cells indicate that Na$^+$ entry is mediated by a 20–30–pS amiloride-sensitive, nonselective, cGMP-gated cation channel in the apical cell membrane (296, 520). The basolateral membrane of IMCD cells contains (Na$^+$, K$^+$)-ATPase, a potassium conductance and a bicarbonate conductance (228, 476).

The results discussed above can be combined into a tentative model for sodium transport in the IMCD (Fig. 7). The model is essentially that described by Koefoed-Johnsen and Ussing for electrogenic sodium transport in the frog skin (267). Sodium entry across the apical membrane occurs down its steep electrochemical gradient through amiloride-sensitive Na$^+$ channels. Sodium is extruded across the basolateral membrane by the (Na$^+$, K$^+$)-ATPase, thereby maintaining a low intracellular Na$^+$ concentration. The basolateral membrane K$^+$ conductance serves to recycle the K$^+$ that enters on the (Na$^+$, K$^+$)-ATPase. The K$^+$ conductance also hyperpolarizes the cell thereby favoring Na$^+$ entry across the apical membrane.

The evidence for additional electroneutral Na$^+$ entry pathways in IMCD cells is controversial. Furosemide and thiazide diuretics both inhibit a portion of Na$^+$ absorption by IMCD segments in vivo (544, 545). In addition, a Na$^+$-K$^+$-2Cl$^-$ cotransporter may be present in isolated rat papillary collecting duct cells (171). Rocha and Kudo (414) also have presented data that support the presence of a Na$^+$-K$^+$-2Cl$^-$ cotransporter in the basolateral membrane of terminal IMCD segments (IMCD2,3). A Na$^+$-K$^+$-2Cl$^-$ cotransporter has been cloned from cultured IMCD cells (86). This cotransporter represents the "secretory" isoform of the Na$^+$-K$^+$-2Cl$^-$ cotransporter (NKCC1 or BSC2) rather than the absorptive isoform present in the apical membrane of the thick ascending

TABLE 11   Electrophysiologic and Transport Properties of Rat IMCD

	V_t (mV) (References)	R_t (Ω-cm^2) (References)	V_{bl} (mV) (References)	fRa (References)	J_{Na} (pmol/mm/min) (References)	J_{Cl} (pmol/mm/min) (References)
Initial IMCD	−2 to 0 (190, 415, 426, 476)	73 (476)	−51 (476)	0.94 (476)	10 (476)	
Terminal IMCD	0 (284, 413, 415)	148 (274)	−81 (274)	0.99 (274)	54–92 (284, 413)	72 (413)

Table from Koeppen BM, Stanton BA. Sodium chloride transport—distal nephron. In: Seldin DW, Giebisch G, eds. *The Kidney: Physiology and Pathophysiology*, 2nd ed. New York: Raven Press; 1992:2003–2039.

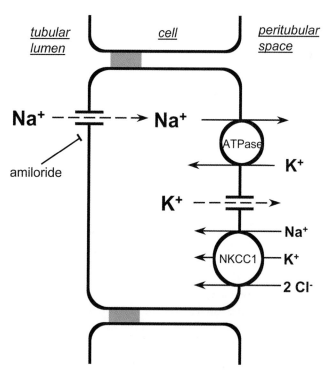

FIGURE 7   A model of Na^+ transport in the inner medullary collecting duct. Apical Na^+ entry proceeds via a nonselective amiloride-sensitive cation channel. Basolateral Na^+-K^+-$2Cl^-$ cotransport may be involved in Na^+ secretion.

limb. This cotransporter appears to participate in NaCl secretion rather than reabsorption. Further work is required to determine what role, if any, electroneutral Na^+ entry pathways play in net Na^+ absorption by the IMCD.

REGULATION OF Na^+ TRANSPORT

The IMCD appears to be the major target site for the potent diuretic hormone, atrial natriuretic peptide (ANP) (473, 576). This hormone, working through cGMP (579) inhibits sodium entry via apical membrane Na^+ channels. In suspensions of rabbit IMCD cells, ANP inhibited O_2 consumption (578) and inhibited conductive $^{22}Na^+$ uptake (577). Light and coworkers (295–297) have examined in detail the effects of ANP on an amiloride-sensitive cation channel in cultured inner medullary cells. In cell-attached patches, both ANP and dibutyryl cGMP inhibited the activity of the cation channel (297). In excised patches cGMP also inhibited the channel. The inhibition by cGMP involves at least two pathways, a phosphorylation-independent pathway and a pathway involving cGMP-dependent protein kinase (295). The latter pathway also involves a pertussis-toxin–sensitive G protein.

Rocha and Kudo (414) have suggested that, in addition to inhibiting Na^+ reabsorption, ANP stimulates Na^+ secretion in the IMCD. In isolated perfused IMCD segments, ANP increased the bath to lumen flux rate of Na^+ and Cl^-. This increase was inhibited by peritubular furosemide and by omission of either counterion leading the authors to propose that ANP stimulated Na^+ secretion via a basolateral

membrane Na^+/K^+/$2Cl^-$ cotransporter (413). Sands et al. (427), however, found no effect of ANP on the Na^+ permeability of the rat IMCD.

In one study, antidiuretic hormone stimulated sodium absorption by terminal IMCD segments perfused in vitro. The stimulation was blocked by luminal amiloride and mediated through a V_1 receptor mechanism (284). Sands et al. (427), however, found no effect of ADH on either transepithelial voltage, transepithelial resistance or on the chloride permeability of rat IMCD segments. If ADH stimulates conductive sodium entry, a decrease in the transepithelial voltage and resistance should have been observed. Likewise, Light et al. (296) failed to find an effect of ADH or cAMP on the amiloride-sensitive cation channel in apical membranes of cultured IMCD cells.

Micropuncture studies by Ullrich et al. demonstrated that mineralocorticoids increased net Na^+ absorption in the terminal IMCD (517). This effect was attributed to a decrease in the passive Na^+ permeability of the tubule leading to a decrease in back-leak of NaCl into the lumen. In support of this hypothesis, Sands et al. (427) have confirmed that mineralocorticoids increase the transepithelial resistance and reduce the passive NaCl permeability of the rat IMCD. Mineralocorticoids may also increase active Na^+ reabsorption in the IMCD. For example, in a recent study of cultured rat IMCD cells, aldosterone produced a threefold to sevenfold stimulation of electrogenic Na^+ transport (217). Likewise, chronic mineralocorticoid exposure in vivo increased the activity of (Na^+, K^+)-ATPase in the IMCD (505).

References

1. Abuladze N, Yanagawa N, Lee I, Jo OD, Newman D, Hwang J, Uyemura K, Pushkin A, Modlin RL, Kurtz I. Peripheral blood mononuclear cells express mutated NCCT mRNA in Gitelman's syndrome: evidence for abnormal thiazide-sensitive NaCl cotransport. *J Am Soc Nephrol* 1998;9:819–826.
2. Adachi S, Uchida S, Ito H, Hata M, Hiroe M, Marumo F, Sasaki S. Two isoforms of a chloride channel predominantly expressed in thick ascending limb of Henle's loop and collecting ducts of rat kidney. *J Biol Chem* 1994;269:17677–17683.
3. Agarwal AK, Mune T, Monder C, White PC. NAD-dependent isoform of 11b-hydroxysteroid dehydrogenase: cloning and characterization of cDNA from sheep kidney. *J Biol Chem* 1994; 269:25959–25962.
4. Aguilar-Bryan L, Nichols CG, Wechsler SW, Clement JP, Boyd AE, Gonzalez G, Herrera-Sosa H, Nguy K, Bryan J, Nelson DA. Cloning of the beta cell high-affinity sulfonylurea receptor: a regulator of insulin secretion. *Science* 1995;268:423–426.
5. Albiston AL, Obeyesekere VR, Smith RE, Krozowski ZS. Cloning and distribution of the human 11b-hydroxysteroid dehydrogenase type 2 enzyme. *Mol Cell Endocrin* 1994;105: R11–R17.
6. Alcorn D, Emslie KR, Boss BD. Selective distal nephron damage during isolated kidney perfusion. *Kidney Int* 1981;19:638–647.
7. Allen GG, Barratt LJ. Effect of aldosterone on the transepithelial potential difference of the rat distal tubule. *Kidney Int* 1981;19:678–686.
8. Allen GG, Barratt LJ. Effect of cisplatin on the transepithelial potential difference of rat distal tubule. *Kidney Int* 1985;27:842–847.
9. Allen GG, Barratt LJ. Origin of positive transepithelial potential difference in early distal segments of rat kidney. *Kidney Int* 1985;27:622–629.
10. Almeida AJ, Burg MB. Sodium transport in the rabbit connecting tubule. *Am J Physiol* 1982;243:F330–F334.
11. Amemiya M, Loffing J, Lotscher M, Kaissling B, Alpern RJ, Moe OW. Expression of NHE-3 in the apical membrane of rat renal proximal tubule and thick ascending limb. *Kidney Int* 1995;48:1206–1215.
12. Amlal H, LeGoff C, Vernimmen C, Soleimani M, Paillard M, Bichara M. ANG II controls Na+-K+(NH+4)-2Cl− cotransport via 20–HETE and PKC in medullary thick ascending limb. *Am J Physiol Cell Physiol* 1998;274:C1047–C1056.
13. Ammala C, Moorhouse A, Gribble F, Ashfield R, Proks P, Smith PA, Sakura H, Coles B, Ashcroft SJ, Ashcroft FM. Promiscuous coupling between the sulphonylurea receptor and inwardly rectifying potassium channels. *Nature* 1996;379:545–548.

14. Ando Y, Asano Y. Luminal prostaglandin E2 modulates sodium and water transport in rabbit cortical collecting ducts. *Am J Physiol* 1995;268:F1093–F1101.
15. International Collaborative Study Group for Bartter-Like Syndrome. Mutations in the gene encoding the inwardly-rectifying renal potassium channel, ROMK, cause the antenatal variant of Bartter syndrome: evidence for genetic heterogeneity. *Hum Mol Genet* 1997;6:17–26 (erratum in *Hum Mol Genet* 1997;6:650).
16. Asher C, Wald H, Rossier BC, Garty H. Aldosterone-induced increase in the abundance of Na+ channel subunits. *Am J Physiol* 1996;271:C605–C611.
17. Ausiello DA, Hall D. Regulation of vasopressin-sensitive adenylate cyclase by calmodulin. *J Biol Chem* 1981;256:9796–9798.
18. Awayda MS, Ismailov, II, Berdiev BK, Fuller CM, Benos DJ. Protein kinase regulation of a cloned epithelial Na+ channel. *J Gen Physiol* 1996;108:49–65.
19. Bachmann S, Velazquez H, Obermuller N, Reilly RF, Moser D, Ellison DH. Expression of the thiazide-sensitive Na-Cl cotransporter by rabbit distal convoluted tubule cells. *J Clin Invest* 1995;96:2510–2514.
20. Bagnasco S, Good D, Balaban R, Burg M. Lactate production in isolated segments of the rat nephron. *Am J Physiol* 1985;248:F522–F526.
21. Bailly C, Imbert-Teboul M, Roinel N, Amiel C. Isoproterenol increases Ca, Mg, and NaCl reabsorption in mouse thick ascending limb. *Am J Physiol* 1990;258:F1224–F1231.
22. Barlet-Bas C, Khadouri C, Marsy S, Doucet A. Enhanced intracellular sodium concentration in kidney cells recruits a latent pool of Na-K-ATPase whose size is modulated by corticosteroids. *J Biol Chem* 1990;265:7799–7803.
23. Barratt LJ, Rector FC Jr, Kokko JP, Tisher CC, Seldin DW. Transepithelial potential difference profile of the distal tubule of the rat kidney. *Kidney Int* 1975;8:368–375.
24. Bayliss JM, Reeves WB, Andreoli TE. Cl^- transport in basolateral renal medullary vesicles. I. Cl^- transport in intact vesicles. *J Membr Biol* 1990;113:49–56.
25. Beaumont K, Vaughn DA, Healy DP. Thiazide diuretic receptors: autoradiographic localization in rat kidney with [3H]metolazone. *J Pharmacol Exp Ther* 1989;250:414–419.
26. Beesley AH, Qureshi IZ, Giesberts AN, Parker AJ, White SJ. Expression of sulphonylurea receptor protein in mouse kidney. *Pflugers Arch Eur J Physiol* 1999;438:1–7.
27. Bencsath P, Szenasi G, Takacs L. Water and electrolyte transport in Henle's loop and distal tubule after renal sympathectomy in the rat. *Am J Physiol* 1985;249:F308–F314.
28. Bennett CM, Brenner BM, Berliner RW. Micropuncture study of nephron function in the Rhesus monkey. *J Clin Invest* 1968;47:203–216.
29. Besseghir K, Trimble ME, Stoner L. Action of ADH on isolated medullary thick ascending limb of the Brattleboro rat. *Am J Physiol* 1986;251:F271–F277.
30. Beutler KT, Masilamani S, Turban S, Nielsen J, Brooks HL, Ageloff S, Fenton RA, Packer RK, Knepper MA. Long-term regulation of ENaC expression in kidney by angiotensin II. *Hypertension* 2003;41:1143–1150.
31. Biner H, Arpin-Bott M, Loffing J, Wang X, Knepper M, Hebert S, Kaissling B. Human cortical distal nephron: distribution of electrolyte and water transport pathways. *J Am Soc Nephrol* 2002;13:836–847.
32. Birkenhager R, Otto E, Schurmann M, Vollmer M, Ruf E, Maier-Lutz I, Beekmann F, Fekete A, Omran H, Feldmann D, Milford D, Jeck N, Konrad M, Landau D, Knoers N, Antignac C, Sudbrak R, Kispert A, Hildebrandt F. Mutation of BSND causes Bartter syndrome with sensorineural deafness and kidney failure. *Nat Genet* 2001;29:310–314.
33. Blazer-Yost BL, Paunescu TG, Helman SI, Lee KD, Vlahos CJ. Phosphoinositide 3-kinase is required for aldosterone-regulated sodium reabsorption. *Am J Physiol* 1999;277:C531–C536.
34. Bleich M, Schlatter E, Greger R. The luminal K^+ channel of the thick ascending limb of Henle's loop. *Pflugers Arch* 1990;415:449–460.
35. Blot-Chabaud M, Jaisser F, Gingold M, Bonvalet JP, Farman N. Na^+-K^+-ATPase-dependent sodium flux in cortical collecting tubule. *Am J Physiol* 1988;255:F605–F613.
36. Boim MA, Ho K, Shuck ME, Bienkowski MJ, Block JH, Slightom JL, Yang Y, Brenner BM, Hebert SC. ROMK inwardly rectifying ATP-sensitive K^+ channel II. Cloning and distribution of alternative forms. *Am J Physiol* 1995;268:F1132–F1140.
37. Deleted in proof.
38. Bonvalet JP, Doignon I, Blot-Chabaud M, Pradelles P, Farman N. Distribution of ^{11}b-hydroxysteroid dehydrogenase along the rabbit nephron. *J Clin Invest* 1990;86:832–837.
39. Boron WF, Sackin H. Measurement of intracellular ionic composition and activities in renal tubules. *Annu Rev Physiol* 1983;45:483–496.
40. Bostonjoglo M, Reeves WB, Reilly RF, Velazquez H, Robertson N, Litwack G, Morsing P, Dorup J, Bachmann S, Ellison DH. 11b-Hydroxysteroid dehydrogenase, mineralocorticoid receptor, thiazide-sensitive Na-Cl cotransporter expression by distal tubules. *J Am Soc Nephrol* 1998;9:1347–1358.
41. Bouby N, Bankir L, Trinh-Trang-Tan M, Minuth WW, Kriz W. Selective ADH-induced hypertrophy of the medullary thick ascending limb in Brattleboro rats. *Kidney Int* 1985; 28:456–466.
42. Bouby N, Trinh-Trang-Tan M, Kriz W, Bankir L. Possible role of the thick ascending limb and of the urine concentrating mechanism in the protein-induced increase in GFR and kidney disease. *Kidney Int* 1987;32:S57–S61.
43. Bouby N, Trinh-Trang-Tan MM, Coutaud C, Bankir L. Vasopressin is involved in renal effects of high-protein diet: study in homozygous Brattleboro rats. *Am J Physiol* 1991;260: F96–100.
44. Boulpaep EL. Recent advances in electrophysiology of the nephron. *Ann Rev Physiol* 1976; 38:20–36.
45. Boyd C, Naray-Fejes-Toth A. Gene regulation of ENaC subunits by serum and glucocorticoid inducible kinase-1 (SGK1). *Am J Physiol Renal Physiol* 200443;866–871.
46. Breuer W. Characterization of chloride channels in membrane vesicles from the kidney outer medulla. *J Membr Biol* 1989;107:35–42.
47. Breyer MD. Feedback inhibition of cyclic adenosine monophosphate-stimulated Na+ transport in the rabbit cortical collecting duct via Na(+)-dependent basolateral Ca++ entry. *J Clin Invest* 1991;88:1502–1510.
48. Breyer MD, Davis L, Jacobson HR, Breyer RM. Differential localization of prostaglandin E receptor subtypes in human kidney. *Am J Physiol* 1996;270:F912–F918.
49. Breyer MD, Fredin D. Effect of vasopressin on intracellular Na+ concentration in cortical collecting duct. *Kidney Int Suppl* 1996;57:S57–S61.
50. Breyer MD, Jacobson HR, Breyer JA. Epidermal growth factor inhibits the hydroosmotic effect of vasopressin in the isolated perfused rabbit cortical collecting tubule. *J Clin Invest* 1988;82:1313–1320.
51. Brezis M, Rosen S, Silva P, Epstein F. Selective vulnerability of the medullary thick ascending limb to anoxia in the isolated perfused rat kidney. *J Clin Invest* 1984;73:182–190.
52. Brezis M, Rosen S, Silva P, Epstein F. Transport activity modifies thick ascending limb damage in the isolated perfused kidney. *Kidney Int* 1984;25:65–72.
53. Brezis M, Rosen S, Spokes K, Silva P, Epstein FH. Substrates induce hypoxic injury to medullary thick limbs of isolated rat kidneys. *Am J Physiol* 1986;251:F710–F717.
54. Brown CDA, Murer H. Characterization of a Na:K:2Cl cotransporter system in the apical membrane of a renal epithelial cell line (LLC-PKV1S). *J Membr Biol* 1985;87:131–139.
55. Brown D, Zhu XL, Sly WS. Localization of membrane-associated carbonic anhydrase type IV in kidney epithelial cells. *Proc Natl Acad Sci U S A* 1990;87:7457–7461.
56. Burg MB, Green N. Function of the thick ascending limb of Henle's loop. *Am J Physiol* 1973;224:659–668.
57. Burg MB, Isaacson L, Grantham JJ, Orloff J. Electrical properties of isolated perfused rabbit renal tubules. *Am J Physiol* 1968;215:788–794.
58. Burnham C, Karlish SJD, Jorgensen PL. Identification and reconstitution of a $Na^+/K^+/Cl^-$ cotransporter and K^+ channel from luminal membranes of renal red outer medulla. *Biochim Biophys Acta* 1985;821:461–469.
59. Canessa CM, Horisberger JD, Rossier BC. Epithelial sodium channel related to proteins involved in neurodegeneration. *Nature* 1993;361:467–470 (see comments).
60. Canessa CM, Merillat A-M, Rossier BC. Membrane topology of the epithelial sodium channel in intact cells. *Am J Physiol* 1994;267:C1682–C1690.
61. Canessa CM, Schild L, Buell G, Thorens B, Gautschi I, Horisberger JD, Rossier BC. Amiloride-sensitive epithelial Na+ channel is made of three homologous subunits. *Nature* 1994;367:463–467 (see comments).
62. Chabardés D, Gagnan-Brunette M, Imbert-Teboul M. Adenylate cyclase responsiveness to hormones in various portions of the human nephron. *J Clin Invest* 1980;65:439–448.
63. Chabardés D, Imbert-Teboul M, Montegut M, Clique A, Morel F. Catecholamine sensitive adenylate cyclase activity in different segments of the rabbit nephron. *Pflugers Arch* 1975;361:9–15.
64. Chamberlin ME, LeFurgey A, Mandel LJ. Suspension of medullary thick ascending limb tubules from the rabbit kidney. *Am J Physiol* 1984;247:F955–F964.
65. Chamberlin ME, Mandel LJ. Substrate support of medullary thick ascending limb oxygen consumption. *Am J Physiol* 1986;251:F758–F763.
66. Chang SS, Grunder S, Hanukoglu A, Rosler A, Mathew PM, Hanukoglu I, Schild L, Lu Y, Shimkets RA, Nelson-Williams C, Rossier BC, Lifton RP. Mutations in subunits of the epithelial sodium channel cause salt wasting with hyperkalaemic acidosis, pseudohypoaldosteronism type 1. *Nat Genet* 1996;12:248–253.
67. Chen L, Reif MC, Schafer JA. Clonidine and PGE2 have different effects on Na+ and water transport in rat and rabbit CCD. *Am J Physiol* 1991;261:F126–F136.
68. Chen L, Williams SK, Schafer JA. Differences in synergistic actions of vasopressin and deoxycorticosterone in rat and rabbit CCD. *Am J Physiol* 1990;259:F147–F156.
69. Chen S-Y, Bhargava A, Mastroberardino L, Meijer OC, Wang J, Buse P, Firestone GL, Verrey F, Pearce D. Epithelial sodium channel regulated by aldosterone-induced protein sgk. *Proc Natl Acad Sci U S A* 1999;96:2514–2519.
70. Chen Z, Vaughn DA, Beaumont K, Fanestil DD. Effects of diuretic treatment and of dietary sodium on renal binding of ^{3}H-metolazone. *J Am Soc Nephrol* 1990;1:91–98.
71. Chen Z, Vaughn DA, Blakely P, Fanestil DD. Adrenocortical steroids increase renal thiazide diuretic receptor density and response. *J Am Soc Nephrol* 1994;5:1361–1368.
72. Chen Z, Vaughn DA, Fanestil DD. Influence of gender on renal thiazide diuretic receptor density and response. *J Am Soc Nephrol* 1994;5:1112–1119.
73. Cheng H-F, Harris RC. Cyclooxygenases, the kidney, and hypertension. *Hypertension* 2004;43:525–530.
74. Choe H, Zhou H, Palmer LG, Sackin H. A conserved cytoplasmic region of ROMK modulates pH sensitivity, conductance, and gating. *Am J Physiol Renal Physiol* 1997;273:F516–F529.
75. Clapp WL, Madsen KM, Verlander JW, Tisher CC. Morphologic heterogeneity along the rat inner medullary collecting duct. *Lab Invest* 1989;60:219–230.
76. Clement JPt, Kunjilwar K, Gonzalez G, Schwanstecher M, Panten U, Aguilar-Bryan L, Bryan J. Association and stoichiometry of K(ATP) channel subunits. *Neuron* 1997;18:827–838.
77. Costanzo LS. Comparison of calcium and sodium transport in early and late rat distal tubules: effects of amiloride. *Am J Physiol* 1984;246:F937–F945.
78. Costanzo LS. Localization of diuretic action in microperfused rat distal tubules: Ca and Na transport. *Am J Physiol* 1985;248:F527–F535.
79. Culpepper RM, Andreoli TE. Interactions among prostaglandin E_2, antidiuretic hormone, cyclic adenosine monophosphate in modulating Cl^- absorption in single mouse medullary thick ascending limbs of Henle. *J Clin Invest* 1983;71:1588–1601.
80. Culpepper RM, Andreoli TE. PGE_2, forskolin, and cholera toxin interactions in modulating NaCl transport in mouse mTALH. *Am J Physiol* 1984;247:F784–F792.
81. de Bermudez L, Windhager EE. Osmotically induced changes in electrical resistance of distal tubules of rat kidney. *Am J Physiol* 1975;229:1536–1546.
82. de la Rosa AD, Coric T, Todorovic N, Shao D, Wang T, Canessa CM. Distribution and regulation of expression of serum- and glucocorticoid-induced kinase-1 in the rat kidney. *J Physiol (Lond)* 2003;551:455–466.
83. de la Rosa AD, Zhang P, Naray-Fejes-Toth A, Fejes-Toth G, Canessa CM. The serum and glucocorticoid kinase sgk increases the abundance of epithelial sodium channels in the plasma membrane of *Xenopus* oocytes. *J Biol Chem* 1999;274:37834–37839.
84. de la Rosa DA, Paunescu TG, Els WJ, Helman SI, Canessa CM. Mechanisms of regulation of epithelial sodium channel by SGK1 in A6 cells. *J Gen Physiol* 2004;124:395–407.

85. DeCoy DL, Snapper JR, Breyer MD. Anti sense DNA down-regulates proteins kinase C-epsilon and enhances vasopressin-stimulated Na+ absorption in rabbit cortical collecting duct. *J Clin Invest* 1995;95:2749–2756.
86. Delpire E, Rauchman MI, Beier DR, Hebert SC, Gullans SR. Molecular cloning and chromosome localization of a putative basolateral Na(+)-K(+)-2C- cotransporter from mouse inner medullary collecting duct (mIMCD-3) cells. *J Biol Chem* 1994;269:25677–25683.
87. deRouffignac C, Elalouf JM. Hormonal regulation of chloride transport in the proximal and distal nephron. *Ann Rev Physiol* 1988;50:123–140.
88. Derst C, Konrad M, Kockerling A, Karolyi L, Deschenes G, Daut J, Karschin A, Seyberth HW. Mutations in the ROMK gene in antenatal Bartter syndrome are associated with impaired K+ channel function. *Biochem Biophys Res Commun* 1997;230:641–645.
89. DiBona GF, Sawin LL. Effect of renal nerve stimulation on NaCl and H_2O transport in Henle's loop of the rat. *Am J Physiol* 1982;243:F576–F580.
90. Dietl P, Good D, Stanton B. Adrenal corticosteroid action on the thick ascending limb. *Semin Nephrol* 1990;10:350–364.
91. Dijkink L, Hartog A, van Os C, Bindels R. The epithelial sodium channel (ENaC) is intracellularly located as a tetramer. *Pflugers Arch* 2002;444:549–555.
92. Dillingham MA, Anderson RJ. Inhibition of vasopressin action by atrial natriuretic factor. *Science* 1986;231:1572–1573.
93. Dixon BS, Breckon R, Fortune J, Sutherland E, Simon FR, Anderson RJ. Bradykinin activates protein kinase C in cultured cortical collecting tubular cells. *Am J Physiol* 1989;257: F808–F817.
94. Djelidi S, Fay M, Cluzeaud F, Escoubet B, Eugene E, Capurro C, Bonvalet JP, Farman N, Blot-Chabaud M. Transcriptional regulation of sodium transport by vasopressin in renal cells. *J Biol Chem* 1997;272:32919–32924.
95. Dobyan DC, Bulger RE. Renal carbonic anhydrase. *Am J Physiol* 1982;243:F311–F324.
96. Doucet A, Katz AI. Mineralocorticoid receptors along the nephron: [^{3}H] aldosterone binding in rabbit tubules. *Am J Physiol* 1981;241:F605–F611.
97. Duarte C, Chomety F, Giebisch G. Effect of amiloride, ouabain, and furosemide on distal tubular function in the rat. *Am J Physiol* 1971;221:632–639.
98. DuBose TDJ, Seldin DW, Kokko JP. Segmental chloride reabsorption in the rat nephron as a function of load. *Am J Physiol* 1978;239:F97–F105.
99. Eaton DC, Becchetti A, Ma H, Ling BN. Renal sodium channels: regulation and single channel properties. *Kidney Int* 1995;48:941–949.
100. Ecelbarger C, Kim G, Wade J, Knepper M. Regulation of the abundance of renal sodium transporters and channels by vasopressin. *Exp Neurol* 2001;171:227–234.
101. Edwards RM, Jackson BA, Dousa TP. Protein kinase activity in isolated tubules of rat renal medulla. *Am J Physiol* 1980;238:F269–F278.
102. El Mernissi G, Doucet A. Short-term effects of aldosterone and dexamethasone on Na-K-ATPase along the rabbit nephron. *Pflugers Arch* 1983;399:147–151.
103. El Mernissi G, Doucet A. Specific activity of Na-K-ATPase after adrenalectomy and hormone replacement along the rabbit nephron. *Pflugers Arch* 1984;402:258–263.
104. Ellison DH, Biemesderfer D, Morrisey J, Lauring J, Desir GV. Immunocytochemical characterization of the high-affinity thiazide diuretic receptor in rabbit renal cortex. *Am J Physiol* 1993;264:F141–F148.
105. Ellison DH, Velazquez H, Wright FS. Adaptation of the distal convoluted tubule of the rat. Structural and functional effects of dietary salt intake and chronic diuretic infusion. *J Clin Invest* 1989;83:113–26.
106. Ellison DH, Velazquez H, Wright FS. Regulation of thiazide diuretic receptors by distal sodium chloride load. *Kidney Int* 1990;37:562 (abstract).
107. Ellison DH, Velazquez H, Wright FS. Thiazide-sensitive sodium chloride cotransport in early distal tubule. *Am J Physiol* 1987;253:F546–F554.
108. Epple HJ, Amasheh S, Mankertz J, Goltz M, Schulzke JD, Fromm M. Early aldosterone effect in distal colon by transcriptional regulation of ENaC subunits. *Am J Physiol Gastro Liver Physiol* 2000;278:G718–G724.
109. Epstein FH, Silva P, Spokes K, Brezis M, Rosen S. Renal medullary Na-K-ATPase and hypoxic injury in perfused rat kidneys. *Kidney Int* 1989;36:768–772.
110. Escalante B, Erlij D, Falck JR, McGiff JC. Effect of cytochrome P450 arachidonate metabolites on ion transport in rabbit kidney loop of Henle. *Science* 1991;251:799–802.
111. Escoubet B, Coureau C, Bonvalet JP, Farman N. Noncoordinate regulation of epithelial Na channel and Na pump subunit mRNAs in kidney and colon by aldosterone. *Am J Physiol* 1997;272:C1482–C1491.
112. Estevez R, Boettger T, Stein V, Birkenhager R, Otto E, Hildebrandt F, Jentsch T. Barttin is a Cl^- channel b-subunit crucial for renal Cl^- reabsorption and inner ear K^+ secretion. *Nature* 2001;414:558–561.
113. Eveloff J, Bayerdorffer E, Silva P, Kinne R. Sodium-chloride transport in the thick ascending limb of Henle's loop. Oxygen consumption studies in isolated cells. *Pflugers Arch* 1981; 389:263–270.
114. Eveloff J, Calamia J. Effect of osmolarity on cation fluxes in medullary thick ascending limb cells. *Am J Physiol* 1986;250:F176–F180.
115. Eveloff J, Kinne R. Sodium-chloride transport in medullary thick ascending limb of Henle's loop: evidence for a sodium-chloride cotransport system in plasma membrane vesicles. *J Membr Biol* 1983;72:173–181.
116. Fanestil DD, Vaughn DA, Blakely P. Dietary NaCl and KCl do not regulate renal density of the thiazide diuretic receptor. *Am J Physiol* 1997;273:R1241–R1245.
117. Farman N, Bonvalet JP. Aldosterone binding in isolated tubules. III. Autoradiography along the rat nephron. *Am J Physiol* 1983;245:F606–F614.
118. Farman N, Oblin ME, Lombes M, Delahaye F, Westphal HM, Bonvalet JP, Gasc JM. Immunolocalization of gluco- and mineralocorticoid receptors in rabbit kidney. *Am J Physiol* 1991;260:C226–C233.
119. Farman N, Vandewalle A, Bonvalet JP. Aldosterone binding in isolated tubules II. An autoradiographic study of concentration dependency in the rabbit nephron. *Am J Physiol* 1982; 242:F69–F77.
120. Figueroa CD, Gonzalez CB, Grigoriev S, Abd Alla SA, Haasemann M, Jarnagin K, Muller-Esterl W. Probing for the bradykinin B2 receptor in rat kidney by anti-peptide and anti-ligand antibodies. *J Histochem Cytochem* 1995;43:137–148.
121. Firsov D, Gautschi I, Merillat AM, Rossier BC, Schild L. The heterotetrameric architecture of the epithelial sodium channel (ENaC). *EMBO J* 1998;17:344–352.
122. Firsov D, Schild L, Gautschi I, Merillat AM, Schneeberger E, Rossier BC. Cell surface expression of the epithelial Na channel and a mutant causing Liddle syndrome: a quantitative approach. *Proc Natl Acad Sci U S A* 1996;93:15370–15375.
123. Forbush B, Palfrey HC. (^{3}H)-bumetanide binding to membranes isolated from dog kidney outer medulla. *J Biol Chem* 1983;258:11787–11792.
124. Friedman PA. Bumetanide inhibition of [CO_2 + HC^*O_3]-dependent and -independent equivalent electrical flux in renal cortical thick ascending limbs. *J Pharmacol Exp Ther* 1986; 238:407–414.
125. Friedman PA, Andreoli TE. CO_2-stimulated NaCl absorption in the mouse renal cortical thick ascending limb of Henle. *J Gen Physiol* 1982;80:683–711.
126. Friedman PA, Andreoli TE. Effects of (CO_2 + HCO_3^-) on electrical conductance in cortical thick ascending limbs. *Kidney Int* 1986;30:325–331.
127. Friedman PA, Hebert SC. Diluting segment in kidney of dogfish shark. I. Localization and characterization of chloride absorption. *Am J Physiol* 1990;258:R398–R408.
128. Frindt G, Burg MB. Effect of vasopressin on sodium transport in renal cortical collecting tubules. *Kidney Int* 1972;1:224–231.
129. Frindt G, Sackin H, Palmer LG. Whole-cell currents in rat cortical collecting tubule: low-Na diet increases amiloride-sensitive conductance. *Am J Physiol* 1990;258:F562–F567.
130. Frindt G, Silver RB, Windhager EE, Palmer LG. Feedback regulation of Na channels in rat CCT. II. Effects of inhibition of Na entry. *Am J Physiol* 1993;264:F565–F574.
131. Fuleihan G-H, Seifter J, Scott J, Brown E. Calcium-regulated renal calcium handling in healthy men: relationship to sodium handling. *J Clin Endocrinol Metab* 1998;83:2366–2372.
132. Funder JW, Pearce PT, Smith R, Smith AI. Mineralocorticoid action: target tissue specificity is enzyme, not receptor, mediated. *Science* 1988;242:583–585.
133. Gallazzini M, Attmane-Elakeb A, Mount DB, Hebert SC, Bichara M. Regulation by glucocorticoids and osmolality of expression of ROMK (Kir 1.1), the apical K channel of thick ascending limb. *Am J Physiol Renal Physiol* 2003;284:F977–F986.
134. Gamba G, Miyanoshita A, Lombardi M, Lytton J, Lee WS, Hediger MA, Hebert SC. Molecular cloning, primary structure, characterization of two members of the mammalian electroneutral sodium-(potassium)-chloride cotransporter family expressed in kidney. *J Biol Chem* 1994;269:17713–17722.
135. Gamba G, Saltzberg SN, Lombardi M, Miyanoshita A, Lytton J, Hediger MA, Brenner BM, Hebert SC. Primary structure and functional expression of a cDNA encoding the thiazide-sensitive, electroneutral sodium-chloride cotransporter. *Proc Natl Acad Sci U S A* 1993; 90:2749–2753.
136. Gapstur SM, Homma S, Dousa TP. cAMP-binding proteins in medullary tubules from rat kidney: effect of ADH. *Am J Physiol* 1988;255:F292–F300.
137. Garg LC, Knepper MA, Burg MB. Mineralocorticoid effects on Na-K-ATPase in individual nephron segments. *Am J Physiol* 1981;240:F536–F544.
138. Garg LC, Narang N, Wingo CS. Glucocorticoid effects on Na-K-ATPase in rabbit nephron segments. *Am J Physiol* 1985;248:F487–F491.
139. Garty H, Edelman IS. Amiloride-sensitive trypsinization of apical sodium channels. *J Gen Physiol* 1983;81:785–803.
140. Garty H, Palmer LG. Epithelial sodium channels: function, structure, and regulation. *Physiol Rev* 1997;77:359–396.
141. Geck P, Pietvgyk C, Burckhardt BC, al. e. Electrically silent cotransport of Na, K, and Cl in Ehrlich cells. *Biochim Biophys Acta* 1980;60:432–447.
142. Gellai M. Modulation of vasopressin antidiuretic action by renal a_2-adrenoceptors. *Am J Physiol* 1990;259:F1–F10.
143. Gesek FA, Friedman PA. Mechanism of calcium transport stimulated by chlorothiazide in mouse distal convoluted tubule cells. *J Clin Invest* 1992;90:429–438.
144. Gesek FA, Friedman PA. On the mechanism of parathyroid hormone stimulation of calcium uptake by mouse distal convoluted tubule cells. *J Clin Invest* 1992;90:749–758.
145. Giebisch G, Hebert S, Wang W. New aspects of renal potassium transport. *Eur J Physiol* 2003;446:289–297.
146. Giebisch G, Klose RM, Windhager EE. Micropuncture study of hypertonic sodium chloride loading in the rat. *Am J Physiol* 1964;206:687–693.
147. Glynn IM, Warner AE. Nature of the calcium dependent potassium lead induced by (+)-propranolol, and its possible relevance to the drug's antiarrhythmic effect. *Br J Pharmacol* 1972;44:271–278.
148. Good DW. Bicarbonate absorption by the thick ascending limb of Henle's loop. *Semin Nephrol* 1990;10:132–138.
149. Good DW. Sodium-dependent bicarbonate absorption by cortical thick ascending limb of rat kidney. *Am J Physiol* 1985;248:F821–F829.
150. Good DW. The thick ascending limb as a site of renal bicarbonate reabsorption. *Semin Nephrol* 1993;13:225–235.
151. Good DW, George T, Wang DH. Angiotensin II inhibits HCO_3^- absorption via a cytochrome P-450–dependent pathway in MTAL. *Am J Physiol Renal Physiol* 1999;276:F726–F736.
152. Good DW, George T, Watts BA 3rd. Basolateral membrane Na+/H+ exchange enhances HCO_3^- absorption in rat medullary thick ascending limb: evidence for functional coupling between basolateral and apical membrane Na+/H+ exchangers. *Proc Natl Acad Sci U S A* 1995;92:12525–12529.
153. Good DW, Knepper MA, Burg MB. Ammonia and bicarbonate transport by thick ascending limb of rat kidney. *Am J Physiol* 1984;247:F35–F44.
155. Good DW, Watts BA 3rd. Functional roles of apical membrane Na+/H+ exchange in rat medullary thick ascending limb. *Am J Physiol* 1996;270:F691–F699.
156. Grantham JJ, Burg MB, Orloff J. The nature of transtubular Na and K transport in isolated rabbit renal collecting tubules. *J Clin Invest* 1970;49:1815–1826.

157. Grantham JJ, Orloff J. Effect of prostaglandin E₁ on the permeability response of the isolated collecting tubule to vasopressin, adenosine 3', 5'-monophosphate, and theophylline. *J Clin Invest* 1968;45:1154–1161.

158. Greger R. Chloride reabsorption in the rabbit cortical thick ascending limb of the loop of Henle. A sodium dependent process. *Pflugers Arch* 1981;390:38–43.

159. Greger R. Chloride transport in thick ascending limb, distal convolution and collecting duct. *Annu Rev Physiol* 1988;50:111–122.

160. Greger R. Coupled transport of Na⁺ and Cl⁻ in the thick ascending limb of Henle's loop of rabbit nephron. *Scand Audiol Suppl* 1981;14:1–14.

161. Greger R, Bleich M, Schlatter E. Ion channels in the thick ascending limb of Henle's loop. *Renal Physiol Biochem* 1990;13:37–50.

162. Greger R, Oberleithner H, Schlatter E, Cassola AC, Weidtke C. Chloride activity in cells of isolated perfused cortical thick ascending limbs of rabbit kidney. *Pflugers Arch* 1983;399:29–34.

163. Greger R, Schlatter E. Presence of luminal K⁺, a prerequisite for active NaCl transport in the cortical thick ascending limb of Henle's loop of rabbit kidney. *Pflugers Arch* 1981;392:92–94.

164. Greger R, Schlatter E. Properties of the basolateral membrane of the cortical thick ascending limb of Henle's loop of rabbit kidney. A model of secondary active chloride transport. *Pflugers Arch* 1983;396:325–334.

165. Greger R, Schlatter E. Properties of the lumen membrane of the cortical thick ascending limb of Henle's loop of rabbit kidney. *Pflugers Arch* 1983;396:315–324.

166. Greger R, Velazquez H. The cortical thick ascending limb and early distal convoluted tubule in the urinary concentrating mechanism. *Kidney Int* 1987;31:590–596.

167. Greger R, Weidtke C, Schlatter E, Wittner M, Gebler B. Potassium activity in cells of isolated perfused cortical thick ascending limbs of rabbit kidney. *Pflugers Arch* 1987;401:52–57.

168. Gross JB, Imai M, Kokko JP. A functional comparison of the cortical collecting tubule and the distal convoluted tubule. *J Clin Invest* 1975;55:1284–1294.

169. Gross JB, Kokko JP. Effects of aldosterone and potassium-sparing diuretics on electrical potential differences across the distal nephron. *J Clin Invest* 1977;59:82–89.

170. Grossman EB, Hebert SC. Modulation of Na-K-ATPase activity in the mouse medullary thick ascending limb of Henle. Effects of mineralocorticoids and sodium. *J Clin Invest* 1988;81:885–892.

171. Grupp C, Pavenstadt-Grupp I, Grunewald RW, Bevan C, Stokes JB, Kinne RKH. A Na-K-Cl cotransporter in isolated rat papillary collecting duct cells. *Kidney Int* 1989;36:201–209.

172. Guan Y, Zhang Y, Breyer RM, Fowler B, Davis L, Hebert RL, Breyer MD. Prostaglandin E2 inhibits renal collecting duct Na+ absorption by activating the EP1 receptor. *J Clin Invest* 1998;102:194–201.

173. Guggino SE, Guggino WB, Green N, Sacktor B. Blocking agents of Ca²⁺-activated K⁺ channels in cultured medullary thick ascending limb cells. *Am J Physiol* 1987;252:C128–C137.

174. Guggino SE, Guggino WB, Green N, Sacktor B. Ca²⁺-activated K⁺ channels in cultured medullary thick ascending limb cells. *Am J Physiol* 1987;252:C121–C127.

175. Guggino WB. Functional heterogeneity in the early distal tubule of the *Amphiuma* kidney: evidence for two modes of Cl⁻ and K⁺ transport across the basolateral cell membrane. *Am J Physiol* 1986;250:F430–F440.

176. Guggino WB, Oberleithner H, Giebisch G. The amphibian diluting segment. *Am J Physiol* 1988;254:F615–F627.

177. Guggino WB, Oberleithner H, Giebisch G, Amiel CM. Relationship between cell volume and ion transport in the early distal tubule of the *Amphiuma* kidney. *J Gen Physiol* 1985;86:31–58.

178. Guinamard R, Chraibi A, Teulon J. A small-conductance Cl⁻ channel in the mouse thick ascending limb that is activated by ATP and protein kinase A. *J Physiol* 1995;485:97–112.

179. Guinamard R, Paulais M, Teulon J. Inhibition of a small-conductance cAMP-dependent Cl⁻ channel in the mouse thick ascending limb at low internal pH. *J Physiol* 1996;490:759–765.

180. Gullans SR, Hebert SC. Metabolic basis of ion transport. In: Brenner BM, ed. *The Kidney.* 5 ed. Philadelphia: WB Saunders; 1996:211–246.

181. Haas M, McManus TJ. Bumetanide inhibits (Na+K+Cl) cotransport at a chloride site. *Am J Physiol* 1983;245:235–240.

182. Haas M, Schmidt WF, McManus TJ. Catecholamine stimulated ion transport in duck red cells: gradient effect in electrically neutral (Na-K-2Cl) cotransport. *J Gen Physiol* 1982;80:125–147.

183. Hall DA, Varney DM. Effect of vasopressin in electrical potential difference and chloride transport in mouse medullary thick ascending limb of Henle's loop. *J Clin Invest* 1980;66:792–802.

184. Hanley MJ, Kokko JP. Study of chloride transport across the rabbit cortical collecting tubule. *J Clin Invest* 1978;62:39–44.

185. Hanley MJ, Kokko JP, Gross JB, Jacobson HR. Electrophysiologic study of the cortical collecting tubule of the rabbit. *Kidney Int* 1980;17:74–81.

186. Hansson JH, Nelson-Williams C, Suzuki H, Schild L, Shimkets R, Lu Y, Canessa C, Iwasaki T, Rossier B, Lifton RP. Hypertension caused by a truncated epithelial sodium channel gamma subunit: genetic heterogeneity of Liddle syndrome. *Nat Genet* 1995;11:76–82.

187. Harding P, Sigmon DH, Alfie ME, Huang PL, Fishman MC, Beierwaltes WH, Carretero OA. Cyclooxygenase-2 mediates increased renal renin content induced by low-sodium diet. *Hypertension* 1997;29:297–302.

188. Harris RC, McKanna JA, Akai Y, Jacobson HR, Dubois RN, Breyer MD. Cyclooxygenase-2 is associated with the macula densa of rat kidney and increases with salt restriction. *J Clin Invest* 1994;94:2504–2510.

189. Hawk CT, Li L, Schafer JA. AVP and aldosterone at physiological concentrations have synergistic effects on Na+ transport in rat CCD. *Kidney Int* 1996;57:S35–41.

190. Hayslett JP, Backman KA, Schon DA. Electrical properties of the medullary collecting duct in the rat. *Am J Physiol* 1980;239:F258–F264.

191. Hayslett JP, Boulpaep EL, Giebisch GH. Factors influencing transepithelial potential difference in mammalian distal tubule. *Am J Physiol* 1978;234:F182–F191.

192. Hayslett JP, Boulpaep EL, Kashgarian M, Giebisch GH. Electrical characteristics of the mammalian distal tubule: comparison of Ling–Gerard and macroelectrodes. *Kidney Int* 1977;12:324–331.

193. Hebert RL, Jacobson HR, Breyer MD. Prostaglandin E2 inhibits sodium transport in rabbit cortical collecting duct by increasing intracellular calcium. *J Clin Invest* 1991;87:1992–1998.

194. Hebert RL, Jacobson HR, Fredin D, Breyer MD. Evidence that separate PGE2 receptors modulate water and sodium transport in rabbit cortical collecting duct. *Am J Physiol* 1993;265:F643–F650.

195. Hebert SC. Hypertonic cell volume regulation in mouse thick limbs. I. ADH dependency and nephron heterogeneity. *Am J Physiol* 1986;250:C907–C919.

196. Hebert SC, Andreoli TE. Effects of antidiuretic hormone on cellular conductance pathways in mouse medullary thick ascending limbs of Henle. II. Determinants of the ADH-mediated increases in transepithelial voltage and in net Cl⁻ absorption. *J Membr Biol* 1984;80:221–233.

197. Hebert SC, Andreoli TE. Ionic conductance pathways in the mouse medullary thick ascending limb of Henle. The paracellular pathway and electrogenic Cl⁻ absorption. *J Gen Physiol* 1986;87:567–590.

198. Hebert SC, Culpepper RM, Andreoli TE. NaCl transport in mouse thick ascending limbs. I. Functional nephron heterogeneity and ADH-stimulated NaCl cotransport. *Am J Physiol* 1981;241:F412–F431.

199. Hebert SC, Culpepper RM, Andreoli TE. NaCl transport in mouse thick ascending limbs. II. ADH enhancement of transcellular NaCl cotransport; origin of transepithelial voltage. *Am J Physiol* 1981;241:F432–F442.

200. Hebert SC, Culpepper RM, Andreoli TE. NaCl transport in mouse thick ascending limbs. III. Modulation of the ADH effect by peritubular osmolality. *Am J Physiol* 1981;241:F443–F451.

201. Hebert SC, Desir G, Giebisch G, Wang W. Molecular diversity and regulation of renal potassium channels. *Physiol Rev* 2005;85:319–371.

202. Hebert SC, Friedman PA. Diluting segment in kidney of dogfish shark. II. Electrophysiology of apical membranes and cellular resistances. *Am J Physiol* 1990;258:R409–R417.

203. Hebert SC, Friedman PA, Andreoli TE. Effects of antidiuretic hormone on cellular conductive pathways in mouse medullary thick ascending limbs of Henle. I. ADH increases transcellular conductance pathways. *J Membr Biol* 1984;80:201–219.

204. Hebert SC, Reeves WB, Molony DA, Andreoli TE. The medullary thick limb: function and modulation of the single-effect multiplier. *Kidney Int* 1987;31:580–589.

205. Helman SI. Determination of electrical resistance of the isolated cortical collecting tubule and its possible anatomical location. *Yale J Biol Med* 1972;45:339–345.

206. Helman SI, Grantham JJ, Burg MB. Effect of vasopressin on electrical resistance of renal cortical collecting tubules. *Am J Physiol* 1971;220:1825–1832.

207. Helms MN, Fejes-Toth G, Naray-Fejes-Toth A. Hormone-regulated transepithelial Na+ transport in mammalian CCD cells requires SGK1 expression. *Am J Physiol Renal Physiol* 2003;284:F480–487.

208. Hierholzer K, Wiederholt M. Some aspects of distal tubular solute and water transport. *Kidney Int* 1976;9:198–213.

209. Hierholzer K, Wiederholt M, Holzgreve H, Giebisch G, Klose RM, Windhager EE. Micropuncture study of renal transtubular concentration gradients of sodium and potassium in adrenalectomized rats. *Pflugers Arch* 1965;285:193–210.

210. Higashihara E, Stokes JB, Kokko JP, Campbell WB, DuBose TD. Cortical and papillary micropuncture examination of chloride transport in segments of the rat kidney during inhibition of prostaglandin production. *J Clin Invest* 1979;64:1277–1287.

211. Hiltunen TPA, Hannila-Handelberg TA, Petajaniemi NA, Kantola IB, Tikkanen IA, Virtamo JC, Gautschi ID, Schild LD, Kontula KA. Liddle's syndrome associated with a point mutation in the extracellular domain of the epithelial sodium channel [gamma] subunit. *J Hypertens* 2002;20:2383–2390.

212. Ho K, Nichols CG, Lederer WJ, Lytton J, Vassilev PM, Kanazirska MV, Hebert SC. Cloning and expression of an inwardly rectifying ATP-regulated potassium channel. *Nature* 1993;362:31–37.

213. Horster M, Schmid H, Schmidt U. Aldosterone in vitro restores nephron Na-K-ATPase of distal segments from adrenalectomized rabbits. *Pflugers Arch* 1980;384:203–206.

214. Hummler E, Barker P, Talbot C, Wang Q, Verdumo C, Grubb B, Gatzy J, Burnier M, Horisberger JD, Beermann F, Boucher R, Rossier BC. A mouse model for the renal salt-wasting syndrome pseudohypoaldosteronism. *Proc Natl Acad Sci U S A* 1997;94:11710–11715.

215. Hunter M, Lopes AG, Boulpaep EL, Giebisch GH. Single channel relationship of calcium-activated potassium channels in the apical membrane of rabbit cortical collecting tubules. *Proc Natl Acad Sci U S A* 1984;81:4237–4239.

216. Hus-Citharel A, Morel F. Coupling of metabolic CO₂ production to ion transport in isolated rat thick ascending limbs and collecting tubules. *Pflugers Arch* 1986;407:421–427.

217. Husted RF, Stokes JB. Separate regulation of Na+ and anion transport by IMCD: location, aldosterone, hypertonicity, TGF-beta 1, and cAMP. *Am J Physiol* 1996;271:F433–F439.

218. Iino Y, Troy JL, Brenner BM. Effects of catecholamines on electrolyte transport in cortical collecting tubule. *J Membr Biol* 1981;61:67–73.

219. Imai M. The connecting tubule: a functional subdivision of the rabbit distal nephron segments. *Kidney Int* 1979;15:346–356.

220. Imai M. Function of the thin ascending limb of Henle of rats and hamsters perfused *in vitro.* *Am J Physiol* 1977;232:F201–F209.

221. Imai M. Functional heterogeneity of the descending limbs of Henle's loop. II.Interspecies defferences among rabbits, rats, and hamsters. *Pflugers Arch* 1984;402:393–401.

222. Imai M, Hayashi M, Araki M. Functional heterogeneity of the descending limbs of Henle's loop. I. Internephron heterogeneity in the hamster kidney. *Pflugers Arch* 1984;402:385–392.

223. Imai M, Kokko JP. Mechanism of sodium and chloride transport in the thin ascending limb of Henle. *J Clin Invest* 1976;58:1054–1060.

224. Imai M, Kokko JP. NaCl, urea, and water transport in the thin ascending limb of Henle: generation of osmotic gradients by passive diffusion of solutes. *J Clin Invest* 1974;53:393–402.

225. Imai M, Kokko JP. Sodium chloride, urea and water transport in the thin ascending limb of Henle. Generation of osmotic gradients by passive diffusion of solutes. *J Clin Invest* 1974; 53:393–402.
226. Imai M, Kusano E. Effect of arginine vasopressin on the thin ascending limb of Henle of hamsters. *Am J Physiol* 1982;243:F167–F172.
227. Imai M, Taniguchi J, Tabei K. Function of thin loops of Henle. *Kidney Int* 1987;31:565–579.
228. Imai M, Yoshitomi K. Electrophysiological study of inner medullary collecting duct of hamsters. *Pflugers Arch* 1990;416:180–188.
229. Inagaki N, Gonoi T, Clement JP IV, Wang C, Aguilar-Bryan L, Bryan J, Seino S. A family of sulfonylurea receptors determines the pharmacological properties of ATP-sensitive K+ channels. *Neuron* 1996;16:1011–1017.
230. Inagaki N, Gonoi T, Clement JP, Namba N, Inazawa J, Gonzalez G, Aguilar-Bryan L, Seino S, Bryan J. Reconstitution of I_{KATP}: an inward rectifier subunit plus the sulfonylurea receptor. *Science* 1995;270:1166–1170.
231. Inagaki N, Gonoi T, Seino S. Subunit stoichiometry of the pancreatic beta-cell ATP-sensitive K+ channel. *FEBS Lett* 1997;409:232–236.
232. Inio Y, Burg MB. Effect of acid–base status in vivo on bicarbonate transport by rabbit renal renal tubules *in vitro*. *Jpn J Physiol* 1981;31:99–107.
233. Ismailov II, McDuffie JH, Benos DJ. Protein kinase A phosphorylation and G protein regulation of purified renal Na+ channels in planar bilayer membranes. *J Biol Chem* 1994; 269:10235–41.
234. Isozaki T, Yoshitomi K, Imai M. Effects of Cl^- transport inhibitors on Cl^- permeability across hamster ascending thin limb. *Am J Physiol* 1989;257:F92–F98.
235. Jacobson HR. Medullary collecting duct acidification. Effects of potassium, HCO_3 concentration and pCO_2. *J Clin Invest* 1984;74:2107–2114.
236. Jacobson HR, Gross JB, Kawamura S, Waters JD, Kokko JP. Electrophysiological study of isolated perfused human collecting ducts. Ion dependency of the transepithelial potential difference. *J Clin Invest* 1976;58:1233–1239.
237. Jamison RL. Micropuncture study of segments of thin loop of Henle in the rat. *Am J Physiol* 1968;215:236–242.
238. Jamison RL, Bennett CM, Berliner RW. Countercurrent multiplication by the thin loops of Henle. *Am J Physiol* 1967;212:357–366.
239. Jeck N, Waldegger P, Doroszewicz J, Seyberth H, Waldegger S. A common sequence variation of the CLCNKB gene strongly activates ClC-Kb chloride channel activity. *Kidney Int* 2004;65:190–197.
240. Jeck N, Waldegger S, Lampert A, Boehmer C, Waldegger P, Lang PA, Wissinger B, Friedrich B, Risler T, Moehle R, Lang UE, Zill P, Bondy B, Schaeffeler E, Asante-Poku S, Seyberth H, Schwab M, Lang F. Activating mutation of the renal epithelial chloride channel ClC-Kb predisposing to hypertension. *Hypertension* 2004;43:1175–1181.
241. Jentsch TJ. Chloride channels: a molecular perspective. *Curr Opin Neurobiol* 1996;6:303–310.
242. Jentsch TJ, Steinmeyer K, Schwarz G. Primary structure of *Torpedo marmorata* chloride channel isolated by expression cloning in *Xenopus* oocytes. *Nature* 1990;348:510–514.
243. Kahle KT, Gimenez I, Hassan H, Wilson FH, Wong RD, Forbush B, Aronson PS, Lifton RP. WNK4 regulates apical and basolateral Cl^- flux in extrarenal epithelia. *Proc Natl Acad Sci U S A* 2004;101:2064–2069.
244. Kahle KT, MacGregor GG, Wilson FH, Van Hoek AN, Brown D, Ardito T, Kashgarian M, Giebisch G, Hebert SC, Boulpaep EL, Lifton RP. Paracellular Cl^- permeability is regulated by WNK4 kinase: Insight into normal physiology and hypertension. *Proc Natl Acad Sci U S A* 2004;101:14877–14882.
245. Kaissling B, Kriz W. Structural analysis of the rabbit kidney. *Embryol Cell Biol* 1979;56: 1–123.
246. Kaissling B, Kriz W. Structural organization of the mammalian kidney. In: Seldin DW, Giebisch G, eds. *The Kidney: Physiology and Pathophysiology*. New York: Raven Press; 1985: 265–306.
247. Kaissling B, LeHir M. Distal tubular segments of the rabbit kidney after adaptation to altered Na^+ and K^+ intake. I. Structural changes. *Cell Tissue Res* 1982;224:469–492.
248. Kaissling B, Stanton BA. Adaptation of distal tubule and collecting duct to increased sodium delivery. I. Ultrastructure. *Am J Physiol* 1988;255:F1256–F1268.
249. Deleted in proof.
250. Kaplan MR, Plotkin MD, Lee WS, Xu ZC, Lytton J, Hebert SC. Apical localization of the Na-K-Cl cotransporter, rBSC1, on rat thick ascending limbs. *Kidney Int* 1996;49:40–47.
251. Deleted in proof.
252. Katz AI, Doucet A, Morel F. Na-K-ATPase activity along the rabit, rat, and mouse nephron. *Am J Physiol* 1979;237:F114–F120.
253. Kellenberger S, Gautschi I, Rossier BC, Schild L. Mutations causing Liddle syndrome reduce sodium-dependent downregulation of the epithelial sodium channel in the *Xenopus* oocyte expression system. *J Clin Invest* 1998;101:2741–2750.
254. Kemendy AE, Kleyman TR, Eaton DC. Aldosterone alters the open probability of amiloride-blockable sodium channels in A6 cells. *Am J Physiol* 1992;263:C825–C837.
255. Khuri RN, Wiederholt M, Streider N, Giebisch G. Effects of graded solute diuresis on renal tubular sodium transport in the rat. *Am J Physiol* 1975;228:1262–1268.
256. Kieferle S, Fong P, Bens M, Vandewalle A, Jentsch TJ. Two highly homologous members of the ClC chloride channel family in both rat and human kidney. *Proc Natl Acad Sci U S A* 1994; 91:6943–6947.
257. Kikeri D, Azar S, Sun A, Zeidel ML, Hebert SC. Na^+-H^+ antiporter and $Na^+(HCO_3^-)_n$ symporter regulate intracellular pH in mouse medullary thick limbs of Henle. *Am J Physiol* 1990;258:F445–F456.
258. Kim G-H, Masilamani S, Turner R, Mitchell C, Wade JB, Knepper MA. The thiazide-ssensitive Na-Cl cotransporter is an aldosterone-induced protein. *Proc Natl Acad Sci U S A* 1998;95:14552–14557.
259. Kimmel PL, Goldfarb S. Effects of isoproterenol on potassium secretion by the cortical collecting tubule. *Am J Physiol* 1984;246:F804–F810.
260. Kinne R, Kinne-Saffran E, Scholermann B. The anion specificity of the sodium-potassium-chloride cotransporter in rabbit outer medulla. Studies on medullary plasma membranes. *Pflugers Arch* 1986;407:168–173.
261. Klaerke DA, Petersen J, Jorgensen PL. Purification of Ca^{2+}-activated K^+ channel protein on calmodulin affinity columns after detergent solubilization of luminal membranes from outer renal medulla. *FEBS Lett* 1987;216:211–216.
262. Klein KL, Wang MS, Torikai S, Davidson WD, Kurokawa K. Substrate oxidation by isolated single nephron segments of the rat. *Kidney Int* 1981;20:29–35.
263. Kleyman TR, Coupaye-Gerald B, Ernst SA. Aldosterone does not alter apical cell-surface expression of epithelial Na^+channels in the amphibian cell line A6'. *J Biol Chem* 1992; 267:9622–9628.
264. Kleyman TR, Cragoe EJ Jr, Kraehenbuhl JP. The cellular pool of Na+ channels in the amphibian cell line A6 is not altered by mineralocorticoids. Analysis using a new photoactive amiloride analog in combination with anti-amiloride antibodies. *J Biol Chem* 1989;264:11995–2000.
265. Knauf F, Yang C, Thomson R, Mentone S, Giebisch G, Aronson P. Idenfification of a chloride-formate exchanger expressed on the brush border membrane of renal proximal tubule cells. *Proc Natl Acad Sci U S A* 2001;98:9425–9430.
266. Knepper M, Kim G-H, Masilamani S. Renal tubule sodium transporter abundance profiling in rat kidney: response to aldosterone and variations in NaCl intake. *Ann NY Acad Sci* 2003;986:562–569.
267. Koefoed-Johnson V, Ussing HH. The nature of the frog skin potential. *Acta Physiol Scand* 1958;42:298–308.
268. Koenig B, Ricapito S, Kinne R. Chloride transport in the thick ascending limb of Henle's loop: potassium dependence and stoichiometry of the NaCl cotransport system in plasma membrane vesicles. *Pflugers Arch* 1983;399:173–179.
269. Koeppen BM. Conductive properties of the rabbit outer medullary collecting duct: inner stripe. *Am J Physiol* 1985;248:F500–F506.
270. Koeppen BM. Conductive properties of the rabbit outer medullary collecting duct: outer stripe. *Am J Physiol* 1986;250:F70–F76.
271. Koeppen BM. Electrophysiological identification of principal and intercalated cells in the rabbit outer medullary collecting duct. *Pflugers Arch* 1987;409:138–141.
272. Koeppen BM. Electrophysiology of collecting duct H^+ secretion: effects of inhibitors. *Am J Physiol* 1989;256:F79–F84.
273. Koeppen BM, Biagi BA, Giebisch GH. Intracellular microelectrode characterization of the rabbit cortical collecting duct. *Am J Physiol* 1983;244:F35–F47.
274. Koeppen BM, Stanton BA. Sodium chloride transport—distal nephron. In: Seldin DW, Giebisch G, eds. *The Kidney: Physiology and Pathophysiology*, 2nd ed. New York: Raven Press; 1992:2003–2039.
275. Kokko JP. Sodium chloride and water transport in the descending limb of Henle. *J Clin Invest* 1970;49:1838–1846.
276. Kokko JP, Rector FC Jr. Countercurrent multiplication system without active transport in inner medulla. *Kidney Int* 1972;2:214–223.
277. Kondo C, Isomoto S, Matsumoto S, Yamada M, Horio Y, Yamashita S, Takemura-Kameda K, Matsuzawa Y, Kurachi Y. Cloning and functional expression of a novel isoform of ROMK inwardly rectifying ATP-dependent K+ channel, ROMK6 (Kir1.1 f). *FEBS Lett* 1996; 399: 122–126.
278. Kondo Y, Yoshitomi K, Imai M. Effect of anion transport inhibitors and ion substitution on Cl transport in the thin ascending limb of Henle's loop. *Am J Physiol* 1987;253:F1206–F1215.
279. Kondo Y, Yoshitomi K, Imai M. Effect of Ca^{2+} on Cl^- transport in thin ascending limb of Henle's loop. *Am J Physiol* 1988;254:F232–F239.
280. Kosari F, Sheng S, Li J, Mak D-OD, Foskett JK, Kleyman TR. Subunit stoichiometry of the epithelial sodium channel. *J Biol Chem* 1998;273:13469–13474.
281. Krapf R. Basolateral membrane $H/OH/HCO_3$ transport in the rat cortical thick ascending limb. Evidence for a electrogenic Na/HCO_3 cotransporter in parallel with a Na/H antiporter. *J Clin Invest* 1988;82:243–241.
282. Kriz W, Kaissling B. Structural organization of the mammalian kidney. In: Seldin DW, Giebisch G, eds. *The Kidney: Physiology and Pathophysiology*, 2nd ed. New York: Raven Press; 1992:707–777.
283. Krozowski Z, Maguire JA, Stein-Oakley AN, Dowling J, Smith RE, Andrews RK. Immunohistochemical localization of the 11b-hydroxysteroid dehydrogenase type II enzyme in human kidney and placenta. *J Clin Endocrinol Metab* 1995;80:2203–2209.
284. Kudo LH, van Baak AA, Rocha AS. Effect of vasopressin on sodium transport across inner medullary collecting duct. *Am J Physiol* 1990;258:F1438–F1447.
285. Kunchaparty S, Palcso M, Berkman J, Velazquez H, Desir GV, Bernstein P, Reilly RF, Ellison DH. Defective processing and expression of thiazide-sensitive Na-Cl cotransporter as a cause of Gitelman's syndrome. *Am J Physiol Renal Physiol* 1999;277:F643–649.
286. Kuo A, Gulbis JM, Antcliff JF, Rahman T, Lowe ED, Zimmer J, Cuthbertson J, Ashcroft FM, Ezaki T, Doyle DA. Crystal structure of the potassium channel KirBac1.1 in the closed state. *Science* 2003;300:1922–1926.
287. Kurokawa K, Yoshitomi K, Ikeda M, Uchida S, Naruse M, Imai M. Regulation of cortical collecting duct function: effect of endothelin. *Am Heart J* 1993;125:582–588.
288. Kyossev Z, Walker PD, Reeves WB. Immunolocalization of NAD-dependent 11b-hydroxysteroid dehydrogenase in human kidney and colon. *Kidney Int* 1996;49:271–281.
289. Laghmani K, Borensztein P, Ambuhl PM, Froissart M, Bichara M, Moe OW, Alpern RJ, Paillard M. Chronic metabolic acidosis enhances NHE-3 protein abundance and transport activity in the rat thick ascending limb by increasing NHE-3 mRNA. *J Clin Invest* 1997; 99:24–30.
290. Lal MA, Proulx PR, Hebert RL. A role for PKC epsilon and MAP kinase in bradykinin-induced arachidonic acid release in rabbit CCD cells. *Am J Physiol* 1998;274:F728–735.
291. Landwehr DM, Klose RM, Giebisch G. Renal tubular sodium and water reabsorption in the isotonic sodium chloride loaded rat. *Am J Physiol* 1967;212:1327–1333.
292. Lauf PK, McManus TJ, Haas M, Forbush B III, Duhm J, Flatman PW, Saier MH, Russell JM. Physiology and biophysics of chloride and cation cotransport across cell membranes. *Fed Proc* 1987;46:2377–2384.

293. LeFurgey A, Tisher CC. Morphology of the rabbit collecting duct. *Am J Anat* 1979;155: 111–123.
294. Leichtweiss HP, Lubbers DW, Weiss C, Baumgarti H, Reschke W. The oxygen supply of the rat kidney: measurements of intrarenal pO2. *Pflugers Arch* 1969;309:328–349.
295. Light DB, Corbin JD, Stanton BA. Dual ion-channel regulation by cyclic GMP and cyclic GMP-dependent protein kinase. *Nature* 1990;344:336–339.
296. Light DB, McCann FV, Keller TM, Stanton BA. Amiloride-sensitive cation channel in apical membrane of inner medullary collecting duct. *Am J Physiol* 1988;255:F278–F286.
297. Light DB, Schwiebert EM, Karlson KH, Stanton BA. Atrial natriuretic peptide inhibits a cation channel in renal inner medullary collecting duct cells. *Science* 1989;243:383–385.
298. Ling BN, Hinton CF, Eaton DC. Amiloride-sensitive sodium channels in rabbit cortical collecting tubule primary cultures. *Am J Physiol* 1991;261:F933–F944.
299. Ling BN, Kokko KE, Eaton DC. Inhibition of apical Na+ channels in rabbit cortical collecting tubules by basolateral prostaglandin E2 is modulated by protein kinase C. *J Clin Invest* 1992;90:1328–1334.
300. Loffing J, Loffing-Cueni D, Hegyi I, Kaplan MR, Hebert SC, Le Hir M, Kaissling B. Thiazide treatment of rats provokes apoptosis in distal tubule cells. *Kidney Int* 1996;50:1180–1190.
301. Loffing J, Pietri L, Aregger F, Bloch-Faure M, Ziegler U, Meneton P, Rossier BC, Kaissling B. Differential subcellular localization of ENaC subunits in mouse kidney in response to high- and low-Na diets. *Am J Physiol Renal Physiol* 2000;279:F252–F258.
302. Lopes AG, Amzel LM, Markakis D, Guggino WB. Cell volume regulation by the thin descending limb of Henle's loop. *Proc Natl Acad Sci U S A* 1988;85:2873–2877.
303. Lu M, Wang T, Yan Q, Wang W, Giebisch G, Hebert SC. ROMK is required for expression of the 70–pS K channel in the thick ascending limb. *Am J Physiol Renal Physiol* 2004;286: F490–495.
304. Lu M, Wang T, Yan Q, Yang X, Dong K, Knepper MA, Wang W, Giebisch G, Shull GE, Hebert SC. Absence of small conductance K+ channel (SK) activity in apical membranes of thick ascending limb and cortical collecting duct in ROMK (Bartter's) knockout mice. *J Biol Chem* 2002;277:37881–37887.
305. Lu M, Zhu Y, Balazy M, Reddy K, Falck J, Wang W. Effect of angiotensin II on the apical K+ channel in the thick ascending limb of the rat kidney. *J Gen Physiol* 1996;108:537–547.
306. MacGregor GG, Dong K, Vanoye CG, Tang L, Giebisch G, Hebert SC. Nucleotides and phospholipids compete for binding to the C terminus of KATP channels. *Proc Natl Acad Sci U S A* 2002;99:2726–2731.
307. MacGregor GG, Xu JZ, McNicholas CM, Giebisch G, Hebert SC. Partially active channels produced by PKA site mutation of the cloned renal K+ channel, ROMK2 (kir1.2). *Am J Physiol Renal Physiol* 1998;275:F415–F422.
308. Malnic G, Giebisch G. Some electrical properties of distal tubular epithelium in the rat. *Am J Physiol* 1972;223:797–808.
309. Malnic G, Klose RM, Giebisch G. Micropuncture study of distal tubular potassium and sodium transport in rat nephron. *Am J Physiol* 1966;211:529–547.
310. Marunaka Y, Eaton DC. Effects of vasopressin and cAMP on single amiloride-blockable Na^+ channels. *Am J Physiol* 1991;260:C1071–C1084.
311. Marver D. Evidence of corticosteroid action along the nephron. *Am J Physiol* 1984;246: F111–F123.
313. Masilamani S, Wang X, Kim G-H, Brooks H, Nielsen J, Nielsen S, Nakamura K, Stokes JB, Knepper MA. Time course of renal Na-K-ATPase, NHE3, NKCC2, NCC, ENaC abundance changes with dietary NaCl restriction. *Am J Physiol Renal Physiol* 2002;283:F648–F657.
314. Matsumura Y, Uchida S, Kondo Y, Miyazaki H, Ko SBH, Hayama A, Morimoto T, Liu W, Sasaki S, Marumo F. Overt nephrogenic diabetes insipidus in mice lacking the CLC-K1 chloride channel. *Nat Genet* 1999;21:95–98.
315. May A, Puoti A, Gaeggeler HP, Horisberger JD, Rossier BC. Early effect of aldosterone on the rate of synthesis of the epithelial sodium channel alpha subunit in A6 renal cells. *J Am Soc Nephrol* 1997;8:1813–22.
316. McCarron D. Diet and blood pressure—the paradigm shift. *Science* 1998;281:933–934.
317. McKinney TD, Davidson KK. Bicarbonate transport in collecting tubules from outer stripe of outer medulla. *Am J Physiol* 1987;253:F816–F822.
318. McNicholas CM, Guggino WB, Schwiebert EM, Hebert SC, Giebisch G, Egan ME. Sensitivity of a renal K+ channel (ROMK2) to the inhibitory sulfonylurea compound glibenclamide is enhanced by coexpression with the ATP-binding cassette transporter cystic fibrosis transmembrane regulator. *Proc Natl Acad Sci U S A* 1996;93:8083–8088.
319. McNicholas CM, Nason MW Jr, Guggino WB, Schwiebert EM, Hebert SC, Giebisch G, Egan ME. A functional CFTR-NBF1 is required for ROMK2-CFTR interaction. *Am J Physiol* 1997;273:F843–F848.
320. McNicholas CM, Wang W, Ho K, Hebert SC, Giebisch G. Regulation of ROMK1 K+ channel activity involves phosphorylation processes. *Proc Natl Acad Sci U S A* 1994;91:8077–8081.
321. McRoberts JA, Erlinger S, Rindler MJ, Saier MH Jr. Furosemide-sensitive salt transport in Madin–Darby canine kidney cell line. Evidence for the cotransport of Na/K/Cl. *J Biol Chem* 1982;257:2260–2266.
322. Mennitt PA, Wade JB, Ecelbarger CA, Palmer LG, Frindt G. Localization of ROMK channels in the rat kidney. *J Am Soc Nephrol* 1997;8:1823–1830.
323. Middleton RE, Pheasant DJ, Miller C. Homodimeric architecture of a ClC-type chloride ion channel. *Nature* 1996;383:337–340 (see comments).
324. Middleton RE, Pheasant DJ, Miller C. Purification, reconstitution, and subunit composition of a voltage-gated chloride channel from *Torpedo electroplax*. *Biochemistry* 1994;33:13189–13198.
325. Misler S, Giebisch G. ATP-sensitive potassium channels in physiology, pathophysiology, and pharmacology. *Curr Opin Nephrol Hypertens* 1992;1:21–33.
326. Miwa T, Imai M. Flow-dependent water permeability of the rabbit descending limb of Henle's loop. *Am J Physiol* 1983;245:F743–F754.
327. Miwa T, Nishimura H. Diluting segment in avian kidney. II. Water and chloride transport. *Am J Physiol* 1986;250:R341–R347.
328. Miyamoto H, Ikehara T, Yamaguchi H, Hosokawa K, Yonezu T, Masuya T. Kinetic mechanism of Na^+, K^+, Cl^--cotransport as studied by Rb^+ influx into HeLa cells: effects of extracellular monovalent ions. *J Membr Biol* 1986;92:135–150.
329. Molony DA, Andreoli TE. Diluting power of thick limbs of Henle. I. Peritubular hypertonicity blocks basolateral Cl^- channels. *Am J Physiol* 1988;255:F1128–F1137.
330. Molony DA, Reeves WB, Andreoli TE. Na^+-K^+-$2Cl^-$ cotransport and the thick ascending limb. *Kidney Int* 1989;36:418–426.
331. Molony DA, Reeves WB, Hebert SC, Andreoli TE. ADH increases apical Na^+-K^+-$2Cl^-$ entry in mouse medullary thick ascending limbs of Henle. *Am J Physiol* 1987;252:F177–F187.
332. Monroy A, Plata C, Hebert SC, Gamba G. Characterization of the thiazide-sensitive Na+-Cl- cotransporter: a new model for ions and diuretics interaction. *Am J Physiol Renal Physiol* 2000;279:F161–F169.
333. Morales MM, Carroll TP, Morita T, Schwiebert EM, Devuyst O, Wilson PD, Lopes AG, Stanton BA, Dietz HC, Cutting GR, Guggino WB. Both the wild type and a functional isoform of CFTR are expressed in kidney. *Am J Physiol Renal Physiol* 1996;270: F1038–F1048.
334. Morel F. Sites of hormone action in the mammalian nephron. *Am J Physiol* 1981;240:F159–F164.
335. Morel F, Chabardes D, Imbert M. Functional segmentation of the rabbit distal tubule by microdetermination of hormone-dependent adenylate cyclase activity. *Kidney Int* 1976;9:264–277.
336. Morel F, Doucet A. Functional segmentation of the nephron. Seldin DW, Giebisch G, eds. *The Kidney: Physiology and Pathophysiology*, 2nd ed. New York: Raven Press; 1992:1049–1086.
337. Morel F, Imbert-Teboul M, Chabardes D. Distribution of hormone-dependent adenylate cyclase in the nephron and its physiological significance. *Ann Rev Physiol* 1981;43:569–581.
338. Morgan T, Berliner RW. Permeability of loop of Henle, vasa recta, and collecting duct to water, urea, and sodium. *Am J Physiol* 1968;215:108–115.
339. Mount DB, Baekgaard A, Hall AE, Plata C, Xu J, Beier DR, Gamba G, Hebert SC. Isoforms of the Na-K-2Cl cotransporter in murine TAL I. Molecular characterization and intrarenal localization. *Am J Physiol Renal Physiol* 1999;276:F347–358.
340. Mune T, Rogerson FM, Nikkila H, Agarwal AK, White PC. Human hypertension caused by mutations in the kidney isozyme of 11b-hydroxysteroid dehydrogenase. *Nat Genet* 1995; 10:394–399.
341. Mune T, White P. Apparent mineralocorticoid excess genotype is correlated with biochemical phenotype. *Hypertension* 1996;27:1193–1199.
342. Munzel PA, Healy DP, Insel PA. Autoradiographic localization of b-adrenergic receptors in rat kidney slices using $[^{125}I]$iodocyanopindolol. *Am J Physiol* 1984;246:F240–F245.
343. Muto S, Furuya H, Tabei K, Asano Y. Site and mechanism of action of epidermal growth factor in rabbit cortical collecting duct. *Am J Physiol* 1991;260:F163–F169.
344. Muto S, Giebisch G, Sansom S. Effects of adrenalectomy on CCD: evidence for differential response of two cell types. *Am J Physiol* 1987;253:F742–F752.
345. Muto S, Yasoshima K, Yoshitomi K, Imai M, Asano Y. Electrophysiological identification of a- and b-intercalated cells and their distribution along the rabbit distal nephron. *J Clin Invest* 1990;86:1829–1839.
346. Na KY, Oh YK, Han JS, Joo KW, Lee JS, Earm J-H, Knepper MA, Kim G-H. Upregulation of Na+ transporter abundances in response to chronic thiazide or loop diuretic treatment in rats. *Am J Physiol Renal Physiol* 2003;284:F133–F143.
347. Nadler SP, Hebert SC, Brenner BM. PGE_2, forskolin, and cholera toxin interaction in rabbit cortical collecting tubule. *Am J Physiol* 1986;250:F127–F135.
348. Nakao A, Allen ML. Regulation of cAMP metabolism by PGE_2 in cortical and medullary thick ascending limb of Henle's loop. *Am J Physiol* 1989;256:C652–C657.
349. Naray-Fejes-Toth A, Canessa C, Cleaveland ES, Aldrich G, Fejes-Toth G. sgk is an aldosterone-induced kinase in the renal collecting duct. Effects on epithelial Na+ channels. *J Biol Chem* 1999;274:16973–16978.
350. Naray-Fejes-Toth A, Fejes-Toth G. Expression cloning of the aldosterone target cell-specific 11b-hydroxysteroid dehydrogenase from rabbit collecting duct cells. *Endocrinology* 1995; 136:2579–2568.
351. Naray-Fejes-Toth A, Fejes-Toth G. Glucocorticoid receptors mediate mineralocorticoid-like effects in cultured collecting duct cells. *Am J Physiol* 1990;259:F672–F678.
352. Naray-Fejes-Toth A, Watlington CO, Fejes-Toth G. 11b-hydroxysteroid dehydrogenase activity in the renal target cells of aldosterone. *Endocrinology* 1991;129:17–21.
353. Nishida M, MacKinnon R. Structural basis of inward rectification: cytoplasmic pore of the G protein-gated inward rectifier GIRK1 at 1.8 A resolution. *Cell* 2002;111:957–965.
354. Nishimura H, Imai M, Ogawa M. Diluting segment in avian kidney. I. Characteristics of transepithelial voltages. *Am J Physiol* 1986;250:R333–R340.
355. Nishimura H, Koseki C, Imai M, Braun EJ. Sodium chloride and water transport in the thin descending limb of Henle of the quail. *Am J Physiol* 1989;257:F994–F1002.
356. Noland TD, Carter CE, Jacobson HR, Breyer MD. PGE2 regulates cAMP production in cultured rabbit CCD cells: evidence for dual inhibitory mechanisms. *Am J Physiol* 1992;263: C1208–C1215.
357. Nonoguchi H, Knepper MA, Manganiello VC. Effects of atrial natriuretic factor on cyclic guanosine monophosphate and cyclic adenosine monophosphate accumulation in microdissected nephron segments from rats. *J Clin Invest* 1987;79:500–507.
358. Nonoguchi H, Sands JM, Knepper MA. ANF inhibits NaCl and fluid absorption in cortical collecting duct of rat kidney. *Am J Physiol* 1989;256:F179–F186.
359. Oberleithner H, Guggino W, Giebisch G. The effect of furosemide on luminal sodium, chloride and potassium transport in the early distal tubule of *Amphiuma* kidney: effects of potassium adaptation. *Pflugers Arch* 1983;396:27–33.
360. Oberleithner H, Guggino W, Giebisch G. Mechanism of distal tubular chloride transport in *Amphiuma* kidney. *Am J Physiol* 1982;242:F331–F339.
361. Oberleithner H, Lang F, Wang W, Giebisch G. Effects of inhibition of chloride transport on intracellular sodium activity in distal amphibian nephron. *Pflugers Arch* 1982;394:55–60.
362. Oberleithner H, Lang F, Wang W, Messner G, Deetzen P. Evidence for an amiloride-sensitive Na^+ pathway in the amphibian diluting segment induced by K^+ adaptation. *Pflugers Arch* 1982;399:166–172.

363. Oberleithner H, Weigt M, Westphale HJ, et al. Aldosterone activates Na+/H+ exchange and raises cytoplasmic pH in target cells of the amphibian kidney. *Proc Natl Acad Sci U S A* 1987; 84:1464–1468.

364. Obermuller N, Bernstein P, Velazquez H, Reilly R, Moser D, Ellison DH, Bachmann S. Expression of the thiazide-sensitive Na-Cl cotransporter in rat and human kidney. *Am J Physiol* 1995;269:F900–F910.

365. Odgaard E, Jakobsen JK, Frische S, Praetorius J, Nielsen S, Aalkjaer C, Leipziger J. Basolateral Na+-dependent HCO₃⁻ transporter NBCn1-mediated HCO₃⁻ influx in rat medullary thick ascending limb. *J Physiol (Lond)* 2004;555:205–218.

366. O'Grady SM, Musch MW, Field M. Stoichiometry and ion affinities of the Na-K-Cl cotransport system in the intestine of the winter flounder (*Pseudopleuronectes americanus*). *J Membr Biol* 1986;91:33–41.

367. Oh Y, Smith PR, Bradford AL, Keeton D, Benos DJ. Regulation by phosphorylation of purified epithelial Na+ channels in planar lipid bilayers. *Am J Physiol* 1993;265:C85–C91.

368. Omata K, Carretero OA, Scicli AG, Jackson BA. Localization of active and inactive kallikrein (kininogenase activity) in the microdissected rabbit nephron. *Kidney Int* 1982; 22: 602–607.

369. O'Neil RG. Aldosterone regulation of sodium and potassium transport in the cortical collecting duct. *Semin Nephrol* 1990;10:365–374.

370. O'Neil RG, Hayhurst RA. Sodium-dependent modulation of the renal Na-K-ATPase: Influence of mineralocorticoids on the cortical collecting duct. *J Membr Biol* 1985;85:169–179.

371. O'Neil RG, Helman SI. Transport characteristics of renal collecting tubules: influences of DOCA and diet. *Am J Physiol* 1977;233:F544–F558.

372. O'Neil RG, Sansom SC. Characterization of apical cell membrane Na⁺ and K⁺ conductances of cortical collecting duct using microelectrode techniques. *Am J Physiol* 1984;247:F14–F24.

373. Ortiz P, Garvin J. Cardiovascular and renal control in NOS-deficient mouse models. *Am J Physiol Regul Integr Comp* 2003;284:R628–R638.

374. Ortiz PA, Garvin JL. Role of nitric oxide in the regulation of nephron transport. *Am J Physiol Renal Physiol* 2002;282:F777–F784.

375. Ortiz PA, Hong NJ, Garvin JL. NO decreases thick ascending limb chloride absorption by reducing Na+-K+-2Cl- cotransporter activity. *Am J Physiol Renal Physiol* 2001;281:F819–F825.

376. O'Shaughnessy K, Karet F. Salt handling and hypertension. *J Clin Invest* 2004;113:1075–1081.

377. Pacha J, Frindt G, Antonian L, Silver RB, Palmer LG. Regulation of Na channels of the rat cortical collecting tubule by aldosterone. *J Gen Physiol* 1993;102:25–42.

378. Palmer LG. Interactions of amiloride and other blocking cations with the apical Na channel in the toad urinary bladder. *J Membr Biol* 1985;87:191–199.

379. Palmer LG, Antonian L, Frindt G. Regulation of the Na-K pump of the rat cortical collecting tubule by aldosterone. *J Gen Physiol* 1993;102:43–57.

380. Palmer LG, Frindt G. Amiloride-sensitive Na channels from the apical membrane of the rat cortical collecting tubule. *Proc Natl Acad Sci U S A* 1986;83:2767–2770.

381. Palmer LG, Li JH, Lindemann B, Edelman IS. Aldosterone control of the density of sodium channels in the toad urinary bladder. *J Membr Biol* 1982;64:91–102.

382. Palmer LG, Sackin H, Frindt G. Regulation of Na+ channels by luminal Na+ in rat cortical collecting tubule. *J Physiol* 1998;509:151–162.

383. Park J, Leong MLL, Buse P, Maiyar AC, Firestone GL, Hemmings BA. Serum and glucocorticoid-inducible kinase (SGK) is a target of the PI 3–kinase-stimulated signaling pathway. *EMBO J* 1999;18:3024–3033.

384. Paulais M, Teulon J. cAMP-activated chloride channel in the basolateral membrane of the thick ascending limb of the mouse kidney. *J Membr Biol* 1990;113:253–260.

385. Payne JA, Forbush B 3rd. Alternatively spliced isoforms of the putative renal Na-K-Cl cotransporter are differentially distributed within the rabbit kidney. *Proc Natl Acad Sci U S A* 1994;91:4544–4548.

386. Payne JA, Xu JC, Haas M, Lytle CY, Ward D, Forbush B 3rd. Primary structure, functional expression, and chromosomal localization of the bumetanide-sensitive Na-K-Cl cotransporter in human colon. *J Biol Chem* 1995;270:17977–17985.

387. Pearce D, Yamamoto KR. Mineralocorticoid and glucocorticoid receptor activities by nonreceptor factors at a composite response element. *Science* 1993;259:1161–1165.

388. Peti-Peterdi J, Komlosi P, Fuson AL, Guan Y, Schneider A, Qi Z, Redha R, Rosivall L, Breyer MD, Bell PD. Luminal NaCl delivery regulates basolateral PGE2 release from macula densa cells. *J Clin Invest* 2003;112:76–82.

389. Peti-Peterdi J, Warnock DG, Bell PD. Angiotensin II directly stimulates ENaC activity in the cortical collecting duct via AT1 receptors. *J Am Soc Nephrol* 2002;13:1131–1135.

390. Petty KJ, Kokko JP, Marver D. Secondary effect of aldosterone on Na-K-ATPase activity in the rabbit cortical collecting tubule. *J Clin Invest* 1981;68:1514–1521.

391. Plata C, Meade P, Hall A, Welch RC, Vazquez N, Hebert SC, Gamba G. Alternatively spliced isoform of apical Na+-K+-Cl[-] cotransporter gene encodes a furosemide-sensitive Na+-Cl[-]cotransporter. *Am J Physiol Renal Physiol* 2001;280:F574–F582.

392. Plata C, Meade P, Vazquez N, Hebert SC, Gamba G. Functional properties of the apical Na+-K+-2Cl- cotransporter isoforms. *J Biol Chem* 2002;277:11004–11012.

393. Plata C, Mount DB, Rubio V, Hebert SC, Gamba G. Isoforms of the Na-K-2Cl cotransporter in murine TAL II. Functional characterization and activation by cAMP. *Am J Physiol Renal Physiol* 1999;276:F359–F366.

394. Plato C, Shesely E, Garvin J. eNOS mediates L-arginine-induced inhibition of thick ascending limb chloride flux. *Hypertension* 2000;35:319–323.

395. Plato CF, Stoos BA, Wang D, Garvin JL. Endogenous nitric oxide inhibits chloride transport in the thick ascending limb. *Am J Physiol Renal Physiol* 1999;276:F159–F163.

396. Plotkin MD, Kaplan MR, Verlander JW, Lee WS, Brown D, Poch E, Gullans SR, Hebert SC. Localization of the thiazide sensitive Na-Cl cotransporter, rTSC1 in the rat kidney. *Kidney Int* 1996;50:174–183.

397. Pollak MR, Delaney VB, Graham RM, Hebert SC. Gitelman's syndrome (Bartter's variant) maps to the thiazide-sensitive cotransporter gene locus on chromosome 16q13 in a large kindred. *J Am Soc Nephrol* 1996;7:2244–2248.

398. Proud D, Nakamura S, Carone FA, Herring PL, Kawamura M, Inagami T, Pisano JJ. Kallikrein-kinin and renin-angiotensin systems in rat renal lymph. *Kidney Int* 1984;25:880–885.

399. Pusch M, Ludewig U, Rehfeldt A, Jentsch TJ. Gating of the voltage-dependent chloride channel ClC-0 by the permeant anion. *Nature* 1995;373:527–531.

400. Rane S, Aperia A. Ontogeny of Na-K-ATPase activity in thick ascending limb and of concentrating capacity. *Am J Physiol* 1985;249:F723–F728.

401. Reeves WB, Andreoli TE. Cl⁻ transport in basolateral renal medullary vesicles. II. Cl⁻ channels in planar lipid bilayers. *J Membr Biol* 1990;113:57–65.s

402. Reeves WB, Andreoli TE. Nephrogenic diabetes insipidus. In: Scriver CR, Beaudet AL, Sly WS, Valle D, eds. *The Metabolic and Molecular Bases of Inherited Disease*, 7th ed. New York: McGraw-Hill; 1995:3045–3072.

403. Reeves WB, Andreoli TE. Tubular sodium transport. In: Schrier RW, ed. *Diseases of the Kidney and Urinary Tract*, 7th ed. Philadelphia: Lippincott Williams & Wilkins; 2001: 135–176.

404. Reeves WB, McDonald GA, Mehta P, Andreoli TE. Activation of K⁺ channels in renal medullary vesicles by cAMP-dependent protein kinase. *J Membr Biol* 1989;109:65–72.

405. Reeves WB, Molony DA. The physiology of loop diuretic action. *Semin Nephrol* 1988;8: 225–233.

406. Reeves WB, Winters CJ, Filipovic DM, Andreoli TE. Cl⁻ channels in basolateral renal medullary vesicles. IX. Channels from mouse MTAL cell patches and medullary vesicles. *Am J Physiol* 1995;269:F621–F627.

407. Reeves WB, Winters CJ, Zimniak L, Andreoli TE. Properties and regulation of medullary thick limb basolateral Cl⁻ channels. *Kidney Int Suppl* 1998;65:S24–S28.

408. Reif MC, Troutman SL, Schafer JA. Sodium transport by rat cortical collecting tubule. Effects of vasopressin and desoxycorticosterone. *J Clin Invest* 1986;77:1291–1298.

409. Reif MC, Troutman SL, Schafer JA. Sustained response to vasopressin in isolated rat cortical collecting tubules. *Kidney Int* 1984;26:725–732.

410. Riccardi D, Hall AE, Chattopadhyay N, Xu JZ, Brown EM, Hebert SC. Localization of the extracellular Ca2+/polyvalent cation-sensing protein in rat kidney. *Am J Physiol* 1998;274: F611–F622.

411. Riccardi D, Lee WS, Lee K, Segre GV, Brown EM, Hebert SC. Localization of the extracellular Ca(2+)-sensing receptor and PTH/PTHrP receptor in rat kidney. *Am J Physiol* 1996;271:F951–F956.

412. Rocha AS, Kokko JP. Sodium chloride and water transport in the medullary thick ascending limb of Henle. *J Clin Invest* 1973;52:612–623.

413. Rocha AS, Kudo LH. Atrial peptide and cGMP effects on NaCl transport in inner medullary collecting duct. *Am J Physiol* 1990;259:F258–F268.

414. Rocha AS, Kudo LH. Factors governing sodium and chloride transport across the inner medullary collecting duct. *Kidney Int* 1990;38:654–667.

415. Rocha AS, Kudo LH. Water, urea, sodium, chloride, potassium transport in the in vitro perfused papillary collecting duct. *Kidney Int* 1982;22:485–491.

416. Rogers PW, Flynn JJ III, Kurtzman NA. The effect of mineralocorticoid deficiency on renal concentrating and diluting capacity. *Proc Soc Exp Biol Med* 1975;148:847–853.

417. Rokaw MD, Wang JM, Edinger RS, Weisz OA, Hui D, Middleton P, Shlyonsky V, Berdiev BK, Ismailov I, Eaton DC, Benos DJ, Johnson JP. Carboxylmethylation of the beta subunit of xENaC regulates channel activity. *J Biol Chem* 1998;273:28746–28751.

418. Rouch AJ, Chen L, Troutman SL, Schafer JA. Na⁺ transport in isolated rat CCD: effects of bradykinin, ANP, clonidine, and hydrochlorothiazide. *Am J Physiol* 1991;260:F86–F95.

419. Ruggles BT, Murayama N, Werness JL, Gapstur SM, Bentley MD, Dousa TP. The vasopressin-sensitive adenylate cyclase in collecting tubules and in thick ascending limb of Henle's loop of human and canine kidney. *J Clin Endocrinol Metab* 1985;60:914–921.

420. Ruknudin A, Schulze DH, Sullivan SK, Lederer WJ, Welling PA. Novel subunit composition of a renal epithelial KATP channel. *J Biol Chem* 1998;273:14165–14171.

421. Rundle SE, Funder JW, Lakshmi V, Monder C. The intrarenal localization of mineralocorticoid receptors and 11 beta-dehydrogenase: immunocytochemical studies. *Endocrinology* 1989;125:1700–1704.

422. Rusvai E, Naray-Fejes-Toth A. A new isoform of 11b-hydroxysteroid dehydrogenase in aldosterone target cells. *J Biol Chem* 1993;268:10717–10720.

423. Sabath E, Meade P, Berkman J, Heros Pdl, Moreno E, Bobadilla NA, Vazquez N, Ellison DH, Gamba G. Pathophysiology of functional mutations of the thiazide-sensitive Na-Cl cotransporter in Gitelman disease. *Am J Physiol Renal Physiol* 2004;287:F195–F203.

424. Saito-Ohara F, Uchida S, Takeuchi Y, Sasaki S, Hayashi A, Marumo F, Ikeuchi T. Assignment of the genes encoding the human chloride channels, CLCNKA and CLCNKB, to 1p36 and of CLCN3 to 4q32–q33 by in situ hybridization. *Genomics* 1996;36:372–374.

425. Sakairi Y, Jacobson HR, Noland TD, Breyer MD. Luminal prostaglandin E receptors regulate salt and water transport in rabbit cortical collecting duct. *Am J Physiol* 1995;269:F257–F265.

426. Sands JM, Knepper MA. Urea permeability of mammalian inner medullary collecting duct system and papillary surface epithelium. *J Clin Invest* 1987;79:138–147.

427. Sands JM, Nonoguchi H, Knepper MA. Hormone effects on NaCl permeability of rat inner medullary collecting duct. *Am J Physiol* 1988;255:F421–F428.

428. Sands JM, Nonoguchi H, Knepper MA. Vasopressin effects on urea and H2O transport in inner medullary collecting duct subsegments. *Am J Physiol* 1987;253:F823–F832.

429. Sansom S, Muto S, Giebisch G. Na-dependent effects of DOCA on cellular transport properties of CCDs from ADX rabbits. *Am J Physiol* 1987;253:F753–F759.

430. Sansom SC, Agulian S, Muto S, Illig V, Giebisch G. K activity of CCD principal cells from normal and DOCA-treated rabbits. *Am J Physiol* 1989;256:F136–F142.

431. Sansom SC, La BQ, Carosi SL. Double-barreled chloride channels of collecting duct basolateral membrane. *Am J Physiol* 1990;259:F46–F52.

432. Sansom SC, O'Neil RG. Effects of mineralocorticoids on transport properties of cortical collecting duct basolateral membrane. *Am J Physiol* 1986;251:F743–F757.

433. Sansom SC, O'Neil RG. Mineralocorticoid regulation of apical cell membrane Na⁺ and K⁺ transport of the cortical collecting duct. *Am J Physiol* 1985;248:F858–F868.

434. Sansom SC, Weinman EJ, O'Neil RG. Microelectrode assessment of chloride conductive properties of cortical collecting duct. *Am J Physiol* 1984;247:F291–F302.

435. Sariban-Sohraby S, Burg M, Wiesmann WP, Chiang PK, Johnson JP. Methylation increases sodium transport into A6 apical membrane vesicles: possible mode of aldosterone action. *Science* 1984;225:745–674.
436. Sariban-Sohraby S, Fisher RS, Abramow M. Aldosterone-induced and GTP-stimulated methylation of a 90-kDa polypeptide in the apical membrane of A6 epithelia. *J Biol Chem* 1993;268:26613–26617.
437. Sasaki S, Imai M. Effects of vasopressin on water and NaCl transport across the in vitro perfused medullary thick ascending limb of Henle's loop of mouse, rat, and rabbit kidneys. *Pflugers Arch* 1980;383:215–221.
438. Sasano H, Fukushima K, Sasaki I, Matsuno S, Nagura H, Krozowski ZS. Immunolocalization of mineralocorticoid receptor in human kidney, pancreas, salivary, mammary and sweat glands: a light and electron microscopic immunohistochemical study. *J Endocrinol* 1992; 132:305–310.
439. Schafer JA, Troutman SL. cAMP mediates the increase in apical membrane Na^+ conductance produced in rat CCD by vasopressin. *Am J Physiol* 1990;259:F823–F831.
440. Schafer JA, Troutman SL, Schlatter E. Vasopressin and mineralocorticoid increase apical membrane driving force for K^+ secretion in rat CCD. *Am J Physiol* 1990;258:F199–F210.
441. Schild L. The epithelial sodium channel: from molecule to disease. *Rev Physiol Biochem Pharmacol* 2004;151:93–107.
442. Schild L, Canessa CM, Shimkets RA, Gautschi I, Lifton RP, Rossier BC. A mutation in the epithelial sodium channel causing Liddle disease increases channel activity in the *Xenopus* laevis oocyte expression system. *Proc Natl Acad Sci U S A* 1995;92:5699–703.
443. Schild L, Lu Y, Gautschi I, Schneeberger E, Lifton RP, Rossier BC. Identification of a PY motif in the epithelial Na channel subunits as a target sequence for mutations causing channel activation found in Liddle syndrome. *EMBO J* 1996;15:2381–237.
444. Schlatter E, Cermak R, Forssmann WG, Hirsch JR, Kleta R, Kuhn M, Sun D, Schafer JA. cGmp-activating peptides do not regulate electrogenic electrolyte transport in principal cells of rat Ccd. *Am J Physiol* 1996;271:F1158–F1165.
445. Schlatter E, Greger R. cAMP increases the basolateral Cl^- conductance in the isolated perfused medullary thick ascending limb of Henle's loop of the mouse. *Pflugers Arch* 1985; 405:367–376.
446. Schlatter E, Greger R, Schafer JA. Principal cells of cortical collecting ducts are not a route of transepithelial Cl^- transport. *Pflugers Arch* 1990;417:317–323.
447. Schlatter E, Schafer JA. Electrophysiological studies in principal cells of rat cortical collecting tubules. ADH increases the apical membrane Na+-conductance. *Pflugers Arch Eur J Physiol* 1987;409:81–92.
448. Schmitt R, Ellison DH, Farman N, Rossier BC, Reilly RF, Reeves WB, Oberbaumer I, Tapp R, Bachmann S. Developmental expression of sodium entry pathways in rat nephron. *Am J Physiol Renal Physiol* 1999;276:F367–F381.
449. Schnermann J, Briggs J, Schubert G. In situ studies of the distal convoluted tubule in the rat. I. Evidence for NaCl secretion. *Am J Physiol* 1982;243:F160–F166.
450. Schuster VL. Mechanism of bradykinin, ADH, cAMP interaction in rabbit cortical collecting duct. *Am J Physiol* 1985;249:F645–F653.
451. Schuster VL, Kokko JP, Jacobson HR. Interactions of lysyl-bradykinin and antidiuretic hormone in the rabbit cortical collecting tubule. *J Clin Invest* 1984;73:1659–1667.
452. Schwalbe RA, Bianchi L, Accili EA, Brown AM. Functional consequences of ROMK mutants linked to antenatal Bartter's syndrome and implications for treatment. *Hum Mol Genet* 1998;7:975–980.
453. Schwartz GJ, Burg MB. Mineralocorticoid effects on cation transport by cortical collecting tubules in vivo. *Am J Physiol* 1978;235:F576–F585.
454. Shanley PF, Johnson GC. Adenine nucleotides, transport activity and hypoxic necrosis in the thick ascending limb of Henle. *Kidney Int* 1989;36:823–830.
455. Shareghi GR, Stoner LC. Calcium transport across segments of the rabbit distal nephron in vitro. *Am J Physiol* 1978;235:F367–F375.
456. Shimizu T, Nakamura M, Yoshitomi K, Imai M. Effects of prostaglandin E2 on membrane voltage of the connecting tubule and cortical collecting duct from rabbits. *J Physiol* 1993; 462:275–289.
457. Shimizu T, Yoshitomi K, Nakamura M, Imai M. Site and mechanism of action of trichlormethiazide in rabbit distal nephron segments perfused in vitro. *J Clin Invest* 1988;82: 721–730.
458. Shimizu T, Yoshitomi K, Taniguchi J, Imai M. Effect of high NaCl intake on Na^+ and K^+ transport in the rabbit distal convoluted tubule. *Pflugers Arch* 1989;414:500–508.
459. Shimkets RA, Warnock DG, Bositis CM, Nelson-Williams C, Hansson JH, Schambelan M, Gill JR Jr, Ulick S, Milora RV, Findling JW, et al. Liddle's syndrome: heritable human hypertension caused by mutations in the beta subunit of the epithelial sodium channel. *Cell* 1994;79:407–414.
460. Silva P, Myers M, Epstein FH. Stoichiometry of sodium chloride transport by rectal gland of Squalus acanthias. *Am J Physiol* 1986;250:516–519.
461. Silver RB, Frindt G, Windhager EE, Palmer LG. Feedback regulation of Na channels in rat CCT. I. Effects of inhibition of Na pump. *Am J Physiol* 1993;264:F557–F564.
462. Simon DB, Bindra RS, Mansfield TA, Nelson-Williams C, Mendonca E, Stone R, Schurman S, Nayir A, Alpay H, Bakkaloglu A, Rodriguez-Soriano J, Morales JM, Sanjad SA, Taylor CM, Pilz D, Brem A, Trachtman H, Griswold W, Richard GA, John E, Lifton RP. Mutations in the chloride channel gene, CLCNKB, cause Bartter's syndrome type III. *Nature Genetics* 1997;17:171–178.
463. Simon DB, Karet FE, Hamdan JM, DiPietro A, Sanjad SA, Lifton RP. Bartter's syndrome, hypokalaemic alkalosis with hypercalciuria, is caused by mutations in the Na-K-2Cl cotransporter NKCC2. *Nat Genet* 1996;13:183–188.
464. Simon DB, Karet FE, Rodriguez-Soriano J, Hamdan JH, DiPietro A, Trachtman H, Sanjad SA, Lifton RP. Genetic heterogeneity of Bartter's syndrome revealed by mutations in the K+ channel, ROMK. *Nat Genet* 1996;14:152–156.
465. Simon DB, Lifton RP. Ion transporter mutations in Gitelman's and Bartter's syndromes. *Curr Opin Nephrol Hypertens* 1998;7:43–47.
466. Simon DB, Nelson-Williams C, Bia MJ, Ellison D, Karet FE, Molina AM, Vaara I, Iwata F, Cushner HM, Koolen M, Gainza FJ, Gitleman HJ, Lifton RP. Gitelman's variant of Bartter's syndrome, inherited hypokalaemic alkalosis, is caused by mutations in the thiazide-sensitive Na-Cl cotransporter. *Nat Genet* 1996;12:24–30.
467. Snyder PM, McDonald FJ, Stokes JB, Welsh MJ. Membrane topology of the amiloride-sensitive epithelial sodium channel. *J Biol Chem* 1994;269:24379–24383.
468. Snyder PM, Olson DR, Thomas BC. Serum and glucocorticoid-regulated kinase modulates Nedd4-2-mediated inhibition of the epithelial Na+ channel. *J Biol Chem* 2002;277:5–8.
469. Snyder PM, Price MP, McDonald FJ, Adams CM, Volk KA, Zeiher BG, Stokes JB, Welsh MJ. Mechanism by which Liddle's syndrome mutations increase activity of a human epithelial Na+ channel. *Cell* 1995;83:969–978.
470. Snyder PM, Steines JC, Olson DR. Relative contribution of Nedd4 and Nedd4-2 to ENaC regulation in epithelia determined by RNA interference. *J Biol Chem* 2004;279:5042–5046.
471. Song J, Hu X, Shi M, Knepper MA, Ecelbarger CA. Effects of dietary fat, NaCl, and fructose on renal sodium and water transporter abundances and systemic blood pressure. *Am J Physiol Renal Physiol* 2004;287:F1204–F1212.
472. Sonnenberg H. Renal tubular effects of atrial natriuretic factor. *Kidney Int* 1985;27:105.
473. Sonnenberg H, Honrath U, Chong CK, Wilson DR. Atrial natriuretic factor inhibits sodium transport in medullary collecting duct. *Am J Physiol* 1986;250:F963–F966.
474. Sonnenberg H, Honrath U, Wilson DR. Effects of amiloride in the medullary collecting duct of rat kidney. *Kidney Int* 1987;31:1121–1125.
475. Stanton B, Janzen A, Klein-Robbenhaar G, DeFronzo R, Giebisch G, Wade J. Ultrastructure of rat initial collecting tubule. Effect of adrenal corticosteroid treatment. *J Clin Invest* 1985;75:1327–1334.
476. Stanton BA. Characterization of apical and basolateral membrane conductances of rat inner medullary collecting duct. *Am J Physiol* 1989;256:F862–F868.
477. Stanton BA. Regulation by adrenal corticosteroids of sodium and potassium transport in loop of Henle and distal tubule of rat kidney. *J Clin Invest* 1986;78:1612–1620.
478. Starremans PGJF, Kersten FFJ, van den Heuvel LPWJ, Knoers NVAM, Bindels RJM. Dimeric architecture of the human bumetanide-sensitive Na-K-Cl co-transporter. *J Am Soc Nephrol* 2003;14:3039–3046.
479. Stephenson JL. Concentration of urine in a central core model of the renal counterflow system. *Kidney Int* 1972;2:85–94.
480. Stockand JD, Edinger RS, Eaton DC, Johnson JP. Toward understanding the role of methylation in aldosterone-sensitive Na^+ transport. *News Physiol Sci* 2000;15:161–165.
481. Stockand JD, Spier BJ, Worrell RT, Yue G, Al-Baldawi N, Eaton DC. Regulation of Na(+) reabsorption by the aldosterone-induced small G protein K-Ras2A. *J Biol Chem* 1999; 274:35449–35454.
482. Stokes JB. Effect of prostaglandin E_2 on chloride transport across the rabbit thick ascending limb of Henle. *J Clin Invest* 1979;64:495–502.
483. Stokes JB. Ion transport by the cortical and outer medullary collecting tubule. *Kidney Int* 1982;22:473–484.
484. Stokes JB. Na and K transport across the cortical and outer medullary collecting tubule of the rabbit: evidence for diffusion across the outer medullary portion. *Am J Physiol* 1982;242: F514–F520.
485. Stokes JB. Pathways of K^+ permeation across the rabbit cortical collecting tubule: effect of amiloride. *Am J Physiol* 1984;246:F457–F466.
486. Stokes JB. Potassium secretion by cortical collecting tubule: relation to sodium absorption, luminal sodium concentration, and transepithelial voltage. *Am J Physiol* 1981;241:F395–F402.
487. Stokes JB, Ingram MJ, Williams AD, Ingram D. Heterogeneity of the rabbit collecting tubule: localization of mineralocorticoid action to the cortical portion. *Kidney Int* 1981;20:340–347.
488. Stokes JB, Kokko JP. Inhibition of sodium transport by prostaglandin E_2 across the isolated, perfused rabbit cortical collecting tubule. *J Clin Invest* 1977;59:1099–1104.
489. Stone DK, Seldin DW, Kokko JP, Jacobson HR. Mineralocorticoid modulation of rabbit medullary collecting duct acidification. *J Clin Invest* 1983;72:77–83.
490. Stoner LC, Burg MB, Orloff J. Ion transport in cortical collecting tubule: effect of amiloride. *Am J Physiol* 1974;227:453–459.
491. Stoner LC, Roch-Ramel F. The effects of pressure on the water permeability of the descending limb of Henle's loop of rabbits. *Pflugers Arch* 1979;382:7–15.
492. Stoos BA, Garcia NH, Garvin JL. Nitric oxide inhibits sodium reabsorption in the isolated perfused cortical collecting duct. *J Am Soc Nephrol* 1995;6:89–94.
493. Summers RJ, Kuhar MJ. Autoradiographic localization of b-adrenoceptors in rat kidney. *Eur J Pharmacol* 1983;91:305–310.
494. Sun A, Grossman EB, Lombardi MJ, Hebert SC. Vasopressin alters the mechanism of apical Cl^- entry from Na^+:Cl^- to Na^+-K^+-$2Cl^-$ cotransport in mouse medullary thick ascending limb. *J Membr Biol* 1991;120:83–94.
495. Sun D, Schafer JA. Dopamine inhibits AVP-dependent Na+ transport and water permeability in rat CCD via a D4-like receptor. *Am J Physiol* 1996;271:F391–400.
496. Takaichi K, Kurokawa K. AVP-sensitive cAMP production is dependent on calmodulin in both MTAL and MCT. *Am J Physiol* 1989;257:F347–F352.
497. Takaichi K, Kurokawa K. High Ca^{2+} inhibits peptide hormone-dependent cAMP production specifically in thick ascending limbs of Henle. *Miner Electrolyte Metab* 1986;12:342–346.
498. Takaichi K, Kurokawa K. Inhibitory guanosine triphosphate-binding protein–mediated regulation of vasopressin action in isolated single medullary tubules of mouse kidney. *J Clin Invest* 1988;255:F834–F840.
499. Takeuchi K, Kato T, Taniyama Y, Tsunoda K, Takahashi N, Ikeda Y, Omata K, Imai Y, Saito T, Ito S, Abe K. Three cases of Gitelman's syndrome possibly caused by different mutations in the thiazide-sensitive Na-Cl cotransporter. *Intern Med* 1997;36:582–485.
500. Takeuchi Y, Uchida S, Marumo F, Sasaki S. Cloning, tissue distribution, and intrarenal localization of ClC chloride channels in human kidney. *Kidney Int* 1995;48:1497–1503.
501. Tamura H, Schild L, Enomoto N, Matsui N, Marumo F, Rossier BC. Liddle disease caused by a missense mutation of beta subunit of the epithelial sodium channel gene. *J Clin Invest* 1996;97:1780–1784.

502. Tanemoto M, Vanoye CG, Dong K, Welch R, Abe T, Hebert SC, Xu JZ. Rat homolog of sulfonylurea receptor 2B determines glibenclamide sensitivity of ROMK2 in *Xenopus* laevis oocyte. *Am J Physiol Renal Physiol* 2000;278:F659–F666.
503. Taniguchi J, Guggino WB. Membrane stretch: a physiological stimulator of Ca^{2+}-activated K^+ channels in thick ascending limb. *Am J Physiol* 1989;257:F347–F352.
504. Taniguchi J, Yoshitomi K, Imai M. K^+ channel currents in basolateral membrane of distal convoluted tubule of rabbit kidney. *Am J Physiol* 1989;256:F246–F254.
505. Terada Y, Knepper MA. Na+-K+-ATPase activities in renal tubule segments of rat inner medulla. *Am J Physiol* 1989;256:F218–F223.
506. Terada Y, Knepper MA. Thiazide-sensitive NaCl absorption in rat cortical collecting duct. *Am J Physiol* 1990;259:F519–F528.
507. Tisher CC, Madsen KM. Anatomy of the kidney. In: Brenner BM, Rector FC Jr, eds. *The Kidney*. Philadelphia: WB Saunders; 1986:3–60.
508. Tomita K, Pisano JJ. Binding of [^{3}H]bradykinin in isolated nephron segments of the rabbit. *Am J Physiol* 1984;246:F732–F737.
509. Tomita K, Pisano JJ, Burg MB, Knepper MA. Effects of vasopressin and bradykinin on anion transport by the rat cortical collecting duct. *J Clin Invest* 1986;77:136–141.
510. Tomita K, Pisano JJ, Knepper MA. Control of sodium and potassium transport in the cortical collecting duct of the rat. Effects of bradykinin, vasopressin, and deoxycorticosterone. *J Clin Invest* 1985;76:132–136.
511. Torikai S, Kurokawa K. Effect of PGE_2 on vasopressin-dependent cell cAMP in isolated single nephron segments. *Am J Physiol* 1983;245:F58–F66.
512. Trinh-Trang-Tan M, Bouby N, Coutaud C, Bankir L. Quick isolation of rat medullary thick ascending limbs: enzymatic and metabolic characterization. *Pflugers Arch* 1986;407:228–234.
513. Turban S, Wang X-Y, Knepper MA. Regulation of NHE3, NKCC2, and NCC abundance in kidney during aldosterone escape phenomenon: role of NO. *Am J Physiol Renal Physiol* 2003;285:F843–F851.
514. Uchida S, Endou H. Substrate specificity to maintain cellular ATP along the mouse nephron. *Am J Physiol* 1988;255:F977–F983.
515. Uchida S, Sasaki S, Furukawa T, Hiraoka M, Imai T, Hirata Y, Marumo F. Molecular cloning of a chloride channel that is regulated by dehydration and expressed predominantly in kidney medulla. *J Biol Chem* 1993;268:3821–3824.
516. Uchida S, Sasaki S, Nitta K, Uchida K, Horita S, Nihei H, Marumo F. Localization and functional characterization of rat kidney–specific chloride channel, ClC-K1. *J Clin Invest* 1995;95:104–113.
517. Ullrich KJ, Papavassiliou F. Sodium reabsorption in the papillary collecting duct of rats. Effect of adrenalectomy, low Na^+ diet, acetazolamide, HCO^--free solutions and of amiloride. *Pflugers Arch* 1979;379:49–52.
518. van Kuijck MA, van Aubel RA, Busch AE, Lang F, Russel FG, Bindels RJ, van Os CH, Deen PM. Molecular cloning and expression of a cyclic AMP-activated chloride conductance regulator: a novel ATP-binding cassette transporter. *Proc Natl Acad Sci U S A* 1996;93:5401–5406.
519. Vandewalle A, Cluzeaud F, Bens M, Kieferle S, Steinmeyer K, Jentsch TJ. Localization and induction by dehydration of ClC-K chloride channels in the rat kidney. *Am J Physiol* 1997; 272:F678–F688.
520. Vandorpe DH, Ciampolillo F, Green RB, Stanton BA. Cyclic nucleotide-gated cation channels mediate sodium absorption by IMCD (mIMCD-K2) cells. *Am J Physiol* 1997;272: C901–C910.
521. Vargas-Poussou R, Feldmann D, Vollmer M, Konrad M, Kelly L, van den Heuvel LP, Tebourbi L, Brandis M, Karolyi L, Hebert SC, Lemmink HH, Deschenes G, Hildebrandt F, Seyberth HW, Guay-Woodford LM, Knoers NV, Antignac C. Novel molecular variants of the Na-K-2Cl cotransporter gene are responsible for antenatal Bartter syndrome. *Am J Hum Genet* 1998;62:1332–13340.
522. Vehaskari VM, Hering-Smith KS, Moskowitz DW, Weiner ID, Hamm LL. Effect of epidermal growth factor on sodium transport in the cortical collecting tubule. *Am J Physiol* 1989;256:F803–F809.
523. Velazquez H, Bartiss A, Bernstein P, Ellison DH. Adrenal steroids stimulate thiazide-sensitive NaCl transport by rat renal distal tubules. *Am J Physiol* 1996;270:F211–F219.
524. Velazquez H, Good DW, Wright FS. Mutual dependence of sodium and chloride absorption by renal distal tubule. *Am J Physiol* 1984;247:F904–F911.
525. Velazquez H, Greger R. Electrical properties of the early distal convoluted tubules of the rabbit kidney. *Renal Physiol* 1986;9:55 (abstract).
526. Velazquez H, Greger R. Influences on basolateral K conductance of cells of early distal convoluted tubule. *Kidney Int* 1986;29:409 (abstract).
527. Velazquez H, Silva T. Cloning and localization of KCC4 in rabbit kidney: expression in distal convoluted tubule. *Am J Physiol Renal Physiol* 2003;285:F49–F58.
528. Verlander JW, Tran TM, Zhang L, Kaplan MR, Hebert SC. Estradiol enhances thiazide-sensitive NaCl cotransporter density in the apical plasma membrane of the distal convoluted tubule in ovariectomized rats. *J Clin Invest* 1998;101:1661–1669.
529. Verrey F, Kraehenbuhl JP, Rossier BC. Aldosterone induces a rapid increase in the rate of Na,K-ATPase gene transcription in cultured kidney cells. *Mol Endocrinol* 1989;3:1369–1376.
530. Vollmer M, Koehrer M, Topaloglu R, Strahm B, Omran H, Hildebrandt F. Two novel mutations of the gene for Kir 1.1 (ROMK) in neonatal Bartter syndrome. *Pediatr Nephrol* 1998;12:69–71.
531. Waldegger S, Jeck N, Barth P, Peters M, Vitzthum H, Wolf K, Seyberth H. Barttin increases surface expression and changes current properties of ClC-K channels. *Eur J Physiol* 2002;444:441–418.
532. Wang T, Agulian SK, Giebisch G, Aronson PS. Effects of formate and oxalate on chloride absorption in rat distal tubule. *Am J Physiol* 1993;264:F730–F736.
533. Wang W. Two types of K^+ channels in thick ascending limb of rat kidney. *Am J Physiol* 1994;267:F599–F605.
534. Wang W, Giebisch G. Dual modulation of renal ATP-sensitive K^+ channel by protein kinases A and C. *Proc Natl Acad Sci U S A* 1991;88:9722–9725.
535. Wang W, Lu M, Balazy M, Hebert SC. Phospholipase A2 is involved in mediating the effect of extracellular Ca2+ on apical K+ channels in rat TAL. *Am J Physiol* 1997;273:F421–F429.
536. Wang WH, Lu M, Hebert SC. Cytochrome P-450 metabolites mediate extracellular Ca(2+)-induced inhibition of apical K+ channels in the TAL. *Am J Physiol* 1996;271:C103–C111.
537. Wang W, White S, Geibel J, Giebisch G. A potassium channel in the apical membrane of rabbit thick ascending limb of Henle's loop. *Am J Physiol* 1990;258:F244–F253.
538. Wangemann P, Wittner M, DiStefano A, Englert HC, Lang HJ, Schlatter E, Greger R. Cl^- channel blockers in the thick ascending limb of the loop of Henle. Structure activity relationship. *Pflugers Arch* 1986;407:S128–S141.
539. Warden DH, Stokes JB. EGF and PGE2 inhibit rabbit CCD Na+ transport by different mechanisms: PGE2 inhibits Na(+)-K+ pump. *Am J Physiol* 1993;264:F670–F677.
540. Watts BA 3rd, Good DW. Apical membrane Na+/H+ exchange in rat medullary thick ascending limb. pH-dependence and inhibition by hyperosmolality. *J Biol Chem* 1994;269: 20250–20255.
541. Whorwood CB, Ricketts ML, Stewart PM. Epithelial cell localization of type 2 11b-hydroxysteroid dehydrogenase in rat and human colon. *Endocrinology* 1994;135:2533–2541.
542. Wiederholt M, Hansen LL. *Amphiuma* kidney as a model for distal tubular transport studies. *Contrib Nephrol* 1980;19:28–32.
543. Wiederholt M, Hansen L, Giebisch G. Dependence of distal peritubular membrane potential on luminal sodium and peritubular potassium. *Pflugers Arch* 1975;355:R55.
544. Wilson DR, Honrath U, Sonnenberg H. Furosemide action on collecting ducts: Effect of prostaglandin synthesis inhibiton. *Am J Physiol* 1983;244:F666–F673.
545. Wilson DR, Honrath U, Sonnenberg H. Thiazide diuretic effect on medullary collecting duct function in the rat. *Kidney Int* 1983;23:711–716.
546. Wilson FH, Disse-Nicodeme S, Choate KA, Ishikawa K, Nelson-Williams C, Desitter I, Gunel M, Milford DV, Lipkin GW, Achard J-M, Feely MP, Dussol B, Berland Y, Unwin RJ, Mayan H, Simon DB, Farfel Z, Jeunemaitre X, Lifton RP. Human hypertension caused by mutations in WNK kinases. *Science* 2001;293:1107–1112.
547. Wilson FH, Kahle KT, Sabath E, Lalioti MD, Rapson AK, Hoover RS, Hebert SC, Gamba G, Lifton RP. Molecular pathogenesis of inherited hypertension with hyperkalemia: The Na-Cl cotransporter is inhibited by wild-type but not mutant WNK4. *Proc Natl Acad Sci U S A* 2003;100:680–684.
548. Wilson RC, Krozowski ZS, Li K, Obeyesekere VR, Razzaghy-Azar M, Harbixon MD, Wei JQ, Shackleton CHL, Funder JW, New MI. A mutation in the HSD11B2 gene in a family with apparent mineralocorticoid excess. *J Clin Endocrinol Metab* 1995;80:2263–2266.
549. Windhager EE. Sodium chloride transport. In: Giebisch G, Tosteson DC, Ussing HH, eds. *Membrane Transport in Biology*. Vol. IV. *Transport Organs*. New York: Springer-Verlag; 1979: 145-214.
550. Windhager EE, Giebisch G. Micropuncture study of renal tubular transfer of sodium chloride in the rat. *Am J Physiol* 1961;200:581–590.
551. Wingo CS. Active and passive chloride transport by the rabbit cortical collecting duct. *Am J Physiol* 1990;258:F1338–F1393.
552. Winters CJ, Reeves WB, Andreoli TE. Cl^- channels in basolateral renal medullary membrane vesicles. IV. Analogous channel activation by Cl^- or cAMP-dependent protein kinase. *J Membr Biol* 1991;122:89–95.
553. Winters CJ, Reeves WB, Andreoli TE. Cl^- channels in basolateral renal medullary membranes. III. Determinants of single channel activity. *J Membr Biol* 1991;118:269–278.
554. Winters CJ, Reeves WB, Andreoli TE. Cl^- channels in basolateral renal medullary vesicles. V. Comparison of basolateral mTALH Cl^- channels with apical Cl^- channels from jejunum and trachea. *J Membr Biol* 1992;128:27–39.
555. Winters CJ, Reeves WB, Andreoli TE. Cl^- channels in basolateral TAL membranes. XIII. Heterogeneity between basolateral MTAL and CTAL Cl^- channels. *Kidney Int* 1998;55: 593–601.
556. Winters CJ, Zimniak L, Reeves WB, Andreoli TE. Cl^- channels in basolateral renal medullary membranes. XII. Anti-rbClC-Ka antibody blocks MTAL Cl(channels. *Am J Physiol* 1997;273:F1030–F1038.
557. Wirz H. The location of antidiuretic action in the mammalian kidney. In: Heller H, ed. *The Neurohypophysis*. New York: Academic Press; 1957:157–182.
558. Wittner M, Di Stefano A, Wangemann P, Nitschke R, Greger R, Bailly C, Amiel C, Roinel N, deRouffignac C. Differential effects of ADH on sodium, chloride, potassium, calcium, and magnesium transport in cortical and medullary thick ascending limbs of mouse nephron. *Pflugers Arch* 1988;412:516–523.
559. Wittner M, Weidtke C, Schlatter E, Di Stefano A, Greger R. Substrate utilization in the isolated perfused cortical thick ascending limb of rabbit nephron. *Pflugers Arch* 1984;402: 52–62.
560. Work J, Galla JH, Booker BB, Schafer JA, Luke RG. Effect of ADH on chloride reabsorption in the loop of Henle of the Brattleboro rat. *Am J Physiol* 1985;249:F698–F703.
561. Work J, Jamison RL. Effect of adrenalectomy on transport in the rat medullary thick ascending limb. *J Clin Invest* 1987;80:1160–1164.
562. Wright FS. Increasing magnitude of electrical potential along the renal distal tubule. *Am J Physiol* 1971;220:624–638.
563. Wulff P, Vallon V, Huang DY, Volkl H, Yu F, Richter K, Jansen M, Schlunz M, Klingel K, Loffing J, Kauselmann G, Bosl MR, Lang F, Kuhl D. Impaired renal Na+ retention in the sgk1-knockout mouse. *J Clin Invest* 2002;110:1263–1268.
564. Xu JZ, Hall AE, Peterson LN, Bienkowski MJ, Eessalu TE, Hebert SC. Localization of the ROMK protein on apical membranes of rat kidney nephron segments. *Am J Physiol* 1997; 273:F739–F748.
565. Xu ZC, Yang Y, Hebert SC. Phosphorylation of the ATP-sensitive, inwardly rectifying K+ channel, ROMK, by cyclic AMP-dependent protein kinase. *J Biol Chem* 1996;271:9313–9319.
566. Yang C-L, Angell J, Mitchell R, Ellison DH. WNK kinases regulate thiazide-sensitive Na-Cl cotransport. *J Clin Invest* 2003;111:1039–1045.
567. Yang T, Huang YG, Singh I, Schnermann J, Briggs JP. Localization of bumetanide- and thiazide-sensitive Na-K-Cl cotransporters along the rat nephron. *Am J Physiol* 1996;271: F931–F939.

568. Yoo D, Flagg TP, Olsen O, Raghuram V, Foskett JK, Welling PA. Assembly and Trafficking of a Multiprotein ROMK (Kir 1.1) Channel Complex by PDZ Interactions. *J Biol Chem* 2004;279:6863–6873.

569. Yoo D, Kim BY, Campo C, Nance L, King A, Maouyo D, Welling PA. cell surface expression of the ROMK (Kir 1.1) channel is regulated by the aldosterone-induced kinase, SGK-1, and protein kinase A. *J Biol Chem* 2003;278:23066–23075.

570. Yoshitomi K, Kondo Y, Imai M. Evidence for conductive Cl⁻ pathways across the cell membranes of the thin ascending limb of Henle's loop. *J Clin Invest* 1988;82:866–871.

571. Yoshitomi K, Koseki C, Taniguchi J, Imai M. Functional heterogeneity in the hamster medullary thick ascending limb of Henle's loop. *Pflugers Arch* 1987;408:600–608.

572. Yoshitomi K, Shimizu T, Imai M. Electrophysiological evidence that trichlormethiazide (TCM) acts on the luminal membrane of the connecting tubule. *Kidney Int* 1989;35:492 (abstract).

573. Yoshitomi K, Shimizu T, Imai M. Functional cellular heterogeneity in the rabbit connecting tubule. *Kidney Int* 1988;33:430 (abstract).

574. Yoshitomi K, Shimizu T, Taniguchi J, Imai M. Electrophysiological characterization of rabbit distal convoluted tubule cell. *Pflugers Arch* 1989;414:457–463.

575. Yun CC, Palmada M, Embark HM, Fedorenko O, Feng Y, Henke G, Setiawan I, Boehmer C, Weinman EJ, Sandrasagra S, Korbmacher C, Cohen P, Pearce D, Lang F. The serum and glucocorticoid-inducible kinase SGK1 and the Na⁺/H⁺ exchange reulating factor NHERF2 synergize to stimulate the renal outer medullary K⁺ channel ROMK1. *J Am Soc Nephrol* 2002;13:2823–2830.

576. Zeidel ML. Renal actions of atrial natriuretic peptide: regulation of collecting duct sodium and water transport. *Annu Rev Physiol* 1990;52:747–759.

577. Zeidel ML, Kikeri D, Silva P, Burrowes M, Brenner BM. Atrial natriuretic peptides inhibit conductive sodium uptake by rabbit inner medullary collecting duct cells. *J Clin Invest* 1988; 82:1067–1074.

578. Zeidel ML, Seifter JL, Lear S, Brenner BM, Silva P. Atrial peptides inhibit oxygen consumption in kidney medullary collecting duct cells. *Am J Physiol* 1986;251:F379–F383.

579. Zeidel ML, Silva P, Brenner BM, Seifter JL. cGMP mediates effects of atrial peptides on medullary collecting duct cells. *Am J Physiol* 1987;252:F551–F559.

580. Zhou H, Tate SS, Palmer LG. Primary structure and functional properties of an epithelial K channel. *Am J Physiol* 1994;266:C809–C824.

581. Zimniak L, Winters CJ, Reeves WB, Andreoli TE. Cl⁻ channels in basolateral renal medullary vesicles. XI. *rbClC-Ka* cDNA encodes basolateral MTAL Cl⁻ channels. *Am J Physiol* 1996;270:F1066–F1072.

582. Zimniak L, Winters CJ, Reeves WB, Andreoli TE. Cl⁻ channels in basolateral renal medullary vesicles. X. Cloning of a Cl⁻ channel from rabbit outer medulla. *Kidney Int* 1995;48: 1828–1836.

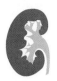

CHAPTER **32**

Mineralocorticoid Action in the Aldosterone-Sensitive Distal Nephron

François Verrey,* Edith Hummler, Laurent Schild, Bernard C. Rossier

Institute of Physiology, University of Zurich, Zurich, Switzerland
University of Lausanne School of Medicine, Lausanne, Switzerland

INTRODUCTION

General Considerations

The kidney of vertebrates plays a major role in the homeostasis of extracellular fluid. Despite large changes in water and salt intake, the kidney is able to maintain the extracellular osmolarity and volume within very narrow margins. Such fine control requires specific factors or hormones. In 1952, Simpson and Tait identified aldosterone as the most potent sodium-retaining factor in mammals. When the sodium-retaining activity of the newly identified steroid hormone was compared to that of cortisol (or corticosterone), aldosterone was found to be 3000-fold more potent in vivo. Aldosterone differs from cortisol (or corticosterone) by the presence of an aldehyde group in position 18 on the second ring. Thus, an apparently minimal change in the structure of the steroid confers on the molecule a strikingly different biological activity (see review in Simpson and Mason [314]). During the evolution of vertebrates, aldosterone appeared about 300 million years ago with amphibia, which were the first vertebrates to adapt to a dry, terrestrial environment. The high degree of conservation of the mechanisms involved in the control of sodium retention points to their biological importance. Comparative studies of physiology, biochemistry, and molecular biology helped in delineating the most significant steps involved. The three most important and conserved functions of aldosterone are to promote sodium reabsorption and to promote potassium and hydrogen secretion across certain "tight" epithelia—that is, epithelia which display high transepithelial electrical resistance and amiloride-sensitive, electrogenic sodium transport. In mammals, such epithelia are found in the distal part of the nephron, bladder, distal part of the intestine (mainly the surface epithelium of distal colon and rectum), and ducts of exocrine glands (salivary, mammary, and sweat glands). In amphibia, the collecting ducts (CDs), colon, urinary bladder, lung, and skin are aldosterone- or corticosteroid-responsive tight epithelia.

The stimulation of potassium secretion by aldosterone is important in the kidney and the colon of mammals but is not found in the amphibian or mammalian bladder or amphibian skin. The hydrogen secretion response has been identified in the reptilian (turtle) bladder and in the amphibian CD. In renal cells, the Na^+ and K^+ responses are localized in principal cells of the mammalian distal nephron or in the granular cell, the principal-cell counterpart in the amphibian bladder. In mammals, sodium and potassium balance can be achieved even in the absence of an intact colon and rectum, while bilateral nephrectomy invariably leads to death, due to the inability of the body to maintain salt and water balances.

Effects of Aldosterone on Transepithelial Sodium Transport Along Nephron and Collecting Duct: Aldosterone-Sensitive Distal Nephron

Figure 1 depicts the major nephron segments involved in salt and water reabsorption. About 90% of the filtered load is reabsorbed across the proximal tubule (PCT and PST), thin limb (TL), thick ascending limb (TAL), and proximal part of the distal convoluted tubule (DCT-1). The final regulation (plus or minus 9% of the filtered load) is hormonally regulated and takes place in the aldosterone-sensitive distal nephron (ASDN) (in yellow), which extends from the distal part of the distal convoluted tubule (DCT-2) to the end of the collecting duct (IMCD) at the papillary duct (219). The ASDN expresses the key molecules involved in the mineralocorticoid signaling pathway, that is, the mineralocorticoid (MR), or glucocorticoid (GR) receptors, 11-βHSD2, Sgk-1, Nedd4-2, ENaC, and Na^+,K^+-ATPase (217). The distribution of apically located sodium and water transport proteins in the distal nephron of rabbits, rats, mice, and humans has been recently reported, allowing anatomo-physiological correlations (34). In mice, the early portion of DCT expresses the sodium thiazide-sensitive chloride cotransporter (NCC). In the more distal part of the DCT (late DCT), there is overlapping expression between NCC and ENaC, whereas CNT is characterized by the lack of NCC expression and the expression of ENaC and aquaporin-2. The morphology of late DCT cells, CNT cells and CCD principal cells differs

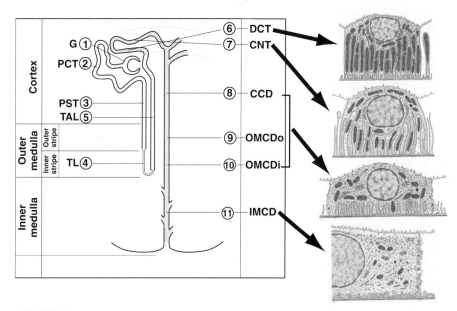

FIGURE 1 Schematic representation of a nephron. On the right (see arrows): DCT cell, a connecting tubule cell, a principal cell of cortical and outer medullary collecting duct, and a principal cell of the inner medullary collecting duct. CCD, cortical collecting duct; CNT, connecting tubule; G, glomerulus; DCT, distal convoluted tubule; IMCD, Inner medullary collecting duct; OMCD, outer medullary collecting duct; PCT, proximal convoluted tubule; PST, proximal straight tubule; TAL, thin ascending limb; TL, thin limb. (Adapted from Kriz RW, Kaissling B. Structural organization of the mammalian kidney. In: Seldin DW, Giebisch G, eds. *The Kidney*, Vol. 1, 3rd ed. Philadelphia: Lippincott Williams & Wilkins; 2000:587–654.)

markedly (196). The DCT cell is characterized by a basal membranous labyrinth, established by cellular interdigitations. The connecting tubule cell (CNT cell) is characterized by a membranous labyrinth established predominantly by infolding of the basal cell membrane. Finally, in the collecting duct of the principal cell, the basal labyrinth is exclusively established by basal infoldings. Membrane infoldings and mitochondrial density progressively decrease from late DCT to CCD, suggesting different metabolic rates. Corresponding to these anatomical features, the rate of sodium transport appears to be quite different between the CNT and CCD. Measurement of sodium fluxes in isolated rabbit CNTs (7, 307) or from rabbit CCDs (339) or rat CCDs (281), indicates at least a 10-fold difference (600–120 vs 0.2–24 pmoles sodium/min/mm in CCD). The rates of sodium transport in OMCD and IMCD are generally low (329), but have been measured only in rabbits (8 vs 1 pmoles/min/mm, respectively). CNT cells are also fully equipped with proteins necessary for responding to aldosterone (MR), 11β-HSD2, Sgk-1, Nedd-4, ENaC, and Na$^+$,K$^+$-ATPase). The CNT cell is also able to secrete potassium (227, 320), and potassium loading induces morphogenetic changes in this cell (177, 320). ROMK is expressed in the apical membrane of DCT, CNT, and CD cells (237, 375). The lack of severe disturbances of sodium and/or potassium and/or water balance in a transgenic mouse model in which ENaC activity was selectively inactivated along the entire CD (290) reemphasized the specific role of the CNT cell in the ASDN to

achieve sodium and potassium balance, even under stressful conditions such as salt restriction and/or salt and water restriction. Whereas CNT cells and CD principal cells are well-characterized target cells for aldosterone action on sodium reabsorption and potassium secretion, the situation is less clear concerning the intercalated cells involved in H/K exchange and H secretion. It is not known whether these cells express MR and 11βHSD2 activity, and the existence of an aldosterone signaling cascade remains to be experimentally demonstrated. The lack of clonal intercalated cell lines has prevented much progress along these lines.

Experimental Models for Studying Aldosterone Action In Vivo and In Vitro

IN VITRO MODELS

The effects of aldosterone on Na$^+$/K$^+$ transport have been extensively studied in vivo in a large variety of species, including rat, rabbit, human, and dog. In many cases, plasma levels of aldosterone can be varied either by steroid injection, by adrenalectomy followed by steroid substitution, or by changing Na$^+$ or K$^+$ intake. The effects of aldosterone or other mineralocorticoid hormones have been studied by a variety of in vivo, ex vivo, and in vitro experimental protocols. A summary of the most relevant references is shown in Table 1. In vivo, Na$^+$/K$^+$ urinary clearances have been performed in nonadrenalectomized and adrenalectomized animals (152, 153) and by micropuncture (127, 254). In nonadrenalectomized mammals, the *acute* effects of aldosterone on Na^+ transport appear to be small and are significant only after 24 hours. Chronic treatment with mineralocorticoids can lead to a large change in cation transport capacity accompanied by important morphological alterations of the target cell, such as membrane amplification (360). By contrast, the adrenalectomized mammals respond to aldosterone in 30–90 minutes, and Na^+ and K^+ transports are strongly regulated by mineralocorticoid hormones. Next, ex vivo organs have been treated in vitro by mineralocorticoid hormones. In 1961, Crabbé (69)

first described the Na^+ transport response in the urinary bladder of the toad in vitro. Since that time, a large number of ex vivo experimental models responsive to aldosterone in vivo or in vitro have been used, namely, toad skin (71), toad lung (96), frog colon (195), hen coprodeum (61), rabbit bladder (205), rabbit colon (145), and rat colon (145). Ex vivo tubules perfused in vitro were taken from in vivo–treated animals. Rabbit CNT (7, 307) and rabbit CCD (330) were first used for methodological reasons, but the studies were extended by the use of rat CCD and more recently mouse CCD (Table 1).

TABLE 1 Experimental Models to Study Aldosterone-Dependent Sodium Transport

	Exposure to Hormone	Measurement	Sodium Transport		References
			Control	Treated	
In Vivo					
Clearance (acute)					
Rat	4 hours (A or DOCA)	FE_{Na}	0.83%	0.067%	152
Ex Vivo					
Isolated organ or tubule					
Toad bladder	4–6 hours (A)	I_{Na}	6 $\mu A/cm^2$	15 μA	69, 270
Toad skin	4–6 hours (A)	I_{sc}	16 μA	43 μA	71
Toad lung	4–5 hours (A)	I_{Na}			96
Hen coprodeum	10 days (LS)	I_{Na}	0 μA	440 μA	61
Rabbit CNT	None	^{22}Na fluxes	20 $pEq.cm^{-1}.sec^{-1}$	7	
		V_T	−5 to −40 mV		
Rabbit CCD	80 minutes (A)	V_T	0 mV	−20 mV	127
Rabbit CCD	11–18 days (DOCA)	V_T	−6.6 mV	−53 mV	254
Rabbit CCD	10–15 days (DOCA)	V_T	−16 mV	−46 mV	304
Rabbit bladder	14 days (LS)	I_{sc}	0.8 μA	2.4 μA	205
Rabbit colon	4 hours (A)	V_T	−13 mV	−26 mV	145
Rat CCD	13–16 days (LS)	N	0	4.5	260
		P_O	0.45	0.4	
Rat CNT	Days (A)	I_{pA}	0 pA/cell	1400 pA/cell	101
Rat colon	8 hours (A)	I_{sc}	230 $\mu A/cm^2$		106, 370
Mouse CCD	Days	I_{pA}	0 pA/cell	1500 pA/cell	264, 289
In Vitro					
Primary cultures					
Mouse CCD	1–8 hours (A)	I_{eq}	10 $\mu A/cm^2$	50 $\mu A/cm^2$	273
Rat IMCD	(A)	I_{sc}	2–6 $\mu A/cm^2$	40 $\mu A/cm^2$	167, 168
Established cell lines					
Amphibian cell lines (spontaneously transformed)					
A6	1–18 hours (A)	I_{SC}	1–2 $\mu A/cm^2$	4 $\mu A/cm^2$	134
TBM,TBc	1–18 hours (A)	I_{SC}	5 $\mu A/cm^2$ 4	50 $\mu A/cm^2$	137
Mammalian cell lines (transformed)					
SV40 (constitutive promotor) transformed mammalian CCD cell lines					
M1 cells	24 hours (D)	I_{SC}	0 $\mu A/cm^2$	70 $\mu A/cm^2$	331
RCCD1		I_{SC}	4 $\mu A/cm^2$	No data	38
RCCD2	0–4 hours (A)	I_{SC}	1–2 $\mu A/cm^2$	6–8 $\mu A/cm^2$	204
SV40 (inducible promotor)					
mpk CCD_{cl14}	0–8 hours (A)	I_{SC}	10 $\mu A/cm^2$	50 $\mu A/cm^2$	27
	1–18 hours (A)				
Mammalian cell lines (spontaneously transformed)					
mCCD clone 1	0–24 hours (A)	I_{SC}	10 $\mu A/cm^2$	50 $\mu A/cm^2$	111
	1–18 hours (A)				

Open tubules are taken from in vivo–treated animals for whole-cell patch clamp, including rat CCD (103, 263, 281), rat CNT (101), mouse CCD (264, 289), and rabbit CCD (142). Other in vitro experiments include primary culture or established cell lines. Cell culture systems have also been very useful in characterizing the aldosterone response in vitro. Primary cultures of adult CCD (76, 155, 200, 328), neonatal rabbit kidney (128), and inner medullary collecting ducts (IMCD) are responsive to aldosterone (169), but the quantity of cells available limits their use for studying the action of aldosterone at the molecular level.

Handler et al. (137) established or characterized cell lines from the *Xenopus laevis* kidney (A6) and from the toad urinary bladder (TBM, TBc). These epithelial cell lines, which can be cloned, differentiate in culture; furthermore, their responses to mineralocorticoids are qualitatively and quantitatively similar to those of the toad bladder (136). Until recently, the culture of mammalian cells responding to aldosterone has been less successful. A cortical collecting duct cell line (M1) has been developed (331). This cell line requires dexamethasone, a synthetic glucocorticoid, to establish a transepithelial amiloride-sensitive transport, but is not sensitive to aldosterone. A rat CCD (RCCD1) cell line was also established, but does not respond to aldosterone (38). In contrast, aldosterone triggers both early nongenomic and late genomic increase in sodium transport in another cell subclone (RCCD2) (77, 204). Another cell line was established by Bens et al. (27) from a transgenic mouse expressing SV40 antigen in the CCD. This cell line conserved a high level of epithelial differentiation and sodium transport is upregulated by a relatively high concentration of aldosterone

(nanomolar range). More recently, the mCCD clonal cell line (mCCDcl1) displays some novel and interesting phenotypes, such as high sensitivity to low concentrations of aldosterone (subnanomolar range), vasopressin-dependent water transport, and ability to secrete potassium (111).

In Vivo Models

Because of the presence of a large number of uncontrollable variables, studies on whole animals are often not convenient for studying the molecular mechanisms of aldosterone action. However, the possibility to produce gene-modified animal models (transgenic mice) has opened the possibility to study the effect of specific molecular defects in vivo and their consequences at the level of aldosterone target cells. In recent years, several mouse models relevant to aldosterone action and the control of blood pressure have been published, and the main data are summarized in Table 2 and at the end of this chapter.

Extent of Na$^+$ Transport Subject to Regulation

According to the well-accepted model of epithelial Na$^+$ transport (189), the two major steps in Na$^+$ reabsorption by renal and other epithelia are (1) facilitated transport—driven by an electrochemical potential difference—across the apical membrane (from urine to cell), and (2) active transport—driven by metabolic energy—across the basolateral membrane (from cell to interstitium). It is now known that the apical-membrane entry step is mediated by Na$^+$-selective amiloride-sensitive ion channels (212), and that the exit step is catalyzed by Na$^+$,K$^+$-ATPase, the ouabain-sensitive Na$^+$ pump (151, 174). These

TABLE 2 Transgenic Mouse Models with Dysfunction in Aldosterone-Dependent Sodium/Potassium Transport

Strain	Phenotype	References
Signaling Cascade		
MR-/-	Severe PHA-1	28, 37
PPARγ	CD-specific-/- blocks thiazolidine dione-induced fluid retention	381
11 β HSD 2-/-	Severe AME	192
Sgk-1-/-	Mild PHA-1	373, 374
CHIF-/-	Mild renal and colon defect in Na/K transport	124
Endothelin receptor	Salt-sensitive hypertension	114w
ENaC		
αENaC-/- αENaC	Alveolar lung clearance failure	162
CD-specific-/- (αENaC$^{lox/lox}$ Hoxb7Cre)	No obvious phenotype	290
Transgenic αENaC-/-Tg	Mild PHA-1	163
Mutation βENaC$^{m/m}$	Mild PHA-1	272
Mutation (βENaC$^{L/L}$)	Liddle's syndrome salt-sensitive hypertension	274
βENaC-/-	Severe PHA-1	234
γENaC-/-	Severe PHA-1	20

two transport mechanisms are the rate-determining steps for transepithelial Na$^+$ transport, and therefore they are the most likely sites of action for aldosterone or for any other hormone that regulates the overall Na$^+$ reabsorption process. In fact, as will be discussed in detail, there is now abundant evidence that both apical and basolateral transport processes are affected by mineralocorticoids.

Various models for studying the response to aldosterone exhibit different maximal transport rates, and different degrees over which transport can be regulated by steroids. In the *toad urinary bladder*, "basal" transport rates measured by the short-circuit current method are around 5–10 μA/cm^2 (118), and aldosterone produces a two- to five-fold increase in transport. In the *rat colon*, in contrast, basal transport rates through amiloride-sensitive channels are lower, while tissues stimulated in vivo by adrenal steroids can have rates of 500–1000 μA/cm^2 (370). Another example of an epithelium whose transport rates can vary over a very large range is the *hen coprodeum*. The short-circuit current is immeasurable when the hens are on a high-Na$^+$ diet and have circulating aldosterone levels of less than 70 pM. However, when aldosterone is elevated to levels exceeding 500 pM by keeping the animals on a low-Na$^+$ diet, currents of over 300 μA/cm^2 are observed (62). Similarly, the *isolated, perfused rat cortical collecting duct* expresses no measurable net Na$^+$ fluxes when the animals are maintained on normal diets. When animals are placed on a low-Na$^+$ diet (to elevate endogenous aldosterone levels) or injected with mineralocorticoids, Na$^+$ reabsorption is as high as 30 pmoles/min/mm, which corresponds to about 100 μA/cm^2 (281, 339). These values match well the recently reported amiloride-sensitive current measured by cell-attached patches of mouse CCD cells (72). Under the standard salt diet, no significant amiloride-sensitive current is observed. Under 12 hours of salt deprivation, the current increases to around 100 pAmps/cell (98) and under chronic salt deprivation (1–2 weeks), the current can reach 400–500 pAmps/cell (72).

Time Course of Response to Aldosterone

Spooner and Edelman (319) first reported that the qualitative effects of aldosterone may depend on time of exposure to the hormone. They measured in the toad bladder, after a latent period lasting approximately 45 minutes, a decrease in transepithelial resistance that was well correlated with the increase in Na$^+$ transport (measured as amiloride-inhibitable short-circuit current) over the first 3 hours of stimulation. After this "early effect," the transport continued to increase during a "late phase" while the resistance remained relatively constant. The "early" and "late" responses to aldosterone can also be distinguished pharmacologically. Both sodium butyrate (342) and thyroid hormone (119) selectively block the late response (>3 hours) to aldosterone. Furthermore, the late response possibly involves the occupancy of a different set of receptors (116, 119). Within the physiological range of aldosterone concentrations, sodium transport is predicted to be

controlled in mCCD cells by MR occupancy during circadian cycles and by MR *and* GR occupancy during salt restriction (Fig. 2) (111).

The initial studies of electrical resistance suggested the possibility that the early response could be mediated by changes in apical Na$^+$ permeability and that the late

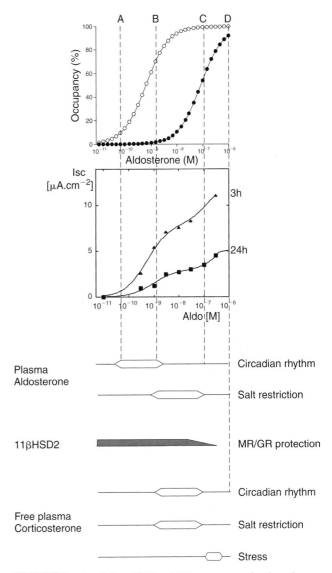

FIGURE 2 Correlation of MR and GR occupancy and early vs. late sodium transport in mCCD cells. Correlation between occupancy of MR versus GR by various agonists and the sodium transport responses I_{sc}. The relative receptor occupancy (percent of maximum binding) of MR (○) and GR (●) was computed according to the binding of MR (○) and GR (●) under binding parameters (upper panel), and sodium transport was measured by I_{sc} at 3 hours (▲) and at 24 hours (■) as shown (middle panel). Plasma aldosterone concentration and free plasma cortisol/corticosterone during circadian rhythm, salt restriction, and stress are indicated to predict receptor occupancy (dashed vertical lines) at different hormonal concentrations. The degree of MR/GR protection by 11β-HSD2 is indicated. GR, glucocorticoid receptors; MR, mineralocorticoid receptors. (In vitro data from Gaeggeler HP, Gonzalez-Rodriguez E, Jaeger NF, Loffing-Cueni D, Norregaard R, Loffing J, Horisberger JD, Rossier BC. Mineralocorticoid versus glucocorticoid receptor occupancy mediating aldosterone-stimulated sodium transport in a novel renal cell line. *J Am Soc Nephrol* 2005;16:878–891.)

response could be mediated by changes in other factors such as the Na^+ pump activity. As discussed in the following, later work has indicated that the situation is not so simple.

In the *adult rat distal colon*, the amount of amiloride-sensitive Na^+ transport is very small under normal conditions (i.e., regular diet but relatively rich in Na^+). An increase in amiloride-sensitive Na^+ transport can be induced in vitro by aldosterone, with a lag period of 2–3 hours (129, 173). Much larger currents can be measured when animals are maintained on a sodium-deficient diet to increase circulating aldosterone or by injection of corticosteroids over a period of days (370). Thus, the amiloride-sensitive short-circuit current was about 60 $\mu A/cm^2$ after 2–3 days on a low-Na^+ diet, and 400 $\mu A/cm^2$ after 30–60 days. Although apical-membrane Na^+ conductance was not measured directly, there was a significant fall in total transepithelial resistance, probably reflecting a decrease in apical resistance.

Similar results were obtained with the *rabbit CCD*. Sansom and O'Neil (296, 297) found that amiloride-sensitive apical-membrane conductance was not maximal even 24 hours after elevation of mineralocorticoids in vivo. They measured a small continued increase between 1 and 14 days after the start of injections. This could indicate that the late phase of hormone action described for the toad bladder can continue to build up the transport rate for more than 24 hours beyond the initial increase in hormone levels. Alternatively, the "very late" effects can be considered as an additional phase of hormone action. This phase may correspond to morphological changes in the cells of the CCD. Wade et al. (360) observed a twofold increase in basolateral surface area in the CCDs from rabbits stimulated with either mineralocorticoids or glucocorticoids for more than one week. The extent of such long-term morphological changes also depends on the Na^+ and K^+ intake (177), indicating that these changes are not uniquely a direct effect of the mineralocorticoid hormone, but also dependent, to some extent, on the apical Na^+ load and the extracellular K^+ level.

While the early effects of the hormone have been more extensively studied, particularly in amphibian model epithelia that can be easily stimulated in vitro, it is not clear which of the early or late response to aldosterone is more physiologically relevant to the regulation of Na^+ reabsorption in the mammalian kidney. Rapid decreases in Na^+ excretion rates in response to injections of mineralocorticoids have been observed in adrenalectomized dogs and rats but not in adrenal-intact animals (19, 152). An early increase in the rate of K^+ excretion was observed in both adrenal-intact and adrenalectomized animals. These findings are of particular interest in the rat, because the isolated CCD from a normal rat does not have any measurable rate of net Na^+ reabsorption, at least when the tubules are perfused in vitro (281, 339). Thus, this segment at least would appear to be poised for stimulation of Na^+ transport. Sansom et al (295) studied the effects of injections of deoxy-corticosterone acetate (DOCA) on the electrical properties of rabbit CCDs isolated and perfused in vitro. They found that in adrenalectomized

animals, increases in transepithelial potential and in apical Na^+ and K^+ conductances could be observed within 3 hours after injection. With adrenal-intact animals, these effects were not evident until 24 hours after the injection (296, 297). It can be hypothesized that the rapid response to mineralocorticoids in adrenalectomized animals corresponds to the early phase of aldosterone action described in amphibian epithelia and that the slower response observed in the adrenal-intact animal corresponds to the "late" response.

In summary, although such lag, early, and/or late phases of aldosterone action have been recognized in most target epithelia, there relative importance and duration can be quite different. For instance, the increase in Na^+ transport during the early response phase is proportional to the pre-existing Na^+ transport. On the other hand, tissues with high baseline transport tend to show no or little late response. This relationship has been verified in many instances in A6 epithelia, and might also be valid for mammalian target epithelia of aldosterone (143, 352).

In vivo, from a physiological or pathophysiological standpoint, the maintenance of sodium and water balance is particularly important under three distinct settings. First, normal day/night circadian regulation imply volume expansion during the day (human) or the night (rodent) and volume contraction during the night (human) or the day (rodent). Circadian variations of plasma renin and plasma aldosterone and thus variations in ENaC activity are well documented (144, 165). Second, variations in daily salt intake will affect blood volume and in turn plasma aldosterone. The earliest well-documented change in plasma aldosterone following 12 hours of salt restriction in rats is a twofold increase in plasma aldosterone and a significant increase of ENaC activity in CCD principal cells (from undetectable level to about 150/pAmp/cell) (98). Long-term salt restriction (1 to 2 weeks) will lead to maximal plasma aldosterone (without changes in plasma cortisol [human] or corticosterone [rodent]) accompanied by maximal ENaC activation (72, 260). Interestingly, the two regulations appear to take place independently of each other and both in kidney and colon. In other words the circadian regulation of sodium transport in distal colon and kidney is *maintained* when salt intake vary over a wide range (363). Finally, under stress (i.e., acute hypovolemia), both plasma aldosterone and cortisol could reach extremely high values, pushing the system to its maximal transport capacity (see discussion in Gaeggeler et al. [111]).

Mechanism for Aldosterone Action: Genomic or Classic Model

In 1964, Porter et al. (270) demonstrated that aldosterone action was dependent on de novo synthesis of RNA and protein. Synthesis of new protein was essential for both early and late mineralocorticoid responses. This original observation led to a general model for the genomic mechanism of action for aldosterone on Na^+ transport that is still accepted today (82, 115, 352). This model is depicted in Fig. 3. Aldosterone diffuses freely across the basolateral membrane and binds to a cytoplasmic receptor. The steroid-receptor complex is transported into the nuclear compartment and binds to specific hormone-responsive elements (HREs) within the promoters of a number of genes that are under aldosterone control. Then, the interaction of the steroid-receptor complex with the transcription machinery leads to an increase in transcription and to the accumulation of the corresponding mRNAs, which are, in turn, translated into their respective proteins, mediators of the Na$^+$ transport response. Four major sites of action for the mineralocorticoid hormones have been proposed and are indicated in the figure: (1) the epithelial amiloride-sensitive Na$^+$ channel or ENaC (site 1), (2) the ouabain-sensitive Na$^+$ pump or Na$^+$,K$^+$-ATPase (site 2), (3) enzymes implicated in ATP synthesis in the mitochondria (site 3), and (4) the tight junctions between the cells (site 4). Sites 1 and 2 have been most extensively studied and will be one of the major focuses of the review.

The main emphasis of this chapter will be on the physiological and molecular mechanisms of aldosterone action on Na$^+$ transport in the principal cell of the mammalian CNT/CCT or the granular cell of the amphibian bladder. We will discuss the following three aspects:

Sodium transport regulation by aldosterone: physiological and biophysical mechanisms. We will review the induced changes in Na$^+$ transport at either of the two limiting barriers, namely the apical membrane and the basolateral membrane. The role of the epithelial Na$^+$ channel and of

the ouabain-sensitive Na$^+$ pump will be emphasized. The effect on K$^+$ secretion will be mentioned only briefly and we will not discuss the mechanism by which aldosterone could promote hydrogen secretion in intercalated cells, because very little is known about the molecular aspects of this regulatory process.

Sodium transport regulation by aldosterone: cellular and molecular mechanisms. The first part will be on the interaction of aldosterone with its classical steroid receptor and its effect on transcription of a set of genes with hormone response elements and also of other inducible/repressible genes. A second important point is the question about how mineralocorticoid specificity can be achieved despite striking similarities between the mineralocorticoid and the glucocorticoid receptors. Furthermore, rapid "nongenomic" effects of corticosteroids (109, 220, 221) have been described in tight epithelia (226, 346, 356) and will be discussed in more details.

The second part will address the question of how transcriptional regulation by aldosterone leads to observed regulatory changes at the transport-protein level. On the one hand, those results obtained by investigating possible mechanisms involved in the regulation of the effectors, namely the epithelial Na$^+$ channel and the Na$^+$ pump, will be analyzed. On the other hand, this information obtained by searching first for aldosterone-regulated gene products, and then asking about their putative role in the physiological response to aldosterone, will be discussed.

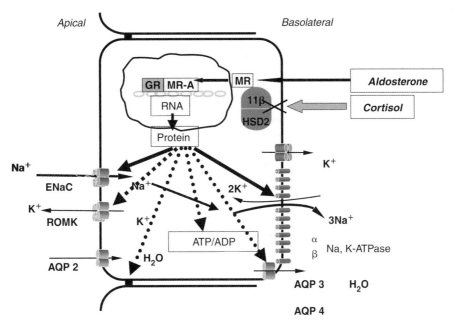

FIGURE 3 Model of the mechanism of aldosterone action in an epithelial target cell. Aldosterone crosses the plasma membrane and binds to its cytosolic receptor. Cortisone is metabolized by the 11β-HSD2 into inactive cortisol with very low affinity for mineralocorticoid receptors. The complex translocates to the nucleus, where it undergoes interaction with promoter regions of target genes, activating or repressing their transcriptional activity. Induced or repressed proteins mediate an increase in transepithelial sodium transport. The effects are produced by the activation of preexisting transport proteins (ENaC, Na,K-ATPase), and the late effect is characterized by an accumulation of further transport proteins and other elements of the sodium transport machinery. Possible effects on ROMK, tight junction proteins, mitochondria, and water transport proteins (AQP 3) are indicated with dotted arrows.

Sodium transport regulation by aldosterone: genetic evidence for the critical role of the aldosterone signaling pathway in humans and mice. We will discuss human and mouse Mendelian diseases affecting various genes involved in sodium transport regulation by aldosterone. These genes define the main limiting steps in aldosterone action and become suitable targets for drug development.

SODIUM TRANSPORT REGULATION BY ALDOSTERONE: HYSIOLOGICAL AND BIOPHYSICAL MECHANISMS

Apical Membrane

CHANGES IN APICAL MEMBRANE IONIC PERMEABILITY

Stimulation of Na^+ transport by aldosterone in vitro was first described in the toad urinary bladder by Crabbé in the early 1960s (69). Many of the early experiments supported the view that an increase in the rate of apical Na^+ entry into toad bladder cells was an important aspect of the response to the hormone (308). This experimental work included the demonstration that polygene antibiotics such as amphotericin B, which are known to form pores in biological membranes, can mimic the effect of aldosterone on the toad bladder, when added to the luminal buffer, suggesting that under nonstimulated conditions the apical entry of Na^+ into the cell was a rate-limiting step for transepithelial Na^+ transport (208). Furthermore, toad bladders treated with amphotericin B did not respond to aldosterone (70). Later it was shown in rabbit descending colon that amphotericin B increased Na^+ transport to levels similar to those measured in aldosterone-treated tissues, but did not increase Na^+ transport in colons previously stimulated by aldosterone (105). The conclusion of these experiments was that the primary effect of both aldosterone and amphotericin was on the apical membrane to promote Na^+ entry into the cell by increasing the membrane conductance to Na^+ ions.

The effect of aldosterone on the apical membrane permeability to Na^+ ions could further be demonstrated by electrophysiological techniques. Combined with tracer flux measurements, these techniques allowed the distinction of conductances through "active transcellular" and "passive paracellular" pathways of the electrical equivalent circuit of the toad bladder, and provided evidences that aldosterone increased conductance of the active transcellular pathway (294). In the rabbit urinary bladder, Lewis and Diamond showed that elevation of the aldosterone level in vivo resulted in an increase of the short-circuit current and a proportional rise in amiloride-sensitive transepithelial conductance in vitro (205). These studies could not distinguish between changes in the conductance of the apical or basolateral membrane. The first clear demonstration of aldosterone effects on the apical membrane Na^+ conductance came from Nagel and Crabbé's work using intracellular mi-

croelectrodes to study the contribution of apical and basolateral resistances to the electrical properties of the whole epithelium of toad skin (245). This approach showed that the resistance of the apical membrane decreases in the presence of aldosterone consistent with an increase in Na^+ entry. This aldosterone-induced increase in an amiloride-sensitive conductance was also confirmed in a cultured renal amphibian cell line A6 (371). Importantly, this conductance increase was not due to an increase in membrane surface area as measured by apical membrane capacitance. Through measurements of intracellular Na^+ activity in rabbit urinary bladder cells, it was shown that aldosterone depolarizes the apical membrane voltage, increases Na^+ transport (as measured by short-circuit current), and increases intracellular Na^+ (81). Therefore, the increase in Na^+ influx across the apical membrane by aldosterone occurred despite a decrease in the electro-chemical driving force for Na^+, implying an increase in the apical membrane permeability to Na^+ ions. Using cable analysis to measure transepithelial, as well as apical and basolateral conductances in the rabbit CCD, Sansom and O'Neil (296) could detect an increase in the apical amiloride-sensitive conductance after mineralocorticoid injection in these animals.

In tight epithelia, measurements of current fluctuations induced by the reversible block of the Na^+ channel with amiloride provided evidence that Na^+ enters the epithelial cells across the apical membrane through Na^+-selective channels (212). This technique performed in a variety of aldosterone-sensitive epithelia including frog skin, toad urinary bladder, hen coprodeum, rabbit descending colon or rabbit urinary bladder indicated that apical Na^+ channels are low in conductance (<5 pS) and carry currents of less than 0.5 pA under short-circuited conditions (265). Applying this technique to the toad urinary bladder, it was shown that aldosterone increased the density of active channels at the cell surface, without affecting the single-channel current. Thus, according to this approach, the effect of the hormone on Na^+ transport is due to an increase in the number of conducting channels in the membrane. Using a similar approach of blocker-induced noise analysis Baxendale et al. reported that aldosterone as well as corticosterone stimulated Na^+ transport by increasing the density of functional channels at the apical membrane in epithelia formed by the A6 cell line (24). In all these cases, the apical amiloride-sensitive channels were found to be highly Na^+ selective with a low conductance (near 5 pS for Na^+ at room temperature) and sensitive to submicromolar concentrations of amiloride.

ALDOSTERONE AND ENaC, THE EPITHELIAL SODIUM CHANNEL

The first resolution of single-channel activity of an amiloride-sensitive Na^+ channel was obtained by patch clamp techniques in cortical collecting tubules of rats maintained on a low-salt diet and in A6 cells (133, 263). As expected from noise analysis, the amiloride-sensitive Na^+ channel in the apical membrane revealed by the patch clamp technique was highly selective for Na^+ over K^+, exhibited a low Na^+ single-channel conductance (5 pS) and a high sensitivity to amiloride block (Ki less than 0.1 μM). No activity of this channel could be detected in the CCD of animals fed a normal Na^+ diet, and channel activity was greatly enhanced in animals that had been Na-depleted. Similar highly selective amiloride-sensitive Na^+ channels were also found in amphibian tight epithelia.

The primary structure of the low-conductance (5 pS), highly Na^+ selective, and amiloride-sensitive Na^+ channel has been quite difficult to establish because of low abundance of the active channel protein in the various aldosterone target epithelia. The amiloride-sensitive epithelial Na^+ channel (ENaC) was cloned from rat distal colon by functional expression in *Xenopus* oocytes (50, 51, 213). The channel is composed of three homologous subunits denoted α, β, and γ ENaC. When coexpressed in *Xenopus laevis* oocytes, the ENaC subunits form a channel with functional characteristics similar to the channel identified by Palmer and coworkers (261) in the rat CCD, a low 5-pS conductance (for Na^+), a high selectivity ratio of Na^+ over K^+ (>20), and a high sensitivity for amiloride with a Ki in the submicromolar range. These functional features strongly suggest identity between the cloned Na^+-channel ENaC and the native aldosterone-sensitive Na^+ channel described in rat CCD. In the *Xenopus* oocyte expression system, the three ENaC subunits are required for maximal expression and activity, and quantification of ENaC subunits expressed at the cell surface indicate that the subunits assemble preferentially in a heterooligomeric αβγ channel complex. This channel, which reproduces the biophysical and pharmacological properties of the native channel, is a heterotetramer made of two α subunits, one β, and one γ subunit in the sequence αβαγ (94).

The tissue distribution of ENaC is compatible with its involvement in Na^+ transport in the aldosterone-sensitive distal nephron (ASDN). Morphological and functional studies on rodent and human kidneys (17, 282) indicated that at least three successive tubule portions, that is, the late portion of the distal convoluted tubule (DCT), the connecting tubule (CNT), and the collecting duct (CD), contribute to the ASDN. Although these segments have distinct structural and functional features (216), they share in common the expression of ENaC, the mineralocorticoid receptor (MR) and the 11-β hydroxysteroid dehydrogenase type II (11-βHSD2) proteins (17).

Experimental evidence from several sources supports the fact that ENaC is the main target for aldosterone action. Rats chronically kept under aldosterone treatment or chronic low-Na diet increase the abundance of αENaC mRNA in the kidney without affecting the mRNAs encoding the β and γ subunits (14, 86, 257). In contrast, the β and γ subunit mRNAs are upregulated in the colon by aldosterone or dexamethasone while the α subunit mRNA is expressed constitutively (14, 86, 283). Coincident increase in the abundance of the αENaC subunit protein was observed (230) in the kidney, indicating that the late response of al-

dosterone is associated with an upregulation of αENaC biosynthesis.

The subcellular localization of ENaC along the ASDN axis changes drastically with the elevation of plasma aldosterone levels in response to changes in the sodium diet (218, 229). In rodents kept under a high dietary sodium intake with low plasma aldosterone levels, ENaC subunits are barely detectable at the luminal membrane and are found almost exclusively at intracellular sites, the identity of which remain to be identified. On a standard dietary sodium intake (European lab chow) with moderate plasma aldosterone levels, alpha, beta, and gamma ENaC subunits are traceable at the luminal membrane of late DCT and early CNT. However, in segments farther downstream (i.e., late CNT and CD), particularly β and γENaC subunits, remain almost exclusively localized at intracellular sites. Under a low dietary sodium intake with high plasma aldosterone levels, ENaC becomes detectable in the luminal membrane along the late DCT, CNT, and CD (218). Nevertheless, the axial gradient for apical ENaC still prevails, and the apical localization of ENaC subunits is more prominent in early ASDN than in late ASDN (218). With the use of real-time RT-PCR and immunofluorescence (Fig. 4) (219), it was shown that an aldosterone injection in adrenalectomized rats acutely induces αENaC subunit expression along the entire ASDN in 2 hours, whereas β- and γENaC are constitutively expressed. In the proximal ASDN portions only, ENaC is shifted toward the apical cellular pole and the apical plasma membrane within 2 and 4 hours, respectively.

Patch clamp techniques made possible studies of aldosterone action on ENaC activity at the apical cell surface of the ASDN. In salt-repleted animals, amiloride-sensitive ENaC currents are barely detectable in cell-attached patches of the apical membrane of rat collecting duct principal cells, ENaC channel activity increased after the animals were kept on a low salt-diet over several days (260) (Fig. 5B). Patch-clamp studies corroborated the immunohistochemically traceable axial gradient of the apical localization of ENaC (104): the ASDN segments isolated from animals kept on a standard US lab chow (that usually contains more sodium than the EC lab chow) exhibited no amiloride-sensitive currents at the single-channel level, whereas CNTs and CDs isolated from rats with elevated plasma aldosterone levels revealed significant single-channel ENaC currents (Fig. 5). In general, amiloride-sensitive currents decreased in the following order: CNT > initial CD > collecting duct (104). These findings on apical ENaC localization and activity are consistent with previous studies on microperfused rat tubules (339) and on isolated rabbit tubules (7) that established several times higher sodium transport rates in early ASDN (i.e., DCT and CNT) than in further downstream ASDN segments (i.e., CD). The axial gradient of ENaC also parallels the progressive decrease of the basolateral Na^+,K^+-ATPase activity along the ASDN (180). Taken together, the data clearly indicate that the aldosterone-dependent adaptation of renal sodium excretion to dietary sodium intake occurs through ENaC, predominantly in the early ASDN while the

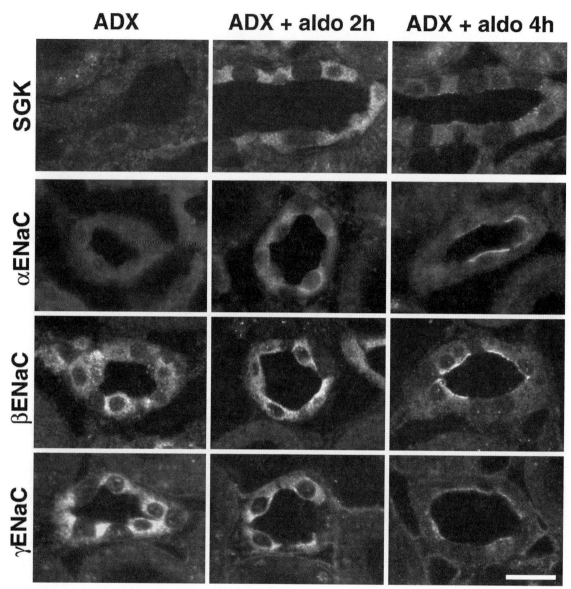

FIGURE 4 CNT profiles in kidney from ADX rats, 2 and 4 hours after aldosterone injection. Immunofluorescence with rabbit antisera against α-, β-, γENaC, and SGK on cryostat sections is shown. Unstained cells in the CNT epithelium are intercalated cells. A strong appearance of the three subunits at the apical pole of principal cells after aldosterone treatment can be observed, accompanied by a strong labeling of SGK, peaking at 2 hours. CNT, connecting tubules. (Adapted from Loffing J, Pietri L, Aregger F, Bloch-Faure M, Ziegler U, Meneton P, Rossier BC, Kaissling B. Differential subcellular localization of ENaC subunits in mouse kidney in response to high- and low-Na diets. *Am J Physiol Renal Physiol* 2000;279:F252–F258.)

late ASDN gets recruited only under high plasma aldosterone levels. The importance of the early ASDN vs. late ASDN for the maintenance of sodium balance was recently highlighted by the development of a mouse model with targeted inactivation of αENaC exclusively in the CD (290). These mice survive well and are able to maintain sodium and potassium balance, even when challenged by salt restriction or potassium loading. It is important to mention that based on ENaC current recordings, the activation ENaC after Na⁺ deprivation can account for the largest part of the reduction in Na⁺ excretion by the kidney, indicating that ENaC represents the major reabsorptive pathway for the renal adaptation to changes in the Na⁺ diet (97, 98).

How aldosterone regulates ENaC during the early and late response has been the topic of intense investigations. The long-term upregulation of ENaC by aldosterone result increase in the abundance of ENaC protein, and from a redistribution of ENaC from a cytosolic pool to the apical membrane as shown by immunohistochemistry studies. During the early response, the effect of aldosterone on ENaC channels is less clear. In vivo ENaC activity can be strongly upregulated without changes in ENaC subunit abundance, suggesting the transfer of a preexisting cytosolic pool of ENaC to the apical membrane during the early phase of the aldosterone response. When ENaC activity was assessed as whole-cell amiloride-sensitive current, 15 hours

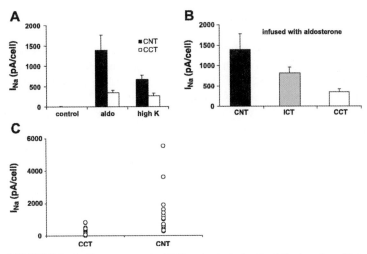

FIGURE 5 Sodium transport in CNT and principal cells of distal nephron (I_{Na}). **A:** I_{Na} in CCT and CNT of control rats fed a normal (control) diet, aldosterone-treated rats fed a normal diet, or rats fed a high-K diet. **B:** I_{Na} in cells of CCT, initial collecting tubule and CNT of aldosterone-treated rats. **C:** Individual values of I_{Na} in CCT and CNT cells of aldosterone-treated rats. CCT, cortical collecting tubules; CNT, connecting tubules. (From Frindt G, Palmer LG. Na channels in the rat connecting tubule. *Am J Physiol* 2004;286:F669–F674 with permission.)

after Na$^+$ deprivation, ENaC activity in rat CCD was drastically increased to a level that corresponded to approximately one-third to one-fourth of the level measured under chronic salt deprivation (97). Interestingly, over this 15-hour period on salt restriction, no detectable changes in the abundance of ENaC mRNA or protein could be detected, suggesting that the increase in ENaC activity does not result during the early response from changes in the biosynthesis of ENaC subunits.

Using a modified method of blocker-induced noise analysis, Helman and colleagues (143) measured the open channel probability (P_o) and the number of active channels N_T during the early phases of aldosterone action in the *Xenopus* A6 kidney cell line and found that the large increase in Na$^+$ transport rates could entirely be attributed to an increase in the number of active channels (N_T). This observation agrees with surface labeling of ENaC in A6 cells, indicating that 6 hours after aldosterone treatment, the abundance of the three ENaC subunits increases by approximately fourfold (8). The relevance of observations made on aldosterone-responding kidney cell lines for our understanding of aldosterone action in vivo remains to be clearly established. As for the kidney and the colon, differences in the modulation of ENaC subunit abundance by aldosterone during the early response exist between the ASDN and amphibian A6 cells (233).

Aldosterone and K$^+$ Secretion

The ASDN of mammals plays also a critical role in the maintenance of K$^+$ homeostasis. In this nephron segment, Na$^+$ reabsorption through ENaC is electrically coupled with K secretion: increasing the Na$^+$ influx depolarizes the apical membrane and increases the driving force for K$^+$ secretion into the lumen and vice a versa (see Fig. 2). Pathophysiological conditions where Na$^+$ absorption is increased in the ASDN (hyperaldosteronism, pseudoaldosteronism) are associated with hypokalemia; conversely, ENaC loss of function in pseudohypoaldosteronism-1 results in a loss of Na$^+$ absorption in the ASDN and a hyperkalemia. Most importantly, inactivation of αENaC along the CD in a mouse model did not impair Na$^+$ and K$^+$ balance or induce a salt-wasting phenotype. It is also well known that aldosterone given exogenously increases renal K$^+$ excretion and decreases plasma K$^+$. The αENaC expression was selectively abolished in CCD but not in the early segments of the ASDN in mice, namely late DCT and CNT (290). These animals survive well and show normal water and Na$^+$ and K$^+$ balance, even when challenged by water deprivation, K$^+$ loading, and salt restriction with plasma aldosterone concentrations similar to those of wild-type mice. We concluded that expression of ENaC in the CCD is not a prerequisite for normal Na$^+$ and K$^+$ balance in mice, which pointed to the importance of ENaC activity in the more proximal nephron segments (290).

In addition, dietary K$^+$ intake modulates K$^+$ secretion—when K$^+$ diet is high, the plasma K$^+$ concentration tends to rise and K$^+$ secretion increases in the collecting duct. A high plasma K$^+$ level not only directly influences K$^+$ excretion by the kidney, but also stimulates aldosterone secretion in adrenal glands. The question is whether aldosterone has a primary effect on K secretion via genomic effects on principal cells of the ASDN.

The K$^+$ secretion in the ASDN is mediated by a K$^+$ conductive pathway in the apical membrane of principal cells. Small conductance inwardly rectifying K$^+$ channels termed SK channels account for most of the apical conductance of principal cells (99, 100, 365). In addition, the number and the conductance of SK channels measured in the CCD can account for the K secretion reported in experiments with isolated and perfused tubules (126). These SK channels have been identified at the molecular level and are the product of the ROMK channel gene. Evidence supporting that SK channels are indeed ROMK came from the similarity of their biophysical properties, and also from the fact that in ROMK knockout mice models, SK channel activity could not be detected in the ASDN (40, 222).

Regarding the possibility that aldosterone directly regulates K^+ secretion, there is no strong evidence that aldosterone at physiological concentrations increases the apical conductance of principal cells in the CCD (262). Rats fed with a low-Na^+ diet have a high plasma level of aldosterone and show a large increase in the density of active ENaC channels in the apical membrane of principal cells, but the density of SK channels remained unchanged (126). Therefore, aldosterone per se without changes in K^+ diet or K^+ plasma levels does not increase SK activity. The activation of ENaC by aldosterone is sufficient to increase the driving force for K^+ secretion leading to an increase in the kaliuresis, without upregulating K channels.

In contrast, a high-K^+ diet increases the density of active SK channels, suggesting the presence of the kaliuretic factor that controls K secretion independently of aldosterone.

Basolateral Membrane

CHANGES IN BASOLATERAL MEMBRANE PERMEABILITY PROPERTIES

Using intracellular microelectrodes on frog skin stimulated with aldosterone, Nagel and Crabbé (245) showed that both apical and basolateral membrane conductances increased. Although the increase in basolateral conductance was low, this effect was well correlated with the increase in short-circuit current. Using the impedance analysis technique to resolve long-term changes in membrane conductances by aldosterone, Wills et al. (371) could not detect significant modifications in the basolateral membrane properties, likely because of substantial background variability. In the rabbit CCD, Sansom and O'Neil (296) observed a doubling in the basolateral membrane conductance after 24 hours of the mineralocorticoid DOCA (deoxy-corticosterone acetate) treatment, which could be accounted for by a rise in basolateral K^+ and Cl^- conductances. It is not clear in these cases whether the mineralocorticoid-induced increase in basolateral membrane conductance is a direct effect of the hormone or secondary to an increase in Na^+ entry into the cell.

An effect of aldosterone on basolateral K^+ channels was also detected in toad bladder TBM cells. In this case, it was shown that the increase in a barium-sensitive K^+ conductance took place during the early phase of the hormone action (1–3 hours) and was not dependent on apical Na^+ influx, since it was not inhibited by apical amiloride (150).

This observation is compatible with the hypothesis that aldosterone acts directly on basolateral K^+ channel function. Subsequently, a similar early aldosterone effect was observed in A6 epithelia. In this case the basolateral K^+ conductance was shown to be volume-activable and quinidine-sensitive (46).

Schultz (303) proposed that apical and basolateral conductances might be closely linked in Na^+-reabsorbing epithelia. These changes in the basolateral membrane conductances may be important to promote not only transcellular Na^+ reabsorption, but also apical potassium secretion. The increase in the rate at which Na^+ is pumped out of the cell, and hence the rate at which K^+ is pumped in, would be matched by an increase in the basolateral K^+ conductance allowing, in the absence of an apical K^+ conductance, all of the extra K^+ influx to be recycled across the basolateral membrane without changes in cell volume. In the CCD of DOCA-treated rabbits, the basolateral-membrane potential can be more negative than the equilibrium potential for K^+, favoring therefore K^+ influx into the cell. This increase in basolateral K^+ conductance could thus augment K^+ efflux across the apical membrane, and therefore promote K^+ secretion in parallel to Na^+ reabsorption.

Morphometric studies have revealed a significant increase in the basal-side surface area of the rabbit CCD principal cells that can be nicely correlated with an increase in single cell capacitance (178, 360). This change in cell surface area could only partially account for the increase in basolateral membrane conductance.

DOES Na^+ PUMP NEED TO BE REGULATED BY ALDOSTERONE?

The rate-limiting step for transcellular Na^+ reabsorption in aldosterone target epithelia is, as described previously, the epithelial Na^+ channel that controls the apical Na^+ influx into the cell. The Na^+ influx via ENaC is determined by the electrochemical driving force for Na^+ and by regulatory factors such as intracellular Na^+ that modulate the activity of Na^+ channels (115). The steady-state intracellular Na^+ concentration depends on the number, functional state, and kinetics (apparent K_m for Na^+, cooperativity) of basolateral Na^+ pumps.

Hence, from the point of view of Na^+ transport, it can be expected that aldosterone, besides regulating Na^+ channels, directly or indirectly might control the number and/or function of Na^+ pumps as well as other factors affecting the driving force for apical Na^+ influx (e.g., basolateral K^+ channels). Correspondingly, it has been shown that the single-channel current of ENaC I_{Na} remains constant over large ranges of transport rates, when the transepithelial transport is increased by aldosterone, indicating that under these conditions, the intracellular Na^+ concentration remains quite stable (35, 125). This suggests a parallel direct regulation of the Na^+ pump function by aldosterone, besides the substrate activation of pumps and the indirect regulation due to changes in

$(Na^+)_i$ produced by the aldosterone-induced increase in apical Na^+ influx. As yet it is not possible to render conclusions on the relative importance of direct regulatory changes induced by aldosterone at the level of the Na^+ pump function versus kinetic and regulatory changes secondary to changes in $(Na^+)_i$ (81).

As mentioned in the following, in the long term (late response), the number of Na^+ pumps is increased by a mechanism that has been shown, in A6 epithelia, to be initiated very early at the level of the transcription of the Na^+,K^+-ATPase genes (354). However, permissive factors, among which the intracellular Na^+ concentration level might play an important role, are certainly required to allow this aldosterone-induced regulation to take place (353).

NA⁺ PUMP

A chapter in this book is dedicated to the structure and the function of Na^+,K^+-ATPase. In brief, the basolaterally restricted Na^+ pump (Na^+,K^+-ATPase) belongs to the family of the P-type ATPases like the Ca^{2+} ATPases of the ER and the plasma membrane. This pump is electrogenic, since it exchanges three intracellular Na^+ for two extracellular K^+, per cycle, and hydrolyzed ATP. The electrogenicity of this transport process results in high transport rates that will contribute to the plasma membrane hyperpolarization, in addition to the K^+ diffusion potential. A technical aspect is that it allows the measurement of the pump function by electrophysiological means.

It appears that the major or only Na^+ pump form expressed in aldosterone target epithelia is of the $\alpha1\beta1$ type. However, a low level of $\beta3$ mRNA has been detected in *Xenopus* A6 cells (47). A small type I transmembrane protein called γ subunit is associated with the enzyme in some tissues such as the kidney. Its function is not yet elucidated, but it might play a role for the control of the K^+ activation of the pumps (26).

Before discussing the regulation of Na^+ pumps by aldosterone, it is useful to briefly mention a few points concerning the possible levels of regulation and how they can be experimentally assessed. Practically, we distinguish the following four general levels at which the actual cellular pump function can be modified:

1. *Modification of the availability of substrates.* The cooperative kinetics of the pump towards intracellular Na^+ and the relatively high apparent Km play an important autoregulatory role, since due to this kinetic behavior, a twofold increase in intracellular Na^+ concentration will lead, in the range of physiologically low intracellular Na^+ concentrations, to an approximately fivefold increase in pump function (30). This dependence of the pumping rate on the intracellular Na^+ concentration implies that the assessment of true regulatory changes requires either to know the intracellular Na^+ concentration or to control it. Limits in the availability of ATP (130) and low extracellular K^+ concentrations

can also limit the function of the Na^+,K^+-ATPase. In general, it has to be emphasized that it is the local concentration of these substrates that is relevant, and therefore, absolute control or measurement is very difficult.

2. *Alteration of the total number of pump units.* Since the number of functional pump units is large in control epithelia (1 to 10×10^6/cell) and the half-life of Na^+ pumps is long (259), it is not possible to increase the relative number of pumps rapidly (353). Technically, the assessment of the number of pumps has long been performed only using (^{3}H)ouabain binding. The interpretation of the results is, however, difficult, since the result will depend on many factors, including the functional state of pumps that need to be in a specific configuration of the reaction cycle (E2P) to bind ouabain. Hence, methods independent of the function, such as the use of antibodies, are more adequate to estimate changes in the total number of pumps, even if no absolute numbers can be derived.

3. *Changing the subcellular localization.* To measure this type of regulation, the quantity of cell surface pumps relative to the total quantity or the intracellular pool has to be evaluated.

4. *Switch between functional state.* For instance, covalent modifications or noncovalent interactions can modify the pump kinetic parameters and may turn off the pump. A general problem with the assessment of this type of regulatory changes is that they are expected to be rapidly reversible and might depend on integrity of the cell structure. This represents a technical difficulty, in particular since intracellular parameters such as the concentrations of substrates (in particular Na^+) have to be controlled or measured at the time pump function assessment to evaluate their functional state.

EARLY EFFECTS OF ALDOSTERONE ON NA⁺ PUMP FUNCTION

Due to the large number of Na^+,K^+-ATPase molecules expressed in unstimulated cells and long half-life, an increase in the rate of synthesis can impact only slowly on their total number. Thus, any major increase in the total number of functional Na^+ pumps observed within few hours has to be due to the activation and/or translocation of pre-existing pumps (353).

Based on this temporal argument, it can be inferred that aldosterone controls the function of existing pumps in cortical collecting ducts of rats. Indeed, in the 1980s, several groups reported that adrenalectomy led to a slow decrease in the CCD Na^+,K^+-ATPase (70%–86% decrease, measured as ATP hydrolysis or ouabain binding), which was reversed within 1 to 3 hours after in vivo or in vitro aldosterone addition (154, 183, 269). Thus, the total pool of pumps must remain relatively stable to allow an early (re)activation by aldosterone. If this hypothesis is correct, we expect that the total number of pumps, as well as the level of mRNA encoding the pump subunits would remain stable after adrenalectomy, despite the major decrease in functional Na^+,K^+-ATPase. Indeed, after adrenalectomy, Na^+,K^+-ATPase protein and mRNA show no change at the level of the kidney cortex and in situ hybridization experiments show only a 30% decrease of $\alpha1$ subunit mRNA and no change in $\beta1$ subunit mRNA in CCD (54, 89).

An early effect on the function of Na^+ pumps has also been observed in *Xenopus* A6 epithelia (30, 31, 268). The production of cell lines expressing an ouabain-resistant $\alpha1$ subunit allowed the electrophysiological measurement of the function of pumps containing this transfected subunit at controlled intracellular Na^+ concentrations (30). Aldosterone increased the activity of endogenous and exogenous pumps in these cells nearly twofold within its early phase of action. It was concluded that this effect could be due to the activation of a small pool of pumps that display a higher affinity to Na^+. Indeed, there was no proportional increase in the number of cell surface pumps and the effect was significant only at (physiologically) low intracellular Na^+ concentrations. No other α subunit isoform than that of the major pump population ($\alpha1$) was involved, since the stimulation was also observed on pumps containing the transfected $\alpha1$ subunit. Experiments with agents interfering with the integrity of the cytoskeleton, with the intracellular Ca^{++} concentration, and with the PKC pathway did not specifically abolish the response of the Na^+,K^+-ATPase to short-term aldosterone (F. Beron and J. Verrey, unpublished data). Thus, it is not yet known how this aldosterone-induced Na^+ pump activation observed in amphibian cells is mediated and how it relates to the reactivation of pumps in adrenalectomized rats described earlier.

An early stimulation of Na^+ pump function measured as ^{86}Rb uptake has also been observed in isolated CCDs of adrenal-intact rats (107). To what extent this effect is similar to the ones already described is also not clear. The partial resistance of this effect to the use of the translation inhibitor cycloheximide might suggest that a nongenomic mechanism played a role.

The aforementioned observations support the hypothesis that aldosterone stimulates Na^+,K^+-ATPase functioning by a pathway that does not depend on an increase in Na^+ influx via ENaC. However, the intracellular concentrations of Na^+ and K^+ are expected to play feedback and/or coregulatory roles. For instance, to maintain intracellular Na^+ within a given concentration range, the effects of intracellular Na^+ on Na^+,K^+-ATPase and ENaC function have to be in opposite directions (and not parallel as in the case of the aldosterone action). Indeed, intracellular Na^+ is known to exert negative feedback regulation on apical ENaC function and to stimulate Na^+,K^+-ATPase function (kinetic effect) and the accumulation of new pumps.

SODIUM TRANSPORT REGULATION BY ALDOSTERONE: CELLULAR AND MOLECULAR MECHANISMS

Nongenomic Actions of Aldosterone

Several studies have demonstrated the existence of rapid, nongenomic actions of aldosterone on intracellular signaling pathways of various animal and human cell types, including some aldosterone target cells (41, 60, 79, 121). These effects are characterized by a short latency of seconds or minutes and have in many cases been shown to involve the activation of a PKC. The postulated plasma membrane receptor with high affinity for aldosterone and low affinity for glucocorticoids has not yet been identified (41, 60).

One of the described nongenomic effects is the stimulation of the Na^+/H^+ exchange in epithelial cells (255, 358). The resulting change in intracellular pH might modulate plasma membrane K^+ and Na^+ conductances, and thus impact transepithelial electrolyte transport by itself or together with classical genomic effects (140). Recently, a nongenomic effect on transepithelial Na^+ transport has been demonstrated in cultured rat cortical collecting duct cells (204). In this case, PKC was shown to be involved and cross-talk with the genomic action of aldosterone was proposed. Another example of nongenomic effect in kidney tubule is the stimulation of the luminal H^+ pump of type-A intercalated cells (372). This effect was characterized by a transient rise in intracellular calcium and a requirement for intact PCK.

Nongenomic effects have been described in several nonepithelial tissues, in particular in the heart and endothelial cells (41, 60). An interesting case of vascular nongenomic aldosterone effect in kidney afferent arterioles has been described recently (345). In this case, the transcription-independent effect appeared to be initiated by binding of aldosterone to the MR and to involve PI-3 kinase, protein kinase B, heat shock protein 90 and NO generation.

Together, the number of different nongenomic effects of aldosterone that have been described, the lack of physiological targets in many cases, as well as the potentially diverse modes of action, do not allow us to draw a unifying conclusion. However, it is likely that nongenomic actions and genomic actions of aldosterone interfere in some instances with each other for the control of physiological functions, including in classical aldosterone target epithelia.

Genomic Actions of Aldosterone

MINERALOCORTICOID AND GLUCOCORTICOID RECEPTORS

The clinical importance of the mineralocorticoid receptors was demonstrated in patients carrying mutations that lead to an autosomal dominant form of pseudohypoaldosteronism, a disease that remits with age (123). Various heterozygous loss-of-function mutations in the human MR (hMR) gene have been identified and characterized, including frameshift, nonsense, and missense mutations, and gene deletions (123, 284, 298, 299, 336, 357). The MR belongs to the nuclear receptor superfamily NR3C2 (66), which includes other steroid hormone receptors such as thyroid hormone, retinoic acid, and vitamin D receptors. Nuclear receptors are modular proteins harboring different conserved domains (228). Some receptor functions are localized to isolated motifs that can be transferred from the receptor to a heterologous protein, whereas other functions require multiple receptor domains. The N-terminus is less conserved among nuclear receptors, both in size and sequence, and represents almost half of the MR protein. This region contains a ligand-independent activation function that is important for interaction with transcriptional coregulators (187, 337) and for intramolecular interactions with the ligand-binding domain (LBD) (286, 287) that lies at the C-terminus (11). This domain is complex, as it harbors regions involved in formation of the ligand-binding pocket, interaction with heat shock proteins, dimerization, and a ligand-dependent activation function 2 that interacts with transcriptional coregulators (228). The centrally located DNA-binding domain (DBD) is the most conserved region of the receptor. It folds into two zinc fingers, in which one zinc atom is tetracoordinated by four cysteines. The core DBD contains two α-helices; the first one, or recognition helix, binds to the major groove of DNA making contacts with specific bases. This domain also contains segments involved in receptor homo- and hetero-dimerization. Putative nuclear localization signals are localized in the C-terminal part of the DBD and the beginning of the hinge region (228). Acting as enhancers or repressors of transcription, steroid receptors target specific DNA sequences; these hormone-responsive elements (HREs) therefore confer inducibility/repressibility to the genes by the corresponding hormone. In the absence of a ligand, the corticosteroid receptors and possibly all other members of the steroid receptor gene family are associated to a heat shock protein complex (147). This maintains the receptors in an inactive but ligand-binding–competent conformation (reviewed by Pratt and Toft [275]). Activation of the receptor by the binding of an agonist or some antagonists results in dissociation of the receptor from that complex, and promotes receptor dimerization. The dimerized receptors can bind to the corresponding hormone-responsive elements and alter transcription of the target gene(s) as do classical sequence-specific transcription factors (for review, see Carson et al. [53]).

The hMR gene spans approximately 400 kb and is composed of 10 exons (378). Two alternative promoters allow for tissue-specific and differential hormonal regulation of hMR expression (203, 377), and multiple hMR isoforms generated through alternative splicing may play a role in modulating mineralocorticoid and glucocorticoid effects in target tissues (379). Mutations within the DNA-binding and ligand-binding domains associated with autosomal dominant or sporadic type-I pseudohypoaldosteronism bind specifically to glucocorticoid-responsive elements but present modified transcriptional properties, which suggest that altered interaction dynamics with DNA as well as modified intracellular localization may be responsible for submaximal transcriptional potency of hMR (298).

There are two types of classical corticosteroid receptors: the high-affinity type 1 or MR (11), and the lower-affinity type 2 or GR (146), which are structurally highly homologous. The glucocorticosteroid hormone cortisol (corticosterone in rodents and toad) binds to MR with a high affinity similar to that of the mineralocorticoid hormone aldosterone (10, 11) and conversely, aldosterone binds to the human GR with a lower affinity quite similar to that of cortisol (292). Cell-specific hormone and receptor specificity-conferring mechanisms discussed later in this chapter are necessary to explain the differences of the response to mineralocorticoid and glucocorticoid hormones at the systemic and organ levels (63, 108, 241). However, the precise role of these two receptors (MR versus GR), the extent of their functional overlap and the role of specificity-conferring mechanism are not yet fully understood, and the analysis of MR/GR-modified animals may help to clarify this issue.

In the 1990s, various splice variants of the gluco- and mineralocorticoid receptors were identified (199, 332, 378). In the case of the GR, a variant has been described that produces an isoform proposed to act as a transdominant inhibitor (18, 85, 146). The general physiological role of this splice variant is not understood, in particular, in view of its species-specific expression (258). An alternatively spliced rat and human mineralocorticoid receptor mRNA causing truncation of the steroid-binding domain was identified, and the deletion variant had the same baseline transactivation activity as the wildtype MR, but did not respond to aldosterone or corticosterone stimulation although a negative regulation of the MR seemed unlikely (382). The differential control of gene expression by the use of alternative promoters might further contribute to the multiplicity and redundancy of these ligand-dependent transcription factors such as GR or MR (300).

Before exposure to steroids, MR and other steroid receptors are associated with a chaperone protein complex anchored by HSP90. Upon binding to the steroid, MR dissociates from its chaperone complex and undergoes a conformational change to an active state that allows for the regulation of specific gene expression in collaboration with a variety of transcriptional coregulatory factors (for review, see Cheung and Smith [58] and Toft [275]). In the absence of ligand, the MR receptor resides both in the cytoplasm and the nucleus. Agonists but not antagonists increase the number of MRs residing in the nucleus and cause aggregation of MRs into distinct clusters that are dependent on both DNA-binding and intact transcriptional activation functions but not on DNA-dependent receptor dimerization (267). The transfer of MR to the nucleus is essentially unidirectional. Recently, a serine/threonine-rich motif was identified that represents one of three nuclear localization signals determining unidirectional transport of the MR to the nucleus (361).

Specific aldosterone-binding, immunochemical staining, and messenger RNA detection have identified MRs in classical mineralocorticoid target tissues such as kidney, gut, and sweat glands, and also in the skin, brain, pituitary, and heart (89, 90). In kidney, aldosterone appears to control sodium reabsorption across the entire distal nephron from the distal convoluted tubule (DCT) to the inner medullary collecting duct (IMCD) (328). Consistent with these physiological data, evidence for the presence of mineralocorticoid receptor in the distal nephron has been demonstrated by hormone binding, RNA analysis, and immunocytochemistry ([89, 353] and references therein). The mineralocorticoid receptor predominates as expected in the distal convoluted tubule and all along the collecting tubule, whereas the glucocorticoid receptor was most abundant in the medullary ascending limbs and distal convoluted tubule (90). The two mRNAs differing in their 5'UTRs (hMRα and hMRβ) have been identified in human distal tubules of the kidney, in cardiomyocytes, in enterocytes of the colonic mucosa, and in keratinocytes and sweat glands (377). In rat kidney, a large prevalence of rat MRα over MRβ mRNA has been reported, whereas both mRNAs were apparently equally expressed in rat hippocampus (199).

MOLECULAR DETERMINANTS OF SPECIFICITY-CONFERRING MECHANISMS AND THE ROLE OF HYDROXYSTEROID DEHYDROGENASE TYPE 2

Aldosterone is present at low concentrations in the extracellular fluid (on the order of 10^{-10}–10^{-8} mol/l). It can diffuse (or eventually be transported) through the plasma membrane of all cells but might encounter a specific receptor only in target cells. The free MRs and GRs are localized mostly in the cytosol (91, 131, 156). At the cellular level, the action of aldosterone is initiated by its binding to the mineralocorticoid receptor. There are, however, other high-affinity ligands for the MR that do not produce the same effects such as progesterone, spironolactone, and other antagonists (292). The working hypothesis to explain this specific differential response follows: (1) agonists bind to and produce a conformational change that fully activates the receptor and elicits the maximal biologic response, (2) partial agonists fully occupy the receptor but afford incomplete activation and thus a partial response, and (3) antagonists fully occupy the receptor, but are not able to induce a conformational change, which is necessary for a crucial functional step, that is, dissociation from the heat shock protein complex, translocation to the nucleus, binding to target DNA, or transactivation/transrepression (88). It has been suggested that, in the absence of ligand, the lower portion of the ligand-binding domain surrounding the ligand-binding cavity is rather dynamic, whereas the binding of agonist ligand compacts the LBD by establishing many polar and hydrophobic contacts, thus stabilizing the C-terminal H12 helix in its active conformation, thereby promoting coactivator binding (see for review Nagy and Schwabe [246]).

More recently, a constitutive active mutation of mineralocorticoid receptor (S810L) has been found in patients with early-onset hypertension that is also markedly exacerbated in pregnancy (122). This mutation alters receptor specificity with progesterone and other steroids lacking 21-hydroxyl groups, normally MR antagonists, thereby becoming potent agonists. Further in vitro transfection experiments revealed that cortisone and 11-dehydrocorticosterone bind and strongly activate the mutant receptor (277, 278). Biochemical studies revealed that S810L mutation induces a change in the receptor conformation and increases stability of the steroid-receptor complex (87). Recent crystallography of the LBD in complexes with progesterone and with deoxycorticosterone (DOC), an agonist of both wildtype and mutant receptors, revealed that the network of contacts created by Leu810 at the A-ring is sufficient to stabilize the progesterone-MR S810L complex in its active state (87) (Fig. 4). The network of contacts created by Leu810 at the A-ring is sufficient to stabilize the progesterone-MR S810L complex and is responsible for the progesterone-induced MR S810L activation. Thereby, DOC adopts a position very similar to that of progesterone (87).

The major glucocorticoid in humans is cortisol. It is synthesized from cholesterol by the cells of the zona fasciculata and zona reticularis and is released into the circulation under the influence of ACTH. In the normal adult in the absence of stress, about 20 mg of cortisol are secreted daily. The rate of secretion changes in a circadian rhythm. In plasma, 95% of the cortisol is bound to plasma proteins, in particular to the corticosteroid-binding globulin (CBG). The plasma level of aldosterone, the main mineralocorticoid hormone, is much lower (2 orders of magnitude) than that of cortisol or corticosterone. Thus, these glucocorticoid hormones, which have a similar high affinity for the MR as aldosterone, would be expected to occupy the high-affinity type I sites (MR). Indeed, even the "effective" free concentration of aldosterone, which in contrast to the natural glucocorticoids has no specific carrier plasma protein, is also quite lower than that of glucocorticoids. However, glucocorticoids normally do not occupy MR nor GR to any significant extent in aldosterone target epithelia. As described in the following, this is essentially due to the expression of a crucial protection mechanism represented by the 11β-hydroxysteroid dehydrogenase type 2. This mechanism hence allows aldosterone to occupy not only the MR but also the GR, such that part of the mineralocorticoid response can be mediated by the GR.

Tissue-specific differences in cortisol-binding proteins (i.e., CBG) could play a role in modulating the local free concentration of glucocorticoids and hence their cellular concentration and availability. Yet another type of mechanism that might influence the binding of aldosterone and glucocorticoids to their receptors is related to the distribution of the hormones between membranes and the more hydrophilic intra and extracellular compartments. Indeed, it has been shown that some steroid hormones are substrates for the membrane transport protein MDR (23). Thus, it could be that the transport into and/or out of target cells influences also the hormone binding to receptors (194).

The question of the hormone specificity of mineralocorticoid versus glucocorticoid hormones is complex for several reasons. First, endogenous mineralocorticoid and glucocorticoid hormones have similar high affinities for the MR and similar low affinities for the GR (10, 292). Second, both nuclear receptors are coexpressed in the classical mineralocorticoid target epithelia. Third, both nuclear corticosteroid receptors can interact with the same regulatory elements of inducible genes and produce similar transactivation in transfection experiments of reporter genes with promoters containing classical HREs (10, 292). And fourth, MR and GR are coexpressed in a variety of tissues in which they mediate distinct physiological effects where specificity can not be attributed to metabolizing enzymes such as 11β-hydroxysteroid dehydrogenase-2 (11β-HSD2) (235, 236). Thus, specificity-conferring mechanisms must exist to explain the difference in physiological action of the mineralocorticoid hormone aldosterone, which is regulated mainly by angiotensin II (AngII) and extracellular potassium, and of glucocorticoid hormones that depend essentially on ACTH. Finally, the various mechanisms causing cell (or tissue) specificity may include, among others, regulation of ligand availability, receptor diversity, and the type of receptor-interacting proteins and of chromatin structure around potential steroid receptor–binding sites on the DNA. An overview of established and putative specificity-conferring mechanisms is given in Table 3.

Despite the fact that the rate of aldosterone synthesis normally is 100- to 1000-fold less than that of glucocorticoids the kidney MRs are selectively occupied by aldosterone. This apparent contradiction can be explained by the colocalization in renal collecting tubules of a cortisol/corticosterone-converting enzyme, 11β-HSD2 with the MR. This enzyme catalyzes the conversion of the active 11-hydroxycorticosteroids (cortisol and corticosterone) to 11-oxocorticosteroids (cortisone or 11-dehydrocorticosterone), which have a much lower affinity for the corticosteroid receptors (110, 184). The tissue distribution of 11β-HSD2 has been examined by enzyme activity assay (NAD-dependent 11-HSD activity), immunocytochemistry and at the RNA level in human, sheep, rat, mice, and rabbits, and essentially parallels that of the MR (2) (5, 64, 181, 313). In fetal mice, 11β-HSD2 has been shown to be more widely expressed starting at embryonic day 9.5 (E9.5). Later, the expression is more restricted, essentially to aldosterone-target tissues, such as the renal distal convoluted tubule and the collecting duct, where it is colocalized with the MR (239, 249). The subcellular localization is thought to be restricted to the endoplasmic reticulum (248). Among tissues that are not classic targets of mineralocorticoids, 11β-HSD2 is often strongly expressed in placenta cells, but with a large variability. It is thought to have a protective function for the fetus by inactivating excess maternal glucocorticoids (197, 207, 306).

The type 1 isoform of 11β-HSD, which functions essentially as a reductase, is expressed in liver, many regions of the brain and other tissues, including the proximal part of the kidney tubule. Findings from the 11β-HSD1 null mice suggest that lack of this enzyme confers protection against metabolic dysfunction (193, 242). Hypersecretion of corticosterone is accompanied by a hypertrophied adrenal. The HPA axis is overcompensating, producing elevated circulating plasma corticosterone levels that might be due to an absence of 11β-HSD1 activity in CNS sites of normal negative feedback sites of glucocorticoids normally tightly regulating their own secretion (148). The generation of a mouse model overexpressing 11β-HSD1 specifically I adipose tissue under control of the adipocyte P2 gene promoter clearly demonstrated the importance of this enzyme

TABLE 3 Established and Putative Specificity-Conferring Mechanisms for Mineralocorticoid versus Glucocorticoid Hormones and Receptors

Ligand availability	Cortisol-binding proteins (e.g., CBG)
	Enzymatic conversion (11-βHSD)
	Network of ligand contacts
	In/out transport of hormones (e.g., through MDR)
Receptor diversity	MR–GR variants
	Synergy control (SC) motifs
DNA vs protein binding	Transcription interference/synergy
	Coactivators, co-repressors
	Chromatin remodeling factors
Dimerization partner	Homodimers/heterodimers
Promoter selection	Chromatin structure/availability
Ligand-independent modulation	Single/tethering/composite HRE
	Promoter architecture
	Promoter-specific functional preference (spacing of HRE)
	Phosphorylation (cross-talk with other signaling pathways)
Coregulator recruitment	Tissue- and cell-specific expression
	Regional distribution of SRCs (steroid receptor coactivators)
Cell and tissue specificity	Differential state of the cell (sensibility, sensitivity)

in adipocyte function and the regulation of metabolism (232). The phenotypic features resemble the disorders in humans that commonly include central obesity, insulin resistance/type 2 diabetes mellitus, dyslipidemia, and hypertension clustered in a single individual. The mice have increased sensitivity to dietary salt and increased plasma levels of angiotensinogen, AngII, and aldosterone. The circulating renin-angiotensin aldosterone system (RAAS) is chronically activated in these mice with increased expression of the renin substrate angiotensinogen in adipocytes, together with elevated plasma levels of renin and the potent vasoconstrictor peptide ANG II driving increased blood pressure (232). Recent data suggest that preventing local regeneration of glucocorticoids by 11-β-hydroxysteroid dehydrogenase type 1 enhances angiogenesis (315).

In contrast, 11β-HSD2, which functions as an oxydase, appears to be expressed only in specific regions of the brain, like the nucleus tractus solitarius, subcommissural organ, or hypothalamus, where it might play an important role in the regulation of MR accessibility for glucocorticoids in cells with aldosterone-specific actions related to blood pressure and salt appetite (288, 305). The crucial role of 11β-HSD2 for preventing the occupancy of the MR by endogenous glucocorticoids is underlined by the fact that the mutations of its gene or the inhibition of its function by licorice (glycyrrhenetic acid) produces a syndrome of apparent mineralocorticoid excess with salt retention and hypertension (244, 326, 368). Genetic manipulation of 11β-HSDs in the mouse has confirmed several hypotheses on the function of these enzymes and elucidated unknown roles, revealing the sensitivity of many intracellular mechanisms to local GC concentration (see for review Paterson et al. [266]). The generation of 11β-HSD2 knockout mice, which closely models AME, allowed analysis of the molecular and cellular changes occurring in the kidney (192). Similar what is observed in human AME, about 50% of the knockout mice die early after birth. The death was preceded by motor weakness and reduced suckling, and intestinal ileus and possible cardiac arrest resulting from severe hypokalemia was suggested (148). The surviving knockouts exhibit hypokalemia, hypochloremia, hypotonic polyuria, and marked hypertension, primarily resulting from unregulated activation of MR by corticosterone although activation may also be involved. They further show striking histological changes, with marked hyperplasia and hypertrophy of the distal nephron consistent with persistent MR activation, leading to electrolyte imbalance and the AME disease phenotype (192). These potentially irreversible structural changes in 11β-HSD2 null mice may also explain why suppression of endogenous GC production does not always reverse the phenotype in human AME (148, 266). 11β-HSD2 is not the unique steroid metabolizing enzyme potentially present in target cells. Conversion of hormones into metabolites by other enzymes takes place in *Xenopus* A6 cells. These metabolites of corticosterone have been shown to be active on Na$^+$ transport (80, 293). Recently, the presence in A6 cells of CYP3A (a member of the cytochrome oxydase P450 family) has been suggested. This enzyme has a 6β-

hydroxylase activity and its inhibition allows apparently corticosterone to act on Na$^+$ transport via the MR, besides its GR-mediated action. This would indicate that CYP3A would normally prevent corticosterone from acting via the MR, in A6 cells (240). An interesting observation is that the action of the 11β-HSD2 might be regulated by hormones that act on Na$^+$ reabsorption. Indeed, AVP was shown at pharmacological concentrations to increase the 11β-HSD2 catalytic activity. This was proposed to be part of the synergy mechanism of AVP and aldosterone on Na$^+$ reabsorption (6).

OTHER SPECIFICITY-CONFERRING MECHANISMS

Two distinct molecular mechanisms are widely accepted to define the actions of nuclear receptors on gene expression: (1) the classic mechanisms involving trans-activation and trans-repression via interaction with cognate DNA-binding sites (e.g., HREs), and (2) mechanisms of transcription interference and synergy mediated by protein–protein interactions between corticosteroid receptors and other trans-acting factors. Transcriptional synergy, functionally defined as a more than additive increase in gene transcription conferred by multiple trans-acting factors or multiple linked cis-acting DNA response elements can result from cooperative binding of trans-acting factors to linked enhancers, cooperative recruitment of transcription initiation complexes and regulation of sequential steps in transcription initiation (292). The distinct capacities for synergy of MR and GR was provided by the observation that the N-terminal domains of MR and GR contain a variable number of synergy control (SC) motifs whose disruption selectively increased GR or MR activity at GRE multimers (171). The synergy motif is a target for modification by the ubiquitin-like modifier SUMO1, which controls the activity and subcellular localization of a variety of proteins. Direct and distinguishable inhibitory roles for SUMO isoforms in the control of transcriptional synergy has been demonstrated (149), although the mechanistic basis for SUMO1 synergy inhibition remains to be determined (see for review Bhargava and Pearce [33] and Stockand [327]).

In addition to the major role played by the prereceptor protective mechanisms, the nature of the cellular responses to aldosterone or glucocorticoid is determined to a large extent by the type and the state of the target cell. Indeed, the set of genes regulated by a given activated receptor is cell specific. This is due to the fact that much more than a single regulatory protein has to bind to a gene to activate its transcription. An intracellular receptor can activate a gene only if an appropriate cell type-specific combination of other gene regulatory proteins is expressed. This opens the possibility of interaction at several levels. As mentioned previously, protein–protein interactions play a central role in the establishment of preinitiation complexes. Thus, the structural differences of the MR and GR, in particular at the level of their amino-terminal domains, certainly allow them to undergo receptor-specific interactions. These interactions, in turn, might selectively modulate the transregulatory action of the receptors, independent of their common DNA-binding properties. Differential expression and regional distribution of steroid receptor coactivators SRC-1 and SRC-2 in brain and pituitary has been found, and two splice variants of the steroid receptor coactivator-1 (SRC-1) 1a and 1e can differ significantly in certain cell populations (235, 236). Thus, each cell might have a specific pattern of coactivators, which in turn may be involved in cell-specific responses to corticosteroids in a promoter- and ligand-dependent way.

Another difference resides in their capability of synergizing with each other on multiple HRE-containing promoters. Indeed, the MR is not capable of synergizing with itself on the multiple HRE promoters on which GR synergizes (292). However, disruption of the dimer formation interface within the DNA-binding domain of the MR allowed multiple MRs to synergize with each other (215). This suggests that synergy of MRs is also possible in vivo but on promoters with a different spacing of the multiple HREs than that allowing the synergy of GRs. A further level of complexity is brought by the fact that MR and GR can interact directly to form heterodimeric complexes. The existence of such complexes has been demonstrated and there transregulatory action shown in cotransfection studies, to differ from those of homodimerized receptors (215, 340). Another prereceptor mechanism that might play a role in selectively modulating the cellular hormone concentration, besides the protective action of 11β-HSD2, is the transmembrane transport of steroid hormones by transport proteins such as MDR (23).

Each ligand interacts somewhat differently with the receptors and, thus, produces a specific conformational change (68). The extreme situation is represented, as mentioned earlier, by antagonists that bind to the receptors, but do not allow them to undergo the normal sequence of events leading to transactivation/repression as do physiological ligands. Progesterone and RU26752 are examples of inactive high-affinity ligands for the MR (88, 108, 292). Similarly, there are qualitative and quantitative differences between the action of receptors bound to different agonists. The classical example is that of the reporter gene experiments using the MMTV promoter, in which MR requires 10 times less aldosterone than cortisol to achieve the maximal level of transactivation, although its binding affinity for both hormones is equal. This phenomenon, which was described by Arriza et al. in 1988 (10), has been termed functional preference. The situation is rendered even more complicated by the fact that this type of difference is certainly also promoter context specific.

Finally, the functional state of receptors can be modulated by covalent modifications or noncovalent interactions (271, 343, 344). In some cases, transactivating activity of sex steroid receptors was demonstrated even in the absence of their steroid ligand upon receptor phosphorylation (252, 271). This type of ligand-dependent and/or independent modulation of the receptor function—for instance, by phosphorylation—provides means of cross-talk with other signaling pathways and could also play a role as hormone/receptor-specificity conferring mecha-

nisms (211, 366). In summary, besides the fact that hormone metabolizing enzymes play an important role in limiting the access of natural glucocorticoids to the corticosteroid receptors of aldosterone target cells, several further specificity conferring mechanisms modulate the action of the different hormones. For instance, each particular hormone-receptor complex can interact with a set of cellular factors. Yet no studies have established the physiological relevance of these factors, particularly their multiplicity and functional redundancy.

PRIMARY VERSUS SECONDARY AND DIRECT VERSUS INDIRECT RESPONSES

The classification of genes regulated by steroid hormones is based on two observations: The requirement for concomitant protein synthesis and the timing of the response. The effects of the steroid hormones on classical primary response genes are mediated through the direct binding of activated receptor complexes to HREs. Thus, the intracellular receptors act in this classical case as sequence-specific transcription factors. The induction of primary response genes is relatively rapid (within 30 minutes) and does not require ongoing protein synthesis.

The structural organization of the HREs on different primary response genes differs considerably. The glucocorticoid receptor (GR) binds, for instance, to at least three types of glucocorticoid response elements (GREs) classified as simple, tethering, or composite (321). It has been suggested that binding of receptors to particular HREs will determine whether the receptor interacts with specific coactivators, corepressors, or transcriptional machinery in a particular cell type (179). Since it has been shown that steroid receptors do also activate certain genes rapidly and independent of ongoing protein synthesis without interacting directly with an HRE (see, for instance, aforementioned effect of GR on β-casein gene), the definition of primary response genes should probably extend to this second type of "HRE-independent primary response genes." The physiological importance of this type of regulatory actions is underlined by the fact that gene modified mice with DNA-binding incompetent GR are viable, in contrast to GR knockout mice (280).

Classical secondary response genes do not bind the receptor complex and their activation depends on the primary response. For instance, a hormone-bound receptor induces directly the synthesis of a protein which itself is a transcription factor or activates a transcription factor which then acts on a secondary response gene. Hence, the time required for this action is longer and the effect depends on protein synthesis. There are many possibilities of secondary responses, even such which might depend rather on nongenomic actions of the steroid receptor. One possibility is that the primary response results in the induction or activation of an mRNA-binding protein, which modulates the mRNA stability and/or translation of secondary response genes (78). Thus, numerous levels of cross-talk between intracellular receptors and other signal transduction pathways exist that contribute to the complexity of gene expression.

Dean and Sanders (73) have proposed a third class of steroid-regulated genes, representing those that bind the hormone-receptor complex but exhibit delayed changes in transcription rates. Such genes, like the α2-globulin gene, appear to be regulated via HREs different from those mediating rapid induction (55). These genes may therefore represent a composite of the pathways involved in the regulation of primary and secondary response genes, since the hormonal response nevertheless requires ongoing protein synthesis. Cloning and identification of the essential proteins may, in the future, resolve this issue for the different steroid receptors.

Physiologists often call a hormonal effect indirect when it is the consequence of a primary physiological effect. In this case, the cascade of events is more complicated than for a secondary response. For instance, the primary effect of a hormone could be the opening of apical Na^+ channels (via any type of signaling cascade). The consequence would be influx of Na^+ into the cell that, in turn, would impact, on the function and the expression of the Na^+ pump. Such an indirect effect involves necessarily many steps and is, thus, susceptible to influence by other parameters (353).

HOW DOES TRANSCRIPTIONAL REGULATION LEAD TO TRANSPORT REGULATION?

This question has interested many scientists over the last four decades. Seminal hypotheses based on a "candidate approach" have been formulated by Edelman and coworkers (82) in the 1960s. The epithelial Na^+ channel (ENaC) and the Na^+ pump (Na^+,K^+-ATPase) are the two main transport proteins mediating sodium reabsorption in the ASDN and thus the main candidates that were further investigated. Starting at the level of Na^+ transport effectors, this approach has permitted to define different phases of the aldosterone action: an early phase characterized by an activation of pre-existing proteins and a late phase during which new structural proteins are accumulated. The second approach to the mechanism of aldosterone action starts from the transcriptional event with the identification of aldosterone-regulated gene products (352). These are then further investigated at the level of their potential involvement in the physiological action of the hormone. Using new powerful techniques to analyze differential gene expression, aldosterone-regulated gene products were identified (discussed in the following). However, it is likely that there are still many important aldosterone-regulated gene products that remain to be identified.

EARLY REGULATORY AND LATE "ANABOLIC" EFFECTS OF ALDOSTERONE

The simplest mechanistic explanation for the transport regulation induced by aldosterone at the transcriptional level would be the transcriptional induction of the involved transport proteins, in particular of ENaC and the Na^+,K^+-ATPase. This would lead to an increase in the number of transporters expressed at the cell surface and to a corresponding change in Na^+ reabsorption. As mentioned previously (and discussed later in the chapter), this type of effect does exist but belongs to the late and very late phases of the physiological response, in particular due to the delay between the change in transcription rate and a measurable physiological effect of the corresponding protein. The duration of the delay depends on the relative change in transcription rate (hence also on the transcription rate before the treatment), the time required for gene transcription, mRNA maturation, mRNA export, translation, protein maturation, routing, and also on RNA and protein half-lives. These times are in the case of many structural proteins and in particular of the Na^+,K^+-ATPase (~1 to 10×10^6 units per principal cell, half-life of ~24 hours [353]) too large, such that transcriptional regulation cannot lead to rapid functional changes but produces slow/late functional (anabolic) responses. The "anabolic" late effect is not limited to transport proteins but is pleiotropic and concerns also other proteins indirectly participating to Na^+ transport (other elements of the transport machinery), such as proteins involved in providing energy for the Na^+ pump function (352).

To explain early functional effects of aldosterone that can be observed long before the "anabolic" effect, one has to assume a functional regulation of preexisting channels and pumps. The working hypothesis is that the activated hormone-receptor complex regulates the transcription of elements of regulatory cascades. Thereby aldosterone modifies the output of the regulatory network that controls the function of ENaC and other transport proteins. As discussed in the following, the identification of early aldosterone-regulated gene products and results of functional experiments support this hypothesis. In contrast to the gene products involved in the late "anabolic" response, the ones involved in the early transport response must have short half-lives at the mRNA and protein levels or be nearly absent at low aldosterone levels such that their quantity can be modified rapidly enough to account for early physiological changes.

ENAC ACTIVATION: TRANSCRIPTIONAL INDUCTION AND REGULATION

Aldosterone directly controls ENaC transcription at the level of the α-subunit gene (238). The mRNA of this subunit was correspondingly shown to increase in ASDN of adrenalectomized rats within 2 hours of aldosterone treatment as well as during long-term treatment (219, 225). This effect can account for the accumulation of α subunit in ASDN cells that was observed also within 2 hours of aldosterone treatment and in the long term (219, 229). Interestingly, at the protein level aldosterone not only increases the amount of αENaC, but also induces a cleavage of γENaC (229). It is likely that this cleavage of γENaC observed in 1999 corresponds to the recently described furin-mediated cleavage of γENaC, a modification at the level of the extracellular loop that appears to be part of the functional maturation of the channel (159, 160, 229). The relationship between the increased cleavage/maturation of ENaC and the action of aldosterone is as yet not clear.

An important aspect in ENaC regulation by aldosterone is the translocation of the channel to the apical pole (Fig. 4). This subcellular shift was observed within 4 hours of an aldosterone treatment, after a long-term aldosterone treatment and after low salt diet (219, 229). This regulation of subcellular channel localization obviously depends also on other factors than only aldosterone, since it is not uniform along the ASDN. Immunofluorescence images show a localization gradient with a strong apical signal in early portions of the ASDN (DCT) and progressively more intracellular labeling along the CNT and CD. The factor(s) that control(s) the axial extension of the apical ENaC translocation appear(s) to depend on sodium status and has not yet been identified.

Although the induction of ENaC is visible as early as 2 hours after the initiation of an aldosterone treatment and its apical translocation within 4 hours, the actual early increase in transepithelial Na$^+$ reabsorption and K$^+$ secretion elicited by an acute aldosterone treatment starts earlier, being measurable within 30 minutes of treatment (152). Thus, the early aldosterone response must also involve the activation of pre-existing but previously silent channels. In this regard, ubiquitylation of ENaC is an important aldosterone-regulated mechanism that has been shown to control the channel surface expression and function. Recent experiments have indicated that the E3 ubiquitin ligase that ubiquitylates ENaC is Nedd4-2 (1, 325). This enzyme binds to a PY motif of the COOH-terminal tails of β- and γENaC via one of its WW domains and ubiquitylates Lys residues in the NH2-terminal tails of ENaC subunits (325). Interestingly, the lack or misense mutations of PY motif in β- and γENaC characteristic of Liddle's syndrome leads to an increase in cell surface ENaC expression and also to an increase in its open probability (P$_o$), a condition leading to Na$^+$ retention, low K$^+$, and hypertension (9, 42, 95, 219). The expression of Nedd4-2 is constitutive but its function is regulated by aldosterone. Indeed, the early aldosterone-induced protein Sgk1, when activated via PDK1 and 2, phosphorylates Nedd4-2 and thereby creates a binding site for 14-3-3 proteins (32, 74, 170, 188). By binding to Nedd4-2, 14-3-3 proteins mask the ENaC interacting motif of Sgk1 and thus prevent ENaC ubiquitylation and downregulation. This mechanism appears to play a central role in the control of ENaC and is the target of the aldosterone-inducible Sgk1. This short cascade represents the first direct link between the aldosterone-regulated transcriptional activity of the MR and the function of ENaC that was demonstrated (Fig. 6) (325).

Besides acting on ENaC expression/function via Nedd4-2, it appears that Sgk1 exerts other effects on ENaC. This kinase has for instance been shown to directly phosphorylate αENaC subunits at the level of its COOH-terminal tail, a post-translational modification that stimulates ENaC function (75). However, the Sgk1-Nedd4-2 pathway is not the only

link between aldosterone and ENaC function. This has been indicated by results of experiments performed with mpkCCD cells expressing Liddle-type ENaC that cannot bind Nedd4-2 and still respond to aldosterone as did gene-modified mice expressing an ENaC β subunit with the Liddle mutation (16, 72). In addition, the C-terminal regions of ENaC β and γ subunits have been shown to be phosphorylated on Ser and Thr residues, and this phosphorylation to be increased after an aldosterone treatment (309–311). The nature of the pathways that link the transcriptional activity of the activated MR to these phosphorylation events and their functional consequences need still to be clarified.

It is possible that ENaC surface expression and/or function is also modulated by aldosterone via its action on intracellular pH, as has been proposed based on observations made in the frog distal tubule, frog skin, toad bladder, and rat CCD (67, 255, 263). An observation that argues against such a possibility is that chronic hyperaldosteronism induced by low-Na$^+$ diet in rats had no effect on the activity of the Na$^+$/H$^+$ exchanger and intracellular pH of CCD cells (260). However, as mentioned previously, it appears that the intracellular pH can be influenced by aldosterone via nongenomic effects on the H$^+$ pump or on Na$^+$/H$^+$ exchange and those effects might in some circumstances play a coregulatory role (79, 223, 224, 372).

A number of data sets that are not easy to reconcile have been generated in amphibian and mammalian epithelia on the putative role of the aldosterone action on lipid metabolism, lipid and protein methylation, protein fatty acylation, and prenylation. The first observations were published in 1978 by Yorio and Bentley (376), suggested that mepacrine, which inhibits phospholipase A, decreases the effect of aldosterone in toad bladder. More recent observations about the role of lipid-based signaling pathways in ENaC regulation have focused on the role of PIP3 (36). Interestingly, these studies establish a link between ENaC and the small G-protein K-Ras that had been previously identified as aldosterone induced in *Xenopus* A6 cells and shown to increase the activity of surface-expressed ENaC in *Xenopus* oocytes (231, 317). It has, for instance, been shown that PIP3 possibly directly increases the P$_o$ of ENaC expressed in CHO cells, and it has been suggested that Ras acts by localizing the PIP3-producing enzyme PI3-K close to the channel (322, 323). Another important role of PIP3 in this context is its role as activator of the PDK kinases that in turn activate aldosterone-inducible Sgk1 (188). This latter aldosterone-induced protein was mentioned previously because of the ENaC-stimulatory effect that it produces by the inhibition of the ubiquitin ligase Nedd4-2 and eventually also by direct phosphorylation of αENaC (75, 325, 355).

NA,K-ATPASE ACTIVATION: TRANSCRIPTIONAL INDUCTION AND REGULATION

The Na$^+$,K$^+$-ATPase α1 and β1 subunit genes have been shown to be regulated by aldosterone in A6 epithelia (354). These are the only genes for which transcriptional regulation

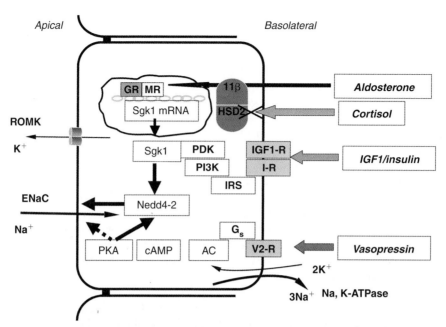

FIGURE 6   Model of the aldosterone-signaling cascade in the principal cells of CCD and interactions with IGF1/insulin- and vasopressin-signaling cascades. Upon binding of the MR-A complex to the promoter of the Sgk1 gene, Sgk1 mRNA increases rapidly and is translated into the Sgk1 protein. Sgk1 is phosphorylated by the PI3/PDK kinases, which are activated upon binding of IGF1 and/or insulin to their cognate receptors (IGF1-R and IR) and activation of the insulin receptor substrate (IRS). The active phosphorylated Sgk1 phosphorylates specific sites on the E3 ubiquitination enzyme Nedd4-2, which, in turn, unbinds from the C-terminus of ENaC β and γ subunits, leading to an increased retention of ENaC channel proteins at the apical membrane. Vasopressin activates adenylate cyclase (AC) through V2R receptors and G_s to increase cAMP and activate PKA, which can phosphorylate Nedd4-2 and/or ENaC (*dotted arrow*). CCD, cortical collecting ducts.

by aldosterone has been formally demonstrated by performing nuclear run-on experiments, in contrast to measuring the level of mRNA accumulation in the presence and absence of a transcription inhibitor (354). The transcription rate of both Na^+,K^+-ATPase subunit genes was increased 15 minutes after hormone addition. Because of the short lag period, this effect has to be direct. However, it was also shown that it depends on the presence of (a) short-lived protein(s), since it was abolished by a 1-hour pretreatment with the translation inhibitor cycloheximide.

This very early transcriptional regulation precedes a relatively slow increase in the mRNA pools. The increase in β1 subunit mRNA starts to be measurable after 1 hour and that of α1 after approximately 3 hours (317, 354). In contrast, the rate of protein synthesis is suggested to be regulated in parallel for both subunits, as measured by pulse-labeling experiments (1-hour pulses) (259). At the levels of protein accumulation, surface expression, and pump function (measured as Na^+ pump current in apically permeabilized cells), the lag period was approximately 5 hours, confirming that despite the early transcriptional events the physiological consequences were "late" (30, 31). This can be explained by the large pre-existing pool of Na^+,K^+-ATPase and the long half-life of the pumps, which is not changed by aldosterone (259). A similar increase in the level of Na^+,K^+-ATPase protein synthesis has been measured in the toad bladder (120). In the

kidney collecting duct, the best-studied aldosterone-sensitive segment of the nephron, two experimental situations have to be considered separately: studies on adrenalectomized animals (ADX) and on adrenal-intact animals. In adrenalectomized rats, the most striking effects of aldosterone on Na^+,K^+-ATPase, measured as hydrolytic activity at V_{max} and by ouabain binding, are too fast to be attributed to changes in the number of pump units and thus have to be considered as regulatory changes at the level of existing pumps. They were described previously in the section titled Early Effects of Aldosterone on Na^+ Pump Function. Studies investigating the Na^+,K^+-ATPase mRNA levels in kidney CCD of adrenalectomized rats have shown that aldosterone complementation compensates the relatively small decrease in the level of Na^+,K^+-ATPase α1-subunit mRNA produced by adrenalectomy (86, 89), is similar to the situation observed for the Na^+ channel in the same kidney tubular segment of adrenalectomized rats, where αENaC is the only regulated subunit. Two groups have demonstrated that an increase in intracellular Na^+ content and/or concentration (corresponding to an increase in cell volume) can trigger in CCD cells the rapid "recruitment" (within minutes) of a latent pool of pumps as large as the pre-existing active pool (measured by ouabain binding or activity assay) (21, 39). Interestingly, the size of this recruitable pool depends on the mineralocorticoid status of the animals and decreases slowly after adrenalectomy. It is only when this pool is "empty" (not any more re-cruitable) that the ouabain-binding sites also start to decrease when measured without prior "recruitment." It is not clear where this pool is located, and the mechanism of activation is not known. It can be postulated that the aldosterone-dependent gene product necessary for the recruitment, and which is slowly decreasing after adrenalectomy, is not a Na^+,K^+-ATPase subunit.

In adrenal-intact animals, aldosterone produces a slow increase in the number of functional Na^+ pumps and Na^+,K^+-ATPase subunits (84, 113, 141, 367). The mechanism underlying this effect has not been studied in CCD and could be similar to the one described previously for the A6 cells. As mentioned earlier, long-term treatments (days) with mineralocorticoid hormone induce a large increase in basolateral surface area (approximately fivefold for principal cells of the CCD) and a parallel increase in Na^+,K^+-ATPase hydrolytic activity (84, 177, 201, 360).

When studying the regulatory action of aldosterone in the context of an organism, it is important to consider the systemic feedback mechanisms that tend to counteract the effect of aldosterone or of low-Na^+ diet at the RNA and transcriptional levels. For instance, in distal colon, Na^+ deprivation and the consecutive increase in aldosterone level increase the level of Na^+,K^+-ATPase mRNA only transiently. The return to baseline (escape) has been shown to be due to a decrease in T3 concentration (369). Furthermore, it has also been shown that the luminal Na^+ influx plays a permissive role for the aldosterone-induced Na^+,K^+-ATPase accumulation in kidney CCD cells (253, 261, 269, 353).

These different observations support the view that mineralocorticoids play an important role in the control of Na^+,K^+-ATPase expression, but that this type of late effect cannot be considered independent of other regulatory networks which operate at the cellular and systemic levels.

Na^+,K^+-ATPase Activation: Early Regulation and Late Accumulation

Aldosterone has been shown to control the transcription of the Na^+,K^+-ATPase genes in A6 epithelia and human 293 cells, an effect that appears to be mediated by a "classical" direct mechanism, that is, binding of the activated MR to cis-acting response elements (190, 354). This action appears to depend, in a Na^+,K^+-ATPase subunit-specific way on the presence of other regulatory factors such as cAMP, T3, and so on (3, 22, 354, 369). This early effect of aldosterone on the transcription of the Na^+,K^+-ATPase genes does not translate into an early physiological effect. Indeed, an increase in the number of functional pumps appears with a delay of more than 3 hours, due to the size of the pump pool and to the long half-life of pump subunit mRNAs and proteins (31).

At the level of its function and/or surface expression, the Na^+,K^+-ATPase has been shown to be directly regulated by aldosterone, that is, independent of the aldosterone-induced Na^+ influx, both in cultured epithelia and rat CCD (22, 334). A puzzling phenomenon induced in CCD by aldoste-rone is a strong increase in maximal pump activity and of the number of Na^+,K^+-ATPase molecules that can be labeled at the cell surface (92, 334). These results indicate that there is a rapid, quantitatively important mechanism of Na^+ pump regulation controlled by aldosterone that has not yet been understood. Interestingly, this aldosterone-induced regulation was observed with Na^+ pumps containing an α1 subunit and not an α2 subunit (333).

Taken together, aldosterone induces a late increase in Na^+,K^+-ATPase expression in the ASDN (>3 hours after hormone addition) that is likely mediated to a large extent by a direct effect of the activated MR on the subunit gene promoters. The complex mechanisms that lead in the long term (chronic treatment over days) to amplification of the basolateral membrane with a further parallel increase in Na^+,K^+-ATPase are not known (353). In addition to this late increase in expression, aldosterone promotes an early activation of the Na^+,K^+-ATPase at the cell surface. The mediators of this Na^+ pump regulation are not known. It might be that in part same mediators trigger the activation of both ENaC and of the Na^+ pump. However, parallel regulation of apical channels and basolateral pumps is not adequate in every physiological situation. For instance, when the intracellular Na^+ concentration increases due to a high Na^+ load, opposite effects on ENaC and on the Na^+,K^+-ATPase are expected. Hence, it could also be that aldosterone controls the key transporters ENaC and the Na^+ pump by affecting the activity of various signaling networks.

Identification of Aldosterone-Regulated RNAs by Gene Expression Profiling

The aim of this section is to mention additional aldosterone-regulated gene products that support the pleiotropic action of aldosterone. Some of these were identified because they were considered as candidates for aldosterone regulation and therefore the impact of the hormone on their expression was directly tested. Others were identified in the context of screening procedures for aldosterone-regulated mRNAs (93, 351). This was the case of the two gene products discussed previously, K-Ras and Sgk1.

Besides ENaC and Na^+,K^+-ATPase, three gene products clearly involved in NaCl reabsorption were identified because they were candidate genes. First, two epithelial transporters were shown to be upregulated in vivo by mineralocorticoids in the long term, the thiazide-sensitive NaCl cotransporter of DCT segment–specific cells and the Cl^-/HCO_3-exchanger pendrin expressed in B intercalated cells (185, 349). Both transporters participate to the NaCl reabsorption and might be upregulated by indirect mechanisms. The third candidate involved in NaCl transport shown to be induced by aldosterone is the regulatory protein WNK1. This latter effect was shown in a cell culture model to be mediated rapidly by activated MR (250). It will be interesting to verify the in vivo regulation of WNK1; its role appears to be control of the balance between the partially overlapping Na^+, K^+ and Cl^- reabsorption (175, 176). The EGF receptor is an additional regulatory protein, the expression of which was shown in kidney cells to be induced by aldosterone. Interestingly, this receptor has been implicated in the signaling of nongenomic actions of aldosterone and might play a role in pathological actions of aldosterone (198).

Molecular biology methods have progressively become available that enabled the identification of regulated gene products. First, Garty and colleagues (15, 117, 335) cloned a cDNA-encoding CHIF, a protein that is induced by aldosterone in the colon and belongs to the FXYD family of small Na^+,K^+-ATPase regulatory proteins. Interestingly, CHIF is also localized to the distal part of the ASDN and increases the apparent affinity of the Na^+,K^+-ATPase for Na^+ (25, 52).

The same group has isolated several cDNA clones encoding mitochondrial proteins that were induced by dexamethasone in rat distal colon (276). This slow, possibly indirect induction of gene products involved in energy metabolism supports the old hypothesis that corticosteroids act on Na^+ transport also by increasing the energy supply to the Na^+,K^+-ATPase. Previously, the activity of citrate synthesis, a nuclear encoded key protein of the citric acid cycle, has been shown to be induced by aldosterone in several, but not all target epithelia (186, 352).

More recently, Spindler and colleagues (317) used a differential display PCR approach to compare cDNA fragments generated from RNA of control and aldosterone-treated A6 epithelia. They showed that only a small proportion of the mRNAs (<0.5%) was significantly regulated within the lag period of aldosterone action, and thus are potentially involved in its early effect. One of the regulated gene products was the A splice variant of a *Xenopus* K-*ras*. Functional experiments in *Xenopus* oocytes showed that this small G-protein activates ENaC at the cell surface (231). The connection of K-Ras with PIP3-mediated ENaC activation has already been described.

Sgk1 has also been mentioned previously as an aldosterone-induced regulatory protein. It was originally identified as corticosteroid-regulated both in *Xenopus laevis* A6 and mouse M1 cells (57, 247). It functions as negative regulator of the ubiquitin ligase Nedd4-2 and thereby stimulates ENaC function (13, 74, 316). Sgk-/- mice have been shown to display under normal diet an increased aldosterone level with a maintained Na^+ balance, whereas they were shown not to retain enough salt under a low-salt diet. This indicates that Sgk1 is involved in the aldosterone-mediated NaCl retention, but that this protein is not the sole mediator of this action (374). Interestingly, Sgk1 has been shown in expression systems to affect the function and/or localization of many other transport proteins, including ROMK and Na^+,K^+-ATPase that are part of the ASDN salt-reabsorption machinery (348). However, regarding K^+ secretion, we should mention that the lower K^+ secretion observed in Sgk1 knockout mice was due to a decrease in driving force and not to a direct effect on ROMK. Whether in vivo Na^+,K^+-ATPase is a target of Sgk1 has not yet been established.

Another aldosterone-regulated gene product that has been identified by subtractive hybridization is NDRG2 (45). Its potential role in the context of sodium transport is not known, but it is mentioned here because its transcriptional regulation was shown to be selective for MR versus GR, unlike that of Sgk1 and others.

Some gene screens were performed by SAGE (serial analysis of gene expression) or gene array analysis on kidney-derived cultured cells (93). The major limitation of these studies was the large number of genes normally repressed in vivo that are expressed in cultured cells and some of which are sensitive to corticosteroids. Nonetheless, some interesting gene products were identified. One of them is the strongly upregulated GILZ, a gene product identified in mpkCCD cells by SAGE analysis (285). Its induction has been verified in kidney, but its functional role has not yet been unraveled (243). In IMCD3 cells, a series of aldosterone-regulated gene products (1-hour treatment) was identified. Sgk1 was one of the most highly regulated ones (132). Intriguingly, two gene products involved in circadian rhythm as well as endothelin-1, a factor recently shown to oppose the action of aldosterone, were identified (4).

The role of the endothelin-B receptor in vascular homeostasis is controversial because the receptor has both pressor and depressor effects in vivo. One potential depressor mechanism of endothelin-B activation is through promotion of natriuresis and diuresis in the renal tubule. In vitro studies suggested that activation of endothelin-B receptors inhibits the activity of ENaC in the renal collecting duct epithelium (112). Rats deficient in endothelin-B exhibit sodium-dependent hypertension due to an absence of tonic inhibition of the epithelial sodium channel in the distal nephron (114). These results suggest that salt-sensitive hypertension is the result of disinhibition of renal ENaC channels.

A more complete list of the gene products regulated by aldosterone in target cells will be useful. We predict that more of them participate in signaling cascades directly affecting the function of cellular machinery for Na^+ reabsorption and K^+ secretion. It is also likely that other gene products implicated in pathways that favor the differentiation of the epithelial cells will be identified as aldosterone induced (318).

Genetically alteration in mice might be applied to other candidate genes (for salt-sensitive hypertension) that have been identified but only tested so far in vitro, such as genes implicated in the insulin pathway such as GILZ (glucocorticoid-induced leucine zipper [285]) or PPARγ (peroxisome proliferator-activated receptor γ [381]), or in ubiquitin/degradation pathway such as Nedd4/Nedd4-2 (see for review Staub et al. [324]) and Nedd4-interacting proteins such as N4WBP5A (191) or NDRG 2 (n-myc downstream-regulated gene 2) (45).

INTERACTIONS WITH OTHER HORMONAL PATHWAYS

The potentiating effect of aldosterone on the action of antidiuretic hormone (ADH) represents another example of the impact of aldosterone on a signaling pathway that regulates ENaC. In A6 cells, an aldosterone pretreatment was shown to massively stimulate ADH-induced cAMP production, by a mechanism involving adenylate cyclase and a more upstream mechanism (352). Furthermore, aldosterone was shown to act synergistically with ADH at the level of ENaC (102, 135, 281, 350). Thus, not only the baseline activity of channels is affected by the pleiotropic action of aldosterone but also its responsiveness to other stimuli. This action depends on the target epithelium as shown for other effects of aldosterone. For instance, cAMP does not increase Na^+ transport in inner medullary collecting duct cells (166).

Insulin also stimulates Na^+ reabsorption in tight epithelia but not via the same pathway as aldosterone (35). The action of both hormones is sensitive to the inhibition of tyrosin phosphorylation and is synergistic, since insulin produces the same relative increase in ENaC in control and in aldosterone-treated A6 cells (279, 380). Synergy can be explained to some extent by the fact that insulin activates Sgk1, whereas aldosterone increases the amount of this kinase that interferes with the Nedd4-2–mediated downregulation of ENaC (12, 362).

There are several other hormones and factors that act on Na^+ reabsorption in aldosterone target cells. For instance, T3 plays different roles by interacting at the transcriptional level and/or downstream in the toad bladder (341), cortical collection duct (22) and colon (369). Other examples are transforming growth factor β and peptide hormones of the atrial natriuretic factor family that have been known to blunt aldosterone action on Na^+ transport (166, 302). Another important factor in Na^+ transport regulation is the apical Na^+ load that also depends on the action of other hormones acting more proximally to aldosterone in excretory organs. The effects of Na^+ influx are multiple and range from the transcription of aldosterone-regulated genes to the regulation of the transport proteins involved in Na^+ reabsorption (see previous discussion and Verrey et al. [353]).

In summary, multiple interactions of aldosterone at the level of signaling pathways of other hormones, and factors acting on Na^+ reabsorption are part of its pleiotropic action. These interactions represent an important element contributing to the stimulatory action of aldosterone on Na^+ transport and to its coordination with other hormones and factors.

HUMAN AND MOUSE DISEASES LINKED TO MR MUTATIONS

Mineralocorticoid Receptor Loss of Function and Gain of Function Mutation

Mice in which the MR was inactivated developed severe symptoms of pseudohypoaldosteronism with failure to thrive, weight loss, severe Na^+ and water loss, and highly stimulated renin-angiotensin system (28) (Fig. 7). At day 10 after birth, these MR-/- mice die since they are not able to compensate for Na^+ loss. Interestingly, amiloride-sensitive Na^+ reabsorption is reduced, but the abundance

of the mRNAs encoding ENaC and Na^+,K^+-ATPase is unchanged in the kidney, indicating that regulation of Na^+ reabsorption via MR may not be achieved by transcriptional control of ENaC and Na^+,K^+-ATPase. In mineralocorticoid receptor knockout mice, expression of the renin-angiotensin system (RAS) is altered, renin being the most stimulated component. Angiotensinogen and AT1 in the liver are also increased, but the other elements of the RAS are not affected (158). The changes in mRNA levels of the components of the RAS in 8-day-old MR-/- mice were not apparent in the heterozygous MR+/- mice. However, these animals have increased urinary sodium loss, a threefold increase in sodium fractional excretion, and modest compensatory stimulation of the circulating RAS, revealed by a threefold increase in renin, AngII, and aldosterone levels compared with those in MR+/+. This suggests a modest neonatal sodium loss, compatible with survival in the MR+/- mice. This mild sodium loss exhibited by these heterozygous mice is somewhat similar to the phenotype observed in patients with autosomal dominant pseudohypoaldosteronism type I (123). In these patients with heterozygous defect in the MR gene, a modest form of neonatal renal salt wasting, with hyperkalemia and acidosis, was observed. The disease remits with age indicating the crucial importance of aldosterone-dependent sodium reabsorption in the postnatal period and its decreasing role with age (29). Daily injections of β methasone, a synthetic glucocorticoid, from day 5 after birth onward prolonged survival of MR-/- mice suggesting that an activated GR can at least partially take over the function of MR, but could not completely replace MR function (28). Daily subcutaneous injections of sodium chloride from day 5 after birth until weaning and continued oral NaCl supply lead to survival of MR knockout mice (37). This NaCl rescue proves that neonatal MR knockout mice die because they are not able to compensate for their renal Na^+ loss. The injections of isotonic NaCl solution enabled the animals to live through a critical phase of life, after which they adapt their salt and water intake to their persistent renal salt wasting. Constitutive hMR overexpression in all MR-expressing tissues, notably the kidney and heart, led to both renal and mild cardiac alterations compatible with hypokalemic nephropathies despite normal potassium serum levels (202).

GR Knockout Mouse

Inactivation of the glucocorticoid receptor in vivo resulted in perinatal death due to respiratory failure (65). Lung maturation was severely retarded and RNA encoding the amiloride-sensitive epithelial sodium channel (ENaC) was diminished. An in vivo mutation in the DNA-binding site that impairs dimerization and prevents direct DNA binding of the GR at HREs resulted in viable mice, clearly demonstrating the in vivo relevance of DNA-binding–independent activities of the GR (280).

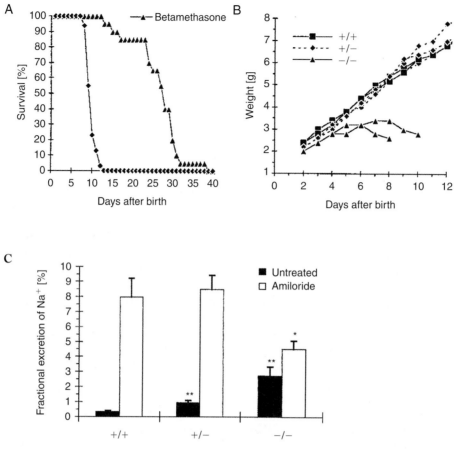

FIGURE 7 **A:** Survival of MR−/− and betamethasone-treated MR−/− mice. Application of betamethasone from day 5 after birth prolonged survival on average by 17 days. **B:** Weight curve of MR−/− mice and their heterozygous (+/−) and wildtype (+/+) litter mates. **C:** Fractional excretion of sodium. At day 8 after birth, the fractional excretion of sodium of untreated (black columns) and amiloride treated (white columns) MR−/−, heterozygous (+/−), and wildtype (+/+) animals are shown. Values of MR-deficient (−/−) or heterozygous (+/−) animals, which are statistically different from wildtype (+/+), are indicated with asterisks. MR, mineralocorticoid receptors. (Adapted from Berger S, Bleich M, Schmid W, Cole TJ, Peters J, Watanabe H, Kriz W, Warth R, Greger R, Schutz G. Mineralocorticoid receptor knockout mice: pathophysiology of Na+ metabolism. *Proc Natl Acad Sci U S A* 1998;95:9424–9429.)

Human and Mouse Diseases Linked to Sgk1 Mutations

The serum- and glucocorticoid-regulated kinase (SGK1) gene has recently been identified as an important aldosterone-induced protein kinase that mediates trafficking of the renal epithelial sodium channel ENaC to the cell membrane. Thus, SGK1 is an attractive candidate for blood pressure regulation and possibly essential hypertension. Indeed, two polymorphisms of the Sgk1 gene that correlate with enhance blood pressure in twin studies have been identified (48). Mice deficient for the serum and glucocorticoid regulated kinase 1 (Sgk1), an aldosterone-induced regulatory protein of ENaC, display modestly higher plasma aldosterone and K+ concentrations (374). This study demonstrates that Sgk1 participates in, but does not fully account for, the mineralocorticoid regulation of ENaC. On a standard NaCl diet, sgk1-/- mice show unaltered renal Na+ excretion, suggesting that the constitutively present isoforms sgk2 and sgk3 might be able to compensate for the loss of Sgk1 expression (see for review Vallon and Lang [348]). However, Sgk1 expression is strongly induced by aldosterone in response to low NaCl intake and under this condition the renal phenotype became evident (Fig. 8) (348, 374). Restriction of dietary NaCl revealed the inability to upregulate NaCl reabsorption despite the presence of excessive plasma aldosterone concentrations and decreased blood pressure and glomerular filtration rate (GFR). Micropuncture experiments revealed compensatory proximal tubular hyper-reabsorption and evidence for a Na+ transport defect. Immunohistochemistry of CNT demonstrated that the kinase is not absolutely necessary for the insertion of ENaC into the apical membrane and ENaC activation, but required for the upregulation of apical membrane ENaC abundance and thereby for Na+ reabsorption in the ASDN (348, 374).

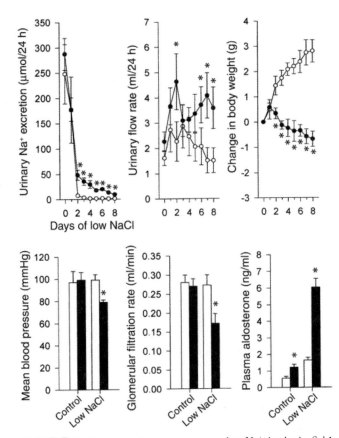

FIGURE 8 Deficient adaptive response to low-Na$^+$ intake in Sgk1 −/− mice. (**Top**) Urinary excretion of Na$^+$ and water, and change in body weight in response to a low-NaCl diet (0 g Na$^+$/kg) assessed in awake mice in metabolic cages (n = 6 each group). (**Bottom**) Shown are mean arterial blood pressure and glomerular filtration rate in anesthetized mice on the control diet and at day 3 after initiating the low-NaC$^+$ diet (0.15 g Na$^+$/kg) (n = 5–6 each group); and plasma aldosterone concentration in mice on control diet and at day 3 after initiating low-NaCl diet (0 g Na$^+$/kg) (n = 8–9 each group). Filled circles and bars indicate Sgk1−/− mice, open circles and bars indicate Sgk1+/+ mice. *P<.05 vs Sgk1+/+ mice. (Adapted from Wulff P, Vallon V, Huang DY, Volkl H, Yu F, Richter K, Jansen M, Schlunz M, Klingel K, Loffing J, Kauselmann G, Bosl MR, Lang F, Kuhl D. Impaired renal Na$^+$ retention in the sgk1-knockout mouse. *J Clin Invest* 2002;110:1263–1268.)

Furthermore, Sgk1-deficient mice show impaired regulation of renal K$^+$ elimination in response to both acute and chronic K$^+$ loading. Reduced ENaC and/or Na$^+$/K$^+$-ATPase activity may account for this effect and enhanced apical abundance of renal outer medullary K$^+$ channel ROMK partly compensated for the defect (157).

Human and Mouse Diseases Linked to ENaC

LIDDLE SYNDROME

Liddle syndrome is a rare disorder (pseudoaldosteronism) described first by G.W. Liddle in a family in which multiple siblings had early onset of severe hypertension associated with hypokalemia (209). Urinary excretion of aldosterone was low in these patients, and no effects of spironolactone on blood pressure could be demonstrated. By contrast, administration

of the Na$^+$-channel blocker, triamterene, together with restriction of salt intake tended to normalize blood pressure. These clinical features suggested that hypertension was due to excessive aldosterone-independent sodium reabsorption in the distal nephron, resulting from the constitutive activation of ENaC. Despite the low plasma aldosterone in these patients, they still responded to aldosterone injections by further decreasing their renal Na$^+$ excretion.

The pedigree of the original kindred described by Liddle was recently extended, clearly demonstrating the autosomal dominant inheritance of the disease (44). A candidate gene approach was used to identify mutations causing this rare Mendelian form of hypertension (312). Complete linkage of Liddle syndrome to a locus encoding the β subunit of ENaC, and analysis of the β gene revealed various mutations in the cytoplasmic C-terminus: deletion or frameshift mutations leading to truncation of a major portion of the C-terminus and missense mutations in a highly conserved proline-rich domain (139, 312, 338). A deletion of the C-terminus in the γ subunit has also been identified as cause of the Liddle's syndrome, whereas no mutations in the α subunit have been linked to this disorder (138). Expression of these β and γ ENaC variants together with α subunits in the *Xenopus* oocyte system revealed a significant increase in ENaC channel activity at the cell surface, consistent with the initial postulate that these hyperactive channel mutants lead to an excessive Na$^+$ reabsorption and hypertension (301).

To elucidate the causal relationship between dietary salt intake, genetically determining salt handling by the kidney, and hypertension, we generated a mouse model for Liddle's syndrome by introducing the R566 stop mutation at the βENaC allele ("knockin" strategy) (Fig. 9) (274). Interestingly, with normal salt diet, the mice carrying the βENaC-mutated L/L allele remain normotensive, despite evidence of hypervolemia and increased Na$^+$ reabsorption in the large intestine. Moreover, plasma pH, Na$^+$, K$^+$, Cl$^-$, or HCO$_3^-$ concentrations were not significantly affected (274). However, the classical Liddle phenotype with higher blood pressure, metabolic alkalosis, and hypokalemia accompanied by cardiac and renal hypertrophy manifests in these mice in response to a high-salt diet (274). Moreover, evidence for impaired ENaC internalization was demonstrated in vivo, as the increase in urinary Na$^+$ excretion upon short 6–12-hour salt repletion following 1 week of low-salt diet is significantly delayed in Liddle mice despite the presence of lower circulating aldosterone concentrations (273). Isolated perfused CCD from Liddle mice exhibit higher transepithelial potential differences, and confluent primary cultures of CCD microdissected from their kidneys exhibit significant lower transepithelial electrical resistance and higher negative potential differences, which is consistent with an overall increased ENaC activity (273). Interestingly, mineralocorticoid upregulation of ENaC expression and function is still maintained in Liddle mice, which show a remarkable high sensitivity to aldosterone in vitro (16) and in vivo (72, 273). Renal CD cells from Liddle mice

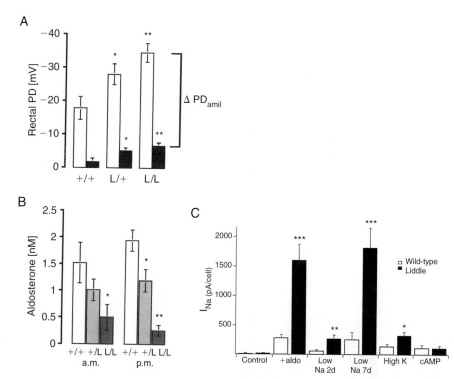

FIGURE 9 **A:** Measurements of sodium transport. In vivo measurements of rectal PD before (white bar) and after (black bar) inhibition by amiloride. Rectal PD was measured in vivo in adult mice (3 to 5 months old) before and after addition of amiloride. The PD_{amil} was determined between 10 A.M. and noon. **B:** Morning and afternoon plasma aldosterone concentrations, wildtype +/+ heterozygous, +/L and L/L mice. (Adapted from Pradervand S, Barker PM, Wang Q, Ernst SA, Beermann F, Grubb BR, Burnier M, Schmidt A, Bindels RJ, Gatzy JT, Rossier BC, Hummler E. Salt restriction induces pseudohypoaldosteronism type 1 in mice expressing low levels of the beta-subunit of the amiloride-sensitive epithelial sodium channel. *Proc Natl Acad Sci U S A* 1999;96:1732–1737.) **C:** Mean values of I_{Na} under various in vivo and in vitro conditions. Open bars represent wildtype mice, and filled bars represent Liddle mice. Control = standard chow, no infusion. +Aldo = standard chow, aldosterone infusion by osmotic minipump for 6–8 days. Low Na = low-Na diet for 2 or 7 days (d). High K = high-K diet for 6–8 days. cAMP = CCTs from mice fed standard chow, without aldosterone infusion treated in vitro with cAMP for 5 to 30 minutes. PD, potential difference. (Adapted from Dahlmann A, Pradervand S, Hummler E, Rossier BC, Frindt G, Palmer LG. Mineralocorticoid regulation of epithelial Na^+ channels is maintained in a mouse model of Liddle's syndrome. *Am J Physiol Renal Fluid Electrolyte Physiol* 2003;285:F310–F318.)

exhibit hyperactive apical vasopressin-regulated CFTR Cl^- conductance that could contribute to the enhance NaCl reabsorption observed in the distal nephron of patients with Liddle's syndrome. In summary, in the Liddle mouse, dysfunction of ENaC in the kidney is demonstrated before onset of arterial hypertension that argues in favor of the kidney hypothesis proposed by Liddle (209).

PHA-1

Another disorder of salt and water metabolism is the pseudohypoaldosteronism type 1 (PHA1), a disease characterized dehydration, hyponatremia, hyperkalemia and metabolic acidosis despite elevated plasma aldosterone concentration and plasma renin activity. The association of renal sodium wasting, hyperkalemia, and failure to respond to mineralocorticoids suggest defective Na^+ reabsorption in the distal nephron. There are two forms of PHA1, an inherited recessive disease characterized by a culminant clinical

presentation in the neonatal period and persisting in adulthood (56, 210) and an autosomal dominant or sporadic form that is milder and remits with age (123). Genetic investigations of kindred with the recessive PHA1 revealed deletion or missense mutations in each of the three ENaC subunits, resulting in decrease channel function when expressed in *Xenopus* oocytes. Linkage of PHA1 to loss of function ENaC variants further support the critical role ENaC in aldosterone regulation of Na^+ reabsorption. Transgenic mice models for recessive PHA1 have been developed (163).

Constitutive gene inactivation studies for all three subunits of ENaC (α, β, and γ, encoded by *Scnn1a*, *Scnn1b*, and *Scnn1g*, respectively) revealed a crucial role for each subunit in survival of the animal (see for review Hummler [161] and Hummler and Horisberger [164]). Constitutive inactivation of the mouse αENaC gene locus demonstrated the crucial role in lung liquid clearance at birth since absence of ENaC function led to respiratory complications and neonatal death (162). The amiloride-sensitive electrogenic Na$^+$ transport in airway epithelia was abolished, indicating that the αENaC is the limiting subunit in the Na$^+$ channel. Mutations that result in ENaC hypofunction in the kidney are expected to induce a salt-wasting syndrome similar to type 1 pseudohypoaldosteronism (43). This renal phenotype was not observed in αENaC knockout mice, because the neonates died too early to manifest electrolyte disturbances. Genetic rescue by reintroducing the αENaC subunit under the control of a heterologous (cytomegalovirus) promoter demonstrated the importance of precise regulation of ENaC (163). These transgenic rescued mice had sufficient basal Na$^+$ absorptive capacity to clear lung liquid and survive the early neonatal period, but developed a severe phenotype similar to PHA1 with salt-wasting, metabolic acidosis, high aldosterone levels, growth retardation, and increased early mortality (163). The same mice present constitutively impaired transepithelial Na$^+$ transport in the lung, which is also found in PHA-1 patients (182), and these mice provide evidence that the defective respiratory transepithelial Na$^+$ transport may facilitate pulmonary edema (83). Moreover, when downregulation of ENaC activity such as observed under hypoxia is imposed on a low constitutive ENaC expression, the resulting reduced Na$^+$ transport rate may become insufficient for airway fluid clearance (256). In comparison, heterozygous mutant mice for αENaC exhibit no obvious lung phenotype and show an intact capacity to maintain blood pressure and Na$^+$ balance, although plasma renin activity did not change when studied in animals on normal and low-NaCl diets. The increased number of AT1 receptors in renal tissues accompanied by an increased vascular responsiveness to exogenous AngII and lowered blood pressure during AngII receptor blockade indicates a compensatory upregulation of AT1 receptors (364). The constitutive inactivation of βENaC and γENaC revealed severe early renal dysfunction that results in early postnatal death (20, 234). Failure to thrive and lethargy are associated with urinary Na$^+$ wasting, K$^+$ retention, and increased plasma aldosterone concentrations, thus reflecting the renal phenotype found in PHA-1 (see for review Bonny and Hummler [42] and Bonny and Rossier [43]). It seems that low residual ENaC activity in these mice is sufficient to circumvent the neonatal lung phenotype, consistent with the assumption that αβ and αγ subunit combinations can establish some ENaC activity in airway epithelia. Inactivation of the γENaC subunit in mice resulted in early death (at 36 hours after birth) of the mice mainly due to disturbed total body electrolyte balance (20). In the course of generating a mouse model for Liddle's syndrome by the insertion of a stop codon corresponding to residue R566 in human βENaC, together with the selection marker neomycin, we obtained mice with a partial disruption of the βENaC gene locus (βENaCm/m) (272). Under a normal salt diet, these mice show a mild PHA1 phenotype with reduced ENaC activity and elevated plasma aldosterone levels, but develop an acute PHA1 with continuous weight loss, hyperkalemia, and de-creased blood pressure when kept under a low-salt diet (272). We concluded that low levels of βENaC subunit mRNA confer sufficient ENaC activity to maintain salt and water homeostasis under normal salt conditions, but are limiting if salt restriction is imposed. The αENaC subunit is important in forming the functional channel, whereas the β- and γENaC subunits are important modulators of ENaC channel function. In lung, β- and γENaC subunits facilitate neonatal lung liquid clearance at birth, whereas in kidney, where Na$^+$ reabsorption is under the control of aldosterone, β- and γENaC subunits are necessary for proper functioning of ENaC.

In summary, although the onset and severity of PHA-1 symptoms vary in these models, the renal phenotype of these mice corresponds well to the human PHA-1 phenotype (with salt-wasting, hyperkalemia, and metabolic acidosis) that reveals the important implication of ENaC in Na$^+$,K$^+$ homeostasis.

Proteolytic Activation of ENaC and CAPs The major part of the ENaC protein faces the extracellular milieu like a receptor, and it was mentioned earlier that furin-mediated cleavage within the extracellular loop appears to be part of the maturation process of α- and βENaC (159, 160). Yet another luminal protease-mediated ENaC activation system has been identified that has been suggested to play an important regulatory role for ENaC function. Originally this hypothesis was formulated when cDNA was identified from the model kidney cell line A6 that encodes a protease that activates upon coexpression ENaC by increasing its P$_o$ (59, 347). This channel-activating protease (CAP-1) and related proteases have been shown to be highly expressed in ENaC-expressing tissues such as kidney and intestine in which protease inhibitors have also been shown to decrease Na$^+$ channel activity (59, 172, 359). The finding that proteolytic events modulate ENaC activity from the extracellular side is supported by the observation made in various cells lines that the application of protease inhibitors decreases and the addition of proteases increases Na$^+$ channel activity (49, 59). As yet the actual mechanism by which this pathway leads to channel activation has not been elucidated. One report suggests that this ENaC activating mechanism is induced by aldosterone. In brief, urinary CAP1/prostasin was augmented by aldosterone in rats and humans (251).

The synergistic activation of ENaC by CAPs and sgk1 in vitro may allow a large dynamic range for ENaC-mediated Na$^+$ regulation crucial for tight control of Na$^+$ homeostasis (359). The constitutive knockout of CAP3 (214) and the tissue-specific knockout of CAP1 (206) already revealed an important role in skin barrier function. The generation of floxed CAP1 mice (i.e., mice in which the CAP1 allele is floxed by loxP sites) currently permit dissection of the role of this positive ENaC regulator in sodium reabsorption in kidney and colon (291).

In summary, the limiting subunit αENaC (in kidney ASDN) is transcriptionally induced by aldosterone relatively quickly. The actual early increase in Na$^+$ transport, however, precedes this effect, and is mediated by aldosterone-induced regulatory proteins. One such regulatory protein is K-Ras, which is induced by aldosterone in *Xenopus* A6 cells, and was shown to stimulate ENaC function via PI3-K. Sgk1, the other known aldosterone-induced regulatory protein, was also shown to be upregulated in ASDN and to regulate ENaC ubiquitylation and function by controlling the activity of ubiquitin ligase Nedd4-2.

PERSPECTIVES: INTEGRATED PHYSIOLOGICAL APPROACH

In Vivo Model to Study Aldosterone Action

Important to our understanding of the in vivo function of genes involved in aldosterone-dependent sodium transport is their analysis by inactivation or modification of these genes in vitro and the study of the consequences of the mutation in vivo. This enables us to dissect complex processes and to draw conclusions about the functional redundancy or absolute requirement of various genes involved in salt reabsorption in the kidney. Thus, the relative importance of each gene defined in the general mechanism of action of aldosterone can now be tested experimentally in animal models. Inactivation of GR, MR, ENaC, and their regulatory proteins, such as 11βHSD2, Sgk1, and CAPs will greatly help our understanding of how and why mineralocorticoid specificity can be achieved in aldosterone target cells. Induced and repressed genes, when defined, should be tested for their physiological relevance in vivo. Finally, the main effectors of sodium transport (Na^+,K^+-ATPase and ENaC) that are regulated by aldosterone can thereby tested in mice models.

CONCLUSIONS

In the future, the identification of all aldosterone-regulated gene products by modern molecular techniques, and the functional investigation of their potential role in the aldosterone action will shed more light onto the cellular regulatory pathways that are relevant for transport regulation by aldosterone. Because of the large number of different pathways acting finally directly or indirectly on the effectors of this transport, in particular on ENaC, it will be necessary to first understand this regulatory action of aldosterone in an experimental system devoid of systemic feedback and coregulatory pathways. The use of gene-modified mouse models is beginning to allow the experimental analysis of specific gene defects in vivo on the whole organism, and also provides the possibility to study the specific defect at the level of target cells. The combination of molecular and physiological approaches using these new models will thus enable us to increase our understanding of complex hormonal action on target cells within the complexity of the organs and the whole body.

References

1. Abriel H, Loffing J, Rebhun JF, Pratt JH, Schild L, Horisberger JD, Rotin D, Staub O. Defective regulation of the epithelial Na+ channel by Nedd4 in Liddle's syndrome. *J Clin Invest* 1999;103:667–673.
2. Agarwal AK, Mune T, Monder C, White PC. NAD (+)-dependent isoform of 11 beta-hydroxysteroid dehydrogenase. Cloning and characterization of cDNA from sheep kidney. *J Biol Chem* 1994;269:25959–25962.
3. Ahmad M, Medford RM. Evidence for the regulation of Na+, K+-ATPase alpha-1 gene expression through the interaction of aldosterone and cAMP-inducible transcriptional factors. *Steroids* 1995;60:147–152.
4. Ahn D, Ge Y, Stricklett PK, Gill P, Taylor D, Hughes AK, Yanagisawa M, Miller L, Nelson RD, Kohan DE. Collecting duct-specific knockout of endothelin-1 causes hypertension and sodium retention. *J Clin Invest* 2004;114:504–511.
5. Albiston AL, Obeyesekere VR, Smith RE, Krozowski ZS. Cloning and tissue distribution of the human 11 beta-hydroxysteroid dehydrogenase type 2 enzyme. *Mol Cell Endocrinol* 1994;105: R11–R17.
6. Alfaidy N, Blotchabaud M, Bonvalet JP, Farman N. Vasopressin potentiates mineralocorticoid selectivity by stimulating 11-beta hydroxysteroid deshydrogenase in rat collecting duct. *J Clin Invest* 1997;100:2437–2442.
7. Almeida AJ, Burg MB. Sodium transport in the rabbit connecting tubule. *Am J Physiol* 1982;243:F330–F334.
8. Alvarez de La Rosa DA, Li H, Canessa CM. Effects of aldosterone on biosynthesis, traffic, and functional expression of epithelial sodium channels in A6 cells. *J Gen Physiol* 2002;119: 427–442.
9. Alvarez de la Rosa DA, Zhang P, Naray-Fejes-Toth A, Fejes-Toth G, Canessa CM. The serum and glucocorticoid kinase sgk increases the abundance of epithelial sodium channels in the plasma membrane of xenopus oocytes. *J Biol Chem* 1999;274:37834–34839.
10. Arriza JL, Simerly RB, Swanson LW, Evans RM. The neuronal mineralocorticoid receptor as a mediator of glucocorticoid response. *Neuron* 1988;1:887–900.
11. Arriza JL, Weinhberger C, Cerelli G, Glaser TM, Handelin BL, Houseman DE, Evans RM. Cloning of human mineralocorticoid receptor complementary DNA: structural and functional knship with the glucocorticoid receptor. *Science* 1987;237:268–275.
12. Arteaga MF, Canessa CM. Functional specificity of Sgk1 and Akt1 on ENaC activity. *Am J Physiol Renal Physiol* 2005;289:F90–F96.
13. Asher C, Sinha I, Garty H. Characterization of the interactions between Nedd4-2, ENaC, and sgk-1 using surface plasmon resonance. *Biochim Biophys Acta* 2003;1612:59–64.
14. Asher C, Wald H, Rossier BC, Garty H. Aldosterone-induced increase in the abundance of Na+ channel subunits. *Am J Physiol* 1996;271:605–611.
15. Attali B, Latter H, Rachamin N, Garty H. A corticosteroid-induced gene expressing an "IsK-like" K+ channel activity in *Xenopus* oocytes. *Proc Natl Acad Sci U S A* 1995;92: 6092–6096.
16. Auberson M, Hoffmann-Pochon N, Vandewalle A, Kellenberger S, Schild L. Epithelial Na+ channel mutants causing Liddle's syndrome retain ability to respond to aldosterone and vasopressin. *Am J Physiol Renal Fluid Electrolyte Physiol* 2003;285:F459–F571.
17. Bachmann S, Bostanjoglo M, Schmitt R, Ellison DH. Sodium transport-related proteins in the mammalian distal nephron—distribution, ontogeny and functional aspects. *Anat Embryol* 1999;200:447–468.
18. Bamberger CM, Bamberger AM, de Castro M, Chrousos GP. Glucocorticoid receptor beta, a potential endogenous inhibitor of glucocorticoid action in humans. *J Clin Invest* 1995;95: 2435–2441.
19. Barger AC, Berlin RD, Tulenko JF. Infusion of aldosterone, 9-alpha-fluorohydrocortisone and antidiuretic hormone into the renal artery of normal and adrenalectomized dogs: effect on electrolyte and water excretion. *Endocrinology* 1958;62:804–815.
20. Barker PM, Nguyen MS, Gatzy JT, Grubb B, Norman H, Hummler E, Rossier B, Boucher RC, Koller B. Role of gammaENaC subunit in lung liquid clearance and electrolyte balance in newborn mice. Insights into perinatal adaptation and pseudohypoaldosteronism. *J Clin Invest* 1998;102:1634–1640.
21. Barlet-Bas C, Khadouri C, Marsy S, Doucet A. Enhanced intracellular sodium concentration in kidney cells recruits a latent pool of Na-K-ATPase whose size is modulated by corticosteroids. *J Biol Chem* 1990;265:7799–7803.
22. Barlet-Bas C, Khadoury C, Marsy S, Doucet A. Sodium-independent in vitro induction of Na+,K+-ATPase by aldosterone in renal target cells: permissive effect of triiodothyronine. *Proc Natl Acad Sci U S A* 1988;85:1707–1711.
23. Barnes KM, Dickstein B, Cutler GB Jr, Fojo T, Bates SE. Steroid treatment, accumulation, and antagonism of P-glycoprotein in multidrug-resistant cells. *Biochemistry* 1996;35:4820–4827.
24. Baxendale-Cox LM, Duncan RL, Liu X, Baldwin K, Els WJ, Helman SI. Steroid hormone-dependent expression of blocker-sensitive ENaCs in apical membranes of A6 epithelia. *Am J Physiol* 1997;273:C1650–C1656.
25. Beguin P, Crambert G, Guennoun S, Garty H, Horisberger JD, Geering K. CHIF, a member of the FXYD protein family, is a regulator of Na,K-ATPase distinct from the gamma-subunit. *EMBO J* 2001;20:3993–4002.
26. Beguin P, Wang X, Firsov D, Puoti A, Claeys D, Horisberger JD, Geering K. The gamma subunit is a specific component of the Na,K-ATPase and modulates its transport function. *EMBO J* 1997;16:4250–4260.
27. Bens M, Vallet V, Cluzeaud F, Pascual-Letallec L, Kahn A, Rafestin-Oblin ME, Rossier BC, Vandewalle A. Corticosteroid-dependent sodium transport in a novel immortalized mouse collecting duct principal cell line. *J Am Soc Nephrol* 1999;10:923–934.
28. Berger S, Bleich M, Schmid W, Cole TJ, Peters J, Watanabe H, Kriz W, Warth R, Greger R, Schutz G. Mineralocorticoid receptor knockout mice: pathophysiology of Na+ metabolism. *Proc Natl Acad Sci U S A* 1998;95:9424–9429.
29. Berger S, Bleich M, Schmid W, Greger R, Schutz G. Mineralocorticoid receptor knockout mice: lessons on Na+ metabolism. *Kidney Int* 2000;57:1295–1298.

30. Beron J, Mastroberardino L, Spillmann A, Verrey F. Aldosterone modulates sodium kinetics of Na,K-ATPase containing an alpha-1 subunit in A6 kidney cell epithelia. *Mol Biol Cell* 1995;6:261–271.
31. Beron J, Verrey F. Aldosterone induces early activation and late accumulation of Na-K-ATPase at surface of A6 cells. *Am J Physiol* 1994;266:C1278–C1290.
32. Bhalla V, Daidie D, Li H, Pao AC, Lagrange LP, Wang J, Vandewalle A, Stockand JD, Staub O, Pearce D. Serum- and glucocorticoid-regulated kinase 1 regulates ubiquitin ligase neural precursor cell-expressed, developmentally down-regulated protein 4-2 by inducing interaction with 14-3-3. *Mol Endocrinol* 2005;19:3073–3084.
33. Bhargava A, Pearce D. Mechanisms of mineralocorticoid action: determinants of receptor specificity and actions of regulated gene products. *Trends Endocrinol Metab* 2004;15:147–153.
34. Biner HL, Arpin-Bott MP, Loffing J, Wang X, Knepper MA, Hebert SC, Kaissling B. Human cortical distal nephron: distribution of electrolyte and water transport pathways. *J Am Soc Nephrol* 2002;13:836–847.
35. Blazer-Yost BL, Liu X, Helman SI. Hormonal regulation of ENaCs: insulin and aldosterone. *Am J Physiol* 1998;274:C1373–C1379.
36. Blazer-Yost BL, Vahle JC, Byars JM, Bacallao RL. Real-time three-dimensional imaging of lipid signal transduction: apical membrane insertion of epithelial Na^+ channels. *Am J Physiol Cell Physiol* 2004;287:C1569–C1576.
37. Bleich M, Warth R, Schmidt-Hieber M, Schulz-Baldes A, Hasselblatt P, Fisch D, Berger S, Kunzelmann K, Kriz W, Schutz G, Greger R. Rescue of the mineralocorticoid receptor knock-out mouse. *Pflugers Arch* 1999;438:245–254.
38. Blot-Chabaud M, Laplace M, Cluzeaud F, Capurro C, Cassingena R, Vandewalle A, Farman N, Bonvalet JP. Characteristics of a rat cortical collecting duct cell line that maintains high transepithelial resistance. *Kidney Int* 1996;50:367–376.
39. Blot-Chabaud M, Wanstok F, Bonvalet J-P, Farman N. Cell sodium-induced recruitment of Na^+-K^+-ATPase pumps in rabbit cortical collecting tubules is aldosterone-dependent. *J Biol Chem* 1990;265:11676–11681.
40. Boim MA, Ho K, Shuck ME, Bienkowski MJ, Block JH, Slightom JL, Yang YH, Brenner BM, Hebert SC. ROMK inwardly rectifying ATP-sensitive K^+ channel. 2. Cloning and distribution of alternative forms. *Am J Physiol Renal Fluid Electrolyte* 1995;37:F1132–F1140.
41. Boldyreff B, Wehling M. Rapid aldosterone actions: from the membrane to signaling cascades to gene transcription and physiological effects. *J Steroid Biochem Mol Biol* 2003;85:375–381.
42. Bonny O, Hummler E. Dysfunction of epithelial sodium transport: from human to mouse. *Kidney Int* 2000;57:1313–1318.
43. Bonny O, Rossier BC. Disturbances of Na/K balance: pseudohypoaldosteronism revisited. *J Am Soc Nephrol* 2002;13:2399–2414.
44. Botero Velez M, Curtis JJ, Warnock DG. Liddles syndrome revisited—a disorder of sodium reabsorption in the distal tubule. *N Engl J Med* 1994;330:178–181.
45. Boulkroun S, Fay M, Zennaro MC, Escoubet B, Jaisser F, Blot-Chabaud M, Farman N, Courtois-Coutry N. Characterization of rat NDRG2 (N-Myc downstream regulated gene 2), a novel early mineralocorticoid-specific induced gene. *J Biol Chem* 2002;277:31506–31515.
46. Broillet M-C, Berger A, Horisberger J-D. Early effects of aldosterone on the basolateral potassium conductance of A6 cells. *Pflügers Arch* 1993;424:91–93.
47. Burgenerkairuz P, Corthesytheulaz I, Merillat AM, Good P, Geering K, Rossier BC. Polyadenylation of Na^+-K^+-ATPase beta (1)-subunit during early development of *Xenopus laevis*. *Am J Physiol* 1994;266:C157–C164.
48. Busjahn A, Aydin A, Uhlmann R, Krasko C, Bahring S, Szelestei T, Feng Y, Dahm S, Sharma AM, Luft FC, Lang F. Serum- and glucocorticoid-regulated kinase (SGK1) gene and blood pressure. *Hypertension* 2002;40:256–260.
49. Caldwell RA, Boucher RC, Stutts MJ. Neutrophil elastase activates near-silent epithelial Na^+ channels and increases airway epithelial Na^+ transport. *Am J Physiol Lung Cell Mol Physiol* 2005;288:L813–L819.
50. Canessa CM, Horisberger JD, Rossier BC. Epithelial sodium channel related to proteins involved in neurodegeneration. *Nature* 1993;361:467–470.
51. Canessa CM, Schild L, Buell G, Thorens B, Gautshi Y, Horisberger J-D, Rossier BC. The amiloride-sensitive epithelial sodium channel is made of three homologous subunits. *Nature* 1994;367:463–467.
52. Capurro C, Coutry N, Bonvalet JP, Escoubet B, Garty H, Farman N. Cellular localization and regulation of CHIF in kidney and colon. *Am J Physiol* 1996;271:C753–C762.
53. Carson-Jurica MA, Schrader WT, O'Malley BW. Steroid receptor family: structure and functions. *Endocr Rev* 1990;11:201–220.
54. Celsi G, Ståhl J, Wang Z-M, Nishi A. Adrenocorticoid regulation of Na^+,K^+-ATPase in adult rat kidney: effects on post-translational processing and mRNA abundance. *Acta Physiol Scand* 1992;145:85–91.
55. Chan GC, Hess P, Meenakshi T, Carlstedt-Duke J, Gustafsson JA, Payvar F. Delayed secondary glucocorticoid response elements. Unusual nucleotide motifs specify glucocorticoid receptor binding to transc-ribed regions of alpha 2u-globulin DNA. *J Biol Chem* 1991;266:22634–22644.
56. Chang SS, Grunder S, Hanukoglu A, Rosler A, Mathew PM, Hanukoglu I, Schild L, Lu Y, Shimkets RA, Nelson-Williams C, Rossier BC, Lifton RP. Mutations in subunits of the epithelial sodium channel cause salt wasting with hyperkalaemic acidosis, pseudohypoaldosteronism type 1. *Nat Genet* 1996;12:248–253.
57. Chen SY, Bhargava A, Mastroberardino L, Meijer OC, Wang J, Buse P, Firestone GL, Verrey F, Pearce D. Epithelial sodium channel regulated by aldosterone-induced protein sgk. *Proc Natl Acad Sci U S A* 1999;96:2514–2519.
58. Cheung J, Smith DF. Molecular chaperone interactions with steroid receptors: an update. *Mol Endocrinol* 2000;14:939–946.
59. Chraibi A, Vallet V, Firsov D, Hess SK, Horisberger JD. Protease modulation of the activity of the epithelial sodium channel expressed in *Xenopus* oocytes. *J Gen Physiol* 1998;111:127–138.
60. Chun TY, Pratt JH. Non-genomic effects of aldosterone: new actions and questions. *Trends Endocrinol Metab* 2004;15:353–354.
61. Clauss W, Arnason SS, Munck BG, Skadhauge E. Aldosterone-induced sodium transport in lower intestine. Effects of varying NaCl intake. *Pflugers Arch* 1984;401:354–360.
62. Clauss W, Durr JE, Guth D, Skadhauge E. Effects of adrenal steroids on Na transport in the lower intestine (coprodeum) of the hen. *J Membr Biol* 1987;96:141–152.
63. Clore J, Schoolwerth A, Watlington CO. When is cortisol a mineralocorticoid? *Kidney Int* 1992;42:1297–1308.
64. Cole TJ. Cloning of the mouse 11 beta-hydroxysteroid dehydrogenase type 2 gene: tissue specific expression and localization in distal convoluted tubules and collecting ducts of the kidney. *Endocrinology* 1995;136:4693–4696.
65. Cole TJ, Blendy JA, Monaghan AP, Krieglstein K, Schmid W, Aguzzi A, Fantuzzi G, Hummler E, Unsicker K, Schütz G. Targeted disruption of the glucocorticoid receptor gene blocks adrenergic chromaffin cell development and severely retards lung maturation. *Gene Dev* 1995;9:1608–1621.
66. Committee NR. A unified nomenclature system for the nuclear receptor superfamily. *Cell* 1999;97:161–163.
67. Cooper GJ, Hunter M. Na^1-H^1 exchange in frog early distal tubule: effect of aldosterone on the set-point. *J Physiol* 1994;479:423–432.
68. Couette B, Fagart J, Jalaguier S, Lombes M, Souque A, Rafestin-Oblin ME. Ligand-induced conformational change in the human mineralocorticoid receptor occurs within its hetero-oligomeric structure. *Biochem J* 1996;315:421–427.
69. Crabbé J. Stimulation of active sodium transport by the isolated toad bladder with aldosterone in vitro. *J Clin Invest* 1961;40:2103–2110.
70. Crabbé J. Suppression by amphotericin B of the effect exerted by aldosterone on active sodium transport. *Arch Int Physiol Biochim* 1967;75:342–345.
71. Crabbé J, Ehrlich EN. Amiloride and the mode of action of aldosterone on sodium transport across toad bladder and skin. *Pflügers Arch* 1968;304:284–296.
72. Dahlmann A, Pradervand S, Hummler E, Rossier BC, Frindt G, Palmer LG. Mineralocorticoid regulation of epithelial Na^+ channels is maintained in a mouse model of Liddle's syndrome. *Am J Physiol Renal Fluid Electrolyte Physiol* 2003;285:F310–F318.
73. Dean DM, Sanders MM. Ten years after: reclassification of steroid-responsive genes. *Mol Endocrinol* 1996;10:1489–1485.
74. Debonneville C, Flores SY, Kamynina E, Plant PJ, Tauxe C, Thomas MA, Munster C, Chraibi A, Pratt JH, Horisberger JD, Pearce D, Loffing J, Staub O. Phosphorylation of Nedd4-2 by Sgk1 regulates epithelial Na ($^+$) channel cell surface expression. *EMBO J* 2001;20:7052–7059.
75. Diakov A, Korbmacher C. A novel pathway of epithelial sodium channel activation involves a serum- and glucocorticoid-inducible kinase consensus motif in the C terminus of the channel's alpha-subunit. *J Biol Chem* 2004;279:38134–38142.
76. Dijkink L, Hartog A, Deen PM, van Os CH, Bindels RJ. Time-dependent regulation by aldosterone of the amiloride-sensitive Na^+ channel in rabbit kidney. *Pflugers Arch* 1999;438:354–360.
77. Djelidi S, Beggah A, Courtois-Coutry N, Fay M, Cluzeaud F, Viengchareun S, Bonvalet JP, Farman N, Blot-Chabaud M. Basolateral translocation by vasopressin of the aldosterone-induced pool of latent Na-K-ATPases is accompanied by alpha1 subunit dephosphorylation: study in a new aldosterone-sensitive rat cortical collecting duct cell line. *J Am Soc Nephrol* 2001;12: 1805–1818.
78. Dodson RE, Shapiro DJ. An estrogen-inducible protein binds specifically to a sequence in the 3' untranslated region of estrogen-stabilized vitellogenin mRNA. *Mol Cell Biol* 1994;14:3130–3138.
79. Doolan CM, Harvey BJ. Modulation of cytosolic protein kinase C and calcium ion activity by steroid hormones in rat distal colon. *J Biol Chem* 1996;271:8763–8767.
80. Duncan RL, Grogan WM, Kramer LB, Watlington CO. Corticosterone's metabolite is an agonist for Na^+ transport stimulation in A6 cells. *Am J Physiol* 1988;255:F736–F748.
81. Eaton DC. Intracellular sodium ion activity and sodium transport in rabbit urinary bladder. *J Physiol (Lond)* 1981;316:527–544.
82. Edelman IS, Bogoroch R, Porter GA. On the mechanism of action of aldosterone on sodium transport: the role of protein synthesis. *Proc Natl Acad Sci U S A* 1963;50:1169–1177.
83. Egli M, Duplain H, Lepori M, Cook S, Nicod P, Hummler E, Sartori C, Scherrer U. Defective respiratory amiloride-sensitive sodium transport predisposes to pulmonary oedema and delays its resolution in mice.*J Physiol (Lond)* 2004;560:857–865.
84. El Mernissi G, Charbades D, Doucet A, Hus-Citharel A, Imbert-Teboul M, Le Bouffant F, Montegut M, Siaume S, Morel F. Changes in tubular basolateral membrane markers after chronic treatment. *Am J Physiol* 1983;245:F100–F109.
85. Encio IJ, Detera-Wadleigh SD. The genomic structure of the human glucocorticoid receptor. *J Biol Chem* 1991;266:7182–7188.
86. Escoubet B, Coureau C, Bonvalet JP, Farman N. Noncoordinate regulation of epithelial Na channel and Na pump subunit mRNAs in kidney and colon by aldosterone. *Am J Physiol* 1997;272: C1482–C1491.
87. Fagart J, Huyet J, Pinon GM, Rochel M, Mayer C, Rafestin-Oblin ME. Cyrstal structure of a mutant mineralocorticoid receptor responsible for hypertension. *Nat Struct Mol Biol* 2005;12:554–555.
88. Fagart J, Wurtz JM, Souque A, Hellal-Levy C, Moras D, Rafestin-Oblin ME. Antagonism in the human mineralocorticoid receptor. *EMBO J* 1998;17:3317–3325.
89. Farman N, Coutry N, Logvinenko N, Blot-Chabaud M, Bourbouze R, Bonvalet JP. Adrenalectomy reduces a1 and not b1 Na^+-K^+-ATPase mRNA expression in rat distal nephron. *Am J Physiol Cell Physiol* 1992;263:C810–C817.
90. Farman N, Oblin ME, Lombes M, Delahaye F, Westphal HM, Bonvalet JP, Gasc JM. Immunolocalization of gluco- and mineralocorticoid receptors in rabbit kidney. *Am J Physiol* 1991;260:C226–C233.
91. Fejestoth G, Pearce D, Narayfejestoth A. Subcellular localization of mineralocorticoid receptors in living cells—effects of receptor agonists and antagonists. *Proc Natl Acad Sci U S A* 1998;95:2973–2978.
92. Feraille E, Mordasini D, Gonin S, Deschenes G, Vinciguerra M, Doucet A, Vandewalle A, Summa V, Verrey F, Martin PY. Mechanism of control of Na,K-ATPase in principal cells of the mammalian collecting duct. *Ann N Y Acad Sci* 2003;986:570–578.
93. Firsov D. Revisiting sodium and water reabsorption with functional genomics tools. *Curr Opin Nephrol Hypertens* 2004;13:59–65.

94. Firsov D, Gautschi I, Merillat AM, Rossier BC, Schild L. The heterotetrameric architecture of the epithelial sodium channel (ENaC). *EMBO J* 1998;17:344–352.
95. Firsov D, Schild L, Gautschi I, Merillat AM, Schneeberger E, Rossier BC. Cell surface expression of the epithelial Na channel and a mutant causing Liddle syndrome: a quantitative approach. *Proc Natl Acad Sci U S A* 1996;93:15370–15375.
96. Fischer F, Clauss W. Regulation of Na^+ channels in frog epithelium: a target tissue for aldosterone action. *Pflugers Arch* 1990;416:62–67.
97. Frindt G, Masilamani S, Knepper MA, Palmer LG. Activation of epithelial Na channels during short-term Na deprivation. *Am J Physiol Renal Physiol* 2001;280:F112–F118.
98. Frindt G, McNair T, Dahlmann A, Jacobs-Palmer E, Palmer LG. Epithelial Na channels and short-term renal response to salt deprivation. *Am J Phys* 2002;283:F717–F726.
99. Frindt G, Palmer LG. Apical potassium channels in the rat connecting tubule. *Am J Physiol Renal Physiol* 2004;287:F1030–F1037.
100. Frindt G, Palmer LG. Low-conductance K channels in apical membrane of rat cortical collecting tubule. *Am J Physiol* 1989;256:F143–F151.
101. Frindt G, Palmer LG. Na channels in the rat connecting tubule. *Am J Physiol* 2004;286: F669–F674.
102. Frindt G, Palmer LG. Regulation of Na channels in the rat cortical collecting tubule: effects of cAMP and methyl donors. *Am J Physiol* 1996;271:F1086–1092.
103. Frindt G, Sackin H, Palmer LG. Whole-cell currents in rat cortical collecting tubule: Low-Na diet increases amiloride-sensitive conductance. *Am J Physiol Renal Fluid Electrolyte Physiol* 1990;258:F562–F567.
104. Frindt G, Silver RB, Windhager EE, Palmer LG. Feedback regulation of Na channels in rat CCT II. Effects of inhibition of Na entry. *Am J Physiol* 1993;264:F565–F574.
105. Frizzell RA, Schultz SG. Effect of aldosterone on ion transport by rabbit colon in vitro. *J Membr Biol* 1978;39:1–26.
106. Fromm M, Schulzke JD, Hegel U. Control of electrogenic Na^+ absorption in rat late distal colon by nanomolar aldosterone added in vitro. *Am J Physiol* 1993;264:E68–E73.
107. Fujii Y, Takemoto F, Katz AI. Early effects of aldosterone on Na-K pump in rat cortical collecting tubules. *Am J Physiol Renal Fluid Electrolyte Physiol* 1990;259:F40–F45.
108. Funder JW. Aldosterone action. *Annu Rev Physiol* 1993;55:115–130.
109. Funder JW. The nongenomic actions of aldosterone. *Endocr Rev* 2005;26:313–321.
110. Funder JW, Pearce PT, Smith R, Smith AI. Mineralocorticoid action: target tissue specificity is enzyme not recpetor mediated. *Science* 1988;242:583–585.
111. Gaeggeler HP, Gonzalez-Rodriguez E, Jaeger NF, Loffing-Cueni D, Norregaard R, Loffing J, Horisberger JD, Rossier BC. Mineralocorticoid versus glucocorticoid receptor occupancy mediating aldosterone-stimulated sodium transport in a novel renal cell line. *J Am Soc Nephrol* 2005;16:878–891.
112. Gallego MS, Ling BN. Regulation of amiloride-sensitive Na^+ channels by endothelin-1 in distal nephron cells. *Am J Physiol Renal Fluid Electrolyte Physiol* 1996;40:F451–F460.
113. Garg LC, Knepper MA, Burg MB. Mineralocorticoid effects on Na-K-ATPase in individual nephron segments. *Am J Physiol* 1981;240:F536–F544.
114. Gariepy CE, Ohuchi T, Williams SC, Richardson JA, Yanagisawa M. Salt-sensitive hypertension in endothelin-B receptor-deficient rats. *J Clin Invest* 2000;105:925–933.
115. Garty H, Palmer L. Epithelial sodium channels: function, structure, and regulation. *Physiol Rev* 1997;77:359–396.
116. Garty H, Peterson-Yantorno K, Asher C, Civan MM. Effects of corticoid agonists and antagonists on apical Na^1 permeability of toad urinary bladder. *Am J Physiol Renal Fluid Electrolyte Physiol* 1994;266:F108–F116.
117. Geering K, Beguin P, Garty H, Karlish S, Fuzesi M, Horisberger JD, Crambert G. FXYD proteins: new tissue- and isoform-specific regulators of Na,K-ATPase. *Ann N Y Acad Sci* 2003;986:388–394.
118. Geering K, Claire M, Gaeggeler H-P, Rossier BC. Receptor occupancy vs induction of Na-K-ATPase and Na^+ transport by aldosterone. *Am J Physiol* 1985;248:C102–C108.
119. Geering K, Gaeggeler HP, Rossier BC. Effects of thyromimetic drugs on aldosterone-dependent sodium transport in the toad bladder. *J Membr Biol* 1984;77:15–23.
120. Geering K, Girardet M, Bron C, Kraehenbühl J-P, Rossier BC. Hormonal regulation of (Na^+,K^+)-ATPase biosynthesis in the toad bladder. Effect of aldosterone and 3,5,3'-triiodo-L-thyronine. *J Biol Chem* 1982;257:10338–10343.
121. Gekle M, Golenhofen N, Oberleithner H, Silbernagl S. Rapid activation of Na^+/H^+ exchange by aldosterone in renal epithelial cells requires $Ca2^+$ and stimulation of a plasma membrane proton conductance. *Proc Natl Acad Sci U S A* 1996;93:10500–10504.
122. Geller DS, Farhi A, Pinkerton N, Fradley M, Moritz M, Spitzer A, Meinke G, Tsai FTF, Sigler PB, Lifton RP. Activating mineralocorticoid receptor mutation in hypertension exacerbated by pregnancy. *Science* 2000;289:119–123.
123. Geller DS, Rodriguez-Soriano J, Vallo Boado A, Schifter S, Bayer M, Chang SS, Lifton RP. Mutations in the mineralocorticoid receptor gene cause autosomal dominant pseudohypoaldosteronism type I. *Nat Genet* 1998;19:279–281.
124. Goldschmidt I, Grahammer F, Warth R, Schulz-Baldes A, Garty H, Greger R, Bleich M. Kidney and colon electrolyte transport in CHIF knockout mice. *Cell Physiol Biochem* 2004;14:113–120.
125. Granitzer M, Mountian I, Vandriessche W. Effect of dexamethasone on sodium channel block and densities in A6 cells. *Pflugers Arch* 1995;430:493–500.
126. Gray DA, Frindt G, Palmer LG. Quantification of K^+ secretion through apical low-conductance K channels in the CCD. *Am J Physiol Renal Physiol* 2005;289:F117–F126.
127. Gross JB, Kokko JP. Effects of aldosterone and potassium-sparing diuretics on electrical potential differences across the distal nephron. *J Clin Invest* 1977;59:82–89.
128. Gross P, Minuth WW, Kriz W, Frömter E. Electrical properties of renal collecting duct principal cell epithelium in tissue culture. *Pflügers Arch* 1986;406:380–386.
129. Grotjohann I, Schulzke JD, Fromm M. Electrogenic Na^+ transport in rat late distal colon by natural and synthetic glucocorticosteroids. *Am J Physiol Gastrointest Liver Physiol* 1999;39: G491–G498.
130. Guerrero ML, Beron J, Spindler B, Groscurth P, Wallimann T, Verrey F. Metabolic support of Na^+ pump in apically permeabilized A6 kidney cell epithelia—role of creatine kinase. *Am J Physiol Cell Physiol* 1997;41:C697–C706.
131. Guiochon-Mantel A, Delabre K, Lescop P, Milgrom E. The Ernst Schering Poster Award. Intracellular traffic of steroid hormone receptors. *J Steroid Biochem Mol Biol* 1996;56:3–9.
132. Gumz ML, Popp MP, Wingo CS, Cain BD. Early transcriptional effects of aldosterone in a mouse inner medullary collecting duct cell line. *Am J Physiol Renal Physiol* 2003;285: 664–F673.
133. Hamilton KL, Eaton DC. Regulation of single sodium channels in renal tissue: a role in sodium homeostasis. *Fed Proc* 1986;45:2713–2717.
134. Handler JS, Perkins FM, Johnson JP. Hormone effects on transport in cultured epithelia with high electrical resistance. *Am J Physiol* 1981;240:C103–C105.
135. Handler JS, Preston AS, Orloff J. Effect of adrenal steroid hormones on the response of the toad's urinary bladder to vasopressin. *J Clin Invest* 1969;48:823–833.
136. Handler JS, Preston AS, Steele RE. Factors affecting the differentiation of epithelial transport and responsiveness to hormones. *Fed Proc* 1984;43:2221–2224.
137. Handler JS, Steele RE, Sahib MK, Wade JB, Preston AS, Lawson NL, Johnson JP. Toad urinary bladder epithelial cells in culture: Maintenance of epithelial structure, sodium transport, and response to hormones. *Proc Natl Acad Sci U S A* 1979;76:4151–4155.
138. Hansson JH, Nelson-Williams C, Suzuki H, Schild L, Shimkets RA, Lu Y, Canessa CM, Iwasaki T, Rossier BC, Lifton RP. Hypertension caused by a truncated epithelial sodium channel g subunit: genetic heterogeneity of Liddle syndrome. *Nat Genet* 1995;11:76–82.
139. Hansson JH, Schild L, Lu Y, Wilson TA, Gautschi I, Shimkets RA, Nelson-Williams C, Rossier BC, Lifton RP. A de novo missense mutation of the beta subunit of the epithelial sodium channel causes hypertension and liddle syndrome, identifying a proline-rich segment critical for regulation of channel activity. *Proc Natl Acad Sci U S A* 1995;92:11495–11499.
140. Harvey BJ, Thomas SR, Ehrenfeld J. Intracellular pH controls cell membrane Na^+ and K^+ conductances and transport in frog skin epithelium. *J Gen Physiol* 1988;92:767–791.
141. Hayhurst RA, O'Neil RG. Time-dependent actions of aldosterone and amiloride on Na^+-K^+-ATPase of cortical collecting duct. *Am J Physiol* 1988;254:F689–F696.
142. Helman SI, Koeppen BM, Beyenbach KW, Baxendale LM. Patch clamp studies of apical membranes of renal cortical collecting ducts. *Pflügers Arch* 1985;405:S71–S76.
143. Helman SI, Liu XH, Baldwin K, Blazeryost BL, Els WJ. Time-dependent stimulation by aldosterone of blocker-sensitive ENaCs in A6 epithelia. *Am J Physiol Cell Physiol* 1998;43: C947–C957.
144. Hilfenhaus M. Circadian rhythm of the renin-angiotensin-aldosterone system in the rat. *Arch Tox* 1976;36:305–316.
145. Hoffmann B, Clauss W. Time-dependent effects of aldosterone on sodium transport and cell membrane resistances in rabbit distal colon. *Pflügers Arch* 1989;415:156–164.
146. Hollenberg SM, Weinberger C, Ong ES, Cerelli G, Oro A, Lebo R, Thompson EB, Rosenfeld MG, Evans RM. Primary structure and expression of a functional human glucocorticoid receptor cDNA. *Nature* 1985;318:635–641.
147. Holley SJ, Yamamoto KR. A role for Hsp90 in retinoid receptor signal transduction. *Mol Biol Cell* 1995;6:1833–1842.
148. Holmes MC, Kotelevtsev Y, Mullins JJ, Seckl JR. Phenotypic analysis of mice bearing targeted deletions of 11beta-hydroxysteroid dehydrogenases 1 and 2 genes. *Mol Cell Endocrinol* 2001;171:15–20.
149. Holmstrom S, Van Antwerp ME, Iniguez-Lluhi JA. Direct and distinguishable inhibitory roles for SUMO isoforms in the control of transcriptional synergy. *Proc Natl Acad Sci U S A* 2003;100:15758–15763.
150. Horisberger J-D. Early effects of aldosterone on the basolateral membrane of tight epithelia. *Renal Physiol Biochem* 1992;15:207.
151. Horisberger J-D. *The Na,K-ATPase: Structure–Function Relationship.* Austin, TX: R.G. Landes Company; 1994.
152. Horisberger J-D, Diezi J. Effects of mineralocorticoids on Na^+ and K^+ excretion in the adrenalectomized rat. *Am J Physiol* 1983;245:F89–F99.
153. Horisberger JD, Diezi J. Inhibition of aldosterone-induced antinatriuresis and kaliuresis by actinomycin D. *Am J Physiol* 1984;246:F201–F204.
154. Horster M, Shmid H, Schmidt U. Aldosterone in vitro restores nephron Na-K-ATPase of distal segments from adrenalectomized rabbits. *Pflügers Arch* 1980;384:203–206.
155. Horster MF, Schmolke M, Gleich R. Expression of pump activity and of transepithelial voltage induced by hormones in cultures cortical collecting tubule cells. *Min Electrolyte Metab* 1989;15:137–143.
156. Htun H, Barsony J, Renyi I, Gould DL, Hager GL. Visualization of glucocorticoid receptor translocation and intranuclear organization in living cells with a green fluorescent protein chimera. *Proc Natl Acad Sci U S A* 1996;93:4845–4850.
157. Huang DY, Wulff P, Volkl H, Loffing J, Richter K, Kuhl D, Lang F, Vallon V. Impaired regulation of renal K^+ elimination in the sgk1-knockout mouse. *J Am Soc Nephrol* 2004;15:885–891.
158. Hubert C, Gasc JM, Berger S, Schutz G, Corvol P. Effects of mineralocorticoid receptor gene disruption on the components of the renin-angiotensin system in 8-day-old mice. *Mol Endocrinol.* 1999;13:297–306.
159. Hughey RP, Bruns JB, Kinlough CL, Harkleroad KL, Tong Q, Carattino MD, Johnson JP, Stockand JD, Kleyman TR. Epithelial sodium channels are activated by furin-dependent proteolysis. *J Biol Chem* 2004;279:18111–18114.
160. Hughey RP, Mueller GM, Bruns JB, Kinlough CL, Poland PA, Harkleroad KL, Carattino MD, Kleyman TR. Maturation of the epithelial Na^+ channel involves proteolytic processing of the alpha- and gamma-subunits. *J Biol Chem* 2003;278:37073–37082.
161. Hummler E. Implication of ENaC in salt-sensitive hypertension. *J Steroid Biochem Mol Biol* 1999;69(Suppl)-:385–390.
162. Hummler E, Barker P, Gatzy J, Beermann F, Verdumo C, Schmidt A, Boucher R, Rossier BC. Early death due to defective neonatal lung liquid clearance in alpha-ENaC-deficient mice. *Nat Genet* 1996;12:325–328.

163. Hummler E, Barker P, Talbot C, Wang Q, Verdumo C, Grubb B, Gatzy J, Burnier M, Horisberger JD, Beermann F, Boucher R, Rossier BC. A mouse model for the renal salt-wasting syndrome pseudohypoaldosteronism. *Proc Natl Acad Sci U S A* 1997;94:11710–11715.
164. Hummler E, Horisberger JD. Genetic disorders of membrane transport. V. The epithelial sodium channel and its implication in human diseases. *Am J Physiol Gastrointest Liver Physiol* 1999;39: G567–G571.
165. Hurwitz S, Cohen RJ, Williams GH. Diurnal variation of aldosterone and plasma renin activity: timing relation to melatonin and cortisol and consistency after prolonged bed rest. *J Appl Physiol* 2004;96:1406–1414.
166. Husted RF, Stokes JB. Separate regulation of Na^+ and anion transport by IMCD: location, aldosterone, hypertonicity, TGF-beta 1 and cAMP. *Am J Physiol* 1996;271:F433–F439.
167. Husted RF, Laplace JR, Stokes JB. Enhancement of electrogenic Na^+ transport across rat inner medullary collecting duct by glucocorticoid and by mineralocorticoid hormones. *J Clin Invest* 1990;86:498–506.
168. Husted RF, Matsushita K, Stokes JB. Induction of resistance to mineralocorticoid hormone in cultured inner medullary collecting duct cells by TGF-beta 1. *Am J Physiol* 1994;267: F767–F775.
169. Husted RF, Takahashi T, Stokes JB. IMCD cells cultured from Dahl S rats absorb more Na^+ than Dahl R rats. *Am J Physiol* 1996;271:F1029–F1036.
170. Ichimura T, Yamamura H, Sasamoto K, Tominaga Y, Taoka M, Kakiuchi K, Shinkawa T, Takahashi N, Shimada S, Isobe T. 14-3-3 proteins modulate the expression of epithelial Na^+ channels by phosphorylation-dependent interaction with Nedd4-2 ubiquitin ligase. *J Biol Chem* 2005;280:13187–13194.
171. Iniguez-Lluhi JA, Pearce D. A common motif within the negative regulatory regions of multipel factors inhibits their transcriptional synergy. *Mol Cell Biol* 2000;20:6040–6050.
172. Iwashita K, Kitamura K, Narikiyo T, Adachi M, Shiraishi N, Miyoshi T, Nagano J, Tuyen do G, Nonoguchi H, Tomita K. Inhibition of prostasin secretion by serine protease inhibitors in the kidney. *J Am Soc Nephrol* 2003;14:11–16.
173. Jorasky D, Cox M, Feldman GM. Differential effects of corticosteroids on Na^+ transport in rat distal colon in vitro. *Am J Physiol* 1985;248:G424–G431.
174. Jorgensen PL. Structure, function and regulation of Na,K-ATPase in the kidney. *Kidney Int* 1986;29:10–20.
175. Kahle KT, Gimenez I, Hassan H, Wilson FH, Wong RD, Forbush B, Aronson PS, Lifton RP. WNK4 regulates apical and basolateral Cl^- flux in extrarenal epithelia. *Proc Natl Acad Sci U S A* 2004;101:2064–2069.
176. Kahle KT, Wilson FH, Lalioti M, Toka H, Qin H, Lifton RP. WNK kinases: molecular regulators of integrated epithelial ion transport. *Curr Opin Nephrol Hypertens* 2004;13:557–562.
177. Kaissling B, Le Hir M. Distal tubular segments of the rabbit kidney after adaptation to altered Na- and K-intake. *Cell Tissue Res* 1982;224:469–492.
178. Kashgarian M, Ardito T, Hirsch DJ, Hayslett JP. Response of collecting tubule cells to aldosterone and potassium loading. *Am J Physiol* 1987;253:F8–F14.
179. Kato S, Sasaki H, Suzawa M, Masushige S, Tora L, Chambon P, Gronemeyer H. Widely spaced, directly repeated PuGGTCA elements act as promiscuous enhancers for different classes of nuclear receptors. *Mol Cell Biol* 1995;15:5858–5867.
180. Katz AI, Doucet A, Morel F. Na-K-ATPase activity along the rabbit, rat, and mouse nephron. *Am J Physiol* 1979;237:114–120.
181. Kenouch S, Alfaidy N, Bonvalet JP, Farman N. Expression of 11 beta-OHSD along the nephron of mammals and humans. *Steroids* 1994;59:100–104.
182. Kerem E, Bistritzer T, Hanukoglu A, Hofmann T, Zhou Z, Bennett W, MacLaughlin E, Barker P, Nash M, Quittell L, Boucher R, Knowles MR. Pulmonary epithelial sodium-channel dysfunction and excess airway liquid in pseudohypoaldosteronism. *N Engl J Med* 1999;341:156–162.
183. Khadouri C, Marsy S, Barlet-Bas C, Doucet A. Short-term effect of aldosterone on NEM-sensitive ATPase in rat collecting tubule. *Am J Physiol* 1989;257:F177–F181.
184. Kim EK, Wood CE, Keller-Wood M. Characterization of 11 beta-hydroxysteroid dehydrogenase activity in fetal and adult ovine tissues. *Reprod Fertil Dev* 1995;7:377–383.
185. Kim G, Masilamani S, Turner R, Mitchell C, Wade J, Knepper M. The thiazide-sensitive Na-Cl cotransporter is an aldosterone-induced protein. *Proc Natl Acad Sci U S A* 1998;95:14552–14557.
186. Kinne R, Kirsten R. Effect of aldosterone on the activity of mitochondrial and cytoplasmic enzymes in the rat kidney. *Pflügers Arch* 1968;300:244–254.
187. Kitagawa H, Yanagisawa J, Fuse H, Ogawa S, Yogiashi Y, Okuno A, Nagasawa H, Nakajima T, Matsumoto T, Kato S. Ligand-selective potentiation of rat mineralocorticoid receptor activation function 1 by a CBP-containing histone acetyltransferase complex. *Mol Cell Biol* 2002;22:3698–3706.
188. Kobayashi T, Cohen P. Activation of serum- and glucocorticoid-regulated protein kinase by agonists that activate phosphatidylinositide 3-kinase is mediated by 3-phosphoinositide-dependent protein kinase-1 (PDK1) and PDK2. *Biochem J* 1999;339:319–328.
189. Koefoed-Johnsen V, Ussing HH. The nature of the frog skin potential. *Acta Physiol Scand* 1958;42:298–308.
190. Kolla V, Litwack G. Transcriptional regulation of the human Na/K ATPase via the human mineralocorticoid receptor. *Mol Cell Biochem* 2000;204:35–40.
191. Konstas AA, Shearwin-Whyatt LM, Fotia AB, Degger B, Riccardi D, Cook DI, Korbmacher C, Kumar S. Regulation of the epithelial sodium channel by N4WBP5A, a novel Nedd4/Nedd4-2-interacting protein. *J Biol Chem* 2002;277:29406–29416.
192. Kotelevtsev Y, Brown RW, Fleming S, Kenyon C, Edwards CR, Seckl JR, Mullins JJ. Hypertension in mice lacking 11beta-hydroxysteroid dehydrogenase type 2. *J Clin Invest* 1999;103: 683–689.
193. Kotelevtsev Y, Holmes MC, Burchell A, Houston PM, Schmoll D, Jamieson P, Best R, Brown RW, Edwards CR, Seckl JR, Mullins JJ. 11beta-hydroxysteroid dehydrogenase type 1 knockout mice show attenuated glucocorticoid-inducible responses and resist hyperglycemia on obesity or stress. *Proc Natl Acad Sci U S A* 1997;94:14924–14929.
194. Kralli A, Yamamoto KR. An FK506-sensitive transporter selectively decreases intracellular levels and potency of steroid hormones. *J Biol Chem* 1996;271:17152–17156.
195. Krattenmacher R, Clauss W. Electrophysiological analysis of sodium-transport in the colon of the frog (*Rana esculenta*). *Pflügers Arch* 1988;411:606–612.
196. Kriz RW, Kaissling B. Structural organization of the mammalian kidney. In: Seldin DW, Giebisch G, eds. *The Kidney*, Vol 1, 3rd ed. Philadelphia: Lippincott Williams & Wilkins; 2000:587–654.
197. Krozowski Z, Maguire JA, Steinoakley AN, Dowling J, Smith RE, Andrews RK. Immunohistochemical localization of the 11 beta-hydroxysteroid dehydrogenase type II enzyme in human kidney and placenta. *J Clin Endocrinol Metab* 1995;80:2203–2209.
198. Krug AW, Grossmann C, Schuster C, Freudinger R, Mildenberger S, Govindan MV, Gekle M. Aldosterone stimulates epidermal growth factor receptor expression. *J Biol Chem* 2003;278:43060–43066.
199. Kwak SP, Patel PD, Thompson RC, Akil H, Watson SJ. 5'-heterogeneity of the mineralocorticoid receptor messenger ribonucleic acid: differential expression and regulation of splice variants within the rat hippocampus. *Endocrinology* 1993;133:2344–2350.
200. Laplace JR, Husted RF, Stokes JB. Cellular responses to steroids in the enhancement of Na^+ transport by rat collecting duct cells in culture. Differences between glucocorticoid and mineralocorticoid hormones. *J Clin Invest* 1992;90:1370–1378.
201. Le Hir M, Kaissling B, Dubach UC. Distal tubular segments of the rabbit kidney after adaptation to altered Na- and K- intake. *Cell Tissue Res* 1982;224:493–504.
202. Le Menuet D, Isnard R, Bichara M, Viengchareun S, Muffat-Joly M, Walker F, Zennaro MC, Lombes M. Alteration of cardiac and renal functions in transgenic mice overexpressing human mineralocorticoid receptor. *J Biol Chem* 2001;276:38911–38920.
203. Le Menuet D, Viengchareun S, Penfornis P, Walker F, Zennaro MC, Lombes M. Targeted oncogenesis reveals a distinct tissue-specific utilization of alternative promoters of the human mineralocorticoid receptor gene in transgenic mice. *J Biol Chem* 2000;75:7878–7886.
204. Le Moellic C, Ouvrard-Pascaud A, Capurro C, Cluzeaud F, Fay M, Jaisser F, Farman N, Blot-Chabaud M. Early nongenomic events in aldosterone action in renal collecting duct cells: PKCalpha activation, mineralocorticoid receptor phosphorylation, and cross-talk with the genomic response. *J Am Soc Nephrol* 2004;5:1145–1160.
205. Lewis SA, Diamond JM. Na^+ transport by rabbit urinary bladder, a tight epithelium. *J Membr Biol* 1976;8:1–40.
206. Leyvraz C, Charles RP, Rubera I, Guitard M, Rotman S, Breiden B, Sandhoff K, Hummler E. The epidermal barrier function is dependent on the serine protease CAP1/Prss8. *J Cell Biol* 2005;70:487–496.
207. Li KX, Smith RE, Ferrari P, Funder JW, Krozowski ZS. Rat 11 beta-hydroxysteroid dehydrogenase type 2 enzyme is expressed at low levels in the placenta and is modulated by adrenal steroids in the kidney. *Mol Cell Endocrinol* 1996;20:67–75.
208. Lichtenstein NS, Leaf A. Effect of amphotericin b on the permeability of the toad bladder. *J Clin Invest* 1965;44:1328–1342.
209. Liddle GW, Bledsoe T, Coppage WS. A familial renal disorder simulating primary aldosteronism but with negligible aldosterone secretion. *Trans Assoc Am Physicians* 1963;76:199–213.
210. Lifton RP. Molecular genetics of human blood pressure variation. *Science* 1996;272:676–680.
211. Lim-Tio SS, Fuller PJ. Intracellular signaling pathways confer specificity of transactivation by mineralocorticoid and glucocorticoid receptors. *Endocrinology* 1998;139:1653–1661.
212. Lindemann B, Van Driessche W. Sodium-specific membrane channels of frog skin are pores: current fluctuations reveal high turnover. *Science* 1977;195:292–294.
213. Lingueglia E, Voilley N, Waldmann R, Lazdunski M, Barbry P. Expression cloning of an epithelial amiloride-sensitive Na^+ channel. *FEBS Lett* 1993;318:95–99.
214. List K, Haudenschild CC, Szabo R, Chen W, Wahl SM, Swaim W, Engelholm LH, Behrendt N, Bugge TH. Matriptase/MT-SP1 is required for postnatal survival, epidermal barrier function, hair follicle development, and thymic homeostasis. *Oncogene* 2002;21:3765–3779.
215. Liu W, Wang J, Yu G, Pearce D. Steroid receptor transcriptional synergy is potentiated by disruption of the DNA-binding domain dimer interface. *Mol Endocrinol* 1996;10:1399–1406.
216. Loffing J, Kaissling B. Sodium and calcium pathways along the mammalian distal nephron: from rabbit to human. *Am J Physiol Renal Physiol* 2003;284:F628–F643.
217. Loffing J, Loffing-Cueni D, Valderrabano V, Klausli L, Hebert SC, Rossier BC, Hoenderop JG, Bindels RJ, Kaissling B. Organization of the mouse distal nephron: distributions of transcellular calcium and sodium transport pathways. *Am J Physiol Renal Physiol* 2001;281:F1021–F1027.
218. Loffing J, Pietri L, Aregger F, Bloch-Faure M, Ziegler U, Meneton P, Rossier BC, Kaissling B. Differential subcellular localization of ENaC subunits in mouse kidney in response to high- and low-Na diets. *Am J Physiol Renal Physiol* 2000;279:F252–F258.
219. Loffing J, Zecevic M, Feraille E, Kaissling B, Asher C, Rossier BC, Firestone GL, Pearce D, Verrey F. Aldosterone induces rapid apical translocation of ENaC in early portion of renal collecting system: possible role of SGK. *Am J Physiol Renal Physiology* 2001;280: F675–F682.
220. Losel R, Schultz A, Wehling M. A quick glance at rapid aldosterone action. *Mol Cell Endocrinol* 2004;217:137–141.
221. Losel RM, Falkenstein E, Feuring M, Schultz A, Tillmann HC, Rossol-Haseroth K, Wehling M. Nongenomic steroid action: controversies, questions and answers. *Physiol Rev* 2003;83:965–1016.
222. Lu M, Wang T, Yan Q, Yang X, Dong K, Knepper MA, Wang W, Giebisch G, Shull GE, Hebert SC. Absence of small conductance K^+ channel (SK) activity in apical membranes of thick ascending limb and cortical collecting duct in ROMK (Bartter's) knockout mice. *J Biol Chem* 2002:277:37881–37887.
223. Lyall V, Biber TUL. Ph modulates cAMP-induced increase in Na^+ transport across frog skin epithelium. *Biochim Biophys Acta Bio-Membr* 1995;1240:65–74.
224. Lyall V, Feldman GM, Biber TUL. Regulation of apical Na^+ conductive transport in epithelia by pH. *Biochim Biophys Acta Bio-Membr* 1995;1241:31–44.
225. MacDonald P, MacKenzie S, Ramage LE, Seckl JR, Brown RW. Corticosteroid regulation of amiloride-sensitive sodium-channel subunit mRNA expression in mouse kidney. *J Endocrinol* 2000;165:25–37.
226. Maguire D, MacNamara B, Cuffe JE, Winter D, Doolan CM, Urbach V, O'Sullivan GC, Harvey BJ. Rapid responses to aldosterone in human distal colon. *Steroids* 1999;64–: 51–63.

227. Malnic G, Muto S, Giebsich G. Regulation of potassium excretion. In: Seldin DW, Giebisch G, eds. *The Kidney*, Vol. 2, 3rd ed. Philadelphia: Lippincott Williams & Wilkins; 2000:1575–1613.
228. Mangelsdorf DJ, Thummel C, Beato M, Herrlich P, Schütz G, Umesono K, Blumberg B, Kastner P, Mark M, Chambon P, Evans RM. The nuclear receptor superfamily: the second decade. *Cell* 1995;83:835–839.
229. Masilamani S, Kim GH, Mitchell C, Wade JB, Knepper MA. Aldosterone-mediated regulation of ENaC alpha, beta, and gamma subunit proteins in rat kidney. *J Clin Invest* 1999;104: R19–R23 (see comment).
230. Masilamani S, Wang X, Kim GH, Brooks H, Nielsen J, Nielsen S, Nakamura K, Stokes JB, Knepper MA. Time course of renal Na-K-ATPase, NHE3, NKCC2, NCC, and ENaC abundance changes with dietary NaCl restriction. *Am J Physiol Renal Fluid Electrolyte Physiol* 2002;283:F648–F657.
231. Mastroberardino L, Spindler B, Forster I, Loffing J, Assandri R, May A, Verrey F. Ras pathway activates epithelial Na^+ channel and decreases its surface expression in *Xenopus* oocytes. *Mol Biol Cell* 1998;9:3417–3427.
232. Masuzaki H, Flier JS. Tissue-specific glucocorticoid reactivating enzyme, 11 beta-hydroxysteroid dehydrogenase type 1 (11 beta-HSD1)—a promising drug target for the treatment of metabolic syndrome. *Curr Drug Targets Immune Endocr Metab Disord* 2003;3:255–262.
233. May A, Puoti A, Gaeggeler HP, Horisberger JD, Rossier BC. Early effect of aldosterone on the rate of synthesis of the epithelial sodium channel alpha subunit in A6 renal cells. *J Am Soc Nephrol* 1997;8:1813–1822.
234. McDonald FJ, Yang B, Hrstka RF, Drummond HA, Tarr DE, McCray PB Jr, Stokes JB, Welsh MJ, Williamson RA. Disruption of the beta subunit of the epithelial Na^+ channel in mice: hyperkalemia and neonatal death associated with a pseudohypoaldosteronism phenotype. *Proc Natl Acad Sci U S A* 1999;96:1727–1731.
235. Meijer OC, Kalkhoven E, Van der Laan S, Steenbergen PJ, Houtman SH, Dijkmans TF, Pearce D, de Kloet ER. Steroid receptor coactivator-1 splice variants differentially affect corticosteroid receptor signaling. *Endocrinology* 2005;146:1438–1448.
236. Meijer OC, Steenbergen PJ, De Kloet ER. Differential expression and regional distribution of steroid receptor coactivators jSRC-1 and SRC-2 in brain and pituitary. *Endocrinology* 2000;141:2192–2199.
237. Mennitt PA, Wade JB, Ecelbarger CA, Palmer LG, Frindt G. Localization of ROMK channels in the rat kidney. *J Am Soc Nephrol* 1997;8:1823–1830.
238. Mick VE, Itani OA, Loftus RW, Husted RF, Schmidt TJ, Thomas CP. The alpha-subunit of the epithelial sodium channel is an aldosterone-induced transcript in mammalian collecting ducts, and this transcriptional response is mediated via distinct cis-elements in the 5'-flanking region of the gene. *Mol Endocrinol* 2001;15:575–588.
239. Monder C, Lakshmi V. Corticosteroid 11 beta-dehydrogenase of rat tissues: immunological studies. *Endocrinology* 1990;126:2435–2443.
240. Morris DJ, Latif SA, Rokaw MD, Watlington CO, Johnson JP. A second enzyme protecting mineralocorticoid receptors from glucocorticoid occupancy. *Am J Physiol Cell Physiol* 1998;43:C1245–C1252.
241. Morris DJ, Souness GW. Protective and specificity-conferring mechanisms of mineralocorticoid action. *Am J Physiol* 1992;263:F759–F768.
242. Morton NM, Paterson JM, Masuzaki H, Holmes MC, Staels B, Fievet C, Walker BR, Flier JS, Mullins JJ, Seckl JR. Novel adipose tissue-mediated resistance to diet-induced visceral obesity in 11 beta-hydroxysteroid dehydrogenase type 1–deficient mice. *Diabetes* 2004;53:931–938.
243. Muller OG, Parnova RG, Centeno G, Rossier BC, Firsov D, Horisberger JD. Mineralocorticoid effects in the kidney: correlation between alphaENaC, GILZ, and Sgk-1 mRNA expression and urinary excretion of Na^+ and K^+. *J Am Soc Nephrol* 2003;14:1107–1115.
244. Mune T, Rogerson FM, Nikkila H, Agarwal AK, White PC. Human hypertension caused by mutations in the kidney isozyme of 11-beta-hydroxysteroid dehydrogenase. *Nat Genet* 1995;10:394–399.
245. Nagel W, Crabbé J. Mechanism of action of aldosterone on active sodium transport across toad skin. *Pflügers Arch* 1980;385:181–187.
246. Nagy L, Schwabe JWR. Mechanism of the nuclear receptor molecular switch. *Trends Biochem Sci* 2004;29:317–324.
247. Naray-Fejes-Toth A, Canessa C, Cleaveland ES, Aldrich G, Fejes-Toth G. sgk is an aldosterone-induced kinase in the renal collecting duct. Effects on epithelial Na^1 channels. *J Biol Chem* 1999;274:16973–16978.
248. Naray–Fejes-Toth A, Fejes-Toth G. Extranuclear localization of endogenous 11beta-hydroxysteroid dehydrogenase-2 in aldosterone target cells. *Endocrinology* 1998;139:2955–2959.
249. Naray–Fejes-Toth A, Fejestoth G. Expression cloning of the aldosterone target cell-specific 11 beta-hydroxysteroid dehydrogenase from rabbit collecting duct cells. *Endocrinology* 1995;136:2579–2586.
250. Naray–Fejes-Toth A, Snyder PM, Fejes-Toth G. The kidney-specific WNK1 isoform is induced by aldosterone and stimulates epithelial sodium channel-mediated Na^+ transport. *Proc Natl Acad Sci U S A* 2004;101:17434–17439.
251. Narikiyo T, Kitamura K, Adachi M, Miyoshi T, Iwashita K, Shiraishi N, Nonoguchi H, Chen L-M, Chai KX, Chao J, Tomita K. Regulation of prostasin by aldosterone in the kidney. *J Clin Invest* 2002;109:401–408.
252. O'Malley BW, Schrader WT, Mani S, Smith C, Weigel NL, Conneely OM, Clark JH. An alternative ligand-independent pathway for activation of steroid receptors. *Recent Prog Horm Res* 1995;50:333–347.
253. O'Neil RG, Hayhurst RA. Sodium-dependent modulation of the renal Na-K-ATPase: Influence of mineralocorticoids on the cortical collecting duct. *J Membr Biol* 1985;85:169–179.
254. O'Neil RG, Helman SI. Transport characteristics of renal collecting tubules: influences of DOCA and diet. *Am J Physiol* 1977;233:F554–F558.
255. Oberleithner H, Weigt M, Westphale H-J, Wang W. Aldosterone activates Na^+/H^+ exchange and raises cytoplasmic pH in target cells of the amphibian kidney. *Proc Natl Acad Sci U S A* 1987;84:1464–1468.
256. Olivier R, Scherrer U, Horisberger JD, Rossier BC, Hummler E. Selected contribution: limiting Na (^{1}) transport rate in airway epithelia from alpha-ENaC transgenic mice: a model for pulmonary edema. *J Appl Physiol* 2002;93:1881–1887.
257. Ono S, Kusano E, Muto S, Ando Y, Asano Y. A low-Na^+ diet enhances expression of mRNA for epithelial Na^1 channel in rat renal inner medulla. *Pflugers Arch* 1997;434: 756–763.
258. Otto C, Reichardt HM, Schutz G. Absence of glucocorticoid receptor-beta in mice. *J Biol Chem* 1997;272:26665–26668.
259. Paccolat MP, Geering K, Gaeggeler HP, Rossier BC. Aldosterone regulation of Na^+ transport and Na^+-K^+-ATPase in A6 cells: role of growth conditions. *Am J Physiol* 1987;252:C468–C476.
260. Pacha J, Frindt G, Antonian L, Silver RB, Palmer LG. Regulation of Na channels of the rat cortical collecting tubule by aldosterone. *J Gen Physiol* 1993;102:25–42.
261. Palmer LG, Antonian L, Frindt G. Regulation of the Na-K pump of the rat cortical collecting tubule by aldosterone. *J Gen Physiol* 1993;102:43–57.
262. Palmer LG, Frindt G. Aldosterone and potassium secretion by the cortical collecting duct. *Kidney Int* 2000;57:1324–1328.
263. Palmer LG, Frindt G. Amiloride-sensitive Na channels from the apical membrane of the rat cortical collecting tubule. *Proc Natl Acad Sci U S A* 1986;83:2767–2770.
264. Palmer LG, Frindt G, Hummler E, Rossier BC. Na channel activity in the collecting duct of a mouse model of Liddle's syndrome. *FASEB J* 2001;15:A430.
265. Palmer LG, Li JHY, Lindemann B, Edelman IS. Aldosterone control the density of sodium channels in the toad urinary bladder. *J Membr Biol* 1982;64:91–102.
266. Paterson JM, Seckl JR, Mullins JJ. Genetic manipulation of 11b-hydroxysteroid dehydrogenases in mice. *Am J Physiol Regul Integr Comp Physiol* 2005;289:R642–R652.
267. Pearce D, Naray-Fejes-Toth A, Fejes-Toth G. Determinants of sub-nuclear organization of mineralocorticoid receptor characterized through analysis of wild type and mutant receptors. *J Biol Chem* 2002;277:1451–1456.
268. Pellanda AM, Gaeggeler HP, Horisberger JD, Rossier BC. Sodium-independent effect of aldosterone on initial rate of ouabain binding in A6 cells. *Am J Physiol* 1992;262:C899–C906.
269. Petty KJ, Kokko JP, Marver D. Secondary effect of aldosterone on Na-K-ATPase activity in the rabbit cortical collecting tubule. *J Clin Invest* 1981;68:1514–1521.
270. Porter GA, Bogoroch R, Edelman IS. On the mechanism of action of aldosterone on sodium transport: the role of RNA synthesis. *Proc Natl Acad Sci U S A* 1964;52:1326–1333.
271. Power RF, Mani SK, Codina J, Conneely OM, O'Malley BW. Dopaminergic and ligand-independent activation of steroid hormone receptors. *Science* 1991;254:1636–1639.
272. Pradervand S, Barker PM, Wang Q, Ernst SA, Beermann F, Grubb BR, Burnier M, Schmidt A, Bindels RJ, Gatzy JT, Rossier BC, Hummler E. Salt restriction induces pseudohypoaldosteronism type 1 in mice expressing low levels of the beta-subunit of the amiloride-sensitive epithelial sodium channel. *Proc Natl Acad Sci U S A* 1999;96:1732–1737.
273. Pradervand S, Vandewalle A, Bens M, Gautschi I, Loffing J, Hummler E, Schild L, Rossier BC. Dysfunction of the epithelial sodium channel expressed in the kidney of a mouse model for Liddle syndrome. *J Am Soc Nephrol* 2003;14:2219–2228.
274. Pradervand S, Wang Q, Burnier M, Beermann F, Horisberger JD, Hummler E, Rossier BC. A mouse model for Liddle's syndrome. *J Am Soc Nephrol* 1999;10:2527–2533.
275. Pratt WB, Toft DO. Steroid receptor interactions with heat shock protein and immunophilin chaperons. *Endocr Rev* 1997;18:306–360.
276. Rachamim N, Latter H, Malinin N, Asher C, Wald H, Garty H. Dexamethasone enhances expression of mitochondrial oxidative phosphorylation genes in rat distal colon. *Am J Physiol Cell Physiol* 1995;38:C1305–C1310.
277. Rafestin-Oblin ME, Fagart J, Souque A, Seguin C, Bens M, Vandewalle A. 11beta-hydroxyprogesterone acts as a mineralocorticoid agonist in stimulating Na^+ absorption in mammalian principal cortical collecting duct cells. *Mol Pharmacol* 2002;62:1306–1313.
278. Rafestin-Oblin ME, Souque A, Bocchi B, Pinon G, Fagart J, Vandewalle A. The severe form of hypertension caused by the activating S810L mutation in the mineralocorticoid receptor is cortisone related. *Endocrinology* 2003;144:528–533.
279. Record RD, Johnson M, Lee S, Blazer-Yost BL. Aldosterone and insulin stimulate amiloride-sensitive sodium transport in A6 cells by additive mechanisms. *Am J Physiol* 1996;271: C1079–C1084.
280. Reichardt HM, Kaestner KH, Tuckermann J, Kretz O, Wessely O, Bock R, Gass P, Schmid W, Herrlich P, Angel P, Schutz G. DNA binding of the glucocorticoid receptor is not essential for survival. *Cell* 1998;93:531–541 (see comment).
281. Reif MC, Troutman SL, Schafer JA. Sodium transport by rat cortical collecting tubule. Effects of vasopressin and desoxycorticosterone. *J Clin Invest* 1986;77:1291–1298.
282. Reilly RF, Ellison DH. Mammalian distal tubule: physiology, pathophysiology, and molecular anatomy. *Physiol Rev* 2000;80:277–313.
283. Renard S, Voilley N, Bassilana F, Lazdunski M, Barbry P. Localization and regulation by steroids of the alpha, beta and gamma subunits of the amiloride-sensitive Na^+ channel in colon, lung and kidney. *Pflügers Arch* 1995;430:299–307.
284. Riepe FG, Krone N, Morlot M, Ludwig M, Sippell WG, Partsch CJ. Identification of a novel mutation in the human mineralocorti-coid receptor gene in a german family with autosomal-dominant pseudohypoaldosteronism type 1: further evidence for marked interindividual clinical heterogeneity. *J Clin Endocrinol Metab* 2003;88:1683–1686.
285. Robert-Nicoud M, Flahaut M, Elalouf JM, Nicod M, Salinas M, Bens M, Doucet A, Wincker P, Artiguenave F, Horisberger JD, Vandewalle A, Rossier BC, Firsov D. Transcriptome of a mouse kidney cortical collecting duct cell line: effects of aldosterone and vasopressin. *Proc Natl Acad Sci U S A* 2001;98:2712–2716.
286. Rogerson FM, Brennan FE, Fuller PJ. Dissecting mineralocorticoid receptor structure and function. *J Steroid Biochem Mol Biol* 2003;85–:389–396.
287. Rogerson FM, Fuller PJ. Interdomain interactions in the mineralocorticoid receptor. *Mol Cell Endocrinol* 2003;200–:45–55.
288. Roland BL, Krozowski ZS, Funder JW. Glucocorticoid receptor, mineralocorticoid receptors, 11 beta-hydroxysteroid dehydrogenase-1 and -2 expression in rat brain and kidney: in situ studies. *Mol Cell Endocrinol* 1995;111:R1–R7.

289. Rubera I, Loffing J, Palmer L, Carroll T, McMahon A, Rossier BC, Hummler E. Renal collecting duct–specific inactivation of alpha ENaC subunit. *J Am Soc Nephrol* 2002;13:277A.
290. Rubera I, Loffing J, Palmer LG, Frindt G, Fowler-Jaeger N, Sauter D, Carroll T, McMahon A, Hummler E, Rossier BC. Collecting duct-specific gene inactivation of alphaENaC in the mouse kidney does not impair sodium and potassium balance. *J Clin Invest* 2003;112:554–565.
291. Rubera I, Meier E, Vuagniaux G, Merillat AM, Beermann F, Rossier BC, Hummler E. A conditional allele at the mouse channel activating protease 1 (Prss8) gene locus. *Genesis* 2002;32:173–176.
292. Rupprecht R, Arriza JL, Spengler D, Reul JM, Evans RM, Holsboer F, Damm K. Transactivation and synergistic properties of the mineralocorticoid receptor: relationship to the glucocorticoid receptor. *Mol Endocrinol* 1993;7:597–603.
293. Sabatini S, Hartsell A, Meyer M, Kurtzman NA, Hierholzer K. Corticosterone metabolism and membrane transport. *Miner Electrolyte Metab* 1993;19:343–350.
294. Saito T, Essig A. Effect of aldosterone on active and passive conductance and ENA in the toad bladder. *J Membr Biol* 1973;13:1–18.
295. Sansom SC, Muto S, Giebisch G. Na-dependent effects of DOCA on cellular transport properties of CCDs from ADX rabbits. *Am J Physiol* 1987;253:F753–F759.
296. Sansom SC, O'Neil RG. Effects of mineralocorticoids on transport properties of cortical collecting duct basolateral membrane. *Am J Physiol* 1986;251:F743–F757.
297. Sansom SC, O'Neil RG. Mineralocorticoid regulation of apical cell membrane Na^+ and K^+ transport of the cortical collecting duct. *Am J Physiol* 1985;248:F858–F868.
298. Sartorato P, Khaldi Y, Lapeyraque AL, Armanini D, Kuhnle U, Salomon R, Caprio M, Viengchareun S, Lombes M, Zennaro MC. Inactivating mutations of the mineralocorticoid receptor in type I pseudohypoaldosteronism. *Mol Cell Endocrinol* 2004;217:119–125.
299. Sartorato P, Lapeyraque AL, Armanini D, Kuhnle U, Khaldi Y, Salomon R, Abadie V, Di Battista E, Naselli A, Racine A, Bosio M, Caprio M, Poulet-Young V, Chabrolle JP, Niaudet P, De Gennes C, Lecornec MH, Poisson E, Fusco AM, Loli P, Lombes M, Zennaro MC. Different inactivating mutations of the mineralocorticoid receptor in fourteen families affected by type I pseudohypoaldosteronism. *J Clin Endocrinol Metab* 2003;88:2508–2517.
300. Schibler U, Sierra F. Alternative promoters in developmental gene expression. *Annu Rev Genet* 1987;21:237–257.
301. Schild L, Canessa CM, Shimkets RA, Gautschi I, Lifton RP, Rossier BC. A mutation in the epithelial sodium channel causing Liddle disease increases channel activity in the *Xenopus laevis* oocyte expression system. *Proc Natl Acad Sci U S A* 1995;92:5699–5703.
302. Schulman G, Lindemeyer R, Barman A, Karnik S, Bastl CP. Atrial natriuretic peptide inhibits mineralocorticoid receptor function in rat colonic surface cells. *J Clin Invest* 1996;98:157–166.
303. Schultz SG. Regulatory mechanisms in sodium-absorbing epithelia. In: Seldin DW, Giebisch G, eds. *The Kidney: Physiology and Pathology*. New York: Raven Press; 1985:189–198.
304. Schwartz GJ, Burg MB. Mineralcorticoid effects on cation trans-port by cortical collecting tubules in vitro. *Am J Physiol* 1978;235:F576–F585.
305. Seckl JR. 11beta-Hydroxysteroid dehydrogenase in the brain: a novel regulator of glucocorticoid action? *Front Neuroendocrinol* 1997;18:49–99.
306. Seckl JR, Benediktsson R, Lindsay RS, Brown RW. Placental 11 beta-hydroxysteroid dehydrogenase and the programming of hypertension. *J Steroid Biochem Mol Biol* 1995;55: 447–455.
307. Shareghi GR, Stoner LC. Calcium transport across segments of the rabbit distal nephron in vitro. *Am J Physiol* 1978;235:F367–375.
308. Sharp GWG, Leaf A. Mechanism of action of aldosterone. *Physiol Rev* 1966;46:593–633.
309. Shi H, Asher C, Chigaev A, Yung Y, Reuveny E, Seger R, Garty H. Interactions of beta and gamma ENaC with Nedd4 can be facilitated by an ERK-mediated phosphorylation. *J Biol Chem* 2002;277:13539–13547.
310. Shi H, Asher C, Yung Y, Kligman L, Reuveny E, Seger R, Garty H. Casein kinase 2 specifically binds to and phosphorylates the carboxy termini of ENaC subunits. *Eur J Biochem* 2002;269:4551–4558.
311. Shimkets RA, Lifton R, Canessa CM. In vivo phosphorylation of the epithelial sodium channel. *Proc Natl Acad Sci U S A* 1998;95:3301–3305.
312. Shimkets RA, Warnock DG, Bositis CM, Nelson-Williams C, Hansson JH, Schambelan M, Gill JR Jr, Ulick S, Milora RV, Findling JW, Canessa CM, Rossier BC, Lifton RP. Liddle's syndrome: heritable human hypertension caused by mutations in the beta subunit of the epithelial sodium channel. *Cell* 1994;79:407–414.
313. Shimojo M, Ricketts ML, Petrelli MD, Moradi P, Johnson GD, Bradwell AR, Hewison M, Howie AJ, Stewart PM. Immunodetection of 11 beta-hydroxysteroid dehydrogenase type 2 in human mineralocorticoid target tissues: evidence for nuclear localization. *Endocrinology* 1997;138:1305–1311.
314. Simpson ER, Mason JI. *Molecular Aspects of the Biosynthesis of Adrenal Steroids*. Oxford: Pergamon; 1979.
315. Small GR, Hadoke PWF, Sharif I, Dover AR, Armour D, Kenyon CJ, Gray GA, Walker BR. Preventing local regeration of glucocorticoids by 11b-hydroxysteroid dehydrogenase type 1 enhances angiogenesis. *Proc Natl Acad Sci U S A* 2005;102:12165–12170.
316. Snyder PM, Olson DR, Thomas BC. SGK modulates Nedd4-2–mediated inhibition of ENaC. *J Biol Chem* 2002;277:5–8.
317. Spindler B, Mastroberardino L, Custer M, Verrey F. Characterization of early aldosterone-induced RNAs identified in A6 kidney epithelia. *Pflugers Arch* 1997;434:323–331.
318. Spindler B, Verrey F. Aldosterone action: induction of p21 (ras) and fra-2 and transcription-independent decrease in myc, jun, and fos. *Am J Physiol Cell Physiol* 1999;45:C1154–C1161.
319. Spooner PM, Edelman IS. Further studies on the effect of ald-oste-rone on electrical resistance of toad bladder. *Biochim Biophys Acta* 1975;406:304–314.
320. Stanton BA, Giebisch G. Mechanism of urinary potassium excretion. *Miner Electrolyte Metab* 1981;5:100–120.
321. Starr DB, Matsui W, Thomas JR, Yamamoto KR. Intracellular receptors use a common mechanism to interpret signaling information at response elements. *Genes Dev* 1996;10: 1271–1283.
322. Staruschenko A, Patel P, Tong Q, Medina JL, Stockand JD. Ras activates the epithelial Na^+ channel through phosphoinositide 3-OH kinase signaling. *J Biol Chem* 2004;279:37771–37778.
323. Staruschenko A, Pochynyuk OM, Tong Q, Stockand JD. Ras couples phosphoinositide 3-OH kinase to the epithelial Na^1 channel. *Biochim Biophys Acta* 2005;1669:108–115.
324. Staub O, Abriel H, Plant P, Ishikawa T, Kanelis V, Saleki R, Horisberger JD, Schild L, Rotin D. Regulation of the epithelial Na^+ channel by Nedd4 and ubiquitination. *Kidney Int* 2000;57: 809–815.
325. Staub O, Verrey F. Impact of Nedd4 proteins and serum and glucocorticoid-induced kinases on epithlial Na^1 transprot in the distal nephron. *J Am Soc Nephrol* 2005;16:3167–3174.
326. Stewart AF, Schutz G. Camptothecin-induced in vivo topoisomerase I cleavages in the transcriptionally active tyrosine aminotransferase gene. *Cell* 1987;50:1109–1117.
327. Stockand JD. New ideas about aldosterone signaling in epithelia. *Am J Physiol Renal Fluid Electrolyte Physiol* 2002;282:F559–F576.
328. Stokes JB. Ion transport by the collecting duct. *Semin Nephrol* 1993;13:202–212.
329. Stokes JB. Ion transport by the cortical and outer medullary collecting tubule. *Kidney Int* 1982;22:473–484.
330. Stoner LC, Burg MB, Orloff J. Ion transport in cortical collecting tubule: effect of amiloride. *Am J Physiol* 1974;227:453–459.
331. Stoos BA, Naray–Fejes-Toth A, Carretero OA, Ito S, Fejes-Toth G. Characterization of a mouse cortical collecting duct cell line. *Kidney Int* 1991;39:1168–1175.
332. Strahle U, Schmidt A, Kelsey G, Stewart AF, Cole TJ, Schmid W, Schutz G. At least three promoters direct expression of the mouse glucocorticoid receptor gene. *Proc Natl Acad Sci U S A* 1992;89:6731–6735.
333. Summa V, Camargo SM, Bauch C, Zecevic M, Verrey F. Isoform specificity of human Na $(^+)$, K $(^+)$-ATPase localization and aldosterone regulation in mouse kidney cells. *J Physiol* 2004;555:355–364.
334. Summa V, Mordasini D, Roger F, Bens M, Martin PY, Vandewalle A, Verrey F, Feraille E. Short term effect of aldosterone on Na,K-ATPase cell surface expression in kidney collecting duct cells. *J Biol Chem* 2001;276:47087–47093.
335. Sweadner KJ, Arystarkhova E, Donnet C, Wetzel RK. FXYD proteins as regulators of the Na,K-ATPase in the kidney. *Ann N Y Acad Sci* 2003;986:382–387.
336. Tajima T, Kitagawa H, Yokoya S, Tachibana K, Adachi M, Nakae J, Suwa S, Katoh S, Fujieda K. A novel missense mutation of mineralocorticoid receptor gene in one Japanese family with a renal form of pseudohypoaldosteronism type 1. *J Clin Endocrinol Metab* 2000;85:4690–4694.
337. Tallec LP, Kirsh O, Lecompte MC, Viengchareun S, Zennaro MC, Dejean A, Lombes M. Protein inhibitor of activated signal transducer and activator of transcription 1 interacts with the N-terminal domain of mineralocorticoid receptor and represses its transscriptional activity: implication of small ubiquitin-related modiefier 1 modification. *Mol Endocrinol* 2003;17:2529–2542.
338. Tamura H, Schild L, Enomoto N, Matsui N, Marumo F, Rossier BC, Sasaki S. Liddle disease caused by a missense mutation of beta subunit of the epithelial sodium channel gene. *J Clin Invest* 1996;97:1780–1784.
339. Tomita K, Pisano JJ, Knepper MA. Control of sodium and potassium transport in the cortical collecting duct of the rat. Effects of bradykinin, vasopressin, and deoxycorticosterone. *J Clin Invest* 1985;76:132–136.
340. Trapp T, Rupprecht R, Castren M, Reul JM, Holsboer F. Heterodimerization between mineralocorticoid and glucocorticoid receptor: a new principle of glucocorticoid action in the CNS. *Neuron* 1994;13:1457–1462.
341. Truscello A, Gäggeler HP, Rossier BC. Thyroid hormone antagonizes an aldosterone-induced protein: a candidate mediator for the late mineralocorticoid response. *J Membr Biol* 1986;89:173–183.
342. Truscello A, Geering K, Gaeggeler HP, Rossier BC. Effects of butyrate on histone deacetylation and aldosterone-dependent Na^+ transport in the toad bladder. *J Biol Chem* 1983;258:3388–3395.
343. Truss M, Beato M. Steroid hormone receptors: interaction with deoxyribonucleic acid and transcription factors. *Endocr Rev* 1993;14:459–479.
344. Tully DB, Allgood VE, Cidlowski JA. Modulation of steroid receptor-mediated gene expression by vitamin B6. *FASEB J* 1994;8:343–349.
345. Uhrenholt TR, Schjerning J, Hansen PB, Norregaard R, Jensen BL, Sorensen GL, Skott O. Rapid inhibition of vasoconstriction in renal afferent arterioles by aldosterone. *Circ Res* 2003;93:1258–1266.
346. Urbach V, Van Kerkhove E, Maguire D, Harvey BJ. Rapid activation of KATP channels by aldosterone in principal cells of frog skin. *J Physiol* 1996;491:111–120.
347. Vallet V, Chraibi A, Gaeggeler HP, Horisberger JD, Rossier BC. An epithelial serine protease activates the amiloride-sensitive sodium channel. *Nature* 1997;389:607–610.
348. Vallon V, Lang F. New insights into the role of serum- and glucocorticoid-inducible kinase SGK1 in the regulation of renal function and blood pressure. *Curr Opin Nephrol Hypertens* 2005;14:59–66.
349. Verlander JW, Hassell KA, Royaux IE, Glapion DM, Wang ME, Everett LA, Green ED, Wall SM. Deoxycorticosterone upregulates PDS (Slc26a4) in mouse kidney: role of pendrin in mineralocorticoid-induced hypertension. *Hypertension* 2003;42:356–362.
350. Verrey F. Antidiuretic hormone action in A6 cells—effect on apical Cl and Na conductances and synergism with aldosterone for NaCl reabsorption. *J Membr Biol* 1994;138: 65–76.
351. Verrey F. Early aldosterone action: toward filling the gap between transcription and transport. *Am J Physiol Renal Fluid Electrolyte Physiol* 1999;46:F319–F327.
352. Verrey F. Transcriptional control of sodium transport in tight epithelial by adrenal steroids. *J Membr Biol* 1995;144:93–110.
353. Verrey F, Beron J, Spindler B. Corticosteroid regulation of renal Na,K-ATPase. *Miner Electrolyte Metab* 1996;22–:279–292.
354. Verrey F, Kraehenbuhl JP, Rossier BC. Aldosterone induces a rapid increase in the rate of Na,K-ATPase gene transcription in cultured kidney cells. *Mol Endocrinol* 1989;3: 1369–1376.

355. Verrey F, Loffing J, Zecevic M, Heitzmann D, Staub O. SGK1: aldosterone-induced relay of Na$^+$ transport regulation in distal kidney nephron cells. *Cell Physiol Biochem* 2003;13: 21–28.

356. Verriere V, Hynes D, Faherty S, Devaney J, Bousquet J, Harvey B. Rapid effects of dexamethasone on intracellular pH and Na^J/H^J exchanger activity in human bronchial epithelial cells. *J Biol Chem* 2005;280:35707–35814.

357. Viemann M, Peter M, Lopez-Siguero JP, Simic-Schleicher G, Sippell WG. Evidence for genetic heterogeneity of pseudohypoaldosteronism type 1: identification of a novel mutation in the human mineralocorticoid receptor in one sporadic case and no mutations in two autosomal dominant kindreds. *J Clin Endocrinol Metab* 2001;86:2056–2059.

358. Vilella S, Guerra L, Helmle KC, Murer H. Aldosterone actions on basolateral Na$^+$/H$^+$ exchange in Madin–Darby canine kidney cells. *Pflugers Arch* 1992;422:9–15.

359. Vuagniaux G, Vallet V, Jaeger NF, Hummler E, Rossier BC. Synergistic activation of ENaC by three membrane-bound channel-activating serine proteases (mCAP1, mCAP2, and mCAP3) and serum- and glucocorticoid-regulated kinase (Sgk1) in *Xenopus* oocytes hormonal regulation of the epithelial sodium channel ENaC: N or P (o)? *J Gen Physiol* 2002;120:191–201.

360. Wade JB, O'Neil RG, Pryor JL, Boulpaep EL. Modulation of cell membrane area in renal collecting tubules by corticosteroid hormones. *J Cell Biol* 1979;81:439–445.

361. Walther RF, Atlas E, Carrigan A, Rouleau Y, Edgecombe A, Visentin L, Lamprecht C, Addicks GC, Haché RJG. A serine/threonine-rich motif is one of three nuclear localization signals that determine unidirectional transport of the mineralocorticoid receptor to the nucleus. *J Biol Chem* 2005;280:17549–17561.

362. Wang J, Barbry P, Maiyar AC, Rozansky DJ, Bhargava A, Leong M, Firestone GL, Pearce D. SGK integrates insulin and mineralocorticoid regulation of epithelial sodium transport. *Am J Physiol Renal Fluid Electrolyte Physiol* 2001;280:F303–F313.

363. Wang Q, Barbry P, Maillard M, Brunner HR, Rossier BC, Burnier M. Salt- and angiotensin II–dependent variations in amiloride-sensitive rectal potential difference in mice. *Clin Exp Pharmacol Physiol* 2000;27:60–66.

364. Wang Q, Hummler E, Maillard M, Nussberger J, Rossier BC, Brunner HR, Burnier M. Compensatory up-regulation of angiotensin II subtype 1 receptors in alpha ENaC knockout heterozygous mice. *Kidney Int* 2001;59:2216–2221.

365. Wang WH, Schwab A, Giebisch G. Regulation of small-conductance K$^+$ channel in apical membrane of rat cortical collecting tubule. *Am J Physiol* 1990;259:F494–F502.

366. Weigel NL. Steroid hormone receptors and their regulation by phosphorylation. *Biochem J* 1996;319:657–667.

367. Welling PA, Caplan M, Sutters M, Giebisch G. Aldosterone-mediated Na/K-ATPase expression is alpha isoform specific in the renal cortical collecting duct. *J Biol Chem* 1993;268:23469–23476.

368. Whorwood CB, Stewart PM. Human hypertension caused by mutations in the 11 beta-hydroxysteroid dehydrogenase gene: a molecular analysis of apparent mineralocorticoid excess. *J Hypertens* 1996;14:S19–S24.

369. Wiener H, Nielsen JM, Klaerke DA, Jorgensen PL. Aldosterone and thyroid hormone modulation of alpha-1- messenger RNA, beta-1-messenger RNA, and Na,K-pump sites in rabbit distal colon epithelium—evidence for a novel mechanism of escape from the effect of hyperaldosteronemia. *J Membr Biol* 1993;133:203–211.

370. Will PC, Cortright RN, DeLisle RC, Douglas JG, Hopfer U. Regulation of amiloride-sensitive electrogenic sodium transport in the rat colon by steroid hormones. *Am J Physiol* 1985;248:G124–G132.

371. Wills NK, Purcell RK, Clausen C, Millinoff LP. Effects of aldosterone on the impedance properties of cultured renal amphibian epithelia. *J Membr Biol* 1993;133:17–27.

372. Winter C, Schulz N, Giebisch G, Geibel JP, Wagner CA. Nongenomic stimulation of vacuolar H$^+$-ATPases in intercalated renal tubule cells by aldosterone. *Proc Natl Acad Sci U S A* 2004;101:2636–2641.

373. Wulff P, Vallon V, Huang DY, Pfaff I, Klingel K, Kauselmann D, Volkl H, Lang F, Kuhl D. Deficient salt retention in the SGK1 knockout mouse. *J Am Soc Nephrol* 2001;12:44A (abstract A0231).

374. Wulff P, Vallon V, Huang DY, Volkl H, Yu F, Richter K, Jansen M, Schlunz M, Klingel K, Loffing J, Kauselmann G, Bosl MR, Lang F, Kuhl D. Impaired renal Na$^+$ retention in the sgk1-knockout mouse. *J Clin Invest* 2002;110:1263–1268.

375. Xu JZ, Hall AE, Peterson LN, Bienkowski MJ, Eessalu TE, Hebert SC. Localization of the ROMK protein on apical membranes of rat kidney nephron segments. *Am J Physiol* 1997;273: F739–F748.

376. Yorio T, Bentley PJ. Phospholipase A and the mechanism of action of aldosterone. *Nature* 1978;271:79–81.

377. Zennaro MC, Farman N, Bonvalet JP, Lombes M. Tissue-specific expression of a and b messenger ribonucleic acid isoforms of the humman mineralocorticoid receptor in normal and pathological states. *J Clin Endocrinol Metab* 1997;82:1345–1352.

378. Zennaro MC, Keightley MC, Kotelevtsev Y, Conway GS, Soubrier F, Fuller PJ. Human mineralocorticoid receptor genomic structure and identification of expressed isoforms. *J Biol Chem* 1995:21016–21020.

379. Zennaro MC, Souque A, Viengchareun S, Poisson E, Lombes M. A new human MR splice variant is a ligand-independent transactivator modulating corticosteroid action. *Mol Endocrinol* 2001;15:1586–1598.

380. Zhang YH, Alvarez de la Rosa D, Canessa CM, Hayslett JP. Insulin-induced phosphorylation of ENaC correlates with increased sodium channel function in A6 cells. *Am J Physiol Cell Physiol* 2005;288:C141–C147.

381. Zhang Z, Zhang A, Kohan D, Nelson R, Gonzalez F, Yand T. Collecting duct-specific deletion of peroxysome prolliferator-activated receptor gamma blocks thiazoldine dione-induced fluid retention. *Proc Natl Acad Sci U S A* 2005;102:9406–9411.

382. Zhou MY, Gomez-Sanchez CE, Gomez-Sanchez EP. An alternatively spliced rat mineralocorticoid receptor mRNA causing truncation of the steroid binding domain. *Mol Cell Endocrinol* 2000;159:125–131.

Chapter **33**

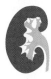

Neural Control of Renal Function

Edward J. Johns and Ulla C. Kopp

University College Cork, Cork, Republic of Ireland
VA Medical Center, Carver College of Medicine, University of Iowa, Iowa City, Iowa, USA

INTRODUCTION

The innervation of the kidney has been a subject of interest even by the earliest investigators and Claude Bernard was one of the first to describe a unilateral diuresis following section of the greater splanchnic nerve in the anesthetized dog. Early in the twentieth century, investigations into the neural control of the kidney were hampered because of Homer Smith (183) who, to a degree, dismissed the renal nerves as contributing little to the physiological regulation of the kidney. However, in the 1960s, as more penetrating methodologies become available, an increasing number of investigators began to reevaluate the potential influences of the renal innervation. Thereafter, over a period of 30–40 years, a great deal of information has been produced that has laid out the basis of current understanding of how the renal sympathetic innervation affects all aspects of renal function. A number of major reviews of the anatomy, physiology, and pharmacology of the sympathetic innervation of the kidney appeared in the 1990s and early 2000s (41, 42, 46), which have brought together the most significant pieces of information about the renal sympathetic nerves at the time. The major focus of this chapter will be to build on these extensive reviews and to highlight major developments over the past few years with the intention of placing the role of sympathetic innervation of the kidney into current perspectives.

NEUROANATOMY, PHARMACOLOGY, AND PHYSIOLOGY

Extrinsic Innervation

The efferent innervation of the kidney comprises preganglionic fibers that arise from spinal segments T_{11}-L_3, although there is variation between both species and individuals within species. These pre-ganglionic fibers traverse to both pre-vertebral (thoraco-lumbar sympathetic chain) and para-vertebral ganglia (aortico-renal, splanchnic, coeliac, superior mesenteric ganglia) that give rise to the post-ganglionic fibers but again, there is great species variation in the overall contribution from the various ganglia; for example, 80% arise from the ipsilateral paravertebral ganglia (T_{11}–L_2) in the rat and hamster, but only 50% in the cat and monkey (T_{11}–L_3) (46). Figure 1 provides a brief outline of these neural pathways. Tracer studies with horseradish peroxidase and herpes virus have been used to demonstrate the neural pathways for sympathetic innervation. The preganglionic sympathetic nerve fibers in the rat are primarily located in the intermediolateral column of the spinal cord, from T_9–T_{13}, suggesting that they descend three to four segments before exiting the spinal column at T_{11}–L_3. A number of nuclei within the central nervous system project to these intermediolateral areas of the spinal cord, including the raphe nuclei, rostral ventrolateral medulla, an A5 group, and the paraventricular hypothalamic nucleus (46). There is a view that descending projections from the supraspinal systems are the primary regulators of sympathetic outflow to the kidney.

Evaluation of the size and type of nerves forming the efferent innervation of the kidney continue. Analyses performed in the rabbit utilizing EM studies in the cortex, have demonstrated that two types of nerve fibers are present that have somewhat different diameters (40, 137). This observation has formed the basis for the view that various functionalities exist within these different nerve populations, that is, they may primarily control hemodynamic function, renin release, or fluid reabsorption. DiBona and Sawin (55) performed a detailed count and diameter evaluation of nerve bundles entering the rat kidney. They found that 96% of the fibers were unmyelinated, but the 4% myelinated had an average diameter of 1.26 ± 0.01 μm with a bimodal distribution of diameters, with 1.1 μm at one end and 1.6 μm at the other. More recently, Fazan and colleagues (67) found that compared to the rat, nerve fibers for the mouse had a similar mean diameter, 0.76 ± 0.02 μm, but the distribution was clearly unimodal. This observation in the mouse would, to a degree, contradict the notion that different nerves innervate specific cell types (vascular, epithelial, or granular) of the renal tissue to control selected functions.

Intrinsic Innervation

The nerves generally traverse from the ganglia, running alongside the renal artery, and enter the hilus of the kidney where they begin to divide, with smaller nerve bundles approximately

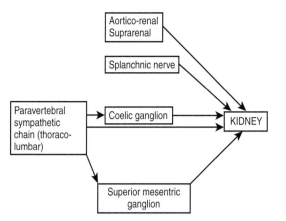

FIGURE 1 Principal ganglia providing sympathetic postganglionic fibers that innervate the kidney.

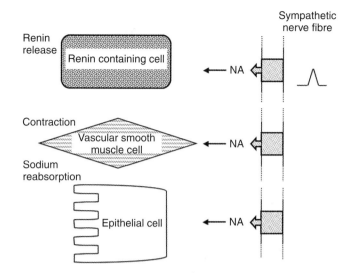

FIGURE 2 Sympathetic fibers have varicosities adjacent to the neuroeffector junctions at the renin-containing cells, the vascular smooth muscle cells (interlobular arteries, afferent and efferent arterioles), and the epithelial cells of the proximal tubule, thick ascending limb of the loop of Henle, and the distal tubule. Noradrenaline (NA) is contained in granules within the varicosities that are exocytosed following passage of an action potential.

following the major divisions of the blood vessels. The sympathetic nerves begin to divide into smaller bundles, which then start to penetrate and form a network throughout the cortical and juxtamedullary areas. In their early studies, Barajas and coworkers (6, 7) demonstrated that discrete neuroeffector junctions are present at the afferent and efferent arterioles, the granular cells of the juxtaglomerular apparatus, the proximal tubules and distal tubules, and the thick limb of the ascending limb of the loop of Henle. This group of investigators, utilizing electron microscopy, went on to show that the sympathetic nerves were typical autonomic fibers in that they had varicosities associated with the neuroeffector junctions that contained dense cored vesicles. Using a tritiated noradrenaline radiographic approach, they (6, 7) clearly showed the presence of noradrenaline, and although there was a suggestion that acetylcholine esterase was present, there was no indication that the fibers were in any way cholinergic. Later more detailed studies indicated that there was variation in the number of neuroeffector junctions along the nephron, with the greatest being at the proximal tubule, less in the thick ascending limb of the loop of Henle and least in the distal tubules and collecting duct (46). Interestingly, when calculated as the density of neuroeffector junctions per unit length, it was found to be greatest in the thick ascending limb of the loop of Henle and progressively less in the distal and proximal tubules (6, 7). There is also a regional variation with the innervation being greatest along the corticomedullary border and becoming less in the outer cortex and deeper regions of the medulla. This regional variation in innervation density is paralleled in both the vascular and tubular structures. Fig. 2 illustrates the cell types where neuroeffector junctions have been described and the functions they may regulate.

Pharmacology

NEUROTRANSMITTERS

There is now a large body of evidence from a range of biochemical and pharmacological studies that indicates the primary neurotransmitter arising from the sympathetic in-

nervation is noradrenaline. Indeed, functional studies have shown that renal denervation, in the initial stages, is associated with a marked decrease in noradrenaline content of some 95% (46), while activation of the renal sympathetic nerves results in an elevation in noradrenaline production or spillover into the renal venous blood (63, 64). The role of dopamine and potential dopaminergic nerve-mediated influences remains unclear, and this is because all adrenergic nerve varicosities contain dopamine as an intermediary in noradrenaline biosynthesis. Thus, although there is evidence that dopamine levels are reduced by renal denervation at a functional level, there is little evidence that dopamine acts as a neurotransmitter (46) in the neural regulation of renal hemodynamic function, renin release, or fluid reabsorption.

ADRENOCEPTORS

It is now clear that multiple types of adrenoceptors are present in the kidney that mediate the actions of noradrenaline released from the nerve varicosities, and that a range of α_1- and α_2-adrenoceptors subtypes exist at both the vasculature and nephrons of the kidney. At a functional level, stimulation of the adrenoceptors cause a vasoconstriction of vascular smooth muscle, reabsorption of fluid at tubular epithelial cells and renin release at the juxtaglomerular granular cells. More recently, a number of molecular biological and cloning investigations have defined α_1-adrenoceptors into α_{1A}-, α_{1B}-, and α_{1D}- subtypes, α_2-adrenoceptors into α_{2A}-, α_{2B}-, and α_{2C}-subtypes and β-adrenoceptors as β_1-, β_2- and β_3-subtypes, all of which are G-protein–coupled receptors comprising a superfamily of membrane proteins that signal the actions of adrenaline and noradrenaline (188). The α_1-

adrenoceptors utilize a range of signaling pathways, including activation of phospholipases A and C, mobilization of intracellular calcium stores as well as opening voltage-dependent and -independent calcium channels (173), which results in a rapid vascular smooth muscle contraction. Interestingly, noradrenaline binding to α_1-adrenoceptors also activates the MAP kinase pathways that, in the longer term, are responsible for regulating growth and hypertrophy of the vascular smooth muscle (200). There are reports that α_{1A}- and α_{1B}-adrenoceptors are present to a similar degree in the cortex and outer stripe of the medulla while in the inner stripe of the medulla the α_{1B}-adrenoceptor subtype appears to predominate (68). However, in terms of hemodynamic functionality, α_{1A}-adrenoceptors are more effective than the α_{1B}-adrenoceptor subtypes in causing renal vasoconstriction.

α-Adrenoceptors are also present on the epithelial cells of the nephron where they modulate fluid reabsorption. At these sites there is evidence, at least in the proximal tubule, that α_1-adrenoceptor stimulation engages both the phospholipase C and MAP kinase (201) pathways, but these signal to different endpoints, that is, to the sodium–hydrogen exchanger (NHE), isoforms-1 and -3, respectively (133). At the more distal sections of the nephron, distal tubule, and collecting duct, α_2-adrenoceptors are the primary subtype, and in this segment their activation results in a decrease in cAMP that blunts the action of other factors signaling through this pathway, such as, for example, AVP (172). β_1-Adrenoceptors are found primarily on the granular renin-containing cells of the afferent arteriole and their activation stimulates adenylyl cyclase, which in turn increases intracellular levels of cAMP. The β_2-adrenoceptors found on the tubules, primarily collecting duct, also utilize cAMP production as the signaling molecule but their function at this site has not been resolved.

Physiology

The end result of activation of the various signaling pathways via ligand binding to the adrenoceptors is an increase in fluid reabsorption at the level of the proximal tubule. There is sound evidence (2) that the catecholamines can stimulate Na, K-ATPase at the basolateral membrane. More recently, it has become evident from cultured proximal tubule cell studies that a further aspect of increased fluid reabsorption is that entry of sodium from the lumen, across the apical membrane into the cell, should be increased, thereby allowing the sodium to be pumped via the Na, K-ATPase out of the cell across the basolateral membrane. There is evidence from micropuncture studies (162), as well as in vitro studies (134), that the NHE is activated, particularly isoform-3, which is the isoform primarily responsible for the regulation of sodium entry into the epithelial at the proximal tubule and loop of Henle (133, 134). The NHE protein in the proximal tubule appears to be present in the microvilli, either incorporated into the plasma membrane (203) where it is likely to be active, or internally in the subendosomal layer or in the endosomes where it is likely to be inactive in terms of a transporting protein. It has been reported that the NHE3 can be translocated from apical to subendosomal regions in response to acute increases in renal perfusion pressure (208). The question arises as to whether this translocation of NHE3 from intracellular compartments into the membrane (149) could be one way in which the catecholamines might increase the level at which sodium and fluid reabsorption takes place across the proximal tubular cells, but acting over a longer timeframe rather than the immediate responses. The situation in the TALH and the distal nephron is even less clear than that of the proximal tubule, but the potential exists for catecholamines to be active at these sites, as well as stimulating fluid reabsorption via NHE3 in the same way.

CONTROL OF RENAL CIRCULATION

Activation of Renal Sympathetic Nerves

The earliest studies involving the renal sympathetic nerves quickly established that they had potent vasoconstrictor properties. Cohnheim and Roy (30), using a renal plethysmograph, demonstrated that renal volume was decreased following asphyxia or when the cut ends of the renal nerves were stimulated. Indeed, these early plethysmographic studies also identified the spinal origin of the vasoconstrictor fibers. Since that time, a range of studies, utilizing both direct electrical stimulation and reflex activation of the renal nerves, have elaborated on these basic observations. With the advent of the modern flow meters to measure renal blood flow dynamically, studies were performed in anesthetized dog, cats, rabbits, and rats (46), which convincingly demonstrated that direct electrical stimulation of the renal nerves caused frequency-related reductions in renal blood flow. Furthermore, reflex activation of the renal sympathetic nerves, either as a consequence of activation of the baroreceptor reflex by reduction in carotid sinus pressure (211) or activation of the somatosensory system (43, 57, 191) resulted in a renal nerve–mediated reduction in renal blood flow. Together, these reports and observations were taken to indicate an action of the renal nerves to cause contraction of the vascular smooth muscle of the resistance vessels, thereby reducing blood flow through the tissue. While the innervation of the afferent arteriole would cause a reduction in renal blood flow because it is the major resistance bed within the kidney, the impact and relative importance of a neurally induced vasoconstriction at the efferent arteriole is less clear-cut in terms of its overall contribution to the reduction in renal blood flow. Indeed, Luff and co-workers (39, 137), when working with the rabbit, were able to identify at the ultrastructural level two types of fibers that were differentially distributed, one type innervating only the afferent arteriole and a second type evenly distributed between afferent and efferent arterioles, which they argued enabled independent regulation of the two resistance vasculatures. However, an alternative view is that because of the differing wall thicknesses and lengths of the afferent and efferent arterioles, even if both vessels constricted to a similar degree, the constriction in the efferent arteriole would have a greater impact on glomerular filtration pressure (38) and hence filtration rate.

It had become apparent from a number of studies that there was a disparity in the magnitudes of the reduction in renal blood flow as against glomerular filtration rate (20). Studies in the anesthetized rabbit (84), cat (101) and rat (80) demonstrated that modest neurally induced reductions in renal blood flow (of 15%–20%) were accompanied by either no change or a small 2%–5% reduction in glomerular filtration. However, if the studies were undertaken when the action of angiotensin II (Ang II) was prevented, either using β-adrenoceptor antagonists to prevent renin release, converting enzyme inhibitors or AT-1 receptor blocking drugs, then the neural impact on glomerular filtration rate became much greater with the magnitude of reductions becoming roughly proportionate with renal blood flow. These reports and observations gave rise to the important concept that the renal nerves, indirectly via locally produced Ang II acting at the efferent arteriole, could ensure that over a modest range of variation in renal blood flow, the glomerular filtration rate, and hence filtered load presented to the nephrons, was maintained at a relatively constant level.

Renal Denervation

A great deal of knowledge has now accumulated as to how the renal nerves control renal hemodynamics with most being derived from experimental studies using anesthetized animals. What remains unclear is whether under basal, unstressed conditions the renal sympathetic nerves do have a tonic influence on basal blood flow through the kidney. The reasons for this uncertainty resides in the manner of the experimental studies, whether anesthetized or conscious preparations were used, if anesthetized the degree of surgical stress and type of anesthesia used may be influential, and, to a degree, the species under study. Thus, in a number of reports in the anesthetized rat, there was very little change in renal blood flow following acute renal denervation (46). However, in these studies there was often a relatively long period of time between basal measurements and surgical manipulation and denervation of the kidney, and postsurgery measurements; consequently, it was difficult to determine whether changes had taken place. In an attempt to resolve this issue, Kompanowska-Jezierska and colleagues (105) devised a study in which there was minimal surgical interference in the areas surrounding the renal artery where the renal nerves usually pass and the denervation process was very rapid. This involved inserting an electrocautery wire around the bulk of the nerves and denervation was undertaken when a current was passed to destroy the neural tissue. Under these conditions,

over the first 10 to 20 minutes an approximate 20% increase in blood perfusing the outer cortex occurred when measured by laser doppler flowmetry. Thus, the data provided support for sufficient activity in the renal nerves to decrease basal renal blood flow. This view was to a degree supported by the reports of Malpas and Evans (143) who found that in conscious rabbits 7 days after renal denervation, renal blood flow was 55%–65% higher in the denervated compared to the innervated kidney, perhaps indicative of greater basal sympathetic outflow in the rabbit.

Recent studies by Yoshimoto and coworkers (210), using the conscious rat, showed that while basal renal blood flow in the groups of animals with either intact or denervated kidneys could not be distinguished, an increase in renal sympathetic nerve activity due to increased motor activity because of grooming and movement caused a proportionate decrease in blood flow to the intact kidneys, whereas the flow to the denervated kidneys was unchanged. The relationship between renal blood flow and stress induced activation of the sympathetic nervous system, was the basis of the study undertaken by Brod (20). The author demonstrated in humans that in the unstressed state, administration of an adrenergic blocking drug, dibenamine, had no effect on PAH clearance, but if the patients were tense, anxious, and/or stressed, then the dibenamine was associated with a rise in PAH clearance (effective renal plasma flow) compatible with the view that a tonic renal nerve–induced reduction in renal blood flow. Thus, it is generally accepted that the degree of tonic influence of the renal sympathetic nerves on basal hemodynamics is dependent on the degree of stress impinging on the subjects, and that in the normal conscious state the renal sympathetic nerves have relatively little impact.

Autocrine and Paracrine Influences on Neurotransmission

It is becoming apparent that the interstitium of the kidney contains a complex milieu of hormones and factors that may vary across the cortex and medulla, but can determine the level of functions, vascular smooth muscle, and renin-containing and epithelial cells. It is recognized that at the neuroeffector junction itself, neuromodulator influences can come into play and influence the amount of noradrenaline released in response to depolarization caused by the passage of an action potential. An outline of potential interactions with various agents is illustrated in Fig. 3.

ADRENOCEPTORS

At an early stage it was recognized that presynaptic α_2-adrenoceptors were able to act in an autoinhibitory fashion, whereby when activated by noradrenaline released into the neuroeffector junction, they decreased neurotransmitter release caused by subsequent depolarizations. There is evidence that this situation pertains to the kidney in that α_2-adrenoceptors have been shown to be present (13, 14), while blockade of α_2-adrenoceptors have been found in the

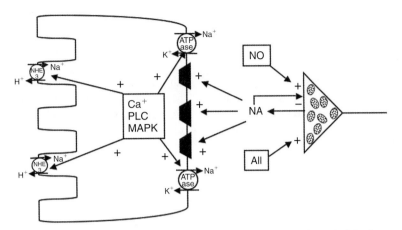

FIGURE 3 NA released into the neuroeffector junction acts on the epithelial cells to activate phospholipase C, increases intracellular calcium (Ca$^+$), which initiates MAP kinase signaling pathways to activate both the NHE3 and the basolateral sodium/potassium ATPase. Noradrenaline itself exerts an autoinhibitory feedback action on further release (−) while NO and AII exert an action (+) to increase the amount of noradrenaline release on the passage of each action potential. AII, angiotensin II; NHE3, apical sodium–hydrogen exchanger isoform 3; NO, nitric oxide; NA noradrenaline.

dog (88) to enhance noradrenaline release and renal nerve–induced vasoconstriction. It would appear that a similar situation exists in the rabbit (85), where blockade of α$_2$-adrenoceptors peripherally had little effect on renal nerve induced vasoconstrictions but potentiated the renal nerve–mediated antidiuresis and antinatriuresis.

ANGIOTENSIN II

A second important neuromodulator is Ang II, high levels of which are found in the renal interstitium (95, 161, 181). Again, it would appear that there are presynaptic AT1 receptors that, when occupied, facilitate the release of noradrenaline. This was first reported by Boke and Malik (16), using the isolated perfused rat kidney, who found that renal nerve–induced catecholamine release into the renal vein was facilitated when Ang II was added to the perfusate. At a functional level, studies in the anesthetized rat using both direct and reflex activation of the renal nerves, at levels having little or no effect on renal hemodynamics, caused decreases in fluid excretion that were blocked in the presence of an angiotensin-converting enzyme inhibitor (80) and restored following administration of exogenous Ang II (99). Similar observations were reported by Veelken and colleagues (194) in the conscious rat where administration of the AT1-receptor antagonist ZD 7155 blunted renal nerve–dependent antidiuresis and antinatriuresis in response to an air-jet stress test. Together, these findings support the view that at both renal vascular and epithelial cell neuroeffector junctions, occupation of presynaptic AT1 receptors enhances neurotransmission. It would seem that these receptors are fully occupied even at low endogenous levels of Ang II (192), and their ability to modulate neurotransmission may not normally become important given the high endogenous levels of the peptide

in the kidney. There may be other interactions at the postsynaptic membrane of the epithelial cells. Recently Quan and Baum (174, 175) demonstrated that the ability of Ang II to stimulate proximal tubule fluid reabsorption was blunted following acute renal denervation, but augmented if the renal sympathetic nerves were stimulated at low levels that did not affect the filtration rate.

NITRIC OXIDE

A third potentially important factor determining noradrenaline release and hence the impact of noradrenaline or functional endpoints is nitric oxide (NO). There are three isoforms of nitric oxide synthase (NOS)—endothelial (eNOS), neuronal (nNOS), and inducible (iNOS)—all of which are found in the kidney. eNOS has been found along the vasculature and glomerular capillaries (5, 147), nNOS has been reported to be present in the renal nerves (135) and at low concentrations along the tubules (19) and high concentrations in the macula densa (203), while iNOS is expressed constitutively in the medulla (106). It is possible that in the environment of the neuroeffector junction, NO may have both presynaptic and postsynaptic actions and this probably contributes to the conflicting findings that have been reported. Thus, in the anesthetized dog, the low-level renal nerve–stimulated noradrenaline output was enhanced following NOS inhibition and suppressed in the presence of an NO donor consistent with an inhibitory presynaptic action (59, 142). In the rat, Tanioka et al. (190), using the isolated perfused rat kidney, observed that NOS blockade suppressed renal nerve–mediated noradrenaline output and renal vasoconstrictor responses, indicative of a facilitating action of NO. To a degree this has been supported in the anesthetized rat (195) where renal nerve-induced vasoconstrictions were blunted at some frequencies following NOS inhibition. In terms of the influence of NO and renal nerve stimulated increases in sodium reabsorption, there is a lack of consistency. It is evident that NOS inhibition increases proximal tubule fluid reabsorption and is decreased by exogenous NO (60, 163), suggesting an inhibitory action of NO on reabsorptive processes. However, this action of NO is only evident if the renal nerves are intact (204); moreover, renal nerve-induced increases in fluid reabsorption are prevented by NOS blockade, consistent with facilitating action of NO (206). In attempting to clarify these differing reports, it is possible that NO could act in two ways: (1) directly within the postsynaptic cell, either vasculature or epithelial cells, where it may blunt the neurally controlled cell function, or (2) indirectly by facilitating neurotransmitter release. The differing balances between these two sites of action may simply reflect how the NO-generating systems may be activated by various experimental conditions of the investigations.

Neural Regulation of Intrarenal Hemodynamics

MEASUREMENT OF INTRARENAL HEMODYNAMICS

The measurement of blood flow through the cortical and medullary regions of the kidney is difficult and fraught with technical limitations. Videomicroscopic techniques have been used to evaluate blood flow in the medulla and papilla (31) but this approach only measures flow through single vasa recta vessels. The rhubidium-86 methodology has been used, but this only provides a single estimation from one kidney (83), while the H2-washout method is to a degree compromised by the accuracy of data curve fitting (3, 4), and trapping labeled microspheres in glomerular arterioles can only provide at most two to three measurements per kidney (28). More recently, there has been greater use of laser-doppler technology, which can be applied relatively easily to allow continuous measurements of blood perfusion through the cortex and medulla of the same kidney. The principal drawback of this technique is that the values recorded are not flow, but rather comprise a flux measurement derived from the product of the velocity as well as the number of red cells moving through the volume of tissue illuminated by the laser. Consequently, the values arising from this technique represent qualitative rather than quantitative evaluations, and therefore conclusions using this approach should be considered with caution.

ACTIVATION OF RENAL NERVES

Nonetheless, with these caveats in mind, a series of investigations addressed how and whether the renal sympathetic nerves may differentially regulate blood flow through the cortex and medulla. Early studies in this area applying the H2-washout approach in the anesthetized dog (3, 4), indicated that adrenergically mediated decreases in flow were of comparable magnitude in both cortical and medullary regions. Similar findings were reported using the rhubidium-

86 methodology (83) in that stimulation of the renal sympathetic nerves caused equivalent decreases in flow through both the cortex and medulla. By contrast, in later reports Rudenstam et al. (176) used laser-doppler flowmetry in the rat and observed a relative resistance of medullary perfusion to decrease in response to renal sympathetic nerve stimulation. Eppel et al. (62) and Leonard et al. (131) used the same technique in the anesthetized rabbit, and evaluated the responsiveness of the cortical and medullary perfusions to a range of stimulation parameters and different patterns of stimulation while incorporating frequency-enhanced signals. This group observed that over most of the stimulation frequency range that reductions of perfusion in the medulla were smaller than those occurring in either the cortex or total renal blood flow. It was evident that the dynamic response to a range of stimulus frequencies was different, with the medullary vasculature being more responsive than the cortex at higher frequencies. This group (77) went on to show that the reduction in perfusion resulting from renal sympathetic nerve stimulation was greater in the cortex than medulla at most stimulus frequencies, but that the magnitude of reduction was similar across the medullary region, irrespective of the depth at which measurements were made (inner or outer medulla). This to a degree contrasts with the findings in the anesthetized rat (195) where the inner medullary perfusion was less responsive than the outer medullary area to renal nerve stimulation. The reasons underlying the differences reported in the sensitivity of the two vascular regions to adrenergic stimulation are unclear; they may reside in the differing characteristics of the afferent and efferent arterioles, possible variations in innervation density, species variation, or the mix of paracrine and autocrine factors residing in the interstitium in these different regions (65).

CONTROL OF RENAL TUBULAR SOLUTE AND WATER TRANSPORT

Renal Denervation

Claude Bernard (12) reported one of the earliest observations that the innervation of the kidney impacted on excretory function; he noted that section of the splanchnic nerve of the anesthetized dog caused an increase in urine flow. In a more modern context, the question was whether the increased fluid excretion was due indirectly to an increase in glomerular filtration rate or whether it was the result of a direct action on the tubular reabsorptive processes of the epithelial cells. A number of attempts were made to analyze this problem, but the early data of Bonjour and colleagues (17) using the anesthetized dog, convincingly demonstrated that the elevated urine flow and sodium excretion subsequent to the section of the renal sympathetic nerves were independent of any changes in glomerular filtration rate, whether as a result of spontaneous changes or perturbations imposed experimentally on the kidney. These authors came to the conclusion that the raised fluid excretion reflected a direct influence of the nerves on tubular function. Thereafter, this view was supported by a series of reports using micropuncture techniques that directly examined reabsorptive rates along accessible segments of the nephron. Bello-Reuss and colleagues (10, 11) made key observations in the anesthetized rat, demonstrating that sectioning of the splanchnic nerves had a minimal effect on the single-nephron glomerular filtration rate but was associated with significant decreases in both absolute and fractional sodium and water reabsorption at the proximal tubule. These conclusions were supported by other investigators at the time using comparable techniques to directly measure tubular function (189, 205, 206).

Renal Nerve Stimulation

Removing the influence of the renal sympathetic nerves represents only one way of illustrating their action, and to fully appreciate their influence a corresponding series of studies were necessary in which they were activated. This was approached by examining how kidney function was altered when the renal nerves were stimulated electrically at different levels and frequencies. In a groundbreaking study, La Grange and coworkers (129), using the anesthetized dog, found that direct electrical stimulation of the nerves at subthreshold levels for changing either renal blood flow or glomerular filtration rate, caused a 30%–40% fall in water and sodium excretion, which was interpreted as a direct action of the renal nerves on tubular fluid reabsorption. A similar situation was observed in the rabbit (84) and rat (102) in that electrical stimulation of the renal nerves at subthreshold levels for decreasing renal blood flow, decreased both urine flow and sodium excretion. These observations were supported by micropuncture studies that more directly evaluated the tubular actions of the nerves. These reports (10, 11) demonstrated that the absolute and fractional sodium and water reabsorption of the proximal tubule was increased by low-frequency direct electrical stimulation of the renal nerves, which had no effect on the single-nephron filtration rate, that is, when the filtered load to the nephron was unchanged. While the majority of investigators focused on the proximal tubule, DiBona and Sawin (51) evaluated the situation farther along the nephron. They observed in the anesthetized rat that low-frequency stimulation of the renal nerves at rates that did not alter renal blood flow or glomerular filtration rate also increased fluid reabsorption at the thick limb of the ascending loop of Henle.

Thus, there is a large body of information substantiating the view that the renal sympathetic nerves, when activated at low rates that have minimal effects on renal hemodynamics, have a direct action on the transport processes of epithelial cells of the proximal tubule and thick ascending limb of the loop of Henle. The situation regarding the distal tubule and the collecting duct has not been investigated in depth, primarily because of technical hurdles required to evaluate reabsorption in these segments in vivo. However, it is likely that at these low-permeability epithelia, the renal innervation may have little effect, as control of fluid reabsorption is exerted primarily via humoral effectors and also because the transporters within these epithelial cells are more specialized in determining the discrete reabsorption of either water or sodium.

NEURAL CONTROL OF RENIN RELEASE

Renin-Containing Cells

RENIN PRODUCTION

The granular cells of the juxtaglomerular apparatus contain renin and these cells are found in the afferent arterioles at increasing density as the vessel approaches the glomerulus (79). The origin of these cells has only recently been clarified in a study by Sequeira Lopez et al. (177), who used single-cell PCR and double immunostaining combined with lineage makers. By transplanting embryonic kidneys between genetic lineage–marked mice containing cells for renin, smooth muscle, and endothelial cells with wildtype mice, they showed two distinct populations of cells expressing either renin or smooth muscle cell markers, but never both in the same cell. As maturation began to occur, the renin cell began to express the smooth muscle cell markers, suggesting that renin cells could progress into smooth muscle cells and, if required, back into renin cells. Importantly, it appears that the transformation the other way around cannot happen, that is, the smooth muscle cells do not transform into renin cells (170, 177). The situation seems to be that when demand for renin is high, for example as a consequence of reduced renal perfusion pressure when the renal artery becomes constricted or if experimental animals are subjected to a low dietary sodium intake, some smooth muscles will transform back into renin-producing cells. Expression of the renin gene generates a specific mRNA that translates into a large protein, pre-prorenin, which then undergoes processing to generate pro-renin (79). The pre-renin then undergoes one of two fates—it can be secreted constitutively in an unchanged form, which represents "inactive" renin reported and investigated in many early studies, or it is incorporated into the secretory granules where it undergoes further modification into mature renin. The secretion of renin occurs when exocytosis of granules is stimulated, and this is regulated by two main intracellular signaling molecules—cAMP, which stimulates renin release, and intracellular calcium ion concentrations (Ca^{2+}), which inhibit renin secretion.

RENIN CELL ELECTROPHYSIOLOGY

It has become evident from a number of patch clamp studies that the membrane potential of granular cells is determined by a variety of ion channels that are also influenced by cAMP and Ca^{2+}. There are large conductance calcium-sensitive voltage-activated channels that are opened by raised intracellular cAMP (BKa), resulting in hyperpolarization and the L-type voltage–dependent calcium channels (Ca$_v$1.2), which when opened inhibit cAMP-mediated exocytosis (69, 70). It would appear that the normal physiological process is one in which the cAMP stimulation of renin granule exocytosis is protected against activation of L-type calcium channel by the hyperpolarization that results from the cAMP induced opening of the BKa. In this way, renin secretion can occur in a regulated way independent of intracellular Ca^{2+}. These relationships and interactions are illustrated in Fig. 4.

Activation of Renal Nerves

The stimulation of renal secretion and the exocytosis of the granules are regulated through three main routes—renal baroreceptor mechanism, macula densa, and renal sympathetic nerves. Many early investigations into the neural control of kidney function utilized either electrical stimulation or reflex activation of the renal sympathetic nerves, and showed that plasma renin activity or renin secretion was increased (46), which was a response that could be prevented by administration of β-adrenoceptor antagonists. Interpretation of these findings was often complicated by concomitant reductions in renal blood flow and glomerular filtration rate, which could have also contributed to the increase in renin release. Finally, studies by Kopp et al. (107a) and Osborn et al. (165), using the anesthetized dog in which they electrically stimulated the renal sympathetic nerves at frequencies having no effect on renal hemodynamics, showed that the increase in renin secretion was blocked by the β$_1$-adrenoceptor antagonist, metoprolol. This view of renin release from the granular

cells caused by a direct action of neurally released noradrenaline has been supported by comparable observations in the rabbit and rat as well as humans (98).

One of the consequences of the neurally induced renin release is now clear—there is an associated rise in renal renin mRNA. This effect becomes measurable at relatively high levels of renal nerve stimulation over ~1 hour, causing large increases in plasma renin activity (157). Interestingly, a number of reports have indicated that cAMP has an important role in stimulating renin gene expression by binding to an enhancer region upstream of the gene (168, 178), as well as in increasing the stability of renin mRNA (171, 180, 197), which may be mediated via cAMP-dependent phosphorylation mediated by ERK kinases (78). Thus, the nerve-mediated increase in cAMP may act in several ways, including (1) to cause an immediate release of renin as a result of exocytosis of the granules, (2) to increase in renin gene expression, and (3) to cause a stabilization and prolongation of the action of renin mRNA, all actions to ensure that sufficient renin is available and stores replenished. It is likely that this is the consequence of a requirement to ensure that the renin content of the granules within the cells is maintained so that sufficient stores of the protein are available for secretion if and when demand for renin secretion increases.

Neural and Non-Neural Interactions and Renin Release

A number of early observations gave rise to the concept that a background level of renal nerve activity was necessary to allow the various renin-releasing mechanisms to operate normally. The initial studies of Stella et al. (185)

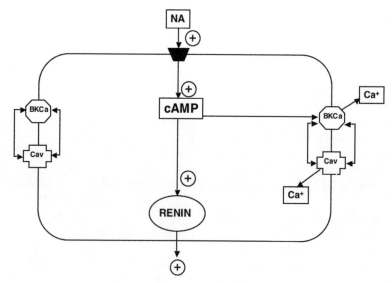

FIGURE 4   Noradrenaline stimulates a β-adrenoceptor on a renin-containing cell to increase intracellular cAMP, which then initiates exocytosis of renin-containing granules that releases renin. At the same time, cAMP acts at the BKCa channel to cause a hyperpolarization, which to a degree suppresses the CaV channel offsetting calcium entry, an effect that tends to inhibit renin secretion.

in the anesthetized cat demonstrated increased renin secretion as a reduction in either renal perfusion pressure, or in renal blood flow, was blunted in the denervated compared to innervated kidneys. Moreover, during reflex activation of the sympathetic nervous system following reduction of perfusion pressure at the carotid sinus, the magnitude of renin release when renal perfusion pressure was reduced was greater in the innervated than denervated kidneys (100). These findings were extended by Holdaas et al. (89) and Osborn et al. (166) using the anesthetized dog who found that furosemide-induced renin release was enhanced when the renal sympathetic nerves were intact compared to that obtained when the kidneys were denervated. Indeed, Kopp and DiBona (118) clearly demonstrated in the dog that the relationship between the magnitude of renin released in response to a particular level of electrical stimulation of the renal nerves was dependent on the prevailing level of renal perfusion pressure. The significance of these observations has remained undefined, but with the recent application of power spectral analysis to renal sympathetic nerve activity, blood pressure, and renal blood flow signals to determine the relationships among them, the possibility arises that this very low level of sympathetic activity impinging on the kidney may be related to determining the sensitivity of vascular components of autoregulation.

INTEGRATION OF RENAL NERVE ACTIVITY AND FUNCTION

Recruitment of Functionalities

An important consideration after having defined the exact mechanisms by which the renal nerves exert their influence on the various endpoints of kidney function, renin release, fluid reabsorption, and renal hemodynamics, is the relationship between the recruitment of these functionalities under normal conditions. This problem has been analyzed by drawing on a variety of reports and observations in anesthetized animals; a consensus formed in which a progressive mobilization of neurally regulated functions is accepted. At low levels of renal nerve stimulation that are subthreshold for changing fluid reabsorption and renal hemodynamics, there is an increase in renin secretion. At somewhat higher levels of renal nerve activation, but again subthreshold for impacting on renal hemodynamics, not only are there larger increases in renin secretion but there are also antidiuresis and antinatriuresis that have been demonstrated in the anesthetized dog, rabbit, and rat (46). It is clear that the renal nerve-induced sodium and water retention under these conditions reflects direct action on proximal tubule reabsorptive processes as described in micropuncture studies using the anesthetized rat (10, 11, 204, 205). At high levels of renal nerve stimulation, the increased renin release and fluid retention are enhanced, but

are now accompanied by reduced renal blood flow and, depending on the actual level of stimulation, a decrease in glomerular filtration rate (46). Indeed, this progressive recruitment of renal functionalities has been shown to occur in humans in an elegant study by Wurzner et al. (207), who used lower-body negative pressure (LBNP) to reflexively activate the sympathetic nervous system. They found that as LBNP was progressively reduced, there were associated proportionate increases in plasma noradrenaline and plasma renin activity, while sodium excretion was only reduced at the lowest LBNP used. During these challenges, renal blood flow and glomerular filtration rate were not changed. The ways in which these functionalities are recruited is illustrated in Fig. 5.

There are two important considerations arising from this pattern of responses. First, at low levels of renal sympathetic nerve activity, the major impact will be on renin release and sodium and water reabsorption. Although at these low levels of activity there will only be small increases in circulating renin (50%–100%) and reductions in sodium excretion of some 20%–40%, if these effects persist over a long period of time, they could have a profound impact on extracellular fluid volume, and thereby the level at which blood pressure is set. Again, it is worth reiterating that these renin-releasing and sodium-retaining responses can occur with little evidence of major reductions in renal hemodynamics.

Secondly, when renal sympathetic nerve activity is raised to high levels by major stressors, for example, emotional challenges or strenuous exercise, then blood flow

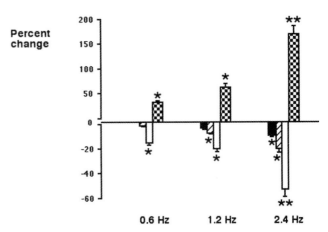

FIGURE 5 At the lowest level of renal nerve stimulation (0.6 Hz), there are significant increases in plasma renin activity (stippled bars) and decreases in sodium excretion (open bars), but no effect on either renal blood flow (hatched bars) or glomerular filtration rate (filled bars). As the frequency of stimulation is increased, there are larger increases in all variables, particularly the decreases in renal haemodynamics become significant. Importantly, the frequency–response relationships are much steeper for plasma renin activity and sodium excretion than for renal blood flow or glomerular filtration rate. (Modified from Hesse IF, Johns EJ. The effect of graded renal nerve stimulation on renal function in the anaesthetized rabbit. *Comp Biochem Physiol A* 1984;79:409–414.)

through the kidney will be markedly reduced. However, it is important to emphasize that these are short-acting events, and therefore they are likely to have only minor influences on overall cardiovascular homeostasis. One caveat may be that, as discussed above, basal renal nerve activity is sufficient to cause a small decrease in renal blood flow, but this could be due to the level of stress experienced by the experimental animals.

Patterns of Electrical Stimulation of Renal Nerves

PATTERNS OF EFFERENT ACTIVITY

The concepts of how the renal nerves influence kidney function have been based largely on experiments in which the sympathetic nerves to the kidney have been dissected out, placed on electrodes, and stimulated using square wave pulses of defined width and voltage at increasing frequencies and constant current delivery. It has been recognized that this pattern of stimulation bears no relation to that passing down the nerves naturally to reach the kidney. Indeed, multifiber nerve recordings have shown the signal to be of a bursting nature, where larger or smaller numbers of fibers fire together in a coordinated or disparate fashion with the result that complex patterns are generated. The question, therefore, arises as to whether the effectiveness or impact of the nerves on one or more functions might be different if they were stimulated in a way more representative of those occurring under natural conditions.

Interestingly, there is a body of information reporting the effect of depolarizing sympathetic fibers using different patterns of electrical stimulation. Lacroix et al. (130) and Nilsson et al. (160), using isolated mesenteric and nasal vessels, demonstrated that larger sympathetically mediated vasoconstrictions were produced using high-frequency bursts of impulses compared to delivery of the same number of impulses as a continuous train. To a degree, this was reinforced by the observations of Hardebo (81), who found that the high-frequency bursting pattern caused a greater release of noradrenaline from cerebral vessels than that achieved with the same number of impulses delivered as a continuous stream. Thus, the amount of neurotransmitters released can be influenced by the exact pattern of stimulation used.

ELECTRICAL ACTIVATION WITH FREQUENCY-ENRICHED STIMULI

Hemodynamics and Function The question arises as to whether the effectiveness or impact of the renal sympathetic nerves could be partially determined by the pattern of stimulation parameters. This was investigated by DiBona and Sawin (49) in the anesthetized rat, using a complex computer-generated stimulus pattern of basically a sine wave in which a randomly generated white-noise signal was embedded. The patterned stimulus was designed to approximate the pattern that the kidney might normally be expected to receive. The authors used two intensity levels, one impacting on renal hemodynamics and one at a lower level that only influenced

excretory function. Importantly, they showed that for the same integrated voltage applied to the nerves, the magnitude of reduction in renal blood flow was greater with the sinusoidal patterned stimulus than with the square-wave stimulus at all frequencies tested. These data are presented in Fig. 6, where there is clearly a shift of the frequency–response curve to the left with the sinusoidal stimuli compared to the square wave stimuli. In a similar way, application of subthreshold stimuli for changing renal hemodynamics had no effect on sodium excretion if delivered in a square wave form, but did cause an antidiuresis and antinatriuresis at the same integrated voltage if the sinusoidal signal was used (Fig. 7). Thus, together these reports serve to emphasize that the way in which the neural signals are delivered into the kidney can determine the impact on end-organ function.

Hemodynamics Malpas and colleagues (75, 144, 145) approached this issue at a different level, using the anesthetized rabbit, in that they investigated whether the bursting pattern of naturally occurring renal nerve activity could in any way determine the dynamic regulation of renal blood flow. Utilizing a similar patterned stimulus, that is, a sine wave of varying voltage within which square wave pulses were embedded, compared to steady square wave pulses, they showed that the frequency of the sine wave could determine the degree of reduction in renal blood flow even though the total current delivered was the same, thereby enhancing tone within the renal vasculature (144). The authors proposed that the low-frequency pulses in renal sympathetic nerve activity were likely to result in an enhanced dynamic gain to allow the renal blood flow to respond rapidly to normal everyday variations in blood pressure. Interestingly, this hypothesis was not supported by an investigation in the rat (52) in which

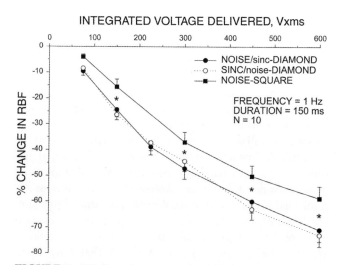

FIGURE 6 This figure demonstrates that delivery of an electrical stimulus as a square wave pulse (NOISE-SQUARE) is less efficient in decreasing RBF at every integrated voltage step compared with stimuli delivered as a sinusoidal wave containing either noise (NOISE/sinc-DIAMOND) or fixed frequency within the sinusoidal wave (SINC/noise-DIAMOND). RBF, renal blood flow. (With permission from Dibona GF, Sawin LL. Functional significance of the pattern of renal sympathetic nerve activation. *Am J Physiol* 1999;277:R346–R353.)

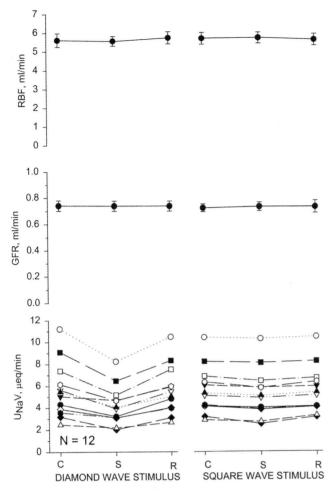

FIGURE 7 Electrical stimulation of renal sympathetic nerves with the diamond wave stimulus, which had no effect on either RBF or GFR and significantly decreased sodium excretive (U_{NaV}), whereas delivery of the same integrated voltage as a square wave stimulus was without effect on any of the measured variables. GFR, glomerular filtration rate; RBF, renal blood flow. (With permission, Dibona GF, Sawin LL. Functional significance of the pattern of renal sympathetic nerve activation. *Am J Physiol* 1999;277: R346–R353.)

the renal nerves were similarly stimulated with sine wave modulation with embedded high-frequency pulses. These investigators found that there were reductions in renal blood flow with superimposed low-frequency oscillations, but that the magnitude of these vasoconstrictor responses was not altered when basal tone was increased by exogenous administration of noradrenaline or Ang II. The reasons for the disparity between these reports are unclear, but may reflect a fundamental difference in the regulation of the renal vasculature in the rabbit versus the rat.

ANALYSIS OF RENAL NERVE ACTIVITY

Interestingly, with the advent of techniques to perform frequency and time domain analyses of physiological signals, it has become possible to resolve frequency and amplitude components, phase relationships, and coherence among renal sympathetic nerve activity, renal blood flow, and blood

pressure. These techniques have been applied recently in an attempt to gain insight as to how low levels of renal sympathetic nerve activity may influence renal function. It is evident from a number of studies in the rabbit, both in conscious and anesthetized studies, that renal sympathetic nerve activity is at a level that tonically reduces renal blood flow (76, 143). Moreover, following power spectral analysis of the renal blood flow signal, it has become apparent that at a spectral frequency range above 0.6 Hz in the renal sympathetic nerve signal, the nerves exert a tonic vasoconstrictor action on the renal vasculature (144). However, the lower-frequency power spectral peaks (<0.6 Hz) cause slow cycles of vasoconstriction and vasodilation, which it has been argued, may enhance the responsiveness of the vasculature to other stimuli to allow renal blood flow and glomerular filtration rate to dynamically adapt to ensure constancy of filtered load and hence fluid processing by the nephron (145). Indeed, it has been emphasized that this role of the renal nerves is integral to the maintenance of cardiovascular homeostasis (9).

The situation in the rat appears somewhat different, as it is clear from many reports (46) that under basal conditions the renal sympathetic nerves do not exert a basal tonic effect on renal blood flow. DiBona and Sawin (50, 54) evaluated the transfer function gain between blood pressure and renal blood flow under a variety of conditions where renal nerve activity was removed or enhanced. There was a characteristic pattern to the transfer gain function under basal conditions; thus, it decreased below zero over the frequency range 0.02–0.06 Hz, which was understood to represent a slower tubuloglomerular feedback mechanism of autoregulation, with a plateau region over the higher frequency range 0.1–0.2 Hz, which reflects the myogenic component of autoregulation. They found (50) that acute denervation had little impact on the overall pattern of transfer function gain over the entire frequency range. By contrast, in two pathophysiological states, congestive heart failure and in the spontaneously hypertensive rat where basal renal sympathetic nerve activity is elevated, transfer function gain was suppressed over both these frequency ranges, but was relatively normalized following acute renal denervation (52). The authors concluded that in rats with elevated renal nerve activity, the coupling between blood pressure and renal blood flow was overridden such that autoregulation of renal blood flow was impaired. These authors went on to show that this effect was mediated via Ang II, as blockade of angiotensin receptors with losartan depressed the transfer function gain in rats fed on low or normal dietary sodium intake, but not a high dietary sodium intake (48, 52). Moreover, this role of Ang II was also evident in the transfer function gain between the pseudorandom stimuli applied electrically and renal blood flow. Indeed, the outcome of these studies indicated that the renin-angiotensin system enhanced the tubuloglomerular feedback component of autoregulation but not the myogenic component and that the elevated Ang II increased the efficiency of transfer of the neural signal to control the renal vasculature.

Reflex Regulation of Renal Nerves

Activity within the renal sympathetic nerves represents an integration of a number of sensory inputs arising from different regions of the body by the central nervous system. The changing output of renal sympathetic nerve activity represents a means by which renal functionalities, that is, renin release, sodium reabsorption, and renal hemodynamics are regulated at an appropriate level. The various sensory systems sending information into the central nervous system are shown in Fig. 8.

CARDIOVASCULAR BARORECEPTORS

High-Pressure Baroreceptors A number of early studies demonstrated that the high-pressure baroreceptors in the carotid sinuses exerted an important influence on the neural regulation of the kidney. Studies undertaken in both the anesthetized and conscious dog in which carotid sinus pressure was reduced mechanically (74, 211) or as a consequence of periods of head-up tilt (43, 152, 153), resulted in increased renal nerve activity, renin secretion, and caused renal nerve–dependent antidiuresis and antinatriuresis with relatively little change in renal hemodynamics. This means that during everyday activity, the baroreflex control of blood pressure will impact on the kidney, but to a greater degree in relation to renin release and sodium and water retention than in regulating vasomotor tone in the kidney. However, what has become evident from a number of conscious rat studies, is that the baroreflex control of renal sympathetic nerve activity is shifted to higher pressure as muscle activity increases, such as during grooming and in response to an exercise load on a treadmill (156, 210).

Low-Pressure Baroreceptors The low-pressure baroreceptors are contained in the cardiopulmonary areas and are stretch receptors embedded in the atria and great veins (superior and inferior venae cavae and pulmonary vein). Activation of these receptors, mechanically by inflation of balloons in the left atria, results in a reflex decrease in renal sympathetic nerve activity associated with an in-

crease in water and sodium excretion (73, 132). While many of these studies were undertaken in anesthetized preparations, DiBona and Sawin (56) demonstrated in the conscious rat that volume expansion decreased and volume depletion increased renal sympathetic nerve activity. These observations correlated with a key report by Miki et al. (152) in the conscious dog showing that during head-out total body water immersion, a maneuver that shifts fluid into the more central compartments of the cardiovascular system caused a reflex renal sympathoinhibition associated with a diuresis and natriuresis. The cardiopulmonary receptors were demonstrated to be essential in this reflex as following chronic cardiac denervation, both the renal sympathoinhibition and excretory responses were markedly blunted when these dogs were subjected to the water immersion challenge (153).

SOMATOSENSORY SYSTEM

A further area of afferent input arises from the somatosensory system. There are mechanoreceptors in the joints and tendons and chemoreceptors within the muscle tissue itself that are sensitive to metabolites (97, 98), while the skin contains nociceptors and thermoreceptors. It is evident that each of these classes of receptors sends important sensory information into the central nervous system to be integrated. At the level of the kidney, an early study by Thames and Abboud (191) demonstrated that sciatic nerve stimulation caused profound reductions in renal blood flow. In a somewhat different scenario in the anesthetized rat, electrical stimulation of the brachial nerves, and application of capsaicin subcutaneously to depolarize afferent nerve endings or inhalation of noxious fumes (35, 36, 212) caused increases in renal sympathetic nerve activity and renal nerve–mediated antidiuresis and antinatriuresis with little change in renal hemodynamics. Interestingly, the magnitude of the renal sympathetic nerve activity responses was to some extent under tonic inhibitory control by the cardiopulmonary receptors, because following their activation, the sympathoexcitatory and antinatriuretic responses were blunted (213). These studies illustrate the point that the somatosensory system provides important input to the brain, but its impact is modulated by input from the cardiovascular baroreceptors.

VISCERAL SYSTEM

Less well studied, but nonetheless important, are the chemo- and mechanoreceptors of the visceral system. In early studies, Weaver and coworkers (198) demonstrated that activation of chemoreceptors in the small intestine of the cat, by bathing with bradykinin, caused a reflex activation of the renal sympathetic nerves. Furthermore, they demonstrated that the effectiveness of this sensory input from the gut was under a tonic inhibitory influence arising from both the low- and high-pressure cardiovascular baroreceptor. For some time, there has been a recognition that important chemo- and mechano-receptors are present within the liver

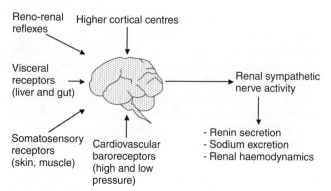

FIGURE 8 This illustration summarizes the input from various sensory systems that are integrated by the central nervous system to determine the degree of renal sympathetic nerve activity to regulate renin secretion, sodium excretion, and renal hemodynamics.

and/or its circulation (86, 127, 155), which when activated, can increase or decrease renal sympathetic nerve activity, and thereby the level of renal nerve-dependent sodium excretion. Again, all these observations point to significant sensory input into the central nervous system from the visceral organs, which is also an important contributory component in determining cardiovascular homeostasis.

HIGHER CORTICAL CENTERS

The role of psychological stress in regulating renal sympathetic nerve outflow and renal function is less clear-cut and far more difficult to study. Nonetheless, chronically instrumented rats have been used and subjected to arousal stimuli, such as the air-jet stress test. This experimental challenge has been found to reflexively increase renal sympathetic nerve activity along with renal nerve–dependent antinatriuresis and antidiuresis (53, 194). However, determining potential control by the cardiovascular baroreceptor of the physiological stresses has been difficult to achieve in studies of conscious subjects. Nonetheless, recent reports have revealed a number of important findings. First, it was apparent that the baroreceptor regulation of renal sympathetic nerve activity was depressed in rapid eye movement sleep, but that there was an adaptation of the baroreflex to function over a higher blood pressure range as the activity of the animal increased (210). Second, during treadmill exercise (154), there was an increased sensitivity of the baroreflex relationship, which the authors interpreted as important in buffering the raised blood pressure under conditions of increased muscular activity. Thus, it is becoming apparent that central command can exert an important modulatory influence on the baroreflex control of renal sympathetic outflow.

REFLEX CONTROL OF SELECTIVE FUNCTIONS

Attention has been focused on whether the renal innervation could selectively regulate either renal hemodynamics, or tubular fluid reabsorption or renin secretion. The findings of Luff et al. in the rabbit (137) and DiBona and Sawin in the rat (55) demonstrated that two types of structurally different nerve fibers exist within the nerve bundles and within the kidney itself. Studies have been undertaken to provide functional support for this hypothesis. Evidence has been produced in the rabbit where glomerular capillary pressure was measured as an indirect estimate of pre- and postglomerular resistances (38–40). Using an Ang II clamp to remove any confounding influences of changes in endogenous Ang II levels, a hypoxic challenge increased glomerular filtration pressure. The authors interpreted these observations as reflecting selective neural regulation of postglomerular vascular resistance, possibly via one of the subtypes of nerve fiber, independent of the renin-angiotensin system.

DiBona and colleagues (41, 55), using the rat, analyzed the strength–duration relationship during direct electrical renal nerve stimulation in relation to renal blood flow and urine flow and sodium excretion, and found a higher stimu-

lation threshold for the nerve fibers involved in regulating renal blood flow compared to those involved in regulating fluid excretion. Moreover, it was found that activity in single sympathetic fibers innervating the kidney could be selectively modified by different reflexes. Thus, arterial baroreceptors, central chemoreceptors, and thermoreceptors could activate a large proportion (88%) of fibers, thereby demonstrating spontaneous activity, whereas only thermoreceptors activated fibers that had no spontaneous activity. In a different series of studies, while examining patterns of renal sympathetic nerve activity by evaluating the peaks of activity and time between peaks, DiBona and colleagues were able to show that recruitment of nerve fibers was comparable to somatosensory (pinch) and heat stimuli, but it was only the heat stimulus that caused a decrease in renal blood flow. The authors suggested that these responses indicate a distinctly different control of sympathetic outflow that could selectively regulate hemodynamic, excretory, or renin secretory activity.

It would seem that there is a small, but persuasive, body of evidence for the view that there may be a degree of selectivity of functional control in the neural control of the kidney. More investigation of this particular topic is needed.

Central Nervous System

CENTRAL PROCESSING

The processing of this sensory information within the central nervous system to generate an appropriate level of sympathetic outflow, not only to the kidney but to other organs, is complex, and attention has been directed towards the cardiovascular baroreceptors, which exert a major influence on autonomic control (34). The sensory information from both the high- and low-pressure baroreceptors passes to the nucleus tractus solitarius (NTS) for initial processing, and subsequently there is output via multiple pathways to the caudal and rostral ventrolateral medulla (CVLM and RVLM) where a complex interaction takes place before the preganglionic fibers are stimulated. The way in which the major sensory inputs feed into these pathways is illustrated and summarized in Fig. 9.

The situation regarding somatosensory and visceral systems and their inputs to areas regulating the autonomic nervous system are much less defined. The somatosensory system appears to have a direct input at three levels—NTS, CVLM, and RVLM (32)—but the actions exerted at each of these sites, whether excitatory or inhibitory, and the neurotransmitters involved, have not been resolved. Interestingly, at a functional level, it has been reported (148) that the RVLM can give rise to activity that is selective for various sympathetically innervated regions, which again underlies the concept of patterned responses to ensure homeostasis. Thus, the exact ways in which information from these sensory systems are integrated to provide an appropriate output of renal sympathetic nerve activity and neural control of renal function remain to be explored.

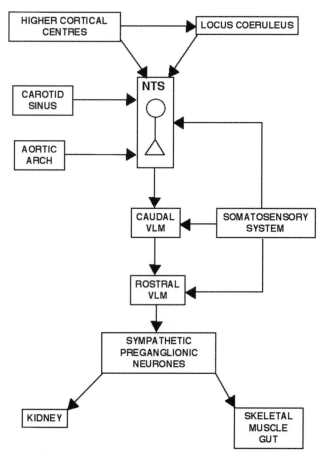

FIGURE 9 This illustration indicates how input from the baroreceptors, somatosensory system, and higher cortical centers act at the nucleus tractus solitarus (NTS), which feeds into the caudal and rostal venterolateral medulla (CVLM and RVLM). This determines the level of excitability of preganglionic neurons and thereby sympathetic outflow to the kidney and other vascular beds.

Brain Angiotensin II

Angiotensin II and Autonomic Pathways There is accumulating evidence that the renin-angiotensin system and Ang II can influence the baroreceptor and somatosensory responses in the sympathetic nerve activity generated by the central nervous system. This can arise in two ways, either via circulating Ang II, or by means of Ang II generated locally within the brain at specific nuclei. Moreover, Ang II receptors have been demonstrated to be present in many regions of the brain, and particularly at nuclei involved with cardiovascular control (1). It is now accepted that in the areas of circumventricular organs, the blood–brain barrier is leaky (151), enabling Ang II to act on nuclei within this region, which have been shown to contain a high density of Ang II receptors. At these sites the peptide is able to influence fluid balance, it stimulates drinking, induces ADH release, and causes an increased sodium reabsorption and renin release (150). The second route whereby Ang II may influence autonomic control is that generated within the brain itself, as all components of the

renin-angiotensin system are present, that is, renin, angiotensinogen converting enzyme, and Ang II receptors (202). It is also necessary to emphasize that immunocytochemical, in situ hybridization studies, and mRNA measurements of Ang II receptors and angiotensinogen have shown them to be present or their genes expressed on those nuclei involved with autonomic control, that is, the NTS, RVLM, and CVLM, and the paraventricular nucleus (PVN) (150), as well as other nuclei of the subfornical organ and the area postrema, which are most likely subject to the action of circulating angiotensin. Neurophysiological studies have shown that local administration of Ang II onto the NTS and RVLM is excitatory and produces a sympathetically mediated pressor response, but when applied to the CVLM, it causes a sympathoinhibition (33, 82); thus, Ang II may have different actions and consequences depending on its site of production and action.

Brain Angiotensin II and Neural Control of Kidney The functional role played by Ang II within the brain in modulating autonomic control, both normally and in pathophysiological states, is only now being elucidated. A number of reports show that the baroreflex control of renal sympathetic nerve activity was suppressed by Ang II, which appeared exaggerated in the spontaneously hypertensive rat (SHR) (90, 128). In terms of the somatosensory reflex, Ang II within the central nervous system is important in that intracerebroventricular-delivered losartan blocked the renal nerve–mediated antinatriuresis and antidiuresis resulting from nociceptor stimulation (92), and that replacing Ang II via the intracerebroventricular (ICV) route restored the renal nerve–dependent functional responses (93), which could be correlated with marked changes in the pattern with which energy was distributed within the renal nerve signal (97, 213). The central issue that arises is to understand what factors could affect the level of Ang II within the central nervous system that would then impact on the degree of autonomic control exerted peripherally and particularly at the kidney.

This very important link between the autonomic control of the cardiovascular system and brain Ang II can be modulated by the level of dietary sodium intake. An early report by Huang and Leenen (91) demonstrated that raised levels of dietary sodium intake in normotensive rats aged 4–8 weeks, led to an increase in baroreflex gain associated with resetting to a higher pressure for renal nerve activity, but not for heart rate. This importance of dietary sodium intake during development has been reinforced by the studies of Osborn and coworkers (21, 164), who showed that in rats fed a high-salt diet, but not a normal low-salt diet, aged 4 to 8 weeks, low-dose infusion of Ang II into the brain (ICV) over 5 days caused a sustained increase in blood pressure associated with a renal nerve–dependent antinatriuresis. This influence of dietary sodium intake on the contribution of Ang II in the brain on central pathways regulating renal sympathetic nerve activity has received some attention. DiBona and coworkers (44, 45) using rats subjected to a low, normal, or high dietary sodium intake for 2 weeks, microinjected an AT-1 receptor antagonist onto the RVLM, and observed a decreased blood pressure and a shift in the baroreflex gain curve for renal nerve activity to a lower pressure in the animals fed a low-sodium diet but not in those animals fed the normal- or high-sodium diets. Furthermore, it was evident that if bicuculline was injected onto the PVN, the increases in blood pressure, heart rate, and renal sympathetic nerve activity were blunted when the AT-1 receptor antagonist was applied to the RVLM. Importantly, the renal sympathetic nerve responses to the bicuculline administration onto the PVN were enhanced in rats subjected to the low-sodium diet but blunted in those fed the high-salt intake.

Together, these findings highlight the importance of Ang II in the brain in determining the sensitivity of neural pathways regulating sympathetic outflow to the kidney. They also emphasize how alterations in dietary sodium intake may impact on these neural control pathways, which may reset kidney function to a level that could predispose the individual to a hypertensive state.

RENORENAL REFLEXES

Afferent Renal Nerves

In the kidney, the majority of afferent renal nerves containing substance P and calcitonin gene–related peptide (CGRP) are located in the renal pelvic wall (110, 117, 136) where their circumferential orientation make them ideally suited for sensing stretch (Fig. 10). Depending on the species, the cell bodies of the afferent renal nerves are located in ipsilateral dorsal root ganglia (DRG) from T_6–L_4, with predomi-

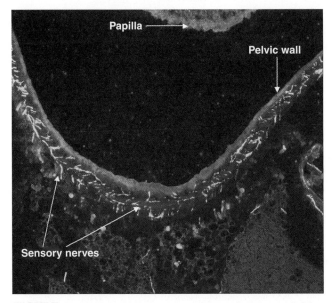

FIGURE 10 Immunofluorescence of renal tissue for substance P. Most nerves containing substance P-like immunoreactivity are found in the subepithelial layer of the pelvic wall with few fibers penetrating into the uroepithelium. (Magnification x240.)

nance in T_{12}–L_3 (58). Viral tracing studies combined with dorsal rhizotomy (DRX) at T_{10}–T_{13} have provided evidence for the afferent renal nerves projecting from the DRG to the ipsilateral dorsal horn mainly in lamina I and II (199). Stimulation of the afferent renal nerves may activate spinal and supraspinal pathways (23, 27, 104, 179). Activation of the afferent renal nerves alters the activity of vasopressin and oxytocin neurons in the paraventricular nucleus of hypothalamus in rats (27), resulting in increases arterial pressure and plasma vasopressin and oxytocin concentrations. These effects were abolished by prior denervation of the stimulated kidney. These data are consistent with a neural circuit involving afferent renal nerves projecting to the neurohypophysis.

Two classes of renal sensory receptors have been identified neurophysiologically: renal mechanoreceptors responding to stretch of the renal pelvic wall and renal chemoreceptors responding to renal ischemia and/or changes in the chemical environment of the renal interstitium. The electrophysiological characteristics of the renal sensory nerves has been previously reviewed extensively (46, 186).

Efferent Plus Afferent Renal Denervation

In healthy normotensive animals, the afferent renal nerves are activated by increases in renal pelvic pressure of magnitude >3 mm Hg, which is commonly seen during high urine flow rate (26, 71, 113), suggesting that the afferent renal nerves are tonically active in conditions of high-sodium diet and/or volume expansion. Supporting this argument are studies in anesthetized volume-expanded rats showing that total (i.e., efferent plus afferent) unilateral renal denervation increases contralateral efferent renal sympathetic nerve activity (ERSNA) and decreases contralateral urinary sodium excretion (i.e., a renorenal reflex response) (29, 47). Because unilateral renal denervation results in an ipsilateral diuresis and natriuresis, total (ipsilateral plus contralateral) urine flow rate and urinary sodium excretion are unchanged. Thus, the afferent renal nerves exert a tonic inhibitory effect on ipsilateral and contralateral ERSNA.

Activation of Renal Mechanosensory Nerves: Physiological Conditions

The inhibitory nature of the afferent renal nerves in healthy normal rats has been further demonstrated in studies examining the functional responses to activation of the afferent renal nerves. Stretching the renal pelvic wall or renal venous wall results in increases in ipsilateral afferent renal nerve activity (ARNA), bilateral decreases in ERSNA, and increases in urinary sodium excretion (122, 125, 141). Ipsilateral renal denervation blocks the increases in urinary sodium excretion, demonstrating that stimulation of renal mechanosensory nerves activates an inhibitory bilateral renorenal reflex mechanism (Fig. 11). The natriuretic nature of the renorenal reflexes would suggest that this reflex mechanism contributes

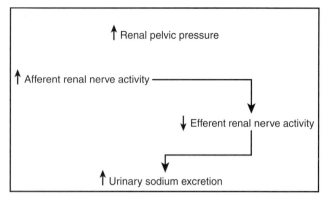

FIGURE 11 Stretching the renal pelvic wall by increasing renal pelvic pressure >3 mm Hg increases afferent renal nerve activity (ARNA), which causes a fall in efferent renal sympathetic nerve activity (ERSNA) and an increase in urinary sodium excretion, that is, a renorenal reflex response.

to total body sodium and fluid volume balance by assisting in the excretion of sodium and water. In this case, it would be expected that this reflex mechanism would be enhanced or upregulated during conditions of sodium and volume loading. Indeed, studies examining the responsiveness of the renal mechanosensory nerves in rats fed various sodium diets showed that in comparison to low dietary sodium intake conditions, high dietary sodium intake enhances the renorenal reflex response (113). At every level of renal pelvic pressure, the increases in both ARNA and urinary sodium

excretion are greater during high dietary sodium intake compared with low dietary sodium intake.

AFFERENT RENAL DENERVATION— DORSAL RHIZOTOMY

The overall importance of this renorenal reflex diuresis and natriuresis can be further evaluated by removing it by DRX at T_9–L_1. Both DRX and sham-DRX rats are able to establish external sodium balance on both a normal dietary sodium intake and a fourfold-higher dietary sodium intake. However, this is achieved at markedly different levels of arterial pressure (112). The process of achieving external sodium balance while consuming an increased dietary sodium intake resulted in a mean arterial pressure in DRX rats that was some 30 mm Hg greater than that in sham-DRX rats (Fig. 12). Importantly, the levels of mean arterial pressure are similar in rats fed either low- or normal-sodium diet (96, 112). Thus, in contrast to sham-DRX rats that were able to excrete a fourfold difference in sodium intake at similar arterial pressure, DRX rats were able to excrete a similar increased sodium intake only at the expense of a marked increase in arterial pressure. Thus, the DRX rats are characterized by impaired pressure natriuresis.

Wang and coworkers (e.g., 196) have presented evidence for salt-sensitive hypertension in rats neonatally treated with capsaicin to destroy the sensory innervation of all organs. The salt-sensitive hypertension in DRX rats would suggest that the lack of intact afferent renal innervation in the cap-

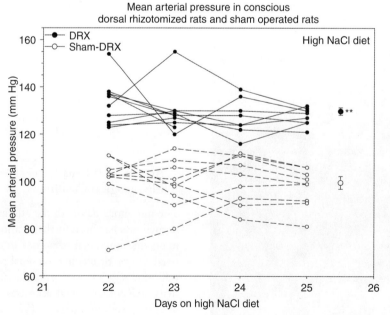

FIGURE 12 Mean arterial pressure measured in conscious rats during 4 consecutive days was 30 mm Hg higher in dorsal rhizotomized (DRX) rats (*solid lines, solid circles*) compared to sham-DRX rats (*dashed lines, open circles*) when both groups were fed a high-sodium diet for 25 days. **$p < .01$ average arterial pressure of 4 days in DRX vs sham-DRX rats. (From Kopp UC, Cicha MZ, Smith LA. Dietary sodium loading increases arterial pressure in afferent renal-denervated rats. *Hypertension* 2003;42:968–973.)

saicin treated rats may contribute to the increased arterial pressure in these rats when fed a high-sodium diet.

MECHANISMS INVOLVED IN ACTIVATION OF RENAL SENSORY NERVES

Isotonic saline volume expansion results in a differential activation of renal mechano- and chemo-sensitive nerves (26). Whereas volume expansion increased the activity of mechanosensitive nerves, it decreased the activity of the chemosensitive nerves, type R2 chemoreceptors. Stretch is associated with an increase in muscle spindle cell membrane sodium permeability resulting in an inward flux of sodium and depolarization (94, 167). The ARNA responses to increased renal pelvic pressure are reduced by renal pelvic administration of amiloride and lidocaine (121, 125), agents known to reduce sodium influx by different mechanisms. Conversely, inhibition of Na^+,K^+-ATPase by ouabain increases the ARNA response to increased renal pelvic pressure (126). These studies suggest that changes in intracellular sodium concentration may modulate the responsiveness of renal pelvic mechanosensitive nerves.

Substance P The presence of substance P containing sensory nerves in the renal pelvic wall (Fig. 10) (117) suggested a role for this neuropeptide in the activation of the renal sensory nerves. Substance P is released from the peripheral renal pelvic sensory nerves by a calcium (Ca^{++})-dependent mechanism requiring influx of Ca_i^{++} via N-type Ca_i^{++} channels in response to prostaglandin E2 (PGE2) (109), a known activator of sensory neurons (e.g., 24, 87, 193). Functional support for a role of substance P in the activation of renal pelvic sensory nerves is derived from in vivo studies showing that activation of renal mechanosensory nerves results in a renal pelvic release of substance P (116, 119, 120). Renal pelvic administration of substance P–receptor antagonists abolishes the renorenal reflex responses to increased renal pelvic pressure (123).

Bradykinin Among the various mechanisms involved in the release of substance P and activation of renal mechanosensory nerves is bradykinin. Bradykinin is a well-known activator of sensory nerve fibers (72). Bradykinin receptors have been localized on sensory nerve fibers (187) and in the lamina propria of the tissue lining the pelvis (146). Bradykinin increases ARNA when administered into the renal pelvis in association with an increased renal pelvic release of PGE2 and substance P and a contralateral natriuresis. Bradykinin 2 (B2) receptor antagonists block the renorenal reflex responses to either bradykinin, per se, or increases in renal pelvic pressure (119, 120). Interestingly, the responses to bradykinin are dependent on the route of administration. In contrast to the inhibitory reflex response elicited by renal pelvic administration of bradykinin (119, 120), administration of bradykinin into the renal artery elicits an excitatory reflex that includes activation of neurosecretory vasopressin cells in the supraoptic nucleus (37), increases in plasma ADH concentration, and increased arterial pressure and vascular resistance in most circulatory beds (184). The sym-

pathoexcitatory effects of intrarenally administered bradykinin were due to activation of afferent renal nerves since they were abolished by denervation of the infused kidney. This reflex has been suggested to be of importance during renal ischemia, which is likely to be associated with increased release of bradykinin.

These findings suggest that bradykinin activates different reflex pathways, one excitatory and one inhibitory, when administered into the renal artery and pelvis, respectively. The physiological or pathophysiological significance of these different reflexes is currently unknown.

Prostaglandin E2 There is considerable evidence for prostaglandins (PGs) enhancing the responsiveness of various sensory nerve fibers (e.g., 158, 169). The kidney, especially the renal medulla, is an active PG-producing tissue (18). A role for PGs in renal sensory receptor activation by reduced renal perfusion pressure was demonstrated by the finding that PG synthesis inhibition reduced the ARNA and reflex pressor responses to reduction in RBF (8, 66). Increasing renal pelvic pressure induces cyclooxygenase 2(COX-2) mRNA in the renal pelvic wall and increases renal pelvic release of prostaglandin E2 (PGE2). Inhibition of COX-2 reduced the renal pelvic release of PGE2 and increase in ARNA produced by increased renal pelvic pressure, suggesting a role for COX-2 in the synthesis of PGE2 in renal pelvic tissue (116). PGE receptors have been classified into four general subtypes, EP1, EP2, EP3, and EP4 based on cloning and pharmacological interventions (15). Immunohistochemical studies together with functional studies have provided evidence for a role of EP4 receptors in the activation of renal pelvic mechanosensory nerves (110).

It is well established that PGE2 activates the cAMP–protein kinase A (PKA) transduction cascade in DRG neurons leading to depolarization of the cell membrane and a release of substance P and CGRP (61, 159, 182). Using various activators and inhibitors of cAMP and PKA it was shown that PGE2 increases the release of substance P and stimulates renal mechanosensory nerves by activating the cAMP/PKA transduction cascade in renal pelvic tissue (115).

The link between bradykinin and increased renal pelvic PGE2 synthesis in the activation of renal mechanosensory nerves is, at least in part, related to activation of the phosphoinositide system via activation of B2 receptors coupled to protein kinase C (119).

Angiotensin II In normal rats, low-sodium diet reduces the responsiveness of renal mechanosensory nerves (113), that is, similar to the well-known reduced responsiveness of carotid baroreceptors in healthy low-sodium diet rats (45, 90). The reduced ARNA response to increased renal pelvic pressure in low-sodium diet rats was associated with impaired PGE2-mediated release of substance P from the isolated renal pelvic wall preparation. These data suggested that the reduced responsiveness of the renal sensory nerves was, at least in part, due to a mechanism at the peripheral sensory nerve endings.

A low-sodium diet is characterized by increased activity of the renin-angiotensin system (44–46). Ang II is present in the renal pelvic wall, the pelvic tissue concentration being similar to that in renal cortex, and modulated by dietary sodium (111). Renal pelvic administration of Ang II reduces and renal pelvic administration of the AT1 receptor antagonist losartan enhances the PGE2-mediated release of substance P and activation of renal mechanosensory nerves (113). Because the effects of losartan on the PGE2-mediated release of substance P was observed in response to acute administration of losartan to the isolated renal pelvic wall preparation, these data suggest that endogenous Ang II exerts its inhibitory effect on renal mechanosensory nerves by a mechanism at the peripheral renal sensory nerve endings. Further studies showed that endogenous Ang II in the renal pelvic tissue reduces the responsiveness of the renal sensory nerves by suppressing the PGE2-mediated activation of cAMP by a pertussis toxin–sensitive mechanism (113).

Activation of Renal Sensory Nerves: Pathological Conditions

Activation of the renal mechanosensory nerves is impaired in rats with congestive heart failure (CHF) (114) and in spontaneously hypertensive rats (SHR) (108, 124). The reduced responsiveness of the renal mechanosensory nerves is related to suppression of the PGE2-mediated release of substance P from the renal sensory nerve endings (114). CHF and SHR are characterized by increased activity of the renin-angiotensin system (46). A role for Ang II in the reduced responsiveness of the renal mechanosensory nerves in CHF rats and SHR was shown by the marked improvement of the responsiveness of these sensory nerves by renal pelvic administration of losartan (108, 114). Studies in renal pelvises from SHR showed the reduced PGE2-mediated release of substance P being at least in part related to Ang II activating a PTX-sensitive mechanism (108). Taken together, these studies suggest that the reduced responsiveness of renal mechanosensory nerves in CHF rats and SHR may contribute to the increased ERSNA and sodium retention prevalent in these pathological models (46). Furthermore, the marked enhancement of the renorenal reflex mechanism produced by AT1 receptor antagonists may contribute to the well-known beneficial effects of inhibiting the renin-angiotensin system in CHF and hypertension.

Suppression of the renorenal reflexes in physiological conditions of sodium retention produced by, for example, low-sodium diet, is an appropriate response. However, in pathological conditions of sodium retention, an impairment of the renorenal reflexes would aggravate the sodium retention.

There are numerous reports on reduced activation of the renal mechanosensory nerves and thus impairment of the inhibitory renorenal reflexes in various renal pathological

conditions. Chen and coworkers (25, 26, 139–141) have presented evidence for reduced natriuretic responses to saline volume expansion in ischemia-induced acute renal failure, obstructive nephropathy, cirrhosis, streptozotocin-induced diabetes, and chronic hypoxia. The impaired natriuretic responses to acute saline volume expansion were associated with reduced increases in ARNA and decreases in ERSNA, suggesting an impairment of the inhibitory renorenal reflexes. This notion was subsequently confirmed by showing impaired ARNA responses and reduced renal pelvic release of substance P and/or activation of NK1 receptors in response to standardized increases in renal pelvic pressure. A role for histamine in suppressing the activation of renal mechanosensory nerves in diabetic rats was suggested by the increased renal pelvic levels of histamine in diabetic rats and restoration of the ARNA responses to increased renal pelvic pressure towards control values following chronic antihistamine treatment.

The depressor effects of (T_9-L_1) DRX observed in rats with one-kidney, one-clip hypertension (103), or 5/6 nephrectomy (22), or in rats exposed to intravenous infusion of cyclosporine (138) would appear to contradict the notion of the afferent renal nerves exerting a tonic inhibitory effect on ERSNA. However, as discussed above, it is likely that different mechanisms are involved in the activation of renal sensory nerves in normal and diseased kidneys. Whereas in normal kidneys, activation of renal sensory nerves elicits inhibitory renorenal reflexes, in diseased kidneys when the inhibitory renorenal reflexes may be impaired, activation of renal sensory nerves may result in excitatory reflexes. In this context, it is interesting that denervation of the ischemic kidney in the two-kidney, one-clip model of hypertension elicits an increase in contralateral urinary sodium excretion, whereas denervation of the nonclipped kidney elicits the expected decrease in contralateral urinary sodium excretion (107). Studies by Katholi and Woods (103) would suggest that adenosine may be one of the mediators involved in the activation of renal sensory nerves in ischemic kidneys. Although there is evidence for an important renal component in the hypertensive process following renal injury produced by intrarenal phenol (209) or 5/6 nephrectomy (22), the mediator(s) at the level of the renal sensory nerve terminal are not known. Data showing that intravenous cyclosporine fails to increase ARNA and arterial pressure in synapsin-deficient mice suggest that the mechanisms causing the sustained increase in ARNA produced by acute intravenous infusion of cyclosporine, a calcineurin inhibitor, involve alterations in synapsin phosphorylation–dephosphorylation in renal sensory nerve terminals (214). The important role of synapsin in the cyclosporine-induced activation of ARNA appears to be unique for cyclosporine because capsaicin, which activates sensory nerves by releasing substance P and/or CGRP, produced similar increases in ARNA in wildtype and synapsin-deficient mice.

SUMMARY

There is considerable evidence for the presence and importance of inhibitory renorenal reflexes contributing to the homeostatic regulation of arterial pressure and sodium balance in normotensive healthy individuals. Activation of the afferent renal nerves and thus the renorenal reflexes is the result of an interaction between PGE2 and Ang II at the peripheral renal sensory nerve endings with PGE2 facilitating and Ang II suppressing the activation (Fig. 13). In conditions of low Ang II activity, including high-sodium diet, the stimulatory effects of PGE2 on adenylyl cyclase will result in activation of renal sensory nerves leading to decreased ERSNA and increased urinary sodium excretion. Conversely, in conditions of high Ang II activity, including low-sodium diet, CHF and spontaneous hypertension, the Ang II–inhibitory influence on adenylyl cyclase would impair the PGE2-mediated activation of renal sensory nerves that would lead to increased ERSNA and sodium retention.

In various renal pathological conditions, activation of the afferent renal nerves and the inhibitory renorenal reflexes are impaired. In these conditions, available data would suggest that excitatory renorenal reflexes prevail and contribute to increased arterial pressure. There is currently little knowledge of the mechanisms involved in activating the excitatory renorenal reflexes.

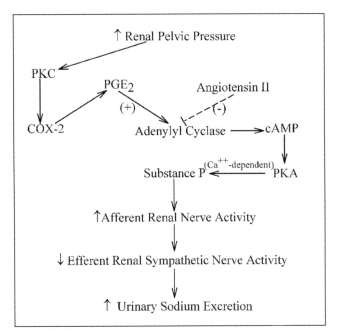

FIGURE 13 In the sequence of events elicited following an increase in the renal pelvic pressure, PGE2 exerts a stimulatory and Ang II an inhibitory effect on the activation of adenylyl cyclase. The interaction between PGE2 and Ang II determines the activation of the renal mechanosensory nerves. In conditions of low endogenous Ang II, there is enhanced activation of the renal mechanosensory nerves, resulting in decreased ERSNA and natriuresis. Conversely, in conditions of high endogenous Ang II, the activation of renal mechanosensory nerves is impaired, which results in increased ERSNA and sodium retention. Ang II, angiotensin II; ERSNA, efferent renal sympathetic nerve activity. (From Kopp UC, Cicha MZ. Impaired substance P release from renal sensory nerves in SHR involves a pertussis toxin-sensitive mechanism. *Am J Physiol Regul Integr Comp Physiol* 2004;286:R326–R333.)

References

1. Allen AM, Moeller I, Jenkins TA, Zhuo J, Aldred GP, Chai SY, Mendelsohn FA. Angiotensin receptors in the nervous system. *Brain Res Bull* 1998;47:17–28.
2. Aperia A, Ibarra F, Svensson LB, Klee C, Greengard P. Calcineurin mediates alpha-adrenergic stimulation of Na+,K+)-ATPase activity in renal tubule cells. *Proc Natl Acad Sci U S A* 1992;89:7394–7397.
3. Aukland K. Hydrogen polarography in measurement of local blood flow: theoretical and empirical basis. *Acta Neurol Scand Suppl* 1965;14:42–45.
4. Aukland K, Bower BF, Berliner RW. Measurement of local blood flow with hydrogen gas. *Circ Res* 1964;14:164–187.
5. Bachmann S, Bosse HM, Mundel P. Topography of nitric oxide synthesis by localizing constitutive NO synthases in mammalian kidney. *Am J Physiol* 1995;268:F885–F898.
6. Barajas L, Liu L, Powers K. Anatomy of the renal innervation: intrarenal aspects and ganglia of origin. *Can J Physiol Pharmacol* 1992;70:735–749.
7. Barajas L, Powers K, Wang P. Innervation of the renal cortical tubules: a quantitative study. *Am J Physiol* 1984;247:F50–F60.
8. Barber JD, Moss NG. Reduced renal perfusion pressure causes prostaglandin-dependent excitation of R2 chemoreceptors in rats. *Am J Physiol* 1990;259:R1243–R1249.
9. Barrett CJ, Navakatikyan MA, Malpas SC. Long-term control of renal blood flow: what is the role of the renal nerves? *Am J Physiol Regul Integr Comp Physiol* 2001;280: R1534–R1545.
10. Bello-Reuss E, Colindres RE, Pastoriza-Munoz E, Mueller RA, Gottschalk CW. Effects of acute unilateral renal denervation in the rat. *J Clin Invest* 1975;56:208–217.
11. Bello-Reuss E, Pastoriza-Munoz E, Colindres RE. Acute unilateral renal denervation in rats with extracellular volume expansion. *Am J Physiol* 1977;232:F26–F32.
12. Bernard C. *Lecons sur les Proprietes Physiologique et les Alterations Pathologique des Liquides de l'Organisme*, Vol. 2. Paris: Bailliere et Fils; 1859.
13. Bohmann C, Schollmeyer P, Rump LC. Alpha 2-autoreceptor subclassification in rat isolated kidney by use of short trains of electrical stimulation. *Br J Pharmacol* 1993;108:262–268.
14. Bohmann C, Schollmeyer P, Rump LC. Effects of imidazolines on noradrenaline release in rat isolated kidney. *Naunyn Schmiedebergs Arch Pharmacol* 1994;349:118–124.
15. Boie Y, Stocco R, Sawyer N, Slipetz DM, Ungrin MD, Neuschafer-Rube F, Puschel GP, Metters KM, Abramovitz M. Molecular cloning and characterization of the four rat prostaglandin E2 prostanoid receptor subtypes. *Eur J Pharmacol* 1997;340:227–241.
16. Boke T, Malik KU. Enhancement by locally generated angiotensin II of release of the adrenergic transmitter in the isolated rat kidney. *J Pharmacol Exp Ther* 1983;226:900–907.
17. Bonjour JP, Churchill PC, Malvin RL. Change of tubular reabsorption of sodium and water after renal denervation in the dog. *J Physiol* 1969;204:571–582.
18. Bonvalet JP, Pradelles P, Farman N. Segmental synthesis and actions of prostaglandins along the nephron. *Am J Physiol* 1987;253:F377–F387.
19. Bosse HM, Bohm R, Resch S, Bachmann S. Parallel regulation of constitutive NO synthase and renin at JGA of rat kidney under various stimuli. *Am J Physiol* 1995;269:F793–F805.
20. Brod J. *The Kidney*. London: Butterworth, 1973.
21. Camara AK, Osborn JL. AT1 receptors mediate chronic central nervous system AII hypertension in rats fed high sodium chloride diet from weaning. *J Auton Nerv Syst* 1998;72:16–23.
22. Campese VM, Kogosov E. Renal afferent denervation prevents hypertension in rats with chronic renal failure. *Hypertension* 1995;25:878–882.
23. Caverson MM, Ciriello J. Effect of stimulation of afferent renal nerves on plasma levels of vasopressin. *Am J Physiol* 1987;252:R801–R807.
24. Chen HI, Chapleau MW, McDowell TS, Abboud FM. Prostaglandins contribute to activation of baroreceptors in rabbits. Possible paracrine influence of endothelium. *Circ Res* 1990;67:1394–1404.
25. Chien CT, Chien HF, Cheng YJ, Chen CF, Hsu SM. Renal afferent signaling diuretic response is impaired in streptozotocin-induced diabetic rats. *Kidney Int* 2000;57:203–214.
26. Chien CT, Fu TC, Wu MS, Chen CF. Attenuated response of renal mechanoreceptors to volume expansion in chronically hypoxic rats. *Am J Physiol* 1997;273:F712–F717.
27. Ciriello J. Afferent renal inputs to paraventricular nucleus vasopressin and oxytocin neurosecretory neurons. *Am J Physiol* 1998;275:R1745–R1754.
28. Clausen G, Tyssebotn I, Kirkebo A, Ofjord ES, Aukland K. Distribution of blood flow in the dog kidney. III. Local uptake of 10 mum and 15 mum microspheres during renal vasodilation and constriction. *Acta Physiol Scand* 1981;113:471–479.
29. Colindres RE, Spielman WS, Moss NG, Harrington WW, Gottschalk CW. Functional evidence for renorenal reflexes in the rat. *Am J Physiol* 1980;239:F265–F270.
30. Cohnheim J, Roy S. Untersuchungen uber die Zirkulation in den Nieren. *Virchows Arch Path Anat Physiol* 1883;92:424–457.
31. Cupples WA, Marsh DJ. Autoregulation of blood flow in renal medulla of the rat: no role for angiotensin II. *Can J Physiol Pharmacol* 1988;66:833–836.
32. Dampney RA. Functional organization of central pathways regulating the cardiovascular system. *Physiol Rev* 1994;74:323–364.
33. Dampney RA, Fontes MA, Hirooka Y, Horiuchi J, Potts PD, Tagawa T. Role of angiotensin II receptors in the regulation of vasomotor neurons in the ventrolateral medulla. *Clin Exp Pharmacol Physiol* 2002;29:467–472.

34. Dampney RA, Horiuchi J, Tagawa T, Fontes MA, Potts PD, Polson JW. Medullary and supramedullary mechanisms regulating sympathetic vasomotor tone. *Acta Physiol Scand* 2003;177:209–218.

35. Davis G, Johns EJ. Effect of somatic nerve stimulation on the kidney in intact, vagotomized and carotid sinus-denervated rats. *J Physiol* 1991;432:573–584.

36. Davis G, Johns EJ. Somatosensory regulation of renal function in the stroke-prone spontaneously hypertensive rat. *J Physiol* 1994;481:753–759.

37. Day TA, Ciriello J. Effects of renal receptor activation on neurosecretory vasopressin cells. *Am J Physiol* 1987;253:R234–R241.

38. Denton KM, Fennessy PA, Alcorn D, Anderson WP. Morphometric analysis of the actions of angiotensin II on renal arterioles and glomeruli. *Am J Physiol* 1992;262:F367–F372.

39. Denton KM, Luff SE, Shweta A, Anderson WP. Differential neural control of glomerular ultrafiltration. *Clin Exp Pharmacol Physiol* 2004;31:380–386.

40. Denton KM, Shweta A, Flower RL, Anderson WP. Predominant postglomerular vascular resistance response to reflex renal sympathetic nerve activation during ANG II clamp in rabbits. *Am J Physiol Regul Integr Comp Physiol* 2004;287:R780–R786.

41. DiBona GF. Nervous kidney. Interaction between renal sympathetic nerves and the renin-angiotensin system in the control of renal function. *Hypertension* 2000;36:1083–1088.

42. DiBona GF. Peripheral and central interactions between the renin-angiotensin system and the renal sympathetic nerves in control of renal function. *Ann N Y Acad Sci* 2001;940:395–406.

43. DiBona GF, Johns EJ. A study of the role of renal nerves in the renal responses to 60 degree head-up tilt in the anaesthetized dog. *J Physiol* 1980;299:117–126.

44. DiBona GF, Jones SY. Sodium intake influences hemodynamic and neural responses to angiotensin receptor blockade in rostral ventrolateral medulla. *Hypertension* 2001;37:1114–1123.

45. DiBona GF, Jones SY, Sawin LL. Effect of endogenous angiotensin II on renal nerve activity and its arterial baroreflex regulation. *Am J Physiol* 1996;271:R361–R367.

46. DiBona GF, Kopp UC. Neural control of renal function. *Physiol Rev* 1997;77:75–197.

47. DiBona GF, Rios LL. Renal nerves in compensatory renal response to contralateral renal denervation. *Am J Physiol* 1980;238:F26–F30.

48. Dibona GF, Sawin LL. Effect of endogenous angiotensin II on the frequency response of the renal vasculature. *Am J Physiol Renal Physiol* 2004;287:F1171–F1178.

49. Dibona GF, Sawin LL. Functional significance of the pattern of renal sympathetic nerve activation. *Am J Physiol* 1999;277:R346–R353.

50. DiBona GF, Sawin LL. Effect of renal denervation on dynamic autoregulation of renal blood flow. *Am J Physiol Renal Physiol* 2004;286:F1209–F1218.

51. DiBona GF, Sawin LL. Effect of renal nerve stimulation on NaCl and H2O transport in Henle's loop of the rat. *Am J Physiol* 1982;243:F576–F580.

52. DiBona GF, Sawin LL. Effect of renal nerve stimulation on responsiveness of the rat renal vasculature. *Am J Physiol Renal Physiol* 2002;283:F1056–F1065.

53. DiBona GF, Sawin LL. Exaggerated natriuresis in experimental hypertension. *Proc Soc Exp Biol Med* 1986;182:43–51.

54. DiBona GF, Sawin LL. Frequency response of the renal vasculature in congestive heart failure. *Circulation* 2003;107:2159–2164.

55. DiBona GF, Sawin LL. Renal hemodynamic effects of activation of specific renal sympathetic nerve fiber groups. *Am J Physiol* 1999;276:R539–R549.

56. DiBona GF, Sawin LL. Renal nerve activity in conscious rats during volume expansion and depletion. *Am J Physiol* 1985;248:F15–F23.

57. DiBona GF, Zambraski EJ, Aguilera AJ, Kaloyanides GJ. Neurogenic control of renal tubular sodium reabsorption in the dog: a brief review and preliminary report concerning possible humoral mediation. *Circ Res* 1977;40:I127–I130.

58. Donovan MK, Wyss JM, Winternitz SR. Localization of renal sensory neurons using the fluorescent dye technique. *Brain Res* 1983;259:119–122.

59. Egi Y, Matsumura Y, Murata S, Umekawa T, Hisaki K, Takaoka M, Morimoto S. The effects of NG-nitro-L-arginine, a nitric oxide synthase inhibitor, on norepinephrine overflow and antidiuresis induced by stimulation of renal nerves in anesthetized dogs. *J Pharmacol Exp Ther* 1994;269:529–535.

60. Eitle E, Hiranyachattada S, Wang H, Harris PJ. Inhibition of proximal tubular fluid absorption by nitric oxide and atrial natriuretic peptide in rat kidney. *Am J Physiol* 1998;274:C1075–C1080.

61. England S, Bevan S, Docherty RJ. PGE2 modulates the tetrodotoxin-resistant sodium current in neonatal rat dorsal root ganglion neurones via the cyclic AMP-protein kinase A cascade. *J Physiol* 1996;495:429–440.

62. Eppel GA, Malpas SC, Denton KM, Evans RG. Neural control of renal medullary perfusion. *Clin Exp Pharmacol Physiol* 2004;31:387–396.

63. Esler M. The sympathetic system and hypertension. *Am J Hypertens* 2000;13:99S–105S.

64. Esler M, Rumantir M, Kaye D, Jennings G, Hastings J, Socratous F, Lambert G. Sympathetic nerve biology in essential hypertension. *Clin Exp Pharmacol Physiol* 2001;28:986–989.

65. Evans RG, Eppel GA, Anderson WP, Denton KM. Mechanisms underlying the differential control of blood flow in the renal medulla and cortex. *J Hypertens* 2004;22:1439–1451.

66. Faber JE. Role of prostaglandins and kinins in the renal pressor reflex. *Hypertension* 1987;10:522–532.

67. Fazan VP, Ma X, Chapleau MW, Barreira AA. Qualitative and quantitative morphology of renal nerves in C57BL/6J mice. *Anat Rec* 2002;268:399–404.

68. Feng F, Pettinger WA, Abel PW, Jeffries WB. Regional distribution of alpha 1-adrenoceptor subtypes in rat kidney. *J Pharmacol Exp Ther* 1991;258:263–268.

69. Friis UG, Jensen BL, Sethi S, Andreasen D, Hansen PB, Skott O. Control of renin secretion from rat juxtaglomerular cells by cAMP-specific phosphodiesterases. *Circ Res* 2002;90:996–1003.

70. Friis UG, Jorgensen F, Andreasen D, Jensen BL, Skott O. Membrane potential and cation channels in rat juxtaglomerular cells. *Acta Physiol Scand* 2004;181:391–396.

71. Genovesi S, Pieruzzi F, Wijnmaalen P, Centonza L, Golin R, Zanchetti A, Stella A. Renal afferents signaling diuretic activity in the cat. *Circ Res* 1993;73:906–913.

72. Geppetti P. Sensory neuropeptide release by bradykinin: mechanisms and pathophysiological implications. *Regul Pept* 1993;47:1–23.

73. Gilmore JP, Echtenkamp S, Wesley CR, Zucker IH. Atrial receptor modulation of renal nerve activity in the nonhuman primate. *Am J Physiol* 1982;242:F592–F598.

74. Gross R, Ruffmann K, Kirchheim H. The separate and combined influences of common carotid occlusion and nonhypotensive hemorrhage on kidney blood flow. *Pflugers Arch* 1979;379:81–88.

75. Guild SJ, Austin PC, Navakatikyan M, Ringwood JV, Malpas SC. Dynamic relationship between sympathetic nerve activity and renal blood flow: a frequency domain approach. *Am J Physiol Regul Integr Comp Physiol* 2001;281:R206–R212.

76. Guild SJ, Barrett CJ, Evans RG, Malpas SC. Interactions between neural and hormonal mediators of renal vascular tone in anaesthetized rabbits. *Exp Physiol* 2003;88:229–241.

77. Guild SJ, Eppel GA, Malpas SC, Rajapakse NW, Stewart A, Evans RG. Regional responsiveness of renal perfusion to activation of the renal nerves. *Am J Physiol Regul Integr Comp Physiol* 2002;283:R1177–R1186.

78. Habelhah H, Shah K, Huang L, Ostareck-Lederer A, Burlingame AL, Shokat KM, Hentze MW, Ronai Z. ERK phosphorylation drives cytoplasmic accumulation of hnRNP-K and inhibition of mRNA translation. *Nat Cell Biol* 2001;3:325–330.

79. Hackenthal E, Paul M, Ganten D, Taugner R. Morphology, physiology, and molecular biology of renin secretion. *Physiol Rev* 1990;70:1067–1116.

80. Handa RK, Johns EJ. Interaction of the renin-angiotensin system and the renal nerves in the regulation of rat kidney function. *J Physiol* 1985;369:311–321.

81. Hardebo JE. Influence of impulse pattern on noradrenaline release from sympathetic nerves in cerebral and some peripheral vessels. *Acta Physiol Scand* 1992;144:333–339.

82. Head GA. Role of AT1 receptors in the central control of sympathetic vasomotor function. *Clin Exp Pharmacol Physiol Suppl* 1996;3:S93–S98.

83. Hermansson K, Kallskog O, Wolgast M. Effect of renal nerve stimulation on the activity of the tubuloglomerular feedback mechanism. *Acta Physiol Scand* 1984;120:381–385.

84. Hesse IF, Johns EJ. The effect of graded renal nerve stimulation on renal function in the anaesthetized rabbit. *Comp Biochem Physiol A* 1984;79:409–414.

85. Hesse IF, Johns EJ. The subtype of alpha-adrenoceptor involved in the neural control of renal tubular sodium reabsorption in the rabbit. *J Physiol* 1984;352:527–538.

86. Hevener AL, Bergman RN, Donovan CM. Hypoglycemic detection does not occur in the hepatic artery or liver: findings consistent with a portal vein glucosensor locus. *Diabetes* 2001;50:399–403.

87. Hintze TH, Kaley G. Ventricular receptors activated following myocardial prostaglandin synthesis initiate reflex hypotension, reduction in heart rate, and redistribution of cardiac output in the dog. *Circ Res* 1984;54:239–247.

88. Hisa H, Araki S, Tomura Y, Hayashi Y, Satoh S. Effects of alpha adrenoceptor blockade on renal nerve stimulation-induced norepinephrine release and vasoconstriction in the dog kidney. *J Pharmacol Exp Ther* 1989;248:752–757.

89. Holdaas H, DiBona GF, Kiil F. Effect of low-level renal nerve stimulation on renin release from nonfiltering kidneys. *Am J Physiol* 1981;241:F156–F161.

90. Huang BS, Leenen FH. Dietary Na and baroreflex modulation of blood pressure and RSNA in normotensive vs. spontaneously hypertensive rats. *Am J Physiol* 1994;266:H496–H502.

91. Huang BS, Leenen FH. Sympathoexcitatory and pressor responses to increased brain sodium and ouabain are mediated via brain ANG II. *Am J Physiol* 1996;270:H275–H280.

92. Huang C, Johns EJ. Role of ANG II in mediating somatosensory-induced renal nerve-dependent antinatriuresis in the rat. *Am J Physiol* 1998;275:R194–R202.

93. Huang C, Johns EJ. Role of brain angiotensin II in the somatosensory induced antinatriuresis in the anaesthetized rat. *Clin Exp Pharmacol Physiol* 2000;27:191–196.

94. Hunt CC, Wilkinson RS, Fukami Y. Ionic basis of the receptor potential in primary endings of mammalian muscle spindles. *J Gen Physiol* 1978;71:683–698.

95. Ichihara A, Kobori H, Nishiyama A, Navar LG. Renal renin-angiotensin system. *Contrib Nephrol* 2004;143:117–130.

96. Janssen BJ, Struijker Boudier HA, Smits JF. Role of afferent renal nerves in renal adaptation to sodium restriction in uninephrectomized rats. *Acta Physiol Scand* 1994;151:395–402.

97. Johns EJ. The autonomic nervous system and pressure-natriuresis in cardiovascular-renal interactions in response to salt. *Clin Auton Res* 2002;12:256–263.

98. Johns EJ. Role of angiotensin II and the sympathetic nervous system in the control of renal function. *J Hypertens* 1989;7:695–701.

99. Johns EJ. The role of angiotensin II in the antidiuresis and antinatriuresis induced by stimulation of the sympathetic nerves to the rat kidney. *J Auton Pharmacol* 1987;7:205–214.

100. Johns EJ. Role of the renal nerves in modulating renin release during pressure reduction at the feline kidney. *Clin Sci (Lond)* 1985;69:185–195.

101. Johns EJ, Lewis BA, Singer B. The sodium-retaining effect of renal nerve activity in the cat: role of angiotensin formation. *Clin Sci Mol Med* 1976;51:93–102.

102. Johns EJ, Manitius J. An investigation into the neural regulation of calcium excretion by the rat kidney. *J Physiol* 1987;383:745–755.

103. Katholi RE, Woods WT. Afferent renal nerves and hypertension. *Clin Exp Hypertens A* 1987;9(Suppl 1):211–226.

104. Knuepfer MM, Akeyson EW, Schramm LP. Spinal projections of renal afferent nerves in the rat. *Brain Res* 1988;446:17–25.

105. Kompanowska-Jezierska E, Walkowska A, Johns EJ, Sadowski J. Early effects of renal denervation in the anaesthetised rat: natriuresis and increased cortical blood flow. *J Physiol* 2001;531:527–534.

106. Kone BC, Baylis C. Biosynthesis and homeostatic roles of nitric oxide in the normal kidney. *Am J Physiol* 1997;272:F561–F578.

107. Kopp UC, Buckley-Bleiler RL. Impaired renorenal reflexes in two-kidney, one clip hypertensive rats. *Hypertension* 1989;14:445–452.

107a. Kopp U, Aurell M, Nilsson IM, Ablad B. The role of beta-1-adrenoceptors in the renin release response to graded renal sympathetic nerve stimulation. *Pfluegers Arch* 1980;387:107–113.

108. Kopp UC, Cicha MZ. Impaired substance P release from renal sensory nerves in SHR involves a pertussis toxin-sensitive mechanism. *Am J Physiol Regul Integr Comp Physiol* 2004;286:R326–R333.
109. Kopp UC, Cicha MZ. PGE2 increases substance P release from pelvis sensory nerves via activation of N-type calcium channels. *Am J Physiol* 1999;276:R1241–R1248.
110. Kopp UC, Cicha MZ, Nakamura K, Nusing RM, Smith LA, Hokfelt T. Activation of EP4 receptors contributes to prostaglandin E2-mediated stimulation of renal sensory nerves. *Am J Physiol Renal Physiol* 2004;287:F1269–F1282.
111. Kopp UC, Cicha MZ, Smith LA. Angiotensin blocks substance P release from renal sensory nerves by inhibiting PGE2-mediated activation of cAMP. *Am J Physiol Renal Physiol* 2003;285:F472–F483.
112. Kopp UC, Cicha MZ, Smith LA. Dietary sodium loading increases arterial pressure in afferent renal-denervated rats. *Hypertension* 2003;42:968–973.
113. Kopp UC, Cicha MZ, Smith LA. Endogenous angiotensin modulates PGE-mediated release of substance P from renal mechanosensory nerve fibers. *Am J Physiol Regul Integr Comp Physiol* 2002;282:R19–R30.
114. Kopp UC, Cicha MZ, Smith LA. Impaired responsiveness of renal mechanosensory nerves in heart failure: role of endogenous angiotensin. *Am J Physiol Regul Integr Comp Physiol* 2003;284:R116–R124.
115. Kopp UC, Cicha MZ, Smith LA. PGE(2) increases release of substance P from renal sensory nerves by activating the cAMP-PKA transduction cascade. *Am J Physiol Regul Integr Comp Physiol* 2002;282:R1618–R1627.
116. Kopp UC, Cicha MZ, Smith LA, Haeggstrom JZ, Samuelsson B, Hokfelt T. Cyclooxygenase-2 involved in stimulation of renal mechanosensitive neurons. *Hypertension* 2000;35:373–378.
117. Kopp UC, Cicha MZ, Smith LA, Hokfelt T. Nitric oxide modulates renal sensory nerve fibers by mechanisms related to substance P receptor activation. *Am J Physiol Regul Integr Comp Physiol* 2001;281:R279–R290.
118. Kopp UC, DiBona GF. Interaction between neural and nonneural mechanisms controlling renin secretion rate. *Am J Physiol* 1984;246:F620–F626.
119. Kopp UC, Farley DM, Cicha MZ, Smith LA. Activation of renal mechanosensitive neurons involves bradykinin, protein kinase C, PGE(2), and substance P. *Am J Physiol Regul Integr Comp Physiol* 2000;278:R937–R946.
120. Kopp UC, Farley DM, Smith LA. Bradykinin-mediated activation of renal sensory neurons due to prostaglandin-dependent release of substance P. *Am J Physiol* 1997;272:R2009–R2016.
121. Kopp UC, Matsushita K, Sigmund RD, Smith LA, Watanabe S, Stokes JB. Amiloride-sensitive Na+ channels in pelvic uroepithelium involved in renal sensory receptor activation. *Am J Physiol* 1998;275:R1780–R1792.
122. Kopp UC, Olson LA, DiBona GF. Renorenal reflex responses to mechano- and chemoreceptor stimulation in the dog and rat. *Am J Physiol* 1984;246:F67–F77.
123. Kopp UC, Smith LA. Effects of the substance P receptor antagonist CP-96,345 on renal sensory receptor activation. *Am J Physiol* 1993;264:R647–R653.
124. Kopp UC, Smith LA, DiBona GF. Impaired renorenal reflexes in spontaneously hypertensive rats. *Hypertension* 1987;9:69–75.
125. Kopp UC, Smith LA, DiBona GF. Renorenal reflexes: neural components of ipsilateral and contralateral renal responses. *Am J Physiol* 1985;249:F507–F517.
126. Kopp UC, Smith LA, Pence AL. Na(+)-K(+)-ATPase inhibition sensitizes renal mechanoreceptors activated by increases in renal pelvic pressure. *Am J Physiol* 1994;267:R1109–R1117.
127. Kostreva DR, Castaner A, Kampine JP. Reflex effects of hepatic baroreceptors on renal and cardiac sympathetic nerve activity. *Am J Physiol* 1980;238:R390–R394.
128. Kumagai H, Averill DB, Ferrario CM. Renal nerve activity in rats with spontaneous hypertension: effect of converting enzyme inhibitor. *Am J Physiol* 1992;263:R109–R115.
129. La Grange RG, Sloop CH, Schmid HE. Selective stimulation of renal nerves in the anesthetized dog. Effect on renin release during controlled changes in renal hemodynamics. *Circ Res* 1973;33:704–712.
130. Lacroix JS, Stjarne P, Anggard A, Lundberg JM. Sympathetic vascular control of the pig nasal mucosa. (I). Increased resistance and capacitance vessel responses upon stimulation with irregular bursts compared to continuous impulses. *Acta Physiol Scand* 1988;132:83–90.
131. Leonard BL, Evans RG, Navakatikyan MA, Malpas SC. Differential neural control of intrarenal blood flow. *Am J Physiol Regul Integr Comp Physiol* 2000;279:R907–R916.
132. Linden RJ, Mary DA, Weatherill D. The nature of the atrial receptors responsible for a reflex decrease in activity in renal nerves in the dog. *J Physiol* 1980;300:31–40.
133. Liu F, Gesek FA. alpha(1)-Adrenergic receptors activate NHE1 and NHE3 through distinct signaling pathways in epithelial cells. *Am J Physiol Renal Physiol* 2001;280:F415–F425.
134. Liu F, Nesbitt T, Drezner MK, Friedman PA, Gesek FA. Proximal nephron Na+/H+ exchange is regulated by alpha 1A– and alpha 1B–adrenergic receptor subtypes. *Mol Pharmacol* 1997;52:1010–1018.
135. Liu GL, Liu L, Barajas L. Development of NOS-containing neuronal somata in the rat kidney. *J Auton Nerv Syst* 1996;58:81–88.
136. Liu L, Barajas L. The rat renal nerves during development. *Anat Embryol (Berl)* 1993;188:345–361.
137. Luff SE, Hengstberger SG, McLachlan EM, Anderson WP. Two types of sympathetic axon innervating the juxtaglomerular arterioles of the rabbit and rat kidney differ structurally from those supplying other arteries. *J Neurocytol* 1991;20:781–795.
138. Lyson T, McMullan DM, Ermel LD, Morgan BJ, Victor RG. Mechanism of cyclosporine-induced sympathetic activation and acute hypertension in rats. *Hypertension* 1994;23:667–675.
139. Ma MC, Huang HS, Chen CF. Impaired renal sensory responses after unilateral ureteral obstruction in the rat. *J Am Soc Nephrol* 2002;13:1008–1016.
140. Ma MC, Huang HS, Chien CT, Wu MS, Chen CF. Temporal decrease in renal sensory responses in rats after chronic ligation of the bile duct. *Am J Physiol Renal Physiol* 2002;283:F164–F172.
141. Ma MC, Huang HS, Wu MS, Chien CT, Chen CF. Impaired renal sensory responses after renal ischemia in the rat. *J Am Soc Nephrol* 2002;13:1872–1883.
142. Maekawa H, Matsumura Y, Matsuo G, Morimoto S. Effect of sodium nitroprusside on norepinephrine overflow and antidiuresis induced by stimulation of renal nerves in anesthetized dogs. *J Cardiovasc Pharmacol* 1996;27:211–217.
143. Malpas SC, Evans RG. Do different levels and patterns of sympathetic activation all provoke renal vasoconstriction? *J Auton Nerv Syst* 1998;69:72–82.
144. Malpas SC, Hore TA, Navakatikyan M, Lukoshkova EV, Nguang SK, Austin PC. Resonance in the renal vasculature evoked by activation of the sympathetic nerves. *Am J Physiol* 1999;276:R1311–R1319.
145. Malpas SC, Leonard BL. Neural regulation of renal blood flow: a re-examination. *Clin Exp Pharmacol Physiol* 2000;27:956–964.
146. Manning DC, Snyder SH. Bradykinin receptors localized by quantitative autoradiography in kidney, ureter, and bladder. *Am J Physiol* 1989;256:F909–F915.
147. Mattson DL, Wu F. Nitric oxide synthase activity and isoforms in rat renal vasculature. *Hypertension* 2000;35:337–341.
148. McAllen RM, May CN. Differential drives from rostral ventrolateral medullary neurons to three identified sympathetic outflows. *Am J Physiol* 1994;267:R935–R944.
149. McDonough AA, Leong PK, Yang LE. Mechanisms of pressure natriuresis: how blood pressure regulates renal sodium transport. *Ann N Y Acad Sci* 2003;986:669–677.
150. McKinley MJ, Albiston AL, Allen AM, Mathai ML, May CN, McAllen RM, Oldfield BJ, Mendelsohn FA, Chai SY. The brain renin-angiotensin system: location and physiological roles. *Int J Biochem Cell Biol* 2003;35:901–918.
151. McKinley MJ, Pennington GL, Oldfield BJ. Anteroventral wall of the third ventricle and dorsal lamina terminalis: headquarters for control of body fluid homeostasis? *Clin Exp Pharmacol Physiol* 1996;23:271–281.
152. Miki K, Hayashida Y, Sagawa S, Shiraki K. Renal sympathetic nerve activity and natriuresis during water immersion in conscious dogs. *Am J Physiol* 1989;256:R299–R305.
153. Miki K, Hayashida Y, Shiraki K. Role of cardiac-renal neural reflex in regulating sodium excretion during water immersion in conscious dogs. *J Physiol* 2002;545:305–312.
154. Miki K, Yoshimoto M, Tanimizu M. Acute shifts of baroreflex control of renal sympathetic nerve activity induced by treadmill exercise in rats. *J Physiol* 2003;548:313–322.
155. Morita H, Nishida Y, Hosomi H. Neural control of urinary sodium excretion during hypertonic NaCl load in conscious rabbits: role of renal and hepatic nerves and baroreceptors. *J Auton Nerv Syst* 1991;34:157–169.
156. Nagura S, Sakagami T, Kakiichi A, Yoshimoto M, Miki K. Acute shifts in baroreflex control of renal sympathetic nerve activity induced by REM sleep and grooming in rats. *J Physiol* 2004;558:975–983.
157. Nakamura A, Johns EJ. Effect of renal nerves on expression of renin and angiotensinogen genes in rat kidneys. *Am J Physiol* 1994;266:E230–E241.
158. Nicol GD, Cui M. Enhancement by prostaglandin E2 of bradykinin activation of embryonic rat sensory neurones. *J Physiol* 1994;480:485–492.
159. Nicol GD, Klingberg DK, Vasko MR. Prostaglandin E2 increases calcium conductance and stimulates release of substance P in avian sensory neurons. *J Neurosci* 1992;12:1917–1927.
160. Nilsson H, Ljung B, Sjoblom N, Wallin BG. The influence of the sympathetic impulse pattern on contractile responses of rat mesenteric arteries and veins. *Acta Physiol Scand* 1985;123:303–309.
161. Nishiyama A, Seth DM, Navar LG. Angiotensin II type 1 receptor-mediated augmentation of renal interstitial fluid angiotensin II in angiotensin II–induced hypertension. *J Hypertens* 2003;21:1897–1903.
162. Nord EP, Howard MJ, Hafezi A, Moradeshagi P, Vaystub S, Insel PA. Alpha 2 adrenergic agonists stimulate Na+–H+ antiport activity in the rabbit renal proximal tubule. *J Clin Invest* 1987;80:1755–1762.
163. Ortiz PA, Garvin JL. Role of nitric oxide in the regulation of nephron transport. *Am J Physiol Renal Physiol* 2002;282:F777–F784.
164. Osborn JL, Camara AK. Renal neurogenic mediation of intracerebroventricular angiotensin II hypertension in rats raised on high sodium chloride diet. *Hypertension* 1997;30:331–336.
165. Osborn JL, DiBona GF, Thames MD. Beta-1 receptor mediation of renin secretion elicited by low-frequency renal nerve stimulation. *J Pharmacol Exp Ther* 1981;216:265–269.
166. Osborn JL, Thames MD, DiBona GF. Role of macula densa in renal nerve modulation of renin secretion. *Am J Physiol* 1982;242:R367–R371.
167. Ottoson D, Shepherd GM. Transducer characteristics of the muscle spindle as revealed by its receptor potential. *Acta Physiol Scand* 1971;82:545–554.
168. Pan L, Black TA, Shi Q, Jones CA, Petrovic N, Loudon J, Kane C, Sigmund CD, Gross KW. Critical roles of a cyclic AMP responsive element and an E-box in regulation of mouse renin gene expression. *J Biol Chem* 2001;276:45530–45538.
169. Pateromichelakis S, Rood JP. Prostaglandin E1-induced sensitization of A delta moderate pressure mechanoreceptors. *Brain Res* 1982;232:89–96.
170. Persson PB. Renin: origin, secretion and synthesis. *J Physiol* 2003;552:667–671.
171. Persson PB, Skalweit A, Thiele BJ. Controlling the release and production of renin. *Acta Physiol Scand* 2004;181:375–381.
172. Pettinger WA, Umemura S, Smyth DD, Jeffries WB. Renal alpha 2-adrenoceptors and the adenylate cyclase-cAMP system: biochemical and physiological interactions. *Am J Physiol* 1987;252:F199–F208.
173. Piascik MT, Perez DM. Alpha1-adrenergic receptors: new insights and directions. *J Pharmacol Exp Ther* 2001;298:403–410.
174. Quan A, Baum M. The renal nerve is required for regulation of proximal tubule transport by intraluminally produced ANG II. *Am J Physiol Renal Physiol* 2001;280:F524–F529.
175. Quan A, Baum M. Renal nerve stimulation augments effect of intraluminal angiotensin II on proximal tubule transport. *Am J Physiol Renal Physiol* 2002;282:F1043–F1048.
176. Rudenstam J, Bergstrom G, Taghipour K, Gothberg G, Karlstrom G. Efferent renal sympathetic nerve stimulation in vivo. Effects on regional renal haemodynamics in the Wistar rat, studied by laser-Doppler technique. *Acta Physiol Scand* 1995;154:387–394.
177. Sequeira Lopez ML, Pentz ES, Robert B, Abrahamson DR, Gomez RA. Embryonic origin and lineage of juxtaglomerular cells. *Am J Physiol Renal Physiol* 2001;281:F345–F356.

178. Sigmund CD, Jones CA, Fabian JR, Mullins JJ, Gross KW. Tissue and cell specific expression of a renin promoter-reporter gene construct in transgenic mice. *Biochem Biophys Res Commun* 1990;170:344–350.

179. Simon JK, Ciriello J. Contribution of afferent renal nerves to the metabolic activity of central structures involved in the control of the circulation. *Can J Physiol Pharmacol* 1989;67:1130–1139.

180. Sinn PL, Sigmund CD. Human renin mRNA stability is increased in response to cAMP in Calu-6 cells. *Hypertension* 1999;33:900–905.

181. Siragy HM, Howell NL, Ragsdale NV, Carey RM. Renal interstitial fluid angiotensin. Modulation by anesthesia, epinephrine, sodium depletion, and renin inhibition. *Hypertension* 1995;25:1021–1024.

182. Smith JA, Davis CL, Burgess GM. Prostaglandin E2-induced sensitization of bradykinin-evoked responses in rat dorsal root ganglion neurons is mediated by cAMP-dependent protein kinase A. *Eur J Neurosci* 2000;12:3250–3258.

183. Smith HW. *The Kidney: Structure and Function in Health and Disease*. New York: Oxford University Press; 1951.

184. Smits JF, Brody MJ. Activation of afferent renal nerves by intrarenal bradykinin in conscious rats. *Am J Physiol* 1984;247:R1003–R1008.

185. Stella A, Calaresu F, Zanchetti A. Neural factors contributing to renin release during reduction in renal perfusion pressure and blood flow in cats. *Clin Sci Mol Med* 1976;51:453–461.

186. Stella A, Zanchetti A. Functional role of renal afferents. *Physiol Rev* 1991;71:659–682.

187. Steranka LR, Manning DC, DeHaas CJ, Ferkany JW, Borosky SA, Connor JR, Vavrek RJ, Stewart JM, Snyder SH. Bradykinin as a pain mediator: receptors are localized to sensory neurons, and antagonists have analgesic actions. *Proc Natl Acad Sci U S A* 1988;85:3245–3249.

188. Summers RJ, Broxton N, Hutchinson DS, Evans BA. The Janus faces of adrenoceptors: factors controlling the coupling of adrenoceptors to multiple signal transduction pathways. *Clin Exp Pharmacol Physiol* 2004;31:822–827.

189. Szenasi G, Bencsath P, Takacs L. Proximal tubular transport and urinary excretion of sodium after renal denervation in sodium depleted rats. *Pflugers Arch* 1985;403:146–150.

190. Tanioka H, Nakamura K, Fujimura S, Yoshida M, Suzuki-Kusaba M, Hisa H, Satoh S. Facilitatory role of NO in neural norepinephrine release in the rat kidney. *Am J Physiol Regul Integr Comp Physiol* 2002;282:R1436–R1442.

191. Thames MD, Abboud FM. Interaction of somatic and cardiopulmonary receptors in control of renal circulation. *Am J Physiol* 1979;237:H560–H565.

192. Tobian L, MacNeill D, Johnson MA, Ganguli MC, Iwai J. Potassium protects against renal tubule lesions in NaCl-fed hypertensive Dahl S rats. *Trans Assoc Am Physicians* 1983;96:417–425.

193. Vasko MR, Campbell WB, Waite KJ. Prostaglandin E2 enhances bradykinin-stimulated release of neuropeptides from rat sensory neurons in culture. *J Neurosci* 1994;14:4987–4997.

194. Veelken R, Hilgers KF, Stetter A, Siebert HG, Schmieder RE, Mann JF. Nerve-mediated antidiuresis and antinatriuresis after air-jet stress is modulated by angiotensin II. *Hypertension* 1996;28:825–832.

195. Walkowska A, Badzynska B, Kompanowska-Jezierska E, Johns EJ, Sadowski J. Effects of renal nerve stimulation on intrarenal blood flow in rats with intact or inactivated NO synthases. *Acta Physiol Scand* 2005;183:99–105.

196. Wang DH, Li J, Qiu J. Salt-sensitive hypertension induced by sensory denervation: introduction of a new model. *Hypertension* 1998;32:649–653.

197. Wang J, Rose JC. Developmental changes in renal renin mRNA half-life and responses to stimulation in fetal lambs. *Am J Physiol* 1999;277:R1130–R1135.

198. Weaver LC, Genovesi S, Stella A, Zanchetti A. Neural, hemodynamic, and renal responses to stimulation of intestinal receptors. *Am J Physiol* 1987;253:H1167–H1176.

199. Weiss ML, Chowdhury SI. The renal afferent pathways in the rat: a pseudorabies virus study. *Brain Res* 1998;812:227–241.

200. Widmann C, Gibson S, Jarpe MB, Johnson GL. Mitogen-activated protein kinase: conservation of a three-kinase module from yeast to human. *Physiol Rev* 1999;79:143–180.

201. Williams NG, Zhong H, Minneman KP. Differential coupling of alpha1-, alpha2-, and beta-adrenergic receptors to mitogen-activated protein kinase pathways and differentiation in transfected PC12 cells. *J Biol Chem* 1998;273:24624–24632.

202. Wright JW, Harding JW. Important role for angiotensin III and IV in the brain renin-angiotensin system. *Brain Res Brain Res Rev* 1997;25:96–124.

203. Wu F, Park F, Cowley AW Jr, Mattson DL. Quantification of nitric oxide synthase activity in microdissected segments of the rat kidney. *Am J Physiol* 1999;276:F874–F881.

204. Wu XC, Harris PJ, Johns EJ. Nitric oxide and renal nerve-mediated proximal tubular reabsorption in normotensive and hypertensive rats. *Am J Physiol* 1999;277:F560–F566.

205. Wu XC, Johns EJ. Interactions between nitric oxide and superoxide on the neural regulation of proximal fluid reabsorption in hypertensive rats. *Exp Physiol* 2004;89:255–261.

206. Wu XC, Johns EJ. Nitric oxide modulation of neurally induced proximal tubular fluid reabsorption in the rat. *Hypertension* 2002;39:790–793.

207. Wurzner G, Chiolero A, Maillard M, Nussberger J, Hayoz D, Brunner HR, Burnier M. Renal and neurohormonal responses to increasing levels of lower body negative pressure in men. *Kidney Int* 2001;60:1469–1476.

208. Yang L, Leong PK, Chen JO, Patel N, Hamm-Alvarez SF, McDonough AA. Acute hypertension provokes internalization of proximal tubule NHE3 without inhibition of transport activity. *Am J Physiol Renal Physiol* 2002;282:F730–F740.

209. Ye S, Zhong H, Yanamadala V, Campese VM. Renal injury caused by intrarenal injection of phenol increases afferent and efferent renal sympathetic nerve activity. *Am J Hypertens* 2002;15:717–724.

210. Yoshimoto M, Sakagami T, Nagura S, Miki K. Relationship between renal sympathetic nerve activity and renal blood flow during natural behavior in rats. *Am J Physiol Regul Integr Comp Physiol* 2004;286:R881–R887.

211. Zambraski EJ, Dibona GF, Kaloyanides GJ. Effect of sympathetic blocking agents on the antinatriuresis of reflex renal nerve stimulation. *J Pharmacol Exp Ther* 1976;198:464–472.

212. Zhang T, Huang C, Johns EJ. Neural regulation of kidney function by the somatosensory system in normotensive and hypertensive rats. *Am J Physiol* 1997;273:R1749–R1757.

213. Zhang T, Johns EJ. Somatosensory influences on renal sympathetic nerve activity in anesthetized Wistar and hypertensive rats. *Am J Physiol* 1997;272:R982–R990.

214. Zhang W, Li JL, Hosaka M, Janz R, Shelton JM, Albright GM, Richardson JA, Sudhof TC, Victor RG. Cyclosporine A-induced hypertension involves synapsin in renal sensory nerve endings. *Proc Natl Acad Sci U S A* 2000;97:9765–9770.

CHAPTER 34

Natriuretic Hormones

David L. Vesely
University of South Florida Cardiac Hormone Center, and James A. Haley Veterans Medical Center, Tampa, Florida, USA

INTRODUCTION

Natriuretic peptide hormones are very important for the maintenance of extracellular fluid volume within a narrow range despite wide variations in dietary sodium intake. This regulation occurs through a complex interplay of the antinatriuretic renin-angiotensin-aldosterone system and the antinatriuretic renal sympathetic system, which help to conserve sodium when sodium intake is low, and the natriuretic hormones, which enhance sodium excretion whenever sodium excess occurs. Several of the natriuretic hormones directly inhibit aldosterone secretion (14, 43, 111, 177, 195, 309, 322) and/or indirectly inhibit aldosterone secretion by inhibiting renin release from the kidney to help regulate extracellular fluid volume (39, 92, 134, 179, 195, 349). This chapter will concentrate on the natriuretic hormones in normal renal physiology, their synthesis, secretion, biologic effects, pathophysiological changes with hypertension and renal diseases, and potential for treating diseases such as acute renal failure.

HISTORY OF ATRIAL NATRIURETIC PEPTIDE HORMONES

In 1628, Harvey (132) first correctly described the heart as a pump, or a muscular organ that contracts in rhythm, pushing blood first to the lungs for oxygenation and then through the peripheral vascular system bringing oxygen and nutrients to every cell in the body. It was another 350 years before the heart was established as an endocrine gland with its main physiologic targets being the kidney and vasculature (313). The history of experimentation leading to defining the natriuretic peptide hormonal system has followed two pathways: physiological and anatomical.

History: Physiological Studies

ASSOCIATION OF HEART AND RENAL FUNCTION

In 1847, Harthshorne suggested that the heart possessed volume receptors capable of sensing the "fullness of bloodstream" induced by whole-body immersion, which he clearly recognized had a diuretic effect (131). This observation received little further notice until 1935, when John Peters of Yale University made the same proposal that "the fullness of the bloodstream may provoke the diuretic response on the part of the kidney" (237). This concept then received experimental verification when it was shown that expansion of blood volume increases urine flow (29, 105, 383). Peters also suggested that the diuretic response was secondary to the ability of the heart or something very near the heart to "sense the fullness of the bloodstream" (237).

BALLOON DISTENTION OF ATRIA

Experimental evidence of an association between cardiac atria and renal function was provided in 1956 by Henry et al. (135), who observed that balloon distention of the left atrium in anesthetized dogs was associated with an increase in urine flow. Because the renal response to left atrial distention could not be elicited after the cervical vagi had been cooled to block nerve conduction, Henry and colleagues (135, 136) concluded that stretch receptors in the left atrium must be present. This finding was later extended to the right atrium (104). In their reports, Henry et al. (135, 136) noted the diuresis but did not investigate whether it was associated with increased salt excretion (natriuresis). It is well established now, however, that balloon distention of the cardiac atrial causes natriuresis as well as diuresis (108, 110, 194). Evidence that animals with denervated hearts or denervated kidneys may also respond to an atrial pressure increase to produce diuresis (191) suggests a hormonal pathway between the heart and the kidney. Part of this hormonal pathway seems to involve atrial natriuretic peptides.

THE "THIRD FACTOR"

With respect to a possible hormonal agent causing natriuresis and diuresis, de Wardener and colleagues (68) demonstrated in 1961 that saline infusion produced an increase in urine flow and sodium excretion in anesthetized dogs independent of changes in glomerular filtration rate (GFR), which was decreased, and even in the presence of high circulating levels of aldosterone. These experiments gave rise to the popular concept that an unidentified "third factor," a term coined by Levinsky and Lalone (188); the other two factors were aldosterone and GFR-affected sodium excretion. The search for this third factor soon focused on a possible hormonal mediator that came to be known as "natriuretic hormone." Although this mediator (or mediators) from plasma or urine of volume-expanded humans or animals that causes natriuresis when injected into animals (37) was never chemically identified, the evidence points toward this third factor having a peptide structure(s) because acid hydrolysis characteristically inactivated this substance (134). The "third factor" that was searched for decades now appears to be a family of peptide hormones termed "atrial natriuretic peptides" (ANPs) since they are found in their highest concentrations in the atria of the heart and have natriuretic properties and are peptides. The third factor(s) also has a property the ability to inhibit Na^+,K^+-ATPase in the kidney (134). Some of the natriuretic peptide hormones synthesized in the heart fill all of the criteria of being the "third factor(s)." Atrial natriuretic peptide (ANP) does not inhibit Na^+,K^+-ATPase (48, 124, 245), so it would not fulfill the criteria of being the "third factor." Three of the other peptide hormones synthesized by the ANP prohormone gene (Fig. 1) namely long-acting natriuretic peptide, vessel dilator, and kaliuretic peptide, however, do inhibit renal Na^+,K^+-ATPase (48, 124) and fill all of the criteria of being the "third factor(s)" that researchers have sought since the 1960s.

History of ANPs: Anatomical Studies

ATRIAL GRANULE STRUCTURE

Shortly before Henry and colleagues (135) reported their observation that balloon distention of atria caused a diuresis, in 1955 Kisch (170), utilizing electron microscopy, described dense granules that were located in the atria but not in the ventricles of mammals. The presence of these dense granules in the cytoplasm of atrial cardiac myocytes but not in the ventricles of the heart was rapidly confirmed by others utilizing electron microscopy (28, 243). Jamieson and Palade (149) demonstrated that such granules are present in cardiocytes of the atria of all mammals, including humans, and were the first, in 1964, to suggest that these granules resemble other granules that release polypeptide hormones (149). These granules are usually adjacent to one or occasionally both poles of the nucleus and are interspersed among the voluminous elements of Golgi complex and within close proximity to the mitochondria (149).

Ultrastructural cytochemistry has shown these granules consist of proteins (141). They incorporate both [^{3}H]-leucine and [^{3}H]-fructose in a pattern identical to other endocrine-secreting cells with protein synthesis occurring in the Golgi complex (140). The ultrastructural features of the specific granules of different species are similar in that they display an amorphous core and a limiting membrane, and generally measure 300–500 nm (65, 149). The size and number of these granules vary among species and generally are inversely related to size. Thus, atrial myocytes from large animals such as cows contain fewer and smaller granules than myocytes from small rodents such as rats (65). In the rat there are up to 600 spherical, electron-opaque granules per cell (65, 149).

EFFECT OF SALT INTAKE ON HEART ATRIAL GRANULES

In 1958, Poche (244) demonstrated that the number of granules present was influenced by changes in food and water intake. The next investigation of the effect of salt and water metabolism on the number of atrial granules occurred only after an 18-year hiatus. Marie et al. (199) demonstrated that the number of granules in the atrial cardiocytes increased when the amount of sodium in an animal's diet was reduced. deBold (63) then performed the corollary experiment of documenting that decreased granularity resulted from sodium loading. Thus, atrial granularity varies inversely with the amount of serum sodium present, which has the implication that the granules must store some substance that is interrelated with sodium balance. These stud-

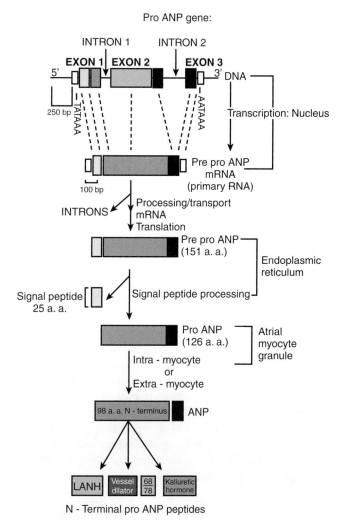

FIGURE 1   Structure of the atrial natriuretic peptide prohormone (proANP) gene. Four peptide hormones (e.g., atrial natriuretic peptide [ANP], long-acting natriuretic peptide [LANP], vessel dilator, and kaliuretic peptide) are synthesized by this gene. Each of these peptide hormones have biological effects, such as natriuresis and diuresis, mediated via the kidney (24, 72, 73, 124, 126, 201, 329, 350, 376). a.a., amino acids; LANH, long-acting natriuretic hormone (a different nomenclature for LANP). (With permission, from Vesely DL. *Atrial Natriuretic Hormones.* Englewood Cliffs, NJ: Prentice Hall; 1992.)

ies led deBold et al. (64) to perform the classic endocrine experiment of infusing cardiac atrial extracts of one group of rats into other rats and monitoring the effect of these extracts on renal function.

ATRIAL EXTRACTS AND NATRIURESIS

In 1922, Banting and Best (20) utilized what is now considered a classic endocrinological technique in their discovery of insulin. They pulverized pancreas with buffer, filtered the crude tissue extract, and found that it produced hypoglycemia in an experimental dog (20). In 1981, deBold and colleagues (64), utilizing a similar approach, infused the supernatants of extracts of rat cardiac atria and rat ventricles into other rats and found that the rat atria extracts, but not the extracts from the rat ventricles, caused dramatic diuresis and natriuresis, with urine flow increasing 10-fold and sodium and chloride excretion increasing 30-fold. This simple but elegant experiment led to the discovery of atrial peptides that have the most potent endogenous natriuretic activity of any substance yet described (305). Atrial natriuretic peptide isolated from these atrial extracts has been found to be a twofold stronger natriuretic producing agent than furosemide (Lasix®), which is one of the most potent natriuretic producing drugs utilized in clinical medicine today (305). Other investigators quickly confirmed this natriuretic action (97), as well as the ability of atrial extracts to cause vasodilation (59, 363). It was rapidly demonstrated that these effects were at least partially due to a peptide(s) that is present in all mammalian atria (64, 305). Further investigation revealed that the atrial extracts have significantly more natriuresis and diuresis than pure synthetic ANP suggesting that other peptide hormones with natriuretic properties were in these atrial extracts (70, 110, 125).

FAMILY OF NATRIURETIC PEPTIDE HORMONES

At first it was thought that a single peptide was found in atrial extracts, but further investigation revealed a sophisticated endocrine system in the atria (and other tissues including the kidney) in which the atrial natriuretic peptide prohormone gene synthesized four peptide hormones (Fig. 1) (23, 315–317) and that two other genes were present as reviewed below. The three other peptide hormones synthesized by the ANP prohormone gene—long-acting natriuretic peptide, vessel dilator, and kaliuretic peptide—were first demonstrated to have biologic effects in 1987 (335), and one of their mechanisms of action, via intracellular messenger cyclic GMP, was also elucidated in 1987 (320). Fifth and sixth members of the natriuretic peptide family were identified in 1988: brain natriuretic peptide (BNP) isolated from a porcine brain cDNA library (295), and urodilatin, a peptide found in urine (187, 216, 282). A seventh member of this family was identified in 1990 in brain tissue and termed C-type natriuretic peptide (CNP) (296). A possible eighth member, DNP, was first described in 1992 (283).

FAMILY OF ATRIAL NATRIURETIC HORMONES: SYNTHESIS OF THREE PROHORMONES

This family of peptide hormones has been designated atrial natriuretic peptides (ANPs), also known as atrial natriuretic hormones (ANHs). These peptide hormones are synthesized by three different genes (85, 103, 187, 197, 216, 262, 369) and then stored as three different prohormones (126–amino acid [a.a.] ANP, 108-a.a. BNP, and 103-a.a. CNP prohormones) (187, 313). In healthy adults, the main site of ANP prohormone synthesis is the atrial myocyte with its mRNA being 30–50-fold higher than that observed in the ventricle (101) but it is also synthesized in a variety of other tissues including the kidney as well (101, 339). The sites of synthesis of the ANPs in approximate order that they contribute to the synthesis of ANPs are listed in Table 1.

PEPTIDE HORMONES ORIGINATING FROM ATRIAL NATRIURETIC PEPTIDE PROHORMONE

Within the 126-a.a. ANP prohormone encoded by a single gene are four peptide hormones (Fig. 1) with blood-pressure lowering, natriuretic, diuretic, and/or kaliuretic (i.e., potassium excreting) properties in both animals (24, 72, 73, 125, 126, 201, 335, 350, 375, 376) and humans (326–329). These peptide hormones, numbered by their a.a. sequences beginning at the N-terminal end of the ANP prohormone consist of the first 30 a.a. of the prohormone (proANP 1–30, long-acting natriuretic peptide [LANP]), a.a. 31–67 (proANP 31–67, vessel dilator); a.a. 79–98 (proANP 79–98, kaliuretic peptide), and a.a. 99–126 (ANP) (Fig. 1). These peptide hormones which were discovered before BNP and CNP were named for their most prominent biologic effects rather than the tissue they were first found because these peptides are synthesized in many tissues (101, 316, 339). Brain natriuretic peptide so named because it was first found in porcine brain cDNA, for example, is actually present in the heart in 10-fold higher concentrations than in the brain (49, 125, 193, 300). Each of the four peptide hormones from the ANP prohormone circulate in healthy humans, with LANP and vessel dilator concentrations in plasma being 15–20-fold higher than ANP and 100-fold higher than BNP (18, 67, 90, 91, 145, 337, 364, 365).

BNP and CNP Prohormones

The BNP and CNP genes, on the other hand, appear to synthesize only one peptide hormone each within their respective prohormones, that is, BNP and CNP (22, 85, 103, 181, 182, 371). The pro BNP gene and its regulation are reviewed in the section on BNP prohormone gene. The biologic effects of BNP and CNP are reviewed in sections on BNP Biologic Effects and CNP: Circulating Concentrations and Biologic Effects.

TABLE 1   Site of Synthesis, Molecular Weight, and Hemodynamic and Natriuretic Properties of Natriuretic Peptides

	Molecular Weight (kD)	Site of Synthesis	MAP	Diuresis	Natriuresis
LANP	3508	Atria, ventricle, GI, lung, kidney, brain, adrenal	↓	↑	↑
Vessel dilator	3878	Atria, ventricle, GI, lung, kidney, brain, adrenal	↓	↑	↑
Kaliuretic peptide	2184	Atria, ventricle, GI, lung, brain, adrenal	↓	↑	—[a]
ANP	3078	Atria, ventricle, GI, lung, kidney, brain, adrenal	↓	↑	↑
Urodilatin	3503	Kidney	↓	↑	↑
BNP	3462	Atria, ventricle, brain, adrenal	↓	↑	↑
CNP	2198	Endothelium, CNS	↓	↑	—
DNP	4191	Atria, ventricle	↓	↑	↑
Adrenomedullin	6029	Adrenal, kidney	↓	↑	↑

Note: The sites of synthesis are listed in approximate order in which they contribute to synthesis.

[a]No significant effect.

ANP, atrial natriuretic peptide; BNP, brain natriuretic peptide; CNP, C-type natriuretic peptide; CNS, central nervous system; DNP, *Dendroaspis* natriuretic peptide; GI, gastrointestinal tract; LANP, long-acting natriuretic peptide; MAP, mean arterial pressure. (With permission, from Vesely DL. Atrial natriuretic peptides in pathophysiological diseases. *Cardiovasc Res* 2001;51: 647–658.)

ORIGINATION OF PEPTIDE HORMONES FROM PROHORMONES

More than one peptide hormone originating from the same prohormone is common with respect to the synthesis of hormones (313). Adrenocorticotropin (ACTH), for example, is derived from a prohormone that contains four known peptide hormones (313). α-MSH, which has natriuretic properties (142, 143), originates from this same prohormone. ACTH, similar to vessel dilator, originates from the middle of its prohormone. The middle of their respective prohormones is the most common origin of hormones with calcitonin, glucagon, vasoactive intestinal peptide, gastrin, cholecystokinin, and substance P as well as ACTH and vessel dilator all originating from the middle of their respective prohormones (313). Several hormones such as vasopressin (antidiuretic hormone [ADH]), oxytocin, pancreatic polypeptide, angiotensin, and gastrin-releasing peptide originate from the N-terminus of their respective prohormones (313) as does long-acting natriuretic peptide (proANF 1–30). The origin of hormones from the C-terminus of their respective prohormones like ANP, BNP, and CNP is less common with somatostatin, inhibin, and parathyroid hormone (PTH) being the only known C-terminal prohormone-derived peptides (313). In the case of PTH, 84 of the 90 a.a. in its prohormone are considered to be the C-terminal "active" hormone; thus, it is not a small C-terminal–derived prohormone peptide, but rather nearly the intact prohormone that serves as the actual peptide hormone.

MOLECULAR BIOLOGY OF NATRIURETIC HORMONAL SYSTEM

ProANP Gene

The gene encoding the synthesis of atrial natriuretic peptide prohormone (proANP) consists of three exon (coding) sequences separated by two intron (intervening) sequences which encode for a mature mRNA transcript approximately 900 bases long (Fig. 1) (121, 155, 156, 220, 227, 286). Translation of human ANP prohormone mRNA results in a 151-a.a. preprohormone (121, 220, 227, 286). Exon 1 encodes the 5′-untranslated region, the hydrophobic signal peptide (leader segment), and the first 16 a.a. of the ANP prohormone (first 16 a.a. of long-acting natriuretic peptide) (119, 121, 220, 227, 286). The signal peptide, which is probably important for the translocation of the precursor peptide from the ribosome into the rough endoplasmic reticulum (220), is cleaved from the preprohormone (151 a.a.) in the endoplasmic reticulum (Fig. 1). The resulting 126-a.a. prohormone is the storage form for the four atrial natriuretic peptide hormones in tissues and the major constituent of the atrial granules (27, 121, 220, 227). The first 16 a.a. of this prohormone encoded by exon 1 are, after proteolytic processing of the ANP prohormone, also the first 16 a.a. of long-acting natriuretic peptide (LANP) (Fig. 1). Exon 3 encodes for the terminal tyrosine (a.a. 126 of the ANP prohormone) in humans, and terminal three a.a. (Try-Arg-Arg) in rat, rabbit, cow, and mouse (119, 121, 220, 227, 286). Deletion of this terminal tyrosine residue encoded by exon 3 does slightly affect the binding of ANP, but does not appear to contribute to biologic activity as there is no apparent decrease in biologic activity when this terminal tyrosine is not present (313). Exon 2 encodes for the rest of the prohormone (a.a. 17–125 in humans) (121, 220, 227, 286).

There is considerable homology in the proANP gene among species, particularly in the encoding and 5′ flanking sequences (227, 351). The homology decreases in the introns of the proANP gene (227). The sequences encoding the atrial natriuretic peptide prohormone are more highly conserved between the human and rodent gene than the intervening sequences or the 5′ and 3′ untranslated sequences (227, 351). Comparison of human, rat, and mouse genomic sequences and dog and rabbit cDNAs demonstrates maximum homology in the regions encoding proANP (93 of the 126 a.a. residues are identical in all five species), whereas in the hydrophobic leader sequence only 5 of the 26 residues are identical (85, 227). The proANP gene has many features common to all eukaryotic genes (33), including a TATTA box (T = thymine, A = adenine), intervening sequences bounded by GT-AG splicing signals (G = guanine), and a consensus sequence found in promoted regions. Also, AATAA polyadenylation addition signals at the three transcription start sites for human (218, 227) and rat (382) proANP mRNAs are located at ~30 base pairs 3′ to the respective TATAA boxes—that is, about 95 base pairs before the initiation codon. The overall size of the proANP transcripts is 950–1050 nucleotides (27, 101, 102). There is a "cap" sequence at the 5′ end of proANP mRNA and a terminal codon (human mRNA only), as in the case of specific mRNA from most eukaryotic cells (250). An interesting feature of the human proANP gene is a consensus sequence for a putative glucocorticoid hormone regulatory element in the second intron (102, 235, 286).

Atrial Natriuretic Peptide: Comparison of Amino Acid Sequences among Species

The amino acid sequence of the whole ANP prohormone synthesized by the above gene is strikingly homologous among many species with differences clustered at the extreme carboxy terminal end of the prohormone as determined from the work of a number of investigators (15, 107, 133, 157, 159, 166, 184, 197, 218, 220, 227, 228, 351, 382). The 28 a.a. in the carboxy terminal end of the ANP prohormone (i.e., ANP) has 93% homology in the following five species: humans, rats, mice, rabbits, and dogs (119, 155, 156). In each species, the C-terminus is distinguished from the rest of the prohormone by forming a 17-a.a. ring structure via the joining by a disulfide bond between two cysteine residues (105 and 121 of the prohormone), as schematically shown in Fig. 2. The ring structure originally was believed to be absolutely necessary for biologic activity (60, 137), but linear forms (same amino acids in linear form) without a ring structure have since been shown also to have biologic activity (30). For full natriuretic and vasorelaxant activity, the Phe-Arg-Tyr (a.a. 124–126) at the COOH terminus (60) and a.a. 99–104 of the

NH$_2$ terminus of ANP are necessary (34). In the dog, it appears that deletion of a.a. 99–102 of prohormone does not affect natriuresis, but deletion of a.a. 103 and 104 (in the ANP N-terminus) decreases natriuretic activity 10-fold (34). The 28-a.a. C-terminal end of the prohormone (ANP) is preceded by the well-conserved dipeptide proline-arginine. Although the presence of Pro-Arg is not a common a cleavage site in prohormones as are a pair of basic amino acids such as Arg-Arg or Lys-Arg, this signal is seen in the processing of gastrin-releasing peptide (262, 313). A single arginine, as found at a.a. 98 of the prohormone, appears to be the proteolytic processing signal in other peptide prohormones also (106, 313).

Except for the addition of the C-terminal Arg-Arg in rodents during synthesis, there is only a single amino acid difference in the mammalian forms of ANP (a.a. 99–126 of prohormone), which is at position 110 of the 126-a.a. prohormone. In rodents (rats, mice, and rabbits), this amino acid is isoleucine, whereas in higher mammals (humans, dogs, pigs, and cows) the amino acid at this position is methionine (15, 85, 86, 106, 158, 227, 286, 351).

LANP: Comparison of Amino Acid Sequences among Species

Twenty of 30 a.a. in long-acting natriuretic peptide (Fig. 2) are exactly the same in the five species, and another six of the remaining 10 amino acids are exactly the same in four out of the five species (15, 85, 86, 106, 286). Of the remaining four amino acids, two are exactly the same in three out of the five species. Thus, only two amino acids (5 and 28 of the prohormone) are not the same in the majority of the species, and these two positions have the same amino acids in at least two of the five species. The LANP amino-acid sequence is thus markedly similar in all five species (15, 85, 86, 106, 286).

Vessel Dilator: Comparison of Amino Acid Sequences among Species

In the same five species, 25 of 37 amino acids in the vessel dilator (Fig. 2) are identical (106, 158, 227, 286, 351). Six of the remaining 12 a.a. are the same in four of the five species, and three of the remaining six a.a. are the same in three out of the five species. Thus, only three a.a. (33, 42, and 43 of the prohormone) are not the same in the majority of the species. The amino acids in these three positions are the same for at least two pair of species (only one out of five does not have an amino acid in this position that is not the same as one of the other species).

Kaliuretic Peptide: Comparison of Amino Acid Sequences among Species

Kaliuretic peptide has highly conserved sequence among the aforementioned five species with 16 of its 20 a.a. (Fig. 2) being the same in all five (15, 85, 86, 106, 158, 286). One of the

Natriuretic Peptides

LANP	Asn-Pro-Met-Tyr-Asn-Ala-Val-Ser-Asn-Ala-Asp-Leu-Met-Asp-Phe-Lys-Asn-Leu-Leu-Asp-His-Leu-Glu-Glu-Lys-Met-Pro-Leu-Glu-Asp
Vessel dilator	Glu-Val-Val-Pro-Pro-Gln-Val-Leu-Ser-Glu-Pro-Asn-Glu-Glu-Ala-Gly-Ala-Ala-Leu-Ser-Pro-Leu-Pro-Glu-Val-Pro-Pro-Trp-Thr-Gly-Glu-Val-Ser-Pro-Ala-Gln-Arg
Kaliuretic peptide	Ser-Ser-Asp-Arg-Ser-Ala-Leu-Leu-Lys-Ser-Lys-Leu-Arg-Ala-Leu-Leu-Thr-Ala-Pro-Arg
ANP	Ser-Leu-Arg-Arg-Ser-Ser-Cys-Phe-Gly-Gly-Arg-Met-Asp-Arg-Ile-Gly-Ala-Gln-Ser-Gly-Leu-Gly-Cys-Asn-Ser-Phe-Arg-Tyr
Urodilatin	Thr-Ala-Pro-Arg-Ser-Leu-Arg-Arg-Ser-Ser-Cys-Phe-Gly-Gly-Arg-Met-Asp-Arg-Ile-Gly-Ala-Gln-Ser-Gly-Leu-Gly-Cys-Asn-Ser-Phe-Arg-Tyr
BNP	Ser-Pro-Lys-Met-Val-Gln-Gly-Ser-Gly-Cys-Phe-Gly-Arg-Lys-Met-Asp-Arg-Ile-Ser-Ser-Ser-Ser-Gly-Leu-Gly-Cys-Lys-Val-Leu-Arg-Arg-His
CNP	Gly-Leu-Ser-Lys-Gly-Cys-Phe-Gly-Leu-Lys-Leu-Asp-Arg-Ile-Gly-Ser-Met-Ser-Gly-Leu-Gly-Cys
DNP	Glu-Val-Lys-Tyr-Asp-Pro-Cys-Phe-Gly-His-Lys-Ile-Asp-Arg-Ile-Asn-His-Val-Ser-Asn-Leu-Gly-Cys-Pro-Ser-Leu-Arg-Asp-Pro-Arg-Pro-Asn-Ala-Pro-Ser-Thr-Ser-Ala
Adrenomedullin	Tyr-Arg-Gln-Ser-Met-Asn-Asn-Phe-Gln-Gly-Leu-Arg-Ser-Phe-Gly-Cys-Arg-Phe-Gly-Thr-Cys-Thr-Val-Gln-Lys-Leu-Ala-His-Gln-Ile-Tyr-Gln-Phe-Thr-Asp-Lys-Asp-Lys-Asp-Asn-Val-Ala-Pro-Arg-Ser-Lys-Ile-Ser-Pro-Gln-Gly-Tyr

FIGURE 2 Amino acid sequences of the natriuretic peptides. Each of the sequences are human sequences except for *Dendroaspis* natriuretic peptide (DNP), whose sequence is only known in the snake. The brackets illustrate the location of cysteine bridges that help to form a ring structure in a number of these peptides. BNP, brain natriuretic peptide; CNP, C-type natriuretic peptide. (With permission, from Vesely DL. Natriuretic peptides and acute renal failure. *Am J Physiol* 2003;285: F167–F177.)

remaining four a.a. is the same in four species, whereas two of the other three a.a. are the same in three of the five species. Thus, only one position in this peptide has an amino acid that is not the same in the majority of the five species. This position (79 of the ANP prohormone) at the N-terminal end of this peptide has the same amino acid in dog and humans (serine), whereas rat and mouse have proline in this position. The amino acid in position 79 of the prohormone is alanine in the rabbit. With only one amino acid not the same in kaliuretic peptide in the majority of the five species tested, this peptide is also remarkably conserved among the species.

This extraordinary conservation among species of LANP, vessel dilator, kaliuretic peptide is not observed in the BNP prohormone where there is a marked difference in amino acid sequence homology among species with respect to species amino acid homology (85, 100, 181, 262, 295).

Tissue-Specific Expression of ProANP Gene

ProANP mRNA transcripts in the atrial myocyte are polyadenylated and are approximately 1050 to 1150 nucleotides long (101). In healthy adult animals and humans, the atrial myocyte is the main site of the ANP prohormone synthesis but it is also synthesized in a variety of other tissues as well (101, 115, 116, 246, 247). ProANP gene expression is 30–50 times higher in the atria of the heart than in extra atrial tissues (101). The expression of

this gene has been found in kidney, gastrointestinal tract (antrum of stomach, small and large intestine), lung, aorta, central nervous system, anterior pituitary and hypothalamus (101, 115, 116, 246, 247). The transcription start site (the 5′ terminus), determined by S1 nuclease and primer extension analysis (101), maps approximately 20 to 25 base pairs downstream from a genomic TATAAAA sequence. This 5′ terminus is thought to dictate the site of transcript initiation by RNA polymerase II (25). A second minor start site is located approximately 80 base pairs farther upstream. This start site lies ~30 base pairs downstream from an AT-rich region that may subserve a primitive promoter function in initiating the latter transcript. Several intermediate transcripts with 5′ terminus between these two start sites also have been identified (101), but it is still unclear if they represent partially processed transcripts from the upstream promoter or transcripts initiated from other occult promoter structures in the vicinity. An example of where the proANP gene synthesized peptides localize in the kidney is illustrated in Fig. 3.

The 3′ terminus of the proANP transcript in polyadenylated RNA from cardiac atria also has been mapped by S_1 nuclease analysis. Two tandemly arranged termini were identified, each of which is positioned ~10 base pairs downstream from an AATAAA sequence, a hexamer that has been shown to function as a cleavage-polyadenylation signal in other systems (249). The two poly(A)$^+$ addition sites

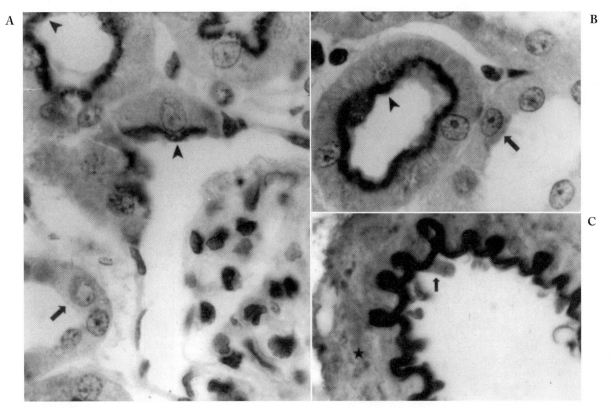

FIGURE 3 Vessel dilator immunoperoxidase staining in the rat kidney reveals strong staining of the sub-brush border of proximal convoluted tubules (*arrowheads* in **A** and **B**), including a proximal tubule in (**A**) originating directly from the top left portion of the glomerulus. The interstitial artery (**C**) had strong proANF (31–67) staining of the elastica with moderate staining of endothelial cells (*arrow*) and media (*). The distal tubules and collecting ducts (*arrows* in **A** and **B**) had weak staining with no demonstrable staining in some of the collecting ducts cells. Magnification x940. (With permission, from Ramirez G, Saba SR, Dietz JR, Vesely DL. Immunocytochemical localization of proANF1-30, proANF 31-67, and atrial natriuretic factor in the kidney. *Kidney Int* 1992;41:334–341.)

appear to be employed with equivalent efficiency both in atrial and extra-atrial proANP transcripts.

Mechanisms of Action of Gene Products of ProANP Gene

Part of the intracellular mechanism of action(s) of the four peptide hormones encoded by the proANP gene is that after they bind to their specific receptors they enhance membrane bound guanylate cyclase to cause an increase in the intracellular messenger cyclic GMP (Fig. 4) (47, 354). Cyclic GMP then stimulates a cyclic GMP-dependent, protein kinase that phosphorylates protein(s) in the cell producing physiologic effects (Fig. 4). The receptors for ANP that mediate ANP biologic effects (e.g., ANP-A and -B receptors) are interesting in that they contain guanylate cyclase and a protein kinase in the receptors themselves (Fig. 5) (77, 176, 316). The NPR-A receptor has a 441-a.a. extracellular portion that binds ANP, which, in turn, activates the catalytic portion of guanylate cyclase in the cell (Fig. 5). The protein kinase in this receptor has an inhibitory influence on guanylate cyclase until this receptor is activated by ANP or BNP (77, 316). There is a 21-a.a. portion of this receptor which attaches this receptor to the membrane (Fig. 5).

PROCESSING OF ATRIAL NATRIURETIC PEPTIDE PROHORMONE IN KIDNEY

ANP prohormone processing is different in the kidney compared to other tissues resulting in an additional four a.a. added to the N-terminus of ANP (proANP 95-126, urodilatin [Fig. 2]), a peptide first identified in urine (282). Thus, in the kidney, the identical four a.a. from the C-terminus of kaliuretic peptide are added to ANP to form the peptide urodilatin (Fig. 2). At first, urodilatin was thought not to circulate (209, 282) and that it was not a hormone. To be defined as a hormone, a given protein has to be synthesized in a tissue or organ, circulate in the bloodstream, and have biologic effects in another tissue or organ (313). With a very sensitive radioimmunoassay, it appears that urodilatin does circulate but in such low concentrations (9–12 pg/ml) that it may not be physiologically relevant (338). Since urodilatin constitutes less than 1% of the circulating natriuretic hormones, it physiologic importance as a circulating hormone is very limited with over 99% of the physiologic natriuretic effects being from the other natriuretic hormones. Urodilatin, however, may have paracrine functions, and may mediate the effects of one of the other natriuretic hormones (ANP) (338). Infusion of ANP increases the circulating concentration of urodilatin

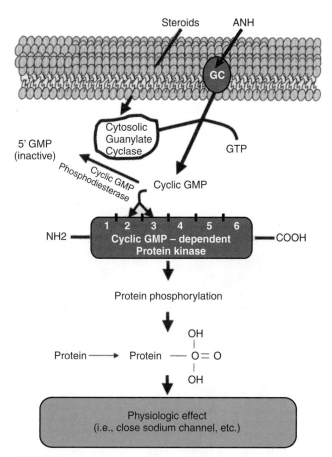

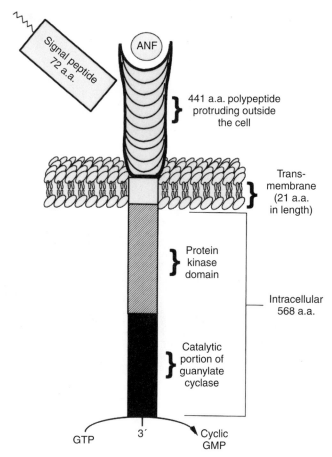

FIGURE 4 Atrial natriuretic hormone (ANH) stimulates a membrane-bound guanylate cyclase. Steroid hormones, on the other hand, diffuse through the cell to enhance the activity of a cytosolic guanylate cyclase. When either membrane-bound or soluble guanylate cyclase is activated, the intracellular messenger, cyclic 3'5' guanosine monophosphate (cyclic GMP) is generated from guanosine triphosphate (GTP). Cyclic GMP then stimulates cyclic GMP-dependent protein kinase, which, in turn, phosphorylates proteins within the cell producing a biologic effect. Cyclic GMP is metabolized to an inactive 5'-GMP within the cell by cyclic GMP phosphodiesterase. (With permission, from Vesely DL. *Atrial Natriuretic Hormones.* Englewood Cliffs, NJ: Prentice Hall; 1992.)

FIGURE 5 Structure of atrial natriuretic peptide (ANP or NPR)-A (active) receptor. The 441 amino-acid (a.a.) extracellular portion of the receptor binds ANP, which activates the catalytic protein of guanylate cyclase within the cell. The protein kinase within this receptor has an inhibitory influence on guanylate cyclase until the receptor is activated by ANP. (With permission, from Vesely DL. *Atrial Natriuretic Hormones.* Englewood Cliffs, NJ: Prentice Hall; 1992.)

suggesting that some ANP effects may be mediated by urodilatin (338). Infusion of long-acting natriuretic peptide, vessel dilator, and kaliuretic peptide, on the other hand, do not affect the circulating concentration of urodilatin in healthy humans (338).

REGULATION OF ATRIAL NATRIURETIC PEPTIDE PROHORMONE GENE

Enhancement of ProANP Gene Expression

STRETCH

Mechanical stretch, or more specifically tension delivered across the atrial wall is a potent activator of proANP gene expression and/or secretion (69, 71, 353). In animals, an increase of sodium intake results in an increase release of the ANP prohormone peptides (73, 75, 348).

THYROID HORMONES

Thyroid hormones thyroxine (T_4) and triiodothyronine (T_3) also regulate proANP gene expression (13, 180). T_3, at concentrations of 10^{-10} to 10^{-9} M, increases proANP mRNA levels twofold in atria and fourfold in ventricular cardiac myocytes in culture (13). The effect of thyroid hormones on proANP mRNA is paralleled by the increase in circulating concentrations of the gene products of this synthesis—vessel dilator, LANP, and ANP—in persons with hypothyroidism treated with thyroid hormone (345).

The effect of thyroid hormones on ANP mRNA levels has also been evaluated by comparing hypothyroid, euthyroid, and hyperthyroid rat proANP mRNA in both atria and ventricles (180). Right atrial proANP mRNA content in hypothyroidism and hyperthyroidism was 41% and 176%, respectively, of euthyroidism (180). Ventricular proANP mRNA content in hypothyroidism and hyperthyroidism was 31% and 178%, respectively, of that in euthyroidism. These changes in proANP mRNA parallel very closely the circulating concentrations of vessel dilator, LANP, and ANP in humans, which are decreased in hypothyroidism and increased in hyperthyroidism (345, 380). In hyperthyroidism, LANP, vessel dilator, and ANP increase threefold, fourfold, and twofold, respectively, in the circulation compared to 54 healthy adults (345). When the hyperthyroid subjects were treated with the antithyroid drug propylthiouracil (PTU) the circulating concentrations of LANP, vessel dilator and ANP decreased 50% after 1 week of treatment with a simultaneous 50% decrease in serum triiodothyronine (T_3) levels (345). In hypothyroidism, the circulating concentrations of LANP and vessel dilator are 50% less and of ANP one-third less than that of healthy adults (345). As discussed previously, the circulating concentrations of these natriuretic hormones return to normal in persons with hypothyroidism after thyroid hormone treatment (345).

GLUCOCORTICOIDS

Dexamethasone, at a dose of 1 mg/day, increases proANP mRNA levels in both atria and ventricles of the rat approximately twofold (102). In cultures of neonatal cardiocytes, dexamethasone increases proANP mRNA three- to fourfold in a dose-dependent fashion (102). This enhancement of proANP mRNA appears to result mainly from transcriptional activation in cells already expressing the gene rather than through recruitment of previously quiescent cells (102). There is negative feedback between cortisol and the gene products of proANP gene expression in that vessel dilator, LANP, kaliuretic hormone, and ANP decrease the circulating concentration of cortisol (344). This decrease in cortisol is due, at least partially, to these ANPs decreasing the circulating concentration of the hypothalamic peptide corticotrophin–releasing hormone (CRH) with a resultant decrease in ACTH, which stimulates the production of cortisol (344).

MINERALOCORTICOIDS

Administration of mineralocorticoids to animals causes transient fluid and sodium retention. Despite continued administration of a mineralocorticoid, animals return to sodium balance within a few days, a phenomenon termed "mineralocorticoid escape." To investigate the role of ANP in mineralocorticoid escape, Ballerman et al. (19) administered DOCA to rats in sodium balance and found plasma ANP levels and atrial proANP mRNA content increased in rats retaining sodium in response to DOCA. After "escape" from the mineralocorticoid-induced sodium retention, plasma ANP levels returned to baseline and relative atrial proANP mRNA content remained moderately elevated (19). This increase in proANP mRNA probably resulted from the secondary cardiovascular effects of the steroids (e.g., increased intravascular volume) rather than from a direct effect of the mineralocorticoids on the ANP-secreting cell, as DOCA has no direct effect on proANP mRNA in an ANP-expressing neonatal cardiocyte preparation (100, 102).

VASOCONSTRICTIVE PEPTIDES

Several vasoconstrictive peptides including endothelin, norepinephrine, and angiotensin II stimulate proANP transcription and secretion (262, 266).

CALCIUM

Primary cultures of neonatal rat cardiocytes exposed for 24 hours to 2 mM $CaCl_2$ in the culture media increase proANP messenger RNA threefold and increase secretion of ANP prohormone into the media threefold (183). When these cardiocytes were treated with the calcium channel-blocking agents diltiazem, nifedipine, or verapamil, both proANP synthesis and secretion decreased to 25%–40% of control values (183).

TRANSGENIC KNOCKOUT AND/OR MICE OVEREXPRESSING ATRIAL NATRIURETIC PEPTIDE PROHORMONE GENE

Transgenic mice with an 11 base-pair deletion in exon 2 of the proANP gene (Fig. 1) have increased blood pressure in homologous (-/-) mice of 8–23 mm Hg compared to wild-type (+/+) mice (152). Exon 2 of the proANP gene encodes for vessel dilator, kaliuretic peptide and ANP (Fig. 2). Exon 2 homozygote mutants have no circulating ANP and they become hypertensive when fed a standard diet (152). Heterozygotes (+/-) with this base pair deletion in exon 2 are salt-sensitive and become hypertensive (systolic blood pressure increases 27 mm Hg) on a high-salt (8%) diet (152). Mice that overexpress the proANP gene, on the other hand, become hypotensive (294).

HUMAN DISEASES WITH UPREGULATION OF ATRIAL NATRIURETIC PEPTIDE PROHORMONE GENE

Cerebrovascular Disease (Stroke and Hypertension)

A genetic linkage study followed 22,071 male physicians, all of whom had no history of stroke, from 1982 to 1999 (265). DNA extracted from peripheral white blood cells of those individuals who had a subsequent stroke revealed that when compared to those without strokes these individuals had a molecular variant in exon 1 of the proANP gene that was associated with a twofold ($p < .01$) increased risk of stroke (265). The individuals who had cerebrovascular accident (stroke) had significantly ($p < .001$) higher systolic and diastolic blood pressures than the persons who did not have a stroke (265). This molecular variant of the proANP gene was found to be an independent risk factor (in addition to hypertension) for a cerebrovascular accident. This molecular variant was found to be responsible for a valine-to-methionine transposition in the peptide hormone synthesized by exon 1, long-acting natriuretic peptide (LANP)

(313). (Exon 1 does not encode for ANP.) In the 16 a.a. of LANP encoded by exon 1 there is only one valine, which is at position 7 of LANP (Fig. 2) (1). Residue #7 (amino acid #7 of the ANP prohormone) is highly conserved among different species (15, 85, 86, 106, 286). In this human study (Physician's Health Study) of cerebrovascular accidents, there was no defect in the structure or expression of the proBNP gene (265). Thus, this large prospective, case-controlled study revealed that carrier status for a mutation in the exon encoding for LANP is associated with a significantly increased (twofold) risk of stroke (265). In humans, blood pressure and the ANPs correlate throughout the 24-hour period in a circadian relationship (292, 293). There is evidence to suggest that long-acting natriuretic peptide reflects salt sensitivity in hypertension-prone individuals even before they develop hypertension (206).

LANP and Stroke

Long-acting natriuretic peptide (LANP) has potent vasodilatory properties in both animals (335) and humans (328, 329). Antisera to LANP (to block the biologic activity of this peptide hormone) results in a significant increase in mean arterial pressure from 112 ± 12 mm Hg to 131 ± 9 mm Hg in normotensive animals and exacerbates hypertension in spontaneously hypertensive rats (SHR) from 140 ± 10 mm Hg to 159 ± 9 mm Hg (74). These antisera data indicate an important physiological role for long-acting natriuretic peptide in the regulation of arterial pressure (74).

In the brain of stroke-prone rats, the expression ANP prohormone gene (which synthesizes LANP) is dramatically reduced (263). Through genotype/phenotype cosegregation analysis of F₂ intercross, from the crossbreeding of stroke-prone and stroke-resistant spontaneously hypertensive rats (SHRs) it was found that a different point mutation in the ANP gene confers a stroke delaying effect (264). This point mutation, which is different from the aforementioned mutation found in humans, results in a serine replacing glycine at amino acid 74 of the ANP prohormone of the stroke-prone rats (264). If a serine replacing glycine in position 74 of the ANP prohormone is important to help prevent strokes, it is of interest that a serine is normally present in position 74 in mice, rabbits, and dogs (313) which may confer some protection from strokes in these species. There were no mutations in the BNP gene and no differences in BNP gene expression between stroke-prone and stroke-resistant animals (263, 264). Thus, these studies in stroke-prone animals suggest that the gene synthesizing the ANP prohormone may be protective against cerebrovascular accidents. These data are consistent with the human data that mutations in one or more portions of this gene (265) can lead to increased incidence of cerebrovascular accidents.

Further evidence of the importance of the peptide hormones synthesized by the ANP prohormone gene derives from studies in mice with the gene knocked out: all develop salt-sensitive hypertension within 1 week leading to stroke

(152). The BNP gene does not upregulate to prevent hypertension and/or stroke when the proANP gene is knocked out (152). Downregulation of the proANP gene in the brain in stroke-prone SHRs has further been found to cosegregate with the occurrence of early strokes in their F₂ descendants (263).

Natriuretic Peptide Hormones and Hypertension

Hypertension is an independent risk factor in addition to mutation in the ANP prohormone gene (265) for a cerebrovascular accident. The original hypothesis for hypertension was that there was a defect in the production of the blood pressure lowering atrial natriuretic peptides (12, 297). Experimental evidence revealed that rather than being decreased these blood pressure lowering peptides are elevated in the circulation in an apparent attempt to overcome the elevated blood pressure (12, 205, 297, 318). ANP increases in essential hypertension (12, 297) and in persons with pheochromocytomas (318). The hypertension associated with pheochromocytomas is characterized by increased circulating concentrations of vessel dilator and long-acting natriuretic peptide (LANP) as well as ANP (319). Each of these blood pressure lowering hormones increase further with surgical manipulation-induced increases in blood pressure, and then these peptides return to normal after surgical removal of the pheochromocytomas and lowering of blood pressure (318, 319). The hypertension of obesity also is associated with increased circulating concentrations of ANP (205) which decreases into the normal range with weight-reduction–induced decrease in high blood pressure.

In a normal pregnancy, atrial natriuretic peptides increase in each trimester with the plasma volume expansion which accompanies a normal pregnancy (207). ANP, vessel dilator and LANP increase dramatically with the hypertension of preeclampsia compared to their circulating concentrations in healthy pregnant women (208). The increased circulating levels of these vasodilatory peptides in hypertension suggest a receptor or postreceptor defect(s) in vasculature is the pathophysiological cause of their increase in hypertension (207, 208). These peptides increase in the circulation in an apparent attempt to "override" the defect (207, 208). This is similar to the negative feedback system of essentially all hormones where a defect in the receptor (or post receptor defect) in the target organ causes an increase in the hormone which stimulates the respective receptor (313). Each of the atrial natriuretic peptides discussed previously has a negative feedback system regulating their own release and that of other natriuretic peptides(328).

If one knocks out the ANP prohormone gene that synthesizes the four atrial natriuretic peptides (Fig. 1), within 1 week the animals develop salt-sensitive hypertension (152) while, on the other hand, transgenic mice overexpressing the ANP prohormone gene develop hypotension (294). In addition to directly vasodilating vasculature, kaliuretic peptide and ANP inhibit the release of the potent vasoconstrictive peptide endothelin which is produced by the vascular endothelium (323). Thus, the ANP prohormone gene and the peptide hormones synthesized by it appear to be very important in blood pressure control in both health and pathology.

Congestive Heart Failure

In congestive heart failure (CHF), proANP gene expression is upregulated (78, 246, 306). The increase in proANP gene expression is, however, not in the atria of the heart, but rather the increase in the proANP gene expression is in the ventricle of the heart (78, 246, 306). Steady state proANP mRNA increases by a factor of 4.3 ± 0.06 in the ventricle of CHF animals compared to sham animals (246). In persons with CHF, there is no defect in the production of these peptides from the ANP prohormone, but rather each are increased in the bloodstream in an attempt by the heart to overcome abnormal sodium and water retention by releasing more of these peptides that cause sodium and water excretion (326, 327, 364). As part of the pathophysiology of CHF, for example, vessel dilator and LANP increase in direct proportion to the severity of CHF as classified by the New York Heart Association (NYHA) (364). The ANP-clearance receptor pathway is not linked to the avid sodium retention and/or to the renal ANP resistance observed in CHF (32).

Cirrhosis with Ascites

Another salt- and water-retaining state, cirrhosis with ascites, is characterized by increased circulating concentration of ANPs and with a 4.1-fold ventricular (but not atrial) increased steady-state proANP messenger RNA (247). Although the liver expresses proANP messenger RNA, there is no upregulation of proANP gene expression in the liver when ascites develops (247). Rather, the upregulation of this gene is only in the ventricle of the heart (247).

LOCALIZATION OF ATRIAL NATRIURETIC PEPTIDE PROHORMONE GENE ON CHROMOSOMES

The proANP gene is located on the distal short arm of chromosome 1 in band 1P36 in humans and on chromosome 4 in mice (313).

ATRIAL NATRIURETIC PEPTIDE PROHORMONE GENE EXPRESSION IN INVERTEBRATES AND PLANTS

In addition to proANP gene being present in mammals and vertebrates, where lower vertebrates such as the frog have an identical proANP gene (268), blue crabs and oysters have been demonstrated to have the proANP gene in their hearts

(248, 314). The proANP gene in oysters and blue crabs can be upregulated by increasing salinity in the external environment, such as when the animal moves from freshwater to seawater (248, 347). This change in environmental salinity also modulates end-product concentrations of this gene expression, that is, the ANPs (232). Environmental salinity also modulates ANP in the teleost fish *Gila atraria* (359). Seawater trout have higher concentrations of ANP, vessel dilator, and LANP than freshwater trout to help them maintain volume homeostasis in a higher salt environment (56). Even the most primitive heart in the animal kingdom contains the atrial natriuretic peptide hormonal system (332). Diving is another modulator of ANP in lower animals, with diving increasing ANP in freshwater diving turtles (16) similar to whole body immersion in humans (336, 337, 342).

Although a gene in the animal kingdom expressing a peptide hormonal system in plants had never been demonstrated previously there is now evidence for a proANP-like gene in plants (346). Southern blots of English ivy (*Hedra helix*) genomic DNA revealed that the proANP gene sequence was present in its roots, stems, and leaves (346). Northern blot analysis of total plant RNA isolated from leaves, roots, and stems of *H. helix* revealed a single 0.85-kilobase proANP transcript in the stems that was similar to the proANP transcript detected in rat heart (346). Semiquantitative analysis suggested that proANP gene expression was less in English ivy compared with that of rat heart atria but similar to the amount found in extra atrial rat tissues when corrected for total RNA and quantitated by two-dimensional scanning (346). In plants, ANPs enhance the flow of water up stems to flowers and leaves, a process that is at least partially due to increasing the rate of transpiration (loss of water from the leaves) via opening the stomatal pores in leaves (333). LANP, vessel dilator, and ANP-like peptides are present in the roots, stems, leaves, and flowers of the more highly developed plants (*Tracheophyta*) and trees (conifers [333]). These peptides are also present in *Bryophyta* (plants without vascular tissue or roots) and even in *Euglena*, a single-cell, flagellated, chlorophyll-containing plant without leaves, stems, or roots (313). The oldest existing trees on Earth, the *Metasequoia*, which exist only in China, contains the ANP prohormone and ANP (370). These peptide hormones are also found in single-cell animals, such as paramecium (331). In single cell organisms, these peptides appear to help maintain the internal volume of the cell (331). ANP-like peptide immunoaffinity purified from English ivy (*H. helix*) and from rose (*Rosa damascena*) leaf extracts induces opening of the stomata of *Tradescantia* sp. in a concentration-dependent manner similar to that observed using rat ANP to open *Tradescantia* sp. stomata allowing water to transpire out of the plant (314). The demonstration of the proANP gene sequences and expression of the ANP-like gene in plants suggests that plants and animals may have evolved much more similarly than previously thought (333).

BRAIN NATRIURETIC PEPTIDE PROHORMONE GENE

The BNP gene is comprised of three exons separated by two introns similar to the proANP gene in Fig. 1 (100, 301). Regulation of the BNP gene is controlled at the transcriptional level by several cis-acting regulatory elements in the proximal promoter and the transcription factors that associate with them (26, 42, 123, 301). The cardiac specific transcription factor GATA 4 plays a major role directing basal activity of the BNP gene promoter (42, 123). GATA 4 is a nuclear mediator of mechanical stretch-activated BNP gene (241) and might function as a central integrator of regulatory activity controlled by other transcription factors such as GATA 6 (42), the neuron restricted silencer element-binding factor (225) and YY1 the embryonic development protein (26). Several of these factors interact synergistically with GATA 4, in both a physical and a functional sense, to stimulate BNP gene transcription (42, 225). Both the pro-ANP and BNP genes are activated in cardiac hypertrophy (100, 123). The GATA 4 transcription factor activates the proANP gene as well as the BNP gene (100, 123, 241).

In healthy animals, cardiac BNP mRNA is mainly of atrial origin, that is, 10–50-fold more abundant than in ventricles (49, 125, 193, 300). In early left ventricular (LV) dysfunction, BNP mRNA markedly increases in the left atrium but remains below or just barely at the level of detection in the ventricles (193). The majority of investigations have found no increase in BNP mRNA in the ventricles in congestive heart failure (125, 193) which is exactly the opposite of ANP prohormone gene expression which increases in the ventricle but not in the atria in sodium and water-retaining states (78, 246, 306). Likewise with streptotocin-induced diabetes BNP mRNA doubles in atria without any change in ventricular myocardium BNP mRNA (49). BNP gene knockout mice do not develop hypertension or hypertrophy (299) as ANP prohormone knockout mice do (152). BNP knockout mice exhibit cardiac fibrosis as the only known effect of the BNP gene being knocked out (299).

SECRETION OF NATRIURETIC PEPTIDES

The main physiological stimulus to secretion of these peptide hormones to control blood volume appears to be a pressure increase in pressure in the atria (69, 71, 239, 266, 267, 353). An increase of 4 to 6 mm Hg in the atria releases the four peptide hormones from the ANP prohormone (71). These peptide hormones, in turn, decrease the volume returning to the heart secondary to their causing a diuresis and natriuresis (71, 201, 350). Rapid heart rates at 125 beats/min and higher release the ANPs into the circulation (223). Both atrial and ventricular arrhythmias with heart rates of 125 beats/min and higher release these peptide hormones and increase the circulating concentrations of these cardiac hormones in humans (222). Hypoxia and a variety of humoral

factors (endothelin, glucocorticoids, acetylcholine, adrenergic agonists) have been suggested as contributing to release but the majority of these humoral factors' effects are to increase ANP prohormone gene synthesis as outlined previously rather than release per se (266, 267). With respect to hyperosmolarity, the threshold for ANP release is as low as 10 mOsmol/kg H_2O and this is regulated by a cross-talk between sarcolemmal L-type Ca^{2+} channel and the sarcoplasmic Ca^{2+} release (151). ANP, vessel dilator, LANP, and kaliuretic peptide have a feedback mechanism whereby they inhibit their own and each other's release (328). CNP also inhibits ANP release (185).

BIOLOGIC EFFECTS OF NATRIURETIC HORMONES AND THEIR MECHANISMS OF ACTION

ANP

VASODILATION

According to the original report by deBold et al. (64) that crude atrial extracts cause diuresis and natriuresis also indicated that these extracts could decrease mean arterial pressure. Crude atrial extracts were then shown to possess vasorelaxant activity in isolated aortic segments (5, 59, 98). The advent of synthetic ANP demonstrated that this pure form of ANP could also cause vasodilation in vitro (99, 280, 321, 363). Both crude (5) and synthetic (94) ANP decrease total peripheral resistance. There is diversity in the ability of ANP to cause vasodilation of preconstricted vessels (98, 173). ANP antagonizes both the contractile response (98, 173) and stimulated calcium entry (313) to norepinephrine and angiotensin II more than to potassium stimulation. There is also variability in relaxing different isolated vasculature preparations by ANP. Thus, large central arteries (aorta and renal) relax, whereas more distal (ear and basilar) arteries are refractory to nanomalor concentrations of ANP (256, 313). Pulmonary, femoral, and iliac arteries are intermediate in their response to ANP (313). One exception to small arteries not responding well upon the addition of ANP is the carotid arteries, which respond well (256). In general, veins do not appear to vasodilate with the addition of ANP as well as arteries do, but ANP has been shown to relax peripheral veins in addition to aortic rings (280).

ANP produces a dose-dependent reduction in systemic blood pressure in humans (357). The immediate hypotensive change of 5.5 mm Hg in 2 minutes with 100-μg ANP intravenously has been associated with a sensation of facial flushing in four of six human subjects, suggesting acute vasodilation of skin (313). ANP elicits greater blood pressure-lowering properties in spontaneously hypertensive rats than in normotensive rats (313). A greater response in hypertensive versus normotensive subjects is also true for most, if not all, antihypertensive agents.

Mechanism of ANP-Induced Vasodilation The vasodilation observed with ANP is endothelium-independent (284, 320, 363). It is mediated by cyclic GMP, which is increased after enhancement of membrane-bound guanylate cyclase by ANP (226, 320, 363). Cyclic GMP itself has been demonstrated to cause vasodilation (255, 284, 363). The vasorelaxation with ANP appears to be independent of calcium (320, 361) and cyclic AMP, with no change in cyclic AMP occurring during the same period of time that cyclic GMP increases (320, 363). With respect to calcium, ANP can both increase cyclic GMP and cause vasodilation with no calcium in the incubation media (226, 320, 354, 363), but possible shifts of calcium that is already in the vasculature are still being debated. The ANP-induced relaxation of contracted vasculature is not blocked by adrenergic antagonists (98), cholinergic antagonists (98), or indomethacin (98), the latter suggesting that this vasodilation is not mediated by prostaglandins.

The fact that ANP-induced relaxation of vasculature is not blocked by adrenergic or cholinergic antagonists (98) suggests that its effects on vasculature are direct, which means without being mediated by the sympathetic nervous system. The ability of ANP to reduce blood pressure, however, may be more complex involving a decrease in cardiac output along with a decrease in total peripheral resistance (200). ANP decreases cardiac output by two different mechanisms. One is by promoting transudation of plasma fluid into the interstitium, which is blood pressure lowering by itself. The transfer of plasma fluid from the vascular to the interstitial compartment mediated by an ANP-induced increase in vascular permeability (231, 362, 372, 381). This effect on vascular permeability is selective and occurs in liver, intestine, and skeletal muscle but not lungs or brain (362, 381). ANP also increases permeability of the glomerular capillary bed, in that protein excretion increases (231, 340, 341). This increase in glomerular permeability has also been observed in patients with nephrotic syndrome, in whom it is thought to occur without any increase in pore size (379). ANP increases the number of small and large pores available to mediate flux (231). The resulting reduction in plasma volume decreases venous return to the heart, which in turn decreases ventricular filling and cardiac output. The ability of ANP to increase permeability in cultured endothelial cells appears to involve cyclic GMP (372). The other mechanism is through suppression of autonomic nerve reflexes. Normally, the decrease in venous return caused by ANP would stimulate reflex cardioacceleration to maintain cardiac output, but, through complex actions in the central nervous system, ANP produces cardioinhibition so that reflex tachycardia does not take place, and cardiac output and blood pressure decrease (103). Inhibition of sympathetic flow to other vascular beds also occurs (103).

NATRIURESIS

In the classic experiment in 1981 by deBold et al. (64), crude atrial cardiac extracts were found to cause marked natriuresis and diuresis. Since that time, purified synthetic ANP has also been found to cause diuresis and natriuresis (8, 93, 234, 290). ANP-induced natriuresis appears to have a dependence on renal vasodilation since ligation of the renal artery eliminates ANP-induced natriuresis (291). ANP has been shown to directly increase renal blood flow in dogs (39). Redistribution of renal blood flow to the proximal (129) and distal (165) tubules has been reported as contributing to the natriuretic effects. The proximal tubule contains guanylate cyclase and cyclic GMP produced by this enzyme increases amiloride-sensitive ^{22}Na uptake in the phosphorylated brush border membranes of the proximal tubule suggesting that the ANP intracellular mediator, cyclic GMP, directly stimulates the Na–H antiporter in the proximal tubule (120).

ANP AND SITE OF ACTION IN KIDNEY

The renal actions of ANP are complex. Hemodynamic effects of pharmacologic doses of exogenous ANP constrict efferent and dilate afferent arterioles (200); the resultant increase in glomerular capillary hydrostatic pressure could increase the glomerular filtration rate (GFR) (53, 93). Physiologic doses of ANP, however, do not increase GFR (93, 234, 290). Soejima et al. (290) infused varying concentrations of ANP from 10- to 230-ng·kg^{-1}·min^{-1}, and found no change in GFR until an infusion rate of 160 ng·kg^{-1}·min^{-1} was obtained. If the increase in GFR is a dose-related phenomenon, physiological levels of ANP would not affect GFR, as the circulating physiological concentration of ANP is below the concentration of ANP that has been found necessary to increase GFR (234, 290). The tubular actions of ANP are also complex. Early micropuncture and microcatheterization studies suggested a late distal nephron site of action but functional studies of ANP in the IMCD indicate that it is a major target site of ANP action in the tubule (375, 377). Binding studies indicated specific binding sites for ANP on inner medullary collecting duct (IMCD) cells (313). ANP increases cGMP accumulation in isolated cells from this segment in a concentration-dependent manner (375). The peptide also inhibits oxygen consumption in IMCD cells, indicative of inhibition of sodium transport (377). This inhibition occurs through a cGMP-mediated effect on an amiloride-sensitive sodium channel (375, 377).

A proximal tubular site of action has been suggested from studies showing that ANP inhibits angiotensin II-stimulated proximal sodium reabsorption at very low concentrations (as low as 10^{-12} mol/L) (96, 130). In the cortical collecting ducts, ANP inhibits tubular water transport by antagonizing the action of vasopressin (76). ANP has been localized by immunoperoxidase and immunofluorescence methods to the sub-brush border of the pars convuluta and pars recta proximal tubule as well as the distal tubule (254, 269). These studies indicate that ANP may have widespread actions on tubular function, and they raise the possibility that other sites, signaling pathways, and actions may be identified in the future. As an example of this, in congestive heart failure there appears to be a renal interaction between sympathetic nerve activity and ANP that has not been observed in healthy animals (238).

ANP INHIBITS RENIN-ALDOSTERONE SYSTEM

Atrial natriuretic peptide has been found to be a potent in vivo and in vitro inhibitor of aldosterone secretion via a direct effect on aldosterone secretion from the zona glomerular cells of adrenal cortex (14, 43, 111, 177, 195, 309, 322) and indirectly through inhibition of renin release from the juxtaglomerular cells of the kidney (39, 92, 134, 179, 195, 349). The mechanism of the inhibition of renin release by ANP appears to involve cyclic GMP as this inhibition is duplicated by permeable analogues of cyclic GMP (134, 179).

LANP, Vessel Dilator, and Kaliuretic Peptide

VASODILATION

LANP, vessel dilator, and kaliuretic peptide cause vasodilation of vasculature that is endothelium independent (320), and similar to ANP endothelium-independent vasodilation of vasculature (284, 321, 363). The amount of vasodilation in vitro with these peptide hormones is similar to that observed with addition of ANP (320). These same peptide hormones have significant blood pressure-lowering effects in vivo (201). When infused over 2 hours at the same 100 ng/kg of body weight·per minute concentration, vessel dilator and ANP were found to decrease blood pressure from an average of 145 to 124 mm Hg ($p <.05$) and from 143 to 123 mm Hg ($p <.05$), respectively (201). Long-acting natriuretic peptide lowered blood pressure from a mean of 138 to 122 mm Hg ($p <.05$), whereas kaliuretic peptide decreased blood pressure from a mean of 155 to 138 mm Hg ($p <.05$) (201). Blood pressure did not change in the control animals throughout the 120-minute pre-experimental period or during the 120-minute experimental period (201). Similar to ANP, the mechanism of vasodilating vasculature for these hormones is mediated by cyclic GMP (320)—the respective mechanism of action involves enhancement of the enzyme guanylate cyclase with resultant increase in the intracellular messenger cyclic GMP (320). The enhancement of guanylate cyclase by these atrial peptides is calcium-independent in vasculature (320).

LANP HORMONE, VESSEL DILATOR, AND KALIURETIC PEPTIDE: NATRIURESIS MECHANISM OF ACTION

Comparison of the relative natriuretic and diuretic potencies of the same dose in 100-ng/kg of body weight per minute of vessel dilator, LANP, and ANP revealed that they have significant natriuretic properties in healthy humans, but kaliuretic peptide enhancement of the urinary sodium excretion rate was not significant (329). The natriuretic properties of vessel dilator are especially impressive in light of the fact that ANP has been found to be a more potent natriuretic and diuretic agent than furosemide (305) and that vessel dilator circulates normally at a 17-fold higher concentration than ANP and 100-fold higher than BNP (67, 90, 91, 113, 145,

336, 337, 364). This 17-fold higher circulating concentration is found both during basal conditions and with release secondary to physiological stimuli such as head-out water immersion where the atria are stretched releasing these peptides (336, 337). It is therefore possible that vessel dilator with its higher concentration in the circulation may contribute more to natriuresis and diuresis that is observed secondary to normal physiological stimuli than does ANP since vessel dilator is 17-fold higher in circulation and its equally potent biologic effects when utilized at the lower circulating concentration of ANP (323, 327, 329). Vessel dilator biologic effects last significantly longer than ANP (6 hours vs 30 minutes) (323, 327, 329). Vessel dilator and ANP, with nearly equal abilities to enhance sodium excretion, are markedly different, however, with respect to potassium excretion (329). Vessel dilator is the only one of the four peptide hormones from the ANP prohormone that does not significantly enhance potassium excretion (201, 329). This potassium-sparing effect of vessel dilator makes it distinctly different from ANP, LANP, and kaliuretic peptide. LANP has similar but more modest diuretic, natriuretic and kaliuretic properties when compared to ANP at the same concentration (329). Kaliuretic peptide does not significantly enhance the fractional excretion of sodium (FE_{Na}), but it is the only natriuretic peptide that significantly enhances the fractional excretion of potassium in healthy humans (FE_k). (Fractional excretion of sodium or potassium is the percentage of glomerular-filtered sodium or potassium that is excreted into the urine [329].) Physiological maneuvers such as head-out-of-water immersion resulting in a central hypervolemia release LANP, vessel dilator, kaliuretic peptide and ANP and produce natriuresis and diuresis (336, 337, 342).

The natriuretic effects of long-acting natriuretic peptide, kaliuretic peptide and vessel dilator have different mechanism(s) of action from ANP in that they inhibit renal Na$^+$,K$^+$-ATPase secondary to their ability to enhance the synthesis of prostaglandin E2 (48, 124) which ANP does not do (48, 124, 245). ANP, BNP, and CNP effects in the kidney are thought to be mediated by cyclic GMP (34, 125, 266, 315).

VESSEL DILATOR AND LANP: SITE OF ACTION IN KIDNEY

Immunohistochemical studies have localized vessel dilator (Fig. 3) and long-acting natriuretic peptide as well as ANP to the sub-brush border of the pars convuluta and pars recta of the proximal tubules of animal (254) and human (269) kidneys. Immunofluorescent studies reveal that each of these peptides has a strong inclination for the perinuclear region in both the proximal and distal tubules (254, 269).

LANP, VESSEL DILATOR, AND KALIURETIC PEPTIDE: RENIN-ALDOSTERONE SYSTEM

Kaliuretic hormone and long-acting natriuretic peptide (LANP) are also potent inhibitors of the circulating concentrations of aldosterone in healthy humans (322). Kaliuretic peptide and LANP effects on decreasing plasma aldosterone levels last for at least 3 hours after their infusions have stopped while ANP no longer has any effect on plasma aldosterone concentrations within 30 minutes of infusion cessation (322). Vessel dilator does not appear to have direct effects on aldosterone synthesis, but is a potent inhibitor (66%) of plasma renin activity (349). Thus, the four peptide hormones from the ANP prohormone gene act as endogenous antagonists of the vasoconstrictor and salt-and-water-retaining systems (e.g., the renin-angiotensin-aldosterone system, vasopressin [76], and endothelin [307, 323]) in the body's defense against blood pressure elevation and plasma volume expansion via direct vasodilator, diuretic, and natriuretic properties. These four peptide hormones' multiple biologic effects are illustrated in Fig. 6. It is important to note in this illustration with respect to the kidney, that these peptide hormones also increase protein excretion (albumin, B2 microglobulin) (204, 340, 341) and phosphate reabsorption (129) as well as cause a natriuresis and diuresis.

Urodilatin

VASODILATION

Urodilatin has vasodilatory effects similar to those of ANP (278, 282). The ANP prohormone post-translational processing is different in the kidney from that which occurs in the heart resulting in an additional four a.a. added to the N-terminus of ANP (proANP 95–126, urodilatin) (Fig. 2) (187, 216, 282). The rest of the amino acids in urodilatin are identical and in the same sequence as those in ANP (Fig. 2). Urodilatin and ANP have identical ring structures formed with cysteine to cysteine bonding (Fig. 2). The four a.a. added to form urodilatin are the same four a.a. present in the C-terminus of kaliuretic peptide in other tissues but in the kidney the prohormone is cleaved between a.a. 94 and 95 rather than between a.a. 98 and 99 to form urodilatin (282). Urodilatin is not formed in the heart or in other tissues except the kidney. This peptide hormone is synthesized by the same gene which synthesizes ANP but in the kidney, as opposed to all other tissues that have been investigated, the ANP prohormone is processed differently resulting in urodilatin rather than ANP being formed (187, 216, 282). Urodilatin at first was thought not to be a hormone in that it was thought that it did not circulate (282) but sensitive assays revealed that it circulates in very low concentrations (9–12 pg/ml) (338). Infusion of ANP increases the circulating concentration of urodilatin suggesting that some ANP effects may be mediated by urodilatin (338). Infusion of long-acting natriuretic peptide, vessel dilator, and kaliuretic peptide, on the other hand, do not affect the circulating concentration of urodilatin in healthy humans (338).

URODILATIN: NATRIURESIS

Urodilatin has natriuretic and diuretic effects similar to ANP (278) and since it has an identical amino acid sequence and ring structure as ANP one would expect it to bind to the same receptors and have similar biologic effects as ANP.

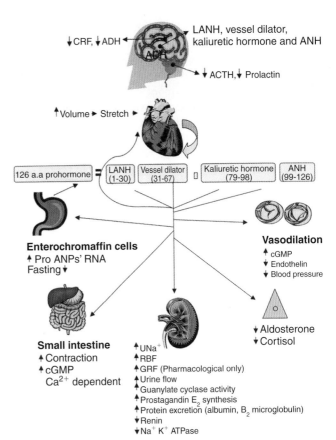

FIGURE 6 Long-acting natriuretic hormone (LANH or LANP), vessel dilator, kaliuretic hormone, and atrial natriuretic hormone (ANH or ANP) are released with increased volume, which causes stretching of the atrium of the heart. The biological effects of these peptide hormones include vasodilation mediated via enhancing guanylate cyclase activity with a resultant increase in the intracellular messenger cyclic GMP and inhibiting the vasoconstrictive peptide endothelin. ANPs cause a natriuresis mediated (except for ANH) by their enhancing the synthesis of prostaglandin E2, which, in turn, inhibits renal Na^+,K^+-ATPase. These peptide hormones also reduce circulating cortisol, aldosterone, and/or plasma renin activity. ANPs decrease corticotrophin-releasing factor (CRF) and antidiuretic hormone (ADH) from the hypothalamus as well as decrease the circulating concentration of adenocorticotropin (ACTH) and prolactin from the anterior pituitary. They increase protein excretion by the kidney (204, 340, 341). (With permission, from Vesely DL. Atrial natriuretic peptide prohormone gene expression: hormones and diseases that upregulate its expression. *IUBMB Life* 2002;53:153–159.)

LOCALIZATION OF URODILATIN IN KIDNEY

Immunohistochemical studies have localized urodilatin to the distal tubule with no evidence of urodilatin in the proximal tubule (254). ANP messenger-RNA studies have confirmed that the ANP prohormone is synthesized in the kidney (122). The amount of the ANP prohormone present in the kidney, however, is only 1/190th of that produced in the atria of the heart (246). These studies taken together suggest that since urodilatin is found mainly in the distal nephron (122, 254, 261) and since it is part of the ANP prohormone (278, 282, 316), synthesis of the ANP prohormone may take place in the distal nephron (122, 254, 261). The ANP prohormone gene is present and can be expressed in the kidney (122, 246). This gene is upregulated within the kidney in early renal failure in diabetic animals (289) and in the remnant kidney of rats with 5/6 reduced renal mass (303). Within the kidney, in addition to urodilatin, the ANP prohormone gene synthesizes LANP, vessel dilator, and a shortened form of kaliuretic peptide, but not ANP per se (117, 316).

URODILATIN AND RENIN-ALDOSTERONE SYSTEM

Urodilatin does not affect renin or aldosterone concentrations (80).

BNP and CNP

BNP: BIOLOGIC EFFECTS

Brain natriuretic peptide (BNP) is a 32-a.a. peptide in humans (45 a.a. in rat) with similar diuretic and natriuretic effects and short half-life as ANP (Fig. 2) (295). BNP half-life is 100-fold shorter than the half-lives of vessel dilator and LANP (4, 181, 295, 296, 313). BNP has remarkable sequence homology to ANP with only four a.a. being different in the 17-a.a. ring structure formed by a disulfide bond common to both peptides (Fig. 2) (181, 182, 262, 266, 295). Although BNP was named (295) for where it was first isolated (porcine brain), the main source of its synthesis and secretion is the heart (10-fold greater than brain) (Table 1) (61, 125, 181, 187, 266, 300). As with ANP, the highest levels of BNP are found in the atria of the heart (125, 300). BNP levels in the atria, however, are less than 1% of ANP levels (300). The immunoreactive level of BNP in the ventricles is only 1% of BNP concentration in the atria; in brief, 99% of BNP is found in the atria (300). BNP, however, has been termed a "ventricular" peptide based on ventricular BNP mRNA levels being similar to those in the atria and the ventricles are much larger than the atria (216).

The 108-a.a. BNP prohormone is processed in the heart to yield a biologic functioning BNP consisting of a.a. 77–108 of the BNP prohormone (in humans) and an N-terminus of the BNP prohormone (a.a. 1–76 of prohormone), both of which circulate (181). BNP circulating concentration is less than 20% of ANPs (125). The sequence homology of BNP differs appreciably across species (both in size and a.a. sequence) (85, 181, 216, 300). The major circulating form varies substantially among species, being 26, 45, and 32 a.a. in pig, rat, and human, respectively (100, 181). The marked sequence variability of BNP explains in part variations in its biologic activity in different species. The peptide hormones from the ANP prohormone, on the other hand, have remarkable homology across different species (15, 85, 86, 103, 106, 286). Mice overexpressing the BNP gene, where the circulating concentration of BNP is 10- to 100-fold higher than in healthy mice, have less glomerular hypertrophy and mesangial expansion with intraglomerular cells than healthy mice 16 weeks after both received renal ablation (163). This mouse model of subtotal

renal ablation, however, also has significantly increased ANP concentrations (230, 303, 378), which may also have contributed to the effects attributed to BNP in the BNP-gene overexpressing mice (163).

CNP: CIRCULATING CONCENTRATIONS AND BIOLOGIC EFFECTS

C-type natriuretic peptide (CNP) is a 22-a.a. peptide with remarkable similarity to ANP and BNP in its amino acid sequence but lacks the carboxy terminal tail of ANP and BNP (Fig. 2) (21, 22, 296). CNP was found originally in the brain but more recent studies suggest that it is also present in the heart (160) and kidney (203, 298). The amount of CNP in the heart, however, is very low and only small amounts are present in plasma (160). Two CNP molecules, 22 and 53 a.a. in length, have been identified in plasma (22, 52). Each is derived from a single CNP prohormone, with the 22-a.a. form contained in the carboxy terminal portion of the 53-a.a. form. The 22-a.a. form predominates in plasma and is more potent than the 53-a.a. form in humans (21, 22, 52, 296). The plasma concentration of CNP is very low with some authors reporting that CNP is not normally detectable but becomes detectable only in renal failure (304) and congestive heart failure (161). CNP is present in the human kidney (203, 298). CNP has been found to have little effect on renal vasoconstriction (373). Although CNP has been reported to have natriuretic effects in some animals, when infused in humans at physiological concentrations and in concentrations that reached four- to 10-fold above those observed in disease states, CNP did not affect renal function (21). Thus, in healthy humans CNP had no effect on renal hemodynamics, systemic hemodynamics, intrarenal sodium handling, sodium excretion, or plasma levels of renin and aldosterone (21). In another study of infusion of CNP in healthy humans, CNP was increased 60-fold in plasma and there were no significant hemodynamic or natriuretic effects (144). The authors of this study concluded that it is unlikely that CNP has any endocrine role in circulatory physiology (144). There is one study in humans where infusion of CNP to increase CNP plasma levels 550-fold above normal caused a $1^1/_2$-fold increase in urine volume and sodium excretion (146). With this very high plasma concentration of CNP, both ANP and BNP also increased 2.4-fold (146), which may have been the cause of the natriuresis and diuresis observed. Each of these studies suggests that CNP does not contribute physiologically to any natriuresis or diuresis in healthy humans (21, 144, 146). The main site of CNP synthesis is vascular endothelium and CNP acts as a paracrine endothelium-derived hyperpolarizing factor (EDHF) via activation of NPR-C receptor and the opening of a G-protein–gated inwardly rectifying K+ channel (GIRK) in mesenteric resistance arteries to mediate vasodilation (44). In conduit vessels, on the other hand, CNP induces relaxation via a cyclic GMP-dependent mechanism (44).

Adrenomedullin and Proadrenomedullin N-Terminal 20 Peptide: Biologic Effects

Adrenomedullin (ADM), a 52-a.a. peptide with one intramolecular disulfide bond (Fig. 2) originally isolated from an extract of a pheochromocytoma (171), also has biologic properties nearly identical to the atrial natriuretic peptides, but these properties are less pronounced than those of the ANPs (Table 1) (154, 171, 172, 271). The C-terminal amino acid, tyrosine, is amidated in ways similar to other biologically active peptides (172). Infusion of ADM lowers blood pressure and produces diuresis and natriuresis (154, 171, 271). Adrenomedullin causes a long-lasting hypotension accompanied by increased heart rate (233). ANP but not LANP, vessel dilator or kaliuretic hormone increases the circulating concentration of adrenomedullin three- to fourfold, suggesting that some of the reported effects of ANP may be mediated via adrenomedullin (321). However, the natriuresis and diuresis secondary to ANP were much larger than has ever been observed with adrenomedullin (321), suggesting that ADM does not mediate all of the natriuretic and diuretic effects of ANP. Adrenomedullin is not produced in the atrium of the heart and therefore is not one of the atrial natriuretic peptides per se as these peptides were so named because they are synthesized in the atria of the heart (Table 1). Adrenomedullin is a larger peptide than any of the atrial natriuretic peptides with its main site of synthesis being in the adrenal (Table 1) but isolated renal cells also have the ability to synthesize adrenomedullin secondary to stimulation by vasopressin via V2 receptors (271, 275). Since vasopressin (antidiuretic hormone, ADH) inhibits a diuresis these findings are opposed to findings that ADM causes a diuresis (154, 171, 271). Adrenomedullin is part of a peptide family that shares structural similarity with calcitonin gene–related peptides and amylin, which share biologic effects and some cross-reactivity between receptors (81, 271, 274). The adrenomedullin prohormone at its N-terminal end contains another biologically active peptide with vasodilating properties known as proadrenomedullin N-terminal 20 peptide (PAMP) (82, 272). The respective secretion of whether more PAMP or adrenomedullin is produced depends on alternate splicing of its prohormone by the enzyme peptidylglycine C-amidating monooxygenase (50, 154, 172, 271, 272). Adrenomedullin exerts its actions through G-protein-coupled membrane receptors linked to adenylate cyclase resulting in an increase in cellular cyclic AMP (271) as opposed to the atrial natriuretic peptides (ANP, BNP, etc.) whose second messenger is cyclic GMP (320, 354, 363). Proadrenomedullin is thought not to act via either cyclic AMP or cyclic GMP but rather via potassium channels, which eventually exert a presympathetic inhibition of sympathetic nerves innervating blood vessels (272).

Dendroaspis Natriuretic Peptide: Biologic Effects

Dendroaspis natriuretic peptide (DNP) is the newest of the natriuretic peptides (Fig. 2). This peptide was isolated from the venom of the green mamba snake *Dendroaspis angusticeps* (283). This venom also contains several polypeptide toxins that block cholinergic receptors to cause paralysis (283). DNP-like peptide has been reported to be present in human plasma and in heart atria (279). In plasma, DNP concentration is very low at 6 pg/ml, which is one-half of 1% of the circulating atrial natriuretic peptides (279). This peptide has a 17-a.a. disulfide ring structure similar to ANP, BNP, and CNP (Fig. 2), and causes a natriuresis, and diuresis in dogs (192). Infusion of DNP does not cause any significant change in the circulating levels of ANP, BNP, or CNP (192).

Richards et al. (259) have questioned whether DNP actually exists in humans and mammals since it has not been characterized by high-pressure liquid chromatography linked to immunoassay, followed by purification and analysis to establish the human amino acid sequence, as has been done with the aforementioned natriuretic peptides. The gene for DNP has not been cloned in the snake or in any mammal as has been done for each of the other natriuretic peptides (259). Richards et al. (259) suggest that DNP may be "snake BNP" since BNP varies markedly in amino acid sequence among species (and the BNP sequence in this snake is unknown). The peptides from the ANP prohormone are markedly conserved among species (15, 85, 86, 103, 106, 286) and one would not suspect that DNP is one of these peptides as their amino-acid sequences are markedly different from DNP. Further experimentation with the studies discussed previously suggested by Richards et al. (259) should give us more insight with respect to this interesting peptide.

Guanylin and Uroguanylin: Biologic Effects

Guanylin, a 15-a.a. peptide (58), and uroguanylin, a 16-a.a. peptide originally isolated from urine (88, 127), are intestinal peptides which are structurally and functionally similar to bacterial heat-stable enterotoxins elaborated by strains of pathogenic *Escherichia coli* intestinal bacteria. Traveler's diarrhea is the result of this enterotoxin interacting with a membrane-bound guanylate cyclase (GC-C receptor) on the luminal surface of enterocytes (77). The resulting increase in cellular cyclic GMP phosphorylates the cystic-fibrosis transmembrane conductance regulator (CFTR) leading to an efflux of chloride into the intestinal lumen (260). Guanylin and uroguanylin have similar structures to this enterotoxin and have their similar mechanism of action via the same GC-C receptor (89). These peptides have been identified in the intestine in different distributions, with guanylin in the colon but not the proximal intestine, and uroguanylin expressed in the proximal intestine but not in the colon (83, 87, 88, 127). These peptides have natriuretic properties (58, 88). The observation of renal expression of guanylin and uroguanylin mRNA (58, 88) suggests renal synthesis and a local action of these peptides in a manner analogous to the ANP prohormone gene products.

The GC-C receptor with which the heart-stable enterotoxin, uroguanylin, and guanylin interact was cloned from intestinal cDNA libraries (77). It exhibits 55% identity to NPR-A and NPR-B receptors in the catalytic region, 39% identity in the protein kinase domain, but only 10% identity in the extracellular region (77). Within the kidneys, heat stable enterotoxin, uroguanylin, and guanylin bind chiefly to apical membranes of proximal tubule cells (83, 89), also a site of CFTR expression (57).

ANP Prohormone System and Expression in Gastrointestinal Tract

Almost 30 years ago it was noted that an oral load of sodium resulted in a natriuresis that was greater than the same amount of sodium chloride given intravenously suggesting that the gastrointestinal tract monitors and responds to oral sodium load (186). Guanylin and uroguanylin may respond to this oral sodium load in the colon and proximal intestine, respectively, but the stomach is an earlier monitor of this sodium load. Immunoreactive ANPs and ANP prohormone mRNA are present in the proximal stomach and antrum (79, 115, 116, 118). ANP prohormone gene expression and gene products LANP and ANP have been localized to the enterochromaffin cells in the lower portion of antropyloric glands of the stomach (116). Fasting for 72 hours in adult rats results in a significant ($p < .05$) decrease in the levels of ANP prohormone messenger RNA, and decrease in immunoreactive long-acting natriuretic peptide and ANP to ~33% of that of fed rats (116). In humans, food intake increases the excretion of LANP, vessel dilator and ANP into the urine suggesting and interaction between the gastrointestinal tract and the kidney (330). A fluid load of Coca-Cola® rapidly (in 15 minutes) decreases the excretion of LANP, vessel dilator, and ANP into the urine allowing more of these peptides which cause a diuresis to be present to respond to the fluid load (330). In the stomach, cholinergic neurons inhibit and pituitary adenylate cyclase-activating polypeptide neurons stimulate ANPs secretion suggesting that there is also neuronal control of their secretion from the stomach (114). ANPs are present not only in stomach but throughout the gastrointestinal tract (small intestine and colon) (109, 339, 352), as opposed to guanylin and uroguanylin, which are present only in specific portions of the gastrointestinal tract (83, 87, 88, 127). Guanylate cyclases A and B which the ANPs interact with are present in the gastrointestinal tract (253) as well as guanylate-C which guanylin and uroguanylin enhance (89). Thus, there appears to be an intricate relationship between the production of natriuretic peptides in the gastrointestinal tract, and their effects on the kidney, which in turn, metabolizes these natriuretic peptides and excretes them into the urine. ANPs also appear to have effects within the gastrointestinal track itself (17). ANP increases the spontaneous phasic contractions of longitudinal muscle two- to fourfold over a concentration range of 10 pm to 1000 mM which was associated with a threefold increase in cyclic GMP (17). Vessel dilator and LANP also increased these spontaneous place contractions which were additive with ANP (17). The ANPs appear to act as neurotransmitters in the gastrointestinal tract to move water and feces through the gastrointestinal tract via increased force of contraction of the longitudinal muscles (17) until feces reaches the anal sphincter which ANP has been shown to relax to expel the contents of the gastrointestinal tract (17, 59).

Melanocyte-Stimulating Hormones

Melanocyte-stimulating hormones (MSHs) are small peptides of three different primary sequences (α-, β-, and γ-MSH) derived from the precursor prohormone proopiomelanocortin (POMC), which also gives rise to ACTH. Thus, MSHs, like ANPs from a prohormone, contain four peptide hormones when proteolytically processed (142, 143). Each of the MSH peptides is natriuretic when infused in experimental animals (46, 142, 143, 229). The mechanisms of action of the MSHs are different from those of the ANPs in that MSH works via intracellular cyclic AMP rather than cyclic GMP (334). The MSH-induced natriuresis does not appear to be a direct effect on the kidney but rather via an interaction with renal nerves to inhibit sodium reabsorption as prior renal denervation completely prevents the natriuresis secondary to MSHs (46).

Ouabain-Like Factors

Ouabain-like factors or "third factors" (factors that circulate and by definition inhibit Na^+,K^+-ATPase) have been searched for decades. As outlined previously, vessel-dilator, long-acting natriuretic peptide, and kaliuretic peptide are circulating peptide hormones (67, 90, 91, 145, 337, 364, 365) that increase in the circulation with volume-expansion which inhibit the ouabain site on renal Na^+,K^+-ATPase (48, 124). ANP does not inhibit renal Na^+,K^+-ATPase (48, 124, 245) and therefore would not be the "third factor" or a ouabain-like factor. Since the other three peptide hormones fulfill all the characteristic of "third factor" they may actually be the "ouabain-like factors" that have been searched for. Utilizing a very sensitive radioimmunoassay to ouabain, EP Gomez-Sanchez et al. determined that ouabain itself does not circulate in human or rat plasma as a peak corresponding to ouabain was not found on high pressure liquid chromatography (112). In most samples, they found only very low levels of a ouabain-like substance was present (112). Since LANP, vessel dilator, and kaliuretic peptide circulate at 100-fold higher levels than this substance, the volume expanded substance(s) that do the majority of inhibiting of Na^+,K^+-ATPase at the ouabain site on the

Na$^+$,K$^+$-ATPase are most likely LANP, vessel dilator, and kaliuretic peptide rather than some substance structurally similar to ouabain, which, if it circulates, is present in extremely low levels in the circulation (112).

NATRIURETIC PEPTIDE RECEPTORS A, B, AND C

Atrial natriuretic peptides, after moving via the circulation to their respective target tissues mediate their action(s) at the cellular level by first binding to high-affinity specific receptors on the cell surface (Fig. 4) which results in the intracellular generation of cyclic GMP via activation of the enzyme guanylate cyclase which resides in the cytosolic domain of these membrane receptors as integral part of these receptors (47, 77, 176). Guanylate cyclase (also termed guanylyl cyclase) catalyzes the formation of the intracellular mediator cyclic 3′, 5′-guanosine monophosphate (cyclic GMP) (320, 354, 363).

The area in the kidney with the most ANP-binding sites is the glomeruli, followed by proximal tubules and then inner medullary collecting ducts (176). With respect to ANP, BNP, and CNP receptors, cDNA cloning has shown three types of natriuretic peptide receptors (NPR): NPR-A, NPR-B, and NPR-C (47, 77, 176, 216). Only NPR-A and NPR-B exhibit the intracellular guanylate cyclase (GC) catalytic domain (Fig. 4), whereas the third cloned receptor, NPR-C, contains no guanylate cyclase domain (77, 176, 216). NPR-A and NPR-B which bind ANP, BNP and CNP, are structurally similar and contain a ligand-binding extracellular domain (176), a protein kinase-like domain, and a guanylate cyclase domain (Fig. 4) (47, 77, 176). Upon ligand biding, a change in receptor conformation allows cytosolic factors to interact with the kinase-like domain leading to activation of guanylate cyclase and the consequent generation of cGMP, the second messenger of the ANPs. The NPR-A receptor binds ANP, BNP, CNP, and urodilatin with a preference for the rank order of selectivity being ANP = urodilatin > BNP > CNP (47, 77, 176, 216). The order is reversed for NPR-B receptor (CNP >> ANP > BNP). NPR-B is structurally similar to the NPR-A receptor with 74% homology at the cytoplasmic domain, but only 44% homology in the extracellular binding domain, which may explain the difference in ligand specificities of the two guanylate cyclase receptors (44, 176).

NPR-A mRNA is expressed mainly in the kidney, in the glomeruli, renal vasculature, proximal tubules, and in the IMCD (19, 47, 176). The distribution of NPR-B overlaps to some extent with that of the NPR-A and is found in the kidney, vasculature, and brain. In vascular endothelium and smooth muscle, the NPR-B is more abundant that NPR-A. Compared to the NPR-A receptor, low levels of the NPR-B receptor are present in the kidney (34, 202).

Number of ANP Receptors per Cell

The number of ANP receptors per cell varies with the cell type (19, 66, 137). Smooth muscle vasculature appears to be the target cell most richly endowed with ANP receptors (137). The reported number of receptors in vascular smooth muscle cells has ranged from 18,400 binding sites per cell to 500,000 (313). Comparison of a variety of cultured cells revealed 310,000, 80,000, 50,000, 14,000, and 3,000 sites per cell for vascular smooth muscle, lung fibroblasts, adrenal cortex, aortic endothelial cells, and Leydig cells of the testis, respectively (313). Twelve thousand ANP-binding sites per cell have been found in kidney glomerular mesangial cells, which is markedly less than in other vascular areas, but the receptors in the mesangial cells exhibited as high affinity as do other vascular areas for ANP (19).

Inverse Relationship of Change in Number of ANP Receptors with Circulating ANP Concentrations

The number of ANP receptors varies with fluid status and inversely with the circulating ANP concentration (313). Deprivation of water decreases the circulating ANP concentration and augments receptor number in both kidney and adrenal gland (313). Rats fed a low-salt diet for 2 weeks exhibit "up regulation" of glomerular ANP receptor density, whereas animals fed a high-salt diet have a decreased receptor density (313). The decrease in total ANP receptors, at least after salt loading, is due exclusively to a decrease in the NPR-C receptor rather than the NPR-A receptor (313).

Structure of NPR-A Receptor

The structure of the NPR-A receptor is illustrated in Fig. 5. This structure was elucidated using complimentary DNA (cDNA) encoding a 115-kD human natriuretic peptide receptor (NPR)-active (A or functional) receptor that possesses guanylate cyclase activity (47, 77, 176). The NPRA receptor has 1029 a.a., a 32-a.a. signal sequence followed by at 441-a.a. extracellular domain (i.e., projecting from the cell) (47, 77, 176). This extracellular portion of the NPR-A receptor is 33% homologous to the 60-kD NPR-C receptor (77, 176). This extracellular portion of the receptor is the binding site for ANP, BNP, and CNP. A 21-a.a. transmembrane portion of the receptor "anchors" the receptor to the membrane. Inside the cell (intracellular domain) there is a 568-a.a. cytoplasmic portion of the receptor with homology (23%) to the protein kinase family (protein kinase domain) being next to the membrane (47, 77, 176), followed by a large guanylate cyclase catalytic portion of the receptor (Fig. 5) that is 42% homologous to cytoplasmic guanylate cyclase (47, 77, 176). The kinase domain binds ATP but lacks true kinase activity. Rather, it functions to inhibit the guanylate cyclase domain. If the kinase domain is "knocked out," guanylate cyclase continuously functions. The molecular weight of this receptor is 114,426 (47).

The guanylate cyclase of human and rat NPR-A receptors are 90% identical throughout their sequences (47, 77). The similar amino acid sequence between the NPR-C receptor (77, 176, 216) and the extracellular portion of the NPR-A receptor reflects a common function shared between them—they both bind ANP, BNP, and CNP.

NPR-C (Clearance) Receptor

Cross-linking studies revealed that in addition to the high-molecular-weight receptors for ANP, BNP, and CNP there was also a low-molecular-weight 60-kD receptor that appeared to be a subunit of the high-molecular-weight receptor (77, 176, 216). This 60-kD receptor was found not to contain guanylate cyclase or to mediate any of the known effects of ANP, such as natriuresis or diuresis (77, 176, 196). Maack et al. (196) have suggested that this low-molecular-weight ANP receptor be called an ANP clearance receptor, based on the observation that administration in vivo of an internally deleted ANP analogue that blocked this receptor resulted in an increase in circulating ANP levels, suggesting that this receptor helps clear ANP from the circulation.

STRUCTURE OF NPR CLEARANCE RECEPTOR

The NPR-C receptor is similar structurally outside the cell to the NPR-A receptor with 496 a.a. compared to the 441 a.a. projecting from the cell for the NPR-A receptor (77, 176, 196). They have a similar single short transmembrane spanning region, but where the two receptors markedly differ is inside the cell. The NPR-C receptor has only a very short 37-a.a. tail into the cytoplasm of the cell as compared to the large 568-a.a. portion in the cell for the NPR-A receptor (47, 77, 176, 196). Neither the protein kinase domain nor the guanylate cyclase catalytic site is present in the NPR-C receptor. The NPR-C receptor is not linked to a second messenger system which explains its inability to cause vasodilation, diuresis, or natriuresis (47, 77, 176, 196). The order of binding to the NPR-C receptor is ANP > CNP > BNP. The NPR-C receptor is the most abundant receptor of the natriuretic receptors, accounting for more than 95% of the total receptor population, and is located at high density in kidney, vascular endothelium, smooth muscle cells, and the heart (77, 176, 196).

Vessel Dilator and LANP Receptors

Vessel dilator and long-acting natriuretic peptide do not bind to the NPR-A, B, or C receptors but rather have their own specific receptors (312, 319, 325, 343). ANP, BNP, and CNP have similar ring structures which are important for binding to the NPR-A, B, and C receptors (47, 77, 176, 196, 216). Vessel dilator, LANP, and kaliuretic peptide, on the other hand, are linear peptide hormones, and one would not expect binding to the above receptors as they do not have the ring structure of the C-terminal prohormone peptides ANP, BNP, and CNP (319, 325).

LANP RECEPTOR

Long-acting natriuretic peptide (LANP) as well as ANP binds specifically to smooth muscle membranes (325), placental membranes (312), distal nephrons (343), proximal tubules (343), and renal cortical and medullary membranes (343). Unlabeled LANP displaces ^{125}I-labeled LANP binding in a concentration-dependent manner (325). ANP and vessel dilator inhibit ^{125}I-labeled LANP binding somewhat at concentrations above which these peptides are known to circulate—that is, 10^{-6} M for ANP and 10^{-7} M for vessel dilator. Similarly, ACTH, growth hormone, and insulin could displace ^{125}I-labeled LANP binding, but only at 10^{-4} M concentrations (i.e., not at their circulating concentrations) (325). Scatchard analysis of the LANP-binding data resulted in a straight line (325), suggesting that these smooth muscle cells contain a single class of high-affinity binding sites for LANP with an equilibrium dissociation constant (K_d) of 0.11 nM. The binding capacity (maximal binding, B_{max}) for LANP was 2.57 fmol/10^6 cells, and the number of binding sites was calculated to be 1548 per cell (325).

VESSEL DILATOR RECEPTOR

Vessel dilator also binds specifically to smooth muscle membranes (325), proximal tubules (343), distal nephrons (343), placental membranes (312), and renal cortical and medullary membranes (343) at a site distinct from the binding of ANP to membranes. The binding of ^{125}I-labeled vessel dilator is competitively inhibited by unlabeled vessel dilator between 10^{-9} and 10^{-11} M (325). The binding of this peptide hormone could be inhibited by concentration (10^{-4} to 10^{-7} M) of ANP, LANP, insulin, and ACTH, which are far in excess of their respective circulating concentrations (325). Scatchard analysis of the vessel dilator–binding data resulted in a straight line (325), suggesting that smooth muscles contain a single class of high-affinity binding sites for vessel dilator with an equilibrium dissociation constant (K_d) of 4 nM. B_{max} for vessel dilator was 59.9 fmol/10^6 cells, and the number of binding sites was calculated to be 36,087 per cell (325).

DEGRADATION OF NATRIURETIC PEPTIDES BY KIDNEY

The inactivation of the ANP, BNP, and CNP occurs via two pathways: binding to clearance receptors and enzymatic degradation. This results in half-life of the ANP, BNP, and CNP in the range of minutes. The clearance receptor (NPR-C) (32, 47, 77, 176, 196) clears the NPs through receptor-mediated uptake, internalization, and lysosomal hydrolysis of ANP, BNP and CNP with rapid and efficient recycling of internalized receptors to the cell surface. Enzymatic degradation of ANP, BNP, and CNP takes place in the lung, liver, and kidney, and the main enzyme responsible for this degradation is neutral endopeptidase (NEP-24.11) (34, 356). NEP, originally referred to as enkephalinase because of its ability to degrade opioid peptides in the brain, was subsequently shown to be identical to a well-characterized zinc metallopeptidase present in the kidney (356). This zinc metalloproteinase hydrolyzes internal peptide bonds of polypeptides rather than those adjacent to their N- or C-terminal ends. NEP has a ubiquitous tissue distribution and multiple functions, sharing structural similarities with various metallopeptidases, including aminopeptidase ACE, and carboxypeptidases A, B, and E (356). NEP is most abundant in the brush borders of the proximal tubules of the kidney where it rapidly degrades filtered ANP, thus preventing ANP from reaching more distal luminal receptors (356). In the case of ANP, NEP-24.11 cleaves the $Cys^{105}–Phe^{106}$ bond to disrupt the ring structure and inactivate the peptide. NEP 24.11 is a nonspecific enzyme that also cleaves enkephalins, endothelin, substance P, kinins, neurotensin, insulin B chain, angiotensin, calcitonin gene–related peptide, and adrenomedullin, as well as ANP, BNP, and CNP. With respect to ANPs in humans, ANP and CNP are preferred substrates for NEP as opposed to BNP with the Cys–Phe bond of human BNP being relatively insensitive to enzymatic cleavage (356).

INFLUENCE OF ACUTE RENAL FAILURE ON CIRCULATING CONCENTRATION OF ATRIAL NATRIURETIC PEPTIDES

Each of the atrial natriuretic peptides from the ANP prohormone (vessel dilator, ANP, LANP, and kaliuretic peptide) (45, 53, 91, 145, 175, 219, 270, 341, 342, 364, 365), BNP (39, 41, 55, 95, 181, 182), and CNP (22, 144, 146, 304) increase in the circulation in salt- and water-retaining states such as renal failure and congestive heart failure, compared to their concentrations in healthy individuals. Thus, in salt- and water-retaining states, there is no decrease in production of these natriuretic and diuretic peptides, but rather there is increased production (mainly from the ventricle of the heart) (78, 102, 246) in an apparent attempt to overcome the salt and water retention via their natriuretic and diuretic properties (326, 327). The disease state associated with the highest circulating concentrations of atrial natriuretic peptides is renal failure (90, 91, 276, 361, 365). One would suspect that atrial natriuretic peptides are higher in renal failure versus Class IV New York Heart Association congestive heart failure patients because of the added pathophysiology of decreased degradation of these peptides with the decreased functioning renal parenchyma (365). Franz et al. (91), however, have shown that there is an increased excretion of ANPs in renal failure and that the increase in vessel dilator excretion occurs even before serum creatinine levels begin to rise. The circulating concentrations of ANPs in chronic renal failure appear to reflect volume status (175, 214, 257, 366). Despite increased circulating ANPs in sodium-retaining disease states, the kidney retains sodium and is hyporesponsive to ANP, LANP, and BNP (35, 181, 251, 308, 326). The mechanism for the attenuated renal response to these natriuretic

peptides is multifactoral and includes renal hypoperfusion, activation of the renin-angiotensin-aldosterone and the sympathetic nervous systems (34, 125, 213).

Influence of Renal Failure on Other Natriuretic Peptides

Adrenomedullin (82, 274, 302), guanylin (169), and uroguanylin (168) increase in renal failure and/or nephrotic syndrome.

HEMODIALYSIS

ANPs

These peptides have been suggested as possible indicators of when to perform dialysis in persons with chronic renal failure (175, 214, 257, 276, 366). Other data, however, suggest that ANPs are not useful to predict when hemodialysis is necessary (29). Hemodialysis lowers the circulating concentration of ANP by 34%–42%, with the amount of decrease appearing to be related to volume status of the patients (175, 361, 366). Hemodialysis does not return the levels of ANP to those of healthy adults (175, 360, 361, 366), and it does not reduce circulating concentrations of vessel dilator and LANP (366). Part of the reason for the difference in hemodialysis effects on ANPs is that less than 1.5% of vessel dilator and LANP cross the dialysis membrane compared to 15% to 25% of ANP crossing hemodialysis membranes (366). Hemodialysis using cellulose-triacetate dialyzers reduces plasma levels of these peptides in ARF more than hemodialysis therapy with polysulfone dialyzers (90).

BNP

Hemodialysis has been reported both to lower (182) and have no effect on circulating BNP levels (49). Before dialysis in persons with chronic renal failure (CRF), plasma BNP levels have no relationship to serum creatinine or mean blood pressure (174). In CRF patients whose plasma BNP levels decrease with dialysis, this decrease correlates with the degree of postural blood pressure drop, but there is no correlation with the fall in serum creatinine (182). In none of the studies of BNP and dialysis (39, 55, 174, 182) has BNP ever returned to its circulating concentration to that of healthy individuals. With volume repletion after hemodialysis there is an exaggerated release of ANP but changes in BNP are small and without any correlation with either atrial or ventricular volume (55).

Adrenomedullin and Proadrenomedullin N-Terminal 20 Peptide

Both adrenomedullin and proadrenomedullin N-terminal 20 peptide (PAMP) increase in chronic renal failure (82, 274, 302). Hemodialysis decreases these peptides to near-control levels with PAMP being 2.17 ± 0.18 fmol/ml versus 1.64 ± 0.12 fmol/ml for controls (302). This is significantly different than for the ANPs as ANPs do not decrease to near that of healthy humans with hemodialysis (175, 360, 361, 366).

Guanylin and Uroguanylin

Both guanylin and uroguanylin are increased in persons with impaired renal function (168, 169). Hemodialysis with EVAL membranes decreases guanylin concentrations after 1 hour of dialysis but the plasma levels after hemodialysis with PC membranes show no change (169).

RENAL TRANSPLANTATION

Successful transplantation of functioning kidneys decreases the markedly elevated circulating levels of atrial natriuretic peptides in persons with ARF to those of healthy individuals (240, 252). Nonfunctioning renal allografts continue to have elevated circulating concentrations of atrial natriuretic peptides (240, 252). Post renal transplant, it takes 7 days for ANP and 10 days for vessel dilator to return to normal (240). This suggests that the allograft kidney does not fully function immediately with respect to clearing these peptides. The half-life of ANP in healthy persons is only 2.5–3.5 minutes (4, 313). If the transplanted kidneys began to function immediately, one would have expected the circulating concentration of ANP to have decreased to the normal range within 24 hours (360 half-lives). Vessel dilator has a 20-fold longer half-life compared to that of ANP (4, 313), which may explain why it takes 3 more days for this peptide hormone to normalize in the circulation after successful renal transplantation. If one gives ANP (via infusion) at the time of renal transplant this does not appear to have any beneficial effect on the outcome of the renal allograft (273). It is important to note that the elevated circulating ANPs in heart failure also normalize with successful heart transplantation (360).

PROTECTIVE AND THERAPEUTIC EFFECTS OF ATRIAL NATRIURETIC PEPTIDES IN ACUTE RENAL FAILURE

ANP and Urodilatin

Acute renal failure (ARF) develops in 2%–5% of all patients admitted to tertiary care hospitals (139, 367). The underlying cause is a renal insult (acute tubular necrosis) in 60% of the patients (139, 367). When dialysis was introduced in the mid-1940s, the mortality resulting from severe ARF was approximately 50% (139). This poor prognosis has not improved, with mortality now in the 40%–80% range in oliguric ARF (9, 31, 62, 138, 139, 277, 367). The occurrence of ARF in the hospital increases the

relative risk of dying by 6.2-fold and the length of hospitalization by 10 days (251).

Several of the atrial peptides have been investigated as possible treatment(s) of ARF. Atrial natriuretic peptide (ANP) had encouraging results in early studies of ARF in animals (54, 190). The infusion of ANP (54, 190, 200, 214, 216, 221, 230, 251, 277, 287) or urodilatin (210, 281, 288) in rat models of ischemic ARF-attenuated renal tissue damage and preserved glomerular filtration rate. Nakamoto et al. (217) and Shaw et al. (287) were able to shorten the course of renal artery cross-clamping–induced ARF in rats with ANP. Conger et al. (54) found marked improvement in GFR in a rat renal artery–clamp model when ANP-III (0.2 μg/kg/min) was given intravenously immediately after clamp release in combination with dopamine sufficient to maintain mean arterial pressure above 100 mm Hg. In the rat, ANP had no effect on GFR when given intravenously but did have a GFR effect when given directly into the renal artery for 4 hours (287). The inability of ANP to increase GFR when given intravenously could be restored if dopamine was given simultaneously (54). In the dog, the improvement in renal perfusion only lasted for a short period after 180-minute infusion of ANP (221). When ANP was given by intra-aortic bolus on days 1 and 2 after the above infusion there was not any significant improvement in renal perfusion on those days (221). Thus, in animals the improvement in renal failure with ANP was only of short duration and depended upon whether ANP was given intravenously or directly into the artery (54, 221, 287).

The administration of 0.2 μg of ANP/kg of body weight^{-1}/min^{-1} for 24 hours to humans with ARF, revealed that ANP did not cause significant improvement and did not reduce the need for dialysis or reduce mortality (7, 189). ANP infusions were associated with decreased survival in the nonoliguric ARF subjects (75% of subjects) (7). The usefulness of ANP for treatment is hampered by its short half-life of 2.5 minutes (4, 313) and by its very short duration of action (54, 190, 195, 201, 251, 329). Of 504 ARF patients treated with ANP, 46% developed hypotension, which would further limit its usefulness in ARF (7). Several of the atrial natriuretic peptides investigated to treat ARF have each resulted in severe hypotension and bradycardia (7, 167). In addition to ANP causing 46% of renal failure patients becoming hypotensive (7), urodilatin has also been associated with severe hypotension and bradycardia, when given as a potential treatment of congestive heart failure (167). ANP is now considered more harmful than helpful with respect to the treatment of acute renal failure (35). ANP has also been investigated in humans with chronic renal failure to determine if it could prevent radiocontrast-induced nephropathy, one cause of hospital-acquired acute renal failure (178). When ANP was given before and during radiocontrast study in 247 patients no beneficial effect was found (178). Urodilatin has been suggested as a possible treatment of renal failure (209, 281, 282) but in double-blind phase II trials in acute renal failure patients, urodilatin has been found to have no beneficial effect (210).

Vessel Dilator

Vessel dilator appears to be one of the ANPs with promising therapeutic potential in ARF. Vessel dilator ($0.3\ \mu g/kg^{-1}/min^{-1}$ via intraperitoneal pump) decreases blood urea nitrogen (BUN) and serum creatinine from 162 ± 4 mg/dl and 8.17 ± 0.5 mg/dl, respectively, to 53 ± 17 mg/dl and 0.98 ± 0.12 mg/dl in acute renal failure animals, where ARF was established for 2 days (after vascular clamping) before vessel dilator was given (51). At day 6 of ARF, mortality decreased to 14% with vessel dilator from 88% without vessel dilator (51). The ARF animals that did not receive vessel dilator had moderate (25%–75% of all tubules involved) to severe (>75% of all tubules necrotic) acute tubular necrosis by day 8 after their ischemic event (Fig. 7B). As shown in Fig. 7B, the tubules of these animals were almost completely destroyed. The destruction of the tubules included both the proximal and distal tubules with the proximal tubules being more severely affected (Fig. 7B). The glomerulus of the ARF animals was spared compared to the renal tubules with glomerulus appearing to be normal in the ARF animals (Fig. 7A and B).

The addition of vessel dilator after renal failure had been present for 2 days resulted in a marked improvement in the renal histology (Fig. 7C) with scores ranging from 0 (no tubular necrosis) to 1+ (<5% of the tubules involved) (51). When the kidneys were examined at day 8 of renal failure, the brush borders of the proximal tubules of the ARF animals treated with vessel dilator were present (Fig. 7C), which was similar to the proximal tubules of healthy animals (Fig. 7A). In the ARF animals not treated with vessel dilator, the brush borders of the tubules were destroyed (Fig. 7B). The glomeruli of vessel dilator-treated ARF animals also appeared normal (Fig. 7C). It should be pointed out that the animals treated with vessel dilator did have severe renal failure before vessel dilator was begun on the second day of renal failure (51). It is important to note that the animals treated with vessel dilator who had a significant increase in survival had nonoliguric renal failure (51). As noted previously, nonoliguric renal failure subjects treated with ANP had a decreased survival and it was the nonoliguric renal failure subjects who did not respond to ANP (7). Vessel dilator, LANP, and kaliuretic peptide, as opposed to ANP, BNP, and urodilatin, have never caused a hypotensive episode when given to either healthy animals or humans (201, 328, 329) or when given to humans with sodium and water retention (219, 326, 327).

The ability of vessel dilator to reverse ischemic ARF is consistent with the important concept, based upon experiments at cellular level and in humans with acute tubular necrosis (ATN), that the pathophysiology of ischemic ARF is due to a sublethal and reversible injury to renal tubular cells (31,

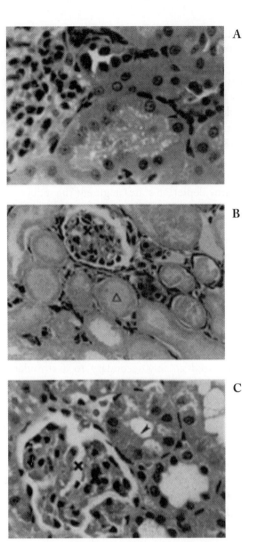

FIGURE 7 Renal histology of healthy Sprague–Dawley rat (**A**) with intact proximal tubular brush border (*arrowhead*). **B:** ARF rat at day 8 with marked tubular necrosis (*open triangle*) and without intact brush border present (>75% of tubules are necrotic). The glomerulus (x) appears to be normal. **C:** ARF rat treated with vessel dilator from days 2 to 5 of ARF with kidney examined after day 8 of ARF reveals brush border to be present in proximal tubule (*arrowhead*). No tubules are necrotic in this ARF animal treated with vessel dilator. The glomerulus (x) is intact. Magnification of hematoxylin and eosin: x426 (A and C) and x320 (B). ARF, acute renal failure. (With permission, from Clark LC, Farghaly H, Saba SR, Vesely DL. Amelioration with vessel dilator of acute tubular necrosis and renal failure established for 2 days. *Am J Physiol* 2000;278:H1555–H1564.)

212). This reversible injury is now thought to contribute more predominately to renal tubular dysfunction than permanent tubular cell necrosis (31, 212). There are pathology similarities between humans and rats with ischemic ATN; in humans, the majority of the injury is to the proximal tubule brush border with predilection for the most severe injury to occur in the proximal straight (S_3 segments) tubules (31, 212). As outlined earlier, it was mainly the proximal tubule brush borders that were regenerated by vessel dilator even when given 2 days after ischemic ATN (51). Part of the improvement by vessel dilator may be due to its ability to cause intrarenal vasodilation as it is a strong vasodilator (335). The reason why vessel dilator has greater beneficial effects than ANP, BNP, CNP, and urodilatin in acute renal failure appears due, at least in part, to its ability to cause the endogenous synthesis of renoprotective prostaglandin E2 (PGE2) which ANP, BNP, CNP, and urodilatin do not do (48, 124).

Prostaglandins have renoprotective effects in ARF (6, 164, 358). An indication that PGE2 is renoprotective (by maintaining glomerular hemodynamics) is the observation that cyclooxygenase inhibitors in congestive heart failure and volume depletion states augment the reduction in RBF and GFR (84, 355). With respect to the mechanism of prostaglandins' protective effects in ARF, there is a dramatic decrease with prostaglandins in the outer medulla perfusion following ischemic injury (162), a region of renal tissue which normally operates "on the verge of ischemia" (36). Prostaglandins have a favorable effect on blood flow distribution to this region (215). In addition, prostaglandins have distinct cytoprotective effects and improve microvascular permeability in ischemic ARF (40, 164). Prostaglandins are not stored in the kidney but rather have to be synthesized acutely secondary to a stimulating agent such as vessel dilator (48, 124) in order for prostaglandins to have a positive beneficial effect in renal failure.

Adrenomedullin

There is evidence that ADM is renoprotective in Dahl salt-sensitive rats in that when perfused for 7 days, the glomerular injury score is 54% less ($p < .05$) than in untreated Dahl salt-sensitive rats (224). The adrenomedullin treated salt-sensitive rats, however, had considerably more ($p < .01$) glomerular sclerosis and anteriolar sclerosis and atrophic tubules after treatment than the control Dahl salt-resistant rats (224).

BNP

BNP has not been investigated as a treatment of acute renal failure but one would expect that BNP, similar to ANP, will have blunted or no effects in ARF compared to its effects in healthy animals (7, 189, 221).

CNP

CNP increases in the circulation in ARF (42) but its effects in acute renal failure are unknown. As discussed above, CNP has no natriuretic effects in healthy humans (21, 44, 146).

DNP

DNP has been evaluated in persons with end-stage renal disease on dialysis and was found not to correlate ($p = .62$) with echocardiographic left ventricular mass index (LVMI), while ANP and BNP did correlate with LVMI of these end-

stage renal patients (41). DNP has not been investigated with respect to its possible therapeutic effects in renal failure.

TREATMENT OF OTHER DISEASES WITH ABNORMAL BLOOD VOLUME

Congestive Heart Failure

As part of the adaptive response to the pathophysiology of congestive heart failure, atrial natriuretic peptides increase in circulation (32, 38, 95, 160, 161, 315, 326, 327, 362). This knowledge has suggested that several of the atrial natriuretic peptides may be useful in the treatment of congestive heart failure (326, 327). The rationale for treatment of the pathophysiology of CHF with atrial peptides (which are already increased in the circulation) is based upon other hormonal systems where if one gives pharmacological rather physiological concentrations of a hormone one often can overcome a defect in the target organ with respect to a particular hormone. In congestive heart failure, the pathophysiology with respect to atrial natriuretic peptides appears to be in the target organ(s)—the kidney has a diminished response to some of the atrial peptides—rather than the heart not producing enough of the respective hormones (313). As outlined previously, the heart actually produces more of these peptide hormones (i.e., the heart does not have a defect in the production of these hormones) in persons with CHF compared to healthy individuals (78, 246, 306). When ANP was investigated for possible treatment of CHF pathophysiology, it was found to have a markedly attenuated natriuretic response (53, 92, 285). The development of edema in nephrotic syndrome has also been suggested to be due to primarily sodium retention secondary to tubular resistance to the natriuretic effect of ANP (231). High-dose administration of ANP produces little or no diuresis or natriuresis in humans with CHF (53). Synthetic brain natriuretic peptide (Nesteride®) in CHF individuals causes a small increase in urine volume (90 ± 38 vs 67 ± 27 ml/hr) (198). Further evaluation indicated that there is no significant natriuresis (3) or diuresis (150, 211) with Nesteride infusion in humans with CHF. In CHF animals, BNP has had no significant natriuretic or diuretic effects (181). BNP can cause significant hypotension, however, in CHF subjects (3, 211) with an incidence of 27% reported with 0.06 µg/kg/min dose (211). Urodilatin infusion in CHF animals, likewise, causes significantly less natriuresis and diuresis compared to healthy animals (1).

One of the other cardiac peptide hormones (vessel dilator), on the other hand, when given intravenously for 60 minutes to NYHA Class III CHF subjects, increases urine flow two- to 13-fold, which is still increased 3 hours after its infusion is stopped (327). In CHF subjects, vessel dilator infusion enhances sodium excretion levels three- to four-fold, and the fractional excretion of sodium (FE_{Na}) sixfold, which are still significantly ($p < .01$) elevated 3 hours later (327). Vessel dilator simultaneously decreases systemic vascular resistance 24%, pulmonary vascular resistance 25%, pulmonary capillary wedge pressure 33%, and central venous pressure 27%, while simultaneously increasing cardiac output 34%, cardiac index 35%, and stroke volume index 24% in individuals with CHF (327). There were no side effects with infusion of vessel dilator in CHF subjects (327). The natriuretic and diuretic effects of vessel dilator to help reverse the pathophysiology of CHF are as potent (not decreased or blunted) in persons with CHF as those observed in healthy persons (327). The ability of vessel dilator to retain its beneficial effects in persons with CHF while the effects of ANP and BNP become blunted appears to be due to the ability of vessel dilator to enhance prostaglandin E2 synthesis in the kidney, which, in turn, inhibits renal Na$^+$,K$^+$-ATPase, resulting in a natriuresis (48, 124). ANP does not enhance the synthesis of prostaglandin E2 or inhibit renal Na$^+$,K$^+$-ATPase (48, 124, 245).

Long-acting natriuretic peptide (LANP) maximally increases urine flow and natriuresis only twofold in persons with CHF (326) compared to four- to fivefold increase in urine flow and three- to eightfold increase in natriuresis in healthy individuals (329). Thus, long-acting effects of natriuretic peptide, like effects of atrial natriuretic peptide in CHF individuals, are blunted compared to effects in healthy individuals (326).

ANTIPROLIFERATIVE AND ANTICANCER PROPERTIES OF ATRIAL NATRIURETIC PEPTIDES

In blood vessels, ANP inhibits smooth muscle cell proliferation (hyperplasia) as well as smooth muscle cell growth (hypertrophy) (2, 147, 148, 374). Atrial natriuretic peptide has growth-regulatory properties in a variety of other tissues including brain, bone, myocytes, red blood cell precursors, and endothelial cells (10, 11, 128, 153, 236, 374). In the kidney, ANP causes antimitogenic and antiproliferative effects in glomerular mesangial cells via inhibiting DNA synthesis (10, 11, 153). The newest discovered property of the ANPs is their ability to inhibit the growth of cancers in vitro and in vivo (310, 311, 324). The first cancer studied both in vitro and in vivo was human pancreatic adenocarcinomas, which have the lowest 5-year survival rate of all common cancers (242, 368). The 5-year survival rate of persons with adenocarcinoma of the pancreas is 1% (242, 368). The median survival is 4 months (242, 368). Current cancer chemotherapy and surgery prolong survival by a few months but the abovementioned survival rates are for persons treated with surgery and/or currently available cancer chemotherapeutic agents (242, 368). Vessel dilator, LANP, kaliuretic peptide, and ANP decrease the number of human pancreatic adenocarcinoma cells in culture by 65%, 47%, 37%, and 34%, respectively, within 24 hours (310). This decrease was sustained without any proliferation of the ad-

enocarcinoma cells occurring in the 3 days following this decrease in number (310). The mechanism resulting in declining cancer cell numbers and antiproliferative effects was an 83% or greater inhibition of DNA synthesis that was not due to enhanced apoptosis (310). Cyclic GMP, one of the known mediators of these peptide hormone mechanism(s) of action, inhibited DNA synthesis in these adenocarcinoma cells by 51%. There was no cytotoxicity to normal cells in these studies (310). Atrial natriuretic peptide has also been reported to reduce the number of hepatoblastoma cells in culture (258).

In vivo, the effects of these peptide hormones as anticancer agents were even more impressive. Vessel dilator (139 ng min^{-1}kg^{-1} of body weight) infused subcutaneously for 14 days completely stopped the growth of human pancreatic adenocarcinomas in athymic mice ($n = 14$) with a decrease in their tumor volume, while the tumor volume increased 69-fold ($p < .001$) in the placebo ($n = 30$)-treated mice (324). When these peptide hormones (each at 1.4 μg min^{-1} kg^{-1} body weight) were infused for 4 weeks, in addition to completely stopping the growth of this aggressive adenocarcinoma, vessel dilator, long-acting natriuretic peptide and kaliuretic peptide decreased human pancreatic adenocarcinoma tumor volume after 1 week by 49%, 28%, and 11%, respectively, with a one- and 20-fold increase in the tumor volume in ANP- and placebo-treated mice (324). Cyclic GMP (2.4 μg min^{-1} kg^{-1} body weight) inhibited after 1 week the growth of this cancer 95% (324).

These four peptide hormones cause a similar decrease in the number of breast adenocarcinoma (311), small-cell lung carcinoma, and squamous-cell lung cancer cells. Within 24 hours, vessel dilator, LANP, kaliuretic peptide, ANP and 8-bromo-cyclic GMP, the cell-permeable analogue of their intracellular mediator cyclic GMP (each at 1 μM), decreased the number of human breast adenocarcinoma cells 60%, 31%, 27%, 40%, and 31%, respectively (311). There was no proliferation in the 3 days following this decrease in breast adenocarcinoma cell number. These same hormones decreased DNA synthesis 69% to 85% in the breast adenocarcinoma cells ($p < .001$). Brain natriuretic peptide and CNP did not decrease the number of breast adenocarcinoma cells or inhibit their DNA synthesis (311).

Cell-cycle progression was directly affected by several of the natriuretic peptides. The majority of the natriuretic peptides had their strongest modification of cell-cycle progression in the synthetic (S) phase of the cell cycle (311). Vessel dilator, long-acting natriuretic peptide, kaliuretic peptide and 8-bromo-cyclic GMP (each at 1 μM) decreased the number of breast cancer cells in the S phase of the cell cycle by 62%, 33%, 50%, and 39%, respectively (all $p < .05$) (311). ANP caused a 40% decrease in the G2-M proliferative phase the cell cycle (311). There was an accumulation of cells in the G0-G1 phase secondary to LANP, vessel dilator, kaliuretic peptide and ANP (311). Vessel dilator, which caused the largest decrease in cells in the S phase, had the largest accumulation of cells in the G0–G1 phase (311).

BNP had no effect on the S phase or any other portion of the cell cycle (311). Western blots revealed that NPR-A and -C receptors were present in the human breast adenocarcinoma cells (311). These peptide hormones anticancer effects in kidney tumors are currently being evaluated.

SUMMARY AND FUTURE DIRECTIONS

Atrial natriuretic peptides are both synthesized in the kidney (117, 246, 303) and have some of their most potent biologic effects, such as natriuresis and diuresis, in the kidney (24, 27, 73, 124, 126, 201, 350, 376). Vessel dilator via its ability to ameliorate acute renal failure and enhance tubule regeneration in acute tubular necrosis (51) may prove useful in the future for the treatment of acute renal failure. BNP and adrenomedullin with their effects in glomerular hypertrophy (163) and glomerular injury (224), respectively, may be useful for the treatment of renal glomerular diseases. Since BNP, ANP, and adrenomedullin do not appear to help tubular diseases such as acute tubular necrosis, the major cause of acute renal failure (139, 367), their therapeutic potential in acute tubular necrosis appears limited. Future studies with these peptide hormones in humans with acute renal failure and/or glomerular diseases are necessary to determine whether the findings in animal models of ARF are applicable to the treatment of humans with acute renal failure.

References

1. Abassi ZA, Powell JR, Golomb E, Keiser HR. Renal and systemic effects of urodilatin in rats with high-output heart failure. *Am J Physiol* 1992;262:F615–F621.
2. Abell TJ, Richards AM, Ikram H, Espiner EA, Yandle T. Atrial natriuretic factor inhibits proliferation of vascular smooth muscle cells stimulated by platelet derived growth factor. *Biochem Biophys Res Commun* 1989;160:1392–1396.
3. Abraham WT, Lowes BD, Ferguson DA, Odom J, Kim JK, Robertson AD, et al. Systemic hemodynamic, neurohormonal, and renal effects of a steady-state infusion of human brain natriuretic peptie in patients with hemodynamically decompensated heart failure. *J Card Fail* 1998;4:37–44.
4. Ackerman BH, Overton RM, McCormick MT, Schocken DD, Vesely DL. Disposition of vessel dilator and long-acting natriuretic peptide in healthy humans after a one-hour infusion. *J Pharmacol Exp Therap* 1997;282:603–608.
5. Ackermann U, Irizawa TG, Milojevie S, Sonnennberg H. Cardiovascular effects of atrial extracts in anesthetized rats. *Can J Physiol Pharmacol* 1984;62:819–826.
6. Agmon Y, Peleg H, Greenfeld Z, Rosen S, Brezis M. Nitric oxide and prostanoids protect the renal outer medulla from radiocontrast toxicity in the rat. *J Clin Invest* 1994;94:1069–1075.
7. Allgren RL, Marbury TC, Rahman SN, Weisberg LS, Fenves AZ, Lafayette RA, et al. Anaritide in acute tubular necrosis. *N Engl J Med* 1997;336:828–834.
8. Anderson JV, Donckier J, Payne NN, Beacham H, Stater JDH, Bloom SR. Atrial natriuretic peptide: evidence as a natriuretic hormone at physiological plasma concentrations in man. *Clin Sci* 1987;72:305–312.
9. Anderson RJ, Schrier RW. Acute renal failure. In: Schrier RW, ed. *Diseases of the Kidney and Urinary Tract*, 7th ed. Philadelphia: Lippincott, Williams & Wilkins; 2001:1093–1136.
10. Appel RG. Growth inhibitory activity of atrial natriuretic factor in rat glomerular mesangial cells. *FEBS Lett* 1988;238:135–138.
11. Appel RG. Growth-regulatory properties of atrial natriuretic factor. *Am J Physiol* 1992;262:F911–F918.
12. Arendt R, Gerbes A, Ritter D, Stangl E, Bach P, Zahringer J. Atrial natriuretic factors in plasma of patients with arterial hypertension, heart failure or cirrhosis of the liver. *J Hypertens* 1986;4(Suppl 2):131–135.
13. Argentin S, Drouin J, Nemer M. Thyroid hormone stimulates rat pro-natriodilatin mRNA levels in primary cardiocyte cultures. *Biochem Biophys Res Commun* 1987;146:1336–1341.
14. Atarashi K, Mulrow PJ, Franco-Saenz R, Snajdar R, Rapp J. Inhibition of aldosterone production by an atrial extract. *Science* 1984;224:992–994.
15. Atlas SA, Kleinert HD, Camargo MJ, Januszewicz A, Sealey JE, Laragh JH, et al. Purification, sequencing and synthesis of natriuretic and vasoactive rat atrial peptide. *Nature* 1984;309:717–719.

16. Baeyens DA, Price E, Winters CJ, Vesely DL. Diving increases atrial natriuretic factor-like peptide in fresh water diving turtles. *Comp Physiol Biochem* 1989;94A:515–518.
17. Baeyens DA, Walters JM, Vesely DL. Atrial Natriuretic factor increases the magnitude of duodenal spontaneous phasic contractions. *Biochem Biophys Res Commun* 1988;155:1437–1443.
18. Baker BJ, Wu WL, Winters CJ, Dinh H, Wyeth R, Sallman AL, et al. Exercise increases the circulating concentration of the N-terminus of the atrial natriuretic factor prohormone in normal humans. *Am Heart J* 1991;122:1395–1402.
19. Ballerman BJ, Bloch KD, Seidman JG, Brenner BM. Atrial natriuretic peptide transcription, secretion and glomerular receptor activity during mineralocorticoid escape in the rat. *J Clin Invest* 1986;78:840–843.
20. Banting FG, Best CH. The internal secretion of the pancreas. *J Lab Clin Med* 1922;7:251–261
21. Barletta G, Lazzeri C, Vecchiarino S, Del Bene R, Messeri G, Dello Sbarba A, et al. Low-dose C-type natriuretic peptide does not affect cardiac and renal function in humans. *Hypertension* 1988;31:802–808.
22. Barr CS, Rhodes P, Struthers AD. C-type natriuretic peptide. *Peptides* 1996;17:1243–1251.
23. Beltowski J, Wojcicka G. Regulation of renal tubular transport by cardiac natriuretic peptides: two decades of research. *Med Sci Monit* 2002;8:RA39–RA52.
24. Benjamin BA, Peterson TV. Effects of proANF-(31-67) on sodium excretion in conscious monkeys. *Am J Physiol Regul Integr Comp Physiol* 1995;269:R1351–R1355.
25. Benoist C, Chambon P. In vivo sequence requirements of the SV40 early promoter region. *Nature* 1981;290:304–310.
26. Bhalla SS, Robitaille L, Nemer M. Cooperative activation by GATA-4 and YY1 of the cardiac B-type natriuretic peptide promoter. *J Biol Chem* 2001;276:11439–11445.
27. Bloch KD, Scott JA, Zisfein JB, Fallon JT, Margolis NN, Seidman CE, et al. Biosynthesis and secretion of proatrial natriuretic factor by cultured rat cardiocytes. *Science* 1985;230:1168–1171.
28. Bompiani GD, Rouiller CH, Hatt PY. Le tissue de conduction du coeur chez le rat. Etude au microscope electronique. I. Le tronc commun du faisceau de His et les cellules claires de L'oreillette droite. *Arch Mal Coeur* 1959;52:1257–1274.
29. Borst JGG. The maintenance of an adequate cardiac output by the regulation of the urinary excretion of water and sodium chloride; an essential factor in the genesis of edema. *Acta Med Scand* 1948;130(Suppl 207):1–71.
30. Bovy PR, O'Neal JM, Olins GM, Patton DR, Mehta PP, McMahon EG, et al. A synthetic linear decapeptide binds to the atrial natriuretic peptide receptors and demonstrates cyclase activation and vasorelaxant activity. *J Biol Chem* 1989;264:20309–20313.
31. Brady HR, Brenner BM, Clarkson MR, Lieberthal W. Acute renal failure. In: Brenner M, ed. *Brenner & Rector's The Kidney*, 6th ed. Philadelphia: WB Saunders; 2000:1201–1262.
32. Brandt RB, Redfield MM, Aarhus LL, Lewicki JA, Burnett JC Jr. Clearance receptor-mediated control of atrial natriuretic factor in experimental congestive heart failure. *Am J Physiol* 1994;266:R936–R943.
33. Breathnach R, Chambon P. Organization and expression of eukaryotic split genes coding for proteins. *Am Rev Biochem* 1981;50:349–383.
34. Brenner BM, Ballermann BJ, Gunning ME, Zeidel ML. Diverse biological actions of atrial natriuretic peptide. *Physiol Rev* 1990;70:665–699.
35. Brenner RM, Chertow GM. The rise and fall of atrial natriuretic peptide for acute renal failure. *Curr Opin Nephrol Hypertens* 1997;6:474–476.
36. Brezis M, Rosen S, Silva P, Epstein FH. Renal ischemia: a new perspective. *Kidney Int* 1984;26:375–383.
37. Bricker NS, Klahr S, Purkerson M, Schultze RG, Avioli LV, Binge SJ. In vitro assay for a humoral substance present during volume expansion and uremia. *Nature* 1968;219:1058–1059.
38. Buckley MG, Sethi D, Markandu ND, Sagnella GA, Singer, DR, MacGregor GA. Plasma concentrations and comparisons of brain natriuretic peptide and atrial natriuretic peptide in normal subjects, cardiac transplant recipients and patients with dialysis-independent or dialysis-dependent chronic renal failure. *Clin Sci* 1992;83:437–444.
39. Burnett JC Jr, Granger JP, Opgenorth TJ. Effects of synthetic atrial natriuretic factor on renal function and renin release. *Am J Physiol* 1984;247:F863–F866.
40. Casey KF, Machiedo GW, Lyons MJ, Slotman GJ, Novak RT. Alteration of postischemic renal pathology by prostaglandin infusion. *J Surg Res* 1980;29:1–10.
41. Cataliotti A, Malatino LS, Jougasaki M, Zoccali C, Castellino P, Giacone G, et al. Circulating natriuretic peptide concentrations in patients with end-state renal disease: role of brain natriuretic peptide as a biomarker for ventricular remodeling. *Mayo Clin Proc* 2001;76:1111–1119.
42. Charron F, Paradis P, Bronchain O, Nemer G, Nemer M. Cooperative interaction between GATA-4 and GATA-6 regulates myocardial gene expression. *Mol Cell Biol* 1999:19:4355–4365.
43. Chartier L, Schiffrin E, Thibault G. Effect of atrial natriuretic factor (ANF)-related peptides on aldosterone secretion by adrenal glomerulosa cells: critical role of the intramolecular disulphide bond. *Biochem Biophys Res Commun* 1984;122:171–174.
44. Chauhan SD, Nilsson H, Ahluwalia A, Hobbs AJ. Release of C-type natriuretic peptide accounts for the biological activity of endothelium-derived hyperpolarizing factor. *Proc Natl Acad Sci U S A* 2003;100:1426–1431.
45. Chen JH, Tsai JH, Lai YH, Hwang SJ. Plasma atrial natriuretic peptide in patients with chronic renal failure. *J Formos Med Assoc* 1990;89:645–650.
46. Chen XW, Ying WZ, Valentin JP, Ling KT, Lin SY, Wiedemann E, et al. Mechanism of the natriuretic action of γ-melanocyte-stimulating hormone. *Am J Physiol* 1997;272:R1946–R1953.
47. Chinkers M, Garbers DL, Chang MS, Lowe DG, Chin HM, Goeddel DV, et al. A membrane form of guanylate cyclase is an atrial natriuretic peptide receptor. *Nature* 1989;338:78–83.
48. Chiou S, Vesely DL. Kaliuretic peptide: The most potent inhibitor of Na^+-K^+-ATPase of the atrial natriuretic peptides. *Endocrinology* 1995;136:2033–2039.
49. Christoffensen C, Goetz JP, Bartles ED, Larsen MD, Ribel U, Rehfeld JF, et al. Chamber-dependent expression of brain natriuretic peptide and its mRNA in normal and diabetic pig heart. *Hypertension* 2002;40:54–60.
50. Chun TH, Itoh H, Ogawa Y, Tamura N, Takaya K, Igaki T, et al. Shear stress augments expression of C-type natriuretic peptide and adrenomedullin. *Hypertension* 1997;29:1296–1302.

51. Clark LC, Farghaly H, Saba SR, Vesely DL. Amelioration with vessel dilator of acute tubular necrosis and renal failure established for 2 days. *Am J Physiol* 2000;278:H1555–H1564.
52. Clavell AL, Stingo AJ, Wei CM, Heublein DM, Burnett JC Jr. C-type natriuretic peptide: a selective cardiovascular peptide. *Am J Physiol* 1993;264:R290–R295.
53. Cody RJ, Atlas SA, Laragh JH, Kubo SH, Covit AB, Ryman KS, et al. Atrial natriuretic factor in normal subjects and heart failure patients: plasma levels and renal, hormonal, and hemodynamic responses to peptide infusion. *J Clin Invest* 1986;78:1362–1374.
54. Conger JD, Falk SA, Yuan BH, Schrier RW. Atrial natriuretic peptide and dopamine in a rat model of ischemic acute renal failure. *Kidney Int* 1989;35:1126–1132.
55. Corboy JC, Walker RJ, Simmonds MB, Wilkins GT, Richards AM, Espiner EA. Plasma natriuretic peptides and cardiac volume during acute changes in intravascular volume in haemodialysis patients. *Clin Sci* 1994;87:679–684.
56. Cousins KL, Farrell AP, Sweeting RM, Vesely DL, Keen JE. Release of atrial natriuretic factor prohormone peptides 1-30, 31-67, and 99-126 from fresh-water and sea-water acclimated perfused trout (*Oncorhynchus mykiss*) hearts. *J Exp Biol* 1997;200:1351–1362.
57. Crawford I, Maloney PC, Zeitlin PL, Guggino WB, Hyde SC, Turley H, et al. Immunocytochemical localization of the cystic fibrosis gene product CFTR. *Proc Natl Acad Sci U S A* 1991;88:9262–9266.
58. Currie MG, Fok KF, Kato J, Moore RJ, Hamra FK, Duffin KL, et al. Guanylin: an endogenous activator of intestinal guanylate cyclase. *Proc Natl Acad Sci U S A* 1992;89:947–951.
59. Currie MG, Geller DM, Cole BR, Boylan JG, Sheng W Yu, Holmberg SW, et al. Bioactive cardiac substances: potent vasorelaxant activity in mammalian atria. *Science* 1983;221:71–73.
60. Currie MG, Geller DM, Cole BR, Siegel NR, Fox KF, Adams SP, et al. Purification and sequence analysis of bioactive atrial peptides. *Science* 1984;223:67–69.
61. Dagnino L, Lavigne JP, Nemer M. Increased transcripts for B-type natriuretic peptide in spontaneously hypertensive rats: quantitative polymerase chain reaction for atrial and brain natriuretic peptide transcripts. *Hypertension* 1992;20:690–700.
62. Davidman M, Olson P, Kohen J, Leither T, Kjellstrand C. Iatrogenic renal disease. *Arch Intern Med* 1991;151:1809–1812.
63. Debold AJ. Heart atria granularity effects changes in water-electrolyte balance. *Proc Soc Exp Biol Med* 1979;161:508–511.
64. Debold AJ, Borenstein HB, Veress AT, Sonnenberg H. A rapid and potent natriuretic response to intravenous injections of atrial myocardial extracts in rats. *Life Sci* 1981;28:89–94.
65. DeBold AJ, Salerno TA. Natriuretic activity of extracts obtained from hearts of different species and from various rat tissues. *Can J Physiol Pharmacol* 1983;61:127–130.
66. De Lean A, Gutkowska J, McNicoll N, Schiller PW, Cantin M, Genest J. Characterization of specific receptors for atrial natriuretic factor in bovine adrenal zona glomerulosa. *Life Sci* 1984;35:2311–2318.
67. De Palo EF, Woloszczuk W, Meneghetti M, DePalo CB, Nielsen HB, Secher NH. Circulating immunoreactive proANP (1-30) and proANP (31-67) in sedentary subjects and athletes. *Clin Chem* 2000;46:843–847.
68. de Wardener HE, Mills IH, Clapham WF, Hayter CJ. Studies on the efferent mechanism of sodium diuresis which follows administration of intravenous saline in the dog. *Clin Sci* 1961; 21:249–258.
69. Dietz JR. Release of natriuretic factor from rat heart–lung preparation by atrial distension. *Am J Physiol* 1984;247:R1093–R1096.
70. Dietz JR, Landon CS, Nazian SJ, Vesely DL, Gower WR Jr. Effects of cardiac hormones on arterial pressure and sodium excretion in NPRa knockout mice. *Exp Biol Med* 2004;229: 813–818.
71. Dietz JR, Nazian SJ, Vesely DL. Release of ANF, proANF 1-98, and proANF 31-67 from isolated rat atria by atrial distention. *Am J Physiol* 1991;260:H1774–H1778.
72. Dietz JR, Scott DY, Landon CS, Nazian SJ. Evidence supporting a physiological role for pro ANP (1-30) in the regulation of renal excretion. *Am J Physiol* 2001;280:R1510–R1517.
73. Dietz JR, Vesely DL, Gower WR Jr, Nazian SJ. Secretion and renal effects of ANF prohormone peptides. *Clin Exp Pharmacol Physiol* 1995;22:115–120.
74. Dietz JR, Vesely DL, Gower WR Jr, Landon CS, Lee S, Nazian SJ. Neutralization of proANP 1-30 exacerbates hypertension in spontaneously hypertensive rat (SHR). *Clin Exp Pharm Physiol* 2003;30:627–631.
75. Dietz JR, Vesely DL, Nazian SJ. The effect of changes in sodium intake on atrial natriuretic factor (ANF) and peptides derived from the N-terminus of the ANF prohormone in the rat. *Proc Soc Exp Biol Med* 1992;200:44–48.
76. Dillingham MA, Anderson RJ. Inhibition of vasopressin action by atrial natriuretic factor. *Science* 1986;250:F963–F966.
77. Drewett JG, Garbers DL. The family of guanylyl cyclase receptors and their ligands. *Endocr Rev* 1994;15:135–162.
78. Edwards BS, Ackerman DM, Lee ME, Reeder GS, Wold LE, Burnett JC. Identification of atrial natriuretic factor within ventricular tissue in hamsters and humans with congestive heart failure. *J Clin Invest* 1988;81:82–86.
79. Ehrenreich H, Sinowatz R, Schulz RM, Arendt RM, Goebel FD. Immunoreactive atrial natriuretic peptide (ANP) in endoscopic biopsies of human gastrointestinal tract. *Res Exp Med* 1989;189:421–425.
80. Elsner D, Muders F, Muntze A, Kromer EP, Forssmann WG, Riegger G. Efficacy of prolonged infusion of urodilatin [ANP 95-126] in patients with congestive heart failure. *Am Heart J* 1995;129:766–773.
81. Entzeroth M, Doods HN, Wieland HA, Wiene W. Adrenomedullin mediates vasodilation via CGRP1 receptors. *Life Sci* 1995;56:PL19–25.
82. Eto T, Washimine H, Kato J, Kitamura K, Yamamoto Y. Adrenomedullin and proadrenalmedullin N-terminal 20 peptide in impaired renal function. *Kidney Int Suppl* 1996;55: S148–S149.
83. Fan X, Hamra FK, Freeman RH, Eber SL, Krause WJ, Lin RW, et al. Uroguanylin: cloning of preprouroguanylin cDNA, mRNA expression in the intestine and heart and isolation of uroguanylin and prouroguanylin from plasma. *Biochem Biophys Res Commun* 1996;219:457–462.
84. Fink MP, Mac Vittie TJ, Casey LC. Effects of nonsteroidal anti-inflammatory drugs on renal function in septic dogs. *J Surg Res* 1984;36:516–525.
85. Flynn TG. Past and current perspectives on the natriuretic peptides. *Proc Soc Exp Biol Med* 1996;98–104.
86. Flynn TG, deBold ML, deBold AJ. The amino acid sequence of an atrial peptide with potent diuretic and natriuretic properties. *Biochem Biophys Res Commun* 1983;117:859–865.
87. Forte LR. Uroguanylin: cloning of preprouroguanylin cDNA, mRNA expression in intestine and heart and isolation of uroguanylin and prouroguanylin from plasma. *Biochem Biophys Res Commun* 1996;219:457–462.
88. Forte LR, Fan S, Hamra FK. Salt and water homeostasis: uroguanylin is a circulating peptide hormone with natriuretic activity. *Am J Kidney Dis* 1996;28:296–304.
89. Forte LR, Krause WJ, Freeman RH. *Escherichia coli* enterotoxin receptors: localization in opossum kidney, intestine, and testis. *Am J Physiol* 1989;257:F874–F881.
90. Franz M, Woloszczuk W, Horl WH. N-terminal fragments of the proatrial natriuretic peptide in patients before and after hemodialysis treatment. *Kidney Int* 2000;58:374–378.
91. Franz M, Woloszczuk W, Horl WH. Plasma concentration and urinary excretion of N-terminal proatrial natriuretic peptides in patients with kidney diseases. *Kidney Int* 2001;59:1928–1934.
92. Freeman RH, David JO, Vari RC. Renal response to atrial natriuretic factor in conscious dogs with caval constriction. *Am J Physiol* 1985;248:R495–R500.
93. Freid TA, Osgood RW, Stein JH. Tubular site(s) of action of atrial natriuretic peptide in rat. *Am J Physiol* 1988;255:F313–F316.
94. Fukioka S, Tamaki T, Fukui K, Ikahara T, Abe Y. Effects of a synthetic human atrial natriuretic polypeptide on regional blood flow in rats. *Eur J Pharmacol* 1985;109:301–304.
95. Fyhrquist F, Tikkanen I, Totterman KJ, Hynynen M, Tikkanen T, Andersson S. Plasma atrial natriuretic peptide in health and disease. *Eur Heart J* 1987;8(Suppl B):117–122.
96. Garcia NH, Garvin JL. ANF and angiotensin II interact via kinases in the proximal straight tubule. *Am J Physiol* 1995;268:F730–F735.
97. Garcia R, Cantin M, Thibault G, Ong H, Genest J. Relationship of specific granules to the natriuretic and diuretic activity of rat atria. *Experientia* 1982;38:1071–1073.
98. Garcia R, Thibault G, Cantin M, Genest J. Effect of a purified atrial natriuretic factor on rat and rabbit vascular strips and vascular beds. *Am J Physiol* 1984;247:R34–R39.
99. Garcia R, Thibault G, Nutt RF, Cantin M, Genest J. Comparative vasoactive effects of native and synthetic atrial natriuretic factor (ANF). *Biochem Biophys Res Commun* 1984;119:685–688.
100. Gardner DG. Natriuretic peptides: markers or modulators of cardiac hypertrophy. *Trends Endo Metab* 2003;14:411–416.
101. Gardner DG, Deschepper CT, Ganong WF, Hane S, Fiddes J, Baxter JD, et al. Extra-atrial expression of the gene for atrial natriuretic factor. *Proc Natl Acad Sci U S A* 1986;83:6697–6701.
102. Gardner DG, Gertz BJ, Deschepper CF, Kim DY. Gene for the rat atrial natriuretic peptide is regulated by glucocorticoids in vitro. *J Clin Invest* 1988;82:1275–1281.
103. Gardner DG, Kovacic-Milivojevic BK, Garmai M. Molecular biology of the natriuretic peptides. In: Vesely DL, ed. *Atrial Natriuretic Peptides.* Trivandrum, India: Research Signpost; 1997:15–38.
104. Gauer OH, Henry JP, Seiker HO. Cardiac receptors and fluid volume control. *Progr Cardiovasc Dis* 1961;4:1–26.
105. Gauer OH, Henry JP. Criculatory basis of fluid volume control. *Physiol Rev* 1963;43:423–481.
106. Geller DM, Currie MG, Siegel NR, Fok KF, Adams SP, Needleman P. The sequence of an atriopeptigen: a precursor of the bioactive atrial peptides. *Biochem Biophys Res Commun* 1984;121:802–807.
107. Geller DM, Currie MG, Wakitani K, Cole BR, Adams SP, Fok KF, et al. Atriopeptins: a family of potent biologically active peptides derived from mammalian atria. *Biochem Biophys Res Commun* 1984;120:333–338.
108. Gillespie DJ, Sandberg RL, Koike TI. Dual effect of left atrial receptors on the excretion of sodium and water in the dog. *Am J Physiol* 1973;255:706–710.
109. Godellas CV, Gower WR Jr, Fabri PJ, Knierim TH, Giordano AT, Vesely DL. Atrial natriuretic factor (ANF)—a possible new gastrointestinal regulatory peptide. *Surgery* 1991;110:1022–1027.
110. Goetz KL, Bond GC, Bloxham DD. Atrial receptors and renal function. *Physiol Rev* 1975;55:157–205.
111. Goodfriend TL, Elliott ME, Atlas SA. Actions of synthetic atrial natriuretic factor on bovine adrenal glomerulosa. *Life Sci* 1984;35:1675–1682.
112. Gomez-Sanchez EP, Foecking MF, Sellers D, Blankenship MS, Gomez-Sanchez CE. Is circulating ouabain-like compound quabain? *Am J Hypertens* 1994;7:647–650.
113. Gower WR Jr, Chiou S, Skolnick K, Vesely DL. Molecular forms of circulating atrial natriuretic peptides in human plasma and their metabolites. *Peptides* 1994;15:861–867.
114. Gower WR, Dietz JR, McCuen RW, Fabri PJ, Lerner EA, Schubert ML. Regulation of atrial natriuretic peptide secretion by cholinergic and PACAP neurons of the gastric antrum. *Am J Physiol* 2003;284:G68–G74.
115. Gower WR Jr, Dietz JR, Vesely DL, Finley CL, Skolnick KA, Fabri PJ, et al. Atrial natriuretic peptide gene expression in the rat gastrointestinal tract. *Biochem Biophys Res Commun* 1994;202:562–570.
116. Gower WR Jr, Salhab KF, Foulis WL, Pillai N, Bund, JR, Vesely DL, et al. Regulation of atrial natriuretic peptide gene expression in gastric antrum by fasting. *Am J Physiol* 2000;278: R770–R780.
117. Gower WR Jr, San Miguel GI, Carter GM, Hassan I, Farese RV, Vesely DL. Atrial natriuretic prohormone gene expression in cardiac and extracardiac tissues of diabetic Goto-Kakizaki rats. *Mol Cell Biochem* 2003;252:263–271.
118. Gower WR Jr, Vesely DL. The gastrointestinal natriuretic peptide system. *Trends Comp Biochem Physiol* 2000;6:125–138.
119. Grammer RT, Fukumi H, Inagami T, Misono KS. Rat atrial natriuretic factor. Purification and vasorelaxant activity. *Biochem Biophys Res Commun* 1983;116:696–703.
120. Green M, Ruiz OS, Kear F, Arruda JA. Dual effect of cyclic GMP on renal brush border Na-H antiporter. *Proc Soc Exp Biol Med* 1991;198:846–851.
121. Greenberg BD, Bencen GH, Seilhamer JJ, Lewicki JA, Fiddes JC. Nucleotide sequence of the gene encoding human ANF precursor. *Nature* 1984;312:656–658.
122. Greenwald JE, Needleman P, Wilkins MR, Schreiner GF. Renal synthesis of atriopeptin-like protein in physiology and pathophysiology. *Am J Physiol* 1991;260:F602–F607.

123. Grepin C, Dagino L, Robitaille L, Haberstroh L, Antakly T, Nemer M. A hormone-encoding gene identifies a pathway for cardiac but not skeletal muscle gene transcription. *Mol Cell Biol* 1994;14:3115–3129.
124. Gunning ME, Brady HR, Otuechere G, Brenner BM, Zeidel ML. Atrial natriuretic peptide (31-67) inhibits Na^+ transport in rabbit inner medullary collecting duct cells: role of prostaglandin E_2. *J Clin Invest* 1992;89:1411–1417.
125. Gunning ME, Brenner BM. Natriuretic peptides and the kidney: current concepts. *Kidney Int* 1992;42(Suppl 38):S127–S133.
126. Habibullah AA, Villarreal D, Freeman RH, Dietz JR, Vesely DL, Simmons JC. Atrial natriuretic peptide fragments in dogs with experimental heart failure. *Clin Exp Pharmacol Physiol* 1995;22:130–135.
127. Hamra FK, Forte LR, Eber SL, Pidhorodeckyj NV, Krause WJ, Freeman RH, et al. Uroguanylin: structure and activity of a second endogenous peptide that stimulates intestinal guanylate cyclase. *Proc Natl Acad Sci U S A* 1993;90:10464–10468.
128. Harma F, Hagiwara H, Inoue A, Yamaguchi A, Yokose S, Furuya M, et al. cGMP produced in response to ANP and CNP regulates proliferation and differentiation of osteoblastic cells. *Am J Physiol* 1996;270:C1311–C1318.
129. Hammond TG, Haramati A, Knox FG. Synthetic atrial natriuretic factor decreases renal tubular phosphate reabsorption in rats. *Am J Physiol* 1985;249:F315–F318.
130. Harris PJ, Thomas D, Morgan TO. Atrial natriuretic peptide inhibits angiotensin-stimulated proximal tubular sodium and water reabsorption. *Nature* 1987;326:697–698.
131. Harthshorne H. *Water versus Hydrotherapy.* Philadelphia: Lloyd P. Smith Press; 1847.
132. Harvey W. *Exercitatio de motu cordis et sanguinis animalibus.* Leake CD (trans.), Francofurti Guilielem Fitzeri, 1628. Springfield, IL: Charles C. Thoma; 1928.
133. Hayashida H, Miyata T. Sequence similarity between epidermal growth factor precursor and atrial natriuretic factor precursor. *FEBS Lett* 1985;185:125–128.
134. Henrich WL. Southwestern Internal Medicine Conference: renal sodium excretion and atrial natriuretic factor. *Am J Med Sci* 1986;291:199–208.
135. Henry JP, Gauer OH, Reeves JL. Evidence of the atrial location of receptors influencing urine flow. *Circ Res* 1956;4:85–90.
136. Henry JP, Pearce JW. The possible role of cardiac atrial stretch receptors in the induction of changes in urine flow. *J Physiol* 1956;131:572–585.
137. Hirata Y, Tomita M, Takada S, Yoshimi H. Vascular receptor binding activities and cyclic GMP responses by synthetic human and rat atrial natriuretic peptides (ANP) and receptor down-regulation by ANP. *Biochem Biophys Res Commun* 1985;128:538–546.
138. Hock R, Anderson RJ. Prevention of drug-induced nephrotoxicity in the intensive care unit. *J Crit Care* 1995;10:33–43.
139. Hou SH, Bushinsky DA, Wish JB, Cohen JJ, Harrington JT. Hospital acquired renal insufficiency: a prospective study. *Am J Med* 1983;74:243–248.
140. Huet M, Benchimol S, Berlinguet JC, Castonguay Y, Cantin M. Cytochimie ultrastructurale des cardiocytes de l'oreillette humaine. IV. Digestion des granules specifiques par less proteases. *J Microsc* 1974;21:147–158.
141. Huet M, Cantin M. Ultrastructural cytochemistry of atrial muscle cells. II. Characterization of the protein content of specific granules. *Lab Invest* 1974;30:525–532.
142. Humphreys MH. Gamma-MSH, sodium metabolism, and salt sensitive hypertension. *Am J Physiol* 2004;286:R417–R430.
143. Humphreys MH, Lin SY. Peptide hormones and the control of sodium excretion. *Hypertension* 1988;11:397–410.
144. Hunt PJ, Richards AM, Espiner EA, Nicholls ME, Yandle TG. Bioactivity and metabolism of C-type natriuretic peptide in normal man. *J Clin Endocrinol Metab* 1994;78:1428–1435.
145. Hunter EFM, Kelly PA, Prowse C, Woods FJ, Lowry PJ. Analysis of peptides derived from pro atrial natriuretic peptide that circulate in man and increase in heart disease. *Scand J Clin Lab Invest* 1998;58:205–216.
146. Igaki T, Itoh H, Suga S, Hama N, Ogawa Y, Komatsu Y, et al. C-type natriuretic peptide in chronic renal failure and its action in humans. *Kidney Int* 1996;49(Suppl 55):S144–S147.
147. Itoh H, Pratt RE, Dzau VJ. Atrial natriuretic polypeptide inhibits hypertrophy of vascular smooth muscle cells. *J Clin Invest* 1990;86:1690–1697.
148. Itoh H, Pratt RE, Ohno M, Dzau VJ. Atrial natriuretic polypeptide as a novel antigrowth factor of endothelial cells. *Hypertension* 1992;19:758–761.
149. Jamieson JD, Palade GE. Specific granules in atrial muscle cell. *J Cell Biol* 1964;23:151–162.
150. Jensen KT, Eiskjaer H, Carstens J, Pedersen EB. Renal effects of brain natriuretic peptide in patients with congestive heart failure. *Clin Sci* 1999;96:5–15.
151. Jin JY, Wen JF, Li D, Cho KW. Osmoregulation of atrial myocytic ANP release: osmotransduction via cross-talk between L-type Ca^{2+} channel and SR Ca^{2+} release. *Am J Physiol* 2004;287:R1101–R1109.
152. John SWM, Krege JH, Oliver PM, Hagaman JR, Hodgkin JB, Pang SC, et al. Genetic decreases in atrial natriuretic peptide and salt-sensitive hypertension. *Science* 1995;267:679–681.
153. Johnson A, Lermioglu F, Garg UC, Morgan-Boyd R, Hassid A. A novel biological effect of atrial natriuretic hormone: inhibition of mesangial cell mitogenesis. *Biochem Biophys Res Commun* 1988;152:893–897.
154. Jougasaki M, Burnett JC Jr. Adrenomedullin: potential in physiology and pathophysiology. *Life Sci* 2000;66:855–872.
155. Kangawa K, Fukuda A, Kubota I, Hayashi Y, Matsuo H. Identification in rat atrial tissue of multiple forms of natriuretic polypeptides of about 3,000 daltons. *Biochem Biophys Res Commun* 1984;121:585–591.
156. Kangawa K, Fukuda A, Matsuo H. Purification and complete amino acid sequence of rat atrial natriuretic polypeptides of 5,000 daltons. *Biochem Biophys Res Commun* 1984;119:933–940.
157. Kangawa K, Fukuda A, Matsuo H. Structural identification of beta- and gamma-human atrial natriuretic polypeptides (β- and γ-ANP). *Nature* 1985;313:397–400.
158. Kangawa K, Matsuo H. Purification and complete amino acid sequence of alpha-human atrial natriuretic polypeptide (alpha-hANP). *Biochem Biophys Res Commun* 1984;118:131–139.
159. Kangawa K, Tawaragi Y, Oikawa S, Mizuno A, Sakuragawa Y, Nakazato M, et al. Identification rat gamma atrial natriuretic polypeptide and characterization of the cDNA encoding its precursor. *Nature* 1984;312:152–155.
160. Karla PR, Anker SD, Struthers AD, Coats AJS. The role of C-natriuretic peptide in cardiovascular medicine. *Eur Heart J* 2001;22:997–1007.
161. Kalra PR, Clague JR, Bolger AP, Anker SD, Poole-Wilson PA, Struthers AD, et al. Myocardial production of C-type natriuretic peptide in chronic heart failure. *Circulation* 2003;107:571–573.
162. Karlberg L, Norlen BJ, Ojteg G, Wolgast M. Impaired medullary circulation in postischemic acute renal failure. *Acta Physiol Scand* 1983;118:11–17.
163. Kasahara M, Mukoyama M, Sugawara A, Makino H, Suganami T, Ogawa Y, et al. Ameliorated glomerular injury in mice over expressing brain natriuretic peptide with renal ablation. *J Am Soc Nephrol* 2000;11:1691–1701.
164. Kaufman RP Jr, Anner H, Kobzik L, Valeri CR, Shepro D, Hechtman, HB. Vasodilator prostaglandins (PG) prevent renal damage after ischemia. *Ann Surg* 1987;205:195–198.
165. Keeler R. Atrial natriuretic factor has a direct, prostaglandin-in-dependent action on kidneys. *Can J Physiol Pharmacol* 1982;60:1078–1082.
166. Kennedy BP, Marsden JJ, Flynn TG, DeBold AJ, Davies PL. Isolation and nucleotide sequence of a cloned cardionatrin cDNA. *Biochem Biophys Res Commun* 1984;122:1076–1082.
167. Kentsch M, Drummer C, Gerzer R, Muller-Esch G. Severe hypotension and bradycardia after continuous intravenous infusion of urodilatin (ANP 95-126) in a patient with congestive heart failure. *Eur J Clin Invest* 1995;25:281–283.
168. Kinoshita H, Fujimoto S, Fukae H, Yokota N, Hisanaga S, Nakazato M, et al. Plasma and urine levels of uroguanylin, a new natriuretic peptide, in nephrotic syndrome. *Nephron* 1999;81:160–164.
169. Kinoshita H, Nakazato M, Yamaguchi H, Matsukura S, Fujimoto S, Eto T. Increased plasma guanylin levels in patients with impaired renal function. *Clin Nephrol* 1997;47:28–32.
170. Kisch B. Studies in comparative electron microscopy of the heart. II. Guinea pig and rat. *Exp Med Surg* 1955;13:404–428.
171. Kitamura K, Kangawa K, Kawamoto M, Ichiki Y, Nakamura S, Matsuo H, et al. Adrenomedullin: a novel hypotensive peptide isolated from human pheochromocytoma. *Biochem Biophys Res Commun* 1993;192:553–560.
172. Kitamura K, Kangawa K, Matsuo H, Eto T. Adrenomedullin: implications for hypertension research. *Drugs* 1995;49:485–495.
173. Kleinert HD, Maack T, Atlas SA, Januszewicz A, Sealey JE, Laragh JH. Atrial natriuretic factor inhibits angiotensin-, norepinephrine-, and potassium-induced vascular contractility. *Hypertension* 1984;6(Suppl I):I143–I147.
174. Kohse KP, Feifel K, Mayer-Wehrstein R. Differential regulation of brain and atrial natriuretic peptides in hemodialysis patients. *Clin Nephrol* 1993;40:83–90.
175. Kojima S, Inoue I, Hirata Y, Kimura G, Saito F, Kawano Y, et al. Plasma concentrations of immunoreactive-atrial natriuretic polypeptide in patients on hemodialysis. *Nephron* 1987;46:45–48.
176. Koller KJ, Goeddel DV. Molecular biology of natriuretic peptides and their receptors. *Circulation* 1992;86:1081–1088.
177. Kudo T, Baird A. Inhibition of aldosterone production in the adrenal glomerulosa by atrial natriuretic factor. *Nature* 1984;312:756–757.
178. Kurnik BR, Allgren RL, Genter FC, Solomon RJ, Bates ER, Weisberg LS. Prospective study of atrial natriuretic peptide for the prevention of radiocontrast-induced nephropathy. *Am J Kidney Dis* 1998;31:674–680.
179. Kurtz A, Della Bruna R, Pfeilschifter J, Taugner R, Bauer C. Atrial natriuretic peptide inhibits renin release from juxtaglomerular cells by cGMP-mediated process. *Proc Natl Acad Sci U S A* 1986;83:4769–4773.
180. Ladenson, PW, Bloch KD, Seidman JG. Modulation of atrial natriuretic factor by thyroid hormone: messenger ribonucleic acid and peptide levels in hypothyroid, euthyroid, and hyperthyroid rat atria and ventricles. *Endocrinology* 1988;123:652–657.
181. Lainchbury J, Richards AM, Nicholls MG. Brain natriuretic peptide in heart failure. In: Vesely DL, ed. *Atrial Natriuretic Peptides.* Trivandrum, India: Research Signpost; 1997:151–158.
182. Lang CC, Choy AM, Henderson IS, Coutie WJ, Struthers AD. Effect of haemodialysis on plasma levels of brain natriuretic peptide in patients with chronic renal failure. *Clin Sci* 1992;82:127–131.
183. La Pointe MC, Deschepper CF, Wu J, Gardner DG. Extracellular calcium regulates expression of the gene for atrial natriuretic factor. *Hypertension* 1990;15:20–28.
184. Lazure C, Seidah NG, Chretien M, Thibault G, Garcia R, Cantin M, et al. Atrial pronatriodilatin: a precursor for natriuretic factor and cardiodilatin. *FEBS Lett* 1984;172:80–86.
185. Lee SJ, Kim SZ, Cui X, Kim SH, Lee KS, Chung YJ, et al. C-type natriuretic peptide inhibits ANP secretion and atrial dynamics in perfused atria: NPR-B-cGMP signaling. *Am Heart J* 2000;278:H208–H221.
186. Lennane RJ, Peart WS, Carey RM, Shaw J. A comparison on natriuresis after oral and intravenous sodium loading in sodium-depleted rabbits: evidence for a gastrointestinal or portal monitor of sodium intake. *Clin Sci Mol Med* 1975;49:433–436.
187. Levin ER, Gardner DG, Samson WK. Natriuretic peptides. *N Engl J Med* 1998;339:321–328.
188. Levinsky NG, Lalone RC. Mechanism of sodium diuresis after saline infusion in the dog. *J Clin Invest* 1963;42:1261–1268.
189. Lewis J, Salem MM, Chertow GM, Weisberg LS, McGrew F, Marbury TC, et al. Atrial natriuretic factor in oliguric acute renal failure. Anaritide Acute Renal Failure Study Group. *Am J Kidney Dis* 2000;36:767–774.
190. Lieberthal W, Sheridan AM, Valeri CR. Protective effect of atrial natriuretic factor and mannitol following renal ischemia. *Am J Physiol* 1990;258:F1266–F1272.
191. Linden RJ, Sreeharan N. Humoral nature of the urine response to stimulation of atrial receptors. *Q J Exp Physiol* 1981;66:431–438.
192. Lisy O, Jougasaki M, Heublein DM, Schirger JA, Chen HH, Wennberg PW, et al. Renal actions of synthetic dendroaspis natriuretic peptide. *Kidney Int* 1999;56:502–508.
193. Luchner A, Stevens TL, Borgeson DD, Redfield M, Wei CM, Porter JG, et al. Differential atrial and ventricular expression of myocardial BNP during evaluation of heart failure. *Am J Physiol* 1998;274:H1684–H1689.
194. Lydtin H, Hamilton WF. Effect of acute changes in left atrial pressure on urine flow in unanesthetized dogs. *Am J Physiol* 1964;207:503–536.

195. Maack T, Marion DN, Camargo MJ, Kleinert HD, Laragh JH, Vaughan ED Jr, et al. Effects of auriculin (atrial natriuretic factor) on blood pressure, renal function, and the renin-aldosterone system in dogs. *Am J Med* 1984;77:1069–1075.
196. Maack T, Suzuki M, Almedida FA, Nussenzveig D, Scarborough RW, McEnroe GA, et al. Physiological role of silent receptors of atrial natriuretic factor. *Science* 1987;238:675–678.
197. Maki M, Takayanagi R, Misono KS, Pandy KN, Tibbetts C, Inagami T. Structure of rat atrial natriuretic factor precursor deduced for cDNA sequence. *Nature* 1984;309:722–724.
198. Marcus LS, Hart D, Packer M, Yushak M, Medina N, Danziger RS, et al. Hemodynamic and renal excretory effects of human brain natriuretic peptide infusions in patients with congestive heart failure. A double-blind, placebo-controlled, randomized crossover trail. *Circulation* 1996;94:3184–3189.
199. Marie JP, Guillemont H, Hatt PY. Le degree de granulation des cardiocytes auriculaires. Etude planimetrique au cours de differents apports d'eau et de sodium chez le rat. *Pathol Biol* 1976;24:549–554.
200. Marin-Grez M, Fleming JT, Steinhausen M. Atrial natriuretic peptide causes pre-glomerular vasodilatation and post-glomerular vasoconstriction in rat kidney. *Nature* 1986;324:473–476.
201. Martin DR, Pevahouse JB, Trigg DJ, Vesely DL, Buerkert JE. Three peptides from the ANF prohormone NH_2-terminus are natriuretic and/or kaliuretic. *Am J Physiol* 1990;258:F1401–F1408.
202. Marttila M, Puhakka J, Luodonpaa M, Vuolteenaho O, Ganten L, Ruskoaho H. Augmentation of BNP gene expression in atria by pressure overload in transgenic rats harboring human renin and angiotensinogen genes. *Blood Press* 1999;8:308–316.
203. Mattingly MT, Brandt RR, Heublein DM, Wei CM, Nir A, Burnett JC Jr. Presence of C-type natriuretic peptide in human kidney and urine. *Kidney Int* 1994;46:744–747.
204. McMurray J, Seidenlin PH, Howey JEA, Balfour DJ, Struthers AD. The effect of atrial natriuretic factor on urinary albumin and beta-2–microglobulin excretion in man. *Hypertension* 1988;6:783–786.
205. McMurray RW, Vesely DL. Weight reduction decreases atrial natriuretic factor and blood pressure in obese patients. *Metabolism* 1989;38:1231–1237.
206. Melander O, Frandsen E, Groop L, Hulthen UL. Plasma proANP 1-30 reflects salt sensitivity in subjects with hereditary for hypertension. *Hypertension* 2002;39:996–999.
207. Merkouris RW, Miller FC, Catanzarite V, Rigg LA, Quirk JG Jr, Vesely DL. Increase in the plasma levels of the N-terminal and C-terminal portions of the prohormone of atrial natriuretic factor in normal pregnancy. *Am J Obstet Gynecol* 1990;162:859–864.
208. Merkouris RW, Miller FC, Catanzarite V, Quirk JG Jr, Rigg LA, Vesely DL. The N-terminal and C-terminal portions of the atrial natriuretic factor prohormone increase during preeclampsia. *Am J Obstet Gynecol* 1991;164:1197–1202.
209. Meyer M, Richter R, Forssmann WG. Urodilatin, a natriuretic peptide with clinical implications. *Eur J Med Res* 1998;3:103–110.
210. Meyer M, Pfarr E, Schirmer G, Uberbacher HJ, Schope K, Bohm E, et al. Therapeutic use of the natriuretic peptide ularitide in acute renal failure. *Ren Fail* 1999;21:85–100.
211. Mills RM, LeJemtel TH, Horton DP, Liang C, Lang R, Silver MA, et al. Sustained hemodynamic effects of an infusion of nesiritide (human b-type natriuretic peptide) in heart failure: a randomized, double-blind, placebo-controlled clinical trail. Natrecor Study Group. *J Am Coll Cardiol* 1999;34:155–162.
212. Molitoris BA, Meyer C, Dahl R, Geerdes A. Mechanism of ischemia-enhanced aminoglycoside binding and uptake by proximal tubule cells. *Am J Physiol* 1993;264:F907–F916.
213. Morgan DA, Peuler JD, Koepke JP, Mark AL, DiBona GF. Renal sympathetic nerves attenuate the natriuretic effects of atrial peptide. *J Lab Clin Med* 1989;114:538–544.
214. Morrissey EC, Wilner KD, Barager RR, Ward DM, Ziegler MG. Atrial natriuretic factor in renal failure and posthemodialytic postural hypotension. *Am J Kidney Dis* 1988;12:510–515.
215. Moskowitz PS, Korobkin M, Rambo ON. Diuresis and improved renal hemodynamics produced by prostaglandin E_1 in the dog with norepinephrine-induced acute renal failure. *Invest Radiol* 1975;10:284–299.
216. Nakao K, Ogawa Y, Suga S, Imura H. Molecular biology and biochemistry of the natriuretic peptide system. I. Natriuretic peptides. *J Hypertens* 1992;10:907–912.
217. Nakamoto M, Shapiro JI, Shanley PF, Chan L, Schrier RW. In vitro and in vivo protective effect of atriopeptin III on ischemic acute renal failure. *J Clin Invest* 1987;80:698–705.
218. Nakayama K, Ohkubo H, Hirose T, Inayama S, Nakanishi S. mRNA sequence for human cardiodilatin-atrial natriuretic factor precursor and regulation of precursor mRNA in rat atria. *Nature* 1984;310:699–701.
219. Nasser A, Dietz JR, Siddique M, Patel H, Khan N, Antwi EK, et al. Effects of kaliuretic peptide on sodium and water excretion in persons with congestive heart failure. *Am J Cardiol* 2001;88:23–29.
220. Nemer M, Chamberland M, Sirois D, Argentin J, Drouin RA, Dixon RA, et al. Gene structure of human cardiac hormone precursor, pronatriodilatin. *Nature* 1984;312:654–656.
221. Neumayer HH, Blossei N, Seherr-Thohs U, Wagner K. Amelioration of postischaemic acute renal failure in conscious dogs by human atrial natriuretic peptide. *Nephrol Dial Transplant* 1990;5:32–38.
222. Ngo L, Bissett JK, Winters CJ, Vesely DL. Plasma prohormone atrial natriuretic peptides 1-98 and 31-67 increase with supraventricular and ventricular arrhytmias. *Am J Med Sci* 1990;300:71–77.
223. Ngo L, Wyeth RP, Bissett JK, Hester WL, Newton MT, Sallman AL, et al. Prohormone atrial natriuretic peptides 1-30, and 99-126 increase in proportion to right ventricular pacing rate. *Am Heart J* 1989;118:893–900.
224. Nishikimi T, Mori Y, Kobayashi N, Tadokoro K, Wang X, Akimoto K, et al. Renoprotective effect of chronic adrenomedullin infusion in Dahl salt-sensitive rats. *Hypertension* 2002; 39:1077–1082.
225. Ogawa E, Saito Y, Kuwahara K, Harada M, Miyamoto Y, Hamana I, et al. Fibronectin signaling stimulates BNP gene transcription by inhibiting neuron-restrictive silencer element–dependent repression. *Cardiovasc Res* 2002;53:451–459.
226. Ohlstein EH, Berkowitz BA. Cyclic guanosine monophosphate mediates vascular relaxation induced by atrial natriuretic factor. *Hypertension* 1985;7:306–310.
227. Oikawa S, Imai M, Inuzuka C, Tawaragi Y, Nakazato H, Matsuo H. Structure of dog and rabbit precursors of atrial natriuretic polypeptides deduced from nucleotide sequence of cloned cDNA. *Biochem Biophys Res Commun* 1985;132:892–899.
228. Oikawa S, Imai M, Ueno A, Tanaka S, Noguchi T, Nakazato H, et al. Cloning and sequence analysis of cDNA encoding a precursor for human atrial natriuretic peptide. *Nature* 1984:309:724–726.
229. Orias R, McCann SM. Natriuresis induced by alpha and beta melanocyte stimulating hormones in rats. *Endocrinology* 1972;90:700–706.
230. Ortola FV, Ballermann BJ, Brenner BM. Endogenous ANP augments fractional excretion of Pi, Ca, and Na in rats with reduced renal mass. *Am J Physiol* 1988;255:F1091–F1097.
231. Palmer BF, Alpern RJ. Pathogenesis of edema formation in the nephrotic syndrome. *Kidney Int* 1997;59:521–527.
232. Palmer PA, Friedl FE, Giordano AT, Vesely DL. Alteration of environmental salinity modulates atrial natriuretic peptides' concentrations in heart, and hemolymph of the oyster, *Crassostrea virginica*. *Comp Biochem Physiol* 1994;108A:589–597.
233. Parkes DG. Cardiovascular actions of adrenomedullin in conscious sheep. *Am J Physiol* 1995;268:H2574–H2578.
234. Paul RV, Kirk KA, Navar LG. Renal autoregulation and pressure natriuresis during ANF-induced diuresis. *Am J Physiol* 1987;253:F424–F431.
235. Payvar F, DeFranco D, Firestone G, Edgar B, Wrange O, O'Kret S, et al. Sequence specific binding of glucocorticoid receptor to MMTV DNA at sites within and upstream of the transcribed region. *Cell* 1983;35:381–392.
236. Pedram A, Razandi M, Hu RM, Levin ER. Vasoactive peptides modulate vascular endothelial cell growth factor production and endothelial cell proliferation and invasion. *J Biol Chem* 1997;272:17097–17103.
237. Peters JP. *Body Water: The Exchange of Fluids in Man*. Springfield, IL: Charles C Thomas; 1935.
238. Pettersson A, Hedner J, Hedner T. Renal interaction between sympathetic activity and ANP in rats with chronic heart failure. *Acta Physiol Scand* 1989;135:487–492.
239. Pettersson A, Hedner J, Ricksten SE, Towle AC, Hedner T. Acute volume expansion as a physiological stimulus for the release of atrial natriuretic peptides in the rat. *Life Sci* 1986;38:1127–1133.
240. Pevahouse JB, Flanigan WJ, Winters CJ, Vesely DL. Normalization of elevated circulating N-terminal and C-terminal atrial natriuretic factor prohormone concentrations by renal transplantation. *Transplantation* 1992;53:1375–1377.
241. Pikkarainen S, Tokola H, Majalahti-Palviainen T, Kerkela R, Hautala N, Bahalla SS, et al. GATA-4 is a nuclear mediator of mechanical stretch–activated hypertrophic program. *J Biol Chem* 2003;278:23807–23816.
242. Pitchumoni CS. Pancreatic disease. In: Stein JH, ed. *Internal Medicine*. St. Louis, MO: Mosby; 1998:2233–2247.
243. Poche R. Electronenmikroskopische untersuchuwgen des liopfuscin im herzmuskel des menschen. *Zbl Allg Path Anat* 1957;96:395.
244. Poche R. Submikroskopische beitrage zur pathologie der herzmuskelzelle bei phosphorvergiftung. Hypertrophie, atrophie und kaliummangel. *Virchows Arch* 1958;331:165–248.
245. Pollock DM, Mullins MM, Banks RO. Failure of atrial myocardial extract to inhibit renal Na^+-K^+-ATPase. *Renal Physiol* 1983;6:295–299.
246. Poulos JE, Gower WR Jr, Sullebarger JT, Fontanet HL, Vesely DL. Congestive heart failure: increased cardiac and extracardiac atrial natriuretic peptide gene expression. *Cardiovasc Res* 1996;32:909–919.
247. Poulos JE, Gower WR Jr, Fontanet HL, Kalmus GW, Vesely DL. Cirrhosis with ascites: increased atrial natriuretic peptide gene expression in rat ventricle. *Gastroenterology* 1995;108:1496–1503.
248. Poulos JE, Gower WR Jr, Friedl FE, Vesely DL. Atrial natriuretic peptide gene expression within invertebratic hearts. *Gen Comp Endocrinol* 1995;100:61–68.
249. Proudfoot N. The end of the message. *Nature* 1982;298:516–517.
250. Proudfoot NT, Brownlee GG. 3' non-coding region sequences in eukaryotic messenger RNA. *Nature* 1976;263:211–214.
251. Rahman SN, Kim GE, Mathew AS, Goldberg CA, Allgren R, Schrier RW, et al. Effects of atrial natriuretic peptide in clinical acute renal failure. *Kidney Int* 1994;45:1731–1738.
252. Raine AE, Anderson JV, Bloom SR, Morris PJ. Plasma atrial natriuretic factor and graft function in renal transplant recipients. *Transplantation* 1989;48:796–800.
253. Rambotti MG, Giambanco I, Spreca A. Detection of guanylate cyclases A and B stimulated by natriuretic peptides in gastrointestinal tract of rat. *Histochem J* 1996;29:117–126.
254. Ramirez G, Saba SR, Dietz JR, Vesely DL. Immunocytochemical localization of proANF1-30, proANF 31-67, and atrial natriuretic factor in the kidney. *Kidney Int* 1992;41:334–341.
255. Rapoport RM. Cyclic guanosine monophosphate inhibition of contraction may be mediated through inhibition of phosphatidylinositol hydrolysis in rat aorta. *Circ Res* 1986;58:407–410.
256. Rapoport RM, Ginsburg R, Waldman SA, Murad F. Effects of atriopeptins on relaxation and cyclic GMP levels in human coronary artery *in vitro*. *Eur J Pharmacol* 1986;124:193–196.
257. Rascher W, Tulassay T, Lang RE. Atrial natriuretic peptide in plasma of volume-overloaded children with chronic renal failure. *Lancet* 1985;2:303–305.
258. Rashed HM, Su H, Patel TB. Atrial natriuretic peptide inhibits growth of hepatoblastoma (HEP G2) cells by means of activation of clearance receptors. *Hepatology* 1993;17:677–684.
259. Richards AM, Lainchbury JG, Nicholls MG, Cameron AV, Yandle TG. *Dendroaspis* natriuretic peptide: endogenous or dubious? *Lancet* 2002;359:5–6.
260. Riordan JR. The cystic fibrosis transmembrane conductance regulator. *Annu Rev Physiol* 1993;55:609–630.
261. Ritter D, Chao J, Needleman P, Tetens E, Greenwald JE. Localization, synthetic regulation, and biology of renal atriopeptin-like prohormone. *Am J Physiol* 1992;263:F503–F509.
262. Rosenzweig A, Seidman CE. Atrial natriuretic factor and related peptide hormones. *Annu Rev Biochem* 1991;60:229–255.
263. Rubattu S, Gilberti R, Ganten U, Volpe M. A differential brain atrial natriuretic peptide expression co-segregates with occurrence of early strokes in the stroke prone phenotype of spontaneously hypertensive rat. *J Hypertens* 1999;17:1849–1852.

264. Rubattu S, Lee-Kirsch MA, DePaolis P, Giliberti R, Gigante B, Lombardi A, et al. Altered structure, regulation, and function of the gene encoding the atrial natriuretic peptide in stroke prone spontaneously hypertensive rat. *Cir Res* 1999;85:900–905.
265. Rubattu S, Ridker P, Stampfer MJ, Volpe M, Henekens CH, Lindpaintner K. The gene encoding atrial natriuretic peptide and the risk of human stroke. *Circulation* 1999;100: 1722–1726.
266. Ruskoaho H. Atrial natriuretic peptide: synthesis, release, and metabolism. *Pharmacol Rev* 1992;44:479–602.
267. Ruskoaho H, Leskinen H, Magga J, Tashinen P, Mantymaa P, Vuolteenaho O, et al. Mechanisms of mechanical load–induced atrial natriuretic peptide secretion: role of endothelin, nitric oxide, and angiotensin II. *J Mol Med* 1997;75:876–885.
268. Ryu H, Cho KW, Kim SH, Kim SZ, Oh SH, Hwang YH, et al. Frog lymph heart synthesizes and stores immunoreactivate atrial natriuretic peptide. *Gen Comp Endocrinol* 1992;87:171–177.
269. Saba SR, Ramirez G, Vesely DL. Immunocytochemical localization of ProANF 1-30, ProANF 31-67, atrial natriuretic factor and urodilatin in the human kidney. *Am J Nephrol* 1993;13:85–93.
270. Sagnella GA, Saggar-Malik AK, Buckley MG, Markandu ND, Eastwood JB, MacGregor GA. Association between atrial natriuretic peptide and cyclic GMP in hypertension and in chronic renal failure. *Clin Chem Acta* 1998;275:9–18.
271. Samson WK. Adrenomedullin and the control of fluid and electrolyte homeostasis. *Annu Rev Physiol* 1999;61:363–389.
272. Samson WK. Proadrenomedullin-derived peptides. *Front Neuroendocrinol* 1998;19:100–117.
273. Sands JM, Neylan JF, Olson RA, O'Brien DP, Whelchel JD, Mitch WE. Atrial natriuretic factor does not improve the outcome of cadaveric renal transplantation. *J Am Soc Nephrol* 1991;1:1081–1086.
274. Sato K, Hirata Y, Imai T, Iwashita M, Mariuo F. Characterization of immunoreactive adrenomedullin in human plasma and urine. *Life Sci* 1995;57:189–194.
275. Sato K, Imai T, Iwashina M, Marumo F, Hirata Y. Secretion of adrenomedullin by renal tubular cell lines. *Nephron* 1998;78:9–14.
276. Saxenhofer H, Gnadinger MP, Weidmann P, Shaw S, Schohn D, Hess C, et al. Plasma levels and dialysance of atrial natriuretic peptide in terminal renal failure. *Kidney Int* 1987;32: 554–561.
277. Schafferhans K, Heidbreder E, Grimm D, Heidland A. Norepinephrine-induced acute renal failure: beneficial effects of atrial natriuretic factor. *Nephron* 1986;44:240–244.
278. Schermuly RT, Weissmann N, Enke B, Ghofrani HA, Forssmann WG, Grimminger F, et al. Urodilatin, a natriuretic peptide stimulating guanylate cyclase, and the phosphodiesterase five inhibitor dipyridamole attenuate experimental pulmonary hypertension. *Am J Respir Cell Mol Biol* 2001;25:219–225.
279. Schirger JA, Heublein DM, Chen HH, Lisy O, Jougasaki M, Wennberg PW, et al. Presence of *Dendroaspis* natriuretic peptide-like immunoreactivity in human plasma and its increase during human heart failure. *Mayo Clin Proc* 1999;74:126–130.
280. Schnermann J, Marin-Grez M, Briggs JP. Filtration pressure response to infusion of atrial natriuretic petides. *Pflugers Arch* 1986;406:237–239.
281. Schramm L, Heidbreder E, Schaar J, Lopau K, Zimmermann J, Gotz R, et al. Toxic acute renal failure in the rat: effects of diltiazem and urodilatin on renal function. *Nephron* 1994;68:454–461.
282. Schulz-Knappe P, Forssmann K, Herbst F, Hock D, Pipkorn R, Forssmann WG. Isolation and structural analysis of 'urodilatin,' a new peptide of the cardiodilatin-(ANP)-family, extracted from human urine. *Klin Wochenschr* 1988;66:752–759.
283. Schweitz H, Vigne P, Moinier D, Frelin C, Lazdunski M. A new member of the natriuretic peptide family is present in the venom of the green mamba (*Dendroaspis augusticeps*). *J Biol Chem* 1992;267:13928–13932.
284. Scivoletto R, Carcalho MHC. Cardionatrin causes vasodilation in vitro which is not dependent on the presence of endothelial cells. *Eur J Pharmacol* 1984;101:143–145.
285. Scriven TA, Burnett JC Jr. Effects of synthetic atrial natriuretic peptide on renal function and renin release in acute experimental heart failure. *Circulation* 1985;72:892–897.
286. Seidman C, Bloch KD, Klein KA, Smith JA, Seidman JG. Nucleotide sequences of the human and mouse atrial natriuretic factor genes. *Science* 1984;226:1206–1209.
287. Shaw SG, Weidmann P, Hodler J, Zimmermann A, Paternostro A. Atrial natriuretic peptide protects against ischemic renal failure in the rat. *J Clin Invest* 1987;80:1232–1237.
288. Shaw SG, Weidmann P, Zimmermann A. Urodilatin, not nitroprusside, combined with dopamine reverses ischemic acute renal failure. *Kidney Int* 1992;42:1153–1159.
289. Shin SJ, Lee YJ, Tan MS, Hsieh TJ, Tsai JH. Increased atrial natriuretic peptide mRNA expression in the kidney of diabetic rats. *Kidney Int* 1997;51:1100–1105.
290. Soejima H, Grekin RJ, Briggs JP, Schnermann J. Renal response of anesthetized rats to low-dose infusion of atrial natriuretic peptide. *Am J Physiol* 1988;255:R449–R455.
291. Sosa RE, Volpe M, Marion DN, Atlas SA, Laragh JH, Vaughn ED Jr, et al. Relationship between renal hemodynamic and natriuretic effects of atrial natriuretic factor. *Am J Physiol* 1986;250:F520–F524.
292. Sothern RB, Vesely DL, Kanabrocki EL, Bremner FW, Third JLAC, Boles MA, et al. Blood pressure and atrial natriuretic peptides correlate throughout the day. *Am Heart J* 1995;129: 907–916.
293. Sothern RB, Vesely DL, Kanabrocki EL, Hermida RC, Bremner FW, Third JLAC, et al. Temporal (circadian) and functional relationship between atrial natriuretic peptides and blood pressure. *Chronobiol Int* 1995;12:106–120.
294. Steinhelper ME, Cochrane KL, Field LJ. Hypotension in transgenic mice expressing atrial natriuretic factor fusion genes. *Hypertension* 1990;16:301–307.
295. Sudoh T, Kangawa K, Minamino W, Matsuo H. A new natriuretic peptide in porcine brain. *Nature* 1988;332:78–81.
296. Sudoh T, Minamino N, Kangawa K, Matsuo H. C-type natriuretic peptide (CNP): a new member of the natriuretic peptide family identified in porcine brain. *Biochem Biophys Res Commun* 1990;168:863–870.
297. Sugawara A, Nakao K, Sakamoto M, Morii N, Yamada T, Itoh H, et al. Plasma concentration of atrial natriuretic polypeptide in essential hypertension. *Lancet* 1985;2:1426–1427.
298. Suzuki E, Hirata Y, Hayakawa H, Omata M, Kojima M, Kangawa K, et al. Evidence for C-type natriuretic peptide production in the rat kidney. *Biochem Biophys Res Commun* 1993;192:532–538.
299. Tamura N, Ogawa Y, Chusho H, Nakamura K, Nakao K, Suda M, et al. Cardiac fibrosis in mice lacking brain natriuretic peptide. *Proc Natl Acad Sci U S A* 2000;97:4239–4244.
300. Tateyama H, Hino J, Minamino N, Kangawa K, Ogihara T, Matsuo H. Characterization of immunoreactive brain natriuretic peptide in human cardiac atrium. *Biochem Biophys Res Commun* 1990;166:1080–1087.
301. Thuerauf DJ, Hanford DS, Glembotski CC. Regulation of rat brain natriuretic peptide transcription. Potential role for GATA-related transcription factors in myocardial gene expression. *J Biol Chem* 1994;269:17772–17775.
302. Tokura T, Kinoshita H, Fujimoto S, Kitamura K, Eto T. Plasma levels of proadrenomedullin N-terminal 20 peptide and adrenomedullin in patients undergoing hemodialysis. *Nephron Clin Pract* 2003;95:C67–C72.
303. Totsune K, Mackenzie HS, Totsune H, Troy JL, Lytton J, Brenner BM. Upregulation of atrial natriuretic peptide gene expression in remnant kidney of rats with reduced renal mass. *J Am Soc Nephrol* 1998;9:1613–1617.
304. Totsune K, Takahashi, Murakami O, Satoh F, Sone M, Mouri T. Elevated plasma C-type natriuretic peptide concentrations in patients with chronic renal failure. *Clin Sci* 1994;87:319–322.
305. Trippodo NC, MacPhee AA, Cole FE, Blakesley HL. Partial chemical characterization of a natriuretic substance in rat atrial heart tissue. *Proc Soc Exp Biol Med* 1982;170:502–508.
306. Tsuchimochi H, Yazaki Y, Ohno H, Takanashi R, Takaku F. Ventricular expression of atrial natriuretic peptide. *Lancet* 1987;2:336–337.
307. Valentin JP, Gardner DG, Wiedemann E, Humphreys MH. Modulation of endothelin effects on blood pressure and hematocrit by atrial natriuretic peptide. *Hypertension* 1991;17:864–869.
308. Valentin JP, Ying WZ, Couser WG, Humphreys MH. Extra renal resistance to atrial natriuretic peptide in rats with experimental nephrotic syndrome. *Am J Physiol* 1998;274:F556–F563.
309. Vari RC, Freeman RH, Davis JO, Villarreal D, Verburg KM. Effect of synthetic atrial natriuretic factor on aldosterone secretion in the rat. *Am J Physiol* 1986;251:R48–R52.
310. Vesely BA, McAfee Q, Gower WR Jr, Vesely DL. Four peptides decrease the number of human pancreatic adenocarcinoma cells. *Eur J Clin Invest* 2003;33:998–1005.
311. Vesely BA, Song S, Sanchez-Ramos J, Fitz SR, Solivan SM, Gower WR Jr, et al. Four peptide hormones decrease the number of human breast adenocarcinoma cells. *Eur J Clin Invest* 2005;35:60–69.
312. Vesely DL. Aprotinin blocks the binding of pro atrial natriuretic peptides 1-30, 31-67, and 99-126 to human placental membranes. *Am J Obstet Gynecol* 1991;165:567–573.
313. Vesely DL. *Atrial Natriuretic Hormones*. Englewood Cliffs, NJ: Prentice Hall; 1992.
314. Vesely DL. Atrial natriuretic peptides within invertebrates and plants. *Trends Comp Biochem Physiol* 1998;4:89–103.
315. Vesely DL. Atrial natriuretic peptides in pathophysiological diseases. *Cardiovasc Res* 2001;51:647–658.
316. Vesely DL. Atrial natriuretic peptide prohormone gene expression: hormones and diseases that upregulate its expression. *IUBMB Life* 2002;53:153–159.
317. Vesely DL. Natriuretic peptides and acute renal failure. *Am J Physiol* 2003;285:F167–F177.
318. Vesely DL, Arnold WC, Winters CJ, Sallman AL, Rico DM. Increased circulating concentration of atrial natriuretic factor in persons with pheochromocytomas. *Clin Exp Hypertens [A]* 1989;11:353–369.
319. Vesely DL, Arnold WC, Winters CJ, Sallman AL, Rico DM. Increased circulating concentration of the N-terminus of the atrial natriuretic prohormone in persons with pheochromocytomas. *J Clin Endocrinol Metab* 1990;71:1138–1146.
320. Vesely DL, Bayliss JM, Sallman AL. Human prepro atrial natriuretic factors 26–55 56–92 and 104–123 increase renal guanylate cyclase activity. *Biochem Biophys Res Commun* 1987;143:186–193.
321. Vesely DL, Blankenship M, Douglass MA, McCormick MT, Rodriguez-Paz G, Schocken DD. Atrial natriuretic peptide increases adrenomedullin in the circulation of healthy humans. *Life Sci* 1996;59:243–254.
322. Vesely DL, Chiou S, Douglass MA, McCormick MT, Rodriguez-Paz G, Schocken DD. Kaliuretic peptide and long acting natriuretic peptide as well as atrial natriuretic factor inhibit aldosterone secretion. *J Endocrinol* 1995;146:373–380.
323. Vesely DL, Chiou S, Douglass MA, McCormick MT, Rodriguez-Paz G, Schocken DD. Atrial natriuretic peptides negatively and positively modulate circulating endothelin in humans. *Metabolism* 1996;45:315–319.
324. Vesely DL, Clark LC, Garces AH, McAfee QW, Soto J, Gower WR Jr. Novel therapeutic approach for cancer using four cardiovascular hormones. *Eur J Clin Invest* 2004;34:674–682.
325. Vesely DL, Cornett LE, McCleod SL, Nash AA, Norris JS. Specific binding sites for prohormone atrial natriuretic peptides 1-30, 31-67, and 99-126. *Peptides* 1990;11:193–197.
326. Vesely DL, Dietz JR, Parks JR, Antwi EA, Overton RM, McCormick MT, et al. Comparison of vessel dilator and long acting natriuretic peptide in the treatment of congestive heart failure. *Am Heart J* 1999;138:625–632.
327. Vesely DL, Dietz JR, Parks JR, Baig M, McCormick MT, Cintron G, et al. Vessel dilator enhances sodium and water excretion and has beneficial hemodynamic effects in persons with congestive heart failure. *Circulation* 1998;98:323–329.
328. Vesely DL, Douglass MA, Dietz JR, Giordano AT, McCormick MT, Rodriguez-Paz G, et al. Negative feedback of atrial natriuretic peptides. *J Clin Endocrinol Metab* 1994;78: 1128–1134.
329. Vesely DL, Douglass MA, Dietz JR, Gower WR Jr, McCormick MT, Rodriguez-Paz G, et al. Three peptides from the atrial natriuretic factor prohormone amino terminus lower blood pressure and produce diuresis, natriuresis, and/or kaliuresis in humans. *Circulation* 1994;90:1129–1140.
330. Vesely DL, Giordano AT. Food intake and body positional change alter the circadian rhythm of atrial natriuretic peptides excretion into human urine. *Chronobiol Int* 1991;8:373–384.
331. Vesely DL, Giordano AT. Atrial natriuretic factor-like peptide and its prohormone within single cell organisms. *Peptides* 1992;13:177–182.

332. Vesely DL, Giordano AT. The most primitive heart in the animal kingdom contains the atrial natriuretic peptide hormonal system. *Comp Biochem Physiol* 1992;101C:325–329.

333. Vesely DL, Gower WRJr, Giordano AT. Atrial natriuretic peptides throughout the plant kingdom: enhancement of solute flow by peptides from the N-terminus of the atrial natriuretic factor prohormone. *Am J Physiol* 1993;265:E465–E477.

334. Vesely DL, Hadley ME. Calcium requirements for melanophore-stimulating hormone action on melanophores. *Science* 1971;173:923–925.

335. Vesely DL, Norris JS, Walters JM, Jespersen RR, Baeyens DA. Atrial natriuretic prohormone peptides 1-30, 31-67 and 79-98 vasodilate the aorta. *Biochem Biophys Res Commun* 1987;148:1540–1548.

336. Vesely DL, Norsk P, Gower WR Jr, Chiou S, Epstein M. Release of kaliuretic peptide during immersion-induced central hypervolemia in healthy humans. *Proc Soc Exp Biol Med* 1995;209:20–26.

337. Vesely DL, Norsk P, Winters CJ, Rico DM, Sallman AL, Epstein M. Increased release of the N-terminal and C-terminal portions of the prohormone of atrial natriuretic factor during immersion-induced central hypervolemia in normal humans. *Proc Soc Exp Biol Med* 1989;192:230–235.

338. Vesely DL, Overton RM, Blankenship M, McCormick MT, Schocken DD. Atrial natriuretic peptide increases urodilatin in the circulation. *Am J Nephrol* 1998;18:204–213.

339. Vesely DL, Palmer PA, Giordano AT. Atrial natriuretic factor prohormone peptides are present in a variety of tissues. *Peptides* 1992;13:165–170.

340. Vesely DL, Perez-Lamboy GI, Schocken DD. Long acting natriuretic peptide, vessel dilator, and kaliuretic peptide enhance urinary excretion of β₂ microglobulin. *Metabolism* 2000;49:1592–1597.

341. Vesely DL, Perez-Lamboy GI, Schocken DD. Long acting natriuretic peptide, vessel dilator, and kaliuretic peptide enhance urinary excretion rate of β₂ microglobulin in congestive heart failure patients. *J Cardiac Failure* 2001;7:55–63.

342. Vesely DL, Preston R, Gower WR Jr, Chiou S, Epstein M. Increased release of kaliuretic peptide during immersion-induced central hypervolemia in cirrhotic humans. *Am J Nephrol* 1996;16:128–137.

343. Vesely DL, Sallman AL, Bayliss JM. Specific binding sites for pro atrial natriuretic factors 1-30, 31-67, and 99-126 on distal nephrons, proximal tubules, renal cortical and medullary membranes. *Renal Physiol Biochem* 1992;15:23–32.

344. Vesely DL, San Miguel GI, Hassan I, Schocken DD. Atrial natriuretic hormone, vessel dilator, long acting natriuretic hormone, and kaliuretic hormone decrease the circulating concentrations of corticotropin releasing hormone, corticotropin and cortisol. *J Clin Endocrinol Metab* 2001;86:4244–4249.

345. Vesely DL, Winters CJ, Sallman AL. Prohormone atrial natriuretic peptides 1-30 and 31-67 increase in hyperthyroidism and decrease in hypothyroidism. *Am J Med Sci* 1989;297:209–215.

346. Vesely MD, Gower WR Jr, Perez-Lamboy GI, Overton RM, Graddy L, Vesely DL. Evidence for an atrial natriuretic peptide-like gene in plants. *Exp Biol Med* 2001;226:61–65.

347. Vesely MD, Vesely DL. Environmental upregulation of atrial natriuretic peptide gene in the living fossil, *Limulus polyphemus*. *Biochem Biophys Res Commun* 1999;254:751–756.

348. Villarreal D, Freeman RH, Reams GP. Natriuretic peptides and salt sensitivity: endocrine cardiorenal integration in heart failure. *Congest Heart Fail* 2002;8:29–36.

349. Villarreal D, Freeman RH, Taraben A, Reams GP. Modulation of renin secretion by atrial natriuretic factor prohormone fragment 31-67. *Am J Med Sci* 1999;318:330–335.

350. Villarreal D, Reams GP, Taraben A, Freeman RH. Hemodynamic and renal effects of pro-ANF 31-67 in hypertensive rats. *Proc Soc Exp Biol Med* 1999;221:166–170.

351. Vlasuk G, Miller J, Beneen G, Lewicki J. Structure and analysis of the bovine atrial natriuretic peptide precursor gene. *Biochem Biophys Res Commun* 1986;136:396–403.

352. Vuolteenaho, O, Arjama O, Vakkuri O, Madsniemi T, Nikkila L, Kangas J, et al. Atrial natriuretic peptide (ANP) in rat gastrointestinal tract. *FEBS Lett* 1988;233:79–82.

353. Vuolteenaho O, Leskinen H, Magga J, Taskinen P, Mantymaa P, Leppaluoto J, et al. Regulation of atrial natriuretic peptide synthesis and secretion. In: Vesely DL, ed. *Atrial Natriuretic Peptides*. Trivandrum, India: Research Signpost; 1997:39–52.

354. Waldman SA, Rapoport RM, Murad F. Atrial natriuretic factor selectively activates particulate guanylate cyclase and elevates cyclic GMP in rat tissues. *J Biol Chem* 1984;259:14332–14334.

355. Walshe JJ, Venuto RC. Acute oliguric renal failure induced by indomethacin: possible mechanism. *Ann Intern Med* 1979;91:47–49.

356. Walter T, Stepan H, Pankow K, Becker M, Schultheiss HP, Sein WE. Biochemical analysis of neutral endopeptidase activity reveals independent catabolism of atrial and brain natriuretic peptide. *J Biol Chem* 2004;385:179–184.

357. Weidmann P, Hasler L, Gnadinger MP, Lang RE, Uehlinger DE, Shaw S, et al. Blood levels and renal effects of atrial natriuretic peptide in normal man. *J Clin Invest* 1986;77:734–742.

358. Werb R, Clark WF, Lindsay RM, Jones EO, Turnbull DI, Linton AL. Protective effect of prostaglandin [PGE₂] in glycerol-induced acute renal failure in rats. *Clin Sci Mol Med* 1978;55:505–507.

359. Westenfelder C, Birch FM, Baranowski RL, Rosenfeld MJ, Shiozawa DK, Kablitz C. Atrial natriuretic factor and salt adaptation in the teleost fish Gila atraria. *Am J Physiol* 1988;255:F1281–F1286.

360. Weston MW, Cintron GB, Giordano AT, Vesely DL. Normalization of circulating atrial natriuretic peptides in cardiac transplant recipients. *Am Heart J* 1994;127:129–142.

361. Wilkins MR, Wood JA, Adu D, Lote CJ, Kendall MJ, Michael J. Change in plasma immunoreactive atrial natriuretic peptide during sequential ultrafiltration and haemodialysis. *Clin Sci* 1986;71:157–160.

362. Williamson JR, Holmberg SW, Chang K, Marvel J, Sutera SP, Needleman P. Mechanisms underlying atriopeptin-induced increases in hematocrit and vascular permeation in rats. *Circ Res* 1989;64:890–899.

363. Winquist RJ, Faison EP, Waldman SA, Schwartz K, Murad F, Rapoport RM. Atrial natriuretic factor elicits an endothelium independent relaxation and activates particulate guanylate cyclase in vascular smooth muscle. *Proc Natl Acad Sci U S A* 1984;81:7661–7664.

364. Winters CJ, Sallman AL, Baker BJ, Meadows J, Rico DM, Vesely DL. The N-terminus and a 4000 molecular weight peptide from the mid portion of the N-terminus of the atrial natriuretic factor prohormone each circulate in humans and increase in congestive heart failure. *Circulation* 1989;80:438–449.

365. Winters CJ, Sallman AL, Meadows J, Rico DM, Vesely DL. Two new hormones: prohormone atrial natriuretic peptides 1-30 and 31-67 circulate in man. *Biochem Biophys Res Commun* 1988;150:231–236.

366. Winters CJ, Vesely DL. Change in plasma immunoreactive N-terminus, C-terminus, and 4000 dalton mid portion of atrial natriuretic factor prohormone with hemodialysis. *Nephron* 1991;58:17–22.

367. Woolf AS, Mansell MA, Hoffbrand BI, Cohen SL, Moult PJ. The effect of low dose intravenous 99-126 atrial natriuretic factor infusion in patients with chronic renal failure. *Postgrad Med J* 1989;65:362–366.

368. Wolff RA, Abbruzzese JL, Evans DB. Neoplasms of the exocrine pancreas. In: Holland JF, Frei E III, eds. *Cancer Medicine*. London: BC Decker Inc.; 2000:1436–1474.

369. Yamanaka M, Greenberg B, Johnson L, Seilhamer J, Brewer M, Friedemann T, et al. Cloning and sequence analysis of the cDNA for the rat atrial natriuretic factor precursor. *Nature* 1984;309:719–722.

370. Yang Q, Gower WR Jr, Li C, Chen P, Vesely DL. Atrial natriuretic-like peptide and its prohormone within *Metasequoia*. *Proc Soc Exp Biol Med* 1999;221:188–192.

371. Yokota N, Bruneau BG, Fernandez BE, Kuroski de Bold ML, Piazza LA, Eid H, et al. Dissociation of cardiac hypertrophy, myosin heavy chain isoform expression, and natriuretic peptide production in DOCA-salt rats. *Am J Hypertens* 1995;8:301–310.

372. Yonemaru M, Ishii K, Murad F, Raffin TA. Atriopeptin-induced increases in endothelial permeability are associated with elevated cGMP levels. *Am J Physiol* 1992;263:L363–L369.

373. Yoshida K, Yamagata T, Tomura Y, Suzuki-Kusaba M, Yoshida M, Hisa H, et al. Effects of c-type natriuretic peptide on vasoconstriction in dogs. *Eur J Pharmacol* 1997;338:131–134.

374. Yu SM, Hung LM, Lin CC. CGMP-elevating agents suppress proliferation of vascular smooth muscle cells by inhibiting the activation of epidermal growth factor signaling pathway. *Circulation* 1997;95:1269–1277.

375. Zeidel ML. Renal actions of atrial natriuretic peptide: Regulation of collecting duct sodium and water transport. *Annu Rev Physiol* 1990;52:747–759.

376. Zeidel ML. Regulation of collecting duct Na⁺ reabsorption by ANP 31-67. *Clin Exp Pharmacol Physiol* 1995;22:121–124.

377. Zeidel ML, Kikeri D, Silva P, Burrowes M, Brenner BM. Atrial natriuretic peptides inhibit conductive sodium uptake by rabbit inner medullary collecting duct cells. *J Clin Invest* 1988;82:1067–1074.

378. Zhang PL, Mackenzie HS, Troy KL, Brenner BM. Effects of natriuretic peptide receptor inhibition on remnant kidney function in rats. *Kidney Int* 1994;46:414–420.

379. Zietse R, Schalekamp MA. Effect of synthetic human atrial natriuretic peptide (102–126) in nephrotic syndrome. *Kidney Int* 1988;34:717–724.

380. Zimmerman RS, Gharib H, Zimmerman D, Heublein D, Burnett JC Jr. Atrial natriuretic peptide in hypothyroidism. *J Clin Endocrinol Metab* 1987;64:353–355.

381. Zimmerman RS, Trippodo NC, MacPhee AA, Martinez AZ, Barbee RW. High-dose atrial natriuretic factor enhances albumin escape from the systemic but not the pulmonary circulation. *Circ Res* 1990;67:461–468.

382. Zivin RA, Condra JH, Dixon R, Seidah NG, Chreitien M, Nemer M, et al. Molecular cloning and characterization of DNA sequences encoding rat and human ANF. *Proc Natl Acad Sci U S A* 1984;81:6325–6329.

383. Zuidema GD, Clarke NP, Reeves JL, Gauer OH, Henry JP. Influence of moderate changes in blood volume on urine flow. *Am J Physiol* 1956;186:89–92.

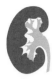

CHAPTER 35

Classical and Novel Hormonal Influences on Renal Tubular Transport, and the Emerging Concept of Intracrine Regulation

Giovambattista Capasso, Edward S. Debnam,* Pedro R. Cutillas,* Nigel J. Brunskill,† and Robert J. Unwin*

Second University of Naples, Naples, Italy
*University College London, London, United Kingdom
†University of Leicester, Leicester, United Kingdom

INTRODUCTION

The major function of the kidney is to maintain a stable extracellular milieu, which is achieved through the processes of filtration at the glomerulus, and reabsorption and secretion along the renal tubule. Various intra- and extra-renal mediators control these processes. The variety of circulating and locally released factors that has been identified to potentially influence renal tubular function in health and disease has increased dramatically in recent years, and their number continues to rise, in part due to the rapid developments in the field of proteomics (364).

In this chapter, we focus on the renal actions of selected classical and some novel "renal" hormones. We begin by describing the nature of each hormone, its main site(s) of production, control of its release and, where known, its cell mechanism of action. Next, we discuss the possible effects of these hormones on whole kidney function, specifically sodium and water handling, and their action at the level of the renal tubular cell, and we end by introducing the concept of a renal "intracrine" regulatory system. Because of functional similarities and shared transport properties of renal and intestinal epithelial cells, and the possibility of a physiologically important enterorenal axis, we also describe the effects of hormones that might act on both cell types.

The classical hormones we consider are glucocorticoids and thyroid hormones, followed by the gut-related hormones glucagon and insulin, and then other and more recently described brain–gut peptide hormones (excluding guanylin and uroguanylin, Chapter 19). We will not discuss the renin-angiotensin-aldosterone system (Chapter 13), prostaglandins, kinins (Chapter 15), catecholamines, or the natriuretic peptides (Chapter 34), which are all covered separately and in detail elsewhere.

CLASSICAL HORMONES

Glucocorticoids

Glucocorticoids, like cortisol, make up over 200 naturally occurring steroids, all synthesized from cholesterol, and they have a characteristic sterane nucleus of five hexane rings and one pentane ring (Fig. 1). The common intermediate in their biosynthesis is pregnenolone. Glucocorticoids are produced in the adrenal cortex under the control of ACTH, and they have important metabolic and anti-inflammatory actions. Cortisol is the main glucocorticoid in humans and it is corticosterone in the rat and mouse.

Originally, the cellular mechanism of action of mineralocorticoids (see Chapter 32) and glucocorticoids was believed to follow a stereotypical sequence: target cell entry, binding to a specific cytosolic receptor, passage into the nucleus with DNA binding, and the initiation of transcription, followed by de novo protein synthesis of still incompletely defined effector molecules (Fig. 2) (374). Differential effects and targets of mineralocorticoids versus glucocorticoids were originally attributed to differences in tissue distribution of specific mineralocorticoid (MR) and glucocorticoid (GR) receptors (141). However, neither receptor is truly specific for its ligand, especially the MR: receptor cloning and expression studies, and comparison of GR and MR, have shown that corticosteroids and aldosterone have equal affinity for MR (140). Cortisol and corticosterone normally circulate in concentrations 10- to 100-fold higher than aldosterone, and so a mechanism must exist to prevent glucocorticoids from causing excessive mineralocorticoid stimulation. Part of the mechanism is the microsomal oxo-reductase enzyme 11β-hydroxysteroid dehydrogenase (11HSD) found in the liver, colon, and kidney (384, 395). This enzyme protects the MR and confers mineralocorticoid specificity by metabolizing cortisol or corticosterone to their inactive metabolites (cortisone and 11-dehydrocorticosterone,

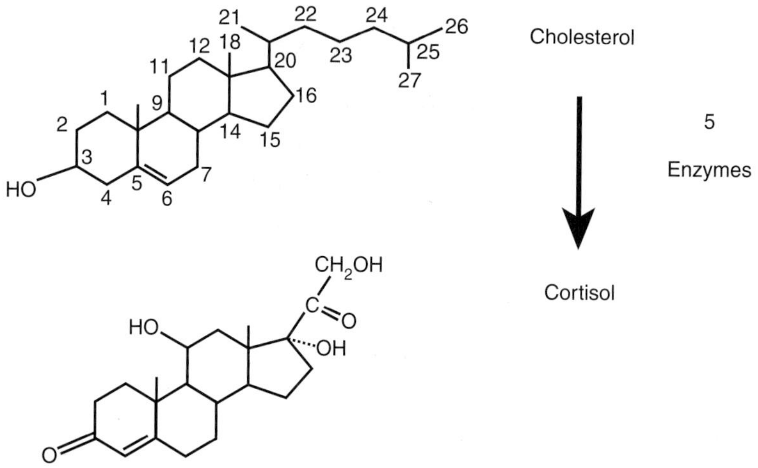

Cholesterol

5
Enzymes

Cortisol

CH$_2$OH

FIGURE 1   Glucocorticoid structure and its precursor. (Courtesy of Dr. J. Honour, Cobbold Laboratories, London, England.)

respectively), which bind only weakly to the MR (and GR) (Fig. 2) (384). Since 11HSD can reduce, as well as oxidize, cortisol and corticosterone (i.e., shuttle between their active and inactive forms), it may also be an important modulator of GR occupancy and activation (395). It could achieve this by controlling local glucocorticoid concentrations in the face of sudden and wide fluctuations in circulating levels. This might be its function in the liver and proximal nephron (259). Broadly, the reductase form of the enzyme, 11HSD1, is found

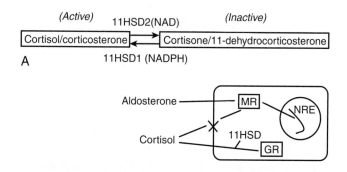

A

B   NRE = Nuclear Response Element

FIGURE 2   **A**: Cortisol–cortisone "shuttle." The microsomal enzyme 11HSD oxidizes active cortisol or corticosterone to its inactive 11-oxo form, but can also reduce its metabolite, depending on isoform and cofactor status. The enzyme that colocalizes with mineralcorticoid receptors in the distal nephron is nicotinamide adenine dinucleotide (NAD)-dependent and probably acts exclusively as an oxidase (11HSD2), whereas the enzyme in the glucorticoid-sensitive proximal tubule and loop of Henle resembles the liver isoforms (11HSD1), is NADP dependent, and may act as a reductase. Carbenoxolone (CS) and glycyrrhetinic acid (GA) inhibit 11HSD, but may differ in isoform specificity. **B**: Circulating glucocorticoids like cortisol and corticosterone (CORTISOL) may be excluded from binding to the unselective mineralocorticoid receptor (MR) by 11HSD enzyme oxidation in mineralocorticoid-selective (aldosterone-sensitive) tissues. Inhibition of 11HSD by the licorice derivative CS and GA could lead to MR overstimulation by glucocorticoids. However, 11HSD present in tissues expressing glucocorticoid receptors (GRs) might restrict (as an oxidase) or enhance (as a reductase) GR activation.

in the proximal nephron, and is the most abundant form in the kidney; and the oxidase form, 11HSD2, is found in the mineralocorticoid-sensitive distal nephron (distal tubule and collecting duct, aldosterone-sensitive distal nephron). Consistent with this is that deletion of the 11HSD2 gene in mice leads to hypertension and hypokalemia, similar to the syndrome of apparent mineralocorticoid excess (AME) in humans (189), in which 11HSD2 mutations have been found (400). In contrast, deletion of 11HSD1 in mice causes a less predictable phenotype, with raised levels of circulating corticosterone and adrenal hyperplasia, presumably a compensatory response to loss of tissue activation of (inactive) 11-dehydrocorticosterone to (active) corticosterone. These animals have impaired gluconeogenesis, but so far there are no reports of any significant changes in their renal function. Interestingly, overexpression of this enzyme in fat cells causes a metabolic syndrome (Syndrome X) in mice consisting of hypertension, visceral obesity, insulin resistance, and dyslipidemia (250). When 11HSD activity was inhibited in vivo in the rat by infusing carbenoxolone, although renal sodium excretion was reduced, micropuncture of the accessible late distal tubule detected no change in sodium reabsorption, but did find increased potassium secretion (48).

Glucocorticoids increase renal blood flow (RBF) and glomerular filtration rate (GFR), largely through improving systemic hemodynamics and enhancing vascular responsiveness to other vasoactive factors, as well as mixed effects on prostaglandin synthesis (39, 351). They also cause an increase in potassium (1, 73, 132) and net acid excretion (397) and ammonia synthesis (393, 394). The effect on potassium excretion may not be directly on the renal tubule, but via an increase in distal tubular flow rate (1), although recently, an action to increase mRNA expression of the potassium channel ROMK in the rat medullary thick ascending limb (TAL) has been described (143). Increased synthesis of ammonia by glucocorticoids is related to stimulation of glutamine uptake and its metabolism (393).

Using specific antibodies against the MR and GR, GR immunostaining is evident along the medullary TAL and distal convoluted tubule, whereas MR immunostaining is seen mainly in the distal convoluted tubule and cortical and medullary collecting ducts (127). The apparent absence of "classical" GR along the proximal tubule is at variance with results of functional studies demonstrating the effects of glucocorticoids on phosphate (137) and bicarbonate (36) reabsorption. However, a nongenomic action of glucocorticoids (and hence no correlation with reported GR distribution) has also been observed that may involve novel and so far unspecified plasma membrane steroid receptors (232), and has been shown to mediate in part the inhibition of phosphate transport (293). Intact nephron, cell suspension, cell culture, and brush border–membrane vesicle studies have all shown inhibition of sodium-phosphate cotransport (136, 300) and stimulation of the sodium–proton ($Na^+–H^+$) exchanger (NHE3) by glucocorticoids (34, 136), as well as a similar response of these transporters to acidosis (8, 57, 210). In the case of NHE3, both glucocorticoids and acidosis activate its gene promoter (74). Isolated tubule studies have demonstrated that glucocorticoids are important in the early postnatal maturation of bicarbonate transport along the rabbit proximal tubule (37), attributable to an increase NHE3 protein abundance (33, 157). Like angiotensin II (147), glucocorticoids can also stimulate bicarbonate exit from proximal tubule cells via the Na^+-HCO_3^- cotransporter (325).

In adrenalectomized rats, sodium, potassium, and bicarbonate reabsorption along the loop of Henle are reduced (352, 373). Physiological replacement of glucocorticoid (as dexamethasone) by osmotic minipump completely restores bicarbonate transport (371), but not absorption of sodium or potassium (352), confirming the importance of GR along the rat loop of Henle. Kunau et al. (unpublished observations) have also found that bicarbonate reabsorption is reduced along the distal tubule following adrenalectomy. In this nephron segment, chronic glucocorticoid administration by osmotic minipump increases thiazide-sensitive sodium-chloride (Na^+-Cl^-) cotransport, which is enhanced when aldosterone is added (373).

Following adrenalectomy, tubular Na^+,K^+-ATPase activity is reduced in the proximal tubule of rabbit and rat (110, 145), in the TAL, distal convoluted tubule, and collecting duct of rabbit (117, 118, 145), and in the collecting duct of rat (269, 270). It is rapidly (within hours) restored by dexamethasone in the rabbit (117, 118, 145), but not in the rat (270), in which it takes several days to recover (269). Stimulation of Na^+,K^+-ATPase activity appears to be direct and not dependent on a change in luminal membrane permeability to sodium and increase in intracellular sodium concentration (236, 237, 316, 401). In proximal tubule cells in culture, increased mRNA expression of the α and β subunits of the amiloride-sensitive epithelial sodium channel (ENaC) is mediated by a protein-dependent pretranslational mechanism (222). In addition to their effects on the transport proteins already mentioned, glucocorticoids have been shown to inhibit sodium-sulfate cotransport in the renal brush border membrane of the chick (318), and to stimulate sulfate secretion via bicarbonate–sulfate exchange in teleost fish (317).

Thyroid Hormones

Thyroid hormones are iodinated amino acids (Fig. 3) that affect a variety of metabolic processes, including the regulation of glucose and lipid metabolism, stimulation of cell growth and maturation, and tissue oxygen consumption (61, 289). They can also influence mineral metabolism and affect the distribution of water and electrolytes between body fluid compartments. Their importance is evident from the clinical disorders of hypo- and hyper-thyroidism.

There are two main thyroid hormones: thyroxine (T_4) and tri-iodothyronine (T_3). Their synthesis requires iodine uptake by the thyroid gland, a process generating a large concentration gradient (up to 500-fold) of iodide between thyroid cells and plasma, leading to the formation of the peptide-bound precursors mono- and di-iodotyrosine. These iodotyrosines undergo oxidative condensation with thyroglobulin (a glycoprotein synthesized in follicular cells) yielding several iodothyronines, including T_4 and T_3 (290). The main secretory product is T_4, which is inactive and only exerts its physiological effect after peripheral deiodination to T_3 by the enzyme thyroxine-5'-deiodinase. Three isoforms of this enzyme have been identified (46): the most important is type I, detected predominantly in the liver and kidneys, which is responsible for the production of two-thirds of total T_3; type II accounts for most of the T_3 found in the pituitary, brain, and in brown fat; type III is involved in reductive deiodination of thyroid hormones and catalyzes the conversion of T_4 to reverse T_3, and conversion of T_3 to 3, 3'-T_2, which are biologically inactive. Type III overexpression can cause "consumptive hypothyroidism." In the blood, T_4 and T_3 are bound to plasma proteins (globulin, prealbumin, and albumin); T_3 is bound less strongly than T_4 and the amount of free T_3 is 8 to 10 times more than T_4—only the free, unbound hormone is active.

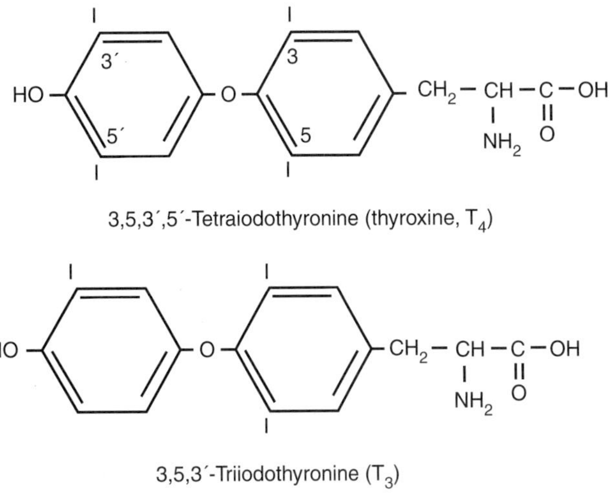

3,5,3',5'-Tetraiodothyronine (thyroxine, T_4)

3,5,3'-Triiodothyronine (T_3)

FIGURE 3 Structure of thyroid hormones.

T_3 enters cells (or is released in the cytoplasm from T_4) and transported to the nucleus, where it binds to specific receptors (Fig. 4). In the kidney and liver, it has been shown that ~85% of nuclear thyroid receptors bind T_3 and ~15% of T_4. T_3 receptors are nuclear receptors that can bind to regulatory gene sequences acting as transcription factors (62). They are members of a large family of hormone-responsive transcription factors that are similar in their structure and mechanism of action. The structure of the receptor includes a COOH-terminal portion that is important for ligand binding, a DNA-binding domain and an NH_4-terminal domain (function unknown) (220). There are two T_3-receptor genes, α and β, located on chromosomes 17 and 13, respectively; each gene has at least two alternative mRNA splice products. There are tissue-specific and developmental patterns of T_3-receptor mRNA expression. In the kidney, there is T_3 mRNA expression of $α_1$, $α_2$, and $β_1$ receptors, but there is little information on the segmental nephron distribution of nuclear binding of thyroid hormones. In development, the $α_1$ T_3 receptor is expressed very early on, especially in the brain; T_3 β receptor mRNA expression increases significantly during development (354). Thyroid status also influences the expression of T_3 receptor mRNA and tissue T_3 receptor protein concentrations. In the rat, injections of T_3 reduce the concentrations of T_3 receptor $α_1$ and T_3 receptor $α_2$ mRNA in the kidney (188).

Understanding the actions of thyroid hormones on renal function is complicated for the following reasons: (1) direct cellular effects can be influenced by changes in renal hemodynamics, (2) heterogeneity of nephron function and variation in thyroid hormone sensitivity, which can offset and mask any segmental nephron effects, and (3) many investigators have used a variety of experimental conditions in which to study thyroid hormone action, especially as the response to thyroid hormones varies according to the duration of hypothyroidism (76). Despite these limitations, chronic hypothyroidism has been shown to reduce RBF and GFR, and to increase urine flow rate and water intake (353). These effects have been attributed to impaired urinary concentration and dilution (121, 257), linked to a reduction in the corticomedullary osmotic gradient (320, 353). Thyroid hormone excess, as in uncomplicated thyrotoxicosis, increases GFR, renal plasma flow (RPF), tubular reabsorption and secretion (135). Hypercalcemia is a recognized feature of hyperthyroidism, but it is usually of modest degree and rarely affects renal function (38); although when severe, as in any case of malignant hypercalcemia, it can reduce urinary concentrating ability (through stimulation of the basolateral TAL calcium receptor (see Chapter 63) and GFR (122).

In humans and animals with hypothyroidism, GFR and RPF are reduced and filtration fraction increased (which would passively enhance proximal tubular fluid reabsorption) (256). After 3 weeks of hypothyroidism, rat single-nephron GFR (SNGFR) is reduced, but administering a competitive angiotensin II antagonist can prevent this (148). This is probably related to a fall in cardiac output in hypothyroidism (77) and associated activation of the renin-angiotensin system, at least at the tissue level, since circulating plasma renin activity seems not to increase. A reduction in GFR might also be explained by a decrease in glomerular surface area, as a result of thyroid hormone deficiency during growth. However, any changes in renal growth related to thyroid hormone action appear to affect the renal tubule more than the glomerulus, as the tubules are relatively short when compared with glomerular surface area (58). Thyroid hormone lack also impairs the renal

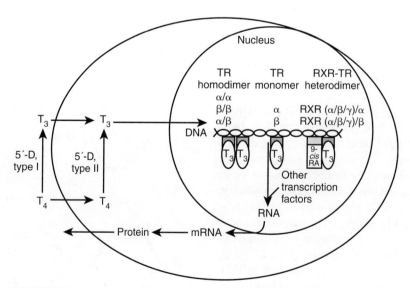

FIGURE 4 Mechanism of thyroid hormone cell action. The enzyme T_4 5'-deiodinase (5'-D) generates T_3 from T_4. T_3 binds to thyroid hormone receptors in the nucleus to form the T_3-receptor complex, which interacts with specific sequences in DNA regulatory regions and modifies gene expression. (With permission, from Brent GA. Mechanisms of disease: the molecular basis of thyroid hormone action. *N Engl J Med* 1994;331:847–853.)

response to unilateral nephrectomy with reduced renal compensatory growth (422).

At the tubular level, hypothyroidism is associated with impaired urinary acidification (246), an aldosterone-independent natriuresis (exaggerated by water ingestion or infusion of mannitol or saline [361]), and a reduction in proximal tubular reabsorption (77). In chronic hypothyroidism there is a significant reduction in proximal tubular sodium reabsorption that cannot be fully explained by the decrease in SNGFR, extracellular volume expansion, or changes in peritubular Starling forces (256). Indeed, a specific defect in sodium-coupled L-histidine transport in hypothyroid rats has been reported, and T_3 administration to hypothyroid rats produces a dose- and time-dependent increase in proximal fluid reabsorption (77). This change is apparent within 24 hours, but even after 6 days of treatment, isotonic fluid reabsorption does not reach normal values, which may be due partly to a lack of tubule growth (Fig. 5).

A direct effect of thyroid hormones on tubular transport has been confirmed by experiments designed to compare the time-course of changes in GFR, filtered sodium load, and specific transport processes. After a single dose of T_3, there is an early increase in cortical Na^+,K^+-ATPase activity before the increase in GFR and sodium load, suggesting a direct tubular effect (Fig. 6) (230). The role of thyroid hormones in regulating sodium pump activity is now well established: activity decreasing in hypothyroidism and increasing following T_3 or T_4 administration (197). However, these early studies were performed on whole kidney tissue. When microdissected single tubules are studied, the response of each nephron segment differs depending on the duration of hypothyroidism. In acute (<2 weeks) experiments in hypothyroid rabbits, a decrease in Na^+,K^+-ATPase activity is found only in the proximal convoluted and straight tubules, and in the cortical and medullary collecting ducts (24). Similarly, in acutely hypothyroid rats, enzyme

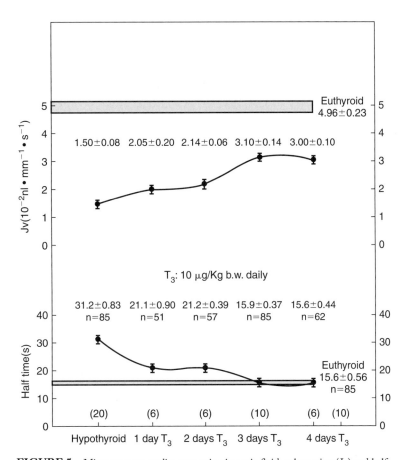

FIGURE 5 Micropuncture studies comparing isotonic fluid reabsorption (Jv) and half-time of reabsorption along the proximal tubules of hypothyroid rats given T_3 (1 μg/100 g body weight^{-1}) and of euthyroid animals. In hypothyroid animals, Jv was reduced compared with that in euthyroid rats. Physiological doses of T_3 significantly increased Jv within 24 hours; however, it did not normalize because the lack of thyroid hormones causes morphological changes, including a reduction of tubule diameter, which is present in hypothyroid rats even after 4 days of T_3. (With permission, from De Santo NG, Capasso G, Kinne R, Moewes B, Carella C, Anastasio P, Giordano C. Tubular transport processes in proximal tubules of hypothyroid rats. Lack of relationship between thyroidal dependent rise of isotonic fluid reabsorption and Na^+-K^+-ATPase activity. *Pflugers Arch* 1982;394:294–301.)

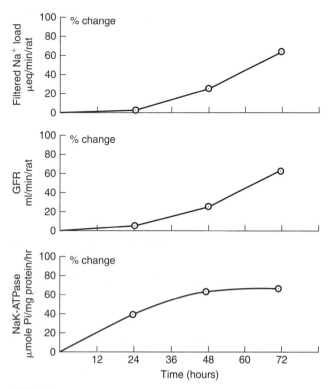

FIGURE 6   Time-course effect of a single injection of T_3 (50 µg/100 g body weight^{-1}) in hypothyroid rats on filtered sodium load, glomerular filtration rate, and renal cortical Na$^+$,K$^+$-ATPase activity. The graph illustrates that the early increase in Na$^+$,K$^+$-ATPase activity precedes the increase in GFR and filtered sodium load, suggesting a direct effect of T_3 on the sodium pump. (With permission, from Lo Cs, Lo TN. Time-course of the renal response to triiodothyronine in the rat. *Am J Physiol* 1979;236:F9–F13.)

activity is decreased only in the proximal convoluted tubule (146), and activity is completely restored within 48 hours following high-dose T_3 administration. In chronically hypothyroid animals all nephron segments of the rabbit show reduced Na$^+$,K$^+$-ATPase activity (25, 26), whereas in the rat only the proximal convoluted and straight tubules are affected (76, 77).

The time-course of restoration in enzyme activity in the rat proximal tubule has been studied in some detail, together with measurements of sodium reabsorption (77). At physiological doses of T_3, Na$^+$,K$^+$-ATPase activity remains low for about 3 days, but after 7 days of treatment enzyme activity reaches ~75% of control. This differs from the time-course of recovery of sodium transport in the same tubule, suggesting an additional effect on tubular transport (Fig. 7). Acute treatment of cells or animals with low doses of T_3 can affect membrane transport processes without de novo synthesis of transport proteins (335). For example, in rat diaphragm and liver cells a single high dose of T_3 given to euthyroid rats increases cell membrane permeability to potassium before any change in Na$^+$,K$^+$-ATPase activity (160). In renal cells, micropuncture studies indicate that potassium permeability is decreased in chronic hypothyroidism, which may be important in the early effect of thyroid

hormones to restore proximal tubular reabsorption (76, 77). It has also been shown that thyroid hormones act on the genes encoding the subunits of Na$^+$,K$^+$-ATPase (62, 253): in primary cultures of rabbit proximal tubule cells exposed to T_3 (10^{-7} M), transcription of the genes for the α and β subunits is activated, and mRNA levels are increased (227).

In addition to effects on Na$^+$,K$^+$-ATPase activity, the effect of thyroid hormones on other sodium transport systems has been studied. Excess thyroid hormone can cause hyperphosphatemia (56): renal brush border–membrane vesicles from hypothyroid rats have a lower capacity for sodium gradient–dependent phosphate uptake compared with hyperthyroid animals (125), a finding confirmed recently and explained by a reduced abundance of the type 2 sodium-phosphate cotransporter (NaPi2) (331). Similarly, in acutely hypothyroid rats high doses of T_3 increase the turnover rate of the sodium-phosphate cotransporter in brush border membranes isolated from proximal straight tubules (420). The effect of thyroid hormones on phosphate transport appears to be age-dependent: in aging rats compared with young rats, sodium-phosphate cotransporter activity is less sensitive to thyroid hormone when levels are reduced or increased (3).

Activity of the Na$^+$–H$^+$ exchanger is also affected by thyroid hormone. In kidney brush border–membrane vesicles from chronically hypothyroid rats, Na$^+$–H$^+$ exchanger activity is reduced compared with control, and is increased in hyperthyroid rats (211). In acutely hypothyroid rats a large dose of T_4 given over 4 days increases Na$^+$–H$^+$ exchanger activity in brush border–membrane vesicles from the outer cortex (mainly proximal convoluted tubules), but not in vesicles from the juxtamedullary cortex (420). This increase in Na$^+$–H$^+$ exchanger activity is independent of GFR and is stimulated in proximal-like opossum kidney cells (OK) without a change in pH$_i$, cell hypertrophy, or tubular hyperplasia (417); it is probably due to stimulation of isoform NHE3 activity (75). In contrast, in another study using brush border–membrane vesicles isolated from kidneys of chronically hypothyroid rats treated for 3 days with low doses of T_3, no significant change was found in amiloride-sensitive Na$^+$ uptake by the Na$^+$–H$^+$ exchanger compared with untreated hypothyroid rats (77). Thus, the effect of thyroid hormone on the Na$^+$–H$^+$ exchanger seems to be dose- and time-dependent; however, when Na$^+$–H$^+$ exchange is measured in brush border–membrane vesicles obtained from euthyroid or chronically hyperthyroid animals under "short-circuit" (conditions with high potassium concentrations on both sides of the vesicle membrane) and in the presence of valinomycin (to permeabilize the membrane to potassium), no difference in electroneutral Na$^+$–H$^+$ exchange is found (238), again supporting a link to an altered membrane permeability for potassium. In a recent study, it has been confirmed that thyroid hormones may alter the expression of several acid-base transport proteins, but only when chronic hypothyroid animals are challenged with an acid load. Under this condition at the level of the

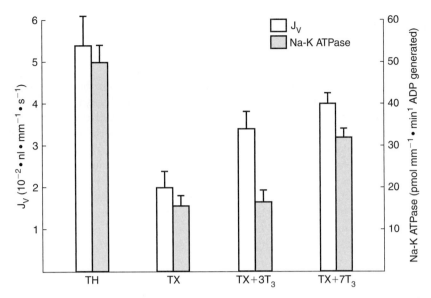

FIGURE 7 Isotonic fluid reabsorption (Jv) and Na$^+$,K$^+$-ATPase activity in late proximal convoluted tubules of euthyroid animals (TH), hypothyroid rats (TX), hypothyroid rats treated for 3 days with 1 μg/100 g body weight^{-1} (TX+T3), hypothyroid rats substituted for 7 days with 1 μg/100 g body weight^{-1}. Note that the hormone replacement induces a significant increase in Jv after 3 days without affecting Na$^+$,K$^+$-ATPase activity. (With permission, data from Capasso G, Lin JT, De Santo NG, Kinne R. Short-term effect of low doses of tri-iodothyronine on proximal tubular membrane Na-K-ATPase and potassium permeability in thyroidectomized rats. *Pflugers Arch* 1985;403:90–96; and Capasso G, Kinne-Saffran E, De Santo NG, Kinne R. Regulation of volume reabsorption by thyroid hormones in the proximal tubule of rat: minor role of luminal sodium permeability. *Pflugers Arch* 1985;403:97–104.)

proximal tubule there is reduced expression of NHE3, the B2 subunit of the H$^+$-ATPase, and of the basolateral Na(+)/HCO3(−) contransporter NBC1, while in the collecting duct there is a higher expression of the acid-secretory type A intercalated cell specific Cl(-)/HCO3(-) exchanger AE1. Therefore, hypothyroidism is associated with a very mild defect in renal acid handling that seems to be located mainly in the proximal tubule, and which is compensated by the distal nephron (257a).

Regarding other transport proteins, one recent study has shown that hypothyroidism is characterized by increased abundance of the bumetanide-sensitive Na$^+$,K$^+$-2Cl$^-$ cotransporter (NKCC2) and aquaporin-2 (AQP2) water channel, probably due to stimulation of vasopressin release by increased levels of hypothalamic thyroid-releasing hormone (TRH), since urinary excretion of vasopressin was elevated (331). On the other hand, the thiazide-sensitive Na$^+$-Cl$^-$ cotransporter, the α, β, and γ subunits of ENaC, and the α$_1$ subunit of Na$^+$,K$^+$-ATPase (see above), all showed a moderate decrease in total kidney protein abundance proportional to the smaller kidney mass in hypothyroid animals. Although these changes were not associated with any obvious disturbance of sodium and water balance, this may become apparent when animals are stressed. Indeed, when hypothyroid rats are challenged by water deprivation (for 36 hours), they maintain significantly higher urine flow rates with reduced urinary and medullary osmolalities compared with controls or thyroid hormone–replaced rats (71). At odds with the former study, western blot

analyses in this study demonstrated decreased protein abundance of several transporters, including Na$^+$,K$^+$-2Cl$^-$, Na$^+$,K$^+$-ATPase, NHE3, AQP2, AQP3, and AQP4, while AQP1 and the urea transporters UTA(1) and UTA(2) were unaffected, making a functional interpretation difficult; however, these findings do seem to indicate a disturbed countercurrent mechanism involving TAL and collecting duct function. In addition, epithelial cell height in the hypothyroid TAL is reduced in its medullary portion and abundance of the TAL-associated Tamm–Horsfall (THP) protein is decreased (330).

Thyroid hormones are also involved in maturational changes in fluid and electrolyte transport (340), an effect linked to their postnatal action to increase Na$^+$–H$^+$ exchanger activity (NHE3) (35), although a compensatory increase in glucocorticoids has also been proposed. In fact, it has been suggested that these two hormones can play a compensatory role for one another: experiments in young rats have shown that lack of both hormones completely abolishes the maturational increase in NHE3 mRNA, protein abundance, and Na$^+$–H$^+$ exchanger activity (158).

In summary, thyroid hormones can modulate renal hemodynamics and tubular transport function. In hypothyroidism, a decrease in GFR, urine concentrating ability and inhibition of sodium reabsorption are now well-documented changes. The effects of thyroid hormones on kidney function are mainly direct and do not depend solely on their known systemic cardiovascular effects.

Glucagon and Related Peptides Secretin and Vasoactive Intestinal Polypeptide

GLUCAGON

Pancreatic glucagon is a catabolic 29–amino acid peptide hormone (molecular weight 3485 Da) secreted from A cells of the pancreas, and it is primarily involved in stimulating liver glycogenolysis and gluconeogenesis to maintain plasma glucose concentrations during the interdigestive period, and in fasting conditions. The glucagon receptor has been cloned; it is a G-protein–coupled receptor with homology to secretin and vasoactive intestinal polypeptide (VIP) receptors (67, 239). High levels of glucagon receptor mRNA expression have been found in liver, kidney, heart, adipose tissue, spleen, pancreatic islets, ovary, and thymus (66, 171, 415).

Glucagon release is stimulated by several hormones, including glucocorticoids (cortisol) and epinephrine, and is inhibited by extracellular glucose, somatostatin, and insulin (370). It is also released following a protein-rich meal, and stimulated by both orally and intravenously administered amino acids, although more effectively by the former route

(286). Glucagon has been implicated in the postprandial and amino acid–induced increase in GFR (Fig. 8) (100), and in the natriuresis of starvation (149, 372). Glucagon is well known to produce renal afferent arteriolar vasodilatation, which was originally thought to account for its hyperfiltering and natriuretic effects (306). Glucagon was later shown to stimulate renal tubular adenylate cyclase through specific receptors, mainly in the distal nephron (70, 260, 304). Thus, the concept of direct tubular effects of glucagon emerged. Glucagon is also known to inhibit proximal tubular sodium and phosphate reabsorption (206), and to increase urate excretion (414). Studies using opposum kidney epithelial (OK) cells show that glucagon chronically (24 hours) activates, but acutely inhibits (1 hour), Na^+-H^+ exchanger (NHE3) activity at the apical membrane via a PKA-dependent pathway (4), indicating that its effects on renal sodium handling are complex. Although early studies were unable to identify glucagon receptors or glucagon-sensitive adenylate cyclase in the proximal tubule (261), recent autoradiographic work has revealed specific binding of radio-iodinated glucagon in both the renal cortex and medulla, and that glucagon-receptor (GR) mRNA is expressed in the proximal tubule, TAL, and

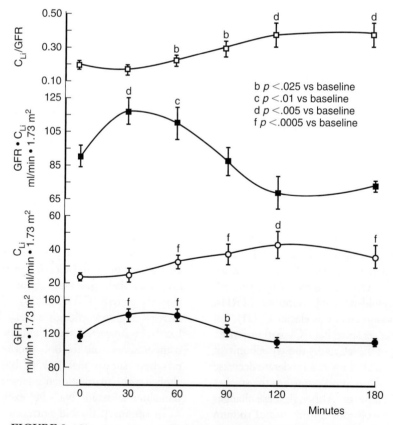

FIGURE 8   Changes in glomerular filtration rate (GFR), lithium clearance (C_{Li}), absolute reabsorption of isotonic fluid along the proximal tubule (GFR-C_{Li}), and fractional excretion of fluid from the proximal tubule (C_{Li}/GFR) in healthy humans following a meat meal. All subjects received a protein load of 2 g/kg body weight^{-1} in the form of cooked red meat. (With permission, from De Santo NG, Capasso G, Anastasio P, et al. Renal handling of sodium after an oral protein load in adult humans. *Renal Physiol Biochem* 1992;15:41–52.)

collecting duct (249), suggesting that glucagon can directly influence tubular cell function.

There is also accumulating evidence that glucagon influences renal function through changes in circulating levels of cAMP. Several studies have remarked that the plasma concentrations of glucagon following a meat meal are insufficient to cause direct renal vasodilatation and the increase in GFR (64, 272). Moreover, the peak rise in plasma levels of glucagon following a meat meal occurs later than the increase in GFR, and levels remain elevated when GFR has fallen to baseline (99, 100) (Figs. 8 and 9). The idea that another circulatory factor related to glucagon might account for this discrepancy comes from studies in which a comparison was made between the renal effects of peripheral and portal vein infusions of glucagon (64, 372). Only after portal vein infusion did glucagon increase GFR and sodium excretion, suggesting a liver-borne factor ("glomerulopressin") as the prime, or comediator, of glucagon's renal effects (2, 218). Recently, Bankir and coworkers have provided evidence that this hepato-renal link could be mediated by glucagon-stimulated, and liver-derived, cAMP (Fig. 10) (21), and disturbances in this axis may explain the renal response to certain pathological states,

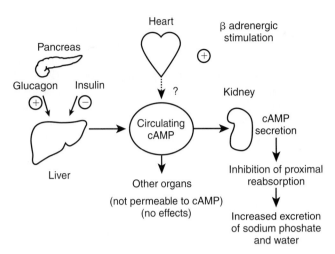

FIGURE 10 Scheme of hypothesis on the role of liver-borne cAMP in control of proximal tubule reabsorption and sodium excretion. Circulating cAMP may represent a physiological hepatorenal link that depends on the insulin/glucagon ratio in portal vein blood. (With permission, from Bankir L, Martin H, Déchaux M, Ahloulay M. Plasma cAMP: a hepatorenal link influencing proximal reabsorption and renal hemodynamics? *Kidney Int* 1997;51:S-50–S-56.)

including the hyperfiltration of diabetes mellitus (20). It has been suggested that cAMP-mediated inhibition of proximal tubular sodium reabsorption, combined with a direct effect of glucagon on sodium reabsorption along the TAL and macula densa region results in inhibition of tubuloglomerular feedback, thus increasing GFR and sodium excretion. But this model requires the existence of renal cAMP receptors that have not yet been identified in mammals, and (presumably) an inhibitory effect of glucagon on sodium transport at the macula densa. However, the effect of glucagon on net sodium excretion seems more variable and depends on the extent to which distal nephron sodium reabsorption may be stimulated (15). As already mentioned, glucagon activates adenylate cyclase along the TAL and collecting duct. Along the TAL, adenylate cyclase stimulation has functionally been linked to increased sodium transport (98, 406), resulting in increased interstitial medullary osmolality (214), possibly due to direct stimulation of the sodium pump (235). More complex is the effect of glucagon on bicarbonate reabsorption along the TAL. In contrast to its stimulatory effect on sodium transport, glucagon acutely reduces bicarbonate reabsorption (150), probably by inhibition of the Na^+–H^+ exchanger; in line with this it also inhibits net urinary acidification and increases urine pH (372).

The importance of pancreatic glucagon in body glucose homeostasis raises the question of whether this hormone influences renal glucose handling. Cyclic AMP and dibutyryl cAMP stimulate proximal renal tubular cell glucose uptake (phloridzin sensitive and SGLT mediated); membrane expression of SGLT1 in *Xenopus* oocytes is enhanced by increased cAMP-dependent PKA activity (412). Interestingly, pancreatic glucagon also promotes phlorizin-insensitive (GLUT-mediated) glucose uptake at the proximal-tubule

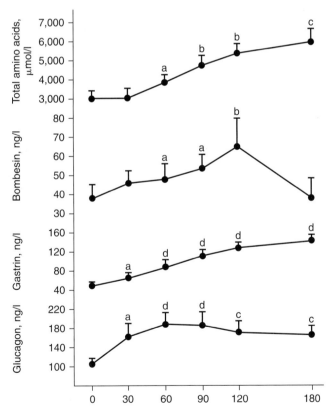

FIGURE 9 Changes in plasma amino acid and hormone concentrations after a meat meal in healthy humans. All the subjects received a protein load of 2 g/kg body weight^{-1} in the form of cooked red meat. $^a p <.05$; $^b p <.01$; $^c p <.005$; $^d p <.001$ versus baseline. (With permission, from De Santo NG, Capasso G, Anastasio P, Coppola S, Bellini L, Lombardi A. Brain–gut peptides and the renal hemodynamic response to an oral protein load: a study of gastrin, bombesin and glucagon in man. *Renal Physiol Biochem* 1992;15:53–56.)

brush border membrane by a process involving PKC activation (Debnam and Marks, unpublished observations). It is possible that the increase in GLUT-mediated glucose transport at the proximal-tubule brush border membrane in experimental type 1 diabetes mellitus (insulinopenic) (248) results from the action of raised levels of plasma glucagon. Surprisingly, SGLT1-mediated glucose transport in the proximal tubule is unchanged in diabetes (248), raising a question over the relationship between glucagon and the PKA signaling pathway in the context of proximal tubular function, especially in diabetes.

In intestinal enterocytes there is evidence that pancreatic glucagon enhances sodium-dependent glucose uptake: exposure of intact intestine (363) or isolated enterocytes (102) to glucagon increases brush border galactose uptake. The response occurs within 30 minutes, indicating that de novo protein synthesis is unlikely to be involved (102). The basis of this rapid response to glucagon is probably a consequence of reduced brush border membrane permeability to sodium, causing membrane hyperpolarization (363). Circumstantial evidence suggests that altered levels of intracellular cAMP are responsible for this permeability change: glucagon elevates enterocyte levels of cAMP (343), and enterocyte exposure to the membrane permeable analog dibutyryl cAMP increases brush border sodium-dependent sugar uptake and membrane potential (156, 343), as well as expression of the glucose transporter SGLT1 (Debnam et al., unpublished observations, 1998).

Does glucagon have a physiological role in regulating whole kidney function? The answer remains speculative, because it is difficult to bring together all the actions of this hormone. Glucagon is a major regulator of normal glucose homeostasis; it increases splanchnic and RBF and GFR; it inhibits proximal sodium and phosphate reabsorption, yet can stimulate glucose uptake; and yet it seems to increase sodium absorption along the distal nephron and decrease urinary acidification. Through its gut and renal effects (mediated largely by cAMP generation) following a meal, glucagon could be important in enhancing glucose conservation, while at the same time promoting excretion of excess dietary sodium. Potentially relevant to the concept of glucagon as an important natriuretic hormone is the report of an increase in frequency of a glucagon receptor missense mutation (which reduces hormone binding and cAMP generation) in essential hypertension (264).

Glucagon-like peptide-1 (GLP-1) and GLP-2 are produced by posttranslational modification of the pre-proglucagon gene product of L-cells of the distal small intestine in response to luminal carbohydrate and fat digestive products. GLP-1 is further processed within the L-cell to GLP-1 (7–36) amide and it is a powerful stimulator of insulin release, as well as being involved in appetite control. Animal studies have reported that GLP-1 has natriuretic and diuretic actions, suggesting a potential role for this peptide in sodium and water homeostasis (262), and infusion studies in humans confirm these actions

(159). GLP-2, like GLP-1, is insulinotrophic, but also influences carbohydrate balance at the intestinal level. Thus, when infused intravenously into rats so as to mimic the postprandial rise in plasma GLP-2 concentration, the peptide enhances facilitated glucose movement across the enterocyte basolateral membrane and sodium-dependent glucose transport (SGLT1) at the brush border (83). Binding sites for GLP-2 have been detected in the villus epithelium (365), suggesting direct intestinal effects of the peptide. Renal GLP-2–binding sites also exist (365) and the peptide is taken up and cleared by the kidney (326). However, the actions of GLP-2 on renal tubular function are unknown.

SECRETIN

Secretin is a 27–amino acid endocrine hormone secreted from the epithelium of the upper small intestine in response to low pH and the presence of nutrient digestive products. Secretin differs from the other two classical gastrointestinal hormones gastrin and cholecystokinin in that its entire amino acid sequence is necessary for its physiological effects. The major function of secretin is to stimulate the secretion of bicarbonate, sodium, and water from the exocrine pancreas in order to maintain an optimum pH for pancreatic enzyme action within the duodenal lumen. Other reported transport effects include increased ion and fluid secretion across the intestinal epithelium (180). The peptide also reduces gastrointestinal motility and transit, resulting from smooth muscle relaxation. In the kidney, arteriolar vasodilatation is probably responsible for the increase in blood flow after secretin administration (88, 382); however, in a micropuncture study secretin has been reported to have a vasoconstrictor effect when perfused directly into peritubular capillaries (323).

Binding sites for secretin have been identified in rat kidney, receptor density being particularly high in the TAL (82); receptor transcript has also been detected in the human kidney (294). These findings are in keeping with many earlier observations that administration of secretin alters urine output and electrolyte excretion. A high-affinity secretin receptor has been identified that is functionally coupled to adenylate cyclase stimulation, and its mRNA has been detected in the kidney (89). The kidney is also a major site of secretin catabolism: renal extraction accounts for some 45% of released secretin (95).

Secretin has been shown to promote sodium excretion in dogs (245). In humans, treatment with secretin increases water and sodium excretion, and RPF (378, 382); these findings are also observed in patients with cystic fibrosis (404). A marked increase in bicarbonate excretion has also been reported in response to secretin (378), suggesting that its postprandial release may explain the transient rise in urinary pH following a meal ("alkaline tide"), although glucagon (see earlier) has also been implicated in this phenomenon. The effects of secretin on transport are independent of changes in GFR, implying that the diuresis is a consequence of reduced tubular sodium reabsorption. In contrast, the micropuncture study referred to earlier found that intraluminal application of secretin in the proximal tubule stimulated fluid reabsorption, while increasing SNGFR (323).

VASOACTIVE INTESTINAL PEPTIDE

VIP is a 28–amino acid peptide originally isolated from the hog small intestine by Said and Mutt (327). VIP is present in both the central and peripheral nervous systems, and is an important physiological modulator, having both neurotransmitter and neurocrine actions. This peptide has some structural homology with secretin and glucagon, which results in some functional overlap; however, it is not considered to be a true (circulating) hormone. Thus, VIP is a vasodilator and may be responsible for hyperemia in salivary and pancreatic tissue during meal-evoked exocrine secretion. Specific endocrine VIP-releasing cells have not been detected in the small intestine; release of supraphysiological levels of VIP in clinical conditions of hyperplasia of VIP-producing neurons (VIPoma) results in increased pancreatic secretion, perhaps reaching levels high enough to cause diarrhea although effects on secretion in the small and large intestine also seem likely.

Available data suggest that VIP has both direct and indirect effects on renal function. Indirect actions may result from release of renin: increased plasma levels of renin have been recorded after VIP infusion in vivo (72, 107) and in vitro (299). In dogs, VIP mediates renin release produced by renal nerve stimulation (299), and its effect on preglomerular blood vessels is almost certainly via adenylate cyclase stimulation (153). There is also evidence that VIP exerts direct actions at a tubular level. Although VIP receptors have not been found on tubular cells, VIP has been shown to stimulate cyclase activity in basolateral membranes isolated from rabbit renal cortex and medulla (152), and human renal membranes (81). These experiments also confirmed receptor specificity: a VIP receptor antagonist reduced the cyclase response to VIP, but not to glucagon (153), and VIP binding to tubular cells increased cAMP levels.

In the isolated perfused rat kidney, VIP increases the excretion of sodium, chloride, potassium, and water (324), a response that was independent of changes in vascular resistance and GFR. In the rabbit in vivo, VIP also increases the excretion of sodium, despite causing a reduction in RPF and GFR (107), results reinforcing the notion of a direct action on tubular ion transport. Interestingly, in this species Duggan and coworkers (176) showed that metabolism of VIP depends on ingested sodium: a chronically low-sodium intake increased VIP's metabolic clearance rate, while acute sodium loading reduced it (176). The same authors also found evidence for a direct natriuretic effect of VIP (113). However, in humans (72) and rats (231), the diuretic and natriuretic effects of intravenous VIP seem to depend on its significant hemodynamic effects.

Addition of VIP to the basolateral surface of an MDCK cell monolayer increases cAMP levels and apical chloride secretion (153). In intestinal enterocytes, which display similar transport properties to tubular cells, VIP binds to specific membrane receptors (5) and it also stimulates fluid and electrolyte secretion (216, 332). A selective blocker of enterocyte VIP receptors has been shown to abolish the secretory effects of VIP (22). Nitric oxide (NO) is involved in the enterocyte secretory response to VIP: NO enhances neuronal release of VIP and potentiates the secretory effect of VIP (268); as in the kidney, the intestinal effects of VIP are mediated by cAMP stimulation (45).

Surprisingly, despite an elevated cellular level of cAMP, VIP reduces enterocyte sugar transport (192). This is in contrast to the stimulatory action of glucagon described earlier. While these conflicting observations suggest that multiple intracellular signaling pathways are involved in the control of nutrient transport, it should be borne in mind that VIP-induced cellular efflux of chloride across the brush border membrane would depolarize this membrane and so diminish the driving force for sodium-dependent sugar uptake. In this context, it is worth noting that cAMP itself stimulates SGLT1-mediated glucose transport in the intestine of cystic fibrosis knockout mice, in which the cAMP-mediated, brush-border chloride conductance is defective (343).

Insulin and Related Peptides, and Amylin

INSULIN

Insulin is an anabolic polypeptide (molecular weight 5734 Da) comprising two chains, A and B, made up of 21 and 30 amino acids, respectively, bound together by two disulfide bridges, as well as a disulfide bridge within the A chain itself. Insulin is synthesized in the β cells of the pancreas and it is the major hormonal regulator of glucose homeostasis. Although several other hormones exert hyperglycemic actions, insulin is the only circulatory hormone to have hypoglycemic effects. Insulin is synthesized as part of a precursor molecule, proinsulin. Cleavage of proinsulin produces insulin and connecting peptide (C-peptide), which are then released from the β cell by exocytosis following appropriate stimuli. C-peptide has several established physiological actions, including stimulation of human and rat renal tubular Na^+,K^+-ATPase activity (287, 367, 424). In the rat medullary TAL, this action is mediated by the PKC signaling pathway (367); studies in human renal tubular cells have also implicated involvement of ERK1 and two MAP kinases (424). In rat proximal tubules, the stimulatory effect of C-peptide on Na^+,K^+-ATPase is enhanced by neuropeptide Y (NPY) (287).

Insulin binds to peripheral insulin receptors causing increased glucose uptake. In the liver, this results in increased glycogenesis, and in adipose tissue fat deposition (221). Insulin also stimulates protein synthesis and acts as a growth factor. There are additional circulating hormones that also promote cell growth, which were formerly known as somatomedins, but are now called insulin-like growth factors (IGF) I and II (421). IGF-I is bound to circulating binding proteins that modulate its action (303). Its main source is the liver, but it is also synthesized in the kidney (glomerulus and distal tubule) (182); IGF-binding proteins and receptor are present in the TAL and other nephron segments (87, 126). Treatment of rats with IGF-I increases kidney size and GFR, decreases renal vascular resistance, and stimulates mesangial cell growth and glomerular matrix production, all of which contribute to the pathogenesis of diabetic renal injury (182, 183, 185). In humans, IGF-I increases RBF and GFR by 25%, and causes sodium retention and extracellular volume expansion (258). There is conflicting evidence over IGF-I's role in the recovery from tubular injury (119). In the proximal tubule, it stimulates phosphate reabsorption (184, 292), vitamin D activation (409), and NHE3 activity (203). Recent studies suggest a dual effect of IGF-I on potassium recycling across the apical TAL cell membrane, since low concentrations of IGF-I stimulate, while high concentrations inhibit, ROMK channel activity: the stimulatory effect of IGF-I is mediated by a MAP kinase-dependent pathway, whereas the inhibitory effect is due to increased activity of tyrosine kinase (391).

IGF-I increases amiloride-sensitive sodium uptake in an MDCK subclone with principal cell-like properties (54). There is growing support for the belief that locally produced IGF-I participates in the development of diabetic glomerular disease and perhaps other forms of progressive glomerular injury. Treatment of diabetic rats with an IGF-I receptor antagonist inhibits early renal hypertrophy and also blocks compensatory renal growth following loss of renal mass (177). IGF-II, like IGF-I, stimulates phosphate absorption in the proximal tubule (124) and both IGF-I and IGF-II can act on the apical and basolateral cell membranes (94, 184, 200).

The insulin receptor, like the receptor for other growth factors, is of the catalytic receptor protein type with a single transmembrane span and coupled to tyrosine kinase (Fig. 11). The liver and kidney are the major sites of insulin breakdown. Insulin is freely filtered at the glomerulus, but is rapidly bound to the proximal-tubule brush border membrane before its uptake, internalization, and degradation within lysosomes of proximal tubule cells (279, 281, 308, 356). Insulin-binding sites (and putative receptors) have been found throughout the nephron, in the glomerulus and proximal tubule (165, 280), and in highest density along the TAL and distal tubule (130, 274). These binding sites and receptor mRNA are reported to be downregulated by a high-sodium diet (333). A closely homologous insulin-like receptor has been found in the kidney and localized to intercalated cells of the collecting duct, but its ligand and function are unknown (31, 251, 291, 315).

The antinatriuretic effect of insulin has been recognized for many years (11, 104, 282, 372), although it has not always been easy to demonstrate, and appears to be independent of any change in GFR (63, 115, 204, 307, 362, 408). Antiphosphaturic and antiuricosuric effects have also been observed (196, 362). However, the data are less clear at the level of the renal tubule. Early free-flow micropuncture

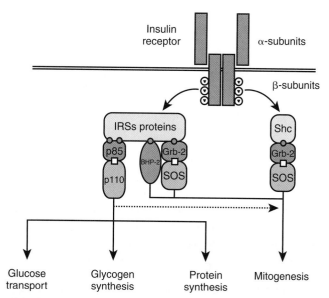

FIGURE 11   The insulin receptor and major signaling pathways for insulin action. The insulin receptor belongs to the large family of receptor proteins with intrinsic tyrosine kinase activity. Following insulin binding to the extracellular domain (α subunits) of the receptor, the protein undergoes autophosphorylation on multiple tyrosine residues. This results in activation of the receptor kinase and tyrosine phosphorylation of a family of insulin receptor substrate (IRS) proteins and Shc, which bind differentially to various downstream signaling proteins. PI3-kinase is critical for metabolic actions of insulin, such as glucose transport, glycogen synthesis, and protein synthesis, whereas the Grb2/SOS complex, which activates the MAP kinase cascade, is critical in the mitogenic response. PI3-kinase probably also modulates the mitogenic response. (Adapted from Virkamäki A, Ueki K, Kahn CR. Protein–protein interaction in insulin signaling and the molecular mechanisms of insulin resistance. *J Clin Invest* 1999;103:931–943.)

experiments suggested inhibition of sodium and fluid reabsorption in rat and dog during insulin and glucose infusion (105), which is consistent with recent findings of lithium clearance studies in hypertensive and diabetic human subjects (115, 204). In contrast, an in vitro study of the isolated perfused rabbit proximal tubule found stimulation of fluid reabsorption by physiological concentrations of insulin (32), and in primary cultures of proximal tubule cells insulin increased Na$^+$–H$^+$ exchanger activity (133). Insulin also stimulates sodium and chloride reabsorption along the loop of Henle (212) and TAL (198, 243), and this is calmodulin-dependent (199). Insulin increases ouabain-sensitive rubidium uptake (a measure of basolateral Na$^+$,K$^+$-ATPase activity) in the proximal tubule (128–130) and cortical collecting duct (131), but it inhibits uptake in the medullary TAL (130). There is still some controversy over whether insulin can directly activate the sodium pump, or if it acts indirectly by increasing sodium transport into cells and stimulates the pump by a rise in intracellular sodium concentration (123, 131, 198, 237, 311, 322, 349). This latter hypothesis is based largely on studies in amphibian A6 cells and toad bladder, and is supported by a recent study reporting ENaC phosphorylation by insulin (423). In A6 cells, insulin-stimulated sodium transport is associated with a rise in intracellular calcium concentration (322), but in the mammalian TAL insulin can enhance sodium transport without altering intracellular calcium concentration (199). In the collecting duct insulin has been shown to augment vasopressin-induced water permeability (although not urea transport) by a mechanism involving increased AQP2 expression (69, 241).

In animal models of insulin-dependent diabetes, studies have reported increases in proximal tubule brush border Na^+–H^+ exchanger (120, 173, 276) and basolateral Na^+,K^+-ATPase (381) activities. Insulin has been shown to be necessary for the normal adaptation and stimulation of sodium-phosphate cotransport activity in response to a low-phosphate diet (336). This occurs through increased transporter insertion into the membrane and synthesis of new transporter protein (336). Insulin also increases gene expression of the sodium-phosphate cotransporter, which can be downregulated by glucagon (226).

Insulin may also modulate angiotensin II and atrial natriuretic peptide (ANP) receptor expression. Reduced angiotensin II–binding and AT1 receptor mRNA levels have been reported in glomeruli (18, 398) and proximal tubules (40, 85) of insulin-deficient diabetic rats, which are restored on administration of insulin. Studies in the rat have also shown that insulin has indirect effects on sodium transport via stimulation of renin release (193). In isolated mesangial cells chloride channel opening in response to angiotensin II is insulin-dependent, which may have implications for glomerular filtration (229). Renal ANP receptors are reduced in this form of diabetes (334), as is the renal response to ANP; however, one study has reported increased mRNA expression for ANP in the kidneys of diabetic rats (346).

Insulin has important effects on renal tubular transport of glucose, most of which occur along the proximal tubule (see Chapter 71). Glucose transporters are classified as either the facilitative (GLUT) family or those coupled to the transmembrane sodium concentration gradient (SGLT1 and SGLT2). GLUT transporters are expressed in all peripheral tissues and are responsible for maintaining appropriate levels of glucose uptake for energy metabolism. They are expressed in a tissue-specific fashion that matches the capacity for glucose transport with its requirement, including in the proximal tubule. Only GLUT4, most abundant in skeletal muscle and adipose tissue, has been clearly shown to be insulin dependent. In kidney and small intestine GLUT transporters are normally expressed at the basolateral membrane, the exception being GLUT5, the fructose transporter, which is located at the apical membrane. GLUT1 is ubiquitous throughout the nephron, while GLUT2 and GLUT5 are found in the proximal tubule; there is some evidence for GLUT4 expression in the glomerulus and TAL (Fig. 12) (86, 87, 103, 247). SGLT1 (the high-affinity, low-capacity isoform) is found at the luminal membrane in the small intestine and throughout the proximal tubule, while SGLT2 appears to be unique to the kidney and is present in the early proximal tubule. SGLT2 has a lower affinity, but a higher capacity for glucose transport, and is suited to the needs of the early proximal tubule where the glucose level is greatest. In chronic insulin-dependent diabetes mellitus, expression of GLUT2 and GLUT5 is increased, but GLUT1 is decreased in experimental type 1 diabetes (86, 111). The normal pattern of expression is restored by administration of IGF-I (10). There is no evidence for altered SGLT1 or SGLT2 protein expression in the kidney in diabetes, but increased Na^+,K^+-ATPase activity in proximal

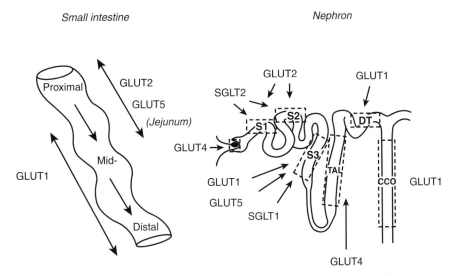

FIGURE 12   Axial distribution of glucose transporters along small intestine and various segments of the nephron. CD, collecting duct; DT, distal tubule; S1, early proximal tubule; S2, convoluted proximal tubule; S3, straight proximal tubule; TAL, thick ascending limb. (With permission, from Debnam ES, Unwin RJ. Hyperglycemia and intestinal and renal glucose transport: implications for diabetic renal injury. *Kidney Int* 1996;50:1101–1109.)

tubule cells occurs (215), and may cause enhanced sodium-dependent glucose uptake.

Confocal studies, and experiments using purified brush border membrane, have shown that type 1 diabetes mellitus in rats causes significant expression of GLUT2 at the renal brush border (248). Increased glucose uptake by this route may be relevant to tubular pathophysiology in diabetes, such as polyol pathway stimulation (265) and activation of protein kinase C, or excessive glycosylation of proteins within the proximal tubule cell (114). It is noteworthy that renal cells do not normally accumulate glycogen, but that diabetes results in considerable glycogen deposition in tubular cells (47, 275), which might be due to increased GLUT2-mediated glucose transport. Interestingly, GLUT2 is also expressed at the intestinal brush border in diabetes (209) and this may contribute to postprandial hyperglycemia, perhaps controlled by increased secretion of GLP-2 (12).

Diabetes reduces GLUT4 expression in renal vascular and glomerular cells, which has been linked to diabetic glomerular hyperfiltration. Insulin administration to diabetic rats restores GLUT4 expression (305). The mechanisms underlying the regulation of renal glucose transporters is still unclear, although both the PKA and PKC signaling pathways are likely to be important in both gut and kidney (209, 412). Recent studies suggest that renal sympathetic nerve activity may control levels of GLUT2 and there appears to be an additive effect of sympathetic hyperactivity and diabetes on GLUT2 expression (329).

A problem in establishing a direct effect of insulin on renal function is that many studies have used a model of insulinopenia, usually streptozotocin-induced. The effect of insulin replacement has then been assumed to indicate the action of insulin itself, rather than being strictly insulin-dependent, since a host of complex metabolic and hormonal changes occur in the absence of insulin. For example, increased secretion of pancreatic glucagon could be responsible for increased GLUT2-mediated glucose uptake in type 1 diabetes (249). However, it is broadly true that many of insulin's actions are counter to those of glucagon; in the kidney, the net effect of insulin on renal function is antinatriuretic.

AMYLIN

Amylin is a 37–amino acid polypeptide co-released with insulin from pancreatic β cells in response to food (93). It acts on skeletal muscle to cause glycogen breakdown and release of lactate, a substrate for hepatic glucose production and glycogen synthesis. It can also inhibit insulin release and is deficient in insulin-dependent diabetes. In excess, amylin mimics non–insulin-dependent type 2 diabetes and circulating levels are high in obesity with insulin resistance. It shares partial homology with NPY, calcitonin gene–related peptide (CGRP), and the hormone calcitonin with which it shares some biological properties, acting via typical G-protein–coupled receptors that stimulate adenylate cyclase (302).

In the rat kidney, amylin-binding sites have been identified exclusively in the proximal tubule; amylin stimulates proximal tubule reabsorption of sodium and causes proliferation of proximal tubule cells in culture (172). The physiological importance of these findings is unclear, but in studies using the SHR rat model of hypertension there appears to be a link between activation of renal amylin receptors and the development of hypertension (411). Supraphysiological plasma levels of amylin in rats enhance sodium excretion, GFR, and RPF (377)—all actions resulting from its vasodilator properties. In contrast to the rat, studies in primate kidney have detected high-affinity binding sites for amylin in the distal nephron and juxtaglomerular apparatus (80). Amylin increases renin release when injected into humans and rats (410), and when infused into the isolated perfused rat kidney (193).

NOVEL BRAIN–GUT PEPTIDES

The following peptide hormones have well-documented effects on the kidney, although their place in the hormonal regulation of renal, and specifically tubular, function remains unclear.

SOMATOSTATIN

Somatostatin (SS), also known as growth hormone (GH)-release inhibiting factor, is a 14–amino acid peptide hormone originally isolated from hypothalamic extracts and found to inhibit the release of GH. During its isolation and purification, several other N-terminal extended homologous peptides were identified: SS-20, SS-25, and SS-28 (a fragment of SS-28 (1-12) is a putative neurotransmitter) (266). SS is found throughout the gastrointestinal tract (in mucosal and neuromuscular layers) and pancreas, and in central and peripheral neurons, often colocalized with norepinephrine (142), and in gut and kidney autonomic nerves (208, 314). Renal SS-like immunoreactivity has been found in some, but not all, species: in toad bladder epithelium and renal tubules (55), in rat glomeruli (139, 217), in human kidney cortex and cultured proximal tubule cells (368), and mesangial cells (369). High-affinity SS-binding sites have been identified in rabbit and human, but not rat, kidney (319, 321). In the human kidney, binding of both octreotide and SS-28 is seen in proximal tubule, vasa recta and collecting ducts, suggesting possible effects of SS on medullary blood flow and tubular transport.

Five genes encoding SS receptors in mice and in humans have been identified (413), of which the type 2 receptor is the most widespread and is linked to a tyrosine phosphatase (106); mRNA for this receptor has been detected in normal kidney (413) and in renal carcinoma tissue (376). More recently, receptor 1 has been found in human collecting duct, and receptor 2 is present in rat and human collecting duct, and glomeruli (19), while in the mouse all 5 receptors are expressed mainly along the proximal tubule (29, 30).

Several studies have demonstrated metabolism of SS by renal tissue, and a transrenal gradient of SS has been found in the rat (341). The metabolic clearance rate of exogenous SS is reduced in chronic renal failure (345), although plasma levels are not increased (234). Renal uptake of Indium-labeled pentetreotide, a synthetic analog of SS used to detect and treat neuroendocrine tumors and lymphomas, has been observed in humans (167), and the analog octreotide competes with native SS for proximal tubule (OK) cell uptake by a megalin/cubilin-mediated endocytic process (28). SS is also inactivated by brush border endopeptidases and after endocytosis by lysosomal enzymes (27); tubular uptake is blocked by lysine infusion, which may be a means of prolonging its action (167). The SS receptors identified in the proximal tubule are not involved in its catabolism.

SS has a paninhibitory effect on the release of most hormones, and its actions were originally defined in the gut. It inhibits pancreatic enzyme secretion, gallbladder contractility, and gastrointestinal motility (7). Circulating plasma concentrations are low and do not change significantly after food (390). Its physiological effects on fluid and electrolyte transport are uncertain, not least because of species and tissue differences. SS has a direct effect on enteroctyes to decrease chloride secretion stimulated by agents that increase intracellular cAMP, such as VIP or prostaglandins (79). Nutrient absorption is strongly inhibited by SS (403) and studies on isolated intestine show that the inhibitory effect is directly on the epithelial cell (9).

In the kidney, depending on the state of water balance, intravenous or intra-arterial SS antagonizes the action of vasopressin, causing diuresis and increased free water clearance (59, 313); except not in humans when given intravenously (383). It does this by blocking (via G_i inhibitory GTP-binding protein stimulation) the vasopressin-induced increase in cAMP along the TAL and collecting duct (195, 405). Its reported effects on renal perfusion are variable and species-dependent. In the dog, it reduces renal perfusion (41) and can cause direct renal vasoconstriction (366); in humans it also decreases RBF (380, 383), while in the cat it causes renal vasodilatation (164). Chronic administration of octreotide prevents the renal hyperfiltration observed in experimental diabetes (16), and SS itself can reduce portal hypertension in cirrhosis (190).

SS antagonizes angiotensin II–induced mesangial cell contraction (144), increases glomerular prostaglandin synthesis (278) and phosphate excretion, and has a biphasic effect on distal nephron water transport (310). Because of its inhibitory effect on the release of several hormones, including glucagon, GH, and insulin, SS has been used to try and elucidate the cause of the postprandial rise in GFR: it has been shown to inhibit the response to an amino acid infusion (272), although how is not known. In addition, SS has been shown to prevent renal hypertrophy in diabetic rats by inhibiting IGF-I synthesis (154, 155), but not the hypertrophy following unilateral nephrectomy (116); it is antiproliferative in OK cells, which express high-affinity SS

receptors (175). As to the physiological role of SS in the kidney, because it does not circulate as a true hormone, and its direct renal vascular or ion transport effects are observed at only pharmacological doses, it is most likely to act as an intrarenal paracrine or autocrine factor, perhaps affecting cell growth and water transport.

PEPTIDE TYROSINE-TYROSINE AND NEUROPEPTIDE Y

Peptide tyrosine-tyrosine (PYY) and NPY are homologous peptides of 36 amino acids, first identified in pig intestine and brain, respectively (360). Early work on the functions of these peptides focused on their gastrointestinal effects, but there is now evidence that both PYY and NPY can affect a variety of tissues, including the kidney. PYY is a gut hormone secreted from endocrine (L) cells present in the epithelium of the (distal) small intestine and colon in response to digestive products of dietary fat (296). It can be classified as a "true" hormone and may be responsible for the so-called ileal brake, which occurs when exposure of the distal intestinal mucosa to dietary lipid inhibits propulsion in the more proximal intestine (296). Unlike PYY, levels of NPY in plasma are low and are not significantly altered by food. However, NPY has a wider distribution as a neuronal peptide in the central and peripheral nervous systems, and is released together with norepinephrine at sympathetic postganglionic nerve endings, where it can have its own direct vasoconstrictor effect, but where it also inhibits norepinephrine release and postsynaptic vasoconstrictive action (233). NPY is also found in neurons within the gut and pancreas; its function in the enteric nervous system may be to modulate epithelial absorptive and secretory function (372). A number of defined physiological roles for NPY have emerged, especially in the central control of appetite (which it stimulates; compare with PYY) and energy balance (255).

PYY and NPY both interact with so-called Y receptors, broadly divided into Y1 and Y2 subclasses, which bind the full-length peptides or their C-terminal portions, respectively, and with high affinity. Y1 receptors mediate the direct vasoconstrictor effect of NPY and, indirectly, its vasodilator effect via NO. Y2 receptors are thought to be mainly presynaptic in the nervous system and suppress neurotransmitter release. A putative Y3 receptor showing specificity for NPY has also been postulated, as well as PYY specific receptors, Y4 and Y5, responsible for appetite suppression. Y receptors are membrane spanning and G-protein coupled, and they inhibit adenylate cyclase. Y2 receptors have been detected in non-neuronal tissue, such as the basolateral membrane of native rabbit proximal tubule (344), and also in cultured proximal tubule cells from a strain of transgenic mouse (379) in which PYY stimulates cell growth. NPY peptide and its receptors are expressed in renal cortical tubules (162).

Intravenous infusion of PYY in humans, simulating the plasma PYY concentrations achieved postprandially, causes decreased GFR and RPF, suppressed levels of renin and aldosterone, and a natriuresis (298). Experimental studies in rats confirm that PYY infusion reduces RBF (49, 53) and plasma renin levels (although not aldosterone), probably via the Y1 receptor, as a Y2 receptor agonist had little effect (49). Natriuresis and diuresis were also observed, mediated by a putative Y5 receptor in the distal nephron (49). Basolateral application of PYY to a mouse medullary collecting duct cell line inhibited electrogenic chloride current, which was likely to be via Y2 receptors (60). The same study showed that PYY inhibits AVP-stimulated cAMP accumulation, which could explain the diuretic action of PYY. Taken together, it is likely that PYY plays a role in the postprandial natriuretic response as part of an entero-renal interaction. In contrast to its effect on fluid and electrolyte transport in the kidney and small intestine, PYY has no effect on colonic epithelium (17).

Like PYY, NPY has also been reported to reduce RBF and increase sodium excretion (49, 53). Because a Y1 antagonist can block the NPY-induced fall in RBF, but not the actions of the peptide on natriuresis and diuresis, various receptor subtypes are likely to be involved in its renal effects. Earlier reports that the natriuretic effect of NPY is mediated by local release of bradykinin (52) have not been confirmed (51); however, intravenous infusion of NPY in rats does increase plasma levels of ANP (23). Renin release is also reduced by NPY, suggesting that downregulation of the RAS system may contribute to the diuresis and natriuresis produced by NPY (161). NPY also causes kaliuresis in rats, an action that involves Y1 receptors and possibly also Y2 (50).

Although NPY is resistant to the action of aminopeptidase N, aminopeptidase W, and angiotensin-converting enzyme, it can be processed at its N-terminus by two proline-preferring amino peptidases, amino peptidase P, and dipeptidyl peptidase IV (255). The latter enzyme generates NPY(3-36), which is a selective Y2 receptor agonist (255). In the renal brush border membranes, neutral endopeptidases and other ectoenzymes hydrolyze NPY and PYY, and breakdown could lead to fragments with differing Y-receptor specificities (254).

Leptin

Leptin is a hormone originating from adipocytes and it has been shown to regulate food intake and energy expenditure. The circulating form of the hormone is a 146–amino acid protein that is encoded by the obesity (ob) gene (91), and is a member of the helical cytokine family (240). Leptin provides one of many signals to the brain via the hypothalamus when there has been a sufficient intake of food to maintain body weight (244). Mice with a mutation in the ob gene, which prevents leptin synthesis, become morbidly obese due to overeating. The human leptin receptor (OB-R) is a member of the class I cytokine receptor family and mediates the weight-regulating effects of leptin (170); mice with a mutation in this gene also become obese (78).

In humans, serum leptin levels correlate with the amount of adipose tissue and are elevated in patients who are obese or have type 2 diabetes (396); proteinuria predicts an increased serum leptin level (138). Obese diabetic (db/db) mice with hyperleptinemia develop glomerular changes similar to human

diabetic nephropathy (92). Serum levels of leptin are also raised in patients with renal failure (342), although it does not seem to correlate with nutritional status (295).

Studies have shown that leptin stimulates proliferation of glomerular endothelial cells and increases the expression of the prosclerotic cytokine transforming growth factor-β1 (TGFβ1) (407). There is growing evidence that increased glucose uptake in cultured glomerular cells is central to the pathophysiology of diabetic nephropathy. Leptin promotes glucose uptake in cultured mesangial cells from diabetic (db/db) mice, and stimulates both TGFβII receptor expression (168) and type 1 collagen production, probably via the PI3 kinase pathway. Leptin-binding sites are present in the kidney, specifically in the inner medulla and corticomedullary regions (339). Immunocytochemical studies have localized leptin receptors to the proximal straight tubule, loop of Henle, distal tubule and collecting duct (163). A truncated form of the leptin receptor (Ob-Ra), though not the full-length receptor (Ob-Rb), is present on mesangial cells of nondiabetic (db/m) and diabetic (db/db) mice (168). Circulating iodinated leptin undergoes glomerular filtration and is taken up by proximal tubule cells via a megalin-mediated and calcium-dependent process (163), and the leptin receptors present along the renal tubule are not involved in leptin metabolism (compare with somatostatin). Various truncated forms of the leptin receptor (Ob-Ra, Ob-Rc, Ob-Rd, Ob-Re) have been identified in many tissues, including the kidney (359). In addition to a direct action on renal cells, leptin may have indirect effects via its inhibition of synthesis and release of NPY (355).

Leptin has very different actions on the renal handling of sodium and water, depending on its mode of administration. Without altering GFR or electrolyte excretion, acute treatment with leptin causes a rapid diuretic and natriuretic effect (42, 43, 339, 342). This natriuretic property of leptin seems to be mediated in part by a reduction in renal medullary Na⁺,K⁺,-ATPase activity (43), and again involves a PI-3 kinase–dependent mechanism (43), In contrast, chronic (7-day) treatment with leptin reduces sodium excretion by stimulating sodium reabsorption, an action that may underlie its hypertensive effect (44). Studies using ob/ob mice have reported raised plasma and urine concentrations of calcium and phosphate, together with enhanced renal expression of the enzymes involved in vitamin D (calcitriol) synthesis (252). These changes can be reversed by treatment with leptin, which suppresses renal 1α-hydroxylase and 24-hydroxylase enzyme activities. However, at present the renal actions of leptin have yet to be fully explored.

Ghrelin

The peptide ghrelin stimulates release of GH from the anterior pituitary and it is one of several hormones affecting appetite and energy balance. Ghrelin is synthesized as a pre-prohormone before being proteolytically cleaved to yield a 28–amino acid peptide. An interesting and unique modification occurs to the hormone during synthesis in the form of an n-octanoic acid bound to one of its amino acids, which is essential for ghrelin biological activity.

Ghrelin is an endogenous ligand for GH secretagogue receptor (GHS-Rs) and regulates pituitary GH secretion. GHS-Rs is found in the hypothalamus and brainstem. Ghrelin affects energy balance in rodents by decreasing fat utilization without significantly changing energy expenditure or physical activity. Daily administration of ghrelin to mice or rats induces weight gain by reducing fat metabolism. Intracerebroventricular administration of ghrelin generates a dose-dependent increase in food intake and body weight. In rats, serum ghrelin concentrations are increased by fasting and reduced by re-feeding or oral glucose, but not by water ingestion.

Synthesis of ghrelin occurs predominantly in epithelial cells lining the fundus of the stomach with smaller amounts produced in other tissues, including the kidney. Evidence for renal expression of the peptide comes from studies in mouse (201, 263) and rat (263) kidneys, and from cultured rat mesangial cells (263). These findings suggest that ghrelin may have a paracrine role in the kidney. Plasma levels of ghrelin are increased in patients with chronic renal failure (295, 418), perhaps due to poor nutrition and reduced calorie intake (295). Clearance of ghrelin during hemodialysis reduces circulating levels toward normal (285, 418). The only published study on the systemic effects of ghrelin has reported that intravenous infusion in humans increases plasma levels of GH and cortisol, but has no effect on sodium or water excretion (271).

Establishing the importance and contribution of these "miscellaneous" peptide hormones expressed in the kidney, and/or having demonstrable renal effects awaits, our technical ability to measure local intrarenal concentrations, including those in tubular fluid (see below). Only then will we be able to assess their physiological relevance to body fluid and electrolyte homeostasis, and normal renal function, and to define more precisely their segmental actions.

CONCEPT OF A RENAL INTRACRINE SYSTEM

Evidence is accumulating that intraluminal factors may play a physiological or pathological role in regulating renal tubular function, so-called "intracrine" regulation. The finding that native fluid withdrawn from the proximal tubule has significant effects on distal tubular function that are not reproduced by artificial tubular fluid of similar electrolyte composition supports the concept that the organic content of tubular fluid might itself influence tubular transport (242). Evidence has also accrued for a variety of apical receptors throughout the nephron that can respond to filtered peptide hormones, or to substances produced within the nephron itself, by altering tubular reabsorption. Several peptide hormones have been identified in normal human urine and in animals (267, 277, 357, 392). The presence of these peptides in urine could be explained by their relatively small size, which would allow them to be present in the glomerular filtrate, and thus the final urine. Renal cells express precursors for at least some of these peptide hormones (205, 277, 305, 357) and their receptors are located on the luminal membrane (101, 134, 166, 207, 301, 348). In the proximal tubule, intraluminal angiotensin II stimulates reabsorption (277), while intraluminal dopamine (312) or nucleotides (13) (see Chapter 18) can reduce it. In the loop of Henle, intraluminal ANP (14) and endothelin (202) inhibit chloride reabsorption, and there is evidence from intracellular Ca^{2+} responses that intraluminal vasopressin may be physiologically active (68). In the distal nephron, intraluminal angiotensin II has been shown to stimulate sodium and water reabsorption in perfused distal tubules (388), intraluminal nucleotides modulate sodium reabsorption in the collecting duct (225, 347), and intraluminal vasopressin can modify ion and water transport (194). It is possible that the enzyme systems present in the brush border membrane of the proximal tubule might normally prevent the downstream effects of filtered bioactive peptides like ANP (399), and/or allow a paracrine action of locally secreted factors (385), as well as having possible implications for tubule dysfunction and progressive renal impairment in proteinuric diseases (284). The possibility that intraluminal peptides can influence tubular function has stimulated the search for analytical methods to measure them. In this context, interest has arisen in the measurement of a range of bioactive peptides in urine as possible markers or causative agents of renal diseases (179, 297). Analyses of the urinary proteome of renal Fanconi syndrome (FS) patients have provided an indirect means to investigate its composition. Genetic defects in inherited forms of this disorder have been mapped to defects in the pathway involved in the reabsorption of peptides from the glomerular filtrate (97). Glomerular function in the FS is not initially compromised and proteinuria is a consequence of defective reabsorption of filtered peptides, including albumin and low-molecular-weight proteins. Thus, it is reasonable to assume that the protein composition of renal Fanconi urine is close to that of normal tubular fluid (although perhaps not identical, because of the action of proteases and luminal membrane-bound enzymes). Immunoassays have detected several bioactive peptides in the urine of Fanconi patients (284), and more recently mass spectrometry has extended the analysis to find several chemokines and cytokines present in Fanconi urine that are not found in normal urine (96). These results indicate that certain cytokines of plasma origin (chiefly, IGF-I and IGF-II) are probably present normally in the glomerular filtrate, a result consistent with previous work (386, 387). Interestingly, precursors for other peptide hormones (namely, EGF and kininogen) are present in normal urine in larger amounts than in Fanconi urine (97), an observation suggesting that the presence of certain peptide hormones in normal urine is a consequence of their secretion along the renal tubule. Indeed, expression of several peptide hormone precursors, including kininogen and EGF, by tubule cells has been reported. Thus, the lumen of the kidney proximal tubule is potentially a dynamic and changing environment. Although it is generally accepted that the control of proximal tubular cell activity occurs primarily as a result of the actions of hormonal effects via specific basolateral (and not luminal) membrane receptors, investigators have known for many years that normal urine contains high-molecular-mass renotropic factors capable of specifically stimulating renal growth (174). The identity of such factors has remained obscure, but as already stated, an increasing number of receptors has been identified in the apical membrane of tubular cells, and there is evidence that the glomerular filtrate contains a variety of molecules capable of cell signaling.

Studies of proximal tubular cell function and urinary composition in disease have begun to illustrate both the range of molecules to which the apical surface of proximal tubule cells is exposed, and the repertoire of responses evoked by their interactions. In glomerular disease, circulating bioactive molecules may leak into the proximal tubule as a result of damage to the glomerular permselective barrier. Alternatively, mediators produced locally by inflamed or diseased glomeruli may translocate into tubular fluid. The result is exposure of the apical surface of the tubular epithelium to unusual molecules in atypical concentrations, and the activation of cell-signaling cascades. For instance, IGF-I is ultrafiltered by nephrotic rats, and is present in proximal tubular fluid at low nanomolar concentrations, whereas in the urine of normal rats, IGF-I is usually undetectable (181). Receptors for IGF-I present in the apical membrane of tubular cells (166) are activated and autophosphorylated following exposure to nephrotic proximal tubular fluid, thus initiating recruitment of PI3 kinase to activated insulin receptor substrate-1 (181, 386). Furthermore, proximal tubule cells are stimulated to divide and secrete collagen types IV and I by the IGF-I present in nephrotic glomerular ultrafiltrate (181). Other growth factors, namely hepatocyte growth factor (HGF) and TGFβ, pass from plasma into tubular fluid in rats with diabetic nephropathy. Again, receptors for both these mediators are present in apical membranes of proximal cells and both HGF and TGFβ induce these cells to synthesize and secrete matrix proteins, such as fibronectin and collagen (386, 387). In addition, activation of tyrosine kinase signaling pathways, including PI3 kinase, by HGF and TGFβ leads to production of proinflammatory agents like MCP1 by proximal tubule cells (386).

In multiple myeloma, excess immunoglobulin light chains are delivered into the proximal tubule and contribute crucially to the development of the myeloma kidney and renal failure. The interaction of these light chains with proximal tubule cells elicits activation of the three major classes of mitogen activated protein kinase, ERK1/2, JNK1/2, and p38. Consequently, activation of NF-κB light chains stimulates proximal cells to produce proinflammatory cytokines (337, 338).

End stage kidney disease is characterized by a common renal histological appearance comprising extensive tubular atrophy with interstitial inflammation and scarring. In the majority of progressive renal diseases, proteinuria is a prominent feature. This common clinical observation in a diverse range of renal diseases has led to the hypothesis that proteinuria per se may play a role in precipitating or perpetuating renal tubulointerstitial inflammation and fibrosis. As a result, many investigators have examined the effects of filtered proteins on proximal tubule cell function and phenotype. Of the filtered proteins, albumin has been studied most. The results of these studies reveal novel and interesting properties of albumin and reinforce the concept that proximal tubular fluid and the apical surface of proximal cells combine to form a signaling environment capable of influencing kidney function in health and disease.

Albumin stimulates activity of a number of signaling pathways in proximal tubule cells: incubation of cells with concentrations of albumin as low as 1–10 μg/ml, well within the conventionally accepted physiological range, strongly activates PI-3 kinase and subsequently the controller of mRNA translation, p70 ribosomal protein S6 kinase (65, 108). At a concentration of 100 μg/ml albumin also activates ERK MAP kinase (109). Indeed, multiple signaling pathways are now known to be involved in proximal cell signaling under conditions of albumin stimulation, including p38 MAP kinase (112), phospholipase C (169), protein kinase C (358), and reactive oxygen species (273, 358). The net result of these albumin effects includes stimulation of proliferation and the secretion of a cocktail of proinflammatory and profibrotic mediators, such as MCP1, RANTES, fractalkine, interleukin-8, endothelin, TGFβ, and fibronectin (6, 112, 273, 358, 389, 416), via activation of several key transcription factors. The secretion of many of these substances is polarized towards the basolateral membrane of the cell. Other phenotypic changes observed in proximal tubule cells following albumin stimulation include proliferation and activation of Na–H exchange (108, 213). Clearly, the machinery exists at the apical surface of proximal tubule cells that allows the translation of messages derived from the glomerulus into signals that may precipitate an inflammatory scarring environment within the tubulointerstitium.

Receptor binding is a prerequisite for proximal tubule cell endocytosis of albumin (see Chapter 74). The enigmatic signaling effects of albumin and the precipitation of proteinuric nephropathy may also be mediated via signaling through a proximal tubule albumin receptor. Recent work demonstrates that binding and endocytosis of albumin by proximal tubule cells requires a co-operative arrangement between two large proteins—megalin and cubilin (90). Cubilin is an entirely extracellular protein and is therefore unlikely to be directly involved in cell signaling. Megalin is a member of the low-density lipoprotein receptor (LDLR) family (191). These receptors share structural and functional properties, interact with a diverse group of ligands, and are transmembrane glycoproteins that contain large extracellular domains and comparatively short intracellular domains (191). Traditionally the LDLR family is regarded solely as endocytic cargo receptors that bind and internalize ligands prior to lysosomal breakdown. This paradigm has recently been challenged (178), with new evidence suggesting novel nonendocytosis-related signaling roles for LDLR.

Megalin is heavily expressed in proximal tubule cells, where it acts as an endocytic receptor for albumin and other macromolecules filtered into the tubular lumen (90). Megalin possesses a longer cytoplasmic tail (megalin-CT) than other LDLR family members with unique sequence motifs (187, 328). Human megalin-CT has three YxNPxY domains acting as coated pit internalization sequences (84) and/or a binding site for phosphotyrosine interaction domains (25), four Src homology-3 (SH3)–binding regions conforming to the XpF-PpXP SH3-binding site consensus recognition motif (419), and one Src homology-2 (SH2) recognition motif for the p85 regulatory subunit of PI3 kinase (350). In addition, there are multiple phosphorylation sites for protein kinase C (PKC), casein kinase II, and cAMP-/cGMP–dependent protein kinase. These findings suggest that megalin may have signaling or trafficking roles in addition to, or distinct from, those of other LDLR family members. Recent evidence posits megalin as a central player in diverse renal diseases (283, 375). Megalin knockout mice exemplify the crucial physiological role of this receptor. Most of these animals die in the perinatal period, displaying a severe developmental brain phenotype, and major abnormalities in proximal tubule cell structure (402). Only 2% survive, but with appreciable albuminuria (224). The severity of these phenotypic changes is difficult to explain on the basis of an endocytic defect alone. Kidney-specific megalin knockout animals are viable, but demonstrate hypocalcemia, osteopathy, and marked proteinuria as a consequence of severely impaired proximal tubular cell endocytosis (223). A variety of signaling proteins have now been shown to interact with megalin-CT (151, 219, 288, 309). Of particular interest are disabled-2 (Dab2), SEMCAP-1, JIP-1, JIP-2, PIP4, 5 kinase homologue, and ANKRA. These proteins are involved in Ras and ERK signaling, GTP-binding protein signaling, JNK scaffold assembly, inositol metabolism, and probable Raf-kinase binding (228), respectively. These proximal tubular cell megalin-CT protein interactions strongly support a role for megalin in signaling, and are likely to be of importance in normal cell and organ function.

Finally, disruption of the hormonal composition of tubular fluid, as in proteinuria, could result in the normal intraluminal regulatory mechanisms being overwhelmed, which in turn could lead to a dysregulation of intracellular signaling pathways and a concomitant alteration in gene expression (183). This may prove to be a generic mechanism to explain the progressive renal dysfunction observed in patients with proteinuria, whatever the initial cause (186) (see Chapter 89).

Acknowledgments

We would like to thank Dr. David Shirley for his help with, and discussion of, the section on the intracrine concept.

References

1. Adam WR, Adams BA, Ellis AG. In vivo estimation of changes in distal tubule flow and their role in dexamethasone-induced kaliuresis in control and potassium-adapted rats. *Clin Exp Pharmacol Physiol* 1987;14:47–57.
2. Ahloulay M, Dechaux M, Laborde K, Bankir L. Influence of glucagon on GFR and on urea and elecytrolyte excretion: direct and indirect effects. *Am J Physiol* 1995;269:F225–F235.
3. Alcalde AI, Sarasa M, Raldua D, Aramayona J, Morales R, Biber J, Murer H, Levi M, Sorribas V. Role of thyroid hormone in regulation of renal phosphate transport in young and aged rats. *Endocrinology* 1999;140:1544–1551.
4. Amemiya M, Kusano E, Muto S, Tabei K, Ando Y, Alpern RJ, Asano Y. Glucagon acutely inhibits and chronically activates NHE3 activity in OKP cells. *Exp Nephrol* 2002;10:26–33.
5. Amiranoff B, Laburthe M, Rosselin G. Differential effects of guanine nucleotides on the first step of VIP and glucagon action in membranes from liver cells. *Biochem Biophys Res Commun* 1980;96:463–468.
6. Arici M, Brown J, Williams M, Harris KP, Walls J, Brunskill NJ. Fatty acids carried on albumin modulate proximal tubular cell fibronectin production: a role for protein kinase C. *Nephrol Dial Transplant* 2002;17:1751–1757.
7. Arnold R, Lankisch PG. Somatostatin and the gastrointestinal tract. *Clin Gastroenterol* 1980; 9:733–753.
8. Arruda JA, Wang LJ, Pahlavan P, Ruiz OS. Glucocorticoids and the renal Na-H antiporter: role in respiratory acidosis. *Regul Pept* 1993;48:329–336.
9. Arruebo MP, Sorribas V, Rodriguez-Yoldi MJ, Murillo MD, Alcalde AI. Effect of VIP on sugar transport in rabbit small intestine in vitro. *Zentralbl Veterinarmed A* 1990;37:123–129.
10. Asada T, Ogawa T, Iwai M, Shimomura K, Kobayashi M. Recombinant insulin-like growth factor I normalizes expression of renal glucose transporters in diabetic rats. *Am J Physiol* 1997;273:F27–F37.
11. Atchley DW, Loeb RF, Richards DW Jr, Benedict EM, Driscoll ME. On diabetic acidosis. *J Clin Invest* 1933;12:297–326.
12. Au A, Gupta A, Schembri P, Cheeseman CI. Rapid insertion of GLUT2 into the rat jejunal brush-border membrane promoted by glucagon-like peptide 2. *Biochem J* 2002;367:247–254.
13. Bailey MA. Inhibition of bicarbonate reabsorption in the rat proximal tubule by activation of luminal P2Y1 receptors. *Am J Physiol Renal Physiol* 2004;287:F789–F796.
14. Bailly C. Effect of luminal atrial natriuretic peptide on chloride reabsorption in mouse cortical thick ascending limb: inhibition by endothelin. *J Am Soc Nephrol* 2000;11:1791–1797.
15. Bailly C, Imbert-Teboul M, Chabardes D, Hus-Citharel A, Montegut J, Clique A, Morel F. The distal nephron of the rat kidney: a target site for glucagon. *Proc Natl Acad Sci U S A* 1980;77:3422–3424.
16. Bak M, Thomsen K, Flyvbjerg A. Effects of the somatostatin analogue octreotide on renal function in conscious diabetic rats. *Nephrol Dial Transplant* 2001;16:2002–2007.
17. Ballantyne GH, Goldenring JR, Fleming FX, Rush S, Flint JS, Fielding LP, Binder HJ, Modlin IM. Inhibition of VIP-stimulated ion transport by a novel Y-receptor phenotype in rabbit distal colon. *Am J Physiol* 1993;264:G848–G854.
18. Ballermann BJ, Skorecki KL, Brenner BM. Reduced glomerular angiotensin II receptor density in early untreated diabetes mellitus in the rat. *Am J Physiol* 1984;247:F110–F116.
19. Balster DA, O'Dorisio MS, Summers MA, Turman MA. Segmental expression of somatostatin receptor subtypes sst(1) and sst(2) in tubules and glomeruli of human kidney. *Am J Physiol Renal Physiol* 2001;280:F457–F465.
20. Bankir L, Ahloulay M, Devreotes PN, Parent CA. Extracellular cAMP inhibits proximal reabsorption: are plasma membrane cAMP receptors involved? *Am J Physiol Renal Physiol* 2002;282:F376–F392.
21. Bankir L, Martin H, Déchaux M, Ahloulay M. Plasma cAMP: a hepatorenal link influencing proximal reabsorption and renal hemodynamics? *Kidney Int* 1997;51:S–50–S–56.
22. Banks MR, Farthing MJ, Robberecht P, Burleigh DE. Antisecretory actions of a novel vasoactive intestinal polypeptide (VIP) antagonist in human and rat small intestine. *Br J Pharmacol* 2005.
23. Baranowska B, Gutkowska J, Lemire A, Cantin M, Genest J. Opposite effects of neuropeptide Y (NPY) and polypeptide YY (PYY) on plasma immunoreactive atrial natriuretic factor (IR-ANF) in rats. *Biochem Biophys Res Commun* 1987;145:680–685.
24. Barlet C, Abdelkhalek B, Doucet A. Sites of thyroid hormone action on Na-K-ATPase along the rabbit nephron. *Pflugers Arch* 1985;405:52–57.
25. Barlet C, Doucet A. Kinetics of triiodothyronine action on Na-K-ATPase in single segments of rabbit nephron. *Pflugers Arch* 1986;407:27–32.
26. Barlet C, Doucet A. Lack of stimulation of kidney Na-K-ATPase by thyroid hormones in long-term thyroidectomized rabbits. *Pflugers Arch* 1986;407:428–431.
27. Barnes K, Doherty S, Turner AJ. Endopeptidase-24.11 is the integral membrane peptidase initiating degradation of somatostatin in the hippocampus. *J Neurochem* 1995;64:1826–1832.
28. Barone R, Van Der SP, Devuyst O, Beaujean V, Pauwels S, Courtoy PJ, Jamar F. Endocytosis of the somatostatin analogue, octreotide, by the proximal tubule–derived opossum kidney (OK) cell line. *Kidney Int* 2005;67:969–976.
29. Bates CM, Kegg H, Grady S. Expression of somatostatin receptors 1 and 2 in the adult mouse kidney. *Regul Pept* 2004;119:11–20.
30. Bates CM, Kegg H, Petrevski C, Grady S. Expression of somatostatin receptors 3, 4, and 5 in mouse kidney proximal tubules. *Kidney Int* 2003;63:53–63.
31. Bates CM, Merenmies JM, Kelly-Spratt KS, Parada LF. Insulin receptor-related receptor expression in non–A intercalated cells in the kidney. *Kidney Int* 1997;52:674–681.
32. Baum M. Insulin stimulates volume absorption in the rabbit proximal convoluted tubule. *J Clin Invest* 1987;79:1104–1109.
33. Baum M, Biemesderfer D, Gentry D, Aronson PS. Ontogeny of rabbit renal cortical NHE3 and NHE1: effect of glucocorticoids. *Am J Physiol* 1995;268:F815–F820.
34. Baum M, Cano A, Alpern RJ. Glucocorticoids stimulate Na$^+$/H$^+$ antiporter in OKP cells. *Am J Physiol* 1993;264:F1027–F1031.
35. Baum M, Dwarkanath V, Alpern RJ, Moe OW. Effects of thyroid hormone on the neonatal renal cortical Na$^+$/H$^+$ antiporter. *Kidney Int* 1998;53:1254–1258.

36. Baum M, Quigley R. Glucocorticoids stimulate rabbit proximal convoluted tubule acidification. *J Clin Invest* 1993;91:110–114.
37. Baum M, Quigley R. Ontogeny of proximal tubule acidification. *Kidney Int* 1995;48: 1697–1704.
38. Baxter JD, Bondy PK. Hypercalcemia of thyrotoxicosis. *Ann Int Med* 1966;65:429–442.
39. Baylis C, Handa R, Sorkin M. Glucocorticoids and control of glomerular filtration rate. *Semin Nephrol* 1990;10:320–329.
40. Becker BN, Kondo S, Cheng HF, Harris RC. Effect of glucose, pyruvate, and insulin on type 1 angiotensin II receptor expression in SV40-immortalized rabbit proximal tubule epithelial cells. *Kidney Int* 1997;52:87–92.
41. Becker RH, Scholtholt J, Jung W, Speht O. A microsphere study on the effects of somatostatin and secretin on regional blood flow in anaesthetized dogs. *Regul Pept* 1982;4:341–351.
42. Beltowski J, Wojcicka W, Gorny D, Marciniak A. Human leptin administered intraperitoneally stimulates natriuresis and decreases renal medullary Na^+, K^+-ATPase activity in the rat—impaired effect in dietary-induced obesity. *Med Sci Monit* 2002;8:BR221–BR229.
43. Beltowski J, Wojcicka G, Jamroz A. Leptin decreases plasma paraoxonase 1 (PON1) activity and induces oxidative stress: the possible novel mechanism for proatherogenic effect of chronic hyperleptinemia. *Atherosclerosis* 2003;170:21–29.
44. Beltowski J, Wojcicka G, Marciniak A, Jamroz A. Oxidative stress, nitric oxide production, and renal sodium handling in leptin-induced hypertension. *Life Sci* 2004;74:2987–3000.
45. Beubler E. Influence of vasoactive intestinal polypeptide on net water flux and cyclic adenosine 3',5'-monophosphate formation in the rat jejunum. *Naunyn Schmiedebergs Arch Pharmacol* 1980;313:243–247.
46. Bianco AC, Salvatore D, Gereben B, Berry MJ, Larsen PR. Biochemistry, cellular and molecular biology, and physiological roles of the iodothyronine selenodeiodinases. *Endocr Rev* 2002;23:38–89.
47. Biava C, Grossman A, West M. Ultrastructural observations on renal glycogen in normal and pathologic human kidneys. *Lab Invest* 1966;15:330–356.
48. Biller KJ, Unwin RJ, Shirley DG. Distal tubular electrolyte transport during inhibition of renal 11beta-hydroxysteroid dehydrogenase. *Am J Physiol Renal Physiol* 2001;280:F172–F179.
49. Bischoff A, Avramidis P, Erdbrugger W, Munter K, Michel MC. Receptor subtypes Y1 and Y5 are involved in the renal effects of neuropeptide Y. *Br J Pharmacol* 1997;120:1335–1343.
50. Bischoff A, Michel MC. Neuropeptide Y enhances potassium excretion by mechanisms distinct from those controlling sodium excretion. *Can J Physiol Pharmacol* 2000;78:93–99.
51. Bischoff A, Neumann A, Dendorfer A, Michel MC. Is bradykinin a mediator of renal neuropeptide Y effects? *Pflugers Arch* 1999;438:797–803.
52. Bischoff A, Rascher W, Michel MC. Bradykinin may be involved in neuropeptide Y-induced diuresis, natriuresis, and calciuresis. *Am J Physiol* 1998;275:F502–F509.
53. Blaze CA, Mannon PJ, Vigna SR, Kherani AR, Benjamin BA. Peptide YY receptor distribution and subtype in the kidney: effect on renal haemodynamics and function in rats. *Am J Physiol* 1977;273:F545–F553.
54. Blazer-Yost BL, Record RD, Oberleithner H. Characterization of hormone-stimulated Na^+ transport in a high-resistance clone of the MDCK cell line. *Pflugers Arch* 1996;432:685–691.
55. Bolaffi JL, Reichlin S, Goodman DBP, Forrest JN Jr. Somatostatin: occurrence in urinary bladder epithelium and renal tubules of the toad, Bufo marinus. *Science* 1980;210:644–646.
56. Bommer J, Bonjour JP, Ritz E, Fleisch H. Parathyroid-independent changes in renal handling of phosphate in hyperthyroid rats. *Kidney Int* 1979;15:117–122.
57. Boross M, Kinsella J, Cheng L, Sacktor B. Glucocorticoids and metabolic acidosis-induced renal transports of inorganic phosphate, calcium, and NH4. *Am J Physiol* 1986;250: F827–F833.
58. Bradley SE, Stephan F, Coelho JF, Reville P. The thyroid and the kidney. *Kidney Int* 1974; 6:346–365.
59. Brautbar N, Levine BS, Coburn JW, Kleeman CR. Interaction of somatostatin with PTH and AVP. Renal effect. *Am J Physiol* 1979;237:E428–E431.
60. Breen CM, Mannon PJ, Benjamin BA. Peptide YY inhibits vasopressin-stimulated chloride secretion in inner medullary collecting duct cells. *Am J Physiol* 1998;275:F452–F457.
61. Brent GA. Mechanisms of disease: the molecular basis of thyroid hormone action. *N Engl J Med* 1994;331:847–853.
62. Brent GA, Moore DD, Larsen PR. Thyroid hormone regulation of gene expression. *Annu Rev Physiol* 1991;53:17–35.
63. Briffeuil P, Huynh Thu T, Kolanowski J. Reappraisal of the role of insulin on sodium handling by the kidney: effect of intrarenal insulin infusion in the dog. *Eur J Clin Invest* 1992;22:523–528.
64. Briffeuil P, Thu TH, Kolanowski J. A lack of direct action of glucagon on kidney metabolism, hemodynamics, and renal sodium handling in the dog. *Metabolism* 1996;45:383–388.
65. Brunskill NJ, Stuart J, Tobin AB, Walls J, Nahorski S. Receptor-mediated endocytosis of albumin by kidney proximal tubule cells is regulated by phosphatidylinositide 3-kinase. *J Clin Invest* 1998;101:2140–2150.
66. Bullock BP, Heller RS, Habener JF. Tissue distribution of messenger ribonucleic acid encoding the rat glucagon-like peptide-1 receptor. *Endocrinology* 1996;137:2968–2978.
67. Burcelin R, Katz EB, Charron MJ. Molecular and cellular aspects of the glucagon receptor: role in diabetes and metabolism. *Diabetes Metab* 1996;22:373–396.
68. Burgess WJ, Balment RJ, Beck JS. Effects of luminal vasopressin on intracellular calcium in microperfused rat medullary thick ascending limb. *Ren Physiol Biochem* 1994;17:1–9.
69. Bustamante M, Hasler U, Kotova O, Chibalin AV, Mordasini D, Rousselot M, Vandewalle A, Martin PY, Feraille E. Insulin potentiates AVP-induced AQP2 expression in cultured renal collecting duct principal cells. *Am J Physiol Renal Physiol* 2005;288:F334–F344.
70. Butlen D, Morel F. Glucagon receptors along the nephron: (^{125}I) glucagon binding in the rat. *Pflugers Arch* 1985;404:348–353.
71. Cadnapaphornchai MA, Kim YW, Gurevich AK, Summer SN, Falk S, Thurman JM, Schrier RW: Urinary concentrating defect in hypothyroid rats: role of sodium, potassium, 2-chloride co-transporter, and aquaporins. *J Am Soc Nephrol* 2003;14:566–574.
72. Calam J, Dimaline R, Peart WS, Singh J, Unwin RJ. Effects of vasoactive intestinal polypeptide on renal function in man. *J Physiol (Lond)* 1983;345:469–75:469–475.
73. Campen TJ, Vaughn DA, Fanestil DD. Mineralo- and glucocorticoid effects on renal excretion of electrolytes. *Pflugers Arch* 1983;399:93–101.
74. Cano A. Characterization of the rat NHE3 promoter. *Am J Physiol* 1996;271:F629–F636.
75. Cano A, Baum M, Moe OW: Thyroid hormone stimulates the renal Na/H exchanger NHE3 by transcriptional activation. *Am J Physiol* 1999;276:C102–C108.
76. Capasso G, De Santo NG, Kinne R. Thyroid hormones and renal transport: cellular and biochemical aspects. *Kidney Int* 1987;32:443–451.
77. Capasso G, De Tommaso G, Pica A, Anastasio P, Capasso J, Kinne R, De Santo NG. Effects of thyroid hormones on heart and kidney functions. *Miner Electrolyte Metab* 1999;25:56–64.
78. Caro JF, Sinha MK, Kolaczynski JW, Zhang PL, Considine RV. Leptin: the tale of an obesity gene. *Diabetes* 1996;45:1455–1462.
79. Carter RF, Bitar KN, Zfass AM, Makhlouf GM. Inhibition of VIP-stimulated intestinal secretion and cyclic AMP production by somatostatin in the rat. *Gastroenterology* 1978;74:726–730.
80. Chai SY, Christopoulos G, Cooper ME, Sexton PM. Characterization of binding sites for amylin, calcitonin, and CGRP in primate kidney. *Am J Physiol* 1998;274:F51–F62.
81. Charlton BG, Neal DE, Simmons NL. Vasoactive intestinal peptide stimulation of human renal adenylate cyclase in vitro. *J Physiol* 1990;423:475–484.
82. Charlton CG, Quirion R, Handelmann GE, Miller RL, Jensen RT, Finkel MS, O'Donohue TL. Secretin receptors in the rat kidney: adenylate cyclase activation and renal effects. *Peptides* 1986;7:865–871.
83. Cheeseman CI. Upregulation of SGLT-1 transport activity in rat jejunum induced by GLP-2 infusion in vivo. *Am J Physiol* 1997;273:R1965–R1971.
84. Chen WJ, Goldstein JL, Brown MS. NPXY, a sequence often found in cytoplasmic tails, is required for coated pit-mediated internalization of the low density lipoprotein receptor. *J Biol Chem* 1990;265:3116–3123.
85. Cheng H–F, Burns KD, Harris RC. Reduced proximal tubule angiotensin II receptor expression in streptozotocin-induced diabetes mellitus. *Kidney Int* 1994;46:1603–1610.
86. Chin E, Zamah AM, Landau D, Gronbcek H, Flyvbjerg A, LeRoith D, Bondy CA. Changes in facilitative glucose transporter messenger ribonucleic acid levels in the diabetic rat kidney. *Endocrinology* 1997;138:1267–1275.
87. Chin E, Zhou J, Bondy C. Anatomical and developmental patterns of facilitative glucose transporter gene expression in the rat kidney. *J Clin Invest* 1993;91:1810–1815.
88. Chou CC, Hsieh CP, Dabney JM. Comparison of vascular effects of gastrointestinal hormones on various organs. *Am J Physiol* 1977;232:H103–H109.
89. Chow BK. Molecular cloning and functional characterization of a human secretin receptor. *Biochem Biophys Res Commun* 1995;212:204–211.
90. Christensen EI, Birn H. Megalin and cubilin: synergistic endocytic receptors in renal proximal tubule. *Am J Physiol Renal Physiol* 2001;280:F562–F573.
91. Chua SC Jr, Chung WK, Wu-Peng XS, Zhang Y, Liu SM, Tartaglia L, Leibel RL. Phenotypes of mouse diabetes and rat fatty due to mutations in the OB (leptin) receptor. *Science* 1996;271:994–996.
92. Cohen MP, Sharma K, Jin Y, Hud E, Wu VY, Tomaszewski J, Ziyadeh FN. Prevention of diabetic nephropathy in db/db mice with glycated albumin antagonists. A novel treatment strategy. *J Clin Invest* 1995;95:2338–2345.
93. Cooper GJ. Amylin compared with calcitonin gene-related peptide: structure, biology, and relevance to metabolic disease. *Endocr Rev* 1994;15:163–201.
94. Cui S, Flyvbjerg A, Nielsen S, Kiess W, Christensen EI. IGF-II/Man-6-P receptors in rat kidney: apical localization in proximal tubule cells. *Kidney Int* 1993;43:796–807.
95. Curtis PJ, Fender HR, Rayford PL, Thompson JC. Catabolism of secretin by the liver and kidney. *Surgery* 1976;80:259–265.
96. Cutillas PR, Norden AG, Cramer R, Burlingame AL, Unwin RJ. Detection and analysis of urinary peptides by on-line liquid chromatography and mass spectrometry: application to patients with renal Fanconi syndrome. *Clin Sci (Lond)* 2003;104:483–490.
97. Cutillas PR, Norden AG, Cramer R, Burlingame AL, Unwin RJ. Urinary proteomics of renal Fanconi syndrome. *Contrib Nephrol* 2004;141:155–169.
98. de Rouffignac C, Elalouf J-M, Roinel N. Physiological control of the urinary concentration mechanism by peptide hormones. *Kidney Int* 1987;31:611–620.
99. De Santo NG, Capasso G, Anastasio P, Coppola S, Bellini L, Lombardi A. Brain–gut peptides and the renal hemodynamic response to an oral protein load: a study of gastrin, bombesin, and glucagon in man. *Renal Physiol Biochem* 1992;15:53.
100. De Santo NG, Capasso G, Anastasio P, Coppola S, De Tommaso G, Coscarella G, Bellini L, Spagnuolo G, Barba G, Lombardi A, Alfieri R, Iacone R, Strazzullo P. Renal handling of sodium after an oral protein load in adult humans. *Renal Physiol Biochem* 1992;15:41–52.
101. Dean R, Murone C, Lew RA, Zhuo J, Casley D, Muller-Esterl W, Alcorn D, Mendelsohn FA. Localization of bradykinin B2 binding sites in rat kidney following chronic ACE inhibitor treatment. *Kidney Int* 1997;52:1261–1270.
102. Debnam ES, Sharp PA. Acute and chronic effects of pancreatic glucagon on sugar transport across the brush border and basolateral membranes of rat jejunal enterocytes. *Exp Physiol* 1993;78:197–207.
103. Debnam ES, Unwin RJ. Hyperglycemia and intestinal and renal glucose transport: Implications for diabetic renal injury. *Kidney Int* 1996;50:1101–1109.
104. DeFronzo RA, Cooke CR, Andres R, Fabona GR, Davies PJ. The effect of insulin on renal handling of sodium, potassium, calcium, and potassium in man. *J Clin Invest* 1975; 55:845–855.
105. DeFronzo RA, Goldberg M, Agus ZS. The effects of glucose and insulin on renal electrolyte transport. *J Clin Invest* 1976;58:83–90.
106. Delesque N, Buscail L, Esteve JP, Rauly I, Zeggari M, Saint-Laurent N, Bell GI, Schally AV, Vaysse N, Susini C. A tyrosine phosphatase is associated with the somatostatin receptor. *Ciba Found Symp* 1995;190:187–96.
107. Dimaline R, Peart WS, Unwin RJ. Effects of vasoactive intestinal polypeptide (VIP) on renal function and plasma renin activity in the conscious rabbit. *J Physiol (Lond)* 1983;344:379–88.
108. Dixon R, Brunskill NJ. Activation of mitogenic pathways by albumin in kidney proximal tubule epithelial cells: implications for the pathophysiology of proteinuric states. *J Am Soc Nephrol* 1999;10:1487–1497.

109. Dixon R, Brunskill NJ. Albumin stimulates p44/p42 extracellular-signal–regulated mitogen-activated protein kinase in opossum kidney proximal tubular cells. *Clin Sci (Lond)* 2000;98: 295–301.
110. Djouadi F, Wijkhuisen A, Bastin J, Vilar J, Merlet-Benichou C. Effect of glucocorticoids on mitochondrial oxidative enzyme and Na-K-ATPase activities in the rat proximal tubule and thick ascending limb of Henle. *Ren Physiol Biochem* 1993;16:249–256.
111. Dominguez JH, Camp K, Maianu L, Feister H, Garvey WT. Molecular adaptations of GLUT1 and GLUT2 in renal proximal tubules of diabetic rats. *Am J Physiol* 1994;266: F283–F290.
112. Donadelli R, Zanchi C, Morigi M, Buelli S, Batani C, Tomasoni S, Corna D, Rottoli D, Benigni A, Abbate M, Remuzzi G, Zoja C. Protein overload induces fractalkine upregulation in proximal tubular cells through nuclear factor kappaB- and p38 mitogen-activated protein kinase-dependent pathways. *J Am Soc Nephrol* 2003;14:2436–2446.
113. Duggan KA, Macdonald GJ. Vasoactive intestinal peptide: a direct renal natriuretic substance. *Clin Sci (Lond)* 1987;72:195–200.
114. Dunlop M. Aldose reductase and the role of the polyol pathway in diabetic nephropathy. *Kidney Int Suppl* 2000;77:S3–S12.
115. Eadington DW, Hepburn DA, Swainson CP. Antinatriuretic action of insulin is preserved after angiotensin I converting enzyme inhibition in normal man. *Nephrol Dial Transplant* 1993;8:29–35.
116. Eiam-ong S, Kurtzman NA, Sabatini S. Renal ATPases twenty-four hours after uninephrectomy: the role of IGF-1. *Miner Electrolyte Metab* 1996;22:234–241.
117. El Mernissi G, Doucet A. Short-term effects of aldosterone and dexamethasone on Na-K-ATPase along the rabbit nephron. *Pflugers Arch* 1983;399:147–151.
118. El Mernissi G, Doucet A. Specific activity of Na-K-ATPase after adrenalectomy and hormone replacement along the rabbit nephron. *Pflugers Arch* 1984;402:258–263.
119. El Nahas AM, Sayed-Ahmed N. Insulin-like growth factor I and the kidney: friend or foe? *Exp Nephrol* 1993;1:205–217.
120. El-Sefi S, Freiberg JM, Kinsella J, Cheng L, Sacktor B. Na^+-H^+ exchange and Na^+-dependent transport systems in streptozotocin diabetic rat kidney. *Am J Physiol* 1987;252:R40–R47.
121. Emmanouel DS, Lindheimar MD, Katz AI. Mechanism of impaired water excretion in hypothyroid rats. *J Clin Invest* 1974;54:926–934.
122. Epstein FH, Friedman LR, Levitin H. Hypercalcemia, nephrocalcinosis and reversible renal insufficiency associated with hyperthyroidism. *N Engl J Med* 1958;258:782–785.
123. Erlij D, De Smet P, Van Driessche W: Effect of insulin on area and Na^+ channel density of apical membrane of cultured toad kidney cells. *J Physiol (Lond)* 1994;481:533–542.
124. Ernest S, Coureau C, Escoubet B. Deprivation of phosphate increases IGF-II mRNA in MDCK cells but IGFs are not involved in phosphate transport adaptation to phosphate deprivation. *J Endocrinol* 1995;145:325–331.
125. Espinosa RE, Keller MJ, Yusufi ANK, Dousa T. Effect of thyroxine administration on phosphate transport across renal cortical brush border membrane. *Am J Physiol* 1984;246: F133–F139.
126. Evan AP, Henry DP, Connors BA, Summerlin P, Lee WH. Analysis of insulin-like growth factors (IGF)-I, and -II, type II IGF receptor and IGF-binding protein-2 mRNA and peptide levels in normal and nephrectomized rat kidney. *Kidney Int* 1995;48: 1517–1529.
127. Farman N. Steroid receptors: Distribution along the nephron. *Semin Nephrol* 1992;12:12–17.
128. Feraille E, Carranza ML, Rousselot M, Favre H. Insulin enhances sodium sensitivity of Na-K-ATPase in isolated rat proximal convoluted tubule. *Am J Physiol* 1994;267:F55–F62.
129. Feraille E, Carranza ML, Rousselot M, Favre H. Modulation of Na^+,$K(^+)$-ATPase activity by a tyrosine phosphorylation process in rat proximal convoluted tubule. *J Physiol (Lond)* 1997;498:99–108.
130. Feraille E, Marsy S, Barlet-Bas C, Rousselot M, Cheval L, Favre H, Doucet A. Insulin unresponsiveness of tubular monovalent cation transport during fructose-induced hypertension in rats. *Clin Sci (Colch)* 1995;88:293–299.
131. Feraille E, Rousselot M, Rajerison R, Favre H. Effect of insulin on Na^+,$K(^+)$-ATPase in rat collecting duct. *J Physiol (Lond)* 1995;488:171–180.
132. Field MJ, Stanton BA, Giebisch G. Differential acute effects of aldosterone, dexamethasone, and hyperkalemia on distal tubular potassium secretion in the rat kidney. *J Clin Invest* 1984; 74:1792–1802.
133. Fine LG, Badie-Dezfooly B, Lowe AG, Hamzeh A, Wells J, Salehmoghaddam S. Stimulation of Na^+/H^+ antiport is an early event in hypertrophy of renal proximal tubular cells. *Proc Natl Acad Sci* 1985;82:1736–1740.
134. Flyvbjerg A, Nielsen S, Sheikh MI, Jacobsen C, Orskov H, Christensen EI. Luminal and basolateral uptake and receptor binding of IGF-I in rabbit renal proximal tubules. *Am J Physiol* 1993;265:F624–F633.
135. Ford RV, Owens JC, Curd GW, Moyer JH, Spurr CL. Kidney function in various thyroid states. *J Clin Endocr Metab* 1961;21:548–553.
136. Freiberg JM, Kinsella J, Sacktor B. Glucocorticoids increase the Na^+-H^+ exchange and decrease the Na^+ gradient-dependent phosphate-uptake systems in renal brush border membrane vesicles. *Proc Natl Acad Sci U S A* 1982;79:4932–4936.
137. Frick A, Durasin I. Proximal tubular reabsorption of inorganic phosphate in adrenalectomized rats. *Pflugers Arch* 1980;385:189–192.
138. Fruehwald-Schultes B, Kern W, Beyer J, Forst T, Pfutzner A, Peters A. Elevated serum leptin concentrations in type 2 diabetic patients with microalbuminuria and macroalbuminuria. *Metabolism* 1999;48:1290–1293.
139. Fujibayashi S, Yamada T, Kurokawa K. Amino acids release somatostatin-like immunoreactivity from isolated glomeruli. *Mol Cell Endocrinol* 1985;41:263–267.
140. Funder JW. Corticosteroid receptors and renal 11 beta-hydroxysteroid dehydrogenase activity. *Semin Nephrol* 1990;10:311–319.
141. Funder JW. Steroid receptors. *Semin Nephrol* 1992;12:6–11.
142. Furness JB, Costa M, Keast JR. Choline acetyltransferase- and peptide immunoreactivity of submucous neurons in the small intestine of the guinea-pig. *Cell Tissue Res* 1984;237: 329–336.
143. Gallazzini M, Attmane-Elakeb A, Mount DB, Hebert SC, Bichara M. Regulation by glucocorticoids and osmolality of expression of ROMK (Kir 1.1), the apical K channel of thick ascending limb. *Am J Physiol Renal Physiol* 2003;284:F977–F986.
144. Garcia-Escribano C, Diez-Marqués M-L, Gonzalez-Rubio M, Rodriguez-Puyol M, Rodriguez-Puyol D. Somatostatin antagonizes angiotensin II effects on mesangial cell contraction and glomerular filtration. *Kidney Int* 1993;43:324–333.
145. Garg LC, Narang N, Wingo CS. Glucocorticoid effects on Na-K-ATPase in rabbit nephron segments. *Am J Physiol* 1985;248:F487–F491.
146. Garg LC, Tisher CC. Effects of thyroid hormone on Na-K-adenosine triphosphatase activity along the rat nephron. *J Lab Clin Med* 1985;106:568–572.
147. Geibel J, Giebisch G, Boron WF. Angiotensin II stimulates both Na^+-H^+ exchange and Na^+-HCO_3^- cotransport in the rabbit proximal tubule. *Proc Natl Acad Sci U S A* 1990;87: 7917–7920.
148. Gillum DM, Falk SA, Hammond WS, Conger JD. Glomerular dynamics in the hypothyroid rat and the role of the renin-angiotensin system. *Am J Physiol* 1987;253:F170–F179.
149. Giordano M, Castellino P, McConnell EL, DeFronzo RA. Effect of amino acid infusion on renal hemodynamics in humans: a dose–response study. *Am J Physiol Renal Fluid Electrolyte Physiol* 1994;267:F703–F708.
150. Good DW. Inhibition of bicarbonate absorption by peptide hormones and cyclic adenosine monophosphate in rat medullary thick ascending limb. *J Clin Invest* 1990;85:1006–1013.
151. Gotthardt M, Trommsdorff M, Nevitt MF, Shelton J, Richardson JA, Stockinger W, Nimpf J, Herz J. Interactions of the low density lipoprotein receptor gene family with cytosolic adaptor and scaffold proteins suggest diverse biological functions in cellular communication and signal transduction. *J Biol Chem* 2000;275:25616–25624.
152. Griffiths NM, Charbades D, Imbert-Teboul M, Siaume-Perez S, Morel F, Simmons NL. Distribution of vasoactive intestinal peptide-sensitive adenylate cyclase activity along the rabbit nephron. *Pflugers Arch* 1988;412:363–368.
153. Griffiths NM, Rugg EL, Simmons NL. Vasoactive intestinal peptide control of renal adenylate cyclase: in vitro studies of canine renal membranes and cultured canine renal epithelial (MDCK) cells. *Q J Exp Physiol* 1989;74:339–353.
154. Gronbaek H, Nielsen B, Frystyk J, Flyvbjerg A, Orskov H. Effect of lanreotide on local kidney IGF-I and renal growth in experimental diabetes in the rat. *Exp Nephrol* 1996;4:295–303.
155. Gronbaek H, Nielsen B, Frystyk J, Orskov H, Flyvbjerg A. Effect of octreotide on experimental diabetic renal and glomerular growth: importance of early intervention. *J Endocrinol* 1995;147:95–102.
156. Grubb BR. Ion transport across the jejunum in normal and cystic fibrosis mice. *Am J Physiol* 1995;268:G505–G513.
157. Guillery EN, Karniski LP, Mathews MS, Page WV, Orlowski J, Jose PA, Robillard JE. Role of glucocorticoids in the maturation of renal cortical Na^+/H^+ exchanger activity during fetal life in sheep. *Am J Physiol* 1995;268:F710–F717.
158. Gupta N, Dwarakanath V, Baum M. Maturation of the Na^+/H^+ antiporter (NHE3) in the proximal tubule of the hypothyroid adrenalectomized rat. *Am J Physiol Renal Physiol* 2004; 287:F521–F527.
159. Gutzwiller JP, Tschopp S, Bock A, Zehnder CE, Huber AR, Kreyenbuehl M, Gutmann H, Drewe J, Henzen C, Goeke B, Beglinger C. Glucagon-like peptide 1 induces natriuresis in healthy subjects and in insulin-resistant obese men. *J Clin Endocrinol Metab* 2004;89: 3055–3061.
160. Haber RS, Loeb JN. Stimulation of potassium efflux in rat liver by a low dose of thyroid hormone: evidence for enhanced cation permeability in the absence of Na,K-ATPase induction. *Endocrinology* 1986;118:207–211.
161. Hackenthal E, Aktories K, Jakobs KH, Lang RE. Neuropeptide Y inhibits renin release by a pertussis toxin-sensitive mechanism. *Am J Physiol* 1987;252:F543–F550.
162. Haefliger JA, Waeber B, Grouzmann E, Braissant O, Nussberger J, Nicod P, Waeber G. Cellular localization, expression and regulation of neuropeptide Y in kidneys of hypertensive rats. *Regul Pept* 1999;82:35–43.
163. Hama H, Saito A, Takeda T, Tanuma A, Xie Y, Sato K, Kazama JJ, Gejyo F. Evidence indicating that renal tubular metabolism of leptin is mediated by megalin but not by the leptin receptors. *Endocrinology* 2004;145:3935–3940.
164. Hamar J, Iripchanov BB, Demchenkeo IT, Dezsi L, Moskalenko JJ. Effect of somatostatin in organ blood flow in anaesthetized cats. *Acta Physiol Hung* 1985;65:47–51.
165. Hammerman MR, Gavin JR. III. Insulin-stimulated phosphorylation and insulin binding in canine renal basolateral membranes. *Am J Physiol* 1984;247:F408–F417.
166. Hammerman MR, Rogers S. Distribution of IGF receptors in the plasma membrane of proximal tubular cells. *Am J Physiol* 1987;253:F841–F847.
167. Hammond PJ, Wade AF, Gwilliam ME, Peters AM, Myers MJ, Gilbey SG, Bloom SR, Calam J. Amino acid infusion blocks renal tubular uptake of an indium-labelled somatostatin analogue. *Br J Cancer* 1993;67:1437–1439.
168. Han DC, Isono M, Chen S, Casaretto A, Hong SW, Wolf G, Ziyadeh FN. Leptin stimulates type I collagen production in db/db mesangial cells: glucose uptake and TGF-beta type II receptor expression. *Kidney Int* 2001;59:1315–1323.
169. Han HJ, Oh YJ, Lee YJ. Effect of albumin on 14C-alpha-methyl-D-glucopyranoside uptake in primary cultured renal proximal tubule cells: involvement of PLC, MAPK, and NF-kappaB. *J Cell Physiol* 2005;202:246–254.
170. Haniu M, Arakawa T, Bures EJ, Young Y, Hui JO, Rohde MF, Welcher AA, Horan T. Human leptin receptor. Determination of disulfide structure and N-glycosylation sites of the extracellular domain. *J Biol Chem* 1998;273:28691–28699.
171. Hansen LH, Abrahamsen N, Nishimura E. Glucagon receptor mRNA distribution in rat tissues. *Peptides* 1995;16:1163–1166.
172. Harris PJ, Cooper ME, Hiranyachattada S, Berka JL, Kelly DJ, Nobes M, Wookey PJ. Amylin stimulates proximal tubular sodium transport and cell proliferation in the rat kidney. *Am J Physiol* 1997;272:F13–F21.
173. Harris RC, Brenner BM, Seifter JL. Sodium–hydrogen exchange and glucose transport in renal microvillus membrane vesicles from rats with diabetes mellitus. *J Clin Invest* 1986; 77:724–733.

174. Harris RH, Hise MK, Best CF. Renotrophic factors in urine. *Kidney Int* 1983;23:616–623.
175. Hatzoglou A, Bakogeorgou E, Papakonstanti E, Stournaras C, Emmanouel DS, Castanas E. Identification and characterization of opioid and somatostatin binding sites in the opossum kidney (OK) cell line and their effect on growth. *J Cell Biochem* 1996;63:410–421.
176. Hawley CM, Duggan KA, Macdonald GJ, Shelley S. Oral sodium regulates extrahepatic metabolism of vasoactive intestinal peptide. *Clin Sci (Lond)* 1991;81:79–83.
177. Haylor J, Hickling H, El Eter E, Moir A, Oldroyd S, Hardisty C, El Nahas AM. JB3, an IGF-I receptor antagonist, inhibits early renal growth in diabetic and uninephrectomized rats. *J Am Soc Nephrol* 2000;11:2027–2035.
178. Herz J, Gotthardt M, Willnow TE. Cellular signalling by lipoprotein receptors. *Curr Opin Lipidol* 2000;11:161–166.
179. Hewitt SM, Dear J, Star RA. Discovery of protein biomarkers for renal diseases. *J Am Soc Nephrol* 2004;15:1677–1689.
180. Hicks T, Turnberg LA. The influence of secretin on ion transport in the human jejunum. *Gut* 1973;14:485–490.
181. Hirschberg R. Bioactivity of glomerular ultrafiltrate during heavy proteinuria may contribute to renal tubulo-interstitial lesions: evidence for a role for insulin-like growth factor I. *J Clin Invest* 1996;98:116–124.
182. Hirschberg R. Insulin-like growth factor I in the kidney. *Miner Electrolyte Metab* 1996;22: 128–132.
183. Hirschberg R, Adler S. Insulin-like growth factor system and the kidney: physiology, pathophysiology, and therapeutic implications. *Am J Kidney Dis* 1998;31:901–919.
184. Hirschberg R, Ding H, Wanner C. Effects of insulin-like growth factor I on phosphate transport in cultured proximal tubule cells. *J Lab Clin Med* 1995;126:428–434.
185. Hirschberg R, Kopple JD. Evidence that insulin-like growth factor I increases renal plasma flow and glomerular filtration rate in fasted rats. *J Clin Invest* 1989;83:326–330.
186. Hirschberg R, Wang S. Proteinuria and growth factors in the development of tubulointerstitial injury and scarring in kidney disease. *Curr Opin Nephrol Hypertens* 2005;14:43–52.
187. Hjalm G, Murray E, Crumley G, Harazim W, Lundgren S, Onyango I, Ek B, Larsson M, Juhlin C, Hellman P, Davis H, Akerstrom G, Rask L, Morse B. Cloning and sequencing of human gp330, a Ca(2+)-binding receptor with potential intracellular signaling properties. *Eur J Biochem* 1996;239:132–137.
188. Hodin RA, Lazar MA, Chin WW. Differential and tissue-specific regulation of the multiple c-erbA messanger RNA species by thyroid hormone. *J Clin Invest* 1990;85:101–105.
189. Holmes MC, Kotelevtsev Y, Mullins JJ, Seckl JR. Phenotypic analysis of mice bearing targeted deletions of 11beta-hydroxysteroid dehydrogenases 1 and 2 genes. *Mol Cell Endocrinol* 2001;171:15–20.
190. Hulagu S, Senturk O, Erdem A, Ozgur O, Celebi A, Karakaya AT, Seyhogullari M, Demirci A. Effects of losartan, somatostatin and losartan plus somatostatin on portal hemodynamics and renal functions in cirrhosis. *Hepatogastroenterology* 2002;49:783–787.
191. Hussain MM, Strickland DK, Bakillah A. The mammalian low-density lipoprotein receptor family. *Annu Rev Nutr* 1999;19:141–72.:141–172.
192. Hyun HS, Onaga T, Mineo H, Kato S. Effect of vasoactive intestinal polypeptide (VIP) on the net movement of electrolytes and water and glucose absorption in the jejunal loop of sheep. *J Vet Med Sci* 1995;57:865–869.
193. Ikeda T, Iwata K, Ochi H. Effect of insulin, proinsulin, and amylin on renin release from perfused rat kidney. *Metabolism* 2001;50:763–766.
194. Inoue T, Nonoguchi H, Tomita K. Physiological effects of vasopressin and atrial natriuretic peptide in the collecting duct. *Cardiovasc Res* 2001;51:470–480.
195. Ishikawa S-E, Saito T, Kuzuya T. Reversal of somatostatin inhibition of AVP-induced cAMP by pertussis toxin. *Kidney Int* 1988;33:536–542.
196. Ishimura E, Nishizawa Y, Emoto M, Maekawa K, Morii H. Effect of insulin on urinary phosphate excretion in type II diabetes mellitus with or without renal insufficiency. *Metabolism* 1996;45:782–786.
197. Ismailbeigi F, Edelman IS. The mechanism of thyroid calorigenesis: role of active sodium transport. *Proc Natl Acad Sci U S A* 1970;67:1071–1078.
198. Ito O, Kondo Y, Takahashi N, Kudo K, Igarashi Y, Omata K, Imai Y, Abe K. Insulin stimulates NaCl transport in isolated perfused MTAL of Henle's loop of rabbit kidney. *Am J Physiol* 1994;267:F265–F270.
199. Ito O, Kondo Y, Takahashi N, Omata K, Abe K. Role of calcium in insulin-stimulated NaCl transport in medullary thick ascending limb. *Am J Physiol* 1995;269:F236–F241.
200. Jacobsen C, Jessen H, Flyvbjerg A. IGF-II receptors in luminal and basolateral membranes isolated from pars convoluta and pars recta of rabbit proximal tubule. *Biochim Biophys Acta* 1995;1235:85–92.
201. Jeffrey IW, Kelly FJ, Duncan R, Hershey JW, Pain VM. Effect of starvation and diabetes on the activity of the eukaryotic initiation factor eIF-2 in rat skeletal muscle. *Biochimie* 1990;72:751–757.
202. Jesus Ferreira MC, Bailly C. Luminal and basolateral endothelin inhibit chloride reabsorption in the mouse thick ascending limb via a Ca(2+)-independent pathway. *J Physiol* 1997;505:749–758.
203. Johnson DW, Brew BK, Poronnik P, Cook DI, Field MJ, Gyory AZ, Pollock CA. Insulin-like growth factor I stimulates apical sodium/hydrogen exchange in human proximal tubule cells. *Am J Physiol* 1997;272:F484–F490.
204. Kageyama S, Yamamoto J, Isogai Y, Fujita T. Effect of insulin on sodium reabsorption in hypertensive patients. *Am J Hypertens* 1994;7:409–415.
205. Kajikawa K, Yasui W, Sumiyoshi H, Yoshida K, Nakayama H, Ayhan A, Yokozaki H, Ito H, Tahara E. Expression of epidermal growth factor in human tissues. Immunohistochemical and biochemical analysis. *Virchows Arch A Pathol Anat Histopathol* 1991;418:27–32.
206. Katz AI, Lindheimer MD. Actions of hormones on the kidney. *Annu Rev Physiol* 1977;39: 97–134.
207. Kaufmann M, Muff R, Stieger B, Biber J, Murer H, Fischer JA. Apical and basolateral parathyroid hormone receptors in rat renal cortical membranes. *Endocrinology* 1994;134:1173–1178.
208. Keast JR, Furness JB, Costa M. Somatostatin in human enteric nerves. Distribution and characterization. *Cell Tissue Res* 1984;237:299–308.
209. Kellett GL. The facilitated component of intestinal glucose absorption. *J Physiol* 2001; 531:585–595.
210. Kinsella J, Cujdik T, Sacktor B. Na^+–H^+ exchange activity in renal brush border membrane vesicles in response to metabolic acidosis: the role of glucocorticoids. *Proc Natl Acad Sci U S A* 1984;81:630–634.
211. Kinsella J, Sacktor B. Thyroid hormones increase Na^+–H^+ exchange activity in renal brush border membranes. *Proc Natl Acad Sci U S A* 1985;82:3606–3610.
212. Kirchner K. Insulin increases loop segment chloride reabsorption in the euglycemic rat. *Am J Physiol* 1988;255:F1206–F1213.
213. Klisic J, Zhang J, Nief V, Reyes L, Moe OW, Ambuhl PM. Albumin regulates the Na^+/H^+ exchanger 3 in OKP cells. *J Am Soc Nephrol* 2003;14:3008–3016.
214. Kompanowska-Jezierska E, Sadowski J, Walkowska A. Glucagon increases medullary interstitial electrolyte concentration in rat kidney. *Can J Physiol Pharmacol* 1995;73:1289–1291.
215. Korner A, Eklof AC, Celsi G, Aperia A. Increased renal metabolism in diabetes. Mechanism and functional implications. *Diabetes* 1994;43:629–633.
216. Krejs GJ, Barkley RM, Read NW, Fordtran JS. Intestinal secretion induced by vasoactive intestinal polypeptide. A comparison with cholera toxin in the canine jejunum in vivo. *J Clin Invest* 1978;61:1337–1345.
217. Kurokawa K, Aponte GW, Fujibayashi S, Yamada T. Somatostatin-like immunoreactivity in the glomerulus of rat kidney. *Kidney Int* 1983;24:754–757.
218. Lang F, Haussinger D, Tschernko E, Capasso G, De Santo NG. Proteins, the liver and the kidney. Hepatic regulation of renal function. *Nephron* 1992;61:1–4.
219. Larsson M, Hjalm G, Sakwe AM, Engstrom A, Hoglund AS, Larsson E, Robinson RC, Sundberg C, Rask L. Selective interaction of megalin with postsynaptic density-95 (PSD-95)-like membrane-associated guanylate kinase (MAGUK) proteins. *Biochem J* 2003; 373:381–391.
220. Lazar MA. Thyroid hormone receptors, multiple forms, multiple possibilities. *Endocr Rev* 1993;14:184–193.
221. Lee J, Pilch PF. The insulin receptor: structure, function, and signaling. *Am J Physiol Cell Physiol* 1994;266:C319–C334.
222. Lee YC, Lin HH, Tang MJ. Glucocorticoid upregulates Na-K-ATPase alpha- and beta-mRNA via an indirect mechanism in proximal tubule cell primary cultures. *Am J Physiol* 1995;268:F862–F867.
223. Leheste JR, Melsen F, Wellner M, Jansen P, Schlichting U, Renner-Muller I, Andreassen TT, Wolf E, Bachmann S, Nykjaer A, Willnow TE. Hypocalcemia and osteopathy in mice with kidney-specific megalin gene defect. *FASEB J* 2003;17:247–249.
224. Leheste JR, Rolinski B, Vorum H, Hilpert J, Nykjaer A, Jacobsen C, Aucouturier P, Moskaug JO, Otto A, Christensen EI, Willnow TE. Megalin knockout mice as an animal model of low molecular weight proteinuria. *Am J Pathol* 1999;155:1361–1370.
225. Lehrmann H, Thomas J, Kim SJ, Jacobi C, Leipziger J. Luminal P2Y2 receptor-mediated inhibition of Na^+ absorption in isolated perfused mouse CCD. *J Am Soc Nephrol* 2002;13:10–18.
226. Li H, Ren P, Onwochei M, Ruch RJ, Xie Z. Regulation of rat Na^+/Pi cotransporter-1 gene expression: the roles of glucose and insulin. *Am J Physiol* 1996;271:E1021–1028.
227. Lin HH, Tang MJ. Thyroid hormone upregulates Na,K-ATPase alpha and beta mRNA in primary cultures of proximal tubule cells. *Life Sci* 1997;60:375–382.
228. Lin JH, Makris A, McMahon C, Bear SE, Patriotis C, Prasad VR, Brent R, Golemis EA, Tsichlis PN. The ankyrin repeat-containing adaptor protein Tvl-1 is a novel substrate and regulator of Raf-1. *J Biol Chem* 1999;274:14706–14715.
229. Ling BN, Seal EE, Eaton DC. Regulation of mesangial cell ion channels by insulin and angiotensin II. Possible role in diabetic glomerular hyperfiltration. *J Clin Invest* 1993;92:2141–2151.
230. Lo CS, Lo TN. Time course of the renal response to triiodothyronine in the rat. *Am J Physiol* 1979;236:F9–F13.
231. Lonergan MA, Field MJ. Renal sodium excretion following systemic infusion of vasoactive intestinal peptide in the rat. *Clin Exp Pharmacol Physiol* 1991;18:819–824.
232. Losel RM, Falkenstein E, Feuring M, Schultz A, Tillmann HC, Rossol-Haseroth K, Wehling M. Nongenomic steroid action: controversies, questions, and answers. *Physiol Rev* 2003;83: 965–1016.
233. Lundberg JM, Terenius L, Hokfelt T, Martling CR, Tatemoto K, Mutt V, Polak J, Bloom S, Goldstein M. Neuropeptide Y (NPY)–like immunoreactivity in peripheral noradrenergic neurons and effects of NPY on sympathetic function. *Acta Physiol Scand* 1982;116:477–480.
234. Lundqvist G, Gustavsson S, Hallgren R. Plasma levels of somatostatin-like immunoreactivity-independence of kidney function. *Clin Endocrinol (Oxf)* 1979;10:489–492.
235. Lynch CJ, McCall KM, Ng YC, Hazen SA. Glucagon stimulation of hepatic Na(+)-pump activity and alpha subunit phosphorylation in rat hepatocytes. *Biochem J* 1996;313: 983–989.
236. Lyoussi B, Crabbe J. Effects of corticosteroids on parameters related to Na^+ transport by amphibian renal distal cells (A6) in culture. *J Steroid Biochem Mol Biol* 1996;59:323–331.
237. Lyoussi B, Crabbe J. Effects of dexamethasone on (Na^+/K^+)-ATPase and other parameters related to transepithelial Na^+ transport by amphibian renal distal cells (A6) in culture. *J Steroid Biochem Mol Biol* 1996;59:333–338.
238. Mackovic-Basic M, Salihagic A, Ries N, Sabolic I. Absence of increased electroneutral Na^+-H^+ exchange in renal cortical brush-border membranes from hyperthyroid rats. *Biochem Pharmacol* 1988;37:1699–1705.
239. MacNeil DJ, Occi JL, Hey PJ, Strader CD, Graziano MP. Cloning and expression of a human glucagon receptor. *Biochem Biophys Res Commun* 1994;198:328–334.
240. Madej T, Boguski MS, Bryant SH. Threading analysis suggests that the obese gene product may be a helical cytokine. *FEBS Lett* 1995;373:13–18.
241. Magaldi AJ, Cesar KR, Yano Y. Effect of insulin on water and urea transport in the inner medullary collecting duct. *Am J Physiol* 1994;266:F394–F399.
242. Malnic G, Berliner RW, Giebisch G. Distal perfusion studies: transport stimulation by native tubule fluid. *Am J Physiol* 1990;258:F1523–F1527.
243. Mandon B, Siga E, Chabardes D, Firsov D, Roinel N, de Rouffignac C. Insulin stimulates Na^+, Cl^-, Ca^{2+}, and Mg^{2+} transports in TAL of mouse nephron: cross-potentiation with AVP. *Am J Physiol* 1993;265:F361–F369.

244. Mantzoros CS. The role of leptin in human obesity and disease: a review of current evidence. *Ann Intern Med* 1999;130:671–680.

245. Marchand GR, Ott CE, Lang FC, Greger RF, Knox FG. Effect of secretin on renal blood flow, interstitial pressure, and sodium excretion. *Am J Physiol* 1977;232:F147–F151.

246. Marcos Morales M, Purchio Brucoli HC, Malnic G, Gil Lopes A. Role of thyroid hormones in renal tubule acidification. *Mol Cell Biochem* 1996;154:17–21.

247. Marcus RG, England R, Nguyen K, Charron MJ, Briggs JP, Brosius FC3. Altered renal expression of the insulin-responsive glucose transporter GLUT4 in experimental diabetes mellitus. *Am J Physiol* 1994;267:F816–F824.

248. Marks J, Carvou NJ, Debnam ES, Srai SK, Unwin RJ. Diabetes increases facilitative glucose uptake and GLUT2 expression at the rat proximal tubule brush border membrane. *J Physiol (Lond)* 2003;553:137–145.

249. Marks J, Debnam ES, Dashwood MR, Srai SK, Unwin RJ. Detection of glucagon receptor mRNA in the rat proximal tubule: potential role for glucagon in the control of renal glucose transport. *Clin Sci (Lond)* 2003;104:253–258.

250. Masuzaki H, Yamamoto H, Kenyon CJ, Elmquist JK, Morton NM, Paterson JM, Shinyama H, Sharp MG, Fleming S, Mullins JJ, Seckl JR, Flier JS. Transgenic amplification of glucocorticoid action in adipose tissue causes high blood pressure in mice. *J Clin Invest* 2003;112:83–90.

251. Mathi SK, Chan J, Watt VM. Insulin receptor-related receptor messenger ribonucleic acid: quantitative distribution and localization to subpopulations of epithelial cells in stomach and kidney. *Endocrinology* 1995;136:4125–4132.

252. Matsunuma A, Kawane T, Maeda T, Hamada S, Horiuchi N. Leptin corrects increased gene expression of renal 25-hydroxyvitamin D3-1 alpha-hydroxylase and -24-hydroxylase in leptin-deficient, ob/ob mice. *Endocrinology* 2004;145:1367–1375.

253. Mcdonough AA, Brown TA, Horowitz B, Chiu R, Schlotterbeck J, Bowen J, Schmitt CA. Thyroid hormone coordinately regulates Na$^+$-K$^+$-ATPase alpha- and beta-subunit mRNA levels in kidney. *Am J Physiol* 1988;254:C323–C329.

254. Medeiros MD, Turner AJ. Processing and metabolism of peptide-YY: pivotal roles of dipeptidylpeptidase-IV, aminopeptidase-P, and endopeptidase-24.11. *Endocrinology* 1994;134:2088–2094.

255. Medeiros MS, Turner AJ. Metabolism and functions of neuropeptide Y. *Neurochem Res* 1996;21:1125–1132.

256. Michael UF, Barenberg EL, Chavez R, Vaamonde CA, Papper S. Renal handling of sodium and water in the hypothyroid rat. *J Clin Invest* 1970;51:1405–1415.

257. Michael UF, Kelley J, Alpert H, Vaamonde CA. Role of distal delivery of filtrate in impaired renal dilution of the hypothyroid rats. *Am J Physiol* 1976;230:699–705.

257a. Mohebbi N, Kovacikova J, Nowik M, Wagner CA. Thyroid hormone deficiency alters expression of acid-base transporters in rat kidney. *Am J Physiol* 2007; April 4.

258. Moller J. Effects of growth hormone on fluid homeostasis. Clinical and experimental aspects. *Growth Horm IGF Res* 2003;13:55–74.

259. Moore CC, Mellon SH, Murai J, Siiteri PK, Miller WL. Structure and function of the hepatic form of 11 beta-hydroxysteroid dehydrogenase in the squirrel monkey, an animal model of glucocorticoid resistance. *Endocrinology* 1993;133:368–375.

260. Morel F. Sites of hormone action in mammalian nephron. *Am J Physiol* 1981;240:F159–F164.

261. Morel F, Doucet A. Hormonal control of kidney function at the cell level. *Physiol Rev* 1986;66:377–468.

262. Moreno C, Mistry M, Roman RJ. Renal effects of glucagon-like peptide in rats. *Eur J Pharmacol* 2002;434:163–167.

263. Mori K, Yoshimoto A, Takaya K, Hosoda K, Ariyasu H, Yahata K, Mukoyama M, Sugawara A, Hosoda H, Kojima M, Kangawa K, Nakao K. Kidney produces a novel acylated peptide, ghrelin. *FEBS Lett* 2000;486:213–216.

264. Morris BJ, Chambers SM. Hypothesis: glucagon receptor glycine to serine missense mutation contributes to one in 20 cases of essential hypertension. *Clin Exp Pharmacol Physiol* 1996;23:1035–1037.

265. Morrisey K, Steadman R, Williams JD, Phillips AO. Renal proximal tubular cell fibronectin accumulation in response to glucose is polyol pathway dependent. *Kidney Int* 1999;55:160–167.

266. Morrison JH, Benoit R, Magistretti PJ, Bloom FE. Immunohistochemical distribution of pro-somatostatin–related peptides in cerebral cortex. *Brain Res* 1983;262:344–351.

267. Mount CD, Lukas TJ, Orth DN. Purification and characterization of epidermal growth factor (beta-urogastrone) and epidermal growth factor fragments from large volumes of human urine. *Arch Biochem Biophys* 1985;240:33–42.

268. Mourad FH, Barada KA, Abdel-Malak N, Bou Rached NA, Khoury CI, Saade NE, Nassar CF. Interplay between nitric oxide and vasoactive intestinal polypeptide in inducing fluid secretion in rat jejunum. *J Physiol* 2003;550:863–871.

269. Mujais SK, Chekal MA, Jones WJ, Hayslett JP, Katz AI. Regulation of renal Na-K-ATPase in the rat. Role of the natural mineralo- and glucocorticoid hormones. *J Clin Invest* 1984;73:13–19.

270. Mujais SK, Chekal MA, Lee SM, Katz AI. Relationship between adrenal steroids and renal Na-K-ATPase. Effect of short-term hormone administration on the rat cortical collecting tubule. *Pflugers Arch* 1984;402:48–51.

271. Nagaya N, Miyatake K, Uematsu M, Oya H, Shimizu W, Hosoda H, Kojima M, Nakanishi N, Mori H, Kangawa K. Hemodynamic, renal, and hormonal effects of ghrelin infusion in patients with chronic heart failure. *J Clin Endocrinol Metab* 2001;86:5854–5859.

272. Nair KS, Pabico RC, Truglia JA, McKenna BA, Statt M, Lockwood DH. Mechanism of glomerular hyperfiltration after a protein meal in humans. Role of hormones and amino acids. *Diabetes Care* 1994;17:711–715.

273. Nakajima H, Takenaka M, Kaimori JY, Hamano T, Iwatani H, Sugaya T, Ito T, Hori M, Imai E. Activation of the signal transducer and activator of transcription signaling pathway in renal proximal tubular cells by albumin. *J Am Soc Nephrol* 2004;15:276–285.

274. Nakamura R, Emmanouel DS, Katz AI. Insulin binding sites in various segments of the rabbit nephron. *J Clin Invest* 1983;72:388–392.

275. Nannipieri M, Lanfranchi A, Santerini D, Catalano C, Van de WG, Ferrannini E. Influence of long-term diabetes on renal glycogen metabolism in the rat. *Nephron* 2001;87:50–57.

276. Nascimento-Gomes G, Gil FZ, Mello-Aires M. Alterations of the renal handling of H$^+$ in diabetic rats. *Kidney Blood Press Res* 1997;20:251–257.

277. Navar LG, Harrison-Bernard LM, Wang CT, Cervenka L, Mitchell KD. Concentrations and actions of intraluminal angiotensin II. *J Am Soc Nephrol* 1999;10(Suppl 11):S189–S195.

278. Nickels D, Schwab N, Poth M. Effects of somatostatin and captopril on glomerular prostaglandin E2 production in normal and diabetic rats. *Prostaglandins* 1993;46:61–73.

279. Nielsen S. Time-course and kinetics of proximal tubular processing of insulin. *Am J Physiol Renal Fluid Electrolyte Physiol* 1992;262:F813–F822.

280. Nielsen S. Sorting and recycling efficiency of apical insulin binding sites during endocytosis in proximal tubule cells. *Am J Physiol* 1993;264:C810–C822.

281. Nielsen S. Endocytosis in renal proximal tubules. Experimental electron microscopical studies of protein absorption and membrane traffic in isolated, in vitro perfused proximal tubules. *Danish Med Bull* 1994;41:243–263.

282. Nizet A, LeFrebre P, Crabbe R. Control by insulin of sodium, potassium and water excretion by the isolated dog kidney. *Pflugers Arch* 1971;323:11–20.

283. Norden AG, Lapsley M, Igarashi T, Kelleher CL, Lee PJ, Matsuyama T, Scheinman SJ, Shiraga H, Sundin DP, Thakker RV, Unwin RJ, Verroust P, Moestrup SK. Urinary megalin deficiency implicates abnormal tubular endocytic function in Fanconi syndrome. *J Am Soc Nephrol* 2002;13:125–133.

284. Norden AG, Lapsley M, Lee PJ, Pusey CD, Scheinman SJ, Tam FW, Thakker RV, Unwin RJ, Wrong O. Glomerular protein sieving and implications for renal failure in Fanconi syndrome. *Kidney Int* 2001;60:1885–1892.

285. Nusken KD, Groschl M, Rauh M, Stohr W, Rascher W, Dotsch J. Effect of renal failure and dialysis on circulating ghrelin concentration in children. *Nephrol Dial Transplant* 2004;19:2156–2157.

286. Ohneda A, Parada E, Eisentraut AM, Unger RH. Characterization of response of circulating glucagon to intraduodenal and intravenous administration of amino acids. *J Clin Invest* 1968;47:2305–2322.

287. Ohtomo Y, Aperia A, Sahlgren B, Johansson BL, Wahren J. C-peptide stimulates rat renal tubular Na$^+$, K$^{(+)}$-ATPase activity in synergism with neuropeptide Y. *Diabetes* 1996;39:199–205.

288. Oleinikov AV, Zhao J, Makker SP. Cytosolic adaptor protein Dab2 is an intracellular ligand of endocytic receptor gp600/megalin. *Biochem J* 2000;347:613–621.

289. Oppenheimer JH, Schwartz HL, Lane JT, Thompson MP. Functional relationship of thyroid hormone-induced lipogenesis, lipolysis, and thermogenesis in the rat. *J Clin Invest* 1991;87:125–132.

290. Oppenheimer JH, Schwartz HL, Mariash CN, Kinlaw WB, Wong NCW, Freake HC. Advance in our understanding of thyroid hormone action at the cellular level. *Endocr Rev* 1987;8:288–308.

291. Ozaki K, Takada N, Tsujimoto K, Tsuji N, Kawamura T, Muso E, Ohta M, Itoh N. Localization of insulin receptor-related receptor in the rat kidney. *Kidney Int* 1997;52:694–698.

292. Palmer G, Bonjour JP, Caverzasio J. Stimulation of inorganic phosphate transport by insulin-like growth factor I and vanadate in opossum kidney cells is mediated by distinct protein tyrosine phosphorylation processes. *Endocrinology* 1996;137:4699–4705.

293. Park S, Taub M, Han H. Regulation of phosphate uptake in primary cultured rabbit renal proximal tubule cells by glucocorticoids: evidence for nongenomic as well as genomic mechanisms. *Endocrinology* 2001;142:710–720.

294. Patel DR, Kong Y, Sreedharan SP. Molecular cloning and expression of a human secretin receptor. *Mol Pharmacol* 1995;47:467–473.

295. Perez-Fontan M, Cordido F, Rodriguez-Carmona A, Peteiro J, Garcia-Naveiro R, Garcia-Buela J. Plasma ghrelin levels in patients undergoing haemodialysis and peritoneal dialysis. *Nephrol Dial Transplant* 2004;19:2095–2100.

296. Pironi L, Stanghellini V, Miglioli M, Corinaldesi R, de Giorgio R, Ruggeri E, Tosetti C, Poggioli G, Morselli Labate AM, Monetti N. Fat-induced ileal brake in humans: a dose-dependent phenomenon correlated to the plasma levels of peptide YY. *Gastroenterology* 1993;105:733–739.

297. Pisitkun T, Shen RF, Knepper MA. Identification and proteomic profiling of exosomes in human urine. *Proc Natl Acad Sci U S A* 2004;101:13368–13373.

298. Playford RJ, Mehta S, Upton P, Rentch R, Moss S, Calam J, Bloom S, Payne N, Ghatei M, Edwards R, Unwin R. Effect of peptide YY on human renal function. *Am J Physiol* 1995;268:F754–F759.

299. Porter JP, Ganong WF. Vasoactive intestinal peptide and renin secretion. *Ann N Y Acad Sci* 1988;527:465–477.

300. Poujeol P, Vandewalle A. Phosphate uptake by proximal cells isolated from rabbit kidney: role of dexamethasone. *Am J Physiol* 1985;249:F74–F83.

301. Poumarat JS, Houillier P, Rismondo C, Roques B, Lazar G, Paillard M, Blanchard A. The luminal membrane of rat thick limb expresses AT1 receptor and aminopeptidase activities. *Kidney Int* 2002;62:434–445.

302. Poyner DR, Sexton PM, Marshall I, Smith DM, Quirion R, Born W, Muff R, Fischer JA, Foord SM. The mammalian calcitonin gene-related peptides, adrenomedullin, amylin, and calcitonin receptors. *Pharmacol Rev* 2002;54:233–246.

303. Price GJ, Berka JL, Edmondson SR, Werther GA, Bach LA. Localization of mRNAs for insulin-like growth factor binding proteins 1 to 6 in rat kidney. *Kidney Int* 1995;48:402–411.

304. Prie D, Friedlander G, Coureau C, Vandewalle A, Cassingena R, Ronco PM. Role of adenosine on glucagon-induced cAMP in a human cortical collecting duct cell line. *Kidney Int* 1995;47:1310–1318.

305. Proud D, Perkins M, Pierce JV, Yates KN, Highet PF, Herring PL, Mark M, Bahu R, Carone F, Pisano JJ. Characterization and localization of human renal kininogen. *J Biol Chem* 1981;256:10634–10639.

306. Pullman TN, Lavender AR, Aho I. Direct effects of glucagon on renal hemodynamics and excretion of inorganic ions. *Metabolism* 1967;16:358–373.

307. Quinones-Galvan A, Ferrannini E. Renal effects of insulin in man. *J Nephrol* 1997;10:188–191.

308. Rabkin R, Hamik A, Yagil C, Hamel FG, Duckworth WC, Fawcett J. Processing of 125I-insulin by polarized cultured kidney cells. *Exp Cell Res* 1996;224:136–142.

309. Rader K, Orlando RA, Lou X, Farquhar MG. Characterization of ANKRA, a novel ankyrin repeat protein that interacts with the cytoplasmic domain of megalin. *J Am Soc Nephrol* 2000;11:2167–2178.

310. Ray C, Carney S, Morgan T, Gillies A. Somatostatin as a modulator of distal nephron water permeability. *Clin Sci (Lond)* 1993;84:455–460.

311. Record RD, Johnson M, Lee S, Blazer-Yost BL. Aldosterone and insulin stimulate amiloride-sensitive sodium transport in A6 cells by additive mechanisms. *Am J Physiol* 1996;271: C1079–:C1084.

312. Reddy S, Gyory AZ, Bostrom T, Cochineas C. Transfer of Na transport inhibition in proximal tubules from saline volume-expanded to nonexpanded rats. *Am J Physiol* 1991;260:F69–F74.

313. Reid IA, Rose JC. An intrarenal effect of somatostatin on water excretion. *Endocrinology* 1977;100:782–785.

314. Reinecke M, Forssmann WG. Neuropeptide (neuropeptide Y, neurotensin, vasoactive intestinal polypeptide, substance P, calcitonin gene-related peptide, somatostatin) immunohistochemistry and ultrastructure of renal nerves. *Histochemistry* 1988;89:1–9.

315. Reinhardt RR, Chin E, Zhang B, Roth RA, Bondy CA. Insulin receptor-related receptor messenger ribonucleic acid is focally expressed in sympathetic and sensory neurons and renal distal tubule cells. *Endocrinology* 1993;133:3–10.

316. Renard S, Voilley N, Bassilana F, Lazdunski M, Barbry P. Localization and regulation by steroids of the alpha, beta and gamma subunits of the amiloride-sensitive Na$^+$ channel in colon, lung and kidney. *Pflugers Arch* 1995;430:299–307.

317. Renfro JL. Adaptability of marine teleost renal inorganic sulfate excretion: evidence for glucocorticoid involvement. *Am J Physiol* 1989;257:R511–R516.

318. Renfro JL, Clark NB, Metts RE, Lynch MA. Glucocorticoid inhibition of Na-SO4 transport by chick renal brush-border membranes. *Am J Physiol* 1989;256:R1176–R1183.

319. Reubi JC, Horisberger U, Studer UE, Waser B, Laissue JA. Human kidney as target for somatostatin: high affinity receptors in tubules and vasa recta. *J Clin Endocrinol Metab* 1993; 77:1323–1328.

320. Reville P, Urban M, Stephan F. Diminution du gradient intrarenal de concentration de l'uree par l'hypothyroidisme chez le rat. *C R Soc Biol* 1965;159:2031–2033.

321. Roca B, Arilla E, Prieto JC. Evidence for somatostatin binding sites in rabbit kidney. *Regul Pept* 1986;13:273–281.

322. Rodriguez–Commes J, Isales C, Kalghati L, Gasalla-Herraiz J, Hayslett JP. Mechanism of insulin-stimulated electrogenic sodium transport. *Kidney Int* 1994;46:666–674.

323. Romano G, Giagu P, Favret G, Bartoli E. Dual effect of secretin on nephron filtration and proximal reabsorption depending on the route of administration. *Peptides* 2000;21:723–728.

324. Rosa RM, Silva P, Stoff JS, Epstein FH. Effect of vasoactive intestinal peptide on isolated perfused rat kidney. *Am J Physiol* 1985;249:E494–E497.

325. Ruiz OS, Wang LJ, Pahlavan P, Arruda JA. Regulation of renal Na-HCO3 cotransporter: III. Presence and modulation by glucocorticoids in primary cultures of the proximal tubule. *Kidney Int* 1995;47:1669–1676.

326. Ruiz-Grande C, Pintado J, Alarcon C, Castilla C, Valverde I, Lopez-Novoa JM. Renal catabolism of human glucagon-like peptides 1 and 2. *Can J Physiol Pharmacol* 1990;68:1568–1573.

327. Said SI, Mutt V. Polypeptide with broad biological activity: isolation from small intestine. *Science* 1970;169:1217–1218.

328. Saito A, Pietromonaco S, Loo AK, Farquhar MG. Complete cloning and sequencing of rat gp330/"megalin," a distinctive member of the low density lipoprotein receptor gene family. *Proc Natl Acad Sci U S A* 1994;91:9725–9729.

329. Schaan BD, Irigoyen MC, Lacchini S, Moreira ED, Schmid H, Machado UF. Sympathetic modulation of the renal glucose transporter GLUT2 in diabetic rats. *Auton Neurosci* 2005; 117:54–61.

330. Schmitt R, Kahl T, Mutig K, Bachmann S. Selectively reduced expression of thick ascending limb Tamm–Horsfall protein in hypothyroid kidneys. *Histochem Cell Biol* 2004;121:319–327.

331. Schmitt R, Klussmann E, Kahl T, Ellison DH, Bachmann S. Renal expression of sodium transporters and aquaporin-2 in hypothyroid rats. *Am J Physiol Renal Physiol* 2003;284: F1097–F1104.

332. Schwartz CJ, Kimberg DV, Sheerin HE, Field M, Said SI. Vasoactive intestinal peptide stimulation of adenylate cyclase and active electrolyte secretion in intestinal mucosa. *J Clin Invest* 1974;54:536–544.

333. Sechi LA, Griffin CA, Schambelan M. Effect of dietary sodium chloride on insulin receptor number and mRNA levels in rat kidney. *Am J Physiol Renal Fluid Electrolyte Physiol* 1994;266: F31–F38.

334. Sechi LA, Valentin J-P, Griffin CA, Lee E, Bartoli E, Humphreys MH, Schambelan M. Receptors for atrial natriuretic peptide are decreased in the kidney of rats with streptozotocin-induced diabetes mellitus. *J Clin Invest* 1995;95:2451–2457.

335. Segal J, Ingbar SH. 3,5,3-tri-iodothyronine enhances sugar transport in rat thymocytes by increasing the intrinsic activity of the plasma membrane sugar transporter. *J Endocr* 1990;124: 133–140.

336. Seifert SA, Hsiao SC, Murer H, Biber J, Kempson SA. Renal endosomal phosphate (Pi) transport in normal and diabetic rats and response to chronic Pi deprivation. *Cell Biochem Funct* 1997;15:9–14.

337. Sengul S, Zwizinski C, Batuman V. Role of MAPK pathways in light chain–induced cytokine production in human proximal tubule cells. *Am J Physiol Renal Physiol* 2003;284:F1245–F1254.

338. Sengul S, Zwizinski C, Simon EE, Kapasi A, Singhal PC, Batuman V. Endocytosis of light chains induces cytokines through activation of NF-kappaB in human proximal tubule cells. *Kidney Int* 2002;62:1977–1988.

339. Serradeil-Le Gal C, Raufaste D, Brossard G, Pouzet B, Marty E, Maffrand JP, Le Fur G. Characterization and localization of leptin receptors in the rat kidney. *FEBS Lett* 1997;404: 185–191.

340. Shah M, Quigley R, Baum M. Maturation of proximal straight tubule NaCl transport: role of thyroid hormone. *Am J Physiol Renal Physiol* 2000;278:F596–F602.

341. Shapiro B, Sheppard M, Kronheim S, Pimstone B. Transrenal gradient of serum somatostatin-like immunoreactivity in the rat. *Horm Metab Res* 1978;10:356.

342. Sharma K, Considine RV, Michael B, Dunn SR, Weisberg LS, Kurnik BR, Kurnik PB, O'Connor J, Sinha M, Caro JF. Plasma leptin is partly cleared by the kidney and is elevated in hemodialysis patients. *Kidney Int* 1997;51:1980–1985.

343. Sharp PA, Debnam ES. The role of cyclic AMP in the control of sugar transport across the brush-border and the basolateral membranes of rat jejunal enterocytes. *Exp Physiol* 1994; 79:203–214.

344. Sheikh SP, Hansen AP, Williams JA. Solubilization and affinity purification of the Y2 receptor for neuropeptide Y and peptide YY from rabbit kidney. *J Biol Chem* 1991;266: 23959–23966.

345. Sheppard M, Shapiro B, Pimstone B, Kronheim S, Berelowitz M, Gregory M. Metabolic clearance and plasma half-disappearance time of exogenous somatostatin in man. *J Clin Endocrinol Metab* 1979;48:50–53.

346. Shin S-J, Lee Y-J, Tan M-S, Hsieh T-J, Tsai J-H. Increased atrial natriuretic peptide mRNA expression in the kidney of diabetic rats. *Kidney Int* 1997;51:1100–1105.

347. Shirley DG, Bailey MA, Unwin RJ. In vivo stimulation of apical P2 receptors in collecting ducts: evidence for inhibition of sodium reabsorption. *Am J Physiol Renal Physiol* 2005;288: F1243–F1248.

348. Siragy HM. AT(1) and AT(2) receptors in the kidney: role in disease and treatment. *Am J Kidney Dis* 2000;36:S4–S9.

349. Smet PD, Erlij D, Van Driessche W. Insulin effects on ouabain binding in A6 renal cells. *Pflugers Arch* 1997;434:11–18.

350. Songyang Z, Shoelson SE, Chaudhuri M, Gish G, Pawson T, Haser WG, King F, Roberts T, Ratnofsky S, Lechleider RJ. SH2 domains recognize specific phosphopeptide sequences. *Cell* 1993;72:767–778.

351. Stanton B, Janzen A, Klein-Robbenhaar G, DeFronzo R, Giebisch G, Wade J. Ultrastructure of rat initial collecting tubule. Effect of adrenal corticosteroid treatment. *J Clin Invest* 1985; 75:1327–1334.

352. Stanton BA. Regulation by adrenal corticosteroids of sodium and potassium transport in loop of Henle and distal tubule of rat kidney. *J Clin Invest* 1986;78:1612–1620.

353. Stephan F, Jahn H, Reville P, Urban M. Action de l'insuffisance thyroidienne chronique sur le débit urinaire et le pouvoir de concentration de rein chez le rat. *Rev Franc Etudes Clin Biol* 1963;8:890–899.

354. Strait KA, Schwartz HL, Perez-Castillo A, Oppenheimer JH. Ralationship of c-erbA mRNA content to tissue triiodothyronine nuclear binding capacity and function in developing and adult rats. *J Biol Chem* 1990;265:10514–10521.

355. Sulyok E, Tulassay T. Natriuresis of fasting: the possible role of leptin-neuropeptide Y system. *Med Hypotheses* 2001;56:629–633.

356. Talor A, Emmanouel DS, Katz AI. Insulin binding and degradation by luminal and basolateral tubular membranes from rabbit kidney. *J Clin Invest* 1982;69:1136–1146.

357. Tang MJ, Lin YJ, Huang JJ. Thyroid hormone upregulates gene expression, synthesis and release of pro-epidermal growth factor in adult rat kidney. *Life Sci* 1995;57:1477–1485.

358. Tang S, Leung JC, Abe K, Chan KW, Chan LY, Chan TM, Lai KN. Albumin stimulates interleukin-8 expression in proximal tubular epithelial cells in vitro and in vivo. *J Clin Invest* 2003;111:515–527.

359. Tartaglia LA. The leptin receptor. *J Biol Chem* 1997;272:6093–6096.

360. Tatemoto K, Mutt V. Chemical determination of polypeptide hormones. *Proc Natl Acad Sci U S A* 1978;75:4115–4119.

361. Taylor RE, Fregly JM. Renal response to propylthiouracil-trated rats to injected mineralcorticoids. *Endocrinology* 1964;75:33–38.

362. Ter Maaten JC, Voorburg A, Heine RJ, Ter Wee PM, Donker AJ, Gans RO. Renal handling of urate and sodium during acute physiological hyperinsulinaemia in healthy subjects. *Clin Sci (Colch)* 1997;92:51–58.

363. Thompson CS, Debnam ES. Hyperglucagonaemia: effects on active nutrient uptake by the rat jejunum. *J Endocrinol* 1986;111:37–42.

364. Thongboonkerd V, Klein JB. Proteomics in Nephrology. Basel: Karger; 2004.

365. Thulesen J, Hartmann B, Orskov C, Jeppesen PB, Holst JJ, Poulsen SS. Potential targets for glucagon-like peptide 2 (GLP–2) in the rat: distribution and binding of i.v. injected (125)I-GLP-2. *Peptides* 2000;21:1511–1517.

366. Toth-Heyn P, Toth M, Tulassay T, Dobi I, Kekesi V, Juhasz-Nagy A. Direct renovascular effect of somatostatin in the dog. *Regul Pept* 1996;67:103–106.

367. Tsimaratos M, Roger F, Chabardes D, Mordasini D, Hasler U, Doucet A, Martin PY, Feraille E. C-peptide stimulates Na$^+$,K$^+$-ATPase activity via PKC alpha in rat medullary thick ascending limb. *Diabetes* 2003;46:124–131.

368. Turman MA, Apple CA. Human proximal tubular epithelial cells express somatostatin: regulation by growth factors and cAMP. *Am J Physiol* 1998;274:F1095–F1101.

369. Turman MA, O'Dorisio MS, O'Dorisio TM, Apple CA, Albers AR. Somatostatin expression in human renal cortex and mesangial cells. *Regul Pept* 1997;68:15–21.

370. Unger RH, Orci L. Physiology and pathophysiology of glucagon. *Physiol Rev* 1976;56: 778–826.

371. Unwin R, Capasso G, Giebisch G. Bicarbonate transport along the loop of Henle. Effects of adrenal steroids. *Am J Physiol* 1995;37:F234–F239.

372. Unwin RJ, Ganz MB, Sterzel RB. Brain–gut peptides, renal function and cell growth. *Kidney Int* 1990;37:1031–1047.

373. Velazquez H, Bartiss A, Bernstein P, Ellisson DH. Adrenal steroids stimulate thiazide-sensitive NaCl transport by rat renal distal tubules. *Am J Physiol* 1996;270:F211–F219.

374. Verrey F, Pearce D, Pfeiffer R, Spindler B, Mastroberardino L, Summa V, Zecevic M. Pleiotropic action of aldosterone in epithelia mediated by transcription and post-transcription mechanisms. *Kidney Int* 2000;57:1277–1282.

375. Verroust PJ, Birn H, Nielsen R, Kozyraki R, Christensen EI. The tandem endocytic receptors megalin and cubilin are important proteins in renal pathology. *Kidney Int* 2002;62:745–756.

376. Vikic-Topic S, Raisch KP, Kvols LK, Vuk-Pavlovic S. Expression of somatostatin receptor subtypes in breast carcinoma, carcinoid tumor, and renal cell carcinoma. *J Clin Endocrinol Metab* 1995;80:2974–2979.

377. Vine W, Smith P, LaChappell R, Blase E, Young A. Effects of rat amylin on renal function in the rat. *Horm Metab Res* 1998;30:518–522.

378. Viteri AL, Poppell JW, Lasater JM, Dyck WP. Renal response to secretin. *J Appl Physiol* 1975;38:661–664.

379. Voisin T, Bens M, Cluzeaud F, Vandewalle A, Laburthe M. Peptide YY receptors in the proximal tubule PKSV-PCT cell line derived from transgenic mice. Relation with cell growth. *J Biol Chem* 1993;268:20547–20554.

380. Vora J, Owens DR, Luzio S, Atifa J, Ryder R, Hayes TM. Renal response to intravenous somatostatin in insulin-dependent diabetic patients and normal subjects. *J Clin Endocrinol Metab* 1987;64:975–979.

381. Wald H, Scherzer P, Popovtzer MM. Enhanced renal tubular ouabain-sensitive ATPase in streptozotocin diabetes mellitus. *Am J Physiol* 1986;251:F164–F170.

382. Waldum HL, Sundsfjord JA, Aanstad U, Burhol PG. The effect of secretin on renal haemodynamics in man. *Scand J Clin Lab Invest* 1980;40:475–478.

383. Walker BJ, Evans PA, Forsling ML, Nelsrop GA. Somatostatin and water excretion in man: An intrarenal action. *Clin Endocrinol* 1985;23:169–174.

384. Walker BR. Defective enzyme-mediated receptor protection: novel mechanisms in the pathophysiology of hypertension. *Clin Sci (Lond)* 1993;85:257–263.

385. Walter M, Unwin R, Nortier J, Deschodt-Lanckman M. Enhancing endogenous effects of natriuretic peptides: inhibitors of neutral endopeptidase (EC.3.4.24.11) and phosphodiesterase. *Curr Opin Nephrol Hypertens* 1997;6:468–473.

386. Wang SN, Lapage J, Hirschberg R. Glomerular ultrafiltration and apical tubular action of IGF-I, TGF-beta, and HGF in nephrotic syndrome. *Kidney Int* 1999;56:1247–1251.

387. Wang SN, Lapage J, Hirschberg R. Glomerular ultrafiltration of IGF-I may contribute to increased renal sodium retention in diabetic nephropathy. *J Lab Clin Med* 1999;134:154–160.

388. Wang T, Giebisch G. Effects of angiotensin II on electrolyte transport in the early and late distal tubule in rat kidney. *Am J Physiol* 1996;271:F143–F149.

389. Wang Y, Rangan GK, Tay YC, Wang Y, Harris DC. Induction of monocyte chemoattractant protein-1 by albumin is mediated by nuclear factor kappaB in proximal tubule cells. *J Am Soc Nephrol* 1999;10:1204–1213.

390. Wass JA, Penman E, Dryburgh JR, Tsiolakis D, Goldberg PL, Dawson AM, Besser GM, Rees LH. Circulating somatostatin after food and glucose in man. *Clin Endocrinol (Oxf)* 1980; 12:569–574.

391. Wei Y, Chen YJ, Li D, Gu R, Wang WH. Dual effect of insulin-like growth factor on the apical 70-pS K channel in the thick ascending limb of rat kidney. *Am J Physiol Cell Physiol* 2004;286:C1258–C1263.

392. Weinberg MS, Oza NB, Levinsky NG. Components of the kallikrein-kinin system in rat urine. *Biochem Pharmacol* 1984;33:1779–1782.

393. Welbourne TC. Glucocorticoid and acid-base homeostasis: effects on glutamine metabolism and transport. *Am J Kidney Dis* 1989;14:293–297.

394. Welbourne TC. Glucocorticoid control of ammoniagenesis in the proximal tubule. *Semin Nephrol* 1990;10:339–349.

395. Whorwood CB, Franklyn JA, Sheppard MC, Stewart PM. Tissue localization of 11 beta-hydroxysteroid dehydrogenase and its relationship to the glucocorticoid receptor. *J Steroid Biochem Mol Biol* 1992;41:21–28.

396. Widjaja A, Stratton IM, Horn R, Holman RR, Turner R, Brabant G. UKPDS 20: plasma leptin, obesity, and plasma insulin in type 2 diabetic subjects. *J Clin Endocrinol Metab* 1997; 82:654–657.

397. Wilcox CS, Cemerikic DA, Giebisch G. Differential effects of acute mineralo- and glucocorticosteroid administration on renal acid elimination. *Kidney Int* 1982;21:546–556.

398. Wilkes BM. Reduced glomerular angiotensin II receptor density in diabetes mellitus in the rat: time-course and mechanism. *Endocrinology* 1987;120:1291–1297.

399. Wilkins MR, Unwin RJ, Kenny AJ. Endopeptidase-24.11 and its inhibitors: potential therapeutic agents for edematous disorders and hypertension. *Kidney Int* 1993;43:273–285.

400. Williams TA, Mulatero P, Filigheddu F, Troffa C, Milan A, Argiolas G, Parpaglia PP, Veglio F, Glorioso N. Role of HSD11B2 polymorphisms in essential hypertension and the diuretic response to thiazides. *Kidney Int* 2005;67:631–637.

401. Willmann JK, Bleich M, Rizzo M, Schmidt-Hieber M, Ullrich KJ, Greger R. Amiloride-inhibitable Na$^+$ conductance in rat proximal tubule. *Pflugers Arch* 1997;434:173–178.

402. Willnow TE, Hilpert J, Armstrong SA, Rohlmann A, Hammer RE, Burns DK, Herz J. Defective forebrain development in mice lacking gp330/megalin. *Proc Natl Acad Sci U S A* 1996;93:8460–8464.

403. Wilson FA, Antonson DL, Hart BL, Warr TA, Cherrington AD, Liljenquist JE. The effect of somatostatin on the intestinal transport of glucose in vivo and in vitro in the rat. *Endocrinology* 1980;106:1562–1567.

404. Windstetter D, Schaefer F, Scharer K, Reiter K, Eife R, Harms HK, Bertele-Harms R, Fiedler F, Tsui LC, Reitmeir P, Horster M, Hadorn HB. Renal function and renotropic effects of secretin in cystic fibrosis. *Eur J Med Res* 1997;2:431–436.

405. Winkler SN, Torakai S, Levine BS, Kurokawa K. Effect of somatostatin on vasopressin-induced antidiuresis and renal cyclic AMP of rats. *Miner Electrolyte Metab* 1982;7:8–14.

406. Wittner M, Distefano A. Effects of antidiuretic hormone, parathyroid hormone and glucagon on transepithelial voltage and resistance of the cortical and medullary thick ascending limb of Henle's loop of the mouse nephron. *Pflugers Arch* 1990;415:707–712.

407. Wolf G, Hamann A, Han DC, Helmchen U, Thaiss F, Ziyadeh FN, Stahl RA. Leptin stimulates proliferation and TGF-beta expression in renal glomerular endothelial cells: potential role in glomerulosclerosis. *Kidney Int* 1999;56:860–872.

408. Wong F, Blendis L, Logan A. Effects of insulin on renal function, sympathetic nervous activity and forearm blood flow in normal human subjects. *Clin Invest Med* 1997;20:344–353.

409. Wong MS, Sriussadaporn S, Tembe VA, Favus MJ. Insulin-like growth factor I increases renal 1,25(OH)2D3 biosynthesis during low-P diet in adult rats. *Am J Physiol* 1997;272:F698–F703.

410. Wookey PJ, Cao Z, Cooper ME. Interaction of the renal amylin and renin-angiotensin systems in animal models of diabetes and hypertension. *Miner Electrolyte Metab* 1998;24:389–399.

411. Wookey PJ, Cooper ME. Amylin: physiological roles in the kidney and a hypothesis for its role in hypertension. *Clin Exp Pharmacol Physiol* 1998;25:653–660.

412. Wright EM, Hirsch JR, Loo DD, Zampighi GA. Regulation of Na$^+$/glucose cotransporters. *J Exp Biol* 1997;200:287–293.

413. Yamada Y, Post SR, Wang K, Tager HS, Bell GI, Seino S. Cloning and functional characterization of a family of human and mouse somatostatin receptors expressed in brain, gastrointestinal tract, and kidney. *Proc Natl Acad Sci U S A* 1992;89:251–255.

414. Yamamoto T, Moriwaki Y, Takahashi S, Tsutsumi Z, Hiroishi K, Yamakita J, Nakano T, Higashino K. Effect of glucagon on renal excretion of oxypurinol and purine bases. *J Rheumatol* 1997;24:708–713.

415. Yamato E, Ikegami H, Takekawa K, Fujisawa T, Nakagawa Y, Hamada Y, Ueda H, Ogihara T. Tissue-specific and glucose-dependent expression of receptor genes for glucagon and glucagon-like peptide-1 (GLP-1). *Horm Metab Res* 1997;29:56–59.

416. Yard BA, Chorianopoulos E, Herr D, van der Woude FJ. Regulation of endothelin-1 and transforming growth factor-beta1 production in cultured proximal tubular cells by albumin and heparan sulphate glycosaminoglycans. *Nephrol Dial Transplant* 2001;16:1769–1775.

417. Yonemura K, Cheng L, Sacktor B, Kinsella JL. Stimulation by thyroid hormone of Na$^+$-H$^+$ exchange activity in cultured opossum kidney cells. *Am J Physiol* 1990;258:F333–F338.

418. Yoshimoto A, Mori K, Sugawara A, Mukoyama M, Yahata K, Suganami T, Takaya K, Hosoda H, Kojima M, Kangawa K, Nakao K. Plasma ghrelin and desacyl ghrelin concentrations in renal failure. *J Am Soc Nephrol* 2002;13:2748–2752.

419. Yu H, Chen JK, Feng S, Dalgarno DC, Brauer AW, Schreiber SL. Structural basis for the binding of proline-rich peptides to SH3 domains. *Cell* 1994;76:933–945.

420. Yusufi ANK, Murayama N, Keller MJ, Dousa T. Modulatory effect of thyroid hormones on uptake of phosphate and other solutes across luminal brush border membrane of kidney cortex. *Endocrinology* 1985;116:2438–2449.

421. Zapf Z, Froescher ER. Insulin-like growth factor/somatomedins: structure, secretion, biological actions and physiologic role. *Hormone Res* 1986;24:121–130.

422. Zechwer IT. Compensatory growth of the kidney after unilateral nephrectomy in thyroidectomized rats. *Am J Physiol* 1946;145:681–684.

423. Zhang YH, Alvarez dlR, Canessa CM, Hayslett JP. Insulin-induced phosphorylation of ENaC correlates with increased sodium channel function in A6 cells. *Am J Physiol Cell Physiol* 2005;288:C141–C147.

424. Zhong Z, Kotova O, Davidescu A, Ehren I, Ekberg K, Jornvall H, Wahren J, Chibalin AV. C-peptide stimulates Na$^+$, K$^+$-ATPase via activation of ERK1/2 MAP kinases in human renal tubular cells. *Cell Mol Life Sci* 2004;61:2782–2790.

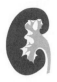

CHAPTER 36

Physiology and Pathophysiology of Sodium Retention and Wastage

Biff F. Palmer, Robert J. Alpern,* and Donald W. Seldin

University of Texas Southwestern Medical Center, Dallas, Texas, USA
*Yale University School of Medicine, New Haven, Connecticut, USA

INTRODUCTION

Extracellular fluid (ECF) volume is determined by the balance between sodium intake and renal excretion of sodium. Under normal circumstances, wide variations in salt intake lead to parallel changes in renal salt excretion, such that ECF volume is maintained within narrow limits. This relative constancy of ECF volume is achieved by a series of afferent sensing systems, central integrative pathways, and renal and extrarenal effector mechanisms acting in concert to modulate sodium excretion by the kidney.

In the major edematous states, effector mechanisms responsible for sodium retention behave in a more or less nonsuppressible manner, resulting in either subtle or overt expansion of ECF volume. In some instances, an intrinsic abnormality of the kidney leads to primary retention of sodium, resulting in expansion of ECF volume. In other instances, the kidney retains sodium secondarily as a result of an actual or sensed reduction in effective circulatory volume.

Renal sodium wastage can be defined as the inability of the kidney to conserve sodium to such an extent that continued loss of sodium into the urine leads to contraction of intravascular volume and hypotension. Renal sodium wastage occurs in circumstances where renal sodium transport is pharmacologically interrupted (administration of diuretics), where the integrity of renal tubular function is breached (tubulointerstitial renal disease), or when mineralocorticoid activity or tubular responsiveness are diminished or absent.

SODIUM INTAKE AND SODIUM BALANCE

Under normal circumstances, renal excretion of sodium is regulated so that balance is maintained between intake and output and ECF volume is stabilized. A subject maintained on a normal sodium diet is in balance when body weight is constant and sodium intake and output are equal. When the diet is abruptly decreased, a transient negative sodium balance ensues. A slight contraction of ECF volume signals activation of sodium-conserving mechanisms, which lead to decreases in urinary sodium excretion. After a few days, sodium balance is achieved and ECF volume and weight are stabilized, albeit at a lower value. If sodium intake is increased to the previous normal values, transient positive sodium balance leads to expansion of ECF volume, thereby suppressing those mechanisms that enhanced sodium reabsorption. A new steady state is reached when ECF volume has risen sufficiently so that sodium excretion now equals intake. In both directions a steady state is achieved whereby sodium intake equals output, while ECF volume is expanded during salt loads and shrunken during salt restriction. The kidney behaves as though ECF volume is the major regulatory element modulating sodium excretion.

The major edematous states—congestive heart failure, cirrhosis of the liver, and nephrotic syndrome—depart strikingly from those constraints. These states are characterized by persistent renal salt retention despite progressive expansion of ECF volume. Unrelenting sodium reabsorption is not the result of diminished sodium intake or even in most cases diminished plasma volume, as dietary salt is adequate and total ECF and plasma volumes are expanded. Renal sodium excretion no longer parallels changes in ECF volume; rather, the kidney behaves as if sensing a persistent low-volume stimulus. Some critical component of ECF volume remains underfilled.

PRIMARY AND SECONDARY EDEMA

A common feature of the major edematous states is persistent renal salt retention despite progressive expansion of both plasma and ECF volume. Two themes have been proposed to explain the persistent salt retention that characterizes the major edematous states: salt retention may be a primary abnormality of the kidney or a secondary response to some disturbance in circulation.

Primary edema (overflow, overfill, nephritic) refers to expansion of ECF volume and subsequent edema formation consequent to a primary defect in renal sodium excretion. Increased ECF volume and expansion of its subcompartments result in manifestations of a well-filled circulation. Hypertension and increased cardiac output are commonly present. The mechanisms normally elicited in response to an underfilled circulation are suppressed (↓ renin-angiotensin-aldosterone, ↓ antidiuretic hormone (ADH), ↓ activity of sympathetic nerves, ↓ circulating catecholamines). Acute poststreptococcal glomerulonephritis and acute or advanced chronic renal failure are examples of primary edema.

Secondary edema (underfill) results from the response of normal kidneys to actual or sensed underfilling of the circulation. In this form of edema, a primary disturbance within the circulation secondarily triggers renal mechanisms for sodium retention. Those systems that normally serve to defend the circulation are activated (↑ renin-angiotensin-aldosterone, ↑ ADH, ↑ activity of sympathetic nerves, ↑ circulating catecholamines). The renal response in underfill edema is similar to that in normal subjects placed on a low-salt diet, that is, low fractional excretion of sodium, increased filtration fraction, and prerenal azotemia. Despite these similarities, a number of critical features distinguish these two states: (1) sodium balance is positive in underfill edema while salt-restricted normal subjects are in balance; and (2) administration of salt to sodium-restricted normals transiently expands ECF volume, after which sodium excretion equals intake, whereas in underfill edema, ECF volume expands progressively consequent to unyielding salt retention; and features of an underfilled circulation persist in underfill edema, while the circulation is normalized in normals.

The circulatory compartment that signals persistent activation of sodium-conserving mechanisms in secondary edema is not readily identifiable. Cardiac output may be high (arteriovenous shunts) or low (congestive heart failure). Similarly, plasma volume may be increased (arteriovenous shunts and heart failure) or decreased (some cases of nephrotic syndrome). The body fluid compartment ultimately responsible for signaling a volume-regulatory reflex leading to renal sodium retention is effective arterial blood volume (EABV). EABV identifies that critical component of arterial blood volume, actual or sensed, that regulates sodium reabsorption by the kidney. In both normal circumstances and the major edematous states, the magnitude of EABV is the major determinant of renal salt and water handling.

CONCEPT OF EFFECTIVE ARTERIAL BLOOD VOLUME

In order to explain adequately persistent sodium retention in underfill edema, two cardinal features must exist. First, there must be a persistent low-volume stimulus sensed by the kidney that is then translated into persistent, indeed often unrelenting, retention of sodium despite adequate salt intake and overexpansion of ECF volume. Second, there must be a disturbance in those forces that partition retained fluid into the various subcompartments of the ECF space, resulting in an inability to terminate the low-volume stimulus. The first

feature can be ascribed to a shrunken EABV, a feature common to all major edematous states. The second feature can be attributed to a disruption in Starling forces, which normally dictate the distribution of fluid within the extracellular compartment. A disturbance in the circulation exists such that retained fluid is unable to restore EABV but rather is sequestered, resulting in edema formation.

Fluctuations in EABV are modulated by two key determinants: (1) filling of the arterial tree (normally determined by venous return and cardiac output), and (2) peripheral resistance (a factor influenced by compliance of the vasculature and degree of arteriolar runoff). A reduction in EABV can be the result of decreased arterial blood volume owing to low cardiac output as in congestive heart failure. Conversely, EABV can be reduced in the face of increased arterial blood volume when there is excessive peripheral runoff as seen in arteriovenous shunting and vasodilation. Increased compliance of the arterial vasculature in which arterial blood volume is reduced relative to the holding capacity of the vascular tree, results in decreased EABV. For example, administration of salt to a subject with a highly compliant or "slack" circulation (as in pregnancy) results in a sluggish natriuretic response, in contrast to a high resistance or "tight" circulation (as in primary aldosteronism or accelerated hypertension) in which salt administration causes prompt natriuresis.

Under normal circumstances, EABV is well correlated with ECF volume. Figure 1 depicts the relationship between subcompartments of ECF volume and renal sodium excretion in both normal and edematous states. Under normal circumstances, subcompartments of ECF volume freely communicate in response to changes in dietary sodium, such that expansion or shrinkage of these compartments occurs in concert (Fig. 1, states 1A and 1B). In steady-state conditions, sodium intake and output are in balance; the set point at which balance is attained is dictated by salt intake.

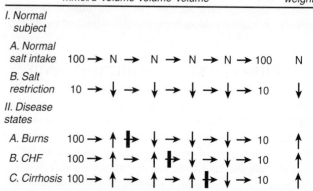

Concept of effective arterial blood volume

	NaCl intake mmol/d	Total ECF volume	Total blood volume	Arterial blood volume	EABV	$U_{Na}V$ mmol/d	Body weight
I. Normal subject							
A. Normal salt intake	100 →	N →	N →	N →	N →	100	N
B. Salt restriction	10 →	↓ →	↓ →	↓ →	↓ →	10	↓
II. Disease states							
A. Burns	100 →	↑ ⊫	↓ →	↓ →	↓ →	10	↑
B. CHF	100 →	↑ →	↑ ⊫	↓ →	↓ →	10	↑
C. Cirrhosis	100 →	↑ →	↑ →	↑ ⊫	↓ →	10	↑

FIGURE 1   Concept of effective arterial blood volume and effect of fluid distributory disturbances on sodium balance and sodium excretion.

By contrast, major edematous states are characterized by a shrunken EABV, which cannot be filled despite expansion of one or more subcompartments. No longer is EABV well correlated with total ECF volume and salt intake. Due to a disturbance in the forces that normally partition fluid into the various subcompartments of ECF space, EABV remains contracted even though total ECF volume is greatly expanded. Activation of sodium-conserving mechanisms persist despite plentiful salt intake. Such derangements in fluid distribution can be categorized as to disturbances in Starling forces within the interstitial space, between interstitial space and vascular tree, and disturbances within the circulation. Types of disturbance are summarized next.

1. *Trapped fluid (Fig. 1, state 2A).* In the first type of disturbance, fluid is trapped within a pathologic compartment such that it cannot contribute to effective extracellular volume, that is, volume capable of filling interstitial and vascular spaces. Decrease in effective extracellular volume leads to decreases in total blood volume, arterial blood volume, and EABV, and renal sodium retention is stimulated. Retention of salt and water cannot reexpand effective extracellular volume as fluid is sequestered into an abnormal fluid compartment behind the "Starling block" within the interstitial space. Such third spacing of fluid into inflamed tissue, vesicles and bullae, peritonitis, necrotizing pancreatitis, rhabdomyolysis, and burns functionally behaves as if lost from the body.

2. *Reduced oncotic pressure.* A reduction in the circulating level of albumin can lead to a second type of fluid maldistribution. Decreased plasma oncotic pressure allows fluid to translocate from the vascular compartment to the interstitial space. Reductions in total blood volume, arterial blood volume, and EABV lead to sodium retention. The retained salt and water, owing to a "Starling block" across the capillary bed, leak into the interstitial space.

3. *Vascular disturbances (Fig. 1, states 2B and 2C).* A third type of fluid distributory disturbance results from abnormalities within the circulation and can be of two types. The prototypical example of the first type is congestive heart failure. A failing ventricle results in decreased cardiac output and high diastolic intraventricular pressures. Venous return is impeded with consequent reductions in arterial blood volume and EABV. Sodium retention is stimulated but arterial blood volume and EABV remain contracted due to a circulatory block across the heart. In consequence, venous volume expands and leads to transudation of fluid into the interstitial space.

The second type of circulatory abnormality that leads to fluid maldistribution is exemplified by arteriovenous shunting (e.g., Paget's disease, beriberi, thyrotoxicosis, anemia, cirrhosis). Widespread shunting through multiple small arteriovenous communications results in increased venous return, thereby augmenting cardiac output and arterial filling. However, arterial runoff and vasodilation lead to underperfusion of some critical area in the microcirculation. The circulatory block lies between the arterial blood volume and EABV.

What distinguishes secondary edematous states from the normal circumstance is an inability to expand EABV owing to Starling or circulatory blocks within the extracellular space. Normally, the system of volume regulation behaves as an open system, such that fluctuations in one compartment are quickly translated into parallel changes in other compartments; total ECF volume and EABV are closely related. In contrast, volume regulation in underfill edema can be regarded as clamped; EABV remains shrunken despite expansion of the subcompartments of the extracellular space. EABV becomes dissociated from total ECF volume; salt retention becomes unrelenting and salt administration cannot reexpand the contracted EABV.

AFFERENT LIMB VOLUME CONTROL

The regulation of extracellular volume by the kidney requires the existence of sensing mechanisms capable of detecting changes in both dietary salt intake and cardiovascular performance (Table 1).

Low-Pressure Baroreceptors

A considerable body of evidence supports the existence of volume receptors located centrally within the thorax, on the venous side of the circulation, capable of sensing contraction and expansion of ECF volume. The great veins and atria are ideally suited for providing a sensitive mechanism to monitor plasma volume by virtue of large capacitance and distensibility. Small changes in central venous pressure lead to large changes in size and wall tension, which are registered by a variety of neural receptors capable of responding to mechanical stretch or transmural pressure. Two such receptors, type A and B, are found in both atria and consist of unencapsulated fibers that run within the vagus nerve (243). Type A receptors may respond to changes in atrial tension but are uninfluenced by atrial volume. In contrast, activity of type B receptors correlates well with atrial size

TABLE 1 Afferent Sensing Mechanisms Involved in Control of Extracellular Fluid Volume

Low-pressure baroreceptors in great veins, atria, lungs
Arterial (high-pressure) baroreceptors in aorta and carotid sinus
Intrarenal sensors
   Cortical mechanoreceptors
   Cortical chemoreceptors
   Myogenic reflex in afferent arteriole
   Tubuloglomerular feedback mechanism
   Juxtaglomerular apparatus
Hepatic volume receptors—osmoreceptors, ionic receptors, baroreceptors
Central nervous system volume sensors—ionic receptors, osmoreceptors

(243). Afferent impulses originating in these low-pressure baroreceptors travel along the vagus nerve and exert a tonic inhibitory effect on central integrative centers in the hypothalamus and medulla, which in turn modulate sympathetic outflow. Diminished atrial distention reduces afferent fiber discharge so that tonic inhibition of the integrative centers is reduced and sympathetic outflow is stimulated (240). Conversely, atrial distention increases afferent impulse trafficking, thereby augmenting inhibition of sympathetic outflow. In addition, changes in atrial distention, probably through similar neural mechanisms, have been shown to alter plasma ADH and renin levels in a direction that parallels sympathetic outflow.

In addition to the atria, there are also receptors with vagal afferents in the lungs, great veins and both ventricles that exert a tonic inhibitory influence over central sympathetic outflow that may play a role in sensing volume. The widespread distribution of these receptors provides for considerable redundancy in the vagal cardiopulmonary reflex such that receptors from one region can likely compensate for the loss of afferent input from another region.

A number of observations suggest that changes in atrial distention can alter urinary sodium excretion through mechanisms that are independent of neural pathways. For example, interruption of the vagus nerve or complete cardiac denervation would be expected to eliminate the renal response to changes in atrial distention. Although such lesions eliminate the diuretic and natriuretic response to atrial balloon inflation or reversible mitral stenosis, they do not eliminate the natriuretic response to volume expansion (147). Similarly, bilateral cervical vagotomy in nonhuman primates, and denervated cardiac allografts in humans fail to alter the normal diuretic and natriuretic response to head-out water immersion (225). Such observations lead to the discovery of natriuretic peptides that are synthesized in the heart and respond to the fullness of the circulation. Atrial natriuretic peptide (ANP) is a peptide synthesized and stored in the cardiac atria. The primary stimulus for its release is atrial distention. Since administration of ANP to human volunteers has been shown to increase the renal excretion of sodium and water, release of this factor is an additional mechanism by which ECF volume is regulated. Maneuvers that lead to distention of the atria and are associated with increased plasma levels of ANP include isotonic volume expansion, head out body water immersion and administration of mineralocorticoids. By contrast, maneuvers that decrease central blood volume such as diuretic administration and lower body negative pressure are associated with a decline in plasma ANP levels.

The cardiac atria are also a source of brain natriuretic peptide (BNP). BNP shares with ANP a high degree of structural homology and biologic activities including vasorelaxation and natriuresis (142). Unlike ANP, however, brain natriuretic peptide is synthesized in and secreted primarily from ventricular myocytes in response to myocardial stretch.

In fact, plasma levels of BNP may be used as a marker of the degree of left ventricular dysfunction (226). The mechanism by which ANP and BNP increase renal salt and water excretion is discussed in the section focused on effector mechanisms.

While sensing mechanisms on the venous side of the circulation clearly play a role in sensing volume in subjects with a normal circulation, they cannot be a major determinant in those edematous states characterized by central venous engorgement in which avid sodium retention persists despite high central venous pressures. In these states, some other component of the circulation is signaling the kidney to retain sodium in a manner that input from the venous side of the circulation is overridden. Analysis of EABV suggests that this sensing system is on the arterial side of the circulation.

Arterial (High-Pressure) Baroreceptors

Baroreceptors in the aorta and carotid sinus participate in the maintenance of ECF volume. In response to changes in arterial pressure, pulse pressure profile, or vascular capacitance, afferent impulses travel along the glossopharyngeal and vagus nerve to an integrative site within the medulla, where central sympathetic outflow is tonically inhibited (195, 264). Reduction in systemic arterial pressure increases sympathetic outflow and results in renal sodium retention. Conversely, increased arterial pressure reduces sympathetic outflow and urinary sodium excretion increases. The renal response to occlusion of an established arteriovenous fistula supports an important role for arterial baroreceptors in modulating renal sodium excretion (91). Closure of a large fistula decreases the runoff of arterial blood into the venous circulation. As a result, diastolic arterial pressure increases. These changes are associated with a prompt increase in renal sodium excretion while renal blood flow and glomerular filtration rate remain constant. By contrast, unloading of the arterial baroreceptors results in activation of several effector mechanisms that lead to renal sodium retention. In humans subjected to lower-body negative pressure sufficient to narrow the pulse pressure, there is activation of the sympathetic nervous system and the renin-angiotensin system as well as increased release of AVP (132). In addition, vascular resistance increases in the forearm, splanchnic, and the renal circulation.

While abundant evidence exists to support an important role for high-pressure baroreceptors in the regulation of ECF volume, some observations suggest that these sensors are not the ultimate determinant of ECF volume. For example, arterial baroreceptor denervation does not diminish the diuretic and natriuretic response to volume expansion. In addition, edematous states can be characterized by persistent renal salt retention even in the setting of increased arterial pressure and increased cardiac output. In these settings, a shrunken EABV must be registered by receptors elsewhere in the arterial circulation.

Intrarenal Sensing Mechanisms

The kidney contains several types of sensing mechanisms capable of detecting alterations in ECF volume. The first type of sensor relates to the rich concentration of sensory neurons in renal cortical structures (223). Using neurophysiologic techniques, two major classes of neural sensory receptors have been identified in the kidney. The first type of receptor is a mechanoreceptor that monitors changes in hydrostatic pressure in the kidney. This receptor is sensitive to changes in arterial perfusion as well as changes in venous and ureteral pressure. The second type of receptor is a chemoreceptor that is responsive to renal ischemia and/or changes in the chemical environment of the renal interstitium. Information registered by both types of receptors is transmitted to the spinal cord and then on to central integrative centers. In this manner, immediate feedback on the function and status of each kidney can be centrally integrated with input from other volume sensors so that body fluid homeostasis can be more precisely regulated.

Renal afferent nerves in one kidney can influence the efferent sympathetic activity in the other kidney in the form of a renalrenal reflex (162). These reflexes have been demonstrated at the ganglionic, spinal and supraspinal level. The nature of the reflex exhibits species difference. In the dog, stimulation of renal mechanoreceptors leads to increased activity of sympathetic nerves in the contralateral kidney resulting in a fall in renal blood flow and urinary sodium excretion (164). By contrast, renal mechanoreceptor or chemoreceptor stimulation in the rat causes a sympathoinhibitory response in the contralateral kidney causing a diuresis and natriuresis (164). In both species, the change in contralateral renal function occurs in the absence of a change in systemic hemodynamics. Further studies in the rat have shown that increasing levels of baseline efferent sympathetic nerve activity exert a facilitory effect on the renalrenal reflex (163). By contrast, inhibition of prostaglandin synthesis, blockade of substance P, and hypoxia all attenuate the reflex (166).

Intrarenal sensing mechanisms enable the kidney to maintain blood flow relatively constant in the setting of varying arterial pressures, a process referred to as autoregulation. Renal autoregulation is accomplished by two mechanisms intrinsic to the kidney: (1) a myogenic reflex intrinsic to the afferent arteriole and (2) tubuloglomerular feedback (TGF). The myogenic reflex describes the ability of the afferent arteriole to either constrict or dilate in response to changes in perfusion pressure. A reduction in pressure elicits a vasodilatory response, while an increase in pressure results in vasoconstriction. The myogenic response is located diffusely within the preglomerular circulation and provides a mechanism to buffer the glomerular capillaries from sudden changes in arterial pressure.

TGF is a second component of renal autoregulation that serves to reinforce the myogenic reflex by responding to changes in distal NaCl concentration (303). The anatomic basis for TGF lies in the juxtaposition of the macula densa cells in the distal nephron to smooth muscle cells in the afferent arteriole. The macula densa cells respond to changes in luminal NaCl concentration by way of a Na,K-2Cl cotransporter located on the apical membrane. A decrease in perfusion pressure causes an initial decline in intraglomerular pressure and glomerular filtration rate resulting in decreased distal delivery of NaCl. The decrease in NaCl concentration is sensed by the macula densa causing a vasodilatory signal to be sent to the afferent arteriole. As a result, intraglomerular pressure and glomerular filtration rate are returned toward normal and distal NaCl delivery increases. The net effect is to stabilize the sodium chloride concentration entering the distal nephron.

A second component of tubuloglomerular feedback is called into play when changes in distal sodium chloride delivery are more pronounced or sustained as occurs when extracellular fluid volume is altered. This component either activates or suppresses renin release from the juxtaglomerular cells. A persistent decrease in delivery of sodium chloride to the macula densa as when ECF volume is contracted stimulates renin release. The subsequent formation of angiotensin II and aldosterone cause renal sodium retention leading to correction of the volume contracted state. A persistent increase in distal sodium chloride delivery reflecting expansion of extracellular fluid volume has the opposite effect. Renin release is also influenced by changes in perfusion pressure at the level of the juxtaglomerular apparatus. Under conditions of decreased renal perfusion, renin release is stimulated independently of any change in glomerular filtration rate or distal sodium delivery. Sympathetic nerve activity is a third mechanism involved in the regulation of renin release. Renal nerve stimulation via activation of beta-adrenergic nerves directly stimulates renin release and this effect can be disassociated from major changes in renal hemodynamics.

Thus, the myogenic reflex and the tubuloglomerular feedback system are components of a sensing mechanism within the kidney that enable changes in volume to be registered. As discussed in more detail below, these systems can alter glomerular hemodynamics in a manner that contributes to the maintenance of a normal ECF volume.

Hepatic and Intestinal Volume Receptors

Several lines of evidence suggest that intrahepatic mechanisms may contribute to the afferent limb of volume control. Located in the portal system, the liver is ideally positioned to monitor dietary sodium intake (168, 222, 233). In this regard, oral sodium loads or infusion of either isotonic or hypertonic saline into the portal vein results in an increase in urinary sodium excretion. The natriuretic response to the intraportal infusion is quantitatively greater than the natriuretic response observed with peripheral infusions. This natriuretic response may be initiated by either osmoreceptors or sodium chloride–sensitive receptors known to be present within the liver. Activation of these receptors leads to decreased renal sympathetic nerve activity, which in turn accounts for the natriuretic response. The afferent limb of this hepatorenal reflex terminates centrally within the nucleus of the solitary tract (222). This reflex can be blocked by hepatic denervation or prior vagotomy. Stimulation of one or both of these receptors may also account for the increased release of plasma AVP from the hypothalamus known to occur with increased concentrations of sodium in the portal circulation. In turn, AVP may play a role in mediating the decrease in renal sympathetic nerve activity at the level of the area postrema (233). A hepatic baroreceptor mechanism has also been identified that can reflexively alter renal sympathetic nerve activity (168). In contrast to stimulation of osmoreceptors and ionic receptors, activation of hepatic baroreceptors leads to increased renal sympathetic nerve activity.

Hepatic and or portal sensing mechanisms can also influence intestinal salt reabsorption through what has been described as a hepatointestinal reflex. The afferent limb of this reflex travels through the vagus nerve and into the nucleus tractus solitarius. Infusion of 9% saline into the portal circulation has been shown to depress jejunal Na absorption through this pathway (222).

A more recently described mechanism by which orally administered Na loads can lead to adjustments in urine Na excretion is through the intestinal release of peptides that regulate cyclic guanosine monophosphate (51, 106). Guanylin and uroguanylin are peptides found throughout the intestine and are released from epithelial cells into both the lumen and the systemic circulation. These peptides exert a natriuretic effect when administered intravenously raising the possibility that they play a physiologic role in adjusting urinary sodium excretion in response to changes in dietary salt intake. The role of hepatic and intestinal sensing mechanisms in the day-to-day regulation of sodium chloride balance remains to be defined.

Central Nervous System Afferent Sensing Mechanisms

While the existence of intracerebral receptors sensitive to changes in osmolality is indisputable, a similar afferent mechanism responsive to changes in sodium balance may also be present. Several lines of evidence suggest the presence of cerebral sodium sensors. For example, infusion of hypertonic saline into the carotid artery results in a quantitatively greater natriuretic effect than that observed with a systemic infusion (313). A natriuretic response is also observed with injection of hypertonic saline into the cerebral ventricles. This later response appears specific to increasing concentrations of sodium chloride rather than increased osmolality since intraventricular infusions of mannitol exert no effect on urinary sodium excretion (65, 206). Other manifestations of central administration of hypertonic saline include a dipsogenic effect, pressor response, increased re-

lease of AVP, and reduction in renin release and renal sympathetic nerve activity. These effects are similar to the pattern of responses elicited by central administration of angiotensin II suggesting that similar neural pathways are involved. In support of this possibility, administration of an angiotensin receptor blocker has been shown to block the pressor response and the natriuresis following the intraventricular infusion of hypertonic saline (206). In addition, receptor blockade significantly reduces the fall in renal sympathetic nerve activity. The role that this sodium sensing system plays in the steady-state control of sodium balance remains to be determined.

RENAL MECHANISMS FOR SODIUM RETENTION

In secondary edema or any state where EABV is consistently contracted, the persistent stimulation of the afferent volume-sensing system described previously leads to the activation of efferent pathways, which signal the kidney to conserve salt. The shrunken EABV promotes the release of catecholamines, activates the renin-angiotensin-aldosterone and sympathetic nervous systems, and stimulates the secretion of ADH. These defenses usually fail to normalize the circulation and renal underperfusion persists. This state of renal underperfusion is characterized by humoral secretions and neurocirculatory reflexes that alter the glomerular and postglomerular circulation and activate various transport systems throughout the nephron (Table 2). The mechanisms of renal sodium handling will now be discussed followed by a discussion of the effector systems that regulate renal salt handling.

Glomerular Filtration Rate

The renal excretion of sodium is ultimately a function of filtered load (calculated as glomerular filtration rate [GFR] times plasma Na concentration) minus the quantity reabsorbed into the peritubular circulation and returned to the systemic circu-

TABLE 2   Effector Mechanisms Regulating Extracellular Fluid Volume

Renal mechanisms for Na retention
Sympathetic nervous system
Renin-angiotensin-aldosterone system
Prostaglandins
Kallikrein-kinin system
Antidiuretic hormone
Endothelin
Nitric oxide
Natriuretic compounds
   Atrial natriuretic peptide
   Brain natriuretic peptide
   C-type natriuretic peptide
   Urodilatin
   Guanylin and uroguanylin

lation. Isolated fluctuations in GFR and hence filtered load of sodium are accompanied by only minor changes in urinary sodium excretion, arguing against a primary role of filtration rate as a regulator of sodium excretion. For example, when GFR is increased by maneuvers other than volume expansion (glucocorticoids, high protein feeding) little change in fractional sodium excretion occurs. Conversely, when the filtered load of sodium is held constant or even reduced, a persistent natriuresis accompanies volume expansion. Near constancy in fractional excretion of sodium in the setting of increases or decreases in GFR is known as glomerular-tubular balance. Changes in GFR are buffered by parallel adaptations in sodium reabsorption by the proximal tubule such that large changes in filtered load of sodium result in only small changes in distal sodium delivery. Given the constraints of glomerulo-tubular balance, it follows that physiologic control of Na excretion involves effector mechanisms operative at the level of the renal tubule.

Proximal Tubule

The proximal tubule reabsorbs approximately 50% of the filtered NaCl, 70%–90% of filtered NaHCO$_3$, and close to 100% of filtered organic solutes. Absorption of these solutes involves both transcellular and paracellular processes. Because the proximal tubule is a very leaky epithelium, paracellular transport occurring by both diffusion and/or convective mechanisms can be significant.

TRANSCELLULAR SOLUTE TRANSPORT

To effect NaHCO$_3$ absorption, H ions are secreted from cell to luminal fluid by an apical-membrane amiloride-sensitive Na/H antiporter and a H ion translocating ATPase. Approximately two-thirds of HCO$_3$ absorption is mediated by the antiporter, while the remainder is accounted for by the H ion pump (266). The energy for H extrusion by the antiporter is derived from the low intracellular Na concentration resulting from the activity of a basolateral Na,K-ATPase. The majority of the base generated in the cell by H efflux exits across the basolateral membrane on the Na/3HCO$_3$ (or equivalently Na/HCO$_3$/CO$_3$) cotransporter (7). The net result of these processes is high rates of acid transport from the peritubular interstitium and blood into the lumen of the proximal tubule. This leads to high rates of NaHCO$_3$ absorption that causes luminal fluid HCO$_3$ concentration to decrease by 60%–80% in the midproximal tubule.

Transcellular NaCl absorption is also mediated by the Na/H antiporter, functioning in parallel with Cl/base exchangers (262). Secretion of H and a negatively charged base at equal rates leads to generation of the neutral acid, HB, which is lipophilic and is thought to recycle across the apical membrane. The nature of the base exchanged with Cl is not totally settled but appears to include OH$^-$, formate$^-$, and oxalate$^-$ (259). With this mode of transport there is no net H secretion and thus no luminal acidification or bicarbonate absorption. Na and Cl enter the cell across the apical membrane at equal rates. The Na exits the cell on the basolateral Na,K-ATPase, while the Cl can exit the cell by one of several possible mechanisms.

Well defined transport systems exist on the apical membrane of the proximal tubule that allow for sodium-coupled transport of a variety of solutes including glucose, amino acids, and inorganic and organic ions. Once again, the driving force for these transporters is a low intracellular Na concentration resulting from the activity of a basolateral Na,K-ATPase. Most of these solutes then exit the basolateral membrane by facilitated diffusion.

PARACELLULAR SOLUTE TRANSPORT

Solutes can also cross the proximal tubule across the paracellular pathway. In general, the major barrier to paracellular solute movement is the tight junction, which in the proximal tubule is highly permeable such that passive fluxes can be significant.

In the early part of the proximal tubule, Na is preferentially reabsorbed with bicarbonate and other nonchloride solutes by transcellular processes. As a result, the concentrations of HCO$_3$ and these other solutes progressively fall along the length of the proximal tubule. Analysis of the fluid in the mid- to late proximal tubule shows a HCO$_3$ concentration of 5–10 mEq/L and virtually no organic solutes. At the same time the chloride concentration progressively increases along the length of the tubule. At the end of the proximal tubule the Cl concentration is 20–40 mEq/L higher than plasma Cl concentrations. The net result of these changes is that driving forces are present for passive paracellular diffusion.

While the driving forces for organic solutes favors back diffusion from the blood and peritubular interstitium into the lumen, the permeability of the late proximal tubule to these solutes is low. As a result, the rates of back diffusion are relatively small. Similarly, the driving force for NaHCO$_3$ favors back diffusion into the proximal tubule lumen. Because of a higher permeability, this back diffusion can be significant, with two-thirds of active HCO$_3$ absorption negated by passive HCO$_3$ back leak in the late proximal tubule (8). Lastly, the high luminal Cl concentration provides a driving force for passive diffusive Cl absorption. Because of the high permeability of the proximal tubule to Cl, fluxes can be large (262). This large paracellular Cl flux generates a lumen-positive voltage in the late proximal tubule that can then provide a driving force for passive Na absorption. Most studies have estimated that one- to two-thirds of NaCl absorption in the late proximal tubule occurs by passive mechanisms (6, 297).

ROLE OF PERITUBULAR STARLING FORCES IN REGULATION OF PROXIMAL TUBULAR SOLUTE TRANSPORT

At any given plasma protein concentration, the magnitude of the protein oncotic force acting along the peritubular capillary will be a function of filtration fraction, that is, fraction of plasma water extracted by the process of glomerular filtration. In turn, filtration fraction is importantly influenced by efferent arteriolar tone. This resistance vessel interposed between the glomerular and peritubular capillary networks importantly influences both glomerular and downstream peritubular hydrostatic pressure.

When a normal individual ingests a high-salt diet, expansion of plasma volume and EABV occurs. As a result, plasma protein concentration is reduced because of hemodilution. In response to expanded EABV, renal plasma flow increases while glomerular filtration rate remains constant or rises only slightly, resulting in decreased filtration fraction. The decline in filtration fraction results in a lower percentage of protein-free ultrafiltrate formation at the glomerulus so that the normal rise in postglomerular protein concentration is less. Peritubular oncotic pressure falls consequent to both systemic dilution and reduced fraction of blood flow undergoing ultrafiltration at the glomerulus. In addition, the lower efferent resistance leads to increased peritubular hydrostatic pressure. Reductions in peritubular colloid osmotic pressure and increases in peritubular hydrostatic pressure lead to decreased uptake of reabsorbate into the peritubular capillary bed. The accumulation of reabsorbate leads to an increase in interstitial pressure, which in turn has been demonstrated to decrease solute and volume absorption across the proximal tubule.

By contrast, salt restriction results in contraction of plasma volume and EABV. Despite the reduction in renal plasma flow, GFR is maintained near normal owing to efferent arteriolar constriction. Filtration fraction increases as a normal amount of protein-free ultrafiltrate is now removed from a decreased volume of blood. The increased fraction of blood flow undergoing ultrafiltration and systemic concentration of albumin lead to a higher concentration of protein in blood leaving the glomerulus and entering the peritubular capillaries. In addition, an increase in efferent arteriolar tone lowers peritubular capillary hydrostatic pressure. Increased peritubular oncotic pressure and decreased peritubular hydrostatic pressure enhance the movement of reabsorbate into peritubular capillaries. Interstitial pressure declines, resulting in less back leak of reabsorbate into the tubular lumen.

Loop of Henle

Mechanisms responsible for regulating renal salt excretion also exist within the loop of Henle. The anatomy of this nephron segment differs according to the originating glomerulus. Superficial glomeruli give rise to loops that are composed of a thin descending limb that extends to the junction of inner and outer medulla and culminates with a thick ascending portion. Glomeruli residing in deeper portions of the renal cortex give rise to a thin descending limb that extends deeper into the inner medulla. From here and in distinction to superficial loops, deep loops possess a thin ascending limb that extends from the bend of Henle's loop to the junction of inner and outer medulla, where the thick

ascending limb arises. The thin descending limb is impermeable to NaCl but has high water permeability. In contrast, the thin ascending limb is impermeable to water but highly permeable to NaCl. The thick ascending limb is also impermeable to water and is characterized by active NaCl reabsorption.

Differential permeabilities for salt and water of each segment within the long loops of Henle provide a mechanism for regulating salt excretion. As water is reabsorbed from the thin descending limb in response to high medullary urea and salt concentrations, the NaCl concentration of fluid entering the thin ascending limb exceeds that within the interstitium. As a consequence, a driving force exists for passive NaCl reabsorption. Conditions that increase medullary blood flow (volume expansion, water diuresis, prostaglandins, ANP) will lead to "washout" of the medullary osmotic gradient and secondarily decrease the driving force for passive NaCl reabsorption. Lower interstitial urea and NaCl concentrations lead to less water extraction from the thin descending limb, resulting in a lower concentration of NaCl entering the thin ascending limb. As a result, NaCl reabsorption is diminished in the thin and thick ascending limbs. The superficial nephron has only a short transit time through the medulla and does not possess a thin ascending limb; thus changes in medullary tonicity have a lesser impact on passive salt efflux in this segment.

The thick ascending limb plays an important role in the regulation of ECF volume by providing mechanisms for the reabsorption of NaCl and NaHCO$_3$. NaCl is transported across the apical membrane by the Na/K/2Cl cotransporter, while a Na/H antiporter initiates the reabsorption of NaHCO$_3$. Salt reabsorption in this segment is regulated by several factors. Prostaglandins have been shown to exert an inhibitory effect on salt absorption in this segment that may be important in the natriuretic response to volume expansion (131). In this setting, enhanced prostaglandin production leads to increased medullary blood flow and a decrease in the medullary interstitial osmolality. As a result, the driving force for passive NaCl absorption is diminished. In addition, micropuncture as well as microperfusion studies have shown that prostaglandins have a direct inhibitory effect on chloride transport in the medullary thick ascending limb (131). In the setting of volume contraction, salt absorption is increased in this segment. This effect is mediated by factors known to be activated in the setting of volume depletion to include renal nerves and AVP.

Cortical Collecting Tubule

The cortical collecting tubule is a low-capacity nephron segment capable of reabsorbing NaCl against steep gradients. As discussed below the principal regulator of Na reabsorption in this segment is aldosterone. Changes in ECF volume through the renin-angiotensin system lead to reciprocal changes in circulating aldosterone levels. Aldosterone stimulates sodium reabsorption by increasing the permeability of the luminal membrane. Both enhanced sodium entry and aldosterone lead to increased Na,K-ATPase activity on the basolateral membrane. Reabsorption of sodium increases the degree of luminal electronegativity that secondarily stimulates chloride reabsorption through the paracellular pathway. AVP has also been shown to increase Na transport in this segment. By contrast, PGE2 and bradykinin inhibit sodium reabsorption in this segment. ANP and brain natriuretic peptide inhibit Na transport in the inner medullary collecting duct.

EFFECTOR MECHANISM REGULATING RENAL SODIUM HANDLING

Sympathetic Nervous System

Postganglionic sympathetic axons originating in the prevertebral celiac and paravertebral ganglia of T6-L4 have been found to innervate cells of afferent and efferent arterioles, the juxtaglomerular apparatus, and the renal tubules. A number of observations suggest that this extensive renal innervation provides the anatomic basis for sympathetic nerves to play an important role in ECF volume regulation (Fig. 2).

Bilateral renal denervation in both anesthetized and conscious animals leads to rapid increases in urinary sodium excretion (31, 277). Conversely, electrical stimulation of renal nerves promptly decreases urinary sodium excretion without alterations in GFR or renal plasma flow (40). Renal nerves also contribute to a reflex arc whereby alterations in sodium handling by one kidney can be adjusted for by the opposite kidney (77).

Sympathetic nerves alter renal salt and water handling by direct and indirect mechanisms. Increased nerve activity indirectly influences proximal sodium reabsorption by altering preglomerular and postglomerular arteriolar tone, thereby effecting changes in filtration fraction. The subse-

quent alterations in peritubular hydrostatic and oncotic forces lead to changes in proximal sodium reabsorption. Renal nerves directly stimulate proximal tubular fluid reabsorption through receptors located on the basolateral membrane of proximal tubular cells (22). In the rabbit proximal tubule, stimulation is mediated by β-adrenergic receptors (22), while in the rat proximal tubule both α- and β-adrenergic receptors play a role (331). Stimulation of α1 and α2 receptors has been shown to increase the activity of the Na/H antiporter (112, 113) and the Na,K-ATPase providing a mechanism by which proximal tubule transport is stimulated. Renal nerve activity also stimulates sodium chloride reabsorption in the loop of Henle and early distal tubule. These indirect and direct effects on renal Na handling are further amplified by the ability of sympathetic nerves to stimulate renin release leading to the formation of angiotensin II and aldosterone.

Renin-Angiotensin-Aldosterone System

The renin-angiotensin-aldosterone system is an important effector mechanism in the control of ECF balance. Physiologic control of this system involves a complex interaction between neural, humoral, and baroreceptor stimuli.

Decreases in renal perfusion provide a direct stimulatory effect for renin release from the juxtaglomerular cells in the afferent arteriole. This baroreceptor-mediated mechanism has been demonstrated in the nonfiltering kidney under conditions of hemorrhagic hypotension or aortic constriction (37). The relationship between changes in perfusion pressure and renin release is defined by a nonlinear curve. Renin release remains relatively constant until pressure falls to a threshold value of 80–90 mm Hg, below which renin release increases in an exponential fashion (153).

Increased sympathetic nerve activity directly stimulates the release of renin from juxtaglomerular cells via activation of renal β1 adrenoreceptors. Sympathetic nerves also have an effect of a modulating baroreceptor-mediated mechanism of renin release by shifting the threshold for renin release to a higher perfusion pressure.

Locally produced prostaglandins stimulate the release of renin. In fact, baroreceptor-stimulated renin release is mediated in part by prostaglandins especially within the autoregulatory range (27). β-adrenergic stimulation of renin release, however, is not mediated by prostaglandins.

Renin release is also influenced by distal tubular sodium chloride concentration by way of the tubuloglomerular feedback mechanism. Sustained increases in delivery of sodium chloride to the macula densa whether from increased single-nephron GFR or decreased absorption of filtrate at more proximal nephron segments suppresses renin release from the juxtaglomerular apparatus. Sustained decreases in distal sodium chloride delivery have the opposite effect. The formation of renin leads to increased circulating angiotensin II (Ang II), which in turn directly affects multiple organ systems involved in blood pressure and volume homeostasis. Ang II

Sympathetic Nervous System in ECF Volume Regulation

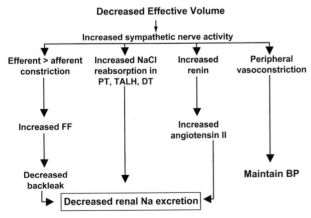

FIGURE 2 Pathways by which sympathetic nerves regulate renal sodium excretion.

serves an important role in stabilizing the circulation by its direct vasoconstrictor activity and by potentiating the vasoconstrictive effects of sympathetic nerves on peripheral neuroeffector junctions. In addition, Ang II is capable of altering renal sodium handling at several sites along the nephron and does so by both indirect and direct mechanisms (Fig. 3).

Ang II preferentially increases the tone of the efferent arteriole so that under conditions of a decreased EABV renal blood flow falls to a greater extent than GFR and filtration fraction increases. As discussed previously, these changes lead to alterations in peritubular Starling forces that favor proximal sodium reabsorption.

Ang II also affects renal Na handling by modulating sympathetic nerve activity. Ang II is capable of increasing sympathetic neurotransmission by facilitating the release of norepinephrine through interactions at the presynaptic junction as well as having stimulatory effects within the central nervous system (69). Ang II also affects sodium balance by enhancing the efficiency of the tubuloglomerular feedback mechanism (214). Increased Ang II levels heighten the responsiveness of the tubuloglomerular mechanism to any given signal delivered by the macula densa.

In addition to these indirect mechanisms, Ang II has direct effects on renal sodium handling. Addition of Ang II to the peritubular capillary has been shown to enhance the rate of volume absorption in the proximal tubule, measured by the split droplet technique (128). In these studies, low concentrations of Ang II stimulate volume absorption, while high concentrations have an inhibitory effect. Similar results have been found in the in vitro perfused proximal convoluted tubule (295). Ang II stimulates HCO_3 absorption in the very early S1 proximal tubule with a lesser effect in the later proximal tubule. This corresponds with the distribution of Ang II receptors in the proximal tubule (82). Ang II has been shown to stimulate the proximal tubule apical membrane Na/H antiporter, and the basolateral membrane $Na/3HCO_3$ symporter in parallel (221). Activation of these transport mechanisms explains the observed increase in $NaHCO_3$ absorption induced by Ang II. Renal sodium handling can be altered by Ang II produced

systemically or by Ang II synthesized locally within the kidney. The proximal tubule possesses all the machinery required for local production of Ang II (215). Indeed, measurement of luminal Ang II concentration have been in the range of 10^{-8} M, which can be compared to systemic concentrations of 10^{-11} to 10^{-10} M (42). These high renal concentrations may allow Ang II to function as an autocrine/paracrine factor. In fact, regulation of renal function by Ang II may be more dependent on regulation of local production than on regulation of systemic production (251, 268).

In addition to effects on the proximal nephron, Ang II enhances distal sodium absorption primarily by stimulating aldosterone release from the adrenal zona glomerulosa. Aldosterone, in turn, increases sodium reabsorption in the cortical collecting tubule. Aldosterone importantly regulates potassium secretion in this nephron segment as well. Enhanced activity of Na,K-ATPase and generation of luminal electronegativity via sodium reabsorption provide a favorable electrochemical gradient for potassium secretion into the tubular lumen. Under conditions in which sodium is reabsorbed more proximally (decreased EABV), however, high levels of aldosterone do not result in potassium loss. Similarly, when distal sodium delivery is plentiful and aldosterone is suppressed (ECF volume expansion) potassium loss is not accelerated. The dependence of K secretion on distal delivery of sodium and aldosterone levels helps to make K excretion independent of changes in extracellular fluid volume.

Prostaglandins

Prostaglandins are compounds derived from metabolism of arachidonic acid that influence both renal blood flow and sodium handling within the kidney. PGI2, synthesized by vascular endothelial cells predominantly within the renal cortex, mediates baroreceptor but not β-adrenergic stimulation of renin release (27). PGE2, produced by interstitial and collecting duct epithelial cells predominantly within the renal medulla, is stimulated by Ang II and has vasodilatory properties. PGF2a is a prostaglandin with vasoconstrictor activity produced from PGE2 by the enzyme PGE2-9-ketoreductase. The activity of this enzyme varies according to salt intake, thus allowing relatively more vasodilation or vasoconstriction depending on the given level of salt balance in the animal.

Under baseline euvolemic conditions prostaglandin synthesis is negligible and as a result these compounds play little to no role in the minute-to-minute maintenance of renal function. Where these compounds come to serve a major role is in the setting of a systemic or intrarenal circulatory disturbance. This interaction is best illustrated when examining renal function under conditions of actual or perceived volume depletion. In this setting, renal blood flow is decreased, and sodium reabsorption, renin release, and urinary concentrating ability are increased. To a large extent, these findings are mediated by the effects of increased circu-

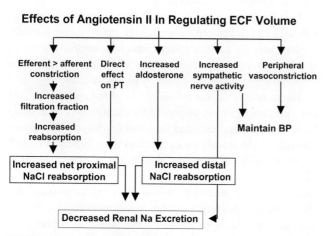

Effects of Angiotensin II In Regulating ECF Volume

FIGURE 3 Pathways by which angiotensin II regulates renal sodium excretion.

lating levels of Ang II, arginine vasopressin (AVP), and catecholamines. At the same time, these hormones stimulate the synthesis of renal prostaglandins, which in turn act to dilate the renal vasculature, inhibit salt and water reabsorption, and further stimulate renin release. Prostaglandin release under these conditions serves to dampen and counterbalance the physiologic effects of the hormones that elicit their production. As a result, renal function is maintained near normal despite the systemic circulation being clamped down. Predictably, inhibition of prostaglandin synthesis will lead to unopposed activity of these hormonal systems resulting in exaggerated renal vasoconstriction and magnified antinatriuretic and antidiuretic effects. In fact, many of the renal syndromes that are associated with the use of NSAIDs can be explained by the predictions of this model.

Prostaglandins predominately exert a natriuretic effect in the kidney. These compounds increase urinary sodium excretion by both indirect and direct mechanisms (Fig. 4). Through their activity as renal vasodilators, prostaglandins may cause an increase in the filtered load of sodium. In addition, these compounds preferentially shunt blood flow to the inner cortical and medullary regions of the kidney. As a result of increased medullary blood flow, there is a fall in the medullary interstitial solute concentration. Processes that reduce the degree of medullary hypertonicity lead to a concomitant reduction in the osmotic withdrawal of water from the normally sodium impermeable thin descending limb of Henle. This, in turn, decreases the sodium concentration of fluid at the hairpin turn. The net effect is less passive reabsorption of sodium across the normally water impermeable thin ascending limb of Henle. Consistent with this mechanism, infusion of PGE1 lowers, and prostaglandin synthesis inhibition raises, sodium chloride and total solute concentration in the medulla (131).

Prostaglandins can also affect sodium reabsorption in the proximal tubule by virtue of their ability to influence the tone of the efferent arteriole. As discussed previously, changes in the tone of this vessel play a central role in determining the Starling forces that govern fluid reabsorption in this nephron segment. By lessening the degree to which the efferent arteriole is constricted, prostaglandins can alter peritubular Starling forces in a manner that leads to a decrease in proximal tubular sodium reabsorption. In a model of high circulating levels of Ang II induced by suprarenal aortic constriction, inhibition of prostaglandin synthesis was found to increase efferent arteriole oncotic pressure and decrease peritubular hydrostatic pressure resulting in a significant increase in proximal fluid reabsorption (244).

In addition to these hemodynamically mediated changes in renal sodium handling, prostaglandins have direct effects on tubular sodium transport. In the isolated perfused tubule, PGE2 has been shown to inhibit sodium transport in the cortical and outer medullary collecting duct (309). Using the same technique, PGE2 has also been shown to decrease NaCl transport in the thick ascending limb of Henle. In vivo studies also support a direct inhibitory effect of prostaglandins on sodium transport in the loop of Henle, distal nephron, and collecting duct (131). The mechanism of this direct inhibitory effect is unclear, but may involve decreased activity of the Na,K-ATPase.

It would at first seem paradoxical that under conditions of volume depletion the kidney would elaborate a compound that has further natriuretic properties. The role of prostaglandins in this setting, however, is to moderate the avid salt retention that would otherwise occur in the setting of unopposed activation of the renin-angiotensin-aldosterone and adrenergic systems. By virtue of their natriuretic properties, prostaglandins play a role in ensuring adequate delivery of filtrate to more distal nephron segments under conditions in which distal delivery is threatened (e.g., renal ischemia, hypovolemia). In addition, diminished NaCl reabsorption in the thick ascending limb of Henle reduces the energy requirements of this segment. This reduction in thick limb workload in conjunction with a prostaglandin-mediated reallocation in renal blood flow help to maintain an adequate oxygen tension in the medulla under conditions that could otherwise have resulted in substantial hypoxic injury.

Kallikrein-Kinin System

Kinins are potent vasodilator peptides found within the kidney but whose physiologic role has yet to be fully defined. Renal kallikrein is a serine protease of high molecular weight produced in the distal tubule. This protease uses the peptide kininogen as a substrate to produce two kinins: bradykinin and lysylbradykinin (also known as kallikrein). These kinins are degraded in the kidney by the same enzyme responsible for conversion of Ang I to Ang II, namely, kininase II (also called angiotensin converting enzyme) (50). Renal kallikrein activity is increased by

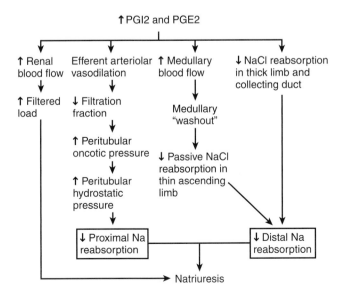

FIGURE 4 Pathways by which renal prostaglandins lead to increased renal sodium excretion.

mineralocorticoids, Ang II, and PGE2 (50). In turn, kinins stimulate renin release and PGE2 production.

Intrarenal infusion of bradykinin increases renal blood flow and sodium excretion without a change in GFR (193). In addition, urinary excretion of bradykinin varies inversely with salt intake (17). Localization of kallikrein in the distal tubule as well as the presence of high-affinity binding sites for bradykinin in the thick ascending limb and cortical and outer medullary collecting ducts support the distal nephron as the site in which kinins affect sodium transport (64). Bradykinin has been found to inhibit net sodium absorption in the in vitro microperfused thick ascending limb and cortical collecting duct (122). In addition, kinins may increase urinary Na excretion by increasing medullary blood flow resulting in a washout of the medullary interstitium (284). Bradykinin can increase renal blood flow either directly or by stimulating the release of vasodilatory prostaglandins (284).

Antidiuretic Hormone

In addition to the well-defined system for osmotic control of vasopressin release, ADH is regulated by an anatomically separate pathway sensitive to changes in EABV. Afferent impulses originating from both low- and high-pressure baroreceptors travel via the vagus nerve to a central integrating center, which modulates ADH release in response to nonosmotic stimuli. Maneuvers that increase pressure in the cardiac atria have a suppressive effect on the release of ADH, while decreased pressure has the opposite effect. A similar relationship exists between ADH release and changes in pressure in the high-pressure baroreceptors located in the carotid artery (292). Baroreceptor-stimulated ADH release leads to increased water absorption by the kidney and in high concentrations may exert a systemic vasoconstrictive effect. ADH can also affect renal sodium handling. Pressor doses of arginine vasopressin have been shown to increase filtration fraction, an effect that secondarily would lead to enhanced proximal NaCl reabsorption. In addition, AVP has a direct tubular effect on solute transport in the thick ascending limb of Henle and the collecting duct. The release of ADH in response to a diminished EABV, along with activation of the renin-angiotensin-aldosterone system and sympathetic nervous system, provides a marker of an underfilled circulation even when edema is widespread.

Endothelin

The endothelins are autocrine/paracrine factors that regulate blood pressure and renal function and may play a role in the regulation of ECF volume. This family of peptides consists of three members called endothelin-1, endothelin-2, and endothelin-3 (ET1, ET2, ET3) (140). These peptides can interact with one of two receptors, termed ETa and ETb. The ETa receptor binds ET1 and ET2 but not ET3, while the ETb receptor can bind all three endothelins with high affinity. Radiolabeled binding and mRNA expression studies suggest that the ETa receptor is primarily expressed in vascular structures, while the ETb receptor is the predominant receptor expressed in the renal tubules both in the proximal and distal nephron. Both ET1 and ET3 are produced locally by kidney tubules and are in an ideal location to bind to ETb receptors located along the nephron.

The effects of endothelin on proximal tubule function have been examined by adding ET1 to the basolateral side of the in vitro perfused proximal straight tubule (107). Low concentrations of ET1–stimulated rates of volume and presumably sodium transport, while high concentrations inhibited transport. The mechanism of this stimulatory effect appears to be mediated by activation of the apical Na/H antiporter through stimulation of the ETb receptor (125).

Nitric Oxide

Nitric oxide is an endothelial derived factor that can function as an effector in the regulation of ECF volume. In particular, nitric oxide has been shown to participate in the natriuretic response to increases in blood pressure or intravenous expansion of ECF volume. An acute increase in arterial pressure normally leads to a natriuretic response, a relationship referred to as pressure natriuresis. Although the exact mechanism of pressure natriuresis is not fully understood, evidence suggests that an increase in renal interstitial hydrostatic pressure and alterations in medullary blood flow may participate in this response. Under conditions of nitric oxide inhibition, an increase in perfusion pressure fails to increase renal interstitial hydrostatic pressure and the natriuretic response is blunted (227). Similarly, inhibition of nitric oxide has been shown to blunt the natriuretic response to intravenous volume expansion (258). These observations suggest that nitric oxide may play a role in augmenting urinary sodium excretion under conditions of volume expansion.

Atrial Natriuretic Peptide and Other Natriuretic Peptides

The synthesis and release of ANP provide a mechanism whereby cardiac atria serve both an afferent and an efferent function in control of ECF volume. This peptide is synthesized by atrial myocytes and is stored as an inactive high-molecular-weight form in granules. Presumably through atrial distention, maneuvers that increase atrial pressure cause release of the active low-molecular-weight form of ANP (78). Acute volume expansion, water immersion, postural changes, and salt feeding all result in increased plasma ANP concentration. Systemic infusion of ANP increases GFR and filtration fraction despite a fall in mean arterial pressure. The increase in GFR may be mediated by increased glomerular capillary hydrostatic pressure resulting from afferent arteriolar dilation and concurrent efferent arteriolar constriction (236). Continuous infusion or bolus injection of ANP produces dramatic increases in renal salt and water excretion. While increased GFR may contribute to increased urinary sodium excretion at high levels of ANP, physiologic concentrations elicit a natriuretic response without a change in GFR, suggesting additional mechanisms whereby sodium excretion is augmented. In this regard, ANP has been found to inhibit sodium reabsorption in the cortical collecting tubule and inner medullary collecting duct (306). In addition, ANP decreases the medullary solute gradient such that passive sodium chloride reabsorption in the thin ascending limb is decreased (63). Finally, ANP reduces renin secretion, blocks aldosterone secretion, and opposes the vasoconstrictive effect of Ang II (Fig. 5).

With the recent discovery of other natriuretic peptides, ANP now appears to be only one member of a family of homologous polypeptide hormones that stimulate diuresis, natriuresis, and vasorelaxation. ANP and brain natriuretic peptide (BNP) are circulating hormones that are primarily synthesized in the cardiac atria and ventricles respectively. C-type natriuretic peptide (CNP) is mainly produced by the vascular endothelium and is thought to act as a local paracrine factor in the control of vascular tone. Studies examining the renal effects of CNP have produced conflicting results but it appears that this peptide is only weakly natriuretic (18, 142, 260). All of the natriuretic peptides mediate their biologic effects through a family of particulate guanylyl cyclase receptors (NPR-A and NPR-B). The affinity of ANP and BNP is greatest for NPR-A, while that of CNP is much higher for NPR-B. All three natriuretic peptides bind to a third receptor (NPR-C), which does not contain guanylyl cyclase and functions predominately as a clearance receptor. Urodilatin is a NH_2 terminal extended form of circulating ANP. However, unlike ANP, this peptide is not found in the systemic circulation, but rather is synthesized in the kidney where it acts as a paracrine factor. Similar to ANP, this peptide exerts a natriuretic effect and presumably participates in the regulation of natriuresis under physiologic conditions (211).

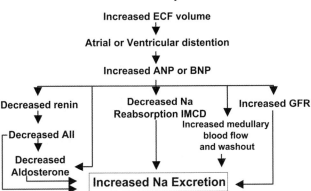

FIGURE 5 Mechanisms by which atrial and brain natriuretic peptide regulate renal sodium excretion.

CONGESTIVE HEART FAILURE

The fundamental abnormality underlying congestive heart failure is an inability of the heart to maintain its function as a pump. As a result, a series of complex compensatory reflexes are initiated that serve to defend the circulation. The renal response to a failing myocardium is retention of salt and water resulting in expansion of ECF volume. If myocardial dysfunction is mild, expansion of ECF volume leads to increased left ventricular end-diastolic volume, which raises cardiac output according to the dictates of the Frank-Starling principle. In this state of compensated congestive heart failure, salt intake and output come into balance but at the expense of an expanded ECF volume. Further deterioration in ventricular function leads to further renal retention of salt and water. There is progressive expansion of ECF volume and features of a congested circulation become manifest: peripheral edema, engorged neck veins, and pulmonary edema. Despite massive overexpansion of ECF volume, the kidneys behave as though they were responding to a low-volume stimulus.

In subsequent sections, a detailed analysis of the afferent and efferent regulatory limbs in congestive heart failure will be provided.

Afferent Sensing Mechanisms in Congestive Heart Failure

LOW-PRESSURE BARORECEPTORS

A characteristic feature in many forms of congestive heart failure is increased stretch and transmural pressure within the cardiac atria. These alterations would normally provide afferent signals that suppress sympathetic outflow and decrease the release of renin and ADH and ultimately result in a diuretic and natriuretic response. In congestive heart failure, this afferent signaling mechanism is markedly perturbed. Despite the presence of venous congestion and elevated cardiac filling pressures sympathetic nervous activity and serum concentrations of renin and ADH are increased and urinary salt excretion is blunted. Several clinical and experimental studies have shown that the responsiveness of the low-pressure baroreflex is diminished.

Greenberg et al. (121) measured afferent signals from pressure-sensitive atrial (type B) receptors in dogs with chronic congestive heart failure induced by tricuspid regurgitation or pulmonary stenosis. In response to saline infusion, receptor firing was markedly decreased as compared to the control dogs. A similar decrease in activity of atrial type B receptors was found in dogs with chronic volume overload and increased cardiac output due to an aortocaval fistula (348). This decrease in sensitivity of atrial mechanoreceptors contributes to the increased and altered regulation of efferent renal sympathetic nerve activity that has been observed in congestive heart failure. Dibner-Dunlap and Thames (66) examined the response of renal sympathetic nerve activity to increases in atrial pressure in a dog model of low-output heart failure induced by rapid ventricular pacing. As compared to controls, there was a markedly impaired reflex reduction of renal sympathetic nerve activity in the heart failure animals when atrial pressure was increased by either volume expansion or by balloon inflation. A similar impairment in atrial mechanoreceptor modulation of renal nerve activity has been described in a rat model of low cardiac–output congestive heart failure (73). In this model, the baroreflex defect was localized to the periphery at the level of the receptor and not the central nervous system (70, 73). In this regard, morphological changes consisting of nerve fiber arborization have been described in the atria of dogs with congestive heart failure (348). Studies in human subjects also suggest that cardiopulmonary mechanoreflexes are impaired in congestive heart failure (216).

HIGH-PRESSURE BARORECEPTORS

The increase in renal sympathetic nerve activity in cardiac failure has also been attributed to impaired arterial baroreceptor function. High-pressure baroreceptors in the carotid sinus and aortic arch normally exert a tonic inhibitory effect on central nervous system sympathetic outflow. A reduction in cardiac output severe enough to reduce mean arterial pressure could lead to reduced activity of the arterial baroreceptors and therefore explain the augmentation in CNS sympathetic outflow and renal salt retention. Although the precise mechanism for the sympathoexcitation is not known, a sustained reduction in arterial pressure is unlikely to be the sole explanation. First, arterial pressure is usually normal in congestive heart failure. Second, arterial baroreceptors adapt to sustained changes in arterial pressure so that afferent activity normalizes despite continued alterations in arterial pressure. Rather, there appears to be an intrinsic abnormality that develops in arterial baroreflex regulation in congestive heart failure (74). Sympathetic function becomes insensitive to manipulations that normally suppress or enhance its activity. For example, infusion of nitroprusside increases both the heart rate and the circulating norepinephrine levels in normal subjects, whereas equivalent hypotensive doses in subjects with congestive heart failure elicit a blunted response (237). Similarly, patients with heart failure show less bradycardia when arterial pressure is raised by infusion of phenylephrine. Such alterations in baroreflex function may result from abnormalities peripherally or alterations in central autonomic regulatory centers.

Several observations suggest that Ang II may contribute to the depressed baroreflex sensitivity in heart failure. As discussed below the renin-angiotensin system is activated in the setting of congestive heart failure. Ang II has been shown to upwardly reset the arterial baroreflex control of heart rate in the rabbit independent of a change in arterial pressure (43). In the rat, increased levels of endogenous Ang II produced by changes in dietary salt intake, tonically increase the basal level of renal sympathetic nerve activity and upwardly reset the arterial baroreflex control of renal sympathetic nerve activity (69). Administration of an Ang II receptor blocker

can reverse these changes in proportion to the degree of activation of the renin-angiotensin system. In a rabbit model of congestive heart failure, administration of an Ang II receptor blocker has been shown to improve the baroreflex control of sympathetic outflow (224). DiBona et al. (68) found that administration of an Ang II receptor blocker decreased efferent renal sympathetic nerve activity and improved the sensitivity of the arterial baroreflex mechanism in rats with congestive heart failure. This improvement was evident when the blocker was administered intravenously or when given directly into the cerebral ventricles. In a subsequent study, these same investigators found that the improved baroreflex regulation of renal sympathetic nerve activity was associated with an improved ability of the kidney to excrete both an acute and a chronic sodium load (71). Interestingly, captopril administered to patients with congestive heart failure restores the normal hemodynamic response to postural tilt and infusion of vasoconstrictive agents (60).

CARDIAC OUTPUT

A reduction in cardiac output has been suggested as the afferent signal that leads to Na retention in heart failure. When cardiac output is reduced by constriction of the abdominal or thoracic vena cava, urinary sodium excretion is typically decreased (267, 294). Restoring cardiac output to normal by autologous blood transfusion ameliorated renal salt retention despite the fact that venous and hepatic pressures were persistently elevated (267). However, other observations question the importance of cardiac output alone as a key sensing mechanism in signaling renal salt retention. For example, using other means to reduce cardiac output comparable to that seen with constriction of the vena cava does not necessarily decrease renal sodium excretion (212). Rats with small to moderate myocardial infarctions have normal capacities to increase cardiac output in response to volume loads but the sodium excretory response in these animals remains blunted. Even when cardiac output is increased above normal as with the creation of an arteriovenous fistula in dogs clinical findings of ascites and peripheral and pulmonary edema develop (348). Despite increased cardiac output, levels of renin, aldosterone, and ANP are high (324). Thus, it is evident that the initiating signal for salt retention in congestive heart failure cannot originate solely from a decrease in cardiac output.

OTHER SENSORS

Other afferent sensing mechanisms potentially active in congestive heart failure include intrahepatic baroreceptors (the evidence for these is controversial) and mechanoreceptors within the kidney. Chemosensitive receptors have been identified within skeletal muscle, heart, and kidney, which by responding to changing levels of metabolic breakdown products may participate in sensing of ECF volume. One such sensing mechanism may relate to the cardiac sympathetic afferent reflex. The reflex begins with sympathetic afferent fibers that respond to changes in cardiac pressure and dimension or substances that may accumulate in ischemia or heart failure. The reflex is excitatory in nature such that activation of the afferent fibers leads to increased central sympathetic outflow. As with the arterial baroreceptor reflex, there is evidence that Ang II plays a modulating role in this reflex (197). Ma et al. (197) found that the cardiac sympathetic afferent reflex is activated in dogs with congestive heart failure and that central Ang II can enhance the degree to which sympathetic outflow is enhanced.

In summary, a contracted EABV serves as the afferent signal that elicits activation of effector mechanisms resulting in sodium retention. As with other edematous disorders, the exact volume compartment that comprises EABV has not been elucidated (Fig. 6).

Effector Mechanisms in Congestive Heart Failure

NEPHRON SITES OF RENAL SODIUM RETENTION

Renal sodium handling in the setting of congestive heart failure is similar to that which occurs in an otherwise normal individual who is volume depleted. Activation of effector mechanisms lead to alterations in renal hemodynamics and tubular transport mechanisms that culminate in renal salt retention.

Renal hemodynamics in congestive heart failure are characterized by reduced renal plasma flow and a well-preserved glomerular filtration rate such that filtration fraction is typically increased. In a rat model of myocardial infarction, Hostetter et al. (135) found a positive correlation between the decline in renal plasma flow and the degree to which left ventricular function was impaired. The glomerular filtration rate remained well preserved as a result of an increased filtration fraction except in the animals with a severely compromised left ventricle. When examined at the level of the single nephron, these hemodynamic changes were found to be the result of a disproportionate increase in efferent arteriolar vasoconstriction and increased glomerular capillary

hydraulic pressure (137). Treatment with an angiotensin-converting enzyme inhibitor caused a decline in filtration fraction and efferent arteriolar resistance suggesting an important role for Ang II in mediating efferent arteriolar constriction. In this regard, changes in glomerular and proximal tubular function seen in states of heart failure are similar to those that result from infusion of Ang II or norepinephrine. Ang II, catecholamines, and renal nerves are all capable of increasing both the afferent and the efferent arteriolar tone but predominantly act on the latter. These changes in glomerular hemodynamics serve to maintain glomerular filtration rate near normal as renal plasma flow declines secondary to impaired cardiac function. As cardiac function progressively declines and the reduction in renal plasma flow becomes severe, the glomerular filtration rate will begin to fall. At this point there is an inadequate rise in filtration fraction because efferent arteriolar vasoconstriction can no longer offset the intense afferent arteriolar constriction. Higher plasma catecholamines and further increases in sympathetic nerve activity acting to provide circulatory stability result in greater constriction of the afferent arteriole such that glomerular plasma flow and transcapillary hydraulic pressure are reduced. In this setting, the glomerular filtration rate becomes dependent on afferent arteriolar flow.

These predictions are consistent with what has been observed in human subjects with varying degrees of left ventricular function (187). As left ventricular function declines, the glomerular filtration rate is initially maintained by an increased filtration fraction. However, in patients with severely depressed left ventricular function a progressive decline in renal blood flow becomes associated with a fall in glomerular filtration rate due to an inadequate rise in filtration fraction. In these patients, administration of an ACE inhibitor can result in a further lowering of the glomerular filtration rate even though systemic arterial pressure remains fairly constant (241).

Both experimental and clinical studies support the proximal nephron as a major site of increased sodium reabsorption in the setting of congestive heart failure. In human subjects, clearance techniques have primarily been employed to demonstrate the contribution of the proximal nephron. For example, infusion of mannitol was shown to increase free-water excretion to a greater extent in patients with congestive heart failure as compared to normal controls. Since mannitol inhibits fluid reabsorption proximal to the diluting segment, it was inferred that enhanced free-water clearance was reflective of augmented delivery of Na to the diluting segment from the proximal tubule (21). A similar conclusion was reached utilizing clearance techniques in the setting of pharmacologic blockade of distal nephron sites (23). In dogs with an arteriovenous fistula, there is a failure to escape from the Na-retaining effects of deoxycorticosterone acetate. In addition, these animals do not develop hypokalemia in contrast to normal controls (144). The failure to develop hypokalemia in the setting of mineralocorticoid excess is best explained by decreased delivery of Na to the distal nephron

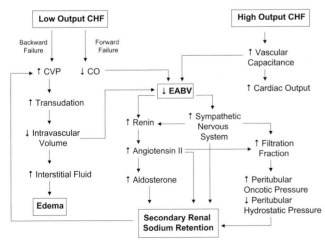

FIGURE 6 Summary of pathways leading to renal sodium retention in low- and high-output congestive heart failure. CO, cardiac output; EABV, effective arterial blood volume; CVP, central venous pressure.

as a result of enhanced proximal Na reabsorption. Alterations in peritubular hydrostatic and oncotic forces as well as direct effects of various neurohormonal effectors account for enhanced proximal sodium and water absorption in this setting (137).

The distal tubule may also importantly contribute to enhanced sodium reabsorption in states of congestive heart failure. Clearance and micropuncture studies have documented enhanced distal nephron sodium reabsorption in various experimental models of heart failure, including arteriovenous fistulas, chronic pericarditis, and chronic partial thoracic vena cava obstruction (14). In dogs with chronic vena cava obstruction (179) and rats with an arteriovenous fistula (310), the loop of Henle was localized as a site of enhanced sodium reabsorption. Similar to the proximal nephron, physical factors influenced by alterations in renal hemodynamics may account for augmented sodium reabsorption in this segment (179).

RENIN-ANGIOTENSIN-ALDOSTERONE SYSTEM

The renin-angiotensin-aldosterone system is activated when the heart fails as a pump (210). Components of this system serve to compensate for decreased cardiac output by stabilizing the circulation and expanding ECF volume.

Several mechanisms known to mediate release of renin are operative in the setting of a failing myocardium. Diminished pressure within the afferent arteriole leads to enhanced renin release via a baroreceptor mechanism, the sensitivity of which is heightened consequent to augmented baseline sympathetic nerve activity (153). Enhanced salt and water reabsorption in the proximal tubule and loop of Henle diminishes sodium chloride concentration at the macula densa providing a stimulatory signal for renin release by way of the tubuloglomerular feedback mechanism. Finally, increased sympathetic nerve activity directly enhances renin release via stimulation of β-adrenergic receptors.

Renin acts on angiotensinogen synthesized in the liver and elsewhere to produce the decapeptide, angiotensin I. Angiotensin I is converted to Ang II by the angiotensin converting enzyme present in the lungs, kidney, and blood vessels throughout the circulation.

Ang II plays a pivotal role in glomerular and proximal tubule function that characterizes most models of congestive heart failure. By selectively increasing efferent arteriolar tone, adjustments in the glomerular and postglomerular circulatory network favor net reabsorption in the proximal tubule. Increased filtration fraction leads to increased peritubular oncotic pressure and in combination with decreased peritubular hydrostatic pressure net sodium reabsorption is enhanced. Ang II also stimulates proximal tubule salt and water reabsorption by a direct mechanism (128, 295). In addition, increased efferent arteriolar resistance tends to increase glomerular capillary hydrostatic pressure, thereby mitigating any fall in GFR that would otherwise occur from decreased renal blood flow. In clinical as well as experimental models of heart failure, administration of ACE inhibitors improves renal

blood flow and increases urinary sodium excretion consistent with important Ang II-mediated effects on the renal microvasculature (85).

Ang II also contributes to renal salt and water retention through effects that lead to increased renal sympathetic nerve activity. Ang II has been shown to depress the sensitivity of the baroreflex mechanism such that a higher pressure is required to decrease central sympathetic outflow. In addition, Ang II directly stimulates sympathetic outflow at the level of the central nervous system. The chronic administration of an ACE inhibitor to patients with congestive heart failure leads to a reduction in central sympathetic outflow and improves the sympathoinhibitory response to baroreflex stimulation (119). Ang II affects renal salt and water handling in the distal nephron through stimulation of aldosterone release by the adrenal gland. Aldosterone acts primarily on the collecting duct to promote tubular reabsorption of sodium. Aldosterone-stimulated sodium reabsorption generates a luminal negative voltage that secondarily enhances excretion of hydrogen and potassium ions. The magnitude of potassium secretion will depend on the volume and composition of filtrate reaching the collecting duct. In this regard, patients with heart failure rarely manifest hypokalemia and alkalosis despite oversecretion of mineralocorticoid unless distal sodium delivery is increased by use of a diuretic. Effector mechanisms acting proximally, including Ang II, sympathetic nerves, and peritubular physical factors, serve to diminish distal delivery of sodium. Thus, although plasma renin and aldosterone levels are frequently elevated in heart failure, there is conflicting data as to the importance of aldosterone in mediating renal salt retention (84, 129, 329).

The conflicting data regarding the importance of the renin-angiotensin-aldosterone system in the generation of cardiac edema is best resolved when analyzed with respect to severity of heart failure. The initial response to constriction of the pulmonary artery or thoracic inferior vena cava in dogs is a reduction in blood pressure and increases in renin and aldosterone levels. These changes are accompanied by nearly complete renal sodium retention (329). Administration of a converting enzyme inhibitor during this acute phase lowers blood pressure further, consistent with an important role of circulating Ang II in the maintenance of blood pressure. Over several days plasma volume and body weight increase, while renin, aldosterone, and sodium balance return to control values. In contrast to the acute setting, administration of a converting enzyme inhibitor during this chronic phase results in no significant hypotension. Animals with more severe impairment of cardiac output have plasma renin and aldosterone levels that remain elevated and these animals remain sensitive to the hypotensive effects of converting enzyme inhibition.

Similar changes in the activation of the renin-angiotensin-aldosterone axis are seen in dogs with an arteriovenous fistula (324). In the early phase of this high-output cardiac failure model, significant elevations in renin and aldosterone levels occur and renal sodium retention is marked. Several days later, after development of peripheral edema and ascites, renin and aldosterone levels returned to baseline and daily sodium excretion begins to match dietary intake.

Studies in humans have shown a similar relationship between the renin-angiotensin-aldosterone system and stage and severity of congestive heart failure (84). This relationship may explain why renal function improves in some patients treated with ACE inhibitors whereas renal function deteriorates in others. Systemic hemodynamcis and plasma renin activity have been compared in such patients (242). In subjects whose renal function worsens after administration of the drug, there is a greater fall in mean right atrial pressure, left ventricular filling pressure, mean arterial pressure, and systemic vascular resistance. In addition, plasma renin activity increases to a greater extent. These changes suggest a more contracted EABV and greater dependency of systemic vascular resistance on circulating Ang II in patients with ACE inhibitor induced renal dysfunction. Maintenance of GFR is critically dependent on Ang II-mediated efferent arteriolar constriction causing an adequate increase in glomerular capillary hydrostatic pressure in order to counterbalances the decrease in renal perfusion.

In summary, during severe decompensated left ventricular failure, decreased EABV elicits release of renin with consequent activation of Ang II and aldosterone. Acutely, increased circulating levels of Ang II serve to maintain systemic blood pressure and contribute to augmented sodium reabsorption through hemodynamic and direct effects on the proximal tubule and enhanced distal sodium reabsorption by stimulating aldosterone release. As ECF volume expands, renin, Ang II, and aldosterone become suppressed, although not necessarily to normal. At this stage, maintenance of systemic blood pressure is more dependent on volume rather than Ang II. Sodium balance is now achieved but at the expense of increased steady-state ECF volume. With further deterioration in cardiac function, persistent activation of the renin-angiotensin-aldosterone system may result, such that systemic blood pressure remains dependent on circulating Ang II despite expansion of ECF volume. In order to predict net renal and hemodynamic effects of converting enzyme inhibition, one has to consider this sequential change in renin to volume dependency of mean arterial blood pressure (311).

SYMPATHETIC NERVOUS SYSTEM

The sympathetic nervous system is activated in congestive heart failure. Plasma norepinephrine levels are elevated and concentrations correlate with degree of left ventricular dysfunction (178). In addition, direct nerve recordings have verified that central sympathetic nerve outflow is increased and this outflow correlates with left ventricular filling pressures (176).

Increased sympathetic tone influences renal reabsorption of salt and water by indirect as well as direct mechanisms. Glomerular hemodynamics are affected in a similar manner to that produced by Ang II. A preferential increase in efferent arteriolar resistance results in increased filtration fraction in patients with decompensated heart failure. Peritubular Starling forces are altered in a manner that enhances proximal salt and water absorption. In addition, sympathetic nerves directly stimulate tubular reabsorption of salt and water in both the proximal and the distal nephron.

Increased sympathetic nerve activity directly stimulates the release of renin from the juxtaglomerular cells and sensitizes the baroreceptor-mediated mechanism of renin release (153). The subsequent formation of Ang II provides a positive feed back loop leading to further increases in sympathetic nerve activity. Increased circulating Ang II sensitizes tissues to the actions of catecholamines and acts synergistically with renal nerves in modulating renal blood flow (248).

The observation that α-adrenergic antagonists and ganglionic blockers abolish sodium retention in dogs with thoracic vena cava constriction supports an important role for renal nerves in mediating salt retention in heart failure (293). In the rat model of cardiac failure due to myocardial infarction, it has been demonstrated that increased activity of renal sympathetic nerves mediates a significant portion of the abnormal renal salt and water retention (72). These animals have an impaired diuretic and natriuretic response to intravenous saline volume loading that is associated with an attenuated inhibition of efferent renal sympathetic nerve activity. The impaired renal excretory response is normalized by prior renal denervation. Renal denervation also normalizes the attenuated diuretic and natriuretic response to ANP in these rats. A similar role for renal nerves in mediating abnormal renal salt and water retention has been shown in a dog model of compensated high-output heart failure (325).

PROSTAGLANDINS

Increased production of prostaglandins plays an important role in maintaining circulatory homeostasis in congestive heart failure. In response to decreases in cardiac output, neurohumoral vasoconstrictor forces (i.e., the renin-angiotensin-aldosterone system, the neurosympathoadrenal axis) participate in the maintenance of systemic arterial pressure and result in increased total peripheral vascular resistance. These same vasoconstrictors stimulate the renal production of vasodilatory prostaglandins such that the rise in renal vascular resistance is less than that seen in the periphery. Vasodilatory prostaglandins function in a counterregulatory role, attenuating the fall in renal blood flow and glomerular filtration rate that would otherwise occur if vasoconstrictor forces were left unopposed (244).

The delicate balance between constrictor and dilator forces upon the renal vasculature is best demonstrated when inhibitors of the cyclooxygenase pathway are given. In a model of congestive heart failure produced by inflation of a balloon in the thoracic inferior vena cava, there is a reduction in cardiac output that is accompanied by a significant rise in systemic vascular resistance, plasma renin activity, and the concentration of norepinephrine. Despite the increase in peripheral vascular resistance, renal vascular resistance does not change and there is only a slight fall in renal blood flow. Administration of indomethacin or meclofenamate in this setting results in a marked decrease in renal blood flow and an increase in renal vascular resistance, suggesting that renal prostaglandins play an important role in the maintenance of renal blood flow under conditions of decreased cardiac output (238).

Renal prostaglandins are also important in moderating the salt and water retention that would otherwise occur in the setting of unopposed activation of effector mechanisms such as angiotensin II, aldosterone, renal sympathetic nerves, and ADH (244). In dogs with chronic pericardial tamponade, the increase in urinary sodium excretion normally seen after pericardiocentesis is attenuated by indomethacin and augmented by infusion of arachidonic acid. Similarly, in humans with decompensated cardiac failure, infusion of prostaglandin E2 results in increased fractional excretion of sodium. In hyponatremic heart-failure patients, administration of indomethacin leads to a decrease in cardiac output and increase in systemic vascular resistance. Prostaglandins play an increasingly important role in modulating renal hemodynamics, sodium excretion, and circulatory homeostasis as the degree of heart failure worsens.

NATRIURETIC PEPTIDES

Circulating levels of ANP are elevated in humans and experimental animals with heart failure. These levels correlate with the severity of disease (59, 271). In patients with varying New York Heart Association functional classes, those of class IV have significantly higher levels than those of class I and class II. These levels vary inversely with left ventricular ejection fraction and decrease as ejection fraction improves during the course of treatment. Since the predominant stimulus for ANP release is atrial stretch, it is noteworthy that both the plasma level and the magnitude of step up across the heart correlates best with atrial pressure (271).

The natriuretic and vasodilatory properties of ANP suggest that this peptide plays an important counterregulatory role in congestive heart failure. In a rat model of heart failure, administration of a monoclonal ANP antibody was found to increase cardiac filling pressure and systemic vascular resistance (81). In this same model, renal blood flow and GFR decreased following the administration of a natriuretic peptide receptor blocker. These hemodynamic changes were accompanied by a reduction in urine flow and urine sodium excretion (203).

Attempts to use ANP therapeutically in congestive heart failure have produced disappointing results (59, 154). ANP infused in patients with heart failure causes only a minimal change in fractional sodium excretion and urine flow rates as compared to the robust response in normal controls (59). The diminished renal responsiveness to ANP is pronounced when considering that baseline endogenous plasma ANP levels are often already elevated five- to sevenfold in heart failure patients. Similarly, inhibition of renin release by ANP is attenuated in heart-failure patients (59).

The mechanism of renal nonresponsiveness in heart failure is not entirely clear. A downregulation of receptors due to sustained exposure to high levels of ANP or altered intrarenal hemodynamics are possibilities. The renal tubules appear to be responsive to ANP since urinary cGMP levels are increased in patients with congestive heart failure (4). One attractive explanation for ANP resistance is decreased delivery of sodium to the distal nephron, that portion of the nephron where ANP normally exerts its direct natriuretic effect. In this regard, administration of an Ang II receptor antagonist, an intervention that would increase distal sodium delivery, can restore the renal responsiveness to ANP (3). Thus, while ANP levels are uniformly elevated in congestive heart failure, potentially beneficial natriuretic properties are overwhelmed by more powerful antinatriuretic effector mechanisms.

Other natriuretic factors have been tested therapeutically in congestive heart failure with mixed results (26). In a double-blind, placebo-controlled trial, infusion of brain natriuretic peptide was associated with a significant reduction in pulmonary capillary wedge pressure, pulmonary artery pressure, right atrial pressure and mean arterial pressure as well as an increase in cardiac index. These hemodynamic benefits were accompanied by a significant increase in urinary volume as well as sodium excretion (201). In a preliminary report, infusion of brain natriuretic peptide was found to have a similar benefit on cardiac filling pressures and systemic vascular resistance, however, in this study only a few patients exhibited an increase in urinary sodium excretion (203). Urodilatin has also been tested in patients with congestive heart failure. A prolonged infusion of this natriuretic factor in 12 patients was reported to lower cardiac preload and to significantly increase urinary sodium excretion (90).

ENDOTHELIN AND NITRIC OXIDE

Circulating levels of endothelin are increased in the setting of congestive heart failure. These levels have been shown to correlate positively with various indices of cardiac dysfunction. Studies in which endothelin antagonists have been administered suggest a possible role for endothelin in the pathophysiology of cardiac failure. In a randomized, double-blind study of human subjects with heart failure, infusion of an ETa and ETb receptor blocker (bosentan) was associated with a reduction in right atrial pressure, pulmonary artery pressure, pulmonary capillary wedge pressure, and mean arterial pressure (152). The effects of administering an antagonist specific for either the ETa or ETb receptor was recently reported in a dog model of congestive heart failure (327). In these animals, ETa blockade alone lead to a reduction in cardiac filling pressures and increased cardiac output. These hemodynamic changes were associated with an increase in GFR and renal plasma flow as well as increased urinary sodium excretion. By contrast, administration of an ETb receptor blocker resulted in an increase in cardiac filling pressures and a decrease in cardiac output. There was no change in GFR however renal plasma flow fell. It was concluded that endogenous endothelins adversely effect cardiac hemodynamics and cause fluid retention primarily through ETa receptors.

Nitric oxide production is increased in congestive heart failure (333). Increased release of nitric oxide from resistance vessels may partly antagonize neurohumoral vasoconstrictor forces. Inhibiting nitric oxide production in heart failure patients causes a significant increase in pulmonary and systemic vascular resistance as well as decline in cardiac output. In the renal vasculature, nitric oxide production is also increased; however, the renal vasodilatory response to nitric oxide is impaired (2). In part, this defect is due to the effects of Ang II since administration of an angiotensin receptor antagonist can restore nitric oxide-mediated renal vasodilation.

ARGININE VASOPRESSIN

Increased circulating levels of AVP is a characteristic finding in patients with congestive heart failure. The nonosmotic release of AVP plays an important role in the development of hyponatremia, which in turn is a well-defined predictor of mortality in heart failure patients. In experimental heart failure, there is upregulation of the mRNA for vasopressin in the hypothalamus (151). In addition, there is increased expression of the mRNA and the protein for the aquaporin-2 water channel (342). In a rat model of heart failure, selective antagonism of the V-2 receptor is associated with a significant improvement in free water clearance (342). Use of a V-2 receptor antagonist to treat hyponatremia in human subjects with heart failure is currently being investigated.

CIRRHOSIS

Renal sodium excretion is normally regulated so that extracellular fluid (ECF) volume is maintained within normal limits. Any maneuver that increases ECF volume will lead to a prompt and sustained natriuresis until the volume returns to normal. In patients with cirrhosis, this homeostatic mechanism becomes deranged such that large increases in ECF volume are accompanied by continued renal salt retention resulting in edema and ascites formation.

Presinusoidal versus Postsinusoidal Obstruction and Ascites Formation

In patients with cirrhosis, the kidneys are normal but are signaled to retain salt in an unrelenting manner. The critical event in the generation of this signal is development of hepatic venous outflow obstruction. In the normal state, the portal circulation is characterized by high flow, low pressure, and low resistance. The imposition of a resistance into this high-flow vasculature will uniformly raise portal pressure, but development of ascites is critically dependent on location of the resistance. Conditions associated with presinusoidal vascular obstruction such as portal vein thrombosis and schistosomiasis raise portal pressure but are not generally associated with ascites. By contrast, hepatic diseases such as Laennec's cirrhosis and Budd Chiari syndrome cause early postsinusoidal vascular obstruction and are associated with marked degrees of salt retention, anasarca, and ascites. Thus, during the development of the cirrhotic process, ascites will accumulate primarily when the pathologic process is associated with hepatic venous outflow obstruction and sinusoidal hypertension.

This distinction between presinusoidal and postsinusoidal obstruction can best be explained by comparing the characteristics of fluid exchange in capillaries of the splanchnic bed versus those in the hepatic sinusoids. The intestinal capillaries are similar to those in the peripheral tissues in that they have continuous membranes with small pores such that a barrier exists preventing plasma proteins from moving into the interstitial space. An increase in capillary hydrostatic pressure will cause the movement of a protein poor fluid to enter the interstitial compartment and decrease the interstitial protein concentration. Interstitial protein concentration is further reduced by an acceleration in lymph flow that is stimulated by the fluid movement. As a result, the interstitial oncotic pressure falls and the plasma oncotic pressure remains unchanged. The net oncotic force therefore rises and offsets the increase in hydrostatic force providing a buffer against excessive fluid filtration. The fall in intestinal lymph protein concentration is maximal at relatively low pressures and is much greater than that observed from the cirrhotic liver (19, 336). Thus, the increase in net oncotic force associated with dilution of the interstitial protein and accelerated lymph flow contribute to the protection against ascites in patients whose only abnormality is portal hypertension.

The situation across the liver sinusoids is quite different. Hepatic sinusoids, unlike capillaries elsewhere in the body, are extremely permeable to protein. As a result, colloid osmotic pressure exerts little influence on movement of fluid. Rather, direction of fluid movement is determined almost entirely by changes in sinusoidal hydraulic pressure. Thus, efflux of protein-rich filtrate into the space of Disse is critically dependent on hepatic venous pressures. Obstruction to hepatic venous outflow will lead to large increments in formation of hepatic lymph and flow through the thoracic duct. Unlike the intestinal capillaries, there is little to no restriction in the movement of protein into the interstitium such that the protein concentration of hepatic lymph will quickly approach that of plasma (118). As a result, no significant oncotic gradient develops between plasma and the interstitium at high sinusoidal pressures and flow.

When sinusoidal pressure increases to such a degree that hepatic lymph formation exceeds the capacity of the thoracic duct to return fluid to the circulation, interstitial fluid weeps off the liver into the peritoneal space and forms ascites. Lymph formation in the setting of cirrhosis can be more than 20-fold greater than that which occurs under normal circumstances (336). Whereas in normal humans

1–1.5 liters/day of lymph are returned to the circulation, subjects with cirrhosis even without ascites may have lymph flow through the thoracic duct as high as 15–20 liters/day (335). The predominance of hepatically produced lymph to overall lymph production is illustrated by studies in experimental animals with cirrhosis. Barrowman and Granger (19) found a 29-fold increase in hepatic lymph flow, while only a threefold increase was noted in the splanchnic lymphatics. Eleven of 19 animals had normal flows of intestinal lymph, while all the cirrhotic animals had increased flows in liver lymph.

Conditions associated with the rapid onset of postsinusoidal obstruction such as acute right sided congestive heart failure and Budd–Chiari syndrome initially give rise to ascitic fluid that has a high protein concentration that may even approach that of plasma. This high protein concentration is reflective of the liver being the predominant source of the ascitic fluid. However, over time the protein content of ascites in these conditions begins to decrease. Witte et al. (337) measured the total protein in ascitic, pleural, and peripheral edema fluid in acute and chronic heart failure patients. In the setting of acute heart failure, the mean concentration of protein in ascitic fluid was approximately 5 g/dl. By contrast, the protein concentration in ascitic fluid of chronic congestive heart failure patients was 2.7 g/dl. A lower protein concentration is also typical of conditions such as Laennec's cirrhosis in which postsinusoidal obstruction develops slowly.

Two phenomena contribute to this change in ascitic fluid protein concentration. If the hepatic sinusoids are subjected to an increased hydrostatic pressure for a long period of time they begin to assume the anatomic and functional characteristics of capillaries found elsewhere in the body, a process referred to as capillarization (289). This change leads to a decrease in albumin permeability such that oncotic forces begin to play some role in hepatic lymph formation. At the same time hypoalbuminemia develops secondary to decreased hepatic synthesis as well as dilution secondary to ECF volume expansion. As a result, the protein content of hepatic lymph, although still high, falls to approximately 50%–55% of plasma values (336).

The second factor contributing to the lower ascitic protein concentration is the superimposition of portal hypertension. Early in the development of portal hypertension when plasma protein concentration is normal only minimal amounts of ascitic fluid is derived from the splanchnic bed due to the buffering effect of increased net oncotic force opposing fluid filtration. Extremely high hydrostatic pressures are required to produce significant amounts of ascitic fluid in the setting of normal plasma protein concentrations. By contrast, less and less hydrostatic pressure is required for the formation of ascitic fluid as the plasma albumin concentration decreases and the net osmotic force declines. In this setting, there is a large contribution of the splanchnic bed to the generation of ascites and the fluid is characterized by a low protein concentration.

The development of portal hypertension is also associated with changes in the splanchnic circulation that secondarily lead to increased lymph production in the splanchnic bed. The importance of the splanchnic lymphatic pool in the generation of ascites is reflected by the fact that in most instances ascitic fluid is transudative and characterized by a protein concentration of <2.5 g/dl. Classically, portal hypertension was considered to be the sole result of increased resistance to portal venous flow. However, studies in experimental models suggest that increased portal venous flow resulting from generalized splanchnic arteriolar vasodilation also plays a role in the genesis of increased portal pressure (40, 326). This vasodilation leads to changes in the splanchnic microcirculation that may predispose to increased filtration of fluid. For example, an acute elevation of venous pressure in the intestine normally elicits a myogenic response that leads to a reduction in blood flow. This decrease in flow is thought to serve a protective role against the development of bowel edema. However, in chronic portal hypertension this myogenic response is no longer present. In this setting, arteriolar resistance is reduced such that capillary pressure and filtration are increased (24). The loss of this autoregulatory mechanism may account for the greater increase in intestinal capillary pressure and lymph flow seen under conditions of chronic portal hypertension when compared to acute increases in portal pressure of the same magnitude (167). The potential causes of splanchnic arteriolar vasodilation are discussed below.

The importance of portal hypertension in the pathogenesis of ascites is highlighted by several observations. First, patients with ascites have significantly higher portal pressures as compared to those without ascites (220). Although the threshold for ascites development is not clearly defined it is unusual for ascites to develop with a pressure below 12 mm Hg. Gines found that only 4 of 99 cirrhotic patients with ascites had a portal pressure <12 mm Hg as estimated by hepatic venous wedged pressure (117). Second, portal pressure correlates inversely with urinary sodium excretion (220). Third, maneuvers designed to reduce portal pressure are known to have a favorable effect on the development of ascites. For example, surgical portosystemic shunts used in the treatment of variceal bleeding reduce portal pressure and are associated with a lower probability of developing ascites during follow up (59). Both side-to-side and end-to-side portocaval anastomosis have been shown effective in the management of refractory ascites in cirrhosis. Recent studies also suggest that reducing portal pressure with a transjugular intrahepatic portasystemic shunt has a beneficial effect on ascites (235).

In summary, ascites develops when the production of lymph from either or both the hepatic sinusoids and the splanchnic circulation exceeds the transport capacity of the lymphatics. In this setting, fluid will begin to weep from the surface of the liver and the splanchnic capillary bed and accumulate as ascites. The final protein concentration measured in the peritoneal fluid is determined by the sum of the two contributing pools of fluid; one relatively high in protein originating in the liver and the other, a low protein filtered across splanchnic capillaries. Hepatic venous outflow obstruction leading to increased sinusoidal pressure and portal hypertension are the major determinants as to whether lymph production will be of a magnitude sufficient for ascitic fluid to accumulate. Increased sinusoidal pressure is also related to the subsequent development of renal salt retention. The mechanism by which sinusoidal hypertension signals the kidney to retain sodium is discussed in the following section.

Afferent Limb of Sodium Retention: Overfill versus Underfill Mechanisms

CLASSICAL UNDERFILL MECHANISM FOR RENAL SALT RETENTION

The mechanism by which hepatic venous outflow obstruction leads to sufficiently high sinusoidal pressures for ascites formation is controversial. The classical (underfill) theory predicts that the degree of hepatic venous outflow obstruction is sufficient in the presence of normal splanchnic perfusion to perturb the balance between rates of hepatic lymph formation and thoracic duct flow, thereby resulting in formation of ascites. Both increased sinusoidal and portal venous pressures in conjunction with hypoalbuminemia cause formation of ascites in the presence of normal splanchnic perfusion. The formation of ascites, however, occurs at the expense of decreased intravascular volume. In consequence, a low venous filling pressure and a low cardiac output activate baroreceptor mechanisms, resulting in renal salt retention. According to this formulation, development of ascites is the primary event that leads to an underfilled circulation and subsequent renal salt retention.

The failure of measured hemodynamic parameters to satisfy predictions of the classical theory has raised questions regarding its validity. As originally conceived, it was predicted that extrasplanchnic plasma volume would be decreased and that cardiac output would be low. When measured, however, these values have rarely been low. In fact, measurements have indicated that total plasma volume is usually elevated in cirrhotic patients. Similarly, cardiac output is rarely low but tends to vary from normal to very high. In addition, studies performed in animal models of cirrhosis have found that sodium retention precedes the formation of ascites, suggesting that salt retention is a cause and not a consequence of ascites formation.

OVERFILL MECHANISM FOR RENAL SALT RETENTION

The incompatibility of measured hemodynamic parameters and timing of renal salt retention with the classical theory of ascites has led others to propose the overflow theory (186). Once again, hepatic disease with venous outflow obstruction is viewed as a prerequisite for development of increased sinusoidal and portal pressures. In contrast to the classical theory, however, normal splanchnic perfusion

fails to raise sinusoidal pressure sufficiently to cause ascites formation. Rather, venous outflow obstruction signals renal sodium retention independent of diminished intravascular volume. Salt retention, in turn, increases plasma volume, cardiac output, and splanchnic perfusion, thus raising sinusoidal and portal pressures sufficiently to culminate in translocation of fluid into the interstitial space and eventually the peritoneum. The combination of portal hypertension and increased arterial volume would lead to overflow ascites formation. This hypothesis is supported by the positive correlation between plasma volume and hepatic venous pressure and the persistence of increased plasma volume after portacaval anastomosis. Moreover, patients with ascites have significantly higher portal pressure than patients without ascites, and portal pressure correlates inversely with urinary sodium excretion (117).

Additional evidence linking hepatic venous outflow obstruction directly to renal sodium retention comes from studies performed in dogs fed the potent hepatotoxin dimethylnitrosamine (183–185). The pathophysiologic disturbances and histologic changes that develop over a 6–8-week period are similar in nature to those seen in Laennec's cirrhosis. In this model, sodium retention and increases in plasma volume precede formation of ascites by about 10 days (183). In order to exclude the possibility that the increase in plasma volume was solely due to an increased splanchnic plasma volume, repeat measurements were obtained after ligation of the superior and inferior mesenteric arteries, the celiac axis, and portal vein. In this way, any contribution of the splanchnic circulation could be excluded. These studies clearly showed that extrasplanchnic plasma volume was elevated at a time when dogs were in positive sodium balance. To further prove that extrasplanchnic plasma volume was increased, end-to-side portacaval shunts were placed prior to inducing cirrhosis (185). This maneuver was designed to prevent any increase in splanchnic plasma volume. In these studies, evidence of salt retention preceded the formation of ascites and was accompanied by a parallel increase in plasma volume.

In another series of studies using this same model, hemodynamic parameters were monitored during control, precirrhotic, and postcirrhotic sodium balance periods (184). Sodium retention was found to precede any detectable change in cardiac output or peripheral vascular resistance. Once ascites developed, plasma volume increased further and this was associated with increased cardiac output and a fall in peripheral vascular resistance. It was concluded that initiation of sodium retention and plasma volume expansion was not dependent on alterations in systemic hemodynamics. This conclusion has been corroborated in the canine model of hepatic cirrhosis induced by bile duct ligation (318) as well as in rats made cirrhotic with carbon tetrachloride inhalation and oral phenobarbital (191).

The pathway by which primary renal sodium retention would be linked to venous outflow obstruction in the overfill theory is not clear. Convincing evidence does exist for the presence of an intrahepatic sensory network composed of osmoreceptors, ionic receptors, and baroreceptors. Studies in which hepatic venous pressure is raised have demonstrated increases in hepatic afferent nerve activity (180, 182, 318). Furthermore, a neural reflex pathway linking hepatic venous congestion and augmented sympathetic nerve activity has been identified (168). In addition, acute constriction of the portal vein in dogs results in renal sodium and water retention in the innervated unilateral kidney, while these effects are abolished in the contralateral denervated kidney (9). In addition to a neural mechanism, there may also be a hormonal system by which the liver and kidney can communicate. Bankir et al. (16) recently suggested that hepatically produced cAMP may be one such hormone. Circulating cAMP is known to inhibit proximal salt and water absorption as well as contribute to the regulation of glomerular filtration rate. According to this hypothesis, decreased circulating cAMP levels as a result of liver disease could secondarily lead to renal salt retention and impaired renal function.

In summary, the overfill hypothesis is supported by a number of observations that indicate sodium retention precedes development of ascites in the absence of hemodynamic factors known to lead to salt retention. Moreover, high cardiac output coupled with increased plasma volume argue strongly for increased arterial blood volume, a finding seemingly incompatible with the underfill theory. Against such an analysis, however, is that mechanisms that sense arterial volume physiologically may be more sensitive than methods used to measure it. It should be noted that while statistically insignificant, there was a fall in blood pressure at the time of positive sodium balance in the dimethylnitrosamine model. This decrease may have been of sufficient magnitude to signal renal salt retention (184). Since cardiac output was unchanged, total peripheral resistance may have decreased. Similarly, patients with hepatic cirrhosis and ascites behave as if they are effectively volume depleted. Despite an increase in cardiac output and plasma volume arterial pressure is typically low. This fall in systemic blood pressure is consistent with an underfilled arterial vascular compartment. Thus, the distinction between classical and overflow theories better rests on the measurement of effective arterial blood volume (EABV).

USE OF EABV TO DISTINGUISH UNDERFILL AND OVERFILL MECHANISMS OF RENAL SALT RETENTION

The classical (underfill) theory predicts that EABV is low in patients with ascites and is the afferent mechanism signaling renal salt retention. The overflow theory predicts that EABV is expanded due to primary salt retention. While EABV cannot be measured directly, assessing the level of activation of neurohumoral effectors known to be regulated by EABV can be considered a measure of it. In this regard, levels of renin, aldosterone, ADH, and norepinephrine can serve as markers reflective of the magnitude of the EABV.

When renin and aldosterone values have been measured in patients with cirrhosis, values have varied from low to high. It is important, however, to consider these levels in the context of whether ascites is present or not. In the absence of ascites, subjects are in sodium balance and renin and aldosterone levels are normal (274). In the presence of ascites, mean renin and aldosterone levels are elevated, but individual values are often still normal (12, 117). This observation seems in conflict with the classical theory as all patients with ascites who are in positive sodium balance should have decreased EABV and high aldosterone levels. However, not all patients with ascites are retaining sodium. In fact, some patients are in balance such that sodium intake equals output. Thus, in examining the mechanism of sodium retention in cirrhosis with ascites, renin and aldosterone levels should be considered with respect to the rate of sodium excretion.

When examined in this fashion, a significant inverse relationship is found between urinary sodium excretion and plasma aldosterone (12, 117). In subjects with ascites who excrete 50–100 mEq of sodium per day, plasma aldosterone concentration is normal (12). As predicted by the classical theory, these patients have normal EABV and thus normal plasma aldosterone concentration. In patients with low rates of urinary sodium excretion, increased plasma aldosterone concentrations are reflective of a contracted EABV. Since aldosterone metabolism is impaired in liver disease, increased plasma concentrations could result from decreased hepatic clearance. When studied, however, increased secretion rate and not impaired metabolism is found to be the major cause of elevated aldosterone levels (279).

Measurement of plasma catecholamines to assess the level of activity of the sympathetic nervous system has been performed in subjects with cirrhosis. Similar to aldosterone, results of these measurements have been conflicting. However, when examined as a function of urinary sodium excretion rate, plasma norepinephrine and urinary sodium excretion are found to vary inversely (36). In addition, plasma norepinephrine is positively correlated with arginine vasopressin (AVP) and plasma renin activity.

Studies have also been performed in which humoral markers reflective of EABV were examined with respect to the ability to excrete water loads (35, 36). In those subjects who excreted less than 80% of a water load over a 5-hour period, plasma concentrations of AVP, renin, aldosterone, and norepinephrine were higher in comparison to those who were able to excrete greater than 80% of the water load (35, 36). In a similar study, cirrhotic patients unable to elaborate a positive free-water clearance after administration of a water load were also shown to have higher levels of AVP, norepinephrine, and plasma renin activity. Furthermore, the impairment in water excretion was found to parallel the clinical severity of disease (228). Thus, in patients with a low urinary sodium concentration or an impaired ability to excrete water loads, measurement of neurohumoral markers suggests the presence of a contracted EABV.

Placement of a peritoneovenous shunt results in a natriuretic response in patients with cirrhosis. This procedure creates direct route for replenishing the intravascular space through mobilization of ascitic fluid. The decrease in plasma renin activity and serum aldosterone levels after peritoneovenous shunting lends further support for a contracted EABV in these patients (39). Similar benefits have been reported in cirrhotic patients treated with the transjugular intrahepatic portal-systemic shunt (235, 269). The observation that large-volume paracentesis without intravenous albumin increases plasma renin activity and impairs renal function in most cirrhotic patients also argues against the overflow theory of ascites (116).

One component of the circulation that appears to be contributing to the overall decrease in EABV is the central circulation. Indirect measurements demonstrate that central blood volume is reduced while noncentral blood volume is expanded (218). In fact, the size of central and arterial blood volume is inversely correlated with sympathetic nervous system activity suggesting that unloading of central arterial baroreceptors is responsible for enhanced sympathetic activity. This conclusion is supported by studies using the technique of head-out water immersion (HWI) (92, 93). In this technique, subjects are seated and immersed in a water bath up to their necks. This technique results in redistribution of ECF volume from the interstitial space into the vasculature with a sustained increase in central blood volume. The central volume expansion is comparable to that induced by infusion of 2 liters of isotonic saline (93). Such a maneuver would be expected to raise both the EABV and the hepatic sinusoidal pressure. The classical theory would predict that HWI would lead to decreases in renin, aldosterone, ADH, and norepinephrine concentrations in response to expansion of EABV. Since renin levels correlate with wedged hepatic vein pressures, the overfill theory would predict further rises in renin and other hormonal systems consequent to initiation of a sinusoidal pressure-sensitive hepatorenal reflex. When HWI was performed in a heterogeneous group of patients with cirrhosis, the natriuretic response was variable, but suppression of renin and aldosterone levels was uniform (97). In a more homogenous group of patients characterized by impaired ability to excrete water and sodium, HWI was shown consistently to suppress plasma AVP, renin, aldosterone, and norepinephrine as well as to increase sodium and water excretion (34, 230).

Taken together, the multiplicity of data support the presence of decreased EABV in patients with decompensated cirrhosis and is most consistent with an underfill mechanism of renal salt retention (Fig. 7). Since blockade of endogenous vasoconstrictor systems in patients with cirrhosis and ascites leads to marked arterial hypotension, activation of these systems function to contribute to the maintenance of arterial pressure. At least one component of the decrease in EABV may be due to an underfilled central circulation. As discussed in the following paragraphs, increased perfusion of arteriovenous communications, systemic vasodilation, and increased perfusion of the splanchnic bed are important factors in the genesis of an underfilled circulation. In addition, these factors play a major role in the hyperdynamic circulation that is typical of patients with chronic liver disease.

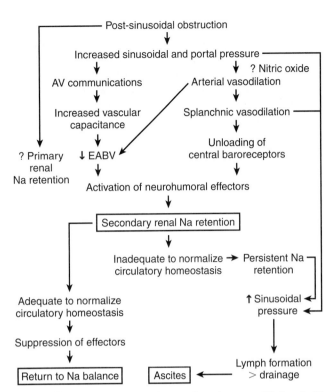

FIGURE 7 Unified theory of ascites formation: a modified underfill mechanism.

Hyperdynamic Circulation in Cirrhosis

ARTERIOVENOUS COMMUNICATIONS

The characteristic circulatory changes observed in animal as well as clinical studies of cirrhosis consist of increased cardiac output, low mean arterial pressures, and low peripheral vascular resistance. The most attractive explanation for a contracted EABV in the setting of such a hyperdynamic circulation assigns a pivotal role to increased vascular capacitance. An increased vascular holding capacity out of proportion to plasma volume results in an underfilled circulation and decreased EABV. One factor that may account for increased vascular capacitance and a hyperdynamic circulation is the formation of widespread arteriovenous communications (32). In cirrhotics, arteriovenous fistula formation has been identified in the pulmonary, mesenteric, and upper and lower extremity circulations. In addition, increased blood flow has been measured in muscle and skin of the upper extremity not attributable to increased oxygen consumption, anemia, or thiamine deficiency (156). Postmortem injection demonstrated intense proliferation of small arteries in the splenic vasculature of patients with cirrhosis (200).

The hemodynamic changes and salt retention that occur with an arteriovenous fistula are reminiscent of what occurs in cirrhotic humans (91). With an open fistula, peripheral vascular resistance falls, cardiac output increases, and diastolic and mean blood pressures fall. The proportionately greater increase in vascular capacitance over cardiac output results in a contracted EABV. Consequent sodium retention expands ECF volume, raises venous filling pressure, and further increases cardiac output until balance is achieved between cardiac output and lowered peripheral resistance. At this point, sodium intake equals excretion, EABV is normalized, and the patient is in balance.

In cirrhosis, a similar imbalance occurs between plasma volume and vascular capacitance such that EABV remains contracted and renal sodium retention is stimulated. In contrast to a simple arteriovenous fistula, however, several factors are present in cirrhosis that makes sodium balance more difficult to achieve. First, these patients often have impaired cardiovascular function (32). Diminished venous return consequent to tense ascites or cardiomyopathy from alcohol or malnutrition may limit increases in cardiac output. Furthermore, depression of left ventricular function in response to increased afterload suggests subclinical cardiac disease despite elevated forward output (188). Second, retained sodium does not remain in the vascular space and lead to increased venous return. Rather, retained sodium becomes sequestered within the abdomen as ascites. Third, increased vascular permeability may further impair ability of retained sodium to expand EABV. Peripheral arterial vasodilation in cirrhotic rats is associated with increased vasopermeability to albumin, electrolytes, and water (49). Examination of interstitial fluid dynamics by means of a subcutaneous plastic capsule reveals substantial increases in interstitial fluid volume early in cirrhosis before appearance of ascites or peripheral edema (287). Such capillary leakage impedes filling of the intravascular compartment and prevents replenishment of a contracted EABV.

PRIMARY ARTERIAL VASODILATION

Arteriovenous fistulas and formation or hyperdynamic perfusion of preexisting capillary beds are changes that develop as cirrhosis progresses. Nevertheless, salt retention occurs early in the cirrhotic process before these anatomic changes are fully established. Since sodium retention antedates the formation of overt ascites and portosystemic shunting, peripheral arterial vasodilation has been proposed to be a primary event in the initiation of sodium and water retention in cirrhosis (291). In this manner, a decreased EABV and increased vascular capacitance could still be the signal for renal salt retention even in the earliest stages of liver injury. The peripheral arterial vasodilation hypothesis is supported by several studies in animal models. In rats with partial ligation of the portal vein, evidence of a reduced systemic vascular resistance precedes the onset of renal salt retention (5). In addition, a direct correlation has been found between the onset of decreased arterial pressure and renal

sodium retention in the spontaneously hypertensive rats with experimental cirrhosis (191). As opposed to the classical underfilling theory, the arterial vascular underfilling would not be the result of a reduction in plasma volume, which in fact is increased, but rather to a disproportionate enlargement of the arterial tree secondary to arterial vasodilation. In the rat with carbon tetrachloride–induced cirrhosis, the fall in peripheral vascular resistance and hyperdynamic circulatory state precede ascites formation suggesting that generalized vasodilation is indeed an early finding with hepatic injury (103).

Perhaps the best evidence to date in support of an underfilled circulation due to arterial vasodilation comes from human studies of HWI accompanied by infusion of a vasoconstrictor. HWI is associated with increased perfusion of the central circulation, however, urinary excretion rates of salt and water improve but do not normalize with this procedure alone (Fig. 4) (34). Since systemic vascular resistance falls during HWI, it was proposed that further vasodilation may prevent complete restoration of EABV in subjects already peripherally vasodilated. Infusion of a vasoconstrictor will increase peripheral vascular resistance but will do little to improve an underfilled central circulation. Predictably, infusion of norepinephrine alone into cirrhotic subjects fails to significantly increase urinary sodium excretion (299). By contrast, when norepinephrine is infused during HWI so as to increase central perfusion and at the same time attenuate the fall in systemic vascular resistance, sodium excretion increases significantly. In six subjects with decompensated cirrhosis, this combined maneuver was found to increase urinary sodium excretion to an amount that when extrapolated over a 24-hr period was greater than sodium intake (299). These results are consistent with the hypothesis that arterial vasodilation causes an abnormal distribution of the total blood volume such that effective central blood volume is reduced.

Splanchnic Arterial Vasodilation As alluded to earlier, arterial vasodilation is particularly marked in the splanchnic arteriolar bed (141, 288, 326). Increasing degrees of splanchnic vasodilation contribute to the fall in mean arterial pressure and unloading of baroreceptors in the central circulation (62). As a result, central afferent sensors signal the activation of neurohumoral effectors, which in turn decrease perfusion of other organs but in particular the kidney. The importance of splanchnic vasodilation in the genesis of renal ischemia has been indirectly illustrated by the response to ornipressin, an analog of AVP that is a preferential splanchnic vasoconstrictor (124, 177). The administration of ornipressin to patients with advanced cirrhosis leads to correction of many of the systemic and renal hemodynamic abnormalities that are present. These include an elevation in mean arterial pressure, reductions in plasma renin activity and norepinephrine concentration, and increases in renal blood flow, glomerular filtration rate, and urinary sodium excretion and volume. Similar benefits have been reported with the combined use of octreotide and midodrine (148).

Role of Nitric Oxide in Arterial Vasodilation The underlying cause of arterial vasodilation particularly in the early
stages of cirrhosis has not been fully elucidated but a great
deal of attention has been focused on humoral factors.
Table 3 lists several vasodilators that have been proposed to
play a role in the hyperdynamic circulation of cirrhosis. Of
these, there is an increasing body of experimental and preliminary human evidence suggesting that increased nitric
oxide production may be an important factor in this process. In both experimental models and in human subjects
with cirrhosis, increased production of nitric oxide can be
demonstrated (278, 304, 330). In the cirrhotic rat, evidence
of increased production is already present when the animals
begin to retain sodium and antedates the appearance of
ascites (23). Administration of nitric oxide synthase inhibitor L-NMMA to cirrhotic human subjects improves the
vasoconstrictor response to noradrenaline suggesting that
overproduction of nitric oxide is an important mediator of
the impaired responsiveness of the vasculature to circulating
vasoconstrictors (48). In addition, this same inhibitor administered in low doses has been shown to correct the hyperdynamic circulation in cirrhotic rats (232). In a more
recent study utilizing this same model, normalization of
nitric oxide production was associated with a marked natriuretic and diuretic response as well as a reduction in the
degree of ascites in cirrhotic rats (202).

The precise mechanism for increased nitric oxide production in cirrhosis is not known but may be mediated at
least in part via the release of tumor necrosis factor-alpha
(189). In experimental models of hepatic disease, for example, the administration of anti-TNF-alpha antibodies or an
inhibitor of nitric oxide synthesis results in increases in
splanchnic and total vascular resistance, an elevation in the
mean arterial pressure, and a reduction in cardiac output
toward or, with nitric oxide inhibition, to normal (189, 232).
Similarly, blocking the signaling events induced by TNF
and nitric oxide production, via inhibition of protein tyrosine kinase, ameliorates the hyperdynamic abnormalities in
rats with cirrhosis and portal hypertension (190). Studies in
cirrhotic humans with an increased cardiac output and systemic vasodilatation have shown evidence of enhanced nitric
oxide production, a finding compatible with the experimental observations.

In patients with cirrhosis, portosystemic shunts and decreased reticuloendothelial cell function allow intestinal
bacteria and endotoxin to enter the systemic circulation.

TABLE 3 Potential Vasodilators in Cirrhosis

Nitric oxide
Glucagon
Calcitonin gene-related peptide
Atrial natriuretic peptide
Brain natriuretic peptide
Prostaglandins
Substance P
Adrenomedullin

Increased circulating endotoxin levels could be a potential
stimulus for tumor necrosis factor-alpha and/or nitric oxide
production. To test this possibility, Chin-Dusting et al. (54)
examined the effect of administering a fluoroquinolone antibiotic on hemodynamics in a group of well-compensated
human cirrhotic patients. It was postulated that the antibiotic would decrease the level of circulating endotoxin and
nitric oxide and improve peripheral hemodynamics. At
baseline patients with cirrhosis had increased basal forearm
blood flow as compared to normal controls. Administration
of the nitric oxide inhibitor, N^G-monomethyl-L-arginine
decreased forearm blood flow both in normals and in cirrhotic patients, but the effect was greater in patients with
cirrhosis. This increased response suggested that nitric oxide
was responsible for peripheral vasodilation in the cirrhotic
patients. Administration of the antibiotic to cirrhotic patients was found to normalize basal forearm blood flow as
well as the response to N^G-monomethyl-L-arginine. This
study is consistent with the notion that bacterial endotoxin
originating in the intestine is an important factor in stimulating nitric oxide production, which in turn contributes to
the arteriolar vasodilation in patients with cirrhosis.

It is not yet known with certainty whether the endothelial (eNOS) or the inducible (iNOS) isoform is primarily
responsible for increased production of nitric oxide. It has
been suggested that the hyperdynamic circulatory state of
cirrhosis may increase shear stress and thereby provide a
stimulus for the upregulation of eNOS (204, 330). Increased
activity of nitric oxide synthase in polymorphonuclear cells
and monocytes (cells that primarily contain iNOS) described in cirrhotic human subjects suggest that the inducible isoform may also play a role in increased production
(204).

In summary, an underfill mechanism appears to explain
the bulk of experimental as well as clinical findings in established cirrhosis (Fig. 7). Less certain are mechanisms responsible for sodium retention that precede the development of ascites. The overfill theory invokes the presence of
a hepatorenal reflex sensitive to subtle rises in intrahepatic
pressure mediating initiation of renal salt retention. However, the finding of decreased peripheral vascular resistance
even at this early stage suggests diminished arterial filling
(184). Early peripheral arterial vasodilation and later formation of anatomic shunts lead to disproportionate increases in
vascular capacitance with subsequent contraction of EABV,
thereby signaling renal salt retention. While it is conceivable
that both overfill mechanisms and underfill mechanisms
may be operative at different stages of disease, the multiplicity of data both clinical and experimental can be assimilated
into an underfill theory.

Concept of Balance in Cirrhosis

In the earliest stages of cirrhosis when arterial vasodilation
is moderate and the lymphatic system is able to return increased lymph production to the systemic circulation, renal

sodium and water retention are sufficient to restore EABV and thereby suppress neurohumoral effectors. Balance is reestablished such that sodium intake equals sodium excretion but at the expense of an increased ECF volume. As liver disease progresses this sequence of arterial underfilling followed by renal salt retention is repeated. As long as the EABV can be restored to near normal levels the activation of effector mechanisms will be moderated and balance will be achieved albeit at ever-increasing levels of ECF volume (Fig. 5). Eventually lymph production will begin to exceed the drainage capacity of the lymphatic system. At this stage of the disease renal salt retention becomes less efficient at restoring EABV as retained fluid is sequestered in the peritoneal cavity as ascites. At the same time arterial underfilling is more pronounced, particularly as splanchnic arteriolar vasodilation becomes more prominent. Activation of neurohumoral effectors is magnified resulting in more intense renal salt retention. Even at this stage of the disease cirrhotic patients with ascites eventually reestablish salt balance. The terminal stages of the cirrhotic process are characterized by extreme arterial underfilling. At this time there is intense and sustained activation of neurohumoral effectors. As a result, renal salt retention is nearly complete as the urine becomes virtually devoid of sodium. The vasoconstrictor input focused in on the kidney is of such a degree that renal failure begins to develop.

Effector Mechanisms in Cirrhosis

NEPHRON SITES OF RENAL SODIUM RETENTION

Salt retention and impaired free-water clearance are characteristic disturbances in renal function in cirrhotic patients. Evidence is available to support an important role for proximal and distal nephron segments in mediating enhanced sodium reabsorption.

Proximal Nephron Indirect evidence supporting enhanced proximal salt reabsorption comes from studies in human cirrhotic subjects in which infusion of mannitol or saline improves free-water clearance (57, 290). Increased proximal tubular salt reabsorption leads to decreased delivery of filtrate to the distal diluting segments, thereby impairing free-water formation. Presumably, by restoring distal delivery of filtrate, mannitol and saline infusions result in increased solute free-water formation. Similar increases in free-water clearance occur when central hypervolemia is induced by HWI. The increase in urine Na is accompanied by increased K excretion, suggesting enhanced distal delivery of sodium. Increased water excretion seen in response to HWI combined with simultaneous infusion of norepinephrine is also consistent with baseline enhanced proximal sodium reabsorption in decompensated cirrhotics (299). Since plasma ADH fell to the same extent in both the combined maneuver and the HWI alone, it was concluded that augmented water excretion during the combined maneuver was attributable to increased distal delivery.

Renal sodium handling has also been assessed in cirrhotic patients with no peripheral edema or ascites (340). Proximal fractional reabsorption of sodium was estimated using clearance techniques in the presence of a hypotonic diuresis. In these patients, proximal fractional sodium reabsorption failed to decrease in response to saline loading. Similar findings were found in studies examining the magnitude of renal sodium absorption that remained after ethacrynic acid and chlorothiazide therapy (86). Diuretic-resistant sodium reabsorption was found to be greater in cirrhotic patients as compared to normal controls, suggesting stimulated proximal salt absorption.

Experimental models of cirrhosis have provided more direct assessment of nephron function. Micropuncture studies in rats made cirrhotic by ligation of the common bile duct demonstrated increases in both the proximal tubule solute reabsorption and the filtration fraction (15). Enhanced proximal reabsorption was attributed to increased peritubular oncotic pressure. The importance of renal hemodynamic factors in abnormal renal handling of salt and water is further highlighted in studies of dogs made cirrhotic by a similar mechanism (207). In those animals chronically ligated, intrarenal administration of the vasodilator acetylcholine was found to ameliorate the blunted natriuretic response to saline infusion. In this model, sodium reabsorption was enhanced in both the proximal and the diluting segments of the nephron (33).

Distal Nephron Clinical and experimental evidence also supports an important role for distal nephron sodium retention in cirrhosis. During hypotonic saline-induced diuresis, renal sodium excretion and solute free-water clearance were measured in order to estimate distal sodium load and distal tubular sodium reabsorption (55). When compared to controls, cirrhotic patients with ascites had similar distal sodium delivery but increased distal fractional sodium reabsorption. In cirrhotic patients manifesting a sluggish natriuretic response to HWI, phosphate clearance was found similar to a group who demonstrated an appropriate increase in urinary sodium excretion (100). Since phosphate clearance was used as a marker of proximal sodium reabsorption, it was concluded that distal sodium reabsorption contributed importantly to renal sodium retention in patients with a sluggish natriuretic response. The results of a prospective, double-blind study comparing the diuretic response of furosemide to spironolactone in cirrhotic patients with ascites suggest that salt absorption in the cortical collecting tubule is enhanced (253). When administered furosemide, only 11 of 21 patients exhibited a diuresis, while 18 of 19 patients responded to spironolactone. Furthermore, 10 patients who failed to respond to furosemide demonstrated a diuretic response to spironolactone. Furosemide inhibits sodium reabsorption in the loop of Henle, thereby increasing delivery to the collecting duct. All patients treated with furosemide had increases in the rate of potassium excretion including the 11 patients who failed to increase urinary sodium excretion. These results, combined with the clinical effectiveness of spironolactone in treatment of cirrhotic ascites, suggest enhanced salt absorption in the aldosterone-sensitive cortical collecting tubule.

In summary, clinical and experimental studies suggest an important role for proximal as well as distal nephron sites mediating renal salt retention in cirrhosis. The relative contribution of different nephron sites to impaired salt and water excretion may depend on the degree to which systemic hemodynamics are altered. With each stage of advancing liver disease there becomes a greater contraction of the EABV. In the earliest stages of liver disease, enhanced proximal reabsorption limits distal delivery of solute in a manner analogous to a nonedematous subject with intravascular volume depletion. If distal delivery can be normalized at this early stage, distal nephron sites may continue to reabsorb sodium avidly and therefore appear as the primary site responsible for ECF volume expansion. With severe reductions in EABV, presumably the proximal nephron becomes the dominate site of fluid reabsorption such that the contribution of the distal nephron becomes much less apparent.

SYMPATHETIC NERVOUS SYSTEM

The sympathetic nervous system has been shown to importantly contribute to abnormalities in body fluid homeostasis in cirrhosis. Studies in rats made cirrhotic by ligating the common bile duct suggest that increased renal nerve activity is a major factor in the progressive salt retention that occurs in these animals (67, 72). In this model, baseline renal nerve activity is increased and fails to decrease appropriately in response to intravenous saline. Renal denervation significantly improves the impaired ability to excrete an oral or intravenous salt load. In addition, renal denervation has been shown to normalize the attenuated diuretic and natriuretic response to the intravenous administration of ANP (155). In chronic metabolic studies, renal denervation also leads to a significant improvement in the positive cumulative sodium balance. The cause of the increased renal nerve activity is multifactorial. Recent studies have demonstrated an impairment in aortic and cardiopulmonary baroreceptor regulation of efferent renal nerve activity (276). In dogs with chronic bile duct ligation, renal nerve activity fails to decrease in response to high NaCl food intake (205). This defect has been attributed to abnormalities in hepatic NaCl-sensitive receptors or their immediate intrahepatic afferent connections.

Studies in human cirrhotic subjects are more indirect but also suggest an important role for the sympathetic nervous system. Levels of norepinephrine in patients with cirrhosis vary from normal to elevated. When measured in decompensated cirrhosis, levels are high and are inversely correlated with urinary sodium excretion (36). Confirming that plasma norepinephrine levels are in fact an index of sympathetic activity and not simply the result of impaired clearance, measurement of hepatic extraction of norepinephrine has been found normal in decompensated cirrhosis (230). In addition, direct measurement of peripheral nerve firing rates

show evidence of increased central sympathetic activity. Patients characterized by impaired ability to excrete water loads have plasma levels of norepinephrine that correlate positively with levels of ADH, aldosterone, and plasma renin activity (36). Decreased EABV leads to baroreceptor-mediated activation of sympathetic nerve activity with subsequent enhancement of proximal salt reabsorption. Renal nerve-mediated decrease in sodium delivery to the diluting segment in addition to nonosmotic release of ADH contributes to the inability to maximally excrete water loads. Furthermore, increased renal nerve activity can indirectly enhance distal sodium reabsorption by stimulating renin release with subsequent formation of aldosterone. If baroreceptor-mediated increases in adrenergic activity are triggered by diminished EABV, then expansion of central blood volume should have a favorable effect in lowering plasma norepinephrine. In addition, decreased levels of norepinephrine should be associated with an improvement in renal salt and water excretion. In this regard, cirrhotic patients subjected to HWI demonstrate significant suppression of plasma norepinephrine levels (230). Moreover, during HWI there is a significant correlation between right atrial pressure, the decrement in plasma norepinephrine, and increase in fractional excretion of sodium (34).

However, other studies have not found a clear cut association between decreased circulating catecholamines and an improved renal excretory response. In a study of patients with decompensated cirrhosis subjected to HWI, there was a striking increase in creatinine clearance and a variable natriuresis that occurred independently of changes in plasma norepinephrine levels (95). Similarly, administration of the α_2 agonist, clonidine, inhibited renal sympathetic nerve activity and increased GFR and urine flow, but did not increase urinary sodium excretion (101). In another study of cirrhotic patients, clonidine was found to decrease the concentration of norepinephrine in the right renal vein but did not change GFR or urinary sodium excretion (280). These studies suggest that while sympathetic nerve activity is increased in cirrhosis, it is not the sole mechanism responsible for impaired salt and water excretion.

In addition to stimulating renal salt and water retention, increased sympathetic tone may also contribute to the renal vasoconstriction that characterizes the cirrhotic state (76, 275). Renal nerves are also likely to be one of several factors responsible for the intense vasoconstriction that characterizes the hepatorenal syndrome (20). Activation of the sympathetic nervous system may serve as a compensatory response to cirrhosis-induced vasodilation. In cirrhotic patients, infusion of the adrenergic blocking agent phentolamine into the renal artery resulted in systemic hypotension (94). The heightened sensitivity of blood pressure to phentolamine infusion is consistent with an important role of sympathetic nerves in maintaining vascular tone.

In summary, the sympathetic nervous system is activated under conditions of decompensated cirrhosis. Overactivity of this system is the result of a contracted EABV.

In addition, there is impaired regulation of sympathetic outflow due to abnormalities in several afferent sensing mechanisms. Increased renal nerve activity contributes to the cumulative salt retention that accompanies advancing liver disease. In addition, activation of sympathetic outflow plays an important compensatory role in maintaining vascular tone in the setting of decreased vascular resistance.

ALDOSTERONE

In patients with cirrhosis and ascites, plasma concentrations of aldosterone are frequently elevated. Although aldosterone metabolism is impaired in liver disease, secretion rates are greatly elevated and are the major cause of elevated levels (279). The relationship between hyperaldosteronism and sodium retention is not entirely clear. Several studies have provided evidence that argues against an important role of aldosterone in mediating salt retention in cirrhosis. For example, patients treated with an aldosterone synthesis inhibitor do not necessarily exhibit a natriuretic response (279). In one study, renal salt excretion and changes in plasma renin and aldosterone levels were examined in 11 patients with ascites subjected to 5 days of high-salt intake. In patients with normal suppression of renin and aldosterone, salt retention and weight gain occurred to the same extent as patients who had persistent hypersecretion of renin and aldosterone (58). In addition, cirrhotic patients in positive sodium balance as compared to controls with matched sodium excretion have increased fractional distal sodium reabsorption despite lower plasma aldosterone levels. In 16 cirrhotic patients subjected to HWI, plasma renin activity and plasma aldosterone levels were found to decrease promptly. Despite suppression of the hormones, however, half of the patients manifested a blunted or absent natriuretic response (97). In another group of cirrhotic patients with ascites and edema, HWI induced a significant natriuresis despite acute administration of desoxycorticosterone, suggesting that enhanced sodium reabsorption can occur independently of increased mineralocorticoid activity.

In contrast, a number of observations support aldosterone as an important factor in the pathogenesis of sodium retention in patients with cirrhosis. For example, adrenalectomy or administration of a competitive inhibitor of aldosterone increases urinary sodium excretion (87). Patients who fail to manifest a diuretic response to furosemide tend to have higher renin and aldosterone levels and lower urinary sodium concentrations prior to treatment (33). Inability of furosemide to increase urinary sodium in these patients may result from reabsorption of delivered sodium in the collecting tubule under the influence of aldosterone. Similarly, patients with the highest renin and aldosterone levels are those who fail to diurese in response to HWI (97, 228). In order to more clearly define the relationship between sodium excretion and plasma aldosterone levels, patients with decompensated cirrhosis were subjected to HWI in combination with infused norepinephrine (229). It was hypothesized that in the setting of decreased EABV, inability to

escape from the sodium-retaining effects of aldosterone results from enhanced proximal sodium reabsorption and therefore decreased distal sodium delivery. Use of HWI combined with norepinephrine so as to maintain peripheral vascular resistance provides the most effective means of increasing central blood volume and restoring EABV (299). In this study, the combined maneuver resulted in the largest negative sodium balance and suppressed plasma renin activity and aldosterone levels to a greater extent than HWI or norepinephrine alone.

As with the conflicting data regarding the role of the proximal and distal nephron in salt retention discussed previously, the degree to which systemic hemodynamics and EABV are impaired may explain some of the conflicting data noted above. It is possible that in patients with the greatest contraction of EABV intense proximal sodium reabsorption limits distal delivery to such an extent that the contribution of aldosterone to increase salt absorption is difficult to detect. By contrast, with less impairment of the EABV, distal delivery is better maintained such that the aldosterone-mediated sodium reabsorption becomes more obvious. In this regard, aldosterone has been shown to contribute to the exaggerated salt retention that occurs in the upright position in patients with early cirrhosis without ascites (30).

PROSTAGLANDINS

The observation that nonsteroidal anti-inflammatory drugs decrease GFR, renal blood flow, and sodium excretion in cirrhotics suggests that prostaglandins may serve a protective role. Ligation of the common bile duct in dogs results in enhanced synthesis of vasodilatory prostaglandins. When prostaglandin synthesis is inhibited with indomethacin, renal blood flow and GFR are reduced significantly (344). A similar protective effect may be present in cirrhotic humans (41). Administration of indomethacin to patients with alcoholic liver disease results in reduced effective renal plasma flow and creatinine clearance. These parameters were corrected when prostaglandin E1 was infused intravenously (41).

Prostaglandins may also importantly influence renal salt and water handling in cirrhosis. Patients pretreated with indomethacin exhibit a blunted natriuretic response to diuretics known to increase renal prostaglandin synthesis (213). In comparison to normal controls, patients with decompensated cirrhosis subjected to HWI demonstrate a threefold greater increase in PGE excretion, which is accompanied by increased creatinine clearance and sodium excretion (98). In subjects with ascites, impaired ability to clear free water is associated with lower urinary PGE2. Intravenous infusion of lysine acetylsalicylate reduced the clearance of free water, while GFR was variably affected. Diminished synthesis of prostaglandins may leave vasopressin-stimulated water reabsorption unopposed, thereby reducing free-water clearance. Prostaglandins may also participate in blood pressure homeostasis. In cirrhotic patients, the pressor response to infused Ang II is impaired. Administration of either indomethacin or ibuprofen results in significant decreases in renin and aldosterone levels and restores pressor sensitivity to infused Ang II (347).

In summary, prostaglandins function in a protective role in decompensated cirrhosis. Similar to other hypovolemic states, prostaglandins act to maintain renal blood flow and GFR by ameliorating pressor effects of Ang II and sympathetic nerves (244). These agents may also serve to mitigate the impairment in free-water clearance that would otherwise occur from unopposed activity of AVP. Administration of prostaglandin inhibitors can partially correct excessive hyperreninemia and hyperaldosteronism and restore the pressor response to Ang II.

KALLIKREIN-KININ SYSTEM

Urinary kallikrein activity is increased in cirrhotic patients with ascites and preserved GFR, while urinary activity decreases in association with impaired renal function (252). The correlation between renal plasma flow and GFR suggests that the renal kallikrein-kinin system may contribute to maintenance of renal hemodynamics in cirrhosis.

At the level of the renal tubule bradykinin has been shown to exhibit a natriuretic effect. However, bradykinin also is a potent peripheral vasodilator and can cause microvascular leakage. In cirrhosis, these later effects could exacerbate an already contracted EABV and cause further salt retention. MacGilchrist et al. (198) studied the effects of kinin inhibition by systemically infusing aprotinin (a strong inhibitor of tissue kallikrein) into a group of patients with cirrhosis. This infusion was associated with a doubling of urinary sodium excretion and an increase in renal plasma flow and GFR. This beneficial effect on renal function in the setting of kinin inhibition was attributed to an improvement in systemic hemodynamics as systemic vascular resistance increased. Similarly, administration of a bradykinin β_2 receptor antagonist to cirrhotic rats normalized renal sodium retention and reduced the activity of the renin-angiotensin-aldosterone system (334). Inhibiting bradykinin-induced microvascular leakage and lessening the degree of vascular underfilling was felt to be the mechanism of the beneficial effect.

NATRIURETIC PEPTIDES

The role of ANP in the pathogenesis of edema in hepatic cirrhosis remains undefined. While atrial ANP content was reduced in cirrhotic rats, most data indicate ANP levels are either normal or elevated in cirrhotic humans (143, 301). Elevated levels are the result of increase cardiac release rather than just impaired clearance. The cause of the high levels is not understood, because atrial pressure is normal and central blood volume is reduced. Stimulating the endogenous release of ANP induces a natriuretic response in some patients with cirrhosis, while other patients are insensitive (301). However, both groups of patients exhibited an increase in urinary cGMP suggesting that the kidney is still capable of responding to ANP even in the absence of a natriuretic effect (301).

Several potential mechanisms may account for ANP resistance in cirrhosis. This resistance could be the result of a defect intrinsic to the kidney or could be the result of altered systemic hemodynamics leading to activation of more potent sodium-retaining mechanisms (199). With regards to the first possibility an altered density of glomerular ANP binding sites has been demonstrated in the bile duct-ligated rat model of cirrhosis (111). In addition, ANP resistance was found in the isolated perfused kidney taken from sodium avid rats with cirrhosis induced by carbon tetrachloride (247). This preparation allows systemic and hormonal factors to be excluded. In the chronic caval dog model of cirrhosis, intrarenal infusion of bradykinin restored ANP responsiveness to previously resistant animals suggesting that an intrarenal deficiency of kinins could be a contributing factor (175).

Other studies have focused on systemic hemodynamics as a cause of ANP resistance. With each stage of advancing liver disease there becomes a greater reduction in EABV. Since ANP resistance tends to occur with more severe and advanced disease it is possible that ANP resistance is directly related to the impairment in EABV. Decreased EABV is associated with enhanced proximal reabsorption of solute. As a result, ANP resistance may be due to decreased delivery of salt to the site where ANP exerts its natriuretic effect. In support of this possibility, ANP resistance could be restored in cirrhotic rats by infusions of vasopressors so as to normalize arterial pressure and presumably improve the decrease in EABV (192). In human cirrhotics, ANP responsiveness can be markedly improved when distal sodium delivery is increased by administration of mannitol (220).

Circulating brain natriuretic peptide (BNP) levels are also increased in patients with cirrhosis (173). Infusion of BNP at a dose that elicits an increase in GFR, renal plasma flow, and urinary sodium excretion in normal controls has no effect in cirrhotic humans. The infusion is associated with an increase in urinary cGMP as well as a fall in plasma aldosterone levels suggesting that the peptide is capable of interacting with its receptor in these patients. As with ANP, the lack of natriuretic response to BNP may be due to overactivity of other antinatriuretic factors as well as decreased delivery of sodium to its tubular site of action.

Adrenomedullin is a peptide with vasodilatory properties that is highly expressed in cardiovascular tissues. Increased circulating levels that correlate with severity of disease have been described in patients with cirrhosis (104). Urodilatin is a natriuretic factor that is exclusively synthesized within the kidney. Unlike other natriuretic factors, levels are not increased in patients with cirrhosis (285).

ENDOTHELIN

Increased circulating levels of endothelin have been reported in cirrhosis (219). The stimulus and pathophysiologic significance of these levels is not known with certainty. The peptide may play a role in the renal vasoconstriction seen in the hepatorenal syndrome (117, 219).

Therapeutic Implications for Treatment of Salt Retention in Cirrhosis

Renal salt retention is the most common abnormality of renal function in chronic liver disease. Whenever urinary sodium excretion falls to an amount less than dietary salt intake ECF volume will begin to expand and eventually lead to the development of ascites and peripheral edema. The approach to the treatment of the cirrhotic patient with ascites is to alter sodium balance in such a way that urinary sodium excretion exceeds dietary salt intake. In this manner, ECF volume will contract. The ultimate goal is to reestablish salt balance at an ECF volume that is clinically associated with the absence of ascites and peripheral edema. The initial step in achieving this goal is to restrict dietary sodium intake. A reasonable starting point is a 88 mEq (2 g) sodium diet (281). Such a regimen can lead to negative salt balance in patients with high levels of baseline urinary sodium excretion (at least >90–100 mEq/day). In such patients, salt restriction alone may lead to resolution of ascites.

DIURETIC THERAPY

In patients with a low level of baseline urinary sodium excretion, dietary salt restriction alone is usually not sufficient to induce negative salt balance. In this situation, diuretic therapy is indicated. Spironolactone is the most commonly used first-line agent for several reasons. First, while normally considered a weak diuretic, spironolactone is oftentimes found to be more clinically effective that loop diuretics in some patients with advanced disease. Under normal circumstances, loop and thiazide diuretics are secreted into the proximal tubular lumen where they travel down stream and exert their natriuretic effect. In the setting of cirrhosis, decreased renal blood flow can limit delivery of these agents to the site of secretion in the proximal nephron. In addition, accumulation of compounds such as bile salts may compete or directly impair the secretory process. The net effect is that there is less delivery of the diuretic to its site of action and the natriuretic effect is limited. By contrast, spironolactone does not require tubular secretion. Rather, this agent enters the cells of the collecting tubule from the blood side. As a result, the efficacy of spironolactone is not impaired with cirrhosis. Second, spironolactone is a potassium sparing diuretic and therefore unlike loop or thiazide diuretics does not cause hypokalemia. The avoidance of hypokalemia is important in the management of cirrhotic patients as potassium depletion can contribute to the development of hepatic encephalopathy. Hypokalemia can lead to increased blood ammonia levels as a result of a stimulatory effect on renal ammonia synthesis as well as increased gastrointestinal absorption of nitrogen secondary to decreased bowel motility.

In patients who fail to develop a significant diuretic response to spironolactone alone, a thiazide diuretic can be added, the dose being determined by the level of renal function. If diuresis is still inadequate, a loop diuretic such as furosemide can be given in combination with the thiazide and spironolactone.

When attempting to initiate diuresis, caution is necessary to avoid excessive volume removal. The rate at which fluid can safely be removed in cirrhosis is dependent upon the presence or absence of peripheral edema. When a diuresis is induced, the fluid is initially lost from the vascular space; the ensuing fall in intravascular pressure then allows the edema fluid to be mobilized to replete the plasma volume. Edema mobilization is relatively rate-unlimited in patients with peripheral edema (263). In comparison, patients who only have ascites can mobilize edema fluid solely via the peritoneal capillaries. The maximum rate at which this can occur is only 300 to 500 ml/day; more rapid fluid removal in the absence of peripheral edema can lead to plasma volume depletion and azotemia.

DIURETIC-RESISTANT PATIENTS

Large-Volume Paracentesis Patients who fail to respond to a combination of dietary salt restriction and diuretic therapy are said to be diuretic resistant. These patients are in a state of persistent positive sodium balance and require a more invasive intervention in order to achieve negative salt balance. Large volume paracentesis is a procedure in which negative salt balance is established acutely by removing some or the entire volume of ascitic fluid. In patients with virtually no sodium in the urine and who are consuming 88 mEq of sodium per day, tense ascites can be avoided in most patients by removing approximately 8 liters of fluid every 2 weeks (282, 283). With some urinary sodium present the time interval required for repeat paracentesis can be extended, while excessive dietary sodium intake will tend to shorten the time interval between procedures.

Large volume paracentesis has been proven to be a safe and effective means to manage cirrhotic patients with tense ascites. In addition to cosmetic and symptomatic benefits, removal of ascites lowers intraabdominal pressure (265). Intrathoracic pressure also falls as a result of increased mobility of the diaphragm. These changes are associated with a reduction in portal pressure, increased cardiac output, decreased activation of neurohumoral effector mechanisms, and a slight improvement in the serum creatinine concentration (194, 265). These effects are transient in nature returning to baseline values by 6 days. Large volume paracentesis has also been shown to reduce intravariceal pressure and variceal wall tension (169).

The need to administer albumin in conjunction with large-volume paracentesis is controversial. The rational for administering albumin would be to minimize effective intravascular volume depletion and renal impairment that could potentially develop as ascitic fluid reaccumulates. Gines et al. (116) studied 105 patients with tense ascites undergoing large-volume paracentesis and randomized the subjects to receive albumin (10 g/liter of ascites removed) or no albumin. Patients not receiving albumin were more likely to show signs of hemodynamic deterioration including an increase in the plasma renin activity; these patients were also much more likely to develop worsening renal function and/or severe hyponatremia (116). More recently, Gines et al. performed total paracentesis in 280 patients with tense ascites and randomized the subjects to replacement with different types of colloid to include albumin, dextran 70, or polygeline (115). Postparacentesis circulatory dysfunction (defined as a >50% increase in plasma renin activity 6 days after the procedure) developed in 85 patients. Of the various replacement fluids, postparacentesis circulatory dysfunction was much less common with albumin administration (19% vs 34% and 38%, respectively). This benefit was limited to patients in whom at least 5 liters of ascitic fluid was removed.

Other studies have shown that large-volume paracentesis can be performed without a deleterious effect on systemic or renal hemodynamics even though albumin has not been given (250, 261). In addition, there is no direct evidence that such replacement therapy impacts on the long term morbidity and mortality of patients with cirrhosis and ascites (217, 282, 283).

Peritoneovenous Shunting Peritoneovenous shunting has been used in the treatment of diuretic-resistant ascites. This procedure allows for ascites to be reinfused into the vascular space by way of the internal jugular vein. In patients with refractory ascites and renal failure due to the hepatorenal syndrome, peritoneovenous shunting has been associated with increased urinary sodium excretion and improved renal function (96, 314). However, the procedure is now rarely performed due to a high complication rate and the lack of survival advantage when compared to medical therapy (114, 308).

Transjugular Intrahepatic Portosystemic Shunt Placement of a transjugular intrahepatic portosystemic shunt (TIPS) is a procedure that lowers intrahepatic and portal pressure. TIPS has primarily been employed as a treatment to control variceal bleeding but also appears to be an effective therapy in refractory ascites. In uncontrolled studies, TIPS has been shown to exert a diuretic effect sufficient enough to reduce and in some cases eliminate the presence of ascites (235, 305). In patients who respond, the dose of diuretics subsequently needed to control ascites can be markedly reduced (235, 305). The maximal benefit on renal function and urinary sodium excretion is often not seen for several weeks following the procedure (338). This delayed natriuretic effect may be related to the increased systemic vasodilation that typically develops immediately after insertion of the shunt (338, 339). This vasodilatory response may be due to increased delivery of vasodilators such as nitric oxide from the splanchnic circulation to the systemic circulation (339). In a small series of patients with hepatorenal syndrome, TIPS was found to improve renal function and reduce the activity of several vasoconstrictor systems (123). Despite the apparent benefit, a recently published randomized controlled trial comparing TIPS to paracentesis found that patient mortality was higher in the TIPS group, particularly in patients with Child-Pugh class C (174). In addition, TIPS placement is associated with a variety of complications that include encephalopathy and stent thrombosis or stenosis (286).

Summary

The sequence in which the various therapies discussed above are instituted can be viewed as a continuum that parallels the severity of the underlying cirrhotic state (Fig. 8). In the earliest stages of the disease, urinary sodium excretion is plentiful and negative salt balance can be achieved by simply

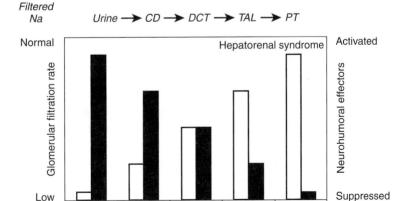

Renal function in cirrhosis: a continuum

FIGURE 8 The fall in glomerular filtration rate (*solid bars*) and activation of neurohumoral effectors (*open bars*) can be viewed as a continuum that varies according to severity of the underlying cirrhotic process. As the disease advances, the urinary Na concentration falls. The filtered load of Na is completely reabsorbed at progressively more proximal sites along the nephron. A patient with hepatorenal syndrome is merely at the end of this continuum when the glomerular filtration rate has fallen sufficiently to cause significant azotemnia.

lowering dietary sodium intake. As the disease advances neurohumoral effectors become more activated initially resulting in more intense renal salt retention and later in a progressive decline in renal function. Eventually the filtered load of sodium becomes completely reabsorbed by the tubule such that the final urine becomes virtually devoid of salt. If some component of the filtered load reaches the collecting duct or beyond, spironolactone will be effective in increasing urinary sodium excretion. Once sodium reabsorption is complete proximal to the collecting duct then thiazides and later loop diuretics will have to be added to spironolactone in order to increase urinary sodium excretion. Eventually the filtered load is completely reabsorbed proximal to the thick ascending loop of Henle. At this point the patient is resistant to the effects of diuretics and requires more invasive procedures such as repetitive large-volume paracentesis in order to remain in salt balance. In the terminal stages of the disease, the glomerular filtration rate falls to such a degree that oliguria, azotemia, and eventually uremia are present and the patient is clinically diagnosed with hepatorenal syndrome. Vasoconstrictive input focused on the kidney is severe. The renal failure is functional in nature, however, since restoration of near normal renal function can be obtained following a liver transplant.

NEPHROTIC SYNDROME

The development of edema is one of the cardinal features of nephrotic syndrome. The mechanism of its formation is not entirely understood. The classical view of edema formation in the nephrotic syndrome describes the process as an underfill mechanism. According to this theory, urinary loss of protein results in hypoalbuminemia and decreased plasma oncotic pressure. As a result, plasma water translocates from the intravascular space into the interstitial space. When the magnitude of this transudation is sufficiently great, clinically detectable edema develops. Reduction in intravascular volume elicits activation of effector mechanisms that signal renal salt and water retention in an attempt to restore plasma volume. The renal response leads to further dilution of plasma protein concentration thereby exaggerating the already reduced plasma oncotic pressure and further enhancing edema formation. In order for this formulation of edema genesis to be true, three critical predictions must be satisfied: (1) blood and plasma volume must be reduced during accumulation of edema; (2) measurement of neurohumoral effectors should reflect activation consequent to contraction of effective arterial blood volume; and (3) maneuvers that increase plasma volume into the normal range should result in a natriuretic response. As discussed below, these predictions are satisfied in some patients, especially those with minimal-change nephrotic syndrome, whereas the majority of nephrotic patients fail to conform to this conceptual model.

Blood and Plasma Volume in Nephrotic Syndrome

The classical view of edema formation assigns a pivotal role to decreased plasma volume serving as the afferent mechanism signaling renal salt and water retention. When measured directly plasma volume has indeed been low in a variable proportion of patients with nephrotic syndrome (171, 209, 319). Even in patients judged to be normovolemic, an exaggerated fall in plasma volume has been observed when nephrotic patients go from the recumbent to standing position (88, 146). This orthostatic reduction in plasma volume can be profound and may, in part, explain the development of acute oliguric renal failure and hypovolemic shock that has been reported in patients with nephrotic syndrome (302).

Most studies, however, have failed to find a consistent reduction in blood and plasma volume in patients with nephrotic syndrome (79, 89, 110, 160). In a survey of 10 studies, plasma volume measurements were analyzed in 217 nephrotic patients (80). In only one-third of patients was plasma volume reduced, whereas it was normal in 42% and increased in 25%. It has been suggested that conflicting measurements of plasma volume in patients with nephrotic syndrome can be reconciled by separating patients according to histologic class (208). In this regard, one study compared the volume status of four patients with minimal change disease to that in five patients with membranous or membranoproliferative lesions (208). In patients with minimal change disease, plasma volume was decreased and plasma renin activity and aldosterone levels were increased. By contrast, plasma volume was either normal or increased and plasma renin activity was suppressed in the latter group. These authors concluded that edema formation in minimal change disease was primarily the result of decreased effective circulatory volume inciting secondary renal salt retention. By contrast, patients with more distorted glomerular architecture were felt to have a primary defect in renal salt excretion leading secondarily to an expanded plasma volume and eventually formation of edema.

Other studies have failed to find such a correlation between histology and plasma volume measurements. Even in patients with untreated minimal change disease, plasma volume has been found to be increased (80). In order to avoid potential methodologic problems, a recent study first established a reference frame for blood volume that was normalized to lean body mass and measured directly from plasma volume and red cell volume in otherwise normal children (328). Blood volume measurements in children with nephrotic syndrome due to minimal change disease as well as other histologic lesions were all found to be within this defined normal range. Following successful therapy with steroids, patients with minimal change disease demonstrate a fall in plasma volume and blood pressure and an increase in plasma renin activity (80). These changes are exactly the opposite of what one would expect if arterial underfilling were the proximate cause of renal salt retention. Finally, a large study of nephrotic patients, including 35 patients with minimal change disease, found virtually all patients have normal or increased plasma and blood volume (109).

Neurohumoral Markers of Effective Circulatory Volume

Measurements of plasma renin activity and aldosterone concentration have been utilized as a method to indirectly differentiate primary sodium retention from an underfill mechanism of edema formation in nephrotic patients. Elevated values would be expected if blood volume was decreased, while suppressed values would occur in the setting of primary renal sodium retention and blood volume expansion. In this regard, plasma renin activity values collated from nine studies were found to be normal or low in 64 of 123 patients investigated (79). Plasma aldosterone levels were also decreased in the majority of these patients. When measured with respect to salt intake or urinary sodium excretion no consistent relationship was found. While some studies have found elevated plasma renin activity and aldosterone concentrations in patients with minimal change diseases others have not (127, 208). In a study examining plasma renin activity with respect to blood volume, no relationship was found in either patients with minimal change disease or those with histologic lesions on light microscopy (110). Although a higher proportion of patients with minimal change disease have elevated plasma renin and aldosterone levels as compared to those with histologic glomerular lesions these values tend to overlap (110, 127). Thus, measurement of various elements of the renin-angiotensin-aldosterone axis suggests that an underfill mechanism may mediate renal sodium retention in some but not all patients with nephrotic syndrome.

Effects of Manipulations to Expand Central Blood Volume

Another approach utilized to investigate the pathogenesis of sodium retention in the nephrotic syndrome has been to examine renal sodium handling and hormonal indices of effective circulatory volume in response to expansion of the intravascular blood volume. This has been primarily achieved by infusing albumin or expanding central blood volume by head-out body water immersion (HWI). The classical view of nephrotic edema would predict that expansion of the intravascular volume should correct renal salt and water retention. In children with minimal change disease, infusion of albumin has been reported to decrease plasma renin activity, arginine vasopressin (AVP), aldosterone, and catecholamines (272, 316). In association with these hormonal changes, there was a significant increase in the glomerular filtration rate, urine flow, and sodium excretion. In a less homogenous group of adult patients with nephrotic syndrome, baseline blood volumes were found to be low when expressed per kilogram wet weight (320). Plasma AVP was inversely correlated with blood volume and failed to decrease in response

to a water load. When blood volume was expanded with 20% albumin, plasma levels of AVP fell accompanied by an augmented water diuresis. It was concluded that a contracted blood volume was responsible for the nonosmotic release of AVP. By contrast, other studies have found either no or only a minimal increase in urinary sodium excretion in response to infusion of albumin. In one study, infusion of hyperoncotic albumin in quantities sufficient to expand blood volume by 35% resulted in only a modest natriuretic response (160). In order to exclude the possibility that the blunted natriuretic response was due to an increase in peritubular colloid osmotic pressure, similar studies have been performed utilizing a prolonged infusion of iso-oncotic albumin. This maneuver was similarly accompanied by only a modest increase in sodium excretion such that the patients remained in positive salt balance (270). Studies utilizing HWI to expand blood volume have likewise produced conflicting results. Expansion of central blood volume by HWI in children with minimal change disease resulted in decreased levels of AVP, aldosterone, noradrenaline and plasma renin activity (272, 273). These changes were accompanied by significant increases in urine flow and sodium excretion. Similarly, adult patients with a variety of histologic lesions subjected to HWI were found to have significant increases in urinary sodium excretion (28, 170). By contrast, a more recent study in 10 patients with a variety of underlying glomerular diseases found only a blunted natriuretic response to HWI (257). While ANP levels rose to the same extent in control and nephrotic subjects suggesting equivalent degrees of volume expansion, peak urinary sodium excretion and urine flow in the nephrotic patients were one-third that in the control group.

A number of other observations also question the pivotal role assigned to hypoalbuminemia and reduced plasma oncotic pressure in the initiation of edema formation (10, 145, 146). For example, reducing plasma protein concentration in humans (10) or experimental animals (145, 146) with plasmapheresis results in either no change or actually increases plasma volume. In addition, patients with congenital analbuminemia demonstrate no disturbance in water and electrolyte balance and do not necessarily develop edema. Despite the reduction in plasma oncotic pressure, these patients exhibit an exaggerated natriuretic response when administered isotonic saline.

In summary, available data would argue for a contracted plasma volume as the afferent mechanism initiating sodium retention in some but not all patients with nephrotic syndrome. Rather, some component of primary renal sodium retention appears to be operative in nephrotic syndrome with histologic glomerular lesions as well as in many patients with minimal change disease (Table 4). Although children with minimal change nephrotic syndrome more often have low blood volume and increased renin-aldosterone profiles, coexistence of a primary impairment in renal sodium excretion cannot be excluded. In this regard, the natriuresis seen in patients recovering from minimal change disease occurs

TABLE 4 Evidence for Primary Renal Sodium Retention in Nephrotic Syndrome

Blood volume is often normal or increased.
Blood pressure is often increased.
Renin activity and aldosterone levels are not uniformly increased.
Onset of natriuresis during recovery precedes rise in plasma protein concentration.
Sodium excretion is modest in response to head-out water immersion or albumin infusion.
Experimental models
  Sodium retention in a unilateral nephrosis model is confined to the diseased kidney.
  Kidneys taken from nephrotic animals and perfused in vitro retain Na.

concurrently with a rise in filtration fraction (157). If an underfill mechanism were operative, one would have expected the baseline filtration fraction to be increased and then to fall with successful treatment. In addition, resolution of salt retention in response to steroid treatment has been shown to occur in the setting of persistent hypoproteinemia (46). Furthermore, the natriuresis and correction of the antinatriuretic neurohumoral profile demonstrated in studies using albumin infusions and HWI may have resulted from central blood volume expansion of a sufficient degree necessary to overcome a primary salt retaining state. Studies in experimental animals are also consistent with a defect intrinsic to the nephrotic kidney as the mechanism responsible for salt retention in the nephrotic syndrome. In the rat model of unilateral proteinuric renal disease induced by infusing puromycin aminonucleoside (PAN) into one kidney, diminished urinary sodium excretion was confined to the proteinuric kidney despite the fact that each kidney shared the same systemic milieu (138). In kidneys taken from rats previously exposed to PAN and then perfused in vitro, less sodium was excreted as compared to kidneys taken from control rats. Utilizing this experimental design, the defect in renal salt excretion was found to be localized to the kidney as systemic and circulating factors were eliminated.

In some patients, both primary salt retention as well as underfill mechanisms of edema formation may coexist. For example, in the earliest stages of a glomerular disease salt retention by the kidney may be primary in origin. As hypoalbuminemia develops and becomes progressively severe, plasma volume may fall and result in an element of superimposed secondary salt retention. The coexistence of these two mechanisms may account for the lack of uniformity in hemodynamic as well as hormonal and neurocirculatory profiles in patients with nephrotic syndrome.

Peripheral Capillary Mechanisms of Edema Formation

The presence of normal or increased plasma volume in the setting of a decreased serum albumin concentration is difficult to reconcile with the classical view of edema formation in the nephrotic syndrome. These findings can best be ex-

plained by examining the alterations that are known to occur in transcapillary exchange mechanisms in the setting of hypoproteinemia.

Fluid movement within the capillary bed between intravascular and interstitial spaces is determined by the balance of Starling forces between these two compartments:

$$J_v = K_f[(P_c - P_i) - (\pi_c - \pi_i)]$$

where J_v is fluid flux along the length of a capillary, K_f is the ultrafiltration coefficient, P_c is capillary hydrostatic pressure, P_i is interstitial hydrostatic pressure, π_c is capillary oncotic pressure, and π_i is interstitial oncotic pressure. On the arterial side of the capillary, the net hydrostatic pressure gradient $P_c - P_i$ (P) exceeds the net colloid osmotic pressure gradient $\pi_c - \pi_i$ (π) resulting in net filtration of fluid into the interstitial space. Due to an axial fall in capillary hydrostatic pressure, the balance of Starling forces at the venous end of the capillary ($\pi > P$) favors net reabsorption of fluid back into the capillary. In some tissues, net hydrostatic pressure exceeds opposing net colloid osmotic pressure throughout the length of the capillary such that filtration occurs along its entire length. Net ultrafiltrate is returned to the circulation via lymphatic flow such that in steady-state conditions total body capillary flux is equal to lymph flow; interstitial and intravascular volume remain stable and edema formation does not occur.

Absence of compensatory mechanisms would predict that small changes in P, π, or K_f would lead to increased fluid transudation and result in clinically detectable edema. However, the poor correlation between plasma albumin concentration and the presence or absence of edema suggests that counterregulatory adjustments do occur in those forces that govern fluid exchange between the intravascular and interstitial space (Table 5). One such factor relates to compliance characteristics of the interstitium (126). Under normal circumstances interstitial pressure ranges from −6 mm Hg to 0 mm Hg. Due to the noncompliant nature of this compartment small increases in interstitial volume result in large increases in interstitial pressure. Such increases in P_i act to oppose further transudation of fluid and provide an initial defense against the formation of edema. Increased interstitial pressure leads to the development of a second factor that also protects against edema formation, namely, increased lymphatic flow. Lymph flow can increase many fold under conditions of augmented net capillary fluid filtration. In patients with edema resulting from heart failure or nephrosis, the disappearance rate of a subcutaneous injection of ^{131}I-albumin is markedly enhanced consistent with increased lymphatic flow (133).

TABLE 5 Edema Defense Mechanisms That Limit Excessive Capillary Fluid Filtration

↑ Interstitial hydrostatic pressure
↑ Lymph flow
↓ Interstitial oncotic pressure
↓ Permeability of the capillary to protein

A third factor that minimizes fluid filtration is a reduction in interstitial oncotic pressure (102). In normal human plasma, colloid oncotic pressure (COP) is about 24 mm Hg and interstitial COP is about 12 mm Hg creating a transcapillary COP gradient of about 12 mm Hg (146). Since transcapillary fluid flux consists primarily of a protein-free ultrafiltrate, interstitial protein concentration tends to become diluted. In addition, increased lymphatic flow removes fluid and protein from the interstitial space and returns both to the vascular compartment thereby further reducing interstitial oncotic pressure. Body albumin pools are redistributed such that a greater fraction than normal is located in the vascular compartment (146). As hypoalbuminemia develops in the nephrotic syndrome, the COP of the interstitial fluid space falls in parallel with the COP of plasma (134, 159, 161). Nephrotic patients studied both in remission and in relapse demonstrate almost equivalent changes in the COP of plasma and the interstitium at all levels of serum albumin (161). The maintenance of the net COP gradient within the normal range mitigates this potential driving force for transudation of fluid into the interstitial space. A final factor that favors decreased fluid filtration is a change in the permeability of the capillary. Under conditions of hypoalbuminemia, the intrinsic permeability of the capillary to protein tends to decrease thereby increasing π_c along the capillary (341).

In summary, the reduction in serum oncotic pressure that accompanies the nephrotic syndrome would be predicted to alter Starling forces in a direction favoring net flux of fluid across the capillary bed. Despite this alteration, however, fluid tends not to accumulate within the interstitium in response to hypoalbuminemia because of the activation of a series of defense mechanisms that serve to oppose those forces favoring fluid movement from the intravascular space. These edema-preventing factors include increased interstitial hydrostatic pressure, accelerated lymphatic flow, a parallel decline in plasma and interstitial oncotic pressure, and decreased capillary permeability to protein. However, in the setting of ongoing primary renal salt retention, these buffering mechanisms become exhausted and clinically apparent edema may become evident. This occurs because salt retention leads to increases in capillary hydrostatic pressure at the very time defense mechanisms normally employed to prevent edema have been maximized. In the hypoproteinemic patient without salt retention, edema-preventing factors may be sufficient to protect against the development of edema. Thus, edema formation in the nephrotic syndrome results from the combined effects of primary salt retention coupled with exhausted defenses against edema (Fig. 9).

The changes in mean arterial pressure and blood volume as a function of varying extracellular fluid volume in hypoalbuminemic nephrotic patients as compared to normoalbuminemic chronic renal-failure patients illustrates these principles (158). In hypoalbuminemic patients with nephrotic syndrome, expansion of the extracellular fluid volume leads to immediate translocation of fluid into the extravascular space as evidenced by little change in mean arterial pressure

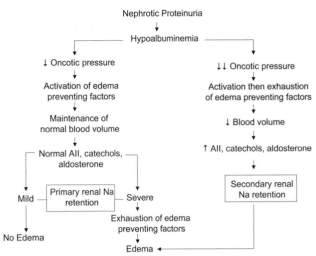

FIGURE 9 The left side of the figure depicts the mechanism of edema formation in most patients with nephrotic syndrome. An important variable that helps to explain the poor correlation between serum albumin concentration and the presence or absence of edema is the degree of primary renal Na retention. With severe Na retention by the kidney, edema-preventing factors become exhausted and edema becomes clinically apparent even when the serum albumin concentration is only mildly depressed. In the setting of mild renal Na retention, these factors remain adequate to prevent edema formation even in the presence of severe hypoalbuminemia. The right side of the figure depicts the classical view of edema formation in which low blood volume serves as the signal for secondary renal Na retention. This mechanism of edema formation is most commonly present in children with minimal change disease. In some patients, both mechanisms of edema formation may be operative. For example, early in the nephrotic syndrome, blood volume is normal and only primary renal Na retention is present. With worsening hypoalbuminemia, blood volume may begin to fall and result in a component of superimposed secondary renal Na retention.

or blood volume. Presumably, factors that serve to prevent edema are already maximized, and are overwhelmed by increases in capillary hydrostatic pressure that occur as a result of extracellular fluid volume expansion. By contrast, normoalbuminemic patients with chronic renal failure develop an increase in mean arterial pressure and blood volume as extracellular fluid volume expands. In these patients, more of the fluid is retained in the vascular tree due to activation of edema preventing factors. At some point of extracellular fluid volume expansion, these factors would also become overwhelmed and clinically detectable edema would develop.

Mechanism of Salt Retention in Nephrotic Syndrome

The intrarenal mechanism responsible for primary sodium retention in nephrotic syndrome has been examined in both experimental studies and clinical studies. A role for reduced GFR contributing to impaired sodium and water excretion was suggested in a study of nine adult patients with nephrotic syndrome due to various causes (298). Baseline inulin clearances were found to be lower in the subset of patients with an impaired capacity to excrete a water load. When these same subjects underwent HWI, increases in sodium and water excretion were found to be correlated with increases in inulin clearance. This improvement was unassociated with a variety of other measured hemodynamic or neurohumoral factors suggesting an important role for GFR. However, other studies show that sodium excretion can be regulated independently from GFR in the nephrotic state. For example, in an animal model of nephrosis, administration of saralasin was found to increase GFR but did not enhance sodium excretion (138). In addition, many patients with nephrotic syndrome have normal or increased GFR and yet avidly retain sodium.

The bulk of experimental and clinical data implicate a tubular mechanism as the primary cause of salt retention in the nephrotic syndrome. Both experimental and clinical studies suggest that proximal reabsorption is decreased and implicate the distal nephron as the site responsible for sodium retention. Utilizing clearance techniques proximal sodium handling was assessed during diuretic-induced distal tubular blockade using chlorothiazide and ethacrynic acid (120). Nephrotic patients exhibited a greater natriuretic response than controls suggesting that distal nephron sites were responsible for enhanced sodium reabsorption. Measurement of tubular glucose handling has been used as a marker of proximal sodium reabsorption (319). In a group of nephrotic patients, glucose titration curves revealed a reduced threshold for glucose reabsorption further suggesting diminished proximal sodium reabsorption. In volume-expanded rats with autologous immune complex nephritis, a model that resembles membranous nephropathy, micropuncture and clearance methodology were used to study the site of sodium retention (29). Absolute proximal sodium reabsorption was decreased in nephrotic rats, while sodium delivery to the late distal tubule of superficial nephrons was comparable in control as well as nephrotic animals. Since fractional excretion of sodium was significantly lower in nephrotic versus control rats, the collecting duct was suggested as a possible site of altered handling of sodium. Enhanced sodium reabsorption in juxtamedullary nephrons not accessible to micropuncture could not be excluded. In the rat model of unilateral proteinuric renal disease induced by infusing PAN into one kidney, diminished urinary sodium excretion was confined to the proteinuric kidney (138). Since sodium delivery to the initial portion of the collecting duct was similar to the control kidney, increased sodium reabsorption at the collecting duct must have been the primary site of salt retention.

Neurohumoral Control of Enhanced Tubular Sodium Excretion

RENIN-ANGIOTENSIN-ALDOSTERONE

Studies demonstrating increased sodium retaining activity in the urine of nephrotic patients lead early investigators to suggest that aldosterone might play an important role in mediating sodium retention in the nephrotic syndrome (196). In rats made nephrotic with PAN, juxtaglomerular cell granularity was found to vary directly with the degree of sodium re-

tention (315). In this same model, prior adrenalectomy prevented sodium retention that otherwise occurred in nephrotic controls with intact capacity to secrete aldosterone (149). When plasma renin activity and aldosterone concentrations were measured in a large group of nephrotic patients placed on a low sodium diet values varied widely although a negative correlation was found between urinary sodium and plasma aldosterone concentration (110). In a study of five nephrotic patients placed on a high salt diet for 8 days, plasma renin activity and plasma aldosterone levels were similar in both nephrotic subjects and control subjects (300). Administration of the aldosterone antagonist, spironolactone, on day 4 of the study resulted in an increase in urinary sodium excretion in the nephrotic patients, while no change was observed in the control group. Since aldosterone exerts salt-retaining effects on the distal nephron, a site implicated in formation of nephrotic edema, excess aldosterone activity is an attractive explanation for observed salt retention. Most data, however, fail to confirm an important role for aldosterone. In patients spontaneously retaining sodium, measurements of plasma renin activity and aldosterone concentration may be either low or high (44, 47). This disassociation is also seen during steroid-induced remission of nephrotic syndrome. In four patients with minimal change disease, plasma renin and aldosterone concentrations fell during steroid induced diuresis but once in remission these hormones returned to the same plasma concentrations observed when edema was present (208). Studies involving administration of either saralasin or converting enzyme inhibitors also fail to support an important role for the renin-angiotensin-aldosterone system in mediating salt retention (45, 47, 83). In nephrotic patients selected for high plasma renin activity, captopril administration also failed to prevent sodium retention despite producing marked reductions in plasma aldosterone (45). In the unilateral model of PAN-induced nephrosis, infusion of saralasin led to substantial increases in total kidney and single-nephron GFR of the perfused kidney, but urinary sodium excretion remained unchanged (138). This observation lends support for an intrarenal mechanism of salt retention independent of changes in GFR or activation of the renin-angiotensin-aldosterone system.

SYMPATHETIC NERVOUS SYSTEM

Increased plasma and urinary catecholamine concentrations have been found in patients with nephrotic syndrome (150, 239). The role of renal sympathetic nerve activity in mediating salt retention in nephrotic syndrome has been studied in rats made nephrotic by injection of adriamycin. An impaired ability to excrete an acute oral or intravenous isotonic saline load was improved by bilateral renal denervation (67). In response to acute infusion of saline, efferent renal sympathetic-nerve activity decreased to a lesser extent than that in control rats. Metabolic balance studies carried out over 26 days revealed an overall decrease in cumulative sodium balance only in those nephrotic rats with bilateral renal denervation (130). It was concluded that renal nerves are an important effector mechanism in the chronic renal sodium retention that characterizes the nephrotic syndrome. Given the evidence for a distal nephron site of sodium reabsorption in nephrotic syndrome, it is noteworthy that beta-adrenergic stimulation of rabbit cortical collecting tubules enhances chloride transport (139). Other studies show that enhanced sodium retention in nephrotic syndrome cannot be entirely explained by sympathetic nervous system activity. In kidneys taken from rats previously exposed to puromycin aminonucleoside and perfused in vitro, less sodium is excreted as compared to kidneys taken from control animals (105). In this preparation, extrinsic neural factors are eliminated. In the adriamycin model of nephrosis, bilateral renal denervation similarly did not correct the blunted volume expansion natriuresis observed in nephrotic rats (322).

ATRIAL NATRIURETIC PEPTIDE

Levels of ANP are reported to be normal or slightly elevated in patients with nephrotic syndrome (316). In animal models of the nephrotic syndrome, renal responsiveness to ANP has generally been found to be blunted (254). In contrast, infusion of synthetic human ANP to nephrotic patients results in increased sodium and water excretion similar to that in normal subjects (346). Infusion of albumin in children with nephrotic syndrome resulted in a rise in ANP levels that closely correlated with urinary sodium excretion. However, other studies have found a blunted natriuretic response to ANP in nephrotic patients (254). It has been proposed that enhanced distal sodium reabsorption in the nephrotic syndrome may, in part, be due to resistance of the collecting duct to the natriuretic actions of ANP (249, 255). The cellular basis of this resistance does not appear to be an abnormality in ANP binding to its receptor. Rather, the mechanism appears to be an inability to generate adequate amounts of the intracellular cGMP as a result of heightened activity of intracellular cGMP phosphodiesterase (323).

In summary, edema formation in the majority of patients with nephrotic syndrome can best be explained by an over-fill mechanism. The maintenance of a normal plasma volume in the setting of hypoalbuminemia is the result of a series of edema preventing factors that act to both oppose fluid filtration across the capillary wall and to return fluid back into the vascular tree. The single most important variable in determining whether these factors are sufficient to prevent edema formation is the degree of renal salt retention. The variability in renal salt retention explains the poor correlation between the presence or absence of edema and the serum albumin concentration. In patients with severe hypoalbuminemia and no edema, renal salt retention is likely to be minimal such that edema preventing factors are sufficient in preventing excessive fluid filtration across the capillary wall. By contrast, edematous patients with near normal serum albumin concentration are more likely to have avid renal salt retention such that the factors opposing fluid filtration become exhausted. The defect in renal salt excretion has not been precisely localized but appears to reside in the distal nephron. The exact mechanism underlying this defect is unknown.

SODIUM WASTAGE

Renal salt wastage may be defined as persistent inappropriate renal loss of sodium from the body sufficient in magnitude to result in shrinkage of extracellular fluid volume causing azotemia, hypotension, and when extreme, circulatory collapse. When evaluating the relationship between urine sodium excretion and dietary intake the initial status of the extracellular fluid volume must be taken into consideration before concluding renal salt wasting is present. For example, renal salt wasting should not be considered present when urine sodium excretion greatly exceeds dietary intake in edematous patients placed on a low-salt diet. In this instance, negative salt balance is an appropriate response to correct the volume expanded state. As extracellular fluid volume normalizes the natriuresis will stop and sodium balance will be reestablished. By contrast, the imposition of a salt restricted diet to a euvolemic patient with chronic kidney disease may result in negative salt balance and contraction of extracellular fluid volume below normal limits. Even though the cumulative amount of sodium lost from the body may be far less than in the diuresing edematous patient, renal salt wasting is considered present since the reduction of extracellular fluid volume has fallen below normal. In this setting, worsening azotemia and hypotension may be present. The critical feature of renal salt wasting is the continued shrinkage of extracellular fluid volume below the lower limit of normal as a result of ongoing natriuresis. Disorders of renal salt wasting can be divided into intrinsic disorders of the kidney and disorders of efferent mechanisms that regulate renal sodium handling.

Intrinsic Renal Disease

CHRONIC KIDNEY DISEASE

Patients with advanced chronic kidney disease may exhibit mild renal salt wastage when subjected to rigid dietary sodium restriction. The pathogenesis of salt wastage is related to the adaptive increase in perfusion of remaining viable nephrons as total nephron mass progressively declines. Accompanying nephron hyperperfusion is a large increase in solute load. This solute load exceeds the reabsorptive capacity of remaining nephrons resulting in increased excretion of salt and water. The nephrons of patients with chronic kidney disease are continuously undergoing an osmotic diuresis of solutes including urea and the sodium salts of acids.

Studies by Coleman et al. (61), support an important role of osmotic diuresis in hyperfiltering nephrons in the genesis of salt wastage in chronic kidney disease. In these experiments, patients with chronic kidney disease are placed on a low sodium diet and then subjected to a water diuresis. As urine volume increases the urine sodium concentration falls to a minimum value and thereafter remains fixed. At this point urine sodium excretion increases in parallel with further increases in urine flow rates. In salt-restricted normal participants subjected to a water diuresis combined with mannitol diuresis, the urine sodium concentration at which flow dependence of urine sodium excretion commences is greater as compared to the level during water diuresis alone. These data indicate that an osmotic diuresis is at least in part responsible for the mild salt wastage observed in patients with chronic kidney disease.

Clinical evidence of salt wastage in most patients with chronic kidney disease is typically only found when dietary salt restriction is extreme. Patients ingesting a dietary sodium of 10–15 mEq/day require a much longer period of time to establish salt balance as compared to normals and in many patients salt balance is never achieved. A persistent negative sodium balance leads to volume depletion, weight loss, relative hypotension, and worsening azotemia. In most instances, these findings are seen during the course of an intercurrent illness when salt intake is abruptly stopped or markedly reduced.

There are several reports in the literature in which renal salt wastage is more severe (53). Most of these cases have been described in patients with what appears to be chronic tubulointerstitial disease accompanied by cystic transformation of the renal medulla. In these unusual cases, urine sodium excretion is of such a magnitude that contraction of extracellular fluid volume develops in the setting of normal salt intake. Medullary cystic disease is an autosomal recessive disorder with cystic changes in corticomedullary and medullary regions of the kidney in which renal salt wastage can be severe.

ACUTE RENAL FAILURE

Transient renal salt wastage is often seen in patients during the recovery phase of acute tubular necrosis. The magnitude of the natriuresis is a function of the amount of salt and water retained as the renal failure developed. Massive salt wasting leading to volume depletion and cardiovascular collapse is not a feature of this disorder. Some degree of salt wastage is often seen following the relief of urinary obstruction. The excretion of retained urea and other solutes contribute to an osmotic diuresis and account for the natriuresis. However, persistent salt wastage after these solutes are cleared does not typically occur.

RENAL TUBULAR DISORDERS

Proximal or type II renal tubular acidosis is associated with renal salt wastage owing to the loss of sodium bicarbonate into the urine. Defective proximal acidification leads to a large increase in distal sodium bicarbonate delivery that is subsequently lost into the urine. The bicarbonaturic effect will continue until the serum bicarbonate concentration falls to a level that matches the reabsorptive capacity of the proximal nephron at which point sodium wastage will cease. As a result, salt wastage is transient in this disorder but nevertheless causes mild volume depletion from inappropriate renal salt loss.

Distal or type I renal tubular acidosis is also characterized by a mild form of renal salt wastage. The defect in distal acidification leads to the development of a hyperchloremic metabolic acidosis. Systemic acidosis impairs proximal salt reabsorption resulting in mild sodium wastage.

Bartter's and Gitelman's syndromes are characterized by renal salt wastage due to genetic defects in ion transporters involved in sodium reabsorption. In Bartter's syndrome impaired salt transport is localized to the thick ascending limb, while in Gitelman's syndrome the defect is localized to the distal convoluted tubule.

A variety of drugs can cause renal salt wastage as a result of tubular injury. This injury can be due to direct toxic effects of the drug as with Cis-platinum, aminoglycosides, and amphotericin B or be the result of acute tubulointerstitial nephritis as reported with methicillin and trimethoprim/sulfamethoxazole.

Disorders of Effector Mechanisms That Regulate Renal Sodium Transport

DECREASED MINERALOCORTICOID ACTIVITY

Mineralocorticoid activity plays an important role in renal sodium conservation. Decreased activity and renal resistance to mineralocorticoids are causes of renal sodium wastage (345). The most clinically relevant form of mineralocorticoid deficiency results from primary diseases of the adrenal cortex. These diseases may either be acquired or congenital in origin. Subnormal aldosterone secretory rates leads to decreased reabsorption of sodium chloride in the cortical collecting tubule of the kidney. The kidney is fundamentally intact and the cortical collecting tubule cell responds normally to exogenously administered mineralocorticoids.

Renal salt wastage is a hallmark of Addison's disease in which patients may demonstrate severe volume depletion and cardiovascular collapse. Addison's disease results from progressive adrenocortical destruction leading to deficiencies in glucocorticoid and mineralocorticoid activity. These patients present with anorexia, vomiting, abdominal pain, weight loss, weakness, and salt craving. Physical examination reveals generalized hyperpigmentation particularly in skin folds and the axillae as well as bluish-grey hyperpigmentation of the lingual and buccal mucosa. Orthostatic hypotension is very common, indicative of volume depletion. Laboratory examination reveals an increased blood urea nitrogen to creatinine ratio characteristic of prerenal azotemia and elevated urinary sodium concentration. Hyponatremia, hyperkalemia and hyperchloremic metabolic acidosis are the characteristic electrolyte abnormalities.

Isolated aldosterone deficiency accompanied by normal glucocorticoid production occurs in association with hyporeninism, as an inherited biosynthetic defect, during protracted heparin administration, and postoperatively following the removal of an aldosterone secreting adenoma. These patients have an inadequate ability to release aldosterone during salt restriction. In severe cases, salt wastage may be present on a normal salt intake.

MINERALOCORTICOID UNRESPONSIVENESS

Defective transport of sodium may also result from abnormalities in tubular responsiveness to aldosterone. Disorders in which there is a resistance to aldosterone have been localized to abnormalities in the mineralocorticoid receptor and to postreceptor defects in the epithelial sodium channel (ENaC) (345).

Pseudohypoaldosteronism type I is an inherited disorder of salt wasting that presents in infancy. The autosomal dominant form of this disease has been linked to functional mutations in the mineralocorticoid receptor. Renal salt wasting in these patients tends to be mild and spontaneously improves as patients age. A second form of the disease is inherited in an autosomal recessive fashion and is caused by inactivating mutations in either the alpha or beta subunits of the epithelial sodium channel in the collecting duct. The clinical manifestations are more severe in this form of the disease. Patients present in infancy with severe unrelenting salt wasting, hyperkalemia, and hyperchloremic metabolic acidosis, and a failure to survive syndrome. In addition to renal manifestations, patients also display frequent respiratory tract illnesses caused by an increase in the volume of airway secretions.

CEREBRAL SALT WASTING

The concept of a CSW syndrome was first introduced by Peters and colleagues in 1950 in a report describing three patients with neurological disorders who presented with hyponatremia, clinical evidence of volume depletion, and renal sodium wasting without an obvious disturbance in the pituitary-adrenal axis (256). These findings were subsequently confirmed in additional patients with widely varying forms of cerebral disease (332). In these initial reports, it was theorized that cerebral disease could lead to renal salt wastage and subsequent depletion of ECF volume by directly influencing nervous input into the kidneys. However, with the subsequent description of SIADH by Schwartz et al. (296), the clinical entity of CSW became viewed as either an extremely rare disorder or a misnomer for what was truly SIADH.

Only in recent years has CSW been thought of as a distinct entity. CSW should be considered in patients with central nervous system disease who develop hyponatremia and otherwise meet the clinical criteria for a diagnosis of SIADH but have a volume status that is inconsistent with that diagnosis. Unlike patients with SIADH who are volume expanded, patients with CSW show evidence of negative salt balance and reductions in plasma as well as total blood volume. The onset of this disorder is typically seen within the first 10 days following a neurosurgical procedure or after a definable event, such as a subarachnoid hemor-

rhage or stroke. CSW has been described in other intracranial disorders, such as carcinomatous or infectious meningitis and metastatic carcinoma.

The mechanism by which cerebral disease leads to renal salt wasting is poorly understood. The most probable process involves disruption of neural input into the kidney and/or central elaboration of a circulating natriuretic factor (Fig. 10). By either or both mechanisms, increased urinary sodium excretion would lead to a decrease in EABV and thus provide a baroreceptor stimulus for the release of AVP. In turn, increased AVP levels would impair the ability of the kidney to elaborate a dilute urine. In this setting, the release of AVP is an appropriate response to the volume depletion. By contrast, release of AVP in SIADH is truly inappropriate, because EABV is expanded.

A probable site for depressed renal sodium absorption in CSW is the proximal nephron. Because this segment normally reabsorbs the bulk of filtered sodium, a small decrease in its efficiency would result in the delivery of large amounts of sodium to the distal nephron and ultimately, into the final urine. Decreased sympathetic input to the kidney would be a probable explanation for impaired proximal reabsorption, because the sympathetic nervous system (SNS) has been shown to alter salt and water handling in this segment through various indirect and direct mechanisms. Because the SNS also plays an important role in the control of renin release, decreased sympathetic tone could explain the failure

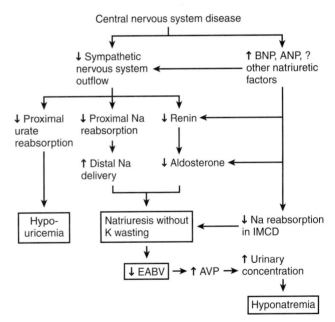

FIGURE 10 The pathophysiology of CSW. Conditions associated with increased urinary sodium excretion in the setting of volume contraction would be expected to result in renal potassium wasting because of increased delivery of sodium to the cortical collecting duct in the setting of increased aldosterone levels. The lack of renal potassium wasting in CSW can be accounted for by the failure of aldosterone to increase in spite of low extracellular fluid volume. ANP, atrial natriuretic peptide; AVP, arginine vasopressin; BNP, brain natriuretic peptide; CSW, cerebral salt wasting; EABV, effective arterial blood volume; IMCD, inner medullary collecting duct.

of circulating renin and aldosterone levels to rise in patients with CSW. The failure of serum aldosterone levels to rise in response to a decreased EABV can account for the lack of renal potassium wasting in spite of large increase in distal delivery of sodium. In this regard, hypokalemia has not been a feature of CSW.

In addition to decreased neural input to the kidney, release of one or more natriuretic factors could also play a role in the renal salt wasting observed in CSW. Atrial natriuretic peptide (ANP) and brain natriuretic peptide (BNP) have several effects that could lead to the clinical syndrome of CSW. For example, infusion of either of these peptides into normal human subjects results in a natriuretic response that is unrelated to changes in blood pressure. The ability of these compounds to increase glomerular filtration rate (GFR) accounts for some of the natriuresis; however, even in the absence of a change in GFR urinary sodium excretion increases because of a direct inhibitory effect on sodium transport in the inner medullary collecting duct. These peptides are also capable of increasing urinary sodium excretion without causing hypokalemia. For example, ANP and BNP are associated with decreased circulating levels of aldosterone because of direct inhibitory effects on renin release in the juxtaglomerular cells of the kidney as well as direct inhibitory effects on aldosterone release in the adrenal gland. In addition, inhibition of sodium reabsorption in the inner medullary collecting duct would not be expected to cause renal potassium wasting, because this segment is distal to the predominant potassium secretory site in the cortical collecting duct. As ECF volume becomes contracted proximal sodium reabsorption would increase resulting in less distal delivery of sodium to the collecting duct. Decreased sodium delivery protects against potassium wasting in the setting of high circulating levels of aldosterone.

ANP and BNP have also been shown to be capable of directly decreasing autonomic outflow through effects at the level of the brain stem. In this manner, natriuretic peptides can act synergistically with CNS disease to decrease neural input to the kidney. The evidence both for and against ANP as well as circulating ouabain-like factor as important factors in the development of CSW has been recently reviewed elsewhere.

For the various natriuretic compounds, Berendes et al. (25) have provided evidence to suggest that BNP might be the more probable candidate to mediate renal salt wasting. The authors compared 10 patients with subarachnoid hemorrhage who underwent clipping of an aneurysm to a control group comprising 10 patients who underwent craniotomy for resection of cerebral tumors. All patients with subarachnoid hemorrhage and none of the control group showed an increase in urine output accompanied by increased urinary sodium excretion that tended to peak 3–4 days following the procedure. Sodium and fluid loss in the urine was matched by intravenous replacement thus preventing the development of hyponatremia. As compared to the control group, significantly greater levels of BNP were found in the subarachnoid hemorrhage patients both before surgery and through postoperative day 8. The BNP concentration was significantly correlated with both urinary sodium excretion as well as intracranial pressure. By contrast, there were no differences in the circulating concentration of ANP or digoxin-like immunoreactive substances between the two groups. Plasma renin concentration was the same in both groups but plasma aldosterone concentrations were suppressed and varied in an opposite direction to that of BNP in the subarachnoid hemorrhage group.

BNP in humans is found primarily found in the cardiac ventricles, but also in the brain. It is not known whether brain or cardiac tissue or both contribute to the increased BNP concentration found in these patients with subarachnoid hemorrhage. Increased release of cardiac BNP could be part of a generalized stress response to the underlying illness, whereas increased intracranial pressure could provide a signal for brain BNP release. In this regard, one could speculate that the development of renal salt wasting and resultant volume depletion in the setting of intracranial disease is a protective measure limiting extreme rises in intracranial pressure. In addition, the vasodilatory properties of these natriuretic peptides might decrease the tendency for vasospasm in disorders such as subarachnoid hemorrhage.

References

1. Aalkjaer C, Frische, S, Leipziger J, et al. Sodium coupled bicarbonate transporters in the kidney, an update. *Acta Physiol Scand* 2004;181:505–512.
2. Abassi ZA, Gurbanov K, Mulroney SE, et al. Impaired nitric oxide–mediated renal vasodilation in rats with experimental heart failure: role of angiotensin II. *Circulation* 1997;96:3655–3664.
3. Abassi ZA, Kelly G, Golomb E, Klein H, Keiser HR. Losartan improves the natriuretic response to ANF in rats with high-output heart failure. *J Pharmacol Exp Ther* 1994;268:224–230.
4. Abraham WT, Hensen J, Kim JK, Durr J, Lesnefsky EJ, Groves BM, Schrier RW. Atrial natriuretic peptide and urinary cyclic guanosine monophosphate in patients with chronic heart failure. *J Am Soc Nephrol* 1992;2:1697–1703.
5. Albillos A, Colombato LA, Groszmann RJ. Vasodilatation and sodium retention in prehepatic portal hypertension. *Gastroenterology* 1992;102:931–935.
6. Alpern RJ, Howlin KJ, Preisig PA. Active and passive components of chloride transport in the rat proximal convoluted tubule. *J Clin Invest* 1985;76:1360–1366.
7. Alpern RJ. Mechanism of basolateral membrane H/OH/HCO3 transport in the rat proximal convoluted tubule: a sodium-coupled electrogenic process. *J Gen Physiol* 1985;86:613–637.
8. Alpern RJ, Cogan MG, Rector FC. Effect of luminal bicarbonate concentration on proximal acidification in the rat. *Am J Physiol* 1982;243:F53–F59.
9. Anderson RJ, Cronin RE, McDonald KM, et al. Mechanisms of portal hypertension-induced alterations in renal hemodynamics, renal water excretion, and renin secretion. *J Clin Invest* 1976;58:964–970.
10. Anderson SB, Rossing N. Metabolism of albumin and G-globulin during albumin infusions and plasmapheresis. *Scand J Clin Lab Invest* 1967;20:183–184.
11. Andrews WHH, Palmer JF. Afferent nervous discharge from the canine liver. *Q J Exp Physiol* 1967;52:269–276.
12. Arroyo V, Bosch J, Mauri M, et al. Renin, aldosterone and renal hemodynamics in cirrhosis with ascites. *Eur J Clin Invest* 1979;9:69–73.
13. Aukland K. Is extracelluar fluid volume regulated? *Acta Physiol Scand Suppl* 1989;36:59–67.
14. Auld RB, Alexander EA, Levinsky NG. Proximal tubular function in dogs with thoracic caval constriction. *J Clin Invest* 1971;50:2150–2158.
15. Bank N, Aynedjian HS. A micropuncture study of renal salt and water retention in chronic bile duct obstruction. *J Clin Invest* 1975;55:994–1002.
16. Bankir L, Martin H, Dechaux M, et al. Plasma cAMP, a hepatorenal link influencing proximal reabsorption and renal hemodynamics? *Kidney Int* 1997;51(Suppl 59):S50–S56.
17. Barabe J, Huberdeau Q, Bernoussi, A. Influence of sodium balance on urinary excretion of immunoreactive kinins in rat. *Am J Physiol* 1988;254:F484–F491.
18. Barletta G, Lazzeri C, Vecchiarino S, et al. Low-dose C-type natriuretic peptide does not affect cardiac and renal function in humans. *Hypertension* 1998;31:802–808.
19. Barrowman JA, Granger DN. Effects of experimental cirrhosis on splanchnic microvascular fluid and solute exchange in the rat. *Gastroenterology* 1984;87:165–172.
20. Bataller R, Gines P, Guevara M, et al. Hepatorenal syndrome. *Semin Liver Dis* 1997;17:233–247.

21. Bell NH, Schedl HP, Bartter FC. An explanation for abnormal water retention and hypoosmolality in congestive heart failure. *Am J Med* 1964;36:351–360.
22. Bello-Reuss E. Effects of catecholamines on fluid reabsorption by the isolated proximal convoluted tubule. *Am J Physiol* 1980;238:F347–F352.
23. Bennett WM, Bagby GC, Antonovic JN, et al. Influence of volume expansion on proximal tubular sodium reabsorption in congestive heart failure. *Am Heart* 1973;85:55–64.
24. Benoit JN, Granger DN. Intestinal microvascular adaptation to chronic portal hypertension in the rat. *Gastroenterology* 1988;94:471–476.
25. Berendes E, Walter M, Cullen P, et al. Secretion of brain natriuretic peptide in patients with aneurysmal subarachnoid haemorrhage. *Lancet* 1997;349:245–249.
26. Berkowitz R. B-type natriuretic peptide and the diagnosis of acute heart failure. *Rev Cardiovasc Med* 2004;5:S3–S16.
27. Berl T, Henrich WL, Erickson AL, et al. Prostaglandins in the beta adrenergic and baroreceptor-mediated secretion of renin. *Am J Physiol*1979;236:F472–F477.
28. Berlyne GM, Sutton J, Brown C, et al. Renal salt and water handling in water immersion in the nephrotic syndrome. *Clin Sci* 1981;61:605–610.
29. Bernard DB, Alexander EA, Couser WG, et al. Renal sodium retention during volume expansion in experimental nephrotic syndrome. *Kidney Int* 1978;14:478–485.
30. Bernardi M, Di Marco C, Trevisani F, et al. Renal sodium retention during upright posture in preascitic cirrhosis. *Gastroenterology* 1993;105:188–193.
31. Berne RM. Hemodynamics and sodium excretion of denervated kidney in anesthetized and unanesthetized dog. *Am J Physiol* 1952;171:148–158.
32. Better O. Renal and cardiovascular dysfunction in liver disease. *Kidney Int* 1986;29: 598–607.
33. Better OS, Massry SG. Effect of chronic bile duct obstruction on renal handling of salt and water. *J Clin Invest* 1972;51:402–411.
34. Bichet DG, Groves BM, Schrier RW. Mechanisms of improvement of water and sodium excretion by immersion in decompensated cirrhotic patients. *Kidney Int* 1983;24:788–794.
35. Bichet DG, Szatalowicz V, Chaimovitz C, et al. Role of vasopressin in abnormal water excretion in cirrhotic patients. *Ann Intern Med* 1982;96:413–417.
36. Bichet DG, Van Putten VJ, Schrier RW. Potential role of increased sympathetic activity in impaired sodium and water excretion in cirrhosis. *N Engl J Med* 1982;307:1552–1557.
37. Blaine EH, Davis JO, Prewitt RL. Evidence for a renal vascular receptor in control of renin secretion. *Am J Physiol* 1971;220:1593–1597.
38. Blantz R. Pathophysiology of pre-renal azotemia. *N Engl J Med* 1998;53:512–523.
39. Blendis LM, Greig PD, Longer B, et al. The renal and hemodynamic effects of the peritoneovenous shunt for intractable hepatic ascites. *Gastroenterology* 1979;77:250–257.
40. Bosch J, Enriquez R, Groszmann RJ, et al. Chronic bile duct ligation in the dog: hemodynamic characterization of a portal hypertensive model. *Hepatology* 1983;3:1002–1007.
41. Boyer TD, Zia P, Reynolds TB. Effect of indomethacin and prostaglandin A1 on renal function and plasma renin activity in alcoholic liver disease. *Gastroenterology* 1979;77:215–222.
42. Braam B, Mitchell KD, Fox J, et al. Proximal tubular secretion of angiotensin II in rats. *Am J Physiol* 1993;264:F891–F898.
43. Brooks VL, Ell KR, Wright RM. Pressure-independent baroreflex resetting produced by chronic infusion of angiotensin II in rabbits. *Am J Physiol* 1993;265:H1275–H1282.
44. Brown EA, Markandu ND, Roulston JE, et al. Is the renin-angiotensin-aldosterone system involved in the sodium retention in the nephrotic syndrome. *Nephron* 1982;32:102–107.
45. Brown EA, Markandu ND, Sagnella GA, et al. Lack of effect of captopril on the sodium retention of the nephrotic syndrome. *Nephron* 1984;37:43–48.
46. Brown EA, Markandu N, Sagnella GA, et al. Sodium retention in nephrotic syndrome is due to an intrarenal defect: evidence from steroid-induced remission. *Nephron* 1985;39:290–295.
47. Brown EA, Sagnella GA, Jones BE, et al. Evidence that some mechanism other than the renin system causes sodium retention in nephrotic syndrome. *Lancet* 1982;2:1237–1239.
48. Campillo B, Chabrier P-E, Pelle G, et al. Inhibition of nitric oxide synthesis in the forearm arterial bed of patients with advanced cirrhosis. *Hepatology* 1995;22:1423–1429.
49. Caramelo C, Fernandez-Munoz D, Santos JC, et al. Effect of volume expansion on hemodynamics, capillary permeability and renal function in conscious, cirrhotic rats. *Hepatology* 1986;6:129–134.
50. Carretero OA, Scicli AG. The renal kallikrein-kinin system. *Am J Physiol* 1980;238:F247–F255.
51. Carrithers SL, Ott CE, Hill MJ, et al. Guanylin and uroguanylin induce natriuresis in mice lacking guanylyl cyclase-C receptor. *Kidney Int* 2004;65:40–55.
52. Castells A, Salo J, Planas R, et al. Impact of shunt surgery for variceal bleeding in the natural history of ascites in cirrhosis: a retrospective study. *Hepatology* 1994;20:584–591.
53. Chagnac A, Zevin D, Weinstein T, et al. Combined tubular dysfunction in medullary cystic disease. *Arch Intern Med* 1986;146:1007–1009.
54. Chin-Dusting J, Rasaratanam B, Jennings G, et al. Effect of fluoroquinolone on the enhanced nitric oxide–induced vasodilation seen in cirrhosis. *Ann Intern Med* 1997;127: 985–988.
55. Chaimovitz C, Szylman P, Alroy G, et al. Mechanism of increased renal tubular sodium reabsorption in cirrhosis. *Am J Med* 1972;52:198–202.
56. Chamberlain MJ, Pringle A, Wrong DM. Oliguric renal failure in the nephrotic syndrome. *Q J Med* 1966;35:215–235.
57. Chiandussi L, Bartoli E, Arras S. Reabsorption of sodium in the proximal renal tubule in cirrhosis of the liver. *Gut* 1978;19:497–503.
58. Chonko AM, Bay WH, Stein J, Ferris TF. The role of renin and aldosterone in the salt retention of edema. *Am J Med* 1977;63:881–889.
59. Cody RJ, Atlas SA, Laragh JH, et al. Atrial natriuretic factor in normal subjects and heart failure patients. *J Clin Invest* 1986;78:1362–1374.
60. Cody RJ, Franklin KW, Kluger J, Laragh JH. Mechanisms governing the postural response and baroreceptor abnormalities in chronic congestive heart failure: effect of acute and long-term converting enzyme inhibition. *Circulation* 1982;66:135–142.
61. Coleman AJ, Arias M, Carter NW, et al. The mechanism of salt wastage in chronic renal disease. *J Clin Invest* 1966;45:1116–1125.
62. Colombato L, Albillos A, Groszmann R. The role of blood volume in the development of sodium retention in portal hypertensive rats. *Gastroenterology* 1996;110:193–198.
63. Davis CL, Briggs JP. Effect of atrial natriuretic peptides on renal medullary solute gradients. *Am J Physiol* 1987;253:F679–F684.
64. Dean R, Murone C, Lew RA, et al. Localization of bradykinin B2 binding sites in rat kidney following chronic ACE inhibitor treatment. *Kidney Int* 1997;52:1261–1270.
65. Denton DA, McKinley MJ, Weisinger RS. Hypothalamic integration of body fluid regulation. *Proc Natl Acad Sci U S A* 1996;93:7397–7404.
66. Dibner-Dunlap ME, Thames MD. Control of sympathetic nerve activity by vagal mechanoreflexes is blunted in heart failure. *Circulation* 1992;86:1929–1934.
67. DiBona GF, Herman PJ, Sawin LL. Neural control of renal function in edema-forming states. *Am J Physiol* 1988;254:R1017–R1024.
68. DiBona GF, Jones SY, Brooks VL. ANG II receptor blockade and arterial baroreflex regulation of renal nerve activity in cardiac failure. *Am J Physiol* 1995;269:R1189–R1196.
69. DiBona GF, Jones SY, Sawin LL. Effect of endogenous angiotensin II on renal nerve activity and its arterial baroreflex regulation. *Am J Physiol* 1996;271:R361–R367.
70. DiBona GF, Jones SY, Sawin LL. Reflex influence on renal nerve activity characteristics in nephrosis and heart failure. *J Am Soc Nephrol* 1997;8:1232–1239.
71. DiBona GF, Jones SY, Sawin LL. Angiotensin receptor antagonist improves cardiac reflex control of renal sodium handling in heart failure. *Am J Physiol* 1998;274:H636–H641.
72. DiBona GF, Sawin LL. Role of renal nerves in sodium retention of cirrhosis and congestive heart failure. *Am J Physiol* 1991;260:R298–R305.
73. DiBona GF, Sawin LL. Reflex regulation of renal nerve activity in cardiac failure. *Am J Physiol* 1994;266:R27–R39.
74. DiBona GF, Sawin LL. Increased renal nerve activity in cardiac failure: arterial vs. cardiac baroreflex impairment. *Am J Physiol* 1995;268:R112–R116.
75. DiBona GF. The functions of renal nerves. *Rev Physiol Biochem Pharmacol* 1982;94:76–157.
76. DiBona GF. Renal neural activity in hepatorenal syndrome. *Kidney Int* 1984;25:841–853.
77. DiBona GF, Rios LL. Renal nerves in compensatory renal response to contralateral renal denervation. *Am J Physiol* 1980;238:F26–F30.
78. Dietz, JR. Release of natriuretic factor from rat heart–lung preparation by atrial distention. *Am J Physiol* 1984;247:R1093–R1096.
79. Dorhout Mees EJ, Geers AB, Koomans HA. Blood volume and sodium retention in the nephrotic syndrome: a controversial pathophysiological concept. *Nephron* 1984;36:201–211.
80. Dorhout Mees EJ, Roos JC, Boer P, et al. Observations on edema formation in the nephrotic syndrome in adults with minimal lesions. *Am J Med* 1979;67:378–384.
81. Drexler H, Hirth C, Stasch H-P, et al. Vasodilatory action of endogenous atrial natriuretic factor in a rat model of chronic heart failure as determined by moncolonal ANF antibody. *Circ Res* 1990;66:1371–1380.
82. Dulin NO, Ernsberger P, Suciu DJ, et al. Rabbit renal epithelial angiotensin II receptors. *Am J Physiol* 1994;267:F776–F782.
83. Dusing R, Vetter H, Kramer HJ. The renin-angiotensin-aldosterone system in patients with nephrotic syndrome: effects of 1-sar-8 ala-angiotensin II. *Nephron* 1980;25:187–192.
84. Dzau VJ, Colucci WS, Hollenberg NK, et al. Relation of the renin-angiotensin-aldosterone system to clinical state in congestive heart failure. *Circulation* 1981;63:645–651.
85. Dzau VJ, Colucci WS, Williams GH, et al. Sustained effectiveness of converting enzyme inhibition in patients with severe congestive heart failure. *N Engl J Med* 1980;302:1373–1379.
86. Earley LE, Martino JA. Influence of sodium balance on the ability of diuretics to inhibit tubular reabsorption. *Circulation* 1970;42:323–334.
87. Eggert RC. Spironolactone diuresis in patients with cirrhosis and ascites. *BMJ* 1970;4: 401–403.
88. Eisenberg, S. Postural changes in plasma volume in hypoalbuminemia. *Arch Intern Med* 1963;112:544–549.
89. Eisenberg S. Blood volume in persons with the nephrotic syndrome. *Am J Med Sci* 1968;255: 320–326.
90. Elsner D, Muders F, Muntze A, et al. Efficacy of prolonged infusion of urodilatin [ANP-(95-126)] in patients with congestive heart failure. *Am Heart J* 1995;29:766–773.
91. Epstein FH, Post RS, McDowell M. The effect of an arteriovenous fistula on renal hemodynamics and electrolyte excretion. *J Clin Invest* 1953;32:233–241.
92. Epstein M. Cardiovascular and renal effects of head-out water immersion in man. *Circ Res* 1976;39:619–628.
93. Epstein M. Deranged sodium homeostasis in cirrhosis. *Gastroenterology* 1979;76:622–635.
94. Epstein M, Berk DP, Hollenberg NK, et al. Renal failure in the patient with cirrhosis. *Am J Med* 1970;49:175–185.
95. Epstein M, Larios O, Johnson G. Effects of water immersion on plasma catecholamines in decompensated cirrhosis. Implications for deranged sodium and water homeostasis. *Miner Electrolyte Metab* 1985;11:25–34.
96 Epstein M. Peritoneovenous shunt in the management of ascites and the hepatorenal syndrome. *Gastroenterology* 1982;82:790–799.
97. Epstein M, Levinson R, Sancho J, et al. Characterization of the renin-aldosterone system in decompensated cirrhosis. *Circ Res* 1977;41:818–829.
98. Epstein M, Lifschitz M, Ramachandran M, et al. Characterization of renal PGE responsiveness in decompensated cirrhosis: implications for renal sodium handling. *Clin Sci* 1983;63:555–563.
99. Epstein M, Pins DS, Schneider N, et al. Determinants of deranged sodium and water homeostasis in decompensated cirrhosis. *J Lab Clin Med* 1976;87:822–839.
100. Epstein M, Ramachandran M, De Nunzio AG. Interrelationship of renal sodium and phosphate handling in cirrhosis. *Miner Electrolyte Metab* 1982;7:305–315.
101. Esler M, Dudley F, Jennings G, et al. Increased sympathetic nervous activity and the effects of its inhibition with clonidine in alcoholic cirrhosis. *Ann Intern Med* 1992;116:446–455.
102. Fadnes HO, Pape JF, Sundsfjord JA. A study on oedema mechanism in nephrotic syndrome. *Scand J Clin Lab Invest* 1986;46:533–538.
103. Fernandez-Munoz D, Caramelo C, Santos JC, et al. Systemic and splanchnic hemodynamic disturbances in conscious rats with experimental liver cirrhosis without ascites. *Am J Physiol* 1985;249:G316–G320.

104. Fernandez-Rodriguez C, Prada I, Prieto J, et al. Circulating adrenomedullin in cirrhosis: relationship to hyperdynamic circulation. *J Hepatol* 1998;98:250–256.
105. Firth JD, Raine AEG, Ledingham JGG. Abnormal sodium handling occurs in the isolated perfused kidney of the nephrotic rat. *Clin Sci* 1989;76:387–395.
106. Forte LR. A novel role for uroguanylin in the regulation of sodium balance. *J Clin Invest* 2003;112:1138–1141.
107. Garcia NH, Garvin JL. Endothelin's biphasic effect on fluid absorption in the proximal straight tubule and its inhibitory cascade. *J Clin Invest* 1994;93:2572–2577.
108. Garnett ES, Webber CE. Changes in blood volume produced by treatment in the nephrotic syndrome. *Lancet* 1967;2:798–799.
109. Geers AB, Koomans HA, Boer P, et al. Plasma and blood volumes in patients with the nephrotic syndrome. *Nephron* 1984;38:170–173.
110. Geers AB, Koomans HA, Roos JC, et al. Functional relationships in the nephrotic syndrome. *Kidney Int* 1984;26:324–330.
111. Gerbes AL, Kollenda MC, Vollmar AM, et al. Altered density of glomerular binding sites for atrial natriuretic factor in bile duct–ligated rats with ascites. *Hepatology* 1991;13:562–566.
112. Gesek FA, Schoolwerth AC. Hormonal interactions with proximal Na+–H+ exchanger. *Amer J Physiol* 1990;258:F514–F521.
113. Gesek FA, Strandhoy JW. Dual interactions between a2-adrenoceptor agonists and the proximal Na+–H+ exchanger. *Am J Physiol* 1990;258:F636–F642.
114. Gines P, Arroyo V, Vargas V, et al. Paracentesis with intravenous infusion of albumin as compared with peritoneovenous shunting in cirrhosis with refractory ascites. *N Engl J Med* 1991;325:829–835.
115. Gines A, Fernandez-Esparrach G, Monescillo A, et al. Randomized trial comparing albumin, dextran 70, and polygeline in cirrhotic patients with ascites treated by paracentesis. *Gastroenterology* 1996;111:1002–1010.
116. Gines P, Tito L, Arroyo V, et al. Randomized comparative study of therapeutic paracentesis with and without intravenous albumin in cirrhosis. *Gastroenterology* 1988;94:1493–1502.
117. Gines P, Fernandez-Esparrach G, Arroyo V, Rodes J. Pathogenesis of ascites in cirrhosis. *Semin Liver Dis* 1997;17:175–189.
118. Granger DN, Miller T, Allen R, et al. Permselectivity of cat liver blood–lymph barrier to endogenous macromolecules. *Gastroenterology* 1979;77:103–109.
119. Grassi G, Cattaneo BM, Seravalle G, et al. Effects of chronic ACE inhibition on sympathetic nerve traffic and baroreflex control of circulation in heart failure. *Circulation* 1997;96: 1173–1179.
120. Grausz H, Lieberman R, Earley LE. Effect of plasma albumin on sodium reabsorption in patients with nephrotic syndrome. *Kidney Int* 1972;1:47–54.
121. Greenberg TT, Richmond WH, Stocking RA, et al. Impaired atrial receptor responses in dogs with heart failure due to tricuspid insufficiency and pulmonary artery stenosis. *Circ Res* 1973;32:424–433.
122. Grider J, Falcone J, Kilpatrick E, Ott C, Jackson B. Effect of bradykinin on NaCl transport in the medullary thick ascending limb of the rat. *Eur J Pharmacol* 1995;287:101–104.
123. Guevara M, Gines P, Bandi J, et al. Transjugular intrahepatic portosystemic shunt in hepatorenal syndrome: effects on renal function and vasoactive systems. *Hepatology* 1998;28:416–422.
124. Guevara M, Gines P, Fernandez-Esparrach G, et al. Reversibility of hepatorenal syndrome by prolonged administration of ornipressin and plasma volume expansion. *Hepatology* 1988; 27:35–41.
125. Guntupalli J, DuBose Jr. TD. Effects of endothelin on rat renal proximal tubule Na+–Pi cotransport and Na+/H+ exchange. *Am J Physiol* 1994;266:F658–F666.
126. Guyton, AC. Interstitial fluid pressure II. Pressure volume curves of the interstitial space. *Circ Res* 1965;16:452–460.
127. Hammond TG, Whitworth JA, Saines D, et al. Renin-angiotensin-aldosterone system in nephrotic syndrome. *Am J Kidney Dis* 1984;4:18–23.
128. Harris PJ, Young JA. Dose-dependent stimulation and inhibition of proximal tubular sodium reabsorption by angiotensin II in the rat kidney. *Pflugers Arch* 1977;367:295–297.
129. Hensen J, Abraham WT, Durr JA, Schrier RW. Aldosterone in congestive heart failure: analysis of determinants and role in sodium retention. *Am J Nephrol* 1991;11:441–446.
130. Herman PJ, Sawin LL, DiBona GF. Role of renal nerves in renal sodium retention of nephrotic syndrome. *Am J Physiol* 1989;256:F823–F829.
131. Higashihara E, Stokes JB, Kokko JP. et al. Cortical and papillary micropuncture examination of chloride transport in segments of the rat kidney during inhibition of prostaglandin production. *J Clin Invest* 1979;64:1277–1287.
132. Hirsch AT, Levenson DJ, Cutler SS, et al. Regional vascular responses to prolonged lower body negative pressure in normal subjects. *Am J Physiol* 1989;257:H219–H225.
133. Hollander W, Reilly P, Burrows BA. Lymphatic flow in human subjects as indicated by the disappearance of 131I-labeled albumin from the subcutaneous tissue. *J Clin Lab Invest* 1989;40:222–223.
134. Hommel E, Mathiesen ER, Aukland K, et al. Pathophysiological aspects of edema formation in diabetic nephropathy. *Kidney Int* 38:1187–1192.
135. Hostetter TH, Pfeffer JM, Pfeffer MA, et al. Cardiorenal hemodynamics and sodium excretion in rats with myocardial infarction. *Am J Physiol* 1983;245:H98–H103.
136. Humphreys MH, Valentin J, Qui C, et al. Underfill and overflow revisited: mechanisms of nephrotic edema. *Trans Am Clin Climatol Assoc* 1992;104:47–59.
137. Ichikawa I, Pfeffer JM, Pfeffer MA, et al. Role of angiotensin II in the altered renal function of congestive heart failure. *Circ Res* 1984;55:669–675.
138. Ichikawa I, Rennke HG, Hoyer JR, et al. Role for intrarenal mechanisms in the impaired salt excretion of experimental nephrotic syndrome. *J Clin Invest* 1983;71:91–103.
139. Iino Y, Troy JL, Brenner, BM. Effects of catecholamines on electrolyte transport in cortical collecting tubule. *J Membr Biol* 1981;61:67–73.
140. Inoue A, Yanagisawa M, Kimura S, et al. The human endothelin family: three structurally and pharmacologically distinct isopeptides predicted by three separate genes. *Proc Natl Acad Sci U S A* 1989;86:2863–2867.
141. Iwao T, Toyonaga A, Sato M, et al. Effect of posture-induced blood volume expansion on systemic and regional hemodynamcis in patients with cirrhosis. *J Hepatol* 1997;27:484–491.
142. Jensen KT, Carstens J, Pedersen EB. Effect of BNP on renal hemodynamics, tubular function and vasoactive hormones in humans. *Am J Physiol* 1998;274:F63–F72.
143. Jimenez W, Martinez-Pardo A, Arroyo V, et al. Atrial natriuretic factor: reduced cardiac content in cirrhotic rats with ascites. *Am J Physiol* 1986;250:F749–F752.
144. Johnston CI, Davis JO, Robb CA, et al. Plasma renin in chronic experimental heart failure and during renal sodium "escape" from mineralocorticoids. *Circ Res* 1968;22: 113–125.
145. Joles JA, Koomans HA, Kortlandt W, et al. Hypoproteinemia and recovery from edema in dogs. *Am J Physiol* 1988;254:F887–F894.
146. Joles J, Rabelink T, Braam B, et al. Plasma volume regulation: defenses against edema formation (with special emphasis on hypoproteinemia). *Am J Nephrol* 1993;13:399–412.
147. Kaczmarczyk G, Drake A, Eisele R, et al. The role of the cardiac nerves in the regulation of sodium excretion in conscious dogs. *Pflugers Arch* 1981;390:125–130.
148. Kalambokis G, Economou M, Fotopoulos A, et al. The effects of chronic treatment with octreotide versus octreotide plus midodrine on systemic hemodynamics and renal hemodynamics and function in nonazotemic cirrhotic patients with ascites. *Am J Gastroenterol* 2004;99:1–7.
149. Kalant N, Das Gupta D, Despointes R, Giroud CJP. Mechanisms of edema in experimental nephrosis. *Am J Physiol* 1962;202:91–96.
150. Kelsch RC, Light GS, Oliver WJ. The effect of albumin infusion upon plasma norepinephrine concentration in nephrotic children. *J Lab Clin Med* 1972;79:516–525.
151. Kim JK, Michel J-B, Soubrier F, et al. Arginine vasopressin gene expression in chronic cardiac failure in rats. *Kidney Int* 1990;38:818–822.
152. Kiowski W, Sutsch G, Hunziker P, et al. Evidence for endothelin-1–mediated vasoconstriction in severe chronic heart failure. *Lancet* 1995;346:732–736.
153. Kirchheim HR, Finke R, Hackenthal E. et al. Baroreflex sympathetic activation increases threshold pressure for the pressure-dependent renin release in conscious dogs. *Pflugers Arch* 1985;405:127–135.
154. Koepke JP, DiBona GF. Blunted natriuresis to atrial natriuretic peptide in chronic sodium-retaining disorders. *Am J Physiol* 1987;252:F865–F871.
155. Koepke JP, Jones S, DiBona GF. Renal nerves mediate blunted natriuresis to atrial natriuretic peptide in cirrhotic rats. *Am J Physiol* 1987;252:R1019–R1023.
156. Kontos HA, Shapiro W, Mauck HP, et al. General and regional circulatory alterations in cirrhosis of the liver. *Am J Med* 1964;37:526–535.
157. Koomans HA, Boer WH, Dorhout Mees EJ. Renal function during recovery from minimal lesions nephrotic syndrome. *Nephron* 1987;47:173–178.
158. Koomans HA, Braam B, Geers AB, et al. The importance of plasma protein for blood volume and blood pressure homeostasis. *Kidney Int* 1986;30:730–735.
159. Koomans HA, Geers AB, Dorhout Mees EJ, et al. Lowered tissue-fluid oncotic pressure protects the blood volume in the nephrotic syndrome. *Nephron* 1986;42:317–322.
160. Koomans HA, Geers AB, Meiracker AH, et al. Effects of plasma volume expansion on renal salt handling in patients with the nephrotic syndrome. *Am J Nephrol* 1984;4:227–234.
161. Koomans HA, Kortlandt W, Geers AB, et al. Lowered protein content of tissue fluid in patients with the nephrotic syndrome: observations during disease and recovery. *Nephron* 1985;40:391–395.
162. Kopp UC. Renorenal reflexes in normotension and hypertension. *Miner Electrolyte Metab* 1989;15:66–73.
163. Kopp UC. Renorenal reflexes: interaction between efferent and afferent renal nerve activity. *Can J Physiol Pharmacol* 1992;70:750–758.
164. Kopp UC, Olson LA, DiBona GF. Renorenal reflex responses to mechano- and chemoreceptor stimulation in the dog and rat. *Am J Physiol* 1984;246:F67–F77.
165. Kopp UC, Smith LA. Inhibitory renorenal reflexes: a role for renal prostaglandins in activation of renal sensory receptors. *Am J Physiol* 1991;261:R1513–R1521.
166. Kopp UC, Smith LA. Effects of the substance P receptor antagonist CP-96,345 on renal sensory receptor activation. *Am J Physiol* 1993;264:R647–R653.
167. Korthuis RJ, Kinden DA, Brimer GE, et al. Intestinal capillary filtration in acute and chronic portal hypertension. *Am J Physiol* 1988;254:G339–G345.
168. Kostreva DR, Castaner A, Kampine JP. Reflex effects of hepatic baroreceptors on renal and cardiac sympathetic nerve activity. *Am J Physiol* 1980;238:R390–R394.
169. Kravetz D, Romero G, Argonz J, et al. Total volume paracentesis decreases variceal pressure, size, and variceal wall tension in cirrhotic patients. *Hepatology* 1997;25:59–62.
170. Krishna GG, Danovitch K, Danovitch GM. Effects of water immersion on renal function in the nephrotic syndrome. *Kidney Int* 1982;21:395–401.
171. Kumagai H, Onoyama K, Iseki K, et al. Role of renin angiotensin aldosterone on minimal change nephrotic syndrome. *Clin Nephrol* 1985;23:229–235.
172. Laragh JH, Cannon PJ, Bentzel CJ, et al. Angiotensin II, norepinephrine, and renal transport of electrolytes and water in normal man and in cirrhosis with ascites. *J Clin Invest* 1963;2: 1179–1192.
173. La Villa G, Riccardi D, Lazzeri C, et al. Blunted natriuretic response to low-dose brain natriuretic peptide infusion in nonazotemic cirrhotic patients with ascites and avid sodium retention. *Hepatology* 1995;22:1745–1750.
174. Lebrec D, Giuily N, Hadengue A, et al. Transjugular intrahepatic portosystemic shunts. Comparison with paracentesis in patients with cirrhosis and refractory ascites: a randomized trial. *J Hepatol* 1996;25:135–144.
175. Legault L, Cernacek P, Levy M, et al. Renal tubular responsiveness to atrial natriuretic peptide in sodium-retaining chronic caval dogs: a possible role for kinins and luminal actions of the peptide. *J Clin Invest* 1992;90:1425–1435.
176. Leimbach WN, Wallin B G, Victor RG, et al. Direct evidence from intraneural recordings for increased central sympathetic outflow in patients with heart failure. *Circulation* 1986; 73: 913–919.
177. Lenz K, Hortnagl H, Druml W, et al. Ornipressin in the treatment of functional renal failure in decompensated liver cirrhosis. *Gastroenterology* 1991;101:1060–1067.
178. Levine TB, Francis GS, Goldsmith SR, et al. Activity of the sympathetic nervous system and renin-angiotensin system assessed by plasma hormone levels and their relation to hemodynamic abnormalities in congestive heart failure. *Am J Cardiol* 49:1659–1666.

179. Levy M. Effects of acute volume expansion and altered hemodynamics on renal tubular function in chronic caval dogs. *J Clin Invest* 1972;51:922–934.

180. Levy M, Wexler MJ. Sodium excretion in dogs with low-grade caval constriction: role of hepatic nerves. *Am J Physiol* 1987;253:F672–F678.

181. Levy M. Sodium retention and ascites formation in dogs with experimental portal cirrhosis. *Am J Physiol* 1977;233:F572–F585.

182. Levy M, Wexler MJ. Hepatic denervation alters first-phase urinary sodium excretion in dogs with cirrhosis. 1987;253:F664–F671.

183. Levy M. Sodium retention and ascites formation in dogs with experimental portal cirrhosis. *Am J Physiol* 233:F572–F585.

184. Levy M, Allotey JB. Temporal relationships between urinary salt retention and altered systemic hemodynamics in dogs with experimental cirrhosis. *J Lab Clin Med* 1978;92:560–569.

185. Levy M, Wexler MJ. Renal sodium retention and ascites formation in dogs with experimental cirrhosis but without portal hypertension or increased splanchnic vascular capacity. *J Lab Clin Med* 1978;91:520–536.

186. Lieberman FL, Denison EK, Reynolds TB. The relationship of plasma volume, portal hypertension, ascites, and renal sodium retention in cirrhosis: the overflow theory of ascites formation. *Ann N Y Acad Sci* 1978;170:202–211.

187. Ljungman S, Laragh JH, Cody RJ. Role of the kidney in congestive heart failure: relationship of cardiac index to kidney function. *Drugs* 1990;39(Suppl 4):10–21.

188. Limas CJ, Guiha NH, Lekagul O, et al. Impaired left ventricular function in alcoholic cirrhosis with ascites. *Circulation* 1974;69:755–760.

189. Lopez-Talavera JC, Merrill WM, Groszmann RJ. Tumor necrosis factor a: a major contributor to the hyperdynamic circulation in prehepatic portal-hypertensive rats. *Gastroenterology* 1995;108:761–767.

190. Lopez-Talavera JC, Levitzki A, Martinez M, et al. Tyrosine kinase inhibition ameliorates the hyperdynamic state and decreases nitric oxide production in cirrhotic rats with portal hypertension and ascites. *J Clin Invest* 1997;100:664–670.

191. Lopez C, Jimenez W, Arroyo V, et al. Temporal relationship between the decrease in arterial pressure and sodium retention in conscious spontaneously hypertensive rats with carbon tetrachloride-induced cirrhosis. *Hepatology* 1991;13:585–589.

192. Lopez C, Jimenez W, Arroyo V, et al. Role of altered systemic hemodynamics in the blunted renal response to atrial natriuretic peptide in rats with cirrhosis and ascites. *J Hepatology* 1989;9:217–226.

193. Lortie M, Regoli D, Rhaleb N-E, Plante G. The role of B1- and B2-kinin receptors in the renal tubular and hemodynamic response to bradykinin. *Am J Physiol* 1992;262:R72–R76.

194. Luca A, Feu F, Garcia-Pagan JC, et al. Favorable effects of total paracentesis on splanchnic hemodynamics in cirrhotic patients with tense ascites. *Hepatology* 1994;20:30–33.

195. Ludbrook J, Ventura S. Roles of carotid baroreceptor and cardiac afferents in hemodynamic responses to acute central hypovolemia. *Am J Physiol* 1996;270:H1538–H1548.

196. Luetscher JA, Johnson BB. Observations on the sodium-retaining corticoid (aldosterone) in the urine of children and adults in relation to sodium balance and edema. *J Clin Invest* 1954;33:1441–1446.

197. Ma R, Zucker IH, Wang W. Central gain of the cardiac sympathetic afferent reflex in dogs with heart failure. *Am J Physiol* 1997;273:H2664–H2671.

198. MacGilchrist A, Craig KJ, Hayes PC, Cumming AD. Effect of the serine protease inhibitor, aprotinin, on systemic haemodynamics and renal function in patients with hepatic cirrhosis and ascites. *Clin Sci* 1994;87:329–335.

199. Maher E, Cernacek P, Levy M. Heterogeneous renal responses to atrial natriuretic factor II. Cirrhotic dogs. *Am J Physiol* 1989;257:R1068–R1074.

200. Manenti F, Williams R. Injection studies of the splenic vasculature in portal hypertension. *Gut* 1966;7:175–180.

201. Marcus LS, Hart D, Packer M, et al. Hemodynamic and renal excretory effects of human brain natriuretic peptide infusion in patients with congestive heart failure: a double-blind, placebo-controlled, randomized crossover trial. *Circulation* 1996;94:3184–3189.

202. Martin P-Y, Ohara M, Gines P, et al. Nitric oxide synthase (NOS) inhibition for one week improves renal sodium and water excretion in cirrhotic rats with ascites. *J Clin Invest* 1998;101:235–242.

203. Martin P-Y, Schrier RW. Sodium and water retention in heart failure: pathogenesis and treatment. *Kidney Int* 1997;51(Suppl 59):S57–S61.

204. Martin P, Gines P, Schrier R. Nitric oxide as a mediator of hemodynamic abnormalities and sodium and water retention in cirrhosis. *N Engl J Med* 1998;339:533–541.

205. Matsuda T, Morita H, Hosomi H, et al. Response of renal nerve activity to high NaCl food intake in dogs with chronic bile duct ligation. *Hepatology* 1996;23:303–309.

206. May CN, McAllen RM. Brain angiotensinergic pathways mediate renal nerve inhibition by central hypertonic NaCl in conscious sheep. *Am J Physiol* 1997;272:R593–R600.

207. Melman A, Massry SG. Role of renal vasodilation in the blunted natriuresis of saline infusion in dogs with chronic bile duct obstruction. *J Lab Clin Med* 1977;89:1053–1065.

208. Meltzer J, Keim HJ, Laragh JH, et al. Nephrotic syndrome: vasoconstriction and hypervolemic types indicated by renin-sodium profiling. *Ann Intern Med* 1979;91:688–696.

209. Metcoff J, Janeway CA. Studies on the pathogenesis of nephrotic edema. *J Pediatr* 1961;58:640–685.

210. Metlauer B, Rouleau JL, Bichet D. et al. Sodium and water excretion abnormalities in congestive heart failure. *Ann Intern Med* 1986;105:161–167.

211. Meyer M, Richter R, Brunkhorst R, et al. Urodilatin is involved in sodium homeostasis and exerts sodium-state–dependent natriuretic and diuretic effects. *Am J Physiol* 1996;271:F489–F497.

212. Migdal S, Alexander A, Levinsky NG. Evidence that decreased cardiac output is not the stimulus to sodium retention during acute constriction of the vena cava. *J Lab Clin Med* 1977;89:809–816.

213. Mirouze D, Zisper RD, Reynolds TB. Effects of inhibitors of prostaglandin synthesis on induced diuresis in cirrhosis. *Hepatology* 1983;3:50–55.

214. Mitchell KD, Navar LG. Enhanced tubuloglomerular feedback during peritubular infusions of angiotensins I and II. *Am J Physiol* 1988;255:F383–F390.

215. Moe OW, Ujiie K, Star RA, et al. Renin expression in renal proximal tubule. *J Clin Invest* 1993;91:774–779.

216. Mohanty PK, Arrowood JA, Ellenbogen KA, et al. Neurohumoral and hemodynamic effects of lower body negative pressure in patients with congestive heart failure. *Am Heart J* 1989;118:78–85.

217. Moller S, Bendtsen F, Henriksen JH. Effect of volume expansion on systemic hemodynamics and central and arterial blood volume in cirrhosis. *Gastroenterology* 1995;109:1917–1925.

218. Moller S, Henriksen JH. Circulatory abnormalities in cirrhosis with focus on neurohumoral aspects. *Semin Nephrol* 1997;17:505–519.

219. Moore K, Wendon J, Frazer M, Karani J, Williams R, Badr K. Plasma endothelin immunoreactivity in liver disease and the hepatorenal syndrome. *N Engl J Med* 1992;327:1774–1778.

220. Morali GA, Tobe SW, Skorecki KL, Blendis LM. Refractory ascites: modulation of atrial natriuretic factor unresponsiveness by mannitol. *Hepatology* 1992;16:42–48.

221. Morduchowicz GA, Sheikh-Hamad D, Dwyer BE, et al. Angiotensin II directly increases rabbit renal brush-border membrane sodium transport: presence of local signal transduction system. *J Membr Biol* 1991;122:43–53.

222. Morita H, Yamashita Y, Nishida Y, et al. Fos induction in rat brain neurons after stimulation of the hepatoportal Na-sensitive mechanism. *Am J Physiol* 1997;272:R913–R923.

223. Moss NG. Electrophysiological characteristics of renal sensory receptors and afferent renal nerves. *Miner Electrolyte Metab* 1989;15:59–65.

224. Murakami H, Liu J-L, Zucker IH. Angiotensin II enhances baroreflex control of sympathetic outflow in heart failure. *Hypertension* 1997;29:564–569.

225. Myers BD, Peterson C, Molina C, et al. Role of cardiac atria in the human renal response to changing plasma volume. *Am J Physiol* 1988;254:F562–F573.

226. Nagaya N, Nishikimi T, Goto Y, et al. Plasma brain natriuretic peptide is a biochemical marker for the prediction of progressive ventricular remodeling after acute myocardial infarction. *Am Heart J* 1998;135:21–28.

227. Nakamura T, Alberola AM, Salazar FJ, et al. Effects of renal perfusion pressure on renal interstitial hydrostatic pressure and Na+ excretion: role of endothelium-derived nitric oxide. *Nephron* 1998;78:104–111.

228. Nicholls KM, Shapiro MD, Groves BS, et al. Factors determining renal response to water immersion in nonexcretor cirrhotic patients. *Kidney Int* 1986 30:417–421.

229. Nicholls KM, Shapiro MD, Kluge R, et al. Sodium excretion in advanced cirrhosis: effect of expansion of central blood volume and suppression of plasma aldosterone. *Hepatology* 1986;6:235–238.

230. Nicholls KM, Shapiro MD, Van Putten VJ, et al. Elevated plasma norepinephrine concentrations in decompensated cirrhosis. *Circ Res* 1985;56:457–461.

231. Niederberger M, Gines P, Tsai P, et al. Increased aortic cyclic guanosine monophosphate concentration in experimental cirrhosis in rats: evidence for a role of nitric oxide in the pathogenesis of arterial vasodilation in cirrhosis. *Hepatology* 1995;21:1625–1631.

232. Niederberger M, Martin P-Y, Gines P, et al. Normalization of nitric oxide production corrects arterial vasodilation and hyperdynamic circulation in cirrhotic rats. *Gastroenterology* 1995;109:1624–1630.

233. Nishida Y, Sugimoto I, Morita H, Murakami H, Hosomi H, Bishop VS. Suppression of renal sympathetic nerve activity during portal vein infusion of hypertonic saline. *Am J Physiol* 1998;274:R97–R103.

234. Noddeland H, Riisnes SM, Fadness HO. Interstitial fluid colloid osmotic and hydrostatic pressures in subcutaneous tissue of patients with nephrotic syndrome. *Scand J Clin Lab Invest* 1982;42:139–146.

235. Ochs A, Rossle M, Haag K, et al. The transjugular intrahepatic portosystemic stent-shunt procedure for refractory ascites. *N Engl J Med* 1995;332:1192–1197.

236. Ohishi K, Hishida A, Honda N. Direct vasodilatory action of atrial natriuretic factor on canine glomerular afferent arterioles. *Am J Physiol* 1988;255:F415–F420.

237. Olivari MT, Levine TB, Cohn JN. Abnormal neurohormonal response to nitroprusside infusion in congestive heart failure. *J Am Coll Cardiol* 1983;2:411.

238. Oliver JA, Sciacia RR, Pinto J, Cannon PJ. Participation of the prostaglandins in the control of renal blood flow during acute reduction of cardiac output in the dog. *J Clin Invest* 1981;67:229–237.

239. Oliver WJ, Kelsch RC, Chandler JP. Demonstration of increased catecholamine excretion in the nephrotic syndrome. *Proc Soc Exp Biol Med* 1967;125:1176–1180.

240. Oren RM, Schobel HP, Weiss RM, Stanford W, Ferguson DW. Importance of left atrial baroreceptors in the cardiopulmonary baroreflex of normal humans. *J Appl Physiol* 1993;74:2672–2680.

241. Packer M, Lee WH, Kessler PD Preservation of glomerular filtration in human heart failure by activation of the renin-angiotensin system. *Circulation* 1986;74:766–774.

242. Packer M, Lee WH, Medina N, et al. Functional renal insufficiency during long-term therapy with captopril and enalapril in severe chronic heart failure. *Ann Intern Med* 1987;106:346–354.

243. Paintal AS. Vagal sensory receptors and their reflex effects. *Physiol Rev* 1973;53:159.

244. Palmer BF. Renal complications associated with use of nonsteroidal anti-inflammatory agents. *J Invest Med* 1995;43:516–533.

245. Palmer BF. Hyponatremia in patients with central nervous system disease: SIADH or CSW. *Trends Endocrinol Metab* 2003;14:182–743.

246. Palmer BF. Renal dysfunction complicating treatment of hypertension. *N Engl J Med* 2002;347:1256–1261.

247. Panos MZ, Gove C, Firth JD, et al. Impaired natriuretic response to atrial natriuretic peptide in the isolated kidney of rats with experimental cirrhosis. *Clin Sci* 1990;79:67–71.

248. Pelayo JC, Ziegler MG, Blantz RC. Angiotensin II in adrenergic-induced alterations in glomerular hemodynamics. *Am J Physiol* 1984;247:F799–F807.

249. Pelayo JC, Ziegler MG, Jose PA et al. Renal denervation in the rat: analysis of glomerular and proximal tubular function. *Am J Physiol* 1983;244:F70–F77.

250. Peltekian KM, Wong F, Liu PP, et al. Cardiovascular, renal, and neurohormonal responses to single large-volume paracentesis in patients with cirrhosis and diuretic-resistant ascites. *Am J Gastroenterol* 1997;92:394–399.

251. Peng Y, Knox FG. Comparison of systemic and direct intrarenal angiotensin II blockade on sodium excretion in rats. *Am J Physiol* 1995;269:F40–F46.
252. Perez-Ayuso RM, Arroyo V, Camps J, et al. Renal kallikrein excretion in cirrhosis with ascites: relationship to renal hemodynamics. *Hepatology* 19844:247–252.
253. Perez-Ayuso RM, Arroyo V, Planas R, et al. Randomized comparative study of efficacy of furosemide versus spironolactone in nonazotemic cirrhosis with ascites. *Gastroenterology* 1983;84:961–968.
254. Perico N, Remuzzi G. Edema of the nephrotic syndrome: the role of the atrial peptide system. *Am J Kidney Dis* 1993;22:355–366.
255. Perico N, Remuzzi G. Renal handling of sodium in the nephrotic syndrome. *Am J Nephrol* 1993;13:413–421.
256. Peters JP, Welt LG, Sims EAH, et al. Salt-wasting syndrome associated with cerebral disease. *Trans Assoc Am Physicians* 1950;63:57–64.
257. Peterson C, Madson B, Perlman A, et al. Atrial natriuretic peptide and the renal response to hypervolemia in nephrotic humans. *Kidney Int* 1988;34:825–831.
258. Peterson TV, Carter AB, Miller RA. Nitric oxide and renal effects of volume expansion in conscious monkeys. *Am J Physiol* 1997;272:R1033–R1038.
259. Petrovic S, Barone S, Weinstin AM, et al. Activation of the apical Na+/H+ exchanger NHE3 by formate: a basis of enhanced fluid and electrolyte reabsorption by formate in the kidney. *Am J Physiol Renal Physiol* 2004;287:F336–F346.
260. Pham I, Sediame S, Maistre G, et al. Renal and vascular effects of C-type and atrial natriuretic peptides in humans. *Am J Physiol* 1997;273:R1457–R1464.
261. Pinto PC, Amerian J, Reynolds TB. Large-volume paracentesis in nonedematous patients with tense ascites: its effect on intravascular volume. *Hepatology* 1988;8:207–210.
262. Planelles G. Chloride transport in the renal proximal tubule. *Pfugers Arch* 2004;448:561–570.
263. Pockros PJ, Reynolds TB. Rapid diuresis in patients with ascites from chronic liver disease: the importance of peripheral edema. *Gastroenterology* 1986;90:1827–1833.
264. Potts JT, Hatanaka T, Shoukas AA. Effect of arterial compliance on carotid sinus baroreceptor reflex control of the circulation. *Am J Physiol* 1996;270:H988–H1000.
265. Pozzi M, Osculati G, Boari G, et al. Time course of circulatory and humoral effects of rapid total paracentesis in cirrhotic patients with tense, refractory ascites. *Gastroenterology* 1994;106:709–719.
266. Preisig PA, Ives HE, Cargoe EJ, et al. The role of the Na–H antiport in rat proximal tubule bicarbonate absorption. *J Clin Invest* 1987;80:970–978.
267. Priebe HJ, Heimann JC, Hedley-White J. Effects of renal and hepatic venous congestion on renal function in the presence of low and normal cardiac output in dogs. *Circ Res* 1980;47: 883–890.
268. Quan A, Baum M. Endogenous production of angiotensin II modulates rat proximal tubule transport. *J Clin Invest* 1996;97:2878–2882.
269. Quiroga J, Sangro B, Nunez M, et al. Transjugular intrahepatic portal-systemic shunt in the treatment of refractory ascites: effect on clinical, renal, humoral, and hemodynamic parameters. *Hepatology* 1995;21:986–994.
270. Rabelink T, Bijlsma J, Koomans H. Iso-oncotic volume expansion in the nephrotic syndrome. *Clin Sci* 1993;84:627–632.
271. Raine AE, Erne P, Burgisser E, et al. Atrial natriuretic peptide and atrial pressure in patients with congestive heart failure. *N Engl J Med* 1986;315:533–537.
272. Rascher W, Tulassay T. Hormonal regulation of water metabolism in children with nephrotic syndrome. *Kidney Int* 1987;32:583–589.
273. Rascher W, Tulassay T, Seyberth HW, et al. Diuretic and hormonal response to head-out water immersion in nephrotic syndrome. *J Pediatr* 1986;109:609–614.
274. Rector WG, Hossack KF. Pathogenesis of sodium retention complicating cirrhosis: is there room for diminished "effective" arterial blood volume? *Gastroenterology* 1988;95:1658–1663.
275. Ring-Larsen H, Henriksen JH, Christensen NJ. Increased sympathetic activity in cirrhosis. *N Engl J Med* 1983;308:1029.
276. Rodriguez-Martinez M, Sawin LL, DiBona GF. Arterial and cardiopulmonary baroreflex control of renal nerve activity in cirrhosis. *Am J Physiol* 1995;268:R117–R129.
277. Rogenes PR, Gottschalk CW. Renal function in conscious rats with chronic unilateral renal denervation. *Am J Physiol* 1982;242:F140–F148.
278. Ros J, Jimenez W, Lamas S, et al. Nitric oxide production in arterial vessels of cirrhotic rats. *Hepatology* 1995;21:554–560.
279. Rosoff L, Zia P, Reynolds T, et al. Studies of renin and aldosterone in cirrhotic patients with ascites. *Gastroenterology* 1975;69:698–705.
280. Roulot D, Moreau R, Gaudin C, et al. Long-term sympathetic and hemodynamic responses to clonidine in patients with cirrhosis and ascites. *Gastroenterology* 1992;102:1309–1318.
281. Runyon BA. Care of patients with ascites. *N Engl J Med* 1994;330:337–342.
282. Runyon BA. Patient selection is important in studying the impact of large-volume paracentesis on intravascular volume. *Am J Gastroenterol* 1997;92:371–373.
283. Runyon BA. Management of adult patients with ascites caused by cirrhosis. *Hepatology* 1998;27:264–272.
284. Saitoh S, Scicli AG, Peterson E, et al. Effect of inhibiting renal kallikrein on prostaglandin E2, water, and sodium excretion. *Hypertension* 1995;25:1008–1013.
285. Salo J, Jimenez W, Kuhn M, et al. Urinary excretion of urodilatin in patients with cirrhosis. *Hepatology* 1996;24:1428–1432.
286. Sanyal AJ, Freedman AM, Luketic VA, et al.: the natural history of portal hypertension after transjugular intrahepatic portosystemic shunts. *Gastroenterology* 1997;112:889–898.
287. Sanz E, Caramelo C, Lopez-Novoa JM. Interstitial dynamics in rats with early stage experimental cirrhosis of the liver. *Am J Physiol* 1989;256:F497–F503.
288. Sato S, Ohnishi K, Sugita S, Okuda K. Splenic artery and superior mesenteric artery blood flow: nonsurgical doppler US measurement in healthy subjects and patients with chronic liver disease. *Radiology* 1987;164:347–352.
289. Schaffner F, Popper H. Capillarization of hepatic sinusoids in man. *Gastroenterology* 1963;44: 239–242.
290. Schedl HP, Bartter FC. An explanation for an experimental correction of the abnormal water diuresis in cirrhosis. *J Clin Invest* 1960;39:248–261.
291. Schrier RW Pathogenesis of sodium and water retention in high-output and low-output cardiac failure, nephrotic syndrome, cirrhosis, and pregnancy. *N Engl J Med* 1988;319:1065–1072, 1127–1134.
292. Schrier RW, Berl T, Anderson RJ. Osmotic and nonosmotic control of vasopressin release. *Am J Physiol* 1979;236:F321–F332.
293. Schrier RW, Humphreys MH. Factors involved in the antinatriuretic effects of acute constriction of the thoracic and abdominal inferior vena cava. *Circ Res* 1971;29:479–489.
294. Schrier RW, Humphreys MH, Ufferman RC. Role of cardiac output and the autonomic nervous system in the antinatriuretic response to acute constriction of the thoracic superior vena cava. *Circ Res* 1971;29:490–498.
295. Schuster VL, Kokko JP, Jacobson HR. Angiotensin II directly stimulates sodium transport in rabbit proximal convoluted tubules. *J Clin Invest* 1984;73:507–515.
296. Schwartz WB, Bennett W, Curelop S, et al. A syndrome of renal sodium loss and hyponatremia probably resulting from inappropriate secretion of antidiuretic hormone. *Am J Med* 1957;13:529–542.
297. Seldin DW, Preisig PA, Alpern RJ. Regulation of proximal reabsorption by effective arterial blood volume. *Semin Nephrol* 1991;11:212–219.
298. Shapiro MD, Nicholls KM, Groves BM, et al. Role of glomerular filtration rate in the impaired sodium and water excretion of patients with the nephrotic syndrome. *Am J Kidney Dis* 1986;8:81–87.
299. Shapiro MD, Nicholls KM, Groves BM, et al. Interrelationship between cardiac output and vascular resistance as determinants of effective arterial blood volume in cirrhotic patients. *Kidney Int* 1985;28:206–211.
300. Shapiro MD, Hasbargen J, Hensen J, et al. Role of aldosterone in the sodium retention of patients with nephrotic syndrome. *Am J Nephrol* 1990;10:44–48.
301. Skorecki KL, Leung WM, Campbell P, et al. Role of atrial natriuretic peptide in the natriuretic response to central volume expansion induced by head-out water immersion in sodium-retaining cirrhotic subjects. *Am J Med* 1988;85:375–382.
302. Smith JD, Hayslett JP. Reversible renal failure in the nephrotic syndrome. *Am J Kidney Dis* 1992;19:201–213.
303. Schnerman J. Juxtaglomerular cell complex in the regulation of renal salt excretion. *Am J Physiol* 1998;274:R263–R279.
304. Sogni P, Garnier P, Gadano A, et al. Endogenous pulmonary nitric oxide production measured from exhaled air is increased in patients with severe cirrhosis. *J Hepatol* 1995;23: 471–473.
305. Somberg KA, Lake JR, Tomlanovich SJ, et al. Transjugular intrahepatic portosystemic shunts for refractory ascites: assessment of clinical and hormonal response and renal function. *Hepatology* 1995;21:709–716.
306. Sonnenberg H, Honrath V, Chong CK, et al. Atrial natriuretic factor inhibits sodium transport in medullary collecting duct. *Am J Physiol* 1986;250:F963–F966.
307. Schnermann J. Juxtaglomerular cell complex in the regulation of renal salt excretion. *Am J Physiol* 1998;274:R263–R279.
308. Stanley MM, Ochi S, Lee KK, et al. Peritoneovenous shunting as compared with medical treatment in patients with alcoholic cirrhosis and massive ascites. *N Engl J Med* 1989;321:1632–1638.
309. Stokes JB, Kokko JP. Inhibition of sodium transport by prostaglandin E2 across isolated, perfused rabbit collecting tubule. *J Clin Invest* 1979;50:1099–1104.
310. Stumpe KO, Solle H, Klein H, et al. Mechanism of sodium and water retention in rats with experimental heart failure. *Kidney Int* 1973;4:309–317.
311. Suki WN. Renal hemodynamic consequences of angiotensin-converting enzyme inhibition in congestive heart failure. *Arch Intern Med* 1989;149:669–673.
312. Taylor AE. Capillary fluid filtration Starling forces and lymph flow. *Circ Res* 1981;49:557–575.
313. Thornborough JR, Passo SS, Rothballer AB. Receptors in cerebral circulation affecting sodium excretion in the cat. *Am J Physiol* 1973;225:138–142.
314. Tobe SW, Morali GA, Greig PD, et al. Peritoneovenous shunting restores atrial natriuretic factor responsiveness in refractory hepatic ascites. *Gastroenterology* 1993;105:202–207.
315. Tobian L, Perry S, Mork J. The relationship of the juxtaglomerular apparatus to sodium retention in experimental nephrosis. *Ann Intern Med* 1962;57:382–388.
316. Tulassay T, Rascher W, Lang RE, et al. Atrial natriuretic peptide and other vasoactive hormones in nephrotic syndrome. *Kidney Int* 1987;31:1391–1395.
317. Uchida Y, Kamisaka K, Ueda H. Two types of renal mechanoreceptors. *Jpn Heart J* 1971;12:233–241.
318. Unikowsky B, Wexler MJ, Levy M. Dogs with experimental cirrhosis of the liver but without intrahepatic hypertension do not retain sodium or form ascites. *J Clin Invest* 1983;72: 1594–1604.
319. Usberti M, Federico S, Cianciaruso B, et al Relationship between serum albumin concentration and tubular reabsorption of glucose in renal disease. *Kidney Int* 1983;16:546–551.
320. Usberti M, Federico S, Meccariello S, et al. Role of plasma vasopressin in the impairment of water excretion in nephrotic syndrome. *Kidney Int* 1984;25:422–429.
321. Usberti M, Gazzotti R, Poiesi C, et al. Considerations on the sodium retention in nephrotic syndrome. *Am J Nephrol* 1995;15:38–47.
322. Valentin J, Qiu C, Muldowney WP, et al. Cellular basis for blunted volume expansion natruresis in experimental nephrotic syndrome. *J Clin Invest* 1992;90:1302–1312.
323. Valentin J, Ying W, Sechi LA, et al. Phosphodiesterase inhibitors correct resistance to natriuretic peptides in rate with Heymann nephritis. *J Am Soc Nephrol* 1996;7:582–593.
324. Villareal D, Freeman RH, Davis JO, et al. Atrial natriuretic factor secretion in dogs with experimental high-output heart failure. *Am J Physiol* 1987;252:H692–H696.
325. Villarreal D, Freeman RH, Johnson RA, et al. Effects of renal denervation on postprandial sodium excretion in experimental heart failure. *Am J Physiol* 1994;266:R1599–R1604.
326. Vorobioff J, Bredfeldt JE, Groszmann RJ. Increased blood flow through the portal system in cirrhotic rats. *Gastroenterology* 1984;87:1120–1126.

327. Wada A, Tsutamoto T, Fukai D, et al. Comparison of the effects of selective endothelin ETA and ETB receptor antagonists in congestive heart failure. *J Am Coll Cardiol* 1997;30:1385–1392.

328. Walle J, Donckerwolcke R, Boer P, et al. Blood volume, colloid osmotic pressure and F-cell ratio in children with the nephrotic syndrome. *Kidney Int* 1996;49:1471–1477.

329. Watkins L, Burton JA, Haber E, et al. The renin-angiotensin-aldosterone system in congestive heart failure in conscious dogs. *J Clin Invest* 1976;57:1606–1617.

330. Weigert AL, Martin P-Y, Schrier RW. Vascular hyporesponsiveness in cirrhotic rats: role of different nitric oxide synthase isoforms. *Kidney Int* 1997;52(Suppl 61):S41–S44.

331. Weinman EJ, Sansom SC, Knight TF, et al. Alpha and beta adrenergic agonists stimulate water absorption in the rat proximal tubule. *J Membr Biol* 1982;69:107–111.

332. Welt LG, Seldin DW, Nelson WP, et al. Role of the central nervous system in metabolism of electrolytes and water. *Arch Intern Med* 1952;90:355–378.

333. Winlaw DS, Smythe GA, Keogh AM, et al. Increased nitric oxide production in heart failure. *Lancet* 1994;344:373–374.

334. Wirth KJ, Bickel M, Hropot M, et al. The bradykinin B2 receptor antagonist Icatibant (HOE 140) corrects avid Na+ retention in rats with CCL4-induced liver cirrhosis: possible role of enhanced microvascular leakage. *Eur J Pharmacol* 1997;337:45–53.

335. Witte MH, Witte CL, Dumont AE. Progress in liver disease: physiological factors involved in the causation of cirrhotic ascites. *Gastroenterology* 1971;61:742–750.

336. Witte MH, Witte CL, Dumont AE. Estimated net transcapillary water and protein flux in the liver and intestine of patients with portal hypertension from hepatic cirrhosis. *Gastroenterology* 1981;80:265–272.

337. Witte CL, Witte MH, Dumont AE, et al. Protein content in lymph and edema fluids in congestive heart failure. *Circulation* 1969;40:623–630.

338. Wong F, Sniderman K, Liu P, et al. The mechanism of the initial natriuresis after transjugular intrahepatic portosystemic shunt. *Gastroenterology* 1997;112:899–907.

339. Wong F, Sniderman K, Liu P, et al. Transjugular intrahepatic portosystemic stent shunt: effects on hemodynamics and sodium homeostasis in cirrhosis and refractory ascites. *Ann Intern Med* 1995;122:816–822.

340. Wood LJ, Massie D, McLean AJ, et al. Renal sodium retention in cirrhosis: tubular site and relation to hepatic dysfunction. *Hepatology* 1988;8:831–836.

341. Wraight EP. Capillary permeability of protein as a factor in the control of plasma volume. *J Physiol* 1974;237:39.

342. Xu D-L, Martin P-Y, Ohara M, et al. Upregulation of aquaporin-2 water channel expression in chronic heart failure rat. *J Clin Invest* 1997;99:1500–1505.

343. Yamauchi H, Hopper J. Hypovolemic shock and hypotension as a complication in the nephrotic syndrome. *Ann Intern Med* 1964;60:242–254.

344. Zambraski EJ, Dunn MJ. Importance of renal prostaglandins in control of renal function after chronic ligation of the common bile duct in dogs. *J Lab Clin Med* 1984;103:549–559.

345. Zennaro M-C, Lombes M. Mineralocorticoid resistance. *Trends Endocrinol Metab* 2004;15:264–270.

346. Zietse R, Schalekamp MA. Effect of synthetic human atrial natriuretic peptide (102–106) in nephrotic syndrome. *Kidney Int* 1988;34:717–724.

347. Zipser RD, Hoefs JC, Speckart PF, et al. Prostaglandins: modulators of renal function and pressor resistance in chronic liver disease. *J Clin Endocrinol Metab* 1979;48:895–900.

348. Zucker IH, Earle AM, Gilmore JP. The mechanism of adaptation of left atrial stretch receptors in dogs with chronic congestive heart failure. *J Clin Invest* 1977;60:323–331.

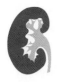

CHAPTER 37

Physiology and Pathophysiology of Diuretic Action

Mark D. Okusa and David H. Ellison

University of Virginia Health System, Charlottesville, Virginia, USA
Oregon Health and Science University, Portland, Oregon, USA

The term *diuretic* derives from the Greek *diouretikos*, meaning "to promote urine." Although infusion of saline or ingestion of water would therefore qualify as being diuretic, the term *diuretic* usually connotes a drug that can reduce the extracellular fluid volume by increasing urinary solute or water excretion (423). The term *aquaretic* (106) has been applied to drugs that increase excretion of solute free water, distinguishing these drugs from traditional diuretics, which enhanced solute with water excretion. The clinical picture of extracellular fluid volume expansion leading to edema or "dropsy" (from the Latin, *hydrops*) has been recognized since the earliest days of recorded history (139). Ancient Egyptians referred to "flooding of the heart" (139) and the Hippocratic Corpus later suggested specific remedies for dropsical patients, although their results are not noted. In 1553, Paracelsus recorded the first truly effective form of therapy for dropsy, inorganic mercury (Calomel [4]). Inorganic mercury remained the mainstay of diuretic treatment until the beginning of this century.

In 1919, the ability of organic mercurial antisyphilitics to affect diuresis was discovered by Vogl, then a medical student (496). This observation led to the development of effective organic mercurial diuretics, drugs that were used commonly until the 1960s. In 1937, the antimicrobial, sulfanilamide, was found to cause metabolic acidosis in patients. Carbonic anhydrase (CA) had been discovered in 1932; it was know that sulfanilamide inhibited this enzyme. Pitts demonstrated that sulfanilamide inhibited sodium (Na) bicarbonate reabsorption in dogs (139) and Schwartz showed that sulfanilamide could induce diuresis in patients with congestive heart failure who were resistant to organic mercurial diuretics (420). Soon, more potent sulfonamide-based carbonic anhydrase inhibitors were developed, but these drugs suffered from side effects and limited potency. Nevertheless, a group at Sharp & Dohme Inc. was stimulated by these developments to explore the possibility that modification of sulfonamide-based drugs could lead to drugs that enhanced Na *chloride* rather than Na *bicarbonate* excretion. The result of this program was the synthesis of chlorothiazide and its marketing in 1957 (32, 33, 34). This drug ushered in the modern era of diuretic therapy and revolutionized the clinical treatment of edema.

The search for more potent classes of diuretics continued, based on the structure of chlorothiazide and sulonamyl derivatives. This led to the development of ethacrynic acid and furosemide in the United States and Germany, respectively (139). The safety and efficacy of these drugs led them to replace the organic mercurials as drugs of first choice for severe and resistant edema. Spironolactone, marketed in 1961, was developed after the properties and structure of aldosterone had been established and steroidal analogues of aldosterone were found to have aldosterone-blocking activity (1). Triamterene was initially synthesized as a folic acid antagonist, but was found to have diuretic and potassium (K)–sparing activity (511).

The availability of safe, effective, and relatively inexpensive diuretic drugs has made it possible to treat edematous disorders and hypertension effectively. Driven by clinical need, however, the development of effective diuretic drugs generated specific ligands that interact with Na and Cl transport proteins in the kidney. In the 1990s, these ligands were used to identify and clone the Na and Cl transport proteins that mediate the bulk of renal Na and Cl reabsorption. The diuretic-sensitive transport proteins that have been cloned include the sodium hydrogen exchanger (NHE) family of proteins (350, 407, 471), the bumetanide-sensitive Na-K-2Cl cotransporters (171, 523), the thiazide-sensitive Na-Cl cotransporter (172), and the epithelial Na channel (77, 78). The information derived from molecular cloning has also permitted identification of inherited human diseases that are caused by mutations in these transport proteins (409). The phenotypes of several of these disorders resemble the manifestations of chronic diuretic administration. The recognition, for example, that Gitelman syndrome results from mutation of the thiazide-sensitive Na-Cl cotransporter (435), has spurred interest in determining how blockade or dysfunction of this transport protein leads to magnesium wasting. Thus, the development of clinically useful diuretics permitted identification and later cloning of specific ion transport pathways. The molecular cloning is now helping to define mechanisms of diuretic action and diuretic side effects. The use of animals in which diuretic-sensitive transport pathways have been "knocked out" should permit a clearer understanding of which diuretic effects result directly or secondarily from actions of the drugs on specific ion transport pathways and which effects result from actions on other pathways or other organ systems.

DIURETIC-SENSITIVE SALT TRANSPORT

In a normal human kidney, approximately 23 M of NaCl are filtered in 150 L of fluid each day. Approximately 6 to 10 g of salt (102–170 mEq NaCl) are consumed each day by individuals on a typical Western diet. To maintain balance, renal NaCl excretion must be approximately 92 to 160 mmol/day (the difference owing to nonrenal losses). Such calculations imply that 99.2% of the filtered NaCl load is reabsorbed by kidney tubules each day (the FE_{Na} is 0.8%). Sodium, chloride, and water reabsorption by the nephron is driven by the metabolic energy in ATP. The ouabain-sensitive Na,K-ATPase is expressed at the basolateral cell membrane of all Na-transporting epithelial cells along the nephron. This pump maintains large ion gradients across the plasma membrane, with the intracellular Na concentration maintained low and the intracellular K concentration maintained high. Because the pump is electrogenic and because it is associated with a K channel, renal epithelial cells have a voltage across the plasma membrane oriented with the inside negative relative to the outside.

The combination of the low intracellular Na concentration and the plasma membrane voltage generates a large electrochemical gradient favoring Na entry from lumen or interstitium. Specific diuretic-sensitive Na transport pathways are expressed at the apical surface of cells along the nephron, permitting vectorial transport of Na from lumen to blood (Fig. 1). Along the proximal tubule, where approximately 50% to 60% of filtered Na is reabsorbed, an isoform of the Na–H exchanger is expressed at the apical membrane (37). Along the thick ascending limb, where approximately 20 to 25 moles of filtered Na is reabsorbed, an isoform of the Na-K-2Cl cotransporter is expressed at the apical membrane (137, 525). Along the distal convoluted tubule, where approximately 5% of filtered Na is reabsorbed, an isoform of the thiazide-sensitive Na-Cl cotransporter is expressed (14, 342). Along the connecting tubule and cortical collecting duct, where approximately 3% of filtered Na is reabsorbed, isoforms of the amiloride-sensitive epithelial Na channel are expressed (131). These apical Na transport pathways form the primary targets for diuretic action.

This chapter will discuss the physiological and pharmacological bases for diuretic action in the kidney. Although some aspects of clinical diuretic usage will be discussed, we have emphasized physiological principles and mechanisms of action. Several recent texts provide detailed discussions of diuretic treatment of clinical conditions (477). Extensive discussions of diuretic pharmacokinetics are also available (54). The influence of renal disease on diuretic drug usage is discussed in the following chapter of this volume.

One classification of diuretic drugs is based on the primary nephron site of action. Such a scheme emphasizes that

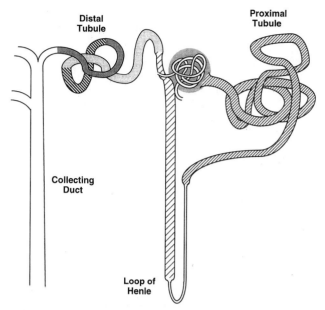

FIGURE 1   Sites of diuretic action along the nephron. Carbonic anhydrase inhibitors reduce Na reabsorption along the proximal tubule (*narrow diagonals*). Loop diuretics inhibit Na and Cl transport along the thick ascending limb of the loop of Henle (*wide diagonals*). Distal convoluted tubule (DCT) diuretics (thiazides and others) inhibit Na and Cl transport along the distal convoluted tubule (along both the DCT-1, *light shading*, and the DCT-2, *cross-hatch*). CCD diuretics inhibit electrogenic Na transport along both the DCT-2 (*cross-hatch*), the connecting tubule (*dark shading*), and the cortical collecting duct (*white*). Thus, sites of action of DCT diuretics overlap with sites of action of CCD diuretics.

drugs of more than one chemical class can affect the same ion transport mechanism. Although most diuretic drugs have actions on more than one nephron segment, most owe their clinical effects primarily to their ability to inhibit Na transport by one particular nephron segment. An exception is the osmotic diuretics. Although these drugs were initially believed to inhibit solute and water flux along the proximal tubule, subsequent studies have revealed effects in multiple segments. Other diuretics, however, will be classified according to their primary site of action.

OSMOTIC DIURETICS

Osmotic diuretics are substances that are freely filtered at the glomerulus, but are poorly reabsorbed (Fig. 2). The pharmacological activity of drugs in this group depends entirely on the osmotic pressure exerted by the drug molecules in solution and not on interaction with specific transport proteins or enzymes. Mannitol is the prototypical osmotic diuretic. Its diuretic effect is not due to interactions with receptors or renal transporters but rather it is due to more complex mechanisms that involve osmotic effects on tubule epithelium and reduction of the medullary interstitial osmolality (30, 279). Because the relationship between the magnitude of effect and concentration of osmotic diuretic

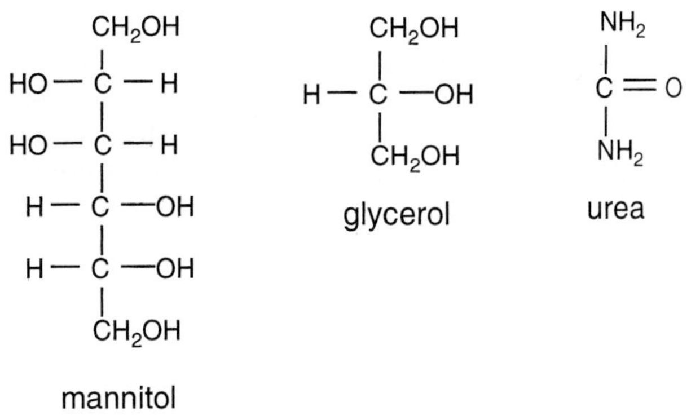

FIGURE 2   Structures of osmotic diuretics.

in solution is linear, all agents used clinically are small molecules. Other agents considered in this class include urea, sorbitol and glycerol.

Urinary Electrolyte Eexcretion

Although osmotic agents do not act directly on transport pathways, the rate of transport of ions is affected. Following the infusion of mannitol, the excretion of sodium, potassium, calcium, magnesium, bicarbonate and chloride is increased (Table 1) (127, 449, 520). The fractional reabsorption rates for sodium and water were reduced by 27% and 12%, respectively, following the infusion of mannitol (421). Reabsorption of magnesium and calcium reabsorption was also reduced in the proximal tubule and loop of Henle, whereas phosphate reabsorption was inhibited slightly in the presence of parathyroid hormone (520).

Mechanism of Action

The functional consequences that result from intravenous infusion of mannitol include an increase in cortical and medullary blood flow, a variable effect on glomerular filtration rate; an increase in excretion of sodium, water, calcium, magnesium, phosphorus, and bicarbonate; and a decrease in medullary concentration gradient. The most pronounced effect observed with mannitol is a brisk diuresis and natriuresis. The mechanisms by which mannitol produces a diuresis are thought to be secondary to (1) an increase in osmotic pressure in the proximal tubule fluid and loop of Henle thereby retarding the passive reabsorption of water and (2) an increase in renal blood flow and washout of the medullary tonicity.

Mannitol is freely filtered at the glomerulus and its presence in the tubule fluid minimizes passive water reabsorption primarily by the proximal tubule and by the thin limbs of the loop of Henle. Normally, within the proximal tubule, sodium reabsorption creates an osmotic gradient for water reabsorption. When an osmotic diuretic is administered, however the osmotic force of the nonreabsorbable solute in the lumen opposes the osmotic force produced by sodium reabsorption (508). Isosmolality of the urine is preserved because molecules of mannitol replace sodium ions reabsorbed. However, sodium reabsorption eventually stops because the luminal sodium concentration is reduced to a point where a limiting gradient is reached and net transport of sodium and water is blocked (421, 520). This view was confirmed by stationary micropuncture studies (516). Quantitatively, mannitol has a greater effect on inhibiting Na and water reabsorption in the loop of Henle than in the proximal tubule. Free-flow micropuncture studies following mannitol infusion in dogs demonstrated a modest decrease in fractional reabsorption of sodium and water by the proximal tubule, but a much larger effect by the loop of Henle (421, 520). Within the loop of Henle the site of action of mannitol appears to be restricted to the thin descending limb resulting in a decrease in reabsorption of Na and water (180). In the thick ascending limb, reabsorption of Na will continue in proportion to its delivery to this segment. The sum of

TABLE 1   Effects of Diuretics on Electrolyte Excretion

	Na	**Cl**	**K**	**Pi**	**Ca**	**Mg**
Osmotic diuretics (35, 36, 524–526)	↑(10–25%)	↑ (15–30%)	↑ (6%)	↑ (5%–10%)	↑ (10–20%)	↑ (>20%)
Carbonic anhydrase inhibitors (74, 157, 255)	↑ (6%)	↑ (4%)	↑ (60%)	↑ (>20%)	↑ or ↑ (<5%)	↑ (<5%)
Loop diuretics (154, 156, 157, 230, 255, 413)	↑ (30%)	↑ (40%)	↑ (60%–100%)	↑ (>20%)	↑ (>20%)	↑ (>20%)
DCT diuretics (154, 230, 252, 255)	↑ (6%–11%)	↑ (10%)	↑ (200%)	↑ (>20%)	↓	↑ (5%–10%)
Na channel blockers (230, 255, 413)	↑ (3%–5%)	↑ (6%)	↑ (8%)	⇔	⇔	↓
Spironolactone (255)	↑ (3%)	↑ (6%)	↓	⇔	⇔	↓

Figures indicate approximate maximal fractional excretions of ions following acute diuretic administration in maximally effective doses. ↑ indicates that the drug increases excretion; ↓ indicates that the drug decreases excretion; ⇔ indicates that the drug has little of no direct effect on excretion. During chronic treatment, effects often wane (Na excretion), may increase (K excretion during DCT diuretic treatment), or may reverse as with uric acid (not shown).

net transport in the thin and thick limbs will determine the net effect of mannitol in the loop of Henle. Further downstream in the collecting duct, mannitol reduces Na and water reabsorption (64).

Renal Hemodynamics

During the administration of mannitol, its molecules diffuse from the blood stream into the interstitial space. In the interstitial space, the increased osmotic pressure draws water from the cells to increase extracellular fluid volume. This effect increases total renal plasma flow (64). Cortical blood flow and medullary blood flow are both increased following mannitol infusion (64), effects seen in both normotensive and hypotensive animals (326). Single-nephron glomerular filtration rate (GFR), on the other hand, increases in cortex and decreases in medulla (180, 467); this action on the medulla washes out the medullary osmotic gradient by reducing papillary sodium and urea content (146, 334). The mechanisms that contribute to the increase in renal blood flow include a decrease in hematocrit and blood viscosity and the release of vasoactive agents. Experimental studies indicate that the osmotic effect of mannitol to increase water movement from intracellular to extracellular space leads to a decrease in hematocrit and in blood viscosity. This fact contributes to a decrease in renal vascular resistance and increase in renal blood flow (334). Both prostacyclin (PGI2) synthesis (234) and atrial natriuretic peptide (524) could mediate the effect of mannitol on renal blood flow. The vasodilatory effect of mannitol is reduced when the recipient is pretreated with indomethacin or meclofenamate suggesting that PGI2 is involved in the vasodilatory effect.

The effect of mannitol on GFR has been variable but most studies indicate that the overall effect of mannitol is to increase GFR (30, 40, 185, 279, 421). Whereas mannitol increased cortical and medullary blood flow, it increased cortical but decreased medullary single-nephron GFR (180, 467). The mechanisms by which mannitol reduces the GFR of deep nephrons are not known, but it has been postulated that mannitol reduces efferent arteriolar pressure. Micropuncture studies examining the determinants of GFR in superficial nephrons have demonstrated that the increase in single-nephron GFR is owing to an increase in single-nephron plasma flow and a decrease in oncotic pressure (40).

Alterations in renal hemodynamics contribute to the diuresis observed following administration of mannitol. An increase in medullary blood flow rate reduces medullary tonicity (146) primarily by decreasing papillary sodium and urea content (187) and increasing urine flow rate (334).

Pharmacokinetics

Mannitol is not readily absorbed from the intestine (30); therefore, it is routinely administered intravenously. Following infusion, mannitol distributes in extracellular fluid with a volume of distribution of approximately 16 l (5); its excretion is almost entirely by glomerular filtration (503). Of the filtered load, less than 10% is reabsorbed by the renal tubule, and a similar quantity is metabolized, probably in the liver. With normal glomerular filtration rate, plasma half-life is approximately 2.2 hours.

Clinical Use

Mannitol is used prophylactically or as treatment for established acute renal failure (30), although the basis for its use in established acute renal failure remains controversial (97, 465). Mannitol improves renal hemodynamics in a variety of situations of impending or incipient acute renal failure. Mannitol (along with hydration and sodium bicarbonate) has been recommended for the early treatment in myoglobinuric acute renal failure (31) and in the prevention of post transplant acute renal failure (194, 269, 480). Although some studies have shown a beneficial effect when used prophylactically in patients at risk for contrast nephropathy (505), most prospective controlled studies have not found mannitol beneficial in preventing acute renal failure and it is not recommended for use in this situation (97, 441).

Mannitol is used for short-term reduction of intraocular pressure (384). By increasing the osmotic pressure, mannitol reduces the volume of aqueous humor and the intraocular pressure by extracting water. Mannitol also decreases cerebral edema and the increase in intracranial pressure associated with trauma, tumors, and neurosurgical procedures (313). Mannitol is used perioperatively in patients undergoing cardiopulmonary bypass surgery. The beneficial effects may be related to its osmotic activity reducing intravenous fluid requirement (227) and its ability to act as a free radical antioxidant (147). Mannitol and other osmotic agents have been used in the treatment of dialysis disequilibrium syndrome (8, 189). This syndrome is characterized acute symptoms immediately following hemodialysis. Most significant symptoms are attributable to disorders of the central nervous system such as: headache, nausea, blurred vision, confusion, seizure, coma and death. Rapid removal of small solutes such as urea during dialysis of patients who are markedly azotemic is associated with the development of an osmotic gradient for water movement into brain cells producing cerebral edema and neurologic dysfunction. Dialysis disequilibrium syndrome can be minimized by slow solute removal and raising plasma osmolality with saline or mannitol.

Adverse Effects

In patients with reduced cardiac output, an increase in extracellular volume induced by mannitol infusion may lead to pulmonary edema. Intravenous administration of mannitol increases cardiac output and pulmonary capillary wedge pressures (5). Acute and prolonged administration of mannitol leads to different electrolyte disturbances. Acute overzealous use or the accumulation of mannitol leads to dilutional metabolic acidosis and hyponatremia (12). Accumulation of mannitol also produces hyperkalemia (301, 325) as a result of an increase in plasma osmolality. An increase in plasma osmolality increases potassium movement from intracellular to extracellular fluid from bulk solute flow and increase in the electrochemical gradient for potassium secretion. Prolonged administration of mannitol can lead to urinary losses of sodium and potassium leading to volume depletion, hypernatremia (as urinary loss of sodium is invariably less than water), and hypokalemia (184). Marked accumulation of mannitol in patients can lead to reversible acute renal failure that appears to be due to vasoconstriction and tubular vacuolization (121, 462, 493). Mannitol-induced acute renal failure usually occurs when large cumulative doses of ~295 g are given to patients with previously compromised renal function (121).

PROXIMAL TUBULE DIURETICS

Carbonic Anhydrase Inhibitors

Through the development of carbonic anhydrase inhibitors, important compounds were discovered that have utility as therapeutic agents and as research tools. Carbonic anhydrase inhibitors have a limited therapeutic role as diuretic agents because of weak natriuretic properties. They are used primarily to reduce intraocular pressure in glaucoma and to enhance bicarbonate excretion in metabolic alkalosis. Carbonic anhydrase inhibitors have been useful in the development of other diuretic agents such as thiazide and loop diuretics and have been instrumental in elucidating transport function in proximal and distal nephron segments. Structures of carbonic anhydrase inhibitors are shown in Fig. 3.

Urinary Electrolyte Excretion

Through their effects on carbonic anhydrase in the proximal tubule, carbonic anhydrase inhibitors increase bicarbonate excretion by 25% to 30% (63, 96, 130, 382). The increase in sodium and chloride excretion is minimal, as most of these ions are reabsorbed by more distal segments (63). However, a residual small but variable amount of sodium is excreted along with bicarbonate ions. Proximal tubule calcium and phosphate reabsorption are blocked by acetazolamide. However, because of distal calcium reabsorption, fractional excretion of calcium does not increase (21). In contrast, phosphate appears to escape distal reabsorption following acetazolamide administration resulting in an increase in fractional excretion of phosphate by ~3% (21, 382). Although proximal tubule magnesium transport is inhibited by carbonic anhydrase inhibitors, fractional excretion is either unchanged or is increased as a result of variable distal reabsorption (382).

Acetazolamide increases potassium excretion (63, 303, 381, 382). Although a direct effect of acetazolamide has not been established, it is likely that several indirect effects could contribute to the observed kaliuresis. Carbonic anhydrase inhibition could block proximal tubule potassium reabsorption and increase delivery to the distal tubule; however, the reported effects of carbonic anhydrase inhibition on proximal tubule transport have been conflicting. Whereas carbonic anhydrase inhibitors decrease proximal tubule sodium, bicarbonate and water absorption during free-flow micropuncture and microperfusion, the effects of carbonic anhydrase inhibitors on proximal tubule potassium transport have been less consistent. In free-flow micropuncture studies carbonic anhydrase inhibition did not affect proximal tubule potassium reabsorption (22); however, in in vivo–perfused proximal tubules carbonic anhydrase inhibition reduced net potassium transport (346). The effect of acetazolamide on the proximal tubule ion transport does however facilitate an increase in tubular fluid flow rate and delivery to the distal nephron of sodium, bicarbonate but not chloride. This effect is thought to increase the concentration of nonreabsorbable anions creating an increase in lumen negative voltage (303) and increase in flow rate (191), factors known to increase potassium secretion by the distal tubule. Acetazolamide can also produce a luminal composition that is low in chloride and high in nonchloride anion. This luminal fluid composition has been demonstrated to stimulate potassium secretion by the distal nephron independent of a change in lumen negative voltage (489).

Mechanism of Action

In the kidney, carbonic anhydrase inhibitors act primarily on proximal tubule cells to inhibit bicarbonate absorption. Carbonic anhydrase, a metalloenzyme containing one zinc atom per molecule, is important in sodium bicarbonate reabsorption and hydrogen ion secretion by renal epithelial cells. The

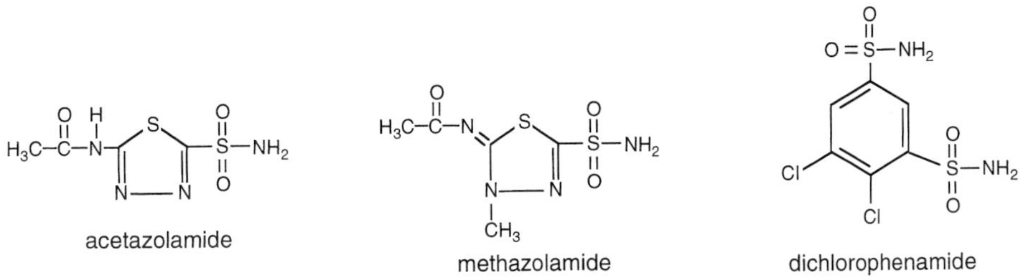

FIGURE 3   Structures of carbonic anhydrase inhibitors.

biochemical, morphological, and functional properties of carbonic anhydrase have been reviewed previously (121, 307, 376). Of the four major isozymes of carbonic anhydrase expressed in mammalian tissues, two appear relevant for luminal acidification in kidney. Type II carbonic anhydrase is distributed widely, comprising more than 95% of the overall activity in kidney and is sensitive to inhibition by sulfonamides (121, 519). Type II carbonic anhydrase is expressed in the cytoplasm and facilitates the secretion of H ions by catalyzing the formation of HCO_3 from OH and CO_2 (Eq. 3). Type IV carbonic anhydrase is bound to renal cortical membranes, comprising up to 5% of the overall activity in kidney, and is sensitive to sulfonamides (150, 309). Type IV carbonic anhydrase, expressed on basolateral and luminal plasma membranes of proximal tubule cells (376, 406, 518) and luminal membrane of intercalated cells (293), catalyzes the dehydration of intraluminal carbonic acid generated from secreted protons (121, 183). Evidence for the physiological importance for carbonic anhydrase is apparent as a deficiency of type II carbonic anhydrase leads to a renal acidification defect resulting in renal tubular acidosis (436). Furthermore, metabolic acidosis leads to an adaptive increase in types II and IV carbonic anhydrase mRNA expression in kidney (472) suggesting the importance of both carbonic anhydrase isoforms in this disorder.

Normally the proximal tubule reabsorbs 80% of the filtered load of sodium bicarbonate and 60% of the filtered load of sodium chloride. Early studies by Pitts et al. (129, 369) and micropuncture studies indicated that hydrogen ion secretion was responsible for bicarbonate absorption and renal acidification (128, 129, 387, 492). The cellular mechanism by which proximal tubules reabsorb bicarbonate is depicted in Fig. 4. The net reaction between filtered HCO_3 and secreted H is occurs by two mechanisms as depicted in Eq. 1 and 2.

Luminal Fluid

$$H^+ + HCO_3^- \rightarrow H_2CO_3 \rightarrow CO_2 + H_2O \qquad (Eq. 1)$$

$$HCO_3^- \xrightarrow{CA} OH^- + CO_2 \qquad (Eq. 2)$$

$$H^+ + OH^- \rightarrow H_2O$$

In the presence of carbonic anhydrase the formation of CO_2 and H_2O occurs predominately by the dissociation of HCO_3 to OH (Eq. 2). However in the absence of carbonic anhydrase the former pathway (Eq. 1) predominates. Luminal carbonic anhydrase prevents H from accumulating in tubule fluid and secondarily permits the continued secretion of H (128). Carbon dioxide rapidly diffuses from the lumen into the cell across the apical membrane. Within the cell, H is secreted into the tubule lumen via Na–H exchange (257, 330, 501) or H-ATPase (59, 255, 256). Following H secretion, OH formed diffuses to the basolateral membrane and combines with CO_2 forming HCO_3, the latter reaction is catalyzed by carbonic anhydrase (Eq. 3).

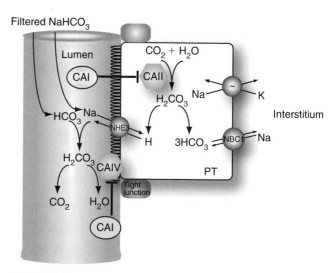

FIGURE 4 Mechanisms of diuretic action in the proximal tubule. Water and CO_2 are catalyzed to form form carbonic acid (H_2CO_3) inside proximal cells. Carbonic anhydrase inside the cell (isoform II, CAII) catalyzes the formation of HCO_3 from OH and CO_2. Bicarbonate leaves the cell via the Na-HCO_3 cotransporter (see text). A second pool of carbonic anhydrase (isoform IV, CAIV) is located in the brush border. This participates in disposing of luminal carbonic acid, formed by the combination of filtered bicarbonate and secreted protons. Both pools of carbonic anhydrase are inhibited by acetazolamide and other carbonic anhydrase inhibitors (see text).

Intracellular Fluid

$$OH^- + CO_2 \xrightarrow{CA} HCO_3^- \qquad (Eq. 3)$$

Bicarbonate ions generated then exit the basolateral membrane via $Na(HCO_3)_3$ cotransport (322). Thus in the early proximal tubule, the net effect of the process described results in the isosmotic reabsorption of $NaHCO_3$. The lumen chloride concentration increases because water of continues to be reabsorbed producing a lumen positive potential (487). These axial changes provide an electrochemical gradient for transport of chloride via paracellular and transcellular pathways. The later pathway for chloride–likely involves a chloride-base exchanger operating in parallel with a Na–H proton exchanger (243, 312). The dual operation of these parallel exchangers results in net NaCl absorption.

Carbonic anhydrase inhibitors act primarily on proximal tubule cells (186) where 60% to 70% of the filtered load of sodium chloride is reabsorbed (99, 282). Despite the magnitude of sodium chloride reabsorption in the proximal tubule segment, the natriuretic potency of carbonic anhydrase inhibitors is relatively weak. This observation is explained by the following: (1) proximal sodium reabsorption is due to carbonic anhydrase as well as noncarbonic anhydrase dependent pathways; (2) any increase in delivery of sodium to distal nephron segments is reabsorbed to a large degree by these distal nephron segments (21, 63, 96); and (3) the development of a hyperchloremic metabolic acidosis results from bicarbonate depletion and renders ineffective subsequent doses of acetazolamide (306). Metabolic acidosis produces resistance of bicarbonate absorption to carbonic anhydrase inhibition (431). Following the induction of metabolic acidosis, the Ki for bicarbonate absorption by membrane impermeant carbonic anhydrase inhibitors was increased by a factor of 100 to 500, suggesting that metabolic acidosis is associated with changes in the physical properties of the carbonic anhydrase protein. For these reasons, carbonic anhydrase inhibitors alone are rarely used as diuretic agents.

Following administration of carbonic anhydrase inhibitors, proximal tubule bicarbonate reabsorption is inhibited variably between 35% and >85% (71, 130, 273, 296, 298, 303, 492). Additional sites of action of carbonic anhydrase inhibitors include proximal straight tubule or loop of Henle (304, 315, 492), distal tubule (183), and collecting and papillary collecting ducts (266, 292, 315, 394, 476). Thus, despite the effect of carbonic anhydrase inhibitors on proximal tubules as well other nephron segments, compensatory reabsorption of bicarbonate at other downstream tubular sites limits net fractional excretion of bicarbonate to ~25% to 30% (96, 130).

The relative contribution of membrane-bound and intracellular carbonic anhydrase to bicarbonate reabsorption has been examined. Both contribute to bicarbonate absorption. The role of membrane-bound carbonic anhydrase was first suggested by Rector, Carter, and Seldin (387). The observation that carbonic anhydrase inhibitors produced an acid disequilibrium pH in the proximal tubule suggested that luminal fluid was normally in contact with carbonic anhydrase. Disequilibrium pH refers to the difference between the pH of tubule fluid in situ (pH_{is}, in this case during infusion of carbonic anhydrase inhibitors) and the pH achieved after the tubule fluid is allowed to reach chemical equilibrium at known PCO_2. Thus in the presence of carbonic anhydrase, the pH measured in situ and at equilibrium should be similar. In the absence of carbonic anhydrase, the dissociation of HCO_3 to OH and CO_2 is slow, allowing H to accumulate in the lumen and reducing pH. The demonstration of an acid disequilibrium pH provided physiological evidence in support of previous histochemical findings that a fraction of enzymatic activity was present in the tubule lumen. Although the cytoplasmic carbonic anhydrase constitutes most enzyme activity in kidney, it is believed that the membrane-bound carbonic anhydrase plays a significant role in bicarbonate reabsorption by the proximal tubule. Studies addressing this question have used carbonic anhydrase inhibitors that differ in their ability to penetrate proximal tubule cell membranes. Benzolamide is charged at normal pH and is relatively impermeant, whereas acetazolamide enters the cell relatively easily (213). Both intravenous (280, 287) and intratubular administration of benzolamide (296) resulted in an acid disequilibrium pH indicating that luminal carbonic anhydrase inhibition contributes to bicarbonate absorption. Furthermore proximal tubular perfusion of benzolamide resulted in 90% inhibition of bicarbonate reabsorp-

tion. Despite near-equal efficacy in inhibiting proximal tubule bicarbonate reabsorption, benzolamide lowered tubular fluid pH, whereas acetazolamide increased tubular fluid pH. These results suggest that the site of action of benzolamide is at the luminal membrane, whereas the site of action of acetazolamide is within the cell. Inhibition of luminal carbonic anhydrase causes lumen pH to decrease because of the continued secretion of hydrogen ions and its accumulation in the tubular lumen. In contrast, acetazolamide does not produce an acid disequilibrium pH (296). The conclusion that tubular fluid was in direct contact with membrane carbonic anhydrase was substantiated by the use of dextran-bound carbonic anhydrase inhibitor (296, 468). In proximal tubules perfused in vivo, Lucci et. al. (297) determined that dextran-bound inhibitors, which inhibit only luminal carbonic anhydrase, decreased proximal tubule bicarbonate absorption by approximately 80% and reduced lumen pH.

Although these studies establish the importance of luminal carbonic anhydrase, they also support a role for intracellular or basolateral carbonic anhydrase. The observation that acetazolamide and benzolamide inhibit proximal tubule bicarbonate reabsorption to a similar degree yet produce opposite effects on tubule fluid pH suggests that intracellular carbonic anhydrase contributes to proximal tubule luminal acidification.

The expression of carbonic anhydrase in the basolateral membrane of proximal tubule cells (406, 518) suggests that this membrane-bound enzyme has an important role in basolateral bicarbonate transport (68, 121). Carbonic anhydrase inhibitors, however, do not directly inhibit the basolateral bicarbonate exit transport system, $Na(HCO_3)$, but rather they inhibit intracellular generation of substrate for the transporter (408, 439).

In the collecting duct, carbonic anhydrase facilitates acid secretion that is mediated by a vacuolar H adenosinetriphosphatase (H-ATPase) (58) and a P-type gastric H,K-ATPase (268, 347, 517). Luminal administration of acetazolamide produced an acid disequilibrium pH in the outer medullary collecting duct suggesting contribution a of luminal carbonic anhydrase (447). In other studies, a membrane-impermeant carbonic anhydrase inhibitor (F-3500; aminobenzolamide coupled to a nontoxic polymer polyoxyethylene) reduced bicarbonate absorption thus confirming the presence of membrane-bound carbonic anhydrase in the outer medullar collecting duct (431). The Ki for inhibition of bicarbonate absorption was 5 μM, consistent with the inhibition of type IV carbonic anhydrase.

Renal Hemodynamics

Inhibition of carbonic anhydrase produces an acute decrease in GFR by activating tubuloglomerular feedback (TGF) (346, 359, 473, 474). Systemic infusion of acetazolamide resulted in a 30% decrease in glomerular filtration rate (GFR). Distally measured single-nephron glomerular filtration rate

(SNGFR) was reduced by 23% during acetazolamide infusion, whereas proximally measured SNGFR was not affected. These results indicated that acetazolamide blocked activated tubuloglomerular feedback, which in turn reduced GFR. Similar results were observed following infusion of benzolamide (473, 474). Sar-ala^8-angiotensin I, an angiotensin II antagonist, prevented the decrease in SGNFR suggesting the involvement of local angiotensin II in response to benzolamide (473).

Pharmacokinetics

Acetazolamide is well absorbed from the gastrointestinal (GI) tract. More than 90% of the drug is plasma-protein bound. The highest concentrations are found in tissues that contain large amounts of carbonic anhydrase (e.g., renal cortex, red blood cells). Renal effects are noticeable within 30 minutes and are usually maximal at 2 hours. Acetazolamide is not metabolized but is excreted rapidly by glomerular filtration and proximal tubular secretion. The half-life is approximately 5 hours and renal excretion is essentially complete in 24 hours (503). In comparison, methazolamide is absorbed more slowly from the GI tract, and its duration of action is long, with a half-life of approximately 14 hours.

Adverse Effects

Generally, carbonic anhydrase inhibitors are well tolerated with infrequent serious adverse effects. Side effects of carbonic anhydrase inhibitors may arise from the continued excretion of electrolytes. Significant hypokalemia and metabolic acidosis may develop (63). In elderly patients with glaucoma treated with acetazolamide (250 to 1000 mg/d), metabolic acidosis was a frequent finding in comparison to a control group (232). Acetazolamide is also associated with nephrocalcinosis and nephrolithiasis due to its effects on urine pH, facilitating stone formation (355). Premature infants treated with furosemide and acetazolamide are particularly susceptible to nephrocalcinosis presumably due to the combined effect of an alkaline urine and hypercalciuria (444). Other adverse effects include drowsiness, fatigue, central nervous system (CNS) depression and parathesias. Bone marrow suppression has been reported (232, 506).

Clinical Use

The popularity of carbonic anhydrase inhibitors as diuretics has waned principally owing to the development of agents that are more effective with fewer toxic side effects. In general, tolerance develops rapidly and renders these drugs less effective. Daily use produces systemic acidemia from an increase in urinary excretion of bicarbonate. Nevertheless, acetazolamide can be administered for short-term therapy usually in combination with other diuretics to patients who are resistant or who do not respond adequately to other agents. The rationale for using a combination of diuretic

agents is based on summation of their effect at different sites along the nephron. In addition to its use as a diuretic agent, carbonic anhydrase inhibitors are used in a number of other clinical situations.

The major indication for the use of acetazolamide as a diuretic agent is in the treatment of patients with metabolic alkalosis that is accompanied by edematous states (376) or chronic obstructive lung disease (17, 318). In patients with cirrhosis, congestive heart failure, or nephrotic syndrome, aggressive diuresis with loop diuretics promotes intravascular volume depletion, secondary hyperaldosteronism, and renal insufficiency, conditions that promote metabolic alkalosis. Administration of sodium chloride to correct the metabolic alkalosis may exacerbate edema. Acetazolamide can improve metabolic alkalosis by decreasing proximal tubule bicarbonate reabsorption thereby increasing the fractional excretion of bicarbonate. An increase in urinary pH (>7.0) indicates enhanced bicarbonaturia. However, it should be noted that potassium depletion should be corrected before acetazolamide use as acetazolamide will increase potassium excretion. The time course of acetazolamide effect is rapid. In critically ill patients on ventilators, following the correction of fluid and electrolyte disturbances, intravenous acetazolamide produced an initial effect within 2 hours and a maximum effect in 15 hours (311).

Acetazolamide is used effectively to treat chronic open-angle glaucoma. The high bicarbonate concentration in aqueous humor is carbonic anhydrase dependent and oral carbonic anhydrase inhibition can be used to reduce aqueous humor formation. Topical formulations are in clinical trials (424, 454) and could prove to be effective without the side effects of orally administered drugs.

Acute mountain sickness usually occurs in sojourners who ascend to heights greater than 2500 to 3000 feet. Symptoms occur within 12 to 72 hours and are characterized by a symptom complex consisting of headache, nausea, dizziness, and breathlessness. Carbonic anhydrase inhibitors improve symptoms and arterial oxygenation (195, 458).

The administration of acetazolamide has been used in the treatment of familial hypokalemic periodic paralysis (195, 393), a disorder characterized by intermittent episodes of muscle weakness and flaccid paralysis. Its efficacy is thought to be related to a decrease in influx of potassium as a result of a decrease in plasma insulin and glucose (230) or to metabolic acidosis. Carbonic anhydrase inhibitors can also be used as an adjunct treatment of epilepsy (391), pseudotumor cerebri (429), and central sleep apnea (430).

By increasing urinary pH, acetazolamide has been used effectively in certain clinical conditions. Acetazolamide is used to treat cystine and uric acid stones by increasing their solubility in urine. Acetazolamide in combination with sodium bicarbonate infusion is also used to treat salicylate toxicity. Salicylates are weak acids (pK$_a$ 3.0) therefore their ionic and nonionic forms exist in equilibrium. They are excreted primarily by the kidney through secretion via the organic anion transport pathway in the proximal tubule. Acetazolamide and sodium bicarbonate infusions increase urinary pH, thereby favoring formation of a nondiffusible nonionic form of salicylate, thus increasing excretion of salicylates (378).

LOOP DIURETICS

The loop diuretics inhibit sodium and chloride transport along the loop of Henle. Although these drugs also impair ion transport by proximal and distal tubules under some conditions, these effects probably contribute little to their action clinically. The loop diuretics available in the United States include furosemide, bumetanide, torsemide and ethacrynic acid (Fig. 5). Organic mercurial diuretics also inhibit ion transport along the loop of Henle, but these drugs are of historical interest, as they are no longer available for clinical use.

Urinary Electrolyte and Water Excretion

Loop diuretics increase the excretion of water, Na, K, Cl, phosphate, magnesium, and calcium (Table 1). The dose response relation between loop diuretic and urinary Na and Cl excretion is sigmoidal (Fig. 6). The steep dose response relation in the therapeutic range has led many to refer to these as "threshold" drugs (54). Loop diuretics have the highest natriuretic and chloriuretic potency of any class of diuretics; they can increase Na and Cl excretion to more than 25% of the filtered load. Following oral water loading the administration of a loop diuretic decreases free water clearance (C_{H_2O}) and increases osmolar clearance, although the urine always remains dilute (135, 186, 422, 455). This effect contrasts with that of osmotic diuretics in which increases in osmolar clearance are associated with increase in C_{H_2O}. During hydropenia, loop diuretics impair the reabsorption of solute free water ($T^C_{H_2O}$). Loop diuretics may induce a "negative" $T^C_{H_2O}$, even during hydropenia. During

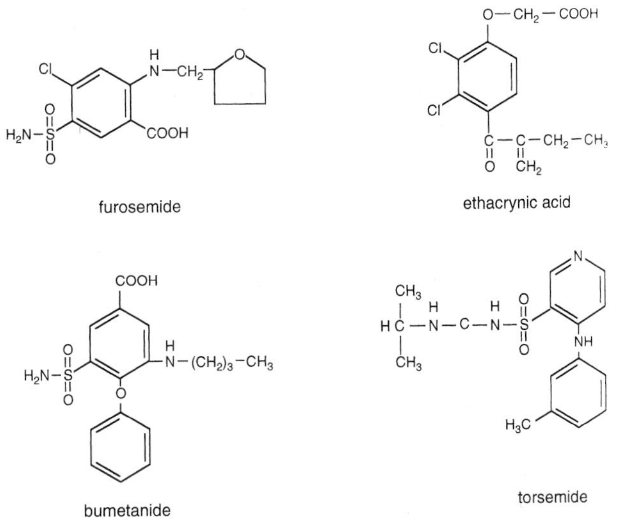

maximal loop diuretic action, the urinary Na concentration is usually between 75 and 100 mM (380). Because urinary K concentrations during furosemide-induced natriuresis remain low, the clearance of electrolyte free water (C_{H_2O}) is increased when loop diuretics are administered during conditions of water diuresis or hydropenia (380). This phenomenon underlies the use of furosemide with normal or hypertonic saline to treat hyponatremia (112).

Mechanisms of Action

SODIUM AND CHLORIDE TRANSPORT

The predominant effect of loop diuretic drugs is to inhibit the electroneutral Na-K-2Cl cotransporter at the apical surface of thick ascending limb cells. The loop of Henle, defined as the region between the last surface proximal segment and the first surface distal segment, reabsorbs from 20% to 50% of the filtered Na and Cl load (250); approximately 10% to 20% is reabsorbed by thick ascending limb cells. The model in Fig. 7 shows key components of Na, K, and Cl transport pathways in a thick ascending limb cell. Although mechanisms of Na and Cl transport have been discussed more thoroughly in other chapters in this volume, some important points deserve emphasis. First, as in other nephron segments, the Na,K-ATPase at the basolateral cell membrane maintains the intracellular Na concentration low (approximately 10-fold lower than interstitial) and the K concentration high (approximately 20-fold higher than interstitial). Potassium channel(s) in the basolateral cell membrane permit K to diffuse out of the cell, rendering the cell membrane voltage oriented with the intracellular surface negative, relative to extracellular fluid (356). A chloride channel in the basolateral cell membrane (481) and a barium-sensitive K-Cl cotransporter permit Cl to exit the cell (117).

The transporter inhibited by loop diuretics is one member of the cation chloride cotransporter family (426). This protein as the Na-K-2Cl cotransporter, second isoform, NKCC2 (or alternatively as the bumetanide-sensitive cotransporter, first isoform [BSC1]), is encoded by the gene SLC12A1. It is a protein with 12 putative membrane-spanning domains that is expressed at the apical membrane of thick ascending limb (241) and macula densa (MD) cells (343). It lies in parallel with a K channel (ROMK, Kir1.1) that permits potassium to recycle from the cell to the lumen (212). The asymmetrical orientation of channels (apical versus basolateral) and the action of the Na,K-ATPase and Na-K-2Cl cotransporter combine to create a transepithelial voltage that is oriented with the lumen positive, with respect to the interstitium. This lumen-positive potential drives absorption of Na, Ca and Mg via the paracellular pathway. The paracellular component of Na reabsorption comprises 50% of the total transepithelial Na transport by thick ascending limb cells (206); it should be noted, however, that both the transcellular and the paracellular components of Na transport are inhibited by loop diuretics, the former directly and the latter indirectly. The thick ascending limb is virtually impermeable to

FIGURE 5   Structures of loop diuretics.

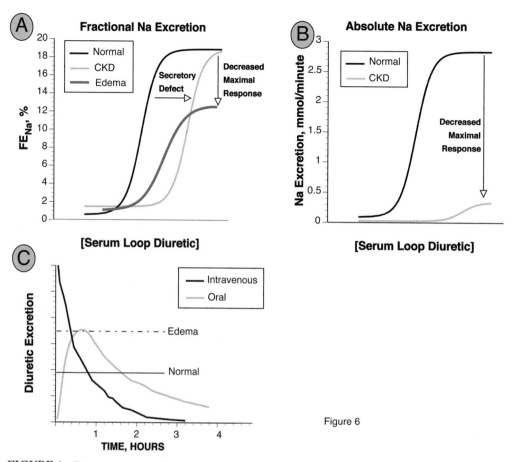

FIGURE 6   Dose response curve for loop diuretics. **A:** The fractional Na excretion (FE$_{Na}$) as a function of loop diuretic concentration. Compared with healthy patients, patients with chronic kidney disease (CKD) show a rightward shift in the curve, owing to impaired diuretic secretion. The maximal response is preserved when expressed as FE$_{Na}$, but when expressed as absolute Na excretion **(B)**, maximal natriuresis is reduced in patients with CKD. Patients with edema demonstrate a rightward and downward shift, even when expressed as FE$_{Na}$ **(A)**. **C:** Comparison of response to intravenous and oral doses of loop diuretics. In a normal individual *(Normal)*, an oral dose may be as effective as an intravenous dose because the time above the natriuretic threshold (indicated by the *"normal" line*) is approximately equal. If the natriuretic threshold increases (as indicated by the *dashed line*, from an edematous patient), the oral dose may not provide a serum level high enough to elicit natriuresis.

water. The combination of solute absorption and water impermeability leads to dilution of tubule fluid.

One model of Na-K-2Cl cotransport, based on the ionic requirements for transport, is shown in Fig. 7 (299). According to this model, the ion-binding sites on the transporter must be occupied sequentially, first by sodium, then by chloride, then by potassium and finally by a second chloride. Loop diuretics are organic anions that bind to the NKCC2 from the luminal surface. Early studies showed that [^{3}H] bumetanide binds to membranes that express the NKCC proteins and that Cl competes for the same binding site on the transport protein (200). More recently, studies using chimeric NKCC molecules have investigated sites of bumetanide binding and interactions with ions by determining effects on ion transport of heterologously expressed NKCC proteins. Using this approach it was shown that changes in amino acids that affect bumetanide binding are not the same as patterns of changes affecting the kinetics of

ion translocation (170, 224). Nevertheless, the second membrane-spanning segment of NKCC2 does appear to participate in both anion and bumetanide affinity (170, 224). A clearer picture of the details of diuretic and ion interaction with the NKCC protein must await a crystal structure.

Although direct inhibition of ion transport is the most important natriuretic action of loop diuretics, other actions may contribute to natriuresis. Thick ascending limb cells have been shown to produce prostaglandin E2 following stimulation with furosemide (320) or low luminal NaCl concentration (363). Blockade of cyclooxygenase reduces the effects of furosemide to inhibit loop segment chloride transport in rats (258); prostaglandin E2, but not I2 can restore this effect (260). Animals defective in PGE2 receptors also demonstrate blunted natriuresis, compared with wild type animals (336), indicating an important role for PGE2 in loop diuretic–induced natriuresis. Increases in

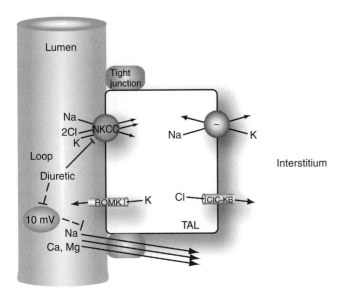

FIGURE 7 Mechanisms of diuretic action along the loop of Henle. Na and Cl are reabsorbed across the apical membrane via the loop diuretic-sensitive Na-K-2Cl cotransporter, NKCC2. Note that the transepithelial voltage along the thick ascending limb is oriented with the lumen positive relative to interstitium. This transepithelial voltage drives a component of Na (and calcium and magnesium) reabsorption via the paracellular pathway (the "tight junction," shown). Loop diuretics block the NKCC2 directly, thereby reducing the magnitude of the transepithelial voltage, and reducing Na, K, Cl, Mg, and Ca reabsorption.

renal prostaglandins may contribute to the hemodynamic effects of loop diuretics, described below.

Calcium and Magnesium Transport

Loop diuretics increase the excretion of the divalent cations, calcium and magnesium. This effect to increase calcium excretion is used to advantage when furosemide is added to saline to treat hypercalcemia (38). Although a component of magnesium and calcium absorption by thick ascending limbs may be active (especially when circulating parathyroid hormone [PTH] levels are high [163]), a large component of their absorption is passive and paracellular, driven by the transepithelial voltage. As described previously, active NaCl transport by thick ascending limb cells leads to a transepithelial voltage, oriented in the lumen positive direction. The paracellular pathway in the thick ascending limb is cation selective; expression of paracellin (claudin 16) appears to play a dominant role (434). The positive voltage in the lumen, relative to interstitium, drives calcium and magnesium absorption through the paracellular pathway (49, 162). Loop diuretics, by blocking the activity of the Na-K-2Cl cotransporter at the apical membrane of thick ascending limb cells, reduce the transepithelial voltage (69, 70, 72, 73). This stops passive paracellular calcium and magnesium absorption.

Renin Secretion

In addition to enhancing Na and Cl excretion, effects that result directly from inhibiting Na and Cl transport, loop diuretics also stimulate renin secretion. A porion of this effect

results from contraction of the extracellular fluid volume (see following section), but loop diuretics also stimulate renin secretion by inhibiting NaCl uptake by macula densa cells. Macula densa cells, which control renin secretion, sense the NaCl concentration in the lumen of the thick ascending limb (416). High luminal NaCl concentrations in the region of the macula densa lead to two distinct but related effects. First they activate the tubuloglomerular feedback response, which suppresses the glomerular filtration rate. Second, they inhibit renin secretion. The relation between these two effects is complex and has been reviewed recently (416), but both appear to be controlled, at least in part, by NaCl movement across the apical membrane (Fig. 8).

The pathways mediating Na and Cl uptake into macula densa cells are similar to to those expressed by adjacent thick ascending limb cells. This includes the loop diuretic–sensitive Na-K-2Cl cotransporter at the apical surface (137, 343). Under normal conditions, an increase in luminal NaCl concentration in the thick ascending limb raises the NaCl concentration inside macula densa cells. Because the activity of the basolateral Na,K-ATPase is lower in macula densa cells than in surrounding thick ascending limb cells (415), the cell NaCl concentration is much more dependent on luminal NaCl concentration in macula densa than in thick ascending limb cells (281). When luminal and macula densa cell NaCl concentrations decline multiple MAP kinases are activated, stimulating COX-2 activity and inducing COX-2 expression. This is followed by the appearance in the juxtaglomerular interstitium of PGE2 and the suppression of adenosine. PGE2 activates EP4 receptors on granular cells, and this results in Gs-mediated adenylate cyclase activation and protein kinase A (PKA)–mediated renin secretory and transcriptional activation (416).

The constitutive (neuronal) isoform of nitric oxide synthase (NOS I) is expressed by macula densa cells, but not by other cells in the kidney. Nitric oxide produced by macula densa cells has a paracrine effect to increase cellular concentrations of cyclic AMP (cAMP) in adjacent juxtaglomerular cells. Cyclic AMP through protein kinase A then stimulates renin secretion. Data suggest that in juxtaglomerular cells, nitric oxide increases cellular concentrations of cGMP which inhibit phosphodiesterase 3 (275). Inhibition of phosphodiesterase-3 permits cAMP accumulation. Several laboratories have reported that furosemide-induced stimulation of renin secretion is dependent on an intact nitric oxide system (84, 231, 388, 418).

The second isoform of cyclooxygenase, COX-2, is highly expressed by macula densa cells; its expression is increased by loop diuretic treatment (204, 267, 305, 363). Blockade of prostaglandin synthesis either by nonspecific cyclooxygenase inhibitors (166) or by specific COX-2 blockers (202) reduces the renin secretory response to loop diuretics. Current views suggest that furosemide, like low luminal NaCl delivery, stimulates renin secretion by macula densa cells by activating COX-2, leading to PGE2 production. PGE2 stimulates EP4 receptors leading to renin synthesis (416).

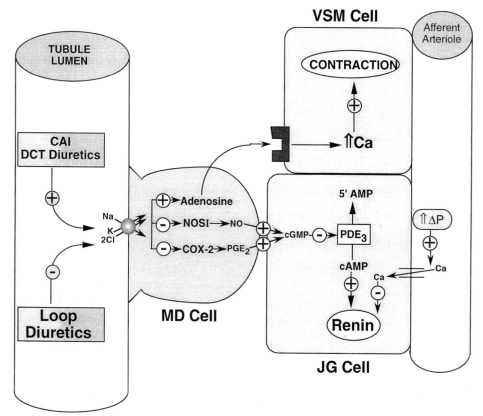

FIGURE 8 Mechanisms of renin secretion and tubuloglomerular feedback. A macula densa (MD) cell is shown expressing the loop diuretic-sensitive Na-K-2Cl cotransporter at its apical surface, in parallel with a K channel. Movement of NaCl into the cell activates production of adenosine. Adenosine interacts with receptors on vascular smooth muscle (VSM) cells, which increase cell calcium causing contraction. This pathway participates importantly in tubuloglomerular feedback. Movement of NaCl across the apical membrane inhibits production of nitric oxide (NO) via nitric oxide synthase I (NOSI). Nitric oxide may diffuse to the extraglomerular mesangium or directly to juxtaglomerular (JG) cells where it increases cGMP. cGMP inhibits phosphodiesterase-3 (PDE3), which metabolizes cAMP to 5′ AMP. cAMP stimulates renin secretion. NaCl uptake across the apical membrane also inhibits cyclooxygenase (COX-2). COX-2 produces prostaglandin E2 (PGE2), which also increases cGMP in juxtaglomerular cells. When loop diuretics inhibit NaCl uptake, renin secretion is stimulated and the tubuloglomerular feedback mechanism is blocked. Carbonic anhydrase inhibitors (CAIs) and distal convoluted tubule (DCT) diuretics increase solute delivery to the macula densa and increase NaCl uptake. These drugs therefore activate tubuloglomerular feedback and may inhibit renin secretion (see text). Increases in hydrostatic pressure in the afferent arteriole inhibit renin secretion primarily by increasing calcium entry.

RENAL HEMODYNAMICS

Most classes of diuretic reduce glomerular filtration; in contrast, loop diuretics tend to preserve glomerular filtration rate and renal blood flow (215), although GFR and renal plasma flow (RPF) can decline if extracellular fluid volume contraction is severe. Loop diuretics reduce renal vascular resistance and increase renal blood flow under experimental conditions (120). This effect is believed to be related in part to the diuretic-induced production of vasoldilatory prostaglandins, although effects on nitric acid production may also occur (101).

Another factor that may contribute to the tendency of loop diuretics to maintain glomerular filtration rate and renal plasma flow despite volume contraction is their effect on the TGF system. The sensing mechanism that activates the

TGF system involves NaCl transport across the apical membrane of macula densa cells by the loop diuretic sensitive Na-K-2Cl cotransporter. Under normal conditions, when the luminal concentration of NaCl reaching the macula densa rises, glomerular filtration rate decreases via TGF. To a large degree, the TGF-mediated decrease in GFR results from afferent arteriolar constriction (416). Although the mechanisms by which ion transport across the apical membrane of macula densa cells translates to afferent arteriolar vasoconstriction are unclear, they appear to involve the production of adenosine (an afferent arteriolar vasoconstrictor) and the increase in mesangial and smooth muscle cell calcium concentrations (416). ATP release from macula densa cells (23) leads to the extracellular formation of adenosine by ecto-5′-nucleotidase (cd73). The fact that TGF is blunted in animals where ecto-5′-nucleotidase and A1 receptors are pharmacologically inhibited and in A1 receptor and ecto-5′-nucleotidase knockout mice strongly support the importance of adenosine formation and activation of adenosine A1 receptors in mediating TGF (61, 456, 466, 479). In a manner analogous to the effects on renin secretion, loop diuretic drugs block tubuloglomerular feedback by blocking the sensing step (522). In the absence of effects on the macula densa, loop diuretics would be expected to suppress GFR and RPF by increasing distal NaCl delivery and activating the TGF system (an effect that is observed during infusion of carbonic anhydrase inhibitors and distal convoluted tubule (DCT) diuretics [346]). Instead, blockade of the TGF permits GFR and RPF to be maintained.

SYSTEMIC HEMODYANAMICS

Acute intravenous administration of loop diuretics increases venous capacitance (119). Most studies suggest that this effect results from stimulation of prostaglandin synthesis by the kidney (50, 329). Other studies, however, suggest that loop diuretics have effects in peripheral vascular beds as well (414), or may stimulate nitric oxide production (101). Pickkers and coworkers examined the local effects of furosemide in the human forearm. Furosemide had no effect on arterial vessels, but did cause dilation of veins, an effect that was dependent on local prostaglandin production (365). Although venodilation and improvements in cardiac hemodynamics frequently result from intravenous therapy with loop diuretics, the hemodynamic response to intravenous loop diuretics may be more complex. Johnston et al. (233) reported that low-dose furosemide increased venous capacitance, but that higher doses did not. It was suggested that furosemide-induced renin secretion may generate angiotensin II–induced vasoconstriction. This vasoconstrictor might overwhelm the prostaglandin-mediated vasodilatory effects in some patients. In two series, 1–1.5-mg/kg furosemide boluses administered to patients with chronic congestive heart failure, resulted in transient *deteriorations* in hemodyanamics (during the first hour), with a decline in stroke volume index, an increase in left ventricular filling pressure (160, 188), and exacerbation of congestive heart failure symptoms. These changes were attributed to activation of the sympathetic nervous system and the renin-angiotensin system by the diuretic drug. Evidence for a role of the renin-angiotensin system in the furosemide-induced deterioration in systemic hemodynamics includes the temporal association between its activation and hemodynamic deterioration (160, 188), and the ability of angiotensin I–converting enzyme inhibitors to prevent much of the pressor effect (160, 188). Other studies have shown that acute loop diuretic administration frequently produces a transient decline in cardiac output; whether diuretic administration increases or decrease left atrial pressure acutely may depend primarily on the state of underlying sympathetic nervous system and renin/angiotensin axis activation.

PHARMACOKINETICS

The three loop diuretics that are used most commonly, furosemide, bumetanide, and torsemide, are absorbed quickly after oral administration, reaching peak concentrations within 0.5 to 2 hours (Fig. 6). Furosemide absorption is slower than the rate of elimination in normal subjects; thus the time to reach peak serum level is slower for furosemide than for bumetanide and torsemide. This phenomenon is called "absorption-limited kinetics" (54). The bioavailability of loop diuretics varies from 50% to 90% (Table 2). When changing a patient from intravenous to oral furosemide, the dose is frequently doubled to account for its limited oral bioavailability (54). The half-lives of the loop diuretics available in the United States vary, but all are relatively short (ranging from approximately 1 hour for bumetanide to 3–4 hours for torsemide). The half-lives of muzolimine, xipamide, and ozolinone, none of which is available in the United States, are 6 to 15 hours.

Loop diuretics are organic anions that circulate tightly bound to albumin (>95%); thus their volumes of distribution are small, except during extreme hypoproteinemia (222). Approximately 50% of an administered dose of furosemide is excreted unchanged into the urine. The remainder appears to be eliminated by glucuronidation, probably by the kidney. Torsemide and bumetanide are eliminated both by hepatic processes and through renal excretion. The differences in metabolic fate mean that the half-life of furosemide is altered by renal failure, whereas this is not true for torsemide and bumetanide.

TABLE 2 Pharmacokinetics of Loop Diuretics

	Bioavailability, % oral dose absorbed	Elimination Half-Life			
		Healthy	Kidney disease	Liver disease	CHF
Furosemide	50% (range, 10%–100%)	1.5–2	2.8	2.5	2.7
Bumetanide	80%–100%	1	1.6	2.3	1.3
Torsemide	80%–100%	3–4	4-5	8	6

CHF, congestive heart failure; h, half-life.

Source: Shankar SS and Brater DC. Loop diuretics: from the Na-K-2Cl transporter to clinical use. *Am J Physiol Renal Physiol* 2003;284: F11–21.

Clinical Use

Loop diuretics are used commonly to treat the edematous conditions, congestive heart failure, cirrhosis of the liver, and nephrotic syndrome. In addition, a variety of other electrolyte, fluid, and acid-base disorders can respond to loop diuretic therapy. Essentials of diuretic treatment of disease are discussed in other reviews. The interested reader is referred to those for details (426, 477).

Loop diuretics are commonly used in the treatment of acute kidney injury. Diuretics may reduce the severity of acute kidney injury by preventing tubule obstruction and decreasing oxygen consumption (210). Their effectiveness in the treatment of acute kidney injury continues to be debated as studies have failed to demonstate convincingly that they impact survival and renal recovery rate of patients with established acute kidney injury (79).

Adverse Effects

There are at least three types of adverse effects of loop diuretics. The first and most common effects result directly from the effects of these drugs on renal electrolyte and water excretion. The second are toxic effects of the drugs that are dose related and predictable. The third are idiosyncratic allergic drug reactions.

Loop diuretics are frequently administered to treat edematous expansion of the extracellular fluid volume. Edema usually results from a decrease in the "effective" arterial blood volume. Thus, zealous diuretic usage or the development of complicating illnesses can lead to excessive contraction of the extracellular fluid volume. This can be manifested by orthostatic hypotension, renal dysfunction, or evidence of sympathetic overactivity. Although patients suffering from congestive heart failure usually require diuretic therapy, the combination of diuretics and angiotensin converting enzyme inhibitors can predispose to renal failure. High diuretic doses or extreme dietary NaCl restriction may predispose to renal dysfunction during therapy with diuretics and angiotensin-converting enzyme (ACE) inhibitors for congestive heart failure (351, 352). In this case, renal failure often abates when the diuretic dose is reduced or the dietary NaCl intake is liberalized, permitting continued administration of the ACE inhibitor.

Other patients at increased risk for relative contraction of the extracellular fluid volume during loop diuretic therapy include elderly patients (437), patients with preexisting renal insufficiency (245), patients with right-sided heart failure or pericardial disease, and concomitant use of nonsteroidal anti-inflammatory drugs.

Disorders of Na and K concentration are among the most frequent adverse effects of loop diuretics. Hyponatremia may be less common with loop diuretics than with DCT diuretics (see following section), but it still may occur. Its pathogenesis is usually multifactorial, but involves the effect of loop diuretics to impair the clearance of solute free water.

Additional factors that may contribute include the nonosmotic release of arginine vasopressin (36), hypokalemia, and hypomagesemia (132). Conversely loop diuretics have been used to treat hyponatremia when combined with hypertonic saline in the setting of the syndrome of inappropriate antidiuretic hormone (SIADH) secretion (201, 419). In constrast, the combination of loop diuretics and angiotensin I-converting enzyme inhibitors has been reported to correct hyponatremia in the setting of congestive heart failure, presumably in part owing to improved cardiac function (134).

Hypokalemia occurs commonly during therapy with loop diuretics, although the magnitude is smaller than the magnitude of hypokalemia induced by diuretics that act in the DCT (loop diuretics, 0.3 mM vs DCT diuretics, 0.5–0.9 mM [354, 385]). Loop diuretics increase the delivery of potassium to the distal tubule because they block potassium reabsorption via the Na-K-2Cl cotransporter. In rats, under control conditions, approximately half the excreted potassium was delivered to the "early" distal tubule. During furosemide infusion, the delivery of potassium to the early distal tubule rose to 28% of the filtered load (216). Thus, it appears that a large component of the effect of loop diuretics to increase potassium excretion acutely reflects their ability to block potassium reabsorption by the thick ascending limb. Nevertheless, during chronic diuretic therapy, the degree of potassium wasting correlates best with volume contraction and serum aldosterone levels (513). These data suggest that, under chronic conditions, the predominant effect of loop diuretics to stimulate potassium excretion results from their tendency to increase mineralocorticoid hormones while simultaneously increasing distal Na and water delivery.

Metabolic alkalosis is very common during chronic treatment with loop diuretics. Loop diuretics cause metabolic alkalosis via several mechanisms. First, they increase the excretion of urine that is bicarbonate free but contains Na and Cl. This leads to contraction of the extracellular fluid around a fixed amount of bicarbonate buffer; a phenomenon known as "contraction alkalosis". This probably contributes only slightly to the metabolic alkalosis that commonly accompanies chronic loop diuretic treatment. Loop diuretics directly inhibit transport of Na and Cl into thick ascending limb cells. In some species, these cells also express an isoform of the Na–H exchanger at the apical surface. When Na entry via the Na-K-2Cl cotransporter is blocked by a loop diuretic, the decline in intracellular Na activity will stimulate H secretion via the Na–H exchanger (190, 263, 340). Loop diuretics stimulate the renin-angiotensin-aldosterone pathway, directly and indirectly, as discussed previously. Aldosterone directly stimulates H secretion by the medullary collecting tubule (452) and increases the magnitude of the transepithelial voltage in the cortical collecting duct. This effect stimulates H secretion via the electrogenic H-ATPase present at the apical membrane of α intercalated cells. Loop diuretics frequently cause hypokalemia, which may contribute to metabolic alkalosis by increasing ammonium production (461), stimulating bicarbonate reabsorption by proximal tubules (439, 440), and increasing the activity of the H,K-ATPase in the distal nephron (517). Finally, contraction of the extracellular fluid volume stimulates Na–H exchange in the proximal tubule and may reduce the filtered load of bicarbonate. All of these factors may contribute to the metabolic alkalosis observed during chronic loop diuretic treatment.

Ototoxicity is the most common toxic effect of loop diuretics that is unrelated to their on the kidney. Deafness, which is usually temporary but can be permanent, was reported shortly after the introduction of loop diuretics (300). It appears likely that all loop diuretics cause ototoxicity, because ototoxicity can occur during use of chemically dissimilar drugs such as furosemide and ethacrynic acid (404). The mechanism of ototoxicity remains unclear, although the stria vascularis, which is responsible for maintaining endolymphatic potential and ion balance (44) appears to be a primary target for toxicity (220). Loop diuretics reduce the striatal potential from $+80$ mV to -10 to -20 mV within minutes of application (404). A characteristic finding in loop diuretic ototoxicity is strial edema. This suggests that toxicity involves inhibition of ion fluxes (220). Ikeda and Morizono (219) detected functional evidence for the presence of a Na-K-2Cl cotransporter in the basolateral membrane of marginal cells. According to the model proposed by these investigators, marginal cells resemble secretory cells in other organ systems, with a Na-K-2Cl cotransporter and Na,K-ATPase at the basolateral cell membrane and channels for K and Cl at the apical surface. According to this model, loop diuretic induced shrinkage of marginal cells results from inhibition of cell Na, K, and Cl uptake across the basolateral cell membrane.

The ototoxic effects of loop diuretics appear to be related to their ability to inhibit the secretory isoform of the Na-K-2Cl cotransporter, NKCC1. This protein has been localized in the lateral wall of the cochlea, using specific antibodies (321) and reverse transcriptase–polymerase chain reaction (RT-PCR) (211). Mice lacking the secretory isoform of the Na-K-2Cl cotransporter are profoundly deaf (113, 158). Loop diuretics cause loss of outer hair cells in the basal turn of the cochlea, rupture of endothelial layers, cystic formation in the stria vascularis, and marginal cell edema in the stria vascularis (404).

Ototoxicity appears to be related to the peak serum concentration of loop diuretic and therefore tends to occur during rapid drug infusion of high doses. This is likely to be related in part to the much lower affinity of the secretory isoform of the Na-K-2Cl cotransporter for loop diuretics (223, 225). For this reason, this complication is most common in patients with uremia (446). It has recommended that furosemide infusion be no more rapid than 4 mg/minute (446). In addition to renal failure, infants, patients with cirrhosis, and patients receiving aminoglycosides or cisplatinum may be at increased risk for ototoxicity (446).

DISTAL CONVOLUTED TUBULE DIURETICS

The first orally active drug that inhibited Na and Cl transport along the DCT was chlorothiazide. Chlorothiazide was developed when chemical modification of sulfonamide based CA inhibitors resulted in substances that increased Na excretion with Cl rather than with HCO_3. This alteration from properties characteristic of CA inhibitors to properties characteristic of DCT diuretics was immediately recognized as clinically significant, because extracellular fluid contains predominantly NaCl rather than $NaHCO_3$ (32, 33, 35), and acidosis limited the effectiveness of CA inhibitors. Subsequent development led to a wide variety of benzothiadiazide (thiazide) diuretics (Fig. 9); all are analogs of 1,2,4-benzothiadiazine-1,

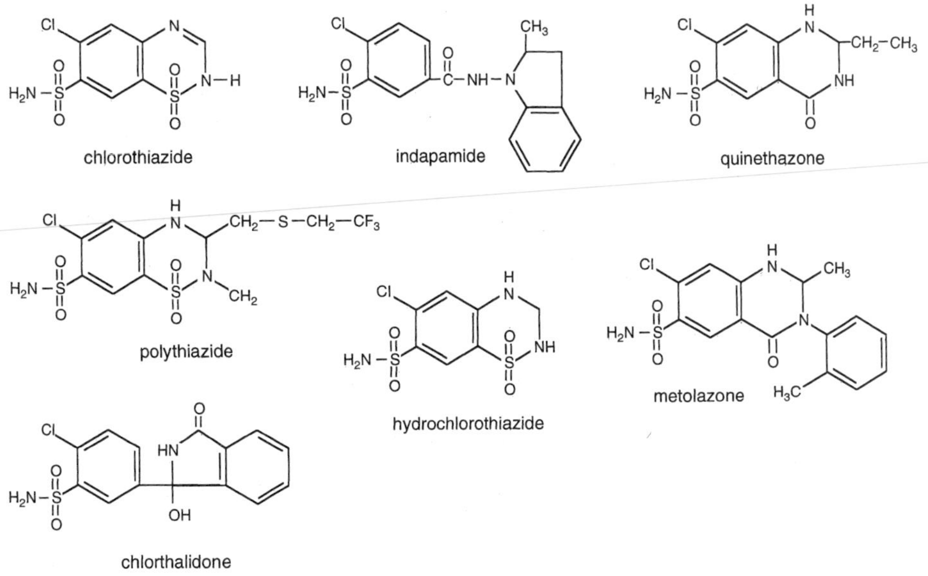

FIGURE 9   Structures of distal convoluted tubule diuretics.

1-dioxide. Other structurally related nonthiazide diuretics include the quinazolinones (such as metolazone) and substituted benzopehenone sulfonamide (such as chlorthalidone). Although the primary site at which these drugs exert their action was a source of confusion (28), molecular identification of their target ion transporter permitted delineation of their predominant site of action as the distal convoluted tubule. Based on the common site at which both true thiazide and "thiazide-like" diuretics inhibit ion transport, it would be reasonable to refer to this class of drugs as *distal convoluted tubule diuretics*.

Urinary Electrolyte and Water Excretion

Acute administration of these drugs increases the excretion of Na, K, Cl, HCO_3, phosphate, and urate (32, 34, 115), although the increases in HCO_3, phosphate, and urate excretion are probably related primarily to CA inhibition (see following section). As such, the effects of DCT diuretics to increase HCO_3, phosphate, and urate excretion may vary, depending on the CA inhibiting potency of the DCT diuretic. Chronically, as contraction of the extracellular fluid volume occurs, uric acid excretion declines and hyperuricemia can occur. Further, any initial excretion of bicarbonate ceases, whereas continuing losses of chloride without bicarbonate and extracellular fluid volume contraction may lead to metabolic alkalosis. In contrast to loop and proximally acting diuretics, DCT diuretics tend to reduce urinary calcium excretion (104, 125). Although the effects on urinary calcium excretion can be variable during acute administration (141), these drugs uniformly lead to calcium retention when administered chronically.

DCT diuretics inhibit the clearance of solute-free water (C_{H_2O}) when administered during water diuresis. This effect is similar to that of loop diuretics and originally led the mistaken inference that they act along the thick ascending limb. In contrast to loop diuretics, however, DCT diuretics do not limit free-water reabsorption during antidiuresis (136).

Mechanism of Action

SODIUM AND WATER TRANSPORT IN THE PROXIMAL TUBULE

DCT diuretics are related chemically to CA inhibitors and most retain significant CA-inhibiting potential (308). As discussed previously, CA inhibitors interfere indirectly with the activity of the apical Na–H exchanger. Although this effect of DCT diuretics may be useful when these drugs are administered acutely (as during intravenous chlorothiazide administration), it probably contributes little to the overall natriuresis during chronic use (274, 298). Yet this effect may play a role in the tendency for DCT diuretics to reduce the glomerular filtration rate and activate the tubuloglomerular feedback mechanism (346). The relative CA-inhibiting potency (shown in parentheses) of some commonly used DCT diuretics is chlorthalidone (67) >benthiazide (50) >polythiazide (40) >chlorothiazide (14) >hydrochlorothiazide (1) >bendroflumethiazide (0.07) (165).

NaCl ABSORPTION IN THE DISTAL NEPHRON

The predominant site at which DCT diuretics inhibit ion transport is the DCT. Although clearance studies had identified one site of thiazide action as the cortical diluting segment (455) and a second site as the proximal tubule (74, 138, 155), micropuncture studies pinpointed the primary site of action as the superficial "distal tubule" (274). This region of the nephron, which lies between the macula densa and the confluence with another nephron to form the cortical collecting duct, is morphologically heterogenous (272). It comprises a short stretch of post–macula densa thick ascending limb, the DCT, the connecting tubule, and the initial portion of the cortical collecting duct. When this morphological heterogeneity became evident, experiments were designed to determine the site of thiazide action more precisely. Microperfusion experiments in rats indicated that thiazide diuretics inhibit Na and Cl transport along the "early" portion of the distal tubule (103, 144), a segment known to contain predominantly DCT cells (390).

Although microperfusion data from rats indicated that thiazide diuretics inhibit Na transport in the DCT, the transition along the distal nephron segments in rats is gradual. For several years, therefore, it was impossible to attribute thiazide-sensitive Na-Cl transport to a specific cell type in the rat (27). In contrast, rabbit distal nephron segments have abrupt transitions. Although early in vitro studies suggested that thiazide-sensitive Na-Cl cotransport is present in connecting tubules instead of DCTs (221, 428), Velázquez and Greger obtained indirect evidence for thiazide-sensitive transport in rabbit DCTs (484). Molecular cloning (172) permitted definitive identification of DCT cells as the only sites of thiazide-sensitive Na-Cl cotransporter expression in both rat and rabbit (14, 342, 371). Friedman and colleagues developed a clonal cell line from immunodissected mouse thick ascending limb and DCT cells that expresses thiazide-sensitive transport (370). Molecular studies identified the DCT as the site of thiazide-sensitive Na-Cl cotransport in this species, as well (76).

In 1984, Velázquez and colleagues reported the mutual dependence of Na and Cl transport in the superficial rat distal tubule (483). The same year, Stokes reported evidence that a directly coupled thiazide-sensitive Na-Cl cotransporter is expressed in the urinary bladder of the winter flounder (451). Gamba et al. (172) cloned this protein and detected a homologous mRNA in mammalian kidney. The same group cloned a rat form of the thiazide-sensitive Na-Cl cotransporter (319). Mouse, human, and rabbit forms were cloned shortly thereafter (45, 435, 485); the gene is *SLC12A3*. This transport protein has been variously called the TSC (thiazide-sensitive cotransporter), the NCCT (sodium chloride cotransporter), and NCC (sodium chloride cotransporter). At the molecular level, the NCC is expressed only by DCT cells in all mammalian species examined. Human, rat, and mouse, expression of NCC extends into a transitional segment, referred to as the DCT-2, which shares properties of the distal convoluted and connecting tubules (76, 342).

Evidence for thiazide action in other nephron segments has also been obtained, however. In vivo catheterization experiments demonstrated a component of thiazide-sensitive Na transport in medullary collecting tubules of rats (515). Some (463), but not other (402) investigators have detected thiazide-sensitive Na-Cl transport in rat cortical collecting ducts perfused in vitro. In those experiments, pretreatment of animals with mineralocorticoid hormones was necessary to elicit the thiazide-sensitive Na and Cl transport. Functional expression of thiazide-sensitive transport activity in the rat cortical and medullary collecting ducts and the rabbit connecting tubule may represent expression of molecularly distinct, but thiazide-sensitive proteins or expression of the NCC at levels below the

limits of detection by in situ hybridization or immunocytochemistry. It should be recalled, however, that thiazides and other related diuretics do inhibit a variety of ion transport proteins and the ability of these drugs to inhibit Na reabsorption in the proximal tubule clearly reflects their actions on proteins distinct from the NCC. A model of NaCl transport by DCT cells is shown in Fig. 10A.

Like loop diuretics, distal convoluted diuretics, including the thiazides, are organic anions that bind to the transport protein from the luminal surface. Results of studies to determine the mechanism by which DCT diuretics interact with the transport protein have varied, depending on the methods used. Before the transport protein was identified at the molecular level, Fanestil and colleagues showed that [³H] metolazone binds avidly to kidney membrane proteins; its binding is inhibited competitively by Cl, suggesting that

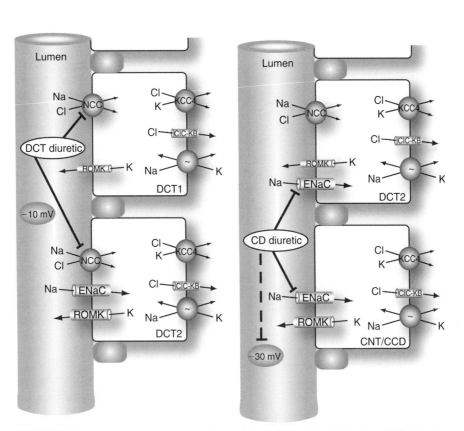

FIGURE 10   Mechanisms of distal convoluted tubule (DCT) and collecting duct (CD) diuretics. **A:** Mechanism of action of DCT diuretics. In rat, mouse, and human, two types of DCT cells have been identified, referred to here as DCT-1 and DCT-2. Na and Cl are reabsorbed across the apical membrane of DCT-1 cells only via the thiazide-sensitive Na-Cl cotransporter. This transport protein is also expressed by DCT-2 cells, where Na can also cross through the epithelial Na channel, ENaC (see text). Thus, the transepithelial voltage along the DCT-1 is close to 0 mV, whereas it is lumen negative along the DCT-2. **B:** Mechanism of action of CD diuretics. The late distal convoluted tubule cells (DCT2 cells) and connecting (CNT) or collecting duct (CD) cells are shown. Na is reabsorbed via the epithelial Na channel (ENaC), which lies in parallel with a potassium channel (ROMK). The transepithelial voltage is oriented with the lumen negative, relative to interstitium (shown by the circled value), generating a favorable gradient for transepithelial K secretion. Drugs that block the epithelial Na value reduce the voltage toward 0 mV (effect indicated by *dashed line*), thereby inhibiting K secretion.

Cl and diuretic compete for the same binding site (18, 470). These results are reminiscent of those that used [³H] bumetanide to study properties of the NKCC proteins and were used to develop a kinetic model for the NCC (87). More recently, Gamba and colleagues have expressed chimeras of the NCC in Xenopus oocytes and determined thiazide affinity based on transport inhibition. The results suggest a more complicated picture. They conclude that thiazide diuretic affinity is conferred by transmembrane segments 8 to 12, whereas transmembrane segments 1 to 7 affect chloride affinity. Both segments are involved in determining Na affinity (323). These data suggest that that the affinity of thiazide diuretics for binding to the transport protein is in a region distinct from that that participates in Cl transport. Resolution of the discrepancies awaits solution of the crystal structure.

CALCIUM AND MAGNESIUM TRANSPORT

When administered chronically, DCT diuretics reduce calcium excretion. This effect has been used clinically to prevention the recurrence of calcium nephrolithiasis (see subsequent sections). As noted previously, acute administration of DCT diuretics has a variable effect on calcium excretion, sometimes leading to increases in calcium excretion (141, 373). This probably reflects the CA-inhibiting capacity of these drugs, because CA inhibitors increase urinary calcium excretion acutely. Ca reabsorption by proximal tubules is functionally coupled to sodium reabsorption (Fig. 11); drugs that inhibit proximal Na reabsorption also inhibit proximal calcium reabsorption (42). During chronic treatment, however, the filtered calcium load decreases, owing to the hemodynamic effects discussed below, and the proximal calcium reabsorption increases, owing to extracellular fluid volume contraction.

Three potential and nonredundant mechanisms have been postulated to account for the hypocalciuric effect of DCT diuretics (143). First, blockade of luminal NaCl entry reduces the tubule cell [Na] sufficiently to enhance the basolateral Na^+–Ca^{2+} exchange (105). A low cellular Na concentration provides part of the driving force for basolateral calcium exit via the 3Na–Ca exchanger. Second, thiazides reduce blockade of luminal NaCl entry reduces cell [Cl⁻]

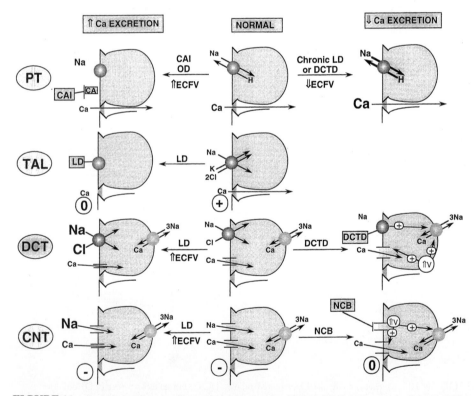

FIGURE 11   Summary of diuretic effects on calcium excretion. Typical cells from the proximal tubule (PT), thick ascending limb (TAL), distal convoluted tubule (DCT), and connecting tubule (CNT) are shown. Normal conditions are shown in the middle. Situations in which calcium excretion increases are shown at left. Situations in which calcium excretion decreases are shown at right. CAI, OD, and ECFV expansion reduce Na reabsorption along the proximal tubule, inhibiting calcium reabsorption secondarily. Chronic diuretic treatment or ECFV contraction increases proximal Ca transport secondarily. LDs inhibit calcium transport by reducing the transepithelial voltage in the thick ascending limb. DCTDs stimulate Ca transport by the DCT via mechanisms discussed in the text. Loop diuretics and ECFV expansion inhibit distal calcium transport by stimulating Na transport along the DCT and the CNT. NCB stimulate distal calcium transport via mechanisms discussed in the text. CAI, carbonic anhydrase inhibitors; OD, osmotic diuretics; ECFV, extracellular fluid volume; LD, loop diuretic; DCTD, distal convoluted tubule diuretic; NCB, Na channel blocking drugs.

concentration, hyperpolarizing the membrane voltage (making the interior of the cell more negative, electrically). Cellular hyperpolarization has at least two effects to enhance calcium absorption. First, as the 3Na–Ca exchanger is electrogenic, increases in cellular negativity stimulate its activity. Second, hyperpolarization increases calcium entry via the transient receptor potential channel subfamily V, member 5 (TRPV5) channel, which is expressed at the apical membrane of DCT and connecting tubule cells (116, 164). The stimulation of calcium uptake into cells and the enhanced calcium exit occur along the distal convoluted tubule, the primary site of thiazide action. An indirect effect of thiazides is that these drugs stimulate proximal reabsorption of Ca^{2+} owing to extracellular volume (ECV) depletion (374). The importance of this proximal effect has been highlighted recently because thiazides reduce Ca^{2+} excretion, even when the TRPV5 channel has been knocked out and the major distal calcium reabsorptive pathway is absent (335). Thiazides produce a sustained reduction in renal Ca^{2+} excretion, which is accompanied by a small rise in serum Ca^{2+} concentration (S_{Ca}).

DCT diuretics increase urinary magnesium chronically and can cause hypomagnesemia (110, 124, 214), although the acute effects of DCT diuretics are more variable. The mechanisms of magnesium transport by DCT cells and their regulation by diuretics are not completely understood. Evidence suggests that an important component of the transepithelial magnesium reabsorptive pathway in the distal nephron comprises the transient receptor potential channel, *TRPM6* (495). Chronic treatment of rats with hydrochlorothiazide reduced the abundance of this transport protein, a finding that was replicated by genetic disruption of the NCC (335). Thus thiazides may induce magnesium wasting, at least in part by reducing the abundance of the apical magnesium reabsorptive channel. These data are consistent with findings from NCC knockout animals. In that model, the DCT1 (early distal convoluted tubule) is atrophic. In as much as this segment normally expresses *TRPM6* at high levels, such atrophy may explain the reduced *TRPM6* expression and magnesium wasting.

Dai et al. (108) proposed that magnesium is transported across the apical membrane of DCT cells by a hyperpolarization-activated magnesium channel. They found that DCT diuretics stimulated magnesium uptake into DCT cells by reducing the intracellular activity of chloride, hyperpolarizing the membrane voltage, and activating magnesium channels. These magnesium channels are sensitive to dihydropyridines but appear to be distinct from calcium channels. Amiloride was found to have similar effects on magnesium uptake (109). Quamme proposed that magnesium wasting in Gitelman syndrome (and by analogy during DCT diuretic treatment) results from hypokalemia and from hyperaldosteronism quamme (383). Ellison suggested that distal magnesium transport may be dependent on the transepithelial voltage. In this case, thiazide diuretics, by increasing aldosterone concentrations and blocking electroneutral Na reabsorption would enhance the luminal negativity. This would inhibit magnesium reabsorption (143).

Renal Hemodynamics

DCT diuretics increase renal vascular resistance and decrease the glomerular filtration rate when given acutely (6, 83, 274). Okusa et al. (346) showed that intravenous chlorothiazide reduced the glomerular filtration rate by 16% when measured as whole-kidney clearance or by micropuncture of a superficial distal tubule. In contrast, however, when flow to the macula densa was blocked and the SNGFR was measured by micropuncture of a proximal tubule, intravenous chlorothiazide had no effect on glomerular filtration rate. These data indicate that diuretic-induced stimulation of the tubuloglomerular feedback system mediates the effect of DCT diuretics on glomerular filtration rate; DCT diuretics are known to increase the concentration of Na in luminal fluid entering the superficial distal tubule. It is assumed that a change in the tubule fluid ion concentration mediates this effect.

During chronic treatment with DCT diuretics, contraction of the extracellular fluid volume develops, thereby increasing solute and water reabsorption by the proximal tubule. This effect reduces the distal Na delivery to levels that are lower than under control conditions. In view of the fact that the initial suppression of glomerular filtration rate resulted from tubuloglomerular feedback, initiated by distal NaCl delivery, the glomerular filtration rate usually returns close to control values during chronic treatment with DCT diuretics (136, 498). Thus, when used chronically, DCT diuretics lead to a state of mild extracellular fluid volume contraction, increased fractional proximal reabsorption, and relatively preserved glomerular filtration.

When administered acutely, the effect of DCT diuretics is variable (314). If urinary NaCl losses are replaced, these drugs tend to suppress renin secretion (62), probably by increasing NaCl delivery to the macula densa (346). In contrast, during chronic administration, renin secretion increases both because solute delivery to the macula densa declines (498) and because volume depletion activates the vascular mechanism for renin secretion.

Pharmacokinetics

DCT diuretics are organic anions that circulate in a highly protein bound state. As with loop diuretics, the amount reaching the tubule fluid by filtration across the glomerular basement membrane is small; the predominant route of entry into tubule fluid is by secretion via the organic anion secretory pathway in the proximal tubule. DCT diuretics are rapidly absorbed, reaching peak concentrations within 1.5 to 4 hours (54). The amount of administered drug that reaches the urine varies greatly (for a review, see 54) as does the half life. Short-acting DCT diuretics include bendroflumethiazide, hydrochlorothiazide, tizolemide, and trichlormethiazide. Medium-acting DCT diuretics include chlorothiazide, hydroflumethiazide, indapamide, and mefruside. Long-acting DCT diuretics include chlorthalidone, metolazone, and polythiazide (54). The clinical effects of the differences in half-life are unclear, except in the incidence of hypokalemia, which is much more common in patients taking the longer acting drugs such as chlorthalidone (385, 433).

Clinical Use

Indications for the use of DCT diuretics are listed in Table 3. DCT diuretics are used most commonly to treat essential hypertension. Despite debate about their potential

TABLE 3   Indications for Diuretic Drugs

I. Indications for osmotic diuretics
  A. Acute or incipient renal failure
  B. To reduce intraocular or intracranial pressure
II. Indications for carbonic anhydrase inhibitors
  A. Glaucoma
  B. Acute mountain sickness
  C. Metabolic alkalosis
  D. Cystinuria
  E. Resistant edema (used in combination with other diuretics)
III. Indications for loop diuretics
  A. Edematous conditions
    1. Congestive heart failure
    2. Cirrhotic ascites
    3. Nephrotic syndrome
  B. Hypercalcemia (with saline)
  C. Hyperkalemia
  D. Hyponatremia (with hypertonic saline)
  E. Hyperkalemic, hyperchloremic metabolic acidosis (type 4 renal tubular acidosis)
  F. Hypermagnesemia
  G. Intoxications
  H. Hypertension
  I. Acute renal failure
IV. Indications for distal convoluted tubule diuretics
  A. Hypertension
  B. Edematous conditions
    1. Congestive heart failure
    2. Cirrhotic ascites
    3. Nephrotic syndrome
  C. Nephrolithiasis
  D. Nephrogenic diabetes insipidus
  E. Osteoporosis
  F. Hypoparathyroidism
  G. Diuretic resistance (used in combination with other diuretics)
V. Indications for collecting duct diuretics
  A. Cirrhotic ascites
  B. Lithium-induced diabetes insipidus
  C. Prevention of hypokalemia (owing to potassium-wasting diuretics)
  D. Prevention of hypomagnesemia (owing to potassium-wasting diuretics)
  E. Diuretic resistance (used in combination with other diuretics)
  F. Congestive heart failure with systolic dysfunction
VI. Indications for aquaretics
  A. Euvolemic hyponatremia
  B. Hypervolemic hyponatremia (experimental)

complications in the setting of essential hypertension, DCT diuretics continue to be recommended as drugs of first choice in the treatment of hypertension (7). DCT diuretics are also used commonly to treat edematous conditions, although they are frequently perceived as being less effective than loop diuretics. Although the maximal effect of loop diuretics to increase urinary Na, Cl, and water excretion is greater than that of DCT diuretics, Leary and colleagues have shown that the cumulative effects of DCT diuretics on urinary Na and Cl excretion are greater than those of once daily furosemide (283). Although these studies were conducted in normal volunteers, they may extend to patients with mild cases of edema. In addition, DCT diuretics have proved useful to treat edematous patients who have become resistant to loop diuretics. In this case, the addition of a DCT diuretic to a regimen that includes a loop diuretic frequently increases urinary Na and Cl excretion dramatically (see following sections).

DCT diuretics have become drugs of choice to prevent the recurrence of kidney stones in patients with idiopathic hypercalciuria. In several controlled and many uncontrolled studies, the recurrence rate for calcium stones has been reduced by up to 80% (149, 277, 526). Relatively high doses are often used for the treatment of nephrolithiasis (57), and some studies suggest that the hypocalciuric effect of DCT diuretics wanes during chronic use in the setting of absorptive hypercalciuria (377). The observation that Gitelman syndrome, an inherited disorder of the thiazide-sensitive Na-Cl cotransporter, may present during adulthood with hypocalciuria suggests that compensatory mechanisms may not exist for the effects of DCT diuretics on calcium transport (240). The ability of DCT diuretics to reduce urinary calcium excretion suggests that these drugs may prevent bone loss. Some (154, 386), but not all (85, 207), epidemiological studies suggested that DCT diuretics reduce the risk of hip fracture and osteoporosis. Clinical trials have confirmed that thiazide diuretics reduce the loss of cortical bone and may prevent hip fraction, although the effect seems modest and does not persist, once the drug has been discontinued (389, 392, 417). Others have indicated that DCT diuretics can be effective in patients with primary hypoparathyroidism, when combined with a low-salt diet (374).

DCT diuretics are also used to treat nephrogenic diabetes insipidus, causing a paradoxical decrease in urinary volume flow rate. This action of DCT diuretics results from the combination of actions. The best studied have included the induction of mild extracellular fluid volume contraction, owing to diuretic-induced natriuresis; suppression of glomerular filtration, owing largely to diuretic-induced activation of the tubuloglomerular feedback; and reduced distal water delivery. Such a mechanism would require depletion of the extracellular fluid volume, a requirement that has been documented in several studies (136, 226). The human distal convoluted tubule, like the thick ascending limb, is nearly impermeable to water (39). Solute reabsorption by the thiazide-sensitive Na-Cl cotransporter therefore contributes directly to urinary dilution; thus blocking Na-Cl cotransport reduces urinary diluting capacity. More recently, DCT diuretics have been shown to alter the abundance of water and salt transport pathways in the distal nephron. Kim and colleagues (252) used a rat model of lithium-induced diabetes insipidus. They showed a lithium-induced decrease in aquaporin expression that could be reversed, partially, by DCT diuretics. Another report showed that DCT diuretics enhance water absorption in inner medullary collecting duct (IMCD) from normal rats (in the absence of antidiuretic hormone [ADH]) and from Brattleboro rats and that the hydrochlorothiazide (HCTZ)–stimulated water permeability was partially blocked by PGE2 (86).

Adverse Effects

Electrolyte disorders, such as hypokalemia, hyponatremia, and hypomagnesemia are common side effects of DCT diuretics. A measurable fall in serum K concentration is nearly universal in patients given DCT diuretics, but most patients do not become frankly hypokalemic (433). In the Antihypertensive and Lipid-Lowering Treatment to Prevent Heart Attack Trial (ALLHAT) study, the largest controlled antihypertensive trial, mean plasma K concentrations were 0.3 mM lower in patients randomized to cholorthalidone, compared with amoldipine (which has little effect on K metabolism): The clinical significance of diuretic-induced hypokalemia continues to be debated (328, 432). Unlike the loop diuretics, DCT diuretics do not influence K transport directly (487, 488). Instead, they increase K excretion indirectly. DCT diuretics increase tubule fluid flow in the connecting tubule and collecting duct, the predominant sites of K secretion along the nephron. Increased flow stimulates K secretion both directly flow and indirectly (372, 504, 521). In addition, DCT diuretic-induced extracellular fluid volume contraction activates the renin-angiotensin-aldosterone system, further stimulating K secretion. Evidence for the central role of aldosterone in diuretic-induced hypokalemia includes the observation that hypokalemia is much more common during treatment with long-acting DCT diuretics, such as chlorthalidone, than with short-acting DCT diuretics, such as hydrochlorothiazide or with the very-short-acting loop diuretics (385). Another reason that DCT diuretics may produce more potassium wasting than loop diuretics is the differences in effects on calcium transport. As discussed previously, loop diuretics inhibit calcium transport by the thick ascending limb, increasing distal calcium delivery. In contrast, DCT diuretics stimulate calcium transport, reducing calcium delivery to sites of potassium secretion. Okusa and colleagues (348, 349) showed that high luminal concentrations of calcium inhibit ENaC in the distal nephron thereby inhibiting potassium secretion. DCT diuretics also increase urinary magnesium excretion and can lead to hypomagnesemia, as discussed above.

Hypomagnesemia may cause or contribute to the hypokalemia observed under these conditions (122, 403). Some studies suggest that maintenance magnesium therapy can prevent or attenuate the development of hypokalemia (123, 344), but this has not been supported universally.

Diuretics have been reported to contribute to more than one half of all hospitalizations for serious hyponatremia. Hyponatremia is especially common during treatment with DCT diuretics, compared with other classes of diuretics, and the disorder is potentially life-threatening (11). Several factors contribute to DCT diuretic–induced hyponatremia. First, as discussed previously, DCT diuretics inhibit solute transport in the terminal portion of the "diluting segment," the distal convoluted tubule. This impairs the ability to excrete free water. Second, DCT diuretics can reduce the GFR, primarily by activating the TGF system. This limits solute delivery to the diluting segment and impairs free-water clearance. Third, DCT diuretics lead to volume contraction, which increases proximal tubule solute and water reabsorption, further restricting delivery to the "diluting segment." Fourth, hyponatremia has been correlated with the development of hypokalemia in patients receiving DCT diuretics (156). Finally, susceptible patients may be stimulated to consume water during therapy with DCT diuretics; although the mechanisms are unclear, this may contribute importantly to the sudden appearance of hyponatremia that can occur during DCT diuretic therapy. Of note, one report suggests that patients who are predisposed to develop hyponatremia during treatment with DCT diuretics will demonstrate an acute decline in serum sodium concentration in response to a single dose of the drug (161). Studies suggest that female gender, advanced age, and low body mass are risk factors for thiazide-induced hyponatremia (93, 94).

DCT diuretics frequently cause metabolic alkalosis. The mechanisms are similar to those described previously for loop diuretics, except that DCT diuretics do not stimulate Na–H exchange in the TAL.

DCT diuretics cause several disturbances of endocrine glands. Glucose intolerance has been a recognized complication of DCT diuretic use since the 1950s. This complication appears to be dose related (80, 203). The pathogenesis of DCT diuretic–induced glucose intolerance remains unclear, but several factors have been suggested to contribute. First, diuretic-induced hypokalemia may alter insulin secretion by the pancreas, via effects on the membrane voltage of pancreatic β cells. When hypokalemia was prevented by oral potassium supplementation, the insulin response to hyperglycemia normalized, suggesting an important role for hypokalemia (208). Hypokalemia may also interfere with insulin-mediated glucose uptake by muscle, but most patients have relatively normal insulin sensitivity (469). Other factors may contribute to glucose intolerance as well. Volume depletion may stimulate catecholamine secretion, but volume depletion during therapy with DCT diuretics is usually very mild. DCT diuretics directly activate calcium-activated potassium channels that are expressed by pancreatic β cells, perhaps contributing to the hyperglycemia (366). Activation of these channels is known to inhibit insulin secretion.

DCT diuretics increase levels of total cholesterol, total triglyceride, and low-density lipoprotein (LDL) cholesterol. These drugs reduce the high-density lipoproteins (HDLs) (469). Definitive information about the mechanisms by which DCT diuretics alter lipid metabolism is not available, but many of the mechanisms that affect glucose homeostasis have been suggested to contribute. Hyperlipidemia, like hyperglycemia, is a dose-related side effect, and one that wanes with chronic diuretic use. In several large clinical studies, the effect of *low-dose* DCT diuretic treatment on serum LDL was not significantly different from that of placebo (193). In the ALLHAT study, mean cholesterol concentrations were higher in the group randomized to chlorthalidone, but the absolute differences at 2 and 4 years were 2 to 3 mg/dl.

CORTICAL COLLECTING TUBULE DIURETICS

Diuretic drugs that act primarily in the cortical collecting tubule (potassium-sparing diuretics) comprise three pharmacologically distinct groups: aldosterone antagonists (spironolactone), pteridines (triamterene), and pyrazinoylguanidines (amiloride) (Fig. 12). The site of action for all diuretics of this class is the cortical collecting duct and the connecting tubule, where they interfere with sodium reabsorption and indirectly potassium secretion. Because of the ability to minimize the normal tendency of diuretic drugs to increase potassium excretion, amiloride (15) and triamterene (196, 199) are considered potassium sparing. Diuretic activity is weak because fractional sodium reabsorption in the collecting tubule usually does not exceed 3% of the filtered load. For this reason, potassium-sparing drugs are ordinarily used in combination with thiazides or loop diuretics, often in a single preparation, to restrict potassium losses and sometimes augment diuretic action. However in certain conditions potassium-sparing diuretics are used as first line agents (Table 3). For example spironolactone is used in the treatment of edema in pa-

tients with cirrhosis (358) and amiloride or triamterene is used as a first-line treatment of Liddle syndrome (82) or Bartter syndrome (345).

Urinary Electrolyte Excretion

Amiloride, triamterene and spironolactone are weak natriuretic agents (Table 1). Their major effect, as described previously, is the ability to diminish potassium excretion. Additionally, these three diuretic agents decrease hydrogen ion excretion by the late distal tubule and collecting ducts. Evidence that spironolactone decreases hydrogen ion excretion comes from the finding of metabolic acidosis associated with mineralocorticoid deficiency (218, 276), and the finding that spironolactone produces metabolic acidosis in patients with cirrhosis who have mineralocorticoid excess (169). In rats, the administration of amiloride and triamterene has been shown to inhibit urinary acidification (15, 199). A common mechanism is likely to be involved in mediating the effects of all three diuretic agents on hydrogen ion secretion. These drugs reduce the lumen negative potential and thus decrease the gradient for hydrogen ion secretion.

Clearance studies in rats have demonstrated that amiloride produces a decrease in calcium excretion (105). In these studies, amiloride produced both a decrease in the calcium clearance/Na clearance ratio (C_{Ca}/C_{Na}), as well as a decrease in the fractional excretion of calcium. The effect of triamterene on clearance of calcium was less clear although, it did decrease the C_{Ca}/C_{Na} ratio. In vivo microperfusion of rat distal tubules showed that the effect of chlorothiazide on calcium absorption was enhanced with amiloride, suggesting that amiloride also increased calcium absorption by the distal tubule (103). Furthermore, in vitro perfusion of connecting tubules has shown that amiloride stimulated calcium absorption (427). Amiloride is believed to stimulate calcium absorption through its ability to block sodium channels, thereby hyperpolarizing apical membrane (163). Hyperpolarization of the apical membrane stimulates calcium entry through epithelial calcium channels TRPV5 (see DCT Diuretics). Amiloride has also been reported to reduce magnesium excretion (66, 124) and to prevent the development of hypomagesemia during therapy with a DCT diuretic (133).

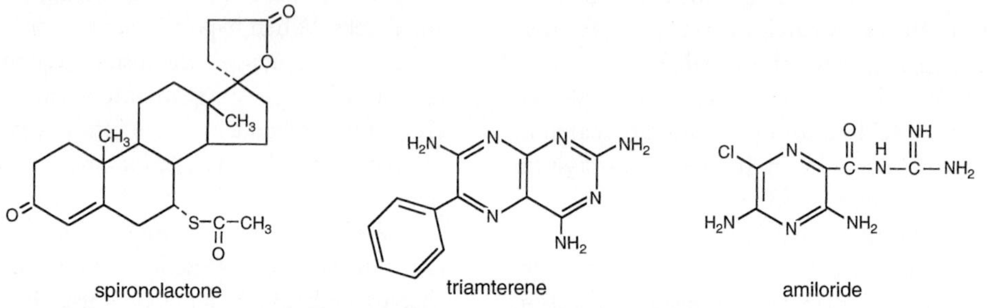

FIGURE 12   Structure of collecting duct diuretics.

Mechanism of Action

The site of action of potassium-sparing diuretics is the distal tubule. In this discussion we define the distal tubule as that region of the nephron located between the macula densa and the junction with another distal tubule to form the collecting duct. This segment is a heterogeneous structure composed of at least four cell types: DCT cells, connecting tubule cells, intercalated cells, and principle cells. The collecting duct is the final site of sodium chloride reabsorption where ~3% of the filtered load is reabsorbed. In addition to actions on the cortical collecting duct, these diuretics inhibit Na and K transport by the connecting tubule, which is an important site of aldosterone stimulated Na absorption and K secretion (13). It is now clear that sites of DCT diuretic action overlap considerably with sites of cortical collecting duct (CCD) diuretic action. Thus, in rat, mouse and human, a transitional segment, with characteristics of both DCT and connecting tubule, is present along the distal tubule (390). This segment, which may form the bulk of the distal tubule in humans, expresses the thiazide-sensitive Na-Cl cotransporter and the amiloride-sensitive epithelial Na channel.

Although the cortical collecting tubule reabsorbs only a small percentage of the filtered Na load, two characteristics render this segment important in the physiology of diuretic action. First, this nephron segment is the primary site of action of the mineralocorticoid, aldosterone, a hormone that controls sodium reabsorption and potassium secretion. Second, virtually all of the potassium that is excreted is due to the secretion of potassium by the collecting tubule. Thus this segment contributes to the hypokalemia seen as a consequence of diuretic action.

The collecting tubule is composed of two cell types that have entirely separate functions. Principle cells are responsible for the transport of sodium, potassium, and water, whereas intercalated cells are primarily responsible for the secretion of hydrogen or bicarbonate ions. The apical membrane of principle cells express separate channels that permit selective conductive transport of sodium and potassium (Fig. 10B). The mechanism by which sodium reabsorption occurs is through conductive sodium channels (for a review, see 411). The low intracellular sodium concentration as a result of the basolateral Na,K-ATPase generates a favorable electrochemical gradient for sodium entry through sodium channels. Because sodium channels are present only in the apical membrane of principle cells, sodium conductance depolarizes the apical membrane resulting in an asymmetric voltage profile across the cell. This effect produces a lumen-negative transepithelial potential difference. The lumen-negative potential difference together with a high-intracellular–to-lumen potassium concentration gradient provides the driving force for potassium secretion.

Sodium is the principle extracellular cation whose conductance across the principle cell of the collecting duct is amiloride sensitive and regulated by the activity and apical membrane expression of epithelial sodium channel (ENaC)

(77, 78). The functional channel comprises at least three homologous subunits, α, β, and γ with a presumed $\alpha_2 \beta_1, \gamma_1$ subunit stoichiometry (157, 270). The biophysical characteristics of ENaC include a low, single-channel conductance of ~5 pS, long open and closed times, a high Na to K^+ selectivity ratio of >100:1, and is inhibited by submicromolar concentrations of amiloride (247). Transcripts encoding the three subunits of ENaC have been identified in classic aldosterone responsive tissues (198). ENaC is the rate-limiting step and a number of factors converge to activate or inhibit its activity. Factors are known to alter the open channel probability, intracellular trafficking, and degradation of ENaC through alterations in gene transcription and posttranslational modification (178, 179, 217, 302, 379). Vasopressin, oxytocin, intracellular signaling elements such as phosphatases, kinases, G-proteins, and cAMP, and intracellular ions are known to regulate its activity (sodium, hydrogen, and calcium) (9, 19, 51, 209). The magnitude of ENaC expression at the apical membrane depends on the equilibrium maintained by the rate of ENaC insertion and the rate of removal from the apical membrane. ENaC internalization and degradation require ubiquitin conjugation of ENaC subunits by a ubiquitin ligase, neural precursor cell–expressed developmentally downregulated protein (Nedd4) (302).

The amount of sodium and potassium present in the final urine is tightly controlled by aldosterone action on principle cells. Extensive studies have demonstrated that in epithelia, aldosterone produces an early increase in sodium conductance (291, 491) followed by a sustained increase in transepithelial sodium transport. As a result, transepithelial sodium transport is increased, an effect that depolarizes the apical membrane. An increase in the lumen negative potential in turn enhances potassium secretion through conductive potassium channels located in the apical membrane. The cellular mechanisms that are responsible for these events have been extensively studied and reviewed (168, 198). The effects of aldosterone are thought to be mediated through classical genomic effect through action on mineralcorticoid receptors and through nongenomic action on mineralocorticoid receptors (168, 198). Genomic actions of aldosterone are initiated by penetration of the hormone through the basolateral membrane of principle cells and attachment to a cytosolic mineralocorticoid receptor, a heterotrimeric 8-9s complex of proteins. This receptor complex includes the steroid binding protein and heat shock proteins (HSPs). Binding of aldosterone to this complex stimulates the release of HSPs leading to the translocation of the receptor-aldosterone complex to the nucleus. The function of HSPs is not clear. It is thought that they facilitate anchoring of unbound steroid receptors to the cytoskeleton maintaining a high-affinity conformation (375). Evidence also indicates that released HSP90 stimulates calcineurin, a protein phosphatase that regulates sodium transport, in a transcription-independent process (475). In the nucleus, aldosterone-induced genes are induced, leading to the production of proteins called aldosterone-induced proteins (AIPs) (490). Newly formed mRNA encoding AIPs leaves the nucleus to direct the production of specific proteins that regulate sodium flux (397). These AIPs proteins regulate channel activity (398, 490) by increasing Na,K-ATPase subunits α, β, and γ of ENaC transcripts (10, 490). In contrast, however, a mineralocorticoid knockout mouse demonstrated essentially normal expression of ENaC subunits in the kidney, suggesting aldosterone regulation ENaC function in a posttranscriptional manner (25). K-ras2A, originally identified in an amphibian kidney-derived cell line (443), is acutely regulated by aldosterone in colon and kidney (396, 397). Serum and glucocorticoid-regulated kinase (sgk), a serine-threonine kinase, is expressed in collecting duct cells (333). Sgk is regulated at the level of transcription by corticosteroids, including aldosterone (88, 333) and in turn is known to phosphorylate Nedd4 ubiquitin ligases (438). Serum and glucocorticoid-regulated kinase modulates Nedd4-2–mediated inhibition of the epithelial Na channel. Nedd4-2 phosphorylation induces serum and glucocorticoid-regulated kinase (SGK) ubiquitination and degradation (527) and prolongs the surface expression and activity of ENaC. N-myc–downstream regulated gene 2 (*NDRG2*) belongs to a new family of differentiation genes that is transcriptionally regulated by aldosterone within 15 minutes (48).

Evidence is accumulating that nongenomic actions of aldosterone target various tissues including kidney, colon, vascular wall, and heart (168). A number of studies have demonstrated a nongenomic effect of aldosterone in kidney from the early in vivo studies (174) to more recent in vitro studies (167, 205, 341). These effects occur rapidly, at subnanomolar concentrations, and are not blocked by protein synthesis inhibitors. In some cases, these nongenomic effects are mediated through classical mineralocorticoid receptors (168).

Spironolactone and Eplerenone

Spirolactones are compounds that have the principle effect of blocking aldosterone action (152, 425). One of the spirolactones, spironolactone (Fig. 12) is an analogue of aldosterone that is extensively metabolized (242, 425). Spironolactone is converted by deacylation to 7α-thiospironolactone or by diethioacetylation to canrenone (152). In the kidney, spironolactone and its metabolites enter target cells from the peritubular side, bind to cytosolic mineralocorticoid receptors and act as competitive inhibitors of the endogenous hormone (100, 286, 312, 401). In studies using radiolabelled spironolactone or aldosterone, [³H]-spironolactone-receptor complexes were found to be excluded from the nucleus. In contrast, [³H]-aldosterone-receptor complexes were detected in the nucleus (312). These results are consistent with the proposal that aldosterone antagonists block the translocation of mineralocorticoid receptors to the nucleus. The mechanism by which aldosterone antagonists block nuclear localization of antagonist-receptor complexes is not known; however, it has been suggested that they destabilize mineralocorticoid receptors facilitating proteolysis (107). As dis-

cussed previously, mineralocorticoid receptors like other steroid receptors contain a steroid-binding unit associated with other cellular components including HSP90, in its inactive state. Steroid binding produces dissociation of HSP90 from the steroid binding unit uncapping the DNA-binding sites. Spironolactone facilitates the release of HSP90 and in combination with rapid dissociation of ligand could lead to degradation of the receptor (107).

A new aldosterone receptor antagonist, eplerenone, is a competitive antagonist of the aldosterone receptor. Replacing the 17α-thoacetyl group of spironolactone with a carbomethoxy group confers improved selectivity for aldosterone receptors and negligible activity at the cytochrome p450 enzyme (114), but 10–20-fold lower affinity for its receptor (111). Eplerenone has a slightly longer half-life of 3.5 hours compared with spironolactone and does not produce important metabolites. In vitro receptor binding studies have revealed that its affinity is approximately 10–20-fold less than spironolactone for the aldosterone receptor.

Spironolactone induces a mild increase in sodium excretion (1%–2%) and a decrease in potassium and hydrogen ion excretion (235, 286). Its effect depends on the presence of aldosterone as spironolactone is ineffective in experimental adrenalectomized animals (286), in patients with Addison's disease (98), and patients on a high-salt diet. In cortical collecting tubules perfused in vitro, spironolactone added to the bath solution reduced the aldosterone-induced, lumen negative transepithelial voltage (196). By blocking sodium absorption in the collecting tubule, a decrease in lumen negative potential reduces the driving force for passive sodium and hydrogen ion secretion (196).

Amiloride and Triamterene

Amiloride and triamterene (Fig. 12) are structurally different but are organic cations that use the same primary site of action (Fig. 10B). Triamterene is an aminopteridine chemically related to folic acid and amiloride is a pyrazinoylguanidine. Systemically administered amiloride results in an increase in sodium excretion and decrease in potassium excretion (15, 65, 216, 382). Their actions on sodium and potassium transport, unlike spironolactone, are independent of aldosterone (65). Systemically administered amiloride produced a small increase in sodium excretion and a much larger decrease in potassium excretion (126, 182, 216). Sampling of tubule fluid from the distal tubule demonstrated an inhibition of the normal rise in the tubule fluid to plasma potassium ratio. These results indicated that amiloride decreased distal tubule potassium secretion. Experiments employing in vivo microperfusion of distal tubules (102, 488) and in vitro perfusion of isolated cortical collecting tubules (450, 453) demonstrated that luminally administered amiloride reduced sodium absorption and potassium secretion. Similar results were obtained following in vivo microperfusion with benazamil (349), a more potent amiloride analogue (285). The mechanism by which amiloride decreases potassium secretion is due to its effect in blocking sodium conductance in the apical membrane of distal tubule and collecting tubule cells (265, 337, 349), thereby decreasing the electrochemical gradient for potassium secretion.

In high concentrations (>100 μM), amiloride interacts nonspecifically with different transporters, enzymes, and receptors, however, at concentrations of 0.05 to 0.5 μM, amiloride interacts specifically with sodium channels (177, 178). Furthermore, aromatic substitutions on the guanidinium moiety render the molecule even more potent (IC$_{50}$ 10–20-fold lower than amiloride) (83, 179). The molecular mechanism by which amiloride blocks sodium channels has been extensively studied and has shed light on structure and functional activity of ENaC (247). In general there is evidence for both ionic block and allosteric inhibition (179). Mutations in all three subunits, αSer-583, βGly-525, and γGly-542, reduced the affinity of amiloride for ENaC (229, 246, 413). Thus, these studies demonstrate contributions to amiloride binding by all three subunits and that amiloride may bind close to the αSer-583 site and may be important in the permeability of Na through ENaC (244).

Clearance and free-flow micropuncture studies using triamterene demonstrated results similar to studies with amiloride (216); however, the mechanism of action is not clearly defined. In earlier studies of rabbit cortical collecting tubules perfused in vitro, triamterene produced a gradual, reversible inhibition of the potential difference after a latent period of 10 minutes (196). Studies, however, suggest that triamterene binds to the epithelial sodium channel and thus has a mechanism of action similar to amiloride (75).

Pharmacokinetics

Spironolactone is poorly soluble in aqueous fluids. Bioavailability of an oral dose is approximately 90% in some commercial preparations. The drug is rapidly metabolized in the liver into a number of metabolites. Canrenone was thought to be the major metabolite of spironolactone (242, 425). This conclusion was based on fluorometric assays. Assays of spironolactone and its metabolites by the use of high-performance liquid chromatography (HPLC), however, demonstrated that fluorometrically measured levels of canrenone overestimated true canrenone levels (317). Using HPLC, the predominant metabolite, 7α-methylspironolactone (175), is responsible for approximately 80% of the potassium-sparing effect. Spironolactone and its metabolites are extensively bound to plasma protein (98%). In normal volunteers, taking spironolactone (100 mg/d) for 15 days, the mean half-lives for spironolactone, canrenone, 7α-thiomethylspironolactone and 6β-hydroxy-7α-thiomethylspironolactone were 1.4, 16.5, 13.8, and 15 hours, respectively. Thus although unmetabolized spironolactone is present in serum, it has a rapid elimination time. The onset of action is extremely slow, with peak response sometimes occurring 48 hours or more after the first dose; effects gradually wane over a period of 48 to 72 hours. Spironolactone is used in cirrhotic patients to induce a natriuresis. In these patients,

pharmacokinetic studies indicate that the half-lives of spironolactone and its metabolites are increased. The half-lives for spironolactone, canrenone, 7α-thiomethylspironolactone and 6β-hydroxy-7α-thiomethylspironolactone are 9, 58, 24, and 126 hours, respectively (457).

Clinical Use

The most common side effect of loop and DCT diuretics is the depletion of body potassium with or without significant lowering of serum K concentration. Hypokalemia of sufficient magnitude may produce nonspecific weakness or may be life threatening. The more severe effects include impairment of neuromuscular function, cardiac dysrhythmia, intestinal disturbances, and partial loss of the ability to concentrate urine. Of particular concern is the potential for cardiac toxicity in patients with congestive heart failure who are maintained on cardiac glycosides. Given these potential problems, it is important to avoid potassium deficit through dietary intake of large amounts of potassium, avoidance of excessive NaCl intake, and monitoring of serum K concentrations. The most effective therapeutic measure is to add a potassium-sparing diuretic to the therapeutic regimen (510), but KCl supplements should be discontinued or plasma K monitored carefully if a potassium-sparing agent is used.

Mineralocorticoid receptor antagonists are most effective in patients with primary (adrenal adenoma or bilateral adrenal hyperplasia) (60) or secondary hyperaldosteronism (congestive heart failure, cirrhosis, nephrotic syndrome) and is ineffective in patients with nonfunctional adrenal gland. These drugs are used for correction of hypokalemia. They are administered alone, with thiazides, or a loop diuretic, to reduce the ECF volume without causing potassium depletion or hypokalemia. Spironolactone is especially appropriate for the treatment of cirrhosis with ascites, a condition invariably associated with secondary hyperaldosteronism. In comparison to loop or thiazide diuretics, spironolactone is equivalent or more effective (278). The reason for this observation could be related to the differences in the mechanism of drug action. Thiazides and loop are highly protein bound and enter the tubule fluid primarily by proximal tubule secretion and not by glomerular filtration. In patients with cirrhosis and ascites, tubular secretion of these agents decreases as a consequence of competition with accumulated toxic organic metabolites. Because thiazide and loop diuretics are luminally acting agents, decreased tubule secretion reduces their effectiveness. In contrast, the activity of spironolactone does not depend on filtration or secretion as they gain access to their cytosolic receptors from the blood side. Thus in patients with cirrhosis and ascites, the effectiveness of spironolactone is unimpaired. A combination of loop diuretic and spironolactone can be used to boost natriuresis when the diuretic effect of spironolactone alone is inadequate.

Although its natriuretic action is weak, mineralocorticoid receptor antagonists lowers blood pressure in patients with mild or moderate hypertension and is frequently prescribed for this purpose. Spironolactone is indicated for the treatment of mineralocorticoid hypertension and recently eplerenone was approved by the FDA for treatment of systemic hypertension (287). Based upon recent clinical trials (367, 368) spironolactone and eplerenone are approved for the treatment of congestive heart failure.

Triamterene or amiloride is generally used in combination with potassium-wasting diuretics (thiazide or loop diuretics), especially when maintenance of normal serum potassium concentrations is clinically important. In addition, amiloride (or triamterene) has also been used as initial therapy in potassium wasting states such as primary hyperaldosteronism (173, 192), Liddle's (46), Bartter's, or Gitelman's syndromes (345). Amiloride has been used in the treatment of lithium-induced nephrogenic diabetes insipidus. The efficacy of amiloride in this disorder relates to the ability of amiloride to block collecting duct sodium channels, a pathway by which lithium uses to gain entry into cells (284, 316).

Adverse Effects

The most serious adverse reaction encountered during therapy with spironolactone and eplerenone is hyperkalemia (368). Serum potassium should be monitored periodically even when the drug is administered with a potassium-wasting diuretic. Patients at highest risk are those with low glomerular filtration rates and those individuals who take potassium supplements concurrently. In patients with cirrhosis and ascites treated with spironolactone, hyperchloremic metabolic acidosis can develop independent of changes in renal function (169). Unwanted antiandrogenic and progestational side effects include gynecomastia in men (400), decreased libido, and impotence. Women may develop menstrual irregularities, hirsutism, or swelling and tenderness of the breast. In subjects receiving eplerenone for heart failure, the incidence of gynecomastia and impotence among men receiving eplerenone was similar to placebo (367), which is in contrast to the effects of spironolactone (368). These differences in side effects are likely related to eplerenone's greater selectivity for the mineralocorticoid receptor versus androgen and progesterone receptors. Spironolactone-induced agranulocytosis has also been reported (509).

Triamterene and amiloride may cause hyperkalemia. The risk of hyperkalemia is highest in patients in patients with limited renal function (e.g., renal insufficiency, diabetes, and elderly patients). Additional complications included elevated serum blood urea nitrogen and uric acid, glucose intolerance, and GI tract disturbances. Triamterene induces crystalluria or cylinduria (151, 357) and may contribute to or initiate formation of renal stones (81) and acute kidney injury when combined with nonsteroidal anti-inflammatory agents (153, 502). The drugs are contraindicated in patients with hyperkalemia, individuals taking potassium supplements in any

form, and in patients with severe renal failure with progressive oliguria.

AQUARETICS (VASOPRESSIN RECEPTOR ANTAGONISTS)

Mechanism of Action

The effects of arginine vasopressin (also called antidiuretic hormone [ADH]) are mediated by two major receptor subtypes: V_1 and V_2. V_1 receptors are expressed in many cell types including vascular smooth muscle (V_{1a}) and adenohypophysis (V_{1b}). V_2-vasopressin receptors are expressed in kidney and seminal vesicle. V_2 receptors have been localized to principle cells of the connecting tubule, cortical and medullary collecting duct (464). Binding of arginine vasopressin to V_2-vasopressin receptors in collecting duct cells results in water reabsorption. Many clinical disorders such as cirrhosis, congestive heart failure, SIADH are associated with high levels of arginine vasopressin that prevent appropriate water excretion resulting in hyponatremia.

A nonpeptide vasopressin receptor antagonist (conivaptan) is now available for clinical use as an intravenous preparation; it is indicated to treat euvolemic hyponatremia. Other antagonists are presently under clinical development. Conivaptan is a benzazepine derivative and the first combined vasopressin $V_{1a}R/V_2R$ antagonist (460). This agent displaced a selective vasopressin $V_{1a}R$ antagonist in a dose-dependent manner from rat liver membranes; the IC_{50} was 2.2 ± 0.1 nmol/l. The agent also caused a concentration-dependent displacement of a vasopressin V_2R antagonist from renal medullary membranes, and the IC_{50} of the binding affinity was 0.4 ± 0.1 nmol/l (353). Oral conivaptan given for 7 days in normotensive rats caused a dose-dependent aquaresis with no effect on specific blood pressure (395). When administered to healthy volunteers orally, conivaptan, effects were observed after 2 hours. Including a sevenfold increase in the urinary flow rate and a decrease in urinary osmolality from 600 mOsm/kg to less than 100 mOsm/kg. Plasma osmolality increased from 283 ± 1.3 mOsm/kg to 289 ± 1.7 mOsm/kg (353).

In double-blind, randomized, placebo-controlled clinical trials, conivaptan was shown to increase serum Na concentrations in a variety of settings (353). Although conivaptan was originally discovered as an orally active V_{1a}/V_2 antagonist, it was developed for intravenous application. In one study it was given intravenously by continuous infusion over 4 days at doses of 40 and 80 mg/d following a loading dose of 20 mg intravenously on the first day. During the study, patients adhered to fluid restriction of 2 l/d. In the group of patients receiving high-dose conivaptan (80 mg/d), the treatment increased the serum sodium concentration significantly from a baseline of 125 mmol/l to 134 mmol/l (353). These data suggest that conivaptan is an efficient therapy of hyponatremia and is safe. Additional information concerning its safety profile, appropriate clinical use, and therapeutic role will certainly become available during the next several years.

GENERAL PRINCIPLES OF DIURETIC ACTION

When a diuretic drug is first administered to a healthy individual, urinary sodium and chloride excretion rates increase. The magnitude of the increase is determined by the nature of the drug, the dose, the gastrointestinal absorption, the delivery to the kidney, entry into tubule fluid (for diuretics that act from the tubule lumen), and the physiological state of the individual. Except for diuretics that act predominantly in the proximal tubule, such as the CA inhibitors, the maximal natriuretic potency of a diuretic can be predicted from its site of action. Table 1 shows that loop diuretics can increase fractional Na excretion to 30%, DCT diuretics can increase it to 9%, and Na channel blockers can increase it to 3% of the filtered load. Because CA inhibitors enhance excretion of Na with bicarbonate rather than chloride, and because they induce adaptive processes that are described more fully in subsequent sections, the maximal natriuretic potency of CA inhibitors is much lower than would be predicted from their site of action. The dose response curve for diuretic action has been best characterized for loop diuretics. In this case the relation is sigmoidal (Fig. 6), when the fractional Na excretion is plotted versus the urinary diuretic concentration (55). Most diuretics act from the luminal surface. Therefore, the best external indicator of diuretic drug concentration at the active site is the urinary diuretic concentration.

The bioavailability of diuretic drugs varies widely, between classes of drugs, between different drugs of the same class, and even between days of the week with the same drug. The bioavailability of loop diuretics ranges from 10% to 100% (mean of 50% for furosemide, 80%–100% for bumetanide and torsemide (Table 2). Limited bioavailability can usually be overcome by appropriate dosing, but some drugs, such as furosemide, are variably absorbed by the same patient on different days making precise titration difficult (55). Although this relation predicts that oral furosemide should be half as potent as intravenous furosemide, the relation is not fixed and depends on the clinical state of the individual. For example, the amount of Na excreted during 24 hours is similar when furosemide is administered to a normal individual by mouth or by vein (Fig. 6). Yet the total amount of furosemide excreted in the urine during the same period is approximately half as great following oral compared with intravenous administration (52, 248). This paradox results from the fact that oral furosemide absorption is slower than its clearance, leading to "absorption-limited" kinetics. Thus, effective serum furosemide concentrations persist longer when the drug is given by mouth because a

reservoir in the gastrointestinal tract continues to supply furosemide to the body. This relation holds for a healthy individual (Fig. 6C), but not necessarily for a patient who suffers from an edematous disorder. In this case, a higher serum drug level may be needed to elicit natriuresis and the lower serum drug level achieved by oral treatment may be inadequate to reach the natriuretic threshold. For this reason, it is customary to double the furosemide dose when changing from intravenous to oral therapy (55). Variations in bioavailability may lead to increased hospitalizations for patients with congestive heart failure treated with furosemide, compared to a drug such as torsemide that is more completely absorbed, but this remains to be established in larger studies (331).

A third factor that determines the maximal natriuresis following diuretic drug administration is drug delivery to its active site. Most diuretics, including the loop diuretics, DCT diuretics, and amiloride, act from the luminal surface. Thus, to be effective, these drugs must be delivered into tubule fluid by glomerular filtration or by tubular secretion. Although diuretics are small molecules, most circulate tightly bound to protein and reach tubule fluid primarily by secretion. When serum albumin concentrations are very low, the volume of diuretic distribution increases (222), but this factor may not be as important in causing diuretic resistance as believed previously (56). Nevertheless, when serum albumin concentrations are less than 2 g/l, reduced diuretic delivery to the kidney may play a role in resistance (41, 159, 181, 332).

Loop and DCT diuretics are organic anions that circulate bound to albumin and reach tubule fluid primarily via the organic anion secretory pathway in the proximal tubule (259). Recent studies have characterized this weak organic anion (OA^-) transport (OAT) process. Four isoforms of an OAT have been cloned and are expressed in the kidney (459, 478). Peritubular uptake by an OAT is a tertiary active process (Fig. 13). Energy derives from the basolateral Na,K^+-ATPase that provides a low intracellular [Na] that drives an uptake of Na coupled to α-ketoglutarate (αKG^-) to maintain a high intracellular level of aKG^-. This in turn drives a basolateral OA^-/aKG^- countertransporter. OAT translocates diuretics into the proximal tubule cell where they can be sequestered in intracellular vesicles. They are secreted across the luminal membrane by a voltage-driven OA^- transporter (271) and by a countertransporter in exchange for urate or OH^-. (459) OAT1 is expressed on the basolateral membrane of the S2 segment of the proximal tubule. Recently, a mouse colony deficient in OAT1 was generated and shown to exhibit dramatically impaired renal organic anion secretion and furosemide resistance (148). Thus, OAT1 plays a central role in mediating loop diuretic secretion by proximal cells. Albumin has been reported to stimulate renal organic anion secretion directly, in a dose-dependent manner, up to a maximum when the concentration reaches 1 g/dl (29).

Endogenous and exogenous substances may compete with diuretics for secretion into tubule fluid and affect

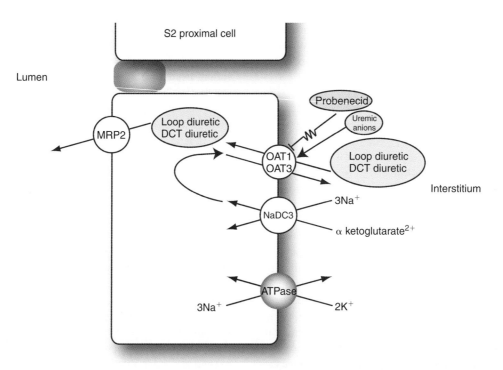

FIGURE 13   Mechanisms of diuretic secretion by proximal tubule cells. Cell diagram of the S2 segment of the proximal tubule showing secretion of anionic diuretic, including loop diuretics and distal convoluted tubule (DCT) diuretics. Peritubular uptake by an organic anion transporter (primarily OAT1, although OAT3 may play a smaller role) is in exchange for α-ketoglutarate. α-ketoglutarate is brought into the cell by the sodium-dependent cation transporter, NaDC3. Luminal secretion can be via a voltage-dependent pathway or in exchange for luminal hydroxyl (OH⁻) or urate. A portion of the luminal transport traverses the multidrug-resistance protein-2 (MRP2) (From Burckhardt BC and Burckhardt G. Transport of organic anions across the basolateral membrane of proximal tubule cells. *Rev Physiol Biochem Pharmacol* 2003;146:95–158, with permission.)

diuretic response. Uremic anions (399), nonsteroidal anti-inflammatory drugs (91), probenecid (53), and penicillins all inhibit loop and DCT diuretic secretion into tubule fluid. Under some conditions, this may predispose to diuretic resistance because the concentration of drug achieved in tubule fluid does not exceed the diuretic threshold. For example, in chronic renal failure, diuretic delivery into the urine is reduced (399). This shifts the diuretic dose response curve to the right, requiring a higher dose to achieve maximal effect (Fig. 6). Surprisingly, however, probenecid *increases* the natriuretic effects of chlorothiazide and furosemide when administered to normal individual (53, 92). This effect results from the probenecid-induced impairment in renal diuretic clearance, which prolongs the effective half-life, permitting diuresis to continue over a longer period of time. Thus, if a dose is sufficient to achieve serum levels that permit rates of diuretic secretion to exceed the diuretic threshold, the effect of an inhibitor will be to increase the natriuretic response. In contrast, in a patient whose dose is near to the diuretic threshold, impairments of secretion can lead to achievement of sub-threshold levels in tubule fluid and to diuretic resistance.

Amiloride and triamterene are organic cations that reach tubule fluid via the organic cation secretory pathway in the proximal tubule. Even though this system is separate from the organic anion transport pathway, probenecid can inhibit this pathway (259). Most data suggest that organic cations are transported across the basolateral membrane by a cation–cation exchange pathway. Movement of cationic diuretics from cell to lumen occurs via an organic cation–H exchanger, which is coupled functionally to the apical Na–H exchanger (259). Creatinine, cimetidine, trimethoprim, quinidine, quinine, atropine, ofloxacin, morphine, and paraquat are all secreted by this pathway (259). Cimetidine has been shown to inhibit the secretion of amiloride (442).

A fourth factor that may influence diuretic effectiveness is protein binding in tubule fluid. Diuretic drugs are normally bound to proteins in the plasma, but not once they are secreted into tubule fluid. This reflects the normally low protein concentrations in tubule fluid. In contrast, when serum proteins such as albumin are filtered in appreciable quantities, diuretic drugs will interact with them (494). This protein-drug interaction appears to inhibit the ability of the diuretic to interact with luminal transport proteins. Kirchner and colleagues (262) showed that adding albumin to diuretic-containing fluid used to perfuse rat loops of Henle reduced the effects of the loop diuretic by approximately 50%. This effect was specific for albumin, since IgG did not mimic it, an effect that could be prevented by perfusing protein-binding inhibitors such as warfarin or sulfisoxizole (261). Yet subsequent studies in proteinuric humans suggest that this mechanism does not play an important role in mediating diuretic resistance in nephrosis (2). Although the reasons for the discrepant results between animal models and humans are unclear, it seems unlikely that urinary albumin binding to diuretics is an important contributor to diuretic resistance.

Patients given diuretic drugs to treat edematous conditions all manifest some diuretic resistance (Fig. 6). This is evident in the shift to the right and downward in the dose response curve for a loop diuretic.

DIURETIC ADAPTATIONS AND DIURETIC RESISTANCE

Although the clinically useful diuretic drugs all increase urinary solute and water excretion, the goal of diuretic therapy of edema is to reduce the extracellular fluid volume. This usually requires an increase in urinary solute and water excretion, but such an increase is not sufficient to effect ECF volume contraction by itself. Furthermore, any initial increase in daily urinary NaCl and water excretion begins to wane after several days of diuretic treatment. That is because of specific renal adaptations that occur during diuretic therapy. Adaptations to diuretic drugs may be classified as immediate, short term, and chronic. When these processes become manifest once the desired extracellular fluid volume has been attained, they are clinically useful and prevent progressive ECF volume contraction. When these same processes develop before achieving the desired ECF volume, they would be viewed as contributing to diuretic resistance. Because specific therapeutic approaches can be devised to overcome these adaptations, an understanding of renal adaptations to diuretic treatment is crucial for understanding diuretic treatment of edema. For the purposes of this discussion, diuretic adaptations will be classified as *immediate*, *short-term*, and *chronic*. Immediate adaptations limit the intrinsic potency of diuretic drugs; these occur during the initial diuretic-induced natriuresis and generally result from intrinsic renal processes. Short term adaptations occur after the initial effect of the diuretic drug has worn off and may result from both systemic and intra-renal processes. Chronic adaptations occur only when diuretic drugs have been administered during a long period (days to weeks). Because diuretic resistance is most commonly observed in patients who have received high doses of diuretic during a long period, these chronic adaptations may be especially relevant to the phenomenon of diuretic resistance in patients.

Immediate Adaptations

About 25 M of sodium are filtered every day by the kidneys in a healthy human. Because dietary salt intake on a Western diet is typically 130 to 260 mmol daily, approximately 3 lb of salt (17 M = 1 kg NaCl) must be reabsorbed every day by the renal tubules to maintain salt balance. As discussed previously, all sodium chloride reabsorption along the mammalian nephron is driven by the action of Na,K-ATPase, which is present along the basolateral cell membrane of most renal epithelial cells. Transepithelial sodium transport occurs because apical transport pathways permit Na to move down its electrochemical gradient from tubule lumen to cell, often coupled to the movement of other ions across the same membrane. Most diuretics drugs act by inhibiting apical Na transport pathways. Because apical Na transport pathways are nephron segment specific, each class of diuretic inhibits Na transport *predominantly* along a single segment of the nephron (Fig. 1). The axial organization of renal tubules and the nephron segment-specific inhibition of salt transport by diuretics means that diuretics have both direct effects and indirect effects on solute transport along the nephron.

When NaCl reabsorption along the thick ascending limb is inhibited by loop diuretics, the NaCl concentration in fluid that enters the distal tubule is greatly increased. In one study, the Na concentration in fluid entering the distal tubule of rats rose from 42 to 140 mM during acute loop diuretic infusion (216). The higher luminal NaCl concentration increased Na absorption along the distal tubule (from 148 to 361 pmol/min) because NaCl transport varies directly with the luminal NaCl concentration. Further, loop diuretics have little or no effect on ion transport along the distal tubule (488). The bulk of the increased NaCl transport along the distal tubule appears to result from enhanced transcellular transport via the thiazide-sensitive Na-Cl cotransporter. In microperfused rat distal tubules, raising the luminal NaCl concentration twofold increased transepithelial Na transport by a factor of 3; this increase could be blocked entirely by luminal chorothiazide (145). The dependence of transepithelial NaCl transport on luminal NaCl concentration probably results from a dependence of the thiazide-sensitive Na-Cl cotransporter on extracellular Na and Cl concentrations (172).

This first level of adaptation to diuretic drugs occurs *during* the period of diuretic-induced natriuresis (521). The *net* effect of acute diuretic administration on urinary Na and Cl excretion, therefore, reflects the sum of effects in the diuretic-sensitive segment (inhibition of NaCl reabsorption) and in diuretic-insensitive segments (secondary stimulation of NaCl reabsorption). Although the most clinically important example of this form of adaptation involves loop diuretics, these compensatory processes occur during administration of most classes of diuretics. The importance of compensatory processes to blunt the acute effects of diuretics is exemplified by CA inhibitors, which inhibit Na transport across cells of the proximal tubule. Because a large portion of the Na that is rejected by the proximal tubule during CA inhibitor administration is reabsorbed along the loop of Henle and distal tubule, only a fraction escapes into the urine. CA inhibitors, therefore, are drugs of only modest potency. Blockade of immediate adaptive processes enhances the effects of the administered diuretic, as when loop diuretics are combined with CA inhibitors, acutely. A similar phenomenon has been observed in animals lacking NHE3, the apical Na–H exchanger of the proximal tubule (295). These animals exhibit minimal salt wasting, owing to compensatory processes.

Short-term Adaptations (Postdiuretic NaCl Retention)

The half-life of most diuretics (especially the loop diuretics) is relatively short. Thus, serum diuretic concentrations are often below the natriuretic threshold during a portion of each day, except when the drugs are infused constantly. This second type of adaptive response to diuretic administration occurs after the peak natriuresis has occurred and is most prominent when the drug concentration in plasma and tubular fluid declines below the diuretic threshold. In this situation, diuretic is no longer present in tubule fluid to inhibit renal Na reabsorption and a period of NaCl retention, often termed "postdiuretic NaCl retention" begins (Fig. 14). The net effect of the diuretic drug during 24 hours, therefore, results from a period of natriuresis (when NaCl transport is inhibited by the diuretic) and a period of antinatriuresis (when the drug concentration is low, before the next dose is given).

Mechanisms that contribute to postdiuretic NaCl retention have been investigated intensively and may be grouped into three classes; *first*, factors that result from changes in extracellular fluid volume; *second*, factors that result from diuretic-induced increases in distal sodium, chloride and fluid delivery; and *third*, factors that result from direct effects of diuretic drugs on tubule transport processes. One signal initiating NaCl retention in the postdiuretic period is the change in extracellular fluid volume and the change in "effective" arterial blood volume. Evidence indicating a central role for changes in ECF volume includes the observation that postdiuretic NaCl retention can be prevented by administering Na, K, and Cl at rates sufficient to equal diuretic induced losses (4). This observation does not, however, exclude a contributory role for mechanisms that occur independent of changes in ECF volume, as will be discussed below.

Diuretic drugs have effects on vascular and ECF volume within minutes of administration, both because of their ability to increase renal Na and Cl excretion and because they have direct vascular effects. These changes activate a number of physiological control systems, which tend to favor NaCl retention and act to attenuate further NaCl loss. Important contributors to ECF volume–dependent NaCl retention have been discussed previously and include changes in the glomerular filtration rate, activation of the renin-angiotensin-aldosterone system, stimulation of efferent renal sympathetic nerves, suppression of atrial natriuretic peptide secretion, and suppression of renal prostaglandin secretion. Postdi-

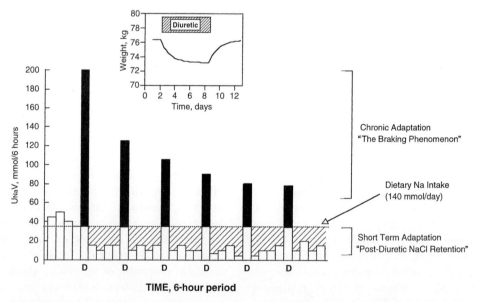

FIGURE 14 Effects of diuretics on urinary Na excretion and extracellular fluid (ECF) volume. **Inset:** Effect of diuretic on body weight, an index of extracellular fluid volume. Note that steady state is reached within 6 to 8 days despite continued diuretic administration. **Main Graph:** Effects of loop diuretic on urinary Na excretion. Bars represent 6-hour periods before (in Na balance) and after doses loop diuretic (D). The dotted line indicates dietary Na intake. The solid portion of bars indicates the amount by which Na excretion exceeds intake during natriuresis. The hatched areas indicate the amount of positive Na balance after the diuretic effect has dissipated. Net Na balance during 24 hours is the difference between the hatched are (postdiuretic NaCl retention) and the solid area (diuretic-induced natriureisis). Chronic adaptation is indicated by progressively smaller peak natriuretic effects (braking phenomenon) and is mirrored by a return to neutral balance, as indicated in the inset, where the solid and hatched areas are equal. As discussed in the text, chronic adaptation requires ECF volume depletion.

uretic NaCl retention has been shown to occur in humans whether dietary NaCl intake is high or low, suggesting that true ECF volume *depletion* may not be essential, but a *decline* in ECF volume was shown to be necessary for secondary NaCl retention during furosemide-induced natriuresis in rats. In rats given furosemide continuously, the secondary decline in NaCl excretion was associated with a 25% decline in glomerular filtration rate suggesting that decreases in filtered NaCl load contribute to short-term adaptations to diuretic treatment (95). In normal humans, changes in glomerular filtration rate were reported to be statistically insignificant during postdiuretic NaCl retention suggesting a decline in filtered Na does not contribute (514). Yet when the data from several subgroups are pooled, a statistically significant decline in GFR can be observed in the postdiuretic period (514); the magnitude of this effect is small, however, and increases in NaCl reabsorption probably play a larger role.

One mechanism that may mediate a decline in GFR after loop diuretic drug concentrations decline may be activation of the tubuloglomerular feedback system. Loop diuretics block this system directly by interfering with Na and Cl uptake by macula densa cells, as discussed above. Thus loop diuretics tend to maintain the GFR higher than would be expected in the absence of diuretic action. When the diuretic concentration declines and the inhibitory effects at the macula densa wane, the tubuloglomerular feedback system is poised to respond again to NaCl delivery and to suppress the GFR thus contributing to postdiuretic NaCl retention.

Diuretic drugs stimulate the renin-angiotensin-aldosterone axis via mechanisms described above and in Fig. 8. The renin-angiotensin-aldosterone axis contributes importantly to renal NaCl homeostasis, but evidence for an important role of these hormones in postdiuretic NaCl retention has been mixed. In healthy volunteers, postdiuretic NaCl retention was unaffected by the angiotensin converting enzyme inhibitor captopril (249) given in doses sufficient to block furosemide-induced changes in angiotensin II and aldosterone levels. Further, in those studies, diuretic-induced changes in blood pressure were similar with or without captopril, suggesting that hypotension did not mediate the NaCl retention in the ACE inhibitor group. These data indicate that postdiuretic NaCl retention *can* occur without activation of the renin-angiotensin-aldosterone system; they do not indicate, however, that stimulation of the renin-angiotensin-aldosterone axis has no role in postdiuretic NaCl retention when it occurs. An important role for the renin-angiotensin-aldosterone axis is implied by comparing the effects of volume removal via loop diuretics and hemofiltration. After diuresis of patients with congestive heart failure, ECF volume rises quickly; after volume removal using ultrafiltration, it does not (3, 310). The patients who received loop diuretics also had a dramatic rise in plasma renin activity, whereas the hemofiltration group did not, suggesting that stimulation of the renin-angiotensin-aldosterone axis contributed to the postdiuretic rebound, under these conditions.

Stimulation of α-adrenergic renal nerves enhances NaCl reabsorption. Petersen et al. (361) showed that systemic α_1 blockade attenuated the secondary reduction in NaCl excretion that occurs during short-term furosemide-induced volume depletion in rats. They concluded that stimulation of α_1 adrenoceptors on proximal tubules contributed to the compensatory response to short-term furosemide infusion. In humans, however, administration of prazosin in doses that block the pressor response to α-adrenergic agonists does not prevent postdiuretic NaCl retention. Even when both prazosin and captopril are administered concurrently, to block both the renin-angiotensin-aldosterone axis and the effects of renal nerve activity, postdiuretic NaCl retention may occur (although in this case, furosemide did reduce mean arterial pressure significantly, which may have contributed to the postdiuretic NaCl retention) (512). Thus, ECF volume dependent stimulation of α_1-adrenergic receptors, especially along the proximal tubule, may contribute to postdiuretic NaCl retention.

Diuretic-induced decrements in ECF volume have been shown to be associated with suppression of atrial natriuretic peptide secretion. These changes occur following diuretic administration in both normal individuals and in patients with nephrotic syndrome (228), chronic glomerulonephritis, and essential hypertension. In some studies, atrial natriuretic peptide concentrations declined before significant changes in extracellular or blood volume occur; in these cases, furosemide-induced changes in venous capacitance may underlie the effect.

The studies discussed in the preceding sections in which postdiuretic NaCl retention occurred despite blockade of several effector mechanisms raise the possibility that changes in ECF volume are not required for postdiuretic NaCl retention to occur. Wilcox and colleagues investigated acute effects of the loop diuretic bumetanide in the absence of extracellular fluid volume depletion. Na, K, Cl, and water were administered to volunteers during loop diuretic administration to balance electrolyte losses completely. When changes in ECF volume were prevented, postdiuretic NaCl retention did not occur, indicating that decrements in ECF volume do play a critical role in postdiuretic NaCl retention. A volume-independent component of adaptation *may also* contribute to NaCl retention, however. When volunteers were challenged with a 100-mmol NaCl load with or without prior diuretic treatment, differences were observed. The NaCl load was excreted fully within 2 days under control conditions; after pretreatment with bumetanide, however, much less of the administered load was excreted during the subsequent two days (4). This result occurred despite complete replacement of water and electrolyte losses induced by the loop diuretic. These results suggest that there are subtle but physiologically significant effects of diuretic administration even in the short term that favor NaCl retention in the absence of changes in ECF volume status (see following sections).

In healthy individuals, diuretic administration strongly activates the control systems discussed previously; in edematous individuals, however, one or more of these control systems may be active at baseline, having contributed to the pathological accumulation of extracellular volume. The role of these control systems in the adaptive response to diuretic may, therefore, be different in healthy and edematous individuals.

One mechanism by which diuretic drugs may increase the tendency for NaCl retention directly without changes in ECF volume involves diuretic-induced *activation* of ion transporters within the diuretic-sensitive nephron segment. The cation chloride cotransporters, such as the Na-K-2Cl cotransporter, are stimulated allosterically by low intracellular chloride concentrations (225); because loop diuretics reduce the Cl concentration in cells of the thick ascending limb, preexisting transporters should be activated, leading to increased NaCl transport capacity. This increase will be unmasked once the luminal concentration of loop diuretic declines. Ecelbarger et al. (137) reported evidence that furosemide administration activates Na-K-2Cl cotransport via more than one mechanism. Five days of furosemide infusion led to a 50% to 100% increase in expression of the Na-K-2Cl cotransporter protein, detected using a polyclonal antibody to the cloned protein, but this treatment also led to an apparent upward mobility shift of 9 kDa in apparent molecular mass. These results were interpreted as suggesting that furosemide blockade of apical NaCl uptake led to both increased expression and "modification" of the Na-K-2Cl cotransporter. As phosphorylation of the Na-K-2Cl cotransporter has been shown to regulate its activity, one possibility is that loop diuretic blockade of the Na-K-2Cl cotransporter activates the transporter via phosphorylation.

A similar mechanism has been reported to occur along the distal tubule during short-term administration of thiazide diuretics. Within 60 minutes of thiazide administration, the number of thiazide-sensitive Na-Cl cotransporters in kidney cortex (measured as the number of [^{3}H]metolazone binding sites) increases substantially (90). The techniques used to estimate the number of transporters in these experiments do not permit determination of whether the increased number reflects insertion of preexisting transporters from a subapical storage pool or activation of transporters that are present but inactive in the apical membrane. Immunocytochemical studies show that a subapical compartment contains thiazide-sensitive Na-Cl cotransporters in DCT cells of rats (371) suggesting that a shuttle system, similar to that proposed to mediate vasopressin induced water permeability in principle cells of the collecting duct, may regulate functional activity of the thiazide-sensitive Na-Cl cotransporter in the distal tubule. This pool has been shown to shuttle to and from the apical membrane in response to physiological perturbation (405). An increase in the number of activated ion transporters at the apical membrane would be expected to increase the transport capacity so that when diuretic concentrations decline, increased Na and Cl transport would result.

Another mechanism by which diuretic drugs may enhance the tendency to NaCl retention directly involves stimulation of transport pathways in nephron segments that lie *distal* to the target of diuretic action (segments that are insensitive to the diuretic drug). For example, the number of thiazide-sensitive Na-Cl transporters in the kidney (and presumably in the DCT) increases within 60 minutes after a loop diuretic has been administered (90). Because thiazide-sensitive transporters are expressed only by nephron segments that *do not* express loop diuretic sensitive pathways, the increased number of thiazide-sensitive Na-Cl cotransporters is believed to result from increases in salt and water delivery to DCT cells (discussed in more detail in the following paragraphs).

Postdiuretic NaCl retention can have major effects on the clinical efficacy of diuretic drugs. The half life of most loop diuretics is short, so that NaCl retention can occur during 18 hours per day, if the drug is administered once daily (Fig. 14). If dietary NaCl intake is low, postdiuretic NaCl retention does not compensate for the drug-induced NaCl losses and NaCl balance becomes negative (the desired therapeutic response). If, on the other hand, dietary NaCl intake is high, then postdiuretic NaCl retention *can* compensate entirely for the initial NaCl losses during the period of drug action. When dietary NaCl intake is high, therefore, salt balance may be neutral, even from the first day of diuretic therapy (43, 514), despite impressive increases in urine volume after each dose of diuretic. This is one reason that dietary NaCl intake is a key determinant of diuretic efficacy, especially for the short-acting loop diuretics.

Chronic Adaptations (The "Braking Phenomenon")

When diuretics reduce ECF volume effectively, NaCl balance gradually returns to neutral despite continued diuretic administration (Fig. 14) (142, 514). This "braking phenomenon" occurs when the magnitude of natriuresis following each diuretic dose declines. Several factors, acting in concert, may participate in chronic adaptation. A critical factor that is necessary for the braking phenomenon to occur is a decline in the ECF volume. Wilcox and coworkers showed that the magnitude of each diuretic-induced natriuresis declined during ECF volume depletion of humans consuming a low NaCl diet. In contrast, when dietary NaCl intake was high, ECF volume depletion did not occur, and the magnitude of diuretic-induced natriuresis did not decline (142, 514). Relative or absolute ECF volume contraction limits NaCl excretion by reducing the amount of NaCl that is filtered and by increasing the amount of NaCl that is reabsorbed. In experimental animals, declines in renal blood flow occur during chronic diuretic treatment. Declines in GFR are usually modest, however, unless volume depletion is extreme or renal perfusion is compromised by drugs or physical factors such as renal artery stenosis. The effects of diuretics on glomerular filtration and renal blood flow are not caused primarily by changes in mean arterial pressure, as the renal autoregulatory response tends to maintain GFR and renal blood flow relatively constant when arterial pressure changes. Instead, ECF volume contraction itself leads to decrements in renal blood flow and glomerular filtration rate; because renal blood flow declines proportionately more than glomerular filtration rate, ECF volume contraction increases the filtration fraction (GFR/RPF).

The role of the proximal tubule in diuretic adaptation has been documented clearly in rats treated chronically with thiazide diuretics and in animals and humans treated with loop diuretics. In the case of thiazide treatment, micropuncture studies showed that hydrochlorothiazide initially inhibited Na and Cl absorption along both the proximal tubule (by inhibiting CA) and the distal tubule (by inhibiting Na-Cl cotransport) of rats (498). After 7 to 10 days of treatment, however, ECF volume contraction led to increases in proximal solute reabsorption, thereby limiting delivery of Na and Cl to the distal sites of thiazide action. During the chronic phase of treatment, inhibition of NaCl transport along the distal nephron (the predominant site of thiazide action) counterbalanced the reduction in distal NaCl delivery; under these conditions, at steady state, urinary NaCl was equal to dietary NaCl intake (498). Loop diuretics such as furosemide have also been shown to inhibit Na and Cl absorption by the proximal tubule, although the mechanism is unclear. But as with DCT diuretics, chronic treatment with loop diuretics leads to ECF volume contraction and enhanced proximal NaCl reabsorption (448). The effects on proximal absorption require decrements in ECF volume was shown by comparing NaCl delivery out of the proximal tubule during furosemide administration with and without volume replacement. Only when the ECF volume was permitted to decline was proximal absorption stimulated (95).

Many of the same effector systems that participate in postdiuretic NaCl retention also may participate in chronic adaptations to diuretic drugs.

PHYSICAL FACTORS

A rise in filtration fraction increases the protein oncotic pressure in peritubular capillaries (more protein-free filtrate is formed per milliliter of blood flow thereby contracting the plasma volume around a constant amount of serum protein). The increased peritubular oncotic pressure increases solute and fluid reabsorption especially in the proximal tubule. ECF volume contraction also enhances proximal solute and fluid reabsorption by decreasing the renal interstitial pressure during chronic diuretic treatment.

SYMPATHETIC RENAL NERVE ACTIVITY

Efferent sympathetic nerves innervate the renal vasculature, the macula densa and essentially all segments of the nephron. Stimulation of sympathetic nerves reduces urinary NaCl excretion by reducing renal blood flow, by stimulating renin release at the macula densa, by stimulating tubule NaCl reabsorption along the nephron, and by interacting with hormonal modulators of NaCl transport (338, 339). Renal nerves may contribute to NaCl retention in edematous disorders, and renal nerve activity is stimulated when furosemide is administered either to normal or volume depleted animals (118). Yet experimental models of chronic diuretic administration have failed to substantiate a central role for renal nerve activity in adaptive processes. Chronic sympathectomy or blockade of α1 receptors inhibits the compensatory increase in proximal NaCl reabsorption that occurs during furosemide induced ECF volume depletion, but these maneuvers did not enhance the natriuretic response to furosemide (362). This indicates that the inhibition of proximal solute reabsorption that occurs secondary to adrenergic blockade is compensated by increased reabsorption distally. Use of systemic pharmacological sympathetic blockade to study the role of renal nerves in diuretic adaptation is limited because of drug-induced systemic hypotension, but Petersen and DiBona (360) showed that even anatomical renal denervation in normal rats does not abrogate the compensatory response to chronic furosemide administration. Although it seems clear that renal nerves do not play a critical role in mediating compensation to chronic diuretic use in normal humans and animals, the consistent observation that diuretics do stimulate renal nerve activity suggests that renal nervous activity may contribute to diuretic adaptation in some patients. In patients suffering from edematous disorders, distal Na reabsorption may already be stimulated; denervation in this situation might lead to significant impairment in adaptation to diuretic drugs.

RENIN-ANGIOTENSIN-ALDOSTERONE

A third factor participating in chronic adaptation to diuretic drugs is the renin-angiotensin-aldosterone system. Renin acts on angiotensinogen to generate angiotensin I, which is converted to angiotensin II by converting enzyme. Angiotensin II stimulates aldosterone secretion from the adrenal cortex; aldosterone stimulates salt reabsorption by the distal nephron. Studies indicate that, in addition to stimulating Na transport by ENaC of the collecting duct, as discussed previously, mineralocorticoid hormones stimulate Na transport by the thiazide-sensitive Na-Cl cotransporter of the DCT (26, 45, 89, 486). In addition, however, angiotensin II directly stimulates Na reabsorption along the proximal and distal tubules by stimulating Na–H exchange activity (499). Thus, diuretic drugs frequently result in stimulation of the renin-angiotensin-aldosterone system and the Na retention that occurs during diuretic treatment may result in part from this. As is the case with renal nerves, it has been difficult to show conclusively that the renin-angiotensin-aldosterone system plays a critical role in chronic adaptation to diuretic drugs. Yet as with renal nerves, the systemic effects of inhibition of the system, either with angiotensin I–converting enzyme inhibitor, angiotensin II receptor blockers, or competitive aldosterone blockers make it difficult to exclude a role for this hormonal system in the compensation to diuretic therapy.

EPITHELIAL HYPERTROPHY AND HYPERPLASIA

Other factors that can enhance renal NaCl reabsorptive capacity are structural and functional changes in the nephron itself. When a diuretic is administered, solute delivery to segments that lie distal to the site of diuretic action increases leading to load dependent increases in solute reabsorption, as discussed above (251). When solute delivery and solute reabsorption increase chronically, epithelial cells undergo hypertrophy and hyperplasia (Fig. 15). Infusion of furosemide into rats continuously for 7 days increased the percentage of renal cortical volume occupied by distal nephron cells. DCT cell volume increased by nearly 100%, with accompanying in-

creases in luminal membrane area per length of tubule, in basolateral membrane area per length of tubule, and in mitochondrial volume per cell (145, 237, 238). Chronic loop diuretic administration increases the Na,K-ATPase activity in the distal convoluted and cortical collecting tubules (Fig. 16) (410, 497), and increases the number of thiazide-sensitive Na-Cl cotransporters, measured as the maximal number of binding sites for [3H] metolazone (89, 342). In one study, chronic furosemide treatment increased expression of mRNA encoding the thiazide-sensitive Na-Cl cotransporter, as detected by in situ hybridization (Fig. 16) (342). In another study, however, mRNA expression of the thiazide-sensitive

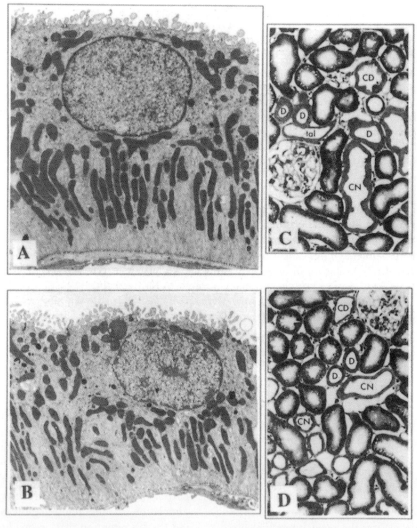

FIGURE 15   Effects of chronic loop diuretic administration on distal convoluted tubule cells of rats. Rats received furosemide continuously for 7 days. **A,B:** Electron micrographs (×10,000) of distal convoluted tubule cells from control and furosemide infused animals respectively. Note that furosemide increases the size of the cell, the size of the nucleus, the amount of mitochondrial volume, and the amount of basolateral membrane area. **C,D:** Photomicrographs of kidney cortices from control and furosemide infused animals respectively (×480). Note thickening of the epithelium in all distal segments. D, distal convoluted tubule; CN, connecting tubule; CD, cortical collecting duct; tal, thick ascending limb. (Photomicrographs are from Ellison DH, Velázquez H, Wright FS. Adaptation of the distal convoluted tubule of the rat: Structural and functional effects of dietary salt intake and chronic diuretic infusion. *J Clin Invest* 1989;83:113–126, with permission.)

A B

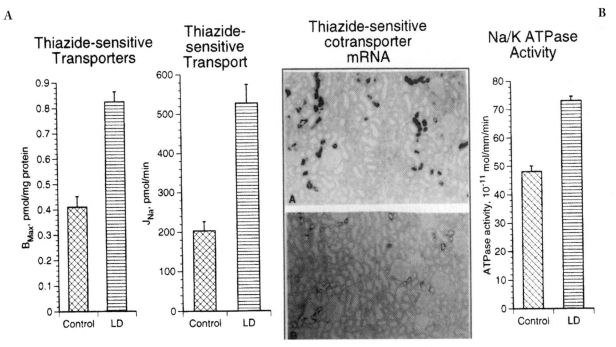

FIGURE 16 Effects of continuous loop diuretic infusion on rat kidney. Loop diuretic infusion increased the number of thiazide-sensitive Na-Cl cotransporters (90), the rate of thiazide-sensitive Na transport along the distal tubule (142), the abundance of thiazide-sensitive Na-Cl cotransporter mRNA (A: Furosemide-treated kidney cortex; B: Control kidney cortex; from Obermüller N, Bernstein PL, Velázquez H, Reilly R, Moser D, Ellison DH, Bachmann S. Expression of the thiazide-sensitive Na-Cl cotransporter in rat and human kidney. *Am J Physiol* 1995;269:F900–F910, with permission), and Na/K ATPase activity along the distal convoluted tubule. (From Scherzer P, Wald H, Popovtzer MM. Enhanced glomerular filtration and Na$^+$,K$^+$-ATPase with furosemide administration. *Am J Physiol* 1987;252:F910–F915, with permission.)

Na-Cl cotransporter, as well as ouabain-sensitive Na,K-ATPase, were not affected by chronic furosemide infusion, when detected by Northern analysis (324). Distal tubule cells that express high levels of transport proteins and are hypertrophic have a higher Na and Cl transport capacity than normal tubules. Compared with tubules from healthy animals, tubules of animals treated chronically with loop diuretics can absorb Na and Cl up to three times more rapidly than control animals, even when salt and water delivery are fixed by microperfusion (Fig. 16). When distal tubules are presented with high NaCl loads, as occurs during loop diuretic administration in vivo, Na and Cl absorption rates approach those commonly observed only in the proximal tubule (145). Chronic treatment of rats with loop diuretics also results in significant *hyperplasia* of cells along the distal nephron. Whereas mitoses of renal tubule epithelial cells are infrequent in adult kidneys, distal tubules from animals treated with furosemide chronically demonstrate prominent mitoses; increased synthesis of DNA in these cells was confirmed by showing increases in labeling of DCT cells with bromodeoxyurindine and proliferating cell nuclear antigen (288).

The diuretic-induced signals that initiate changes in distal nephron structure and function are poorly understood (251). Several factors, acting in concert, may contribute to these changes; these include diuretic induced increases in Na and Cl delivery to distal segments, effects of ECF volume depletion on systemic hormone secretion and renal nerve activity, and local effects of diuretics on autocrine and paracrine secretion. Increased production of angiotensin II or increased secretion of aldosterone resulting from increases in renin activity may contribute to hypertrophy and hyperplasia. Angiotensin is a potent mitogen; angiotensin II receptors have not been localized definitively to DCT cells but functional studies suggest that DCT cells express angiotensin II receptors (500). Beck et al. (20) showed that angiotensin I–converting enzyme inhibitors do not prevent loop diuretic-induced hypertrophy of DCT cells. Yet the hypertrophy during angiotensin I–converting enzyme inhibition is one that results from lengthening of kidney tubules; in their absence the hypertrophy results from thickening of the tubular cells.

Aldosterone also promotes growth of responsive tissues under some circumstances (239); when salt delivery to the collecting duct is increased in the presence of high levels of circulating aldosterone, principle cell hypertrophy develops; when salt delivery is high in the absence of aldosterone secretion, hypertrophy is absent. This indicates that aldosterone plays a permissive role in the development of cellular hypertrophy in this aldosterone responsive renal epithelium. Aldosterone does affect ion transport by cells of the DCT (45, 253, 482, 485), and aldosterone almost certainly contributes to adaptations along the cortical collecting tubule. Yet hypertrophy of DCT cells has been shown to occur during chronic loop diuretic infusion even when changes in circulating mineralocorticoid, glucocorticoid and vasopressin levels are prevented (238).

One intriguing hypothesis is that cellular ion concentrations regulate epithelial cell growth directly (445). Increases in Na uptake across the apical plasma membrane precede cell growth in the TAL during treatment with ADH (47), in principle cells of the CCT during treatment with mineralocorticoid hormones (236, 364), and in the DCT during treatment with loop diuretics (145, 239). Although the cause of the increased Na uptake varies, changes in the intracellular Na concentration appear to precede growth in each example. This hypothesis predicts that blockade of apical Na entry would lead to atrophy of epithelial cells. Chronic treatment of rats with DCT diuretics reduces activity of Na,K-ATPase and Na transport capacity of DCT segments (176, 327), but these experiments are complicated by other structural effects of chronic DCT diuretic treatment, discussed below. Regardless of the proximate stimulus for DCT cell growth, recent experiments have shown that immunoreactivity for insulin-like growth factor-1 (IGF-1) and for an IGF-binding protein (IGFBP-1) increases during chronic treatment of rats with loop diuretics (264). The changes in IGF-1 expression appeared not to result from changes in IGF-1 mRNA expression, but rather appeared to reflect posttranscriptional events. IGFBP-1 mRNA was increased by threefold 18 hours after loop diuretic treatment was initiated. IGF-1 has been shown to participate in regeneration of injured or ischemic renal tissue and promotes cell proliferation and differentiation in vitro. Whether these changes in IGF expression mediate the effects of diuretics on distal nephron structure remains to be established.

Morphological changes in the distal nephron during loop diuretic administration are not restricted to Na-reabsorbing cells. Chronic diuretic infusion stimulates selective hypertrophy of type B intercalated cells (254). Type B intercalated cells secrete bicarbonate and express apical Cl–HCO$_3$ exchangers and basolateral H-ATPase pumps; chronic bumetanide infusion increased the number of apical microvilli in type B cells, increased the basolateral cell membrane area and led to marked cytoplasmic and basolateral labeling for H-ATPase. Type A cells, which normally mediate acid secretion, were small; H-ATPase was distributed primarily within intracellular tubulovesicles in the tubules of treated animals. The authors concluded that the structural changes in intercalated cells resulted from increased distal chloride delivery because serum pH and electrolyte concentrations were not affected by the diuretic treatment. Increased distal chloride delivery might be expected to enhance Cl–HCO$_3$ exchange, increasing transepithelial solute transport, stimulating cell growth via mechanisms similar to those discussed previously.

Chronic diuretic administration has structural effects not only on nephron segments that lie distal to the site of diuretic action, but also on the nephron segments that are directly inhibited by the drugs themselves. Within hours of furosemide administration to rats, autophagocytic vacuoles develop in thick ascending limb cells (16). Following 7 days of furosemide treatment of rats, the cell height of thick ascending limb cells was significantly reduced (145). Chronic treatment of rabbits with loop diuretics decreased Na,K-ATPase activity in medullary thick ascending limb cells by approximately one third (197). These results are consistent with an effect of transepithelial ion transport to stimulate "work hypertrophy" and blockade of transepithelial transport to stimulate "disuse atrophy." When DCT diuretics are administered chronically, Na,K-ATPase activity in the DCT is reduced (176), and the capacity of DCT cells to reabsorb Na and Cl declines (327). Yet chronic administration of DCT diuretics, like genetic disruption of the thiazide-sensitive Na-Cl cotransporter (290), to rats leads to profound changes in cellular morphology; the DCT epithelium becomes disorders, DCT cells undergo apoptosis and necrosis, and interstitial fibrosis occurs (Fig. 17). Chronic treatment also leads to the disappearance of normal polarization of thiazide-sensitive Na-Cl cotransporter proteins. Under normal conditions, immunoreactivity for the thiazide-sensitive Na-Cl cotransporter is restricted to the apical membrane and to a small subapical pool of vesicles (Fig. 17B). During chronic treatment with DCT diuretics, the protein is distributed uniformly throughout the cell. Surprisingly, based on the severe morphological degenerative changes in tubular morphology, chronic thiazide administration results in an *increase* in the density of [³H]metolazone binding sites (functional thiazide-sensitive transporters) in kidney cortex (176) despite a decline in mRNA expression for the transporter (288). These results demonstrate that chronic thiazide administration regulates the thiazide-sensitive transporter in a complex way. Further studies are necessary to determine the mechanisms involved.

Although experimental data concerning structural and functional responses of the distal nephron to chronic treatment with diuretic drugs come predominantly from studies using experimental animals, Loon et al. (294) reported that chronic treatment with loop diuretics in humans enhanced ion transport rates in the distal tubule. They estimated the transport capacity of the DCT as the portion of Na and Cl reabsorption that could be inhibited by thiazide diuretics. When furosemide was administered to volunteers for 1 month, the enhancement in sodium excretion that occurred resulted from dose of a thiazide diuretic was significantly larger. Although these data are necessarily indirect, they are entirely consistent with the data derived from experimental animals given loop diuretics chronically. The ECF volume-independent component of NaCl retention that occurs following loop diuretic administration (4) may also reflect changes in distal nephron structure and function.

Acknowledgments

Work in the authors' laboratories has been supported by grants from the Department of Veterans Affairs (D.H.E.), and American Heart Association and the National Institutes of Health (D.H.E. and M.D.O.).

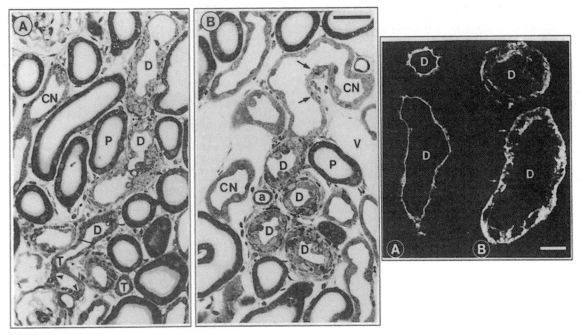

FIGURE 17   Effects of continuous distal convoluted tube (DCT) diuretic treatment on the structure of DCTs. **A,B:** Left side shows photomicrograph of kidney cortex from animals treated chronically with thiazide diuretics; note extreme hyperplasia and dysmorphology of distal segments (compare normal DCTs in Fig. 16). T, thick ascending limb; D, distal convoluted tubule; CN, connecting tubule; CD, collecting duct; P, proximal tubule; a, is arteriole. Double arrow indicates transition from thick ascending limb to distal convoluted tubule; note normal morphology of the thick ascending limb. Magnification ~ 360. **A,B:** Right side shows immunostaining for the thiazide-sensitive Na-Cl cotransporter from control rats **(A)** and rats infused with a thiazide continuously for 10 days **(B)**. Note that the normal apical localization of the transporter immunoreactivity **(A)** is distributed throughout the cytoplasm in animals exposed to diuretics chronically **(B)**. Magnification ~610, bar ~20 μm. (From Loffing J, Loffing-Cueni D, Hegyi I, Kaplan MR, Hebert SC, Le Hir M, Kaissling B. Thiazide treatment of rats provokes apoptosis in distal tubule cells. Kidney Int 1996;50:1180–1190, with permission.)

References

1. Ackerman DM, Hook, JB. Historical background, chemistry, and classification. In: Eknoyan G, Martinez-Maldonado M, eds. *The Physiological Basis of Diuretic Therapy in Clinical Medicine.* Orlando, FL: Grune & Stratton; 1986:1–25.

2. Agarwal R, Gorski JC, Sundblad K, Brater DC.Urinary protein binding does not affect response to furosemide in patients with nephrotic syndrome. *J Am Soc Nephrol* 2000;11:1100–1105.

3. Agostoni P, Marenzi G, Lauri G, Perego G, Schianni M, Sganzerla P, Guazzi MD. Sustained improvement in functional capacity after removal of body fluid with isolated ultrafilration in chronic cardiac insufficiency: Failure of furosemide to provide the same result. *Am J Med* 1994;96:191–199.

4. Almeshari K, Ahlstrom NG, Capraro FE, Wilcox CS. A volume-independent component to postdiuretic sodium retention in humans. *J Am Soc Nephrol* 1993;3:1878–1883.

5. Anderson P, Boreus L, Gordon E, Lagerkranser M, Rudehill A, Lindquist C, Ohman G. Use of mannitol during neurosurgery: interpatient variability in the plasma and CSF levels. *Eur J Clin Pharmacol* 1988;35:643–649.

6. Aperia AC. Tubular sodium rabsorption and the regulation of renal hemodynamics. The effect of chlorothiazide on renal vascular resistance. *Acta Physiol Scand* 1969;75:360–369.

7. Appel LJ. The verdict from ALLHAT: thiazide diuretics are the preferred initial therapy for hypertension. *JAMA* 2002;288:3039–3042.

8. Arieff AI. Dialysis disequilibrium syndrome: Current concepts on pathogenesis and prevention. *Kidney Int* 1994;45:629–620.

9. Arteaga MF, Canessa CM. Functional specificity of Sgk1 and Akt1 on ENaC activity. *Am J Physiol Renal Physiol* 2005;289:F90–96.

10. Asher C, Wald H, Rossier BC, Garty H. Aldosterone-induced increase in the abundance of Na channel subunits. *Am J Physiol Cell Physiol* 1996;271:C605–C611.

11. Ashraf N, Locksley R, Arieff A. Thiazide-induced hyponatremia associated with death or neurologic damage in outpatients. *Am J Med* 1981;70:1163–1168.

12. Aviram A, Pfau A, Czackes JW, Ullman TD. Hyperosmolality with hyponatremia caused by inappropriate administration of mannitol. *Am J Med* 1967;42:648–640.

13. Bachmann S, Bostanjoglo M, Schmitt R, Ellison DH. Sodium transport-related proteins in the mammalian distal nephrons: distribution, ontogeny and functional aspects. *Anat Embryol (Berl)* 1999;200:447–468.

14. Bachmann S, Velázquez H, Obermüller N, Reilly RF, Moser D, Ellison DH. Expression of the thiazide-sensitive Na-Cl cotransporter by rabbit distal convoluted tubule cells. *J Clin Invest* 1995;96:2510–2514.

15. Baer J, Jones C, Spitzer S, Russo H. The potassium sparing and natriuretic activity of N-amidino-3,4- diamino-6-chloropyrazinecarboxamide hydrochloride dihydrate (amiloride hydrochloride). *J Pharmacol Exp Ther* 1967;157:472–485.

16. Bahro M, Gertig G, Pfeifer U. Short-term stimulation of cellular autophagy by furosemide in the thick ascending limb of Henle's loop in the rat kidney. *Cell Tissue Res* 1988;253:625–629.

17. Bear R, Goldstein M, Phillipson M, Ho M, Hammeke M, Feldman R, Handelsman S, Halperin M. Effect of metabolic alkalosis on respiratory function in patients with chronic obstructive lung disease. *Can Med Assoc J* 1977;117:900–903.

18. Beaumont K, Vaughn DA, Fanestil DD. Thiazide diuretic drug receptors in rat kidney: Identification with [3H] Metolazone. *Proc Natl Acad Sci U S A* 1988;85:2311–2314.

19. Becchetti A, Malik B, Yue G, Duchatelle P, Al-Khalili O, Kleyman TR, Eaton DC. Phosphatase inhibitors increase the open probability of ENaC in A6 cells. *Am J Physiol Renal Physiol* 2002;283:F1030–1045.

20. Beck FX, Ohno A, Muller E, Seppi T, Pfaller W. Inhibition of angiotensin-converting enzyme modulates structural and functional adaptation to loop diuretic-induced diuresis. *Kidney Int* 1997;51:36–43.

21. Beck LH, Goldberg M. Effects of acetazolamide and parathyroidectomy on renal transprot of sodium, calcium and phosphate. *Am J Physiol* 1973;224:1136–1142.

22. Beck LH, Senesky D, Goldberg M. Sodium-independent active potassium reabsorption in proximal tubule of the dog. *J Clin Invest* 1973;52:2641–2645.

23. Bell PD, Lapointe JY, Sabirov R, Hayashi S, Peti-Peterdi J, Manabe K, Kovacs G, Okada Y. Macula densa cell signaling involves ATP release through a maxi anion channel. *Proc Natl Acad Sci U S A* 2003;100:4322–4327.

24. Benabe JE, Martinez-Maldonado M. Effects on divalent ion excretion. In: G Eknoyan and M. Martinez-Maldonado, eds. *The Physiological Basis of Diuretic Therapy in Clinical Medicine.* Orlando, FL: Grune & Stratton, Inc.;1986:109–124.

25. Berger S, Bleich M, Schmid W, Cole TJ, Peters J, Watanabe H, Kriz W, Warth R, Greger R, Schutz G. Mineralocorticoid receptor knockout mice: pathophysiology of Na metabolism. *Proc Natl Acad Sci U S A* 1998;95:9424–9429.

26. Bernstein PL, Velázquez H, Bartiss A, Reilly RF, Desir GV, Kunchaparty S, Ellison DH. Adrenal steroids stimulate thiazide-sensitive Na-Cl cotransport by rat distal tubules. *J Am Soc Nephrol* 1994. 282.

27. Berry CA, Rector FC, Jr. Renal transport of glucose, amino acids, sodium, chloride, and water. In: Brenner BM, Rector FC Jr, eds. *The Kidney.* Philadelphia: WB Saunders; 1991:245–282.

28. Berry CA, Ives HE, Rector FC, Jr. Renal transport of glucose, amino acids, sodium, chloride, and water. In: Brenner BM, Rector FC Jr, eds. *The Kidney.* Philadelphia: WB Saunders; 1996:334–370.

29. Beseghir K, Mosig D, Roch-Ramel F. Facilitation by serum albumin of renal tubular secretion of organic anions. *Am J Physiol* 1989;256:F475–F484.
30. Better OS, Rubinstein I, Winaver JM, Knochel JP. Mannitol therapy revisited (1940-1997). *Kidney Int* 1997;51:886–894.
31. Better OS, Stein JH. Early management of shock and prophylaxis of acute renal failure in traumatic rhabdomyolysis. *N Engl Med* 1990;322:825–829.
32. Beyer KH, Jr. Lessons from the discovery of modern diuretic therapy. *Perpect Biol Med* 1976;19:500–508.
33. Beyer KH, Jr. The mechanism of action of chlorothiazide. *Ann NY Acad Sci* 1958;71: 363–379.
34. Beyer KH, Jr, Baer J. The site and mode of action of some sulfonamide-derived diuretics. *Med Clin North Am* 1975;59.
35. Beyer KHJ. Discovery of the thiazides: where biology and chemistry meet. *Perspect Biol Med* 1977;20:410–420.
36. Bichet DG, Van Putten VJ, Schrier RW. Potential role of increased sympathetic activity in impaired sodium and water excretion in cirrhosis. *N Engl Med* 1982;307:1552–1557.
37. Biemesderfer D, Pizzonia J, Abu-Alfa A, Exner M, Reilly R, Igarashi P, Aronson PS. NHE3: A Na/H^+ exchanger isoform of the brush border. *Am J Physiol* 1993;265:F736–F742.
38. Bilezikian JP. Management of hypercalcemia. *J Clin Endocrin Metab* 1993;77:1445–1449.
39. Biner HL, Arpin-Bott MP, Loffing J, Wang X, Knepper M, Hebert SC, Kaissling B. Human cortical distal nephron: distribution of electrolyte and water transport pathways. *J Am Soc Nephrol* 2002;13:836–847.
40. Blantz RC. Effect of mannitol on glomerular ultrafiltration in the hydropenic rat. *J Clin Invest* 1974;54:1135–1143.
41. Blendis L, Wong F. Apr. Intravenous albumin with diuretics: protean lessons to be learnt? [editorial; comment]. *J Hepatol* 1999;30:727–730.
42. Bomsztyk K, George JP, Wright FS. Effects of luminal fluid anions on calcium transport by proximal tubule. *Am J Physiol* 1984;246:F600–F608.
43. Bosch JP, Goldstein MH, Levitt MF, Kahn T. Effect of chronic furosemide administration on hydrogen and sodium excretion in the dog. *Am J Physiol* 1977;232:F397–F404.
44. Bosher SK. The nature of ototoxicity actions of ethacrynic acid upon the mammalian endolymph system. I. Functional aspects. *Acta Otolaryngol* 1980;89:407–418.
45. Bostanjoglo M, Reeves WB, Reilly RF, Velázquez H, Robertson N, Litwack G, Morsing P, Dørup J, Bachmann S, Ellison DH. 11b-hydroxysteroid dehydrogenase, mineralocorticoid receptor and thiazide-sensitive Na-Cl cotransporter expression by distal tubules. *J Am Soc Nephrol* 1998;9:1347–1358.
46. Botero-Velez M, Curtis JJ, Warnock DG. Brief Report: Liddle's syndrome revisited-a disorder of sodium reabsorption in the distal tubule. *N Engl Med* 1994;174:178–8078.
47. Bouby N, Bankir L, Trinh-Trang-Tan MM, Minuth WW, Kriz W. Selective ADH-induced hypertrophy of the medullary thick ascending limb in Brattleboro rats. *Kidney Int* 1985;28:456–466.
48. Boulkroun S, Fay M, Zennaro MC, Escoubet B, Jaisser F, Blot-Chabaud M, Farman N, Courtois-Coutry N. Characterization of rat NDRG2 (N-Myc downstream regulated gene 2), a novel early mineralocorticoid-specific induced gene. *J Biol Chem* 2002;277: 31506–31515.
49. Bourdeau JE, Hellstrom-Stein RJ. Voltage-dependent calcium movement across the cortical collecting duct. *Am J Physiol* 1982; 242:F285–F292.
50. Bourland WA, Day DK, Williamson HE. The role of the kidney in the early nondiuretic action of furosemide to reduce elevated left atrial pressure in the hypervolemic dog. *J Pharmacol Exp Ther* 1977;202:221–229.
51. Boyd C, Naray-Fejes-Toth A. Gene regulation of ENaC subunits by serum- and glucocorticoid-inducible kinase-1. *Am J Physiol Renal Physiol* 2005;288:F505–512.
52. Branch RA, Roberts CJC, Homeida M, Levine D. Determinants of response to frusemide in normal subjects. *Br J Clin Pharmacol* 1977;4:121–127.
53. Brater DC, Chalasani N, Gorski JC, Horlander JCS, Craven R, Hoen H, Maya J. Effect of albumin-furosemide mixtures on response to furosemide in cirrhotic patients with ascites. *Trans Am Clin Climatol Assoc* 2001;112:108–115; discussion 116.
54. Brater DC. Diuretic pharmacokinetics and pharmacodynamics. In: Seldin DW, Gebisch G, eds. *Diuretic Agents: Clinical Physiology and Pharmacology*. San Diego: Academic Press;1997: 189-208.
55. Brater DC. Diuretic therapy. *N Engl Med* 1998;339:387–395.
56. Brater DC. Increase in diuretic effect of chlorothiazide by probenecid. *Clin Pharmacol Ther* 1978;23:259–265.
57. Breslau NA. Use of diuretics in disorders of calcium metabolism. In: Seldin DW, Gebisch G, eds. *Diuretic Agents: Clinical Physiology and Pharmacology*. San Diego: Academic Press;1997: 495–512.
58. Brown D, Hirsch S, Gluck S. An H^+-ATPase in opposite plasma membrane domains in kidney epithelial cell subpopulations. *Nature* 1988;331:622–624.
59. Brown D, Hirsch S, Gluck S. Localization of a proton-pumping ATPase in rat kidney. *J Clin Invest* 1988;82:2114–2126.
60. Brown JJ, Davies DL, Ferriss JB, Fraser R, Haywood E, Lever AF, JI. R. Comparison of surgery and prolonged spironolactone therapy in patients with hypertension, aldosterone excess, and low plasma renin. *B M J* 1972;2:729–720.
61. Brown R, Ollerstam A, Johansson B, Skott O, Gebre-Medhin S, Fredholm B, Persson AE. Abolished tubuloglomerular feedback and increased plasma renin in adenosine A1 receptor-deficient mice. *Am J Physiol Regul Integr Comp Physiol* 2001;281:R1362–1367.
62. Brown TC, Davis JO, Johnston CI. Acute response in plasma renin and aldosterone secretion to diuretics. *Am J Physiol* 1966;211:437–441.
63. Buckalew VM, Jr, Walker BR, Puschett JB, Goldberg M. Effects of increased sodium delivery on distal tubular sodium reabsorption with and without volume expansion in man. *J Clin Invest* 1970;49:2336–2344.
64. Buerkert J, Martin D, Prasad J, Trigg D. Role of deep nephrons and the terminal collecting duct in a mannitol-induced diuresis. *Am J Physiol* 1981;240:F411–F422.
65. Bull MB and Laragh JH. Amiloride. A potassium-sparing natriuretic agent. *Circulation* 1968;37:45–53.
66. Bundy JT, Connito D, Mahoney MD, Pontier PJ. Treatment of idiopathic renal magesium wasting with amiloride. *Am J Nephrol* 1995;15:75–77.
67. Burckhardt BC, Burckhardt G. Transport of organic anions across the basolateral membrane of proximal tubule cells. *Rev Physiol Biochem Pharmacol* 2003;146:95–158.
68. Burckhardt BC, Sato K, Frömter E. Electrophysiological analysis of bicarbonate permeation across the peritubular cell membrane of rat kidney proximal tubule. I. Basic observations. *Pflügers Arch* 1874;401:34–42.
69. Burg MB, Green N. Bicarbonate transport by isolated perfused rabbit proximal convoluted tubules. *Am J Physiol* 1977;233:F307–F314.
70. Burg MB, Green N. Effect of ethacrynic acid on the thick ascending limb of Henle's loop. *Kidney Int* 1973; 4:301–308.
71. Burg MB, Isaacson L, Grantham JJ, Orloff J. Electrical properties of isolated perfused rabbit renal tubules. *Am J Physiol* 1968;215:788–794.
72. Burg MB, Stoner L, Cardinal J, Green N. Furosemide effect on isolated perfused tubules. *Am J Physiol* 1973;225:119–124.
73. Burg MB. Tubular chloride transport and the mode of action of some diuretics. *Kidney Int* 1976;9:189–197.
74. Burke TJ, Marshall WH, Clapp JR, Robinson RR. Renal hemodynamic determinants of chlorothiazide effectiveness. *Clin Res* 1972;88.
75. Busch AE, Suessbrich H, Kunzelmann K, Hipper A, Greger R, Waldegger Mutschler E, Lindemann B, Lang F. Blockade of epithelial Na channels by triamterene-underlying mechanisms and molecular basis. *Pflügers Arch* 1996;432:760–766.
76. Campean V, Kricke J, Ellison D, Luft FC, Bachmann S. Localization of thiazide-sensitive Na(+)-Cl(-) cotransport and associated gene products in mouse DCT. *Am J Physiol Renal Physiol* 2001;281:F1028–1035.
77. Canessa CM, Horisberger J-D, Rossier BC. Epithelial sodium channel related to proteins involved in neurodegeneration. *Nature* 1993;361:467–470.
78. Canessa CM, Schild L, Buell G, Thorens B, Gatuschi I, Horisberger J-D, Rossier BC. Amiloride-sensitive epithelial Na channel is made of three homologous subunits. *Nature* 1994;367:463–467.
79. Cantarovich F, Rangoonwala B, Lorenz H, Verho M, Esnault VL. High-dose furosemide for established ARF: a prospective, randomized, double-blind, placebo-controlled, multicenter trial. *Am J Kidney Dis* 2004;44:402–409.
80. Carlsen JE, Kober L, Torp-Pedersen C, Johansen P. Relation between dose of bendrofluazide, antihypertensive effect, and adverse biochemical effects. *BMJ* 1990;300:975–978.
81. Carr MC, Prien EL, Jr, Babayan, RK. Triamterene nephrolithiasis: Renewed attention is warranted. *J Urol* 1990;144:1339–1340.
82. Casavola V, Guerra L, Reshkin SJ, Jacobson KA, Verrey F, Murer H. Effect of adenosine on Na and Cl curents in A6 monolayers. Receptor localization and messenger involvement. *J Membrane Biol* 1996;151:237–245.
83. Cassin S, Vogh B. Effect of Hydrochlorothiazide on renal blood flow and clearance of para-aminohippurate and creatinine. *Proc Soc Exp Biol Med* 1966;122:970–973.
84. Castrop H, Schweda F, Mizel D, Huang Y, Briggs J, Kurtz A, Schnermann J. Permissive role of nitric oxide in macula densa control of renin secretion. *Am J Physiol Renal Physiol* 2004;286: F848–857.
85. Cauley JA, Cummings SR, Seeley DG, Black D, Browner W, Kuller LH, Nevitt, MC. Effects of thiazide diuretic therapy on bone mass, fractures, and falls. *Ann Intern Med* 1993;118:666–673.
86. Cesar KR, Magaldi AJ. Thiazide induces water absorption in the inner medullary collecting duct of normal and Brattleboro rats. *Am J Physiol* 1999;277:F756–760.
87. Chang H, Fujita T. A kinetic model of the thiazide-sensitive Na-Cl cotransporter. *Am J Physiol* 1999;276.
88. Chen SY, Bhargava A, Mastroberardino L, Meijer OC, Wang J, Buse P, Firestone GL, Verrey F, Pearce D. Epithelial sodium channel regulated by aldosterone-induced protein sgk. *Proc Natl Acad Sci U S A* 1999;96:2514–2519.
89. Chen Z, Vaughn DA, Blakeley P, Fanestil DD. Adrenocortical steroids increase renal thiazide diuretic receptor density and response. *J Am Soc Nephrol* 1994;5:1361–1368.
90. Chen ZF, Vaughn DA, Beaumont K, Fanestil DD. Effects of diuretic treatment and of dietary sodium on renal binding of 3H-metolazone. *J Am Soc Nephrol* 1990;1:91–98.
91. Chennavasin P, Seiwell R, Brater DC, Liang WM. Pharmacodynamic analysis of the furosemide-probenecid interaction in man. *Kidney Int* 1979;16:187–195.
92. Chennavasin P, Seiwell R, Brater DC. Pharmacokinetic- dynamic analysis of the indomethacin-furosemide interaction in man. *J Pharmacol Exp Ther* 1980;215:77–81.
93. Chow KM, Kwan BC, Szeto CC. Clinical studies of thiazide-induced hyponatremia. *J Natl Med Assoc* 2004;96:1305–1308.
94. Chow KM, Szeto CC, Wong TY, Leung CB, Li PK. Risk factors for thiazide-induced hyponatraemia. *Qjm* 2003;96:911–917.
95. Christensen S, Steiness E, Christensen H. Tubular sites of furosemide natriuresis in volume-replaced and volume-depleted conscious rats. *J Pharmacol Exp Ther*1986; 239:211–218.
96. Cogan MG, Maddox DA, Warnock DG, Lin ET, Rector FC, Jr. Effect of acetazolamide on bicarbonate reabsorption in the proximal tubule of the rat. *Am J Physiol* 1979;237:F447–F454.
97. Conger JD. Interventions in clinical acute renal failure: What are the data? *Am J Kid Dis* 1995;26:565–576.
98. Coppage WS, Liddle GW. Mode of action and clinical usefulness of aldosterone antagonists. *Ann NY Acad Sci* 1960;88:815–810.
99. Cortney MA, Mylle M, Lassiter WE, Gottschalk CW. Renal tubular transport of water, solute, and PAH in rats loaded with isotonic saline. *Am J Physiol* 1965;1199:1205–1200.
100. Corvol P, Claire M, Oblin ME, Geering K, Rossier B. Mechanism of the antimineralocorticoid effects of spironolactones. *Kidney Int* 1981;20:1–6.
101. Costa MA, Loria A, Elesgaray R, Balaszczuk AM, Arranz C. Role of nitric oxide pathway in hypotensive and renal effects of furosemide during extracellular volume expansion. *J Hypertens* 2004;22:1561–1569.
102. Costanzo LS, Weiner IM. On the hypocalciuric action of chlorothiazide. *J Clin Invest* 1974;54:628–637.

103. Costanzo LS, Windhager EE. Calcium and sodium transport by the distal convoluted tubule of the rat. *Am J Physiol* 1978;235:F492–F506.
104. Costanzo LS. Comparison of calcium and sodium transport in early and late rat distal tubules: effect of amiloride. *Am J Physiol* 1984;246:F937–F945.
105. Costanzo LS. Localization of diuretic action in microperfused rat distal tubules: Ca and Na transport. *Am J Physiol* 1985;248:F527–F535.
106. Costello-Boerrigter LC, Boerrigter G, Burnett JC, Jr. Revisiting salt and water retention: new diuretics, aquaretics, and natriuretics. *Med Clin North Am* 2003;87:475–491.
107. Couette B, Lombes M, Baulieu E-E, Rafestin-Oblin M-E. Aldosterone antagonists destablilize the mineralocorticoid receptor. *Biochem J* 1992;282:697–702.
108. Dai LJ, Friedman PA, Quamme GA. Cellular mechanisms of chlorothiazide and potassium depletion on $Mg2^+$ uptake in mouse distal convoluted tubule cells. *Kidney Int* 1997;51:1008–1017.
109. Dai LJ, Friedman PA, Quamme GA. Mechanisms of amiloride stimulation of $Mg2^+$ uptake in immortalized mouse distal convoluted tubule cells. *Am J Physiol* 1997;F249:F256.
110. Dai LJ, Ritchie G, Kerstan D, Kang HS, Cole DE, Quamme GA. Magnesium transport in the renal distal convoluted tubule. *Physiol Rev* 2001;81:51–84.
111. de Gasparo M, Joss U, Ramjoue HP, Whitebread SE, Haenni H, Schenkel L, Kraehenbuehl C, Biollaz M, Grob J, Schmidlin J, et al. Three new epoxy-spirolactone derivatives: characterization in vivo and in vitro. *J Pharmacol Exp Ther* 1987;240:650–656.
112. Decaux G, Waterlot Y, Genette F, Mockel J. Treatment of the syndrome of inappropriate antidiuretic hormone with furosemide. *N Engl Med* 1981;304:329–330.
113. Delpire E, Lu J, England R, Dull C, Thorne T. Deafness and imbalance associated with inactivation of the secretory Na-K-2Cl co-transporter. *Nat Genet* 1999; 22:192–195.
114. Delyani JA. Mineralocorticoid receptor antagonists: the evolution of utility and pharmacology. *Kidney Int* 2000;57:1408–1411.
115. Demartini FE, Wheaton EA, Healy LA, Laragh JH. Effect of chlorothiazide on the renal excretion of uric acid. *Am J Med* 1962;32:572–577.
116. den Dekker E, Hoenderop JG, Nilius B, Bindels RJ. The epithelial calcium channels, TRPV5 & TRPV6: from identification towards regulation. *Cell Calcium* 2003;33:497–507.
117. di Stefano A, Greger R, Desfleurs E, De Rouffignac C, Wittner M. A Ba(2+)-insensitive K^+ conductance in the basolateral cell membrane of rabbit cortical thick ascending limb cells. *Cell Physiol Biochem* 1998;8:89–105.
118. DiBona GF, Sawin LL. Renal nerve activity in conscious rats during volume expansion and depletion. *Am J Physiol* 1985;248:F15–F23.
119. Dikshit K, Vyden JK, Forrester JS, Chatterjee K, Prakash R, Swan HJC. Renal and extrarenal hemodynamic effects of furosemide in congestive heart failure after acute myocardial infarction. *N Engl Med* 1973;288:1087–1090.
120. Dluhy RG, Wolf GL, Lauler DP. Vasodilator properties of ethacrynic acide in the perfused dog kidney. *Clin Sci* 1970;38:347–357.
121. Dobyan DC, Bulger RE. Renal carbonic anhydrase. *Am J Physiol* 1982;243:F311–F324.
122. Dorup I, Skajaa K, Thybo NK. Oral magnesium supplementation restores the concentrations of magnesium, potassium and sodium-potassium pumps in skeletal muscle of patients receiving diuretic treatment. *J Intern Med* 1993;233:117–123.
123. Dorup I. Magnesium and potassium deficiency. Its diagnosis, occurrence and treatment in diuretic therapy and its consequences for growth, protein synthesis and growth factors. *Acta Physiol Scand* 1994;150 (Suppl):7–55.
124. Douban S, Brodsky MA, Whang DD. Significance of magnesium in congestive heart failure. *Am Heart J* 1996;132:664–671.
125. Duarte CG, Bland JH. Calcium, phosphorous and uric acid clearances after intravenous administration of chorothiazide. *Metabolism* 1965;14:211–219.
126. Duarte CG, Chomety G, Giebisch G. Effect of amiloride, ouabain, and furosemide on distal tubular function in the rat. *Am J Physiol* 1971;221:632–639.
127. Duarte CG, Watson JF. Calcium reabsorption in proximal tubule of the dog nephron. *Am J Physiol* 1967;212:1355–1360.
128. DuBose TD, Lucci MS. Effect of carbonic anhydrase inhibition on superficial and deep nephron bicarbonate reabsorption inthe rat. *J Clin Invest* 1983;71:55–65.
129. DuBose TD, Jr., Pucacco LR, Carter NW. Determination of disequilibrium pH in the rat kidney in vivo. Evidence for hydrogen ion secretion. *Am J Physiol* 1981;240:F138–F146.
130. DuBose TD, Jr., Pucacco LR, Seldin DW, Carter NW, Kokko JP. Microelectrode determination of pH and PCO2 in rat proximal tubule after benzolamide: Evidence for hydrogen ion secretion. *Kidney Int* 1979;15:624–629.
131. Duc C, Farman N, Canessa CM, Bonvalet J-P, Rossier BC. Cell-specific expression of epithelial sodium channel a, b, and g subunits in aldosterone-responsive epithelia from the rat: Localization by in situ hybridization and immunocytochemistry. *J Cell Biol* 1994;127:1907–1921.
132. Dyckner T, Webster PO. Magnesium treatment of diuretic-induced hyponatremia with a preliminary report on a new aldosterone antagonist. *J Am Coll Nutr* 1982;1:149–153.
133. Dyckner T, Wester P-O, Widman L. Amiloride prevents thiazide-induced intracellular potassium and magnesium losses. *Acta Med Scand* 1988;224:25–30.
134. Dzau VJ, Hollenberg NK. Renal response to captopril in severe heart failure: role of furosemide in natriuresis and reversal of hyponatremia. *Ann Intern Med* 1984;100:777–782.
135. Earley LE, Friedler RM. Renal tubular effects of ethacrynic acid. *J Clin Invest* 1964;43:1495.
136. Earley LE, Orloff J. The mechanism of antidiuresis associated with the administration of hydrochlorothiazide to patients with vasopressin-resistant diabetes insipidus. *J Clin Invest* 1962;41:1988–1997.
137. Ecelbarger CA, Terris J, Hoyer JR, Nielsen S, Wade JB, Knepper MA. Localization and regulation of the rat renal Na-K^+-2Cl cotransporter, BSC-1. *Am J Physiol Renal Physiol* 1996;271:F619–F628.
138. Edwards BR, Baer PG, Sutton RAL, Dirks JH. Micropuncture study of diuretic effects on sodium and calcium reabsorption in the dog nephron. *J Clin Invest* 1973;52:2418–2427.
139. Eknoyan G, Sawa H, Hyde S, Wood JM, Schwartz A, Suki W. Effect of diuretics on oxidative phosphorylation of dog kidney mitochondria. *J Pharmacol Exp Ther* 1975;194:614–623.
140. Eknoyan G, Suki WN, Martinez-Maldonado M. Effect of diuretics on urinary excretion of phosphate, calcium, and magnesium in thyroparathyroidectomized dogs. *J Lab Clin Med* 1970;76:257–266.
141. Eknoyan G. A history of diuretics. In: Seldin DW, Gebisch G, eds. *Diuretic Agents: Clinical Physiology and Pharmacology*. San Diego: Academic Press; 1997:3–27.
142. Ellison DH, Velázquez H, Wright FS. Adaptation of the distal convoluted tubule of the rat: Structural and functional effects of dietary salt intake and chronic diuretic infusion. *J Clin Invest* 1989;83:113–126.
143. Ellison DH, Velázquez H, Wright FS. Thiazide sensitive sodium chloride cotransport in the early distal tubule. *Am J Physiol* 1987;253:F546–F554.
144. Ellison DH. Diuretic resistance: physiology and therapeutics. *Semin Nephrol* 1999;19:581–597.
145. Ellison DH. Divalent cation transport by the distal nephron: insights from Bartter's and Gitelman's syndromes. *Am J Physiol Renal Physiol* 2000;279:F616–625.
146. Elpers MJ, Selkurt EE. Effects of albumin infusion on renal function in the dog. *Am J Physiol* 1920;153:161–160.
147. England MD, Cavarocchi NC, O'Brien JF, Solis E, Pluth JR, Orszulak TA, Kaye MP, Schaff HV. Influence of antioxidants (mannitol and allopurinol) on oxygen free radical generation during and after cardiopulmonary bypass. *Circulation* 1986;74:134–137.
148. Eraly SA, Vallon V, Vaughn DA, Gangoiti JA, Richter K, Nagle M, Monte JC, Rieg T, Truong DM, Long JM, et al. Decreased renal organic anion secretion and plasma accumulation of endogenous organic anions in OAT1 knock-out mice. *J Biol Chem* 2006;281:5072–5083.
149. Ettinger B, Citron JT, Livermore B, Dolman LI. Chlorthalidone reduces calcium oxalate calculous recurrence but magnesium hydroxide does not. *J Urol* 1988;39:679–684.
150. Eveloff J, Swenson ER, Maren TH. Carbonic anhydrase activity of brush border and plasma membraens prepared from rat kidney cortex. *Biochemical Pharmacol* 1979;28:1434–1437.
151. Fairley KF, Woo KT, Birch DF, Leaker BR, Ratnaike S. Triamtrene-induced crystalluria and cylinduria: clinical and experimental studies. *Clin Nephrol* 1986;26:169–173.
152. Fanestil DD. Mechanism of action of aldosterone blockers. *Sem Nephrol* 1988;8:249–263.
153. Favre L, Glasson P, Vallotton MB. Reversible acute renal failure from combined triamterene and indomethacin: a study in healthy subjects. *Ann Intern Med* 1982;96:317–320.
154. Felson DT, Sloutskis D, Anderson JJ, Anthony JM, Kiel DP. Thiazide diuretics and the risk of hip fracture. Results from the Framingham study. *JAMA* 1991;265:370–373.
155. Fernandez PC, Puschett JB. Proximal tubular actions of metolazone and chlorothiazide. *Am J Physiol* 1973;225:954–961.
156. Fichman MP, Vorherr H, Kleeman CR, Telfer N. Diuretic-induced hyponatremia. *Ann Intern Med* 1971;75:853–863.
157. Firsov D, Gautschi I, Merillat AM, Rossier BC, Schild L. The heterotetrameric architecture of the epithelial sodium channel (ENaC). *EMBO J* 1998;17:344–352.
158. Flagella M, Clarke LL, Miller ML, Erway LC, Giannella RA, Andringa A, Gawenis LR, Kramer J, Duffy JJ, Doetschman T, et al. Mice lacking the basolateral Na-K-2Cl cotransporter have impaired epithelial chloride secretion and are profoundly deaf. *J Biol Chem* 1999;274:26946–26955.
159. Fliser D, Zurbruggen I, Mutschler E, Bischoff I, Nussberger J, Franek E, Ritz E. Coadministration of albumin and furosemide in patients with the nephrotic syndrome *Kidney Int* 1999;55:629–634.
160. Francis GS, Siegel RM, Goldsmith SR, Olivari MT, Levine B, Cohn JN. Acute vasoconstrictor response to intravenous furosemide in patients with chronic congestive heart failure. *Ann Intern Med* 1985;103:1–6.
161. Friedman E, Shadel M, Halkin H, Farfel Z. Thiazide-induced hyponatremia: Reproducibility by single dose rechallenge and an analysis of pathogenesis. *Ann Intern Med* 1989;110:24–30.
162. Friedman PA, Hebert SC. *Site and Mechanism of Diuretic Action*. San Diego: Academic Press, 1997:75–111.
163. Friedman PA. Basal and hormone-activated calcium absorption in mouse renal thick ascending limbs. *Am J Physiol* 1988;254:F62–F70.
164. Friedman PA. Calcium transport in the kidney. *Curr Opin Nephrol Hypertens* 1999;8:589–595.
165. Friedman PA. Codependence of renal calcium and sodium transport. *Annu Rev Physiol* 1998;60:179–197.
166. Frölich JC, Hollifield JW, Dormois JC, Frölich BL, Seyberth H, Michelakis AM, Oates JA. Suppression of plasma renin activity by indomethacin in man. *Circ Res* 1976;39: 447–452.
167. Fujii Y, Takemoto F, Katz AI. Early effects of aldosterone on Na-K pump in rat cortical collecting tubules. *Am J Physiol* 1990;259:F40–45.
168. Funder JW. The nongenomic actions of aldosterone. *Endocr Rev* 2005;26:313–321.
169. Gabow PA, Moore S, Schrier RW. Spironolactone-induced hyperchloremic acidosis in cirrhosis. *Ann Intern Med* 1979;90:338–340.
170. Gagnon E, Bergeron MJ, Brunet GM, Daigle ND, Simard CF, Isenring P. Molecular mechanisms of Cl transport by the renal $Na(^+)$-$K(^+)$-Cl cotransporter. Identification of an intracellular locus that may form part of a high affinity Cl(-)-binding site. *J Biol Chem* 2004;279:5648–5654.
171. Gamba G, Miyanoshita A, Lombardi M, Lytton J, Lee WS, Hediger MA, Hebert SC. Molecular cloning, primary structure, and characterization of two members of the mammalian electroneutral sodium-(potassium)-chloride cotransporter family expressed in kidney. *J Biol Chem* 1994;269:17713–17722.
172. Gamba G, Saltzberg SN, Lombardi M, Miyanoshita A, Lytton J, Hediger MA, Brenner BM, Hebert SC. Primary structure and functional expression of a cDNA encoding the thiazide-sensitive, electroneutral sodium-chloride cotransporter. *Proc Natl Acad Sci U S A* 1993;90: 2749–2753.
173. Ganguly A, Weinberger MH. Triamteren-thiazide combination:alternative therapy for primary aldosteronism. *Clin Pharmacol Ther* 1981;30:246–250.
174. Ganong WF, Mulrow PJ. Rate of change in sodium and potassium excretion after injection of aldosterone into the aorta and renal artery of the dog. *Am J Physiol* 1958;195:337–342.
175. Gardiner P, Schrode K, Quinlan D, Martin BK, Boreham DR, Rogers MS, Stubbs K, Smith M, Karim A. Spironolactone metabolism: steady-state serum levels of the sulfur-containing metabolites. *J Clin Pharmacol* 1989;29:342–347.
176. Garg LC, Narang N. Effects of hydrochlorothiazide on Na-K-ATPase activity along the rat nephron. *Kidney Int* 1987;31:918–922.

177. Garty H, Benos D. Characteristics and regulatory mechanisms of the amiloride-blockable Na channel. *Physiol Rev* 1988;68:309–373.
178. Garty H. Mechanisms of aldosterone action in tight epithelia. *J Membrane Biol* 1986;90: 193–205.
179. Garty H. Molecular properties of epithelial, amiloride-blockable Na channels. *FASEB J* 1994;8:522–528.
180. Gennari FJ, Kassirer JP. Oct 3. Osmotic diuresis. *N Engl J Med* 1974;291:714–720.
181. Gentilini P, Casini-Raggi V, Di Fiore G, Romanelli RG, Buzzelli G, Pinzani M, La Villa G, Laffi G. Albumin improves the response to diuretics in patients with cirrhosis and ascites: results of a randomized, controlled trial. *J Hepatol* 1999;30:639–645.
182. Giebisch G, Malnic G, DeMello GB, DeMello-Aires M. Kinetics of luminal acification in cortical tubules of the rat kidney. *J Physiol* 1977;267:571–599.
183. Giebisch G. Amiloride effects on distal nephron function. In: Straub RW, Bolis L, eds. *Cell Membrane Receptors for Drugs and Hormones: A Multidisciplinary Approach*. New York: Raven Press; 1978:337–342.
184. Gipstein RM, Boyle JD. Hypernatremia complicating prolonged mannitol diuresis. *N Engl Med* 1965;272:1116–v1110.
185. Goldberg AH, Lilienfield LS. Effects of hypertonic mannitol on renal vascular resistance. *Proc Soc Exp Biol Med* 1965;119:635-–642.
186. Goldberg M, Ramirez MA. Effects of saline and mannitol diuresis on the renal concentrating mechanism in dogs: alterations in renal tissue solutes and water. *Clin Sci* 1967;32:475–493.
187. Goldberg M. The renal physiology of diuretics. In: Orloff JJ, Berliner RW, eds. *Handbook of Physiology, Section 8, Renal Physiology*. Washington, DC: American Physiologic Society; 1973:1003–1031.
188. Goldsmith SR, Francis G, Cohn JN. Attenuation of the pressor response to intravenous furosemide by angiotensin converting enzyme inhibition in congestive heart failure. *Am J Cardiol* 1989;64:1382–1385.
189. Gong G, Lindberg J, Abrams J, Whitaker WR, Wade CE, Gouge S. Comparison of hypertonic saline solutions and dextran in dialysis-induced hypotension. *J Am Soc Nephrol* 1993;3:1808–1812.
190. Good DW, Wright FS. Luminal influences on potassium secretion: sodium concentration and fluid flow rate. *Am J Physiol* 1979;236:F192–F205.
191. Good DW. Sodium-dependent bicarbonate absorption by cortical thick ascending limb of rat kidney. *Am J Physiol* 1985;248:F821–F829.
192. Griffing GT, Cole AG, Aurecchia SA, Sindler BH, Komanicky P, Melby JC. Amiloride for primary hyperaldosteronism. *Clin Pharmacol Ther* 1982;31:56–61.
193. Grimm RH, Jr, Flack JM, Granditis, GA. Treatment of Mild Hypertension Study (TOMHS) Research Group. Long-term effects on plasma lipids of diet and drugs to treat hypertension. *JAMA* 1996;75:1549–1556.
194. Grino JM, Miravitlles R, Castelao AM. Flush solution with mannitol in the prevention of post-transplant renal failure. *Transplant Proc* 1987;19:4140–4142.
195. Grissom CK, Roach RC, Sarnquist FH, Hackett PH. Acetazolamide in the treatment of acute mountain sickenss: clinical efficacy and effect on gas. *Ann Intern Med* 1992;116: 461–465.
196. Gross JB, Kokko JP. Effects of aldosterone and potassium-sparing diuretics on electrical potential differences across the distal nephron. *J Clin Invest* 1977;59:82–89.
197. Grossman EB, Hebert SC. Modulation of Na-K-ATPase activity in the mouse medullary thick ascending limb of Henle: Effects of mineralocorticoids and sodium. *J Clin Invest* 1988;81:885–892.
198. Gründer S, Rossier BC. A reappraisal of aldosterone effects on kidney: new insights provided by epithelial sodium channel cloning. *Curr Opin Nephrol Hypertension* 1997;6:35–39.
199. Guignard JP, Peters G. Effects of triamterene and amiloride on urinary acidification and potassium excretion in the rat. *Eur J Pharmacol* 1970;110:255–267.
200. Haas M, McManus TJ. Bumetanide inhibits (Na $^+$ K $^+$ 2Cl) co-transport at a chloride site. *Am J Physiol* 1983;245:C235–C240.
201. Hantman D, Rossier B, Zohlman R, Schrier RW. Rapid correction of hyponatremia in the syndrom of inappropriate secretion of antidiuretic hormone: An alternative treatment to hypertonic saline. *Ann Intern Med* 1973;78:870–875.
202. Harding P, Sigmon DH, Alfie ME, Huang PL, Fishman MC, Beierwaltes WH, Carretero OA. Cyclooxygenase-2 mediates increased renal renin content induced by low-sodium diet. *Hypertension* 1997;29:297–302.
203. Harper R, Ennis CN, Heaney AP, Sheridan B, Gormley M, Atkinson AB, Johnston GD, Bell PM. A comparison of the effects of low- and conventional-dose thiazide diuretic on insulin action in hypertensive patients with NIDDM. *Diabetologia* 1995;38:853–859.
204. Harris RC, McKanna JA, Akai Y, Jacobson HR, Dubois RN, Breyer MD. Cyclooxygenase-2 is associated with the macula densa of rat kidney and increases with salt restriction. *J Clin Invest* 1994;94:2504–2510.
205. Harvey BJ, Higgins M. Nongenomic effects of aldosterone on $Ca2^+$ in M-1 cortical collecting duct cells. *Kidney Int* 2000;57:1395–1403.
206. Hebert SC, Reeves WB, Molony DA, Andreoli TE. The medullary thick limb: function and modulation of the single-effect multiplier. *Kidney Int* 1987;31:580–588.
207. Heidrich FE, Stergachis A, Gross KM. Diuretic drug use and the risk for hip fracture. *Ann Intern Med* 1991;115:1–6.
208. Helderman JH, Elahi D, Andersen DK, Raizes GS, Tobin JD, Shocken D, Andres R. Prevention of the glucose intolerance of thiazide diuretics by maintenance of body potassium. *Diabetes* 1983;32:106–111.
209. Helms MN, Yu L, Malik B, Kleinhenz DJ, Hart CM, Eaton DC. Role of SGK1 in nitric oxide inhibition of ENaC in Na-transporting epithelia. *Am J Physiol Cell Physiol* 2005;289: C717–726.
210. Heyman SN, Rosen S, Epstein FH, Spokes K, Brezis ML. Loop diuretics reduce hypoxic damage to proximal tubules of the isolated perfused rat kidney. *Kidney Int* 1994;45:981–985.
211. Hidaka H, Oshima T, Ikeda K, Furukawa M, Takasaka T. The Na-K-Cl cotransporters in the rat cochlea: RT-PCR and partial sequence analysis. *Biochem Biophys Res Comm* 1996;220: 425–430.
212. Ho K, Nichols CG, Lederer WJ, Lytton J, Vassilev PM, Kanazirska MV, Hebert SC. Cloning and expression of an inwardly rectifying ATP-regulated potassium channel. *Nature* 1993;362:31–38.
213. Holder LB, Hayes SL. Diffusion of sulfonamides in aqueous buffers and into red cells. *Mol Pharmacol* 1965;1:266–279.
214. Hollifield JW. Thiazide treatment of systemic hypertension: Effects on serum magnesium and ventricular ectopy. *Am J Cardiol* 1989;63:22G–25G.
215. Hook JB, Blatt AH, Brody MJ, Williamson HE. Effects of several saluretic-diuretic agents on renal hemodynamics. *J Pharmacol Exp Ther* 1966;154:667–673.
216. Hropot M, Fowler NB, Karlmark B, Giebisch G. Tubular action of diuretics: distal effects on electrolyte transport and acidification. *Kidney Int* 1985;28:477–489.
217. Hughey RP, Bruns JB, Kinlough CL, Harkleroad KL, Tong Q, Carattino MD, Johnson JP, Stockand JD, Kleyman TR. Epithelial sodium channels are activated by furin-dependent proteolysis. *J Biol Chem* 2004;279:18111–18114.
218. Hulter HN, Ilnicki LP, Harbottle JA, Sebastian A. Impaired renal H^+ secretion and NH3 production in mineralocorticoid-deficient glucocorticoid replete dogs. *Am J Physiol* 1977;232: F136–F146.
219. Ikeda K, Morizono T. Electrochemical profiles for monvalent ions in the stria vascularis: cellular model of ion transport mechanisms. *Hear Res* 1989;39:279–286.
220. Ikeda K, Oshima T, Hidaka H, Takasaka T. Molecular and clinical implications of loop diuretic ototoxicity. *Hear Res* 1997;107:1–8.
221. Imai M, Nakamura R. Function of distal convoluted and connecting tubules studied by isolated nephron fragments. *Kidney Int* 1982;22:465–472.
222. Inoue M, Okajima K, Itoh K, Ando Y, Watanabe N, Yasaka T, Nagase S, Morino Y. Mechanism of furosemide resistance in analbuminemic rats and hypoalbuminemic patients. *Kidney Int* 1987;32:198–203.
223. Isenring P, Forbush B. Ion transport and ligand binding by the Na-K-Cl cotransporter, structure-function studies. *Comp Biochem Physiol A Mol Integr Physiol* 2001;130:487–497.
224. Isenring P, Jacoby SC, Chang J, Forbush B. Mutagenic mapping of the Na-K-Cl cotransporter for domains involved in ion transport and bumetanide binding. *J Gen Physiol* 1998;112:549–558.
225. Isenring P, Jacoby SC, Payne JA, Forbush B, III. Comparison of Na-K-Cl cotransporters. *J Biol Chem* 1998;273:11295–11301.
226. Janjua NR, Jonassen TE, Langhoff S, Thomsen K, Christensen S. Role of sodium depletion in acute antidiuretic effect of bendroflumethiazide in rats with nephrogenic diabetes insipidus. *J Pharmacol Exp Ther* 2001;299:307–313.
227. Jenkins IR, Curtis AP. The combination of mannitol and albumin in the priming solution reduces positive intraoperative fluid balance during cardiopulmonary bypass. *Perfusion* 1995;10:301–305.
228. Jespersen B, Jensen L, Sorensen SS, Pedersen EB. Atrial natriuretic factor, cyclic 3',5'-guanosine monophosphate and prostaglandin E2 in liver cirrhosis: Relation to blood volume and changes in blood volume after furosemide. *Eur J Clin Invest* 1990;20:632–641.
229. Ji HL, Bishop LR, Anderson SJ, Fuller CM, Benos DJ. The role of Pre-H2 domains of alpha- and delta-epithelial Na channels in ion permeation, conductance, and amiloride sensitivity. *J Biol Chem* 2004;279:8428–8440.
230. Johnsen T. Effect upon serum insulin, glucose and potassium concentrations of acetazolamide during attacks of familial periodic hypokalemic paralysis. *Acta Neurol Scand* 1977;56:533–541.
231. Johnson RA, Freeman RH. Renin release in rats during blockade of nitric oxide synthesis. *Am J Physiol Regul Integr Comp Physiol* 1994;266:R1723–R1729.
232. Johnson T, Kass MA. Hematologic reactions to carbonic anhydrase inhibitors. *Am J Opthal* 1986;101:410–418.
233. Johnston GD, Nicholls DP, Leahey WJ. The dose-response characteristics of the acute non-diuretic peripheral vascular effects of frusemide in normal subjects. *Br J Clin Pharmacol* 1984;18:75–81.
234. Johnston PA, Bernard DB, Perrin NS, Levinsky NG. Prostaglandins mediate the vasodilatory effect of mannitol in the hypoperfused rat kidney. *J Clin Invest* 1981;68:127–133.
235. Kagawa CM. Blocking the renal electrolyte effects of mineralocorticoids with an orally active steroidal spirolactone. *Endocrinology* 1960;65:125–132.
236. Kaissling B, Stanton BA. Adaptation of distal tubule and collecting duct to increased sodium delivery. I. Ultrastructure. *Am J Physiol* 1988;255:F1256–F1268.
237. Kaissling B, Stanton BA. Structure-function correlation in electrolyte transporting epithelia. In: Seldin DW, Giebisch G, eds. *The Kidney: Physiology and Pathophysiology*. New York: Raven Press; 1992:779–801.
238. Kaissling B, Bachmann S, Kriz W. Structural adaptation of the distal convoluted tubule to prolonged furosemide treatment. *Am J Physiol* 1985;248:F374–F381.
239. Kaissling B. Structural adaptation to altered electrolyte metabolism by cortical distal segments. *Fed Proc* 1985;44:2710–2716.
240. Kamel KS, Oh MS, Halperin ML. Bartter's, Gitelman's, and Gordon's syndromes. From physiology to molecular biology and back, yet still some unanswered questions. *Nephron* 2002;92 Suppl 1:18–27.
241. Kaplan MR, Plotkin MD, Lee WS, Xu ZC, Lytton J, Hebert SC. Apical localization of the Na-K-Cl cotransporter, rBSC1, on rat thick ascending limbs. *Kidney Int* 1996;49:40–47.
242. Karim A. Spironolactone: disposition, metabolism, pharmacodynamics and bioavailability. *Drug Metab Rev* 1978;8:151–188.
243. Karniski LP, Aronson PS. Chloride/formate exchange with formic acid recycling: A mechanism of active chloride transport across epithelial membranes. *Proc Natl Acad Sci* 1985;82:6362–6365.
244. Kashlan OB, Sheng S, Kleyman TR. On the interaction between amiloride and its putative alpha-subunit epithelial Na channel binding site. *J Biol Chem* 2005 l280:26206–26215.
245. Kaufman AM, Levitt MF. The effect of diuretics on systemic and renal hemodynamics in patients with renal insufficiency. *Am J Kidney Dis* 1985;5:A71–A78.
246. Kellenberger S, Schild L. Epithelial sodium channel/degenerin family of ion channels: a variety of functions for a shared structure. *Physiol Rev* 2002;82:735–767.

247. Kellenberger S, Gautschi I, Schild L. Mutations in the epithelial Na channel ENaC outer pore disrupt amiloride block by increasing its dissociation rate. *Mol Pharmacol* 2003;64:848–856.
248. Kelly MR, Cutler RE, Forrey AW, Kimpel BM. Pharmacokinetics of orally administered furosemide. *Clin Pharmacol Ther* 1973;15:178–186.
249. Kelly RA, Wilcox CS, Mitch WE, Meyer TW, Souney PF, Rayment CM, Friedman PA, Swartz SL. Response of the kidney to furosemide, II: effect of captopril on sodium balance. *Kidney Int* 1983;24:233–239.
250. Khuri RN, Wiederholt M, Strieder N, Giebisch G. Effects of graded solute diuresis on renal tubular sodium transport in the rat. *Am J Physiol* 1975;228:1262–1268.
251. Kim GH, Lee JW, Oh YK, Chang HR, Joo KW, Na KY, Earm JH, Knepper MA, Han JS. Antidiuretic effect of hydrochlorothiazide in lithium-induced nephrogenic diabetes insipidus is associated with upregulation of aquaporin-2, Na-Cl co-transporter, and epithelial sodium channel. *J Am Soc Nephrol* 2004;15:2836–2843.
252. Kim GH, Masilamani S, Turner R, Mitchell C, Wade JB, Knepper MA. The thiazide-sensitive Na-Cl cotransporter is an aldosterone-induced protein. *Proc Natl Acad Sci U S A* 1998;95: 14552–14557.
253. Kim GH. Long-term adaptation of renal ion transporters to chronic diuretic treatment. *Am J Nephrol* 2004;24:595–605.
254. Kim J, Welch WJ, Cannon JK, Tisher CC, Madsen KM. Immunocytochemical response of type A and type B intercalated cells to increased sodium chloride delivery. *Am J Physiol Renal Fluid Electrolyte Physiol* 1992;262:F288–F302.
255. Kinne-Saffran E, Kinne R. Presence of bicarbonate stimulated ATPase in the brush border microvillus membranes of the proximal tubule. *Proc Soc Exp Biol Med* 1974;146:751–753.
256. Kinne-Saffran E, Beauwens R, Kinne R. An ATP-driven proton pump in brush-border membranes from rat renal cortex. *J Membrane Biol* 1982;64:67–76.
257. Kinsellar JL, Aronson PS. Properties of the Na-H^+ exchanger in renal microvillus membrane vesicles. *Am J Physiol* 1980;238:F461–F469.
258. Kirchner KA, Martin CJ, Bower JD. Prostaglandin E2 but not I2 restores furosemide response in indomethacin-treated rats. *Am J Physiol* 1986;250:F980–F985.
259. Kirchner KA, Voelker JR, Brater DC. Binding inhibitors restore furosemide potency in tubule fluid containing albumin. *Kidney Int* 1991;40:418–424.
260. Kirchner KA. Impairment of diuretic secretion. In: Seldin DW, Giebisch G, eds. *Diuretic Agents: Clinical Physiology and Pharmacology*. San Diego: Academic Press; 1997:259–270.
261. Kirchner KA. Prostaglandin inhibitors alter loop segment chloride uptake during furosemide diuresis. *Am J Physiol* 1985;248:F698–F704.
262. Kirchner, KA Voelker JR, Brater DC. Intratubular albumin blunts the response to furosemide-A mechanism for diuretic resistance in the nephrotic syndrome. *J Pharmacol Exp Ther* 1990;252:1097–1101.
263. Knepper MA, Good DW, Burg MB. Ammonia and bicarbonate transport by rat cortical collecting ducts perfused in vitro. *Am J Physiol* 1985;249:F870–F877.
264. Kobayashi S, Clemmons DR, Nogami H, Roy AK, Venkatachalam MA. Tubular hypertrophy due to work load induced by furosemide is associated with increses of IGF-1 and IGFBP-1. *Kidney Int* 1995;47:818–828.
265. Koeppen BM, Helman SI. Acidifcation of luminal fluid by the rabbit cortical collecting tubule perfused in vitro. *Am J Physiol* 1982;242:F521–F531.
266. Koeppen BM, Biagi BA, Giebisch G. Intracellular microelectrode charcterization of the rabbit cortical collecting duct. *Am J Physiol* 1983;244:F35–F47.
267. Komhoff M, Jeck ND, Seyberth HW, Grone HJ, Nusing RM, Breyer MD. Cyclooxygenase-2 expression is associated with the renal macula densa of patients with bartter-like syndrome. *Kidney Int* 2000;58:2420–2424.
268. Kone BC. Renal H,K-ATPase: structure, function and regulation. *Min Electrol Metab* 1996;22:349–365.
269. Koning OH, Ploeg RJ, van Bockel JH, Groenewegen M, van der Woude FJ, Persijn GG, Hermans J. Risk factors for delayed graft function in cadaveric kidney transplantion : a prospective study of renal function and graft survival after preservation with University of Wisconsin solution in multi-organ donors. European Multicenter Study Group. *Transplantation* 1963;63:1620–1628.
270. Kosari F, Sheng S, Li J, Mak DO, Foskett JK, Kleyman TR. Subunit stoichiometry of the epithelial sodium channel. *J Biol Chem* 1998;273:13469–13474.
271. Krick W, Wolff NA, Burckhardt G. Voltage-driven p-aminohippurate, chloride, and urate transport in porcine renal brush-border membrane vesicles. *Pflugers Arch* 2000;441: 125–132.
272. Kriz W, Kaissling B. Structural organization of the mammalian kidney. In: Seldin DW, Giebisch G, eds. *The Kidney: Physiology and Pathophysiology*. New York: Raven Press; 1992:779–802.
273. Kunau RT, Jr. The influence of carbonic anhydrase inhibitor, Benzolamide (Cl11,366), on the reabsorption of chloride, sodium, and bicarbonate in the proximal tubule of the rat. *J Clin Invest* 1972;51:294–306.
274. Kunau RT, Jr., Weller DR, Webb HL. Clarification of the site of action of chlorothiazide in the rat nephron. *J Clin Invest* 1975;56:401–407.
275. Kurtz A, Gotz KH, Hamann M, Wagner C. Stimulation of renin secretion by nitric oxide is mediated by phosphodiesterase 3. *Proc Natl Acad Sci U S A* 1998;95:4743–4747.
276. Kurtzman NA, White MG, Rogers PW. Aldosterone deficiency and renal bicarbonate reabsorption. *J Lab Clin Med* 1971;77:931–940.
277. Laerum E and Larsen S. Thiazide prophylaxis of urolithiasis. A double-blind study in general practice. *Acta Med Scand* 1984;215:383–389.
278. Laffi G, La Villa G, Carloni V, Foschi M, Bartoletti L, Quartini M, Gentilini P. Loop diuretic therapy in liver cirrhosis with ascites. *J Cardiovasc Pharmacol* 1993;22 (Suppl 3): S51–S58.
279. Lang F, Quehenberger P, Greger R, Oberleithner H. Effect of benzolamide on luminal pH in proximal convoluted tubules of the rat kidney. *Pflügers Arch* 1978;375:39–43.
280. Lang F. Osmotic diuresis. *Renal Physiol* 1987;59:173–170.
281. Lapointe J-Y, Laamarti A, Hurst AM, Fowler BC, Bell PD. Activation of Na:2Cl:K cotransport by luminal chloride in macula densa cells. *Kidney Int* 1995;47:752–757.
282. Lassiter WE, Gottschalk CW, Mylle M. Micropuncture study of net transtubular movement of water and urea in nondiuretic mammalian kidney. *Am J Physiol* 1961;200:1139–1146.
283. Leary WP, Reyes AJ. Renal excretory actions of diuretics in man: Correction of various current errors and redefinition of basic concepts. In: Reyes AJ, Leary WP, eds. *Clinical Pharmacology and Therapeutic Uses of Diuretics*. Stuttgart: Gustav Fischer Verlag; 1988:153–166.
284. Leblanc G. The mechanism of lithium accumulation in the isolated frog skin epithelium. *Pflügers Arch* 1972;337:1–18.
285. Li JH-Y, Cragoe EJ, Jr., Lindemann B. Structure-activity relationship of amiloride analogs as blockers of epithelial Na channels: II. Side-chain modifications. *J Membrane Biol* 1987;95:171–185.
286. Liddle GW. Aldosterone antagonists and triamterene. *Ann NY Acad Sci* 1966;134:466–460.
287. Liew D, Krum H. Aldosterone receptor antagonists for hypertension: what do they offer? *Drugs* 2003;63:1963–1972.
288. Loffing J, Le Hir M, Kaissling B. Modulation of salt transport rate affects DNA synthesis in vivo in rat renal tubules. *Kidney Int* 1995;47:1615–1623.
289. Loffing J, Loffing-Cueni D, Hegyi I, Kaplan MR, Hebert SC, Le Hir M, Kaissling B. Thiazide treatment of rats provokes apoptosis in distal tubule cells. *Kidney Int* 1996;50:1180–1190.
290. Loffing J, Vallon V, Loffing-Cueni D, Aregger F, Richter K, Pietri L, Bloch-Faure M, Hoenderop JG, Shull GE, Meneton P, et al. Altered renal distal tubule structure and renal Na(+) and Ca(2+) handling in a mouse model for Gitelman's syndrome. *J Am Soc Nephrol* 2004;15:2276–2288.
291. Loffing J, Zecevic M, Feraille E, Kaissling B, Asher C, Rossier BC, Firestone GL, Pearce D, Verrey F. Aldosterone induces rapid apical translocation of ENaC in early portion of renal collecting system: possible role of SGK. *Am J Physiol Renal Physiol* 2001;280:F675–682.
292. Lombard WE, Kokko JP, Jacobson HR. Bicarbonate transport in cortical and outer medullary collecting tubules. *Am J Physiol* 1983;244:F289–F296.
293. Lonnerholm G, Wistrand PJ. Membrane-bound carbonic anhydrase CA IV in the human kidney. *Acta Physiol Scand* 1991;141:231–234.
294. Loon NR, Wilcox CS, Unwin RJ. Mechanism of impaired natriuretic response to furosemide during prolonged therapy. *Kidney Int* 1989;36:682–689.
295. Lorenz JN, Schultheis PJ, Traynor T, Shull GE, Schnermann J. Micropuncture analysis of single-nephron function in NHE3-deficient mice. *Am J Physiol* 1999;277:F447–453.
296. Lucci MS, Pucacco LR, DuBose TD, Jr., Kokko JP, Carter NW. Direct evaluation of acidification by rat proximal tubule: role of carbonic anhydrase. *Am J Physiol* 1980;238:F372–F379.
297. Lucci MS, Tinker JP, Weiner I, DuBose TD, Jr. Function of proximal tubule carbonic anhydrase defined by selective inhibition. *Am J Physiol* 1983;245:F443–F449.
298. Lucci MS, Warnock DG, Rector FC, Jr. Carbonic anhydrase-dependent reabsorption in the rat proximal tubule. *Am J Physiol* 1979;236:F58–F65.
299. Lytle C, McManus TJ, Haas M. A model of Na-K-2Cl cotransport based on ordered ion binding and glide symmetry. *Am J Physiol* 1998;274:C299–C309.
300. Maher JF, Schreiner GF. Studies on ethacrynic acid in patients with refractory edema. *Ann Intern Med* 1965;62:15–29.
301. Makoff DL, DaSilva JA, Rosenbaum BJ. On the mechanism of hyperkalemia due to hyperosomotic expansion with saline or mannitol. *Clin Sci* 1971;41:383–380.
302. Malik B, Price SR, Mitch WE, Yue Q, Eaton DC. Regulation of epithelial sodium channels by the ubiquitin-proteasome proteolytic pathway. *Am J Physiol Renal Physiol* 2006;290: F1285–1294.
303. Malnic G, Klose RM, Giebisch G. Micropuncture study of distal tubular potassium and sodium transport in rat nephron. *Am J Physiol* 1966;211:529–547.
304. Malnic G, Mello Aires M, Giebisch G. Micropunture study of renal tubular hydrogen ion transport in the rat. *Am J Physiol* 1972;222:147–158.
305. Mann B, Hartner A, Jensen BL, Kammerl M, Kramer BK, Kurtz A. Furosemide stimulates macula densa cyclooxygenase-2 expression in rats. *Kidney Int* 2001;59:62–68.
306. Maren TH. Carbonic anhydrase inhibition. IV; The effects of metabolic acidosis on the response to Diamox. *Bull Johns Hopkins Hosp* 1956;98:159–183.
307. Maren TH. Carbonic anhydrase: Chemistry, physiology, and inhibition. *Pharmacol Rev* 1967;47:597–781.
308. Maren TH. Current status of membrane-bound carbonic anhydrase. 1980;341:246-258.
309. Maren TH. Relations between structure and biological activity of sulfonamides. *Annu Rev Pharmacol Toxicol* 1976;16:309–327.
310. Marenzi G, Lauri G, Grazi M, Assanelli E, Campodonico J, Agostoni P. Circulatory response to fluid overload removal by extracorporeal ultrafiltration in refractory congestive heart failure. *J Am Coll Cardiol* 2001;38:963–968.
311. Marik PE, Kussman BD, Lipman J, Kraus P. Acetazolamide in the treatment of metabolic alkalosis in critically ill patients. *Heart Lung* 1991;20:455–459.
312. Marver D, Stewart J, Funder JW, Feldman D, Edelman IS. Renal aldosterone receptors: Studies with [3H]adlosterone and the antimineralocorticoid [3H]spirolactone (SC26304). *Proc Natl Acad Sci U S A* 1974;71:1431–1435.
313. McGraw CP, Howard G. Effect of mannitol on increased intracranial pressure. *Neurosurgery* 1983;13:269–271.
314. McGuffin WL, Jr, Gunnells JC. Intravenously administered chlorothiazide in diagnostic evaluation of hypertensive disease. *Arch Intern Med* 1969;123:124–130.
315. McKinney TD, Burg M. Bicarbonate and fluid absorption by renal proximal straight tubule. *Kidney Int* 1977;12:1–8.
316. Mehta PK, Sodhi B, Arruda JAL, Kurtzman NA. Interaction of amiloride and lithium on distal urinary acidification. *J Lab Clin Med* 1979;93:983–993.
317. Merkus FWHM, Overdiek JWPM, Cilissen J, Zuidema J. Pharmacokinetics of spironolactone after a single dose: evaluation of the true canrenone serum concentrations during 24 hours. *Clin Exp Hypertens* 1983;5:249–269.
318. Miller PD, Berns AS. Acute metabolic alkalosis perpetuating hypercarbia: a role for acetazolamide in chronic obstructive pulmonary disease. *JAMA* 1977;238:2400–2401.
319. Miyanoshita A, Gamba G, Lytton J, Lombardi M, Brenner BM, Hebert SC. Primary structure and functional expression of the rat renal thiazide-sensitive Na:Cl cotransporter. *Proceedings of the 12th International Congress of Nephrology*. 1993;110.

320. Miyanoshita A, Terada M, Endou H. Furosemide directly stimulates prostaglandin E2 production in the thick ascending limb of Henle's loop. *J Pharmacol Exp Ther* 1989;251:1155–1159.
321. Mizuta K, Adachi M, Iwasa KH. Ultrastructural localization of the Na-K-Cl cotransporter in the lateral wall of the rabbit cochlear duct. *Hear Res* 1997;106:154–162.
322. Moe OW, Preisig PA, and Alpern AJ. Cellular model of proximal tubule NaCl and $NaHCO_3$ absorption. *Kidney Int* 1990;38:605-611.
323. Moreno E, San Cristobal P, Rivera M, Vazquez N, Bobadilla NA, Gamba G. Affinity defining domains in the Na-Cl cotransporter: different location for Cl and thiazide binding. *J Biol Chem* 2006;281:17266–17275.
324. Moreno G, Merino A, Mercado A, Herrera JP, Gonzalez-Salazar J, Correa-Rotter R, Hebert SC, Gamba G. Electroneutral Na-coupled cotransporter expression in the kidney during variations of NaCl and water metabolism. *Hypertension* 1998;31:1002–1006.
325. Moreno M, Murphy C, Goldsmith C. Increase in serum potassium resulting from the administration of hypertonic mannitol and other solutions. *J Lab Clin Med* 1969;73:291–290.
326. Morris CR, Alexander EA, Bruns FJ, Levinsky NG. Restoration and maintenance of glomerular filtration by mannitol during hypoperfusion of the kidney. *J Clin Invest* 1972;51:1555–1564.
327. Morsing P, Velázquez H, Wright FS, Ellison DH. Adaptation of distal convoluted tubule of rats, II: effects of chronic thiazide infusion. *Am J Physiol* 1991;261:F137–F143.
328. Moser M. Diuretics should continue to be one of the preferred initial therapies in the management of hypertension: the argument for. *J Clin Hypertens (Greenwich)* 2005;7:111–116; quiz 121–112.
329. Mukherjee SK, Katz MA, Michael UF, Ogden DA. Mechanisms of hemodynamic actions of furosemide: differentiation of vascular and renal effects on blood pressure in functionally anephric hypertensive patients. *Am Heart J* 1981;101:313–318.
330. Murer H, Hopfer U, Kinne R. Sodium/proton antiport in brush-border membrane vesicles isolated from rat small intestine and kidney. *Biochem J* 1976;154:597–604.
331. Murray MD, Deer MM, Ferguson JA, Dexter PR, Bennett SJ, Perkins SM, Smith FE, Lane KA, Adams LD, Tierney WM, et al. Open-label randomized trial of torsemide compared with furosemide therapy for patients with heart failure. *Am J Med* 2001;111:513–520.
332. Na KY, Han JS, Kim YS, Ahn C, Kim S, Lee JS, Bae KS, Jang IJ, Shin SG, Huh W, et al. Does albumin preinfusion potentiate diuretic action of furosemide in patients with nephrotic syndrome? *J Korean Med Sci* 2001;16:448–454.
333. Naray-Fejes-Toth A, Canessa C, Cleaveland ES, Aldrich G, Fejes-Toth G. sgk is an aldosterone-induced kinase in the renal collecting duct. Effects on epithelial Na channels. *J Biol Chem* 1999; 274:16973–16978.
334. Nashat FS, Scholefield FR, Tappin JW, Wilcox CS. The effect of acute changes in haematocrit in the anaesthetized dog on the volume and character of the urine. *J Physiol* 1969;205:305–316.
335. Nijenhuis T, Vallon V, van der Kemp AW, Loffing J, Hoenderop JG, Bindels RJ. Enhanced passive $Ca2^{+}$ reabsorption and reduced $Mg2^{+}$ channel abundance explains thiazide-induced hypocalciuria and hypomagnesemia. *J Clin Invest* 2005;115:1651–1658.
336. Nusing RM, Treude A, Weissenberger C, Jensen B, Bek M, Wagner C, Narumiya S, Seyberth HW. Dominant role of prostaglandin E2 EP4 receptor in furosemide-induced salt-losing tubulopathy: a model for hyperprostaglandin E syndrome/antenatal Bartter syndrome. *J Am Soc Nephrol* 2005;16:2354–2362.
337. Oates JA, Fitzgerald GA, Branch RA, Jackson EK, Knapp HR, Roberts LJ. Clinical implications of prostaglandin and thromboxane A2 formation (first of two parts). *N Engl Med* 1988;319:689–698.
338. Oates JA, Fitzgerald GA, Branch RA, Jackson EK, Roberts LJ. Clinical implications of prostaglandin and thromboxane A2 formation (second of two parts). *N Engl Med* 1988;319: 761–768.
339. Oberleithner H, Lang F, Messner G, Wang W. Mechanism of hydrogen ion transport in the diluting segment of frog kidney. *Pflügers Arch* 1984;402:272–280.
340. Oberleithner H, Weigt M, Westphale H-J, Wang W. Aldosterone activates Na/H^{+} exchange and raises cytoplasmic pH in target cells of the amphibian kidney. *Proc Natl Acad Sci U S A* 1987;84:1464–1468.
341. Obermüller N, Bernstein PL, Velázquez H, Reilly R, Moser D, Ellison DH, Bachmann S. Expression of the thiazide-sensitive Na-Cl cotransporter in rat and human kidney. *Am J Physiol* 1995;269:F900–F910.
342. Obermüller N, Kunchaparty S, Ellison DH, Bachmann S. Expression of the Na-K-2Cl cotransporter by macula densa and thick ascending limb cells of rat and rabbit nephron. *J Clin Invest* 1996;98:635–640.
343. Odvina CV, Mason RP, Pak CY. Prevention of thiazide-induced hypokalemia without magnesium depletion by potassium-magnesium-citrate. *Am J Ther* 2006;13:101–108.
344. Okusa MD, Bia MJ. Bartter's Syndrome. In *Endocrinology and Metabolism*. PP Foa and MP Cohen, editors. New York: Springer-Verlag. 231–263, 1987.
345. Okusa MD, Erik A, Persson G, Wright FS. Chlorothiazide effect on feedback-mediated control of glomerular filtration rate. *Am J Physiol* 1989;257:F137–F144.
346. Okusa MD, Unwin RJ, Velázquez H, Giebisch G, Wright FS. Active potassium absorption by the renal distal tubule. *Am J Physiol Renal Physiol* 1992;262:F488–F493.
347. Okusa MD, Velazquez H, Ellison DH, Wright FS. Luminal calcium regulates potassium transport by the renal distal tubule. *Am J Physiol* 1990;258:F423–428.
348. Okusa MD, Velazquez H, Wright FS. Effect of Na-channel blockers and lumen Ca on K secretion by rat renal distal tubule. *Am J Physiol* 1991;260:F459–465.
349. O'Neil RG, Sansom SC. Characterization of apical cell membrane Na and K^{+} conductances of cortical collecting duct using microelectrode techniques. *Am J Physiol* 1984;247:F14–F24.
350. Orlowski J, Kandasamy FA, Shull GE. Molecular cloning of putative members of the Na/H exchanger gene family. *J Biol Chem* 1992;267:9331–9339.
351. Packer M, Lee WH, Medina N, Yushak M, Kessler PD. Functional renal insufficiencey during long-term therapy with captopril and enalapril in severe congestive heart failure. *Ann Intern Med* 1987;106:346–354.
352. Packer M. Identification of risk factors predisposing to the development of functional renal insufficiency during treatment with converting-enzyme inhibitors in chronic heart failure. *Cardiology* 1989;76(Suppl 2):50–55.
353. Palm C, Pistrosch F, Herbrig K, Gross P. Vasopressin antagonists as aquaretic agents for the treatment of hyponatremia. *Am J Med* 2006;119:S87–92.
354. Palmer BF. Potassium disturbances associated with the use of diuretics. San Diego: Academic Press;1997:571–583.
355. Parfitt AM. Acetazolamide and sodium bicarbonate induced nehrocalcinosis and nephrolithiasis; relationship to citrate and calcium excretion. *Arch Intern Med* 1969;124:736–740.
356. Paulais M, Lachheb S, Teulon J. A Na- and Cl -activated K^{+} channel in the thick ascending limb of mouse kidney. *J Gen Physiol* 2006;127:205–215.
357. Perazella MA. Crystal-induced acute renal failure. *Am J Med* 1999;106:459–465.
358. Perez-Ayuso RM, Arroyo V, Planas R, Gaya J, Bory F, Rimola A, Rivera F, Rodes J. Randomized comparative study of efficacy of furosemide versus spironolactone in nonazotemic cirrhosis with ascites. Relationship between the diuretic response an the activity of the renin-aldosterone system. *Gastroenterology* 1983;84:961–968.
359. Persson AEG, Wright FS. Evidence for feedback mediated reduction of glomerular filtration rate during infusion of acetazolamide. *Acta Physiol Scand* 1982;114:1–7.
360. Petersen JS, DiBona GF. Effects of renal denervation on sodium balance and renal function during chronic furosemide administration in rats. *J Pharmacol Exp Ther* 1992;262:1103–1109.
361. Petersen JS, Shalmi M, Abildgaard U, Christensen S. Alpha-1 blockade inhibits compensatory sodium reabsorption in the proximal tubules during furosemide-induced volume contraction. *J Pharmacol Exp Ther* 1991;258:42–48.
362. Petersen JS, Shalmi M, Lam HR, Christensen S. Renal response to furosemide in conscious reats: Effects of acute instrumentation and peripheral sympathectomy. *J Pharmacol Exp Ther* 1991;258:1–7.
363. Peti-Peterdi J, Komlosi P, Fuson AL, Guan Y, Schneider A, Qi Z, Redha R, Rosivall L, Breyer MD, Bell PD. Luminal NaCl delivery regulates basolateral PGE2 release from macula densa cells. *J Clin Invest* 2003;112:76–82.
364. Petty KJ, Kokko JP, Marver D. Secondary effect of aldosterone on Na-K ATPase activity in the rabbit cortical collecting tubule. *J Clin Invest* 1981;68:1514–1521.
365. Pickkers P, Dormans TP, Russel FG, Hughest AD, Thien T, Schaper N, Smits P. Direct vascular effects of furosemide in humans. *Circulation* 1997;96:1847–1852.
366. Pickkers P, Schachter M, Hughes AD, Feher MD, Sever PS. Thiazide-induced hyperglycaemia: A role for calcium-activated potassium channels? *Diabetologia* 1996;39:861–864.
367. Pitt B, Remme W, Zannad F, Neaton J, Martinez F, Roniker B, Bittman R, Hurley S, Kleiman J, Gatlin M. Eplerenone, a selective aldosterone blocker, in patients with left ventricular dysfunction after myocardial infarction. *N Engl J Med* 2003;348:1309–1321.
368. Pitt B, Zannad F, Remme WJ, Cody R, Castaigne A, Perez A, Palensky J, Wittes J. The effect of spironolactone on morbidity and mortality in patients with severe heart failure. Randomized Aldactone Evaluation Study Investigators. *N Engl J Med* 1999;341:709–717.
369. Pitts RF, Alexander RS. The nature of renal tubular mechanism for acidifying the urine. *Am J Physiol* 1945;144:239–254.
370. Pizzonia JH, Gesek FA, Kennedy SM, Coutermarsh BA, Bacskai BJ, Friedman PA. Immunomagnetic separation, primary culture, and characterization of cortical thick ascending limb plus distal convoluted tubule cells from mouse kidney. *In Vitro Cell Dev Biol* 1991;27A:409–416.
371. Plotkin MD, Kaplan MR, Verlander JW, Lee W-S, Brown D, Poch E, Gullans SR, Hebert SC. Localization of the thiazide sensitive Na-Cl cotransporter, rTSC1, in the rat kidney. *Kidney Int* 1996;50:174–183.
372. Pluznick JL, Wei P, Grimm PR, Sansom SC. BK-{beta}1 subunit: immunolocalization in the mammalian connecting tubule and its role in the kaliuretic response to volume expansion. *Am J Physiol Renal Physiol* 2005;288:F846–854.
373. Popovtzer MM, Subryan VL, Alfrey AC, Reeve EB, Schier RW. The acute effect of chlorothiazide on serum-ionized calcium. Evidence for a parathyroid hormone-dependent mechanism. *J Clin Invest* 1975;55:1295–1302.
374. Porter RH, Cox BG, Heaney D, Hostetter TH, Stinebaugh BJ, Suki WN. Treatment of hypoparathyroide patients with chlorthalidone. *N Engl Med* 1978;298:577–581.
375. Pratt WB. The role of heat shock proteins in regulating the function, folding, and trafficking of the glucocorticoid receptor. *J Biol Chem* 1993;268:21455–21458.
376. Preisig PA, Toto RD, Alpern RJ. Carbonic anhydrase inhibitors. *Renal Physiol* 1987;10: 136–159.
377. Preminger GM, Pak CYC. Eventual attenuation of hypocalciuric response to hydrochlorothiazide in absorptive hypercalciuria. *J Urol* 1987;137:1104–1109.
378. Prescott LF, Balali-Mood M, Critchley JA, Johnstone AF, Proudfoot AT. Diuresis or urinary alkalinization for salicylate poisoning? *B M J* 1982;285:1383–1386.
379. Prince LS and Welsh MJ. Cell surface expression and biosynthesis of epithelial Na channels. *Biochem J* 1998;336 (Pt 3):705–710.
380. Puschett JB, Goldberg M. The acute effects of furosemide on acid and electrolyte excretion in man. *J Lab Clin Med* 1968;71:666–677.
381. Puschett JB, Rastegar A. Comparative study of the effects of metolazone and other diuetics on potassium excretion. *Clin Pharmacol Ther* 1973;15:397–405.
382. Puschett JB, Winaver J. Efects of diuretics on renal function. In: Windhager EE, ed. *Handbook of Physiology. Section 8: Renal Physiology*. New York: Oxford University Press; 1992:2335–2406.
383. Quamme GA. Renal magnesium handling: New insights in undertsanding old problems. *Kidney Int* 1997;52:1180–1195.
384. Quon DK, Worthen DM. Dose response of intravenous mannitol on the human eye. *Ann Opthalmol* 1981;13:1392–1393.
385. Ram CV, Garrett BN, Kaplan NM. Moderate sodium restriction and various diuretics in the treatment of hypertension. *Arch Intern Med* 1981;141:1015–1019.
386. Ray WA, Griffin MR, Downey W, Melton LJ, III. Long-term use of thiazide diuretics and risk of hip fracture. *Lancet* 1989;1:687–690.
387. Rector FC, Jr., Carter NW, Seldin DW. The mechanism of bicarbonate reabsorption in the proximal and distal tubules of the kidney. *J Clin Invest* 1965;44:278–290.
388. Reid IA, Chou L. Effect of blockade of nitric oxide synthesis on the renin secretory response to frusemide in concious rabbits. *Clin Sci* 1995;88:657–663.

389. Reid IR, Ames RW, Orr-Walker BJ, Clearwater JM, Horne AM, Evans MC, Murray MA, McNeil AR, Gamble GD. Hydrochlorothiazide reduces loss of cortical bone in normal postmenopausal women: a randomized controlled trial. *Am J Med* 2000;109:362–370.
390. Reilly RF, Ellison DH. Mammalian distal tubule: physiology, pathophysiology, and molecular anatomy. *Physiol Rev* 2000;80:277–313.
391. Reiss WG, Oles KS. Acetazolamide in the treatment of seizures. *Ann Pharmacother* 1996;30:514–519.
392. Rejnmark L, Vestergaard P, Pedersen AR, Heickendorff L, Andreasen F, Mosekilde L. Dose-effect relations of loop- and thiazide-diuretics on calcium homeostasis: a randomized, double-blinded Latin-square multiple cross-over study in postmenopausal osteopenic women. *Eur J Clin Invest* 2003;33:41–50.
393. Resnick JS, Engle WK, Griggs RC, Stam AC. Acetazolamide prophylaxis in hypokalemic periodic paralysis. *N Engl Med* 1968;278:582–586.
394. Richardson RMA, Kunau RT, Jr. Bicarbonate reabsorption in the papillary collecting duct: effect of acetazolamide. *Am J Physiol* 1982;243:F74–F80.
395. Risvanis J, Naitoh M, Johnston CI, Burrell LM. In vivo and in vitro characterisation of a nonpeptide vasopressin V(1A) and V(2) receptor antagonist (YM087) in the rat. *Eur J Pharmacol* 1999;381:23–30.
396. Rogerson FM, Brennan FE, Fuller PJ. Dissecting mineralocorticoid receptor structure and function. *J Steroid Biochem Mol Biol* 2003;85:389–396.
397. Rogerson FM, Brennan FE, Fuller PJ. Mineralocorticoid receptor binding, structure and function. *Mol Cell Endocrinol* 2004;217:203–212.
398. Rokaw MD, Benos DJ, Palevsky PM, Cunningham SA, West ME, Johnson JP. Regulation of a sodium channel-associated G-protein by aldosterone. *J Biol Chem* 1996;271:4491–4496.
399. Rose H, O'Malley K, Pruitt A. Depression of renal clearance of furosemide in man by azotemia. *Clin Pharmacol Ther* 1976;21:141–146.
400. Rose LI, Underwood RH, Newmark SR, Kisch ES, Williams GH. Pathophysiology of spironolactone-induced gynecomastia. *Ann Intern Med* 1977;87:398–403.
401. Rossier BC, Wilce PA, Edelman SI. Spironolactone antagonism of aldosterone action on Na transport andRNA metabolism in toad bladder epithelium. *J Membrane Biol* 1977;32:177–170.
402. Rouch AJ, Chen L, Troutman SL, Schafer JA. Na transport in isolated rat CCD: Effects of bradykinin, ANP, clonidine, and hydrochlorothiazide. *Am J Physiol Renal Fluid Electrolyte Physiol* 1991;260:F86–F95.
403. Rude RK. Physiology of magnesium metabolism and the important role of magnesium in potassium deficiency. *Am J Cardiol* 1989;63:31G–34G.
404. Rybak LP. Ototoxicity of loop diuretics. *Otolaryngol Clin Nortle Am* 1993;26:829–844.
405. Sandberg MB, Maunsbach AB, McDonough AA. Redistribution of distal tubule Na-Cl cotransporter (NCC) in response to a high-salt diet. *Am J Physiol Renal Physiol* 2006;291: F503–508.
406. Sanyal G, Pessah NI, Maren TH. Kinetics and inhibition of membrane-bound carbonic anhydrase from canine renal cortex. *Biochimica et Biophysica Acta* 1965;1981:128–137.
407. Sardet C, Franchi A, Pouysségur J. Molecular cloning, primary structure, and expression of the human growth factor-activatable Na/H^+ antiporter. *Cell* 1989;56:271–280.
408. Sasaki S, Marumo F. Effects of carbonic anhydrase inhibitors on basolateral base transport of rabbit proximal straight tubule. *Am J Physiol* 1989;257:F947–F952.
409. Scheinman SJ, Guay-Woodford LM, Thakker RV, Warnock DG. Mechanisms of Disease: Genetic Disorders of Renal Electrolyte Transport. *N Engl J Med* 1999;340:1177–1187.
410. Scherzer P, Wald H, Popovtzer MM. Enhanced glomerular filtration and $Na-K^+$-ATPase with furosemide administration. *Am J Physiol* 1987;252:F910–F915.
411. Schild L, Giebisch G, Karniski LP, Aronson PS. Effect of formate on volume reabsorption in the rabbit proximal tubule. *J Clin Invest* 1987;79:32–38.
412. Schild L, Schneeberger E, Gautschi I, Firsov D. Identification of amino acid residues in the a, b and g subunits of the epithelial sodium channel (ENaC) involved in amiloride block and ion permeation. *J Gen Physiol* 1997;109:15–26.
413. Schild L. The epithelial sodium channel: from molecule to disease. *Rev Physiol Biochem Pharmacol* 2004;151:93–107.
414. Schmieder RE, Messerli FH, deCarvalho JGR, Husserl FE. Immediate hemodynamic response to furosemide in patients undergoing chronic hemodialysis. *Am J Kidney Dis* 1987;9:55–59.
415. Schnermann J. Homer W Smith Award lecture. The juxtaglomerular apparatus: from anatomical peculiarity to physiological relevance. *J Am Soc Nephrol* 2003;14:1681–1694.
416. Schnermann J. Juxtaglomerular cell complex in the regulation of renal salt excretion. *Am J Physiol* 1998;274:R263–R279.
417. Schoofs MW, van der Klift M, Hofman A, de Laet CE, Herings RM, Stijnen T, Pols HA, Stricker BH. Thiazide diuretics and the risk for hip fracture. *Ann Intern Med* 2003;139: 476–482.
418. Schricker K, Hamann M, Kurtz A. Nitric oxide and prostaglandins are involved in the macula densa control of renin system. *Am J Physiol* 1995;269:F825–F830.
419. Schrier RW. New treatments for hyponatremia. *N Engl Med* 1978;298:214–215.
420. Schwartz WB. The effect of sulfanilamide on salt and water excretion in congestive heart failure. *N Engl Med* 1949;240:173–177.
421. Seely JF, Dirks JH. Micropuncture study of hypertonic mannitol diuresis in the proximal and distal tubule of the dog kidney. *J Clin Invest* 1969;48:2330–2339.
422. Seldin DW, Eknoyan G, Suki WN, Rector FC, Jr. Localization of diuretic action from the pattern of water and electrolyte excretion. *Ann NY Acad Sci* 1966;139:328–343.
423. Seldin DW, Giebisch G. Preface. In: Seldin DW, Giebisch G, eds. *Diuretic Agents: Clinical Physiology and Pharmacology*. San Diego: Academic Press;1997:xiii–xvii.
424. Serle JB. Pharmacological advances in the treatment of glaucoma. *Drugs Aging* 1994;5: 156–170.
425. Shackleton CR, Wong NLM, Sutton RA. Distal (potassium-sparing) diuretics. In: Dirks JH, Sutton RAL, eds. *Diuretics Physiology, Pharmacology and Clinical Use*. Philadelphia: WB Saunders; 1986:117–134.
426. Shankar SS, Brater DC. Loop diuretics: from the Na-K-2Cl transporter to clinical use. *Am J Physiol Renal Physiol* 2003;284:F11–21.
427. Shimizu T, Nakamura M, Yoshitomi K, Imai M. Interaction of trichlormethiazide or amiloride with PTH in stimulating $Ca2^+$ absorption in rabbit CNT. *Am J Physiol* 1991;261: F36–F43.
428. Shimizu T, Yoshitomi K, Nakamura M, Imai M. Site and mechanism of action of trichlormethiazide in rabbit distal nephron segments perfused in vitro. *J Clin Invest* 1988;82: 721–730.
429. Shoeman JF. Childhood pseudotumor cerebri: clinical and intracranial pressure response to acetazolamide and furosemide treatment in a case series. *J Child Neurol* 1994; 9:130–134.
430. Shore ET, Millman EP. Central sleep apnea and acetazolamide therapy. *Arch Intern Med* 1983;143:1278–1270.
431. Shuichi T, Schwartz GJ. HCO_3 absorption in rabbit outer medullary collecting duct: role of luminal carbonic anhydrase. *Am J Physiol* 1998;274:F139–F147.
432. Sica DA. Diuretics should continue to be one of the preferred initial therapies in the management of hypertension: the argument against. *J Clin Hypertens (Greenwich)* 2005;7:117–120; quiz 121–112.
433. Siegel D, Hulley SB, Black DM, Cheitlin MD, Sebastian A, Seeley DG, Hearst N, Fine R. Diuretics, serum and intracellular electrolyte levels, and ventricular arrhythmias in hypertensive men. *JAMA* 1992;267:1083–1089.
434. Simon DB, Lu Y, Choate KA, Velazquez H, Al-Sabban E, Praga M, Casari G, Bettinelli A, Colussi G, Rodriguez-Soriano J, et al. Paracellin-1, a renal tight junction protein required for paracellular $Mg2^+$ resorption [see comments]. *Science* 1999;285:103–106.
435. Simon DB, Nelson-Williams C, Bia MJ, Ellison D, Karet FE, Molina AM, Vaara I, Iwata F, Cushner HM, Koolen M, et al. Gitelman's variant of Bartter's syndrome, inherited hypokalemic alkalosis, is caused by mutations in the thiazide-sensitive Na-Cl cotransporter. *Nat Genet* 1996;12:24–30.
436. Sly WS, Whyte MP, Sundaram V, Tashian RE, Hewett-Emmett D, Guibaud P, Vainsel M, Baluarte HJ, Gruskin A, Al-Mosawi M, et al. Carbonic anhydrase II deficiency in 12 families with the autosomal recessive syndrome of osteopetrosis with renal tubular acidosis and cerebral calcification. *N Engl Med* 1985;313:139–145.
437. Smith WE, Steele TH. Avoiding diuretic related complications in older patients. *Geriatrics* 1983;38:117–119.
438. Snyder PM, Olson DR, Thomas BC. Serum and glucocorticoid-regulated kinase modulates Nedd4-2-mediated inhibition of the epithelial Na channel. *J Biol Chem* 2002;277:5–8.
439. Soleimani M, Aronson PS. Effects of acetazolamide on Na-HCO-3 cotransport in basolateral membrane vesicles isolated from rabbit renal cortex. *J Clin Invest* 1989;83:945–951.
440. Soleimani M, Aronson PS. Ionic mechanism of Na-HCO-3 cotransport in rabbit renal basolateral membrane vesicles. *J Biol Chem* 1989;264:18302–18308.
441. Solomon R, Werner C, Mann D, D'Elia J, Silva P. Effects of saline, mannitol, and furosemide on acute decreases in renal function induced by radiocontrast agents *N Engl Med* 1994;331:1416–1420.
442. Somogyi AA, Hovens CM, Muirhead MR, Bochner F. Renal tubular secretion of amiloride and its inhibition by cimetidine in humans and in an animal model. *Drug Metab Dispos* 1989;17:190–196.
443. Spindler B, Mastroberardino L, Custer M, Verrey F. Characterization of early aldosterone-induced RNAs identified in A6 kidney epithelia. *Pflugers Arch* 1997;434:323–331.
444. Stafstrom CE, Gilmore HE, Kurtin PS. Nephrocalcinosis complicating medical treatment of posthemorrhagic hydrocephalus. *Pediatr Neurol* 1992;8:179–182.
445. Stanton BA, Kaissling B. Regulation of renal ion transport and cell growth by sodium. *Am J Physiol* 1989;257:F1–F10.
446. Star RA, Burg MB, Knepper MA. Luminal disequilibrium pH and ammonia transport in outer medullary collecting duct. *Am J Physiol* 1987;29984:26980–28021.
447. Star RA. *Ototoxicity*. San Diego: Academic Press; 1997:637–642.
448. Stein JH, Osgood RW, Boonjarern S, Cox JW, Ferris TF. Segmental sodium reabsorption in rats with mild and severe volume depletion. *Am J Physiol* 1974;227:351–359.
449. Stinebaugh BJ, Bartow SA, Eknoyan G, Martinez-Maldonado M, Suki WN. Renal handling of bicarbonate: effect of mannitol diuresis. *Am J Physiol* 1971;220:1271–1274.
450. Stokes JB. Ion transport by the cortical and outer medullary collecting tubule. *Kidney Int* 1982;22:473–484.
451. Stokes JB. Sodium chloride absorption by the urinary bladder of the winter flounder: a thiazide-sensitive electrically neutral transport system. *J Clin Invest* 1984;74:7–16.
452. Stone DK, Seldin DW, Kokko JP, Jacobson HR. Mineralocorticoid modulation of rabbit medullary collecting duct acidification. *J Clin Invest* 1983;72:77–83.
453. Stoner LC, Burg MB, Orloff J. Ion transport in cortical collecting tubule; effect of amiloride. *Am J Physiol* 1974;227:453–459.
454. Stroupe KT, Forthofer MM, Brater DC, Murray MD. Healthcare costs of patients with heart failure treated with torasemide or furosemide. *Pharmacoeconomics* 2000;17(5):429–440.
455. Suki W, Rector FC, Jr., Seldin DW. The site of action of furosemide and other sulfonamide diuretics in the dog. *J Clin Invest* 1965;44:1458–1469.
456. Sun D, Samuelson LC, Yang T, Huang Y, Paliege A, Saunders T, Briggs J, Schnermann J. Mediation of tubuloglomerular feedback by adenosine: evidence from mice lacking adenosine 1 receptors. *Proc Natl Acad Sci U S A* 2001;98:9983–9988.
457. Sungaila I, Bartle WR, Walker SE, DeAngelis C, Uetrecht J, Pappas C, Vidins E. Spironolactone pharmacokinetics and pharmacodynamics in patients with cirrhotic ascites. *Gastroenterology* 1992;102:1680–1685.
458. Sutton JR, Houston CS, Mansell AL, McFadden MD, Hackett PM, Rigg JR, Powles AC. Effect of acetazolamide on hypoxemia during sleep at high altitude. *N Engl Med* 1979;301: 1329–1331.
459. Sweet DH, Bush KT, Nigam SK. The organic anion transporter family: from physiology to ontogeny and the clinic. *Am J Physiol Renal Physiol* 2001;281:F197–205.
460. Tahara A, Tomura Y, Wada KI, Kusayama T, Tsukada J, Takanashi M, Yatsu T, Uchida W, Tanaka A. Pharmacological profile of YM087, a novel potent nonpeptide vasopressin V1A and V2 receptor antagonist, in vitro and in vivo. *J Pharmacol Exp Ther* 1997;282:301–308.
461. Tannen RL. The effect of uncomplicated potassium depletion on urine acidification. *J Clin Invest* 1970;49:813–827.

462. Temes SP, Lilien OM, Chamberlain W. A direct vasoconstrictor effect of mannitol on the renal artery. *Surg Gynecol Obstet* 1975;141:223–226.

463. Terada Y, Knepper MA. Thiazide-sensitive NaCl absorption in rat cortical collecting duct. *Am J Physiol Renal Physiol* 1990;259:F519–F528.

464. Terada Y, Tomita K, Nonoguchi H, Yang T, Marumo F. Different localization and regulation of two types of vasopressin receptor messenger RNA in microdissected rat nephron segments using reverse transcription polymerase chain reaction. *J Clin Invest* 1993;92:2339–2345.

465. Thadhani R, Pascual M, Bonventre JV. Acute renal failure. *N Engl J Med* 1996;334:1448–1460.

466. Thomson S, Bao D, Deng A, Vallon V. Adenosine formed by 5′-nucleotidase mediates tubuloglomerular feedback. *J Clin Invest* 2000;106:289–298.

467. Thurau K. Renal hemodynamics. *Am J Med* 1964;36:698–719.

468. Tinker JP, Coulson R, Weiner IM. Dextran-bound inhibitors of carbonic anhydrase. *J Pharmacol Exp Ther* 1981;218:600–607.

469. Toto RA. Metabolic derangements associated with diuretic use: Insulin resistance, dyslipidemia, hyperuricemia, and anti-adronergic effects. In: Seldin DW, Giebisch G, eds. *Diuretic Agents: Clinical Physiology and Pharmacology*. San Diego: Academic Press; 1997:621–636.

470. Tran JM, Farrell MA, Fanestil DD. Effect of ions on binding of the thiazide-type diuretic metolazone to kidney membrane. *Am J Physiol* 1990;258:F908–F915.

471. Tse C-M, Brant SR, Walker S, Pouyssegur J, Donowitz M. Cloning and sequenceing of a rabbit cDNA encoding an intestinal and kidney-specific Na/H⁺ exchanger isoform (NHE-3). *J Biol Chem* 1992;267:9240–9346.

472. Tsuruoka S, Kittelberger AM, Schwartz GJ. Carbonic anhydrase II and IV mRNA in rabbit nephron segments: stimulation during metabolic acidosis. *Am J Physiol* 1998;274:F259–267.

473. Tucker BJ, Blantz RC. Studies on the mechanism of reduction in glomerular filtration rate after benzolamide. *Pflügers Arch* 1980;388:211–216.

474. Tucker BJ, Steiner RW, Gushwa L, Blantz RC. Studies on the tubuloglomerular feedback system in the rat: The mechanism of reduction in filtration rate with benzolamide. *J Clin Invest* 1978;62:993–1004.

475. Tumlin JA, Lea JP, Swanson CE, Smith CL, Edge SS, Someren JS. Aldosterone and dexamethasone stimulate calcineurin activity through a transcription-independent mechanism involving steroid receptor-associated heat shock proteins. *J Clin Invest* 1997;99:1217–1223.

476. Ullrich KJ, Papavassiliou. Bicarbonate reabsorption in the papillary collecting duct of rats. *Pflügers Arch* 1981;389:271–275.

477. Unwin R, Capasso G, Wilcox CS. Therapeutic Use of Diuretics. In: Brady HR, Wilcox CS, eds. *Therapy in Nephrology and Hypertension*. Philadelphia: WB Saunders; 1999:654–665.

478. Uwai Y, Saito H, Hashimoto Y, Inui KI. Interaction and transport of thiazide diuretics, loop diuretics, and acetazolamide via rat renal organic anion transporter rOAT1. *J Pharmacol Exp Ther* 2000;295:261–265.

479. Vallon V, Richter K, Huang DY, Rieg T, Schnermann J. Functional consequences at the single-nephron level of the lack of adenosine A1 receptors and tubuloglomerular feedback in mice. *Pflugers Arch* 2004;448:214–221.

480. Van Valenberg PLJ, Hoitsma AJ, Tiggeler RGWL. Mannitol as an indispensable constituent of an intraoperative hydation protocol for the prevention of acute renal failure after renal cadaveric transplantation. *Transplantation* 1987;784:788–1987.

481. Vandewalle A, Cluzeaud F, Bens M, Kieferle S, Steinmeyer K, Jentsch TJ. Localization and induction by dehydration of ClC-K chloride channels in the rat kidney. *Am J Physiol* 1997;272:F678–688.

482. Velázquez H, Greger R. Electrical properties of the early distal convoluted tubules of the rabbit kidney. *Renal Physiol* 1986;55.

483. Velázquez H, Wright FS. Control by drugs of renal potassium handling. *Ann Rev Pharmacol Toxicol* 1986;26:293–309.

484. Velázquez H, Wright FS. Effects of diuretic drugs on Na, Cl, and K transport by rat renal distal tubule. *Am J Physiol* 1986;250:F1013–F1023.

485. Velázquez H, Bartiss A, Bernstein PL, Ellison DH. Adrenal steroids stimulate thiazide-sensitive NaCl transport by the rat renal distal tubule. *Am J Physiol* 1996;270:F211–F219.

486. Velázquez H, Good DW, Wright FS. Mutual dependence of sodium and chloride absorption by renal distal tubule. *Am J Physiol* 1984;247:F904–F911.

487. Velázquez H, Naray-Fejes-Toth A, Reilly RF, Ellison DH. NaCl cotransporter and 11-b-hydroxysteroid dehydrogenase are coexpressed in rabbit distal convoluted tubule. *FASEB J* 1996;A368.

488. Velázquez H, Náray-Fejes-Tóth A, Silva T, Andújar E, Reilly RF, Desir GV, Ellison DH. The distal convoluted tubule of the rabbit coexpresses NaCl cotransporter and 11b-hydroxysteroid dehydrogenase. *Kidney Int* 1998;54:464–472.

489. Velázquez H, Wright FS, Good DW. Luminal influences on potassium secretion: chloride replacement with sulfate. *Am J Physiol* 1982;242:F46–F55.

490. Verrey F, Pearce D, Pfeiffer R, Spindler B, Mastroberardino L, Summa V, Zecevic M Pleiotropic action of aldosterone in epithelia mediated by transcription and post-transcription mechanisms. *Kidney Int* 2000;57:1277–1282.

491. Verrey F. Transcriptional control of sodium transport in tight epithelia by adrenal steroids. *J Membrane Biol* 1995;144:93–110.

492. Vieira FL, Malnic G. Hydrogen ion secretion by rat renal cortical tubule as studied by an antimony microelectrode. *Am J Physiol* 1968;214:710–718.

493. Visweswaran P, Massin EK, Dubose TDJ. Mannitol-induced acute renal failure. *J Am Soc Nephrol* 1997;8:1028–1033.

494. Voelker JR, Jameson DM, Brater DC. In vitro evidence that urine composition affects the fraction of active furosemide in the nephrotic syndrome. *J Pharmacol Exp Ther* 1989;250:772–778.

495. Voets T, Nilius B, Hoefs S, van der Kemp AW, Droogmans G, Bindels RJ, Hoenderop JG. TRPM6 forms the Mg²⁺ influx channel involved in intestinal and renal Mg²⁺ absorption. *J Biol Chem* 2004;279:19–25.

496. Vogl A. The discovery of the organic mercurial diuretics. *Am Heart J* 1950;39:881–883.

497. Wald H, Scherzer P, Popovtzer MM. Na,K-ATPase in isolated nephron segments in rats with experimental heart failure. *Circ Res* 1991;68:1051–1058.

498. Walter SJ, Shirley DG. The effect of chronic hydrochlorothiazide administration on renal function in the rat. *Clin Sci (Lond)* 1986;70:379–387.

499. Wang T, Giebisch G. Angiotensin II regulates bicarbonate and fluid transport in the early and late distal tubule in rat kidney. *J Am Soc Nephrol* 1994;673.

500. Wang T, Giebisch G. Effects of angiotensin II on electrolyte transport in the early and late distal tubule in rat kidney. *Am J Physiol Renal Fluid Electrolyte Physiol* 1996;271:F143–F149.

501. Warnock DG, Reenstra WW, Yee VJ. Na/H⁺ antiporter of brush border vesicles: studies with acridine orange uptake. *Am J Physiol* 1982;242:F733–F739.

502. Weinberg MS, Quigg RJ, Salant DJ, Bernard DB. Anuric renal failure precipitated by indomethacin and triamterene. *Nephron* 1985;40:216–218.

503. Weiner IM. Diuretics and other agents employed in the mobilization of edema fluid. In: Gilman AG, Rall TW, Nies AS, Taylor AS, eds. *The Pharmacological Basis of Therapeutics*. New York: Pergamon Press;1990:713–742.

504. Weinstein AM. A mathematical model of rat distal convoluted tubule, II: potassium secretion along the connecting segment. *Am J Physiol Renal Physiol* 2005;289:F699–720.

505. Weisberg LS, Kurnick PB, Kurnik BR. Risk of radiocontrast in patients with and without diabetes mellitus. *Kidney Int* 1994; 45:259–250.

506. Werblin TP, Pollack IP, Liss RA. Blood dyscrasias in patients suing methazolamide (Neptazane) for glaucoma. *Opthalmology* 1980;87:350–354.

507. Wesson LG, Jr., Anslow WP. Excretion of sodium and water during osmotic diuresis in the dog. *Am J Physiol* 1948;153:465–474.

508. Wesson LG. Magnesium, calcium and phosphate excretion during osmotic diuresis in the dog. *J Lab Clin Med* 1967;60:422–432.

509. Whitling AM, Pergola PE, Sang JL, Talbert RL. Spironolactone-induced agranulocytosis. *Ann Pharmacother* 1997;31:582–585.

510. Widmer P, Maibach R, Kunzi UP, Capaul R, Mueller U, Galeazzi R, Hoigne R. Diuretic-related hypokalaemia: the role of diuretics, potassium supplements, glucocorticoids and beta 2-adrenoceptor agonists. Results from the comprehensive hospital drug monitoring programme, berne (CHDM). *Eur J Clin Pharmacol* 1995;49:31–36.

511. Wiebelhaus VD, Weinstock J, Maass AR, Brennan FT, Sosnowski G, Larsen T. The diuretic and natruretic activity of triamterene and several related pteridnes in the rat. *J Pharmacol Exp Ther* 1965;149:397–403.

512. Wilcox CS, Guzman NJ, Mitch WE, Kelly RA, Maroni BJ, Souney PF, Rayment CM, Braun L, Colucci R, Loon NR. Na,K⁺ and BP homeostasis in man during furosemide: Effects of prozosin and captopril. *Kidney Int* 1987;31:135–141.

513. Wilcox CS, Mitch WE, Kelly RA, Freidman PA, Souney PF, et al. Factors affecting potassium balance during frusemide administration. *Clin Sci* 1984;67:195–203.

514. Wilcox CS, Mitch WE, Kelly RA, Skorecki K, Meyer TW, Friedman PA, Souney PF. Response of the kidney to furosemide, I: effects of salt intake and renal compensation. *J Lab Clin Med* 1983;102:450–458.

515. Wilson DR, Honrath U, Sonnenberg H. Thiazide diuretic effect on medullary collecting duct function in the rat. *Kidney Int* 1983;23:711–716.

516. Windhager EE, Whittembury G, Oken DE, Schatzmann HJ, Solomon AK. Single proximal tubules of the necturus kidney, III: dependence of H2O movement on NaCl concentration. *Am J Physiol* 1959;197:313–318.

517. Wingo CS, Straub SG. Active proton secretion and potassium absorption in the rabbit outer medullary collecting duct. Functional evidence for proton-potassium-activated adenosine triphosphatase. *J Clin Invest* 1989;84:361–365.

518. Wistrand PJ and Kinne R. Carbonic anhydrase activity of isolated brush border and basal-lateral membranes of renal tubular cells. *Pflügers Arch* 1977;370:121–126.

519. Wistrand PJ, Wahlstrand T. Rat renal and erythrocyte carbonic anhydrases: Purification and properties. *Biochimica et Biophysica Acta* 1977;481:712–721.

520. Wong NLM, Quamme GA, Sutton RAL, Dirks JH. Effects of mannitol on water and electrolyte transport in dog kidney. *J Lab Clin Med* 1979;94:683–692.

521. Wright FS, Schnermann J. Interference with feedback control of glomerular filtration rate by furosemide, triflocin, and cyanide. *J Clin Invest* 1974;53:1695–1708.

522. Wright FS. Flow-dependent transport processes: filtartion, absorption, secretion. *Am J Physiol* 1982;243:F1–F11.

523. Xu J-C, Lytle C, Zhu T, Payne JA, Benz E, Jr., Forbush B, III. Molecular cloning and functional expression of the bumetanide-sensitive Na-K-Cl cotransporter. *Proc Natl Acad Sci U S A* 1994;92:2201–2205.

524. Yamasaki Y, Nishiuchi T, Kojima A, Saito H, Saito S. Effects of an oral water load and intravenous administration of isotonic glucose, hypertonic saline, mannitol and furosemide on the release of atrial natriuretic peptide in men. *Acta Endocrinol (Copenh)* 1988;119:269–278.

525. Yang TX, Huang YNG, Singh I, Schnermann J, Briggs JP. Localization of bumetanide- and thiazide-sensitive Na-K-Cl cotransporters along the rat nephron. *Am J Physiol Renal Physiol* 1996;271:F931–F939.

526. Yendt ER, Cohanim M. Prevention of calcium stones with thiazides. *Kidney Int* 1978;13:397–409.

527. Zhou R, Snyder PM. Nedd4-2 phosphorylation induces serum and glucocorticoid-regulated kinase (SGK) ubiquitination and degradation. *J Biol Chem* 2005;280:4518–4523.

CHAPTER **38**

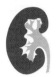

Aquaporin Water Channels in Mammalian Kidney

Søren Nielsen, Tae-Hwan Kwon,* Henrik Dimke, and Jørgen Frøkiær[†]

University of Aarhus, Aarhus, Denmark
*Kyungpook National University, Taegu, Korea
[†]Aarhus University Hospital-Skejby, Aarhus, Denmark

Water is the most abundant component of all cells, and the ability to absorb and release water is considered a fundamental process of life. Plasma membranes serve as selective barriers that control the solute composition of the cell and regulate the entry of ions, small uncharged solutes, and water. Epithelial tissues have apical and basolateral plasma membranes that constitute serial barriers that regulate the transepithelial movement of solutes and water, thereby contributing to the homeostasis of multicellular organisms. Identification and characterization of the molecular entities responsible for the function of biologic membranes have been longstanding goals of physiologists; however, the molecular identity of water transporters remained unknown until less than two decades ago.

Because water can slowly diffuse through lipid bilayers, all biologic membranes exhibit some degree of water permeability. Nevertheless, observations made in multiple laboratories indicated that specialized membrane water-transport molecules must exist in tissues with distinctively high water permeability (see review [69]). For example, the water permeability of red cell membranes is higher than that of many other cell types or artificial lipid bilayers, and the activation energy of this process is equivalent to the diffusion of water in solution, E_a <5 kcal/mol (264). In addition, reversible inhibition by $HgCl_2$ and a subset of organomercurials suggested that the water transporter is a membrane protein (see review [177]). Further evidence that a membrane protein is involved in water transport was provided by the observation that some epithelial tissues exhibit changes in water permeability on a time scale that is not compatible with changes in lipid composition.

Kidneys are the major determinant of body water and electrolyte composition. Thus comprehending the mechanisms of water transport is essential to understanding mammalian kidney physiology and water balance. Because of its importance to human health, water permeability has been particularly well characterized in the mammalian kidney (see review [141]). Approximately, 180 l/day of glomerular filtrate is generated in an average adult human, most of this is reabsorbed by the highly water permeable proximal tubules and descending thin limbs of Henle's loop. The ascending thin limbs and thick limbs are relatively impermeable to water and empty into renal distal tubules and ultimately into the collecting ducts. The collecting ducts are extremely important clinically in water-balance disorders, because they are the chief site of regulation of water reabsorption. Basal epithelial water permeability in collecting duct principle cells is low, but the water permeability can become exceedingly high when stimulated with vasopressin (also known as ADH, antidiuretic hormone). In this regard, the toad urinary bladder behaves like the collecting duct, and it has served as an important model of vasopressin-regulated water permeability. Stimulation of this epithelium with vasopressin produces an increase in water permeability in the apical membrane, which coincides with the redistribution of intracellular particles to the cell surface (21, 23, 124, 292). These particles were believed to contain water channels.

DISCOVERY OF AQP1

The molecular identity of membrane water channels long proved elusive. Attempts to purify water channel proteins from native tissues, or to isolate water channel cDNAs by expression cloning, were unproductive (see review [6]). This may be explained by the physical characteristics of water, a simple molecule not amenable to chemical modification such as introduction of chemical cross-linking groups or labels. In addition, $HgCl_2$ was known to inhibit membrane water channels, a property potentially useful in identification of the water channel proteins. However, because the agent reacts with free sulfhydryls in other proteins, its inhibitory effect on water channels is not specific. This circumstance led to the mistaken identification of the band 3 anion exchanger as a molecular water channel (265). In addition, the diffusional permeability of all biologic membranes results in high background permeability and frustrated efforts to clone cDNAs for water channels by functional expression.

The recognized characteristics of membrane water channels led to chance identification of the first known water channel. In the process of isolating the 32-kD bilayer-spanning polypeptide component of the red cell Rh blood group antigen (7), a 28-kD polypeptide was partially copurified (50). Initial studies demonstrated that the 28-kD polypeptide comprises hydrophobic amino acids and exhibits an unusual detergent solubility, which facilitated purification and biochemical characterization. The 28-kD polypeptide was found to exist as an oligomeric protein with physical dimensions of a tetramer; a unique N-terminal amino acid sequence was identified (259) that permitted cDNA cloning (232). Also of note, radiation inactivation studies of water permeability by renal vesicles yielded a target size of 30 kD (283). Because the 28-kD polypeptide was found to be abundant in red cells, renal proximal tubules, and descending thin limbs (50), it was suggested that this protein might be the sought-after water channel. Although this protein was first known as "CHIP28" (channellike integral protein of 28 kDa), the need for a functionally relevant name was recognized. The name "aquaporin" was coined. After recognition of related proteins with similar functions, this name was formally proposed for the emerging family of water channels now known as the aquaporins (8). Thus CHIP28 was designated aquaporin-1 (AQP1). The Human Genome Nomenclature Committee has embraced this nomenclature for all related proteins (3), and 13 such related proteins have been identified in mammals.

The measurement of the movement of water across cell membranes poses a unique experimental challenge. Unlike ion conductances, which may be measured electrophysiologically, or solute transport, which may be measured with radioactive substrates, transmembrane water movement in cells relies on determination of changes in cell volume in response to an osmotic driving force. The *Xenopus laevis* oocyte expression system was used to search for water channel RNAs, because these cells are known to exhibit remarkably low membrane water permeability (70, 325). Oocytes injected with cRNA encoding AQP1 exhibit remarkably high osmotic water permeability ($P_f \sim 200 \times 10^{-4}$ cm/sec),

causing the cells to swell rapidly and eventually rupture in hyposmotic buffer (233). In contrast, control oocytes not injected with AQP1 cRNA exhibited less than one-tenth of this permeability.

Oocyte studies demonstrated that AQP1 behaves like the water channels in native cell membranes (233). Osmotically induced swelling of oocytes expressing AQP1 occurs with low activation energy and is reversibly inhibited by $HgCl_2$. Moreover, AQP1 oocytes fail to demonstrate any measurable increase in membrane current. Although these early studies demonstrated only swelling of oocytes, it was predicted that the direction of water flow through AQP1 is determined by the orientation of the osmotic gradient. Thus AQP1 oocytes swell in hyposmolar buffers but shrink in hyperosmolar buffers (195).

To confirm that the interpretation of the oocyte studies was correct, highly purified AQP1 protein from human red cells was reconstituted with pure phospholipids into proteoliposomes, which were compared with simple vesicles (liposomes) by rapid transfer to hyperosmolar buffer (317). These studies permitted determination of the unit water permeability, which had an astonishingly high value ($p_f \sim 3 \times 10^9$ water molecules subunit^{-1} sec^{-1}). Moreover, the water permeability is reversibly inhibited by $HgCl_2$ and exhibits low activation energy. Several of these studies have been confirmed by using red cell membranes partially depleted of other proteins (284), and attempts to demonstrate permeation by other small solutes or even protons showed that AQP1 is water selective (318). Together, these studies indicated that AQP1 is both necessary and sufficient to explain the well-recognized membrane water permeability of the red cell, and suggested that AQP1 or similar proteins could be the long-sought-after epithelial water channels of the nephron and collecting ducts.

STRUCTURE AND FUNCTION OF AQUAPORINS

General Structure of AQP1

The availability of pure AQP1 protein in milligram quantities and the simple functional assay in oocytes led to rapid advances in the understanding of the molecular structure of AQP1. Hydropathy analysis of the deduced amino acid sequence of AQP1 predicted that the protein resides primarily within the lipid bilayer (232), a feature in agreement with initial studies of red cell AQP1 (50, 259). As previously described for the homologue major intrinsic protein from lens (MIP, now referred to as AQP0), the polypeptide contains an internal repeat (Fig. 1), with the N- and the C-terminal halves being sequence-related and each containing the signature motif Asn-Pro-Ala (NPA) (226, 301), suggesting ancestral gene duplication (232). When evaluated by hydropathy analysis, six bilayer-spanning domains, five connecting loops (A–E) and intracellular N and C termini are predicted. Attenuated total reflection-FTIR (Fourier transform infrared spectroscopy) of

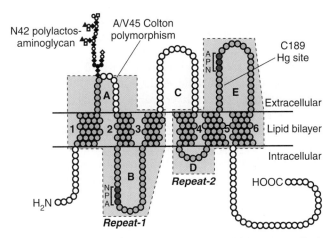

FIGURE 1 Proposed membrane topology of AQP1 subunit. Each molecule subunit spans the plasma membrane six times with the N and C termini in the cytoplasmic space. Extracellular and intracellular loops are labeled *A* through *E* (122). Loop A contains attachment site for a polylactosaminoglycan at asparagine-42 and the Co blood group polymorphism at alanine/valine-45 (261). The aquaporin signature motif asparagine-proline-alanine (NPA) is present in the loops band E. Loop E also contains the site of mercury inhibition at cysteine-189. The amino acid sequences of C termini of the known aquaporins are not conserved and sufficiently immunogenic to permit preparation of specific polyclonal antibodies to each aquaporin (see text). (From Heymann, J B, Agre, P, Engel, A, Progress on the structure and function of aquaporin 1. *J Struct Biol* 1998;121:191–206, with permission.)

highly purified red cell AQP1 reconstituted into membrane crystals demonstrated a lack of β structure in AQP1, indicating the existence of tilted α helices (25).

The two homologues domains equivalent to the N and C termini halves of the protein consist of three transmembrane helices, which are thought to be orientated oppositely in the lipid bilayer (237). A system was adapted for analyzing the structure of AQP1 after minimally perturbing the molecule by adding peptide epitopes at various sites. It was important that the epitope did not destroy function and could be localized to intracellular or extracellular sites with antibodies and by selective proteolysis of intact membranes or inside-out membrane vesicles. These studies demonstrated that loop C resides at the extracellular surface of the oocytes and the intracellular location of loop D as well as the N and C termini. Moreover, the obverse symmetry of the N and C termini halves of the molecule was confirmed (Fig. 1) (234).

Loops B and E

Loops B and E encompass the two NPA motifs and are the most conserved regions in the major intrinsic protein family. The loops exhibit significant hydrophobicity, suggesting association with the lipid bilayer (232). Subsequent studies implicated loops B and E as a structural component of the aqueous pathway. Experiments expressing AQP1 in *Xenopus* oocytes led to the observations that Cys[189] in loop E is the site of mercurial inhibition (235, 324). Site-directed mutagenesis experiments in oocytes

revealed that substitution of Cys[189] with a serine residue eliminates $HgCl_2$ sensitivity and increases osmotic water permeability, while substitution with larger amino acids residues prevents facilitated water transport (235). These results suggest that water transport and selectivity in AQP1 is somehow dependent on the steric properties of Cys[189]. In accordance with the internal repeat theory, Ala[73] located in loop B, the equivalent to Cys[189] in loop E was investigated. By creating double mutants expressing Cys[189] as a serine and Ala[73] as a cysteine, the $HgCl_2$ sensitivity and osmotic water permeability were restored (122). These results suggested that loops B and E were arranged in a symmetrical fashion and underlined that these loops were functionally essential for water permeability. This line of inquiry led to the "hourglass" model (122) in which these domains overlap midway between the leaflets of the bilayer, creating a constitutively open, narrow aqueous pathway (Fig. 2).

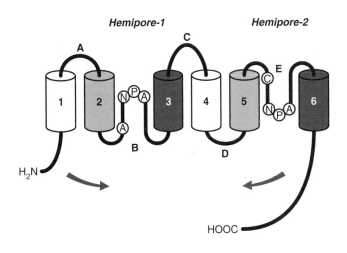

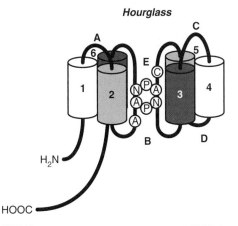

FIGURE 2 Hourglass model of aquaporin-1 (AQP1) structure. Bilayer spans 1–3 (*Repeat-1*) and spans 4–6 (*Repeat-2*) are sequence related and are oriented in obverse symmetry. Loop B and loop E are believed to dip into the bilayer and emerge from the same side **(top)**. When folded together, loops Band E form a single aqueous pathway (the "hourglass") flanked by the site of mercury inhibition at cysteine-189 **(bottom)**. (From Jung JS, Preston GM, Smith BL, Guggino WB, Agre P. Molecular structure of the water channel through aquaporin CHIP: the hourglass model. *J Biol Chem* 1994;269:14648–14654, with permission.)

Tetrameric Organization

Early biophysical characterization of AQP1 suggested that the protein formed multisubunit oligomers (259). Rotary and unidirectionally shadowed freeze-fracture electron microscopic analyses of AQP1 protein from human red cell membranes reconstituted in proteoliposomes provided detailed molecular insights. AQP1 had an oligomeric structure, consisting of a four subunits surrounding a central depression. These tetrameric structures were also seen in highly water-permeable nephron segments expressing native AQP1 (288). Although the oligomerization of AQP1 is still not understood in detail, all studies indicate that the protein is a tetramer composed of functionally independent aqueous pores (122, 235, 256, 283).

Structural Analyses and Molecular Dynamics of Aquaporins

By reconstituting the highly purified red cell AQP1 into membranes under controlled conditions, membrane crystals were produced with AQP1 in highly uniform lattices. These membranes appeared as flat sheets or as large, resealed vesicles in which the AQP1 protein was found to fully retain water permeability (296). Thus the opportunity to define the structure of AQP1 in a biologically active state became possible. Electron microscopic studies by multiple groups permitted the elucidation of the protein at increasing levels of resolution. By performing high-resolution electron microscopic evaluation of negatively stained membranes at a series of tilts, a three-dimensional view was obtained (295). Image projections revealed the presence of multiple bilayer-spanning domains, and atomic force microscopy further defined the orientation and extramembranous dimensions of AQP1 (297). Electron crystallographic analysis of cryopreserved specimens has been undertaken at tilts of up to 60 degrees. These analyses revealed the three-dimensional structure of AQP1 at increasing resolutions, down to 3.8 Å (29, 116, 163, 163, 196, 197, 206, 238, 239, 294). X-ray crystallographic analysis has added further information about the structure of AQP1. Using the previously described method, the structure of AQP1 has been determined down to a resolution of 2.2 Å (270). In contrast to the previous studies, the high resolution enables observation of water molecules in transit trough the channel. Based on the combined efforts, a detailed picture of AQP1's tertiary structure could be formed

As earlier studies indicated, the AQP1 monomers form a tetrameric cluster. The model shows an extension of the tetramer from the extracellular plane, while the intracellular surfaces form a shallow depression. The N termini from one monomer is closely situated near the C termini of the neighboring monomer. The gap formed by the four monomers narrows from 8.5 Å down to 3.5 Å. The residues surrounding the gab are hydrophobic, suggesting an interaction with a hydrophobic molecule (206). So despite the monomeric formation of a central cavity, the tetrameric structure does

not support the transport of water. This is in concert with earlier observations, suggesting that each monomer is capable of facilitating water transport.

The dimensions of each monomer are 40 Å across and 60 Å long as reported by Sui et al. (Fig. 3) (270). The monomer is composed of six bilayer-spanning α helices surrounding a central density. The C loop located on the extracellular surface connects the N and C termini halves of the protein. Part of the central density represents the B and E loops, which appears as two short α-helix structures not permeating the membrane (Fig. 3) (197). This organization is strikingly similar to the proposed hourglass arrangement of the B and E loops (122). The NPA containing loops are located on opposite sides of the membrane, juxtapositional to each other, interacting trough their NPA motifs. The central density is composed of an extracellular and intracellular vestibule, separated by a narrow pore. The extracellular vestibule is approximately 15 Å at its widest (270). Following the extracellular vestibule toward the lipid bilayer, a decrease in diameter occurs and the pore becomes exceedingly small (206, 270). The constriction site (also referred to as the aromatic/arginine constriction) is located 20 Å from the beginning of the extracellular vestibule and is composed of several highly conserved residues in conventional aquaporins. The constriction site is approximately 2.8 Å wide, about the diameter of a water molecule (270). After the constriction site the pore continues for 20 Å, a region termed the "selectivity filter" (270). The selectivity filter is slightly wider and part of the region is formed by the helical loops B and E (206, 270). This situates the asparagine residues in the NPA motifs within the selectivity filter (206, 270). Additionally, Cys[189] in loop E protrudes into the pore, confirming earlier studies, suggesting that $HgCl_2$ sensitivity was due to steric hindrance of water movement trough the pore (122, 206, 270). Following the pore toward the intracellular vestibule, the diameter increases again reaching 15 Å again (Fig. 3) (270).

Using molecular dynamic simulations, de Groot and Grubmüller (44) obtained time-resolved, atomic-resolution models of water transport trough AQP1 (44). From the extracellular vestibule, water molecules enter the constriction site, composed of side chains from the aromatic Phe[56] and His[180], and the charged Arg[195]. This conformation situates the water molecule, allowing hydrogen bonding with the polar residues, thereby reducing hydrogen bonding between water molecules. In addition, electrostatic repulsion by Arg[195] suggests that the constriction site is the main site for exclusion of protons (hydronium ions) and other ions (44). This is further supported by mutagenic analysis of the residues in the constriction site, showing permeation of urea, glycerol, and ammonia in AQP1 when altered. Moreover, replacing Arg[195] with a valine residue appears to facilitate proton transport (18). Now passing onward trough the hydrophobic selectivity filter, exposed polar moieties mainly consisting of backbone carbonyls, lead the water molecules toward the NPA motifs. The water molecule transiently reorients to bond with the two asparagines residues of the

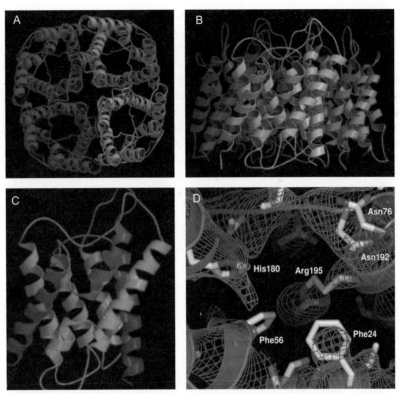

FIGURE 3 A,B: Structure of the human AQP1 tetramer, viewed from the top **(A)** and side **(B). C:** Structure of the human AQP1 monomer. **D:** Model of the central pore region of human AQP1-EM3 structure (pdb code 1H6I [42]) together with the 3.8 Å resolution EM potential map rendered at 1.0s (206). Several residues critical for AQP1-facilitated water transport are marked. (From de Groot BL, Engel A, Grubmuller H. The structure of the aquaporin-1 water channel. a comparison between cryo-electron microscopy and x-ray crystallography. *J Molecul Biol* 2003;325:485–493, with permission.) See color insert.

NPA motifs and is led out of the selectivity filter toward the intracellular vestibule, again by hydrogen bonding with a few selected backbone carbonyls. Hence, the selectivity filter encompassing the highly conserved NPA motifs appears to serve mainly as a filter for size (44), while the ar/R constriction is a major checkpoint for solute and ion permeability. The *Escherichia coli* aquaglyceroporin (GlpF) selectively facilitates glycerol transport over that of water (193). Evaluation of differences between AQP1 and GlpF using molecular dynamic simulations revealed a larger selectivity filter in GlpF. Moreover, the preference for glycerol could be explained by what de Groot and Grubmüller describe as a glycerol-mediated "induced fit" gating motion (i.e, glycerol transport serves as the prime mechanism for water exclusion) (44).

Structural characterizations of crystallized human AQP2 in two-dimensional protein-lipid arrays by atomic force microscopy and electron crystallography have revealed the structure of AQP2 at a resolution of 4.5 Å in the membrane plane (250). As AQP1, AQP2 is found in a tetrameric assembly in the lipid bilayer (250, 300). The AQP2 monomer shows structural features similar to those earlier reported for AQP1 (250), while structural variation is found around the tetramers axis (75, 250).

The structure of AQP0 has also been determined down to a resolution of 2.2 Å (86, 94). The water conductance of AQP0 is much lower than that reported for AQP1 (204), possibly due to highly conserved tyrosine residues in AQP0s, imposing further constriction on the channel (94). The constriction site is smaller than that in AQP1 and the selectivity filter is also more narrow (86, 94). Molecular dynamics studies suggest that water movement is facilitated by AQP0 due to thermal motions of certain side chains, although this builds up a free-energy barrier, possibly contributing to the lower permeability in AQP0 (90). The extensive analyses of the structure of various AQP isoforms have provided detailed insight into the molecular basis for transmembrane water transport. Future studies aimed at defining the distinct structure of other members, including aquaglyceroporins like AQP7 and AQP9 that appear to be involved in metabolism rather than water transport may provide further insights. It should also be indicated that several studies have been aimed at identifying novel aquaporin blockers. Although some progress has been reported, only few compounds, including related tetra-ammonium compounds, have shown selective effects on AQPs (22, 51, 289). Also copper (320) and nickel (321), significantly blocks aquaporins.

DISTRIBUTION OF AQP1 IN KIDNEY AND OTHER TISSUES

Well before recognition of its function, the red cell AQP1 protein was known to be expressed at high levels in the proximal convoluted tubules and descending thin limbs of kidney (50). This was confirmed with polyclonal rabbit antiserum (247) and was defined in rat and human kidney with affinity-purified immunoglobulin specific for the N and C terminal domains of AQP1 (192, 216). In all studies, AQP1 was demonstrated to be constitutively present in the apical plasma membranes (i.e., the brush borders) and in basolateral membranes of S2 and S3 segment proximal tubules (Fig. 4). Quantitative immunoblotting indicated that AQP1 makes up 0.9% of total membrane protein from rat renal cortex and 4% of brush-border proteins (216). Enzyme-linked immunosorbent assay (ELISA) measurements of microdissected tubules revealed that proximal tubules contain approximately 20 million copies of AQP1 per cell (179). Additionally, AQP1 is found in the plasma membrane of glomerular mesangial cells in humans, although not in rats (17, 192, 216). Other immunohistochemical and immunogold electron microscopic studies have demonstrated AQP1 in multiple capillary endothelia throughout the body (132, 217, 253), including the renal vasa

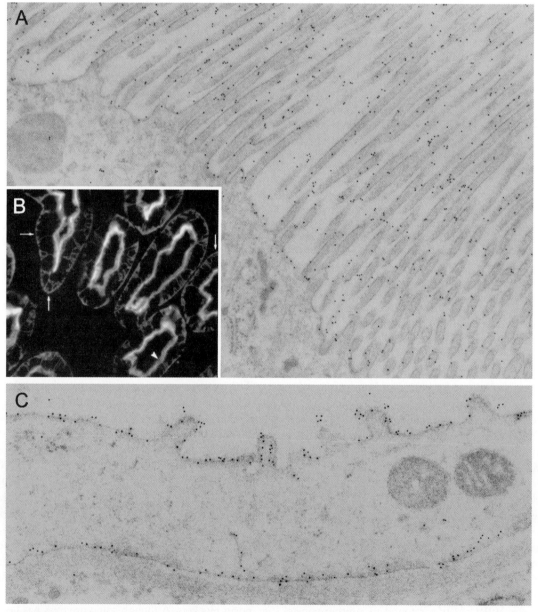

FIGURE 4   Distribution of aquaporin-1 (AQP1) in kidney. Ultrathin cryosections of. rat renal cortex and inner medulla stained with anti-immunogold AQP1. **A:** Strong labeling is present over the apical brush border of S3 section of proximal tubule. **B:** Strong labeling is present over apical and basolateral membrane of thin descending limb of Henle's loop. (From Nielsen S, Smith B, Christensen EI, Knepper MA, Agre P. CHIP28 water channels are localized in constitutively water-permeable segments of the nephron. *J Cell Biol* 1993;120:371–383, with permission.) See color insert.

recta (224). AQP1 also is abundant in peribronchiolar capillary endothelium, where expression is induced by glucocorticoids (132, 133) apparently acting through the classic glucocorticoid response elements in the *AQP1* gene (198). In addition, AQP1 has been defined in multiple water-permeable epithelia including choroid plexus; peritoneal mesothelial cells (156); fetal membranes (182); at multiple locations in eye, including ciliary epithelium, lens epithelium, and corneal endothelium (96, 217, 266); and in hepatobiliary epithelium (243), pancreatic interlobular ducts (144), heart and skeletal muscle (13), gall bladder (27), salvary glands (89), inner ear (106), and several other organs including the nervous system (see review [271]). AQP1 has also been localized in tumor cells and their vasculature (63). Developmental expression of AQP1 is complex: transient expression occurs in some tissues before birth; expression in other tissues is subsequent to birth; constitutive life-long expression is found in other tissues (20, 133, 260).

AQP1 DEFICIENCY

Humans have been identified who totally lack the AQP1 protein. The human *AQP1* gene was localized to chromosome 7p14, and the Co blood group antigens were previously linked to 7p, suggesting a molecular relationship. It was determined that the Co blood group antigen results from an Ala/Val polymorphism at the extracellular surface of red cell AQP1 (261) (Fig. 1). Although the International Blood Group Referencing Laboratory in Bristol, England, has detailed phenotyping information on millions of donors worldwide, only six individuals had been shown to lack Co. Most of these Co-null individuals are women who developed anti-Co during pregnancy. Three of these Co-null individuals were found to have mutations in the *AQP1* gene (236). Although the exceedingly rare blood group phenotype makes them impossible to match for blood transfusion, it was surprising that none of them exhibited any other obvious severe clinical phenotype. The extreme rarity of the Co-null state may reflect an important developmental role, resulting in reduced fetal survival; however, the frequency of the heterozygous state is unknown. Detailed studies of the urinary concentrating ability of Co-null individuals revealed a marked inability of the individuals to concentrate urine to more than 400 mOsm/l even in the presence of dehydration or 1-desamino-8-D-arginine vasopressin (dDAVP) treatment, revealing a significant urinary concentrating defect (134). Moreover Co-null individuals display reduced pulmonary vascular permeability (135).

The development of *AQP1* gene knockout mice has provided further insights into the role of AQP1 in renal water homeostasis. AQP1-null (AQP1$^{-/-}$) mice appeared moderately polyuric under basal conditions. However, AQP1$^{-/-}$ animals exhibited an extreme degree of polyuria and polydipsia when undergoing water deprivation, including rapid hyperosmolar extracellular fluid volume depletion (172). Additionally, AQP1$^{-/-}$ mice failed to respond appropriately to vasopressin, suggesting that renal water conservation and

urinary concentration is highly dependent on AQP1 protein (172). Detailed classic in vivo and in vitro physiological evaluation of proximal tubules from the AQP1$^{-/-}$ mice established that transepithelial water permeability was reduced by 80% and led to approximate 50% decrease in proximal tubule fluid reabsorption (252). The apparent differences in transepithelial water permeability and proximal tubule fluid reabsorption is likely dependant on the generation of a hypotonic filtrate in proximal tubules of AQP1$^{-/-}$ mice (282). Despite these observations, distal fluid delivery in AQP1$^{-/-}$ remained unchanged due to a compensatory reduction in single-nephron glomerular filtration (252). When blunting the tubuloglomerular feedback (TGF) response and thereby the compensatory reduction in glomerular filtration observed in AQP1$^{-/-}$ mice, ambient urine osmolalities and urinary flow rates appeared indifferent from normal AQP1$^{-/-}$ mice, probably due to distal tubular compensatory mechanisms (98). The impaired proximal fluid reabsorption observed in AQP1$^{-/-}$ mice, albeit with normal distal fluid delivery, suggests that the polyuric phenotype largely depends on a concentrating defect, impairing collecting duct water reabsorption.

Studies using isolated perfused thin descending limbs have revealed that the osmotic water permeability of the type II thin descending limbs (outer medullary thin descending limbs from long-loop nephron) is decreased by 90% relative to wildtype values in kidneys from AQP1 knockout mice (35). Additionally, earlier observations using freeze-fracture electron microscopic techniques showed a remarkably high density of intramembrane particles in the thin descending limb of rat, which has been attributed to the tetrameric assembled AQP1 subunits (288). In the thin descending limb of AQP1$^{-/-}$ mice, the abundance and size of these intramembrane particles was markedly reduced (35). Moreover, the distribution of AQP1 in the vasa recta suggests a role in microvascular exchange, hence affecting urinary concentration. The distribution of AQP1 in the vasa recta suggests a role in microvascular exchange, hence affecting urinary concentration. In the presence of a NaCl gradient, osmotic water permeability was almost eliminated in the descending vasa recta of AQP1$^{-/-}$ mice, leading to a predicted reduction in medullary interstitial osmolality and likely an impairment of countercurrent multiplication (225). Additional studies using adenoviral gene delivery restored AQP1 protein expression in the proximal tubule epithelia and renal microvessels of AQP1$^{-/-}$ knockout mice, albeit not in the descending thin limbs. The adenovirus treated mice showed slight restoration of the concentrating defect during water deprivation, probably due to reinsertion of AQP1 water channels in the vasa recta, although urinary concentrating ability still was highly insufficient in comparison to wildtype mice (307). In conclusion, the severe concentrating defect seen in the AQP1$^{-/-}$ mice, primarily results from impaired water absorption in the thin descending limb, underlining the necessity for a constitutively high water permeability in this segment, for a functional countercurrent multiplication system.

ADDITIONAL FUNCTIONS OF AQP1

AQP1 is generally believed to be a constitutively active, water-selective pore. Nonetheless, some observations contradict this. A small degree of permeation by glycerol has been seen in oocytes and may represent opening of an unidentified leak pathway (1), and the biologic significance remains unclear (195). Forskolin was reported to induce a cation current in AQP1-expressing oocytes (315), but multiple other scientific groups have failed to reproduce this effect (5). Although small changes in water permeability by oocytes expressing a bovine homologue of AQP1 have also been ascribed to vasopressin and atrial natriuretic peptide, the significance is uncertain (227). Likewise, secretin-induced membrane trafficking has been noted in isolated cholangiocytes (183, 184); however, this awaits confirmation by immunoelectron microscopy. Permeation of AQP1 by CO_2 has also been evaluated. Rates of pH change are about 40% higher in oocytes expressing AQP1 (207) than in control oocytes. Although the background permeation of lipid bilayers by CO_2, as well as oxygen, ammonia, nitric oxide, and other gases, may be high (240), the potential physiological relevance of AQP1 permeation by gases warrants more study (see review [[41]]). Additionally, AQP1 appears to play a role in cell migration (245). AQP1$^{-/-}$ mice implanted with tumor cells show reduced tumor vascularity and growth, thus leading to improved survival, in comparison to wildtype mice. Moreover, in vitro analysis of endothelial cells isolated from AQP1$^{-/-}$ mice, showed marked impairment in cell migration (245). In primary cultures of proximal tubule cells from AQP1$^{-/-}$ mice, in vitro cell migration was impaired compared to AQP1$^{+/+}$ mice. Furthermore, in an ischemia–reperfusion model of acute renal tubular injury, AQP1$^{-/-}$ mice showed more severe pathological changes including more prominent tubule degeneration (93). Thus, although the evidence that AQP1 functions as a water channel is incontrovertible, the possibility of yet undiscovered transport functions cannot be excluded.

AQUAPORINS IN KIDNEY

The first functional definition of one member of a protein family often prompts a search for related proteins. This has certainly been the case for the aquaporins, and the homology cloning approach has been undertaken by multiple laboratories whose combined efforts have expanded the aquaporin family membership list. Homology cloning has most frequently been undertaken by using polymerase chain amplification with degenerate oligonucleotide primers (4). Thirteen mammalian aquaporins are now known, and they form at least two subgroups: water-selective channels (orthodox aquaporins) and channels permeated by water, glycerol, and other small molecules (aquaglyceroporins). Given the large potential for confusion, the Human Genome Organization has established an Aquaporin Nomenclature System (3), accessible on the Internet (http://www.gene.ucl.ac.uk/nomenclature). Of the known aquaporins, eight are expressed in mammalian kidney (Table 1). Soon after AQP1 was discovered to be a water channel, AQP2 was identified in renal collecting duct (84), where it is regulated by vasopressin and is involved in multiple clinical disorders (Table 2). AQP3 was identified in kidney and other tissues and was found to be permeated by glycerol and water (59, 112, 169). AQP4, an $HgCl_2$-insensitive water channel, is most abundantly expressed in brain and is present in kidney collecting duct in the basolateral plasma membrane of principle and inner

TABLE 1   Aquaporins in Kidney

AQP	Localization (renal)	Subcellular Distribution	Regulation	Localization (extrarenal)
AQP1	S2, S3 segments of proximal tubules	Apical and basolateral plasma membranes	Glucocorticoids (peribronchiolar capillary endothelium)	Multiple tissues, including capillary endothelia, choroids plexus, ciliary and lens epithelium, etc.
AQP2	Collecting duct principal cells	Intracellular vesicles, apical plasma membrane	Vasopressin stimulates short-term exocytosis long-term biosynthesis	Epididymis
AQP3	Collecting duct principal cells	Basolateral plasma membrane	Vasopressin stimulates long-term biosynthesis	Multiple tissues, including airway basal epithelia, conjunctiva, colon
AQP4	Collecting duct principal cells	Basolateral plasma membrane	Dopamine, protein kinase C	Multiple tissues, including central nervous system astroglia, ependyma, airway surface epithelia
AQP6	Collecting duct intercalated cells	Intracellular vesicles	Rapidly gated	Unknown
AQP7	S3 proximal tubules	Apical plasma membrane	Insulin (adipose tissue)	Multiple tissues, including adipose tissue, testis, and heart
AQP8	Proximal tubule, collecting duct cells	Intracellular domains	Unknown	Multiple tissues, including gastrointestinal tract, testis, and airways
AQP11	Proximal tubule	Intracellular domains	Unknown	Multiple tissues, including liver, testes, and brain

AQP, aquaporin.

TABLE 2   Water-balance Disorders Associated with Aquaporin Abnormalities

Congenital defects
Central diabetes insipidus
Mutation in gene encoding vasopressin (Brattleboro rat)
Nephrogenic diabetes insipidus
Mutations in gene encoding V_2 receptor (human, X-linked)
Mutations in gene encoding aquaporin-2 (human, dominant and
    recessive)
Partial concentration defects
Targeted disruption of gene encoding aquaporin-1 (mouse)
Targeted disruption of gene encoding aquaporin-4 (mouse)
Acquired defects
Lithium treatment
Hypokalemia
Hypercalcemia
Postobstructive nephropathy, unilateral or bilateral
Conditions with water retention
Congestive heart failure
Hepatic cirrhosis
Nephritic syndrome
Pregnancy
Other conditions
Syndrome of inappropriate vasopressin secretion
Primary polydipsia
Chronic renal failure
Acute renal failure
Low-protein diet
Age-induced reduction in renal concentration

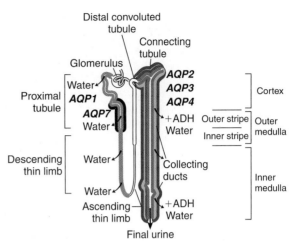

FIGURE 5   Sites of aquaporin (AQP1) expression in kidney and segmental water-transport function. Proximal nephron: AQP1 is present in apical and basolateral plasma membranes of proximal tubules and thin descending limbs. AQP6 is present in intracellular vesicles of collecting duct intercalated cells. AQP7 is present in proximal tubules. Distal nephron: aquaporins are not present in ascending limbs. Collecting duct: AQP2 is present in intracellular vesicles and apical plasma membranes of principle cells; AQP3 and AQP4 are present in basolateral membranes. AQP6 is present in intracellular vesicles in type A intercalated cells.

medullary collecting duct (IMCD) cells and is also present in other tissues but is not inhibited by mercury (97, 121). AQP6 was identified at the cDNA level and found to be localized in intracellular vesicles in the collecting duct intercalated cells in the kidney (170, 173, 313). AQP7 is permeated by water and glycerol (111, 147). First cloned from testis (111), AQP7 is present in segment 3 proximal tubule brush-border membranes where it facilitates glycerol and water transport (262). AQP8 is an $HgCl_2$-sensitive water channel found in intracellular domains of proximal tubule and collecting duct cells (62, 174); however, its function remains unclear. AQP11 is found in the cytoplasm of renal proximal tubule cells (201). The exact function is not established, although deletion of the *AQP11* gene produces a severe phenotype with renal vacuolization and cyst formation (201).

Localization and Function of AQP2, AQP3, AQP4, AQP6, AQP7, AQP8, and AQP11 in Kidney

The amino acid sequences of the N and C termini of the different aquaporins are not closely related, and specific polyclonal antibodies can be raised in rabbits immunized with synthetic peptides conjugated to carrier proteins such as keyhole limpet hemocyanin. As with AQP1, these antibodies have permitted localization of the other aquaporins in kidney by immunocytochemistry, immunoelectron microscopy, and single-tubule microdissection combined with ELISA (Fig. 5).

Three aquaporins (AQP2, AQP3, and AQP4) are expressed in the collecting duct principle cells and the connecting tubule segment, sites where vasopressin regulates epithelial water permeability. AQP2 is located in the apical plasma membrane and small intracellular vesicles of collecting duct principle cells (Fig. 6) (211). ELISA measurements of microdissected rat collecting ducts have revealed that AQP2 is an extremely abundant protein in the collecting duct, with more than 6 million copies per cell throughout the collecting duct system (137). Additional studies using the single-tubule ELISA method and immunocytochemistry demonstrated colocalization of AQP2 and V_2 vasopressin receptor expression on connecting tubule arcades, suggesting that regulated water transport may occur in the arcades of the cortical labyrinth in addition to the collecting duct (40, 137). Additionally, AQP2 has been identified in the basolateral membranes of connecting tubules and inner medullary collecting ducts (38).

The apical plasma membrane is the rate-limiting barrier for transepithelial water transport across the collecting duct principle cell and is the site where vasopressin regulates water permeability (71). Localization of AQP2 in the apical plasma membrane suggested that it is the target for vasopressin-regulated collecting duct water permeability (Fig. 6). This conclusion was firmly established by multiple studies. A direct correlation between AQP2 expression and collecting duct water permeability has been demonstrated in Brattleboro rats, which lack circulating vasopressin owing to a mutation in the gene encoding vasopressin precursor protein (53). Likewise, human patients with mutations in the *AQP2* gene manifest severe vasopressin-resistant nephrogenic diabetes insipidus (49), demonstrating the requirement for AQP2 in collecting duct water transport. Lack of functional AQP2 expression in mice, by generation of *AQP2* gene knockouts, produces a severe concentration defect, resulting in early postnatal death

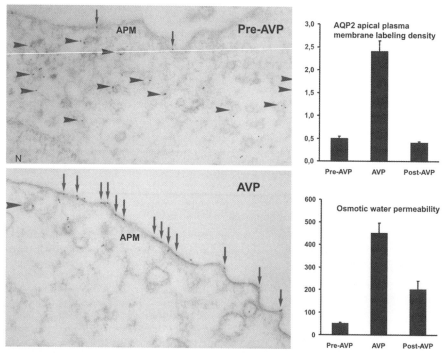

FIGURE 6   Vasopressin-induced trafficking of aquaporin-2 (AQP2) in isolated, perfused rat collecting duct and resulting changes in water permeability. Anti-AQP2 immunogold electron microscopy of ultrathin cryosections of isolated rat collecting duct fixed before exposure to arginine vasopressin (pre-AVP, **top left**) and after exposure (AVP, **bottom left**). Note intracellular AQP2 (*arrowheads*) and plasma membrane AQP2 (*small arrows*). Quantification of AQP2 labeling density before, during, or after vasopressin exposure (**top right**). Quantification of osmotic water permeability of isolated collecting duct (**bottom right**). N, nucleus; M, mitochondrion. Magnification, ×50,000. (From Nielsen S, Chou CL, Marples D, Christensen EI, Kishore BK, Knepper MA. Vasopressin increases water permeability of kidney collecting duct by inducing translocation of aquaporin-CD water channels to plasma membrane. *Proc Natl Acad Sci U S A* 1995;92:1013–1017, with permission.)

(244, 305). Moreover, morphological changes, including renal medullary atrophy and dilation of the collecting ducts, are observed in these mice (244, 305). Generation of AQP2$^{-/-}$ knockouts selectively in the collecting ducts, but not in the connecting tubule segments, rescues mice from the lethal phenotype, however body weight, urinary production, and the response to water deprivation is still severely impaired (244). Additionally, in a tamoxifen-inducible mouse model of *AQP2* gene deletion, adult mice presents with severe polyuria, a marked urinary concentration defect, and develop mild renal damage (309). Together these studies demonstrate the pivotal role of AQP2 in urinary concentration.

AQP3 is localized in a large variety of organs and highly expressed in the kidney. AQP3 was originally cloned from rat kidney (59, 112, 169) and when expressed in *Xenopus* oocytes it facilitated glycerol transport (discussed in subsequent sections) and increased HgCl$_2$-sensitive osmotic water permeability (175, 308, 323). Moreover, channel gating is regulated by protons and copper (320, 323). AQP4 was found to be expressed in several tissues with high abundance in the brain. In oocyte expression studies, the protein increased osmotic water permeability in an HgCl$_2$-insensitive manner (97, 308).

AQP3 and AQP4 are also present in the connecting tubule and collecting duct principle cells; however, the sites where they are expressed do not overlap with the expression of AQP2 in most portions of the collecting duct (40, 58, 77, 275). AQP3 and AQP4 are restricted to the basolateral plasma membranes of collecting duct principle cells, where they are presumed to permit water entry into the interstitium. Although both are basolateral water channels, they are distributed differently along the collecting duct system, with the greatest abundance of AQP3 in cortical and outer medullary collecting ducts and the greatest abundance of AQP4 in IMCDs (275). AQP4 is also found in basolateral membranes of proximal tubule S3 segments, although only in mice (285). Using freeze-fracture electron microscopy, orthogonal arrays of intramembrane particles (OAPs) were demonstrated in the basolateral membranes of the proximal tubule S3 segment in AQP4$^{+/+}$, but not in AQP4$^{-/-}$ mice (285). AQP4 is expressed in two splice isoforms, the M1 and M23 splice variants. The M23-AQP4 appears to be the OAP-forming water channel when expressed in LLC-PK1 cells. When organized in OAPs a significantly higher single-channel water permeability coefficient is observed in comparison to the non–AOP-forming M1-AQP4 (38, 258). Shuttling of AQP3 or AQP4 is not expected to occur as the predominant fraction is found in the plasma membrane (short- and long-term regulation of these aquaporins will be discussed later). Sodium restriction or aldosterone infusion in normal and Brattleboro rats greatly increases the abundance of AQP3, while AQP3 abundance is markedly reduced during aldosterone deficiency, suggesting a direct effect of aldosterone on collecting duct AQP3 expression (155). AQP4 appears to be regulated by protein kinase C (PKC) and dopamine, where stimulation by these factors decreases water permeability in AQP4-transfected cells (322).

Deletion of the *AQP3* gene induces polyuria and polydipsia and a marked reduction in osmotic water permeability in the basolateral plasma membrane of the cortical collecting duct (175). Moreover, urinary osmolality is reduced in $AQP3^{-/-}$ mice and they fail to respond appropriately to dDAVP, thus presenting with a urinary concentrating defect (175). Targeted disruption of AQP4 in mice results in a 75% reduction in the osmotic water permeability of the inner medullary collecting duct (32). However, phenotypically the $AQP4^{-/-}$ mice appeared grossly normal, presenting with a very mild urinary concentrating defect (176). In double $AQP3^{-/-}/AQP4^{-/-}$ knockout mice concentrating ability was only slightly more impaired than in the $AQP3^{-/-}$ mice (175). It should be noted that the localization of AQP2 in basolateral membranes in the connecting tubule and inner medullary collecting duct raises the possibility, that the observed effect is partly compensated by this mechanism (38).

AQP6 vesicles reside in subapical vesicles within intercalated cells of collecting duct, where it is coexpressed with the V-type H^+-ATPase (311, 313). AQP6 appears functionally distinct from other known aquaporins. Oocyte expression studies have revealed low water permeability of AQP6 during basal conditions, while in the presence of $HgCl_2$ a rapid increase in water permeability and ion conductance is observed. Additionally, reductions in pH (<5.5) quickly and reversibly increase anion conductance and water permeability in AQP6-expressing oocytes (311). Subsequent studies have shown that the channel is permeable to halides, with the highest permeability to NO_3^- (107, 311), while the ionic selectivity becomes less specific after the addition of $HgCl_2$ (101). Moreover, when Asn^{60}, a residue unique in mammalian AQP6, is converted to glycine, a highly conserved residue in other mammalian aquaporins, anionic permeability is abolished and osmotic water permeability is increased during basal conditions (166).

AQP7 is a member of the aquaglyceroporin family and was originally cloned from rat testis (111). Additionally, AQP7 is expressed in several organs including adipose tissue and kidney (111, 136). In the kidney, AQP7 localizes to the brush-border membrane of the proximal tubule S3 segment (110, 208). Expression of AQP7 in *Xenopus* oocytes showed that AQP7 facilitated the transport of glycerol and urea in addition to water (111). The development of AQP7 knockout mice has aided in understanding the physiology role of AQP7. Glycerol excretion is markedly increased in $AQP7^{-/-}$ mice, suggesting a role for AQP7 in facilitating proximal tubular glycerol transport and possibly renal gluconeogenesis (discussed in subsequent sections) (262). In terms of water transport, $AQP7^{-/-}$

mice experience only a slight reduction in proximal tubule membrane water permeability, and AQP7/AQP1 double-knockout mice showed only a slightly more severe urinary concentrating defect than the $AQP1^{-/-}$ mice during water deprivation (262). Additionally, evaluation of the channels permeability to urea in $AQP7^{-/-}$ mice revealed no change in urinary urea excretion or urea accumulation in the papilla, indicating a less prominent physiological role in urea transport (262). Expression of AQP7 in *Xenopus* oocytes increases the permeability to arsenite, thereby providing a possible route for arsenite uptake in mammalian cells (167). The physiological role of these observations waits further investigation.

Cloning of the murine AQP8 water channel (114, 146, 174), revealed its presence in many organs, including the kidney (62, 114, 146, 174). In kidney, AQP8 localizes to intracellular domains of proximal tubule and collecting duct cells (62). Expression of AQP8 in *Xenopus* oocytes increased $HgCl_2$-sensitive osmotic water permeability. Additionally, oocyte expression of AQP8 showed permeability to urea (174). Targeted deletion of the *AQP8* gene produced a mild phenotype in the $AQP8^{-/-}$ mice with no obvious changes in renal parameters (306). Subsequent studies have suggested that AQP8 facilitates NH_3 transport in *Xenopus* oocytes (104, 165) and in ammonia transport deficient yeast (115). In $AQP8^{-/-}$ mice, ammonia loading mildly reduced hepatic ammonia accumulation and increased renal ammonia excretion (310), indicating that AQP8 does not play a significant physiological role in facilitated NH_3 transport.

Recently a new aquaporin was cloned from rat testis: AQP11 (114). This AQP has only one NPA motif and shares low similarity with the conventional aquaporins. AQP11 is most abundantly expressed in the testis, kidney, and liver (114). In the kidney, the AQP11 protein localizes to the cytoplasm of the renal proximal tubules (201). While lack of plasma membrane expression of the AQP11 protein in *Xenopus* oocytes greatly impaired measurements of transport (201), targeted deletion of the *AQP11* gene in mice resulted in a severe phenotype with vacuolization and cyst formation in the proximal tubule. The $AQP11^{-/-}$ mice died of renal failure, and kidneys were polycystic. The cyst epithelia contained vacuoles and the $AQP11^{-/-}$ mice also presented with a proximal tubular endosomal acidification defect (201).

AQUAGLYCEROPORINS

AQP3, AQP7, and AQP9 constitute a subgroup of aquaporins with a broader permeation range that includes glycerol, hence the name "aquaglyceroporins." AQP3, which transports water and glycerol, were cloned by three groups at the same time (59, 112, 169). The distribution at multiple sites, including the kidney collecting duct principle cells, airway epithelia, skin, urinary bladder, and secretory glands, suggests several functions (58, 77, 220). AQP3-null mice exhibit a nephrogenic diabetes insipidus phenotype; however, human mutants have not yet been reported. AQP7 is also permeated by water and glycerol and is localized to the apical brush border of the proximal tubules, especially to the S3 segment. Recent studies have indicated that AQP7 may play a role for glycerol metabolism by showing adaptation to fasting by glycerol transport through AQP7 in adipose tissue (178). AQP7$^{-/-}$ mice have a significant lower plasma glycerol concentration than wildtype mice and impaired adipocytic glycerol release in response to a β3-receptor stimulation (178). Moreover, AQP7$^{-/-}$ mice experience severe hypoglycemia but show normal hepatic gluconeogenesis during fasting, indicative of defective adipocytic glycerol transport in these mice (178). Glycerol excretion is also markedly increased in AQP7$^{-/-}$ mice, suggesting a role for AQP7 in facilitating proximal tubular glycerol transport (262). AQP9, which is expressed in the liver but not in kidney (113, 143, 279), is permeated by a range of solutes including glycerol and urea (278). It has been demonstrated that expression of AQP9 in liver was induced up to 20-fold in rats fasted for 24 to 96 hours and that AQP9 levels gradually declined after refeeding (28). This indicates that the liver takes up glycerol for gluconeogenesis through AQP9 during starvation.

VASOPRESSIN REGULATION OF KIDNEY AQUAPORINS

Of all the aquaporins, AQP2 has evoked the largest interest by nephrologists, because it is expressed in principle cells of renal collecting duct, where it is the primary target for short-term regulation of collecting duct water permeability (210, 246, 304). AQP2 and AQP3 also are regulated either directly or indirectly by vasopressin through long-term effects that alter the abundance of these water-channel proteins in collecting duct cells (53, 58, 158, 211, 276).

Short- and Long-Term Regulation of Water Permeability in the Collecting Duct

Two modes of vasopressin-mediated regulation of water permeability have been identified in the renal collecting duct. Both involve regulation of the AQP2 water channel. Short-term regulation is the widely recognized process by which vasopressin rapidly increases water permeability of principle cells by binding to vasopressin V_2 receptors at the basolateral membranes, a response measurable within 5 to 30 minutes after increasing the peritubular vasopressin concentration (150, 293). It is believed that vasopressin, acting through a cyclic adenosine monophosphate (cAMP) cascade, causes intracellular AQP2 vesicles to fuse with the apical plasma membrane, which increases the number of water channels in the apical plasma membrane (Figs. 6 and 7). Long-term regulation of collecting duct water permeability is seen when circulating vasopressin levels are increased for 24 hours or more, resulting in an increase in the maximal water permeability of the collecting duct epithelium (158). This response is a consequence of an increase in the abundance of AQP2 water

channels per cell in the collecting duct (53, 211), apparently due to increased transcription of the *AQP2* gene (Fig. 7).

Short-Term Regulation of AQP2 by Vasopressin-Induced Trafficking

The final concentration of the urine depends on the medullary osmotic gradient built up by the loop of Henle, and the water permeability of the collecting ducts through the cortex and medulla (see review [219]). Collecting duct water permeability is regulated by vasopressin, and it has been suspected for many years on the basis of indirect biophysical evidence that the vasopressin-induced increase in water permeability depended on the appearance of specific water channels in the apical plasma membrane of the vasopressin-responsive cells. Molecular actions of vasopressin to increase epithelial water permeability were first demonstrated in the 1950s and early 1960s in skin and urinary bladder of amphibia (100, 145). Direct demonstrations that vasopressin rapidly increases water permeability of isolated collecting ducts were made during the next few years (88, 200). These studies undertaken with in vitro preparations showed that vasopressin applied to the basolateral aspect of the collecting duct cells directly increased transepithelial water permeability within minutes. Kinetic studies in isolated perfused inner medullary collecting ducts revealed an increase in osmotic water permeability after only 40 seconds of incubation at 37°C, and half of the maximal water permeability was reached within 10 minutes (212, 293). cAMP has been implicated in the regulatory process, because direct application of cAMP analogues to the collecting duct was found to mimic the short-term effects of vasopressin (88).

Multiple studies with affinity-purified polyclonal antibodies to AQP2 have unequivocally established that AQP2 is specifically involved in the vasopressin-induced increases of renal collecting duct water permeability. Soon after isolation of the AQP2 cDNA and generation of specific antibodies (84), immunoperoxidase microscopy and immunoelectron microscopy clearly demonstrated that principle cells within renal collecting ducts contain abundant AQP2 in the apical plasma membranes and in subapical vesicles (53, 211). These studies strongly supported the "shuttle hypothesis" originally proposed more than a decade earlier (145). This hypothesis proposed that water channels can shuttle between an intracellular reservoir in subapical vesicles and the apical plasma membrane and that vasopressin alters water permeability by regulating the shuttling process (292). Shuttling of AQP2 was directly demonstrated in isolated perfused tubule studies (210). In these studies, water permeability of isolated perfused collecting ducts was measured before or after stimulation with vasopressin, and the tubules were fixed directly for immunoelectron microscopic examination (Fig. 6). Vasopressin stimulation resulted in a markedly decreased immunogold labeling of intracellular AQP2 accompanied by a fivefold increase in the appearance of AQP2 immunogold particles in the apical plasma membrane. This redistribution was associated with an increase in osmotic

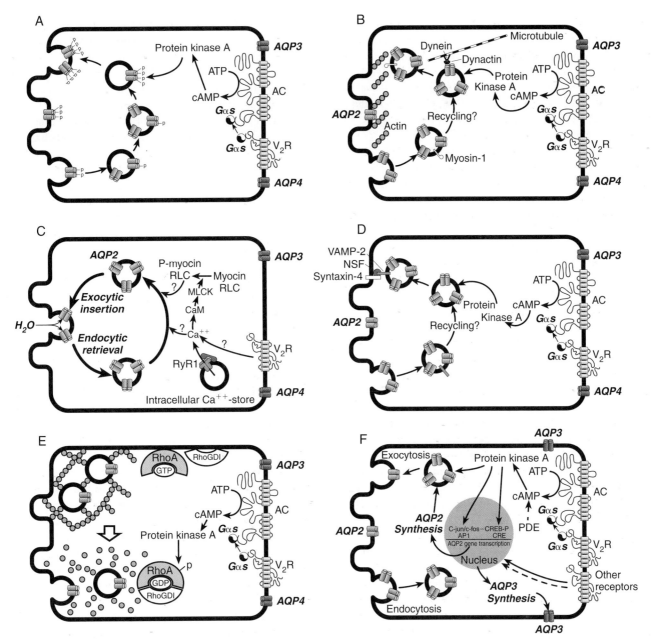

FIGURE 7 Regulation of aquaporin (AQP)2 trafficking (**A–E**) and expression (**F**) in collecting duct principle cells. **A:** Vasopressin binding to basolateral G-protein-linked V$_2$ receptor stimulates adenylyl cyclase (AC); cyclic adenosine monophosphate (cAMP) activates protein kinase A to phosphorylate AQP2 in intracellular vesicles; phosphorylated AQP2 is exocytosed to the apical plasma membrane, resulting in increased apical membrane water permeability. **B:** Overview of cytoskeletal elements, which may be involved in AQP2 trafficking. AQP2-containing vesicles may be transported along microtubules by dynein/dynactin. The cortical actin web may act as a barrier to fusion with the plasma membrane. **C:** Intracellular calcium signalling and AQP2 trafficking. Increases in intracellular Ca^{2+} concentration may arise from stimulation of the V$_2$ receptor. The existence and potential role of other receptors and pathways (e.g., VACM1) in Ca^{2+} mobilization is still uncertain. The downstream targets of the calcium signal are unknown and conflicting data exist on the importance of a rise in intracellular Ca^{2+} for the hydroosmotic response to vasopressin. **D:** Vesicle targeting receptors and AQP2 trafficking. AQP2 vesicles dock at the apical membrane by association of VAMP2 with syntaxin-4 targets in the presence of NSF. The role of these remains to be established. **E:** Changes in the actin cytoskeleton associated with AQP2 trafficking to the plasma membrane. Inactivation of RhoA by phosphorylation and increased formation of RhoARhoGDI complexes seem to control the dissociation of actin fibres seen after vasopressin stimulation. **F:** cAMP participates in the long-term regulation of AQP2 by increasing the levels of the catalytic subunit of PKA in the nuclei, which is thought to phosphorylate transcription factors such as CREB-P (cyclic AMP responsive element–binding protein) and C-Jun/c-Fos. Binding of these factors are thought to increase gene transcription of AQP2 resulting in synthesis of AQP2 protein, which in turn enters the regulated trafficking system. In parallel, AQP3 and AQP4 synthesis and trafficking to the basolateral plasma membrane takes place. Importantly AQP2 regulation can be modified by a number of hormones including dopamine, ANP, prostaglandin E2 (PGE2), and adrenergic hormones. See text for details. AC, adenylyl cyclase; cAMP, cyclic AMP; PKA, protein kinase A; V2R, vasopressin V$_2$ receptors. (From Nielsen S, Frokiar J, Marples D, Kwon TH, Agre P, Knepper MA. Aquaporins in the kidney: from molecules to medicine. *Physiol Rev* 2002;82:205–244, with permission.)

water permeability of similar magnitude. These findings were reproduced in vivo by injecting rats with vasopressin, which also caused redistribution of AQP2 to the plasma membrane of collecting duct principle cells (188, 246). In contrast to the effect of vasopressin treatment, removal of vasopressin led to a reappearance of AQP2 in intracellular vesicles and a decline in osmotic water permeability in the isolated perfused collecting duct system (Fig. 6) (210). Moreover, the offset response to vasopressin has been examined in vivo by acute treatment of rats with vasopressin-V_2 receptor antagonist (37, 99) or acute water loading (to reduce endogenous vasopressin levels [248]). These treatments (both reducing vasopressin action) resulted in a prominent internalization of AQP2 from the apical plasma membrane to intracellular subapical vesicles, further underscoring the role of AQP2 trafficking in the regulation of collecting duct water permeability and the reversibility of AQP2 trafficking to the plasma membrane.

The quantity of AQP2 in the apical plasma membrane is determined by the relative rates of exocytosis and endocytosis. Both processes occur continuously, and their relative rates are regulated to effect changes in water permeability. Kinetic evidence indicates that vasopressin regulates both endocytosis and exocytosis of apical water channels (140, 212). These conclusions are supported by multiple earlier experiments with fluid-phase markers, which assessed rates of internalization of the apical plasma membrane (24, 159, 268). Intravenous injection of horseradish peroxidase was followed by uptake of the material into intracellular vesicles and multivesicular bodies by collecting duct principle cells (24). When compared with normal rats, the rate of uptake by vasopressin-deficient Brattleboro rats was much lower; however, this difference was lost after administration of vasopressin, presumably reflecting an effect of vasopressin to accelerate exocytosis, followed by a secondary increase in the rate of endocytosis to reestablish the steady state. These observations were supported by studies with fluorescein-labeled dextrans (159), which confirmed that vasopressin enhances the rate of endocytosis of the apical plasma membrane under steady-state conditions. In apparent contrast, removal of vasopressin from isolated perfused rabbit cortical collecting ducts also was accompanied by increased endocytosis of horseradish peroxidase from the lumen, and it was suggested that water channels also would be internalized at an increased rate (268). Similar results were obtained in isolated rat inner medullary collecting duct, which showed that vasopressin washout was associated with increased appearance of albumin-gold or cationic ferritin in small apical vesicles and multivesicular bodies (215). Presumably this response reflects a direct effect of vasopressin to decrease the intrinsic rate of endocytosis and is reversed on vasopressin removal. Therefore it appears that two factors affect the rate of endocytosis of the apical plasma membrane of collecting duct principle cells: (1) vasopressin directly decelerates endocytosis by unknown mechanisms, and (2) vasopressin indirectly accelerates the rate of endocytosis by stimulating

exocytosis and increasing the total amount of apical plasma membrane. The latter effect is believed to be slower than the former, resulting in a biphasic decline in water permeability on vasopressin removal (140, 212). Other studies have demonstrated that apical endocytosis is most rapid at about 3 to 5 minutes after vasopressin washout from isolated perfused inner medullary collecting ducts (215), corresponding to the period of the most rapid decrease in transepithelial water permeability (140, 212). Thus these results strongly suggest that vasopressin directly regulates endocytosis and exocytosis of AQP2. Presumably the net increase in water permeability seen in response to vasopressin is due to direct stimulation of exocytosis and direct inhibition of endocytosis.

Several groups have now successfully reconstituted the AQP2 delivery system using cultured cells transfected with either wildtype AQP2 or AQP2 tagged with a marker protein or a fluorescent protein (48, 126–128, 281). The studies have recently been reviewed (78). Using such cultured cells stably transfected with AQP2, it has been shown that AQP2 trafficking occurs from vesicles to the plasma membrane, albeit in some cases to the basolateral membrane, as well as retrieval and subsequent trafficking back to the surface upon repeated stimulation. This recycling of AQP2 also occurs in LLC-PK1 cells in the continued presence of cycloheximide preventing de novo AQP2 synthesis. Despite remaining uncertainties, a working model for collecting duct water permeability permits molecular insight into this process (Fig. 7). The short-term effects of vasopressin-enhanced water permeability are explained by the redistribution of AQP2 to the apical plasma membrane in collecting duct principle cells. Acting through the V_2 receptor, vasopressin stimulates adenylyl cyclase; the elevated levels of intracellular cAMP activates protein kinase A (PKA), causing a redistribution of AQP2 from intracellular vesicles to the apical plasma membrane by inducing exocytosis of AQP2 vesicles and by inhibiting endocytosis of AQP2 from the apical membrane. The net increase of AQP2 in the apical plasma membrane increases the water permeability. In the preantidiuretic state, the apical membrane is the rate-limiting barrier for transepithelial water transport, because AQP3 and AQP4 are abundant in the basolateral plasma membrane. Thus increasing the water permeability of the apical plasma membrane by insertion of AQP2 water channels results in an increase in the transepithelial osmotic water permeability. Whereas the general model is now well established, the molecular details explaining how an elevation in intracellular cAMP levels regulates trafficking of AQP2 to the apical plasma membrane and back remain uncertain. Serine at position 256, in the carboxyl terminal tail of AQP2, is apparently a substrate for PKA, and regulation of exocytosis and endocytosis of AQP2 is expected to involve phosphorylation and dephosphorylation of AQP2 (127, 149, 157) and of ancillary proteins involved in the trafficking processes. This question will likely be a major focus of future research.

Signal Transduction Pathways Involved in Vasopressin Regulation of AQP2 Trafficking

The signal transduction pathways have been described thoroughly in previous reviews (139, 219). cAMP levels in collecting duct principle cells are increased by binding of vasopressin to V_2 receptors (60, 148). The synthesis of cAMP by adenylate cyclase is stimulated by a V_2-receptor–coupled heterotrimeric GTP-binding protein, G_s. G_s interconverts between an inactive GDP-bound form and an active GTP-bound form, and the vasopressin-V_2–receptor complex catalyzes the exchange of GTP for bound GDP on the α subunit of G_s. This causes release of the α subunit, $G_s\alpha$-GTP, which subsequently binds to adenylate cyclase thereby increasing cAMP production. PKA is a multimeric protein that is activated by cAMP and consists in its inactive state of two catalytic subunits and two regulatory subunits. When cAMP binds to the regulatory subunits, these dissociate from the catalytic subunits, resulting in activation of the kinase activity of the catalytic subunits.

AQP2 contains a consensus site for PKA phosphorylation (RRQS) in the cytoplasmic COOH terminus at Ser256 (84). Studies using ^{32}P labeling or using an antibody specific for phosphorylated AQP2 showed a very rapid phosphorylation of AQP2 (within 1 minute) in response to vasopressin treatment of slices of the kidney papilla (221). This is compatible with the time course of vasopressin-stimulated water permeability of kidney collecting ducts (293). As described previously, PKA-induced phosphorylation of AQP2 apparently does not change the water conductance of AQP2 significantly. Importantly, it was demonstrated that vasopressin or forskolin treatment failed to induce translocation of AQP2 when Ser256 was substituted by an alanine (S256A) in contrast to a significant regulated trafficking of wildtype AQP2 in LLC-PK1 cells (127). A parallel study by Sasaki and colleagues demonstrated the lack of cAMP-mediated exocytosis of mutated (S256A) AQP2 transfected into LLC-PK1 cells (83). Thus, these studies indicate a specific role of PKA-induced phosphorylation of AQP2 for regulated trafficking. To explore this further an antibody was designed that exclusively recognizes AQP2 that is phosphorylated in the PKA consensus site (serine 256). In normal rats phosphorylated AQP2 is present in intracellular vesicles and apical plasma membranes, whereas in Brattleboro rats phosphorylated AQP2 is mainly located in intracellular vesicles as shown by immunocytochemistry and immunoblotting using membrane fractionation (36). Importantly, dDAVP treatment of Brattleboro rats caused a marked redistribution of phosphorylated AQP2 to the apical plasma membrane, which is in agreement with an important role of PKA phosphorylation in this trafficking (36). Conversely, treatment with V_2-receptor antagonist induced a marked decrease in the abundance of phosphorylated AQP2 (36) likely due to reduced PKA activity and/or increased dephosphorylation of AQP2 (e.g., by increased phosphatase activity). Moreover, the necessity for the Ser256 phosphorylation in the AQP2-regulated urine concentration is underlined by the recent identification of this

site as being spontaneously mutated in congenital progressive hydronephrosis (CPH) (194). The spontaneous conversion of the serine phospho site to leucine in the cytoplasmic tail of the AQP2 protein in CPH mice prevents its phosphorylation at Ser256 and inhibits the subsequent accumulation of AQP2 on the apical membrane of the collecting duct principle cells. This causes polydipsia, polyuria, and severe urinary concentration defect leading to hydronephrosis and obstructive nephropathy in these mice. Three previously unknown phosphorylation sites in the C terminus of AQP2 was identified (S261, S264, and S269) using liquid chromatography coupled with mass spectrometry neutral loss scanning (103). During basal conditions, AQP2 phosphorylated on Ser261 is approximately 24-fold more abundant than Ser256-phosphorylated AQP2. During administration of dDAVP a striking decrease in Ser261 phosphorylation was observed, while AQP2 phosphorylated on both Ser256 and Ser261 as well as Ser256 phosphorylated AQP2 increased (103).

Prostaglandin E2 (PGE2) has been known to inhibit vasopressin-induced water permeability by reducing cAMP levels. Zelenina et al. (319) investigated the effect of PGE_2 on PKA phosphorylation of AQP2 in rat kidney papilla and the results suggest that the action of prostaglandins are associated with retrieval of AQP2 from the plasma membrane, but that this appears to be independent of AQP2 phosphorylation by PKA (319).

Phosphorylation of AQP2 by other kinases (e.g., protein kinase C or casein kinase II) may potentially participate in regulation of AQP2 trafficking. Angiotensin II–induced activation of protein kinase C could be, at least in part, involved in the AQP2 trafficking/expression (154). Phosphorylation of other cytoplasmic or vesicular regulatory proteins may also be involved. These issues remain to be investigated directly.

Involvement of the Cytoskeleton and Ca^{2+} in AQP2 Trafficking

The cytoskeleton has been shown to be involved in the AQP2 trafficking in kidney collecting duct. In particular, the microtubular network has been implicated in this process, since chemical disruption of microtubules inhibits the increase in permeability both in the toad bladder and in the mammalian collecting duct (230, 231). Thus, AQP2 vesicles may be transported along microtubules on their ways to the apical plasma membrane. The microtubule based motor protein dynein and the associated protein Arp1, which is part of the protein complex dynactin, was found by immunoblotting to be among the proteins associated with AQP2 vesicles from rat inner medulla. Immunoelectron microscopy further supported the presence of both AQP2 and dynein on the same vesicles (189). Moreover, both vanadate (nonspecific inhibitor of ATPases) and EHNA (specific inhibitor of dynein) inhibit the antidiuretic response in toad bladder (45, 185) and kidney collecting duct (255). Thus, it is likely that dynein may drive the microtubule-dependent delivery of AQP2-containing vesicles to the apical plasma membrane.

Actin filaments are also involved in the hydrosmotic response (52, 54, 123, 205, 228, 290). Evidence was provided that the myosin light chain kinase (MLCK) pathway, through calmodulin-mediated calcium activation of MLCK, leads to phosphorylation of myosin regulatory light chain and non–muscle myosin 2 motor activity (34). Studies in isolated perfused rat IMCDs showed the MLCK-inhibitors ML-7 and ML-9 reduce the vasopressin-induced increase in water permeability (34), indicating that MLCK may be a downstream target for the vasopressin-induced Ca^{2+} signal.

The intracellular Ca^{2+} concentration has been shown to increase on stimulation of isolated perfused rat IMCDs with vasopressin or dDAVP (267). These observations have been followed by a number of studies of the role of Ca^{2+} in the vasopressin-induced increase in water permeability. Vasopressin or 8-4-chlorophenylthio–cAMP induced a marked increase in intracellular $[Ca^{2+}]$ in isolated perfused IMCD, and BABTA blocked the rise in intracellular $[Ca^{2+}]$ and cocontaminantly led to inhibition of the vasopressin-induced increase in tubular water permeability (33). Moreover blocking calmodulin with W7 or trifluoperazine also inhibited the effect of vasopressin on tubular water permeability and inhibited the vasopressin-induced AQP2 plasma membrane targeting in primary cultured IMCD cells (33). Removing Ca^{2+} from both bath and lumen in isolated perfused tubules did not affect the vasopressin-induced Ca^{2+} signal, indicating that Ca^{2+} was released from an intracellular source. This was further supported by the observations that ryanodine inhibited the Ca^{2+} signal in perfused IMCDs and inhibited AQP2 accumulation in the plasma membrane in primary cultured IMCD cells. In addition, RyR1 ryanodine receptor was localized to rat IMCD by immunohistochemistry (33). Ryanodine receptors are generally known to mediate a positive feedback and release Ca^{2+} from intracellular stores in response to an initial rise in intracellular $[Ca^{2+}]$. Thus, it is likely that another mechanism is responsible for the initialization of the rise in intracellular $[Ca^{2+}]$. Further studies revealed that vasopressin or dDAVP elicited oscillations in intracellular $[Ca^{2+}]$ in isolated perfused rat IMCDs (314). The results on isolated perfused IMCDs indicate that an intracellular increase in $[Ca^{2+}]$ is an obligate component of the vasopressin response leading to increased AQP2 expression in the apical plasma membrane. However, there is a discrepancy between the results from primary cultured IMCD cells (168) and isolated perfused IMCD tubules (33) with regard to the role of intracellular $[Ca^{2+}]$ in vasopressin-induced AQP2 trafficking. Consistent with this, Lorenz et al. (168) demonstrated that AQP2 shuttling is evoked neither by AVP-dependent increase of $[Ca^{2+}]$ nor AVP-independent increase of $[Ca^{2+}]$ in primary cultured IMCDs cells from rat kidney, although clamping of intracellular $[Ca^{2+}]$ below resting levels inhibits AQP2 exocytosis. Further studies are required to clarify this discrepancy, which may be related to altered expression levels of vasopressin receptors and/or AQP2, or other elements in the AQP2 trafficking system.

Mechanism of AQP2 Trafficking by Targeting Receptors

The mechanism by which AQP2 vesicles are targeted to the apical plasma membrane and the mechanism by which cAMP controls docking and fusion of vesicles is a current area of active investigation. Considerable insight into this problem has been obtained from studies of regulated exocytosis of synaptic vesicles, which involve the actions of multiple proteins (14, 263). Vesicle-targeting receptors (often referred to as "SNAREs") are believed to induce specific interaction of vesicles with membrane sites. Vesicle-targeting receptors associated chiefly with translocating vesicles are known as "VAMPs" (vesicle-associated membrane proteins, also referred to as synaptobrevins) and "synaptotagmins." Two other families of membrane proteins are believed to serve as receptors in target membranes: the "syntaxins" and SNAP-25 homologues. Several of these SNAREs have been found in renal collecting ducts (76, 95, 109, 138, 164, 180, 181, 214).

Syntaxins are 30–40-kD integral membrane proteins. Syntaxins have a one-bilayer–spanning domain near the C-terminus, so the majority of the protein resides in the cytoplasm. Syntaxins are widely distributed among mammalian tissues. It has been established that syntaxin-4 is expressed in the mammalian collecting duct by studies using polyclonal antibodies raised to conjugated peptides specific for individual syntaxins, and this has been confirmed by reverse transcription–polymerase chain reaction (180). Immunolocalization studies have demonstrated that syntaxin-4 is predominantly located in the apical plasma membrane of collecting duct principle cells, where AQP2 is targeted in response to vasopressin.

VAMPs are believed to induce specific docking of vesicles by interacting directly with syntaxins in the target plasma membrane (Fig. 7). Although their primary amino acid sequences are not related to syntaxins, VAMPs also have a single-bilayer–spanning domain near the C-terminus, and most of the protein resides in the cytoplasm. Three VAMP isoforms were initially identified (269): VAMP-1, VAMP-2, and VAMP-3 (also referred to as "cellubrevin"), and subsequently several additional homologues have been cloned (2). VAMP-2 and VAMP-3 have been localized in principle cells of renal collecting duct (76, 95, 109, 138, 164, 180, 181, 214). Double-labeling immunoelectron microscopy revealed that AQP2 and VAMP-2 reside in the same intracellular vesicles in collecting duct principle cells (214). Furthermore, AQP2 vesicles isolated by differential centrifugation were found to contain VAMP-2 (95, 164).

At this time, several putative vesicle-targeting proteins are known to reside in collecting duct principle cells. VAMP-2 resides in AQP2 intracellular vesicles, and syntaxin-4 resides in the apical plasma membrane. In vitro binding assays have documented that VAMP-2 binds syntaxin-4 with high affinity, but VAMP-2 has not been shown to interact with syntaxin-3 or syntaxin-2 (26, 229). Thus VAMP-2 and syntaxin-4 are likely participants in the targeting of AQP2 vesicles to the apical plasma membrane; however, a functional role for these targeting proteins remains to be formally demonstrated. A third SNARE protein, SNAP-23, has also been identified in principle cells of the collecting duct (109). Although considered a target-membrane SNARE (t-SNARE), SNAP-23 is present in AQP2-containing vesicles and in the apical plasma membrane of principle cells. VAMP-2, syntaxin-4, and SNAP-23 may potentially form a complex with the N-ethylmaleimide–sensitive factor (NSF). Finally, synaptotagmin VIII, a calcium-insensitive homologue, was identified in collecting duct principle cells (138) and may potentially play a role in vesicle targeting.

Recently, LC-MS/MS–based proteomic analysis of immunoisolated AQP2-containing intracellular vesicles from rat IMCD revealed that AQP2-containing vesicles are heterogeneous and that intracellular AQP2 resides chiefly in endosomes, trans-Golgi network, and rough endoplasmic reticulum (15). Vasopressin-stimulated exocytosis of AQP2 vesicles involves several steps including (1) translocation of vesicles from a diffuse distribution throughout the cell to the apical region of the cell, (2) translocation of AQP2 across the apical part of the cell composed of a dense filamentous actin network, (3) priming of vesicles for docking, (4) docking of vesicles, and (5) fusion of vesicles with the apical plasma membrane. Theoretically, each of these steps could be targeted for regulation by vasopressin. If the SNARE proteins are involved in the vasopressin-induced trafficking of AQP2 to the apical plasma membrane, the regulatory mechanism might involve selective phosphorylation of one of the SNARE proteins or an ancillary protein that binds to them, possibly via PKA or calmodulin-dependent kinase II. Although the SNARE proteins are recognized as potential targets for phosphorylation (74, 241, 257), there is no evidence for the phosphorylation in the collecting duct. As noted previously, however, AQP2 appears to be a target for PKA-mediated phosphorylation at a serine in position 256 (149). The phosphorylation does not modify the single-channel water permeability of AQP2 (157) and instead the phosphorylation is believed to play a critical role in regulation of AQP2 trafficking to the plasma membrane (83, 127). The establishment of a role for these SNARE proteins in regulated trafficking of AQP2 will most likely depend on the preparation of targeted knockouts for each of these genes in the collecting duct.

Long-Term Regulation of Aquaporin Expression

It has been known for more than 40 years that urinary concentrating ability is regulated through a long-term conditioning effect of sustained increases in vasopressin levels exerted over a period of days (120). The physiological and molecular basis for long-term conditioning of urinary concentrating ability is still being investigated. Water restriction causes a large, stable increase in water permeability of IMCDs dissected from rat kidneys and perfused in vitro (158). Thus water permeability of the tubules from water-restricted rats became fivefold greater than that measured in

well-hydrated rats by a mechanism independent of the short-term action of vasopressin. Other studies confirmed that water restriction enhances the vasopressin-independent water permeability of collecting ducts (91, 291) and increases vasopressin-stimulated water permeability (72). This contrasts with the lack of an observed increase in urea permeability in water-restricted rats (158). These studies provided the firm conclusion that restriction of water intake for 24 hours or longer leads to marked increase in the water-reabsorbing capacity of the renal collecting duct epithelium.

Further studies with antipeptide antibodies have documented that the conditioned increase in water permeability is associated with increased expression of aquaporin proteins in collecting duct principle cells. Specifically, the increased water permeability that occurs in response to water restriction is accompanied by significant increases in the levels of AQP2 and AQP3 proteins in rat collecting ducts (58, 211, 212). Water restriction for 24 to 48 hours resulted in an approximately fivefold increase in AQP2 protein in the rat renal inner medulla when measured by immunoblotting (211, 212) and by immunostaining (99). This increase paralleled the increase in water permeability in response to water restriction (158).

A direct role for vasopressin in AQP2 expression has been established by multiple studies. Continuous infusion of arginine vasopressin into Brattleboro rats for 5 days resulted in a threefold increase in AQP2 expression and a threefold increase in water permeability of IMCDs (53). When the time course of AQP2 expression in inner medullary collecting duct was studied, it was found that 5 days of vasopressin infusion was required to reach maximal AQP2 levels in Brattleboro rats (137).

Vasopressin is believed to be essential for evoking AQP2 expression, because Brattleboro rats totally lack circulating vasopressin and fail to exhibit increased expression of AQP2 protein after long-term water restriction (31). Moreover, administration of a selective V_2-receptor antagonist blocked the increase in AQP2 expression normally seen with thirsting in normal rats (99), whereas administration of the V_2-selective agonist dDAVP to rats elicited a large increase in renal AQP2 mRNA (82) and AQP2 protein abundance (57). The question of hyperosmolar induction of AQP2 during thirsting has been raised; however, 5-day infusion of arginine vasopressin increased AQP2 comparably in renal cortex and medulla. This indicates that the vasopressin-induced expression of AQP2 is not critically dependent on increased osmolality or ionic strength in the tissue surrounding the collecting ducts (276). Thus it has been clearly established that the major increase in AQP2 water channel expression elicited by restriction of water intake is due to vasopressin binding to the V_2 receptor in collecting duct principle cells. However, studies of the mechanism of escape from the antidiuretic effects of vasopressin (56, 57) makes it clear that AQP2 expression is regulated by other factors in addition to vasopressin (see later).

AQP3 protein expression also has been found to parallel AQP2 expression. A marked increase in AQP3 protein expression was observed in rats in response to restriction of water intake (58) and after a 5-day infusion of arginine vaso-pressin (276). These conditions did not lead to observed changes in AQP1 or AQP4 protein expression (275, 276). Thus it is concluded that long-term circulation of high vaso-pressin levels is associated with an adaptive increase in maximal water permeability in collecting ducts, apparently due a selective increase in the expression of both AQP2 and AQP3 in the principle cells of the collecting duct.

The adaptive changes in AQP2 and AQP3 expression are believed to be due to transcriptional regulation of these genes. Increased AQP2 mRNA was found in the inner medullas of water-restricted rats (171) and in response to infusion of dDAVP (57, 82). All of these studies indicate that the long-term upregulation of AQP2 expression in the rat kidney is due to elevation of the levels of AQP2 mRNA. Vasopressin-induced increase in AQP2 mRNA expression could reflect either increased gene transcription or reduced transcript degradation. Examination of the 3′-untranslated region of the AQP2 mRNA has not revealed the presence of recognizable mRNA stabilization motifs, and it is presumed that vasopressin directly increases *AQP2* gene transcription; however, no direct evidence supports this presumption. Transcriptional regulation would most likely occur through the vasopressin-induced increases in intracellular cyclic AMP that activates protein kinase A in collecting duct cells. Examination of the 5′-flanking region of the *AQP2* gene revealed a putative cAMP-response element (CRE), which may play a role in the vasopressin-induced increase in AQP2 expression (280). Attempts to demonstrate expression of AQP2 promoter-luciferase reporter constructs have been undertaken in cultured renal epithelial cells and suggest that the putative CRE can drive increased expression of the *AQP2* gene; however, the inability of the cell line to express AQP2 protein limits the interpretation (105, 191, 312).

As with AQP2, AQP3 mRNA levels were induced by infusion with the selective V_2-agonist dDAVP (57). Examination of the 5′-flanking DNA of AQP3 failed to reveal a CRE; however, Sp1 and AP2 cis-regulatory elements are present (108), and these are known to be associated with cyclic AMP-mediated transcriptional regulation of other genes.

DYSREGULATION OF RENAL AQUAPORINS IN WATER BALANCE DISORDERS

In a variety of conditions renal water handling is disturbed. Over the past decade, the role of changes in the expression and/or function of aquaporins has been investigated in a range of these conditions, including genetic defects or acquired defects showing a decreased renal responsiveness to vasopressin (acquired nephrogenic diabetes insipidus). The importance of aquaporins playing an essential role for regulation of renal water balance has been established (Table 2) and the following represents extracted and updated information reported in previous reviews by the authors or other investigators (9, 213, 219, 242).

URINARY CONCENTRATING DEFECTS

Inherited Diabetes Insipidus

There are two significant inherited forms of diabetes insipidus (DI): central and nephrogenic. In central (or neurogenic) DI, there is a defect of vasopressin production. Central DI (CDI) is rarely hereditary in humans, but usually occurring as a consequence of head trauma or diseases in the hypothalamus or pituitary gland. The Brattleboro rat provides an excellent model of this condition. These animals have a total or near-total lack of vasopressin production (251). Consequently, Brattleboro rats have substantially decreased expression levels of vasopressin-regulated AQP2 compared with the parent strain (Long Evans), and the AQP2 deficit was reversed by chronic vasopressin infusion, suggesting that patients lacking vasopressin are likely to have decreased AQP2 expression (53). The subsequent work showing that expression of AQP3 is also regulated by vasopressin implies that the expression levels of these water channels will also be decreased in patients with CDI. The most important denominator is the deficiency of AQP2 trafficking to the apical membrane. These deficits are likely to be the most important causes of the polyuria from which these patients suffer, which will be reversed by the desmopressin treatment. The second form of DI is called nephrogenic DI (NDI), and is caused by the inability of the kidney to respond to vasopressin stimulation. The most commonly hereditary cause (95% of the cases) is an X-linked disorder associated with mutations of the V_2-vasopressin receptor making the collecting duct cells insensitive to vasopressin (19). Although there is no direct evidence, it is likely that this form of NDI will be associated with decreased expression of AQP2, since the cells are unable to respond to circulating vasopressin. This will compound the lack of AQP2 trafficking. Consistent with this, urinary AQP2 levels are very low in patients with X-linked NDI (47, 125). However, since the amount of AQP2 in the urine appears to be determined largely by the response of the collecting duct cells to vasopressin (299) rather than their content of AQP2, the data must be interpreted with caution with respect to predicting AQP2 expression levels. More rarely (5% of the cases), congenital diabetes insipidus (CNDI) is inherited in an autosomal recessive fashion which is not due to mutations in the gene encoding the V_2 vasopressin receptor, but these patients have been found to possess mutations in alleles of the *AQP2* gene, and the sites of point mutations were observed at functionally important sites in the water transport pathway (49, 203, 223, 286). Since these patients manifest a particularly severe form of DI, the critical role of AQP2 in renal water conservation was established. It is believed that these mutations lead to abnormal intracellular routing of the expressed protein (46). More than 155 mutations in the vasopressin receptor gene have been recognized to cause CNDI. Functional analysis has been carried out for over 79 (199) of these mutations (199). The analyses have revealed four types of mutant receptors. The most common being impaired intracellular trafficking, which is seen in up to 70% of cases (199). The remaining types include reduced ligand binding capacity, failure to generate cAMP, and defects in the synthesis of stable mRNA (142). Of the 155 known mutations, only five cause partial CNDI (D85N, R104C, G201D, P322S, and S329R). A different kindred was identified with a dominant form of NDI, and biochemical evaluations revealed that the mutation in the cytoplasmic C-terminus block the trafficking of AQP2 vesicles to the cell surface (202). Thus, intracellular trafficking of vesicles containing products of the mutant allele and the product of the normal allele may be misdirected. It is not known if these individuals suffer a more or less severe clinical defect.

Acquired Nephrogenic Diabetes Insipidus

Acquired abnormalities of AQP2 expression has been implicated in multiple clinical disorders associated with abnormal water balance (Table 2). The role of vasopressin-regulated AQP2 has been established in a number of rat models with acquired NDI. In many of these conditions the kidney is unable to handle water due to an impaired responsiveness to vasopressin and in the following the most important of these conditions are described.

Lithium-Induced NDI

Lithium is a major therapeutic agent used to treat bipolar disorder (also referred to as "manic depressive disease"), which affects approximately 1% of the U.S. population (277). However, lithium treatment is associated with a variety of renal side effects including (i.e., a pronounced vasopressin-resistant polyuria and inability to concentrate urine) (153, 186), increased urinary sodium excretion (39), and distal renal tubular acidosis (131). Patients who have been treated with lithium manifest a slow recovery of urinary concentrating ability when treatment is discontinued. In rats treated with lithium for 4 weeks, AQP2 and AQP3 levels were progressively reduced to approximately 5% of levels in control rats (153, 186). AQP2 downregulation was paralleled by a progressive development of severe polyuria (153, 186). Quantitative immunoelectron microscopy of AQP2 labeling in the inner IMCD principle cells showed that there was a reduction of AQP2 in the apical plasma membrane, basolateral plasma membrane, and intracellular vesicles. Reduction in AQP2 (and AQP3) expression may be induced by a lithium-dependent impairment in the production of cAMP in collecting duct principle cells (39), indicating that inhibition of cAMP production may in part be responsible for the reduction in AQP2 expression as well as the inhibition of targeting to the plasma membrane in response to lithium treatment. This is consistent with the presence of a cAMP-responsive element in the 5′-untranslated region of the *AQP2* gene (105, 191) and with the demonstration that mice with inherently low cAMP levels have low expression of AQP2 (DI$^{+/+}$ severe mouse) (81). Lithium treatment is also associated with a concomitant increase in

urinary sodium excretion, which is likely to play a role in polyuria. A study demonstrated that chronic lithium treatment induces a marked decrease in protein abundance of epithelial sodium channel β- and γENaC in the cortex and outer medulla, whereas the other renal sodium transporters upstream from the connecting tubule are unchanged (209). This was also revealed by immunocytochemistry showing an almost complete absence of βENaC and γENaC labeling in cortical and outer medullary collecting duct. This suggests a reduced responsiveness to aldosterone and vasopressin in these specific renal tubule segments and that dysregulation of ENaC subunits is likely to play a role in the development of natriuresis and partly in the decreased urinary concentrating ability in rats with lithium-induced NDI.

Hypokalemia and Hypercalcemia

Hypokalemia and hypercalcemia are also associated with polyuria due to a vasopressin-resistant urinary concentrating defect. Rat models of these conditions are valuable tools to study the molecular defects. Treating rats with a potassium-deficient diet for 4 days induced a significant hypokalemia that was associated with downregulation of AQP2 expression and polyuria (187). Likewise hypercalcemia induced in rats by orally treatment for 7 days with dihydrotachysterol produced a urinary concentrating defect and polyuria that was also associated with downregulation of AQP2 (55, 249). Thus, both hypokalemia and hypercalcemia are associated with downregulation of AQP2 expression and immunolocalization studies of AQP2 demonstrated similar features In addition to the downregulation of AQP2, expression of Na-K-2Cl cotransporter in the thick ascending limb was decreased in both conditions (61, 298), suggesting that reduced sodium and chloride reabsorption in the thick ascending limb and hence decreased medullary hyperosmolality could also partly contribute to the polyuria and decreased urinary concentration in hypokalemia and hypercalcemia. Thus, these studies in part describe the underlying molecular defects involved in the development of the polyuria in these conditions.

Urinary Tract Obstruction

Another serious condition seen in both children and adults is urinary tract obstruction, which is associated with complex changes in renal function involving marked alterations in both glomerular and tubular function and bilateral urinary tract obstruction (BUO) may result in long-term impairment in the ability to concentrate urine (316). BUO for 24 hours in rats is associated with markedly reduced expression of AQP2, -3, -4, and -1 (80, 129, 162). In addition, BUO is associated with marked downregulation of key sodium transporters and urea transporters (161). Following release of the obstruction, there is a marked polyuria during which AQP2 and AQP3 levels remain downregulated up to 2 weeks after release providing an explanation at the molecular level for the observed postobstructive polyuria. In a number of studies, BUO has been demonstrated to be associated with COX2 induction and cellular infiltration of the renal medulla (30, 222). Using specific COX2 inhibition to rats subjected to BUO it was demonstrated that this treatment prevents downregulation of AQP2 and several sodium transporters located at the proximal tubule and mTAL (30, 222). Moreover, specific inhibition of the AT1 receptor to rats subjected to BUO prevented downregulation of NaPi2 in the PT, BSC1 in the mTAL and AQP2 in the CD 3 days after release of BUO (117), confirming that the renin-angiotensin system plays an important role for the pathophysiological changes in urinary tract obstruction.

In contrast to BUO conditions, unilateral ureteral obstruction is not associated with changes in the absolute excretion of sodium and water since the nonobstructed kidney compensates for the reduced ability of the obstructed kidney to excrete solutes (79, 161). These studies demonstrated a profound downregulation of AQP1, -2, -3, and -4 and pAQP2 levels in the obstructed kidney, suggesting that local factors play a major role.

Renal Failure

Renal failure, both acute and chronic, is associated with polyuria and a urinary concentrating defect and in both cases there is a wide range of glomerular and tubular abnormalities that contribute to the overall renal dysfunction. Ischemia and reperfusion (I/R)–induced experimental acute renal failure (ARF) in rats is a model that is widely used. In this model there are structural alterations in renal tubule, in association with an impaired urinary concentration.

ARF is associated with defects in collecting duct water and proximal tubule water reabsorption and defects in solute handling (92, 273, 287). Using the isolated tubule microperfusion model, it was demonstrated that water reabsorption in the proximal tubule and cortical collecting duct was significantly reduced following ischemia (92) and no differences in either basal or vasopressin-induced cAMP levels in outer or inner medulla in rats with ARF were demonstrated (10), supporting the view that there are defects in collecting duct water reabsorption. Consistent with these findings, it was demonstrated that AQP2 and AQP3 expression in the collecting duct as well as AQP1 expression in the proximal tubule are significantly reduced in response to ARF (66, 151). The decreased levels of aquaporins were associated with impaired urinary concentration in rats with oliguric or nonoliguric ARF. The reduced expression of AQP1, AQP2, and AQP3 and the reduced urinary concentration capacity was significantly prevented by co-treatment with alpha-melanocyte-stimulating hormone (α-MSH), which is an anti-inflammatory cytokine that inhibits both neutrophil and nitric oxide pathways (151). This finding indicates that decreased levels of aquaporins in the proximal tubule and collecting duct in postischemic kidneys may play a significant role in the impaired urinary concentration. It was also demonstrated that hemorrhagic shock-

induced ARF is associated with decreased expression of collecting duct water channel AQP2 and AQP3 (87) and that erythropoietin treatment (single or combined with α-MSH) in rats with I/R-induced ARF, which is known to prevent caspase-3, -8, and -9 activation in vivo and reduces apoptotic cell death (254), prevents or reduces the urinary concentrating defects and downregulation of AQPs expression levels (87). Patients with advanced chronic renal failure (CRF) have urine that remains hypotonic to plasma despite the administration of supramaximal doses of vasopressin (272). This vasopressin-resistant hyposthenuria specifically implies abnormalities in collecting duct water reabsorption in patients with CRF. Recent observations demonstrated virtual absence of V_2-receptor mRNA in the inner medulla of CRF rat kidneys (274) providing evidence for significant defects in the collecting duct water permeability. Consistent with these observations, it has shown both decreased collecting duct water channel AQP2 and AQP3 expression and a vasopressin-resistant downregulation of AQP2 in a 5/6 nephrectomy-induced CRF rat model (152).

WATER RETENTION

Congestive Heart Failure

Retention of sodium and water is a common and clinically important complication of congestive heart failure (CHF). Two studies have examined the changes in renal AQP expression in rats with CHF induced by ligation of the left coronary artery (218, 303) to test if upregulation of AQP2 expression and targeting may play a role in the water retention in CHF. Both studies demonstrated that renal water retention in severe CHF in rats is associated with dysregulation of AQP2 in the renal collecting duct principle cells involving both an increase in the AQP2 expression and a marked redistribution of AQP2 to the apical plasma membrane (218, 303). Rats with severe CHF had significantly elevated left ventricular end-diastolic pressures (LVEDPs) and had reduced plasma sodium concentrations (218). Immunoblotting revealed a threefold increase in AQP2 expression compared with sham-operated animals. These changes were associated with elevated LVEDP or hyponatremia, since animals with normal LVEDP and plasma sodium levels did not have increased AQP2 levels compared with sham-operated controls (218). Furthermore, this study showed an increased plasma membrane targeting, providing an explanation for the increased permeability of the collecting duct and an increase in water reabsorption. This may provide an explanation for excess free-water retention in severe CHF and the development of hyponatremia. In parallel, the other study showed upregulation of AQP2 protein and AQP2 mRNA levels in kidney inner medulla and cortex in rats with CHF (303). These rats had significantly decreased cardiac output and, importantly, increased plasma vasopressin levels. Furthermore, in this study administration of V$_2$-antagonist OPC 31260 was associated with a significant increase in diuresis, a decrease in urine osmolality, a rise in plasma osmolality, and a significant reduction in AQP2 protein and AQP2 mRNA levels compared with untreated rats with CHF. Consistent with this, treatment of V$_2$-receptor antagonist in human patients with heart failure is associated with a dose-related increase in water excretion and a decrease in urinary AQP2 excretion (190).

Hepatic Cirrhosis

Hepatic cirrhosis is another chronic condition associated with water retention. It has been suggested that an important pathophysiological factor in the impaired ability to excrete water could be increased levels of plasma vasopressin. However, unlike CHF, the changes in expression of AQP2 protein levels vary considerably between different experimental models of hepatic cirrhosis. Several studies have examined the changes in renal AQP expression in rats with cirrhosis induced by common bile duct ligation (CBDL) (68, 118, 119). The rats displayed impaired vasopressin-regulated water reabsorption despite normal plasma vasopressin levels. Consistent with this, semiquantitative immunoblotting showed a significant decrease in AQP2 expression in rats with hepatic cirrhosis (68, 118). In addition, the expression levels of AQP3 and AQP4 were downregulated in CBDL rats. This may predict a reduced water permeability of the collecting duct in this model (68), hence renal water reabsorption in the collecting duct is decreased in rats with compensated liver cirrhosis. In contrast, Fujita et al. (82) demonstrated that hepatic cirrhosis induced by intraperitoneal administration of carbon tetrachloride (CCl$_4$) was associated with a significant increase in AQP2 protein levels and AQP2 mRNA expression. Interestingly, AQP2 mRNA expression correlated with the amount of ascites, suggesting that AQP2 may play a role in the abnormal water retention followed by the development of ascites in hepatic cirrhosis (12). In a different model of CCl$_4$-induced cirrhosis, using CCl$_4$ inhalation, AQP2 expression was not increased (67). There was, however, evidence for increased trafficking of AQP2 to the plasma membrane, consistent with the presence of elevated levels of vasopressin in the plasma. Interestingly, there was a marked increase in AQP3 expression that is likely due to increased vasopressin levels. The pattern of increased AQP3 expression without upregulation of AQP2 is consistent with previous findings observed in the vasopressin escape (56), suggesting that the lack of increase in AQP2 expression could be a result of a normal compensatory response related to the escape phenomenon. Although the explanation for the differences between cirrhosis induced by CBDL and CCl$_4$ administration remains to be determined, it is well known that the dysregulation of body water balance depends on the severity of cirrhosis (85, 130, 302). CBDL results in a compensated cirrhosis characterized by peripheral vasodilation and increased cardiac output, whereas cirrhosis induced by 12 weeks of CCl$_4$ administration may be associated with the late state of decompensated liver cirrhosis char-

acterized by sodium retention, edema, and ascites (85, 130, 160). Thus the downregulation of AQP2 observed in milder forms of cirrhosis (i.e., in a compensated stage without water retention) may represent a compensatory mechanism to prevent development of water retention. In contrast, the increased levels of vasopressin seen in severe "noncompensated" cirrhosis with ascites may induce an inappropriate upregulation of AQP2 that would in turn participate in the development of water retention.

Experimental Nephrotic Syndrome

The nephrotic syndrome is characterized by extracellular volume expansion with excessive renal salt and water reabsorption. The underlying mechanisms of salt and water retention are poorly understood; however, they can be expected to be associated with dysregulation of solute transporters and water channels (130). In contrast to CHF and liver cirrhosis, a marked downregulation of AQP2 and AQP3 expression was demonstrated in rats with PAN-induced and adriamycin-induced nephrotic syndromes (11, 64, 65). The reduced expression of collecting duct water channels could represent a physiologically appropriate response to extracellular volume expansion. The signal transduction involved in this process is not clear, but circulating vasopressin levels are high in rats with PAN-induced nephrotic syndrome. Thus, the marked downregulation of AQP2 in experimental nephrotic syndrome may share similarities with the downregulation of AQP2 in water-loaded dDAVP-treated rats that escape from the action of vasopressin (56, 57).

Syndrome of Inappropriate Antidiuretic Hormone Secretion and Vasopressin Escape

Hyponatremia, defined as a serum sodium less than 135 mmol/l, is one of the most commonly encountered electrolyte disorders of clinical medicine (73). The predominant cause of hyponatremia is an inappropriate secretion of vasopressin relative to serum osmolality or the "syndrome of inappropriate antidiuretic hormone secretion" (SIADH) (16). SIADH occurs most frequently in association with vascular, infectious, or neoplastic abnormalities in the lung or central nervous system. In an experimental rat model of SIADH, it was shown that AQP2 mRNA expression and AQP2 protein expression were increased in the collecting duct (82). Thus, increased expression of AQP2 in the collecting duct accounts for the water retention and hyponatremia in SIADH.

The degree of the hyponatremia is limited by a process that counters the water retaining action of vasopressin, namely "vasopressin escape." Vasopressin escape is characterized by a sudden increase in urine volume with a decrease in urine osmolality independent of high circulating vasopressin levels. The onset of escape coincides temporally with a marked decrease in renal AQP2 protein as measured by immunoblotting as well as decreased mRNA expression, as assessed by Northern blotting (56). In contrast to AQP2, there are no decreases in renal expression of AQP1, AQP3, and AQP4 (56). These results suggest that escape from vasopressin-induced antidiuresis is attributable, at least in part, to a selective vasopressin-independent decrease in AQP2 expression in the renal collecting duct.

Acknowledgments

Support for this chapter was partially provided by funds from the Danish National Research Foundation, The European Commission, the Danish Medical Research Council, Novo Nordic Foundation, Karen Elise Jensen Foundation and the National Institutes of Health. Portions of the text were previously published in abridged form and are reproduced and modified with permission (4). Moreover the authors gratefully acknowledge the major contributions from Peter Agre and Mark Knepper, who together with Søren Nielsen, authored the previous version of this chapter.

References

1. Abrami L, Tacnet F, Ripoche P, Evidence for a glycerol pathway through aquaporin 1 (CHIP28) channels. *Pflugers Arch* 1995;430:447–458.
2. Advani RJ, Bae HR, Bock JB, Chao DS, Doung YC, Prekeris R, Yoo JS, Scheller RH. Seven novel mammalian SNARE proteins localize to distinct membrane compartments. *J Biol Chem* 1998;273:10317–10324.
3. Agre P. Molecular physiology of water transport: aquaporin nomenclature workshop. Mammalian aquaporins. *Biol Cell* 1997;89:255–257.
4. Agre P, Bonhivers M, Borgnia MJ. The aquaporins, blueprints for cellular plumbing systems. *J Biol Chem* 1998;273:14659–14662.
5. Agre P, Lee MD, Devidas S, Guggino WB. Aquaporins and ion conductance. *Science* 1997;275:1490.
6. Agre P, Preston GM, Smith BL, Jung JS, Raina S, Moon C, Guggino WB, Nielsen S. Aquaporin CHIP: the archetypal molecular water channel. *Am J Physiol* 1993;265:F463–F476.
7. Agre P, Saboori AM, Asimos A, Smith BL. Purification and partial characterization of the Mr 30,000 integral membrane protein associated with the erythrocyte Rh(D) antigen. *J Biol Chem* 1987;262:17497–17503.
8. Agre P, Sasaki S, Chrispeels MJ. Aquaporins: a family of water channel proteins. *Am J Physiol* 1993;265:F461.
9. Agre P, King LS, Yasui M, Guggino WB, Ottersen OP, Fujiyoshi Y, Engel A, Nielsen S. Aquaporin water channels - from atomic structure to clinical medicine. *J Physiol* 2002;542:3–6.
10. Anderson RJ, Gordon JA, Kim J, Peterson LM, Gross PA. Renal concentration defect following nonoliguric acute renal failure in the rat. *Kidney Int* 1982;21:583–591.
11. Apostol E, Ecelbarger CA, Terris J, Bradford AD, Andrews P, Knepper MA. Reduced renal medullary water channel expression in puromycin aminonucleoside—induced nephrotic syndrome. *J Am Soc Nephrol* 1997;8:24.
12. Asahina Y, Izumi N, Enomoto N, Sasaki S, Fushimi K, Marumo F, Sato C. Increased gene expression of water channel in cirrhotic rat kidneys. *Hepatology* 1995;21:169–173.
13. Au CG, Cooper ST, Lo HP, Compton AG, Yang N, Wintour EM, North KN, Winlaw DS. Expression of aquaporin 1 in human cardiac and skeletal muscle. *J Mol Cell Cardiol* 2004;36:655–662.
14. Bajjalieh SM, Scheller RH. The biochemistry of neurotransmitter secretion. *J Biol Chem* 1995;270:1971–1974.
15. Barile M, Pisitkun T, Yu MJ, Chou CL, Verbalis MJ, Shen RF, Knepper MA. Large scale protein identification in intracellular aquaporin-2 vesicles from renal inner medullary collecting duct. *Mol Cell Proteomics* 2005;4:1095–1106.
16. Bartter FC, Schwartz WB. The syndrome of inappropriate secretion of antidiuretic hormone. *Am J Med* 1967;42:790–806.
17. Bedford JJ, Leader JP, Walker RJ. Aquaporin expression in normal human kidney and in renal disease. *J Am Soc Nephrol* 2003;14:2581–2587.
18. Beitz E, Wu B, Holm LM, Schultz JE, Zeuthen T. Point mutations in the aromatic/arginine region in aquaporin 1 allow passage of urea, glycerol, ammonia, and protons. *Proc Natl Acad Sci U S A* 2006;103:269–274.
19. Bichet DG. Vasopressin receptors in health and disease. *Kidney Int* 1996;49:1706–1711.
20. Bondy C, Chin E, Smith BL, Preston GM, Agre P. Developmental gene expression and tissue distribution of the CHIP28 water-channel protein. *Proc Natl Acad Sci U S A* 1993;90:4500–4504.
21. Bourguet J, Chevalier J, Hugon JS. Alterations in membrane-associated particle distribution during antidiuretic challenge in frog urinary bladder epithelium. *Biophs J* 1976;16:627–639.
22. Brooks HL, Regan JW, Yool AJ. Inhibition of aquaporin-1 water permeability by tetraethylammonium. Involvement of the loop E pore region. *Mol Pharmacol* 2000;57:1021–1026.

23. Brown D, Orci L. Vasopressin stimulates formation of coated pits in rat kidney collecting ducts. *Nature* 1983;302:253–255.
24. Brown D, Weyer P, Orci L. Vasopressin stimulates endocytosis in kidney collecting duct principal cells. *Eur J Cell Biol* 1988;46:336–341.
25. Cabiaux V, Oberg KA, Pancoska P, Walz T, Agre P, Engel A. Secondary structures comparison of aquaporin-1 and bacteriorhodopsin. a Fourier transform infrared spectroscopy study of two-dimensional membrane crystals. *Biophs J* 1997;73:406–417.
26. Calakos N, Bennett MK, Peterson KE, Scheller RH. Protein-protein interactions contributing to the specificity of intracellular vesicular trafficking. *Science* 1994;263:1146–1149.
27. Calamita G, Ferri D, Bazzini C, Mazzone A, Botta G, Liquori G, Paulmichl M, Portincasa P, Meyer G, Svelto M. Expression and subcellular localization of the AQP8 and AQP1 water channels in the mouse gall-bladder epithelium. *Biol Cell* 2005;97(6):415–423.
28. Carbrey JM, Gorelick-Feldman DA, Kozono D, Praetorius J, Nielsen S, Agre P. Aquaglyceroporin AQP9. Solute permeation and metabolic control of expression in liver. *Proc Natl Acad Sci U S A* 2003;100:2945–2950.
29. Cheng A, Van Hoek AN, Yeager M, Verkman AS, Mitra AK. Three-dimensional organization of a human water channel. *Nature* 1997;387:627–630.
30. Cheng X, Zhang H, Lee HL, Park JM. Cyclooxygenase-2 inhibitor preserves medullary aquaporin-2 expression and prevents polyuria after ureteral obstruction. *J Urol* 2004;172(6 Pt 1):2387–2390.
31. Chou CL, DiGiovanni SR, Mejia R, Nielsen S, Knepper MA. Oxytocin as an antidiuretic hormone. I. Concentration dependence of action. *Am J Physiol* 1995;269:F70–F77.
32. Chou CL, Ma T, Yang B, Knepper MA, Verkman AS. Fourfold reduction of water permeability in inner medullary collecting duct of aquaporin-4 knockout mice. *Am J Physiol* 1998;274:C549–C554.
33. Chou CL, Yip KP, Michea L, Kador K, Ferraris JD, Wade JB, Knepper MA. Regulation of aquaporin-2 trafficking by vasopressin in the renal collecting duct. Roles of ryanodine-sensitive Ca2+ stores and calmodulin. *J Biol Chem* 2000;275:36839–36846.
34. Chou CL, Christensen BM, Frische S, Vorum H, Desai RA, Hoffert JD, de Lanerolle P, Nielsen S, Knepper MA. Non-muscle myosin II and myosin light chain kinase are downstream targets for vasopressin signaling in the renal collecting duct. *J Biol Chem* 2004;279:49026–49035.
35. Chou CL, Knepper MA, Hoek AN, Brown D, Yang B, Ma T, Verkman AS. Reduced water permeability and altered ultrastructure in thin descending limb of Henle in aquaporin-1 null mice. *J Clin Invest* 1999;103:491–496.
36. Christensen BM, Zelenina M, Aperia A, Nielsen S. Localization and regulation of PKA-phosphorylated AQP2 in response to V(2)-receptor agonist/antagonist treatment. *Am J Physiol Renal Physiol* 2000;278:F29–F42.
37. Christensen BM, Marples D, Jensen UB, Frokiaer J, Sheikh-Hamad D, Knepper M, Nielsen S. Acute effects of vasopressin V2-receptor antagonist on kidney AQP2 expression and subcellular distribution. *Am J Physiol Renal Physiol* 1998;275:F285–F297.
38. Christensen BM, Wang W, Frokiar J, Nielsen S. Axial heterogeneity in basolateral AQP2 localization in rat kidney. effect of vasopressin. *Am J Physiol Renal Physiol* 2003;284:F701–F717.
39. Christensen S, Kusano E, Yusufi AN, Murayama N, Dousa TP. Pathogenesis of nephrogenic diabetes insipidus due to chronic administration of lithium in rats. *J Clin Invest* 1985;75:1869–1879.
40. Coleman RA, Wu DC, Liu J, Wade JB. Expression of aquaporins in the renal connecting tubule. *Am J Physiol Renal Physiol* 2000;279:F874–F883.
41. Cooper GJ, Zhou Y, Bouyer P, Grichtchenko II, Boron WF. Transport of volatile solutes through AQP1. *J Physiol* 2002;542:17–29.
42. de Groot BL, Engel A, Grubmuller H. A refined structure of human aquaporin-1. *FEBS Lett* 2001;504:206–211.
43. de Groot BL, Engel A, Grubmuller H. The structure of the aquaporin-1 water channel. A comparison between cryo-electron microscopy and x-ray crystallography. *J Mol Biol* 2003;325:485–493.
44. de Groot BL, Grubmuller H. Water permeation across biological membranes. Mechanism and dynamics of aquaporin-1 and GlpF. *Science* 2001;294:2353–2357.
45. de Sousa RC, Grosso A. Vanadate blocks cyclic AMP-induced stimulation of sodium and water transport in amphibian epithelia. *Nature* 1979;279:803–804.
46. Deen PM, Croes H, van Aubel RA, Ginsel LA, van Os CH. Water channels encoded by mutant aquaporin-2 genes in nephrogenic diabetes insipidus are impaired in their cellular routing. *J Clin Invest* 1995;95:2291–2296.
47. Deen PM, van Aubel RA, Van Lieburg AF, van Os CH. Urinary content of aquaporin 1 and 2 in nephrogenic diabetes insipidus. *J Am Soc Nephrol* 1996;7:836–841.
48. Deen PM, van Aubel RA, Van Lieburg AF, van Os CH. Urinary content of aquaporin 1 and 2 in nephrogenic diabetes insipidus. *J Am Soc Nephrol* 1996;7:836–841.
49. Deen PM, Verdijk MA, Knoers NV, Wieringa B, Monnens LA, van Os CH, van Oost BA. Requirement of human renal water channel aquaporin-2 for vasopressin-dependent concentration of urine. *Science* 1994;264:92–95.
50. Denker BM, Smith BL, Kuhajda FP, Agre P. Identification, purification, and partial characterization of a novel Mr 28,000 integral membrane protein from erythrocytes and renal tubules. *J Biol Chem* 1988;263:15634–15642.
51. Detmers FJM, de Groot BL, Muller EM, Hinton A, Konings IBM, Sze M, Flitsch SL, Grubmuller H, Deen PMT. Quaternary ammonium compounds as water channel blockers. specificity, potency and site of action. *J Biol Chem* 2006;281:14207–14214.
52. Dibona DR. Cytoplasmic involvement in ADH-mediated osmosis across toad urinary bladder. *Am J Physiol* 1983;245:C297–C307.
53. DiGiovanni SR, Nielsen S, Christensen EI, Knepper MA. Regulation of collecting duct water channel expression by vasopressin in Brattleboro rat. *Proc Natl Acad Sci U S A* 1994;91:8984–8988.
54. Ding GH, Franki N, Condeelis J, Hays RM. Vasopressin depolymerizes F-actin in toad bladder epithelial cells. *Am J Physiol* 1991;260:C9–16.

55. Earm JH, Christensen BM, Frokiaer J, Marples D, Han JS, Knepper MA, Nielsen S. Decreased aquaporin-2 expression and apical plasma membrane delivery in kidney collecting ducts of polyuric hypercalcemic rats. *J Am Soc Nephrol* 1998;9:2181–2193.
56. Ecelbarger CA, Chou CL, Lee AJ, DiGiovanni SR, Verbalis JG, Knepper MA. Escape from vasopressin-induced antidiuresis: role of vasopressin resistance of the collecting duct. *Am J Physiol* 1998;274:F1161–F1166.
57. Ecelbarger CA, Nielsen S, Olson BR, Murase T, Baker EA, Knepper MA, Verbalis JG. Role of renal aquaporins in escape from vasopressin-induced antidiuresis in rat. *J Clin Invest* 1997;99:1852–1863.
58. Ecelbarger CA, Terris J, Frindt G, Echevarria M, Marples D, Nielsen S, Knepper MA. Aquaporin-3 water channel localization and regulation in rat kidney. *Am J Physiol* 1995;269: F663–F672.
59. Echevarria M, Windhager EE, Tate SS, Frindt G. Cloning and expression of AQP3, a water channel from the medullary collecting duct of rat kidney. *Proc Natl Acad Sci U S A* 1994;91:10997–11001.
60. Edwards RM, Jackson BA, Dousa TP. ADH-sensitive cAMP system in papillary collecting duct. effect of osmolality and PGE2. *Am J Physiol* 1981;240:F311–F318.
61. Elkjar ML, Kwon TH, Wang W, Nielsen J, Knepper MA, Frokiar J, Nielsen S. Altered expression of renal NHE3, TSC, BSC-1, and ENaC subunits in potassium-depleted rats. *Am J Physiol Renal Physiol* 2002;283:F1376–F1388.
62. Elkjar ML, Nejsum LN, Gresz V, Kwon TH, Jensen UB, Frokiar J, Nielsen S. Immunolocalization of aquaporin-8 in rat kidney, gastrointestinal tract, testis, and airways. *Am J Physiol Renal Physiol* 2001;281:F1047–F1057.
63. Endo M, Jain RK, Witwer B, Brown D. Water channel (aquaporin 1) expression and distribution in mammary carcinomas and glioblastomas. *Microvas Res* 1999;58:89–98.
64. Fernandez-Llama P, Andrews P, Ecelbarger CA, Nielsen S, Knepper M. Concentrating defect in experimental nephrotic syndrone. altered expression of aquaporins and thick ascending limb Na+ transporters. *Kidney Int* 1998;54:170–179.
65. Fernandez-Llama P, Andrews P, Nielsen S, Ecelbarger CA, Knepper MA. Impaired aquaporin and urea transporter expression in rats with adriamycin-induced nephrotic syndrome. *Kidney Int* 1998;53:1244–1253.
66. Fernandez-Llama P, Andrews P, Turner R, Saggi S, Di Mari J, Kwon T-H, Nielsen S, Safirstein R, Knepper MA. Role of collecting duct aquaporins in polyuria of post-ischemic acute renal failure in rats. *J Am Soc Nephrol* 1999;10:1658–1668.
67. Fernandez-Llama P, Jimenez W, Bosch-Marce M, Arroyo V, Nielsen S, Knepper MA. Dysregulation of renal aquaporins and Na-Cl cotransporter in CCl4-induced cirrhosis. *Kidney Int* 2000;58:216–228.
68. Fernandez-Llama P, Turner R, Dibona G, Knepper MA. Renal expression of aquaporins in liver cirrhosis induced by chronic common bile duct ligation in rats. *J Am Soc Nephrol* 1999;10:1950–1957.
69. Finkelstein A. *Water Movement Through Lipid Bilayers, Pores, and Plasma Membranes. Theory and Reality.* New York: John Wiley & Sons; 1987.
70. Fischbarg J, Kuang KY, Vera JC, Arant S, Silverstein SC, Loike J, Rosen OM. Glucose transporters serve as water channels. *Proc Natl Acad Sci U S A* 1990;87:3244–3247.
71. Flamion B, Spring KR. Water permeability of apical and basolateral cell membranes of rat inner medullary collecting duct. *Am J Physiol* 1990;259:F986–F999.
72. Flamion B, Spring KR, Abramow M. Adaptation of inner medullary collecting duct to dehydration involves a paracellular pathway. *Am J Physiol* 1995;268:F53–F63.
73. Flear CT, Gill GV, Burn J. Hyponatraemia: mechanisms and management. *Lancet* 1981;2: 26–31.
74. Foster LJ, Yeung B, Mohtashami M, Ross K, Trimble WS, Klip A. Binary interactions of the SNARE proteins syntaxin-4, SNAP23, and VAMP-2 and their regulation by phosphorylation. *Biochemistry* 1998;37:11089–11096.
75. Fotiadis D, Suda K, Tittmann P, Jeno P, Philippsen A, Muller DJ, Gross H, Engel A. identification and structure of a putative Ca2+-binding domain at the C Terminus of AQP1. *J Mol Biol* 2002;318:1381–1394.
76. Franki N, Macaluso F, Schubert W, Gunther L, Hays RM. Water channel-carrying vesicles in the rat IMCD contain cellubrevin. *Am J Physiol* 1995;269:C797–C801.
77. Frigeri A, Gropper MA, Turck CW, Verkman AS. Immunolocalization of the mercurial-insensitive water channel and glycerol intrinsic protein in epithelial cell plasma membranes. *Proc Natl Acad Sci U S A* 1995;92:4328–4331.
78. Frische S, Kwon TH, Frokiaer J, Nielsen S. Aquaporin-2 trafficking. In: Boles E, Kramer R, eds. *Molecular Mechanisms Controlling Transmembrane Transport.* Berlin: Springer; 353–377.
79. Frokiaer J, Christensen BM, Marples D, Djurhuus JC, Jensen UB, Knepper MA, Nielsen S. Downregulation of aquaporin-2 parallels changes in renal water excretion in unilateral ureteral obstruction. *Am J Physiol* 1997;273:F213–F223.
80. Frokiaer J, Marples D, Knepper MA, Nielsen S. Bilateral ureteral obstruction downregulates expression of vasopressin-sensitive AQP-2 water channel in rat kidney. *Am J Physiol* 1996;270:F657–F668.
81. Frokiaer J, Marples D, Valtin H, Morris JF, Knepper MA, Nielsen S. Low aquaporin-2 levels in polyuric DI +/+ severe mice with constitutively high cAMP-phosphodiesterase activity. *Am J Physiol Renal Physiol* 1999;276:F179–F190.
82. Fujita N, Ishikawa SE, Sasaki S, Fujisawa G, Fushimi K, Marumo F, Saito T. Role of water channel AQP-CD in water retention in SIADH and cirrhotic rats. *Am J Physiol* 1995;269: F926–F931.
83. Fushimi K, Sasaki S, Marumo F. Phosphorylation of serine 256 is required for cAMP-dependent regulatory exocytosis of the aquaporin-2 water channel. *J Biol Chem* 1997;272: 14800–14804.
84. Fushimi K, Uchida S, Hara Y, Hirata Y, Marumo F, Sasaki S. Cloning and expression of apical membrane water channel of rat kidney collecting tubule. *Nature* 1993;361: 549–552.
85. Gines P, Berl T, Bernardi M, Bichet DG, Hamon G, Jimenez W, Liard JF, Martin PY, Schrier RW. Hyponatremia in cirrhosis. from pathogenesis to treatment. *Hepatology* 1998;28:851–864.
86. Gonen T, Sliz P, Kistler J, Cheng Y, Walz T. Aquaporin-0 membrane junctions reveal the structure of a closed water pore. *Nature* 2004;429:193–197.
87. Gong H, Wang W, Kwon TH, Jonassen T, Frokiaer J, Nielsen S. Reduced renal expression of AQP2, p-AQP2 and AQP3 in haemorrhagic shock-induced acute renal failure. *Nephrol Dial Transplant* 2003;18:2551–2559.
88. Grantham JJ, Burg MB. Effect of vasopressin and cyclic AMP on permeability of isolated collecting tubules. *Am J Physiol* 1966;211:255–259.
89. Gresz V, Kwon TH, Hurley PT, Varga G, Zelles T, Nielsen S, Case RM, Steward MC. Identification and localization of aquaporin water channels in human salivary glands. *Am J Physiol Gastrointest Liver Physiol* 2001;281:G247–G254.
90. Han BG, Guliaev AB, Walian PJ, Jap BK. Water Transport in AQP0 aquaporin. Molecular dynamics studies. *J Mol Biol* 2006;360:285–296.
91. Han JS, Maeda Y, Ecelbarger C, Knepper MA. Vasopressin-independent regulation of collecting duct water permeability. *Am J Physiol* 1994;266:F139–F146.
92. Hanley MJ. Isolated nephron segments in a rabbit model of ischemic acute renal failure. *Am J Physiol* 1980;239:F17–F23.
93. Hara-Chikuma M, Verkman AS. Aquaporin-1 facilitates epithelial cell migration in kidney proximal tubule. *J Am Soc Nephrol* 2006;17:39–45.
94. Harries WEC, Akhavan D, Miercke LJW, Khademi S, Stroud RM. The channel architecture of aquaporin 0 at a 2.2-A resolution. *Proc Natl Acad Sci U S A* 2004;101:14045–14050.
95. Harris HW Jr, Zeidel ML, Jo I, Hammond TG. Characterization of purified endosomes containing the antidiuretic hormone-sensitive water channel from rat renal papilla. *J Biol Chem* 1994;269:11993–12000.
96. Hasegawa H, Lian SC, Finkbeiner WE, Verkman AS. Extrarenal tissue distribution of CHIP28 water channels by in situ hybridization and antibody staining. *Am J Physiol* 1994;266:C893–C903.
97. Hasegawa H, Ma T, Skach W, Matthay MA, Verkman A S. Molecular cloning of a mercurial-insensitive water channel expressed in selected water-transporting tissues. *J Biol Chem* 1994;269:5497–5500.
98. Hashimoto S, Huang Y, Mizel D, Briggs J, Schnermann J. Compensation of proximal tubule malabsorption in AQP1-deficient mice without TGF-mediated reduction of GFR. *Acta Physiol Scand* 2004;181:455–462.
99. Hayashi M, Sasaki S, Tsuganezawa H, Monkawa T, Kitajima W, Konishi K, Fushimi K, Marumo F, Saruta T. Expression and distribution of aquaporin of collecting duct are regulated by vasopressin V2 receptor in rat kidney. *J Clin Invest* 1994;94:1778–1783.
100. Hays RM, LEAF A. Studies on the movement of water through the isolated toad bladder and its modification by vasopressin. *J Gen Physiol* 1962;45:905–919.
101. Hazama A, Kozono D, Guggino WB, Agre P, Yasui M. Ion permeation of AQP6 water channel protein. single-channel recordings after Hg2+ activation. *J Biol Chem* 2002;277:29224–29230.
102. Heymann JB, Agre P, Engel A. Progress on the structure and function of aquaporin 1. *J Struct Biol* 1998;121:191–206.
103. Hoffert JD, Pisitkun T, Wang G, Shen RF, Knepper MA. Quantitative phosphoproteomics of vasopressin-sensitive renal cells. Regulation of aquaporin-2 phosphorylation at two sites. *Proc Natl Acad Sci U S A* 2006;103:7159–7164.
104. Holm LM, Jahn TP, Moller AL, Schjoerring JK, Ferri D, Klaerke DA, Zeuthen T. NH3 and NH4+ permeability in aquaporin-expressing Xenopus oocytes. *Pflugers Arch* 2005;450:4428.
105. Hozawa S, Holtzman EJ, Ausiello DA. cAMP motifs regulating transcription in the aquaporin 2 gene. *Am J Physiol* 1996;270:C1695–C1702.
106. Huang D, Chen P, Chen S, Nagura M, Lim DJ, Lin X. Expression patterns of aquaporins in the inner ear. evidence for concerted actions of multiple types of aquaporins to facilitate water transport in the cochlea. *Hear Res* 2002;165:85–95.
107. Ikeda M, Beitz E, Kozono D, Guggino WB, Agre P, Yasui M. Characterization of aquaporin-6 as a nitrate channel in mammalian cells. requirement of pore-lining residue threonine 63. *J Biol Chem* 2002;277:39873–39879.
108. Inase N, Fushimi K, Ishibashi K, Uchida S, Ichioka M, Sasaki S, Marumo F. Isolation of human aquaporin 3 gene. *J Biol Chem* 1995;270:17913–17916.
109. Inoue T, Nielsen S, Mandon B, Terris J, Kishore BK, Knepper MA. SNAP-23 in rat kidney: colocalization with aquaporin-2 in collecting duct vesicles. *Am J Physiol* 1998;275:F752–F760.
110. Ishibashi K, Imai M, Sasaki S. Cellular localization of aquaporin 7 in the rat kidney. *Nephron Exp Nephrol* 2000;8:252–257.
111. Ishibashi K, Kuwahara M, Gu Y, Kageyama Y, Tohsaka A, Suzuki F, Marumo F, Sasaki S Cloning and functional expression of a new water channel abundantly expressed in the testis permeable to water, glycerol, and urea. *J Biol Chem* 1997;272:20782–20786.
112. Ishibashi K, Sasaki S, Fushimi K, Uchida S, Kuwahara M, Saito H, Furukawa T, Nakajima K, Yamaguchi Y, Gojobori T. Molecular cloning and expression of a member of the aquaporin family with permeability to glycerol and urea in addition to water expressed at the basolateral membrane of kidney collecting duct cells. *Proc Natl Acad Sci U S A* 1994;91:6269–6273.
113. Ishibashi K, Kuwahara M, Gu Y, Tanaka Y, Marumo F, Sasaki S. Cloning and functional expression of a new aquaporin (AQP9) abundantly expressed in the peripheral leukocytes permeable to water and urea, but not to glycerol. *Biochem Biophys Res Commun* 1998;244:268–274.
114. Ishibashi K, Kuwahara M, Kageyama Y, Tohsaka A, Marumo F, Sasaki S. Cloning and functional expression of a second new aquaporin abundantly expressed in testis. *Biochem Biophys Res Commun* 1997;237:714–-718.
115. Jahn TP, Moller ALB, Zeuthen T, Holm LM, Klaerke DA, Mohsin B, Kuhlbrandt W, Schjoerring JK. Aquaporin homologues in plants and mammals transport ammonia. *FEBS Lett* 2004;574:31–36.
116. Jap BK, Li H. Structure of the osmo-regulated H2O-channel, AQP-CHIP, in projection at 3.5 A resolution. *J Mol Biol* 1995;251:413–420.
117. Jensen AM, Li C, Praetorius HA, Norregaard R, Frische S, Knepper MA, Nielsen S, Frokiaer J. Angiotensin II mediates downregulation of aquaporin water channels and key renal sodium transporters in response to urinary tract obstruction. *Am J Physiol Renal Physiol* 2006;291: F1021–1032.

118. Jonassen TE, Nielsen S, Christensen S, Petersen JS. Decreased vasopressin-mediated renal water reabsorption in rats with compensated liver cirrhosis. *Am J Physiol* 1998;275:F216–F225.
119. Jonassen TE, Promeneur D, Christensen S, Petersen JS, Nielsen S. Decreased vasopressin-mediated renal water reabsorption in rats with chronic aldosterone-receptor blockade. *Am J Physiol Renal Physiol* 2000;278:F246–F256.
120. Jones RV, De Wardener HE. Urine concentration after fluid deprivation or pitressin tannate in oil. *B M J* 1956;271–274.
121. Jung JS, Bhat RV, Preston GM, Guggino WB, Baraban JM, Agre P. Molecular characterization of an aquaporin cDNA from brain: candidate osmoreceptor and regulator of water balance. *Proc Natl Acad Sci U S A* 1994;91:13052–13056.
122. Jung JS, Preston GM, Smith BL, Guggino WB, Agre P. Molecular structure of the water channel through aquaporin CHIP: the hourglass model. *J Biol Chem* 1994;269:14648–14654.
123. Kachadorian WA, Ellis SJ, Muller J. Possible roles for microtubules and microfilaments in ADH action on toad urinary bladder. *Am J Physiol* 1979;236:F14–F20.
124. Kachadorian WA, Wade JB, DiScala VA. Vasopressin. induced structural change in toad bladder luminal membrane. *Science* 1975;190:67–69.
125. Kanno K, Sasaki S, Hirata Y, Ishikawa S, Fushimi K, Nakanishi S, Bichet DG, Marumo F. Urinary excretion of aquaporin-2 in patients with diabetes insipidus. *N Engl J Med* 1995; 332:1540–1545.
126. Katsura T, Ausiello DA, Brown D. Direct demonstration of aquaporin-2 water channel recycling in stably transfected LLC-PK1 epithelial cells. *Am J Physiol Renal Physiol* 1996;270: F548–F553.
127. Katsura T, Gustafson CE, Ausiello DA, Brown D. Protein kinase A phosphorylation is involved in regulated exocytosis of aquaporin-2 in transfected LLC-PK1 cells. *Am J Physiol* 1997;272:F817–F822.
128. Katsura T, Verbavatz J, Farinas J, Ma T, Ausiello DA, Verkman AS, Brown D. Constitutive and regulated membrane expression of aquaporin 1 and aquaporin 2 water channels in stably transfected LLC-PK1 epithelial cells. *Proc Natl Acad Sci U S A* 1995;92:7212–7216.
129. Kim SW, Cho SH, Oh BS, Yeum CH, Choi KC, Ahn KY, Lee J. Diminished renal expression of aquaporin water channels in rats with experimental bilateral ureteral obstruction. *J Am Soc Nephrol* 2001;12:2019–2028.
130. Kim SW, Schou UK, Peters CD, de Seigneux S, Kwon TH, Knepper MA, Jonassen TEN, Froki J, Nielsen S. Increased apical targeting of renal epithelial sodium channel subunits and decreased expression of type 2 11beta-hydroxysteroid dehydrogenase in rats with CCl4-induced decompensated liver cirrhosis. *J Am Soc Nephrol* 2005;16:3196–3210.
131. Kim YH, Kwon TH, Christensen BM, Nielsen J, Wall SM, Madsen KM, Frokiaer J, Nielsen S. Altered expression of renal acid-base transporters in rats with lithium-induced NDI. *Am J Physiol Renal Physiol* 2003;285:F1244–F1257.
132. King LS, Nielsen S, Agre P. Aquaporin-1 water channel protein in lung: ontogeny, steroid-induced expression, and distribution in rat. *J Clin Invest* 1996;97:2183–2191.
133. King LS, Nielsen S, Agre P. Aquaporins in complex tissues, I: developmental patterns in respiratory and glandular tissues of rat. *Am J Physiol* 1997;273:C1541–C1548.
134. King LS, Choi M, Fernandez PC, Cartron JP, Agre P. Defective urinary concentrating ability due to a complete deficiency of aquaporin-1. *N Engl J Med* 2001;345:175–179.
135. King LS, Nielsen S, Agre P, Brown RH. Decreased pulmonary vascular permeability in aquaporin-1-null humans. *Proc Natl Acad Sci U S A* 2002;99:1059–1063.
136. Kishida K, Kuriyama H, Funahashi T, Shimomura I, Kihara S, Ouchi N, Nishida M, Nishizawa H, Matsuda M, Takahashi M, Hotta K, Nakamura T, Yamashita S, Tochino Y, Matsuzawa Y. Aquaporin adipose, a putative glycerol channel in adipocytes. *J Biol Chem* 2000;275:20896–20902.
137. Kishore BK, Terris JM, Knepper MA. Quantitation of aquaporin-2 abundance in microdissected collecting ducts: axial distribution and control by AVP. *Am J Physiol* 1996;271:F62–F70.
138. Kishore BK, Wade JB, Schorr K, Inoue T, Mandon B, Knepper MA. Expression of synaptotagmin VIII in rat kidney. *Am J Physiol* 1998;275:F131–F142.
139. Knepper M, Nielsen S, Chou CL, DiGiovanni SR. Mechanism of vasopressin action in the renal collecting duct. *Sem Nephrol* 14:302–321.
140. Knepper MA, Nielsen S. Kinetic model of water and urea permeability regulation by vasopressin in collecting duct. *Am J Physiol* 1993;265:F214–F224.
141. Knepper MA, Wade JB, Terris J, Ecelbarger CA, Marples D, Mandon B, Chou CL, Kishore BK, Nielsen S. Renal aquaporins. *Kidney Int* 1996;49:1712–1717.
142. Knoers NV, van Os CH. Molecular and cellular defects in nephrogenic diabetes insipidus. *Curr Opin Nephrol Hypertens* 1996;5:353–358.
143. Ko SB, Uchida S, Naruse S, Kuwahara M, Ishibashi K, Marumo F, Hayakawa T, Sasaki S. Cloning and functional expression of rAOP9L a new member of aquaporin family from rat liver. *Biochem Mol Biol Int* 1999;47:309–318.
144. Ko SBH, Naruse S, Kitagawa M, Ishiguro H, Furuya S, Mizuno N, Wang Y, Yoshikawa T, Suzuki A, Shimano S, Hayakawa T. Aquaporins in rat pancreatic interlobular ducts. *Am J Physiol Gastrointest Liver Physiol* 2002;282:G324–G331.
145. Koefoed-Johnsen V, Ussing HH. The contributions of diffusion and flow to the passage of D2O through living membranes; effect of neurohypophyseal hormone on isolated anuran skin. *Acta Physiol Scand* 1953;28:60–76.
146. Koyama Y, Yamamoto T, Tani T, Nihei K, Kondo D, Funaki H, Yaoita E, Kawasaki K, Sato N, Hatakeyama A. Expression and localization of aquaporins in rat gastrointestinal tract. *Am J Physiol* 1999;276:C621–C627.
147. Kuriyama H, Kawamoto S, Ishida N, Ohno I, Mita S, Matsuzawa Y, Matsubara K, Okubo K. Molecular cloning and expression of a novel human aquaporin from adipose tissue with glycerol permeability. *Biochem Biophy Res Commun* 1997;241:53–58.
148. Kurokawa K, Massry SG. Interaction between catecholamines and vasopressin on renal medullary cyclic AMP of rat. *Am J Physiol* 1973;225:825–829.
149. Kuwahara M, Fushimi K, Terada Y, Bai L, Marumo F, Sasaki S. cAMP-dependent phosphorylation stimulates water permeability of aquaporin-collecting duct water channel protein expressed in Xenopus oocytes. *J Biol Chem* 1995;270:10384–10387.
150. Kuwahara M, Verkman AS. Pre-steady-state analysis of the turn-on and turn-off of water permeability in the kidney collecting tubule. *J Membr Biol* 1989;110:57–65.
151. Kwon T-H, Frokiaer J, Fernandez-Llama P, Knepper MA, Nielsen S. Reduced abundance of aquaporins in rats with bilateral ischemia-induced acute renal failure. prevention by alpha-MSH. *Am J Physiol* 1999;277:F413–F427.
152. Kwon T-H, Frokiaer J, Knepper MA, Nielsen S. Reduced AQP1, -2, and -3 levels in kidneys of rats with CRF induced by surgical reduction in renal mass. *Am J Physiol* 1998;275:F724–F741.
153. Kwon T-H, Laursen UH, Marples D, Maunsbach AB, Knepper MA, Frokiaer J, Nielsen S. Altered expression of renal AQPs and Na(+) transporters in rats with lithium-induced NDI. *Am J Physiol Renal Physiol* 2000;279:F552–F564.
154. Kwon TH, Nielsen J, Knepper MA, Frokiaer J, Nielsen S. Angiotensin II AT1 receptor blockade decreases vasopressin-induced water reabsorption and AQP2 levels in NaCl-restricted rats. *Am J Physiol Renal Physiol* 2005;288:F673–F684.
155. Kwon TH, Nielsen J, Masilamani S, Hager H, Knepper MA, Frokiar J, Nielsen S. Regulation of collecting duct AQP3 expression. Response to mineralocorticoid. *Am J Physiol Renal Physiol* 2002;283:F1403–F1421.
156. Lai KN, Li FK, Yui Lan HAO, Tang SYDN, Tsang AWL, Chan DTM, Leung JC. Expression of aquaporin-1 in human peritoneal mesothelial cells and its upregulation by glucose in vitro. *J Am Soc Nephrol* 2001;12:1036–1045.
157. Lande MB, Jo I, Zeidel ML, Somers M, Harris HW Jr. Phosphorylation of aquaporin-2 does not alter the membrane water permeability of rat papillary water channel-containing vesicles. *J Biol Chem* 1996;271:5552–5557.
158. Lankford SP, Chou CL, Terada Y, Wall SM, Wade JB, Knepper MA. Regulation of collecting duct water permeability independent of cAMP-mediated AVP response. *Am J Physiol* 1991;261:F554–F566.
159. Lencer WI, Brown D, Ausiello DA, Verkman AS. Endocytosis of water channels in rat kidney. cell specificity and correlation with in vivo antidiuresis. *Am J Physiol* 1990;259:C920–C932.
160. Levy M, Wexler MJ. Hepatic denervation alters first-phase urinary sodium excretion in dogs with cirrhosis. *Am J Physiol* 1987;253:F664–F671.
161. Li C, Wang W, Knepper MA, Nielsen S, Frokiar J. Downregulation of renal aquaporins in response to unilateral ureteral obstruction. *Am J Physiol Renal Physiol* 2003;284:F1066–F1079.
162. Li C, Wang W, Kwon TH, Isikay L, Wen JG, Marples D, Djurhuus JC, Stockwell A, Knepper MA, Nielsen S, Frokiar J. Downregulation of AQP1, -2, and -3 after ureteral obstruction is associated with a long-term urine-concentrating defect. *Am J Physiol Renal Physiol* 2001;281: F163–F171.
163. Li H, Lee S, Jap BK. Molecular design of aquaporin-1 water channel as revealed by electron crystallography. *Nat Struct Mol Biol* 1997;4:263–265.
164. Liebenhoff U, Rosenthal W. Identification of Rab3-, Rab5a- and synaptobrevin II-like proteins in a preparation of rat kidney vesicles containing the vasopressin-regulated water channel. *FEBS Lett* 1995;365:209–213.
165. Liu KF, Nagase HF, Huang CG, Fau C, Calamita GF, Agre P. Purification and functional characterization of aquaporin-8. *Biol Cell* 2006;98:153–161.
166. Liu K, Kozono D, Kato Y, Agre P, Hazama A, Yasui M. From the cover: conversion of aquaporin 6 from an anion channel to a water-selective channel by a single amino acid substitution. *Proc Natl Acad Sci U S A* 2005;102:2192–2197.
167. Liu Z, Shen J, Carbrey JM, Mukhopadhyay R, Agre P, Rosen BP. Arsenite transport by mammalian aquaglyceroporins AQP7 and AQP9. *Proc Natl Acad Sci U S A* 2002;99:6053–6058.
168. Lorenz D, Krylov A, Hahm D, Hagen V, Rosenthal W, Pohl P, Maric K. Cyclic AMP is sufficient for triggering the exocytic recruitment of aquaporin-2 in renal epithelial cells. *EMBO Rep* 2003;4:88–93.
169. Ma T, Frigeri A, Hasegawa H, Verkman AS. Cloning of a water channel homolog expressed in brain meningeal cells and kidney collecting duct that functions as a stilbene-sensitive glycerol transporter. *J Biol Chem* 1994;269:21845–21849.
170. Ma T, Frigeri A, Skach W, Verkman AS. Cloning of a novel rat kidney cDNA homologous to CHIP28 and WCH-CD water channels. *Biochem Biophy Res Commun* 1993;197:654–659.
171. Ma T, Hasegawa H, Skach WR, Frigeri A, Verkman AS. Expression, functional analysis, and in situ hybridization of a cloned rat kidney collecting duct water channel. *Am J Physiol* 1994;266:C189–C197.
172. Ma T, Yang B, Gillespie A, Carlson EJ, Epstein CJ, Verkman AS. Severely impaired urinary concentrating ability in transgenic mice lacking aquaporin-1 water channels. *J Biol Chem* 1998;273:4296–4299.
173. Ma T, Yang B, Kuo WL, Verkman AS. cDNA cloning and gene structure of a novel water channel expressed exclusively in human kidney: evidence for a gene cluster of aquaporins at chromosome locus 12q13. *Genomics* 1996;35:543–550.
174. Ma T, Yang B, Verkman AS. Cloning of a novel water and urea-permeable aquaporin from mouse expressed strongly in colon, placenta, liver, and heart. *Biochem Biophy Res Commun* 1997;240:324–328.
175. Ma T, Song Y, Yang B, Gillespie A, Carlson EJ, Epstein CJ, Verkman AS. Nephrogenic diabetes insipidus in mice lacking aquaporin-3 water channels. *Proc Natl Acad Sci U S A* 2000;97:4386–4391.
176. Ma T, Yang B, Gillespie A, Carlson EJ, Epstein CJ, Verkman AS. Generation and phenotype of a transgenic knockout mouse lacking the mercurial-insensitive water channel aquaporin-4. *J Clin Invest* 1997;100:957–962.
177. Macey RI. Transport of water and urea in red blood cells. *Am J Physiol* 1984;246:C195–C203.
178. Maeda N, Funahashi T, Hibuse T, Nagasawa A, Kishida K, Kuriyama H, Nakamura T, Kihara S, Shimomura I, Matsuzawa Y. Adaptation to fasting by glycerol transport through aquaporin 7 in adipose tissue. *Proc Natl Acad Sci U S A* 2004;101:17801–17806.
179. Maeda Y, Smith BL, Agre P, Knepper MA. Quantification of aquaporin-CHIP water channel protein in microdissected renal tubules by fluorescence-based ELISA. *J Clin Invest* 1995;95:422–428.
180. Mandon B, Chou CL, Nielsen S, Knepper MA. Syntaxin-4 is localized to the apical plasma membrane of rat renal collecting duct cells: possible role in aquaporin-2 trafficking. *J Clin Invest* 1996;98:906–913.
181. Mandon B, Nielsen S, Kishore BK, Knepper MA. Expression of syntaxins in rat kidney. *Am J Physiol* 1997;273:F718–F730.

182. Mann SE, Ricke EA, Yang BA, Verkman AS, Taylor RN. Expression and localization of aquaporin 1 and 3 in human fetal membranes. *Am J Obstet Gynecol* 2002;187:902–907.
183. Marinelli RA, Pham L, Agre P, LaRusso NF. Secretin promotes osmotic water transport in rat cholangiocytes by increasing aquaporin-1 water channels in plasma membrane: evidence for a secretin-induced vesicular translocation of aquaporin-1. *J Biol Chem* 1997;272:12984–12988.
184. Marinelli RA, Tietz PS, Pham LD, Rueckert L, Agre P, LaRusso NF. Secretin induces the apical insertion of aquaporin-1 water channels in rat cholangiocytes. *Am J Physiol Gastrointest Liver Physiol* 1999;276:G280–G286.
185. Marples D, Barber B, Taylor A. Effect of a dynein inhibitor on vasopressin action in toad urinary bladder. *J Physiol* 1996;490(Pt 3):767–774.
186. Marples D, Christensen S, Christensen EI, Ottosen PD, Nielsen S. Lithium-induced downregulation of aquaporin-2 water channel expression in rat kidney medulla. *J Clin Invest* 1995;95:1838–1845.
187. Marples D, Frokiaer J, Dorup J, Knepper MA, Nielsen S. Hypokalemia-induced downregulation of aquaporin-2 water channel expression in rat kidney medulla and cortex. *J Clin Invest* 1996;97:1960–1968.
188. Marples D, Knepper MA, Christensen EI, Nielsen S. Redistribution of aquaporin-2 water channels induced by vasopressin in rat kidney inner medullary collecting duct. *Am J Physiol* 1995;269:C655–C664.
189. Marples D, Schroer TA, Ahrens N, Taylor A, Knepper MA, Nielsen S. Dynein and dynactin colocalize with AQP2 water channels in intracellular vesicles from kidney collecting duct. *Am J Physiol* 1998;274:F384–F394.
190. Martin PY, Abraham WT, Lieming X, Olson BR, Oren RM, Ohara M, Schrier RW. Selective V2-receptor vasopressin antagonism decreases urinary aquaporin-2 excretion in patients with chronic heart failure. *J Am Soc Nephrol* 1999;10:2165–2170.
191. Matsumura Y, Uchida S, Rai T, Sasaki S, Marumo F. Transcriptional regulation of aquaporin-2 water channel gene by cAMP. *J Am Soc Nephrol* 1997;8:861–867.
192. Maunsbach AB, Marples D, Chin E, Ning G, Bondy C, Agre P, Nielsen S. Aquaporin-1 water channel expression in human kidney. *J Am Soc Nephrol* 1997;8:1–14.
193. Maurel C, Reizer J, Schroeder JI, Chrispeels MJ, Saier MH Jr. Functional characterization of the *Escherichia coli* glycerol facilitator, GlpF, in Xenopus oocytes. *J Biol Chem* 1994;269:11869–11872.
194. McDill BW, Li SZ, Kovach PA, Ding L, Chen F. Congenital progressive hydronephrosis (cph) is caused by an S256L mutation in aquaporin-2 that affects its phosphorylation and apical membrane accumulation. *Proc Natl Acad Sci U S A* 2006;103:6952–6957.
195. Meinild AK, Klaerke DA, Zeuthen T. Bidirectional water fluxes and specificity for small hydrophilic molecules in aquaporins 0-5. *J Biol Chem* 1998;273:32446–32451.
196. Mitra AK, Van Hoek AN, Wiener MC, Verkman AS, Yeager M. The CHIP28 water channel visualized in ice by electron crystallography. *Nat Struct Biol* 1995;2:726–729.
197. Mitsuoka K, Murata K, Walz T, Hirai T, Agre P, Heymann JB, Engel A, Fujiyoshi Y. The structure of aquaporin-1 at 4.5-a resolution reveals short [alpha]-helices in the center of the monomer. *J Struct Biol* 1999;128:34–43.
198. Moon C, King LS, Agre P. Aqp1 expression in erythroleukemia cells: genetic regulation of glucocorticoid and chemical induction. *Am J Physiol* 1997;273:C1562–C1570.
199. Morello JP, Salahpour A, Petaja-Repo UE, Laperriere A, Lonergan M, Arthus MF, Nabi IR, Bichet DG, Bouvier M. Association of calnexin with wild type and mutant AVPR2 that cause nephrogenic diabetes insipidus. *Biochemistry* 2001;40:6766–6775.
200. Morgan T, Berliner RW. Permeability of the loop of Henle, vasa recta, and collecting duct to water, urea, and sodium. *Am J Physiol* 1968;215:108–115.
201. Morishita Y, Matsuzaki T, Hara-chikuma M, Andoo A, Shimono M, Matsuki A, Kobayashi K, Ikeda M, Yamamoto T, Verkman A, Kusano E, Ookawara S, Takata K, Sasaki S, Ishibashi K. Disruption of aquaporin-11 produces polycystic kidneys following vacuolization of the proximal tubule. *Mol Cell Biol* 2005;25:7770–7779.
202. Mulders SM, Bichet DG, Rijss JP, Kamsteeg EJ, Arthus MF, Lonergan M, Fujiwara M, Morgan K, Leijendekker R, van der SP, van Os CH, Deen PM. An aquaporin-2 water channel mutant which causes autosomal dominant nephrogenic diabetes insipidus is retained in the Golgi complex. *J Clin Invest* 1998;102:57–66.
203. Mulder SM, Knoers NV, Van Lieburg AF, Monnens LA, Leumann E, Wuhl E, Schober E, Rijss JP, van Os CH, Deen PM. New mutations in the AQP2 gene in nephrogenic diabetes insipidus resulting in functional but misrouted water channels. *J Am Soc Nephrol* 1997;8:242–248.
204. Mulders SM, Preston GM, Deen PMT, Guggino WB, Os CH, Agre P. Water channel properties of major intrinsic protein of lens. *J Biol Chem* 1995;270:9010–9016.
205. Muller J, Kachadorian WA. Aggregate-carrying membranes during ADH stimulation and washout in toad bladder. *Am J Physiol* 1984;247:C90–C98.
206. Murata K, Mitsuoka K, Hirai T, Walz T, Agre P, Heymann JB, Engel A, Fujiyoshi Y. Structural determinants of water permeation through aquaporin-1. *Nature* 2000;407:599–605.
207. Nakhoul NL, Davis BA, Romero MF, Boron WF. Effect of expressing the water channel aquaporin-1 on the CO2 permeability of Xenopus oocytes. *Am J Physiol* 1998;274:C543–C548.
208. Nejsum LN, Elkjaer M-L, Hager H, Frokiaer J, Kwon TH, Nielsen S. Localization of aquaporin-7 in rat and mouse kidney using RT-PCR, immunoblotting, and immunocytochemistry. *Biochem Biophys Res Commun* 2000;277:164–170.
209. Nielsen J, Kwon TH, Praetorius J, Kim YH, Frokiaer J, Knepper MA, Nielsen S. Segment-specific ENaC downregulation in kidney of rats with lithium-induced NDI. *Am J Physiol Renal Physiol* 2003;285:F1198–F1209.
210. Nielsen S, Chou CL, Marples D, Christensen EI, Kishore BK, Knepper MA. Vasopressin increases water permeability of kidney collecting duct by inducing translocation of aquaporin-CD water channels to plasma membrane. *Proc Natl Acad Sci U S A* 1995;92:1013–1017.
211. Nielsen S, DiGiovanni SR, Christensen EI, Knepper MA, Harris HW. Cellular and subcellular immunolocalization of vasopressin- regulated water channel in rat kidney. *Proc Natl Acad Sci U S A* 1993;90:11663–11667.
212. Nielsen S, Knepper MA. Vasopressin activates collecting duct urea transporters and water channels by distinct physical processes. *Am J Physiol* 1993;265:F204–F213.
213. Nielsen S, Knepper MA, Kwon T-H, Frokiaer J. Regulation of water balance. Urine concentration and dilution. In: Schrier RW, ed. *Diseases of the Kidney and Urinary Tract.* Philadelphia: Lippincott Williams & Wilkins; 2004:109–134.
214. Nielsen S, Marples D, Birn H, Mohtashami M, Dalby NO, Trimble M, Knepper M. Expression of VAMP-2-like protein in kidney collecting duct intracellular vesicles. Colocalization with Aquaporin-2 water channels. *J Clin Invest* 1995;96:1834–1844.
215. Nielsen S, Muller J, Knepper MA. Vasopressin- and cAMP-induced changes in ultrastructure of isolated perfused inner medullary collecting ducts. *Am J Physiol* 1993;265:F225–F238.
216. Nielsen S, Smith B, Christensen EI, Knepper MA, Agre P. CHIP28 water channels are localized in constitutively water-permeable segments of the nephron. *J Cell Biol* 1993;120:371–383.
217. Nielsen S, Smith BL, Christensen EI, Agre P. Distribution of the aquaporin CHIP in secretory and resorptive epithelia and capillary endothelia. *Proc Natl Acad Sci U S A* 1993;90:7275–7279.
218. Nielsen S, Terris J, Andersen D, Ecelbarger C, Frokiaer J, Jonassen T, Marples D, Knepper MA, Petersen JS. Congestive heart failure in rats is associated with increased expression and targeting of aquaporin-2 water channel in collecting duct. *Proc Natl Acad Sci U S A* 1997;94:5450–5455.
219. Nielsen S, Frokiar J, Marples D, Kwon TH, Agre P, Knepper MA. Aquaporins in the kidney: from molecules to medicine. *Physiol Rev* 2002;82:205–244.
220. Nielsen S, King LS, Christensen BM, Agre P. Aquaporins in complex tissues, II: subcellular distribution in respiratory and glandular tissues of rat. *Am J Physiol Cell Physiol* 1997;273:C1549-C1561.
221. Nishimoto G, Zelenina M, Li D, Yasui M, Aperia A, Nielsen S, Nairn AC. Arginine vasopressin stimulates phosphorylation of aquaporin-2 in rat renal tissue. *Am J Physiol* 1999;276:F254–F259.
222. Norregaard R, Jensen BL, Li C, Wang W, Knepper MA, Nielsen S, Frokiaer J. COX-2 inhibition prevents downregulation of key renal water and sodium transport proteins in response to bilateral ureteral obstruction. *Am J Physiol Renal Physiol* 2005;289:F322–F333.
223. Oksche A, Moller A, Dickson J, Rosendahl W, Rascher W, Bichet DG, Rosenthal W. Two novel mutations in the aquaporin-2 and the vasopressin V2 receptor genes in patients with congenital nephrogenic diabetes insipidus. *Hum Genet* 1996;98:587–589.
224. Pallone TL, Kishore BK, Nielsen S, Agre P, Knepper MA. Evidence that aquaporin-1 mediates NaCl-induced water flux across descending vasa recta. *Am J Physiol* 1997;272:F587–F596.
225. Pallone TL, Edwards A, Ma T, Silldorff EP, Verkman AS. Requirement of aquaporin-1 for NaCl-driven water transport across descending vasa recta. *J Clin Invest* 2000;105:2222.
226. Pao GM, Wu LF, Johnson KD, Hofte H, Chrispeels MJ, Sweet G, Sandal NN, Saier MH Jr. Evolution of the MIP family of integral membrane transport proteins. *Mol Microbiol* 1991;5:33–37.
227. Patil RV, Saito I, Yang X, Wax MB. Expression of aquaporins in the rat ocular tissue. *Exp Eye Res* 1997;64:203–209.
228. Pearl M, Taylor A. Actin filaments and vasopressin-stimulated water flow in toad urinary bladder. *Am J Physiol* 1983;245:C28–C39.
229. Pevsner J, Hsu SC, Braun JE, Calakos N, Ting AE, Bennett MK, Scheller RH. Specificity and regulation of a synaptic vesicle docking complex. *Neuron* 1994;13:353–361.
230. Phillips ME, Taylor A. Effect of nocodazole on the water permeability response to vasopressin in rabbit collecting tubules perfused in vitro. *J Physiol* 1989;411:529–544.
231. Phillips ME, Taylor A. Effect of colcemid on the water permeability response to vasopressin in isolated perfused rabbit collecting tubules. *J Physiol* 1992;456:591–608.
232. Preston GM, Agre P. Isolation of the cDNA for erythrocyte integral membrane protein of 28 kilodaltons. member of an ancient channel family. *Proc Natl Acad Sci U S A* 1991;88:11110–11114.
233. Preston GM, Carroll TP, Guggino WB, Agre P. Appearance of water channels in Xenopus oocytes expressing red cell CHIP28 protein. *Science* 1992;256:385–387.
234. Preston GM, Jung JS, Guggino WB, Agre P. Membrane topology of aquaporin CHIP. Analysis of functional epitope-scanning mutants by vectorial proteolysis: *J Biol Chem* 1994;269:1668–1673.
235. Preston GM, Jung JS, Guggino WB, Agre P. The mercury-sensitive residue at cysteine 189 in the CHIP28 water channel. *J Biol Chem* 1993;268:17–20.
236. Preston GM, Smith BL, Zeidel ML, Moulds JJ, Agre P. Mutations in aquaporin-1 in phenotypically normal humans without functional CHIP water channels. *Science* 1994;265:1585–1587.
237. Reizer J, Reizer A, Saier MH Jr. The MIP family of integral membrane channel proteins. sequence comparisons, evolutionary relationships, reconstructed pathway of evolution, and proposed functional differentiation of the two repeated halves of the proteins. *Crit Rev Biochem Mol Biol* 1993;28:235–257.
238. Ren G, Cheng A, Reddy V, Melnyk P, Mitra AK. Three-dimensional fold of the human AQP1 water channel determined at 4 A resolution by electron crystallography of two-dimensional crystals embedded in ice. *J Mol Biol* 2000;301:369–387.
239. Ren G, Reddy VS, Cheng A, Melnyk P, Mitra AK. Visualization of a water-selective pore by electron crystallography in vitreous ice. *Proc Natl Acad Sci U S A* 2001;98:1398–1403.
240. Reuss L. Focus on "Effect of expressing the water channel aquaporin-1 on the CO2 permeability of Xenopus oocytes". *Am J Physiol* 1998;274:C297–C298.
241. Risinger C, Bennett MK. Differential phosphorylation of syntaxin and synaptosome-associated protein of 25 kDa (SNAP-25) isoforms. *J Neurochem* 1999;72:614–624.
242. Robben JH, Knoers NVAM, Deen PMT. Cell biological aspects of the vasopressin type-2 receptor and aquaporin 2 water channel in nephrogenic diabetes insipidus. *Am J Physiol Renal Physiol* 2006;291:F257–F270.
243. Roberts SK, Yano M, Ueno Y, Pham L, Alpini G, Agre P, LaRusso NF. Cholangiocytes express the aquaporin CHIP and transport water via a channel-mediated mechanism. *Proc Natl Acad Sci U S A* 1994;91:13009–13013.
244. Rojek A, Fuchtbauer EM, Kwon TH, Frokiar J, Nielsen S. Severe urinary concentrating defect in renal collecting duct-selective AQP2 conditional-knockout mice. *Proc Natl Acad Sci U S A* 2006;103:6037–6042.
245. Saadoun S, Papadopoulos MC, Hara-Chikuma M, Verkman AS. Impairment of angiogenesis and cell migration by targeted aquaporin-1 gene disruption. *Nature* 2005;434:786–792.

246. Sabolic I, Katsura T, Verbavatz JM, Brown D. The AQP2 water channel: effect of vasopressin treatment, microtubule disruption, and distribution in neonatal rats. *J Membr Biol* 1995; 143:165–175.

247. Sabolic I, Valenti G, Verbavatz JM, Van Hoek AN, Verkman AS, Ausiello DA, Brown D. Localization of the CHIP28 water channel in rat kidney. *Am J Physiol* 1992;263:C1225–C1233.

248. Saito T, Ishikawa SE, Sasaki S, Fujita N, Fushimi K, Okada K, Takeuchi K, Sakamoto A, Ookawara S, Kaneko T, Marumo F, Saito T. Alteration in water channel AQP-2 by removal of AVP stimulation in collecting duct cells of dehydrated rats. *Am J Physiol Renal Physiol* 1997;272:F183–F191.

249. Sands JM, Flores FX, Kato A, Baum MA, Brown EM, Ward DT, Hebert SC, Harris HW. Vasopressin-elicited water and urea permeabilities are altered in IMCD in hypercalcemic rats. *Am J Physiol Renal Physiol* 1998;274:F978–F985.

250. Schenk AD, Werten PJL, Scheuring S, de Groot BL, Muller SA, Stahlberg H, Philippsen A, Engel A. The 4.5 A structure of human AQP2. *J Mol Biol* 2005;350:278–289.

251. Schmale H, Ivell R, Breindl M, Darmer D, Richter D. The mutant vasopressin gene from diabetes insipidus (Brattleboro) rats is transcribed but the message is not efficiently translated. *EMBO J* 1984;3(13):3289–3293.

252. Schnermann J, Chou CL, Ma T, Traynor T, Knepper MA, Verkman AS. Defective proximal tubular fluid reabsorption in transgenic aquaporin-1 null mice. *Proc Natl Acad Sci U S A* 1998;95:9660–9664.

253. Schnitzer JE, Oh P. Aquaporin-1 in plasma membrane and caveolae provides mercury-sensitive water channels across lung endothelium. *Am J Physiol* 1996;270:H416–H422.

254. Sharples EJ, Patel N, Brown P, Stewart K, Mota-Philipe H, Sheaff M, Kieswich J, Allen D, Harwood S, Raftery M, Thiemermann C, Yaqoob MM. Erythropoietin protects the kidney against the injury and dysfunction caused by ischemia-reperfusion. *J Am Soc Nephrol* 2004;15:212–224.

255. Shaw S, Marples D. N-ethylmaleimide causes aquaporin-2 trafficking in the renal inner medullary collecting duct by direct activation of protein kinase A. *Am J Physiol Renal Physiol* 2005;288:F832–F839.

256. Shi LB, Skach WR, Verkman AS. Functional independence of monomeric CHIP28 water channels revealed by expression of wildtype mutant heterodimers. *J Biol Chem* 1994;269:10417–10422.

257. Shimazaki Y, Nishiki TI, Omori A, Sekiguchi M, Kamata Y, Kozaki S, Takahashi M. Phosphorylation of 25-kDa synaptosome-associated protein: possible involvement in protein kinase C-mediated regulation of neurotransmitter release. *J Biol Chem* 1996;271:14548–14553.

258. Silberstein C, Bouley R, Huang Y, Fang P, Pastor-Soler N, Brown D, van Hoek AN. Membrane organization and function of M1 and M23 isoforms of aquaporin-4 in epithelial cells. *Am J Physiol Renal Physiol* 2004;287:F501–F511.

259. Smith BL, Agre P. Erythrocyte Mr 28,000 transmembrane protein exists as a multisubunit oligomer similar to channel proteins. *J Biol Chem* 1991;266:6407–6415.

260. Smith BL, Baumgarten R, Nielsen S, Raben D, Zeidel ML, Agre P. Concurrent expression of erythroid and renal aquaporin CHIP and appearance of water channel activity in perinatal rats. *J Clin Invest* 1993;92:2035–2041.

261. Smith BL, Preston GM, Spring FA, Anstee DJ, Agre P. Human red cell aquaporin CHIP. I. Molecular characterization of ABH and Colton blood group antigens. *J Clin Invest* 1994;94:1043–1049.

262. Sohara E, Rai T, Miyazaki JI, Verkman AS, Sasaki S, Uchida S. Defective water and glycerol transport in the proximal tubules of AQP7 knockout mice. *Am J Physiol Renal Physiol* 2005;289:F1195–F1200.

263. Sollner T, Whiteheart SW, Brunner M, Erdjument-Bromage H, Geromanos S, Tempst P, Rothman JE. SNAP receptors implicated in vesicle targeting and fusion. *Nature* 1993;362:318–324.

264. Solomon AK. Characterization of biological membranes by equivalent pores. *J Gen Physiol* 1968;51(5):Suppl:335S.

265. Solomon AK, Chasan B, Dix JA, Lukacovic MF, Toon MR, Verkman AS. The aqueous pore in the red cell membrane: band 3 as a channel for anions, cations, nonelectrolytes, and water. *Ann N Y Acad Sci* 1983;414:97–124.

266. Stamer WD, Snyder RW, Smith BL, Agre P, Regan JW. Localization of aquaporin CHIP in the human eye. implications in the pathogenesis of glaucoma and other disorders of ocular fluid balance. *Invest Ophthalmol Vis Sci* 1994;35:3867–3872.

267. Star RA, Nonoguchi H, Balaban R, Knepper MA. Calcium and cyclic adenosine monophosphate as second messengers for vasopressin in the rat inner medullary collecting duct. *J Clin Invest* 1988;81:1879–1888.

268. Strange K, Willingham MC, Handler JS, Harris HW JR. Apical membrane endocytosis via coated pits is stimulated by removal of antidiuretic hormone from isolated, perfused rabbit cortical collecting tubule. *J Membr Biol* 1988;103:17–28.

269. Sudhof TC, De CP, Niemann H, Jahn R. Membrane fusion machinery: insights from synaptic proteins. *Cell* 1993;75:1–4.

270. Sui H, Han BG, Lee JK, Walian P, Jap BK. Structural basis of water-specific transport through the AQP1 water channel. *Nature* 2001;414:872–878.

271. Takata K, Matsuzaki T, Tajika Y. Aquaporins: water channel proteins of the cell membrane. *Prog Histochem Cytochem* 2004;39:1–83.

272. Tannen RL, Regal EM, Dunn MJ, Schrier RW. Vasopressin-resistant hyposthenuria in advanced chronic renal disease. *N Engl J Med* 1969;280:1135–1141.

273. Tanner GA, Sloan KL, Sophasan S. Effects of renal artery occlusion on kidney function in the rat. *Kidney Int* 1973;4:377–389.

274. Teitelbaum I, McGuinness S. Vasopressin resistance in chronic renal failure. Evidence for the role of decreased V2 receptor mRNA. *J Clin Invest* 1995;96:378–385.

275. Terris J, Ecelbarger CA, Marples D, Knepper MA, Nielsen S. Distribution of aquaporin-4 water channel expression within rat kidney. *Am J Physiol* 1995;269:F775–F785.

276. Terris J, Ecelbarger CA, Nielsen S, Knepper MA. Long-term regulation of four renal aquaporins in rats. *Am J Physiol* 1996;271:F414–F422.

277. Timmer RT, Sands JM. Lithium intoxication. *J Am Soc Nephrol* 1999;10:666–674.

278. Tsukaguchi H, Shayakul C, Berger UV, Mackenzie B, Devidas S, Guggino WB, van Hoek AN, Hediger MA. Molecular Characterization of a broad selectivity neutral solute channel. *J Biol Chem* 1998;273:24737–24743.

279. Tsukaguchi H, Weremowicz S, Morton CC, Hediger MA. Functional and molecular characterization of the human neutral solute channel aquaporin-9. *Am J Physiol Renal Physiol* 1999;277:F685–F696.

280. Uchida S, Sasaki S, Fushimi K, Marumo F. Isolation of human aquaporin-CD gene. *J Biol Chem* 1994;269:23451–23455.

281. Valenti G, Frigeri A, Ronco PM, D'Ettorre C, Svelto M. Expression and functional analysis of water channels in a stably AQP2-transfected human collecting duct cell line. *J Biol Chem* 1996;271:24365–24370.

282. Vallon V, Verkman AS, Schnermann J. Luminal hypotonicity in proximal tubules of aquaporin-1-knockout mice. *Am J Physiol Renal Physiol* 2000;278:F1030–F1033.

283. Van Hoek AN, Hom ML, Luthjens LH, de, J, Dempster JA, van Os CH. Functional unit of 30 kDa for proximal tubule water channels as revealed by radiation inactivation. *J Biol Chem* 1991;266:16633–16635.

284. Van Hoek AN, Verkman AS. Functional reconstitution of the isolated erythrocyte water channel CHIP28. *J Biol Chem* 1992;267:18267–18269.

285. van Hoek AN, Ma T, Yang B, Verkman AS, Brown D. Aquaporin-4 is expressed in basolateral membranes of proximal tubule S3 segments in mouse kidney. *Am J Physiol Renal Physiol* 2000;278:F310–F316.

286. Van Lieburg AF, Verdijk MA, Knoers VV, van Essen AJ, Proesmans W, Mallmann R, Monnens LA, van Oost BA, van Os CH, Deen PM. Patients with autosomal nephrogenic diabetes insipidus homozygous for mutations in the aquaporin 2 water-channel gene. *Am J Hum Genet* 1994;55:648–652.

287. Venkatachalam MA, Bernard DB, Donohoe JF, Levinsky NG. Ischemic damage and repair in the rat proximal tubule. differences among the S1, S2, and S3 segments. *Kidney Int* 1978;14:31–49.

288. Verbavatz JM, Brown D, Sabolic I, Valenti G, Ausiello DA, Van Hoek AN, Ma T, Verkman AS. Tetrameric assembly of CHIP28 water channels in liposomes and cell membranes. a freeze-fracture study. *J Cell Biol* 1993;123:605–618.

289. Verkman AS. Applications of aquaporin inhibitors. *Drug News Perspect* 2001;14(7):412–420.

290. Wade JB, Kachadorian WA. Cytochalasin B inhibition of toad bladder apical membrane responses to ADH. *Am J Physiol* 1988;255:C526–C530.

291. Wade JB, Nielsen S, Coleman RA, Knepper MA. Long-term regulation of collecting duct water permeability: freeze-fracture analysis of isolated perfused tubules. *Am J Physiol* 1994;266:F723–F730.

292. Wade JB, Stetson DL, Lewis SA. ADH action: evidence for a membrane shuttle mechanism. *Ann N Y Acad Sci* 1981;372:106–117.

293. Wall SM, Han JS, Chou CL, Knepper MA. Kinetics of urea and water permeability activation by vasopressin in rat terminal IMCD. *Am J Physiol* 1992;262:F989–F998.

294. Walz T, Hirai T, Murata K, Heymann JB, Mitsuoka K, Fujiyoshi Y, Smith BL, Agre P, Engel A. The three-dimensional structure of aquaporin-1. *Nature* 1997;387:624–627.

295. Walz T, Smith BL, Agre P, Engel A. The three-dimensional structure of human erythrocyte aquaporin CHIP. *EMBO J* 1994;13:2985–2993.

296. Walz T, Smith BL, Zeidel ML, Engel A, Agre P. Biologically active two-dimensional crystals of aquaporin CHIP. *J Biol Chem* 1994;269:1583–1586.

297. Walz T, Tittmann P, Fuchs KH, Muller DJ, Smith BL, Agre P, Gross H, Engel A. Surface topographies at subnanometer-resolution reveal asymmetry and sidedness of aquaporin-1. *J Mol Biol* 1996;264:907–918.

298. Wang W, Li C, Kwon TH, Miller RT, Knepper MA, Frokiaer J, Nielsen S. Reduced expression of renal Na+ transporters in rats with PTH-induced hypercalcemia. *Am J Physiol Renal Physiol* 2004;286:F534–F545.

299. Wen HUA, Frokiaer J, Kwon TH, Nielsen S. Urinary excretion of aquaporin-2 in rat is mediated by a vasopressin-dependent apical pathway. *J Am Soc Nephrol* 1999;10:1416–1429.

300. Werten PJL, Hasler L, Koenderink JB, Klaassen CHW, de Grip WJ, Engel A, Deen PMT. Large-scale purification of functional recombinant human aquaporin-2. *FEBS Lett* 2001;504:200–205.

301. Wistow GJ, Pisano MM, Chepelinsky AB. Tandem sequence repeats in transmembrane channel proteins. *Trends Biochem Sci* 1991;16:170–171.

302. Wood LJ, Massie D, McLean AJ, Dudley FJ. Renal sodium retention in cirrhosis: tubular site and relation to hepatic dysfunction. *Hepatology* 1988;8:831–836.

303. Xu DL, Martin PY, Ohara M, St JJ, Pattison T, Meng X, Morris K, Kim JK, Schrier RW. Upregulation of aquaporin-2 water channel expression in chronic heart failure rat. *J Clin Invest* 1997;99:1500–1505.

304. Yamamoto T, Sasaki S, Fushimi K, Ishibashi K, Yaoita E, Kawasaki K, Marumo F, Kihara I. Vasopressin increases AQP-CD water channel in apical membrane of collecting duct cells in Brattleboro rats. *Am J Physiol Cell Physiol* 1995;268:C1546–C1551.

305. Yang B, Gillespie A, Carlson EJ, Epstein CJ, Verkman AS. Neonatal Mortality in an Aquaporin-2 Knock-in Mouse Model of Recessive Nephrogenic Diabetes Insipidus. *J Biol Chem* 2001;276:2775–2779.

306. Yang B, Song Y, Zhao D, Verkman AS. Phenotype analysis of aquaporin-8 null mice. *Am J Physiol Cell Physiol* 2005;288:C1161–C1170.

307. Yang B, Tonghui Dong JY, Verkman AS. Partial correction of the urinary concentrating defect in aquaporin-1 null mice by adenovirus-mediated gene delivery. *Hum Gene Ther* 2000; 11:567–575.

308. Yang B, Verkman AS. Water and glycerol permeabilities of aquaporins 1-5 and MIP determined quantitatively by expression of epitope-tagged constructs in Xenopus oocytes. *J Biol Chem* 1997;272:16140–16146.

309. Yang B, Zhao D, Qian L, Verkman AS. Mouse model of inducible nephrogenic diabetes insipidus produced by floxed aquaporin-2 gene deletion. *Am J Physiol Renal Physiol* 2006;291:F465–472.

310. Yang B, Zhao D, Solenov E, Verkman AS. Evidence from knockout mice against physiologically significant aquaporin 8 facilitated ammonia transport. *Am J Physiol Cell Physiol* 2006;291:C417–423.

311. Yasui M, Hazama A, Kwon TH, Nielsen S, Guggino WB, Agre P. Rapid gating and anion permeability of an intracellular aquaporin. *Nature* 1999;402:184–187.

312. Yasui M, Zelenin SM, Celsi G, Aperia A. Adenylate cyclase-coupled vasopressin receptor activates AQP2 promoter via a dual effect on CRE and AP1 elements. *Am J Physiol* 1997;272:F443–F450.

313. Yasui M, Kwon TH, Knepper MA, Nielsen S, Agre P. Aquaporin-6. An intracellular vesicle water channel protein in renal epithelia. *Proc Natl Acad Sci U S A* 1999;96:5808–5813.

314. Yip KP. Coupling of vasopressin-induced intracellular Ca2+ mobilization and apical exocytosis in perfused rat kidney collecting duct. *J Physiol* 2002;538:891–899.

315. Yool AJ, Stamer WD, Regan JW. Forskolin stimulation of water and cation permeability in aquaporin 1 water channels. *Science* 1996;273:1216–1218.

316. Zeidel M, Pirtskhalaishvili G. Urinary tract obstruction. In: Brenner BM, ed. *The Kidney*. Philadelphia: Saunders; 2004:1867–1894.

317. Zeidel ML, Ambudkar SV, Smith BL, Agre P. Reconstitution of functional water channels in liposomes containing purified red cell CHIP28 protein. *Biochemistry* 1992;31:7436–7440.

318. Zeidel ML, Nielsen S, Smith BL, Ambudkar SV, Maunsbach AB, Agre P. Ultrastructure, pharmacologic inhibition, and transport selectivity of aquaporin channel-forming integral protein in proteoliposomes. *Biochemistry* 1994;33:1606–1615.

319. Zelenina M, Christensen BM, Palmer J, Nairn AC, Nielsen S, Aperia A. Prostaglandin E(2) interaction with AVP: effects on AQP2 phosphorylation and distribution. *Am J Physiol Renal Physiol* 2000;278:F388–F394.

320. Zelenina M, Tritto S, Bondar AA, Zelenin S, Aperia A. Copper inhibits the water and glycerol permeability of aquaporin-3. *J Biol Chem* 2004;279:51939–51943.

321. Zelenina M, Bondar AA, Zelenin S, Aperia A. Nickel and extracellular acidification inhibit the water permeability of human aquaporin-3 in lung epithelial cells. *J Biol Chem* 2003;278:30037–30043.

322. Zelenina M, Zelenin S, Bondar AA, Brismar H, Aperia A. Water permeability of aquaporin-4 is decreased by protein kinase C and dopamine. *Am J Physiol Renal Physiol* 2002;283:F309–F318.

323. Zeuthen T, Klaerke DA. Transport of water and glycerol in aquaporin 3 is gated by H+. *J Biol Chem* 1999;274:21631–21636.

324. Zhang R, Van Hoek AN, Biwersi J, Verkman AS. A point mutation at cysteine 189 blocks the water permeability of rat kidney water channel CHIP28k. *Biochemistry* 1993;32:2938–2941.

325. Zhang RB, Logee KA, Verkman AS. Expression of mRNA coding for kidney and red cell water channels in Xenopus oocytes. *J Biol Chem* 1990;265:15375–15378.

CHAPTER **39**

Thirst and Vasopressin

Gary L. Robertson
Feinberg Medical School of Northwestern University, Chicago, Illinois, USA

Thirst and the antidiuretic hormone, arginine vasopressin, form the principle elements of a powerful and precise homeostatic system that acts to maintain the "effective" osmotic pressure of body fluids. The latter variable, also known as tonicity, is determined by the concentration in body water of solutes such as sodium, potassium, and chloride that do not equilibrate freely across cell membranes. It is obviously of vital importance since mechanisms to control it are found throughout the animal kingdom and significant disturbances in the normal level cause clinical disability in humans. However, the reason for its importance is less clear and it may be that regulating the *tonicity* of body fluids is mainly an indirect way to minimize changes in the *volume* of water within cells, particularly those of the brain.

Water is by far the largest component of the body. In a healthy adult, it makes up 55% to 60% of body weight and is divided between the intracellular and extracellular compartments in a ratio of about 2:1. Extracellular fluid is subdivided further between the interstitial and intravascular (plasma) compartments in a ratio of about 3:1. Thus, a human weighing 70 kg contains about 39 liters of water of which 26 liters is intracellular, 10 liters is interstitial fluid, and 3 liters is plasma. The *distribution* of water between the intracellular and extracellular compartments is determined by the relative amount of osmotically effective solute they contain because most cell membranes are freely permeable to water and cannot withstand an osmotic gradient. Thus, a change in the tonicity of one compartment results in a rapid redistribution of water with the other compartment until osmotic equilibrium is reestablished. However, the concentration of particular solutes in each compartment differs markedly due to active uptake or exclusion by specific transport systems in cell membranes. In extracellular fluid (ECF), sodium and its anions normally make up 95% of all solutes and nearly 100% of osmotically effective solute. Therefore, the measurement of plasma osmolality by a freezing point or vapor pressure method approximates closely the tonicity of body fluids. Urea and glucose contribute little if anything because, ordinarily, they are present in relatively low molar concentrations and enter cells very rapidly. In the absence of insulin, however, glucose becomes osmotically effective because it enters cells much more slowly. In intracellular fluid (ICF), the major solutes are potassium and its anions but other as yet unidentified solutes are also present and must contribute significantly to tonicity. Thus, an increase in body sodium or decrease in potassium expands ECF at the expense of ICF whereas a decrease in body sodium or increase in potassium expands ICF at the expense of ECF. On the other hand, a gain or loss of body water with no change in solute is distributed rapidly and evenly across all compartments in equal proportion to their size.

Body water also exchanges with the environment at highly variable rates depending on several external and internal influences that are not altogether controlled by thirst or vasopressin. Water is continuously lost by evaporation. The rate can vary markedly depending on ambient temperature and physical activity (2) but is at least 10 to 20 ml/kg a day (0.7 to 1.4 liters in a 70-kg human) even at rest in a comfortably cool environment. Urine output is tightly regulated by vasopressin but, in humans, cannot be reduced below a certain minimum required to excrete the load of sodium, chloride, potassium, urea, and other surplus or waste solutes derived from the diet and metabolism. Thus, at a normal solute load 600 to 1200 mOsm/d), urine output is at least 10 to 20 ml/kg a day (0.7 to 2.1 l/day in a 70-kg human) even when it is maximally concentrated under the action of vasopressin. The combined minimal daily water loss in a healthy adult is, therefore, at least 20 to 40 ml/kg (1.4 to 2.8 liters in a 70-kg human) and may be much more at times depending on changes in diet, activity, and temperature. Normally, this loss does not result in dehydration because it is replaced by an equivalent intake of water. Part of the intake (7 to 14 ml/kg or 0.5 to 1.0 liters in a 70-kg human) comes from the diet and metabolism of fat. Most if not all of the rest is drunk with meals probably in response to the slight increase in tonicity and thirst induced by adsorption of sodium and other solutes in food. Water ingested in excess of homeostatic need (e.g., as a result of social, cultural, medical, or psychological influences) is quickly offset by a commensurate increase in urine output mediated by a decrease in urine concentration (see subsequent sections).

VASOPRESSIN AND RELATED PEPTIDES

Chemistry

Arginine vasopressin, the antidiuretic hormone of humans and most other mammals (54, 40), is a nonapeptide containing an intrachain disulfide bridge and a tripeptide tail on which the terminal carboxyl is amidated (Fig. 1). Substitution of lysine for arginine in position 8 yields lysine vasopressin (LVP), the antidiuretic hormone found exclusively in pigs and other members of the suborder Suina (118). Vasopressin is structurally similar to oxytocin (Fig. 1), another nonapeptide hormone found in the posterior pituitary of all mammals (118). Oxytocin differs chemically from vasopressin by the substitution of isoleucine for phenylalanine at position three and of leucine for arginine at position eight.

Anatomy

Vasopressin and oxytocin are produced by the hypothalamic neurohypophyseal tract (Fig. 2). It is composed of magnocellular neurons that arise bilaterally in the supraoptic and paraventricular nuclei of the hypothalamus, project medially to merge in the pituitary stalk, and continue into the sella turcica where they form the posterior lobe of the pituitary (60,135,137,143,178). Microscopically, the posterior pituitary appears as a densely interwoven network of capillaries, pituicytes, and large nonmyelinated neurons containing many electron-dense secretory granules. The neurons terminate as bulbous enlargements on capillary networks at many different levels throughout the stalk and body of the neurohypophysis. On a T1-weighted magnetic resonance image (MRI), the posterior pituitary usually appears as a hyperintense signal or "bright spot" (40). The origin of this signal is still unknown but it appears to be closely related to the content or turnover of vasopressin (80) and is almost invariably absent not only in patients with the pituitary form of diabetes insipidus (43) but

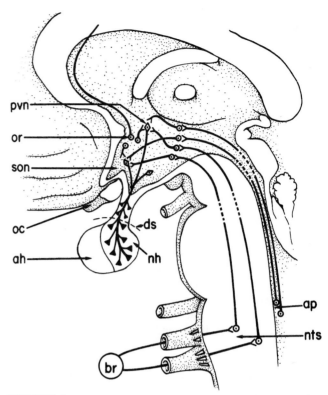

FIGURE 2 Anatomy of the neurohypophysis and principle regulatory afferents. Structures are abbreviated as follows: nh, neurohypophysis; ah, adenohypophysis; ds, diaphragm sella; oc, optic chiasm; son, supraoptic nucleus; pvn, paraventricular nucleus; or, osmoreceptors; br, baroreceptors; nts, nucleus tractus solitarius; ap, area postrema. (Adapted from Robertson GL. Diseases of the posterior pituitary. In: Felig P, Baxter J, Broadus A, et al, eds. *Endocrinology and Metabolism*, 2nd Edition, New York: McGraw-Hill, 1987:338–385, with permission.)

also in many of those with nephrogenic diabetes insipidus (Robertson GL, 2000, unpublished data). Vasopressin immunoactivity is also present in the suprachiasmatic nucleus and many other areas of the brain (137, 143,178).

The hypothalamic neurohypophyseal tract is supplied with blood by branches of the superior and inferior hypophyseal arteries that arise from the posterior communicating and intracavernous portions of the internal carotids (60). In the body of the neurohypophysis, the arterioles break up into the aforementioned capillary networks that drain directly into the jugular vein by way of the sellar, cavernous, and lateral venous sinuses. In the stalk or infundibulum, the primary capillary networks coalesce into another system, the portal veins, which perfuse the anterior pituitary before discharging into the systemic circulation. Because of its high blood supply, the normal neurohypophysis also emits a strongly enhanced MRI signal within 5 to 20 seconds of infusing a contrast agent (130).

Biosynthesis

Like most peptides, vasopressin is synthesized as part of a protein precursor that has a molecular mass of approximately 21,000 Da (81,108). This precursor is composed of a signal

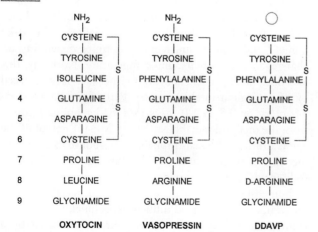

POSITION

	OXYTOCIN	VASOPRESSIN	DDAVP
	NH₂	NH₂	○
1	CYSTEINE	CYSTEINE	CYSTEINE
2	TYROSINE	TYROSINE	TYROSINE
3	ISOLEUCINE	PHENYLALANINE	PHENYLALANINE
4	GLUTAMINE	GLUTAMINE	GLUTAMINE
5	ASPARAGINE	ASPARAGINE	ASPARAGINE
6	CYSTEINE	CYSTEINE	CYSTEINE
7	PROLINE	PROLINE	PROLINE
8	LEUCINE	ARGININE	D-ARGININE
9	GLYCINAMIDE	GLYCINAMIDE	GLYCINAMIDE

FIGURE 1 Primary structure of arginine vasopressin and related peptides.

peptide at its amino terminus, vasopressin, the vasopressin-binding protein, neurophysin, and a glycosylated peptide, copeptin, at its carboxyl terminus (Fig. 3). During or after translocation to the endoplasmic reticulum, the signal peptide is removed and the N terminus of the vasopressin moiety binds to a pocket in the neurophysin moiety. The prohormone then folds, forms a number of intrachain disulfide bridges, and dimerizes (22) before moving through the Golgi and into the neurosecretory granules where it is transported down the axon and further processed to yield amidated vasopressin, neurophysin, and copeptin (23). Vasopressin and neurophysin are stored in nerve terminals as insoluble complexes that dissociate completely after release into the systemic circulation (21). Biosynthesis of vasopressin appears to be accelerated by stimuli, such as dehydration or hypertonic saline infusion (127), which increase secretion. However, this compensatory response develops slowly and may not completely offset the increased rate of release because pituitary stores of the hormone are severely depleted by a strong, sustained secretory stimulus such as prolonged water deprivation (97).

The gene encoding the vasopressin–neurophysin precursor in humans is located distally on the short arm of chromosome 20 (20p13) (109). It contains three exons that code for (1) the signal peptide, vasopressin, a dipeptide link, and the N-terminal variable portion of neurophysin; (2) the middle, highly conserved part of neurophysin; and (3) the C-terminal variable portion of neurophysin, a peptide link, and the glycopeptide, copeptin (Fig. 3) (131). The 5'-untranslated region upstream of the transcription start site

also has many conserved sequences, suggesting a possible role in gene regulation (108). The gene in rats (64), cows (125), and mice (59) is similar to that in humans but has several substitutions at either end of the highly conserved central portion of the neurophysin moiety. The vasopressin and oxytocin genes are closely linked with an intergenic region of only 11 kb (94,131). However, they are transcribed from opposite DNA strands, implying a tail-to-tail orientation, differ significantly in putative regulatory regions (108), and are expressed in mutually exclusive sets of neurons (93). The oxytocin gene also differs significantly from the vasopressin gene in that it does not contain a copeptin encoding sequence in exon-3 (108).

Effects

The principle action of vasopressin is to decrease urine output by increasing urine concentration. This antidiuretic effect is achieved by binding to G-protein–coupled V_2 receptors (20) located on the basal surface of principle cells in the distal and collecting tubules of the kidney. These receptors increase intracellular cyclic AMP (cAMP) (37) thereby inducing phosphorylation and translocation of preformed aquaporin-2 (AQP2) water-conducting channels into the apical (luminal) surface of the cell. In the absence of vasopressin stimulation, these channels are stored in intracellular vesicles and the luminal surfaces of the distal and collecting tubules including the tight junctions between cells are impermeable to water. Therefore, the large volume of dilute filtrate that normally issues from the ascending limb of

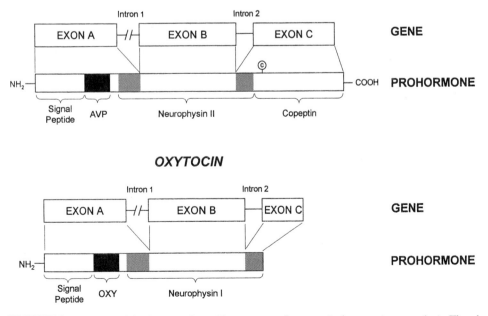

FIGURE 3 Structure of the human polypeptide precursors of vasopressin (vasopressin–neurophysin II) and oxytocin (oxytocin–neurophysin I) and the genes that encode them. (From Richter D. Molecular events in expression of vasopressin and oxytocin and their cognate receptors. *Am J Physiol* 1988;255:F207, with permission.)

Henle's loop passes unmodified through the distal tubules and collecting ducts, resulting in the excretion of very large volumes of maximally dilute urine (flow > 10 ml/min, osmolality <60 mOsm/kg). This condition is known as a *water diuresis*. In the presence of vasopressin stimulation, translocation and insertion of the AQP2 water channels into the luminal surface of tubular cells allow water in the dilute tubular fluid to be reabsorbed down the osmotic gradient into the cell and then out into the hypertonic renal medulla through AQP3 and AQP4 water channels located on the basolateral surface (78). Since water is reabsorbed without solute, the fluid that remains is decreased in volume and increased in concentration before it is excreted as urine. The magnitude of this antidiuretic effect is exquisitely sensitive to the concentration of plasma vasopressin. It reaches a maximum corresponding to a urine flow of about 0.5 ml/min and an osmolality around 1200 mOsm/kg at a plasma vasopressin level of only about 4 to 5 pg/ml (Fig. 4). Vasopressin also influences the activity of a urea transporter (UTA1) in the inner medullary collecting duct by binding to V_2 receptors and increasing cAMP (172). By replenishing the concentration of urea in the renal medulla, this transporter may enhance urinary concentrating capacity by increasing the hypertonic gradient that drives vasopressin dependent reabsorption of water.

At higher concentrations, vasopressin and its V_2 receptor selective analogue, des-amino-D-arginine vasopressin (desmopressin) can also stimulate release of factor VIII and other clotting factors from vascular endothelium (7). This effect has no known physiologic role but has been exploited pharmacologically to control bleeding during surgery in patients with hemophilia and other disorders. Vasopressin also binds to two other types of receptors known as V_{1a} and V_{1b} (95, 148). They act via stimulating phospholipase C and are expressed in blood vessels and many areas of the brain, including the large vasopressin-producing cells in the supraoptic nucleus (63, 157). Their role in human physiology/pathophysiology has not yet been defined but they may have some effects on blood pressure or pituitary adrenal function.

The principle physiologic action of oxytocin appears to be to facilitate nursing by contracting smooth muscle in mammary glands. These effects are mediated by oxytocin-specific receptors (180). Oxytocin also has a weak antidiuretic effect, which is mediated via the V_2 receptor (27). Several other variations on the vasopressin–oxytocin molecule have been identified in amphibians and fish, where they may play a similar role in the regulation of salt and water balance (1, 133).

The actions of vasopressin can be mimicked or blocked by a variety of peptides and nonpeptides that bind to its receptors The first to be developed was desmopressin (Fig. 1), a peptide analogue that selectively activates V_2 receptors at plasma concentrations at least as low as the native hormone (159). Desmopressin also has a longer duration of antidiuretic action than vasopressin because it is degraded less rapidly. It also does not constrict blood vessels or other smooth muscles presumably because it does not bind as well to V_1 receptors. It has now replaced vasopressin as the treatment of choice for patients with the pituitary (vasopressin deficient) form of diabetes insipidus. An analogue of desmopressin antagonizes selectively the antidiuretic action of vasopressin in rats (134) but it is ineffective in primates where it behaves as a partial agonist (3). More recently, several nonpeptide, V_1 and/or V_2 receptor antagonists have been used experimentally to treat patients with hyponatremia due to osmotically inappropriate secretion of vasopressin in congestive heart failure, cirrhosis, and the syndrome of inappropriate antidiuretic hormone (103, 104, 128, 170, 140)

Quantitation

The assay of vasopressin at physiologic levels presents an unusual combination of pitfalls and problems requiring exceptional effort to circumvent them (112). One problem is the unusually low concentrations at which the hormone normally circulates and acts. In healthy, normally hydrated, recumbent humans, the plasma vasopressin concentration is usually between 0.5 and 2.5 pg/ml ($\sim 10^{-13}$ M). This level is at least one order of magnitude lower than most other hormones yet it is sufficient to concentrate the urine (Fig. 4). Basal levels in other mammals are similar. Moreover, plasma also contains oxytocin, a nonpeptide that is structurally similar to vasopressin but has different biologic effects. Therefore, the assay used must be specific and sensitive. The only method now available that can meet both requirements is radioimmunoassay. However, it too presents unusual problems because vasopressin is relatively small and weakly antigenic. To complicate matters, most if not all the vasopressin antisera that have been generated are susceptible to nonspecific interference by one or more as yet unidentified components of plasma. Therefore, vasopressin must be extracted from plasma even if the antiserum used is sensitive enough to detect the hormone at physiologic concentrations. Moreover, there is no one extraction method that works with all assays because each antiserum differs as to the

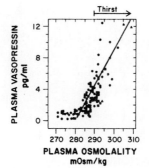
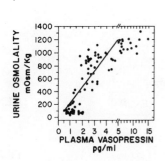

FIGURE 4   Relationship of plasma vasopressin to plasma and urine osmolalities in healthy adults. The arrow indicates the level of plasma osmolality at which thirst begins (Adapted from Robertson GL, Athar S, Shelton RL. Osmotic control of vasopressin function. In: Andreoli TE, Grantham JJ, Rector RC Jr (eds.). *Disturbances in body fluid osmolality*. Bethesda, MD: American Physiological Society, 1977:125–148, with permission.)

amount and type of interference to which it is susceptible. Therefore, the extraction method must be selected and tailored for the particular antiserum being used. For example, acetone extraction eliminates all the interference "seen" by one antiserum but not another (112). A third problem is the lack of a universal reference standard. Judging from the advertised biologic potency, those available vary by as much as twofold in purity and unknown values usually are not corrected for these differences. Therefore, unless the purity or potency of the standards is specified, it is impossible to compare absolute values reported by different laboratories even if they use the same antiserum and extraction technique.

The radioimmunoassay of vasopressin in urine would appear to be much easier than plasma because the concentrations are usually much higher and interference by other substances is much less. However, urine samples must usually be diluted or concentrated to a constant solute concentration (preferably hypotonic) because some antisera are affected by high concentrations of salt or urea. Also, to adjust for the effect of changes in antidiuresis per se, the total amount of vasopressin in a urine sample must be expressed as a function of the length of time over which the sample was collected or of the amount of a solute such as creatinine that is excreted at a relatively constant rate. Finally, the effect of changes in glomerular filtration or solute clearance on urinary vasopressin clearance must always be kept in mind (vide infra).

REGULATION OF SECRETION

Osmotic

The most important determinant of vasopressin secretion under physiologic conditions is the "tonicity" or effective osmotic pressure of body water (112, 117). Its effect is mediated by a group of cells known collectively as osmoreceptors (161). Their exact location is uncertain, but a great variety of indirect evidence indicates that they are concentrated in the anterior hypothalamus near to, but separate from, the supraoptic nucleus (Fig. 2) (52, 69, 86, 105, 113, 115, 155, 158). This area receives its blood supply from small perforating branches of the anterior cerebral or communicating arteries (60). Interruption of these vessels eliminates the osmoregulation of thirst and vasopressin without affecting the neurohypophysis or its response to nonosmotic stimuli (113).

The functional properties of the osmoregulatory mechanism resemble those of a discontinuous or "set point" receptor (Fig. 4). Thus, when plasma osmolality is below a certain minimum or threshold levels, plasma vasopressin is suppressed to very low or undetectable concentrations (<0.5 pg/ml). Above that set point, plasma vasopressin increases steeply in direct proportion with the increase in plasma osmolality. The slope of the line describing this relationship indicates that, on average, a rise in plasma osmolality of 1% increases plasma vasopressin by 1 pg/ml, an amount suffi-

cient to significantly alter urinary concentration and flow (Fig. 4). This extraordinary sensitivity confers on the osmoreceptor the primary role in mediating the antidiuretic response to changes in water balance.

The sensitivity of the osmoregulatory system can vary from person to person by as much as 10-fold (121). In some, a change in plasma vasopressin sufficient to significantly alter antidiuresis can be induced by a change in plasma osmolality as little as 0.5 mOsm/kg (0.17%), which is too small to be detected by laboratory osmometers. At the other extreme of normal, a comparable change in plasma vasopressin may require a change in plasma osmolality of as much as 5 mOsm/kg (1.7%). These individual differences in osmoregulatory sensitivity are constant over prolonged periods of time and appear to be determined largely by unknown genetic factors (Fig. 5) (175). However, the sensitivity of the osmoregulatory system is not immutable because the slope of the line describing the plasma vasopressin–osmolality relationship can be altered by a variety of conditions and drugs including hypovolemia, angiotensin, glucopenia, insulinopenia, lithium, gender and aging (vide infra).

The osmotic threshold for vasopressin secretion also varies from person to person (121). In healthy adults, it corresponds to a plasma osmolality that averages 280 mOsm/kg but can range anywhere from 275 to 290 mOsm/kg. These individual differences also are reproducible over time and appear to be determined by unknown genetic factors (Fig. 5) (175). However, they too can be altered by changes in blood pressure or effective blood volume, pregnancy, the menstrual cycle, chorionic gonadotrophin, and estrogen (vide infra).

It is uncertain whether the threshold concept accurately represents the operation of the osmoreceptor at its most fundamental level (96, 122, 167). Moreover, there is reason to think that vasopressin secretion reflects the balance of inhibitory as well as stimulatory inputs from a bimodal osmoregulatory system because patients and animals with adipsic hypernatremia due to destruction of the osmoreceptors may lose the capacity to osmotically suppress as well as to stimulate vasopressin secretion (113–115). If so, the inhibitory and stimulatory osmoreceptors probably have a common set or null point that corresponds closely to the normal basal tonicity of body fluids. As a practical matter, however, the concept of an osmotic threshold remains, for the present, a valid and useful way of describing many aspects of normal and abnormal osmoregulatory function in the intact animal.

It is also uncertain whether vasopressin is secreted continuously or episodically in response to osmotic stimulation. When nonosmotic stimuli such as posture, activity, and blood pressure are controlled, infusion of hypertonic saline in humans almost always produces a smooth progressive increase in systemic venous plasma vasopressin that correlates very closely with the increase in plasma osmolality (11, 46, 112, 145, 163, 175). However, samples obtained from

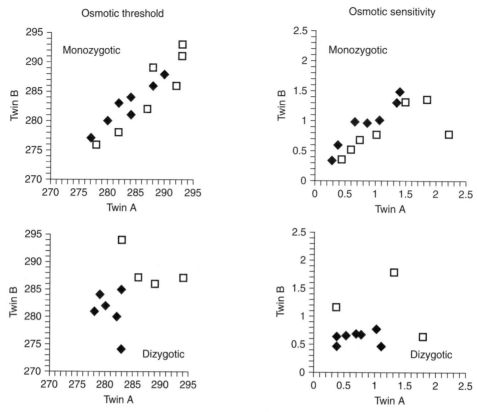

FIGURE 5   Genetic basis of individual variation in the osmoregulation of vasopressin secretion and thirst. The threshold and sensitivity for the osmotic stimulation of vasopressin secretion and thirst were determined by regression analysis of measurements made during hypertonic saline infusion in seven monozygotic and six dizygotic twin pairs. Each point indicates the value found in one twin as a function of the value found in the other member of the pair. The threshold values for vasopressin (*closed diamonds*) and thirst (*open squares*) are shown on the left. The sensitivities or slopes of the same two responses are shown on the right. The findings in monozygotes are shown in the two top panels; those in dizygotes in the two bottom panels. Note that both the threshold and the sensitivity of vasopressin and thirst responses showed considerable individual variation and these differences correlated closely within monozygotic but not dizygoptic twin pairs. (Redrawn from Zerbe RL, Miller JZ, Robertson GL. The reproducibility and heritability of individual differences in osmoregulatory function in normal humans. *J Lab Clin Med* 1991;117:51–59, with permission.)

experimental animals nearer the source of the hormone, for example, from the internal jugular vein, exhibit large fluctuations in plasma vasopressin during osmotic stimulation (168). Whether these fluctuations reflect an intrinsic property of the neurohypophysis or the osmoreceptors or are artifacts of the experimental conditions is unknown. Irregular phasic firing of the neurosecretory neurons has been observed by unit recording techniques, but this activity is unlikely to be related to episodic fluctuations in plasma vasopressin, because the discharge cycles have a much shorter periodicity and are not synchronized from cell to cell.

The sensitivity of the osmoregulatory mechanism is not the same for all solutes (Fig. 6) (88, 154, 176). Sodium and its anions, which normally account for nearly all of the effective osmotic pressure of plasma and interstitial fluid, are the most potent solutes known in stimulating vasopressin release. However, certain sugars, such as mannitol and sucrose, are also effective when infused intravenously. Indeed, particle for particle, mannitol appears to be just as potent

as sodium chloride (176). In this respect, therefore, the control mechanism behaves as though it were a true osmoreceptor. However, an increase in plasma osmolality produced by infusion of urea or glucose causes little or no increase in plasma vasopressin in healthy adults (88, 154, 176) probably because these solutes can penetrate cell membranes very rapidly. These differences are independent of any recognized nonosmotic influence, indicating that they are probably a property of the osmoreceptors themselves.

The basic mechanism by which osmoreceptors sense and respond to changes in the tonicity of body fluids has not been completely established. On the basis of studies in dogs, Verney proposed that the osmoreceptor is stimulated when its intracellular volume is reduced by an osmotically driven efflux of water (Fig. 7) (161). If that is true, the stimulatory potency of a solute would be a function of the rate at which it enters the osmoreceptor cell. Solutes that enter slowly would be "effective" because they create an

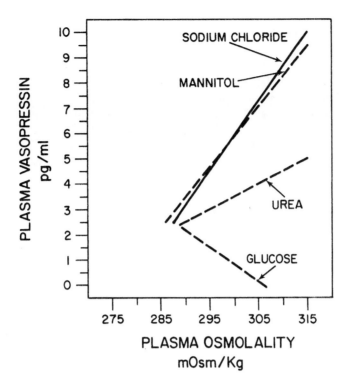

FIGURE 6   Solute specificity of the osmoreceptor. The lines represent the relationships of plasma vasopressin to plasma osmolality in healthy adults during intravenous infusion of hypertonic solutions of different solutes.

osmotic gradient that draws water from the cell; whereas those that penetrate rapidly would be ineffective because they would not create a hydro-osmotic gradient. This theory is consistent with the observations that hypertonic

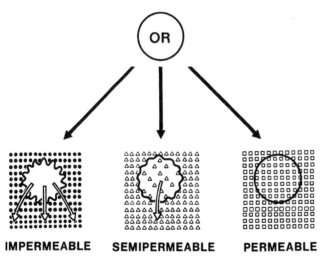

FIGURE 7   Hypothetical mechanism for solute specificity of osmoreceptors. Each of the three figures represents schematically the solute and water contents of an osmoreceptor cell exposed to a different hypertonic solution. Arrows indicate the direction and volume of net water flow. Stimulation of the osmoreceptor presumably is proportional to the level of dehydration. Note that at comparable extracellular concentrations, impermeable solutes create a larger osmotic gradient and extract more water than semipermeable solutes, whereas freely permeable solutes produce no gradient or net water flow across the cell membrane.

sodium and mannitol, which are excluded from cells, are potent stimulants whereas hypertonic glucose, which enters cells rapidly in the presence of insulin, does not increase vasopressin secretion. However, because mannitol does not cross the blood brain barrier, these observations are also consistent with the theory that the osmoreceptors are actually sodium receptors located on the brain side of the blood brain barrier (88, 102). However, the sodium receptor theory is not consistent with the relatively small rise in plasma vasopressin produced by an acute rise in plasma urea (150, 176) because it also crosses the blood–brain barrier slowly, reducing brain water and raising the concentration of sodium in brain ECF as a result. This singular disparity indicates that most, if not all, of the osmoreceptors are probably located on the somatic side of the blood-brain barrier and that another factor, most likely the solute permeability of the osmoreceptor cell itself, determines the specificity of the system. This concept is also consistent with the observations that (1) a severe deficiency of insulin sensitizes the osmoreceptors to stimulation by hyperglycemia presumably by decreasing its permeability to glucose (162); and (2) the osmoreceptors appear to be located in or near the organum vasculosum lamina terminalis of the anterior hypothalamus a region that is known to lack a blood–brain barrier.

Because of the solute specificity of the osmoreceptors, laboratory measurements of plasma osmolality over-estimate the true osmotic stimulus of vasopressin when ineffective solutes such as urea or glucose are elevated. In that situation, plasma vasopressin must be assessed in relation to the "effective" plasma osmolality (ePos). This value can be estimated in any of several ways. One is the formula:

$$ePos = 2 \times Pna$$

in which Pna is the plasma sodium concentration in mmol/l. This approach assumes that sodium and its anions are the only effective solute present and is probably justified if insulin is not deficient. However, it could underestimate stimulus strength in the presence of unmeasured idiogenic solute(s) that is/are osmotically effective. Another way to estimate ePos is to subtract from measured plasma osmolality (mPos) the molar contributions of the elevations in urea and glucose using the formula

$$ePos = mPos - [U + G - 7.5]$$

in which *U* and *G* area the measured concentrations of urea and glucose in mmol/l. This approach is probably also justified if insulin is present but could over-estimate stimulus strength in the presence of some unmeasured solute(s) that is/are *not* osmotically effective. When insulin is severely deficient, however, a different approach must be used because glucose then becomes about half as potent as sodium on a molar basis (162, 234). In that situation, a satisfactory approximation of the effective osmotic stimulus can be calculated by changing the formula above to

$$ePos = mPos - [U + G/2 - 7 - 5]$$

Hemodynamic

Secretion of vasopressin is also affected by changes in blood volume or pressure (39, 50, 112, 161, 164, 174). The functional properties of this baroregulatory system are exemplified in Fig. 7. In healthy adult humans, monkeys, and rats, acutely lowering blood pressure in any of several ways increases plasma vasopressin by an amount that is roughly proportional to the degree of hypotension induced. However, the stimulus-response relationship follows a distinctly exponential pattern (Fig. 8). Thus, small decreases in blood pressure of the order of 5% to 10% usually have little or no perceptible effect on plasma vasopressin, whereas decreases of 20% to 30% result in plasma hormone levels many times those required to produce maximum antidiuresis. An acute reduction in blood volume has a qualitatively and quantitatively similar effect (Fig. 8). Thus, plasma vasopressin does not rise appreciably until blood volume falls by at least 6% to 8%. Beyond that point, it begins to rise at a much faster rate and usually reaches levels 20 to 30 times normal when blood volume is reduced 20% to 30%. Chronic or sustained hypovolemia seems have even less effect on vasopressin, at least in rats. If blood volume is reduced more than 10% for 12 to 32 hours, plasma vasopressin is not elevated even though pituitary stores of the hormone and the response to acute osmotic or hypotensive stimuli are undiminished (65). Thus, attenuation of the vasopressin response appears to be

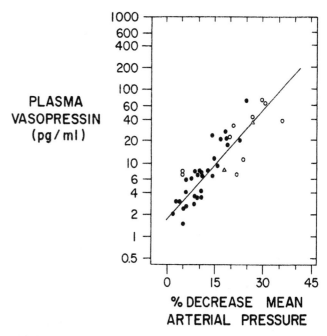

FIGURE 8   Relationship between plasma vasopressin and percentage decrease in arterial pressure in healthy adults. Hypotension was produced by infusion of a ganglionic blocker (*filled symbols*) or phlebotomy followed by orthostasis (*open symbols*). Note that plasma vasopressin is plotted on a log scale. (From Robertson GL. The role of osmotic and hemodynamic variables in regulating vasopressin secretion. In: James VHT (ed.). *Proceedings of the Fifth International Congress of Endocrinology*, Vol. 1. Excerpta Medica International Congress Series No. 402. Amsterdam: Excerpta Medica, 1977:126–130, with permission.)

due to selective desensitization of the volume control mechanism. The effect on vasopressin of acute and chronic changes in blood volume has not been as thoroughly investigated in other species but seems to be similar in dogs (8, 173) and humans (57, 111, 112). Thus, acutely reducing blood volume by as much as 7% has little or no effect on plasma vasopressin in recumbent healthy adults. Acute orthostasis, which decreases effective blood volume by 10% to 15%, usually doubles plasma vasopressin while hypovolemia of more than 20% results in much larger increases. Chronic hypovolemia caused by a deficiency of aldosterone also increases vasopressin secretion in humans (118).

The effect of acute hypovolemia on vasopressin secretion appears to be mediated largely by neuronal afferents that arise in pressure sensitive receptors in the left side of the heart (54, 84) and project by way of the vagus and glossopharyngeal nerves to primary synapses on the nuclei of the solitary tracts in the medulla. From there, signals ascend to the hypothalamus via postsynaptic pathways that appear to be mediated in part by a highly selective opioid neurotransmitter of the kappa subclass in the lateral parabrachial nucleus (66–68, 120). The vasopressin response to acute hypotension is mediated by neurogenic afferents that arise in high-pressure receptors in the aorta and carotid sinus and project via the vagus and glossopharyngeal nerves, presumably, to the nuclei of the solitary tracts (77, 84). From there, pathways that are at least partly noradrenergic (132) ascend to the hypothalamus. At least for part of their length, these ascending pathways are separate from those that mediate the vasopressin response to hypovolemia because they are not blocked by opioid antagonists that abolish the response to hypovolemia (66, 67, 120).

An acute increase in blood volume or pressure appears to inhibit vasopressin secretion (17, 19, 70, 141). This effect is relatively small and requires a large increase to cause the inhibition (Fig. 8). The pathways that mediate the hemodynamic suppression of vasopressin secretion are unknown. They may exert a tonic inhibitory effect on vasopressin under basal, normovolemic, and normotensive conditions because interruption of primary vagal afferents results in an acute rise in secretion (136, 151). If so, the stimulatory effect of acute hypovolemia or hypotension may be mediated at least in part by removal of this tonic hemodynamic inhibition. The influence on vasopressin of *chronic* increases in blood volume or pressure also is largely undefined. The osmoregulation of vasopressin secretion appears to be normal in patients with uncomplicated essential hypertension (6, 119) but the set point may be elevated in primary hyperaldosteronism (51) suggesting that chronic hypervolemia has an effect opposite to that of hypovolemia.

The different stimulus–response patterns of the osmoregulatory and baroregulatory systems have important implications for their role in the physiology and pathophysiology of vasopressin secretion. (Fig. 9). Because day-to-day variations in total body water rarely exceed 2% to 3%, their effect on vasopressin secretion must be mediated largely, if not exclusively, by the more sensitive osmoregulatory system. This explains why patients with selective destruction of the osmoreceptor exhibit a markedly subnormal vasopressin response to changes in water balance, even though their baroregulatory mechanisms appear to be completely intact (113, 118). However, the baroregulatory system probably mediates many pharmacologic and pathologic effects on vasopressin secretion (Table 1).

Changes in blood volume or pressure large enough to affect vasopressin secretion do not interfere with osmoregulation of the hormone. Instead, they appear to act by shifting the set of the system in such a way as to increase or decrease the effect on vasopressin of a given osmotic stimulus (Fig. 10) (39, 98, 107, 116, 117, 147, 165). Thus, vasopressin secretion can still be fully suppressed if plasma osmolality falls below the new, lower set point. This feature of the interaction is important, because it preserves the capacity to limit changes in tonicity of body fluids even when the primary mission of osmoregulation is compromised slightly to help defend blood volume or pressure. It also means that the osmoregulatory and baroregulatory systems, although different in location and function, ultimately converge and act upon the same population of neurosecretory neurons (72, 117).

TABLE 1 Variables that Influence Vasopressin Secretion

Osmotic
  Plasma osmolality
    Changes in water balance
    Infusion of hypertonic, hypotonic solutions
Hemodynamic
  Blood volume (total or effective)
    Posture
    Hemorrhage
    Aldosterone deficiency or excessive
    Gastroenteritis
    Congestive failure
    Cirrhosis
    Nephrosis
    Positive-pressure breathing
    Diuretics
  Blood pressure
    Orthostatic hypotension
    Vasovagal reaction
    Drugs (isoproterenol, norepinephrine, nicotine, nitroprusside, trimethaphan, histamine, bradykinin)
Emetic
  Nausea
  Drugs (apomorphine, morphine, nicotine, cholecystokinin)
  Motion sickness
Glucopenic
  Intracellular hypoglycemia
    Drugs (insulin, 2-deoxyglucose)
Other
  Stress
  Temperature
  Angiotensin
  PCO_2, PO_2, pH
Drugs and hormones (see Table 2)

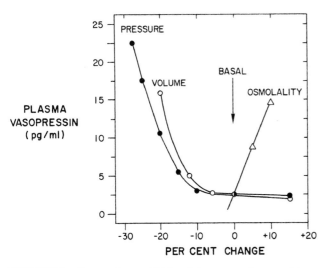

FIGURE 9 Comparative sensitivities of the osmoregulatory and baroregulatory systems. Note that vasopressin secretion is more sensitive to small changes in blood osmolality than to small changes in blood volume or pressure. (Adapted from Robertson GL. Diseases of the posterior pituitary. In: Felig P, Baxter J, Broadus A, et al, eds. *Endocrinology and Metabolism*, 2nd Edition, New York: McGraw-Hill, 1987:338–385, with permission.)

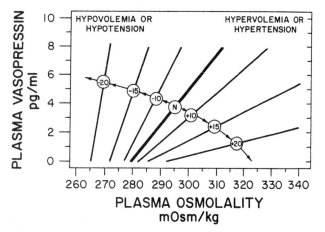

FIGURE 10 Effects of hemodynamic variables on the osmoregulation of vasopressin. Each line depicts the relationship of plasma vasopressin to plasma osmolality in the presence of varying levels of acute hypovolemia or hypotension (*left*) or hypervolemia or hypertension (*right*). Note that hemodynamic influences do not disrupt osmoregulation of vasopressin but raise or lower the set of the mechanism in proportion to the magnitude of the change in blood volume or pressure. Some change in the slope or sensitivity of the osmotic response may also occur, although this effect is less consistent. (From Robertson GL, Shelton RL, Athar S. The osmoregulation of vasopressin. *Kidney Int* 1976;10:25–37.)

Emetic

Nausea is an extremely potent stimulus for vasopressin secretion in humans (123). The pathways that mediate this effect have not been defined but they probably involve the chemoreceptor trigger zone in the area postrema of the medulla. The effect on vasopressin is instantaneous and

extremely potent (Fig. 11). Increases of 100 to 500 times basal levels are not unusual, even when the nausea is transient and unaccompanied by vomiting or changes in blood pressure. Pretreatment with fluphenazine, haloperidol, or promethazine in doses sufficient to prevent nausea completely abolishes the vasopressin response (123). The inhibitory effect of these dopamine antagonists is specific for emetic stimuli, because they do not alter the vasopressin response to osmotic or hemodynamic stimuli. Water loading blunts, but does not abolish, the effect of nausea on vasopressin release, suggesting that osmotic and emetic influences interact in a manner similar to osmotic and hemodynamic pathways. The effect of emetic stimuli is also species dependent. Whereas emetics such as apomorphine, cholecystokinin, lithium chloride, and copper sulfate stimulate the secretion of vasopressin but not oxytocin in humans (90, 123) and monkeys (160), they increase the secretion of oxytocin but have little effect on vasopressin in rodents (87).

Emetic stimuli probably mediate many pharmacologic and pathologic effects on vasopressin secretion. These include not only apomorphine (123), but also high doses of morphine (33, 38), nicotine (25), alcohol (123), cholecystokinin (90, 160) and motion sickness (47). They may also be responsible, at least in part, for the increases in vasopressin secretion that have been observed with intravenous cyclophosphamide (36, 146) acute hypoxia (62), diabetic ketoacidosis (177), vasovagal syncope (169), and hyperemesis gravidarum (29). Because nausea and vomiting are frequent side effects of many other drugs and diseases, additional examples of nausea-induced vasopressin

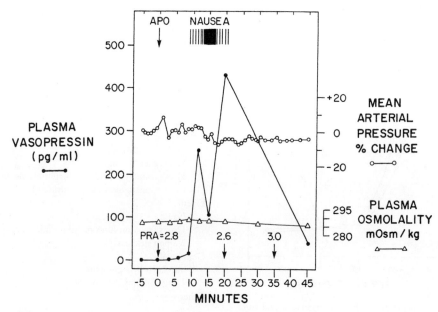

FIGURE 11 Effect of nausea on vasopressin secretion. Apomorphine was injected at the point indicated by the vertical arrow. Note that the increase in plasma vasopressin coincided with the occurrence of nausea and was not associated with detectable changes in plasma osmolality or blood pressure. (From Robertson GL. Vasopressin function in health and disease. *Recent Prog Horm Res* 1977;33: 333–385, with permission.)

secretion doubtlessly will be observed. The potency and ubiquity of emetic stimuli create special problems for research studies of vasopressin secretion in animals and unconscious subjects, because the occurrence of nausea is difficult to ascertain except by verbal report.

Glucopenia

Acute hypoglycemia is an equally consistent but less potent stimulus for vasopressin release (10, 13, 15). The receptor and pathway that mediate this effect are unknown. However, they seem to be separate from those of other recognized stimuli, because hypoglycemia stimulates vasopressin secretion in patients who have lost selectively the capacity to respond to osmotic, hemodynamic, or emetic stimuli (15). The effect of hypoglycemia is not due to nonspecific stress, because it can occur in the absence of symptoms and is more pronounced in rats (13), a species in which vasopressin secretion appears to be unaffected by pain and other noxious stimuli. The variable that actually triggers the release of vasopressin may be an intracellular deficiency of glucose or one of its metabolites because 2-deoxyglucose is also an effective stimulus (12,153). The stimulus-response relationship to hypoglycemia appears to be exponential (Fig. 12). Thus, in healthy adults, an acute decrease of plasma glucose of as much as 10% to 20% usually has little or no effect, whereas a decrease of 50% increases plasma vasopressin by about threefold. The rate of decrease in glucose is probably the critical determinant, however, because the increase in plasma vasopressin is not sustained even when the hypoglycemia persists (13). In addition, the vasopressin response is accentuated by dehydration and abolished by water loading (13). Thus, glucopenic stimuli probably act in concert with osmotic influences even though the osmoreceptors per se are unnecessary for the response.

Angiotensin

The renin-angiotensin system has also been implicated in the control of vasopressin secretion (99). The precise site and mechanism of action have not been defined, but one or more central receptors seem likely, because angiotensin II is most effective when injected directly into brain ventricles or cranial arteries (75, 99). The levels of plasma renin or angiotensin required to stimulate vasopressin release have not been determined but probably are quite high. When given intravenously, pressor doses of angiotensin II increase plasma vasopressin by only about twofold to fourfold (99). The magnitude of the vasopressin response may depend on the concurrent osmotic stimulus, because angiotensin has been observed to increase the sensitivity without significantly altering the set of the osmoregulatory system (142, 171). Hence, the effect of angiotensin on vasopressin may be imperceptible when plasma osmolality is depressed and exaggerated when plasma osmolality is high.

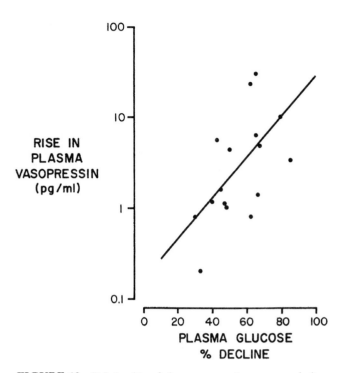

FIGURE 12 Relationship of plasma vasopressin to percent decline in plasma glucose in healthy adults. Hypoglycemia was produced by intravenous injection of insulin. Note that plasma vasopressin is plotted on a log scale. (From Baylis PH, Heath DA. Plasma-arginine-vasopressin response to insulin-induced hypoglycemia. *Lancet* 1977;11:428–430, with permission.)

This dependence on osmotic influences resembles that seen with moderate hypovolemic or glucopenic stimuli and may account for the failure of some investigators to demonstrate stimulation by peripherally administered angiotensin (24). Countervailing responses of the baroregulatory system to the increase in blood pressure may also inhibit the vasopressin response. It is not known if the endogenous renin-angiotensin system of plasma or the isorenins of brain and spinal fluid play any role in the regulation of vasopressin in health or disease.

Other Influences

STRESS

Nonspecific stress caused by pain, emotion, or physical exercise has long been thought to release vasopressin (126). However, it has never been determined whether this effect is mediated by a specific pathway or is due simply to secondary stimuli, such as the hypotension or nausea, which often accompanies the vasovagal reaction to pain or emotional stress. In rats and humans, a variety of stresses capable of activating the pituitary adrenal axis and sympathetic nervous system do not stimulate vasopressin secretion unless they also lower blood pressure or alter blood volume (41, 74, 112). Whether other species are more susceptible to noxious stimuli per se is unknown. The marked increase in plasma vasopressin elicited by manipulation of the abdominal viscera in anesthetized dogs has been attributed to nociceptive influences (156), but mediation by emetic or other known pathways cannot be excluded in this setting.

TEMPERATURE

Temperature can also influence vasopressin secretion (139, 149). In healthy adults, exposure to cold for a relatively short period of time depresses plasma vasopressin and heat has the opposite effect. These changes are independent of changes in plasma osmolality, but they cannot as yet be divorced from changes in effective blood volume or blood pressure. Thus, it is unclear whether there is a distinct thermoregulatory system for vasopressin secretion.

HYPOXIA

Acute hypoxia can also stimulate release of vasopressin (4), but this effect is inconstant (14, 28) and, in conscious humans at least, occurs only if hypotension or nausea develops (62). Therefore, hypoxia per se may not be a primary or direct stimulus for vasopressin.

OROPHARYNX

Vasopressin secretion is also inhibited by drinking per se (32, 53, 52). This occurs before there is a detectable decrease in plasma osmolality or sodium concentration and does not depend on the water reaching the stomach. It is unrelated to changes in blood pressure or blood volume but may depend on the volume or temperature of the fluid ingested because, in humans at least, small volumes of water (100 ml) at room temperature are less inhibitory than larger volumes (700–1200 ml) or small amounts of ice. Thus, the inhibition may be mediated by neural afferents that originate in taste, temperature, or other sensory receptors in the oropharynx. Inhibition of vasopressin by these oropharyngeal receptors is not only rapid but of very short duration. This may explain why the early-phase oropharyngeal inhibition of vasopressin is not associated with a concurrent decrease in urine concentration. However, the most curious aspect of the opharyngeal effect is the rapidity of the fall in plasma vasopressin. Reductions of more than 50% within 5 minutes are reported even though plasma vasopressin is cleared metabolically with a half-time of 10 to 30 minutes (see subsequent sections). This raises the question of whether the subjects were in an unsteady state of vasopressin secretion immediately before drinking; or whether activation of oropharyngeal receptors briefly accelerates the clearance of vasopressin or produces something that interferes with its assay.

AGE

Normal aging also appears to alter the osmoregulation of vasopressin secretion in humans but the nature of the change is controversial (18, 61, 83, 92). Some find that the vasopressin response to an osmotic stimulus is enhanced but others report no change or a decreased response.

These differences are unexplained and may represent individual variation in the neuronal control systems impacted by the aging process. Histologic studies of the human brain show no decrease in the number of large cell bodies in the supraoptic and paraventricular nucleus (138) but MRI studies indicate that the posterior pituitary bright spot is diminished or absent more often in the elderly (150). The latter is consistent with either a decrease or an increase in vasopressin secretion since diminution of the pituitary bright spot can be due to atrophy of the gland or to more rapid turnover of vasopressin. The ability to osmotically suppress vasopressin secretion and dilute the urine does not seem to change appreciably with age but the capacity to excrete a water load diminishes markedly due apparently to the large age related reduction in glomerular filtration rate (30). Oropharyngeal inhibition of vasopressin secretion appears to be slowed in the elderly (106) but this does not seem to significantly impair the overall rate of urinary water excretion once plasma osmolality begins to fall. The capacity to maximally concentrate the urine also diminishes with age but this is also due largely to renal factors (124).

GENDER, PREGNANCY, THE MENSTRUAL CYCLE, AND GONADAL HORMONES

The effects of gender on the osmoregulation of vasopressin secretion are complex and somewhat unsettled. There does not appear to be any significant difference between adult human males and non-gravid females (175) but pregnancy results in a relatively large reduction in the osmotic threshold for vasopressin release in rats as well as humans (9, 85). Downward resetting of the osmostat also occurs during the luteal phase of the human menstrual cycle (144, 163) but the difference is much smaller than in pregnancy and is smaller even than the range of individual differences in men and non-gravid women (175). Hence, it is unlikely to affect mean values in a population containing women in various phases of menstruation. The cause of the resetting is uncertain but may be mediated by relaxin (85), an increase in estrogens (145) or chorionic gonadotropin (46) since they also lower the set of the osmostat in humans. Progesterone appears to have no affect (26). In rats, large doses of estrogen seem to have a different effect than in humans since they enhance the slope or sensitivity of the vasopressin response to plasma osmolality but do not significantly alter its set point (9).

DRUGS AND OTHER HORMONES

Many drugs and hormones also influence vasopressin secretion (Table 2). Those that stimulate such as histamine, bradykinin, prostaglandin, α-endorphin, and high doses of morphine have not been studied sufficiently to define their mechanisms of action but most if not all probably work by decreasing blood pressure or producing nausea. Vincristine may have a direct toxic effect on the neurohypophysis or peripheral neurons involved in the regulation of vasopressin secretion. Lithium, which antagonizes the antidiuretic

TABLE 2   Drugs and Hormones That Affect Vasopressin Secretion

Stimulatory	Inhibitory
Acetycholine	Fluphenazine
Morphine (high doses)	Haloperidol
Epinephrine	Promethazine
Histamine	Oxilorphan
Bradykinin	Butorphanol
Prostaglandins	Opiods (κ and δ agonists)
β-Endorphin	Morphine (low doses)
Cyclophosphamide	Alcohol
Vincristine	Carbamazepine
Lithium	? Glucocorticoids
? Chlorpropamide	? Phenytoin
? Clofibrate	
? Corticotropin-releasing factor	

effect of vasopressin, also increases secretion of the hormone. This effect is independent of changes in water balance and appears to result from an increase in sensitivity of the osmoregulatory system (56). The stimulatory effects of chlorpropamide and clofibrate are still controversial and a mechanism of action has not been proposed. In high doses, vasopressin can also stimulate its own secretion (44). The mechanism of this feedback effect is unknown, but it appears to be totally independent of any of the other recognized osmotic and nonosmotic stimulus. It is probably of little physiologic significance because sodium depletion and large doses of the hormone are required to consistently elicit this response.

Inhibitors such as the dopaminergic antagonists fluphenazine, haloperidol, and promethazine probably act by suppressing the emetic center because they inhibit the vasopressin response to nausea but not to osmotic or hemodynamic stimuli. Many opiates are also inhibitory. They include oxilorphan and butorphanol, the κ-agonists U50488 (100), leu-morphin, and U62066E, as well as low doses of morphine. In the case of morphine and butorphanol, the inhibition is due to an increase in the osmotic threshold for vasopressin release and is independent of changes in blood volume or pressure (71, 91). The mechanism of the resetting has not been completely defined. However, it would appear to be due to the agonist properties of these opiates because it can be blocked by naloxone (58, 71). The inhibitory effect of alcohol may also be mediated in part by endogenous opiates because it is also due to upward resetting of the osmostat and can be partly reversed by treatment with naaloxone (101). Carbamazepine inhibits vasopressin secretion by diminishing the sensitivity of the osmoregulatory system (55). This effect is not dependent on changes in blood volume, blood pressure, or blood glucose and suggests that the ability of carbamazepine to produce antidiuresis in patients with neurogenic (pituitary) diabetes insipidus is due to an independent action on the kidney.

DISTRIBUTION AND CLEARANCE

The plasma vasopressin concentration is a function of the rate of secretion, volume of distribution and rate of clearance. After release into the systemic circulation, vasopressin appears to distribute quickly into a space equal to extracellular fluid volume (82, 112). In healthy adults, equilibration between the vascular and extravascular compartments is largely complete within 10 minutes. The rapidity with which vasopressin diffuses across capillary membranes is consistent with its relatively small size and lack of binding to neurophysin or other macromolecular components of plasma. The rapid decline during the mixing phase is followed by a second, slower decline that presumably reflects the metabolic or irreversible phase of clearance (82, 112). It has a half-life of 10 to 30 minutes. Thus, the total clearance rate of vasopressin ranges from about 10 to 20 ml/kg body weight per minute. The metabolic clearance rate increases markedly during pregnancy, reaching a level three- to fourfold greater than normal by the third trimester (31). Smaller animals such as rats also clear vasopressin much more rapidly because their cardiac output is much higher relative to body weight and surface area (82).

Although many tissues have the capacity to inactivate vasopressin in vitro, most metabolism in vivo appears to occur in liver and kidney (82). In pregnancy, vasopressin is also degraded by a vasopressinase produced by the placenta (31, 83).

Some vasopressin is excreted intact in the urine. The amount can vary considerably depending on the overall rate of solute excretion (112) but it is never more than a fraction of total irreversible clearance. In healthy, normally hydrated adults, the urinary clearance of vasopressin ranges from 0.1 to 0.6 ml/kg/min. The mechanisms involved in the excretion of vasopressin have not been defined but it is probably filtered at the glomerulus and variably reabsorbed at one or more sites along the tubule. The latter process seems to be influenced by the reabsorption of sodium and chloride in the proximal nephron, because the urinary clearance rate of vasopressin varies by as much as 20-fold in direct relationship to the clearance rate of total solute (112). Thus, changes in urinary vasopressin excretion do not provide a reliable guide to changes in plasma vasopressin if glomerular filtration or solute clearance is inconstant or abnormal.

THIRST

The regulation of fluid intake is an indispensable part of the homeostatic system that serves to maintain the tonicity of body fluids. Because the water lost through evaporation and urination cannot be reduced below the minimum needed for cooling and urinary excretion of dietary waste, it is essential to ensure that this obligatory loss is always replaced. Some of the requisite water comes from food and the metabolism of fat but the amounts are limited and often inadequate especially when evaporative loss rises due to an increase in ambient temperature or physical activity. The additional intake needed to offset this deficiency is provided by the thirst mechanism. Its importance is dramatically illustrated by the episodes of severe and sometimes fatal hypertonic dehydration that occur in patients who lack the sensation of thirst (115). The opposite risk—that of hypotonic overhydration—is not as great because the mechanisms for excreting excess water can normally offset all but the most pathologically extreme polydipsia. However, the capacity of this aquaretic safety valve can be reduced severely by a decrease in urinary solute load or a nonosmotic stimulus to vasopressin secretion. Thus, a backup mechanism for inhibiting water intake could also be of value to defend against overhydration. This antidipsic mechanism appears to operate by producing a sense of satiation or distaste for water.

Definition

Thirst may be defined as the subjective sensation of a desire or need for water. It is sometimes associated with feelings of dry mouth, headache, or irritability but these symptoms are not specific to thirst since they also have other causes. It must also be distinguished from cultural, social, psychological, medical, and other motivations to drink. The opposite of thirst is the feeling of satiation. It is not simply the absence of thirst but a conscious aversion to drinking that can make unflavored fluids taste unpleasant. It may be associated with other less specific symptoms such as fullness or even nausea, particularly if a large amount of water is drunk within a short space of time.

Anatomy

The parts of the brain that mediate the conscious awareness of thirst and satiation have not been fully defined. Studies using functional magnetic resonance imaging or positron emission tomography of the brain in healthy adults have shown that thirst is associated with activation in several areas including the anterior wall of the third ventricle, anterior cingulate cortex, parahippocampal gyrus, inferior and middle frontal gyrus, insula, and cerebellum (42). Drinking to satiation suppresses the activity in the anterior cingulate cortex (Brodmann area [BA] 32) before there is a decrease in plasma sodium or the activity in the anterior hypothalamus. This suggests that BA 32 is directly involved in the awareness of thirst and can be suppressed by pathways not involving the osmoreceptors. The difficulty with such findings, however, is that the sensation of thirst probably activates many brain areas involved in secondary feelings, thoughts or responses such as anxiety, discomfort or physical movement induced by feelings of thirst. To differentiate these secondary areas of arousal from those that mediate the consciousness of thirst per se, it will be necessary to employ a variety of other unpleasant stimuli as controls (48) or study the effect of discrete strokes or other ablative lesions in different brain areas.

Effects

Thirst induces the ingestion of water or other fluids unless there is some physical impediment to drinking. If intense, it may drive an animal to drink sea water or even urine even though these fluids are markedly hypertonic and only aggravate the underlying problem. Within 30 to 45 minutes of drinking, water is absorbed from the gastrointestinal tract and is carried by blood throughout the body, distributing rapidly between ECF and ICF in a ratio of about 1:2. Thus, it dilutes all body fluid equally, restoring tonicity toward normal. The total amount of fluid drunk at one time, commonly referred to as a "bout" of drinking, is roughly proportional to the elevation in plasma osmolality. It is also remarkably close to the volume needed to restore tonicity to normal even though the amount absorbed by the end of the bout is insufficient to normalize plasma osmolality and sodium. This pause in drinking may due to rapid inhibition of thirst by neural pathways arising in oropharyngeal receptors (see subsequent section). However, the inhibition is of short duration (10–15 minutes) and soon gives way to a return of thirst and drinking until enough water is absorbed to lower plasma osmolality to basal levels. These bouts may be repeated two or three times for up to 2 to 3 hours until the hypertonicity is completely eliminated.

Satiation aids in the defense against hypotonicity by producing a conscious aversion to drinking water. In humans, it occurs less often and less strongly than the sensation of thirst but seems to result in negative "thirst" ratings and a marked reduction of spontaneous fluid intake after induction of plasma hypotonicity either by water loading or repeat administration of high doses of the V_2 agonist, desmopressin (79).

Quantitation

Thirst cannot be measured objectively at present. However, changes in its intensity can be estimated by subjective report and scoring on a visual analog scale (175). The volume of spontaneous fluid intake can also be taken as an indirect measure of thirst but these findings should be interpreted with caution because of the many other motivations to drink. Satiation can also be estimated on a visual analog scale or monitoring reductions in spontaneous fluid intake.

Regulation

OSMOTIC

Like the secretion of vasopressin, thirst is influenced by a number of variables. Probably the most important under physiologic conditions is the tonicity or effective osmotic pressure of body fluids (115). Its effect is also mediated via hypothalamic osmoreceptors that are anatomically distinct from but intermingled with those that regulate vasopressin (5, 45, 89). Their functional properties are also similar to that of the vasopressin osmoreceptors except that the threshold for thirst seems to be set slightly higher. In healthy adults, the level of plasma osmolality at which thirst begins averages about 295 mOsm/kg and ranges from 289 to 307 mOsm/kg. It is almost always from 5 to 15 mOsm/kg higher than the osmotic threshold for vasopressin release (112, 115, 175). In most people, therefore, thirst is not experienced until plasma osmolality rises to a level at which plasma vasopressin is high enough to maximally concentrate the urine. In other respects, the thirst osmoreceptors behave much like those for vasopressin secretion. They have the same solute specificity since increases in plasma osmolality produced by infusion of hypertonic saline or mannitol are dipsogenic, whereas those resulting from infusions of hypertonic urea or glucose are not (154, 176). Their sensitivity—that is, the intensity of the thirst produced by a given rise in plasma osmolality, and their set points differ significantly from person to person. These differences also appear to be genetically determined (Fig. 5) (175). However, one or both properties also can be altered by changes in blood volume (166), pregnancy (85), the menstrual cycle (144, 163), and human chorionic gonadotrophin (46). Estrogen apparently does not alter the osmoregulation of thirst in humans (145).

Other Influences

HEMODYNAMIC

Anecdotal evidence indicates that thirst can also be stimulated by severe reductions in blood volume or blood pressure. The pathways that mediate this effect have not been defined but are probably the same as those that mediate the effects on vasopressin (see previous section). In rats, a hypovolemia-induced increase in angiotensin II may also play an important role (see subsequent section) but such an effect has not been convincingly documented in humans. Also like vasopressin, moderate reductions in blood volume lower the osmotic threshold for thirst but do not otherwise interfere with continued operation of the osmoregulatory system (166).

ANGIOTENSIN

In rats and some other animals, angiotensin II stimulates water intake particularly when injected into the lateral ventricles or other areas of brain (89). Presumably, the increased intake is due to thirst although some other type of inducement cannot be excluded. In humans, the dipsogenic effect of angiotensin II has not been investigated. However, it is probably unimportant under physiologic conditions because its suppression by hypertonic saline infusion does not prevent the marked increase in thirst induced by a relatively small rise in plasma osmolality (176).

GLUCOPENIA

Although anecdotal evidence suggests that thirst can also be induced by acute, insulin-induced hypoglycemia, controlled studies are lacking (Fig. 12). However, it is clear that an intracellular deficiency of glucose produced by adminis-

tration of 2-deoxyglucose stimulates thirst as well as vasopressin release (153). Neither effect is likely to play a role in the physiology or pathophysiology of water balance.

OROPHARYNX

Like vasopressin secretion, thirst is also inhibited rapidly and transiently by the act of drinking per se (49). The characteristics of this effect are similar to those for vasopressin (see previous section). They appear to be independent of osmotic and hemodynamic influences as well as the solute content of the fluid but may be influenced by its volume or temperature. The inhibition of thirst is extremely rapid and nearly complete, decreasing the sensation to near zero in a matter of minutes. However, it is also transient, lasting no more than 10 to 15 minutes, well short of the time required to absorb enough water to begin reducing the osmotic stimulus. Thus, thirst begins to increase again before undergoing a second decline due to absorption of the water and lowering of plasma osmolality. This timing is consistent with the temporal dissociation between the drinking induced decrease of positron emission tomography (PET) and MRI activity in the anterior cingulated cortex and the anterior hypothalamus (lamina terminalis) (42). It may also explain why drinking in response to a strong osmotic stimulus often occurs in 2 or more bouts separated by 15 to 30 minutes.

EATING

It is common knowledge documented by observational studies that most of the water ingested each day is drunk in association with meals (Fig. 13) (34). The finding that the amount of liquid drunk with each meal correlates with its estimated protein and carbohydrate content and not with its estimated sodium content lead to a theory that eating per se is a major independent stimulus to thirst unrelated to osmotic stimulation (35). However, in healthy adults allowed to eat, drink, and ambulate at will, there appears to be slight increases in plasma osmolality and decreases in plasma protein during meals (Fig. 14). Thus, it is not yet certain if drinking with meals is due to osmotically induced thirst or to some other stimulus such as taste or cultural habit.

AGING

In contrast to vasopressin secretion, the sensation of thirst and the drinking response to dehydration is diminished among the elderly (76). The reason, however, is controversial. One theory holds that the sensitivity of the response is decreased due to loss of the potentiating effect of the mild volume depletion that occurs during dehydration. Others find that the decrease in thirst is due largely to upward resetting of the thirst osmostat with little or no decrease in sensitivity. Compared to healthy young adults, however, there does not appear to be any change in the amount of fluid consumed in response to a given level of thirst or in the rapidity and extent of thirst suppression by oropharyngeal influences.

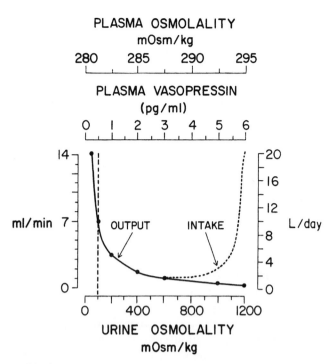

FIGURE 13   Relationship of water intake and urine output to plasma osmolality, plasma vasopressin and urine osmolality in a typical healthy adult. The calculated urine output (*solid line*) assumes an average solute load of 600 mOsm/day and an insensible loss of 1 l/day. The estimated water intake (*dashed line*) assumes a basal rate (food, metabolism, and meals) of 2 l/day. (Adapted from Robertson GL. Diseases of the posterior pituitary. In: Felig P, Baxter J, Broadus A, et al, eds. *Endocrinology and Metabolism*, 2nd Edition, New York: McGraw-Hill, 1987:338–385, with permission.)

ROLE OF VASOPRESSIN AND THIRST IN OSMOREGULATION

Vasopressin and thirst act in concert to control the tonicity of body fluids by raising or lowering body water to keep the concentration of osmotically effective solutes within a very narrow range. The upper and lower limits of this range correspond to the osmotic thresholds for thirst and vasopressin secretion, respectively, because the large increase in water intake or excretion that normally occurs at these thresholds prevents any further increase or decrease in the tonicity of body fluid (Fig. 13). Thus, even patients with a severe polyuria due to a deficiency of vasopressin maintain tonicity within normal limits simply by drinking more while those with severe polydipsia do the same by increasing urine output. Because the level of plasma osmolality at which the thirst and vasopressin osmostats are "set" differs appreciably from person to person (Fig. 5) (175), the absolute level at which tonicity is maintained in different people also differs by as much as 10 to 15 mOsm/L (3%–5%). Within each person, however, the level of tonicity is maintained very tightly about halfway between his or her osmotic threshold for thirst and vasopressin secretion. From that midpoint, even a tiny increase or decrease in tonicity resulting from a change in water or sodium balance elicits

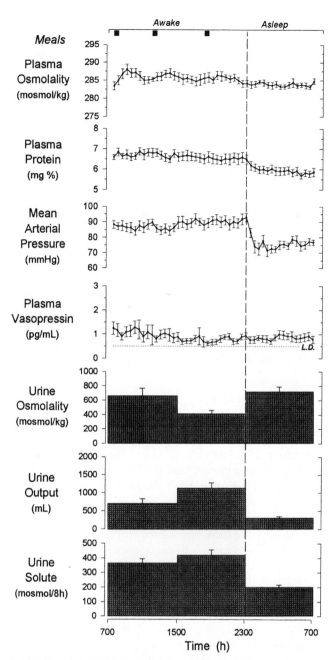

FIGURE 14   Circadian variations in antidiuretic function and related variables in healthy young adults. Each value is the mean ± SEM of nine subjects (four females and five males) on ad libitum intake of food and water. The three closed squares at the top indicate meals. Fluid intake, which is not shown, averaged 3.1 l/day. It occurred in equal amounts during the two periods of the day (7 AM to 3 PM and 3 PM to 11 PM), usually with meals. (From Robertson GL, Rittig S, and Kovacs L, unpublished, 1993).

a prompt change in vasopressin secretion and urine production as well as in thirst and water intake. The resultant increase decrease in body water rapidly restores tonicity to the equilibrium level. Consequently, within each person, the osmolality of plasma and other body fluids rarely deviates by more than 3 to 5 mOsm/kg (1%–1.5%) even in the face of large variations in insensible water loss and dietary solute load.

In humans, at least, the operation of this elegant osmoregulatory system is subject to a continuous barrage of hemodynamic stimuli induced by changes in posture, physical activity and sleep (Fig. 14). However, these changes in blood volume and pressure have a minor effect on osmoregulation probably because they are not large enough to get beyond the relatively flat portion of the exponential, stimulus-response curve (Fig. 9). In addition, they sometimes act in opposing ways. During sleep, for example, mean arterial pressure falls dramatically but plasma volume increases and plasma vasopressin does not change (Fig. 14). Thus, the decrease in urine output and increase in urine osmolality that normally occurs at night in healthy young adults is due largely if not totally to a reduction in solute load (Fig. 14). In healthy children, however, plasma vasopressin is reported to increase at night (110), suggesting that there may be an age-dependent circadian variation in the hormone.

References

1. Acher R, Chauvet J, Rouille Y. Adaptive evolution of water homeostasis regulation in amphibians. *Biol Cell* 1997;89:283–291.
2. Adolph EF, et al. In: Visscher MB, Bronk DW, Landis EM, et al., eds. *Physiology of Man in the Desert*. New York: Hafner; 1969.
3. Allison NL, Albrightson-Winslow CR, Brooks, et al. Species heterogeneity and antidiuretic hormone antagonists: what are the predictors? In: Cowley AW, Liard JF, Ausiello DA, eds. *Vasopressin: Cellular and Integrative Functions*. New York: Raven Press; 1988:207–214.
4. Anderson RJ, Pluss RG, Berns AS, et al. Mechanism of effect of hypoxia on renal water function. *J Clin Invest* 1978;62:769–777.
5. Andersson B. Regulation of water intake. *Physiol Rev* 1978;58:582–603.
6. Ando T, Shimamoto K, Nakahashi Y, et al. Plasma antidiuretic hormone levels in patients with normal and low renin essential hypertension and secondary hypertension. *Endocrinol Jpn* 1983;30:567–570.
7. Argenti D, Jensen BK, Heald D. The pharmacokinetics and pharmacodynamics of desmopressin: effect on plasma factor VIII: C and von Willebrand factor. *Am J Therap* 1997;41: 3–8.
8. Arndt JO. Diuresis induced by water infusion into the carotid loop and its inhibition by small hemorrhage. *Pflugers Arch* 1965;282: 313–322.
9. Barron WM. Water metabolism and vasopressin secretion during pregnancy. *Baillieres Clin Obstet Gynaecol* 1987;1:853–871.
10. Baylis PH, Heath DA. Plasma-arginine-vasopressin response to insulin-induced hypoglycemia. *Lancet* 1977;11: 428–430.
11. Baylis PH, Robertson GL. Plasma vasopressin response to hypertonic saline infusion to assess posterior pituitary function. *J Roy Soc Med* 1980;73:255–260.
12. Baylis PH, Robertson GL. Vasopressin response to 2-deoxy-d-glucose in the rat. *Endocrinology* 1980;107:1970–1974.
13. Baylis PH, Robertson GL. Rat vasopressin response to insulin induced hypoglycemia. *Endocrinology* 1980;107:1975–1979.
14. Baylis PH, Stockley RA, Heath DA. Effect of acute hypoxaemia on plasma arginine vasopressin in conscious man. *Clin Sci Mol Med* 1977;53:401–404.
15. Baylis PH, Zerbe RL, Robertson GL. Arginine vasopressin response to insulin-induced hypoglycemia in man. *J Clin Endocrinol Metab* 1981;53:935–940.
16. Beck LH. The aging kidney: defending a delicate balance of fluid and electrolytes. *Geriatrics* 2000;55:26–28, 31–32.
17. Berl T, Cadnapaphornachai P, Harbottle JA, et al. Mechanism of suppression of vasopressin during alpha-adrenergic stimulation with norepinephrine. *J Clin Invest* 1974;53:219–227.
18. Bevilacqua M, Norbiato G, Chebat E, et al. Osmotic and nonosmotic control of vasopressin release in the elderly: effect of metoclopramide. *J Clin Endocrinol Metab* 1987;65:1243–1247.
19. Billman GE, Keyl MJ, Dickey DT, et al. Hormonal and renal response to plasma volume expansion in the primate Macaca mulatta. *Am J Physiol* 1983;244:H201–205.
20. Birnbaumer M, Seibold A, Gilbert S, et al. Molecular cloning of the receptor for human antidiuretic hormone. *Nature* 1992;357:333–335.
21. Breslow E. The neurophysins. *Adv Enzymol* 1974;40:271–333.
22. Breslow E. The conformation and functional domains of neurophysins. In: Gross P, Richter D, Robertson GL, eds. *Vasopressin*. Paris: John Libbey Eurotext; 1993:143–155.
23. Brownstein MJ, Russell JT, Gainer H. Synthesis, transport and release of posterior pituitary hormones. *Science* 1980;207:373–378.
24. Cadnapaphornachai P, Boykin J, Harbottle JA, et al. Effect of angiotensin II on renal water excretion. *Am J Physiol* 1975;228:155–159.
25. Cates JE, Garrod O. The effect of nicotine on urinary flow in diabetes insipidus. *Clin Sci* 1951;10:145–160.
26. Calzone WL, Silva C, Keefe DL, Stachenfeld NS, et al. Progesterone does not alter osmotic regulation of AVP. *Am J Physiol* 2001;281:R2011–2020.
27. Chou CL, DiGiovanni SR, Luther A, et al. Oxytocin as an antidiuretic hormone. II: role of V2 vasopressin receptor. *Am J Physiol* 1995;269:F78–F85.
28. Claybaugh JR, Hansen JE, Wozniak DB. Response of antidiuretic hormone to acute exposure to mild and severe hypoxia in man. *J Endocrinol* 1978;77:157–160.
29. Coutinho EM. Oxytocic and antidiuretic effects of nausea in women. *Am J Obstet Gynecol* 1969;105:127–131.
30. Crowe MJ, Forsling ML, Rolls BJ, et al. Altered water excretion in healthy elderly men. *Age Ageing* 1987;16:285–293.
31. Davison JM, Sheills EA, Barron WM, et al. Changes in the metabolic clearance of vasopressin and in plasma vasopressinase throughout human pregnancy. *J Clin Invest* 1989;83:1313–1318.
32. Davison JM, Shiells EA, Philips PR, et al. Suppression of AVP release by drinking despite hypertonicity during and after gestation. *Am J Physiol* 1988;254:F588–F592.
33. deBodo RC. The antidiuretic action of morphine and its mechanism. *J Pharmacol Exp Ther* 1944;82:74–85.
34. DeCastro JM. A microregulatory analysis of spontaneous fluid intake by humans: evidence that the amount of fluid ingestion and its timing is governed by feeding. *Physiol Behav* 1988; 43:705–714.
35. DeCastro JM. The relation of spontaneous macronutrient and sodium intake with fluid ingestion and thirst in humans. *Physiol Behav* 1991;49:513–519.
36. DeFronzo RA, Braine H, Colvin OM, et al. Water intoxication in man after cyclophosphamide therapy: time course and relation to drug activation. *Ann Intern Med* 1973;78:861–869.
37. Do US. ATP: Cyclic nucleotides in renal pathophysiology. In: Brenner BM, Stein JH, eds. *Hormonal Function and the Kidney*. New York: Churchill Livingstone; 1979:251–285.
38. Duke HN, Pickford M, Watt JA. The antidiuretic effect of morphine: its site and mode of action in the hypothalamus of the dog. *Q J Exp Physiol* 1951;36:149–158.
39. Dunn FL, Brennan TJ, Nelson AE, et al. The role of blood osmolality and volume in regulating vasopressin secretion in the rat. *J Clin Invest* 1973;52:3212–3219.
40. Du Vigneaud V. Hormones of the posterior pituitary gland: oxytocin and vasopressin. In: Du Vigneaud V, Bing RJ, Oncley JL, et al., eds. *The Harvey Lectures* 1954–55. Orlando, FL: Academic Press; 1956:1–24.
41. Edelson JT, Robertson GL. The effect of the cold pressor test on vasopressin secretion in man. *Psychoneuroendocrinology* 1986;11:307–316.
42. Egan G, Silk T, Zamarripa F, et al, Neural correlates of the emergence of consciousness of thirst. *Proc Nat Acad Sci U S A* 2003;100:15241–15246.
43. Elster AD. Modern imaging of the pituitary. *Radiology* 1993;187:1–14.
44. Engel P, Rowe J, Minaker K, et al. Effect of exogenous vasopressin on vasopressin release. *Am J Physiol* 1984;249:E202–E207.
45. Erickson S, Simon-Oppermann C, Simon E, et al. Occlusion of rostroventral 3rd ventricle abolishes drinking but not AVP release in response to central osmotic stimulation. *Brain Res* 1988;448:121–127.
46. Evbuomwan IO, Davison JM, Baylis PH, Murdoch AP. Altered osmotic thresholds for arginine vasopressin secretion and thirst during superovulation and in the ovarian hyperstimulation syndrome (OHSS): relevance to the pathophysiology of OHSS. *Fertil Steril* 2001;75: 933–941.
47. Eversmann T, Guttsmann M, Uhlich E, et al. Increased secretion of growth hormone, prolactin, antidiuretic hormone and cortisol induced by the stress of motion sickness. *Aviat Space Environ Med* 1978;49:53–57.
48. Farrel MJ, Egan GF, Zamarripa F, et al, Unique, common and interacting cortical correlates of thirst and pain. *Proc Soc Nat Acad Sci U S A* 2006;103:2416–2421.
49. Figaro MK and Mack GW. Control of fluid intake in dehydrated humans; role of oropharyngeal stimulation. *Am J Physiol* 1997;272:R1740–46.
50. Fumoux F, Czernichow P, Arnauld E, et al. Effect of hypotension induced by sodium nitrocyanoferrate (III) on the release of arginine vasopressin in the unanaesthetized monkey. *J Endocrinol* 1978;78:449–450.
51. Ganguly A, Robertson GL. Elevated threshold for vasopressin release in primary aldosteronism. *Clin Res* 1980;28:330A.
52. Gardiner TW, Verbalis JG, Stricker EM. Impaired secretion of vasopressin and oxytocin in rats after lesions of nucleus medianus. *Am J Physiol* 1985;249:R681–R688.
53. Geelen G, Keil LC, Kravik SE, et al. Inhibition of plasma vasopressin after drinking in dehydrated humans. *Am J Physiol* 1984;247: R968–R971.
54. Goetz KL, Wang Be, Sundet WD. Comparative effects of cardiac receptors and sinoaortic baroreceptors on elevations of plasma vasopressin and renin activity elicited by haemorrhage. *J Physiol (Lond)* 1984;879:440–445.
55. Gold PW, Robertson GL, Ballenger JC, et al. Carbamazepine diminishes the sensitivity of the plasma arginine vasopressin response to osmotic stimulation. *J Clin Endocrinol Metab* 1983;57:952–957.
56. Gold PW, Robertson GL, Post RM, et al. The effect of lithium on the osmoregulation of arginine vasopressin secretion. *J Clin Endocrinol Metab* 1983;56:295–299.
57. Goldsmith SR, Francis GS, Crowley AW, et al. Response of vasopressin and norepinephrine to lower body negative pressure in humans. *Am J Physiol* 1982;243:H970–H973.
58. Greidanus TB, Thody TJ, Verspaget H, et al. Effects of morphine and ß endorphin on basal and elevated plasma levels of alpha-MSH and vasopressin. *Life Sci* 1979;24:579–586.
59. Hara Y, Battey J, Gainer H. Structure of mouse vasopressin and oxytocin genes. *Mol Brain Res* 1990;8:319–324.
60. Haymaker W. Hypothalamo-pituitary neural pathways and the circulatory systems of the pituitary. In: Haymaker W, et al, eds. *The Hypothalamus*. Springfield, IL: Charles C Thomas; 1969:219.

61. Helderman JH, Vestal RE, Rowe JW, et al. The response of arginine vasopressin to intravenous ethanol and hypertonic saline in man: the impact of aging. *J Gerontol* 1978;33:39–47.
62. Heyes M, Farber MO, Manfredi F, et al. Acute effects of hypoxia on renal and endocrine function in normal man. *Am J Physiol* 1982;243:R265–R270.
63. Hurbin A, Boisson-Agasse L, Orcel H, et al. The VIa and VIb but not the V2 vasopressin receptor genes are expressed in the supraoptic nucleus of the rat hypothalamus and the transcripts are essentially colocalized in the vasoptessinergic magnocellular neurons. *Endocrinology* 1988;139:4701–4707.
64. Ivell R, Richter D. Structure and comparison of the oxytocin and vasopressin genes from rat. *Proc Nat Acad Sci U S A* 1984;81:2006–2010.
65. Iwasaki Y, Gaskill MB, Robertson GL. Adaptive resetting of the volume control of vasopressin secretion during susrained hypovolemia. *Am J Physiol* 1995;268: R349–357.
66. Iwasaki Y, Gaskill MB, Robertson GL. The effect of selective opioid antagonists on vasopressin secretion in the rat. *Endocrinology* 1994;134:55–62.
67. Iwasaki Y, Gaskill MB, Boss CA, et al. The effect of the non-selective opioid antagonist diprenorphine on vasopressin secretion in the rat. *Endocrinology* 1994;134:48–54.
68. Iwasaki Y, Gaskill MB, Fu R, et al. Opioid antagonist diprenorphine microinjected in parabrachial nucleus selectively inhibits vasopressin response to hypovolemic stimuli in the rat. *J Clin Invest* 1993;92: 2230–2239.
69. Jewell PA, Verney EB. An experimental attempt to determine the site of the neurohypophyseal osmoreceptors in the dog. *Philos Trans R Soc Lond (Biol)* 1957;240:197–324.
70. Jhamandas JH, Renaud LP. Neurophysiology of a central baroreceptor pathway projecting to hypothalamic vasopressin neurons. *Can J Neurol Sci* 1987;14:17–24.
71. Kamoi K, White K, Robertson GL. Opiates elevate the osmotic threshold for vasopressin (VP) release in rats. *Clin Res* 1979;27:254A.
72. Kannan H, Yagi K. Supraoptic neurosecretory neurons: evidence for the existence of converging inputs both from carotid baroreceptors and osmoreceptors. *Brain Res* 1978;145:385–390.
73. Kaufmann JE and Vischer UM. Cellular mechanisms of the hemostatic effects of desmopressin. *J Thromb Hemostasis* 2003;1:682–689.
74. Keil LC, Severs WE. Reduction of plasma vasopressin levels of dehydrated rats following acute stress. *Endocrinology* 1977;100:30–38.
75. Keil Le, Summy-Long J, Severs WE. Release of vasopressin by angiotensin II. *Endocrinology* 1975;96:1063–1065.
76. Kenney WL, Chiu P. Influence of age on thirst and fluid intake. *Med Sci Sports Exerc* 2001;33:1524–1532.
77. Kirchheim HR. Systemic arterial baroreceptor reflexes. *Physiol Rev* 1976;56:100–176.
78. Knepper M. Molecular physiology of urinary concentrating mechanism: regulation of aquaporin-2 water channels by vasopressin. *Am J Physiol* 1997;272:F3–F12.
79. Kovacs L, Rittig S, Robertson GL. Effects of sustained antidiuretic treatment on plasma sodium concentration and body water homeostasis in healthy humans on ad libitum fluid intake. *Clin Res* 1991;40:165A..
80. Kurokawa H, Fujisawa I, Nakano Y, et al. Posterior lobe of the pituitary gland: correlation between signal intensity on T-1 weighted MR images and vasopressin concentration. *Radiology* 1988;207:79–83.
81. Land H, Schutz G, Schmale H, et al. Nucleotide sequence of cloned cDNA encoding bovine arginine vasopressin neurophysin II precursor. *Nature* 1982;295:299–303.
82. Lausen HD. Metabolism of the neurohypophysial hormones. In: Geige SR, ed. *Handbook of Physiology, Section 7. Endocrinology. Vol. IV, Part 1.* Bethesda, MD: American Physiological Society; 1974:287–393.
83. Ledingham JGG, Crowe MJ, Forsling ML, et al. Effects of aging on vasopressin secretion, water excretion and thirst in man. *Kidney Int J* 1987;32(Suppl 2):S90–S92.
84. Lee M, Thrasher TN, Keil LC, et al. Cardiac receptors, vasopressin, and corticosteroid release during arterial hypotension in dogs. *Am J Physiol* 1986;251:R614–R620.
85. Lindheimer MD, Davison JM. Osmoregulation, the secretion of arginine vasopressin and its metabolism during pregnancy. *Eur J Endocrinol* 1995;132:133–143.
86. Mangiapane ML, Thrasher TN, Keil LC, et al. Deficits in drinking and vasopressin secretion after lesions of the nucleus medianus. *Neuroendocrinology* 1983;37:73–77.
87. McCann MJ, Verbalis JG, Stricker EM. LiCl and CCK inhibit gastric emptying and feeding and stimulate OT secretion in rats. *Am J Physiol* 1989;256:R463–R468.
88. McKinley MJ, Denton DA, Weisinger RS. Sensors for antidiuresis and thirst-osmoreceptors or CSF sodium detectors? *Brain Res* 1978;141:89–103.
89. McKinley MJ, Cairns MJ, Denton DA, et al. Physiological and pathophysiological influences on thirst. *Physiol Behav* 2004;81:795–803.
90. Miaskiewicz SL, Stricker EM, Verbalis JG. Neurohypophyseal secretion in response to cholecystokinin but not meal-induced gastric distension in humans. *J Clin Endocrinol Metab* 1989;68;837–843.
91. Miller M. Role of endogenous opioids in neurohypophyseal function of man. *J Clin Endocrinol Metab* 1980;50:1016–1020.
92. Miller M. Fluid and electrolyte homeostasis in the elderly: physiological changes of ageing and clinical consequences. *Baillieres Clin Endocrinol Metab* 1997;11:367–387.
93. Mohr E, Bahnsen U, Kiessling C, et al. Expression of the vasopressin and oxytocin genes in rats occurs in mutually exclusive sets of hypothalamic neurons. *FEBS Lett* 1988;242:144–148.
94. Mohr E, Schmitz E, Richter D. A single rat genomic DNA fragment encodes both the oxytocin and vasopressin genes separated by 11 kilobases and oriented in opposite transcriptional directions. *Biochimie* 1988;70:649–654.
95. Morel A, O'Carrol AM, Brownstein MJ, et al. Molecular cloning and expression of a rat VIa arginine vasopressin receptor. *Nature* 356:523–526, 1992.
96. Moses AM. Is there an osmotic threshold for vasopressin release? *Am J Physiol* 1978;234: E339–E340.
97. Moses AM, Miller M. Accumulation and release of pituitary vasopressin in rats heterozygous for hypothalamic diabetes insipidus. *Endocrinology* 1970;86:34–41.
98. Moses AM, Miller M, Streeten DHP. Quantitative influence of blood volume expansion on the osmotic threshold for vasopressin release. *J Clin Endocrinol Metab* 1967;27:655–662.
99. Mouw D, Bonjour JP, Malvin RL, et al. Central action of angiotensin in stimulating ADH release. *Am J Physiol* 1971;220:239–242.
100. Oiso Y, Iwasaki Y, Kondo K, et al. Effect of the opioid kappa-receptor agonist U50488H on the secretion of arginine vasopressin. *Neuroendocrinology* 1988;48:658–662.
101. Oiso Y, Robertson GL. Role of endogenous opiates in mediating ethanol-induced suppression of vasopressin. *Endocrinology* 1982;751: 267(abstr).
102. Olsson K, Kolmodin R. Dependence of basic secretion of antidiuretic hormone on cerebrospinal fluid (Na). *Acta Physiol Scand* 1974;91: 286–288.
103. Onishi A, Orita Y, Okahara R, et al. Potent aquaretic agent. A novel, nonpeptide selective vasopressin 2 antagonist (OPC-31260) in men. *J Clin Invest* 1993;92:2653–2659.
104. Onishi A, Ko Y, Fujihara H, et al. Pharmacokinetics, safety and pharmacologic effects of OPC-21268, a non-peptide, orally active vasopressin VI receptor antagonist, in humans. *J Clin Pharmacol* 1993;33: 230–238.
105. Peck JW, Blass EM. Localization of thirst and antidiuretic osmoreceptors by intracranial injections in rats. *Am J Physiol* 1975;228:1501–1509.
106. Phillips PA, Bretherton J, Risvanis D, et al. Effects of drinking on thirst and vasopressin in dehydrated elderly men. *Am J Physiol* 1993;264:R877–881.
107. Quillen EW, Crowley AW. Influence of volume changes in osmolality-vasopressin relationships in conscious dogs. *Am J Physiol* 1983;244:H73–H79.
108. Richter D. Molecular events in expression of vasopressin and oxytocin and their cognate receptors. *Am J Physiol* 1988;255:F207.
109. Rao VV, Loffler C, Battey J, et al. The human gene for oxytocin neurophysin I (OXT) is physically mapped to chromosome 20p13 by in situ hybridization. *Cytogenet Cell Genet* 1992; 61:271–271.
110. Rittig S, Knudsen DB, Norgaard JP, et al. Abnormal diurnal rhythm of plasma vasopressin and urinary output in patients with enuresis. *Am J Physiol* 1989;256:F664–F671.
110a. Robertson GL. Diseases of the posterior pituitary. In: Felig P, Baxter J, Broadus A, et al, eds. *Endocrinology and Metabolism*, 2nd Edition, New York: McGraw-Hill, 1987:338–385.
111. Robertson GL. The role of osmotic and hemodynamic variables in regulating vasopressin secretion. In: James VHT, ed. *Proceedings of the Fifth International Congress of Endocrinology,* Vol. 1. Excerpta Medica International Congress Series No. 402. Amsterdam: Excerpta Medica; 1977:126–130.
112. Robertson GL. Vasopressin function in health and disease. *Recent Prog Horm Res* 1977;33: 333–385.
113. Robertson GL. Physiopathology of ADH secretion. In: Tolis G, Labrie F, Martin JB, et al, eds. *Clinical Neuroendocrinology: A Pathophysiological Approach.* New York: Raven Press; 1979:2260.
114. Robertson GL. Physiology of ADH secretion. *Kidney Int* 1987;32:S20–S26.
115. Robertson GL. Disorders of thirst in man. In: Ramsay, D, ed. *Thirst: Physiological and Psychological Aspects.* London: Springer-Verlag; 1991:453–475.
116. Robertson GL, Athar S. The interaction of blood osmolality and blood volume in regulating plasma vasopressin in man. *J Clin Endocrinol Metab* 1976;42:613–620.
117. Robertson GL, Athar S, Shelton RL. Osmotic control of vasopressin function. In: Andreoli TE, Grantham JJ, Rector RC Jr, eds. *Disturbances in Body Fluid Osmolality.* Bethesda, MD: American Physiological Society; 1977:125–148.
118. Robertson GL, Aycinena P. Neurogenic disorders of osmoregulation. *Am J Med* 1982;72: 339–353.
119. Robertson GL, Ganguly A. Osmoregulation and baroregulation of plasma vasopressin in essential hypertension. *J Cardiovasc Pharmacol* 1986;8:S87–S91.
120. Robertson GL, Oiso Y, Vokes TP, et al. Diprenorphine inhibits selectively the vasopressin response to hypovolemic stimuli. *Trans Assoc Am Physicians* 1985;98:322–333.
121. Robertson GL, Shelton RL, Athar S. The osmoregulation of vasopressin. *Kidney Int* 1976; 10:25–37.
122. Rodbard D, Munson PJ. Editorial comment. *Am J Physiol* 1978;234:E340–E342.
123. Rowe JW, Shelton RL, Helderman JH, et al. Influence of the emetic reflex on vasopressin release in man. *Kidney Int* 1979;16:729–735.
124. Rowe JW, Andres R, Tobin JD, Norris AH, Shock NW. The effect of age on creatinine clearance in men : a cross-sectional and longitudinal study. *J Geront* 1976;31:155–163.
125. Ruppert S, Scherer G, Schutz G. Recent gene conversion involving bovine vasopressin and oxytocin precursor genes suggested by the nucleotide sequence. *Nature* 1984;308:554–557.
126. Rydin H, Verney EB. The inhibition of water-diuresis by emotional stress and by muscular exercise. *Q J Exp Physiol* 1938;27:373–374.
127. Sachs H, Fawcett P, Takabatake Y, et al. Biosynthesis and release of vasopressin and neurophysin. *Recent Prog Horm Res* 1969;25:484–491.
128. Saito T, Ishikawa S, Abe K, et al. Acute aquaresis by the nonapeptide arginine vasopressin (AVP) antagonist OPC-312260 improves hypo-natremia in patients with syndrome of inappropriate secretion of antidiuretic hormone (SIADH). *J Clin Endocrinol Metab* 1997;82: 1054–1057.
129. Sands JM, Mammalian urea transporters. *Ann Rev Physiol* 2003;65:543–566.
130. Sato N, Ishizaka H, Yagi H, et al. Posterior lobe of the pituitary in diabetes insipidus: dynamic MR imaging. *Radiology* 1993;186:357–360.
131. Sausville E, Carney D, Battey J. The human vasopressin gene is linked to the oxytocin gene and is selectively expressed in a cultured lung cancer cell line. *J Biol Chem* 1985;260:10236–10241.
132. Sawchenko PE, Swanson LW. Central noradrenergic pathways for the integration of hypothalamic neuroendocrine and autonomic responses. *Science* 1981;214:685–687.
133. Sawyer W. Evolution of antidiuretic hormones and functions. *Am J Med* 1967;42:678–686.
134. Sawyer WH, Manning M. The development of potent and specific vasopressin antagonists. *Kidney Int* 1988;34(Suppl 26):S34–S37.
135. Scharrer E, Scharrer B. Hormones produced by neurosecretory cells. *Recent Prog Horm Res* 1954;10:183–240.
136. Schrier RW, Bed T, Harbottle JA. Mechanism of the antidiuretic effect associated with interruption of parasympathetic pathways. *J Clin Invest* 1972;51:2613–2620.
137. Schwaab DE Neurohypophysial peptides in the human hypothalamus in relation to development, sexual differentiation, aging and disease. *Regul Pept* 1993;45:143–147.

138. Schwaab DE Aging of the human hypothalamus. *Horm Res* 1995;43:8–11.

139. Segar WE, Moore WW. The regulation of antidiuretic hormone release in man. *J Clin Invest* 1968;47:2143–2151.

140. Serradeil-Le Gal C, Wagnon J, Valette G, et al. Nonpeptide vasopressin receptor antagonists: development of selective and orally active V1a, V2 and V1b receptor ligands. *Prog Brain Res* 2002;139:197–210.

141. Shimamoto K, Miyahara M. Effect of norepinephine infusion on plasma vasopressin levels in normal human subjects. *Clin Endocrinol Metab* 1976;43:201–204.

142. Shimizu K, Share L, Claybaugh JR. Potentiation of angiotensin II of the vasopressin response to an increasing plasma osmolality. *Endocrinology* 1973;93:42–50.

143. Sofroniew MY, Weindl A, Schrell U, et al. Immunohistochemistry of vasopressin, oxytocin and neurophysin in the hypothalamus and extrahypothalamic regions of the human and primate brain. *Acta Histochemica* 1981;34 Suppl:79–95.

144. Spruce BA, Baylis PH, Burd J, et al. Variation of osmoregulation of arginine vasopressin during the human menstrual cycle. *Clin Endocrinol* 1985;22:37–42.

145. Stachenfeld NS, Keefe DL. Estrogen effects on osmotic regulation of AVP and fluid balance. *Am J Physiol* 2002;283(4):E711–21.

146. Steele TH, Serpick AA, Block JB. Antidiuretic response to cyclophosphamide in man. *J Pharmacol Exp Ther* 1973;185:245–253.

147. Stricker EM, Verbalis JG. Interaction of osmotic and volume stimuli in regulation of neurohypophyseal secretion in rats. *Am J Physiol* 1986;250:R267–R275.

148. Sugimoto T, Saito M, Mochizuki S, et al. Molecular cloning and functional expression of a cDNA encoding the human V1b vasopressin receptor. *J Biol Chem* 1994;269:270–288.

149. Takamata A, Mack GW, Stachenfelcl MS, et al. Body temperature modification of osmotically induced vasopressin secretion and thirst in humans. *Am J Physiol* 1995;269:R874–R880.

150. Terano T, Seya A, Tamura Y, et al. Characteristics of the pituitary gland in elderly subjects from magnetic resonance images: relationship to pituitary hormone secretion. *Clin Endocrinol* 1996;45:273–279.

151. Thames MD, Schmid PG. Cardiopulmonary receptors with vagal afferents tonically inhibit ADH release in the dog. *Am J Physiol* 1979;237:H299–H304.

152. Thompson CJ, Burd JM, Baylis PH. Acute suppression of plasma vasopressin and thirst after drinking in hypernatremic humans. *Am J Physiol* 1987;252:RI138–RI142.

153. Thompson DA, Cambell RG, Lilavivat U, et al. Increased thirst and plasma arginine vasopressin levels during 2-deoxy-D-glucose-induced glucoprivation in humans. *J Clin Invest* 1981;67:1083–1093.

154. Thrasher TN, Brown CJ, Keil LC, et al. Thirst and vasopressin release in the dog: an osmoreceptor or sodium receptor mechanism? *Am J Physiol* 1980;238:R333–R339.

155. Thrasher TN, Keil LC. Regulation of drinking and vasopressin secretion: role of organum vasculosum lamina terminalis. *Am J Physiol* 1987;253:RI08–RI20.

156. Ukai M, Moran WH, Zimmerman B. The role of visceral afferent pathways on vasopressin secretion and urinary excretory patterns during surgical stress. *Ann Surg* 1968;168:16–28.

157. Vaccari C, Lolait S, Ostrowski NL. Comparative distribution of vasopressin VI b and oxytocin receptor messenger ribonucleic acids in brain. *Endocrinology* 1998;139:5015–5033.

158. Van Germert M, Miller M, Carey RJ, et al. Polyuria and impaired ADH release following medial preoptic lesioning in the rat. *Am J Physiol* 1975;228:1293–1297.

159. Vavra I, Machova A, Holecek Y, et al. Effect of a synthetic analogue of vasopressin in animals and in patients with diabetes insipidus. *Lancet* 1968;1:948–952.

160. Verbalis JG, Richardson DW, Stricker EM. Vasopressin release in response to nausea-producing agents and cholecystokinin in monkeys. *Am J Physiol* 1987;252:R749–R753.

161. Verney EB. The antidiuretic hormone and the factors which determine its release. *Proc R Soc Lond (Biol)* 1947;135:25–106.

162. Vokes T, Aycinena PR, Robertson GL. Effect of insulin on osmoregulation of vasopressin. *Am J Physiol* 1987;252:E538–E548.

163. Vokes TJ, Weiss NM, Schreiber J, et al. Osmoregulation of thirst and vasopressin during normal menstrual cycle. *Am J Physiol* 1988;254: R641–R647.

164. Wade CE, Keil LC, Ramsay DJ. Role of volume and osmolality in the control of plasma vasopressin in dehydrated dogs. *Neuroendocrinology* 1983;37:349–353.

165. Wang BC, Sundet WD, Hakumaki MOK, et al. Cardiac receptor influences on the plasma osmolality-plasma vasopressin relationship. *Am J Physiol* 1984;246(15):H360–H368.

166. Weiss NM, Conder ML, Robertson GL. The effect of hypovolemia on the osmoregulation of thirst and AVP. *Clin Res* 1984;32:786A.

167. Weitzman RE, Fisher DA. Log-linear relationship between plasma arginine vasopressin and plasma osmolality. *Am J Physiol* 1977;233:E37–E40.

168. Weitzman RE, Fisher DA, DiStefano JH III, et al. Episodic secretion of arginine vasopressin. *Am J Physiol* 1977;233:E32–E36.

169. Wiggins RC, Basar I, Slater JDH, et al. Vasovagal hypotension and vasopressin release. *Clin Endocrinol* 1977;6:387–393.

170. Wong LL, Verbalis JG. Vasopressin V2 receptor antagonists. *Cardiovas Res* 2001;51:391–402.

171. Yamaguchi K, Koike M, Hama H. Plasma vasopressin response to peripheral administration of angiotensin in conscious rats. *Am J Physiol* 1985;248:R249–R256.

172. Yang B, Bankir L. Urea and urine concentrating ability: new insights from studies in mice. *Am J Physiol* 2005;288:F881–896.

173. Zehr JE, Hawe A, Tsakiris AG, et al. ADH levels following nonhypotensive hemorrhage in dogs with chronic mitral stenosis. *Am J Physiol* 1971;221:312–317.

174. Zerbe RL, Henry D, Robertson GL. Vasopressin response to orthostatic hypotension: etiological and clinical implications. *Am J Med* 1983;74:265–271.

175. Zerbe RL, Miller JZ, Robertson GL. The reproducibility and heritability of individual differences in osmoregulatory function in normal humans. *J Lab Clin Med* 1991;117:51–59.

176. Zerbe RL, Robertson GL. Osmoregulation of thirst and vasopressin secretion in human subjects: effect of various solutes. *Am J Physiol* 1983;224:E607–E614.

177. Zerbe RL, Vinicor F, Robertson GL. Plasma vasopressin in uncontrolled diabetes mellitus. *Diabetes* 1979;28:503–508.

178. Zimmerman EA. The organization of oxytocin and vasopressin pathways. In: Martin JB, Reichlin S, Bick KL, eds. *Neurosecretion and Brain Peptides.* New York: Raven Press; 1981:63–75.

179. Zingg H, Lefebvre D, Almazan G. Regulation of vasopressin gene expression in rat hypothalamic neurons. *J Biol Chem* 1986;12956–12959.

180. Zingg HH, LaPorte SA. The oxytocin receptor. *Trends Endocrinol Metab* 2003;14:222–227.

CHAPTER **40**

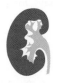

The Urine Concentrating Mechanism and Urea Transporters

Jeff M. Sands and Harold E. Layton

Emory University School of Medicine, Atlanta, Georgia, USA
Duke University, Durham, North Carolina, USA

The ability to vary water excretion is essential for mammals, which generally do not have continuous access to water but must maintain a nearly constant blood plasma osmolality. Mammals, therefore, need a mechanism that allows them to regulate water loss to closely match water intake. In addition, because sodium and its anions are the principle osmotic constituents of blood plasma, and plasma sodium concentration must be kept nearly constant, water loss must be regulated by a mechanism that decouples water and sodium. These critical regulatory capabilities are provided by the kidney's urine concentrating mechanism: when water intake is large enough to dilute blood plasma, a urine more dilute than plasma is produced to concentrate the plasma; when water intake is so small that blood plasma is concentrated, a urine more concentrated than plasma is produced to dilute the plasma. In both cases, the rate of sodium excretion is small and varies little; indeed the total solute excretion rate varies little (Fig. 1).

Urine osmolality varies widely in response to changes in water intake. Following a prolonged period without water intake, such as occurs when an individual sleeps, human urine osmolality may rise to ~1200 mOsm/kg H$_2$O, about four times plasma osmolality (~290 mOsm/kg H$_2$O). However, following the ingestion of large quantities of water, such as commonly occurs at breakfast, urine osmolality may decrease rapidly. Humans (and other mammalian species) are able to dilute their urine to ~50 mOsm/kg H$_2$O. Such large and rapid changes in osmolality require that the cells of the inner medulla have adaptive mechanisms (e.g., osmolytes) to protect them from osmotic damage.

Maximum urine osmolality varies widely among mammalian species. The long-nosed bat *Leptonycteris sanborni* can concentrate only to about 350 mOsm/kg H$_2$O, while the Australian hopping mouse *Notomys alexis* can concentrate to nearly 9400 mOsm/kg H$_2$O (22). Primates can typically concentrate their urines from ~1000 to 2000 mOsm/kg H$_2$O (22, 354, 355). Beluga whales and bottle-nosed dolphins, which have access only to hypertonic ocean water (~1000 mOsm/kg H$_2$O), can concentrate urine up to ~1800 mOsm/kg H$_2$O (23). Most laboratory data relevant to the

urine concentrating mechanism have been obtained from rabbits or rodents that can achieve higher maximum urine osmolalities than humans: rabbits can concentrate to ~1400 mOsm/kg H$_2$O, rats to ~3000 mOsm/kg H$_2$O, mice and hamsters to ~4000 mOsm/kg H$_2$O, and chinchillas to ~7600 mOsm/kg H$_2$O (22, 23, 149).

Regardless of maximum concentrating ability, the kidneys of all mammals maintain an osmotic gradient that increases from the corticomedullary boundary to the tip of the medulla (papillary tip). This osmotic gradient is sustained even in diuresis, although it is diminished in magnitude relative to antidiuresis (88, 157). The major constituent of the osmotic gradient in the outer medulla is NaCl; in the inner medulla, the major constituents are NaCl and urea (88, 157). The cortex is nearly isotonic to plasma, while the papillary tip is hypertonic to plasma and, in antidiuresis, has osmolality similar to urine (149). The major urinary solutes are sodium and potassium accompanied by univalent anions and by urea; urea is the predominant solute in urine during antidiuresis (88, 157). The sodium, potassium, and urea concentrations in rat plasma, papillary tissue, and urine, during both diuresis and antidiuresis, are given in Table 1.

The mechanisms responsible for the separate control of water and sodium excretion are largely located in the renal medulla, where the nephron segments and vasa recta are arranged in complex but specific anatomic relationships, both in terms of which segments connect to which segments and in terms of three-dimensional configuration. The production of concentrated urine involves complex interactions among the nephron segments and vasculature. In the outer medulla, thick ascending limbs of the loop of Henle actively absorb NaCl, diluting the luminal fluid and providing NaCl to increase the osmolality of the medullary interstitium, pars recta, descending limbs, collecting ducts, and vasculature. The countercurrent configuration of nephron segments and vessels allows the generation of a medullary osmolality gradient along the corticomedullary axis. In the inner medulla, osmolality continues to increase, but the source of the concentrating effect remains controversial. However, the most widely accepted mechanism remains passive absorption of

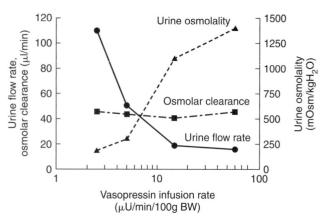

FIGURE 1 *Independent control of water and solute excretion. Rats were infused with exogenous vasopressin and given a water load (4% of body weight) to suppress endogenous vasopressin secretion. Vasopressin infusion causes a significant decrease in urine flow rate (left axis, circles) and increase in urine osmolality (right axis, triangles) but has little effect on osmolar clearance (left axis, squares). Figure is modified, with permission, from Knepper MA, Rector FC, Jr. Urinary concentration and dilution. In: Brenner BM, ed. The Kidney, 5th ed. Philadelphia: WB Saunders; 1996:532–570, using data from Atherton JC, Green R, Thomas S. Influence of lysine-vasopressin dosage on the time course of changes in renal tissue and urinary composition in the conscious rat. J Physiol 1971;213:291–309.*

NaCl, in excess of solute secretion, from thin ascending limbs of the loops of Henle (162, 324).

KIDNEY STRUCTURE

The structural organization of the mammalian kidney is discussed in detail elsewhere in Chapter 20. This section, based in large measure on key studies (167, 171, 189), summarizes features that are pertinent to the urine concentrating mechanism.

The kidney generally contains short-looped and long-looped nephrons; both have loops of Henle that are arranged in a hairpin configuration (Fig. 2). They differ in two important aspects: The loops of short-looped nephrons turn near the inner-outer medullary border and lack a thin ascending limb, whereas the loops of long-looped nephrons extend into the inner medulla and contain a thin ascending limb. Thin ascending limbs are found only in the inner medulla and their transition to thick ascending limbs defines the inner-outer medullary border. Thus, only thick ascending limbs are found in the outer medulla, regardless of the type of loop. Some mammalian kidneys (e.g., human kidneys) have a sub-population of nephrons whose loops of Henle do not reach into the medulla; these nephrons are called cortical nephrons. Tubular fluid flows from thick ascending limbs of both short- and long-looped nephrons to distal convoluted tubules. Several distal tubules merge to form cortical collecting ducts that descend through the cortex and then become medullary collecting ducts that pass through the outer medulla. The collecting ducts merge along the entire length of the inner medulla, ultimately forming the ducts of Bellini, which open into the renal pelvis at the papillary tip.

Small mammals, such as rodents, have unipapillate kidneys. In these mammals, the papilla is an inverted pyramid-shaped portion of the innermost inner medulla; the papilla descends into the renal pelvis. Larger mammals (including humans) have multipapillate kidneys in which each papilla descends into a renal calyx. The renal pelvis is formed from the merging of these calyces. In all mammals, urine exits through the ducts of Bellini into the renal pelvis. The pelvis, which connects to the ureter, is bounded by two epithelia: the papillary surface epithelium lining the surface of the papilla and a ureteral-type epithelium extending from the ureter up into the renal pelvic fornices (137, 175, 287, 316).

TABLE 1 Plasma, Papilla, and Urine Composition During
Diuresis and Antidiuresis in Rats

A. Diuresis (urine flow/animal = 192 ml/min)

Component	Plasma	Papilla	Urine
Na^+ (mEq/l)	138	159	5.4
K^+ (mEq/l)	6.0	66.0	5.9
Urea (mM)	4.5	34.1	22.6
Osmolality (mOsm/kg H_2O)	304	572	59

B. Antidiuresis (urine flow/animal = ~5 μl/min)

Component	Plasma	Papilla	Urine
Na^+ (mEq/l)	145	417	148
K^+ (mEq/l)	6.7	102	140
Urea (mM)	4.4	605	946
Osmolality (mOsm/kg H_2O)	314	1832	1805

Sources: Atherton JC, Hai MA, Thomas S. Acute effects of lysine vasopressin injection (single and continuous) on urinary composition in the conscious water diuretic rat. *Pflügers Arch* 1969;310:281–296; Atherton JC, Hai MA, Thomas S. The time course of changes in renal tissue composition during water diuresis in the rat. *J Physiol* 1968;197:429–443; Hai MA, Thomas S. The time-course of changes in renal tissue composition during lysine vasopressin infusion in the rat. *Pflügers Arch* 1969;310:297–319.

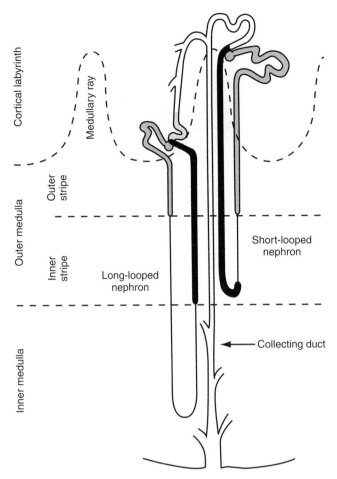

FIGURE 2 Basic structure of mammalian kidney. The major kidney regions are shown on the left. The diagram shows both a long-looped and a short-looped nephron. Glomeruli are shown as circles, proximal tubules are hatched, thin limbs of Henle's loop are lines, thick ascending limbs of Henle's loops are solid, distal convoluted tubules are stippled, and the collecting duct system is open. (From Knepper MA, Rector FC, Jr. Urinary concentration and dilution. In: Brenner BM, ed. *The Kidney,* 5th ed. Philadelphia: WB Saunders; 1996:532–570, with permission.)

The descending and ascending vasa recta, which provide the blood supply for the medulla, are arranged roughly in parallel. Although their configuration is similar to the hairpin configuration of the loops of Henle, there is an important anatomic difference: the tubular segments that make up the loops of Henle are contiguous, whereas the descending and ascending vasa recta are separated by capillary plexuses. Blood enters the medulla through descending vasa recta, passes through capillary plexuses located at various depths within the medulla, then enters ascending vasa recta. Vascular bundles, which are aggregations of both descending and ascending vasa recta, form in the outer stripe but become much more prominent in the inner stripe. Lemley and Kriz have proposed using the vascular bundle (see detail, Fig. 3) as the histotopographical core around which the various outer medullary tubule structures are arranged (167, 169, 171, 189).

Studies of inner medullary structure by Kriz and coworkers (167, 169, 171, 189), and studies by Pannabecker and

Dantzler (250, 252), found that the inner medullary connecting ducts (IMCDs) in the inner medullary base form clusters that coalesce along the corticomedullary axis. In the base of the inner medulla, thin descending limbs are predominantly present at the periphery of these clusters and appear to form an asymmetric ring around each collecting duct cluster. In contrast, thin ascending limbs are distributed relatively uniformly amongst collecting ducts and thin descending limbs. In Munich-Wistar rats, Pannabecker and Dantzler (252) identified three population groups of loops of Henle, distinguished by thin ascending limb position at the base of the inner medulla and by differing loop length. Group 1 loops, having thin ascending limbs that are interposed between collecting ducts, reach a mean length of ~700 μm into the inner medulla; group 2 loops, having thin ascending limbs that are adjacent to just one collecting duct, reach ~1500 μm; and group 3 loops, having thin ascending limbs that lie more than one-half tubule diameter from a collecting duct, reach ~2200 μm. As collecting ducts coalesce and shorter loops disappear, the originating portions of longer thin ascending limbs run alongside the collecting ducts for substantial distances.

Distinct types of interstitium are found in the vascular bundle in the outer medulla, in the interbundle region of the outer medulla, and in the inner medulla (189). These interstitia may play an important role in medullary solute and water transfer, especially in the inner medulla, where interstitial cells are interspersed in a gelatinous matrix of acid mucopolysaccharides, which is largely devoid of any capillary plexuses, laterally flowing capillaries, or lymphatics (124, 170, 189). Thus, the inner medullary interstitium should greatly slow lateral bulk flow of solutes and water.

The number of nephrons found in mammals, and thus the number of loops of Henle, varies over many orders of magnitude, increasing sub-linearly with increasing body mass (275). The mouse has about 12,400 nephrons per kidney (275); rat, 30,000 to 40,000 (152, 275); rabbit, 230,000 (152, 275); human, 0.3 to 1.4 million (236, 239); elephant, 7.5 million (275); and fin whale, 192 million (239). In contrast, medullary thickness in mammals varies from 3 to 25 mm, thus indicating that maximum loop of Henle length varies over about an order of magnitude (23); proximal tubule diameter changes little from rat to fin whale, increasing by a factor of about 1.3 (40, 239).

Although loops of Henle of variable length are found in all mammals, most mammals are thought to have both short- and long-looped nephrons. Exceptions include the dog, with all long loops (320), and the mountain beaver *Aplodontia rufa*, which has thick ascending limbs only and has a renal medulla that corresponds to the outer medulla of other mammals (258). Generally, however, there are more short-looped than long-looped nephrons, and the long-looped nephrons tend to exhibit substantial variation in the depth reached within the inner medulla. Measurements in the rabbit (295) and rat (90, 152) indicate that the decrease in loop of Henle and collecting duct population in the inner

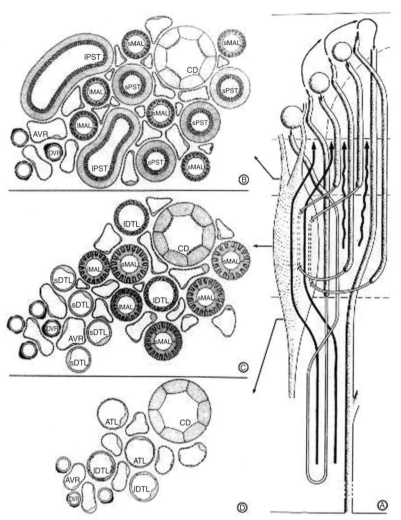

FIGURE 3   Organization of the rat renal medulla as represented by Lemley and Kriz. Shown are a schematic longitudinal section **(A)** and cross-sections through the outer stripe of the outer medulla **(B)**, inner stripe of the outer medulla **(C)**, and the inner medulla (IM) **(D)**. **A:** One long and two short loops of Henle, collecting duct, and a vascular bundle (shown in three-dimensional solid form). The vascular bundle contains ascending vasa recta (AVR) originating from the inner medulla (AVRIM; *long, bold-face arrows*) and the descending limbs of the short-looped nephrons (sDTL). Ascending vasa recta originating from the inner stripe (AVRIS; *bold, wavy arrows*) ascend directly within the interbundle region. In the cross-sections **(B–D)**, the relationships of four short and two long loops of Henle are shown with collecting duct (CD) and vasa recta. **B:** In the outer stripe, the proximal straight tubules (PST) and medullary thick ascending limbs of long-looped nephrons (lMAL) are located among the AVRIM near the vascular bundle. Located at a distance from the vascular bundle are the collecting ducts (CD) and the PSTs and thick ascending limbs from short-looped nephrons (sMAL). These structures are surrounded by AVRIS and the true capillaries (smaller unlabeled structures). **C:** In the inner stripe, the core of a vascular bundle contains AVR and descending vasa recta (DVR), whereas sDTL are found among the AVRIM in the periphery. In the interbundle region, the thin descending limbs of long-looped nephrons (lDTL) and CD run together with thick ascending limbs of short-looped nephrons (sMAL); the lMAL are found bordering the vascular bundle. **D:** In this section through the upper IM, a vascular bundle is still discernible, but AVR are already present throughout the cross-section. The CD is distant from the vascular bundle. Between the bundle and the CD are lDTL (with different wall structures corresponding to upper and lower part epithelia) and ascending limbs of long-looped nephrons (ATL). AVR and DVR, ascending and descending vasa recta; CD, collecting duct; DTL, descending thin limb; MAL, medullary thick ascending limb; PST, proximal straight tubule (pars recta); s and l, short-looped and long-looped nephrons, respectively; OS, IS, and IM, outer and inner stripe of the outer medulla and inner medulla, respectively. (From Lemley KV, Kriz W. Cycles and separations: The histotopography of the urinary concentrating process. *Kidney Int* 1987;31:538–548, with permission.)

medulla is approximately exponential, with most loops of Henle turning back in the outer portion of the inner medulla and with collecting ducts converging to a few ducts of Bellini. A similar pattern is seen in the medullary cones of the avian kidney (41), which, like the mammalian kidney, is able to produce concentrated urine, though only to osmolalities of about twice that of blood plasma (382).

The pattern of decrease in the tubule populations of the rat renal medulla (90, 152) is portrayed in Fig. 4, which gives curves approximating loop and collecting duct population as a function of normalized medullary depth. About 38,000 loops and 7,300 collecting ducts extend through most of the outer medulla (152). About 28% to 33% of the loops of Henle in rat have thin ascending limbs and reach into the inner medulla (167, 320). The populations of loops of Henle and collecting ducts both decline rapidly, but the loop population decreases more rapidly so that the loop and collecting duct populations are more nearly equal in the papilla. In human, about one of seven of the loops of Henle reaches into the inner medulla (239).

Figure 4 also portrays the concentration of urea, the sum of the concentrations of sodium and its anions, and the osmolality, as a function of medullary depth, as determined in tissue slices harvested from vasopressin-treated Wistar rats (6, 8, 88). The experimental data points, indicated in Fig. 4, are connected by natural cubic splines which generate smooth curves; these curves have shapes supported by other studies in rat (60, 159). Osmolality increases by a factor of about 2 in the outer medulla and by an additional factor of 3 in the inner medulla, where urea makes a substantive contribution. As can be inferred from the values for urine (U) in Fig. 4, sodium is largely carried by flow in the loops of Henle and vasculature, while urea makes up a large portion of the solute in collecting duct flow. Potassium has a tissue concentration of about 80 to 100 mM along the medulla, but it makes a larger contribution (~150 mM) to urine (6, 88).

The osmolality increase along the outer medulla arises from the vigorous transepithelial transport of NaCl from thick ascending limbs into the surrounding interstitium. This effect is augmented by a process of countercurrent multiplication, described in a subsequent section (vide infra). However, as shown in Fig. 4, the osmolality gradient is largest in the papilla, even though only a small fraction of the loops, tubules, and vasa recta reach into the papilla, and even though the population of tubules and vessels is rapidly decreasing there. The remarkable capacity for generating high osmolalities in so small a volume (~0.5% of total kidney volume [124]) has thus far resisted a generally satisfactory explanation.

TRANSPORT PROPERTIES OF INDIVIDUAL NEPHRON SEGMENTS

This section will review the water, urea, and sodium permeability values measured in isolated perfused tubules in nephron segments involved in producing concentrated or dilute

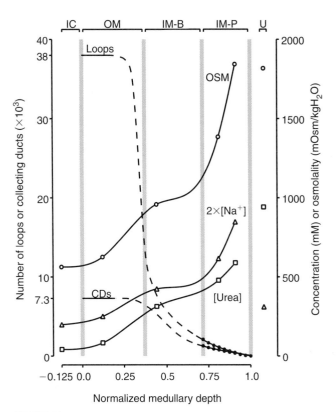

FIGURE 4 Loop of Henle and collecting duct population in rat (scale at left) as a function of normalized medullary depth; also, tissue osmolality, concentration of urea, and concentration of sodium plus its anion (scale at right). Loop of Henle and collecting duct populations decrease in inner medulla because loops turn back and collecting ducts merge. The osmolality gradient is larger in the outer medulla and papilla than in the outer part of the inner medulla. The gradient is largest in the papilla, where the osmolality and concentration profiles appear to increase exponentially. The shape of the sodium profile has been corroborated by electron microprobe measurements (159). IC, inner cortex; OM, outer medulla; IM, outer part (base) of inner medulla; P, papilla or inner part (tip) of inner medulla; U, urine. Figure based on published data. Curves connecting data points are natural cubic splines, computed by standard algorithms (261). Dashed curve segments are interpolations without supporting measurements. Tubule populations in papilla are from reference (90); tubule populations in outer medulla are based on estimates in reference (152). Concentrations and osmolalities are from tissue slices and urine samples collected 4.5 hours after onset of vasopressin infusion at 15 μU/min per 100 g body weight. Data are from Fig. 5 in reference (6) and Figures 1, 3, 9 in reference (88); slice locations were given in reference (8). The osmolality reported in the inner cortex seems high relative to the reported plasma concentration of 314 mOsm/kg H₂O. The osmolality and concentration profiles, as drawn in reference (88), apparently do not take into account relative distances between tissue sample sites.

urine. Thin limb segments are difficult to perfuse and most measurements involving different species have been made by different laboratories. Thus, some caution must be used in comparing these values. Tables 2 through 5 contain values obtained from animals receiving food and water ad libitum; representative values were chosen since space does not permit citing every original manuscript.

In the past decade, many of the proteins that mediate water, urea, and sodium transport in nephron segments important for urinary concentration and dilution have been

TABLE 2   Permeability Properties in Thin Descending Limb Nephron Segments[a]

	Chinchilla	Rat	Rabbit	Hamster
Thin descending limb type I				
Na[b]	0–2 (1, 160, 271)[c]	4.8 (108)		
Urea[b]	13 (220)[c]	1-2 (161, 341)[c]	8 (108)	
Water[d]	2295 (106)[c]	2420 (160)[c]	3257 (108)	
Na$^+$,K$^+$-ATPase[e]	2–5 (134, 345)[c]	2–4 (134)[c]		
Thin descending limb type II				
Na[b]	1 (1, 160, 271)[c]	23–66 (108, 111)		
Urea[b]	3 (47)	0 (247)	1 (161, 341)[c]	3 (108, 111)
Water[d]	2600 (45, 49) 2295 (106)[c]	2315 (160)[c]	5378 (108)	
Na$^+$,K$^+$-ATPase[e]	2–5 (134, 345)[c]	2–4 (134)[c]		
Thin descending limb type III				
Na[b]	29 (47)	4 (111)		
Urea[b]	17–29 (47, 187)	13 (220)[c]	13 (111)	
Water[d]	1550 (45, 49)	2295 (106)[c]	1693 (111)	
Na$^+$,K$^+$-ATPase[e]	3 (345)			
Thin descending limb type III distal (Papillary subsegment)				
Na[b]	74 (47)			
Urea[b]	48 (47)			
Water[d]	60 (45, 49)			

[a] References are in parenthesis.

[b] Units: 10^{-5} cm/sec

[c] Subsegment not specified, thus cannot differentiate between thin descending limb subtypes.

[d] Units: μm/sec.

[e] Units: pmol/mm/min.

cloned (Fig. 5). The water channels (called aquaporins) and sodium transporters are discussed in detail elsewhere in Chapters 31 and 38. The urea transport proteins and their role in the long-term regulation of the urine concentrating mechanism are discussed later in this chapter.

In general, the water, urea, and sodium transport proteins are highly specific. Reflection coefficients are not included in Tables 2 through 5 since the specificity of these transport proteins appears to eliminate a molecular basis for solvent drag and suggests that the reflection coefficients should be 1. Despite the lack of a molecular basis for solvent drag, models for urinary concentration that are based on reflection coefficients that are less than 1 are briefly discussed, for completeness, later in this chapter.

Thin Descending Limb

Thin descending limbs are conventionally divided into types I, II, and III: Types I and II are located in the outer medulla in short- and long-looped nephrons, respectively, while type III limbs are located in the inner medulla (110, 168). The chinchilla has an additional subsegment (type III distal) in the deepest 20% of the inner medulla of the longest loops of Henle (49). The osmotic water permeability of all thin descending limb subtypes is extremely high in all species studied (Table 2) due to the presence of aquaporin-1 (AQP1) water channels (262) in both the

apical and basolateral plasma membranes (49, 227, 228, 276). AQP1, a constitutively active water channel, is present in sufficient abundance to account for the measured rates of transepithelial water transport (206). Transgenic mice lacking the AQP1 channel (which is also found in proximal tubule and descending vasa recta) were found to have greatly impaired urine concentrating capability, which was attributed in large measure to defective water absorption from the proximal tubules and descending limbs, which may lead to an overloading of available concentrating capacity (201, 306). The chinchilla type III distal thin descending limb is the only subsegment that has a low osmotic water permeability (45, 49). Although functional studies of a similar prebend thin descending limb subsegment are not available in other species, anatomic studies show that the rat thin descending limb lumen becomes significantly larger 100 to 400 μm before the bend of the loop (158) and that avian loops of Henle contain a prebend segment (30). The prebend segment could be functionally important as a site of solute absorption (179, 185–187).

Urea permeability varies in different portions of the thin descending limb (Table 2). Urea permeability is relatively low in types I and II thin descending limbs (47, 108, 111, 161, 247, 341). Urea permeability is higher in type III thin descending limbs (47, 111, 187, 220) and is quite high in the chinchilla type III distal thin descending limb (47). The

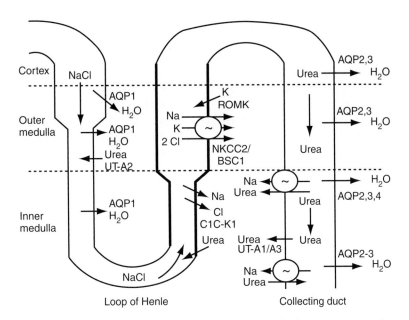

FIGURE 5 Location and identities of the water, urea, and sodium transport proteins involved in the passive mechanism hypothesis for countercurrent multiplication in the inner medulla (162, 324). The major kidney regions are shown on the left. NaCl is actively absorbed across the thick ascending limb by the apical membrane Na^+-K^+-$2Cl^-$ cotransporter (NKCC2, BSC1), and the basolateral membrane Na^+,K^+-ATPase (not shown). K^+ is recycled through an apical membrane ROMK channel. Water is absorbed across the descending limb by AQP1 water channels in both apical and basolateral plasma membranes. In the presence of vasopressin, water is absorbed across the apical plasma membrane of the collecting duct by AQP2 water channels. Water is absorbed across the basolateral plasma membrane by AQP3 water channels in the cortical and outer medullary collecting duct and by both AQP3 and AQP4 water channels in the inner medullary collecting duct (IMCD). Urea is concentrated within the collecting duct lumen (by water absorption) until it reaches the terminal IMCD where it is absorbed by the UT-A1 and UT-A3 urea transporters. According to the passive mechanism hypothesis (see text), the tubular fluid that enters the thin ascending limb from the contiguous thin descending limb has a higher NaCl and a lower urea concentration than the inner medullary interstitium, resulting in passive NaCl absorption and dilution of the tubular fluid within the thin ascending limb. Also shown are two active urea transport pathways: a sodium–urea countertransporter is expressed in the terminal IMCD of normal rats and is upregulated by water diuresis (132); a sodium–urea cotransporter is expressed in the initial IMCD of hypercalcemic rats or rats fed a low-protein diet but not from rats fed a normal protein diet (116, 117, 133). AQP, aquaporin; UT, urea transporter.

reflection coefficient for urea is close to 1 in thin descending limbs (108, 160).

Sodium permeability is relatively low in rabbit types I and II (1, 160, 271) and hamster types I and III thin descending limbs (108, 111), but is relatively high in hamster type II and chinchilla types III and III distal thin descending limbs (47, 108, 111). Na^+,K^+-ATPase activity is very low in all thin descending limb segments in which it has been measured (134, 345). Rabbit types I and II thin descending limbs have a NaCl reflection coefficient that is close to 1 (160). However, the measured NaCl reflection coefficient is heterogeneous in hamster: 0.83 in type II and 0.99 in type III thin descending limbs (108, 342).

The perfused tubule studies reviewed above provide important information about the transport properties of the individual nephron segments comprising the descending limb of the loop of Henle. In contrast, micropuncture studies provide in vivo information about the concentrations of solute within the portions of the descending limb that are accessible to micropuncture: comparisons are made between the composition of tubular fluid near the ends of those proximal convoluted tubules that are accessible on the cortical surface and the composition of fluid in the bends of the longest loops of Henle near the papillary tip. Since proximal tubules on the surface of the kidney originate from superficial glomeruli and the loops of Henle, which reach the papillary tip, generally originate from juxtamedullary nephrons, it is not possible, currently, to compare fluid samples taken from cortical and medullary sites in a single nephron. Thus, the validity of this comparison depends on the assumption that the composition and delivery of solute and water to the beginning of the superficial and juxtamedullary descending limbs are similar. In addition, papillary micropuncture requires the removal of the ureter, which also reduces maximum urinary concentrating ability by a mechanism that is not completely understood (85, 100, 256). Thus, micropuncture studies are limited to studies performed during moderate, not maximal, antidiuretic conditions.

In the rat, osmolality increases along the length of the descending limb. Water removal accounts for 90% of this increase in osmolality in Brattleboro rats that are not treated with vasopressin (123). When Brattleboro rats are treated with vasopressin, there is an increase in the osmotic pressure of the descending limb fluid and in the volume of water absorbed from the descending limb (123). This rise in descending limb fluid osmolality results from water extraction (60%) and from urea addition (40%) (123, 256). The delivery of urea to the end of the thin descending limb averages 550% of the filtered load of urea (256). Thus, urea is either secreted into the descending limb fluid (15) or there is a major difference between the filtered load of urea in superficial versus juxtamedullary glomeruli. When urea is infused into rats fed a low-protein diet, both water extraction from the descending limb and urinary concentrating ability are significantly increased (257).

In the hamster, ~65% of the osmotically active solute in fluid obtained near the bend of the loop of Henle is due to sodium (plus a univalent anion) while ~20% is due to urea (85). Since only ~10% of the filtered load of water reaches the bend of the loop of Henle, the high luminal fluid sodium concentration results primarily from water extraction from the descending limb (85). Both sodium and inulin concentrations increase along the length of the hamster descending limb, showing that water is extracted from the descending limb fluid (208, 209). As in the rat, significant amounts of urea are added to the descending limb fluid.

Psammomys obesus, a desert rodent, feeds on halophilic plants that provide water along with large quantities of NaCl. In these animals, tubular fluid flow rate decreases by 1.7-fold along the descending limb while osmotic pressure increases fourfold (60, 118). Water removal accounts for 40% of the increase and solute addition accounts for 60% under moderate NaCl loading conditions (60). Unlike the rat, NaCl is the principle solute added to descending limb fluid (60); urea is added but is much less important than in the rat. In *Psammomys* producing more highly concentrated urine (though still less concentrated than can be achieved by the intact animal), NaCl addition accounts for nearly 80% of the rise in osmolality (60).

Thin Ascending Limb

The thin ascending limb (Table 3) has extremely low osmotic water permeability in all species studied (45, 49, 106, 109) and no aquaporin proteins have been detected (reviewed in 225). Although the thin ascending limb has a urea permeability that is lower than its NaCl permeability (47, 106, 165, 220), it is significantly higher than the value that mathematical models indicate is required for the effective operation of the hypothesized passive mechanism (vide in-

fra). While this is true in all species, it is especially true in chinchilla (47, 187).

The thin ascending limb has a very low level of Na$^+$,K$^+$-ATPase activity (134, 345) that would not support a significant rate of active sodium transport (163). However, some in vivo studies have found evidence for active sodium transport in thin ascending limbs (209, 256). The thin ascending limb has a high passive NaCl permeability (47, 106, 109, 165, 220). Chloride transport occurs transcellularly via the ClC-K1 chloride channel, which is present in both the apical and basolateral plasma membranes (364). Vasopressin increases chloride transport in thin ascending limbs (344) and water deprivation increases the mRNA abundance of ClC-K1 (363). Transgenic mice lacking the ClC-K1 transporter were found to have greatly reduced urine concentrating capability, which was attributed to defective chloride transport in thin ascending limb (2). Sodium transport is thought to occur paracellularly since no apical plasma membrane sodium transport pathway has been demonstrated (166, 343).

When rabbit thin ascending limbs are perfused in vitro with concentration gradients of NaCl and urea that simulate in vivo conditions (NaCl gradient from lumen-to-bath and a urea gradient from bath-to-lumen), they are able to dilute their luminal fluid by purely passive means. Perfusing rabbit thin ascending limbs in vitro with solutions whose osmolality is increased from 290 to 600 mOsm/kg H$_2$O by adding NaCl to the perfusate and urea to the bath (to mimic the higher concentration of NaCl in the tubule lumen and the higher urea concentration in the medullary interstitium) reduces collected fluid osmolality to 70% of perfusate osmolality, suggesting that it may be possible to dilute the luminal fluid within thin ascending limbs without active transport in vivo (109).

Heterogeneity in Thin Limbs of Long Loops

Pannabecker et al. (250) investigated inner medullary functional structure in Munich-Wistar rats by means of computer-assisted three-dimensional reconstructions of cross-sections in which tubules were identified and labeled by direct immunofluorescence of antibodies raised against specific transport proteins. The reconstructions indicate that thin descending limbs of Henle's loops that have bends within the first millimeter below the outer-inner medullary boundary lack the water transporter AQP1. Thin descending limbs of loops that have bends beyond the first millimeter express AQP1 for about the first 40% of their length below the outer-inner medullary boundary, but beyond that point lack AQP1 expression. Expression of ClC-K1 chloride channels begins abruptly with a prebend segment of length ~165 μm, and ClC-K1 expression continues uniformly along the entire length of thin ascending limbs. Colocalization of AQP1 and ClC-K1 was not found in any loop of Henle segment. Preliminary sections show no evidence of expression of the urea transporters UT-A1, UT-A2, or UT-A4 in thin limbs below

TABLE 3 Permeability Properties in Ascending Limb Nephron Segments[a]

	Chinchilla	Rat	Rabbit	Mouse
Thin ascending limb				
Na[b]	238 (47)	80 (106)	26 (109)	55–88 (106, 165)
Urea[b]	171 (47)	14–23 (106, 220)	7 (109)	19 (106)
Water[c]	0–8 (45, 49)	25 (106)	13 (109)	29 (106)
Na$^+$,K$^+$-ATPase[d]	2–4 (134, 345)	3 (134)		
Medullary thick ascending limb				
Na[b]	6 (272)	2 (94)		
Cl[b]	1 (272)	1 (94)		
Urea[b]	1.4 (outer stripe) (148) 0.6–0.9 (inner stripe) (148)	1 (273)		
Water[c]	0 (272)	23 (89)		
K[b]	1 (309)			
PD[e]	2–3 (235)	3–7 (107, 272, 338)		
Na$^+$,K$^+$-ATPase[d]	41–139 (outer stripe) (81) 260 (inner stripe) (81)	41-124 (134)	62 (134)	
Cortical thick ascending limb				
Na[b]	1 (211)	3 (34)		
Cl[b]	1 (211)	1 (34)		
Urea[b]	1.5 (148)	2 (147)		
Water[c]	0 (272)	23 (89)		
PD[e]	3–7 (34, 35)			
Na$^+$,K$^+$-ATPase[d]	83–133 (81)	16–31 (134)	61 (134)	

[a] References are in parenthesis.

[b] Units: 10^{-5} cm/sec.

[c] Units: μm/sec.

[d] Units: pmol/mm/min.

[e] PD, transepithelial potential difference, mV.

the first millimeter of the inner medulla (179). These observations are generally consistent with expression patterns indicated in other immunocytochemical studies in rat (227, 370). However, Mejia and Wade (214) found in Sprague-Dawley rats that ~30% of thin descending limbs that reached deep into the papilla labeled for AQP1 (in Brattleboro rats, ~11%); and Wade et al. (370) found colabeling of a UT-A urea transport protein and AQP1 in thin descending limbs in the base of the inner medulla of Brattleboro rats (these limbs may correspond to the longer population identified by Pannabecker et al. [250]).

Previously, Pannabecker et al. (251) found in inner medulla (of Munich-Wistar rats, Sprague-Dawley rats, ICR mice, and New Zealand white rabbits) that a large fraction of thin limbs of loops of Henle exhibit regions of alternating segment types usually associated solely with descending limbs (labeling for AQP1 and UT-A2) or with ascending limbs (labeling for ClC-K1). The mixed-type limbs appear to be mostly located away from the central portions of the cross sections of the inner medulla on which the three-dimensional reconstructions described above were based (250, 252).

Thick Ascending Limb

Both the medullary and cortical portions of the thick ascending limb (Table 3) have osmotic water permeabilities that are essentially zero, and neither subsegment expresses aquaporin proteins (reviewed in 225). Thus, the primary mechanism for diluting the luminal fluid in thick ascending limbs is net absorption of solute, particularly NaCl. NaCl is actively absorbed by the Na$^+$-K$^+$-2Cl$^-$ cotransporter (NKCC2, BSC1) in the apical plasma membrane and the sodium pump (Na$^+$,K$^+$-ATPase) in the basolateral plasma membrane. The thick ascending limb from short-looped nephrons can lower the concentration of NaCl in the fluid from ~300 mM at loop bend tubular to ~117 to 140 mM at the corticomedullary border (35, 99), while the cortical thick ascending limb can lower the concentration of NaCl to ~32 mM (272). However, the medullary portion has the capacity to absorb more NaCl than the cortical portion, as evidenced by the higher Na$^+$,K$^+$-ATPase activity in the medullary thick ascending limb (81, 134). The regulation of NaCl absorption in the thick ascending limb is discussed in detail in Chapter 31.

Vasopressin increases NaCl absorption in medullary and cortical thick ascending limbs in mouse (217, 384). This response is consistent with vasopressin's role in urinary concentration and suggests that vasopressin can increase or maintain concentrating ability by increasing NaCl absorption across thick ascending limbs. However, vasopressin does not increase NaCl absorption in human and canine, and only weakly stimulates absorption in rabbit medullary thick ascending limbs (217).

Urea permeability in the medullary thick ascending limb is lower than in the cortical thick ascending limb (148, 273). In rat, the transition to higher urea permeability occurs between the inner and outer stripe portions of the medullary thick ascending limb, while in rabbit it occurs between outer medulla and cortex (148). Urea permeability in the thick ascending limb could permit dilution of tubular fluid by passive urea absorption.

Cortical Collecting Duct

The cortical collecting duct has an extremely low osmotic water permeability (Table 4) in the absence of vasopressin (86, 268, 290). Vasopressin significantly increases the osmotic water permeability by a factor of 10 to 100 in rat (268, 290) and rabbit (86). Arachidonic acid metabolites, produced by cytochrome P450, inhibit vasopressin-stimulated osmotic water permeability by a post–cyclic AMP (cAMP) mechanism (9). The mechanism by which vasopressin increases osmotic water permeability is discussed in detail in Chapter 38.

The cortical collecting duct has a low urea permeability that is unaffected by vasopressin (148, 286). Thus, vasopressin-induced water absorption will increase the urea concentration within the lumen of the cortical collecting duct, and also the osmolality, provided that there is no significant net absorption of solutes.

The cortical collecting duct is the major site for aldosterone-mediated sodium absorption and potassium secretion (87). Vasopressin also stimulates sodium absorption in the cortical collecting duct (357). Sodium is actively absorbed via the epithelial sodium channel (ENaC) in the apical plasma membrane of principle cells (248) and is responsible for the generation of a lumen-negative voltage (87). Sodium exits the principle cell via Na^+,K^+-ATPase in the basolateral plasma membrane (81, 134). Chloride is transported by both paracellular and transcellular pathways. Chloride absorption is primarily passive in rabbit, although some evidence for chloride absorption against an electrochemical gradient exists (91). Active chloride absorption occurs in rat and is stimulated by vasopressin and inhibited by bradykinin (356).

OUTER MEDULLARY COLLECTING DUCT

Few permeability measurements exist for the rat outer medullary collecting duct (Table 4). In rabbit, the outer medullary collecting duct has a low osmotic water permeability which is increased 20- to 30-fold by vasopressin (102, 273). The urea permeability is low in the outer medullary collecting duct in both rat and rabbit (148, 273).

TABLE 4   Permeability Properties in Cortical and Outer Medullary Collecting Duct Segments[a]

	Rat	Rabbit
Cortical collecting duct		
Na[b]	0.1 (340)	
K[b]	1–2 (337, 340)	
Cl[b]	2–5 (91, 340)	
Urea[b] ±[c] AVP	1 (148, 286)	0–1 (86, 297)
Water[d] −AVP	17–43 (268, 290)	4–13 (3, 174, 296)
+AVP	389–994 (234, 268, 290)	166–280 (3, 174, 196, 296)
Na^+,K^+−ATPase[e]	13–81 (81, 134, 345)	12–23 (80, 134, 135, 237, 298)
Outer medullary collecting duct		
Na[b]	0.39 (337)	
K[b]	0.59 (337)	
Cl[b]	0.5 (339)	
Urea[b]	3.5 (290)	0.3 (273)
Water[d] −AVP	14 (102, 273)	
+AVP	445 (102, 273)	
Na^+,K^+−ATPase[e]	11–41 (81, 345)	8–19 (80, 134, 135, 298)

[a] References are in parenthesis.

[b] Units: 10^{-5} cm/sec.

[c] ±AVP: value unchanged by AVP, −AVP: no vasopressin, +AVP: with vasopressin

[d] Units: μm/sec.

[e] Units: pmol/mm/min.

INNER MEDULLARY COLLECTING DUCT

The IMCD was originally divided into three subsegments: $IMCD_1$, $IMCD_2$, and $IMCD_3$ (205). Subsequent studies showed that the inner medullary collecting duct could generally be viewed as consisting of two morphologically and functionally distinct subsegments: the initial IMCD (corresponding to the $IMCD_1$) and the terminal IMCD (corresponding to the $IMCD_2$ and $IMCD_3$) (54, 55, 286, 290). However, some studies have found functional differences between the $IMCD_2$ and $IMCD_3$ (130, 132). Histologically, the rat initial IMCD (or $IMCD_1$) contains 90% principle cells and 10% intercalated cells (55); the rat terminal IMCD (or $IMCD_2$ and $IMCD_3$) contains a unique cell type, the IMCD cell (54). Most of the permeability values available for IMCD subsegments are from the rat (Table 5).

In the absence of vasopressin, the initial IMCD has a low osmotic water permeability, which is increased 10- to 30-fold by vasopressin (112, 289, 290). Urea permeability is low in the initial IMCD and is unaffected by vasopressin (112, 117, 130, 286, 290). The initial IMCD from normal rats does not show any active urea transport (83, 117, 132).

The terminal IMCD has a higher basal (no vasopressin) osmotic water permeability than other portions of the collecting duct (112, 289, 290). Vasopressin can rapidly increase osmotic water permeability by a factor of 10 (289, 290). The terminal IMCD also has a higher basal urea permeability than other portions of the collecting duct (112, 130, 164, 286, 290). Vasopressin and hypertonicity can each increase urea permeability by a factor of 4-6, and together they can increase urea permeability by a factor of 10 (83, 112, 164,

TABLE 5 Permeability Properties in Inner Medullary Collecting Duct Subsegments[a]

	Rat	Rabbit	Hamster
Initial inner medullary collecting duct ($IMCD_1$)			
Urea[b] $\pm$[c]AVP	2−5 (117, 130, 286, 290)	1 (286)	8−9 (112)
Sodium−Urea[d]	0 (117, 132)		
Water[e] −AVP	16−81 (176, 289, 290)		
+AVP	148−460 (176, 289, 290)	534 (112)	
Na^+,K^+−ATPase[f]	18−42 (345)		
Terminal inner medullary collecting duct ($IMCD_2$)			
Na[b]	1 (291)	2 (112)	
K[b]	4 (274)		
Cl[b]	1−2 (274, 291)		
Urea[b] −AVP	15−46 (130, 164, 176, 286, 290)	12 (286)	12 (112)
+AVP	69−93 (130, 164, 290)	32 (112)	
+Hypertonic bath:	120−143 (83, 292)		
+Hypertonic bath and AVP:	163−190 (83, 292)		
Sodium−Urea[g]	0−1 (117, 132)		
Water[e] −AVP	70-333 (176, 289, 290)		
+AVP	208−749 (176, 289, 290)	646 (112)	
Na^+,K^+-ATPase[f]	12−40 (345)		
Terminal inner medullary collecting duct ($IMCD_3$)			
Na[b]	1 (291)		
Urea[b] −AVP	39−49 (130, 286)	13 (286)	
+AVP	110 (130)		
Sodium−urea[g]	−9 (132)		
Water[e] −AVP	43−145 (289, 290)		
+AVP	389−749 (289, 290)		
Na^+,K^+−ATPase[f]	8-17 (345)		
Papillary surface epithelium			
Chloride[b] $\pm$AVP	2-3 (244)		
Urea[b] $\pm$AVP	1 (286)		
Water[d] $\pm$AVP	14 (244)		

[a] References are in parenthesis.

[b] Units: 10^{-5} cm/sec.

[c] $\pm$AVP: value unchanged by AVP, −AVP: no vasopressin, +AVP: with vasopressin.

[d] Sodium−urea cotransport, units: pmol/mm/min.

[e] Units: μm/sec.

[f] Units: pmol/mm/min.

[g] Sodium−urea countertransport, units: pmol/mm/min; +, urea absorption; −, urea secretion.

290, 292). Although early studies suggested a urea reflection coefficient of less than 1, more recent studies which remeasured the urea reflection coefficient and explicitly measured the dissipation of the imposed urea gradient showed that the urea reflection coefficient is one (50, 156). The $IMCD_2$ subsegment from normal rats does not show any active urea transport (117, 132). However, active urea secretion, which is completely dependent upon luminal sodium, is present in the $IMCD_3$ from normal rats, suggesting that sodium absorption may be coupled to urea secretion (132).

Sodium and chloride permeabilities are low in the terminal IMCD (112, 274, 291). It is controversial as to whether active NaCl absorption occurs in the IMCD since micropuncture studies show substantial rates of active NaCl absorption but perfused tubule studies were unable to detect it (291, 365, 377).

PAPILLARY SURFACE EPITHELIUM

Only a few permeability coefficients have been measured across the papillary surface epithelium and these have been measured only in rabbit (Table 5). The urea and osmotic water permeabilities are low and unaffected by vasopressin (244, 286). The basal chloride permeability is higher than that of the terminal IMCD and is inhibited by vasopressin (244). The apical membrane of the papillary surface epithelial cell expresses a $Na^+-K^+-Cl^-$ cotransporter that is stimulated by vasopressin and inhibited by bumetanide (287). The basolateral membrane contains a potassium conductive pathway in rat and rabbit (267, 285).

GENERAL FEATURES OF URINARY CONCENTRATION AND DILUTION

Countercurrent Multiplication

Countercurrent multiplication is the process by which a small osmolality difference between fluid flows in ascending and descending limbs, at each level of the outer medulla, is multiplied by the countercurrent flow configuration to establish a large axial osmolality difference. This axial difference, distributed along the corticomedullary axis, is frequently referred to as the corticomedullary osmolality gradient. The principle of countercurrent multiplication is illustrated i n Fig. 6. The loop shown in the figure panels may be identified with a short loop of Henle; the left channel is analogous to the descending limb while the right channel is analogous to the thick ascending limb. The channels are separated by a water-impermeable barrier. Vertical arrows indicate flow down the left channel and flow up the right channel. Left-directed horizontal arrows indicate active transport of solute from the right channel to the left channel. The numbers within channels indicate local fluid osmolality. Successive panels represent the time course of the multiplication process.

Panel A of Fig. 6 illustrates a loop with isosmolar fluid throughout. In panel B, an active transport mechanism has

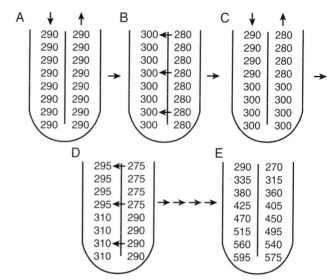

FIGURE 6 Countercurrent multiplication of a single effect. **A:** Process begins with isosmolar fluid throughout both channels. **B:** Active solute transport establishes a 20-mOsm/kg H_2O transverse gradient (single effect) across the boundary separating the channels. **C:** Fluid flows half way down the descending limb and up the ascending limb. **D:** Active transport reestablishes a 20-mOsm/kg H_2O transverse gradient. Note that the luminal fluid near the bend of the loop achieves a higher osmolality than loop-bend fluid in **B**. **E:** As the processes in **C** and **D** are repeated, the bend of the loop achieves a progressively higher osmolality so that the final axial osmotic gradient far exceeds the transverse 20-mOsm/kg H_2O gradient generated at any level.

pumped enough solute to establish a 20 mOsm/kg H_2O osmolality difference between the ascending and descending flows at each level. This small difference, transverse to the flow, is called the "single effect." Panel C illustrates the osmolality values after the fluid has convected the solute half way down the left channel and half way up the right channel. In panel D, the active transport mechanism has re-established a 20-mOsm/kg H_2O osmolality difference, and the luminal fluid near the bend of the loop has attained a higher osmolality than in panel A. By successive iterations of this process, a progressively higher osmolality is attained at the loop bend, and a large osmolality difference is generated along the flow direction. This is illustrated in panel E, where the osmolality at the loop bend is ~300 mOsm/kg H_2O above the osmolality of the fluid entering the loop. Thus, the "single effect" of a 20-mOsm/kg H_2O difference has been multiplied axially down the length of the loop by the process of countercurrent multiplication.

The process of countercurrent multiplication in the short loops of Henle is similar to the process shown in Fig. 6. The tubular fluid of the proximal tubule that enters the outer medulla is isotonic to plasma (about 290 mOsm/kg H_2O). That fluid is concentrated as it passes through the pars recta and on into the thin descending limb. At the bend of the loop of Henle, the tubular fluid osmolality attains an osmolality about twice that of blood plasma. The fluid is then diluted as it flows up the medullary thick ascending limb, so that the fluid emerging from this nephron segment is hypo-osmotic to plasma. The thick ascending limb is nearly impermeable to water and it has a low permeability to NaCl, but its epithelium vigorously transports NaCl from the tubular lumen by an active transport mechanism.

However, countercurrent multiplication in the loops of Henle differs in important ways from the process shown in Fig. 6. The descending and thick ascending limbs do not abut one another; therefore solute is not directly transported from ascending limbs to descending limbs. Rather, NaCl is pumped from thick ascending limbs to the interstitium, raising the osmolality of the interstitial fluid and the blood flowing through the vasa recta and capillaries. The increased interstitial osmolality withdraws water from thin descending limbs, and some NaCl may diffuse into thin descending limbs, thus raising the osmolality of descending limb fluid. The NaCl absorbed from ascending limbs and the water absorbed from descending limbs is carried to the cortex by the vasa recta, which, somewhat like the loops of Henle, are arranged in a countercurrent configuration. Thus, a large axial osmolality difference, from the corticomedullary boundary to the boundary of the inner and outer medulla, is established in the loops of Henle, the vasculature, and the interstitium.

In addition, Fig. 6 does not represent the flow in the collecting ducts. Some of the water and solute in thick ascending limb tubular fluid delivered to the cortex re-enters the outer medulla in the collecting ducts, and in the presence of vasopressin, sufficient water is absorbed from the collecting ducts, as a consequence of the hyper-osmotic medullary interstitium, to bring collecting duct flow to near osmotic equilibrium with the surrounding interstitium. Thus, a large axial osmolality difference, similar to that in the thin descending limb, is established in collecting duct fluid.

Finally, the discrete, sequential process represented in Fig. 6 does not arise under normal physiologic conditions. Rather, the axial osmolality difference, or gradient, is sustained in near steady-state, much as indicated in panel E, with a bend osmolality that is limited primarily by the rate of active transport, the diffusive back-leak of NaCl into the ascending limb, the length of the loop, the rate of water absorption from collecting duct flow, and the dissipative effects of the vasculature.

The axial osmolality gradient in the inner medulla is also believed to be generated by the countercurrent multiplication of a small transverse osmolality difference, presumably between thin ascending and thin descending limbs. However, evidence for significant active transport from thin ascending limbs is lacking, and experiments indicate that the thin ascending limbs are highly permeable to both NaCl and urea. Thus, the inner medullary single effect must arise from a mechanism different from that found in the outer medulla. The roles of the vasculature and collecting duct are considered below; a more detailed treatment of countercurrent multiplication, and in particular, the concentrating mechanism of the inner medulla, is given in a subsequent section (vide infra).

Countercurrent Exchange

The descending and ascending vasa recta are arranged in a counter-flow configuration connected by a capillary plexus. Vasa recta are freely permeable to water, sodium, and urea, and achieve osmotic equilibration through a combination of water absorption and solute secretion (399). Descending vasa recta gain solute and loose water while ascending vasa recta loose solute and gain water. The exchange of solute and water between the descending and ascending vasa recta and the surrounding interstitium is called "countercurrent exchange."

Efficient countercurrent exchange is essential for producing concentrated urine because hypotonic fluid carried into the medulla and hypertonic fluid carried away from the medulla tend to dissipate the work of countercurrent multiplication. Thus, to minimize wasted work, fluid flowing through the vasa recta must achieve near-osmotic equilibrium with the surrounding interstitium at each medullary level, and fluid entering the cortex from the ascending vasa recta must have an osmolality close to that of blood plasma. Conditions that decrease medullary blood flow, such as volume depletion, improve the efficiency of countercurrent exchange and urine concentrating ability by allowing more time for blood in the ascending vasa recta to loose solute and achieve osmotic equilibration (399). Conversely, conditions which increase medullary blood flow, such as osmotic diuresis, impair the efficiency of countercurrent exchange and decrease urine concentrating ability (399). For a detailed treatment of countercurrent exchange, see Chapters 9 and 23 on renal circulation and lymphatics.

Role of the Collecting Duct

The collecting duct, under the control of vasopressin and other factors, is the nephron segment responsible for final control of water excretion. Whereas countercurrent multiplication in the loops of Henle generates a corticomedullary osmotic gradient, and countercurrent exchange in the vasa recta minimizes the dissipative effect of vascular flow, the excretion of water requires another structural component, the collecting duct system, which starts in the cortex and ends at the papillary tip. In the absence of vasopressin, the cortical, outer medullary, and initial inner medullary portions of the collecting duct are nearly water impermeable. (The terminal IMCD has a moderate water permeability even in the absence of vasopressin [vide supra].) Since the fluid that leaves the thick ascending limb and enters the cortical collecting duct is dilute relative to plasma, excretion of dilute urine only requires that not much water be absorbed nor much solute be secreted along the collecting duct.

In the presence of vasopressin, the entire collecting duct becomes highly water permeable. This process takes place in the following way. Plasma osmolality increases when a person or an animal becomes water depleted. Osmoreceptors in the hypothalamus, which can sense an increase of only 2 mOsm/kg H_2O, stimulate vasopressin secretion from the posterior pituitary. Vasopressin binds to V2 receptors in the basolateral plasma membrane of principal and IMCD cells in the collecting duct, stimulates adenylyl cyclase to produce cAMP, activates protein kinase A, phosphorylates aquaporin-2 (AQP2) at serine 256, inserts water channels into the apical membrane, and increases water absorption across the collecting duct (225). This regulated trafficking of AQP2 between subapical vesicles and the apical plasma membrane is the major mechanism for acute regulation of water absorption by vasopressin (225). Wade and colleagues originally proposed the "membrane shuttle hypothesis," which proposes that water channels are stored in vesicles and inserted exocytically into the apical plasma membrane in response to vasopressin (371). Since the cloning of AQP2, the shuttle hypothesis has been proven experimentally in rat inner medulla (225). Subsequent studies have elucidated several signal transduction pathways that are involved in regulating AQP2 trafficking (insertion and retrieval of AQP2) and the role of vesicle targeting proteins (SNAP/SNARE system) and the cytoskeleton (225); these processes are discussed in more detail in Chapter 38.

Vasopressin-induced water permeability allows water to be absorbed across the collecting ducts at a sufficiently high rate for collecting duct tubular fluid to attain near-osmotic equilibration with the hyperosmotic medullary interstitium; the absorbed water is returned to the systemic circulation via the ascending vasa recta. Most water is absorbed from collecting ducts in the cortex and outer medulla. Although the inner medulla has a higher osmolality than the outer medulla, its role in absorbing water from the collecting duct is important only when maximal water conservation is required. More water is actually absorbed across the IMCD during diuresis than antidiuresis, owing to the large transepithelial osmolality difference (122).

COUNTERCURRENT MULTIPLICATION: HISTORY AND THEORY

Overview

The conceptual history of the urine concentrating mechanism may be divided into three periods. The first period, extending from 1942 through 1971, was inaugurated by the publication of a study by Kuhn and Ryffel (173), who proposed that concentrated urine is produced by the countercurrent multiplication of a "single effect," and who constructed a working apparatus that exemplified the principles of countercurrent multiplication. During this first period, the theory of the countercurrent multiplication hypothesis was developed further and experimental evidence accumulated that supported the hypothesis as the explanation for the concentrating mechanism of the outer medulla. In particular, active transport of NaCl from thick ascending limbs was identified as the source of the outer medullary single effect (272, 367).

The second period of conceptual history, extending from 1972 through 1992, was inaugurated by the simultaneous publication, by Kokko and Rector and by Stephenson, of papers proposing that a "passive mechanism" provides the single effect for countercurrent multiplication in the inner medulla (162, 324). According to the passive mechanism hypothesis, a net solute efflux from thin ascending limbs results from favorable transepithelial NaCl and urea gradients; these gradients arise from the separation of NaCl and urea, which is largely driven by the outer medullary concentrating mechanism. Although initially much experimental evidence appeared to support the passive mechanism, findings from many subsequent studies are difficult to reconcile with this hypothesis (48, 70, 124). Moreover, mathematical models incorporating measured transepithelial permeabilities failed to predict a significant inner medullary concentrating effect (187, 216, 379). The discrepancy between the consistently negative results from mathematical modeling studies and the very effective inner medullary concentrating effect has persisted through more than three decades. The discrepancy has helped to stimulate research on the transport properties of the renal tubules of the inner medulla and to the formulation of several highly sophisticated mathematical models (notably, 378), but no model study has resolved the discrepancy to the general satisfaction of experimentalists and modelers.

In the early 1990s, new hypotheses for the inner medullary concentrating mechanism began to receive serious consideration, and a third period of conceptual thought may be considered to have begun in 1993: in that year, Knepper and colleagues proposed a key role for the peristalsis of the papilla (48, 150), and in 1994 Jen and Stephenson (125) examined the principle of "externally driven" countercurrent multiplication, arising (e.g., by the net production of osmotically active particles in the interstitium). At about the same time, perfused tubule studies in chinchilla, which can produce very highly concentrated urine, provided evidence that the passive mechanism, as originally proposed, cannot explain the inner medullary concentrating mechanism (47). Studies have sought to further develop hypotheses involving peristalsis (155) and the potential generation of osmotically active particles, especially lactate (97, 349). In 2004, evidence suggesting an absence of significant urea transport proteins in loops of Henle reaching deep into the medulla led to a reconsideration of hypotheses related to the passive mechanism (179).

Countercurrent Multiplier Hypothesis

In 1942, Kuhn and Ryffel proposed that urine is concentrated by means of multiplication (or augmentation) of a single effect ("Vervielfältigung des Einzeleffektes") (173). More precisely, they suggested that a small osmotic pressure difference between flows in parallel renal tubules (the single effect) was multiplied, by means of the countercurrent principle ("Gegenstromprinzip"), resulting in a large increase in osmotic pressure along the corticomedullary axis (vide supra: Fig. 6 and accompanying discussion). Kuhn and Ryffel, however, made no specific conjectures regarding which tubules or what transport properties were involved. To test their hypothesis, Kuhn and Ryffel constructed an apparatus that, by embodying the countercurrent principle, and using phenol and sucrose solutions separated by selectively permeable membranes, was able to increase the concentration of the sucrose solution by a factor of 3.5. This apparatus suggested that three fundamental components are needed for a physiologically plausible mechanism for generating concentrated urine: (1) countercurrent flow; (2) a source of energy to sustain a single effect (in this case, potential energy in the form of the differing solutions); and (3) specific membrane permeability characteristics.

In a 1951 study, Hargitay and Kuhn (92) proposed the basic framework for the modern conception of the urine concentrating mechanism. They hypothesized that the loop of Henle is a biological realization of a hair-pin counterflow system, that the loops of Henle would generate a corticomedullary osmolality gradient, and that final urine concentration would be achieved by the osmotic withdrawal of water from collecting ducts. Their study, which included a working apparatus and a mathematical model, confirmed that countercurrent multiplication could generate a significant axial concentration gradient. However, their apparatus relied on the transport of water across the separating membrane, and they used a mechanical pressure as a driving force to sustain the single effect. The pressure required for a significant axial gradient (estimated at 550 mm Hg) was judged by the authors to far exceed a pressure likely to be found in vivo (~120 mm Hg). They proposed, as an alternative, a single effect arising from water transport driven by a process of electro-osmosis ("electroosmose"), which was hypothesized to arise from metabolic processes in epithelial cells. In 1959, a mathematical analysis by Kuhn and Ramel showed that active NaCl transport from ascending limbs could serve to provide the required single effect (369).

The countercurrent multiplier hypothesis was bolstered by a 1951 study in which Wirz, Hargitay, and Kuhn used slices of renal tissue from hydropenic rats to demonstrate an osmotic pressure gradient, starting at approximately the corticomedullary boundary, and increasing along the corticomedullary axis to the papillary tip. In subsequent experimental studies, active transport of NaCl from thick ascending limbs was established as the driving force required to sustain the transepithelial osmolality difference needed for countercurrent multiplication in the outer medulla (272, 367), and the osmotic absorption of water from collecting ducts into the hypertonic interstitium was established as the ultimate process by which collecting duct fluid is concentrated in antidiuresis (218). However, investigation of the inner medullary renal tubules revealed no active transport process that could generate a significant transepithelial osmolality difference (220, 319).

Concentrating Mechanism of the Outer Medulla

In the presence of vasopressin, the outer medullary concentrating mechanism is believed to operate as follows. Transepithelial active transport of NaCl, from the tubular fluid of thick ascending limbs and into the surrounding interstitium, raises the osmolality of interstitial fluid and promotes the osmotic absorption of water from the tubular fluid of descending limbs and collecting ducts. Because of the absorption of fluid from descending limbs, the fluid delivered to the ascending limbs has a high NaCl concentration that favors the transepithelial transport of NaCl from ascending limb fluid. (There may also be some diffusion of NaCl into descending limb fluid.) NaCl transport dilutes the tubular fluid of thick ascending limbs, so that at each medullary level the fluid osmolality is less than that in the other tubules and in the vessels, and so that the fluid delivered to the cortex is dilute relative to blood plasma. The ascending limb fluid that enters the cortex is further diluted by active NaCl transport from cortical thick ascending limbs, so that its osmolality is generally less than the osmolality of blood plasma. In cortical collecting ducts, which are water-permeable in the presence of vasopressin, sufficient water is absorbed to return the fluid to isotonicity with blood plasma. This water absorption greatly reduces the load that is placed on the concentrating mechanism by the fluid that re-enters the medulla. In the absence of vasopressin, the collecting duct system, both in the cortex and outer medulla, is much less water permeable, and even though some water is absorbed due to the very large osmotic pressure gradient, fluid that is dilute relative to plasma is delivered by the collecting ducts to the border of the outer and inner medulla.

This modern conceptual formulation of the outer medullary concentrating mechanism (which is very similar to the proposal of Hargitay and Kuhn as modified by Kuhn and Ramel [92, 369]) is supported by mathematical modeling studies using parameters compatible with micropuncture and perfused tubule experiments (187, 332, 333, 374). In particular, the osmotic gradients in the outer medulla predicted by simulations are consistent with the gradients reported in tissue slice experiments, where osmolality is increased by a factor of 2 to 3 (60, 204).

Mass Balance in the Renal Medulla

For the outer medullary gradient to be sustained in a steady state, the water and solute flows in the tubules and vessels of the outer medulla, and therefore, the spatial distribution of water and solute, must remain nearly fixed (provided there are no significant metabolic solute sources or sinks). Thus, for any transverse slice of the medulla, say of a thickness extending from axial location X_1 to X_2, the directed sum of water flow rates in all tubules and vessels at X_1 must equal that at level X_2, and the directed sum of solute flow rates in all tubules and vessels at level X_1 must equal that at level X_2. This is the principle of steady-state mass balance (for an explicit mathematical formulation see 157).

Global mass balance for the outer medulla is thought to be preserved as follows (the relatively small effects of long-looped nephrons, of vasa recta reaching into the inner medulla, and of solutes other than NaCl are ignored here for simplicity). At the corticomedullary boundary, the water flowing in ascending vasa recta exceeds that flowing in descending vasa recta, owing to water absorption from thin descending limbs and collecting ducts. In contrast, the water flow emerging from thick ascending limbs is about half that entering descending limbs at the corticomedullary boundary. The directed sum of these flows, plus flow entering collecting ducts, results in a small net flow from the cortex into the outer medulla that nearly equals collecting duct water flow at the inner-outer medullary boundary.

Similarly, solute flows must be balanced. At the corticomedullary boundary, the solute emerging from ascending vasa recta exceeds that flowing in descending vasa recta, owing to NaCl absorption from thick ascending limbs. In contrast, the solute flow emerging from thick ascending limbs is reduced (relative to flow entering descending limbs) by a larger fraction than is thick ascending limb fluid flow, say, by somewhat more than half. The directed sum of these solute flows at the corticomedullary boundary, plus solute flow entering collecting ducts, results in a small net solute flow that is nearly equal to collecting duct solute flow at the inner-outer medullary boundary.

The ratio of NaCl to water in net flow across the corticomedullary boundary, and the ratio of NaCl to water in collecting duct flow at the inner-outer medullary boundary, both depend on whether the animal is in a diuretic or antidiuretic state. In either case, a greater fraction of loop of Henle solute flow is absorbed, relative to water flow, in the outer medulla, and consequently, a greater fraction of water is delivered to the cortex, relative to solute. Consequently, dilute fluid is delivered by the thick ascending limbs to the cortex, and this fluid is further diluted by NaCl transport from the cortical thick ascending limb.

In diuresis, little water is absorbed from the cortical collecting ducts. Consequently, the net fluid absorbed into the cortical circulation (taking into account NaCl absorption from cortical thick ascending limbs) is concentrated relative to blood plasma, and the fluid re-entering the outer medulla in collecting ducts remains dilute, relative to blood plasma. The low water permeability of the outer medullary collecting duct in diuresis will prevent any significant dilution of vasa recta flow and thus prevent any significant reduction in the concentrating capacity of the countercurrent mechanism. Thus, combined with slightly concentrated flow from ascending vasa recta, the ultimate effect of fluid absorbed in the cortex will be to raise the osmolality of the systemic circulation. Moreover, owing to the dominating effect of hypotonic fluid flowing from the cortical collecting ducts into the outer medullary collecting ducts, the net fluid flow from the cortex to the outer medulla will be dilute, relative to systemic plasma, and as a consequence of mass balance, the net flow of collecting duct fluid across the in-ner-outer medullary boundary will be dilute, relative to blood plasma.

In antidiuresis, much water is absorbed from the water-permeable cortical collecting ducts. Consequently the net fluid absorbed in the cortex, from fluid entering the cortex via the thick ascending limbs, is dilute, relative to plasma, and its diluting effect on the cortex outweighs the concentrating effect of slightly hypertonic ascending vasa recta flow. Collecting duct fluid entering the outer medulla is isotonic to blood plasma, and relative to the case of diuresis, reduced in flow rate, so that the fluid absorbed from the now-permeable outer medullary collecting duct does not significantly reduce the concentrating capacity of the countercurrent mechanism. Thus, the ultimate effect of dilute fluid absorbed from the cortical collecting duct is to lower the osmolality of the systemic circulation. Moreover, owing to the dominating effect of dilute fluid emerging from the outer medullary thick ascending limbs into the cortex, the net flow from the cortex to the outer medulla will be concentrated, relative to systemic blood plasma, and as a consequence of mass balance, the net flow of collecting duct fluid across the inner-outer medullary boundary will be concentrated, relative to blood plasma.

Because the inner medullary concentrating effect remains elusive, and because the net generation of osmotically active molecules has been suggested as a possible source of the single effect for the inner medulla (97, 125, 351), the role of the inner medullary concentrating mechanism has been ignored in our description of mass balance. However, a mass balance analysis similar to that given above for the outer medulla would apply to the inner medulla separately, and thus also to the whole medulla, according to most hypotheses for the inner medullary concentrating mechanism. (In the presence of oscillations in tubular flow mediated by the tubuloglomerular feedback mechanism [98], or in the presence of peristalsis of the papilla [269], mass balance would have to be reformulated for time-averaged flows.) In any case, the overall effect of mass balance in the renal medulla, in diuresis, is that systemic blood plasma is concentrated by the production of a urine that is dilute, relative to plasma; in antidiuresis, blood plasma is diluted by the production of a urine that is concentrated, relative to plasma.

The Passive Mechanism Hypothesis for the Inner Medulla

While the hypothesis of countercurrent multiplication for the outer medulla was being established, with active NaCl transport from thick ascending limbs generating the single effect, isolated perfused tubule experiments in rabbits demonstrated that the thin ascending limb had no significant active NaCl transport (220, 272) but instead had relatively high permeabilities to sodium and urea while being impermeable to water (109). The inner medullary thin descending limb, in contrast, was found to be highly water permeable, but to have low sodium and urea permeabilities (160, 161). Moreover, evidence from some species showed that urea tended to accumulate in the inner medulla, with concentrations similar to those of NaCl (88), and it had long been known that urea administration enhances maximum urine concentration in protein-deprived rats and humans (78). Several models were published that sought to explain the inner medullary concentrating mechanism (191, 230-232, 259), but they failed to gain general acceptance.

In 1972, independent papers by Kokko and Rector and by Stephenson (appearing in the same volume of *Kidney International*) proposed that the single effect in the inner medulla arises from a "passive mechanism" (162, 324). The key components of the passive mechanism are represented in Fig. 5. Active absorption of NaCl from the thick ascending limb and the subsequent absorption of water from the cortical and outer medullary collecting ducts work together to increase the urea concentration of collecting duct fluid. Urea diffuses down its concentration gradient from the highly urea permeable terminal IMCD into the inner medullary interstitium; urea is trapped in the inner medulla by countercurrent exchange in the vasa recta (vide supra). The fluid entering the thin ascending limb has a high NaCl concentration relative to urea, and the thin ascending limb is hypothesized to have a high NaCl permeability, relative to urea. In addition, due to accumulation of urea in the interstitium, the NaCl concentration in the thin ascending limb exceeds the NaCl concentration in the interstitium, and consequently NaCl diffuses down its concentration gradient into the interstitium. If the thin ascending limb has sufficiently low urea permeability, the rate of NaCl efflux from the ascending limb will exceed the rate of urea influx, resulting in the dilution of thin ascending limb fluid and the flow of relatively dilute fluid up the thin ascending limb at each level and into the thick ascending limb. Thus, dilute fluid is removed from the inner medulla, and mass balance requires that the osmolality of the inner medulla be progressively elevated along the tubules of the inner medulla. The elevated osmolality will draw water from the thin descending limbs, thus raising the NaCl concentration of the descending limb flow that enters thin ascending limbs. In addition, the elevated osmolality of the inner medulla will draw water from the water-permeable IMCD, raising the concentration of urea in collecting duct flow; accumulation of NaCl in the interstitium will tend to sustain a transepithelial urea concentration gradient favorable to urea absorption from the terminal IMCD.

Several matters are worthy of note. First, this process, described previously in step-wise fashion, should be thought of as a continuous, steady-state process. Second, although the mechanism is characterized as "passive," it depends on the separation of NaCl and urea that is sustained by the active absorption of NaCl by thick ascending limbs. The separated high-concentration flows of NaCl (in the loop of Henle) and of urea (in the collecting duct) constitute a source of potential energy that is used to effect a net transport of solute from the thin ascending limb. Thus, the laws of thermodynamics are not violated. Third, the description speaks loosely of NaCl and urea as solutes having equal

standing, but the atoms of NaCl are nearly completely dissociated so that each NaCl molecule has nearly twice the osmotic effect of each urea molecule. This distinction must be represented in formal mathematical descriptions. Fourth, the passive mechanism hypothesis is similar to the concentrating mechanism of the outer medulla, inasmuch as it depends on net solute absorption from the thin ascending limb to dilute thin ascending limb fluid and raise the osmolality of adjacent flows and structures. Finally, the concentrating effect is balanced, as in the outer medulla, by the dissipative effects of vascular flows and by the production of a small amount of highly concentrated urine. These dissipative effects limit the achievable urine osmolality.

The passive mechanism hypothesis, as described previously, closely follows the Kokko and Rector formulation (162), which made use of key ideas set forth by Kokko in a largely experimental study (161). Kokko and Rector acknowledged Niesel and Rosenbleck (231) for the proposal that urea absorbed from the IMCD contributes to the inner medullary osmolality gradient. Kokko and Rector presented the passive mechanism hypothesis conceptually, and although it was accompanied by a plausible set of solute fluxes, concentrations, and fluid flow rates that are consistent with the requirements of mass balance, their presentation did not include a mathematical treatment, and it did not demonstrate that measured loop of Henle permeabilities were consistent with the hypothesis. Stephenson's presentation of the passive hypothesis (324) included a more mathematical treatment and it introduced the highly influential central core assumption (vide infra), but it also did not contain a mathematical reconciliation of tubular transport properties with the hypothesis.

The crucial test needed to confirm the passive mechanism hypothesis was an adequate mathematical representation of all the major components of the hypothesized mechanism, including tubular and vascular flows, transepithelial transport, tubular and vascular interactions, and medullary anatomy. The mathematical representation was needed to show that the magnitudes and distributions of the flow rates, transport rates, interactions, and structures, could produce a medullary gradient consistent with tissue slice experiments and measured urine osmolalities.

The Central Core Assumption

In the same paper that set forth the passive mechanism hypothesis (324), Stephenson introduced the central core assumption, in which the interstitium and the vasculature are merged into a single compartment through which the renal tubules interact. Stephenson argued that if the vasa recta were sufficiently permeable to solutes and water, the vasa recta would serve as a nearly perfect countercurrent exchanger, in nearly complete osmotic equilibrium with each other, and with the interstitium, at each medullary level. In such case a very substantial simplification in conceptual and mathematical analysis could be obtained: the central core could be treated very much as an additional species of tubule, but serving a special role as the medium through which other tubules interact. Using the central core assumption, Stephenson was able to derive simplified mathematical expressions that not only aided the model analysis of the passive mechanism but which were general enough to permit extensive analysis in terms of fundamental quantities (323-327).

The central core assumption, as illustrated by Stephenson, is represented in Fig. 7. The upper panel depicts the interaction of the renal tubules with the central core. The lower panels show that the central core may be conceptualized as a single tubule through which the other tubules interact. The central core may be considered to carry, from the medulla to the cortex, the net water and solutes absorbed from the tubules.

The central core assumption has been examined in several theoretical studies (126, 136, 330), all of which concluded that the assumption is a good approximation provided that vasa recta permeabilities are sufficiently high; experiments on vasa recta have tended to confirm the high permeabilities that are required for nearly ideal countercurrent exchange (see Chapters 9 and 23). The central core assumption has been used in a number of mathematical models and computer simulations (75, 167, 169–171, 179, 180, 185, 187, 189, 330, 333). However, models based on the central core assumption cannot incorporate the effects of the radial organization of medullary structures with respect to the vascular bundles, because that organization is likely to result in differing solute concentrations in the various interstitial spaces and vascular flows as a function of their positions with respect to the bundles (189, 378).

Computer Simulations

Computer simulations of the urine concentrating mechanism are based on detailed mathematical models; the models consist of differential equations and algebraic relations that embody transepithelial transport processes and the requirements of water and solute mass balance. The degree of sophistication of these models has varied substantially in the number of molecular species represented, the degree of detail in the formulation of epithelial transport, the numbers of loops of Henle and collecting ducts, the representation of the vasculature, and the representation of three-dimensional connectivity. Because the mathematical models involve a large number of nonlinear equations, explicit solutions in terms of elementary functions cannot be obtained, and approximate solutions must be found by the methods of numerical analysis. Owing to the very large permeabilities measured in some renal tubules and to orders-of-magnitude changes in the water and solute flow rates along the nephron, model solutions are difficult to approximate, and consequently a large amount of effort has been expended in the development of suitable numerical methods (see, e.g., 178, 188, 213, 348, 381). For comprehensive reviews of models and simulations of the concentrating mechanism, including substantial mathematical detail (see references 181 and 328).

The passive mechanism hypothesis was developed at about the same time that it was becoming practical to perform large-scale simulations on digital computers. Indeed, a computer simulation by Stewart and collaborators (335, 336) appeared in the same issue of *Kidney International* that contained the papers that set forth the passive mechanism hypothesis (162, 324). In the absence of active NaCl transport from thin ascending limbs, a significant inner medullary osmolality gradient was generated when loop urea permeabilities were set to 0.1×10^{-5} cm/sec. But the gradient was greatly diminished when thin descending limb urea permeability was increased to 0.3×10^{-5} cm/sec, a small value compared with measurements in all species examined (Table 2). Thus, the addition of a small amount of urea to thin descending limb fluid resulted in a marked decrease in the inner medullary gradient. Moreover, the

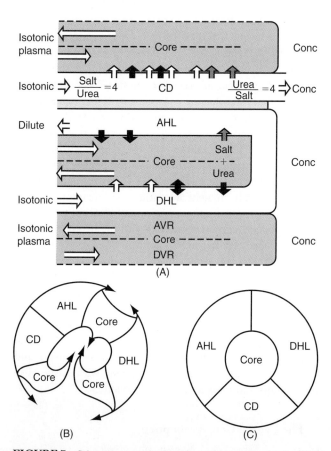

FIGURE 7 Schematic representation of central core assumption, in which the interstitium and vasa recta (AVR, DVR) are merged into a single compartment (CORE). Upper panel **(A)** shows interaction of tubules with CORE. Vertical arrows indicate transepithelial fluxes of NaCl (*black*), urea (*hatched*), and water (*white*); horizontal arrows indicate relative fluid flow. Water is absorbed from descending limb of Henle (DHL) into CORE, urea enters DHL from CORE, and NaCl may move in either direction. NaCl is absorbed from ascending limb of Henle (AHL) into CORE, while urea enters AHL. Water, NaCl, and urea are absorbed from collecting duct (CD) into CORE; as a result of differential absorption, salt/urea concentration reverses. **B:** CORE from **(A)** being consolidated into a final cross-section **(C)**, in which a single CORE compartment interacts with AHL, DHL, and CD. (From Stephenson JL. Concentration of urine in a central core model of the renal counterflow system. *Kidney Int* 1972;2:85–94, with permission.)

authors reported that "Computer simulation confirmed that low sodium or high urea permeability in ascending limb, or high sodium or urea permeability in descending limb, singly or in combination, virtually abolished the osmotic gradient in the inner medulla." These results were difficult to reconcile with experiments that had shown significant net urea addition to both thin descending and ascending limbs in the hamster (208).

This early simulation immediately cast doubt on the passive mechanism hypothesis, and it reported a result that was confirmed in many subsequent simulations: the addition of urea to the loops of Henle reaching into the inner medulla tends to dissipate the transepithelial NaCl and urea gradients that are required for the successful operation of the passive mechanism (see 18, 42, 75, 180, 216, 379). If the thin descending limb is significantly urea-permeable, so that osmotic equilibration of descending limb fluid with the interstitium is accomplished in significant measure by the net secretion of urea, then the NaCl concentration difference between descending limb fluid and interstitial fluid is diminished. Consequently, the gradient favoring NaCl diffusion from thin ascending limb fluid into the interstitium is diminished. (This gradient can also be diminished by the diffusion of NaCl from descending limbs, which raises the relative urea concentration in descending limb fluid.) If the thin ascending limb is significantly urea permeable, diffusion of urea from the interstitium into thin ascending limb fluid counterbalances the diluting effect of the diffusion of NaCl from ascending limb fluid into the interstitium. Consequently, fluid in the ascending limb tends to osmotic equilibrium with respect to surrounding interstitial fluid. Because thin ascending limb fluid is not dilute relative to fluid in tubules and vessels at the same level, there is no inner medullary single effect to be multiplied through the countercurrent flow configuration.

Figure 8, based on data from a simulation published in 1996 (187), shows results that are representative of most simulation studies. Medullary osmolality and concentrations of electrolytes and urea are given as flow-weighted averages, taken across all tubules at each medullary level. Figure 8 has been drawn so that it may be easily compared with Fig. 4. The simulation used loop and collecting duct distributions that are similar to those displayed in Fig. 4, and the flow-weighted profiles in Fig. 8 are roughly comparable to the tissue-slice profiles in Fig. 4, although it must be kept in mind that Fig. 4 includes the effects of intracellular fluid.

Panel A in Fig. 8 shows results obtained using NaCl and urea permeabilities based on values measured in inner medullary thin descending and ascending limbs of chinchilla (Tables 2 and 3). Owing to the significant entry of urea into descending and ascending limbs, no inner medullary gradient is generated. Moreover, the profile labeled as $2 \times [\text{Elec}^+]$, arising mostly from sodium and its anions, fails to show an exponential rise as it does in Fig. 4 and in electron microprobe experiments (357). Parameter studies showed that loop urea permeabilities and descending limb NaCl permeability

must all be reduced to the range of 1 to 5×10^{-5} cm/sec to elicit a significant concentrating effect (187).

Panel B in Fig. 8 shows profiles obtained when loop urea permeability and descending limb NaCl permeability were reduced to 1×10^{-5} cm/sec. Ascending limb NaCl permeability remains high, 294×10^{-5} cm/sec. With these parameters, simulation profiles are remarkably similar to those reported for the rat in Fig. 4. However, the greatly reduced permeabilities used for urea and NaCl in descending limbs, and for urea in ascending limbs, are much smaller than those measured in rat (Tables 2 and 3), and the urine osmolality obtained, 1922 mOsm/kg H_2O, is far smaller than the maximum urine osmolality obtained in chinchilla, 7600 mOsm/kg H_2O (22, 23, 149).

Mathematical simulations of the urine concentrating mechanism have become increasingly comprehensive and sophisticated in the representation of tubular transport (e.g., 332, 333, 351) and medullary architecture (e.g., 185, 187, 350, 375, 378). This evolution is a consequence of the increasing body of experimental knowledge, faster computers with increased computational capacity, and the sustained failure of simulations to exhibit a significant inner medullary concentration gradient.

Stephenson and collaborators reexamined the passive mechanism hypothesis in a two-nephron central core model, in which the electrolyte concentrations for sodium, potassium, and chloride were represented along with urea (333). In a simulation using transport parameters from rabbit inner medulla, a significant inner medullary gradient could only be obtained when the urea permeabilities in both descending and ascending limbs had been reduced to less than 10^{-6} cm/sec. For permeability values obtained from hamster, urea and electrolyte permeabilities had to be greatly reduced, especially in thin descending limbs. Although it has been frequently suggested that a reduction in the urea reflection coefficient for the collecting duct epithelium could augment collecting duct osmolality by retaining urea in excess of fluid (vide infra), this study showed that such a reduction was ineffective without a mechanism for generating a salt gradient in the core.

Layton and collaborators, in a series of papers, have sought to elucidate the role of the distributed loops of Henle (180, 182–185, 187). These studies employ a model representation of the loops of Henle that allows the simulation of loops turning back at all levels of the inner medulla while also representing the fluid flow and concentrations in individual loops (184). Previously, models had typically used a small number of discrete loops (e.g., 213) or had employed shunts between a merged descending and ascending flow to represent the decreasing number of loops of Henle as a function of inner medullary depth (e.g., 216).

The distributed loop representation has been used to obtain several theoretical results. If solute is mostly absorbed near loop bends, then the loop distribution may allow a cascade effect that tends to increase the achievable concentration, provided, of course, that a net solute absorption can

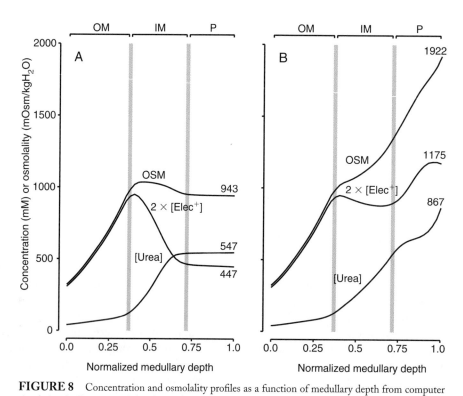

FIGURE 8   Concentration and osmolality profiles as a function of medullary depth from computer simulation by Layton et al. (187). Profiles represent flow-weighted averages across all tubules. Cation concentration [$Elec^+$] arose from Na^+, except in collecting ducts, where both Na^+ and K^+ were represented. Urine values are given at right of each panel. Profiles in A were computed from loop of Henle permeabilities based on measurements in chinchilla (see Tables 2 and 3) (47). The nonincreasing osmolality profile in the inner medulla is similar to that computed with lower permeability values from rabbit, rat, and hamster in a number of model studies (e.g., 18, 75, 180, 216, 379).

Profiles in **B** were obtained when urea permeability ($\times 10^{-5}$ cm/sec) was reduced from 16.8 to 1 in inner medullary descending limbs and from 170 to 1 in thin ascending limbs. Resulting profiles compare favorably with data from rat (Fig. 4), but despite greatly reduced urea permeabilities, model urine osmolality falls far short of 7600 mOsm/kg H_2O, the maximum concentrating capability of chinchilla (22). Note that while tubular electrolytes (primarily Na^+ and accompanying anions) account for most of the simulated osmolality in the outer medulla (**A** and **B**), the experimental results in Fig. 4 show a large osmotic gap; this gap is mostly accounted for by large intracellular concentrations of K^+. (The profiles in **A** and **B** were computed from data generated for cases designated V and I, respectively, in ref. 187.)

be obtained (184, 185). The concentrating effect can be further enhanced if solute is absorbed from a short, prebend segment of the descending limb with low water permeability (185), as has been detected in chinchilla (49), and which may be present in other species (vide supra). Layton hypothesized that a cascade effect could allow the generation of an inner medullary osmolality gradient, despite large loop urea permeabilities, provided that the passive mechanism could operate near loop bends (180, 183). Average flow, taken over all thin ascending limbs at each medullary level, would be hypo-osmotic relative to the flows in the surrounding tubules and vessels, due to the effect of more and more loops turning, as one proceeds from the papillary tip to the outer medulla. However, simulations using reported permeabilities in rat or chinchilla failed to support this hypothesis (180, 187).

Studies by Wexler and collaborators have sought to assess the role of preferential interactions among tubules and

vessels (351, 374–376, 378, 380). Wexler, Kalaba, and Marsh introduced what has become known as the WKM model (378, 380), which was based on the organization of tubules around vascular bundles (Fig. 3), and which therefore allowed both axial and radial concentration gradients. The preferential interaction of collecting ducts with both thick and thin ascending limbs was proposed as the key principle that allowed the generation of an inner medullary osmolality gradient. The preferential interaction with thick ascending limbs allowed highly concentrated collecting duct fluid to pass from the outer medulla to the inner medulla. The preferential interaction with thin ascending limbs allowed the passive mechanism to operate, since a urea-rich environment could be sustained around thin ascending limbs, and dissipative interaction of collecting ducts with thin descending limbs was diminished.

The WKM model drew criticism for some of its structural and transport assumptions (90, 126, 329, 331).

Subsequent studies responded to these criticisms (with modified model assumptions) and acknowledged that preferential interactions are not sufficient to explain the inner medullary concentrating effect in the papilla (351, 374, 376). Nonetheless, results from the WKM model and its successors have provided persuasive evidence that preferential interactions can be a significant factor in the degree of the outer and inner medullary concentrating effects. Moreover, the model structure permits sensitivity testing as a function of interaction strength, and compared to other model studies, it allows for a more accurate assessment of solute and water recycling pathways.

Two hypotheses closely related to the passive mechanism have been proposed by Layton et al. (179); these hypotheses were motivated by implications of studies in rat by Pannabecker et al. (250, 252). One hypothesis is based directly on the principles of the passive mechanism: low urea permeabilities in thin limbs of Henle were assumed because no significant labeling for urea transport proteins was found in loops reaching deep into the inner medulla (179). A second, more innovative hypothesis assumed very high urea loop of Henle permeabilities, but limited NaCl permeability and zero water permeability in thin descending limbs reaching deep into the inner medulla. Thus, in the innermost inner medulla, tubular fluid urea concentration in loops of Henle would nearly equilibrate with the local interstitial urea concentration; thin descending limb fluid osmolality would be raised by urea secretion; and substantial NaCl absorption would occur in the prebend segment and early thin ascending limb. Both hypotheses emphasize the role of the decreasing loop of Henle population, which facilitates a spatially distributed NaCl absorption, along the inner medulla, from prebend segments and early thin ascending limbs. A distinctive aspect of both hypotheses is an emphasis on NaCl transport from the IMCDs as an important active transport process that separates NaCl from tubular fluid urea and that indirectly drives water and urea absorption from the collecting ducts. Computer simulations for both hypotheses predicted urine osmolalities, flow, and concentrations consistent with urine from moderately antidiuretic rats. The critical dependence of the first hypothesis on low loop urea permeabilities is subject to the criticism that urea transport may be paracellular rather than transepithelial: that hypothesis depends on more conclusive experiments to determine urea transport properties in rat. The second hypothesis may contribute to understanding the concentrating mechanism in chinchilla in which high loop urea permeabilities have been measured (47).

Steady-State Alternatives to the Passive Mechanism

The passive mechanism hypothesis is a comprehensive explanation for a large body of experimental findings, including the dilution of thin ascending limb fluid without active transport (109, 120, 121), a role for urea in the concentrating mechanism (78), and the NaCl and urea permeabilities

measured in loops of Henle from rabbit inner medulla (Tables 2 and 3). However, the larger permeabilities measured in rat, hamster, and chinchilla, in conjunction with the results of numerous simulation studies, have provided little support for the hypothesis. Significant concentrations of urea measured in long loops of rat and hamster (123, 208, 256) are generally consistent with studies reporting high loop urea permeabilities. In addition, some animals with high urine concentrating ability (e.g., the *Psammomys*) generate a medullary gradient that depends mostly on NaCl, with little medullary urea accumulation (61), a result that suggests that, at least in some species, a mechanism differing from the passive mechanism is involved. Thus, while the passive mechanism hypothesis remains highly influential in experimental and theoretical research, the accumulated evidence, from experimental and mathematical studies, indicates that crucial elements are missing in our understanding of the inner medullary concentrating effect.

Alternatives to the original passive mechanism hypothesis have taken three forms. First, many simulation studies have attempted to show that a better representation of transepithelial transport, or of medullary anatomy, is required for the effective operation of the passive mechanism; some of these studies were summarized in the preceding section. Second, a number of steady-state mechanisms involving a single effect generated in either thin descending limbs or collecting ducts have been proposed. Third, several hypotheses that depend on the peristaltic contractions of the pelvic wall, and their impact on the papilla, have been proposed. The steady-state alternatives involving descending limbs or collecting ducts are considered directly below, within a general context of possible steady-state mechanisms; mechanisms involving peristalsis are considered in the subsequent subsection.

On the basis of the principle of mass balance, Knepper and colleagues have provided a systematic classification of possible steady-state concentrating models for the inner medulla (150, 157). The classification shows that a single effect for countercurrent multiplication can exist in any structure having axial flow. Thus, a single effect could be present in thin descending limbs, thin ascending limbs, collecting ducts, descending vasa recta, or ascending vasa recta. The classification also shows that a concentrating single effect in an upward flowing stream (toward the cortex) would require a tubular fluid osmolality less than that of the surrounding interstitium, whereas a single effect in a downward flowing stream would require a tubular fluid osmolality exceeding that of the interstitium. Thus, for example, the active transport of NaCl from the thick ascending limbs of the outer medulla lowers the osmolality of the upward flowing tubular fluid relative to the surrounding interstitium; similarly the passive mechanism hypothesis proposes that diffusion of NaCl from thin ascending limbs renders tubular fluid hypo-osmotic relative to the interstitium.

Several investigators have proposed a single effect in descending limbs arising from flow that is hyperosmotic relative to the interstitium. Bonventre and Lechene (27) proposed that the equilibration of descending limb flow with a compartment rendered hyperosmotic by active NaCl transport from ascending limbs, or active secretion of solute into descending limb, produces a relatively hyperosmotic descending flow from the outer medulla into the inner medulla. In a mathematical simulation, Lory (197) showed that an inwardly directed NaCl transport combined with a loop of Henle cascade could produce a significant concentrating effect (197). Jen and Stephenson (125) performed a general mathematical analysis of mechanisms involving a hyperosmotic descending limb flow and concluded that such mechanisms, in theory, could generate a potent single effect. Their claim was supported by a subsequent simulation study by Thomas and Wexler (351), which represented an external osmotic driving force to extract water from descending limbs and collecting ducts; the driving force was hypothesized to arise from the accumulation of osmotically active particles in local vessels or capillaries as a consequence of osmolyte production. Layton and colleagues (187) suggested that a descending limb single effect is consistent with the high NaCl and urea permeabilities of chinchilla ascending limb: the ascending limb could function as an equilibrating segment, in which high permeabilities reduce dissipative osmotic lag. However, despite the attractive features of a descending limb single effect, experimental support for a relatively hypertonic descending limb is lacking. Moreover, in most species examined, the NaCl and urea permeabilities in thin descending limbs are too high to sustain a significant transepithelial osmolality gradient in the papilla, where the concentrating effect is most pronounced.

A single effect in the IMCD would require that the osmolality of luminal flow exceed the osmolality of the surrounding interstitium. Rabinowitz (265) proposed such a single effect based on the assumption that the urea reflection coefficient for the collecting duct is significantly less than unity. He showed that the resulting reduction in the osmotic effect of urea in the collecting duct could, in theory, result in a water flux from collecting duct to interstitium that would significantly raise the osmolality of collecting duct fluid. A number of investigators have proposed or analyzed this hypothesis, including Sanjana et al. (294), Bonventre and Lechene (27), Chandhoke et al. (43), and Imai et al. (110). However, experimental studies indicate that the urea reflection coefficient in rat does not differ significantly from unity (50, 156).

Thomas (349) and Hervy and Thomas (97) have investigated the hypothesis that the concentrating mechanism of the inner medulla may be driven or aided by lactate accumulation in the rat papilla. Anaerobic glycolysis in the hypoxic inner medulla is a net source of osmoles, because two lactates are produced for each glucose molecule; however, the rate of production may not be sufficient to produce a general concentrating effect. However, modeling studies (97) indicate that lactate produced from glucose by anaerobic glycolysis could concentrate tubular fluid in thin descending limbs and collecting ducts (thus producing descending flows in these tubules that are relatively hyperosmotic to flows in other structures at each medullary level), provided that the descending limbs and collecting ducts are impermeable to lactate, as appears to be the case from low lactate levels in urine. However, several conditions require experimental verification: sufficient lactate production, impermeability of thin descending limbs to lactate, and sufficient intra-medullary lactate cycling by vascular countercurrent exchange. The lactate-based mechanism is attractive because it appears to be insensitive to thin descending limb urea permeability and independent of a necessary role for urea. However, modeling results for this mechanism appear to produce sub-physiological urine flow and do not explain the experimentally observed urea gradient in rat.

Hypotheses Based on the Peristalsis of the Papilla

Regular, sustained peristaltic contractions of the smooth muscles of the renal pelvic wall have been observed in a number of mammalian species. In the unipapillate kidneys of hamsters and rats, peristaltic contractions are propagated from the fornices to the lower pelvis and continue in synchrony down the ureter. In the multi-papillate kidneys of both humans and pigs, peristaltic contractions pass from the fornices down the calyces surrounding each papilla, but contractions in calyces are not synchronized with each other or with the peristalsis of the ureter. For a comprehensive review of the anatomy, physiology, and peristalsis of the renal pelvic region, see reference 301.

In hamsters and rats, the rates of pelvic contractions are about 13 and 25 per minute, respectively (269, 302). The contractions interrupt fluid flow by forcing the collecting ducts, loops of Henle, and capillaries of the papilla to collapse. In hamster, the contractions induce bolus flow down the papillary collecting duct, with a bolus speed of about 1.6 mm/sec. At the low urine flow rates characteristic of antidiuresis, boluses are so short that, 1 mm from the papillary tip, collecting ducts may be collapsed up to 94% of the time (269). Even so, large quantities of urea, electrolytes, and, especially, water are absorbed in the final millimeters of the collecting duct system. Indeed, about 50% of the water in a bolus passing through the final millimeter of the collecting duct is absorbed (305).

The blood in the capillaries of the papilla undergoes complicated motion during a pelvic contraction (302). As a peristaltic wave approaches, blood is trapped in the capillaries closest to the papillary tip, which are full and expanded. As the wave passes over, the capillaries empty, with blood moving up both the descending and ascending vasa recta; after the wave has passed, the capillaries refill. The fluid motion in the loops of Henle is much like that of blood in the capillaries: fluid is trapped at the turns of the loops, and may move retrograde up the descending limbs as the peristaltic wave passes (303). A net orthograde flow through the capillaries and loops of Henle is ensured by glomerular filtration pressure.

During the rising urine flow rates that accompany the onset of diuresis, the peristalsis in hamsters and rats induces refluxes of urine over the papilla and up into the fornices (302). These refluxes, called full refluxes, may bathe the papillary surface epithelium with urine that is hypo-osmotic and that has a low urea concentration, relative to the medullary structures; thus water may diffuse into the medulla, and urea may diffuse out. Experiments in hamsters suggest that full refluxes accelerate the transition to the diuretic state (300). When urine flow is constant or decreasing, refluxes are sporadic and limited to the lower 50 to 100 μm of the papilla (302).

Experiments have shown that the excision of the pelvic wall results in a substantial reduction in urine osmolality (53, 240, 307); the reduction has been attributed to the disruption of pelvic urea recycling (26, 28, 307) or to the dissipative effect of medullary blood flow, increased by continuous flow (269), or by prostaglandin release (53). However, no significant change in osmolality was found in urine samples from rats 5 to 40 minutes after the smooth muscles of the pelvic wall were paralyzed with a topical application of verapamil and dimethylsulfoxide (240). In the same study, the excision of the pelvic wall dramatically reduced the osmolality gradient in the papilla, and the gradient was substantially reduced when the ureter was severed just beyond the papillary tip, a procedure that preserved pelvic peristalsis (and intermittent urine flow) but eliminated urine reflux (240). These results were interpreted to mean that while an intact pelvic wall, continuous with the ureter, is required for the production of maximally concentrated urine, the pelvic contractions are not. However, some experiments suggest that the peristaltic contractions do play a direct role in the concentrating mechanism. When the pelvic wall in rats was removed, causing a 10% decrease/hour in urine osmolality, and peristalsis then simulated by a mechanical system, the decrease was reduced to 5%/hour (270). When the muscles of the pelvic wall in hamster were paralyzed by cauterization or by xylocaine, urine osmolality was reduced by about 20% after 1 hour (304), through a reduction in papillary sodium content.

Several studies have provided evidence of solute and water transport across the papillary surface epithelium. When the papillae of rats and gerbils were bathed in a solution containing ^{14}C-urea and ^{3}H-water, there was a marked tissue label for urea, increasing from cortex to inner medulla, and a smaller effect for water (253). When the papilla was bathed in vivo with artificial solutions containing varying concentrations of urea, higher concentration of urea in the superfusate led to a higher osmolality in the urine that was collected as it emerged from the terminal IMCD (26). Fluid collected from small catheters inserted far up into the fornices of the rat pelvis extracted fluid with concentrations of inulin and total solutes that were significantly lower than the concentrations in urine collected at the papillary tip (17).

Recycling of urea from urine across the papillary surface epithelium has been proposed as a component of the inner medullary concentrating mechanism (27, 198). However, a comparison of ureteral urine and urine collected from the ducts of Bellini of hydropenic hamsters showed no significant differences in filtered water and urea (210), and an analysis based on measured urea permeability and papillary surface area in rabbits suggests that urea transport across the papillary surface epithelium is negligible (286).

The lack of a satisfactory explanation for the inner medullary concentrating effect has led to the formulation of hypotheses based on the peristaltic contractions of the smooth muscles of the pelvic wall. Layton proposed that the NaCl and urea concentrations in the tubular cells and interstitium undergo oscillations in tandem with the contractions (183). Urea absorbed from boluses advancing down the collecting duct system would transiently, and substantially, increase urea concentration in collecting duct cells and in the interstitium. Immediately following passage of the peristaltic wave, NaCl absorbed from restored orthograde loop of Henle flow would significantly raise the interstitial NaCl concentration. The very large urea concentration encountered by loop flow would, perhaps, be sufficient to result in the transient operation of the passive mechanism near loop bends, raising interstitial osmolality. Consequently, water, in excess of solute, would be absorbed from the next bolus passing down the collecting duct, and a large urea gradient, resulting from increased interstitial NaCl, would favor urea absorption. However, as in the case of the steady-state formulation of the passive mechanism, the large permeabilities measured in chinchilla (47) suggest that rapid equilibration of NaCl and urea concentrations across thin ascending limbs would compromise this hypothesis.

Knepper and collaborators proposed that water may be driven out of thin descending limbs by the advancing peristaltic wave, thus concentrating tubular fluid and generating a single effect in descending limbs (48, 150). A sufficient net water flux might be achieved if the compliance of the papillary surface epithelium exceeds that of the thin descending limb and if large enough pressures are attained by the compression wave. After the passage of the wave, solute would be absorbed in the relatively water-impermeable pre-bend segment and in the early portion of the thin ascending limb, where NaCl and urea permeabilities are high. This hypothesis provides no explanation for the special role of urea in the production of high urine concentrations (78).

Schmidt-Nielsen (299) proposed that the contraction-relaxation cycle creates negative pressures in the interstitium that act to transport water, in excess of solute, from the collecting duct system. According to this hypothesis, the compression wave would raise hydrostatic pressure in the collecting duct lumen, promoting a water flux into collecting duct cells. Because pressure would induce water flow through aquaporin water channels, without a commensurate solute flux, the remaining luminal fluid would be concentrated, relative to the contents of collecting duct cells and the surrounding interstitium. After the peristaltic wave had passed, the collecting ducts would be collapsed. The papilla, transiently lengthened and narrowed by the wave, would rebound and a negative hydrostatic pressure would develop in the elastic interstitium, which is rich in glycosamine glycans and hyaluronic acid. The negative pressure would withdraw water from the collecting duct cells (through aquaporins) and into the vasa recta, which reopen during the relaxation phase of the contraction and carry reabsorbate toward the cortex. This hypothesis appears to provide no role for long loops of Henle, and it does not explain the large NaCl gradient generated in the papilla (88, 357) or the special role of urea in producing concentrated urine (78).

Knepper et al. (155) hypothesized that hyaluronic acid, which is plentiful in the interstitium of the rat papilla, could serve as a mechano-osmotic transducer (i.e., that the intrinsic visco-elastic properties of hyaluronic acid could be used to transform the mechanical work of papillary peristalsis into osmotic work that could be used to concentrate urine). Three distinct concentrating mechanisms arising from peristalsis are proposed: (1) In the contraction phase, interstitial sodium activity would be reduced through the immobilization of cations by their pairing with fixed negative charges on hyaluronic acid. This would result in a lowered NaCl concentration in fluid that can be expressed from the interstitium, and that relatively dilute fluid would enter the ascending vasa recta. In the relaxation phase, water would be absorbed from descending thin limbs; (2) as a result of decreased interstitial pressure (previously proposed by Knepper and coworkers [48, 150]); and (3) as a result of elastic forces exerted by the expansion of the elastic interstitial matrix arising from hyaluronic acid. If water is so absorbed, without proportionate solute, then the descending limb tubular fluid would be relatively concentrated relative to other flows.

All of the hypotheses involve complex, highly coordinated cycles, with critical combinations of permeabilities, flow rates, compliances, pressures, and frequencies of peristalsis. Moreover, a determination of the adequacy of these hypotheses would appear to require a comprehensive knowledge of the physical properties of the renal papilla and a demonstration that the energy input of the contractions, plus any other sources of harnessed energy, is sufficient to account for the osmotic work performed. Thus the evaluation of these hypotheses, whether by means of experiments or mathematical models, presents a daunting technical challenge.

OSMOPROTECTIVE OSMOLYTES

Since the osmolality in the renal medulla is able to vary rapidly over a wide range, medullary cells must be able to adapt to this unusual osmotic environment in order to survive (27, 389). One way for medullary cells to achieve osmotic balance would be for these cells to accumulate intracellularly the major osmotically active compounds (osmolytes) that are found extracellularly in the medullary interstitium and urine (i.e., NaCl and urea) (153). The problem with this approach is that NaCl and urea can perturb protein function (389). If medullary cells accumulated such perturbing osmolytes to

achieve osmotic balance, then it is likely that these cells would need to develop special mechanisms that would allow their proteins to function over a wide range of intracellular ionic compositions and/or in high concentrations of urea.

An alternative mechanism would be for medullary cells to accumulate osmotically active substances that do not alter protein function (i.e., nonperturbing osmolytes) (33, 36, 389). This second approach is used by medullary cells (Fig. 9). Medullary cells accumulate nonperturbing or "organic" osmolytes such as sorbitol, glycerophosphocholine, betaine, inositol, and taurine (11, 79, 153, 280, 387). These organic osmolytes are divided into two general categories: compatible and counteracting osmolytes. Sorbitol, inositol, and taurine are the major compatible osmolytes and have no effect on protein function. They are accumulated intracellularly to osmotically balance extracellular NaCl (79, 280, 386). Glycerophosphocholine and betaine are the major counteracting osmolytes: in addition to being osmotically active, they have stabilizing effects on protein function and counteract the destabilizing effects of urea when they are accumulated intracellularly at a ratio of 1 M of counteracting osmolyte to 2 M of urea (33, 36, 386, 388–390).

In the medulla, organic osmolytes are regulated to respond to prolonged periods without water ingestion followed by short periods in which water is ingested (79). During periods of antidiuresis, medullary cells maintain high intracellular concentrations of organic osmolytes to match

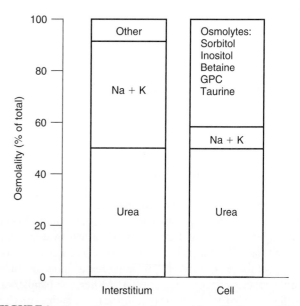

FIGURE 9   Comparison of osmotic composition of the inner medullary interstitium and of cells in the inner medulla. Sodium and potassium salts in the interstitium are balanced by compatible osmolytes (sorbitol, inositol, taurine). The denaturing effect of urea is balanced by counteracting osmolytes (betaine, glycerophosphocholine [GPC]). Data from Beck F, Dorge A, Rick R, Thurau K. Intra- and extracellular element concentrations of rat renal papilla in antidiuresis. *Kidney Int* 1984;25:397–403; and Beck F, Dorge A, Rick R, Thurau K. Osmoregulation of renal papillary cells. *Pflugers Arch* 1985;405(Suppl 1):S28–S32. (From Knepper MA, Rector FC, Jr. Urinary concentration and dilution. In: Brenner BM, ed. *The Kidney*, 5th ed. Philadelphia: WB Saunders; 1996:532–570, with permission.)

extracellular osmolality. When water is ingested, these cells respond by rapidly losing osmolytes into the urine by increasing their cell membrane permeability to these osmolytes, thus decreasing intracellular osmolality (79, 280). However, the medullary cells continue osmolyte production during these short periods of diuresis. Although this continued osmolyte production may appear inefficient, it enables the cell to respond rapidly to the cessation of water ingestion. When water ingestion ceases, the cell's permeability to osmolyte efflux decreases, and intracellular osmolyte concentration is rapidly restored since osmolyte production is maintained (79, 280). However, if the diuresis is prolonged (days), then osmolyte production is decreased in addition to the increase in cell permeability (79, 280). In this case, osmolyte concentration cannot be restored rapidly since the upregulation of osmolyte production requires an increase in the transcription of osmolyte genes and new protein synthesis (79).

ROLE OF UREA

Urea plays a unique role in the urinary concentrating mechanism. Its importance to the generation of concentrated urine has been appreciated since 1934 when Gamble and colleagues (78) described "an economy of water in renal function referable to urea." Several studies show that maximal urine concentrating ability is decreased in protein-deprived animals and humans and is restored by urea infusion (59, 66, 78, 96, 142, 193, 254, 257). This is the mechanism that has been proposed to explain why protein-restricted and malnourished humans are unable to concentrate their urine maximally. A UT-A1/UT-A3 knockout mouse (70) and a UT-B knockout mouse (146, 391, 392) were each shown to have urine concentrating defects. Thus, any solution to the question of how the inner medulla concentrates urine needs to take into account some effect derived from urea.

Facilitated Urea Transporters

Several early studies in dog and rat suggested that vasopressin could increase urea permeability across the IMCD (119, 219–221). Direct evidence was obtained in the 1980s when three groups showed that vasopressin could increase passive urea permeability in isolated perfused rat IMCDs (164, 274, 290). A specific facilitated or carrier-mediated urea transport process in rat and rabbit terminal IMCDs was first proposed in 1987 (290). The physiologic studies provided a functional characterization for a vasopressin-regulated urea transporter (reviewed in references 10, 278, 279, 281, 310). Two urea transporter genes have been cloned: the UT-A (*Scl14A2*) gene encodes six protein and nine cDNA isoforms; the UT-B (*Scl14A1*) gene encodes a single isoform (Table 6). The UT-A gene was initially cloned from rat (222), then from human and mouse (12, 71). It has two promoter elements: Promoter I is upstream of exon 1 and drives the transcription of UT-A1, UT-A1b, UT-A3, UT-A3b, and UT-A4; promoter II is located within intron 12 and drives the transcription of UT-A2 and UT-A2b (13, 222).

UT-A1 is the largest UT-A protein and is expressed in the apical plasma membrane of cells in the IMCD (12, 140, 229). Urea transport by UT-A1 is stimulated by cAMP when expressed in *Xenopus* oocytes (73, 264, 312) and by vasopressin when stably expressed in UT-A1-MDCK cells (76). Western blots of inner medullary tip proteins show bands at both 117 and 97 kDa; both bands represent glycosylated versions of a nonglycosylated 84-kDa UT-A1 protein (29). UT-A1 protein is most abundant in the inner medullary tip; only the 97-kDa protein is detected in the inner medullary base, and it is not detected in outer medulla or cortex (229, 282, 283). UT-A3 is also expressed in the IMCD (128), although its location varies between species: it is expressed in the apical membrane in rat (347) but in the basolateral membrane in mouse (334). Urea transport by UT-A3 is stimulated by cAMP analogues when expressed in human embryonic kidney (HEK) 293 cells or

TABLE 6 Cloned Mammalian Urea Transporters

Gene	Isoform	Tissue Localization
Slc14A1	UT-B	Red blood cells, endothelial cells, descending vasa recta
Slc14A2	UT-A1/UT-A1b	Inner medullary collecting duct - apical membrane
	UT-A2/UT-A2b	Thin descending limb (also heart and liver)
	UT-A3/UT-A3b	Inner medullary collecting duct Apical membrane in rat Basolateral membrane in mouse
	UT-A4	Rat medulla (not detected in mouse)
	UT-A5	Testis (not expressed in kidney)
	UT-A6	Colon (not expressed in kidney)

The original references can be found in the following reviews: 10, 278, 281, 310, 398.

Xenopus oocytes in three studies (73, 128, 318) but not in a fourth (313).

UT-A2 was actually the first cloned urea transporter (396) and is expressed in thin descending limbs (140, 229, 370). Urea transport by UT-A2 is not stimulated by cAMP analogues when expressed in either *Xenopus* oocytes or HEK-293 cells (4, 128, 264, 311, 312, 317, 396). UT-A4 is expressed in rat kidney medulla, although its exact location is unknown, and it has not been detected in mouse kidney (71, 73, 146). Urea transport by UT-A4 is stimulated by cAMP analogues when expressed in HEK-293 cells (128). UT-A5 and UT-A6 are expressed in testis and colon, respectively, but not in kidney (72, 318). In addition, there are three UT-A cDNA variants with alternative 3'-untranslated regions but no difference in coding region: UT-A1b, UT-A2b, and UT-A3b (13).

The UT-B cDNA was initially cloned from a human erythroid cell line (243), then from rodents (58, 293, 362, 391). UT-B protein is the Kidd antigen (in humans) and several mutations of the UT-B/Kidd antigen gene exist (199, 200, 241, 242, 314); red blood cells from these individuals also lack phloretin-sensitive facilitated urea transport (141). The human UT-B gene encodes a single cDNA and a single protein (199); both the N and C termini are located intracellularly (200). However in rat, two cDNA sequences (UT-B1, UT-B2) that differ by only a few nucleotides at their 3' end have been reported (58, 362). Whether the two cDNAs truly represent different rat UT-B isoforms, a polymorphism, or a sequencing artifact is uncertain since humans have only a single isoform. UT-B protein is detected as a broad band between 45 and 65 kDa in human red blood cells and 35 to 55 kDa in rodent red blood cells and kidney medulla (352, 360, 391). UT-B protein and phloretin-inhibitable urea transport are present in descending vasa recta (103, 245–247, 352, 360, 385, 391).

Several studies have addressed the question of whether UT-B transports urea only, or water and urea (315, 391, 393). Although red blood cells from a UT-B/AQP1 double-knockout mouse show that UT-B can function as a water channel, the amount of water transported through UT-B under physiologic conditions is small (in comparison with AQP1) and is probably not physiologically significant to the urine concentrating mechanism (392).

Rapid Regulation of Facilitated Urea Transport

The primary method for investigating the rapid regulation of urea transport has been perfusion of rat IMCDs. This method provides physiologically relevant functional data, although it cannot determine which urea transporter isoform is responsible for a specific functional effect in rat terminal IMCDs since both UT-A1 and UT-A3 are expressed in this nephron segment. Functional studies show that phloretin-inhibitable urea transport is present in both the apical and basolateral plasma membranes, with the apical membrane being the rate-limiting barrier for vasopressin-

stimulated urea transport (321). As discussed previously, it is unclear whether UT-A3 is the basolateral membrane urea transporter (334, 347).

Vasopressin (acting through cAMP) increases urea permeability within minutes of its addition to the bath fluid in rat terminal IMCDs (226, 290, 292, 322), suggesting that vasopressin acts by binding to V2 receptors, stimulating adenylyl cyclase and generating cAMP, and ultimately increasing transepithelial urea transport. Oxytocin also increases urea permeability by binding to V2 receptors and increasing cAMP production in rat terminal IMCDs (44). The acute stimulation of urea permeability by vasopressin occurs by an increase in the number of functional urea transporters (V_{max}) without a change in the transporter's affinity (K_m) for urea (46). Adding vasopressin to the lumen of a perfused rat terminal IMCD also increases urea permeability by binding to luminal V2 receptors (233). However, when vasopressin is first added to the bath, adding vasopressin to the lumen inhibits urea permeability, suggesting that luminal vasopressin is a negative modulator of basolateral vasopressin on urea permeability in rat terminal IMCDs (233).

One mechanism for rapid regulation is a vasopressin-stimulated increase in UT-A1 phosphorylation (397). The deduced amino acid sequence for UT-A1 contains several consensus sites for phosphorylation by PKA, as well as by protein kinase C (PKC) and tyrosine kinase (128). Vasopressin increases the phosphorylation of both the 117- and 97-kDa UT-A1 proteins within 2 minutes in rat IMCD suspensions, consistent with the time course for vasopressin-stimulated urea transport in perfused rat terminal IMCDs (226, 322, 372, 397). A selective V2-receptor agonist (dDAVP [1-desamino-8-D-arginine vasopressin], desmopressin) also increases UT-A1 phosphorylation, and PKA inhibitors block the phosphorylation of UT-A1 by vasopressin (397). These findings strongly suggest that vasopressin rapidly increases urea transport in rat terminal IMCDs by increasing UT-A1 phosphorylation. Vasopressin also increases urea flux and UT-A1 phosphorylation in stably transfected UT-A1-MDCK cells (76).

Another mechanism by which vasopressin could rapidly increase urea transport is regulated trafficking or redistribution of UT-A1 between an intracellular compartment and the apical plasma membrane. However, the single study that has examined this mechanism did not find evidence for regulated trafficking of UT-A1 in Brattleboro rats, which lack vasopressin (114).

Increasing osmolality to high physiological values, either by adding NaCl or mannitol, in the absence of vasopressin, acutely increases urea permeability in rat terminal IMCDs (83, 172, 292), suggesting that hyperosmolality is an independent stimulator of urea transport. When osmolality is increased and vasopressin is present, they have additive stimulatory effects on urea permeability (51, 83, 172, 292). Hyperosmolality-stimulated urea permeability is inhibited by phloretin and the urea analogue thiourea (83). Kinetic studies show that hyperosmolality, like vasopressin, stimulates urea permeability by increasing V_{max} rather than K_m (83). However, hyperosmolality stimulates urea permeability via increases in intracellular calcium and activation of PKC (84, 129) while vasopressin stimulates urea permeability via increases in adenylyl cyclase (322). Thus, both hyperosmolality and vasopressin increase urea permeability by increasing V_{max}, but they do so via different second messenger pathways.

Active Urea Transporters

Functional evidence exists for two types of active urea transport in the rat collecting duct: sodium–urea cotransport and sodium–urea countertransport (reviewed in 278, 279). Although no sodium-dependent active urea transporter has been cloned, several sodium-coupled cotransporters (rabbit sodium–glucose cotransporters 1 and 3, human sodium–chloride–γ-minobutyric acid [GABA] cotransporter 1) behave as urea channels when expressed in *Xenopus* oocytes (190, 249).

LONG-TERM REGULATION OF UREA TRANSPORTERS

Vasopressin

Administering vasopressin to Brattleboro rats (which lack vasopressin) for 5 days decreases UT-A1 protein abundance in the inner medulla (138, 346). However, administering vasopressin for 12 days increases UT-A1 protein abundance (138). This delayed increase in UT-A1 protein is consistent with the time course for the increase in inner medullary urea content in Brattleboro rats following vasopressin administration (93). In normal rats, suppressing endogenous vasopressin levels by 2 weeks of water diuresis also decreases UT-A1 protein abundance (138). This time course may be explained by analysis of UT-A promoter I since the 1.3 kb that has been cloned does not contain a cAMP response element (CRE) and cAMP does not increase promoter activity (222, 223). However, promoter I does contain a tonicity enhancer (TonE) element and hyperosmolality increases promoter activity (222, 223). Thus, vasopressin may increase UT-A1 indirectly after directly increasing the transcription of other genes, such as the Na-K-2Cl cotransporter NKCC2/BSC1, which begins to increase inner medullary osmolality (105, 395). Consistent with this hypothesis, water-restricting rats with primary polydipsia results in an increase in plasma vasopressin but no increase in medullary osmolality or UT-A1 protein abundance (38).

In Brattleboro rats, UT-A2 mRNA increases at 4 and 72 hours after administering dDAVP, while UT-A1 mRNA is unchanged (32). The dDAVP-stimulated increase in UT-A2 mRNA is consistent with the presence of a CRE in UT-A promoter II and the stimulation of promoter II activity by cAMP (222).

Administering vasopressin or dDAVP for 6 hours reduces UT-B mRNA abundance in the outer and inner medullas of Brattleboro rats (263). In contrast, administering vasopressin or dDAVP for 5 days increases UT-B mRNA abundance in the inner stripe of the outer medulla and the inner medullary base, while it is still decreased in the inner medullary tip (263). Administering dDAVP for 7 days to normal rats decreases UT-B protein abundance in the inner medulla (360).

Other Factors Regulating Urea Transporter Abundance

Feeding rats a low-protein diet for at least 2 weeks results in a decrease in the fractional excretion of urea (254), induces the functional expression of vasopressin-stimulated urea permeability in the initial IMCD (4, 115, 117), increases basal urea permeability in the $IMCD_3$ (133), and increases the abundance of the 117-kDa glycoprotein form of UT-A1 in the inner medulla (346). The low-protein diet induced vasopressin-stimulated urea permeability in the initial IMCD is stimulated by hyperosmolality and inhibited by phloretin and thiourea (4, 117). Thus, it has the same functional characteristics as the vasopressin-stimulated urea permeability that is normally expressed in the terminal IMCD (4). Whether the mRNA abundance of UT-A1 or UT-A2 changes in the inner medulla of low-protein fed rats is controversial (4, 104, 317). Varying dietary protein between 10% and 40% has no effect on UT-B mRNA abundance in any portion of the medulla in either normal or Brattleboro rats (104).

Glucocorticoids (dexamethasone) increase the fractional excretion of urea (151) and decrease UT-A promoter I activity, UT-A1 and UT-A3 mRNA abundances, UT-A1 protein abundance, and facilitated urea transport (82, 224, 255). Mineralocorticoids (aldosterone) also decrease UT-A1 protein abundance in the inner medulla of adrenalectomized rats, and this decrease can be blocked by spironolactone, a mineralocorticoid-receptor antagonist (82). In contrast, spironolactone does not block the decrease due to dexamethasone (82), indicating that each steroid hormone works through its own receptor. Aldosterone-induced volume expansion (with a high NaCl diet) decreases both UT-A1 and UT-A3 protein abundances (373).

Dahl salt-sensitive rats have increased abundances of UT-A1 and UT-A3 proteins in the inner medulla, and of facilitated urea transport in the terminal IMCD (69). They also have an increased level of the corticosterone-inactivating enzyme 11β-hydroxysteroid dehydrogenase type II (69). Inactivating glucocorticoids by increasing 11β-hydroxysteroid dehydrogenase type II would lessen the repression of UT-A promoter I activity, thereby increasing UT-A1 and UT-A3 transcription and abundance.

Uncontrolled diabetes mellitus (induced by streptozotocin) causes an osmotic diuresis and increases urea excretion, corticosterone production, and plasma vasopressin levels (31, 215, 359). UT-A1 protein abundance decreases at 3 to

5 days after inducing diabetes mellitus in the rat inner medulla, but not in adrenalectomized, diabetic rats (139, 144). The decrease in UT-A1 protein abundance is restored by giving dexamethasone to adrenalectomized diabetic rats, indicating that glucocorticoids mediate the decrease in UT-A1 protein (144).

In contrast, UT-A1 mRNA and protein are increased 10 to 21 days after diabetes mellitus is induced in normal rats (16, 139). UT-A1 protein did not increase in diabetic Brattleboro rats, indicating that vasopressin is necessary for this increase in UT-A1 (138). In addition, vasopressin did not increase UT-A1 phosphorylation in either Brattleboro rats or diabetic Brattleboro rats, indicating that vasopressin is necessary for the increase in UT-A1 protein abundance and phosphorylation that occurs at 10 to 21 days after diabetes is induced (138).

Angiotensin II does not affect basal (no vasopressin) facilitated urea permeability in rat terminal IMCDs (129). However, it increases vasopressin-stimulated urea permeability and UT-A1 phosphorylation via a PKC-mediated effect (129). Thus, angiotensin II may play a physiologic role in the urinary concentrating mechanism by augmenting the maximal urea permeability response to vasopressin. In the inner medulla of mice that lack tissue angiotensin converting enzyme, and hence lack angiotensin II, UT-A1 protein abundance is decreased to 25% of the level in wildtype mice (67, 145). Administering angiotensin II to these mice for 2 weeks did not correct the reduction in UT-A1 protein or in urine concentrating ability (145).

Hypercalcemia or hypokalemia reduces urine concentrating ability (77, 127, 192, 283). Basal urea permeability is increased in terminal IMCDs from hypercalcemic rats compared with normocalcemic control rats (283). Consistent with this functional increase, the abundance of UT-A1 protein is also increased (283). These changes may be regulated by a calcium-sensing receptor in the apical plasma membrane of cells in the terminal IMCD (288). A low-potassium diet reduces the abundance of UT-A1, UT-A3, and UT-B proteins in the inner medulla, but increases UT-A2 protein abundance in the outer medulla (127).

Hypothyroidism reduces urine concentrating ability but does not alter UT-A1 or UT-A2 protein abundance in rats (37). Water restricting hypothyroid rats does not alter either UT-A1 or UT-A2 abundance (37).

Urine concentrating ability is reduced in normal aging (reviewed in 277). UT-A1, UT-A3, and UT-B proteins are reduced in kidneys of aged rats (57, 260, 361). A supraphysiologic dose of dDAVP increases UT-A1 and UT-B protein abundances and urine osmolality in aged rats, but not to the levels observed in younger rats (56).

UT-A1, UT-A3, and UT-B protein abundances are reduced by bilateral or unilateral ureteral obstruction in rat inner medulla (194). The abundance of all three urea transporters remained reduced at 2 weeks after release of bilateral ureteral obstruction (194).

Lithium causes nephrogenic diabetes insipidus and an inability to concentrate urine (reviewed in 353). Lithium-treated rats have a marked reduction in inner medullary interstitial osmolality, AQP2 protein, UT-A1 and UT-B proteins, and vasopressin-stimulated UT-A1 phosphorylation (52, 143, 207, 238).

Genetic Knockout of Urea Transporters

Humans with genetic loss of Kidd antigen (UT-B) are unable to concentrate their urine above 800 mOsm/kg H_2O, even following overnight water deprivation and exogenous vasopressin administration (284). Mice with a genetic knockout of UT-B also have mildly reduced urine concentrating ability, which is not improved by urea loading (14, 391). UT-A1 and UT-A3 abundances are unchanged in UT-B knockout mice, but UT-A2 protein abundance is increased (146). Since UT-A2 mediates urea recycling through the thin descending limb, it may be upregulated to partially compensate for the loss of urea recycling through UT-B, thereby contributing to the mild phenotype observed in humans lacking UT-B/Kidd antigen and in UT-B knockout mice.

Mathematical models of microcirculatory exchange between the descending and ascending vasa recta predict that the absence of UT-B will decrease the efficiency of small solute trapping within the renal medulla, thereby decreasing the efficiency of countercurrent exchange and urine concentrating ability (64, 65). Thus, UT-B protein expression in red blood cells and/or descending vasa recta is necessary for the production of maximally concentrated urine (14, 64, 65, 202, 203, 284).

Genetic knockout of both UT-A1 and UT-A3 in mice results in reduced urine concentrating ability, reduced inner medullary interstitial urea content, and a lack vasopressin-stimulated or phloretin-inhibitable urea transport in their IMCD (70). However, these mice are able to concentrate their urine almost as well as wildtype mice when both are fed a low-protein diet (70), which supports the hypothesis that IMCD urea transport contributes to urine concentrating ability by preventing urea-induced osmotic diuresis (21). After water restriction, inner medullary tissue urea content was markedly reduced, but there was no measurable difference in NaCl content between UT-A1/UT-A3 knockout mice and wildtype mice (70). While this latter finding appears to be inconsistent with the predictions of the passive mechanism for urinary concentration (162, 324), the design of this aspect of the study (70) probably prevents a definitive conclusion of there being no difference in NaCl content, because the measurements were based on the whole inner medulla rather than the papilla. It is in the papilla where NaCl concentrations have been found to rise to high levels, but even there it is increasing to the highest values near the very tip of the papilla. Thus, the averaging of tissue from the entire inner medulla may have masked any increase at the papillary tip.

Active Urea Transport

When urine concentrating ability is reduced, there are changes in active urea transport that follow one of two patterns (115–117, 131–133). The first pattern, which occurs in response to water diuresis, is upregulation of active urea secretion in the $IMCD_3$ and its induction in the $IMCD_2$. This increase in urea secretion will directly decrease urea content in the deep inner medulla. The second pattern, which occurs in response to a low-protein diet, hypercalcemia, and furosemide, is induction of active urea absorption in the $IMCD_1$ and inhibition of active urea secretion in the $IMCD_3$. This second pattern will increase urea delivery to the inner medullary base, thereby decreasing urea delivery to the inner medullary tip; the accompanying inhibition of active urea secretion in the $IMCD_3$ may prevent an even greater reduction in urea content in the deep inner medulla.

UREA RECYCLING

Several urea recycling pathways are believed to contribute to high urea concentrations within the inner medulla (21, 154, 177). The major recycling pathway involves urea absorption from the terminal IMCD, mediated by UT-A1 and UT-A3, and secretion into the thin descending limb and, especially, the thin ascending limb (Fig. 10). Collecting ducts and thin ascending limbs are virtually contiguous within the inner medulla (189). The urea that enters the thin ascending limb is carried distally as the luminal fluid moves through several nephron segments having very low urea permeability until it reaches the urea-permeable terminal IMCD. Thus, urea is recycled from the terminal IMCD through the interstitium into the thin ascending limb and back to the terminal IMCD.

Two other pathways for urea recycling may exist in the kidney (154). One pathway is urea absorption from terminal IMCDs through ascending vasa recta and secretion into thin descending limbs of short-looped nephrons (368), mediated by UT-A2 (370), or into descending vasa recta, mediated by UT-B. The other pathway is urea absorption from cortical thick ascending limbs and secretion into proximal straight tubules (154). All three urea recycling pathways would limit urea dissipation from the inner medulla where it is needed to increase interstitial osmolality (154).

It must be emphasized that the terminal IMCD is the only portion of the collecting duct in which vasopressin increases urea permeability, even though the entire collecting duct is permeable to water when vasopressin is present. Water absorption from the cortical, outer medullary, and initial inner medullary collecting ducts concentrates urea within the collecting duct lumen. When the luminal fluid finally reaches the urea-permeable terminal IMCD, the luminal urea concentration is very high and exceeds that in vasa recta (113, 256, 257, 366), allowing urea to be rapidly absorbed into the deepest portion of the inner medullary interstitium, where, in many studied mammals, it is needed to concentrate urine maximally (42, 290). This pattern of urea and water permeabilities separates the primary sites of urea and water absorption (Fig. 5); water is primarily absorbed in the cortex and outer medulla where there is extensive vascularization with high blood flow and the absorbed water can be returned to the circulation without diluting the deep inner medulla. Urea is primarily absorbed in the deep inner medulla (42, 290).

Urea serves a second function in the medulla: it is the major source for excretion of nitrogenous waste; large quantities of urea need to be excreted daily. The kidney's ability to concentrate urea reduces the need to excrete water simply to remove nitrogenous waste. In addition, a high interstitial urea concentration is able to osmotically balance urea within the collecting duct lumen. If interstitial urea were unavailable to offset the osmotic effect of luminal urea destined for excretion, then the interstitial NaCl concentration would have to be much higher (21, 70).

DEVELOPMENT OF URINE CONCENTRATING ABILITY

Newborn mammals and birds are unable to concentrate their urine (39, 63, 195, 308, 383). Rats and rabbits do not develop the ability to concentrate their urine maximally until 14 to 21 days after birth (68, 74, 95, 212, 308). In rats, the increase in urine osmolality is paralleled by an increase in both medullary sodium and urea content (266). In 10-day-old rats, neither urea nor NaCl loading enhances urine concentrating ability (358). However, in 20-day-old rats, urea loading significantly

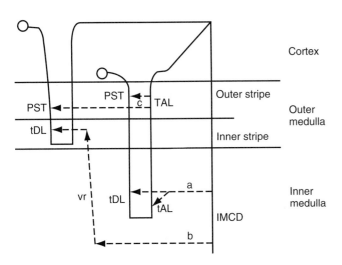

FIGURE 10 Urea recycling pathways in mammalian kidney. Diagram shows a short-looped nephron (**left**) and a long-looped nephron (**right**). Dotted lines labeled *a, b,* and *c* show urea recycling pathways. PST, proximal straight tubule; tDL, thin descending limb of Henle's loop; tAL, thin ascending limb of Henle's loop; TAL, thick ascending limb of Henle's loop; IMCD, inner medullary collecting duct; and vr, vasa recta. (From Knepper MA, Roch-Ramel F. Pathways of urea transport in the mammalian kidney. *Kidney Int* 1987;31:629–633, with permission.)

increases urine osmolality following water deprivation; NaCl loading has no effect (358). The development of urine concentrating ability can be hastened by giving glucocorticoids to 10- to 17-day-old rats, but not to older rats (266, 394). Conversely, adrenalectomizing 16-day-old rats slows the development of urine concentrating ability and abolishes the increase in inner medullary sodium and urea concentrations that normally occurs at this age (266).

In 1-day-old rats, the thin descending limb, thin ascending limb, and IMCD are all nearly water impermeable (195). At day 4, AQP1 mRNA is detected in the thin descending limb and water permeability increases, however, it does not reach adult levels until day 14 (195). Even though AQP2 protein is detected starting at day 1, water permeability remains low in the IMCD at day 7, but reaches adult levels at day 14 (25, 144, 195). However, AQP2 trafficking in the immature kidney responds normally to vasopressin (25) and AQP2 mRNA and protein levels increase 24 hours after a single dose of betamethasone (394).

In fetal rat kidney, UT-A protein is not detected and UT-B protein is weakly detected at embryonic age 20 days (140). In 1-day-old rats, UT-A1, UT-A2, and UT-B proteins appear (140), but the IMCD has a low urea permeability that is not stimulated by vasopressin (195). At day 14, urea permeability becomes vasopressin-stimulatable and UT-A1 mRNA is detected, although the values are only one third of adult levels (195). UT-A1, UT-A2, and UT-B proteins increase progressively until adult levels are achieved at 21 days of age (140). Thus, the time course for the increases in UT-A1, UT-A2, and UT-B proteins coincides with the development of urine concentrating ability. On the basis of the functional implications of these findings, Lui et al. (195) proposed that the concentrating mechanism in newborn rats is similar to that in the avian kidney, which has very low descending limb water permeability, does not use urea, and can concentrate urine to only moderate levels; however, within about 14 days, the neonatal rat kidney more closely resembles the adult rat kidney.

In rabbits, the sodium concentration in cortex and medulla is similar regardless of age (74). However, the medullary/cortical urea concentration ratio increases markedly between 14 and 21 days of age, coincident with the development of concentrated urine (74). This increase in medullary/cortical urea concentration is primarily due to a reduction in cortical urea concentration, rather than an increase in medullary urea content (74). However, in dogs, the developmental increase in urinary concentrating ability is due predominantly to an increase in the medullary sequestration of urea (101).

Newborn humans also have an inability to concentrate their urine (62). Infants fed a high protein diet are able to increase their urine osmolality following water deprivation; infants given a diet in which the extra protein is replaced by NaCl achieve a lower urine osmolality (62). Thus, even in infants, urea has a special role in the production of concentrated urine (62, 78).

Aldose reductase enzyme activity is absent in IMCDs from newborn rat pups (<12 hours old) but is present in 3-day-old pups and increases progressively up to 20 days of age; enzyme activity then decreases to adult levels (308). Consistent with these functional measurements, aldose reductase mRNA cannot be detected, even by reverse transcriptase–polymerase chain reaction, in inner medullas from newborn rats (<12 hours old) but can be detected in 3-day-old pups (308). Aldose reductase mRNA abundance peaks between 8 and 20 days after birth, then decreases to levels found in adult rats (24, 308). Thus, aldose reductase mRNA and enzyme activity are induced prior to urine concentrating ability during development.

SUMMARY

Concentrated urine is produced in the renal medulla through the generation of an osmotic gradient extending from the corticomedullary boundary to the papillary tip. In the outer medulla, this gradient is generated by the countercurrent multiplication of a comparatively small transepithelial difference in osmotic pressure. This small difference, called a single effect, arises from the active transport of NaCl from thick ascending limbs, which dilutes ascending limb flow relative to flow in vessels and other tubules. The gradient in the inner medulla may also be generated by the countercurrent multiplication of a single effect, but the single effect has not been definitively identified. Although the passive mechanism, proposed by Kokko and Rector (162) and by Stephenson (324), remains the most widely accepted hypothesis for the inner medullary single effect, much of the evidence from perfused tubule and micropuncture studies, and from the UT-A1/UT-A3 knockout mouse (70) is inconclusive or at variance with the passive mechanism. Moreover, the passive mechanism has not been supported by mathematical simulations using measured transepithelial transport parameters.

Nonetheless, there have been important advances in the understanding of key components of the urine concentrating mechanism, notably the identification and localization of key transport proteins for water, urea, and sodium, and the elucidation of the role and regulation of osmoprotective osmolytes. Continued experimental investigation of transepithelial transport and its regulation, both in normal animals and in genetically engineered mice, and incorporation of the resulting information into mathematical simulations, may help to more fully elucidate the inner medullary concentrating mechanism.

Acknowledgments

This work was supported by National Institutes of Health grants R01-DK41707 and R01-DK63657 (J.M.S.), P01-DK61521 (J.M.S.), and R01-DK42091 (H.E.L.).

References

1. Abramow M, Orci L. On the "tightness" of the rabbit descending limb of the loop of Henle-physiological and morphological evidence. *Int J Biochem* 1980;12:23–27.
2. Akizuki N, Uchida S, Sasaki S, Marumo F. Impaired solute accumulation in inner medulla of *Clcnk1 -/-* mice kidney. *Am J Physiol Renal Physiol* 2001;280:F79–F87.
3. Ando Y, Jacobson HR, Breyer MD. Phorbol myristate acetate, dioctanoylglycerol, and phosphatidic acid inhibit the hydroosmotic effect of vasopressin on rabbit cortical collecting tubule. *J Clin Invest* 1987;80:590–593.
4. Ashkar ZM, Martial S, Isozaki T, Price SR, Sands JM. Urea transport in initial IMCD of rats fed a low-protein diet: functional properties and mRNA abundance. *Am J Physiol Renal Physiol* 1995;268:F1218–F1223.
5. Atherton JC, Green R, Thomas S. Influence of lysine-vasopressin dosage on the time course of changes in renal tissue and urinary composition in the conscious rat. *J Physiol* 1971;213:291–309.
6. Atherton JC, Hai MA, Thomas S. Acute effects of lysine vasopressin injection (single and continuous) on urinary composition in the conscious water diuretic rat. *Pflugers Arch* 1969; 310:281–296.
7. Atherton JC, Hai MA, Thomas S. The time course of changes in renal tissue composition during water diuresis in the rat. *J Physiol* 1968;197:429–443.
8. Atherton JC, Hai MA, Thomas S. The time course of changes in renal tissue composition during mannitol diuresis in the rat. *J Physiol* 1968;197:411–428.
9. Badr KF. Kidney and endocrine system, 1: eicosanoids. In: Massry SG, Glassock RJ, eds. *Textbook of Nephrology,* 3rd ed. Baltimore: Williams and Wilkins; 1995:182–191.
10. Bagnasco SM. Gene structure of urea transporters. *Am J Physiol Renal Physiol* 2003;284: F3–F10.
11. Bagnasco SM, Balaban RS, Fales HM, Yang YM, Burg MB. Predominantly osmotically active organic solutes in rat and rabbit renal medullas. *J Biol Chem* 1986;261:5872–5877.
12. Bagnasco SM, Peng T, Janech MG, Karakashian A, Sands JM. Cloning and characterization of the human urea transporter UT-A1 and mapping of the human *Slc14a2* gene. *Am J Physiol Renal Physiol* 2001;281:F400–F406.
13. Bagnasco SM, Peng T, Nakayama Y, Sands JM. Differential expression of individual UT-A urea transporter isoforms in rat kidney. *J Am Soc Nephrol* 2000;11:1980–1986.
14. Bankir L, Chen K, Yang B. Lack of UT-B in vasa recta and red blood cells prevents urea-induced improvement of urinary concentrating ability. *Am J Physiol Renal Physiol* 2004;286: F144–F151.
15. Bankir L, Trinh-Trang-Tan M-M. Urea and the kidney. In: Brenner BM, ed. *Brenner and Rector's The Kidney,* 6th ed. Philadelphia: Saunders; 2000:637–679.
16. Bardoux P, Ahloulay M, Le Maout S, Bankir L, Trinh-Trang-Tan MM. Aquaporin-2 and urea transporter-A1 are up-regulated in rats with type I diabetes mellitus. *Diabetologia* 2001;44:637–645.
17. Bargman J, Leonard SL, McNuly E, Robertson CR, Jamison RL. Examination of transepithelial exchange of water and solute in the rat renal pelvis. *J Clin Invest* 1984;74:1860–1870.
18. Barrett GL, Packer JS, Davies JM. Sodium chloride, water and urea handling in the rat renal medulla: a computer simulation. *Renal Physiol* 1986;9:223–240.
19. Beck F, Dorge A, Rick R, Thurau K. Intra- and extracellular element concentrations of rat renal papilla in antidiuresis. *Kidney Int* 1984;25:397–403.
20. Beck F, Dorge A, Rick R, Thurau K. Osmoregulation of renal papillary cells. *Pflugers Arch* 1985;405(Suppl 1):S28–S32.
21. Berliner RW, Levinsky NG, Davidson DG, Eden M. Dilution and concentration of the urine and the action of antidiuretic hormone. *Am J Med* 1958;24:730–744.
22. Beuchat CA. Body size, medullary thickness, and urine concentrating ability in mammals. *Am J Physiol Regul Integr Comp Physiol* 1990;258:R298–R308.
23. Beuchat CA. Structure and concentrating ability of the mammalian kidney: correlations with habitat. *Am J Physiol Regul Integr Comp Physiol* 1996;271:R157–R179.
24. Bondy CA, Lightman SL. Developmental and physiological regulation of aldose reductase mRNA expression in renal medulla. *Mol Endocrinol* 1989;3:1409–1416.
25. Bonilla-Felix M, Jiang W. Aquaporin-2 in the immature rat: expression, regulation, and trafficking. *J Am Soc Nephrol* 1997;8:1502–1509.
26. Bonventre JV, Karnovsky MJ, Lechene CP. Renal papillary epithelial morphology in antidiuresis and water diuresis. *Am J Physiol Renal Physiol* 1978;235:F69–F76.
27. Bonventre JV, Lechene C. Renal medullary concentrating process: an integrative hypothesis. *Am J Physiol Renal Physiol* 1980;239:F578–F588.
28. Bonventre JV, Roman RJ, Lechene C. Effect of urea concentration of pelvic fluid on renal concentrating ability. *Am J Physiol Renal Physiol* 1980;239:F609–F618.
29. Bradford AD, Terris J, Ecelbarger CA, et al. 97 and 117 kDa forms of the collecting duct urea transporter UT-A1 are due to different states of glycosylation. *Am J Physiol Renal Physiol* 2001;281:F133–F143.
30. Braun EJ, Reimer PR. Structure of avian loop of Henle as related to countercurrent multiplier system. *Am J Physiol Renal Physiol* 1988;255:F500–F512.
31. Brooks DD, Nutting DF, Crofton JT, Share L. Vasopressin in rats with genetic and streptozotocin-induced diabetes. *Diabetes* 1989;38:54–57.
32. Brooks HL, Ageloff S, Kwon TH, et al. cDNA array identification of genes regulated in rat renal medulla in response to vasopressin infusion. *Am J Physiol Renal Physiol* 2003;284: F218–F228.
33. Burg MB. Role of aldose reductase and sorbitol in maintaining the medullary intracellular milieu. *Kidney Int* 1988;33:635–641.
34. Burg MB, Bourdeau JE. Function of the thick ascending limb of Henle's loop. In: Vogel HG, Ullrich KJ, eds. *New Aspects of Renal Function.* Amsterdam: Excerpta Medica; 1978:91–102.
35. Burg MB, Green N. Function of the thick ascending limb of Henle's loop. *Am J Physiol* 1973;224:659–668.
36. Burg MB, Kador PF. Sorbitol, osmoregulation, and the complications of diabetes. *J Clin Invest* 1988;81:635–640.
37. Cadnapaphornchai MA, Kim Y-W, Gurevich AK, et al. Urinary concentrating defect in hypothyroid rats: role of sodium, potassium, 2-chloride co-transporter, and aquaporins. *J Am Soc Nephrol* 2003;14:566–574.
38. Cadnapaphornchai MA, Summer SN, Falk S, Thurman JM, Knepper MA, Schrier RW. Effect of primary polydipsia on aquaporin and sodium transporter abundance. *Am J Physiol Renal Physiol* 2003;285:F965–F971.
39. Calcagno PL, Rubin MI, Weintraub DH. Studies on the renal concentrating and diluting mechanisms in the premature infant. *J Clin Invest* 1954;33:91–96.
40. Calder WAI, Braun EJ. Scaling of osmotic regulation in mammals and birds. *Am J Physiol Regul Integr Comp Physiol* 1983;244:R601–R606.
41. Casotti G, Lindberg KK, Braun EJ. Functional morphology of the avian medullary cone. *Am J Physiol Regul Integr Comp Physiol* 2000;279:R1722–R1730.
42. Chandhoke PS, Saidel GM. Mathematical model of mass transport throughout the kidney. Effects of nephron heterogeneity and tubular-vascular organization. *Ann Biomed Eng* 1981;9:263–301.
43. Chandhoke PS, Saidel GM, Knepper MA. Role of inner medullary collecting duct NaC1 transport in urinary concentration. *Am J Physiol Renal Physiol* 1985;18:F688–F697.
44. Chou C-L, DiGiovanni SR, Luther A, Lolait SJ, Knepper MA. Oxytocin as an antidiuretic hormone. II. Role of V_2 vasopressin receptor. *Am J Physiol Renal Physiol* 1995;269:F78–F85.
45. Chou C-L, Knepper MA. In vitro perfusion of chinchilla thin limb segments: segmentation and osmotic water permeability. *Am J Physiol Renal Physiol* 1992;263:F417–F426.
46. Chou C-L, Knepper MA. Inhibition of urea transport in inner medullary collecting duct by phloretin and urea analogues. *Am J Physiol Renal Physiol* 1989;257:F359–F365.
47. Chou C-L, Knepper MA. In vitro perfusion of chinchilla thin limb segments: urea and NaCl permeabilities. *Am J Physiol Renal Physiol* 1993;264:F337–F343.
48. Chou C-L, Knepper MA, Layton HE. Urinary concentrating mechanism: the role of the inner medulla. *Semin Nephrol* 1993;13:168–181.
49. Chou C-L, Nielsen S, Knepper MA. Structural-functional correlation in chinchilla long loop of Henle thin limbs: A novel papillary subsegment. *Am J Physiol Renal Physiol* 1993;265: F863–F874.
50. Chou C-L, Sands JM, Nonoguchi H, Knepper MA. Urea-gradient associated fluid absorption with $\sigma_{urea}=1$ in rat terminal collecting duct. *Am J Physiol Renal Physiol* 1990;258: F1173–F1180.
51. Chou C-L, Sands JM, Nonoguchi H, Knepper MA. Concentration dependence of urea and thiourea transport pathway in rat inner medullary collecting duct. *Am J Physiol Renal Physiol* 1990;258:F486–F494.
52. Christensen S, Kusano E, Yusufi ANK, Murayama N, Dousa TP. Pathogenesis of nephrogenic diabetes insipidus due to chronic administration of lithium in rats. *J Clin Invest* 1985;75:1869–1879.
53. Chuang EL, Reineck HJ, Osgood RW, Kunau RT, Stein JH. Studies on the mechanism of reduced urinary osmolality after exposure of the renal papilla. *J Clin Invest* 1978;61:633–639.
54. Clapp WL, Madsen KM, Verlander JW, Tisher CC. Morphologic heterogeneity along the rat inner medullary collecting duct. *Lab Invest* 1989;60:219–230.
55. Clapp WL, Madsen KM, Verlander JW, Tisher CC. Intercalated cells of the rat inner medullary collecting duct. *Kidney Int* 1987;31:1080–1087.
56. Combet S, Geffroy N, Berthonaud V, et al. Correction of age-related polyuria by dDAVP: molecular analysis of aquaporins and urea transporters. *Am J Physiol Renal Physiol* 2003;284: F199–F208.
57. Combet S, Teillet L, Geelen G, et al. Food restriction prevents age-related polyuria by vasopressin-dependent recruitment of aquaporin-2. *Am J Physiol Renal Physiol* 2001;281: F1123–F1131.
58. Couriaud C, Ripoche P, Rousselet G. Cloning and functional characterization of a rat urea transporter: Expression in the brain. *Biochim Biophys Acta Gene Struct Expression* 1996;1309: 197–199.
59. Crawford JD, Doyle AP, Probst H. Service of urea in renal water conservation. *Am J Physiol* 1959;196:545–548.
60. de Rouffignac C. The urinary concentrating mechanism. In: Kinne RKH, ed. *Urinary Concentrating Mechanisms: Comparative Physiology.* Basel: Karger; 1990:31–102.
61. de Rouffignac C, Morel F. Micropuncture study of water, electrolytes and urea movements along the loop of Henle in *Psammomys. J Clin Invest* 1969;48:474–486.
62. Edelmann CM, Jr., Barnett HL, Troupkou V. Renal concentrating mechanisms in newborn infants. Effect of dietary protein and water content, role of urea, and responsiveness to antidiuretic hormone. *J Clin Invset* 1960;39:1062–1069.
63. Edelmann CM, Jr., Barnett HL, Troupkou V. Renal concentrating mechanisms in newborn infants. Effect of dietary protein and water content, role of urea, and responsiveness to antidiuretic hormone. *J Clin Invest* 1960;39:1062–1069.
64. Edwards A, Pallone TL. Facilitated transport in vasa recta: Theoretical effects on solute exchange in the medullary microcirculation. *Am J Physiol Renal Physiol* 1997;272:F505–F514.
65. Edwards A, Pallone TL. A multiunit model of solute and water removal by inner medullary vasa recta. *Am J Physiol Heart Circ Physiol* 1998;274:H1202–H1210.
66. Epstein FH, Kleeman CR, Pursel S, Hendrikx A. The effect of feeding protein and urea on the renal concentrating process. *J Clin Invest* 1957;36:635–641.
67. Esther CR, Jr., Marrero MB, Howard TE, et al. The critical role of tissue angiotensin-converting enzyme as revealed by gene targeting in mice. *J Clin Invset* 1997;99:2375–2385.
68. Falk G. Maturation of renal function in infant rats. *Am J Physiol* 1955;181:157–170.
69. Fenton RA, Chou C-L, Ageloff S, Brandt W, Stokes III JB, Knepper MA. Increased collecting duct urea transporter expression in Dahl salt-sensitive rats. *Am J Physiol Renal Physiol* 2003;285:F143–F151.
70. Fenton RA, Chou C-L, Stewart GS, Smith CP, Knepper MA. Urinary concentrating defect in mice with selective deletion of phloretin-sensitive urea transporters in the renal collecting duct. *Proc Natl Acad Sci U S A* 2004;101:7469–7474.
71. Fenton RA, Cottingham CA, Stewart GS, Howorth A, Hewitt JA, Smith CP. Structure and characterization of the mouse UT-A gene (*Slc14a2*). *Am J Physiol Renal Physiol* 2002;282: F630–F638.

72. Fenton RA, Howorth A, Cooper GJ, Meccariello R, Morris ID, Smith CP. Molecular characterization of a novel UT-A urea transporter isoform (UT-A5) in testis. *Am J Physiol Cell Physiol* 2000;279:C1425–C1431.

73. Fenton RA, Stewart GS, Carpenter B, et al. Characterization of the mouse urea transporters UT-A1 and UT-A2. *Am J Physiol Renal Physiol* 2002;283:F817–F825.

74. Forrest JN, Jr., Stanier MW. Kidney composition and renal concentrating ability in young rabbits. *J Physiol* 1966;187:1–4.

75. Foster DM, Jacquez JA. Comparison using central core model of renal medulla of the rabbit and rat. *Am J Physiol Renal Physiol* 1978;234:F402–F414.

76. Fröhlich O, Klein JD, Smith PM, Sands JM, Gunn RB. Urea transport in MDCK cells that are stably transfected with UT-A1. *Am J Physiol Cell Physiol* 2004;286:C1264–C1270.

77. Galla JH, Booker BB, Luke RG. Role of the loop segment in the urinary concentrating defect of hypercalcemia. *Kidney Int* 1986;29:977–982.

78. Gamble JL, McKhann CF, Butler AM, Tuthill E. An economy of water in renal function referable to urea. *Am J Physiol* 1934;109:139–154.

79. Garcia-Perez A, Burg MB. Renal medullary organic osmolytes. *Physiol Rev* 1991;71:1081–1115.

80. Garg LC, Knepper MA, Burg MB. Mineralocorticoid effects on Na-K-ATPase in individual nephron segments. *Am J Physiol Renal Physiol* 1981;240:F536–F544.

81. Garg LC, Mackie S, Tisher CC. Effect of low potassium-diet on Na-K-ATPase in rat nephron segments. *Pflugers Arch* 1982;394:113–117.

82. Gertner R, Klein JD, Bailey JL, et al. Aldosterone decreases UT-A1 urea transporter expression via the mineralocorticoid receptor. *J Am Soc Nephrol* 2004;15:558–565.

83. Gillin AG, Sands JM. Characteristics of osmolarity-stimulated urea transport in rat IMCD. *Am J Physiol Renal Physiol* 1992;262:F1061–F1067.

84. Gillin AG, Star RA, Sands JM. Osmolarity-stimulated urea transport in rat terminal IMCD: role of intracellular calcium. *Am J Physiol Renal Physiol* 1993;265:F272–F277.

85. Gottschalk CW, Mylle M. Micropuncture study of composition of loop of Henle fluid in desert rodents. *Am J Physiol* 1959;204:532–535.

86. Grantham JJ, Burg MB. Effect of vasopressin and cyclic AMP on permeability of isolated collecting tubules. *Am J Physiol* 1966;211:255–259.

87. Grantham JJ, Burg MB, Orloff J. The nature of transtubular Na and K transport in isolated rabbit renal collecting tubules. *J Clin Invest* 1970;49:1815–1826.

88. Hai MA, Thomas S. The time-course of changes in renal tissue composition during lysine vasopressin infusion in the rat. *Pflugers Arch* 1969;310:297–319.

89. Hall DA, Varney DM. Effect of vasopressin in electrical potential differences and chloride transport in mouse medullary thick ascending limb of Henle. *J Clin Invest* 1980;66:792–802.

90. Han JS, Thompson KA, Chou C-L, Knepper MA. Experimental tests of three-dimensional model of urinary concentrating mechanism. *J Am Soc Nephrol* 1992;2:1677–1688.

91. Hanley MJ, Kokko JP. Study of chloride transport across the rabbit cortical collecting tubule. *J Clin Invest* 1978;62:39–44.

92. Hargitay B, Kuhn W. Das Multiplikationsprinzip als Grundlage der Harnkonzentrierung in der Niere. *Z Elektrochem* 1951;55:539–558.

93. Harrington AR, Valtin H. Impaired urinary concentration after vasopressin and its gradual correction in hypothalamic diabetes insipidus. *J Clin Invest* 1968;47:502–510.

94. Hebert SC, Culpepper RM, Andreoli TE. NaCl transport in mouse medullary thick ascending limbs. I. Functional nephron heterogeneity and ADH-stimulated NaCl cotransport. *Am J Physiol Renal Physiol* 1981;241:F412–F431.

95. Heller H. Effects of dehydration on adult and newborn rats. *J Physiol* 1949;108:303–314.

96. Hendrikx A, Epstein FH. Effect of feeding protein and urea on renal concentrating ability in the rat. *Am J Physiol* 1958;195:539–542.

97. Hervy S, Thomas SR. Inner medullary lactate production and urine-concentrating mechanism: a flat medullary model. *Am J Physiol Renal Physiol* 2003;284:F65–F81.

98. Holstein-Rathlou N-H, Marsh DJ. Oscillations of tubular pressure, flow, and distal chloride concentration in rats. *Am J Physiol Renal Physiol* 1989;256:F1007–F1014.

99. Horster M. Loop of Henle functional differentiation: In vitro perfusion of the isolated thick ascending segment. *Pflugers Arch* 1978;378:15–24.

100. Horster M, Thurau K. Micropuncture studies on the filtration rate of single superficial and juxtamedullary glomeruli in the rat kidney. *Pflugers Arch* 1968;301:162–181.

101. Horster M, Valtin H. Postnatal development of renal function: micropuncture and clearance studies in the dog. *J Clin Invest* 1971;50:779–795.

102. Horster MF, Zink H. Functional differentiation of the medullary collecting tubule: Influence of vasopressin. *Kidney Int* 1982;22:360–365.

103. Hu MC, Bankir L, Michelet S, Rousselet G, Trinh-Trang-Tan M-M. Massive reduction of urea transporters in remnant kidney and brain of uremic rats. *Kidney Int* 2000;58:1202–1210.

104. Hu MC, Bankir L, Trinh-Trang-Tan MM. mRNA expression of renal urea transporters in normal and Brattleboro rats: effect of dietary protein intake. *Exp Nephrol* 1999;7:44–51.

105. Igarashi P, Whyte DA, Nagami GT. Cloning and kidney cell-specific activity of the promoter of the murine renal Na-K-Cl cotransporter gene. *J Biol Chem* 1996;271:9666–9674.

106. Imai M. Function of the thin ascending limbs of Henle of rats and hamsters perfused in vitro. *Am J Physiol Renal Physiol* 1977;232:F201–F209.

107. Imai M. Effect of bumetanide and furosemide on the thick ascending limb of Henle's loop of rabbits and rats perfused in vitro. *Eur J Pharmacol* 1977;41:409–416.

108. Imai M, Hayashi M, Araki M. Functional heterogeneity of the descending limbs of Henle's loop. I. Internephron heterogeneity in the hamster kidney. *Pflugers Arch* 1984;402:385–392.

109. Imai M, Kokko JP. Sodium, chloride, urea, and water transport in the thin ascending limb of Henle. *J Clin Invest* 1974;53:393–402.

110. Imai M, Taniguchi J, Tabei K. Function of thin loops of Henle. *Kidney Int* 1987;31:565–579.

111. Imai M, Taniguchi J, Yoshitomi K. Transition of permeability properties along the descending limb of long-loop nephron. *Am J Physiol Renal Physiol* 1988;254:F323–F328.

112. Imai M, Taniguchi J, Yoshitomi K. Osmotic work across inner medullary collecting duct accomplished by difference in reflection coefficients for urea and NaCl. *Pflugers Arch* 1988;412:557–567.

113. Imbert M, de Rouffignac C. Role of sodium and urea in the renal concentrating mechanism in Psammomys obesus. *Pflugers Arch* 1976;361:107–114.

114. Inoue T, Terris J, Ecelbarger CA, Chou C-L, Nielsen S, Knepper MA. Vasopressin regulates apical targeting of aquaporin-2 but not of UT1 urea transporter in renal collecting duct. *Am J Physiol Renal Physiol* 1999;276:F559–F566.

115. Isozaki T, Gillin AG, Swanson CE, Sands JM. Protein restriction sequentially induces new urea transport processes in rat initial IMCDs. *Am J Physiol Renal Physiol* 1994;266:F756–F761.

116. Isozaki T, Lea JP, Tumlin JA, Sands JM. Sodium-dependent net urea transport in rat initial IMCDs. *J Clin Invest* 1994;94:1513–1517.

117. Isozaki T, Verlander JW, Sands JM. Low protein diet alters urea transport and cell structure in rat initial inner medullary collecting duct. *J Clin Invest* 1993;92:2448–2457.

118. Ito M, Oiso Y, Murase T, et al. Possible involvement of inefficient cleavage of preprovasopressin by signal peptidase as a cause for familial central diabetes insipidus. *J Clin Invest* 1993;91:2565–2571.

119. Jaenike JR. The influence of vasopressin on the permeability of the mammalian collecting duct to urea. *J Clin Invest* 1961;40:144–151.

120. Jamison RL. Micropuncture study of segments of thin loop of Henle in the rat. *Am J Physiol* 1968;215:236–242.

121. Jamison RL, Bennett CM, Berliner RW. Countercurrent multiplication by the thin loops of Henle. *Am J Physiol* 1967;212:357–366.

122. Jamison RL, Buerkert J, Lacy FB. A micropuncture study of collecting tubule function in rats with hereditary diabetes insipidus. *J Clin Invest* 1971;50:2444–2452.

123. Jamison RL, Buerkert J, Lacy FB. A micropuncture study of Henle's thin loop in Brattleboro rats. *Am J Physiol* 1973;224:180–185.

124. Jamison RL, Kriz W. *Urinary Concentrating Mechanism. Structure and Function.* New York: Oxford University Press; 1982.

125. Jen JF, Stephenson JL. Externally driven countercurrent multiplication in a mathematical model of the urinary concentrating mechanism of the renal inner medulla. *Bull Math Biol* 1994;56:491–514.

126. Jen JF, Wang H, Tewarson RP, Stephenson JL. Comparison of central core and radially separated models of renal inner medulla. *Am J Physiol Renal Physiol* 1995;268:F693–F697.

127. Jung J-Y, Madsen KM, Han K-H, et al. Expression of urea transporters in potassium-depleted mouse kidney. *Am J Physiol Renal Physiol* 2003;285:F1210–F1224.

128. Karakashian A, Timmer RT, Klein JD, Gunn RB, Sands JM, Bagnasco SM. Cloning and characterization of two new mRNA isoforms of the rat renal urea transporter: UT-A3 and UT-A4. *J Am Soc Nephrol* 1999;10:230–237.

129. Kato A, Klein JD, Zhang C, Sands JM. Angiotensin II increases vasopressin-stimulated facilitated urea permeability in rat terminal IMCDs. *Am J Physiol Renal Physiol* 2000;279:F835–F840.

130. Kato A, Naruse M, Knepper MA, Sands JM. Long-term regulation of inner medullary collecting duct urea transport in rat. *J Am Soc Nephrol* 1998;9:737–745.

131. Kato A, Sands JM. Active sodium-urea counter-transport is inducible in the basolateral membrane of rat renal initial inner medullary collecting ducts. *J Clin Invest* 1998;102:1008–1015.

132. Kato A, Sands JM. Evidence for sodium-dependent active urea secretion in the deepest subsegment of the rat inner medullary collecting duct. *J Clin Invest* 1998;101:423–428.

133. Kato A, Sands JM. Urea transport processes are induced in rat IMCD subsegments when urine concentrating ability is reduced. *Am J Physiol Renal Physiol* 1999;276:F62–F71.

134. Katz AI. Distribution and function of classes of ATPases along the nephron. *Kidney Int* 1986;29:21–31.

135. Katz AI, Doucet A, Morel F. Na-K-ATPase activity along the rabbit, rat and mouse nephron. *Am J Physiol Renal Physiol* 1979;237:F114–F120.

136. Kellogg RB. Some singular perturbation problems in renal models. *J Math Anal Appl* 1987;128:214–240.

137. Khorshid MR, Moffat DB. The epithelia lining the renal pelvis in the rat. *J Anat* 1974;118:561–569.

138. Kim D-U, Sands JM, Klein JD. Role of vasopressin in diabetes mellitus-induced changes in medullary transport proteins involved in urine concentration in Brattleboro rats. *Am J Physiol Renal Physiol* 2004;286:F760–F766.

139. Kim D-U, Sands JM, Klein JD. Changes in renal medullary transport proteins during uncontrolled diabetes mellitus in rats. *Am J Physiol Renal Physiol* 2003;285:F303–F309.

140. Kim Y-H, Kim D-U, Han K-H, et al. Expression of urea transporters in the developing rat kidney. *Am J Physiol Renal Physiol* 2002;282:F530–F540.

141. Kimoto Y, Constantinou CE. Effects of [1-desamino-8-D-arginine]vasopressin and papaverine on rabbit renal pelvis. *Eur J Pharmacol* 1990;175:359–362.

142. Klahr S, Alleyne GAO. Effects of chronic protein-calorie malnutrition on the kidney. *Kidney Int* 1973;3:129–141.

143. Klein JD, Gunn RB, Roberts BR, Sands JM. Down-regulation of urea transporters in the renal inner medulla of lithium-fed rats. *Kidney Int* 2002;61:995–1002.

144. Klein JD, Price SR, Bailey JL, Jacobs JD, Sands JM. Glucocorticoids mediate a decrease in the AVP-regulated urea transporter in diabetic rat inner medulla. *Am J Physiol Renal Physiol* 1997;273:F949–F953.

145. Klein JD, Quach DL, Cole JM, et al. Impaired urine concentration and the absence of tissue ACE: the involvement of medullary transport proteins. *Am J Physiol Renal Physiol* 2002;283:F517–F524.

146. Klein JD, Sands JM, Qian L, Wang X, Yang B. Upregulation of urea transporter UT-A2 and water channels AQP2 and AQP3 in mice lacking urea transporter UT-B. *J Am Soc Nephrol* 2004;15:1161–1167.

147. Knepper MA. Urea transport in nephron segments from medullary rays of rabbits. *Am J Physiol Renal Physiol* 1983;244:F622–F627.

148. Knepper MA. Urea transport in isolated thick ascending limbs and collecting ducts from rats. *Am J Physiol Renal Physiol* 1983;245:F634–F639.

149. Knepper MA. Measurement of osmolality in kidney slices using vapor pressure osmometry. *Kidney Int* 1982;21:653–655.

150. Knepper MA, Chou C-L, Layton HE. How is urine concentrated by the renal inner medulla? *Contrib Nephrol* 1993;102:144–160.

151. Knepper MA, Danielson RA, Saidel GM, Johnston KH. Effects of dietary protein restriction and glucocorticoid administration on urea excretion in rats. *Kidney Int* 1975;8:303–315.

152. Knepper MA, Danielson RA, Saidel GM, Post RS. Quantitative analysis of renal medullary anatomy in rats and rabbits. *Kidney Int* 1977;12:313–323.

153. Knepper MA, Rector FC, Jr. Urinary concentration and dilution. In: Brenner BM, ed. *The Kidney*, 5th ed. Philadelphia: WB Saunders; 1996:532–570.

154. Knepper MA, Roch-Ramel F. Pathways of urea transport in the mammalian kidney. *Kidney Int* 1987;31:629–633.

155. Knepper MA, Saidel GM, Hascall VC, Dwyer T. Concentration of solutes in the renal inner medulla: interstitial hyaluronan as a mechano-osmotic transducer. *Am J Physiol Renal Physiol* 2003;284:F433–F446.

156. Knepper MA, Sands JM, Chou C-L. Independence of urea and water transport in rat inner medullary collecting duct. *Am J Physiol* Renal Physiol 1989;256:F610–F621.

157. Knepper MA, Stephenson JL. Urinary concentrating and diluting processes. In: Andreoli TE, Hoffman JF, Fanestil DD, Schultz SG, eds. *Physiology of Membrane Disorders*, 2nd ed. New York: Plenum; 1986:713–726.

158. Koepsell H, Kriz W, Schnermann J. Pattern of luminal diameter changes along the descending and ascending thin limbs of the loop of Henle in the inner medullary zone of the rat kidney. *Z Anat Entwickl Gesch* 1972;138:321–328.

159. Koepsell H, Nicholson WAP, Kriz W, Hohling HJ. Measurements of exponential gradients of sodium and chlorine in the rat kidney medulla using the electron microprobe. *Pflugers Arch* 1974;350:167–184.

160. Kokko JP. Sodium chloride and water transport in the descending limb of Henle. *J Clin Invest* 1970;49:1838–1846.

161. Kokko JP. Urea transport in the proximal tubule and the descending limb of Henle. *J Clin Invest* 1972;51:1999–2008.

162. Kokko JP, Rector FC. Countercurrent multiplication system without active transport in inner medulla. *Kidney Int* 1972;2:214–223.

163. Kondo Y, Abe K, Igarashi Y, Kudo K, Tada K, Yoshinaga K. Direct evidence for the absence of active Na⁺ reabsorption in hamster ascending thin limb of Henle's loop. *J Clin Invest* 1993;91:5–11.

164. Kondo Y, Imai M. Effects of glutaraldehyde fixation on renal tubular function, I: preservation of vasopressin-stimulated water and urea pathways in rat papillary collecting duct. *Pflugers Arch* 1987;408:479–483.

165. Kondo Y, Imai M. Effect of glutaraldehyde on renal tubular function, II: selective inhibition of Cl⁻ transport in the hamster thin ascending limb of Henle's loop. *Pflugers Arch* 1987;408:484–490.

166. Koyama S, Yoshitomi K, Imai M. Effect of protamine on ion conductance of ascending thin limb of Henle's loop from hamsters. *Am J Physiol Renal Physiol* 1991;261:F593–F599.

167. Kriz W. Der architektonische und funktionelle Aufbau der Rattenniere. *Z Zellforsch* 1967;82:495–535.

168. Kriz W, Bankir L. A standard nomenclature for structures of the kidney. *Am J Physiol Renal Physiol* 1988;254:F1–F8.

169. Kriz W, Bankir L. Structural organization of the renal medullary counterflow system. *Fed Proc* 1983;42:2379–2385.

170. Kriz W, Lever AF. Renal countercurrent mechanisms: structure and function. *Am Heart J* 1969;78:101–118.

171. Kriz W, Schnermann J, Koepsell H. The position of short and long loops of Henle in the rat kidney. *Z Anat Entwicklungsgesch* 1972;138:301–319.

172. Kudo LH, César KR, Ping WC, Rocha AS. Effect of peritubular hypertonicity on water and urea transport of inner medullary collecting duct. *Am J Physiol Renal Physiol* 1992;262:F338–F347.

173. Kuhn W, Ryffel K. Herstellung konzentrierrter Lösungen aus verdünnten durch blosse Membranwirkung: Ein Modellversuch zur Funktion der Niere. *Hoppe-Seylers Z Physiol Chem* 1942;276:145–178.

174. Kuwahara M, Berry CA, Verkman AS. Rapid development of vasopressin-induced hydroosmosis in kidney collecting tubules measured by a new fluorescence technique. *Biophys J* 1988;54:595–602.

175. Lacy ER, Schmidt-Nielsen B. Anatomy of the renal pelvis in the hamster. *Am J Anat* 1979;154:291–320.

176. Lankford SP, Chou C-L, Terada Y, Wall SM, Wade JB, Knepper MA. Regulation of collecting duct water permeability independent of cAMP-mediated AVP response. *Am J Physiol Renal Physiol* 1991;261:F554–F566.

177. Lassiter WE, Gottschalk CW, Mylle M. Micropuncture study of net transtubular movement of water and urea in nondiuretic mammalian kidney. *Am J Physiol* 1961;200:1139–1146.

178. Layton AT, Layton HE. An efficient numerical method for distributed-loop models of the urine concentrating mechanism. *Math Biosci* 2003;118:111–132.

179. Layton AT, Pannabecker TL, Dantzler WH, Layton HE. Two modes for concentrating urine in rat inner medulla. *Am J Physiol Renal Physiol* 2004;287:F816–F839.

180. Layton HE. Urea transport in a distributed loop model of the urine-concentrating mechanism. *Am J Physiol Renal Physiol* 1990;258:F1110–F1124.

181. Layton HE. Mathematical models of the mammalian urine concentrating mechanism. In: Layton HE, Weinstein AM, eds. *The IMA Volumes in Mathematics and Its Applications, Vol. 129, Membrane Transport and Renal Physiology*. New York: Springer-Verlag; 2002:233–272.

182. Layton HE. Distributed loops of Henle in a central core model of the renal medulla: where should the solute come out? *Math Comput Modelling* 1990;14:533–537.

183. Layton HE. Concentrating urine in the inner medulla of the kidney. *Comments Theor Biol* 1989;1:179–196.

184. Layton HE. Distribution of Henle's loops may enhance urine concentrating capability. *Biophys J* 1986;49:1033–1040.

185. Layton HE, Davies JM. Distributed solute and water reabsorption in a central core model of the renal medulla. *Math Biosci* 1993;116:169–196.

186. Layton HE, Davies JM, Casotti G, Braun EJ. Mathematical model of an avian urine concentrating mechanism. *Am J Physiol Renal Physiol* 2000;279:1139–1160.

187. Layton HE, Knepper MA, Chou C-L. Permeability criteria for effective function of passive countercurrent multiplier. *Am J Physiol Renal Physiol* 1996;270:F9–F20.

188. Layton HE, Pitman EB, Knepper MA. A dynamic numerical method for models of the urine concentrating mechanism. *SIAM J Appl Math* 1995;55:1390–1418.

189. Lemley KV, Kriz W. Cycles and separations: The histotopography of the urinary concentrating process. *Kidney Int* 1987;31:538–548.

190. Leung DW, Loo DDF, Hirayama BA, Zeuthen T, Wright EM. Urea transport by cotransporters. *J Physiol (Lond)* 2000;528:251–257.

191. Lever AF. The vasa recta and countercurrent multiplication. *Acta Med Scand* 1965;178:1–43.

192. Levi M, Peterson L, Berl T. Mechanism of concentrating defect in hypercalcemia. Role of polydipsia and prostaglandins. *Kidney Int* 1983;23:489–497.

193. Levinsky NG, Berliner RW. The role of urea in the urine concentrating mechanism. *J Clin Invest* 1959;38:741–748.

194. Li C, Klein JD, Wang W, et al. Altered expression of urea transporters in response to ureteral obstruction. *Am J Physiol Renal Physiol* 2004;286:F1154–F1162.

195. Liu W, Morimoto T, Kondo Y, Iinuma K, Uchida S, Imai M. "Avian-type" renal medullary tubule organization causes immaturity of urine-concentrating ability in neonates. *Kidney Int* 2001;60:680–693.

196. Lorenzen M, Frindt G, Taylor A, Windhager EE. Quinidine effect on hydrosmotic response of collecting tubules to vasopressin and cAMP. *Am J Physiol Renal Physiol* 1987;252:F1103–F1111.

197. Lory P. Effectiveness of a salt transport cascade in the renal medulla: computer simulations. *Am J Physiol Renal Physiol* 1987;252:F1095–F1102.

198. Lory P, Gilg A, Horster M. Renal countercurrent system: role of collecting duct convergence and pelvic urea predicted from a mathematical model. *J Math Biol* 1983;16:281–304.

199. Lucien N, Sidoux-Walter F, Olivès B, et al. Characterization of the gene encoding the human Kidd blood group urea transporter protein: evidence for splice site mutations in Jk_null individuals. *J Biol Chem* 1998;273:12973–12980.

200. Lucien N, Sidoux-Walter F, Roudier N, et al. Antigenic and functional properties of the human red blood cell urea transporter hUT-B1. *J Biol Chem* 2002;277:34101–34108.

201. Ma TH, Yang BX, Gillespie A, Carlson EJ, Epstein CJ, Verkman AS. Severely impaired urinary concentrating ability in transgenic mice lacking aquaporin-1 water channels. *J Biol Chem* 1998;273:4296–4299.

202. Macey RI. Transport of water and urea in red blood cells. *Am J Physiol Cell Physiol* 1984;246:C195–C203.

203. Macey RI, Yousef LW. Osmotic stability of red cells in renal circulation requires rapid urea transport. *Am J Physiol Cell Physiol* 1988;254:C669–C674.

204. Macri P, Breton S, Marsolais M, Lapointe JY, Laprade R. Hypertonicity decreases basolateral K⁺ and Cl⁻ conductances in rabbit proximal convoluted tubule. *J Membr Biol* 1997;155:229–237.

205. Madsen KM, Tisher CC. Structural-functional relationship along the distal nephron. *Am J Physiol Renal Physiol* 1986;250:F1–F15.

206. Maeda Y, Smith BL, Agre P, Knepper MA. Quantification of aquaporin-CHIP water channel protein in microdissected renal tubules by fluorescence-based ELISA. *J Clin Invest* 1995;95:422–428.

207. Marples D, Christensen S, Christensen EI, Ottosen PD, Nielsen S. Lithium-induced downregulation of aquaporin-2 water channel expression in rat kidney medulla. *J Clin Invest* 1995;95:1838–1845.

208. Marsh DJ. Solute and water flows in thin limbs of Henle's loop in the hamster kidney. *Am J Physiol* 1970;218:824–831.

209. Marsh DJ, Azen SP. Mechanism of NaCl reabsorption by hamster thin ascending limb of Henle's loop. *Am J Physiol* 1975;228:71–79.

210. Marsh DJ, Martin CM. Lack of water or urea movement from pelvic urine to papilla in hydropenic hamsters. *Miner Electrolyte Metab* 1980;3:81–86.

211. Mason J, Gutsche H-U, Moore L, Müller-Suur R. The early phase of experimental acute renal failure. IV. The diluting ability of the short loops of Henle. *Pflugers Arch* 1979;379:11–18.

212. McCrory WW, Jr. *Developmental Nephrology*. Cambridge, MA: Harvard University Press; 1972:123–161.

213. Mejia R, Stephenson JL. Solution of a multinephron, multisolute model of the mammalian kidney by Newton and continuation methods. *Math Biosci* 1984;68:279–298.

214. Mejia R, Wade JB. Immunomorphometric study of rat renal inner medulla. *Am J Physiol Renal Physiol* 2002;282:F553–F557.

215. Mitch WE, Bailey JL, Wang X, Jurkovitz C, Newby DN, Price SR. Evaluation of signals activating ubiquitin-proteasome proteolysis in a model of muscle wasting. *Am J Physiol Cell Physiol* 1999;276:C1132–C1138.

216. Moore LC, Marsh DJ. How descending limb of Henle's loop permeability affects hypertonic urine formation. *Am J Physiol Renal Physiol* 1980;239:F57–F71.

217. Morel F, Imbert-Teboul M, Chabardes D. Distribution of hormone-dependent adenylate cyclase in the nephron and its physiologic significance. *Annual Rev Physiol* 1981;43:569–581.

218. Morel F, Mylle M, Gottschalk CW. Tracer microinjection studies of effect of ADH on renal tubular diffusion of water. *Am J Physiol* 1965;209:179–187.

219. Morgan T. Permeability of the nephron to urea. In: Schmidt-Nielsen B, Kerr DWS, eds. *Urea and the Kidney*. Amsterdam: Excerpta Medica Foundation; 1970:186–192.

220. Morgan T, Berliner RW. Permeability of the loop of Henle, vasa recta, and collecting duct to water, urea, and sodium. *Am J Physiol* 1968;215:108–115.

221. Morgan T, Sakai F, Berliner RW. In vitro permeability of medullary collecting duct to water and urea. *Am J Physiol* 1968;214:574–581.

222. Nakayama Y, Naruse M, Karakashian A, Peng T, Sands JM, Bagnasco SM. Cloning of the rat Slc14a2 gene and genomic organization of the UT-A urea transporter. *Biochim Biophys Acta* 2001;1518:19–26.

223. Nakayama Y, Peng T, Sands JM, Bagnasco SM. The TonE/TonEBP pathway mediates tonicity-responsive regulation of UT-A urea transporter expression. *J Biol Chem* 2000; 275:38275–38280.
224. Naruse M, Klein JD, Ashkar ZM, Jacobs JD, Sands JM. Glucocorticoids downregulate the rat vasopressin-regulated urea transporter in rat terminal inner medullary collecting ducts. *J Am Soc Nephrol* 1997;8:517–523.
225. Nielsen S, Frokiaer J, Marples D, Kwon ED, Agre P, Knepper M. Aquaporins in the kidney: from molecules to medicine. *Physiol Rev* 2002;82:205–244.
226. Nielsen S, Knepper MA. Vasopressin activates collecting duct urea transporters and water channels by distinct physical processes. *Am J Physiol Renal Physiol* 1993;265:F204–F213.
227. Nielsen S, Pallone T, Smith BL, Christensen EI, Agre P, Maunsbach AB. Aquaporin-1 water channels in short and long loop descending thin limbs and in descending vasa recta in rat kidney. *Am J Physiol Renal Physiol* 1995;268:F1023–F1037.
228. Nielsen S, Smith BL, Christensen EI, Knepper MA, Agre P. CHIP28 water channels are localized in constitutively water-permeable segments of the nephron. *J Cell Biol* 1993;120:371–383.
229. Nielsen S, Terris J, Smith CP, Hediger MA, Ecelbarger CA, Knepper MA. Cellular and subcellular localization of the vasopressin-regulated urea transporter in rat kidney. *Proc Natl Acad Sci U S A* 1996;93:5495–5500.
230. Niesel W, Röskenbleck H. Moglichkeiten der Konzentrierung von Stoffen biologischen Gegenstromsystemen. *Pflugers Arch* 1963;276:555–567.
231. Niesel W, Röskenbleck H. Konzentrierung von Lösungen unterschiedlicher Zusammensetzung durch alleinige Gegenstromdiffusion und Geggenstromosmose als möglicher Mechanismus der Harnkonzentrierung. *Pflugers Arch* 1965;283:230–241.
232. Niesel W, Röskenbleck H, Hanke P, Specht N, Heure L. Die gegenseitige Beeinflussung von Harnstoff, NaCl, KCl und Harnfluss bei der Bildung eines maximal konzentrierten Harns. *Pflugers Arch* 1970;315:308–320.
233. Nonoguchi H, Owada A, Kobayashi N, et al. Immunohistochemical localization of V_2 vasopressin receptor along the nephron and functional role of luminal V_2 receptor in terminal inner medullary collecting ducts. *J Clin Invest* 1995;96:1768–1778.
234. Nonoguchi H, Sands JM, Knepper MA. Atrial natriuretic factor inhibits NaCl and fluid absorption in cortical collecting duct of rat kidney. *Am J Physiol Renal Physiol* 1989;256:F179–F186.
235. Nonoguchi H, Tomita K, Marumo F. Effects of atrial natriuretic peptide and vasopressin on chloride transport in long- and short-looped medullary thick ascending limbs. *J Clin Invest* 1992;90:349–357.
236. Nyengaard JR, Bendtsen TF. Glomerular number and size in relation to age, kidney weight, and body surface in normal man. *Anat Rec* 1992;232:194–201.
237. O'Neil RG, Dubinsky WP. Micromethodology for measuring ATPase activity in renal tubules: mineralocorticoid influence. *Am J Physiol Cell Physiol* 1984;247:C314–C320.
238. Okusa MD, Crystal LJT. Clinical manifestations and management of acute lithium intoxication. *Am J Med* 1994;97:383–389.
239. Oliver J. *Nephrons and Kidneys: A Qualitative Study of Development and Evolutionary Mammalian Renal Architecture.* New York: Harper and Row, 1968.
240. Oliver RE, Roy DR, Jamison RL. Urinary concentration in the papillary collecting duct of the rat. *J Clin Invest* 1982;69:157–164.
241. Olivès B, Martial S, Mattei MG, et al. Molecular characterization of a new urea transporter in the human kidney. *FEBS Lett* 1996;386:156–160.
242. Olivès B, Mattei M-G, Huet M, et al. Kidd blood group and urea transport function of human erythrocytes are carried by the same protein. *J Biol Chem* 1995;270:15607–15610.
243. Olives B, Neau P, Bailly P, et al. Cloning and functional expression of a urea transporter from human bone marrow cells. *J Biol Chem* 1994;269:31649–31652.
244. Packer RK, Sands JM, Knepper MA. Chloride and osmotic water permeabilities of isolated rabbit renal papillary surface epithelium. *Am J Physiol Renal Physiol* 1989;257:F218–F224.
245. Pallone TL. Characterization of the urea transporter in outer medullary descending vasa recta. *Am J Physiol Regul Integr Comp Physiol* 1994;267:R260–R267.
246. Pallone TL, Nielsen S, Silldorff EP, Yang S. Diffusive transport of solute in the rat medullary microcirculation. *Am J Physiol Renal Physiol* 1995;269:F55–F63.
247. Pallone TL, Work J, Myers RL, Jamison RL. Transport of sodium and urea in outer medullary descending vasa recta. *J Clin Invest* 1994;93:212–222.
248. Palmer LG, Frindt G. Amiloride-sensitive Na channels from the apical membrane of the rat cortical collecting tubule. *Proc Natl Acad Sci U S A* 1986;83:2767–2770.
249. Panayotova-Heiermann M, Wright EA. Mapping the urea channel through the rabbit Na^+-glucose cotransporter SGLT1. *J Physiol (Lond)* 2001;535:419–425.
250. Pannabecker TL, Abbott DE, Dantzler WH. Three-dimensional functional reconstruction of inner medullary thin limbs of Henle's loop. *Am J Physiol Renal Physiol* 2004;286:F38–F45.
251. Pannabecker TL, Dahlmann A, Brokl OH, Dantzler WH. Mixed descending- and ascending-type thin limbs of Henle's loop in mammalian renal inner medulla. *Am J Physiol Renal Physiol* 2000;278:F202–F208.
252. Pannabecker TL, Dantzler WH. Three-dimensional lateral and vertical relationships of inner medullary loops of Henle and collecting ducts. *Am J Physiol Renal Physiol* 2004;287: F767–F774.
253. Paxton WG, Runge M, Horaist C, Cohen C, Alexander RW, Bernstein KE. Immunohistochemical localization of rat angiotensin II AT_1 receptor. *Am J Physiol Renal Physiol* 1993;264: F989–F995.
254. Peil AE, Stolte H, Schmidt-Nielsen B. Uncoupling of glomerular and tubular regulations of urea excretion in rat. *Am J Physiol Renal Physiol* 1990;258:F1666–F1674.
255. Peng T, Sands JM, Bagnasco SM. Glucocorticoids inhibit transcription and expression of the rat UT-A urea transporter gene. *Am J Physiol Renal Physiol* 2002;282:F853–F858.
256. Pennell JP, Lacy FB, Jamison RL. An in vivo study of the concentrating process in the descending limb of Henle's loop. *Kidney Int* 1974;5:337–347.
257. Pennell JP, Sanjana V, Frey NR, Jamison RL. The effect of urea infusion on the urinary concentrating mechanism in protein-depleted rats. *J Clin Invest* 1975;55:399–409.
258. Pfeiffer EW, Nungesser WC, Iverson DA, Wallerius JF. The renal anatomy of the primitive rodent, *Aplodontia rufa*, and a consideration of its functional significance. *Anat Rec* 1960;137:227–235.
259. Pinter GG, Shohet JL. Origin of sodium concentration profile in the renal medulla. *Nature* 1963;200:955–958
260. Preisser L, Teillet L, Aliotti S, et al. Downregulation of aquaporin-2 and-3 in aging kidney is independent of V_2 vasopressin receptor. *Am J Physiol Renal Physiol* 2000;279:F144–F152.
261. Press WH, Teukolsky SA, Vetterling WT, Flannery BP. *Numerical Recipes in FORTRAN: The Art of Scientific Computing,* 2nd ed. New York: Cambridge University Press; 1992,pp107–110.
262. Preston GM, Carroll TP, Guggino WB, Agre P. Appearance of water, channels in *Xenopus* oocytes expressing red cell CHIP28 protein. *Science* 1992:256:385–387.
263. Promeneur D, Bankir L, Hu MC, Trinh-Trang-Tan M-M. Renal tubular and vascular urea transporters: influence of antidiuretic hormone on messenger RNA expression in Brattleboro rats. *J Am Soc Nephrol* 1998;9:1359–1366.
264. Promeneur D, Rousselet G, Bankir L, et al. Evidence for distinct vascular and tubular urea transporters in the rat kidney. *J Am Soc Nephrol* 1996;7:852–860.
265. Rabinowitz L. Discrepancy between experimental and theoretical urine-to-papilla osmotic gradient. *J Appl Physiol* 1970;29:389–390.
266. Rane S, Aperia A, neroth P, Lundin S. Development of urinary concentrating capacity in weaning rats. *Pediatr Res* 1985;19:472–475.
267. Reeves WB. Conductive properties of papillary surface epithelium. *Am J Physiol Renal Physiol* 1994;266:F259–F265.
268. Reif MC, Troutman SL, Schafer JA. Sustained response to vasopressin in isolated rat cortical collecting tubule. *Kidney Int* 1984;26:725–732.
269. Reinking LN, Schmidt-Nielsen B. Peristaltic flow of urine in the renal papillary collecting ducts of hamsters. *Kidney Int* 1981;20:55–60.
270. Reinking LN, Veale MC. Mechanical stimulation of renal pelvic wall peristalsis in the rat. *Experientia* 1984;40:540–541.
271. Rocha AS, Kokko JP. Membrane characteristics regulating potassium transport out of the isolated perfused descending limb of Henle. *Kidney Int* 1973;4:326–330.
272. Rocha AS, Kokko JP. Sodium chloride and water transport in the medullary thick ascending limb of Henle. Evidence for active chloride transport. *J Clin Invest* 1973;52:612–623.
273. Rocha AS, Kokko JP. Permeability of medullary nephron segments to urea and water: Effect of vasopressin. *Kidney Int* 1974;6:379–387.
274. Rocha AS, Kudo LH. Water, urea, sodium, chloride, and potassium transport in the in vitro perfused papillary collecting duct. *Kidney Int* 1982;22:485–491.
275. Rytand DA. The number and size of mammalian glomeruli as related to kidney and body weight, with methods for their enumeration and measurement. *Am J Anat* 1938;62:507–520.
276. Sabolic I, Valenti G, Verbavatz J-M, et al. Localization of the CHIP28 water channel in rat kidney. *Am J Physiol Cell Physiol* 1992;263:C1225–C1233.
277. Sands JM. Urine-concentrating ability in the aging kidney. *Sci Aging Knowledge Environ* 2003;24:pe15.
278. Sands JM. Mammalian urea transporters. *Annu Rev Physiol* 2003;65:543–566.
279. Sands JM. Molecular mechanisms of urea transport. *J Membr Biol* 2003;191:149–163.
280. Sands JM. Regulation of intracellular polyols and sugars in response to osmotic stress. In: Strange K, ed. *Cellular and Molecular Physiology of Cell Volume Regulation.* Boca Raton, FL: CRC Press; 1994:133–144.
281. Sands JM. Renal urea transporters. *Curr Opin Nephrol Hypertens* 2004;13:525–532
282. Sands JM. Urea transport: It's not just "freely diffusible" anymore. *News Physiol Sci* 1999;14:46–47.
283. Sands JM, Flores FX, Kato A, et al. Vasopressin-elicited water and urea permeabilities are altered in the inner medullary collecting duct in hypercalcemic rats. *Am J Physiol Renal Physiol* 1998;274:F978–F985.
284. Sands JM, Gargus JJ, Fröhlich O, Gunn RB, Kokko JP. Urinary concentrating ability in patients with Jk(a-b-) blood type who lack carrier-mediated urea transport. *J Am Soc Nephrol* 1992;2:1689–1696.
285. Sands JM, Ivy EJ, Beeuwkes III R. Transmembrane potential difference of renal papillary epithelial cells. Effect of urea and DDAVP. *Am J Physiol Renal Physiol* 1985;248:F762–F766.
286. Sands JM, Knepper MA. Urea permeability of mammalian inner medullary collecting duct system and papillary surface epithelium. *J Clin Invest* 1987;79:138–147.
287. Sands JM, Knepper MA, Spring KR. Na-K-Cl cotransport in apical membrane of rabbit renal papillary surface epithelium. *Am J Physiol Renal Physiol* 1986;251:F475–F484.
288. Sands JM, Naruse M, Baum M, et al. An apical extracellular calcium/polyvalent cation-sensing receptor regulates vasopressin-elicited water permeability in rat kidney inner medullary collecting duct. *J Clin Invest* 1997;99:1399–1405.
289. Sands JM, Naruse M, Jacobs JD, Wilcox JN, Klein JD. Changes in aquaporin-2 protein contribute to the urine concentrating defect in rats fed a low-protein diet. *J Clin Invest* 1996;97:2807–2814.
290. Sands JM, Nonoguchi H, Knepper MA. Vasopressin effects on urea and H_20 transport in inner medullary collecting duct subsegments. *Am J Physiol Renal Physiol* 1987;253:F823–F832.
291. Sands JM, Nonoguchi H, Knepper MA. Hormone effects on NaCl permeability of rat inner medullary collecting duct subsegments. *Am J Physiol Renal Physiol* 1988;255:F421–F428.
292. Sands JM, Schrader DC. An independent effect of osmolality on urea transport in rat terminal IMCDs. *J Clin Invest* 1991;88:137–142.
293. Sands JM, Timmer RT, Gunn RB. Urea transporters in kidney and erythrocytes. *Am J Physiol Renal Physiol* 1997;273:F321–F339.
294. Sanjana VF, Robertson CR, Jamison RL. Water extraction from the inner medullary collecting tubule system: a role for urea. *Kidney Int* 1976;10:139–148.
295. Sasaki Y, Takahashi T, Suwa N. Quantitative structural analysis of the inner medulla of rabbit kidney. *Tohoku J Exp Med* 1969;98:21–32.
296. Schafer JA, Andreoli TE. Cellular constraints to diffusion. The effect of antidiuretic hormone on water flows in isolated mammalian collecting tubules. *J Clin Invest* 1972;51:1264–1278.
297. Schafer JA, Andreoli TE. The effect of antidiuretic hormone on solute flows in mammalian collecting tubules. *J Clin Invest* 1972;51:1279–1286.
298. Schmidt U, Horster M. Na-K-activated ATPase: Activity maturation in rabbit nephron segments dissected in vitro. *Am J Physiol Renal Physiol* 1977;233:F55–F60.

299. Schmidt-Nielsen B. The renal concentrating mechanism in insects and mammals: a new hypothesis involving hydrostatic pressures. *Am J Physiol Regul Integr Comp Physiol* 1995;268: R1087–R1100.
300. Schmidt-Nielsen B. The renal pelvis. *Kidney Int* 1987;31:621–628.
301. Schmidt-Nielsen B. Function of the pelvis. In: Kinne RKH, ed. *Urinary Concentrating Mechanisms.* Basel: Karger; 1990:103–140.
302. Schmidt-Nielsen B, Churchill M, Reinking LN. Occurrence of renal pelvic refluxes during rising urine flow rate in rats and hamsters. *Kidney Int* 1980;18:419–431.
303. Schmidt-Nielsen B, Graves B. Changes in fluid compartments in hamster renal papilla due to peristalsis in the pelvic wall. *Kidney Int* 1982;22:613–625.
304. Schmidt-Nielsen B, Graves B, MacDuffie H. Effect of peristaltic contractions of the renal papilla in hamsters, *Misocricetus auratus. Bull MDIBL* 1985;25:70–72.
305. Schmidt-Nielsen B, Reinking LN. Morphometry and fluid reabsorption during peristaltic flow in hamster renal papillary collecting ducts. *Kidney Int* 1981;20:789–798.
306. Schnermann J, Chou CL, Ma TH, Traynor T, Knepper MA, Verkman AS. Defective proximal tubular fluid reabsorption in transgenic aquaporin-1 null mice. *Proc Natl Acad Sci U S A* 1998;95:9660–9664.
307. Schütz W, Schnermann J. Pelvic urine composition as a determinant of inner medullary solute concentration and urine osmolality. *Pflugers Arch* 1972;334:154–166.
308. Schwartz GJ, Zavilowitz BJ, Radice AD, Garcia-Perez A, Sands JM. Maturation of aldose reductase expression in the neonatal rat inner medulla. *J Clin Invest* 1992;90:1275-1283.
309. Shareghi GR, Agus ZS. Magnesium transport in the cortical thick ascending limb of Henle's loop of the rabbit. *J Clin Invest* 1982;69:759–769.
310. Shayakul C, Hediger MA. The SLC14 gene family of urea transporters. *Pflugers Arch* 2004; 447:603–609.
311. Shayakul C, Knepper MA, Smith CP, DiGiovanni SR, Hediger MA. Segmental localization of urea transporter mRNAs in rat kidney. *Am J Physiol Renal Physiol* 1997;272:F654–F660.
312. Shayakul C, Steel A, Hediger MA. Molecular cloning and characterization of the vasopressin-regulated urea transporter of rat kidney collecting ducts. *J Clin Invest* 1996;98:2580–2587.
313. Shayakul C, Tsukaguchi H, Berger UV, Hediger MA. Molecular characterization of a novel urea transporter from kidney inner medullary collecting ducts. *Am J Physiol Renal Physiol* 2001;280:F487–F494.
314. Sidoux-Walter F, Lucien N, Nissinen R, et al. Molecular heterogeneity of the Jk_{null} phenotype: expression analysis of the Jk(S291P) mutation found in Finns. *Blood* 2000;96:1566–1573.
315. Sidoux-Walter F, Lucien N, Olivès B, et al. At physiological expression levels the Kidd blood group/urea transporter protein is not a water channel. *J Biol Chem* 1999;274:30228–30235.
316. Silverblatt FJ. Ultrastructure of the renal pelvic epithelium of the rat. *Kidney Int* 1974;5: 214–220.
317. Smith CP, Lee W-S, Martial S, et al. Cloning and regulation of expression of the rat kidney urea transporter (rUT2). *J Clin Invest* 1995;96:1556–1563.
318. Smith CP, Potter EA, Fenton RA, Stewart GS. Characterization of a human colonic cDNA encoding a structurally novel urea transporter, UT-A6. *Am J Physiol Cell Physiol* 2004;287: C1087–C1093.
319. Smith HW. The fate of sodium and water in the renal tubules. *Bull NY Acad Med* 1959; 35:293–316.
320. Sperber I. Studies on the mammalian kidney. *Zool Bidrag Uppsala* 1944;22:249-437.
321. Star RA. Apical membrane limits urea permeation across the rat inner medullary collecting duct. *J Clin Invest* 1990;86:1172–1178.
322. Star RA, Nonoguchi H, Balaban R, Knepper MA. Calcium and cyclic adenosine monophosphate as second messengers for vasopressin in the rat inner medullary collecting duct. *J Clin Invest* 1988;81:1879–1888.
323. Stephenson JL. Concentrating engines and the kidney. IV. Mass balance in a single stage of a multistage model of the renal medulla. *Math Biosci* 1981;55:265–278.
324. Stephenson JL. Concentration of urine in a central core model of the renal counterflow system. *Kidney Int* 1972;2:85–94.
325. Stephenson JL. Concentrating engines and the kidney. I. Central core model of the renal medulla. *Biophys J* 1973;13:512–545.
326. Stephenson JL. Concentrating engines and the kidney. III. Canonical mass balance equation for multinephron models of the renal medulla. *Biophys J* 1976;16:1273–1286.
327. Stephenson JL. Concentrating engines and the kidney. II. Multisolute central core systems. *Biophys J* 1973;13:546–567.
328. Stephenson JL. Urinary concentration and dilution: models. In: Windhager EE, ed. *Handbook of Physiology: Renal Physiology.* Bethesda: American Physiological Society; 1992:1349–1408.
329. Stephenson JL, Jen JF, Wang H, Tewarson RP. Convective uphill transport of NaCl from ascending thin limb of loop of Henle. *Am J Physiol Renal Physiol* 1995;268:F680–F692.
330. Stephenson JL, Tewarson RP, Mejia R. Quantitative analysis of mass and energy balance in non-ideal models of the renal counterflow system. *Proc Natl Acad Sci U S A* 1974;71:1618–1622.
331. Stephenson JL, Wang H, Tewarson RP. Effect of vasa recta flow on concentrating ability of models of renal inner medulla. *Am J Physiol Renal Physiol* 1995;268:F698–F709.
332. Stephenson JL, Zhang Y, Eftekhari A, Tewarson RP. Electrolyte transport in a central core model of the renal medulla. *Am J Physiol Renal Physiol* 1989;253:F982–F997.
333. Stephenson JL, Zhang Y, Tewarson RP. Electrolyte, urea, and water transport in a two-nephron central core model of the renal medulla. *Am J Physiol Renal Physiol* 1989;257:F388–F413.
334. Stewart GS, Fenton RA, Wang W, et al. The basolateral expression of mUT-A3 in the mouse kidney. *Am J Physiol Renal Physiol* 2004;286:F979–F987.
335. Stewart J, Luggen ME, Valtin H. A computer model of the renal countercurrent system. *Kidney Int* 1972;2:253–263.
336. Stewart J, Valtin H. Computer simulation of osmotic gradient without active transport in renal inner medulla. *Kidney Int* 1972;2:264–270.
337. Stokes JB. Sodium and potassium transport across the cortical and outer medullary collecting tubule of the rabbit: Evidence for diffusion across the outer medullary portion. *Am J Physiol Renal Physiol* 1982;242:F514–F520.
338. Stokes JB. Effect of prostaglandin E_2 on chloride transport across the rabbit thick ascending limb of Henle. *J Clin Invest* 1979;64:495–502.
339. Stokes JB, Ingram MJ, Williams AD, Ingram D. Heterogeneity of the rabbit collecting tubule: Localization of mineralocorticoid hormone action to the cortical portion. *Kidney Int* 1981;20:340–347.
340. Stoner LC, Burg MB, Orloff J. Ion transport in cortical collecting tubule effect of amiloride. *Am J Physiol* 1974;227:453–459.
341. Stoner LC, Roch-Ramel F. The effects of pressure on the water permeability of the descending limb of Henle's loops of rabbits. *Pflugers Arch* 1979;382:7–15.
342. Tabei K, Imai M. K transport in upper portion of descending limbs of long-loop nephron from hamster. *Am J Physiol Renal Physiol* 1987;252:F387–F392.
343. Takahashi N, Kondo Y, Fujiwara I, Ito O, Igarashi Y, Abe K. Characterization of Na^+ transport across the cell membranes of the ascending thin limb of Henle's loop. *Kidney Int* 1995;47:789–794.
344. Takahashi N, Kondo Y, Ito O, Igarashi Y, Omata K, Abe K. Vasopressin stimulates Cl^- transport in ascending thin limb of Henle's loop in hamster. *J Clin Invest* 1995;95:1623–1627.
345. Terada Y, Knepper MA. Na^+ -K^+-ATPase activities in renal tubule segments of rat inner medulla. *Am J Physiol Renal Physiol* 1989;256:F218–F223.
346. Terris J, Ecelbarger CA, Sands JM, Knepper MA. Long-term regulation of collecting duct urea transporter proteins in rat. *J Am Soc Nephrol* 1998;9:729–736.
347. Terris JM, Knepper MA, Wade JB. UT-A3: localization and characterization of an additional urea transporter isoform in the IMCD. *Am J Physiol Renal Physiol* 2001;280:F325–F332.
348. Tewarson RP, Wang H, Stephenson JL, Jen JF. Efficient computer algorithms for kidney modeling. *Math Modelling Sci Computing* 1993;1:164–171.
349. Thomas SR. Inner medullary lactate production and accumulation: a vasa recta model. *Am J Physiol Renal Physiol* 2000;279:F468–F481.
350. Thomas SR. Cycles and separations in a model of the renal medulla. *Am J Physiol Renal Physiol* 1998;275:F671–F690.
351. Thomas SR, Wexler AS. Inner medullary external osmotic driving force in a 3D model of the renal concentrating mechanism. *Am J Physiol Renal Physiol* 1995;269:F159–F171.
352. Timmer RT, Klein JD, Bagnasco SM, et al. Localization of the urea transporter UT-B protein in human and rat erythrocytes and tissues. *Am J Physiol Cell Physiol* 2001;281:C1318–C1325.
353. Timmer RT, Sands JM. Lithium intoxication. *J Am Soc Nephrol* 1999;10:666–674.
354. Tisher CC. Relationship between renal structure and concentrating ability in the rhesus monkey. *Am J Physiol* 1971;220:1100–1106.
355. Tisher CC, Schrier RW, McNeil JS. Nature of urine concentrating mechanism in the macaque monkey. *Am J Physiol* 1972;223:1128–1137.
356. Tomita K, Pisano JJ, Burg MB, Knepper MA. Effects of vasopressin and bradykinin on anion transport by the rat cortical collecting duct. Evidence for an electroneutral sodium chloride transport pathway. *J Clin Invest* 1986;77:136–141.
357. Tomita K, Pisano JJ, Knepper MA. Control of sodium and potassium transport in the cortical collecting duct of the rat. Effects of bradykinin, vasopressin, and deoxycorticosterone. *J Clin Invest* 1985;76:132–136.
358. Trimble ME. Renal response to solute loading in infant rats: relation to anatomical development. *Am J Physiol* 1970;219:1089–1097.
359. Trinder D, Phillips PA, Stephenson JM, et al. Vasopressin V_1 and V_2 receptors in diabetes mellitus. *Am J Physiol Endocrinol Metab* 1994;266:E217–E223.
360. Trinh-Trang-Tan M-M, Bouby N, Kriz W, Bankir L. Functional adaptation of thick ascending limb and internephron heterogeneity to urine concentration. *Kidney Int* 1987;31:549–555.
361. Trinh-Trang-Tan MM, Geelen G, Teillet L, Corman B. Urea transporter expression in aging kidney and brain during dehydration. *Am J Physiol Regul Integr Comp Physiol* 2003;285: R1355–R1365.
362. Tsukaguchi H, Shayakul C, Berger UV, Tokui T, Brown D, Hediger MA. Cloning and characterization of the urea transporter UT3. Localization in rat kidney and testis. *J Clin Invest* 1997;99:1506–1515.
363. Uchida S, Sasaki S, Furukawa T, et al. Molecular cloning of a chloride channel that is regulated by dehydration and expressed predominantly in kidney medulla. *J Biol Chem* 1993;268:3821–3824.
364. Uchida S, Sasaki S, Nitta K, et al. Localization and functional characterization of rat kidney-specific chloride channel, ClC-K1. *J Clin Invest* 1995;95:104–113.
365. Ullrich KJ, Papavassiliou F. Sodium reabsorption in the papillary collecting ducts of rats. *Pflugers Arch* 1979;379:49–52.
366. Ullrich KJ, Rumrich G, Schmidt-Nielsen B. Urea transport in the collecting duct of rats on normal and low protein diet. *Pflugers Arch* 1967;295:147–156.
367. Ullrich KJ, Schmidt-Nielsen B, O'Dell R, et al. Micropuncture study of composition of proximal and distal tubular fluid in rat kidney. *Am J Physiol* 1963;204:527–531.
368. Valtin H. Structural and functional heterogeneity of mammalian nephrons. *Am J Physiol Renal Physiol* 1977;233:F491–F501.
369. Vehaskari VM, Hering-Smith KS, Moskowitz DW, Weiner ID, Hamm LL. Effect of epidermal growth factor on sodium transport in the cortical collecting tubule. *Am J Physiol Renal Physiol* 1989;256:F803–F809.
370. Wade JB, Lee AJ, Liu J, et al. UT-A2: a 55 kDa urea transporter protein in thin descending limb of Henle's loop whose abundance is regulated by vasopressin. *Am J Physiol Renal Physiol* 2000;278:F52–F62.
371. Wade JB, Stetson DL, Lewis SA. ADH action: evidence for a membrane shuttle mechanism. *Annals NY Acad Sci* 1981;372:106–117.
372. Wall SM, Suk Han J, Chou C-L, Knepper MA. Kinetics of urea and water permeability activation by vasopressin in rat terminal IMCD. *Am J Physiol Renal Physiol* 1992;262:F989–F998.
373. Wang X-Y, Beutler K, Nielsen J, Nielsen S, Knepper MA, Masilamani S. Decreased abundance of collecting duct urea transporters UT-A1 and UT-A3 with ECF volume expansion. *Am J Physiol Renal Physiol* 2002;282:F577–F584.
374. Wang X, Thomas SR, Wexler AS. Outer medullary anatomy and the urine concentrating mechanism. *Am J Physiol Renal Physiol* 1998;274:F413–F424.

375. Wang X, Wexler AS, Marsh DJ. The effect of solution non-ideality on membrane transport in three-dimensional models of the renal concentrating mechanism. *Bull Math Biol* 1994; 56:515–546.

376. Wang XQ, Wexler AS. The effects of collecting duct active NaCl reabsorption and inner medulla anatomy on renal concentrating mechanism. *Am J Physiol Renal Physiol* 1996;270: F900–F911.

377. Weinstein AM. A mathematical model of the inner medullary collecting duct of the rat: pathways for Na and K transport. *Am J Physiol Renal Physiol* 1998;274:F841–F855.

378. Wexler AS, Kalaba RE, Marsh DJ. Three-dimensional anatomy and renal concentrating mechanism. I. Modelling results. *Am J Physiol Renal Physiol* 1991;260:F368–F383.

379. Wexler AS, Kalaba RE, Marsh DJ. Passive, one-dimensional countercurrent models do not simulate hypertonic urine formation. *Am J Physiol Renal Physiol* 1987;253:F1020–F1030.

380. Wexler AS, Kalaba RE, Marsh DJ. Three-dimensional anatomy and renal concentrating mechanism. II. Sensitivity results. *Am J Physiol Renal Physiol* 1991;260:F384–F394.

381. Wexler AS, Marsh DJ. Numerical methods for three-dimensional models of the urine concentrating mechanism. *Appl Math Comput* 1991;45:219–240.

382. Williams JB, Pacelli MM, Braun EJ. The effect of water deprivation on renal function in conscious unrestrained Gambel's quail (*Callipepla gambelli*). *Physiol Zool* 1991;64:1200–1216.

383. Winberg J. Determination of renal concentrating capacity in infants and children without renal disease. *Acta Paediatr* 1959;48:318–328.

384. Wittner M, Di Stefano A, Mandon B, Roinel N, de Rouffignac C. Stimulation of NaCl reabsorption by antidiuretic hormone in the cortical thick ascending limb of Henle's loop of the mouse. *Pflugers Arch* 1991;419:212–214.

385. Xu Y, Olives B, Bailly P, et al. Endothelial cells of the kidney vasa recta express the urea transporter HUT11. *Kidney Int* 1997;51:138–146.

386. Yancey PH. Osmotic effectors in kidneys of xeric and mesic rodents: corticomedullary distribution and changes with water availability. *J Comp Physiol B* 1988;158:369–380.

387. Yancey PH, Burg MB. Distribution of major organic osmolytes in rabbit kidneys in diuresis and antidiuresis. *Am J Physiol Renal Physiol* 1989;257:F602–F607.

388. Yancey PH, Burg MB. Counteracting effects of urea and betaine in mammalian cells in culture. *Am J Physiol Regul Integr Comp Physiol* 1990;258:R198–R204.

389. Yancey PH, Clark ME, Hand SC, Bowlus RD, Somero GN. Living with water stress: evolution of osmolyte systems. *Science* 1982;217:1214–1222.

390. Yancey PH, Somero GN. Methylamine osmoregulatory solutes of elasmobranch fishes counteract urea inhibition of enzymes. *J Exp Zool* 1980;212:205–213.

391. Yang B, Bankir L, Gillespie A, Epstein CJ, Verkman AS. Urea-selective concentrating defect in transgenic mice lacking urea transporter UT-B. *J Biol Chem* 2002;277:10633–10637.

392. Yang B, Verkman AS. Analysis of double knockout mice lacking aquaporin-1 and urea transporter UT-B. *J Biol Chem* 2002;277:36782–36786.

393. Yang BX, Verkman AS. Urea transporter UT3 functions as an efficient water channel - Direct evidence for a common water/urea pathway. *J Biol Chem* 1998;273:9369–9372.

394. Yasui M, Marples D, Belusa R, et al. Development of urinary concentrating capacity: Role of aquaporin-2. *Am J Physiol Renal Physiol* 1996;271:F461–F468.

395. Yasui M, Zelenin SM, Celsi G, Aperia A. Adenylate cyclase-coupled vasopressin receptor activates AQP2 promoter via a dual effect on CRE and AP1 elements. *Am J Physiol Renal Physiol* 1997;272:F443–F450.

396. You G, Smith CP, Kanai Y, Lee W-S, Stelzner M, Hediger MA. Cloning and characterization of the vasopressin-regulated urea transporter. *Nature* 1993;365:844–847.

397. Zhang C, Sands JM, Klein JD. Vasopressin rapidly increases the phosphorylation of the UT-A1 urea transporter activity in rat IMCDs through PKA. *Am J Physiol Renal Physiol* 2002;282:F85–F90.

398. Zhao HY, Tian W, Cohen DM. Rottlerin inhibits tonicity-dependent expression and action of TonEBP in a PKCδ-independent fashion. *Am J Physiol Renal Physiol* 2002;282:F710–F717.

399. Zimmerhackl BL, Robertson CR, Jamison RL. The medullary microcirculation. *Kidney Int* 1987;31:641–647.

CHAPTER **41**

Hyponatremia

Richard H. Sterns and Stephen M. Silver

University of Rochester School of Medicine and Dentistry, Rochester, New York, USA

THE PLASMA SODIUM CONCENTRATION AND BODY FLUID TONICITY

Sodium and its accompanying anions are the principle osmotically active solutes in extracellular fluid (71, 92). When extracellular osmolality is low, intracellular osmolality is equally low. Therefore, although there are exceptions (Table 1), hyponatremia is usually associated with hypoosmolality and dilution of all body fluids (71, 72, 92).

When (as is usually the case) the concentration of nonpermeant extracellular solutes other than sodium is very low, the plasma sodium concentration is a function of three variables as indicated by the following equation:

$$\text{Plasma } [Na^+] \cong \frac{\text{Exchangeable } Na^+ + \text{Exchangeable } K^+}{\text{Total body water}}$$

(Eq. 1)

Only the exchangeable fractions of sodium and potassium are included in the equation because one third of body sodium is bound to bone and osmotically inactive (71). This relationship, which has been validated empirically (72), indicates that the plasma (or serum) sodium concentration can be reduced by depletion of body cations, by an increase in body water, or by a combination of these processes (220). It has been emphasized that the original equation describing the relationship between the plasma sodium concentration, exchangeable sodium, exchangeable potassium, and total body water has an intercept that can be explained theoretically (189). The simplified form of the relationship (Eq. 1), which omits the intercept, is useful conceptually, but should not be considered a completely accurate basis for predicting the effect of therapy on the plasma sodium concentration.

It is intuitively obvious that the extracellular sodium concentration should be proportional to the body's content of water and soluable sodium. The sodium concentration falls when the body retains water (without solute) or when there are net external losses of sodium (without water). The importance of intracellular potassium stores to the plasma sodium concentration is less obvious (99, 190). In potassium depletion, sodium ions move intracellularly as intracellular potassium is lost, bal-

ancing negative charges on intracellular macromolecules. Thus, external loss of exchangeable potassium causes an internal loss of extracellular sodium. Similarly, when intracellular potassium is replaced by hydrogen ions, rather than sodium, or when it is lost with phosphate (an intracellular anion), the loss of osmotically active intracellular solute causes a redistribution of water from the intracellular to the extracellular fluid compartments, diluting extracellular sodium ions.

PHYSIOLOGIC CONTROL OF WATER EXCRETION

Osmotic Regulation

Controlled by changes in water intake, vasopressin secretion, and water excretion, the plasma sodium concentration is normally prevented from rising above 142 mEq/l or falling below 135 mEq/l. When the plasma sodium concentration changes by as little as 1% (with a corresponding change in plasma osmolality), cell volume receptors ("osmoreceptors") in the hypothalamus respond, relaying signals to vasopressin-secreting neurons located in the supraoptic and paraventricular nuclei whose axons terminate in secretory bulbs in the neurohypophysis (8, 19, 215). The antidiuretic hormone, arginine vasopressin, which is released into the systemic circulation by the neurohypophysis, controls water excretion by the kidneys. The hormone activates V2 receptors on the basolateral membrane of principle cells in the renal collecting duct, initiating a cyclic AMP–dependent process that culminates in increased production of water channels (aquaporin-2) and their insertion into the cells' luminal membranes (145, 154). The effect of vasopressin on water flow is inhibited by locally produced prostaglandin E2, which is stimulated by vasopressin action on V1 receptors (211). Vasopressin's short half-life in the circulation and continuous shuttling of aquaporins between the collecting duct's cell membrane and cytosol allow rapid changes in urinary water excretion in response to changes in body fluid tonicity.

Vasopressin levels are normally unmeasurable when the plasma sodium concentration falls to approximately

TABLE 1   Causes of Nonhypotonic Hyponatremia

Plasma Osmolality	Disorder	Pathogenesis
Normal	Pseudohyponatremia Hyperlipidemia Multiple myeloma	Excess nonaqueous material decreases plasma water content; no change in ECF or ICF volume
	Exogenous solutes Isotonic intravenous mannitol Irrigant absorption	Expansion of ECF volume with nonsodium solutes and water; no change in ICF volume
Increased	Hyperglycemia, hypertonic intravenous mannitol, and maltose containing immunoglobulin G solutions	Initial expansion of ECF volume and shift of water out of cells; decrease in ICF volume

ECF, extracellular fluid; ICF, intracellular fluid.

135 mEq/l. Low levels of the hormone allow the excretion of large volumes of a maximally dilute urine ($\oplus$50 mOsm/kg), which reduces body water content and restores the plasma sodium concentration to normal. At higher plasma sodium levels, plasma vasopressin is directly related to the plasma sodium concentration, reaching levels that are high enough to promote the excretion of maximally concentrated urine ($\oplus$1200 mOsm/kg) at a plasma sodium concentration of approximately 142 mEq/l. A rising plasma sodium concentration also stimulates thirst. Ingested water is retained, returning the plasma sodium concentration back towards normal.

Hemodynamic Regulation

Under day-to-day conditions, vasopressin secretion, urinary free-water excretion, and thirst respond primarily to changes in body fluid tonicity. Under pathologic conditions, osmotic control of vasopressin secretion and thirst can be overridden by hemodynamic stimuli (216). In addition to input from osmoreceptors, the hypothalamic neurons that secrete vasopressin also receive neural input from baroreceptors in the great vessels and volume receptors in the atria. When these receptors are stimulated by hypotension or by a major reduction in plasma volume, impulses are carried via cranial nerves IX and X to the hypothalamus. The thirst center in the hypothalamus responds to similar nonosmotic stimuli. Vasopressin and thirst responses to hypovolemia and hypotension lead to water retention despite hypotonicity of body fluids. These hemodynamic responses can be regarded as back-up systems that serve to maintain arterial blood volume under emergency conditions, sacrificing tonicity to tissue perfusion. Although high levels of vasopressin occur in response to hypovolemia, under experimental conditions, a rather large stimulus is required; while plasma vasopressin is measurably increased by a 1% change in plasma osmolality, a 10% change in extracellular fluid volume is required to elicit the same response. However, these experimental findings are difficult to reconcile with clinical observations

suggesting that nonosmotic vasopressin secretion occurs with more subtle volume depletion.

HYPOTONIC HYPONATREMIA: CLASSIFICATION AND PATHOGENESIS

Traditionally, patients with hyponatremia are divided into categories according to their body sodium content and/or intravascular volume: low body sodium content (volume depletion), high body sodium content (edematous conditions), or normal body sodium content (euvolemic hyponatremia or syndrome of inappropriate antidiuretic hormone secretion [SIADH]) (183). Although this time-honored approach is often helpful to clinicians, intravascular volume and body sodium content do not always change in parallel (e.g., self-induced water intoxication), and some causes of hyponatremia (e.g., diuretic induced and cerebral salt wasting) may be difficult to classify by intravascular volume. Moreover, physiologic responses to extracellular volume expansion and contraction often create ambiguities in volume status. Thus, secondary water retention in response to volume depletion and secondary natriuresis in response to water overload may ultimately yield similar values for total body sodium and water (Fig. 1).

Table 2 classifies hyponatremia by the physiologic mechanism underlying the electrolyte disturbance. As the plasma sodium concentration is proportional to the ratio of exchangeable cations and total body water, it follows that changes in sodium concentration are related to external balances of sodium, potassium and water. However, because the plasma sodium concentration is normally maintained within a narrow physiologic range by control systems which regulate water balance, hypotonic hyponatremia can only occur if water excretion is impaired or overwhelmed. The various causes of hyponatremia are therefore divided according to the status of urinary water excretion. Disordered water balance is often accompanied by changes in cation balance, which also play a pivotal role in the pathogenesis of hyponatremia.

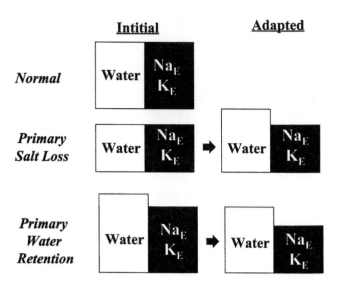

FIGURE 1 Body water and cation content in hyponatremia. When the primary disturbance is loss of salt water (*middle*), compensatory mechanisms are triggered—hemodynamically mediated thirst and vasopressin secretion—which result in secondary water retention. When the primary disturbance is pathologic secretion of vasopressin and water retention (*bottom*), compensatory mechanisms are triggered—increased secretion of atrial natriuretic peptide, decreased secretion of aldosterone, and pressure natriuresis—which result in secondary salt loss. Because of these adaptations, primary salt loss and primary water retention both result in near normal values for total body water and decreased body cation stores.

TABLE 2 Pathophysiologic Classification of Hypotonic Hyponatremia

Urine Diluting Ability	Cause of Hyponatremia
Unimpaired	Psychotic polydipsia
	Beer potomania
	Infantile water intoxication
Impaired: vasopressin-independent	Oliguric renal failure
	Tubular interstitial renal disease
	Diuretics
	Nephrogenic syndrome of antidiuresis[a]
Impaired: vasopressin-dependent	Hemodynamically mediated
	Volume depletion
	Spinal cord disease
	Congestive heart failure
	Cirrhosis
	Addison's disease[b]
	Cerebral salt wasting[b]
	Syndrome of inappropriate antidiuretic hormone secretion (see Table 3)

[a]Hereditary disorder of the V2 receptor with clinical features of syndrome of inappropriate antidiuretic hormone secretion but with undetectable plasma vasopressin levels.

[b]Disorders with both hemodynamic and nonhemodynamic bases for vasopressin release.

WATER INTOXICATION WITH MAXIMALLY DILUTE URINE

Pathophysiology

Rarely, fluid intake can overwhelm normal mechanisms for water excretion. In the absence of vasopressin, urine osmolality falls to approximately 50 mOsm/kg. A typical American diet provides a daily load of 600 to 900 mOsm of solute (electrolytes and urea) that must be excreted. At this rate of solute excretion, the volume of maximally dilute urine equals 12 to 18 liters per day, or 500 to 750 ml/hour. Water intake can occasionally exceed this large excretory capacity. Patients with severe acute water intoxication are truly "water logged" and susceptible to pulmonary edema due to retained water.

Self-Induced Water Intoxication in Psychotic Polydipsia

Polydipsia and polyuria are extremely common among institutionalized patients with mental illness (53, 126, 137, 176, 214). Many patients with polydipsia have frequent episodes of hyponatremia, which may present with seizures. About half the reported cases have had maximally dilute urine (urine osmolalities below 100 mOsm/kg) at presentation. In others, inappropriately concentrated urine was present immediately following seizures or in association with nausea (137) but the rate of correction of hyponatremia indicates that the urine became dilute soon afterwards.

In most psychotic water drinkers, hyponatremia can be ascribed to a generalized dilution of body solutes by retained water; thus, body weight increases in proportion to the severity of hyponatremia. Patients gain weight and become hyponatremic during the course of the day and then spontaneously diurese, normalizing their plasma sodium concentration and body weight during the night. Caregivers in psychiatric hospitals routinely monitor weight changes in patients who are habitual water drinkers to determine when access to water must be rigidly restricted to avoid severe symptomatic hyponatremia.

Agents that interfere with the ability to maximally dilute the urine (e.g., diuretics or carbamazepine) should be avoided in polydipsic patients as they can precipitate a rapid onset of life-threatening hyponatremia (24, 140).

Water Intoxication in Infants

Acute water intoxication is common among infants who are given excessively dilute formula (33, 138, 223). The hungry infant ingests large volumes of fluid leading to water retention despite the excretion of maximally dilute urine. Once water is restricted, the plasma sodium concentration self-corrects as large volumes of urine are excreted.

Beer Drinkers' Potomania

Alcoholics who eat little and subsist on large volumes of beer may also become hyponatremic while excreting maximally dilute urine (80, 112, 280). Beer's low protein content and the protein sparing effect of its carbohydrate result in profoundly reduced blood urea nitrogen concentrations and urinary urea excretion. The total daily excretion of urinary solute may be only 200 to 300 mOsm. Thus, even at a urine osmolality of 50 mOsm/kg, urine output is limited to 4 to 6 liters per day, an amount that fails to match the enthusiastic beer drinker's intake of electrolyte-free water. A similar phenomenon has been reported in nonbeer drinkers with a large fluid and low-protein intake (27, 264, 280). Volume depletion from gastrointestinal losses and transient vasopressin release caused by nausea or alcohol withdrawal may further limit the beer drinker's ability to excrete free water, contributing to the development and persistence of hyponatremia (277).

VASOPRESSIN-INDEPENDENT DEFECTS IN WATER EXCRETION

Pathophysiology

Maximal free-water excretion depends on adequate delivery of glomerular filtrate to the renal diluting segments (the ascending limb of the loop of Henle and the distal tubule), reabsorption of salt without water by the diluting segments to create hypotonic fluid within the tubular lumen, and a collecting duct that is relatively impermeable to water so that the dilute tubular fluid formed "upstream" can be eliminated in the final urine. Hyponatremia occurs when water is taken in at a time when these mechanisms are not functioning normally.

Renal Failure

The most obvious cause of impaired water excretion is oliguric renal failure. Even when nonoliguric, patients with advanced renal failure have fixed isosthenuria and are unable to excrete dilute urine despite normally suppressed vasopressin secretion. In the absence of renal failure, urinary dilution can still be impaired despite low levels of vasopressin by two mechanisms: (1) enhanced proximal reabsorption of the glomerular filtrate, limiting fluid delivery to the renal diluting segments (as in volume depletion, congestive heart failure [CHF], and cirrhosis) (111); (2) impaired sodium reabsorption in the renal diluting segments (by diuretics or tubular interstitial disease) (164).

Diuretic-induced Hyponatremia

Thiazides and loop diuretics interfere with the ability to maximally dilute the urine (21). Thus both classes of diuretic can lead to water intoxication in patients who habitually ingest extremely large volumes of water. Diuretics are one of the most important causes of hyponatremia (1, 42, 102, 104, 123, 148, 247, 266). Most cases are caused by thiazide or thiazide-like agents; loop diuretics are implicated much less commonly. Thiazides may be the sole factor responsible for causing hyponatremia and they may also exacerbate hyponatremia in patients with disorders associated with SIADH (101, 184, 266). The mechanism of thiazide-induced hyponatremia remains somewhat unclear; however, as for all causes of hyponatremia, water retention and/or cation depletion must be responsible.

Most cases of thiazide-induced hyponatremia have occurred in elderly, small women who have been prescribed diuretics for the treatment of hypertension (1, 43, 48, 83, 102, 247). Healthy elderly people do not excrete water as efficiently as do younger ones and the impairment of renal diluting ability caused by thiazides is more pronounced in elderly people, especially those who have previously experienced thiazide-induced hyponatremia (45). The predisposition of elderly women to severe hyponatremia may be explained by body size: Small changes in body water and electrolyte content can lead to marked changes in serum sodium.

One of the most remarkable features of thiazide-induced hyponatremia is the rapidity with which it can occur. In susceptible individuals, the serum sodium may fall within hours of diuretic ingestion and severe hyponatremia can develop in less than 2 days (1, 12, 83, 89). In most reported cases, the duration of thiazide use has been less than 2 weeks. On the other hand, in some cases thiazides had been used chronically without incident until, for some reason, water intake increased, dietary salt and protein intake decreased, or an intercurrent illness led to "inappropriate" antidiuretic hormone secretion (1, 29, 42). Mild hyponatremia often persists for a few weeks when diuretic therapy is withdrawn from patients with diuretic-induced hyponatremia (108), apparently reflecting temporary "resetting" of the osmostat (57), or alternatively, slow restoration of depleted cation stores.

Although thiazide diuretics do not inhibit the ability to concentrate the urine, they do impair diluting ability in several ways (68, 164, 246, 260, 276): inhibition of electrolyte transport at the cortical diluting sites; direct stimulation of vasopressin release; reduction of glomerular filtration; and enhancement of fractional proximal water reabsorption, reducing delivery to diluting sites.

Several investigators have documented positive water balance during the onset of thiazide-induced hyponatremia and negative balance during its correction (12, 89, 124, 140). Some patients with thiazide-induced hyponatremia have low serum uric acid levels and high uric acid clearances (markers of volume expansion), which return to normal as the serum sodium normalizes (248, 266). Similarly, fractional urea excretion may be higher during hyponatremia, than after correction of the electrolyte disturbance (1). Water retention is not associated with a decrease in urine volume. Most affected patients drink large amounts of water and the superimposed diuretic prevents urine output from keeping pace with water intake (1, 12).

Although increased total body water often contributes to the pathogenesis of thiazide-induced hyponatremia, there are many cases in which body weight decreased or remained the same during the fall in serum sodium (83, 90, 117, 134). In others, direct measurements of total body water in affected patients have been normal (83). In these cases, other explanations for hyponatremia must be sought.

Negative cation balance plays a major role in the pathogenesis of diuretic-induced hyponatremia. Rejected cations may be excreted at a total concentration which exceeds that of plasma directly "desalinating" the plasma even in the absence of water intake (12). Potassium depletion is an important factor in many cases; treatment of hypokalemia has been shown to increase the plasma sodium concentration with no change in body weight (83). One study suggested that magnesium repletion can act similarly, presumably through an effect on skeletal muscle Na,K-ATPase (66). Surprisingly, despite negative cation balance, many patients appear to be euvolemic. Apparently, enough water is retained to offset the initial tendency toward hypovolemia. Once diuretics are withdrawn, urinary sodium excretion falls to very low levels (83, 89).

VASOPRESSIN-DEPENDENT DEFECTS IN WATER EXCRETION

Pathophysiology

Normally, in response to hypotonicity, vasopressin secretion is suppressed, the collecting duct is impermeable to water, and a maximally dilute urine is formed. In two large surveys of hospitalized patients with hyponatremia, over 90% of cases were associated with elevated vasopressin levels (7, 105). Vasopressin levels are rarely elevated into pathologic ranges even in cases associated with ectopic secretion by tumors. Rather, vasopressin levels are inappropriately high relative to the plasma osmolality. Nonosmotic vasopressin secretion may be an adaptive response driven by hemodynamic stimuli or it may be "inappropriate" and independent of any of the usual physiologic mechanisms which regulate water excretion. Persistent vasopressin secretion despite hypo-osmolality allows ingested or infused free water to be retained, causing hypotonic hyponatremia. Vasopressin-mediated hyponatremia is characterized by urine which is more concentrated (usually much more) than 100 mOsm/kg and which becomes more dilute after administration of a V2 receptor antagonist (see Treatment of Hypotonic Hyponatremia).

Patients with inappropriate vasopressin secretion must take in water to become hyponatremic. In some cases, hyponatremia develops when electrolyte-free water is administered parenterally. More commonly, patients become hyponatremic while ingesting water. Theoretically, osmotic inhibition of thirst should prevent water ingestion when the ability to ex-

crete water is impaired. However, patients with SIADH continue to drink despite plasma osmolalities below the normal osmotic threshold for thirst. Formal testing has shown that there is downward resetting of the osmotic threshold for thirst in SIADH but that thirst responds to osmotic stimulation and is suppressed by drinking around the lowered set point (242).

Escape From Vasopressin-Induced Water Retention

Experimentally, after several days of constant vasopressin infusion and constant water intake, there is an escape from the antidiuretic effect of vasopressin. With the onset of vasopressin escape, the urine becomes less concentrated, allowing water balance to be reestablished at a new steady state in which the plasma sodium concentration stabilizes at a level lower than normal. It has been suggested that this escape is in part due to pressure induced natriuresis and diuresis. More recently, vasopressin escape has been attributed to a vasopressin-independent decrease in aquaporin-2 water channel expression in the renal collecting duct triggered by water loading. In rats, escape has been shown to coincide temporally with a marked decrease in renal aquaporin-2 protein, accompanied by suppression of aquaporin-2 mRNA levels (Fig. 2) (70). Shuttling of aquaporin water channels from intracellular vesicles to the plasma membrane remains intact. Studies examining the mechanisms underlying the decrease in AQP2 have shown reduced V2-receptor mRNA expression and binding, and a decrease in c-AMP production in response to vasopressin in collecting duct suspension (69). Rats undergoing vasopressin escape show an increase in plasma and urine aldosterone and mean arterial pressure; thiazide-sensitive Na-Cl cotransporter and ENaC proteins known to be upregulated by aldosterone are increased in abundance in the distal nephron, attenuating renal sodium losses (245). Inhibition of nitric oxide synthase or prostaglandin synthesis synergistically inhibits the escape phenomenon, supporting a role for nitric oxide and prostaglandins in mediating vasopressin escape (182).

In conditions characterized by vasopressin-mediated water retention, (e.g., SIADH, CHF), renal escape from vasopressin-induced antidiuresis (along with decreased water intake in some cases) permits patients with vasopressin-mediated hyponatremic states to manifest a relatively stable level of hyponatremia, despite continued water intake and continued presence of vasopressin.

HEMODYNAMIC CAUSES OF VASOPRESSIN-MEDIATED HYPONATREMIA

Pathophysiology

Hypovolemia, heart failure, and cirrhosis are the most common nonosmotic stimuli for antidiuretic hormone secretion (225). In a series of 100 consecutive hospitalized

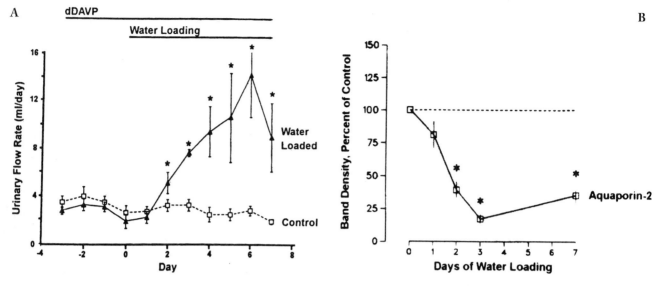

FIGURE 2   Vasopressin escape (70). **A:** The gradual increase in urine flow rate (accompanied by a decrease in urine osmolality) that occurs when rats treated continuously with 1-desamino-8-D-arginine vasopressin are made hyponatremic with water loading. The escape from the antidiuretic effect of vasopressin begins on the second day of water loading. **B:** Levels of aquaporin-2 protein levels from kidney homogenates taken on each day of water lowing. Levels of aquaporin-2 protein decrease despite continued administration of vasopressin, and correlate with changes in urine volume.

patients with hypotonic hyponatremia, volume contraction (29%), advanced heart failure (25%), and liver cirrhosis (16%) were identified as the cause of hyponatremia in a high percentage of cases (105). The hemodynamic abnormalities that stimulate vasopressin release in these conditions also promote sodium reabsorption by the renal tubules (mediated by aldosterone, increased sympathetic nervous system activity, peritubular Starling forces, etc.), causing both sodium and water retention. In volume depletion, sodium retention serves to replace a sodium deficit; in heart failure and cirrhosis, sodium retention serves to compensate for the circulatory abnormality but it also causes edema.

Volume Depletion

Sodium and potassium losses associated with gastrointestinal fluids (or with urinary losses caused by osmotic or loop diuretics) do not directly lower the plasma sodium concentration because these fluids are either hypotonic or isotonic. However, the intravascular volume depletion caused by such losses is a hemodynamic stimulus for thirst and vasopressin secretion; as a result, ingested water is retained, lowering the plasma sodium concentration. Thus, hyponatremia in these conditions is associated with a reduced content of both total body cations and water. However, in many patients, compensatory water retention makes it difficult to detect the underlying volume depletion. Laboratory clues, including a low urine sodium concentration and elevated serum uric acid levels can be helpful diagnostically (44).

Spinal Cord Disease

Hyponatremia is very common after spinal cord injury, particularly among patients with complete quadriplegia (208, 231). Contributing factors include a large water intake (reflecting physician recommendations, angiotensin II–mediated thirst, loss of pharyngeal and gastric satiety signals), and baroreceptor-mediated vasopressin release. One study showed normal osmoregulation of vasopressin secretion and excretion of a water load when subjects were supine, but with the subjects in a sitting position, there was a reduced osmotic threshold and increased sensitivity for vasopressin release, and urine diluting ability and free water clearance were markedly impaired (311).

Edematous Conditions

Severe hyponatremia can occur despite increased body sodium content if retained sodium is offset by a disproportionate increase in body water.

CONGESTIVE HEART FAILURE

Hyponatremia in heart failure stems from reduced cardiac output and blood pressure, which stimulate vasopressin, catecholamines, and the renin-angiotensin-aldosterone axis (198, 224, 225, 230). Increased vasopressin levels have even been documented in patients with impaired left ventricular function before the onset of symptomatic heart failure (85). Hyponatremic patients with CHF have higher levels of plasma renin activity, norepinephrine, and epinephrine and lower renal and hepatic plasma flows than normonatremic patients with an apparently similar degree of heart disease. Hyponatremia in heart failure is associated with a poor prognosis (202).

HEPATIC CIRRHOSIS

Cirrhosis is characterized by a hyperdynamic circulation with low blood pressure, low systemic vascular resistance, and high cardiac output (169). Systemic vasodilatation causes relative underfilling of the arterial vascular compartment and neurohumoral responses similar to those that occur in response to a low cardiac output (170). Activation of the renin-angiotensin-aldosterone axis and the sympathetic system combined with nonosmotic release of vasopressin results in renal water and sodium retention (75, 95). Escape from the sodium-retaining effect of aldosterone does not occur and there is renal resistance to atrial natriuretic peptide. Although the pathogenesis of the peripheral arterial vasodilatation is incompletely understood, increased vascular nitric oxide by the endothelium may play a role. In a rat model of cirrhosis, normalization of vascular nitric oxide production with a nitric oxide synthetase inhibitor corrects the hyperdynamic circulation, improves sodium and water excretion, and decreases neurohumoral activation (169).

Peritoneovenous shunting of hyponatremic cirrhotic patients with refractory ascites improves cardiac output, renal plasma flow, and creatinine clearance and results in an immediate diuresis and natriuresis with a decrease in urine osmolality and an increase in plasma sodium concentration associated with a small but significant decrease in plasma vasopressin levels (169).

INAPPROPRIATE VASOPRESSIN SECRETION

Pathophysiology

DEFINITIONS

Nonosmotic release of vasopressin without a hemodynamic stimulus to account for it is considered "inappropriate" (226). When Bartter and Schwarz first described SIADH, they defined clinical criteria for the disorder which are still generally accepted: hypo-osmolality and clinical euvolemia with a sodium-containing urine (>30 mmol/l) that is less than maximally dilute (>100 mOsm/kg) without recent diuretic use or impaired renal function. Schwarz and Bartter also excluded endocrine disorders—primary and secondary adrenal insufficiency and hypothyroidism—from this designation. We have not made this exclusion because patients with undiagnosed endocrine disturbances may present with all the clinical features of SIADH. Indeed, the discovery of SIADH is often the presenting feature of a clinically important systemic disease. Abnormal vasopressin secretion may be caused by ectopic production of the hormone by tumors, disordered secretion by the neurohypophysis, or increased sensitivity to the hormone (Table 3).

Patients with the SIADH retain ingested water but they have no evidence of volume depletion and no tendency to form edema. Because of water retention, SIADH causes mild, subclinical volume expansion, which is reflected by high uric acid clearance, a low plasma uric acid concentration, and urine sodium excretion which matches or exceeds sodium intake (20, 167). Clinicians make use of these characteristics to distinguish SIADH from hyponatremia caused by volume depletion. The recently described syndrome of nephrogenic inappropriate antidiuresis is discussed in this section because it exhibits clinical features of SIADH; in physiological terms, however, it is a cause of hyponatremia that is independent of vasopressin as plasma vasopressin levels are undetectable (Table 2) (79).

PATTERNS OF VASOPRESSIN SECRETION

In most patients with SIADH, vasopressin secretion has followed one of two basic patterns: "reset osmostat" or "vasopressin leak" (215, 318). In the reset osmostat variant of SIADH, seen in patients with chronic, debilitating illness and in normal pregnancy, the urine can be diluted maximally, but at a lower set point than normal (57). Such patients are thus mildly hyponatremic, but unlike other patients with SIADH, their plasma sodium concentration is stable, and they do not require dietary water restriction or other measures used to treat chronic hyponatremia. In the vasopressin-leak variant, the basal level of vasopressin is elevated and unresponsive to osmotic stimuli when the plasma osmolality is low, but the levels increase appropriately when the plasma osmolality increases above a threshold level. Less commonly, patients exhibit erratic vasopressin secretion, which is unrelated to osmotic stimuli. In about 10% of patients with typical clinical manifestations of SIADH, plasma vasopressin levels are at a low basal level that fails to increase as plasma osmolality increases. Such a pattern would be expected if an antidiuretic factor other than vasopressin were produced or if the collecting tubules were hypersensitive to normal hormone levels.

INTERPLAY OF WATER RETENTION AND CATION DEPLETION IN SIADH

In SIADH, increased intravascular volume decreases renin secretion and increases release of atrial natriuretic peptide. These volume and hormonal changes promote sodium excretion despite a low serum sodium concentration. Natriuresis in SIADH blunts the increase in extracellular volume caused by water retention (Fig. 1) (167, 315) but it also exacerbates hyponatremia (Eq. 1). Balance studies in a group of patients with SIADH showed that during a period of high water and low sodium intake, the plasma sodium concentration decreased by 8 mEq/l with no gain in weight and no increase in chloride space (a measure of extracellular fluid volume) (50). Negative sodium and potassium balances accounted for the stability of extracellular volume and for more than 80% of the calculated solute loss. During a period of high sodium intake, more than 600 mEq of sodium was retained (with only a small increase in weight and chloride space), fully accounting for the 11-mEq/l increase in serum

TABLE 3   Causes of Syndrome of Inappropriate Antidiuretic Hormone Secretion

Major Classification	Common Examples
Tumors	Small cell lung cancer
	Head and neck tumors
Lung diseases	Pulmonary infection
	Hypoxia and hypercarbia
	Severe asthma
Neurologic disorders	Subarachnoid hemorrhage[a]
	Guillain-Barrè syndrome[a]
	Central nervous system infections
	Cerebral hemorrhage and infarction
	Brain tumors
Endocrine diseases	Hypothyroidism[a]
	Hypopituitarism
	Isolated adrenocorticotropic hormone deficiency
Medications	Arginine vasopressin and desmopressin acetate
	Amiodarone
	Chlorpropamide
	Carbamazepine and oxcarbazepine
	Cyclophosphamide
	Nonsteroidal anti-inflammatory agents
	Serotonin reuptake inhibitors
	Tricyclic antidepressants
	Vincristine
	3,4-methylenedioxymethamphetamine (ecstasy)
Hereditary	Nephrogenic syndrome of antidiuresis[b]
Miscellaneous, transitory causes	Surgery
	Pain and stress
	Nausea
	Alcohol withdrawal

[a]Disorders with both hemodynamic and nonhemodynamic bases for vasopressin release.

[b]Hereditary disorder of the V2 receptor with clinical features of syndrome of inappropriate antidiuretic hormone secretion but with undetectable plasma vasopressin levels.

sodium concentration (50). In this study, there was a strong negative correlation between water intake and sodium balance and between water intake and aldosterone secretory rate. Similar findings have been reported in studies in which pituitary extract was administered chronically to healthy subjects (133, 158, 315).

In an experimental model of SIADH produced by DDAVP and half-isotonic saline in the rat, hyponatremia was caused exclusively by negative balances of sodium and potassium; water balance, which was slightly negative, did not contribute to the decrease in sodium concentration (98). Despite negative balances for sodium, chloride, and water, the extracellular volume (measured by inulin space) was not contracted, suggesting that water shifted from the intracellular to the extracellular space in response to the loss of intracellular solute (potassium and phosphate).

Similarly, direct measurements of body composition in a rat model of chronic SIADH showed that after 14 days of severe hyponatremia, body water content had returned to control levels (Fig. 3) (294). Body sodium and chloride levels were reduced after 1 day of hyponatremia and were

sustained for 14 days, and body potassium was significantly decreased after 7 days. Acutely, water retention was the major cause of hyponatremia, but solute depletion was primarily responsible when the electrolyte disturbance was sustained.

Urinary losses can directly lower the plasma sodium concentration when the concentration of sodium plus potassium in the urine is higher than the plasma sodium concentration. This can occur when high vasopressin levels (which concentrate the urine) and high rates of sodium and potassium excretion occur together. The excretion of hypertonic urine generates free water, in essence, "desalinating" the plasma (263).

SERUM BICARBONATE CONCENTRATION IN SIADH

In SIADH, the serum sodium and chloride concentrations are lowered by dilution, but the serum bicarbonate concentration is typically normal (56, 100). This finding has been explained by a direct effect of hyponatremia on the adrenal gland to increase aldosterone secretion which then augments renal net acid excretion (49). Patients with hyponatremia due to hypopituitarism have many features in

A

B

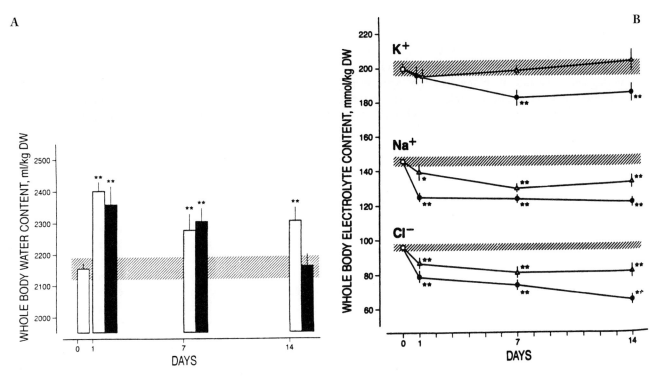

FIGURE 3 Body water content in experimental syndrome of inappropriate antidiuretic hormone secretion (SIADH) (294). **A:** Measurements of body water content in rats made hyponatremic with 1-desamino-8-D-arginine vasopressin (dDAVP) and a liquid diet. The open bar at the far left of the figure represents measurements obtained in normonatremic controls given no dDAVP. The black bars represent measurements obtained in animals made severely hyponatremic (plasma sodium 106 to 112 mmol/l) by giving dDAVP at 5 ng/h; the gray bars represent measurements obtained in animals made less hyponatremic (plasma sodium 119 to 124 mmol/l) by giving dDAVP at 1 ng/hr. Body water content initially increases after the first day of hyponatremia at both doses of dDAVP, but falls to control levels after 14 days of severe hyponatremia. **B:** Whole-body Na, K, and Cl measurements in the same experiment. Cation and chloride losses occur, beginning on the first day of hyponatremia and are more severe in animals given the higher dose of dDAVP (with lower plasma sodium levels). Depletion of Na and Cl most likely represent adaptive responses to extracellular fluid volume expansion caused by retained water. Depletion of body K most likely represents a cell volume adaptive response.

common with patients with nonendocrine SIADH, but their serum bicarbonate concentrations are about 5 mmol/l lower. Consistent with the hypothesis that hyponatremia-induced hyperaldosteronism is responsible for the normal serum bicarbonate in classic SIADH, aldosterone levels are much lower in patients with ACTH deficiency than in patients with nonendocrine SIADH (56).

Common Causes of SIADH

TUMORS

The first cases of SIADH were described in patients with lung cancer (226). Small cell carcinoma of the lung remains a common cause of the syndrome; approximately 10% to 15% of these patients present with SIADH, whereas fewer than 1% of patients with non–small cell lung cancer become hyponatremic (162, 249). Ectopic production of vasopressin appears to be responsible for most cases hyponatremia associated with small cell carcinoma (135, 181). Arginine vasopressin, oxytocin, and neurophysins have been found by radioimmunoassay in tumors and are produced by the vast majority of small cell lung cancers; the quantity of vasopressin peptide is closely cor-

related with the presence of hyponatremia (159, 172, 194). Atrial natriuretic peptide mRNA has also been detected in a high percentage of cell lines from patients with small cell cancer (28, 37, 103, 159). Hyponatremia develops in approximately 3% to 7% of patients with head and neck cancer (81, 249, 278); the mechanism for SIADH associated with these tumors is unknown. Although a number of other tumors can produce vasopressin, there are very few reports of hyponatremia associated with them (249).

PULMONARY DISEASE

Mild hyponatremia has long been recognized in patients with tuberculosis (122, 238). The mechanism for vasopressin release has not been determined, but hormone levels fall in response to water loading, reflecting the reset osmostat variant of SIADH. Hyponatremia resolves within days to weeks of antituberculous therapy. Plasma vasopressin levels are typically elevated on admission in patients with bacterial pneumonia and fall rapidly during treatment (65). Hyponatremia is common (139, 282) and usually self-corrects relatively rapidly after a few days (64). Abnormal vasopressin secretion in simple pneumonia is not attributable to hypovolemia, hypotension, or abnormal PO_2 or PCO_2. An antidiuretic decapeptide ("pneumadin"), which rapidly increases arginine vasopressin levels, has been isolated from rat and human lung (18, 149, 302). Further study is needed to determine if the decapeptide mediates SIADH associated with pneumonia and other lung disorders. Acute respiratory failure (hypoxia and hypercarbia) and severe asthma are also associated with SIADH (78, 229, 290).

ENDOCRINE DISEASE

Hyponatremia is present in up to 88% of patients with Addison disease and in 28% of patients with isolated ACTH deficiency (292). In Addison disease, vasopressin is released in response to volume depletion caused by mineralocorticoid deficiency and altered hemodynamics caused by glucocorticoid deficiency. Glucocorticoids may also directly inhibit vasopressin release. Unlike Addison disease, impaired water excretion in hypopituitarism is not associated with hyperkalemia and does not respond to volume replacement with isotonic saline so that hyponatremia in this condition has all the features of SIADH (30, 58, 195, 196). However, hyponatremia in patients with hypopituitarism is associated with a lower serum bicarbonate concentration than in patients with hyponatremia from other causes of SIADH (56). Impaired water excretion in hypopituitarism and in adrenalectomized mineralocorticoid replaced subjects is associated with elevated vasopressin levels; administration of a vasopressin V2 receptor antagonist normalizes urinary water excretion in adrenalectomized mineralocorticoid replaced rats (128). Inhibitory glucocorticoid receptors have been identified in the magnocellular neurons which secrete vasopressin and these receptors are markedly increased under hypo-osmolar conditions (25, 141, 206). Hyponatremia with clinical features of SIADH has been described frequently in hypothyroidism; impaired water excretion can be corrected rapidly by the administration of thyroid hormone. However, it is unclear whether hemodynamic or intrarenal factors, rather than vasopressin, are responsible for impaired water excretion in this condition (109, 132).

NONDIURETIC DRUGS

Arginine vasopressin used therapeutically in the treatment of gastrointestinal bleeding or in the management of septic shock and the vasopressin analogue, desmopressin acetate (DDAVP), a pure V2 receptor agonist used to treat diabetes insipidus, enuresis, and von Willebrand disease, may cause hyponatremia (35, 150). In addition, a growing number of drugs that are unrelated to vasopressin have been reported to cause hyponatremia. Most published reports involve thiazide and thiazide-like diuretics, chlorpropamide, carbamazepine, oxcarbantipsychotics, antidepressants, and nonsteroidal anti-inflammatory drugs (31, 41, 291). Carbamazepine, vincristine, and vinblastine increase vasopressin release by unknown mechanisms, and hyponatremia associated with these agents is dose related (31). Carbamazepine most commonly causes hyponatremia when it is given to subjects who habitually drink large volumes of water (291, 317).

Several drugs associated with hyponatremia appear to increase the response of the collecting duct to circulating vasopressin (31, 180). Chlorpropamide has been the most thoroughly studied (306). In addition to augmenting release of vasopressin from the neurohypophysis, chlorpropamide increases the number of vasopressin receptors on collecting tubule cells (120) and inhibits renal medullary synthesis of prostaglandin E2, an agent that blunts the hydro-osmotic effect of vasopressin by diminishing adenylate cyclase activity (175, 304, 319). Inhibition of PGE2 permits increased cAMP formation, enhancing the effect of the hormone. Nonsteroidal anti-inflammatory agents increase the hydro-osmotic effect of vasopressin by a similar mechanism. Hyponatremia attributable solely to nonsteroidals has been rarely reported, but these commonly used drugs may exacerbate other causes of hyponatremia (47, 210). Hyponatremia caused by cyclophosphamide and carbamazepine may also be due to enhanced vasopressin action, but the mechanism for this effect has not yet been elucidated (291). Cyclophosphamide's antidiuretic effect is delayed with a time course that parallels excretion of active metabolites of the drug (261). Cyclophosphamide's antidiuretic effect may be enhanced by indomethacin (303). There are many reports of SIADH associated with psychotropic drugs, including phenothiazines, monoamine oxidase inhibitors, and tricyclic antidepressants; causality has been most convincingly demonstrated with tricyclics (259). More recently a large number of cases of SIADH have been reported in patients taking serotonin reuptake inhibitors (163, 258, 314). Prospective series in elderly patients have shown that 12% to 40% became hyponatremic within 2 weeks of starting therapy with paroxetine (76, 77, 314). All of these agents act centrally and could conceivably affect vasopressin release directly. The recreational drug, 3,4-methylenedioxymethamphetamine ("ecstasy") has been associated with severe, and sometimes fatal, acute hyponatremia (113). Ecstasy induces vasopressin secretion, and users of the drug who become hyponatremic typically manifest marked polydipsia (34, 119). In four case reports, SIADH has been noted during amiodarone-loading (13).

POSTOPERATIVE SIADH

Vasopressin levels are elevated after operative procedures and remain elevated for several days (281). Administration of hypotonic fluid during this period of antidiuresis causes acute hyponatremia with potentially disastrous consequences.

Urinary cation loss has been shown to play an important role in the pathogenesis of hyponatremia in patients with postoperative SIADH. In the postoperative period, it is common for physicians to infuse several liters of isotonic or hypotonic saline solutions, exceeding the intended replacement of third-space and external losses and actually causing extracellular fluid volume expansion. A balance study in women undergoing uncomplicated gynecologic surgery showed that sodium and potassium concentrations in the urine peaked at 295 ± 9 mEq/l and remained hypertonic to plasma for the first 16 hours after induction of anesthesia (Fig. 4) (263). Because of the action of vasopressin and the natriuretic

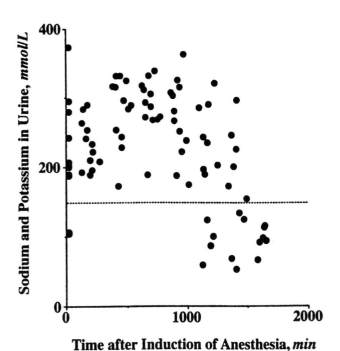

FIGURE 4 Urine electrolytes in postoperative syndrome of inappropriate antidiuretic hormone secretion (SIADH) (263). The figure depicts the sum of urine sodium and potassium concentrations obtained postoperatively in 22 women undergoing uncomplicated gynecologic surgery and receiving infusions of 0.9% saline (sodium concentration 154 mmol/l) or lactated Ringers solution (sodium concentration 130 mmol/l). The dotted line represents a urine cation concentration of 150 mmol/l, isotonic to normal plasma water. During the first 1000 minutes after the induction of anesthesia, urine cation concentrations were uniformly hypertonic to plasma, contributing to the genesis of hyponatremia. In samples obtained after 1000 minutes (from 16 to 24 hours), the urine remained hypertonic in some patients and became hypotonic in others. Hypotonic urine (below the dotted line) contributes to the correction of hyponatremia.

response to saline-induced volume expansion, electrolyte-free water was generated, lowering the plasma sodium concentration despite infusion of isotonic saline. The infused saline was, in effect, "desalinated." A similar phenomenon occurs when patients with subarachnoid hemorrhage and "cerebral salt wasting" are given large volumes of isotonic saline to protect cerebral perfusion (63).

NEUROLOGIC DISORDERS AND CEREBRAL SALT WASTING

An association between hyponatremia and intracranial disease has been recognized since the 1950s, and hyponatremia has been reported in a variety of systemic diseases involving the central nervous system (CNS), including systemic lupus erythematosus, Guillain-Barrè syndrome, meningitis, encephalitis, brain tumors, and brain abscesses (205). Noting increased urinary sodium excretion in hyponatremic patients with neurologic disorders, Peters referred to the condition as "cerebral salt wasting" (209). Once it was recognized that high rates of urinary sodium excretion could be caused by unregulated secretion of antidiuretic hormone,

most investigators ascribed hyponatremia in brain disease to SIADH, a syndrome that has been associated with an array of CNS disorders, consistent with the multiple anatomic pathways leading to vasopressin secretion by hypothalamic neurons (Table 3) (151).

Cerebral salt wasting was generally a forgotten term until the early 1980s, when a more concerted effort was made to understand the pathogenesis of hyponatremia in patients with intracranial disease (especially subarachnoid hemorrhage) (185, 186). Reduced blood and plasma volume were found in most patients with intracranial disease who were presumed to have hyponatremia secondary to SIADH (166, 168, 187, 244, 316). Prospective studies of patients with subarachnoid hemorrhage given maintenance fluids documented negative sodium balance, decreasing plasma volume, and increasing blood urea nitrogen (BUN) levels among patients who became hyponatremic within a week of presentation (153, 186, 309). A course consistent with cerebral salt wasting was also observed in patients with head injury, brain metastases, and hydrocephalus (91, 200, 279).

The diagnosis of cerebral salt wasting has important clinical implications, especially in subarachnoid hemorrhage, where volume depletion and fluid restriction have been reported to predispose to cerebral ischemia and infarction (115, 308). This finding, and evidence that volume expansion protects against cerebral ischemic events in subarachnoid hemorrhage, has led to a general acceptance of "hypertensive, hypervolemic, hemodilutional" therapy for the disorder (199, 241, 243, 289). When such treatment is given, a high urine sodium concentration and hyponatremia are not reliable indicators of salt wasting because hyponatremia may be due to SIADH, and the natriuresis may be a response to iatrogenic volume expansion. In one study, a positive balance for sodium could be documented in most patients believed to have cerebral salt wasting when calculations included all infusions from the time of first contact with medical or paramedical personnel (38). High levels of catecholamines, which are often associated with brain injury, decrease venous capacitance and raise blood pressure, potentially increasing "effective arterial blood volume" and promoting a physiological natriuresis (239).

As in patients with SIADH, plasma vasopressin levels are increased and urine sodium concentrations are elevated, but the increased vasopressin secretion in cerebral salt wasting has been attributed to volume depletion caused by the primary salt wasting. Investigation into the pathogenesis of cerebral salt wasting has focused primarily on the relative roles of natriuretic hormones and vasopressin after subarachnoid hemorrhage (59–62, 173, 228). Atrial natriuretic peptide (ANP) and brain natriuretic peptide (BNP) are both derived from cardiac tissue and have natriuretic and aldosterone inhibiting properties. Though BNP has been localized to the hypothalamus, it is primarily of cardiac origin. Cardiac release of ANP and BNP is regulated in part by the CNS, and brain injury may induce their release from cardiac tissue. Plasma ANP levels generally correlate with the presence and severity of blood in the ventricles and increased intracranial pressure (62). In one study, however, plasma levels of BNP but not ANP or vasopressin were correlated with urinary sodium excretion (23) and in a rat model of cerebral salt wasting, ANP levels decreased and BNP levels did not change (147). It is thus unclear whether elevated natriuretic peptide levels are responsible for natriuresis in subarachnoid hemorrhage, and other factors, such as altered sympathetic tone, depressed aldosterone levels and ouabain-like compound, and endothelin may contribute (60, 205, 307, 316). In fact, several studies have indicated that fludrocortisone may be effective in the treatment of cerebral salt wasting (40, 114, 129, 313).

Regardless of the pathogenesis of renal salt wasting in patients with subarachnoid hemorrhage, hyponatremia appears to be caused by vasopressin release that is independent of volume depletion and is thus "inappropriate." In a large prospective study of acute aneurysmal subarachnoid hemorrhage treated aggressively with isotonic saline (between 3 and 8 liters daily), hyponatremia developed in one third of the patients within 4 to 6 days, despite positive fluid balance, increased blood volume, and suppressed plasma renin and aldosterone levels (63). Plasma vasopressin was measured at concentrations of 1 to 4 pg/ml despite plasma osmolality levels at which the hormone should have been undetectable. Although plasma ANP levels were also increased in most patients, they did not correlate with serum sodium concentration. Thus, it is likely that both salt loss and SIADH contribute in varying degrees to the pathogenesis of hyponatremia after subarachnoid hemorrhage.

Nephrogenic Syndrome of Inappropriate Antidiuresis

Two infants have been described who presented with clinical and laboratory evaluations typical of SIADH with undetectable plasma vasopressin levels (79). DNA sequencing of each patient's vasopressin receptor V2R gene identified missense mutations in both, with resultant changes in codon 137 from arginine to cysteine or leucine. These novel mutations cause constitutive activation of the vasopressin receptor, analogous to loss-of-function mutations found in patients with X-linked nephrogenic diabetes insipidus. The new syndrome has been named "nephrogenic syndrome of inappropriate antidiuresis" (79).

ADAPTATIONS TO HYPOTONIC HYPONATREMIA

Organic Osmolytes and Cell Volume Regulation

The osmotic challenges faced by hyponatremic patients are analogous to those faced by invertebrate organisms when they are exposed to a hypotonic environment. Throughout nature, cells respond to water stress in a similar manner. Water crosses cell membranes in response to osmotic forces equalizing the activities of intracellular and extracellular

solute. Cell volume is determined by the amount and concentration of intracellular solute. Since at equilibrium intracellular and extracellular osmolalities are equal, the relationship between cell volume and extracellular osmolality can be described by the following equation:

$$\text{Cell Water} = \frac{\text{Cell solute content}}{\text{Extracellular osmolality}} \qquad \text{(Eq. 2)}$$

Hypotonicity causes cells to swell initially as water diffuses into them, equalizing the osmolality of intracellular and extracellular fluids. Almost immediately, however, most cells begin to adjust their volume back toward normal (174, 275). This "volume regulatory decrease," is explained by reductions in cell solute content. The first response to osmotic stress is a loss of potassium. With time, loss of organic solutes dominates the response.

Most cells maintain relatively high concentrations of small, osmotically active organic molecules known as "organic osmolytes." The major organic osmolytes found in nature are limited to a few classes of compounds—polyols, methylamines, and free amino acids—that are shared by diverse species. Organic osmolytes are nonperturbing solutes; unlike sodium and potassium, their intracellular concentrations may vary widely without affecting tertiary protein structure. Cells accumulate organic osmolytes under hypertonic conditions and lose them when confronted with hypotonicity. Several organic osmolytes are exported from swollen cells through a common channel, the volume-sensitive organic osmolyte/anion channel (VSOAC) (74, 275). Osmolytes are transported into the cell by specific transporters such as the sodium-myoinositol transporter (SMIT) (125) and the taurine transporter (TAUT) (22).

Cell volume control mechanisms could modify the relationship between the plasma sodium concentration and body water, sodium, and potassium content shown in Eq. 1. For example, if the intracellular fluid compartment were to lose 15% of its solute (exclusive of potassium) in response to cell swelling, the amount of water needed to lower the plasma sodium concentration would be reduced by one-third. Some balance studies in patients with very low plasma sodium concentrations have failed to fully account for the severity of hyponatremia, a finding that would be expected if there were substantial losses of organic osmolytes from body cells.

Brain Adaptations to Hyponatremia

The need for cell volume regulation is greatest in the brain, where the rigid calvarium limits the degree of tissue swelling that can be tolerated (106, 152). An increase in brain water content of more than about 5% to 10% is incompatible with life. Although the capillary endothelium that forms the blood–brain barrier has a limited permeability to ions and other solutes, it allows relatively rapid water movement into the brain. Therefore, an osmotic gradient between the brain and plasma can exist only transiently, and it is dissipated by water movement in less than one hour. Hydraulic conductivity of the capillaries which form the blood–brain barrier decreases in response to hypotonicity (197). However, because the brain and plasma must eventually come into osmotic equilibrium, this adaptation can only postpone brain swelling. The brain's interstitial fluid compartment communicates with the spinal fluid through a series of extracellular channels. Bulk flow of fluid between the brain's interstitial space and the cerebrospinal fluid provides a rapid defense against osmotic brain swelling. Ultimately, protection against lethal cerebral edema depends on the ability of brain cells to reduce their solute content.

In experimental hyponatremia in the rat, depletion of brain sodium, potassium, and chloride accounts for about two thirds of the adaptive decrease in brain osmolality, while approximately one third is contributed by organic osmolyte losses. Within 24 hours of the onset of hyponatremia, diminished brain concentrations of myoinositol, glutamate, creatine/phosphocreatine, and taurine can be detected (270). During sustained hyponatremia, these compounds plus glycerophosphorylcholine and glutamine continue to be lost from the brain for approximately 3 days (283–285, 296). Reduced concentrations of these solutes persist when animals are kept severely hyponatremic for as long as 2 weeks. The loss of organic osmolytes contributes substantially to the early and late adaptations to hyponatremia. In rats whose serum sodium concentrations were reduced to 96 mmol/l in 1 day, brain water content increased by less than 5%; it was estimated that the increase would have been 11% had there been no losses of organic osmolytes (270). After 3 days of hyponatremia, additional losses of brain solute further decrease the severity of brain edema; animals exhibit minimal neurologic findings despite serum sodium concentrations of 95 to 100 mmol/l (274).

Magnetic resonance spectroscopy has provided evidence of reduced concentrations of organic osmolytes in the brains of patients with hyponatremia (301). One study showed that the peak associated with inositol remained depressed for at least 2 weeks after correction of hyponatremia (Fig. 5) (116). An adaptive response of the brain is evident among patients with chronic hyponatremia. Computed axial tomography and magnetic resonance images do not show evidence of brain edema and neurologic symptoms may be subtle, even in patients with serum sodium concentrations less than 110 mEq/l. Most patients with hyponatremia of this severity survive, and the few neurologic sequelae that occur appear to be caused by overzealous correction of hyponatremia rather than the electrolyte disturbance itself (266, 272).

In contrast to chronic hyponatremia, patients who become severely hyponatremic in less than 48 hours develop headaches, vomiting, agitated delirium, and eventually stupor, seizures, and coma. The clinical syndrome in humans and experimental animals is associated with cerebral edema,

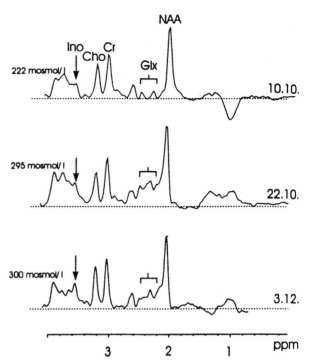

FIGURE 5 Brain organic osmolytes in human hyponatremia (116). The figure depicts the results of magnetic resonance spectroscopy of the brain of a single patient before and after treatment of severe hyponatremia (plasma sodium 101 mmol/l, plasma osmolality 222 mOsm/kg). The spectroscopy tracings were obtained on three different dates. The top tracing, taken on October 10, when the plasma osmolality was 222 mOsm/l shows an extremely low inositol peak (*arrow*). The middle tracing, taken on October 22, 10 days after treatment of hyponatremia when the plasma osmolality was 295 mOsm/l, shows an inositol peak that is still depressed. The bottom tracing taken on December 3, 7 weeks after correction of hyponatremia shows a much higher inositol peak.

which can be reversed by the administration of hypertonic saline. On occasion, acute hyponatremia can lead to respiratory arrest, transtentorial herniation, and death (4, 9, 10, 14, 17). When large volumes of water are retained in a short time, the arterial sodium concentration (to which the brain is exposed) may be up to 4 mmol/l lower than the venous concentration (which is most commonly sampled for clinical sodium measurements) (227).

Age and Sex and the Adaptation to Hyponatremia

A single group of investigators have reported on over 100 previously healthy patients who became hyponatremic 1 to 2 days after routine elective surgery and subsequently died or suffered permanent brain damage. Individual patients had serum sodium concentrations as high as 129 mEq/l when they developed respiratory arrest and brain herniation (10, 14, 17). The most recent reports emphasize the frequent association of hyponatremic encephalopathy with neurogenic pulmonary edema (14) and terminal diabetes insipidus (86). Remarkably, virtually all of the reported patients were women, usually of child-bearing age (17), or prepubescent children (10). These findings led these authors to suggest that sex hormones alter the adaptive mechanisms that protect against brain edema in hyponatremia.

The same investigators have used experimental models to test their hypothesis that hyponatremia causes more severe brain swelling in females than in males. The results of these studies are inconclusive. The investigators initially found that mortality from hyponatremia was markedly increased in adult female rats (87) (a finding that has not been reproduced by other laboratories) (293). They attributed excess mortality in females to lower levels of brain Na,K-ATPase (and thus a decreased ability to extrude brain sodium) and to increased susceptibility to

vasopressin-induced vasoconstriction of the cerebral vasculature. In vitro studies showed that estrogens inhibit volume regulation in rat brain astrocyte culture (88). However, measurements of brain water and solutes in whole brain by these and other investigators show comparable responses to hyponatremia in male and female animals (Fig. 6) (293)

Arieff and coworkers reported that although brain water and electrolyte contents in hyponatremic adult male and female rats do not differ, the brains of newborn rats paradoxically accumulate excess sodium in response to hyponatremia unless the animals are pretreated with testosterone (11). Silver and coworkers were unable to reproduce this provocative finding (234).

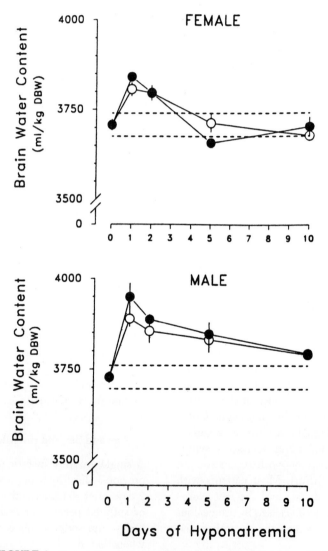

FIGURE 6   Brain water content in hyponatremic male and female rats (293). The figure depicts measurements of brain water content obtained in male and female rats made hyponatremic with a liquid diet and either arginine vasopressin (*solid circles*) or 1-desamino-8-D-arginine vasopressin (*open circles*). Brain water contents are comparable in the two sexes, returning to or toward control values after 10 days of hyponatremia.

Hypoxia and the Adaptation to Hyponatremia

Some investigators have emphasized the adverse effects of hypoxia in hyponatremic patients. According to this view, when brain damage complicates symptomatic hyponatremia an hypoxic episode can usually be implicated (146). Although, it is likely that hypoxia is an important factor among patients with acute hyponatremia who die of cerebral edema, the role of hypoxia in the demyelinating brain lesions which complicate the treatment of chronic hyponatremia has not been proven (253). Despite recurrent episodes of acute hyponatremia, hyponatremic seizures, respiratory arrests requiring endotracheal intubation, and rapid correction of hyponatremia (due to spontaneous diuresis), infants, and psychotic patients with acute water intoxication rarely develop neurologic sequelae (272).

Hyponatremic animals are more likely to die when exposed to hypoxia than normonatremic animals, and ischemic brain injury impairs the adaptive loss of brain sodium that protects against brain swelling in hyponatremia (300). In addition, hyponatremia has been shown to lower levels of the antioxidants taurine, glutathione, and ascorbate in brain tissue, which could predispose to oxidant injury when a period of hypoxia is followed by reoxygenation (46, 240).

RAPID CORRECTION OF HYPONATREMIA AND OSMOTIC DEMYELINATION

Biochemical Effects of Rapid Correction of Hyponatremia

Adaptations that protect against brain swelling also predispose to injury when sustained hypotonicity is suddenly corrected. When the plasma sodium is returned to normal, cellular solutes lost in the adaptive phase must be recovered to prevent cellular dehydration. Electrolytes and glutamate quickly return to the brain after correction, but reaccumulation of other organic osmolytes requires several days because it requires upregulation of sodium-dependent transport proteins (161, 257). After rapid correction of hyponatremia, solute-depleted brain cells are initially dehydrated. Brain electrolyte content then "overshoots" increasing to supernormal levels, possibly in compensation for the deficit in organic osmolyte content (Fig. 7) (255, 297).

Clinical Effect of Rapid Correction of Hyponatremia

In humans, correction of severe chronic hyponatremia by more than 10 to 12 mEq/l in 24 hours or 18 mEq/l in less than 48 hours is associated with a distinctive clinical disorder known as the "osmotic demyelination syndrome" (4, 32, 136, 157, 171, 273). In typical cases of the syndrome, improvement of hyponatremic symptoms during correction of hyponatremia is followed within one to several days by gradual neurologic deterioration. Behavioral disturbances,

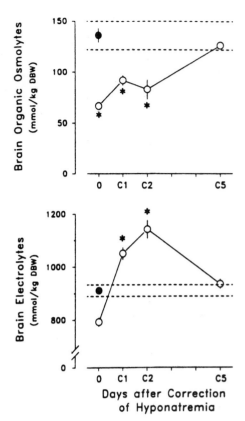

FIGURE 7 Brain organic osmolytes and brain electrolytes after rapid correction of experimental hyponatremia (297). The figure depicts measurements of brain organic osmolytes (**top panel**) and brain electrolytes (**bottom panel**) made in rats made hyponatremic with 1-desamino-8-D-arginine vasopressin (dDAVP) and a liquid diet and then corrected by withdrawal of dDAVP. Brain organic osmolytes remain significantly below normonatremic control levels (*solid circle* and *dotted lines*) on the first 2 days after correction (C1 and C2) and have not reached normal levels until 5 days after correction (C5). During the first 2 days after correction, brain electrolyte content "overshoots," exceeding control levels.

seizures, movement disorders, or akinetic mutism may emerge and severe cases develop clinical features of a pontine disorder (pseudobulbar palsy, quadriparesis, and pseudocoma).

The clinical symptoms are associated with demyelinating brain lesions that can be demonstrated by magnetic resonance images (177, 221). The most characteristic lesions are located in the center of the pons ("central pontine myelinolysis") (2, 188, 192), but histologically similar lesions are often found in a symmetrical distribution in extrapontine areas of the brain in which there is a close admixture of gray and white matter (157). The lesions are distinctly different from those caused by hypoxia, and the lesions may develop without a preceding hypoxic insult (171, 271–273).

Patients with acute hyponatremia (e.g., infants and psychotic patients) usually tolerate rapid correction of hyponatremia without developing complications and patients with liver disease (a disorder characterized by low levels of brain myoinositol [213]), alcoholism, malnutrition, and potassium depletion (165) seem to be particularly susceptible to osmotic demyelination.

Experimental Models of Osmotic Demyelination

The osmotic demyelination syndrome has been reproduced in animal models in three different species by multiple laboratories (15, 16, 127, 143, 144, 156, 193, 274, 299). These studies have confirmed the strong clinical impression that the disorder is caused by treatment of hyponatremia rather than hyponatremia itself. Osmotic demyelination does not develop in animals with uncorrected or slowly corrected hyponatremia. Rapid correction of chronic (3 days) but not acute hyponatremia produces a delayed onset of neurologic symptoms and brain lesions that are histologically similar to those seen in the human disease. Neurologic deterioration and histologic brain damage are preceded by pathologic evidence of blood-brain barrier disruption that can be demonstrated ultrastructurally as early as 3 hours and by magnetic resonance imaging one day after rapid correction of hyponatremia (3, 217, 218). After excessive correction of chronic hyponatremia, reinduction of hyponatremia when neurologic findings begin to appear improves survival and prevents the subsequent appearance of myelinolysis in rats; this strategy has been successfully used in isolated clinical case reports (201, 251, 254).

Depletion of brain organic osmolytes is felt to play a key role in the blood–brain barrier disruption and demyelination that occurs after rapid correction of hyponatremia. In rats, measurements of organic osmolyte content in different areas of the brain after rapid correction of hyponatremia has shown that areas with the most severe demyelinating lesions are those with the least recovery of organic osmolytes (160). It has been suggested that blood–brain barrier disruption can be explained by loss of organic osmolytes from brain capillary endothelial cells during the adaptation to hyponatremia with subsequent endothelial cell shrinkage after rapid correction. Blood–brain barrier disruption permits complement and possibly other toxic plasma constituents to enter the brain, which may explain the occurrence of progressive myelinolysis even after blood–brain integrity is restored (3).

Hyponatremic animals with uremia are relatively tolerant of rapid correction, with a lower incidence and severity of myelinolysis than nonuremic animals (252, 255). Resistance to myelinolysis in uremia is associated with more rapid reuptake of organic osmolytes, in particular myoinositol, following rapid correction of hyponatremia. In addition, rapidly corrected uremic animals do not exhibit the "overshoot" in brain sodium content seen in nonuremic animals. Normalization of brain myoinositol can be accelerated in nonuremic hyponatremic rats by administering myoinositol exogenously during rapid correction of the electrolyte disturbance (235). Exogenous myoinositol improves survival and reduces mortality from rapid correction of chronic hyponatremia in rats (236).

TREATMENT OF HYPOTONIC HYPONATREMIA

Treatment Modalities

WATER RESTRICTION

Even with maximally concentrated urine, evaporative water losses from the skin and lungs will lead to negative water balance and gradual correction of hyponatremia regardless of the cause of the electrolyte disturbance. In patients whose ability to dilute the urine is intact (e.g., self-induced water intoxication) or can be restored to normal (e.g., by saline infusion in volume-depleted subjects) restriction of free water leads to a steady and sometimes rapid increase in the plasma sodium concentration. In patients with persistent defects in water excretion (e.g., SIADH caused by tumors), water restriction alone increases the plasma sodium concentration extremely slowly.

SODIUM CHLORIDE

Assuming that free-water intake is restricted, sodium chloride solutions increase the plasma sodium concentration as long as the electrolyte concentration of the solution exceeds that of the urine. As urine cation concentrations rarely exceed 400 mEq/l, 3% sodium chloride (513 mEq/l) is always an effective treatment for hyponatremia. Isotonic saline itself does little to increase the plasma sodium concentration unless it provokes a water diuresis by eliminating a hemodynamic stimulus for vasopressin secretion caused by volume depletion. In fact, large volumes of isotonic saline can exacerbate hyponatremia in patients with SIADH who excrete highly concentrated urine (263).

POTASSIUM CHLORIDE

Given the relationship between the plasma sodium concentration and exchangeable sodium and potassium (72, 190), it follows that potassium repletion of hypokalemic hyponatremic subjects should increase the plasma sodium concentration. There is a limited published experience validating this expectation in patients with diuretic-induced hyponatremia (83), and in the authors' experience (unpublished observations) potassium effectively corrects hyponatremia regardless of the cause of potassium depletion.

LOOP DIURETICS

By blocking sodium reabsorption in the ascending limb of the loop of Henle, loop diuretics impair the ability to maximally concentrate the urine, even in the presence of high levels of plasma vasopressin. Used alone, or in combination with angiotensin-converting enzyme inhibitors, loop diuretics are effective in treating hyponatremia associated with edematous conditions (67, 73, 203, 310). In patients with SIADH, loop diuretics can be combined with 3% saline for the treatment of hyponatremic emergencies (110). Traditionally, in this maneuver, urinary sodium losses are matched with infused saline. However, given the adaptive loss of sodium that occurs in SIADH, it may be more appropriate to allow sodium intake to exceed urinary losses. In patients with SIADH who require chronic outpatient therapy, loop diuretics combined with oral salt tablets and potassium replacement (or concurrent therapy with a potassium sparing diuretic) are effective.

DEMECLOCYCLINE

Demeclocycline is a tetracycline antibiotic that blocks the effect of vasopressin in the collecting duct. After a few days of therapy, demeclocycline induces a state of nephrogenic diabetes insipidus which resolves within several days when the drug is stopped (54). This side effect of the antibiotic has been exploited in the long-term treatment of SIADH (84, 286). Demeclocycline is nephrotoxic in patients with heart failure and liver disease (178, 207).

UREA

Urea, administered orally in a daily dose of 0.5 g/kg body weight per day, increases urinary electrolyte free-water losses, allowing liberalized fluid intake in patients with chronic hyponatremia due to SIADH and other disorders such as CHF (39, 55). However, it tastes poorly and is contraindicated in liver and renal failure. Intravenous urea has also been effective in treating acute hyponatremia (212). In experimental models, Soupart and Decaux have demonstrated that acute correction of chronic hyponatremia with urea decreases the risk of myelinolysis (256). Although the mechanism of this protection is unknown, it has been speculated that urea enters the brain and then is cleared from the plasma more slowly than it is cleared from brain tissue (232, 237), thereby protecting against brain cell

shrinkage after rapid correction. Experience with urea is much more extensive in Europe than the United States.

V2-RECEPTOR ANTAGONISTS

Sustained hyponatremia is usually mediated by excessive vasopressin secretion. Therefore, specific V2 antagonists have long been sought to provide a specific and predictable means of treating hyponatremia (142).

The first peptide vasopressin antagonists, developed in the 1980s, were nonselective and inactive if taken orally (295). More recently, selective nonpeptide antagonists have been developed and tested in laboratory animals and humans; they are likely to be approved for clinical use in the near future. These agents induce a dose-related water diuresis lasting approximately 6 hours without a significant increase in urinary sodium or potassium excretion; therefore, vasopressin receptor antagonists are sometimes called "aquaretics" (Fig. 8) (51, 222, 295).

Tolvaptan (OPC-41061), lixivaptan (VPA-985), and conivaptan (YM-087) are currently being tested in clinical trials. Tolvaptan and lixivaptan are selective for the vasopressin-2 (V2) receptor responsible for the antidiuretic actions of arginine vasopressin, conivaptan is active at both the V2 receptor and the V1a receptor responsible for the vasoconstricting properties of arginine vasopressin. Both selective V2 antagonists have been shown to be effective in correcting hyponatremia due to SIADH, cirrhosis, and heart failure in humans (93, 94, 312). Conivaptan corrects hyponatremia in animal models of cirrhosis (82), but it may be contraindicated in the human disease, because blockade of the V1a receptor may potentially provoke the hepatorenal syndrome. However, the dual-receptor activity may be particularly

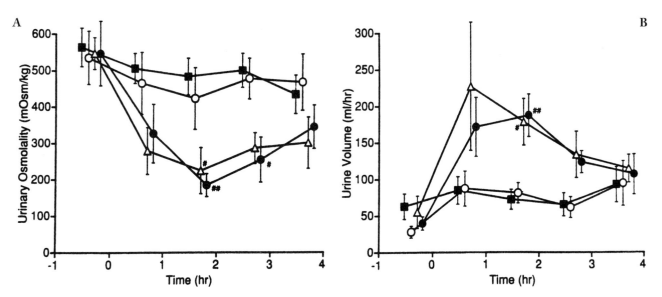

FIGURE 8   Response to V2 receptor blocker in patients with syndrome of inappropriate antidiuretic hormone secretion (SIADH) (222). The figure depicts urine osmolality **(A)** and volume **(B)** in control subjects (*closed squares*) and in patients with SIADH given OPC-31260 intravenously in three doses: 0.1 mg/kg (*open circles*), 0.25 mg/kg (*open triangles*), and 0.5 mg/kg (*closed circles*). The urine osmolality falls significantly below control values and urine volume increases significantly above control values after 1 hour at the two higher doses of the drug.

useful in patients with CHF because of afterload reduction from V1a receptor blockade combined with reduced cardiac preload and increased sodium concentrations induced by V2-receptor antagonism (96, 288).

Because these agents cause a brisk and relatively prolonged water diuresis, V2-receptor antagonists may risk overly rapid correction and osmotic demyelinization if they are used to treat severe chronic hyponatremia. Indeed, in an experimental model of chronic hyponatremia, increasing the plasma sodium concentration with a V2-receptor antagonist was comparable to hypertonic saline in causing osmotic demyelination (298).

Therapeutic Guidelines

The proper treatment of hyponatremia is a controversial topic that has been extensively reviewed (4, 26, 250, 265, 267-269). There is a general consensus that the dangers of cerebral edema and seizures mandate prompt and definitive treatment with one of the previously described modalities to ensure that the plasma sodium concentration begins to return to normal. Initial therapy in patients with acute hyponatremia or severe symptoms should probably begin with a bolus infusion of 1 to 2 ml/kg body weight of 3% saline, aiming for an increase of 1 to 2 mEq/l (121). Therapy in all patients should be limited to avoid iatrogenic injury. Many investigators argue that correction should not exceed 10 mEq/l in a single day or 18 mEq/l in 2 days because these rates are sometimes harmful in susceptible patients and have no proven advantage over more limited correction. All investigators agree that correction should not exceed 20 mEq/l in a single day or 25 mEq/L in 2 days because these rates of correction are associated with a high incidence of severe and permanent brain damage. It should be emphasized that these are limits and not therapeutic goals; given the risks of severe neurological injury, and the danger of inadvertently "overshooting the mark" owing to an unexpected water diuresis, therapeutic regimens should be targeted at an increase of 8 mEq/l/day, with adjustments based on frequent measurements of the serum sodium concentration (4).

NONHYPOTONIC HYPONATREMIA

Pseudohyponatremia

Plasma is normally 93% water. Thus, a sodium concentration of 143 mEq/l in a sample of whole plasma reflects a sodium concentration of 154 mEq/l in plasma water (143/0.93 = 154). Physiologic saline solutions (for example, 0.9% NaCl) were designed to reproduce the sodium concentration in plasma water.

Pseudohyponatremia is an exaggeration of the physiologic dilution of plasma sodium by nonaqueous material. High concentrations of intravascular protein (as in multiple myeloma) or lipid "dilute" the plasma sodium concentration, but do not alter the solute concentrations of the intracellular

or interstitial fluid compartments. Because the "diluent" in these conditions is nonaqueous, the sodium concentration of the aqueous portion of a plasma sample, as determined by an ion-specific electrode in undiluted serum or plasma, is normal (287, 305). Plasma osmolality, as measured by an osmometer, is also normal. Thus, hyponatremia associated with hyperlipidemia or hyperproteinemia, can be considered artifactual, and is called "pseudo-hyponatremia." Laboratory determinations which depend on a diluting step yield artifactually low sodium concentrations in samples taken from patients with severe hyperlipidemia or plasma cell dyscrasias even if the instrument uses an ion-specific electrode (155, 287). In these disorders, the plasma aliquot obtained for dilution contains less plasma water (and therefore less sodium) than normal; the sodium concentration in the diluted sample is thus artifactually reduced.

Hypertonic and Isotonic Hyponatremia

PATHOPHYSIOLOGY

If nonpermeant solutes other than sodium salts accumulate in the extracellular space, the extracellular fluid volume expands, reducing the concentration of the sodium normally present in this fluid compartment. Plasma osmolality varies, depending on the cause of the syndrome.

Retention of a sodium-free isotonic solution (e.g., infusion of isotonic mannitol in a patient with renal insufficiency who excretes the solute slowly) causes isotonic hyponatremia. Mannitol, a solute that is unable to permeate cell membranes, is confined to the extracellular space; the fluid infused with the solute is similarly confined (191). Thus, the extracellular fluid expands, and the intracellular compartment is unaffected. Sodium-free hypotonic solutions containing impermeant solutes can be considered isotonic solutions to which water has been added; hyponatremia caused by these solutions is primarily extracellular, but plasma osmolality is slightly reduced and the intracellular compartment is slightly diluted.

Retention of a sodium-free hypertonic solution (e.g., infusion of hypertonic mannitol) causes hypertonic hyponatremia. In this case, intracellular water is osmotically drawn to the extracellular fluid compartment, compounding the dilution of extracellular sodium caused by the infused diluent. Thus, the sodium concentration of the extracellular space is reduced while the osmolality of both extracellular and intracellular fluid compartments is increased (262). A similar phenomenon has been described after administration of IgG solutions containing maltose or sucrose (204).

HYPERGLYCEMIA

Glucose normally contributes only 5 mOsm/l to plasma osmolality. The osmotic importance of glucose increases dramatically in patients with diabetic hyperglycemia. As glucose cannot permeate most cell membranes without insulin, hyperglycemia attracts intracellular water to the extracellular space, causing hyponatremia despite hyperosmolality of both extracellular and intracellular fluid compartments. Several correction factors have been offered to quantify this relationship (219). However, a precise correction factor is probably unobtainable because in practice, hyperglycemia develops, in part, from the ingestion of glucose with water and resolves, in part, from the urinary excretion of glucose with water (52). As a rough estimate, assume that the serum sodium concentration is lowered by 2 mEq/l for every 100-mg/dl increase in blood glucose.

IRRIGANT ABSORPTION SYNDROME

Until recently, fluid used to irrigate the operative field during transurethral resection of the prostate (TURP) and hysteroscopy had to be electrolyte free (130). To avoid hemolysis, isosmotic to slightly hypo-osmotic solutions of mannitol, sorbitol, or glycine have been used. Several liters of irrigant may be absorbed systemically during these procedures, causing profound hyponatremia (97, 107, 118). There are fundamental differences between irrigant absorption hyponatremia and postoperative hypotonic hyponatremia.

The most commonly used irrigant is 1.5% (200 mOsm/ kg) glycine. Unlike patients dying of water intoxication, cerebral edema is not a prominent finding after systemic absorption of glycine irrigant, and, in contrast to water intoxication, plasma osmolality is only mildly decreased despite severe hyponatremia (5, 36). Glycine and its metabolites, primarily serine and glucose, remain in the plasma for hours after absorption, contributing to plasma osmolality (5, 6).

Studies in experimental animals indicate that isosmotic (2.2%) glycine is initially confined to the extracellular space, markedly diluting the plasma sodium concentration without changing plasma osmolality (233). As the amino acid enters skeletal muscle cells, carrying water with it, the plasma sodium concentration increases, but plasma osmolality remains constant owing to increased plasma levels of glycine, serine and other amino acids, urea, and glucose; in the absence of hypo-osmolality, brain water content increased only slightly because glycine did not enter the brain (Fig. 9) (233). Toxicity from glycine or its metabolites, rather than hyponatremia, may contribute to the neurologic symptoms that develop after irrigant absorption. Glycine is a major inhibitory transmitter in retina, and visual hallucinations and transient blindness may occur even in the absence of hyponatremia after prostatectomy using glycine irrigant (179). Plasma ammonia levels increase in glycine infused animals and in humans who have absorbed glycine irrigant (5, 131). In brain, ammonia is metabolized by glutamine synthase to form glutamine which may serve to protect the brain from the effects of hyperammonemia in liver failure (213). In animals infused with isosmotic glycine, increased brain glutamine may contribute to the small increase in brain water content occurs (233). Levels of ammonia, a major metabolite of glycine, have correlated with neurologic symptoms in some but not all studies.

New resectoscopes that permit endoscopic surgery using isotonic saline have become available. As their use becomes more widespread, it is likely that irrigant absorption

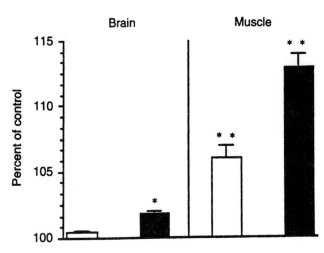

FIGURE 9 Muscle and brain water contents in experimental irrigant absorption syndrome (233). The figure depicts measurements of brain and skeletal muscle tissue water contents, expressed as a percentage of normonatremic controls, made in ureter-ligated rats, 2 hours after infusion of intravenous infusion of isotonic mannitol (open bars) or glycine (black bars). Brain water content is only slightly higher after infusion of glycine than after infusion of mannitol (reflecting minimal but statistically significant penetration of the blood-brain barrier by glycine), and muscle water content is markedly higher in glycine infused animals, reflected the diffusion of glycine into muscle cells.

syndromes, though fascinating, will be relegated to historical interest (130).

HYPEROSMOLALITY WITHOUT HYPONATREMIA

Increased concentrations of permeant solutes like urea or ethanol do not affect the distribution of water in body fluid compartments and do not cause hyponatremia. However, these solutes increase the plasma osmolality and may cause diagnostic confusion if they are present in patients with hypotonic hyponatremia from other causes.

References

1. Abramow M, Cogan E. Clinical aspects and pathophysiology of diuretic-induced hyponatremia. *Adv Nephrol Necker Hosp* 1984;13:1–28.
2. Adams RD, Victor M, Mancall EL. Central pontine myelinolysis: a hitherto undescribed disease occurring in alcoholic and malnourished patients. *AMA Arch Neurol Psychiatry* 1959;81:154–172.
3. Adler S, Martinez J, Williams DS, Verbalis JG. Positive association between blood brain barrier disruption and osmotically-induced demyelination. *Mult Scler* 2000;6:24–31.
4. Adrogue HJ, Madias NE. Hyponatremia. *N Engl J Med* 2000;342:1581–1589.
5. Agarwal R, Emmett M. The post-transurethral resection of prostate syndrome: therapeutic proposals. *Am J Kidney Dis* 1994;24:108–111.
6. Agraharkar M, Agraharkar A. Posthysteroscopic hyponatremia: evidence for a multifactorial cause. *Am J Kidney Dis* 1997;30:717–719.
7. Anderson RJ, Chung HM, Kluge R, Schrier RW. Hyponatremia: a prospective analysis of its epidemiology and the pathogenetic role of vasopressin. *Ann Intern Med* 1985;102:164–168.
8. Antunes-Rodrigues J, de Castro M, Elias LL, McCann SM. Neuroendocrine control of body fluid metabolism. *Physiol Rev* 2004;84:169–208.
9. Arieff AI. Hyponatremia, convulsions, respiratory arrest, and permanent brain damage after elective surgery in healthy women. *N Engl J Med* 1986;314:1529–1535.
10. Arieff AI, Ayus JC, Fraser CL. Hyponatraemia and death or permanent brain damage in healthy children. *BMJ* 1992;304:1218–1222.
11. Arieff AI, Kozniewska E, Roberts TP, Vexler ZS, Ayus JC, Kucharczyk J. Age, gender, and vasopressin affect survival and brain adaptation in rats with metabolic encephalopathy. *Am J Physiol* 1995;268(Pt 2):R1143–1152.

12. Ashraf N, Locksley R, Arieff AI. Thiazide-induced hyponatremia associated with death or neurologic damage in outpatients. *Am J Med* 1981;70:1163–1168.
13. Aslam MK, Gnaim C, Kutnick J, Kowal RC, McGuire DK. Syndrome of inappropriate antidiuretic hormone secretion induced by amiodarone therapy. *Pacing Clin Electrophysiol* 2004;27(Pt 1):831–832.
14. Ayus JC, Arieff AI. Pulmonary complications of hyponatremic encephalopathy. Noncardiogenic pulmonary edema and hypercapnic respiratory failure. *Chest* 1995;107:517–521.
15. Ayus JC, Krothapalli RK, Armstrong DL. Rapid correction of severe hyponatremia in the rat: histopathological changes in the brain. *Am J Physiol* 1985;248(Pt 2):F711–719.
16. Ayus JC, Krothapalli RK, Armstrong DL, Norton HJ. Symptomatic hyponatremia in rats: effect of treatment on mortality and brain lesions. *Am J Physiol* 1989;257(Pt 2):F18–22.
17. Ayus JC, Wheeler JM, Arieff AI. Postoperative hyponatremic encephalopathy in menstruant women. *Ann Intern Med* 1992;117:891–897.
18. Batra VK, Mathur M, Mir SA, Kapoor R, Kumar MA. Pneumadin: a new lung peptide which triggers antidiuresis. *Regul Pept* 1990;30:77–87.
19. Baylis PH, Thompson CJ. Osmoregulation of vasopressin secretion and thirst in health and disease. *Clin Endocrinol (Oxf)* 1988;29:549–576.
20. Beck LH. Hypouricemia in the syndrome of inappropriate secretion of antidiuretic hormone. *N Engl J Med* 1979;301:528–530.
21. Beermann B. Thiazides and loop-diuretics therapeutic aspects. *Acta Med Scand Suppl* 1986; 707:75–78.
22. Benrabh H, Bourre JM, Lefauconnier JM. Taurine transport at the blood-brain barrier: an in vivo brain perfusion study. *Brain Res* 1995;692:57–65.
23. Berendes E, Walter M, Cullen P, Prien T, Van Aken H, Horsthemke J, Schulte M, von Wild K, Scherer R. Secretion of brain natriuretic peptide in patients with aneurysmal subarachnoid haemorrhage. *Lancet* 1997;349:245–249.
24. Beresford HR. Polydipsia, hydrochlorothiazide, and water intoxication. *JAMA* 1970;214: 879–883.
25. Berghorn KA, Knapp LT, Hoffman GE, Sherman TG. Induction of glucocorticoid receptor expression in hypothalamic magnocellular vasopressin neurons during chronic hypoosmolality. *Endocrinology* 1995;136:804–807.
26. Berl T. Treating hyponatremia: damned if we do and damned if we don't. *Kidney Int* 1990; 37:1006–1018.
27. Blaustein DA, Schwenk MH. "Beer potomania" in a non-beer drinker. *Clin Nephrol* 1997;48:203–204.
28. Bliss DP, Jr., Battey JF, Linnoila RI, Birrer MJ, Gazdar AF, Johnson BE. Expression of the atrial natriuretic factor gene in small cell lung cancer tumors and tumor cell lines. *J Natl Cancer Inst* 1990;82:305–310.
29. Booker JA. Severe symptomatic hyponatremia in elderly outpatients: the role of thiazide therapy and stress. *J Am Geriatr Soc* 1984;32:108–113.
30. Boykin J, DeTorrente A, Erikson A, Robertson G, Schrier R. Role of vasopressin in impaired water excretion of glucocorticoid deficiency. *J Clin Invest* 1978;62:738–744.
31. Brater DC. Drug-induced electrolyte disorders and use of diuretics. In: Kokko JP, Tannen RL, eds. *Fluids and Electrolytes,* 3rd ed. Philadelphia: WB Saunders; 1996:693–728.
32. Brown WD. Osmotic demyelination disorders: central pontine and extrapontine myelinolysis. *Curr Opin Neurol* 2000;13:691–697.
33. Bruce RC, Kliegman RM. Hyponatremic seizures secondary to oral water intoxication in infancy: association with commercial bottled drinking water. *Pediatrics* 1997;100:E4.
34. Brvar M, Kozelj G, Osredkar J, Mozina M, Gricar M, Bunc M. Polydipsia as another mechanism of hyponatremia after 'ecstasy' (3,4 methyldioxymethamphetamine) ingestion. *Eur J Emerg Med* 2004;11:302–304.
35. Callreus T, Ekman E, Andersen M. Hyponatremia in elderly patients treated with desmopressin for nocturia: a review of a case series. *Eur J Clin Pharmacol* 2005;61:281–284.
36. Campbell HT, Fincher ME, Sklar AH. Severe hyponatremia without severe hypoosmolality following transurethral resection of the prostate (TURP) in end-stage renal disease. *Am J Kidney Dis* 1988;12:152–155.
37. Campling BG, Sarda IR, Baer KA, Pang SC, Baker HM, Lofters WS, Flynn TG. Secretion of atrial natriuretic peptide and vasopressin by small cell lung cancer. *Cancer* 1995;75:2442–2451.
38. Carlotti AP, Bohn D, Rutka JT, Singh S, Berry WA, Sharman A, Cusimano M, Halperin ML. A method to estimate urinary electrolyte excretion in patients at risk for developing cerebral salt wasting. *J Neurosurg* 2001;95:420–424.
39. Cauchie P, Vincken W, Decaux G. Urea treatment for water retention in hyponatremic congestive heart failure. *Int J Cardiol* 1987;17:102–104.
40. Celik US, Alabaz D, Yildizdas D, Alhan E, Kocabas E, Ulutan S. Cerebral salt wasting in tuberculous meningitis: treatment with fludrocortisone. *Ann Trop Paediatr* 2005;25:297–302.
41. Chan TY. Drug-induced syndrome of inappropriate antidiuretic hormone secretion. Causes, diagnosis and management. *Drugs Aging* 1997;11:27–44.
42. Chow KM, Kwan BC, Szeto CC. Clinical studies of thiazide-induced hyponatremia. *J Natl Med Assoc* 2004;96:1305–1308.
43. Chow KM, Szeto CC, Wong TY, Leung CB, Li PK. Risk factors for thiazide-induced hyponatraemia. *QJM* 2003;96:911–917.
44. Chung HM, Kluge R, Schrier RW, Anderson RJ. Clinical assessment of extracellular fluid volume in hyponatremia. *Am J Med* 1987;83:905–908.
45. Clark BA, Shannon RP, Rosa RM, Epstein FH. Increased susceptibility to thiazide-induced hyponatremia in the elderly. *J Am Soc Nephrol* 1994;5:1106–1111.
46. Clark EC, Thomas D, Baer J, Sterns RH. Depletion of glutathione from brain cells in hyponatremia. *Kidney Int* 1996;49:470–476.
47. Clive DM, Stoff JS. Renal syndromes associated with nonsteroidal anti-inflammatory drugs. *N Engl J Med* 1984;310:563–572.
48. Cogan E, Abramow M. Diuretic-induced hyponatraemia in elderly hypertensive women. *Lancet* 1983;2:1249.
49. Cohen JJ, Hulter HN, Smithline N, Melby JC, Schwartz WB. The critical role of the adrenal gland in the renal regulation of acid-base equilibrium during chronic hypotonic expansion. Evidence that chronic hyponatremia is a potent stimulus to aldosterone secretion. *J Clin Invest* 1976;58:1201–1208.
50. Cooke CR, Turin MD, Walker WG. The syndrome of inappropriate antidiuretic hormone secretion (SIADH): pathophysiologic mechanisms in solute and volume regulation. *Medicine (Baltimore)* 1979;58:240–251.
51. Costello-Boerrigter LC, Smith WB, Boerrigter G, Ouyang J, Zimmer CA, Orlandi C, Burnett JC Jr. Vasopressin-2 receptor antagonism augments water excretion without changes in renal hemodynamics or sodium and potassium excretion in human heart failure. *Am J Physiol Renal Physiol* 2006;290:F273–F278.
52. Davids MR, Edoute Y, Stock S, Halperin ML. Severe degree of hyperglycaemia: insights from integrative physiology. *QJM* 2002;95:113–124.
53. de Leon J. Polydipsia—a study in a long-term psychiatric unit. *Eur Arch Psychiatry Clin Neurosci* 2003;253:37–39.
54. De Troyer A. Demeclocycline. Treatment for syndrome of inappropriate antidiuretic hormone secretion. *JAMA* 1977;237:2723–2726.
55. Decaux G, Genette F. Urea for long-term treatment of syndrome of inappropriate secretion of antidiuretic hormone. *Br Med J (Clin Res Ed)* 1981;283:1081–1083.
56. Decaux G, Musch W, Penninckx R, Soupart A. Low plasma bicarbonate level in hyponatremia related to adrenocorticotropin deficiency. *J Clin Endocrinol Metab* 2003;88:5255–5257.
57. DeFronzo RA, Goldberg M, Agus ZS. Normal diluting capacity in hyponatremic patients. Reset osmostat or a variant of the syndrome of inappropriate antidiuretic hormone secretion. *Ann Intern Med* 1976;84:538–542.
58. Diederich S, Franzen NF, Bahr V, Oelkers W. Severe hyponatremia due to hypopituitarism with adrenal insufficiency: report on 28 cases. *Eur J Endocrinol* 2003;148:609–617.
59. Diringer M, Ladenson PW, Stern BJ, Schleimer J, Hanley DF. Plasma atrial natriuretic factor and subarachnoid hemorrhage. *Stroke* 1988;19:1119–1124.
60. Diringer MN. Neuroendocrine regulation of sodium and volume following subarachnoid hemorrhage. *Clin Neuropharmacol* 1995;18:114–126.
61. Diringer MN, Kirsch JR, Ladenson PW, Borel C, Hanley DF. Cerebrospinal fluid atrial natriuretic factor in intracranial disease. *Stroke* 1990;21:1550–1554.
62. Diringer MN, Lim JS, Kirsch JR, Hanley DF. Suprasellar and intraventricular blood predict elevated plasma atrial natriuretic factor in subarachnoid hemorrhage. *Stroke* 1991;22:577–581.
63. Diringer MN, Wu KC, Verbalis JG, Hanley DF. Hypervolemic therapy prevents volume contraction but not hyponatremia following subarachnoid hemorrhage. *Ann Neurol* 1992;31: 543–550.
64. Dixon BS, Anderson RJ. Pneumonia and the syndrome of inappropriate antidiuretic hormone secretion: don't pour water on the fire. *Am Rev Respir Dis* 1988;138:512–513.
65. Dreyfuss D, Leviel F, Paillard M, Rahmani J, Coste F. Acute infectious pneumonia is accompanied by a latent vasopressin-dependent impairment of renal water excretion. *Am Rev Respir Dis* 1988;138:583–589.
66. Dyckner T, Wester PO. Effects of magnesium infusions in diuretic induced hyponatraemia. *Lancet* 1981;1(Pt 1):585–586.
67. Dzau VJ, Hollenberg NK. Renal response to captopril in severe heart failure: role of furosemide in natriuresis and reversal of hyponatremia. *Ann Intern Med* 1984;100:777–782.
68. Earley LE, Kahn M, Orloff J. The effects of infusions of chlorothiazide on urinary dilution and concentration in the dog. *J Clin Invest* 1961;40:857–866.
69. Ecelbarger CA, Murase T, Tian Y, Nielsen S, Knepper MA, Verbalis JG. Regulation of renal salt and water transporters during vasopressin escape. *Prog Brain Res* 2002;139:75–84.
70. Ecelbarger CA, Nielsen S, Olson BR, Murase T, Baker EA, Knepper MA, Verbalis JG. Role of renal aquaporins in escape from vasopressin-induced antidiuresis in rat. *J Clin Invest* 1997;99:1852–1863.
71. Edelman IS, Leibman J. Anatomy of body water and electrolytes. *Am J Med* 1959;27:256–277.
72. Edelman IS, Leibman J, O'Meara MW, Birkenfeld LW. Interrelations between serum sodium concentrations, serum osmolality and total exchangeable sodium, total exchangeable potassium and total body water. *J Clin Invest* 1958;37:1236–1256.
73. Elisaf M, Theodorou J, Pappas C, Siamopoulos K. Successful treatment of hyponatremia with angiotensin-converting enzyme inhibitors in patients with congestive heart failure. *Cardiology* 1995;86:477–480.
74. Emma F, McManus M, Strange K. Intracellular electrolytes regulate the volume set point of the organic osmolyte/anion channel VSOAC. *Am J Physiol* 1997;272(Pt 1):C1766–1775.
75. Epstein M. Derangements of renal water handling in liver disease. *Gastroenterology* 1985;89: 1415–1425.
76. Fabian TJ, Amico JA, Kroboth PD, Mulsant BH, Corey SE, Begley AE, Bensasi SG, Weber E, Dew MA, Reynolds CF 3rd, Pollock BG. Paroxetine-induced hyponatremia in older adults: a 12-week prospective study. *Arch Intern Med* 2004;164:327–332.
77. Fabian TJ, Amico JA, Kroboth PD, Mulsant BH, Reynolds CF 3rd, Pollock BG. Paroxetine-induced hyponatremia in the elderly due to the syndrome of inappropriate secretion of antidiuretic hormone (SIADH). *J Geriatr Psychiatry Neurol* 2003;16:160–164.
78. Farber MO, Weinberger MH, Robertson GL, Fineberg NS, Manfredi F. Hormonal abnormalities affecting sodium and water balance in acute respiratory failure due to chronic obstructive lung disease. *Chest* 1984;85:49–54.
79. Feldman BJ, Rosenthal SM, Vargas GA, Fenwick RG, Huang EA, Matsuda-Abedini M, Lustig RH, Mathias RS, Portale AA, Miller WL, Gitelman SE. Nephrogenic syndrome of inappropriate antidiuresis [see comment]. *N Engl J Med* 2005;352:1884–1890.
80. Fenves AZ, Thomas S, Knochel JP. Beer potomania: two cases and review of the literature. *Clin Nephrol* 1996;45:61–64.
81. Ferlito A, Rinaldo A, Devaney KO. Syndrome of inappropriate antidiuretic hormone secretion associated with head neck cancers: review of the literature. *Ann Otol Rhinol Laryngol* 1997;106(Pt 1):878–883.
82. Fernandez-Varo G, Ros J, Cejudo-Martin P, Cano C, Arroyo V, Rivera F, Rodes J, Jimenez W. Effect of the V1a/V2-AVP receptor antagonist, Conivaptan, on renal water metabolism and systemic hemodynamics in rats with cirrhosis and ascites. *J Hepatol* 2003;38:755–761.
83. Fichman MP, Vorherr H, Kleeman CR, Telfer N. Diuretic-induced hyponatremia. *Ann Intern Med* 1971;75:853–863.

84. Forrest JN, Jr., Cox M, Hong C, Morrison G, Bia M, Singer I. Superiority of demeclocycline over lithium in the treatment of chronic syndrome of inappropriate secretion of antidiuretic hormone. *N Engl J Med* 1978;298:173–177.

85. Francis GS, Benedict C, Johnstone DE, Kirlin PC, Nicklas J, Liang CS, Kubo SH, Rudin-Toretsky E, Yusuf S. Comparison of neuroendocrine activation in patients with left ventricular dysfunction with and without congestive heart failure. A substudy of the Studies of Left Ventricular Dysfunction (SOLVD). *Circulation* 1990;82:1724–1729.

86. Fraser CL, Arieff AI. Fatal central diabetes mellitus and insipidus resulting from untreated hyponatremia: a new syndrome. *Ann Intern Med* 1990;112:113–119.

87. Fraser CL, Kucharczyk J, Arieff AI, Rollin C, Sarnacki P, Norman D. Sex differences result in increased morbidity from hyponatremia in female rats. *Am J Physiol* 1989;256(Pt 2): R880–885.

88. Fraser CL, Swanson RA. Female sex hormones inhibit volume regulation in rat brain astrocyte culture. *Am J Physiol* 1994;267(Pt 1):C909–914.

89. Friedman E, Shadel M, Halkin H, Farfel Z. Thiazide-induced hyponatremia. Reproducibility by single dose rechallenge and an analysis of pathogenesis. *Ann Intern Med* 1989;110: 24–30.

90. Fuisz RE, Lauler DP, Cohen P. Diuretic-induced hyponatremia and sustained antidiuresis. *Am J Med* 1962;33:783–791.

91. Ganong CA, Kappy MS. Cerebral salt wasting in children. The need for recognition and treatment. *Am J Dis Child* 1993;147:167–169.

92. Gennari FJ. Current concepts. Serum osmolality. Uses and limitations. *N Engl J Med* 1984;310:102–105.

93. Gerbes AL, Gulberg V, Gines P, Decaux G, Gross P, Gandjini H, Djian J. Therapy of hyponatremia in cirrhosis with a vasopressin receptor antagonist: a randomized double-blind multicenter trial. *Gastroenterology* 2003;124:933–939.

94. Gheorghiade M, Gattis WA, O'Connor CM, Adams KF, Jr., Elkayam U, Barbagelata A, Ghali JK, Benza RL, McGrew FA, Klapholz M, Ouyang J, Orlandi C. Effects of tolvaptan, a vasopressin antagonist, in patients hospitalized with worsening heart failure: a randomized controlled trial. *JAMA* 2004;291:1963–1971.

95. Gines P, Berl T, Bernardi M, Bichet DG, Hamon G, Jimenez W, Liard JF, Martin PY, Schrier RW. Hyponatremia in cirrhosis: from pathogenesis to treatment. *Hepatology* 1998; 28:851–864.

96. Goldsmith SR. Current treatments and novel pharmacologic treatments for hyponatremia in congestive heart failure. *Am J Cardiol* 2005;95:14B–23B.

97. Gonzales R, Brensilver JM, Rovinsky JJ. Posthysteroscopic hyponatremia. *Am J Kidney Dis* 1994;23:735–738.

98. Gowrishankar M, Chen CB, Cheema-Dhadli S, Steele A, Halperin ML. Hyponatremia in the rat in the absence of positive water balance. *J Am Soc Nephrol* 1997;8:524–529.

99. Gowrishankar M, Chen CB, Mallie JP, Halperin ML. What is the impact of potassium excretion on the intracellular fluid volume: importance of urine anions. *Kidney Int* 1996;50:1490–1495.

100. Graber M, Corish D. The electrolytes in hyponatremia. *Am J Kidney Dis* 1991;18:527–545.

101. Grantham JJ, Brown RW, Schloerb PR. Asymptomatic hyponatremia and bronchogenic carcinoma: the deleterious effect of diuretics. *Am J Med Sci* 1965;249:273–279.

102. Greenberg A. Diuretic complications. *Am J Med Sci* 2000;319:10–24.

103. Gross AJ, Steinberg SM, Reilly JG, Bliss DP, Jr., Brennan J, Le PT, Simmons A, Phelps R, Mulshine JL, Ihde DC, et al. Atrial natriuretic factor and arginine vasopressin production in tumor cell lines from patients with lung cancer and their relationship to serum sodium. *Cancer Res* 1993; 53:67–74.

104. Gross P, Ketteler M, Hausmann C, Reinhard C, Schomig A, Hackenthal E, Ritz E, Rascher W. Role of diuretics, hormonal derangements, and clinical setting of hyponatremia in medical patients. *Klin Wochenschr* 1988;66:662–669.

105. Gross PA, Pehrisch H, Rascher W, Schomig A, Hackenthal E, Ritz E. Pathogenesis of clinical hyponatremia: observations of vasopressin and fluid intake in 100 hyponatremic medical patients. *Eur J Clin Invest* 1987;17:123–129.

106. Gullans SR, Verbalis JG. Control of brain volume during hyperosmolar and hypoosmolar conditions. *Annu Rev Med* 1993;44:289–301.

107. Hahn RG. The transurethral resection syndrome. *Acta Anaesthesiol Scand* 1991;35:557–567.

108. Hamburger S, Koprivica B, Ellerbeck E, Covinsky JO. Thiazide-induced syndrome of inappropriate secretion of antidiuretic hormone. Time course of resolution. *JAMA* 1981;246: 1235–1236.

109. Hanna FW, Scanlon MF. Hyponatraemia, hypothyroidism, and role of arginine-vasopressin. *Lancet* 1997;350:755–756.

110. Hantman D, Rossier B, Zohlman R, Schrier R. Rapid correction of hyponatremia in the syndrome of inappropriate secretion of antidiuretic hormone. An alternative treatment to hypertonic saline. *Ann Intern Med* 1973;78:870–875.

111. Harrington AR. Hyponatremia due to sodium depletion in the absence of vasopressin. *Am J Physiol* 1972;222:768–774.

112. Harrow AS. Beer potomania. *South Med J* 1995;88:602.

113. Hartung TK, Schofield E, Short AI, Parr MJ, Henry JA. Hyponatraemic states following 3,4-methylenedioxymethamphetamine (MDMA, 'ecstasy') ingestion. *QJM* 2002;95:431–437.

114. Hasan D, Lindsay KW, Wijdicks EF, Murray GD, Brouwers PJ, Bakker WH, van Gijn J, Vermeulen M. Effect of fludrocortisone acetate in patients with subarachnoid hemorrhage. *Stroke* 1989;20:1156–1161.

115. Hasan D, Wijdicks EF, Vermeulen M. Hyponatremia is associated with cerebral ischemia in patients with aneurysmal subarachnoid hemorrhage. *Ann Neurol* 1990;27:106–108.

116. Haussinger D, Laubenberger J, vom Dahl S, Ernst T, Bayer S, Langer M, Gerok W, Hennig J. Proton magnetic resonance spectroscopy studies on human brain myo-inositol in hypo-osmolarity and hepatic encephalopathy. *Gastroenterology* 1994;107:1475–1480.

117. Heinemann H, Demartini F, Laragh JH. The effect of chlorothiazide on renal excretion of electrolytes and free water. *Am J Med* 1959;26:853–861.

118. Henderson DJ, Middleton RG. Coma from hyponatremia following transurethral resection of prostate. *Urology* 1980;15:267–271.

119. Henry JA, Fallon JK, Kicman AT, Hutt AJ, Cowan DA, Forsling M. Low-dose MDMA ("ecstasy") induces vasopressin secretion. *Lancet* 1998;351:1784.

120. Hensen J, Haenelt M, Gross P. Water retention after oral chlorpropamide is associated with an increase in renal papillary arginine vasopressin receptors. *Eur J Endocrinol* 1995;132:459–464.

121. Hew-Butler T, Almond C, Ayus JC, Dugas J, Meeuwisse W, Noakes T, Reid S, Siegel A, Speedy D, Stuempfle K, Verbalis J, Weschler L. Consensus statement of the 1st International Exercise-Associated Hyponatremia Consensus Development Conference, Cape Town, South Africa 2005. *Clin J Sport Med* 2005;15:208–213.

122. Hill AR, Uribarri J, Mann J, Berl T. Altered water metabolism in tuberculosis: role of vasopressin. *Am J Med* 1990;88:357–364.

123. Hochman I, Cabili S, Peer G. Hyponatremia in internal medicine ward patients: causes, treatment and prognosis. *Isr J Med Sci* 1989;25:73–76.

124. Horowitz J, Keynan A, Ben-Ishay D. A syndrome of inappropriate ADH secretion induced by cyclothiazide. *J Clin Pharmacol New Drugs* 1972;12:337–341.

125. Ibsen L, Strange K. In situ localization and osmotic regulation of the Na(+)-myo-inositol cotransporter in rat brain. *Am J Physiol* 1996;271(Pt 2):F877–885.

126. Illowsky BP, Kirch DG. Polydipsia and hyponatremia in psychiatric patients. *Am J Psychiatry* 1988;145:675–683.

127. Illowsky BP, Laureno R. Encephalopathy and myelinolysis after rapid correction of hyponatraemia. *Brain* 1987;110(Pt 4):855–867.

128. Ishikawa S, Schrier R. Effect of arginine vasopressin antagonist on renal water excretion in glucocorticoid and mineralocorticoid deficient rats. *Kidney Int* 1982;22:587–593.

129. Ishikawa SE, Saito T, Kaneko K, Okada K, Kuzuya T. Hyponatremia responsive to fludrocortisone acetate in elderly patients after head injury. *Ann Intern Med* 1987;106:187–191.

130. Issa MM, Young MR, Bullock AR, Bouet R, Petros JA. Dilutional hyponatremia of TURP syndrome: a historical event in the 21st century. *Urology* 2004;64:298–301.

131. Istre O, Jellum E, Skajaa K, Forman A. Changes in amino acids, ammonium, and coagulation factors after transcervical resection of the endometrium with a glycine solution used for uterine irrigation. *Am J Obstet Gynecol* 1995;172:939–945.

132. Iwasaki Y, Oiso Y, Yamauchi K, Takatsuki K, Kondo K, Hasegawa H, Tomita A. Osmoregulation of plasma vasopressin in myxedema. *J Clin Endocrinol Metab* 1990;70:534–539.

133. Jaenike JR, Waterhouse C. The renal response to sustained administration of vasopressin and water in man. *J Clin Endocrinol Metab* 1961;21:231–242.

134. Januezewicz W, Heinemann H, Demartini F, Laragh J. A clinical study of the effects of hydrochlorothiazide on the renal excretion of electrolytes and free water. *N Engl J Med* 1959;261:264–269.

135. Johnson BE, Chute JP, Rushin J, Williams J, Le PT, Venzon D, Richardson GE. A prospective study of patients with lung cancer and hyponatremia of malignancy. *Am J Respir Crit Care Med* 1997;156:1669–1678.

136. Karp BI, Laureno R. Pontine and extrapontine myelinolysis: a neurologic disorder following rapid correction of hyponatremia. *Medicine (Baltimore)* 1993;72:359–373.

137. Kawai N, Baba A, Suzuki T, Shiraishi H. Roles of arginine vasopressin and atrial natriuretic peptide in polydipsia-hyponatremia of schizophrenic patients. *Psychiatry Res* 2001;101:39–45.

138. Keating JP, Schears GJ, Dodge PR. Oral water intoxication in infants. An American epidemic. *Am J Dis Child* 1991;145:985–990.

139. Kennedy PG, Mitchell DM, Hoffbrand BI. Severe hyponatraemia in hospital inpatients. *Br Med J* 1978;2:1251–1253.

140. Kennedy RM, Earley LE. Profound hyponatremia resulting from a thiazide-induced decrease in urinary diluting capacity in a patient with primary polydipsia. *N Engl J Med* 1970;282: 1185–1186.

141. Kiss JZ, Van Eekelen JA, Reul JM, Westphal HM, De Kloet ER. Glucocorticoid receptor in magnocellular neurosecretory cells. *Endocrinology* 1988;122:444–449.

142. Kitiyakara C, Wilcox CS. Vasopressin V2-receptor antagonists: panaceas for hyponatremia? *Curr Opin Nephrol Hypertens* 1997;6:461–467.

143. Kleinschmidt-DeMasters BK, Norenberg MD. Neuropathologic observations in electrolyte-induced myelinolysis in the rat. *J Neuropathol Exp Neurol* 1982;41:67–80.

144. Kleinschmidt-DeMasters BK, Norenberg MD. Rapid correction of hyponatremia causes demyelination: relation to central pontine myelinolysis. *Science* 1981;211:1068–1070.

145. Knepper MA, Verbalis JG, Nielsen S. Role of aquaporins in water balance disorders. *Curr Opin Nephrol Hypertens* 1997;6:367–371.

146. Knochel JP. Hypoxia is the cause of brain damage in hyponatremia. *JAMA* 1999;281 (24):2342–2343.

147. Kojima J, Katayama Y, Moro N, Kawai H, Yoneko M, Mori T. Cerebral salt wasting in subarachnoid hemorrhage rats: model, mechanism, and tool. *Life Sci* 2005;76:2361–2370.

148. Kone B, Gimenez L, Watson AJ. Thiazide-induced hyponatremia. *South Med J* 1986;79: 1456–1457.

149. Kosowicz J, Miskowiak B, Konwerska A, Tortorella C, Nussdorfer GG, Malendowicz LK. Tissue distribution of pneumadin immunoreactivity in the rat. *Peptides* 2003;24:215–220.

150. Kristeller JL, Sterns RH. Transient diabetes insipidus after discontinuation of therapeutic vasopressin. *Pharmacotherapy* 2004;24:541–545.

151. Kroll M, Juhler M, Lindholm J. Hyponatraemia in acute brain disease. *J Intern Med* 1992;232:291–297.

152. Kuncz A, Doczi T, Bodosi M. The effect of skull and dura on brain volume regulation after hypo- and hyperosmolar fluid treatment. *Neurosurgery* 1990;27:509–514; discussion 514–515.

153. Kurokawa Y, Uede T, Ishiguro M, Honda O, Honmou O, Kato T, Wanibuchi M. Pathogenesis of hyponatremia following subarachnoid hemorrhage due to ruptured cerebral aneurysm. *Surg Neurol* 1996;46:500–507; discussion 507–508.

154. Kwon TH, Hager H, Nejsum LN, Andersen ML, Frokiaer J, Nielsen S. Physiology and pathophysiology of renal aquaporins. *Semin Nephrol* 2001;21:231–238.

155. Ladenson JH, Apple FS, Koch DD. Misleading hyponatremia due to hyperlipemia: a method-dependent error. *Ann Intern Med* 1981;95:707–708.

156. Laureno R. Central pontine myelinolysis following rapid correction of hyponatremia. *Ann Neurol* 1983;13:232–242.

157. Laureno R, Karp BI. Myelinolysis after correction of hyponatremia. *Ann Intern Med* 1997;126:57–62.
158. Leaf A, Bartter FC, Santos RF, Wrong O. Evidence in man that urinary electrolyte loss induced by pitressin is a function of water retention. *J Clin Invest* 1953;32:868–878.
159. Legros JJ, Geenen V, Carvelli T, Martens H, Andre M, Corhay JL, Radermecker M, Zangerle PF, Sassolas G, Gharib C, et al. Neurophysins as markers of vasopressin and oxytocin release. A study in carcinoma of the lung. *Horm Res* 1990;34:151–155.
160. Lien YH. Role of organic osmolytes in myelinolysis. A topographic study in rats after rapid correction of hyponatremia. *J Clin Invest* 95:1579–1586, 1995.
161. Lien YH, Shapiro JI, Chan L. Study of brain electrolytes and organic osmolytes during correction of chronic hyponatremia. Implications for the pathogenesis of central pontine myelinolysis. *J Clin Invest* 1991;88:303–309.
162. List AF, Hainsworth JD, Davis BW, Hande KR, Greco FA, Johnson DH. The syndrome of inappropriate secretion of antidiuretic hormone (SIADH) in small-cell lung cancer. *J Clin Oncol* 1986;4:1191–1198.
163. Liu BA, Mittmann N, Knowles SR, Shear NH. Hyponatremia and the syndrome of inappropriate secretion of antidiuretic hormone associated with the use of selective serotonin reuptake inhibitors: a review of spontaneous reports. *CMAJ* 1996;155:519–527.
164. Loffing J. Paradoxical antidiuretic effect of thiazides in diabetes insipidus: another piece in the puzzle[comment]. *J Am Soc Nephrol* 2004;15:2948–2950.
165. Lohr JW. Osmotic demyelination syndrome following correction of hyponatremia: association with hypokalemia. *Am J Med* 1994;96:408–413.
166. Lolin Y, Jackowski A. Hyponatraemia in neurosurgical patients: diagnosis using derived parameters of sodium and water homeostasis. *Br J Neurosurg* 1992;6:457–466.
167. Maesaka JK, Batuman V, Yudd M, Salem M, Sved AF, Venkatesan J. Hyponatremia and hypouricemia: differentiation from SIADH. *Clin Nephrol* 1990;33:174–178.
168. Maroon JC, Nelson PB. Hypovolemia in patients with subarachnoid hemorrhage: therapeutic implications. *Neurosurgery* 1979;4:223–226.
169. Martin PY, Gines P, Schrier RW. Nitric oxide as a mediator of hemodynamic abnormalities and sodium and water retention in cirrhosis. *N Engl J Med* 1998;339:533–541.
170. Martin PY, Schrier RW. Pathogenesis of water and sodium retention in cirrhosis. *Kidney Int Suppl* 1997;59:S43–49.
171. Martin RJ. Central pontine and extrapontine myelinolysis: the osmotic demyelination syndromes. *J Neurol Neurosurg Psychiatry* 2004;75(Suppl 3):iii22–28.
172. Maurer LH, O'Donnell JF, Kennedy S, Faulkner CS, Rist K, North WG. Human neurophysins in carcinoma of the lung: relation to histology, disease stage, response rate, survival, and syndrome of inappropriate antidiuretic hormone secretion. *Cancer Treat Rep* 1983;67: 971–976.
173. McGirt MJ, Blessing R, Nimjee SM, Friedman AH, Alexander MJ, Laskowitz DT, Lynch JR. Correlation of serum brain natriuretic peptide with hyponatremia and delayed ischemic neurological deficits after subarachnoid hemorrhage. *Neurosurgery* 2004;54:1369-73; discussion 1373–1374.
174. McManus ML, Churchwell KB, Strange K. Regulation of cell volume in health and disease. *N Engl J Med* 1995;333:1260–1266.
175. Mendoza SA, Brown CFJ. Effect of chlorpropamide on osmotic water flow across toad bladder and the response to vasopressin, theophylline and cyclic AMP. *J Clin Endocrinol Metab* 1974;38:883–889.
176. Mercier-Guidez E, Loas G. Polydipsia and water intoxication in 353 psychiatric inpatients: an epidemiological and psychopathological study. *Eur Psychiatry* 2000;15:306–311.
177. Miller GM, Baker HL, Jr., Okazaki H, Whisnant JP. Central pontine myelinolysis and its imitators: MR findings. *Radiology* 1988;168:795–802.
178. Miller PD, Linas SL, Schrier RW. Plasma demeclocycline levels and nephrotoxicity. Correlation in hyponatremic cirrhotic patients. *JAMA* 1980;243:2513–2515.
179. Mizutani AR, Parker J, Katz J, Schmidt J. Visual disturbances, serum glycine levels and transurethral resection of the prostate. *J Urol* 1990;144:697–699.
180. Moses AM, Miller M. Drug-induced dilutional hyponatremia. *N Engl J Med* 1974;291: 1234–1239.
181. Moses AM, Scheinman SJ. Ectopic secretion of neurohypophyseal peptides in patients with malignancy. *Endocrinol Metab Clin North Am* 1991;20:489–506.
182. Murase T, Tian Y, Fang XY, Verbalis JG. Synergistic effects of nitric oxide and prostaglandins on renal escape from vasopressin-induced antidiuresis. *Am J Physiol Regul Integr Comp Physiol* 2003;284:R354–362.
183. Narins RG, Jones ER, Stom MC, Rudnick MR, Bastl CP. Diagnostic strategies in disorders of fluid, electrolyte and acid-base homeostasis. *Am J Med* 1982;72:496–520.
184. Neafsey PJ. Thiazides and selective serotonin reuptake inhibitors can induce hyponatremia. *Home Healthc Nurse* 2004;22:788–790.
185. Nelson PB, Seif S, Gutai J, Robinson AG. Hyponatremia and natriuresis following subarachnoid hemorrhage in a monkey model. *J Neurosurg* 1984;60:233–7.
186. Nelson PB, Seif SM, Maroon JC, Robinson AG. Hyponatremia in intracranial disease: perhaps not the syndrome of inappropriate secretion of antidiuretic hormone (SIADH). *J Neurosurg* 1981;55:938–941.
187. Nelson RJ. Blood volume measurement following subarachnoid haemorrhage. *Acta Neurochir Suppl (Wien)* 1990;47:114–121.
188. Newell KL, Kleinschmidt-DeMasters BK. Central pontine myelinolysis at autopsy; a twelve year retrospective analysis. *J Neurol Sci* 1996;142:134–139.
189. Nguyen MK, Kurtz I. New insights into the pathophysiology of the dysnatremias: a quantitative analysis. *Am J Physiol Renal Physiol* 2004;287:F172–180.
190. Nguyen MK, Kurtz I. Role of potassium in hypokalemia-induced hyponatremia: lessons learned from the Edelman equation. *Clin Exp Nephrol* 2004;8:98–102.
191. Nissenson AR, Weston RE, Kleeman CR. Mannitol. *West J Med* 1979;131:277–284.
192. Norenberg MD, Leslie KO, Robertson AS. Association between rise in serum sodium and central pontine myelinolysis. *Ann Neurol* 1982;11:128–135.
193. Norenberg MD, Papendick RE. Chronicity of hyponatremia as a factor in experimental myelinolysis. *Ann Neurol* 1984;15:544–547.
194. North WG, Friedmann AS, Yu X. Tumor biosynthesis of vasopressin and oxytocin. *Ann N Y Acad Sci* 1993;689:107–121.
195. Oelkers W. Hyponatremia and inappropriate secretion of vasopressin (antidiuretic hormone) in patients with hypopituitarism. *N Engl J Med* 1989;321:492–496.
196. Olchovsky D, Ezra D, Vered I, Hadani M, Shimon I. Symptomatic hyponatremia as a presenting sign of hypothalamic-pituitary disease: a syndrome of inappropriate secretion of antidiuretic hormone (SIADH)-like glucocorticosteroid responsive condition. *J Endocrinol Inves* 2005;28:151–156.
197. Olson JE, Banks M, Dimlich RV, Evers J. Blood-brain barrier water permeability and brain osmolyte content during edema development. *Acad Emerg Med* 1997;4:662–673.
198. Oren RM. Hyponatremia in congestive heart failure. *Am J Cardiol* 2005;95:2B–7B.
199. Oropello JM, Weiner L, Benjamin E. Hypertensive, hypervolemic, hemodilutional therapy for aneurysmal subarachnoid hemorrhage. Is it efficacious? No. *Crit Care Clin* 1996;12:709–730.
200. Oster JR, Perez GO, Larios O, Emery WE, Bourgoignie JJ. Cerebral salt wasting in a man with carcinomatous meningitis. *Arch Intern Med* 1983;143:2187–2188.
201. Oya S, Tsutsumi K, Ueki K, Kirino T. Reinduction of hyponatremia to treat central pontine myelinolysis. *Neurology* 2001;57:1931–1932.
202. Packer M, Lee WH, Kessler PD, Gottlieb SS, Bernstein JL, Kukin ML. Role of neurohormonal mechanisms in determining survival in patients with severe chronic heart failure. *Circulation* 1987;75(Pt 2):IV80–92.
203. Packer M, Medina N, Yushak M. Correction of dilutional hyponatremia in severe chronic heart failure by converting-enzyme inhibition. *Ann Intern Med* 1984;100:782–789.
204. Palevsky PM, Rendulic D, Diven WF. Maltose-induced hyponatremia. *Ann Intern Med* 1993;118:526–528.
205. Palmer BF. Hyponatremia in patients with central nervous system disease: SIADH versus CSW. *Trends Endocrinol Metab* 2003;14:182–187.
206. Papanek PE, Sladek CD, Raff H. Corticosterone inhibition of osmotically stimulated vasopressin from hypothalamic-neurohypophysial explants. *Am J Physiol* 1997;272(Pt 2):R158–162.
207. Perez-Ayuso RM, Arroyo V, Camps J, Jimenez W, Rodamilans M, Rimola A, Gaya J, Rivera F, Rodes J. Effect of demeclocycline on renal function and urinary prostaglandin E2 and kallikrein in hyponatremic cirrhotics. *Nephron* 1984;36:30–37.
208. Peruzzi WT, Shapiro BA, Meyer PR, Jr., Krumlovsky F, Seo BW. Hyponatremia in acute spinal cord injury. *Crit Care Med* 1994;22:252–258.
209. Peters JP, Welt LG, Sims EA, Orloff J, Needham J. A salt-wasting syndrome associated with cerebral disease. *Trans Assoc Am Physicians* 1950;63:57–64.
210. Petersson I, Nilsson G, Hansson BG, Hedner T. Water intoxication associated with non-steroidal anti-inflammatory drug therapy. *Acta Med Scand* 1987;221:221–223.
211. Raymond KH, Lifschitz MD. Effect of prostaglandins on renal salt and water excretion. *Am J Med* 1986;80:22–33.
212. Reeder RF, Harbaugh RE. Administration of intravenous urea and normal saline for the treatment of hyponatremia in neurosurgical patients. *J Neurosurg* 1989;70:201–206.
213. Restuccia T, Gomez-Anson B, Guevara M, Alessandria C, Torre A, Alayrach ME, Terra C, Martin M, Castellvi M, Rami L, Sainz A, Gines P, Arroyo V. Effects of dilutional hyponatremia on brain organic osmolytes and water content in patients with cirrhosis. *Hepatology* 2004;39:1613–1622.
214. Riggs AT, Dysken MW, Kim SW, Opsahl JA. A review of disorders of water homeostasis in psychiatric patients. *Psychosomatics* 1991;32:133–48.
215. Robertson GL, Aycinena P, Zerbe RL. Neurogenic disorders of osmoregulation. *Am J Med* 1982;72:339–353.
216. Robertson GL, Ganguly A. Osmoregulation and baroregulation of plasma vasopressin in essential hypertension. *J Cardiovasc Pharmacol* 1986;8(Suppl 7):S87–91.
217. Rojiani AM, Cho ES, Sharer L, Prineas JW. Electrolyte-induced demyelination in rats. 2. Ultrastructural evolution. *Acta Neuropathol (Berl)* 1994;88:293–299.
218. Rojiani AM, Prineas JW, Cho ES. Electrolyte-induced demyelination in rats. 1. Role of the blood-brain barrier and edema. *Acta Neuropathol (Berl)* 1994;88:287–292.
219. Roscoe JM, Halperin ML, Rolleston FS, Goldstein MB. Hyperglycemia-induced hyponatremia: metabolic considerations in calculation of serum sodium depression. *Can Med Assoc J* 1975;112:452–453.
220. Rose BD. New approach to disturbances in the plasma sodium concentration. *Am J Med* 1986;81:1033–1040.
221. Ruzek KA, Campeau NG, Miller GM. Early diagnosis of central pontine myelinolysis with diffusion-weighted imaging. *AJNR Am J Neuroradiol* 2004;25:210–213.
222. Saito T, Ishikawa S, Abe K, Kamoi K, Yamada K, Shimizu K, Saruta T, Yoshida S. Acute aquaresis by the nonpeptide arginine vasopressin (AVP) antagonist OPC-31260 improves hyponatremia in patients with syndrome of inappropriate secretion of antidiuretic hormone (SIADH). *J Clin Endocrinol Metab* 1997;82:1054–1057.
223. Schaeffer AV, Ditchek S. Current social practices leading to water intoxication in infants. *Am J Dis Child* 1991;145:27–28.
224. Schrier RW. Pathogenesis of sodium and water retention in high-output and low-output cardiac failure, nephrotic syndrome, cirrhosis, and pregnancy (2). *N Engl J Med* 1988;319: 1127–1134.
225. Schrier RW, Gurevich AK, Cadnapaphornchai MA. Pathogenesis and management of sodium and water retention in cardiac failure and cirrhosis. *Semin Nephrol* 2001;21:157–172.
226. Schwartz WB, Bennett W, Curelop S, Bartter FC. A syndrome of renal sodium loss and hyponatremia probably resulting from inappropriate secretion of antidiuretic hormone. *Am J Med* 1957;23:529–5242.
227. Shafiee MA, Charest AF, Cheema-Dhadli S, Glick DN, Napolova O, Roozbeh J, Semenova E, Sharman A, Halperin ML. Defining conditions that lead to the retention of water: the importance of the arterial sodium concentration. *Kidney Int* 2005;67:613–621.
228. Shimoda M, Yamada S, Yamamoto I, Tsugane R, Sato O. Atrial natriuretic polypeptide in patients with subarachnoid haemorrhage due to aneurysmal rupture. Correlation to hyponatremia. *Acta Neurochir (Wien)* 1989;97:53–61.
229. Shimura N, Arisaka O. Urinary arginine vasopressin in asthma: consideration of fluid therapy. *Acta Paediatr Jpn* 1990;32:197–200.

230. Sica DA. Hyponatremia and heart failure-pathophysiology and implications. *Congest Heart Fail* 2005;11:274–277.
231. Sica DA, Midha M, Zawada E, Stacy W, Hussey R. Hyponatremia in spinal cord injury. *J Am Paraplegia Soc* 1990;13:78–83.
232. Silver SM, DeSimone JA, Jr., Smith DA, Sterns RH. Dialysis disequilibrium syndrome (DDS) in the rat: role of the "reverse urea effect." *Kidney Int* 1992;42:161–166.
233. Silver SM, Kozlowski SA, Baer JE, Rogers SJ, Sterns RH. Glycine-induced hyponatremia in the rat: a model of post-prostatectomy syndrome. *Kidney Int* 1995;47:262–268.
234. Silver SM, Schroeder BM, Bernstein P, Sterns RH. Brain adaptation to acute hyponatremia in young rats. *Am J Physiol* 1999;276(Pt 2):R1595–1599.
235. Silver SM, Schroeder BM, Sterns RH. Brain uptake of myoinositol after exogenous administration. *J Am Soc Nephrol* 2002;13:1255–12560.
236. Silver SM, Schroeder BM, Sterns RH, Rojiani A. Myoinositol administration improves survival and reduces myelinolysis after rapid correction of hyponatremia in rats. *J Neuropathol Exp Neurol* 2006;65:1–8.
237. Silver SM, Sterns RH, Halperin ML. Brain swelling after dialysis: old urea or new osmoles? *Am J Kidney Dis* 1996;28:1–13.
238. Sims EA, Welt LG, Orloff J, Needham JW. Asymptomatic hyponatremia in pulmonary tuberculosis. *J Clin Invest* 1950;29:1545–1557.
239. Singh S, Bohn D, Carlotti AP, Cusimano M, Rutka JT, Halperin ML. Cerebral salt wasting: truths, fallacies, theories, and challenges. *Crit Care Med* 2002;30:2575–2579.
240. Siushansian R, Dixon SJ, Wilson JX. Osmotic swelling stimulates ascorbate efflux from cerebral astrocytes. *J Neurochem* 1996;66:1227–1233.
241. Sivakumar V, Rajshekhar V, Chandy MJ. Management of neurosurgical patients with hyponatremia and natriuresis. *Neurosurgery* 1994;34:269–274; discussion 274.
242. Smith D, Moore K, Tormey W, Baylis PH, Thompson CJ. Downward resetting of the osmotic threshold for thirst in patients with SIADH. *Am J Physiol Endocrinol Metab* 2004;287: E1019–1023.
243. Solomon RA, Fink ME, Lennihan L. Early aneurysm surgery and prophylactic hypervolemic hypertensive therapy for the treatment of aneurysmal subarachnoid hemorrhage. *Neurosurgery* 1988;23:699–704.
244. Solomon RA, Post KD, McMurtry JG 3rd. Depression of circulating blood volume in patients after subarachnoid hemorrhage: implications for the management of symptomatic vasospasm. *Neurosurgery* 1984;15:354–361.
245. Song J, Hu X, Khan O, Tian Y, Verbalis JG, Ecelbarger CA. Increased blood pressure, aldosterone activity, and regional differences in renal ENaC protein during vasopressin escape. *Am J Physiol Renal Physiol* 2004;287:F1076–1083.
246. Sonnenblick M, Algur N, Rosin A. Thiazide-induced hyponatremia and vasopressin release. *Ann Intern Med* 1989;110:751.
247. Sonnenblick M, Friedlander Y, Rosin AJ. Diuretic-induced severe hyponatremia. Review and analysis of 129 reported patients. *Chest* 1993;103:601–606.
248. Sonnenblick M, Rosin AJ. Significance of the measurement of uric acid fractional clearance in diuretic induced hyponatraemia. *Postgrad Med J* 1986;62:449–452.
249. Sorensen JB, Andersen MK, Hansen HH. Syndrome of inappropriate secretion of antidiuretic hormone (SIADH) in malignant disease. *J Intern Med* 1995;238:97–110.
250. Soupart A, Decaux G. Therapeutic recommendations for management of severe hyponatremia: current concepts on pathogenesis and prevention of neurologic complications. *Clin Nephrol* 1996;46:149–169.
251. Soupart A, Ngassa M, Decaux G. Therapeutic relowering of the serum sodium in a patient after excessive correction of hyponatremia. *Clin Nephrol* 1999;51:383–386.
252. Soupart A, Penninckx R, Stenuit A, Decaux G. Azotemia (48 h) decreases the risk of brain damage in rats after correction of chronic hyponatremia. *Brain Res* 2000;852:167–172.
253. Soupart A, Penninckx R, Stenuit A, Decaux G. Lack of major hypoxia and significant brain damage in rats despite dramatic hyponatremic encephalopathy. *J Lab Clin Med* 1997;130: 226–231.
254. Soupart A, Penninckx R, Stenuit A, Perier O, Decaux G. Reinduction of hyponatremia improves survival in rats with myelinolysis-related neurologic symptoms. *J Neuropathol Exp Neurol* 1996;55:594–601.
255. Soupart A, Silver S, Schrooeder B, Sterns R, Decaux G. Rapid (24-hour) reaccumulation of brain organic osmolytes (particularly myo-inositol) in azotemic rats after correction of chronic hyponatremia. *J Am Soc Nephrol* 2002;13:1433–1441.
256. Soupart A, Stenuit A, Perier O, Decaux G. Limits of brain tolerance to daily increments in serum sodium in chronically hyponatraemic rats treated with hypertonic saline or urea: advantages of urea. *Clin Sci (Lond)* 1991;80:77–84.
257. Spector R, Lorenzo AV. Myo-inositol transport in the central nervous system. *Am J Physiol* 1975;228:1510–1518.
258. Spigset O. Adverse reactions of selective serotonin reuptake inhibitors: reports from a spontaneous reporting system. *Drug Saf* 1999;20:277–287.
259. Spigset O, Hedenmalm K. Hyponatremia in relation to treatment with antidepressants: a survey of reports in the World Health Organization data base for spontaneous reporting of adverse drug reactions. *Pharmacotherapy* 1997;17:348–352.
260. Spital A. Diuretic-induced hyponatremia. *Am J Nephrol* 1999;19:447–452.
261. Spital A, Ristow S. Cyclophosphamide induced water intoxication in a woman with Sjogren's syndrome. *J Rheumatol* 1997;24:2473–2475.
262. Spital A, Sterns RH. The paradox of sodium's volume of distribution. Why an extracellular solute appears to distribute over total body water. *Arch Intern Med* 1989;149:1255–1257.
263. Steele A, Gowrishankar M, Abrahamson S, Mazer CD, Feldman RD, Halperin ML. Postoperative hyponatremia despite near-isotonic saline infusion: a phenomenon of desalination. *Ann Intern Med* 1997;126:20–25.
264. Steiner RW. Physiology of beer or non-beer potomania. *Am J Kidney Dis* 1998;32:1123.
265. Sterns RH. Severe hyponatremia: the case for conservative management. *Crit Care Med* 1992; 20:534–539.
266. Sterns RH. Severe symptomatic hyponatremia: treatment and outcome. A study of 64 cases. *Ann Intern Med* 1987;107:656–64.
267. Sterns RH. The management of hyponatremic emergencies. *Crit Care Clin* 1991;7:127–142.
268. Sterns RH. The management of symptomatic hyponatremia. *Semin Nephrol* 1990;10:503–514.
269. Sterns RH. The treatment of hyponatremia: first, do no harm. *Am J Med* 1990;88:557–560.
270. Sterns RH, Baer J, Ebersol S, Thomas D, Lohr JW, Kamm DE. Organic osmolytes in acute hyponatremia. *Am J Physiol* 1993;264(Pt 2):F833–836.
271. Sterns RH, Cappuccio JD, Silver SM, Cohen EP. Neurologic sequelae after treatment of severe hyponatremia: a multicenter perspective. *J Am Soc Nephrol* 1994;4:1522–1530.
272. Sterns RH, Clark EC, Silver SM. Clinical consequences of hyponatremia and its correction. In: Seldin DW, Giebisch G, eds. *The Kidney: Clinical Disorders of Water Metabolism*. New York: Raven Press; 1993:225–236.
273. Sterns RH, Riggs JE, Schochet SS, Jr. Osmotic demyelination syndrome following correction of hyponatremia. *N Engl J Med* 1986;314:1535–1542.
274. Sterns RH, Thomas DJ, Herndon RM. Brain dehydration and neurologic deterioration after rapid correction of hyponatremia. *Kidney Int* 1989;35:69–75.
275. Strange K. Cellular volume homeostasis. *Adv Physiol Educ* 2004;28:155–159.
276. Szatalowicz VL, Miller PD, Lacher JW, Gordon JA, Schrier RW. Comparative effect of diuretics on renal water excretion in hyponatraemic oedematous disorders. *Clin Sci (Lond)* 1982;62:235–238.
277. Taivainen H, Laitinen K, Tahtela R, Kilanmaa K, Valimaki MJ. Role of plasma vasopressin in changes of water balance accompanying acute alcohol intoxication. *Alcohol Clin Exp Res* 1995;19:759–762.
278. Talmi YP, Hoffman HT, McCabe BF. Syndrome of inappropriate secretion of arginine vasopressin in patients with cancer of the head and neck. *Ann Otol Rhinol Laryngol* 1992;101:946–949.
279. Tanneau RA, Pennec YL, Jouquan J, Le Menn G. Cerebral salt wasting in elderly persons. *Ann Intern Med* 1987;107:120.
280. Thaler SM, Teitelbaum I, Berl T. "Beer potomania" in non-beer drinkers: effect of low dietary solute intake. *Am J Kidney Dis* 1998;31:1028–1031.
281. Thomas TH, Morgan DB. Post-surgical hyponatraemia: the role of intravenous fluids and arginine vasopressin. *Br J Surg* 1979;66:540–2.
282. Thomas TH, Morgan DB, Swaminathan R, Ball SG, Lee MR. Severe hyponatraemia. A study of 17 patients. *Lancet* 1978;1:621–624.
283. Thurston JH, Hauhart RE. Brain amino acids decrease in chronic hyponatremia and rapid correction causes brain dehydration: possible clinical significance. *Life Sci* 1987;40: 2539–2542.
284. Thurston JH, Hauhart RE, Nelson JS. Adaptive decreases in amino acids (taurine in particular), creatine, and electrolytes prevent cerebral edema in chronically hyponatremic mice: rapid correction (experimental model of central pontine myelinolysis) causes dehydration and shrinkage of brain. *Metab Brain Dis* 1987;2:223–241.
285. Thurston JH, Sherman WR, Hauhart RE, Kloepper RF. Myo-inositol: a newly identified nonnitrogenous osmoregulatory molecule in mammalian brain. *Pediatr Res* 1989;26:482–485.
286. Trump DL. Serious hyponatremia in patients with cancer: management with demeclocycline. *Cancer* 1981;47:2908–2912.
287. Turchin A, Seifter JL, Seely EW. Clinical problem-solving. Mind the gap. *N Engl J Med* 2003;349:1465–1469.
288. Udelson JE, Smith WB, Hendrix GH, Painchaud CA, Ghazzi M, Thomas I, Ghali JK, Selaru P, Chanoine F, Pressler ML, Konstam MA. Acute hemodynamic effects of conivaptan, a dual V(1A) and V(2) vasopressin receptor antagonist, in patients with advanced heart failure. *Circulation* 2001;104:2417–2423.
289. Ullman JS, Bederson JB. Hypertensive, hypervolemic, hemodilutional therapy for aneurysmal subarachnoid hemorrhage. Is it efficacious? Yes. *Crit Care Clin* 1996;12:697–707.
290. Valli G, Fedeli A, Antonucci R, Paoletti P, Palange P. Water and sodium imbalance in COPD patients. *Monaldi Arch Chest Dis* 2004;61:112–116.
291. Van Amelsvoort T, Bakshi R, Devaux CB, Schwabe S. Hyponatremia associated with carbamazepine and oxcarbazepine therapy: a review. *Epilepsia* 1994;35:181–188.
292. Verbalis J. Hyponatremia: endocrinologic causes and consequences of therapy. *Trends Endocrinol Metab* 1992;3:1–7.
293. Verbalis JG. Hyponatremia induced by vasopressin or desmopressin in female and male rats. *J Am Soc Nephrol* 1993;3:1600–1606.
294. Verbalis JG. Pathogenesis of hyponatremia in an experimental model of the syndrome of inappropriate antidiuresis. *Am J Physiol* 1994;267(Pt 2):R1617–1625.
295. Verbalis JG. Vasopressin V2 receptor antagonists. *J Mol Endocrinol* 2002;29:1–9.
296. Verbalis JG, Gullans SR. Hyponatremia causes large sustained reductions in brain content of multiple organic osmolytes in rats. *Brain Res* 1991;567:274–282.
297. Verbalis JG, Gullans SR. Rapid correction of hyponatremia produces differential effects on brain osmolyte and electrolyte reaccumulation in rats. *Brain Res* 1993;606:19–27.
298. Verbalis JG, Martinez AJ. Determinants of brain myelinolysis following correction of chronic hyponatremia in rats. In: Jamison RL, Jaid S, eds. *Vasopressin*. Paris: John Libby; 1991: 539–547.
299. Verbalis JG, Martinez AJ. Neurological and neuropathological sequelae of correction of chronic hyponatremia. *Kidney Int* 1991;39:1274–1282.
300. Vexler ZS, Ayus JC, Roberts TP, Fraser CL, Kucharczyk J, Arieff AI. Hypoxic and ischemic hypoxia exacerbate brain injury associated with metabolic encephalopathy in laboratory animals. *J Clin Invest* 1994;93:256–264.
301. Videen JS, Michaelis T, Pinto P, Ross BD. Human cerebral osmolytes during chronic hyponatremia. A proton magnetic resonance spectroscopy study. *J Clin Invest* 1995;95: 788–793.
302. Watson JD, Jennings DB, Sarda IR, Pang SC, Lawson B, Wigle DA, Flynn TG. The antidiuretic effect of pneumadin requires a functional arginine vasopressin system. *Regul Pept* 1995;57:105–114.
303. Webberley MJ, Murray JA. Life-threatening acute hyponatraemia induced by low dose cyclophosphamide and indomethacin. *Postgrad Med J* 1989;65:950–952.
304. Webster B, Bain J. Antidiuretic effect and complications of chlorpropamide therapy in diabetes insipidus. *J Clin Endocrinol Metab* 1970;30:215–227.
305. Weisberg LS. Pseudohyponatremia: a reappraisal. *Am J Med* 1989;86:315–318.

306. Weissman PN, Shenkman L, Gregerman RI. Chlorpropamide hyponatremia: drug-induced inappropriate antidiuretic-hormone activity. *N Engl J Med* 1971;284:65–71.

307. Wijdicks EF, Schievink WI, Burnett JC, Jr. Natriuretic peptide system and endothelin in aneurysmal subarachnoid hemorrhage. *J Neurosurg* 1997;87:275–280.

308. Wijdicks EF, Vermeulen M, Hijdra A, van Gijn J. Hyponatremia and cerebral infarction in patients with ruptured intracranial aneurysms: is fluid restriction harmful? *Ann Neurol* 1985; s17:137–140.

309. Wijdicks EF, Vermeulen M, ten Haaf JA, Hijdra A, Bakker WH, van Gijn J. Volume depletion and natriuresis in patients with a ruptured intracranial aneurysm. *Ann Neurol* 1985;18:211–216.

310. Wilcox CS, Guzman NJ, Mitch WE, Kelly RA, Maroni BJ, Souney PF, Rayment CM, Braun L, Colucci R, Loon NR. Na+, K+, and BP homeostasis in man during furosemide: effects of prazosin and captopril. *Kidney Int* 1987;31:135–141.

311. Williams HH, Wall BM, Horan JM, Presley DN, Crofton JT, Share L, Cooke CR. Nonosmotic stimuli alter osmoregulation in patients with spinal cord injury. *J Clin Endocrinol Metab* 1990;71:1536–1543.

312. Wong F, Blei AT, Blendis LM, Thuluvath PJ. A vasopressin receptor antagonist (VPA-985) improves serum sodium concentration in patients with hyponatremia: a multicenter, randomized, placebo-controlled trial. *Hepatology* 2003;37:182–191.

313. Woo MH, Kale-Pradhan PB. Fludrocortisone in the treatment of subarachnoid hemorrhage-induced hyponatremia. *Ann Pharmacother* 1997;31:637–639.

314. Woo MH, Smythe MA. Association of SIADH with selective serotonin reuptake inhibitors. *Ann Pharmacother* 1997;31:108–110.

315. Wrong O. The relationship between water retention and electrolyte excretion following administration of anti-diuretic hormone. *Clin Sci (Lond)* 1956;15:401–418.

316. Yamaki T, Tano-oka A, Takahashi A, Imaizumi T, Suetake K, Hashi K. Cerebral salt wasting syndrome distinct from the syndrome of inappropriate secretion of antidiuretic hormone (SIADH). *Acta Neurochir (Wien)* 1992;115:156–162.

317. Yassa R, Iskandar H, Nastase C, Camille Y. Carbamazepine and hyponatremia in patients with affective disorder. *Am J Psychiatry* 1988;145:339–342.

318. Zerbe R, Stropes L, Robertson G. Vasopressin function in the syndrome of inappropriate antidiuresis. *Annu Rev Med* 1980;31:315–327.

319. Zusman RM, Keiser HR, Handler JS. Inhibitiion of vasopressin-stimulated prostaglandin E biosynthesis by chlorpropamide in the toad urinary bladder. Mechanism of enhancement of vasopressin-stimulated water flow. *J Clin Invest* 1977;60:1348–1353.

CHAPTER 42

Hypernatremic States

Christopher J. Rivard, Wei Wang, and Laurence Chan
University of Colorado Health Sciences Center, Denver, Colorado, USA

Hypernatremia can occur with normal, increased, or decreased total-body sodium content. In healthy individuals and in normal conditions, the plasma concentration of sodium ranges between 136 and 143 mEq/l of plasma despite large individual variations in the intake of salt and water. The concentration is maintained at constant levels because of the homeostatic mechanism in the body. Claude Bernard was the first to appreciate that higher animals "have really two environments: a *milieu exterieur* in which the organism is situated, and a *milieu interieur* in which the tissue element live." The latter is the extracellular fluid (ECF) that bathes the cells of the body (186, 210, 222). Maintenance of this consistency of plasma sodium and solute activity is the function of the thirst-neurohypophyseal-renal axis (207, 213). Thirst and urinary concentration are the main defenses against hyperosmolality and hence hypernatremia. Hypernatremia is a relatively common problem with prevalence in hospitalized patients of 0.5% to 2%. It is defined as plasma Na^+ concentration ($[Na^+]$) greater than 145 mEq/l. It can be produced by the administration of hypertonic sodium solutions or, in almost all cases, by the loss of free water. Since $[Na^+]$ is an effective osmole, the increase in the plasma osmolality (P_{osm}) induced by hypernatremia creates an osmotic gradient that results in water movement out of the cells into the ECF. It is this cellular dehydration particularly in the brain that is primarily responsible for the neurologic symptoms associated with hypernatremia. A similar syndrome can be produced when the plasma osmolality is elevated by hyperglycemia. However, when hyperosmolality is due to the accumulation of cell-permeable solute such as urea or ethanol, there is no water shift in the steady state because osmotic equilibrium is reached by solute entering the cell.

REGULATION OF WATER HOMEOSTASIS

Significance of the Plasma Sodium Concentration

The total-body water (about 60% of body weight in males, and 50% in females) is distributed between the intracellular fluid (ICF, 60% of body water) and extracellular fluid (ECF, 40% of body water) spaces (1, 19, 20, 86). Flame photometry

has made the plasma sodium concentration one of the simplest and most frequently measured constituents of the body fluids. It is not always appreciated that a given concentration of the plasma sodium may be consistent with different functional states (53, 65). The plasma sodium is simply a concentration term and as such reflects only the relative amounts of sodium and water present in the sample. The concentration is not a measure of total-body sodium content (87). It is determined empirically by the following relationship:

$$Plasma\ [Na^+] = \frac{Total\text{-}body\ Na^+ + Total\text{-}body\ K^+}{Total\text{-}body\ water} \qquad (Eq.\ 1)$$

The relationship indicates the fact that hypernatremia can occur as a consequence of a decrease total-body water, an increase in total-body sodium, or a combination of these events. It gives no information regarding replacement or removal of sodium. When flame spectrophotometer is used to measure the amount of sodium in a plasma sample, substances such as plasma proteins, abnormally high glucose, and lipid can occupy a large fraction of the plasma volume and underestimate the actual sodium concentration. The ionic composition of the plasma is measured as milliequivalents per liter of plasma. Only about 930 ml of each liter of plasma is water. The remaining 70 ml is occupied by the plasma proteins and to lesser degree lipids. In the presence of hyperlipidemia or hyperproteinemia, the plasma water content may be less than 93%.

Generation of Hypernatremia

Since Na^+ and its accompanying anions are the major effective ECF osmoles, hypernatremia is a state of hyperosmolality. As a result of the fixed number of ICF particles, maintenance of osmotic equilibrium in hypernatremia results in ICF volume contraction. The increase in the plasma osmolality induced by hypernatremia creates an osmotic gradient that results in water movement out of the cells into the ECF. A similar syndrome can be produced when plasma osmolality is elevated by hyperglycemia. When hyperosmolality is due to the accumulation of a cell-permeable solute such as urea or ethanol, there is no water shift because osmotic equilibrium is reached by solute entry into cells. Therefore, both urea and ethanol are ineffective osmoles. Plasma osmolality can be measured directly by determining freezing point depression or vapor pressure (69, 88). Variable changes in the plasma sodium concentration occur with hyperglycemia. Since glucose enters cells slowly, an increase in the plasma glucose concentration raises effective plasma osmolality and causes water to move from the cells into the ECF. By dilution, this lowers the plasma Na^+ concentration. In theory, every 62-mg/dl increment in the plasma glucose concentration should draw enough water out of the cells to reduce the plasma Na^+ concentration 1 mEq/l (219, 223).

The number of particles per gram of water determines the osmolality of a solution. Since sodium salts (particularly NaCl and $NaHCO_3$), glucose, and urea are primary extracellular osmoles, the plasma osmolality can be approximated from

Plasma osmolality (P_{osm}) =

$$2 \times \text{Plasma } [Na^+] + \frac{[\text{Glucose}]}{18} + \frac{\text{BUN}}{2.8} \quad \text{(Eq. 2)}$$

where 2 reflects the osmotic contribution of the anion accompanying Na^+ and 18 and 2.8 represent the conversion of the plasma glucose concentration and blood urea nitrogen (BUN) from units of milligrams per deciliter (mg/dl) into millimoles per liter (mmol/l).

Although urea contributes to the absolute value of the P_{osm}, it does not act to hold water within the extracellular space because of its membrane permeability. Therefore, urea is an ineffective osmole and does not contribute to the effective P_{osm}.

In general, the effective plasma osmolality can be calculated from

Effective plasma osmolality =

$$\text{Measured plasma osmolality} - \frac{\text{BUN}}{2.8}$$

or estimated from

Effective plasma osmolality = $2 \times \text{Plasma } [Na^+] + \dfrac{[\text{Glucose}]}{18}$

$$\text{(Eq. 3)}$$

Under normal circumstances, glucose and urea contributes less than 10 mOsm/kg H_2O, and the plasma Na^+ concentration is the main determinant of the plasma osmolality, the osmolality of body fluids can be estimated to be twice the plasma sodium concentration (88).

The major ECF particles are Na^+ and its accompanying anions Cl^- and HCO_3^-, a high plasma sodium concentration is always associated with a high osmolality. This indicates that water is needed to restore isotonicity. The water deficit can be estimated from the plasma sodium level. The percentage increase in sodium concentration approximates the percentage decrease in total-body water. The water deficit can be estimated by the equation

$$\text{Water deficit} = \text{Total-body Water} \times \left(\frac{\text{Plasma } [Na^+]}{140} - 1 \right)$$

$$\text{(Eq. 4)}$$

Total-body water varies with body size and fat content. It is approximately 60% of body weight in young men, 50% of body weight in old men and young women, and only 40% in elderly women.

DEFENSE MECHANISMS AGAINST WATER DEPLETION

Two primary mechanisms defend the body against water depletion and hyperosmolality of extracellular fluid space. These two defense mechanisms are the capacity of the kidney to excrete a concentrated urine and stimulation of thirst to increase water intake. Each pathway is very effective and disturbance of urinary concentrating mechanism alone generally does not cause hyperosmolality if the thirst mechanism is intact.

Control of ADH Secretion

Hypernatremia results in the stimulation of both the antidiuretic hormone (ADH) release and thirst by the hypothalamic osmoreceptors (Fig. 1). Argenine vasopressin is the ADH in humans. Argenine vasopressin binds to specific receptors on collecting ducts (V2 receptors), which are coupled to cyclic AMP (cAMP) formation. The regulation of ADH release from the posterior pituitary is dependent primarily on two mechanisms: osmotic and nonosmotic pathways (Fig. 2). The osmotic regulation of ADH is dependent on osmoreceptor cells in the anterior hypothalamus (89). These cells, most likely by altering their volume, recognize changes in ECF osmolality. Cell volume is decreased readily by substances that are restricted to the ECF, such as hypertonic saline or hypertonic mannitol. These substances are effective in stimulating ADH release. In contrast, urea moves readily into cells and therefore does not alter cell volumes and does not effectively stimulate ADH release. A similar response pattern is evident when vasopressin release is studied in the hypothalamo–neurohypophyseal complex in organ culture. Specifically, sodium chloride, sucrose, and mannitol at 310 mOsm/kg H_2O cause a threefold increase in argenine vasopressin release, while urea and glucose fail to stimulate vasopressin. These studies also support the view that the receptor response to changes in osmolality rather than sodium. The effects of increased osmolality on vasopressin release are associated with a measurable increase in vasopressin precursor messenger RNA (mRNA) in the hypothalamus (150, 236) and salt-loading increases vasopressin RNA in the pituitary (93, 172). Vasopressin release can also occur in the absence of changes in plasma osmolality

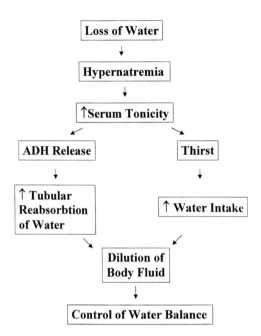

FIGURE 1 Regulation of water homeostasis: feedback loop for the stimulation of antidiuretic hormone (ADH) release and thirst. Hypernatremia results in an increase in the plasma osmolality, which enhances ADH secretion and thirst, resulting in water retention and a reduction in the plasma osmolality toward normal.

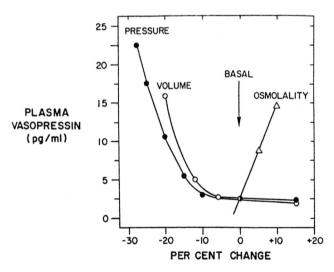

FIGURE 2 Osmotic and nonosmotic stimulation of arginine vasopressin release. (From Robertson GL, Berl T. Pathophysiology of water metabolism. In: Brenner BM, Rector FC Jr, eds. *The Kidney*, 4th ed. Philadelphia: WB Saunders; 1991:883.)

(252). Physical pain, emotional stress, hypoglycemia, and a decrease in blood pressure or blood volume are important nonosmotic stimuli for vasopressin release. A 7% to 10% decrement in blood pressure or blood volume causes the prompt release of vasopressin (Fig. 2). Although there are considerable genetically determined individual variations in both the threshold and sensitivity, a close correlation

between argenine vasopressin and plasma osmolality has been demonstrated in subjects with various states of hydration (Fig. 3).

The secretion of ADH generally begins when the plasma osmolality exceeds 275 to 285 mOsm/kg H_2O. The threshold for thirst appears to be approximately 10 mOsm/kg H_2O above that of vasopressin release. Prevention of a total-body water deficit is thus largely dependent on water intake as modulated by thirst. The thirst center appears to be closely associated anatomically with the osmoreceptors in the region of the hypothalamus. Defects in thirst response may involve either organic or generalized central nervous system lesions and can lead to severe water deficit even in the presence of a normal concentrating mechanism. The water deficit will occur more promptly if renal concentrating ability is also impaired (137).

Thirst and the Maintenance of Hypernatremia

Thirst is in fact so effective that even patients with complete diabetes insipidus avoid hypernatremia by fluid intake in excess of 10 l/day (6, 79, 78). Hypernatremia supervenes therefore only when hypotonic fluid losses occur in combination with a disturbance in water intake. This is most commonly seen in the aged with an alteration in level of consciousness, in the very young with inadequate access to water, or in a rare subject with a primary disturbance in thirst (189, 190). Prevention of a total-body water deficit is thus largely dependent on water intake as modulated by thirst. The thirst center appears to be closely associated anatomically with the osmoreceptors in the region of the hypothalamus. Defects in thirst response may involve either organic or generalized central nervous system lesions and can lead to severe water deficit even in the presence of a normal concentrating mechanism.

In summary, persistent hypernatremia does not occur in normal subjects, because the ensuing rise in plasma osmolality stimulates both the releases of ADH; thereby

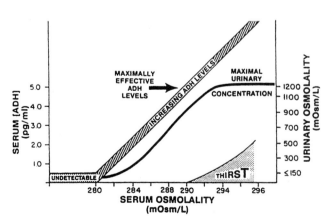

FIGURE 3 Antidiuretic hormone (ADH) levels, urinary osmolality, and thirst as functions of serum osmolality. (From Narins RG, Krishna GC. Disorders of water balance. In: Stein JH, ed. *Internal Medicine.* Boston: Little, Brown; 1990:836.)

minimizing further water loss and, more importantly, thirst. The associated increase in water intake then lowers the plasma sodium concentration back to normal. This regulatory system is so efficient that the plasma osmolality is maintained within a range of 1% to 2% despite wide variations in sodium and water intake. Even patients with diabetes insipidus, who often have marked polyuria due to diminished ADH effect, maintain a near-normal plasma sodium concentration by appropriately increasing water intake. The net effect is that hypernatremia primarily occurs in those patients who cannot express thirst normally: infants and adults with impaired mental status (182). The latter most often occurs in the elderly, who also appear to have diminished osmotic stimulation of thirst. A patient with a plasma sodium concentration of 150 mEq/l or more who is alert but not thirsty has, by definition, a hypothalamic lesion affecting the thirst center.

CELLULAR RESPONSE TO HYPERNATREMIA

Volume Regulation

When exposed to a change in extracellular osmolality, a cell shrinks or swells and subsequently exhibits either a regulatory volume increase or a regulatory volume decrease (98, 141, 142). When exposed to hypertonicity, a cell loses water until the intracellular and extracellular osmolality are equal. Recovery of water is mediated by accumulation of inorganic and organic solutes known as osmolytes (98, 104). The principle inorganic osmolytes are Na^+, K^+, and Cl^-. The principle organic osmolytes may be classified into three general groups: polyols, methylamines, and amino acids (77). A comparison of major and minor organic osmolytes for the kidney and brain are depicted in Table 1.

While hypernatremia in mammals affects all tissues, the greatest potential for harm is to the brain and kidney. Of these two organs, even modest changes in serum osmolality can have severe consequences to the brain, resulting in volume changes. In the brain, acute hypernatremia is associated with a rapid decrease in water content and a corresponding increase in solute concentration (141). In a study of rats by Cserr and coworkers (47, 48), acute hypernatremia (plasma $Na^+ = 180$ mEq/l) was accompanied by a prompt decrease (7%) in total-brain water content. The fall in water content was less than expected for simple osmotic behavior, indicating significant volume regulation had occurred. Moreover, the decrease in total brain water was the result of a fall in extracellular volume. Intracellular volume was not significantly changed at 30 and 90 minutes. The rapid regulatory volume increase was mediated by increases in Na^+, K^+, and Cl^- (48). Most of these ions were derived from bulk flow of NaCl from cerebral spinal fluid (CSF). There was also a lesser contribution of electrolytes from the blood. During experimental hypernatremia in rabbits, intracellular brain water content also decreased by 12% at 1 hour and by 17% at 4 hours, accompanied by a corresponding increase in intracellular osmolality (12). Most of the acute increase in brain osmolality was due to an increase in intracellular sodium and potassium concentrations (198). Although a substantial component of the increase in electrolyte concentration resulted from transcellular water loss, whole-brain electrolyte content also increased with the sodium content increasing from 268 ± 9 mm/kg dry weight in control animals to 321 ± 19 mmol/kg dry weight after 4 hours of hypernatremia. After sustained hypernatremia of 7 days' duration, brain water and volume values were restored to normal. More prolonged hypernatremia results in accumulation of organic osmolytes to restore total brain water content to normal levels (37, 109, 113).

In the kidney, the general mechanism for cellular osmoregulation in the face of hypertonic conditions involves the accumulation of organic rather than inorganic osmolytes. This strategy for the transport of organic rather than inorganic osmolytes across the cellular membrane has been explained in at least three hypothesized mechanisms as detailed in Table 2. However, before mounting a coordinated osmoresponse, cells experience a "molecular mayhem" (192) due to the initial decrease in cellular volume resulting in crowding of macromolecules and an increase in ionic osmolytes. These early changes in the cellular status as well as the loss of water which can affect a variety of biochemical processes can result in a variety of deleterious effects on normal cellular functions and viability as depicted in Table 3.

Osmolytes

Organic molecules serve an important biologic function in the process of cellular osmoregulation (206). When extracellular osmolality increases, organic molecules accumulate in the cells, thus maintaining cell volume and counteracting the perturbation of enzyme function and protein structure by high concentrations of inorganic ions and other molecules

TABLE 1 Organic Osmolytes in Kidney and Brain

Organic Osmolyte	Kidney (127)	Brain (141,142)
Major	Glutamate	Glutamate
	Glutamine	Glutamine
	Taurine	Taurine
	Myo-inositol	Myo-inositol
	Urea	Urea
	Alanine	Alanine
	Sorbitol	Aspartate
	GPC	Glycine
	Betaine	GABA
Minor	Val/Leu/Isoleu	Theonine
	Phosphocreatine	GPC
	Creatine	Betaine
		Choline
		Phosphocreatine
		Lysine
		Serine

GABA, γ-aminobutyric acid; GPC, glycerophosphory choline.

TABLE 2   Proposed hypothesis for cellular osmoregulation in the kidney

Name	Details	Reference
Compatible osmolyte principle	Cells accumulate high levels of polyols or certain amino acids that do not affect protein function in contrast to NaCl or KCl	(33)
Counteracting osmolyte principle	Cells accumulate methylamines (i.e., GPC or betaine) to attenuate the destabilizing effect of urea on protein structure	(32, 249)
Constant transmembrane gradient	Cells maintain constant transmembrane gradients for sodium and potassium thus the driving force for sodium gradient-coupled transport systems for organic and inorganic solutes	(95,96)

TABLE 3   Effect of early hypertonic stress on kidney cell function

General function	Reference
DNA – Damage, inhibition of repair, dissociation of protein from chromatin	(57, 58, 136, 192)
Metabolism, Cell Growth – Disruption of mitochondria function, cell cycle arrest, growth factor-dependent signaling inhibition, alteration in cytoskeletal structure, inhibition of protein translation	(2, 18, 45, 56, 58, 67, 83, 161, 169, 173)
Secondary stress, Apoptosis – Induction of secondary oxidative stress, apoptosis	(45, 58, 253)

such as urea (250). Lien and his coworkers (141) studied the effect of varying degrees and duration of hypernatremia on the concentrations of substances believed to be important idiogenic brain osmoles in rats using conventional biochemical assays, nuclear magnetic resonance spectroscopy, and high performance liquid chromatography. Idiogenic osmoles have been postulated to develop in the brain cells of patients suffering from chronic elevations in the osmolality of ECF. Moreover, the rapid correction of the osmolality of such patients is associated with the development of cerebral edema.

It has been known for more than 30 years that changes in intracellular brain sodium and potassium concentrations cannot account for all of the observed changes in brain osmolality that occur during chronic exposure to extracellular hypernatremia. The solutes that develop to maintain equality between extracellular and intracellular brain osmolality during this adaptation to hyperosmotic stress have been investigated by several groups. Arieff and his associates (7, 8) have demonstrated that osmoles accumulated in the brain of chronic hypernatremic but not in acute hypernatremic rabbits. Other investigators have shown that the level of amino acids and their derivatives such as glutamine, taurine, and urea rise in the brain of chronic hypernatremic animals, and account for about half of the increment of brain osmoles (234). However, many of the idiogenic osmoles have not yet been characterized in brain tissue. Polyols and trimethylamines accumulate intracellularly in marine animals, plants, and bacteria when extracellular or environmental osmolality is significantly increased. In this study, it was found that the inorganic osmolytes account for 50% to 60% of the increase in solute content, whereas organic osmolytes account for the remainder during adaptation to chronic hypernatremia (Fig. 4).

Recovery from chronic hypernatremia involves a small transient rise in brain water, which is restored to normal within 48 hours. With the exception of myoinositol, all the electrolytes and organic osmoles fall to normal levels within 24 to 48 hours. The cellular mechanisms responsible for the loss of intracellular organic osmolytes are poorly understood. In vitro studies of brain tissue found that cell swelling causes rapid loss of electrolytes and organic osmolytes. The losses of cellular K^+ and Cl^- are likely mediated by swelling activated ion channels. Characterization of the organic osmolyte efflux pathways suggest that they represent pores or channels in the membrane that are permeable to Cl^- as well as small organic salts. Roy and Banderali described a chloride channel that can transport small organic solute such as taurine and amino acids (213). No specific inhibitors of the pathways are known. However, inhibitors of arachidonic acid metabolism are able to prevent activation of the efflux pathway, implicating eicosanoids in the signal transduction mechanism.

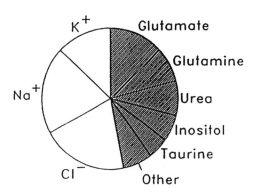

FIGURE 4   Relative changes in brain osmolytes in chronic hypernatremia. (From Lien YH, Shapiro JI, Chan L. Effects of hypernatremia on organic brain osmoles. *J Clin Invest* 1990;85:1427–1435, with permission.)

TABLE 4   Published Experimental Models of Animals with Hypernatremia

| Duration | Animal Species | Changes of Osmolality (mmol/kg) | Contribution to Osmolality Change | | | | |
			Na⁺	K⁺	Cl⁺	Other Solutes	Reference
Acute hypernatremia (hours)							
1	Rat	139	24	24	ND	Amino acids Urea	Chan et al.
1	Rabbit	60	38	32	18	ND	Arieff et al.
2	Rat	101	ND	ND	ND	Urea	Lien et al.
3	Rat	117	30	19	30	ND	Holliday et al.
4	Rat	55	ND	ND	ND	Amino acids	Lockwood
4	Rabbit	96	21	26	24	Amino acids	Arieff et al.
9	Rabbit	118	29	19	25	ND	Sotos et al.
Chronic hypernatremia (days)							
3	Rat	74	ND	ND	ND	Polyols	Lohr et al.
4	Rat	83	ND	ND	ND	Amino acids	Lockwood et al.
4	Mouse	80	19	26	ND	Amino acids Urea	Thurston et al.
5	Rat	50	ND	ND	ND	Amino acids Methylamines polyols	Heilig et al.
7	Rat	80	25	1	25	ND	Holliday et al.
7	Rabbit	80	8	5	15	Amino acids	Arieff et al.
		58	28	21	19	ND	
7	Rat	102	ND	ND	ND	Amino acids Methylamines Polyols urea	Lien et al.

ND, no data.

Lien et al. (141, 142) reviewed previous studies to estimate the percentage of the osmolality that is still idiogenic. The contributions of electrolytes and other solutes to the changes in brain osmolality for various durations and degrees of hypernatremia were reported in different studies (Table 4).

As a group, amino acids represent the major pool of brain organic osmolytes (20%–30%); polyols and methylamines represent 7% to 10%. Taurine, a sulfonated amino acid, appears to be very important in neonatal brain volume regulation. Urea (8%–9%), unlike other osmolytes, is not preferentially accumulated intracellularly. Therefore, the vast majority of the total change in brain osmolality can be accounted for by changes in the concentrations of measured solutes. In other words, there are no significant idiogenic brain osmoles (225, 226).

Response to hypertonic conditions in the kidney depends on the cell type as determined by presence along the nephron. Microdissection of kidney nephron segments for study is difficult; however, data may be obtained from in vitro studies of stable cell lines derived from specific nephron segments. An example of the heterogeneous nature of osmolyte accumulation in response to hypertonic stress in cells along the nephron is depicted in Fig. 5.

While these data only summarize the changes in selected organic osmolytes, the data indicate that different cells accumulate different osmolytes when challenged to increasing extracellular tonicity. Proximal and distal tubule cells accumulate more myoinositol as compared with inner medullary collecting duct cells and the reverse is true for glycerophosphoryl choline (GPC) in collecting duct cells. The cells located in the inner medullary collecting duct (IMCD) cells

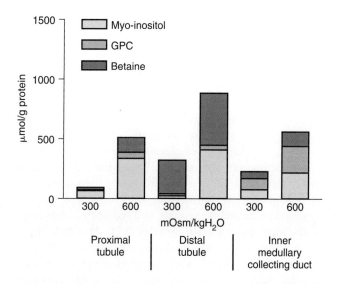

FIGURE 5   Comparison of typical organic osmolytes accumulated in cell lines derived from the proximal tubule (LLC-PK1), distal tubule (thick ascending loop of Henle [TALH]), and inner medullary collecting duct (IMCD). (From Grunewald RW, Kinne RK. Osmoregulation in the mammalian kidney: the role of organic osmolytes. *J Exp Zool* 1999;283:708–724; and Nakanishi T, Balaban RS, Burg MB. Survey of osmolytes in renal cell lines. *Am J Physiol* 1988;255:C181–191, with permission.)

are exposed to the greatest range in tonicity and are therefore valuable in studying the effects of chronic hypertonicity on cellular accumulation of organic osmolytes. Figure 6 demonstrates that IMCD$_3$ cells accumulate varying amounts of different organic osmolytes in response to increasing levels of tonicity.

Of interest in these cells is the substantial accumulation of sorbitol at substantially high hypertonic conditions. Sorbitol plays an important role in the osmotic response, especially at high tonicity, because it is not required to be transported across the membrane in the face of a substantial concentration gradient but rather is metabolized from glucose by the cellular protein aldose reductase (AR). Thus within the same cell line of the kidney, substantial changes in the accumulation of specific osmolytes occurs with increasing tonicity. In the kidney, further metabolism of sorbitol by sorbitol dehydrogenase (SDH) produces fructose (polyol pathway). Studies show that IMCD$_3$ cells chronically adapted to increasing levels of tonicity increase AR message while at the same time decreasing message for SDH (Fig. 7). This allows cells to accumulate the organic osmolyte sorbitol. During a reduction in tonicity, cells can export sorbitol from the cell via sorbitol permease or by upregulation of SDH, thereby converting sorbitol to fructose with eventual recycling to glucose in the cell.

Accumulations of minor organic osmolytes in the kidney are similar to major organic osmolytes in demonstrating differential accumulation with increasing levels of hypertonicity. Figure 8 shows that similar to major organic osmolytes, IMCD cells accumulate various amino acids as minor organic osmolytes to different levels in response to increasing extracellular tonicity. Glutamate and glutamine constitute the greatest level of accumulation.

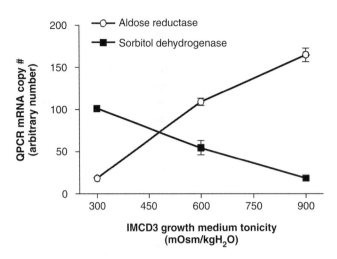

FIGURE 7   Changes in cellular message levels for aldose reductase and sorbitol dehydrogenase in IMCD$_3$ cells in response to chronic adaptation to increasing tonicity.

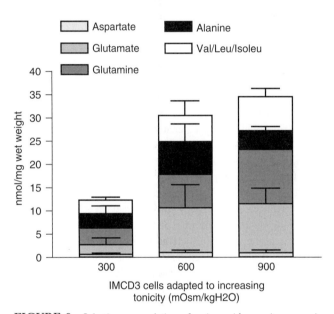

FIGURE 8   Selective accumulation of amino acids as minor organic osmolytes in inner medullary collecting duct cells at increasing extracelluar tonicity. (From Klawitter J, Rivard CJ, Capasso JM, et al. Metabolnomic analysis of the effects of adaptation to hypertonicity in inner medullary collecting duct (IMCD3) cells. *J Am Soc Nephrol* 2004;15:90A.)

Regulation of Transcription in Response to Hypertonicity

Hypertonicity-induced stimulation of transcription plays an important role in the adaptation of renal cells to hypertonicity (165, 166). The regulatory sequence element named tonicity-responsive enhancer (TonE) has been found in the promoter region of a large number of osmotic response genes identified in Table 5. TonE binding proteins (TonEBPs) mediate the transcriptional stimulation in response to hypertonicity. These sequences have been found in the 5′ flanking region of the aldose reductase gene in several species suggesting a common mechanism by which

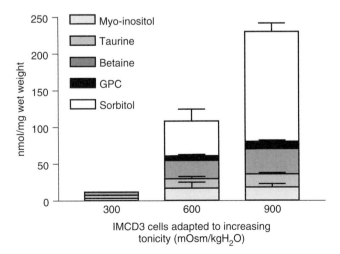

FIGURE 6   Comparison of relative changes in common organic osmolyte concentration in IMCD$_3$ cells chronically adapted to increasing tonicity. (From Klawitter J, Rivard CJ, Capasso JM, et al. Metabolnomic analysis of the effects of adaptation to hypertonicity in inner medullary collecting duct (IMCD3) cells. *J Am Soc Nephrol* 2004;15:90A.)

TABLE 5   Tonicity enhancer binding protein (TonEBP) target genes

Target Gene			
Gene Name	**Abbreviation**	**Function**	**Reference**
Aldose reductase	AR	Conversion of glucose to sorbitol	(131, 148)
Sodium/myo-inositol contransporter	SMIT	Transports myo-inositol	(148, 201)
Sodium/chloride/betaine cotransporter	BGT1	Transport betaine	(148, 166)
Urea transporter	UT-A	Vasopressin-regulated urea transporter	(175)
Taurine transporter	TauT	Specific amino acid transporter	(117)
Heat shock protein 70	HSP70-2	Molecular chaperone	(90, 247)
Sodium-coupled neutral amino acid transporter-2	ATA2, SNAT2	Neutral amino acid transporter	(235)
Osmotic stress protein 94	Osp94	Putative molecular chaperone	(132)
Aquaporin 2	AQP2	Water channel	(122, 148)

tonicity response genes are regulated (165, 166). In general little is understood about the mechanism by which mammalian cells recognize hypertonicity and how the signal is transmitted to TonE.

Nuclear Magnetic Resonance Spectroscopy

Nuclear magnetic resonance (NMR) is a physical phenomenon of atomic nuclei that has many biochemical and biophysical applications (35, 36, 212). The methodologies derived from NMR imaging enable the chemical identification of different molecules, kinetic analysis of suitable chemical reactions, studies of secondary and tertiary protein structure, and analysis of receptor–ligand interactions. It is this latter application that has become an important clinical tool. The application of spectroscopy in concert with different imaging methods ultimately may prove even more valuable than imaging alone in our understanding of the pathogenesis of different diseases. Bloch and Purcell first demonstrated NMR as a physical phenomenon, independently, in 1946. The fundamental basis of the NMR phenomenon is that nuclei have a quantum characteristic called spin, which because of the charged nature of the nucleus results in these nuclei having magnetic moments and the net biologic samples having magnetic moment in the direction of an applied external magnetic field (Bo). Transitions between the spin state aligned with and against the Bo field can be induced by a radiofrequency pulse and samples by radiofrequency antenna as free induction decay (FID). The FID can be transformed from a plot of magnetization versus time to a plot of magnetization versus frequency, also called an NMR spectrum, by a mathematical manipulation called a Fourier transformation. The frequency of the FID (ν) can be predicted by the knowledge of the nucleus under study and its gyromagnetic ratio (τ), and the magnitude of the Bo field by the following relationship:

$$\nu = \tau Bo/2\pi \qquad \text{(Eq. 5)}$$

The area under the resultant spectral peak is directly proportional to the quantity of nuclei existing free in solution in the sample being studied. This, in fact, is the basis of NMR imaging experiments. Spectroscopic methodologies make use of the fact that the chemical environment of a given nucleus placed in a Bo field will affect the effective magnetic field of a given nucleus (B_{eff}). This can be described by the chemical environment of a nucleus defining the density of the electron cloud about that nucleus, which tends to appose the Bo field. We can, therefore, describe a shielding constant σ that results from this electron cloud apposing the Bo field in the following equation:

$$B_{eff} = Bo\,(1 - \sigma) \qquad \text{(Eq. 6)}$$

The magnitude of σ is usually small, and it is expressed in the dimensionless term of parts per million (ppm). This means that the spectrum acquired from a sample, containing the same nucleus in different chemical environments, will have multiple spectral peaks corresponding to these different chemical environments, allowing for chemical identification on the basis of the shielding constants of these nuclei, also known as chemical shift. Chemical shift, expressed in parts per million, is independent of the strength of the Bo field. Although other physical phenomena may be used in chemical identification (e.g., spin coupling, nuclear Overhauser effect), chemical shift is the primary method of chemical identification that has been used in NMR of living tissues (35, 36).

Figure 9 shows the H-1 NMR spectra of brain extract from normal and hypetnatremic rats. The most prominent peaks represent N-acetylaspartate (2.02 ppm) and phosphocreatine (3.03 and 3.93 ppm). The peaks in the range of 2.0 to 2.5 ppm represent primarily amino acids, which have not been completely characterized yet. But it was evident that the peak area was larger in severe chronic hypernatremia than normal rat. The major peaks of polyols and trimethylamines were located between 3.1 and 3.9 ppm; GPC, 3.23; betaine, 3.26; myoinositol, 3.27, 3.57, 3.59, 3.61, and 4.06; and sorbitol, 3.85 ppm. We observed the increase of GPC, betaine, and myoinositol in severe chronic hypernatremia compared with normal rats. Sorbitol peak was not visualized in normal rats with severe chronic hypernatremia.

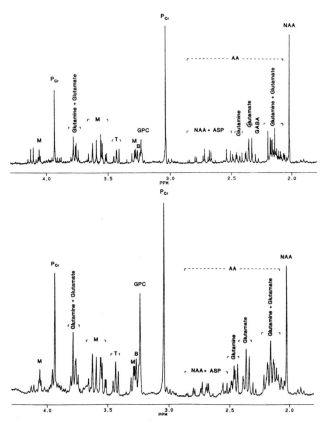

FIGURE 9 Proton nuclear magnetic resonance (NMR) spectra of brain extracts from normal rat **(A)** and severe chronic hypernatremic rat **(B)**. These spectra are the sum of 128 transients and are referenced to trimethylsilylpropprionate (TSP). Only peaks derived from glycerophosphoryl choline (GPC), betaine (7), myoinositol (M), amino acids (AA), phosphocreatine (PCr), and N-acetylaspartate (NAA) have been labeled. (From Lien YH, Shapiro JI, Chan L. Effects of hypernatremia on organic brain osmoles. *J Clin Invest* 1990;85:1427–1435, with permission.)

The spectra of brain extracts from acute hypernatremia were similar to those of normal rats and thus are not shown (141).

Using clinical magnetic resonance imaging (MRI) and spectroscopy, Lee and his coworkers (138) examined an 18-month-old girl with severe dehydration and hypernatremia (plasma sodium concentration 195 mEq/l). A conventional 1.5-Tesla (1.5 T) Sigma General Electric magnetic resonance scanner was used. After MRI, quantitative proton NMR spectroscopy was performed in the parietal and occipital regions of the patient's cerebral cortex, revealing primarily white matter and gray matter, respectively. Spectra from the same regions in 50 healthy infants were also acquired. MRI revealed partial haloprosencephaly. Proton NMR spectroscopy of occipital gray matter and parietal white matter revealed several striking abnormalities (Fig. 10). The principle abnormality was a reversal of the normal ratio of peak intensities between the neuronal metabolite N-acetylaspartate and the putative osmolyte *myoinositol*. The principle change was in the concentration of myoinositol, which was three times normal, whereas that of

N-acetylaspartate was normal. Concentrations of choline and glutamine (plus glutamate) were also increased. The sequential spectra obtained during correction of the dehydration are shown (Fig. 10).

The calculated concentrations of the five principle metabolites shown in the spectra of the infant's brain on days 4 to 36 are shown in Table 6. The direct determination of patterns of disordered cerebral organic osmolytes by proton NMR spectroscopy may be valuable in guiding therapy (138, 216).

NMR analyses of metabolic changes in the kidney in response to hypertonic stress have focused on specific cell

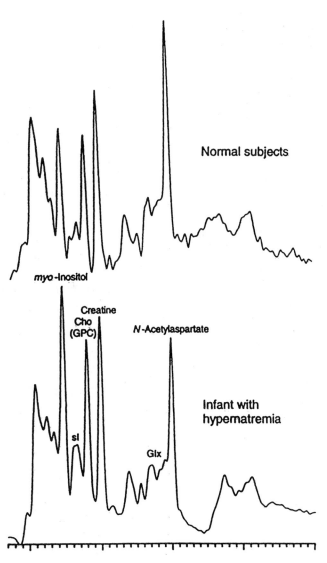

FIGURE 10 Short–echo-time proton nuclear magnetic resonance (NMR) spectrum of cortical gray matter in an infant with severe dehydration. The striking differences from normal in this patient were the apparent increase in *myo*-inositol and the decrease in N-acetylaspartate. The increase in *myo*-inositol was accompanied by increases in the concentrations of its stereoisomer, scyllo-inositol (sl), and choline-containing compounds (ho), especially glycerophosphoryl choline (GPC), glutamine plus glutamate (Glx), and creatine. (From Lee JH, Arcinue E, Ross BD. Brief report: organic osmolytes in the brain of an infant with hypernatremia. *N Engl J Med* 1994;331:439–442, with permission.)

TABLE 6   Results of Clinical Proton NMR Specteroscopy for Cerebral Osmometry
of the Brain of an Infant with Hypernatremia and Normal Subjects

| Metabolite | Normal Subjects | Day 4 | Study Patients (mmol) | | | |
			Day 7	Day 11	Day 22	Day 36
Myo-inositol	6	18	13	13	11	10
Choline	1.5	3.3	2.6	2.7	2.7	2.5
Creatine	8	10	8	9	8	8
Glutamine plus glutamate	15	18	15	15	15	10
N-acetylaspartate	8	6	6	7	7	7
Total	38.5	55.3	44.6	46.7	43.7	37.5
Excess metabolite	0	+16.8	+6.1	+8.2	+5.2	−1.0

Peak areas were converted to concentrations as previously described (56). The T1 and T2 relaxation times of water and each metabolite were within the normal range given in that report except for myoinositol, for which the value obtained in this study was 209 msec. As compared with a mean (± SD) of 301 ± 33 in the study by Ernst et al. (56). From Lee JH, Arcinue E, Ross BD. Brief report: organic osmolytes in the brain of an infant with hypernatremia (see comments). *N Engl J Med* 1994;331:439–442, with permisssion.

lines and, in particular, the inner medullary collecting duct. Analysis of changes in organic osmolytes with respect to chronic adaptation of IMCD₃ cells to increasing tonicity from 300 to 900 mOsm/kg H₂O were studied by proton NMR as shown in Fig. 11. Gross examination of NMR spectra demonstrates profound changes in nearly all organic osmolytes. Analysis of phosphorylated compounds can be determined by ³¹P NMR as shown in Fig. 12. In a similar fashion, initial refection indicates a substantial increase in GPC with more minor changes in GPE and PCr. While ³¹P NMR has been used for analysis of nucleotide triphosphates (NTPs) possibly improved techniques involving HPLC-MS appears to provide for higher sensitivity, greater reproducibility and throughput for analytical measurements.

ETIOLOGY OF HYPERNATREMIC STATES

Hypernatremia may be due to primary Na⁺ gain or water deficit (Table 7). The two components of an appropriate response to hypernatremia are increased water intake stimulated by thirst and the excretion of the minimum volume of maximally concentrated urine reflecting ADH secretion in response to an osmotic stimulus (184, 204). Most cases of hypernatremia result from the loss of water. Since water is distributed between the ICF and the ECF in a 2:1 ratio, a given amount of solute-free water loss will result in a twofold greater reduction in the ICF compartment than the ECF compartment. Sodium overload will result in hypernatremia with an increase in total-body sodium and

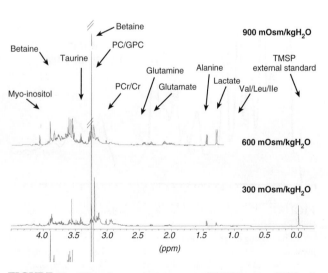

FIGURE 11   ¹H–nuclear magnetic resonance (NMR) spectra of PCA cell extracts. These spectra show the differences between cells cultivated in media containing 300 (**bottom**), 600 (**middle**), and 900 mOsm/kg H₂O (**upper spectrum**). GPC, glycerophosphocholine; PC, phosphocholine; Cr, creatine; PCr, phosphocreatine; TMSP, trimethylsilyl propionic-2,2,3,3,-d4 acid.

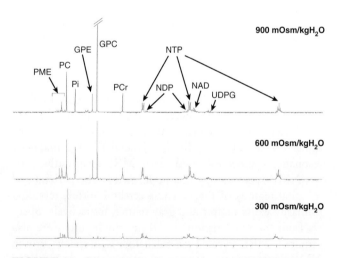

FIGURE 12   ³¹P–nuclear magnetic resonance (NMR) spectra of PCA cell extracts. These spectra show the differences between cells cultivated in media containing 300 (**bottom**), 600 (**middle**), and 900 mOsm/kg H₂O (**upper spectrum**). PME, phosphomonoester; PC, phophocholine; Pi, inorganic phosphate; GPE, glycerophophoethanolamine; GPC, glycerophophocholine; PCr, phosphocreatine; NTP, nucleotide triphosphates; NDP, nucleotide diphosphates; NAD, nicotinamide adenine dinucleotide; UDPG, uridine diphosphate glucose.

TABLE 7   Etiology of Hypernatremic States

Water loss
   Insensible
      Increased sweating
      Burns
      Respiratory infections
   Renal
      Central diabetes insipidus
      Nephrogenic diabetes insipidus
      Osmotic diuresis
   Gastrointestinal
      Osmotic diarrhea
   Hypothalamic
      Primary hypodipsia
      Reset osmostat due to volume expansion in primary mineralocorticoid excess
   Water loss into cells
   Seizures or severe exercise
   Rhabdomyoluiss
Sodium overload
   Administration of hypertonic NaCl or NaHCO$_3$
   Ingestion of sodium

the patient will have an increase in ECF. Water deficit however may occur with low or normal total-body sodium.

Water deficit in excess of sodium deficit is associated with hypovolemic hypernatremia and the patient will have low total-body sodium. When hypernatremia is caused by pure water loss, the patient is euvolemic and the total-body sodium remains normal. The causes of water losses in both of these settings may be renal or extrarenal. Renal losses of water may be a consequence of diabetes insipidus or osmotic diuresis. Diabetes insipidus will be discussed in more detail later in this chapter in hypernatremia associated with normal total-body sodium.

In the absence of increased water losses, hypernatremia can still develop (with normal total-body sodium) if there is primary hypothalamic disease impairing thirst (called *hypodipsia*). Two different syndromes have been described, which are most often due to tumors, granulomatous diseases (such as sarcoidosis), or vascular disease. In the first, there is a defect in thirst, with or without concomitant diabetes insipidus. In this disorder, forced water intake is usually sufficient to maintain a normal plasma sodium concentration (202, 203). Other hypodipsic patients will not respond to water loading, as the excess water will be excreted in the urine with little change in the plasma sodium concentration (123, 156).

Transient hypernatremia (in which the plasma sodium concentration can rise by 10 to 15 mEq/l within a few minutes) can be induced by severe exercise or seizures, which are also associated with the development of lactic acidosis. In this setting, the breakdown of glycogen into smaller, more osmotically active molecules (such as lactate) can increase the cell osmolality, thereby causing the osmotic movement of water into the cells. The plasma sodium concentration returns to normal within 5 to 15 minutes after the cessation of exertion.

CLASSIFICATION OF HYPERNATREMIA BASED ON TOTAL-BODY SODIUM:

Another clinical approach to the hypernatremic patient is based on the assessment of the ECF volume status and the total-body sodium.

Hypernatremia in Patients with Low Total-Body Sodium

Patients who sustain losses of both sodium and water but with a relatively greater loss of water are classified as having hypernatremia with low total-body sodium. Signs of hypovolemia include orthostatic hypotension, tachycardia, flat neck veins, poor skin turgor, and dry mucous membranes are usually present. Isotonic sodium chloride should be given until systemic hemodynamics is stabilized.

The sources of free-water loss that can lead to hypernatremia if intake is not increased include insensible water loss from the skin by evaporation and sweat are dilute fluids, the loss of which is increased by fever, exercise, and exposure to high temperatures. Burns and infections will also increase the water loss. Some gastrointestinal losses, particularly osmotic diarrheas, will promote the development of hypernatremia because the sodium plus potassium concentration is less than that in the plasma (218). Although primarily recognized in children, lactulose-induced diarrhea leading to hypernatremia appears to be common. Since the renal water- and sodium-conserving mechanisms operate normally in these patients, urinary osmolality is high (usually >800 mOsm/kg H$_2$O) and urinary sodium concentration is low (<10 mEq/l). An elevation in the plasma sodium concentration with diarrhea illness is particularly common in infants in whom fluid replacement with a relatively dilute solution can minimize the risk of hypernatremia. Decreased release of ADH or renal resistance to its effect causes the excretion of relatively dilute urine (191, 205). Most of these patients have a normal thirst mechanism. As a result, they typically present with polyuria and polydipsia, and at most a high-normal plasma sodium concentration. However, marked and symptomatic hypernatremia can occur if a central lesion impairs both ADH release and thirst, thereby preventing replacement of the urinary water losses.

An osmotic diuresis due to glucose, mannitol, or urea causes an increase in urine output in which the sodium plus potassium concentration is well below that in the plasma because of the presence of the nonreabsorbed organic solute. Patients with diabetic ketoacidosis or nonketotic hyperglycemia typically present with marked hyperosmolality, although the plasma sodium concentration may not be elevated due to hyperglycemia-induced water movement out of the cells. Hypotonic losses can also occur by the renal route during a loop diuretic-induced hypotonic diuresis or an osmotic diuresis with mannitol, glucose, glycerol, or, more rarely, urea. Elderly patients with partial urinary tract obstruction can excrete large volumes of hypotonic urine (239). The urine in these cases is hypotonic or isotonic, and the urinary sodium concentration is greater than 20 mEq/l. Since glucose and mannitol enhance osmotic water movement from the intracellular fluid to the ECF compartment, some of these patients may have a normal or even low serum sodium concentration in spite of serum hypertonicity.

Hypernatremia in Patients with Normal Total-Body Sodium

When hypernatremia is caused by pure water loss, total-body sodium remains normal. Patients are usually euvolemic. The extrarenal sources of such water losses are the skin and the respiratory tract. A high environmental temperature as well as a febrile or hypermetabolic state can cause considerable water losses. If such hypotonic losses are not accompanied by appropriate water intake, hypernatremia supervenes. Urine osmolality is very high, reflecting an intact osmoreceptor-vasopressin-renal response. Urinary sodium concentration will vary according to the patient's sodium intake. This kind of hypernatremia has been reported in hepatic failure (244). It was believed to occur due to total-body water loss. The possible mechanisms include increased insensible losses, decreased access to water secondary to hepatic encephalopathy and increased hypotonic losses in stool secondary to osmotic cathartics used for treatment of encephalopathy. Chronic alcoholic subjects with end stage liver disease who present with fulminant liver failure and hepatic encephalopathy have a high mortality rate (128, 244). Patients with liver disease who develop hypernatremia are particularly susceptible to the development of cerebral demyelinating lesions.

Diabetes insipidus is a polyuric disorder characterized by high rates of electrolyte free water excretion (42). When these are not appropriately replaced hypernatremia supervenes. The causes of central neurogenic diabetes insipidus are listed in Table 8. If the thirst mechanism is intact and water is available, patients with central diabetes insipidus do not develop hypernatremia and thus have no symptoms except for the inconvenience associated with the marked polyuria and polydipsia. With concomitant hypodipsia, no access to water, or an illness that precludes adequate water intake, however, severe and even life-threatening hypernatremia can supervene.

Hypernatremia secondary to nonosmotic urinary water loss is usually due to central or neurogenic diabetes insipidus characterized by impaired argenine vasopressin secretion, or nephrogenic diabetes insipidus resulting from end-organ (renal) resistance to the actions of AVP. The most common cause of central diabetes insipidus is destruction of the neurohypophysis. This may occur as a result of trauma, neurosurgery, granulomatous disease, neoplasms, vascular accidents,

TABLE 8 Causes of Central Diabetes Insipidus (CDI)

Hereditary
  Autosomal dominant
  Autosomal recessive (Wolfram syndrome)
Acquired
  Head trauma, skull fracture, and orbital trauma
  Posthypophysectomy
  Suprasellar and intrasellar tumors
    Primary (suprasellar cyst, craniopharyngioma, pinealoma, meningioma, and glioma)
    Metastatic (breast or lung cancer, leukemia, and lymphomas)
Granulomas
  Sarcoid
  Wegener granulomatosis
  Tuberculosis
  Syphilis
Histiocytosis
  Eosinophilic granuloma
  Hand-Schuller-Christian disease
Infections
  Encephalitis
  Meningitis
  Guillain-Barre syndrome
Vascular
  Cerebral aneurysm
  Cerebral thrombosis or hemorrhage
  Sickle cell disease
  Postpartum necrosis (Sheehan syndrome)
  Pregnancy (transient)

or infection. In many cases, central diabetes insipidus is idiopathic and may occasionally be hereditary. The familial form of the disease is inherited in an autosomal dominant fashion and has been attributed to mutations in the propressophysin (argenine vasopressin precursor) gene (26, 125, 157, 159, 167). Nephrogenic diabetes insipidus may be either inherited or acquired. Congenital nephrogenic diabetes insipidus I is an X-linked recessive trait due to mutations in the V2 receptor gene (24, 38, 114, 115, 119, 129, 130, 211). Mutations in the autosomal aquaporin-2 gene may also result in NDI (9, 27, 51, 120, 154, 178). The aquaporin-2 gene encodes the water channel protein whose membrane insertion is stimulated by AVP. The causes of sporadic nephrogenic diabetes insipidus are numerous and include drugs (especially lithium) (15, 29, 41, 43, 60, 81, 91, 243), hypercalcemia, hypokalemia, and conditions that impair medullary hypertonicity (e.g., papillary necrosis or osmotic diuresis) (21, 99, 124, 139, 187). Pregnant women, in the second or third trimester, may develop nephrogenic diabetes insipidus as a result of excessive elaboration of vasopressinase by the placenta (14, 221).

Congenital nephrogenic diabetes insipidus is a rare hereditary disorder in which the renal tubule is insensitive to vasopressin (209). The disease manifests itself in the complete clinical form only in males and in a subclinical form in females suggesting a sex-linked dominant inheritance with variable penetrance in the female. The gene responsible for the defect has, in fact, been mapped to region 28 on the long arm of the X chromosome (Xq28). Although the disease is most probably inborn, the diagnosis is usually not made until the infant has hyposmolar urine with severe dehydration, hypernatremia, vomiting, and fever. Unlike some of the females, who have partial responsiveness to vasopressin, the male with the full-blown complete form of this disorder will not have hypertonic urine even in the face of severe dehydration. The impaired growth and occasional mental retardation that supervene in these cases are most likely due to repeated episodes of dehydration and hypernatremia rather than being integral components of the disease. Hydronephrosis is also common in these patients, perhaps because of voluntary retention of large volumes of urine, with subsequent vesicoureteral reflux (34).

Neither vasopressin nor other pharmacologic agents that potentiate its action or stimulate its release, such as chlorpropamide, are effective in concentrating the urine of patients with nephrogenic diabetes insipidus. An intact thirst mechanism is therefore indispensable for the maintenance of good hydration in children with this disorder, as is careful monitoring of fluid balance. Since the excretion of solute requires further water losses, children with this disorder who need rehydration should receive hypotonic (2.5%) rather than isotonic (5%) glucose solutions. Glucosuria may occur with the latter solution and thus aggravate fluid losses.

Limitation of oral solute intake (low-sodium diet) may also lead to a decrease in urine flow in patients with nephrogenic diabetes insipidus. Thiazide diuretics, which inhibit sodium reabsorption in the cortical diluting segment of the nephron, have met with some success in the management of these patients. The ability of thiazides to diminish sodium reabsorption in this water-impermeable portion of the nephron would itself decrease C_{H_2O} but not urine flow. It seems most likely that the decrease in urine flow is secondary to the sodium loss and ECF volume contraction. ECF volume depletion in turn decreases glomerular filtration rate (GFR) and increases proximal tubular sodium and water reabsorption. These secondary effects of the diuretic agent then decrease urine flow. The ECF volume contraction can be maintained with a low sodium intake after discontinuance of the diuretic, so that the therapy still remains effective. The addition of amiloride to hydrochlorothiazide may provide added benefit (4, 126, 133, 183). Nonsteroidal anti-inflammatory agents have been found to be effective.

The acquired form of nephrogenic diabetes insipidus is much more common than the congenital form of the disease, but it is rarely severe (23). While maximal concentrating ability is impaired in this disorder, the ability to elaborate a hypertonic urine is usually preserved. Nocturia, polyuria, and polydipsia may occur in this acquired form of nephrogenic diabetes insipidus, but the urine volumes are generally less (<3–4 l/day) than those observed with complete central diabetes insipidus, psychogenic water-drinking, or congenital nephrogenic central diabetes insipidus. The more common causes of acquired nephrogenic diabetes insipidus are listed in Table 9.

TABLE 9 Causes of Acquired Nephrogenic Diabetes Insipidus (NDI)

Chronic renal disease
  Polycystic disease
  Medullary cystic disease
  Ureteral obstruction
  Amyloidosis
  Advanced renal failure of any etiology
Electrolyte disorders
  Hypokalemia
  Hypercalcemia
Drugs
  Alcohol
  Lithium
  Demeclocycline
  Glyburide
  Amphotericin
  Foscarnet
Sickle cell disease
Dietary abnormalities
  Excessive water intake
  Decreased sodium chloride intake
  Decreased protein intake
Miscellaneous
  Gestational diabetes insipidus

A defect in renal concentrating capacity is a consistent accompaniment of most forms of advanced renal failure (230, 232). Thus, chronic renal failure constitutes a form of acquired nephrogenic diabetes insipidus. Advanced renal insufficiency of any cause can cause a vasopressin resistance associated with hypotonic urine. In some forms of kidney disease vasopressin unresponsiveness can occur at a stage when GFR is not markedly diminished. The occurrence of a profound diuresis in association with a concentrating defect in glomerular diseases of the kidney is rare, and in general, a close correlation exists between GFR and maximal urinary osmolality. The causes of the defect in renal concentrating capacity associated with chronic renal failure are probably multiple (73, 74, 85). These include (1) a disruption of inner medullary structures or local alterations in medullary blood flow as is seen in tubulointerstitial diseases, sickle cell disease (31, 227), and analgesic nephropathy; (2) impairment in sodium chloride transport out of the thick ascending limb of Henle's loop, a process that limits maximal interstitial tonicity; and (3) increase in solute excretion in the remaining few functioning nephrons, an adaptive response to the need to excrete the same solute load as the normal kidney.

Hypokalemia has long been known to cause polyuria as a consequence of a vasopressin resistant renal concentrating defect (198). A direct effect of hypokalemia on the collecting tubule is supported by studies in the toad bladder which show a decrease in cyclic AMP and vasopressin-stimulated water flow when potassium is removed from the bathing solution (75). These findings suggest both a precyclic AMP and postcyclic AMP defect. The hypokalemia induced resistance to vasopressin is associated with decreased cyclic

AMP accumulation apparently due to decreased adenylyl cyclase activity. Hypokalemia from any cause, such as diarrhea, chronic diuretic use, or primary aldosteronism, may be associated with a urinary concentrating defect. The defect is generally reversible but requires a longer time (1–3 months) than would be expected from a purely functional defect.

Hypercalcemia is another well-recognized cause of impaired urinary concentrating ability (16, 92, 144). A decrement in medullary interstitial tonicity is clearly present with hypercalcemia, which may be related to diminished solute reabsorption in the thick ascending limb. This defect is associated with a decrement in AVP-stimulated adenylate cyclase in this nephron segment. The concentrating defect is, however, multifactorial as the elaboration of hypotonic urine implies an intrinsic defect in the collecting tubule. In this regard, studies in isolated toad bladders as well as papillary collecting ducts reveal a decreased response to vasopressin in hypercalcemia.

Various pharmacologic agents have been found to impair the renal capacity to concentrate urine (Table 9). Ethanol and phenytoin (Dilantin) seem to exert their action by a central effect on vasopressin release (84). Some hypoglycemic agents cause a diuresis by a mechanism probably unrelated to suppression of vasopressin release. The renal toxicity of amphotericin can manifest in the form of a concentrating defect (59). Foscarnet, an agent increasingly employed in the treatment of cytomegalovirus (CMV) infection in patients with acquired immune deficiency syndrome (AIDS), has been described to cause a nephrogenic diabetes insipidus (68, 123).

The drugs most commonly associated with nephrogenic diabetes insipidus are demeclocycline and lithium (15, 29, 40, 43, 60, 91). Since it was first recognized as a cause of nephrogenic diabetes insipidus, demeclocycline has become the drug of choice for the treatment of the syndrome of inappropriate ADH secretion (SIADH). It has yet to be determined if demeclocycline reduces argenine vasopressin secretion. It is clear, however, that demeclocycline induces dose-dependent decreases in human renal medullary adenylate cyclase activity. Since the drug decreases not only vasopressin but also cyclic AMP–stimulated water flow, a postcyclic AMP defect may be operant (193).

Lithium is the most common cause of nephrogenic diabetes insipidus. There is no evidence that lithium impairs vasopressin release. In terms of the mechanism of its renal action, lithium does not interfere with accumulation of medullary solutes. Thus, an intrinsic tubular defect is postulated. In this regard, lithium decreases vasopressin-stimulated water transport in the perfused cortical collecting duct. An inhibition in adenylate cyclase or in cyclic AMP generation is observed in human tissue and cultured cells exposed to the cation as well as animals chronically treated with lithium. More recently a downregulation of the vasopressin regulated water channel (aquaporin) has been

described in lithium-treated rats (121). It is of interest that the urinary aquaporin levels remained low after removal of lithium in line with the slow recovery of concentrating ability seen in man.

A renal concentrating defect is a common accompaniment of sickle cell anemia and sickle cell trait (10, 31, 188). Sickling of red blood cells in the hypertonic medullary interstitium with occlusion of the vasa recta appears to cause inner medullary and papillary damage. Microradioangiographic studies have failed to demonstrate vasa recta blood flow in patients with sickle cell disease. The resultant medullary ischemia may impair sodium chloride transport in the ascending limb and thus diminish medullary tonicity. Transfusions of normal blood have been shown to restore renal concentrating capacity in children, thus indicating that the sickled red blood cells have a role in the defect. With more prolonged disease, medullary infarcts occur, and the concentrating defect is no longer reversible with transfusions.

The syndrome of essential hypernatremia and hypodipsia has been described in patients with normal total-body sodium. A partial list of causes of this hypodipsia-hypernatremia syndrome is shown in Table 10. These patients exhibit persistent hypernatremia not explained by any volume loss. There is absence or attenuation of thirst. The patient may also have partial diabetes insipidus and a normal renal response to ADH. This is due to a primary hypothalamic disease impairing thirst (called *hypodipsia*). Two different syndromes have been described, which are most often due to tumors, granulomatous diseases (such as sarcoidosis), or vascular disease. In the first, there is a defect in thirst, with or without concomitant diabetes insipidus. In this disorder, forced water intake is usually sufficient to

TABLE 10   Causes of the Hypodipsia-Hypernatremia Syndrome

Ectopic pinealoma
Dysgerminoma/germinoma
Craniopharyngioma
Teratoma
Meningioma
Metastatic bronchial carcinoma
Eosinophilic granuloma
Hand-Schuller-Christian disease
Ganulomatous tumor
Hypothalamic neuronal degeneration
Subarachnoid hemorrhage
Posttraumatic carotid cavernous fistula
Microcephaly
Occult hydrocephalus
Head trauma
Aneurysectomy (anterior communicating artery)
Sarcoidosis

From Levi M, Berl T. Water metabolism In: Gonick HC, ed. *Current Nephrology*, Vol 5. Chicago: Year Book Medical; 1982:37.

maintain a normal plasma sodium concentration (202, 203). Other hypodipsic patients will not respond to water loading, as the excess water will be excreted in the urine with little change in the plasma sodium concentration (123, 156). It had been postulated that these patients had a reset osmostat upward (called *essential hypernatremia*), so that the new high plasma sodium concentration was recognized as normal (111, 112). Thus, giving water will decrease ADH release and the excess water will be excreted in dilute urine. It is now clear, however, that these patients have selective injury to the osmoreceptors, with ADH secretion being primarily governed by changes in volume (100). Thus, the suppression of ADH release by water loading in this setting is due to the associated mild volume expansion, rather than a fall in plasma osmolality. True resetting of the osmostat upwards has been described only in patients with primary mineralocorticoid excess (such as primary hyperaldosteronism). The plasma sodium concentration in these patients is usually between 143 and 147 mEq/l. It is presumed that the suppressive effect of chronic mild volume expansion on ADH release is responsible for the resetting. This appears to be due to a specific osmoreceptor defect resulting in nonosmotic regulation of argenine vasopressin release. These patients are characterized by persistent hypernatremia not explained by any apparent extracellular volume loss with a normal response to AVP. It has been proposed that these patients have a "resetting" of the osmoreceptor, since these patients tend to concentrate and dilute urine at inappropriately high levels of plasma osmolality (30, 54, 55, 101, 163, 168). However, using the regression analysis of plasma argenine vasopressin level versus plasma osmolality, it has been shown that in some of these patients the tendency to concentrate and dilute urine at inappropriately high levels of plasma osmolality is due solely to a marked reduction in sensitivity or gain of the osmoregulatory mechanism. In other patients, however, plasma argenine vasopressin levels fluctuate in a random manner bearing no apparent relationship to changes in plasma osmolality. Such patients frequently display large swings in serum sodium concentration. It appears that most patients with essential hypernatremia fit one of these two patterns (204, 233).

Hypodipsia can also occur in elderly patients without overt hypothalamic lesions and can culminate in severe hypernatremia (163, 220). It has been suggested that a decrement in angiotensin II-mediated thirst existed in the elderly (190, 248).

Hypernatremia in Patients with Increased Total-Body Sodium

Hypernatremia with increased total-body sodium is the least common type of hypernatremia and is usually due to exogenous administration of hypertonic sodium containing solutes (Table 11) (69). Acute and often marked hypernatremia (in which the plasma sodium concentration can exceed 175–200 mEq/l) can be induced by the administration of hypertonic sodium-containing solutions. Hypernatremia supervenes during resuscitative efforts with hypertonic sodium bicarbonate (7, 155), inadvertent intravascular infusion of hypertonic saline in therapeutic abortions, inadvertent dialysis against a high sodium concentration dialysate, sea water drowning, and even after ingestion of large quantities of sodium chloride tablets (66, 158, 197, 214, 246). Accidental or nonaccidental salt poisoning has been reported in infants and young children and in patients taking highly concentrated saline emetic or gargle (3, 66, 185). The hypernatremia in this setting will correct spontaneously if renal function is normal, since the excess sodium will be rapidly excreted in the urine. This process can be facilitated by inducing a sodium and water diuresis with a loop diuretic and then replacing the urine output with water. Too rapid correction should be avoided if the patient is asymptotic. Since the hypernatremia is generally very acute with little time for cerebral adaptation. These patients are less likely to develop cerebral edema during correction (116, 118). The degree of hyperosmolality is typically mild unless the thirst mechanism is abnormal or access to water is limited. This occurs in infants, the physically handicapped, patients with impaired mental status, in the postoperative state, and in patients on ventilators. Patients with primary hyperaldosteronism and Cushing syndrome have slight, clinically unimportant elevations in serum sodium concentration. As expected, patients

TABLE 11   Therapeutic Hypertonic Solutions

Solute	Molecular Weight	Concentration (mg/dL%)	Osmolality (mosm/kg water)	Typical Container Size (ML)	Use
Sodium chloride	58.5	3	1026	500	Emergency teatment of hypotonic states; intraamniotic instillation for therapeutic abortion
		5	1711	500	
		20	6845	250	
Sodium bicarbonate	84.0	5	1190	500	Treatment of metaboliuc acidosis, hyperkalemia, cardiopulmonary arrest
		7.5	1786	50	

From Morrison G, Singer L. Hyperosmolal states. In: Narins RG, ed. *Clinical Disorders of Fluid and Electrolyte Metabolism.* New York: McGraw-Hill; 1994:646.

with hypernatremia and high total-body sodium excrete generous quantities of the cation in the urine.

CLINICAL FEATURES IN HYPERNATREMIA

A complete history and physical examination will often provide clues as to the underlying cause of hypernatremia (143, 199). Relevant symptoms and signs include the absence or presence of thirst, diaphoresis, diarrhea, polyuria, and the features of ECF volume contraction (164, 171, 176, 177). The major symptoms of hypernatremia are neurologic and include altered mental status, weakness, neuromuscular irritability, focal neurologic deficits, and occasionally coma or seizures (Table 12). As a consequence of hypertonicity, water shifts out of cells, leading to a contracted ICF volume. A decreased brain cell volume is associated with an increased risk of subarachnoid or intracerebral hemorrhage (5, 71, 76, 134). Patients may also complain of polyuria or thirst. For unknown reasons, patients with polydipsia from CDI tend to prefer ice-cold water. The signs and symptoms of volume depletion are often present in patients with a history of excessive sweating, diarrhea, or an osmotic diuresis (14, 61, 64, 80, 143, 245, 251).

The severity of the clinical manifestations is related to the acuity and magnitude of the rise in plasma Na^+ concentration. Chronic hypernatremia is generally less symptomatic as a result of adaptive mechanisms designed to defend cell volume. Brain cells initially take up Na^+ and K^+ salts, later followed by accumulation of organic osmolytes such as inositol. This serves to restore the brain ICF volume towards normal.

The signs and symptoms of hypernatremia are most likely related to a variety of anatomic derangements. The most prominent manifestations of hyperosmolar disorders are of a neurologic nature (103, 105, 108, 152, 153, 200, 231). The loss of volume and the shrinkage of brain cells associated with the hyperosmolar states cause tearing of cerebral vessels. In addition to these gross anatomic changes, the brain sustains alterations in the composition of water and solutes that may be of great importance in the pathophysiology of the symptoms of hypernatremia. These are responses designed to regulate volume and restore cell size.

TABLE 12   Signs and Symptoms of Hypernatremia

Intense thirst
Irritability
Signs of volume depletion (variable)
Nausea or vomiting
Depression of sensorium
Seizures (unusual in adults)
Focal neurologic deficits
Muscle spasticity (unusual in adults)
Fever
Labored respiration

Thus, the water losses are not as severe as would be predicted. In the early phase, the entry of sodium and chloride into brain cells greatly mitigates the loss of water that would otherwise occur from ideal osmotic behavior. After 7 days of hypernatremia, brain water has returned to control levels as brain osmolality remains elevated. At this time idiogenic osmoles account for as much as 60% of the increase in intracellular osmolality. It now seems possible that some of these idiogenic osmoles are due to an increase in intracellular amino acids, particularly taurine. In addition, accumulation of osmolytes such as urea, glutamine, glycerolphosphorylcholine, and myoinositol has been documented in hypernatremic rats as well as in human using NMR spectroscopy.

Measurement of urine volume and osmolality are essential in the evaluation of hypernatremia. The appropriate renal response to hypernatremia is the excretion of the minimum volume (500 ml/d) of maximally concentrated urine (urine osmolality greater than 800 mOsm/kg H_2O). These findings suggest extrarenal or remote renal water loss or administration of hypertonic Na^+ salt solutions. The presence of a primary Na^+ excess can be confirmed by the presence of ECF volume expansion and natriuresis (urine Na^+ concentration usually greater than 100 mmol/l). Many causes of hypernatremia are associated with polyuria and a submaximal urine osmolality. The product of the urine volume and osmolality, i.e., the solute excretion rate, is helpful in determining the basis of the polyuria. To maintain a steady state, total solute excretion must equal solute production. Individuals eating a normal diet generate approximately 600 mOsm/d. Therefore, daily solute excretion in excess of 750 mOsm/d defines an osmotic diuresis. This can be confirmed by measuring the urine glucose and urea. In general, both CDI and NDI present with polyuria and hypotonic urine (urine osmolality less than 250 mOsm/kg H_2O). The degree of hypernatremia is usually mild unless there is an associated thirst abnormality.

THERAPY FOR HYPERNATREMIA

The therapeutic goals are to stop ongoing water loss by treating the underlying cause and to correct the water deficit. The specific approach depends on the patient's ECF volume (Table 13). Reversal of hypernatremic state must be undertaken slowly to prevent neurological complications. Rapid correction may result in cerebral edema, seizure, and death (52, 143, 160, 162, 228, 229, 237, 238).

When the patient has low total-body sodium, as evidenced by circulatory manifestations (e.g., orthostatic hypotension), isotonic sodium chloride should be given until systemic hemodynamics are stabilized. Thereafter, the hypernatremia can be treated with 0.45% sodium chloride or 5% dextrose. When the patient is hypervolemic and hypernatremic, the removal of excess sodium is the goal, which can be achieved either by administration of diuretics along

TABLE 13   Diagnosis and Therapeutic Approach to the Hypernatremic Patient

		Urinary		
	Causes	Tonicity	Na$^+$ (mEq/L)	Therapies

Hypovolemia
Low total-body Na$^+$
Na$^+$, H$_2$O loss
	Renal loss
	  Osmotic or loop diuretics
	    Postobstruction
	    Intrinsic renal disease
		Iso-
		Hypo-
			>20	Hypotonic saline

	Extrarenal loss
	  Dermal
	    Sweating
	    Burns
	  Gastrointestinal
	    Diarrhea
	    Fistulas
		Hyper-	<10	

Euvolemia
Normal total-body Na$^+$
H$_2$O loss
	Renal loss
	  Diabetes insipidus
	    Nephrogenic
	    Central
	    Partial
	    Gestational
	  Hypodispsia
		Hypo-
		Iso-
		Hyper-
			Variable	Water replacement

	Extrarenal loss
	  Insensible losses
	    Respiratory
	    Dermal
		Hyper-	Variable	

Hypervolemia Increased total-body Na$^+$ Na$^+$ addition	Primary hyperaldosteronism Cushing syndrome Hypertonic dialysate Hypertonic sodium bicarbonate Sodium chloride tablets	Iso- Hyper-	>20	Diuretics and water replacement

with 5% dextrose or, if renal function is impaired, by dialysis. The euvolemic hypernatremic patient who has sustained pure water losses requires water replacement as a 5% dextrose infusion.

The water deficit in this setting can be calculated based on the current sodium concentration and body weight, using the assumption that total-body water is approximately 50% or 60% of body weight

$$\text{Water deficit} = \text{Total-body water} \times \left(\frac{\text{Plasma } [\text{Na}^+] - 140}{140} \right)$$

$$\text{(Eq. 7)}$$

In addition to replacing the calculated water deficit, ongoing fluid losses should be replaced. In acute hypernatremia, repletion of the water deficit may be faster. The electrolytes accumulate in the brain during hypernatremia are rapidly extruded into the extracellular space during treatment, minimizing the risk of cerebral edema (160). In contrast, rapid correction in chronic hypernatremia is potentially dangerous. In this case, a sudden decrease in osmolality could potentially cause a rapid shift of water into cells that have undergone osmotic adaptation. This would result in swollen brain cells and increase the risk of seizures or permanent neurologic damage (110). A

slower rate of correction probably can prevent this sequence of events by allowing idiogenic osmoles time to be dissipated.

The plasma Na$^+$ concentration should be lowered by 0.5 mmol/L per hour and by no more than 12 mmol/L over the first 24 hours. The safest route of administration of water is by mouth or via a nasogastric tube (or other feeding tube). Alternatively, 5% dextrose in water or half-isotonic saline can be given intravenously. The patient's neurological status should be monitored carefully throughout treatment. Deterioration of neurological status after an initial improvement suggests the development of cerebral edema and mandates temporary discontinuation or slowing the rate of water replacement.

In patients with essential hypernatremia and the elderly with hypodipsia, 1 to 2 liters of water per day may need to be administered as a prescription. Chlorpropamide itself augments thirst and its use with desmopressin in patients with adipsia has been proposed.

Patients with central diabetes insipidus do not develop hypernatremia if the thirst mechanism is intact and that water is available. Hormonal replacement and pharmacologic agents are available for the treatment of central diabetes insipidus. In acute settings, such as after hypophysectomy, the aqueous vasopressin (Pitressin) preparation is preferable. Its short duration of action allows for more careful monitoring and decreases the likelihood of complications such as water intoxication. In chronic settings, vasopressin tannate in oil (Pitressin Tannate) is potent and effective for 24 to 72 hours. It requires a deep subcutaneous or intramuscular injection by a fairly large-gauge needle because of the viscosity of the oil vehicle. This material can cause sterile abscesses in some subjects and on occasion be associated with resistance due to development of antibodies (215, 217, 240). A modification of the natural vasopressin molecule to form desmopressin acetate (dDAVP) has resulted in a compound with prolonged antidiuretic activity (6–24 hours) and virtual elimination of vasopressor activity (antidiuretic to pressor ratio of approximately 2000:1) as compared with the natural hormone argenine vasopressin (duration of action of 2–4 hours and antidiuretic to pressor ratio of 1:1; 102, 170, 195, 196, 208). Substitution of D-argenine for L-argenine at position 8 resulted in a peptide DAVP with diminished vasopressor activity, and deamination of the hemicysteine at position 1 gave rise to a second peptide, with enhanced antidiuretic to pressor activity and prolonged duration of action. dDAVP is administered intranasally in the dosage ranging from 10 to 20 μg every 8 to 12 hours (25, 49). Intranasal dDAVP is now the treatment of choice for central diabetes insipidus.

In some patients with partial central diabetes insipidus, drugs that stimulate argenine vasopressin secretion or enhance its action on the kidney have been useful. These include chlorpropamide, clofibrate, carbamazepine, and nonsteroidal anti-inflammatory drugs (NSAIDs) (17, 63, 82, 242). Since with very dilute urine of fixed osmolality the urine volume is determined by the solute load requiring excretion, a reduction of salt and protein in the diet will reduce the major urinary solutes and thus the volume of urine necessary to accommodate their excretion (88). A number of pharmacologic agents with antidiuretic properties are also used. Chlorpropamide (Diabinese) is the most commonly used. Its antidiuretic effects are manifested only if some vasopressin is present and is therefore useful only in partial diabetes insipidus. In Brattleboro rats with diabetes insipidus, chlorpropamide augmented the antidiuretic responses to dDAVP. A trial of 250 mg every day or twice a day may be offered to patients with partial central diabetes insipidus and at least 7 days allowed for an effect to occur. The anticonvulsant carbamazepine (Tegretol) has also caused antidiuresis in subjects with diabetes insipidus. A combination of chlorpropamide and carbamazepine has been found to provide an effect that could be synergistic (179, 194). Clofibrate also has been used to treat partial central diabetes insipidus.

In patients with nephrogenic diabetes insipidus, the concentrating defect may be reversible by treating the underlying disorder or eliminating the offending drug. Symptomatic polyuria can be treated with a low-sodium diet and thiazide diuretics (4). This induces mild volume depletion, which leads to enhanced proximal reabsorption of salt and water and decreased delivery to the site of action of AVP, the collecting duct. By impairing renal prostaglandin synthesis, NSAIDs potentiate argenine vasopressin action and thereby increase urine osmolality and decrease urine volume (140). Amiloride may be useful in patients with nephrogenic diabetes insipidus who need to be on lithium (72, 243). The nephrotoxicity of lithium requires the drug to be taken up into collecting duct cells via the amiloride-sensitive Na$^+$ channel.

CLINICAL STUDIES AND OUTCOME

The clinical outcome of patients with hypernatremia depends on the age of the patient and the rapidity with which the hypernatremic state was attained (70, 180, 181). Acute hypernatremia is associated with a 40% mortality, whereas the mortality for chronic hypernatremia is about 10%. In children, the mortality of acute hypernatremia ranges between 10% and 70%, with a mean of approximately 45%. Unfortunately, even in survivors neurologic sequelae are common, affecting as many as two thirds of the children (39, 44, 46, 62, 182). In adults, acute elevation of serum sodium above 160 mEq/l is associated with a 75% mortality, while the mortality in chronic cases is approximately 60%. Note, however, that in the adult, hypernatremia frequently occurs in the setting of serious underlying diseases, which may be the primary cause of the high mortality (13, 59, 94, 241).

Table 14 summarizes clinical studies of hypernatremia in adults that have been published over the past two decades. From these varied studies (22, 50, 106, 147, 149, 180, 181, 224), it is apparent that hypernatremia is a common disturbance with an incidence ranging from less than 1% to more than 3%. The variation in incidence is in part a function of the populations at risk and the definition of hypernatremia used in various studies. The patient groups at increased risk for development of severe hypernatremia are listed in Table 15. Hypernatremia developing in nonhospitalized adults is predominantly a disease of the elderly (11, 28, 135, 149, 151), is commonly a manifestation of underlying infection, and may reflect inadequate nursing care of patients in chronic care facilities. However, hospital-acquired hypernatremia occurs in a wider range of patients with an age distribution more similar to the general hospitalized population. The main factor contributing to the development of hypernatremia is the inability to control water intake in the setting of increased water losses. Pure water loss from diabetes insipidus rarely contributes to its development; more common etiologies of water loss include diuretic administration, solute diuresis, enteral fluid loss, and fever. The results from these clinical series support the recommendation that the serum sodium concentration be corrected promptly but gradually over 48 to 72 hours.

TABLE 14 Published Clinical Series of Patients with Hypernatremia

Series (reference)	Definition ([Na], mmol/L)	N	Incidence	Age (years, mean ± SD)	Etiologic Factors	Mortality
Daggett et al.	>154	20	0.12%	N/A	Diabetes mellitus (40%) CNS disease (40%)	40%
Mahowald and Himmelstein	>150	23	N/A	72±12	Infection (74%)	52%
Himmelstein et al.	>150	56	0.65–2.25	73±15	Infection (77%) Nursing home care (52%)	46%
Snyder et al.	>148 (age >60 years)	162	1.1%	78±9	Febrile illness infirmity Nutritional supplementa-tion postoperative state	42%
Bhatnagar and Weinkove	>160	27	N/A	71.4	Poor intake (38%) Increased insensible losses Diuresis (29%) Increased GI losses (25%)	79%
Long et al.	>150	160	0.3%	76 (median)	Diuretics (72%) Depressed sensorium (71%) Febrile illness (60%) Mechanical ventilation (28%)	54%
Borra et al.	>150	111	3.5%	On admission 83 ± 11 Hospital-acquired 76 ± 15	Infection (65%) Malignancy (12%) Diabetes mellitus (7%)	49%
Palevsky	>150	103	On admission 0.2% Hospital-acquired 1.0%	On admission 77 ± 17 Hospital-acquired 59 ± 19	On admission infection (83%) Hospital-acquired fever (56%) Mechanical ventilation (49%) Enteral fluid loss (40%) Mental status changes (36%)	41%

CNS, central nervous system; GI, gastrointestinal.

TABLE 15 Patient Groups at Increased Risk for Development of Severe Hypernatremia

Elderly patients
Hospitalized patients
 Hypertonic infusions
 Tube feedings
 Osmotic diuretics
 Lactulose
 Mechanical ventilation
 Patients with decreased baseline levels of consciousness
Patients with uncontrolled diabetes
Patients with underlying polyuric disorders

References

1. Abraham WT, Schrier RW. Body fluid volume regulation in health and disease. *Adv Intern Med* 1994;39:23–47.
2. Alexander MR, Tyers M, Perret M, et al. Regulation of cell cycle progression by Swe1p and Hog1p following hypertonic stress. *Mol Biol Cell* 2001;12:53–62.
3. Allerton JP, Strom JA. Hypernatremia due to repeated doses of charcoal-sorbitol. *Am J Kidney Dis* 1991;17:581–584.
4. Alon U, Chan JC. Hydrochlorothiazide-amiloride in the treatment of congenital nephrogenic diabetes insipidus. *Am J Nephrol* 1985;5:9–13.
5. AlOrainy IA, O'Gorman AM, Decell MK. Cerebral bleeding, infarcts, and presumed extrapontine myelinolysis in hypernatraemic dehydration. *Neuroradiology* 1999;41:144–146.
6. Anderson B. Regulation of water intake. *Physiol Rev* 1978;58:582.
7. Arieff AI, Guisado R. Effects on the central nervous system of hypernatremic and hyponatremic states. *Kidney Int* 1976;10:104–116.
8. Arieff AI, Guisado R, Lazarowitz VC. The pathophysiology of hyperosmolar states. In: Andreoli TE, Grantham JJ, Rector FC, eds. *Disturbances in Body Fluid Osmolality*. Baltimore: Williams & Wilkins; 1977:227.
9. Asai T, Kuwahara M, Kurihara H, et al. Pathogenesis of nephrogenic diabetes insipidus by aquaporin-2 C-terminus mutations. *Kidney Int* 2003;64:2–10.
10. Ataga KI, Orringer EP. Renal abnormalities in sickle cell disease. *Am J Hematol* 2000;63:205–211.
11. Ayus JC, Arieff AI. Abnormalities of water metabolism in the elderly. *Semin Nephrol* 1996;16:277–288.
12. Ayus JC, Armstrong DL, Arieff AI. Effects of hypernatraemia in the central nervous system and its therapy in rats and rabbits. *J Physiol* 1996;492(Pt 1):243–255.
13. Bacic A, Gluncic I, Gluncic V. Disturbances in plasma sodium in patients with war head injuries. *Mil Med* 1999;164:214–217.
14. Barron WM, Cohen LH, Ulland LA, et al. Transient vasopressin-resistant diabetes insipidus of pregnancy. *N Engl J Med* 1984;310:442–444.
15. Baylis PH, Heath DA. Water disturbances in patients treated with oral lithium carbonate. *Ann Intern Med* 1978;88:607–609.
16. Beck N, Singh H, Reed SW, et al. Pathogenic role of cyclic AMP in the impairment of urinary concentrating ability in acute hypercalcemia. *J Clin Invest* 1974;54:1049–1055.
17. Becker DJ, Foley TP, Jr. 1-deamino-8-D-argenine vasopressin in the treatment of central diabetes insipidus in childhood. *J Pediatr* 1978;92:1011–1015.
18. Belli G, Gari E, Aldea M, et al. Osmotic stress causes a G1 cell cycle delay and downregulation of Cln3/Cdc28 activity in Saccharomyces cerevisiae. *Mol Microbiol* 2001;39:1022–1035.
19. Berl T. The cAMP system in vasopressin-sensitive nephron segments of the vitamin D-treated rat. *Kidney Int* 1987;31:1065–1071.
20. Berl T, Anderson RJ, McDonald KM, et al. Clinical disorders of water metabolism. *Kidney Int* 1976;10:117–132.
21. Berl T, Linas SL, Aisenbrey GA, et al. On the mechanism of polyuria in potassium depletion. The role of polydipsia. *J Clin Invest* 1978;60:620–625.

22. Bhatnagar D, Weinkove C. Serious hypernatraemia in a hospital population. *Postgrad Med J* 1988;64:441–443.

23. Bichet DG. Nephrogenic diabetes insipidus. *Am J Med* 1998;105:431–442.

24. Bichet DG, Birnbaumer M, Lonergan M, et al. Nature and recurrence of AVPR2 mutations in X-linked nephrogenic diabetes insipidus. *Am J Hum Genet* 1994;55:278–286.

25. Bichet DG, Razi M, Lonergan M, et al. Hemodynamic and coagulation responses to 1-desamino[8-D-argenine] vasopressin in patients with congenital nephrogenic diabetes insipidus. *N Engl J Med* 1988;318:881–887.

26. Birnbaumer M. The V2 vasopressin receptor mutations and fluid homeostasis. *Cardiovasc Res* 2001;51:409–415.

27. Boccalandro C, De Mattia F, Guo DC, et al. Characterization of an aquaporin-2 water channel gene mutation causing partial nephrogenic diabetes insipidus in a Mexican family: evidence of increased frequency of the mutation in the town of origin. *J Am Soc Nephrol* 2004;15: 1223–1231.

28. Borra SI, Beredo R, Kleinfeld M. Hypernatremia in the aging: causes, manifestations, and outcome. *J Natl Med Assoc* 1995;87:220–224.

29. Boton R, Gaviria M, Batlle DC. Prevalence, pathogenesis, and treatment of renal dysfunction associated with chronic lithium therapy. *Am J Kidney Dis* 1987;10:329–345.

30. Brezis M, Weiler-Ravell D. Hypernatremia, hypodipsia and partial diabetes insippidus: a model for defective osmoregulation. *Am J Med Sci* 1980;279:37–45.

31. Buckalew VM, Jr., Someren A. Renal manifestations of sickle cell disease. *Arch Intern Med* 1974;133:660–669.

32. Burg MB. Coordinate regulation of organic osmolytes in renal cells. *Kidney Int* 1996;49: 1684–1685.

33. Burg MB. Molecular basis of osmotic regulation. *Am J Physiol* 1995;268: F983–996.

34. Carter RD, Goodman AD. Nephrogenic diabetes insipidus accompanied by massive dilatation of the kidneys, ureters and bladder. *J Urol* 1963;89:366–369.

35. Chan L. The current status of magnetic resonance spectroscopy—basic and clinical aspects. *West J Med* 1985;143:773–781.

36. Chan L, Shapiro JI. Contributions of nuclear magnetic resonance to study of acute renal failure. *Ren Fail* 1989;11:79–89.

37. Chan PH, Fishman RA. Elevation of rat brain amino acids, ammonia and idiogenic osmoles induced by hyperosmolality. *Brain Res* 1979;161:293–301.

38. Chan Seem CP, Dossetor JF, Penney MD. Nephrogenic diabetes insipidus due to a new mutation of the argenine vasopressin V2 receptor gene in a girl presenting with non-accidental injury. *Ann Clin Biochem* 1999;36(Pt 6):779–782.

39. Chilton LA. Prevention and management of hypernatremic dehydration in breast-fed infants. *West J Med* 1995;163:74–76.

40. Christensen S. Acute and chronic effects of vasopressin in rats with lithium-polyuria. *Acta Pharmacol Toxicol (Copenh)* 1976;38:241–253.

41. Christensen S, Kusano E, Yusufi AN, et al. Pathogenesis of nephrogenic diabetes insipidus due to chronic administration of lithium in rats. *J Clin Invest* 1985;75:1869–1879.

42. Chu HI, Liu SH, Yu TF. Water and electrolyte metabolism in diabetes insipidus. *Proc Soc Exp Biol Med* 1941;46:682.

43. Cogan E, Abramow M. Inhibition by lithium of the hydroosmotic action of vasopressin in the isolated perfused cortical collecting tubule of the rabbit. *J Clin Invest* 1986;77:1507–1514.

44. Cooper WO, Atherton HD, Kahana M, et al. Increased incidence of severe breastfeeding malnutrition and hypernatremia in a metropolitan area. *Pediatrics* 1995;96:957–960.

45. Copp J, Wiley S, Ward MW, et al. Hypertonic shock inhibits growth factor receptor signaling, induces caspase-3 activation, and causes reversible fragmentation of the mitochondrial network. *Am J Physiol Cell Physiol* 2005;288: C403–415.

46. Crook M, Robinson R, Swaminathan R. Hypertriglyceridaemia in a child with hypernatremia due to a hypothalamic tumour. *Ann Clin Biochem* 1995;32(Pt 2):226–228.

47. Cserr HF, DePasquale M, Patlak CS. Regulation of brain water and electrolytes during acute hyperosmolality in rats. *Am J Physiol* 1987;253:F522–529.

48. Cserr HF, DePasquale M, Patlak CS. Volume regulatory influx of electrolytes from plasma to brain during acute hyperosmolality. *Am J Physiol* 1987;253: F530–537.

49. Cunnah D, Ross G, Besser GM. Management of cranial diabetes insipidus with oral desmopressin (DDAVP). *Clin Endocrinol (Oxf)* 1986;24:253–257.

50. Daggett P, Deanfield J, Moss F, et al. Severe hypernatraemia in adults. *Br Med J* 1979;1: 1177–1180.

51. de Mattia F, Savelkoul PJ, Kamsteeg EJ, et al. Lack of argenine vasopressin-induced phosphorylation of aquaporin-2 mutant AQP2-R254L explains dominant nephrogenic diabetes insipidus. *J Am Soc Nephrol* 2005;16:2872–2880.

52. De Petris L, Luchetti A, Emma F. Cell volume regulation and transport mechanisms across the blood-brain barrier: implications for the management of hypernatraemic states. *Eur J Pediatr* 2001;160:71–77.

53. De Wardener HE, Herxheimer A. The effect of a high water intake on the kidney's ability to concentrate the urine in man. *J Physiol* 1957;139:42.

54. DeRubertis FR, Michelis MF, Beck N, et al. "Essential" hypernatremia due to ineffective osmotic and intact volume regulation of vasopressin secretion. *J Clin Invest* 1971;50:97–111.

55. DeRubertis FR, Michelis MF, Davis BB. "Essential" hypernatremia. Report of three cases and review of the literature. *Arch Intern Med* 1974;134:889–895.

56. Desai BN, Myers BR, Schreiber SL. FKBP12-rapamycin-associated protein associates with mitochondria and senses osmotic stress via mitochondrial dysfunction. *Proc Natl Acad Sci U S A* 2002;99:4319–4324.

57. Dmitrieva NI, Cai Q, Burg MB. Cells adapted to high NaCl have many DNA breaks and impaired DNA repair both in cell culture and in vivo. *Proc Natl Acad Sci U S A* 2004;101: 2317–2322.

58. Dmitrieva NI, Michea LF, Rocha GM, et al. Cell cycle delay and apoptosis in response to osmotic stress. *Comp Biochem Physiol A Mol Integr Physiol* 2001;130:411–420.

59. Douglas JB, Healy JK. Nephrotoxic effects of amphotericin B, including renal tubular acidosis. *Am J Med* 1969;46:154–162.

60. Dousa TP. Interaction of lithium with vasopressin-sensitive cyclic AMP system of human renal medulla. *Endocrinology* 1974;95:1359–1366.

61. Dunger DB, Broadbent V, Yeoman E, et al. The frequency and natural history of diabetes insipidus in children with Langerhans-cell histiocytosis. *N Engl J Med* 1989;321:1157–1162.

62. Dunn K, Butt W. Extreme sodium derangement in a paediatric inpatient population. *J Paediatr Child Health* 1997;33:26–30.

63. Durr JA, Hensen J, Ehnis T, et al. Chlorpropamide upregulates antidiuretic hormone receptors and unmasks constitutive receptor signaling. *Am J Physiol Renal Physiol* 2000;278: F799–808.

64. Durr JA, Hoggard JG, Hunt JM, et al. Diabetes insipidus in pregnancy associated with abnormally high circulating vasopressinase activity. *N Engl J Med* 1987;316:1070–1074.

65. Edelman IS, Leibman J, O'Meara MP, et al. Interrelations between serum sodium concentration, serum osmolarity and total exchangeable sodium, total exchangeable potassium and total body water. *J Clin Invest* 1958;37:1236–1256.

66. Ellis RJ. Severe hypernatremia from sea water ingestion during near-drowning in a hurricane. *West J Med* 1997;167:430–433.

67. Escote X, Zapater M, Clotet J, et al. Hog1 mediates cell-cycle arrest in G1 phase by the dual targeting of Sic1. *Nat Cell Biol* 2004;6:997–1002.

68. Farese RV, Jr., Schambelan M, Hollander H, et al. Nephrogenic diabetes insipidus associated with foscarnet treatment of cytomegalovirus retinitis. *Ann Intern Med* 1990;112: 955–956.

69. Feig PU, McCurdy DK. The hypertonic state. *N Engl J Med* 1978;297:1444–1454.

70. Finberg L. Hypernatremic (hypertonic) dehydration in infants. *N Engl J Med* 1973;289: 196–198.

71. Finberg L, Luttrell C, Redd H. Pathogenesis of lesions in the nervous system in hypernatremic states. II. Experimental studies of gross anatomic changes and alterations of chemical composition of the tissues. *Pediatrics* 1959;23:46–53.

72. Finch CK, Kelley KW, Williams RB. Treatment of lithium-induced diabetes insipidus with amiloride. *Pharmacotherapy* 2003;23:546–550.

73. Fine LG, Salehmoghaddam S. Water homeostasis in acute and chronic renal failure. *Semin Nephrol* 1984;4:289.

74. Fine LG, Schlondorff D, Trizna W, et al. Functional profile of the isolated uremic nephron. Impaired water permeability and adenylate cyclase responsiveness of the cortical collecting tubule to vasopressin. *J Clin Invest* 1978;61:1519–1527.

75. Finn AL, Handler JS,Orloff J. Relation between toad bladder potassium content and permeability response to vasopressin. *Am J Physiol* 1966;210:1279–1284.

76. Fiordalisi I. Central nervous system complications during hypernatremia and its repair. *Arch Pediatr Adolesc Med* 1994;148:539–540.

77. Fishman RA, Chan PH. Changes in ammonia and amino acid metabolism induced by hyperosmolality in vivo and in vitro. *Trans Am Neurol Assoc* 1976;101:34–39.

78. Fitzsimons JT. Angiotensin, thirst, and sodium appetite: retrospect and prospect. *Fed Proc* 1978,37:2669-2675.

79. Fitzsimons JT. Thirst. *Physiol Rev* 1972;52:468.

80. Ford SM, Jr. Transient vasopressin-resistant diabetes insipidus of pregnancy. *Obstet Gynecol* 1986;68:288–289.

81. Forrest JN, Jr., Cohen AD, Torretti J, et al. On the mechanism of lithium-induced diabetes insipidus in man and the rat. *J Clin Invest* 1974;53:1115–1123.

82. Froyshov I, Haugen HN. Chlorpropamide treatment in diabetes insipidus. *Acta Med Scand* 1968,183:397–400.

83. Fumarola C, La Monica S, Guidotti GG. Amino acid signaling through the mammalian target of rapamycin (mTOR) pathway: Role of glutamine and of cell shrinkage. *J Cell Physiol* 2005;204:155–165.

84. Gabow PA. Ethylene glycol intoxication. *Am J Kidney Dis* 1988;11:277–279.

85. Gabow PA, Kaehny WD, Johnson AM, et al. The clinical utility of renal concentrating capacity in polycystic kidney disease. *Kidney Int* 1989;35:675–680.

86. Gamble JL. *Chemical Anatomy, Physiology, and Pathology of Extracellular Fluid.* Cambridge, MA: Harvard University Press; 1944.

87. Gault MH, Dixon ME, Doyle M, et al. Hypernatremia, azotemia, and dehydration due to high-protein tube feeding. *Ann Intern Med* 1968;68:778–791.

88. Gennari FJ. Current concepts. Serum osmolality. Uses and limitations. *N Engl J Med* 1984;310:102–105.

89. Gines P, Abraham WT, Schrier RW. Vasopressin in pathophysiological states. *Semin Nephrol* 1994;14:384–397.

90. Go WY, Liu X, Roti MA, et al. NFAT5/TonEBP mutant mice define osmotic stress as a critical feature of the lymphoid microenvironment. *Proc Natl Acad Sci U S A* 2004;101: 10673–10678.

91. Goldberg H, Clayman P, Skorecki K. Mechanism of Li inhibition of vasopressin-sensitive adenylate cyclase in cultured renal epithelial cells. *Am J Physiol* 1988;255:F995–1002.

92. Goldfarb S, Agus ZS. Mechanism of the polyuria of hypercalcemia. *Am J Nephrol* 1984;4: 69–76.

93. Goldsmith C, Beasley HK, Whalley PJ, et al. The effect of salt deprivation on the urinary concentrating mechanism in the dog. *J Clin Invest* 1961;40:2043–2052.

94. Gowrishankar M, Sapir D, Pace K, et al. Profound natriuresis, extracellular fluid volume contraction, and hypernatremia with hypertonic losses following trauma. *Geriatr Nephrol Urol* 1997;7:95–100.

95. Grunewald JM, Grunewald RW, Kinne RK. Ion content and cell volume in isolated collecting duct cells: effect of hypotonicity. *Kidney Int* 1993;44:509–517.

96. Grunewald JM, Grunewald RW, Kinne RK. Regulation of ion content and cell volume in isolated rat renal IMCD cells under hypertonic conditions. *Am J Physiol* 1994;267:F13–19.

97. Grunewald RW, Kinne RK. Osmoregulation in the mammalian kidney: the role of organic osmolytes. *J Exp Zool* 1999;283:708–724.

98. Gullans SR, Verbalis JG. Control of brain volume during hyperosmolar and hypoosmolar conditions. *Annu Rev Med* 1993;44:289–301.

99. Gutsche HU, Peterson LN, Levine DZ. In vivo evidence of impaired solute transport by the thick ascending limb in potassium-depleted rats. *J Clin Invest* 1984;73:908–916.
100. Halter JB, Goldberg AP, Robertson GL, et al. Selective osmoreceptor dysfunction in the syndrome of chronic hypernatremia. *J Clin Endocrinol Metab* 1978;44:609–616.
101. Hammond DN, Moll GW, Robertson GL, et al. Hypodipsic hypernatremia with normal osmoregulation of vasopressin. *N Engl J Med* 1986;315:433–436.
102. Harris AS. Clinical experience with desmopressin: efficacy and safety in central diabetes insipidus and other conditions. *J Pediatr* 1989;114:711–718.
103. Hartfield DS, Loewy JA, Yager JY. Transient thalamic changes on MRI in a child with hypernatremia. *Pediatr Neurol* 1999;20:60–62.
104. Heilig CW, Stromski ME, Blumenfeld JD, et al. Characterization of the major brain osmolytes that accumulate in salt-loaded rats. *Am J Physiol* 1989;257: F1108–1116.
105. Hilliard TN, Marsh MJ, Malcolm P, et al. Radiological case of the month. Sagittal sinus thrombosis in hypernatremic dehydration. *Arch Pediatr Adolesc Med* 1998;152:1147; discussion, 1148.
106. Himmelstein DU, Jones AA, Woolhandler S. Hypernatremic dehydration in nursing home patients: an indicator of neglect. *J Am Geriatr Soc* 1983;31:466–471.
107. Ho SN. Intracellular water homeostasis and the mammalian cellular osmotic stress response. *J Cell Physiol* 2006;206:9–15.
108. Hochstenbach SL, Ciriello J. Effects of plasma hypernatremia on nucleus tractus solitarius neurons. *Am J Physiol* 1994;266: R1916–1921.
109. Hochstenbach SL, Ciriello J. Plasma hypernatremia induces c-fos activity in medullary catecholaminergic neurons. *Brain Res* 1995;674:46–54.
110. Hogan GR, Dodge PR, Gill SR, et al. The incidence of seizures after rehydration of hypernatremic rabbits with intravenous or ad libitum oral fluids. *Pediatr Res* 1984;18: 340–345.
111. Hollenberg NK. Set point for sodium homeostasis: surfeit, deficit, and their implications. *Kidney Int* 1980;17:423–429.
112. Hollenberg NK. Surfeit, deficit, and the set point for sodium homeostasis. *Kidney Int* 1982;21:883–884.
113. Holliday MA, Kalayci MN, Harrah J. Factors that limit brain volume changes in response to acute and sustained hyper- and hyponatremia. *J Clin Invest* 1968,47:1916–1928.
114. Holtzman EJ, Harris HW, Jr., Kolakowski LF, Jr., et al. Brief report: a molecular defect in the vasopressin V2-receptor gene causing nephrogenic diabetes insipidus. *N Engl J Med* 1993;328:1534–1537.
115. Holtzman EJ, Kolakowski LF, Jr., Geifman-Holtzman O, et al. Mutations in the vasopressin V2 receptor gene in two families with nephrogenic diabetes insipidus. *J Am Soc Nephrol* 1994; 5:169–176.
116. Ishikawa S, Sakuma N, Fujisawa G, et al. Opposite changes in serum sodium and potassium in patients in diabetic coma. *Endocr J* 1994;41:37–43.
117. Ito T, Fujio Y, Hirata M, et al. Expression of taurine transporter is regulated through the TonE (tonicity-responsive element)/TonEBP (TonE-binding protein) pathway and contributes to cytoprotection in HepG2 cells. *Biochem J* 2004;382:177–182.
118. Kahn T. Hypernatremia with edema. *Arch Intern Med* 1999;159:93–98.
119. Kambouris M, Dlouhy SR, Trofatter JA, et al. Localization of the gene for X-linked nephrogenic diabetes insipidus to Xq28. *Am J Med Genet* 1988;29:239–246.
120. Kamsteeg EJ, Bichet DG, Konings IB, et al. Reversed polarized delivery of an aquaporin-2 mutant causes dominant nephrogenic diabetes insipidus. *J Cell Biol* 2003;163:1099–1109.
121. Kanno K, Sasaki S, Hirata Y, et al. Urinary excretion of aquaporin-2 in patients with diabetes insipidus. *N Engl J Med* 1995;332:1540–1545.
122. Kasono K, Saito T, Tamemoto H, et al. Hypertonicity regulates the aquaporin-2 promoter independently of argenine vasopressin. *Nephrol Dial Transplant* 2005;20:509–515.
123. Keuneke C, Anders HJ, Schlondorff D. Adipsic hypernatremia in two patients with AIDS and cytomegalovirus encephalitis. *Am J Kidney Dis* 1999;33:379–382.
124. Kim JK, Summer SN, Berl T. The cyclic AMP system in the inner medullary collecting duct of the potassium-depleted rat. *Kidney Int* 1984;26:384–391.
125. Kinoshita K, Miura Y, Nagasaki H, et al. A novel deletion mutation in the argenine vasopressin receptor 2 gene and skewed X chromosome inactivation in a female patient with congenital nephrogenic diabetes insipidus. *J Endocrinol Invest* 2004;27:167–170.
126. Kirchlechner V, Koller DY, Seidl R, et al. Treatment of nephrogenic diabetes insipidus with hydrochlorothiazide and amiloride. *Arch Dis Child* 1999;80:548–552.
127. Klawitter J, Rivard CJ, Capasso JM, et al. Metabolnomic analysis of the effects of adaptation to hypertonicity in inner medullary collecting duct (IMCD3) cells. *J Am Soc Nephrol* 2004;15:90A.
128. Kleeman CR, Rubini ME, Lamdin E, et al. Studies on alcohol diuresis, II: the evaluation of ethyl alcohol as an inhibitor of the neurohypophysis. *J Clin Invest* 1955;34:448–455.
129. Knoers N, Monnens LA. A variant of nephrogenic diabetes insipidus: V2 receptor abnormality restricted to the kidney. *Eur J Pediatr* 1991;150:370–373.
130. Knoers N, van der Heyden H, van Oost BA, et al. Nephrogenic diabetes insipidus: close linkage with markers from the distal long arm of the human X chromosome. *Hum Genet* 1988;80:31v38.
131. Ko BC, Ruepp B, Bohren KM, et al. Identification and characterization of multiple osmotic response sequences in the human aldose reductase gene. *J Biol Chem* 1997;272: 16431–16437.
132. Kojima R, Randall JD, Ito E, et al. Regulation of expression of the stress response gene, Osp94: identification of the tonicity response element and intracellular signalling pathways. *Biochem J* 2004;380:783–794.
133. Konoshita T, Kuroda M, Kawane T, et al. Treatment of congenital nephrogenic diabetes insipidus with hydrochlorothiazide and amiloride in an adult patient. *Horm Res* 2004;61: 63–67.
134. Korkmaz A, Yigit S, Firat M, et al. Cranial MRI in neonatal hypernatraemic dehydration. *Pediatr Radiol* 2000;30:323–325.
135. Kugler JP, Hustead T. Hyponatremia and hypernatremia in the elderly. *Am Fam Physician* 2000;61:3623–3630.
136. Kultz D, Chakravarty D. Hyperosmolality in the form of elevated NaCl but not urea causes DNA damage in murine kidney cells. *Proc Natl Acad Sci U S A* 2001;98:1999–2004.
137. Kumar S, Berl T. Sodium. *Lancet* 1998;352:220–228.
138. Lee JH, Arcinue E, Ross BD. Brief report: organic osmolytes in the brain of an infant with hypernatremia. *N Engl J Med* 1994;331:439–442.
139. Levi M, Peterson L, Berl T. Mechanism of concentrating defect in hypercalcemia. Role of polydipsia and prostaglandins. *Kidney Int* 1983;23:489–497.
140. Libber S, Harrison H, Spector D. Treatment of nephrogenic diabetes insipidus with prostaglandin synthesis inhibitors. *J Pediatr* 1986;108:305–311.
141. Lien YH, Shapiro JI, Chan L. Effects of hypernatremia on organic brain osmoles. *J Clin Invest* 1990;85:1427–1435.
142. Lien YH, Shapiro JI, Chan L. Study of brain electrolytes and organic osmolytes during correction of chronic hyponatremia. Implications for the pathogenesis of central pontine myelinolysis. *J Clin Invest* 1991;88:303–309.
143. Lin M, Liu SJ, Lim IT. Disorders of water imbalance. *Emerg Med Clin North Am* 2005;23: 749-770, ix.
144. Lins LE. Renal function in hypercalcemia. A clinical and experimental study. *Acta Med Scand Suppl* 1979;632:1–46.
145. Lockwood AH. Acute and chronic hyperosmolality. Effects on cerebral amino acids and energy metabolism. *Arch Neurol* 1975;32:62–64.
146. Lohr JW, McReynolds J, Grimaldi T, et al. Effect of acute and chronic hypernatremia on myoinositol and sorbitol concentration in rat brain and kidney. *Life Sci* 1988;43: 271–276.
147. Long CA, Marin P, Bayer AJ, et al. Hypernatraemia in an adult in-patient population. *Postgrad Med J* 1991;67:643–645.
148. Lopez-Rodriguez C, Antos CL, Shelton JM, et al. Loss of NFAT5 results in renal atrophy and lack of tonicity-responsive gene expression. *Proc Natl Acad Sci U S A* 2004;101:2392–2397.
149. Mahowald JM, Himmelstein DU. Hypernatremia in the elderly: relation to infection and mortality. *J Am Geriatr Soc* 1981;29:177–180.
150. Majzoub JA, Rich A, van Boom J, et al. Vasopressin and oxytocin mRNA regulation in the rat assessed by hybridization with synthetic oligonucleotides. *J Biol Chem* 1983;258: 14061–14064.
151. Mandal AK, Saklayen MG, Hillman NM, et al. Predictive factors for high mortality in hypernatremic patients. *Am J Emerg Med* 1997;15:130–132.
152. Manelfe C, Louvet JP. Computed tomography in diabetes insipidus. *J Comput Assist Tomogr* 1979;3:309–316.
153. Marks SL, Taboada J. Hypernatremia and hypertonic syndromes. *Vet Clin North Am Small Anim Pract* 1998;28:533–543.
154. Marr N, Bichet DG, Hoefs S, et al. Cell-biologic and functional analyses of five new Aquaporin-2 missense mutations that cause recessive nephrogenic diabetes insipidus. *J Am Soc Nephrol* 2002;13:2267–2277.
155. Mattar JA, Weil MH, Shubin H, et al. Cardiac arrest in the critically ill, II: hyperosmolal states following cardiac arrest. *Am J Med* 1974;56:162–168.
156. McIver B, Connacher A, Whittle I, et al. Adipsic hypothalamic diabetes insipidus after clipping of anterior communicating artery aneurysm. *Br Med J* 1991;303:1465–1467.
157. McLeod JF, Kovacs L, Gaskill MB, et al. Familial neurohypophyseal diabetes insipidus associated with a signal peptide mutation. *J Clin Endocrinol Metab* 1993;77:599A–599G.
158. Meadow R. Non-accidental salt poisoning. *Arch Dis Child* 1993;68:448–452.
159. Merendino JJ, Jr., Speigel AM, Crawford JD, et al. Brief report: a mutation in the vasopressin V2-receptor gene in a kindred with X-linked nephrogenic diabetes insipidus. *N Engl J Med* 1993;328:1538–1541.
160. Meyers A. Fluid and electrolyte therapy for children. *Curr Opin Pediatr* 1994;6:303–309.
161. Michea L, Ferguson DR, Peters EM, et al. Cell cycle delay and apoptosis are induced by high salt and urea in renal medullary cells. *Am J Physiol Renal Physiol* 2000;278:F209–218.
162. Miller NL, Finberg L. Peritoneal dialysis for salt poisoning. Report of a case. *N Engl J Med* 1960,263:1347–1350.
163. Miller PD, Krebs RA, Neal BJ, et al. Hypodipsia in geriatric patients. *Am J Med* 1982;73: 354–356.
164. Milles JJ, Spruce B, Baylis PH. A comparison of diagnostic methods to differentiate diabetes insipidus from primary polyuria: a review of 21 patients. *Acta Endocrinol (Copenh)* 1983;104: 410–416.
165. Miyakawa H, Woo SK, Chen CP, et al. Cis- and trans-acting factors regulating transcription of the BGT1 gene in response to hypertonicity. *Am J Physiol* 1998;274:F753–761.
166. Miyakawa H, Woo SK, Dahl SC, et al. Tonicity-responsive enhancer binding protein, a rel-like protein that stimulates transcription in response to hypertonicity. *Proc Natl Acad Sci U S A* 1999;96:2538–2542.
167. Miyakoshi M, Kamoi K, Murase T, et al. Novel mutant vasopressin-neurophysin II gene associated with familial neurohypophyseal diabetes insipidus. *Endocr J* 2004;51:551–556.
168. Moder KG, Hurley DL. Fatal hypernatremia from exogenous salt intake: report of a case and review of the literature. *Mayo Clin Proc* 1990;65:1587–1594.
169. Morley SJ, Naegele S. Phosphorylation of eukaryotic initiation factor (eIF) 4E is not required for de novo protein synthesis following recovery from hypertonic stress in human kidney cells. *J Biol Chem* 2002;277:32855–32859.
170. Moses AM, Coulson R. Augmentation by chlorpropamide of 1-deamino-8-D-argenine vasopressin-induced antidiuresis and stimulation of renal medullary adenylate cyclase and accumulation of adenosine 3',5'-monophosphate. *Endocrinology* 1980;106:967–972.
171. Moses AM, Streeten DH. Differentiation of polyuric states by measurement of responses to changes in plasma osmolality induced by hypertonic saline infusions. *Am J Med* 1967;42: 368–377.
172. Murphy D, Levy A, Lightman S, et al. Vasopressin RNA in the neural lobe of the pituitary: dramatic accumulation in response to salt loading. *Proc Natl Acad Sci U S A* 1989;86: 9002–9005.
173. Naegele S, Morley SJ. Molecular cross-talk between MEK1/2 and mTOR signaling during recovery of 293 cells from hypertonic stress. *J Biol Chem* 2004;279:46023–46034.

174. Nakanishi T, Balaban RS, Burg MB. Survey of osmolytes in renal cell lines. *Am J Physiol* 1988;255:C181–191.

175. Nakayama Y, Peng T, Sands JM, et al. The TonE/TonEBP pathway mediates tonicity-responsive regulation of UT-A urea transporter expression. *J Biol Chem* 2000;275:38275–38280.

176. Narins RG, Krishna GC. Disorders of water balance. In: Stein JH. *Internal Medicine*. Boston: Little, Brown; 1987:794.

177. Narins RG, Riley LJ, Jr. Polyuria: simple and mixed disorders. *Am J Kidney Dis* 1991;17:237–241.

178. Nielsen S, Frokiaer J, Marples D, et al. Aquaporins in the kidney: from molecules to medicine. *Physiol Rev* 2002;82:205–244.

179. Orloff J, Burn MB. Vasopressin-resistant diabetes insipidus. In: Stanbury J, Wyngaarden JB, Frederickson NS, eds. *The Metabolic Basis of Inherited Disease*, 3rd ed. New York: McGraw-Hill; 1972:1567.

180. Palevsky PM. Hypernatremia. *Semin Nephrol* 1998;18:20–30.

181. Palevsky PM, Bhagrath R, Greenberg A. Hypernatremia in hospitalized patients. *Ann Intern Med* 1996;124:197–203.

182. Papadimitriou A, Kipourou K, Manta C, et al. Adipsic hypernatremia syndrome in infancy. *J Pediatr Endocrinol Metab* 1997;10:547–550.

183. Pattaragarn A, Alon US. Treatment of congenital nephrogenic diabetes insipidus by hydrochlorothiazide and cyclooxygenase-2 inhibitor. *Pediatr Nephrol* 2003;18:1073–1076.

184. Perez GO, Oster JR, Robertson GL. Severe hypernatremia with impaired thirst. *Am J Nephrol* 1989;9:421–434.

185. Peskind ER, Jensen CF, Pascualy M, et al. Sodium lactate and hypertonic sodium chloride induce equivalent panic incidence, panic symptoms, and hypernatremia in panic disorder. *Biol Psychiatry* 1998;44:1007–1016.

186. Peters JP. Water exchange. *Physiol Rev* 1944;24:491–531.

187. Peterson LN. Vitamin D-induced chronic hypercalcemia inhibits thick ascending limb NaCl reabsorption in vivo. *Am J Physiol* 1990;259: F122–129.

188. Pham PT, Pham PC, Wilkinson AH, et al. Renal abnormalities in sickle cell disease. *Kidney Int* 2000;57:1–8.

189. Phillips PA, Bretherton M, Johnston CI, et al. Reduced osmotic thirst in healthy elderly men. *Am J Physiol* 1991;261: R166–171.

190. Phillips PA, Rolls BJ, Ledingham JG, et al. Reduced thirst after water deprivation in healthy elderly men. *N Engl J Med* 1984;311:753–759.

191. Pollock AS, Arieff AI. Abnormalities of cell volume regulation and their functional consequences. *Am J Physiol* 1980;239: F195–205.

192. Proft M, Struhl K. MAP kinase-mediated stress relief that precedes and regulates the timing of transcriptional induction. *Cell* 2004;118:351–361.

193. Quintanilla AP. Pathophysiology of renal concentrating defects. *Ann Clin Lab Sci* 1981;11:300–307.

194. Rado JP. Combination of carbamazepine and chlorpropamide in the treatment of "hyporesponder" pituitary diabetes insipidus. *J Clin Endocrinol Metab* 1974;38:1–7.

195. Rado JP, Marosi J, Borbely L, et al. Individual differences in the antidiuretic response induced by DDAVP in diabetes insipidus. *Horm Metab Res* 1976;8:155–156.

196. Redmond GP, Rothner AD, Hahn JF, et al. Combined desmopressin (DDAVP) and chlorpropamide therapy for diabetes insipidus with absent thirst. *Cleve Clin Q* 1983;50:351–352.

197. Reid DE, Frigoletto FJ, Goodlin RC. Hypernatremia from intravascular saline infusion during therapeutic abortion. *JAMA* 1972;220:1749.

198. Relman AS, Schwartz WB. The kidney in potassium depletion. *Am J Med* 1958;24:764–773.

199. Richman RA, Post EM, Notman DD, et al. Simplifying the diagnosis of diabetes insipidus in children. *Am J Dis Child* 1981;135:839–841.

200. Riggs JE. Neurologic manifestations of electrolyte disturbances. *Neurol Clin* 2002;20:227–239, vii.

201. Rim JS, Atta MG, Dahl SC, et al. Transcription of the sodium/myo-inositol cotransporter gene is regulated by multiple tonicity-responsive enhancers spread over 50 kilobase pairs in the 5'-flanking region. *J Biol Chem* 1998;273:20615–20621.

202. Robertson G. Disorders of thirst in man. In: Ramsay D, Booth D, eds. *Thirst: Physiological and Psychological Aspects*. London: Springer-Verlag; 1991:453.

203. Robertson G. Pathophysiology of water metabolism. In: Brenner B, ed. *The Kidney*. Philadelphia: WB Saunders; 1996:873–928.

204. Robertson G. The physiopathology of ADH secretion. In: Tolis G, Labrie F, Martin J, eds. *Clinical Neuroendocrinology: A Pathophysiological Approach*. New York: Ravens Press; 1979:247.

205. Robertson GL. Antidiuretic hormone. Normal and disordered function. *Endocrinol Metab Clin North Am* 2001;30:671–694, vii.

206. Robertson GL, Aycinena P, Zerbe RL. Neurogenic disorders of osmoregulation. *Am J Med* 1982;72:339–353.

207. Robertson GL, Berl T. Pathophysiology of water metabolism. In: Brenner BM, Rector FCJ, eds. *The Kidney*, 4th ed. Philadelphia: WB Saunders; 1991:677.

208. Robertson GL, Harris A. Clinical use of vasopressin analogues. *Hosp Pract (Off Ed)* 1989;24:114–118, 126–118, 133 passim.

209. Robertson GL, McLeod JF, Zerbe RL, et al. Vasopressin function in heritable forms of diabetes insipidus. In: Gross P, Richter D, Robertson GL, eds. *Vasopressin*. Paris: John Libbey Eurotext; 1993:493–502.

210. Rose BD. New approach to disturbances in the plasma sodium concentration. *Am J Med* 1986;81:1033–1040.

211. Rosenthal W, Seibold A, Antaramian A, et al. Molecular identification of the gene responsible for congenital nephrogenic diabetes insipidus. *Nature* 1992;359:233–235.

212. Ross B, Freeman D, Chan L. Contributions of nuclear magnetic resonance to renal biochemistry. *Kidney Int* 1986;29:131–141.

213. Roy G, Banderali U. Channels for ions and amino acids in kidney cultured cells (MDCK) during volume regulation. *J Exp Zool* 1994;268:121–126.

214. Sanderson NA, Katz MA. The fate of hypertonic saline administered during hemodialysis. *Anna J* 1994;21:162–169; discussion 170.

215. Scherbaum WA, Bottazzo GF. Autoantibodies to vasopressin cells in idiopathic diabetes insipidus: evidence for an autoimmune variant. *Lancet* 1983;1:897–901.

216. Schulman M. Organic osmolytes in the brain of an infant with hypernatremia. *N Engl J Med* 1994;331:1776–1777.

217. Seckl JR, Dunger DB. Diabetes insipidus. Current treatment recommendations. *Drugs* 1992;44:216–224.

218. Shiau YF, Feldman GM, Resnick MA, et al. Stool electrolyte and osmolality measurements in the evaluation of diarrheal disorders. *Ann Intern Med* 1985;102:773–775.

219. Shoker AS. Application of the clearance concept to hyponatremic and hypernatremic disorders: a phenomenological analysis. *Clin Chem* 1994;40:1220–1227.

220. Silver AJ. Aging and risks for dehydration. *Cleve Clin J Med* 1990;57:341–344.

221. Siristatidis C, Salamalekis E, Iakovidou H, et al. Three cases of diabetes insipidus complicating pregnancy. *J Matern Fetal Neonatal Med* 2004;16:61–63.

222. Smith HW. *From Fish to Philosopher: The Story of Our Internal Environment*. Boston: Little, Brown; 1953.

223. Smithline N, Gardner KD, Jr. Gaps: anionic and osmolal. *JAMA* 1976;236:1594–1597.

224. Snyder NA, Feigal DW, Arieff AI. Hypernatremia in elderly patients. A heterogeneous, morbid, and iatrogenic entity. *Ann Intern Med* 1987;107:309–319.

225. Sotos JF, Dodge PR, Talbot NB. Studies in experimental hypertonicity, II: hypertonicity of body fluids as a cause of acidosis. *Pediatrics* 1962,30:180–193.

226. Soupart A, Penninckx R, Namias B, et al. Brain myelinolysis following hypernatremia in rats. *J Neuropathol Exp Neurol* 1996;55:106–113.

227. Statius van Eps LW, Pinedo-Veels C, de Vries GH, et al. Nature of concentrating defect in sickle-cell nephropathy. Microradioangiographic studies. *Lancet* 1970;1:450–452.

228. Sterns RH, Baer J, Ebersol S, et al. Organic osmolytes in acute hyponatremia. *Am J Physiol* 1993;264:F833–836.

229. Sterns RH, Riggs JE, Schochet SS, Jr. Osmotic demyelination syndrome following correction of hyponatremia. *N Engl J Med* 1986;314:1535–1542.

230. Tannen RL, Regal EM, Dunn MJ, et al. Vasopressin-resistant hyposthenuria in advanced chronic renal disease. *N Engl J Med* 1969;280:1135–1141.

231. Tareen N, Martins D, Nagami G, et al. Sodium disorders in the elderly. *J Natl Med Assoc* 2005;97:217–224.

232. Teitelbaum I, McGuinness S. Vasopressin resistance in chronic renal failure. Evidence for the role of decreased V2 receptor mRNA. *J Clin Invest* 1995;96:378–385.

233. Thompson CJ, Baylis PH. Thirst in diabetes insipidus: clinical relevance of quantitative assessment. *Q J Med* 1987;65:853–862.

234. Thurston JH, Hauhart RE, Dirgo JA. Taurine: a role in osmotic regulation of mammalian brain and possible clinical significance. *Life Sci* 1980;26:1561–1568.

235. Trama J, Go WY, Ho SN. The osmoprotective function of the NFAT5 transcription factor in T cell development and activation. *J Immunol* 2002;169:5477–5488.

236. Uhl GR, Zingg HH, Habener JF. Vasopressin mRNA in situ hybridization: localization and regulation studied with oligonucleotide cDNA probes in normal and Brattleboro rat hypothalamus. *Proc Natl Acad Sci U S A* 1985;82:5555–5559.

237. Verbalis JG, Gullans SR. Rapid correction of hyponatremia produces differential effects on brain osmolyte and electrolyte reaccumulation in rats. *Brain Res* 1993;606:19–27.

238. Vexler ZS, Ayus JC, Roberts TP, et al. Hypoxic and ischemic hypoxia exacerbate brain injury associated with metabolic encephalopathy in laboratory animals. *J Clin Invest* 1994;93:256–264.

239. Visser L, Devuyst O. Physiopathology of hypernatremia following relief of urinary tract obstruction. *Acta Clin Belg* 1994;49:290–295.

240. Vokes TJ, Gaskill MB, Robertson GL. Antibodies to vasopressin in patients with diabetes insipidus. Implications for diagnosis and therapy. *Ann Intern Med* 1988;108:190–195.

241. Vullo-Navich K, Smith S, Andrews M, et al. Comfort and incidence of abnormal serum sodium, BUN, creatinine and osmolality in dehydration of terminal illness. *Am J Hosp Palliat Care* 1998;15:77–84.

242. Wales JK. Treatment of diabetes insipidus with carbamazepine. *Lancet* 1975;2:948–951.

243. Walker RG. Lithium nephrotoxicity. *Kidney Int Suppl* 1993;42:S93–98.

244. Warren SE, Mitas JA, Swerdlin AH. Hypernatremia in hepatic failure. *JAMA* 1980;243:1257–1260.

245. Weiss NM, Robertson GL. Water metabolism in endocrine disorders. *Semin Nephrol* 1984;4:303.

246. Williams DJ, Jugurnauth J, Harding K, et al. Acute hypernatraemia during bicarbonate-buffered haemodialysis. *Nephrol Dial Transplant* 1994;9:1170–1173.

247. Woo SK, Lee SD, Na KY, et al. TonEBP/NFAT5 stimulates transcription of HSP70 in response to hypertonicity. *Mol Cell Biol* 2002;22:5753–5760.

248. Yamamoto T, Harada H, Fukuyama J, et al. Impaired argenine-vasopressin secretion associated with hypoangiotensinemia in hypernatremic dehydrated elderly patients. *JAMA* 1988;259:1039–1042.

249. Yancey PH, Burg MB. Counteracting effects of urea and betaine in mammalian cells in culture. *Am J Physiol* 1990;258:R198–204.

250. Yancey PH, Clark ME, Hand SC, et al. Living with water stress: evolution of osmolyte systems. *Science* 1982;217:1214–1222.

251. Yap HY, Tashima CK, Blumenschein GR, et al. Diabetes insipidus and breast cancer. *Arch Intern Med* 1979;139:1009–1011.

252. Zerbe RL, Robertson GL. A comparison of plasma vasopressin measurements with a standard indirect test in the differential diagnosis of polyuria. *N Engl J Med* 1981;305:1539–1546.

253. Zhang Z, Dmitrieva NI, Park JH, et al. High urea and NaCl carbonylate proteins in renal cells in culture and in vivo, and high urea causes 8-oxoguanine lesions in their DNA. *Proc Natl Acad Sci U S A* 2004;101:9491–9496.

CHAPTER 43

Polyuria and Diabetes Insipidus

Daniel G. Bichet

Hôpital du Sacré-Coeur de Montréal, Montréal, Québec, Canada

Diabetes insipidus is a disorder characterized by the excretion of abnormally large volumes (>30 ml/kg body weight/day for an adult patient) of dilute urine (<250 mmol/kg). Four basic defects can be involved. The most common, a deficient secretion of the antidiuretic hormone (ADH) arginine vasopressin (AVP), is referred to as *neurogenic* (or central, neurohypophyseal, cranial, or hypothalamic) diabetes insipidus. Diabetes insipidus can also result from renal insensitivity to the antidiuretic effect of AVP, which is referred to as *nephrogenic* diabetes insipidus (NDI). Excessive water intake can result in polyuria, which is referred to as *primary polydipsia*: It can be due to an abnormality in the thirst mechanism, referred to as dipsogenic diabetes insipidus; it can also be associated to a severe emotional cognitive dysfunction, referred to as *psychogenic polydipsia*. Finally, increased metabolism of vasopressin during pregnancy is referred to as *gestational* diabetes insipidus.

ARGININE VASOPRESSIN

Synthesis

Nonapeptides of the vasopressin family are the key regulators of water homeostasis in amphibia, reptiles, birds, and mammals. Since these peptides reduce urinary output, they are also referred to as antidiuretic hormones. Oxytocin and AVP (Fig. 1) are synthesized in separate populations of magnocellular neurons of the supraoptic and paraventricular nuclei (151). Oxytocin is most recognized for its key role in parturition and milk letdown in mammals (199). The axonal projections of AVP- and oxytocin-producing neurons from supraoptic and paraventricular nuclei reflect the dual function of AVP and oxytocin as hormones and as neuropeptides, in that they project their axons to several brain areas and to the neurohypophysis. Another pathway from parvocellular neurons to the hypophysial portal system transports high concentration of AVP to the anterior pituitary gland. AVP produced by this pathway together with the corticotropin-releasing hormone are two major hypothalamic secretagogues regulating the secretion of adrenocorticotropic hormone by the anterior pituitary (90).

AVP and its corresponding carrier protein, neurophysin II, are synthesized as a composite precursor by the magnocellular and parvocellular neurons described previously. The precursor is packaged into neurosecretory granules and transported axonally in the stalk of the posterior pituitary (34). On route to the neurohypophysis, the precursor is processed into the active hormone. Prepro-vasopressin has 164 amino acids and is encoded by the 2.5-kb *AVP* gene located in chromosome region 20p13 (148). The *AVP* gene (coding for AVP and neurophysin II) and the *OXT* gene (coding for oxytocin and neurophysin I) are located in the same chromosome region, at a very short distance from each other (12 kb in humans) in head-to-head orientation. Data from transgenic mouse studies indicate that the intergenic region between the *OXT* and the *AVP* genes contains the critical enhancer sites for cell-specific expression in the magnocellular neurons (34). It is phylogenetically interesting to note that *cis* and *trans* components of this specific cellular expression have been conserved between the *Fugu* isotocin (the homolog of mammalian oxytocin) and rat oxytocin genes (188). Exon 1 of the *AVP* gene encodes the signal peptide, AVP, and the NH_2-terminal region of NPII. Exon 2 encodes the central region of NPII, and exon 3 encodes the COOH-terminal region of NPII and the glycopeptide. Pro-vasopressin is generated by the removal of the signal peptide from prepro-vasopressin and the addition of a carbohydrate chain to the glycopeptide. Additional posttranslation processing occurs within neurosecretory vesicles during transport of the precursor protein to axon terminals in the posterior pituitary, yielding AVP, NPII, and glycopeptide (Fig. 2). The AVP-NPII complex forms tetramers that can self-associate to form higher oligomers (Fig. 3) (36).

In the posterior pituitary, AVP is stored in vesicles. Exocytotic release is stimulated by minute increases in serum osmolality (hypernatremia, osmotic regulation) and by more pronounced decreases of extracellular fluid (hypovolemia, nonosmotic regulation). Oxytocin and neurophysin I are released from the posterior pituitary by the suckling response in lactating females. The neuropeptides oxytocin and vasopressin are involved in new fascinating studies of the neurobiology of attachment (81) and central vasopressin and oxytocin receptors may regulate the autonomic expression of fear (79).

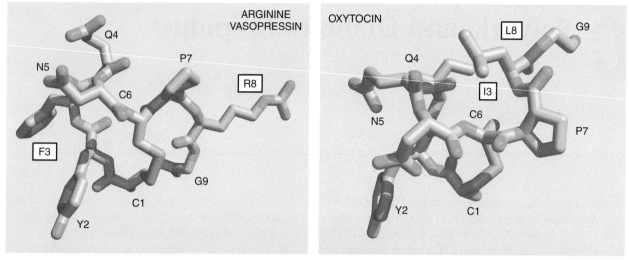

FIGURE 1 Contrasting structures of arginine-vasopressin (AVP) and oxytocin (OT). The peptides differ only by two amino acids (F3 → I3 and R8 → L8 in AVP and OT, respectively). The conformation of AVP was obtained from Mouillac B, Chini B, Balestre MN, et al. The binding site of neuropeptide vasopressin V1a receptor. Evidence for a major localization within transmembrane regions. *J Biol Chem* 1995;270:25771–25777; and the conformation of OT was obtained from the Protein Data Bank (PDB Id 1XY1).

Osmotic and Nonosmotic Stimulation

The regulation of AVP release from the posterior pituitary is dependent primarily on two mechanisms involving the osmotic and nonosmotic pathways (160). The osmotic regulation of AVP is dependent on osmoreceptor cells. Although magnocellular neurons are themselves osmosensitives, they require input from the lamina terminalis to respond fully to osmotic challenges. Neurons in the lamina terminalis are also osmosensitive and because the subfornical organ (SFO) and the organum vasculosum of the lamina terminalis (OVLT) lie outside the blood–brain barrier, they can integrate this information with endocrine signals borne by circulating hormones, such as angiotensin

II (ANG II), relaxin, and atrial natriuretic peptide (ANP). While circulating ANG II and relaxin excite oxytocin and vasopressin magnocellular neurons, ANP inhibits vasopressin neurons. In addition to an angiotensinergic path from the SFO, the OVLT and the median preoptic nucleus provide direct glutaminergic and GABAergic projections to the hypothalamo-neurohypophysial system. Nitric oxide and apelin may also modulate neurohormone release (50).

In magnocellular neurons, stretch-inactivating cationic channels transduce osmotically evoked changes in cell volume and results in functionally relevant changes in membrane potential; hypertonicity will trigger a membrane depolarization of these cells and AVP secretion (29,

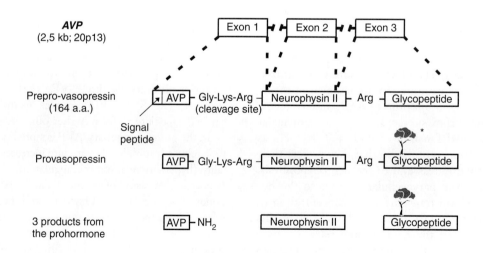

*addition of a carbohydrate chain

FIGURE 2 Structure of the human vasopressin (AVP) gene and prohormone.

30). Recent studies demonstrate that a variant of the transient receptor potential vanilloid type-1 (Trpv1) channel is expressed in osmosensitive neurons of the SON. Knockout mice ($Trpv1^{-/-}$) showed a pronounced serum hyperosmolality under basal conditions and abnormal AVP responses to osmotic stimulation in vivo. These results suggest that the $Trpv1$ gene encodes a central component of the osmoreceptor (175).

Cell volume is decreased most readily by substances that are restricted to the extracellular fluid, such as hypertonic saline or hypertonic mannitol, which not only enhance osmotic water movement from the cells but also very effectively stimulate AVP release. In contrast, hypertonic urea, which moves rapidly into the cells, neither readily alters cell volume nor effectively stimulates AVP

release (207). The osmoreceptor cells are very sensitive to changes in extracellular fluid osmolality. With fluid deprivation a 1% increase in extracellular fluid osmolality stimulates AVP release, whereas with water ingestion a 1% decrease in extracellular fluid osmolality suppresses AVP release.

AVP release can also be caused through a nonosmotic mechanism (Fig. 4). Large decrements in blood volume or blood pressure (>10%) sensed by stretch and baroreceptors in the central venous and arterial system stimulate AVP release. A variety of hypothalamic neurotransmitters, including monoamines and neuropeptides, are involved in the control of AVP release (105). Noradrenaline in the supraoptic nuclei, as well as in the paraventricular nuclei, has a primary excitatory effect on AVP release, most probably mediated through α_1-adrenergic receptors (146). ANG II is also a potent stimulant of AVP release (59). It is of note that knockout mice with loss-of-function of angiotensinogen (a precursor peptide of ANG II) or of the angiotensin receptor type 1A, do not demonstrate obvious alterations in thirst or in water balance (83, 135, 179). Mice that lack the gene encoding the angiotensin receptor type 2 have a mild impairment in drinking response to water deprivation (74). β-adrenergic receptors (105) and opioid receptors (157) may be involved in the inhibition of AVP release.

The osmotic stimulation of AVP release by dehydration or hypertonic saline infusion, or both, is regularly used to test the AVP secretory capacity of the posterior pituitary. This secretory capacity can be assessed directly by comparing the plasma AVP concentration measured sequentially during a dehydration procedure with the normal values and then correlating the plasma AVP with the

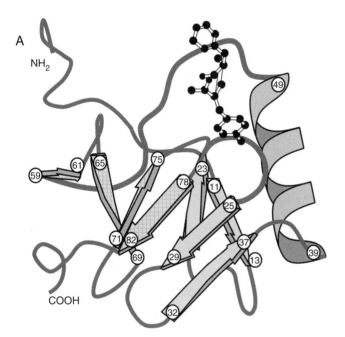

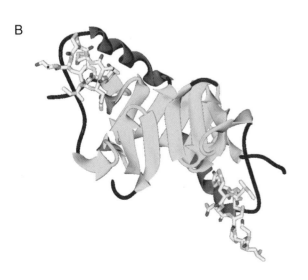

FIGURE 3   A: Three-dimensional structure of a bovine peptide–neurophysin monomer complex. The structure of each chain is 12% helix and 40% β sheet. The chain is folded into two domains as predicted by disulfide-pairing studies. The amino-terminal domain begins in a long loop (residues 1–10), then enters a four-stranded (residues 11–13, 19–23, 25–29, and 32–37) antiparallel β sheet *(sheet I; four shaded arrows)*, followed by a three-turn 3_{10}-helix (residues 39–49) and another loop (residues 50–58). The carboxyl-terminal domain is shorter, consisting of only a four-stranded (residues 59–61, 65–69, 71–75, and 78–82) antiparallel β sheet *(sheet II; four cross-hatched arrows)* (36). The arginine-vasopressin molecule *(balls and sticks model)* is shown in the peptide-binding pocket of the neurophysin monomer. The strongest interactions in this binding pocket are salt bridge interactions between the αNH_3^+ group of the peptide, the γ-COO^- group of Glu^{NP47} (residue number 47 of the neurophysin molecule), and the side chain of Arg^{NP8}. The γ-COO^- group of Glu^{NP47} plays a bifunctional role in the peptide-binding pocket: (a) it directly interacts with the hormone; (b) it interacts with other neurophysin residues to establish the correct, local structure of the peptide-neurophysin complex. Arg^{NP8} and Glu^{NP47} are conserved in all neurophysin sequences from mammals to invertebrates. **B:** Ribbon drawing (Midas) of the dimer neurophysin-oxytocin. The bound oxytocin sits in binding pockets located at the end of a three-turn 3_{10}-helix. (From Rose JP, Wu CK, Hsiao CD, et al. Crystal structure of the neurophysin-oxytocin complex. *Nat Struct Biol* 1996;3:163–169, with permission.) See color insert.

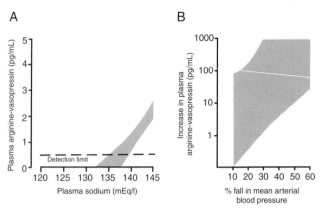

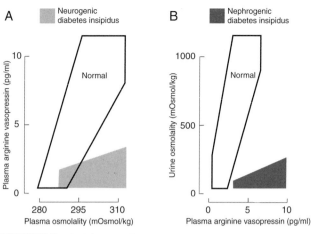

FIGURE 4   Osmotic and nonosmotic stimulation of arginine-vasopressin (AVP). **A:** The relationship between plasma AVP (P_{AVP}) and plasma sodium (P_{Na}) in 19 healthy subjects is described by the gray area, which includes the 99% confidence limits of the regression line P_{Na}/P_{AVP}. The osmotic threshold for AVP release is about 280 to 285 mmol/kg or 136 mEq of sodium per liter. AVP secretion should be abolished when plasma sodium is lower than 135 mEq/l (15). **B:** Increase in plasma AVP during hypotension. Note that a large diminution in blood pressure in healthy humans induces large increments in AVP. (From Vokes T, Robertson GL. Physiology of secretion of vasopressin. In: Czernichow P, Robinson AG, eds. *Diabetes Insipidus in Man.* Basel: S. Karger; 1985:127–155, with permission.)

FIGURE 5   **A:** Schematic diagram of the relationship between plasma arginine-vasopressin (AVP) and plasma osmolality during hypertonic saline infusion. In patients with neurogenic diabetes insipidus, plasma AVP is almost always subnormal relative to plasma osmolality. In contrast, patients with primary polydipsia or nephrogenic diabetes insipidus (NDI) have values within the normal range *(light gray area).* **B:** Relationship between urine osmolality and plasma AVP during a dehydration test. Patients with NDI have hypotonic urine despite high plasma AVP. In contrast, patients with neurogenic diabetes insipidus or primary polydipsia have values within the normal range *(dark gray area).* (From Zerbe RL, Robertson GL. Disorders of ADH. *Med North Am* 1984;13:1570–1574, with permission.)

urinary osmolality measurements obtained simultaneously (Fig. 5) (206).

The AVP release can also be assessed indirectly by measuring plasma and urine osmolalities at regular intervals during the dehydration test (125). The maximum urinary osmolality obtained during dehydration is compared with the maximum urinary osmolality obtained after the administration of vasopressin or 1-desamino-8-D-arginine vasopressin (dDAVP; Pitressin: 5 units subcutaneously [SQ] in adults; 1 unit SQ in children; or dDAVP 1-4 μg intravenously during 5 to 10 minutes).

The nonosmotic stimulation of AVP release can be used to assess the vasopressin secretory capacity of the posterior pituitary in a rare group of patients with the essential hyponatremia and hypodipsia syndrome. Although some of these patients may have partial central diabetes insipidus, they respond normally to nonosmolar AVP release signals such as hypotension, emesis, and hypoglycemia (19). In all other cases of suspected central diabetes insipidus, these nonosmotic stimulation tests will not give additionnal clinical information (10).

Cellular Actions of Vasopressin

The neurohypophyseal hormone AVP has multiple actions, including the inhibition of diuresis, contraction of smooth muscle, platelet aggregation, stimulation of liver glycogenolysis, modulation of adrenocorticotropic hormone release from the pituitary, and central regulation of somatic and higher functions (thermoregulation, blood pressure, autonomic expression of fear, neurobiology of attachment) (79, 81, 88). These multiple actions of AVP could be explained by the interaction of AVP with at least three types of

G-protein–coupled receptors: The V1a (vascular hepatic) and V1b (anterior pituitary) receptors act through phosphatidylinositol hydrolysis to mobilize calcium (130), and the V2 (kidney) receptor is coupled to adenylate cyclase (88).

The first step in the action of AVP on water excretion is its binding to V2 receptors on the basolateral membrane of the collecting duct cells (Fig. 6). The human V2 receptor gene, *AVPR2*, is located in chromosome region Xq28 and has three exons and two small introns (26, 172). The sequence of the complementary DNA (cDNA) predicts a polypeptide of 371 amino acids with a structure typical of guanine-nucleotide (G) protein–coupled receptors with seven transmembrane, four extracellular, and four cytoplasmic domains (Fig. 7) (194). The activation of the V2 receptor on renal collecting tubules stimulates adenylyl cyclase by the way of the stimulatory G-protein (G_s) and promotes the cyclic adenosine monophosphate (cAMP)–mediated incorporation of the water channels aquaporin-2 (AQP2) into the luminal surface of these cells. This process is the molecular basis of the vasopressin-induced increase in the osmotic water permeability of the apical membrane of the collecting tubule. The human AQP2 gene is located in chromosome region 12q13 and has four exons and three introns (51, 52, 168). It is predicted to code for a polypeptide of 271 amino acids that is organized into two repeats oriented at 180 degrees to each other and has six membrane-spanning domains, both terminal ends located intracellularly, and conserved Asn-Pro-Ala boxes (Fig. 8). These features are characteristic of the major intrinsic protein family (168). AQP2 is detectable in urine, and changes in urinary excretion of this protein can be used as an index of the action of

Outer and inner medullary collecting duct

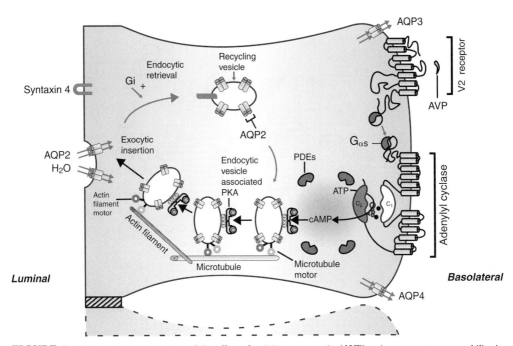

FIGURE 6   Schematic representation of the effect of arginine-vasopressin (AVP) to increase water permeability in the principle cells of the collecting duct. AVP is bound to the V2 receptor (a G-protein–linked receptor) on the basolateral membrane. The basic process of G-protein–coupled receptor signaling consists of three steps: A hepta-helical receptor that detects a ligand (in this case, AVP) in the extracellular milieu, a G-protein ($G_{\alpha s}$) that dissociates into α subunits bound to GTP and $\beta\gamma$ subunits after interaction with the ligand-bound receptor, and an effector (in this case, adenylyl cyclase) that interacts with dissociated G-protein subunits to generate small-molecule second messengers. AVP activates adenylyl cyclase, increasing the intracellular concentration of cAMP. The topology of adenylyl cyclase is characterized by two tandem repeats of six hydrophobic transmembrane domains separated by a large cytoplasmic loop and terminates in a large intracellular tail. The dimeric structure (C_1 and C_2) of the catalytic domains is represented. Conversion of ATP to cAMP takes place at the dimer interface. Two aspartate residues (in C_1) coordinate two metal cofactors (Mg^{2+} or Mn^{2+}, *small black circles*), which enable the catalytic function of the enzyme (183). Adenosine is the large open circle and the three phosphate groups (ATP) are the three small open circles. Protein kinase A (PKA) is the target of the generated cAMP. The binding of cAMP to the regulatory subunits of PKA induces a conformational change, causing these subunits to dissociate from the catalytic subunits. These activated subunits (C) as shown here are anchored to an aquaporin-2 (AQP2)–containing endocytic vesicle via san A-kinase anchoring protein (AKAP). The local concentration and distribution of the cAMP gradient is limited by phosphodiesterase (PDE). Cytoplasmic vesicles carrying the water channel proteins (represented as homotetrameric complexes) are fused to the luminal membrane in response to AVP, thereby increasing the water permeability of this membrane. The dissociation of AKAP from the endocytic vesicle is not represented. Microtubules and actin filaments are necessary for vesicle movement toward the membrane. When AVP is not available, AQP2 water channels are retrieved by an endocytic process, and water permeability returns to its original low rate. AQP3 and AQP4 water channels are expressed constitutively at the basolateral membrane. From (25), with permission.

vasopressin on the kidney (93). AQP2 is exclusively present in principle cells of inner medullary collecting duct cells and is diffusely distributed in the cytoplasm in the euhydrated condition, whereas apical staining of AQP2 is intensified in the dehydrated condition or after vasopressin administration (65, 133, 134).

AVP also increases the water reabsorptive capacity of the kidney by regulating the urea transporter variants UT-A1/3, which are present in the inner medullary collecting duct, predominantly in its terminal part (57). AVP also increases the permeability of principle collecting duct cells to sodium. In summary, as stated elegantly by Ward and colleagues (192), in the absence of AVP stimulation, collecting duct epithelia exhibit very low permeabilities to sodium urea and

water. These specialized permeability properties permit the excretion of large volumes of hypotonic urine formed during intervals of water diuresis. In contrast, AVP stimulation of the principle cells of the collecting ducts leads to selective increases in the permeability of the apical membrane to water (P_f), urea (P_{urea}), and Na (P_{Na}).

These actions of vasopressin in the distal nephron are possibly modulated by prostaglandins E2 and by the luminal calcium concentration. High levels of E-prostanoid (EP3) receptors are expressed in the kidney. However, mice lacking EP3 receptors for prostaglandin E2 were found to have quasinormal regulation of urine volume and osmolality in response to various physiological stimuli (60). An apical calcium/polycation receptor protein expressed in the terminal portion of the inner

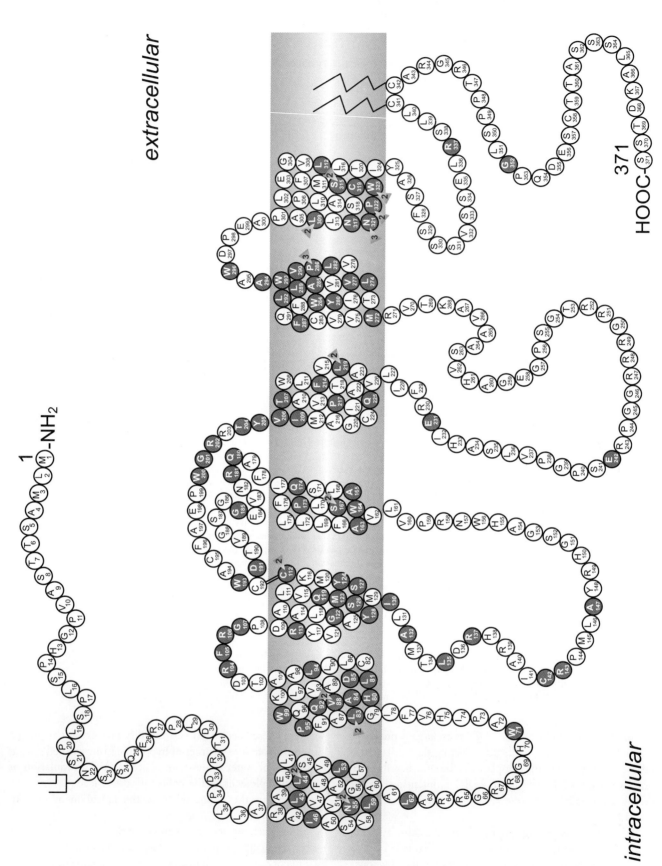

FIGURE 7 Schematic representation of the V2 receptor and identification of 184 putative disease-causing *AVPR2* mutations. Predicted amino acids are given as the one-letter amino-acid code. Solid symbols indicate missense or nonsense mutations; a number indicates more than one mutation in the same codon; other types of mutations are not indicated on the figure. The extracellular, transmembrane, and cytoplasmic domains are defined according to Mouillac B, Chini B, Balestre MN, et al. The binding site of neuropeptide vasopressin V1a receptor. Evidence for a major localization within transmembrane regions. *J Biol Chem* 1995;270:25771–25777. There are 90 missense, 18 nonsense, 45 frameshift deletion or insertion, seven in-frame deletion or insertions, four splice sites, 19 large deletion mutations, and one complex mutation. See http://www.medicine.mcgill.ca/nephros for a list of mutations.

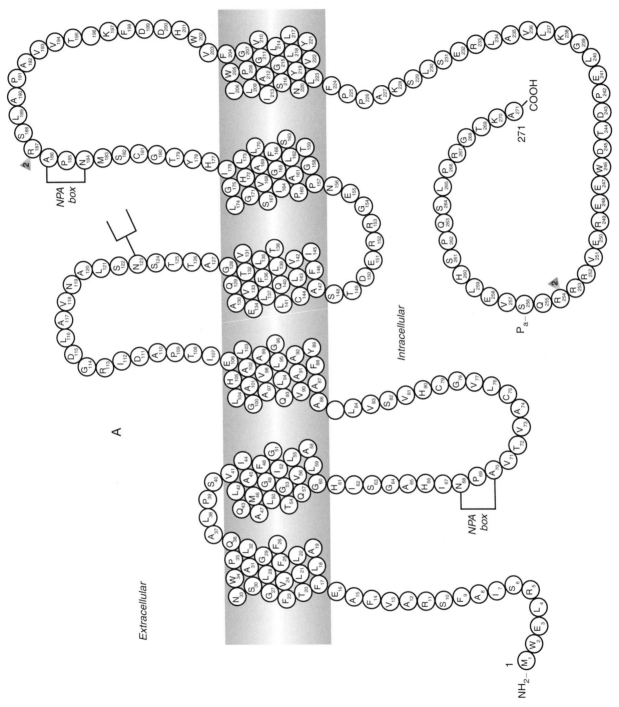

FIGURE 8 **A:** Schematic representation of aquaporin-2 (AQP2) and identification of 38 putative disease-causing AQP2 mutations. Solid symbols indicate missense or nonsense mutations; a number indicates more than one mutation in the same codon; other types of mutations are not indicated on the figure. The locations of the NPA boxes (Asparagine, N; Proline, P; Alanine, A) and the protein kinase A phosphorylation site (Pa) are indicated. The extracellular, transmembrane, and cytoplasmic domains are defined according to Deen PMT, Verdijk MAJ, Knoers NVAM, et al. Requirement of human renal water channel aquaporin-2 for vasopressin-dependent concentration of urine. *Science* 1994;264:92–95. Solid symbols indicate the location of the missense or nonsense mutations. There are 28 missense, two nonsense, six frameshift deletion or insertion, and two splice-site mutations.

medullary collecting duct of the rat has been shown to reduce AVP-elicited osmotic water permeability when luminal calcium concentration rises (165). This possible link between calcium and water metabolism may play a role in the pathogenesis of renal stone formation (165).

THE BRATTLEBORO RAT WITH AUTOSOMAL RECESSIVE NEUROGENIC DIABETES INSIPIDUS

The classical animal model for studying diabetes insipidus has been the Brattleboro rat with autosomal recessive neurogenic diabetes insipidus. *di/di* rats are homozygous for a 1-bp deletion (G) in the second exon, which results in a frameshift mutation in the coding sequence of the carrier neurophysin II (NPII) (Fig. 9) (169). The polyuric symptoms are also observed in heterozygous *di/n* rats. Homozygous Brattleboro rats may still demonstrate some V2 antidiuretic effect since the administration of a selective nonpeptide V2 antagonist (SR121463A, 10 mg/kg intraperitoneal) induced a further increase in urine flow rate (200 to 354 ± 42 ml/24 hours) and a decline in urinary osmolality (170 to 92 ± 8 mmol/kg) (173). Oxytocin, which is present at enhanced plasma concentrations in Brattleboro rats, may be responsible for the antidiuretic activity observed (5, 40). Oxytocin is not stimulated by increased plasma osmolality in humans. The Brattleboro rat model is therefore not strictly comparable with the rarely observed human cases of autosomal recessive neurogenic diabetes insipidus (45, 198).

KNOCKOUT MICE WITH URINARY CONCENTRATION DEFECTS

A useful strategy to establish the physiological function of a protein is to determine the phenotype produced by pharmacological inhibition of protein function or by gene disruption. Transgenic knockout mice deficient in AQP1, AQP2, AQP3,

AQP4, AQP3 and AQP4, CLCNK1, NKCC2, NFAT5, AVPR2, or AGT have been engineered (39, 109–112, 122, 139, 180, 202, 205). Angiotensinogen (AGT)–deficient mice are characterized by both concentrating and diluting defects secondary to a defective renal papillary architecture (139).

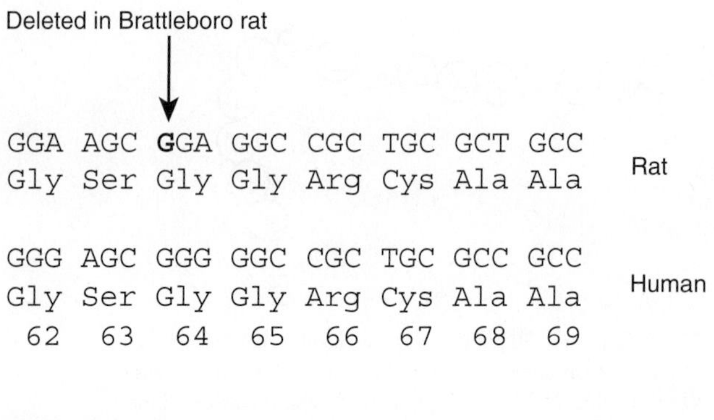

As reviewed by Rao and Verkman (147) extrapolation of data in mice to humans must be made with caution. For example, the maximum osmolality of mouse (< 3000 mOsm/kg H_2O) is much greater than that of human urine (1000 mOsmol/kg H_2O) and normal serum osmolality in mice is 330 to 345 mOsmol/kg H_2O, substantially greater than that in humans (280–290 mOsm/kg H_2O). Protein expression patterns and thus the interpretation of phenotype studies may also be species-dependent. For example, AQP4 is expressed in both proximal tubule and collecting duct in mouse but only in collecting duct in rat and human (147).

The *Aqp3*, *Aqp4*, *Clcnk1* and *Agt* knockout mice have no identified human counterparts. Of interest, *AQP1*-null humans have no obvious symptoms (145). Knockout mice deficient in AVPR2, AQP2, NKCC2, or ROMK suffer from severe dehydration and die during their first week of life. Adult conditional and tissue-specific AQP2-knockout mice survived (161, 203).

Ethylnitrosourea-mutagenized mice heterozygous for the F204V mutation in the *Aqp2* gene have been described (107) and mice from the Jackson Laboratory with congenital progressive hydronephrosis bear the S256L mutation in *Aqp2* which affects its phosphorylation and apical membrane accumulation (123).

QUANTITATING RENAL WATER EXCRETION

Diabetes insipidus is characterized by the excretion of abnormally large volumes of hypo-osmotic urine (< 250 mmol/kg). This definition excludes osmotic diuresis, which occurs when excess solute is being excreted, as with glucose in the polyuria of diabetes mellitus. Other agents that produce osmotic diuresis are mannitol, urea, glycerol, contrast media, and loop diuretics. Osmotic diuresis should be considered when solute excretion exceeds 60 mmol/hour. The quantification of water excretion (free-water clearance, osmolar clearance, free electrolyte water reabsorption, effective water clearance) is described elsewhere in this textbook.

Deleted in Brattleboro rat

↓

```
GGA AGC GGA GGC CGC TGC GCT GCC
Gly Ser Gly Gly Arg Cys Ala Ala    Rat


GGG AGC GGG GGC CGC TGC GCC GCC
Gly Ser Gly Gly Arg Cys Ala Ala    Human
 62  63  64  65  66  67  68  69
```

FIGURE 9 Neurophysin II genomic and amino acid sequence showing the 1-bp (G) deleted in the Brattleboro rat. The human sequence (GenBank entry M11166) is also shown. It is almost identical to the rat prepro sequence. In the Brattleboro rat, G1880 is deleted with a resultant frameshift after 63 amino acids (amino acid-1 is the first amino acid of neurophysin II).

CLINICAL CHARACTERISTICS OF DIABETES INSIPIDUS DISORDERS

Neurogenic Diabetes Insipidus

COMMON FORMS

Failure to synthesize or secrete vasopressin normally limits maximal urinary concentration and, depending on the severity of the disease, causes varying degrees of polyuria and polydipsia. Experimental destruction of the vasopressin-synthesizing areas of the hypothalamus (supraoptic and paraventricular nuclei) causes a permanent form of the disease. Similar results are obtained by sectioning the hypophyseal hypothalamic tract above the median eminence. Sections below the median eminence, however, produce only transient diabetes insipidus. Lesions to the hypothalamic-pituitary tract are frequently associated with a three-stage response in experimental animals and in humans (189): (1) An initial diuretic phase lasting from a few hours to 5 to 6 days; (2) a period of antidiuresis unresponsive to fluid administration. This antidiuresis is probably due to vasopressin release from injured axons and may last from a few hours to several days (because urinary dilution is impaired during this phase, continued water administration can cause severe hyponatremia); and (3) a final period of diabetes insipidus. The extent of the injury determines the completeness of the diabetes insipidus and, as already discussed, the site of the lesion determines whether the disease will be permanent.

Twenty-five percent of patients studied after transsphenoidal surgery developed spontaneous isolated hyponatremia, 20% developed diabetes insipidus, and 46% remained normonatremic. Normonatremia, hyponatremia, and diabetes insipidus were associated with increasing degrees of surgical manipulation of the posterior lobe and pituitary stalk during surgery (140). Central diabetes insipidus observed after transphenoidal surgery is often transient and only 2% of patients need a long-term treatment with dDAVP (131).

The causes of central diabetes insipidus in adults and in children are listed in Table 1 (47, 71, 114, 128). Rare causes of central diabetes insipidus include leukemia, thrombotic thrombocytopenic purpura, pituitary apoplexy, sarcoidosis (58) and Wegener granulomatosis, xanthoma

disseminatum (137), septooptico dysplasia and agenesis of the corpus callosum (121), metabolic (anorexia nervosa), lymphocytic hypophysitis (80), necrotizing infundibulo-hypophysitis (2). Maghnie et al. (114) studied 79 patients with central diabetes insipidus. Additional deficits in anterior pituitary hormones were documented in 61% of patients, a median of 0.6 years (range, 01–18.0 years) after the onset of diabetes insipidus. The most frequent abnormality was growth hormone deficiency (59%), followed by hypothyroidism (28%), hypogonadism (24%), and adrenal insufficiency (22%). Seventy-five percent of the patients with Langerhans cell histiocytosis had an anterior pituitary hormone deficiency that was first detected a median of 3.5 years after the onset of diabetes insipidus (114). None of the patients with central diabetes insipidus secondary to AVP mutations developed anterior pituitary hormone deficiencies

RARE FORMS

Autosomal Dominant and Recessive Neurogenic Diabetes Insipidus

Lacombe (100) and Weil (195) described a familial non–X-linked form of diabetes insipidus without any associated mental retardation. The descendants of the family described by Weil were later found to have autosomal dominant neurogenic diabetes insipidus (35, 55, 196). Neurogenic diabetes insipidus (OMIM 125700) (141) is a well-characterized entity, secondary to mutations in AVP (OMIM 192340) (141). Patients with autosomal dominant neurogenic diabetes insipidus retain some limited capacity to secrete AVP during severe dehydration, and the polyuropolydipsic symptoms usually appear after the first year of life (152) when the

TABLE 1 Etiology of Hypothalamic Diabetes Insipidus in Children and Adults

	Children (%)	Children and young adults (%)	Adults (%)
Primary brain tumor[a]	49.5	22	30
Before surgery	33.5		13
After surgery	16		17
Idiopathic (isolated or familial)	29	58	25
Histiocytosis	16	12	-
Metastatic cancer[b]	-		8
Trauma[c]	2.2	2.0	17
Postinfectious disease	2.2	6.0	-

Data from Czernichow P, Pomarede R, Brauner R, Rappaport R. Neurogenic diabetes insipidus in children. In: Czernichow P, Robinson AG (eds.). *Frontiers of Hormone Research*. Basel, Switzerland: S. Karger, 1985:190–20; Greger NG, Kirkland RT, Clayton GW, Kirkland JL. Central diabetes insipidus. 22 years' experience. *Am J Dis Child* 1986;140:551–554; Moses AM, Blumenthal SA, Streeten DHP. Acid-base and electrolyte disorders associated with endocrine disease: pituitary and thyroid. In: Arieff AI, de Fronzo RA (eds.). *Fluid, Electrolyte and Acid-Base Disorders*. New York: Churchill Livingstone, 1985:851–892; Maghnie M, Cosi G, Genovese E, et al. Central diabetes insipidus in children and young adults. *N Engl J Med* 2000;343:998–1007.

[a]Primary malignancy: craniopharyngioma, dysgerminoma, meningioma, adenoma, glioma, astrocytoma. [b]Secondary: metastatic from lung or breast, lymphoma, leukemia, dysplastic pancytopenia. [c]Trauma could be severe or mild.

infant's demand for water is more likely to be understood by adults.

More than 50 *AVP* mutations segregating with autosomal dominant or autosomal recessive neurohypophyseal diabetes insipidus have been described (41) (see http://www.medicine.mcgill.ca/nephros for a list of mutations). The mechanisms by which a mutant allele causes neurohypophyseal diabetes insipidus could involve the induction of magnocellular cell death as a result of the accumulation of AVP precursors within the endoplasmic reticulum (84, 164, 176). This hypothesis could account for the delayed onset of the disease. In addition to the "misfolding neurotoxicity" caused by mutant AVP precursors, the interaction between the wildtype and the mutant precursors suggests that a dominant-negative mechanism may also contribute to the pathogenesis of autosomal dominant diabetes insipidus (85). The absence of symptoms in infancy in autosomal dominant neurohypophyseal diabetes insipidus is in sharp contrast with NDI secondary to mutations in *AVPR2* or in *AQP2,* in which the polyuropolydipsic symptoms are present during the first week of life.

Of interest, errors in protein folding represent the underlying basis for many inherited diseases (44, 185, 197) and are also pathogenic mechanisms for *AVP, AVPR2,* and *AQP2* mutants. Why AVP-misfolded mutants are cytotoxic to AVP-producing neurons is an unresolved issue. Protein misfolding, an "unfolded protein response" in cells, and the accumulation of excess misfolded protein leading to apoptotic cell death are well documented for autosomal dominant retinitis pigmentosa (94).

Three families with autosomal recessive neurohypophyseal diabetes insipidus in which the patients were homozygous or compound heterozygotes for *AVP* mutations have been identified (45, 198). Two of these families are characterized phenotypically by severe and early onset (in the first 3 months of life) with polyuria, polydipsia, and dehydration. As a consequence, early hereditary diabetes insipidus can be neurogenic or nephrogenic.

Wolfram Syndrome

Wolfram syndrome, also known as DIDMOAD, is an autosomal recessive neurodegenerative disorder accompanied by insulin-dependent diabetes mellitus and progressive optic atrophy. The acronym DIDMOAD describes the following clinical features of the syndrome: *d*iabetes *i*nsipidus, *d*iabetes *m*ellitus, *o*ptic *a*trophy, and sensorineural *d*eafness. An unusual incidence of psychiatric symptoms has also been described in patients with this syndrome. These included paranoid delusions, auditory or visual hallucinations, psychotic behavior, violent behavior, organic brain syndrome typically in the late or preterminal stages of their illness, progressive dementia, and severe learning disabilities or mental retardation or both. Patients with Wolfram syndrome develop diabetes mellitus and bilateral optical atrophy mainly in the first decade of life, the diabe-

tes insipidus is usually partial and of gradual onset, and the polyuria can be wrongly attributed to poor glycemic control. Furthermore, a severe hyperosmolar state can occur if untreated diabetes mellitus is associated with an unrecognized posterior pituitary deficiency. The dilatation of the urinary tract observed in the DIDMOAD syndrome may be secondary to chronic high urine flow rates and, perhaps, to some degenerative aspects of the innervation of the urinary tract. The gene responsible for Wolfram syndrome located in chromosome region 4p16.1, encodes a putative 890–amino acid transmembrane protein referred as *wolframin*. Wolframin is an endoglycosidase H–sensitive glycoprotein, which localizes primarily in the endoplasmic reticulum of a variety of neurons including neurons in the supraoptic nucleus and neurons in the lateral magnocellular division of the paraventricular nucleus (53, 181). Disruption of the *Wfs1* gene in mice cause progressive β cell loss and impaired stimulus-secretion coupling in insulin secretion but central diabetes insipidus is not observed in $Wfs^{-/-}$ mice (82).

SYNDROME OF HYPERNATREMIA AND HYPODIPSIA

Some patients with the hypernatremia and hypodipsia syndrome may have partial central diabetes insipidus. These patients also have persistent hypernatremia that is not due to any apparent extracellular volume loss, absence or attenuation of thirst, and a normal renal response to AVP. In almost all the patients studied, the hypodipsia has been associated with cerebral lesions in the vicinity of the hypothalamus. It has been proposed that in these patients there is a "resetting" of the osmoreceptor because their urine tends to become concentrated or diluted at inappropriately high levels of plasma osmolality. However, using the regression analysis of plasma AVP concentration versus plasma osmolality, it has been shown that in some of these patients the tendency to concentrate and dilute urine at inappropriately high levels of plasma osmolality is due solely to a marked reduction in sensitivity or a gain in the osmoregulatory mechanism (78). This finding is compatible with the diagnosis of partial central diabetes insipidus. In other patients, however, plasma AVP concentrations fluctuate in a random manner, bearing no apparent relationship to changes in plasma osmolality. Such patients frequently display large swings in serum sodium concentration and frequently exhibit hypodipsia. It appears that most patients with "essential hypernatremia" fit one of these two patterns (Fig. 10). Both of these groups of patients consistently respond normally to nonosmolar AVP release signals, such as hypotension, emesis, hypoglycemia, or all three. These observations suggest that (1) the osmoreceptor may be anatomically as well as functionally separate from the nonosmotic efferent pathways and neurosecretory neurons for vasopressin and a hypothalamic lesion may impair the osmotic release of AVP while the nonosmotic re-

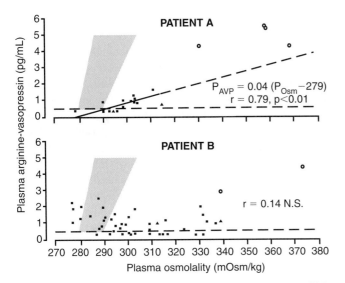

FIGURE 10 Plasma arginine vasopressin (PAVP) as a function of "effective" plasma osmolality (P_{Osm}) in two patients with adipsic hypernatremia. Open circles indicate values obtained on admission; filled squares indicate those obtained during forced hydration; filled triangles indicate those obtained after 1 to 2 weeks of ad libitum water intake; gray areas indicate range of normal values. (From Robertson GL. The physiopathology of ADH secretion. In: Tolis G, Labrie F, Martin JB, Naftolin F, eds. *Clinical Neuroendocrinology: A Pathophysiological Approach.* New York: Raven Press; 1979:247–260, with permission).

lease of AVP remains intact; and (2) the osmoreceptor neurons that regulate vasopressin secretion are not totally synonymous with those that regulate thirst, although they appear to be anatomically close if not overlapping.

Nephrogenic Diabetes Insipidus

In NDI, the kidney is unable to concentrate urine despite normal or elevated concentrations of the antidiuretic hormone arginine vasopressin. In congenital NDI, the obvious clinical manifestations of the disease, that is polyuria and polydipsia, are present at birth and need to be immediately recognized to avoid severe episodes of dehydration. It is clinically useful to distinguish two types of hereditary NDI: A "pure" type characterized by loss of water only and a complex type characterized by loss of water and ions. Patients who have congenital NDI and mutations in the *AVPR2* or *AQP2* genes have a pure NDI phenotype with loss of water but normal conservation of sodium, potassium, chloride, and calcium. Patients with inactivating mutations in genes (*SLC12A1*, *KCNJ1*, *CLCNKB*, *CLCNKA* and *CLCNKB* in combination, or *BSND*) that encode the membrane proteins of the thick ascending limb of the loop of Henle have a complex polyuropolydipsic syndrome with loss of water, sodium, chloride, calcium, magnesium, and potassium. Most (> 90%) of pure congenital NDI patients have mutations in the *AVPR2* gene, the Xq28 gene coding for the vasopressin V2 (antidiuretic) receptor. In less than 10% of the families studied, congenital NDI has an autosomal recessive inheritance and mutations have been identified in the *AQP2* gene located in chromo-

some region 12q13, that is, the vasopressin-sensitive water channel. When studied in vitro, most *AVPR2* mutations lead to receptors that are trapped intracellularly and are unable to reach the plasma membrane. A minority of the mutant receptors reaches the cell surface but are unable to bind AVP or to trigger an intracellular cAMP signal. Similarly, *AQP2* mutant proteins are trapped intracellularly and cannot be expressed at the luminal membrane. AVPR2 and AQP2-trafficking defects are correctable by chemical chaperones

LOSS-OF-FUNCTION MUTATIONS OF *AVPR2*

X-linked NDI (OMIM 304800) (141) is secondary to *AVPR2* mutations, which result in a loss of function or dysregulation of the V2 receptor (64). Males who have an *AVPR2* mutation have a phenotype characterized by early dehydration episodes, hypernatremia, and hyperthermia as early as the first week of life. Dehydration episodes can be so severe that they lower arterial blood pressure to a degree that is not sufficient to sustain adequate oxygenation to the brain, kidneys, and other organs. Mental and physical retardation and renal failure are the classical "historic" consequences of a late diagnosis and lack of treatment. Heterozygous females exhibit variable degrees of polyuria and polydipsia because of skewed X chromosome inactivation (4, 136).

Clinical Characteristics

The historic clinical characteristics include hypernatremia, hyperthermia, mental retardation, and repeated episodes of dehydration in early infancy (46, 61, 193, 200). Mental retardation, a consequence of repeated episodes of dehydration, was prevalent in the Crawford and Bode study (46), in which only nine (11%) of 82 patients had normal intelligence. Early recognition and treatment of X-linked NDI with an abundant intake of water allows a normal lifespan with normal physical and mental development (132). Two characteristics suggestive of X-linked NDI are the familial occurrence and the confinement of mental retardation to male patients. It is then tempting to assume that the family described in 1892 by McIlraith (124) and discussed by Reeves and Andreoli (150) was an X-linked NDI family.

Crawford and Bode (46) clearly describe the early symptoms of the nephrogenic disorder and its severity in infancy. The first manifestations of the disease can be recognized during the first week of life. The infants are irritable, cry almost constantly, and, although eager to suck, will vomit milk soon after ingestion unless prefed with water. The history given by the mothers often include persistent constipation, erratic unexplained fever, and failure to gain weight. Although the patients characteristically show no visible evidence of perspiration, increased water loss during fever or in warm weather exaggerates the symptoms. Unless the condition is recognized early, children experience frequent bouts of hypertonic dehydration, sometimes complicated by convulsions or death; mental retardation is a frequent consequence of these episodes. The intake of large quantities of water, combined with the patient's voluntary restriction of dietary salt and protein intake, lead to hypocaloric dwarfism beginning in infancy. Frequently, lower urinary tract dilatation and obstruction, probably secondary to the large volume of urine produced (178), develop in affected children. Dilatation of the lower urinary tract is also seen in primary polydipsic patients and in patients with neurogenic diabetes insipidus (31, 66). Chronic renal insufficiency may occur by the end of the first decade of life and could be the result of episodes of dehydration with thrombosis of the glomerular tufts (46).

History

In 1989, we observed that the administration of dDAVP, a V2-receptor agonist, increased plasma cAMP concentrations in healthy subjects but had no effect in 14 male patients with X-linked NDI (17). Intermediate responses were observed in obligate carriers of the disease, corresponding to half of the normal receptor response. On the basis of these results, we predicted that the defective gene in these patients with X-linked NDI was likely to code for a defective V2 receptor (17). Since that time, a number of experimental results have confirmed our hypothesis: (1) The NDI locus was mapped to the distal region of the long arm of the X chromosome Xq28 (18, 91, 95, 186); (2) the V2 receptor was identified as a candidate gene for NDI (87); (3) the human V2 receptor was cloned (26); and (4) 184 putative disease-causing mutations have now been identified in the V2 receptor and the list of mutations is still expanding (Fig. 7).

Population Genetics of *AVPR2* Mutations

X-linked NDI is generally a rare disease in which the affected male patients do not concentrate their urine after administration of AVP (22). Because this form is a rare, recessive X-linked disease, female individuals are unlikely to be affected, but heterozygous female individuals can exhibit variable degrees of polyuria and polydipsia because of skewed X chromosome inactivation. In Quebec, the incidence of this disease among male individuals was estimated to be approximately 8.8 in 1,000,000 male live births (4). A founder effect of two particular *AVPR2* mutations (20), one in Ulster Scot immigrants (the Hopewell mutation, W71X) and one in a large Utah kindred (the Cannon pedigree), result in an elevated prevalence of X-linked NDI in their descendants in certain communities in Nova Scotia, Canada, and Utah, United States (20). These founder mutations have now spread all over the North American continent. We have identified the W71X mutation in 42 affected male individuals who reside predominantly in the Maritime Provinces of Nova Scotia and New Brunswick and the L312X mutation in eight affected males who reside in the central United States. We know of 98 living affected male individuals of the Hopewell kindred and 18 living affected male individuals of the Cannon pedigree.

To date, 184 putative disease-causing *AVPR2* mutations have been published in 287 NDI families (Fig. 7).

We propose that all families with hereditary diabetes insipidus should have their molecular defect identified. The molecular identification underlying X-linked NDI is of immediate clinical significance because early diagnosis and treatment of affected infants can avert the physical and mental retardation that results from repeated episodes of dehydration. Affected premature male infants may experience less severe polyuric symptoms and may need only increased hydration during their first week without a need for hydrochlorothiazide treatment. Water should be offered every 2 hours day and night, and temperature, appetite, and growth should be monitored. Admission to hospital may be necessary for continuous gastric feeding. The voluminous amounts of water kept in patients' stomachs will exacerbate physiological gastrointestinal reflux in infants and toddlers, and many affected boys frequently vomit. These young patients often improve with the absorption of an H$_2$ blocker and with metoclopramide (which could induce extrapyramidal symptoms) or with domperidone, which seems to be better tolerated and efficacious. As mentioned previously, all polyuric states (whether neurogenic, nephrogenic, or psychogenic) can induce large dilatations of the urinary tract and bladder (31, 46, 66), and bladder function impairment has been well documented in patients who bear *AVPR2* or *AQP2* mutations (174, 184). Of interest, in mice with congenital progressive hydronephrosis (cph) homozygote for the S266L mutation (*Aqp2*) the congenital obstructive uropathy is likely a result of the polyuria (123). Chronic renal failure secondary to bilateral hydronephrosis has been observed as a long-term complication in these patients. Renal and abdominal ultrasound should be done annually, and simple recommendations, including frequent urination and "double voiding" could be important to prevent these consequences.

Expression Studies

Classification of the defects of naturally occurring mutant human V2 receptors can be based on a similar scheme to that used for the LDL receptor. Mutations have been grouped according to the function and subcellular localization of the mutant protein whose cDNA has been transiently transfected in a heterologous expression system (77). Using this classification, type 1 mutant V2 receptors reach the cell surface but display impaired ligand binding and are consequently unable to induce normal cAMP production. The presence of mutant V2 receptors on the surface of transfected cells can be determined pharmacologically. By carrying out saturation binding experiments using tritiated AVP, the number of cell surface mutant V2 receptors and their apparent binding affinity can be compared with that of the wildtype receptor. In addition, the presence of cell surface receptors can be assessed directly by using immunodetection strategies to visualize epitope-tagged receptors in whole-cell immunofluorescence assays.

Type 2 mutant receptors have defective intracellular transport. This phenotype is confirmed by carrying out, in parallel, immunofluorescence experiments on cells that are intact (to demonstrate the absence of cell surface receptors) or permeabilized (to confirm the presence of intracellular receptor pools). In addition, protein expression is confirmed by Western blot analysis of membrane preparations from transfected cells. It is likely that these mutant type 2 receptors accumulate in a pre-Golgi compartment, because they are initially glycosylated but fail to undergo glycosyl-trimming maturation.

Type 3 mutant receptors are ineffectively transcribed and lead to unstable mRNA, which are rapidly degraded. This subgroup seems to be rare, since Northern blot analysis of cells expressing mutant V2 receptors showed mRNA of normal quantity and molecular size.

Most of the *AVPR2* mutants that we and other investigators have tested are type 2 mutant receptors. They did not reach the cell membrane and were trapped in the interior of the cell (12, 75, 127, 201). Other mutant G-protein–coupled receptors (170) and gene products that cause genetic disorders are also characterized by protein misfolding. Mutations that affect the folding of secretory proteins; integral plasma membrane proteins; or enzymes destined to the endoplasmic reticulum, Golgi complex, and lysosomes results in loss-of-function phenotypes irrespective of their direct impact on protein function because these mutant proteins are prevented from reaching their final destination (162). Folding in the endoplasmic reticulum is the limiting step: Mutant proteins which fail to correctly fold are retained initially in the endoplasmic reticulum and subsequently often degraded. Key proteins involved in the urine countercurrent mechanisms are good examples of this basic mechanism of misfolding. *AQP2* mutations responsible for autosomal recessive NDI are characterized by misrouting of the misfolded mutant proteins and are trapped in the endoplasmic reticulum (182). Mutants that encode other renal membrane proteins that are responsible for Gitelman syndrome (98), Bartter syndrome (73, 143), and cystinuria (38) are also retained in the endoplasmic reticulum.

The *AVPR2* missense mutations are likely to impair folding and to lead to rapid degradation of the misfolded polypeptide and not to the accumulation of toxic aggregates (as is the case for AVP mutants), because the other important functions of the principle cells of the collecting duct (where *AVPR2* is expressed) are entirely normal. These cells express the epithelial sodium channel (ENac). Decreased function of this channel results in a sodium-losing state (27). This has not been observed in patients with *AVPR2* mutations. By contrast, another type of conformational disease is characterized by the toxic retention of the misfolded protein. The relatively common Z mutation in α_1-antitrypsin deficiency not only causes retention of the mutant protein in the endoplasmic reticulum but also affects the secondary structure by insertion of the reactive center loop of one molecule into a destabilized β sheet of a second molecule (108). These polymers clog up the endoplasmic reticulum of hepatocytes and lead to cell death and juvenile hepatitis, cirrhosis, and hepatocarcinomas in these patients (103).

If the misfolded protein/traffic problem that is responsible for so many human genetic diseases can be overcome and the mutant protein transported out of the endoplasmic reticulum to its final destination, these mutant proteins could be sufficiently functional (44). Therefore, using pharmacological chaperones or pharmacoperones to promote escape from the endoplasmic reticulum is a possible therapeutic approach (11, 162, 185). We used selective nonpeptide V2 and V1 receptor antagonists to rescue the cell-surface expression and function of naturally occurring misfolded human V2 receptors (127). Because the beneficial effect of nonpeptide V2 antagonists could be secondary to prevention and interference with endocytosis, we studied the R137H mutant previously reported to lead to constitutive endocytosis (6). We found that the antagonist did not prevent the constitutive β-arresting-promoted endocytosis (12). These results indicate that as for other *AVPR2* mutants, the beneficial effects of the treatment result from the action of the pharmacological chaperones. In clinical studies, we administered a nonpeptide vasopressin antagonist SR49059 to five adult patients who have NDI and bear the del62-64, R137H, and W164S mutations. SR49059 significantly decreased urine volume and water intake and increased urine osmolality whereas sodium, potassium, and creatinine excretions and plasma sodium levels were constant throughout the study (13). This new therapeutic approach could be applied to the treatment of several hereditary diseases resulting from errors in protein folding and kinesis (44, 185).

Because most human gene-therapy experiments using viruses to deliver and integrate DNA into host cells are potentially dangerous (68), other treatments are being actively pursued. Schöneberg and colleagues (167) used aminoglycoside antibiotics because of their ability to suppress premature termination codons (116). They demonstrated that geneticin, a potent aminoglycoside antibiotic, increased AVP-stimulated cAMP in cultured collecting duct cells prepared from E242X mutant mice. The urine concentrating ability of heterozygous mutant mice was also improved.

LOSS-OF-FUNCTION MUTATIONS OF *AQP2* (OMIM 222000, 125800, 107777)

On the basis of desmopressin infusion studies and phenotypic characteristics of both male and female individuals who are affected with NDI, a non–X-linked form of NDI with a postreceptor (post-cAMP) defect was suggested (32, 96, 101, 141). A patient who presented shortly after birth with typical features of NDI but who exhibited normal coagulation and normal fibrinolytic and vasodilatory responses to desmopressin was shown to be a compound heterozygote for two missense mutations (R187C and S217P) in the *AQP2* gene (51). To date, 38 putative disease-causing *AQP2* mutations have been identified in 40 NDI families (Fig. 8). The oocytes of the African clawed frog (*Xenopus laevis*) have provided a most useful experimental system for studying the function of many channel proteins. This convenient expression system was key to the discovery of AQP1 by Agre (1) because frog oocytes have very low permeability and survive even in freshwater ponds. Control oocytes are injected with water alone; test oocytes are injected with various quantities of synthetic transcripts from AQP1 or AQP2 DNA (cRNA). When subjected to a 20-mOsm osmotic shock, control oocytes have exceedingly low water permeability but test oocytes become highly permeable to water. These osmotic water permeability assays demonstrated an absence or very low water transport for all of the cRNA with *AQP2* mutations. Immunofluorescence and immunoblot studies demonstrated that these recessive mutants were retained in the endoplasmic reticulum.

AQP2 mutations in autosomal recessive NDI, which are located throughout the gene result in misfolded proteins that are retained in the endoplasmic reticulum. In contrast, the dominant mutations reported to date are located in the region that codes for the carboxyl terminus of AQP2 (92, 99, 120). Dominant AQP2 mutants form heterotetramers with wildtype AQP2 and are misrouted.

COMPLEX POLYUROPOLYDIPSIC SYNDROME

In contrast to a pure NDI phenotype, with loss of water but normal conservation of sodium, potassium, chloride, and calcium, in Bartter syndrome, patients' renal wasting starts prenatally and polyhydramnios often leads to prematurity. Bartter syndrome (OMIM 601678, 241200, 607364, and 602522) refers to a group of autosomal recessive disorders caused by inactivating mutations in genes (*SLC12A1*, *KCNJ1*, *CLCNKB*, *CLCNKA* and *CLCNKB* in combination, or *BSND*) that encode membrane proteins of the thick ascending limb of the loop of Henle (for review see 23, 24). Although Bartter syndrome and Bartter mutations are commonly used as a diagnosis, it is likely, as explained by Jeck et al. (89), that the two patients with a mild phenotype originally described by Dr. Bartter had Gitelman syndrome, a thiazide-like, salt-losing tubulopathy with a defect in the distal convoluted tubule (89). As a consequence, salt-losing tubulopathy of the furosemide type is a more physiologically appropriate definition.

Thirty percent of the filtered sodium chloride is reabsorbed in the thick ascending limb of the loop of Henle through the apically expressed sodium-potassium-chloride cotransporter NKCC2 (encoded by the *SLC12A1* gene), which uses the sodium gradient across the membrane to transport chloride and potassium into the cell. The potassium ions must be recycled through the apical membrane by the potassium channel ROMK (encoded by the *KCNJ1* gene). In the large experience of Seyberth and colleagues (142), who studied 85 patients with a hypokalemic salt-losing tubulopathy, all 20 patients with *KCNJ1* mutations (except one) and all 12 patients with *SLC12A1* mutations were born as preterm infants after severe polyhydramnios.

Of note, polyhydramnios is never seen during a pregnancy that leads to infants bearing *AVPR2* or *AQP2* mutations. The most common causes of increased amniotic fluid include maternal diabetes mellitus, fetal malformations and chromosomal aberrations, twin-to-twin transfusion syndrome, rhesus incompatibility, and congenital infections (117). Postnatally, polyuria was the leading symptom in 19 of the 32 patients. Renal ultrasound revealed nephrocalcinosis in 31 of these patients. These patients with complex polyuropolydipsic disorders are often poorly recognized and may be confused with pure NDI. As a consequence, congenital polyuria does not suggest automatically *AVPR2* or *AQP2* mutations, and polyhydramnios, salt wasting, hypokalemia, and nephrocalcinosis are important clinical and laboratory characteristics that should be assessed. In patients with Bartter syndrome (salt-losing tubulopathy/furosemide type), the dDAVP test will only indicate a partial type of NDI. The algorithm proposed by Peters et al. (142) is useful since most mutations in *SLC12A1* and *KCNJ1* are found in the carboxyl terminus or in the last exon and, as a consequence, are amenable to rapid DNA sequencing.

ACQUIRED NEPHROGENIC DIABETES INSIPIDUS

Acquired NDI is much more common than congenital NDI but it is rarely as severe. The ability to produce hypertonic urine is usually preserved even though there is inadequate concentrating ability of the nephron. Polyuria and polydipsia are therefore moderate (3–4 l/d).

The more common causes of acquired NDI are listed in Table 2. Lithium administration has become the most frequent cause; 54% of 1105 unselected patients on chronic lithium therapy, NDI developed (28). Nineteen percent of these patients had polyuria, as defined by a 24-hour urine output exceeding 3 l. The mechanism whereby lithium causes polyuria has been extensively studied. Lithium inhibits adenylyl cyclase in a number of cell types including renal epithelia (42, 43). The concentration of lithium in urine of patients on well-controlled lithium therapy (i.e., 10–40 mOsmol/l) is sufficient to exert this effect. Measurement of adenylyl cyclase activity in membranes isolated from a cultured pig kidney cell line (LLC-PK$_1$) revealed that lithium in the concentration range of 10 mOsmol/l interfered with the hormone-stimulated guanyl nucleotide regulatory unit (G$_s$) (69). The effect of chronic lithium therapy has been studied in rat kidney membranes prepared from the inner medulla. It caused a marked downregulation of AQP2, only partially reversed by cessation of therapy, dehydration, or dDAVP treatment, consistent with clinical observations of slow recovery from lithium-induced urinary concentrating defects (118). Downregulation of AQP2 has also been shown to be associated with the development of severe polyuria resulting from other causes of acquired NDI (hypokalemia) (119), release of bilateral ureteral obstruction (63), and hypercalciuria (166)). Thus,

TABLE 2   Causes of Nephrogenic Diabetes Insipidus

Narrow definition of NDI: water permeability of the collecting duct not increased by AVP
Congenital (idiopathic)
Hypercalcemia
Hypokalemia
Drugs:
    Lithium
    Nonpeptide vasopressin receptor (V_2) antagonists
    Demeclocycline
    Amphotericin B
    Methoxyflurane
    Diphenylhydantoin
    Nicotine
    Alcohol
Broad definition of NDI: defective medullary countercurrent function
Renal failure, acute or chronic (especially interstitial nephritis or obstruction)
Medullary damage:
    Sickle-cell anemia and trait
    Amyloidosis
    Sjögren syndrome
    Sarcoidosis
    Hypercalcemia
    Hypokalemia
    Protein malnutrition
    Cystinosis

(Modified from Magner PO, Halperin ML. Polyuria-a pathophysiological approach. *Med North America* 1987;15:2987–2997, with permission).

AQP2 expression is severely downregulated in both congenital (93) and acquired NDI. More studies will be needed to determine whether nonpeptide vasopressin agonists, permeable cAMP-like compounds or other signaling molecules will be able to restore AQP2 expression and function (106). For patients on long-term lithium therapy, amiloride has been proposed to prevent the uptake of lithium in the collecting ducts, thus preventing the inhibitory effect of intracellular lithium on water transport (9).

Primary Polydipsia

Primary polydipsia is a state of hypotonic polyuria secondary to excessive fluid intake. Primary polydipsia was extensively studied by Barlow and de Wardener in 1959 (7); however, the understanding of the pathophysiology of this disease has made little progress. Barlow and de Wardener (7) described seven women and two men who were compulsive water drinkers; their ages ranged from 48 to 59 years, except for one patient was 24 years old. Eight of these patients had histories of previous psychological disorders, which ranged from delusions, depression, and agitation to frank hysterical behavior. The other patient appeared normal. The consumption of water fluctuated irregularly from hour to hour or from day to day; in some patients, there were remissions and relapses lasting several months or longer. In eight of the patients, the mean plasma osmolality was significantly lower than normal. Vasopressin tannate in oil made most of these patients feel ill; in one, it caused overhydration. In four patients, the fluid in-

take returned to normal after electroconvulsive therapy or a period of continuous narcosis; the improvement in three was transient, but in the fourth it lasted 2 years. Polyuric female subjects might be heterozygous for de novo or previously unrecognized *AVPR2* mutations, may bear *AQP2* mutations and may be classified as compulsive water drinkers (158). Therefore, the diagnosis of compulsive water drinking must be made with care and may represent our ignorance of yet undescribed pathophysiological mechanisms. Robertson (158) has described under the name "dipsogenic diabetes insipidus" a selective defect in the osmoregulation of thirst. Three studied patients had, under basal conditions of ad libitum water intake, thirst, polydipsia, polyuria, and high-normal plasma osmolality. They had a normal secretion of AVP, but osmotic threshold for thirst was abnormally low. These dipsogenic diabetes insipidus cases might represent up to 10% of all patients with diabetes insipidus (158).

Diabetes Insipidus and Pregnancy

PREGNANCY IN A PATIENT KNOWN TO HAVE DIABETES INSIPIDUS

An isolated deficiency of vasopressin without a concomitant loss of hormones in the anterior pituitary does not result in altered fertility, and with the exception of polyuria and polydipsia, gestation, delivery, and lactation are uncomplicated (3). Patients may require increasing dosages of dDAVP. The increased thirst may be due to a resetting of the thirst osmostat (49).

Increased polyuria also occurs during pregnancy in patients with partial NDI (86). These patients may be obligatory carriers of the NDI gene (62) or may be homozygotes, compound heterozygotes, or may have dominant AQP2 mutations.

SYNDROMES OF DIABETES INSIPIDUS THAT BEGIN DURING GESTATION AND REMIT AFTER DELIVERY

Barron et al. (8) described three pregnant women in whom transient diabetes insipidus developed late in gestation and subsequently remitted postpartum. In one of these patients, dilute urine was present despite of high plasma concentrations of AVP. Hyposthenuria in all three patients was resistant to administered aqueous vasopressin. Because excessive vasopressinase activity was not excluded as a cause of this disorder, Barron et al. labeled the disease vasopressin resistant rather than NDI.

A well-documented case of enhanced activity of vasopressinase has been described in a woman in the third trimester of a previously uncomplicated pregnancy (54). She had massive polyuria and markedly elevated plasma vasopressinase activity. The polyuria did not respond to large intravenous doses of AVP but responded promptly to dDAVP, a vasopressinase-resistant analogue of AVP. The polyuria disappeared with the disappearance of the vasopressinase. It is suggested that pregnancy may be associated with several different forms of diabetes insipidus, including central, nephrogenic, and vasopressinase mediated (33, 76, 86).

INVESTIGATION OF A PATIENT WITH POLYURIA

Plasma sodium and osmolality are maintained within normal limits (136–143 mOsmol/l for plasma sodium; 275–290 mOsmol/kg for plasma osmolality) by a thirst-AVP-renal axis. Thirst and AVP release, both stimulated by increased osmolality, is a "double-negative" feedback system (104). Even when the AVP component of this double-negative regulatory feedback system is lost, the thirst mechanism still preserves the plasma sodium and osmolality within the normal range, but at the expense of pronounced polydipsia and polyuria. Thus, the plasma sodium concentration or osmolality of an untreated patient with diabetes insipidus may be slightly greater than the mean normal value, but these small increases have no diagnostic significance.

Theoretically, it should be relatively easy to differentiate between neurogenic diabetes insipidus, NDI, and primary polydipsia by comparing the osmolality of urine obtained during dehydration with that of urine obtained after the administration of dDAVP. Patients with neurogenic diabetes insipidus should reveal a rapid increase in urinary osmolality, whereas it should increase normally in response to moderate dehydration in patients with primary polydipsia. However, for several reasons, these distinctions may not be as clear as one might expect (156). First, chronic polyuria resulting from any cause interferes with the maintenance of the medullary concentration gradient and this "wash-out" effect diminishes the maximum concentrating ability of the nephron. The extent of the blunting varies in direct proportion to the severity of the polyuria. Hence, for any given basal urine output, the maximum urine osmolality achieved in the presence of saturating concentrations of AVP is depressed to the same extent in patients with primary polydipsia, neurogenic diabetes insipidus or NDI (Fig. 11). Second, most patients with neurogenic diabetes insipidus maintain a small, but detectable, capacity to secrete AVP during severe dehydration, and urinary osmolality may then increase to greater than the plasma osmolality. Third, patients referred to as partial diabetes insipidus (either neurogenic or nephrogenic) and patients with acquired NDI have an incomplete response to AVP and are able to concentrate their urine to varying degrees in a dehydration test. Finally, all polyuric states (whether neurogenic, nephrogenic or psychogenic) can induce large dilatations of the urinary tract and bladder (31, 66). As a consequence, the urinary bladder of these patients has an increased residual capacity and changes in urinary osmolality induced by diagnostic maneuvers might be difficult to demonstrate.

Indirect Tests for Diabetes Insipidus

The measurement of urinary osmolality after dehydration and dDAVP administration is usually referred to as "indirect testing" because AVP secretion is indirectly assessed through changes in urinary osmolalities (125). The patient is main-

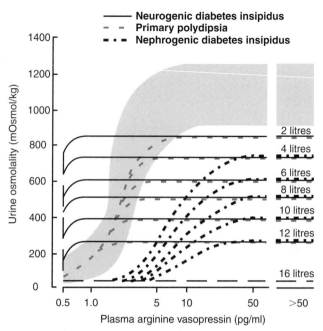

FIGURE 11 Schematic diagram of the relationship between urine osmolality and plasma vasopressin in patients with polyuria of diverse cause and severity. The shaded area represents the normal range. For each of the three categories of polyuria, the relationship is described by a family of sigmoid curves that differ in height. These differences in height reflect differences in maximum concentrating capacity due to "wash-out" of the medullary concentration gradient. They are proportional to the severity of the underlying polyuria (indicated in litres at the right-handed side of each plateau) and are largely independent of the cause. The three categories of diabetes insipidus differ principally in the submaximal or ascending portion of the dose-response curve. In patients with neurogenic diabetes insipidus, this part of the curve lies to the left of normal, reflecting increased sensitivity to the antidiuretic effects of very low concentrations of plasma vasopressin. In contrast, in patients with neurogenic diabetes insipidus, this part of the curve lies to the right of normal, reflecting decreased sensitivity to the antidiuretic effects of normal concentrations of plasma vasopressin. In primary polydipsia, this relationship is relatively normal. (From Robertson GL. Diagnosis of diabetes insipidus. In: Czernichow P, Robinson AG (eds.). *Frontiers of Hormone Research.* Basel: Karger, 1985:176–189, with permission.)

tained on a complete fluid-restriction regimen until urinary osmolality reaches a plateau, as indicated by an hourly increase of less than 30 mOsmol/kg for at least 3 successive hours. After measuring the plasma osmolality, 2 μg dDAVP are administered subcutaneously. Urinary osmolality is measured 30 and 60 minutes later. The last urinary osmolality value obtained before the dDAVP injection and the highest value obtained after the injection are compared. In patients with severe neurogenic diabetes insipidus, urinary osmolality after dehydration is usually low (<200 mOsmol/kg) and increases more than 50% after dDAVP administration. In patients with severe NDI, urinary osmolality after dehydration is also low (<200 mOsmol/kg) but does not increase after dDAVP administration (<20%). Urinary osmolality increases to variable degrees (10% to 50%) after dDAVP administration to patients with partial neurogenic or partial nephrogenic diabetes insipidus. In patients with primary polydipsia, maximum urinary osmolality will be obtained after dehydration (>295 mOsmol/kg) and does not increase after dDAVP administration (<10%).

Alternatively, plasma sodium and plasma and urinary osmolalities can be measured at the beginning of the dehydration procedure and at regular intervals (usually hourly) thereafter depending on the severity of the polyuria (14). For example, an 8-year-old patient (body weight 31 kg) with a clinical diagnosis of congenital NDI (later found to bear an *AVPR2* mutation) continued to excrete large volumes of urine (300 ml/h) during a short 4-hour dehydration test. During this time, the patient suffered from severe thirst, his plasma sodium was 155 mOsmol/l, plasma osmolality was 310 mOsmol/kg, and urinary osmolality was 85 mOsmol/kg. The patient received 1 μg of dDAVP intravenously and was allowed to drink water. Repeated urinary osmolality measurements demonstrated a complete urinary resistance to dDAVP. It would have been dangerous and unnecessary to prolong the dehydration further in this young patient. Thus, the usual prescription of overnight dehydration should not be used in patients, and especially children, with severe polyuria and polydipsia (more than 30 ml/kg body weight per day). Great care should be taken to avoid any severe hypertonic state, arbitrarily defined as plasma sodium greater than 155 mOsmol/l.

Direct Tests of Diabetes Insipidus

The two approaches of Zerbe and Robertson are used (206), although they are expensive, time-consuming, and difficult to do on young patients. In the first approach, during the dehydration test, plasma is collected hourly and assayed for AVP. The results are plotted on a nomogram depicting the normal relationship between plasma sodium or osmolality and plasma AVP in normal individuals (Fig. 5A). If the relationship goes below the normal range, the disorder is diagnosed as neurogenic diabetes insipidus.

In the second approach: NDI can be differentiated from primary polydipsia by analyzing the relationship between plasma AVP and urinary osmolality at the end of the dehydration period (Fig. 5B). However, definitive differentiation might be impossible because a normal or even supranormal AVP response to increased plasma osmolality occurs in polydipsic patients. None of the patients with psychogenic or other forms of severe polydipsia studied by Robertson showed any evidence of pituitary suppression (156).

In a comparison of diagnoses based on indirect versus direct tests of AVP function in 54 patients with polyuria of diverse cause, Robertson (156) found that the indirect test was reliable only for patients with severe defects. Three patients with severe NDI and 16 of 17 patients with severe neurogenic diabetes insipidus were accurately diagnosed. However, the error rate of the indirect test was about 50% in diagnosing partial neurogenic diabetes insipidus, partial NDI, or primary polydipsia in patients who were able to concentrate their urine to varying degrees when water deprived. The benefits of combined direct and indirect testing of AVP function have been discussed by Stern and Valtin (177). The diagnosis of primary polydipsia remains one of exclusion and the cause could be psychogenic (7) or inappropriate thirst (158, 159). Psychiatric patients with polydipsia and hyponatremia have unexplained defects in urinary dilution, the osmoregulation of water intake or the secretion of vasopressin (70).

Therapeutic Trial of dDAVP

In selected patients with an uncertain diagnosis, a closely monitored therapeutic trial of dDAVP (10 μg intranasally twice a day for 2 to 3 days) may be used to distinguish partial NDI from partial neurogenic diabetes insipidus or primary polydipsia. If dDAVP at this dosage causes a significant antidiuretic effect, NDI is effectively excluded. If polydipsia and polyuria are abolished and plasma sodium does not go below the normal range, the patient probably has neurogenic diabetes insipidus. Conversely, if dDAVP causes a reduction in urine output without reduction in water intake and hyponatremia appears, the patient probably has primary polydipsia. Since fatal water intoxication is a remote possibility, the dDAVP trial should be closely monitored.

The methods of differential diagnosis of diabetes insipidus are described in Table 3.

Carrier Detection, Perinatal Testing, and Early Treatment

The identification of mutations in the genes that cause hereditary diabetes insipidus allows the early diagnosis and management of at-risk members of families with identified mutations. We encourage physicians who follow families with autosomal neurogenic, X-linked and autosomal NDI to recommend mutation analysis before the birth of an infant because early diagnosis and treatment can avert the physical and mental retardation associated with episodes of dehydration. Diagnosis of X-linked NDI was accomplished by mutation testing of cultured amniotic cells (*n* = 6), chorionic villus samples (*n* = 7), or cord blood obtained at birth (*n* = 31) in 44 of our patients. Twenty-one males were found to bear mutant sequences, 16 males were not affected, and five females were not carriers. These affected patients were immediately given abundant water intake, a low-sodium diet, and hydrochlorothiazide. They never experienced episodes of dehydration, and their physical and mental development is normal. Gene analysis is also important for the identification of nonobligatory female carriers in families with X-linked NDI. Most females heterozygous for a mutation in the V2 receptor do not have clinical symptoms: Few are severely affected (4, 138, 187). Mutation detection in families with inherited neurogenic diabetes insipidus provides a powerful clinical tool for early diagnosis and management of subsequent cases, especially in early childhood, when diagnosis is difficult and the clinical risks are the greatest (126).

TABLE 3   Differential Diagnosis of Diabetes Insipidus

1. Measure plasma osmolality and/or sodium concentration under conditions of *ad libitum* fluid intake. If plasma osmolality is >295 mOsmol/kg and sodium is >143 mOsmol/l, the diagnosis of primary polydipsia is excluded and the work-up should proceed to step (5) and/or (6) to distinguish between NDI and neurogenic diabetes insipidus. *Otherwise:*
2. Perform a dehydration test. If urinary concentration does not occur before plasma osmolality reaches 295 mOsmol/kg and/or sodium reaches 143 mOsmol/l, the diagnosis of primary polydipsia is again excluded and the work-up should proceed to step (5) and/or (6). *Otherwise:*
3. Determine the ratio of urine to plasma osmolality at the end of the dehydration test. If it is <1.5, the diagnosis of primary polydipsia is again excluded and the work-up should proceed to step (5) and/or (6). *Otherwise:*
4. Perform a hypertonic saline infusion with measurement of plasma AVP and osmolality at intervals during the procedure. If the relationship between these two variables falls below the normal range, the diagnosis of neurogenic diabetes insipidus is established (Fig. 51-5A). *Otherwise:*
5. Perform a dDAVP infusion test. If urine osmolality increases by <150 mOsmol/kg above the value obtained at the end of the dehydration test, the diagnosis of NDI is established. *Alternatively:*
6. Measure urine osmolality and plasma AVP at the end of the dehydration test. If the relationship falls below the normal range, the diagnosis of NDI is established (Fig. 51-5B).

Data from Robertson GL. Differential diagnosis of polyuria. *Annu Rev Med* 1988;39:425–442.

Neurogenic diabetes insipidus (central or Wolfram) is easily treated with dDAVP (21). All complications of congenital NDI are prevented by an adequate water intake. Thus, patients should be provided with unrestricted amounts of water from birth to ensure normal development. In addition to a low-sodium diet, the use of diuretics (thiazides) or indomethacin may reduce urinary output. This advantageous effect has to be weighed against the side effects of these drugs (thiazides: electrolyte disturbances; indomethacin: reduction of the glomerular filtration rate and gastrointestinal symptoms).

RADIOIMMUNOASSAY OF AVP AND OTHER LABORATORY DETERMINATIONS

Radioimmunoassay of AVP

Three developments were basic to the elaboration of a clinically useful radioimmunoassay for plasma AVP (153, 154): (1) the extraction of AVP from plasma with petrol-ether and acetone and the subsequent elimination of nonspecific immunoreactivity; (2) the use of highly specific and sensitive rabbit antiserum; and (3) the use of a tracer (^{125}I-AVP) with high specific activity. These same extraction procedures are still widely used (15, 16, 48, 191), and commercial tracers (^{125}I-AVP) and antibodies are available. AVP can also be extracted from plasma by using Sep-Pak C18 cartridges (72, 102, 204).

Blood samples collected in chilled 7-ml lavender-stoppered tubes containing ethylenediaminetetraacetic acid are centrifuged at 4°C, 1000 g (3000 rpm in a usual laboratory centrifuge), for 20 minutes. This 20-minute centrifugation is mandatory for obtaining platelet-poor plasma samples because a large fraction of the circulating vasopressin is associated with the platelets in humans (16, 144). The tubes may be kept for 2 hours on slushed ice before centrifugation. Plasma is then separated, frozen at −20°C and extracted within 6 weeks of sampling. Details for sample preparation (Table 4) and assay procedure (Table 5) can be found in writings by Bichet and colleagues (15, 16). An AVP radioimmunoassay should be validated by demonstrating (1) a good correlation between plasma sodium or osmolality and plasma AVP during dehydration and infusion of hypertonic saline solution (Fig. 4); and (2) the inability to obtain detectable values of AVP in patients with severe central diabetes insipidus. Plasma AVP immunoreactivity may be elevated in patients with diabetes insipidus following hypothamic surgery (171).

In pregnant patients, the blood contains high concentrations of cystine aminopeptidase, which can (in vitro) inactivate enormous quantities (ng $\times$ mL^{-1} $\times$ min^{-1}) of AVP. However, phenanthrolene effectively inhibits these cystine aminopeptidases (Table 6).

Aquaporin-2 Measurements

Urinary AQP2 excretion could be measured by radioimmunoassay (93) or quantitative Western analysis (56) and could provide an additional indication of the responsiveness of the collecting duct to AVP.

Plasma Sodium, Plasma, and Urine Osmolality

Measurements of plasma sodium, plasma, and urinary osmolality should be immediately available at various intervals during dehydration procedures. Plasma sodium is easily measured by flame photometry or with a sodium-specific electrode (113). Plasma and urinary osmolalities are also reli-

TABLE 4   Arginine Vasopressin Measurements: Sample Preparation

4 °C – Blood in EDTA tubes
Centrifugation 1,000 g $\times$ 20 min.
Plasma frozen -20°C
Extraction:
    2 mL acetone + 1 mL plasma
    1,000 g x 30 min 4° C
    Supernatant + 5 mL of petrol-ether
    1,000 g $\times$ 20 min 4°C
    Freeze -80° C
    Throw nonfrozen upper phase
    Evaporate lower phase to dryness
    Store desiccated samples at -20° C

TABLE 5   Arginine Vasopressin Measurements: Assay Procedure

Day 1	Assay set-up 400 μL/tube (200 μL sample or standard + 200 μL of antiserum or buffer) Incubation 80 hours, 4°C
Day 4	^{125}I-AVP 100 μL/tube 1,000 cpm/tube Incubation 72 hours, 4°C
Day 7	Separation dextran + charcoal

ably measured by freezing point depression instruments with a coefficient of variation at 290 mmol/kg of less than 1%.

At variance with published data (16, 206), we have found that plasma and serum osmolalities are equivalent (i.e., similar values are obtained). Blood taken in heparinized tubes is easier to handle because the plasma can be more readily removed after centrifugation. The tube used (green-stoppered tube) contains a minuscule concentration of lithium and sodium, which does not interfere with plasma sodium or osmolality measurements. Frozen plasma or urinary samples can be kept for further analysis of their osmolalities because the results obtained are similar to those obtained immediately after blood sampling, except in patients with severe renal failure. In the latter patients, plasma osmolality measurements are increased after freezing and thawing but the plasma sodium values remain unchanged.

Plasma osmolality measurements can be used to demonstrate the absence of unusual osmotically active substances (e.g., glucose and urea in high concentrations, mannitol, ethanol) (67). With this information, plasma or serum sodium measurements are sufficient to assess the degree of dehydration and its relationship to plasma AVP. Nomograms describing the normal plasma sodium/plasma AVP relationship (Fig. 4) are equally as valuable as classic nomograms describing the relationship between plasma osmolality and effective osmolality (i.e., plasma osmolality minus the contribution of "ineffective" solutes: glucose and urea).

MAGNETIC RESONNANCE IMAGING IN PATIENTS WITH DIABETES INSIPIDUS

Magnetic resonance imaging (MRI) permits visualization of the anterior and posterior pituitary glands and the pituitary stalk. The pituitary stalk is permeated by numerous capillary loops of the hypophyseal–portal blood system.

TABLE 6   Measurements of Arginine Vasopressin Levels in Pregnant Patients

1,10-phenanthroline monohydrate (Sigma) solubilized with several drops of glacial acetic acid
0.1 mL/10 mL of blood

Data from Davison JM, Gilmore EA, Durr J, et al. Altered osmotic thresholds for vasopressin secretion and thirst in human pregnancy. *Am J Physiol* 1984;246:F105–109.

This vascular structure also provides the principle blood supply to the anterior pituitary lobe, because there is no direct arterial supply to this organ. In contrast, the posterior pituitary lobe has a direct vascular supply. Therefore, the posterior lobe can be more rapidly visualized in a dynamic mode after administration of a gadolinium (gadopentate dimeglumine) as contrast material during MRI. The posterior pituitary lobe is easily distinguished by a round, high-intensity signal (the posterior pituitary "bright spot") in the posterior part of the sella turcica on T1-weighted images. This round, high-intensity signal is usually absent in patients with central diabetes insipidus, but a systemic evaluation of well-characterized patients with autosomal dominant central diabetes insipidus has not been done. MRI is reported to be the best technique with which to evaluate the pituitary stalk and infundibulum in patients with idiopathic polyuria. A thickening or enlargement of the pituitary stalk may suggest an infiltrative process destroying the neurohypophyseal tract (149).

TREATMENT

In most patients with complete hypothalamic diabetes insipidus, the thirst mechanism remains intact. Thus, hypernatremia does not develop in these patients and they suffer only from the inconvenience associated with marked polyuria and polydipsia. If hypodipsia develops or access to water is limited, then severe hypernatremia can supervene. The treatment of choice for patients with severe hypothalamic diabetes insipidus is dDAVP, a synthetic, long-acting vasopressin analogue, with minimal vasopressor activity but a large antidiuretic potency. The usual intranasal daily dose is between 5 and 20 μg. To avoid the potential complication of dilutional hyponatremia, which is exceptional in these patients as a result of an intact thirst mechanism, dDAVP can be withdrawn at regular intervals to allow the patients to become polyuric. Aqueous vasopressin (Pitressin) or dDAVP (4.0 μg/1-ml ampule) can be used intravenously in acute situations such as after hypophysectomy or for the treatment of diabetes insipidus in the brain-dead organ donor. Pitressin tannate in oil and nonhormonal antidiuretic drugs are somewhat obsolete and now rarely used. For example, chlorpropamide (250–500 mg daily) appears to potentiate the antidiuretic action of circulating AVP, but troublesome side effects of hypoglycemia and hyponatremia do occur.

The treatment of congenital NDI has been reviewed by Knoers and Monnens (97). An abundant unrestricted water intake should always be provided, and affected patients should be carefully followed during their first years of life. Water should be offered every 2 hours day and night, and temperature, appetite, and growth should be monitored. The parents of these children easily accept setting their alarm clock every 2 hours during the night. Hospital admission may be necessary to allow continuous gastric feeding. A low-osmolar and low-sodium diet, hydrochlorothiazide (1–2 mg/kg/d) alone or with amiloride, and indomethacin (0.75–1.5 mg/kg) substantially reduce water excretion and are helpful in the treatment of children. Many adult patients receive no treatment.

Acknowledgments

The author work cited in this chapter was supported by the Canadian Institutes of Health Research, the Kidney Foundation of Canada, and the Fonds de la Recherche en Santé du Québec. D.G.B. holds a Canada Research Chair in Genetics of Renal Diseases. We thank our coworkers, Marie-Françoise Arthus, Joyce Crumley, Mary Fujiwara, Michèle Lonergan, and Kenneth Morgan; and many colleagues who contributed families and ideas to our work. Typing and computer graphics expertise have been done by Danielle Binette.

References

1. Agre P. Aquaporin water channels (Nobel Lecture). *Angew Chem Int Ed Engl* 2004;43: 4278–4290.
2. Ahmed SR, Aiello DP, Page R, et al. Necrotizing infundibulo-hypophysitis: a unique syndrome of diabetes insipidus and hypopituitarism. *J Clin Endocrinol Metab* 1993;76:1499–1504.
3. Amico JA. Diabetes insipidus and pregnancy. In: Czernichow P, Robinson AG, eds. *Frontiers of Hormone Research*. Basel, Switzerland: Karger; 1985: 266–277.
4. Arthus M-F, Lonergan M, Crumley MJ, et al. Report of 33 novel *AVPR2* mutations and analysis of 117 families with X-linked nephrogenic diabetes insipidus. *J Am Soc Nephrol* 2000;11:1044–1054.
5. Balment RJ, Brimble MJ, Forsling ML. Oxytocin release and renal actions in normal and Brattleboro rats. *Ann N Y Acad Sci* 1982;394:241–253.
6. Barak LS, Oakley RH, Laporte SA, Caron MG. Constitutive arrestin-mediated desensitization of a human vasopressin receptor mutant associated with nephrogenic diabetes insipidus. *Proc Natl Acad Sci U S A* 2001;98:93–98.
7. Barlow ED, de Wardener HE. Compulsive water drinking. *Q J Med New Series* 1959;28: 235–258.
8. Barron WM, Cohen LH, Ulland LA, et al. Transient vasopressin-resistant diabetes insipidus of pregnancy. *N Engl J Med* 1984;310:442–444.
9. Batlle DC, von Riotte AB, Gaviria M, Grupp M. Amelioration of polyuria by amiloride in patients receiving long-term lithium therapy. *N Engl J Med* 1985;312:408–414.
10. Baylis PH, Gaskill MB, Robertson GL. Vasopressin secretion in primary polydipsia and cranial diabetes insipidus. *Q J Med* 1981;50:345–358.
11. Bernier V, Lagace M, Bichet DG, Bouvier M. Pharmacological chaperones: potential treatment for conformational diseases. *Trends Endocrinol Metab* 2004;15:222–228.
12. Bernier V, Lagace M, Lonergan M, et al. Functional rescue of the constitutively internalized V2 vasopressin receptor mutant R137H by the pharmacological chaperone action of SR49059. *Mol Endocrinol* 2004;18:2074–2084.
13. Bernier V, Morello JP, Zarruk A, et al. Pharmacologic chaperones as a potential treatment for X-linked nephrogenic diabetes insipidus. *J Am Soc Nephrol* 2006;17:232–243.
14. Bichet D. Nephrogenic diabetes insipidus. In: Davison A, Cameron J, Grünfeld J, et al., eds. *Oxford Textbook of Clinical Nephrology*. New York: Oxford University Press; 1998: 1095–1109.
15. Bichet DG, Kortas C, Mettauer B, et al. Modulation of plasma and platelet vasopressin by cardiac function in patients with heart failure. *Kidney Int* 1986;29:1188–1196.
16. Bichet DG, Arthus M-F, Barjon JN, et al. Human platelet fraction arginine-vasopressin. *J Clin Invest* 1987;79:881–887.
17. Bichet DG, Razi M, Arthus MF, et al. Epinephrine and dDAVP administration in patients with congenital nephrogenic diabetes insipidus. Evidence for a pre-cyclic AMP V2 receptor defective mechanism. *Kidney Int* 1989;36:859–866.
18. Bichet DG, Hendy GN, Lonergan M, et al. X-linked nephrogenic diabetes insipidus: From the ship Hopewell to restriction fragment length polymorphism studies. *Am J Hum Genet* 1992;51:1089–1102.
19. Bichet DG, Kluge R, Howard RL, Schrier RW. Hyponatremic states. In: Seldin DW, Giebisch G, eds. *The Kidney: Physiology and Pathophysiology*. New York: Raven Press; 1992: 1727–1751.
20. Bichet DG, Arthus M-F, Lonergan M, et al. X-linked nephrogenic diabetes insipidus mutations in North America and the Hopewell hypothesis. *J Clin Invest* 1993;92:1262–1268.
21. Bichet DG. Nephrogenic and central diabetes insipidus. In: Schrier RW, Gottschalk CW, eds. *Diseases of the Kidney*. New York: Little, Brown; 1997: 2429–2449.
22. Bichet DG, Fujiwara TM. Nephrogenic diabetes insipidus. In: Scriver CR, Beaudet AL, Sly WS, et al., eds. *The Metabolic and Molecular Bases of Inherited Disease*. New York: McGraw-Hill; 2001: 4181–4204.
23. Bichet DG. Nephrogenic diabetes insipidus: New developments. *Nephrol Self-Assessment Progr* 2004;3:187–191.
24. Bichet DG, Fujiwara TM. Reabsorption of sodium chloride—lessons from the chloride channels. *N Engl J Med* 2004;350:1281–1283.
25. Bichet DG. Editorial: Lithium, cyclic AMP signaling, A-kinase anchoring proteins and aquaporin-2. *J Am Soc Nephrol* 2006;17:920–922.
26. Birnbaumer M, Seibold A, Gilbert S, et al. Molecular cloning of the receptor for human antidiuretic hormone. *Nature* 1992;357:333–335.
27. Bonnardeaux A, Bichet DG. Inherited disorders of the renal tubule. In: Brenner BM, ed. *Brenner & Rector's The Kidney*. Philadelphia: Saunders; 2004: 1697–1741.
28. Boton R, Gaviria M, Batlle DC. Prevalence, pathogenesis, and treatment of renal dysfunction associated with chronic lithium therapy. *Am J Kidney Dis* 1987;10:329–345.
29. Bourque CW, Oliet SHR, Richard D. Osmoreceptors, osmoreception, and osmoregulation. *Front Neuroendocrinol* 1994;15:231–274.
30. Bourque CW, Oliet SHR. Osmoreceptors in the central nervous system. *Annu Rev Physiol* 1997;59:601–619.
31. Boyd SD, Raz S, Ehrlich RM. Diabetes insipidus and nonobstructive dilatation of urinary tract. *Urology* 1980;16:266–269.
32. Brenner B, Seligsohn U, Hochberg Z. Normal response of factor VIII and von Willebrand factor to 1-deamino- 8D-arginine vasopressin in nephrogenic diabetes insipidus. *J Clin Endocrinol Metab* 1988;67:191–193.
33. Brewster UC, Hayslett JP. Diabetes insipidus in the third trimester of pregnancy. *Obstet Gynecol* 2005;105:1173–1176.
34. Burbach JP, Luckman SM, Murphy D, Gainer H. Gene regulation in the magnocellular hypothalamo-neurohypophysial system. *Physiol Rev* 2001;81:1197–1267.
35. Camerer JW. Eine ergänzung des Weilschen diabetes-insipidus-stammbaumes. *Archiv für Rassenund Gesellschaftshygiene Biologie* 1935;28:382–385.
36. Chen L, Rose JP, Breslow E, et al. Crystal structure of a bovine neurophysin II dipeptide complex at 2.8 Angström determined from the single-wave length anomalous scattering signal of an incorporated iodine atom. *Proc Natl Acad Sci U S A* 1991;88:4240–4244.
37. Cheng A, van Hoek AN, Yeager M, et al. Three-dimensional organization of a human water channel. *Nature* 1997;387:627–630.
38. Chillaron J, Estevez R, Samarzija I, et al. An intracellular trafficking defect in type I cystinuria rBAT mutants M467T and M467K. *J Biol Chem* 1997;272:9543–9549.
39. Chou C-L, Knepper MA, van Hoek AN, et al. Reduced water permeability and altered ultrastructure in thin descending limb of Henle in aquaporin-1 null mice. *J Clin Invest* 1999;103:491–496.
40. Chou CL, DiGiovanni SR, Luther A, et al. Oxytocin as an antidiuretic hormone II. Role of V2 vasopressin receptor. *Am J Physiol* 1995;269(1pt2):F78–F85.
41. Christensen JH, Rittig S. Familial neurohypophyseal diabetes insipidus—an update. *Semin Nephrol* 2006;26:209–223.
42. Christensen S, Kusano E, Yusufi AN, et al. Pathogenesis of nephrogenic diabetes insipidus due to chronic administration of lithium in rats. *J Clin Invest* 1985;75:1869–1879.
43. Cogan E, Svoboda M, Abramow M. Mechanisms of lithium-vasopressin interaction in rabbit cortical collecting tubule. *Am J Physiol* 1987;252:F1080–1087.
44. Cohen FE, Kelly JW. Therapeutic approaches to protein-misfolding diseases. *Nature* 2003;426:905–909.
45. Couture Y, Arthus M-F, Fujiwara TM, et al. Severe early-onset autosomal recessive familial neurohypophyseal diabetes insipidus secondary to novel AVP mutations. Submitted.
46. Crawford JD, Bode HH. Disorders of the posterior pituitary in children. In: Gardner LI, ed. *Endocrine and Genetic Diseases of Childhood and Adolescence*. Philadelphia: WB Saunders; 1975:126–158.
47. Czernichow P, Pomarede R, Brauner R, Rappaport R. Neurogenic diabetes insipidus in children. In: Czernichow P, Robinson AG, eds. *Frontiers of Hormone Research*. Basel, Switzerland: S. Karger; 1985:190–209.
48. Davison JM, Gilmore EA, Durr J, et al. Altered osmotic thresholds for vasopressin secretion and thirst in human pregnancy. *Am J Physiol* 1984;246:F105–109.
49. Davison JM, Shiells EA, Philips PR, Lindheimer MD. Serial evaluation of vasopressin release and thirst in human pregnancy. Role of human chorionic gonadotrophin in the osmoregulatory changes of gestation. *J Clin Invest* 1988;81:798–806.
50. De Mota N, Reaux-Le Goazigo A, El Messari S, et al. Apelin, a potent diuretic neuropeptide counteracting vasopressin actions through inhibition of vasopressin neuron activity and vasopressin release. *Proc Natl Acad Sci U S A* 2004;101:10464–10469.
51. Deen PMT, Verdijk MAJ, Knoers NVAM, et al. Requirement of human renal water channel aquaporin-2 for vasopressin-dependent concentration of urine. *Science* 1994;264:92–95.
52. Deen PMT, Weghuis DO, Sinke RJ, et al. Assignment of the human gene for the water channel of renal collecting duct aquaporin 2 (AQP2) to chromosome 12 region q12->q13. *Cytogenet Cell Genet* 1994;66:260–262.
53. Domenech J, Gomez-Zaera M, Nunes V. Study of the WFS1 gene and mitochondrial DNA in Spanish Wolfram syndrome families. *Clin Genet* 2004;65:463–469.
54. Durr JA, Hoggard JG, Hunt JM, Schrier RW. Diabetes insipidus in pregnancy associated with abnormally high circulating vasopressinase activity. *N Engl J Med* 1987;316:1070–1074.
55. Dölle W. Eine weitere ergänzung des Weilschen diabetes-insipidus-stammbaumes. *Zeitschrift für Menschliche Vererbungsund Konstitutionslehre* 1951;30:372–374.
56. Elliot S, Goldsmith P, Knepper M, et al. Urinary excretion of aquaporin-2 in humans: a potential marker of collecting duct responsiveness to vasopressin. *J Am Soc Nephrol* 1996;7: 403–409.
57. Fenton RA, Shodeinde A, Knepper MA. UT-A urea transporter promoter, UT-Aalpha, targets principal cells of the renal inner medullary collecting duct. *Am J Physiol Renal Physiol* 2006;290:F188–195.
58. Fery F, Plat L, van de Borne P, et al. Impaired counterregulation of glucose in a patient with hypothalamic sarcoidosis. *N Engl J Med* 1999;340:852–856.
59. Fitzsimons JT. Angiotensin, thirst, and sodium appetite. *Physiol Rev* 1998;78:583–686.
60. Fleming EF, Athirakul K, Oliverio MI, et al. Urinary concentrating function in mice lacking EP3 receptors for prostaglandin E2. *Am J Physiol* 1998;275:F955–961.

61. Forssman H. On the mode of hereditary transmission in diabetes insipidus. *Nordisk Medicine* 1942;16:3211–3213.

62. Forssman H. On hereditary diabetes insipidus, with special regard to a sex-linked form. *Acta Med Scand* 1945;159:1–196.

63. Frokiaer J, Marples D, Knepper MA, Nielsen S. Bilateral ureteral obstruction downregulates expression of vasopressin-sensitive AQP-2 water channel in rat kidney. *Am J Physiol* 1996; 270:F657–F668.

64. Fujiwara TM, Bichet DG. Molecular biology of hereditary diabetes insipidus. *J Am Soc Nephrol* 2005;16:2836–2846.

65. Fushimi K, Sasaki S, Yamamoto T, et al. Functional characterization and cell immunolocalization of AQP-CD water channel in kidney collecting duct. *Am J Physiol* 1994;267:F573–582.

66. Gautier B, Thieblot P, Steg A. Mégauretère, mégavessie et diabète inspide familial. *Semin Hop* 1981;57:60–61.

67. Gennari FJ. Current concepts. Serum osmolality. Uses and limitations. *N Engl J Med* 1984;310:102–105.

68. Glover DJ, Lipps HJ, Jans DA. Towards safe, non-viral therapeutic gene expression in humans. *Nat Rev Genet* 2005;6:299–310.

69. Goldberg H, Clayman P, Skorecki K. Mechanism of Li inhibition of vasopressin-sensitive adenylate cyclase in cultured renal epithelial cells. *Am J Physiol* 1988;255:F995–1002.

70. Goldman MB, Luchins DJ, Robertson GL. Mechanisms of altered water metabolism in psychotic patients with polydipsia and hyponatremia. *N Engl J Med* 1988;318:397–403.

71. Greger NG, Kirkland RT, Clayton GW, Kirkland JL. Central diabetes insipidus. 22 years' experience. *Am J Dis Child* 1986;140:551–554.

72. Hartter E, Woloszczuk W. Radioimmunological determination of arginine vasopressin and human atrial natriuretic peptide after simultaneous extraction from plasma. *J Clin Chem Clin Biochem* 1986;24:559–563.

73. Hayama A, Rai T, Sasaki S, Uchida S. Molecular mechanisms of Bartter syndrome caused by mutations in the BSND gene. *Histochem Cell Biol* 2003;119:485–493.

74. Hein L, Barsh GS, Pratt RE, et al. Behavioural and cardiovascular effects of disrupting the angiotensin II type-2 receptor gene in mice. *Nature* 1995;377:744–747.

75. Hermosilla R, Oueslati M, Donalies U, et al. Disease-causing V(2) vasopressin receptors are retained in different compartments of the early secretory pathway. *Traffic* 2004;5: 993–1005.

76. Hiett AK, Barton JR. Diabetes insipidus associated with craniopharyngioma in pregnancy. *Obstet Gynecol* 1990;76:982–984.

77. Hobbs HH, Russell DW, Brown MS, Goldstein JL. The LDL receptor locus in familial hypercholesterolemia: mutational analysis of a membrane protein. *Annu Rev Genet* 1990; 24: 133–170.

78. Howard RL, Bichet DG, Schrier RW. Hypernatremic and polyuric states. In: Seldin DW, Giebisch G, eds. *The Kidney: Physiology and Pathophysiology*. New York: Raven Press; 1992:753–1778.

79. Huber D, Veinante P, Stoop R. Vasopressin and oxytocin excite distinct neuronal populations in the central amygdala. *Science* 2005;308:245–248.

80. Imura H, Nakao K, Shimatsu A, et al. Lymphocytic infundibuloneurohypophysitis as a cause of central diabetes insipidus. *N Engl J Med* 1993;329:683–689.

81. Insel TR, Young LJ. The neurobiology of attachment. *Nat Rev Neurosci* 2001;2:129–136.

82. Ishihara H, Takeda S, Tamura A, et al. Disruption of the WFS1 gene in mice causes progressive beta-cell loss and impaired stimulus-secretion coupling in insulin secretion. *Hum Mol Genet* 2004;13:1159–1170.

83. Ito M, Oliverio MI, Mannon PJ, et al. Regulation of blood pressure by the type 1A angiotensin II receptor gene. *Proc Natl Acad Sci U S A* 1995;92:3521–3525.

84. Ito M, Jameson JL, Ito M. Molecular basis of autosomal dominant neurohypophyseal diabetes insipidus. Cellular toxicity caused by the accumulation of mutant vasopressin precursors within the endoplasmic reticulum. *J Clin Invest* 1997;99:1897–1905.

85. Ito M, Yu RN, Jameson JL. Mutant vasopressin precursors that cause autosomal dominant neurohypophyseal diabetes insipidus retain dimerization and impair the secretion of wild-type proteins. *J Biol Chem* 1999;274:9029–9037.

86. Iwasaki Y, Oiso Y, Kondo K, et al. Aggravation of subclinical diabetes insipidus during pregnancy. *N Engl J Med* 1991;324:522–526.

87. Jans DA, van Oost BA, Ropers HH, Fahrenholz F. Derivatives of somatic cell hybrids which carry the human gene locus for nephrogenic diabetes insipidus (NDI) express functional vasopressin renal V2-type receptors. *J Biol Chem* 1990;265:15379–15382.

88. Jard S, Elands J, Schmidt A, Barberis C. Vasopressin and oxytocin receptors: an overview. In: Imura H, Shizume K, eds. *Progress in Endocrinology*. Amsterdam: Elsevier Science; 1988: 1183–1188.

89. Jeck N, Schlingmann KP, Reinalter SC, et al. Salt handling in the distal nephron: lessons learned from inherited human disorders. *Am J Physiol Regul Integr Comp Physiol* 2005;288: R782–795.

90. Kalogeras KT, Nieman LN, Friedman TC, et al. Inferior petrosal sinus sampling in healthy human subjects reveals a unilateral corticotropin-releasing hormone-induced arginine vasopressin release associated with ipsilateral adrenocorticotropin secretion. *J Clin Invest* 1996;97: 2045–2050.

91. Kambouris M, Dlouhy SR, Trofatter JA, et al. Localization of the gene for X-linked nephrogenic diabetes insipidus to Xq28. *Am J Med Genet* 1988;29:239–246.

92. Kamsteeg E-J, Bichet DG, Konings IBM, et al. Reversed polarized delivery of an aquaporin-2 mutant causes dominant nephrogenic diabetes insipidus. *J Cell Biol* 2003;163: 1099–1109.

93. Kanno K, Sasaki S, Hirata Y, et al. Urinary excretion of aquaporin-2 in patients with diabetes insipidus. *N Engl J Med* 1995;332:1540–1545.

94. Kennan A, Aherne A, Humphries P. Light in retinitis pigmentosa. *Trends Genet* 2005;21: 103–110.

95. Knoers N, van der Heyden H, van Oost BA, et al. Three-point linkage analysis using multiple DNA polymorphic markers in families with X-linked nephrogenic diabetes insipidus. *Genomics* 1989;4:434–437.

96. Knoers N, Monnens LA. A variant of nephrogenic diabetes insipidus: V2 receptor abnormality restricted to the kidney. *Eur J Pediatr* 1991;150:370–373.

97. Knoers N, Monnens LA. Nephrogenic diabetes insipidus: clinical symptoms, pathogenesis, genetics and treatment. *Pediatr Nephrol* 1992;6:476–482.

98. Kunchaparty S, Palcso M, Berkman J, et al. Defective processing and expression of thiazide-sensitive Na-Cl cotransporter as a cause of Gitelman's syndrome. *Am J Physiol* 1999;277: F643–649.

99. Kuwahara M, Iwai K, Ooeda T, et al. Three families with autosomal dominant nephrogenic diabetes insipidus caused by aquaporin-2 mutations in the C-terminus. *Am J Hum Genet* 2001;69:738–748.

100. Lacombe UL. De la polydipsie. In: *Imprimerie et Fonderie de Rignoux*. Paris; 1841:87.

101. Langley JM, Balfe JW, Selander T, et al. Autosomal recessive inheritance of vasopressin-resistant diabetes insipidus. *Am J Med Genet* 1991;38:90–94.

102. LaRochelle FT, Jr., North WG, Stern P. A new extraction of arginine vasopressin from blood: the use of octadecasilyl-silica. *Pflugers Arch* 1980;387:79–81.

103. Lawless MW, Greene CM, Mulgrew A, et al. Activation of endoplasmic reticulum-specific stress responses associated with the conformational disease Z alpha 1-antitrypsin deficiency. *J Immunol* 2004;172:5722–5726.

104. Leaf A. Neurogenic diabetes insipidus. *Kidney Int* 1979;15:572–580.

105. Leibowitz SF. Impact of brain monoamines and neuropeptides on vasopressin release. In: Cowley AWJ, Liard JF, Ausiello DA, eds. *Vasopressin. Cellular and Integrative Functions*. New York: Raven; 1988:379–388.

106. Li Y, Shaw S, Kamsteeg E-J, et al. Development of lithium-induced nephrogenic diabetes insipidus is dissociated from adenylyl cyclase activity. *J Am Soc Nephrol* 2006;17:1063–1072.

107. Lloyd DJ, Hall FW, Tarantino LM, Gekakis N. Diabetes insipidus in mice with a mutation in aquaporin-2. *PLoS Genet* 2005;1:e20.

108. Lomas DA, Evans DL, Finch JT, Carrell RW. The mechanism of Z alpha 1-antitrypsin accumulation in the liver. *Nature* 1992;357:605–607.

109. Lopez-Rodriguez C, Antos CL, Shelton JM, et al. Loss of NFAT5 results in renal atrophy and lack of tonicity-responsive gene expression. *Proc Natl Acad Sci U S A* 2004;101: 2392–2397.

110. Ma T, Yang B, Gillespie A, et al. Generation and phenotype of a transgenic knockout mouse lacking the mercurial-insensitive water channel aquaporin-4. *J Clin Invest* 1997;100: 957–962.

111. Ma T, Yang B, Gillespie A, et al. Severely impaired urinary concentrating ability in transgenic mice lacking aquaporin-1 water channels. *J Biol Chem* 1998;273:4296–4299.

112. Ma T, Song Y, Yang B, et al. Nephrogenic diabetes insipidus in mice lacking aquaporin-3 water channels. *Proc Natl Acad Sci U S A* 2000;97:4386–4391.

113. Maas AH, Siggaard-Andersen O, Weisberg HF, Zijlstra WG. Ion-selective electrodes for sodium and potassium: a new problem of what is measured and what should be reported. *Clin Chem* 1985;31:482–485.

114. Maghnie M, Cosi G, Genovese E, et al. Central diabetes insipidus in children and young adults. *N Engl J Med* 2000;343:998–1007.

115. Magner PO, Halperin ML. Polyuria—a pathophysiological approach. *Med North Am* 1987;15:2987–2997.

116. Mankin AS, Liebman SW. Baby, don't stop! *Nat Genet* 1999;23:8–10.

117. Marek S, Tekesin I, Hellmeyer L, et al. [Differential diagnosis of a polyhydramnion in hyperprostaglandin e syndrome: a case report]. *Z Geburtshilfe Neonatol* 2004;208: 232–235.

118. Marples D, Christensen S, Christensen EI, et al. Lithium-induced downregulation of aquaporin-2 water channel expression in rat kidney medulla. *J Clin Invest* 1995;95:1838–1845.

119. Marples D, Frokiaer J, Dorup J, et al. Hypokalemia-induced downregulation of aquaporin-2 water channel expression in rat kidney medulla and cortex. *J Clin Invest* 1996;97:1960–1968.

120. Marr N, Bichet DG, Lonergan M, et al. Heteroligomerization of an aquaporin-2 mutant with wild-type aquaporin-2 and their misrouting to late endosomes/lysosomes explains dominant nephrogenic diabetes insipidus. *Hum Mol Genet* 2002;11:779–789.

121. Masera N, Grant DB, Stanhope R, Preece MA. Diabetes insipidus with impaired osmotic regulation in septo-optic dysplasia and agenesis of the corpus callosum. *Arch Dis Child* 1994;70:51–53.

122. Matsumura Y, Uchida S, Kondo Y, et al. Overt nephrogenic diabetes insipidus in mice lacking the CLC-K1 chloride channel. *Nat Genet* 1999;21:95–98.

123. McDill BW, Li SZ, Kovach PA, et al. Congenital progressive hydronephrosis (cph) is caused by an S256L mutation in aquaporin-2 that affects its phosphorylation and apical membrane accumulation. *Proc Natl Acad Sci U S A* 2006;103:6952–6957.

124. McIlraith CH. Notes on some cases of diabetes insipidus with marked family and hereditary tendencies. *Lancet* 1892;2:767–768.

125. Miller M, Dalakos T, Moses AM, et al. Recognition of partial defects in antidiuretic hormone secretion. *Ann Intern Med* 1970;73:721–729.

126. Miller WL. Molecular genetics of familial central diabetes insipidus. *J Clin Endocrinol Metab* 1993;77:592–595.

127. Morello JP, Salahpour A, Laperrière A, et al. Pharmacological chaperones rescue cell-surface expression and function of misfolded V2 vasopressin receptor mutants. *J Clin Invest* 2000; s105:887–895.

128. Moses AM, Blumenthal SA, Streeten DHP. Acid-base and electrolyte disorders associated with endocrine disease: pituitary and thyroid. In: Arieff AI, de Fronzo RA, eds. *Fluid, Electrolyte and Acid-Base Disorders*. New York: Churchill Livingstone; 1985:851–892.

129. Mouillac B, Chini B, Balestre MN, et al. The binding site of neuropeptide vasopressin V1a receptor. Evidence for a major localization within transmembrane regions. *J Biol Chem* 1995;270:25771–25777.

130. Nathanson MH, Moyer MS, Burgstahler AD, et al. Mechanisms of subcellular cytosolic Ca2+ signaling evoked by stimulation of the vasopressin V1a receptor. *J Biol Chem* 1992;267: 23282–23289.

131. Nemergut EC, Zuo Z, Jane JA, Jr., Laws ER, Jr. Predictors of diabetes insipidus after transsphenoidal surgery: a review of 881 patients. *J Neurosurg* 2005;103:448–454.
132. Niaudet P, Dechaux M, Trivin C, et al. Nephrogenic diabetes insipidus: Clinical and pathophysiological aspects. *Adv Nephrol Necker Hosp* 1984;13:247–260.
133. Nielsen S, DiGiovanni SR, Christensen EI, et al. Cellular and subcellular immunolocalization of vasopressin-regulated water channel in rat kidney. *Proc Natl Acad Sci U S A* 1993;90:11663–11667.
134. Nielsen S, Chou C-L, Marples D, et al. Vasopressin increases water permeability of kidney collecting duct by inducing translocation of aquaporin-CD water channels to plasma membrane. *Proc Natl Acad Sci U S A* 1995;92:1013–1017.
135. Nimura F, Labosky P, Kakuchi J, et al. Gene targeting in mice reveals a requirement for angiotensin in the development and maintenance of kidney morphology and growth factor regulation. *J Clin Invest* 1995;96:2947–2954.
136. Nomura Y, Onigata K, Nagashima T, et al. Detection of skewed X-inactivation in two female carriers of vasopressin type 2 receptor gene mutation. *J Clin Endocrinol Metab* 1997;82:3434–3437.
137. Odell WD, Doggett RS. Xanthoma disseminatum, a rare cause of diabetes insipidus. *J Clin Endocrinol Metab* 1993;76:777–780.
138. Oksche A, Dickson J, Schülein R, et al. Two novel mutations in the vasopressin V2 receptor gene in patients with congenital nephrogenic diabetes insipidus. *Biophys Biochem Res Com* 1994;205:552–557.
139. Okubo S, Niimura F, Matsusaka T, et al. Angiotensinogen gene null-mutant mice lack homeostatic regulation of glomerular filtration and tubular reabsorption. *Kidney Int* 1998;53: 617–625.
140. Olson BR, Gumowski J, Rubino D, Oldfield EH. Pathophysiology of hyponatremia after transsphenoidal pituitary surgery. *J Neurosurg* 1997;87:499–507.
141. Online Mendelian Inheritance in Man, OMIM. McKusick-Nathans Institute for Genetic Medicine, Johns Hopkins University (Baltimore, MD) and National Center for Biotechnology Information, National Library of Medicine (Bethesda, MD). Available at: http://www.ncbi.nlm.nih.gov/omim/.
142. Peters M, Jeck N, Reinalter S, et al. Clinical presentation of genetically defined patients with hypokalemic salt-losing tubulopathies. *Am J Med* 2002;112:183–190.
143. Peters M, Ermert S, Jeck N, et al. Classification and rescue of ROMK mutations underlying hyperprostaglandin E syndrome/antenatal Bartter syndrome. *Kidney Int* 2003;64: 923–932.
144. Preibisz JJ, Sealey JE, Laragh JH, et al. Plasma and platelet vasopressin in essential hypertension and congestive heart failure. *Hypertension* 1983;5:I129–138.
145. Preston GM, Smith BL, Zeidel ML, et al. Mutations in aquaporin-1 in phenotypically normal humans without functional CHIP water channels. *Science* 1994;265:1585–1587.
146. Randle JC, Mazurek M, Kneifel D, et al. Alpha 1-adrenergic receptor activation releases vasopressin and oxytocin from perfused rat hypothalamic explants. *Neurosci Lett* 1986;65: 219–223.
147. Rao S, Verkman AS. Analysis of organ physiology in transgenic mice. *Am J Physiol Cell Physiol* 2000;279:C1–C18.
148. Rao VV, Loffler C, Battey J, Hansmann I. The human gene for oxytocin-neurophysin I (OXT) is physically mapped to chromosome 20p13 by in situ hybridization. *Cytogenet Cell Genet* 1992;61:271–273.
149. Rappaport R. Magnetic resonance imaging in pituitary disease. *Growth Genetics & Hormones* 1995;11:1–5.
150. Reeves WB, Andreoli TE. Nephrogenic diabetes insipidus. In: Scriver CR, Beaudet AL, Sly WS, Valle D, eds. *The Metabolic and Molecular Bases of Inherited Disease.* New York: McGraw-Hill; 1995:3045–3071.
151. Richter D. Molecular events in the expression of vasopressin and oxytocin and their cognate receptors. *Am J Physiol* 1988;255:F207–F219.
152. Rittig R, Robertson GL, Siggaard C, et al. Identification of 13 new mutations in the vasopressin-neurophysin II gene in 17 kindreds with familial autosomal dominant neurohypophyseal diabetes insipidus. *Am J Hum Genet* 1996;58:107–117.
153. Robertson GL, Klein LA, Roth J, Gorden P. Immunoassay of plasma vasopressin in man. *Proc Natl Acad Sci U S A* 1970;66:1298–1305.
154. Robertson GL, Mahr EA, Athar S, Sinha T. Development and clinical application of a new method for the radioimmunoassay of arginine vasopressin in human plasma. *J Clin Invest* 1973;52:2340–2352.
155. Robertson GL. The physiopathology of ADH secretion. In: Tolis G, Labrie F, Martin JB, Naftolin F, eds. *Clinical Neuroendocrinology: A Pathophysiological Approach.* New York: Raven Press; 1979:247–260.
156. Robertson GL. Diagnosis of diabetes insipidus. In: Czernichow P, Robinson AG, eds. *Frontiers of Hormone Research.* Basel: Karger; 1985:176–189.
157. Robertson GL, Oiso Y, Vokes TP, Gaskill MB. Diprenorphine inhibits selectively the vasopressin response to hypovolemic stimuli. *Trans Assoc Am Physicians* 1985;98:322–333.
158. Robertson GL. Dipsogenic diabetes insipidus: a newly recognized syndrome caused by a selective defect in the osmoregulation of thirst. *Trans Assoc Am Physicians* 1987;100:241–249.
159. Robertson GL. Differential diagnosis of polyuria. *Annu Rev Med* 1988;39:425–442.
160. Robertson GL, Berl T. Pathophysiology of water metabolism. In: Brenner BM, Rector FC, eds. *The Kidney.* Philadelphia: WB Saunders; 1996:873–928.
161. Rojek A, Fuchtbauer EM, Kwon TH, et al. Severe urinary concentrating defect in renal collecting duct-selective AQP2 conditional-knockout mice. *Proc Natl Acad Sci U S A* 2006;103: 6037–6042.
162. Romisch K. A cure for traffic jams: small molecule chaperones in the endoplasmic reticulum. *Traffic* 2004;5:815–820.
163. Rose JP, Wu CK, Hsiao CD, et al. Crystal structure of the neurophysin-oxytocin complex. *Nat Struct Biol* 1996;3:163–169.
164. Russell TA, Ito M, Yu RN, et al. A murine model of autosomal dominant neurohypophyseal diabetes insipidus reveals progressive loss of vasopressin-producing neurons. *J Clin Invest* 2003;112:1697–1706.
165. Sands JM, Naruse M, Baum M, et al. Apical extracellular calcium/polyvalent cation-sensing receptor regulates vasopressin-elicited water permeability in rat kidney inner medullary collecting duct. *J Clin Invest* 1997;99:1399–1405.
166. Sands JM, Flores FX, Kato A, et al. Vasopressin-elicited water and urea permeabilities are altered in IMCD in hypercalcemic rats. *Am J Physiol* 1998;274:F978–985.
167. Sangkuhl K, Schulz A, Rompler H, et al. Aminoglycoside-mediated rescue of a disease-causing nonsense mutation in the V2 vasopressin receptor gene in vitro and in vivo. *Hum Mol Genet* 2004;13:893–903.
168. Sasaki S, Fushimi K, Saito H, et al. Cloning, characterization, and chromosomal mapping of human aquaporin of collecting duct. *J Clin Invest* 1994;93:1250–1256.
169. Schmale H, Richter D. Single base deletion in the vasopressin gene is the cause of diabetes insipidus in Brattleboro rats. *Nature* 1984;308:705–709.
170. Schoneberg T, Schulz A, Biebermann H, et al. Mutant G-protein-coupled receptors as a cause of human diseases. *Pharmacol Ther* 2004;104:173–206.
171. Seckl JR, Dunger DB, Bevan JS, et al. Vasopressin antagonist in early postoperative diabetes insipidus. *Lancet* 1990;355:1353–1356.
172. Seibold A, Brabet P, Rosenthal W, Birnbaumer M. Structure and chromosomal localization of the human antidiuretic hormone receptor gene. *Am J Hum Genet* 1992;51:1078–1083.
173. Serradeil-Le Gal C, Lacour C, Valette G, et al. Characterization of SR 121463A, a highly potent and selective, orally active vasopressin V2 receptor antagonist. *J Clin Invest* 1996; 98:2729–2738.
174. Shalev H, Romanovsky I, Knoers NV, et al. Bladder function impairment in aquaporin-2 defective nephrogenic diabetes insipidus. *Nephrol Dial Transplant* 2004;19:608–613.
175. Sharif Naeini R, Witty MF, Seguela P, Bourque CW. An N-terminal variant of Trpv1 channel is required for osmosensory transduction. *Nat Neurosci* 2006;9:93–98.
176. Siggaard C, Rittig S, Corydon TJ, et al. Clinical and molecular evidence of abnormal processing and trafficking of the vasopressin preprohormone in a large kindred with familial neurohypophyseal diabetes insipidus due to a signal peptide mutation. *J Clin Endocrinol Metab* 1999;84:2933–2941.
177. Stern P, Valtin H. Verney was right, but [editorial]. *N Engl J Med* 1981;305:1581–1582.
178. Streitz JMJ, Streitz JM. Polyuric urinary tract dilatation with renal damage. *J Urol* 1988;139:784-–785.
179. Sugaya T, Nishimatsu S, Tanimoto K, et al. Angiotensin II type 1a receptor-deficient mice with hypotension and hyperreninemia. *J Biol Chem* 1995;270:18719–18722.
180. Takahashi N, Chernavvsky DR, Gomez RA, et al. Uncompensated polyuria in a mouse model of Bartter's syndrome. *Proc Natl Acad Sci U S A* 2000;97:5434–5439.
181. Takeda K, Inoue H, Tanizawa Y, et al. WFS1 (Wolfram syndrome 1) gene product: predominant subcellular localization to endoplasmic reticulum in cultured cells and neuronal expression in rat brain. *Hum Mol Genet* 2001;10:477–484.
182. Tamarappoo BK, Verkman AS. Defective aquaporin-2 trafficking in nephrogenic diabetes insipidus and correction by chemical chaperones. *J Clin Invest* 1998;101:2257–2267.
183. Tesmer JJ, Sunahara RK, Gilman AG, Sprang SR. Crystal structure of the catalytic domains of adenylyl cyclase in a complex with Gsalpha.GTPgammaS. *Science* 1997;278:1907–1916.
184. Ulinski T, Grapin C, Forin V, et al. Severe bladder dysfunction in a family with ADH receptor gene mutation responsible for X-linked nephrogenic diabetes insipidus. *Nephrol Dial Transplant* 2004;19:2928–2929.
185. Ulloa-Aguirre A, Janovick JA, Brothers SP, Conn PM. Pharmacologic rescue of conformationally-defective proteins: implications for the treatment of human disease. *Traffic* 2004;5: 821–837.
186. van den Ouweland AM, Knoop MT, Knoers VV, et al. Colocalization of the gene for nephrogenic diabetes insipidus (DIR) and the vasopressin type 2 receptor gene (AVPR2) in the Xq28 region. *Genomics* 1992;13:1350–1352.
187. van Lieburg AF, Verdijk MAJ, Schoute F, et al. Clinical phenotype of nephrogenic diabetes insipidus in females heterozygous for a vasopressin type 2 receptor mutation. *Hum Genet* 1995;96:70–78.
188. Venkatesh B, Si-Hoe SL, Murphy D, Brenner S. Transgenic rats reveal functional conservation of regulatory controls between the Fugu isotocin and rat oxytocin genes. *Proc Natl Acad Sci U S A* 1997;94:12462–12466.
189. Verbalis JG, Robinson AG, Moses AM. Postoperative and post-traumatic diabetes insipidus. In: Czernichow P, Robinson AG, eds. *Frontiers of Hormone Research.* Basel, Switzerland: S. Karger; 1985:247–265.
190. Vokes T, Robertson GL. Physiology of secretion of vasopressin. In: Czernichow P, Robinson AG, eds. *Diabetes Insipidus in Man.* Basel: S. Karger; 1985: 27–155.
191. Vokes TP, Aycinena PR, Robertson GL. Effect of insulin on osmoregulation of vasopressin. *Am J Physiol* 1987;252:E538–548.
192. Ward DT, Hammond TG, Harris HW. Modulation of vasopressin-elicited water transport by trafficking of aquaporin-2-containing vesicles. *Annu Rev Physiol* 1999;61:683–697.
193. Waring AG, Kajdi L, Tappan V. Congenital defect of water metabolism. *Am J Dis Child* 1945;69:323–325.
194. Watson S, Arkinstall S. *The G Protein Linked Receptor Factsbook.* London: Academic Press; 1994.
195. Weil A. Ueber die hereditare form des diabetes insipidus. *Archives fur Pathologische Anatomie und Physiologie and fur Klinische Medicine (Virchow's Archives)* 1884;95:70–95.
196. Weil A. Ueber die hereditare form des diabetes insipidus. *Deutches Archiv fur Klinische Medizin* 1908;93:180–290.
197. Welch WJ, Howard M. Commentary: Antagonists to the rescue. *J Clin Invest* 2000;105: 853–854.
198. Willcutts MD, Felner E, White PC. Autosomal recessive familial neurohypophyseal diabetes insipidus with continued secretion of mutant weakly active vasopressin. *Hum Mol Genet* 1999;8:1303–1307.
199. Williams PD, Pettibone DJ. Recent advances in the development of oxytocin receptor antagonists. *Curr Pharm Design* 1996;2:41–58.
200. Williams RM, Henry C. Nephrogenic diabetes insipidus transmitted by females and appearing during infancy in males. *Ann Int Med* 1947;27:84–95.

201. Wuller S, Wiesner B, Loffler A, et al. Pharmacochaperones post-translationally enhance cell surface expression by increasing conformational stability of wild-type and mutant vasopressin V2 receptors. *J Biol Chem* 2004;279:47254–47263.

202. Yang B, Gillespie A, Carlson EJ, et al. Neonatal mortality in an aquaporin-2 knock-in mouse model of recessive nephrogenic diabetes insipidus. *J Biol Chem* 2001;276:2775–2779.

203. Yang B, Zhou D, Verkman AS. Mouse model of inducible nephrogenic diabetes insipidus produced by floxed aquaporin-2 gene deletion. *Am J Physiol Renal Physiol* 2006;291:F465–572.

204. Ysewijn-Van Brussel KA, De Leenheer AP. Development and evaluation of a radioimmunoassay for Arg8-vasopressin, after extraction with Sep-Pak C18. *Clin Chem* 1985;31:861–863.

205. Yun J, Schoneberg T, Liu J, et al. Generation and phenotype of mice harboring a nonsense mutation in the V2 vasopressin receptor gene. *J Clin Invest* 2000;106:1361–1371.

206. Zerbe RL, Robertson GL. A comparison of plasma vasopressin measurements with a standard indirect test in the differential diagnosis of polyuria. *N Engl J Med* 1981;305:1539–1546.

207. Zerbe RL, Robertson GL. Osmoregulation of thirst and vasopressin secretion in human subjects: effect of various solutes. *Am J Physiol* 1983;244:E607–614.

208. Zerbe RL, Robertson GL. Disorders of ADH. *Med Clin North Am* 1984;13:1570–1574.

Regulation and Disorders of Potassium Homeostasis

CHAPTER **44**

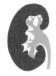

The Molecular Biology of Renal Potassium Channels

WenHui Wang and Steven C. Hebert

New York Medical College, Valhalla, New York, USA
Yale University School of Medicine, New Haven, Connecticut, USA

The regulation of urinary potassium excretion depends on the coordinated function of potassium transporters (cotransporters and exchangers), ion pumps and specialized channels in apical and basolateral membranes of distinct cell types along the distal nephron of the mammalian kidney. Potassium channels are key members of this integrated transport system in renal epithelial cells. First, renal K^+ channels participate in generating cell membrane potential; since numerous transport processes are electrogenic, changes in cell membrane potential could alter the transport rate of a given substance. Second, renal K^+ channels are involved in the volume regulation that is essential for preventing cell swelling or shrinking in the hypotonic or hypertonic environment. Third, renal K^+ channels play an important role in K^+ recycling which is essential for maintaining the function of several transport proteins such as Na^+,K^+-ATPase. Finally, renal K^+ channels are extremely involved in K^+ secretion in the cortical collecting duct. Figure 1 shows a scheme providing an overview regarding the role of K channels in different renal segments.

Since K^+ channels play such an important role in kidney function, understanding the structure and regulation of renal K^+ channels is essential to gaining insights into the molecular mechanisms of kidney potassium handling. In the past decade, the development of molecular biology and the patch-clamp techniques has had a significant impact on exploration of the molecular identity of some renal K^+ channels. We are, however, only at the beginning of this molecular adventure.

This chapter summarizes our current understanding of the molecular identity of renal K^+ channels, and will specifically focus on the ROMK ($K_{IR}1$) channel. We will discuss similarities, as well as certain differences, in the properties of cloned K^+ channels compared to native K^+ channels expressed in the different nephron segments.

THE MOLECULAR BIOLOGY OF ROMK ($K_{IR}1$), A DISTAL K^+ SECRETORY CHANNEL

ROMK Channel Structure and Isoforms

The K^+ channel, *ROMK* ($K_{IR}1$) (72), belongs to a growing family of inwardly rectifying K^+ (K_{IR}) channels (144) that are functionally characterized by high potassium selectivity and by weak or strong inward rectification. ROMK, like all K_{IR} channels, has a predicted structural topology consisting of two membrane spanning segments on either side of an amphipathic region with high homology to the pore-forming H5 segment of voltage-gated K^+ channels (Fig. 2) (76, 86, 100). This topology corresponds to the C-terminal half of the voltage-gated K^+ channels suggesting a common ancestral origin (84, 85, 87). Both N- and C-terminal ends are predicted to face the cytosol and provide regulatory domains (Fig. 2) that can be phosphorylated by kinases (220) and that interact with protons (33, 53, 132), nucleotides (135), and phosphoinositides (74, 77).

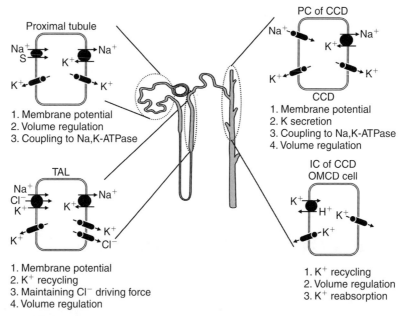

FIGURE 1   Cell model demonstrating the role of K channels in different renal segments.

Although this simple topology model has been challenged (175), X-ray crystallographic structure of a K⁺ channel from *Streptomyces lividans* (48) is consistent with the originally proposed model for ROMK (76) and the molecular model developed by Guy (68), each containing two membrane spanning segments and cytoplasmic N and C termini. This model has been confirmed and extended based on the Xray crystal structures for two inward rectifiers, Girk1 (Kir3) (145) and KirBac (101), the prokaryotic ortholog of the mammalian inward rectifiers like ROMK. In both structures the N and C termini interact. While in Girk1 the N–C interaction is formed within each subunit, in KirBac the N terminus of one

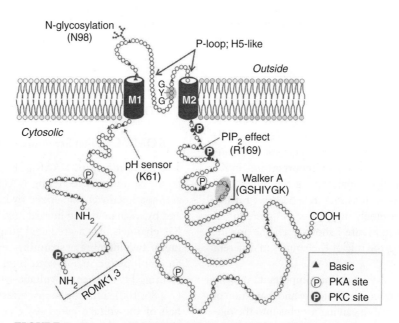

FIGURE 2   Topology of ROMK (K$_{IR}$1.1) K1 channel. M1 and M2 represent the two membrane-spanning domains characterizing the inward-rectifier family of potassium channel. Some important functional sites are indicated. A short amphipathic segment in the M1-M2 linking segment in ROMK is homologous to the pore-forming (P-loop) or H5 region of classic voltage-gated Shaker K⁺ channels cloned from the fruit fly. See text for discussion. The canonical G-Y-G amino acid sequence found in all K⁺ channels is shown in the H5 segment.

subunit interacts with the C terminus of the adjacent subunit. This intermolecular N–C interaction is thought to be involved in channel gating (67). Biochemical analyses have also supported this model. Using Fourier transform infrared (FTIR) and circular dichroism (CD) spectroscopy, Brazier and coworkers analyzed the secondary structure of a synthetic peptide containing the two membrane spanning segments, M1 and M2 (Fig. 2), and the flanking H5-like region (22). Their analyses indicate that both M1 and M2 segments adopt a α-helical structure in phospholipids, also consistent with our original model for ROMK (76). Moreover, Minor and coworkers (138) employed a yeast genetic screening technique to analyze the packing structure of the M1 and M2 domains. Their analysis suggests that M2 segments line the pore and are surrounded by M1 segments that also participate in subunit-subunit interactions in the tetrameric channel complex (Fig. 3A) (see [34] for a brief review). Consistent with this view, both M2 and the proximal C terminus determine both homo- and heteromultimerization on K_{IR} channels (122, 186, 192, 216, 216, 222).

The segment linking the M1 and M2 transmembrane α-helices is extracellular as it contains an N-linked glycosylation site (see Fig. 1) (76, 176). A short amphipathic segment in the M1-M2 linker in ROMK is homologous to the pore-forming H5 region of classic voltage-gated *Shaker* K^+ channels cloned from the fruit fly, *Drosophilia melanogaster*

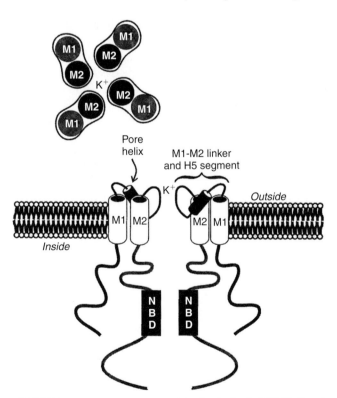

FIGURE 3 Multimeric structure of the K_{IR} family. **A:** ROMK, like all K_{IR} channels, is formed from a tetrameric assembly of subunits. M2 segments line the channel pore and are surrounded by M1 segments that also participate in subunit–subunit interactions in the tetrameric channel complex. **B:** Two of the four subunits forming the tetrameric ROMK channel are depicted. The nucleotide binding domain on the channel C terminus is shown.

(27, 86). This suggests that ROMK and voltage (as well as cyclic nucleotide)–gated channels evolved from a common ancestral gene and supports an important role for the H5 region in forming the channel pore (63, 69, 86, 128, 229, 231). In addition, this H5-like region contains the Gly-Try-Gly triplet (Fig. 2) that is conserved in channels with high K^+ selectivity (73, 85). The role of the segment linking M1 and M2 in formation of the channel pore is also supported by mutations in this region altering channel block by cations (Fig. 3B) (167, 224, 234). The molecular model of a cation channel from *Streptomyces lividans* has confirmed the important role of both the H5 loop, as well as the segment linking the first membrane helix with the H5 segment, in forming the selectivity barrier of the channel pore (127).

Analogous to the voltage-gated K^+ (Kv) channels (70), the predicted model analysis supports a tetrameric structure for K_{IR} channels (36, 42, 52, 223). In this model each subunit of the tetramer contributes to the ion permeation pathway and selectivity barrier (Fig. 2).

While specific amino acid residues critical for assembly of ROMK subunits into tetramers have not been identified, multiple interactions in N and C termini and in the M1-H5-M2 core appear to be needed (98). The latter is consistent with the intermolecular interactions of N- and C-termini seen in the Kirbac1.1 structure (101). While the functional ROMK tetramers permit rapid permeation of K^+ ions, a study performed in *Xenopus laevis* oocytes expressing ROMK channels indicates that H_2O movement through the pore is negligible (166). This is consistent with the high expression of ROMK in K^+ secretion low water permeability epithelia in the loop of Henle, distal tubule and collecting duct (see ROMK Protein Localization). Although no molecular images of ROMK protein have been achieved to deduce further the structure of the channel, height fluctuations have been observed using the atomic force microscope and the molecular sandwich technique when the channel is exposed to agents modifying gating (e.g., pH and PKA phosphorylation) (147). Since these latter molecular fluctuations occurred under conditions that activate ROMK channels (e.g., ATP, protein kinase A and pH), ROMK tetramers may change shape with alterations in channel activity.

ROMK Channel Isoforms

Following the cloning of ROMK1 (K_{IR}1.1a) from rat kidney (76), three additional alternatively spliced forms of this channel were isolated (Figs. 2 and 4) and named ROMK2 (K_{IR}1.1b), ROMK3 (K_{IR}1.1c) (20, 234), and ROMK6 (K_{IR}1.1d) (96). The encoded ROMK proteins differ at the beginning of the N terminus: ROMK2 (also rat ROMK6, which has the same amino acid sequence as ROMK2); Fig. 4 (96) has the shortest N terminus and splicing adds 19 or 26 amino acids for ROMK1 or ROMK3, respectively (see Figs. 2 and 4). Relative ROMK mRNA abundance measured by competitive PCR has shown that ROMK2 and ROMK3 are much more abundant than ROMK1 or

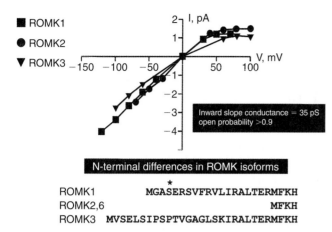

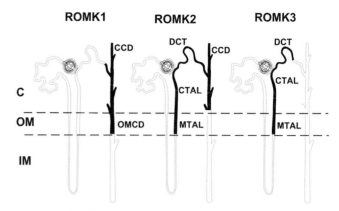

FIGURE 4 The ROMK splice variants. Current-voltage relationships for ROMK1, 2, and 3 are shown. Each of these variants has a similar I-V curve and calculated single-channel conductance of ~35 pS. The open probability of these three channels is also similar and greater than 0.9. ROMK1, 2, 3, and 6 N-terminal amino-acid sequences are shown using the single-letter notation for residues. ROMK2 and 6 have an identical amino acid sequence. ROMK1 and ROMK3 have 19 and 26 additional N-terminal amino acids, respectively, compared with ROMK2 or ROMK6. The asterisk in the ROMK1 sequence indicated a functional PKC phosphorylation site.

ROMK6 in rat kidney (16). A novel set of ROMK proteins, about one third the size of native ROMK, has been suggested to be formed from alternative splicing of the ROMK core exon (17). The significance of these putative smaller channel proteins remains unclear. Six splice variants (19, 179, 227) have been identified in the human ROMK gene, *KCNJ1*, located on chromosome 11q24 (19). These six human transcripts apparently encode only three distinct polypeptides, two of which are similar to rat ROMK1 and ROMK2 (19)). A rat homologue of the third human ROMK isoform has not been identified. Two ROMK homologues have also been cloned from human kidney but their roles in renal function are unknown (180).

ROMK Channel Localization

Rat ROMK1-3 is differentially expressed along the nephron from the thick ascending limb of Henle, TAL, to the outer medullary collecting duct (OMCD); (Fig. 5) (20, 104). The rat TAL and distal convoluted tubule, DCT, express ROMK2 and ROMK3 messenger RNA while principle cells in the cortical collecting duct (CCD), express ROMK1 and ROMK2 transcripts (Fig. 5). The outer medullary collecting duct cells appear to express only ROMK1 transcripts. The general single-channel properties of the ROMK1, 2 and 3 isoforms are similar (e.g., single-channel conductance and open probability) (Fig. 4). Although the specific functional/regulatory consequences of the different isoforms have not been fully elucidated, a serine at the fourth position in the extended N-terminus in ROMK1 has been shown to be required for sensitivity to arachidonic acid (Figs. 2 and 4) (125) and protein kinase C (126) (see ROMK Function). Thus ROMK1 may add distinct functional characteristics to ROMK channels. No

FIGURE 5 The distribution of the ROMK1, 2, and 3 isoforms along the rat nephron. The shaded regions indicate the localization of ROMK transcripts and protein. CCD, cortical collecting duct; CTAL, cortical thick ascending limb; DCT, distal convoluted tubule; MTAL, medullary thick ascending limb; OMCD, outer medullary collecting duct. In the CCD and OMCD, ROMK is expressed only in principle cells.

specific role for the extended N terminus of ROMK3 has been identified. Whether tetrameric ROMK channels are formed of different subunits (e.g., heterotetramers of ROMK2 and ROMK1 in the cortical collecting duct) or exist only as homo-tetramers is not known. Finally, ROMK transcripts are present in some other tissues (76) including the early gravid uterus (123). Roles for ROMK in these tissues have not been determined.

Antibody generated to sequences of ROMK shared by all isoforms has demonstrated an apical pattern of channel protein expression in rat TAL (including macula densa cells), distal collecting duct (DCT), and early CNT cells, and principle cells of the CCD and OMCD (95, 136, 153, 219). This localization is consistent with the ROMK channel providing a K⁺ secretory pathway in these renal epithelia.

ROMK Channel Properties Are Similar to the Distal (SK) K⁺ Secretory Channel

The single-channel characteristics and regulatory properties of ROMK channels expressed in *X. laevis* frog oocytes are virtually identical to those of the native ATP-sensitive, small conductance (SK) channels in TAL cells (Fig. 6) (204, 209) and principle cells in the CCD (Fig. 7) (59, 139, 171, 205–207, 210). Similar kinetic characteristics of K^+, NH_4^+, and Tl^+ have been observed in the native secretory K^+ channel in the rat CCD and ROMK2 channels expressed in *X. laevis* oocytes (30, 155), leading Palmer and coworkers to conclude that the native SK and cloned ROMK channels were identical.

A further characteristic of the low conductance secretory K^+ channel found in principle cells is a lack of sensitivity to external TEA⁺ (58, 59, 206–208). This organic cation also has no effect on K^+ secretion by this nephron segment. ROMK isoforms when expressed in *X. laevis* oocytes share this lack of TEA⁺ sensitivity (76).

The general properties of ROMK channels expressed in *Xenopus* oocytes include (1) weak inward rectification

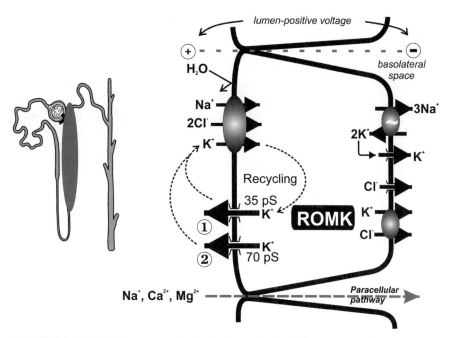

FIGURE 6 Model for ion transport in the thick ascending limb. The two types of apical K+ channels are shown: 35-pS (also called the small K+ or SK channel) and 70-pS channels. ROMK and SK functional and regulatory characteristics are essentially identical. It has been proposed that the 70-pS channel is also formed by ROMK in association with another channel subunit, but this remains to be demonstrated.

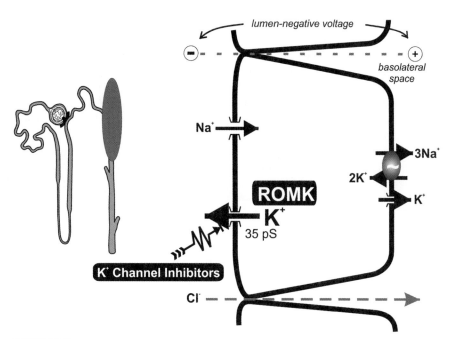

FIGURE 7 Model for ion transport by the principle cell in the collecting duct. The apical K+ secretory channel in this cell is ROMK.

(Fig. 4) that is dependent on the binding of cytosolic Mg^{2+} or other polyvalent cations to the channel pore (45, 56, 116, 122, 143, 216); (2) activation by protein kinase A–dependent phosphorylation processes (124, 134, 219, 220); (3) inhibition by high concentrations of MgATP (135); (4) inhibition by slight reductions in cytosolic pH (105, 193); and (5) inhibition by arachidonic acid and protein kinase C (125, 126). When coupled with the gene expression and protein localization studies, these functional similarities strongly suggest that ROMK makes up the pore-forming subunit of the renal distal SK potassium channel (155, 206).

Characteristics of the ROMK Channel Pore

Channel kinetics. ROMK channel are characterized by a high open probability (*Po*) of greater than 0.9 (30, 32, 76, 124). The high open probability results from one open state and two closed states. One closed state is very short (~1 millisecond; 99% frequency) and the other is longer (~40 milliseconds) but very infrequent (~1%) (32, 124). The infrequent closed state is due to blocking by divalent cations as it can be abolished by EDTA (32). Choe and coworkers (32) have also suggested that the closed state of ROMK results from K^+ ions transiently blocking its own pathway. Such a model would not require large molecular motions, but rather small molecular oscillations.

Channel rectification. One of the fundamental characteristics of ROMK, as well as all K_{IR}, channels is inward rectification, the property of passing current easier in the inward than in the outward direction (Fig. 4). Although this seems to be contrary to the role of ROMK in K^+ secretion, the inward rectification observed with ROMK, and with the kidney K^+ secretory channel, is "weak." The term "weak" rectification refers to the ability of ROMK to actually pass outward current, albeit to a lesser extent than inward current. Many of the other K_{IR} channels are "strong" rectifiers and characteristically pass little to no outward current. The very high open probability of the ROMK channel, usually greater than 0.9, may help make up for the rectification effect on K^+ secretion. In other words, although the outward conductance (ease of passing K^+ secretory current) is less than the inward conductance, the channels are open most of the time and thus able to secrete large amounts of K^+. We know that inward rectification of ROMK is due to blocking of the inner mouth of the channel pore by Mg^{2+} (143) or cytosolic polyamines like spermine or spermidine (56, 116). Thus, it is possible that variations in the cytosolic concentrations of these inorganic and organic cations could provide an important mechanism regulating outward (i.e., K^+ secretory) current.

Kinetic studies of inward rectification by Mg^{2+} and polyamines indicate that the effect is voltage-dependent, depends on the concentration of K^+ on both sides of the membrane, and varies with the K^+ reversal potential (32, 143, 148, 184). These latter investigators have interpreted these observations to suggest both an interaction between permeant and blocking ions and the presence of a variable energy well within the channel pore. The latter may relate to movement of a flexible selectivity filter into and out of the pore (32), a model consistent with alterations in the height of ROMK protein with channel activating agents observed by atomic force microscopy (147). Consistent with the role of M2 in channel gating and rectification, Choe and coworkers (31) have also shown that differences in M2 and the extracellular loop between M1 and M2 could account for the distinct channel kinetics of weak (ROMK2; $K_{IR}1.1$) versus strong (IRK1; $K_{IR}2.1$) inward rectifier channels.

While the H5-like region appears to contribute to the channel pore and selectivity filter of K_{IR} channels, several laboratories have demonstrated the importance of the M2 segment and COOH-termini in determining the inward rectifying characteristics of inwardly rectifying K^+ channels (122, 186, 216, 222). This is consistent with channel models of K_{IR} where the M2 segment lines the channel pore (Fig. 3) (138). Two residues appear to be particularly important in determining whether the rectification is strong or weak. In strong inward rectifiers like IRK1 ($K_{IR}2.1$) (100) a negatively charged residue, aspartic acid (D172 in IRK1), in the M2 membrane segment has been shown to be critical for strong inward rectification (122, 216). In ROMK the aspartate residue is replaced by asparagine (Fig. 8; IR Site #1, N171 in ROMK1), consistent with the weak rectification of this channel. A second residue located in the C terminus has also been shown to be an important contributor to strong rectification in IRK1 (222). This glutamate residue (E224 in IRK1) is replaced by a glycine residue in ROMK (Fig. 8; IR Site #2). This C-terminal glycine residue in ROMK is a part of the Walker A site that contributes to the nucleotide binding interactions (see Fig. 1 and IR Site #2 in Fig. 8) in the nucleotide-binding domain (NBD) (Fig. 3B), and thus serves a different gating function in ROMK. As expected from this model, exchange of the ROMK C terminus with that on IRK1 produces strong rectification in oocytes injected with the mutant ROMK channel (186).

Finally, two different extracts of venoms have been suggested to specifically inhibit ROMK channels (80, 88). The snake toxin, δ-dendrotoxin (80), and the honey bee venom extract, teriapin, and the modified compound, tertiapin-Q (88, 168) appear to block ROMK activity by interacting with channel pore. Observation, however, indicates that tertiapin-Q can also block Maxi-K (or BK, *hSlo1*) Ca^{2+}-activated K^+ channels (91) so that its utility in defining ROMK activity in nephron segments expressing both ROMK and Maxi-K channels is questionable.

Regulation of the ROMK K+ Channel

ROMK channel activity, like that of the native SK channel in TAL and principle cells, is regulated by a variety of factors that either activate or inhibit channel activity (Fig. 9). The molecular mechanisms for these alterations in channel function are rapidly being identified.

PHOSPHORYLATION BY PROTEIN KINASE A

Protein kinase A (PKA)–dependent phosphorylation processes activated by receptor-mediated events or alterations in cytosolic second messengers (e.g., cyclic AMP [cAMP]) play important roles in regulating the native SK channel in principle cells of the CCD (Fig. 10) (205–207, 210, 211). Phosphorylation–dephosphorylation processes also modulate the activity of the cloned ROMK K^+ channel (124–126, 134, 220). K^+ channel activity in excised inside-out patches of oocytes expressing ROMK requires activation by PKA-dependent phosphorylation processes (134). Rundown, or

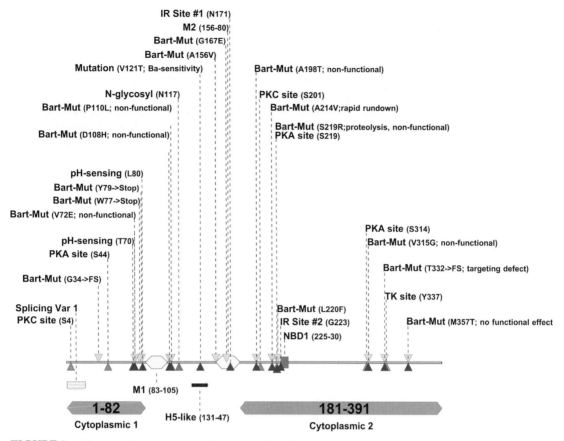

FIGURE 8 The major functional and regulatory sites and the Bartter syndrome mutations are shown in this schematic representation of ROMK1, K_{IR}1.1a. See text for discussion.

loss of ROMK channel activity in these patches, occurs whenever phosphatase-mediated dephosphorylation activity is greater than PKA-mediated phosphorylation.

The critical PKA phosphorylation sites are on the channel protein itself (Fig. 2). This has been demonstrated by several observations. First, ROMK protein expressed in HEK-293 cells can be phosphorylated by PKA (220). Phosphopeptide analysis and mapping have shown three serine residues phosphorylated by PKA (one residue on the N terminus [serine 25 in ROMK2] and two residues on the C terminus [serine 200 and serine 294 in ROMK2]). Mutation of any single PKA phosphorylation site on ROMK2 reduces whole-cell K^+ currents by 35% to 40% in oocytes; mutation of two or more of the three sites produces nonfunctional channels (220). This is

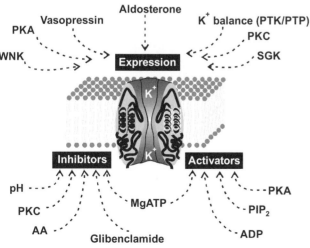

FIGURE 9 The major identified regulators of ROMK channels.

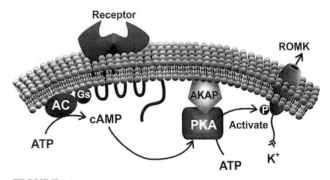

FIGURE 10 Activation of ROMK channels by Gs-coupled receptors requires a protein kinase A (PKA) anchoring protein or A kinase anchoring protein (AKAP). Activation of the receptor generated cyclic AMP (cAMP) that, in turn, activates PKA. PKA then phosphorylates ROMK at the three known PKA sites. The latter increases the channel open probability or increases the number of active channels in the membrane.

consistent with the critical role of PKA phosphorylation in channel activation. Second, at the single-channel level, the N-terminal and C-terminal PKA phosphorylation sites alter the channel activity, albeit differently (124). None of the mutations with serine residues replaced by alanine alters the single-channel conductance. Each of the C-terminal PKA phosphorylation site mutations, however, reduces open probability (P_o) by about 40% due to the appearance of a new long, closed state. This reduction in P_o is sufficient to account for the observed reduction in whole oocyte currents (220). Replacing the N-terminal serine with alanine does not change P_o, but does reduce by about 60% the probability of finding functioning channels. The mechanism for this latter reduction in active channels is not known. The mechanism by which PKA increases ROMK channel activity may include stimulation of surface expression and enhance the effect of PIP2 on ROMK channels. It has been shown that stimulation of PKA increases the sensitivity of ROMK channels to PIP2 in *Xenopus* oocytes (115). A study demonstrates that mutation of serine residue 44 to aspartate increases the surface delivery of ROMK channels (146). One of the fundamental characteristics of SK channels in principle cells and in the TAL is their activation by G_s-coupled receptors or by the addition of cAMP (206). However, channel activation requires more than PKA holoenzyme and ROMK. Wang and coworkers have shown that ROMK1 channels expressed in *X. laevis* oocytes could not be activated by cAMP unless expressed with A kinase anchoring protein (AKAP) (4). AKAPs are *A-kinase anchoring proteins* that bind PKA holoenzyme (catalytic plus regulatory subunits) and maintain the enzyme at specific intracellular sites (55, 159). Since stages V to VI *X. laevis* oocytes used in these experiments appeared to lack AKAPs (4), expression of an AKAP (e.g., AKAP79) appears to be required to direct the PKA holoenzyme to the plasma membrane in oocytes in a manner similar to that shown in HEK 293 cells (159). In AKAP79 + ROMK1 coexpressing oocytes, cAMP plus forskolin gives rise to a 35% increase in whole-cell K^+ current and cAMP + MgATP reverses rundown in inside-out excised membrane patches (4). At least two issues remain unanswered by these studies: (1) What AKAP is mediating the PKA effect in specific renal tubules?; and (2) What site(s) is(are) being phosphorylated by PKA to mediate the increased channel activity? Implicit in the latter is the question of whether a specific PKA phosphorylation site on ROMK is mediating the cyclic AMP/forskolin effect shown by Wang and coworkers (4). Regarding the former, several novel AKAPs have recently been cloned from mouse (43). One of these, AKAP-KL, is expressed in kidney tubules at apical borders.

EFFECT OF ARACHIDONIC ACID

Like the native SK channel in the CCD (64), ROMK1 channels expressed in *Xenopus* oocytes are sensitive to arachidonic acid (AA) (125, 126). The effect of AA is specific since other fatty acids failed to mimic the effect of AA (125). However, AA has little to no effect on the other two ROMK family members, ROMK2 and ROMK3 (126).

Since the amino acid sequences of the ROMK channels are identical, with the exception of the N terminus, the role of the N terminus in mediating the effect of AA is strongly suggested. This is supported by the demonstration that deletion of the initial 37 AAs of ROMK1 abolished the effect of AA. Moreover, a serine residue at the fourth position within the N terminus of ROMK1 has been shown to play a crucial role in the AA-mediated inhibition of ROMK1 since mutation of this serine residue to alanine abolished the effect of AA (Figs. 1 and 3) (126). Since this serine residue is a putative protein kinase C (PKC) phosphorylation site (76) and AA has been shown to activate PKC, the effect of AA may depend on stimulation of a membrane-bound PKC.

PHOSPHORYLATION BY PROTEIN KINASE C

Activation of prophosphorylation processes inhibits the apical SK channel in the CCD (210). ROMK1, which is exclusively expressed in collecting ducts, has three potential PKC phosphorylation sites involving serine residues; one on the N terminus and two on the C-terminal end. ROMK2 and ROMK3 only have the two C-terminal PKC phosphorylation sites (Figs. 2 and 4). Using in vitro phosphorylation assays it was observed that serine residue 4 in the N terminus and serine residue 201 in the C terminus are two major PKC-induced phosphorylation sites. The effect of PKC on ROMK channels is a complex. It was demonstrated that phosphorylation of serine residue 4 or 201 is essential for ROMK1 export to the plasma membrane (111). On the other hand, stimulation of PKC in vivo has been shown to inhibit ROMK channel activity. The N-terminal serine residue at the fourth position appears to be most important to PKC-mediated K^+ channel inhibition of ROMK1. Interestingly this is the same residue critical for the inhibitory effect of arachidonic acid (Fig. 4) (1). However, it is possible that PKC-induced inhibition of ROMK channels may be indirect resulting from a decrease in PIP2 content. Stimulation of PKC decreases the PIP2 level in the plasma membrane (233). Because PIP2 is essential for maintaining ROMK channels in the open state, decreases in PIP2 levels may contribute to the PKC-induced inhibition.

PHOSPHORYLATION OF ROMK BY PROTEIN TYROSINE KINASE

The ROMK channel is a substrate of protein tyrosine kinase (PTK) and tyrosine residue 337 in the C terminus of ROMK1 has been demonstrated to be a PTK phosphorylation site (140). Tyrosine phosphorylation of ROMK is regulated by dietary K^+ intake: a low K^+ intake increases, whereas a high K^+ intake decreases tyrosine phosphorylation (112). The regulation of tyrosine phosphorylation of ROMK by K^+ diet is partially achieved by modulating the expression of Src family PTK in response to a dietary K^+ intake. Low K^+ increases whereas a high K^+ suppresses the expression of Src family PTK (214). Immunostaining has also demonstrated that c-Src, the most ubiquitously distributed member of Src family PTK, is present in the thick ascending limb, connecting tubule, and cortical collecting duct (114). Although the fate of tyrosine phosphorylated ROMK is not completely understood, the stimulation of tyrosine phosphorylation of ROMK1 facilitates channel internalization (Fig. 11) (140). Because ROMK1 is exclusively expressed in the connecting tubule and CCD, this mechanism should play an important role in K^+ balance during K^+ restriction. Tyrosine phosphorylation of ROMK is regulated by an aldosterone-independent mechanism because low K^+ intake suppresses the aldosterone level while stimulating the expression of PTK. The mechanism by which low K^+ intake stimulates Src family PTK is not completely understood. However, two lines of evidence indicates that superoxide is a mediator of the effect of K^+ diet on the Src family PTK: (1) low K^+ intake stimulates superoxide anion levels and (2) incubation of M1 cells, a cultured mouse CCD principle cells, with hydrogen peroxide increases the expression of c-Src (11). The notion that superoxide anion could serve as a second messenger of low K^+ intake on the Src family PTK is also supported by the finding that suppression of superoxide anion attenuates the effect of low K^+ intake on c-Src expression and diminishes the tyrosine phosphorylation of ROMK. Thus, superoxide and PTK-pathway play important roles in maintaining K homeostasis.

REGULATION BY WNK; "WITH NO LYSINE (K)" KINASE

WNK4 is a serine-threonine kinase and has been identified in both distal convoluted tubule (DCT) and the CCD. Wildtype WNK4 has been shown to suppress the expression of the Na-Cl cotransporter in the plasma membrane of the DCT and accordingly, to inhibit Na absorption (221). The gene product encoding the inactivated WNK4 causes pseudohypoaldosteronism type II, a disease with characteristics of hypertension and low aldosterone levels. WNK4 is also expressed in the CCD and expression of WNK4 in oocytes decreased the expression of ROMK1 (89). However, the inhibitory effect of WNK4 on ROMK1 does not require the kinase activity because co-expression of the inactivated

WNK4 also resulted in inhibiting expression of ROMK1 in *Xenopus* oocytes (Fig. 11). The physiological role of WNK4 may be that the WNK4 serves as a switch between Na transport and K^+ secretion. The WNK4-induced inhibition of Na^+ transport in the DCT is expected to increase Na^+ delivery to the CCD and enhance the Na^+ absorption, which leads to augmentation of the driving force for K^+ secretion. However, because WNK4 inhibits ROMK channel activity, increases in electrochemical gradient for K^+ secretion would have a diminished effect on renal K^+ secretion. Mutation of WNK4 would release the inhibition of Na-Cl cotransporter and leads to stimulation of Na^+ transport in the DCT. Moreover, inactivated WNK4 further decreases the surface expression of ROMK, reduces K^+ secretion in the CCD and causes hyperkalemia.

REGULATION BY UBIQUITINATION

Ubiquitination plays an important role in the regulation of protein degradation and recycling by attaching ubiquitin molecules to lysine residue of substrate protein. Ubiquitination can further be classified into monoubiquitination by adding only one or two ubiquitin molecules to the substrate protein or polyubiquitination by attaching more than four ubiquitin molecules. The polyubiquitinated protein is subjected to degradation whereas monoubiquitinated proteins are targeted to internalization and possibly recycling to the cell membrane. Recently, it has been shown that ROMK1 channel activity could be regulated by monoubiquitination and the ubiquitin binding site is on lysine residue 22 on the N-terminus of ROMK1 (Fig. 11) (113). The physiological importance of monoubiquitination in the regulation of ROMK channel is still not clear. Because ROMK channel activity in the CCD decreases in response to stimulation of PTK, it would be interesting to determine whether monoubiquitination is required for the PTK-induced internalization of ROMK1 in the CCD.

REGULATION BY SERUM AND GLUCOCORTICOID-INDUCIBLE KINASE-1

Several separate studies have demonstrated that serum and glucocorticoid-inducible kinase-1 (SGK1) can increase the activity of ROMK in the presence of Na/H exchange regulating factor (NHERF) (230, 232). It is possible that NHERF is served as a scaffold protein required for the stimulatory effect of SGK1 on ROMK (Fig. 11). The mechanism of the SGK1 effect may be through stimulation of the serine phosphorylation of ROMK1. Confocal microscopy and cell-surface antibody-binding assay have further shown that stimulation of SGK-induced phosphorylation increases the expression of ROMK1 channels in plasma membrane. The phosphorylation site of ROMK1 induced by SGK is located on serine residue 44 in the N terminus, which is also a putative PKA-phosphorylation site because mutation of serine 44 to alanine abolished the effect of SGK. The role of SGK on K secretion is also demonstrated in SGK null mice

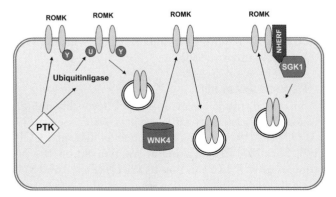

FIGURE 11   Cell model demonstrating the regulation of ROMK1 channel in the cortical collecting duct by PTK, WNK4, ubiquitination, and SGK.

in which renal K secretion is impaired. However, it is not known whether the stimulatory effect of SGK on renal K^+ secretion is the result of increased ENaC activity, which in turn augments the electrochemical gradient for K^+ secretion, or due to a direct stimulation of ROMK channel insertion. ROMK expression in the apical membrane of the TAL and CCD is actually increased rather than decreased in SGK null mice (78). This suggests that the role of SGK in stimulating ROMK insertion may not be essential or can be replaced by other kinases such as cAMP-dependent protein kinase A. A possible role of SGK is to regulate renal K^+ secretion in response to a daily dietary K^+ intake. It has been shown that a high dietary K^+ intake for 12 hours stimulates SGK expression in the kidney (156). Interestingly, ROMK channel activity significantly increased in the CCD from rats on a high K^+ diet for only 6 hours. Thus, SGK may regulate ROMK channel activity in the CT and CCD in response to a daily variation of dietary K^+ intake.

REGULATION BY NUCLEOTIDES AND INTERACTIONS WITH THE CYSTIC FIBROSIS TRANSMEMBRANE CONDUCTANCE REGULATOR

MgATP both activates and inhibits ROMK channels (Fig. 9) with the net effect of nucleotide action being the integration of these opposite and complex events. Activation occurs by stimulation of PKA-mediated phosphorylation (see previous section) or by altering the generation of phosphatidylinositol 4,5-bisphosphate (PIP2) (77 and see section on regulation by PIP2). These processes modulate channel gating or plasma membrane channel density (e.g., by regulating trafficking of the channel to the apical plasma membrane for the endoplasmic reticulum) (146). Inhibition of the SK secretory channel in CCD by MgATP (205) identifies this channel as belonging to a subgroup of K_{IR} channels, referred to as ATP-sensitive or K_{ATP} channels (the classical K_{ATP} channels, Kir6.x and Kir1.1, or ROMK channels) (6, 139). The renal SK or K_{ATP} channel is somewhat less sensitive to ATP than the pancreatic β cell, or other, K_{ATP} channels. As observed with other K_{ATP} channels (6, 90), addition of MgADP to MgATP inhibited ROMK channels relieves the ATP block (135). Thus, changes in the cytosolic MgATP concentration, or in the MgATP/ADP ratio, as may occur with alterations in the activity of Na^+,K^+-ATPase, could modulate ROMK channel activity. This may provide one mechanism for coupling basolateral Na^+-pump activity with apical K^+ secretion in the principle cells of the CCD.

Channel inhibition by Mg-ATP is incompletely understood; however, the mechanism likely involves both direct binding of MgATP to the ROMK protein at an unconventional nucleotide binding site (NBD) (Fig. 2B) and interaction with cystic fibrosis transmembrane conductance regulator (CFTR). The direct binding of ATP to K_{ATP} channels is supported by cross-linking of azido-ATP compounds to the channel proteins (45, 188, 189). In addition, biochemical observations using fluorescent ATP analogues have shown

that Mg-ATP can bind directly to K_{ATP} channels including ROMK (44, 45, 196). Both N- and C-terminal segments form the nucleotide-binding site, which is situated at a region modeled to be involved in channel gating (39, 45, 47). The crucial N–C terminal interaction occurs between adjacent subunits; in other words, the nucleotide binding site is intermolecular. As observed with other K_{ATP} channels (6, 90), addition of ADP to ATP inhibited ROMK channels relieved the ATP block (135).

Only a few studies have found that ATP can inhibit ROMK when expressed alone in *X. laevis* oocytes (132, 135, 165), suggesting that direct binding of MgATP to ROMK is insufficient for channel inhibition. CFTR has been proposed to be the critical protein that is required for transduction of nucleotide binding to channel gating (Fig. 12B) (75, 165). A characteristic of K_{ATP} channels including the renal SK channel is their sensitivity to inhibition by sulfonylureas like glibenclamide (Glyburide) (6, 7). The pancreatic β-cell K_{ATP} channel is formed by two subunits; a pore-forming polypeptide, $K_{IR}6.2$, and the sulfonylurea-binding protein, SUR1 (an ABC [ATP-binding cassette] protein family member like CFTR [2, 10, 25] in a 4:4 ratio [Fig. 12A] [36, 81, 117]). $K_{IR}6.2$ provides the K^+ channel permeation pathway and ATP binding-inhibition site, while SUR is required for sulfonylurea binding and for certain aspects of regulation by nucleotides (e.g., ADP effects) (1, 10, 137). In the kidney, glibenclamide induces natriuresis in rats (35, 129) and patch-clamp experiments have shown that 200 μM glibenclamide inhibits the apical SK channel in the rat TAL by about 60% to 70% (203, 204). The sensitivity of the SK channel in TAL to sulfonylureas is, however, much less than in other K_{ATP} channels (139). Thus the ability of glibenclamide to inhibit the K^+ secretory channels in renal distal tubule suggests that a SUR-like protein is associated with this channel and is involved in the sulfonylurea effect (Fig. 12C). CFTR is expressed in the same apical regions as ROMK channels in the CTAL and CCD (38) and a functional truncated hemi-CFTR is also expressed in the MTAL (141). Consistent with ROMK-CFTR interactions, glibenclamide- and Mg-ATP–sensitive whole-cell K^+ currents in *X. laevis* oocytes are only observed when ROMK is coexpressed with CFTR (131, 165). Moreover, a functional nucleotide binding domain, NBD1, on CFTR is required for glibenclamide sensitivity of ROMK K^+ currents (133).

REGULATION BY pH

Small reductions in cytosolic pH reversibly inhibit ROMK channel activity expressed in *X. laevis* oocytes (33, 53, 132, 172, 193) and the SK channel in TAL and CCD (170, 205, 207, 210). Lysine at position 80 on the N-terminus of ROMK1 (K61 on ROMK2) (Figs. 2 and 8) is primarily responsible for conferring this pH sensitivity as mutation of this residue abolished pH dependency (33, 53). Other residues on the N terminus of ROMK have

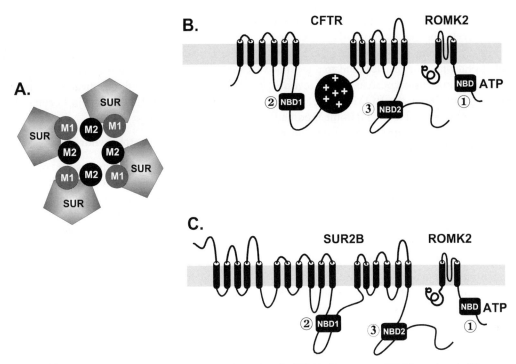

FIGURE 12 Assembly of KATP and ROMK channels with ATP binding cassette (ABC) proteins. **A:** The proposed hetero-octameric complex forming ATP-sensitive (KATP) channels with four K_{IR} subunits and four sulfonylurea receptor (SUR) subunits. The M1 and M2 membrane segment arrangement is as shown in Figure 2 with the M2 membrane segments lining the channel pore. **B:** The topology of CFTR and ROMK channels proposed to form kidney KATP channels. A single nucleotide-binding domain (NBD, *1*) is present on the C-terminus of ROMK while two NBDs (*2* and *3*) are found on CFTR. **C:** The topology of the sulfonylurea receptor, SUR2B, and ROMK proposed to form kidney KATP channels.

also been shown to modulate sensitivity to pH (33), consistent with the internal pH sensor being on N-terminal domain of the channel protein. Studies have also suggested that pH-dependent gating of ROMK1 is associated with conformational changes in both N and C termini (172). pH-dependent gating of ROMK is rapidly reversible so long as the exposure to low pH (6.0–7.0) is short. Longer exposure to low pH results in "irreversibility." Schulte and coworkers have provided an explanation for the latter. The pH-dependent conformational change in ROMK apparently exposes N- and C-terminal cysteine residues forming disulfide bridges that lock the protein in a closed conformation. The disulfide bridges can be broken by DTT (dithiothreitol) resulting in channel reopening.

Cytosolic pH can also alter ROMK channel activity in another way. The $K_{1/2}$ for inhibition of ROMK channel activity is not fixed but can be modulated by altering cytosolic side pH. McNicholas and coworkers (132) found that decreasing the pH from 7.4 to 7.2 on the cytosolic face of excised patches from oocytes expressing ROMK2 reduced the $K_{1/2}$ for MgATP inhibition from about 2.5 mM to less than 0.5 mM, almost a 10-fold increase in affinity with this small acidification. This effect appears to be independent of the lysine residue implicated in pH-dependent regulation of ROMK channel activity (33, 53)

indicating that another pH sensor may be present on ROMK. Thus reductions in cytosolic pH within the physiological range can affect ROMK channel activity in an ATP-independent and ATP-dependent manner. Interestingly, a histidine residue in $K_{IR}6.2$ (H216) (Fig. 2) (15) in a region corresponding to the Walker A site in ROMK has been shown to mediate pH-dependent modulation of polyamine block of this K_{ATP} channel. A negatively charged glutamic acid residue in this C-terminal region (e.g., E224 in $K_{IR}2$) has also been shown to modulate block by Mg^{2+} or polyamines (222). Thus, this region of the C-terminus of K_{IR} channels is involved in a variety of different gating functions (ATP, pH, polyamines).

REGULATION BY PHOSPHOINOSITIDES

Phospholipids, particularly PIP2 (phosphatidylinositol 4,5-bisphosphate), have been shown to modulate K_{ATP} channels including ROMK1 (14, 74, 77). Exposure of inside-out patches from oocytes expressing $K_{IR}6.2$ to PIP2 reduces of the ATP-sensitivity of this K_{ATP} channels apparently by reducing the probability of ATP binding to its receptor site (14). Consequently, increasing concentrations of PIP2 increase K_{ATP} channel activity. PIP2 interacts with the K_{IR} pore-forming subunit rather than the SUR subunit of K_{ATP} channels since PIP2 modifies the ATP sensitivity of the C-terminal truncated $K_{IR}6.2$ channel in the absence of SUR1 (14). ROMK, like many K_{IR} channels, contains a high density of positively charged amino acids just C terminal to M2 (Fig. 2). Huang and coworkers (77) have shown that labeled phospholipid vesicles bind to a recombinant ROMK1 C terminal fusion protein. These investigators implicated arginine 186 in the ROMK1 C terminus (Fig. 2) as a mutation of this residue to glutamine modified PIP2 effects. Since PIP2 is generated by ATP-dependent lipid kinases, Huang and coworkers have suggested that the stimulatory effect of ATP may be due to the generation of PIP2 (77). Thus, alterations in PIP2 generation consequent to activation of G protein–coupled receptors would provide a mechanism for modulating the activity of K_{ATP} channel including ROMK.

REGULATION OF ROMK EXPRESSION IN KIDNEY

Since K^+ homeostasis is mainly controlled by aldosterone and the potassium load, is not surprising that ROMK mRNA expression in rat kidney is regulated by aldosterone, K^+ adaptation and vasopressin (Fig. 9). It is well established that rats fed a high-K diet adapt by upregulating renal K^+ secretion and excretion (130). This results, at least in part, from an increase in the SK channel density in CCD (154). Wald and coworkers (200) found that K^+ deficiency reduces ROMK mRNA expression in both cortex and medulla, while K^+ loading increases ROMK transcript slightly only in medulla. The specific ROMK isoforms that changed with potassium were not assessed. Moreover, Frindt and coworkers (60) found that ROMK transcript abundance by in situ hybridization in the CCD was not affected by a high K^+ diet. Thus the high K^+ diet induced increase in density of active SK channels in principle cells in the CCD is not due to increased abundance of ROMK mRNA. Rather changes in ROMK protein abundance, channel activation, or ROMK channel translocation to the membrane are potential mechanisms to account for the high-K^+ adaptation effect on SK channels in the principle cells.

Mineralocorticoids also regulate ROMK abundance. Adrenalectomy decreased ROMK mRNA abundance in cortex but increased transcript abundance in the medulla (200). In this latter study, K^+ deficiency in adrenalectomized rats reduced ROMK mRNA to control levels suggesting that the hyperkalemia associated with adrenalectomy was the cause for the increased ROMK message in medulla. In another study, White and colleagues (16) showed that aldosterone administration by minipump to adrenal intact rats increased ROMK transcripts in whole kidney. In the latter study, the ROMK2, 3, and 6 isoforms were increased by the mineralocorticoid. This latter study would be consistent with mineralocorticoid-mediated regulation of ROMK mRNA abundance in cortex.

Vasopressin, via cyclic AMP, stimulates K^+ secretion in principle cells (207) and activates the apical K^+ channels in TAL cells (162, 204) (Fig. 6). Although the activation of PKA by camp would phosphorylate ROMK (or the SK

channel), it remains to be shown whether this is sufficient to account for the stimulation of K^+ channel activity or whether additional mechanisms, such as channel insertion into the membrane, are required. As discussed previously, PKA-anchoring proteins appear to be required for camp activation of ROMK currents in oocytes (Fig. 10) (4).

Lessons from Bartter Syndrome

Bartter syndrome (13) comprises a set of autosomal recessive renal tubulopathies characterized by hypokalemic metabolic alkalosis, salt wasting, hyperreninemia, and hyperaldosteronsim (8, 66, 92, 164). Antenatal Bartter syndrome is the most severe form of the inherited disorders and is characterized by hyperprostaglandinemia (prostaglandin E2 [PGE2]). Antenatal Bartter syndrome is genetically heterogeneous resulting from mutations in one of five genes (71). Three of the Bartter genes encode the major Na^+, K^+, Cl^- transporters in the TAL: the *SLC12A1* gene encoding the apical Na-K-2Cl cotransporter (182, 197), the *CLCKB* basolateral Cl^- channel (181), and the *KCNJ1* apical K^+ recycling channel, ROMK (see mutations in Fig. 8) (93, 183, 199). Mutations in two other genes also produce the Bartter phenotype: barttin and the extracellular calcium-sensing receptor (CaSR). Barttin is a membrane protein that is required for trafficking of the ClCKb channel to the basolateral membrane of TAL cells and loss-of-function mutations in barttin result in the absence of basolateral Cl^- channel activity (51). Gain-of function mutations in the CaSR result in inhibition of Na,K-ATPase, NKCC2, and apical 70-pS K-channel activity (71, 198, 212).

The effect of loss-of-function mutations in ROMK on TAL function can be understood since apical K^+ recycling is crucial both to supplying K^+ to the Na-K-2Cl cotransporter and to generation of the lumen positive transepithelial voltage that drives 50% of the reabsorbed sodium through the paracellular pathway (18, 65). ROMK channels with some of the Bartter mutations express no or little function in *X. laevis* oocytes (41, 173), consistent mutations in *KCNJ1* in Bartter syndrome resulting with ROMK loss-of-function. Based on the location of the amino acid residue altered with certain KCNJ1 mutations (e.g., at or near phosphorylation sites or the nucleotide binding site), the resultant ROMK channels would be expected to exhibit altered gating (see previous discussion, Regulation of the ROMK K^+ Channel). A ROMK-deficient mouse has been developed and exhibits a Bartter-like phenotype (118, 121).

While both human and mouse studies clearly demonstrate the importance of ROMK in TAL function, several questions regarding the resulting Bartter phenotype remained. First, two types of apical K^+ channels have been observed in the rat TAL (204), an SK channel with characteristics typical of ROMK and an intermediate conductance (~70 pS) channel that is similar only in some properties with ROMK. In rat TAL cells, however, the 70-pS channel predominates so that mutations in the ROMK gene that generates inactive SK channels would only be expected to have minimal effect on the apical K^+ conductance of TAL cells. This has suggested that the intermediate conductance channel requires ROMK for function (e.g., as a subunit or as a regulator). This possibility has been established by the absence of 70-pS K^+ channels in the TAL from ROMK-null mice (120). Second, ROMK comprises the apical K^+ secretory channel in principle cells of the CCD. Yet, Bartter individuals with *KCNJ1* mutations are hypokalemic. This suggests that these Bartter individuals adopt alternative mechanisms for K^+ secretion. Elucidation of these mechanisms will likely provide important insights to potassium handling by distal nephron segments including the collecting duct.

OTHER RENAL POTASSIUM CHANNELS

Several other K^+ channels have been cloned from kidney-derived cell lines or are found in mammalian kidney (Fig. 13). Physiological roles for these channels are less defined than that for ROMK.

The 6-TM Renal K Channels

KCNQ1 CHANNEL

KCNQ1 forms a small conductance (2–10 pS) Kv channel in kidney, existing as a heteromultimeric complex with KCNE1 (minK). MinK has a single-transmembrane segment and is highly expressed at the apical membrane.

KCNQ1 and KCNE1 have been extensively characterized in the heart, where they play crucial roles in cardiac repolarization (12, 169, 202). Mutations of these genes cause long QT syndrome. Both KCNQ1/KCNE1 are abundantly expressed in the kidney, where they may prevent the membrane depolarization that occurs following stimulation of electrogenic Na^+-coupled transport of glucose or amino acids (195). Accordingly, KCNE1-deficient mice exhibit a reduction in glucose and amino acid uptake by the proximal tubule. However, additional Kv channels, such as Maxi-K^+ and KCNA10, may also participate in stabilizing proximal tubule membrane potential during electrogenic Na^+ uptake.

KCNA10 CHANNEL

KCNA10 is found at the apical membrane of the proximal tubule (228). The *KCNA10* gene is located on 1p11-13 and transcripts are expressed in kidney, heart, and aorta. KCNA10 has 58% amino acid identity with Kv1.3, which also resides at 1p11-13 (151). The predicted secondary structure is identical to that of other Shaker-related K^+ channels, including intracellular N and C termini, six transmembrane segments, a voltage sensor (S4), and a pore (P) region. Unlike Shaker proteins, however, KCNA10 contains a putative cyclic nucleotide (CN) binding domain at the C terminus suggesting that protein function is regulated by cyclic nucleotides.

Kv1.3 CHANNEL

Kv1.3 is intronless and its longest open reading frame (1539 nucleotides) encodes a 513–amino-acid protein. Hydropathy analysis indicates that rabKv1.3 has six

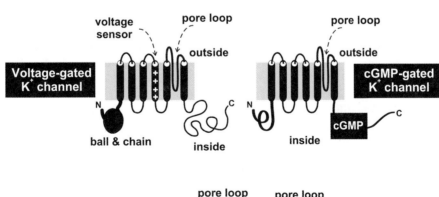

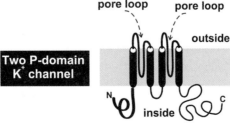

FIGURE 13 Proposed topologies of the voltage-gated, cyclic nucleotide-gated, and two P-domain K^+ channel expressed in mammalian kidney. The pore loops are indicated in each channel. Note the two pore loops for the two-P channel.

transmembrane domains, S1–S6, and a pore region. Kv1.3 contains consensus sequences for a protein kinase C site (PKC) between S4 and S5, a tyrosine kinase phosphorylation site at the amino terminus, and an N-glycosylation site between S1 and S2. Several recent findings support the notion that Kv1.3 participates in distal tubular Na^+ reabsorption and K^+ secretion.

MAXI-K^+ CHANNEL

Maxi-K^+ channels are another type of 6-TM K^+ channels believed to play a significant role in renal solute transport. Large Ca^{2+}-activated K^+ currents have been detected at the apical membrane of the principle cells of the CCD (79). Their contribution to K^+ secretion was deemed uncertain in light of their very low open probability. Two studies highlight the role of these K^+ channels in flow-dependent potassium secretion both in the connecting tubule (191) and in the cortical collecting duct (217).

The 2-TM Renal K^+ Channel (Non-ROMK)

$K_{IR}2.3$ CHANNEL

In cortical collecting duct principle cells the maintenance of the negative membrane potential depends, at least in part, on the activity of an inwardly rectifying 18-pS K^+ channel. This basolateral K^+ channel has been suggested to be the inwardly rectifying K^+ channel, $K_{IR}2.3$ (215). The kidney $K_{IR}2.3$ was cloned from a mouse CCD cell line and its expression in kidney confirmed by Northern analysis (215). When the MDCK cells were transfected with $K_{IR}2.3$, the channel was expressed in the basolateral membrane (102) and a basolateral sorting signal was identified at the COOH-terminal tail (103, 149). $K_{IR}2.3$ shares some biophysical properties with the native 18-pS K^+ channel such as high open probability and channel conductance, 14.5 pS (215).

$K_{IR}4.1/4.2$ AND $K_{IR}5.1$ CHANNELS

Evidence suggests that heteromeric $K_{IR}4.0/K_{IR}5.1$ channels form the basolateral small-conductance K^+ channel in distal nephron segments (119). The inward rectifier K^+ channel, $K_{IR}4.1$, was originally identified from rat brain and exhibits 53% amino acid identity to ROMK1 (21, 187). The kidney also expresses $K_{IR}4.1$ mRNA and the channel protein has been immunolocalized to the basolateral membrane of distal nephron segments (DCT, CNT, and ICD) (83). Internal protons decrease $K_{IR}4.1$ K^+ current by reducing open probability, however, internal protons also increase channel conductance (225). Mice with deletion of the $K_{IR}4.1$ gene (*KCNJ10*) have been generated (94) but a specific renal phenotype, to our knowledge, has not been identified.

$K_{IR}4.2$ was originally cloned from human kidney and called $K_{IR}1.3$ (180). While this study reported that $K_{IR}4.2$ channels are not functional in *X. laevis* oocytes (180), subsequent studies have shown that this protein forms inward rectifying K^+ channels that are inhibited by protein kinase C and internal protons (119, 160). $K_{IR}4.2$ mRNA is found in human (180) and mouse (119) kidney, and in the latter species, specifically in the DCT.

The inward rectifier K^+ channel, $K_{IR}5.1$, was also cloned from rat brain but does not form functional K^+ channels by itself when expressed in *X. laevis* oocytes (also known as BIR9) (21). $K_{IR}5.1$ mRNA is present in kidney (21, 190), and channel protein is abundantly expressed in PT and in DCT and CCD segments (194) where $K_{IR}4.1$ is also expressed (83). Studies have demonstrated that $K_{IR}4.1$ or $K_{IR}4.2$ with $K_{IR}5.1$ forms heteromeric inward rectifying K^+ channels with distinct properties in both heterologous expression systems (97, 119, 190) and native kidney (190). The heteromeric interaction of $K_{IR}5.1$ with other K_{IR} K^+ channels is specific for $K_{IR}4.x$ channels and requires a small region in the proximal COOH-terminus of $K_{IR}4.1$ (97). A study showed that the basolateral small-conductance K^+ channel in distal nephron segments is most similar to heteromeric $K_{IR}4.1(K_{IR}4.2)/K_{IR}5.1$ channels (119). The most dramatic and specific effect of the $K_{IR}4.x$-$K_{IR}5.1$ assembly on K^+ channel function is the shift in the pKa for inhibition by internal protons from 6.0 to the physiologically relevant pKa of 7.4 (161, 190, 194, 218). Internal pH sensitivity of $K_{IR}4.1$-$K_{IR}5.1$ is modulated by PIP2 (226) similarly to $K_{IR}1.1$ (ROMK) (110).

$K_{IR}6.1$ CHANNEL

$K_{IR}6.1$ (previously known as uK_{ATP}-1) was originally cloned from a rat pancreatic islet cell cDNA library using $K_{IR}3.1$ as a probe (82) and belongs to the $K_{IR}6.0$ (ATP-sensitive; K_{ATP}) subfamily of inwardly rectifying K^+ channels (144, 177). Exogenous expression of $K_{IR}6.1$ channels in *X. laevis* oocytes forms ATP-sensitive channels only when coexpressed with a sulfonylurea receptor protein (26, 177). Although this inward rectifier is predominantly found in brain, heart, and vascular tissue, expression in kidney has been documented (50, 82). $K_{IR}6.1$ has been localized to both mitochondria (185) and plasma membranes (24, 185). Upregulation of $K_{IR}6.1$ mRNA has been observed following ischemic injury in rat kidney consistent with the proposed role of K_{ATP} channel activation in protection from ischemic damage (e.g., in the heart) (3). $K_{IR}6.1$ was cloned from rabbit proximal tubule cDNA library and expression of $K_{IR}6.1$, SUR2A and SUR2B in rabbit proximal tubule conformed by polymerase chain reaction (PCR) (24). Functional studies in *X. laevis* oocytes suggested that $K_{IR}6.1$ may form the basolateral ATP- and taurine-sensitive K^+ channel involved in the basolateral K^+ conductance of proximal tubules (24). Adenylate kinase, which promotes phosphoryl transfer between ATP and ADP and associates with K_{ATP} channels (28), has been cloned from the rabbit proximal tubule library (23) and may associate with $K_{IR}6.1$ in these cells to promote metabolic sensing.

$K_{IR}7.1$ CHANNEL

The inward rectifier K^+ channel, $K_{IR}7.1$, was originally cloned from human brain cDNA libraries after searching the GenBank expressed sequence tag (EST) database using $K_{IR}1.1$ and $K_{IR}6.2$ (99, 157). The $K_{IR}7.1$ K^+ channel displays unusual K^+ permeation properties with a low single-channel conductance of 50 fS, low sensitivity to blocking by external Ba^{2+} or Cs^+, and very low dependence of conductance on external K^+ (46, 99, 157). PCR and Western blot analyses have identified $K_{IR}7.1$ transcripts and protein in rat, guinea pig, and human kidney (40, 99, 150, 157). Expression of $K_{IR}7.1$ along the rat nephron was demonstrated by Western blots of microdissected nephron segments (150) and showed K^+ channel protein in TAL, DCT, CNT, CCD, OMCD, and IMCD cells (150). Immunostaining localized $K_{IR}7.1$ to basolateral membranes of DCT and principle cells (150). In the guinea pig, $K_{IR}7.1$ protein is expressed in basolateral membranes of proximal tubule and TAL cells (40). In the CCD, $K_{IR}7.1$ is expressed in principle cells, but not intercalated cells. The unique pore properties of $K_{IR}7.1$ and its localization close to Na,K-ATPase suggested that this K^+ channel may be functionally coupled to Na,K-ATPase and involved in K^+ recycling across basolateral membranes (142, 150).

Channel Inducing Factor

Channel inducing factor (CHIF) is a single-membrane–spanning protein that was originally identified in a rat colonic cDNA library and is most similar to the γ subunit of Na,K-ATPase (9). However, a minK (IsK)–like K^+ channel activity was found when CHIF was expressed in *X. laevis* oocytes (9). Subsequently, CHIF was shown to be expressed at basolateral membranes of the OMCD and IMCD (54, 178) where it functions as a regulator of Na,K-ATPase activity, similar to the pump γ subunit (61). CHIF mRNA is suppressed by a low K^+ diet, independently of aldosterone, while a high K^+ diet increases CHIF transcripts in an aldosterone-dependent manner (201). In a ischemic reperfusion injury model in rats, both CHIF and ROMK were downregulated, and thereby, could contribute to the hyperkalemia of acute renal failure (62).

The Two-Pore K^+ Channels

The most recently discovered class of K^+ channels is characterized by a topology containing two pores or P-loops. These channels are also appropriately referred to as the "two-pore domain" (or K_t, two-P, TWIK-related) K^+ channels (see [163]). K_t channels exhibit four membrane-spanning domains consisting of two K_{IR}-like domains that are linked in a single subunit (Fig. 11) (5, 29, 37, 106, 152, 163). Structurally similar channels have been identified in the *C. elegans* genome project and represent the most abundant class of K^+ channels in this species (213). The TWIK-related channels, including TWIK1 (5, 37, 106–108, 152, 163), TWIK2 (29), TREK1 (57, 109, 163), TASK1 (49,

163) and TASK2 (163) are all expressed in mammalian kidney (163).

TWIK1 (106) and TWIK2 (29) express weakly inward-rectifying K^+ channels that are inhibited by intracellular acidification. Transcripts for TWIK1 are expressed in rabbit cortical TAL and collecting duct (152) and TWIK1 protein has been localized to the brush border of proximal convoluted tubules, intracellular and apical borders of intercalated cells in the CCD, and in cortical and medullary TAL cells (37). TREK1 gives rise to mechanosensitive outward-rectifying K^+ currents that are activated by arachidonic acid and are inhibited by protein kinases A and C (57, 158). TASK channels exhibit noninactivating outward-rectifying K^+ currents that are very sensitive to external pH (49, 163). While the properties of TWIK-related K^+ channels do not fit with any of the known native K^+ channels in kidney, their widespread expression in mammalian and other organisms (e.g., *C. elegans*) suggests either that they have been missed in patch clamp recording or that they associate with other (unidentified to date) subunits to produce pores with native channel properties.

SUMMARY AND CONCLUSIONS

Although we have gained significant insights into the structural diversity of K^+ channels expressed in the mammalian kidney, many new channels will likely be identified in the near future. Likewise electrophysiological studies continue to expand our database of physiologically and pharmacologically distinct K^+ channels. The exciting challenge is to identify which channel genes encode which native channels. Given that many K^+ channels are probably composed of more than one subunit (e.g., the K_{ATP} channels), this challenge is somewhat daunting and will require many more years of investigation. Finally, we expect that new inherited disorders due to mutations in some of these channel genes (channelopathies) will be identified. These channelopathies will not only provide new insights into the physiological roles of K^+ channels but will likely raise new questions as it has for ROMK mutations in Bartter syndrome.

Acknowledgments

W.H.W is supported by DK47402 and DK54983 and S.C.H. is supported by DK54999 and DK17433 from the National Institutes of Health.

References

1. Aguilar-Bryan L, Clement JP, Gonzalez G, Kunjilwar K, Babenko A, Bryan J. Toward understanding the assembly and structure of K_{ATP} channels. *Physiol Rev* 1998;78:227–245.

2. Aguilar-Bryan L, Nichols CG, Wechsler SW, Clement JP, IV, Boyd AE, III, González G, Herrera-Sosa H, Nguy K, Bryan J, Nelson DA. Cloning of the b cell high-affinity sulfonylurea receptor: a regulator of insulin secretion. *Science* 1995;268:423–426.

3. Akao M, Otani H, Horie M, Takano M, Kuniyasu A, Nakayama H, Kouchi I, Murakami T, Sasayama S. Myocardial ischemia induces differential regulation of K_{ATP} channel gene expression in rat hearts. *J Clin Invest* 1997;100:3053–3059.

4. Ali S, Chen X, Lu M, Xu J-C, Lerea KM, Hebert SC, Wang W. A kinase anchoring protein (AKAP) is required for mediating the effect of PKA on ROMK1. *Proc Natl Acad Sci U S A* 1998;95:10274–10278.
5. Arrighi I, Lesage F, Scimeca J-C, Carle GF, Barhanin J. Structure, chromosome localization, and tissue distribution of the mouse *twik* K$^+$ channel gene. *FEBS Lett* 1998;425:310–316.
6. Ashcroft SJH, Ashcroft FM. Properties and functions of ATP-sensitive K-channels. *Cell Signal* 1990;2:197–214.
7. Ashcroft SJH, Ashcroft FM. The sulfonylurea receptor. *Biochim Biophys Acta* 1992; 1175:45–59.
8. Asteria C. Molecular basis of Bartter's syndrome: new insights into correlation between genotype and phenotype. *Eur J Endocrinol* 1997;137:613–615.
9. Attali B, Latter H, Rachamim N, Garty H. A corticosteroid-induced gene expressing an "IsK-like" K$^+$ channel activity in *Xenopus* oocytes. *Proc Natl Acad Sci U S A* 1995;92: 6092–6096.
10. Babenko AP, Aguilar-Bryan L, Bryan J. A view of sur/KIR6.X, K_{ATP} channels. *Ann Rev Physiol* 1998;60:667–687.
11. Babilonia E, Wei Y, Sterling H, Kaminski P, Wolin MS, Wang WH. Superoxide anions are involved in mediating the effect of low K intake on c-Src expression and renal K secretion in the cortical collecting duct. *J Biol Chem* 2005;280:10790–10796.
12. Barhanin J, Lesage F, Guillemare E, Fink M, Lazdunski M, Romey G. KvLQT1 and IsK (minK) proteins associate to form the I_{ks} cardiac potassium current. *Nature* 1996;384:78–80.
13. Bartter FC, Pronove P, Gill JR, Jr., MacCardle RC, Diller E. Hyperplasia of the juxtaglomerular complex with hyperaldosteronoism and hypokalemic alkalosis. *Am J Med* 1962;33:811–828.
14. Baukrowitz T, Schulte U, Oliver D, Herlitze S, Krauter T, Tucker SJ, Ruppersberg JP, Fakler B. PIP_2 and PIP as determinants for ATP inhibition of K_{ATP} channels. *Science* 1998;282:1141–1144.
15. Baukrowitz T, Tucker SJ, Schulte U, Benndorf K, Ruppersberg JP, Fakler B. Inward rectification in K_{ATP} channels: a pH switch in the pore. *EMBO J* 1999;18:847–853.
16. Beesley AH, Hornby D, White SJ. Regulation of distal nephron K$^+$ channels (ROMK) mRNA expression by aldosterone in rat kidney. *J Physiol* 1998;509:629–634.
17. Beesley AH, Ortega B, White SJ. Splicing of a retained intron within ROMK K$^+$ channel RNA generates a novel set of isoforms in rat kidney. *Am J Physiol Cell Physiol* 1999;276: C585–C592.
18. Bleich M, Schlatter E, Greger R. The luminal K$^+$ channel of the thick ascending limb of Henle's loop. *Pflügers Arch* 1990;415:449–460.
19. Bock JH, Shuck ME, Benjamin CW, Chee M, Bienkowski MJ, Slightom JL. Nucleotide sequence analysis of the human KCNJ1 potassium channel locus. *Gene* 1997;188:9–16.
20. Boim MA, Ho K, Shuck ME, Bienkowski MJ, Block JH, Slightom JL, Yang Y, Brenner BM, Hebert SC. ROMK inwardly rectifying ATP-sensitive K$^+$ channel. II. Cloning and distribution of alternative forms. *Am J Physiol* 1995;268:F1132–F1140.
21. Bond CT, Pessia M, Xia XM, Lagrutta A, Kavanaugh MP, Adelman JP. Cloning and expression of a family of inward rectifier potassium channels. *Recep Chan* 1994;2:183–191.
22. Brazier SP, Ramesh B, Haris PI, Lee DC, Srai SK. Secondary structure analysis of the putative membrane-associated domains of the inward rectifier K$^+$ channel ROMK1. *Biochem J* 1998;335:375–380.
23. Brochiero E, Coady MJ, Klein H, Laprade R, Lapointe JY. Activation of an ATP-dependent K$^+$ conductance in *Xenopus* oocytes by expression of adenylate kinase cloned from renal proximal tubules. *Biochim Biophys Acta* 2001;1510:29–42.
24. Brochiero E, Wallendorf B, Gagnon D, Laprade R, Lapointe JY. Cloning of rabbit Kir6.1, SUR2A, and SUR2B: possible candidates for a renal K_{ATP} channel. *Am J Physiol Renal Physiol* 2002;282:F289–F300.
25. Bryan J, Aguilar-Bryan L. The ABCs of ATP-sensitive potassium channels: more pieces of the puzzle. *Curr Opin Cell Biol* 1997;9:553–559.
26. Bryan J, Aguilar-Bryan L. Sulfonylurea receptors: ABC transporters that regulate ATP-sensitive K$^+$ channels. *Biochim Biophys Acta* 1999;1461:285–303.
27. Butler A, Wei A, Baker K, Salkoff L. A family of putative potassium channel genes in *Drosophila*. *Science* 1989;243:943–947.
28. Carrasco AJ, Dzeja PP, Alekseev AE, Pucar D, Zingman LV, Abraham MR, Hodgson D, Bienengraeber M, Puceat M, Janssen E, Wieringa B, Terzic A. Adenylate kinase phosphotransfer communicates cellular energetic signals to ATP-sensitive potassium channels. *Proc Natl Acad Sci U S A* 2001;98:7623–7628.
29. Chavez RA, Gray AT, Zhao BB, Kindler CH, Mazurek MJ, Mehta Y, Forsayeth JR, Yost CS. TWIK-2, a new weak inward rectifing member of the tandem pore domain potassium channel family. *J Biol Chem* 1999;274:7887–7892.
30. Chepilko S, Zhou H, Sackin H, Palmer LG. Permeation and gating properties of a cloned renal K$^+$ channel. *Am J Physiol* 1995;268:C389–C401.
31. Choe H, Palmer LG, Sackin H. Structural determinants of gating in inward-rectifier K$^+$ channels. *Biophys J* 1999;76:1988–2003.
32. Choe H, Sackin H, Palmer LG. Permeation and gating of an inwardly rectifying potassium channel. Evidence for a variable energy well. *J Gen Physiol* 1998;112:433–446.
33. Choe H, Zhou H, Palmer LG, Sackin H. A conserved cytoplasmic region of ROMK modulates pH sensitivity, conductance, and gating. *Am J Physiol Renal Physiol* 1997;273:F516–F529.
34. Clapham DE. Unlocking family secrets: K$^+$ channel transmembrane domains. *Cell* 1999;97: 547–550.
35. Clark MA, Humphrey SJ, Smith MP, Ludens JH. Unique natriuretic properties of the ATP-sensitive K$^+$ channel blocker glyburide in concious rats. *J Pharmacol Exp Ther* 1993;165: 933–937.
36. Clement JP, Kunjilwar K, Gonzalez G, Schwanstecher M, Panten U, Aguilar-Bryan L, Bryan J. Association and stoichiometry of K_{ATP} channel subunits. *Neuron* 1997;18:827–838.
37. Cluzeaud F, Reyes R, Escoubet B, Fay M, Lazdunski M, Bonvalet JP, Lesage F, Farman N. Expression of TWIK-1, a novel weakly inward rectifying potassium channel in rat kidney. *Am J Physiol Cell Physiol* 1998;275:C1602–C1609.
38. Crawford I, Maloney PC, Zeitlin PL, Guggino WB, Hyde SC, Turley H, Gatter KC, Harris A, Higgins CF. Immunocytochemical localization of the cystic fibrosis gene product CFTR. *Proc Natl Acad Sci U S A* 1991;88:9262–9266.
39. Dabrowski M, Tarasov A, Ashcroft FM. Mapping the architecture of the ATP-binding site of the KATP channel subunit Kir6.2. *J Physiol* 2004;557:347–354.
40. Derst C, Hirsch JR, Preisig-Muller R, Wischmeyer E, Karschin A, Doring F, Thomzig A, Veh RW, Schlatter E, Kummer W, Daut J. Cellular localization of the potassium channel Kir7.1 in guinea pig and human kidney. *Kidney Int* 2001;59:2197–2205.
41. Derst C, Konrad M, Köckerling A, Karschin A, Daut J, Seyberth HW. Mutations in the ROMK gene in antenatal Bartter syndrome are associated with impaired K$^+$ channel function. *Biochem Biophys Res Comm* 1997;230:641–645.
42. Doi T, Fakler B, Schultz JH, Ehmke H, Brandle U, Zenner HP, Sussbrich H, Lang F, Ruppersberg JP, Busch AE. Subunit-specific inhibition of inward-rectifier K$^+$ channels by quinidine. *FEBS Lett* 1995;375:193–196.
43. Dong F, Feldmesser M, Casadevall A, Rubin CS. Molecular characterization of a cDNA that encodes six isoforms of a novel murine A kinase anchor protein. *J Biol Chem* 1998;273:6533–6541.
44. Dong K, Tang L, MacGregor GG, Hebert SC. Localization of the ATP/phosphatidylinositol 4,5 diphosphate-binding site to a 39-amino acid region of the carboxyl terminus of the ATP-regulated K$^+$ channel Kir1.1. *J Biol Chem* 2002;277:49366–49373.
45. Dong K, Tang L, MacGregor GG, Leng Q, Hebert SC. Novel nucleotide-binding sites in ATP-sensitive potassium channels formed at gating interfaces. *EMBO J* 2005;24:1318–1329.
46. Doring F, Derst C, Wischmeyer E, Karschin C, Schneggenburger R, Daut J, Karschin A. The epithelial inward rectifier channel Kir7.1 displays unusual K$^+$ permeation properties. *J Neurosci* 1998;18:8625–8636.
47. Doyle DA. Structural changes during ion channel gating. *Trends Neurosci* 2004;27:298–302.
48. Doyle DA, Cabral JM, Pfuetzner RA, Kuo A, Gulbis JM, Cohen SL, Chait BT, MacKinnon R. The structure of the potassium channel: molecular basis of K$^+$ conduction and selectivity. *Science* 1998;280:69–77.
49. Duprat F, Lesage F, Fink M, Reyes R, Heurteaux C, Lazdunski M. TASK, a human background K$^+$ channel to sense external pH variations near physiological pH. *EMBO J* 1997;16:5464–5471.
50. Erginel-Unaltuna N, Yang WP, Blanar MA. Genomic organization and expression of KCNJ8/Kir6.1, a gene encoding a subunit of an ATP-sensitive potassium channel. *Gene* 1998;211:71–78.
51. Estevez R, Boettger T, Stein V, Birkenhager R, Otto E, Hildebrandt F, Jentsch TJ. Barttin is a Cl$^-$ channel b-subunit crucial for renal Cl$^-$ reabsorption and inner ear K$^+$ secretion. *Nature* 2001;414:558–561.
52. Fakler B, Bond CT, Adelman JP, Ruppersberg JP. Heterooligomeric assembly of inward-rectifier K$^+$ channels from subunits of different subfamilies: $K_{ir}2.1$ (IRK1) and $K_{ir}4.1$ (BIR10). *Pflug Arch Eur J Physiol* 1996;433:77–83.
53. Fakler B, Schultz JH, Yang J, Schulte U, Brändle U, Zenner HP, Jan LY, Ruppersberg JP. Identification of a titratable lysine residue that determines sensitivity of kidney potassium channels (ROMK) to intracellular pH. *EMBO J* 1996;15:4093–4099.
54. Farman N, Fay M, Cluzeaud F. Cell-specific expression of three members of the FXYD family along the renal tubule. *Ann N Y Acad Sci* 2003;986:428–436.
55. Faux MC, Scott JD. Molecular glue: kinase anchoring and scaffold proteins. *Cell* 1996;85:9–12.
56. Ficker E, Taglialatela M, Wible BA, Henley CM, Brown AM. Spermine and spermidine as gating molecules for inward rectifier K$^+$ channels. *Science* 1994;266:1068–1072.
57. Fink M, Duprat F, Lesage F, Reyes R, Romey G, Heurteaux C, Lazdunski M. Cloning, functional expression and brain localization of a novel unconventional outward rectifier K$^+$ channel. *EMBO J* 1996;15:6854–6862.
58. Frindt G, Palmer LG. Ca-activated K channels in apical membrane of mammalian CCT, and their role in K secretion. *Am J Physiol Renal Fluid Electrolyte Physiol* 1987;252–21:F458–F467.
59. Frindt G, Palmer LG. Low-conductance K channels in apical membrane of rat cortical collecting tubule. *Am J Physiol Renal Fluid Electrolyte Physiol* 1989;256-25:F143–F151.
60. Frindt G, Zhou H, Sackin H, Palmer LG. Dissociation of K channel density and ROMK mRNA in rat cortical collecting tubule during K adaptation. *Am J Physiol* 1998;274: F525–F531.
61. Fuzesi M, Goldshleger R, Garty H, Karlish SJ. Defining the nature and sites of interaction between FXYD proteins and Na,K-ATPase. *Ann N Y Acad Sci* 2003;986:532–533.
62. Gimelreich D, Popovtzer MM, Wald H, Pizov G, Berlatzky Y, Rubinger D. Regulation of ROMK and channel-inducing factor (CHIF) in acute renal failure due to ischemic reperfusion injury. *Kidney Int* 2001;59:1812–1820.
63. Goulding EH, Tibbs GR, Liu D, Siegelbaum SA. Role of H5 domain in determining pore diameter and ion permeation through cyclic nucleotide-gated channels. *Nature* 1993;364:61–64.
64. Grantham JJ, Lowe CM, Dellasega M, Cole BR. Effect of hypotonic medium on K and Na content of proximal renal tubules. *Am J Physiol Renal Fluid Electrolyte Physiol* 1977;232: F42–F49.
65. Greger R, Bleich M, Schlatter E. Ion channels in the thick ascending limb of Henle's loop. *Renal Physiol Biochem* 1990;13:37–50.
66. Guay-Woodford LM. Molecular insights into the pathogenesis of inherited renal tubular disorders. *Curr Opin Nephrol Hyperten* 1995;4:121–129.
67. Gulbis JM, Doyle DA. Potassium channel structures: do they conform? *Curr Opin Struct Biol* 2004;14:440–446
68. Guy HR, Durell SR. Developing three-dimensional models of ion channel proteins. *Ion Channels* 1996;4:1–40.
69. Hartmann HA, Kirsch GE, Drewe JA, Taglialatela M, Joho RH, Brown AM. Exchange of conduction pathways between two related K$^+$ channels. *Science* 1991;251:942–944.
70. Hebert SC. General principles of the structure of ion channels. *Am J Med* 1998;104:87–98.

71. Hebert SC. Bartter syndrome. *Curr Opin Nephrol Hypertens* 2003;12:527–532.

72. Hebert SC, Wang W-H. Structure and function of the low conductance K_{ATP} channel, ROMK. *Wien Klin Wochenschr* 1997;109:471–476.

73. Heginbotham L, Abramson T, MacKinnon R. A functional connection between the pores of distantly related ion channels as revealed by mutant K^+ channels. *Science* 1992; 258:1152–1155.

74. Hilgemann DW, Ball R. Regulation of cardiac Na^+-Ca^{2+} exchange and K_{ATP} potassium channels by PIP_2. *Science* 1996;273:956–959.

75. Ho K. The ROMK-cystic fibrosis transmembrane conductance regulator connection: new insights into the relationship between ROMK and cystic fibrosis transmembrane conductance regulator channels. *Curr Opin Nephrol Hypertens* 1998;7:49–58.

76. Ho K, Nichols CG, Lederer WJ, Lytton J, Vassilev PM, Kanazirska MV, Hebert SC. Cloning and expression of an inwardly rectifying ATP-regulated potassium channel. *Nature* 1993;362:31–38.

77. Huang C-L, Feng S, Hilgemann DW. Direct activation of inward rectifier potassium channels by PIP_2 and its stabilization by Gbg. *Nature* 1998;391:803–806.

78. Huang DY, Wulff P, Volkl H, Loffing J, Richter K, Kuhl D, Lang F, Vallon V. Impaired regulation of renal K elimination in the sgk1-knockout mouse. *J Am Soc Nephrol* 2004;15:885–891.

79. Hunter M, Lopes AG, Boulpaep EL, Giebisch G. Single channel recordings of calcium-activated potassium channels in the apical emmbrane of rabbit cortical collecting tubules. *Proc Natl Acad Sci U S A* 1984;81:4237–4239.

80. Imredy JP, Chen C, MacKinnon R. A snake toxin inhibitor of inward rectifier potassium channel ROMK1. *Biochemistry* 1998;37:14867–14874.

81. Inagaki N, Gonoi T, Seino S. Subunit stoichiometry of the pancreatic b-cell ATP-sensitive K^+ channel. *FEBS Lett* 1997;409:232–236.

82. Inagaki N, Tsuura Y, Namba N, Masuda K, Gonoi T, Horie M, Seino Y, Mizuta M, Seino S. Cloning and functional characterization of a novel ATP-sensitive potassium channel ubiquitously expressed in rat tissues, including pancreatic islets, pituitary, skeletal muscle, and heart. *J Biol Chem* 1995;270:5691–5694.

83. Ito M, Inanobe A, Horio Y, Hibino H, Isomoto S, Ito H, Mori K, Tonosaki A, Tomoike H, Kurachi Y. Immunologicalization of an inwardly rectifying K^+ channel, K_{AB}-2 (Kir4.1), in the basolateral membrane of renal distal tubular epithelia. *FEBS Lett* 1996;388:11–15.

84. Jan LY, Jan YN. Tracing the roots of ion channels. *Cell* 1992;715:715–718.

85. Jan LY, Jan YN. Potassium channels and their evolving gates. *Nature* 1994;371:119–122.

86. Jan LY, Jan YN. Cloned potassium channels from eukaryotes and prokaryotes. *Ann Rev Neurosci* 1997;20:91–123.

87. Jan LY, Jan YN. Voltage-gated and inwardly rectifying potassium channels. *J Physiol* 1997;505:267–282.

88. Jin W, Lu Z. A novel high-affinity inhibitor for inward-rectifier K^+ channels. *Biochemistry* 1998;37:13291–13299.

89. Kahle KT, Wilson FH, Leng Q, Lalioti MD, O'Connell AD, Dong K, Rapson AK, MacGregor GG, Giebisch G, Hebert SC, Lifton RP. WNK4 regulates the balance between renal NaCl reabsorption and K^+ secretion. *Nat Genet* 2003;35:372–376.

90. Kakei M, Kelly RP, Ashcroft SJH, Ashcroft FM. The ATP-sensitivity of K^+ channels in rat pancreatic B-cells is modulated by ADP. *FEBS Lett* 1986;208:63–66.

91. Kanjhan R, Coulson EJ, Adams DJ, Bellingham MC. Tertiapin-Q blocks recombinant and native large conductance K channels in a use-dependent manner. *J Pharmacol Exp Ther* 2005; 314:1353–1361.

92. Karolyi L, Koch MC, Grzeschik KH, Seyberth HW. The molecular genetic approach to "Bartter's syndrome." *J Mol Med* 1998;76:317–325.

93. Karolyil L, Konrad M, Kockerling A, Ziegler A, Zimmermann DK, Roth B, et al. Mutations in the gene encoding the inwardly-rectifying renal potassium channel, ROMK, cause the antenatal variant of Bartter syndrome: evidence for genetic heterogeneity. *Human Mol Gen* 1997;6:17–26.

94. Kofuji P, Ceelen P, Zahs KR, Surbeck LW, Lester HA, Newman EA. Genetic inactivation of an inwardly rectifying potassium channel (Kir4.1 subunit) in mice: phenotypic impact in retina. *J Neurosci* 2000;20:5733–5740.

95. Kohda Y, Ding W, Phan E, Housini I, Wang J, Star RA, Huang CL. Localization of the ROMK potassium channel to the apical membrane of distal nephron in rat kidney. *Kidney Int* 1998;54:1214–1223.

96. Kondo C, Isomoto S, Matsumoto S, Yamada M, Horio Y, Yamashita S, Takemura-Kameda K, Matsuzawa Y, Kurachi Y. Cloning and functional expression of a novel isoform of ROMK inwardly rectifying ATP-dependent K^+ channel, ROMK6 (Kir1.1f). *FEBS Lett* 1996;399:122–126.

97. Konstas AA, Korbmacher C, Tucker SJ. Identification of domains which control the heteromeric assembly of Kir5.1/Kir4.0 potassium channels. *Am J Physiol Cell Physiol* 2003;284:C910–C917.

98. Koster JC, Bentle KA, Nichols CG, Ho K. Assembly of ROMK1 (Kir1.1a) inward rectifier K^+ channel subunits involves multiple interaction sites. *Biophys J* 1998;74:1821–1829.

99. Krapivinsky G, Medina I, Eng L, Krapivinsky L, Yang Y, Clapham DE. A novel inward rectifier K^+ channel with unique pore properties. *Neuron* 1998;20:995–1005.

100. Kubo Y, Baldwin TJ, Jan YN, Jan LY. Primary structure and functional expression of a mouse inward rectifier potassium channel. *Nature* 1993;362:127–133.

101. Kuo A, Gulbis JM, Antcliff JF, Rahman T, Lowe ED, Zimmer J, Cuthbertson J, Ashcroft FM, Ezaki T, Doyle DA. Crystal structure of the potassium channel KirBac1.1 in the closed state. *Science* 2003;300:1922–1926.

102. Le Maout S, Brejon M, Olsen O, Merot J, Welling PA. Basolateral membrane targeting of a renal-epithelial inwardly rectifying potassium channel from the cortical collecting duct, CCD- IRK3, in MDCK cells. *Proc Natl Acad Sci U S A* 1997;94:13329–13334.

103. Le Maout S, Welling PA, Brejon M, Olsen O, Merot J. Basolateral membrane expression of a K^+ channel, Kir 2.3, is directed by a cytoplasmic COOH-terminal domain. *Proc Natl Acad Sci U S A* 2001;98:10475–10480.

104. Lee W-S, Hebert SC. The ROMK inwardly rectifying ATP-sensitive K^+ channel. I. Expression in rat distal nephron segments. *Am J Physiol Renal Fluid Electrolyte Physiol* 1995;268: F1124–F1131.

105. Leipziger J, MacGregor GG, Cooper GJ, Xu J, Hebert SC, Giebisch G. PKA site mutations of ROMK2 channels shift the pH dependence to more alkaline values. *Am J Physiol Renal Physiol* 2000;279:F919–F926.

106. Lesage F, Guillemare E, Fink M, Duprat F, Lazdunski M, Romey G, Barhanin J. TWIK-1, a ubiquitous human weakly inward rectifying K^+ channel with a novel structure. *EMBO J* 1996; 15:1004–1011.

107. Deleted in proof.

108. Lesage F, Lauritzen I, Duprat F, Reyes R, Fink M, Heurteaux C, Lazdunski M. The structure, function and distribution of the mouse TWIK-1 K^+ channel. *FEBS Lett* 1997;402:28–32.

109. Lesage F, Lazdunski M. Mapping of human potassium channel genes TREK-1 (*KCNK2*) and TASK (*KCNK3*) to chromosomes 1q41 and 2p23. *Genomics* 1998;51:478–479.

110. Leung YM, Zeng WZ, Liou HH, Solaro CR, Huang CL. Phosphatidylinositol 4,5-bisphosphate and intracellular pH regulate the ROMK1 potassium channel via separate but interrelated mechanisms. *J Biol Chem* 2000;275:10182–10189.

111. Lin DH, Sterling H, Lerea KM, Giebisch G, Wang WH. Protein kinase C (PKC)-induced phosphorylation of ROMK1 is essential for the surface expression of ROMK1 channels. *J Biol Chem* 2002;277:44332–44338.

112. Lin DH, Sterling H, Lerea KM, Welling P, Jin L, Giebisch G, Wang WH. K depletion increases the protein tyrosine-mediated phosphorylation of ROMK. *Am J Physiol Renal Physiol* 2002;283:F671–F677.

113. Lin DH, Sterling H, Wang Z, Babilonia E, Yang B, Dong K, Hebert SC, Giebisch G, Wang WH. ROMK1 channel activity is regulated by monoubiquitination. *Proc Natl Acad Sci U S A* 2005;102:4306–4311.

114. Lin DH, Sterling H, Yang B, Hebert SC, Giebisch G, Wang WH. Protein tyrosine kinase is expressed and regulates ROMK1 location in the cortical collecting duct. *Am J Physiol Renal Physiol* 2004;286:F881–F892.

115. Liou HH, Zhou SS, Huang CL. Regulation of ROMK1 channel by protein kinase A via a phosphatidylinositol 4,5-bisphosphate-dependent mechanism. *Proc Natl Acad Sci U S A* 1999; 96:5820–5825.

116. Lopatin AN, Makhina EN, Nichols CG. Potassium channel block by cytoplasmic polyamines as the mechanism of intrinsic rectification. *Nature* 1994;372:366–369.

117. Lorenz E, Alekseev AE, Krapivinsky GB, Carrasco AJ, Clapham DE, Terzic A. Evidence for direct physical association between a K^+ channel (Kir6.2) and ATP-binding cassette protein (SUR1) which affects cellular distribution and kinetic behavior of an ATP-sensitive K^+ channel. *Mol Cell Biol* 1998;18:1652–1659.

118. Lorenz JN, Baird NR, Judd LM, Noonan WT, Andringa A, Doetschman T, Manning PA, Liu LH, Miller ML, Shull GE. Impaired renal NaCl absorption in mice lacking the ROMK potassium channel, a model for type II Bartter's syndrome. *J Biol Chem* 2002;277:37871–37880.

119. Lourdel S, Paulais M, Cluzeaud F, Bens M, Tanemoto M, Kurachi Y, Vandewalle A, Teulon J. An inward rectifier K^+ channel at the basolateral membrane of the mouse distal convoluted tubule: similarities with Kir4-Kir5.1 heteromeric channels. *J Physiol* 2002;538:391–404.

120. Lu M, Wang T, Yan Q, Wang W, Giebisch G, Hebert SC. ROMK is required for expression of the 70pS K channel in the thick ascending limb. *Am J Physiol Renal Physiol* 2004;286: F490–F495.

121. Lu M, Wang T, Yan Q, Yang X, Dong K, Knepper MA, Wang W, Giebisch G, Shull GE, Hebert SC. Absence of small-conductance K^+ channel (SK) activity in apical membranes of thick ascending limb and cortical collecting duct in ROMK (Bartter's) knockout mice. *J Biol Chem* 2002;277:37881–37887.

122. Lu Z, MacKinnon R. Electrostatic tuning of Mg^{2+} affinity in an inward-rectifier K^+ channel. *Nature* 1994;371:243–246.

123. Lundgren DW, Moore JJ, Chang SM, Collins PL, Chang AS. Gestational changes in the uterine expression of an inwardly rectifying K^+ channel, ROMK. *Proc Soc Exp Biol Med* 1997;216:57–64.

124. MacGregor GG, Xu J, McNicholas CM, Giebisch G, Hebert SC. Partially active channels produced by PKA site mutation of the cloned renal K^+ channel ROMK2. *Am J Physiol Renal Physiol* 1998;275:F415–F422.

125. Macica CM, Yang Y, Hebert SC, Wang W-H. Arachidonic acid inhibits the activity of the cloned renal K^+ channel, ROMK1. *Am J Physiol Renal Fluid Electrolyte Physiol* 1996;40: F588–F594.

126. Macica CM, Yang Y, Lerea K, Hebert SC, Wang W. Role of the NH_2 terminus of the cloned renal K^+ channel, ROMK1, in arachidonic acid-mediated inhibition. *Am J Physiol Renal Physiol* 1997;274:F175–F181.

127. MacKinnon R, Cohen SL, Kuo A, Lee A, Chait BT. Structural conservation in prokaryotic and eukaryotic potassium channels. *Science* 1998;280:106–109.

128. MacKinnon R, Yellen G. Mutations affecting TEA blockade and ion permeation in voltage-activated K^+ channels. *Science* 1990;250:276–279.

129. Makita K, Takahashi K, Kerara A, Jacobson HR, Falck JR, Capdevila JH. Experimental and/or genetically controlled alterations of the renal microsomal cytochrome P450 epoxygenase induce hypertension in rats fed a high salt diet. *J Clin Invest* 1994;94:2414–2420.

130. Malnic G, Klose R, Giebisch G. Micropuncture study of renal potassium excretion in the rat. *Am J Physiol* 1964;206:674–686.

131. McNicholas CM, Guggino WB, Schwiebert EM, Hebert SC, Giebisch G, Egan ME. Sensitivity of a renal K^+ channel (ROMK2) to the inhibitory sulfonylurea compound, glibenclamide, is enhanced by co-expression with the ATP-binding cassette transporter cystic fibrosis transmembrane regulator. *Proc Natl Acad Sci U S A* 1996;93:8083–8088.

132. McNicholas CM, MacGregor GG, Islas LD, Yang Y, Hebert SC, Giebisch G. pH-dependent modulation of the cloned renal K^+ channel, ROMK. *Am J Physiol Renal Physiol* 1998;275:F972–F981.

133. McNicholas CM, Nason MW, Guggino WB, Schwiebert EM, Hebert SC, Giebisch G, Egan ME. A functional CFTR-NBF1 is required for ROMK2-CFTR interaction. *Am J Physiol Renal Physiol* 1997;273:F843–F848.

134. McNicholas CM, Wang W, Ho K, Hebert SC, Giebisch G. Regulation of ROMK1 K^+ channel activity involves phosphorylation processes. *Proc Natl Acad Sci U S A* 1994;91:8077–8081.

135. McNicholas CM, Yang Y, Giebisch G, Hebert SC. Molecular site for nucleotide binding on an ATP-sensitive renal K⁺ channel (ROMK2). *Am J Physiol Renal Fluid Electrolyte Physiol* 1996;271:F275–F285.

136. Mennitt PA, Wade JB, Ecelbarger CA, Palmer LG, Frindt G. Localization of ROMK channels in the rat kidney. *J Am Soc Nephrol* 1997;8:1823–1830.

137. Mikhailov MV, Proks P, Ashcroft FM, Ashcroft SJ. Expression of functionally active ATP-sensitive K-channels in insect cells using baculovirus. *FEBS Lett* 1998;429:390–394.

138. Minor DL, Masseling SJ, Jan YN, Jan LY. Transmembrane structure of an inwardly rectifying potassium channel. *Cell* 1999;97:879–891.

139. Misler S, Giebisch G. ATP-sensitive potassium channels in physiology, pathophysiology, and pharmacology. *Curr Opin Nephrol Hypertens* 1992;1:21–33.

140. Moral Z, Dong K, Wei Y, Sterling H, Deng H, Ali S, Gu R, Huang XY, Hebert SC, Giebisch G, Wang WH. Regulation of ROMK1 channels by protein-tyrosine kinase and -tyrosine phosphatase. *J Biol Chem* 2001;276:7156–7163.

141. Morales MM, Carroll TP, Morita T, Schwiebert EM, Devuyst O, Wilson PD, Lopes AG, Stanton BA, Dietz HC, Cutting GR, Guggino WB. Both the wild type and a functional isoform of CFTR are expressed in kidney. *Am J Physiol Renal Fluid Electrolyte Physiol* 1996;270:F1038–F1048.

142. Nakamura N, Suzuki Y, Sakuta H, Ookata K, Kawahara K, Hirose S. Inwardly rectifying K⁺ channel Kir7.1 is highly expressed in thyroid follicular cells, intestinal epithelial cells and choroid plexus epithelial cells: implication for a functional coupling with Na⁺,K⁺-ATPase. *Biochem J* 1999;342(Pt 2):329–336.

143. Nichols CG, Ho K, Hebert SC. Mg²⁺-dependent inward rectification of ROMK1 potassium channels expressed in *Xenopus* oocytes. *J Physiol* 1994;476:399–409.

144. Nichols CG, Lopatin AN. Inward rectifier potassium channels. *Ann Rev Physiol* 1997;59: 171–191.

145. Nishida M, MacKinnon R. Structural basis of inward rectification. cytoplasmic pore of the G protein-gated inward rectifier GIRK1 at 1.8 Å resolution. *Cell* 2002;111:957–965.

146. O'Connell AD, Leng Q, Dong K, MacGregor GG, Giebisch G, Hebert SC. Phosphorylation regulated ER retention signal in the ROMK potassium channel. *Proc Natl Acad Sci U S A* 2005;102:9954–9959.

147. Oberleithner H, Schneider SW, Henderson RM. Structural activity of a cloned potassium channel (ROMK1) monitored with the atomic force microscope: The "molecular-sandwich" technique. *Proc Natl Acad Sci U S A* 1997;94:14144–14149.

148. Oliver D, Hahn H, Antz C, Ruppersberg JP, Fakler B. Interaction of permeant and blocking ions in cloned inward-rectifier K⁺ channels. *Biophys J* 1998;74:2318–2326.

149. Olsen O, Liu H, Wade JB, Merot J, Welling PA. Basolateral membrane expression of the Kir 2.3 channel is coordinated by PDZ interaction with Lin-7/CASK complex. *Am J Physiol Cell Physiol* 2002;282:C183–C195.

150. Ookata K, Tojo A, Suzuki Y, Nakamura N, Kimura K, Wilcox CS, Hirose S. Localization of inward rectifier potassium channel Kir7.1 in the basolateral membrane of distal nephron and collecting duct. *J Am Soc Nephrol* 2000;11:1987–1994.

151. Orias M, Bray-Ward P, Curran ME, Keating MT, Desir GV. Genomic localization of the human gene for KCNA10, a cGMP-activated K channel. *Genomics* 1997;42:33–37.

152. Orias M, Velazquez H, Tung F, Lee G, Desir GV. Cloning and localization of a double-pore K channel, KCNK1: exclusive expression in distal nephron segments. *Am J Physiol* 1997;273: F663–F666.

153. Palmer LG. Potassium secretion and the regulation of distal nephron K channels. *Am J Physiol* 1999;277:F821–F825.

154. Palmer LG, Antonian L, Frindt G. Regulation of apical K and Na channels and Na/K pumps in rat cortical collecting tubule by dietary K. *J Gen Physiol* 1994;104:693–710.

155. Palmer LG, Choe H, Frindt G. Is the secretory K channel in the rat CCT ROMK? *Am J Physiol Renal Fluid Electrolyte Physiol* 1997;273:F404–F410.

156. Palmer LG, Frindt G. Regulation of apical K channels in rat cortical collecting tubule during changes in dietary K intake. *Am J Physiol* 1999;277:F805–F812.

157. Partiseti M, Collura V, Agnel M, Culouscou JM, Graham D. Cloning and characterization of a novel human inwardly rectifying potassium channel predominantly expressed in small intestine. *FEBS Lett* 1998;434:171–176.

158. Patel AJ, Honore E, Maingret F, Lesage F, Fink M, Duprat F, Lazdunski M. A mammalian two pore domain mechano-gated S-like K⁺ channel. *EMBO J* 1998;17:4283–4290.

159. Pawson T, Scott JD. Signaling through scaffold, anchoring, and adaptor proteins. *Science* 1997;278:2075–2080.

160. Pearson WL, Dourado M, Schreiber M, Salkoff L, Nichols CG. Expression of a functional Kir4 family inward rectifier K⁺ channel from a gene cloned from mouse liver. *J Physiol* 1999;514(Pt 3):639–653.

161. Pessia M, Imbrici P, D'Adamo MC, Salvatore L, Tucker SJ. Differential pH sensitivity of Kir4.1 and Kir4.2 potassium channels and their modulation by heteropolymerisation with Kir5.1. *J Physiol* 2001;532:359–367.

162. Reeves WB, McDonald GA, Mehta P, Andreoli TE. Activation of K⁺ channels in renal medullary vesicles by cAMP-dependent protein kinase. *J Membr Biol* 1989;109:65–72.

163. Reyes R, Duprat F, Lesage F, Fink M, Salinas M, Farman N, Lazdunski M. Cloning and expression of a novel pH-sensitive two pore domain K⁺ channel from human kidney. *J Biol Chem* 1998;273:30863–30869.

164. Rodriguez-Soriano J. Bartter and related syndromes: the puzzle is almost solved. *Pediatr Nephrol* 1998;12:315–327.

165. Ruknudin A, Schulze DH, Sullivan SK, Lederer WJ, Welling PA. Novel subunit composition of a renal epithelial K_ATP channel. *J Biol Chem* 1998;273:14165–14171.

166. Sabirov RZ, Morishima S, Okada Y. Probing the water permeability of ROMK1 and amphotericin B channels using *Xenopus* oocytes. *Biochim Biophys Acta* 1998;1368:19–26.

167. Sabirov RZ, Tominaga T, Miwa A, Okada Y. A conserved arginine residue in the pore region of an inward rectifier K channel (IRK1) as an external barrier for cationic blockers. *J Gen Physiol* 1997;110:665–677.

168. Sackin H, Vasilyev A, Palmer LG, Krambis M. Permeant cations and blockers modulate pH gating of ROMK channels. *Biophys J* 2003;84:910–921.

169. Sanguinetti MC, Curran ME, Zou A, Shen J, Spector PS, Atkinson DL, Keating MT. Coassembly of K_vLQT1 and minK (IsK) proteins to form cardiac I_Ks potassium channel. *Nature* 1996;384:80–83.

170. Schlatter E, Bleich M, Hirsch J, Greger R. pH-sensitive K⁺ channels in the distal nephron. *Nephrol Dial Transpl* 1993;8:488–490.

171. Schlatter E, Lohrmann E, Greger R. Properties of the potassium conductances of principal cells of rat cortical collecting ducts. *Pflügers Arch* 1992;420:39–45.

172. Schulte U, Hahn H, Wiesinger H, Ruppersberg JP, Fakler B. pH-dependent gating of ROMK (K_ir1.1) channels involves conformational changes in both N and C termini. *J Biol Chem* 1998;273:34575–34579.

173. Schwalbe RA, Bianchi L, Accili EA, Brown AM. Functional consequences of ROMK mutants linked to antenatal Bartter's syndrome and implications for treatment. *Hum Mol Genet* 1998;7:975–980.

174. Deleted in proof.

175. Schwalbe RA, Bianchi L, Brown AM. Mapping the kidney potassium channel ROMK1. Glycosylation of the pore sequence and the COOH terminus. *J Biol Chem* 1997;272:25217–25223.

176. Schwalbe RA, Wang Z, Bianchi L, Brown AM. Novel sites of N-glycosylation in ROMK1 reveal the putative pore-forming segment H5 as extracellular. *J Biol Chem* 1996;271:24201–24206.

177. Seino S. ATP-sensitive potassium channels: a model of heteromultimeric potassium channel/receptor assemblies. *Ann Rev Physiol* 1999;61:337–362.

178. Shi H, Levy-Holzman R, Cluzeaud F, Farman N, Garty H. Membrane topology and immunolocalization of CHIF in kidney and intestine. *Am J Physiol Renal Physiol* 2001;280: F505–F512.

179. Shuck ME, Block JH, Benjamin CW, Tsai T-D, Lee KS, Slightom JL, Bienkowski MJ. Cloning and characterization of multiple forms of the human kidney ROM-K potassium channel. *J Biol Chem* 1994;269:24261–24270.

180. Shuck ME, Piser TM, Block JH, Slightom JL, Lee KS, Bienkowski MJ. Cloning and characterization of two K⁺ inward rectifier (K_ir) 1.1 potassium channel homologs from human kidney (K_ir1.2 and K_ir1.3). *J Biol Chem* 1997;272:586–593.

181. Simon DB, Bindra RS, Mansfield TA, Nelson-Williams C, Mendonça E, Stone R, et al. Mutations in the chloride channel gene, CLCNKB, cause Bartter's syndrome type III. *Nat Genet* 1997;17:171–178.

182. Simon DB, Karet FE, Hamdan JM, DiPietro A, Sanjad SA, Lifton RP. Bartter's syndrome, hypokalaemic alkalosis with hypercalciuria, is caused by mutations in the Na-K-2Cl cotransporter NKCC2. *Nat Genet* 1996;13:183–188.

183. Simon DB, Karet FE, Rodriguez-Soriano J, Hamdan JH, DiPietro A, Trachtman H, Sanjad SA, Lifton RP. Genetic heterogeneity of Bartter's syndrome revealed by mutations in the K⁺ channel, ROMK. *Nat Genet* 1996;14:152–156.

184. Spassova M, Lu Z. Coupled ion movement underlies rectification in an inward-rectifier K⁺ channel. *J Gen Physiol* 1998;112:211–221.

185. Suzuki M, Kotake K, Fujikura K, Inagaki N, Suzuki T, Gonoi T, Seino S, Takata K. Kir6.1: a possible subunit of ATP-sensitive K⁺ channels in mitochondria. *Biochem Biophys Res Commun* 1997;241:693–697.

186. Taglialatela M, Wible BA, Caporaso R, Brown AM. Specification of pore properties by the carboxyl terminus of inwardly rectifying K⁺ channels. *Science* 1994;264:844–847.

187. Takumi T, Ishii T, Horio Y, Morishige K, Takahashi N, Yamada M, Yamashita T, Kiyama H, Sohmiya K, Nakanishi S, Kurachi Y. A novel ATP-dependent inward rectifier potassium channel expressed predominantly in glial cells. *J Biol Chem* 1995;270:16339–16346.

188. Tanabe K, Tucker SJ, Ashcroft FM, Proks P, Kioka N, Amachi T, Ueda K. Direct photoaffinity labeling of Kir6.2 by (g-³²P)ATP-(g)4- azidoanilide. *Biochem Biophys Res Commun* 2000;272:316–319.

189. Tanabe T, Tucker SJ, Matsuo M, Proks P, Ashcroft FM, Seino S, Amachi T, Ueda K. Direct photoaffinity labeling of the Kir6.2 subunit of the ATP-sensitive K⁺ channel by 8-azido-ATP*. *J Biol Chem* 1999;274:3931–3933.

190. Tanemoto M, Kittaka N, Inanobe A, Kurachi Y. *In vivo* formation of a proton-sensitive K⁺ channel by heteromeric subunit assembly of Kir5.1 with Kir4.1. *J Physiol* 2000;525(Pt 3): 587–592.

191. Taniguchi J, Imai M. Flow-dependent activation of maxi K⁺ channels in apical membrane of rabbit connecting tubule. *J Membr Biol* 1998;164:35–45.

192. Tinker A, Jan YN, Jan LY. Regions responsible for the assembly of inwardly rectifying potassium channels. *Cell* 1996;87:857–868.

193. Tsai TD, Shuck ME, Thompson DP, Bienkowski MJ, Lee KS. Intracellular H⁺ inhibits a cloned rat kidney outer medulla K⁺ channel expressed in *Xenopus* oocytes. *Am J Physiol* 1995; 268:C1173–C1178.

194. Tucker SJ, Imbrici P, Salvatore L, D'Adamo MC, Pessia M. pH dependence of the inwardly rectifying potassium channel, Kir5.1, and localization in renal tubular epithelia. *J Biol Chem* 2000;275:16404–16407.

195. Vallon V, Grahammer F, Richter K, Bleich M, Lang F, Barhanin J, Volkl H, Warth R. Role of KCNE1-dependent K⁺ fluxes in mouse proximal tubule. *J Am Soc Nephrol* 2001;12: 2003–2011.

196. Vanoye CG, MacGregor GG, Dong K, Tang L, Buschmann AE, Hall AE, Lu M, Giebisch G, Hebert SC. The carboxyl termini of K_ATP channels bind nucleotides. *J Biol Chem* 2002; 277:23260–23270.

197. Vargas-Poussou R, Feldmann D, Vollmer M, Konrad M, Kelly L, van den Heuvel LP, et al. Novel molecular variants of the Na-K-2Cl cotransporter gene are responsible for antenatal Bartter syndrome. *Am J Hum Genet* 1998;62:1332–1340.

198. Vargas-Poussou R, Huang C, Hulin P, Houillier P, Jeunemaitre X, Paillard M, Planelles G, Dechaux M, Miller RT, Antignac C. Functional characterization of a calcium-sensing receptor mutation in severe autosomal dominant hypocalcemia with a Bartter-like syndrome. *J Am Soc Nephrol* 2002;13:2259–2266.

199. Vollmer M, Koehrer M, Topaloglu R, Strahm B, Omran H, Hildebrandt F. Two novel mutations of the gene for Kir 1.1 (ROMK) in neonatal Bartter syndrome. *Pediatr Nephrol* 1998; 12:69–71.

200. Wald H, Garty H, Palmer LG, Popovtzer MM. Differential regulation of ROMK expression in kidney cortex and medulla by aldosterone and potassium. *Am J Physiol* 1998;275:F239–F245.

201. Wald H, Popovtzer MM, Garty H. Differential regulation of CHIF mRNA by potassium intake and aldosterone. *Am J Physiol* 1997;272:F617–F623.

202. Wang Q, Curran ME, Splawski I, Burn TC, Millholland JM, VanRaay TJ, Shen J, Timothy KW, Vincent GM, de Jager T, Schwartz PJ, Toubin JA, Moss AJ, Atkinson DL, Landes GM, Connors TD, Keating MT. Positional cloning of a novel potassium channel gene: KLQT1 mutations cause cardiac arrhythmias. *Nat Genet* 1996;12:17–23.

203. Wang T, Wang W-H, Klein-Robbenhaar G, Giebisch G. Effects of glyburide on renal tubule transport and potassium-channel activity. *Renal Physiol Biochem* 1995;18:169–182.

204. Wang WH. Two types of K$^+$ channel in TAL of rat kidney. *Am J Physiol Renal Fluid Electrolyte Physiol* 1994;267:F599–F605.

205. Wang WH, Giebisch G. Dual effect of adenosine triphosphate on the apical small conductance K$^+$ channel of the rat cortical collecting duct. *J Gen Physiol* 1991;98:35–61.

206. Wang WH, Hebert SC, Giebisch G. Renal K$^+$ channels: structure and function. *Ann Rev Physiol* 1997;59:413–436.

207. Wang WH, Sackin H, Giebisch G. Renal potassium channels and their regulation. *Annu Rev Physiol* 1992;54:81–96.

208. Wang WH, Schwab A, Giebisch G. Regulation of small-conductance K$^+$ channel in apical membrane of rat cortical collecting duct. *Am J Physiol Renal Fluid Electrolyte Physiol* 1990;259:F494–F502.

209. Wang WH, White S, Geibel J, Giebisch G. A potassium channel in the apical membrane of rabbit thick ascending limb of Henle's loop. *Am J Physiol Renal Fluid Electrolyte Physiol* 1990; 258-27:F244–F253.

210. Wang WH, Giebisch G. Dual modulation of renal ATP-sensitive K$^+$ channel by protein kinases A and C. *Proc Natl Acad Sci U S A* 1991;88:9722–9725.

211. Wang WH, Giebisch G. The role of potassium and sodium channels in renal tubule electrolyte transport. *Nippon Jinzo Gakkai Shi* 1991;33:448–462.

212. Watanabe S, Fukumoto S, Chang H, Takeuchi Y, Hasegawa Y, Okazaki R, Chikatsu N, Fujita T. Association between activating mutations of calcium-sensing receptor and Bartter's syndrome. *Lancet* 2002;360:692–694.

213. Wei A, Jegla T, Salkoff L. Eight potassium channel families revealed by the *C. elegans* genome project. *Neuropharmacology* 1996;35:805–829.

214. Wei Y, Bloom P, Lin DH, Gu RM, Wang WH. Effect of dietary K intake on the apical small-conductance K channel in the CCD: Role of protein tyrosine kinase. *Am J Physiol Renal Physiol* 2001;281:F206–F212.

215. Welling PA. Primary structure and functional expression of a cortical collecting duct K$_{ir}$ channel. *Am J Physiol* 1997;273:F825–F836.

216. Wible BA, Taglialatela M, Ficker E, Brown AM. Gating of inwardly rectifying K$^+$ channels localized to a single negatively charged residue. *Nature* 1994;371:246–249.

217. Woda CB, Bragin A, Kleyman TR, Satlin LM. Flow-dependent K$^+$ secretion in the cortical collecting duct is mediated by a maxi-K channel. *Am J Physiol Renal Physiol* 2001;280: F786–F793.

218. Xu H, Cui N, Yang Z, Qu Z, Jiang C. Modulation of kir4.1 and kir5.1 by hypercapnia and intracellular acidosis. *J Physiol* 2000;524(Pt 3):725–735.

219. Xu JZ, Hall AE, Peterson LN, Bienkowski MJ, Eessalu TE, Hebert SC. Localization of the ROMK protein on apical membranes of rat kidney nephron segments. *Am J Physiol Renal Physiol* 1997;273:F739–F748.

220. Xu ZC, Yang Y, Hebert SC. Phosphorylation of the ATP-sensitive, inwardly rectifying K$^+$ channel, ROMK, by cyclic AMP-dependent protein kinase. *J Biol Chem* 1996;271:9313–9319.

221. Yang C-L, Angell J, Mitchell R, Ellison DH. WNK kinases regulate thiazide-sensitive Na-Cl cotransport. *J Clin Invest* 2003;111:947–950.

222. Yang J, Jan YN, Jan LY. Control of rectification and permeation by residues in two distinct domains in an inward rectifier K$^+$ channel. *Neuron* 1995;14:1047–1054.

223. Yang J, Jan YN, Jan LY. Determination of the subunit stoichiometry of an inwardly rectifying potassium channel. *Neuron* 1995;15:1441–1447.

224. Yang J, Yu M, Jan YN, Jan LY. Stabilization of ion selectivity filter by pore loop ion pairs in an inwardly rectifying potassium channel. *Proc Natl Acad Sci U S A* 1997;94:1568–1572.

225. Yang Z, Jiang C. Opposite effects of pH on open-state probability and single channel conductance of kir4.1 channels. *J Physiol* 1999;520(Pt 3):921–927.

226. Yang Z, Xu H, Cui N, Qu Z, Chanchevalap S, Shen W, Jiang C. Biophysical and molecular mechanisms underlying the modulation of heteromeric Kir4.1-Kir5.1 channels by CO$_2$ and pH. *J Gen Physiol* 2000;116:33–45.

227. Yano H, Philipson LH, Kugler JL, Tokuyama Y, Davis EM, Le Beau MM, Nelson DJ, Bell GI, Takeda J. Alternative splicing of human inwardly rectifying K$^+$ channel ROMK1 mRNA. *Mol Pharmacol* 1994;45:854–860.

228. Yao X, Tian S, Chan H-Y, Biemesderfer D, Desir GV. Expression of KCNA10, a voltage-gated K channel, in glomerular endothelium and at the apical membrane of the renal proximal tubule. *J Am Soc Nephrol* 2002;13:2831–2839.

229. Yellen G, Jurman ME, Abramson T, MacKinnon R. Mutations affecting internal TEA blockade identify the probable pore-forming region of a K$^+$ channel. *Science* 1991;251: 939–942.

230. Yoo D, Kim BY, Campo C, Nance L, King A, Maouyo D, Welling PA. Cell surface expression of the ROMK (Kir 1.1) channel is regulated by the aldosterone-induced kinase, SGK-1, and protein kinase A. *J Biol Chem* 2003;278:23066–23075.

231. Yool AJ, Schwarz TL. Alteration of ionic selectivity of a K$^+$ channel by mutation of the H5 region. *Nature* 1991;349:700–704.

232. Yun CC, Palmada M, Embark HM, Fedorenko O, Feng Y, Henke G, Setiawan I, Boehmer C, Weinman EJ, Sandrasagra S, Korbmacher C, Cohen P, Pearce D, Lang F. The serum and glucocorticoid-inducible kinase SGK1 and the Na$^+$/H$^+$ exchange regulating factor NHERF2 synergize to stimulate the renal outer medullary K$^+$ channel ROMK1. *J Am Soc Nephrol* 2002; 13:2823–2830.

233. Zeng WZ, Li XJ, Hilgemann DW, Huang CL. Protein kinase C inhibits ROMK1 channel activity via a phosphatidylinositol 4,5-bisphosphate-dependent mechanism. *J Biol Chem* 2003;278:16852–16856.

234. Zhou H, Chepilko S, Schutt W, Choe H, Palmer LG, Sackin H. Mutations in the pore region of ROMK enhance Ba^{2+} block. *Am J Physiol* 1996;271:C1949–C1956.

CHAPTER **45**

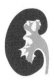

Expression, Function, and Regulation of H$^+$,K$^+$-ATPase in the Kidney

Carsten A. Wagner and John P. Geibel

University of Zurich, Zurich, Switzerland
Yale University School of Medicine, New Haven, Connecticut, USA

Three types of ATPases have been identified in prokaryotes and eukaryotes: F-type, V-type and P-type ATPases. F-type ATPases are found in bacteria, plants, and in the inner membrane of mitochondria using the proton gradient to synthesize ATP. V-type ATPases reverse this process by generating H$^+$ gradients across membranes when hydrolyzing ATP. V-type ATPases are found in many intracellular organelles and in some specialized cells in the plasma membrane. The structure and function of V-type H$^+$-ATPases have been extensively reviewed (56, 57, 72). P-type ATPases comprise a large family of ATPases that couple the hydrolysis of ATP to the movement of ions across membranes and undergo phosphorylation during this process. A variety of cations is transported by P-type ATPases such as: Na$^+$, K$^+$, H$^+$, Ca^{2+}, Cu^{2+}, or Mg^{2+} in a unidirectional and bidirectional manner. Thus, P-type ATPases provide for energy-dependent movement of ions over membranes. This chapter will focus on the function and regulation of H$^+$,K$^+$-ATPases mediating the cellular uptake of K$^+$ against H$^+$ excretion. Another member of this important family of P-type ATPases, Na$^+$,K$^+$-ATPase, will be reviewed in another chapter of this book (Chapter 3).

In contrast to F-type and V-type ATPases, in mammals P-type ATPases consist of only two heteromeric subunits; an α subunit that is mainly involved in ion translocation and ATP-hydrolysis and a β subunit that appears essential for membrane targeting and protein stability. Two isoforms of α and β subunits have been identified in mammals, the gastric alpha (ATP4α) and β (ATP4β) subunits, and the nongastric α (ATP12α, formerly known as ATP1AL1) that most likely associates with the β1 subunit of the Na$^+$,K$^+$-ATPase (for nomenclature and former aliases see http://www.gene.ucl.ac.uk/nomenclature/).

Besides their expression in kidney, H$^+$,K$^+$-ATPases have been found in numerous other tissues including stomach, colon, skin, and urinary bladder. In the stomach the H$^+$,K$^+$-ATPase is essential for gastric acid secretion, in the colon an isoform of this protein is involved in K$^+$ absorption. In the kidney, as discussed below, both of these subtypes of

H$^+$,K$^+$-ATPases are expressed and appear to be mainly involved in K$^+$-absorption under conditions of systemic potassium depletion. Several aspects of H$^+$,K$^+$-ATPase biology have been reviewed elsewhere (11, 26, 38, 67, 78, 80).

FUNCTIONAL PROPERTIES, PHARMACOLOGY, AND PHYSIOLOGY

Three Types of H$^+$,K$^+$-ATPase Activity

On the basis of functional and pharmacological properties, at least three types of H$^+$,K$^+$-ATPase activity have been identified and distinguished in renal tubules. These subtypes differ in their (1) sensitivity to the inhibitors Sch 28080 and ouabain, (2) specificity for K$^+$ versus Na$^+$ ions, (3) response to dietary K$^+$ intake, and (4) cellular localization. Table 1 summarizes the main features of these subtypes (7, 67).

The term "H$^+$,K$^+$-ATPase" implies that the exchange of potassium and protons is the only or at least major transport mode of this class of ATPases. Heterologous expression of H$^+$,K$^+$-ATPase α and β subunits, as well as experiments with renal and colonic tissues, strongly suggests that besides the experimental substrate rubidium (Rb), that Na$^+$ and NH$_4^+$ may also be (physiological) substrates (19, 20). The functional significance of these observations, however, is not clear. The sensitivity against the model inhibitors SCH 28080 (a potassium competitive inhibitor), ouabain (a Na$^+$,K$^+$-ATPase inhibitor that inhibits the colonic H$^+$,K$^+$-ATPase isoform) and omeprazole (a specific inhibitor of gastric H$^+$,K$^+$-ATPase isoform) appears to differ between species and depends on the combinations of α and β subunits coexpressed (15, 17, 38, 48).

An Associated K$^+$ Conductance

In the luminal membrane of gastric parietal cells, H$^+$,K$^+$-ATPase activity depends on the recycling of K$^+$ ions across the apical membrane providing luminal K$^+$ for pump activity (81, 82). In the cortical and outer medullary

TABLE 1 Types of H$^+$,K$^+$-ATPase Activity

	Type I	Type II	Type III
Ion specificity	K$^+$	K$^+$	Na$^+$ and K$^+$
Inhibitors	Sch 28080	Sch 28080	Sch 28080
	(IC$_{50}$ ~ 0.3 μM)	(IC$_{50}$ ~ 2 μM)	(IC$_{50}$ ~ 1 μM)
	Ouabain	Ouabain	Ouabain
	(Not sensitive)	(IC$_{50}$ ~ 6 μM)	(IC$_{50}$ ~ 20 μM)
Response to dietary K	Active during normal K	Reduced during low K	Present during low K
Localization	Type A-IC (CCD and OMCD) Type B-IC (CCD)	Proximal tubule, TAL	PC (CCD and OMCD) Type A-IC (OMCD)
Type	Gastric	Nongastric/noncolonic	Colonic

CCD, cortical collecting duct; OMCD, outer medullary collecting duct; PC, principle cell; TAL, thick ascending limb of the loop of Henle; type A-IC, type A intercalated cell; type B-IC, type B intercalated cell.

collecting duct, an increase in ambient CO$_2$ stimulates bicarbonate absorption, this stimulation is sensitive to the H$^+$,K$^+$-ATPase inhibitor Sch 28080 and barium, an inhibitor of luminal K$^+$-secretory channels (4, 87). Interestingly, this response is different in animals on a normal-K$^+$ and low-K$^+$ diet along with dietary K$^+$ depletion, which abolishes Ba^{2+} sensitivity (86). These data indicate that luminal H$^+$,K$^+$-ATPase activity under standard conditions requires a parallel K$^+$ conductance, possibly localized in neighboring principle cells (87). During K$^+$ depletion H$^+$,K$^+$-ATPase functions independent from this apical K$^+$ conductance but can be inhibited by basolateral Ba^{2+} application pointing to an additional K$^+$ conductance that may participate in K$^+$ reabsorption via H$^+$,K$^+$-ATPases (84). The apical K$^+$ conductance in principle cells is most likely represented by the small-conductance K$^+$ channel identified as ROMK channel based on the sensitivity to low pH and Ba^{2+}. Experiments using in vitro–perfused outer medullary collecting ducts (OMCDs) prepared from ROMK-deficient mice demonstrate that H$^+$,K$^+$-ATPase activity is reduced when insufficient levels of luminal K$^+$ are present. Furthermore there is an increase in H$^+$,K$^+$-ATPase activity in ROMK-deficient mice that have been on a low-K$^+$ diet demonstrating the ability of the H$^+$,K$^+$-ATPase activity to act as a K$^+$-loading mechanism (J. Kakboson, S. Hebert, G. Giebisch, and J. Geibel, unpublished observations, 2005).

EXPRESSION IN THE KIDNEY

The presence of H$^+$,K$^+$-ATPases in the kidney has been demonstrated on several levels using functional measurements and investigations of the distribution of mRNA and protein along the nephron. Presently, four genes are known in humans that encode subunits of H$^+$,$^+$-ATPases, two genes for gastric α and β subunits (ATP4α and ATP4β), and two genes encoding an nongastric α subunit (ATP12α) and a β subunit (ATP1β1) that can associate with Na$^+$,K$^+$-ATPases or ATP12α (Table 2). In rat, three splice variants of ATP12α have been identified and termed HKα$_{2a}$, HKα$_{2b}$, and HKα$_{2c}$ (11).

Distribution of mRNAs Encoding H$^+$,K$^+$-ATPase Subunits

Various techniques such as polymerase chain reaction (PCR), in situ hybridization, and transgenic expression of reporter genes have been used to map the distribution of mRNAs encoding H$^+$,K$^+$-ATPase subunits in rat, mouse, and rabbit kidneys. However, the results are highly controversial and it is unclear if only species- and technique-related differences can account for these differences.

THE α SUBUNITS

The presence of the gastric H$^+$,K$^+$-ATPase subunit in kidney has remained controversial. Several groups have identified mRNA by Northern blot in rat and mouse kidney (25, 52–54). In situ hybridization demonstrated reactivity in intercalated cells, and with a lower intensity in principle cells of the entire collecting system (1). However, other groups failed to detect significant amounts of its mRNA in rat kidney by PCR (13). Similarly, we failed to detect the gastric alpha subunit in mouse kidney (unpublished results). mRNA levels of the nongastric H$^+$,K$^+$-ATPase α subunit have been detected by many groups with its abundance being low in cortex, higher in medulla (2, 14, 25, 40, 52, 55, 61), and increased during potassium restriction as discussed in subsequent sections. The distribution of mRNA of the nongastric H$^+$,K$^+$-ATPase α subunit HKcα was also investigated by PCR in rat kidney and found to be present in low copy numbers in the cortical thick ascending limb, cortical collecting ducts (CCDs), and outer medullary collecting ducts (49). In rabbit kidney, PCR revealed HKcα mRNA only in CNT, CCD, and OMCD. Furthermore, PCR showed HKcα in type A and B intercalated cells and in principle cells (32). However, cells were obtained by immunosorting, a process that was not evaluated for its

TABLE 2 Genes Encoding Human Gastric and Nongastric H$^+$,K$^+$-ATPase Subunits

Name	Subunit	Chromosomal Localization	Acc. No.
ATP4A (HKα$_1$, HKgα)	Gastric α	19q13.1	NM_000704
ATP4B (HKgβ)	Gastric β	13q34	M75110
ATP12A (HKα$_4$, ATP1AL1, HKcα)	Nongastric	13q11-q12.1	NP_001667
ATP1β1 (ATP1B, HKcβ)	β$_1$ Na$^+$,K$^+$-ATPase	1q22-q25	P05026

quality on RNA level. In one report, in situ hybridization failed to detect the nongastric α subunit in normal rat kidney (39), whereas another report detected this subunit in kidneys from normal and K$^+$-depleted rats. In this latter study, signals were found in intercalated and principle cells (weaker) in the CNT, CCD, OMCD and inner medullary collecting duct (IMCD). The signal in OMCD and IMCD increased during K$^+$ restriction (2).

T HE **β** SUBUNI TS

In situ hybridization for the gastric β subunit (HKgβ) produced signals in rat and rabbit kidney in intercalated like cells in the distal convoluted tubule, CNT, CCD, and outer-stripe OMCD. Most cells in the inner stripe of the outer medulla as well as in the IMCD were strongly positive. A few positive cells were found in the proximal tubule and a weak signal in the cortical thick ascending limb (9). Another approach used transgenic mice expressing a transgene containing the promoter region of the gastric β subunit linked to X-gal and found X-gal staining in the entire collecting duct system with most cells being positive. However, it also appeared that the transgene had not been transmitted to all acid-secretory cells in the stomach and thus the pattern of expression has to be taken with caution (8).

Evidence for H$^+$,K$^+$-ATPase Protein Localization

The results coming from antibody-based studies attempting to localize H$^+$,K$^+$-ATPase subunits in kidney are not unequivocal. Immunoreactivity for the gastric HKgα subunit was detected in human kidney in intercalated and principle cells in cortical and medullary collecting duct. The staining was diffusely cytoplasmic and intracellular (42). In contrast, another study using monoclonal anti-HKgα antibodies detected immunoreactivity only in intercalated cells in rat and rabbit kidney. The staining was also mainly cytoplasmic and a subgroup of intercalated cells was not stained (79). Immunoreactivity for the nongastric HKcα subunit was detected in cortical and medullary intercalated cells and with a lower intensity in principle cells (42). The rat HKα$_{2c}$ subunit, homologous to the human HKcα subunit, was detected in rabbit kidney in intercalated cells in the cortex and medulla and more weakly in principle cells and in the

cortical thick ascending limb. In all cells, staining was predominantly apically distributed (71). An additional study described HKα2 staining only in a cell population that appeared to be principle cells in the outer medullary collecting duct (61); however, the lack of details left questions as to the localization of the protein.

Functional Mapping of H$^+$,K$^+$-ATPase Expression

H$^+$,K$^+$-ATPase activity has been detected in several nephron segments including the proximal tubule, the thick ascending limb of the loop of Henle, and the cortical and the medullary collecting ducts (45, 67, 83). The first functional evidence for H$^+$,K$^+$-ATPase activity was obtained by measuring K$^+$-activated, Na$^+$-independent ATPase activity, not sensitive to ouabain and inhibited by Sch 28080 and found in the CNT, CCD, and OMCD (24, 34). However, as discussed previously, subsequent studies with cloned and heterologously expressed H$^+$,K$^+$-ATPases as well as more detailed studies in renal tissues revealed that these criteria were not sufficient and that H$^+$,K$^+$-ATPase isoforms exist that are also Na$^+$-activated and ouabain sensitive (20, 45, 83).

Type III H$^+$,K$^+$-ATPase activity (i.e., Na$^+$-activated, ouabain and Sch 28080 sensitive) was detected in the proximal convoluted and straight tubule and in cortical and medullary portions of the thick ascending limb, but not in the cortical and medullary collecting duct under normal conditions (83). During dietary K$^+$ deprivation, type III H$^+$,K$^+$-ATPase activity disappears from the proximal tubule and TAL and is now detected in the cortical and medullary collecting duct (83). In addition to measuring ATPase activity, intracellular pH measurements and CO$_2$ fluxes were used to map H$^+$,K$^+$-ATPase activity. The intracellular pH recovery from an acid load is reduced by Sch 28080 in isolated rat inner medullary thin limbs of the loop of Henle (58). In mouse-isolated CCD, OMCD, and IMCD, a fraction of the Na$^+$-independent H$^+$ extrusion from intercalated cells is not sensitive to concanamycin, an inhibitor of vacuolar H$^+$-ATPases and may reflect H$^+$,K$^+$-ATPase activity (73). Acid secretion in the terminal rat IMCD is Sch 28080 sensitive during metabolic acidosis. However, unphysiological conditions of high luminal HCO$_3$ were used (75). CO$_2$ fluxes in rat OMCD and initial IMCD but not CCD are partly Sch

28080 sensitive (36). In rat IMCD, CO_2 absorption during K^+ depletion is sensitive to Sch 28080 and ouabain, whereas ouabain is without effect in normal rats (52). K^+ depletion increases total and Sch 28080–sensitive bicarbonate absorption in the terminal rat IMCD. However, about 50% of this bicarbonate absorption is insensitive to ouabain and Sch 28080 (74).

REGULATION

Regulation of H^+,K^+-ATPase function and expression has been reported for several conditions. Experiments and interpretation of data are hampered by the fact that several isoforms of H^+,K^+-ATPases may underlie the observed activity and the distinction between these isoforms has been difficult. In general, regulation of H^+,K^+-ATPases has been observed on several levels (function and abundance) and in different settings (animal studies vs cell culture models). Many of these studies have been summarized in various reviews (25, 26, 38, 67).

Mechanisms of Regulation

Regulation of H^+,K^+-ATPase activity has been observed on several levels. Changes in mRNA were found during K^+ deprivation as well as parallel alterations of protein abundance. However, no specific transcription factors or proteins interacting with H^+,K^+-ATPases increasing or decreasing protein life time have been reported as in the case of other renal transporters and channels.

INTERNALIZATION AND RECYCLING

An interesting feature of the gastric H^+,K^+-ATPase is the regulation of activity by insertion, retrieval, and recycling of H^+,K^+-ATPases to and from the membrane. This has been studied extensively in the gastric acid–secretory parietal cell. There, insertion of H^+,K^+-ATPases containing tubulovesicular structures into the apical membrane is initiated by several hormones triggering phospholipase C, Ca^{2+}, and protein kinase C–dependent pathways as well as cAMP and protein kinase A–dependent cascades (82). In addition, a number of proteins involved in connecting the cytoskeleton to intracellular vesicles such as ezrin have been implicated in the insertion process (82). Activity of luminal H^+,K^+-ATPases, however, is also determined by the rate of retrieval from the membrane. The β subunit of the gastric H^+,K^+-ATPase contains a tyrosine-based internalization motif (Y-motif) that has been shown in a transgenic mouse model expressing a β subunit lacking the Y-motif to be important for retrieval of active pumps from the membrane (21). These animals suffer from excessive gastric acid secretion and stomach ulcers. The same mouse model also showed increased renal gastric type H^+,K^+-ATPase protein abundance associated with higher plasma K^+ concentrations and lower urinary fractional potassium excretion (76).

Acid-base status and other parameters were not altered. Internalization of H^+,K^+-ATPases in gastric parietal cells may also be regulated by the CD63 glycoprotein, a member of the so-called tetraspanin family (27). In gastric parietal cells, CD63 colocalizes with H^+,K^+-ATPases and promotes in transfected cells their internalization, a process depending on the presence of adaptor protein complexes (27). CD63 is also expressed in kidney (41, 51); however, its cellular distribution has not been reported. A yeast two-hybrid screen identified CD63 interactions with the carboxy-terminus of the nongastric H^+,K^+-ATPase α subunit but not with the α subunits of gastric H^+,K^+-ATPase or Na^+,K^+-ATPases (16). RNA interference experiments in HEK 293 cells demonstrated that the reduction in CD63 expression did not affect H^+,K^+-ATPase abundance but enhanced its surface expression and associated Rb^+ fluxes. Thus, it appears that H^+,K^+-ATPase activity in the kidney is regulated by internalization, that the Y-motif is involved in internalization, and that the tetraspanin CD63 could participate in this process.

HORMONAL REGULATION

Little is known about acute and chronic regulation of H^+,K^+-ATPase expression and activity by hormones. Stimulation of H^+,K^+-ATPase activity through β-adrenergic receptors, V2 vasopressin receptors, and glucagon and calcitonin receptors has been demonstrated (45, 46). Stimulation through β receptors (using isoproterenol) and calcitonin receptors occurs in type A and B intercalated cells in the CCD of rats kept on a normal potassium diet and affected mainly type I H^+,K^+-ATPase activity (45), whereas after 2 weeks of a low-potassium diet the isoproterenol- and calcitonin-mediated stimulation was abolished. Vasopressin stimulates, in contrast, type III H^+,K^+-ATPase activity in principle cells in the CCD and OMCD and in type A intercalated cells only in the OMCD (45). Stimulation of type III H^+,K^+-ATPase activity was only seen in animals kept on a chronic low-potassium diet.

All hormonal stimulators signal through an elevation of intracellular cAMP and protein kinase A (PKA) activity. Isoproterenol stimulates H^+,K^+-ATPase activity in the CCD through a pathway that depends on G_s proteins activating an adenylate cyclase and PKA with subsequent stimulation of G_i proteins, Ras, Raf1, and ERK1/2 kinases (46). In contrast, stimulation by calcitonin in type A intercalated cells is mediated by cAMP and downstream activation of a PKA-dependent pathway and a pathway involving the cAMP-activated guanine-nucleotide exchange factor (EPAC I), Rap1, RafB, and ERK1/2 (47).

Regulation During Changes in Electrolyte Intake and Status

Several lines of evidence suggest that H^+,K^+-ATPase abundance and activity are regulated by dietary intake and urinary excretion of Na^+ and K^+.

H$^+$,K$^+$-ATPASE IS INCREASED DURING POTASSIUM DEPLETION

Because of its ability to mediate K$^+$ reabsorption and the ability of the kidney to prevent urinary K$^+$ loss during K$^+$ deprivation, regulation of H$^+$,K$^+$-ATPases by dietary K$^+$ intake has received much attention. A decrease in dietary K$^+$ intake or increased loss of K$^+$ from the body is associated with an increase in H$^+$,K$^+$-ATPase activity and abundance of some of its subunits (12, 14, 24, 40, 49, 74, 83), whereas hyperkalemia causes a decrease in H$^+$,K$^+$-ATPase activity (35).

Evidence indicates that hypokalemia increases H$^+$,K$^+$-ATPase activity in the cortical, outer, and inner medullary collecting ducts (7, 12, 24, 43, 44, 52, 55, 74, 75, 83). This activity is Sch 28080 and ouabain sensitive, suggesting that it is mediated by type III H$^+$,K$^+$-ATPases (83). Type III H$^+$,K$^+$-ATPase activity in the proximal tubule and cTAL is decreased during K$^+$ deprivation (83).

On the molecular level, the information is more controversial. In rat kidney, K$^+$ deprivation causes an increase in the nongastric HKcα mRNA in the CCD and OMCD as detected by PCR (49) and Northern blot (25, 40, 55, 61). The induction of HKcα mRNA is not modulated or dependent on aldosterone or cortisol (40). Regulation of the HKcβ mRNA and protein has not been reported for kidney but shown to be induced in colon during K$^+$ deprivation (60). In the case of the gastric H$^+$,K$^+$-ATPase subunits, an increase in HKgα mRNA has been reported on the basis of findings from Northern blots (52), PCR, and in situ hybridization (3); however, it appears that the abundance of HKgα mRNA was very low if even present. DuBose et al. (25) found no change in HKgα mRNA during K$^+$ depletion, whereas Cheval and Doucet (13) could not detect any significant HKgα transcript numbers by PCR in dissected rat nephron segments from normal and K$^+$-deprived rats.

The signal initiating the upregulation of H$^+$,K$^+$-ATPases during K$^+$ deprivation has not been identified. Because the increase in H$^+$,K$^+$-ATPase expression precedes the development of systemic hypokalemia, it has been suggested that cellular hypokalemia may act as a trigger (77). A role for pituitary hormones has been suggested on the basis of observation that upregulation is diminished in hypophysectomized rats despite hypokalemia (77).

Urinary acidification is increased during hypokalemia and has been mainly attributed to a stimulation of H$^+$-secretory and bicarbonate salvage mechanisms leading to metabolic alkalosis (5, 10, 31, 63). Stimulation of Na$^+$,H$^+$-exchanger NHE3 as well of vacuolar H$^+$-ATPases in the distal tubule and cortical collecting duct was demonstrated. The relative contribution of these transport pathways and H$^+$,K$^+$-ATPases is unknown. This question was addressed in a rat model and in a cell line derived from the initial outer medullary collecting duct of mice where incubation in a low K$^+$ medium increased Sch 28080–sensitive H$^+$,K$^+$-ATPase activity but not vacuolar H$^+$-ATPase activity. In contrast, incubation in acid medium stimulated only vacuolar H$^+$-ATPases (37). In the rat model, chronic hypokalemia for 7 days increased Sch 28080–sensitive ATPase activity in CCD and OMCD segments, whereas bafilomycin-sensitive ATPase activity decreased in both segments (29). These results are in clear contrast and further experiments are needed to resolve the question of the relative regulation and contribution of both enzymes to urinary acidification and bicarbonate absorption during hypokalemia.

Increasing ambient CO$_2$ levels cause a stimulation of H$^+$,K$^+$-ATPase activity in the CCD and OMCD (84, 85, 87). The underlying mechanism has been further characterized in potassium-restricted rabbits and shown to be dependent on intracellular carbo-anhydrase activity, intracellular Ca^{2+}, calmodulin-dependent kinases, and the requirement of an intact microtubular network (85).

The overall contribution of H$^+$,K$^+$-ATPases to renal potassium-salvaging mechanisms, however, has been challenged by a mouse model deficient for the nongastric H$^+$,K$^+$-ATPase α subunit (HKcα) where no renal defect in K$^+$ retention was found under normal and potassium restriction. Only fecal K$^+$ loss caused hypokalemia (50). Unfortunately, the gastric isoform was not investigated in this mouse model. A second mouse model deficient for the gastric α subunit appears to have no abnormality in systemic acid-base and electrolyte homeostasis, suggesting that loss of the renal expression of this subunit may be either compensated or not needed during normal conditions. A detailed analysis of the renal phenotype of this mouse under various conditions is missing (69).

SODIUM CHLORIDE RESTRICTION STIMULATES H$^+$,K$^+$-ATPASE

A chronic NaCl-depleted diet in rat cortical collecting duct intercalated cells sstimulated a Sch 28080–sensitive H$^+$,K$^+$-ATPase and induced additional Sch 28080–insensitive, ouabain-sensitive H$^+$,K$^+$-ATPase activity (64). This stimulatory effect is most likely not due to increased aldosterone levels as treatment of rats with aldosterone does not stimulate H$^+$,K$^+$-ATPase (29, 64). At least for the HKcα subunit it has been shown that there is no change in mRNA and protein abundance during Na$^+$ depletion (61).

Regulation During Acid-Base Disturbances

As indicated previously, the role and contribution of H$^+$,K$^+$-ATPases to renal acid excretion and systemic acid-base homeostasis are unclear. Several authors have addressed the question of whether H$^+$,K$^+$-ATPases are regulated by acid-base status and could participate in acid secretion during acidosis. Fejes-Toth et al. (33) reported an increase in the relative mRNA abundance of the nongastric α subunit in cortical collecting ducts prepared from rabbits subjected to a short-term acid or alkali load using a semi-quantitative PCR approach. Despite a large scattering of data, the authors assumed a role of nongastric H^+,K^+-ATPases at the basolateral side of type B intercalated cells contributing to bicarbonate secretion during alkalosis (33). In contrast, other studies found no evidence for regulation of HKgα and HKcα on protein or mRNA levels during metabolic acidosis (14, 25).

A two- to threefold stimulation of luminal H^+,K^+-ATPase activity was found in peanut-lectin–positive type B intercalated cells in rabbit cortical collecting duct after 8 to 14 days of a mild metabolic acidosis. Interestingly, this increase was observed without a significant change in blood and muscle K^+ content. H^+,K^+-ATPase in control and acidotic animals was completely inhibited by Sch 28080 (65, 66). Thus, this study suggests that an apical H^+,K^+-ATPase contributes to acid excretion from type B intercalated cells during chronic metabolic acidosis.

Increased H^+,K^+-ATPase activity was observed in the collecting duct from rats with chronic respiratory acidosis whereas acute and chronic respiratory alkalosis reduced H^+,K^+-ATPase activity. As the ATPase measurements were performed with ouabain present, these data suggest that a type I or II H^+,K^+-ATPase was affected (30).

Developmental Regulation and Expression

Renal excretion of potassium is low in newborns and growing children, a fact that may reflect the requirement of potassium for growth and cell division (6, 23). Two factors appear to contribute to the kidneys ability to retain potassium early in life, the low expression of the K^+-secretory ROMK channel (23, 62) and an already high Sch 28080–sensitive H^+,K^+-ATPase activity in the luminal membrane of neonatal peanut-lectin–positive intercalated cells (i.e., type B intercalated cells) (18). The molecular identity underlying this H^+,K^+-ATPase activity has not been elucidated.

OTHER FUNCTIONS OF RENAL H^+,K^+-ATPases

In the cortical collecting duct from rabbits on a K^+Cl^--containing diet, basolateral ouabain stimulates chloride absorption that is inhibited by Sch 28080. Bicarbonate secretion is sensitive to Sch 28080 under this condition. Apical Sch 28080–sensitive Na^+-absorption was observed. Thus, it has been proposed that type B intercalated cells in the CCD can mediate Na^+ and Cl^- absorption through the parallel action of an apical $H^+,Na^+(K^+)$-ATPase and a Cl^-/HCO_3^- exchanger (88). This apical Cl^-/HCO_3^- is most likely represented by pendrin, which, however, is downregulated by K^+Cl^- (59). More experiments are required to resolve this question.

ASSOCIATED DISEASES

At least three diseases have been associated with dysfunctional H^+,K^+-ATPases, a rare case of distal renal tubular acidosis with hypokalemia due to potassium wasting, and two syndromes that may be caused by toxic effects of lithium and vanadate.

Lithium treatment for bipolar mood disorders is often associated with a renal acidification defect leading to distal renal tubular acidosis. Chronic lithium treatment of rats induces an inhibition of H^+-ATPase activity, stimulation of H^+,K^+-ATPase activity in the CCD, and inhibition in the OMCD (28). The functional significance remains to be established.

A high incidence of distal renal tubular acidosis (dRTA) has been noted in some rural areas of Northeastern Thailand (70). This type of dRTA occurs mainly during summer months and is associated with hypokalemia, low urinary citrate excretion, and decreased red blood cell Na^+,K^+-ATPase activity. In addition, many patients have decreased gastric acid secretion. Particularly high vanadium concentrations have been detected in the drinking water in these areas, and high concentrations of vanadium were found in the urine of patients. Inhibition of H^+,K^+-ATPases and Na^+,K^+-ATPases are among many biological processes affected by vanadium. The inhibition of gastric acid secretion together with decreased urinary acidification have been taken as evidence that vanadium primarily affects H^+,K^+-ATPase activity in stomach and kidney and that decreased H^+,K^+-ATPase activity underlies this syndrome of dRTA. In a rat model, treated with vanadate over 10 days, hypokalemic/hyperchloremic metabolic acidosis with a mildly elevated urinary pH was found. In the cortical and medullary collecting ducts, H^+,K^+-ATPase and Na^+,K^+-ATPase activity were reduced, whereas H^+-ATPase activity remained unaltered (22). However, in view of the mild or not-existing renal phenotype of H^+,K^+-ATPase–deficient mice it remains to be determined whether the renal problems seen in these patients can be sufficiently explained with decreased H^+,K^+-ATPase activity.

In 2001, Simpson and Schwartz (68) reported the case of a child with severe hypokalemia, metabolic acidosis, and hypomagnesaemia probably caused by renal and probable fecal potassium wasting, dRTA, and mild urinary magnesium wasting. Gastric acid secretion was apparently normal. On the basis of these findings, the authors proposed a possibly inborn defect in the colonic H^+,K^+-ATPase isoform. However, the subsequent sequencing did not reveal any obvious genetic abnormalities in the genes encoding the colonic isoform.

SUMMARY

H^+,K^+-ATPase activity is present in various nephron segments and appears to mediate cellular uptake of potassium in exchange for H^+ extrusion. On the basis of functional and pharmacological inhibitor profiles, at least three different subtypes can be distinguished. Their molecular correlate has not been firmly established and awaits complete identification. H^+,K^+-ATPase function and expression correlate best with dietary K^+ intake and are stimulated during K^+ deprivation. However, it appears that at least the nongastric H^+,K^+-ATPase is dispensable for the K^+-saving function of the kidney. The correlation between H^+,K^+-ATPase function and expression and acid-base status and transport is weak. Thus, the primary role of H^+,K^+-ATPases may be to participate in K^+ saving during chronic K^+ deprivation. The signals initiating H^+,K^+-ATPase activity during K^+ depletion are currently unknown. The elucidation of associated proteins that may contribute to H^+,K^+-ATPase polar expression and regulation has only begun.

References

1. Ahn KY, Kone BC. Expression and cellular localization of mRNA encoding the "gastric" isoform of H^+-K^+-ATPase alpha-subunit at rat kidney. *Am J Physiol* 1995;268:F99–109.

2. Ahn KY, Park KY, Kim KK, Kone BC. Chronic hypokalemia enhances expression of the H^+-K^+-ATPase alpha 2-subunit gene in renal medulla. *Am J Physiol* 1996;271:F314–321.

3. Ahn KY, Turner PB, Madsen KM, Kone BC. Effects of chronic hypokalemia on renal expression of the "gastric" H^+-K^+-ATPase alpha-subunit gene. *Am J Physiol* 1996;270:F557–566.

4. Armitage FE, Wingo CS. Luminal acidification in K-replete $OMCD_i$: inhibition of bicarbonate absorption by K removal and luminal Ba. *Am J Physiol* 1995;269:F116–124.

5. Bailey MA, Fletcher RM, Woodrow DF, Unwin RJ, Walter SJ. Upregulation of H^+-ATPase in the distal nephron during potassium depletion: structural and functional evidence. *Am J Physiol* 1998;275:F878–884.

6. Baum M, Quigley R, Satlin L. Maturational changes in renal tubular transport. *Curr Opin Nephrol Hypertens* 2003;12:521–526.

7. Buffin-Meyer B, Younes-Ibrahim M, Barlet-Bas C, Cheval L, Marsy S, Doucet A. K depletion modifies the properties of Sch-28080-sensitive K-ATPase in rat collecting duct. *Am J Physiol* 1997;272:F124–131.

8. Callaghan JM, Tan SS, Khan MA, Curran KA, Campbell WG, Smolka AJ, Toh BH, Gleeson PA, Wingo CS, Cain BD, et al. Renal expression of the gene encoding the gastric H^+-K^+-ATPase beta-subunit. *Am J Physiol* 1995;268:F363–374.

9. Campbell-Thompson ML, Verlander JW, Curran KA, Campbell WG, Cain BD, Wingo CS, McGuigan JE. In situ hybridization of H-K-ATPase beta-subunit mRNA in rat and rabbit kidney. *Am J Physiol* 1995;269:F345–354.

10. Capasso G, Jaeger P, Giebisch G, Guckian V, Malnic G. Renal bicarbonate reabsorption in the rat. II. Distal tubule load dependence and effect of hypokalemia. *J Clin Invest* 1987;80:409–414.

11. Caviston TL, Campbell WG, Wingo CS, Cain BD. Molecular identification of the renal H^+,K^+-ATPases. *Semin Nephrol* 1999;19:431–437.

12. Cheval L, Barlet-Bas C, Khadouri C, Feraille E, Marsy S, Doucet A. K^+-ATPase-mediated Rb^+ transport in rat collecting tubule: modulation during K^+ deprivation. *Am J Physiol* 1991;260:F800–805.

13. Cheval L, Elalouf JM, Doucet A. Re-evaluation of the expression of the gastric H,K-ATPase alpha subunit along the rat nephron. *Pflugers Arch* 1997;433:539–541.

14. Codina J, Delmas-Mata JT, DuBose TD Jr. Expression of HKalpha2 protein is increased selectively in renal medulla by chronic hypokalemia. *Am J Physiol* 1998;275:F433–440.

15. Codina J, Kone BC, Delmas-Mata JT, DuBose TD Jr. Functional expression of the colonic H^+,K^+-ATPase alpha-subunit. Pharmacologic properties and assembly with X^+,K^+-ATPase beta-subunits. *J Biol Chem* 1996;271:29759–29763.

16. Codina J, Li J, Dubose TD Jr. CD63 Interacts with the carboxy-terminus of the colonic H^+,K^+-ATPase to increase plasma membrane localization and Rb^+-uptake. *Am J Physiol Cell Physiol* 2005;288(6):C1279–1286.

17. Codina J, Wall SM, DuBose TD Jr. Contrasting functional and regulatory profiles of the renal H^+,K^+-ATPases. *Semin Nephrol* 1999;19:399–404.

18. Constantinescu A, Silver RB, Satlin LM. H-K-ATPase activity in PNA-binding intercalated cells of newborn rabbit cortical collecting duct. *Am J Physiol* 1997;272:F167–177.

19. Cougnon M, Bouyer P, Jaisser F, Edelman A, Planelles G. Ammonium transport by the colonic H^+-K^+-ATPase expressed in Xenopus oocytes. *Am J Physiol* 1999;277:C280–287.

20. Cougnon M, Bouyer P, Planelles G, Jaisser F. Does the colonic H,K-ATPase also act as an Na,K-ATPase? *Proc Natl Acad Sci U S A* 1998;95:6516–6520.

21. Courtois-Coutry N, Roush D, Rajendran V, McCarthy JB, Geibel J, Kashgarian M, Caplan MJ. A tyrosine-based signal targets H/K-ATPase to a regulated compartment and is required for the cessation of gastric acid secretion. *Cell* 1997;90:501–510.

22. Dafnis E, Spohn M, Lonis B, Kurtzman NA, Sabatini S. Vanadate causes hypokalemic distal renal tubular acidosis. *Am J Physiol* 1992;262:F449–453.

23. Delgado MM, Rohatgi R, Khan S, Holzman IR, Satlin LM. Sodium and potassium clearances by the maturing kidney: clinical-molecular correlates. *Pediatr Nephrol* 2003;18:759–767.

24. Doucet A, Marsy S. Characterization of K-ATPase activity in distal nephron: stimulation by potassium depletion. *Am J Physiol* 1987;253:F418–423.

25. DuBose TD Jr, Codina J, Burges A, Pressley TA. Regulation of H^+-K^+-ATPase expression in kidney. *Am J Physiol* 1995;269:F500–507.

26. DuBose TD Jr, Gitomer J, Codina J. H^+,K^+-ATPase. *Curr Opin Nephrol Hypertens* 1999;8:597–602.

27. Duffield A, Kamsteeg EJ, Brown AN, Pagel P, Caplan MJ. The tetraspanin CD63 enhances the internalization of the H,K-ATPase beta-subunit. *Proc Natl Acad Sci U S A* 2003;100:15560–15565.

28. Eiam-Ong S, Dafnis E, Spohn M, Kurtzman NA, Sabatini S. H-K-ATPase in distal renal tubular acidosis: urinary tract obstruction, lithium, and amiloride. *Am J Physiol* 1993;265:F875–880.

29. Eiam-Ong S, Kurtzman NA, Sabatini S. Regulation of collecting tubule adenosine triphosphatases by aldosterone and potassium. *J Clin Invest* 1993;91:2385–2392.

30. Eiam-ong S, Laski ME, Kurtzman NA, Sabatini S. Effect of respiratory acidosis and respiratory alkalosis on renal transport enzymes. *Am J Physiol* 1994;267:F390–399.

31. Elkjar ML, Kwon TH, Wang W, Nielsen J, Knepper MA, Frokiar J, Nielsen S. Altered expression of renal NHE3, TSC, BSC-1, and ENaC subunits in potassium-depleted rats. *Am J Physiol Renal Physiol* 2002;283:F1376–F1388.

32. Fejes-Toth G, Naray-Fejes-Toth A, Velazquez H. Intrarenal distribution of the colonic H,K-ATPase mRNA in rabbit. *Kidney Int* 1999;56:1029–1036.

33. Fejes-Toth G, Rusvai E, Longo KA, Naray-Fejes-Toth A. Expression of colonic H-K-ATPase mRNA in cortical collecting duct: regulation by acid/base balance. *Am J Physiol* 1995;269:F551–557.

34. Garg LC, Narang N. Ouabain-insensitive K-adenosine triphosphatase in distal nephron segments of the rabbit. *J Clin Invest* 1988;81:1204–1208.

35. Garg LC, Narang N. Suppression of ouabain-insensitive K-ATPase activity in rabbit nephron segments during chronic hyperkalemia. *Ren Physiol Biochem* 1989;12:295–301.

36. Gifford JD, Rome L, Galla JH. H^+-K^+-ATPase activity in rat collecting duct segments. *Am J Physiol* 1992;262:F692–695.

37. Guntupalli J, Onuigbo M, Wall S, Alpern RJ, DuBose TD Jr. Adaptation to low-K^+ media increases H^+-K^+-ATPase but not H^+-ATPase-mediated pH_i recovery in $OMCD_1$ cells. *Am J Physiol* 1997;273:C558–571.

38. Jaisser F, Beggah AT. The nongastric H^+-K^+-ATPases: molecular and functional properties. *Am J Physiol* 1999;276:F812–824.

39. Jaisser F, Coutry N, Farman N, Binder HJ, Rossier BC. A putative H^+-K^+-ATPase is selectively expressed in surface epithelial cells of rat distal colon. *Am J Physiol* 1993;265:C1080–1089.

40. Jaisser F, Escoubet B, Coutry N, Eugene E, Bonvalet JP, Farman N. Differential regulation of putative K^+-ATPase by low-K^+ diet and corticosteroids in rat distal colon and kidney. *Am J Physiol* 1996;270:C679–687.

41. Kennel SJ, Lankford PK, Foote LJ, Davis IA. Monoclonal antibody to rat CD63 detects different molecular forms in rat tissue. *Hybridoma* 1998;17:509–515.

42. Kraut JA, Helander KG, Helander HF, Iroezi ND, Marcus EA, Sachs G. Detection and localization of H^+-K^+-ATPase isoforms in human kidney. *Am J Physiol Renal Physiol* 2001;281:F763–768.

43. Kuwahara M, Fu WJ, Marumo F. Functional activity of H-K-ATPase in individual cells of OMCD: localization and effect of K^+ depletion. *Am J Physiol* 1996;270:F116–122.

44. Laroche-Joubert N, Doucet A. Collecting duct adaptation to potassium depletion. *Semin Nephrol* 1999;19:390–398.

45. Laroche-Joubert N, Marsy S, Doucet A. Cellular origin and hormonal regulation of K^+-ATPase activities sensitive to Sch-28080 in rat collecting duct. *Am J Physiol Renal Physiol* 2000;279:F1053–1059.

46. Laroche-Joubert N, Marsy S, Luriau S, Imbert-Teboul M, Doucet A. Mechanism of activation of ERK and H-K-ATPase by isoproterenol in rat cortical collecting duct. *Am J Physiol Renal Physiol* 2003;284:F948–954.

47. Laroche-Joubert N, Marsy S, Michelet S, Imbert-Teboul M, Doucet A. Protein kinase A-independent activation of ERK and H,K-ATPase by cAMP in native kidney cells: role of Epac I. *J Biol Chem* 2002;277:18598–18604.

48. Li J, Codina J, Petroske E, Werle MJ, Willingham MC, DuBose TD Jr. The effect of beta-subunit assembly on function and localization of the colonic H^+,K^+-ATPase alpha-subunit. *Kidney Int* 2004;66:1068–1075.

49. Marsy S, Elalouf JM, Doucet A. Quantitative RT-PCR analysis of mRNAs encoding a colonic putative H, K-ATPase alpha subunit along the rat nephron: effect of K^+ depletion. *Pflugers Arch* 1996;432:494–500.

50. Meneton P, Schultheis PJ, Greeb J, Nieman ML, Liu LH, Clarke LL, Duffy JJ, Doetschman T, Lorenz JN, Shull GE. Increased sensitivity to K^+ deprivation in colonic H,K-ATPase-deficient mice. *J Clin Invest* 1998;101:536–542.

51. Miyamoto H, Homma M, Hotta H. Molecular cloning of the murine homologue of CD63/ME491 and detection of its strong expression in the kidney and activated macrophages. *Biochim Biophys Acta* 1994;1217:312–316.

52. Nakamura S, Amlal H, Galla JH, Soleimani M. Colonic H^+-K^+-ATPase is induced and mediates increased HCO_3^- reabsorption in inner medullary collecting duct in potassium depletion. *Kidney Int* 1998;54:1233–1239.

53. Nakamura S, Amlal H, Schultheis PJ, Galla JH, Shull GE, Soleimani M. HCO_3^- reabsorption in renal collecting duct of NHE-3-deficient mouse: a compensatory response. *Am J Physiol* 1999;276:F914–921.

54. Nakamura S, Amlal H, Soleimani M, Galla JH. Pathways for HCO₃⁻ reabsorption in mouse medullary collecting duct segments. *J Lab Clin Med* 2000;136:218–223.

55. Nakamura S, Wang Z, Galla JH, Soleimani M. K⁺ depletion increases HCO₃⁻ reabsorption in OMCD by activation of colonic H⁺-K⁺-ATPase. *Am J Physiol* 1998;274:F687–692.

56. Nelson N, Harvey WR. Vacuolar and plasma membrane proton-adenosinetriphosphatases. *Physiol Rev* 1999;79:361–385.

57. Nishi T, Forgac M. The vacuolar (H+)-ATPases—nature's most versatile proton pumps. *Nat Rev Mol Cell Biol* 2002;3:94–103.

58. Pannabecker TL, Brokl OH, Kim YK, Abbott DE, Dantzler WH. Regulation of intracellular pH in rat renal inner medullary thin limbs of Henle's loop. *Pflugers Arch* 2002;443: 446–457.

59. Quentin F, Chambrey R, Trinh-Trang-Tan MM, Fysekidis M, Cambillau M, Paillard M, Aronson PS, Eladari D. The Cl⁻/HCO₃⁻ exchanger pendrin in the rat kidney is regulated in response to chronic alterations in chloride balance. *Am J Physiol Renal Physiol* 2004; 287:F1179–1188.

60. Sangan P, Kolla SS, Rajendran VM, Kashgarian M, Binder HJ. Colonic H-K-ATPase beta-subunit: identification in apical membranes and regulation by dietary K depletion. *Am J Physiol* 1999;276:C350–360.

61. Sangan P, Rajendran VM, Mann AS, Kashgarian M, Binder HJ. Regulation of colonic H-K-ATPase in large intestine and kidney by dietary Na depletion and dietary K depletion. *Am J Physiol* 1997;272:C685–696.

62. Satlin LM. Postnatal maturation of potassium transport in rabbit cortical collecting duct. *Am J Physiol* 1994;266:F57–65.

63. Silver RB, Breton S, Brown D. Potassium depletion increases proton pump (H⁺-ATPase) activity in intercalated cells of cortical collecting duct. *Am J Physiol Renal Physiol* 2000;279: F195–202.

64. Silver RB, Choe H, Frindt G. Low-NaCl diet increases H-K-ATPase in intercalated cells from rat cortical collecting duct. *Am J Physiol* 1998;275:F94–102.

65. Silver RB, Frindt G, Mennitt P, Satlin, LM. Characterization and regulation of H-K-ATPase in intercalated cells of rabbit cortical collecting duct. *J Exp Zool* 1997;279:443–455.

66. Silver RB, Mennitt PA, Satlin LM. Stimulation of apical H-K-ATPase in intercalated cells of cortical collecting duct with chronic metabolic acidosis. *Am J Physiol* 1996;270:F539–547.

67. Silver RB, Soleimani M. H⁺-K⁺-ATPases: regulation and role in pathophysiological states. *Am J Physiol* 1999;276:F799–811.

68. Simpson AM, Schwartz G J. Distal renal tubular acidosis with severe hypokalaemia, probably caused by colonic H⁺/K⁺-ATPase deficiency. *Arch Dis Child* 2001;84:504–507.

69. Spicer Z, Miller ML, Andringa A, Riddle TM, Duffy JJ, Doetschman T, Shull GE. Stomachs of mice lacking the gastric H,K-ATPase alpha-subunit have achlorhydria, abnormal parietal cells, and ciliated metaplasia. *J Biol Chem* 2000;275:21555–21565.

70. Tosukhowong P, Tungsanga K, Eiam-Ong S, Sitprija V. Environmental distal renal tubular acidosis in Thailand: an enigma. *Am J Kidney Dis* 1999;33:1180–1186.

71. Verlander JW, Moudy RM, Campbell WG, Cain BD, Wingo CS. Immunohistochemical localization of H-K-ATPase alpha₂ᶜ-subunit in rabbit kidney. *Am J Physiol Renal Physiol* 2001;281:F357–365.

72. Wagner CA, Finberg KE, Breton S, Marshansky V, Brown D, Geibel JP. Renal vacuolar H⁺-ATPase. *Physiol Rev* 2004;84:1263–1314.

73. Wagner CA, Lukewille U, Valles P, Breton S, Brown D, Giebisch GH, Geibel JP. A rapid enzymatic method for the isolation of defined kidney tubule fragments from mouse. *Pflugers Arch* 2003;446:623–632.

74. Wall SM, Mehta P, DuBose TD Jr. Dietary K⁺ restriction upregulates total and Sch-28080-sensitive bicarbonate absorption in rat tIMCD. *Am J Physiol* 1998;275:F543–549.

75. Wall SM, Truong AV, DuBose TD Jr. H⁺-K⁺-ATPase mediates net acid secretion in rat terminal inner medullary collecting duct. *Am J Physiol* 1996;271:F1037–1044.

76. Wang T, Courtois-Coutry N, Giebisch G, Caplan MJ. A tyrosine-based signal regulates H-K-ATPase-mediated potassium reabsorption in the kidney. *Am J Physiol* 1998;275: F818–826.

77. Wang Z, Baird N, Shumaker H, Soleimani M. Potassium depletion and acid-base transporters in rat kidney: differential effect of hypophysectomy. *Am J Physiol* 1997;272:F736–743.

78. Wingo CS, Cain BD. The renal H-K-ATPase: physiological significance and role in potassium homeostasis. *Annu Rev Physiol* 1993;55:323–347.

79. Wingo CS, Madsen KM, Smolka A, Tisher CC. H-K-ATPase immunoreactivity in cortical and outer medullary collecting duct. *Kidney Int* 1990;38:985–990.

80. Wingo CS, Smolka, A J. Function and structure of H-K-ATPase in the kidney. *Am J Physiol* 1995;269:F1–16.

81. Wolosin JM, Forte JG. Stimulation of oxyntic cell triggers K⁺ and Cl⁻ conductances in apical H⁺-K⁺-ATPase membrane. *Am J Physiol* 1984;246: C537–545.

82. Yao X, Forte JG. Cell biology of acid secretion by the parietal cell. *Annu Rev Physiol* 2003;65: 103–131.

83. Younes-Ibrahim M, Barlet-Bas C, Buffin-Meyer B, Cheval L, Rajerison R, Doucet A. Ouabain-sensitive and -insensitive K-ATPases in rat nephron: effect of K depletion. *Am J Physiol* 1995;268:F1141–1147.

84. Zhou X, Lynch IJ, Xia SL, Wingo CS. Activation of H⁺-K⁺-ATPase by CO₂ requires a basolateral Ba²⁺-sensitive pathway during K restriction. *Am J Physiol Renal Physiol* 2000;279: F153–160.

85. Zhou X, Nakamura S, Xia SL, Wingo CS. Increased CO₂ stimulates K/Rb reabsorption mediated by H-K-ATPase in CCD of potassium-restricted rabbit. *Am J Physiol Renal Physiol* 2001;281:F366–373.

86. Zhou X, Wingo CS. Mechanisms of rubidium permeation by rabbit cortical collecting duct during potassium restriction. *Am J Physiol* 1992;263:F1134–1141.

87. Zhou X, Wingo CS. Stimulation of total CO₂ flux by 10% CO₂ in rabbit CCD: role of an apical Sch-28080- and Ba-sensitive mechanism. *Am J Physiol* 1994;267:F114–120.

88. Zhou X, Xia SL, Wingo CS. Chloride transport by the rabbit cortical collecting duct: dependence on H,K-ATPase. *J Am Soc Nephrol* 1998;9:2194–2202.

CHAPTER 46

Extrarenal Potassium Metabolism

Robert M. Rosa and Franklin H. Epstein

The Feinberg School of Medicine, Northwestern University, Chicago, Illinois, USA
Beth Israel Deaconess Medical Center, Harvard Medical School, Boston, Massachusetts, USA

Internal potassium homeostasis is defined as the regulation of potassium distribution between the intracellular and extracellular fluid compartments, as distinct from the net gain or loss of potassium from the body. While the kidney plays the predominant role in maintaining external potassium balance, nonrenal tissues, especially muscle and liver, are quantitatively the most important organs involved in the regulation of internal potassium balance.

The ratio of potassium between intracellular and extracellular fluids is critically important not only to the behavior of electrically excitable cells, such as muscle and nerve, but also to the vital processes of all living cells. The reason for this is that a major regulator of cell function is the transmembrane potential. The determinants of this membrane potential are described by the Goldman-Hodgkin-Katz equation, the most important term of which is the logarithm of the ratio of internal to external ionic activity of potassium.

Of the 3500 mEq of potassium found in the body of a 70-kg human, about 98% is confined to intracellular water (Fig. 1). Of this, 80% is contained in muscle cells, at a concentration of about 150 mEq/l. The remaining 2% of total body potassium (about 70 mEq) is located in the extracellular fluid (about 14 L), where the normal concentration is 3.5 to 5.5 mEq/l. The chief biological mechanism responsible for maintaining this 30-fold potassium gradient between cell water and extracellular fluid is the Na,K-ATPase pump, situated in the plasma membrane of all animal cells. A minor role is played by the inward transport of potassium coupled with sodium and chloride, via the Na,K-2Cl transporter in the plasma membrane of some cells. Transcellular distribution of potassium is also modulated by hormonal factors such as insulin and catecholamines, by hydrogen ion balance, plasma osmolality, intracellular potassium content, and by factors that affect the passive movement of potassium through membrane channels, such as the level of intracellular calcium and pH (Table 1). Some of these factors, such as the activity of Na,K-ATPase and the distribution of hydrogen ions, may concurrently affect the potassium content of cells of the distal nephron and thereby influence the external balance of potassium.

From a practical standpoint, a key determinant of transmembrane potential is the plasma potassium. Since the concentration of potassium inside cells far exceeds extracellular concentration, percentile changes in intracellular potassium are relatively small even during extreme degrees of total body potassium surfeit, deficit, or internal redistribution. The changes in extracellular potassium seen in diseased states are therefore much more likely to alter the membrane potential of cells than are concomitant changes in intracellular potassium. For this reason, a variety of mechanisms have evolved to preserve the extracellular concentration of potassium within the normal range.

If a moderate load of potassium (0.5 mEq/kg) is administered intravenously over 1 hour, about 40% of it is excreted into the urine at the end of that time. Within 3 hours, renal excretion is complete and the serum potassium, which initially increases by about 0.6 mEq/l, returns to baseline (310, 412). The response of the normal human kidney to an oral load of potassium is more sluggish; while potassium excretion increases six- to 10-fold within a few hours (201, 202, 414), only about half of the load is excreted during the first 3 to 6 hours after it is ingested (47, 157, 200, 290, 414).

Consumption of only 35 mEq of potassium by a 70-kg adult during an average meal (an amount equivalent to 1% of total body potassium) would, if confined exclusively to the extracellular space, raise the plasma potassium by 2.5 mEq/l—enough to have pronounced effects on neuromuscular function. It is well established, however, that a potassium load given to a healthy human or dog has an apparent volume of distribution of 70% to 80% of body weight, somewhat greater than total body water (47, 415), instead of the 20% that represents extracellular fluid. In other words, only a small portion (about one fourth) of the 35 mEq of ingested potassium will normally remain in the extracellular compartment, raising the concentration of potassium in plasma by only about 0.6 mEq/l. In contrast, a similar load of potassium administered to patients with deranged extrarenal potassium homeostasis may produce serious hyperkalemia (288).

The cells also buffer plasma potassium during potassium depletion. In states of progressive potassium deficiency, as depletion worsens, a greater amount of potassium is lost from within cells to lessen the fall in external concentration and to minimize the alteration in its intracellular to extracellular ratio.

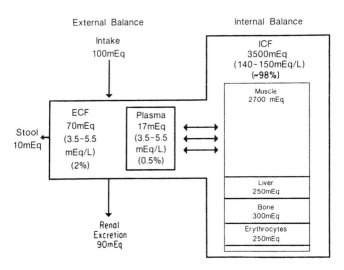

FIGURE 1 Internal potassium homeostasis in a 70-kg person. The potassium concentration in the extracellular fluid (ECF) depends on both the external balance (intake and output) and the internal balance (distribution between extracellular and intracellular fluid [ICF]). Factors affecting internal balance are listed in Table 1. Note that the large ICF pool exists at a far greater K concentration than the small ECF pool; the ECF pool will therefore change more dramatically with changes in total body K or K distribution.

TABLE 1 Factors Affecting Internal Potassium Homeostasis

Factor	Effect on Potassium
Insulin	Enhanced cell uptake
β-Catecholamines	Enhanced cell uptake
α-Catecholamines	Impaired cell uptake
Acidosis	Impaired cell uptake and enhanced efflux[a]
Alkalosis	Enhanced cell uptake and reduced efflux[a]
External potassium balance	Loose correlation
Drugs	See text
Hyperosmolality	Enhance cell efflux

[a]Degree varies with disturbance.

These examples of potassium surfeit or deficit emphasize the critical role of internal potassium homeostasis in mitigating potentially dangerous changes in the plasma potassium. Disorders of the factors that mediate this adjustment thus may have substantial clinical importance and are the primary topic of this chapter.

POTASSIUM DEPLETION AND REPLETION

In many conditions, such as vomiting, diabetic ketoacidosis, and chronic renal failure, abnormalities of internal and external potassium homeostasis coexist. Just as internal potassium homeostasis can affect potassium uptake and excretion by the kidney, so changes in external potassium balance, by altering cellular potassium content, can independently influence internal potassium homeostasis.

Potassium Depletion

The idealized curvilinear relationship between total body potassium and the serum potassium concentration illustrated in Fig. 2 is derived from several measurements in hypokalemic patients with positive potassium balance during replacement therapy (255, 262, 330) and from unpublished data on hyperkalemic humans and animals (332). In the early stages of depletion, extracellular potassium loss is proportionately greater than the loss of cellular potassium (206). Nonetheless, since only a small fraction of total body potassium is extracellular, the quantity of potassium lost from the extracellular compartment is much smaller than that lost from inside cells.

In the early phases of hypokalemia (>2.5 mEq/l), patients tend to display an almost linear relationship between total body potassium and the serum potassium concentration. It has been observed that a change of 100 to 200 mEq in total body potassium (about 5%) is required to lower the serum potassium by 1.0 mEq/l (332). In such a situation, the extracellular potassium concentration would be expected to fall proportionately more (e.g., 4.0 to 3.0 mEq/l) than the intracellular concentration (e.g., 140 to 133 mEq/l). Because of the relationship of cell membrane potentials to the ratio of internal to external ionic activity of potassium, excessive extracellular potassium loss would be expected to hyperpolarize cells (resting membrane potential is increased). This expectation has been confirmed in studies of early potassium deficiency in both dogs (41) and humans (303).

When potassium depletion becomes more severe, so that serum levels fall below about 2.5 mEq/l, a further 1.0-mEq/l fall will represent a much larger 200- to 400-mEq decrement

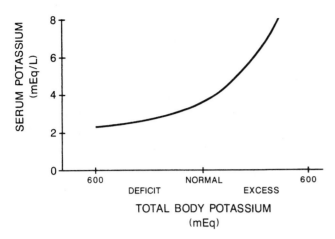

FIGURE 2 Idealized relationship between the serum potassium concentration and the body potassium content. (From Saris S, Lowenthal DT, Affrime MB, Rosenthal L, Swartz G. Lack of effect of nonsteroidal anti-inflammatory drugs on exercise-induced hyperkalemia. *N Engl J Med* 1982; 307:559–560, with permission.)

in total body potassium (greater than 10%), reflecting a greater degree of potassium loss from within the cells (133, 332) than occurred in the early phases of depletion. Decreased cell potassium content has, in fact, been observed in several tissues during severe hypokalemia (31, 262, 282).

In severe potassium depletion cells tend to depolarize (resting membrane potential is decreased), at least in dogs (41), which, like humans, then develop weakness and muscle paralysis.

Potassium Repletion

During potassium repletion for severe hypokalemia, cellular potassium uptake is enhanced both in animals (249, 356) and in humans (360); the administered potassium has an increased volume of distribution. As potassium is gained by the body and the stores become higher, the cellular uptake of potassium decreases. In anuric humans, for example, the cellular uptake of a potassium load decreases as total body potassium increases (360). Extracellular potassium then tends to rise and membrane potential decreases (408). The important therapeutic caveat in the late phases of correction of potassium depletion is that less potassium administration is required than in earlier phases to increase serum potassium, which may rise suddenly to unexpected, dangerously hyperkalemic levels (56).

As reviewed extensively by Sterns et al. (360), the serum potassium alone is, at best, an extremely rough guide for estimating potassium replacement therapy, presumably because other factors, such as acid-base status, influence it. A low serum potassium value (e.g., 3.0 mEq/l) may be associated with a range of total body deficits spanning a few hundred milli-equivalents (Fig. 2).

The exact mechanisms that produce this curvilinear relationship are uncertain. They may stem in part from impair-

ment of the electrogenic sodium pump (41, 95, 223). During potassium depletion in rats, skeletal muscle potassium loss is associated with a reduced capacity for Na-K pumping and a reversible decrease in the number of ^{3}H-ouabain binding sites (273). A possible mechanism for suppression of the Na-K pump during potassium depletion is enhanced stimulation of α-adrenoreceptors (10) (see Catecholamines).

INSULIN

The effect of insulin on potassium homeostasis was first demonstrated two years after its purification by Banting and Best. Harrop and Benedict (171) and Briggs and Koechig (52) described the fall in serum potassium coincident with lowering of blood sugar when insulin was administered to diabetic patients as well as in the nondiabetic human, dog, and rabbit. Later, there were reports of severe hypokalemia in insulin-treated patients with ketoacidosis who developed paralysis (180).

Cellular Mechanism

The hypokalemic action of insulin derives from its capacity to cause net potassium uptake in skeletal muscle (82, 144, 426), adipose tissue, and hepatic cells (30, 60, 217), as well as other extrarenal sites (160). This effect was formerly assumed to occur to preserve electrical neutrality when insulin-mediated glucose uptake produced intracellular anionic sugars (164, 257) and deposited potassium as an accompaniment of glycogen in the liver (134).

This classical hypothesis did not explain the clinical observation that sudden lowering of serum potassium could precede the fall in blood sugar in insulin-treated diabetic coma. Zierler (427) first noted that insulin's effect on potassium movement in rat muscle occurred even in the absence of glucose; its known effect to increase sodium efflux in vitro also occurred without glucose (94). Furthermore, enhancement of potassium disposal in the intact animal was separable temporally from glucose uptake (21, 203) and occurred at plasma insulin concentrations having no measurable influence on uptake of glucose in vivo (429). Different receptor mechanisms for potassium and glucose transport appear to exist (257).

In vitro, insulin is known to stimulate both potassium uptake (159, 238) and sodium efflux (82, 256) in frog and rat muscle preparations. Similar effects have been reported in rat adipose tissue (302), hepatocytes (132), and other cells (105). Considerable evidence (257) suggests that following binding to cell surface receptors (96), insulin accelerates monovalent cation transport by stimulating Na,K-ATPase, the sodium–potassium pump. Most convincing is the fact that both insulin-stimulated net sodium efflux and potassium influx are blocked by ouabain (82, 159, 162, 256). In vitro, addition of insulin to purified plasma membrane of skeletal muscle increases the activity of the Na,K-ATPase

(150). Little evidence is currently available on whether insulin affects potassium permeability or potassium channels in skeletal muscle cells. Insulin activation of sodium–hydrogen exchange sensitive to amiloride (258) does not appear to be important to sodium-pump–mediated potassium uptake (80). In adipocytes, insulin-stimulated uptake of K^+ and Rb^+ is inhibited by bumetanide and by removal of Cl^- from the extracellular fluid, suggesting a primary action of insulin on the Na-K-2Cl cotransporter (319). On the other hand, in skeletal muscle insulin does not appear to activate the cotransport of K^+ with Na^+ and Cl^- (158).

Stimulation of active sodium–potassium transport by Na,K-ATPase could be due to a de novo increase in the number of sodium pump sites or to allosteric activation of existing sites. The latter theory is consistent with the rapid activation of transport that occurs (301) as well as with the lack of new ouabain binding sites (81, 129) after exposure to insulin in vitro.

At least three molecular forms of the Na,K-ATPase catalytic subunit have been identified, designated $\alpha 1$, $\alpha 2$, and $\alpha 3$. The $\alpha 2$ (or $\alpha +$) subunit, present in muscle cells and adipocytes but not liver, is activated by insulin (233). In liver, on the other hand, the effect of insulin can be entirely accounted for by increased intracellular sodium concentration (132). Insulin also activates a KCl cotransporter uptake system in a cultured cell line resembling skeletal muscle (396).

It should be noted that insulin is known to produce hyperpolarization of cellular membranes not only in skeletal muscle (425, 428) but in a variety of other tissues (29, 216). This rapid effect appears to precede measurable increases in intracellular potassium (426). Although stimulation of Na,K-ATPase could account for insulin's hyperpolarizing effect (259), failure of ouabain to block it, at least in some studies, suggests that changes in ion permeability may be responsible. The role of hyperpolarization in mediating insulin effects on cation transport is uncertain. The effect of insulin to stimulate active sodium and potassium transport in skeletal muscle is mimicked by insulin-like growth factor 1 (IGF-1) (117).

In Vivo Effects

Abundant evidence therefore exists that insulin increases net uptake of potassium ions by several tissues in vitro. Since skeletal muscle is well documented to respond to insulin and is the major body reservoir for potassium, it is the most likely dominant site for insulin-stimulated extrarenal potassium disposal in vivo. Human forearm muscle (and adipose tissue) increases potassium uptake during arterial infusion (429) of insulin.

Wilde (407) noted that injected potassium rapidly disappeared from the blood of cats but was followed by a secondary rise in serum potassium. Recent investigation suggests that, at least during insulin infusion, hepatic disposal plays an important role in potassium homeostasis in the first hour of exposure to insulin in humans (109). Splanchnic uptake accounted for two thirds of the fall in plasma potassium dur-

ing euglycemic hyperinsulinemia. In the second hour, net splanchnic uptake reversed, and peripheral tissues became the dominant site of potassium disposal.

That the effect of insulin on extrarenal potassium homeostasis is dose related is well established (Fig. 3) (36, 93). In normal subjects, neither intramuscular nor subcutaneous administration of insulin, which achieved plasma insulin levels of about 50 μU/ml, decreased the plasma potassium (167). Intravenous insulin injection, by comparison, produced 40-fold greater insulin levels, which were accompanied by steady-state reduction in plasma potassium, with a maximal effect of about 30% occurring 50 minutes after insulin injection. On the other hand, much smaller increments of insulin, about threefold above basal values, during constant venous (109, 251) or intra-arterial infusion (21, 140, 429), also appear capable of augmenting potassium uptake in vivo (360). In rats, short-term potassium depletion prevents the hypokalemic effect of insulin (74).

Clinical Implications

The relevance of these findings to a given clinical situation will depend on the magnitude of potassium load requiring disposal and the elevation of insulin accompanying it. Following carbohydrate feeding, for example, increased liver uptake of potassium occurs (134). Since peripheral venous insulin levels for 2 hours following oral glucose loading are elevated fivefold (417), well within the range capable of augmenting potassium uptake, it seems likely that insulin contributes to the transient decrease in potassium that occurs after feeding (418). Even basal circulating insulin levels may be essential to disposal of an acute potassium load, since disposal is impaired when basal levels are decreased 50% by somatostatin (111). The effect of carbohydrate meals to blunt or prevent hyperkalemia may be particularly important in anuric patients dependent on extracorporeal dialysis (16).

During exogenous potassium challenge, the importance of insulin to potassium disposal by the intact organism deprived of endogenous insulin (179, 294, 318, 338) or resistant to the actions of insulin (107) is well established. As expected, supraphysiologic doses of exogenous insulin are capable of improving potassium tolerance (318). Thus, for emergency treatment of hyperkalemia, the administration of insulin together with glucose is indicated even if the patient is not diabetic, since higher plasma levels of insulin can be achieved than with glucose alone.

The ability of potassium loading to stimulate the release of pancreatic insulin directly, in amounts sufficient to contribute to disposal of that potassium, is less clear. In pancreatic B cells, ATP-sensitive K channels link cellular membrane potential to hormone secretion (106). These channels control the transmembrane potential and thereby the calcium channels that trigger glucose-induced insulin secretion (292). Depolarization of the cell membrane (as expected with hyperkalemia) induces an increase in insulin secretion (103). In humans (115) and intact dogs (101, 178, 295), minor

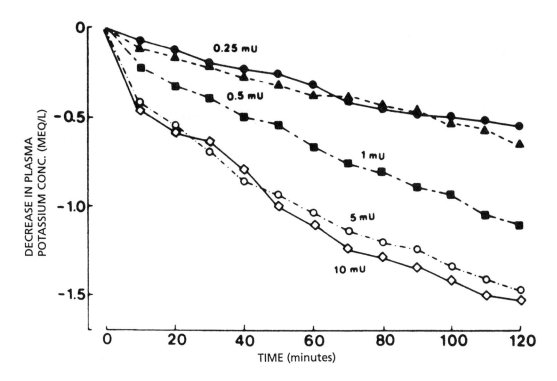

FIGURE 3 Dose-related effect of euglycemic hyperinsulinemia on plasma potassium concentration. Infusion of insulin at the doses shown produced plasma insulin levels of approximately 25, 50, 100, 500, and 1000 μ/ml above basal values. (From Bia M, DeFronzo R. The medullary collecting duct (MCD) does not play a primary role in potassium (K) adaptation following decreased GFR. *Clin Res* 1978;26:457A, with permission.)

increments in blood potassium appear capable of triggering pancreatic insulin secretion. Since elevations in portal venous insulin far exceed those in the peripheral circulation when insulin release is stimulated (6, 43, 178), it seems reasonable to conclude that, under conditions of significant hyperkalemia, induction of insulin release to promote potassium uptake does constitute a homeostatic feedback control system.

GLUCAGON

The effect of glucagon on extrarenal potassium disposal has been difficult to isolate, because the hormone also influences the secretion of insulin, epinephrine, and aldosterone. Administration of glucagon to cats does appear to mobilize potassium from the liver and produce a transient rise in arterial potassium levels (416). In humans, the hyperkalemic response to the hormone appears to be only partly due to an epinephrine-like effect of glucagon to increase liver glycogenolysis (242).

For example, aortic injection of glucagon in humans, which results in hepatic vein glucagon levels within the pathophysiologic range, causes a transient increment in hepatic vein potassium concentrations, but this precedes the slow rise in glucose in hepatic venous blood (241). The specific source of the modest rise in hepatic venous potassium

under these conditions has not been determined. Previous in vitro investigations using perfused rat liver suggest that glucagon releases potassium directly from the liver (60, 138). The effect would not appear to be due to diminished Na-K pump–mediated potassium uptake, since isolated rat hepatocytes exposed to glucagon actually undergo stimulation of this cation pump (232).

Systemic infusion of glucagon to physiologic levels tends to elevate plasma potassium slightly by an extrarenal mechanism, at least when glucagon-induced insulin secretion is suppressed by somatostatin, both in normal subjects (242) and in diabetic subjects (64). It is unclear whether hyperglucagonemia, which occurs in decompensated diabetes mellitus (265), uremia (40), and exhausting exercise (207), affects potassium homeostasis. In the dog, potassium-stimulated insulin release appears to be accompanied by a modest rise in circulating glucagon (207, 318).

CATECHOLAMINES

The observation of D'Silva (97) in 1934 that epinephrine lowers the serum potassium in cats has since acquired important physiologic and clinical relevance (76, 128, 364). Although D'Silva emphasized the rapid rise in the serum potassium that followed a bolus injection of epinephrine (now believed to be a consequence of transient hepatic discharge of potassium by α-adrenergic stimulation) (85, 98, 379), of greater significance was the sustained "after-fall" in serum potassium that he observed. This secondary decrease in potassium was found to persist throughout a 1-hour infusion of epinephrine (380).

Since epinephrine inhibited the renal excretion of potassium (197, 348), its late hypokalemic action was attributed to net uptake of potassium by extrarenal tissues. Indeed, in vivo limb studies in dogs (297) and humans (104, 163) as well as tissue analysis and ion flux studies supported accelerated uptake of potassium, primarily in skeletal muscle (386), but also in liver (386) and heart (153), in response to epinephrine. In vitro, epinephrine was demonstrated to stimulate potassium uptake as well as sodium efflux by isolated skeletal muscle in both rats (26, 79) and humans (26). A similar effect was present in rat diaphragm (130), cat cardiac muscle (230), and frog sartorius muscle (173).

Because epinephrine may influence insulin secretion, it was necessary to show that its hypokalemic effect was independent of insulin (112, 293). Independence from renin-mediated aldosterone release was established by the lowering of potassium despite nephrectomy (38, 274). Since extrarenal potassium disposal was impaired when nephrectomized rats were subjected to adrenalectomy or to chemical sympathectomy (338), both circulating adrenomedullary epinephrine as well as peripheral sympathetic nervous activity appeared to be important sources of sympathetic influence on potassium.

β-Adrenergic Effects

Epinephrine stimulates both α- and β-adrenergic receptors (9). The conclusion that its hypokalemic action was a result of β-adrenergic stimulation derived from experiments many years later using β-agonists and β-antagonists (297, 379). Isoproterenol, a nonspecific β-agonist, reproduced the prolonged hypokalemia earlier observed by D'Silva, and this effect was reversed by the β-adrenergic antagonist propranolol; likewise, epinephrine's effects on cation flux were blocked by β-antagonists (76, 310).

β-agonists and antagonists have been used to establish that the stimulating effect of catecholamines on potassium uptake is mediated by the β₂-receptor subtype (37, 374). Epinephrine's effect on potassium is prevented by the presence of nonselective β-antagonists such as propranolol (108, 228, 230, 297, 310, 387, 388) and timolol (365) as well as by the nonspecific α-β-blocker labetalol (395). Less reversal occurs with the partially β₁-selective antagonists metoprolol (78) and atenolol (365). No effect on potassium appears to be produced by the more specific β₁-antagonist practolol (229, 230). In addition, the selective β₂-antagonists butoxamine (37, 370) and ICI-118551 (54, 363) are able to block the hypokalemic action of β-agonists.

Numerous studies of β-agonists have revealed that several β₂-agonists, including salbutamol (172, 222, 345, 346,

376), terbutaline (48, 183, 260, 274), fenoterol (168), and ritodrine (48) lower potassium levels, unlike the β₁-agonist ITP (230), which has no effect. These pharmacologic studies therefore provide strong support for β₂ mediation of adrenergic effects to enhance potassium disposal.

Mechanism of Action

The specific cellular mechanism by which cell surface β₂-receptor stimulation augments transcellular potassium uptake in affected tissues has been evaluated in detail. Compelling evidence now exists to support the proposal of Clausen (76) that β₂ stimulation initiates cyclic AMP formation (185), which leads to activation of the sodium pump (Na,K-ATPase) and therefore electrogenic sodium efflux accompanied by potassium uptake (77). β-receptors are known to stimulate adenylate cyclase (73, 144, 185), enhancing conversion of intracellular ATP to cyclic AMP (63). Linkage of β-receptors and cyclic AMP is supported by the ability of theophylline to potentiate the effect of epinephrine on cation transport and membrane potential (76), as well as by the increase in membrane potential that dibutyryl cyclic AMP and theophylline produce in rat diaphragm muscle (50). Epinephrine, in stimulating cation transport, is well known to produce hyperpolarization of membranes in skeletal muscle (76).

The sodium pump of muscle cells and lipocytes is activated by cyclic AMP. For example, Na,K-ATPase activity in smooth muscle membrane fragments is enhanced by exposure to cyclic AMP (323). The most compelling evidence that catecholamine-mediated potassium influx involves the β-adrenergic system through activation of the sodium pump, however, are the demonstrations in a series of experiments that potassium influx occurs as active movement of the cation against its electrochemical gradient (322); ouabain blocks the ability of epinephrine to promote potassium influx in rat soleus muscle (79); epinephrine markedly increases the ouabain-sensitive ^{22}Na efflux by stimulating the Na-K pump in frog skeletal muscle and this effect is blocked by propranolol (194); epinephrine produces membrane hyperpolarization and transient decreases in extracellular potassium and intracellular sodium, which is blocked by ouabain, in isolated rat soleus muscle and human intercostal muscle (26); and isoproterenol directly stimulates the Na-K pump in isolated rabbit myocytes (113). While the specific sequence of events linking β-adrenergic stimulation to sodium pump activity has not been delineated, phosphorylation of some portion of the sodium pump after β₂-receptor stimulation is presumably involved (322). β-adrenergic agents also stimulate the cellular uptake of potassium via the Na-K-2Cl transporter in the skeletal muscle membrane of rats (158).

There are numerous clinical examples showing that enhanced exogenous or endogenous β-adrenergic stimulation augments extrarenal potassium uptake in humans. Whether high potassium levels can stimulate secretion of endogenous adrenomedullary epinephrine and thereby form a homeostatic feedback loop remains unresolved. Supraphysiologic levels of potassium in vitro can cause the release of catecholamines from isolated chromaffin cells (119) and perfused adrenal glands (25), possibly related to the membrane depolarizing effect of a high potassium level. Induction of tyrosine hydroxylase, the rate-limiting enzyme in catecholamine biosynthesis (337), by extremely high levels of potassium has also been observed. Reports that intra-arterial injections of KCl augment catecholamine release in cats (389) and in the dogfish shark (275) suggest a potential role for potassium as a catecholamine secretagogue in vivo.

Although specific stimulation of catecholamine release by potassium is not established, it is clear that physiologic elevations of endogenous catecholamines do enhance potassium uptake. Similar to the pharmacologic doses of epinephrine used in earlier animal reports of its protective effect during potassium loading (177, 230, 380) as well as of its ability to lower basal potassium (243), relatively small doses (108, 310) have also been shown to enhance extrarenal disposal of an acute potassium load. It has also been established that ambient potassium may be lowered when sustained epinephrine infusions (Fig. 4) (55) elevate plasma concentrations of epinephrine to levels no higher than those observed in stressful conditions such as myocardial infarction (196), surgical stress (169), and diabetic ketoacidosis (75). By comparison, acute β blockade does not appear to elevate fasting potassium levels (55), suggesting that basal β-adrenergic tone plays a limited role in potassium homeostasis in healthy, fasted individuals at rest.

It has been appreciated, however, that there are two common physiologic circumstances in which endogenous catecholamines could act to defend against increments in extracellular potassium concentration. The first of these is postprandial disposal of dietary potassium. Feeding is now known to be associated with stimulation of the sympathetic nervous system (219). Since only half of the potassium ingested in a meal is normally excreted within 6 hours (157), enhanced β-adrenergic–mediated extrarenal potassium disposal may help to limit elevations of serum potassium in the immediate postprandial period. In conjunction with enhanced potassium uptake due to insulin release, this mechanism would be particularly important in subjects at risk for hyperkalemia for any reason.

The second circumstance is the dramatic effect of catecholamine release during vigorous exertion to moderate the acute physiologic hyperkalemia of exercise. Catecholamines circulate at high levels during vigorous exercise and the associated short-term elevation of potassium that is released into the circulation from working muscles is exaggerated by β blockade (Fig. 5) (70, 410), suggesting that endogenous β-adrenergic activity does protect against extreme hyperkalemia during exhaustive exercise.

α-Adrenergic Effects

The fact that opposing α- and β-adrenergic influences have in the past been reported on smooth muscle tone (218), glucoregulatory hormones (184), presynaptic membrane receptors (400), and changes in intracellular second

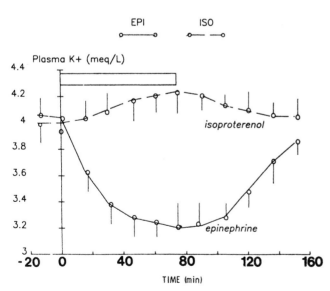

FIGURE 4 Effect of epinephrine and isoproterenol infusions (long box) on the plasma potassium concentration. The contrasting effects of the two β agonists probably are due to the relative β2 selectivity of epinephrine at the dose given. Plasma epinephrine concentrations achieved by infusion were similar to those known to occur in myocardial infarction and other disorders. (From Brown MJ. Hypokalemia from beta 2-receptor stimulation by circulating epinephrine. *Am J Cardiol* 1985;56:3D–9D, with permission.)

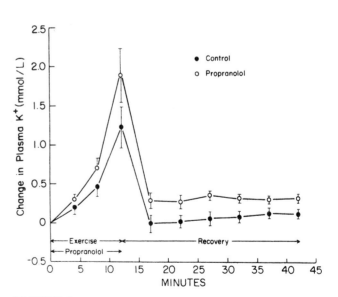

FIGURE 5 Effect of adrenergic blockade on the plasma potassium concentration during vigorous exercise and recovery. β blockade with propranolol potentiated the rise of plasma potassium at peak exercise and prolonged its elevation during recovery. In the same subjects, α blockade with phentolamine was shown to lower the peak plasma potassium level as well as the overall potassium curve. (From Watson KR, O'Kell RT. Lack of relationship between Mg2+ and K+ concentrations in serum. *Clin Chem* 1980;26:520–521, with permission.)

messengers (185, 189) suggests the role of α-adrenergic agonists in potassium homeostasis. As noted previously, the early rise in extracellular potassium emphasized by D'Silva in 1934 (97) was later attributed to α-mediated hepatic potassium release, by the mixed α- and β-agonist epinephrine (379). This initial rise in potassium could be prevented by α blockade (379). In addition, phenylephrine, a pure α-agonist, was observed to cause a sustained increase in potassium in dogs (191, 379).

When phenylephrine was infused into normal human subjects who were challenged with an intravenous potassium load, the overall rise in plasma potassium was augmented by about 50% (412) despite no change in insulin, renin, aldosterone, or urinary potassium. In separate studies, addition of the α-antagonist phentolamine blocked the phenylephrine effect on potassium disposal. Neither α stimulation nor blockade appeared to affect the concentration of potassium in the absence of potassium loading.

Other evidence suggests that the α effect might directly contribute to potassium homeostasis in certain circumstances. α-Receptor stimulation during vigorous exercise contributes to the acute rise in potassium that is maximal at peak exercise and limits the dramatic fall due to potassium reuptake during recovery (410). Furthermore, during potassium depletion in rats, the sodium–potassium pump of skeletal muscle is suppressed by an increase in α-adrenergic activity mediated by nerves, an action that would mitigate the expected fall in plasma potassium concentration (10). It is therefore speculated that enhanced α-agonist activity might act to preserve potassium similarly during a variety of acute illnesses, such as myocardial infarction (55) or delirium tremens (392), where catecholamine stimulation of both β- and α-receptors may coexist. Unopposed stimulation of α-receptors may contribute to the impairment of potassium disposal caused by β-receptor blockade.

Dopamine

The infusion of dopamine is known to augment glomerular filtration rate, renal plasma flow, osmolar clearance, sodium excretion (246), and potassium excretion (247) in healthy humans and animals. Levodopa, the metabolic precursor of dopamine, has also been reported to enhance renal potassium excretion (141, 161), and an increase in endogenous dopamine produced by protein feeding has been associated with augmented kaliuresis (409). On the other hand, the dopamine antagonist metoclopramide also increases potassium excretion, an action ascribed to its blockade of tonic dopaminergic inhibition of aldosterone release (69). Whether the dopaminergic system plays a role in extrarenal potassium homeostasis remains uncertain. Both dopamine and dobutamine lower plasma potassium when infused into anesthetized dogs, but only by a few tenths of a milliequivalent per liter (44). While some studies demonstrate enhanced extrarenal potassium uptake into cells following administration of metoclopramide (34, 315, 421), others demonstrate no

such effect of either metoclopramide (68, 298, 352) or the dopamine agonist bromocriptine (68, 298, 406). The discrepancy between these studies may be attributed, at least in part, to the fact that metoclopramide is a nonspecific antagonist of dopamine (375). The determination of the role, if any, of the dopaminergic system in extrarenal potassium homeostasis must await studies employing specific dopamine antagonists.

Clinical Implications

The clinical significance of epinephrine-induced hypokalemia is underscored by reports of hypokalemia occurring during acute illnesses, such as myocardial infarction, as well as during medical treatment with β-agonists (1). Struthers et al. (365) discovered that when epinephrine infusion produced circulating epinephrine levels similar to those found after myocardial infarction, the serum potassium fell from 4.06 to 3.22 mEq/l in healthy volunteers. This ability of small doses of epinephrine to diminish potassium levels was confirmed by Brown et al. (55). In this context, the frequency of hypokalemia during acute myocardial infarction has been observed to be 8% to 30% (116, 234, 309, 377). Concomitant therapy with diuretics may further increase the frequency of hypokalemia during myocardial infarction (192, 271) as it appears to do in normal subjects who are experimentally infused with epinephrine (366).

Because several studies have suggested that hypokalemia is an independent risk factor for cardiac arrhythmias in patients with acute myocardial infarction, these observations may have clinical relevance. A higher incidence of atrial fibrillation (121) and ventricular arrhythmias are reported in hypokalemic compared with normokalemic patients during infarction (234, 270). In one report (309), ventricular tachycardia or fibrillation increased threefold (to 35%) and hospital mortality doubled in hypokalemic patients with myocardial infarction.

It must be appreciated, however, that the hypokalemia reported during earlier studies of epinephrine infusion occurred when high concentrations of plasma epinephrine were sustained by infusion. Whether elevations of plasma epinephrine during acute myocardial infarction are similarly sustained, rather than transient (196), is uncertain. The contribution of circulating epinephrine to the hypokalemia that may occur during this form of acute illness therefore remains hypothetical. Nonetheless, pharmacologic data suggest that such acutely ill patients may be protected from the hypokalemia that is sometimes associated with myocardial infarction by the use of β-blockers (272, 387, 388). Whether the beneficial effect of β blockade reported in this setting is due to diminution in hypokalemia-related arrhythmias is not known. That hypokalemia is not more prevalent in the setting of acute myocardial infarction may, in part, be a consequence of a simultaneous elevation in plasma norepinephrine, suggesting α-receptor stimulation that might antagonize the effect of epinephrine on potassium homeostasis.

Transient lowering of potassium levels has also been reported in other acute medical conditions (20, 89, 248, 263) in which catecholamines might stimulate β-adrenergic receptors capable of increasing cellular uptake of potassium. Pharmacologic therapy using β₂-agonists such as terbutaline, ritodrine and salbutamol to prevent premature labor (48, 172, 260, 344, 376) may produce a substantial degree of hypokalemia. Administration of salbutamol and albuterol in the treatment of bronchospasm (308, 345) may also produce unwanted hypokalemia. In this context, it is important to appreciate that administration of inhaled β₂-agonists to healthy volunteers in doses similar to those used by asthmatic patients during an acute attack has produced decrements of the plasma potassium of as much as 0.9 mEq/l (168). These observations raise the disturbing possibility that such usage of these agents may be the explanation for the high incidence of sudden death in adolescent asthmatics (312). Hypokalemia in this setting might be further exaggerated by the concomitant use of theophylline (413) or other methylxanthines (143, 227). Theophylline not only increases the level of circulatory catecholamines but also enhances catechol stimulation of adenylate cyclase by blocking inhibitory adenosine receptors.

The clinical significance of the adrenergic nervous system in potassium balance is also evident in the well-established effect of β-antagonists to elevate extracellular potassium concentration. An example is the acute effect of propranolol to exaggerate the hyperkalemia of vigorous exercise (410). Some (283, 284, 390), but not all (27, 358), investigators have reported a 10% to 15% increase in ambient plasma potassium during chronic β blockade with nonselective agents. In addition, one study suggests that the serum potassium may rise above 6 mEq/l in patients on nonselective β blockers at the time of open heart surgery (291). Transient hyperkalemia has been reported after cyclosporine administration in patients on β-blocking agents, but not when these are omitted (285). Patients receiving succinylcholine anesthesia may also be at risk for the development of hyperkalemia (244). Patients with end-stage renal failure on dialysis, moreover, regularly exhibit an increase in predialysis potassium of about 1 mEq/l when treated with propranolol (24). Despite the clinical relevance of these studies describing an increase in extracellular potassium concentration in a variety of clinical conditions in patients receiving β blockers, it is important to realize that β blockers are unlikely to produce any significant increment in potassium concentration in subjects in whom the other mechanisms of potassium homeostasis are intact.

Since some studies do substantiate the anticipated absence of effect on potassium of cardioselective β₁-antagonists (23, 231, 291), selected groups of patients at risk for hyperkalemia might be protected from significant elevations in potassium due to β blockade by the use of such selective agents. Such patients include those with diabetes mellitus, hypoaldosteronism, and renal failure.

THYROID

Thyroid hormones enhance the activity of Na,K-ATPase in muscle cells (186), accelerating the extrarenal disposal of potassium (214). A portion of this effect can be ascribed to upregulation of β-adrenergic receptors and an increase in β-adrenergic responsiveness, but there appears to be a direct effect on cellular Na,K-ATPase as well (214). Hypokalemic paralysis occasionally complicates thyrotoxicosis; in such cases urinary excretion of potassium is always low, reinforcing the hypothesis that the low serum potassium reflects a shift of potassium from the extracellular to the intracellular compartment rather than urinary losses of potassium. The hypokalemia and paralysis respond to the administration of β-adrenergic blocking agents (226). This syndrome has been reported many times in Asians but is extremely rare in whites and blacks. It is not, moreover, associated with the inherited mutations in the calcium and sodium ion channels reported to cause familial hypokalemic periodic paralysis but may in some cases be associated with a mutation in a channel mediating potassium efflux (114). Hyperkalemia has been reported in hypothyroid dogs after exercise but not in humans with hypothyroidism (321).

ACID-BASE

Although acid-base balance affects potassium excretion by the kidney, shifts of potassium in and out of body cells are the initial way in which acid-base disturbances alter serum potassium. These movements are influenced by a variety of factors, including the changes in extracellular and intracellular pH, the degree of cellular buffering, the nature of the anion accompanying H^+, and the associated changes in hormonal and neural regulators of potassium uptake, including insulin and catecholamines.

The concentration of potassium in plasma tends to vary in the same direction as that of free hydrogen ions (136, 221, 360, 372), so that acidosis promotes hyperkalemia and alkalosis promotes hypokalemia. Since approximately 40% of the acid buffering capacity of the body is provided by intracellular proteins, largely in muscle cells (329), and since potassium is the chief intracellular cation of muscle, the release of intracellular potassium is to be expected as a consequence of the intracellular buffering of hydrogen ions. Conversely, with repair of acidosis, or during alkalosis, potassium will tend to move into cells. This exchange of K^+ for H^+ is not necessarily equimolar and the routes across the plasma membrane that are responsible for such transfers have not been completely delineated. A simple reciprocal exchange of K^+ and H^+ via a single plasma membrane transporter has not been described in muscle cells.

Hydrogen Ion

The importance of pH in affecting internal potassium distribution during acidosis was demonstrated in early studies (59, 152, 306, 339). Fenn and Cobb (136) reported in 1934 that potassium exited from skeletal muscle in vitro when the bath pH was lowered and moved into the tissue when blood at physiologic pH was substituted for acidic medium. They invoked the Donnan equilibrium to account for similarity in the intracellular to extracellular ratios of hydrogen and potassium ions, so that a decrease in that ratio produced by acidosis would be associated with a decrease in the ratio for potassium—that is, an increase in extracellular K^+. In vivo as well, an approximately linear relationship appears to exist between the potassium gradient and the pH gradient across muscle cell membranes, as predicted by the Donnan effect (53, 391). Nevertheless, the shifts in potassium observed in experimental situations are not always fully explained, either by the Donnan effect or by changes in membrane potential (8, 391).

Since the ratio of K^+ concentration inside cells to that outside cells (Ki/Ke), for skeletal muscle is approximately 30, the maintenance of a similar hydrogen ion ratio between intracellular and extracellular fluid would require an intracellular pH of approximately 5.92. However, intracellular pH is actually in the range of 6.9 to 7.0, so that the intracellular to extracellular proton ratio is only approximately 3 rather than 30. The major reason for this is the operation of the amiloride-sensitive Na^+-H^+ antiporter, which transports H^+ out of cells by a secondary active mechanism that ultimately derives its energy from ATP via the Na,K-ATPase of plasma membranes.

Moreover, the direction of the movement of potassium during acute acid-base disorders is not uniform among various tissues (8). During acute respiratory acidosis, potassium moves out of the cells in muscle and liver, but into cardiac muscle. Yet, in both skeletal and cardiac muscle, the ratio of intracellular to extracellular hydrogen ion concentration falls. As will be seen subsequently, powerful evidence has been adduced under both in vitro and in vivo conditions suggesting that in some circumstances the ionic ratios of hydrogen and potassium can be dissociated and transmembrane fluxes of potassium change in the face of a stable pH gradient.

Inhibition of the sodium-potassium pump of plasma membranes by an acid pH contributes importantly to the relationship between acidosis and plasma potassium. In every case in which it has been measured, an increase in plasma potassium associated with systemic acidosis is accompanied by a fall in intracellular potassium. The optimal pH for mammalian Na,K-ATPase is 7.5 to 7.6, whereas intracellular pH of muscle is 6.9 to 7.2 (343). The effect of pH on the activity of the sodium–potassium pump is exerted from the intracellular, rather than the extracellular, side of the membrane (51, 122). In bladder epithelial cells, for example, a reduction of intracellular pH by 0.3 units, from pH 7.2 to 6.9, reduced pump activity to about 70% of that at pH 7.2. On the other hand, alkalinizing the cell interior to pH 7.5 led to a 35% increase in sodium pump activity (122).

In addition to a direct effect of pH on the sodium–potassium transport enzyme, an indirect mechanism might involve the linked operation of the Na^+-H^+ antiporter and the Na,K-ATPase. An attractive mechanism to explain the shift of potassium out of cells that occurs in acidosis involves the linked operation of these two transporters. Both of these transporters are present in the plasma membranes of most cells including skeletal muscle. Acidification of the extracellular fluid would be expected to slow the rate at which hydrogen ions leave the cell and sodium ions enter, via the Na^+-H^+ antiporter. The resultant decrease in intracellular sodium concentration would slow the Na-K pump, reduce active uptake of potassium by cells, and increase the concentration of potassium in extracellular fluid. A prediction of this hypothesis is that amiloride, which blocks the Na-H antiporter, would prevent the hyperkalemia produced by acidosis. It is not yet known whether this is the case, but amiloride does block the extracellular acidosis produced by KCl infusions (18).

Finally, intracellular acidosis appears to open ATP-sensitive potassium channels in skeletal muscle by reducing the degree of channel inhibition by ATP, an action that might accelerate efflux of K^+ from muscle cells during anoxia or extreme acidosis (102).

Mineral Acids

Acute mineral acidosis, produced by infusing HCl or NH4Cl, elevated plasma potassium by an average of 0.7 mEq/l per 0.1 unit decrease in blood pH, in 14 different studies summarized by Adrogue and Madias (8). The results of these studies were extremely variable, however, ranging from 0.24 to 1.67 mEq/l per 0.1 pH unit.

One reason for the variability in these reports is that the effect of mineral acid infusions on plasma potassium depends on the duration of the acidosis (236, 278, 339, 360). Immediately following an acute acid infusion there is a marked fall in extracellular pH and bicarbonate, followed by a gradual rise over the next 2 hours or so, as tissue buffering and respiratory compensation moderate the initial changes in blood pH (278, 329, 339, 372). Plasma potassium begins to rise early in the course of the infusion and increases progressively as buffering takes place, so that its concentration does not change in parallel with the change in pH. Late in the course of an acute acid load, when cell buffers have been exhausted and intracellular pH drops sharply, plasma potassium rises more steeply.

It might be expected that the hyperkalemic response to an acid load would be influenced by the state of muscle potassium. Experimental potassium depletion induced by deoxycorticosterone acetate (DOCA) (mean plasma K^+ 1.9 mEq/l) did indeed attenuate the increase in plasma potassium produced by metabolic acidosis but did not prevent it, and the percentage rise in plasma potassium from baseline induced by NH_4Cl acid loading was not significantly different from that of controls (384).

Clinical observations on the endogenous mineral acidosis of uremia, due to retention of sulfate and phosphate, suggest that the change in potassium that is observed when acidosis is corrected is of the magnitude expected in experimental mineral acidosis (331, 332).

Organic Acids

That changes in acidity are not the sole determinant of the kalemic response to acidosis is indicated by the disparate effects which mineral acidosis and nonmineral acidosis have on potassium. In humans and animals, infusion of organic acids such as acetic, lactic, or β-hydroxybutyric acid produces far smaller elevations of potassium than does hydrochloric acid (33, 199, 277, 278, 378). The prevailing hypothesis is that the anions of organic acids, either by readily penetrating the intracellular compartment (8), by entering cells as intact molecules (307), or by being formed endogenously within cells (146), minimize the necessity for potassium cations to leave cells in exchange for hydrogen ions (289). The addition of HCl to rat diaphragms in vitro results in a loss of potassium from the muscle (306), whereas when extracellular pH is lowered by addition of acetic acid, β-hydroxybutyric acid, or lactic acid, no shift of potassium out of the cell is observed (307).

For similar degrees of clinical severity, less elevation of serum potassium occurs with endogenous organic acidosis encountered in ill patients than with mineral acidosis, although the correlation of pH and serum potassium in clinical states of organic acidosis is further complicated by prior total body potassium depletion, oliguric renal failure, hypercatabolism, and other factors (289). Ketone acids, for example, stimulate the secretion of insulin by the normal pancreas, while suppressing the secretion of glucagon. Infusions of hydrochloric acid, on the other hand, do not stimulate insulin secretion but enhance plasma glucagon (6), which in turn tends to elevate the serum potassium. The sympathoadrenal system, which is strongly activated in most clinical states accompanied by organic acidosis (e.g., diabetic or alcoholic ketoacidosis, and the lactic acidosis of circulatory shock), plays an important role in minimizing hyperkalemia, because of the hypokalemic action of β-adrenergic stimulation. Moderately severe potassium depletion (as occurs in diabetic ketoacidosis) itself attenuates the increase in plasma potassium induced by metabolic acidosis (384).

Untreated severe diabetic ketoacidosis is characterized by marked deficits (200–300 mEq) in total body potassium (211), owing primarily to coincident potassium losses from the gastrointestinal tract or kidneys. Despite these losses, hypokalemia is uncommon, present in only 4% of episodes in one series (28), probably because of concomitant acidosis. Serum potassium is usually normal or elevated at presentation (86), but falls during successful treatment. Hypokalemia during recovery from diabetic ketoacidosis is most prominent in patients who initially received sodium bicarbonate.

Since insulin plays a significant role in cellular shifts of potassium, insulin lack is presumably important in promoting hyperkalemia during diabetic ketoacidosis (7), as it is in patients with hyperosmolar nonketotic coma, who may have severe hyperkalemia without acidosis (22).

Similar to uncontrolled diabetes, several factors in lactic acidosis complicate the effect of acidemia per se on serum potassium. These include volume depletion, prerenal azotemia, hypercatabolism, concomitant diabetes, catecholamine effects, and external potassium imbalance (235). Although severe hyperkalemia is unusual in lactic acidosis, Perez et al. (289) have pointed out the absence of detailed studies on potassium in this varied disorder. In experimental lactic acid infusion in animals (378) and in uncomplicated postseizure lactic acidosis in humans (146, 276, 305), potassium does not increase with the appearance of acidosis. However, in other forms of lactic acidosis, such as those earlier encountered due to phenformin therapy in diabetes (86)) and other forms not associated with tissue hypoxia, mild elevation of potassium may occur (146). Renal insufficiency may be a contributing factor in such patients.

Most patients with alcoholic ketoacidosis have a normal extracellular potassium concentration (92, 224), although there is significant variability.

The effects of rarer forms of organic acidosis on internal potassium homeostasis have been reviewed elsewhere in detail (289).

Respiratory Acidosis

The effect of acute respiratory acidosis to elevate plasma potassium is, in general, smaller in magnitude than that of metabolic acidosis, though some effect can usually be detected (5, 53, 221, 328). A rise varying from 0.06 to 0.3 mEq K^+/liter per 0.1 pH unit was detected in 22 studies of mild to moderate respiratory acidosis (8). More severe experimental acidosis, provoked by inhaled concentrations of CO_2 as high as 30%, induce more pronounced hyperkalemia (8). In anephric dogs, the initial effect on potassium is small but after 2 hr of respiratory acidosis may increase to the range observed in metabolic acidosis (360). On the other hand, in in vitro experiments, when the extracellular medium bathing isolated rat diaphragms was acidified by raising the ambient CO_2 from 2% to 10%, no shift in potassium was observed (307), consistent with the ability of carbonic acid to permeate cells, as do other organic acids. Chronic respiratory acidosis produced in dogs was not attended by hyperkalemia (328).

The increase in serum potassium induced by severe respiratory acidosis in intact rats could be roughly approximated from the decrease in $(H^+)i/(H^+)o$ and was attributed to the importance of the Donnan effect in producing these changes (53). In addition, it is very likely that sympathoadrenal stimulation plays a major role in modulating serum potassium during respiratory acidosis in vivo since it is well established that acute hypercapnia results in an intense sympathetic discharge and an increase in the plasma concentration of epinephrine (8, 267). Glycogenolysis induced by epinephrine probably contributes to the initial release of glucose and potassium from the liver with hypercapnia, noted by Fenn and Asano (135), and the hypokalemic effect of β-adrenergic stimulation is likely to blunt the movement of potassium out of skeletal muscle that would otherwise accompany acidosis. Probably for this reason, mild respiratory acidosis induced acutely in anesthetized patients was not found to elevate the plasma potassium (268), although β-adrenergic blockade produced marked hyperkalemia in hypercapneic animals (373).

Bicarbonate

It has been suggested that the serum bicarbonate concentration, even at constant or "isohydric" pH, alters extrarenal potassium distribution and might account in part for the weak correlation between pH and serum potassium in many studies. Under conditions of constant blood pH, infusion of sodium bicarbonate appears to lower serum potassium (2, 8, 204), and during acidosis in rats, potassium may correlate better with serum bicarbonate than with blood pH (131). A similar correlation can be found in patients with hyperkalemia of diverse etiologies (145), as well as in experimental acute ammonium chloride acidosis (61). This has been taken to indicate that bicarbonate therapy, in addition to beneficially raising pH, corrects hyperkalemia directly, perhaps via intracellular transfer with the potassium cation.

Another explanation of the same data is that it is the quantity of acid buffered by cells rather than the arterial pH that governs the release of intracellular potassium. This would account for the fact that extracellular bicarbonate, rather than arterial pH, sometimes seems to exert an independent controlling influence on extracellular potassium. Effective buffering of an acid load by intracellular and extracellular buffers, so as to produce a low serum bicarbonate and a normal arterial pH, involves the liberation of substantial amounts of potassium cations from intracellular proteins (411).

It can be inferred from the foregoing that alkali treatment of hyperkalemia should be most effective when the plasma bicarbonate is low and acidosis marked, and less so when plasma bicarbonate and pH are normal; this is indeed the case (45). This result is also inherent in the finding that the changes in plasma potassium produced by metabolic alkalosis are smaller than those seen in metabolic acidosis.

Alkalosis

Metabolic and respiratory alkalosis are commonly associated with hypokalemia. In both, renal losses are important in initiating and perpetuating hypokalemia, but extrarenal adjustments are also involved. Acute alkalosis induced by infusions of sodium bicarbonate usually leads to a decrement in plasma potassium concentrations. The delta(K)p/delta

pH slope is usually smaller than that commonly observed in acute mineral acidosis, though the reported range is wide, from −0.09 to −0.42 mEq/l per 0.1 pH unit (8, 264, 340). The initial change is not attributable to kaliuresis. Acute respiratory alkalosis produces a comparable decrease in plasma potassium, although during voluntary overbreathing this fall may be counteracted by an increase in circulating norephinephrine, which, as noted earlier, tends to increase plasma potassium (210). It should be pointed out that most studies of extrarenal effects of metabolic alkalosis have involved the infusion of hypertonic solutions of sodium bicarbonate. Since hypertonicity itself promotes a rise in plasma potassium, this would tend to counteract any hypokalemic effect of alkalosis per se.

An intuitively appealing explanation for the extrarenal effect of alkalosis is replacement of H^+ associated with cellular buffers by potassium, in the reverse of the sequence discussed earlier by which acidosis releases intracellular potassium ions. Enhanced exchange of intracellular H^+ for extracellular Na^+ via the amiloride-sensitive Na^+-H^+ antiporter would accelerate cellular potassium accumulation by stimulating the Na,K-ATPase pump. In addition, intracellular alkalosis probably stimulates the sodium-potassium pump directly, as discussed earlier.

The combined effects of respiratory alkalosis on renal and extrarenal potassium handling commonly produce mild hypokalemia (around 3.0 mEq/l) resistant to potassium replacement, in hypocapneic patients who are artificially ventilated. Extreme hypocapneic alkalosis and hypokalemia, as seen in recently intubated patients who are overventilated, may produce serious cardiac arrhythmias (125).

ALDOSTERONE

In addition to its action on the kidney to increase potassium excretion, aldosterone enhances potassium secretion into intestinal fluids and saliva. In that sense, its effect on serum potassium can be said to have an extrarenal component. Aldosterone also has an independent action to accelerate renal acid excretion, and the consequent alkalosis itself has a secondary effect on cellular uptake of potassium. Apart from these mechanisms, there is no convincing evidence for a direct action of aldosterone to increase potassium uptake by muscle cells. For example, incubation of isolated rat diaphragms with aldosterone results in a loss, rather than a gain, of intracellular potassium (4, 225).

An extrarenal action of aldosterone has been suggested in the past because of several lines of evidence. First, in experimental animals, hyperkalemia after adrenalectomy seemed not to be entirely accounted for by a positive balance of potassium (110). Furthermore, the fall in plasma potassium accompanying the administration of mineralocorticoids was not necessarily associated with an increase in potassium excretion (280, 419, 420). Interpretation of such data is complicated because of the effect of adrenal medullary hormones on extrarenal potassium uptake and the renal action of mineralocorticoids to retain sodium and excrete acid, resulting in expansion of extracellular fluid volume and alkalosis, both of which might secondarily lower serum potassium.

Long-term treatment of dogs by Young and Jackson (420) with high doses of aldosterone altered the relationship between plasma potassium and total body exchangeable potassium, so that at any level of exchangeable potassium, plasma potassium was lower than in untreated animals. In these experiments, however, mean plasma bicarbonate was significantly higher in aldosterone-treated dogs than in controls, leaving open the possibility that aldosterone-induced alkalosis influenced potassium distribution.

Bia et al. (38) gave intravenous potassium loads to adrenalectomized and nephrectomized rats and found that the acute administration of aldosterone prior to infusing potassium blunted the hyperkalemia. The differences they observed, however, were small and could have been completely accounted for by a modest increase in the potassium concentration of gastrointestinal secretions (e.g., an increase of 20 mEq/l in 1 ml of intestinal fluid) caused by the known action of aldosterone to increase intestinal potassium secretion.

The role of mineralocorticoids in the disposition of an oral potassium load was studied in anephric humans by Sugarman and Brown (367). Anephric patients were given 0.5 mEq/kg of KCl after 72 hours of mineralocorticoid treatment (10 mg DOCA daily) or spironolactone (300 mg daily). The rise in serum potassium was delayed by DOCA, but the difference from control experiments with spironolactone was most marked at 1 hr, much less pronounced at 2 and 3 hours, and not present at 24 hours, suggesting that the mineralocorticoid had delayed absorption of potassium from the gastrointestinal tract. Chronic administration of high doses of mineralocorticoids is said to diminish serum potassium slightly in anuric patients, perhaps because of an increase in stool potassium (341).

Finally, Alexander and Levinsky (12) reported that chronic potassium loading improved extrarenal disposal of an acute potassium load given after a night's fast, an effect abolished by adrenalectomy and restored by chronic (but not acute) high-dose mineralocorticoid replacement. They postulated that chronic hyperaldosteronism acts directly by enhancing cellular uptake of an acute potassium load (12). Another interpretation was offered by Spital and Sterns (356). These investigators showed that when dietary potassium is withdrawn from rats previously fed a high-potassium diet, high rates of potassium excretion persist and "overshoot," causing these animals to become progressively more depleted of potassium than controls. This "paradoxical potassium depletion" is responsible, at least in part, for extrarenal potassium adaptation, by creating a sink of potassium-hungry cells that avidly take up potassium and thereby blunt the increment in plasma potassium after an acute potassium load. Hyperaldosteronism magnifies urinary potassium losses during fasting and thus promotes potassium deple

tion, which in turn facilitates the uptake into muscle of an acute potassium load (355).

In summary, aldosterone and other mineralocorticoid hormones do accelerate the extrarenal disposal of potassium, but probably not by a direct effect on muscle. The changes observed can be accounted for by the known actions of aldosterone on the renal and gastrointestinal transport of sodium and potassium, and the separate action of aldosterone to produce systemic alkalosis by enhancing acid excretion.

RENAL FAILURE

In states of mild to moderate chronic renal failure, the ability to excrete potassium is well maintained by an adaptive increase in the rate of fractional potassium excretion to levels near the maximal for subjects with normal renal function (327, 333). As renal function declines further, however, so does the ability to excrete potassium in a timely manner (126). With advanced renal failure, potassium is retained longer (414) and dependence on extrarenal disposal becomes more critical.

Whether extrarenal potassium disposal is enhanced, normal, or impaired in the setting of uremia remains controversial (316). Studies in which an oral potassium load was given found that patients with chronic renal failure excreted only one fourth (290) to one half (157, 200) the amount of potassium excreted by subjects with normal renal function over a comparable period of time. Nonetheless, an exaggerated rise in serum potassium did not always occur (157, 290). Reports of impaired extrarenal disposal of an oral potassium load in patients with chronic renal failure might be criticized either because the patients had higher basal serum potassium concentrations or might have been more acidotic than the control subjects (137, 200, 361). Another study that concluded that extrarenal potassium disposal was impaired in patients with chronic renal failure involved chronic rather than acute potassium loading (193). A more general criticism of studies administering oral potassium that might account for some of the discrepant conclusions, however, is the inherent difficulty of estimating the rate of gastrointestinal absorption of potassium in the setting of renal failure.

With intravenous potassium loading, however, most (35, 38, 295), but not all (383), animal studies appear to show a discernible defect in extrarenal potassium disposal in the setting of renal failure. With rare exceptions, however (35, 154), these studies examined extrarenal potassium homeostasis immediately after acute nephrectomy rather than in the uremic state.

If extrarenal potassium disposal is impaired in uremia, it cannot be a consequence of increased cellular potassium content or high total body potassium, since both are normal or low in this state (3, 32, 39, 253, 326, 354). There does not appear to be peripheral resistance to insulin-mediated potassium uptake (19), despite the known resistance to the action of insulin on glucose metabolism in renal failure (399). The chronic hyperinsulinemia of end-stage renal failure may afford some protection against hyperkalemia. Renin production, which might be expected to be suppressed in patients with end-stage renal disease, is normal or elevated in many patients. Furthermore, both hyperkalemia (91, 360) and salt restriction (325) appear to stimulate aldosterone production adequately in the setting of chronic renal failure (in patients who do not have hyporeninemic hypoaldosteronism) and a lowering of the plasma potassium suppresses aldosterone secretion normally (90).

Catecholamines circulate at increased levels in most (65, 174), but not all (46), patients with renal failure. While it is likely that much, if not all, of this increase is a consequence of decreased renal excretion, the pressor and pulse responses to norepinephrine infusion have been reported to be impaired in renal failure (46, 65). Both intravenous (254) and inhaled (17) albuterol appear, however, to be effective and rapid therapeutic modalities to treat hyperkalemia in patients with advanced renal failure. If β-adrenergic–mediated extrarenal potassium homeostasis is blunted in renal failure when compared with healthy subjects (359), it may well be in those whose endogenous plasma epinephrine levels are chronically elevated (240) or who are more acidemic. Contrariwise, it should be appreciated that the administration of drugs that possess β2-antagonist properties can produce significant hyperkalemia in patients with renal failure on dialysis (24).

Impaired extrarenal disposal of potassium in uremia might conceivably be caused by high circulating levels of parathyroid hormone. Infusion of parathyroid hormone appears to impair extrarenal disposition of a potassium load in nephrectomized rats (369), an action ascribed to the enhancement of potassium efflux from cells produced by increasing intracellular calcium. Potassium tolerance in partially nephrectomized rats with chronic renal failure is improved by parathyroidectomy and by administration of the calcium channel blocker verapamil (349).

Metabolic acidosis can impair cellular potassium uptake (see Acid-Base) and alkalinization has been demonstrated to reverse this effect in anuric patients (361). Part of this effect of acidosis may be to diminish the activity of Na,K-ATPase, which has a pH optimum in the range of 7.5 to 7.6 in mammalian tissue (343).

That the activity of the Na-K pump is impaired in the erythrocytes of some uremic subjects has been well established (188, 209, 213, 393, 398, 422, 423). The impairment is correlated with an increase in intracellular sodium of red blood cells. Also, the diminished pump activity is reversed when the red blood cells of uremic patients are incubated in normal plasma (209) or when the patients are dialyzed (188, 213, 299, 422), and the impairment is reproduced when normal erythrocytes are incubated in uremic plasma (88, 209). These studies suggest the presence of a circulating inhibitor of the Na-K pump in some uremics. Other investigators have reported a decrease in the number of pump sites, estimated by ouabain binding, rather than in the activity of the pump

(defined as the ion turnover rate per pump site) in the red blood cells of certain uremic patients (72, 195). Experimental uremia in rats decreases the Na, K-ATPase activity of skeletal muscle (120), an effect reproduced by incubating normal muscle cells with uremic serum(120). The excessive rise in plasma potassium exhibited by patients with chronic renal failure undergoing exercise is consistent, moreover, with an impairment in skeletal muscle Na,K-ATPase in humans with this condition (317).

MAGNESIUM

In a variety of clinical states, potassium depletion accompanies magnesium depletion. Among patients with hypokalemia, the coincidence of magnesium deficiency may range from less than 10% (394) to over 40% (401, 404). Clinical conditions with a high incidence of combined deficiencies in potassium and magnesium, such as diuretic administration, alcoholism, and diabetic ketoacidosis, generally involve a defect in renal conservation of potassium. Along with interest in the relationship between extrarenal magnesium and potassium balances (350) has come information on the relationship of their movements in and out of cells (313).

Because potassium and magnesium are the principal intracellular cations, it is not surprising that an important physiologic relationship might exist between them. For each, reduced intracellular concentrations may exist in certain states of depletion, out of proportion to the reduction in serum levels (13, 215). Furthermore, a high correlation is found between magnesium and potassium concentrations in extrarenal tissues, such as skeletal muscle (14). A deficiency of magnesium evokes potassium depletion in animals and humans. In rats, however, serum potassium remains normal (239), whereas in human subjects, hypokalemia is often observed (13, 401).

A specific effect of magnesium depletion on potassium homeostasis can be deduced from experimental magnesium deficiency states in which magnesium deficiency is associated with renal potassium wasting (336). One proposed mechanism is of importance to their internal homeostasis, insofar as it would involve a direct effect of magnesium depletion on the ability of both renal and extrarenal cells to preserve their potassium (350, 402).

It is known that experimental dietary magnesium depletion in rats results in loss of cellular potassium in cardiac as well as skeletal muscle (314). Furthermore, during magnesium depletion in both animals (405) and humans (336), the intracellular deficiency of potassium cannot be restored by provision of potassium alone; correction of the magnesium deficiency is required. Clinical combined depletion may play a role in cardiac arrhythmias seen in patients with alcoholism or on diuretics (401, 403), underscoring the importance of magnesium replacement in the correction of refractory hypokalemia and cellular potassium depletion.

Two extrarenal mechanisms have been suggested: reduced Na,K-ATPase activity, and increased cell membrane permeability to potassium. Cellular potassium depletion due to diminished active potassium uptake mediated by Na,K-ATPase might occur because this cation pump requires cellular magnesium (343). Animal studies have shown that magnesium depletion is associated with a reduced concentration of Na-K pump units in rat skeletal muscle (205). Reduced ouabain binding, indicative of a decreased number of Na-K pumps, has also been found in humans treated with diuretics who developed low muscle potassium concentrations associated with hypomagnesemia (118). Additional data suggest that magnesium depletion may also exert its effect on intracellular potassium through an impairment of the activity of the sodium-potassium pump per se, rather than on the number of pump sites per cell (142).

The second proposed mechanism of potassium loss would involve effects of magnesium on membrane potassium channels. In mammalian heart cells and in a cultured insulin-secreting cell line investigated by the patch-clamp technique, physiologic concentrations of intracellular magnesium block outward current by inhibiting the opening of ATP-sensitive potassium channels (139, 181). Magnesium may therefore play an important role in the low conductance of the outward potassium current through these channels (385) under normal conditions. Such a direct effect of magnesium on potassium channels might result in cellular potassium depletion during magnesium deficiency.

DRUGS

Medications are the primary etiologic factor in as many as one third of cases of clinically significant hyperkalemia (66, 279, 286, 296) and are contributing factors in more than 60% of hyperkalemic episodes in hospitalized adults (304). Potassium supplements, angiotensin-converting enzyme inhibitors, angiotensin II–receptor antagonists, potassium-sparing diuretics, trimethoprim, pentamidine, heparin, and prostaglandin-suppressing drugs that induce hyporeninemic hypoaldosteronism account for most of these cases; relative to those, hyperkalemia due to drugs that alter internal potassium distribution would appear to be uncommon (279, 335). As is true for drug-induced hyperkalemia in general, the risk of significant hyperkalemia is substantially increased in patients with diabetes mellitus, renal insufficiency, and hypoaldosteronism and in the elderly. In most other cases, the rise in potassium is mild (279).

Impaired Extrarenal Disposal

Hyperkalemia due to β-adrenergic blockers, the most common medications that elevate potassium by extrarenal mechanisms, was discussed in an earlier section. A small, transient increase in serum potassium usually occurs in patients given depolarizing muscle relaxants such as succinylcholine (49,

165, 187, 362). Exaggerated increments, however, may occur in patients with central nervous system diseases, spinal cord injury, increased intracranial pressure, and a variety of other ailments (296). Because potassium efflux from muscle end plates occurs during normal depolarization, massive efflux of the cation from sensitized muscle can account for the hyperkalemia noted in patients with neurologic motor deficits, tetanus, or muscle damage (397), or complicating the neuroleptic malignant syndrome (151) and skeletal muscle metastasis of a rhabdomyosarcoma (212).

Why burn patients and those with intracranial lesions not involving upper motor neurons (187) are also at risk is not clear. One possible mechanism would be proliferation of muscle end plates (165) in such patients. In patients at risk, succinylcholine should be used with caution and in the smallest dose possible, and with pretreatment by nondepolarizing muscle relaxants (397).

Muscle cell breakdown may also result in hyperkalemia in patients who develop myositis due to the HMG-CoA reductase inhibitor, lovastatin (123). Such reactions are more likely when lovastatin is administered in combination with gemfibrozil, cyclosporine, and nicotinic acid (166). HMG-CoA reductase inhibitors are commonly used in patients already predisposed to hyperkalemia due to diabetes mellitus or renal insufficiency.

Arginine HCl, in doses used for correction of metabolic alkalosis, may increase serum potassium (11). When this cationic amino acid is taken up by cells, potassium is displaced into the extracellular fluid. Hyperkalemia is more likely in patients with renal failure (175), who are unable to excrete this endogenous potassium load, and in those with liver failure, who are unable to metabolize the administered arginine normally (62). The magnitude of potassium rise in normal subjects is under 1 mEq/l (11); it is not closely correlated with pH and may occur in patients before correction of the alkalosis is accomplished (62). Lysine HCl may also increase serum potassium levels. The antifibrinolytic agent epsilon aminocaproic acid (Amicar) has been reported to cause hyperkalemia as well (287), although the mechanism underlying this effect is unclear.

Trivial increments in potassium may also occur at therapeutic or mildly toxic levels of cardiac glycosides (124, 324). Blockade of Na,K-ATPase–mediated potassium uptake with normal doses of digitalis has minimal effect on the serum potassium, since glycoside binding to skeletal muscle, the major body reservoir of potassium, is limited. At toxic concentrations of digitalis, however, such as following massive overdose, hyperkalemia is well described and indicates a poor prognosis (42, 347). The toxic concentration of digitalis also prevents standard treatment of the hyperkalemia with calcium. Although no significant effect to retard potassium disposal in normal subjects with therapeutic digitalis levels has been published, it is likely that such an effect may exacerbate hyperkalemia in patients at risk. In patients with renal failure, for example, even modest digoxin toxicity resulting from therapeutic doses is reported to cause hyperkalemia

(281). In fact, of drugs known to induce hyperkalemia, digoxin was the most frequently encountered among patients with hyperkalemic episodes (304), and nearly one fourth of these had toxic digoxin levels.

Nonsteroidal anti-inflammatory drugs produce hyperkalemia best attributed to their antikaliuretic effect, which results in positive potassium balance (84, 149). No impairment of extrarenal potassium homeostasis has been directly demonstrated (83, 304, 320).

Lithium intoxication in animals is associated with a progressive elevation in serum potassium and electrocardiogram abnormalities characteristic of hyperkalemia. However, only at concentrations of plasma lithium (>10 mEq/l) many times the therapeutic lithium levels (1 mEq/l) attained in manic-depressive patients (170) do these changes occur. Increments in serum potassium of less than 1 mEq/l have been reported during chronic lithium therapy (245), but frank hyperkalemia is rarely observed (155). Lithium may displace intracellular potassium from human red blood cells and from skeletal muscle (245).

Enhanced Extrarenal Disposal

Drug-induced lowering of serum potassium by exogenous insulin and β-adrenergic agonists was described in detail earlier. Increased circulating catecholamine levels as well as enhancement of catechol stimulation of adenylate cyclase also appear to mediate in part the effect of methylxanthine derivatives such as theophylline. Hypokalemia due to β-adrenergic stimulation may occur with severe theophylline toxicity (198) in humans. Propranolol is reported to block hypokalemia due to theophylline toxicity in the dog (198). Whether therapeutic levels of aminophylline are important in acutely lowering serum potassium in humans is unclear (424). Other methylxanthines such as caffeine might also be expected to decrease potassium concentrations (227), not only by stimulating release of catecholamines but also by their blockade of high-affinity (A1) adenosine receptors, which normally act to inhibit adenylate cyclase.

Several clinical studies have reported minor decreases in serum potassium levels in patients treated with calcium antagonists, sometimes associated with increased urinary potassium losses (381). Severe hypokalemia with heart block may complicate overdosage of verapamil (252). Enhanced extrarenal potassium disposal has been demonstrated with the calcium channel blockers verapamil, nifedipine, and nitrendipine (100, 250, 368). In one study (368), pretreatment with either verapamil or nifedipine reduced by about 40% the increment in plasma potassium produced over 1 hour by the infusion of KCl in nephrectomized rats. The effect was not mediated by changes in pH, bicarbonate, insulin, aldosterone, or the α- or β-adrenergic systems. Diltiazem has been shown to reduce the interdialytic rate of increase in plasma potassium in patients with end-stage renal disease (351). Diminished calcium-mediated potassium efflux from cells may be responsible, since increased intracellular calcium enhances potassium permeability in vitro (the Gardos effect) (148) in erythrocytes and other cells (58). While this action would lower plasma potassium, the net effect of calcium channel blockers in clinical practice is complicated by the fact that these agents also inhibit secretion of aldosterone (67, 266), which in turn would tend to produce potassium retention.

OTHER FACTORS

Two other factors that may clinically elevate serum potassium levels by affecting extrarenal potassium homeostasis are hyperosmolarity and cellular necrosis. Less well described are the effects of barium, cesium, and body hypothermia to lower serum potassium levels by extrarenal shifts. A sudden increase in cell mass produced by rapid proliferation may sequester potassium intracellularly and result in hypokalemia.

Hyperosmolarity

Hypertonic potassium-free solutions administered to normal human subjects fail to lower plasma potassium, despite expanding the extracellular fluid compartment (334). This observation suggests that plasma potassium is maintained during the infusion by movement of potassium out of cells, impelled by an increase in its intracellular concentration, because of contraction of the intracellular volume. Potassium levels are maintained even when dilutional acidosis is prevented by incorporating bicarbonate into the hypertonic infusion (237).

A modest rise in plasma potassium concentration (0.3–0.6 mEq/l) can be produced in normal subjects by moderate increases in tonicity (10 mOsm/kg) (261). The effect is of clinical importance chiefly in diabetics, in whom plasma tonicity can be raised by 40 to 50 mOsm/kg during hyperglycemia, and who lack insulin-mediated potassium uptake. Glucose-induced hyperkalemia is more pronounced in diabetics deficient in aldosterone secretion (156), or during treatment with captopril (300), but it may also be observed in diabetics with normal aldosterone responses. The standard 100-g oral glucose tolerance test produced an average increment of 1.3 mEq/l in plasma potassium in four such patients (269). The effect of hyperosmolarity on potassium homeostasis may also be present in patients with cerebral edema or with renal insufficiency when treated with large quantities of hypertonic mannitol.

Cellular Necrosis

When renal excretion and extrarenal disposal of potassium are exceeded, release of intracellular potassium into the extracellular compartment during cellular necrosis will result in hyperkalemia. The most common sources are muscle, tumor cells, and erythrocytes.

Traumatic muscle injury, due to motor vehicle collisions, alcoholism, cocaine abuse (342), or other etiologies, may produce life-threatening hyperkalemia, usually during rhabdomyolytic renal failure. Catabolic states, such as sepsis, compound fractures, burns, major surgery, or overwhelming infections, result in protein breakdown to meet increased energy demands. Skeletal muscle, the source of protein loss, may release sufficient potassium to cause severe hyperkalemia, if renal excretory mechanisms are compromised.

Accelerated breakdown of a large leukemic tumor burden, especially during induction of chemotherapy, produces kaliuresis and may cause symptomatic hyperkalemia. Burkitt lymphoma, a rapidly growing neoplasm, while not causing hyperkalemia even in azotemic patients prior to chemotherapy (87), may result in hyperkalemia within hours of treatment, even in the absence of renal insufficiency. Fatal hyperkalemia has also been reported after initial tumor lysis therapy in acute lymphocytic leukemia, chronic lymphocytic leukemia, and lymphosarcoma. The tumor lysis syndrome is only rarely reported after treatment of nonlymphomatous solid tumors (71). Intensive supportive therapy probably accounts for the absence of hyperkalemia reported in some series (382).

Transient hyperkalemia, in the absence of renal failure, occasionally occurs during hemolytic states such as congenital or acquired hemolytic anemia, hemoglobinopathy, or transfusion reactions. Conversely, plasma potassium may fall during the rapid proliferation of erythrocytes and their precursors when severe pernicious anemia is successfully treated (176, 190, 220).

Barium

Barium is a well-known inhibitor of potassium exit channels in muscle at concentrations of 1 to 5 mM (353). In vitro, Ba^{2+}-treated muscle develops flaccid paralysis and depolarization secondary to this change in potassium permeability (147). Hypokalemia is therefore a feature of barium poisoning, as are cardiac arrhythmias and skeletal muscle paralysis (311), associated with depolarization of muscle fibers (353). Barium poisoning is thought to be responsible for Pa Ping paralysis reported in Chinese patients who had eaten salt or drunk wine with a high content of barium salts (15, 182).

Cesium

Cesium chloride has been marketed as part of an alternative therapy for malignancy. Cesium appears in the periodic table below rubidium and potassium with a positive valence of 1; its salts are extremely toxic, causing hypokalemia, cardiac arrhythmias, prolonged Q-T interval, and torsade de pointes, probably like barium, by blocking potassium exit channels (99).

Hypothermia

Acute transient hypokalemia has been described in patients with hypothermia associated with accidental trauma or following surgery (57, 208). When body temperature returns to normal, the hypokalemia disappears. Postoperative hypothermia (<36.5°C) was found in 40% of patients undergoing gastrointestinal and vascular surgery. Low serum potassium levels coincided with postoperative hypothermia in over half of these, whereas no patients with normothermia became hypokalemic. Urinary potassium losses did not account for the differences (57). The hypokalemia of experimental hypothermia is not prevented by β-adrenergic blockade (357). It may be related to the alkalosis that regularly accompanies hypothermia because of the effect of lowered temperature to reduce the dissociation of carbonic acid (127).

Race

The extrarenal disposal of an intravenous load of KCl is delayed in normal young blacks as compared with whites, perhaps attributable to a racial tendency to lower Na,K-ATPase activity in the cells of black individuals (371).

References

1. [No author.] Adrenaline and potassium: everything in flux. *Lancet* 1983;2:1401–1403.
2. Abrams WB, Lewis DW, Bellet S. The effect of acidosis and alkalosis on the plasma potassium concentration and the electrocardiogram of normal and potassium depleted dogs. *Am J Med Sci* 1951;222:506–515.
3. Adesman J, Goldberg M, Castleman L, Friedman IS. Simultaneous measurement of body sodium and potassium using Na22 and K42. *Metabolism* 1960;9:561–569.
4. Adler S. An extrarenal action of aldosterone on mammalian skeletal muscle. *Am J Physiol* 1970;218:616–621.
5. Adler S, Fraley DS. Potassium and intracellular pH. *Kidney Int* 1977;11:433–442.
6. Adrogue HJ, Chap Z, Ishida T, Field JB. Role of the endocrine pancreas in the kalemic response to acute metabolic acidosis in conscious dogs. *J Clin Invest* 1985;75:798–808.
7. Adrogue HJ, Lederer ED, Suki WN, Eknoyan G. Determinants of plasma potassium levels in diabetic ketoacidosis. *Medicine (Baltimore)* 1986;65:163–172.
8. Adrogue HJ, Madias NE. Changes in plasma potassium concentration during acute acid-base disturbances. *Am J Med* 1981;71:456–467.
9. Ahlquist R. A Study of the adrenotropic receptors. *Am J Physiol* 1948;153:586–600.
10. Akaike N. Sodium pump in skeletal muscle: central nervous system-induced suppression by alpha-adrenoreceptors. *Science* 1981;213:1252–1254.
11. Alberti KG, Johnston H, Lauler D. The effect of arginine and its derivatives on potassium metabolism in the dog. *Clin Res* 1967;15:476.
12. Alexander EA, Levinsky NG. An extrarenal mechanism of potassium adaptation. *J Clin Invest* 1968;7:740–748.
13. Alfrey AC. Disorders of magnesium metabolism. In: Seldin DWG, ed. *The Kidney: Physiology and Pathophysiology.* New York: Raven Press; 1985:1281–1295.
14. Alfrey AC, Miller NL, Butkus D. Evaluation of body magnesium stores. *J Lab Clin Med* 1974;84:153–162.
15. Allen AS. Pa Ping, or Kiating paralysis. *Chinese Med J* 1943;61:296–301.
16. Allon M, Dansby L, Shanklin N. Glucose modulation of the disposal of an acute potassium load in patients with end-stage renal disease. *Am J Med* 1993;94:475–482.
17. Allon M, Dunlay R, Copkney C. Nebulized albuterol for acute hyperkalemia in patients on hemodialysis. *Ann Intern Med* 1989;110:426–429.
18. Altenberg GA, Aristimuno PC, Amorena CE, Taquini AC. Amiloride prevents the metabolic acidosis of a KCl load in nephrectomized rats. *Clin Sci (Lond)* 1989;76:649–652.
19. Alvestrand A, Wahren J, Smith D, DeFronzo RA. Insulin-mediated potassium uptake is normal in uremic and healthy subjects. *Am J Physiol* 1984;246(Pt 1):E174–80.
20. Amin DN, Henry JA. Propranolol administration in theophylline overdose. *Lancet* 1985;1:520–521.
21. Andres R, Baltzan MA, Cader G, Zierler KL. Effect of insulin on carbohydrate metabolism and on potassium in the forearm of man. *J Clin Invest* 1962;41:108–115.
22. Arieff AI, Carroll HJ. Nonketotic hyperosmolar coma with hyperglycemia: clinical features, pathophysiology, renal function, acid-base balance, plasma-cerebrospinal fluid equilibria and the effects of therapy in 37 cases. *Medicine (Baltimore)* 1972;51:73–94.
23. Arrizabalaga P, Montolio J, Martinez-Vea A, Andreu L, Lopez-Pedret J, Revert L. Increase in serum potassium caused by beta-2 adrenergic blockade in terminal renal failure: Absence of mediation by insulin or aldosterone. *Kidney Int* 1983;24:427.
24. Arrizabalaga P, Montoliu J, Martinez Vea A, Andreu L, Lopez Pedret J, Revert L. Increase in serum potassium caused by beta-2 adrenergic blockade in terminal renal failure: absence of mediation by insulin or aldosterone. *Proc Eur Dial Transplant Assoc* 1983;20:572–576.
25. Baker PF, Rink TJ. Catecholamine release from bovine adrenal medulla in response to maintained depolarization. *J Physiol* 1975;253:593–620.
26. Ballanyi K, Grafe P. Changes in intracellular ion activities induced by adrenaline in human and rat skeletal muscle. *Pflugers Arch* 1988;411:283–288.

27. Bauer JH. Effects of propranolol therapy on renal function and body fluid composition. *Arch Intern Med* 143:927–931.
28. Beigelman PM. Potassium in severe diabetic ketoacidosis. *Am J Med* 1973;54:419–420.
29. Beigelman PM, Hollander PB. Effects of hormones Upon adipose tissue membrane electrical potentials. *Proc Soc Exp Biol Med* 1964;116:31–35.
30. Berg T, Iversen JG. K+ transport in isolated rat liver cells stimulated by glucagon and insulin in vitro. *Acta Physiol Scand* 1976;97:202–208.
31. Bergstrom J, Alvestrand A, Furst P, Hultman E, Sahlin K, Vinnars E, Widstrom A. Influence of severe potassium depletion and subsequent repletion with potassium on muscle electrolytes, metabolites and amino acids in man. *Clin Sci Mol Med Suppl* 1976;51:589–599.
32. Bergstrom J, Alvestrand A, Furst P, Hultman E, Widstam-Attorps U. Muscle intracellular electrolytes in patients with chronic uremia. *Kidney Int Suppl* 1983;16:S153–160.
33. Bettice JA, Gamble JL, Jr. Skeletal buffering of acute metabolic acidosis. *Am J Physiol* 1975;229:1618–1624.
34. Bevilacqua M, Norbiato G, Raggi U, Micossi P, Baggio E, Prandelli M. Dopaminergic control of serum potassium. *Metabolism* 1980;29:306–310.
35. Bia M, DeFronzo R. The medullary collecting duct (MCD) does not play a primary role in potassium (K) adaptation following decreased GFR. *Clin Res* 1978;26:457A.
36. Bia MJ, DeFronzo RA. Extrarenal potassium homeostasis. *Am J Physiol* 1981;240:F257–268.
37. Bia MJ, Lu D, Tyler K, De Fronzo RA. Beta adrenergic control of extrarenal potassium disposal. A beta-2 mediated phenomenon. *Nephron* 1986;43:117–122.
38. Bia MJ, Tyler KA, DeFronzo RA. Regulation of extrarenal potassium homeostasis by adrenal hormones in rats. *Am J Physiol* 1982;242:F641–644.
39. Bilbrey GL, Carter NW, White MG, Schilling JF, Knochel JP. Potassium deficiency in chronic renal failure. *Kidney Int* 1973;4:423–430.
40. Bilbrey GL, Faloona GR, White MG, Knochel JP. Hyperglucagonemia of renal failure. *J Clin Invest* 1974;53:841–847.
41. Bilbrey GL, Herbin L, Carter NW, Knochel JP. Skeletal muscle resting membrane potential in potassium deficiency. *J Clin Invest* 1973;52:3011–3018.
42. Bismuth C, Gaultier M, Conso F, Efthymiou ML. Hyperkalemia in acute digitalis poisoning: prognostic significance and therapeutic implications. *Clin Toxicol* 1973;6:153–162.
43. Blackard WG, Nelson NC. Portal and peripheral vein immunoreactive insulin concentrations before and after glucose infusion. *Diabetes* 1979;19:302–306.
44. Blevins RD, Whitty AJ, Rubenfire M, Maciejko JJ. Dopamine and dobutamine induce hypokalemia in anesthetized dogs. *J Cardiovasc Pharmacol* 1989;13:662–666.
45. Blumberg A, Weidmann P, Shaw S, Gnadinger M. Effect of various therapeutic approaches on plasma potassium and major regulating factors in terminal renal failure. *Am J Med* 1988;85: 507–512.
46. Botey A, Gaya J, Montoliu J, Torras A, Rivera F, Lopez-Pedret J, Revert L. Postsynaptic adrenergic unresponsiveness in hypotensive haemodialysis patients. *Proc Eur Dial Transplant Assoc* 1981;18:586–591.
47. Bourdillon J. Distribution in body fluids and excretion of ingested ammonium chloride, potassium chloride, and sodium chloride. *Am J Physiol* 1937;120:411–419.
48. Braden GL, von Oeyen PT, Germain MJ, Watson DJ, Haag BL. Ritodrine- and terbutaline-induced hypokalemia in preterm labor: mechanisms and consequences. *Kidney Int* 1997;51:1867–1875.
49. Brass EP, Thompson WL. Drug-induced electrolyte abnormalities. *Drugs* 1982;24: 207–28.
50. Bray JJ, Hawken MJ, Hubbard JI, Pockett S, Wilson L. The membrane potential of rat diaphragm muscle fibres and the effect of denervation. *J Physiol* 1976;255:651–667.
51. Breitwieser GE, Altamirano AA, Russell JM. Effects of pH changes on sodium pump fluxes in squid giant axon. *Am J Physiol* 1987;253(Pt 1):C547–554.
52. Briggs A, Koechig I. Some changes in the composition of blood due to the injection of insulin. *J Biol Chem* 1924;8:721–730.
53. Brown EB, Jr., Goott B. Intracellular hydrogen ion changes and potassium movement. *Am J Physiol* 1963;204:765–770.
54. Brown MJ. Hypokalemia from beta 2-receptor stimulation by circulating epinephrine. *Am J Cardiol* 1985;56:3D–9D.
55. Brown MJ, Brown DC, Murphy MB. Hypokalemia from beta2-receptor stimulation by circulating epinephrine. *N Engl J Med* 1983;309:1414–1419.
56. Brown RS. Extrarenal potassium homeostasis. *Kidney Int* 1986;30:116–127.
57. Bruining HA, Boelhouwer RU. Acute transient hypokalemia and body temperature. *Lancet* 1982;2:1283–1284.
58. Burgess GM, Claret M, Jenkinson DH. Effects of quinine and apamin on the calcium-dependent potassium permeability of mammalian hepatocytes and red cells. *J Physiol* 1981; 317:67–90.
59. Burnell JM, Scribner BH, Uyeno BT, Villamil MF. The effect in humans of extracellular pH change on the relationship between serum potassium concentration and intracellular potassium. *J Clin Invest* 1956;35:935–939.
60. Burton SD, Mondon CE, Ishida T. Dissociation of potassium and glucose efflux in isolated perfused rat liver. *Am J Physiol* 1967;212:261–266.
61. Bushinsky DA, Coe FL. Hyperkalemia during acute ammonium chloride acidosis in man. *Nephron* 1985;40:38–40.
62. Bushinsky DA, Gennari FJ. Life-threatening hyperkalemia induced by arginine. *Ann Intern Med* 1978;89(Pt 1):632–634.
63. Buur T, Clausen T, Holmberg E, Johansson U, Waldeck B. Desensitization by terbutaline of beta-adrenoceptors in the guinea-pig soleus muscle: biochemical alterations associated with functional changes. *Br J Pharmacol* 1982;76:313–317.
64. Cagliero E, Martina V, Massara F, Molinatti GM. Glucagon-induced increase in plasma potassium levels in type 1 (insulin-dependent) diabetic subjects. *Diabetologia* 1983;24:85–87.
65. Campese VM, Romoff MS, Levitan D, Lane K, Massry SG. Mechanisms of autonomic nervous system dysfunction in uremia. *Kidney Int* 1981;20:246–253.
66. Cannon-Babb ML, Schwartz AB. Drug-induced hyperkalemia. *Hosp Pract (Off Ed)* 1986;21: 99–107, 111, 114–127.
67. Capponi AM, Lew PD, Jornot L, Vallotton MB. Correlation between cytosolic free Ca2+ and aldosterone production in bovine adrenal glomerulosa cells. Evidence for a difference in the mode of action of angiotensin II and potassium. *J Biol Chem* 1984;259:8863–8869.
68. Carey RM, Thorner MO, Ortt EM. Dopaminergic inhibition of metoclopramide-induced aldosterone secretion in man. Dissociation of responses to dopamine and bromocriptine. *J Clin Invest* 1980;66:10–18.
69. Carey RM, Thorner MO, Ortt EM. Effects of metoclopramide and bromocriptine on the renin-angiotensin-aldosterone system in man. Dopaminergic control of aldosterone. *J Clin Invest* 1979;63:727–735.
70. Carlsson E, Fellenius E, Lundborg P, Svensson L. beta-Adrenoceptor blockers, plasma-potassium, and exercise. *Lancet* 1978;2:424–425.
71. Cech P, Block JB, Cone LA, Stone R. Tumor lysis syndrome after tamoxifen flare. *N Engl J Med* 1986;315:263–264.
72. Cheng JT, Kahn T, Kaji DM. Mechanism of alteration of sodium potassium pump of erythrocytes from patients with chronic renal failure. *J Clin Invest* 1984;74:1811–1120.
73. Cheng LC, Rogus EM, Zierler K. Catechol, a structural requirement for (Na+ + K+)-ATPase stimulation in rat skeletal muscle membrane. *Biochim Biophys Acta* 1977;464: 338–346.
74. Choi CS, Thompson CB, Leong PK, McDonough AA, Youn JH. Short-term K(+) deprivation provokes insulin resistance of cellular K(+) uptake revealed with the K(+) clamp. *Am J Physiol Renal Physiol* 2001;280:F95–F102.
75. Christensen NJ. Plasma norepinephrine and epinephrine in untreated diabetics, during fasting and after insulin administration. *Diabetes* 1974;23:1–8.
76. Clausen T. Adrenergic control of Na+-K+-homoeostasis. *Acta Med Scand Suppl* 1983;672: 111–115.
77. Clausen T, Everts ME. Regulation of the Na-K-pump in skeletal muscle. *Kidney Int* 1989; 35:1–13.
78. Clausen T, Flatman JA. Beta 2-adrenoceptors mediate the stimulating effect of adrenaline on active electrogenic Na-K-transport in rat soleus muscle. *Br J Pharmacol* 1980;68:749–755.
79. Clausen T, Flatman JA. The effect of catecholamines on Na-K transport and membrane potential in rat soleus muscle. *J Physiol* 1977;270:383–414.
80. Clausen T, Flatman JA. Effects of insulin and epinephrine on Na+-K+ and glucose transport in soleus muscle. *Am J Physiol* 1987;252(Pt 1):E492–9.
81. Clausen T, Hansen O. Active Na-K transport and the rate of ouabain binding. The effect of insulin and other stimuli on skeletal muscle and adipocytes. *J Physiol* 1977;270:415–430.
82. Clausen T, Kohn PG. The effect of insulin on the tran sport of sodium and potassium in rat soleus muscle. *J Physiol* 1977;265:19–42.
83. Clive DM, Gurwitz J, Williams M, Rossetti R. Nonsteroidal antiinflammatory drugs (NSAID) do not impair potassium metabolism in normal humans. In: 10th International Congress of Nephrology.
84. Clive DM, Stoff JS. Renal syndromes associated with nonsteroidal antiinflammatory drugs. *N Engl J Med* 1984;310:563–572.
85. Coats RA. Effects of apamin on alpha-adrenoceptor-mediated changes in plasma potassium in guinea-pigs. *Br J Pharmacol* 1983;80:573–580.
86. Cohen AS, Vance VK, Runyan JW, Jr., Hurwitz D. Diabetic acidosis: an evaluation of the cause, course and therapy of 73 cases. *Ann Intern Med* 1960;52:55–86.
87. Cohen LF, Balow JE, Magrath IT, Poplack DG, Ziegler JL. Acute tumor lysis syndrome. A review of 37 patients with Burkitt's lymphoma. *Am J Med* 1980;68:486–491.
88. Cole CH, Balfe JW, Welt LG. Induction of a ouabain-sensitive ATPase defect by uremic plasma. *Trans Assoc Am Physicians* 1968;81:213–220.
89. Conci F, Procaccio F, Boselli L. Hypokalemia from beta2-receptor stimulation by epinephrine. *N Engl J Med* 1984;310:1329.
90. Cooke CR, Horvath JS, Moore MA, Bledsoe T, Walker WG. Modulation of plasma aldosterone concentration by plasma potassium in anephric man in the absence of a change in potassium balance. *J Clin Invest* 1973;52:3028–3032.
91. Cooke CR, Ruiz-Maza F, Kowarski A, Migeon CJ, Walker WG. Regulation of plasma aldosterone concentration in anephric man and renal transplant recipients. *Kidney Int* 1973;3: 160–166.
92. Cooperman MT, Davidoff F, Spark R, Pallotta J. Clinical studies of alcoholic ketoacidosis. *Diabetes* 1974;3:433–439.
93. Cox M, Sterns RH, Singer I. The defense against hyperkalemia: the roles of insulin and aldosterone. *N Engl J Med* 1978;299:525–532.
94. Creese R. Sodium fluxes in diaphragm muscle and the effects of insulin and serum proteins. *J Physiol* 1968;197:255–278.
95. Cumberbatch M, Morgan DB. Erythrocyte sodium and potassium in patients with hypokalaemia. *Clin Sci (Lond)* 1983;64:167–176.
96. Czech MP. Molecular basis of insulin action. *Annu Rev Biochem* 1977;46:359–384.
97. D'Silva JL. The action of adrenaline on serum potassium. *J Physiol* 1934;82:393–398.
98. D'Silva JL. Action of adrenaline on the perfused liver. *J Physiol* 1936;87:181–188.
99. Dalal AK, Harding JD, Verdino RJ. Acquired long QT syndrome and monomorphic ventricular tachycardia after alternative treatment with cesium chloride for brain cancer. *Mayo Clin Proc* 2004;79:1065–1069.
100. Davidovics Y, Peer G, Cabili S, Blum M, Serban I, Wollman Y, Iaina A. Effect of verapamil on disposition of intravenous potassium in diabetic anephric uremic rats. *Miner Electrolyte Metab* 1993;19:99–102.
101. Davidson MB, Hiatt N. Effect of KCl administration on insulin secretion in dogs. *Isr J Med Sci* 1972;8:752–754.
102. Davies NW, Standen NB, Stanfield PR. The effect of intracellular pH on ATP-dependent potassium channels of frog skeletal muscle. *J Physiol* 1992;445:549–568.
103. Dawson CM, Lebrun P, Herchuelz A, Malaisse WJ, Goncalves AA, Atwater I. Effect of temperature upon potassium-stimulated insulin release and calcium entry in mouse and rat islets. *Horm Metab Res* 1986;18:221–224.
104. De La Lande IS, Manson J, Parks VJ, Sandison AG, Skinner SL, Whelan RF. The local metabolic action of adrenaline on skeletal muscle in man. *J Physiol* 1961;157:177–184.

105. De Luise MA, Harker M. Insulin stimulation of Na+-K+ pump in clonal rat osteosarcoma cells. *Diabetes* 1988;37:33–37.

106. de Weille JR, Fosset M, Mourre C, Schmid-Antomarchi H, Bernardi H, Lazdunski M. Pharmacology and regulation of ATP-sensitive K+ channels. *Pflugers Arch* 1989;414(Suppl 1): S80–87.

107. DeFronzo RA. Obesity is associated with impaired insulin-mediated potassium uptake. *Metabolism* 1988;37:105–108.

108. DeFronzo RA, Bia M, Birkhead G. Epinephrine and potassium homeostasis. *Kidney Int* 1981;20:83–91.

109. DeFronzo RA, Felig P, Ferrannini E, Wahren J. Effect of graded doses of insulin on splanchnic and peripheral potassium metabolism in man. *Am J Physiol* 1980;238:E421–427.

110. DeFronzo RA, Lee R, Jones A, Bia M. Effect of insulinopenia and adrenal hormone deficiency on acute potassium tolerance. *Kidney Int* 1980;17:586–594.

111. DeFronzo RA, Sherwin RS, Dillingham M, Hendler R, Tamborlane WV, Felig P. Influence of basal insulin and glucagon secretion on potassium and sodium metabolism. Studies with somatostatin in normal dogs and in normal and diabetic human beings. *J Clin Invest* 1978;61: 472–479.

112. Deibert DC, DeFronzo RA. Epinephrine-induced insulin resistance in man. *J Clin Invest* 1980;65:717–721.

113. Desilets M, Baumgarten CM. Isoproterenol directly stimulates the Na+-K+ pump in isolated cardiac myocytes. *Am J Physiol* 1986;251(Pt 2): H218–225.

114. Dias Da Silva MR, Cerutti JM, Arnaldi LA, Maciel RM. A mutation in the KCNE3 potassium channel gene is associated with susceptibility to thyrotoxic hypokalemic periodic paralysis. *J Clin Endocrinol Metab* 2002;87:4881–4884.

115. Dluhy RG, Axelrod L, Williams GH. Serum immunoreactive insulin and growth hormone response to potassium infusion in normal man. *J Appl Physiol* 1972;33:22–26.

116. Donnelly T, Gray H, Simpson E, Rodger JC. Serum potassium in acute myocardial infarction. *Scottish Med J* 1980;25:176.

117. Dorup I, Clausen T. Insulin-like growth factor I stimulates active Na(+)-K+ transport in rat soleus muscle. *Am J Physiol* 1995;268(Pt 1):E849–857.

118. Dorup I, Skajaa K, Clausen T, Kjeldsen K. Reduced concentrations of potassium, magnesium, and sodium-potassium pumps in human skeletal muscle during treatment with diuretics. *Br Med J (Clin Res Ed)* 1988;296:455–458.

119. Douglas WW. Stimulus-secretion coupling: the concept and clues from chromaffin and other cells. *Br J Pharmacol* 1968;34:453–474.

120. Druml W, Kelly RA, May RC, Mitch WE. Abnormal cation transport in uremia. Mechanisms in adipocytes and skeletal muscle from uremic rats. *J Clin Invest* 1988;81:1197–1203.

121. Dyckner T, Helmers C, Lundman T, Wester PO. Initial serum potassium level in relation to early complications and prognosis in patients with acute myocardial infarction. *Acta Med Scand* 1975;197:207–210.

122. Eaton DC, Hamilton KL, Johnson KE. Intracellular acidosis blocks the basolateral Na-K pump in rabbit urinary bladder. *Am J Physiol* 1984;247(Pt 2):F946–954.

123. Edelman S, Witztum JL. Hyperkalemia during treatment with HMG-CoA reductase inhibitor. *N Engl J Med* 1989;320:1219–1220.

124. Edner M, Ponikowski P, Jogestrand T. The effect of digoxin on the serum potassium concentration. *Scand J Clin Lab Invest* 1993;53:187–189.

125. Edwards R, Winnie AP, Ramamurthy S. Acute hypocapneic hypokalemia: an iatrogenic anesthetic complication. *Anesth Analg* 1977;56:786–792.

126. Elkinton JR, Tarail R, Peters JP. Transfers of potassium in renal insufficiency. *J Clin Invest* 1949;27:378–388.

127. Ellis RJ, Hoover E, Gay WA, Ebert PA. Metabolic alterations with profound hypothermia. *Arch Surg* 1974;109:659–663.

128. Epstein FH, Rosa RM. Adrenergic control of serum potassium. *N Engl J Med* 1983;309: 1450–1451.

129. Erlij D, Grinstein S. The number of sodium ion pumping sites in skeletal muscle and its modification by insulin. *J Physiol* 1976;259:13–31.

130. Evans RH, Smith JW. Mode of action of catecholamines on skeletal muscle. *J Physiol* 1973;232:81P–82P.

131. Farley DS, Adler S. Isohydric regulation of plasma potassium by bicarbonate in the rat. *Kidney Int* 1976;9:333–343.

132. Fehlmann M, Freychet P. Insulin and glucagon stimulation of (Na+-K+)-ATPase transport activity in isolated rat hepatocytes. *J Biol Chem* 1981;256:7449–7453.

133. Feig PU, Shook A, Sterns RH. Effect of potassium removal during hemodialysis on the plasma potassium concentration. *Nephron* 1981;27:25–30.

134. Fenn WO. The deposition of potassium and phosphate with glycogen in rat livers. *J Biol Chem* 1939;128:297–307.

135. Fenn WO, Asano T. Effects of carbon dioxide inhalation on potassium liberation from the liver. *Am J Physiol* 1956;185:567–576.

136. Fenn WO, Cobb DM. The potassium equilibrium in muscle. *J Gen Physiol* 1934;17: 629–656.

137. Fernandez J, Oster JR, Perez GO. Impaired extrarenal disposal of an acute oral potassium load in patients with endstage renal disease on chronic hemodialysis. *Miner Electrolyte Metab* 1986;12:125–129.

138. Finder AG, Boyme T, Shoemaker WC. Relationship of hepatic potassium efflux to phosphorylase activation induced by glucagon. *Am J Physiol* 1964;206:738–742.

139. Findlay I. The effects of magnesium upon adenosine triphosphate-sensitive potassium channels in a rat insulin-secreting cell line. *J Physiol* 1987;391:611–629.

140. Fineberg SE, Merimee TJ. Effects of comparative perfusions of equimolar, single component insulin and proinsulin in the human forearm. *Diabetes* 1973;22:676–686.

141. Finlay GD, Whitsett TL, Cucinell EA, Goldberg LI. Augmentation of sodium and potassium excretion, glomerular filtration rate and renal plasma flow by levodopa. *N Engl J Med* 1971;284:865–870.

142. Fischer PW, Giroux A. Effects of dietary magnesium on sodium-potassium pump action in the heart of rats. *J Nutr* 1987;117:2091–2095.

143. Flack JM, Ryder KW, Strickland D, Whang R. Metabolic correlates of theophylline therapy: a concentration-related phenomenon. *Ann Pharmacother* 1994;28:175–179.

144. Flatman JA, Clausen T. Combined effects of adrenaline and insulin on active electrogenic Na+-K+ transport in rat soleus muscle. *Nature* 1979;281:580–581.

145. Fraley DS, Adler S. Correction of hyperkalemia by bicarbonate despite constant blood pH. *Kidney Int* 1977;12:354–360.

146. Fulop M. Serum potassium in lactic acidosis and ketoacidosis. *N Engl J Med* 1979;300:1087–1089.

147. Gallant EM. Barium-treated mammalian skeletal muscle: similarities to hypokalaemic periodic paralysis. *J Physiol* 1983;335:577–590.

148. Gardos G. The function of calcium in the potassium permeability of human erythrocytes. *Biochim Biophys Acta* 1958;30:653–654.

149. Garella S, Matarese RA. Renal effects of prostaglandins and clinical adverse effects of nonsteroidal anti-inflammatory agents. *Medicine (Baltimore)* 1984;63:165–181.

150. Gavryck WA, Moore RD, Thompson RC. Effect of insulin upon membrane-bound (Na+ + K+)-ATPase extracted from frog skeletal muscle. *J Physiol* 1975;252:43–58.

151. George AL, Jr., Wood CA, Jr. Succinylcholine-induced hyperkalemia complicating the neuroleptic malignant syndrome. *Ann Intern Med* 1987;106:172.

152. Giebisch G, Berger L, Pitts RF. The extrarenal response to acute acid-base disturbances of respiratory origin. *J Clin Invest* 1955;34:231–245.

153. Glitsch HG, Haas HG, Trautwein W. The effect of adrenaline on the K and Na fluxes in the frog's atrium. *Naunyn Schmiedebergs Arch Exp Pathol Pharmakol* 1965;250:59–71.

154. Goecke IA, Bonilla S, Marusic ET, Alvo M. Enhanced insulin sensitivity in extrarenal potassium handling in uremic rats. *Kidney Int* 1991;39:39–43.

155. Goggans FC. Acute hyperkalemia during lithium treatment of manic illness. *Am J Psychiatry* 1980;137:860–861.

156. Goldfarb S, Cox M, Singer I, Goldberg M. Acute hyperkalemia induced by hyperglycemia: hormonal mechanisms. *Ann Intern Med* 1976;84:426–432.

157. Gonick HC, Kleeman CR, Rubini ME, Maxwell MH. Functional impairment in chronic renal disease. 3. Studies of potassium excretion. *Am J Med Sci* 1971;261:281–290.

158. Gosmanov AR, Thomason DB. Insulin and isoproterenol differentially regulate mitogen-activated protein kinase-dependent Na(+)-K(+)-2Cl(-) cotransporter activity in skeletal muscle. *Diabetes* 2002;51:615–623.

159. Gourley DR. Separation of insulin effects on K content and O2 consumption of frog muscle with cardiac glycosides. *Am J Physiol* 1961;200:1320–1326.

160. Gourley DR, Bethea MD. Insulin effect on adipose tissue sodium and potassium. *Proc Soc Exp Biol Med* 1964;115:821–823.

161. Granerus AK, Jagenburg R, Svanborg A. Kaliuretic effect of L-dopa treatment in parkinsonian patients. *Acta Med Scand* 1977;201:291–297.

162. Grinstein S, Erlij D. Insulin unmasks latent sodium pump sites in frog muscle. *Nature* 1974; 251:57–58.

163. Grob D, Liljestrand A, Johns RJ. Potassium movement in normal subjects: effect on muscle function. *Am J Med* 1957;23:340–355.

164. Groen J, Willebrands A, Kamminga E, Van Schothorst H, Godfried E. De invloed van toediening van glycose op het kaliumgehalte van het bloedserum bij normale personen en bijniet-diabetische patienten. *Nederlands Militair Geneeskundig Tijdschrift* 1950;94:2187–2201.

165. Gronert GA, Theye RA. Pathophysiology of hyperkalemia induced by succinylcholine. *Anesthesiology* 1975;43:89–99.

166. Grundy SM. HMG-CoA reductase inhibitors for treatment of hypercholesterolemia. *N Engl J Med* 1988;319:24–33.

167. Guerra SM, Kitabchi AE. Comparison of the effectiveness of various routes of insulin injection: insulin levels and glucose response in normal subjects. *J Clin Endocrinol Metab* 1976;42: 869–874.

168. Haalboom JR, Deenstra M, Struyvenberg A. Hypokalaemia induced by inhalation of fenoterol. *Lancet* 1985;1:1125–1127.

169. Halter JB, Pflug AE, Porte D, Jr. Mechanism of plasma catecholamine increases during surgical stress in man. *J Clin Endocrinol Metab* 1977;45:936–944.

170. Hariharasubramanian N, Devi D, Rao A. Serum potassium levels during lithium therapy of manic depressive psychosis. In: Johnson FN, Johnson S, eds. *Lithium in Medical Practice*. Baltimore: University Press; 1978:205–208.

171. Harrop G, Benedict E. The role of phosphate and potassium in carbohydrate metabolism following insulin administration. *Proc Soc Exp Biol Med* 1923;20:430–431.

172. Hastwell G, Lambert BE. The effect of oral salbutamol on serum potassium and blood sugar. *Br J Obstet Gynaecol* 1978;85:767–769.

173. Hays ET, Dwyer TM, Horowicz P, Swift JG. Epinephrine action on sodium fluxes in frog striated muscle. *Am J Physiol* 1974;227:1340–1347.

174. Henrich WL, Katz FH, Molinoff PB, Schrier RW. Competitive effects of hypokalemia and volume depletion on plasma renin activity, aldosterone and catecholamine concentrations in hemodialysis patients. *Kidney Int* 1977;12:279–284.

175. Hertz P, Richardson JA. Arginine-induced hyperkalemia in renal failure patients. *Arch Intern Med* 1972;130:778–780.

176. Hesp R, Chanarin I, Tait CE. Potassium changes in megaloblastic anaemia. *Clin Sci Mol Med* 1975;49:77–79.

177. Hiatt N, Chapman LW, Davidson MB. Influence of epinephrine and propranolol on transmembrane K transfer in anuric dogs with hyperkalemia. *J Pharmacol Exp Ther* 1979;209:282–286.

178. Hiatt N, Davidson MB, Bonorris G. The effect of potassium chloride infusion on insulin secretion in vivo. *Horm Metab Res* 1972;4:64–68.

179. Hiatt N, Yamakawa T, Davidson MB. Necessity for insulin in transfer of excess infused K to intracellular fluid. *Metabolism* 1974;23:43–49.

180. Holler J. Potassium deficiency occurring during the treatment of diabetic acidosis. *JAMA* 1946;131:1186–1189.

181. Horie M, Irisawa H, Noma A. Voltage-dependent magnesium block of adenosine-triphosphate-sensitive potassium channel in guinea-pig ventricular cells. *J Physiol* 1987;387:251–272.

182. Huang K-W. Pa Ping (transient paralysis simulating family periodic paralysis). *Chinese Med J* 1943;61:305–312.

183. Hurlbert BJ, Edelman JD, David K. Serum potassium levels during and after terbutaline. *Anesth Analg* 1981;60:723–725.

184. Imura H, Kato Y, Ikeda M, Morimoto M, Yawata M. Effect of adrenergic-blocking or -stimulating agents on plasma growth hormone, immunoreactive insulin, and blood free fatty acid levels in man. *J Clin Invest* 1971;50:1069–1079.

185. Insel PA. Identification and regulation of adrenergic receptors in target cells. *Am J Physiol* 1984;247(Pt 1):E53–58.

186. Ismail-Beigi F, Edelman IS. Effects of thyroid status on electrolyte distribution in rat tissues. *Am J Physiol* 1973;225:1172–1177.

187. Iwatsuki N, Kuroda N, Amaha K, Iwatsuki K. Succinylcholine-induced hyperkalemia in patients with ruptured cerebral aneurysms. *Anesthesiology* 1980;53:64–67.

188. Izumo H, Izumo S, DeLuise M, Flier JS. Erythrocyte Na-K pump in uremia. Acute correction of a transport defect by hemodialysis. *J Clin Invest* 1984;74:581–588.

189. Jakobs KH, Saur W, Schultz G. Reduction of adenylate cyclase activity in lysates of human platelets by the alpha-adrenergic component of epinephrine. *J Cyclic Nucleotide Res* 1976;2:381–392.

190. James GW, Abbott LD, Jr. Metabolic studies in pernicious anemia. I. Nitrogen and phosphorus metabolism during vitamin B12-induced remission. *Metabolism* 1952;1:259–270.

191. Jauchem JR, Vick RL. Phenylephrine-induced hyperkalemia: role of the liver. *Proc Soc Exp Biol Med* 1980;163:478–481.

192. Johansson BW, Dziamski R. Malignant arrhythmias in acute myocardial infarction. Relationship to serum potassium and effect of selective and non-selective beta-blockade. *Drugs* 1984;28(Suppl 1):77–85.

193. Kahn T, Kaji DM, Nicolis G, Krakoff LR, Stein RM. Factors related to potassium transport in chronic stable renal disease in man. *Clin Sci Mol Med* 1978;54:661–666.

194. Kaibara K, Akasu T, Tokimasa T, Koketsu K. Beta-adrenergic modulation of the Na+-K+ pump in frog skeletal muscles. *Pflugers Arch* 1985;405:24–28.

195. Kaji D, Thomas K. Na+-K+ pump in chronic renal failure. *Am J Physiol* 1987;252(Pt 2):F785–793.

196. Karlsberg RP, Cryer PE, Roberts R. Serial plasma catecholamine response early in the course of clinical acute myocardial infarction: relationship to infarct extent and mortality. *Am Heart J* 1981;102:24–29.

197. Katz LD, D'Avella J, DeFronzo RA. Effect of epinephrine on renal potassium excretion in the isolated perfused rat kidney. *Am J Physiol* 1984;247(Pt 2):F331–338.

198. Kearney TE, Manoguerra AS, Curtis GP, Ziegler MG. Theophylline toxicity and the beta-adrenergic system. *Ann Intern Med* 1985;102:766–769.

199. Keating RE, Weichselbaum TE, Alanis M, Margraf HW, Elman R. The movement of potassium during experimental acidosis and alkalosis in the nephrectomized dog. *Surg Gynecol Obstet* 1953;96:323–330.

200. Keith NM, Osterberg AE. The tolerance for potassium in severe renal insufficiency. *J Clin Invest* 1947;26:773–783.

201. Keith NM, Osterberg AE, Burchell HB. Some effects of potassium salts in man. *Ann Intern Med* 1942;16:879–892.

202. Keith NM, Osterberg AE, E. KH. The excretion of potassium by the normal and diseased kidney. *Trans Assoc Am Physicians* 1940;55:219–222.

203. Kestens PJ, Haxhe JJ, Lambotte L, Lambotte C. The effect of insulin on the uptake of potassium and phosphate by the isolated perfused canine liver. *Metabolism* 1963;12:941–50.

204. Kim WG, Brown EB, Jr. Potassium transfer with constant extracellular pH. *J Lab Clin Med* 1968;71:678–685.

205. Kjeldsen K, Norgaard A. Effect of magnesium depletion on 3H-ouabain binding site concentration in rat skeletal muscle. *Magnesium* 1987;6:55–60.

206. Knochel JP. Neuromuscular manifestations of electrolyte disorders. *Am J Med* 1982;72:521–535.

207. Knochel JP. Role of glucoregulatory hormones in potassium homeostasis. *Kidney Int* 1977;11:443–452.

208. Koht A, Cane R, Cerullo LJ. Serum potassium levels during prolonged hypothermia. *Intensive Care Med* 1983;9:275–277.

209. Kramer HJ, Gospodinov D, Kruck F. Functional and metabolic studies on red blood cell sodium transport in chronic uremia. *Nephron* 1976;16:344–358.

210. Krapf R, Caduff P, Wagdi P, Staubli M, Hulter HN. Plasma potassium response to acute respiratory alkalosis. *Kidney Int* 1995;47:217–224.

211. Kreisberg RA. Diabetic ketoacidosis: new concepts and trends in pathogenesis and treatment. *Ann Intern Med* 1978;88:681–695.

212. Krikken-Hogenberk LG, de Jong JR, Bovill JG. Succinylcholine-induced hyperkalemia in a patient with metastatic rhabdomyosarcoma. *Anesthesiology* 1989;70:553–555.

213. Krzesinski JM, Rorive G. Sodium-lithium countertransport in red cells. *N Engl J Med* 1983;309:987–988.

214. Kubota K, Ingbar SH. Influences of thyroid status and sympathoadrenal system on extrarenal potassium disposal. *Am J Physiol* 1990;258(Pt 1):E428–435.

215. Ladefoged K, Hagen K. Correlation between concentrations of magnesium, zinc, and potassium in plasma, erythrocytes and muscles. *Clin Chim Acta* 1988;177:157–166.

216. LaManna VR, Ferrier GR. Electrophysiological effects of insulin on normal and depressed cardiac tissues. *Am J Physiol* 1981;240:H636–644.

217. Lambotte L, Shoemaker W. Effect of insulin on hepatic K movements as influenced by hypothermia, barbiturate, and dibenzyline. *Physiologist* 1964;7:184A.

218. Lands AM, Arnold A, McAuliff JP, Luduena FP, Brown TG, Jr. Differentiation of receptor systems activated by sympathomimetic amines. *Nature* 1967;214:597–598.

219. Landsberg L, Young JB. Fasting, feeding and regulation of the sympathetic nervous system. *N Engl J Med* 1978;298:1295–1301.

220. Lawson DH, Murray RM, Parker JL. Early mortality in the megaloblastic anaemias. *Q J Med* 1972;41:1–14.

221. Leibman J, Edelman IS. Interrelations of plasma potassium concentration, plasma sodium concentration, arterial pH and total exchangeable potassium. *J Clin Invest* 1959;38:2176–2188.

222. Leitch AG, Clancy LJ, Costello JF, Flenley DC. Effect of intravenous infusion of salbutamol on ventilatory response to carbon dioxide and hypoxia and on heart rate and plasma potassium in normal men. *Br Med J* 1976;1:365–367.

223. Levin ML, Rector FC, Jr., Seldin DW. Effects of potassium and ouabain on sodium transport in human red cells. *Am J Physiol* 1968;214:1328–1332.

224. Levy LJ, Duga J, Girgis M, Gordon EE. Ketoacidosis associated with alcoholism in nondiabetic subjects. *Ann Intern Med* 1973;78:213–219.

225. Lim VS, Webster GD. The effect of aldosterone on water and electrolyte composition of incubated rat diaphragms. *Clin Sci* 1967;33:261–270.

226. Lin SH, Lin YF. Propranolol rapidly reverses paralysis, hypokalemia, and hypophosphatemia in thyrotoxic periodic paralysis. *Am J Kidney Dis* 2001;37:620–623.

227. Lindinger MI, Graham TE, Spriet LL. Caffeine attenuates the exercise-induced increase in plasma [K+] in humans. *J Appl Physiol* 1993;74:1149–1155.

228. Ljunghall S, Joborn H, Rastad J, Akerstrom G. Plasma potassium and phosphate concentrations—influence by adrenaline infusion, beta-blockade and physical exercise. *Acta Med Scand* 1987;221:83–93.

229. Lockwood RH, Lum BK. Effects of adrenalectomy and adrenergic antagonists on potassium metabolism. *J Pharmacol Exp Ther* 1977;203:103–111.

230. Lockwood RH, Lum BK. Effects of adrenergic agonists and antagonists on potassium metabolism. *J Pharmacol Exp Ther* 1974;189:119–129.

231. Lundborg P. The effect of adrenergic blockade on potassium concentrations in different conditions. *Acta Med Scand Suppl* 1983;672:121–126.

232. Lynch CJ, Bocckino SB, Blackmore PF, Exton JH. Calcium-mobilizing hormones and phorbol myristate acetate mediate heterologous desensitization of the hormone-sensitive hepatic Na+/K+ pump. *Biochem J* 1987;248:807–813.

233. Lytton J, Lin JC, Guidotti G. Identification of two molecular forms of (Na+,K+)-ATPase in rat adipocytes. Relation to insulin stimulation of the enzyme. *J Biol Chem* 1985;260:1177–1184.

234. Madias JE, Shah B, Chintalapally G, Chalavarya G, Madias NE. Admission serum potassium in patients with acute myocardial infarction: its correlates and value as a determinant of in-hospital outcome. *Chest* 2000;118:904–913.

235. Madias NE. Lactic acidosis. *Kidney Int* 1986;29:752–774.

236. Magner PO, Robinson L, Halperin RM, Zettle R, Halperin ML. The plasma potassium concentration in metabolic acidosis: a re-evaluation. *Am J Kidney Dis* 1988;11:220–224.

237. Makoff DL, Da Silva JA, Rosenbaum BJ. On the mechanism of hyperkalaemia due to hyperosmotic expansion with saline or mannitol. *Clin Sci* 1971;41:383–393.

238. Manery JF, Dryden EE, Still JS, Madapallimattam G. Enhancement (by ATP, insulin, and lack of divalent cations) of ouabain inhibition of cation transport and ouabain binding in frog skeletal muscle; effect of insulin and ouabain on sarcolemmal (Na + K)MgATPase. *Can J Physiol Pharmacol* 1977;55:21–33.

239. Manitius A, Epstein FH. Some observations on the influence of a magnesium-deficient diet on rats, with special reference to renal concentrating ability. *J Clin Invest* 1963;42:208–215.

240. Martinez Vea A, Montoliu J, Andreu L, Torras A, Gaya J, Lopez-Pedret J, Revert L. Beta adrenergic modulation of extrarenal potassium disposal in terminal uraemia. *Proc Eur Dial Transplant Assoc* 1983;19:756–760.

241. Massara F, Cagliero E, Maccario M, Orzan F, Carini G. Pathophysiological doses of glucagon cause a transient increase of the hepatic vein potassium concentration in man. *Miner Electrolyte Metab* 1986;12:142–146.

242. Massara F, Martelli S, Cagliero E, Camanni F, Molinatti GM. Influence of glucagon on plasma levels of potassium in man. *Diabetologia* 1980;19:414–417.

243. Massara F, Tripodina A, Rotunno M. Propranolol block of epinephrine-induced hypokaliaemia in man. *Eur J Pharmacol* 1970;10:404–407.

244. McCammon RL, Stoelting RK. Exaggerated increase in serum potassium following succinylcholine in dogs with beta blockade. *Anesthesiology* 1984;61:723–725.

245. McCusick V. The effect of lithium on the electrocardiogram of animals and relation of this effect to the ratio of the intracellular and extracellular concentrations of potassium. *J Clin Invest* 1954;33:598–610.

246. McDonald RH, Jr., Goldberg LI, McNay JL, Tuttle EP, Jr. Effect of dopamine in man: augmentation of sodium excretion, glomerular filtration rate, and renal plasma flow. *J Clin Invest* 1964;43:1116–1124.

247. Meyer MB, McNay JL, Goldberg LI. Effects of dopamine on renal function and hemodynamics in the dog. *J Pharmacol Exp Ther* 1967;156:186–192.

248. Mikhailidis DP, Dandona P. Adrenaline and potassium. *Lancet* 1984;1:170–171.

249. Miller H, Darrow D. Relation of muscle electrolyte to alteration in serum potassium and to the toxic effects of injected potassium chloride. *Am J Physiol* 1940;130:747–758.

250. Mimran A, Ribstein J, Sissmann J. Effects of calcium antagonists on adrenaline-induced hypokalaemia. *Drugs* 1993;46(Suppl 2):103–107.

251. Minaker KL, Rowe JW. Potassium homeostasis during hyperinsulinemia: effect of insulin level, beta-blockade, and age. *Am J Physiol* 1982;242:E373–377.

252. Minella RA, Schulman DS. Fatal verapamil toxicity and hypokalemia. *Am Heart J* 1991;121(Pt 1):1810–1812.

253. Mitch WE, Wilcox CS. Disorders of body fluids, sodium and potassium in chronic renal failure. *Am J Med* 1982;72:536–550.

254. Montoliu J, Lens XM, Revert L. Potassium-lowering effect of albuterol for hyperkalemia in renal failure. *Arch Intern Med* 1987;147:713–717.

255. Moore FD, Boling EA, Ditmore HB, Jr., Sicular A, Teterick JE, Ellison AE, Hoye SJ, Ball MR. Body sodium and potassium. V. The relationship of alkalosis, potassium deficiency and surgical stress to acute hypokalemia in man; experiments and review of the literature. *Metabolism* 1955;4:379–402.

256. Moore RD. Effect of insulin upon the sodium pump in frog skeletal muscle. *J Physiol* 1973;232:23–45.

257. Moore RD. Effects of insulin upon ion transport. *Biochim Biophys Acta* 1983;737:1–49.

258. Moore RD. Stimulation of Na: H exchange by insulin. *Biophys J* 1981;33:203–210.
259. Moore RD, Rabovsky JL. Mechanism of insulin action on resting membrane potential of frog skeletal muscle. *Am J Physiol* 1979;236:C249–254.
260. Moravec MA, Hurlbert BJ. Hypokalemia associated with terbutaline administration in obstetrical patients. *Anesth Analg* 1980;59:917–920.
261. Moreno M, Murphy C, Goldsmith C. Increase in serum potassium resulting from the administration of hypertonic mannitol and other solutions. *J Lab Clin Med* 1969;73:291–298.
262. Morgan DB, Cumberbatch M, Swaminathan R. The relation between plasma, erythrocyte and total body potassium in patients with hypokalemia. *Miner Electrolyte Metab* 1981;5:233–239.
263. Morgan DB, Young RM. Acute transient hypokalaemia: new interpretation of a common event. *Lancet* 1982;2:751–752.
264. Mostellar ME, Tuttle EP, Jr. Effects of alkalosis on plasma concentration and urinary excretion of inorganic phosphate in man. *J Clin Invest* 1964;43:138–149.
265. Muller WA, Faloona GR, Unger RH. Hyperglucagonemia in diabetic ketoacidosis. Its prevalence and significance. *Am J Med* 1973;54:52–57.
266. Nadler JL, Hsueh W, Horton R. Therapeutic effect of calcium channel blockade in primary aldosteronism. *J Clin Endocrinol Metab* 1985;60:896–899.
267. Nahas GG, Steinsland OS. Increased rate of catecholamine synthesis during respiratory acidosis. *Respir Physiol* 1968;5:108–117.
268. Natalini G, Seramondi V, Fassini P, Foccoli P, Toninelli C, Cavaliere S, Candiani A. Acute respiratory acidosis does not increase plasma potassium in normokalaemic anaesthetized patients. A controlled randomized trial. *Eur J Anaesthesiol* 2001;18:394–400.
269. Nicolis GL, Kahn T, Sanchez A, Gabrilove JL. Glucose-induced hyperkalemia in diabetic subjects. *Arch Intern Med* 1981;141:49–53.
270. Nordrehaug JE. Malignant arrhythmia in relation to serum potassium in acute myocardial infarction. *Am J Cardiol* 1985;56:20D–23D.
271. Nordrehaug JE, Johannessen KA, von der Lippe G. Serum potassium concentration as a risk factor of ventricular arrhythmias early in acute myocardial infarction. *Circulation* 1985; 71:645–649.
272. Nordrehaug JE, Johannessen KA, von der Lippe G, Sederholm M, Grottum P, Kjekshus J. Effect of timolol on changes in serum potassium concentration during acute myocardial infarction. *Br Heart J* 1985;53:388–393.
273. Norgaard A, Kjeldsen K, Clausen T. Potassium depletion decreases the number of 3H-ouabain binding sites and the active Na-K transport in skeletal muscle. *Nature* 1981;293:739–741.
274. Olsson A, Persson S, Schroder R. Effects of terbutaline and isoproterenol on hyperkalemia in nephrectomized rabbits. *Scand J Urol Nephrol* 1977;12:35–38.
275. Opdyke DF, Carroll RG, Keller NE. Systemic arterial pressor responses induced by potassium in dogfish, Squalus acanthias. *Am J Physiol* 1981;241:R228–232.
276. Orringer CE, Eustace JC, Wunsch CD, Gardner LB. Natural history of lactic acidosis after grand-mal seizures. A model for the study of an anion-gap acidosis not associated with hyperkalemia. *N Engl J Med* 1977;297:796–769.
277. Oster JR, Perez GO, Castro A, Vaamonde CA. Plasma potassium response to acute metabolic acidosis induced by mineral and nonmineral acids. *Miner Electrolyte Metab* 1980;4:28–36.
278. Oster JR, Perez GO, Vaamonde CA. Relationship between blood pH and potassium and phosphorus during acute metabolic acidosis. *Am J Physiol* 1978;235:F345–351.
279. Paice B, Gray JM, McBride D, Donnelly T, Lawson DH. Hyperkalaemia in patients in hospital. *Br Med J (Clin Res Ed)* 1983;286:1189–1192.
280. Pan YJ, Young DB. Experimental aldosterone hypertension in the dog. *Hypertension* 1982; 4:279–287.
281. Papadakis MA, Wexman MP, Fraser C, Sedlacek SM. Hyperkalemia complicating digoxin toxicity in a patient with renal failure. *Am J Kidney Dis* 1985;5:64–66.
282. Patrick J, Bradford B. A comparison of leucocyte potassium content with other measurements in potassium-depleted rabbits. *Clin Sci* 1972;42:415–421.
283. Pedersen EB, Kornerup HJ. Relationship between plasma aldosterone concentration and plasma potassium in patients with essential hypertension during alprenolol treatment. *Acta Med Scand* 1976;200:263–267.
284. Pedersen G, Pedersen A, Pedersen EB. Effect of propranolol on total exchangeable body potassium and total exchangeable body sodium in essential hypertension. *Scand J Clin Lab Invest* 1979;39:167–170.
285. Pei Y, Richardson R, Greenwood C, Wong PY, Baines A. Extrarenal effect of cyclosporine A on potassium homeostasis in renal transplant recipients. *Am J Kidney Dis* 1993;22:314–319.
286. Perazella MA. Drug-induced hyperkalemia: old culprits and new offenders. *Am J Med* 2000; 109:307–314.
287. Perazella MA, Biswas P. Acute hyperkalemia associated with intravenous epsilon-aminocaproic acid therapy. *Am J Kidney Dis* 1999;33:782–785.
288. Perez GO, Oster JR, Pelleya R, Caralis PV, Kem DC. Hyperkalemia from single small oral doses of potassium chloride. *Nephron* 1984;36:270–271.
289. Perez GO, Oster JR, Vaamonde CA. Serum potassium concentration in acidemic states. *Nephron* 1981;27:233–243.
290. Perez GO, Pelleya R, Oster JR, Kem DC, Vaamonde CA. Blunted kaliuresis after an acute potassium load in patients with chronic renal failure. *Kidney Int* 1983;24:656–662.
291. Petch MC, McKay R, Bethune DW. The effect of beta, adrenergic blockade on serum potassium and glucose levels during open heart surgery. *Eur Heart J* 1981;2:123–126.
292. Petersen OH, Dunne MJ. Regulation of K+ channels plays a crucial role in the control of insulin secretion. *Pflugers Arch* 1989;414(Suppl 1):S115–20.
293. Pettit GW, Vick RL. An analysis of the contribution of the endocrine pancreas to the kalemotropic actions of catecholamines. *J Pharmacol Exp Ther* 1974;190:234–242.
294. Pettit GW, Vick RL. Contribution of pancreatic insulin to extrarenal potassium homeostasis: a two-compartment model. *Am J Physiol* 1974;226:319–324.
295. Pettit GW, Vick RL, Swander AM. Plasma K plus and insulin: changes during KCl infusion in normal and nephrectomized dogs. *Am J Physiol* 1975;228:107–109.
296. Ponce SP, Jennings AE, Madias NE, Harrington JT. Drug-induced hyperkalemia. *Medicine (Baltimore)* 1985;64:357–370.
297. Powell WJ, Jr., Skinner NS, Jr. Effect of the catecholamines on ionic balance and vascular resistance in skeletal muscle. *Am J Cardiol* 1966;18:73–82.
298. Pratt JH, Ganguly A, Parkinson CA, Weinberger MH. Stimulation of aldosterone secretion by metoclopramide in humans: apparent independence of renal and pituitary mediation. *Metabolism* 1981;30:129–134.
299. Quarello F, Boero R, Guarena C, Rosati C, Giraudo G, Giacchino F, Piccoli G. Acute effects of hemodialysis on erythrocyte sodium fluxes in uremic patients. *Nephron* 1985;41:22–25.
300. Rado JP. Glucose-induced hyperkalemia during captopril treatment. *Arch Intern Med* 1983; 143:389.
301. Resh MD. Insulin activation of (Na+,K+)-adenosinetriphosphatase exhibits a temperature-dependent lag time. Comparison to activation of the glucose transporter. *Biochemistry* 1983; 22:2781–2784.
302. Resh MD, Nemenoff RA, Guidotti G. Insulin stimulation of (Na+,K+)-adenosine triphosphatase-dependent 86Rb+ uptake in rat adipocytes. *J Biol Chem* 1980. 255:10938–10945.
303. Riecker G, Bolte HD, Rohl D. Hypokaliamie and membranpotential. *Reanimation et Organes Artificiels* 1954;1:41–50.
304. Rimmer JM, Horn JF, Gennari FJ. Hyperkalemia as a complication of drug therapy. *Arch Intern Med* 1987;147:867–869.
305. Rodgrove HJ, Alabaster S. Lactic acidosis in seizures. *N Engl J Med* 1977;297:1352.
306. Rogers TA. Tissue buffering in rat diaphragm. *Am J Physiol* 1957;191:363–366.
307. Rogers TA, Wachenfeld AE. Effect of physiologic acids on electrolytes in rat diaphragm. *Am J Physiol* 1958;193:623–626.
308. Rohr AS, Spector SL, Rachelefsky GS, Katz RM, Siegel SC. Efficacy of parenteral albuterol in the treatment of asthma. Comparison of its metabolic side effects with subcutaneous epinephrine. *Chest* 1986;89:348–351.
309. Rolton H, Simpson E, Donnelly T, Rodger JC. Plasma potassium in acute myocardial infarction. *Eur Heart J* 1981;2(Suppl A):21A.
310. Rosa RM, Silva P, Young JB, Landsberg L, Brown RS, Rowe JW, Epstein FH. Adrenergic modulation of extrarenal potassium disposal. *N Engl J Med* 1980;302:431–434.
311. Roza O, Berman LB. The pathophysiology of barium: hypokalemic and cardiovascular effects. *J Pharmacol Exp Ther* 1971;177:433–439.
312. Rubinstein S, Hindi RD, Moss RB, Blessing-Moore J, Lewiston NJ. Sudden death in adolescent asthma. *Ann Allergy* 1984;53:311–318.
313. Ryan MP. Interrelationships of magnesium and potassium homeostasis. *Miner Electrolyte Metab* 1993;19:290–295.
314. Ryan MP, Whang R, Yamalis W, Aikawa JK. Effect of magnesium deficiency on cardiac and skeletal muscle potassium during dietary potassium restriction. *Proc Soc Exp Biol Med* 1973; 143:1045–1047.
315. Sager PT, DeFronzo RA. Dopaminergic regulation of extrarenal potassium metabolism. *Miner Electrolyte Metab* 1987;13:385–392.
316. Salem MM, Rosa RM, Batlle DC. Extrarenal potassium tolerance in chronic renal failure: implications for the treatment of acute hyperkalemia. *Am J Kidney Dis* 1991;18:421–440.
317. Sangkabutra T, Crankshaw DP, Schneider C, Fraser SF, Sostaric S, Mason K, Burge CM, Skinner SL, McMahon LP, McKenna MJ. Impaired K+ regulation contributes to exercise limitation in end-stage renal failure. *Kidney Int* 2003;63:283–290.
318. Santeusanio F, Faloona GR, Knochel JP, Unger RH. Evidence for a role of endogenous insulin and glucagon in the regulation of potassium homeostasis. *J Lab Clin Med* 1973;81:809–817.
319. Sargeant RJ, Liu Z, Klip A. Action of insulin on Na(+)-K(+)-ATPase and the Na(+)-K(+)-2Cl- cotransporter in 3T3-L1 adipocytes. *Am J Physiol* 1995;269(Pt 1):C217–225.
320. Saris S, Lowenthal DT, Affrime MB, Rosenthal L, Swartz G. Lack of effect of nonsteroidsal anti-inflammatory drugs on exercise-induced hyperkalemia. *N Engl J Med* 1982;307:559–560.
321. Schaafsma IA, van Ernst MG, Kouistra HS, Verklej CB, Peeters ME, Boer P, Rijnberk A, Everts ME. Exercise-induced hyperkalemia in hypothyroid dogs. *Domest Anim Endocrinol* 2003;22:113–225.
322. Scheid CR, Fay FS. Beta-adrenergic stimulation of 42K influx in isolated smooth muscle cells. *Am J Physiol* 1984;246(Pt 1):C415–421.
323. Scheid CR, Honeyman TW, Fay FS. Mechanism of beta-adrenergic relaxation of smooth muscle. *Nature* 1979;277:32–36.
324. Schmidt TA, Bundgaard H, Olesen HL, Secher NH, Kjeldsen K. Digoxin affects potassium homeostasis during exercise in patients with heart failure. *Cardiovasc Res* 1995;29:506–511.
325. Schrier RW, Regal EM. Influence of aldosterone on sodium, water and potassium metabolism in chronic renal disease. *Kidney Int* 1972;1:156–168.
326. Schultze G, Koeppe P, Molzahn M. Restoration of total body potassium in the course of long-term hemodialysis treatment. *Miner Electrolyte Metab* 1981;6:139–145.
327. Schwartz WB. Potassium and the kidney. *N Engl J Med* 1955;253:601–608.
328. Schwartz WB, Brackett NC, Jr., Cohen JJ. The response of extracellular hydrogen ion concentration to graded degrees of chronic hypercapnia: the physiologic limits of the defense of pH. *J Clin Invest* 1965;44:291–301.
329. Schwartz WB, Orning KJ, Porter R. The internal distribution of hydrogen ions with varying degrees of metabolic acidosis. *J Clin Invest* 1957;36:373–382.
330. Schwartz WB, Relman AS. Metabolic and renal studies in chronic potassium depletion resulting from overuse of laxatives. *J Clin Invest* 1953;32:258–271.
331. Schwarz KC, Cohen BD, Lubash GD, Rubin AL. Severe acidosis and hyperpotassemia treated with sodium bicarbonate infusion. *Circulation* 1959;19:215–220.
332. Scribner BH, Burnell JM. Interpretation of the serum potassium concentration. *Metabolism* 1956;5:468–479.
333. Seldin DW, Carter NW, Rector FC, Jr. Consequences of renal failure and their management. In: Strauss MB, Welt LG, eds. *Diseases of the Kidney*. Boston: Little, Brown; 1963:173–217.
334. Seldin DW, Tarail R. Effect of hypertonic solutions on metabolism and excretion of electrolytes. *Am J Physiol* 1949;159:160–174.
335. Shemer J, Modan M, Ezra D, Cabili S. Incidence of hyperkalemia in hospitalized patients. *Isr J Med Sci* 1983;19:659–661.
336. Shils ME. Experimental human magnesium depletion. *Medicine (Baltimore)* 1969;48:61–85.

337. Silberstein SD, Lemberger L, Klein DC, Axelrod J, Kopin IJ. Induction of adrenal tyrosine hydroxylase in organ culture. *Neuropharmacology* 1972;11:721–726.
338. Silva P, Spokes K. Sympathetic system in potassium homeostasis. *Am J Physiol* 1981;241: F151–155.
339. Simmons DH, Avedon M. Acid-base alterations and plasma potassium concentration. *Am J Physiol* 1959;197:319–36.
340. Singer RB, Clark JK, Barker ES, Crosley AP, Jr., Elkinton JR. The acute effects in man of rapid intravenous infusion of hypertonic sodium bicarbonate solution. I. Changes in acid-base balance and distribution of the excess buffer base. *Medicine (Baltimore)* 1955;34:51–95.
341. Singhal PC, Desroches L, Mattana J, Abramovici M, Wagner JD, Maesaka JK. Mineralocorticoid therapy lowers serum potassium in patients with end-stage renal disease. *Am J Nephrol* 1993;13:138–141.
342. Singhal PC, Rubin RB, Peters A, Santiago A, Neugarten J. Rhabdomyolysis and acute renal failure associated with cocaine abuse. *J Toxicol Clin Toxicol* 1990;28:321–330.
343. Skou JC. Enzymatic basis for active transport of Na+ and K+ across cell membrane. *Physiol Rev* 1965;45:596–617.
344. Smith SK, Thompson D. The effect of intravenous salbutamol upon plasma and urinary potassium during premature labour. *Br J Obstet Gynaecol* 1977;84:344–347.
345. Smith SR, Kendall MJ. Inhaled bronchodilators and hypokalaemia. *Lancet* 1983;2:218.
346. Smith SR, Ryder C, Kendall MJ, Holder R. Cardiovascular and biochemical responses to nebulised salbutamol in normal subjects. *Br J Clin Pharmacol* 1984;18:641–644.
347. Smith TW, Willerson JT. Suicidal and accidental digoxin ingestion. Report of five cases with serum digoxin level correlations. *Circulation* 1971;44:29–36.
348. Smythe CM, Nickel JF, Bradley SE. The effect of epinephrine (USP), l-epinephrine, and l-norepinephrine on glomerular filtration rate, renal plasma flow, and the urinary excretion of sodium, potassium, and water in normal man. *J Clin Invest* 1952;31:499–506.
349. Soliman AR, Akmal M, Massry SG. Parathyroid hormone interferes with extrarenal disposition of potassium in chronic renal failure. *Nephron* 1989;52:262–267.
350. Solomon R. The relationship between disorders of K+ and Mg+ homeostasis. *Semin Nephrol* 1987;7:253–262.
351. Solomon R, Dubey A. Diltiazem enhances potassium disposal in subjects with end-stage renal disease. *Am J Kidney Dis* 1992;19:420–426.
352. Sowers JR, Brickman AS, Sowers DK, Berg G. Dopaminergic modulation of aldosterone secretion in man is unaffected by glucocorticoids and angiotensin blockade. *J Clin Endocrinol Metab* 1981;52:1078–1084.
353. Sperelakis N, Schneider MF, Harris EJ. Decreased K+ conductance produced by Ba++ in frog sartorius fibers. *J Gen Physiol* 1967;50:1565–1583.
354. Spergel G, Bleicher SJ, Goldberg M, Adesman J, Goldner MG. The effect of potassium on the impaired glucose tolerance in chronic uremia. *Metabolism* 1967;16:581–585.
355. Spital A, Sterns RH. Extrarenal potassium adaptation: the role of aldosterone. *Clin Sci (Lond)* 1989;76:213–219.
356. Spital A, Sterns RH. Paradoxical potassium depletion: a renal mechanism for extrarenal potassium adaptation. *Kidney Int* 1986;30:532–537.
357. Sprung J, Cheng EY, Gamulin S, Kampine JP, Bosnjak ZJ. Effects of acute hypothermia and beta-adrenergic receptor blockade on serum potassium concentration in rats. *Crit Care Med* 1991;19:1545–1551.
358. Steiness E. Negative potassium balance during beta-blocker treatment of hypertension. *Clin Pharmacol Ther* 1982;31:691–694.
359. Stemmer CL, Perez GO, Oster JR. Impairment of beta 2-adrenoceptor-stimulated potassium uptake in end-stage renal disease. *J Clin Pharmacol* 1987;20:628–631.
360. Sterns RH, Cox M, Feig PU, Singer I. Internal potassium balance and the control of the plasma potassium concentration. *Medicine (Baltimore)* 1981;60:339–354.
361. Sterns RH, Feig PU, Pring M, Guzzo J, Singer I. Disposition of intravenous potassium in anuric man: a kinetic analysis. *Kidney Int* 1979;15:651–660.
362. Striker T, Morrow A. Effect of succinylcholine on the level of serum potassium in man. *Anesthesiology* 1968;29:214–215.
363. Struthers AD, Reid JL. Adrenaline causes hypokalaemia in man by beta 2 adrenoceptor stimulation. *Clin Endocrinol (Oxf)* 1984;20:409–414.
364. Struthers AD, Reid JL. The role of adrenal medullary catecholamines in potassium homoeostasis. *Clin Sci (Lond)* 1984;66:377–382.
365. Struthers AD, Reid JL, Whitesmith R, Rodger JC. The effects of cardioselective and non-selective beta-adrenoceptor blockade on the hypokalaemic and cardiovascular responses to adrenomedullary hormones in man. *Clin Sci (Lond)* 1983;65:143–147.
366. Struthers AD, Whitesmith R, Reid JL. Prior thiazide diuretic treatment increases adrenaline-induced hypokalaemia. *Lancet* 1983;1:1358–13561.
367. Sugarman A, Brown RS. The role of aldosterone in potassium tolerance: studies in anephric humans. *Kidney Int* 1988;34:397–403.
368. Sugarman A, Kahn T. Calcium channel blockers enhance extrarenal potassium disposal in the rat. *Am J Physiol* 1986;250(Pt 2):F695–701.
369. Sugarman A, Kahn T. Parathyroid hormone impairs extrarenal potassium tolerance in the rat. *Am J Physiol* 1988;254(Pt 2):F385–390.
370. Sugarman A, Kaji DM, Stein RM, Kahn T. Extrarenal potassium transport and the beta 2-adrenergic system. *J Lab Clin Med* 1984;103:912–921.
371. Suh A, DeJesus E, Rosner K, Lerma E, Yu W, Young JB, Rosa RM. Racial differences in potassium disposal. *Kidney Int* 2004;66:1076–1081.
372. Swan RC, Pitts RF. Neutralization of infused acid by nephrectomized dogs. *J Clin Invest* 1955;34:205–212.
373. Takahashi T, Kato A, Miura Y, Karube T, Sakai M, Amagasa S. [The effect of beta-adrenergic blockade on the plasma potassium elevation induced by acute respiratory acidosis during halothane or fentanyl anesthesia]. *Masui* 1994;43:479–486.
374. Tannen RL. Potassium disorders. In: Kokko JP, Tannen RL, eds. *Fluids and Electrolytes.* Philadelphia: Saunders; 1986:150–228.
375. Taylor P. Cholinergic agonists. In: Goodman AG, Goodman LS, Rall TW, Murad F, eds. *The Pharmacological Basis of Therapeutics*, 7th ed. New York: MacMillan; 1985:108.
376. Thomas DJ, Dove AF, Alberti KG. Metabolic effects of salbutamol infusion during premature labour. *Br J Obstet Gynaecol* 1977;84:497–499.
377. Thomas R, Hicks S. Myocardial infarction: Ventricular arrhythmias associated with hypokalemia. *Clin Sci* 1981;61:32.
378. Tobin RB. Varying role of extracellular electrolytes in metabolic acidosis and alkalosis. *Am J Physiol* 1958;195:685–692.
379. Todd EP, Vick RL. Kalemotropic effect of epinephrine: analysis with adrenergic agonists and antagonists. *Am J Physiol* 1971;220:1964–1969.
380. Todd EP, Vick RL, Bonner FM, Leudke DW. The influence of the rate of infusion on the kalemotropic effect of epinephrine. *Arch Int Physiol Biochim* 1969;77:33–45.
381. Trost BN, Weidmann P. Metabolic effects of calcium antagonists in humans, with emphasis on carbohydrate, lipid, potassium, and uric acid homeostases. *J Cardiovasc Pharmacol* 1988; 12(Suppl 6): S86–92.
382. Tsokos GC, Balow JE, Spiegel RJ, Magrath IT. Renal and metabolic complications of undifferentiated and lymphoblastic lymphomas. *Medicine (Baltimore)* 1981;60:218–229.
383. Tuck ML, Davidson MB, Asp N, Schultze RG. Augmented aldosterone and insulin responses to potassium infusion in dogs with renal failure. *Kidney Int* 1986;30:883–890.
384. Vaamonde CA, Oster JR, Alpert HC, Rodriguez GR. Effect of potassium depletion on acidosis-induced changes in plasma potassium concentration. *Miner Electrolyte Metab* 1985;11:381–388.
385. Vandenberg CA. Inward rectification of a potassium channel in cardiac ventricular cells depends on internal magnesium ions. *Proc Natl Acad Sci U S A* 1987;84:2560–2564.
386. Vick RL, Todd EP, Luedke DW. Epinephrine-induced hypokalemia: relation to liver and skeletal muscle. *J Pharmacol Exp Ther* 1972;181:139–146.
387. Vincent HH, Boomsma F, Man in't Veld AJ, Derkx FH, Wenting GJ, Schalekamp MA. Effects of selective and nonselective beta-agonists on plasma potassium and norepinephrine. *J Cardiovasc Pharmacol* 1984;6:107–114.
388. Vincent HH, Man in't Veld AJ, Boomsma F, Schalekamp MA. Prevention of epinephrine-induced hypokalemia by nonselective beta blockers. *Am J Cardiol* 1985;56:10D–14D.
389. Vogt M. The secretion of the denervated adrenal medulla of the cat. *Br J Pharmacol* 1952; 7:325–330.
390. Waal-Manning HJ. Metabolic effects of beta-adrenoreceptor blockers. *Drugs* 1976;11(Suppl 1):121–126.
391. Waddell WJ, Bates RG. Intracellular pH. *Physiol Rev* 1969;49:285–329.
392. Wadstein J, Skude G. Does hypokalaemia precede delirium tremens? *Lancet* 1978;2:549–550.
393. Walter U, Becht E. Red blood cell sodium transport and phosphate release in uremia. *Nephron* 1983;34:35–41.
394. Watson KR, O'Kell RT. Lack of relationship between Mg2+ and K+ concentrations in serum. *Clin Chem* 1980;26:520–521.
395. Weidmann P, De Chatel R, Ziegler WH, Flammer J, Reubi F. Alpha and beta adrenergic blockade with orally administered labetalol in hypertension. Studies on blood volume, plasma renin and aldosterone and catecholamine excretion. *Am J Cardiol* 1978;41:570–576.
396. Weil-Maslansky E, Gutman Y, Sasson S. Insulin activates furosemide-sensitive K+ and Cl- uptake system in BC3H1 cells. *Am J Physiol* 1994;267(Pt 1):C932–939.
397. Weintraub HD, Heisterkamp DV, Cooperman LH. Changes in plasma potassium concentration after depolarizing blockers in anaesthetized man. *Br J Anaesth* 1969;41:1048–1052.
398. Welt LG, Sachs JR, McManus TJ. An ion transport defect in erythrocytes from uremic patients. *Trans Assoc Am Physicians* 1964;77:169–181.
399. Westervelt FB, Jr. Uremia and insulin response. *Arch Intern Med* 1970;126:865–869.
400. Westfall TC. Local regulation of adrenergic neurotransmission. *Physiol Rev* 1977;57: 659–728.
401. Whang R. Magnesium and potassium interrelationships in cardiac arrhythmias. *Magnesium* 1986;5:127–133.
402. Whang R, Flink EB, Dyckner T, Wester PO, Aikawa JK, Ryan MP. Magnesium depletion as a cause of refractory potassium repletion. *Arch Intern Med* 1985;145:1686–1689.
403. Whang R, Oei TO, Aikawa JK, Ryan MP, Watanabe A, Chrysant SG, Fryer A. Magnesium and potassium interrelationships, experimental and clinical. *Acta Med Scand Suppl* 1981;647: 139–144.
404. Whang R, Oei TO, Hamiter T. Frequency of hypomagnesmia associated with hypokalemia in hospitalized patients. *Am J Clin Pathol* 1979;71:610.
405. Whang R, Welt LG. Observations in experimental magnesium depletion. *J Clin Invest* 1963; 42:305–313.
406. Whitfield L, Sowers JR, Tuck ML, Golub MS. Dopaminergic control of plasma catecholamine and aldosterone responses to acute stimuli in normal man. *J Clin Endocrinol Metab* 1980;51:724–729.
407. Wilde W. The distribution of potassium in the cat after intravascular injection. *J Biol Chem* 1939;128:309–317.
408. Williams JA, Withrow CD, Woodbury DM. Effects of nephrectomy and KC1 on transmembrane potentials, intracellular electrolytes, and cell pH of rat muscle and liver in vivo. *J Physiol* 1971;212:117–128.
409. Williams M, Young JB, Rosa RM, Gunn S, Epstein FH, Landsberg L. Effect of protein ingestion on urinary dopamine excretion. Evidence for the functional importance of renal decarboxylation of circulating 3,4-dihydroxyphenylalanine in man. *J Clin Invest* 1986;78:1687–1693.
410. Williams ME, Gervino EV, Rosa RM, Landsberg L, Young JB, Silva P, Epstein FH. Catecholamine modulation of rapid potassium shifts during exercise. *N Engl J Med* 1985;312: 823–827.
411. Williams ME, Rosa RM, Epstein FH. Hyperkalemia. *Adv Intern Med* 1986;31:265–291.
412. Williams ME, Rosa RM, Silva P, Brown RS, Epstein FH. Impairment of extrarenal potassium disposal by alpha-adrenergic stimulation. *N Engl J Med* 1984;311:145–149.
413. Wilson JD, Sutherland DC, Thomas AC. Has the change to beta-agonists combined with oral theophylline increased cases of fatal asthma? *Lancet* 1981;1:1235–1237.
414. Winkler AW, Hoff HE, Smith PK. The toxicity of orally administered potassium salts in renal insufficiency. *J Clin Invest* 1941;20:119–126.
415. Winkler AW, Smith PK. The apparent volume of distribution of potassium injected intravenously. *J Biol Chem* 1938;124:589–598.

416. Wolfson S, Ellis S. Effects of glucagon on plasma potassium. *Proc Soc Exp Biol Med* 1958;91: 226–228.

417. Yalow RS, Berson SA. Immunoassay of endogenous plasma insulin in man. *J Clin Invest* 1960;39:1157–1175.

418. Young DB. Analysis of long-term potassium regulation. *Endocr Rev* 1985;6:24–44.

419. Young DB. Quantitative analysis of aldosterone's role in potassium regulation. *Am J Physiol* 1988;255(Pt 2):F811–22.

420. Young DB, Jackson TE. Effects of aldosterone on potassium distribution. *Am J Physiol* 1982;243:R526–530.

421. Zanella MT, Bravo EL. In vitro and in vivo evidence for an indirect mechanism mediating enhanced aldosterone secretion by metoclopramide. *Endocrinology* 1982;111:1620–1625.

422. Zannad F, Kessler M, Royer RJ, Robert J. Effect of hemodialysis on red blood cell Na+-K+-ATPase activity in terminal renal failure. *Nephron* 1985;40:127–128.

423. Zannad F, Royer RJ, Kessler M, Huriet B, Robert J. Cation transport in erythrocytes of patients with renal failure. *Nephron* 1982;32:347–350.

424. Zantvoort FA, Derkx FH, Boomsma F, Roos PJ, Schalekamp MA. Theophylline and serum electrolytes. *Ann Intern Med* 1986;104:134–135.

425. Zierler K, Rogus EM. Rapid hyperpolarization of rat skeletal muscle induced by insulin. *Biochim Biophys Acta* 1981;640:687–692.

426. Zierler KL. Effect of insulin on membrane potential and potassium content of rat muscle. *Am J Physiol* 1959;197:515–523.

427. Zierler KL. Effect of insulin on potassium efflux from rat muscle in the presence and absence of glucose. *Am J Physiol* 1960;198:1066–1070.

428. Zierler KL. Increase in resting membrane potential of skeletal muscle produced by insulin. *Science* 1957;126:1067–1080.

429. Zierler KL, Rabinowitz D. Effect of very small concentrations of insulin on forearm metabolism. persistence of its action on potassium and free fatty acids without its effect on glucose. *J Clin Invest* 1964;43:950–962.

CHAPTER 47

Regulation of Potassium Excretion

Gerhard Malnic, Shigeaki Muto, and Gerhard Giebisch

Universidade de São Paulo, São Paulo, Brazil
Jichi Medical School, Shimotsuke Tochigi, Japan
Yale University School of Medicine, New Haven, Connecticut, USA

OVERVIEW OF POTASSIUM DISTRIBUTION AND EXCRETION: INTERNAL AND EXTERNAL BALANCE

As the most abundant cation in intracellular fluid, potassium plays an important role in a variety of cell functions. The high K^+ concentration in cells and the low K^+ concentration in extracellular fluid are essential to many of the electrical properties of cell membranes in both excitable (nerve, muscle) and nonexcitable tissues (transporting epithelia) (273, 454). Cell potassium also contributes importantly to the effective osmolality of intracellular fluid and thus to the regulation of cell volume (273, 453, 454, 517). Changes in cell potassium tend to modify intracellular acidity, and thus potassium can indirectly influence a variety of metabolic processes by altering cytosolic hydrogen ion activity (2, 270). These important functions depend on the coordinated action of a variety of regulation mechanisms that serve to maintain constant total-body potassium content (50-55 mmol/kg body weight) and appropriate partition of potassium between extracellular and intracellular fluid (2, 151, 270, 296, 349, 398).

INTERNAL POTASSIUM BALANCE

Figures 1A and 1B schematically shows several features of the distribution of potassium in the body and the transporters involved. More than 98% of body potassium is inside cells, principally in skeletal muscle. Maintenance of a healthy steady state requires stabilizing the plasma concentration of potassium at low levels and safeguarding balance between intake and excretion of potassium. These rates are approximately 100 mmol/day in healthy people, although individual variations in diet may result in rates that are 50% higher or lower. Potassium enters the extracellular fluid by reabsorption from the small intestine, a process not subject to specific regulation (231). Since the total potassium content of extracellular fluid is approximately equal to the daily intake, potassium must temporarily be taken up by cells to prevent dangerous fluctuations of plasma potassium levels. Figure 2

summarizes the factors acutely modulating the distribution of potassium between extra- and intracellular fluid and maintaining internal potassium balance (77, 366, 386, 437). Chronic factors modulating ATP pump density and extrarenal potassium deposition include such factors as thyroid hormone, exercise, and cell growth that increases cell potassium intake whereas diabetes, chronic potassium deficiency, and chronic renal failure impair potassium transfer into cells (77, 366). Racial differences in potassium distribution have also been reported (437).

High concentrations of potassium in the cell depend on the regulated interplay between active uptake by Na^+,K^+-ATPase and passive backleak through potassium channels and carrier-mediated transport processes (152, 453, 454). When potassium enters the extracellular fluid, active, pump-mediated Na^+,K^+-ATPase-dependent potassium uptake into cells occurs rapidly, constitutes a first line of defense, and prevents or ameliorates dangerous fluctuations of potassium in the extracellular fluid. Because of the efficiency of cell uptake, plasma K^+ concentration is kept remarkably constant in the range from 3.5 to 5.0 mM (2, 45-47, 84, 85, 89, 90, 91, 422-424). Variations in potassium intake are matched within hours by parallel adjustments in potassium excretion. The kidney is responsible for most potassium excretion and for most of the variation in excretion when adaptive adjustments are made (44, 144, 148, 149, 415, 530). The colon is also able to excrete potassium and to respond to stimuli calling for greater or lesser excretion (27, 51, 176, 231, 286, 459); however, its contribution is overshadowed by that of the kidney.

EXTERNAL POTASSIUM BALANCE: THE ROLE OF THE KIDNEY

Renal regulation of body potassium balance requires that the kidneys excrete most of the potassium gained each day from food. To accomplish excretion of this variable quantity of potassium, the kidney must extract potassium from blood in which potassium circulates at a rather low concentration. Even though dietary potassium intake is approximately

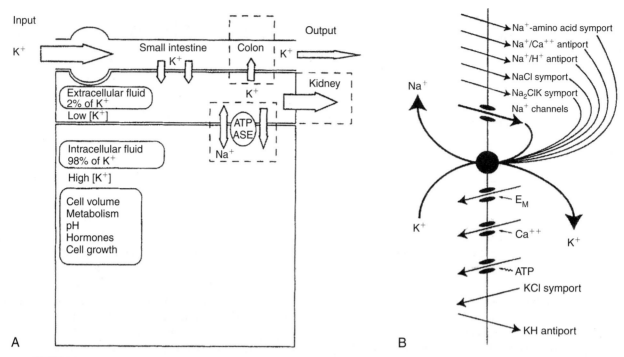

FIGURE 1   A: Distribution of K^+ in the body and pathways of K^+ entry and exit. **B:** Transporters involved in the distribution of K^+ and Na^+ across cell membranes. The activity of the Na^+,K^+-ATPase in cell membranes is opposed by several symporters, antiporters and ion channels. (From Giebisch G. A trail of research on potassium. *Kidney Int* 2002;62:1498–1512, with permission.)

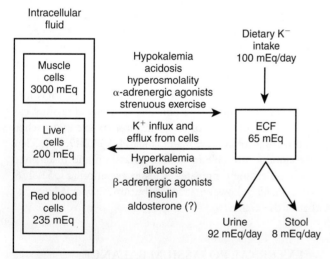

FIGURE 2   Distribution of K^+ between the intracellular and extracellular (ECF) fluid compartments. Only $\oplus 2\%$ of the total body K^+ is present in the ECF, with most of the remainder in intracellular fluid, here represented by three of the largest cellular compartments. The distribution of K^+ represents a balance between active uptake into cells by the Na^+,K^+-ATPase and the passive leak of K^+ out of cells. This balance is influenced by the K^+ concentration of the ECF as well as by the factors listed above and below the two arrows. A typical daily K^+ intake of 100 mmol is matched by the sum of a small excretion in the stool and the regulated excretion of K^+ by the kidneys. (From Giebisch G. A trail of research on potassium. *Kidney Int* 2002;62:1498–1512, with permission.)

equal to sodium intake (80–120 mM/day), the concentration of potassium in plasma, and therefore the rate at which potassium is filtered by glomeruli, is only one thirtieth of that of sodium. Nevertheless, the glomerular filtration rate (GFR) of normal kidneys is high enough that potassium could conceivably be excreted by filtration alone. Since two human kidneys together filter approximately 180 l/day, filtration of plasma containing potassium at 4 mM could remove up to 720 mmol/day. However, if the GFR were reduced to 10% to 15% of normal, as it may be in a variety of disease states, filtration alone would not be able to keep up with the normal dietary intake. Even if the GFR were reduced only by half, because not all filtered potassium can escape reabsorption, it is likely that renal excretion would be inadequate and potassium would be retained. Furthermore, even when GFR is normal, an excretion mechanism relying solely on filtration would have a limited capacity for adaptive increase and could not achieve the 20-fold increase in potassium excretion that has been observed in animals exposed to increased intake of potassium by diets high in potassium or parenteral infusions containing potassium. Indeed, glomerular filtration is not the only route traveled by potassium on its way into the urine. It has been known since the 1940s that the kidney does possess secretory mechanisms enabling it to transfer potassium from plasma to tubule fluid (40–42, 44, 288, 306–308, 525). Table 1 summarizes the conclusions based on such studies. Clearance experiments established the ability of renal tubules to either secrete or reabsorb potassium, that these transport processes

TABLE 1 Main Features of Potassium Transport, Based on Clearance Experiments

1. K^+ secreted by renal tubules (excreted K^+ > filtered K^+)
2. K^+ excretion can be dissociated form the rate of glomerular filtration
3. Reabsorption of K^+ along the nephron precedes K^+ secretion
4. Secretion of K^+ occurs by exchange for Na^+
5. K^+ tolerance: Increased K excretion at relatively low K^+ in plasma
6. Reciprocal relation between urinary excretion of K^+ and H^+, carbonic anhydrase inhibitors induce kaliuresis
7. Adrenal steroids stimulate K^+ secretion

occurred simultaneously and that they are distributed to specific sites in the nephron.

A simplified but generally adequate view of the arrangement of the renal processes involved in potassium excretion is that proximal nephron segments between the glomerulus and the distal convoluted tubule (DCT) reabsorb a rather fixed fraction (80%–90%) of the filtered potassium, whereas distal tubules and collecting ducts either secrete a variable quantity of potassium into tubule fluid (91, 144, 148, 149, 152, 184, 281, 282, 416, 532) or effectively reabsorb potassium (281, 282, 326, 526). The secretory transfer of potassium is accomplished by certain specialized cells in distal tubules and collecting ducts. Although these cells constitute only a minute fraction of the body's intracellular fluid volume, the fact that excreted potassium enters the urine principally by this secretory route is emphasized in Fig. 1, where excreted potassium is shown as being derived from an intracellular pool. By varying the rate and even the direction of potassium transport, the distal nephron is also able to respond homeostatically to changes in dietary potassium intake or to changes in extracellular potassium caused by other gains (parenteral administration, release from cellular pools) or losses (from the gastrointestinal [GI] tract or skin). In people ingesting potassium at 80 to 120 mmol/day, the usual rate of potassium excretion in the postabsorptive period between meals is approximately 10% of the rate of potassium filtration. In the hours following meals, or ingestion or infusion of supplementary potassium salts, the rate of urinary excretion of potassium can increase greatly to approach or even exceed the rate at which it is filtered. Most evidence indicates that such increments in potassium excretion can be attributed to an increase in the quantity secreted by distal nephron segments. Increased secretion may not entirely account for increases in potassium excretion in all cases however, and variations in reabsorption by tubule segments, either proximal or distal to the main secretory sites, may become important in some circumstances.

If potassium intake is reduced or eliminated (or if the body is depleted of potassium by prior renal or nonrenal losses), urinary potassium excretion declines rapidly as the deficit in total-body potassium increases. Within a few days potassium excretion can be reduced to very low levels (263, 281, 282, 338), but potassium conservation is less complete than that of sodium in many clinical situations when subjects are ill or stressed (112).

General Aspects of Potassium Transport Along the Nephron

The generalization that filtered potassium is largely reabsorbed by proximal nephron segments and that excreted potassium is secreted by distal segments provides a useful framework for integrating information about renal handling of potassium, but a closer look at the cytologically distinct subdivisions of the nephron and the way each handles potassium reveals a more complicated picture. Potassium is not continuously reabsorbed from all tubule segments proximal to the secretory sites in the distal tubules and collecting ducts. The rather constant fractional delivery of potassium (10%–20% of the filtered quantity) that has been found by collecting and analyzing samples of fluid from the earliest portion of the superficial DCT accessible to micropuncture is probably achieved by a sequence of reabsorption, secretion, and reabsorption as the glomerular filtrate travels through the proximal tubule and the loop of Henle (147, 150–152, 281, 282, 415, 530, 531, 534). At present, secretion of potassium into loops of Henle has been documented only for the juxtamedullary nephron population (94, 211–214, 531); however, it seems likely that the more superficial nephrons behave similarly.

Figures 3 and 4 represent a schematic representation of the renal elements responsible for potassium excretion. The location and naming of the subdivisions generally follow the scheme outlined by Kriz and Bankir (243). Some features that distinguish superficial and deep nephrons are pictured. Potassium is filtered and reabsorbed from proximal convoluted tubules (PCTs) of superficial and deep nephrons. As the proximal straight tubule (PST) enters the outer medulla, the direction of potassium transport reverses and potassium is secreted into the third proximal segment (S3) and into the thin descending limb of the loop of Henle (211–214). Higher potassium concentrations are attained in loops of deeper nephrons that penetrate further into the inner medulla.

Potassium can be reabsorbed by thick ascending limbs (TALs) and net reabsorption probably occurs in both medullary and cortical TALs of both deep and superficial nephrons (165, 178, 179). The portion of the distal tubule beyond the macula densa segment where each ascending limb contacts its parent glomerulus (a term often used to describe results for micropuncture and microperfusion experiments) comprises several segments that are cytologically distinguishable. The DCT, extending approximately 1 mm beyond the macula densa, is functionally distinct from the TAL segment and probably contributes modestly to potassium excretion.

The next segment of the distal tubule—the connecting tubule (CNT), and the segment following it, the cortical collecting duct (CCD)—are the major sites of potassium

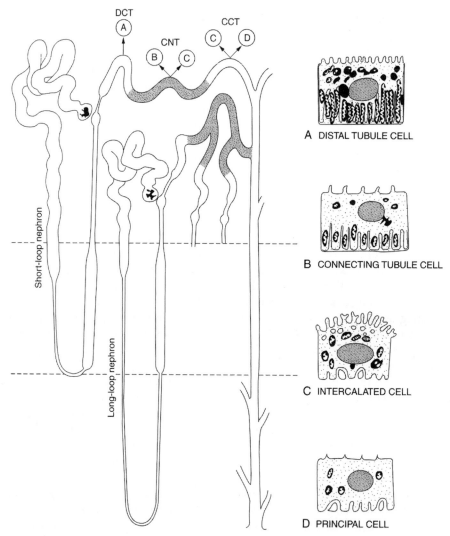

FIGURE 3   Schematic illustration of the distal nephron segments. CCT, cortical collecting tubule; CNT, connecting tubule; DCT, distal convoluted tubule. (From Imai M, Nakamura R. Function of distal convoluted and connecting tubules studied by isolated nephron fragments. *Kidney Int* 1982;22:465–472, with permission.)

secretion. In superficial nephrons, epithelium characteristic of the CCD appears some distance proximal to the first confluence of two distal tubules. This region has also been referred to as the late distal tubule, or the initial collecting tubule (ICT). In deeper nephrons, the CNTs frequently join to form arcades before flowing into the collecting duct. The separate segments of the distal tubule are discussed subsequently in more detail. Potassium is secreted into the collecting duct throughout the cortex and probably in the outer stripe of the outer medulla as well (430, 431). In the inner stripe of the outer medulla, potassium reabsorption appears once again and contributes to potassium accumulation in the medullary interstitium. Both secretion and reabsorption of potassium have been described along the terminal portions of the inner medullary collecting duct (365, 367, 369, 395, 407, 409, 429–433).

POTASSIUM TRANSPORT BY INDIVIDUAL NEPHRON SEGMENTS

Glomerulus

Potassium ions that are free in plasma water pass across the glomerular capillary membrane in the filtrate with little hindrance. Nonfilterable proteins in plasma may bind a small fraction of potassium (257) and restrict filtration. The net negative charge on these plasma proteins tends to reduce potassium concentration in glomerular filtrate relative to plasma water (Donnan equilibrium), but the concentration of potassium in plasma is approximately 6% lower than in plasma water. These factors tend to cancel each other and the concentrations of potassium in glomerular filtrate and in plasma, or serum, are approximately equal.

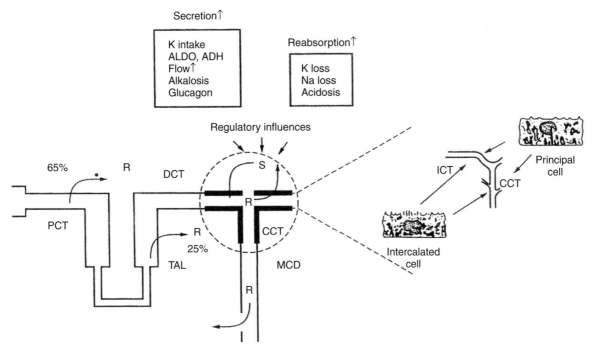

FIGURE 4 Overview of K$^+$ transport along the nephron. Secretion (S) largely determines the excretion of K$^+$ during normal and high K$^+$ intake; reabsorption (R) determines the excretion of K$^+$ in K$^+$ depletion. Note the cell heterogeneity in the distal nephron (see Fig. 3). ADH, antidiuretic hormone; ALDO, aldosterone; CCT, cortical collecting tubule; DCT, distal convoluted tubule; MCD, medullary collecting duct; PCT, proximal convoluted tubule; TAL, thick ascending limb of Henle. (From Giebisch G. A trail of research on potassium. *Kidney Int* 2002;62:1498–1512, with permission.)

Although variations in GFR do cause proportional variations in the rate of potassium filtration, they do not usually result in large changes in potassium excretion because mechanisms promoting glomerulotubular balance tend to stabilize the rate of potassium delivery out of the proximal tubule and the loop of Henle. In the 1950s, when renal clearance methods were first applied systematically to the study of potassium regulation by the kidney, it was observed that rates of glomerular filtration and final potassium excretion could be varied independently of one another (44, 87). However, if GFR is reduced enough to decrease sodium and water excretion, the rate of potassium excretion will also decrease (87).

Proximal Convoluted Tubule: Direction, Magnitude, and Mechanism of Transport

Information about the direction and magnitude of potassium transport processes along the nephron was obtained in the 1960s by micropuncture techniques applied to the intact kidneys in anesthetized animals. Collections of fluid samples from superficial proximal tubules showed that about 50% of filtered potassium reaches the last accessible surface segment of the PCT (282). Collections from proximal sites close to the glomerulus showed that reabsorption of potassium may be preceded by a small leak of potassium into the lumen (458), but reabsorption occurs along the remainder of the accessible length of this nephron segment (53, 144, 146,

147, 150, 151, 277, 281, 282, 284, 361, 503, 530, 531). The reabsorption of potassium, like that of sodium, generally proceeds without developing a large concentration difference across the proximal tubule wall. Thus, roughly similar fractions of water, sodium, and potassium are absorbed as fluid flows along the proximal tubule. Although potassium concentration has been reported to increase (38) or to remain unchanged (95) along the proximal tubule, a few studies have provided suggestive evidence that in some circumstances proximal reabsorption of potassium can proceed against an electrochemical gradient and that potassium concentration may decline (by about 10%) between early and late proximal segments in rat kidneys (55, 235).

Three mechanisms participate in potassium reabsorption by the proximal tubule: solvent drag, diffusion, and apparent active transport. First, the consistently observed association between potassium transport and fluid transport suggests that a fraction of proximal potassium absorption depends on the simultaneous rate of fluid absorption. Addition of increasing amounts of mannitol to perfusion solutions otherwise resembling fluid reaching the late proximal tubule causes net fluid and potassium transport to decrease and then reverse direction (55). This dependence of potassium transport on net fluid transport and the finding of low reflection coefficients of potassium (500) indicate direct coupling of potassium and fluid through the same transport pathway: a solvent drag mechanism.

Second, diffusion of potassium from luminal to peritubular fluid may also occur because fluid absorption raises potassium concentration in the proximal tubule and thus creates a concentration difference favoring potassium absorption. This mechanism would require the proximal tubule to be sufficiently permeable to potassium to allow rather modest passive driving forces to effect absorptive transport. In vivo microperfusion experiments show that proximal potassium transport is sensitive to changes in luminal potassium concentration and transepithelial voltage (55, 56, 500). The apparent potassium permeability is higher in the proximal tubule (237) than in the distal tubule (280), and the dependence of potassium transport on the transepithelial electrochemical potential difference evident in these experiments is consistent with diffusive movement through a paracellular pathway. As pointed out, such paracellular movement of potassium is importantly affected by the concurrent rate of net fluid transport. However, the finding that barium, a potent potassium channel blocker, slows the reabsorption of potassium suggests that a transcellular route of potassium transport is also present (237, 471). Little is known about this transport pathway.

Third, evidence supporting a contribution of apparent active potassium absorption is based on the direction of the electrochemical driving force of potassium in at least part of the proximal tubule and by the special micro-environment of the paracellular compartment between proximal tubule cells. Movement of potassium ions against an electrochemical potential gradient in the early proximal tubule is implied by experimental findings demonstrating both a concentration of potassium in the tubule lumen below that in arterial plasma and a lumen-negative transepithelial potential (131, 133, 284). Dissociation between sodium-driven fluid movement and potassium transport has also, albeit rarely, been observed (38). These findings suggest a transport mode other than solvent drag and diffusion. Direct measurements of the electrochemical driving force for potassium across the apical cell membrane in amphibian proximal tubules also support active potassium reabsorption (13, 133).

A cell model summarizing the major mechanisms involved in proximal tubular potassium transport is pictured in Fig. 5. It includes a sodium-potassium exchange pump (Na$^+$,K$^+$-ATPase) in the basolateral membrane, a potassium conductance in the apical membrane, and a pathway for potassium transport between cells. Two pathways for potassium exit across the basolateral membrane are shown: a conductive channel and a K-Cl cotransporter (18, 501). Note also that the transepithelial potential along the tubule changes from lumen-negative values in the early PCT to lumen-positive values in the late PCT (131).

Evidence for a component of active potassium reabsorption is strongest in early segments of the proximal convoluted tubule. At the beginning of the proximal tubule the transepithelial electrical potential is oriented with the lumen negative (131) and the luminal potassium concentration may be lower than in plasma (55, 56). The apical membrane has a potassium conductance and permits potassium ions to leak continuously from cell to lumen (13, 235) but potassium reabsorption exceeds such potassium fluxes further downstream. Weinstein (510) has suggested that the apparent movement of potassium against an electrochemical driving force does not require an active, directly energy-driven reabsorptive mechanism for potassium in the apical cell membrane. Given that Na$^+$,K$^+$-ATPase-driven uptake of potassium does occur in the cell membranes lining the paracellular compartment between cells, such transport could deplete this compartment of potassium, particularly if the diffusion resistance to potassium across the basolateral exit was low. A situation could then develop as illustrated in Fig. 5, in which the luminal fluid equilibrates with the low-potassium fluid in the interspace and effectively decreases the potassium concentration in the lumen below peritubular plasma levels. Exit of potassium ions from the interspace into the peritubular fluid would be driven, according to Weinstein, by bulk movement of fluid and potassium along the hydrostatic pressure gradient that normally develops along the interspace from its luminal to basolateral end.

In the later part of the PCT, the transepithelial potential difference becomes lumen positive (131) and provides for an additional favorable driving force for net potassium reab-

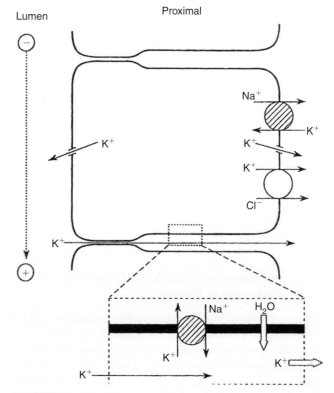

FIGURE 5   Model of proximal tubule cell. Transepithelial voltage is lumen negative in S1 and becomes lumen positive in S2. Enlargement of lateral membrane and the intercellular and extracellular space illustrates postulated mechanism permitting absorption of potassium against a concentration gradient. (From Weinstein AM. Modeling the proximal tubule: complications of the paracellular pathway. *Am J Physiol Renal* 1988;254: F297–F305, with permission.)

sorption. It is likely that potassium movement is driven by the transepithelial voltage occurs through the paracellular shunt pathway. Potassium movement is also affected by net fluid movement. Experiments using in vivo microperfusion (55, 56) have shown that the direction of net potassium transport depends on that of net fluid movement when the latter was changed by varying tubule fluid osmolarity (addition of mannitol). Previous observations had already shown that maneuvers inhibiting proximal sodium and water transport (extracellular volume expansion) also block potassium reabsorption (53, 145, 417, 530–534). This effect is consistent with the notion that sodium-dependent fluid reabsorption entrains potassium ions.

A careful investigation of transepithelial electrochemical gradients of K^+ demonstrates the effect of changes in the electrical potential difference on tubule K^+ concentration (401). Marked differences were observed between potassium-replete and potassium-depleted animals; whereas a lumen-positive potential was recorded in replete animals, the transepithelial potential difference was reversed in K^+-depleted animals and the potassium concentration ratio across the late proximal tubule significantly elevated. These data support the view that diffusion along an electrochemical gradient plays a critical role in transport of potassium across the proximal tubule.

In proximal tubule cells, as in other cells in the body, steady-state levels of cell potassium depend on the balance between *active* uptake from interstitial fluid, and *passive* leakage from the cytosol either to the interstitium or to the tubule lumen. Potassium ions are actively taken up by the ATP-driven sodium-potassium exchange pump located in the basolateral membranes. Several lines of evidence establish the active nature of potassium uptake. Microelectrode measurements of basolateral membrane voltage and of potassium activities show that the electrical potential difference across cell membranes of both amphibian and mammalian tubule cells is too small to account for the measured intracellular potassium activity by passive distribution. Also, inhibitor studies indicate that ATPase-driven accumulation of potassium is responsible for high cell potassium concentrations. Inhibition of Na^+,K^+-ATPase activity reduces intracellular K^+ concentrations and content (48, 49, 72, 108, 191, 246, 317, 370, 371, 453, 454).

The basolateral sodium-potassium pump operates in an electrogenic mode: the rate at which sodium ions are pumped out of the cell exceeds the rate at which potassium ions are taken in. The contribution of such an electrogenic cation exchange to the steady-state voltage across the basolateral membrane is probably small; however, sudden activation of the pump, by raising cell sodium, increasing extracellular potassium from low levels, or warming tubules previously cooled, leads to rapid hyperpolarization of the basolateral cell membrane to levels that can exceed the equilibrium potential that could be generated by passive diffusion of potassium ions (48, 49, 72, 108, 191, 196, 317, 355, 370, 371).

Figure 6 illustrates additional transporters in the apical and basolateral membranes of proximal tubule cells. Potassium channels are present in both cell membranes and serve several functions. They generate the cell-negative electrical potential which constitutes an important driving force for the entry of positively charged solutes and the basolateral exit of negatively charged solutes (144, 147, 148, 151, 152, 181). Sodium-coupled electrogenic glucose and amino acid transport across the apical membrane of proximal tubule cells is facilitated by the cell-negative potential. Chloride diffusion, electrogenic Na^+-HCO_3^- and Ca^{2+}-Na^+ exchange are also modulated by the magnitude of the potassium-dependent basolateral membrane potential. Potassium channels are also involved in volume regulation of proximal tubule cells (372). Both apical and basolateral potassium channels are activated by cell swelling, directly by stretching of the membrane or indirectly by volume-dependent calcium entry through nonselective cation channels (125, 347, 372). Apical potassium channels are also sensitive to changes in membrane voltage with depolarization leading to increased activity. This is an important mechanism that tends to stabilize the cell-negative potential, especially during activation of positively charged electrogenic cotransport. Basolateral potassium channels are inhibited by an increase in cell ATP, by a fall in pH, by cyclic AMP and taurine (181), and they have been implicated in renal cell damage by hypoxia (362). Molecular cloning of several potassium channels has demonstrated their expression in the membranes of proximal tubule cells (see Chapter 44).

Coupling Between Sodium Transport and Basolateral Potassium Channels

Many observations indicate that the constancy of intracellular potassium in the presence of large changes in transepithelial net sodium transport does depend on appropriate modulations of the basolateral potassium conductance (509). Because a major pathway for sodium reabsorption is transcellular and involves the basolateral sodium-potassium exchange pump, large changes in the rate of sodium extrusion necessarily cause large changes in potassium uptake. However, by varying the magnitude of the leak conductance in proportion to changes in pump rate, cells in renal (36, 37, 198, 252, 287, 491, 509, 512) and other transporting epithelia (158, 406) are able to maintain cytosolic potassium activity, and cell volume, within narrow limits. Possible mechanisms involved in the coupling between active sodium extrusion across the basolateral membrane and apical and basolateral potassium conductances are depicted in Fig. 7. Changes in cell volume and pH have a significant effect on potassium channels, alkalosis increasing and acidosis decreasing the open probability (34, 168, 245, 249, 318, 325, 389, 491, 492). During substrate-induced stimulation of proximal sodium transport, cell pH rises with a time course that matches the observed increase in basolateral potassium conductance (34, 318, 492). Although the effect is most

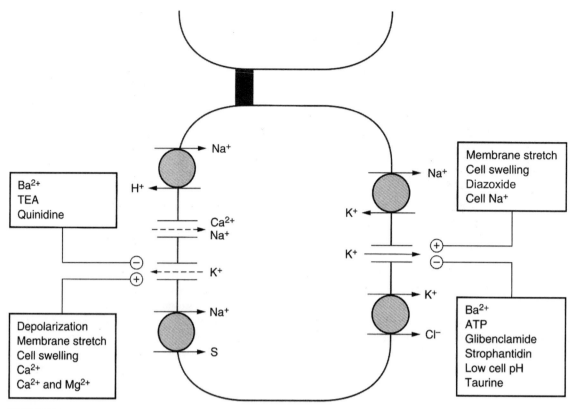

FIGURE 6 Model of a proximal tubule cell, including the main transport pathways and the apical and basolateral K⁺ channels. ATP, adenosine triphosphate; TEA, tetraethylammonium. (From Malnic G, Bailey MA, Giebisch G. Control of renal potassium excretion. In: Brenner B, ed. *The Kidney,* 7th ed., Vol. 1. Philadelphia: WB Saunders; 2004:453–496, with permission.)

pronounced in the thick ascending limb of Henle's loop and in the collecting duct, the finding that aldosterone stimulates sodium-hydrogen exchange and elevates cell pH is also consistent with a role of pH in the homeostatic regulation of potassium channel activity (34, 181, 318). Changes in the concentration of calcium in tubule cells, especially those correlated with fluctuations in cell volume and nitric oxide may also couple basolateral Na⁺,K⁺-ATPase activity to potassium permeability. Moreover, alterations in basolataeral cell potential have also been implicated, since stimulation of electrogenic Na⁺-K⁺ pump activity hyperpolarizes tubule cells. Such membrane voltage changes are known to activate voltage-sensitive potassium channels (497).

A marked sensitivity of renal potassium channel activity to alterations in the cell ATP/ADP ratio has been observed. Whereas small amounts of ATP are required for the activity of some potassium channels in the renal tubule, millimolar concentrations of ATP inhibit channel activity, an effect that can be reversed by ADP (181, 486). Renal potassium channels sensitive to the inhibitory action of ATP include potassium channels in the basolateral membrane of proximal tubule cells (198, 446). It appears that transport-related changes in cell ATP levels modify cell potassium conductance. Observations in which stimulation of sodium transport in proximal tubules resulted in a significant fall in cell ATP, and other studies in which inhibition of sodium trans-

port elevated ATP levels in several tubule segments (35–37, 446), point to the possible involvement of the ATP/ADP ratio in the control of potassium channel activity. Figure 8 provides an illustration of the effects of transport stimulation on basolateral potassium channel activity and a cell model with a proposed "cross-talk" mechanism involving changes in cell ATP levels (198, 446, 512).

Thus, a transport-related change in the basolateral membrane potential of tubule cells may be involved in coupling the potassium conductance to the pump activity. Measurements of the basolateral conductance of tubule cells of the proximal tubule (197, 232) and the collecting duct (191), as well as patch-clamp studies, in which the open probability of basolateral potassium channels was examined as a function of the membrane potential (197, 251, 497) show an increase in potassium conductance of potassium channel open probability with cell hyperpolarization. To the extent that stimulation of basolateral ATPase activity elevates the cell-negative potential, potassium conductance would also be expected to increase.

Schultz has drawn attention to an additional relationship between transport events in the luminal and basolateral membrane of epithelial cells that involves changes in pump-related potassium conductance (396, 397). In leaky epithelia, such as the proximal tubule, stimulation of cotransport of sodium ions with organic solutes such as glucose or amino acids augments

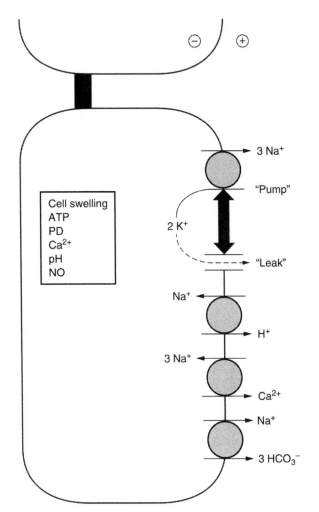

FIGURE 7   Relationship between the activity of basolateral Na$^+$,K$^+$-ATPase and the leak through K$^+$ channels. The *two-headed arrow* indicates linkage between the pump and K$^+$ channels; as K$^+$ uptake increases, permeability to K$^+$ increases, and vice versa. The *inset* includes factors that could mediate the pump-leak coupling. Basolateral transporters that may alter these variables are also shown. ATP, adenosine triphosphate; NO, nitric oxide; PD, potential difference. (From Malnic G, Bailey MA, Giebisch G. Control of renal potassium excretion. In: Brenner B, ed. *The Kidney*, 7th ed., Vol. 1. Philadelphia: WB Saunders; 2004:453–496, with permission.)

sodium entry across the apical membrane. Since the cotransporter carries positive current into the cell, the cell-negative electrical potential is reduced (59, 252, 277). In tight epithelia, such as the cortical collecting duct (CCD), mineralocorticoids increase apical sodium conductance and thus bring about depolarization of the apical cell membrane (59, 239, 240, 333, 335, 382). An essential feature of these effects in both cell types is that the very maneuvers that increase sodium transport tend to curtail further sodium entry because the depolarization of the apical cell membrane reduces the electrochemical driving force for sodium transport into the cell. Stated differently, sodium transport mechanisms that carry current do not increase sodium entry as much as they could *if* they did not carry current that acts to depolarize the apical cell membrane when the sodium transport rate is increased.

It appears that the increase in potassium conductance that occurs with stimulation of sodium pumping across the basolateral membrane provides an important transport-sustaining feedback loop. The rise in potassium conductance hyperpolarizes the basolateral membrane. This increase in the voltage across the basolateral membrane changes the transepithelial voltage and causes current to flow through the intercellular spaces. This current flow through the paracellular shunt pathway tends to increase the luminal membrane voltage and thus to restore the driving force for sodium entry across the luminal membrane. Evidence for the operation of such a mechanism has been obtained by means of microelectrode measurements in cells not only of the PCT (59, 252), but also of the cortical collecting tubule (239, 240, 333, 382), the small intestine (158, 169), and the epithelium of the trachea (406, 513).

It may be concluded from these considerations that the linkage between the active sodium-potassium pump and the passive potassium-leak pathways in the basolateral membrane of renal tubule cells serves to maintain cell potassium constant during fluctuations of sodium-potassium pump activity and during cell volume changes. In addition, pump-induced alterations of potassium conductance initiate a sequence of electrophysiological events that stabilize the voltage across the apical membrane and thereby maintain optimal electrochemical driving forces for sodium entry during stimulation of net sodium transport.

Loop of Henle: Potassium Recycling, Direction, Magnitude, and Mechanism of Transport

Free-flow micropuncture and microperfusion studies show net reabsorption of potassium between the last accessible segment of surface proximal tubules and the first accessible segment of surface distal tubules (88, 213, 282, 449, 450, 452, 530, 531). As shown in Fig. 3, this portion of the nephron comprises several morphologically and functionally distinct segments: the second and third segments of the proximal tubule (S2 and S3), the thin descending and thin ascending limbs, and the medullary and cortical thick ascending limbs. The contributions of each of these segments to the overall absorption that reduces the delivery of potassium to the distal tubule to approximately 10% to 15% of the filtered quantity cannot be assessed separately by sampling only surface segments of proximal and distal tubules.

Following up on earlier observations by de Rouffignac and Morel (88) and Diezi et al. (94), Jamison et al. (211–214) demonstrated that the K$^+$ concentration in the loop of Henle fluid near the tip of the papilla could be as much as 10 times higher than the K$^+$ concentration in systemic plasma. de Rouffignac and Morel (88) suggested that potassium is added to tubule fluid along the descending limb after being absorbed from the ascending limb and collecting duct and thus recognized the phenomenon of potassium recycling. Jamison and coworkers showed that the rate of potassium delivery to the end of the descending limb of deep nephrons was equal to the

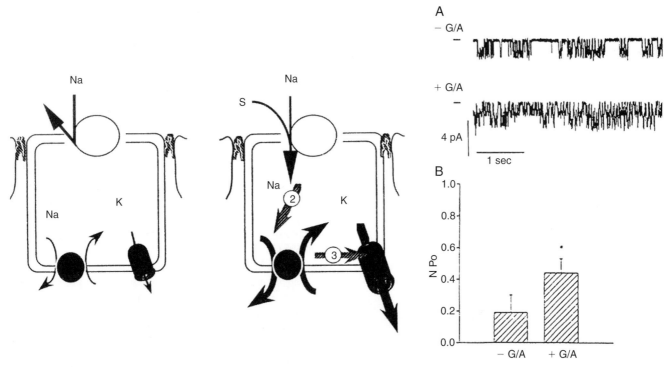

FIGURE 8   Left: Coupling between Na$^+$,K$^+$-ATPase activity and K$^+$ recycling in the basolateral membrane of proximal tubule cells (36, 37, 198, 512). Net rate of sodium transport was stimulated by addition of organic substrates (S; i.e., glucose or amino acid) to the lumen. Thus (*1*) apical Na entry via Na-dependent substrate cotransporters is stimulated in the presence of substrates. (*2*) The Na$^+$, K$^+$-ATPase subsequently revs up so that active efflux of Na into the interstitium matches passive apical sodium entry. (*3*) Ensuring that the increased active uptake of K$^+$ via the Na$^+$,K$^+$-ATPase will be efficiently recycled back across the basolateral membrane, K$^+$ channel activation ensues. (*Kidney Int* 1995;48:1017–1023.) **Right: A:** Patch-clamp analysis of basolateral K$^+$ channel activity in isolated perfused proximal tubule. Data for experiments before ($-$) and during ($+$) perfusion of glucose and alanine (G/A). Horizontal bars indicate zero current. **B:** Effect of luminal addition of glucose and alanine on single-K channel open probability (NPo). $p < .02$. (*Am J Physiol Renal* 1993;264:F760–764.)

rate of potassium filtration in normal rats (212) and exceeded it in rats either fed a high-potassium diet (28) or infused acutely with potassium (17). The observation that isolated thin limbs of Henle lack a mechanism of active potassium secretion (203, 204) supports the view that potassium enters the descending limb passively. If potassium is also secreted into the proximal straight tubule of superficial nephrons (502, 529), and the delivery of potassium to the distal convoluted tubule of deep nephrons is substantially less than the filtered quantity, then potassium must be reabsorbed by ascending limbs in both populations of nephrons. Thus, potassium is trapped in the medulla by countercurrent exchange between the ascending and descending limbs of the loop of Henle. Studies of isolated thick ascending limbs perfused in vitro show that these segments are capable of absorbing potassium (69).

As originally postulated by Jamison et al. (214) and shown in Fig. 9, one pathway by which potassium can be brought to the renal medulla is absorption from the medullary collecting duct. Stokes (428, 430, 431) has shown that the outer medullary collecting duct is adequately permeable to both sodium and potassium and therefore could permit potassium reabsorption to occur passively. Potassium secretion by cells of the distal tubule and the cortical collecting duct provide the source of potassium that accumulates in the

renal medulla. Accordingly, more potassium recycles with stimulation of secretion, whereas suppression of secretion attenuates the deposition of potassium in the renal medulla (96, 110, 111, 171, 185, 214, 436).

Recognizing, as pictured in Fig. 9, that potassium is secreted into tubule fluid in (at least) two sites along the nephron, first into a proximal part of the nephron (the end-proximal tubule and descending limb) and second into a more distal region (the connecting tubule and cortical collecting duct segments), we might ask whether secretion at both of these sites contributes to total potassium excretion. For instance, when potassium intake is suddenly increased after a period of potassium deprivation, renal potassium excretion, distal potassium secretion, and potassium recycling (96, 110, 111, 171, 185, 214, 436) all increase. Jamison and coworkers (214) concluded that potassium secretion into descending limbs might contribute to final potassium excretion. Considering the effect of medullary recycling of potassium on renal potassium excretion, Stokes also proposed that rising medullary K$^+$ concentrations contribute to increasing potassium excretion. They suggested that higher luminal and interstitial K$^+$ concentrations inhibit NaCl and water absorption by the loop of Henle and thus increase the flow rate and sodium concentration in fluid entering the distal tubule, providing optimum conditions for the distal

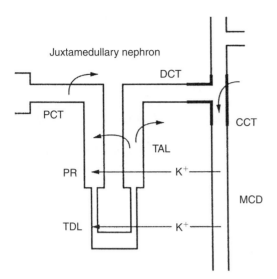

Juxtamedullary nephron

FIGURE 9 Sites of K$^+$ movement into and out of the nephron. The diagram emphasizes the movement of K$^+$ from the collecting ducts to the descending limbs of the loop of Henle via the medullary interstitium. CCT, cortical collecting tubule; DCT, distal convoluted tubule; MCD, medullary collecting duct; PCT, proximal convoluted tubule; PR, pars recta; TAL, thick ascending limb; TDL, thin descending limb. (Field MJ, Giebisch G. Mechanisms of segmental potassium reabsorption and secretion. In: Seldin DW, Giebisch G, eds. *The Regulation of Potassium Balance*. New York: Raven Press; 1989:139–156, with permission.)

segments to secrete potassium maximally (428). Although these results were not confirmed by Sufit and Jamison (436), they did, however, observe that fractional delivery of potassium to the distal tubule increased to higher levels than seen in many other conditions, although the levels were not as high in the final urine. Sufit and Jamison concluded that the renal response to a sudden increase in total body potassium includes inhibition of net K$^+$ reabsorption by the loop of Henle and thus participation by the loop in the increase in renal potassium excretion (436).

One way that potassium recycling and the decrease of potassium reabsorption by the loop of Henle following potassium loading contribute to the increase in urinary potassium excretion is by redistributing the relative amounts of potassium secretion along the tubule. To maintain a given rate of potassium excretion, the rate of "distal" secretion of potassium must be lower in the presence of recycling than in its absence because recycling allows the amount of potassium lost from the medullary collecting duct to be partly preserved for excretion by entering the descending limb of Henle's loop. Were it not for recycling of potassium, secretion would have to increase by the amount of potassium lost from the medullary collecting duct and carried into the systemic circulation. To prevent potassium excretion from declining, plasma potassium or other factors stimulating potassium secretion would have to increase. Stated differently, recycling of potassium in the medulla allows the kidney to compensate for the inefficiency of the medullary collecting duct. It does so by effectively preserving the excretion of all the potassium secreted by the distal tubule and cortical col-

lecting duct. However, this contribution of the loop of Henle should not be considered independent and additional to the potassium contributed by the distal secretory segments. The increase in potassium recycling accompanies, but does not add to, the increase in distal potassium secretion that occurs in response to an acute potassium infusion.

A second way that medullary potassium recycling may serve renal potassium excretion is by establishing conditions that make it possible for the distal nephron to excrete potassium in a variety of physiological circumstances (465). Because the rate of urine flow is determined mainly by considerations of water balance, a constant rate of potassium excretion must be associated with a wide range of urinary concentrations of potassium. When rats are deprived of dietary potassium for a few days and are permitted free access to water, urinary K$^+$ concentrations are 20 to 30 mM and medullary K$^+$ concentrations are 5 to 10 mM. When rats are continuously ingesting diets with moderate or high-potassium content and are permitted free access to water, urinary K$^+$ concentrations are 200 to 300 mM and medullary K$^+$ concentrations are 35 to 40 mM (214). These rates may be more than 10-fold higher than when rats are deprived of potassium. When water intake is low and potassium intake is high, tubule fluid K$^+$ concentrations in the medullary collecting duct must be maintained in excess of 200 mM. It is likely that the effect of the recycling process to increase medullary interstitial potassium to the 35- to 40-mM range may allow the urine K$^+$ concentration to rise to the high levels necessary to permit the ingested potassium to be excreted in relatively small urine volumes. Thus, as potassium secretion by cortical segments increases, some of the secreted potassium is lost to the medullary interstitium. However, enough of this potassium is trapped in the medulla so that the K$^+$ concentration in the medullary interstitium increases to a level sufficient to diminish K$^+$ reabsorption from the collecting duct.

Thick Ascending Limb Cell Transport Mechanisms

Studies on the isolated mammalian thick ascending limb (TAL) of the loop of Henle and of the amphibian (*Amphiuma*) early distal tubule have provided remarkably similar results that have allowed insight into the mechanisms for potassium transport in these nephron segments. A cell model picturing potassium movement in the TAL is presented in Fig. 10. The primary driving force for net potassium reabsorption is ATP-driven active Na$^+$-K$^+$ exchange across the basolateral membrane. It is this transport operation that generates the steep sodium gradient that provides the energy for the entry of Na$^+$ across the apical cell membrane. Entry of each Na$^+$ is coupled to the entry of one K$^+$ and two Cl$^-$ (67–69, 157, 161, 165, 177, 319, 387). This Na$^+$-2Cl$^-$-K$^+$ cotransport mechanism is the site of action of the potent "loop" diuretics. Also present in the apical membrane is a second pathway for sodium entry into cells via Na-H exchange (not shown in Fig. 10). Conductive pathways are

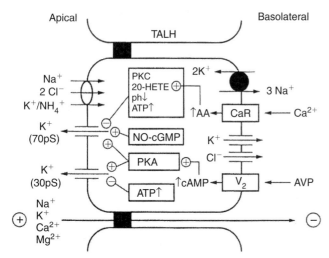

FIGURE 10 Model of a thick ascending limb cell, including the main transport pathways and the apical and basolateral ion channels. Potassium may also leave the cell across the basolaterall membrane by KCl cotransport (not shown). Note that the lumen-positive transepithelial potential difference drives cation reabsorption through the paracellular pathway. AA, arachidonic acid; ATP, adenosine triphosphate; CaR, extracellular calcium-sensing receptor; cGMP, cyclic guanonine monophosphate; 20-HETE, 20-hydroxyeicosatetraenoic acid; NO, nitric oxide; PKA, protein kinase A; PKC, protein kinase C; TALH, thick ascending limb of Henle; V_2, receptor for arginine vasopressin. (From Malnic G, Bailey MA, Giebisch G. Control of renal potassium excretion. In: Brenner B, ed. *The Kidney*, 7th ed., Vol. 1. Philadelphia: WB Saunders; 2004:453–496, with permission.)

shown in the apical and basolateral membranes (162–164, 177–179, 319, 321, 322). The K^+ concentration gradient across the apical membrane favors diffusion of potassium from cell to lumen and allows local recycling of potassium ions back to the tubule lumen. This back-diffusion provides a continuous luminal supply of potassium ions for cotransport with sodium and chloride. The K^+ leak in the luminal membrane is also responsible for net potassium secretion under those conditions in which the activity of the reabsorptive cotransport mechanism has been impaired.

Evidence pointing to the operation of the Na^+-$2Cl^-$-K^+ cotransporter in the apical membrane includes the mutual dependence of these ions for transport. Net reabsorption of ions (Na^+, K^+, and Cl^-) and the lumen-positive potential are abolished in the absence, from the lumen, of any of the three ions (165, 168, 177, 319). In addition, luminal application of furosemide also eliminates transport of all three ions and the transepithelial potential (69, 165, 168, 177, 387). Interference with the cotransport system, by appropriate luminal ion substitution or administration of furosemide, also affects the cellular ion activities. Inhibition of the luminal Na^+-$2Cl^-$-K^+ cotransporter lowers cellular chloride and sodium activities, thereby supporting the view that the cotransport system is the main pathway for entry of sodium and chloride ions into the cell across the apical membrane (160, 177, 322–324).

Two aspects of potassium transport across the TAL deserve mention. These concern both morphological and functional heterogeneity of the cells lining this nephron segment. First, comparison between the morphology and electrophysiological properties of TAL cells suggests the presence of at least two cell types with different permeability properties of the apical and basolateral cell membranes (9, 204). The potassium permeability of the apical membrane of one cell population exceeds that of the basolateral membrane in one cell population, that of the cortical thick ascending limb, whereas the opposite relation was observed in the medullary thick ascending limb. These permeability differences may be associated with functional disparities, potassium secretion being the prevalent transport mode in the cortical TAL, and reabsorption in the medullary TAL (204, 447).

Another difference between the transport modes of cortical and medullary TAL concerns the potassium sensitivity of the apical cotransporter to potassium (352). Figure 11 shows two cell models that indicate that vasopressin switches the apical sodium chloride transporter from a potassium-insensitive mode to one that depends critically on the presence of potassium in the tubule lumen. Alternative splicing of the transporter gene has been suggested as the molecular mechanism for the functional differences. In the presence of vasopressin, both apical Na^+-$2Cl^-$-K^+ transport and apical potassium recycling are expected to be stimulated. As a consequence, NaCl transport is maximally stimulated and results in optimal salt accumulation in the medullary interstitium. The situation is different during water diuresis. With the decline of extracellular fluid tonicity, tubule cells swell and apical sodium chloride operates in a potassium-independent mode (352). The mechanism of switching between the two transport modes is not known. Additional evidence that the supply of potassium is needed to safeguard Na^+-$2Cl^-$-K^+ cotransport in the cortical TAL is the observation that sodium reabsorption decreases sharply following the depletion of potassium from the lumen or following the administration of potassium channel blockers (484). These maneuvers also attenuate tubuloglomerular feedback (457).

Patch-clamp techniques have identified at least two potassium channels in the *apical* membrane that mediate potassium recycling. Some of their properties are summarized in Fig. 10 (52, 199, 200, 201, 485, 487, 490). The open probability of these apical potassium channels is high, and they are inhibited by barium, low cell pH, millimolar concentration of ATP, and protein kinase C (PKC). Cell alkalinization and cyclic AMP and NO and cyclic GMP stimulate potassium channels. Apical potassium channels are also activated by furosemide, a process mimicking the effects of aldosterone (318, 319). The latter, in amphibian early distal tubules, enhances apical Na-H exchange and alkalinizes cell pH. When furosemide is given, apical sodium entry is blocked and the intracellular sodium concentration decreases. As a consequence, the driving force for apical Na-H exchange increases and alkalinizes the cytoplasm. Because apical potassium channels are stimulated by cell alkalinization, their activity increases (318). This sequence of events

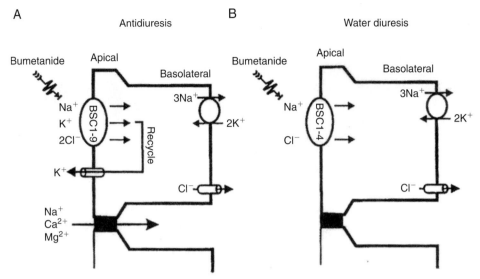

FIGURE 11 Proposed model for thick ascending limb (TAL) function. **A:** Operation during water conservation. **B:** Operation during maximal water diuresis. (*Am J Physiol Renal* 2001;280:F574–F582.)

explains why the full expression of the aldosterone effect on potassium permeability depends on an intact Na-H exchange in the apical cell membrane.

An interesting effect concerns the sequences of events following an increase in peritubular calcium which has been shown to inhibit both apical potassium channels and Na^+-$2Cl^-$-K^+ cotransport (181). Patch-clamp studies have demonstrated that these inhibitory effects of calcium are mediated through activation of P450 and PKC (494).

The *basolateral* membrane of TAL cells permits diffusion of both potassium and chloride; however, the chloride conductance is dominant (163, 165, 177, 181, 487). The potassium conductance provides one exit pathway and the K^+-Cl^- cotransport and an identified $KHCO_3^-$ cotransport mechanism provide additional pathways for K^+ movement from cell to interstitium. The Cl^- concentration gradient across the basolateral membrane favors diffusion of chloride from interstitium into the cell. Thus, both the luminal K^+ conductance and the basolateral Cl^- conductance tend to generate diffusion potentials oriented with the cell interior negative to the extracellular fluids. Because the K^+ concentration gradient across the apical membrane exceeds the Cl^- concentration gradient across the basolateral membrane, the voltage across the apical membrane exceeds the voltage across the basolateral membrane. These unequal electrical potential differences arranged in series generate the lumen-positive transepithelial voltage. This voltage gradient provides a driving force for reabsorption of potassium (and sodium) by passive diffusion through the paracellular shunt pathway.

Overall potassium reabsorption along the loop of Henle is the result of two opposing events: secretion into the descending limb of Henle's loop as a consequence of potassium recycling (see Fig. 9), and secondary active potassium reabsorption along the TAL of Henle's loop. Stimulation of po-

tassium secretion into the descending limb and enhanced delivery to the tip of Henle's loop have been demonstrated during potassium loading by puncture of juxtamedullary nephrons (211–214).

Several factors modulate potassium reabsorption along the loop of Henle (449, 450). Potassium reabsorption is enhanced by restricting dietary potassium intake, provided a constant load of fluid and potassium is delivered into the loop of Henle; administration of a high-potassium diet has the opposite effect (449). Reabsorptive transport of potassium in perfused loops of Henle is sensitive to aldosterone, which stimulates potassium reabsorption (411, 449). However, no reduction in the rate of potassium transport was observed in studies with perfused thick ascending limbs isolated from adrenalectomized animals (528). Several factors have been identified to modulate potassium recycling and then affect its delivery into the distal tubule. Recycling of potassium between the collecting duct and the descending limb of Henle's loop is enhanced following aldosterone administration in adrenalectomized animals (185). Calcitonin reduced medullary recycling by inhibition of potassium secretion into the distal tubule (111), whereas vasopressin had the opposite effect (110). Urea recycling is a significant factor that increases delivery of fluid to principle tubule cells and thus has been shown to stimulate potassium secretion (171). Because ammonium ions may substitute for potassium ions on the apical Na^+-$2Cl^-$-K^+ cotransport site, hyperkalemia may inhibit ammonium accumulation in the renal medulla and impede its translocation into the collecting tubule (107, 156).

The effects of mineralocorticoids have also been studied in the *amphibian* diluting segment, a portion of the nephron that shares many functions with the mammalian thick ascending limb (168). The amphibian diluting segment normally reabsorbs potassium, but it may secrete potassium following potassium loading (320), administration of loop diuretics (319, 321), alkalinization of the peritubular fluid (382), or administration of aldosterone (492, 516). Aldosterone stimulates both cell potassium uptake and release into the lumen, an effect that is reversed by exposure to amiloride (516). Acidosis inhibits the Na-K pump as well as the basolateral potassium channel (196, 199, 209). In contrast, alkalosis stimulates both pump-mediated uptake of potassium into cells and passive potassium efflux from the cells of the diluting segment. Apical K^+ channel activity also increases with cell volume (168, 201).

Reversal of the direction of potassium transport, from reabsorption to secretion, frequently follows administration of loop diuretics. Free-flow micropuncture and loop perfusion studies (168, 192, 310, 303, 450) in the mammalian kidney, as well as perfusion of the amphibian diluting segment, show sharply reduced rates of potassium reabsorption or reversal to net potassium secretion following the inhibition of the apical Na^+-$2Cl^-$-K^+ cotransporter by loop diuretics such as furosemide (68, 387, 466), torasemide (451), ethacrinic acid (67), and bumetanide (451, 463). The secretion of potassium is the consequence of unopposed potassium diffusion from the cell into the lumen.

Several experimental studies show that vasopressin enhances net sodium, chloride, and potassium transport across the thick ascending limb of Henle (177-179). Vasopressin action increases basolateral chloride permeability and accelerates chloride extrusion into the peritubular fluid. Vasopressin also enhances the affinity of the apical cotransporter for potassium (179) and augments the apical potassium permeability (178, 179). This increase in permeability speeds up apical membrane recycling of potassium and stimulates Na^+-$2Cl^-$-K^+ cotransport. The inhibitory effect of peritubular elevation of Ca^{2+} on apical potassium channel activity has already been mentioned (181, 494). Studies show that loss-of-function mutations of the apical ROMK channels can lead to Bartter syndrome. Interference with recycling of potassium ions in the apical membrane accounts for diminished sodium and potassium reabsorption and explain the loss of sodium and potassium, hypokalemia and high levels of aldosterone (21, 181).

Figure 12 illustrates two mechanisms by which inhibition (or absence) of apical potassium channels curtails sodium chloride and potassium reabsorption in the TAL (21). First, diminished potassium recycling across the apical membrane lowers the turnover rate of Na^+-$2Cl^-$-K^+ cotransport. Second, the drastic reduction of the lumen-positive potential compromises the main driving force for passive movement of potassium through the paracellular pathway. Moreover, absence of the apical potassium conductance also abolishes current flow across the paracellular pathway as well as current flow across the basolateral membrane. The latter is largely carried by chloride ions which normally leave the cell along a favorable electrochemical gradient through chloride channels. Interference with such chloride exit from the cell is expected to increase its cell concentration and diminish apical activity of Na^+-$2Cl^-$-K^+ cotransport.

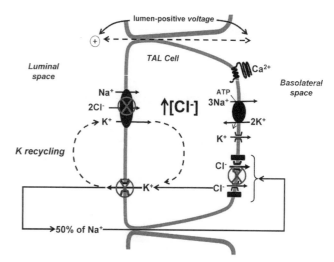

FIGURE 12   Dual role of apical K^+ channel in function of TAL. Note recycling of K^+ across the apical membrane and its contribution to current flow along the paracellular pathway. Potassium current across the apical membrane and the paracellular pathway is normally balanced by chloride current across the basolateral membrane. (From Bailey MA, Cantone A, Yan Q, MacGregor GG, Leng Q, Amorim JBO, Wang T, Hebert SC, Giebisch G, Malnic G. Maxi-K channels contribute to urinary potassium excretion in the ROMK-deficient mouse model of type II Bartter's syndrome and in adaptation to a high K diet. *Kidney Int* 2006;70:51–59, with permission.)

Distal Convoluted Tubule Cell: Direction, Magnitude, and Mechanism of Transport

Pathways contributing to potassium transport by DCT cells are shown in Fig. 13. Again, the Na^+,K^+-ATPase pump in the basolateral membrane is responsible for sodium extrusion and potassium uptake. Two conductive pathways in the basolateral membrane allow for K^+ and Cl^- exit. Potassium is also able to move from the cell across the apical membrane. Experimental evidence suggests that this movement occurs primarily through a K^+-Cl^- cotransporter, although in some preparations there is also evidence for barium-sensitive K^+ channels (540). The predominant path for sodium entry from the lumen is a Na-Cl cotransporter that differs from the Na^+-$2Cl^-$-K^+ mechanism in the thick ascending limb: the Na-Cl cotransporter in the DCT is blocked by thiazide diuretics but not inhibited by bumetanide (81, 116, 463, 466–468). Some evidence indicates that amiloride-sensitive sodium channels may also be present in the apical membrane (540). The junctional complexes between cells are cation-selective and permit diffusion of Na^+ and K^+ through the paracellular pathway from interstitium to lumen.

Evidence for the apical K^+-Cl^- cotransporter has come largely from microperfusion studies with rats (114, 115, 462, 464). Potassium secretion in this segment is increased when the luminal concentration of either potassium or chloride is decreased. This increase in K^+ secretion occurs without a change in transepithelial voltage and is not blocked by barium. Recirculation of chloride ions across the apical membrane is an important element of the mechanism of potassium secretion in the distal convoluted tubule, particularly

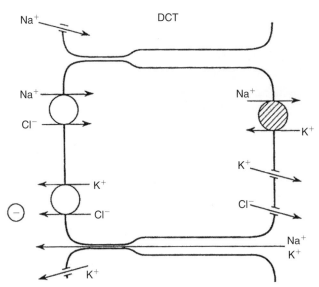

FIGURE 13 Model of distal convoluted tubule (DCT) cell. Some observations point to a lack of conductive pathways (channels) in the apical membrane; other studies have found evidence for Na and K conductances.

when chloride concentrations are kept low by the administration of poorly reabsorbable anions like SO_4 (464). Under such conditions, thiazide diuretics, by blocking apical chloride entry via NaCl cotransport, inhibit potassium secretion. This would be expected if potassium ions were entering the tubule by an electroneutral K^+-Cl^- cotransport mechanism.

Connecting Tubule and Cortical Collecting Duct Cells: Direction, Magnitude, and Mechanism of Transport

Two cell types—principle cells and intercalated cells—are involved in regulating renal potassium excretion. The *principle* cells are the most numerous cells in the ICD and the CCD. Principle cells are able to secrete potassium (144, 148, 149, 151, 152, 281, 282, 415, 431, 465, 530, 531, 534) and are the cells subject to the most important regulatory influences. A second, *intercalated* cell type, less numerous, has been shown to actively reabsorb potassium. This is accomplished by an active, ATP-dependent electroneutral exchange process in which hydrogen ion secretion is coupled to potassium reabsorption (101, 210, 241, 402, 403, 405, 522).

POTASSIUM SECRETION

Investigations have provided strong evidence that nephron segments upstream of the cortical collecting tubule, such as the TAL, late distal convoluted tubule, and connecting tubule, play a role in potassium homeostasis (205, 294, 369, 508). Based on experiments in mice, it has been suggested that under most experimental conditions, aldosterone-sensitive sodium reabsorption and potassium secretion are achieved along the connecting tubule. The collecting tubule's contribution to potassium secretion would emerge and become important whenever transport in the connecting tubule is compro-

mised, or its transport capacity challenged and thus insufficient, for instance, during ingestion of a high-potassium diet. Theoretical analysis, based on known morphology (tubule length) and transport parameters has also supported the importance of connecting tubule-mediated potassium transport in maintaining potassium homeostasis. Inspection of Fig. 14 shows that the requisite transport processes as well as their regulatory proteins are shared by the late distal convoluted tubule, connecting tubule and CCD (294). Experimental evidence suggests that there are no major differences in the basic transport properties of principle cells in connecting tubules and collecting ducts.

Figure 15 summarizes the main transport processes mediating potassium secretion in principle cells. Potassium uptake across the basolateral membrane is coupled to active sodium extrusion by the Na^+,K^+-ATPase. This sodium-potassium exchange pump is responsible for high cellular potassium activities. It responds to several stimuli known to modulate net potassium transport (acid-base disturbances, changes in plasma potassium, and variations in circulating levels of mineralocorticoid hormones) (144, 148, 149, 151, 152, 240, 313, 314, 333, 377, 382). The pump also provides for coupling between sodium reabsorption and potassium secretion. From the rapid depolarization of the basolateral membrane voltage caused by addition of ouabain to the peritubular bathing solution, it has been concluded that the sodium-potassium exchange pump operates in an electrogenic fashion, particularly following stimulation by desoxycorticosterone (DOC) treatment (239, 240, 375, 376, 382). Figure 15 also indicates a potassium conductance in the basolateral membrane. This K^+ channel permits the high cell potassium to drive outwardly directed diffusion that is largely responsible for the cell negativity. A comparison of the modes of renal transport of potassium and rubidium shows that potassium is more effectively secreted and reabsorbed than rubidium (31–33).

The apical membrane has both sodium and potassium conductances. The sodium concentration gradient from lumen to cell favors diffusion of sodium ions into the cells; this diffusion reduces the cell-negative voltage across the apical membrane relative to the voltage across the basolateral membrane. This asymmetrical electrical polarization of the apical and basolateral membranes favors diffusive movement of potassium from cell to lumen and is the source of the lumen-negative transepithelial potential difference and permits diffusive movement of potassium from cell to lumen (144, 147, 151, 152, 181, 279, 281, 282). Sodium channels (see Chapter 28) play an important role in regulating apical potassium transport by their effect on the apical membrane potential (125). The apical membrane voltage is reduced following administration of mineralocorticoids (152, 332–335). In contrast, the inhibitory effect of amiloride upon potassium secretion is associated with hyperpolarization of the apical membrane, and thus reduction of the lumen-negative transepithelial voltage (239, 240, 330, 331). This apical hyperpolarization is the consequence

Sodium and potassium transport in the DCT, CNT, and CCD

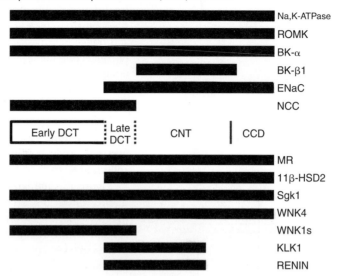

FIGURE 14   Expression patterns of sodium and potassium transport systems and of their regulatory proteins along the distal convoluted tubule (DCT), connecting tubule (CNT), and cortical collecting duct (CCD). In rat, mouse, and human, the sodium-chloride cotransporter (NCC) characterizes the DCT and colocalizes in the late DCT with the epithelial sodium channel (ENaC), which is also expressed in the CNT and CCD. The inwardly rectifying potassium channel (ROMK) and Na,K-ATPase are localized, respectively, in the apical and basolateral membrane along the aldosterone-sensitive distal nephron. Note that the expression of some regulatory proteins is restricted to the DCT and CNT and does not extend to the CCD. MR, mineralocorticoid receptor; 11β-HSD2, 11β-hydroxysteroid dehydrogenase type 2; Sgk1, serum and glucocorticoid-inducible kinase; WNK4, with no lysine kinase 4; WNK1s, kidney-specific form with no lysine kinase 1; KLK1, tissue kallikrein. (From Meneton P, Loffing J, Warnock DG. Sodium and potassium handling by the aldosterone-sensitive distal nephron; the pivotal role of the distal and connecting tubule. *Am J Physiol Renal* 2004;287:F593–F601; and Pluznick JL, Wei P, Grimm PR, Sansom SC. BK-ß1 subunit: immunolocalization in the mammalian connecting tubule and its role in the kaliuretic response to volume expansion. *Am J Physiol Renal* 2005;288:F846–F854, with permission.)

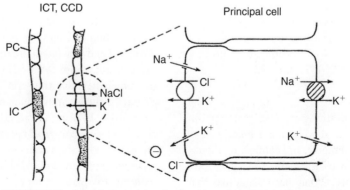

FIGURE 15   Model of principle cell, connecting tubule, initial collecting tubule (ICT), and cortical collecting duct (CCD). Transcellular Na absorption proceeds through apical Na$^+$ channels and the basolateral Na$^+$-K$^+$ pump. K$^+$ secretion depends on K$^+$ uptake by Na$^+$-K$^+$ pump and movement through apical K$^+$ channels or K$^+$-Cl$^-$ cotransporter. (From Giebisch G. A trail of research on potassium. *Kidney Int* 2002;62:1498–1512, with permission.)

of the drug-induced decrease in apical sodium conductance. The potassium conductance of the apical membrane is variable and has been found to be increased by adaptation to high-potassium intake (313, 320), by administration of mineralocorticoid hormones (239, 240, 314, 333, 335, 377, 382), and by vasopressin (383, 384, 391, 392). On the other hand, potassium conductance is reduced by acidification of the luminal, peritubular, and cellular fluids. Either lowering bicarbonate or elevating PCO_2 reduces the potassium conductance of the luminal membrane (314, 417, 439). This effect is consistent with the potassium-sparing effect of acute acidosis as demonstrated in perfusion studies of the distal tubule (414). Coupling between basolateral Na^+, K^+-ATPase activity and apical potassium and sodium channels has also been observed (312).

Renal Potassium Channels

The apical sodium as well as apical and basolateral potassium channels have been extensively studied by applying the patch-clamp technique to cultured amphibian kidney cells and to cells of isolated mammalian collecting ducts (128, 130, 144, 146–148, 150–152, 180, 181, 290, 341, 344, 347, 348, 485, 487, 493, 498) (see Chapter 44). Figures 16 to 18 summarize our present state of knowledge about apical and basolateral potassium channels of principle tubule cells. Figure 16 provides information of the properties and factors modulating the activity of the low-conductance secretory potassium channel but the apical membrane is also the site of stretch-sensitive, Ca^{2+}-activated maxi-potassium channels.

The apical low-conductance potassium channels are highly potassium selective and have a high open probabil-

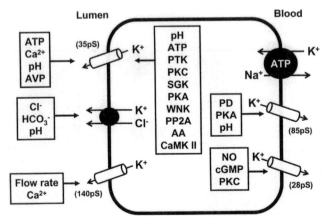

FIGURE 16 Model of principle cell including apical and basolateral transport pathways involved in potassium secretion. AA, arachidonic acid; ATP, adenosine triphosphate; AVP, arginine vasopressin; cGMP, cyclic guanosine monophosphate; NO, nitric oxide; PD, potential difference; PIP2, phosphatidylinositol 4,5-bisphosphate; PKA, protein kinase A; PKC, protein kinase C; PTK, protein tyrosine kinase; SGK, serum glucocorticoid-inducible kinase 1; WNK, with no lysine kinase; CaMK, Ca-calmodulin kinase. (From Malnic G, Bailey MA, Giebisch G. Control of renal potassium excretion. In: Brenner B, ed. *The Kidney,* 7th ed., Vol. 1. Philadelphia: WB Saunders; 2004:453–496, with permission.)

ity. They are stimulated by low concentrations of ATP and cyclic AMP-dependent protein kinase A, as well as by alkalinization of the cytoplasm. They are inhibited by barium, arachidonic acid (495) calcium-calmodulin kinase II, millimolar concentrations of ATP, calcium-dependent protein kinase C, and acidification of the cell fluid. The channel is sensitive to phosphorylation processes as evidenced by the observation that protein phosphatase (PP) inhibitors prevent channels "run-down," (i.e., the decline of channel activity frequently following excision of channel-containing membrane patches). The open probability of the secretory potassium channel is not markedly voltage dependent; calcium ions do not directly affect channel activity in excised membrane patches. Increased channel activity is often reflected by recruitment of channels into the active pool (181).

The potassium channel mediating potassium secretion has been extensively investigated, and found to be identical to a cloned, inwardly rectifying, low-conductance, ATP-regulated potassium channel (ROMK, Kir1) that shares many properties with native potassium channels in the apical membrane of principle tubule cells (180, 181, 344, 348). Figure 17 summarizes the known structure of this channel and factors modulating its activity. Important characteristics of this channel include high single-channel open probability, significant sensitivity to inhibition by low cytosolic pH and protein kinase C, and stimulation by protein kinase A. Channel density increases with high-potassium intake (130, 341, 487, 489, 491, 496). Several additional factors have been identified to modify ROMK activity. SGK (serum and glucocorticoid-inducible kinase 1), (194, 250, 456, 458, 539) and phosphoinositides (186, 193) stimulate ROMK whereas WINK (with no lysine kinase) decreases channel activity (216, 519). Ubiquitination has also been shown to be involved in channel retrieval from the apical membrane (262). Both AKAP (A-kinase anchoring protein (8) and NHERF (Na/H exchange regulating factor) (538) are necessary for optimal expression of K^+ channels in principle cells.

An important feature of the secretory, low-conductance potassium channel (ROMK) is its sensitivity to ATP. Both the native as well as the cloned potassium channel are dependent on phosphorylation processes which depend on low concentrations of ATP and cyclic AMP, whereas the channel is markedly inhibited by mM concentrations of ATP (486). Three serine sites on ROMK channels can be phosphorylated, and their inactivation by mutagenesis significantly reduces channel activity (180, 244, 272, 292, 293, 535).

An additional phosphorylation site involves a specific tyrosine residue on ROMK (482, 488). Interestingly, such tyrosine phosphorylation is regulated by potassium intake, and involves modulation of Src-related protein tyrosine kinases. A key element of this control mechanism involves channel endocytosis that is sensitive to the balance between tyrosine-kinase and tyrosinase phosphatase activity (489). Thus, low-potassium intake enhances expression of cSrk,

Regulatory Sites on the ROMK K⁺ Channel

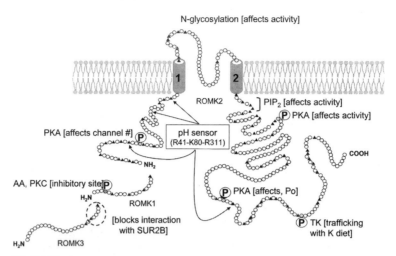

FIGURE 17 Structure of a cloned renal low-conductance K⁺ channel. Note two membrane-spanning domains and several potential binding sites for protein kinase A (PKA) and protein kinase C (PKC), as well as a PO_4^{3-} binding loop. AA, arachidonic acid; ATP, adenosine triphosphate; PIP_2, phosphatidyl inositol 4,5-biphosphate; TK, tyrosine kinase. (From Hebert SC. An ATP-regulated, inwardly rectifying potassium channel from rat kidney (ROMK). *Kidney Int* 1995;48:1010–1016; and Hebert SC, Desir G, Giebisch G, and Wang WH. Molecular diversity and regulation of renal potassium channels. *Physiol Rev* 2005;85:319–371, with permission.)

ROMK phosphorylation, and endocytotic removal of apical potassium channels. The opposite effects take place by high-potassium intake. Evidence has implicated superoxide as a mediator of the dietary effects on ROMK expression, because suppression of superoxide production abolished the effects of changes in potassium diet on apical potassium channels in principle cells (302).

The ROMK channel can also form associations with other proteins: coexpression with CFTR restores the sensitivity of cloned potassium channels to the inhibitory action of glibenclamide (290) and of ATP (267). A nucleotide binding site has also been identified on ROMK channels and may be responsible for channel regulation by ATP (460). The importance of ROMK channels for K⁺ secretion is underscored by a comparison between potassium secretion measured in perfused rat cortical collecting tubules and ROMK channel properties assessed in patch clamp studies (channel density and single-channel conductance). Such an analysis shows that this apical potassium channel can fully account for the observed potassium movement in a variety of experimental conditions. Model calculations included analysis of the stimulating effects of aldosterone and high-potassium diets (159).

Inspection of Fig. 16 indicates that a second potassium channel is present in the apical membrane of principle cells. The channel's topology is shown in Fig. 18, and its properties differ significantly from ROMK (181, 304, 353). These maxi-potassium channels are present in both principle and intercalated cells (128, 130, 166, 181, 195, 339, 341, 344, 347, 348, 353), and their open-probability, as defined in

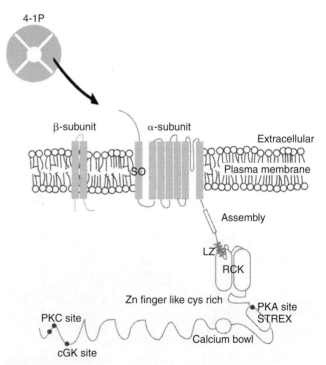

FIGURE 18 Structure of the maxi-potassium channel, a member of the voltage-dependent potassium channel family, with an extra transmembrane domain (SO) and domain/motifs conferring calcium sensitivity. LZ, leucine zipper; RCK, regulating conductance of potassium; ZN, finger-like cysteine rich; PKA, protein kinase A; STREX, stress axis regulated exon; cGK, cGMP protein kinase; PKC, protein kinase C. (From Morita T, Hanaoka K, Morales MM, Montrose-Rafizadeh C, Guggino WB. Cloning and characterization of maxi K⁺ channel a-subunit in rabbit kidney. *Am J Physiol Renal* 1997;273:F615–F624, with permission.)

split-open, isolated connecting tubules and cortical collecting tubules, is quite low although their single-channel conductance is about five times that of ROMK. Moreover, their activity increases with high cell calcium and membrane depolarization. Another distinguishing feature includes the channel's sensitivity to membrane stretch. Strong evidence implicates this potassium channel in mediating an important fraction of potassium secretion during high lumen flow rates in connecting and collecting ducts (526), during kaliuresis following potassium loading (21, 315, 354), and during application of vasopressin to the lumen fluid (11, 12). It has been suggested that high flow rate along connecting and collecting tubules activates apical calcium channels which in turn stimulate Ca-sensitive maxi-potassium channels (265).

An unresolved problem concerns the contribution of Ca^{2+}-sensitive maxi-potassium channels to potassium secretion under physiological conditions. Single-channel analysis by patch-clamp techniques is limited to "split-open" tubules in the absence of membrane surface stretch. Thus, it is difficult to evaluate maxi-potassium channel activity in conditions that represent physiological flow conditions in vivo.

The *basolateral* K^+ channels, shown in Fig. 16, are also potassium selective, some are activated by membrane hyperpolarization, and are inhibited by barium. It is apparent from inspection of Fig. 16 that basolateral potassium channels are characterized by several factors that distinguish them from their apical homologues (187, 188, 268, 269, 388, 393). First, a subpopulation of basolateral potassium channels responds to hyperpolarization by increased activity (496). This mechanism contributes to the observed enhancement of potassium conductance with stimulation of electrogenic Na^+,K^+-ATPase activity (497). Second, basolateral potassium channels are stimulated by NO and cGMP (187, 188, 268, 269). The evidence for the involvement of NO is the decline in basolateral potassium channel activity by inhibiting nitric oxide synthase whereas donors of exogenous NO stimulate these channels. Application of cGMP analogues also activate basolateral potassium channels, and hyperpolarize the basolateral membrane. This induces an increase in the apical membrane potential through current flow via the paracellular pathway and stimulates sodium entry across the apical membrane of principle cells (268). Features shared by these channels are their lack of inhibition by ATP and a biphasic effect of changes in cell calcium: whereas low concentrations stimulate basolateral potassium channels (via activation of cGMP), high levels of Ca^{2+} inhibit potassium channels (187, 188, 268, 388).

Attention should also be drawn to a cloned, inwardly-rectifying potassium channel (Kir2.3) that was obtained from a mouse cell line, and which is expressed in the basolateral membrane of MDCK cells (511). The channel may be involved in stabilizing the basolateral membrane potential and shares some properties with potassium channels identified by patch-clamp techniques. Another inward-rectifying potassium channel (Kir7.1) has also been located in the basolateral

membrane of the distal nephron (336). This activity is modulated by changes in dietary potassium intake and may thus play a role in the control of potassium transport.

Apical Cotransport of Potassium Chloride

Microperfusion studies of superficial distal tubules in the rat and of isolated rabbit CCDs have provided evidence that a neutral cotransport mechanism in the apical membrane couples potassium and chloride movement from cell to lumen (10, 114, 115, 462, 464, 534). This K-Cl cotransport mechanism is also shown in Fig. 16. The key evidence for an electroneutral K-Cl cotransport mechanism is that potassium secretion into the distal tubule is stimulated when the lumen is perfused with a solution having a low chloride concentration. This stimulation of potassium transport occurs without changes in the transepithelial voltage across the distal tubule wall and persists in the presence of barium. K-Cl cotransport is not a major secretory pathway under physiological conditions, but may contribute substantially to potassium secretion when the concentration of chloride in the lumen declines. This may occur with the delivery of poorly reabsorbable anions such as sulfate, phosphate, and especially bicarbonate into the distal tubule (10, 264).

POTASSIUM REABSORPTION

Intercalated Cells

Intercalated cells (Figs. 4, 5, and 19) are scattered among the principle cells of the cortical and outer medullary collecting duct and also among the cells of the distal tubule (infrequently in the distal convoluted tubule, and more commonly in the connecting tubule and initial collecting tubule) (86, 221, 274). Several types of intercalated cells have been recognized: A-type cells are able to secrete hydrogen ions, and B-type cells secrete bicarbonate ions. A third, "mixed" type, containing Cl^--HCO_3^- exchangers in both the apical and basolateral membrane has also been described (506).

The A-type cells may also be responsible for potassium reabsorption, as shown in Fig. 19. Several important differences between intercalated cells and principle cells should be noted. The Na^+,K^+-ATPase in basolateral membranes of intercalated cells has a much lower activity than in principle cells. This difference has been shown both by immunocytochemistry (227) and by measurements of rubidium uptake from peritubular fluid by single cells (31). Intercalated cells also have low ion conductances of the apical membrane. Microelectrode measurements make it unlikely that Na channels are present in the apical membrane of intercalated cells. Instead, potassium enters these cells largely through a K-H exchanger, the K^+,H^+-ATPase. Evidence for a basolateral barium-sensitive exit pathway has also become available (271, 522).

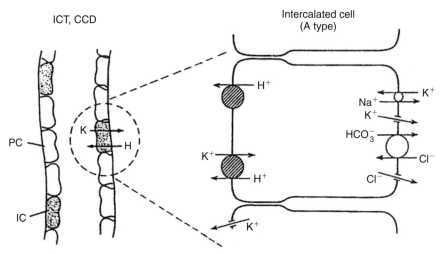

FIGURE 19   Model of acid secreting (A-type) intercalated cells in the ICT and CCD. These cells are the site of potassium absorption via an H,K-ATPase. Proton secretion is also driven by an H-ATPase (From Giebisch G. A trail of research on potassium. *Kidney Int* 2002;62:1498–1512, with permission.)

Several isoforms of K^+,H^+-ATPase, distinguished by different K^+-Na^+ selectivity of the exchange processes, and by different sensitivities to inhibitors such as gastric K^+-H^+ blockers and ouabain, are responsible for active K^+ absorption in intercalated cells (4, 82, 93, 100, 101, 106, 139, 210, 255, 297, 402, 403, 506, 522, 524, 549). Thus, two types of K^+,H^+-ATPase have been described in rat and mouse cortical and outer medullary collecting tubules, and they have been shown to be structurally identical to isoforms of K^+,H^+-ATPases cloned from gastric mucosa and colonic mucosa. Their importance is suggested by numerous functional studies (15, 65, 78, 93, 101). However, a study based on experiments in gastric and colonic K^+,H^+-ATPase knockout mice has provided strong evidence for an as yet unidentified additional transport mechanism for linked potassium reabsorption and hydrogen ion secretion that is distinct from known K^+,H^+-ATPases (93). The importance of this transporter is underscored by its demonstrated ability to compensate effectively for the loss of function of both gastric and colonic K^+,H^+-ATPase (93). Similar results have also been reported using the mouse cortical collecting tubule (351). Thus, the contribution of individual K^+,H^+-ATPases and other unidentified transporters to the maintenance of potassium and hydrogen ion balance is not fully understood.

Two inhibitors of the gastric K^+,H^+-ATPase, omeprazole and Sch 28080, decrease both potassium absorption and hydrogen secretion in the distal tubule and the outer medullary collecting duct. K^+-H^+ exchange has been found increased during metabolic acidosis (404), experimental potassium depletion (15, 64, 100, 101, 106, 189, 208, 209, 248, 254, 405, 541) and during administration of a low-sodium diet (402, 405). Increased sensitivity to potassium depletion was reported in "knockout" mice lacking the colonic isoform of K^+,H^+-ATPase. Surprisingly, however, the ability of renal potassium conservation was quite well

preserved and most of the loss of potassium occurred by fecal excretion (295). Active potassium absorption occurs in several epithelia, including the turtle urinary bladder (202) and the intestinal mucosa (126, 518).

Morphological studies of the apical cell membrane of *intercalated* cells in potassium-depleted rats have shown changes in fine structure, such as an increase in the number of rod-shaped particles and amplification of the microplicae (222, 224, 225, 425). These alterations in membrane structure are specific for the luminal membrane of intercalated cells. Intercalated cells also undergo marked morphological amplification of their apical membranes following acidification. These changes suggest that potassium reabsorption and hydrogen ion secretion are functionally linked.

Medullary Collecting Duct Cells

Several sections of the medullary collecting ducts have been distinguished on the basis of morphological and functional differences. The *outer medulla* can be grossly separated into outer and inner stripes and the *inner medulla* can be subdivided into outer and inner halves. The inner medullary collecting duct is separated into corresponding initial and terminal segments. Most of these collecting duct segments participate in the regulation of potassium excretion.

The medullary collecting duct in the *outer stripe* resembles the cortical collecting duct. Potassium secretion and sodium reabsorption continue (427, 429, 430), and the cells lining this segment have morphological and functional properties similar to principle and intercalated cells (221).

The collecting duct in the *inner stripe* is characterized by a different transport pattern. Available evidence strongly suggests both passive and active transport mechanisms (523, 524). Potassium secretion is absent when isolated tubule segments are perfused with symmetrical solutions. The lack of a significant potassium conductance in the apical cell membrane supports this view (419). However, when appropriate transepithelial potassium gradients are applied, significant potassium movement occurs, presumably via the paracellular transport route (523, 524). Potassium depletion increases the passive potassium permeability (419). Changes in the lumen potassium concentration are thus likely to induce passive transepithelial potassium movement, either in the secretory or reabsorptive direction. The generation of electrical potentials also activates passive potassium movement. For instance, a lumen-positive potential, generated by electrogenic hydrogen ion secretion, induces significant potassium reabsorption (266). This coupling between potassium and hydrogen movement may explain why augmented proton secretion is frequently associated with enhanced potassium reabsorption.

An active potassium-hydrogen exchange mechanism has also been detected in collecting ducts isolated from the *inner stripe* of the outer medulla in potassium-depleted rabbits (524). Activation of this transporter also contributes to the stimulation of potassium reabsorption and hydrogen ion secretion that is observed in potassium depletion.

Both reabsorption and secretion of potassium ions have been observed in the *inner medullary* collecting duct. Fig. 20 summarizes some of the known transport properties of inner medullary collecting duct cells (367). Patch-clamp studies have demonstrated the presence of an ATP-sensitive K^+-selective channel in cultured cells of the inner medullary collecting duct (373). Another important feature of inner medullary collecting duct cells is a nonspecific cation channel in the apical membrane (260). Depending on the apical transmembrane electrochemical driving forces, this channel may mediate both sodium reabsorption and potassium secretion. At very high lumen potassium concentrations, passive reabsorption of potassium may also take place. The presence of a furosemide-sensitive Na^+-$2Cl^-$-K^+ cotrans-

porter in the basolateral membrane of inner medullary collecting duct cells has also been reported (167, 367, 548).

CONTROL OF RENAL POTASSIUM TRANSPORT

Proximal Tubule

The proximal tubule is the main site of potassium reabsorption but does not appear to play an important role in the regulation of potassium excretion. Potassium transport is largely dependent on sodium and fluid movement. Accordingly, potassium reabsorption usually changes with variations of proximal tubule sodium and fluid transport. Increased delivery of potassium into the loop of Henle may thus be expected in conditions of osmotic diuresis or other conditions of inhibition of proximal tubule sodium and fluid transport.

Potassium entry into the proximal straight tubule (S3 in Fig. 9) has also been reported (211, 213, 214). Such secretory transport has been demonstrated in vitro (211, 213, 229, 230, 385), but it is likely that modest potassium secretion also occurs in vivo. Given the increase in medullary potassium concentration along the corticomedullary axis, potassium ions may enter the tubule lumen by diffusion as part of the process of medullary recycling (211, 213, 385).

Thick Ascending Limb of Henle, Distal Convoluted Tubule, Connecting and Collecting Tubules

Available information is insufficient to evaluate the separate contributions of each of these segments to the regulation of renal potassium excretion. The TAL normally reabsorbs a significant fraction of filtered and recycled potassium. However, reabsorption may be significantly reduced, or even replaced by net secretion, following direct inhibition of Na-2Cl-K cotransport or interference with apical potassium recycling (21, 181, 451). Diminished reabsorption of potassium in the TAL may contribute to enhanced urinary excretion whenever TAL function is compromised (21, 192). Modest rates of potassium secretion have been observed along the mammalian distal convoluted tubule (114, 394), but the effects upon this nephron segments of those factors known to modulate potassium transport at other nephron sites have not been fully explored. Changes in tubule flow rate and dietary potassium intake do not affect potassium secretion (394). In vivo micropuncture and microperfusion experiments indicate that the DCT is the main site of action of thiazide diuretics (81, 463, 466–468). An interesting relationship between sodium chloride and potassium transport has been observed in microperfusion experiments. When apical sodium entry was stimulated by raising the Na^+ concentration in the tubule lumen, potassium secretion increased. It is likely that enhanced chloride entry increased cell chloride and stimulated K-Cl cotransport from cell to

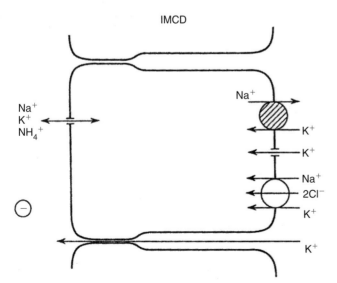

FIGURE 20 Model of inner medullar collecting duct (IMCD) cell. Apical cation channels are equally permeable to Na^+ and K^+.

lumen (464). Thus, recycling of chloride appears to play a significant role in potassium secretion in distal convoluted tubule cells.

The ICT ("late distal" tubule), the CNTs, and the CCDs are the main nephron sites that control potassium excretion (144, 149, 151, 152, 236, 415, 530, 531). Information on the transport function of the initial collecting tubule has been obtained by either free-flow or in vivo microperfusion studies. The CCD has been investigated by in vitro microperfusion techniques. Both tubule segments are distinguished by marked cell heterogeneity, and net transport of potassium, either in the secretory or reabsorptive direction, results from varying rates of potassium secretion (through principle cells) and potassium reabsorption (through intercalated cells).

Figure 21 summarizes several factors that affect potassium secretion by cells of the distal tubule and CCD (152, 327, 328). Luminal factors include both the flow rate and the composition of fluid entering the distal tubule or cortical collecting duct. Peritubular factors include changes in specific ion concentrations and hormones. The most important systemic changes that affect these factors include potassium intake, adrenal steroids, salt and water balance, and acid-base balance.

Potassium Intake

Both increases and decreases in potassium intake, as well as acute loading with potassium-containing fluids, initiate appropriate adjustments in renal K^+ excretion. Increases in potassium intake tend to raise plasma K^+ concentration (253). Not only does elevated plasma K^+ concentration affect the kidney directly, but it also stimulates the adrenal glands to secrete aldosterone (60, 103, 134). Decreases in potassium intake, or losses of potassium that exceed intake, tend to reduce total-body potassium content, plasma K^+ concentration, and aldosterone secretion.

POTASSIUM LOADING

Potassium excretion and potassium secretion along the initial collecting tubule rise sharply with parenteral administration of potassium-containing solutions (148, 151, 152, 253, 281, 282, 350, 532). The stimulation of potassium secretion after acute potassium loading has been demonstrated both in free-flow and microperfusion studies. Factors contributing to increased rates of potassium secretion include increases in plasma potassium (416, 544), aldosterone levels (60, 103, 120, 121, 134, 135, 432, 543), and distal flow rate (120, 121, 155, 236, 247, 278). The independent and separate effects of these variables have been explored in microperfusion experiments in which flow rate, luminal ion concentrations, and the levels of mineralocorticoids and glucocorticoids were controlled (121, 123, 154, 155, 416, 533). Significant stimulation of distal potassium secretion followed an increase in either plasma potassium, plasma aldosterone, or luminal flow rate, whereas dexamethasone had no direct effect on potassium transport.

Chronic potassium loading increases the secretory capacity of the distal nephron so that at a given plasma potassium level, renal potassium excretion is significantly accelerated (1, 41–44, 409, 410, 412, 416, 420). Figure 22 illustrates relationships between plasma potassium concentration and either renal potassium excretion or distal potassium secretion in control animals and in animals fed a high-potassium diet for 4 weeks. Pretreatment with the high-potassium diet led to powerful stimulation of potassium secretion and a more rapid onset of kaliuresis (532). This stimulation of potassium secretion at normal or only slightly elevated plasma K^+ levels following chronic elevation of potassium intake is a clear example of an adaptive change in renal function. Adaptation to a high alimentary intake of potassium may occur even when the plasma aldosterone concentration is kept constant (313). Full adaptation, though, does require an increase in mineralocorticoid levels (120–123, 341–343, 345). Along with an enhanced rate of potassium uptake by nonrenal cells (7, 45), the increased secretory capacity of distal tubule cells promotes potassium tolerance: the ability of animals fed a high-potassium diet to survive an acute

Thick Ascending Limb Cell – Potassium Reabsorption

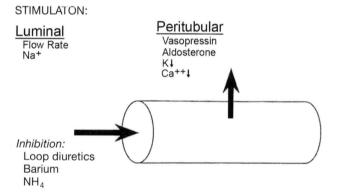

STIMULATION:

Luminal
Flow Rate
Na$^+$

Peritubular
Vasopressin
Aldosterone
K↓
Ca^{++}↓

Inhibition:
Loop diuretics
Barium
NH$_4$

Principal Tubule Cell – Potassium Secretion

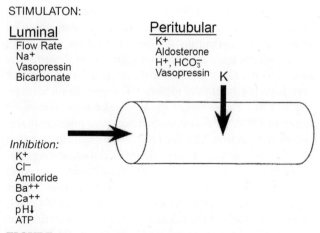

STIMULATION:

Luminal
Flow Rate
Na$^+$
Vasopressin
Bicarbonate

Peritubular
K$^+$
Aldosterone
H$^+$, HCO$_3^-$
Vasopressin   K

Inhibition:
K$^+$
Cl$^-$
Amiloride
Ba^{++}
Ca^{++}
pH↓
ATP

FIGURE 21 Summary of factors affecting K^+ reabsorption in thick ascending limb and K^+ secretion by principle cells.

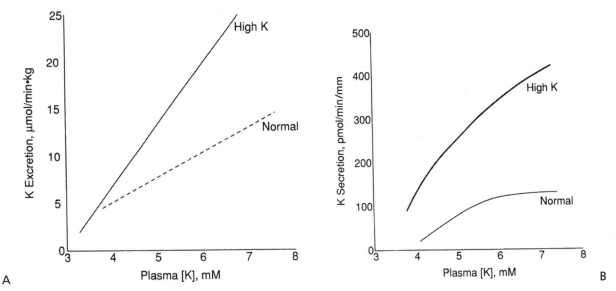

FIGURE 22   Relation between plasma K$^+$ concentration and renal K$^+$ excretion, **A**, and distal tubule K$^+$ secretion, **B**. (From Stanton BA, Giebisch G. Renal potassium transport. In: Windhager EE, ed. *Handbook of Physiology: Renal Physiology.* New York: Oxford University Press; 1991:813–874; and Stanton BA, Giebisch GH. Potassium transport by the renal distal tubule: Effect of potassium loading. *Am J Physiol Renal* 1982;243:F487–F493, with permission.)

potassium load that would otherwise be fatal. A striking example of potassium adaptation is the ability of a reduced number of nephrons—such as in chronic renal failure—to sharply increase potassium secretion and to maintain potassium balance (142).

The adaptive increase in secretory capacity has clear morphological and biochemical correlates in the distal tubule and CCD (222, 224, 225, 412, 413, 420). Proliferation of the basolateral cell membrane is highly significant in potassium-adapted animals and closely associated with a sharp increase of Na$^+$,K$^+$-ATPase (97, 98, 132, 222, 224, 225, 258, 309). Hyperkalemia and mineralocorticoids independently initiate the amplification of the basolateral membrane and the attendant increase in ATPase activity (410). Thus, changes in basolateral membrane area, Na$^+$,K$^+$-ATPase content, and potassium secretory rates are tightly coupled (412, 413, 420). Morphological changes are apparent after 24 hours of increased K$^+$ intake and increase for about another week before a plateau is reached (420). Increased potassium excretion may continue beyond cessation of a high-potassium intake (311).

Stimulation of principle cell basolateral membrane amplification also occurs with increased delivery of fluid and sodium ions to the potassium secretory site of the initial collecting tubule (113, 220, 223, 224, 258, 360, 547). The underlying mechanism appears to be stimulation of sodium reabsorption, which is linked to potassium secretion. Thus, chronic administration of furosemide to animals, in which fluctuations of aldosterone and changes in electrolyte balance were prevented, led to a sharp increase of potassium secretion and sodium reabsorption (408). Membrane amplification and a state of potassium adaptation at the single nephron level have also been observed in unilaterally ne-

phrectomized animals in which potassium balance is maintained by redistribution of Na$^+$ reabsorption from proximal to distal nephron sites and increased delivery of fluid into the distal nephron of the remaining nephron population (408). Again, the morphological changes of basolateral membrane amplification occur predominantly in the principle cell population.

Figure 23 shows a cell model including the main known factors that coordinate the activation of several mechanisms in response to a high-potassium intake. An important response to a surfeit of potassium is the increase in aldosterone, whose main effect on K$^+$ transport in principle cells involves stimulation of apical Na$^+$ channels and the basolateral Na$^+$,K$^+$-ATPase. High-potassium feeding also increases the pool of active ROMK in principle cells by diminishing apical removal of channels by endocytosis (302, 488, 489, 496). Moreover, a high-potassium diet may not only diminish K$^+$ reabsorption by lowering H-K exchange but also by enhancing apical recycling of potassium in intercalated cells, possibly by maxi-potassium channels. However, direct evidence for the latter mechanism has not yet been obtained.

POTASSIUM DEPRIVATION

Renal potassium excretion drops sharply after withdrawal of potassium from the diet. At the same time, distal tubule potassium secretion is markedly depressed or disappears altogether (118, 141, 143, 282). Aldosterone secretion is suppressed. Net secretion of potassium may cease and be replaced by net reabsorption along the initial collecting duct when rats were fed a low-K diet for 1 week (326) or when potassium-depleted rats were also given amiloride, a known blocker of potassium secretion by principle cells. Potassium reabsorption appears to involve both active and passive

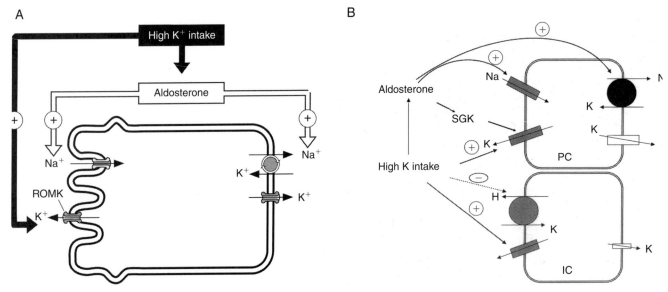

FIGURE 23   Models of high-potassium intake in principle cells. **A:** Model of principle cell in the cortical collecting duct (CCD) illustrating the mechanism by which high-K⁺ diet increases K⁺ secretion. High K⁺ intake stimulates aldosterone secretion, which in turn activates epithelial sodium channels (ENaCs) and Na⁺,K⁺-ATPase. Increased ENaC activity augments the driving force for K⁺ secretion, whereas stimulation of Na⁺,K⁺-ATPase can indirectly activate ROMK channel activity by a cross-talk mechanism. In addition, high K⁺ intake can directly increase the ROMK channel activity. **B:** Cell models showing the coordinated interaction of K⁺ transporters in principle and intercalated cells during high K⁺ intake. (*Ann Rev Physiol* 2004;66:547–569.)

transport mechanisms. Active K-H exchange is significantly increased in cortical and medullary collecting tubule segments in which potassium reabsorption is stimulated (64, 100, 102, 106, 522, 541). Passive potassium reabsorption in the outer medullary collecting duct occurs in states of potassium depletion. Thus, an increase of passive potassium permeability in the outer medullary collecting duct has been reported and could favor accelerated potassium retrieval from the lumen (524).

Figure 24 provides an overview of the transport changes that take place following administration of a low-potassium diet (302, 488, 496). Shown on the left is the sequence of events involving tyrosine phosphorylation of ROMK by Src which initiates the endocytotic removal of apical K⁺ channels. Specific tyrosine phosphorylation on the C terminus of ROMK in the apical membrane of principle tubule cells from animals fed a low-potassium diet is critical, but it is presently unresolved how principle tubule cells sense small

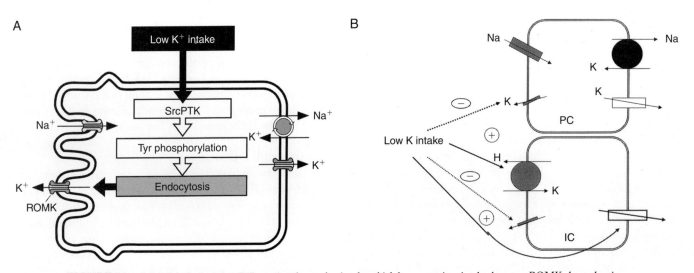

FIGURE 24   **A:** Model of principle cell illustrating the mechanism by which low-potassium intake decreases ROMK channel activity. Low-potassium intake increases protein tyrosine kinase (PTK) activity and tyrosine phosphorylation of ROMK. As a consequence, ROMK channels are internalized. **B:** Cell models showing the coordinated interaction of K⁺ transporters in principle and intercalated cells during K⁺ retention. (*Ann Rev Physiol* 2004;66:547–569.)

changes in extracellular potassium concentration. It has already been mentioned that superoxide production is closely associated with the low-potassium response (19). It should be noted that the response of apical potassium channel density to potassium intake is independent of aldosterone and supports previous findings that increased potassium excretion persists in tubules from animals fed a high-potassium diet in which changes in mineralocorticoid concentration were prevented (313).

Upregulation of Na^+,K^+-ATPase activity has also been observed in tubules following potassium-depletion (62, 109, 206). The original idea that such ATPase activity involves relocation to the apical membrane (175) was not supported by immunological studies (63). It should be noted that reduced net secretion of potassium during potassium depletion in the presence of enhanced Na^+,K^+-ATPase-mediated potassium uptake across the basolateral membrane would have to involve increased backleak through basolateral potassium channels (63). It is well established that potassium depletion stimulates renal growth (444), a condition in which Na^+,K^+-ATPase might be expected to increase, but

the relationship between K^+-depletion, renal growth factors and basolateral Na^+,K^+-ATPase activity remains to be further explored.

Potassium depletion has also been shown to involve changes in the distribution of H,K-ATPases in cortical and outer medullary collecting ducts (14, 189). As shown in Fig. 25, the ouabain-insensitive isoform of H,K-ATPase is down-regulated in potassium depletion and replaced by an isoform that is sensitive to inhibition by ouabain and less selective for potassium compared to sodium (189). Whereas normally H,K-ATPases have been localized to alpha-intercalated cells, remodeling of H,K-ATPases in potassium depletion involves their targeting to principle cells (254). The presence of significant amounts of H,K-ATPases in proximal tubules and segments of the loop of Henle is of interest, but its functional implications are not known.

Since ammonium can substitute for potassium on both Na,K-ATPase and Na-2Cl-K transporters, changes in extracellular potassium exert a significant effect on acid excretion (476, 477-481). The interactions between potassium and ammonium are summarized in Fig. 26 (277).

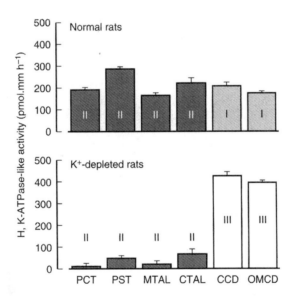

Subtypes of H^+,K^+-ATPase-like activity along the rat nephron

	I	II	III
Pharmacologic profile (IC$_{50}$)			
Sch 28080	0.2 μM	1.5 μM	0.5 μM
Ouabain	Insensitive	5 μM	10 μM
Cation selectivity	K^+	K^+	K^+ or Na^+

IC$_{50}$, 50% inhibitory concentration.
Subtype I is similar to the gastric isoform. Subtypes II and III include the colonic isoform.

FIGURE 25   Distribution of three subtypes of H^+,K^+-ATPase–like activities, defined in the lower panel, along the nephron of normal rats and potassium-depleted rats. (From Horisberger JD, Doucet A. Renal ion translocating ATPases: the P type family 139. In: Seldin DW, Giebisch G, eds. *The Kidney: Physiology and Pathophysiology*, 3rd ed. Philadelphia: Lippincott Williams & Wilkins; 2002:139–170, with permission.)

Under conditions of potassium depletion, the interstitial concentration of potassium declines, and carrier and pump-mediated uptake of ammonium in inner and outer medullary collecting ducts increases. Enhancement of cell hydrogen ion supply stimulates apical hydrogen ion secretion, in part through the H-K exchange mechanism thus enhancing potassium reabsorption. Net potassium secretion decreases further by the inhibition of apical potassium channels by tubule trapping of ammonium which blocks ROMK (172, 173). Hyperkalemia has the opposite effect. Potassium ions replace ammonium on Na^+,K^+-ATPase and the Na^+-K^+-$2Cl^-$ cotransporter, which leads to diminished cell acidification and hydrogen ion availability for apical secretion. As a consequence, hyperkalemia may induce metabolic acidosis (480).

Changes in aldosterone modulate, but are not fully responsible for, the renal response to potassium deprivation.

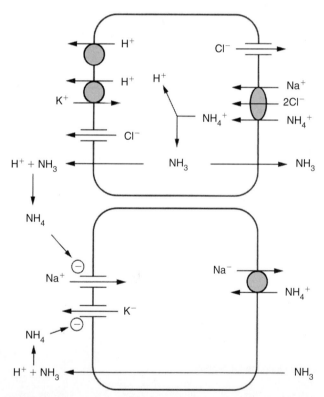

FIGURE 26 Active K^+ reabsorption in the intercalated cell of the outer medullary collecting duct (OMCD) during K^+ depletion. Note that NH_4^+ can bind to the extracellular K^+ site of basolateral Na^+,K^+-ATPase and the Na^+-$2Cl^-$-K^+ cotransporter and thereby stimulate H^+ secretion and K^+ reabsorption. Diffusion trapping of NH_4^+ in the tubule lumen directly inhibits K^+ secretion. CCD, cortical collecting duct; CTAL, cortical thick ascending limb of Henle; MTAL, medullary thick ascending loop of Henle; PCT, proximal convoluted tubule; PST, proximal straight tubule. (From Malnic G, Bailey MA, Giebisch G. Control of renal potassium excretion. In: Brenner B (ed.). The Kidney, 7th ed., Vol. 1. Philadelphia: WB Saunders, 2004:453–496 and Wall SM. Impact of K^+ Homeostasis on net acid secretion in rat terminal inner medullary collecting duct: Role of the Na-K-ATPase. *Am J Kidney Dis* 2000;36: 1079–1088, with permission.)

This mineralocorticoid has been shown to attenuate the urinary loss of potassium, but potassium excretion continues to diminish when animals are put on a low-potassium diet despite the prevention of a decrease in circulating aldosterone (310, 337, 338, 461).

Ultrastructural changes in medullary collecting ducts during potassium depletion are confined to the intercalated cell population and include a marked increase in the length of the apical cell membrane, an increase in the number of rod-shaped particles in the apical membrane, and a fall in the number of subapical cytoplasmic vesicles (425). These morphological observations suggest an increase in the number of apical potassium transporters, most likely the K, H-ATPase. The fact that similar morphological changes have been observed in intercalated cells of acidotic animals (275) supports the view that potassium reabsorption and acid excretion are functionally linked.

Adrenal Steroids

Mineralocorticoids have long been known to stimulate sodium reabsorption and, under appropriate conditions, enhance potassium secretion. Figure 27 demonstrates the effects of aldosterone treatment on potassium excretion (544). Results from experiments in which mineralocorticoids were administered for prolonged periods of time, until a steady state was reached, are shown. Aldosterone significantly enhanced the efficiency of potassium excretion as evidenced by the fact that, at each plasma potassium concentration, more potassium was excreted by animals with higher aldosterone levels. Expressed differently, as the aldosterone level rises, the same amount of potassium can be excreted at progressively lower plasma potassium levels. The direct stimulatory effect of mineralocorticoids on potassium secretion by the distal tubule and CCD has been amply demonstrated (46, 80, 120–123, 183, 333, 335). Enhanced uptake of potassium into extrarenal tissues has also been reported (45, 47, 453).

The effects of mineralocorticoids, closely related to potassium metabolism, on the transport mechanisms of principle collecting duct cells are summarized in Fig. 28A and 28B. Shown are the changes of apical and basolateral ion conductances and the basolateral Na^+-K^+ pump. The effects of mineralocorticoids depend on the antecedent hormonal condition, the duration of hormone treatment, and the modifying effects of sodium ions on potassium transport (120). Key aldosterone-sensitive transport mechanisms of principle cells include the basolateral Na^+-K^+ exchange pump, apical Na^+ channels, and K^+ channels in both apical and basolateral membranes. Mineralocorticoid hormone action occurs in several serial steps summarized in Fig. 28B. They include binding of aldosterone (A) to cytoplasmic receptors to form the aldosterone-receptor complex (RA), activation of the gene to initiate transcription, synthesis of new aldosterone-induced proteins (AIPs), and actions on apical and basolateral transport

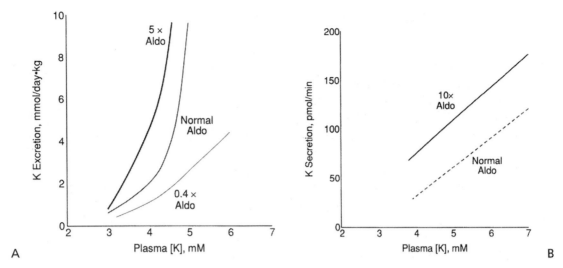

FIGURE 27   The relation between plasma K⁺ concentration and renal K⁺ excretion (**A**) (from ref. 415), and distal K⁺ secretion (**B**) (from ref. 416) is affected by circulating aldosterone. Effects of increased and decreased aldosterone are shown with respect to normal levels.

operations. This process can be divided into early and late phases.

In the *early* phase, mineralocorticoids activate the apical sodium conductance and thus stimulate sodium entry. With this increase in sodium entry and cell sodium activity, the basolateral pump turnover increases and potassium secretion rises (99, 228, 335, 376, 377, 381). It has also been shown that enhanced sodium entry per se leads to rapid

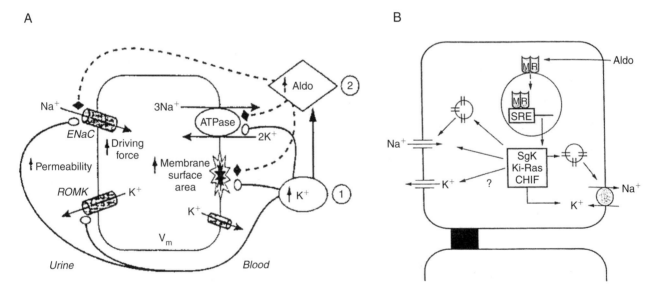

FIGURE 28   **A:** Factors involved in the regulation of K⁺ transport by aldosterone and peritubular K⁺. (*1*) Changes in peritubular K⁺ increase apical K⁺ and Na⁺ channel activity, stimulate Na⁺,K⁺-ATPase activity, and augment the basolateral membrane area. High K⁺ also activates the release of aldosterone. (*2*) Changes in aldosterone stimulate apical Na channels but enhance K⁺ channel activity only during chronic hyperkalemia. Similar to high K⁺, aldosterone stimulates Na⁺,K⁺-ATPase activity and increases the basolateral membrane area and Na⁺,K⁺-ATPase activity. (From Giebisch G. A trail of research on potassium. *Kidney Int* 2002;62:1498–1512, courtesy of S. Hebert.) **B:** Simplified summary of the early genomic effects of aldosterone (Aldo) on mechanisms of Na⁺ and K⁺ transport in collecting duct principle cells. Aldosterone binds the mineralocorticoid receptor (MR), and the complex interacts directly with genomic DNA via a steroid response element (SRE). *Trans*-activation of gene expression leads to transcription of the aldosterone-induced proteins SgK (serum and glucocorticoid-inducible kinase), Ki-Ras (Kirsten-Ras), and CHIF (corticosteroid hormone-induced factor). These proteins increase the activity of Na⁺,K⁺-ATPase by increasing pump turnover and recruiting latent ATPase to the basolateral membrane. Similarly, increased permeability of the apical membrane to Na⁺ may relate to both direct effects on existing channels and insertion of channel-laden vesicles. Aldosterone also increases the permeability of the apical membrane to K⁺. Whether this process reflects a direct action of an early-response protein on ROMK or an indirect effect of increased Na⁺ reabsorption is uncertain. During the late phase of aldosterone action (>6 hours), expression of the transport proteins themselves is increased. (From Booth RE, Johnson JP, Stockand JD. Aldosterone. *Adv Physiol Educ* 2002;26:8–20, with permission.)

insertion of Na⁺,K⁺-ATPase units into the basolateral membrane from an enzyme pool whose magnitude depends on the pre-existing aldosterone levels (25, 26, 54, 153, 309, 438, 472). Thus, the acute effects of aldosterone include significant stimulation of Na⁺,K⁺-ATPase. These early phase effects on Na⁺-K⁺ exchange involve an increase in pump activity with insertion of additional pump units (99, 228). Continued exposure to elevated mineralocorticoid levels results in *late*-phase changes including an additional increase in both potassium and sodium transport rates, insertion of additional basolateral Na-K pump units, and further enhancement of the apical sodium and potassium conductances (240, 276, 332, 333, 376, 377, 469).

The electrophysiological consequences of chronic mineralocorticoid administration are shown in Fig. 29. The basolateral membrane voltage may hyperpolarize and the direction of passive potassium transport reverses (240, 377). The mineralocorticoid-induced increase in the basolateral electrogenic Na⁺-K⁺ exchange and basolateral potassium conductance (which is strongly inward-rectifying) account for the rise of the membrane potential *above* the potassium equilibrium potential. The increase in membrane voltage provides a driving force for potassium uptake into principle cells. This sequence of events suppresses the backflux of potassium from cell to peritubular fluid and increases the efficiency of potassium secretion.

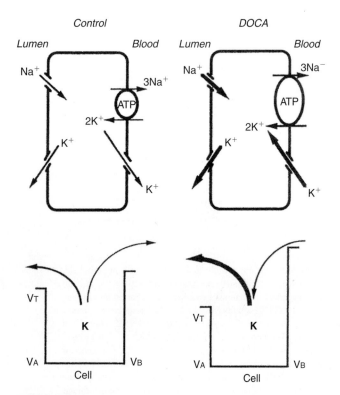

FIGURE 29   Schema of cortical collecting tubule cell with key site of potassium transport. Depending on the magnitude of the electrical potential difference across the basolateral cell membrane, potassium ions may either leave the cell (recycle) **(top)** or be taken up into the cell in parallel with pump-mediated potassium transport **(bottom)**.

Measurements of cell potassium levels in tubules harvested from chronically mineralocorticoid-treated animals do not show an increase in cell potassium content or activity (377). This observation attests to the precise adjustments of basolateral pump activity to apical potassium conductance. Possible mechanisms of this interaction between basolateral and apical transport mechanisms could be activated are mineralocorticoid-induced changes in cell ATP, Ca⁺⁺ and pH levels. Were the stimulation of basolateral Na⁺-K⁺ exchange to reduce cell ATP concentrations, apical potassium channels would be released from inhibition. Such a mechanism has been demonstrated in the proximal tubule (512). It is also possible that aldosterone activates basolateral Na-H exchange, alkalinizes the cytoplasm, and activates the apical secretory potassium channels. Principle cells have been observed to extrude hydrogen ions across the basolateral membrane by Na-H exchange (73), and because aldosterone accelerates Na-H exchange in cells of the diluting segment (318, 325), this mechanism is an attractive possibility. Finally, cell Ca⁺⁺ changes could also be involved owing to the effects of pump-induced alterations of cell sodium concentrations that affect Na⁺-Ca⁺⁺ exchange (440).

Sodium ions importantly modify the stimulating effect of mineralocorticoids on potassium secretion. Thus, the kaliuretic effect of chronic DOC treatment is effectively abolished by a low-sodium diet and is amplified by a high-sodium intake (399). Studies on single cortical collecting tubules have confirmed the importance of an intact apical sodium entry mechanism and an adequate lumen sodium supply for the full stimulation of Na⁺,K⁺-ATPase activity that follows mineralocorticoid administration (285, 474, 475). As pointed out above, switching from a low- to a high-sodium environment induces a rapid increase of ATPase activity (25, 26, 83). This prompt activation is consistent with a permissive role for Na ions in mineralocorticoid action mediated by the stimulating effect of sodium to insert pump units from a latent cytoplasmic pool into the basolateral membrane. Such experiments have shown that raising intracellular sodium concentrations enhances the cell surface expression of Na,K-ATPase α subunit in mammalian cortical collecting duct principle cells. This process involves cAMP-dependent and cAMP-independent pathways (25, 26, 54, 153, 438, 472). Moreover, such activation of Na,K-ATPase is modulated by aldosterone, since cortical collecting ducts from aldosterone-depleted animals have a greatly diminished response to the change in ambient sodium, implying that the size of the cell sodium pool is strongly influenced by mineralocorticoids. In tubules from DOC-treated animals, amiloride significantly attenuates pump stimulation (332, 377). These results support the view that apical sodium entry into principle cells is necessary to allow full expression of mineralocorticoid stimulation of Na⁺,K⁺-ATPase activity.

The efficacy of aldosterone-induced kaliuresis is also affected by urine flow rate (121, 123). Microperfusion experiments have shown that direct effects of aldosterone on potassium transport are modified by simultaneous modulation or urine flow rate. Thus, even when aldosterone enhances potassium secretion in perfused single distal tubules, the antidiuretic effect of aldosterone may result in a decline of urinary potassium excretion. On the other hand, dexamethasone does not increase potassium secretion in tubules perfused at a constant rate, but elicits kaliuresis through its effect on enhancing urine flow rate (121–123).

It has been shown that aldosterone may act on renal distal nephron ion transport in less than 10 minutes by a short-term mechanism that starts action, which is not affected by actinomycin D or spironolactones and thus independent of protein synthesis (58, 298, 470). This nongenomic effect of aldosterone does not involve action on the cell nucleus and the transcription and translation processes. The initial data on the nongenomic effect of aldosterone demonstrated primarily stimulation of Na^+-H^+ exchange. These effects are thought to be mediated by membrane receptors for aldosterone. Membrane binding sites of very low (0.1 nM) dissociation constant (kd) for aldosterone, which modulated Na^+-H^+ exchange were first described in human polymorphonuclear leucocytes. Such sites had no affinity for dexamethasone, corticosterone, ouabain, amiloride, and 18-hydroxyprogesterone (140, 505). Similar receptors for aldosterone were also found in pig kidney, but these had higher values of kd for desoxycorticosterone acetate and corticosterone (75). These membrane receptors are different from the classical cytoplasmic mineralocorticoid receptors (MRs), since MR knockout mice still display the nongenomic effect of aldosterone (174). Activation of the nongenomic mechanism via membrane receptors includes a signaling path involving G protein, inositol triphosphate, Ca^{2+} and protein kinase C, as well as MAP-Kinase (140, 276, 470). It has been demonstrated that current through epithelial sodium channels (ENaCs) of isolated rabbit cortical collecting duct principle cells are stimulated by nongenomic action of aldosterone (550). Inasmuch as these nongenomic actions involve apical sodium channels, they could also have significant indirect effects on potassium secretion.

Also occurring in the late phase of mineralocorticoid administration are significant morphological changes in principle cells (411, 418, 420, 474, 475). Mineralocorticoids have a direct effect on basolateral membrane amplification independent of changes in potassium balance and plasma potassium levels (410). Sodium ions are required for full mineralocorticoid effects: morphological changes fail to develop fully during administration of a low-sodium diet (418). In contrast to the changes observed in principle and connecting tubule cells, significant changes in basolateral membrane area fail to occur in *intercalated* cells during either diet- or hormone-induced stimulation of tubular potassium secretion (313, 409, 420).

The effects of *glucocorticoids* on potassium transport in the distal nephron are indirect and depend on increased flow rate past those tubule segments endowed with the ability to secrete potassium ions (46, 120–123). No direct effect of glucocorticoids has been seen when tubules are perfused at a constant flow rate (123). It is thought that glucocorticoids act by enhancing flow rate—increasing glomerular filtration rate (29, 30) and decreasing the water permeability of distal tubules (121)—and thus indirectly increase potassium excretion.

Attention should be drawn to an important mechanism that regulates the interaction between gluco- and mineralocorticoids in principle cells. Target specificity of aldosterone receptors is strongly modulated by the activity of the enzyme 11-β-hydroxysteroid-dehydrogenase, type 2 (11β-HSD2). The enzyme degrades cortisol, but not aldosterone to inactive metabolites. Thereby, it protects the fairly unspecific aldosterone receptor from being flooded by the relatively high cortisol concentrations (119, 135). Micropuncture studies have underscored the importance of 11 β-HSD2 by demonstrating that inhibition of the enzyme increases distal tubule potassium secretion and sodium reabsorption (22, 50, 400). Inactivating mutations of the gene for 11 β-HSD2 have been shown to cause a clinical syndrome of apparent mineralocorticoids excess with sodium retention, hypertension and potassium depletion, and a mouse knockout model of the enzyme displays hypertension and hypokalemia (242, 426). It is also of interest that a high-potassium diet decreases the activity of 11β-HSD2. Thus, the augmented access of glucocorticoids to mineralocorticoid receptors may participate in the renal adaptation to dietary changes in potassium and sodium (443).

Salt and Water Balance

Potassium excretion generally changes in association with changes in sodium excretion. On one hand, interventions that increase salt and water excretion—high-salt intake, extracellular volume expansion, saline infusion, administration of diuretics acting upstream of the initial collecting tubule, and infusion of sodium salts of poorly reabsorbable anions—all stimulate potassium excretion (16, 53, 144, 145, 151, 192, 236, 361, 415, 463, 466–468, 533, 534). On the other hand, maneuvers that diminish sodium excretion—rapid reduction of glomerular filtration rate, sodium depletion, and volume contraction—all decrease potassium excretion. It is thus well established that distal secretion of potassium depends importantly on the delivery of sodium and tubule fluid to the sites of potassium secretion.

Fig. 30 illustrates the effect of different levels of sodium intake on the steady-state relationship between plasma potassium and urinary potassium excretion at clamped aldosterone levels (542). Potassium excretion at a given plasma K^+ level is stimulated by augmenting sodium intake. A given rate of potassium excretion occurs at lower plasma potassium levels when sodium intake is elevated. This enhancement of potassium excretion is thought to depend on increased delivery of fluid and sodium into the distal tubule and CCD.

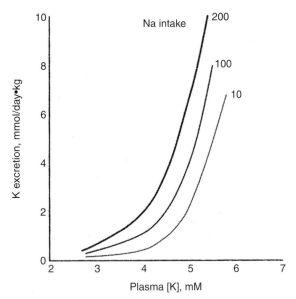

FIGURE 30 The relation between plasma K⁺ concentration and renal K⁺ excretion is affected by dietary Na intake. (From Young DB, Jackson TE, Tipayamontri U, et al. Effects of sodium intake on steady-state potassium excretion. *Am J Physiol Renal* 1984;246:F772–F778, with permission.)

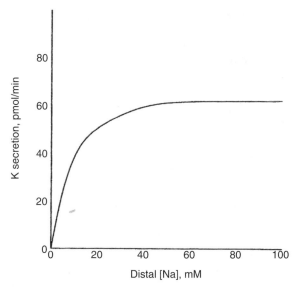

FIGURE 32 Distal K⁺ secretion requires that luminal Na⁺ concentration exceed approximately 25 to 35 mM (From Good DW, Wright FS. Luminal influences of potassium secretion: sodium concentration and fluid flow rate. *Am J Physiol Renal* 1979;236:F192–F205, with permission.)

Studies on single tubules, using micropuncture (236, 247) and microperfusion (117, 154, 155, 278) techniques, have confirmed that tubule fluid flow rate and luminal sodium concentration independently affect potassium secretion. Figures 31 and 32 summarize the effects of flow rate and of tubule fluid sodium concentrations on potassium secretion along the distal tubule. Increasing the flow rate of fluid delivered to the distal tubule invariably stimulates potassium secretion. For a given flow rate, potassium secretion is augmented in animals with a high-potassium intake (236, 278)

or after mineralocorticoid administration (123, 183); it is decreased in animals on a low-potassium diet (236).

Two separate mechanisms underlie the increase of distal potassium secretion with enhanced flow rate (415). The first involves linkage between sodium absorption and potassium secretion. Increasing luminal sodium concentration augments sodium absorption (234), and potassium secretion is stimulated by accelerated turnover of the normally unsaturated basolateral Na⁺,K⁺-ATPase. This view is based on the following observations: (1) Increasing fluid delivery into the distal tubule usually increases the sodium concentration in the lumen, depolarizes the apical cell membrane, and thus creates a more favorable electrochemical gradient for potassium secretion. This effect is of greatest importance when luminal Na concentration shifts from low to high levels (117, 155, 278, 433). (2) Enhanced sodium entry from the lumen into principle cells during augmented delivery of fluid also stimulates the basolateral Na,K-ATPase and accelerates potassium translocation into cells from the peritubular fluid. Thus, as long as basolateral pump activity is able to respond to increased lumen delivery of sodium with increased Na⁺-K⁺ exchange, potassium secretion continues at a high enough rate to either prevent (in the lower range of lumen flow rates) or to curtail (in the higher range of lumen flow rates) a decline of the concentration of potassium in the tubule lumen. If potassium concentrations decline less than flow rate increases, potassium secretion rates increase. Experimental conditions in which lumen potassium concentrations remain constant during diuretic conditions (192), and in which the concentration difference between cell interior and lumen remain unaltered despite marked stimulation of potassium secretion (see Table 24 in ref. 415), underscore the importance

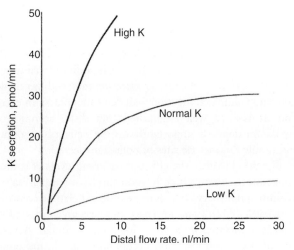

FIGURE 31 The relation between flow rate of tubule fluid in distal tubule and distal K⁺ secretion is affected by dietary K⁺ intake: normal K⁺ diet; low-K⁺ diet; high-K⁺ diet. (From Khuri RN, Wiederholt M, Strieder N, et al. Effects of flow rate and potassium intake on distal tubular potassium transfer. *Am J Physiol Renal* 1975;228:1249–1261, with permission.)

of accelerated and coupled potassium and sodium transport. By "clamping" the potassium concentration in the lumen to fairly constant levels over the range of low physiological levels (~5 nl/min), the connecting and collecting tubule emerges as the major control site of potassium excretion (415).

A second mechanism that links changes in luminal flow to distal K$^+$ secretion is a flow-dependent fall of lumen potassium concentration with increasing delivery of fluid to the distal tubule (155). Evidence from microperfusion studies shows that potassium secretion may rise with flow rate in association with decreasing potassium concentration in the lumen (155). The flow-dependent increase of the potassium concentration gradient across the apical cell membrane provides an increased driving force for potassium secretion. This mechanism linking potassium secretion to flow rate is able to increase potassium secretion under conditions in which increased sodium delivery into the distal tubule fails to stimulate basolateral sodium and potassium exchange. Diminished apical sodium uptake and low lumen potassium concentrations would be expected to hyperpolarize the apical membrane potential and thus tend to reduce the electrochemical driving force favoring potassium secretion. It appears safe to conclude that the functional state of the basolateral Na$^+$,K$^+$-ATPase transport system determines the extent to which increased fluid delivery is able to stimulate potassium secretion.

Although apical sodium channels are a key pathway for entry of sodium into principle cells, potassium excretion appears not to be entirely dependent on apical sodium supply. Animals maintained on a low-sodium diet do respond with kaliuresis to acute potassium loading (350), and potassium excretion increases in animals given amiloride, a potent apical sodium channel blocker (537). Moreover, humans very well tolerate a diet high in potassium and low in sodium (329). An explanation for the apparent dissociation between apical sodium supply and maintained ability for potassium secretion may be the presence of at least two additional sodium entry pathways in principle tubule cells. These are located in the basolateral membrane and include sodium-hydrogen and sodium-calcium exchange (73, 440). Activity of these basolateral entry pathways may, at least in part, replace apical sodium supply and maintain potassium secretion under conditions of low distal fluid and sodium delivery, especially under conditions of elevated levels of plasma potassium (142).

The ability of the distal tubule and cortical collecting duct to maintain a fairly constant potassium concentration in the lumen over the physiological range of flow rates has two important consequences. First, the marked flow dependence of potassium secretion in the distal tubule and CCD endows the process of potassium secretion with great sensitivity to changes in the delivery of sodium and fluid. This tubule segment is thus responsible for the enhanced rate of potassium excretion that follows inhibition of sodium and fluid reabsorption upstream of the distal tubule and collecting duct (192) (see Diuretics section). Second, the ability of the distal nephron segments to "clamp" the potassium concentration has implications for the physiological importance of those components of potassium secretion that occur upstream during potassium recycling. Potassium secreted upstream of the initial collecting tubule determines the amount of potassium secreted along the distal convoluted and initial collecting tubule as the tubule fluid approaches the "late" distal tubule epithelium. Hence, with stimulation of medullary potassium recycling, the concentration of potassium in the early distal tubule rises and approaches the clamped concentration of the initial collecting tubule. A smaller fraction of excreted potassium is then contributed by distal secretion. Conversely, when medullary recycling of potassium is minimal and the concentration of potassium in the fluid entering the distal tubule is low, a larger fraction of excreted potassium has to be secreted by the distal tubule and the CCD. A noninvasive method for evaluation of the transtubule gradient of potassium in the cortical collecting duct ("cortical distal nephron") has been described (514, 515). Such estimates have been used to evaluate in patients the effects of hormones, diuretics, and acid-base disturbances. The method allows distinction between modulation of urine potassium excretion by changes in either flow rate and/or alteration brought about by direct effects on potassium secretion in principle tubule cells. This approach has also shown that urea recycling, by enhancing flow rate in the cortical collecting tubule, provides a mechanism for aiding potassium excretion (171).

Chronic enhancement of sodium delivery into the distal nephron, for instance, during treatment with loop diuretics, leads to both functional and morphological adjustments in the downstream tubule segments. These changes involve increased capacity for sodium absorption and potassium secretion, and marked basolateral membrane amplification, in cells of the distal convoluted, connecting, and initial collecting tubules (83, 113, 223, 256, 258, 408, 420). Prolonged increased entry of sodium into cells of the distal tubule must be responsible for transport stimulation because the functional and morphological changes persist when plasma aldosterone, vasopressin, and potassium are held constant (408). Increased transport in collecting duct segments following treatment with diuretics that act on the loop of Henle or the distal convoluted tubule may curtail sodium excretion as well as promote potassium secretion (305). An increase in amiloride-sensitive potassium secretion has been observed following uninephrectomy, and is linked to an initial increase in plasma potassium concentration and increased distal tubule fluid delivery (6).

Nonchloride sodium salts also affect urinary potassium excretion. Thus, the kaliuretic effects of sulfate, phosphate, and bicarbonate are well established (23). Prolonged fasting and the enhanced excretion of short-chain fatty acids and organic acid radicals also promote potassium loss (226, 261). Interestingly, infusion of sodium bicarbonate is more kaliuretic than similar amounts of sulfate (70). It is generally assumed that the stimulating effect of poorly reabsorbable anions on potassium secretion is mediated by their effects on the lumen-negative potential (76, 280). Although there is evidence that the transepithelial potential difference effectively alters potassium secretion (138), it is unlikely that the effects of poorly reabsorbable anions are solely mediated by changing the transepithelial potential, because sulfate-induced enhancement has been shown to continue in the presence of effective blockade of sodium and potassium channels (464). This suggests that stimulation of potassium secretion in the presence of sulfate is mediated by low tubule chloride which stimulates electroneutral potassium chloride cotransport (464). Perfusion studies also provide support for the notion that lumen alkalinization and bicarbonate directly stimulate potassium secretion through augmenting potassium chloride cotransport (10).

Acid-Base Balance

Acid-base derangements have long been known to affect the excretion of potassium, and losses of potassium, particularly in states of alkalosis, are well documented (41, 43, 44, 141, 148, 150–152, 279, 283). Figure 33 shows the striking dependence of renal potassium excretion and distal potassium secretion on blood pH (414, 415). It is apparent that alkalosis stimulates and acidosis depresses potassium excretion.

Clearance, stop-flow, micropuncture, and microperfusion studies indicate that the distal tubule and cortical collecting duct are the main nephron sites where acid-base changes affect potassium secretion. The right-side panel of Fig. 33 shows results of a microperfusion study in which tubule flow rate and solute composition of luminal fluid were kept constant. Metabolic acidosis, produced by gavage of 3 to 4 mmol NH₄Cl 1 hour before the measurements, caused distal potassium secretion to decrease. Metabolic alkalosis, produced by intravenous infusion of 3 to 4 mmol sodium bicarbonate 1 hour before the measurements, caused distal potassium secretion to increase. Direct effects of acid-base disorders on potassium transport in these nephron segments can be distinguished from indirect effects that include changes of (1) distal flow rate, (2) composition of fluid reaching the distal tubule, and (3) aldosterone levels (414). Changes in plasma potassium cannot be held directly responsible for acid-base–related changes in potassium excretion because hyperkalemia is frequently associated with acidosis, whereas hypokalemia is commonly observed in alkalosis (2, 43, 141, 279).

The direct effects of acid-base disorders, summarized in Fig. 34, involve modifications of both basolateral and apical transport functions. With regards to the *basolateral* membrane, alkalosis stimulates active potassium uptake (92) and increases the permeability to potassium ions Acidosis has the opposite effect, including direct inhibition of basolateral Na⁺,K⁺-ATPase activity (314). The permeability increase in alkalosis shifts the membrane potential close toward the potassium equilibrium potential and minimizes potassium loss from cells into the peritubular fluid. Acid-base–related changes in the *apical* cell membrane are also observed and involve a striking sensitivity of both potassium and sodium channel activity upon cytosolic pH (439). Over a narrow and physiological intracellular pH range, acidosis (pH 7.0) suppresses and alkalosis (pH 7.4) stimulates sodium and potassium channel activity (180, 181, 346, 491). Figure 35 shows relevant results (491). Summarized is the relation between channel open probability and cytosolic pH of the low-conductance apical potassium channel. Patch-clamp studies have also demonstrated that the inhibition of apical ROMK channels by ATP is enhanced after lowering cytosolic pH (291). Alkalosis has the opposite effect; it increases

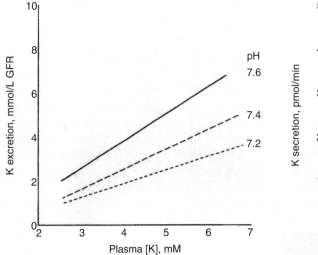

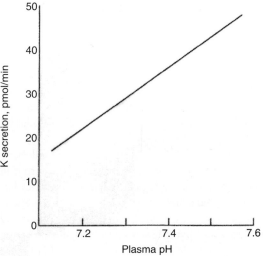

FIGURE 33   **A:** The relation between plasma K⁺ concentration and renal K1 excretion is affected by plasma pH. (From Stanton BA, Giebisch G. Renal potassium transport. In: Windhager EE, ed. *Handbook of Physiology: Renal Physiology.* New York: Oxford University Press; 1991;813–874, with permission.) **B:** Distal K⁺ secretion is affected by plasma pH. (From Stanton BA, Giebisch G. Effects of pH on potassium transport by renal distal tubule. *Am J Physiol Renal* 1982;242:F544–F551, with permission.)

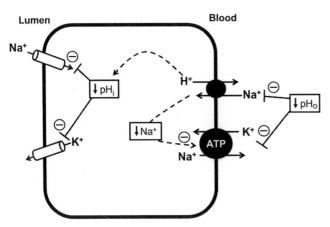

FIGURE 34   Cell model of the effects of metabolic acidosis on apical cell basolateral potassium transport.

open probability and causes insertion of additional potassium channels. It has also been shown that potassium channels in the frog's early distal tubule are activated during alkalinization by the appearance of new potassium channels in the apical membrane (199).

Additional stimuli modulating potassium secretion in acid-base disturbances involve the delivery in metabolic alkalosis of tubule fluid with high bicarbonate and low chloride concentrations to the distal nephron. Several effects are noteworthy: bicarbonate and other poorly permeant anions act as osmotic diuretics and increase distal tubule flow rate, and low lumen chloride concentration stimulates neutral

K-Cl secretion across the apical membrane in distal convoluted and principle cells (114, 462, 464). It has also been shown that bicarbonate ions appear to activate potassium excretion directly (10, 70, 261). Figure 36 shows results of in vivo microperfusion experiments in which luminal chloride was replaced with sulfate Reducing luminal Cl^- concentration below 20 mM stimulates potassium secretion into the distal tubule without changing the transepithelial voltage. Unidirectional flux measurements show that the increase in K^+ secretion occurs because the cell to lumen flux is enhanced. This enhanced secretory flux is not blocked by barium in the lumen (114).

The effects of acid-base changes on potassium reabsorption should also be mentioned. Potassium transport across the outer medullary collecting duct is affected by changes in electrogenic hydrogen ion transport. Acidosis enhances electrogenic hydrogen pumping and tends to increase the lumen-positive potential, whereas alkalosis has the opposite effect. Passive potassium reabsorption would thus be increased during acidosis and depressed in alkalosis. Independent of these indirect effects, metabolic acidosis has been shown to stimulate the activity of the apical K^+,H^+-ATPase in isolated rabbit CCDs (404).

The effects on potassium excretion of metabolic acidosis depend on the duration of the acid-base disturbance. When flow rate along single distal tubules is kept constant, acidosis depresses potassium secretion (414), but in free-flow conditions in intact tubules, potassium secretion may rise as a consequence of increased fluid flow rate thought to result from inhibition of proximal transport during acidosis (16,

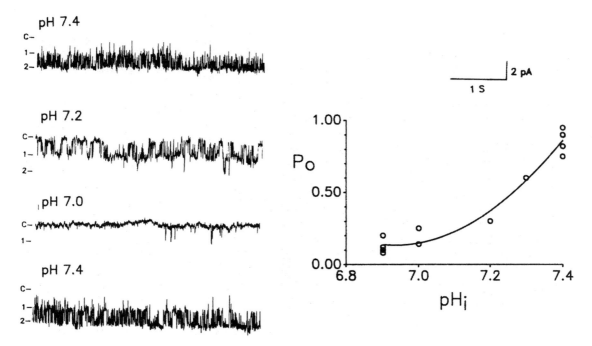

FIGURE 35   **Left:** Effect of changes in cytosolic pH or K^+ channel activity in principle tubule cell. Closed states are indicated by C. **Right:** Relationship between intracellular pH (pH$_i$) and open probability of channel (P$_o$). Note the high sensitivity of open probability of the K^+ channel to pH in the range 7.0 to 7.4. (From Wang W, Geibel J, Giebisch G. Regulation of the small conductance K channels in the apical membrane of rat cortical collecting tubule. *Am J Physiol Renal* 1990;259:F494–F502, with permission.)

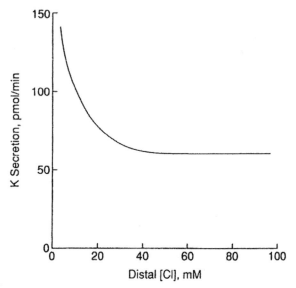

FIGURE 36   Distal K$^+$ secretion is inhibited by presence of Cl$^-$ in the tubule lumen and is stimulated when Cl$^-$ concentration falls below 20 mM. (From Velazquez H, Ellison DH, Wright FS. Chloride-dependent potassium secretion in early and late distal tubules. *Am J Physiol Renal* 1987;253: F555–562, with permission.)

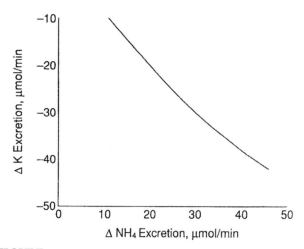

FIGURE 37   Changes in renal potassium excretion are negatively correlated with changes in ammonium excretion. (From Tannen RL. Effect of potassium on renal acidification and acid-base homeostasis. *Semin Nephrol* 1987;7:263–272; and Tannen RL. Potassium and acid-base balance. In: Giebisch G, ed. *Current Topics in Membranes and Transport*, Vol 28. Orlando, FL: Academic Press; 1987:207–223, with permission.)

415). Such an increase in distal fluid and sodium delivery stimulate potassium secretion during loading with ammonium chloride, in diabetic acidosis and in proximal tubular acidosis. Taken together, it is clear that the effects of acid-base disturbances on potassium excretion are mediated by two major components, direct effects related to pH and secondary effects having to do with modification of the rate of distal tubule flow and its composition, with aldosterone release and acid-base–induced changes in ammonium metabolism.

Changes of aldosterone secretion also play a significant role in modulating kaliuresis during chronic metabolic acidosis. Evidence supporting the view that elevated hormone levels, possibly related to extracellular volume depletion, contribute importantly to potassium loss during chronic metabolic acidosis supports observations that potassium excretion is reduced in acidosis when aldosterone levels are not allowed to increase (415).

Renal production of ammonium is important not only to renal acid excretion, and therefore to maintenance of acid-base balance, but also to renal potassium excretion. Tannen has drawn attention to the inverse relationship between urinary potassium and ammonium excretion shown in Fig. 37 (441, 442). Studies in in vivo and isolated perfused kidneys have demonstrated that potassium excretion is depressed when ammonium excretion is enhanced, an effect that has been localized in micropuncture studies to tubule sites beyond the initial collecting tubule (207). Studies of isolated perfused kidneys have excluded systemic acid-base and endocrine factors (78). The cell mechanism of the inhibitory effect of ammonium on potassium excretion is not known. It is possible that competition between potassium and ammo-

nium at the potassium binding site of the Na$^+$,K$^+$-ATPase in the basolateral membrane of principle tubule cells is involved (476-479).

Other Hormones

VASOPRESSIN

Vasopressin stimulates the secretion of potassium ions across the distal tubule (124) and cortical collecting duct (121, 124, 383, 384, 392, 393, 445). In vivo perfusion studies and electrophysiological exploration of the cell mechanisms underlying the action of vasopressin on potassium transport in principle cells indicate that activation of potassium secretion is caused by an increase of the apical sodium permeability. Apical membrane depolarization and basolateral pump activation follow and promote enhanced potassium entry into the tubule lumen (391–393). Besides this effect on the driving force of potassium, patch-clamp studies have shown that vasopressin also increases the density of potassium channels in the apical membrane of principle tubule cells (71). The effects of vasopressin on potassium secretion in cortical collecting ducts are sharply augmented by mineralocorticoid pretreatment (383).

It has also been shown that luminal vasopressin has the ability to stimulate K$^+$ secretion via activation of V1 receptors (11). This luminal effect of vasopressin differs from the basolateral action of vasopressin by not involving cyclic AMP-PKA but, as shown in Fig. 38, the phospholipase-IP3, Ca-PKC signaling pathway. A key role of Ca was established by showing that chelators such as Bapta abolished the luminal effects of vasopressin (12). These observations strongly suggest that Ca^{2+}-sensitive maxi-potassium channels mediate the luminal effects of vasopressin. In contrast,

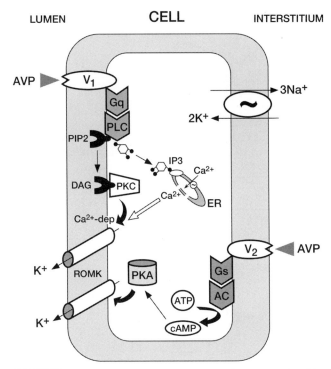

FIGURE 38 Signaling mechanisms of luminal (V1 receptors) and basolateral (V2 receptors) action of AVP (arginine vasopressin). PLC, phospholipase C; ER, endoplasmic reticulum. (From Amorim JB, Musa-Aziz R, Mello-Aires M, Malnic G. Signaling path of the action of AVP on distal K⁺ secretion. *Kidney Int* 2004;66:696–704, with permission.)

the basolateral effects of vasopressin are due to stimulation of V2 receptors and involve modulation of ROMK channels (71). The inhibitory effects on potassium secretion of angiotensin and prostaglandins are similarly mediated by the phospholipase A–arachidonic acid pathway (181).

Catecholamines and Glucagon

Both α- and β-adrenergic agonists affect potassium transport by distal nephron segments. Care must be taken, however, to distinguish direct tubule effects from extrarenal effects because epinephrine activates potassium uptake in liver and muscle and lowers plasma potassium levels (45, 47, 89, 91). Nevertheless, when plasma potassium levels are prevented from declining after epinephrine administration by infusion of potassium-containing fluids, renal potassium excretion still falls. The epinephrine effect to suppress potassium secretion, or to enhance potassium reabsorption, has been localized to nephron sites beyond the initial collecting tubule (91). Treatment with adrenergic agonists has been shown to reduce the lumen-negative voltage and chloride absorption in cortical collecting ducts (215).

Insulin

This hormone plays an important role in the regulation of extrarenal potassium homeostasis (45, 90), and its renal effects are modest and complex. Insulin administration has been observed to reduce potassium excretion (90), but

the role of changes of plasma potassium and other hormone levels have proved difficult to control. In one clearance study, in which efforts were made to maintain constant potassium levels in the blood, insulin modestly increased potassium excretion (368). In contrast, in another microperfusion study of isolated CCDs, insulin reduced potassium secretion (136). *Glucagon* has also been shown to have a significant effect on potassium excretion. Its infusion induces a prompt increase in potassium excretion, and it has been suggested that the enhanced excretion of potassium following food intake may be related to glucagon release (3).

Diuretics

Diuretic drugs, used primarily to promote excretion of salt and water, also affect renal potassium excretion (116, 145, 148, 152, 192, 306, 364, 463, 466–468). Study of diuretic actions has provided important information concerning potassium transport mechanisms. Figure 39 illustrates the primary renal sites of action of compounds representative of three classes of diuretic drugs that act from the luminal side of tubule cells (364). Loop diuretics, such as furosemide, act mainly on the Na-K-2Cl cotransporter in the apical membrane of thick ascending limb cells (67–69, 161, 165, 387). Thiazide diuretics have their primary action on an Na-Cl cotransporter in cells of the distal convoluted tubule (81, 468). Loop and thiazide diuretics are both capable of increasing potassium excretion. Potassium-sparing diuretics, exemplified by amiloride and triamterene, block Na channels in principle cells of the ICT and CCD (20, 104, 190, 330).

Because renal potassium excretion depends primarily on secretion by principle cells in the CNT, ICT, and CCD, the action of amiloride can be considered to be direct in the sense that it targets these cells. The diffusion of Na ions from lumen to cell through the Na-selective channels of principle cells depolarizes the apical membrane and creates a favorable electrochemical driving force for K⁺ secretion. Amiloride blockade of these channels increases the cell-negative voltage across the apical membrane and opposes K⁺ secretion. These changes in apical membrane voltage are reflected in opposite changes in the lumen-negative transepithelial voltage: amiloride blockade decreases the transepithelial potential difference. Luminal Ca²⁺ also blocks Na channels and has similar inhibitory effects on potassium secretion (327, 328).

Loop diuretics increase renal K⁺ excretion, in part by direct effects on TAL cells, and also by secondary effects on principle cells in the CNT, ICT and CCD. Furosemide inhibition of the Na-K-2Cl cotransporter leaves the cell to lumen flux through apical potassium channels unopposed, resulting in either greatly reduced K⁺ absorption or even reversal to produce net K⁺ secretion, along the TAL (161, 303, 451, 452). The inhibition of Na and Cl absorption in the TAL also reduces medullary interstitial

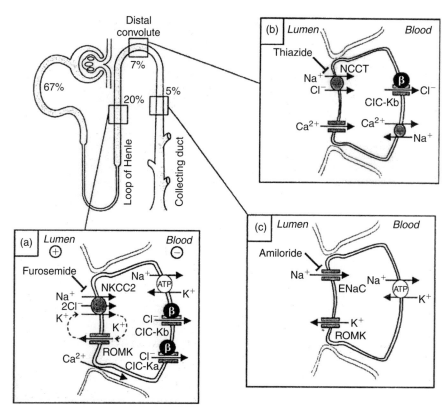

FIGURE 39   Distribution of NKCC2, ROMK, the ClC-β-subunit Barttin, ClC-Kb, and NCCT along the nephron and site of action of the classic diuretic agents (*a*) furosemide, (*b*) thiazide, and (*c*) amiloride. (From Reinalter SC, Jeck N, Peters M, Seyberth HW. Pharmacotyping of hypokalaemic salt-losing tubular disorders. *Acta Physiol Scand* 2004;181:513–521, with permission.)

osmolality and results in decreased fluid absorption along the descending limb. Thus, loop diuretics not only decrease potassium reabsorption in the thick ascending limb but, in addition, increase the rate of fluid delivery out of the loop of Henle and provide a flow-rate stimulus to K^+ secretion along the distal tubule and collecting duct (192, 236). It should be noted that different degrees of kaliuresis have been observed in animal studies with furosemide and piretanide. The latter is less potent in promoting loss of potassium owing to stimulation of bradykinin production which curtails sodium entry into collecting duct principle cells (66).

Thiazide diuretics also promote renal potassium excretion; however, they do not do so by their action on DCT cells. These cells supply a fraction of total K^+ excretion, apparently largely via an apical K-Cl cotransporter; however, the direct action of thiazides would be expected to reduce cell Cl concentration and would therefore serve to reduce chloride-dependent K^+ secretion (116, 463, 466, 468). Indeed, a decline in potassium excretion has been reported following the administration of thiazides during infusion of sodium sulfate which lowers the concentration of chloride and would thus upregulate potassium secretion by potassium-chloride cotransport (464, 466, 467). One likely explanation for the effect of thiazides to promote potassium excretion rather than diminish it focuses on the increase in distal sodium and fluid delivery through inhibition of sodium chloride cotransport. By inhibiting carbonic anhydrase-dependent sodium and bicarbonate reabsorption in the proximal tubule, thiazides also tend to increase the flow rate of fluid into the distal nephron (192).

Osmotic diuretics exert their kaliuretic action largely by increasing fluid and sodium delivery into the distal tubule following proximal tubule transport inhibition. Poorly permeant anions such as sulfate, phosphate bicarbonate, ferrocyanide and hippurate not only augment distal fluid and sodium delivery, but also facilitate potassium secretion by stimulating potassium-chloride cotransport because they lower the chloride concentration in the lumen (10, 115). It should be noted though that with increased fluid loads delivered to the distal nephron, larger fractions of potassium also enter the distal nephron. Additional mechanisms favoring potassium loss during administration of diuretic agents also involve hormonal effects. As extracellular volume shrinks owing to urinary loss of sodium chloride, aldosterone and vasopressin release stimulate potassium secretion.

Maturation of Potassium Transport

A condition essential for adequate growth is the effective conservation of potassium in the newborn (379, 380). Perfusion studies in rabbits show absence of potassium secretion during the first 3 weeks of life. An analysis of apical potassium channel activity in principle cells indicates reduced activity, whereas potassium reabsorption via H^+,K^+-ATPase exchange in intercalated cells is highly active (39, 79, 527). Potassium retention in the newborn is thus mediated by diminished or even absent potassium secretion and H^+,K^+-ATPase–mediated potassium absorption. Changes in the number of apical potassium channels play an important role in limiting potassium secretion in the neonatal kidney. Low GFR and low distal flow rates may be an additional component favoring potassium retention. The coordination of these factors contributes to the potassium retention that is characteristic of the neonatal kidney (380).

Circadian Rhythm

Renal potassium excretion varies during the 24-hour day (299, 300). Some of this variation occurs because of spacing between meals or other episodes of potassium intake. However, even when potassium ingestion is spread evenly throughout the day and night, a pattern of lower rates of K^+ excretion at night and in the morning, and higher rates in the afternoon emerges (299, 300, 357, 358). Figure 40 shows the response of human subjects to an intravenous K^+ load, given either starting at midnight or midday (301). The relation between plasma concentration and rate of renal K^+ excretion at different times of the day-night cycle is also summarized. It is apparent that the kaliuretic response was significantly diminished at night. Thus, higher concentrations of potassium were required at night to effect potassium excretion.

These daily fluctuations of K^+ excretion have not been fully explained. As with other circadian rhythms, the periodicity is related to the light-dark cycle and depends on a pacemaker in the central nervous system (299, 300). Also, it is likely that the changes in potassium excretion are produced by changes in distal secretion. It has been reported that changes in aldosterone are not required (357, 358, 359) but that the higher K^+ excretions during daytime may be related to enhanced bicarbonate loss in the urine (421).

Integrated Regulation of Potassium Homeostasis

Renal potassium excretion is regulated by multiple factors acting at several transport sites in response to influences originating outside the kidney. The final rate of excretion of potassium is determined by the net effect of mechanisms that may be cooperating or competing. In some situations the individual regulatory factors may act together, while in other cases they may change in directions that tend to cancel one another. Reasonable predictions of the rate of potassium excretion can be derived from knowledge of expected changes of individual factors (545).

Model calculations of tubule potassium transport have provided interesting insights between water and potassium transport. It was suggested that the increase in potassium concentration along both the water-permeable connecting and collecting tubule was not only mediated by net secretion

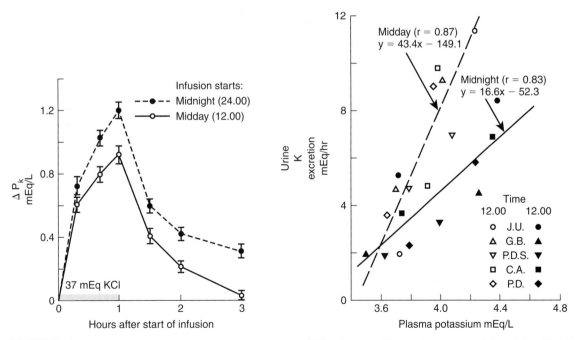

FIGURE 40   **Left:** Response of plasma potassium concentration (PK) in human subjects to intravenous infusion of 37 mEq of potassium chloride solution in 250 ml of water provided over 1 hour either starting at midnight (*dashed line*) or midday (*solid line*). **Right:** Relationship between plasma potassium concentration and rate of renal potassium excretion in human subject at midnight (*solid line*) or midday (*dashed line*). (From Moore-Ede MC. Physiology of the circadian timing system: predictive versus reactive homeostasis. *Am J Physiol* 1986;250:R735–R752, with permission.)

in principle cells, but also by vasopressin-dependent fluid equilibration (434, 435, 507, 508). Indeed, it becomes apparent that the final potassium concentration in both nephron segments may reach such high concentrations that they exceed the maximal transepithelial potassium gradient that can be achieved by potassium secretion in principle cells. As a consequence, both the CNT and CCD can become sites of modest, albeit significant, reabsorption of potassium. Calculations based on these cell models also allowed an assessment of the interactions between axial flow rate along the CNT and CCD, the sodium load, transepithelial potential difference and water permeability. It has also made possible an analysis of the factors leading to the typical kaliuresis produced by thiazides (508).

An example of *cooperative* factors modulating potassium transport is seen in the renal response to a high-potassium intake. As noted previously, the increase in plasma K^+ concentration promotes potassium uptake by potassium-secreting cells (92). It also stimulates the adrenal gland to secrete aldosterone (60, 103, 134), which in turn promotes potassium secretion by cells of the distal nephron. Increased plasma K^+ concentration also inhibits sodium and fluid reabsorption by the proximal tubule (61) and thus increases flow rate into the distal nephron.

Evidence of the involvement of such factors in response to a change in K^+ intake was also obtained in a careful study using human subjects (356). Dietary potassium was increased from 100 to 400 mmol/day. Renal potassium excretion progressively increased so that external K^+ balance was restored within 3 days. During the first 2 hours after each meal, plasma K^+ rose by approximately 0.5 mM and then subsided, returning to the normal range before the next meal. Plasma aldosterone also increased after meals. The changes in plasma aldosterone (from 400 to 900 pM) were proportionately larger than the 10% to 20% increase in plasma K^+. Evidence that distal flow and sodium delivery increased after meals as well came from the observation that sodium excretion increased from 50 to 200 μmol/min. Thus, the concerted actions of multiple regulatory mechanisms improve the defense against the danger of hyperkalemia.

The effectiveness of aldosterone to stimulate potassium secretion is modulated by SGK1 (serum- and glucocorticoid-regulated kinase-1; 504). This kinase affects several renal transport processes. Inspection of Fig. 41 shows that that the stimulation of apical sodium and potassium channels, as well as of basolateral Na^+,K^+-ATPase through aldosterone, involves participation of SGK (74, 250, 316). Formation of SGK is upregulated by aldosterone (182, 456), and coexpression experiments in heterologous expression systems of SGK with Na^+ or K^+ channels, and with Na^+,K^+-ATPase, indicates increased activity of these transporters. It is significant that the reabsorption of sodium and the secretion of potassium are impaired in SGK knockout mice (194). Impaired upregulation of urinary potassium excretion during chronic potassium loading was also demonstrated by maintenance of potassium balance, but at elevated aldosterone levels (194). SGK has been

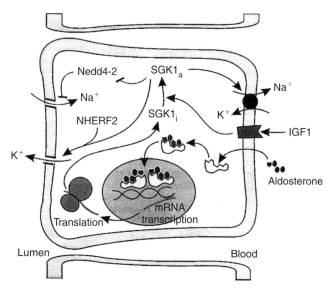

FIGURE 41   Role of SGK1 in the regulation of Na^+ reabsorption and K^+ secretion in principle cells of the collecting duct. Aldosterone stimulates the transcription and expression of SGK1. The inactive $SGK1_i$ requires activation to $SGK1_a$, e.g., by insulin-like growth factor (IGF)1. $SGK1_a$ then enhances the activity of the epithelial sodium channel (ENaC) and K^+ channel ROMK1 in the luminal cell membrane and of the Na^+,K^+ATPase in the basolateral cell membrane. The regulation of ENaC is accomplished by inhibition of the ubiquitin ligase Nedd4-2, the regulation of ROMK1 requires the cooperation with the Na^+-H^+ exchange regulating factor NHERF2. (From Vallon V, Wulff P, Huang DY, Loffing J, Völkl H, Kuhl D, Lang F. Role of Sgk1 in salt and potassium homeostasis. *Am J Physiol* 2004;288:R4–R10, with permission.)

shown to enhance abundance of ROMK in the membrane of oocytes, a process that also involves the cooperative effect of NHERF (Na-H exchange regulating factor). Increased activity of ROMK is also mediated by a significant shift in pH-sensitivity of the channel (250, 340).

Derangements in the regulation of aldosterone regulation can have important consequences concerning the maintenance of potassium balance. The hypokalemia that appears in primary hyperaldosteronism has long been recognized (141, 143). Experimental administration of excess mineralocorticoid hormone (DOC) or aldosterone produces the effects seen in patients with adrenal overproduction of aldosterone. Sodium excretion falls initially, but within a few days it then increases until balance between intake and output is restored. Plasma sodium concentration does not change; however, arterial blood pressure is increased. The "escape" from the sodium-retaining effect of mineralocorticoid excess has been attributed to inhibition of Na reabsorption by factors related to extracellular fluid volume expansion (170, 238), and thiazide-sensitive Na-Cl cotransport has been defined as the key tubule transport that is downregulated during mineralocorticoid escape (448, 499). In contrast to sodium, potassium excretion rises to levels exceeding K^+ intake, continues for a longer period, and results in hypokalemia. This continued stimulation of distal potassium secretion appears to be related to the same volume-related inhibition of sodium reabsorption that limits the period of sodium retention. Inhibition of proximal sodium and fluid absorption leads to increased distal delivery of sodium and fluid and therefore to a *flow-rate* stimulus to potassium secretion. Protective mechanisms, activated by the progressively increasing potassium depletion involves stimulation of potassium reabsorption by H^+,K^+-ATPase activation which progressively restrains further potassium loss.

It should be noted that some investigators are not satisfied that all stimuli acting to promote increased K^+ excretion have been identified. Rabinowitz and his coworkers have argued that increases in K^+ excretion after ingestion of potassium are not fully explained by changes in plasma K, circulating aldosterone, or distal delivery of fluid and sodium. It has also been suggested that sensors in the liver or the brain may be involved in regulating potassium homeostasis (5, 303a, 359). A hepatic potassium sensor would explain the observation that a potassium load given by infusion into the portal vein is more kaliuretic compared to the same amount of potassium injected intravenously into the systemic circulation (73a). Moreover, by restricting the initial rise of potassium to the hepatic circulation, kaliuresis could be induced without larger and potentially harmful fluctuations of potassium in the general circulation (73a, 303a). Hepatic afferent nerve activity has been reported to increase with potassium injection into the portal vein, but these mechanisms modulating potassium transport during different potassium intake need further exploration.

When potassium intake is restricted, reductions in plasma K^+ and circulating aldosterone withdraw the stimulus to potassium secretion and renal potassium excretion tends to fall. However, in some circumstances the integrated actions of all factors, because of competing priorities, fail to maintain potassium balance. For example, if potassium intake is being restricted along with other food because an individual has just undergone an abdominal operation, stress-related stimulation of aldosterone secretion may put high aldosterone levels in competition with low plasma K^+ levels and cause the rate of potassium excretion to exceed the rate of intake. Furthermore, if saline infusions are maintaining extracellular fluid volume and urine flow, a high flow rate of tubule fluid may further compromise the ability of the kidney to retain potassium.

In other circumstances, competition among the regulatory factors may actually serve the cause of potassium homeostasis. Changes in sodium intake are a relevant example. Although changes in sodium intake lead to changes in circulating aldosterone and extracellular fluid volume, they do not result in important deviations from potassium balance. Lack of sodium enhances proximal fluid reabsorption, may decrease distal flow rate and diminish potassium excretion. However, the simultaneous stimulation of the renin-angiotensin-aldosterone system acts to promote potassium excretion. Similarly, with deprivation of water alone, competition among regulatory factors may also act to stabilize potassium excretion. The potassium-retaining influence of low luminal flow rate is opposed by the stimulatory influence on potassium secretion of increased circulating vasopressin.

The relation between potassium secretion and sodium reabsorption is also affected by a family of protein kinases. They have been designated as WNK (owing to the absence of lysine in the kinase subdomain) and immunohistochemical studies demonstrated their predominant localization in the distal convoluted tubule and collecting ducts (219, 536). Functional studies of WNK4 have defined three interdependent mechanisms of action summarized in Fig. 42. These include inhibition of both the thiazide-sensitive NaCl cotransporter in the connecting tubule and the apical secretory ROMK channel in the apical membrane of principle cells (216, 219). In addition, WNK4 upregulates paracellular chloride permeability in MDCK cells, an in vitro distal tubule transport model (217). Presence of wildtype WNK4, by its inhibitory action upon Na-Cl cotransport, favors delivery of sodium to potassium-secretory nephron sites, yet the simultaneous inhibitory action upon ROMK activity provides a break on potassium secretion. Of interest are mutations of WINK4 in patients with hypertension and hyperkalemia: these are characterized by loss of function of WINK4, which stimulates sodium reabsorption. At the same time, these mutations of WNK4 lead to a gain of function of ROMK and interference of effective potassium secretion (218, 473). Moreover, the observed gain-of-function of paracellular chloride function further favors sodium retention. Taken together, these derangements of WNK4 function suggest its critical role in the genesis of pseudohyperaldosteronism type II (PHA-II) (57, 259, 520, 521).

Finally, in some acid-base disturbances, the net result of several influences on potassium secretion may cause the kidney to excrete potassium at rates exceeding potassium intake and thus to deplete body potassium. In metabolic alkalosis, plasma K^+ concentration tends to be low because cell uptake of potassium is enhanced (127). Aldosterone levels are often elevated and also tend to promote potassium secretion. Increased distal delivery of bicarbonate, associated with increased distal flow, and high luminal bicarbonate concentration permits distal Cl concentration to fall to low levels and thus further favors potassium secretion of KCl cotransport.

In acute metabolic acidosis, decreased uptake of potassium by distal cells tends to reduce potassium secretion. However, as acidosis proceeds, proximal fluid absorption is increasingly inhibited and distal flow rate begins to increase (16, 141). An additional factor favoring potassium secretion is the elevation of aldosterone that has been observed in chronic metabolic acidosis (233). Taken together, it is important to recognize that renal potassium excretion has multiple determinants and that they may not always be responding only to changes in potassium balance.

Acknowledgments

We are grateful to Dr. Fred Wright, who was a major contributor and co-author of previous chapters in the earlier editions. We are also indebted to Drs. S. Hebert and

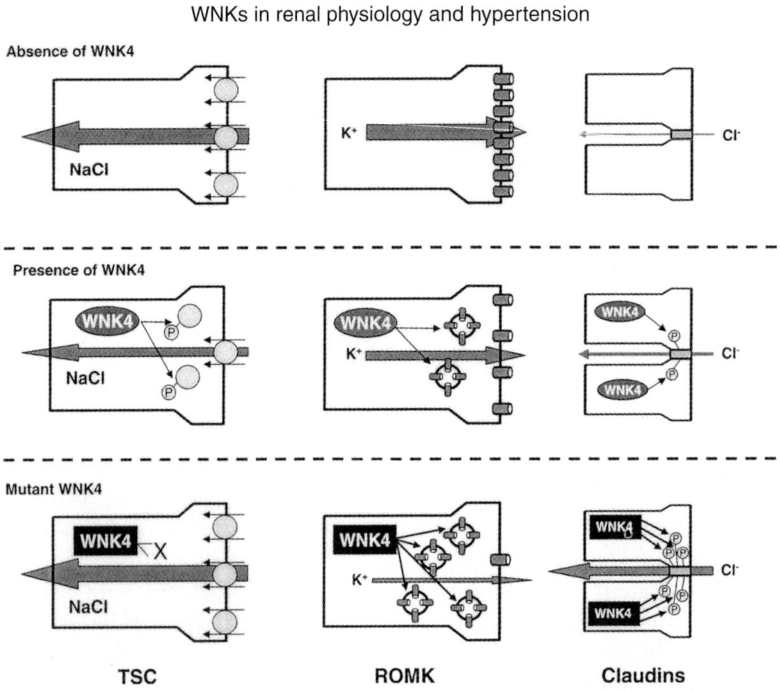

WNKs in renal physiology and hypertension

FIGURE 42   Schematic representation of distal nephron ion transport pathways and the effect of wildtype WNK4 and pseudohyperaldosteronism type II (PHA-II)–type mutations. **Top:** Transport model for thiazide-sensitive Na⁺-Cl⁻ cotransporter (TSC) in the distal convoluted duct (DCT), ROMK K⁺ channel in the collecting duct (CD), and paracellular Cl⁻ transport in the CD. **Middle:** Effect of wildtype WNK4 in which TSC activity is reduced, due to a phosphorylation-dependent mechanism, ROMK activity is reduced, due to a clathrin-dependent endocytosis mechanism that appears to require no phosphorylation, and paracellular Cl⁻ transport is increased in association with claudin phosphorylation. **Bottom:** Effect of PHA-II–type mutations in WNK4. Loss-of-function behavior is seen in TSC, whereas gain-of-function behavior is observed in ROMK and paracellular Cl⁻ transport. (From Gamba G. Role of WNK kinases in regulating tubular salt and potassium transport and in the development of hypertension. *Am J Physiol Renal* 2005;288:245–252, with permission.)

W. Wang, who have shared over many years with us their knowledge and insights into renal potassium transport. Drs. J. Pluznick and F. Beck, Ms. Leah Sanders, and R. M. Klose have also contributed by careful editing of the manuscript. Mr. Mark Saba also helpful preparing the illustrations.

References

1. Adam WR, Dawborn JK. Potassium tolerance in rats. *Aust J Exp Biol Med Sci* 1972;50: 757–786.
2. Adler S, Fraley DS. Potassium and intracellular pH. *Kidney Int* 1977;11:433–442.
3. Ahloulay M, Dechaux M, Laborde K, et al. Influence of glucagon on GFR and on urea and electrolyte excretion: direct and indirect effects. *Am J Physiol Renal* 1995;269:F225–F235.
4. Ahn KY, Kone BE. Expression and cellular localization of mRNA encoding the "gastric" isoform of H⁺-K⁺-ATPase a-subunit in rat kidney. *Am J Physiol Renal* 1995;268:F99–F109.
5. Aizman RI, Finkinshtein YaD, Turner AYa. Reflex mechanism of potassium homeostasis regulation. *Nefrologia* 1985;V:103–108.
6. Aizman RI, Rabinowitz L, Mayer-Harnisch C. Early effects of uninephrectomy on K homeostasis in unanesthetized rats. *Am J Physiol* 1996;270:R434–R442.
7. Alexander EA, Levinsky NG. An extrarenal mechanism for potassium adaptation. *J Clin Invest* 1968;47:740–748.
8. Ali S, Chen X, Lu M, Xu JC, Lerea KM, Hebert SC, Wang W. A kinase anchoring protein (AKAP) is required for mediating the effect of PKA on ROMK1. *Proc Natl Acad Sci U S A* 1998;95:10274–10278.
9. Allen F, Tisher CC. Morphology of the ascending thick limb of Henle. *Kidney Int* 1976;9:8.
10. Amorim JB, Bailey MA, Musa-Aziz R, et al. Role of luminal anion and pH in distal tubule potassium secretion. *Am J Physiol Renal* 2003;284:F381–F388.
11. Amorim JB, Malnic G. V1 receptors in luminal action of vasopressin on distal K⁺ secretion. *Am J Physiol Renal* 2000;278:F809–F816.
12. Amorim JB, Musa-Aziz R, Mello-Aires M, Malnic G. Signaling path of the action of AVP on distal K⁺ secretion. *Kidney Int* 2004;66:696–704.
13. Anagnostopoulos T, Planelles G. Cell and luminal activities of chloride, potassium, sodium and protons in the late distal tubule of Necturus kidney. *J Physiol (London)* 1987;393:73–89.
14. Antes LM, Kujubu DA, Fernandez PE. Hypokalemia and the pathology of ion transport molecules. *Semin Nephrol* 1998;18:31–45.
15. Armitage FE, Wingo CS. Luminal acidification in K-replete OMCDi: contributions of H-K-ATPase and bafilomycin-A1-sensitive H-ATPase. *Am J Physiol Renal* 1994;267:F450–F458.
16. Aronson PS, Giebisch G. Mechanisms of chloride transport in the proximal tubule. *Am J Physiol Renal* 1997;273:F179–F192.
17. Arrascue JF, Dobyan DC, Jamison RL. Potassium recycling in the renal medulla: effects of acute potassium chloride administration to rats fed a potassium-free diet. *Kidney Int* 1981;20: 348–352.
18. Avison MJ, Gullans SR, Ogino T, et al. Na⁺ and K⁺ fluxes stimulated by Na⁺-coupled glucose transport: evidence for a Ba²⁺-insensitive K⁺ efflux pathway in rabbit proximal tubules. *J Membr Biol* 1988;105:197–205.
19. Babilonia E, Wei Y, Sterling H, Kaminski P, Wolin MS, Wang WH. Superoxide anions are involved in mediating the effect of low K intake on c-Src expression and renal K secretion in the cortical collecting duct. *J Biol Chem* 2005;280:10790–10796.
20. Baer JE, Jones CB, Spitzer SA, et al. The potassium sparing and natriuretic activity of N-amindino-3.4-diamino-6-chloro-pytazine-carboxyamide hydrochloride dihydrate (amiloride hydrochloride). *J Pharmacol Exp Ther* 1967;157:472–485.
21. Bailey MA, Cantone A, Yan Q, MacGregor GG, Leng Q, Amorim JBO, Wang T, Hebert SC, Giebisch G, Malnic G. Maxi-K channels contribute to urinary potassium excretion in the ROMK-deficient mouse model of type II Bartter's syndrome and in adaptation to a high K diet. *Kidney Int* 2006;70:51–59.
22. Bailey MA, Unwin RJ, Shirley DG. In vivo inhibition of renal 11 beta-hydroxysteroid dehydrogenase in the rat stimulates collecting duct sodium reabsorption. *Clin Sci (Lond)* 2001;101: 195–198.

23. Bank N, Aynedjian HS. A micropuncture study of potassium excretion by the remnant kidney. *J Clin Invest* 1973;52:1480–1490.
24. Bank N, Schwartz WE. The influence of anion penetrating ability on urinary acidification and the excretion of titratable acid. *J Clin Invest* 1960;39:1516–1525.
25. Barlet-Bas C, Cheval L, Feraille E, et al. Regulation of tubular Na-K ATPase. In: Hatano M, ed. *Nephrology, Proceedings of the XIth International Congress of Nephrology*. Berlin: Springer; 1991:419–434.
26. Barlet-Bas C, Khadouri C, Marsy S, et al. Enhanced intracellular sodium concentration in kidney cells recruits a latent pool of Na^+-K^+ATPase whose size is modulated by corticosteroids. *J Biol Chem* 1990;265:7799–7803.
27. Bastl C, Hayslett JP, Binder H. Increased large intestinal secretion of potassium in renal insufficiency. *Kidney Int* 1977;12:9–16.
28. Battilana CA, Bhattacharya J, Lacy FB, et al. Effect of chronic potassium loading on potassium secretion by the pars recta or descending limb of the juxtamedullary nephron in the rat. *J Clin Invest* 1978;62:1093–1103.
29. Baylis C, Brenner BM. Mechanism of the glucocorticoid-induced increase in glomerular filtration rate. *Am J Physiol Renal* 1978;234:F166.
30. Baylis C, Handa RK, Sorkin M. Glucocorticoids and control of glomerular filtration rate. *Semin Nephrol* 1990;10:320.
31. Beck FX, Dörge A, Blumner E, et al. Cell rubidium uptake: a method for studying functional heterogeneity in the nephron. *Kidney Int* 1988;33:642–651.
32. Beck F-X, Dörge A, Giebisch G, Thurau K. Studies on the mechanism of rubidium-induced kaliuresis. *Kidney Int* 1989;36:175–182.
33. Beck F-X, Giebisch G, Thurau K. Effect of K depletion on renal K and Rb excretion: Evidence for activation of K reabsorption. *Kidney Int* 1992;42:272–278.
34. Beck JS, Breton S, Giebisch G, et al. Potassium conductance regulation by pH in rabbit proximal convoluted tubules. *Am J Physiol Renal* 1992;263:F453–F458.
35. Beck JS, Breton S, Mairbaurl H, et al. Relationship between sodium transport and intracellular ATP in isolated perfused rabbit proximal convoluted tubule. *Am J Physiol Renal* 1991; 261:F634–F639.
36. Beck JS, Hurst AM, Lapointe JV, et al. Regulation of basolateral K^+ channels in proximal tubule studied during continuous microperfusion. *Am J Physiol Renal* 1994;264: F496–F501.
37. Beck JS, Laprade R, Lapointe J-Y. Coupling between transepithelial Na^+ transport and basolateral K^+ conductance in renal proximal tubule. *Am J Physiol Renal* 1994;266:F517 –F527.
38. Beck LH, Senesky D, Goldberg M. Sodium-independent active potassium reabsorption in proximal tubule of the dog. *J Clin Invest* 1973;52:2641–2645.
39. Benchimol C, Zavilowitz B, Satlin LM. Developmental expression of ROMK mRNA in rabbit cortical collecting duct. *Pediatr Res* 2000;47:46–52.
40. Berliner RW, Kennedy TJ Jr, Hilton G. Renal mechanisms for excretion of potassium. *Am J Physiol Renal* 1950;162:348–367.
41. Berliner RW, Kennedy TJ, Orloff J. Relationship between acidification of the urine and potassium metabolism. *Am J Med* 1951;11:274–282.
42. Berliner RW, Kennedy TJ. Renal tubular secretion of potassium in the dog. *Proc Soc Exp Biol Med* 1948;67:542–545.
43. Berliner RW. Renal secretion of potassium and hydrogen ions. *Fed Proc* 1952;11:695–700.
44. Berliner RW. Renal mechanisms for potassium excretion. *Harvey Lect* 1961;55:141–171.
45. Bia MJ, DeFronzo RA. Extrarenal potassium homeostasis. *Am J Physiol Renal* 1981;240: F257–F268.
46. Bia MJ, Tyler K, DeFronzo RA. The effect of dexamethasone on renal electrolyte excretion in the adrenalectomized rat. *Endocrinology* 1981;III:882–888.
47. Bia MJ, Tyler KA, DeFronzo RA. Regulation of extrarenal potassium homeostasis by adrenal hormones in rats. *Am J Physiol Renal* 1981;242:F461–F468.
48. Biagi B, Kubota T, Sohtell M, et al. Intracellular potentials in rabbit proximal tubules perfused in vitro. *Am J Physiol Renal* 1981;240:F200–F21O.
49. Biagi B, Sohtell M, Giebisch G. Intracellular potassium activity in the rabbit proximal straight tubule. *Am J Physiol Renal* 1981;241:F677–F686.
50. Biller KJ, Unwin RJ, Shirley DG. Distal tubular electrolyte transport during inhibition of renal 11 beta-hydroxysteroid dehydrogenase. *Am J Physiol Renal* 2001;280:F172.
51. Binder HJ, Sandle GI. Electrolyte transport in the mammalian colon. In: Johnson LR, ed. *Physiology of the Gastrointestinal Tract*, 3rd ed. New York: Raven Press; 1994:2133–2172.
52. Bleich M, Schlatter E, Greger R. K^+ channel of the thick ascending limb of Henle's loop. *Pflügers Arch* 1990;415:449–460.
53. Bloomer HA, Rector FC Jr, Seldin DW. The mechanism of potassium reabsorption in the proximal tubule of the rat. *J Clin Invest* 1963;42:277–285.
54. Blot-Chabaud M, Wanstock F, Bonvalet J-P, Farman N. Cell-sodium-induced recruitment of Na^+/K^+-ATPase pumps in rabbit collecting tubules is aldosterone-dependent. *J Biol Chem* 1990;265:11676–11681.
55. Bomsztyk K, Wright FS. Dependence of ion fluxes on fluid transport by rat proximal tubule. *Am J Physiol Renal* 1986;250:F680–F689.
56. Bomsztyk K, Wright FS. Effect of luminal potassium concentration and transepithelial voltage on potassium transport by the renal proximal tubule. *Fed Proc* 1983;42:304.
57. Bonny O, Rossier BC. Disturbances of Na/K balance: Pseudohypoaldosteronism revisited. *J Am Soc Nephrol* 2002;13:2399–2414.
58. Booth RE, Johnson JP, Stockand JD. Aldosterone. *Adv Physiol Educ* 2002;26:8–20.
59. Boulpaep EL, Sackin H. Equivalent electrical circuit analysis and rheogenic pumps in epithelia. *Fed Proc* 1979;38:2030–2036.
60. Boyd JE, Mulrow PJ. Further studies of the influence of potassium upon aldosterone production in the rat. *Endocrinology* 1972;90:299–301.
61. Brandis M, Keyes J, Windhager EE. Potassium-induced inhibition of proximal tubular fluid reabsorption in rats. *Am J Physiol Renal* 1972;222:421–427.
62. Buffin-Meyer B, Marsy S, Barlet-Bas C, et al. Regulation of renal Na^+-K^+-ATPase in rat thick ascending limb during K^+ depletion: evidence for modulation of Na^+ affinity. *J Physiol (London)* 1996;490:623–632.
63. Buffin-Meyer B, Verbatz JM, Cheval L, et al. Regulation of Na^+, K^+ ATPase in the rat outer medullary collecting duct during potassium depletion. *J Am Soc Nephrol* 1998;9:538–550.
64. Buffin-Meyer B, Younes-Ibrahim M, Barlet-Bas C, Cheval L, Marsy S, Doucet A. K depletion modifies the properties of Sch-28080-sensitive K-ATPase in rat collecting duct. *Am J Physiol Renal* 1997;272:F124–F131.
65. Buffin-Meyer B, Younes-Ibrahim M, Barlet-Bas C, et al. K depletion modifies the properties of Sch-28080-sensitive K-ATPase in rat collecting duct. *Am J Physiol Renal* 1997;272:F124.
66. Buffin-Meyer B, Younes-Ibrahim M, El Mernissi G, Cheval L, Marsy S, Grima M, Girolami J-P, Doucet A. Differential regulation of collecting duct Na^+-K^+-ATPase and K^+ excretion by furosemide and piretanide: Role of bradykinin. *J Am Soc Nephrol* 2004;15:876–884.
67. Burg MB, Green N. Effect of ethacrynic acid on the thick ascending limb of Henle's loop. *Kidney Int* 1973;4:301–308.
68. Burg MB, Stoner L, Cardinal J, et al. Furosemide effect on isolated perfused tubules. *Am J Physiol Renal* 1973;225:119–124.
69. Burg MB. Thick ascending limb of Henle's loop. *Kidney Int* 1982;22:454–464.
70. Carlisle EJ, Donnelly SM, Ethier JH, et al. Modulation of the secretion of potassium by accompanying anions in humans. *Kidney Int* 1991;39:1206.
71. Cassola AC, Giebisch G, Wang W. Vasopressin increases the density of apical low-conductance K^+ channels in rat CCD. *Am J Physiol Renal* 1993;264:F502–F509.
72. Cemerikic D, Wilcox CS, Giebisch G. Intracellular potential and K^+ activity in rat kidney proximal tubular cells in acidosis and K^+ depletion. *J Membr Biol* 1982;69:159–165.
73. Chaillet JR, Lopes AG, Boron WE. Basolateral Na-H exchange in the rabbit cortical collecting tubule. *J Gen Physiol* 1985;86:785–812.
73a. Chen P, Guzman JP, Leong PKK, Yang LE, Perianayagam A, Babilonia E, Ho JS, Youn JH, Wang WH, McDonough AA. Modest dietary K^+ restriction provokes insulin resistance of cellular K^+ uptake and phosphorylation of renal outer medulla K^+ channel without fall in plasma K^+ concentration. *Am J Physiol* 2006;290:C1355–C1363.
74. Chen SY, Bhargava A, Mastroberardino L, Meijer OC, Wang J, Buse P, Firestone GL, Verrey F, Pearce D. Epithelial sodium channel regulated by aldosterone-induced protein sgk. *Proc Natl Acad Sci U S A* 1999;96:2514–2519.
75. Christ M, Sippel K, Eisen C, Wehling M. Non-classical receptors for aldosterone in plasma membranes from pig kidneys. *Mol Cell Endocrinol* 1994;99:R31–R34.
76. Clapp JR, Rector FC, Seldin DW. Effect of unreabsorbed anion on proximal and distal transtubular potentials in the rat. *Am J Physiol* 1962;202:781.
77. Clausen T. Long- and short-term regulation of the Na^+-K^+ pump in skeletal muscle. *News Physiol Sci* 1996;11:24–30.
78. Codina J, Kone BC, Delmas-Mata JT, DuBose TD Jr. Functional expression of the colonic H^+, K^+-ATPase a subunit. Pharmacologic properties and assembly with X^+-K^+-ATPase ß subunits. *J Biol Chem* 1996;271:29759–29763.
79. Constantinescu A, Silver RB, Satlin LM. H-K-ATPase activity in PNA-binding intercalated cells of newborn rabbit cortical collecting duct. *Am J Physiol Renal* 1979;272:F167–F177.
80. Cortney MA. Renal tubular transfer of water and electrolytes in adrenalectomized rats. *Am J Physiol Renal* 1969;216:589.
81. Costanzo LS. Localization of diuretic action in microperfused rat distal tubules: Ca and Na transport. *Am J Physiol Renal* 1985;248:F197–F211.
82. Cougnon M, Bouyer P, Planelles G, Jaisser F. Does the colonic H-K-ATPase also act as an Na-K-ATPase *Proc Natl Acad Sci U S A* 1998;95:6516–6520.
83. Coutry N, Blot-Chabaud M, Mateo P, et al. Time course of sodium induced Na^+-K^+-ATPase recruitment in rabbit cortical collecting tubule. *Am J Physiol* 1992;263:C61–C68.
84. Cox JR, Platts MM, Horn ME, et al. The effect of aldosterone on sodium and potassium distribution in man. *J Endocrinol* 1966;36:103–114.
85. Cox M, Sterns RH, Singer I. The defense against hyperkalemia: the roles of insulin and aldosterone. *N Engl J Med* 1978;299:525–532.
86. Crayen M, Thoenes W Architektur und cytologische Charakterisierung des distalen Tubulus der Rattenniere. *Fortschr Zool* 1975;23:279–288.
87. Davidson DG, Levinsky NG, Berliner RW. Maintenance of potassium excretion despite reduction of glomerular filtration during sodium diuresis. *J Clin Invest* 1958;37:548–555.
88. De Rouffignac C, Morel E. Micropuncture study of water, electrolytes and urea movements along the loops of Henle in Psammomys. *J Clin Invest* 1969;48:474–486.
89. DeFronzo RA, Bia M, Birkhead G. Epinephrine and potassium homeostasis. *Kidney Int* 1981;20:83–91.
90. DeFronzo RA, Goldberg M, Agus Z. The effects of glucose and insulin on renal electrolyte transport. *J Clin Invest* 1976;58:83–90.
91. DeFronzo RA, Stanton B, Klein-Robbenhaar G, et al. Inhibitory effect of epinephrine on renal potassium secretion: a micropuncture study. *Am J Physiol Renal* 1983;245:F303–F311.
92. deMello-Aires M, Giebisch G, Malnic G, et al. Kinetics of potassium transport across single distal tubules of rat kidney. *J Physiol (London)* 1973;232:47–70.
93. Dherbecourt O, Cheval L, Bloch-Faure M, Meneton P, Doucet A. Molecular identification of Sch28080-sensitive K-ATPase activities in the mouse kidney. *Pflüger Arch* 2006;451: 769–775.
94. Diezi J, Michoud P, Aceves J, Giebisch G. Micropuncture study of electrolyte transport across papillary collecting duct of the rat. *Am J Physiol Renal* 1973;224:623–634.
95. Diezi J, Michaud P, Grandchamp A, et al. Effects of nephrectomy on renal salt and water transport in the remaining kidney. *Kidney Int* 1976;10:450–462.
96. Dobyan DC, Lacy FB, Jamison RL. Suppression of potassium-recycling in the renal medulla by short-term potassium deprivation. *Kidney Int* 1979;16:704–709.
97. Doucet A, Katz AI, Morel F. Determination of Na-K-ATPase activity in single segments of the mammalian nephron. *Am J Physiol Renal* 1979;237:F105–F113.
98. Doucet A, Katz AI. Renal potassium adaptation: Na-K-ATPase activity along the nephron after chronic potassium loading. *Am J Physiol Renal* 1980;238:F380–F386.
99. Doucet A, Katz AI. Short-term effect of aldosterone on Na-K-ATPase in single nephron segments. *Am J Physiol Renal* 1981;241:F273–F278.
100. Doucet A, Marsy S. Characterization of K-ATPase activity in distal nephron: stimulation by potassium depletion. *Am J Physiol Renal* 1987;253:F418–F423.

101. Doucet A. H^+, $K(^+)$-ATPase in the kidney: localization and function in the nephron. *Exp Nephrol* 1997;5:271–276.
102. Doucet A. Functional control of Na-K-ATPase in single nephron segments of the mammalian kidney. *Kidney Int* 1998;34:749–760.
103. Douglas JG. Effects of high potassium diet on angiotensin II receptors and angiotensin-induced aldosterone production in rat adrenal glomerulosa cells. *Endocrinology* 1980;106: 983–990.
104. Duarte CG, Chomety F, Giebisch G. Effect of amiloride, ouabain, and furosemide on distal tubular function in the rat. *Am J Physiol Renal* 1971;221:F632–F639.
105. DuBose TD Jr, Caflisch CR. Effect of selective aldosterone deficiency on acidification in nephron segments of the rat inner medulla. *J Clin Invest* 1988;82:1624–1632.
106. DuBose TD Jr, Codina J, Burges A, Pressley TA. Regulation of $H(^+)$-$K(+)$-ATPase expression in kidney. *Am J Physiol Renal* 1995;269:F500–F507.
107. DuBose TD Jr. Hyperkalemic hyperchloremic metabolic acidosis: pathophysiologic insights. *Kidney Int* 1997;51:591–602.
108. Edelman A, Curci S, Samarzija I, et al. Determination of intracellular K^+ activity in rat kidney proximal tubular cells. *Pflügers Arch* 1978;378:37–45.
109. Eiam-Ong S, Kurtzman NA, Sabatini S. Regulation of collecting tubule adenoside triphosphatases by aldosterone and potassium. *J Clin Invest* 1993;91:2385.
110. Elalouf J-M, Roinel N, de Rouffignac C. Effects of DAVP on rat juxtamedullary nephrons: stimulation of medullary K recycling. *Am J Physiol Renal* 1985;249:F291–F298.
111. Elalouf J-M, Roinel N, de Rouffignac C. Effects of human calcitonin on water and electrolyte movements in rat juxtamedullary nephrons: inhibition of medullary K recycling. *Pflugers Arch* 1986;406:502–508.
112. Elkinton JR, Danowski TS. *The Body Fluids.* Baltimore: Williams & Wilkins; 1955.
113. Ellison DH, Velazquez H, Wright FS. Adaptation of the distal convoluted tubule of the rat: structural and functional effects of dietary salt intake and chronic diuretic infusion. *J Clin Invest* 1989;83:113–126.
114. Ellison DH, Velazquez H, Wright FS. Mechanisms of sodium, potassium and chloride transport by the renal distal tubule. *Miner Electrolyte Metab* 1987;13:422–432.
115. Ellison DH, Velazquez H, Wright FS. Stimulation of distal potassium sectetion by low lumen chloride in the presence of barium. *Am J Physiol Renal* 1985;248:F638–F649.
116. Ellison DH, Velazquez H, Wright FS. Thiazide-sensitive sodium chloride cotransport in early distal tubule. *Am J Physiol Renal* 1987;253:F546–F554.
117. Engbretson BG, Stoner LC. Flow-dependent potassium secretion by rabbit cortical collecting tubule in vitro. *Am J Physiol Renal* 1987;253:F896–F903.
118. Ethier JH, Kamel KS, Magner PO, et al. The transtubular potassium concentration in patients with hypokalemia and hyperkalemia. *AmJ Kidney Dis* 1990;15:309–315.
119. Farman N. Steroid receptors: Distribution along the nephron. *Semin Nephrol* 1992;12:12.
120. Field M, Giebisch G. Steroid effects on renal function. In: Laragh JH, Brenner BM, eds. *Hypertension: Pathophysiology, Diagnosis and Management.* New York: Raven Press; 1990:1273–1285.
121. Field MJ, Giebisch G. Hormonal control of renal potassium excretion. *Kidney Int* 1985;27: 379–387.
122. Field MJ, Giebisch G. Mechanisms of segmental potassium reabsorption and secretion. In: Seldin DW, Giebisch G, eds. *The Regulation of Potassium Balance.* New York: Raven Press; 1989:139–156.
123. Field MJ, Stanton BA, Giebisch GH. Differential acute effects of aldosterone, dexamethasone and hyperkalemia on distal tubular potassium secretion in the rat kidney. *J Clin Invest* 1984;74:1792–1802.
124. Field MJ, Stanton BA, Giebisch GH. Influence of ADH on renal potassium handling: a micropuncture and microperfusion study in Brattleboro rats. *Kidney Int* 1984;25:502–511.
125. Filipovic D, Sackin H. A calcium-permeable stretch-activated cation channel in renal proximal tubule. *Am J Physiol Renal* 1991;260:F119–F129.
126. Foster ES, Sandle GI, Hayslett JP, et al. Dietary potassium modulates active potassium absorption and secretion in rat distal colon. *Am J Physiol* 1986;251:G619–G626.
127. Fraley DS, Adler S, Isohydric regulation of plasma potassium by bicarbonate in the rat. *Kidney Int* 1976;9:333–343.
128. Frindt G, Palmer LG. Apical potassium channels in the rat connecting tubule. *Am J Physiol Renal* 2004;287:F1030–F1037.
129. Frindt G, Palmer LG. Na channels in the rat connecting tubule. *Am J Physiol Renal* 2004;286: F669–F674.
130. Frindt G, Palmer LG. Low-conductance K channels in apical membrane of rat cortical collecting tubule. *Am J Physiol Renal* 1989;256:F143–F151.
131. Frömter E, Gessner K. Free flow potential profile along rat kidney proximal tubule. *Pflugers Arch* 1974;351:69–84
132. Fujii Y, Mujais SK, Katz AI. Renal potassium adaptation: role of the Na-K-ATP pump in rat cortical collecting tubules. *Am J Physiol Renal* 1989;256:F279–F284.
133. Fujimoto M, Kubota I, Kotera K. Electrochemical profile of K and CI ions across the proximal tubule of bullfrog kidneys. *Contrib Nephrol* 1977;6:114–123.
134. Funder JW, Blair-West JR, Coughlan JP, et al. Effect of plasma (K^+) on the secretion of aldosterone. *Endocrinology* 1969;85:381–384.
135. Funder JW. Aldosterone action. *Annu Rev Physiol* 1993;55:115.
136. Furuya H, Tabei K, Muto S, et al. Effect of insulin on potassium secretion in the rabbit cortical collecting tubule. *Am J Physiol Renal* 1991;262:F30–F35.
137. Gamba G. Role of WNK kinases in regulating tubular salt and potassium transport and in the development of hypertension. *Am J Physiol Renal* 2005;288:245–252.
138. Garcia-Filho E, Malnic G, Giebisch G. Effects of changes in electrical potential difference on tubular potassium transport. *Am J Physiol Renal* 1980;238:F235.
139. Garg LC, Narang N. Ouabain-insensitive K-adenosine triphosphatase in distal nephron segments of the rabbit. *J Clin Invest* 1988;81:1204–1208.
140. Gekle M, Freudinger R, Mildenberger S, Schenk K, Marschitz I, Schramek H. Rapid activation of Na^+/H^+-exchange in MDCK cells by aldosterone involves MAP-kinase ERK1/2. *Pflugers Arch* 2001;441:781–786.
141. Gennari FJ, Cohen JJ. Role of the kidney in potassium homeostasis: lessons from acid-base disturbances. *Kidney Int* 1975;8:1–5.
142. Gennari FJ, Segal AS. Hyperkalemia: an adaptive response in chronic renal insufficiency. *Kidney Int* 2002;62:1–9.
143. Gennari FJ. Hypokalemia. *N Engl J Med* 1998;339:451–459.
144. Giebisch G, Wang W. Potassium transport: from clearance to channels and pumps. *Kidney Int* 1995;49:1624–1631.
145. Giebisch G. Effects of diuretics on renal transport of potassium. *Methods Pharmacol* 1976;4A:121–164.
146. Giebisch G. Recent advances in the field of renal potassium excretion: what can we learn from potassium channels? *Yale J Biol Med* 1998;70:311–322.
147. Giebisch G. Renal potassium channels: an overview. *Kidney Int* 1995;48:1004–1009.
148. Giebisch G. Renal potassium transport. In: Giebisch G, Tosteson DC, Ussing HH, eds. *Membrane Transport in Biology*, Vol. IVA. Berlin: Springer-Verlag; 1978:215–298.
149. Giebisch G. Some reflections on the mechanism of renal tubular potassium transport. *Yale Biol Med* 1975;48:315–336.
150. Giebisch G. A trail of research on potassium. *Kidney Int* 2002;62:1498–1512.
151. Giebisch, G. Challenges to potassium metabolism: Internal distribution and external balance. *Wiener Klinische Wochenschrift* 2004;116/11–12:353–366.
152. Giebisch, G. Renal potassium transport: Mechanisms and regulation. *Am J Physiol Renal* 1998;274:F817–833.
153. Gonin S, Deschenes G, Roger F, Bens M, Martin PY, Carpentier JL, Vandewalle A, Doucet A, Feraille E. Cyclic AMP increases cell surface expression of functional Na-K-ATPase units in mammalian cortical collecting duct principal cells. *Mol Biol Cell* 2001;13:255–264.
154. Good DW, Velazquez H, Wright FS. Luminal influences on potassium secretion: low sodium concentration. *Am J Physiol Renal* 1984;246:F609–F619.
155. Good DW, Wright FS. Luminal influences of potassium secretion: sodium concentration and fluid flow rate. *Am J Physiol Renal* 1979;236:F192–F205.
156. Good DW. Effects of potassium on ammonium transport by medullary thick ascending limb of the rat. *Am J Physiol Renal* 1987;80:1358–1365.
157. Good DW. Sodium-dependent bicarbonate absorption by cortical thick ascending limb of rat kidney. *Am J Physiol Renal* 1985;248:F821–F829.
158. Grasset E, Gunter-Smith P, Schultz SG. Effects of Na-coupled alanine transport on intracellular K activities and the K conductance of the basolateral membranes of Necturus small intestine. *J Membr Biol* 1983;71:89–94.
159. Gray DA, Frindt G, Palmer LG. Quantification of K^+ secretion through apical low-conductance K channels in the CCD. *Am J Physiol Renal* 2005;289:F117–F126.
160. Greger R, Oberleithner H, Schlatter E, et al. Chloride activity in cells of isolated perfused cortical thick ascending limbs of rabbit kidney. *Pflugers Arch* 1983;399:29–41.
161. Greger R, Schlatter E. Cellular mechanism of the action of loop diuretics on the thick ascending limb of Henle's loop. *Klin Wochenschr* 1983;61:1019–1027.
162. Greger R, Schlatter E. Presence of luminal K, a prerequisite for active NaCl transport in the cortical thick ascending limb of Henle's loop of rabbit kidney. *Pflugers Arch* 1981;392: 92–94.
163. Greger R, Schlatter E. Properties of the basolateral membrane of the cortical thick ascending limb of Henle's loop of rabbit kidney. A model for secondary active chloride transport. *Pflugers Arch* 1983;396:325–334.
164. Greger R, Schlatter E. Properties of the lumen membrane of the cortical thick ascending limb of Henle's loop of rabbit kidney. *Pflugers Arch* 1983;396:315–324.
165. Greger R. Ion transport mechanisms in thick ascending limb of Henle's loop of mammalian nephrons. *Physiol Rev* 1985;65:760–797.
166. Grunnet M, Hay-Schmidt A, Klaerke DA. Quantification and distribution of big conductance Ca^{2+}-activated K^+ channels in kidney epithelia. *Biochim Biophys Acta* 2005;1714: 114–124.
167. Grupp C, Pavenstadt-Grupp R, Grunewald W, et al. A Na-K-CI cotransporter in isolated rat papillary collecting duct cells. *Kidney Int* 1989;36:201–209.
168. Guggino WE, Oberleithner H, Giebisch G. The amphibian diluting segment. *Am J Physiol Renal* 1988;254:F615–F627.
169. Gunter-Smith PJ, Grasset E, Schultz SG. Sodium-coupled amino acid and sugar transport by Necturus small intestine. An equivalent circuit analysis of a rheogenic cotransport system. *J Membr Biol* 1982;66:25–39.
170. Hall JE, Granger JP, Smith MJ, et al. Role of renal hemodynamics and arterial pressure in aldosterone "escape." *Hypertension* 1984;6(suppl 1):183–192.
171. Halperin ML, Gowrishankar M, Mallie JP, et a1. Urea recycling: an aid to the excretion of potassium during antidiuresis. *Nephron* 1996;72:507–511.
172. Hamm LL, Gillespie C, Klahr S. Ammonium chloride inhibits Na^+ and K^+ transport in the cortical collecting tubule. *Contrib Nephrol* 1985;47:125.
173. Hamm LL, Gillespie C, Klahr S. NH_4Cl inhibition of transport in the rabbit cortical collecting tubule. *Am J Physiol Renal* 1985;248:F631.
174. Haseroth K, Gerdes D, Berger S, Feuring M, Gunther A, Herbst C, Christ M, Wehling M. Rapid nongenomic effects of aldosterone in mineralocorticoid-receptor-knockout mice. *Biochem Biophys Res Commun* 1999;266:257–261.
175. Hayashi M, Katz AI. The kidney in potassium depletion. I. Na^+-K-ATPase activity and (^{3}H)ouabain binding in MCT. *Am J Physiol Renal* 1987;252:F437.
176. Hayslett JP, Halevy J, Pace PE, et al. Demonstration of net potassium absorption in mammalian colon. *Am J Physiol* 1982;242:G209–G214.
177. Hebert SC, Andreoli TE. Control of NaCl transport in the thick ascending limb. *Am J Physiol Renal* 1984;246:F745–F756.
178. Hebert SC, Andreoli TE. Effects of antidiuretic hormone on cellular conductive pathways in mouse medullary thick ascending limbs of Henle: II. Determinants of the ADH-mediated increases in transepithelial voltage and in net Cl- absorption. *J Membr Biol* 1984;80:221–233.
179. Hebert SC, Friedman PA, Andreoli TE. Effects of antidiuretic hormone on cellular conductive pathways in mouse medullary thick ascending limbs of Henle: 1. ADH increases transcellular conductance pathways. *J Membr Biol* 1984;80:201–209.

180. Hebert SC. An ATP-regulated, inwardly rectifying potassium channel from rat kidney (ROMK). *Kidney Int* 1995;48:1010–1016.
181. Hebert SC, Desir G, Giebisch G, Wang WH. Molecular diversity and regulation of renal potassium channels. *Physiol Rev* 2005;85:319–371.
182. Henke G, Setiawan I, Böhmer C, Lang F. Activation of Na^+-K^+-ATPase by the serum and glucocorticoid dependent kinase (SGK) isoforms. *Kidney Blood Press Res* 2002;25:370–374.
183. Hierholzer K, Wiederholt M, Holzgreve H, et al. Micropuncture study of renal transtubular concentration gradients of sodium and potassium in adrenalectomized rats. *Pflugers Arch* 1965;285:193–210.
184. Hierholzer K. Secretion of potassium and acidification in collecting ducts of mammalian kidney. *Am J Physiol Renal* 1961;201:318–324.
185. Higashihara E, Kokko JP. Effects of aldosterone on potassium recycling in the kidney of adrenalectomized rats. *Am J Physiol Renal* 1985;248:F219–F227.
186. Hilgemann DW, Feng S, Nasuhoglu C. The complex and intriguing lives of PIP2 with ion channels and transporters. *Sci STKE* 2001;RE19.
187. Hirsch J, Schlatter E. K channels in the basolateral membrane of rat cortical collecting duct are regulated by a cGMP-dependent protein kinase. *Pflugers Arch* 1995;429:338–344.
188. Hirsch J, Schlatter E. K channels in the basolateral membrane of rat cortical collecting duct. *Kidney Int* 1995;48:1036–1046.
189. Horisberger JD, Doucet A. Renal ion translocating ATPases: the P type family 139. In: Seldin DW, Giebisch G, eds. *The Kidney: Physiology and Pathophysiology,* 3rd ed. Philadelphia: Lippincott Williams & Wilkins; 2002:139–170.
190. Horisberger J-D, Giebisch G. Potassium-sparing diuretics. *Renal Physiol* 1987;10:198–200.
191. Horisberger J-D, Giebisch G. Voltage dependence of the basolateral membrane conductance in the Amphiuma collecting tubule . *J Membr Biol* 1988;105:257–263.
192. Hropot M, Fowler N, Karlmark B, et al. Tubular action of diuretics: distal effects on electrolyte transport and acidification. *Kidney Int* 1985;28:477–489.
193. Huang CL, Feng S, Hilgemann DW. Direct activation of inward rectifier potassium channels by PIP2 and its stabilization by Gß. *Nature* 1998;391:803–806.
194. Huang DY, Wulff P, Völkl H, Loffing J, Richter K, Kuhl D, Lang F, Vallon V. Impaired regulation of renal K^+ elimination in the sgk1-knockout mouse. *J Am Soc Nephrol* 2004;15: 885–891.
195. Hunter M, Lopes A, Boulpaep E, et al. Regulation of single K-channels from apical membrane of rabbit collecting tubule. *Am J Physiol Renal* 1986;251:F725–F733.
196. Hunter M, Oberleithner H, Henderson RM, et al. Whole cell potassium currents in single early distal tubule cells. *Am J Physiol Renal* 1988;255:F699–F703.
197. Hunter M. Potassium-selective channels in the basolateral membrane of single proximal tubule cells of frog kidney. *Pflugers Arch* 1991;418:26–34.
198. Hurst AM, Beck JS, Laprade R, et al. Na^+ pump inhibition down regulates an ATP-sensitive K^+ channel in rabbit proximal convoluted tubule. *Am J Physiol Renal* 1993;264:F760–F764.
199. Hurst AM, Hunter M. Acute changes in channel density of amphibian diluting segment. *Am J Physiol* 1990;259:C1005–C1009.
200. Hurst AM, Hunter M. Apical membrane potassium channels in frog diluting segment. Stimulation by furosemide. *Am J Physiol Renal* 1992;262:F606–F614.
201. Hurst AM, Hunter M. Stretch-activated channels in single early distal tubule cells of the frog. *J Physiol (London)* 1990;430:13–24.
202. Husted RF, Steinmetz. Mechanisms of K^+ transport in isolated turtle urinary bladder. *J Clin Invest* 1982;70:832–834.
203. Imai M, Nakamura R. Function of distal convoluted and connecting tubules studied by isolated nephron fragments. *Kidney Int* 1982;22:465–472.
204. Imai M, Tsuruoka S, Yoshitomi K, et al. Morphological and functional heterogeneity of the thick ascending limb of Henle's loop. *Clin Exp Nephrol* 1999;1:9.
205. Imai M. The connecting tubule: a functional subdivision of the rabbit distal nephron segments. *Kidney Int* 1979;15:346–356.
206. Imbert-Teboul M, Doucet A, Marsy S, Siaume-Perez S. Alteration of enzymatic activities along rat collecting tubule in potassium depletion. *Am J Physiol Renal* 1987;253:F408.
207. Jaeger P, Karlmark B, Giebisch G. Ammonium transport in rat cortical tubule: relationship to potassium metabolism. *Am J Physiol Renal* 1983;245:F593–F600.
208. Jaisser F, Beggah AT. The nongastric H+-K+-ATPases: molecular and functional properties. *Am J Physiol Renal* 1999;276:F812–F824.
209. Jaisser F, Escoubet B, Coutry N, Eugene E, Bonvalet JP, Farman N. Differential regulation of putative K^+-ATPase by low-K^+ diet and corticosteroids in rat distal colon and kidney. *Am J Physiol* 1996;270:C679–C687.
210. Jaisser F, Horisberger JD, Geering K, et al. Mechanisms of urinary K^+ and H^+ excretion: primary structure and functional expression of a novel H-K-ATPase. *J Cell Biol* 1993;123: 1421–1429.
211. Jamison R, Muller-Suur R. Potassium recycling. In: Giebisch G, ed. *Current Topics in Membranes and Transport*, Vol. 28. Orlando, FL: Academic Press; 1987:115–131.
212. Jamison RL, Lacy FB, Pennell JP, et al. Potassium secretion by the descending limb of pars recta of the juxtamedullary nephron in vivo. *Kidney Int* 1976;9:323–332.
213. Jamison RL, Work J, Schafer JA. New pathways for potassium transport in the kidney. *Am J Physiol Renal* 1982;242:F297–F312.
214. Jamison RL. Potassium recycling. *Kidney Int* 1987;31:695–703.
215. Jino Y, Troy JL, Brenner BM. Effects of catecholamines on electrolyte transport in cortical collecting tubules. *J Membr Biol* 1981;61:67–73.
216. Kahle KT, Wilson FH, Leng Q, et al. WNK4 regulates the balance between renal NaCl reabsorption and K^+ secretion. *Nat Genet* 2003;35:302–303.
217. Kahle KT, MacGregor GG, Wilson FH, Van Hoek AN, Brown D, Ardito T, Kashgarian M, Giebisch G, Hebert SC, Boulpaep EL, Lifton RP. Paracellular Cl- permeability is regulated by WNK4 kinase: Insight into normal physiology and hypertension. *Proc Natl Acad Sci* 2004;101:14877–14882.
218. Kahle KT, Wilson FH, Leng Q, Lalioti MD, O'Connell AD, Dong K, Rapson A, MacGregor GG, Giebisch G, Hebert SC, Lifton RP. WNK4 regulates the balance between renal NaCl reabsorption and K^+ secretion. *Nat Genet* 2003;35(4):372–376.
219. Kahle KT, Wilson FH, Lifton RP. Regulation of diverse ion transport pathways by WNK4 kinase: a novel molecular switch. *Trends Endocrinol Metabol* 2005;16(3):98–103.
220. Kaissling B, Bachmann S, Kriz W. Structural adaptation of the distal convoluted tubule to prolonged furosemide treatment. *Am J Physiol Renal* 1985;248:F374–F381.
221. Kaissling B, Kriz W. *Structural Analysis of Rabbit Kidney*. Berlin: Springer; 1979.
222. Kaissling B, Le Hir M. Distal tubular segments of the rabbit kidney after adaptation to altered Na- and K-intake. I. Structural changes. *Cell Tissue Res* 1982;224:469–492.
223. Kaissling B, Stanton BA. Adaptation of distal tubule and collecting duct to increased sodium delivery. 1. Ultrastructure. *Am J Physiol Renal* 1988;255:F1256–F1268.
224. Kaissling B. Structural adaptation to altered electrolyte metabolism by cortical distal segments. *Fed Proc* 1985;44:2710–2716.
225. Kaissling B. Structural aspects of adaptive changes in renal electrolyte excretion. *Am J Physiol Renal* 1982;224:469–492.
226. Kamel SK, Lin SH, Cheema-Dhadli S, et al. Prolonged total fasting: A feast for the integrative physiologist. *Kidney Int* 1998;53:531.
227. Kashgarian M, Biemesderfer D, Caplan M, et al. Monoclonal antibody to Na, K-ATPase: immunocytochemical localization along nephron segments. *Kidney Int* 1985;28:899–913.
228. Katz AI. Renal Na-K-ATPase: its role in tubular sodium and potassium transport. *Am J Physiol Renal* 1982;242:F207–F219.
229. Kaufman JS, Hamburger RJ. Passive potassium transport in the isolated proximal convoluted tubule. *Am J Physiol Renal* 1985;248:F228–F232.
230. Kaufman JS, Hamburger RJ. Potassium transport in the isolated proximal convoluted tubule. *Am J Physiol Renal* 1982;244:F297–F313.
231. Kaunitz JD, Barrett KE, McRoberts JA. Electrolyte secretion and absorption: Small intestine and colon. In: Yamada T, ed. *Textbook of Gastroenterology*, Vol 1, 2nd ed. Philadelphia: JB Lippincott; 1995:316–361.
232. Kawahara K, Hunter M, Giebisch G. Potassium channels in Necturus proximal tubule. *Am J Physiol Renal* 1987;253:F488–F494.
233. Khadouri C, Marsy S, Barlet-Bas C, Cheval L, Doucet A. Effect of metabolic acidosis and alkalosis on NEM-sensitive ATPase in rat nephron segments. *Am J Physiol Renal* 1992;262: F583–F590.
234. Khuri R, Wiederholt M, Strieder N, et al. Effects of graded solute diuresis on renal tubular sodium transport in the rat. *Am J Physiol Renal* 1975;228:1261–1268.
235. Khuri RN, Agulian SK, Bogharian K. Electrochemical potentials of potassium in proximal renal tubule of rat. *Pflügers Arch* 1974;346:319–326
236. Khuri RN, Wiederholt M, Strieder N, et al. Effects of flow rate and potassium intake on distal tubular potassium transfer. *Am J Physiol Renal* 1975;228:1249–1261.
237. Kibble JD, Wareing M, Wilson RXI, et al. Effect of barium on potassium diffusion across the proximal convoluted tubule of the anesthetized rat. *Am J Physiol Renal* 1995;268:F778–F783.
238. Knox FG, Romero JE. Mechanism for escape from the sodium retaining effects of mineralocorticoids. In: Kaufman XI, Wambach G, Helber A, Meuer KA, eds. *Mineralocorticoids and Hypertension*. Berlin: Springer-Verlag; 1983:81–100.
239. Koeppen BM, Biagi BA, Giebisch GH. Intracellular microelectrode characterization of the rabbit cortical collecting duct. *Am J Physiol Renal* 1983;244:F35–F47.
240. Koeppen BM, Giebisch G. Mineralocorticoid regulation of sodium and potassium transport by the cortical collecting duct. In: Graves S, ed. *Regulation and Development of Membrane Transport Processes*. New York: Wiley; 1983:89–104.
241. Kone BE. Renal H-K-ATPase: structure, function, and regulation. *Miner Electrolyte Metab* 1996;22:349–365.
242. Kotelevtsev Y, Brown RW, Fleming S, et al. Hypertension in mice lacking 11 beta-hydroxysteroid dehydrogenase type 2. *J Clin Invest* 1999;103:683.
243. Kriz XI, Bankir L. A standard nomenclature for structures of the kidney. *Am J Physiol Renal* 1988;254:FI-F8.
244. Kubokawa M, McNicholas C, Higgins MA, et al. Regulation of ATPsensitive K^+ channel by membrane-bound protein phosphatases in rat principal cell. *Am J Physiol Renal* 1995;269: F355–F362.
245. Kubokawa M, Mori Y, Fujimoto K, et al. Basolateral pH-sensitive K^+ channels mediate membrane potential of proximal tubule cells in bullfrog kidney. *Jpn J Physiol* 1998;48:1–8.
246. Kubota T, Biagi BA, Giebisch G. Intracellular potassium activity measurements in single proximal tubules of Necturus kidney. *J Membr Biol* 1983;73:51–60.
247. Kunau RT, Webb ML, Botman SE. Characteristics of the relationship between the flow rate of tubular fluid and potassium transport in the distal tubule of the rat. *J Clin Invest* 1974;54: 1488–1495.
248. Kuwahara M, Fu WJ, Marumo F. Functional activity of H-K-ATPase in individual cells of OMCD: localization and effect of K^+ depletion. *Am J Physiol Renal* 1996;270: F116–F122.
249. Kuwahara M, Ishibashi K, Krapf R, et al. Effect of lumen pH on cell pH and cell potential in rabbit proximal tubules. *Am J Physiol Renal* 1989;256:F1075–F1083.
250. Lang F, Henke G, Embark HM, Waldegger S, Palmada M, Bohmer C, Vallon V. Regulation of channels by the serum and glucocorticoid-inducible kinase: implications for transport, excitability and cell proliferation. *Cell Physiol Biochem* 2003;13:41–50.
251. Lang F, Messner G, Rehwald W. Electrophysiology of sodium-coupled transport in proximal renal tubules. *Am J Physiol Renal* 1986;250:F953–F962.
252. Lapointe JY, Garneau L, Bell PD, et al. Membrane crosstalk in the mammalian proximal tubule during alterations in transepithelial sodium transport. *Am J Physiol Renal* 1990;258: F339–F345.
253. Laragh JH, Capeci NE. Effect of administration of potassium chloride on serum sodium and potassium concentration. *Am J Physiol Renal* 1955;180:539–544.
254. Laroche-Joubert N, Marsy S, Doucet A. Cellular origin and hormonal regulation of K^+-ATPase activities sensitive to Sch-28080 in rat collecting duct. *Am J Physiol Renal* 2000;279: F1053–F1059.
255. Laroche-Joubert N, Marsy S, Michelet S, Imbert-Teboul M, Doucet A. Protein kinase A-independent activation of ERK and H-K-ATPase by cAMP in native kidney cells: role of Epac 1. *J Biol Chem* 2002;277:18598–18604.

256. Le Hir M, Kaissling B, Dubach UC. Distal tubular segments of the rabbit kidney after adaptation to altered Na- and K-intake. II. Changes in Na-K-ATPase activity. *Cell Tissue Res* 1982;224:493–504.
257. LeGrimellec C, Poujeol P, de Rouffignac E. ^{3}H-inulin and electrolyte concentrations in Bowman's capsule in rat kidney. *Pflügers Arch* 1975;354:117–131.
258. LeHir M, Kaissling B, Dubach UE. Distal tubular segments of the rabbit kidney after adaptation to altered Na- and K-intake. II. Changes in Na-K-ATPase activity. *Cell Tissue Res* 1982;224:493–504.
259. Leng Q, Kahle KT, Rinehart J, MacGregor GG, Wilson FH, Canessa CM, Lifton RP, Hebert SC. WNK3, a kinase related to genes mutated in hereditary hypertension with hyperkalaemia, regulates the K^+ channel ROMK1 (Kir1.1). *J Physiol* 2006;571(2):275–286.
259a. Leviel F, Borenstein B, Honillier P, Paillard M, Bichara M. Electroneutral K^+/HCO_3^- cotransport in cells of medullary thick ascending limb of rat kidney. *J Clin Invest* 1992;90: 869–878.
260. Light DB, McCann FV, Keller TM, et al. Amiloride-sensitive cation channel in apical membrane of inner medullary collecting duct. *Am J Physiol Renal* 1988;255:F278–F285.
261. Lin SH, Cheema-Dhadli S, Gowrishankar M, et al. Control of excretion of potassium: Lessons from studies during prolonged total fasting in human subjects. *Am J Physiol Renal* 1997;273:F796.
262. Lin D-H., Sterling H, Wang Z, Babilonia E, Yang B, Dong K, Hebert SC, Giebisch G, Wang W-H. ROMK1 channel activity is regulated by monoubiquitination. *Proc Nat Acad Sci U S A* 2005;102:4306–4311.
263. Linas SL, Peterson LN, Anderson RJ, et al. Mechanism of renal potassium conservation in the rat. *Kidney Int* 1979;15:601–611.
264. Lindinger MI, Franklin TW, Lands LC, Pedersen PK, Welsh DG, Heigenhauser GJ. $NaHCO_3$ and $KHCO_3$ ingestion rapidly increases renal electrolyte excretion in humans. *J Appl Physiol* 2000;88:540–550.
265. Liu W, Xu S, Woda C, Kim P, Weinbaum S, Satlin LM. Effect of flow and stretch on the $[Ca^{2+}]$i response of principal and intercalated cells in cortical collecting duct. *Am J Physiol Renal* 2003;285:F998–F1012.
266. Lombard WE, Kokko JP, Jacobson HR. Bicarbonate transport in cortical and outer medullary collecting tubules. *Am J Physiol Renal* 1983;244:F289–F296.
267. Lu M, Leng Q, Egan ME, Caplan MJ, Boulpaep EL, Giebisch GH, Hebert SC. CFTR is required for PKA-regulated ATP sensitivity of Kir1.1 potassium channels in mouse kidney. *J Clin Sci* 2006;116:797–807.
268. Lu M, Wang WH. Nitric oxide regulates the low-conductance K channel in the basolateral membrane of the cortical collecting duct. *Am J Physiol* 1996;270:C1336–C1342.
269. Lu M, Wang WH. Protein kinase C stimulates the small-conductance K channel in the basolateral membrane of the collecting duct of the rat kidney. *Am J Physiol Renal* 1996;271: F1045–F1051.
270. Lubin M. Cell potassium and the regulation of protein synthesis. In: Hoffman JF, ed. *The Cellular Functions of Membrane Ttransport.* Englewood Cliffs, NJ: Prentice-Hall; 1964: 193–211.
271. Lynch IJ. Basolateral Ba abolishes stimulation of H-K-ATPase by 10% CO2 in cortical collecting duct (CCD) of K-restricted rabbits. *J Am Soc Nephrol* 1998;9:9A.
272. MacGregor GG, Xu J, McNicholas CM, Giebisch G, Hebert SC. Partially active channels produced by PKA site mutation of the cloned renal K^+ channel ROMK2. *Am J Physiol Renal* 1998;275:F415–F422.
273. MacKnight ADC, Leaf A. Regulation of cellular volume. In: Andreoli TA, Hoffman JF, Fanestil DD, eds. *Physiology of Membrane Disorders.* New York: Plenum; 1978:315–334.
274. Madsen KM, Tisher C. Structural-functional relationships along the distal nephron. *Am J Physiol Renal* 1986;250:F1–F15.
275. Madsen KM, Tisher CE. Cellular response to acute respiratory acidosis in rat medullary collecting duct. *Am J Physiol Renal* 1983;245:F670–F679.
276. Maguire D, MacNamara B, Cuffe JE, Winder D, Doolan CM, Urbach V, O'Sullivan GC, Harvey BJ. Rapid responses to aldosterone in human distal colon. *Steroids* 1999;64:51–63.
277. Malnic G, Bailey MA, Giebisch G. Control of renal potassium excretion. In: Brenner B, ed. *The Kidney*, 7th ed., Vol. 1. Philadelphia: WB Saunders; 2004:453–496.
278. Malnic G, Berliner RW, Giebisch G. Flow dependence of K^+ secretion in cortical distal tubules of the rat. *Am J Physiol Renal* 1989;256:F932–F941.
279. Malnic G, De Mello-Aires M, Giebisch G. Potassium transport across renal distal tubules during acid-base disturbances. *Am J Physiol Renal* 1971;221:1192–1208.
280. Malnic G, Giebisch G. Some electrical properties of distal tubular epithelium in the rat. *Am J Physiol Renal* 1972;223:797–808.
281. Malnic G, Klose RM, Giebisch G. Microperfusion study of distal tubular potassium and sodium transfer in rat kidney. *Am J Physiol Renal* 1966;211:548–599.
282. Malnic G, Klose RM, Giebisch G. Micropuncture study of renal potassium excretion in the rat. *Am J Physiol Renal* 1964;206:674–686.
283. Malvin RL, Wilde WS, Sullivan LP. Localization of nephron transport by stop-flow analysis. *Am J Physiol Renal* 1958;194:135–142.
284. Marsh DJ, Ullrich KJ, Rumrich G. Micropuncture analysis of the behavior of potassium ions in rat renal cortical tubules. *Pflügers Arch* 1963;277:107–119.
285. Marver D, Kokko JP. Renal target sites and the mechanism of action of aldosterone. *Miner Electrolyte Metab* 1983;9:1–18.
286. Mathialahan T, Maclennan KA, Sandle LN, Verbeke C, Sandle GI. Enhanced large intestinal potassium permeability in end-stage renal disease. *J Pathol* 2005;206:46–51.
287. Matsumura Y, Cohen B, Guggino WE, et al. Regulation of the basolateral potassium conductance of the Necturus proximal tubule. *J Membr Biol* 1984;79:153–161.
288. McCance RA, Widdowson EM. Alkalosis with disordered kidney function. *Lancet* 1937; 2:247–249.
289. McDonough AA, Thompson CB, Youn JH. Skeletal muscle regulates extracellular potassium. *Am J Physiol Renal* 2002;282:F967–F974.
290. McNicholas CM, Guggino WE, Schwiebert EM, et al. Sensitivity of a tenal K^+ channel (ROMKI) to the inhibitory sulfonylurea compound glibencamide is enhanced by coexpression with the ATP-binding cassette transporter cystic fibrosis transmembrane regulator. *Proc Natl Acad Sci U S A* 1996;93:8083–8088.
291. McNicholas CM, MacGregor GG, Islas LD, Yang Y, Hebert SC, Giebisch G. pH-dependent modulation of the cloned renal K^+ channel, ROMK. *Am J Physiol Renal* 1998;275:F971–F981.
292. McNicholas CM, Wang W, Ho K, et al. Regulation of ROMKI K^+ channel activity involves phosphorylation processes. *Proc Natl Acad Sci U S A* 1994;91:8077–8081.
293. McNicholas CM, Yang Y, Giebisch G, et al. Molecular site for nucleotide binding on an ATP-sensitive renal K^+ channel (ROMKI). *Am J Physiol Renal* 1996;271:F275–F285.
294. Meneton P, Loffing J, Warnock DG. Sodium and potassium handling by the aldosterone-sensitive distal nephron;the pivotal role of the distal and connecting tubule. *Am J Physiol Renal* 2004;287:F593–F601.
295. Meneton P, Schultheis PJ, Greeb J, Nieman ML, Liui LH, Clarke LL, Duffy JJ, Doetschman T, Lorenz JN, Shull GE. Increased sensitivity to K^+ deprivation in colonic H-K-ATPase-deficient mice. *J Clin Invest* 1998;101:536–542.
296. Miller CE, Remenchik AP. Problems involved in accurately measuring the K content of the human body. *Ann NY Acad Sci* 1963;110:175–188.
297. Modyanov NN, Mathews PM, Grishin AV, et al. Human ATPIALI gene encodes a ouabain-sensitive H-K-ATPase. *Am J Physiol* 1995;269:C992–C997.
298. Moellic CL, Ouvrard-Pascaud A, Capurro C, Cluzeaud F, Fay M, Jaisser F, Farman N, Blot-Chabaud M. Early nongenomic events in aldosterone action in renal collecting duct cells: PKCa activation, mineralocorticoid receptor phosphorylation, and cross-talk with the genomic response. *J Am Soc Nephrol* 2004;15:1145–1160.
299. Moore-Ede MC, Herd JA. Renal electrolyte circadian rhythms: independence from feeding and activity patterns. *Am J Physiol Renal* 1977;232:FI28–FI35.
300. Moore-Ede MC. Physiology of the circadian timing system: predictive versus reactive homeostasis. *Am J Physiol* 1986;250:R735–R752.
301. Moore-Ede MD, Meguid MM, Fitzpatrick GF, et al. Circadian variation in response to potassium infusion. *Clin Pharmacol Ther* 1978;23:218–227.
302. Moral Z, Deng K, Wei Y, Sterling H. Deng H, Ali S, Gu RM, Huang XY, Hebert SC, Giebisch G, Wang WH. Regulation of ROMK1 channels by protein tyrosine kinase and tyrosine phosphatase. *J Biol Chem* 2001;276:7156–7163.
303. Morgan TO, Tadokoro M, Martin D, et al. Effect of furosemide on Na^+ and K^+ transport studied by microperfusion of the rat nephron. *Am J Physiol Renal* 1970;218:292–297.
303a. Morita H, Fujiki N, Miyahara T, Lee K, Tanaka K. Hepatoportal bumetanide-sensitive K^+-sensor mechanism controls urinary K^+ excretion. *Am J Physiol* 2000;278:R1134–R1139.
304. Morita T, Hanaoka K, Morales MM, Montrose-Rafizadeh C, Guggino WB. Cloning and characterization of maxi K^+ channel a-subunit in rabbit kidney. *Am J Physiol Renal* 1997;273: F615–F624.
305. Morsing P, Velazquez H, Wright FS, et al. Adaptation of the distal convoluted tubule of the rat. 11. Effect of chronic thiazide infusion. *Am J Physiol Renal* 1991;261:F137–F143.
306. Mudge GH, Ames A, Foulks J, et al. Effects of drugs on renal secretion of potassium in the dog. *Am J Physiol Renal* 1950;161:F151–F158.
307. Mudge GH, Foulks J, Gilman A. Renal secretion of potassium in the dog during cellular dehydration. *Am J Physiol Renal* 1950;161:F159–F166.
308. Mudge GH, Foulks J, Gilman A. The renal excretion of potassium. *Proc Soc Exp Biol Med* 1948;67:545–547.
309. Mujais SK, Chekal MA, Jones WJ, et al. Regulation of renal Na-K ATPase in the rat: role of the natural mineralo- and glucocorticoid hormones. *J Clin Invest* 1984;73:13–19.
310. Mujais SK, Chen Y, Nora NA. Discordant aspects of aldosterone resistance in potassium depletion *Am J Physiol Renal* 1992;262:F972–F979.
311. Mujais WK. Renal memory after potassium adaptation: role of Na^+-K^+-ATPase. *Am J Physiol Renal* 1988;254:F845.
312. Muto S, Asano Y, Seldin D, et al. Basolateral Na^+ pump modulates apical Na^+ and K^+ conductances in rabbit cortical collecting ducts. *Am J Physiol Renal* 1999;276:F143–F158.
313. Muto S, Sansom SC, Giebisch G. Effects of high K^+ diet on the electrical properties of cortical collecting ducts from adrenalectomized rabbits. *J Clin Invest* 1988;81:376–380.
314. Muto S. Potassium transport in the mammalian collecting duct. *Physiol Rev* 2001;81: 85–116.
315. Najjar F, Zhou H, Morimoto E et al. Dietary K^+ regulates apical membrane expression of maxi-K channels in rabbit cortical collecting duct. *Am J Physiol Renal* 2005;289:F922–F932.
316. Náray-Fejes-Tóth A, Canessa C, Cleaveland ES, Aldrich G, Fejes-Tóth G. Sgk is an aldosterone-induced kinase in the renal collecting duct. Effects on epithelial Na^+ channels. *J Biol Chem* 1999;274:16973–16978.
317. Nelson JA, Nechay RB. Interaction of ouabain and K in vivo with respect to renal adenosine triphosphatase activity and Na reabsorption. *J Pharmacol Exp Ther* 1971;176:558–562.
318. Oberleithner H, Dietl P, Munich G, et al. Relationship between luminal Na^+H^+ exchange and luminal K^+ conductance in diluting segment of frog kidney. *Pflügers Arch* 1985;405: 5110–5114.
319. Oberleithner H, Giebisch G, Lang F, et al. Cellular mechanism of the furosemide sensitive transport system in the kidney. *Klin Wochenschr* 1982;60:1173–1179.
320. Oberleithner H, Guggino W, Giebisch G. Potassium transport in the distal tubule of Amphiuma kidney: effects of potassium adaptation. *Pflügers Arch* 1983;396:185–191.
321. Oberleithner H, Guggino W, Giebisch G. The effect of furosemide on luminal sodium, chloride and potassium transport in the early distal tubule of Amphiuma kidney: effects of potassium adaptation. *Pflügers Arch* 1983;396:27–33.
322. Oberleithner H, Lang F, Greger R, et al. Effect of luminal potassium transport on cellular sodium activity in the early distal tubule of Amphiuma kidney. *Pflugers Arch* 1983;396: 34–40.
323. Oberleithner H, Lang F, Wang W, et al. Effects of inhibition of chloride transport on intracellular sodium activity in distal amphibian nephron. *Pflugers Arch* 1982;394:55–60.
324. Oberleithner H, Ritter M, Lang F, et al. Anthracene-9-carboxylic acid inhibits renal chloride reabsorption. *Pflugers Arch* 1983;398:172–174.

325. Oberleithner H, Weight M, Westphale HD, et al. Aldosterone activates Na/H exchange and raises cytoplasmic pH in target cells of the amphibian kidney. *Proc Natl Acad Sci U S A* 1987; 84:1464–1488.
326. Okusa MD, Unwin RJ, Velazquez H, et al. Active potassium absorption by the renal distal tubule. *Am J Physiol Renal* 1992;31:F488.
327. Okusa MD, Velazquez H, Ellison DH, et al. Luminal calcium regulates potassium transport by the renal distal tubule. *Am J Physiol Renal* 1990;258:F423–F428.
328. Okusa MD, Velazquez H, Wright FS. Effect of Na-channel blockers and lumen Ca on K secretion by rat renal distal tubule. *Am J Physiol Renal* 1991;260:F459–F465.
329. Oliver WJ, Cohen EL, Neel JV. Blood pressure, sodium intake, and sodium related hormones in the Yanomamo Indians, a "no-salt" culture. *Circulation* 1975;52:146.
330. O'Neil RG, Boulpaep EL. Effect of amiloride on the apical cell membrane cation channels of a sodium-absorbing, potassium-secreting renal epithelium. *J Membr Biol* 1979;50:365–387.
331. O'Neil RG, Boulpaep EL. Ionic conductive properties and electrophysiology of the rabbit cortical collecting tubule. *Am J Physiol Renal* 1982;243:F81–F95.
332. O'Neil RG, Hayhurst RA. Sodium-dependent modulation of the renal Na-K-ATPase: influence of mineralocorticoids on the cortical collecting duct. *J Membr Biol* 1985;85: 169–179.
333. O'Neil RG, Helman S1. Transport characteristics of renal collecting tubules: influences of DOCA and diet. *Am J Physiol Renal* 1977;233:F544–F558.
334. O'Neil RG, Sansom SE. Characterization of apical cell membrane Na^+ and K^+ conductances of cortical collecting duct using microelectrode techniques. *Am J Physiol Renal* 1984;247: F14–F24.
335. O'Neil RG. Aldosterone regulation of sodium and potassium transport in the cortical collecting tubule. *Semin Nephrol* 1990;10:365–374.
336. Ookata K, Tojo A, Suzuki Y, Nakamura N, Kimura K, Wilcox CS, Hirose S. Localization of inward rectifier potassium channel Kir7.1 in the basolateral membrane of distal nephron and collecting duct. *J Am Soc Nephrol* 2000;11:1987–1994.
337. Ornt DB, Radke KJ, Scandling JD. Effect of aldosterone on renal potassium conservation in the rat. *Am J Physiol* 1996;270:E1003–E1008.
338. Ornt DB, Tannen RL. Demonstration of an intrinsic renal adaptation for K^+ conservation in short-term K^+ depletion. *Am J Physiol Renal* 1983;245:F329–F338.
339. Pacha J, Frindt G, Sackin H, et al. Apical maxi K channels in intercalated cells of cortical collecting tubule. *Am J Physiol Renal* 1991;261:F696–F705.
340. Palmada M, Embark HM, Wyatt AW, Böhmer C, Lang F. Negative charge at the consensus sequence for the serum- and glucocorticoid-inducible kinase, SGK1, determines pH sensitivity of the renal outer medullary K^+ channel, ROMK1. *Biochem Biophys Res Comm* 2003;307: 967–972.
341. Palmer L. Potassium secretion and the regulation of distal nephron K channels. *Am J Physiol Renal* 1999;277:F821–F825.
342. Palmer LG, Frindt G. Alosterone and potassium secretion by the cortical collecting duct. *Kidney Int* 2000;547:1324–1328.
343. Palmer LG, Antonian L, Frindt G. Regulation of apical K and Na channels and Na/K pumps in rat cortical collecting tubule by dietary K. *J Gen Physiol* 1994;104:693–710.
344. Palmer LG, Choe H, Frindt G. Is the secretory K channel in the rat CCT ROMK? *Am J Physiol Renal* 1997;273:F404–F410.
345. Palmer LG, Frindt G. Regulation of apical K channels in rat cortical collecting tubule during changes in dietary K intake. *Am J Physiol Renal* 1999;277:F805–F812.
346. Palmer LG, Frindt G. Effects of cell Ca and pH on Na channels from rat cortical collecting tubule. *Am J Physiol Renal* 1987;253:F333–F339.
347. Palmer LG, Sackin H. Regulation of renal ion channels. *FASEB J* 1988;2:3061–3065.
348. Palmer LG. Potassium secretion and the regulation of distal nephron K channels. *Am J Physiol Renal* 1999;277:F821–F825.
349. Patrick J. Assessment of body potassium stores. *Kidney Int* 1977;11:476–490.
350. Peterson LN, Wright FS. Effect of sodium intake on renal potassium excretion. *Am J Physiol Renal* 1977;233:F225–F234.
351. Petrovic S, Spicer Z, Greeley T, Shull GE, Soleimani M. Novel Schering and ouabain-insensitive potassium-dependent proton secretion in the mouse cortical collecting duct. *Am J Physiol Renal* 2002;282:F133–F143.
352. Plata C, Meade P, Hall A, Welch RC, Vazquez N, Hebert SC, Gamba G. Alternatively spliced isoform of apical Na^+-K^+-Cl^- cotransporter gene encodes a furosemide-sensitive Na^+-Cl^- cotransporter. *Am J Physiol Renal* 2001;280:F574–F582.
353. Pluznick JL, Sansom SC. BK channels in the Kidney: Role in K^+ secretion and localization of molecular components. *Am J Physiol* 2006;291:F517–F529.
354. Pluznick JL, Wei P, Grimm PR, Sansom SC. BK-ß1 subunit: immunolocalization in the mammalian connecting tubule and its role in the kaliuretic response to volume expansion. *Am J Physiol Renal* 2005;288:F846–F854.
355. Proverbio F, Whittembury G. Cell electrical potential during enhanced Na extrusion in guinea-pig cortex slices. *J Physiol (London)* 1975;50:559–578.
356. Rabelink TJ, Koomans HA, Hene J, et al. Early and late adjustment to potassium loading in humans. *Kidney Int* 1990;38:942–947.
357. Rabinowitz L, Berlin R, Yamauchi H. Plasma potassium and diurnal cyclic potassium excretion in the rat. *Am J Physiol Renal* 1987;253:F1178–F1181.
358. Rabinowitz L, Wydner CJ, Smith KM, et al. Diurnal potassium excretory cycles in the rat. *Am J Physiol Renal* 1986;250:F930–F941.
359. Rabinowitz L. Homeostatic regulation of potassium exctetion. *J Hypertens* 1989;7:433–442.
360. Rastegar A, Biemesderfer D, Kashgarian M, et al. Changes in membrane surfaces of collecting duct cells in potassium adaptation. *Kidney Int* 1980;18:293–301.
361. Rector FC Jr, Bloomer HA, Seldin DW. Proximal tubular reabsorption of potassium during mannitol diuresis in rats. *J Lab Clin Med* 1964;63:100–105.
362. Reeves WE, Shah SV. Activation of potassium channels contributes to hypoxic injury in proximal tubules. *J Clin Invest* 1994;94:2289–2294.
363. Reeves WE, Winters Q, Zimniak L, et al. Medullary thick limbs: renal concentrating segments. *Kidney Int* 1996;50:S154–S164.
364. Reinalter SC, Jeck N, Peters M, Seyberth HW. Pharmacotyping of hypokalaemic salt-losing tubular disorders. *Acta Physiol Scand* 2004;181:513–521.
365. Reineck HJ, Osgood RW, Stein JH. Net potassium addition beyond the superficial distal tubule of the rat. *Am J Physiol Renal* 1978;235:F104–F110.
366. Rhee MS, Perianayagam A, Chen P, Youn JH, McDonough AA. Dexamethasone treatment causes resistence to insulin-stimulated cellular potassium uptake in the rat. *Am J Physiol Cell Physiol* 2004;287;C1229–C1237.
367. Rocha AS, Kudo LH. Water, urea, sodium, chloride, and potassium transport in the in vitro isolated perfused papillary collecting duct. *Kidney Int* 1982;22:485–491.
368. Rosetti L, Robbenhaar GK, Giebisch G, et al. Effect of insulin on renal potassium metabolism. *Am J Physiol Renal* 1987;252:F60–F64.
369. Rubert I, Loffing J, Palmer LG, Frindt G, Fowler-Jaeger N, Sauter D, Carroll T, McMahon A, Hummler E, Rossier BC. Collecting duct-specific gene inactivation of aENaC in the mouse kidney does not impair sodium and potassium balance. *J Clin Invest* 2003;112: 554–565.
370. Sackin H, Boulpaep EL. Isolated perfused salamander proximal tubule. II. Monovalent ion replacement and rheogenic transport. *Am J Physiol Renal* 1981;241:F540–F555.
371. Sackin H, Boulpaep EL. Rheogenic transport in the renal proximal tubule. *J Physiol (London)* 1983;82:819–851.
372. Sackin H. Stretch-activated potassium channels in renal proximal tubule. *Am J Physiol Renal* 1987;241:F540–F555.
373. Sansom SC, Mougouris T, Ono S, et al. ATP-sensitive K^+-selective channels of inner medullary collecting duct cells. *Am J Physiol Renal* 1994;267:F489–F496.
374. Sansom SC, O'Neil RG. Mineralocorticoid regulation of apical cell membrane Na^+ and K^+ transport of the cortical collecting duct. *Am J Physiol Renal* 1985;248:F858–F868.
375. Sansom SE, Agulian S, Muto S, et al. K activity of CCD principal cells from normal and DOCA-treated rabbits. *Am J Physiol Renal* 1989;256:F136–F142.
376. Sansom SE, Muto S, Giebisch G. Na-dependent effects of DOCA on cellular transport properties of CCDs from ADX rabbits. *Am J Physiol Renal* 1987;253:F753–F759.
377. Sansom SE, O'Neil RG. Effects of mineralocorticoids on transport properties of cortical collecting duct basolateral membrane. *Am J Physiol Renal* 1986;241:F743–F757.
378. Sastrasinh S, Tannen RL. Effect of potassium on renal NH3 production. *Am J Physiol Renal* 1983;244:F383–F391.
379. Satlin LM. Postnatal maturation of potassium transport in rabbit cortical collecting duct. *Am J Physiol Renal* 1994;266:F57–F65.
380. Satlin LM. Regulation of potassium transport in the maturing kidney. *Semin Nephrol* 1999;19(2):155–165.
381. Sauer M, Flemmer A, Thurau K, Beck FX. Sodium entry routes in principal and intercalated cells of the isolated perfused cortical collecting duct. *Pflugers Arch* 1990;416:88–93.
382. Schafer C, Westphale HJ, Oberleithner H. Contrasting action of H^+ and Ca^{2+} on K^+-transport in diluting segment of frog kidney. *Cell Physiol Biochem* 1991;1:286–293.
383. Schafer JA, Troutman SL, Schlatter E. Vasopressin and mineralocorticoid increase apical membrane driving force for K^+ secretion in rat CCD. *Am J Physiol Renal* 1990;258: F199–F210.
384. Schafer JA, Troutman SL. Effect of ADH on rubidium transport in isolated perfused rat cortical collecting tubule. *Am J Physiol* 1986;250:F1063–F1072.
385. Schafer JA, Work J. Transport properties of the pars recta. *Nephrology* 1985;1:186–195.
386. Schafer J. Renal regulation of potassium, calcium and magnesium. In: Johnson CR, ed. *Essential Medical Physiology*, 3rd ed. San Diego, CA: Elsevier Academic Press; 2003:437–446.
387. Schlatter E, Greger R, Widtke C. Effect of "high ceiling" diuretics on active salt transport in the cortical thick ascending limb of Henle's loop of rabbit kidney. Correlation of chemical structure and inhibitory potency. *Pflügers Arch* 1983;396:210–217.
388. Schlatter E, Haxelmans S, Ankorina I. Correlation between intracellular activities of Ca^{2+} and Na^+ in rat cortical collecting duct: a possible coupling mechanism between Na^+-K^+-ATPase and basolateral K conductance. *Kidney Blood Press Res* 1996;19:24–31.
389. Schlatter E, Haxelmans S, Hirsch J, et al. pH dependence of K conductances of rat cortical collecting duct principal cells. *Pflügers Arch* 1994;428:631–640.
390. Schlatter E, Lohrmann E, Greger R. Properties of the potassium conductances of principal cells of rat cortical collecting ducts. *Pflügers Arch* 1992;420:39–45.
391. Schlatter E, Schafer JA. Electrophysiological studies in principal cells of rat cortical collecting tubules. ADH increases the apical membrane Na^+-conductance. *Pflugers Arch* 1987;409: 81–92.
392. Schlatter E. Antidiuretic hormone regulation of electrolyte transport in the distal nephron. *Renal Physiol Biochem* 1989;12:65–84.
393. Schlatter E. Regulation of ion channels in the cortical collecting duct. *Renal Physiol Biochem* 1993;16:21-36.
394. Schnermann J, Steipe B, Briggs JP. *In situ* studies of distal convoluted tubule in rat. II. K secretion. *Am J Physiol Renal* 1987;252:F970–F976.
395. Schon DA, Backman KA, Hayslett JP. Role of the medullary collecting duct in potassium excretion in potassium-adapted animals. *Kidney Int* 1981;20:655–662.
396. Schultz SG. Homocellular regulatory mechanisms in sodium-transporting epithelia: avoidance of extinction by "flush-through." *Am J Physiol Renal* 1981;21:F579–F590.
397. Schultz SG. Homocellular regulatory mechanisms in sodium-transporting epithelia: an extension of the Koefoed-Johnsen-Ussing model. *Semin Nephrol* 1982;2:343–347.
398. Sejersted OM, Sjøgaard, G. Dynamics and consequences of potassium shifts in skeletal muscle and heart during exercise. *Physiol Rev* 2000;80:1411–1481.
399. Seldin DW, Welt LG, Cart JH. The role of sodium salts and adrenal steroids in the production of hypokalemic alkalosis. *Yale J Biol Med* 1956;29:229–247.
400. Sewell KJ, Shirley DG, Michael AE, Thompson A, Norgate DP, Unwin RJ. In vivo inhibition of renal 11b-hydroxysteroid dehydrogenase by carbenoxolone in the rat and its relationship to sodium excretion. *Clin Sci* 1998;95:435–443.
401. Shirley DG, Walter SJ, Folkerd EJ, et al. Transepithelial electrochemical gradient in the proximal convoluted tubule during potassium depletion in the rat. *J Physiol (London)* 1998;513:551–557.

402. Silver RB, Frindt G, Mennitt P, et al. Characterization and regulation of H-K-ATPase in intercalated cells of rabbit cortical collecting duct. *J Exp Zool* 1997;279:443–455.
403. Silver RB, Frindt G. Functional identification of H^+/K^+-ATPase in intercalated cells of cortical collecting tubule. *Am J Physiol Renal* 1993;264:F259–F266.
404. Silver RB, Mennitt PA, Sadin LM. Stimulation of apical H-K-ATPase in intercalated cells of cortical collecting duct with chronic metabolic acidosis. *Am J Physiol Renal* 1996;270:F539.
405. Silver RB, Soleimani M. H^+-K^+-ATPases: regulation and role in pathophysiological states. *Am J Physiol Renal* 1999;276:F799–F811.
406. Smith PL, Frizzell RA. Chloride secretion by canine tracheal epithelium: IV: Basolateral membrane K permeability parallels secretion rate. *J Membr Biol* 1984;77:187–199.
407. Sonnenberg H. Medullary collecting duct function in antidiuretic and in salt- or water-diuretic rats. *Am J Physiol Renal* 1974;226:F501–F506.
408. Stanton B, Kaissling B. Adaptation of distal tubule and collecting duct to increased sodium delivery. II. Na^+ and K^+ transport. *Am J Physiol Renal* 1988;255:F1269–F1275.
409. Stanton B, Klein-Robbenhaar G, Wade J, et al. Effects of adrenalectomy and chronic adrenal corticosteroid replacement on potassium transport in rat kidney. *J Clin Invest* 1985;75: 1317–1326.
410. Stanton B, Pan L, Deetjen P, et al. Independent effects of aldosterone and potassium on induction of potassium adaptation in rat kidney. *Clin Invest* 1987;79:198–206.
411. Stanton B. Regulation by adrenal corticosteroids of sodium and potassium transport in loop of Henle and distal tubule of rat kidney. *J Clin Invest* 1986;78:1612–1620.
412. Stanton B. Renal potassium adaptation: cellular mechanisms and morphology. In: Giebisch G, ed. *Current Topics in Membranes and Transport*, Vol. 28. Orlando, FL: Academic Press; 1987:225–267.
413. Stanton BA, Biemesderfer D, Wade JB, et al. Structural and functional study of the rat distal nephron: effects of potassium adaptation and potassium depletion. *Kidney Int* 1981;19:36–48.
414. Stanton BA, Giebisch G. Effects of pH on potassium transport by renal distal tubule. *Am J Physiol Renal* 1982;242:F544–F551.
415. Stanton BA, Giebisch G. Renal potassium transport. In: Windhager EE, ed. *Handbook of Physiology: Renal Physiology*. New York: Oxford University Press; 1991;813–874.
416. Stanton BA, Giebisch GH. Potassium transport by the renal distal tubule: effect of potassium loading. *Am J Physiol Renal* 1982;243:F487–F493.
417. Stanton BA, Guggino WB, Giebisch G. Acidification of the basolateral solution reduces potassium conductance of the apical membrane. *Ped Proc* 1982;41:1006.
418. Stanton BA, Janzen A, Wade J, et al. Ultrastructure of rat initial collecting tubule: effect of adrenal corticosteroid treatment. *J Clin Invest* 1985;75:1327–1334.
419. Stanton BA. Characterization of apical and basolateral membrane conductances of rat inner medullary collecting duct. *Am J Physiol Renal* 1989;256:F862–F868.
420. Stanton BA. Renal potassium transport: morphological and functional adaptations. *Am J Physiol* 1989;257:R989–R997.
421. Steele A, deVeber H, Quaggin SE, et al. What is responsible for the diurnal variation in potassium excretion? *Am J Physiol* 1994;267:R554–R560.
422. Sterns RH, Cox M, Feig PU, et al. Internal potassium balance and the control of the plasma potassium concentration. *Medicine (Baltimore)* 1981;60:339–354.
423. Sterns RH, Feig PU, Pring M, et al. Disposition of intravenous potassium in anuric man: a kinetic analysis. *Kidney Int* 1979;15:651~660.
424. Sterns RH. Oscillations of plasma K^+ and insulin during K^+ infusion in awake anephric dogs. *Am J Physiol Renal* 1982;243:F44–F52.
425. Stetson DL, Wade JB, Giebisch G. Morphologic alterations in the rat medullary collecting duct following potassium depletion. *Kidney Int* 1980;17:45–56.
426. Stewart PM, Krozowski ZS, Gupta A, et al. Hypertension in the syndrome of apparent mineralocorticoid excess due to mutation of the 11 beta-hydroxysteroid dehydrogenase type 2 gene. *Lancet* 1996;247:88.
427. Stokes JB, Ingram MJ, Williams AD, et al. Heterogeneity of the rabbit collecting tubule: localization of mineralocorticoid hormone action to the cortical portion. *Kidney Int* 1981;20:340–347.
428. Stokes JB. Consequences of potassium recycling in the renal medulla. Effects on ion transport by the medullary thick ascending limb of Henle's loop. *J Clin Invest* 1982;70: 219–229.
429. Stokes JB. Ion transport by the collecting duct. *Semin Nephrol* 1993;13:202–212.
430. Stokes JB. Ion transport by the cortical and outer medullary collecting tubule. *Kidney Int* 1982;22:473–484.
431. Stokes JB. Na and K transport across the cortical and outer medullary collecting tubule of the rabbit: evidence for diffusion across the outer medullary portion. *Am J Physiol Renal* 1982;242:F514–F520.
432. Stokes JB. Potassium intoxication: pathogenesis and treatment. In: Seldin DW, Giebisch G, eds. *The Regulation of Potassium Balance*. New York: Raven Press; 1989:269–302.
433. Stokes JB. Potassium secretion by cortical collecting tubule: relation to sodium absorption, luminal sodium concentration, and transepithelial voltage. *Am J Physiol Renal* 1981;241: F395–F402.
434. Strieter J, Stephenson JL, Giebisch G, Weinstein AM. A mathematical model of the rabbit cortical collecting tubule. *Am J Physiol Renal* 1992;F1063–F1075.
435. Strieter J, Weinstein AM, Giebisch G, Stephenson JL. Regulation of K transport in a mathematical model of the cortical collecting tubule. *Am J Physiol Renal* 1992;263:F1076–F1086.
436. Sufit CR, Jamison RL. Effect of acute potassium load on reabsorption in Henle's loop in the rat. *Am J Physiol Renal* 1983;245:F569–F576.
437. Suh A, DeJesus E, Rosner K, Lerma E, Yu W, Young JB, Rosa RM. Racial differences in potassium disposal. *Kidney Int* 2004;66:1076–1081.
438. Summa V, Mardasini D, Roger F, Bens M, Martin PY, Vandewalle A, Verry F, Feraille E. Short term effect of aldosterone on Na-K-ATPase cell surface expression in kidney collecting duct cells. *J Biol Chem* 2001;276:47087–47093.
439. Tabei K, Muto S, Furuya H, Sakairi Y, Ando Y, Asano Y. Potassium secretion is inhibited by metabolic acidosis in rabbit cortical collecting ducts in vitro. *Am J Physiol Renal* 1995;268: F490–F495.
440. Taniguchi S, Marchetti J, Morel F. Na/Ca exchangers in collecting cells of rat kidney. A single tubule fura-2 study. *Pflugers Arch* 1989;415:191–197.
441. Tannen RL. Effect of potassium on renal acidification and acid-base homeostasis. *Semin Nephrol* 1987;7:263–272.
442. Tannen RL. Potassium and acid-base balance. In: Giebisch G, ed. *Current Topics in Membranes and Transport*, Vol 28. Orlando, FL: Academic Press; 1987:207–223.
443. Thompson A, Bailey MA, Michael AE, Unwin RJ. Effects of changes in dietary intake of sodium and potassium and of metabolic acidosis on 11beta-hydroxysteroid dehydrogenase activities in rat kidney. *Exp Nephrol* 2000;8:44–51.
444. Toback FG, Ordonez NG, Bortz SL, Spargo B. Zonal changes in renal structure and phospholipids metabolism in potassium-deficient rats. *Lab Invest* 1976;34:115–124.
445. Tomita K, Pisano J, Knepper MA. Control of sodium and potassium transport in the cortical collecting duct of the rat. Effects of bradykinin, vasopressin, and deoxycorticosterone. *J Clin Invest* 1985;76:132–136.
446. Tsuchiya K, Wang W, Giebisch G, et al. ATP is a coupling modulator of parallel Na^+/K^+ ATPase-K^+ channel activity in the renal proximal tubule. *Proc Natl Acad Sci U S A* 1992; 89:6418–6422.
447. Tsuruoka S, Koseki C, Muto S, et al. Axial heterogeneity of potassium transport across hamster thick ascending limb of Henle's loop. *Am J Physiol Renal* 1994;267:F121.
448. Turban S, Wang XY, Knepper MA. Regulation of NHE3 NKCC2, and NCC abundance in kidney during aldosterone escape phenomenon: role of NO. *Am J Physiol Renal Physiol* 2003;285:F843–F851.
449. Unwin R, Capasso G, Giebisch G. Potassium and sodium transport along the loop of Henle: effects of altered dietary potassium intake. *Kidney Int* 1994;46:1092–1099.
450. Unwin RJ, Capasso G, Giebisch G, et al. Loop of Henle (LOH) potassium transport and the urinary concentrating mechanism. In: DeSanto NG, Capasso G, eds. *Acid-base and Electrolyte Balance*. Naples: Institute Italy Pere Gli Studi Filosofici; 1995:243–256.
451. Unwin RJ, Walter SJ, Giebisch G, Capasso G, Shirley DG. Localisation of diuretic effects along the loop of Henle in vivo. *Clin Sci* 2000;98:481–488.
452. Unwin, RJ, Capasso G, Giebisch G, Shirley DG Walter SJ. Loop of Henle (LOH) potassium transport and the urinary concentrating mechanism. In: *Acid-Base and Electrolyte Balance*, DeSanto and Capasso, eds. Proc 2nd Borelli Congress, July 1995:243–256. Inst. Ital. Per gli Studi Filosofici; 1995.
453. Ussing HH, Leaf A. Transport across multimembrane systems. In: Giebisch G, Tosteson DC, Ussing HH, ed. *Membrane Transport in Biology*, Vol. 3. New York: Springer-Verlag; 1978:1.
454. Ussing HH. The alkali metal ions in isolated systems and tissues. In: *Handbuch der experimentellen Pharmakologie*. Heidelberg: Springer-Verlag; 1960:1–195.
455. Vallon V, Grahammer F, Völkl H, Sandu CD, Richter K, Rexhepaj R, Gerlach U, Rong Q, Pfeifer K, Lang F. KCNQ1 dependent transport in renal and gastrointestinal epithelia. *Proc Natl Acad Sci U S A* 2005;102:17864–17869.
456. Vallon V, Lang F. New insights into the role of serum- and glucocorticoid-inducible kinase SGK1 in the regulation of renal function and blood pressure. *Curr Opin Nephrol Hypertens* 2005;14:59–66.
457. Vallon V, Osswald H, Blantz RC, et al. Potential role of luminal potassium in tubuloglomerular feedback. *J Am Soc Nephrol* 1997;8:1831–1837.
458. Vallon V, Wulff P, Huang DY, Loffing J, Völkl H, Kuhl D, Lang F. Role of Sgk1 in salt and potassium homeostasis. *Am J Physiol* 2004;288:R4–R10.
459. Van Ypersele de Strihou C. Potassium homeostasis in renal failure. *Kidney Int* 1997;11: 491–504.
460. Vanoye CG, MacGregor GG, Dong K, Tang L, Hall AE, Lu M, Giebisch G, Hebert SC. The carboxy-termini of KATP channels form functional tetramers that bind TNP-ATP with negative cooperativity. *J Biol Chem* 2002;277:23260–23270.
461. Vasuvattakul S, Quaggin SE, Scheich AM, Bayoumi A, Goguen JM, Cheema-Dhadli S, Halperin ML. Kaliuretic response to aldosterone: Influence of the content of potassium in the diet. *Am J Kidney Dis* 1993;21:152–160.
462. Velazquez H, Ellison DH, Wright FS. Chloride-dependent potassium secretion in early and late distal tubules. *Am J Physiol Renal* 1987;253:F555–562.
463. Velazquez H, Giebisch G. Effects of diuretics on specific transport systems. *Semin Nephrol* 1988;8:295–304.
464. Velazquez H, Wright FS, Good DW. Luminal influences on potassium secretion: chloride replacement with sulfate. *Am J Physiol Renal* 1982;242:F46--F55.
465. Velazquez H, Wright FS. Tubular Potassium Transport. In: *Diseases of the Kidney and Urinary Tract*. Schrier RW, ed, 7th ed. Philadelphia: Lippincott, Williams & Wilkins; 2001.
466. Velazquez H, Wright FS. Control by drugs of renal potassium handling. *Annu Rev Pharmacol Toxicol* 1986;26:293–309.
467. Velazquez H, Wright FS. Effects of diuretic drugs on Na, Cl, and K transport by rat renal distal tubule. *Am J Physiol Renal* 1986;250:FI013–FI023.
468. Velazquez H. Thiazide diuretics. *Renal Physiol* 1987;10:184–197.
469. Verrey F, Loffing J, Zecevic M, Heitzmann D. SGK1: Aldosterone-induced relay of Na^+ transport regulation in distal kidney nephron cells. *Cell Physiol Biochem* 2003;13:21–28.
470. Verrey F. Early aldosterone effects. *Exp Nephrol* 1998;6:294–301.
471. Vestri S, Malnic G. Mechanism of potassium transport across proximal tubule epithelium in the rat. *Braz J Med Biol Res* 1990;23:1195–1199.
472. Vinciguerra M, Deschenes G, Hasler U, Mardasini D, Rousselot M, Doucet A, Vandewalle A, Martin P-Y, Feraille E. Intracellular Na^+ control cell surface expression of Na, K-ATPase via a camp-independent PKA pathway in mammalian kidney collecting duct cells. *Mol Biol Cell* 2003;14:2677–2688.
473. Wade JB, Fang L, Liu J, Li D, Yang C-L, Subramanya AR, Maouyo D, Mason A, Ellison DH, Welling PA. WNK1 kinase isoform switch regulates renal potassium excretion. *Proc Natl Acad Sci U S A* 2006;103:8558–8563.
474. Wade JB, O'Neil RG, Pryor JL, et al. Modulation of cell membrane area in renal collecting tubules by corticosteroid hormones. *J Cell Biol* 1979;81:439–445.
475. Wade JB, Stanton BA, Field MJ, et al. Morphological and physiological responses to aldosterone: time course and sodium dependence. *Am J Physiol Renal* 1990;259:F88–F94.

476. Wall SM, Davis BS, Hassell KA, et al. In rat tIMCD, NH4$^+$ uptake by Na^+-K^+-ATPase is critical to net acid secretion during chronic hypokalemia. *Am J Physiol Renal* 1999;277: F866.
477. Wall SM, Fischer MP, Kim GH, et al. In rat inner medullary collecting duct, NH uptake by the Na-K-ATPase is increased during hypokalemia. *Am J Physiol Renal* 2002;282:F91.
478. Wall SM, Fischer MP. Contribution of the Na^+-K^+-2Cl^- cotransporter (NKCC11) to transepithelial transport of H^+, NH4$^+$, K^+ and Na^+ in rat outer medullary collecting duct. *J Am Soc Nephrol* 2002;13:827.
479. Wall SM, Koger LM. NH4$^+$ transport mediated by Na^+-K^+-ATPase in rat inner medullary collecting duct. *Am J Physiol Renal* 1994;267:F660.
480. Wall SM. Impact of K^+ homeostasis on net acid secretion in rat terminal inner medullary collecting duct: Role of the Na-K-ATPase. *Am J Kidney Dis* 2000;36:1079.
481. Wall SM. Impact of K^+ homeostasis on net acid secretion in rat terminal inner medullary collecting duct: Role of the Na-K-ATPase. *Am J Kidney Dis* 2000;36:1079–1088.
482. Wang W, Lerea KM, Chan M, Giebisch G. Protein tyrosine kinase regulates the number of renal secretory K channels. *Am J Physiol Renal* 2000;278:F165–F171.
483. Wang T, Wang W, Klein-Robbenhaar G, et al. Effects of a novel KATP channel blocker on renal tubule function and K channel activity. *J Pharmacol Exp Ther* 1995;273:1382–1389.
484. Wang T, Wang W, Klein-Robbenhaar G, et al. Effects of glyburide on renal tubule transport and potassium-channel activity. *Renal Physiol Biochem* 1995;18:169–182.
485. Wang W, Geibel J, Giebisch G. Potassium channels in apical membrane of rat thick ascending limb of Henle's loop. *Am J Physiol Renal* 1990;258:F244–F253.
486. Wang W, Giebisch G. Dual effect of adenosine triphosphate on the apical small conductance K^+ channel of rat cortical collecting duct. *J Gen Physiol* 1991;98:1–27.
487. Wang W, Hebert SC, Giebisch G. Renal K^+ channels: structure and function. *Annu Rev Physiol* 1997;59:413–416.
488. Wang W, Lerea KM, Chan M, Giebisch G. Protein tyrosine kinase regulates the number of renal secretory K^+ channels. *Am J Physiol Renal* 2000;278:F165–F171.
489. Wang W. Regulation of renal K transport by dietary K intake. *Ann Rev Med* 2003;66: 547–569.
490. Wang W. Two types of potassium channels in thick ascending limb of rat kidney. *Am J Physiol Renal* 1994;267:F599–F605.
491. Wang W, Geibel J, Giebisch G. Regulation of the small conductance K channels in the apical membrane of rat cortical collecting tubule. *Am J Physiol Renal* 1990;259:F494–F502.
492. Wang W, Henderson RM, Geibel J, et al. Mechanism of aldosteroneinduced increase of K^+ conductance in early distal renal tubule cells of the frog. *J Membr Biol* 1989;111:277–289.
493. Wang WH, Geibel J, Giebisch G. Mechanism of apical K^+ channel modulation in principal renal tubule cells. *J Gen Physiol* 1993;101:673–694.
494. Wang WH, Lu M, Hebert SC. P450 metabolites mediate extracellular Ca^{2+}-induced inhibition of apical K^+ channels in the thick ascending limb of the rat kidney. *Am J Physiol Renal* 1996;266:F813–F822.
495. Wang WH, Lu M. Effect of arachidonic acid on activity of the apical K channel in the thick ascending limb of the rat kidney. *J Gen Physiol* 1995;106:727–743.
496. Wang WH. Regulation of renal K^+ transport by dietary K^+ intake. *Ann Rev Physiol* 2004;66:547–569.
497. Wang WH. Regulation of the hyperpolarization-activated K^+ channel in the lateral membrane of the cortical collecting duct. *J Gen Physiol* 1995;106:25–43.
498. Wang WH. View of K^+ secretion through the apical K channel of cortical collecting duct. *Kidney Int* 1995;48:1024–1030.
499. Wang XY, Masilamani S, Nielsen J, Kwon TH, Brooks HL, Nielsen S, Knepper MA. The renal thiazide-sensitive Na-Cl cotransporter as mediator of the aldosterone-escape phenomenon. *J Clin Invest* 2001;108:215–222.
500. Wareing M, Wilson RW, Kibble JD, et al. Estimated potassium reflection coefficient in perfused proximal convoluted tubules of the anaesthetized rat in vivo. *J Physiol (London)* 1995;488.1:153–161.
501. Warnock DG, Eveloff J. K-Cl cotransport systems. *Kidney Int* 1989;36:412–417.
502. Wasserman AG, Agus ZS. Potassium secretion in the rabbit proximal straight tubule. *Am J Physiol Renal* 1983;245:F167–F174.
503. Watson JF, Clapp IR, Berliner RW. Micropuncture study of potassium concentration in proximal tubule of dog and rat Necturus. *J Clin Invest* 1964;43:595–605.
504. Webster MK, Goya L, Ge Y, Maiyar AC, Firestone GL. Characterization of sgk, a novel member of the serine/threonine protein kinase gene family which is transcriptionally induced by glucocorticoids and serum. *Mol Cell Biol* 1993;13:2031–2040.
505. Wehling M, Christ M, Theisen K. Membrane receptors for aldosterone: a novel pathway for mineralocorticoid action. *Am J Physiol* 1992;263:E974–E979.
506. Weiner ID, Milton AE. H^+-K^+-ATPase in rabbit cortical collecting duct B-type intercalated cell. *Am J Physiol Renal* 1996;270:F518–F530.
507. Weinstein AM. A mathematical model of rat cortical collecting duct: determinants of the transtubular potassium gradient. *Am J Physiol Renal* 2001;280:F1072–F1092.
508. Weinstein AM. A mathematical model of rat distal convoluted tubule. II. Potassium secretion along the connecting segment. *Am J Physiol Renal* 2005;289:F721–F741.
509. Weinstein AM. Coupling of entry to exit by peritubular K^+ permeability in a mathematical model of rat proximal tubule. *Am J Physiol Renal* 1996;271:F158–F168.
510. Weinstein AM. Modeling the proximal tubule: complications of the paracellular pathway. *Am J Physiol Renal* 1988;254:F297–F305.
511. Welling PA. Primary structure and functional expression of a cortical collecting duct Kir channel. *Am J Physiol Renal* 1997;273:F825–F836.
512. Welling PA. "Cross-talk" and the role of KATP channels in the proximal tubule. *Kidney Int* 1995;48:1017–1023.
513. Welsh MI, McCann JD. Intracellular calcium regulates basolateral potassium channels in a chloride secreting epithelium. *Proc Natl Acad Sci U S A* 1985;82:8823–8826.
514. West ML, Bendz O, Chen CB. et al. Development of a test to evaluate the transtubular potassium concentration gradient in the cortical collecting duct in vivo. *Miner Electrolyte Metab* 1986;12:226–233.
515. West ML, Marsden PA, Richardson RMA, et al. New clinical approach to evaluate disorders of potassium excretion. *Miner Electrolyte Metab* 1986;12:234–238.
516. Westphale HI, Schafer C, Oberleithner H. Aldosterone stimulates cellular K^+ uptake and K^+ release in the diluting segment of the frog kidney. *Cell Physiol Biochem* 1991;1:89–97.
517. Whittembury G, Grantham RR. Cellular aspects of renal sodium transport and cell volume regulation. *Kidney Int* 1976;9:103–120.
518. Wills NK, Biagi B. Active potassium transport by rabbit descending colon epithelium. *J Membr Biol* 1982;64:195–203.
519. Wilson FH, Kahle K, Sabath E, et al. Molecular pathogenesis of inherited hypertension with hyperkalemia: the Na-Cl cotransporter is inhibited by wild-type but not mutant WNK4. *Proc Natl Acad Sci U S A* 2003;100:680–684.
520. Wilson FH, Disse-Nicodème, Choate KA, Ishikawa K, Nelson-Williams C, Desitter I, et al. Human hypertension caused by mutations in WNK kinases. *Science* 2001;293:1107–1112.
521. Wilson FH, Kahle KT, Sabath E, Lalioti MD, Rapson AK, Hoover RS, Hebert SC, Gamba G, Lifton RP. Molecular pathogenesis of inherited hypertension with hyperkalemia: The Na-Cl cotransporter is inhibited by wild-type but not mutant WNK4. *Proc Natl Acad Sci U S A* 2003;100:680–684.
522. Wingo CS, Cain BD. The renal H-K-ATPase; physiological significance and role in potassium homeostasis. *Annu Rev Physiol* 1993;55:323–347.
523. Wingo CS. Potassium secretion by the cortical collecting tubule: effect of Cl gradients and ouabain. *Am J Physiol Renal* 1989;256:F306–F313.
524. Wingo CS. Potassium transport by the medullary collecting tubule of the rabbit: effects of variation in K intake. *Am J Physiol Renal* 1987;253:F1136–F1141.
525. Wirz H. Untersuchungen ueber die Nierenfinktion in adrenalektomierten Katzen. *Relv Physiol Pharmacol Acta* 1945;3:589.
526. Woda CB, Bragin A, Kleyman TR, Satlin LM. Flow-dependent K^+ secretion in the cortical collecting duct is mediated by a maxi-K channel. *Am J Physiol Renal* 2001;280:F786–F793.
527. Woda CB, Miyawaki N, Ramalakshmi S, Ramkumar M, Rojas R, Zavilowitz B, Kleyman TR, Satlin LM. Ontogeny of flow-stimulated potassium secretion in rabbit cortical collecting duct: functional and molecular aspects. *Am J Physiol Renal* 2003;285:F629–-F639.
528. Work I, Jamison RL. Effect of adrenalectomy on transport in the rat medullary thick ascending limb. *J Clin Invest* 1987;80:1160–1164.
529. Work I, Troutman SL, Schafer JA. Transport of potassium in the rabbit pars recta. *Am J Physiol Renal* 1982;242:F226–F237.
530. Wright FS. Renal potassium handling. *Semin Nephrol* 1987;7:174–184.
531. Wright FS, Giebisch G. Renal potassium transport: contributions of individual nephron segments and populations. *Am J Physiol Renal* 1978;235:F515–F527.
532. Wright FS, Strieder N, Fowler NB, et al. Potassium secretion by distal tubule after potassium adaptation. *Am J Physiol Renal* 1971;221:F437–F448.
533. Wright FS. Flow dependent transport processes: filtration, absorption, secretion. *Am J Physiol Renal* 1982;243:F1–Fl1.
534. Wright FS. Sites and mechanisms of potassium transport along the renal tubule. *Kidney Int* 1977;11 :415–432.
535. Xu Z-C, Yang Y, Hebert SC. Phosphorylation of the ATP-sensitive, inwardly-rectifying K^+ channel, ROMK, by cyclic AMP-dependent protein kinase. *J Biol Chem* 1996;271: 9313–9319.
536. Yang C-L, Angell J, Mitchell R, Ellison DH. WNK kinases regulate thiazide-sensitive Na-Cl cotransport. *J Clin Invest* 2003;111:1039–1045.
537. Yeyati NL, Etcheverry JC, Adrogue HJ. Kaliuretic response to potassium loading in amiloride-treated dogs. *Ren Physiol Biochem* 1990;13:190–199.
538. Yoo D, Flagg TP, Olsen O, Raghuram V, Foskett JK, Welling PA. Assembly and trafficking of a multiprotein ROMK (Kir1.1) channel complex by PDZ interactions. *J Biol Chem* 2004;279:6863–-6973.
539. Yoo D, Kim BY, Campo C, Nance L, King A, Maouyo D, Welling PA. Cell surface expression of the ROMK (Kir 11) channel is regulated by the aldosterone-induced kinase, SGK-1, and protein kinase. *J Biol Chem* 2003;278:23066–23075.
540. Yoshitomi K, Shimizu T, Taniguchi I, et al. Electrophysiological characterization of rabbit distal convoluted tubule cell. *Pflugers Arch* 1989;414:457–463.
541. Younes-Ibrahim M, Barlet-Bas C, Buffin-Meyer B, Cheval L, Rajerison R., Doucet A. Ouabain-sensitive and -insensitive K-ATPases in rat nephron: effect of K depletion. *Am J Physiol Renal* 1995;268:F1141–F1147.
542. Young DB, Jackson TE, Tipayamontri U, et al. Effects of sodium intake on steady-state potassium excretion. *Am J Physiol Renal* 1984;246:F772–F778.
543. Young DB. Quantitative analysis of aldosterone role in potassium regulation. *Am J Physiol Renal* 1988;255:Fl269–Fl275.
544. Young DB. Relationship between plasma potassium concentration and renal potassium excretion. *Am J Physiol Renal* 1982;242:F599–F603.
545. Young DB. *Role of Potassium in Preventive Cardiovascular Medicine.* Norwell, MA: Kluwer; 2001.
546. Yun CC, Palmada M, Embark HM, Feng Y, Henke G, Setiawan I, Boehmer C, Weinmann EJ, Korbmacher C, Cohen P, Pearce D, Lang F. The serum and glucocorticoid inducible kinase SGK1 and the Na^+/H^+ exchange regulating factor NHERF2 synergize to stimulate the renal outer medullary K^+ channel ROMK1. *J Am Soc Nephrol* 2002;13:2823–2830.
547. Zalups RK, Stanton BA, Wade JB, et al. Structural adaptation in initial collecting tubule following reduction in renal mass. *Kidney Int* 1985;27:636–642.
548. Zeidel ML, Seifter JL, Leor S, et al. Atrial peptides inhibit oxygen consumption in kidney medullary collecting duct cells. *Am J Physiol Renal* 1986;251:F379–F383.
549. Zhou X, Wingo CS. H-K-ATPase enhancement of Rb efflux by cortical collecting duct. *Am J Physiol Renal* 1992;263:F43–F48.
550. Zhou ZH, Bubien JK. Nongenomic regulation of ENaC by aldosterone. *Am J Physiol Cell Physiol* 2001;281:C1118–C1130.

CHAPTER 48

Potassium Deficiency

Salim K. Mujais and Adrian I. Katz

Northbrook, Illinois, USA
University of Chicago, Chicago, Illinois, USA

Potassium deficiency is one of the most common electrolyte disorders (Table 1) encountered in clinical medicine. Its significance varies from the marginal abnormality of minimal clinical relevance, to the life threatening arrhythmogenic emergencies. Patients undergoing cardiac surgery with extracorporeal circulation are at high risk for potassium depletion, despite high levels of supplementation (208). Extremes of both potassium surfeit and deficit trigger aggressive diagnostic and therapeutic interventions. Potassium depletion, however, tends to have a more protracted course, and may consequently have wide reaching effects on multiple organ systems. A rational approach to the diagnosis and management of potassium depletion should be based on a clear understanding of the determinants of potassium balance and the myriad consequences of potassium depletion. The diagnosis of potassium depletion presents an additional challenge to the clinician because the skewed distribution of this cation between the intracellular and extracellular fluid compartments (98% of total body potassium is intracellular) makes plasma potassium levels only an approximate index of total body potassium stores. The assessment of potassium deficiency or excess is further complicated by the frequent occurrence of intercompartmental shifts: given the disparity between the size of the potassium pool in the two compartments, it is easy to visualize why the quantitative estimate of potassium deficit (or its very detection when it is subtle) from plasma potassium levels is often inadequate. The picture is rendered more complex by the fact that the elements known to influence internal and external potassium balance are themselves subject to alterations secondary to potassium deficit. The development of potassium depletion may lead to renal changes that worsen the negative balance of the cation thus creating a vicious cycle. As will be discussed in detail, potassium depletion impairs sodium chloride absorption in the thick ascending limb of Henle's loop with an increase in distal sodium delivery, which may enhance urinary K loss. This chapter reviews clinical aspects of potassium deficiency but focuses on the pathophysiology of renal functional and morphologic alterations that characterize this condition, including the renal effects of systemic changes produced by potassium deficiency.

ETIOLOGY OF POTASSIUM DEFICIENCY

The prevalence and severity of the different etiologic groups of potassium depletion mirror the importance of the mechanisms involved in the maintenance of external potassium balance. Thus renal losses represent the most frequent cause of potassium depletion, in concordance with the renal route being the principle regulator of external balance of this cation. In addition, the mechanisms of potassium depletion can be understood as an accentuation of physiologic processes aimed at avoiding total body potassium excess. Because a detailed analysis of the mechanism of potassium depletion in each of the many categories listed in Table 2 would be repetitive and superfluous, the following discussion is limited to illustration of the basic principles mentioned previously.

Nephrogenic Potassium Deficiency

Nephrogenic potassium depletion results from a pathologic amplification of the normal kaliuretic mechanisms. Frequently, several kaliuretic mechanisms are activated simultaneously and their additive effects accentuate the kaliuresis (Table 3). Most diuretics, for example, increase luminal flow and sodium delivery to the potassium secretory segment. The negative sodium balance engendered increases mineralocorticoid levels, which in turn enhance the activity of the Na-K pump in the cortical collecting tubule (183), and the concurrent metabolic alkalosis increases anion delivery to this tubular site as well. The combined effect of these changes is to enhance potassium secretion. It is therefore evident that a process that induces decreased NaCl and K transport in the thick ascending limb leads to activation of cooperative factors (flow, sodium delivery, mineralocorticoid effect, and transepithelial potential difference) that conspire to increase potassium excretion.

The initiating alteration can stimulate directly kaliuretic mechanisms or activate them secondarily. The enhanced kaliuresis of diuretic use is secondary to impaired sodium reabsorption proximal to the tubular potassium secretory site. Mineralocorticoid excess, however, acts primarily on kaliuretic mechanisms. In this condition, secondary changes also contribute to enhancement of the primary kaliuretic

TABLE 1   Prevalence of Hypokalemia

Population	Criterion	Total	%	Reference
General hospital	<3.5	58,167	21	203
	<3.0	58,167	5.2	
Hospitalized general	<3.0	33,426	3.52	122
Hospitalized geriatric	<3.0	1418	5	244
Hospitalized acquired immunodeficiency syndrome	<3.5	99	23.1	165
Outpatient eating disorder	<3.5	945	4.6	94
Intestinal bypass outpatient	<3.5	475	28	246

effect, because the increased distal NaCl delivery that develops during the escape from mineralocorticoid excess further promotes the kaliuresis.

The development of potassium depletion may lead to renal changes that worsen the negative balance of the cation, thus creating a vicious cycle. As will be discussed in detail, potassium depletion impairs sodium chloride absorption in the thick ascending limb, an alteration that mimics the ef-

fect of a loop diuretic. Sodium delivery increases, with ensuing hyperreninemia and hyperaldosteronism leading to persistent potassium loss.

The occurrence of potassium depletion activates renal kaliferic (potassium-conserving) mechanisms, which on balance are less efficient than kaliuretic mechanisms. The contrast between kaliuretic and kaliferic mechanisms is best illustrated by examining the consequences of dietary manipulations leading to either potassium excess or deficiency. With dietary potassium excess, total body potassium surfeit does not develop in the presence of normal kidneys and potassium balance is maintained (182). In contrast, with a potassium-deficient diet, potassium depletion develops (107, 108). It is clear that kaliferic mechanisms are less rigorous than kaliuretic factors in maintaining the constancy of the internal environment in regard to this cation. While kaliferic mechanisms are not well defined, it appears that potassium depletion is rarely due to failure of kaliferic mechanisms but rather to excessive kaliuretic effect. The converse, however, is not true:

TABLE 2   Etiologies of Potassium Depletion

Nephrogenic potassium deficiency	Fanconi syndrome
Diuretics	Idiopathic
Mineralocorticoid excess	Cystinosis
Primary aldosteronism	With idiopathic nephrotic syndrome
Adrenal adenoma	Postobstructive disease
Bilateral adrenal hyperplasia	Diuretic phase of acute tubular necrosis
Glucocorticoid-suppressible adrenal hyperplasia	Magnesium depletion
Secondary aldosteronism	Drug nephrotoxicity: gentamicin, cisplatin, amphotericin,
Renal artery stenosis	capreomycin, rifampin, viomycin
Accelerated and malignant hypertension	Nonreabsorbable anion
Reninoma	Drugs: penicillin, nafcillin, carbenicillin, ticarcillin
Juxtaglomerular tumor	Diabetic ketoacidosis
Ovarian Sertoli cell tumor	Alkali loading
Ovarian stromal cell tumor	**Enterogenic potassium deficiency**
Pulmonary carcinoma	Diarrhea
Renal clear cell carcinoma	Congenital chloride-losing diarrhea
Retroperitoneal leiomyosarcoma	VIP-producing tumors
Orbital hemangiopericytoma	Generalized juvenile polyposis coli
L-Dopa treatment	Laxative abuse
Nonaldosterone mineralocorticoid excess	Intestinal bypass for morbid obesity
Adrenal deoxycorticosterone production	Inflammatory bowel disease
17-α-Hydroxylase deficiency	Colonic villous adenoma
11-β-Hydroxylase deficiency	Geophagia
Adrenocorticotropic hormone excess (pituitary or ectopic)	Excessive enemas
Adrenal carcinoma	**Mixed disorders**
Licorice (glycyrrhizic acid) or carbenoxolone ingestion	Gastric alkalosis
Gossypol	**Miscellaneous**
Glucocorticoid excess	Dietary deficiency
Congenital potassium-wasting disorders	Eating disorders
Bartter syndrome	Prolonged exercise in hot environment
Non–Bartter congenital syndrome	Lysozymuria of leukemia
Liddle syndrome	Alcoholism
Intrinsic renal disease	Thyrotoxicosis
Renal tubular acidosis: types I and II	Postresuscitation
Tubular interstitial disease	Drug induced
Sjögren syndrome	Betamimetics, theophylline
Toluene or paint sniffing	
α Chain disease	

VIP, vasoactive intestinal polypeptide

TABLE 3 Factors Influencing Distal Nephron Potassium Secretion and Their Modification by Diuretics

Factor	Effect of Diuretics
Plasma potassium	−
Luminal flow rate	+
Luminal sodium (concentration and delivery rate)	+
Transepithelial potential difference	+
Luminal anions	+
Hormones	
Mineralocorticoids	+
Glucocorticoids	0
Antidiuretic hormone	0
Acid-base status	
Arterial pH	+
Ammonia excretion	0

+, promote; 0, no effect; −, reduce.

that is, hyperkalemia is probably never due to excess kaliferic effect. Aging does not seem to impair either kaliuretic or kaliferic mechanisms (60).

With the development of potassium depletion, a "braking" phenomenon occurs: Intrinsic kaliferic mechanisms are activated pari passu with attenuation of kaliuretic factors. Potassium depletion will reduce aldosterone secretion. The developing hypokalemia may alter basolateral potassium transport in the cortical collecting tubule (and consequently potassium secretion), and intracellular potassium depletion will reduce its gradient across the luminal membrane.

Genetic Syndromes

Advances in the molecular biology of three genetic syndromes associated with hypokalemia deserve examinations, namely Bartter syndrome, Gitelman syndrome, and Liddle syndrome. While these syndromes in their pure forms are rare and the nephrologist is likely to encounter but a handful of cases with Bartter (22) or Gitelman syndromes (and even fewer cases with Liddle syndrome), the examination of these syndromes offers invaluable insight into the pathogenesis of potassium depletion.

BARTTER AND GITELMAN SYNDROMES

Among the different forms of hereditary renal tubulopathies associated with hypokalemia, metabolic alkalosis and normotension, two main types of disorders have been identified: Gitelman disease, which appears to be a homogeneous post–Henle's loop disorder, and Bartter syndrome, a heterogeneous Henle loop disorder. The term *Bartter syndrome* has been used to describe a spectrum of inherited renal tubular disorders featuring hypokalemic metabolic alkalosis and additional clinical and biochemical features. Its pathogenesis remained uncertain until recent molecular genetic approaches demonstrated that mutations in genes encoding specific ion transporters produce distinct clinical and physiologic findings exhibiting hypokalemic alkalosis (240).

A specific gene has been found responsible for Gitelman disease, encoding the thiazide-sensitive Na-Cl cotransporter (TSC) of the distal convoluted tubule. From a phenotypic point of view the characteristic findings of this disease are hypocalciuria, hypomagnesemia and tetanic crises appearing during childhood or later. Many subjects are asymptomatic.

Molecular Biology of Bartter Syndrome The pathogenesis of Bartter syndrome has been elucidated by the identification of specific molecular lesions that disturb tubular transport in the thick ascending limb of Henle's loop (TAL) to lead to the full constellation of clinical findings characteristic of the syndrome. These molecular defects, however, are far from simple or uniform. Recent reports have suggested that the phenotype-genotype correlation in Bartter syndrome is complex. Five genes have been identified as causing Bartter syndrome (types I–V), with the unifying pathophysiology being the loss of salt transport by the thick ascending limb. Phenotypic differences in Bartter types I to V relate to the specific physiological roles of the individual genes in the kidney and other organ systems (109).

At least five different genes have been shown to be responsible for Bartter syndrome, characterized by mutations in the proteins encoding respectively the bumetanide-sensitive Na-K-2Cl cotransporter (type I), the inwardly-rectifying renal potassium channel (type II), a renal chloride channel (type III), a chloride channel regulator, Barttin (type IV) and a calcium sensing receptor (type V), all located in the ascending limb of Henle's loop. Mutations in the first two transport proteins have been demonstrated in patients with the hypercalciuric forms of Bartter syndrome associated with nephrocalcinosis (respectively, Bartter syndrome types I and II), who were often born after pregnancies complicated by polyhydramnios and premature delivery. Mutations in the gene encoding a renal chloride channel were recently recognized in patients with a Henle tubular defect not associated with nephrocalcinosis (Bartter syndrome type III). Most of the latter group of patients was normohypercalciuric and developed dehydration and life-threatening hypotension in the first year of life (34).

Simon et al. (239) demonstrated linkage of Bartter syndrome to the renal Na-K-2Cl cotransporter gene *NKCC2*, and identified frameshift or nonconservative missense mutations of this gene that co-segregate with the disease. These findings demonstrated the molecular basis of Bartter syndrome, and suggested potential phenotypes in heterozygous carriers of *NKCC2* mutations (Bartter type I). *NKCC2* mutations, however, can be excluded in some Bartter kindreds, prompting examination of regulators of cotransporter activity. One regulator is believed to be ROMK, an ATP-sensitive K-channel that "recycles" reabsorbed K back to the tubule lumen. Examination of the *ROMK* gene in four Bartter kindreds revealed mutations that cosegregate with the disease and disrupt ROMK function (Bartter type II) (238). A variety of mutations of the ROMK protein that can affect channel function continue to be reported (50, 148). Structurally and functionally distinct from other channel families, inwardly rectifying potassium (Kir) channels are ubiquitously expressed and serve functions as diverse as regulation of resting membrane potential, maintenance of K homeostasis, control of heart rate, and hormone secretion. In humans, persistent hyperinsulinemic hypoglycemia of infancy, a disorder affecting the function of pancreatic β cells, and Bartter syndrome, characterized by hypokalemic alkalosis, hypercalciuria, increased serum aldosterone, and plasma renin activity, are the two major diseases linked so far to mutations in a Kir channel or associated protein (4). Early postnatal hyperkalemia, sometimes severe, may complicate antenatal Bartter syndrome associated with ROMK mutations. Its association with hyponatremia and hyperreninemic hyperaldosteronism may erroneously suggest the diagnosis of pseudohypoaldosteronism type I. The expression of ROMK in both the thick ascending limb and cortical collecting duct (CCD) may explain this apparently tubular maturation phenomenon (72). Several different mutations in the basolateral chloride channel CLCNKB have been described. The clinical characterization revealed a highly variable phenotype ranging from episodes of severe volume depletion and hypokalemia during the neonatal period to almost asymptomatic patients diagnosed during adolescence. Interestingly, the phenotype elicited by CLCNKB mutations occasionally includes a Gitelman-like phenotype (139). Barttin is a β subunit that is required for the trafficking of CLC-K (ClC-Ka and ClC-Kb) channels to the plasma membrane in both the thick ascending limb and the marginal cells in the scala media of the inner ear that secrete potassium ion-rich endolymph. Loss-of-function mutations in barttin thus cause Bartter syndrome with sensorineural deafness (Bartter type IV) (233). In addition, severe gain-of-function mutations in the extracellular calcium ion–sensing receptor can result in a Bartter phenotype because activation of this G-protein–coupled receptor inhibits salt transport in the thick ascending limb (a furosemide-like effect) (Bartter type V).

Characterization of the clinical features associated with each mutation in a large cohort of genetically defined patients suggest that *ROMK* and *NKCC2* mutations usually have uniform clinical presentations, whereas mutations in ClC-Kb occasionally lead to phenotypic overlaps with the NCCT or, less commonly, with the ROMK/NKCC2 cohort (205).

The phenotype has also been reported in other dysfunctions affecting the TAL such as case of mitochondriopathy combined with tubule functional disturbances compatible with Bartter syndrome and definitive sensorineural blindness (174). It is assumed that the disruption of cellular energetics may have been responsible for the transport abnormality. Nephropathy has been induced in animal models of mitochondriopathies (269). It is therefore likely that the list of types of Bartter syndrome may expand with future identifications of abnormalities capable of disrupting tubular transport in the TAL.

Molecular Biology of Gitelman Syndrome Gitelman syndrome, the hypokalemic-hypomagnesemic variant with hypocalciuria, was linked to the gene encoding the thiazide-sensitive Na-Cl cotransporter (TSC) located on chromosome 16q. This linkage has been observed by several investigators. Karolyi et al. (133) performed linkage analysis in 17 families

with clinical manifestations consistent with the syndrome with four highly polymorphic chromosome 16 DNA markers closely linked to the TSC gene. Linkage of Gitelman syndrome to the TSC locus was confirmed in all families, and no linkages were observed at this locus in families with classic Bartter syndrome and hyperprostaglandin E syndrome (133).

Additional linkage analysis was done by Lemmink et al. (152). Based on the localization of a 2.6 cDNA encoding the human TSC to chromosome 16q13, polymorphic markers spanning the region from 16p12 to 16q21 were tested for linkage to the Gitelman syndrome locus in three Dutch families with autosomal recessive inheritance of this disorder with positive results (152). Subsequently they tested the group of Gitelman patients for mutations in the human TSC gene, and identified two mutations in three Gitelman families (152).

Simon et al. (241) also demonstrated complete linkage of Gitelman syndrome to the locus encoding the renal thiazide-sensitive Na-Cl cotransporter, and identified a wide variety of nonconservative mutations, consistent with loss-of-function alleles, in affected subjects. They speculated that these mutant alleles lead to reduced sodium chloride reabsorption in the more common heterozygotes. Mastroianni et al. (169) cloned the cDNA coding for the human Na-Cl thiazide-sensitive cotransporter. They observed 12 mutations consistent with a loss of function of the Na-Cl cotransporter in Gitelman syndrome. Two missense replacements, R209W and P349L, were also found in the study of Simon et al. (241) and could represent ancient mutations. The other mutations include three deletions, two insertions, and six missense mutations. When all mutations from both studies are considered, missense mutations seem to be more frequently localized within the intracellular domains of the molecule, rather than in its transmembrane or extracellular domains.

Takeuchi et al. (252, 253) also observed a multitude of mutations in Japanese patients with the syndrome. Using polymerase chain reaction (PCR) amplification and direct sequencing, they identified in one kindred a novel nonconservative missense mutation at amino acid 623 position, which substitutes proline for leucine (L623P), and creates an Nci I restriction site in exon 15. The mutation was not detected in healthy subjects. Nci I digestion of PCR-amplified exon 15 DNA fragments from individuals in the family indicated the autosomal recessive inheritance of the disorder (253). This mutation was not detected in two additional kindreds they studied (252). In molecular genetic analysis of additional patients, seven different mutations of the *NCCT* gene were identified consisting of three missense, one splice site, and three silent mutations. Four of these mutations were novel (287). These results support the view that Gitelman syndrome is caused by a variety of mutations in the thiazide-sensitive Na-Cl cotransporter.

The apparent homogeneity of Gitelman syndrome (GS) is not without challenge. Jeck et al. (123) have described three patients whose profile does not fit the model of only mutations in a single gene encoding the thiazide-sensitive Na-Cl cotransporter as the molecular basis of GS. They described three unrelated patients presenting with the typical laboratory findings of Gitelman syndrome. Mutational analysis in these patients revealed no abnormality in the Na-Cl transporter gene. Instead, all patients were found to carry previously described mutations in the *CLCNKB* gene, which encodes the kidney-specific chloride channel ClC-Kb, raising the possibility of genetic heterogeneity. Review of the medical histories revealed manifestation of the disease within the first year of life in all cases. Clinical presentation included episodes of dehydration, weakness, and failure to thrive, much more suggestive of classic Bartter syndrome than of GS. The coexistence of hypomagnesemia and hypocalciuria was not present from the beginning. In the follow-up, however, a drop of both parameters below normal range was a consistent finding reflecting a transition from Bartter to GS phenotype. The phenotypic overlap may indicate a physiologic cooperation of the apical thiazide-sensitive Na-Cl cotransporter and the basolateral chloride channel for salt reabsorption in the distal convoluted tubule (123). Recent studies suggest that in kindred with the CLCNKB R438H mutation, there is significant intrafamilial heterogeneity, namely the presence of Gitelman syndrome and Bartter syndrome phenotypes. This implies that Gitelman can be caused by a mutation in a gene other than Na-Cl transporter gene (289).

Pathogenic Mechanisms in Bartter and Gitelman Syndromes The cellular pathways underlying the pathogenesis of some types of Bartter and Gitelman syndromes are illustrated in Figs. 1 and 2, respectively, and comparisons to specific diuretic effects shown in Tables 4 and 5. Defective NaCl reabsorption in the TAL secondary to any of the transporter protein mutations will lead to increased Na delivery to more distal segments that are not equipped to handle the increased Na load. This will lead to salt wasting and hypovolemia. The latter will activate the renin-angiotensin system and aldosterone secretion, which will tend to enhance Na absorption along the nephron. Angiotensin II (Ang II) enhances proximal salt reabsorption and aldosterone acts at the

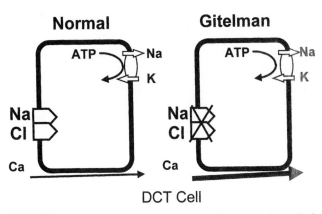

FIGURE 2 Cellular mechanisms underlying Gitelman syndrome. **Left panel:** Normal distal cortical tubule cell. **Right panel:** Consequences of a loss-of-function mutation in the Na-Cl cotransporter.

TABLE 4 Comparison of Bartter Syndrome and Effects of Loop Diuretics

Loop Diuretics	Bartter Syndrome
Salt wasting	Salt wasting
Hypokalemia	Hypokalemia
Alkalosis	Alkalosis
Hypercalciuria	Hypercalciuria
High-plasma renin activity and aldosterone	High-plasma renin activity and aldosterone
Na-K-Cl inhibition	Na-K-Cl mutation

TABLE 5 Comparison of Gitelman Syndrome and Effects of Thiazide Diuretics

Thiazide Diuretics	Gitelman Syndrome
Salt wasting	Salt wasting
Hypokalemia	Hypokalemia
Alkalosis	Alkalosis
Hypocalciuria	Hypocalciuria
High-plasma renin activity and aldosterone	High-plasma renin activity and aldosterone
Na-Cl inhibition	Na-Cl mutation

level of the collecting duct. The net effect of aldosterone would be to stimulate the Na-K pump and enhance CCT Na reabsorption. These mechanisms will simultaneously favor K secretion by this segment and the increased Na delivery to this segment will conspire to maximize this effect. Ultimately hypokalemia will ensue along with its consequences which become part of the constellation of findings of this syndrome. The pathways for Gitelman syndrome are similar with the distinction that because the transport capacity of the DCT is lower than that of the TAL, the amount of salt wasting is milder, hence the late manifestation of the syndrome. The consequences to downstream nephron segments, however, would be qualitatively similar to those of Bartter syndrome. Comparison of the two syndromes is detailed in Table 6.

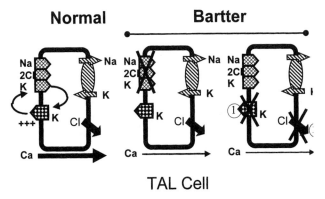

FIGURE 1 Cellular mechanisms underlying two types of Bartter syndrome: left panel shows the operation of a normal thick ascending loop cell; the middle panel shows a Na-K-2Cl transporter loss-of-function mutation; the right panel illustrates the effects of a K channel loss-of-function mutation (see text).

TABLE 6   Comparison of Bartter Syndrome
and Gitelman Syndrome

Bartter Syndrome	Gitelman Syndrome
Salt wasting	Salt wasting
Hypokalemia/alkalosis	Hypokalemia/alkalosis
Childhood	Adulthood
Hypercalciuria	Hypocalciuria
High-plasma renin activity and aldosterone	High-plasma renin activity and aldosterone
Na-K-Cl inhibition	Na-Cl mutation

LIDDLE SYNDROME

Liddle syndrome (pseudoaldosteronism) is an autosomal dominant form of human hypertension characterized by a constellation of findings suggesting constitutive activation of the amiloride-sensitive distal renal epithelial sodium channel (71, 227, 273, 274). The syndrome is a monogenic form of hypertension characterized metabolically by hypokalemia and suppressed levels of aldosterone as well as attenuation of the activity of the renin-angiotensin system (272). The hypertension is of the salt-sensitive type and the syndrome has been identified in various ethnic groups including whites, Asians, and blacks (84). Examination of large kindreds (71) demonstrates variability in the severity of hypertension and hypokalemia in this disease, raising the possibility that this disease may be underdiagnosed among patients with essential hypertension.

Molecular Biology of Liddle Syndrome The amiloride-sensitive epithelial Na channel is formed by the assembly of three homologous subunits, α, β, and γ. The channel is characterized by its sensitivity to amiloride and to some amiloride derivatives, by its high selectivity for lithium and sodium, and by its slow kinetics (20, 158). The subunits proteins contain a large extracellular loop, located between two transmembrane α-helices. The NH$_2$ and COOH terminal segments are cytoplasmic and contain potential regulatory segments that are able to modulate the activity of the channel (20, 158). In Liddle syndrome mutations within the cytoplasmic COOH terminal of the β- and γ-chains of the epithelial Na channel lead to hyperactivity of the channel (228). Epithelial Na channel activity is tightly controlled by several distinct hormonal systems, including corticosteroids and vasopressin (20, 158). In the kidney, aldosterone is the major sodium-retaining hormone, acting by stimulation of Na reabsorption through the epithelium. Renal RNA levels of the three subunits, however, are not altered by aldosterone, suggesting that other mechanisms control Na channel activity in the kidney (20, 158).

The expression level of each of the subunits is markedly different in various Na absorbing epithelia raising the possibility that channels with different subunit composition may function in vivo (172). The functional properties of channels formed by the association of α with β and of α with γ in the *Xenopus* oocyte expression system reveal some interesting differences (172). α-β channels differ from α-γ

channels in expressing larger Na than Li currents whereas α-γ channels expressed smaller Na than Li currents, and by differential sensitivity to amiloride, the half-inhibition constant (Ki) of amiloride being 20-fold larger for α-β channels than for α-γ channels (172). This finding may have relevance to different clinical responses to amiloride observed in patients with Liddle syndrome (vide infra)

Genetics The genes encoding epithelial sodium channel (ENaC) have been identified and revealed a heteromultimeric structure of the protein composed of three homologous αβγ subunits. Analysis of these genes from patients affected by Liddle syndrome identified mutations in the carboxy-terminus of ENaC subunits causing channel hyperactivity, consistent with increased sodium reabsorption in the distal nephron.

Most of the mutations reported are either nonsense mutations or frame shift mutations, which would truncate the cytoplasmic carboxyl terminus of the β or γ subunits of the channel, suggesting that these domains are important for the normal regulation of this channel (86, 104, 119, 191). Shimkets et al. (234) demonstrated complete linkage of the gene encoding the β subunit of the epithelial sodium channel to Liddle syndrome in Liddle's original kindred. Analysis of this gene revealed a premature stop codon that truncates the cytoplasmic carboxyl terminus of the encoded protein in affected subjects. Examination of subjects with Liddle syndrome from four additional kindreds demonstrated either premature termination or frameshift mutations in this same carboxy-terminal domain in all four (234).

Schild et al. (227) have studied the functional consequences of the mutation identified in the original kindred described by Liddle, which introduces a premature stop codon in the channel β subunit, resulting in a deletion of almost all of the C terminus of the encoded protein. Coexpression of the mutant β subunit with wildtype α and γ subunits in *Xenopus laevis* oocytes resulted in an approximately threefold increase in the amiloride-sensitive Na current (INa) compared with the wildtype channel. This change in INa reflected an increase in the overall channel activity characterized by a higher number of active channels in membrane patches. The truncation mutation in the β subunit of epithelial Na channel did not alter the biophysical and pharmacological properties of the channel—including unitary conductance, ion selectivity, or sensitivity to amiloride block (227). Tamura et al. (254), like others (227, 234) found a missense mutation in β subunit which correlated with the clinical manifestations in the studied kindred. Functional expression studies in the *Xenopus* oocytes revealed constitutive activation of the mutant indistinguishable from that observed for the deletion mutant identified in the original pedigree of Liddle (227, 234). Jeunemaitre and colleagues (125) identified a deletion of 32 nucleotides that had modified the open reading frame and introduced a stop codon at position 582. Expression of this β mutant caused more than a threefold increase in the amiloride-sensitive sodium current, without modification of the unitary properties of the channel. Kellenberger et al. (134) have shown that while wildtype ENaC is downregulated by intracellular Na, Liddle mutants decrease the channel sensitivity to inhibition by intracellular Na. This event results at high intracellular Na activity in 1.2- to 2.4-fold higher cell surface expression and 2.8- to 3.5-fold higher average current per channel in Liddle mutants compared with the wild type. In addition, while a rapid increase in the intracellular Na activity induces downregulation of the activity of wildtype ENaC, it does not in Liddle mutant oocytes (134).

Mutations of the γ subunit have also been identified (105). Hansson et al. (105) demonstrated that the syndrome can also result from a mutation truncating the carboxy terminus of the γ subunit of this channel; this truncated subunit also activates channel activity. These findings demonstrate genetic heterogeneity of Liddle syndrome, and indicate independent roles of β and γ subunits in the negative regulation of channel activity.

Expression of truncated β and γ hENaC subunits increases Na current (242). However, truncation does not alter single-channel conductance or open state probability, suggesting there are more channels in the plasma membrane. Moreover, truncation of the C-terminus of the β subunit increases apical cell-surface expression of hENaC in a renal epithelium (242). Thus, by deleting a conserved motif, Liddle mutations increase the number of Na channels in the apical membrane, which increases renal Na absorption and creates a predisposition to hypertension.

Pathogenesis of Liddle Syndrome While genetic linkage studies have identified gain-of-function mutations linking Liddle disease to a locus on chromosome 16 encoding the β-subunit of an amiloride-sensitive Na channel (ASSC), and expressions of the mutant gene have manifested increase Na channel activity, definitive proof requires measurements of increase Na channel activity in patients with the syndrome. Peripheral blood lymphocytes (PBLs) express ASSC that are functionally indistinguishable from those expressed by Na reabsorbing renal epithelial cells. Bubien et al. (38) examined the amiloride-sensitive Na conductance in PBL from affected and unaffected individuals from the original Liddle pedigree using whole cell patch clamp. Typically, the basal Na currents in cells from affected individuals were maximally activated. Basal Na currents in cells from unaffected individuals were minimal and could be maximally activated by superfusion with agonists. Affected cells could not be further stimulated. Superfusion with a supermaximal concentration of amiloride inhibited both the cAMP-activated Na conductance in unaffected cells and the constitutively activated inward conductance in affected cells. Cytosolic addition of a peptide identical to the terminal 10 amino acids of the truncated β-subunit normalized the cAMP-mediated but not the pertussis toxin-induced regulation of the mutant ASSC (38). The findings show that lymphocyte ASSC are constitutively activated in affected individuals, that a mutation of the β-subunit alters ASSC responsiveness to specific regulatory effectors, and that the cellular mechanism responsible for the pathophysiology of Liddle syndrome is abnormal regulation of Na channel activity.

A mouse model carrying a premature stop codon corresponding to the mutation (L) found in the original pedigree that recapitulates to a large extent the human disease has been developed. In vivo, on 6 to 12 hours of salt repletion, after 1 week of low-salt diet, the L/L mice show a delayed urinary sodium excretion, despite a lower aldosterone secretion as compared with controls. After 6 hours of salt of repletion, the ENaC γ subunit is rapidly removed from the apical plasma membrane in wildtype mice, whereas it is retained at the apical membrane in L/L mice. Ex vivo, isolated perfused cortical collecting duct (CCD) from L/L mice exhibit higher transepithelial potential differences than perfused CCD isolated from +/+ mice. In vitro, confluent primary cultures of CCD microdissected from L/L kidneys grown on permeable filters exhibit significant lower transepithelial electrical resistance and higher negative potential differences than their cultured L/+ and +/+ CCD counterparts. The equivalent short-circuit current (I(eq)) and the amiloride-sensitive I(eq) was approximately twofold higher in cultured L/L CCD than in +/+ CCD. Thus, this study brings three independent lines of evidence for the constitutive hyperactivity of ENaC in CCD from mice harboring the Liddle mutation (210).

The consequences of increased Na reabsorption at the level of the cortical collecting tubule are functionally indistinguishable from the alterations in the principle cells induced by hyperaldosteronism (Figs. 3 and 4). These include an increased in luminal Na reabsorption leading to stimulation of the basolateral Na-K pump. At the luminal level, enhanced Na reabsorption is paralleled by increased potassium secretion. This constellation of changes in the CCT principle cells leads to volume expansion, hypertension, and suppression of the renin-angiotensin system and aldosterone secretion (Table 7). While an escape akin to mineralocorticoid escape likely occurs, the hypertension and metabolic consequences persist.

Treatment Based on its pathogenesis, the rational treatment of the syndrome is aimed at inhibition of the enhanced activity of the sodium channel in the collecting duct. This sodium channel is amiloride sensitive and the drug is successful in controlling the hypertension as well as correcting the metabolic abnormalities. Resolution of the hypokalemia can be observed in most cases in response to treatment. The dose of amiloride required for therapeutic success varies, with some patients requiring more than 20 mg per day, and in the occasional patient either additional antihypertensive therapy, or a small dose of potassium supplements may be required for full normalization of the clinical and metabolic profiles. It is interesting to speculate that the differential therapeutic response to amiloride in patients with Liddle syndrome may be related to differential mutations of β versus γ subunits, as these mutations may confer different sensitivities to the drug (172).

Normal   Liddle

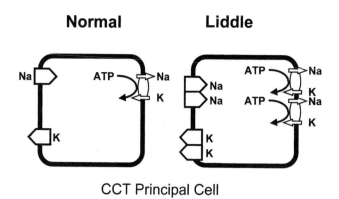

CCT Principal Cell

FIGURE 3   Cellular mechanisms underlying Liddle syndrome. **Left panel:** Normal cortical collecting tubule (CCT) cell. **Right panel:** Consequences of a gain-of-function mutation in the Na channel.

Normal   Hyperaldo

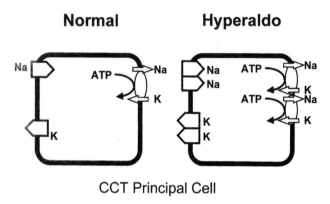

CCT Principal Cell

FIGURE 4   Cellular mechanisms in hyperaldosteronism. **Left panel:** Normal cortical collecting tubule (CCT) cell. **Right panel:** Effects of hyperaldosteronism, which are similar at the cellular level to Liddle syndrome.

TABLE 7   Comparison of Hyperaldosteronism and Liddle Syndrome

Hyperaldosteronism	Liddle Syndrome
Salt retention	Salt retention
Hypokalemia	Hypokalemia
Hypertension	Hypertension
High aldosterone	Low aldosterone
Low-plasma renin activity	Low-plasma renin activity
High CCT function	Na channel mutation

Enterogenic Potassium Deficiency

The electrolyte concentration profile along the intestinal tract clearly indicates that the colon is the main site of gastrointestinal potassium secretion, accounting for the high concentration of the cation in stools (Table 8). It is increasingly evident from physiologic studies that potassium secretion in the colon bears a large degree of similarity to potassium secretion in the renal collecting tubule, being enhanced by similar factors, notably aldosterone levels, plasma potassium, and sodium reabsorption (76–78, 102, 221, 251). The last characteristic is responsible for the limited increase in potassium excretion compared to the dramatic losses of sodium during diarrheal states (75). Because colonic potassium secretion depends on a lumen-negative electrical potential generated by active, electrogenic sodium reabsorption, potassium losses are limited in large-volume diarrheal states, in which the colon is unable to lower the high luminal sodium effectively. Despite this limiting factor, potassium losses through this route can reach up to 100 mEq/day in severe diarrheal states (75).

This volume-limited ability to excrete potassium in the colon contrasts with the effects of flow on potassium excretion in the collecting tubule (164). Furthermore, this characteristic may explain the greater potassium depletion observed during diarrheal states in which stool volume is smaller and with chronic diarrheal syndromes (177, 236). In those conditions, the chronic hypovolemia activates the renin-angiotensin system and the resulting increase in aldosterone levels stimulates

TABLE 8   Composition of Intestinal Fluid

Site[a]	Flow Rate (ml/day)	Ion Concentrations			
		Na (mEq/l)	K (mEq/l)	Cl (mEq/l)	HCO_3 (mEq/l)
Duodenum	9000	60	15	60	15
Jejunum	3000	140	6	100	30
Ileum	1000	140	8	60	70
Colon	100	40	90	15	30

the colon to reabsorb more sodium by increasing both luminal sodium channels and basolateral Na-K pump activity (212). With moderate diarrheal volume, sodium absorption may be sufficient to generate a transepithelial potential difference that promotes potassium excretion. This explains the profound potassium depletion encountered in patients with chronic diarrhea or laxative abuse.

When enteric potassium loss is induced by administration of exchange resins, renal conservation develops early and is manifested by a sharp decline in renal potassium excretion (177). The braking phenomenon may be less apparent in hypokalemic states caused by diarrhea as the accompanying metabolic acidosis (177) may limit the initial drop in plasma potassium by inducing intercompartmental shifts. Since potassium excretion by the colon is directly related to plasma potassium, the delay in plasma level decline may help sustain the colonic potassium loss. In diarrheal states, the resultant metabolic acidosis and hyperaldosteronism may delay or blunt compensatory renal potassium conservation.

The etiology of hypokalemia in a rare but often dramatic diarrheal state, villous adenoma of the colon or rectum, is linked to the secretory product of the tumor cells. Dense villous projections of mucus-secreting epithelial cells can produce up to several liters of fluid daily, with a potassium concentration ranging from 15 to 107 mEq/l (177). Separate from any other process, this output by the tumor is capable of inducing significant negative potassium balance.

Mixed Disorders

Potassium depletion developing as a result of gastric fluid loss has a composite etiology. Gastric fluid contains approximately 10 mEq K/l, and chronic vomiting or nasogastric suction would result in only modest direct potassium losses. In parallel, however, renal potassium losses induced by the developing alkalosis and hyperaldosteronism compound the total body deficit of the cation. During its initiation phase, the metabolic alkalosis leads to increased delivery of sodium bicarbonate to the cortical collecting tubule, while the volume depletion stimulates aldosterone secretion. This combination (gastric alkalosis) can lead to renal losses reaching 100 to 200 mEq/day (177).

Numerous other causes of potassium depletion are listed in Table 2.

SYSTEMIC CHANGES RELEVANT TO RENAL FUNCTION

Systemic Hemodynamics

EFFECT ON BLOOD PRESSURE AND ITS DETERMINANTS

Potassium depletion has been shown to decrease arterial blood pressure in animal studies and has had a variable effect in human studies (144, 146, 264), which are limited in number and have not evaluated systemic hemodynamics specifically. In normotensive subjects, Krishna et al. (144, 146) have shown that short-term potassium restriction leads to a modest elevation in blood pressure on a usual sodium intake (120–200 mEq/day) (146), but not when dietary sodium is restricted to 35 mEq/day (144). Patients with primary hypertension respond to potassium depletion with a decline in blood pressure paradoxically associated with a positive sodium balance (264). Potassium supplementation, however, lowers blood pressure in hypertensives with diuretic-induced hypokalemia (131).

A more extensive evaluation of the effects of potassium depletion on systemic hemodynamics has been done in experimental animals. Potassium depletion leads to a reduction in arterial blood pressure in normotensive rats (163, 154, 276 188) and dogs (2, 17, 85), although in the latter species the response is not uniform. In most studies, the decline in blood pressure was related to a decrease in peripheral vascular resistance with a normally maintained cardiac output (17, 85, 154). This systemic vasodilator effect similarly develops in animals with a variety of experimental forms of hypertension, including rats with Grollman hypertension (177), two-kidney one-clip Goldblatt hypertension (29, 73), and spontaneous hypertension (155). The reduction of blood pressure in renovascular hypertension was related to a decrease in peripheral vascular resistance to levels below those in normotensive rats and a simultaneous increase in cardiac output (29). Blood pressure lowering by potassium depletion was effective in prevention of the development of renovascular hypertension and in its reversal once established (29). The sum of the evidence therefore indicates a broad hypotensive effect of potassium depletion. The mechanisms of this hypotensive effect are not clear, and many of the blood pressure determinants have not been examined systematically. Plasma volume, for example, is increased in normotensive, potassium-depleted rats (154), dogs (85), and humans (177) but is normal when renovascular hypertension is induced in potassium-depleted rats (29). The role of the expanded extracellular fluid volume in the systemic hemodynamic changes has not been elucidated, although inferential evidence suggests that it may contribute to the generation of the high cardiac output. Why an autoregulatory increase in vascular resistance does not follow the high flow rate is not clear.

Studies in humans, however, have suggested that the development of hypokalemia has a prohypertensive effect at least against the background of preexisting hypertension. Dietary K depletion in hypertensive and normotensive humans leads to a rise in blood pressure and an exaggerated response to salt loading (55, 145, 146). K depletion secondary to diuretic therapy is thought to contribute to any residual elevation in blood pressure that is observed and K supplementation is purported to mitigate against this effect (131). Epidemiologic data suggest that potassium intake and blood pressure are correlated inversely. In normotensive subjects, those who are salt sensitive or who have a family history of hypertension appear to benefit most from the hypotensive effects of potassium supplementation. The greatest hypotensive effect of potassium supplementation occurs in patients with severe hypertension. This effect is pronounced with prolonged potassium supplementation. The antihypertensive effect of increased potassium intake appears to be mediated by several factors, which include enhancing natriuresis, modulating baroreflex sensitivity, direct vasodilation, or lowering cardiovascular reactivity to norepinephrine or Ang II (21).

Recent studies have focused on whether hypokalemia that occurs with low-dose diuretics is associated with a reduced benefit on cardiovascular events from blood pressure control. Analysis of the Systolic Hypertension in the Elderly Program (SHEP), a 5-year randomized, placebo-controlled clinical trial of chlorthalidone-based treatment of isolated systolic hypertension in older persons has shown that after 1 year of treatment, 7.2% of the participants randomized to active treatment had a serum potassium below 3.5 mmol/l compared with 1% of the participants randomized to placebo (p <.001). After adjustment for known risk factors and study drug dose, the participants who received active treatment and who experienced hypokalemia had a similar risk of cardiovascular events, coronary events, and stroke as those randomized to placebo. Within the active treatment group, the risk of these events was 51%, 55%, and 72% lower, respectively, among those who had normal serum potassium levels compared with those who experienced hypokalemia (p <.05). The participants who had hypokalemia after 1 year of treatment with a low-dose diuretic did not experience the reduction in cardiovascular events achieved among those who did not have hypokalemia (82).

The effect of potassium depletion on the L-arginine–nitric oxide pathway in arterial tissues has been evaluated in K-depleted New Zealand white rabbits. Carotid arterial ring contractile response to norepinephrine was enhanced, and relaxation in response to the endothelium-dependent vasodilators acetylcholine and calcium ionophore A-23187 was attenuated, in rabbits fed low-potassium diet (all p <.01 compared with responses in rabbits fed control diet). Both the enhanced contraction and attenuated relaxation were abolished by treatment of arterial rings with superoxide dismutase but not by treatment with L-arginine or indomethacin. Carotid artery rings from rabbits fed the low-potassium diet showed approximately 100% greater superoxide anion formation than those from rabbits fed control diet (p <.01), whereas plasma and urinary nitrite levels were similar in both groups of rabbits. These observations indicate that low-potassium diet enhances the sensitivity of the carotid artery to vasoconstrictor stimuli and reduces the sensitivity to endothelium-dependent stimuli. Attenuation of endothelium-dependent relaxation appears to be secondary to increased free radical generation, which may degrade nitric oxide. Altered vasoreactivity may underlie the genesis of hypertension in populations consuming diets low in potassium (286).

RESISTANCE TO PRESSOR HORMONES

Alterations in the systemic responses to pressor hormones occur in potassium depletion (29, 43, 73, 85, 188, 204), and may be an important factor in its effect on blood pressure. Pressor resistance to Ang II (156, 204) and vasopressin (188) has been observed, but the response to norepinephrine has been variable and mostly normal (73, 156, 204). Resistance to Ang II appears to be due to a postreceptor defect, since it occurred despite increased binding of Ang II to vascular smooth muscle receptors (156, 204). In the dog, the decreased angiotensin sensitivity is partially restored by indomethacin administration and is associated with a parallel decrease in plasma renin activity (PRA) (85). The mechanism of the resistance to vasopressin has not been elucidated (188).

CARDIAC CONSEQUENCES

Experimental studies of potassium depletion reveal significant alterations in myocardial function. In potassium-depleted rats, a modest decline in myocardial K occurs indicating that the myocardium is relatively protected from major K loss (41). The decline in intracellular K is paralleled by an upregulation of the myocardial Na-K pump pool (41).

Evaluation of the cardiac implications of chronic potassium depletion in humans has been limited and likely confounded by the effects of treatment. A study in patients with Gitelman syndrome has identified a very high prevalence of prolonged QT interval consistent with the expectation that potassium and magnesium depletion tend to prolong the duration of the action potential of the cardiomyocyte (74). These studies, however, were done in patients receiving appropriate supplementations and may be worsened under conditions of noncompliance (288) or of simultaneous intake of drugs known to affect the QT interval, thus making these patients at increased risk of arrhythmogenic events (74). No evidence was found of any alterations in myocardial structure by echocardiography or predisposition to cardiac ischemia by stress testing (74).

One cardiovascular aspect that remains unresolved is the approach to arrhythmias in normotensive-hypokalemic tubulopathies (54, 288). As indicated previously, potassium and magnesium depletion prolong the duration of the action potential of the cardiomyocyte, which predisposes to ventricular arrhythmias. In addition, potassium or magnesium depletion might impair cardiac performance. The QT interval is often prolonged in primary renal hypokalemia-hypomagnesaemia. Results of continuous ambulatory electrocardiography, exercise testing and echocardiography from small studies are reassuring. Nonetheless, it would be prudent to assume that dangerous cardiac arrhythmias may occur in patients with very severe hypokalemia, during medication with drugs that prolong the QT interval or in the context of short-term nonadherence to the recommended regimen of care (74).

Hormonal Changes

ALDOSTERONE

A decrease in aldosterone levels or excretion is generally observed with potassium depletion (36, 64, 177). Small changes in serum potassium concentration can influence aldosterone secretion (36), and a reduction of 0.5 mEq/l led to a 46% decrement in plasma aldosterone levels (111). Hypokalemia directly inhibits aldosterone secretion in vivo and in vitro (36, 177), but whether plasma potassium level or potassium concentration in glomerulosa cells is more important in this effect has not been determined. Decreased intracellular potassium when Na,K-ATPase is inhibited with ouabain in vitro diminishes the stimulation of aldosterone production by potassium, as well as by ACTH and cAMP (173). Dietary sodium intake also modulates the effects of potassium on aldosterone (142). In animals fed a high-NaCl diet, potassium depletion had no demonstrable effect on plasma aldosterone (142) despite the relative elevation of PRA, suggesting altered adrenal responsiveness to angiotensin. Conversely, sodium loading in potassium-deficient rats leads to a further reduction in the adrenal conversion of corticosterone to aldosterone, the same mechanism responsible for the decline in aldosterone secretion in potassium depletion (187). Potassium depletion suppresses the aldosterone response to low-NaCl diet in rats (142) and humans (111) but does not completely abolish it (142). Furthermore, the response to exogenous Ang II is also maintained (187). In addition to the direct effects of the ion, potassium depletion is associated with alkalosis, which might by itself contribute to the inhibition of aldosterone production.

VASOPRESSIN RELEASE

Urine concentrating ability is impaired in potassium depletion (see subsequent discussion). This defect is associated with increased thirst (whether the increased thirst is due to increased Ang II levels has not been resolved) and may be, as suggested by some aberrant observations in clinical potassium depletion (177), partially responsive to vasopressin. This has suggested an abnormality in the neurohypophyseal system that may lead to diminished vasopressin release (219). In a longitudinal study in which potassium depletion was induced in dogs by a combination of initial intestinal resin and subsequent maintenance on a potassium-deplete diet, Rutecki et al. (219) have demonstrated a blunted response of vasopressin secretion in response to hypertonic saline with the development of potassium depletion. While baseline vasopressin values were normal, the slope of vasopressin level versus plasma sodium concentrations was greatly decreased. This blunted response was partly corrected with indomethacin administration (219). The mechanism of the defect in vasopressin release at the osmoreceptor level in potassium depletion is unclear, and the correction after inhibition of prostaglandin synthesis is not readily explainable. When hypokalemia was induced by deoxycorticosterone acetate (DOCA) administration in the dog, a different profile was observed: the slope of the regression line was not different, but the threshold for vasopressin release was increased (99). This observation was related to the increased extracellular volume and is similar to the finding in patients with primary aldosteronism; it may not, however, be the sole explanation, because extracellular volume is also increased in dietary potassium depletion (85, 154). In contrast to these controlled experimental observations, Jespersen et al. (124) reported an exaggerated vasopressin response to 24-hour water deprivation in two patients with Bartter-like syndrome and hypokalemia. The disparity may be related to volume depletion occurring in these two patients (124).

CATECHOLAMINES

Sympathoadrenal activity is increased in hypokalemic states due to Bartter syndrome and dietary depletion (97, 98). The increase involves both the release of norepinephrine from nerve terminals and epinephrine from the adrenals. This is likely a compensatory response to the peripheral resistance to catecholamines or may be mediated by elevated levels of vasodilator prostaglandins, as it is attenuated by indomethacin administration (97).

RENIN-ANGIOTENSIN

Chronic potassium depletion is associated with elevated plasma renin activity in the rat (142, 162, 187), dog (85, 219), and human (177). In the rat, the increase in PRA is paralleled by an increase in renal renin content (162), suggesting that renal renin biosynthesis (as distinct from renin release) is also increased by potassium depletion. The increased PRA is not suppressed by acute NaCl infusion (162) or dietary NaCl loading (Fig. 3) (142) [except if the animals have undergone simultaneous potassium and sodium depletion (187)] nor is it stimulated by acute, selective chloride depletion as occurs in potassium-replete rats (162). This is consistent with impaired macula densa control of renin release, which may relate to the impaired chloride transport in the loop of Henle in potassium depletion. The latter may also explain the baseline hyperreninemia in potassium depletion, if one postulates that the macula densa exhibits a tonic inhibitory influence over renin release under normal conditions. A normal response to hypotensive hemorrhage and anesthesia was observed, however, in potassium depletion (162). The intact baroreceptor response to hemorrhage suggests that both afferent baroreceptor stimulus and renin release mechanisms function normally in potassium depletion, and the response to anesthesia suggest that efferent stimuli also function normally. Potassium depletion did not interfere with the suppression of PRA by albumin-induced volume expansion (142) and it augmented the response to chronic NaCl deprivation (142), the latter being probably related to the greater negative sodium balance observed in potassium-depleted rats on a low-salt diet. Indomethacin administration leads to a decrease in PRA (85). This response, however, is nonspecific, because indomethacin reduces the hyperreninemia that develops after diuretic administration or use of converting enzyme inhibitors.

In hyperprostaglandin E syndrome (HPGES) and classic Bartter syndrome (cBS), tubular salt and water losses stimulate renin secretion, which is dependent on enhanced cyclooxygenase-2 (COX-2) enzymatic activity. In contrast to other renal COX metabolites, only prostaglandin E2 (PGE2) is selectively up-regulated in these patients. To determine the intrarenal source of PGE2 synthesis, the expression of microsomal PGE2 synthase (mPGES), whose product PGE2 has been shown to stimulate renin secretion in vitro, was evaluated in renal tissue obtained from various groups of patients. Expression of mPGES was analyzed by immunohistochemistry in eight patients with HPGES, in two patients with cBS, and in six control subjects. Expression of mPGES immunoreactive protein was observed in cells of the macula densa in five of eight HPGES patients and in one of two cBS patients. Expression of mPGES immunoreactive protein was not observed in cells associated with the macula densa in kidneys from control subjects without a history consistent with activation of the renin angiotensin system. Co-induction of COX-2 and mPGES in cells of the macula densa suggests that PGE2 activates renin secretion in these patients (138).

Inhibition of stimulated PGE2 formation with indomethacin results in a significant improvement of clinical symptoms and is therefore part of standard therapy. The role of COX-2 selective inhibitors has been recently evaluated. In patients with Bartter syndrome, both indomethacin and rofecoxib ameliorated clinical symptoms, the typical laboratory findings, and significantly suppressed PGE2 and PGE-M excretion to normal values. Rofecoxib suppressed hyperreninemia to a similar extent as indomethacin suggesting that in patients with HPS/aBS, excessive PGE2 synthesis and hyperreninemia is dependent on COX-2 activity (217).

Pulmonary Changes

The metabolic alkalosis generated by potassium depletion in the rat is associated with a rise in the partial pressure of carbon dioxide in arterial blood (92, 93). This hypercapnia is due to reduced ventilation (93) rather than increased metabolic production, because the basal metabolic rate in potassium depletion tends to decrease (193). The compensatory change appears to be due to a decrease in respiratory frequency without any change in tidal volume (93). The decreased frequency is related to prolonged duration of expiration (93, 192) and leads to a decrease in minute ventilation; prolongation of inspiratory time (192) has not been consistently observed (93). These changes are well established after the third week of potassium depletion in the rat and are progressive when it is continued (93). Lengthening of the expiratory phase could be due either to upper airway resistance or to altered neural control of postinspirational diaphragm movement. The latter is a more likely cause as tracheostomy fails to correct the change

in expiratory duration (192). The contribution of a lower metabolic rate and body temperature are unlikely explanations, as potassium-depleted rats maintain a slower ventilatory rate compared to animals matched for metabolic rate and body temperature (193). The altered breathing pattern persists despite vagotomy (192) and has been likened to that observed with chronic pneumotaxic center lesions (194) and catecholamine depletion with reserpine treatment (194). Although increased sympathoadrenal function has been observed in potassium depletion (see previous discussion), tissue studies reveal impaired catecholamine release (143). Finally, there is the possibility that potassium depletion may alter the regulation of cerebrospinal fluid bicarbonate levels, which may contribute to changes in ventilatory rate (194).

Disorders of acid-base homeostasis due to alterations in urine acidification are discussed in a subsequent section of this chapter.

RENAL CHANGES IN POTASSIUM DEFICIENCY

Morphology

EXPERIMENTAL STUDIES

Renal hypertrophy is a universal finding in studies of potassium depletion since the early report by Schraeder et al. in 1937 (177). This renal growth has distinct morphologic characteristics. The increase in kidney mass is not uniform, being more prominent in the outer medulla, as reflected in the relative contribution of the different zones to total kidney weight in potassium-depleted rats described by Ordonez et al. (199). In such animals total outer medulla dry weight comprises 27% of renal dry weight compared to 11.8% in control animals; in contrast, total cortical weight was 70.3% compared to 86%, and the percentage of papillary weight was unchanged. Thus growth of the outer medulla is disproportionately great compared to that of cortex or papilla in potassium-depleted rats. The growth process consists of both hyperplastic and hypertrophic components. The increase in kidney mass is associated with increments in total protein, RNA and DNA content, protein/DNA, and RNA/DNA, and in incorporation of infused radiolabeled amino acids, observations that indicate cell growth as well as formation of new cells (100). The renal proteins increased by this process are myriad, including membrane components as well as a host of cell enzymes. In addition to enzymes involved in ammoniagenesis and transport, to be discussed later, increases in renal pyruvate kinase, glucose-6-phosphate dehydrogenase, and 6-phosphogluconate dehydrogenase have been observed (61, 177).

The increase in membrane synthesis involves all three components, namely, proteins, cholesterol, and phospholipids. Toback and colleagues (199, 258, 260) have provided evidence for increased biosynthesis of phosphatidylcholine, the major phospholipid of renal cell membranes, preceding the appearance of new organelles and surface structures, and the onset of cell division (260). Increased phosphatidylcholine synthesis was observed in the papilla as early as 18 hours after initiation of a potassium-deficient diet, followed at 36 hours by similar changes in the inner stripe of the outer medulla and the inner cortex (260). The enhanced synthesis paralleled the lysosome biogenesis in the papilla (see later discussion) and the hyperplasia and hypertrophy in the other renal zones (260). The increased biosynthesis is coupled to unchanged turnover rate (258, 260). During repletion, biosynthesis is reduced, turnover rate is increased, and resolution of the morphologic alterations is observed (199).

The growth-promoting effect of potassium depletion is not limited by the state of the organ for it occurs in intact as well as in previously damaged kidneys. Peterson et al. (207) have shown that institution of potassium depletion in a model of remnant kidney (5/6 nephrectomy) led to an increase in renal mass and RNA content beyond what is expected of the surgical ablation alone.

The collecting duct is the principle nephron site where morphologic alterations occur in potassium depletion. Glomerular and vascular lesions have rarely been observed in pure potassium deficiency and changes in proximal convoluted tubules have been limited to vacuolar degeneration. While most studies agree on the morphologic changes in individual collecting duct cells, conflicting statements have been made regarding the proportion of cell types and cell number. Hansen et al. (104) and Stetson et al. (247) observed extensive swelling of the epithelium of the collecting duct involving both principle and intercalated cells that was generally confined to the outer medullary segment of the collecting duct (MCT). No changes were observed in either principle or intercalated cells of the initial collecting tubule (245). Intercalated cells in the MCT segment develop extensive microplicae over the entire luminal surface with increased luminal surface boundary length (104), whereas no change was observed in basolateral membrane length or in the luminal or basolateral aspects of principle cells (247). There was no alteration in the proportion of intercalated and principle cells in any part of the collecting duct (104), and no actual increase in cell number when examined in cross section or any increase in mitotic figures (104, 247). In contrast, Evan et al. (70) and Ordonez and Spargo (Ordonez and Spargo 1976) have reported an increased proportion of intercalated cells particularly in the inner stripe of the outer medulla. Furthermore, proliferative changes in this nephron segment to the point of adenomatous occlusion of the tubular lumen have been observed (98). The reasons for these divergent findings are not clear, since similar durations and degrees of depletion have been used. The weight of the evidence favors the view that morphologic changes in individual cells as well as an increase in cell number do develop. At the nephron segment level the cell swelling is manifested by a striking increase in the diameter and volume of MCT. These changes are apparent by the end of the first week and are progressive (117) (Figs. 5–8). This hypertrophic response

occurs in adrenalectomized and in thyroidectomized animals as well, albeit to a lesser absolute degree, reflecting partial dependence on trophic effects of these two hormonal systems. The growth is partially attenuated by inhibition of angiotensin converting enzyme suggesting a role for the hyperreninemia of K depletion in the promotion of this dysregulated growth (180, 184, 220).

The occurrence of these structural changes in growing organisms has been evaluated by Ray et al. (213). Potassium-depleted animals had significant growth retardation and increased RAS activity, manifested by high plasma renin activity, recruitment of renin-producing cells along the afferent arterioles, and down-regulation of Ang II receptors in renal glomeruli and ascending vasa rectae. Potassium-depleted kidneys also showed tubulointerstitial injury with tubular cell proliferation, osteopontin expression, macrophage infiltration, and early fibrosis. These changes were associated with induction of salt sensitivity (213).

Among the various morphologic changes that occur in potassium depletion, the most remarkable is the accumulation of cytoplasmic droplets in medullary cells. These start in the epithelial cells of the collecting duct at the tip of the papilla and extend upward into the outer medulla until the corticomedullary junction (223). The extension is dependent on the duration of potassium depletion. This droplet accumulation involves not only the epithelial cells but also interstitial and other cells in the medulla and results in considerable enlargement of cell volume. The droplets occupy most of the cytoplasm of the papillary cells and lead to a reduction of other cellular organelles such as mitochondria and Golgi apparatus (223). With potassium repletion these changes are reversed, with a decrease in droplets and an increase in the number of mitochondria and a more elaborate Golgi apparatus (223), paralleled by the appearance of empty membrane-bound vacuoles (223). The droplets are believed to be the consequence of disturbed phospholipid homeostasis (260), and their lysosomal nature is suggested by their content of hydrolytic enzymes (11). Thus Aithal et al. (11) have shown a parallel increase in the activities of five hydrolytic enzymes typical of lysosomes and the number and size of droplets observed during progressive potassium depletion. With repletion, the activities of the enzymes return to normal at a rate dependent on the duration of the preceding potassium deficiency (11). The decrease in enzyme activities is associated with a concomitant disappearance of the droplets from medullary cells (11).

Ureteral ligation in potassium-deficient rats is followed by resolution of droplets presumably because of increased renal medullary potassium content (224). The severity of droplet formation depends on the method of induction of potassium depletion with minimal droplet formation developing with DOCA-induced compared with dietary deficiency (222).

Tubular and interstitial apoptosis are observed during potassium depletion. Apoptotic cells are located mainly in the outer medulla. Bcl-2 protein distributed in the tubules

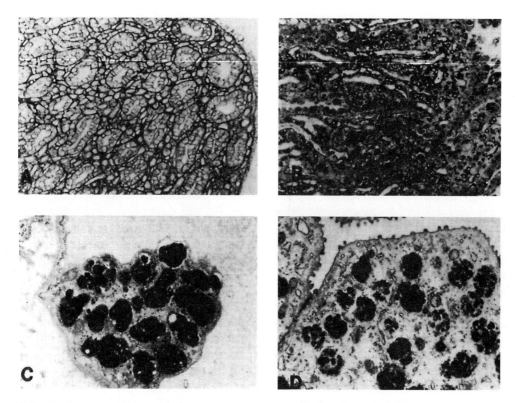

FIGURE 5   Light and electron microscopic changes in the papillary tip of potassium-depleted rats. **A:** Normal appearance of the papilla ($\times$ 145). **B:** Contrasting appearance of the same area with potassium depletion ($\times$ 145). **C:** Transmission electron microscopy showing capillary endothelial cell with massive cytoplasmic accumulation of the characteristic particulate structures ($\times$ 13,300). **D:** Large osmophilic densities in the cytoplasm of cells of the terminal collecting tubule ($\times$ 7200). (From Toback FG, Ordonez NG, et al. Zonal changes in renal structure and phospholipid metabolism in potassium-deficient rats. *Lab Invest* 1976;34:115–124, with permission.)

of the outer medulla is significantly decreased in potassium-depleted rats, while immunoreactivity for Bax protein tends to increase above control levels. There is a significant decrease in levels of bcl2 mRNA in potassium-depleted rats relative to those in controls. Expression of Bax mRNA in potassium-depleted tended to increase, while ratios of bcl2 mRNA to Bax mRNA significantly decreased. These results suggest that apoptosis is associated with progression of cellular proliferation in hypokalemic nephropathy, and a decrease in bcl2 may be involved in promoting this apoptotic process (136).

HUMAN STUDIES

Unlike experimental studies where potassium depletion can be induced selectively, clinical observations are frequently based on complex conditions where potassium deficiency is accompanied by numerous other alterations in sodium balance and acid-base homeostasis. Such heterogeneity in etiologic categories is compounded by variability in disease duration and therapeutic interventions, besides intrinsic variability of the disease prior to obtaining the pathologic specimen. It is possible that associated abnormalities of sodium and hydrogen ion balance, as well as the duration and therapy of potassium depletion, may alter its

histopathologic manifestations in humans. Elucidation of this condition is further complicated by clinical reports where separation into etiologic categories and discrimination between confounding variables have not been undertaken. More importantly, clinical material is usually limited to cortical biopsies, and sampling of medullary and papillary structures may be lacking. The following description is limited to the more common clinical derangements in which, with the previously mentioned caveats, relatively adequate material is available. A sobering observation comes from autopsy studies in healthy adults in Thailand. Potassium depletion prevails among the healthy population of northeast Thailand. In an autopsy study of hypokalemic healthy adult Thai subjects who died of vehicular accidents, none of the patients had renal histopathological change compatible with a diagnosis of focal or diffuse interstitial nephritis and there was minimal renal tubulointerstitial change (151).

Degenerative changes in proximal tubule cells have been a consistent finding in human studies of potassium depletion. While such changes, in general, lack specificity, close examination frequently reveals characteristics of these lesions that make them diagnostic. For example, electron microscopic studies have shown that the vacuolar degeneration

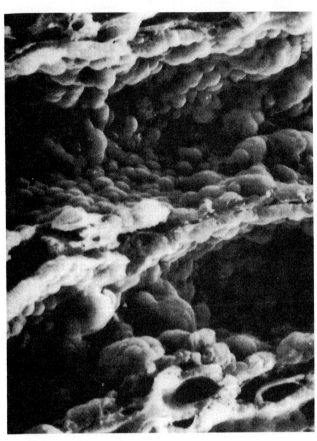

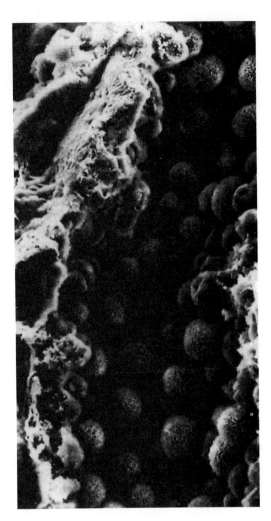

FIGURE 6 Tufts of reactive medullary collecting tubule cells of a potassium-depleted rat extend into the alternately narrowed and widened lumina. Scanning electron microscopy, × 450. (From Polderman KH, Girbes AR. Severe electrolyte disorders following cardiac surgery: a prospective controlled observational study. *Crit Care* 2004;8:R459–466, with permission.)

FIGURE 8 Scanning electron microscopy of the inner zone of the outer medulla of a potassium-depleted rat, depicting hypertrophy of intercalated cells (× 1500). (From Mujais S, Katz AI. Potassium deficiency. In: Seldin DW, Giebisch G, eds. *The Kidney: Physiology and Pathophysiology*. Philadelphia: Lippincott, Williams & Wilkins; 2000:1615–1646, with permission.)

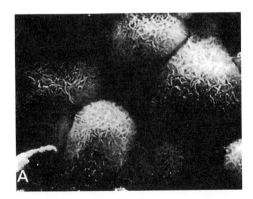
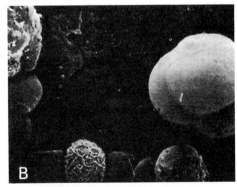

FIGURE 7 Scanning electron microscopy of the inner zone of the outer medulla of a potassium-depleted rat. **A:** Intercalated cells increased in number and have prominent microvilli (× 1280). **B:** Papillary projections into the lumen (× 1280). (From Toback FG, Ordonez NG, et al. Zonal changes in renal structure and phospholipid metabolism in potassium-deficient rats. *Lab Invest* 1976;34:115–124, with permission.)

associated with potassium depletion is located predominantly between the cells and the tubular basement membrane, differing from that caused by osmotic diuretics and contrast media, which is exclusively intracellular.

BARTTER SYNDROME

The renal pathology in Bartter syndrome shares many of the alterations observed with potassium depletion (Table 9), such as vacuolization of proximal tubules (271), hyperplasia of renal medullary interstitial cells (81, 271), and periodic acid Schiff (PAS)–positive granules in cells of the medullary collecting tubule and the loop of Henle (80, 81, 271). In addition, this syndrome manifests a striking hyperplasia and hypergranularity of cells of the juxtaglomerular apparatus with a parallel prominence of the macula densa (52, 177). However, studies in children and adults with Bartter syndrome (81, 262, 275) have convincingly shown that cytoplasmic granules develop in all cell types of the renal papilla and regress after potassium supplementation (262). These findings emphasize the similarity of the morphologic changes in the renal medulla of potassium-depleted humans and experimental animals (Table 9). The lack of awareness of this concordance may be due to the sampling problem of renal biopsy specimens, or to the fact that the clinical material was obtained after various therapeutic interventions.

BEHAVIORAL DISORDERS

Under this heading are included behavioral abnormalities relating mostly to body image or somatization of psychological conflict manifesting as anorexia nervosa, bulimia nervosa, and laxative and diuretic abuse. The obvious existence of confounding variables makes it difficult to assign all the morphologic changes to potassium depletion, yet the similarities with experimental changes, and the presence of potassium depletion as the unifying mechanism of the disparate etiologies, make a strong argument for a pathophysiologic role of potassium deficit.

Riemenschneider and Bohle (218) have reported the largest single series of 40 patients with long-standing hypokalemia due to abuse of laxatives, diuretics, anorexia nervosa, or chronic vomiting. Their findings are consistent with most other reports in the literature describing far fewer cases (177) and can be considered as relatively representative of the lesions found in this group of patients.

Glomerular changes consisted mostly of a reduction in capillary surface and Bowman capsule areas, and an increase in the mesangial space. The glomerular shrinkage was not associated with any alterations in cellular constitution of the tuft (218). Of note is the increase in juxtaglomerular complex size in many of the patients to levels comparable to, or even exceeding, those observed in Bartter syndrome. Such findings underscore the nonspecificity of this change, which is likely secondary to defective chloride absorption in the thick ascending limb rather than a characteristic feature of Bartter syndrome. Tubule vacuolization was not a frequent or pathognomonic observation (218), although it was considered characteristic by Conn and Johnson (177), who coined the term kaliopenic nephropathy in 1956. More important for the prognosis of these patients is the occurrence of degenerative changes such as tubular atrophy, dilatation, epithelial flattening, and thickening of the basement membrane (11). Again, these alterations are nonspecific and reflect evidence of chronic injury. Increased interstitial surface area and lymphocytic cellular infiltration were frequent. PAS-positive granules have been observed in some of these patients in all medullary cells when biopsy material of those deeper regions was available (218).

Taken together, these observations suggest that many of the renal changes seen in potassium-depleted animals have their counterparts in clinical cases. Many are found uniformly across different diagnostic categories and are thus not peculiar to any single clinical etiology of potassium depletion. The significance of these findings is in the grave prognostic outlook that they portend. Some of these changes (glomerular shrinkage, tubular atrophy, interstitial fibrosis) are evidence of irreversible renal damage, and the occurrence of renal insufficiency in this group of patients has been convincingly demonstrated (56, 177). Indeed, in some unfortunate young women the condition has led to end-stage renal disease (3).

TABLE 9   Comparison of Bartter Syndromes and Dietary Potassium Depletion

Parameter	Bartter Syndrome	Dietary	Concordance
Hypokalemia	Present	Present	Yes
Pressor resistance	Present	Present	Yes
Proximal tubulopathy	Present	Present	Yes
Papillary inclusions	Present	Present	Yes
Juxtaglomerular hyperplasia	Present	Present	Yes
Hyperadrenergic state	Present	Present	Yes
Alkalosis	Present	Present	Yes
Thick ascending limb chloride reabsorption	Reduced	Reduced	Yes
Blood pressure	Reduced	Reduced	Yes
Prostaglandins	Increased	Increased	Yes
Plasma rennin	Increased	Increased	Yes
Aldosterone	Increased	Reduced	No
Kaliuresis	Increased	Reduced	No

Primary Aldosteronism

A confounding element in the renal pathology of this condition is the coexistence of changes secondary to hypertension and potassium depletion. Furthermore, the systemic consequences of increased aldosterone production, notably hypertension, may lead to its early diagnosis and thus limitation of renal damage. In addition, the prevalent practice of prescribing potassium supplementation for many hypertensive patients on diuretic therapy, or to patients with primary aldosteronism preoperatively, may attenuate the severity of the potassium deficit.

The apparently additive insults of hypertension and potassium deficiency are illustrated in the study of 18 patients with primary aldosteronism by Danforth et al. (59). Moderate to severe hypertensive changes (fibrous thickening of small vessels and glomerular hyalinization) and kaliopenic lesions (vacuolization and degeneration of tubular epithelia) were observed in 14 (78%) and 16 (89%) patients, respectively. The hypertensive changes appeared to be more severe in this group than in subjects with primary hypertension of similar severity, suggesting a possible synergistic effect of potassium depletion.

Renal Hormonal Systems

An additional role of local induction of the components of the renin-angiotensin system relate to the participation of this system in renal injury. Angiotensin-converting enzyme (ACE) or kininase II has a pivotal role determining the local activity of the renin angiotensin and kallikrein kinin systems. Pertinent to tubulointerstitial injury, where infiltration and proliferation of macrophages and fibroblast occur, ACE also regulates the levels of the natural hemoregulatory peptide, N-acetyl-seryl-aspartyl-lysyl-proline (Ac-SDKP). ACE activity increases in proximal tubules from hypokalemic rats as well as other models of renal injury. ACE, in addition to Ang II generation, may play a pathogenic role through the hydrolysis of BK and Ac-SDKP. Thus, local increase in ACE can be a novel mechanism involved in tubulointerstitial renal injury, providing a pathological basis for the putative deleterious effect of ACE in the diseased kidneys, and the beneficial effect of ACE inhibition (267).

In rats with hypokalemic nephropathy tubulointerstitial injury with macrophage infiltration, interstitial collagen type III deposition, and an increase in osteopontin expression (a tubular marker of injury) are observed. The renal injury was associated with increased cortical ACE expression and continued cortical Ang II generation despite systemic suppression of the renin-angiotensin system, an increase in renal endothelin-1, a decrease in renal kallikrein, and a decrease in urinary nitrite/nitrates and PGE2 excretion. These alterations in vasoactive mediators favor intrarenal vasoconstriction and an ischemic pattern of renal injury (250).

The role of the elevation in renal endothelin-1 (ET-1) in mediating hypokalemic renal injury can be explored by the blockade of ET-A receptors (ETAs) and ET-B receptor (ETB). Rats on a low-potassium diet developed tubulointerstitial injury with an elevation of renal prepro–ET-1 mRNA level. There was an increase in tubular osteopontin expression, macrophage infiltration, collagen accumulation, and tubular cell hyperplasia. ETA blockade significantly ameliorated all parameters for renal injury in the cortex without suppressing local ET-1 and ETA expression. By contrast, ETB blockade significantly reduced local ET-1 and ETA expression and improved the injury to a similar extent in the cortex. In the medulla, ETA or ETB blockade only partially blocked renal injury. These results indicate that ET-1 can mediate hypokalemic renal injury in two different ways: by directly stimulating ETA and by locally promoting endogenous ET-1 production via ETB. Thus, ETA as well as ETB blockade may be renoprotective in hypokalemic nephropathy (249).

Another hormonal system that may play a role in K depletion is the insulin-like growth factor (IGF-I). IGF-I mRNA decreases in potassium-deficient rats, whereas mRNA for IGF binding protein-1 (IGFBP-1), a collecting duct-associated protein, increases (263, 266). These findings are consistent with a sustained role for IGF-I in promoting the exaggerated renal growth of K-depletion and appear to be mediated through local trapping of IGF-I by the overexpressed IGFBP-1, which together with IGF-I can promote renal growth. The selective localization of transforming growth factor-β to hypertrophied nonhyperplastic nephron segments containing IGF-I raises the possibility that transforming growth factor-β may be serving to convert the mitogenic action of IGF-I into a hypertrophic response in these segments. It is also conceivable that transforming growth factor-β may be a cause of the tubulointerstitial infiltrate. Finally, the low circulating IGF-I levels likely contribute to the impaired body growth (263).

Renal Hemodynamics

In contrast to the peripheral vasodilatation described previously, potassium depletion in experimental animals, with few exceptions (85), was found to lead to a decrease in renal blood flow related to increased renal vascular resistance (1, 2, 154, 206, 278). In normotensive humans, modest potassium restriction is associated with a significant reduction in renal blood flow (112). This contrast between the effects of potassium depletion on peripheral and renal resistance is likely related to the operation of intrarenal hormonal factors contributing to the renal vasoconstriction. Increased intrarenal Ang II secondary to the hyperreninemia of potassium depletion no doubt contributes, as evidenced by the partial restitution of renal blood flow toward normal when the renin-angiotensin system is interrupted by either a converting enzyme inhibitor or an Ang II antagonist (154). Further evidence for a role of Ang II is the blunted renal vasoconstrictor response to exogenous Ang II in potassium-restricted normotensive humans, presumably because of receptor occupancy by elevated endogenous Ang II (112). Furthermore, the increased renal generation of thromboxane is an additional factor because renal blood flow also increases in response to inhibition of cyclooxygenase (154, 206) and thromboxane synthetase (154). The use of combined angiotensin antagonists and cyclooxygenase inhibitors leads to complete normalization of renal blood flow in the potassium-depleted rat (154).

Examination of regional renal blood flow has been undertaken because of the possibility that reduced blood flow to the inner medulla may influence the development of the concentrating defect observed in potassium depletion. Peterson (206) has shown, however, that the concentration defect occurs earlier than the decrement in inner medullary plasma flow, and that the latter phenomenon is a late occurrence that is not readily reversed by indomethacin.

A modest reduction in GFR has often been reported in experimental potassium depletion (2, 101, 160, 163, 177, 206, 276) although some studies have failed to demonstrate it (44, 45, 85, 126, 132). When measured, single-nephron glomerular filatration rate (SNGFR) was reduced to the same extent as whole-kidney GFR (177). Part of the discrepancy in observations related to GFR may be due to the reference index used. Potassium depletion is associated with renal hypertrophy but reduced body weight gain, and therefore use of these indices to normalize GFR measurements will give divergent results. In humans, modest K depletion (K deficit of 200 mEq) is associated with reduction in GFR that is worsened by indomethacin (6), but unaffected by angiotensin converting enzyme inhibition (6). Others, however, have found no changes in renal blood flow or GFR under similar conditions (144, 145).

Tubular Function

A heterogeneous pattern of structural involvement occurs along the nephron with sparing of the glomerulus and progressive pathology from proximal to distal segments, particularly the medullary components of the latter. Structural–functional relationships have not been rigorously examined, and the direction of functional change cannot always be predicted from the structural alteration. For example, increased proton secretion occurs in both the proximal and distal nephron, whereas the structural changes at these sites are qualitatively and quantitatively different. Within-segment heterogeneity also develops, as evident from the enhanced potassium reclamation in the collecting duct which develops simultaneously with impaired responsiveness to vasopressin.

PROXIMAL CONVOLUTED TUBULE

Sodium Chloride Studies of sodium chloride transport in this segment are of two kinds: acute alterations in peritubular potassium under controlled experimental conditions and micropunture studies in animals chronically K depleted. The effects of reduced bath potassium on NaCl transport in isolated perfused proximal tubules have been described by several investigators (40, 46). Reduction of bath potassium

concentration below 2.5 mM inhibits NaCl transport in the rabbit PCT (40, 46). Similar results have been obtained in more distal segments such as the thick ascending limb (vide infra). Decrements in NaCl reabsorption, as evidenced by decreased net fluid absorption by this segment, have also been observed during capillary microperfusion with hypokalemic solutions (49).

Studies in potassium-depleted animals show a different pattern of alterations in transport. Walter et al. (270) performed micropuncture studies on anaesthetized rats which had been kept on a potassium-deficient diet for 2 weeks. In these animals, total glomerular filtration rate (GFR) and single-nephron filtration rate were significantly lower than in controls. Fractional reabsorption by the proximal convoluted tubule was enhanced and end-proximal fluid delivery was markedly reduced. They suggested that the reduction in Na delivery to the loop of Henle (arising from the changes in filtration rate and proximal tubular reabsorption) might contribute to the reduced medullary osmotic concentration observed during K depletion. These observations of enhanced proximal reabsorption are in keeping with other studies showing reduced fractional excretion of lithium in K depletion (236), presumably a surrogate measurement for enhanced proximal sodium reabsorption.

Hormonal mechanisms operative at this nephron site to enhance Na reabsorption show increased expression of their receptors. Huang et al. (114) have shown that K depletion leads to an increase in the expression of the adrenergic receptor α_{2B}, the most abundant α_2-adrenergic receptor in rat kidney, which is exclusively located in the proximal nephron. Similarly, K depletion leads to an increase in Ang II receptors at this site (vide infra) (83). The parallelism between the behavior of two agonist hormones receptors and the expected physiologic response observed in potassium-depleted animals underscores the limitations and nonrepresentative nature of acute studies with acute alterations in extracellular K manipulations.

Bicarbonate Chronic potassium depletion augments fractional (45, 147, 177) and absolute (45, 49) bicarbonate reabsorption along the proximal tubule of the rat as determined by free-flow micropuncture and microperfusion studies. In contrast, acute exposure of proximal tubules to hypokalemia (K = 2 mM) in capillary microperfusion experiments had no effect on bicarbonate reabsorption but significantly reduced net volume reabsorption by PCT (49). The mechanism of this enhanced bicarbonate reabsorption is not completely unraveled, although several elements have been clarified. It is likely that increased cellular acidification plays an important role (49). This is suggested by the significant hyperpolarization of proximal tubule cells in rats developing metabolic alkalosis with potassium depletion (236). This hyperpolarization appears to be due to a proportionally lesser fall in cell potassium as compared to extracellular potassium concentration and may accelerate basolateral bicarbonate exit, thereby lowering intracellular pH. The latter change would enhance luminal hydrogen ion secretion through activation of the luminal Na-H exchanger and lead, in turn, to enhanced bicarbonate reabsorption. Support for this construct is derived from data showing a decrease in renal intracellular pH and an increase in luminal Na-H exchanger activity with potassium depletion (177). The decrease in intracellular pH is greater than that observed with chronic metabolic acidosis and is rapidly reversible by acute administration of KCl. The contrast in the effects of chronic versus acute hypokalemia on bicarbonate transport is paralleled by opposing effects on cell polarization. While in chronic potassium depletion the proximal tubular cell hyperpolarizes (48), acute reduction of peritubular potassium leads to sharp depolarization in the rabbit (35) proximal tubules. The changes in chronic depletion are probably related to differential changes in plasma and cell potassium concentrations. Beck et al. (24) reported a 54% decline in plasma potassium (from 4.4 to 2 mEq/l) compared with a 22% decrement in proximal tubular cell potassium (from 150.1 to 117.7 mEq/kg wet weight). Finally, Soleimani et al. (243) using basolateral and luminal vesicles from rat renal cortex demonstrated that potassium depletion increases luminal Na^+-H^+ exchange and basolateral Na-CO_3-HCO_3 cotransport in rat renal cortex.

Increased levels of Ang II are capable of promoting proximal tubule Na-H exchanger activity (159) by interacting with specific receptors found in this nephron segment (186). Recent work in experimental animals and tissue culture suggests that K depletion leads to an increase in AT1 Ang II receptors in the proximal tubule. Burns and Smith (42) observed an increase in mRNA expression of proximal tubule AT1 Ang II receptors with K depletion in rabbits. In cell cultures, a low extracellular K had the same effect. These findings may help explain the enhanced bicarbonate reabsorption observed in the setting of K depletion. K depletion increases both the ambient Ang II concentration and the expression of the receptor for the hormone in the proximal tubule. This combination of changes can readily be envisaged to stimulate the Na-H antiporter and consequently enhance bicarbonate reabsorption in this segment. Such a sequence of events would enhance proximal Na reabsorption. A limiting secondary change that could offset these stimulating influences is the development of alkalemia that reduces proximal bicarbonate reabsorption (14). The failure of metabolic alkalosis to develop in the rabbit, the species in which the increases in Ang II receptors have been described, may be related to the development of mineralocorticoid deficiency with its associated metabolic acidosis (171).

It is surprising that the increase in bicarbonate reabsorption, presumed to be due to an increase in Na-H antiporter activity, is not paralleled by an increased expression of this protein in the kidney of potassium-depleted animals. Wang et al. (271) found no change in the expression of Na/H exchanger-3 (NHE3) mRNA and its cognate protein after 6 and 14 days in rats on a low-potassium diet. The mRNA levels for NHE1, NHE2, and NHE4 also remained unchanged at 6 and 14 days of the low-potassium diet. Further work is required to reconcile these apparent inconsistencies.

An additional factor that would contribute to the acid-base balance and reflect changes in proximal tubule transport is the effect of K depletion on citrate reabsorption in this nephron segment. Chronic K depletion causes hypocitraturia. Levi et al. (153) have shown in brush border membranes obtained from K-depleted rats an increase in the V_{max} of the proximal tubule apical membrane Na-citrate cotransporter.

Phosphate The regulation of an important component of proximal tubular function, namely, phosphate reclamation, seems to be abnormal in potassium-depleted rats. Under basal conditions, phosphate balance as reflected in plasma phosphate levels and urinary phosphate excretion is normal. The phosphaturic response to parathyroid hormone (PTH) and dibutyryl cyclic AMP infusions, however, is reduced, as is urinary cyclic AMP excretion in response to PTH (26). In addition to these changes in urinary excretion, presumably representing altered proximal nephron function, studies in isolated tubules show that PTH-sensitive adenylate cyclase in rabbit pars recta is also affected (215). These results suggest pre- and postcyclic AMP generation defects. Their detailed exploration, in a manner analogous to the evaluation of vasopressin-sensitive adenylate cyclase (see later discussion), has not been undertaken, but it appears that in potassium depletion there is a generalized impairment of the adenylate cyclase system and its responses to various hormones along the nephron.

Hypokalemia has also been invoked in contributing to the range of proximal tubular dysfunctions observed in children with primary distal renal tubular acidosis. Low-molecular-weight (LMW) proteinuria, phosphaturia, and generalized aminoaciduria have been described with resolution after metabolic correction (274).

LOOP OF HENLE

Eknoyan et al. (69) were the first to suggest that a defect in sodium transport by the thick ascending limb (TAL) could explain the concentrating defect of potassium depletion. Renal chloride wasting has been described with potassium depletion in rats (161, 177), although in humans the response has varied with the severity of the potassium depletion: enhanced chloride conservation was observed with moderate, short-term potassium depletion (126), and chloride wasting with severe potassium depletion (88). Luke et al. (160, 163) have shown in balance studies impaired chloride conservation in potassium-depleted rats, and with micropuncture and microperfusion studies they found diminished net chloride reabsorption between the latest proximal and earliest distal segment, as well as increased luminal chloride concentration at the latter site (160). These findings were consistent with impaired TAL absorption, and the defect was only partially corrected with indomethacin (160). Gutsche et al. (101), using the micro stop-flow technique, have provided evidence for defective sodium transport in the TAL of potassium-depleted rats. The severity of the defect correlated with the decrease in plasma potassium concentration and was rapidly reversed with acute potassium administration. Acute administration of potassium also increases outer medullary heat production (presumably reflecting the metabolic energy expenditure of transport) in the potassium-depleted dog (176). In addition, net NaCl transport is inhibited by reduction in bath potassium concentration in isolated perfused TAL (95).

More recent work has uncovered the molecular basis of the observed defects in electrolyte reabsorption in the TAL. Amlal et al. (15) have shown downregulations of chloride-absorbing transporters with potassium depletion. Feeding potassium deficient (KD) diet to rats resulted in decreases in mRNA levels for the apical Na-K-2Cl cotransporter in the medulla by 56% and 51% at 6 and 14 days of KD diet, respectively. Functional studies in tubular suspensions from medullary TAL demonstrated that the Na-K-2Cl cotransporter activity decreased by approximately 45% and approximately 37% at 6 and 14 days of KD diet, respectively. mRNA levels for the thiazide-sensitive Na-Cl cotransporter also decreased by 57% and 64% at 6 and 14 days of KD diet. Decreased expression of the apical Na-Cl and the Na-K-2Cl cotransporters became evident at 48 and 72 hours of KD, respectively. These changes in transport expression were paralleled by functional changes in chloride reabsorption.

Changes in the activity of the Na-K pump in this nephron segment have been explored by Buffin-Meyer et al. (39). Within 2 weeks of K depletion, Na-K-ATPase activity and [^{3}H]ouabain binding increased by 30% to 50% in the medullary thick ascending limb (MTAL), confirming previous findings in this model (107). Despite this increase in the number of Na-K-ATPase units, the transport capacity of the Na-K pump, determined by ouabain-sensitive Rb uptake in the presence of an extracellular concentration of Rb mimicking the kalemia determined in K depleted rats (2.3 mM Rb), was reduced in MTAL from LK rats. Inhibition of the Na-K pump was not accounted for by changes in either extracellular K or intracellular Na concentrations, but by a decrease in the pump affinity for Na (39).

It is important to highlight this defective NaCl reabsorption in the TAL in view of the notion advocated by Gill and Bartter, and reinforced by the molecular biology of the syndrome, that defective tubular reabsorption of chloride in the TAL is a unique feature of Bartter syndrome (90). Their thesis was based on the assumption that this abnormality has not been observed in other clinical forms of hypokalemia, such as chronic vomiting (90) or diuretic abuse (209). Studies in experimental animals subjected to dietary potassium depletion have reproduced many of the features of the clinical syndrome, including the "characteristic" defective chloride reabsorption in the TAL (Table 9). The pathogenesis of Bartter syndrome has been recently elucidated by elegant genetic studies showing that mutations in either the Na-K-2Cl transporter or the K channel are responsible for the impaired NaCl reabsorption in TAL (vide supra).

Impaired chloride reabsorption may secondarily enhance potassium secretion in the distal tubule. As the handling of the cation in the latter segment is chloride responsive, this would accentuate kaliuretic mechanisms and lead to a self-magnifying vicious circle.

Basolateral and apical Na-H exchangers (NHEs) in TAL are involved in NH_4^+ and HCO_3^- absorption, respectively. The NH_4^+ absorption rate in Henle's loop is increased in potassium depletion, which may be secondary to the increased NH_4^+ concentration in luminal fluid and/or to an increased NH_4^+ absorptive capacity of TAL. HCO_3^- absorptive capacity in Henle's loop is unchanged in KD despite the presence of metabolic alkalosis. The effects of K-depletion on the expression of basolateral NHE-1 and the expression of apical NHE-3 in TAL have been examined by Laghmani et al. (150). NHE-1 protein abundance was similarly increased (approximately 90%) at 2 and 5 weeks of K-depletion, while NHE-1 mRNA amount in TAL cells was increased at 2 weeks and returned to normal values by 5 weeks. NHE-3 protein abundance remained unchanged in 2 and 5 weeks of K-depletion, while NHE-3 mRNA was unchanged by 2 weeks and reduced by approximately 50% at 5 weeks. In potassium depletion, the increased NHE-1 expression may support an increased TAL NH_4^+ absorptive capacity. The lack of change in NHE-3 expression despite the presence of metabolic alkalosis is in agreement with the unchanged HCO_3^- absorptive capacity of Henle's loop (150).

DISTAL TUBULE

While significant bicarbonate reabsorption normally takes place along the distal tubule, this is achieved with very little change in tubular bicarbonate concentration (45). The rate of bicarbonate absorption is not altered in potassium depletion, despite a lower delivery rate and the presence of a greater lumen-to-plasma bicarbonate concentration difference due to the higher plasma levels and lower luminal levels achieved (45). That distal tubules of potassium-depleted rats have an enhanced capacity to absorb bicarbonate, as proximal tubules do, was shown in experiments in which delivery rates of bicarbonate were increased to levels similar to those in controls, and bicarbonate reabsorption was higher than in the potassium-replete animals (44). In the distal tubule bicarbonate reabsorption is relatively insensitive to peritubular alkalinization and the systemic alkalosis present does not affect acid secretion (44). The mechanism therefore is not self-limiting, and no "braking" of the enhanced bicarbonate reabsorption occurs. This is due to enhanced electrogenic proton secretion (H^+-ATPase) as demonstrated in in vivo microperfusion of the superficial distal tubule in potassium depleted animals (18).

Potassium secretion in the accessible portion of distal nephron, which consists in part of distal convoluted and in part initial collecting tubule, is reduced to near zero in potassium depletion (245). This occurs despite the increased delivery of chloride, suggesting that kaliferic changes, perhaps the decrement in plasma and cell potassium (24), are effective at this site. Considering, however, the small contribution of this segment to net external potassium balance, this adaptive response is not sufficient to prevent the continuing potassium deficit.

COLLECTING DUCT

This segment is the site of major structural changes in potassium depletion, and the alterations in its transport functions are primarily responsible for some of the principle manifestations of potassium deficiency, namely, metabolic alkalosis and defective urinary concentrating ability.

Bicarbonate Studies in collecting duct obtained from potassium-depleted animals have been limited and are subject to species variations. Although bicarbonate transport has been studied in rabbit collecting tubules (171), it should be noted that the findings in this species are difficult to reconcile with observations in rats and humans, because the rabbit develops a metabolic acidosis in response to potassium depletion. McKinney and Davidson (171) found that the potential difference was less lumen-negative in the isolated perfused CCT from potassium-depleted rabbits and less lumen-positive in the MCT. In the latter segment, bicarbonate absorption (or, conversely, hydrogen ion secretion) was decreased (171).

Insight into alterations in hydrogen ion secretion at this nephron site in the rat can nevertheless be gleaned from clearance studies examining titration of specific buffers. Kornandakieti and Tannen (141) have examined distal hydrogen ion secretion in isolated perfused kidneys using a design that controlled for alterations in ammonia production by excluding glutamine from the perfusate, and in proximal bicarbonate reclamation by using a very low filtered load of bicarbonate. Distal nephron (alternatively collecting duct) contribution to urinary acidification was ascertained by providing a surfeit of creatinine as a urinary buffer. Under these conditions, titratable acidity to pH 6.0 reflects the acid secretory capacity of a defined functional nephron segment, namely, the collecting duct. At comparable buffer loads, kidneys from potassium-depleted rats had a lower urinary pH and a higher titratable acid excretion compared to control rats (140, 141), both changes reflecting the increased hydrogen ion secretory capacity of the collecting duct. The alteration with potassium depletion was similar to that observed in chronic metabolic acidosis. Considering that metabolic alkalosis suppresses distal acidification as assessed by this method (140), the stimulation by potassium depletion becomes more remarkable in the face of the alkalemic state of the animals. Potassium deficiency thus exerts a primary, aldosterone- and sodium-independent, stimulatory effect on collecting duct hydrogen ion secretion, likely at the level of the putative proton pump. A biochemical counterpart of this functional observation is provided by the observation of increased *N*-ethylmaleimide–sensitive ATPase in medullary collecting tubules from potassium-depleted rats (177), assuming that the measured enzyme reflects the activity of a proton-translocating ATPase.

Pendrin belongs to a superfamily of Cl⁻-anion exchangers and has been localized to the apical side of non–type A intercalated cells of the cortical collecting duct, and reduced bicarbonate secretion was demonstrated in a pendrin knockout mouse model. In chronic potassium depletion, known to elicit a metabolic alkalosis, pendrin protein levels are decreased and pendrin expression is shifted to an intracellular pool with the relative number of pendrin positive cells reduced. These results are in agreement with a potential role of pendrin in bicarbonate secretion and regulation of acid-base transport in the cortical collecting duct (268).

Potassium Potassium transport in this segment is altered in a direction that favors potassium conservation. In the cortical collecting tubule (CCT) obtained from potassium-depleted animals, net potassium transport is reduced to zero, whereas in control states net secretion is observed (229). In the inner stripe of the outer medullary collecting tubule, Wingo (280) has observed ut the apparent potassium permeability is physiologically regulated and increases during dietary potassium restriction. The inner medullary collecting duct also contributes to potassium conservation (62, 103). Diezi et al. (62) demonstrated active potassium reabsorption in the papillary collecting tubule of potassium-depleted rats by micropuncture sampling at different levels of the segment. Backman and Hayslett (16), using microcatheterization techniques, have examined potassium handling in the inner medullary collecting duct following short-term potassium deprivation. Although under control conditions there was little net transport of potassium along the inner medullary collecting duct, significant potassium absorption (90% of the delivered load) occurred in potassium-depleted animals. This topic is discussed in further detail in subsequent sections of this chapter.

Urea Reabsorption The concentrating defect of potassium depletion occurs in association with decrements in the concentration of solutes in the medullary interstitium (177), which result in a decreased osmotic gradient for water reabsorption from the collecting duct during antidiuresis. Decreased inner medullary osmolarity may be related to impaired urea delivery to the papilla from juxtamedullary nephrons, or to diminished urea absorption in the renal medulla and impairment of urea recirculation. Urea absorption in the papillary duct, however, was found to be normal (276), as was water absorption in the accessible portion of the papillary duct. These results suggest that terminal papillary duct water and urea reabsorption are preserved in potassium depletion and the defect in urinary concentration is proximal to the accessible portion of the papillary duct: that is, it is not due to impaired urea absorption in the terminal portions of the nephron (see also following section). However, recent experimental evidence in mice suggests that this may not be completely true. Urea transport in the kidney is mediated by a family of transporter proteins that include the renal urea transporter (UT-A) and the erythrocyte urea transporter (UT-B). Potassium depletion was associated with reduced expression of UT-A1, UT-A3, and UT-B but increased expression of UT-A2 suggesting that reduced expression of urea transporters may play a role in the impaired urine-concentrating ability associated with potassium deprivation (128).

Integrated Renal Functions

Renal Concentrating Ability

The concentrating defect of potassium depletion is manifest primarily as a limitation of maximal urinary concentrating ability rather than persistent hyposthenuria. Several factors appear to contribute to its genesis and these are discussed later. It is important to note that potassium depletion also results in polydypsia, thus accentuating polyuria independent of the urinary concentrating defect (30). In humans, thirst is a prominent symptom of experimental potassium depletion (87). In the rat, the increased water intake precedes the development of the urinary concentrating defect (30) and restriction of fluid intake in the initial phase attenuates the polyuria, although it does not prevent the ultimate development of the urinary concentrating defect (30). Primary polydypsia is thus a major contributing factor to the early polyuria in potassium depletion. This may explain the observation that the polyuria of hypokalemic subjects is often in excess of the urine volume obligated by their concentrating defect.

In humans, the concentrating defect has been observed in pathologic and experimental potassium depletion. A quantitative relationship between the degree of potassium deficiency and the urinary concentrating defect is provided by the elegant study of Rubini (177) in normal adult men subjected to experimental potassium depletion. A depression of maximal osmolality was observed when the negative potassium balance exceeded 200 mEq, and with a deficit of over 350 mEq, maximal osmolality was reduced to a mean of 340 mOsm/kg.

In the rabbit, the polyuria and decreased urinary osmolarity are well established by the end of 1 week of potassium depletion and persist thereafter (117). The rat, however, is still capable of generating a maximally concentrated urine by the end of 1 week (30), but by 2 weeks the concentrating defect is fully established and stable (206).

The concentrating defect seen in the potassium-depleted rabbit is resistant to vasopressin in vivo, and there is decreased hydrosmotic response to vasopressin in isolated CCT (214), which is normalized by inhibition of prostaglandin synthesis or addition of pertussis toxin in vitro (216). A normal hydrosmotic response of potassium depleted rabbit CCT to an analog of 3′-5′-cyclic monophosphate (cAMP), and persistence of the abnormal vasopressin response in the presence of a phosphodiesterase inhibitor provide indirect evidence of a cellular defect in vasopressin-sensitive adenylate cyclase (214). Indeed, such a decrease in vasopressin stimulation of adenylate cyclase activity has been observed in CCT of potassium-depleted rabbits (215). This defect in adenylate cyclase paralleled and was equal in magnitude to the abnormal hydrosmotic response observed in this segment (215). It should be noted that this abnormality was observed when the tubular segment was obtained without the use of collagenase pretreatment and it was abolished by the use of proteases, a finding that prompted Raymond et al. (215) to suggest that the defect induced by potassium depletion was protease sensitive. The fact that pertussis toxin normalizes the hydrosmotic response of the CCT to vasopressin suggests that the defect in vasopressin-sensitive adenylate cyclase is mediated by the inhibitory guanine nucleotide-binding regulatory component (Ni) of adenylate cyclase (216). The tubular defect induced by potassium depletion was not restricted to the CCT but also affected the PTH-sensitive adenylate cyclase in the rabbit pars recta (215). The impairment of distinct hormone-sensitive adenylate cyclases localized to different nephron segments suggests a generalized modulating effect of potassium depletion on plasma membrane function in renal epithelial cells.

The findings in the rat are divergent in regard to vasopressin-sensitive adenylate cyclase but similar as far as water permeability. Carney et al. (47) have shown that basal diffusional water permeability was not different in potassium-depleted and control animals, whereas the response to vasopressin was significantly diminished (Fig. 9). Vasopressin-sensitive adenylate cyclase activity was found to be normal in potassium-depleted rat CCT (117), increased in outer medullary collecting tubule (MCTo) (117, 135), and decreased or unchanged (117) in inner medullary collecting tubules. Of note, both studies that observed increased activity in the MCT found it to be decreased in the medullary thick ascending limb (MAL) (117, 135). The reasons for this intranephron heterogeneity and for the divergence between investigators are unclear. (Both studies [117, 135] used collagenase-treated tubules.) The difference between rat and rabbit CCT is less puzzling as species differences in the inhibitory modulation of vasopressin responsiveness in the CCT have been reported (177). Thus prostaglandin E2 inhibits AVP-stimulated osmotic water permeability in rabbit CCT but not in that of the rat (177). An additional difficulty in interpreting studies of rat tubules is the variance between these studies and results obtained from medullary slices that unequivocally show an impairment of AVP-dependent cyclic AMP system in potassium-deficient rats (28).

Hypokalemia results in a decrease in aquaporin-2 (AQP2) expression in principle cells of rat collecting ducts (cortical and medullary), in parallel with the development of polyuria, and the degree of downregulation is consistent with the level of polyuria induced. Potassium repletion is associated with normalization of AQ2 expression and urine output (166).

Regulation of AVP-sensitive adenylate cyclase by alterations in extracellular potassium has been explored in rat renal papillary collecting tubule cells in culture (118). Exposure of these cells to a potassium-free medium for more than 24 hours was associated with an attenuated cellular cAMP

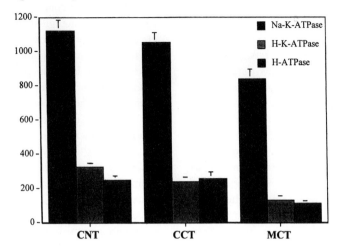

FIGURE 9 In control rats on a normal K diet, H,K-ATPase activity was present throughout the rat collecting duct with a hierarchy of CNT>CCT> MCT. This hierarchy of enzyme activity is similar to that observed for other transport ATPases such as Na,K-ATPase and NEM-sensitive ATPase (H-ATPase). CNT, connecting tubule; CCT, cortical collecting tubule; MCT, medullary collecting tubule. Reference (181).

response to both vasopressin and forskolin. These in vitro data (118) coupled to the above results from fresh tissue suggest that reduced extracellular potassium leads to changes in cell responsiveness to vasopressin by altering the adenylate cyclase system.

The observation that prostaglandin synthesis may be increased in potassium depletion and that PGs exert an antagonistic effect on the renal action of vasopressin prompted examination of their role in mediating the renal concentrating defect. Inhibition of prostaglandin formation failed to improve the renal concentrating defect in the dog with dietary potassium depletion, although urinary excretion of prostaglandin E was increased (219). Partial correction of the concentrating defect was observed in dogs depleted of potassium by exogenous mineralocorticoid excess (68, 99) when treated with indomethacin, which restored the renal response to vasopressin (99). In the rabbit, the reduction in maximal concentrating ability was related temporally to a significant increase in urinary prostaglandin E excretion, and treatment with prostaglandin synthesis inhibitors partially corrected the concentrating defect (216). The partial correction occurred in rabbits depleted of potassium for 2 weeks, whereas with shorter potassium depletion (1 week), indomethacin led to complete correction of the concentrating defect (216). In the potassium-depleted rat, however, indomethacin failed to alter the concentrating defect despite effective inhibition of medullary tissue prostaglandin synthesis (30). These variations in the response to prostaglandin inhibition are paralleled by variations in the rate of PG synthesis. In the dog PGE2 excretion is increased by dietary potassium de-

pletion and DOCA administration (68, 85, 99, 219), and urinary PGE2 is also increased in the rabbit (215). A more detailed picture of PG changes is available in the rat, in which neither PGE2 excretion (96, 113) nor papillary tissue content (27, 30) is altered by potassium depletion. In contrast, thromboxane B2 content and synthesis increased in papilla from potassium-depleted rats (27).

The concentrating defect in potassium depletion is likely multifactorial with several of the contributing mechanisms acting in complementary fashion. Impaired NaCl reabsorption in the TAL limits the establishment of a hypertonic interstitium. The defect in this first prerequisite for urine concentration may be amplified by the polydypsia and the consequent medullary washout. To this is added an aberration in the second prerequisite for effective urinary concentration, namely, an impaired response to vasopressin in parts of the collecting duct. Diminished interstitial osmotic drive for water extraction coupled to subnormal vasopressin-permeabilization of the otherwise water-impermeable collecting duct epithelium conspire to produce the defect in urine concentration. There is also evidence in potassium depletion for a decrease in inner medullary organic osmolytes which might precede the renal concentrating defect. Aldose reductase (an osmoregulatory protein) mRNA abundance was reduced in potassium depletion (189, 190).

The resistance to vasopressin is not restricted to its osmotic effect, but extends to other cellular actions of the hormone. Vasopressin is known to enhance Na reabsorption in the CCT and secondarily enhance Na-K pump activity. In K-depleted rats both the hydroosmotic effect and the Na-K pump stimulatory effects are blunted (184).

As alluded to previously, the renal concentrating defect typical for chronic potassium depletion may also be related to inadequate accumulation of osmolytes. Papillary interstitial ionic strength (sum of Na, Cl, and K) in antidiuretic low-potassium rats is significantly reduced compared with antidiuretic normal-potassium rats. The lower interstitial ionic strength in antidiuretic low potassium is associated with a lower total content of organic osmolytes in the inner medulla (25).

Urine Acidification

Species Differences Potassium is capable of modulating several acidification mechanisms including proximal bicarbonate reabsorption, distal hydrogen ion secretion, renal ammonia production, and aldosterone levels, yet the role of potassium depletion in inducing and sustaining metabolic alkalosis has been the subject of debate. This can be attributed to the divergent responses of different species. In the dog, potassium depletion results in hyperchloremic metabolic acidosis due to a decline in renal acid excretion secondary to mineralocorticoid deficiency (87, 115, 270). In this species, administration of aldosterone prevents the development of the metabolic acidosis (115). Similar results have been obtained in the rabbit fed a potassium-deficient, high-protein diet (171). The metabolic acidosis in these animals was related to (45) a decline in collecting tubule acid secretion and was also corrected by mineralocorticoid administration (171). In contrast to these two species, the potassium-depleted rat develops a metabolic alkalosis (44, 45, 87, 92, 93). In humans, moderate potassium depletion results in modest elevation of plasma bicarbonate (126). The small change in plasma bicarbonate level has cast doubt on whether clinically significant metabolic alkalosis can be accounted for solely on the basis of potassium depletion, or whether other factors need to be considered. Two observations, however, lend credence to an important role for potassium depletion in the generation of metabolic alkalosis in humans. The first is provided by cases of severe potassium depletion with metabolic alkalosis, chloride wasting, and no mineralocorticoid excess, where the alkalosis is corrected by replenishing potassium stores (88). The second observation derives from the work of Hernandez et al. (110), who demonstrated that development of metabolic alkalosis is dependent on the level of concomitant sodium intake during induction of dietary potassium depletion. A significant increase in plasma bicarbonate was observed when sodium intake was restricted to mitigate the positive sodium balance that develops during potassium depletion (110, 126, 144, 177), and expansion of extracellular fluid volume could attenuate a developing metabolic alkalosis (149). Indeed, studies in rats show that salt loading prevents the development of metabolic alkalosis with potassium depletion (92). Finally, the metabolic alkalosis in rats is reversed with refeeding a potassium-replete diet, which leads to normalization of pH and bicarbonate concentrations within 3 days of refeeding (79).

Ammonia Chronic potassium depletion is a potent stimulus for renal NH_3 production (79, 120, 225, 256, 258), and the augmented renal ammoniagenesis is believed to have important physiological and pathophysiological roles. Increased urinary ammonia excretion secondary to enhanced renal ammonia production is associated with potassium conservation (see later discussion), and the higher rate of ammonium excretion increases the capacity of the kidney to excrete acid, thereby contributing to the metabolic alkalosis.

A modest increase in renal cortical mitochondrial ammonia production is observed as early as 3 days after initiation of dietary potassium depletion in rats and reaches a plateau at the end of 2 weeks (225). This results from increases in both glutamine deamidation and glutamate deamination (225). The increment in phosphate-dependent glutaminase (PDG) activity antedates the increase in ammonia production and continues even after ammonia production has leveled off (225). The dissociation between PDG and ammonia production may be related to limitation of the latter by either mitochondrial glutamine uptake or inhibition of the enzyme by the produced glutamate. Potassium repletion leads to prompt decreases in both ammonia production (225) and PDG activity (87, 171), but these parameters do not normalize in parallel with replenishment of renal stores (79, 225). The mechanism and effects of this delayed recovery are not entirely clear, particularly since ammonium excretion returns to normal levels (79). The potassium-depleted rat responds appropriately to acid loading by further increasing both phosphate-dependent glutaminase and ammonia excretion (79). Changes in other enzyme systems related to glutamine metabolism occur as well: an increase in glutamine transaminase activity and decrease in omega deamidase activity, two enzymes that constitute the glutaminase II pathway (transamination of glutamine followed by deamidation of α-ketoglutarate) (79), have been reported. In addition, an increase in phosphoenolypyruvate carboxykinase (PEPCK) has also been observed. This enzyme, located primarily in the cytosol, is essential for removal of α-ketoglutarate (79).

The tubular sites of increased ammonia production have been examined by Nonoguchi et al. (196) in microdissected tubules of a rat model of potassium depletion. Potassium depletion led to a threefold increase in ammonia production in the S1 segment of the proximal tubule, and a doubling of ammonia production in the S2 segment and in both the cortical and medullary portions of the collecting tubule (196). No changes in ammonia production were observed in the S3 segment (pars recta) or in the thick ascending limb or distal convoluted tubule. The increase in ammonia production in S1 occurred in both superficial and juxtamedullary nephrons, although the change was greater in the former (196). This increased ammoniagenesis was paralleled by increased gluconeogenesis from glutamine and pyruvate occurring mostly in S1 and to a lesser degree in S2 (285).

**H-K-ATPase
(pmol/mm/h)**

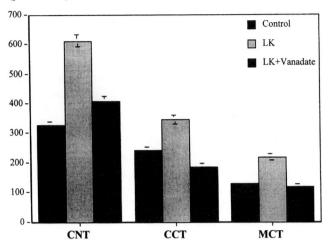

FIGURE 10 Chronic potassium depletion (low potassium [LK], 3 weeks) led to a generalized increase in H,K-ATPase activity, with the greater increments occurring in segments of higher basal activity, CNT> CCT>MCT. Chronic vanadate administration (LK + vanadate) obliterated the effect of K depletion. CNT, connecting tubule; CCT, cortical collecting tubule; MCT, medullary collecting tubule. (From Mujais SK. Transport enzymes and renal tubular acidosis. *Semin Nephrol* 1998;18:74–82, with permission.)

The primary mechanism by which potassium depletion stimulates renal ammonia production is not precisely known. Increased renal ammonia production and excretion despite the simultaneous presence of metabolic alkalosis suggest that intracellular factors rather than the requirements of extracellular acid-base homeostasis dictate renal ammonia metabolism in this condition. The intracellular acidosis that occurs in potassium depletion may initiate the adaptive response in ammoniagenesis, but other pathways may also contribute. Studies using renal slices have suggested that the increase in renal ammonia production may be limited to the cortex without any changes in the medulla (256). Insight into the specific tubular sites where ammonia handling is altered can be gleaned from a micropuncture study by Jaeger et al. (120), in which late proximal and early distal tubular ammonium concentrations and delivery rates were increased in potassium depletion. It appears that the proximal tubule is the major site of ammonium secretion, as no alteration in ammonium was observed between early and late distal sites and the amount of ammonia delivered to the latter could account for the majority of ammonium excretion (120).

Relevance of Increased Ammonia Production It has been suggested that increased ammonia production may contribute to the renal morphological changes in potassium depletion (197). This suggestion is based on observations dating as far back as 1890, when Heinz observed vacuolation of nucleated cells by ammonia (177). This alteration has been shown to be due to trapping of ammonia as ammonium in acidic lysosomes, leading to their osmotic swelling and vacuolization (lysosomotropic amine) (230). Ammonia effects on cells

include vacuolization of lysosomes and inhibition of endocytosis and protein degradation by lysosomes (secondary to an increase in lysosomal pH and consequent inhibition of acid hydrolase). Ammonia decreases the number of receptors for many cell-surface ligands such as insulin (167) and epidermal growth factor (170), due to trapping of the receptor-ligand complex in lysosomes and interruption of receptor recycling leading to depletion of surface receptors. These events could explain the vacuolization observed in proximal and collecting duct cells, the tubular proteinuria and enzymuria (197), and resistance to the effects of hormones that require internalization of receptor-ligand complex.

Many of these ammonia-induced lysosomal changes find their morphologic and functional counterpart in potassium depletion. What has not been resolved, however, is whether these changes, which are usually corrected with potassium repletion, are responsible for the irreversible damage with progression to end-stage renal disease seen with prolonged potassium depletion in the rat (177) and in clinical cases in humans. Furthermore, it has not been determined whether prevention of the increase in ammonia production abolishes or ameliorates these changes. Partial answers to these questions have been offered by Tolins et al. (261), who used alkali loading to suppress renal ammonia production. Bicarbonate supplementation reduced the renal hypertrophy produced by potassium depletion, histologic evidence of tubular injury, and peritubular deposition of the third component of complement (261). The latter phenomenon may be related to activation of complement by ammonia, a concept first proposed in 1959 by Beeson and Rowley (177).

The sum of evidence indicates that increased renal ammonia production is maladaptive in that it is capable of activating mechanisms of renal injury, and that its suppression may ameliorate the tubulointerstitial lesions of potassium depletion.

Integration of Changes in Urinary Acidification Titratable acid excretion is reduced in hypokalemic rats and net acid output appears to be largely mediated by the enhanced ammonium excretion (132). The fall in titratable acidity is likely due to diminished urinary phosphate (132). This is compensated for by the provision of ammonia as a dominant urinary buffer accounting for the increased urinary pH observed in this condition. The hypervolemia and alkalemia of potassium depletion do not appear to diminish proximal bicarbonate reclamation. The net result of the various changes in renal acidification in the rat is to promote the development and maintenance of metabolic alkalosis by coupling increased proximal bicarbonate reclamation, distal proton secretion, and generation of urinary buffer (ammonia), all these effects apparently representing alterations in the normal regulatory mechanisms operating in the potassium-replete kidney.

RENAL TRANSPORT ENZYMES

Under normal dietary potassium intake, most of the filtered potassium is reabsorbed before the end of the distal convoluted tubule and urinary potassium is derived primarily from its secretion beyond this point, that is, in the collecting tubule (284). Animals depleted of potassium, in contrast, conserve this cation by elaborating a nearly potassium-free urine, accomplished by drastically reducing or abolishing potassium secretion in the cortical collecting tubule and increasing its reabsorption in the inner stripe of the outer medullary collecting tubule and in the papillary collecting duct (16, 103, 157, 280, 284). Although it was known for some time that in potassium-depleted animals the reabsorption of potassium across the luminal membrane of certain nephron segments, including the medullary collecting tubule, must proceed against an unfavorable gradient (248), enquiries into the biochemical mechanisms involved in active potassium transport have begun more recently with attempts to define the role of several transport ATPases in this process (63, 89, 107, 117, 281).

Na,K-ATPase Active translocation of potassium across cell membranes is mediated chiefly by Na,K-ATPase, the biochemical expression of the Na-K pump. For example, potassium secretion in the CCT first requires its active uptake by the basolateral membrane Na-K pump (284), and chronic increments in dietary potassium intake lead to enhanced ability to secrete potassium associated with an adaptive increase in Na,K-ATPase in this nephron segment (179, 182). Conversely, one would anticipate renal Na,K-ATPase to be decreased in potassium-depleted animals, but the few studies that examined this issue surprisingly found an increase in enzyme activity in kidney homogenates from rats and dogs fed a potassium-deficient diet (57, 157). Furthermore, both acute and long-term exposure to low ambient potassium leads to substantial increments in the number and/or activity of Na-K pumps in several cultured cell lines (209, 211, 277). Combined with earlier reports that potassium absorption from the rat (65, 248) and *Amphiuma* (279) tubular lumen is inhibited by ouabain, these observations suggested the possibility that Na-K pumps might be found on the apical membrane of certain nephron segments, where they could energize potassium reabsorption. To test this hypothesis, Hayashi and Katz (107) examined the effect of low-potassium diet on Na,K-ATPase from various segments of the rat nephron.

Potassium depletion produced a striking, time-dependent increase in Na,K-ATPase activity selectively in the inner stripe of outer medullary collecting tubules (MCTi.s.). After 3 weeks on a potassium-free diet, enzyme activity in MCTi.s. was over fourfold higher than in control animals. An even more impressive increment in Na,K-ATPase activity in this segment (sevenfold) after 5 weeks of potassium depletion was subsequently reported by Imbert-Teboul et al. (117); in both studies the increase in enzyme activity exceeded by a substantial margin that in tubular volume (117) or protein content (107), indicating that it is not merely a reflection of the concomitant hypertrophy observed in this region of the nephron. Na,K-ATPase activity returned to baseline after 7 days of potassium repletion (107). The induction of Na,K-ATPase synthesis by K depletion is observed in adrenal intact as well as adrenalectomized rats

(184) and is not prevented by thyroidectomy (220). Although both of these hormonal ablative interventions diminish the absolute quantitative increase, relative changes continue to occur unaffected by the absence of the trophic hormones. The increase in enzyme activity (and the structural hypertrophic changes) in the collecting duct of adrenalectomized rats can be partially attenuated by administration of angiotensin converting enzyme inhibitors, suggesting a role for the hyperreninemia of K depletion in the development of the morphologic and enzymatic changes (180) in addition to its contributions to hemodynamic alterations.

At the level of the thick ascending limb, an apparent paradox emerges. NaCl reabsorption along the loop of Henle is reduced in K-depleted rats, yet K depletion is known to induce an upregulation of Na,K-ATPase in most tissues including the thick ascending limbs of the loop of Henle. This was examined by Buffin-Meyer et al. (39). Within 2 weeks of K depletion, Na,K-ATPase activity and [^{3}H]-ouabain binding were increased by 30% to 50% in the medullary portion of the thick ascending limb (MTAL). Despite this increase in the number of Na,K-ATPase units, the transport capacity of the Na-K pump, determined by ouabain-sensitive Rb$^+$ uptake was reduced in MTAL from K depleted rats. Inhibition of the Na-K pump was not accounted for by changes in either extracellular K or intracellular Na concentrations, but by a decrease in the pump affinity for Na (39).

Because MCTi.s. plays an important role in potassium reabsorption and the maximum increment in pump activity coincided with the virtual elimination of potassium from the urine, it has been postulated that the enhanced Na,K-ATPase activity may be involved in potassium reabsorption, which predicates its location in the luminal membrane. Further supporting this hypothesis, the binding of [^{3}H]-ouabain to intact tubules, which reflects the number of enzyme units in the basolateral membrane, was similar in potassium-depleted and control animals. By contrast, when tubules were permeabilized by hypotonic lysis and freeze-thawing, there was an increase in ouabain binding in potassium-depleted tubules that roughly paralleled that in Na,K-ATPase activity. As this procedure exposes pump units otherwise inaccessible in intact cells, the results suggest that these additional pumps were located either intracellularly or on the luminal membrane, where they could be involved in potassium reabsorption.

The hypothesis that the increased number of Na-K pumps in potassium-depleted animals may be involved in potassium reabsorption was further tested in renal function experiments (107). The authors compared the response to ouabain of isolated perfused kidneys from 3-week potassium-depleted and control rats, based on the assumption that if the increased Na,K-ATPase activity in the former group represents even in part a potassium-absorptive pump, ouabain ought to increase potassium excretion. This prediction was indeed confirmed, as ouabain increased potassium excretion by potassium-depleted kidneys at each concentration of potassium in the perfusate.

The combined results of the studies summarized above suggest the operation of a ouabain-sensitive, potassium-absorptive pump in the medullary collecting tubule of potassium-depleted rats. While the concept of a luminal Na-K pump seems at odds with the prevailing view on the location of Na,K-ATPase predominantly in the basolateral membrane, it has been proposed before to explain potassium absorption by another epithelium: Husted and Steinmetz (116) described a potassium-absorptive pump at the luminal membrane of the turtle urinary bladder that was inhibited by removal of sodium or by mucosal (but not serosal) ouabain; that is, it displayed the characteristics of a Na,K-ATPase. Apical localization of Na,K-ATPase has also been demonstrated in pathologic models, namely, ischemic renal injury (175). If the enzyme in the MCT were only in the basolateral membrane, it is hard to visualize why it would increase so strikingly during potassium depletion and how this could promote maximal potassium conservation; rather, such an event would probably enhance potassium secretion and therefore be maladaptive. In an attempt to explain this paradox Buffin-Meyer et al. (40) suggested that the marked increase in Na,K-ATPase in the MCT (which they located at the basolateral membrane) promotes enhanced *sodium* reabsorption in this segment, although no data were provided. The authors further hypothesized that the increased urinary potassium excretion that would of necessity occur in this model is prevented by K recycling across the basolateral membrane. Clearly, a satisfactory understanding of this intriguing adaptation will require further study.

Regulation of Na,K-ATPase in K Depletion The alterations in Na,K-ATPase in K depletion are not limited to increased expression, but also extend to the response of the enzyme to regulatory hormones.

Aldosterone resistance, defined as absent kaliuretic response to exogenous hormone, has been described in K depletion. It is not clear whether the absent kaliuresis is due to activation of K-conserving mechanisms or to failure of activation of the Na-K pump in cortical collecting tubules (CCT) by mineralocorticoids. Mujais et al. (184) examined the response to aldosterone in adrenalectomized male Sprague-Dawley rats allocated to either a normal or a low-K diet. Na-K pump activity in microdissected CCT and medullary collecting tubules (MCT, inner stripe of the outer medulla) was determined at 7 or 21 days after allocation to the dietary groups before and after exogenous aldosterone. K depletion led to progressive hypertrophic changes in the CCT and MCT manifest in increased baseline Na-K pump activity. In both K repletion and short-term K depletion (7 days), aldosterone led to the expected increase in CCT Na-K pump activity. With long-term K depletion, however, the CCT Na-K pump response to aldosterone was blunted. In the MCT, where under normal conditions the Na-K pump is aldosterone unresponsive, an increasingly aberrant responsiveness to the mineralocorticoid was observed with progressive K depletion. These results suggest that apparent aldosterone resistance in short-term K depletion is likely due to activation of K-conserving mechanisms with early preservation of the CCT biochemical response to the hormone. With long-term K depletion, a blunted biochemical response to aldosterone may contribute to the absent kaliuretic response. In the MCT, K depletion led to the development of aberrant responsiveness to aldosterone.

Resistance to the hydrosmotic effects of vasopressin has been described in K depletion, but it was not clear whether other effects of vasopressin, notably its effects on the Na-K pump in the collecting duct, were similarly affected. In adrenalectomized Sprague-Dawley rats allocated to either a normal K (NK) or low-K (LK) diet, Mujais et al. (185) measured Na-K pump activity in cortical collecting duct (CCD) and medullary collecting duct (MCD) 21 days after allocation to the dietary groups before and after exogenous vasopressin. In animals on NK diet, vasopressin (AVP) led to a doubling of Na-K pump activity in the CCD. In K-depleted animals, which had a higher baseline Na-K pump activity, an increase was also observed, but this increase was quantitatively less than in K-replete rats. The findings in the MCD were similar; in rats on a NK diet, vasopressin led to a significant increase in Na-K pump activity. With K depletion, this directional change was preserved, but was quantitatively smaller than in K-replete rats.

Potassium-Stimulated ATPases It has also been proposed that potassium reabsorption in the distal nephron may be mediated by a ouabain-insensitive, potassium-stimulated ATPase, similar to, or identical with, the H,K-ATPase responsible for the coupled countertransport of these two ions in gastric mucosa (63, 89, 281). This concept is based on both morphologic and functional measurements in collecting tubules of potassium-depleted animals.

Morphologic studies, reviewed in preceding sections of this chapter, consistently demonstrated a marked hypertrophy of the medullary collecting tubule of potassium-deficient animals, especially in the inner stripe (70, 104, 247, 260). Cell growth was prominent in intercalated (dark) cells (70, 104, 260) and was characterized by striking enlargement of luminal microplicae (104) and boundary length of the luminal membrane, whereas the basolateral membrane was unaffected (247). These cells display rod-shaped particles (studs) on the cytoplasmic aspect of the luminal membrane that increase in number in potassium-deficient animals at the expense of similar particles present on subapical vesicles, presumably due to the fusion of the latter with the plasmalemma (247). Such studies have led naturally to the suggestion that intercalated cells are responsible for potassium reabsorption in the MCT, and to intriguing questions—still unsolved—about the nature of the rod-shaped particles on their apical membrane.

Profile of H,K-ATPase Along the Nephron H,K-ATPase is present along the entire length of the collecting duct from the early connecting tubule to the inner medullary collecting duct (9, 64, 66, 89, 121, 184, 185, 220). In control rats on a normal K diet, we identified H,K-ATPase activity throughout the collecting duct with a hierarchy of CNT>CCT>MCT (Fig. 9) (181). This hierarchy of enzyme activity *under baseline conditions* is similar to that observed for other transport ATPases such as Na,K-ATPase (184, 185) and NEM-sensitive ATPase (H-ATPase) (178). The activity of H,K-ATPase is quantitatively similar to that of H-ATPase (178), and both enzymes display a much lower activity than Na,K-ATPase (Fig. 9). This profile has been amply documented in studies showing both HK1 (gastric) and HK2 (colonic) isoforms of the enzyme with overlapping segmental distribution along the collecting duct (9, 66, 67). This hierarchical distribution implies that a *kaliferic* (potassium conserving) transporter shares its locale with *kaliuretic* processes. Indeed the highest activity of the K-*conserving* ATPase is in segments traditionally thought to be major sites of K *secretion*.

This segmental distribution may appear counterintuitive in view of the traditional concept of K conservation being a medullary function. This disquieting observation is further magnified by the profile during K depletion. In our studies chronic K depletion (3 weeks) led to a generalized increase in H,K-ATPase activity, with the greater increments occurring in segments of higher basal activity, CNT>CCT>MCT (Fig. 10). This is in contrast to the morphologic changes that occur in the collecting duct with K depletion which display a hypertrophic response with the hierarchy: MCT>CCT>CNT (107, 178, 184, 185), and is also divergent from the changes observed in other transport ATPases with K depletion such as Na,K-ATPase and H-ATPase which follow in their directional changes the morphologic alterations (180–185). Such a pattern may appear incongruous if one considers that active K conservation is predominantly a function of the medullary segments of the collecting duct. It should be remembered, however, that a dominant aspect of K conservation is attenuation of K secretion (177). As such, teleological reasoning would allow that the enhancement of H,K-ATPase activity in the cortical segments may contribute to K conservation by attenuating the net effect of K secretion in those segments.

The possibility that different isoforms may behave differently under inducing conditions is familiar in the ATPases area. While the concept has not been successfully validated for Na,K-ATPase because in renal tubules the α_1 isoform is overwhelmingly predominant, some findings with H,K-ATPase are intriguing (7–9, 121). Ahn et al. (7, 8) using in situ hybridization and competitive poly-

merase chain reaction found modest enhancement of the gastric isoform (HKα1) with potassium depletion that was confined to cortical segments, whereas HKα2 was more abundant after K depletion in the medullary portions of the collecting duct. Such differential induction has been reported by others (Table 10), except for Marsy et al. (168) who reported a uniform induction of HKα2 in both cortical and medullary segments of the collecting duct. These findings would imply that enzymatic measurements in tubular segments reflect predominantly the gastric isoform, and that the increase in the colonic isoform follows the general pattern of medullary $>>$ cortical hypertrophy observed in K depletion (177). Such an increase in HKα2 can not be considered adaptive as the hyperplastic/hypertrophic response of the collecting duct in K depletion is generalized (177). The medullary collecting duct undergoes dysregulated growth in K depletion with generalized increase in all transport ATPases (180–185). Whether these changes are functionally significant or simply nonspecific remains to be determined.

Effects of H,K-ATPase inhibitors The role of the transporter can be defined either by examination of adaptive changes in response to inducing conditions (acidosis or potassium depletion, see subsequent sections) or by examining the consequences of inhibition of baseline activity. In control rats on a normal K diet, chronic administration of vanadate (an inhibitor of some ATPases) inhibited H,K-ATPase activity in all segments of the collecting duct (Fig. 11) without the development of K wasting. Vanadate administration with potassium depletion obliterated the increment in H,K-ATPase activity expected with potassium deficiency (Fig. 10) without, however, impairing K conservation. Vanadate had no effect on H-ATPase activity along the collecting duct (Fig. 12), but did lead to a major inhibition of Na,K-ATPase activity in these nephron segments (Fig. 13).

In control rats on a normal K diet, chronic administration of Sch 28080 (a purported specific inhibitor of H,K-ATPase) inhibited H,K-ATPase activity in all segments of the collecting duct (Fig. 11). Sch 28080 had no effect on H-ATPase activity along the collecting duct (Fig. 12), but did lead to a major inhibition of Na,K-ATPase activity at these nephron segments (Fig. 13), a finding not previously recognized based on in vitro work. These observations imply that the consequences of the use of these inhibitors in vivo are not specific to the target transporter since simultaneous inhibition of Na,K-ATPase can alter K and H ion handling in the collecting duct.

TABLE 10 Profile of H,K-ATPase Isoform Induction by K Depletion

Investigator (Ref)	Species	Isoform	Location
Ahn et al. (9)	Rat	HKα1	Cortical
Ahn et al. (8)	Rat	HKα2	Medullary
Marsy et al. (168)	Rat	HKα2	Cortical and medullary

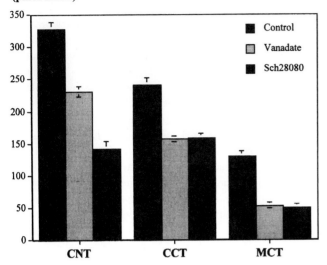

H-K-ATPase
(pmol/mm/h)

FIGURE 11 In control rats on a normal-potassium diet, chronic administration of vanadate and Sch 28080 inhibited H,K-ATPase activity in all segments of the collecting duct. (From Mujais SK. Transport enzymes and renal tubular acidosis. *Semin Nephrol* 1998;18:74–82, with permission.)

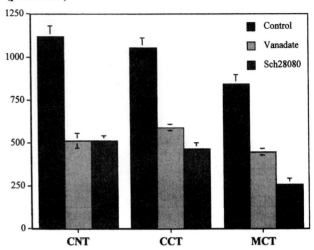

Na-K-ATPase
(pmol/mm/h)

FIGURE 13 In control rats on a normal-potassium diet, chronic administration of vanadate and Sch 28080 led to a major inhibition of Na-K-ATPase activity along the collecting duct. (From Mujais SK. Transport enzymes and renal tubular acidosis. *Semin Nephrol* 1998;18:74–82, with permission.)

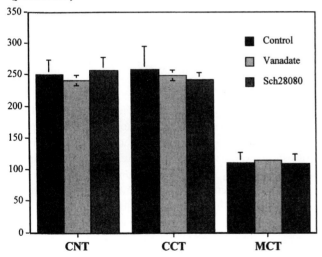

H-ATPase
(pmol/mm/h)

FIGURE 12 In control rats on a normal-potassium diet, chronic administration of vanadate and Sch 28080 had no effect on H-ATPase activity along the collecting duct. (From Mujais SK. Transport enzymes and renal tubular acidosis. *Semin Nephrol* 1998;18:74–82, with permission.)

Role of H,K-ATPase in K Conservation Biochemical and transport studies have implicated H,K-ATPase in K-reabsorptive activity and H+ secretion in the collecting tubule (282, 283). The enzyme is presumed to play a K-conserving role, hence its activity is expected to adapt to K balance. This postulate, however, should not be construed to imply that K conservation is of necessity dependent on such an adaptive

change in enzyme activity, for two main reasons: First, the role of the adaptive increase in enzyme activity has not been shown in vivo or at the level of overall renal K handling to be determinative of K or H balance; and second, one should always evaluate critically enzymatic changes in the collecting duct in K deprivation because of the striking hypertrophic response observed in this segment (177). If a defect in H,K-ATPase is to produce a hypokalemic RTA, then the enzyme must be crucial to K conservation and inhibition of the enzyme should impair homeostatic response to K depletion.

In the rat, K conservation develops rapidly (Fig. 14) and before any observable changes in H,K-ATPase activity are observed (Fig. 15). We observed the attainment of the lowest urinary K excretion in the absence of any measurable changes in enzyme activity. Inhibition of the enzyme with either vanadate or Sch 28080 does not lead to potassium wasting in normal rats, nor does it lead to impairment of potassium conservation during potassium depletion when the inhibitors are given before initiation of the KD diet and concurrently with it (Fig. 14). The profile of potassium conservation was identical whether the rats received either inhibitor or were left untreated showing a similar time course for the achievement of minimal potassium excretion and similar steady-state plasma and urinary potassium. Results with inhibitor studies, however, must be interpreted with caution as these inhibitors when given in vivo may not be specific and indeed both vanadate and Sch 28080 in our hands also inhibited Na,K-ATPase, perhaps reflecting the extensive homology of the two transporters. This latter effect would attenuate K secretory mechanisms and possibly balance the loss of a kaliferic role of H,K-ATPase.

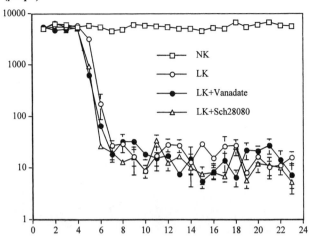

Urinary K excretion (μEq/d)

NK
LK
LK+Vanadate
LK+Sch28080

FIGURE 14 Institution of a low-potassium diet (on the 5th day of metabolic balance studies) in the rat was followed by a rapid development of K conservation that reached steady state by the third day on the low-potassium diet. Chronic administration of vanadate or Sch 28080 had no effect on this adaptive pattern (*n* = 10–12 for each group). (From Mujais SK. Transport enzymes and renal tubular acidosis. *Semin Nephrol* 1998;18: 74–82, with permission.)

A low basal activity of H,K-ATPase such as in hypothyroidism (220) does not impair K conservation even though the enzyme level is much lower than euthryroid animals. There is reason to believe that the role assigned to H,K-ATPase in the K conservation of K depletion has been exag-

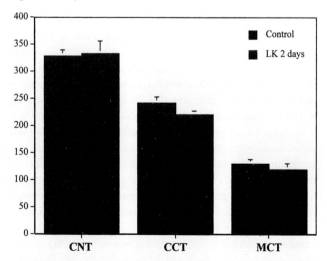

H-K-ATPase (pmol/mm/h)

Control
LK 2 days

CNT   CCT   MCT

FIGURE 15 Potassium conservation with the institution of a low-potassium (LK) diet develops without any measurable changes in the activity of H,K-ATPase in the collecting duct (*n* = 8 for each diet). (From Mujais SK. Transport enzymes and renal tubular acidosis. *Semin Nephrol* 1998;18:74–82, with permission.)

gerated at the expense of the role played by other renal changes that contribute to K conservation.

H-ATPases H-ATPase has been identified in various segments of the mammalian nephron by a variety of methods. Its activity in the collecting duct appears to be the highest and it is at this site that it manifests adaptive changes in response to altered electrolytes, hormonal and acid-base conditions (23). The effects of dietary potassium depletion on the activity and distribution of the H-ATPase in the distal nephron of the Sprague-Dawley rat and H-ATPase activity were assessed by Bailey et al. (18). Dietary potassium depletion increased electrogenic H-ATPase activity in the rat distal tubule that was associated with increased insertion of pumps into the apical membrane (19). These findings were confirmed and expanded by Silver et al. (237). The rate of pH(i) recovery in intercalated cells (ICs) in response to an acute acid load, a measure of plasma membrane H-ATPase activity, was increased after K-depletion to almost three times that of controls. This was associated with a change in the distribution of membrane-bound proton pumps in the IC population of cortical collecting duct from potassium-depleted rats. Immunocytochemical analysis of collecting ducts from control and K-depleted rats showed that potassium depletion increased the number of ICs with tight apical H-ATPase staining and decreased the number of cells with diffuse or basolateral H-ATPase staining. Taken together, these data indicate that chronic potassium depletion induces a marked increase in plasma membrane H-ATPase activity in individual ICs (237).

Renal Potassium Conservation

CHARACTERISTICS

Dietary potassium restriction results in a decrease in urinary potassium excretion of variable magnitude depending on the species. In all species, however, the decline in potassium excretion does not match the reduced intake and a persistently negative potassium balance is observed. In humans subjected to short-term dietary potassium deprivation (intake less than 1 mEq/day), urinary potassium excretion declines but never approaches intake (177), the adaptation being gradual and not reaching a maximum until 5 to 7 days (Fig. 16). With less stringent dietary restriction (potassium intake of 10–15 mEq/day), potassium conservation does not become maximal until 10 to 14 days (177). Similarly, when a negative potassium balance is induced by the administration of potassium binding resins, renal excretion diminishes but continues to contribute to the negative potassium balance (177). The slow onset of potassium conservation manifested during persistent renal and fecal losses results in a progressive negative potassium balance.

The efficiency of potassium conservation appears to be greater in other species. In the rat subjected to dietary potassium deprivation, urinary potassium excretion falls promptly and parallels intake by 72 to 96 hours after institution of

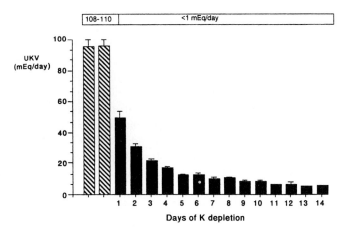

FIGURE 16 Potassium balance in humans. (From Mujais SK. Transport enzymes and renal tubular acidosis. *Semin Nephrol* 1998;18:74–82, with permission.)

potassium-deficient diet (157). This more efficient adaptation does not develop, however, until tissue depletion of potassium has occurred (157). Hayashi and Katz (107) reported that after 3 days of potassium deprivation rats excreted 5% of the prediet daily urinary potassium, and after 3 weeks only about 1%, but the urine never became totally potassium-free.

The conservation of potassium can be conceived as being due to attenuation of kaliuretic mechanisms, in part by resistance to normally kaliuretic influences, and in part by activation of kaliferic ones. Both phenomena need to be examined in the context of the renal and systemic changes that occur with potassium depletion, considering the likelihood that factors of major importance early in potassium deficiency may be supplemented or supplanted by alterations developing during prolonged potassium depletion.

MECHANISMS

Potassium secretion in the CCT is markedly attenuated but may not cease even with profound degrees of potassium depletion (164, 282). The reduced level of potassium secretion is accompanied by a decrease in the responsiveness to established kaliuretic factors. Malnic et al. (164) have shown that potassium-depleted rats maintain their ability to increase potassium secretion in response to increments in tubular flow, albeit at a much diminished level. Linas et al. (157) have also demonstrated that the response to increased distal delivery of sodium by infusion of sodium chloride or sodium sulfate is attenuated, but not abolished. Similar findings have been observed in the isolated perfused kidney of potassium-depleted rats, indicating the intrinsic renal character of this adaptive mechanism, which persists in the absence of systemic influences (202, 255). Ornt (200) has shown that isolated perfused kidneys from potassium-depleted rats displayed an attenuated kaliuretic response to increased perfusate potassium concentration, and Tannen and Gerrits (255) observed a diminished kaliuresis in iso-

lated perfused kidneys from potassium-depleted rats when the perfusate was alkalinized or upon the addition of sodium sulfate. Finally, potassium-depleted humans seem to be resistant to the kaliuretic influence of water and osmotic diuresis, and of metabolic alkalosis (177).

It has been suggested that an "escape" from kaliuretic influences may occur in states of potassium depletion, a concept analogous to that of escape from the sodium-retaining effects of chronic mineralocorticoid administration. Thus no kaliuretic response is observed in rats when DOCA is administered 72 hours after initiation of potassium depletion (157). In contrast, resistance to the kaliuretic effects of mineralocorticoids does not develop in short-term (7–10 days) potassium-depleted humans (177), in whom administration of DOCA is associated with a kaliuresis despite the presence of hypokalemia and a large negative potassium balance (177).

The decline in aldosterone levels that accompanies potassium depletion contributes to renal potassium conservation. When mineralocorticoid activity is maintained constant early in potassium depletion by exogenous administration, a more profound negative potassium balance is observed (157). Moreover, adrenalectomized rats on fixed aldosterone replacement achieve maximal potassium conservation after a time interval that is directly proportional to the level of aldosterone replacement: the lower the ambient aldosterone level the shorter the time to maximal conservation and the lesser the negative potassium balance (201).

Studies in experimental animals and humans have suggested that increased urinary ammonium excretion accompanying increased ammonia production reduces potassium excretion, hence the proposed role for increased ammonia production in potassium conservation (120, 226, 257). Jaeger et al. (120) observed a decrease in absolute and fractional urinary potassium excretion after primary stimulation of ammonium excretion by acute glutamine loading. The decline in potassium excretion appears to be due to enhanced potassium reabsorption beyond the late distal tubule, because fractional potassium delivery to this site was unchanged. Sastrasinh and Tannen (226) have shown that this potassium-sparing effect of glutamine administration is directly related to the increase in urinary ammonium excretion and not to changes in renal ammonia production: when ammonium excretion following glutamine was curtailed by urinary alkalinization, the attenuating effect of glutamine loading on potassium excretion was markedly reduced. Since enhanced hydrogen ion secretion plays a role in the potassium-sparing effect of glutamine, it could be hypothesized that alkalinization of collecting duct fluid by increased ammonia delivery would facilitate hydrogen ion secretion. If the latter process were mediated by H,K-ATPase, the augmented hydrogen ion secretion might be coupled to enhanced potassium reabsorption.

The previous observations of enhanced renal potassium conservation with primary augmentation of ammoniagenesis have provided the background for the suggestion that the increased ammoniagenesis of potassium depletion contributes to the activation of kaliferic processes. Examination of the temporal profile of the two phenomena, however, shows a clear dissociation between the early decrease in urinary potassium excretion that follows dietary restriction of potassium and the delayed increase in ammonia production and ammonium excretion (225). In fact, potassium excretion reaches its nadir prior to any substantial increase in renal ammoniagenesis. This temporal dissociation suggests that renal ammonia production does not play a significant role in the early renal conservation of potassium, but does not exclude the possibility that increased ammoniagenesis contributes to potassium conservation during the chronic phase of potassium depletion.

Miscellaneous

MITOCHONDRIAL ENERGY PRODUCTION

Defective transport function in the TAL looms as an important central abnormality in potassium depletion. It likely contributes to the impaired urinary concentrating ability, hyperreninemia, and hyperchloruria of the kaliopenic kidney in some species. Defective Na-K pump activity may contribute to the defective transport at this nephron site. A reduced number of Na-K pumps, a regulatory abnormality of pump in situ turnover rate, or a reduced supply of energy substrate may all contribute to the observed abnormal Na-K pump function.

Impairment of renal medullary energy metabolism, involving oxidative processes that predominate as the energy supply of this region, has long been recognized in potassium depletion (130). Furthermore, in vitro studies show that 72-hour exposure of renal papillary cells in culture to potassium-free medium is associated with a decline in cellular ATP content (259).

Aithal et al. (10, 11) have examined the mechanism underlying the abnormal energy supply in renal mitochondria

isolated from potassium-deficient rats. Their studies show a dual defect in aerobic metabolism consisting of decreased electron flow through the mitochondrial respiratory chain and reduced oxidative phosphorylation. This dual perturbation was limited to the inner stripe of the outer medulla and seems to be related to the reduced mitochondrial potassium content as it is completely reversed by potassium repletion in vivo and in vitro. The in vivo reversibility of decreased mitochondrial ATP formation is reminiscent of the correction of the transport defect in TAL by potassium administration discussed previously. It appears likely therefore that a reduced supply of energy substrate underlies the defective sodium chloride absorption in TAL which initiates a cascade of secondary renal abnormalities.

DIVALENT CATION METABOLISM

The clinical syndromes of potassium deficiency can be associated with simultaneous alterations in divalent cation metabolism. These alterations are not necessarily due to potassium depletion per se, but may result from the convergence of pathophysiologic factors. The interrelatedness of these abnormalities is complex and requires multipronged interventions. To wit, magnesium supplementation alone in patients with Gitelman syndrome while significantly increasing plasma and intracellular magnesium and plasma calcium, fails to affect blood levels of parathyroid hormone and calcitriol and plasma and intracellular potassium (33) in some studies while succeeding in others (51). Further, magnesium supplementation can lead to normalization of the transtubular K concentration gradient in most patients with Gitelman (129). The lack of universal normalization suggests a degree of heterogeneity in the phenotype or a confounding effect of other variables such as chronicity of the hypomagnesemia. In diuretic-induced magnesium deficiency, magnesium repletion consistently improves the parallel hypokalemia (53).

The independent effects of potassium depletion can be ascertained only from experimental studies where potassium deficiency is the primary and only alteration induced. In such conditions, potassium depletion alters divalent cation metabolism in nonuniform fashion. Hypercalciuria is observed in rats (64) and humans (126) in the face of normocalcemia, suggesting impaired renal handling of calcium. This is readily understandable in view of the defect in NaCl absorption in the TAL, which aborts the favorable conditions for calcium reabsorption, a condition akin to the hypercalciuria produced by loop diuretics. Overall calcium balance as judged by tissue levels does not appear to be altered. This finding, however, should be evaluated in the context of impaired growth and reduced weight gain of potassium-deficient animals, as the stunted growth may be masking an abnormality in calcium balance.

Reciprocal changes in potassium and magnesium balance develop with potassium depletion. Hypermagnesemia, magnesuria, and a positive magnesium balance have been observed in rats subjected to dietary potassium depletion

(64). A decrement in tissue magnesium content was also observed. The net effect is an increase in total body magnesium with shift of the ion into the extracellular space. The hypermagnesemia is likely the cause of hypermagnesuria, although defective renal handling of the cation secondary to impaired loop transport as a contributing factor cannot be excluded. Additionally, changes at the level of the DCT cell may be operative. Dai et al. (58) have shown that Mg uptake was diminished in potassium depleted DCT cells. Hyperpolarization of the plasma membrane with the cell permeant anion, SCN^-, corrected Mg uptake in potassium depleted cells, suggesting that the basis for diminished uptake may, in part, be due to depolarization of the membrane voltage. Correction of hypermagnesemia by DOCA administration (64) is not conclusive evidence of aldosterone deficiency being responsible for impaired magnesium homeostasis, because the mineralocorticoid in that study was administered in large doses.

SUSCEPTIBILITY TO NEPHROTOXIC AND ISCHEMIC INJURY

Potassium depletion markedly enhances the nephrotoxicity of gentamicin in several species (37, 137). Renal impairment is observed earlier than in potassium-replete animals and is of greater severity (37,137). The mechanism by which potassium depletion enhances the susceptibility of the kidney to gentamicin-induced injury is unknown. It is possible that the renal hemodynamic and hormonal changes observed with potassium depletion may be contributory. Reduction in renal blood flow, increased thromboxane B2 production (137) and decreased PGE2 synthesis may each contribute to this enhanced susceptibility. Captopril appears to enhance aminoglycoside nephrotoxicity in part because of kinin-stimulated renal thromboxane B2 production (137). Aminoglycosides are also capable of inducing reversible tubular damage in the absence of any change in the renal function, such as a hypokalemic metabolic alkalosis associated with hypomagnesemia (13).

Hypokalemia and potassium depletion are frequent complications of amphotericin B therapy. As in the case of gentamicin-induced renal failure, amphotericin B nephrotoxicity is potentiated by potassium depletion (32). Potassium depletion, however, does not influence the acute renovascular effects of amphotericin B but potentiates its tubular toxicity. While selective distal tubular epithelial toxicity seems to be responsible for the profound potassium wasting observed with amphotericin administration, this does not preclude maintained responsiveness to kaliferic interventions. Ural et al. (265) have recently shown that administration of spironolactone concomitantly with amphotericin resulted in higher plasma potassium levels and lower requirements for supplementations to maintain plasma potassium within normal limits.

Hypokalemia and hypomagnesemia are frequently encountered in patients with acquired immunodeficiency syndrome (AIDS). The antiretroviral drugs zidovudine (AZT) and didanosine (ddI) are widely used in these patients and data suggest that the presence of potassium depletion may uncover untoward renal consequences. In hypokalemic rats, both drugs produce a decrease in GFR and in renal blood flow consequent to renal vasoconstriction and associated with alterations in tubular function (characterized by an increased fractional excretion of sodium). Hypomagnesemia induced a decrease in glomerular filtration rate and in renal blood flow only in AZT-treated rats. Hypokalemia appears to predispose to AZT and ddI nephrotoxicity, while hypomagnesemia predisposes only to AZT nephrotoxicity. Thus, chronic AZT and ddI administration may produce acute renal failure in patients with AIDS with hypokalemia and/or hypomagnesemia (231). Similarly, Seguro et al. (232) have shown that potassium depletion also enhances the tubular damage from ischemic insults. It is clear from this variety of studies that potassium depletion causes a general predisposition to greater renal injury.

TREATMENT OF CLINICAL POTASSIUM DEFICIENCY: GENERAL PRINCIPLES

The treatment of potassium deficiency should address interruption or attenuation of kaliuretic mechanisms and correction of the potassium deficit. Attention to both components is crucial because simple supplementation may be only partially effective in conditions other than dietary deficiency. The limited success of supplementation alone in primary aldosteronism, for example, is related to the fact that this modality reinforces already operative kaliuretic mechanisms and attenuates kaliferic processes: By increasing plasma potassium, supplementation will favor potassium secretion and reduce potassium reabsorption in the collecting duct. Attention to the mechanisms operative in the individual patient will result in greater therapeutic success at a lower cost. It is the delay in recognizing the persistence of kaliuretic mechanisms that often leads to frustrating instances where potassium supplementation alone fails.

Attenuation of kaliuretic mechanisms needs to be addressed in the context of their etiology. Reversal of the initiating event is an obvious recommendation for nonrenal mechanisms. In nephrogenic potassium depletion attention to factors that promote kaliuresis is paramount (e.g., high-salt intake in a patient receiving diuretics). Pharmacologic interventions such as provision of potassium-sparing agents (amiloride, triamterene) may be useful temporizing measures if the disease is potentially amenable to cure (primary aldosteronism due to an adrenal adenoma) or may serve as chronic therapy directed at the specific etiology (Liddle syndrome) or when cure is not readily achievable (bilateral adrenal hyperplasia). In some conditions such as Bartter syndrome, additive modalities need to be used (potassium supplementation, indomethacin, converting enzyme inhibitors, etc.) and even then success is limited. In even the most difficult cases, however, a systematic attempt at understanding the causes of potassium loss as the basis on which to devise a rational intervention will reduce waste and undesirable side effects while ensuring a reasonable modicum of success.

References

1. Abbrecht PH. Effects of potassium deficiency on renal function in the dog. *J Clin Invest* 1969;48:432–442.
2. Abbrecht PH. Cardiovascular effects of chronic potassium deficiency in the dog. *Am J Physiol* 1972;223:555–560.
3. Abdel-Rahman EM, Moorthy AV. End-stage renal disease (ESRD) in patients with eating disorders. *Clin Nephrol* 1997;47:106–111.
4. Abraham MR, Jahangir A, et al. Channelopathies of inwardly rectifying potassium channels. *FASEB J* 1999;13:1901–1910.
5. Agnoli GC, Borgatti R, et al. Effects of experimental potassium depletion on renal function and urinary prostanoid excretion in normal women during hypotonic polyuria. *Clin Physiol* 1990;10:345–362.
6. Agnoli GC, Borgatti R, et al. Effects of angiotensin-converting enzyme inhibition on renal dysfunction induced by moderate potassium depletion in healthy women. *Clin Physiol* 1994; 14:205–222.
7. Ahn KY, Kone BC. Expression and cellular localization of mRNA encoding the gastric isoform of H(+)-K(+)-ATPase alpha-subunit in rat kidney. *Am J Physiol* 1995;268(Pt 2): F99–109.
8. Ahn KY, Park KY, et al. Chronic hypokalemia enhances expression of the H(+)-K(+)-ATPase alpha 2-subunit gene in renal medulla. *Am J Physiol* 1996;271(Pt 2):F314–321.
9. Ahn KY, Turner PB, et al. Effects of chronic hypokalemia on renal expression of the gastric H(+)-K(+)-ATPase alpha-subunit gene. *Am J Physiol* 1996;270(Pt 2):F557–566.
10. Aithal HN, Toback FG. Defective mitochondrial energy production during potassium depletion nephropathy. *Lab Invest* 1998;39:186–192.
11. Aithal HN, Toback FG, et al. Formation of renal medullary lysosomes during potassium depletion nephropathy. *Lab Invest* 1977;36:107–113.
12. Aithal HN, Toback FG, et al. Functional defects in mitochondria of renal inner red medulla during potassium depletion nephropathy. *Lab Invest* 1977;37:423–429.
13. Alexandridis G, Liberopoulos E, et al. Aminoglycoside-induced reversible tubular dysfunction. *Pharmacology* 2003;67:118–120.
14. Alpern RJ, Cogan MG, et al. Effect of luminal bicarbonate concentration on proximal acidification in the rat. *Am J Physiol* 1982;243:F53–59.
15. Amlal H, Wang Z, et al. Potassium depletion downregulates chloride-absorbing transporters in rat kidney. *J Clin Invest* 1998;101:1045–1054.
16. Backman KA, Hayslett JP. Role of the medullary collecting duct in potassium conservation. *Pflugers Arch* 1983;396:297–300.
17. Bahler RC, Rakita L. Cardiovascular function in potassium-depleted dogs. *Am Heart J* 1971; 81:650–657.
18. Bailey M, Capasso G, et al. The relationship between distal tubular proton secretion and dietary potassium depletion: evidence for up-regulation of H+ -ATPase. *Nephrol Dial Transplant* 1999;14:1435–1440.
19. Bailey MA, Fletcher RM, et al. Upregulation of H+-ATPase in the distal nephron during potassium depletion: structural and functional evidence. *Am J Physiol* 1998;275(Pt 2):F878–884.
20. Barbry P, Hofman P. Molecular biology of Na+ absorption. *Am J Physiol* 1997;273(Pt 1): G571–585.
21. Barri YM, Wingo CS. The effects of potassium depletion and supplementation on blood pressure: a clinical review. *Am J Med Sci* 1997;314:37–40.
22. Bartter FC, Pronove P, et al. Hyperplasia of the juxtaglomerular complex with hyperaldosteronism and hypokalemic alkalosis. A new syndrome. *J Am Soc Nephrol* 1998;9:516–528.
23. Bastani B. Immunocytochemical localization of the vacuolar H(+)-ATPase pump in the kidney. *Histol Histopathol* 1997;12:769–779.
24. Beck FB, Dorge A, et al. Element concentrations of renal and hepatic cells under potassium depletion. *Kidney Int* 1982;22:250–256.
25. Beck FX, Muller E, et al. Inner-medullary organic osmolytes and inorganic electrolytes in K depletion. *Pflugers Arch* 2000;439:471–476.
26. Beck N, Davis BB. Impaired renal response to parathyroid hormone in potassium depletion. *Am J Physiol* 1975;228:179–183.
27. Beck N, Shaw JO. Thromboxane B2 and prostaglandin E2 in the K+-depleted rat kidney. *Am J Physiol* 1981;240:F151–157.
28. Beck N, Webster SK. Impaired urinary concentrating ability and cyclic AMP in K+-depleted rat kidney. *Am J Physiol* 1976;231:1204–1208.
29. Benedetti RG, Linas SL. Effect of potassium depletion on two-kidney, one-clip renovascular hypertension in the rat. *Kidney Int* 1985;28:621–628.
30. Berl T, Aisenbrey GA, et al. Renal concentrating defect in the hypokalemic rat is prostaglandin independent. *Am J Physiol* 1980;238:F37–41.
31. Berl T, Linas SL, et al. On the mechanism of polyuria in potassium depletion. The role of polydipsia. *J Clin Invest* 1977;60:620–625.
32. Bernardo JF, Murakami S, et al. Potassium depletion potentiates amphotericin-B-induced toxicity to renal tubules. *Nephron* 1995;70:235–241.
33. Bettinelli A, Basilico E, et al. Magnesium supplementation in Gitelman syndrome. *Pediatr Nephrol* 1999;13:311–314.
34. Bettinelli A, Vezzoli G, et al. Genotype-phenotype correlations in normotensive patients with primary renal tubular hypokalemic metabolic alkalosis. *J Nephrol* 1998;11:61–69.
35. Biagi B, Kubota T, et al. Intracellular potentials in rabbit proximal tubules perfused in vitro. *Am J Physiol* 1981;240:F200–210.

36. Boyd JE, Palmore WP, et al. Role of potassium in the control of aldosterone secretion in the rat. *Endocrinology* 1971;88:556–565.
37. Brinker KR, Bulger RE, et al. Effect of potassium depletion on gentamicin nephrotoxicity. *J Lab Clin Med* 1981;98:292–301.
38. Bubien JK, Ismailov II, et al. Liddle's disease: abnormal regulation of amiloride-sensitive Na+ channels by beta-subunit mutation. *Am J Physiol* 1996;270(Pt 1):C208–213.
39. Buffin-Meyer B Marsy S, et al. Regulation of renal Na+,K(+)-ATPase in rat thick ascending limb during K+ depletion: evidence for modulation of Na+ affinity. *J Physiol* 1996;490 (Pt 3):623–632.
40. Buffin-Meyer B, Verbavatz JM, et al. Regulation of Na+, K(+)-ATPase in the rat outer medullary collecting duct during potassium depletion. *J Am Soc Nephrol* 1998;9:538–550.
41. Bundgaard H. Potassium depletion improves myocardial potassium uptake in vivo. *Am J Physiol Cell Physiol* 2004;287:C135–141.
42. Burns KD, Smith IB. Potassium depletion stimulates mRNA expression of proximal tubule AT1 angiotensin II receptors. *Nephron* 1998;78:73–81.
43. Campbell WB, Schmitz JM. Effect of alterations in dietary potassium on the pressor and steroidogenic effects of angiotensins II and III. *Endocrinology* 1978;103:2098–2104.
44. Capasso G, Jaeger P, et al. Renal bicarbonate reabsorption in the rat. II. Distal tubule load dependence and effect of hypokalemia. *J Clin Invest* 1987;80:409–414.
45. Capasso G, Kinne R, et al. Renal bicarbonate reabsorption in the rat, I: effects of hypokalemia and carbonic anhydrase. *J Clin Invest* 1986;78:1558–1567.
46. Cardinal J, Duchesneau D. Effect of potassium on proximal tubular function. *Am J Physiol* 1978;234:F381–385.
47. Carney S, Rayson B, et al. A study in vitro of the concentrating defect associated with hypokalaemia and hypercalcaemia. *Pflugers Arch* 1976;366:11–17.
48. Cemerikic D, Wilcox CS, et al. Intracellular potential and K+ activity in rat kidney proximal tubular cells in acidosis and K+ depletion. *J Membr Biol* 1982;69:159–165.
49. Chan YL, Biagi B, et al. Control mechanisms of bicarbonate transport across the rat proximal convoluted tubule. *Am J Physiol* 1982;242:F532–543.
50. Cho JT, Guay-Woodford LM. Heterozygous mutations of the gene for Kir 1.1 (ROMK) in antenatal Bartter syndrome presenting with transient hyperkalemia, evolving to a benign course. *J Korean Med Sci* 2003;18:65–68.
51. Cho YJ, Park GT, et al. Renal potassium wasting and hypocalciuria ameliorated with magnesium repletion in Gitelman's syndrome. *J Korean Med Sci* 1997;12:157–159.
52. Christensen JA, bader H, et al. The structure of the juxtaglomerular apparatus in Addison's disease, Bartter's syndrome, and in Conn's syndrome: a comparative, morphometric, light microscopic study on serial secions. *Virchows Arch A Pathol Anat Histol* 1976;370:103–112.
53. Cohen N, Alon I, et al. Metabolic and clinical effects of oral magnesium supplementation in furosemide-treated patients with severe congestive heart failure. *Clin Cardiol* 2000;23:433–436.
54. Cortesi C, Foglia PE, et al. Prevention of cardiac arrhythmias in pediatric patients with normotensive-hypokalemic tubulopathy. Current attitude among European pediatricians. *Pediatr Nephrol* 2003;18:729–730.
55. Coruzzi P, Brambilla L, et al. Potassium depletion and salt sensitivity in essential hypertension. *J Clin Endocrinol Metab* 2001;86:2857–2862.
56. Cremer W, Bock KD. Symptoms and course of chronic hypokalemic nephropathy in man. *Clin Nephrol* 1977;7:112–119.
57. Cronin RE, Nix KL, et al. Renal cortex ion composition and Na-K-ATPase activity in gentamicin nephrotoxicity. *Am J Physiol* 1982;242:F477–483.
58. Dai LJ, Friedman PA, et al. Cellular mechanisms of chlorothiazide and cellular potassium depletion on Mg2+ uptake in mouse distal convoluted tubule cells. *Kidney Int* 1997;51:1008–1017.
59. Danforth DN Jr, Orlando MM, et al. Renal changes in primary aldosteronism. *J Urol* 1977; 117:140–144.
60. de Araujo M, De BM, et al. Renal potassium handling in aging rats. *Kidney Blood Press Res* 1998;21:425–431.
61. Dies F, Lotspeich WD. Hexose monophosphate shunt in the kidney during acid-base and electrolyte imbalance. *Am J Physiol* 1967;212:61–71.
62. Diezi J, Michoud P, et al. Micropuncture study of electrolyte transport across papillary collecting duct of the rat. *Am J Physiol* 1973;224:623–634.
63. Doucet A, Marsy S. Characterization of K-ATPase activity in distal nephron: stimulation by potassium depletion. *Am J Physiol* 1987;253(Pt 2):F418–423.
64. Duarte CG. Magnesium metabolism in potassium-depleted rats. *Am J Physiol* 1978;234: F466–471.
65. Duarte CG, Chomety F, et al. Effect of amiloride, ouabain, and furosemide on distal tubular function in the rat. *Am J Physiol* 1971;221:632–640.
66. DuBose TD Jr, Codina J. H,K-ATPase. *Curr Opin Nephrol Hyperten* 1996;5:411–416.
67. DuBose TD Jr, Codina J, et al. Regulation of H(+)-K(+)-ATPase expression in kidney. *Am J Physiol* 1995;269(Pt 2):F500–507.
68. Dusing R, Gill JR Jr, et al. The role of prostaglandins in diabetes insipidus produced by desoxycorticosterone in the dog. *Endocrinology* 1982;110:644–649.
69. Eknoyan G, Martinez-Maldonado M, et al. Renal diluting capacity in the hypokalemic rat. *Am J Physiol* 1970;219:933–937.
70. Evan A, Huser J, et al. The effect of alterations in dietary potassium on collecting system morphology in the rat. *Lab Invest* 1980;42:668–675.
71. Findling JW, Raff H, et al. Liddle's syndrome: prospective genetic screening and suppressed aldosterone secretion in an extended kindred. *J Clin Endocrinol Metab* 1997;82: 1071–1074.
72. Finer G, Shalev H, et al. Transient neonatal hyperkalemia in the antenatal (ROMK defective) Bartter syndrome. *J Pediatr* 2003;142:318–323.
73. Fisher ER, Funckes AJ. Effects of potassium deficiency on experimental renovascular hypertension. *Lab Invest* 1967;16:539–549.
74. Foglia PE, Bettinelli A, et al. Cardiac work up in primary renal hypokalaemia-hypomagnesaemia (Gitelman syndrome). *Nephrol Dial Transplant* 2004;19:1398–1402.
75. Fordtran JS. Speculations on the pathogenesis of diarrhea. *Fed Proc* 1967;26:1405–1414.

76. Foster ES, Hayslett JP, et al. Mechanism of active potassium absorption and secretion in the rat colon. *Am J Physiol* 1984;246(Pt 1):G611–617.

77. Foster ES, Jones WJ, et al. Role of aldosterone and dietary potassium in potassium adaptation in the distal colon of the rat. *Gastroenterology* 1985;88(Pt 1):41–46.

78. Foster ES, Sandle GI, et al. Dietary potassium modulates active potassium absorption and secretion in rat distal colon. *Am J Physiol* 1986;251(Pt 1):G619–626.

79. Fraley DS, Adler S, et al. Relationship of phosphate-dependent glutaminase activity to ammonia excretion in potassium deficiency and acidosis. *Miner Electrolyte Metab* 1985;11:140–149.

80. France R, Gray ME, et al. Intracellular granules of the renal medulla in a case of potassium depletion due to renal potassium wasting. Electron microscopic comparison with renal medullary granules in the potassium-depleted rat. *Am J Pathol* 1978;91:299–312.

81. France R, Shelley WM, et al. Abnormal intracellular granules of the renal papilla in a child with potassium depletion (Bartter's syndrome) and renal tuberous sclerosis. *Johns Hopkins Med J* 1974;135:274–285.

82. Franse LV, Pahor M, et al. Hypokalemia associated with diuretic use and cardiovascular events in the Systolic Hypertension in the Elderly Program. *Hypertension* 2000;35:1025–1030.

83. Fryer JN, Burns KD, et al. Effect of potassium depletion on proximal tubule AT1 receptor localization in normal and remnant rat kidney. *Kidney Int* 2001;60:1792–1799.

84. Gadallah MF, Abreo K, et al. Liddle's syndrome, an underrecognized entity: a report of four cases, including the first report in black individuals. *Am J Kidney Dis* 1995;25:829–835.

85. Galvez OG, Bay WH, et al. The hemodynamic effects of potassium deficiency in the dog. *Circ Res* 1977;40Suppl 1:I11–16.

86. Gao PJ, Zhang KX, et al. Diagnosis of Liddle syndrome by genetic analysis of beta and gamma subunits of epithelial sodium channel-a report of five affected family members. *J Hypertens* 2001;19:885–889.

87. Garella S, Chang B, et al. Alterations of hydrogen ion homeostasis in pure potassium depletion: studies in rats and dogs during the recovery phase. *J Lab Clin Med* 1979;93:321–331.

88. Garella S, Chazan JA, et al. Saline-resistant metabolic alkalosis or chloride-wasting nephropathy. Report of four patients with severe potassium depletion. *Ann Intern Med* 1970;73:31–38.

89. Garg LC, Narang N. Ouabain-insensitive K-adenosine triphosphatase in distal nephron segments of the rabbit. *J Clin Invest* 1988;81:1204–1208.

90. Gill JR Jr, Bartter FC. Evidence for a prostaglandin-independent defect in chloride reabsorption in the loop of Henle as a proximal cause of Bartter's syncrome. *Am J Med* 1978;65:766–772.

91. Girard P, Brun-Pascaud M, et al. Selective dietary potassium depletion and acid-base equilibrium in the rat. *Clin Sci* 1985;68:301–309.

92. Girard P, Brun-Pascaud M, et al. Development of the respiratory compensation to progressive metabolic alkalosis resulting from potassium depletion in conscious rats. *Clin Sci* 1983;64:497–504.

93. Girard P, Polianski J, et al. Ventilatory adaptation to metabolic alkalosis in adult awake potassium restricted rats. *Respir Physiol* 1984;57:23–30.

94. Greenfeld D, Mickley D, et al. Hypokalemia in outpatients with eating disorders. *Am J Psychiatry* 1995;152:60–63.

95. Greger R. Cation selectivity of the isolated perfused cortical thick ascending limb of Henle's loop of rabbit kidney. *Pflugers Arch* 1981;390:30–37.

96. Gullner HG, Bartter FC. The role of urinary prostaglandin E and cyclic AMP in the polyuria of hypokalemia in rats. *Prostaglandins Med* 1980;4:13–19.

97. Gullner HG, Gill JR Jr, et al. Correction of increased sympathoadrenal activity in Bartter's syndrome by inhibition of prostaglandin synthesis. *J Clin Endocrinol Metab* 1980;50:857–861.

98. Gullner HG, Lake CR, et al. Hypokalemia stimulates plasma epinephrine and norepinephrine in the rat. *Arch Int Pharmacodyn Ther* 1982;260:78–82.

99. Gullner HG, West D, et al. Diabetes insipidus with renal resistance to vasopressin in the desoxycorticosterone-treated dog: a possible role for prostaglandins. *Ren Physiol* 1987;10:40–46.

100. Gustafson AB, Shear L, et al. Protein metabolism in vivo in kidney, liver, muscle, and heart of potassium-deficient rats. *J Lab Clin Med* 1973;82:287–296.

101. Gutsche HU, Peterson LN, et al. In vivo evidence of impaired solute transport by the thick ascending limb in potassium-depleted rats. *J Clin Invest* 1984;73:908–9016.

102. Halevy J, Budinger ME, et al. Role of aldosterone in the regulation of sodium and chloride transport in the distal colon of sodium-depleted rats. *Gastroenterology* 1981;291:1227–1233.

103. Halperin ML, Honrath U, et al. Effects of chronic hypokalaemia and adrenalectomy on potassium transport by the medullary collecting duct of the rat. *Clin Sci (Lond)* 1989;76:189–194.

104. Hansen GP, Tisher CC, et al. Response of the collecting duct to disturbances of acid-base and potassium balance. *Kidney Int* 1980;17:326–337.

105. Hansson JH, Nelson-Williams C, et al. Hypertension caused by a truncated epithelial sodium channel gamma subunit: genetic heterogeneity of Liddle syndrome. *Nat Genet* 1995;11:76–82.

106. Hansson JH, Schild L, et al. A de novo missense mutation of the beta subunit of the epithelial sodium channel causes hypertension and Liddle syndrome, identifying a proline-rich segment critical for regulation of channel activity. *Proc Natl Acad Sci U S A* 1995;92:11495–11499.

107. Hayashi M, Katz AI. The kidney in potassium depletion. I. Na+-K+-ATPase activity and [3H]ouabain binding in MCT. *Am J Physiol* 1987;252(Pt 2):F437–446.

108. Hayashi M, Katz AI. The kidney in potassium depletion. II. K+ handling by the isolated perfused rat kidney. *Am J Physiol* 1987;252(Pt 2):F447–452.

109. Hebert SC. Bartter syndrome. *Curr Opin Nephrol Hypertens* 2003;12:527–532.

110. Hernandez RE, Schambelan M, et al. Dietary NaCl determines severity of potassium depletion-induced metabolic alkalosis. *Kidney Int* 1987;31:1356–1367.

111. Himathongkam T, Dluhy RG, et al. Potassim-aldosterone-renin interrelationships. *J Clin Endocrinol Metab* 1975;41:153–159.

112. Hollenberg NK, Williams G, et al. The influence of potassium on the renal vasculature and the adrenal gland, and their responsiveness to angiotensin II in normal man. *Clin Sci Mol Med* 1975;49:527–534.

113. Hood VL, Dunn MJ. Urinary excretion of prostaglandin E2 and prostaglandin F2alpha in potassium-deficient rats. *Prostaglandins* 1978;15:273–280.

114. Huang L, Wei YY, et al. Alpha 2B-adrenergic receptors: immunolocalization and regulation by potassium depletion in rat kidney. *Am J Physiol* 1996;270(Pt 2):F1015–1026.

115. Hulter HN, Sebastian A, et al. Pathogenesis of renal hyperchloremic acidosis resulting from dietary potassium restriction in the dog: role of aldosterone. *Am J Physiol* 1980;238:F79–91.

116. Husted RF, Steinmetz PR. Potassium absorptive pump at the luminal membrane of turtle urinary bladder. *Am J Physiol* 1981;241:F315–321.

117. Imbert-Teboul M, Doucet A, et al. Alterations of enzymatic activities along rat collecting tubule in potassium depletion. *Am J Physiol* 1987;253(Pt 2):F408–417.

118. Ishikawa S, Saito T, et al. Role of potassium in vasopressin-induced production of cyclic AMP in rat renal papillary collecting tubule cells in culture. *J Endocrinol* 1987;113:199–204.

119. Jackson SN, Williams B, et al. The diagnosis of Liddle syndrome by identification of a mutation in the beta subunit of the epithelial sodium channel. *J Med Genet* 1998;35:510–512.

120. Jaeger P, Karlmark B, et al. Ammonium transport in rat cortical tubule: relationship to potassium metabolism. *Am J Physiol* 1983;245(Pt 1):F593–600.

121. Jaisser F. [Molecular and functional diversity of NA,K-ATPase and renal H,K-ATPases]. *Nephrologie* 1996;17:401–408.

122. Janko O, Seier J, et al. [Hypokalemia-incidence and severity in a general hospital]. *Wien Med Wochenschr* 1992;142:78–81.

123. Jeck N, Konrad M, et al. Mutations in the chloride channel gene, CLCNKB, leading to a mixed Bartter-Gitelman phenotype. *Pediatr Res* 2000;48:754–758.

124. Jespersen B, Danielsen H, et al. Effect of chronic hypokalaemia on renal concentrating ability and secretion of arginine vasopressin. *Scand J Clin Lab Invest* 1987;47:5–9.

125. Jeunemaitre X, Bassilana F, et al. Genotype-phenotype analysis of a newly discovered family with Liddle's syndrome. *J Hypertens* 1997;15:1091–1100.

126. Jones JW, Sebastian A, et al. Systemic and renal acid-base effects of chronic dietary potassium depletion in humans. *Kidney Int* 1982;21:402–410.

127. Deleted in proof.

128. Jung JY, Madsen KM, et al. Expression of urea transporters in potassium-depleted mouse kidney. *Am J Physiol Renal Physiol* 2003;285:F1210–1224.

129. Kamel KS, Harvey E, et al. Studies on the pathogenesis of hypokalemia in Gitelman's syndrome: role of bicarbonaturia and hypomagnesemia. *Am J Nephrol* 1998;18:42–49.

130. Kannegiesser H, Lee JB. Role of outer renal medullary metabolism in the concentrating defect of K depletion. *Am J Physiol* 1971;220:1701–1707.

131. Kaplan NM, Carnegie A, et al. Potassium supplementation in hypertensive patients with diuretic-induced hypokalemia. *N Engl J Med* 1985;312:746–749.

132. Karlmark B, Jaeger P, et al. Luminal buffer transport in rat cortical tubule: relationship to potassium metabolism. *Am J Physiol* 1983;245(Pt 1):F584–592.

133. Karolyi L, Ziegler A, et al. Gitelman's syndrome is genetically distinct from other forms of Bartter's syndrome. *Pediatr Nephrol* 1996;10:551–554.

134. Kellenberger S, Gautschi I, et al. Mutations causing Liddle syndrome reduce sodium-dependent downregulation of the epithelial sodium channel in the Xenopus oocyte expression system. *J Clin Invest* 1998;101:2741–2750.

135. Kim JK, Jackson BA, et al. Effect of potassium depletion on the vasopressin-sensitive cyclic AMP system in rat outer medullary tubules. *J Lab Clin Med* 1982;99:29–38.

136. Kimura T, Nishino T, et al. Expression of Bcl-2 and Bax in hypokalemic nephropathy in rats. *Pathobiology* 2001;69:237–248.

137. Klotman PE, Boatman JE, et al. Captopril enhances aminoglycoside nephrotoxicity in potassium-depleted rats. *Kidney Int* 1985;2 8:118–127.

138. Komhoff M, Reinalter SA, et al. Induction of microsomal prostaglandin E2 synthase in the macula densa in children with hypokalemic salt-losing tubulopathies. *Pediatr Res* 2004;55:261–266.

139. Konrad M, Vollmer M, et al. Mutations in the chloride channel gene CLCNKB as a cause of classic Bartter syndrome. *J Am Soc Nephrol* 2000;11:1449–1459.

140. Kornandakieti C, Grekin R, et al. Hydrogen ion secretion by the rat distal nephron: adaptation to chronic alkali and acid ingestion. *Am J Physiol* 1983;245:F349–358.

141. Kornandakieti C, Tannen RL. Hydrogen ion secretion by the distal nephron in the rat: effect of potassium. *J Lab Clin Med* 1984;104:293–303.

142. Kotchen TA, Guthrie GP Jr, et al. Effects of NaCl on renin and aldosterone responses to potassium depletion. *Am J Physiol* 1983;244:E164–169.

143. Krakoff LR. Potassium deficiency and cardiac catecholamine metabolism in the rat. *Circ Res* 1972;30:608–615.

144. Krishna GG, Chusid P, et al. Mild potassium depletion provokes renal sodium retention. *J Lab Clin Med* 1987;109:724–730.

145. Krishna GG, Kapoor SC. Potassium depletion exacerbates essential hypertension. *Ann Intern Med* 1991;115:77–83.

146. Krishna GG, Miller E, et al. Increased blood pressure during potassium depletion in normotensive men. *N Engl J Med* 1989;320:1177–1182.

147. Kunau RT Jr, Frick A, et al. Micropuncture study of the proximal tubular factors responsible for the maintenance of alkalosis during potassium deficiency in the rat. *Clin Sci* 1968;34:223–231.

148. Kunzelmann K, Hubner M, et al. A Bartter's syndrome mutation of ROMK1 exerts dominant negative effects on K(+) conductance. *Cell Physiol Biochem* 2000;10:117–124.

149. Kurtzman NA. Regulation of renal bicarbonate reabsorption by extracellular volume. *J Clin Invest* 1970;49:586–595.

150. Laghmani K, Richer C, et al. Expression of rat thick limb Na/H exchangers in potassium depletion and chronic metabolic acidosis. *Kidney Int* 2001;60:1386–1396.

151. Lelamali K, Khunkitti W, et al. Potassium depletion in a healthy north-eastern Thai population: no association with tubulo-interstitial injury. *Nephrology (Carlton)* 2003;8:28–32.

152. Lemmink HH, van den Heuvel LP, et al. Linkage of Gitelman syndrome to the thiazide-sensitive sodium-chloride cotransporter gene with identification of mutations in Dutch families. *Pediatr Nephrol* 1996;10:403–407.

153. Levi M, McDonald LA, et al. Chronic K depletion stimulates rat renal brush-border membrane Na-citrate cotransporter. *Am J Physiol* 1991;261(Pt 2):F767–773.

154. Linas SL, Dickmann D. Mechanism of the decreased renal blood flow in the potassium-depleted conscious rat. *Kidney Int* 1982;21:757–64.

155. Linas SL, Marzec-Calvert R. Potassium depletion ameliorates hypertension in spontaneously hypertensive rats. *Hypertension* 1986;8:990–996.

156. Linas SL, Marzec-Calvert R, et al. Mechanism of the antihypertensive effect of K depletion in the spontaneously hypertensive rat. *Kidney Int* 1988;34:18–25.

157. Linas SL, Peterson LN, et al. Mechanism of renal potassium conservation in the rat. *Kidney Int* 1979;15:601–611.

158. Lingueglia E, Voilley N, et al. Molecular biology of the amiloride-sensitive epithelial Na+ channel. *Exp Physiol* 1996;81:483–492.

159. Liu FY, Cogan MG. Angiotensin II stimulation of hydrogen ion secretion in the rat early proximal tubule. Modes of action, mechanism, and kinetics. *J Clin Invest* 1988;82: 601–607.

160. Luke RG, Booker BB, et al. Effect of potassium depletion on chloride transport in the loop of Henle in the rat. *Am J Physiol* 1985;248(Pt 2):F682–687.

161. Luke RG, Levitin R. Impaired renal conservation of chloride and the acid-base changes associated with potassium depletion in the rat. *Clin Sci* 1976;32:511–526.

162. Luke RG, Lyerly RH, et al. Effect of potassium depletion on renin release. *Kidney Int* 1982; 21:14–19.

163. Luke RG, Wright FS, et al. (1978). Effects of potassium depletion on renal tubular chloride transport in the rat. *Kidney Int* 1978;14:414–427.

164. Malnic G, Berliner RW, et al. Flow dependence of K+ secretion in cortical distal tubules of the rat. *Am J Physiol* 1989;256(Pt 2):F932–941.

165. Manfro RC, Stumpf AG, et al. [Hydroelectrolyte, acid-base, and renal function changes in patients with acquired immunodeficiency syndrome]. *Rev Assoc Med Bras* 1993;39:43–47.

166. Marples D, Frokiaer J, et al. Hypokalemia-induced downregulation of aquaporin-2 water channel expression in rat kidney medulla and cortex. *J Clin Invest* 1996;97:1960–1968.

167. Marshall S, Green A, et al. Evidence for recycling of insulin receptors in isolated rat adipocytes. *J Biol Chem* 1981;256:11464–11470.

168. Marsy S, Elalouf JM, et al. Quantitative RT-PCR analysis of mRNAs encoding a colonic putative H, K-ATPase alpha subunit along the rat nephron: effect of K+ depletion. *Pflugers Arch* 1996;432:494–500.

169. Mastroianni N, Bettinelli A, et al. Novel molecular variants of the Na-Cl cotransporter gene are responsible for Gitelman syndrome. *Am J Hum Genet* 1996;59:1019–10126.

170. McKanna JA, Haigler HT, et al. Hormone receptor topology and dynamics: morphological analysis using ferritin-labeled epidermal growth factor. *Proc Natl Acad Sci U S A* 1979;76:5689–5693.

171. McKinney TD, Davidson KK. Effect of potassium depletion and protein intake in vivo on renal tubular bicarbonate transport in vitro. *Am J Physiol* 1987;252(Pt 2):F509–516.

172. McNicholas CM, Canessa CM. Diversity of channels generated by different combinations of epithelial sodium channel subunits. *J Gen Physiol* 1997;109:681–692.

173. Mendelsohn FA, Mackie C. Relation of intracellular K+ and steroidogenesis in isolated adrenal zona glomerulosa and fasciculata cells. *Clin Sci Mol Med* 1975;49:13–26.

174. Menegon LF, Amaral TN, et al. Renal sodium handling study in an atypical case of Bartter's syndrome associated with mitochondriopathy and sensorineural blindness. *Ren Fail* 2004;26: 195–197.

175. Molitoris BA, Falk SA, et al. Ischemia-induced loss of epithelial polarity. Role of the tight junction. *J Clin Invest* 1989;84:1334–1339.

176. Monclair T, Sejersted OM, et al. Influence of plasma potassium concentration on the capacity for sodium reabsorption in the diluting segment of the kidney. *Scand J Clin Lab Invest* 1980;40:27–36.

177. Mujais S, Katz AI. Potassium deficiency. In: Seldin DW, Giebisch G, eds. *The Kidney: Physiology and Pathophysiology.* Philadelphia: Lippincott, Williams & Wilkins; 2000:1615–1646.

178. Mujais SK. Effects of aldosterone on rat collecting tubule N-ethylmaleimide-sensitive adenosine triphosphatase. *J Lab Clin Med* 1987;109:34–39.

179. Mujais SK. Renal memory after potassium adaptation: role of Na+-K+-ATPase. *Am J Physiol* 1988;254(Pt 2):F845–850.

180. Mujais SK. Collecting duct changes in potassium depletion: effects of ACE inhibition. *Am J Physiol* 1994;266(Pt 2):F419–424.

181. Mujais SK. Transport enzymes and renal tubular acidosis. *Semin Nephrol* 1998;18:74–82.

182. Mujais SK, Chekal MA, et al. Regulation of renal Na+-K+-ATPase in the rat: role of increased potassium transport. *Am J Physiol* 1986;251(Pt 2):F199–207.

183. Mujais SK, Chekal MA, et al. Modulation of renal sodium-potassium-adenosine triphosphatase by aldosterone. Effect of high physiologic levels on enzyme activity in isolated rat and rabbit tubules. *J Clin Invest* 1985;76:170–176.

184. Mujais SK, Chen Y, et al. Discordant aspects of aldosterone resistance in potassium depletion. *Am J Physiol* 1992;262(Pt 2):F972–979.

185. Mujais SK, Chen Y, et al. Vasopressin resistance in potassium depletion: role of Na-K pump. *Am J Physiol* 1992;263(Pt 2):F705–710.

186. Mujais SK, Kauffman S, et al. Angiotensin II binding sites in individual segments of the rat nephron. *J Clin Invest* 1986;77:315–318.

187. Muller J, Hofstetter L, et al. Role of the renin-angiotensin system in the regulation of late steps in aldosterone biosynthesis by sodium intake of potassium-deficient rats. *Endocrinology* 1984;115:350–356.

188. Murray BM, Paller MS. Pressor resistance to vasopressin in sodium depletion, potassium depletion, and cirrhosis. *Am J Physiol* 1986;51(Pt 2):R525–530.

189. Nakanishi T, Nishihara F, et al. NaCl and/or urea infusion fails to increase renal inner medullary myo-inositol in protein-deprived rats. *Am J Physiol* 1996;271(Pt 2):F1255–1263.

190. Nakanishi T, Yamauchi A, et al. Potassium depletion modulates aldose reductase mRNA in rat renal inner medulla. *Kidney Int* 1996;50:828–834.

191. Nakano Y, Ishida T, et al. A frameshift mutation of beta subunit of epithelial sodium channel in a case of isolated Liddle syndrome. *J Hypertens* 2002;20:2379–2382.

192. Nattie EE. Breathing patterns in the awake potassium-depleted rat. *J Appl Physiol* 1977;43: 1063–1074.

193. Nattie EE, Melton JE. Breathing in the potassium depleted rat: the role of metabolic rate and body temperature. *Respir Physiol* 1979;38:223–233.

194. Nattie EE, Tenney SM. Effect of potassium depletion on cerebrospinal fluid bicarbonate homeostasis. *Am J Physiol* 1976;231:579–587.

195. Nattie EE, Tenney SM. Effects of potassium depletion on control of breathing in awake rats. *Am J Physiol* 1976;231:588–592.

196. Nonoguchi H, Takehara Y, et al. Intra- and inter-nephron heterogeneity of ammoniagenesis in rats: effects of chronic metabolic acidosis and potassium depletion. *Pflugers Arch* 1986;407: 245–251.

197. O'Reilly DS. Increased ammoniagenesis and the renal tubular effects of potassium depletion. *J Clin Pathol* 1984;37:1358–1362.

198. Ordonez NG, Spargo BH. The morphologic relationship of light and dark cells of the collecting tubule in potassium-depleted rats. *Am J Pathol* 1976;84:317–326.

199. Ordonez NG, Toback FG, et al. Zonal changes in renal structure and phospholipid metabolism during reversal of potassium depletion nephropathy. *Lab Invest* 1977;6:33–47.

200. Ornt DB. Effect of potassium concentration and ouabain on the renal adaptation to potassium depletion in isolated perfused rat kidney. *Can J Physiol Pharmacol* 1986;64:1427–1233.

201. Ornt DB, Radke KJ, et al. Effect of aldosterone on renal potassium conservation in the rat. *Am J Physiol* 1996;270(Pt 1):E1003–1008.

202. Ornt DB, Tannen RL. Demonstration of an intrinsic renal adaptation for K+ conservation in short-term K+ depletion. *Am J Physiol* 1983;245:F329–338.

203. Paice BJ, Paterson KR, et al. Record linkage study of hypokalaemia in hospitalized patients. *Postgrad Med J* 1986;62:187–191.

204. Paller MS, Douglas JG, et al. Mechanism of decreased vascular reactivity to angiotensin II in conscious, potassium-deficient rats. *J Clin Invest* 1984;73:79–86.

205. Peters M, Jeck N, et al. Clinical presentation of genetically defined patients with hypokalemic salt-losing tubulopathies. *Am J Med* 2002;112:183–190.

206. Peterson LN. Time-dependent changes in inner medullary plasma flow rate during potassium-depletion. *Kidney Int* 1984;25:899–905.

207. Peterson LN, Carpenter B, et al. Potassium depletion enhances renal compensatory hypertrophy in the nephrectomized rat. *Miner Electrolyte Metab* 1987;13:57–62.

208. Polderman KH, Girbes AR. Severe electrolyte disorders following cardiac surgery: a prospective controlled observational study. *Crit Care* 2004;8:R459–466.

209. Pollack LR, Tate EH, et al. Na+, K+-ATPase in HeLa cells after prolonged growth in low K+ or ouabain. *J Cell Physiol* 1981;106:85–97.

210. Pradervand S, Vandewalle A, et al. Dysfunction of the epithelial sodium channel expressed in the kidney of a mouse model for Liddle syndrome. *J Am Soc Nephrol* 2003;14:2219–2228.

211. Pressley TA, Haber RS, et al. Stimulation of Na,K-activated adenosine triphosphatase and active transport by low external K+ in a rat liver cell line. *J Gen Physiol* 1986;87:591–606.

212. Rajendran VM, Kashgarian M, et al. Aldosterone induction of electrogenic sodium transport in the apical membrane vesicles of rat distal colon. *J Biol Chem* 1989;264:18638–18644.

213. Ray PE, Suga S, et al. Chronic potassium depletion induces renal injury, salt sensitivity, and hypertension in young rats. *Kidney Int* 2001;59:1850–1858.

214. Raymond KH, Davidson KK, et al. In vivo and in vitro studies of urinary concentrating ability in potassium-depleted rabbits. *J Clin Invest* 1985;76:561–566.

215. Raymond KH, Holland SD, et al. Protease effects on adenylate cyclase in potassium-depleted rabbit kidney. *Am J Physiol* 1988;255(Pt 2):F1033–1039.

216. Raymond KH, Lifschitz MD, et al. Prostaglandins and the urinary concentrating defect in potassium-depleted rabbits. *Am J Physiol* 1987;253(Pt 2):F1113–1119.

217. Reinalter SC, Jeck N, et al. Role of cyclooxygenase-2 in hyperprostaglandin E syndrome/antenatal Bartter syndrome. *Kidney Int* 2002;62:253–260.

218. Riemenschneider T, Bohle A. Morphologic aspects of low-potassium and low-sodium nephropathy. *Clin Nephrol* 1983;19:271–279.

219. Rutecki GW, Cox JW, et al. Urinary concentrating ability and antidiuretic hormone responsiveness in the potassium-depleted dog. *J Lab Clin Med* 1982;100:53–60.

220. Salem MM, Chen Y, et al. Potassium adaptation in hypothyroidism: changes in transport adenosinetriphosphatases. *Am J Physiol* 1993;264(Pt 2):F31–36.

221. Sandle GI, Foster ES, et al. The electrical basis for enhanced potassium secretion in rat distal colon during dietary potassium loading. *Pflugers Arch* 1985;403:433–439.

222. Sarkar K, Levine DZ. Minimal medullary droplets in DOCA-induced potassium depletion of rats. *Invest Urol* 1978;15:280–283.

223. Sarkar K, Levine DZ. Ultrastructural changes in the renal papillary cells of rats during maintenance and repair of profound potassium depletion. *Br J Exp Pathol* 1979;60:120–129.

224. Sarkar K, Nash LA, et al. Effects of ureteral ligation on renal medullary lesions of potassium depletion. *Br J Exp Pathol* 1983;64:677–683.

225. Sastrasinh S, Sastrasinh M. Renal mitochondrial glutamine metabolism during K+ depletion. *Am J Physiol* 1986;250(Pt 2):F667–673.

226. Sastrasinh S, Tannen RL. Mechanism by which enhanced ammonia production reduces urinary potassium excretion. *Kidney Int* 1981;20:326–331.

227. Schild L. The ENaC channel as the primary determinant of two human diseases: Liddle syndrome and pseudohypoaldosteronism. *Nephrologie* 1996;17:395–400.

228. Schild L, Lu Y, et al. Identification of a PY motif in the epithelial Na channel subunits as a target sequence for mutations causing channel activation found in Liddle syndrome. *EMBO J* 1996;15:2381–2387.

229. Schwartz GJ, Burg MB. Mineralocorticoid effects on cation transport by cortical collecting tubules in vitro. *Am J Physiol* 1978;235:F576–585.

230. Seglen PO. Inhibitors of lysosomal function. *Methods Enzymol* 1983;96:737–764.

231. Seguro AC, De Araujo M, et al. Effects of hypokalemia and hypomagnesemia on zidovudine (AZT) and didanosine (ddI) nephrotoxicity in rats. *Clin Nephrol* 2003;59:267–272.

232. Seguro AC, Shimizu MH, et al. Effect of potassium depletion on ischemic renal failure. *Nephron* 1989;51:350–354.

233. Shalev H, Ohali M, et al. The neonatal variant of Bartter syndrome and deafness: preservation of renal function. *Pediatrics* 2003;112(Pt 1):628–633.

234. Shimkets RA, Warnock DG, et al. Liddle's syndrome: heritable human hypertension caused by mutations in the beta subunit of the epithelial sodium channel. *Cell* 1994;79: 407–414.

235. Shirley DG, Walter SJ. Renal tubular lithium reabsorption in potassium-depleted rats. *J Physiol* 1997;501(Pt 3):663–670.

236. Shirley DG, Walter SJ, et al. Transepithelial electrochemical gradients in the proximal convoluted tubule during potassium depletion in the rat. *J Physiol* 1998;513(Pt 2):551–557.

237. Silver RB, Breton S, et al. Potassium depletion increases proton pump (H(+)-ATPase) activity in intercalated cells of cortical collecting duct. *Am J Physiol Renal Physiol* 2000;279:F195–202.

238. Simon DB, Karet FE, et al. Bartter's syndrome, hypokalaemic alkalosis with hypercalciuria, is caused by mutations in the Na-K-2Cl cotransporter NKCC2. *Nat Genet* 1996;13:183–188.

239. Simon DB, Karet FE, et al. Genetic heterogeneity of Bartter's syndrome revealed by mutations in the K+ channel, ROMK. *Nat Genet* 1996;14:152–156.

240. Simon DB, Lifton RP. The molecular basis of inherited hypokalemic alkalosis: Bartter's and Gitelman's syndromes. *Am J Physiol* 1996;271(Pt 2):F961–966.

241. Simon DB, Nelson-Williams C, et al. Gitelman's variant of Bartter's syndrome, inherited hypokalaemic alkalosis, is caused by mutations in the thiazide-sensitive Na-Cl cotransporter. *Nat Genet* 1996;12:24–30.

242. Snyder PM, Price MP, et al. Mechanism by which Liddle's syndrome mutations increase activity of a human epithelial Na+ channel. *Cell* 1995;83:969–978.

243. Soleimani M, Bergman JA, et al. Potassium depletion increases luminal Na+/H+ exchange and basolateral Na+:CO3=:HCO3̄ cotransport in rat renal cortex. *J Clin Invest* 1990;86:1076–1083.

244. Sorensen IJ, Matzen LE. [Serum electrolytes and drug therapy of patients admitted to a geriatric department]. *Ugeskr Laeger* 1993;155:3921–3924.

245. Stanton BA, Biemesderfer D, et al. Structural and functional study of the rat distal nephron: effects of potassium adaptation and depletion. *Kidney Int* 1981;19:36–48.

246. Starkloff GB, Donovan JF, et al. Metabolic intestinal surgery. Its complications and management. *Arch Surg* 1975;110:652–657.

247. Stetson DL, Wade JB, et al. Morphologic alterations in the rat medullary collecting duct following potassium depletion. *Kidney Int* 198017:45–56.

248. Strieder N, Khuri R, et al. Studies on the renal action of ouabain in the rat. Effects in the non-diuretic state. *Pflugers Arch* 1974;349:91–107.

249. Suga S, Yasui N, et al. Endothelin A receptor blockade and endothelin B receptor blockade improve hypokalemic nephropathy by different mechanisms. *J Am Soc Nephrol* 2003;14:397–406.

250. Suga SI., Phillips MI, et al. Hypokalemia induces renal injury and alterations in vasoactive mediators that favor salt sensitivity. *Am J Physiol Renal Physiol* 2001;281:F620–9.

251. Sweiry JH, Binder HJ. Characterization of aldosterone-induced potassium secretion in rat distal colon. *J Clin Invest* 1989;83:844–851.

252. Takeuchi K, Kato T, et al. Three cases of Gitelman's syndrome possibly caused by different mutations in the thiazide-sensitive Na-Cl cotransporter. *Intern Med* 1997;36:582–585.

253. Takeuchi K, Kure S, et al. Association of a mutation in thiazide-sensitive Na-Cl cotransporter with familial Gitelman's syndrome. *J Clin Endocrinol Metab* 1996;81:4496–4499.

254. Tamura H, Schild L, et al. Liddle disease caused by a missense mutation of beta subunit of the epithelial sodium channel gene. *J Clin Invest* 1996;97:1780–1784.

255. Tannen RL, Gerrits L.). Response of the renal K+-conserving mechanism to kaliuretic stimuli: evidence for a direct kaliuretic effect by furosemide. *J Lab Clin Med* 1986;107:176–184.

256. Tannen RL, Kunin AS. Effect of potassium on ammoniagenesis by renal mitochondria. *Am J Physiol* 1976;231:44–51.

257. Tannen RL, Terrien T. Potassium-sparing effect of enhanced renal ammonia production. *Am J Physiol* 1975;228:699–705.

258. Toback FG. Phosphatidylcholine metabolism during renal growth and regeneration. *Am J Physiol* 1984;246(Pt 2):F249–259.

259. Toback FG, Aithal HN, et al. Altered bioenergetics in proliferating renal cells during potassium depletion. *Lab Invest* 1979;41:265–267.

260. Toback FG, Ordonez NG, et al. Zonal changes in renal structure and phospholipid metabolism in potassium-deficient rats. *Lab Invest* 1976;34:115–124.

261. Tolins JP, Hostetter MK, et al. Hypokalemic nephropathy in the rat. Role of ammonia in chronic tubular injury. *J Clin Invest* 1987;79:1447–1458.

262. Toyoshima H, Watanabe T. . Rapid regression of renal medullary granular change during reversal of potassium depletion nephropathy. *Nephron* 1988;48:47–53.

263. Tsao T, Fawcett J, et al. Expression of insulin-like growth factor-I and transforming growth factor-beta in hypokalemic nephropathy in the rat. *Kidney Int* 2001;59:96–105.

264. Ullian ME, Linas SL. Hemodynamic effects of potassium. *Semin Nephrol* 1987;7:239–252.

265. Ural AU, Avcu F, et al. Spironolactone: is it a novel drug for the prevention of amphotericin B-related hypokalemia in cancer patients? *Eur J Clin Pharmacol* 2002;57:771–773.

266. van Neck JW, Flyvbjerg A, et al. IGF, type I IGF receptor and IGF-binding protein mRNA expression in kidney and liver of potassium-depleted and normal rats infused with IGF-I. *J Mol Endocrinol* 1997;19:59–66.

267. Vio CP, Jeanneret VA. Local induction of angiotensin-converting enzyme in the kidney as a mechanism of progressive renal diseases. *Kidney Int Suppl* 2003;86:S57–63.

268. Wagner CA, Finberg KE, et al. Regulation of the expression of the Cl-/anion exchanger pendrin in mouse kidney by acid-base status. *Kidney Int* 2002;62:2109–2117.

269. Wallace DC. Mouse models for mitochondrial disease. *Am J Med Genet* 2001;106:71–93.

270. Walter SJ, Shore AC, et al. Effect of potassium depletion on renal tubular function in the rat. *Clin Sci (Lond)* 1988;75:621–628.

271. Wang Z, Baird N, et al. Potassium depletion and acid-base transporters in rat kidney: differential effect of hypophysectomy. *Am J Physiol* 1997;272(Pt 2):F736–743.

272. Warnock DG. Liddle syndrome: an autosomal dominant form of human hypertension. *Kidney Int* 1998;53:18–24.

273. Warnock DG. Liddle syndrome: genetics and mechanisms of Na+ channel defects. *Am J Med Sci* 2001;322:302–307.

274. Watanabe T. Proximal renal tubular dysfunction in primary distal renal tubular acidosis. *Pediatr Nephrol* 2005;20:86–88.

275. Watanabe T, Toyoshima H. Intracytoplasmic granules of the inner medulla and papilla of the potassium depleted human kidney. *Virchows Arch A Pathol Anat Histol* 1981;392:309–319.

276. Webster SK, Reineck HJ, et al. Urea reabsorption along the papillary collecting duct in potassium-deficient rats. *Proc Soc Exp Biol Med* 1985;179:96–100.

277. Werdan K, Schneider G, et al. Chronic exposure to low K+ increases cardiac glycoside receptors in cultured cardiac cells: different responses of cardiac muscle and non muscle cells from chicken embryos. *Biochem Pharmacol* 1984;33:1161–1164.

278. Whinnery MA, Kunau RT Jr. Effect of potassium deficiency on papillary plasma flow in the rat. *Am J Physiol* 1979;237:F226–231.

279. Wiederholt M, Sullivan WJ, et al. Potassium and sodium transport across single distal tubules of Amphiuma. *J Gen Physiol* 1971;57:495–525.

280. Wingo CS. Potassium transport by medullary collecting tubule of rabbit: effects of variation in K intake. *Am J Physiol* 1987;253(Pt 2):F1136–1141.

281. Wingo CS. Active proton secretion and potassium absorption in the rabbit outer medullary collecting duct. Functional evidence for proton-potassium-activated adenosine triphosphatase. *J Clin Invest* 1989;84:361–365.

282. Wingo CS, Seldin DW, et al. Dietary modulation of active potassium secretion in the cortical collecting tubule of adrenalectomized rabbits. *J Clin Invest* 1982;70:579–586.

283. Wingo CS, Smolka AJ. Function and structure of H-K-ATPase in the kidney. *Am J Physiol* 1995;269(Pt 2):F1–16.

284. Wright FS, Giebisch G. Regulation of potassium excretion. In: Seldin DW, Giebisch G, eds. *The Kidney: Physiology and Pathophysiology.* New York: Raven Press; 1985:1223–1249.

285. Yamada H, Nakada J, et al. Intra- and inter-nephron heterogeneity of gluconeogenesis in the rat: effects of chronic metabolic acidosis and potassium depletion. *Pflugers Arch* 1986;407:1–7.

286. Yang BC, Li DY, et al. Increased superoxide anion generation and altered vasoreactivity in rabbits on low-potassium diet. *Am J Physiol* 1998;274(Pt 2):H1955–1961.

287. Yoo TH, Lee SH, et al. Identification of novel mutations in Na-Cl cotransporter gene in a Korean patient with atypical Gitelman's syndrome. *Am J Kidney Dis* 2003;42:E11–16.

288. Zanolari Calderari M, Vigier RO, et al. Electrocardiographic QT prolongation and sudden death in renal hypokalemic alkalosis. *Nephron* 2002;91:762–763.

289. Zelikovic I, Szargel R, et al. A novel mutation in the chloride channel gene, CLCNKB, as a cause of Gitelman and Bartter syndromes. *Kidney Int* 2003;63:24–32.

CHAPTER 49

Clinical Disorders of Hyperkalemia

Kamel S. Kamel, Shih-Hua Lin,* and Mitchell L. Halperin

University of Toronto, Toronto, Ontario, Canada
*National Defense Medical Center, Taipei, Taiwan

Hyperkalemia is a common electrolyte disorder that may have detrimental effects, the most serious of which is a cardiac arrhythmia (44). This threat and th e absolute concentration of potassium (K^+) in plasma (P_K), however, are not tightly correlated. The basis of hyperkalemia will be a shift of K^+ out of cells if the time course for its development is short and/or if there is little K^+ intake. On the other hand, chronic hyperkalemia implies that there is a defect in the regulation of K^+ excretion by the kidney.

Basic Concept for the Movement of Potassium Ions Across Cell Membranes

K^+ is the principal cation in cells. The movement of K^+ ions across cell membranes has two requirements; first, there must be a driving force; second there must be a K^+ ion channel in that membrane (Fig. 1).

DRIVING FORCE

Potassium is kept inside the cell by an electrical force; the cell interior has a negative voltage. It follows that an increase in the negative cell voltage is required to shift K^+ inside the cells. There are two options to make the interior of cells more negative, import of anions or export of cations; the usual mechanism is the export of cations. The cation is usually sodium (Na^+) because of its abundance and the presence of a means to cause its transmembrane movement.

The negative voltage in cells is generated by the activity of the electrogenic cation pump, the Na^+,K^+-ATPase. This pump exports three Na^+ ions while importing only two K^+ ions; hence there is an export of one third of a positive charge per Na^+ exit from that cell (Fig. 2). Because Na^+ movement is much greater than that of impermeable ICF anions (macromolecular phosphates such as RNA, DNA, and phospholipids), a negative intracellular voltage is generated.

There are three ways to increase ion pumping by the Na,K-ATPase: first, a rise the concentration of its rate-limiting substrate-Na^+ in cells (this can occur very quickly); second, a higher Na,K-ATPase activity caused by activation of existing Na,K-ATPase units in cell membranes by phosphorylation (this too can occur relatively quickly); third, an increase in the number of active Na,K-ATPase pump units in cell membranes by recruitment or synthesis of new units (this takes more time to occur).

The driving force for the secretion of K^+ by principal cells in the cortical collecting duct (CCD) is a lumen-negative voltage. This lumen-negative voltage is generated by the electrogenic reabsorption of Na^+ in that nephron segment (reabsorption of Na^+ faster than its accompanying anion, chloride (Cl^-) (Fig. 3).

ION CHANNELS FOR POTASSIUM

Several different types of channels permit the diffusion of K^+ through cell membranes (2). Some of these channels are regulated by voltage, others by ligands such as calcium ions (Ca^{2+}), and yet others by metabolites such as adenosine diphosphate (ADP); the latter are called K_{ATP} channels. Because K^+ ions do *not* reach diffusion equilibrium, control of the open probability of K^+ channel regulates this voltage.

The major K^+ ion channel that adjusts the intracellular voltage is the K^+_{ATP} channel. This is a misnomer because these K^+_{ATP} channels are not regulated by the concentration of ATP that exists in cells as it never falls sufficiently to result in opening of these channels. The signal to open K^+_{ATP} channels may be related to a change in the concentration of a related nucleotide, ADP. When the concentration of ADP rises, this channel will open; conversely, when the ADP concentration falls, K^+_{ATP} channels will close. This regulation of K^+_{ATP} channels adjusts the negative voltage in cells, which can regulate or gate other ion channels. The best example is the voltage-gated Ca^{2+} channel, which is opened by a less negative voltage in cells. By modulating the concentration of ionized Ca^{2+} in cells, many other functions are controlled because ionized Ca^{2+} is a major signal for regulation of intracellular processes.

Example: Regulation of the K^+_{ATP} channel by ADP plays a critical role in the release of insulin. When the concentration of glucose in plasma ($P_{Glucose}$) is high, a metabolic signal is generated in β cells of the pancreas to cause the release of insulin. This signal—a fall in the (ADP)—is generated when the rate of oxidation of glucose rises in β cells. This lower ADP causes the K^+_{ATP} channels to close and thus the

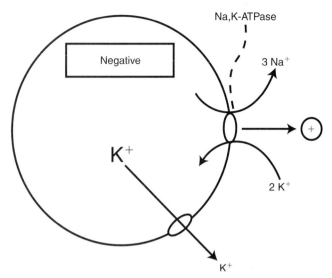

FIGURE 1 Movement of potassium across cell membranes. The circle represents a cell membrane. There is a much higher [K$^+$] in cells than in the extracellular fluid (ECF) compartment. This high intracellular fluid (ICF) [K$^+$] is the result of having a negative voltage inside cells. This negative voltage is generated by the electrogenic export of more Na$^+$ ions than the import of K$^+$ by Na,K-ATPase. In addition, for the passive movement of K$^+$, there must be open K$^+$ channels in the cell membrane. To cause a redistribution of K$^+$ across the ECF–ICF interface, there must be either a change in the magnitude of the electrical driving force and/or the conductance of K$^+$ channels because the latter do not normally permit K$^+$ to diffuse to electrochemical equilibrium across cell membranes.

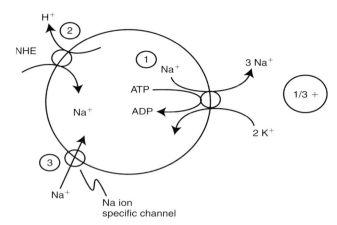

FIGURE 2 Na,K-ATPase activity and the export of positive voltage. Na,K-ATPase generates the electrical driving force for K$^+$ entry into cells providing that the source of Na$^+$ pumped was either Na$^+$ that existed in cells (*site 1*) or Na$^+$ that entered cells in an electroneutral fashion via Na$^+$-H$^+$ exchanger (NHE), (*site 2*). If the source of Na$^+$ pumped were Na$^+$ that entered cells via the Na$^+$-specific ion channel (*site 3*), the voltage in cells would become less negative. K$^+$ channel conductance limits the rate of K$^+$ exit. (From Halperin ML. *The ACID Truth and BASIC Facts—With a Sweet Touch, an enLYTEnment,* 5th ed. Toronto: RossMark Medical Publishers; 2004, with permission.)

Mg^{2+}. In the CCD, ROMK channels are the main ones responsible for K$^+$ entry into the lumen of this nephron segment (39,77,78,110).

REGULATION OF POTASSIUM HOMEOSTASIS

Regulation of K$^+$ homeostasis has two important aspects. First, the control of the transcellular distribution of K$^+$ is vital for survival because it acts to limit acute changes in the P$_K$. Second, the regulation of K$^+$ excretion by the kidney maintains overall K$^+$ balance; nevertheless, this is a much slower process.

ACUTE CONTROL OF THE P$_K$

DISTRIBUTION OF K$^+$ BETWEEN EXTRACELLULAR AND INTRACELLULAR FLUID COMPARTMENTS

A shift of K$^+$ into cells requires an increase in the negative voltage inside cells. The components of this process are described below.

Na,K-ATPase The activity of Na,K-ATPase is higher when the concentration of Na$^+$ rises in cells. The impact of this increase in pump activity on the net voltage, however, depends on whether the Na$^+$ entry step into cells is electroneutral or electrogenic.

Electroneutral Entry of Sodium into Cells This occurs when Na$^+$ ions enter cells in exchange for hydrogen ions (H$^+$) via the Na$^+$-H$^+$ exchanger (NHE) (Fig. 6, left side) (22). The NHE is normally *inactive* in cell membranes as can be deduced from the fact that the concentrations of its substrates (Na$^+$ in the extracellular fluid [ECF] and H$^+$ in the

intracellular fluid (ICF) compartment becomes less negative because fewer K$^+$ (positive charges) exit β cells (Fig. 4). This less negative ICF voltage increases the conductance of voltage-gated Ca^{2+} channels and hence the intracellular ionized Ca^{2+} concentration rises: This is the final signal to release insulin from β cells.

A similar logic can be used to deduce how the blood flow to exercising muscle may be controlled using intracellular Ca^{2+} as the signal (Fig. 5). During a sprint, L-lactic acid is released from skeletal muscle cells. When lactic acid enters vascular smooth muscle cells, H$^+$ and/or lactate lead to opening of the K$^+$$_{ATP}$ channels. As a result, K$^+$ ions exit and the voltage in these cells becomes more negative. This causes closure of voltage-gated Ca^{2+} channels and less entry of Ca^{2+} into cells and hence vasodilation (for review, see reference [23]).

Although many types of K$^+$ channel have been identified in the kidney, the location of these K$^+$ channels along the nephron and their exact function is largely unknown with the exception of the rat outer medullary K$^+$ (ROMK) channels. In the loop of Henle, ROMK channels play a key role that permit K$^+$ to recycle across the apical membrane of the cells of its thick ascending limb, which is an essential step for NaCl reabsorption in this nephron segment. Moreover, this K$^+$ recycling produces a lumen-positive transepithelial potential difference that drives the paracellular absorption of Na$^+$, Ca^{2+}, and

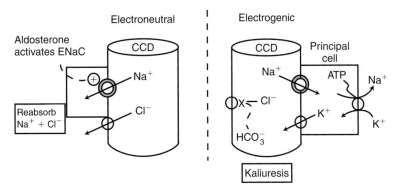

FIGURE 3 Electrogenic and electroneutral reabsorption of Na^+ in the cortical collecting duct. The barrel-shaped structures represent the cortical collecting duct (CCD) and the rectangles represent principal cells. Na^+ is reabsorbed via epithelial Na^+ channel (ENaC); this reabsorption is increased by aldosterone (the shaded enlarged circle). Net secretion of K^+ occurs through its specific ion channel (rat outer medullary K^+ [ROMK]). Electroneutral reabsorption of Na^+ is shown on the left and an example of electrogenic reabsorption of Na^+ (HCO_3^- or an alkaline luminal pH decreasing the apparent permeability for Cl^- in the CCD) is shown to the right of the dashed vertical line. (From Halperin ML. *The ACID Truth and BASIC Facts—With a Sweet Touch, an enLYTEnment*, 5th ed. Toronto: RossMark Medical Publishers; 2004, with permission.)

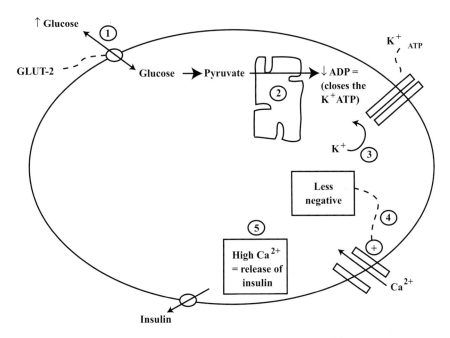

FIGURE 4 Signal system to release insulin from β cells of the pancreas. The large oval represents a β cell of the pancreas. When the $P_{Glucose}$ rises, the intracellular fluid glucose ($ICF_{Glucose}$) rises to the same extent because of the type of glucose transporter (GLUT-2, *site 1*) in these cells. The adenosine diphosphate (ADP) level falls when glucose is oxidized (*site 2*) and this permits K_{ATP} channels to be closed. The ICF compartment becomes less negative when K^+_{ATP} channels close (*site 3*). This opens voltage-gated Ca^{2+} channels and raises the ionized Ca^{2+} concentration in the cytosol (*site 4*). A higher ionized Ca^{2+} in these cells causes the release of insulin (*site 5*).

ICF compartment) are considerably higher than that of its products (Na^+ in the ICF and H^+ in the ECF compartment) in steady state. The two major activators of NHE are insulin (70) and a higher concentration of H^+ in the ICF compartment (22).

Electrogenic Entry of Sodium into Cells The Na^+ channel in cell membranes is normally gated by voltage. When open, one cationic charge enters the cell per Na^+ transported. Since only one third of a charge exits per Na^+ ion pumped via the Na,K-ATPase (Fig. 2), this diminishes

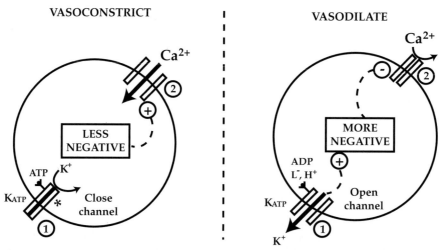

FIGURE 5 Vasomotor tone in vascular smooth muscle cells. The circles represent vascular smooth muscle cells. When the intracellular fluid (ICF) has a less negative voltage because its K^+_{ATP} channel is closed, the voltage-gated Ca^{2+} channel can be maintained in an open configuration permitting a sustained rise in the ICF (Ca^{2+}). Hence there will be vasoconstriction (shown to the left of the dashed vertical line). In contrast, when an increase in blood flow is needed, K^+_{ATP} channels will open because of a high concentration of L-lactate anions (L^-) and H^+. This will lead to a more negative ICF voltage and closure of their voltage-gated Ca^{2+} channels and thereby, vasodilation.

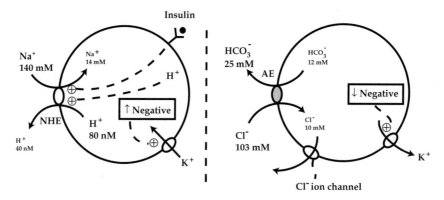

FIGURE 6 Role of Na^+-H^+ exchanger (NHE) and anion exchanger (AE) in the shift of K^+ across cell membranes. The circle represents a cell membrane. NHE and the AE are normally *inactive* in cell membranes. As shown on the left, there are two major activators of NHE, insulin and a higher concentration of H^+ in the intracellular fluid (ICF) compartment. As Na^+ exit via the Na,K-ATPase, the net effect is a more negative intracellular voltage and the entry of K^+ into cells. As shown on the right, HCO^{3-} will be exported and Cl^- will enter cells when the AE is activated. The rise in $[Cl^-]$ in cells allows the intracellular negative voltage to drive the exit of Cl^- ions through their specific Cl^- ion channel. This latter step will lead to the export of negative voltage and the subsequent exit of K^+ from cells.

the degree of intracellular negative voltage that leads to net *exit* of K^+ and hence, a rise in the P_K. This could explain the development of hyperkalemia in patients with hyperkalemic periodic paralysis (36).

HORMONES THAT AFFECT THE DISTRIBUTION OF POTASSIUM

Catecholamines β_2-adrenergic agonists cause a shift of K^+ into cells due to activation of the Na,K-ATPase via a cyclic-AMP–dependent mechanism that phosphorylates this ion pump (19). This leads to the export of pre-existing intracellular Na^+ (Fig. 2). An acute shift of K^+ into cells and hypokalemia

are seen in conditions associated with a surge of catecholamines (e.g., patients with a subarachnoid hemorrhage, myocardial ischemia, and/or an extreme degree of anxiety) (85).

β_2 agonists are used to shift of K^+ into cells in patients with emergency hyperkalemia. Nonspecific ß blockers are being used for therapy of the subtype of hypokalemic periodic paralysis associated with hyperthyroidism (21, 62).

Insulin The effect of insulin to shift K^+ into cells is due primarily to an augmentation of the electroneutral entry of Na^+ into cells via NHE (6, 25, 118). This, in conjunction with stimulating the electrogenic Na,-K-ATPase, causes the voltage in cells to become more negative (Fig. 2). This effect of insulin has been used clinically in the emergency treatment of patients with hyperkalemia. In contrast, a lack of actions of insulin will result in a shift of K^+ out of cells and the development of hyperkalemia in patients with diabetic ketoacidosis despite having a total-body K^+ deficit.

Acid–Base Influences When an acid is added to the body, most of the H^+ are buffered in the ICF compartment (100). Monocarboxylic acids enter cells via a specific transporter. This is an electroneutral process, and it does not cause K^+ to shift out of cells (50). A possible mechanism to explain how K^+ may shift out of cells in other types of metabolic acidosis is illustrated in Fig. 6 (right side). Activation of the Cl^-/HCO_3^- anion exchanger (AE) will cause HCO_3^- to exit cells and Cl^- to enter cells (5). Since cells have Cl^- channels in their membrane (109), the rise in the concentration of Cl^- in the ICF in conjunction with the usual negative voltage forces Cl^- to exit cells. As this exit of Cl^- is electrogenic, it causes a less negative voltage in cells and K^+ will exit from cells (26).

Several clinical implications follow from this analysis. First, if hyperkalemia is present in a patient with metabolic acidosis due to a monocarboxylic organic acid, causes for hyperkalemia other than the acidosis should be sought (e.g., lack of insulin in patients with diabetic ketoacidosis, tissue injury, and a lack of ATP to drive the Na,K-ATPase in patients with L-lactic acidosis due to hypoxia [73]). Second, although inorganic acidosis (addition of HCl) causes a shift of K^+ out of cells, patients with chronic hyperchloremic metabolic acidosis (e.g., patients with chronic diarrhea or renal tubular acidosis [RTA]) usually have a low P_K because of excessive loss of K^+ in the diarrhea fluid (33) or the urine (91).

Respiratory acid-base disorders, on the other hand, cause only small changes in the P_K as there is little movement of Na^+ or Cl^- across cell membranes in these disorders (1, 10).

Tissue Catabolism Hyperkalemia may be seen with crush injury and the tumor lysis syndrome (6). In these patients, factors that compromise the kidney's ability to excrete K^+ are usually present as well. In patients with diabetic ketoacidosis, there is a total-body K^+ depletion (101) but hyperkalemia due to a shift of K^+ from cells secondary to a lack of insulin (118). The corollary is that during therapy, complete replacement of the deficit of K^+ must await the provision of cellular constituents (phosphate, amino acids, magnesium, etc.) and the presence of anabolic signals.

Long-Term Regulation of Potassium Homeostasis

Control of the renal excretion of K^+ maintains overall daily K^+ balance. Although the usual intake of K^+ in adults eating a typical Western diet is close to 1 mmol/kg body weight, the rate of excretion of K^+ can match an intake of more than 200 mmol/day with only a minor rise in the P_K (105).

Control of K^+ secretion occurs primarily in the late distal convoluted tubule, the connecting tubule, and the CCD (39). Two factors influence the rate of excretion of K^+; the flow rate in the terminal CCD (Eq. 1) and the net secretion of K^+ by principal cells in the CCD, which raises the luminal concentration of K^+ ($[K^+]_{CCD}$).

$$K \text{ excretion} = \text{Flow rate}_{CCD} \times [K^+]_{CCD} \quad \text{(Eq. 1)}$$

There is an interplay between the magnitudes of the flow rate in the CCD and the $[K^+]_{CCD}$ that permits the kidney to excrete all the K^+ that was ingested in steady state. The most important setting for this interplay is in a patient who may develop hyperkalemia. For example, if the flow rate in the CCD were to decline (vide infra), each remaining liter would have to have a higher $[K^+]_{CCD}$ in order to excrete this daily K^+ load. This can pose a problem for K^+ homeostasis if there is a large K^+ load to excrete, a limited ability to generate a lumen-negative voltage in the CCD, and/or a diminished number of open ROMK channels in the luminal membrane of principal cells in this nephron segment.

FLOW RATE IN THE CORTICAL COLLECTING DUCT

When vasopressin acts and the late distal nephron is permeable to water, the flow rate in the CCD is determined by the rate of delivery of osmoles because the osmolality of fluid in the terminal CCD is equal to the plasma osmolality (P_{osm}) (Eq. 2). Since vasopressin acts throughout the 24-hour cycle (92), a minimum estimate of the flow rate in the terminal CCD is obtained by dividing the rate of excretion of osmoles by the osmolality of its luminal fluid (or the P_{osm}) (Fig. 7).

While the rate of flow in the CCD is high during a water diuresis, the rate of excretion of K^+ need not be elevated, even when mineralocorticoids act (30), because vasopressin must be present to have high rates of K^+ secretion through ROMK channels (34).

$$\text{Flow rate}_{CCD} = (U_{osm} \times \text{Urine flow rate})/P_{osm} \quad \text{(Eq. 2)}$$

POTASSIUM SECRETION IN THE LUMEN OF THE CORTICAL COLLECTING DUCT

The secretory process for K^+ in principal cells has two elements. First, a lumen-negative voltage must be generated via electrogenic reabsorption of Na^+ by epithelial Na^+ channels (ENaC). Second, open ROMK channels must be present in the luminal membrane of principal cells (4).

Aldosterone actions lead to an increase the activity of ENaC (38). The steps involved include binding of aldosterone to its receptor in the cytoplasm of principal cells, entry of this hormone-receptor complex into the nucleus, and then the synthesis of new proteins including serum and glucocorticoid regulated kinase (SGK) (for review, see [32, 35]). SGK increases the apical membrane expression of ENaC. The mechanism seems to be related to the effect of SGK to phosphorylate the ubiquitin ligase Nedd4-2, which reduces its interaction with ENaC. Inhibition of the Nedd4-2–induced endocytosis of ENaC leads to increased expression of ENaC in the luminal

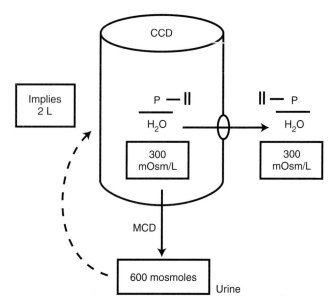

FIGURE 7 Noninvasive estimate of the flow rate in the terminal cortical collecting duct. The barrel-shaped structure represents the cortical collecting duct (CCD). When vasopressin acts, the P_{osm} and the osmolality in the luminal fluid of the terminal CCD are equal (represented as 300 mOsm/kg H_2O for easy math). For example, if 600 mOsm are excreted in a given time, the minimum flow rate to the CCD would be 2 l. (From Halperin ML. *The ACID Truth and BASIC Facts—With a Sweet Touch, an enLYTEnment*, 5th ed. Toronto: RossMark Medical Publishers; 2004, with permission.)

membrane and increased Na^+ transport (104). Another mechanism by which aldosterone activates ENaC involves proteolytic cleavage of the channel by serine proteases. Aldosterone induces production of "channel activating proteases" (CAPs 1–3) (108). These proteases activate ENaC by increasing its open probability, rather than by increasing expression at the cell surface.

Under most circumstances, variations in the luminal Na^+ concentration in the CCD do not regulate the net secretion of K^+ (107). The reabsorption of Na^+ in the CCD can be electroneutral or electrogenic depending on whether Cl^- is reabsorbed as fast as Na^+ (electroneutral) or slower than Na^+ (electrogenic) (Fig. 3). The pathway(s) for the reabsorption of Cl^- in the CCD is(are) not well defined, but it is likely that paracellular pathways play an important role (98, 115). The concentration of HCO_3^- and/or an alkaline luminal fluid pH seem to increase the activity of K^+ secretion in the CCD. Although the mechanism has not been fully validated, it was suggested that this may be due to a decrease in the apparent permeability of Cl^- (16) and/or an increase in ROMK open probability in this nephron segment. If Na^+ is not reabsorbed faster than Cl^- in the CCD, an appreciably lumen-negative voltage cannot develop (115, 117). The hyperkalemia in patients with type II pseudohypoaldosteronism (Gordon syndrome) may be an example for this pathophysiology. Two factors are important to achieve this near-equal rate of ion transport in the CCD (Fig. 8, right panel). First, low delivery of Na^+ and Cl^- to the CCD occurs because the reabsorption of Na^+ and Cl^- was augmented in the distal convoluted tubule

because of increased activity of Na^+-Cl^- cotransporter (NCC) (115). Second, ECF volume expansion suppresses the release of aldosterone; this leads to less open ENaC. Hence the rate of reabsorption of Cl^- in the CCD may match that of Na^+.

Dietary K^+ intake is an important regulator of ROMK channels. Low K^+ intake decreases, whereas a high K^+ intake increases the number of ROMK channels in the luminal membrane of principal cells (for review, see [111]). Several lines of evidence suggest that protein tyrosine kinase mediates the effect of low K^+ intake on ROMK channels (60). K^+ depletion increases the expression and activity of protein tyrosine kinase and tyrosine phosphorylation of ROMK channels results in their endocytosis. K^+ channels are abundant and have a high open probability on a potassium-rich diet (77, 78). In rats ROMK channels do not seem to be rate limiting for net secretion of K^+ unless the P_K falls to the mid–3-mM range (17).

CLINICAL TOOLS TO ASSESS THE CONTROL OF THE RENAL EXCRETION OF POTASSIUM

Examine the Rate of Excretion of Potassium

There is no normal rate of K^+ excretion. Healthy subjects in steady state excrete all the K^+ they eat and absorb from the gastrointestinal (GI) tract. Therefore we use the expected rate of K^+ excretion in healthy subjects who were given a K^+ load to assess the renal response in a patient with hyperkalemia. They can augment the rate of excretion of K^+ to greater than 200 mmol/day, which was achieved with only a minor increase in P_K (101, 105). Therefore, a patient with chronic hyperkalemia and a rate of excretion of K^+ that is higher than the "usual" but less than 200 mmol/day has a defect in renal K^+ excretion; in addition, a higher rate of K^+ intake is contributing to the degree of hyperkalemia in this patient.

To assess the rate of excretion of K^+, a 24-hour urine collection is not necessary. One can use the ratio of the concentrations of K^+ and creatinine in a spot urine sample ($U_K/U_{Creatinine}$) despite the diurnal variation in K^+ excretion (96). This analysis is predicated on the fact that creatinine is excreted at a near-constant rate throughout the day (20). Moreover, a $U_K/U_{Creatinine}$ in a spot urine provides more relevant information because the stimulus to drive K^+ excretion (e.g., P_K) can be known at that time. The expected value in a patient with hyperkalemia is > 15 mmol K^+/mmol creatinine (> 150 mmol K^+/g creatinine).

Estimate the Flow Rate in the Terminal Cortical Collecting Duct

As discussed previously, the flow rate in the terminal CCD is directly proportional to the number of osmoles delivered to the terminal CCD (Fig. 7; Eq. 2). For example, in the time period during which 300 mOsm were excreted, at least 1 l of fluid traversed the terminal CCD because the osmolality of fluid in the terminal CCD is close to 300 mOsm/

Usual delivery of Na & Cl to CCD | Cl approximateses Na reabsorption in the CCD

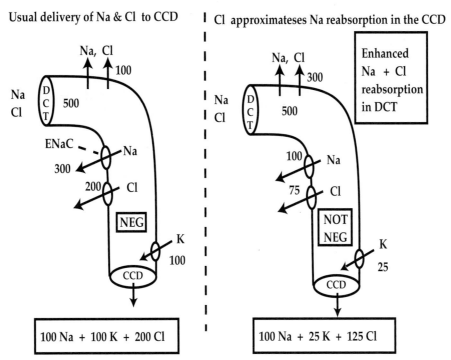

FIGURE 8 Secretion of K^+ in the cortical collecting duct. The early portion structure represents the distal convoluted tubule (DCT) and the lower part represents the cortical collecting duct (CCD); the numbers are provided for illustrative purposes only. Under normal conditions (shown to the left of the vertical line), Na^+ is reabsorbed faster than Cl^-, which creates a negative luminal voltage and thereby provides the driving force to secrete all ingested K^+. As shown in the right portion of the figure, a low delivery of Na^+ and Cl^- to the CCD has occurred, but hyperkalemia has not yet developed. In this setting, the reabsorption of NaCl is stimulated in the DCT. Accordingly, Na^+ and Cl^- can only be reabsorbed at near-equivalent rates because there is a lower ENaC activity due to ECFV expansion, which suppresses the release of aldosterone, and as a result, a lumen-negative voltage cannot be generated.

kg H_2O (equal to the P_{osm}). Because most people excrete at least iso-osmolar urine over virtually the entire 24-hour period (92), the rate of excretion of osmoles provides a minimum estimate of the flow rate in the terminal CCD.

The "usual" rate of osmole excretion is close to 0.5 mOsm/min or 720 mOsm/day. The major osmoles in the terminal CCD are urea and Na^+ plus Cl^- which are present in equi-osmolar amounts. A low flow rate in the terminal CCD could be due to a low rate of delivery of urea (low intake of proteins) and/or of Na^+ and Cl^- (low effective circulating volume, low intake of salt).

Estimate the $[K^+]_{CCD}$

A reasonable approximation of the $[K^+]_{CCD}$ can be obtained by adjusting the U_K for the amount of water reabsorbed in the medullary collecting duct. This is done by dividing the U_K by the $(U/P)_{osm}$ (the P_{osm} equals the osmolality of the fluid in the terminal CCD when vasopressin acts) (Fig. 7) (Eq. 3). The assumption here (reasonable in most circumstances) is that only a small proportion of K^+ delivered to the medullary collecting duct was secreted or reabsorbed in this nephron segment (7).

$$[K^+]_{CCD} = [K^+]_{urine}/(U/P)_{osm} \quad \text{(Eq. 3)}$$

TRANSTUBULAR POTASSIUM GRADIENT

To calculate the transtubular potassium gradient (TTKG), divide the $[K^+]_{CCD}$ by the P_K (Fig. 9; Eq. 4). Although a number of assumptions are made in the calculation of the TTKG, it provides a reasonable semiquantitative reflection of the driving force for K^+ secretion in the terminal CCD. The expected value for the TTKG in a healthy subject given a K^+ load is above 7 (31).

$$TTKG = [K^+]_{CCD}/P_K \quad \text{(Eq. 4)}$$

ESTABLISH THE BASIS FOR THE ABNORMAL $[K^+]_{CCD}$

There are two bases for a low value for the $[K^+]_{CCD}$ in a patient with hyperkalemia. First, even if a lumen-negative voltage could be generated, the secretion of K^+ might still be low if there were too few ROMK channels with a high open probability in the luminal membrane of the CCD. Although no diseases have been directly attributed to this pathophysiology, we must still include it in the differential diagnosis of a lower than expected $[K^+]_{CCD}$.

The most common explanation for a lower-than-expected $[K^+]_{CCD}$ is a less negative voltage in the lumen of the CCD due to a lower electrogenic reabsorption of Na^+ in the CCD (Fig. 3). There are two main causes for this low lumen-negative voltage. In the first, there is a

Potassium issues   Water issues

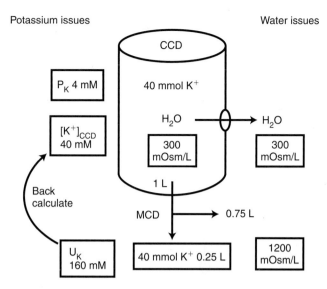

FIGURE 9 The transtubular K⁺ concentration gradient. The barrel-shaped structure represents the cortical collecting duct (CCD) and the arrow below the CCD is the medullary collecting duct (MCD). In this example, the luminal K⁺ concentration is 40 mM or 10-fold larger than the peritubular K⁺ concentration of 4 mM. Consider what happens when 1 L of fluid traverses the MCD where 75% of the water is reabsorbed. In this example, no K⁺ is reabsorbed or secreted in the MCD. Therefore the concentration of K⁺ in a spot urine sample (U_K) is fourfold higher (40–160 mM) as is the U_{osm} (300–1200 mOsm/kg H_2O). This should be taken into account in assessing the U_K. (From Halperin ML. *The ACID Truth and BASIC Facts—With a Sweet Touch, an enLYTEnment*, 5th ed. Toronto: RossMark Medical Publishers; 2004, with permission.)

slower rate of Na⁺ reabsorption of Na⁺ in the CCD. The basis for this defect is a low quantity of ENaC in the luminal membrane (e.g., adrenal insufficiency, blockers of the aldosterone receptor in principal cells), molecular defects diminishing the number of ENaC units in the luminal membrane of the CCD, or the presence of cationic compounds in the lumen of the CCD that block ENaC (e.g., K⁺-sparing diuretics or trimethoprim). These patients will have a low ECF volume and an inappropriately higher-than-expected rate of excretion of Na⁺ and Cl⁻ in this setting.

The second category includes disorders that lead to a rate of reabsorption of Cl⁻ that matches that of Na⁺ in the CCD. This may be due to an increased permeability for Cl⁻ in the CCD, the so-called Cl⁻-shunt disorder (87). On the other hand, the site of the lesion might be in the distal convoluted tubule where there is an enhanced electroneutral reabsorption of Na⁺ and Cl⁻ via a Na⁺-Cl⁻ cotransporter (NCC). In this latter setting, the delivery of Na⁺ and Cl⁻ to the CCD will not be sufficiently large to permit the rate of reabsorption of Na⁺ to appreciably exceed the rate of reabsorption of Cl⁻ in the CCD (Fig. 8, left side). In addition, the activity may be lower due to a reduced level of aldosterone caused by the expanded ECF volume. Independent of the site of the lesion, these patients will have an expanded ECF volume and a very low plasma renin activity, but they will retain the ability to excrete Na⁺ and Cl⁻-poor urine

when the ECF volume is contracted (e.g., after giving a diuretic plus a low-salt diet).

CLINICAL APPROACH TO THE PATIENT WITH HYPERKALEMIA

It is imperative to recognize when hyperkalemia represents a medical emergency because therapy must take precedence over diagnosis. A step-by-step approach to diagnosis of hyperkalemia is illustrated in Flow Chart 1 where the emphasis is to seek answers to the following questions.

Are There Laboratory or Technical Problems?

Hemolysis, megakaryocytosis, fragile tumor cells, a K⁺ channel disorder in red blood cells (47), and excessive fist-clenching during blood sampling (28) should be excluded. Pseudohyperkalemia can be present in cachectic patients because the normal T-tubule architecture in skeletal muscle may be disturbed. This permits more K⁺ to be released into venous blood, even without excessive fist-clenching during blood sampling. The presence of electrocardiogram (ECG) changes due to hyperkalemia means that this electrolyte disorder is electrically important, even if there are reasons for pseudohyperkalemia.

Is Hyperkalemia Acute and/or Is Potassium Intake Very Low?

If the answer is yes, there is a shift of K⁺ out of cells, proceed to an analysis of factors that could destroy cells or decrease the magnitude of the intracellular negative voltage (86). If hyperkalemia was mainly due to a shift of K⁺ out of cells (e.g., patients with disorders leading to low insulin levels, patients with hyperkalemic periodic paralysis, and hyperkalemia due to exhaustive exercise), aggressive measures to remove a large quantity of K⁺ from the body (e.g., dialysis) should not be undertaken. Rather, if there are alarming changes in the ECG, the emphasis for therapy is to antagonize the electrical effects of a high P_K, increase the magnitude of the intracellular negative voltage to induce a shift of K⁺ into cells, and excrete just enough K⁺ to minimize the cardiac risk.

What Is the Rate of Potassium Excretion?

If the urinary excretion of K⁺ is considerably less than 200 mmol/day or less than 15 mmol K⁺/mmol creatinine (<150 mmol K⁺/g creatinine), it is inappropriately low in the presence of hyperkalemia and its basis should be examined by asking the following questions (Flow Chart 2).

What Is the Reason for the Low Potassium Excretion?

The two components of the K⁺ excretion formula need to be interpreted in terms of events in the terminal CCD (Eq. 1).

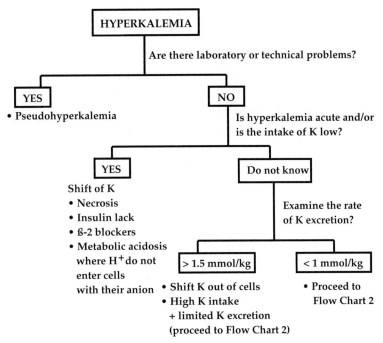

FLOW CHART 1   Initial steps in the patient with hyperkalemia. The steps are illustrated and the final diagnostic categories are preceded by a bullet symbol. In the absence of an emergency that demands urgent therapy, proceed with this diagnostic algorithm. Rates of K^+ excretion are in mmol/kg body weight/day. (From Halperin ML. *The ACID Truth and BASIC Facts—With a Sweet Touch, an enLYTEnment*, 5th ed. Toronto: RossMark Medical Publishers, 2004, with permission.)

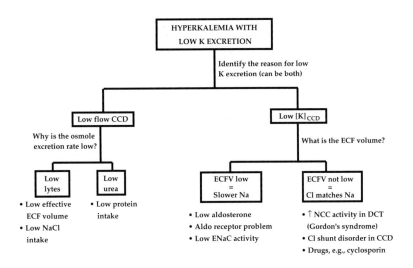

FLOW CHART 2   Renal causes for hyperkalemia and a low rate of excretion of potassium. For details, see text. Lytes, electrolytes. (From Halperin ML. *The ACID Truth and BASIC Facts—With a Sweet Touch, an enLYTEnment*, 5th ed. Toronto: RossMark Medical Publishers; 2004, with permission.)

IS THE FLOW RATE IN THE TERMINAL CORTICAL COLLECTING DUCT LOW?

This can be examined when vasopressin is acting ($U_{osm} > P_{osm}$) by determining the osmole excretion rate (Eq. 3). The usual rate of excretion of osmoles is close to 0.5 mOsm/min. A low rate of excretion of osmoles could be due to a low rate of excretion of NaCl and/or urea.

WHY IS THE $[K^+]_{CCD}$ ABNORMALLY LOW?

Seek the basis for a diminished negative luminal voltage in the CCD: disorders that cause the reabsorption of Na^+ to be particularly low in this nephron segment or disorders that lead to a rate of reabsorption of Cl^- that does not differ appreciably in magnitude from that of Na^+ in this location (Fig. 8, right side).

SLOWER SODIUM TYPE OF LESION

These patients have a low effective ECF volume that may be obvious clinically or by finding a high plasma renin activity. Notwithstanding the plasma renin activity will be low in the presence of a low ECF volume in patients with a defect in renin release from the juxtaglomerular apparatus. If the concentration of Na^+ in the urine (U_{Na}) is not very low in a patient with a low effective ECF volume, a renal defect in the reabsorption of Na^+ is present. A slower Na^+-type of defect due to a low level of aldosterone in plasma is suspected if there is a rise in the $[K^+]_{CCD}$ about 2 hours after the administration of a physiologic equivalent dose of an exogenous mineralocorticoid (100 μg of fludrocortisone). In addition, the U_{Na} and concentration of Cl^- in the urine (U_{Cl}) should fall to very low values. This diagnosis is confirmed by measuring the concentration of aldosterone in plasma.

On the other hand, if the patient did not respond to exogenous mineralocorticoids, the presumptive diagnosis would be a slower Na^+ lesion that is due to blockade of the aldosterone receptor (e.g., drugs such as spironolactone) or a reduced activity of ENaC in principal cells (blockade by cationic drugs such as amiloride or trimethoprim, or an inherited disorder such as type I pseudohypoaldosteronism).

CHLORIDE IS REABSORBED AT A SIMILAR RATE TO SODIUM IN THE CORTICAL COLLECTING DUCT

One probable mechanism is a reduced delivery of Na^+ and Cl^- to the CCD because of excessive reabsorption of Na^+ and Cl^- in the distal convoluted tubule (117). The ECF volume should be high, plasma renin activity low, and the concentration of aldosterone in plasma low considering that hyperkalemia is present. The patients with this disorder exhibit an unusually large fall in blood pressure when thiazide diuretics are given (65). A rise in $[K^+]_{CCD}$ is expected under conditions of increased Na^+ and Cl^- delivery to the CCD along with open ENaC.

The disorder in some patients may be due to an increased permeability for Cl^- in the CCD (Cl^--shunt disorder [87]). The clinical picture is similar to that described in the paragraph above. A rise in the $[K^+]_{CCD}$ with the induction of bicarbonaturia (but not with the administration of exogenous mineralocorticoids alone) supports this diagnosis.

SPECIFIC CAUSES OF HYPERKALEMIA

A list of the causes of hyperkalemia based on their possible underlying pathophysiology is provided in Table 1 and a list of drugs that may cause hyperkalemia is shown in Table 2.

Chronic Renal Insufficiency

Hyperkalemia occurs frequently in patients with advanced, chronic kidney disease and it is due to a diminished ability to excrete K^+. Applying the principles of physiology outlined earlier in this chapter [K^+ exiting the CCD = (Flow rate)$_{CCD}$

TABLE 1 Causes of Hyperkalemia

- High intake of K^+
  - Only if combined with low excretion of K^+
- Shift of K^+ out of cells
  - Cell necrosis
  - Lack of insulin
  - Use of nonselective β blockers (small effect if only factor)
  - Metabolic acidosis where the anion is largely restricted to the ECF compartment
  - Rare causes (e.g., hyperkalemic periodic paralysis)
- Diminished K^+ loss in the urine
  - Low flow rate in CCD (low osmole excretion rate)
  - Low $[K^+]_{CCD}$ (diminished electrogenic reabsorption of Na^+ in the CCD)
  - Primary decrease in flux of Na^+ through ENaC
  - Very low delivery of Na^+ to the CCD
  - Low levels of aldosterone (e.g., Addison disease)
  - Blockade of the aldosterone receptor (e.g., spironolactone)
- Low ENaC activity (type I pesudohypoaldosteronism)
- Blockade of ENaC (e.g., amiloride, triamterene, trimethoprim)
  - Cl^- reabsorbed at a similar rate as Na^+
  - Increased reabsorption of Na^+ and Cl^- in the distal convoluted tubule (e.g., Gordon syndrome [WNK kinase-4 and/or kinase-1 mutations])
  - Possible Cl^- shunt in the CCD (e.g., some of the causes of hyporeninemic hypoalosteronism, diabetic nephropathy, drugs, e.g., cyclosporin)

CCD, cortical collecting duct; ECF, extracellular fluid; ENaC, epithelial Na^+ channel.

× $[K^+]_{CCD}$], there are two major reasons that lead to a diminished rate of excretion of K^+. First, a low flow rate in the CCD, which depends primarily on the diet of an individual patient with this chronic condition rather than on the glomerular filtration rate (GFR) per se. In more detail, because the flow rate in the terminal CCD is directly related to the rate of excretion of osmoles when vasopressin acts (96), this low flow rate is due to a diminished rate of excretion of the

TABLE 2 Drugs That Can Cause Hyperkalemia

- Drugs containing potassium (only increase P_K if K^+ excretion is compromised)
  - KCl, table salt substitutes
- **Drugs causing a K shift from ICF to ECF**
  - Drug causing depolarization such as succinylcholine
  - Drugs causing cell necrosis such as chemotherapy causing tumor lysis
  - Drugs impairing insulin release from β cells such as α-adrenergic agonists
  - $β_2$-adrenergic receptor blockers
- **Drugs that interfere with K excretion in the urine**
  - Drugs that cause acute renal failure or interstitial nephritis
  - Drugs that inhibit the release of aldosterone (e.g., heparin)
  - Drugs that interfere with the renin-angiotensin II axis (e.g., angistensin II converting enzyme inhibitors and angiotensin II receptor blockers)
  - Aldosterone receptor blockers (e.g., spironolactone)
  - Drugs that block ENaC in the CCD (e.g., amiloride, trimethopim)
  - Drugs the interfere with activation of ENaC via proteolytic cleavage (e.g., nafamostat mesylate)

CCD, cortical collecting duct; ECF, extracellular fluid; ENaC, epithelial Na^+ channel; ICF, intracellular fluid.

two major urine osmoles, urea (low-protein diet) and Na^+ plus Cl^- (salt-restricted diet). Second, to have the same rate of K^+ excretion when the flow rate in the CCD is decreased, each liter traversing the CCD must have a higher $[K^+]_{CCD}$. Two factors contribute to the inability to raise the $[K^+]_{CCD}$ in this setting. Although the flow rate in the CCD may only be modestly decreased, there is a very large reduction in the number of residual CCD segments in this group of patients. Hence the flow rate through each remaining CCD segment will be very high. When the flow rate per CCD is high, the ability to reabsorb Na^+ much faster than Cl^- in the CCD is diminished and the lumen-negative voltage will not be high enough to raise the $[K^+]_{CCD}$ sufficiently. This limited capacity to excrete K^+ will be much worse when the intake of K^+ is particularly high due to an excessive intake of salt substitutes that contain KCl or the ingestion of a large volume of fruit juice (71). In addition, these patients may be taking drugs that compromise the ability to secrete K^+ in the CCD. Prominent on the list are drugs that diminish the secretion of aldosterone (angiotensin-converting enzyme [ACE] inhibitors or angiotensin II receptor blockers) and aldosterone receptor blockers (e.g., spironolactone).

Addison's Disease

The most common cause of this disorder used to be bilateral adrenal destruction due to tuberculosis, but now autoimmune adrenalitis accounts for most cases (74). Additional causes include other infectious diseases (disseminated fungal infection), adrenal replacement by metastatic carcinoma or lymphoma, adrenal hemorrhage or infarction.

Patients with chronic primary adrenal insufficiency may have chronic malaise, fatigue, anorexia, generalized weakness, and weight loss. Salt craving is a distinctive feature in certain patients. Hyperpigmentation is evident in nearly all patients. In most patients, the blood pressure is low and postural symptoms of dizziness and syncope are common. The P_K is usually close to 5.5 mM unless a significant degree of intravascular volume depletion diminishes the flow rate in CCD. Nevertheless, hyperkalemia is not seen on presentation in approximately one third of the cases (reviewed in [37]). Other possible abnormal laboratory findings include hyponatremia, hyperchloremic metabolic acidosis, hypoglycemia, and eosinophilia. Some patients may present with acute adrenal crisis and shock.

The diagnosis can be established by finding low plasma aldosterone and cortisol levels, high plasma renin activity, and a blunted cortisol response to the administration of adrenocorticotrophic hormone (ACTH). Adrenal crisis is an emergency that requires immediate restoration of the intravascular volume (intravenous saline) and correction of the cortisol deficiency (administer dexamethasone or hydrocortisone). Beware of raising the P_{Na} too rapidly if hyponatremia is present because of the risk of osmotic demyelination in a catabolic patient (reviewed in [61]) and because administration of cortisol can lead, indirectly, to a

fall in the circulating level of vasopressin (84). Therefore we prefer to give 1-desamino-8-D-arginine vasopressin (dDAVP) at the outset of intravenous therapy to avoid a large water diuresis that could result in a sudden and excessive rise in the P_{Na} with the development of the osmotic demyelination syndrome.

Patients with chronic adrenal insufficiency should receive replacement therapy with both a glucocorticoid and a mineralocorticoid. For the former, 25 mg of hydrocortisone (15 mg in the morning and 10 mg in the afternoon) is usually given. For mineralocorticoid replacement, fludrocortisone in a single dose of 50 to 200 μg is usually used. Dose adjustments are made based on patients' symptoms, ECF volume status, blood pressure measurements and P_K.

Hyperkalemia Due to Inherited Disorders of Aldosterone Biosynthesis

The inherited enzyme deficiencies involved in aldosterone biosynthesis include 21-hydroxylase, 3-hydroxysteroid dehydrogenase, cholesterol desmolase, and aldosterone synthetase deficiencies. Except for aldosterone synthetase deficiency, the other three disorders (also called congenital adrenal hyperplasia) are combined with glucocorticoid deficiency because the cortisol biosynthesis is also affected in these three disorders (112). Salt wasting, hyponatremia, hyperkalemia, and hypotension are common features. 21-hydrolyase deficiency is the most common and more easily recognized in affected females who usually have masculine-type genitalia at birth due to excess secretion of fetal adrenal androgen. The diagnosis is confirmed by the finding of an elevated serum 17-hydroxyprogesterone, the substrate for the absent enzyme. Patients with 3-hydroxysteroid dehydrogenase and cholesterol desmolase deficiencies usually have the signs of sex steroid deficiency and are distinguishable from the androgen excess in 21-hydrolyase deficiency. In aldosterone synthetase defects, aldosterone synthesis is decreased but corticosterone secretion is enhanced and its serum concentration is elevated. Aldosterone synthetase defect can be divided into two types: type I corticosterone methyl oxidase (COM-I) defect and type II corticosterone methyl oxidase (COMI-I) defect (113). Serum 18-hydroxycorticosterone is deficient in patients with COM-I defect, but increased in COMI-I defect.

Pseudohypoaldosteronism Type I

The underlying pathophysiology is a "closed" ENaC in the CCD (Fig. 10). There are two different forms of this disorder with different modes of inheritance.

AUTOSOMAL RECESSIVE FORM

Most mutations are frame-shift or premature stop codon defects in the α subunit of ENaC (88). Clinically, the disease is permanent and involves all aldosterone target organs. Patients usually present in the neonatal period with renal salt

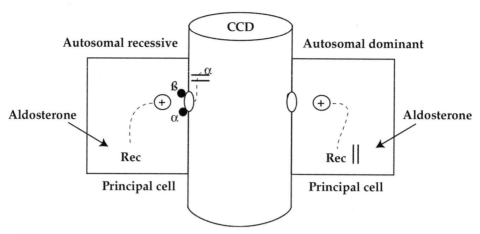

FIGURE 10   Molecular basis of pseudohypoaldosteronism type I. For details, see text. The site of the lesion is in the α subunit of epithelial Na⁺ channel (ENaC) in the autosomal recessive form of the disorder (shown in the cell on the left). This leads to an absence of the Na⁺ channel per se. In contrast, the molecular defect is in the aldosterone receptor (Rec) in the autosomal dominant defect (shown in the cell on the right). (From Halperin ML. *The ACID Truth and BASIC Facts—With a Sweet Touch, an enLYTEnment*, 5th ed. Toronto: RossMark Medical Publishers, 2004, with permission.)

wasting, hyperkalemia, metabolic acidosis, failure to thrive, and weight loss. ENaC activity is also impaired in the lung, and this leads to excessive airway fluid and lower respiratory tract infections.

AUTOSOMAL DOMINANT FORM

This is due to mutations involving the mineralocorticoid receptor (13). The clinical disorder is usually mild and may remit with time. Patients fail to respond to exogenous mineralocorticoids and their plasma aldosterone levels and plasma renin activity are markedly elevated. Treatment includes supplementation with NaCl and inducing the loss of K^+ through the GI tract. Dialysis may be required for treatment of life-threatening hyperkalemia.

Syndrome of Hyporeninemic Hypoaldosteronism

Patients in this arbitrary diagnostic category represent a heterogeneous group with regard to the pathophysiology of their disorder.

GROUP WITH LOW CAPABILITY OF PRODUCING RENIN

The basis of this group of disorders may be destruction of, or a biosynthetic defect in the juxtaglomerular apparatus, which leads to hyporeninemia and thereby to a low plasma aldosterone level. Accordingly, there is a relatively "slower" reabsorption of Na^+ in the CCD. Hyperkalemia will develop if there is a sufficiently large intake of K^+ such that a rise in the P_K must be present to permit the kidneys to excrete this K^+ load at the appropriate rate because of the chronic low aldosterone levels. The ECF volume will tend to be low with clinical features that were described earlier. Patients with this disorder are expected to have a significant rise in their $[K^+]_{CCD}$ with the administration of exogenous mineralocorticoids.

GROUP WITH LOW STIMULUS TO PRODUCE RENIN

There are two subtypes in this group of patients. The first has an enhanced reabsorption of Na^+ and Cl^- in the distal convoluted tubule due to an abnormal regulation of the signal system that affects the distribution of the Na^+-Cl^- cotransporter (NCC) which leads to more active units in the luminal membrane (115); it is discussed in the section on pseudohypoaldosteronism type II. This enhanced upstream reabsorption of Na^+ and Cl^- results in a low delivery of Na^+ and Cl^- to the CCD, which compromises the ability of this nephron segment to reabsorb Na^+ faster than Cl^-, and thereby leads to a diminished excretory capacity for K^+. ECF volume expansion is a hallmark of the pathophysiology and it results in hyporeninemia and thus a lower-than-expected plasma aldosterone level given the hyperkalemia. Accordingly, these patients do not have an appreciable rise in their $[K^+]_{CCD}$ with exogenous mineralocorticoids, but their $[K^+]_{CCD}$ should rise when thiazide diuretics are given (higher Na^+ and Cl^- delivery to the CCD) if ENaCs are open.

The second subtype in this group of patients has similar clinical findings to those described previously, but there is no known molecular lesion. This syndrome is most commonly seen in patients with diabetic nephropathy. The basis of the disorder remains to be established. It is possible that the reabsorption of Na^+ and Cl^- may be augmented in the distal convoluted tubule or these patients may have a "Cl shunt" disorder in the CCD (53, 80, 87). Patients with a Cl^- shunt have a significant increase in their $[K^+]_{CCD}$ with the induction of bicarbonaturia (inhibition of the reabsorption of Cl^- in the CCD) (52).

Differentiation between these two groups of patients with hyporeninemic hypoaldosteronism has implications for therapy. The use of exogenous mineralocorticoids (9 α-fludrocortisone) is of benefit for the group of patients who cannot produce enough renin as it results in kaliuresis and re-expansion of the ECF volume due to retention of Na^+. Diuretic therapy poses a threat to these patients because it would cause a more severe ECF volume contraction. In the group with a low stimulus to produce renin due to an expanded ECF volume, mineralcorticoids may aggravate the degree of hypertension. In the subgroup of patients with an increased activity of NCC, the administration of a thiazide diuretic should enhance the kaliuresis and lower the blood pressure. In the subgroup with a Cl^- shunt, the administration of diuretics might help lower blood pressure and increase rate of K^+ by increasing the flow rate in the CCD. The activity of K^+ secretion may be increased by bicarbonaturia; HCO_3^- loss may have to be replaced to avoid the development of metabolic acidosis.

Pseudohypoaldosteronism Type II (Gordon Syndrome)

The term "pseudohypoaldosteronism type II" is misleading from a physiologic perspective because patients with this syndrome have salt retention and hypertension, findings associated with more rather than less aldosterone activity.

The basis for increased reabsorption of Na^+ and Cl^- in the distal convoluted tubule in this disorder has been clarified recently (115). Major deletions in the genes encoding for WNK kinase-1 and WNK kinase-4 (WNK stands for with no lysine [K is the abbreviation for lysine]) were reported in these patients. Both of these kinases are found in the distal convoluted tubule and in the CCD. WNK kinase-1 is cytoplasmic, whereas WNK kinase-4 is present primarily in tight junctions in the distal convoluted tubule and in the cytoplasm and tight junctions in the CCD. WNK kinase-4 normally causes a decrease in luminal NCC activity (Fig. 11) (117). Therefore, if WNK kinase-4 were deleted, reabsorption of Na^+ and Cl^- by NCC in the distal convoluted tubule will be augmented.

The role of WNK kinase-1 is to inactivate WNK kinase-4. As a result, there will be more NCC units located in the luminal membrane of the distal convoluted tubule. The molecular defect in WNK kinase-1 is a removal of intron bases that leads to its activation (gain of function).

The higher activity of the thiazide-sensitive NCC observed by Yang et al. (117) could explain the hypertension, hyperkalemia, and suppressed plasma renin activity that are common features in this disorder. Because angiotensin II levels are low, the release of aldosterone is decreased and plasma aldosterone levels are inappropriately low with hyperkalemia. This, together with decreased delivery of Na^+ and Cl^- to the CCD permits Cl^- reabsorption to match that of Na^+ (diminished ENaC activity due to the low aldosterone). The overall result is to cause low luminal negative voltage in the CCD and the development of hyperkalemia. The increased NCC activity in these patients accounts for the marked fall in blood pressure in these patients treated with thiazide diuretics (65).

WNK4 Effect; Less NCC   **WNK1 Effect; More NCC**

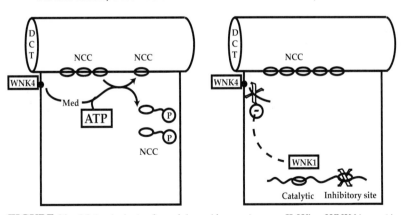

FIGURE 11 Molecular basis of pseudohypoaldosteronism type II. When WNK kinase-4 is active, a message is delivered by an unknown mediator (Med) to decrease the number of active Na^+-Cl^- cotransporter (NCC) units in the luminal membrane of the distal convoluted tubule. As a result, reabsorption of Na^+ and Cl^- is diminished (a thiazide-like effect, left portion of the figure). As shown in the right portion of the figure, mutations in the gene encoding for WNK kinase-4 that *decrease* its activity should lead to more active NCC units in the luminal membrane of this nephron segment and thereby more NaCl reabsorption in the distal convoluted tubule (Gordon syndrome). When WNK kinase-1 is active, it leads to inhibition of WNK kinase-4. Mutations in the gene encoding for WNK kinase-1 cause a major deletion of its inhibitory region and this leads to *gain* of function, so WNK kinase-4 is inhibited. As a result, there is an enhanced NCC activity, which diminishes the rate of electrogenic reabsorption of Na^+ in the CCD. (From Halperin ML. *The ACID Truth and BASIC Facts—With a Sweet Touch, an enLYTEnment*, 5th ed. Toronto: RossMark Medical Publishers; 2004, with permission.)

Hyperkalemic Periodic Paralysis

This syndrome has an autosomal dominant inheritance and is the result of a mutation in the gene encoding for the α–subunit of the skeletal muscle tetrodotoxin sensitive Na^+ channel (36). When the muscle is stimulated to contract, Na^+ influx depolarizes the cell. As the resting membrane potential approaches -50 mV, normal Na^+ channels close. In patients with hyperkalemic periodic paralysis, these defective Na^+ channels fail to close, causing the cells to have less negative resting membrane potential. Depending on the absolute voltage, lesser changes may result in myotonia, while larger changes can cause paralysis. Treatment of the acute attack is with measures to cause K^+ to shift into cells. Excessive excretion of K^+ should be avoided. Acetozolamide seems to be effective, though its mechanism of action is not clear.

Drugs Associated with Hyperkalemia

With respect to many of the drugs that are associated with hyperkalemia, the mechanisms for the defect in K^+ excretion have not been studied in sufficient detail to draw unequivocal conclusions about how each agent causes hyperkalemia in a given patient. This assessment requires measurement of the rate of excretion of K^+ and its two components in terms of events in the CCD. The cause of an inappropriately low $[K^+]_{CCD}$ is further examined with an assessment of the ECF volume (measure the U_{Na} and U_{Cl} and the renin activity and aldosterone levels in plasma), the response to physiological doses of exogenous mineralocorticoids [expect a rise in the $[K^+]_{CCD}$ if the defect is one of low aldosterone] as well as the response to increasing the flow rate in the CCD with the administration of a diuretic [expect a rise in the $[K^+]_{CCD}$ if the defect is one of a Cl^- shunt disorder]. It is possible that this information could lead to more specific modes of therapy in individual patients.

In general, drugs that cause hyperkalemia can be classified into those that affect the shift of K^+ into cells and those that impair its the renal excretion.

DRUGS THAT AFFECT CELLULAR REDISTRIBUTION OF POTASSIUM

Nonselective β-adrenergic blockers may diminish the $β_2$-adrenergic mediated shift of K^+ into cells (24). In general, only a minor rise in the P_K is observed. Nevertheless, more significant degrees of hyperkalemia may develop after vigorous exercise (114) or if there is an underlying disease or the intake of drugs that may impair the excretion of K^+ by the kidney.

Digitalis overdose may be accompanied by hyperkalemia as a result of the inhibition of the Na,K-ATPase pump (95, 116). The use of depolarizing agents such as succinylcholine during anesthesia may cause a shift of K^+ from cells and cause hyperkalemia (41). Arginine hydrochloride used in the treatment of hepatic coma and severe metabolic alkalosis (14, 27) and ε-aminocaproic acid (79), a synthetic amino acid structurally similar to lysine and arginine used to treat severe hemorrhage also causes an efflux of K^+ from cells, resulting in life-threatening hyperkalemia, especially in patients with impaired renal function.

· Impaired K^+ redistribution via the activation of K^+ channel by fluoride poisoning (9, 66) leads to life-threatening hyperkalemia and may be ameliorated by the administration of quinidine and amidarone (99).

DRUGS THAT INTERFERE WITH RENAL POTASSIUM EXCRETION

Drugs That Inhibit the Release of Renin; Nonsteroidal Anti-inflammatory Drugs and COX-2 Inhibitors Secretion of renin by cells in the afferent glomerular arterioles and by cells of the macula densa in the early distal tubule appears to be mediated in part by locally produced prostaglandins (46). As a result, prostaglandin synthesis inhibition can lead to low plasma renin activity and low levels of aldosterone in plasma. COX-2 inhibitors produce identical effects. The rise in the P_K is very small in healthy subjects, but a significant degree of hyperkalemia may develop in the presence of certain diseases or with the intake of drugs that may impair the renal excretion of K^+.

DRUGS THAT INTERFERE WITH THE RENIN-ANGIOTENSIN-ALDOSTERONE AXIS

ACE Inhibitors and Angiotensin II Receptor Blockers The two major stimuli for the release of aldosterone are angiotensin II and an increase in the P_K. The effect of hyperkalemia to stimulate the release of aldosterone acts in concert with angiotensin II that is generated locally within the adrenal glomerulosa (56). Blocking both of these actions with an ACE inhibitor is expected to reduce aldosterone secretion and thereby impair the renal excretion of K^+. Of note, however, aldosterone levels are not fully suppressed in patients on chronic therapy with ACE inhibitors (102). Furthermore, there are no reported studies that examined the effect of exogenous mineralocorticiods on the renal excretion of K^+ in patients who develop hyperkalemia while on ACE inhibitors. While it is estimated that the overall incidence of hyperkalemia is approximately 10% in patients taking this class of drugs (76), the rise in the P_K is less than 0.5 mEq/l in patients with relatively normal renal function. In contrast, more severe hyperkalemia may be seen in patients with renal insufficiency, concurrent use of a drug that impairs renal K^+ excretion such as a potassium-sparing diuretic or a nonsteroidal anti-inflammatory drug or among the elderly.

Limited evidence suggests that increases in the P_K may be less pronounced with an angiotensin II receptor blocker than with an ACE inhibitor (0.12 vs 0.28 mEq/l) in patients with a reduced GFR (8). There are no data, however, to suggest that patients who developed significant hyperkalemia on ACE inhibitors can be safely treated with angiotensin II receptor blockers.

Drugs That Inhibit Aldosterone Synthesis: Heparin Aldosterone synthesis is selectively reduced in patients who are treated with heparin (75, 93, 94). This seems to be due to an effect of heparin that leads to a reduction in the number and affinity of adrenal angiotensin II receptors. Even low-dose heparin (5000 units twice daily) can lead to a reduction in plasma aldosterone concentrations. Nevertheless, the degree of decrease in plasma aldosterone may not be of sufficient magnitude to affect the renal excretion of K^+ in many patients who receive this drug. It has been estimated that a greater than normal P_K occurs in 7% of patients; severe hyperkalemia occurs only if some other impairment in K^+ excretion is present such as renal insufficiency or treatment with an ACE inhibitor or a potassium-sparing diuretic. Hyperkalemia has also been noted in patients receiving low-molecular-weight heparin (15).

Antifungal Agents Certain drugs in this class such as ketoconazole (103) and possibly fluconazole may cause hyperkalemia because they impair the synthesis of adosterone.

Aldosterone Receptor Antagonists: Spironolactone and Eplerenone Hyperkalemia is a potential problem in patients on the nonspecific mineralocorticoid receptor antagonist, spironolactone (51), or the selective mineralocorticoid receptor antagonist eplerenone (81). The incidence of hyperkalemia is dose dependent with detectable effects even at doses of 25 mg spironolactone per day (82). At higher doses, the risk of severe hyperkalemia increases. Of special concern is the rise in the use of these drugs after the demonstrated improved survival with the use of aldosterone antagonists in patients with congestive heart failure in both the Randomized Aldosterone Evaluation Study (RALES) trial with spironolactone (82) and the Eplerenone Post AMI Heart Failure Survival Study (EPHESUS) trial with eplerenone (81). This was illus-

trated in a population-based study of computerized drug prescription records and hospitalizations in Ontario, Canada, from 1994 to 2001, an interval that includes the date of publication of the results of RALES in 1999 (51). The frequency with which spironolactone was prescribed to patients with heart failure who were taking an ACE inhibitor rose significantly after the publication of RALES (from 30 prescriptions per 1000 patients in early 1999 to 149 prescriptions per 1000 patients by late 2001). Over the same interval, there were significant increases among these patients in the rates of hospital admissions for hyperkalemia (from 4.0 to 11.0 per 1000) and of in-hospital death from hyperkalemia (from 0.7 to 2.0 per 1000)

Drugs That Block ENaC: Trimethoprim and Pentamidine The cationic form of trimethoprim and pentamidine causes hyperkalemia and salt wasting by blocking ENaC in the lumen of the CCD (Fig. 12) (90). Patients with HIV and *Pneumocystis carinii* pneumonia treated with trimethoprim not infrequently develop hyperkalemia (18, 40, 106). Although this was attributed to the use of high doses of trimethoprim in these patients, trimethoprim may cause a rise in P_K when used in conventional doses. Another factor that may explain the high incidence of hyperkalemia in patients treated with trimethoprim is the low flow rate in the terminal CCD. Because the dietary intake in this group of patients is very poor, the rate of excretion of osmoles (urea and NaCl) is low and the flow rate in the terminal CCD is also low. There is another, more important effect of this reduced flow rate in the CCD. Not only can this diminish the rate of excretion of K^+ (Eq. 2), but it also increases the concentration of trimethoprim in the lumen of the CCD for a given rate of excretion of this drug (same quantity of trimethoprim is now in a smaller volume) (Fig. 12). Hence the ability of trimethoprim to block the ENaCs in principal cells in the CCD will be enhanced (89).

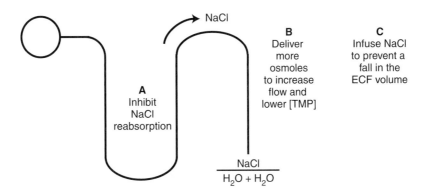

FIGURE 12 Method to lower the concentration of trimethoprim in the cortical collecting duct (CCD). The concentration of trimethoprim will fall in the lumen of the CCD when the number of osmoles delivered to this nephron segment rises (*point B*). To achieve this aim, inhibit the reabsorption of Na^+ and Cl^- in the loop of Henle (*point A*). To avoid further contraction of the extracellular fluid volume, the patient must receive more NaCl than is excreted in the urine (*point C*). (From Halperin ML. *The ACID Truth and BASIC Facts—With a Sweet Touch, an enLYTEnment,* 5th ed. Toronto: RossMark Medical Publishers; 2004, with permission.)

Patients with HIV infections also have other problems that make them prone to develop hyperkalemia. For example, a shift of K^+ from cells may occur due to suppression of insulin release by α-adrenergics released in response to ECF volume contraction (83). Thus, the blockade of ENaC causes the hyperkalemia not only by diminishing the rate of secretion of K^+ in the CCD, but also by an indirect effect that leads to a shift of K^+ out of cells.

With regard to therapy, loop diuretics may help by lowering the concentration of trimethoprim in the luminal fluid in the CCD. Enough NaCl must be given to defend the ECF volume. Because only the protonated form of trimethoprim blocks ENaC (90), increasing the urine pH should cause less trimethoprim to be in its cationic form and hence its antikaliuretic effect should be minimized. Inducing bicarbonaturia with acetazolamide is a rationale therapeutic option when continuation of trimethoprim is necessary and blockade of ENaC is likely. Enough alkali would need to be given to avoid the development of metabolic acidosis.

Drugs That Cause a Chloride Shunt–type Disorder: Calcineurine Inhibitors (Cyclosporin, FK 506) Hyperkalemia develops in some patients receiving cyclosporin or FK 506 following organ transplantation. The pathophysiology of hyperkalemia and the clinical signs in these patients resembles that of Gordon syndrome (52, 87). The finding that inducing bicarbonaturia leads to an increase in the TTKG is consistent with the hypothesis of Kamel et al. (52) that the defect is an increased permeability for Cl^- in the CCD.

Drugs That Interfere with Activation of ENaC via Proteolytic Cleavage: Nafamostat Mesylate Nafamostat mesylate is a potent serine protease inhibitor that has been widely used in Japan for the treatment of acute pancreatitis and disseminated intravascular coagulation and as an anticoagulant in hemodialysis (48). It can cause hyperkalemia primarily by the decreased urinary K^+ excretion (58). The mechanism is related to the metabolites of nafamostat that inhibit the aldosterone-inducible, membrane-associated, channel-activating proteases such as CAP1 (i.e., prostasin) (72). A novel mechanism by which aldosterone activates ENaC involves proteolytic cleavage of the channel by serine proteases. These proteases activate ENaC by increasing the open probability of the channel rather than by increasing expression at the cell surface. Inhibition of CAP1 by nafamostat diminishes the activity of ENaC and may lead to hyperkalemia.

THERAPY OF HYPERKALEMIA

Medical Emergencies

The major danger of a severe degree of hyperkalemia is a cardiac arrhythmia. Because mild ECG changes may progress rapidly to a dangerous arrhythmia, any patient with an ECG abnormality related to hyperkalemia should be considered as a potential medical emergency. In certain circumstances, we treat patients with a P_K above 7.0 mM aggressively, even in the absence of ECG changes—the exceptions include those who develop hyperkalemia after extreme exercise (e.g., the ultramarathon) (67), most patients on chronic hemodialysis, and infants.

ANTAGONIZE THE CARDIAC EFFECTS OF HYPERKALEMIA

Ca^{2+} is the best agent and its effects should be evident within minutes. It is usually given as 20 to 30 ml of a 10% calcium gluconate solution (two to three ampules) or 10 ml of 10% $CaCl_2$ (one ampule). This dose can be repeated in 5 minutes if ECG changes persist. The effect usually lasts 30 to 60 minutes. Extreme caution should be exerted in patients on digitalis because hypercalcemia may aggravate digitalis toxicity.

INDUCE A SHIFT OF POTASSIUM INTO THE INTRACELLULAR FLUID

Insulin A number of studies support the use of insulin to treat acute hyperkalemia (2, 4, 12, 57, 59). Large doses of insulin (20 units of regular insulin) are needed to have the supraphysiological levels of insulin in plasma that are required for a maximal shift of K^+ into cells. Monitoring the $P_{Glucose}$ and giving glucose as needed can minimize the risk of developing hypoglycemia.

$\beta2$-Adrenergic Agonists β_2-adrenergic stimulation lowers the P_K in patients with renal failure (2, 3, 58, 59, 63, 64, 68, 69). Allon et al. (3) used 10 and 20 mg of nebulized albuterol and observed a decline in the P_K that was sustained for at least 2 hours. The maximum decrease in P_K was 0.6 and 1.0 mM with the 10- and the 20-mg doses, respectively. There was a minimal increase in heart rate and a notable absence of cardiovascular side effects. However, since 20% to 40% of patients are resistant to this therapy, and it is not possible to predict nonresponders, we do not recommend it as a sole emergency therapy. Moreover, we are concerned about the safety of these drugs in the doses used for the treatment of hyperkalemia, which are four to eight times that prescribed for the treatment of acute asthma. The combination of nebulized β_2 agonists and insulin was reported to produce a greater fall in P_K (1.2 mM) compared with either drug alone (~ 0.65 mM) (2). One should note however that only 10 units of regular insulin was given in this study and the magnitude of the fall in P_K was lower than that observed in other studies using higher doses of insulin (12). Thus, it remains uncertain whether β_2 agonists would have a P_K lowering effect additive to that of higher doses of insulin.

Sodium Bicarbonate A number of studies have found $NaHCO_3$ therapy to be ineffective as the sole treatment of hyperkalemia (12, 43, 11). It is noteworthy that these studies were performed in stable hemodialysis patients who did not have significant acidosis (i.e., NHE was presumably inactive). Studies that examined the combined use of $NaHCO_3$ with insulin also have conflicting results

(4, 57). Thus the question remains as to whether $NaHCO_3$ would be effective in patients with a more significant degree of acidosis. There are no data in the literature to answer this question definitively (for review, see [54]). Given this uncertainty, we only use $NaHCO_3$ in addition to other therapies to treat emergency hyperkalemia in patients with a significant degree of acidosis. Caution is warranted because an excessive administration of $NaHCO_3$ has the risk of inducing hypernatremia, ECF volume expansion, carbon dioxide retention, and hypocalcemia.

No Medical Emergency

REMOVAL OF POTASSIUM FROM THE BODY

It is important to appreciate that very much less K^+ loss is needed to lower the P_K from 7.0 to 6.0 mM than to lower it from 6.0 to 5.0 mM (97). Hence creating a small K^+ loss can be very important when there is a severe degree of hyperkalemia.

ENHANCING THE EXCRETION OF POTASSIUM IN THE URINE

If K^+ excretion is low because of a low urine volume, but with a high U_K, a loop diuretic may induce kaliuresis by increasing the flow rate in the CCD. One can avoid unwanted ECF volume contraction by replacing the $NaCl$ lost in the urine. This $NaCl$ should be given at the same tonicity as the urine to avoid creating a dysnatremia. If the U_K is unduly low, giving a mineralocorticoid (100 μg florinef) and possibly inducing bicarbonaturia with a carbonic anhydrase inhibitor may cause a substantial kaliuresis. HCO_3^- lost in the urine might need to be replaced.

CATION EXCHANGE RESINS

A cation exchange resin can exchange bound Na^+ (kayexalate) or Ca^{2+} (calcium resonium) for cations including K^+. Kayexalate contains 4 mEq of Na^+ per gram, but only a small amount of exchange of Na^+ for K^+ occurs in the gastrointestinal tract (29). The only favorable location for the exchange of Na^+ for K^+ is in the lumen of the colon, but a number of factors limit the magnitude of this process. Based on data obtained from patients with ileostomy, the amount of K^+ delivered to the colon that would be available for this exchanger is close to only 5 mEq/day. Cations other than K^+ such as NH_4^+, Ca^{2+}, and Mg^{2+} may exchange for resin-bound Na^+. One possible theoretical benefit to the use of cation exchange resins is if they were to lower the K^+ concentration in luminal water, thereby enhancing the net secretion of K^+ by the rectosigmoid colon. Even if K^+ were secreted in the colon, the low stool volume would limit the total K^+ loss. For example, if the lumen-negative transepithelial voltage were −90 mV, and the P_K were 5 mM, the concentration of K^+ in stool water would be 100 mM. With a usual stool volume of 125 ml of which 75% is water, only 10 mmol of K^+ would be lost by this route. Thus, there

is little if any benefit of using resins for the treatment of acute hyperkalemia (42) and little benefit of adding resins to cathartics in the setting of chronic hyperkalemia (54).

DIALYSIS

Hemodialysis is more effective than peritoneal dialysis for removing K^+. Removal rates of K^+ can approximate 35 mmol/hr with a dialysate bath K^+ concentration of 1 to 2 mM. A glucose-free dialysate is preferable to avoid the glucose-induced release of insulin and the subsequent shift of K^+ into cells, lessening the removal of K^+.

References

1. Adrogue HJ, Madias NE. Changes in plasma potassium concentration during acute acid-base disturbances. *Am J Med* 1981;71:456–467.
2. Allon M, Copkney C. Albuterol and insulin for treatment of hyperkalemia in hemodialysis patients. *Kidney Int* 1990;38:869–872.
3. Allon M, Dunlay R, Copkney C. Nebulized albuterol for acute hyperkalemia in patients on hemodialysis. *Ann Intern Med* 1989;110:426–429.
4. Allon M, Shanklin N. Effect of bicarbonate administration on plasma potassium in dialysis patients: interactions with insulin and albuterol. *Am J Kidney Dis* 1996;28:508–514.
5. Alper S. The band 3-related anion exchanger (AE) gene family. *Ann Rev Physiol* 1991;53:549–564.
6. Arrambide K, Toto RD. Tumor lysis syndrome. *Sem Nephrol* 1993;13:273–280.
7. Backman KA, Hayslett JP. Role of the medullary collecting duct in potassium conservation. *Pflugers Arch* 1983;396:297–300.
8. Bakris GL, et al. ACE inhibition or angiotensin receptor blockade: impact on potassium in renal failure. *Kidney Int* 2000;58:2084.
9. Baltazar RF, Mower MM, Reider R, Funk M, Salomon J. Acute fluoride poisoning leading 000to fatal hyperkalemia. *Chest* 1980;78:660–663.
10. Bercovici M, Chen C, Goldstein M, Stinebaugh B, Halperin M. Effect of acute changes in the PaCO2 on acid-base parameters in normal dogs and dogs with metabolic acidosis or alkalosis. *Can J Physiol Pharmacol* 1983;61:166–173.
11. Blumberg A, Weidmann P, Ferrari P. Effect of prolonged bicarbonate administration on plasma potassium in terminal renal failure. *Kidney Int* 1992;41:369–374.
12. Blumberg A, Weidmann P, Shaw S, Gnadinger M. Effect of various therapeutic approaches on plasma potassium and major regulating factors in terminal renal failure. *Am J Med* 1988;85:507–512.
13. Bonny O, Rossier BC. Disturbances of Na/K balance: Pseudohypoaldosteronism revisted. *J Am Soc Nephrol* 2002;13:2399–2414.
14. Bushinsky DA, Gennari FJ. Life-threatening hyperkalemia induced by arginine. *Ann Int Med* 1978;89:632–634.
15. Canova CR, et al. Effect of low molecular weight heparin on serum potassium. *Lancet* 1997;349:1447.
16. Carlisle EJF, Donnelly SM, Ethier J, Quaggin SE, Kaiser U, Vasuvattakul S, Kamel KS, Halperin ML. Modulation of the secretion of potassium by accompanying anions in humans. *Kidney Int* 1991;39:1206–1212.
17. Cheema-Dhadli S, Lin S-H, Chong CK, Kamel KS, Halperin ML. Requirements for a high rate of potassium excretion in rats consuming a low electrolyte diet. *J Physiol* 2006;572:493–501.
18. Choi MJ, Fernandez PC, Patnaik A, Coupaye-Gerard B, D'Andrea D, Zerlip H, Kleyman TR. Trimethoprim induced hyperkalemia in a patient with AIDS. *N Engl J Med* 1993;328:703–706.
19. Clausen T. Regulation of active Na^+-K^+ transport in skeletal muscle. *Physiol Rev* 1986;66:542–580.
20. Cockcroft DW, Gault MH. Prediction of creatinine clearance from serum creatinine. *Nephron* 1976;16:31–41.
21. Conway MJ, Seibel JA, Eaton RP. Thyrotoxicosis and hypokalemic periodic paralysis: Improvement with beta blockade. *Ann Int Med* 1974;81:332–336.
22. Counillon LL, Pouyssegur RJ. The members of the Na+/H+ exchanger gene family: their structure, function, expression, and regulation. In: Seldin DW, Giebisch G, eds. *The Kidney: Physiology & Pathophysiology*. Philadelphia: Lippincott Williams & Wilkins; 2000:223–234.
23. Davids MR, Edoute Y, Jungas RL, Halperin ML. Facilitating an understanding of integrative physiology: Emphasis on the compositon of body fluid compartments. *Can J Physiol Pharmacol* 2002;80:835–850.
24. DeFronzo RA, Bia M, Birkhead G. Epinephrine and potassiun homeostasis. *Kidney Int* 1981;20:83.
25. DeFronzo RA, Sherwin RS, Dillingham M, Hendler R, Tamborlane WV, Felig P. Influence of basal insulin and glucagon secretion on potassium and sodium metabolism: studies with somatostatin. *J Clin Invest* 1978;61:472–479.
26. DeMars C, Hollister K, Tomassoni A, Himmelfarb J, Halperin ML. Citric acidosis: A life-threatening cause of metabolic acidosis. *Ann Emerg Med* 2001;38:588–591.
27. Dickerman HW, Walker WG. Effect of cationic amino acid infusion on potassium metabolism in vivo. *Am J Physiol* 1964;206:403–408.

28. Don BR, Sebastian A, Cheitlin M, Christiansen M, Schambelan M. Pseudohyperkalemia caused by fist clenching during phlebotomy. *N Engl J Med* 1990;322:1290–1292.
29. Emmett M, Hootkins RE, Fine KD. Effect of three laxatives and a cation exchange resin on fecal sodium and potassium excretion. *Gastroenterology* 1995;108:752–760.
30. Ethier JH, Honrath U, Veress A, Sonnenberg H, Halperin ML. Nephron site responsible for the reduced kaliuretic response to mineralocorticoids during hypokalemia in rats. *Kidney Int* 1990;38:812–817.
31. Ethier JH, Kamel KS, Magner PO, Lemann JJ, Halperin ML. The transtubular potassium concentration in patients with hypokalemia and hyperkalemia. *Am J Kidney Dis* 1990;15: 309–315.
32. Farman N, Boulkroun S, Courtois-Coutry N. SGK: an old enzyme revisited. *J Clin Invest* 2002;110:1233–1234.
33. Field M. Intestinal transport and the pathophysiology of diarrhea. *J Clin Invest* 2003;111: 931–943.
34. Field MJ, Giebisch GJ. Hormonal control of renal potassium excretion. *Kidney Int* 1985;27: 379–387.
35. Flores SY, Debonneville C, Staub O. The role of Nedd4/Nedd4-like dependant ubiquity-lation in epithelial transport processes. *Pflugers Arch* 2003;446:334–338.
36. Fontaine B, Khurana TS, Hoffman EP, et al. Hyperkalemic periodic paralysis and the adult muscle sodium channel alpha-subunit gene. *Science* 1990;250:1000–1002.
37. Gagnon RF, Halperin ML. Possible mechanisms to explain the absence of hyperkalemia in a patient with Addison's disease. *Nephrol Dial Transplant* 2001;16:1280–1284.
38. Garty H. Regulation of the epithelial Na^+ channel by aldosterone: Open questions and emerging answers. *Kidney Int* 2000;57:1270–1276.
39. Giebisch G: Renal potassium transport: mechanisms and regulation. *Am J Physiol* 1998;274: F817–F833.
40. Greenberg S, Reiser IW, Chou S-Y, Porush JG. Trimethoprim-sulfamethoxazole induces reversible hyperkalemia. *Ann Intern Med* 1993;119:291–295.
41. Gronert GA, Theye RA. Pathophysiology of hyperkalemia induced by succinylcholine. *Anesthesiology* 1975;43:89–99.
42. Gruy-Kapral C, Emmett M, Santa Ana CA. Effect of single dose resin-cathartic therapy on serum potassium concentration in patients with end-stage renal disease. *J Am Soc Nephrol* 1998;9:1924–1930.
43. Guttierez R, Schlessinger F, Oster JR, Rietberg B, Perez GO. Effect of hypertonic versus isotonic sodium bicarbonate on plasma potassium concentration in patients with end-stage renal disease. *Miner Electrolyte Metab* 1991;17:297–302.
44. Halperin ML, Kamel KS. Potassium. *Lancet* 1998;352:135–142.
45. Halperin ML. *The ACID Truth and BASIC Facts—With a Sweet Touch, an enLYTEnment*, 5th ed. Toronto: RossMark Medical Publishers; 2004:
46. Harris RZ. Cyclooxygenase-2 in the kidney. *J Am Soc Nephrol* 2000;42:2387–2394.
47. Iolascon A, Stewart GW, Ajetunmobi JF, Perrotta S, Delaunay J, Carella M, Zelante L, Gasparini P. Familial pseudohyperkalemia maps to the same locus as dehydrated hereditary stomatocytosis (hereditary xerocytosis). *Blood* 1999;93:3120–3123.
48. Iwashita K, Kitamura K, Narikiyo T, Adachi M, Shiraishi N, Miyoshi T, Nagano J, Tuyendo G, Nonoguchi H, Tomita K. Inhibition of prostasin secretion by serine protease inhibitors in the kidney. *J Am Soc Nephrol* 2003;14:11–16.
49. Jiang Q, Wang D, MacKinnon R. Electron microscopic analysis of KcAP voltage-dependent K+channels in an open conformation. *Nature* 2004;430:806–810.
50. Juel C, Halestrap AP. Lactate transport in skeletal muscle-role and regulation of the mono-carboxylate transporter. *J Physiol* 1999;517:633–642.
51. Juurlink DN, Mamdani MM, Lee DS, Kopp A, Austin PC, Laupacis A, Redelmeier DA. Rates of hyperkalemia after publication of the Randomized Aldactone Evaluation Study. *N Engl J Med* 2004;351:543–551.
52. Kamel K, Ethier JH, Quaggin S, Levin A, Albert S, Carlisle EJF, Halperin ML. Studies to determine the basis for hyperkalemia in recipients of a renal transplant who are treated with cyclosporin. *J Am Soc Nephrol* 1992;2:1279–1284.
53. Kamel KS, Quaggin S, Scheich A, Halperin ML. Disorders of potassium homeostasis: an approach based on pathophysiology. *Am J Kidney Dis* 1994;24:597–613.
54. Kamel KS, Wei C. Controversial issues in treatment of hyperkalemia. *Nephrol Dialysis Transpl* 2003;18:2215–2218.
55. Kemper MJ, Harps E, Muller-Wiefel DE. Hyperkalemia: therapeutic options in acute and chronic renal failure. *Clin Nephrol* 1995;46:67–69.
56. Kifor I, et al. Potassium stimulated angiotensin release from adrenal capsules and enzymati-cally digested cells of the zona gloerulosa. *Endocrinology* 1991;129:823.
57. Kim HJ. Combined effect of bicarbonate and insulin with glucose in acute therapy of hyper-kalemia in end-stage renal disease patients. *Nephron* 1996;72:476–482.
58. Kitagawa H, Chang H, Fujita T. Hyperkalemia due to nafamostat mesylate. *N Engl J Med* 1995;332:687.
59. Lens XM, Montoliu J, Cases A, Campistol JM, Revert L. Treatment of hyperkalemia in renal failure: salbutamol v. insulin. *Nephrol Dial Transplant* 1989;4:228–232.
60. Lin DH, Sterling H, Yang B, Hebert SC, Giebisch G, Wang WH. Protein tyrosine kinase is expressed and regulates ROMK1 location in the cortical collecting duct. *Am J Physiol* 2004;286:F881–F892.
61. Lin SH, Hsu Y-J, Chiu J-S, Chu S-J, Davids MR, Halperin ML. Osmotic demyelination syndrome: A potentially avoidable disaster. *Q J Med* 2003;96:935–947.
62. Lin SH, Lin YF. Propranolol rapidly reverses paralysis, hypokalemia and hypophosphatemia in thyrotoxic periodic paralysis. *Am J Kidney Dis* 2001;37:620–624.
63. Liou HH, Chiang SS, Wu SC, et al. Hypokalemic effects of intravenous infusion or nebuliza-tion of salbutamol in patients with chronic renal failure. *Am J Kidney Dis* 1994;23:266–270.
64. Mandelberg A, Krupnik Z, Houri S. Salbutamol metered-dose inhaler with spacer for hyper-kalemia: how fast? how safe? *Chest* 1999;115:617–622.
65. Mayan H, Vered I, Mouallem M, Tzadok-Witkon M, Pauzner R, Farfel Z. Pseudohypoaldo-steronism type II: marked sensitivity to thiazides, hypercalciuria, normomagnesemia, and low bone mineral density. *J Clin Endocrinol Metab* 2002;87:3248–3254.
66. McIvor ME, Cummings CE, Mower MM, Wenk RE, Lustgarten JA, Baltazar RF, Salomon J. Sudden cardiac death from acute fluoride intoxication: the role of potassium. *Ann Emerg Med* 1987;16:777–781.
67. McKechnie JK, Leary WP, Joubert SM. Some electrocardiographic and biochemical changes recorded in marathon runners. *S Afr Med J* 1967;41:722–725.
68. Montoliu J, Almirall J, Ponz E, Campistol JM, Revert L. Treatment of hyperkalemia in renal failure with salbutamol inhalation. *J Intern Med* 1990;228:35–37.
69. Montoliu J, Lens XM, Revert L. Potassium-lowering effect of albuterol for hyperkalemia in renal failure. *Arch Intern Med* 1987;147:713–717.
70. Moore RD. Stimulation of Na:H exchange by insulin. *Biophys J* 1981;33:203–210.
71. Mueller BA, Scott MK, Sowinski KM, Prag KA. Noni juice (morinda citrifolia): Hidden potential for hyperkalemia? *Am J Kidney Dis* 2000;35:310–312.
72. Muto S, Imai M, Asano Y. Mechanisms of the hyperkalemia caused by nafamostat mesilate: effects of its two metabolites on Na^+ and K^+ transport properties in the rabbit cortical col-lecting duct. *Br J Pharmacol* 1994;111:173–178.
73. Orringer CE, Eustace JC, Wunsch CD, Gardner LB. Natural history of lactic acidosis after Grand-Mal seizures. *N Engl J Med* 1977;297:796–799.
74. Orth DN, Kovacs WJ. The adrenal cortex. In: Wilson JD, Foster DW, Kronenberg HM, Larsen PR, eds. *Williams Textbook of Endocrinology*, 9th ed. Philadelpha: WB Saunders; 1998:550.
75. Oster JR, Singer I, Fisherman LM. Heparin-induced aldosterone suppression and hyperka-lemia. *Am J Med* 1995;98:575–586.
76. Palmer BF. Managing hyperkalemia caused by inhibitors of the renin-angiotension-aldosterone system. *N Engl J Med* 2004;351:585–592.
77. Palmer L, Antonian J, Frindt G. Regulation of the apical K and Na channels and Na/K pumps in the rat cortical collecting tubule by dietary K. *J Gen Physiol* 1994;105:693–710.
78. Palmer L, Frindt G. Regulation of the apical K channels in the rat cortical collecting tubule during changes in K intake. *Am J Physiol* 1999;277:F805–F812.
79. Perazella MA, Biswas P. Acute hyperkalemia associated with intravenous epsilon-aminocaproic acid therapy. *Am J Kidney Dis* 1999;33:782–785.
80. Phelps KR, Lieberman RL, Oh MS, Carroll HJ. Pathophysiology of the syndrome of hypo-reninemic hypoaldosteronism. *Metabolism* 1980;29:186–199.
81. Pitt B, Remme W, Zannad F, Neaton J, Martinez F, Roniker B, Bittman RSH, Kleiman J, Gatlin M. Eplerenone Post-Acute Myocardial Infarction Heart Failure Efficacy and Survival Study Investigators. Eplerenone, a selective aldosterone blocker, in patients with left ven-tricular dysfunction after myocardial infarction. *N Engl J Med* 2003;348:1309–1321.
82. Pitt B, Zannad F, Remme WJ, Cody R, Castaigne A, Perez A, Palensky J, Wittes J. The effect of spironolactone on morbidity and mortality in patients with severe heart failure. *N Engl J Med* 1999;341:709–717.
83. Porte DJ. Sympathetic regulation of insulin secretion. *Arch Intern Med* 1969;123:252–260.
84. Raff H. Glucocorticoid inhibition of neurohypophysial vasopressin secretion. *Am J Physiol* 1987;252:R635–R644.
85. Rosa RM, Silva P, Young JB, Landsberg L, Brown RS, Rowe JW, Epstein FH. Adrenergic modulation of extrarenal potassium disposal. *N Engl J Med* 1980;302:431–434.
86. Rosa RM, Williams ME, Epstein FH. Extrarenal potassium metabolism. In: Seldin DW, Giebisch G, eds. *The Kidney: Physiology and Pathophysiology*, 2nd ed. New York: Raven Press; 1992:2165–2190.
87. Schambelan M, Sebastian A, Rector FC Jr. Mineralocorticoid-resistant renal hyperkalemia without salt wasting (type II pseudohypoaldosteronism): Role of increased renal chloride reabsorption. *Kidney Int* 1981;19:716–727.
88. Schild L. The ENaC channel as the primary determinant of two human diseases: Liddle's syndrome and pseudohypoaldosteronism. *Neprhologie* 1996;17:395–400.
89. Schreiber M, Halperin ML. Urea excretion rate as a contributor to trimethoprim-induced hyperkalemia. *Ann Int Med* 1994;120:166–167.
90. Schreiber MS, Chen C-B, Lessan-Pezeshki M, Halperin ML, Schlanger LE, Patnaik A, Ling BN, Kleyman TR. Antikaliuretic action of trimethoprim is minimized by raising urine pH. *Kidney Int* 1996;49:82–87.
91. Sebastian A, McSherry E, Morris RC Jr. Renal potassium wasting in renal tubular acidosis (RTA): its occurrence in types 1 and 2 RTA despite sustained correction of systemic acidosis. *J Clin Invest* 1971;50:667–678.
92. Shafiee MA, Bohn D, Hoorn EJ, Halperin ML. How to select optimal maintenance intra-venous fluid therapy. *Q J Med* 2003;96:601-610.
93. Sherman RA, et al. Suppression of aldosterone production by low-dose heparin. *Am J Nephrol* 1986;6:165.
94. Siebels M, Andrassy K, Vecsei P, Seelig HP, Back T, Nawroth P, Weber E. Dose dependent suppression of mineralocorticoid metabolism by different heparin fractions. *Thromb Res* 1992;66:467–473.
95. Smith TW, Willerson JT. Suicidal and accidental digoxin ingestion. Report of five cases with serum digoxin level correlations. *Circulation* 1971;44:29–36.
96. Steele A, deVeber H, Quaggin SE, Scheich A, Ethier J, Halperin ML. What is responsible for the diurnal variation in potassium excretion? *Am J Physiol* 1994;36:R554–R560.
97. Sterns RH, Guzzo J, Feig PU, Singer I. Internal potassium balance and the control of the plasma potassium concentration. *Medicine* 1981;60:339–354.
98. Stokes JB. Ion transport by the collecting duct. *Sem Nephrol* 1993;13:202–212.
99. Su M, Chu J, Howland MA, Nelson LS, Hoffman RS. Amiodarone attenuates fluoride-induced hyperkalemia in vitro. *Acad Emerg Med* 2003;10:105–109.
100. Swan RC, Pitts RF. Neutralization of infused acid by nephrectomized dogs. *J Clin Invest* 1955;34:205–212.
101. Talbott JH, Schwab RS. Recent advances in the biochemistry and therapeutics of potassium salts. *N Engl J Med* 1940;222:585–590.
102. Textor SC, Bravo EL, Tarazi RC. Hyperkalemia in azotemic patients during angiotensin-converting enzyme inhibition and aldosterone reduction with captopril. *Am J Med* 1982;158: 26–32.
103. Tucker WSJ, Snell BB, Island DP, Gregg CR. Reversible adrenal insufficiency induced by ketoconazole. *JAMA* 1985;253:2413–2414.

104. Vallon V, Lang F. New insights into the role of serum- and glucocorticoid-inducible kinase SGK1 in the regulation of renal function and blood pressure. *J Am Soc Nephrol* 2005;14: 59–66.

105. van Buren M, Rabelink TJ, van Rijn HJM, Koomans HA. Effects of acute NaCl, KCl and KHCO₃ loads on renal electrolyte excretion in humans. *Clin Sci* 1992;83:567–574.

106. Velazquez H, Perazella MA, Wright FS, Ellison DH. Renal mechanism of trimethoprim-induced hyperkalemia. *Ann Intern Med* 1993;119:295–301.

107. Velazquez H, Wright FS, Good DW. Luminal influences on potassium secretion: chloride replacement with sulfate. *Am J Physiol* 1982;242:F46–F55.

108. Vuagniaux G, Vallet V, Jaeger NF, Hummler E, Rossier BC. Synergistic activation of ENaC by three membrane-bound channel-activating serine proteases (mCAP1, mCAP2, and mCAP3) and serum- and glucocorticoid-regulated kinase (Sgk1) in Xenopus oocytes. *J Gen Physiol* 2002;120:191–201.

109. Waldegger S, Jentsch TJ. From tonus to tonicity: physiology of ClC chloride channels. *J Am Soc Nephrol* 2000;11:1331–1339.

110. Wang WH, Hebert SC. The molecular biology of renal K⁺ channels. In: Seldin DW, Giebisch G, eds. *The Kidney: Physiology & Pathophysiology.* Philadelphia: Lippincott Williams & Wilkins; 2000:235–249.

111. Wang WH. Regulation of renal K transport by dietary K intake. *Annu Rev Physiol* 2004;66:547–569.

112. White PC, Speiser PW. Congenital adrenal hyperplasia. *Endocrine Rev* 2000;21:245–291.

113. White PC: Disorders of aldosterone biosynthesis and action. *Mol Cell Endocrinol* 2004;217: 81–87.

114. Williams ME, Gervino EV, Rosa RM, Landsberg L, Young JB, Silva P, Epstein FH. Catecholamine modulation of rapid potassium shifts during exercise. *N Engl J Med* 1985;312: 823–827.

115. Wilson FH, Disse-Nocodeme S, Choate KA, Ishikawa K, Nelson-Williams C, Desitter I, et al. Human hypertension caused by mutations in WNK kinases. *Science* 2001;293: 1107–1112.

116. Woolf AD, Wenger T, Smith TW, Lovejoy FHJ. The use of digoxin-specific Fab fragments for severe digitalis intoxication in children. *N Engl J Med* 1992;326:1739–1744.

117. Yang C-L, Angell J, Mitchell R, Ellison DH. WNK kinases regulate thiazide-sensitive Na-Cl cotransport. *J Clin Invest* 2003;111:1039–1045.

118. Zierler KL, Rabinowitz D. Effect of very small concentrations of insulin on forearm metabolism: persistence of its action on potassium and free fatty acids without its effect on glucose. *J Clin Invest* 1963;43:950–962.

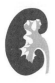

CHAPTER 50

The Effects of Electrolyte Disorders on Excitable Membranes

Daniel I. Levy and Steve A. N. Goldstein

University of Chicago, Chicago, Illinois, USA

THE NATURE OF EXCITABILITY

In 1902, Julius Bernstein (9) hypothesized that cells were bounded by membranes selectively permeable to K^+ ions at rest and permeable to other ions when excited. Over the past 50 years, we have learned this hypothesis to be correct in its essentials, and the agents of such permeation are transmembrane proteins called ion channels (51). Ion channels are present in all membranes. They underlie minute biological events such as the response of a single rod cell to a photon of light, degranulation of an activated mast cell, and proliferation of a T cell in response to a specific antigen. Ion channels also mediate spectacular events like heart beats, fluid and electrolyte homeostasis, intestinal peristalsis, and memories. Today, identification of genes for ion channels and their regulatory subunits has been combined with sensitive methods that allow characterization of channel function at remarkable resolution; the behavior of single molecules can be evaluated in real time. In this chapter, we will discuss the key elements of how ion channels participate in maintaining the cellular membrane potential as well as how excitable cells are activated. We also present advances in our understanding of ion channel structure and modulation of ion channel activity. In terms of these fundamental principles, we will explain how electrolyte disturbances can lead to serious dysfunction of nerve, muscle, and the heart.

Selective Permeability, Membrane Potentials, and Ionic Gradients

Electrical signals are the fastest means of communication in the body. The flow of electricity provides a rapid way for the dendritic tree of a neuron to integrate inputs from a finger placed on a hot stove, initiate reflex withdrawal of the painful appendage, inform the brain of the developing situation, and coordinate synchronized contraction of the heart in the finger's startled owner. In clinical settings, these events can be monitored by extracellular recordings such as electrocardiograms (ECGs), electroencephalograms (EEGs) and electromyograms (EMGs), which mea-sure small signals (typically microvolts) due to electric currents that are generated by excitable cells. Such signals are a distant reflection of what is happening at the cell membrane where neurotransmitter release, contraction, and excitability itself are unfolding. To understand excitability (and how it gives rise to the extracellular signals our clinical tools detect) we must consider what is learned from intracellular recordings.

A microelectrode is a glass tube (usually ~1 mm wide with a tip drawn down to ~0.5 μm) that is used to penetrate a cell membrane with minimal damage so the membrane can reseal tightly around the glass. Consider two such electrodes in a salt solution bathing a cell (Fig. 1A). The electrodes are filled with a conducting solution (e.g., 150 mM KCl) and connected through a voltmeter by a silver wire that serves to establish electric continuity between the solutions. The voltmeter reads zero since the system is at equilibrium. If one of the electrodes is advanced across a cell membrane into a living cell, the voltmeter registers an abrupt change revealing an electrical potential difference between the two electrodes; this is the membrane potential (Fig. 1B), which is set up by the motions of ions across the membrane and represents a balance of chemical and electrical forces. How this develops is most readily understood if we first consider just the major cations (K^+ and Na^+) and anion (Cl^-) in cells and serum.

Active transport systems, such as the Na^+-K^+ pump, keep cytosolic K^+ levels high and Na^+ levels low (Table 1). Pumps are slow (maximal turnover rates of 60–100 Na^+ ions each second), but are present in cells at high abundance (10^5–10^7 per cell) and serve to couple the use of cellular energy (hydrolysis of adenosine triphosphate [ATP]) to each transport event. This establishes an ionic gradient across the membrane which serves as a reservoir of chemical energy due to the decreased entropy. The cell is now poised to use this stored energy by opening ion channel pathways through the membrane. Ion channels are fast (transporting 10^6–10^8 ions each second), low-abundance proteins (10–1000 per cell) that dissipate ionic gradients by opening a water-filled pathway across the membrane to allow free diffusion of selected

A

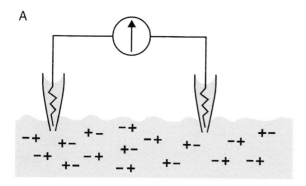

B

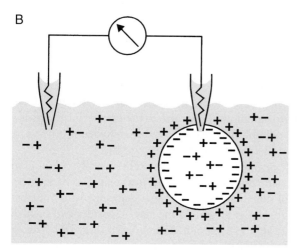

FIGURE 1 Schematic representation of a voltmeter and mammalian cell in serum. **A:** The voltmeter measures no potential difference when both electrodes are outside the cell in the bath solution. **B:** The voltmeter registers a negative membrane potential when one electrode moves into the cell. Excess negative charge inside the cell at equilibrium represents a small fraction of the total number of charged ions in the cell. The unbalanced charges accumulate at the membrane.

TABLE 1 Typical Ionic Composition of Muscle Cells and Serum and Equilibrium Potential

Ion (X)	Cell (mM)	Serum (mM)	$E_{rev} = \dfrac{RT}{zF} \ln \dfrac{[X]ext}{[X]in}$
Sodium (Na$^+$)	12	145	+67
Potassium (K$^+$)	155	4	−97
Chloride (Cl$^-$)	4	125	−93
Calcium (Ca^{2+})	<0.0001	1.5	>100
Magnesium (Mg^{2+})	1–15	1	–

Source: Hille B. *Ion Channels of Excitable Membranes*, 3rd ed. Sunderland, MA: Sinauer; 2001; and Dyckner T, Wester PO. The relation between extra- and intracellular electrolytes in patients with hypokalemia and/or diuretic treatment. *Acta Med Scand* 1978;204:269–282.

brane, the Nernst potential is the same as the equilibrium potential for K$^+$ ions, E$_K$, and is expressed as:

$$E_K = \frac{RT}{zF} \ln \frac{K_{ext}}{K_{in}} \qquad \text{(Eq. 1)}$$

where R is the gas constant, T is the temperature in degrees Kelvin, z is the charge of the ion, F is the Faraday constant, and K_{ext} and K_{in} the concentrations of K$^+$ in the extracellular and intracellular compartments, respectively. For K$^+$ ions at physiological temperature (37°C), RT/zF is ~27 mV and E$_K$ is, ~ −97 mV. The Nernst potentials of Na$^+$, K$^+$, Cl$^-$, and Ca^{2+} for a typical cell in serum are given in Table 1. Mammalian cells have resting potentials of −60 to −90 mV because K$^+$ ions are not the only ions that cross cell membranes at rest. Thus, pathways for transmembrane Na$^+$ flux allow these ions to flow down their chemical and electrical gradients into the cell and shift the membrane potential toward the Nernst potential for Na$^+$ (E$_{Na}$ ≈ +67 mV). The resting membrane potential of a cell (E$_m$) results from the permeability and concentration gradients of all ions in the system. Resting potentials are close to E$_K$ because more K$^+$ selective pathways are open in resting cells than those for other ions.

Definitions, Nomenclature, and Why Electrical Signals Are So Fast

A brief foray into the units and measures of excitation is needed to make the biology of excitation accessible. Net flow of charge is called current (abbreviated, I). Conductance (G) is a measure of the ease with which current flows between two points. The potential difference (ΔV) is defined as the work required to move a unit of charge from one point to another. These three measures are related by the second key relationship of cellular electrophysiology, Ohm's law:

$$I = G\Delta V \qquad \text{(Eq. 2)}$$

This equation indicates that the current (measured in amperes, A) is equal to the product of the conductance (measured in siemens, S) and the potential difference across the

ions down their electrochemical gradients. Thus, an open K$^+$ channel allows K$^+$ ions to diffuse out of a cell down the K$^+$ concentration gradient, leaving behind negative counterions. The excess of negative charge inside the cell constitutes an electrical energy that is registered on the voltmeter as a negative membrane potential (Fig. 1B). Although this electrical energy can be large, the imbalance of charge reflects a miniscule fraction of the total number of ions within the cell (see next section).

If the channel stays open, K$^+$ ions continue to flow until the chemical energy favoring outward K$^+$ movement (down the concentration gradient) is balanced by the electrical energy favoring movement of the positively charged ions into the negative cell interior (down the electrical gradient). At equilibrium, the forces are equal, efflux equals influx, and there is no net movement of K$^+$ ions across the membrane. The Nernst potential is the membrane potential that yields equilibrium for transport of a particular ionic species across a membrane (and is one of two key relationships central to cellular electrophysiology). For a purely K$^+$ selective mem-

conductor (measured in volts, V); by convention, positive current flows in the direction of movement of positive charges. Ohm's law can also be written in terms of resistance (R) to current flow (measured in ohms):

$$R = \frac{I}{\Delta V} \qquad \text{(Eq. 3)}$$

When 1 V is applied across a 1-ohm resistor or a 1-S conductor, a current of 1 A flows. Ion channels in the cell membrane act as conductors that span an insulator. When an insulator is interposed between two conducting solutions, it acts as a capacitor. The capacitance (C, measured in farads, F) of the insulator arises from the attraction of separated charges across the barrier and depends on its geometry and dielectric constant (ε). The specific capacitance of human cell membranes is ~ 1 $\mu F/cm^2$ and is a measure of how much charge (Q) must be moved from one side to the other to set up a given potential difference:

$$C = \frac{Q}{\Delta V} \qquad \text{(Eq. 4)}$$

It is now possible to understand why electrical signals are so rapid. Reconsider the small cell in Fig. 1 with a diameter of 12 μm and a resting membrane potential of -100 mV. This cell has a capacitance of 10^{-11} F and, therefore, 6 million positive charges left the cell (Eq. 4) to produce the resting potential. While this sounds significant, it represents less than 1/10,000 of the total cations in the cell (a volume of 10^{-12} L with 150 mM cations indicates 10^{11} total cations before the exodus). Figure 1B emphasizes two salient features. First, almost all ions in the cell and the external solution have balancing counter-ions; in contrast, unbalanced charges are at the membrane boundary. This is because unbalanced charges repel each other and move apart until their movement is limited. Second, unbalanced charges at the membrane are not necessarily the same as those produced initially by charge separation. Because ions are always in motion, they often exchange places. Thus, an unbalanced ion in the center of the cell will repel its neighbors, causing them to repel their neighbors, and so on until the unbalanced charge resides at the bounding membrane surface. This process (which is simply the conduction of electricity in an ionic solution) is much faster than diffusion. That is, it would take much longer for the original ion to diffuse to the membrane than it actually takes for its electrical influence to be felt. This is the fundamental mechanism that makes electrical signals fast.

By convention, the current across a membrane is taken as positive when positive charges are moving outward. Current is equal to the change in charge over time, $dQ/dt = I$. Combining this with Eq. 4 gives the relationship between changes in membrane voltage and time, assuming the capacitance change is negligible:

$$\frac{d\Delta V}{dt} = -\frac{I}{C} \qquad \text{(Eq. 5)}$$

The effect of opening one channel with a typical current of 1 pA (6×10^6 charges/sec) in our 12-μm cell is to cause the membrane voltage to change at a rate of -100 mV each second (6×10^6 charges/sec divided by 6×10^7 charges/V). As K^+ ions are moving toward their equilibrium condition, the voltage is shifting toward E_K. If two channels were to open at once, the membrane potential would change at twice the rate.

Voltage-Clamp Technique and Ionic Currents

Much of what we understand about electrical signals comes from application of voltage-clamp technique. Developed by Cole and Marmont in the 1940s, it was applied shortly thereafter to studies of the ionic basis for action potentials, notably by Hodgkin and Huxley (53–55). In voltage-clamp technique, the membrane voltage is controlled by the experimentalist and the current that flows to maintain the commanded voltage is measured. It is common to make voltage-clamp measurements on a small patch of membrane isolated on the tip of a glass pipette with a high-resistance (gigaohm) seal (Fig. 2). In on-cell

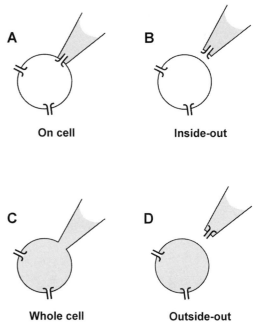

FIGURE 2 Schematic representation of the modes of voltage-clamp analyses. First, a high-resistance seal is formed between the electrode glass and the cell membrane (on-cell mode, **A**); the membrane patch can then be pulled off the cell, exposing its cytoplasmic face to the bath solution (inside-out mode, **B**). Alternatively, the on-cell seal can be broken so that the pipette solution is in free communication with the cell interior (whole-cell mode, **C**); from whole-cell mode, the pipette can be withdrawn to form an excised membrane patch with the extracellular membrane face exposed to the bath (outside-out mode, **D**). (For methodologic detail, see Kettenmann H, Grantyn R. *Practical Electrophysiological Methods.* New York: Wiley-Liss; 1992:249–299.)

mode, channels in the patch maintain continuity with the intracellular contents (and thus regulatory influences). The patch can be excised from the cell in inside-out or outside-out configuration allowing the experimentalist to control solution composition on both sides of the membrane. If the cell-attached patch is broken while the pipette maintains tight contact with the cell membrane, the voltage of the entire cell can be controlled and whole-cell currents from the composite activity of all channels in the cell are measured.

The recorded activity of a single K$^+$-selective ion channel in an on-cell membrane patch is shown in Fig. 3. The opening of this one channel allows 5×10^7 K$^+$ ions to cross the membrane each second when the membrane is clamped to -120 mV. Channels are characterized by their single-channel conductance (γ, measured in picosiemens, pS) and unitary current (i, measured in picoamperes, pA) as distinguished from G and I, the conductance and current of a population of channels. Graphing the single-channel current amplitude against membrane voltage gives a current-voltage relation or i-V curve (Fig. 3). Applying Ohm's law (Eq. 3) to the single-channel data ($\gamma = i/\Delta V$) shows that the slope of the i-V relation is the single-channel conductance and the intercept with the voltage axis is the reversal potential at which no current flows. The reversal potential for the channel in Fig. 3 is close to E_K determined by the Nernst relation (Eq. 1), as expected for a K$^+$ channel.

Sodium and Potassium Channels and Action Potentials

Voltage-gated channels open (activate) in response to changes in membrane potential because the electric field acts on the channel to change its protein conformation (or state). It is voltage-gated sodium (Na$^+$) channels that initiate action potentials and voltage-gated K$^+$ channels that cause them to end. Action potentials are large depolarizations (positive movements) of membrane potential associated with neural signals and muscular contraction (Fig. 4). In excitable cells, basal efflux of K$^+$ ions keeps the cell potential at negative (or polarized) values near E_K. An initial depolarization causes Na$^+$ channels to open, allowing positive Na$^+$ ions to flow into the cell down their concentration gradient and shifting the membrane potential in the positive direction. At some potential, Na$^+$ influx is greater than K$^+$ efflux and net current is inward. At this threshold, the membrane begins to move regeneratively to positive potentials as more and more Na$^+$ channels open and the membrane potential rushes toward E_{Na}. The threshold is set by a balance of K$^+$ and Na$^+$ channel activity and is thus controlled by regulation of channel gene expression, protein turnover rates, and modulation of channel activity by accessory molecules and second messengers.

The explosive phase of the action potential slows first because voltage-gated Na$^+$ channels close after opening (in

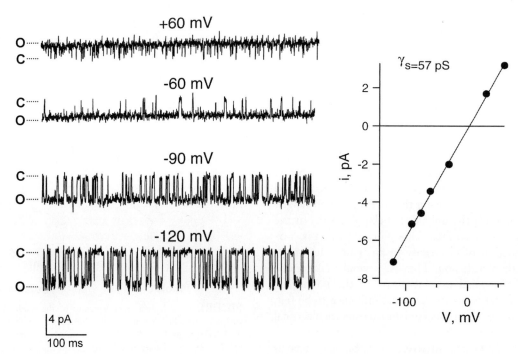

FIGURE 3   Single-channel currents through the *Drosophila melanogaster* open-rectifier K$^+$ channel (ORK1) expressed in *Xenopus laevis* oocytes and studied in an on-cell membrane patch. The channel has an open probability close to 1.0 during bursts and is shown here in the presence of a blocker, Ba^{2+} (5 mM), to reveal the open (O) and closed (C) state levels (filtered at 1 kHz). The plot shows a unitary slope conductance (γ_s) of 57 pS under these conditions: pipette solution has 140 mM KCl so that E_K is ≈ 0 mV. (From Goldstein SA, Wang KW, Ilan N, et al. Sequence and function of the two P domain potassium channels: implications of an emerging superfamily. *J Mol Med* 1998;76:13–20, with permission.)

A

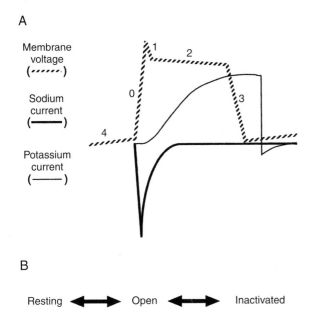

Membrane
voltage
($\cdots\cdots$)

Sodium
current
(—)

Potassium
current
(—)

B

Resting ⟷ Open ⟷ Inactivated

C

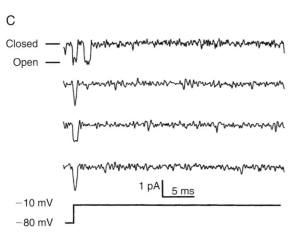

Closed —

Open —

1 pA | 5 ms

−10 mV

−80 mV

FIGURE 4   Representation of a cardiac action potential with Na^+ and K^+ currents. **A:** Diagram of the phases of a cardiac Purkinje cell action potential with currents through two contributing channels superimposed. (From Fozzard H. *Ion Channels in the Cardiovascular System: Function and Dysfunction.* Armonk, NY: Futura Publishing; 1994:81–99, with permission.) Channel currents associated with the five phases of the action potential: phase 0, rapid depolarization (I_{Na}, I_{Ca}); phase 1, fast repolarization (I_{to}); phase 2, plateau (I_{Ca}); phase 3, delayed repolarization (I_{Kr}, I_{Ks}); and phase 4, pacemaker depolarization (I_{IR}, I_f). **B:** Scheme for gating of an inactivating voltage-gated channel. **C:** Single-channel recordings from a cardiac voltage-gated Na^+ channel. In response to a change in voltage from −80 mV to −10 mV, the channel moves from resting to open conformation and then to an inactive state.

a process called inactivation) despite maintained depolarization (Figs. 4B and 4C). The membrane repolarizes to its negative resting potential when K^+ channels open after a delay; the delay prevents overlap of repolarizing K^+ currents and the initial depolarizing phase of the action potential. Thus, inward Na^+ currents move the membrane potential positively toward E_{Na}, whereas subsequent outward K^+ currents return the cell to rest near E_K. Because it takes some

milliseconds for Na^+ channels to recover from inactivation, time during which they do not pass current, the membrane is temporarily inexcitable. This interval is called the refractory period.

The initial movement to threshold comes either from another part of the cell or results from activity of other ion channels. For example, acetylcholine released from a motor nerve crosses the neuromuscular junction to bind to nicotinic acetylcholine receptor channels on the postsynaptic membrane; these channels produce inward cation currents that depolarize the muscle membrane to threshold, initiating an action potential and muscular contraction.

ION CHANNELS

The Ion Conduction Pathway

Before the structure of any integral membrane protein had been determined, ion channels were known to pass ions by forming water-filled holes across cell membranes. First suggested by Hodgkin and Keynes (55) in 1955 and elegantly rendered by Miller (94) in 1987, the porelike structure of ion channels can be divined from four basic attributes. The first we have already considered—high unitary transport rates. Single-channel currents are enormous compared with the turnover rates of other transport proteins. This difference in speed is based on their disparate mechanisms. Non-channel transport events involve the physical movement of the protein with each turnover event. Every translocation requires exposure of a binding site on one side of a membrane, binding of the permeant species, occlusion of the site, a conformational change to allow exposure of the ion on the opposite side of the membrane, and, finally, ion release. Each step must then be carried out in reverse to achieve a complete transport cycle. It is easy to imagine that less time and energy would be spent if opening a passageway permitted diffusion of millions of ions without the need for further conformation changes. The fastest transporters are three orders of magnitude slower than ion channels; the Cl^-/HCO_3^- exchanger, band 3, moves 10^4 chloride ions per second at room temperature.

The second attribute of ion channels that demands a pore structure is their low temperature coefficient for function. The influence of temperature on Na^+ and K^+ currents in the squid axon was studied by Hodgkin, Huxley, and Katz (53) and found to be small ($Q_{10} \approx 1.3$, corresponding to an enthalpic energy barrier of ~5 kcal/mol). This was indistinguishable from the value determined for unrestricted diffusion of the ions in aqueous solution. Since increasing the temperature provides thermal energy to drive protein movements, a low Q_{10} argues against the coupling of any large conformational changes in protein structure to individual ion transport events. Enzymes and carrier-type transporters show a significantly higher enthalpic barrier ($Q_{10} \approx 3$, corresponding to ~18 kcal/mol).

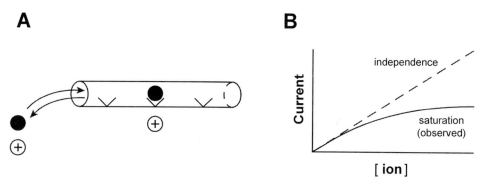

FIGURE 5   A: Model of a multi-ion pore. Ions entering a channel may find it occupied and be unable to traverse the membrane. For this reason, ions do not move through multi-ion channels independently but show saturating velocity **(B)** at high substrate concentration. (See Hille B. *Ion Channels of Excitable Membranes*, 3rd ed. Sunderland, MA: Sinauer; 2001; and Hodgkin AL, Keynes RD. The potassium permeability of a giant nerve fibre. *J Physiol* 1955;128:61–88.)

A third attribute of channel function that supports a pore structure is ion–ion flux coupling. Ions crossing the membrane through channels do not act independently. That is, ion flux is not directly proportional to ion concentration because sometimes an ion enters the channel only to find it is occupied and impassable (Fig. 5A). Whether by repulsion between charged ions or mechanical obstruction, increasing ion concentration leads to current saturation (Fig. 5B) just as an enzyme reaches a saturating velocity at high substrate concentration (V_{max} in the Michaelis-Menten model of enzyme kinetics). Ion–ion flux coupling occurs when one ion sweeps another with it through the channel. Experimentally, this is assessed by studying how voltage alters inward and outward ion flux. In squid axons, K^+ ions behave as if they carry a charge of +2 or +3 because they traverse the membrane with one or two other K^+ ions (8, 55).

The fourth phenomenon that argues for a pore structure is ion–water flux coupling. Ion channels contain water in addition to ions. The pore is too narrow to allow the water molecules to pass each other or the ions. This means that if water is forced to flow by hydrostatic or osmotic pressure, it will drag ions across the membrane even if there is no chemical or electrical gradient acting on the ions. A voltage can be applied to reduce the ion current to zero and the value of this voltage (the "streaming potential") can be used to determine the number of water molecules lined up in single file within the pore (93, 109).

High unitary transport rates, low temperature coefficients, ion–ion flux coupling, and ion–water flux coupling are observed in ion channels. These four behaviors have also been demonstrated for gramicidin A, a small-peptide antibiotic known to form a pore in membranes (34). Using x-ray crystallography of ion channels, MacKinnon and colleagues have solved atomic-resolution structures of ion channels, directly showing their pores to be transmembrane pathways filled with water and conducting ions (28, 62, 63, 75). Similar pore structures for voltage-gated Na and ligand-gated channels have been supported by electron microscopy (95, 112).

Ion Permeation: How Channels Are Fast and Specific

In biology, high specificity is typically associated with tight binding as exemplified by antigen-antibody interactions. However, K^+ channels show high specificity (greater than 1000:1 for K^+ over Na^+) and high throughput (10^7 K^+ ions per second) (136). How this is thought to transpire can be understood by considering the structure of the *Streptomyces lividans* K^+ channel, KcsA (Fig. 6). To move across the membrane, K^+ ions must exchange a shell of stabilizing water molecules for new interactions with the channel protein. Na^+ ions do not readily occupy a K^+ pore site as they bind their hydrating waters more tightly, and are too large to enter the pore while hydrated. When dehydrated, Na^+ ions are ≈ 0.4 Å smaller than K^+ ions so that channel residues optimally positioned to coordinate K^+ appear to be too distant to stabilize a naked Na^+ ion. High-resolution structures (96, 141) of the KcsA channel reveal that two dehydrated K^+ ions are held within the pore by 16 hydrogen bonds that make up the selectivity sequence. The entry of a third K^+ ion to one side of the pore apparently destabilizes the coordination of the resident K^+ ions and causes a repositioning of hydrogen bonding such that the K^+ ion at the opposite side leaves the pore. The three-ion configuration is assumed to be a high-energy transitional state. It is not observed experimentally, but is presumed to underlie the remarkably high throughput of ion conduction in a K^+ channel. A similar mechanism is likely to also operate in Ca^{2+} and Na^+ channels (16, 18).

Channel Proteins and Domain Function: P Loops, Voltage Sensors, and Gates

Ion channels are named for the ions they permit to traverse the membrane. Cloning of genes for voltage-gated Na^+, Ca^{2+}, and K^+ channels made clear their membership in an extended molecular superfamily marked by similarities in primary sequence and predicted membrane topology (60).

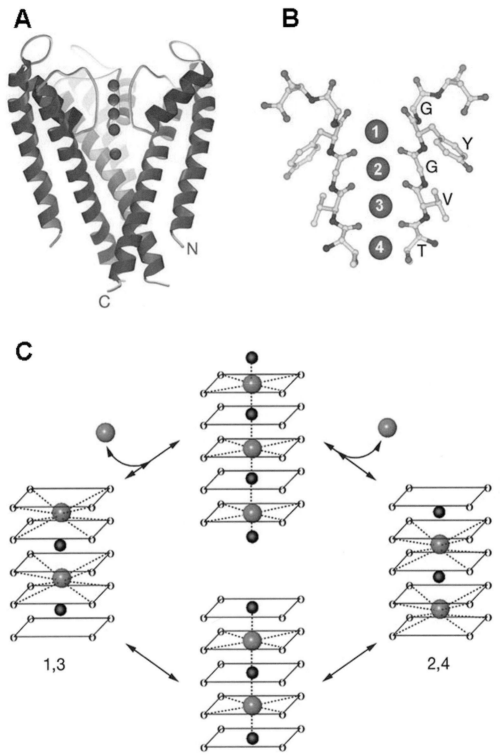

FIGURE 6   Crystal structure of the KcsA K$^+$ channel. The channel, cloned from *Streptomyces lividans*, was analyzed by x-ray crystallography to a resolution of 2.0 Å. Images reveal four identical subunits forming a transmembrane pore filled with K$^+$ ions and water molecules. **A:** A ribbon representation of the KcsA channel tetramer viewed from a side view, with the subunit closest to the viewer removed. The selectivity filter is shown as thinner rods and the locations of K$^+$ binding are seen as spheres. **B:** A close-up view of the selectivity filter, using a ball-and-stick representation, with front and back subunits removed. This narrow region is 12 Å long and lined by main-chain carbonyl oxygen atoms; the K$^+$ binding sites are numbered, with position 1 closest to the extracellular face. **C:** A schematic of the throughput cycle of K$^+$ ions through the channel's pore, with K$^+$ ions and water molecules shown as large and small spheres, respectively. Dotted lines represent hydrogen bonds, and the binding configurations noted as 1,3 and 2,4 are considered to be relatively stable, low-energy states (3 o'clock and 9 o'clock positions). Ion throughput occurs as a new K$^+$ ion is partially dehydrated and stabilized by hydrogen bonds within the selectivity filter (12 o'clock position). Because this transition is a high-energy state, one of the two peripheral K$^+$ ions quickly exits the pore. The 6 o'clock position shows an alternative transitional state allowing a switch of ions from the 1,3 to the 2,4 configuration, and vice-versa. (From Morais-Cabral JH, Zhou Y, MacKinnon R. Energetic optimization of ion conduction rate by the K$^+$ selectivity filter. *Nature* 2001;414:37–42, with permission.)

Once cloned, the protein domains that participate in specific channel functions were identified by site-directed mutation, and a crude idea of the molecular architecture of ion channel pores emerged that was later seen in the solved structures for bacterial K$^+$ channels: hourglass in shape with a short tight selectivity filter (Figs. 6A and 6B). Na$^+$ and Ca^{2+} channels contain four homologous domains, each with six predicted membrane-spanning segments (Fig. 7A). Voltage-gated K$^+$ channel subunits are similar in size and topology to a single Na$^+$ channel domain (Fig. 7B). These channels share an overall tetrameric anatomy like that found for KcsA and other crystallized channels. A single conduction pore is formed either through pseudosymmetric folding of four homologous domains or aggregation of four independent subunits (45, 83). The residues linking every fifth and sixth membrane-spanning segment contribute to pore formation (P domains) and are arrayed centrally as four "pore loops" (84). Some K$^+$ channel subunits contain one P loop and two transmembrane segments, such as the KcsA channel (Fig. 7C); others have two P loops and four or more transmembrane stretches (Figs. 7D and 7E) (38).

THE PORE

The first clue to the location of the pore came from studies of inhibition of the *Shaker* K$^+$ channel of *Drosophila melanogaster* by the scorpion neurotoxin charybdotoxin (81). Prior studies indicated that the toxin inhibited by physically binding in the ion conduction pathway and that binding involved negatively-charged channel sites (5, 80, 92). Systematic point mutation of negative channel residues revealed that a glutamate in the region linking transmembrane segments 5 and 6 (S5, S6) was a toxin interaction site and suggested the channel pore was nearby (81). Residues across this S5–S6 linker region were subsequently shown to be critical to toxin binding (39, 40, 79) and to contain sites mediating pore blockade by agents applied from both the extracellular and intracellular solution as expected if the residues span the membrane (82, 135). Comparison of sequences of cloned K$^+$ channels allowed identification of a "signature sequence" of eight highly conserved residues in the P domains of all K$^+$-selective ion channels (TMTTV-GYG in *Shaker* K$^+$ channels) (47, 48). These residues coordinate K$^+$ ions in the KcsA channel (Figs. 6A and 6B).

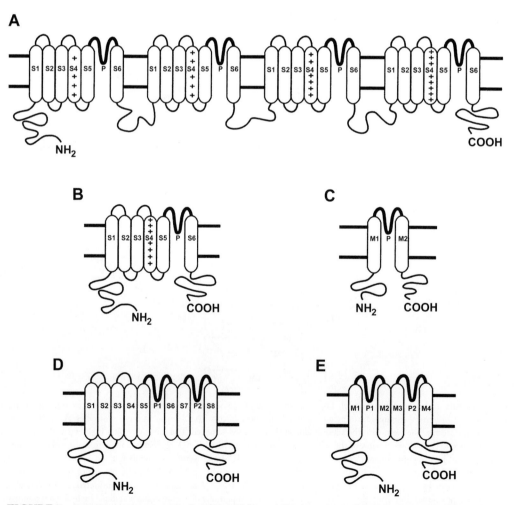

FIGURE 7   Probable membrane topologies of Na$^+$, Ca^{2+}, and K$^+$ channel pore-forming subunits. **A:** Voltage-gated Na$^+$ and Ca^{2+} channels. **B:** Voltage-gated K$^+$ channels. **C:** Inward rectifier K$^+$ channels, KcsA, and epithelial Na$^+$ channels. **D:** A two–P-domain outward rectifier K$^+$ channel. **E:** A two P-domain open rectifier K$^+$ channel.

THE S4 DOMAIN AND VOLTAGE SENSING

In 1952, Hodgkin and Huxley (53) first proposed that changes in voltage might cause movement of charged "gating particles" within nerve membranes to turn Na^+ and K^+ conductances on and off. After cloning revealed the primary sequences of the voltage-gated channels, residues in the fourth predicted transmembrane segment (S4) of each subunit or domain became the leading candidates for these voltage sensing charges (Figs. 7A and 7B) (100). S4 segments are marked by positively-charged arginine or lysine residues at every third or fourth position, a motif unique to voltage-sensing ion channels. Extensive evaluation of the effects of S4 mutagenesis on voltage-gated channel opening and direct evidence that the segment moves in response to changes in transmembrane voltage strongly supports the idea that S4 is a major part of the voltage sensor. Additionally, acidic countercharges are distributed in transmembrane stretches 2 and 3 of K^+ channels and these interact with the positive S4 charges to contribute to voltage sensing (10). The S4 segment appears to be at the periphery of the channel, with its charged residues facing centrally, based on studies of archaeal (25) and mammalian (75, 76) K^+ channels. At present, the movements of the voltage sensor are a topic of intense investigation.

LIGAND GATING

Other channels are activated or closed by the binding of small molecules. Thus, two acetylcholine (ACh) molecules bind to the external face of the nicotinic ACh receptor channel of neuromuscular junctions leading to the opening of its cation-selective pore. In the heart, binding of ACh to muscarinic receptors liberates $G\beta\gamma$ in sinoatrial and atrioventricular nodal cells; the G-protein binds directly to cardiac K^+ channels leading to their activation. This explains the response of the heart to ACh released by the vagus nerve, which opens K^+ channels and allows an efflux of K^+ ions to shift the membrane to more negative potentials. This slows the heart rate by protracting the rise of membrane potential to the threshold for Na^+-channel activation (65). In neurons, there are myriad ligand-gated ion channels that respond to a variety of neurotransmitters to allow specific ion flux (i.e., a single ionic species) or nonselective cation or anion flux. Another mechanism by which ion channels can be modulated by ligand binding is via pore blockade. For example, intracellular Mg^{2+} and polyamines enter the pores of inwardly rectifying (IR) K^+ channels and physically interfere with ion permeation until the membrane voltage is negative to E_K and external K^+ ions can move into the pore to dislodge the blockers (77) (see discussion of cardiac action potentials in subsequent sections).

ACTIVATION AND INACTIVATION GATES

The location and movement of the gates that close pores and move away during channel activation are not yet known for all ion channels. However, a comparison of structural data between KcsA and a bacterial calcium-gated K^+ channel (MthK) that was crystallized in the open configuration supports a mechanism by which the helices following the P domain form a gate by making an "inverted teepee" that blocks intracellular side of the selectivity filter (the inner vestibule). In the open state, these helices open the gate by bending at a glycine "hinge" to allow for ionic access to the pore (62). In other K^+ channels where this glycine residue is conserved, it is believed that this gating mechanism is also used. There is also experimental evidence to support a gate that blocks off the inner vestibule in voltage-gated K^+ channels (74). In K2P background channels, the activation gating appears to occur in the outer vestibule (142). Structural data from nicotinic ACh channels, suggests a third picture for channel opening: the binding of ligand to the extracellular region of the channel allows for conduction of cations by inducing a widening of the pore itself (126).

Fast inactivation of voltage-gated channels has been well delineated. Inactivation, as occurs in the Na^+ channels that initiate action potentials and many K^+ channels, is relatively voltage-insensitive and results from internal channel residues moving into the pore after the channel has opened (37, 57). It is by this mechanism that the regenerative activity of Na^+ channels is controlled (Fig. 4).

Modifying Channel Function

A DIVERSITY OF CHANNEL SUBUNITS

Most channels form by the association of multiple pore-forming subunits; this provides a mechanism for functional diversity: altered subunit composition (17). Thus, voltage-gated Cl^- channels are dimeric, ATP-gated 2PX receptor channels trimeric (or possibly hexameric, see [101]), voltage-gated K^+ channels tetrameric, and nicotinic acetylcholine receptor channels pentameric. Functional diversity can be generated by formation of heteromers of nonidentical channel subunits. For example, three of the four isoforms of G-protein–regulated inward-rectifier K^+ channels (GIRK2-4, or Kir3.2-3.4) can exist as homotetramers in the brain, but GIRK1 appears to complex with GIRK2 in mammalian cerebellar neurons. Also, GIRK1/4 heteromers underlie the I_{KACh} current of the heart (85). Similarly, the profile of K^+-channel currents from Kv1 (*Shaker*) family potassium channels in the brain is expanded by forming tetramers of one, two, or four different isoforms per tetramer (23).

ACCESSORY SUBUNITS

An even greater assortment of functional channels can be achieved by assembly of channel complexes with pore-forming and accessory subunits. All major classes of voltage-gated ion channels have been shown to stably interact with accessory subunits, which are often referred to as "β subunits." This growing list of accessory subunits includes soluble cytosolic proteins, type I and type II single transmembrane-spanning proteins, and subunits that span the membrane 2, 4, and even 17 times. Many of these proteins are depicted in Fig. 8.

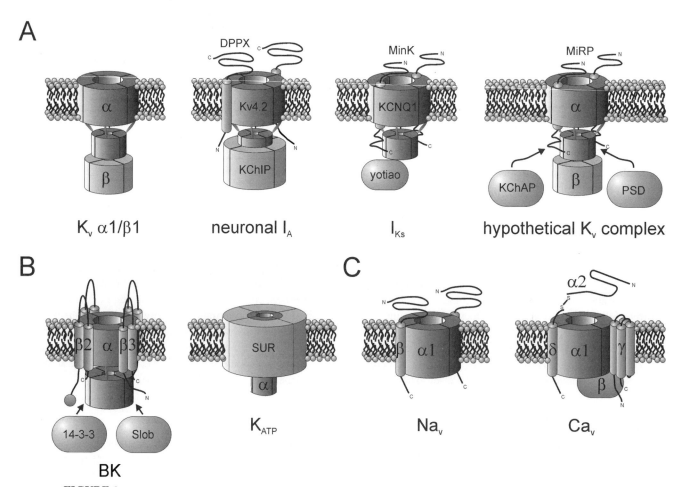

FIGURE 8 Some examples of ion channel accessory subunits. **A:** Cartoons representing K+ channel complexes and native current correlate where known, showing pore-forming α and ancillary β subunits in relation to the plasma membrane. Left to right: A cytoplasmic β subunit ($K_v\beta1$) subunit tetramer docks tightly with the cytoplasmic N-terminal domains of an voltage-gated K+ channel ($K_v\alpha1$) tetramer to form a $K_v\alpha1$-$K_v\beta1$ channel complex; four cytoplasmic K+ channel interacting proteins (KChIPs) co-assemble with a Kv4.2 α-subunit tetramer and associated DPPX subunits, underlying the neuronal A-type (I_A) potassium current; a KCNQ1 α-subunit tetramer associated with 2 MinK subunits and the protein kinase A-protein phosphatase-1 targeting protein, yotiao, underlying the cardiac slowly activating delayed-rectifiers (I_{Ks}) potassium current; a hypothetical K_v channel complex comprising a tetramer of a subunits plus MinK-related peptides (MiRPs), K+ channel associated protein (KChAP) and postsynaptic density protein (PSD). **B:** Ca^{2+} (BK) and ATP (K_{ATP}) sensitive K+ channel complexes and their accessory subunits. BK channel α subunits can associate with transmembrane (TM) β subunits designated β1-4 and also interact with cytoplasmic Slob protein and the ubiquitous regulatory protein, 14-3-3. K_{ATP} channels co-assemble from four TM α subunits and four TM sulfonylurea receptors (SUR). **C:** Voltage-gated Na^+ (Na_v) and Ca^{2+} (Ca_v) channel complexes and their associated δ subunits. Na_v α subunits associate with TM β subunits; Ca_v channels comprise a complex assembly of a single TM β subunit linked by a disulfide bond to an extracellular α2 subunit, a four TM-domain γ subunit, and a cytoplasmic β subunit. (From McCrossan ZA, Abbott GW. The MinK-related peptides. *Neuropharmacology* 2004;47:787–821, with permission.)

One family of accessory subunits, MinK and the MinK-related peptides (MiRPs), are single transmembrane-spanning proteins that play a fundamental role in controlling K+-channel gating kinetics, conductance, pharmacology, and trafficking (2, 87). The physiologic relevance of these proteins is exemplified by the association of clinical disorders with their mutation leading to congenital long QT syndrome, predisposition to drug-induced arrhythmia, sensorineural deafness, and periodic paralysis (1, 29, 114, 118). MinK, for example, endows the KCNQ1 channel with the unique biophysical properties—including slower activation and inactivation and a more depolarized threshold for activation—that allow it to op-

erate the normal cardiac slow delayed rectifier current (I_{Ks}) (115, 118); and as a short-circuit K+ conductance of proximal-tubule brush border that facilitates solute-coupled Na^+ transport (127). MiRP1 establishes the cardiac rapid delayed rectifier (I_{Kr}) current by assembly with the hERG K+ channel (3) and may also complex with Kv4 and hyperpolarization-activated cation (HCN) channels in the heart that underlie the transient outward (I_{to}) (27, 139) and pacemaker (I_f) (26, 138) currents, respectively. In distinction to the effects of MinK on KCNQ1, the association of MiRP2 with KCNQ1 creates a noninactivating "leak" channel thought to function in the gastrointestinal tract (113). MiRP2 also partners with the predominate skeletal muscle K$^+$ channel, Kv3.4, to lower the threshold for channel activation (1) and with Kv2.1 and Kv3.1 in brain to slow gating kinetics (88).

Another family of integral membrane proteins, KCNMB, has four family members, all of which alter the properties of the calcium- and voltage-gated K$^+$ channel, BK (also called MaxiK or K$_{Ca}$). BK is a widely expressed potassium channel that can attenuate Ca^{2+} influx from voltage-gated Ca^{2+} channels by hyperpolarizing the cell membrane in response to local elevations of Ca^{2+}. In vascular smooth muscle, BK channels co-associate with KCNMB1 (β1), which greatly increases their calcium sensitivity (89). This enables tight control of vascular tone in response to a rising [Ca^{2+}], as demonstrated in a mouse model of hypertension, produced by a knockout of the *KCNMB1* gene (13). Rat adrenal chromaffin cells release catecholamines in response to electrical stimulation; a subset expressing KCNMB2 lack the ability to fire rapidly, while those expressing BK alone maintain a relatively hyperpolarized membrane potential to allow for repetitive firing (132). Splice variants of KCNMB3 expressed in spleen, liver, kidney, and pancreas endow BK with different degrees of inactivation (125), KCNMB4 is found predominately in the central nervous system, where it alters calcium-sensitivity and slows activation of BK (12).

To illustrate the rich variety of channel behaviors that can be produced by accessory subunits, consider the Kv4 family of voltage-gated K$^+$ channels that underlie rapidly activating and inactivating neuronal currents (A-type or I$_{SA}$) and more slowly inactivating, transient outward currents in the heart (I$_{to}$). In dog heart, expression of Kv4.3 mRNA is stable from the endocardium to the epicardium, even though I$_{to}$ current amplitude is greater—and shows faster recovery from inactivation—in epicardial myocytes. The gradient of I$_{to}$ parallels the expression of the soluble K$^+$-channel interacting protein 2 (KChIP2) that enhances surface expression and speeds recovery from inactivation of Kv4 channels (108). The surface expression, gating, and pharmacology of myocardial Kv4.3 can also be modulated by other soluble accessory proteins such as K$^+$-channel associated protein (KChAP) (67) and Kvβ (68, 133). In the brain, Kv4.3 channels interact in some cells with the integral membrane protein, dipeptidyl-aminopeptidase–like protein 6 (DPPX), leading to dramatically enhanced rates of activation, inactivation, and recovery from inactivation (99), whereas it associates in some interneurons with KChIP1 protein (105), These are examples of cellular "tuning" of the biophysical properties of one channel by accessory subunits to achieve different functions.

POSTTRANSLATIONAL MODIFICATION

Ion channel properties can also be altered by posttranslational modifications such as glycosylation, palmitoylation, sumoylation, and partial proteolysis. The effects of N-linked glycosylation on channels are somewhat variable. For example, glycosylation can affect gating of Kv1.1 potassium channels (122) and Na$^+$ channels (140); whereas it increases surface expression/stability of the nicotinic ACh receptor (91), purinergic (P2X) receptors (124), and the hERG K$^+$ channel (42).

Palmitoylation involves a reversible attachment of the long-chain fatty-acid, palmitate, to modify protein–lipid interactions and target proteins to specific microdomains of the plasma membrane. The Kv1.1 potassium channel appears to be palmitoylated at the cytoplasmic linker between the S2 and S3 transmembrane segments to speed the channel's activation kinetics (44). The γ subunit of GABA$_A$ (γ-aminobutyric acid) receptor/channels are also palmitoylated, enabling clustering at the neuronal synapses (104).

Sumoylation involves the covalent modification with small ubiquitin-related modifier (SUMO) proteins that have generally been thought to mediate nuclear trafficking. However, sumoylation is now known to silence the background potassium channel, K2P1, of brain, heart, and kidney, while it resides in the plasma membrane (102). Another recently recognized modification is furin proteolysis of the α and γ subunits during maturation of the epithelial Na$^+$ channel, ENaC, which appears to be necessary for normal channel gating (59).

SECOND-MESSENGER REGULATION

Like many other cellular proteins, ion channels are subject to regulation by a panoply of second messengers including kinases, phosphatases, nucleotides, phosphoinositides and other fatty acids, calcium ions, protons (pH), and reactive-oxygen species including nitric oxide. Consider again the calcium- and voltage-gated K$^+$ channel BK, which has multiple consensus sites for phosphorylation: BK channels may show increased or decreased activity when modulated by protein kinase A or protein kinase C, depending on the splice variant expressed. The channel can also be regulated by the cellular redox state, eicosanoids, nitric oxide, the heme molecule, and intracellular pH (121, 129). This is, of course, in addition to modulation of gating by cytosolic Ca^{2+}.

DRUGS THAT ACT ON ION CHANNELS

Many drugs act on ion channels to modify their function. Some simply occlude the ion conduction pore while others alter channel activity by changing the opening or closing process. Lidocaine blocks Na$^+$ channels only when they are open. This is called use-dependent blockade. After application of the drug, the first depolarization elicits a nearly normal current indicating that little block has occurred; subsequent depolarizations show progressively smaller currents as the drug binds incrementally and does not unbind at rest (123). Conversely, the alkaloid batrachotoxin keeps Na$^+$ channels open on a time scale of hours while pinacidil, and diazepam, are examples of drugs that act to increase the open probability of ATP-sensitive K$^+$ channels and GABA-activated chloride channels, respectively. Since ion channels are in all cells, drugs can cause unintended side effects by action outside the target organ.

Indeed, most drugs act on more than one channel population. Quinidine blocks not only cardiac Na$^+$ channels but many K$^+$ channels and side effects are a major consideration when choosing antiarrhythmic therapies. Other drugs act to alter secondary messenger systems. In this way, epinephrine acts via G-protein–coupled receptors of the heart to increase cyclic adenosine monophosphate (cAMP) levels, protein kinase A activity, and phosphorylation of cardiac Ca^{2+} and K$^+$ channels, thus leading to increased activity of both channel types. The result is greater contractility (due to increased intracellular Ca^{2+}) and faster heart rate (due to increased K$^+$ flux and a shortened cardiac action potential).

EXCITABLE TISSUES

Impulse Propagation in Nerves

One of the key features of electrical signals is the speed at which they spread from one part of a cell to another (even in a long muscle fiber or nerve axon). Membrane potentials can extend passively by electrotonic spread; this mechanism is like the conduction of electricity through a wire. However, cells do not make good "wires" and conduction in this fashion has a limited range. Conversely, action potentials can spread without attenuation over long distances because of the regenerative action of voltage-gated ion channels. Both mechanisms operate in excitable cells.

Electrotonic spread is inefficient as membrane potential differences dissipate along the length of a cell because current flows not only axially within the cell but also escapes across its membrane through ion channels. How far an electrical signal can travel in this fashion depends on how much current flows in each pathway. The channels that establish the resting potential determine the membrane resistance (r$_m$) such that more open channels will reduce r$_m$, allowing more current to leak out of the cell and therefore dissipate a depolarized membrane potential. The length of propagation of an action potential is a function of the r$_m$ and the axial resistance (r$_{ax}$, which is determined by the cross-sectional area and the resistivity of the axonal cytoplasm) such that an increased r$_m$ will allow for longer propagation but greater r$_{ax}$ will reduce this distance. With about 10^5 open K$^+$ channels over a 1-cm length of a typical 10-μm nonmyelinated axon, the membrane resistance is about 100-fold smaller than the axial resistance, and most of the current will flow out of the membrane. Different strategies allow electrical signals to travel farther distances. These include increasing axon diameter (which will reduce r$_{ax}$ by more than r$_m$) and by insulating regions of the axonal membrane with myelin to increase r$_m$.

Consider how action potential propagation occurs in a myelinated axon. In this case, Na$^+$ channels are restricted to nodes of Ranvier spaced roughly 1 mm apart. When a nodal membrane is depolarized by Na$^+$ entry the peak of the action potential is many times larger than threshold. This means that despite substantial attenuation of the signal due to the electrotonic decay (1/e, that is ~one third, of the signal remains for each millimeter traveled), an adjacent node will easily be brought above threshold, causing Na$^+$ channels in this node to open and the wave of depolarization to move along the fiber. Although the passive cable properties of the axon allow conduction of the depolarization to occur in both directions, the Na$^+$ channels of the recently depolarized nodes are inactivated and therefore regeneration and propagation of the action potential proceeds only in the forward direction.

Conduction in an unmyelinated fiber happens in the same general way except that Na$^+$ channels are distributed evenly along the cell and propagation occurs as a continuous process. Factors that affect conduction velocity include axon size (larger diameter axons have relatively less drop of the potential across the membrane), membrane capacitance (the capacitance per unit area of all cell membranes is essentially the same; however, a myelin sheath increases r$_m$, decreases capacitance and boosts conduction velocity 10- to 100-fold), Na$^+$ channel density (increased channel number decreases threshold and increases peak currents to increase conduction velocity) and Na$^+$ channel activity (diminished by drugs such as lidocaine and by temperature extremes, which slow opening or speed inactivation).

Electromechanical Coupling in Skeletal Muscle

When an action potential travels down a motor neuron from the spinal cord it reaches nerve terminals on a number of muscle fibers that compose its motor unit. The action potential depolarizes the presynaptic nerve terminal causing its voltage-sensitive Ca^{2+} channels to open. An influx of Ca^{2+} ions from the extracellular space leads synaptic vesicles to fuse with the cell membrane, releasing their stored ACh into the synaptic cleft (characteristically ~100 vesicles fuse, each containing ~1000 ACh molecules). The ACh molecules traverse the cleft and bind to ACh receptors (AChRs) on the muscle membrane (or sarcolemma) at localized regions, the motor end plates.

ACh binding causes AChRs to open and cations to flow; this depolarizes the muscle membrane, bringing its Na$^+$ channels to threshold and initiating an action potential. Continuous with the sarcolemma is a network of transverse tubules (T-tubules) that penetrate the entire cross-section of the muscle fiber. The function of the network is to propagate the action potential from the sarcolemma to the muscle center. The need for such a system is apparent if one considers the time course for most natural transduction processes that involve second messengers. Because muscle fibers are large (50–100 μm in diameter) diffusion of a soluble mediator from the surface membrane to the fiber center would take ~1 second. Electrical conduction transmits the stimulus to the contractile apparatus in milliseconds. Moreover, under normal conditions, the amount of ACh released is so great that every nerve action potential results in a muscle action potential and contraction of the motor unit.

Signals from T-tubules are transmitted by a unique channel gating mechanism (Fig. 9). Action potentials travel from the sarcolemma to the T-tubular membrane where voltage-dependent L-type Ca^{2+} channels called dihydropyridine (DHP) receptors sense the depolarization. The signal then crosses to ryanodine receptors (also called Ca^{2+}-release channels) in the sarcoplasmic reticulum (SR); the SR is an intracellular membrane system that surrounds the muscles' contractile filament bundles called myofibrils. A high concentration of Ca^{2+} (~1 mM) is maintained inside the SR by an ATP-driven Ca^{2+} pump (the Ca^{2+}-ATPase) and it is Ca^{2+} release that allows muscle contraction; binding of Ca^{2+} to troponin shifts the position of tropomyosin on the actin filament, allowing myosin heads to interact with actin to generate force. The signal from the T-tubule travels through its DHP receptors by a direct mechanical linkage to the ryanodine receptors in the SR terminal cisternae to cause their opening and release of Ca^{2+} ions.

To control muscular movement, the termination of the response must also be rapid. This is achieved by three mechanisms. The primary event is re-uptake of Ca^{2+} into the SR. This is mediated by the Ca^{2+}-ATPase which is present at high density (>10,000 molecules/μm^2) and the Ca^{2+} buffering protein of the SR, calsequestrin, which can bind ~40 Ca^{2+} ions per molecule. Second, ACh in the synaptic cleft is rapidly hydrolyzed by acetylcholinesterase; it is choline that is taken back up into the nerve termini. Finally, repolarization of the T-tubule leads to closure of the ryanodine receptor halting release of Ca^{2+} from the SR. When no longer stimulated, the muscular action potential ends by the usual processes of Na^+ channel inactivation and opening of K^+ channels.

A single motor nerve axon may branch extensively and innervate many muscle fibers. Each muscle fiber, however, has only one endplate and therefore receives input from only one axon. The group of fibers innervated by a single neuron is called a motor unit. Weak contractions in a muscle group involve activity in small motor units with only a few fibers. To elicit larger forces, larger motor units are recruited. Thus, the small motor units in the extraocular muscles contain only three to six muscle fibers, whereas large motor units in the gastrocnemius can contain more than 1000.

Contraction can be blocked at each step by toxins and drugs. Thus, some Ca^{2+} channel blockers and botulinum toxin block release of ACh from nerve termini. Curare and snake toxins can block the ACh receptor. Most local anesthetics and tetrodotoxin block Na^+ channels. Dihydropyridines block the voltage-sensing action of the DHP receptor, whereas dantrolene blocks opening of the ryanodine receptor.

Smooth Muscle

Although smooth muscle controls the resistance of blood vessels, digestion of food, and uterine contraction (among many examples), it is much less well understood than skeletal or cardiac muscle. Like them, smooth muscles contract due to actin-myosin interactions; however, control of contraction and the geometry of smooth muscle filaments are unique. Smooth muscles are sensitive to a wide variety of mediators including hormones, peptides, and diffusible messengers like nitric oxide (NO). Thus, vascular smooth muscles relax in response to ACh, epinephrine, NO, atrial natriuretic peptide, and prostaglandin I; they contract to norepinephrine, angiotensin II, and in response to mechanical stretch.

Smooth muscle cells are smaller (2–10 μm in diameter, 100–500 μm in length) than skeletal muscle fibers and have no T-tubules. They do have a small SR compartment that stores Ca^{2+} ions. Although Ca^{2+} activates contraction in smooth muscle cells, it is by a different mechanism than in skeletal muscle. Here, the primary control of contraction is phosphorylation of myosin, which allows it to interact with actin. The phosphorylation is catalyzed by the myosin light-chain kinase, an enzyme activated by Ca^{2+} through the binding of a Ca^{2+}-calmodulin complex. Smooth muscle cells are sometimes electrically coupled to allow waves of electrical activity as seen in the gastrointestinal tract or uterus.

Some interesting types of channels observed in smooth muscle include BK channels, which are opened by depolarization and/or rises in intracellular Ca^{2+}; stretch-activated cation channels; receptor-operated Ca^{2+} channels that do not require membrane depolarization to activate; and ATP-sensitive K^+ channels that are normally held closed by the

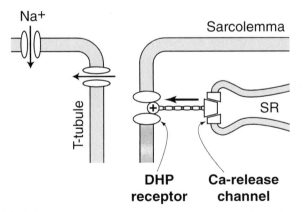

FIGURE 9 Schematic of skeletal muscle activation. Acetylcholine molecules bind to receptors in the motor end plates of the sarcolemma, causing these channels to open and initiating an action potential (Na^+ flux is indicated). This leads to depolarization of the T-tubule membrane network that penetrates the muscle fiber and contains voltage-gated Na^+ channels that propagate the signal rapidly and with high fidelity. Specialized junctions are present between T-tubules and the terminal cisternae of the sarcoplasmic reticulum (SR) called triads: In the T-tubule are dihydropyridine (DHP) receptors that sense depolarization and, apparently via a direct mechanical linkage, cause Ca^{2+}-release channels to open, leading to contraction. These Ca^{2+} channels (also known as ryanodine receptors) are large protein complexes formed by four 400-kD subunits that traverse the space between the T-tubule and SR membranes.

presence of intracellular ATP and function primarily under ischemic conditions when ATP levels fall.

Cardiac Action Potentials

Unlike skeletal muscle, the heart beats by itself. Innervation of the heart by the autonomic nervous system serves to modulate the rate and strength of contractions. Pacemaking in the heart is provided by specialized myocardial nodal cells that produce rhythmic action potentials. The timing of action potential propagation in the heart from sinus node to Purkinje fiber to working muscle is uniquely important for its effective function as a pump. Although cardiac myocytes are striated muscle cells, they differ from skeletal myocytes in that calcium influx from L-type Ca^{2+} channels (DHP receptors) play a much greater role in triggering Ca^{2+} release from the ryanodine receptors (so-called "Ca^{2+}-induced Ca^{2+} release").

The action potential in working muscle and Purkinje fibers is similar to that in axons, in that voltage-gated Na^+ and K^+ channels play a central role. These cells exhibit a pattern of cyclical excitability with five phases (Fig. 4). Phase 0 is an explosive rise in membrane potential due to a rush of Na^+ into the cell (down its concentration gradient) through voltage-gated Na^+ channels that open with membrane depolarization; these channels then rapidly inactivate. Phase 1 is a brief repolarization step mediated by voltage-gated K^+ channels that open with depolarization and, like phase 0 Na^+ channels, rapidly inactivate. Because outward flow of K^+ (down its concentration gradient) makes the cell interior more negative, opening K^+ channels shifts the cell toward more negative potentials. Phase 2, the plateau in the action potential, is coincident with myocardial contraction and results from the cumulative activity of a number of channel and carrier-type transporters. The duration of phase 2 is determined by the activity of voltage-gated Ca^{2+} channels, as well as K^+ channels that open with a delay in response to membrane depolarization and remain open until the membrane is again hyperpolarized. These delayed outward K^+ currents return the membrane to its resting potential during phase 3 and allow the heart to relax. Phase 4, the pacemaker potential, is a slow rise in membrane potential attributed to closing of other K^+ channels and the slow opening of hyperpolarization-activated cation channels and instigates the next cycle of excitation and contraction. In broad outline, cardiac excitation results from rapid, voltage-dependent gating of Na^+ channels; delayed, voltage-dependent gating of K^+ channels; and the ability of both channel types to discriminate between Na^+ and K^+ ions.

The heart differs from other excitable tissues in having a longer action potential duration (APD) and a longer refractory period that lasts several hundred milliseconds. During the refractory period, the muscle is unresponsive to electrical stimuli and will not conduct action potentials. The long duration of cardiac action potentials is largely due to the action of Ca^{2+} channels. Ca^{2+} channels are much like Na^+ channels: They are activated by depolarization and they inactivate. However, both processes are much slower in Ca^{2+} channels, so that if subjected to a long depolarization, Ca^{2+} currents are maintained. This allows the membrane to sustain its depolarized status during plateau. Moreover, these channels are essential for Ca^{2+} entry into the myocardial cells to produce contraction. Thus, Ca^{2+} channel blockers decrease the height and duration of the cardiac action potential as well as the force of contraction. These differences between Ca^{2+} and Na^+ channels explain the behavior of pacemaking tissue of the heart (sinoatrial and atrioventricular nodes) when compared with the conduction system (His bundle and Purkinje fibers) and working myocardium. Na^+ channels support rapid conduction in the His-Purkinje system and working muscle, but are inactive in nodal tissue. Ca^{2+} channels generate the slow upstroke characteristic of nodal cells and are responsible for supporting a prolonged plateau phase in the His-Purkinje system and working muscle.

The resting potential of cardiac muscle cells is quite negative. This suggests that a powerful K^+ current is active at rest. These currents are mediated by inward rectifier (IR) K^+ channels, which open when the membrane is hyperpolarized below E_K but close above this potential. The IR channels hold the potential near E_K, but do not interfere with action potential development because they do not pass current at the depolarized voltages where Ca^{2+} or Na^+ channels initiate the upstroke. A rectifier is an electronic device that allows current to pass only in one direction. Analogously, the IR channels cannot pass K^+ ions when current flow becomes outward. The mechanism underlying this behavior is remarkably simple (Fig. 10). At potentials positive to E_K, the outflow of ions is impeded because intracellular Mg^{2+} and polyamines are driven into the pore and physically occlude the conduction pathway. At potentials more negative than E_K, K^+ ions entering the pore from the outside electrostatically "knock" the blocking ions out of the pore to open it for inward ion flux. This mechanism can explain a paradoxical result that can be found in cells that greatly depend on IR channels to maintain the resting membrane potential: although the Nernst relation (Eq. 1) would predict that lowering serum K^+ should make cells more negative by lowering E_K, fewer K^+ ions outside will allow IR channels to remain blocked, and the membrane potential can become more positive as other ionic conductances become predominant.

Pacemaking nodal cells of the heart have relatively few IR K^+ channels to keep resting membrane potential near E_K and express a nonselective cation current (I_f) that activates during the hyperpolarized phase 4 of the cardiac cycle to cause a progressive depolarization. As a result, resting membrane potential is more positive and voltage-gated Na^+ channels are largely inactivated, whereas voltage-gated Ca^{2+} channels remain able to open. These slowly activating Ca^{2+} channels produce the shallow phase 0 upstroke characteristic of cardiac nodal pacemaking cells.

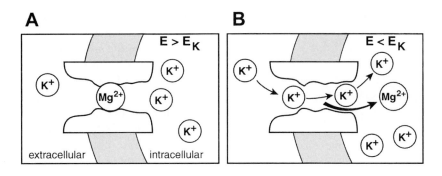

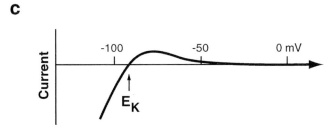

FIGURE 10 Inward rectifier K^+ channels are active near resting membrane potential. A rectifier is a device that allows current to pass in only one direction; inward rectifier K^+ channels allow inward currents but shut down as flux becomes outward. The mechanism is elegantly simple: at potentials positive to the Nernst equilibrium for K^+ ($E > E_K$), the outward flow of ions allows blocking ions (cytoplasmic Mg^{2+} and polyamines) to be driven into the pore where they bind with high affinity and block ion flow (**A**). At potentials that are negative to E_K ($E < E_K$), K^+ ions entering from the outside sweep the blocking ions out of the pore and keep it open for K^+ influx (**B**). The potassium current through these channels is shown in **C**, emphasizing why these channels are called inward rectifiers.

DISORDERED EXCITABILITY

Diseases of Ion Channels

As the molecular basis for ion channel function has been revealed, so has the basis for an increasing number of ion channel-mediated diseases. Because of the critical participation of ion channels in cellular physiology, diseases of these channels affect not only excitable cells but also non-excitable tissue such as lung, bone, pancreas, and of course, the kidney. "Channelopathies" may represent either inherited or acquired loss or gain of channel function and have provided physiologists with a great deal of insight into normal physiology, ion-channel structure and function, mechanisms of inter- and intracellular signaling, and the bases of bulk electrolyte transport. Well over 50 channelopathies have been described and many are reviewed by Hübner and Jentsch (58). In addition, channelopathies of renal salt transport are discussed in Chapter 36.

Mutations that lead to loss of function can be due to low levels of channel protein in the membrane. Thus, the most common variant of cystic fibrosis is marked by inherent instability of the CFTRΔ508 Cl^- channel protein leading to its rapid intracellular degradation. Mutation of barttin, an accessory subunit involved in the normal surface expression of CLC chloride channels in the inner ear and in the nephron's thick ascending limb, can cause salt wasting and deafness (Bartter syndrome type IV) (31, 32). Autoantibodies mediate channel degradation in myasthenia gravis, Lambert-Eaton syndrome and one form of acquired myotonia. Alternatively, loss-of-function disorders can be seen when channels reach the membrane and have a normal turn-over rate but show decreased activity. Examples in humans include persistent hyperinsulinemic hypoglycemia of infancy (PHHI) and the inherited congenital myotonias (Thomsen and Becker syndromes) in which channels open poorly or stay open for only a short time. Other loss-of-function disorders are the result of decreased single-channel conductance, inappropriate down-regulation, decreased agonist affinity, and blockade by drugs or poisons.

Disorders resulting from gain of function include hyperkalemic periodic paralysis (HYPP) in which channels open too readily and paramyotonia congenita (PC) in which they inactivate too slowly. Liddle syndrome is effectively a disorder of apparent mineralocorticoid excess that is largely mediated by reduced turnover at the cell surface of mutant epithelial Na^+ channel (ENaC) subunits. Other gain-of-function diseases are due to channels that have an abnormally high open probability due to mutations or exogenous activation by drugs or poisons. The pathophysiology of neuronal cell death in stroke appears to involve dysfunctional up-regulation of N-methyl-D-aspartate (NMDA) receptors (glutamate-activated Na^+ and Ca^{2+} channels).

In addition to rare diseases, there are common polymorphisms of ion channels that can predispose individuals to disease, such as a variant ENaC subunit that is associated with sodium-sensitive hypertension (7) or the T8A polymorphism of MiRP1 (KCNE2) that increases susceptibility to sulfamethoxazole-related long QT syndrome (114).

Electrolyte and pH Abnormalities

The central role of K^+ in setting cellular resting potential explains why abnormal serum K^+ levels produce the most common and prominent signs and symptoms referable to altered excitability. Abnormalities of calcium, magnesium, and pH can also affect neuromuscular excitability and cardiac pacemaking; and such manifestations will be exacerbated by potassium disturbances. Whereas hypo- and hypernatremia can disturb neurologic function, this is largely the result of movement of water with subsequent altered intracranial pressure (6). The clinical manifestations and management of these electrolyte disorders are discussed in greater detail elsewhere in this text; here, we consider the situations in which altered ionic and acid-base composition produce electrophysiologic effects. Each can be understood in terms of the basic concepts we have presented.

POTASSIUM

Rate of change of Kext and symptoms: As described previously, it is the ratio of K^+ concentration in the intracellular and extracellular fluids that determines membrane excitability. Since K^+ is primarily restricted to the intracellular fluid, the ratio K_{in}/K_{ext} is influenced predominantly by the relatively small K^+ concentration in the extracellular compartment. As a result, minor shifts of K^+ into or out of cells can produce large and potentially lethal changes in K_{ext}. One can generalize that changes in K_{ext} will produce effects by altering resting membrane potential; that hypokalemia tends to produce hyperpolarization; and, conversely, that hyperkalemia leads to depolarization. However, the effects of altered K^+ also depend on the speed at which K^+ levels change. Thus, acute hypokalemia, as seen in severe diarrhea, leads a greater decrease in extracellular than intracellular K^+ levels. From the Nernst relation (Eq. 1) we calculate that E_K under normal ionic conditions (155 K_{in}, 4.0 K_{ext}) is −97 mV while it is −114 mV in acute hypokalemia (145 K_{in}, 2.0 K_{ext}). Hyperpolarization moves the membrane potential away from threshold leading to decreased excitability and symptoms of weakness or paralysis. With a slower depletion of body potassium stores, intracellular K^+ of skeletal muscle can fall as much as 30% (119), shifting E_K to only −107mV (112 K_{in}, 2.0 K_{ext}), minimizing symptoms. Similarly, hyperkalemia that develops rapidly, as seen in tumor lysis syndrome, can shift E_K to −68 mV (160 K_{in}, 12.5 K_{ext}) producing paralysis and arrhythmias secondary to Na^+-channel inactivation and conduction failure. Conversely, chronic hyperkalemia with compensation is more likely to produce partial depolarization (170 K_{in}, 8 K_{ext}, E_K = −82 mV) (106) and a lower risk for adverse sequelae.

Hyperkalemia: a medical emergency: Hyperkalemia rarely elicits extracardiac manifestations until serum levels rise above 8.0 mEq/L, at which point an ascending muscular weakness may occur that can progress to a flaccid paralysis (130) or diaphragmatic paresis (36). The initial—and most worrisome—toxic effects of hyperkalemia are cardiac and include complete heart block, ventricular fibrillation, and cardiac arrest. In the heart, elevated extracellular K^+ tends to depolarize excitable cells and lead to Na^+ channel inactivation. This produces an attenuated ventricular action potential upstroke (now carried largely by inward Ca^{2+} currents) and slowed propagation of excitation across the myocardium (Fig. 11). An additional effect of the high K_{ext} is increased amplitude of the delayed rectifier K^+ current, apparently effected by enhanced recovery from inactivation of I_{Kr} (11, 134). The increased K^+ current steepens the slope of phase 3 of the cardiac action potential, thereby speeding myocardial repolarization. The ECG with hyperkalemia is notable for a dampening of P waves (due to pronounced attenuation of the action potential in atrial cells), T waves that are large and peaked (due to accelerated repolarization), and— with severe hyperkalemia—a widening of the QRS complex (due to slow propagation of excitation) (120).

These ECG changes signify a profound derangement of the myocardial conductances, explaining why this scenario can rapidly degenerate to ventricular fibrillation. Potassium intoxication occurs with renal failure, hemolysis, tissue necrosis, adrenal failure, drugs that interfere with K^+ excretion, and excessive K^+ supplementation. Hypocalcemia, hyponatremia, and acidosis all exacerbate the effects of hyperkalemia.

Hyperkalemia is a genuine electrolyte emergency. Current recommendations include urgent care for any patient with evidence of hyperkalemia on a surface electrocardiogram or serum levels above 6 or 6.5 mEq/L. Treatments are aimed toward antagonizing the effects of hyperkalemia on membrane potential, rapidly lowering serum K^+ by shifting it from the extracellular compartment into cells, and removing K^+ from the body. Treating the disorder that led to hyperkalemia and minimizing other factors that increase K_{ext} are also appropriate. Specific measures include the administration of intravenous calcium, which can reverse electrocardiogram changes in minutes by directly antagonizing the effects of hyperkalemia on membrane potential (see following section on calcium). Shifting K_{ext} into cells is favored by administration of insulin (along with glucose, to prevent hypoglycemia). If the patient is acidemic, sodium bicarbonate is also effective. Finally, inhalation of 10 to 20 mg of the β_2-selective catecholamine albuterol is to be considered (4, 73), as stimulation of the β_2 receptors can activate the Na^+,K^+-ATPase via cAMP to move K^+ into cells (15, 20). Insulin might similarly stimulate the Na^+, K^+-ATPase (22), or perhaps the ATPase is secondarily activated by a rise of intracellular Na^+ caused by activation of Na^+-H^+ countertransport (110). If a metabolic acidosis

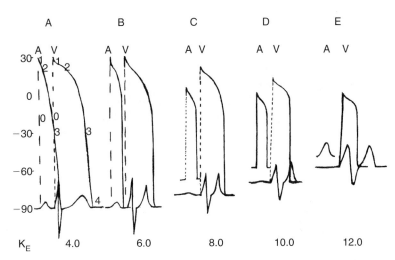

FIGURE 11 Electrophysiologic recordings of atrial (A) and ventricular (V) action potentials (AP) from isolated rabbit hearts, superimposed on the electrocardiogram. The y-axis shows the transmembrane potential in millivolts; and the extracellular K^+ (K_E, in mEq/L) concentration is noted below each set of tracings. In tracings **A** and **B**, the resting membrane potential (RMP) is -90 mV and the total amplitude of the AP is 120 mV. Note how increasing K_{ext} leads to a rise of the RMP and a reduced amplitude of the AP; with a greater effect seen in the atrium. Also note the shorter duration of the AP, and the significantly accelerated phase 3 hyperpolarization. The slope of phase 3 correlates with the downslope of the T-wave on the electrocardiogram, causing a "peaking" effect. (From Surawicz B. Relationship between electrocardiogram and electrolytes. *Am Heart J* 1967;73:814–834, with permission.)

exists, then administration of bicarbonate will buffer serum protons and promote Na^+-H^+ exchange, and subsequently activate Na^+,K^+-ATPase activity (46). Removing K^+ from the body is achieved with the use of diuretics or oral/rectal administration of cation exchange resin. Often critical in those with significant renal impairment, hemodialysis can lower K_{ext} much more rapidly. It should be noted that digoxin therapy and left ventricular hypertrophy are risk factors for complex ventricular arrhythmias when dialysate K^+ is as low as 2.0 mEq/L (97).

High external K^+ levels seen in healthy subjects during exercise are not associated with arrhythmia. Elevated levels of circulating catecholamines appear to be an important protective factor as they increase Ca^{2+} currents and counteract the effects of hyperkalemia. Catechols increase the upstroke and duration of cardiac action potentials and decrease the tendency toward arrhythmia associated with slow impulse propagation and shortened refractory period.

Hypokalemia: Hypokalemia produces a variety of clinical disturbances including drowsiness, fatigue, anorexia, constipation, weakness, and flaccid paralysis. At extremely low levels (< 1.5 mEq/L), muscle necrosis can occur as well as ascending paralysis with eventual impairment of respiratory function (130). The electrocardiogram is notable for long QT intervals and flattened T waves. Since ventricular action potentials lengthen more than those in the atria, atrioventricular block can develop. Cardiac rhythm disturbances are rare in patients without underlying disease. However, those taking digoxin and those with cardiac ischemia, heart failure, or left-ventricular hypertrophy are at risk for development of arrhyth-

mias even with mild to moderate hypokalemia (86). This may be partly mediated by a downregulation of cardiac potassium channels with these conditions (98). In addition, other causes for prolonged QT interval, including medications or congenital and acquired channelopathies, will also increase the risk of hypokalemia-associated arrhythmia (107).

Hypokalemia is most often the result of K^+ depletion due to abnormal losses but rarely is due to abrupt shifts from the extracellular to intracellular compartment. K^+ loss through the kidney secondary to chronic use of diuretics or in the stool as a result of diarrhea are most common. Some other causes of hypokalemia include renal tubular defects, starvation, vomiting, diabetic ketoacidosis, and hyperaldosteronism.

A rare cause of hypokalemia is intoxication with barium salts, which indirectly causes a profound shift of serum K^+ into cells. Barium effectively blocks background ("leak") potassium channels, but does not alter Na^+,K^+-ATPase activity (21, 116). Thus, K^+ is pumped into cells but does not leak out; the intracellular accumulation of K^+ can lead to a life-threatening hypokalemia (72).

Potassium depletion will increase systolic and diastolic blood pressure when sodium intake is not restricted (24, 66) and potassium supplementation can have a mild salutary effect on systemic blood pressure (131); although low serum K^+ levels do not clearly correlate the development of hypertension in the general population (128). In addition, potassium supplementation may reduce the risk of stroke in some populations (33, 43, 117). The hypertensive effect of hypokalemia may be due to increased contraction of vascular smooth muscle by reduced activity of Na^+,K^+-ATPase, raising Na^+_{in} and causing cellular depolarization. The increased Na^+_{in} will inhibit Na^+/Ca^{2+} exchange and also promote smooth-muscle contraction by raising Ca^{2+}_{in} (19). In addition hypokalemia may also promote cardiovascular disease by stimulating smooth-muscle proliferation and platelet aggregation (137).

CALCIUM

Hypocalcemia: Approximately 45% of serum Ca^{2+} is bound to protein, primarily albumin. Bound Ca^{2+} is in equilibrium with the soluble ionized fraction that influences membrane excitation. The most common cause of reduced total serum Ca^{2+} is hypoalbuminemia, however, ionized Ca^{2+} is normal in this condition. The ratio of bound and free Ca^{2+} is altered by acid-base status and this can influence excitation: acidosis increases the ionized fraction while alkalosis decreases it. Common causes of true hypocalcemia include vitamin D deficiency, acute pancreatitis, magnesium deficiency, hypophosphatemia, hypoparathyroidism, pseudohypoparathyroidism, and renal tubular acidosis. Common symptoms are tetany, confusion, and seizures. Hyperkalemia and hypomagnesemia potentiate the cardiac and neuromuscular irritability produced by hypocalcemia, and vice versa.

Hypercalcemia and membrane stabilization: Hypercalcemia is caused by hyperparathyroidism, neoplastic disorders, vitamin D intoxication, sarcoidosis and other pulmonary granulomatous diseases, milk-alkali syndrome, immobilization, hyperthyroidism, and acute adrenal insufficiency. Symptoms include nausea, vomiting, constipation, polyuria, psychosis, and coma. Serious arrhythmias from hypercalcemia are relatively rare, although the length of the QT interval is inversely proportional to the serum Ca^{2+} concentration.

Increased extracellular Ca^{2+} is said to stabilize excitable cells, rendering them less responsive; low pH has the same effect. At first, this effect appears to be paradoxical. Inward Ca^{2+} currents are associated with excitation and are, in fact, seen to increase when external Ca^{2+} concentration is elevated. The stabilization is instead due to the strong effect of Ca^{2+} on the voltage sensitivity of voltage-gated channels, especially Na^+ channels. Membrane proteins can have fixed negative charges near their extracellular surfaces, contributed by polar amino acids and/or carbohydrates. These sites will preferentially bind divalent cations in the extracellular milieu. Channels in the membrane experience not only to the potential difference across the membrane (E_m) but also from these charges, and they respond to a local potential difference across the interior of the membrane (ψ). While ψ_i follows E_m, the channel senses the more positive local potential ψ_i. Thus, at -50 mV, where Na^+ channels begin to activate, ψ_i is close to 0 mV. As external Ca^{2+} is raised it binds with fairly high affinity to the local binding sites. As a result, ψ_i is no longer so positive, and from the point of view of the Na^+ channel the local environment is more hyperpolarized. Thus, it takes a greater depolarization to achieve activation threshold. Hydrogen ions have the same effect: titrating acidic groups on the surface neutralizes negative

surface charges and moves Na^+ channels away from their threshold for activation. This simplified explanation is more fully discussed in Chapter 20 of (51).

MAGNESIUM

Critical to a variety of cellular functions, especially those that use ATP, disturbances in magnesium can affect many organs including the heart and neuromuscular system. Magnesium balance depends on intake and renal excretion which is regulated in the distal nephron. Depletion of body Mg^{2+} may be caused by renal tubular wasting from congenital disorders or agents such as diuretics or nephrotoxins, or may follow reduced intake from malnutrition or enteropathies. Negative balance results in decreased serum and intracellular levels, while renal failure may allow for rapid elevation of serum Mg^{2+} As discussed in Chapter 61, hypomagnesemia can cause neuromuscular irritability and increase the risk of cardiac arrhythmia. In some respects, Mg^{2+} and Ca^{2+} have similar mechanisms of action in that reduced extracellular concentrations will effectively lower the threshold for action potentials (49) (see previous discussion of hypercalcemia). While these divalents may share some extracellular binding sites, the fact that isolated hypomagnesemia or isolated hypocalcemia can promote neuronal excitability suggests that there are also sites that selectively bind one cation over the other.

With respect to cardiac excitability, hypomagnesemia (like hypocalcemia) acts to exacerbate hypokalemic and digitalis toxicity and increase the risk for ventricular arrhythmia. This may be partly related to surface-potential effects, but low Mg^{2+}_{ext} also enhances activation of hERG (I_{Kr}) (52), leading to abnormally fast repolarization. Further, a reduction of intracellular Mg^{2+} concentration can increase outward K^+ currents from IR channels, hyperpolarizing cardiomyocytes (Fig. 10). Because potassium-sparing diuretics minimize Mg^{2+} depletion, they should be considered in patients at high risk for arrhythmia (56).

In vascular smooth muscle, Ca^{2+} and Mg^{2+} have antagonistic effects, such that hypomagnesemia actually promotes smooth-muscle contractility. This appears to be related to lowered intracellular Mg^{2+}, as Mg^{2+} acts as an inhibitor of IP_3-mediated (70) and calcium-mediated (71, 90) Ca^{2+} release from the sarcoplasmic reticulum. In contrast to smooth muscle, cardiac myocytes respond to hypomagnesemia with a slight decrease of contractility (69, 103); although the mechanism of this phenomenon is less well understood. Taken together, this explains improved blood pressure with moderate Mg^{2+} levels due to improved cardiac contractility (69, 103), and vasodilatation-associated hypotension seen with boluses of Mg^{2+} salts for treatment of preterm labor.

ACID-BASE STATUS AND EXCITABILITY

Each of the four primary acid-base disturbances (as well as mixed disorders) gives rise to secondary compensatory responses. Thus, respiratory acidosis induces a secondary increase in HCO_3^- to return blood pH toward normal. In general, acidemia (increased extracellular H^+) will inhibit

Na^+-H^+ countertransport, leading to reduced intracellular Na^+ and therefore increased extracellular K^+. This can lead to hyperkalemia with its attendant cardiovascular risks. Conversely, alkalemia (decreased extracellular H^+) leads to increased inward K^+ and Na^+ flux and may produce hypokalemia. Serum Na^+ is rarely altered significantly by changes in pH due to its normally high serum level.

There are also specific effects of protons on ion channels. For example, H^+ ions can bind to negative charges on the external face of Na^+ channels, to shift the surface potential in the same fashion as Ca^{2+} or Mg^{2+} ions (50 and therefore reduce Na^+-channel activity. However, there seems to be a converse effect on cardiac pacemaker channels (14), so that acidemia can actually potentiate cardiac irritability.

THE BIG PICTURE: RESPONSE TO ELECTROLYTE DISORDERS HAS MANY MITIGATING FACTORS

Based on our understanding of the many factors involved in membrane excitability, we can begin to understand why one patient may transiently tolerate a serum K^+ level of 8.0 mEq/L and another may suffer sudden death related to a K^+ of 7.0 mEq/L. The response of excitable tissue will be dependent upon the chronicity of the hyperkalemia (affecting intracellular levels, and therefore membrane potential); the state of the autonomic nervous system, affecting levels of ACh and catecholamines on the heart; the presence of any drugs that can alter intracellular calcium concentration or cardiac ion channel activity; levels of other electrolytes or protons in the serum; and genetic polymorphisms in ion channel pore-forming and accessory subunits and other proteins. Further, it seems reasonable to speculate that derangements of electrolytes may lead to compensatory second-messenger modulation of ion channels or altered expression of ion channels and/or their accessory subunits, as demonstrated in failing hearts (61, 78, 98, 111)

SUMMARY

Ion channels mediate the electrical activity of all cells. Their function in excitable tissues like nerves and muscles is particularly relevant to clinical medicine. These proteins are characterized by their finely timed opening and closing, high throughput, and high selectivity. Ion channels form transmembrane water-filled pores with multiple ion binding sites in tandem. Disorders of electrolytes affect cellular function through altered excitability. Numerous common medications and several ion-channel polymorphisms influence ion channel activity and may exacerbate the effects of electrolyte disorders on the function of nerve, muscle, and heart. The mechanism underlying most channel-mediated disorders is yet to be discerned, and some diseases have yet to be recognized as due to ion-channel dysfunction. However, rapid progress has been made over the last 15 years, enhancing our understanding of basic mechanisms and our capacity to treat disorders of membrane excitability.

References

1. Abbott GW, Butler MH, Bendahhou S, et al. MiRP2 forms potassium channels in skeletal muscle with Kv3.4 and is associated with periodic paralysis. *Cell* 2001;104:217–231.
2. Abbott GW, Goldstein SA. A superfamily of small potassium channel subunits: form and function of the MinK-related peptides (MiRPs). *Q Rev Biophys* 1998;31:357–398.
3. Abbott GW, Sesti F, Splawski I, et al. MiRP1 forms I_{Kr} potassium channels with HERG and is associated with cardiac arrhythmia. *Cell* 1999;97:175–187.
4. Allon M, Shanklin N. Effect of albuterol treatment on subsequent dialytic potassium removal. *Am J Kidney Dis* 1995;26:607–613.
5. Anderson CS, MacKinnon R, Smith C, et al. Charybdotoxin block of single Ca^{2+}-activated K^+ channels. Effects of channel gating, voltage, and ionic strength. *J Gen Physiol* 1988;91:317–333.
6. Arieff AI, Llach F, Massry SG. Neurological manifestations and morbidity of hyponatremia: correlation with brain water and electrolytes. *Medicine* 1976;55:121–129.
7. Baker EH, Dong YB, Sagnella GA, et al. Association of hypertension with T594M mutation in ß subunit of epithelial sodium channels in black people resident in London. *Lancet* 1998;351:1388–1392.
8. Begenisich T, De Weer P. Potassium flux ratio in voltage-clamped squid giant axons. *J Gen Physiol* 1980;76:83–98.
9. Bernstein J. Untersuchungen zur thermodynamik der bioelektrischen ströme. Erster thiel. *Pflugers Arch* 1902;92:521–562.
10. Bezanilla F. The voltage sensor in voltage-dependent ion channels. *Physiol Rev* 2000;80:555–592.
11. Bouchard R, Clark RB, Juhasz AE, et al. Changes in extracellular K^+ concentration modulate contractility of rat and rabbit cardiac myocytes via the inward rectifier K^+ current IK1. *J Physiol* 2004;556:773–790.
12. Brenner R, Jegla TJ, Wickenden A, et al. Cloning and functional characterization of novel large conductance calcium-activated potassium channel β subunits, hKCNMB3 and hKC-NMB4. *J Biol Chem* 2000;275:6453–6461.
13. Brenner R, Peréz GJ, Bonev AD, et al. Vasoregulation by the β1 subunit of the calcium-activated potassium channel. *Nature* 2000;407:870–876.
14. Brown RH, Jr., Noble D. Displacement of activator thresholds in cardiac muscle by protons and calcium ions. *J Physiol* 1978;282:333–343.
15. Caswell AH, Baker SP, Boyd H, et al. β-adrenergic receptor and adenylate cyclase in transverse tubules of skeletal muscle. *J Biol Chem* 1978;253:3049–3054.
16. Catterall WA. From ionic currents to molecular mechanisms: the structure and function of voltage-gated sodium channels. *Neuron* 2000;26:13–25.
17. Catterall WA. Structure and function of voltage-gated ion channels. *Annu Rev Biochem* 1995;64:493–531.
18. Catterall WA. Structure and regulation of voltage-gated Ca^{2+} channels. *Annu Rev Cell Dev Biol* 2000;16:521–555.
19. Chen WT, Brace RA, Scott JB, et al. The mechanism of the vasodilator action of potassium. *Proc Soc Exp Biol Med* 1972;140:820–824.
20. Clausen T, Everts ME. Regulation of the Na,K-pump in skeletal muscle. *Kidney Int* 1989;35:1–13.
21. Clausen T, Overgaard K. The role of K^+ channels in the force recovery elicited by Na^+-K^+ pump stimulation in Ba^{2+}-paralysed rat skeletal muscle. *J Physiol* 2000;527(Pt 2):325–332.
22. Clausen T. Na^+-K^+ pump regulation and skeletal muscle contractility. *Physiol Rev* 2003;83:1269–1324.
23. Coleman SK, Newcombe J, Pryke J, et al. Subunit composition of Kv1 channels in human CNS. *J Neurochem* 1999;73:849–858.
24. Coruzzi P, Brambilla L, Brambilla V, et al. Potassium depletion and salt sensitivity in essential hypertension. *J Clin Endocrinol Metab* 2001;86:2857–2862.
25. Cuello LG, Cortes DM, Perozo E. Molecular architecture of the KvAP voltage-dependent K^+ channel in a lipid bilayer. *Science* 2004;306:491–495.
26. Decher N, Bundis F, Vajna R, et al. KCNE2 modulates current amplitudes and activation kinetics of HCN4: influence of KCNE family members on HCN4 currents. *Pflugers Arch* 2003;446:633–640.
27. Deschenes I, Tomaselli GF. Modulation of Kv4.3 current by accessory subunits. *FEBS Lett* 2002;528:183–188.
28. Doyle DA, Morais-Cabral J, Pfuetzner RA, et al. The structure of the potassium channel: molecular basis of K^+ conduction and selectivity. *Science* 1998;280:69–77.
29. Duggal P, Vesely MR, Wattanasirichaigoon D, et al. Mutation of the gene for IsK associated with both Jervell and Lange-Nielsen and Romano-Ward forms of long-QT syndrome. *Circulation* 1998;97:142–146.
30. Dyckner T, Wester PO. The relation between extra- and intracellular electrolytes in patients with hypokalemia and/or diuretic treatment. *Acta Med Scand* 1978;204:269–282.
31. Embark HM, Böhmer C, Palmada M, et al. Regulation of CLC-Ka/barttin by the ubiquitin ligase Nedd4-2 and the serum- and glucocorticoid-dependent kinases. *Kidney Int* 2004;66:1918–1925.
32. Estévez R, Boettger T, Stein V, et al. Barttin is a Cl^- channel β-subunit crucial for renal Cl^- reabsorption and inner ear K^+ secretion. *Nature* 2001;414:558–561.
33. Fang J, Madhavan S, Alderman MH. Dietary potassium intake and stroke mortality. *Stroke* 2000;31:1532–1537.
34. Finkelstein A, Andersen OS. The gramicidin A channel: a review of its permeability characteristics with special reference to the single-file aspect of transport. *J Membr Biol* 1981;59:155–171.
35. Fozzard H. *Ion Channels in the Cardiovascular System: Function and Dysfunction.* Armonk, NY: Futura Publishing; 1994:81–99.
36. Freeman SJ, Fale AD. Muscular paralysis and ventilatory failure caused by hyperkalaemia. *Br J Anaesth* 1993;70:226–227.
37. Goldin AL. Mechanisms of sodium channel inactivation. *Curr Opin Neurobiol* 2003;13:284–290.

38. Goldstein SA, Bockenhauer D, O'Kelly I, et al. Potassium leak channels and the KCNK family of two-P-domain subunits. *Nat Rev Neurosci* 2001;2:175–184.

39. Goldstein SA, Miller C. A point mutation in a *Shaker* K⁺ channel changes its charybdotoxin binding site from low to high affinity. *Biophys J* 1992;62:5–7.

40. Goldstein SA, Pheasant DJ, Miller C. The charybdotoxin receptor of a *Shaker* K⁺ channel: peptide and channel residues mediating molecular recognition. *Neuron* 1994;12:1377–1388.

41. Goldstein SA, Wang KW, Ilan N, et al. Sequence and function of the two P domain potassium channels: implications of an emerging superfamily. *J Mol Med* 1998;76:13–20.

42. Gong Q, Anderson CL, January CT, et al. Role of glycosylation in cell surface expression and stability of HERG potassium channels. *Am J Physiol Heart Circ Physiol* 2002;283:H77–84.

43. Green DM, Ropper AH, Kronmal RA, et al. Serum potassium level and dietary potassium intake as risk factors for stroke. *Neurology* 2002;59:314–320.

44. Gubitosi-Klug RA, Mancuso DJ, Gross RW. The human Kv1.1 channel is palmitoylated, modulating voltage sensing: Identification of a palmitoylation consensus sequence. *Proc Natl Acad Sci U S A* 2005;102:5964–5968.

45. Guy HR, Seetharamulu P. Molecular model of the action potential sodium channel. *Proc Natl Acad Sci U S A* 1986;83:508–512.

46. Halperin ML, Kamel KS. Potassium. *Lancet* 1998;352:135–140.

47. Heginbotham L, Abramson T, MacKinnon R. A functional connection between the pores of distantly related ion channels as revealed by mutant K⁺ channels. *Science* 1992;258:1152–1155.

48. Heginbotham L, Lu Z, Abramson T, et al. Mutations in the K⁺ channel signature sequence. *Biophys J* 1994;66:1061–1067.

49. Hille B, Woodhull AM, Shapiro BI. Negative surface charge near sodium channels of nerve: divalent ions, monovalent ions, and pH. *Philos Trans R Soc Lond B Biol Sci* 1975;270:301–318.

50. Hille B. Charges and potentials at the nerve surface: Divalent ions and pH. *J Gen Physiol* 1968;51:221–236.

51. Hille B. *Ion Channels of Excitable Membranes*, 3rd ed. Sunderland, MA: Sinauer; 2001.

52. Ho WK, Kim I, Lee CO, et al. Voltage-dependent blockade of HERG channels expressed in Xenopus oocytes by external Ca²⁺ and Mg²⁺. *J Physiol* 1998;507(Pt 3):631–638.

53. Hodgkin AL, Huxley AF, Katz B. Measurement of current-voltage relations in the membrane of the giant axon of Loligo. *J Physiol* 1952;116:424–448.

54. Hodgkin AL, Huxley AF. A quantitative description of membrane current and its application to conduction and excitation in nerve. *J Physiol* 1952;117:500–544.

55. Hodgkin AL, Keynes RD. The potassium permeability of a giant nerve fibre. *J Physiol* 1955;128:61–88.

56. Hollifield JW. Magnesium depletion, diuretics, and arrhythmias. *Am J Med* 1987;82:30–37.

57. Hoshi T, Zagotta WN, Aldrich RW. Biophysical and molecular mechanisms of *Shaker* potassium channel inactivation. *Science* 1990;250:533–538.

58. Hübner CA, Jentsch TJ. Ion channel diseases. *Hum Mol Genet* 2002;11:2435–2445.

59. Hughey RP, Bruns JB, Kinlough CL, et al. Epithelial sodium channels are activated by furin-dependent proteolysis. *J Biol Chem* 2004;279:18111–18114.

60. Jan LY, Jan YN. Tracing the roots of ion channels. *Cell* 1992;69:715–718.

61. Jiang M, Zhang M, Tang DG, et al. KCNE2 protein is expressed in ventricles of different species, and changes in its expression contribute to electrical remodeling in diseased hearts. *Circulation* 2004;109:1783–1788.

62. Jiang Y, Lee A, Chen J, et al. The open pore conformation of potassium channels. *Nature* 2002;417:523–526.

63. Jiang Y, Lee A, Chen J, et al. X-ray structure of a voltage-dependent K⁺ channel. *Nature* 2003;423:33–41.

64. Kettenmann H, Grantyn R. *Practical Electrophysiological Methods*. New York: Wiley-Liss; 1992:249–299.

65. Krapivinsky G, Gordon EA, Wickman K, et al. The G-protein-gated atrial K⁺ channel I_KACh is a heteromultimer of two inwardly rectifying K⁺-channel proteins. *Nature* 1995;374:135–141.

66. Krishna GG, Miller E, Kapoor S. Increased blood pressure during potassium depletion in normotensive men. *N Engl J Med* 1989;320:1177–1182.

67. Kuryshev YA, Gudz TI, Brown AM, et al. KChAP as a chaperone for specific K⁺ channels. *Am J Physiol Cell Physiol* 2000;278:C931–941.

68. Kuryshev YA, Wible BA, Gudz TI, et al. KChAP/Kvβ1.2 interactions and their effects on cardiac Kv channel expression. *Am J Physiol Cell Physiol* 2001;281:C290–299.

69. Kyriazis J, Kalogeropoulou K, Bilirakis L, et al. Dialysate magnesium level and blood pressure. *Kidney Int* 2004;66:1221–1231.

70. Laurant P, Touyz RM. Physiological and pathophysiological role of magnesium in the cardiovascular system: implications in hypertension. *J Hypertens* 2000;18:1177–1191.

71. Laver DR, Baynes TM, Dulhunty AF. Magnesium inhibition of ryanodine-receptor calcium channels: evidence for two independent mechanisms. *J Membr Biol* 1997;156:213–229.

72. Layzer RB. Periodic paralysis and the sodium-potassium pump. *Ann Neurol* 1982;11:547–552.

73. Liou HH, Chiang SS, Wu SC, et al. Hypokalemic effects of intravenous infusion or nebulization of salbutamol in patients with chronic renal failure: comparative study. *Am J Kidney Dis* 1994;23:266–271.

74. Liu Y, Holmgren M, Jurman ME, et al. Gated access to the pore of a voltage-dependent K⁺ channel. *Neuron* 1997;19:175–184.

75. Long SB, Campbell EB, Mackinnon R. Crystal structure of a mammalian voltage-dependent Shaker family K⁺ channel. *Science* 2005;309:897–903.

76. Long SB, Campbell EB, Mackinnon R. Voltage sensor of Kv1.2: structural basis of electromechanical coupling. *Science* 2005;309:903–908.

77. Lopatin AN, Makhina EN, Nichols CG. Potassium channel block by cytoplasmic polyamines as the mechanism of intrinsic rectification. *Nature* 1994;372:366–369.

78. Lundquist AL, Manderfield LJ, Vanoye CG, et al. Expression of multiple KCNE genes in human heart may enable variable modulation of IKs. *J Mol Cell Cardiol* 2005;38:277–287.

79. MacKinnon R, Heginbotham L, Abramson T. Mapping the receptor site for charybdotoxin, a pore-blocking potassium channel inhibitor. *Neuron* 1990;5:767–771.

80. MacKinnon R, Miller C. Mechanism of charybdotoxin block of the high-conductance, Ca²⁺-activated K⁺ channel. *J Gen Physiol* 1988;91:335–349.

81. MacKinnon R, Miller C. Mutant potassium channels with altered binding of charybdotoxin, a pore-blocking peptide inhibitor. *Science* 1989;245:1382–1385.

82. MacKinnon R, Yellen G. Mutations affecting TEA blockade and ion permeation in voltage-activated K⁺ channels. *Science* 1990;250:276–279.

83. MacKinnon R. Determination of the subunit stoichiometry of a voltage-activated potassium channel. *Nature* 1991;350:232–235.

84. MacKinnon R. Pore loops: an emerging theme in ion channel structure. *Neuron* 1995;14:889–892.

85. Mark MD, Herlitze S. G-protein mediated gating of inward-rectifier K⁺ channels. *Eur J Biochem* 2000;267:5830–5836.

86. Materson BJ. Diuretics, potassium, and ventricular ectopy. *Am J Hypertens* 1997;10:68S–72S.

87. McCrossan ZA, Abbott GW. The MinK-related peptides. *Neuropharmacology* 2004;47:787–821.

88. McCrossan ZA, Lewis A, Panaghie G, et al. MinK-related peptide 2 modulates Kv2.1 and Kv3.1 potassium channels in mammalian brain. *J Neurosci* 2003;23:8077–8091.

89. McManus OB, Helms LM, Pallanck L, et al. Functional role of the β subunit of high conductance calcium-activated potassium channels. *Neuron* 1995;14:645–650.

90. Meissner G, Darling E, Eveleth J. Kinetics of rapid Ca²⁺ release by sarcoplasmic reticulum. Effects of Ca²⁺, Mg²⁺, and adenine nucleotides. *Biochemistry* 1986;25:236–244.

91. Merlie JP, Sebbane R, Tzartos S, et al. Inhibition of glycosylation with tunicamycin blocks assembly of newly synthesized acetylcholine receptor subunits in muscle cells. *J Biol Chem* 1982;257:2694–2701.

92. Miller C. Competition for block of a Ca²⁺-activated K⁺ channel by charybdotoxin and tetraethylammonium. *Neuron* 1988;1:1003–1006.

93. Miller C. Coupling of water and ion fluxes in a K⁺-selective channel of sarcoplasmic reticulum. *Biophys J* 1982;38:227–230.

94. Miller C. *Neuromodulation: The Biochemical Control of Neuronal Excitability*. New York: Oxford University Press; 1987:39–63.

95. Miyazawa A, Fujiyoshi Y, Unwin N. Structure and gating mechanism of the acetylcholine receptor pore. *Nature* 2003;423:949–955.

96. Morais-Cabral JH, Zhou Y, MacKinnon R. Energetic optimization of ion conduction rate by the K⁺ selectivity filter. *Nature* 2001;414:37–42.

97. Morrison G, Michelson EL, Brown S, et al. Mechanism and prevention of cardiac arrhythmias in chronic hemodialysis patients. *Kidney Int* 1980;17:811–819.

98. Näbauer M, Kääb S. Potassium channel down-regulation in heart failure. *Cardiovasc Res* 1998;37:324–334.

99. Nadal MS, Ozaita A, Amarillo Y, et al. The CD26-related dipeptidyl aminopeptidase-like protein DPPX is a critical component of neuronal A-type K⁺ channels. *Neuron* 2003;37:449–461.

100. Noda M, Shimizu S, Tanabe T, et al. Primary structure of *Electrophorus electricus* sodium channel deduced from cDNA sequence. *Nature* 1984;312:121–127.

101. North RA. Molecular physiology of P2X receptors. *Physiol Rev* 2002;82:1013–1067.

102. Rajan S, Plant LD, Rabin ML, et al. Sumoylation silences the plasma membrane leak K⁺ channel K2P1. *Cell* 2005;121:37–47.

103. Rasmussen HS, Videbaek R, Melchior T, et al. Myocardial contractility and performance capacity after magnesium infusions in young healthy persons: a double-blind, placebo-controlled, cross-over study. *Clin Cardiol* 1988;11:541–545.

104. Rathenberg J, Kittler JT, Moss SJ. Palmitoylation regulates the clustering and cell surface stability of GABA_A receptors. *Mol Cell Neurosci* 2004;26:251–257.

105. Rhodes KJ, Carroll KI, Sung MA, et al. KChIPs and Kv4 α subunits as integral components of A-type potassium channels in mammalian brain. *J Neurosci* 2004;24:7903–7915.

106. Robertson WV, Dunihue FW. Water and electrolyte distribution in cardiac muscle. *Am J Physiol* 1954;177:292–298.

107. Roden DM. Drug-induced prolongation of the QT interval. *N Engl J Med* 2004;350:1013–1022.

108. Rosati B, Pan Z, Lypen S, et al. Regulation of KChIP2 potassium channel ß subunit gene expression underlies the gradient of transient outward current in canine and human ventricle. *J Physiol* 2001;533:119–125.

109. Rosenberg PA, Finkelstein A. Interaction of ions and water in gramicidin A channels: streaming potentials across lipid bilayer membranes. *J Gen Physiol* 1978;72:327–340.

110. Rosic NK, Standaert ML, Pollet RJ. The mechanism of insulin stimulation of Na⁺,K⁺-ATPase transport activity in muscle. *J Biol Chem* 1985;260:6206–6212.

111. Saito J, Niwano S, Niwano H, et al. Electrical remodeling of the ventricular myocardium in myocarditis: studies of rat experimental autoimmune myocarditis. *Circ J* 2002;66:97–103.

112. Sato C, Ueno Y, Asai K, et al. The voltage-sensitive sodium channel is a bell-shaped molecule with several cavities. *Nature* 2001;409:1047–1051.

113. Schroeder BC, Waldegger S, Fehr S, et al. A constitutively open potassium channel formed by KCNQ1 and KCNE3. *Nature* 2000;403:196–199.

114. Sesti F, Abbott GW, Wei J, et al. A common polymorphism associated with antibiotic-induced cardiac arrhythmia. *Proc Natl Acad Sci U S A* 2000;97:10613–10618.

115. Sesti F, Goldstein SA. Single-channel characteristics of wild-type IKs channels and channels formed with two minK mutants that cause long QT syndrome. *J Gen Physiol* 1998;112:651–663.

116. Sjodin RA, Ortiz O. Resolution of the potassium ion pump in muscle fibers using barium ions. *J Gen Physiol* 1975;66:269–286.

117. Smith NL, Lemaitre RN, Heckbert SR, et al. Serum potassium and stroke risk among treated hypertensive adults. *Am J Hypertens* 2003;16:806–813.

118. Splawski I, Tristani-Firouzi M, Lehmann MH, et al. Mutations in the hminK gene cause long QT syndrome and suppress IKs function. *Nat Genet* 1997;17:338–340.

119. St. George S, Freed SC, Rosenman RH, et al. Influence of potassium deprivation and adrenalectomy on potassium concentration of the myocardium. *Am J Physiol* 1955;181:550–552.

120. Surawicz B. Relationship between electrocardiogram and electrolytes. *Am Heart J* 1967;73: 814–834.

121. Tang XD, Santarelli LC, Heinemann SH, et al. Metabolic regulation of potassium channels. *Annu Rev Physiol* 2004;66:131–159.

122. Thornhill WB, Wu MB, Jiang X, et al. Expression of Kv1.1 delayed rectifier potassium channels in Lec mutant Chinese hamster ovary cell lines reveals a role for sialidation in channel function. *J Biol Chem* 1996;271:19093–19098.

123. Tomaselli GF, Feldman AM, Yellen G, et al. Human cardiac sodium channels expressed in *Xenopus* oocytes. *Am J Physiol* 1990;258:H903–906.

124. Torres GE, Egan TM, Voigt MM. N-Linked glycosylation is essential for the functional expression of the recombinant P2X2 receptor. *Biochemistry* 1998;37:14845–14851.

125. Uebele VN, Lagrutta A, Wade T, et al. Cloning and functional expression of two families of β-subunits of the large conductance calcium-activated K+ channel. *J Biol Chem* 2000;275: 23211–23218.

126. Unwin N. Acetylcholine receptor channel imaged in the open state. *Nature* 1995; 373:37–43.

127. Vallon V, Grahammer F, Richter K, et al. Role of KCNE1-dependent K+ fluxes in mouse proximal tubule. *J Am Soc Nephrol* 2001;12:2003–2011.

128. Walsh CR, Larson MG, Vasan RS, et al. Serum potassium is not associated with blood pressure tracking in the Framingham Heart Study. *Am J Hypertens* 2002;15:130–136.

129. Weiger TM, Hermann A, Levitan IB. Modulation of calcium-activated potassium channels. *J Comp Physiol A Neuroethol Sens Neural Behav Physiol* 2002;188:79–87.

130. Weiner M, Epstein FH. Signs and symptoms of electrolyte disorders. *Yale J Biol Med* 1970;43:76–109.

131. Whelton PK, He J, Cutler JA, et al. Effects of oral potassium on blood pressure. Meta-analysis of randomized controlled clinical trials. *JAMA* 1997;277:1624–1632.

132. Xia XM, Ding JP, Lingle CJ. Molecular basis for the inactivation of Ca2+- and voltage-dependent BK channels in adrenal chromaffin cells and rat insulinoma tumor cells. *J Neurosci* 1999;19:5255–5264.

133. Yang EK, Alvira MR, Levitan ES, et al. Kvβ subunits increase expression of Kv4.3 channels by interacting with their C termini. *J Biol Chem* 2001;276:4839–4844.

134. Yang T, Roden DM. Extracellular potassium modulation of drug block of I$_{Kr}$. Implications for torsade de pointes and reverse use-dependence. *Circulation* 1996;93:407–411.

135. Yellen G, Jurman ME, Abramson T, et al. Mutations affecting internal TEA blockade identify the probable pore-forming region of a K+ channel. *Science* 1991;251:939–942.

136. Yellen G. Ionic permeation and blockade in Ca2+-activated K+ channels of bovine chromaffin cells. *J Gen Physiol* 1984;84:157–186.

137. Young DB, Lin H, McCabe RD. Potassium's cardiovascular protective mechanisms. *Am J Physiol* 1995;268:R825–837.

138. Yu H, Wu J, Potapova I, et al. MinK-related peptide 1: A beta subunit for the HCN ion channel subunit family enhances expression and speeds activation. *Circ Res* 2001;88:E84–87.

139. Zhang M, Jiang M, Tseng GN. MinK-related peptide 1 associates with Kv4.2 and modulates its gating function: potential role as beta subunit of cardiac transient outward channel? *Circ Res* 2001;88:1012–1019.

140. Zhang Y, Hartmann HA, Satin J. Glycosylation influences voltage-dependent gating of cardiac and skeletal muscle sodium channels. *J Membr Biol* 1999;171:195–207.

141. Zhou Y, Morais-Cabral JH, Kaufman A, et al. Chemistry of ion coordination and hydration revealed by a K+ channel-Fab complex at 2.0 Å resolution. *Nature* 2001;414:43–48.

142. Zilberberg N, Ilan N, Goldstein SA. KCNKO: opening and closing the 2-P-domain potassium leak channel entails "C-type" gating of the outer pore. *Neuron* 2001;32:635–648.

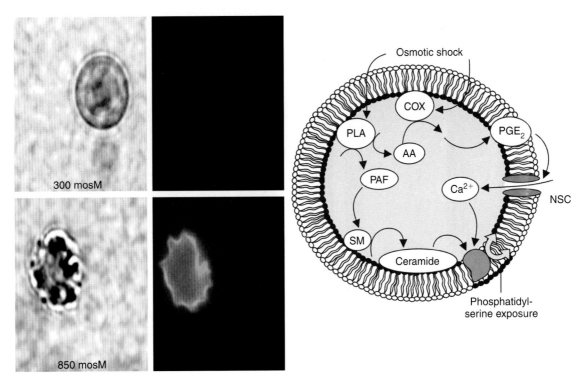

FIGURE 6–7.

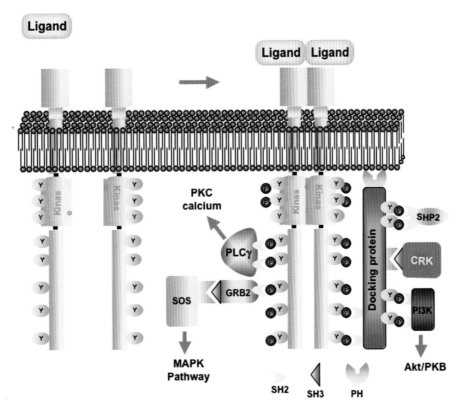

FIGURE 11–3.

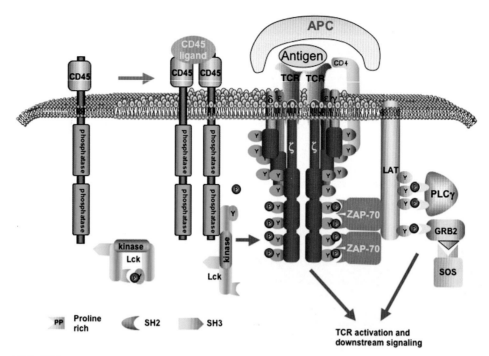

FIGURE 11–5.

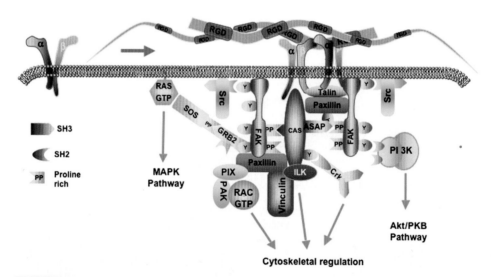

FIGURE 11–7.

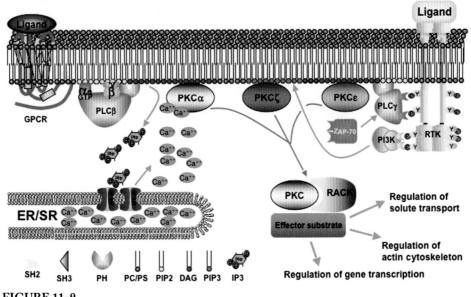

FIGURE 11–9.

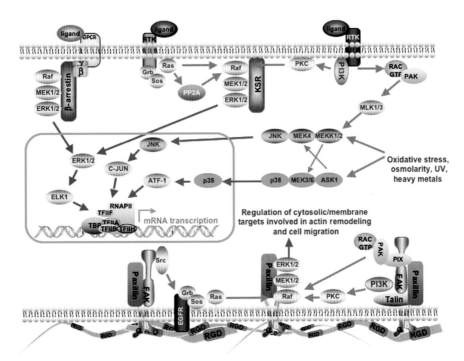

FIGURE 11–10.

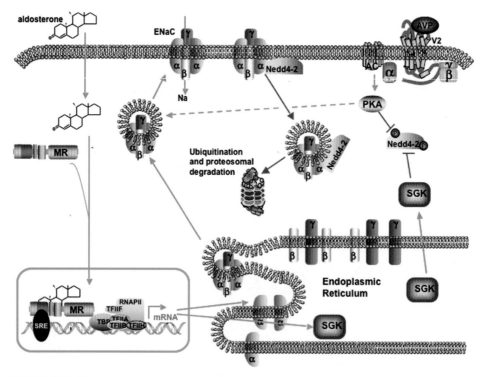

FIGURE 11–13.

A

	$(X\text{-}P_{-2}\text{-}X\text{-}P_0)$
Type I	X-S/T-X-Φ-COOH
Type II	X-Φ-X-Φ-COOH
Type III	X-X-C-COOH

B

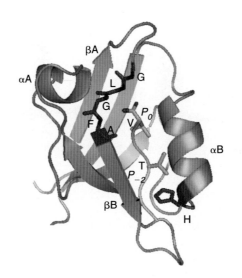

FIGURE 12–1.

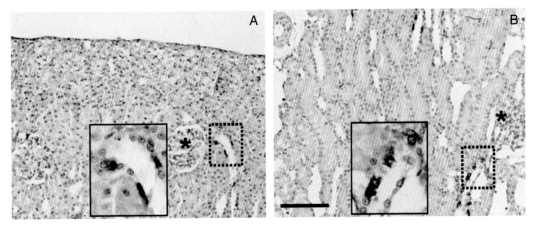

FIGURE 14–5.

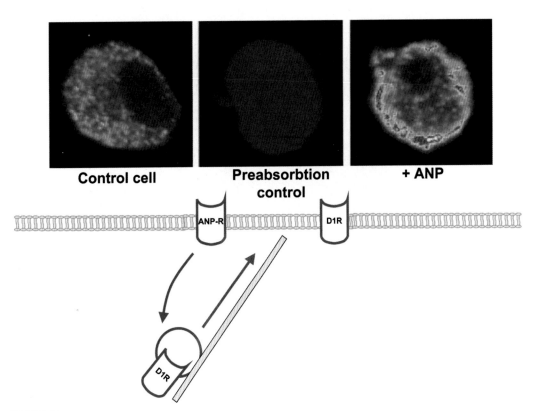

FIGURE 18–9.

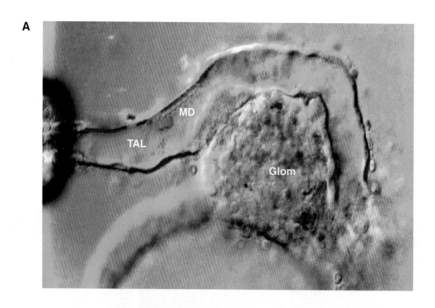

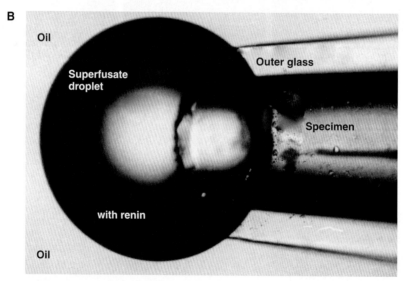

FIGURE 22–12.

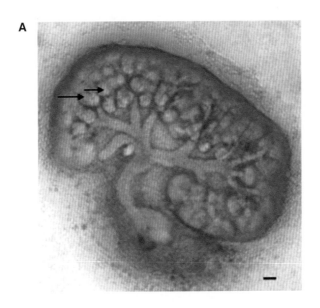

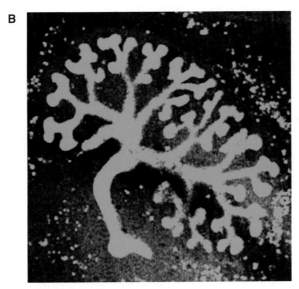

FIGURE 24–4.

A

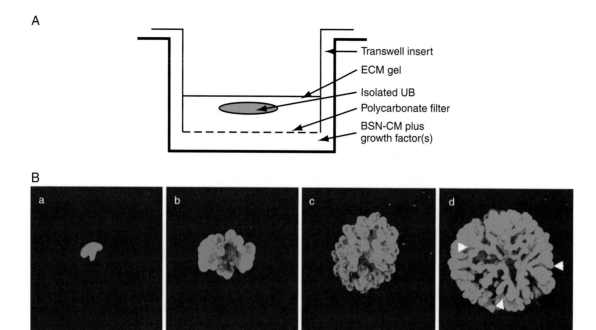

FIGURE 24–5.

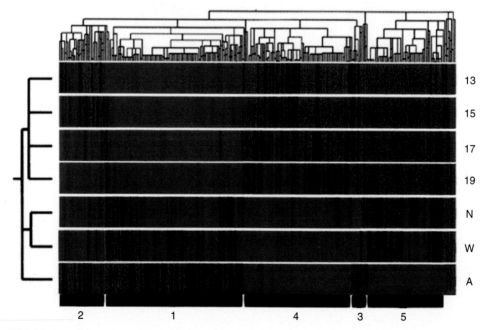

FIGURE 24–6.

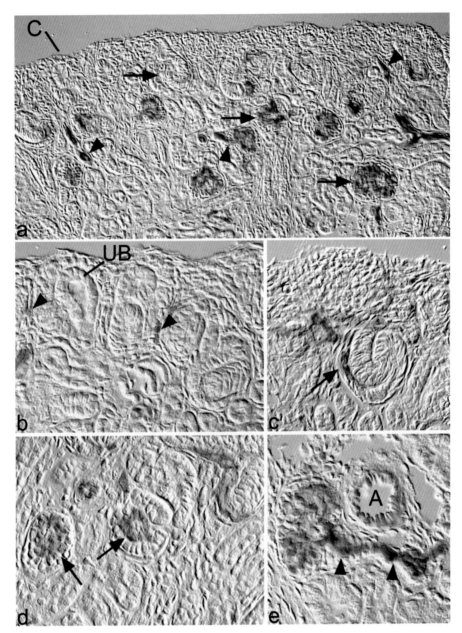

FIGURE 25–1.

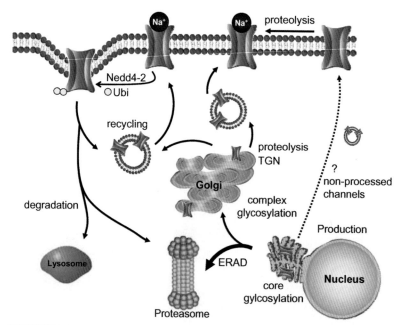

FIGURE 28–4.

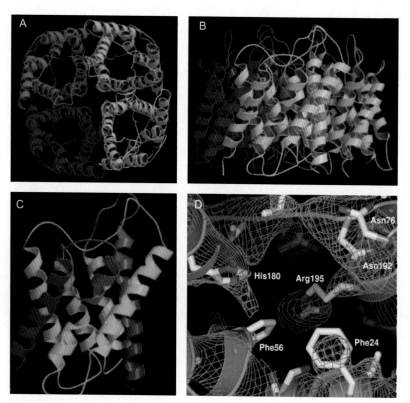

FIGURE 38–3.

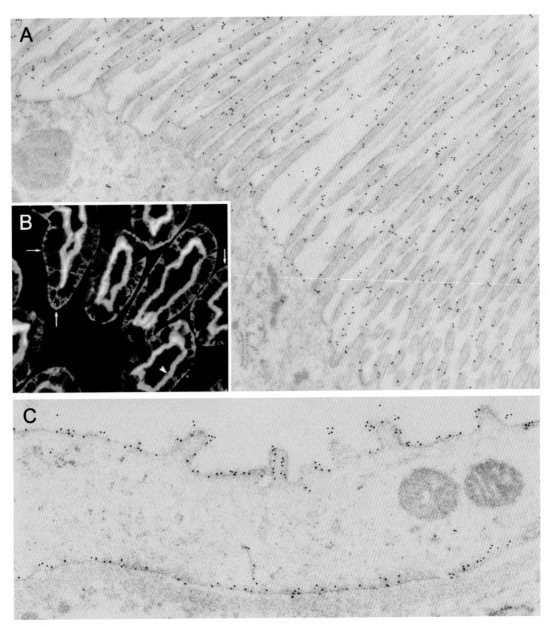

FIGURE 38–4.

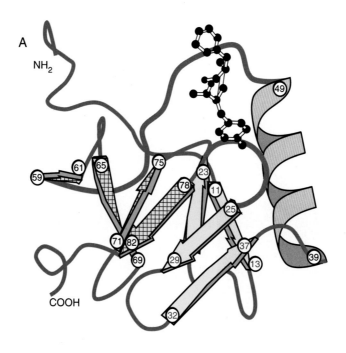

A

NH₂

COOH

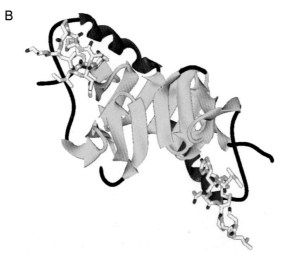

B

FIGURE 43–3.